The 5-Minute Clinical Consult Premium 2017

Premium

2017

25th EDITION

The 5-Minute Clinical Consult Premium
2017

25th EDITION

1-Year Enhanced Online Access + Print

Editor-in-Chief

Frank J. Domino, MD
Professor and Director of Predoctoral Education
Department of Family Medicine and Community Health
University of Massachusetts Medical School
Worcester, Massachusetts

Associate Editors

Robert A. Baldor, MD, FAAFP
Professor and Senior Vice-Chairman
Department of Family Medicine and Community Health
University of Massachusetts Medical School
Worcester, Massachusetts

Jeremy Golding, MD, FAAFP
Professor of Family Medicine and Obstetrics & Gynecology
University of Massachusetts Medical School
Quality Officer
Department of Family Medicine and Community Health
University of Massachusetts Memorial Health Care
Hahnemann Family Health Center
Worcester, Massachusetts

Mark B. Stephens, MD, MS, FAAFP, CAPT, MC, USN
Professor and Chair
Department of Family Medicine
Uniformed Services University
Bethesda, Maryland

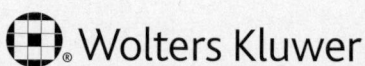

Philadelphia • Baltimore • New York • London
Buenos Aires • Hong Kong • Sydney • Tokyo

5MinuteConsult

Acquisitions Editor: Rebecca Gaertner
Product Development Editor: Leanne Vandetty
Marketing Manager: Rachel Mante Leung
Production Project Manager: Priscilla Crater
Design Coordinator: Holly McLaughlin
Manufacturing Coordinator: Beth Welsh
Prepress Vendor: Absolute Service, Inc.

25th edition

9 8 7 6 5 4 3 2 1

Printed in China

Library of Congress Cataloging-in-Publication Data available from the Publisher upon request.

ISBN-13: 978-14963-3997-3
ISBN-10: 1-4963-3997-5

LWW.com

Deciding how to apply medical data to an individual requires us to develop an approach, a method, to delivering a population-based science to an individual. We learned this method from someone, a wise mentor, in our past. In medical school, my mentor was a pediatric surgeon; in my current world, my mentors are my good friends and colleagues. We sit around a coffee or meal and challenge each other's approaches and absorb some of their vision in the process.

This year's 5-Minute Clinical Consult is dedicated to our mentors in medicine. Our mentors in life deserve our gratitude for our personal development. Our mentors in medicine deserve our gratitude every time we sit with a patient.

A very good friend (and mentor) has a saying, "Don't wait for the eulogy." Not tomorrow, but today, give your medical mentor a call, or drop a note (ideally on paper, but email if you must), and say thanks. Thanks for their influence on you, and thanks from your patients for helping them get the great care you provide.

Now pay it forward. Expand your role as a mentor. Take a learner in your office, be it a medical, NP, or PA student. Do it every year. Your knowledge may not be as current as theirs, but your wisdom on how to deliver care is exceptional. This is the gift of the mentor, and it cannot be taught by book, video, or televised debate. The Hippocratic Oath challenges us to "teach them my art." "Doctor" literally means teacher. Give thanks to your mentors, and give the gift of being one in return.

FRANK J. DOMINO, MD

PREFACE

> "There can be no happiness if the things we believe are different from the things we do."
>
> **–FREYA STARK**

A colleague was recently overheard describing all that was wrong with health care—the electronic record, ICD-10 and the new billing rules, conflicting guidelines, and the loss of the "old days." Delivering health care has always required learning what is new and juggling a variety of needs. Delivering personalized health care is an even greater challenge.

Medicine is also the most rewarding of careers and it is the best "job." We collaborate with others who share a mission to help people live better and partner with patients to meet their goals and provide care as they suffer through their illnesses.

We are so incredibly fortunate to have a job where we deliver, on a daily basis, care which is congruent with our belief that we can make the world better, one patient at a time. Consider your friends outside of medicine, can they say their daily work is consistent with making the world a better place? I suspect it is far greater a challenge for them to find happiness.

We picnic in summer, despite the mosquitoes, and we endure the cold to ski (or, at least enjoy a place by the fireplace with a good book). The annoyances should never prevent us from seeing the incredible good we do and from missing the happiness it provides.

Welcome to the 2017 edition of *The 5-Minute Clinical Consult*. This is a book of diseases, diagnostic methods, and treatment recommendations. Much of the work provided by primary care providers is focused on helping the patients help themselves to be healthier. Diet, exercise, safety, and prevention are the interventions that provide the greatest number of people with the greatest return on longevity and its enjoyment.

In our role, we do more than diagnose and treat disease. Yet, when you listen to patients' stories, or touch them, their burden is in some way lifted. We are a place for patients to turn when they are in need, sometimes when they have no place else to turn.

Our role is more than preventing and treating illness. We are leaders. Asking a recently widowed person how he or she will get through tomorrow is more than a condolence, it is a therapeutic intervention. Prompting an "at-risk" teen to use contraception, avoid drugs, or consider higher education are all therapeutic interventions. Dropping an email to your state legislator about a pressing issue affecting your patient population and stating publicly your opinion about important community issues are all components of your position and role and more valued than you probably imagine.

This year's *The 5-Minute Clinical Consult* is here to assist in fulfilling our role as a health care provider. In each patient interaction, in addition to bringing your clinical expertise, remember how others view you, as a leader, and the power of your words and actions. Encourage them to dream more, learn more, do more, and to be more.

Our editorial team has collaborated with hundreds of authors so that you may deliver your patients the best care. Each topic provides you with quick answers you can trust, where and when you need them most, either in print or online at www.5MinuteConsult.com.

This highly organized content provides you with the following:
- Differential diagnosis support from our expanded collection of algorithms
- Current evidence-based designations highlighted in each topic
- 570+ commonly encountered diseases in print, with an additional 1,400 online topics, including content from *The 5-Minute Pediatric Consult* and *Rosen & Barkin's 5-Minute Emergency Medicine Consult*
- FREE point-of-care CME and CE: 1/2 hour credit for every digital search
- Thousands of images to help support visual diagnosis of all conditions
- Video library of procedures, treatment, and physical therapy
- A to Z drug database from Facts & Comparisons®
- Laboratory test interpretation from *Wallach's Interpretation of Diagnostic Tests*
- More than 3,000 patient handouts in English and Spanish
- ICD-10 codes and *DSM-5* criteria; additionally, SNOMED codes are available online.

Our website, www.5MinuteConsult.com, delivers quick answers to your questions. It is an ideal resource for patient care. Integrating *The 5-Minute Clinical Consult* content into your workflow is easy and fast. And our patient education handouts can assist in helping you meet meaningful use compliance.

If you purchased the Premium Edition, your access includes 1 year FREE; the Standard Edition includes a free 10-day trial! The site promises an easy-to-use interface, allowing smooth maneuverability between topics, algorithms, images, videos, and patient education materials as well as more than 1,400 online-only topics.

Evidence-based health care is the integration of the best medical information with the values of the patient and your skill as a clinician. We have updated our EBM content so you can focus on how to best apply it in your practice.

We have solved the health maintenance challenge by including the link to the U.S. Preventive Services Task Force calculator. Enter a patient's gender and age and you are presented with the best recommendations to keep that specific patient healthy.

The algorithm section includes both diagnostic and treatment algorithms. This easy-to-use graphic method helps you evaluate an abnormal finding and prioritize treatment. They are also excellent teaching tools, so share them with the learners in your office.

In our role as clinicians, caring for those who are ill or helping to prevent illness, we use tests and prescribe treatments, hoping they improve outcomes. More important, our words and actions, even a shared smile, can make a huge difference. Thank you for being a leader in your practice and community.

The 5-Minute Clinical Consult editorial team values your observations, so please share your thoughts, suggestions, and constructive criticism through our website, www.5MinuteConsult.com.

FRANK J. DOMINO, MD
JANUARY 31, 2016

EVIDENCE-BASED MEDICINE

WHAT IS EVIDENCE-BASED MEDICINE?

Remember when we used to treat every otitis media with antibiotics? These recommendations came about because we applied logical reasoning to observational studies. If bacteria cause an acute otitis media, then antibiotics should help it resolve sooner, with less morbidity. Yet, when rigorously studied (via a systematic review), we found little benefit to this intervention.

The underlying premise of evidence-based medicine (EBM) is the evaluation of medical interventions and the literature that supports those interventions, in a systematic fashion. EBM hopes to encourage treatments proven to be effective and safe. And when insufficient data exists, it hopes to inform you on how to safely proceed.

EBM uses end points of real patient outcomes, morbidity, mortality, and risk. It focuses less on intermediate outcomes (bone density) and more on patient conditions (hip fractures).

Implementing EBM requires three components: the best medical evidence, the skill and experience of the provider, and the values of the patients. Should this patient be screened for prostate cancer? It depends on what is known about the test, on what you know of its benefits and harms, your ability to communicate that information, and that patient's informed choice.

This book hopes to address the first EBM component, providing you access to the best information in a quick format. Although not every test or treatment has this level of detail, many of the included interventions here use systematic review literature support.

The language of medical statistics is useful in interpreting the concepts of EBM. Below is a list of these terms, with examples to help take the confusion and mystery out of their use.

Prevalence: *proportion of people* in a population who have a disease (in the United States, 0.3% [3 in 1,000] people >50 years have colon cancer)

Incidence: How many *new cases of a disease* occur in a population during an interval of time; for example, "the estimated incidence of colon cancer in the United States is 104,000 in 2005."

Sensitivity: Percentage of people with disease who test positive; for mammography, the sensitivity is 71–96%.

Specificity: Percentage of people without disease who test negative; for mammography, the specificity is 94–97%.

Suppose you saw ML, a 53-year-old woman, for a health maintenance visit, ordered a *screening* mammogram, and the report demonstrates an irregular area of microcalcifications. She is waiting in your office to receive her test results, what can you tell her?

Sensitivity and specificity refer to characteristics of people who are *known to have disease* (sensitivity) or those who are *known not to have disease* (specificity). But, what you have is an abnormal test result. To better explain this result to ML, you need the positive predictive value.

Positive predictive value (PPV): Percentage of *positive* test results that are truly positive; the PPV for a woman aged 50 to 59 years is approximately 22%. That is to say that only 22% of abnormal screening mammograms in this group truly identified cancer. The other 78% are false positives.

You can tell ML only one out of five abnormal mammograms correctly identify cancer; the four are false positives, but the only way to know which mammogram is correct is to do further testing.

The corollary of the PPV is the negative predictive value (NPV), which is the percentage of negative test results that are truly negative.

The PPV and NPV tests are population-dependent, whereas the sensitivity and specificity are characteristics of the test, and have little to do with the patient in front of you. So when you receive an abnormal lab result, especially a screening test such as mammography, understand their limits based on their PPV and NPV.

Treatment information is a little different. In discerning the statistics of randomized controlled trials of interventions, first consider an example. The Scandinavian Simvastatin Survival Study (4S) (*Lancet.* 1994;344[8934]:1383–1389) found using simvastatin in patients at high risk for heart disease for 5 years resulted in death for 8% of simvastatin patients versus 12% of those on placebo; this results in a relative risk of 0.70, a relative risk reduction of 33%, and a number needed to treat of 25.

There are two ways of considering the benefits of an intervention with respect to a given outcome. The absolute risk reduction is the difference in the percentage of people with the condition before and after the intervention. Thus, if the incidence of myocardial infarction (MI) was 12% for the placebo group and 8% for the simvastatin group, the absolute risk reduction is 4% (12% − 8% = 4%).

The relative risk reduction reflects the improvement in the outcome as a percentage of the original rate and is commonly used to exaggerate the benefit of an intervention. Thus, if the risk of MI were reduced by simvastatin from 12% to 8%, then the relative risk reduction would be 33% (4%/12% = 33%); 33% sounds better than 4%, but the 4% is the absolute risk reduction and reflects the true outcome.

Absolute risk reduction is usually a better measure of *clinical* significance of an intervention. For instance, in one study, the treatment of mild hypertension has been shown to have relative risk reduction of 40% over 5 years (40% fewer strokes in the treated group). However, the absolute risk reduction was only 1.3%. Because mild hypertension is not strongly associated with strokes, aggressive treatment of mild hypertension yields only a small clinical benefit. Don't confuse relative risk reduction with relative risk.

Absolute (or attributable) risk (AR): the percentage of people in the placebo or intervention group who reach an end point; in the simvastatin study, the absolute risk of death was 8%.

Relative risk (RR): the risk of disease of those treated or exposed to some intervention (i.e., simvastatin) divided by those in the placebo group or who were untreated

– If RR is <1.0, it reduces risk—the smaller the number, the greater the risk reduction.

– If RR is >1.0, it increases risk—the greater the number, the greater the risk increase.

Relative risk reduction (RRR): the relative decrease in risk of an end point compared to the percentage of that end point in the placebo group

If you are still confused, just remember that the RRR is an overestimation of the actual effect.

Number needed to treat (NNT): This is the number of people who need to be treated by an intervention to prevent one adverse outcome. A "good" NNT can be a large number (>100) if risk of serious outcome is great. If the risk of an outcome is not that dangerous, then lower (<25) NNTs are preferred.

The NNT should be compared to a similar statistic, the number needed to harm (NNH). This is the number of people who have to be given treatment before one excess side effect or harm occurs. When the NNT is compared to the NNH, you and the patient can judge whether the benefit of the intervention is great enough to outweigh the risk of harm.

EVIDENCED-BASED GRADING

To help you interpret diagnostic and treatment recommendations within *The 5-Minute Clinical Consult*, we have graded the best information within the text and highlighted this content.

An "A" grade means the reference is from the highest quality resource, such as a systematic review. A *systematic review* is a summary of the medical literature on a given topic that uses strict, explicit methods to perform a thorough search of the literature and then provides a critical appraisal of individual studies, concluding in a recommendation. The most prestigious collection of systematic reviews is from the Cochrane Collaboration (www.cochrane.org).

A "B" grade means the data referenced comes from high-quality randomized controlled trials performed to minimize bias in their outcome. Bias is anything that interferes with the truth; in the medical literature, it is often unintentional, but it is much more common than we appreciate. In short, always assume some degree of bias exists in any research endeavor.

A "C" grade implies the reference used does not meet the A or B requirements; they are often treatments recommended by consensus groups (such as the American Cancer Society). In some cases, they may be the standards of care. But implicit in a group's recommendation is the bias of the author or the group that supports the reference. For example, the American Urological Society's recommendation around screening for prostate cancer may be motivated by their narrow scope and financial benefit. Compare this to the recommendations of the U.S. Preventive Services Task Force (www.ahrq.gov), which recommends against screening for prostate cancer.

BIAS

Bias is anything that interferes with the truth. There are many types of bias that should be considered by the publishers of medical information. Below describes a number of bias types that often affect our care without us knowing it is present.

Publication bias occurs when research is not published; this is often when a study finds data that does *not* support an intervention. The motivation to publish information that "didn't work" is low. It is estimated that up to 40% of all medical research never gets published. When you read of an effective intervention, wonder if other studies did not show benefit and went unpublished.

Comparator bias occurs when research compares an intervention to placebo, when placebo is not the standard of care. Knowing a new antibiotic is more effective than placebo for treating a condition is not helpful if you typically use a drug or procedure. Why not release research comparing the new drug to the standard of care? Sometimes the new treatment is no better than the current standard. And if a study was done to see if the new is better than the old and not published, you have an example of publication bias.

Selection bias involves choosing study populations that might be different than the average patient or just reporting a just subset of study participants from a study. Either will result in the data being skewed because it can only be applied to small subset of people.

Attrition bias and the concept of intention to treat. Attrition bias is when researchers do not fully acknowledge and address how a study deals with participants who do not adhere to the research protocol or drop out completely. Intention to treat analysis hopes to diminish attrition bias by statistically considering the nonadhering or dropped out patients as unsuccessfully benefiting from the intervention.

Commercial (funder) bias involves who paid for the research being done, and do they have a vested interest in the outcome. If the developer of a new drug does a large study, or a researcher has a personal financial interest in seeing a study succeed, they may consciously or unconsciously alter what is reported in a study. The data may be accurate, but until this is studied by less vested interests, some feel its outcome cannot be clinically applied.

Have you been annoyed how one week you learn of a randomized controlled trial that supports a treatment, to be followed the next week with a contradictory article? Statisticians have figured out how to resolve this using something called a systematic review.

A systematic review gathers all the literature on a topic, say using antibiotics to treat otitis media, and combines the data to determine if the sum of all the trials tells a different story than any single trial. The large number of participants in this type of research results in a much more statistically (and clinically) significant conclusion than any single paper. Want more? Check this out: http://community.cochrane.org/about-us/evidence-based-health-care.

A meta-analysis is a quantitative systematic review and demonstrates its outcomes in the form of a forest plot. The bottom line with interpretation of a forest plot is to look for the diamond on the bottom. If it is to LEFT of the vertical line, it means risk of an outcome was reduced by the intervention. If it is fully to the RIGHT, then risk of that outcome was increased. And if the diamond touches the vertical line, it means there was no statistical influence of the intervention on the outcome.

We hope this brief introduction to EBM has been informative, clear, and helpful. If any of the information above seems unclear, or if you have a question, please contact us via www.5MinuteConsult.com.

ACKNOWLEDGMENTS

This is the 25th edition of *The 5-Minute Clinical Consult*, a comprehensive point-of-care tool to assist in the care of patients. From beginning to end, one cannot find a more current and easy-to-use collection of clinically useful content.

Developing and maintaining a book and website of this magnitude requires an equally broad effort from its supporting team. I wish to thank the dedication and tireless efforts of many: executive editor, Rebecca Gaertner; product development editor, Leanne Vandetty; marketing manager, Rachel Mante Leung; and publisher, Lisa McAllister.

This 2017 edition is the direct result of the dedication and insights of our associate editors. I wish to thank Drs. Robert Baldor, Jeremy Golding, and Mark Stephens for their hard work and overwhelming commitment to *The 5-Minute Clinical Consult*. And to Dr. Jill Grimes for her continued support while away.

I wish to especially thank my wife, Sylvia, and my daughter, Molly, who have given greatly for this book.

The challenge of completing a book covering this broad a spectrum of medicine requires insights and skills far beyond my own. Many thanks to my mentors Bob Baldor and Mark Quirk who have been an enormous support—always there to encourage, reassure, and impart wisdom.

Many in the academic and health care worlds are due thanks for support, insight, and friendship: Daniel Lasser, Alan Churnan, Michele Pugnaire, Karen Rayla, Phil Fournier, Erik Garcia, Jeff Stovall, Jim Comes, Len Levin, Judy Norberg, J. Herb Stevenson, Robert Jenal, Michael Kidd, Zainab Nawab, Sanjiv and Amita Chopra, Vasilios (Bill) Chrisostomidis, James (Jay) Broadhurst, Danuta Antkowiak, Atreyi Chakrabarti, Kerry Morse, Kate Peasha, the staff of Shrewsbury Family Medicine, Mark Powicki, Steve Messineo, and the faculty and amazing students of the University of Massachusetts Medical School.

Medicine is a challenge I have fortunately not had to meet alone. Thanks to my parents, Frank and Angela (Jean); my brother, John and his family, Marylou, Cate, and Jane; Frank, Mary Anne, Diane, and David Christian; the Diana and Hymie Lipschitz family; and the Bob and Ruth Pabreza family; they are responsible for who I am and my success in life.

I am blessed with the best of friends; without them, I would not be a physician. Thanks to Bob Bacic, Ron Jautz, Richard Onorato, John Horcher, Auguste Turnier, Bob Smith, Paul Saivetz, Bob and Nancy Gallinaro, Drew and Jill Grimes, Louay Toma, Laurie, Alan, Daniel, Jenny and Matt Bugos, Alan Ehrlich, Andy Jennings, Bill Demianiuk, Mark Steenbergen, John and Kathleen Polanowicz, Phil and Carol Pettine, Mark Shelton, Steve Bennett, Vicki Triolo, and Michael Bernatchez.

—FRANK J. DOMINO, MD

CONTRIBUTING AUTHORS

Adil Abdalla, MD
Department of Gastroenterology
CHI Health
Omaha, Nebraska

Basmah Abdalla, MD†
Clinical Instructor
Kidney Transplant Program
Department of Medicine
David Geffen School of Medicine at UCLA
Los Angeles, California

Thomas L. Abell, MD
Arthur M. Schoen, MD Chair in
    Gastroenterology
Department of Gastroenterology
University of Louisville
Louisville, Kentucky

Alain Michael P. Abellada, MD
Medical Director
Family Medicine Hospitalist Service
Blanchfield Army Community Hospital
Fort Campbell, Kentucky

George M. Abraham, MD, MPH
Associate Chief of Medicine
Saint Vincent Hospital
Professor of Medicine
University of Massachusetts Medical School
Worcester, Massachusetts

Mohammed Abunada, MD
Colorectal Surgeon
Hamad Medical Corporation
Doha, Qatar

Anne Claire Adams, MD
Family Medicine Resident
Department of Family Medicine
The Christ Hospital
University of Cincinnati College of
    Medicine
Cincinnati, Ohio

Rae Adams, MD
Associate Professor of Family and
    Community Medicine
Texas A&M Health Science Center
    College of Medicine
Bryan, Texas

Faraz Ahmad, MD
Family Medicine Resident
Preventative Medicine Resident
Family Medicine Residency Program
Department of Family Medicine and
    Community Health
University Hospitals Case Medical Center
Cleveland, Ohio

Nadir Ahmad, MD, FACS
Division Head
Otolaryngology–Head & Neck Surgery
Associate Professor
Director
Head & Neck Cancer Program
Cooper University Health Care
MD Anderson at Cooper Cancer Center
Cooper Medical School of Rowan University
Camden, New Jersey

Shahla Ahmad, MD
Family and Community Medicine Resident
Department of Family and Community
    Medicine
Penn Slate Milton S. Hershey Medical
    Center
Penn State College of Medicine
Hershey, Pennsylvania

Sumera R. Ahmad, MD†
Pulmonary and Critical Care Fellow
Department of Pulmonary and Critical
    Care
University of Massachusetts Memorial
    Medical Center
Worcester, Massachusetts

Yasir Ahmed, MD
Resident
Penn State Hershey Eye Center
Penn State College of Medicine
Hershey, Pennsylvania

Jowhara Al-Qahtani, MD
General Surgery Resident
Maimonides Medical Center
Brooklyn, New York

Bedoor Alabbas, MD
George Washington University Hospital
Washington, DC

Gillian Alex, MD
Surgery Resident
Rush University Medical Center
Chicago, Illinois

Andrew G. Alexander, MD
Assistant Clinical Professor of Family
    Medicine
University of California, Riverside School
    of Medicine
Riverside, California

Mohammed Algodi, MD
Clinical Study Supervisor
Cardiology
Montefiore Medical Center
Bronx, New York

Fozia Akhtar Ali, MD†
Assistant Professor/Clinical
Department of Family and Community
    Medicine
University of Texas Health Science
    Center at San Antonio
San Antonio, Texas

Jason B. Alisangco, DO, FAAFP†
Sports Medicine Fellow
Fort Belvoir Community Hospital
Fort Belvoir, Virginia

Shahriar Alizadegan, MD
Medical College of Wisconsin
Milwaukee, Wisconsin

Andrew S. Allegretti, MD
Fellow in Nephrology
Division of Nephrology
Brigham and Women's Hospital
Massachusetts General Hospital
Harvard Medical School
Boston, Massachusetts

J. Aaron Allgood, DO
Assistant Professor
Clinical Medicine and Public Health
A.T. Still University School of Osteopathic
    Medicine
Mesa, Arizona

Richard W. Allinson, MD
Associate Professor
Department of Surgery
The Texas A&M University System Health
    Sciences Center
Senior Staff Physician
Baylor Scott & White Clinic
Waco, Texas

Ziad Alnabki, MD
Fellow
University of Louisville
Louisville, Kentucky

Melanie Dawn Altizer, MD
Assistant Professor
Department of Obstetrics and Gynecology
Carilion Clinic
Roanoke, Virginia

Angelic M. Alvarez, MD
Resident
Universidad Central del Este College of
    Medicine
San Pedro de Macoris, Dominican
    Republic

Felix N. Alvarez, MD
Internal Medicine Hospitalist
Yuma Regional Medical Center
Yuma, Arizona

Crystal Amadi, MD[†]
Resident Physician
Department of Family and Community
    Medicine
University of Texas Health Science
    Center at San Antonio
San Antonio, Texas

David L. Anderson, MD[†]
Resident Physician
Department of Family Medicine
Dwight D. Eisenhower Army Medical
    Center
Augusta, Georgia

Garland Edward Anderson, II, MD
Clinical Instructor of Family Medicine
Rural Family Medicine Program
Louisiana State University
Our Lady of the Angels Hospital
Bogalusa, Louisiana

Jennifer Anderson, PharmD[†]
Oncology Pharmacy Resident
University of Illinois at Chicago College
    of Pharmacy
Chicago, Illinois

Roger Allan Anderson, MD[†]
Staff Ophthalmologist
Department of Ophthalmology
Madigan Army Medical Center
Tacoma, Washington

Adam Anglyn, DO
Campbell University College of
    Osteopathic Medicine
Lumberton, North Carolina

Tanya E. Anim, MD
Fellow in Women's Health with Obstetrics
    Focus
Florida Hospital Family Medicine
    Residency Program
Winter Park, Florida

Shari Anthony, MD
Resident
Department of Family Medicine
Bayfront Family Health Center
St. Petersburg, Florida

Tad Antognini, MD
University of Massachusetts Medical
    School
Worcester, Massachusetts

Kashif S. Anwar, MD
Physician
Department of Family Medicine
University Hospitals Portage Medical
    Center
Ravenna, Ohio

Michael Apostolis, MD
Department of Pulmonology
St. Elizabeth Youngstown Hospital
Youngstown, Ohio

Paul M. Arguin, MD[†]
Captain
United States Public Health Service
Chief, Domestic Unit
Malaria Branch
Center for Global Health
Centers for Disease Control and Prevention
Atlanta, Georgia

Michael Argyle, DO
Resident
David Grant USAF Medical Center
Travis Air Force Base, California

Forest W. Arnold, DO, MSc
Associate Professor and Hospital
    Epidemiologist
Division of Infectious Diseases
University of Louisville School of Medicine
Louisville, Kentucky

James J. Arnold, DO, FAAFP[†]
Senior Associate Program Director
National Capital Consortium Family
    Medicine Residency
Fort Belvoir Community Hospital
Fort Belvoir, Virginia

Michael Arnold, MD, CDR, MC[†]
Department Head, Branch Health Clinic
United States Naval Hospital
United States Navy
Naples, Italy

Aneel A. Ashrani, MD, MS
Assistant Professor
Division of Hematology
Department of Internal Medicine
Mayo Clinic
Rochester, Minnesota

Anne R. Atalig, MD, CPT[†]
Department of Family Medicine
Dwight D. Eisenhower Army Medical
    Center
Fort Gordon, Georgia

Patricia Ruth Atchinson, DO
Emergency Medicine Resident
Dartmouth Hitchcock Medical Center
Lebanon, New Hampshire

Carlos Atore, MD
Dell Medical School, University of Texas
    at Austin
Austin, Texas

Maximos Attia, MD
Clinical Assistant Professor
Guthrie/Robert Packer Hospital Family
    Medicine Residency Program
Medical Director
Walk-in Clinic and Anti-coagulation
    Clinics
Sayre, Pennsylvania

Stephen E. Auciello, MD
Resident Physician
Family Medicine Residency Program
OhioHealth Riverside Methodist Hospital
Columbus, Ohio

Sudeep K. Aulakh, MD, FACP, FRCPC
Director of Ambulatory Education
Baystate Internal Medicine Residency
Co-Director of Baystate Primary Care
    Residency
Assistant Professor of Medicine
Baystate Health Medical Center
Tufts University School of Medicine
Springfield, Massachusetts

Gerard P. Aurigemma, MD
Professor of Medicine and Radiology
University of Massachusetts Medical School
Director, Noninvasive Cardiology
University of Massachusetts Memorial
    Medical Center
Worcester, Massachusetts

Philip H. Aurigemma, MD
Orthopedic Surgery Resident
Department of Orthopedic Surgery and
    Rehabilitation
University of Massachusetts Medical School
Worcester, Massachusetts

Swati Avashia, MD, FAAP[†]
Assistant Professor of Medicine
Department of Internal Medicine/
    Pediatrics/Integrative and Holistic
    Medicine
Family Medicine Residency Program
Dell Medical School, University of Texas
    at Austin
Austin, Texas

Nida S. Awadallah, MD
Assistant Clinical Professor
Department of Family Medicine
Rose Family Medicine Residency
University of Colorado
Denver, Colorado

Jennifer L. Ayres, PhD
Director of Behavioral Health Services
Assistant Professor of Medicine
Dell Medical School, University of Texas
    at Austin
Austin, Texas

Holly L. Baab, MD
Assistant Director
Bayfront Family Medicine Residency
St. Petersburg, Florida

Sultan M. Babar, MD
Sports Medicine Fellow
Cabarrus Sports Medicine
Concord, North Carolina

Franklyn C. Babb, MD, FAAFP
Assistant Professor and Clerkship Director
Department of Family and Community
    Medicine
Texas Tech University Health Sciences
    Center School of Medicine
Lubbock, Texas

Megan Babb, DO
Resident
Mercy Family Health Center
Sacramento, California

Kavita Babu, MD
Associate Professor
Department of Emergency Medicine
Division of Medical Toxicology
University of Massachusetts Memorial
    Medical Center
Worcester, Massachusetts

Elisabeth L. Backer, MD
Clinical Associate Professor
Department of Family Medicine
University of Nebraska Medical Center
Omaha, Nebraska

Melissa Badowski, PharmD[†]
Clinical Assistant Professor
University of Illinois at Chicago College of
    Pharmacy
Chicago, Illinois

Shaun Baker, DO
ENT Resident Physician
Philadelphia College of Osteopathic
    Medicine
Philadelphia, Pennsylvania

Robert A. Baldor, MD, FAAFP
Professor and Senior Vice-Chairman
Department of Family Medicine and
    Community Health
University of Massachusetts Medical School
Worcester, Massachusetts

Andrew Baldwin, MD, MPH[†]
Family Medicine Residency Staff
Fort Belvoir Community Hospital
Fort Belvoir, Virginia

Jonathan R. Ballard, MD, MPH, MPhil
Medical Director of Ambulatory Services
Assistant Professor
Department of Family and Community
    Medicine
University of Kentucky College of Medicine
Lexington, Kentucky

Rahul Banerjee, MD
Department of Internal Medicine
Hospital of the University of Pennsylvania
Philadelphia, Pennsylvania

Vigyan Bang, MD
Department of Internal Medicine
Lahey Hospital & Medical Center
Burlington, Massachusetts

Arham K. Barakzai, MD
Resident
Department of Internal Medicine -
    Crittenton
Wayne State University School of Medicine
Detroit, Michigan

Brent J. Barber, MD
Associate Professor, Pediatric Cardiology
University of Arizona College of Medicine
Tucson, Arizona

Anne M. Barnard, MD[†]
Group Health Cooperative Family
    Medicine Residency
Group Health Cooperative
Seattle, Washington

Elise J. Barney, DO[†]
Assistant Professor of Clinical Medicine
Department of Internal Medicine
Arizona College of Osteopathic Medicine
    Midwestern University
Glendale, Arizona

Wendy Brooks Barr, MD, MPH, MSCE
Associate Residency Director
Lawrence Family Medicine Residency
Assistant Professor of Family Medicine
Tufts University School of Medicine
Lawrence, Massachusetts

John P. Barrett, MD, MPH, MS, FAAFP[†]
Colonel of Medical Corps, U.S. Army
Uniformed Services University of the
    Health Sciences
Bethesda, Maryland

Michael C. Barros, PharmD, BCPS,
    BCACP
Clinical Assistant Professor of Pharmacy
    Practice
Temple University School of Pharmacy
Clinical Pharmacy Specialist of
    Ambulatory Care
Temple University, Heart and Vascular
    Center/Medicine Group Practice/
    Endocrinology
Philadelphia, Pennsylvania

Krithika Baskaran, DDS
Assistant Professor
Department of Restorative Dentistry
School of Dental Medicine
University of Colorado Anschutz Medical
    Campus
Aurora, Colorado

Jonathan S. Bassett, MD[†]
Faculty Physician
Eglin Family Medicine Residency
Eglin Air Force Base
Valparaiso, Florida

Erin Bassett-Novoa, MD
Lawrence Family Medicine Residency
Greater Lawrence Family Health Center
Lawrence, Massachusetts

Brian D. Bates, MD
Family Medicine Resident
Department of Family Medicine
Boston University Medical Campus
Boston, Massachusetts

Brian P. Bateson, DO
General Surgery Resident
Department of Surgery
Georgia Regents University
Augusta, Georgia

Trevor J. Batty, DO
Arizona College of Osteopathic Medicine,
  Midwestern University
Glendale, Arizona

Kay A. Bauman, MD, MPH
Medical Director
New Mexico Department of Corrections
Professor
Department of Family and Community
  Medicine
University of New Mexico School of
  Medicine
Albuquerque, New Mexico

Dennis J. Baumgardner, MD
Clinical Adjunct Professor of Family
  Medicine
University of Wisconsin School of
  Medicine and Public Health
Director of Research
Aurora University of Wisconsin Medical
  Group
Associate Director
Center for Urban Population Health
Milwaukee, Wisconsin

Hillery Bavani, DO, CPT, USA[†]
Family Medicine Resident
Martin Army Community Hospital
Fort Benning, Georgia

Jeffrey Baxter, MD
Assistant Professor
Department of Family Medicine and
  Community Health
University of Massachusetts Medical School
Worcester, Massachusetts

Cheryl Bayart, MD, MPH
Department of Dermatology
Cleveland Clinic Foundation
Cleveland, Ohio

Sheryl Beard, MD, FAAFP
Senior Associate Program Director
Via Christi Family Medicine Residency
  Program
Clinical Assistant Professor
University of Kansas School of Medicine–
  Wichita
Wichita, Kansas

Patricia Beauzile, MD[†]
Resident Physician
Department of Obstetrics and
  Gynecology
Virginia Tech Carilion School of Medicine
Roanoke, Virginia

Joshua R. Beer, DO[†]
Resident
Department of Family Medicine
Naval Hospital Jacksonville
Jacksonville, Florida

Adriane E. Bell, MD[†]
Faculty
Family Medicine Residency Program
Department of Family Medicine
Tripler Army Medical Center
Honolulu, Hawaii

Hershey S. Bell, MD, MS, FAAFP
Professor
Vice President of Academic Affairs and
  Dean
Lake Erie College of Osteopathic
  Medicine School of Pharmacy
Eric, Pennsylvania and Bradenton, Florida

Paul P. Belliveau, PharmD, RPh
Professor of Pharmacy Practice
Massachusetts College of Pharmacy and
  Health Sciences University
Worcester, Massachusetts

Sheldon Benjamin, MD
Professor of Psychiatry and Neurology
Department of Psychiatry
University of Massachusetts Medical
  School
Worcester, Massachusetts

Terrell Benold, MD[†]
Assistant Clinical Professor
Dell Medical School, University of Texas
  at Austin
Austin, Texas

Jennifer Bepko, MD[†]
Faculty of Family Medicine
Family Medicine Residency
Davis Grant Medical Center
Travis Air Force Base, California

Jasmine S. Beria, DO, MPH[†]
Resident Physician
Department of Internal Medicine
Mount Sinai St. Luke's Roosevelt Hospital
New York, New York

Louis J. Berk, MD
Chief Resident and Assistant Clinical
  Instructor
Department of Family Medicine
SUNY Downstate Medical Center
Brooklyn, New York

Jamie L. Berkes, MD
Assistant Professor of Medicine
Department of Internal Medicine
Loyola University
Maywood, Illinois

Bettina Bernstein, DO
Clinical Assistant Professor of
  Psychiatry
Philadelphia College of Osteopathic
  Medicine
Philadelphia, Pennsylvania

John F. Bertagnolli, Jr., DO
Associate Professor of Family Medicine
Director of Pain and Palliative Care
Rowan University School of Osteopathic
  Medicine
Stratford, New Jersey

Neela Bhajandas, PharmD
Clinical Assistant Professor of
  Pharmacy
Temple University School of Pharmacy
Philadelphia, Pennsylvania

Varun Kumar Bhalla, MD
Pediatric Surgical Critical Care Fellow
Children's National Health System
Washington, DC

Nirmanmoh Bhatia, MD
Clinical Fellow
Department of Medicine
Vanderbilt University School of Medicine
Nashville, Tennessee

Ghazaleh Bigdeli, MD, FCCP
Pulmonary Rehab Associates
Youngstown, Ohio

Stephanie J. Billings, MD
Family Medicine Doctor
Holyoke Health
Holyoke, Massachusetts

Barton L. Blackorby, MD[†]
Resident Ophthalmologist
Department of Ophthalmology
Madigan Army Medical Center
Tacoma, Washington

James D. Blake, MD[†]
Hoover Family Medicine
MedCenter Hoover
Hoover, Alabama

Lewis S. Blevins, Jr., MD
Professor of Neurological Surgery
    and Medicine
Director
California Center for Pituitary Disorders
    at University of California San
    Francisco
San Francisco, California

David Bode, MD[†]
Dwight D. Eisenhower Army Medical
    Center
Fort Gordon, Georgia

Aaron R. Bolduc, MD
Surgery Department
Georgia Regents University
Augusta, Georgia

Kimberly Bombaci, MD
UMass Memorial Health Care
Worcester, Massachusetts

Brandon W. Bonds, MD
Resident
West Kendall Baptist Hospital
Miami, Florida

Katrina A. Booth, MD
Assistant Professor
Department of Medicine
Division of Gerontology, Geriatrics, and
    Palliative Care
University of Alabama at Birmingham
Birmingham, Alabama

Azra Borogovac, MD
Department of Medicine
University of Massachusetts Medical
    School
Worcester, Massachusetts

Marie L. Borum, MD, EdD, MPH
Professor of Medicine
Director
Division of Gastroenterology and Liver
    Diseases
George Washington University
Washington, DC

Emily Bouley, MD
University of Massachusetts Medical
    School
Worcester, Massachusetts

Andrew Boylan, MD
Urology Resident
University of Connecticut School of
    Medicine
Farmington, Connecticut

Rachel Bramson, MD
Associate Professor
Department of Family and Community
    Medicine
Texas A&M Health Science Center
    College of Medicine
Bryan, Texas

Jay A. Brieler, MD[†]
Assistant Professor
Department of Family and Community
    Medicine
Saint Louis University School of Medicine
St. Louis, Missouri

Jacob Michael Bright, DO[†]
Captain of Medical Corps, U.S. Army
Family Medicine Residency Program
Dwight D. Eisenhower Army Medical Center
Fort Gordon, Georgia

Emma Brooks, MD
Assistant Professor
Department of Family Medicine
Oregon Health & Science University
Portland, Oregon

Christine M. Broszko, MD[†]
Resident Physician
Department of Family Medicine
University of Nebraska Medical Center
Omaha, Nebraska

Benjamin P. Brown, MD
Resident
Department of Obstetrics and Gynecology
University of Chicago Medical Center
Chicago, Illinois

Matthew C. Brown, MD[†]
Family Medicine Resident
Department of Family Medicine
David Grant Medical Center
Travis Air Force Base, California

Michael L. Brown, MD
Psychiatrist
Christus St. Patrick Hospital
Lake Charles, Louisiana

Theodore R. Brown, DO, MPH, FAAFP[†]
Lieutenant Colonel of Medical Corps,
    U.S. Army
Health Fitness Directorate
National Defense University
Fort Lesley J. McNair
Washington, DC

Karen Browning, MD
Obstetrics and Gynecology Resident
Women & Infants Hospital
Brown University
Providence, Rhode Island

Karen Brubaker, MD
Resident
Department of Emergency Medicine
University of Pittsburgh Medical Center
Pittsburgh, Pennsylvania

Darren S. Bryan, MD
General Surgery Resident
Department of Surgery
University of Chicago
Chicago, Illinois

Matthew E. Bryant, MD[†]
Family Practice Physician
Dwight D. Eisenhower Army Medical
    Center
Fort Gordon, Georgia

Carl Bryce, MD, Capt, USAF[†]
Nellis Family Medicine Residency
Nellis Air Force Base
Las Vegas, Nevada

Merima Bucaj, DO[†]
Family Medicine Attending Physician
Family Medicine Residency Program
David Grant Medical Center
Travis Air Force Base, California

Andrew D. Buchan, DO
Internal Medical Resident
Southeastern Regional Medical Center
Lumberton, North Carolina

Nitin Budhwar, MD
Associate Professor
Department of Family and Community
    Medicine
University of Texas Southwestern Medical
    Center
Dallas, Texas

Han Q. Bui, MD, MPH[†]
Naval Medical Clinic Quantico
Quantico, Virginia

Christopher W. Bunt, MD, FAAFP[†]
Assistant Professor
Department of Family Medicine
Uniformed Services University of the
    Health Sciences
Bethesda, Maryland

Tiffany Burca, DO
Family Medicine Residency
University of Nebraska Medical Center
Omaha, Nebraska

Kristina Burgers, MD, FAAFP[†]
Family Medicine Physician
Womack Army Medical Center
Fort Bragg, North Carolina

John R. Burk, MD
Texas Pulmonary and Critical Care
    Consultants, PA
Fort Worth, Texas

Harold J. Bursztajn, MD
Associate Clinical Professor of Psychiatry
Cofounder, Program in Psychiatry and
    the Law
Beth Israel Deaconess Medical Center
Psychiatry of Harvard Medical School
President of the American Unit of the
    UNESCO Bioethics Chair
Boston, Massachusetts

David C. Bury, DO[†]
Family Medicine Physician
Camp Casey U.S. Army Health Clinic
Dongducheon, South Korea

Jason N. Butler, DO, MS[†]
Womack Family Medicine Resident
Womack Army Medical Center
Fort Bragg, North Carolina

Nancy Byatt, DO, MBA, FAPM
Assistant Professor of Psychiatry and
    Obstetrics & Gynecology
UMass Memorial Medical Center/UMass
    Medical School
Worcester, Massachusetts

Stephen D. Cagle, Jr., MD, Capt,
    USAF, MC[†]
Nellis Air Force Base
Las Vegas, Nevada

Mitchell A. Cahan, MD, MBA, FACS
Associate Professor of Surgery
University of Massachusetts Medical
    School
Worcester, Massachusetts

Boris E. Calderon, DO
Internal Medicine Resident
Southeastern Health
Campbell University School of
    Osteopathic Medicine
Lumberton, North Carolina

Daniel Callaway, MD
Fellow
Hasbro Children's Hospital
Providence, Rhode Island

Ryan J. Callery, MD
Assistant Professor
Department of Obstetrics and
    Gynecology
UMass Memorial Medical Center
Worcester, Massachusetts

Carolyn Cammarano, PharmD, RPh
Fellow
School of Pharmacy
Massachusetts College of Pharmacy and
    Health Sciences University
Boston, Massachusetts

Maya Campara, PharmD, BCPS
Clinical Assistant Professor
Clinical Pharmacist
Transplant Department of Pharmacy
    Practice
University of Illinois at Chicago
Chicago, Illinois

Christinne D. Canela, MD
Assistant Professor
Department of Obstetrics and Gynecology
Carilion Clinic
Virginia Tech Carilion School of Medicine
Roanoke, Virginia

Patrick M. Carey, DO[†]
Department of Family and Sports Medicine
Dwight D. Eisenhower Army Medical
    Center
Fort Gordon, Georgia

Samuel B. Carli, MD
Physician, Internal Medicine
PeaceHealth Southwest Medical Center
Vancouver, Washington

Robert Thomas Carlisle, MD, MPH[†]
Faculty Physician
Department of Family Medicine
Tripler Army Medical Center
Honolulu, Hawaii

Amanda M. Carnes, MD[†]
Family Medicine Physician
Department of Family Medicine
Bassett Army Community Hospital
Fort Wainwright, Alaska

Rachel Marinch Carpenter, MD[†]
Chief Resident
Exempla Saint Joseph Family Medicine
    Resident
Denver, Colorado

Jewell P. Carr, MD
Family Medicine
Carolinas HealthCare System
Charlotte, North Carolina

Noel J.M. Carrasco, MD, FAAP[†]
Professor of Pediatrics, Neonatal-
    Perinatal Medicine
A.T. Still University School of Osteopathic
    Medicine
Mesa, Arizona

Dana G. Carroll, PharmD, BCPS, CDE
Associate Clinical Professor
Pharmacy Practice Department
Auburn University Harrison School of
    Pharmacy
Department of Family Medicine
University of Alabama College of
    Community Health Sciences
Tuscaloosa, Alabama

Kevin A. Carter, DO, FAASM
Associate Professor of Family Medicine
Ohio University Heritage College of
    Osteopathic Medicine
Athens, Ohio

Merle A. Carter, MD, FACEP
Faculty
Emergency Medicine Residency Program
Einstein Medical Center
Philadelphia, Pennsylvania

Marissa T. Casagrande, PharmD
Pharmacy Resident
Temple University Health System
Philadelphia, Pennsylvania

Casandra Cashman, MD, FAAFP
Assistant Director
Community East Family Medicine
    Residency Program
Indianapolis, Indiana

Mary Cataletto, MD, FAAP, FCCP[†]
Professor of Clinical Pediatrics
SUNY at Stony Brook
Clinical Campus at Winthrop University
    Hospital
Stony Brook, New York

Rodrigo Cavallazi, MD
Assistant Professor of Medicine
Division of Pulmonary, Critical Care and
    Sleep Disorders Medicine
University of Louisville Hospital
Louisville, Kentucky

Lorena Ceci, MD
University of Massachusetts Medical School
Worcester, Massachusetts

Jan Cerny, MD, PhD[†]
Assistant Professor in Medicine
University of Massachusetts
Department of Medicine
Division of Hematology/Oncology
Bone Marrow Transplantation
Director, Leukemia Program
University of Massachusetts Medical School
Associate Director, Cancer Research
  Office
UMass Memorial Cancer Center
Worcester, Massachusetts

Olga M. Cerón, MD
Assistant Professor
University of Massachusetts Medical
  School
UMass Memorial Eye Center
Department of Ophthalmology
UMass Memorial Medical Center,
  Hahnemann Campus
Worcester, Massachusetts

Rachel L. Cetta, DO
Traditional Rotating Intern
Beaumont South Shore Hospital
Trenton, Michigan

Elie Chalhoub, MD
Fellow
Department of Hematology & Medical
  Oncology
Tulane University School of Medicine
New Orleans, Louisiana

Justin D. Chaltry, DO[†]
Family Medicine Resident Physician
Martin Army Community Hospital
Fort Benning, Georgia

Cindy J. Chambers, MD, MAS, MPH
Department of Dermatology
UC Davis Health System
Sacramento, California

Ronald G. Chambers, Jr., MD, FAAFP
Program Director
Methodist Family Medicine Residency
  Program
Sacramento, California

Matthew Chandler, MD
Division of Gastroenterology and Liver
  Diseases
George Washington University Hospital
Washington, DC

Aditya Chandrasekhar, MD, MPH
Instructor in Medicine
Harvard Medical School
Boston, Massachusetts

Felix B. Chang, MD, DABMA, FAAMA
Clinical Associate Professor
Department of Family Medicine and
  Community Health
University of Massachusetts Medical
  School
Director of Inpatient Service
UMass Fitchburg Family Medicine
  Residency Program
UMass Memorial Health Alliance Hospital
Academic Hospital Medicine
UMass Memorial Medical Group
Leominster, Massachusetts

Jennifer G. Chang, MD[†]
Family Medicine Faculty Physician
Ehrling Bergquist Family Medicine
  Residency Clinic
Offutt Air Force Base, Nebraska

Joann Y. Chang, MD
Resident Physician
Memorial Family Medicine
Long Beach Memorial Medical Center
Long Beach, California

Millicent King Channell, DO, MA, FAAO
Associate Professor
Departments of Family Medicine and
  Osteopathic Manipulative Medicine
Rowan University School of Osteopathic
  Medicine
Stratford, New Jersey

Jason Chao, MD, MS
Professor
Department of Family Medicine &
  Community Health
University Hospitals Case Medical Center
Case Western Reserve University
Cleveland, Ohio

Arka Chatterjee, MD[†]
Chief Fellow
Division of Cardiovascular Disease
University of Alabama at Birmingham
Birmingham, Alabama

Sarah H. Cheeseman, MD[†]
Professor of Medicine, Pediatrics,
  and Microbiology and Physiological
  Systems
University of Massachusetts Medical
  School
Division of Infectious Diseases and
  Immunology
UMass Memorial Medical Center
Worcester, Massachusetts

Amy Chen, MD, PhD
Assistant Professor
Department of Neurology
University of Rochester
Rochester, New York

Anthony M. Cheng, MD
Resident Physician
Department of Family Medicine
Oregon Health & Science University
Portland, Oregon

Moses H. Cheng, MAJ, MC, USA[†]
Department of Family Medicine
Naval Hospital Camp Pendleton
Camp Pendleton, California

Suma Chennubhotla, MD
Department of Internal Medicine
University of Louisville
Louisville, Kentucky

Karina I. Chiari, MD
Resident
Creighton University Medical Center
Omaha, Nebraska

Sonia Nagy Chimienti, MD[†]
Associate Dean for Student Affairs
Clinical Associate Professor
Department of Medicine, Division of
  Infectious Diseases
University of Massachusetts Medical
  School
Worcester, Massachusetts

Shideh Chinichian, MD[†]
Resident
Dignity Health Methodist Hospital of
  Sacramento
Sacramento, California

Alia Chisty, MD, MS, FACP[†]
Assistant Professor
Lewis Katz School of Medicine at
  Temple University
Philadelphia, Pennsylvania

Tayseer Husain Chowdhry, MD, MA
General Surgery Resident
Department of Surgery
Georgia Regents University
Augusta, Georgia

Vasilios Chrisostomidis, DO
Assistant Professor
Department of Family Medicine and
  Community Health
University of Massachusetts Medical
  School
Worcester, Massachusetts

Felicia Chu, MD
Assistant Professor
Department of Neurology
University of Massachusetts Medical
    School
Worcester, Massachusetts

Annise Chung, DO
Resident
Philadelphia College of Osteopathic
    Medicine
Philadelphia, Pennsylvania

Peter I. Chung, MD
Resident
Department of Internal Medicine
University of Massachusetts Medical Center
North Worcester, Massachusetts

Lee T. Church, MD[†]
Nellis Air Force Base
Las Vegas, Nevada

Brian Ciampa, MD
Gastroenterology Fellow
Department of Gastroenterology
George Washington University Hospital
Washington, DC

Daniel A. Cieslak, MD[†]
Resident Physician
Nellis Family Medicine Residency
Mike O'Callaghan Federal Medical Center
Nellis Air Force Base
Las Vegas, Nevada

S. Lindsey Clarke, MD, FAAFP
Medical University of South Carolina
    Area Health Education Consortium
    Professor—Greenwood/Family
    Medicine
Self Regional Healthcare Family
    Medicine Residency Program
Greenwood, South Carolina

Roselyn Jan Wuthrich Clemente-
    Fuentes, MD[†]
Faculty
Family Medicine Residency
Eglin Air Force Base
Valparaiso, Florida

Lisa Clemons, MD
Blackstock Family Health Center
Austin, Texas

David M. Clive, MD
Professor of Medicine
Department of Medicine
University of Massachusetts Medical
    School
Worcester, Massachusetts

Kara M. Coassolo, MD
Clinical Associate Professor
University of South Florida
Morsani College of Medicine
Tampa, Florida
Department of Obstetrics and
    Gynecology
Division of Maternal-Fetal Medicine
Lehigh Valley Health Network
Allentown, Pennsylvania

Jason E. Cohn, DO, MS[†]
Resident Physician
Department of Otolaryngology–Facial
    Plastic Surgery
Philadelphia College of Osteopathic
    Medicine
Philadelphia, Pennsylvania

Caroline A. Coicou, MD
Clinical Assistant Instructor
Department of Family Medicine
SUNY Downstate Medical Center
Brooklyn, New York

Timothy J. Coker, MD[†]
Assistant Program Director
Ehrling Bergquist Family Medicine
    Residency Program
Offutt Air Force Base, Nebraska

Brian R. Coleman, MD
Associate Professor
Department of Family Medicine
University of Oklahoma
Oklahoma City, Oklahoma

Sarah Coles, MD
Clinical Educator
Family Medicine Residency
Banner University Medical Center
Director of Longitudinal Patient Care
    Course
Department of Family, Community and
    Preventive Medicine
University of Arizona College of
    Medicine—Phoenix
Phoenix, Arizona

Irene C. Coletsos, MD
Associate Professor of Psychiatry
University of Massachusetts Medical School
Worcester, Massachusetts

Rebecca Collins, DO, MPH, FAAFP
Medical Director, Core Faculty, and
    Assistant Professor
NYMC Phelps Family Medicine
    Residency Program
New York Medical College
Sleepy Hollow, New York

Miguel Concepcion, MD[†]
Clinical Instructor
Tufts School of Medicine
Department of Family Medicine
Carney Hospital
Boston, Massachusetts

Stephen J. Conner, MD[†]
Chief of Family Medicine Maternal-
    Newborn Service
Dwight D. Eisenhower Army Medical
    Center
Fort Gordon, Georgia

Stephanie L. Conway, PharmD, RPh
Assistant Professor of Pharmacy Practice
Massachusetts College of Pharmacy and
    Health Sciences University
Worcester, Massachusetts

Stephen L. Cook, MD[†]
Resident Physician
Nellis Family Medicine Residency
Mike O'Callaghan Federal Medical Center
Las Vegas, Nevada

Anna Cooley, MD
UMass Memorial Children's Medical
    Center
Worcester, Massachusetts

Bryce L. Coombs, DO[†]
Resident Physician
Nellis Family Medicine Residency
Nellis Air Force Base
Las Vegas, Nevada

Maryann R. Cooper, PharmD, BCOP
Assistant Professor of Pharmacy Practice
Massachusetts College of Pharmacy and
    Health Sciences University
Manchester, New Hampshire

Jennifer M. Cornwell, DO[†]
Resident
Department of Family Medicine
    Residency
Martin Army Community Hospital
Fort Benning, Georgia

Macario C. Corpuz, MD, MBA, FAAFP
Medical Staff
St. Vincent Medical Group
Worcester, Massachusetts

Mathew J. Cosenza, DO, RPh
Adena ENT and Allergy
Adena Regional Medical Center
Chillicothe, Ohio

Erica F. Crannage, PharmD, BCPS, BCACP
Assistant Professor
Department of Pharmacy Practice
St. Louis College of Pharmacy
St. Louis, Missouri

Nathaniel D. Cranney, DO
Resident
Family Medicine Residency Program
Carl R. Darnalll Army Medical Center
Fort Hood, Texas

Paul Crawford, MD[†]
Program Director
Nellis Family Medicine Residency
Nellis Air Force Base
Las Vegas, Nevada

Dustin Creech, MD
Air Force Medicine-Scott
Belleville Family Medicine Clinic
Belleville, Illinois

Alan Cropp, MD, FCCP
Department of Pulmonary Medicine
St. Elizabeth Hospital Health Center
Youngstown, Ohio

Steven J. Crosby, MA, BSP, RPh, FASCP
Assistant Professor of Pharmacy Practice
Massachusetts College of Pharmacy and Health Sciences University
Boston, Massachusetts

Jason E. Cross, PharmD[†]
Associate Professor of Pharmacy Practice
Massachusetts College of Pharmacy and Health Sciences University
Worcester, Massachusetts
Assistant Director
Pharmacy Residency
Baystate Health Medical Center
Springfield, Massachusetts

Mary Anne de la Cruz Estacio, DO
Family Medicine Resident
University of Texas Health Science Center at San Antonio
San Antonio, Texas

Hongyi Cui, MD, PhD
Assistant Professor of Surgery
Associate Director, Acute Care Surgery
Department of Genera and Laparoscopic Surgery
University of Massachusetts Medical School
UMass Memorial Medical Center
Worcester, Massachusetts

Emily M. Culliney, MD, FAAFP[†]
Assistant Professor and Staff Physician
Family Medicine Residency
Mike O'Callaghan Federal Medical Center
Nellis Air Force Base
Las Vegas, Nevada

Luma Dababneh, MD
Family Practice Resident
Department of Family Medicine
Summa Barberton Hospital
Barberton, Ohio

William Dabbs, MD
Clinical Educator
Family Medicine
Banner Good Samaritan Family Medicine Residency
Phoenix, Arizona

Heather A. Dalton, MD[†]
Family Medicine Resident
David Grant Medical Center
Travis Air Force Base, California

Anthony Dambro, MD[†]
Assistant Program Director
Camp Lejeune Family Medicine Residency
Naval Hospital Camp Lejeune
Camp Lejeune, North Carolina

Joanne Dannenhoffer, MD
Resident
University of Massachusetts Medical School
Worcester, Massachusetts

Lisa M. Dapuzzo, MD[†]
Obstetrician-Gynecologist
Lehigh Valley Health Network
Clinical Assistant Professor
University of South Florida
Morsani College of Medicine
Allentown, Pennsylvania

Daniela Darrah, MD
Associate Professor
Department of Anesthesiology
Division of Critical Care Anesthesiology
Columbia University Medical Center
New York, New York

Akhil Das, MD, FACS
Assistant Professor
Department of Urology
Thomas Jefferson University
Philadelphia, Pennsylvania

Amy M. Davis, MD[†]
Associate Program Director
Family Medicine Residency Program
David Grant Medical Center
Travis Air Force Base, California

Jessica Davis, MD
Assistant Clinical Professor of Medicine
Department of Internal Medicine
George Washington University
Washington, DC

Oksana Davydov, MD
Assistant Professor of Medicine
Department of Endocrinology and Metabolism
Mount Sinai St. Luke's Roosevelt Hospital
New York, New York

Courtney Dawley, DO
Department of Adult Medicine/Family Medicine
Vacaville Medical Center
Vacaville, California

Robert C. Day, MD
Obstetrics and Gynecology
Kaiser Permanente
Santa Clara, California

Sondra M. De Antonio, MD
Adjunct Assistant Professor
Department of Internal Medicine
Rowan University School of Osteopathic Medicine
Stratford, New Jersey

Garreth C. Debiegun, MD, FACEP, FAWM
Clinical Assistant Professor
Department of Emergency Medicine
Maine Medical Center
Tufts University School of Medicine
Portland, Maine

Alec DeCastro, MD
Director of Trident Family Medicine Residency Program
Chief of Primary Care Sports Medicine
Department of Family Medicine
Medical University of South Carolina
Charleston, South Carolina

Alexei DeCastro, MD
Assistant Professor
CAQ Sports Medicine
Department of Family Medicine/Sports Medicine
Medical University of South Carolina
Charleston, North Carolina

Danielle Defoe, MS, DO
New York Institute of Technology College of Osteopathic Medicine
Old Westbury, New York

Jeremy D. DeFoe, DO[†]
Resident
Department of Family Medicine
Dwight D. Eisenhower Army Medical
    Center
Fort Gordon, Georgia

Konstantinos E. Deligiannidis, MD, MPH,
    FAAFP
Assistant Professor
Department of Family Medicine and
    Community Health
University of Massachusetts Medical
    School
Worcester, Massachusetts

John Delzell, Jr., MD, MSPH
Herbert Wertheim College of Medicine
Florida International University
Miami, Florida

Deborah M. DeMarco, MD, FACP[†]
Senior Associate Dean of Clinical
    Affairs
Associate Dean of Graduate Medical
    Education
Professor of Medicine
Division of Rheumatology
University of Massachusetts Medical
    School
Worcester, Massachusetts

LeeAnne Denny, MD
Clinical Educator
Banner Good Samaritan Hospital
Phoenix, Arizona

David DeNofrio, MD
Associate Professor of Medicine
Department of Medicine
Tufts University School of Medicine
Boston, Massachusetts

Richard F. DeSouza, MD
Clinical Instructor of Medicine
Yale School of Medicine
Attending Physician/Hospitalist
Yale-New Haven Hospital
New Haven, Connecticut

Sara M. DeSpain, MD[†]
Chief Resident
Family Medicine Residency
Offutt Air Force Base
University of Nebraska Medical Center
Omaha, Nebraska

Richard D. Detheridge, MD[†]
Staff Provider
Brian Allgood Army Community Hospital
U.S. Army MEDDAC-Korea

Mathew J. Devine, DO[†]
Associate Medical Director and Assistant
    Professor
Department of Family Medicine
University of Rochester
Rochester, New York

William W. Dexter, MD, FACSM
Sports Medicine Program
Maine Medical Center
Portland, Maine

Lisa M. Diaz, DO
Osteopathic Physician
South Miami, Florida

Michelle DiBetta, MD[†]
Family Medicine Resident
Bayfront Family Health Center
St. Petersburg, Florida

Daniel R. DiBlasi, DO[†]
Flight Surgeon
Department of Primary Care
Evans Army Community Hospital
Fort Carson, Colorado

Howard Dickey-White, MD, FACEP
Chief Medical Officer
4M Medical Management
Akron, Ohio

Caleb Dickison, DO
Family Medicine Residency
Carl R. Darnall Army Medical Center
Fort Hood, Texas

Aimee L. Dietle, PharmD
Assistant Professor of Pharmacy Practice
Massachusetts College of Pharmacy and
    Health Sciences University
Worcester, Massachusetts

Michael Dietz, DO
HealthSource of Ohio
New Richmond, Ohio

Mary DiGiulio, DO[†]
Family Medicine Residency Program
Dwight D. Eisenhower Army Medical
    Center
Fort Gordon, Georgia

Robert J. Dimeff, MD
Professor of Orthopedic Surgery and
    Family & Community Medicine
Medical Director of Sports Medicine
University of Texas Southwestern Medical
    Center
Dallas, Texas

John M. Doan, DO
Traditional Rotating Intern
St. Petersburg General Hospital
St. Petersburg, Florida

Jason E. Domagalski, MD, FAAFP
Assistant Professor and Associate
    Program Director
Family Medicine Residency
University of California Riverside
Palm Springs, California

Rebecca S. Domalski, DO
New York Institute of Technology College
    of Osteopathic Medicine
Old Westbury, New York

Frank J. Domino, MD
Professor and Director of Predoctoral
    Education
Department of Family Medicine and
    Community Health
University of Massachusetts Medical School
Worcester, Massachusetts

Kathleen M. Donahue, DO[†]
Department of Family Medicine-
    Obstetrics
Naval Hospital Camp Lejeune
Camp Lejeune, North Carolina

Tammy Donoway, DO, FAAFP[†]
Assistant Residency Program Director
Department of Family Medicine
Womack Army Medical Center
Fort Bragg, North Carolina

Kristin D'Orsi, DO
Resident Physician
Department of Obstetrics and Gynecology
University of Massachusetts Medical School
Worcester, Massachusetts

Hobie Dotson, PsyD
Clinical Psychologist and Assistant
    Professor
Department of Family and Community
    Medicine
North Fork Valley Community Health Center
University of Kentucky
Hazard, Kentucky

Mark S. Douglas, MD, FAAD[†]
Staff Dermatologist
Naval Hospital Jacksonville
Jacksonville, Florida

Drew-Anne Drapala, MD
Resident Physician
Methodist Hospital Family Medicine
    Residency
Sacramento, California

Scott A. Drummond, Jr., DO, DABR[†]
Chief of Radiology
Bassett Army Community Hospital
Fort Wainwright, Alaska

Anahita Dua, MD
Postdoctoral Fellow
Center for Translational Injury Research
Houston, Texas

Nerissa P. Duchin, MD
Resident in Psychiatry
Harvard Longwood Psychiatry Residency
    Training Program
Boston, Massachusetts

Maurice Duggins, MD
Clinical Associate Professor
Department of Family and Community
    Medicine
Kansas University School of Medicine–
    Wichita
Associate Director, Via Christi Family
    Medicine Residency Program
Wichita, Kansas

Kaelen C. Dunican, PharmD
Associate Professor
Department of Pharmacy Practice
Massachusetts College of Pharmacy and
    Health Sciences University
Worcester, Massachusetts

Noel Dunn, MD[†]
Family Medicine Resident
Madigan Army Medical Center
Tacoma, Washington

Maegen Dupper, MD
Assistant Clinical Professor
Department of Family Medicine
University of California, Riverside
Riverside, California

Cheryl Durand, PharmD
Associate Professor of Pharmacy Practice
Massachusetts College of Pharmacy and
    Health Sciences University
Worcester, Massachusetts/Manchester,
    New Hampshire

Amber Durani, PA
Physician Assistant
Plano, Texas

William Jerry Durbin, MD
Professor of Pediatrics and Internal
    Medicine
University of Massachusetts Medical School
Worcester, Massachusetts

Allison Durica, MD
Medical Director of Outpatient Resident
    High Risk Obstetrics & Gynecology
    Clinic
Chief, Division of Maternal-Fetal Medicine
Assistant Professor, Obstetrics and
    Gynecology
Carilion Clinic Obstetrics & Gynecology
Clinical Faculty, Carilion Clinic Maternal
    Fetal Medicine
Carilion Clinic
Virginia Tech Carilion School of Medicine
Roanoke, Virginia

Virginia Van Duyne, MD
Assistant Professor
Associate Residency Director of
    Women's Health Education
Department of Family Medicine and
    Community Health
University of Massachusetts Worcester
    Family Medicine Residency Program
Family Health Center of Worcester
Worcester, Massachusetts

Danielle M. Eagan, DO, RD, LSN
Internal Medicine Resident
Southeastern Health
Lumberton, North Carolina

John Scott Earwood, MD[†]
Associate Professor of Family Medicine
Department of Family and Community
    Medicine
Dwight D. Eisenhower Army Medical
    Center
Fort Gordon, Georgia

Joshua L. Eaton, MD, FAWM[†]
Staff Physician
Eglin Family Medicine Residency
Eglin Air Force Base
Valparaiso, Florida

Phillip Marks Ecker, MD
Dermatologist
Minnesota Dermatology, PA
Plymouth, Minnesota

Samuel Ecker, DO
Dermatology Resident
Larkin Community Hospital
Miami, Florida

Elizabeth A. Egitto, DO[†]
Resident
Dwight D. Eisenhower Army Medical
    Center
Fort Gordon, Georgia

Alan M. Ehrlich, MD
Assistant Professor of Family Medicine
University of Massachusetts Medical School
Worcester, Massachusetts

Jordan Eisenstock, MD
Departments of Neurology and
    Psychiatry
University of Massachusetts Memorial
    Healthcare
Assistant Professor
University of Massachusetts Medical School
Director of Neurorehabilitation
Fairlawn Rehabilitation Hospital
Worcester, Massachusetts

William G. Elder, PhD
Professor
Family and Community Medicine
University of Kentucky
Lexington, Kentucky

Erynn E. Elleby, MD
Family Medicine Resident
Saint Louis University Family Medicine
    Residency Program
Belleville, Illinois

Taiwona Elliot, DO[†]
Director of Osteopathic Student Medical
    Education
Osteopathic Program Director
Southern Regional Area Health
    Education Center
Fayetteville, North Carolina

Carrie Lynn Ellis, DVM, MS
Associate Veterinarian
Animal Hospital on Mt. Lookout Square
Cincinnati, Ohio

Robert Ellis, MD
Associate Professor
Department of Family and Community
    Medicine
University of Cincinnati
Cincinnati, Ohio

Pamela Ellsworth, MD
Professor of Urology
Chief of Division of Pediatric Urology
Vice-Chairman of Department of Urology
UMass Memorial Medical Center
University of Massachusetts Medical
    School
Worcester, Massachusetts

Christina Emanuel, MD
Resident
Summa Akron City Hospital
Akron, Ohio

Todd J. Endicott, DO[†]
Comprehensive Ophthalmologist
Naval Hospital Jacksonville
Jacksonville, Florida

Lauren Engelmann, MD
Chief Resident in Family Medicine
Dell Medical School, University of Texas
    at Austin
Austin, Texas

Katelin Engerer, MD
Resident
Dartmouth-Hitchcock Medical Center
Lebanon, New Hampshire

Deborah R. Erlich, MD, MMedEd
Assistant Clerkship Director
Department of Family Medicine
Tufts University School of Medicine
Boston, Massachusetts

Justin Thomas Ertle, BS, MD
Internal Medicine
George Washington University
Washington, DC

Alicia D. Evans, MD[†]
Family Medicine Resident
Dwight D. Eisenhower Army Medical
    Center
Fort Gordon, Georgia

Emily Evans-Hoeker, MD
Assistant Professor of Obstetrics and
    Gynecology
Virginia Tech Carilion School of Medicine
Physician, Reproductive Endocrinology
    and Infertility
Department of Obstetrics and
    Gynecology
Carilion Clinic
Adjunct Assistant Professor
Reproductive Endocrinology and Infertility
Department of Obstetrics and
    Gynecology
University of North Carolina
Roanoke, Virginia

John T. Ewing, DO[†]
Faculty Physician
Department of Family Medicine
Naval Hospital Camp Lejeune
Camp Lejeune, North Carolina

William A. Fabricius, MD[†]
Hematology-Oncology Fellow
Division of Hematology and Oncology
Department of Medicine
University of Massachusetts Medical School
Worcester, Massachusetts

Stephen C. Fabry, MD
Lahey Hospital & Medical Center
Burlington, Massachusetts
Associate Clinical Professor of Medicine
Tufts University School of Medicine
Boston, Massachusetts

Margaret Fairhurst, DO
Internal Medicine Resident
University Hospitals–Regional Medical
    Center
Richmond Heights, Ohio

Pang-Yen Fan, MD
Professor of Medicine
Division of Renal Medicine
University of Massachusetts Medical School
Worcester, Massachusetts

John P. Fardal, DO
Resident
University of Texas Austin DMS Family
    Medicine Residency Program
Austin, Texas

Matthew V. Fargo, MD, MPH[†]
Director
Family Medicine Residency Program
Dwight D. Eisenhower Army Medical
    Center
Fort Gordon, Georgia

William Farkas, DO, CPT, MC, USA[†]
Resident Physician
Womack Family Medicine Residency
    Center
Fort Bragg, North Carolina

Kara C. Farley, MD[†]
Family Medicine Residency Program
Naval Hospital Jacksonville
Jacksonville, Florida

Edwin A. Farnell, IV, MD[†]
Associate Program Director
Family Medicine Residency
Dwight D. Eisenhower Army Medical
    Center
Fort Gordon, Georgia

Geoffrey Strider Farnsworth, MD[†]
Flight Physician
Mike O'Callaghan Federal Medical Center
Las Vegas, Nevada

Umer Farooq, MD, MBBS[†]
Addiction Psychiatrist
Clinical Assistant Professor
Michigan College of Human Medicine
Grand Rapids, Michigan

Olusola Fasusi, MD
Categorical Surgery Resident
Georgia Regents University
Augusta, Georgia

Rhonda A. Faulkner, PhD
Director of Behavioral Medicine
Department of Family Medicine
Saint Joseph Hospital
University of Illinois at Chicago Master
    Affiliate
Chicago, Illinois

Kinder K. Fayssoux, MD[†]
Core Faculty
Eisenhower Family Medicine Residency
    Program
La Quinta, California

Jeffrey P. Feden, MD, FACEP
Assistant Professor
Department of Emergency Medicine
The Warren Alpert Medical School of
    Brown University
Providence, Rhode Island

Ryan B. Feeney, PharmD[†]
Pharmacy Practice Resident
Department of Pharmacy Services
Temple University Hospital
Philadelphia, Pennsylvania

Neil J. Feldman, DPM, FACFAS
Owner
Central Massachusetts Podiatry, PC
Worcester, Massachusetts

Edward Feller, MD, FACP, FACG
Clinical Professor of Medicine and Health
    Service, Policy and Practice
The Warren Alpert Medical School of
    Brown University
Providence, Rhode Island

Chris-Gerald Ferguson, MD[†]
Resident
Department of Family Medicine
SUNY Downstate Medical Center
Brooklyn, New York

Kathleen Ferrer, MD, AAHIVS
Assistant Professor of Pediatrics
Division of Infectious Disease, Special
    Immunology Section
Division of Hospitalist Medicine
Children's National Health System
George Washington University School of
    Medicine
Washington, DC

William Fiden, MD[†]
Family Medicine Residency
Patient Centered Medical Home
Womack Army Medical Center
Fort Bragg, North Carolina

Andreas Filippaios, MD[†]
Internal Medicine Resident
Department of Internal Medicine
Lahey Hospital & Medical Center
Burlington, Massachusetts

Sara J. Fine, MD
University of Massachusetts Medical School
Worcester, Massachusetts

Stanley Fineman, MD
Adjunct Associate Professor of Pediatrics
Atlanta Allergy & Asthma
Emory University School of Medicine
Atlanta, Georgia

Jonathon M. Firnhaber, MD
Associate Professor
Department of Family Medicine
Brody School of Medicine at East
  Carolina University
Greenville, North Carolina

Casey Fisher, DO
Philadelphia College of Osteopathic
  Medicine
Philadelphia, Pennsylvania

Daniel J. Fisher, MD
Assistant Director
Community East Family Medicine
  Residency
Indianapolis, Indiana

Timothy P. Fitzgibbons, MD, PhD
Assistant Professor of Medicine
Cardiovascular Division
University of Massachusetts Medical
  School
Worcester, Massachusetts

Theodore B. Flaum, DO, FACOFP[†]
Assistant Professor
Department of Osteopathic Manipulative
  Medicine
New York Institute of Technology College
  of Osteopathic Medicine
Old Westbury, New York

Joseph A. Florence, MD[†]
Professor
Director of Rural Programs
East Tennessee State University
James H. Quillen College of Medicine
Johnson City, Tennessee

Emily K. Flores, PharmD, BCPS
Associate Professor of Pharmacy
  Practice
Bill Gatton College of Pharmacy
Adjunct Faculty
Department of Family Medicine
James H. Quillen College of Medicine
East Tennessee State University
Johnson City, Tennessee

Kendra Flores, MS, CGC
Licensed Genetic Counselor
Division of Genetics
Clinical Instructor of Pediatrics
Department of Pediatrics
University of Massachusetts Medical
  School
Worcester, Massachusetts

Harry W. Flynn, Jr., MD
Bascom Palmer Eye Institute
Miami, Florida

Jay Fong, MD
Assistant Professor
Department of Pediatrics
University of Massachusetts Medical
  Center
Worcester, Massachusetts

Joao C.S. Fontoura, Jr., MD
Resident Physician
Internal Medicine and Pediatrics
University of South Florida
Tampa, Florida

William Fosmire, MD
Medical Director
Bruner Family Medicine Center
Saint Joseph Family Medicine Residency
Denver, Colorado

Phillip Fournier, MD[†]
Clinical Professor of Family Medicine and
  Community Health
University of Massachusetts Medical
  School
Worcester, Massachusetts

Robert L. Frachtman, MD, FACG
Austin Gastroenterology, PA
Austin, Texas

Mony Fraer, MD, FACP, FASN
Assistant Professor
Internal Medicine and Nephrology
University of Iowa Hospital and Clinics
Iowa City, Iowa

C. Jack Fraim, MD
Assistant Professor
Department of Neurology
Dell Medical School, University of Texas
  at Austin
Austin, Texas

Brian Frank, MD
Assistant Professor
Family Medicine
Oregon Health and Science University
Portland, Oregon

Jason K. Frankel, MD
Resident Physician
Division of Urology
University of Connecticut Health Center
Farmington, Connecticut

Charles Fredericks, MD
Surgical Resident
Department of General Surgery
Rush University Medical School
Chicago, Illinois

Minjin Fromm, MD[†]
Assistant Professor
Department of Orthopedics and Physical
  Rehabilitation
University of Massachusetts Medical
  School
Worcester, Massachusetts

Melissa J. Fullerton, MD
Assistant Professor
Department of Family Medicine
University of Virginia Health System
Charlottesville, Virginia

Noah D. Futterman, DO[†]
Emergency Medicine Resident
Department of Emergency Medicine
Rutgers-Robert Wood Johnson Medical
  School
New Brunswick, New Jersey

Heidi L. Gaddey, MD[†]
Program Director
Family Medicine Residency
Ehrling Bergquist Clinic
Offutt Air Force Base, Nebraska

Steven W. Gale, MD[†]
Family Medicine Resident
Offutt Air Force Base
University of Nebraska Medical Center
Omaha, Nebraska

Rodolfo J. Galindo, MD
Assistant Professor of Medicine
Division of Endocrinology, Diabetes and
   Bone Diseases
Icahn School of Medicine at Mount Sinai
New York, New York

Curtis L. Galke, DO
Assistant Professor
Family and Community Medicine
The University of Texas Health Science
   Center at San Antonio
Associate Program Director, Family
   Medicine Residency
University of Texas Health Science
   Center at Antonio-Rio Grande Valley-
   Doctors Hospital at Renaissance
Edinburg, Texas

Sumanth Gandra, MD, MPH
Postdoctoral Fellow
Center for Disease Dynamics, Economics
   & Policy
Washington, DC

Jennifer J. Gao, MD[†]
Medical Oncology Fellow
National Cancer Institute
National Institutes of Health
Bethesda, Maryland

Andrew Gara, MD
University of Massachusetts Medical
   School
Worcester, Massachusetts

Luis T. Garcia, MD
Program Director
Family Medicine Residency
Presence Saint Joseph Hospital
Chicago, Illinois

Bruce Jay Gardner, MD[†]
Assistant Professor of Family Medicine
Department of Family and Community
   Medicine
Saint Louis University School of Medicine
St. Louis, Missouri

Thomas P. Garigan, MD, MA[†]
Faculty
Family Medicine Residency
Department of Family and Community
   Medicine
Dwight D. Eisenhower Army Medical
   Center
Fort Gordon, Georgia

William T. Garrison, PhD[†]
Professor of Pediatrics
University of Massachusetts Medical
   School
Worcester, Massachusetts

Anette Galang Gawelko, DO[†]
Clinical Assistant Professor of Clinical
   Education
Department of Family Medicine
Arizona College of Osteopathic Medicine,
   Midwestern University
Glendale, Arizona

Gerald Gehr, MD
Assistant Professor of Medicine
Dartmouth Medical School
Hanover, New Hampshire

Felix Geissler, MD, PhD
Vice-President, Regional Medical Officer
   for JPAC
Medical Affairs Sanofi KK
Tokyo, Japan

Barry C. Gentry, MD[†]
Naval Hospital Camp Lejeune
Camp Lejeune, North Carolina

Shari L. Gentry, MD[†]
Naval Hospital Camp Lejeune
Camp Lejeune, North Carolina

Paul George, MD, MHPE
Associate Professor of Family
   Medicine
Director of the Year II Curriculum and
   Primary Care-Population Medicine
   Program
The Warren Alpert Medical School of
   Brown University
Providence, Rhode Island

Travis C. Geraci, MD[†]
General Surgery Resident
The Warren Alpert Medical School of
   Brown University
Providence, Rhode Island

Fereshteh Gerayli, MD, FAAFP
Professor, Family Medicine
Johnson City Family Medicine Residency
   Program
East Tennessee State University
James H. Quillen College of Medicine
Johnson City, Tennessee

Tiana M. Germann, MD
Resident Physician
Department of Family Medicine
SUNY at Stony Brook
Stony Brook, New York

Amaninderapal S. Ghotra, MD
Department of Internal Medicine
Division of General Internal Medicine
Palliative Medicine and Medical
   Education
University of Louisville
Louisville, Kentucky

Lawrence M. Gibbs, MD, MSEd[†]
Assistant Professor
Family Medicine Residency Program
Scott Air Force Base
Saint Louis University
Belleville, Illinois

Jonathan Giordano, DO, MSc
Department of Emergency Medicine
Maimonides Medical Center
Brooklyn, New York

Joseph Gladwell, MD
Family Medicine Resident
OhioHealth Riverside Methodist Hospital
Columbus, Ohio

Gerald Gleich, MD
Adjunct Professor of Internal Medicine
   and Pediatrics
Research Professor of Dermatology
University of Utah
Salt Lake City, Utah

Cody B. Godfrey, DO
Resident Physician
University Medical Center Brackenridge
Austin, Texas

Ankur Goel, MD
Department of General Surgery
Georgia Regents University
Augusta, Georgia

Sujan Gogu, DO[†]
Resident
Department of Family Medicine
University of Texas Health Science
   Center at San Antonio
San Antonio, Texas

Jeremy Golding, MD, FAAFP
Professor of Family Medicine and
    Obstetrics & Gynecology
University of Massachusetts Medical
    School
Quality Officer
Department of Family Medicine and
    Community Health
University of Massachusetts Memorial
    Health Care
Hahnemann Family Health Center
Worcester, Massachusetts

Rayna Goldstein, MD
Mount Sinai Hospital
New York, New York

Walter K. Goljan, MD
Webster Square Medical Center
Worcester, Massachusetts

Mercedes E. Gonzalez, MD, FAAD
Pediatric Dermatology of Miami
Miami, Florida

Herbert P. Goodheart, MD[†]
Associate Clinical Professor
Department of Dermatology
Mount Sinai College of Medicine in
    New York City
New York, New York
Director of Dermatology
Elmhurst Hospital Center
Queens, New York

Geetha Gopalakrishnan, MD
Director
Hallett Center of Diabetes and
    Endocrinology
East Providence, Rhode Island
Associate Professor of Medicine
The Warren Alpert Medical School of
    Brown University
Providence, Rhode Island

Dónal Kevin Gordon, MD
Residency Program Director
Cedar Rapids Family Medicine
    Residency
Cedar Rapids, Iowa

Fredric D. Gordon, MD, AGAF
Associate Professor of Medicine
Tufts University School of Medicine
Director of Hepatology
Lahey Hospital & Medical Center
Burlington, Massachusetts

Edward A. Gotfried, DO, FACOS[†]
Director
New York Institute of Technology Center
    for Global Health
Associate Professor
Department of Osteopathic Manipulative
    Medicine
New York Institute of Technology College
    of Osteopathic Medicine
Old Westbury, New York

Parag Goyal, MD
Division of Cardiology
Department of Medicine
New York Presbyterian Hospital
Weill Cornell Medical Center
New York, New York

Shami Goyal, MD
University of Pittsburgh Physicians
Department of Family Medicine
University of Pittsburgh Medical Center
    Matilda Theiss Health Center
Pittsburgh, Pennsylvania

Jane M. Grant-Kels, MD
Professor of Dermatology, Pathology, and
    Pediatrics
Chairman of Department of Dermatology
Director of Dermatopathology
Director of the Cutaneous Oncology
    Program and Melanoma Center
Dermatology Residency Director
Assistant Dean of Clinical Affairs
University of Connecticut Health Center
Farmington, Connecticut

Anthony W. Gray, Jr., MD[†]
Associate Professor of Medicine
Tufts University School of Medicine
Pulmonary and Critical Care Medicine
Lahey Hospital & Medical Center
Burlington, Massachusetts

Meredith Gray, MD
Resident
Department of Obstetrics and
    Gynecology
Virginia Tech Carilion
Roanoke, Virginia

Michael J. Gray, MD, MA, MS, ATC
Attending Physician
Emergency Care Center
Harrington Hospital
Southbridge, Massachusetts

Robert H. Gray, MD, MS[†]
Resident
Family Medicine Residency
Eglin Air Force Base, Florida

Whitney A. Gray, CRNP[†]
Adult/Gerontology Nurse Practitioner
Division of Gerontology, Geriatrics and
    Palliative Care
University of Alabama at Birmingham
    Hospital
Birmingham, Alabama

Jonathan Green, MD
General Surgery Resident
Department of General Surgery
University of Massachusetts Medical
    School
Worcester, Massachusetts

Ellen M. Greenblatt, BSc, MDCM
Medical Director
Centre for Fertility and Reproductive
    Health
Mount Sinai Hospital
Associate Professor
University of Toronto
Toronto, Ontario, Canada

David A. Greenwald, MD
Associate Division Director
Division of Gastroenterology
Montefiore Medical Center
Professor of Clinical Medicine
Albert Einstein College of Medicine
Bronx, New York

Heather O'Connor Greer, MD
Assistant Professor
Department of Obstetrics and
    Gynecology
Carilion Clinic
Roanoke, Virginia

Simon B. Griesbach, MD
Instructor
Department of Family and Community
    Medicine
Medical College of Wisconsin
Milwaukee, Wisconsin

Charles K. Grigsby, MD
Resident, Surgery
Georgia Regents University
Augusta, Georgia

Andrew Grimes, MD
Medical Director
Capitol Anesthesiology Association
Austin, Texas

Jill Ann Grimes, MD
UHS Urgent Care Physician
University of Texas at Austin
Austin, Texas
Clinical Instructor
Department of Family Medicine and
    Community Health
University of Massachusetts Medical
    School
Worcester, Massachusetts

Kristin Grindstaff, DO
Family Medicine Residency
Community Health Network
Indianapolis, Indiana

Matthew K. Griswold, MD
Fellow in Medical Toxicology
Division of Medical Toxicology
Department of Emergency Medicine
University of Massachusetts Medical School
Worcester, Massachusetts

Scott P. Grogan, DO, MBA, FAAFP[†]
Associate Residency Director
Family Medicine Residency Program
Dwight D. Eisenhower Army Medical
    Center
Fort Gordon, Georgia

Janet Grotticelli, DO, MBA, CHSE[†]
Clinical Assistant Professor
Department of Primary Care
Director of Medical Simulation
Primary Care Skills & OSCE
Touro College of Osteopathic Medicine
New York, New York

Alma M. Guerrero, MD
Resident in Internal Medicine
Department of Medicine
Brown University
Providence, Rhode Island

John A. Guisto, MD, FACEP
Professor of Emergency Medicine
Department of Emergency Medicine
University of Arizona College of Medicine
Tucson, Arizona

Neena R. Gupta, MD[†]
Medical Director and Assistant Professor
Pediatric Kidney Transplant Program
Department of Pediatrics Division of
    Pediatric Nephrology
University of Massachusetts Medical
    School
UMass Memorial Children's Medical
    Center
Worcester, Massachusetts

Sergey G. Gurevich, MD
Internal Medicine Resident
New York Presbyterian Hospital
Weill Cornell Medical College
New York, New York

Emily E. Gutgsell, MD
Family Medicine Resident
Rose Family Medicine Residency
Denver, Colorado

Reem Hadi, MD
Family Medicine
The University of Texas Health Science
    Center at San Antonio
San Antonio, Texas

David Haight, MD[†]
Fort Campbell, Kentucky

Ildiko Halasz, MD
VA Boston Healthcare System
Primary Care Clinic
West Roxbury, Maryland

P. Benson Ham, III, MD, MS
General Surgery Resident
Department of Surgery
Georgia Regents University
Augusta, Georgia

Shadi Hamdeh, MD
Department of Internal Medicine
Creighton University School of Medicine
Omaha, Nebraska

Jennifer L. Hamilton, MD, PhD, FAAFP
Assistant Professor
Department of Family, Community, and
    Preventive Medicine
Drexel University College of Medicine
Philadelphia, Pennsylvania

Dalia Hammoud, MD
Fellow
Department of Hematology/Oncology
Tulane Medical Center
New Orleans, Louisiana

Marissa Hamrick, MD
Instructor of Family Medicine
Boston University School of Medicine
Boston, Massachusetts

Ihab Hamzeh, MD, FACC
Division of Cardiology
Department of Medicine
Baylor College of Medicine
Houston, Texas

Jessica Handel, DO
Associate Program Director
St. Elizabeth Family Medicine Residency
St. Elizabeth Health Center
Youngstown, Ohio

Richard Haney, DO[†]
Resident
Dwight D. Eisenhower Army Medical
    Center
Fort Gordon, Georgia

Fariah Hanna, MBBS
General Physician
Pakistan

David Hardy, MD, RPVI
Assistant Professor of Vascular Surgery
Department of Surgery
Georgia Regents University
Augusta, Georgia

Allison Hargreaves, MD
Assistant Professor
University of Massachusetts Medical School
Associate Director, Family Medicine
    Residency Program
UMass Memorial Medical Center
Worcester, Massachusetts

Dausen J. Harker, MD[†]
Group Practice Manager
Carl R. Darnall Army Medical Center
Fort Hood, Texas

Lisa M. Harris, DO[†]
Family Medicine Faculty
Womack Army Medical Center
Fort Bragg, North Carolina

Ayesha Hasan, MD
Department of Obstetrics and Gynecology
Akron General Medical Center
Akron, Ohio

Robert M. Hasty, DO, FACOI, FACP
Vice President of Medical Education
Southeastern Health
Associate Dean for Postgraduate Affairs
Campbell University School of
    Osteopathic Medicine
Lumberton, North Carolina

Robyn M. Hatley, MD
Professor of Surgery and Pediatrics
Department of Surgery
Children's Hospital of Georgia
Georgia Regents Health System
Augusta, Georgia

Fern R. Hauck, MD, MS
Spencer P. Bass MD Twenty-First
  Century Professor of Family Medicine
Professor of Public Health Sciences
Director, International Family Medicine
  Clinic
Department of Family Medicine
University of Virginia
Charlottesville, Virginia

Aaron Hauptman, MD
Resident
The University of Texas Southwestern
  Austin
Austin, Texas

Matthew Kendall Hawks, MD[†]
Resident Physician
Family Medicine
Nellis Air Force Base
Las Vegas, Nevada

Beverly N. Hay, MD
Associate Professor
University of Massachusetts Medical School
Chief of Division of Pediatric Genetics
UMass Memorial Medical Center
Worcester, Massachusetts

Munawar Hayat, MD
Resident
University of Texas Southwestern
  Medical Center
Dallas, Texas

Kevin Heaton, DO[†]
Primary Care Sports Medicine
Access Sports Medicine and Orthopaedics
Exeter, New Hampshire

Brandon David Hecht, DO[†]
Captain of Medical Corps, U.S. Army
Department of Primary Care
Blanchfield Army Community Hospital
Fort Campbell, Kentucky

Robyn Heidenreich, MD
Family Medicine Resident
Loma Linda University School of
  Medicine
Loma Linda, California

Andrew S. Hellenga, MD
Department of Family and Community
  Medicine
Saint Louis University School of Medicine
St. Louis, Missouri

Scott T. Henderson, MD
Director of Medical Services
Student Health Center
University of Missouri
Columbia, Missouri

Michelle I. Henne, MD
Family Practice Resident
Bayfront Family Health Center
St. Petersburg, Florida

Jaroslaw T. Hepel, MD
Assistant Professor
Department of Radiation Oncology
Rhode Island Hospital
Brown University
Providence, Rhode Island
Department of Radiation Oncology
Tufts Medical Center, Tufts University
Boston, Massachusetts

Christina R. Hermos, MD[†]
Assistant Professor of Pediatrics
Department of Pediatrics, Division of
  Pediatric Immunology and Infectious
  Diseases
University of Massachusetts Medical
  School
UMass Memorial Children's Medical
  Center
Worcester, Massachusetts

David N. Herrmann, MBBCh
Professor of Neurology and Pathology
University of Rochester
Rochester, New York

Lee J. Herskowitz, DO, MBA
Associate Professor
A.T. Still University School of Osteopathic
  Medicine Arizona
Mesa, Arizona

Brian Hertz, MD[†]
Internal Medicine
Kaiser Permanente
San Rafael, California

Mary Annette Hess, PhD, FNP-BC,
  CNS[†]
Assistant Professor/Nurse Practitioner
Acute, Chronic and Continuing Care
School of Nursing
Birmingham, Alabama

David L. Heymann, MD, DTMH
Professor of Infectious Disease
  Epidemiology
London School of Hygiene & Tropical
  Medicine
London, United Kingdom

David G. Hicks, MD
Professor
Department of Pathology and Laboratory
  Medicine
Director
Surgical Pathology Unit
University of Rochester Medical Center
Rochester, New York

John Hill, DO
Professor and Director of Primary Care
  Sports Medicine Fellowship
Department of Family Medicine
School of Medicine
University of Colorado Anschutz Medical
  Campus
Aurora, Colorado

H. Anh Hinshaw, MD[†]
Resident Physician in Health Outcomes
  International
Ehrling Berquist Family Medicine
  Residency
Department of Family Medicine
University of Nebraska Medical Center
Omaha, Nebraska

Matthew Hinton, PharmD
Clinical Pharmacy Specialist
Department of Emergency Medicine
Temple University Hospital
Philadelphia, Pennsylvania

Michael P. Hirsh, MD
Professor of Surgery and Pediatrics
University of Massachusetts Medical
  School
Surgeon-in-Chief
UMass Memorial Children's Medical
  Center
Worcester, Massachusetts

Crystal L. Hnatko, DO[†]
Director of Sports Medicine
Napa Solano Family Medicine Residency
Kaiser Permanente Vallejo Medical
  Center
Vallejo, California
Adjunct Faculty Physician of U.S. Air
  Force Reserve
Family Medicine Residency
David Grant Medical Center
Travis Air Force Base, California

Brandi Hoag, DO
Director
St. Vincent Ambulatory Care Center
Worcester, Massachusetts

Abigail Weil Hoffman, MD
General Surgery Resident
Georgia Regents University
Augusta, Georgia

Thomas S. Hoke, MD
Primary Care
Sports Medicine Fellow
Maine Medical Center
Portland, Maine

N. Wilson Holland, MD, FACP, AGSF[†]
Associate Chief of Staff for Education
Atlanta Veterans Affairs Medical Center
Associate Professor of Medicine
General Medicine and Geriatrics
Department of Medicine
Emory University School of Medicine
Atlanta, Georgia

Roger P. Holland, MD, PhD[†]
Family Medicine Residency
Dwight D. Eisenhower Army Medical Center
Fort Gordon, Georgia

Megan Hollis, MD
Medical Director
Conway Health and Resource Center
Washington, DC

Katherine Holmes, MD
Assistant Professor of Medicine
Department of Family Medicine
SUNY Upstate Medical University
Syracuse, New York

Steven B. Holsten, Jr., MD, FACS
Associate Professor of Surgery
Georgia Regents University
Augusta, Georgia

Laurie A.M. Hommema, MD[†]
Program Director
Riverside Family Medicine Residency
OhioHealth Riverside Methodist Hospital
Columbus, Ohio

Amer Homsi, MD
General Surgery Resident
Department of Surgery
The Brooklyn Hospital Center
Brooklyn, New York

J. David Honeycutt, MD, FAAFP, FAWM[†]
Predoctoral Coordinator and Associate
    Program Director
Nellis Family Medicine Residency
Mike O'Callaghan Federal Medical Center
Nellis Air Force Base
Las Vegas, Nevada

Stanton C. Honig, MD
Clinician in Urology
Clinical Professor of Urology
Director of Yale Men's Health Program
Yale School of Medicine
New Haven, Connecticut

Maeve K. Hopkins, MA, MD[†]
Resident Physician
Department of Obstetrics & Gynecology
Duke University Hospital
Durham, North Carolina

Michael P. Hopkins, MD, MEd
Chairman and Professor
Department of Obstetrics and Gynecology
Northeast Ohio Medical University
Rootstown, Ohio
Program Director
Department of Obstetrics and Gynecology
Aultman Hospital
Canton, Ohio

James M. Horowitz, MD, FACC
Assistant Professor of Medicine
Associate Director of Cardiac Care Unit
Co-Director of Pulmonary Embolism
    Advanced Care
Department of Medicine
Weill Cornell Medical College
New York, New York

Robert W. Hostoffer, DO, FACOP, FAAP,
    FACOI
Associate Professor of Pediatrics
Case Western Reserve University
Cleveland, Ohio

James E. Hougas, III, MD, Maj,
    USAF, MC[†]
Family Medicine Residency Faculty
Assistant Professor
Uniformed Services University of the
    Health Sciences
Bethesda, Maryland
Nebraska Family Medicine Residency
    Faculty
55th Medical Operations Squadron
Offutt Air Force Base
Adjunct Assistant Professor
University of Nebraska Medical Center
Omaha, Nebraska

Antoun Houranieh, RPh, MS, PhD
Pharmaceutical Services
VA Boston Healthcare System
Boston, Massachusetts

Steven A. House, MD, FAAFP, FAAHPM,
    HMDC
Associate Professor
University of Louisville
Department of Family and Geriatric
    Medicine
Program Director
University of Louisville/Glasgow Family
    Medicine Residency Program
Glasgow, Kentucky

Alex P. Houser, DO[†]
Womack Family Medicine Residency
    Clinic
Womack Army Medical Center
Fort Bragg, North Carolina

Kattie Hoy, MD[†]
Attending Physician
Family Medicine Residency Clinic
Eglin Air Force Base
Valparaiso, Florida

Amanda Hu, MD, FRCSC
Assistant Professor
Department of Otolaryngology–Head &
    Neck Surgery
Drexel University College of Medicine
Philadelphia, Pennsylvania

Chi-Cheng Huang, MD
Adjunct Assistant Professor of
    Pediatrics
Boston University School of Medicine
Boston, Massachusetts
Assistant Professor of Medicine
Tufts University School of Medicine
Department of Hospital Medicine
Lahey Hospital & Medical Center
Burlington, Massachusetts

Garrett W. Huck, MD, Capt, USAF[†]
Nellis Air Force Base Family Medicine
    Residency
Nellis Air Force Base
Las Vegas, Nevada

Heather J. Hue, MD, MPH[†]
Hematology & Medical Oncology
Lone Tree, Colorado

Dennis E. Hughes, DO, FACEP
Department of Emergency Services
CoxHealth
Branson, Missouri

Karen A. Hughes, MD, FAAFP
Associate Director
Family Medicine Residency Program
North Mississippi Medical Center
Tupelo, Mississippi

Karen A. Hulbert, MD
Associate Professor
Department of Family and Community
 Medicine
Medical College of Wisconsin
Milwaukee, Wisconsin

Jennifer L. Hunt, MD†
Resident in Aerospace/Occupational
 Medicine
Naval Aerospace Medical Institute
Pensacola, Florida

John C. Huscher, MD
Associate Professor and Associate
 Program Director
Family Medicine Residency, Rural
 Training Track
University of Nebraska Medical School
Norfolk, Nebraska

Zeeshan Hussain, MD
Resident
Internal Medicine
University of Louisville
Louisville, Kentucky

Carol Hustedde, PhD
Assistant Professor
Department of Family and Community
 Medicine
University of Kentucky College of
 Medicine
Lexington, Kentucky

Jeremy Wade Hutson, DO
Family Medicine Resident
Department of Medical Education
Southeastern Regional Medical Center
Lumberton, North Carolina

Benjamin Hyatt, MD
Assistant Professor of Medicine
Division of Gastroenterology
University of Massachusetts Medical
 School
Worcester, Massachusetts

Robert J. Hyde, MD, MA, NRP, FACEP
Assistant Professor of Medicine/
 Emergency Medicine
Department of Medicine
Geisel School of Medicine at Dartmouth
Hanover, New Hampshire

Mary Iaculli, DO
Resident
Department of Family Medicine
Boston Medical Center
Boston, Massachusetts

Brenda W. Iddins, DNP, FNP-BC
University of Alabama at Birmingham
Birmingham, Alabama

Wajiha Illyas, MD†
Volunteer Research Assistant
Heart of the City Health Center
Grand Rapids, Michigan

P. Charles Inboriboon, MD, MPH,
 FACEP†
Assistant Professor and Associate
 Program Director
Department of Emergency Medicine
University of Missouri–Kansas City
Kansas City, Missouri

Byron M. Ingram, DO
Internal Medicine Resident
Southeastern Regional Medical Center
Lumberton, North Carolina

Jamal Islam, MD, MS†
Associate Professor and Assistant
 Director of Residency Program
Department of Family Medicine
University of Texas Medical Branch
Galveston, Texas

Pablo I. Hernandez Itriago, MD, MS,
 FAAFP
Boston University Medical Campus
Boston, Massachusetts

Tatiana P. Ivan, MD
Family Medicine
Baptist Health Primary Care
Miami, Florida

Khalid A. Jaboori, MD, MPH†
Interim Director
Family Medicine Residency
Madigan Army Medical Center
Tacoma, Washington

Christine K. Jacobs, MD, FAAFP†
Professor and Residency Program
 Director
Department of Family and Community
 Medicine
Saint Louis University School of Medicine
St. Louis, Missouri

Quratulanne H. Jan, MD
Department of Family Medicine
Henry Ford Health System
Southfield, Michigan

Kyu K. Jana, MD
Assistant Professor
University of Texas Medical Branch
Galveston, Texas

Maissaa Janbain, MD
Fellow
Tulane University School of Medicine
New Orleans, Louisiana

Adam J. Janicki, MD†
Department of Emergency Medicine
The Warren Alpert Medical School of
 Brown University
Providence, Rhode Island

Elizabeth Janopaul-Naylor, MD
Department of Psychiatry
Cambridge Health Alliance
Harvard Medical School
Boston, Massachusetts

Lisa N. Jarnagin, MBBCh, BAO
Resident
Department of Internal Medicine
Lahey Hospital & Medical Center
Burlington, Massachusetts

Courtney I. Jarvis, PharmD
Associate Professor
Department of Pharmacy Practice
Massachusetts College of Pharmacy and
 Health Sciences University
Worcester, Massachusetts

Salmaan Jawaid, MD
Pediatric Resident
Department of Internal Medicine
University of Massachusetts Medical Center
Worcester, Massachusetts

Cynthia Jeremiah, MD
Assistant Professor
Department of Family Medicine
UMass Memorial Medical Center
Worcester, Massachusetts

Pim Jetanalin, MD
Assistant Professor
Department of Medicine/Rheumatology
University of Missouri–Kansas City
Kansas City, Missouri

Zaiba Jetpuri, DO, MBA
Assistant Professor
Department of Family Medicine
University of Texas Southwestern Medical
 Center
Dallas, Texas

Anub G. John, MD
Resident
Division of Internal Medicine
University of Louisville
Louisville, Kentucky

Brett Johnson, DO[†]
Family Medicine
Mike O'Callaghan Federal Medical Center
Nellis Air Force Base
Las Vegas, Nevada

Isaiah Johnson, MD
Department of Obstetrics and
    Gynecology
Carilion Clinic
Roanoke, Virginia

Jessica Johnson, MD, MPH
Chief Resident
Department of Family Medicine
Oregon Health and Science University
Portland, Oregon

Julia V. Johnson, MD
Professor and Chair
Department of Obstetrics and Gynecology
University of Massachusetts Medical School
Worcester, Massachusetts

Kassie S. Johnson, MD
Fellow
Primary Care Sports Medicine
Christus Santa Rosa Health System
San Antonio, Texas

Leigh D. Johnson, MD
Assistant Professor
Department of Family Medicine Johnson
    City Residency
East Tennessee State University
Johnson City, Tennessee

Julie Ann Johnston, MD
Faculty
Lawrence Family Medicine Residency
Lawrence, Massachusetts
Clinical Instructor
Department of Family Medicine
Tufts University School of Medicine
Boston, Massachusetts

Daniel L. Jones, MD
Fellow
Primary Care Sports Medicine
University of Massachusetts Medical
    School
Worcester, Massachusetts

Marci D. Jones, MD
Associate Professor
Department of Orthopedic Surgery
University of Massachusetts
Worcester, Massachusetts

Rachel M. Jones, DO[†]
Department of Family Medicine
    Residency
Martin Army Community Hospital
Fort Benning, Georgia

Stacy Jones, MD
Capitol Anesthesiology Association
Austin, Texas

Melody A. Jordahl-Iafrato, MD
Program Director
South Campus Family Medicine
    Residency
Assistant Professor
Department of Family and Community
    Medicine
University of Arizona College of Medicine
Tucson, Arizona

Arjun S. Joshi, MD
Associate Professor of Surgery
Ear, Nose & Throat Center
George Washington University Medical
    Faculty Associates
George Washington University
Washington, DC

Maurice F. Joyce, MD, EdM
Resident
Department of Anesthesiology
Tufts Medical Center
Boston, Massachusetts

Patrick Wakefield Joyner, MD, MS,
    LCDR[†]
Bone & Joint/Sports Medicine Institute
Naval Medical Center Portsmouth
Portsmouth, Virginia

Tya-Mae Y. Julien, MD
Department of Gastroenterology and
    Hepatology
Baylor/Richardson Medical Center
Richardson, Texas

Tipsuda Junsanto-Bahri, MD
Chairman
Basic Biomedical Sciences
Assistant Professor
Internal Medicine and Pathology
Course Director, Pathology
Touro College of Osteopathic Medicine
New York, New York

Jenna Kahn, MD
Radiation Oncology Resident
Department of Radiation Oncology
Virginia Commonwealth University
Richmond, Virginia

Gregory Kainz, DO
Department of Obstetrics and
    Gynecology
Lehigh Valley Health Network
Allentown, Pennsylvania

Achyut B. Kamat, MD
Clinical Associate Professor
Department of Emergency Medicine
The Warren Alpert School of Medicine at
    Brown University
Providence, Rhode Island

Amar Kapur, DO, CPT, MC, USA[†]
Medical Director
JBER–Soldier Centered Medical Home
Fort Richardson, Alaska

Rahul Kapur, MD, CAQSM
Associate Professor
Family Medicine and Sports Medicine
University of Pennsylvania
Department of Family Medicine and
    Community Health
Penn Sports Medicine Center
Philadelphia, Pennsylvania

Atil Y. Kargi, MD
Fellowship Program
Associate Professor of Medicine
Division of Endocrinology, Diabetes, and
    Metabolism
University of Miami Miller School of
    Medicine
Miami, Florida

Anilkumar Katta, MD
Department of Allergy and Immunology
Lahey Hospital & Medical Center
Burlington, Massachusetts

Anubhav Kaul, MD
Associate Professor
Department of Family Medicine
Loma Linda University School of Medicine
Loma Linda, California

Viren Kaul, MD
Chief Resident
Department of Internal Medicine
Lahey Hospital & Medical Center
Burlington, Massachusetts

Neha Kaushik, MD[†]
Resident Physician
Department of Family Medicine
Penn State Milton S. Hershey Medical
    Center
Hershey, Pennsylvania

Clara M. Keegan, MD
Assistant Professor
Department of Family Medicine
University of Vermont Medical Center
Burlington, Vermont

Jennifer Tickal Keehbauch, MD
Associate Professor
Department of Family Medicine
Loma Linda University School of Medicine
Loma Linda, California

Brian P. Keene, DO[†]
Resident
Martin Army Community Hospital
Fort Benning, Georgia

Chad Robert Keller, DO
Department of Otolaryngology–Head &
    Neck Surgery
Doctors Hospital
Columbus, Ohio

Amanda Martin Kelley, MD, MPH&TM[†]
University of Rochester Medical Center
Rochester, New York

Christina Kelly, MD, FAAFP
Faculty
Family Medicine Residency
Carl R. Darnall Army Medical Center
Fort Hood, Texas

Matthew C. Kelly, MD[†]
Family Medicine Residency Clinic
U.S. Army Medical Corps
Carl R. Darnall Army Medical Center
Fort Hood, Texas

Jeremy R. Kenison, DO[†]
Naval Hospital Bremerton
Bremerton, Washington

Robert M. Kershner, MD, MS, FACS[†]
Eye Physician and Surgeon
Professor and Chairman
Department of Ophthalmic Medical
    Technology
Palm Beach State College
President and CEO
Ophthalmic Consulting
Jupiter, Florida

Tarun Kewalramani, MD
Department of Hematology and
    Oncology
Lahey Hospital & Medical Center
Burlington, Massachusetts

Anila Khaliq, MD
Faculty
Family Medicine Residency Program
St. Elizabeth Medical Center
Utica, New York
Hospitalist
Rome Memorial Hospital
Rome, New York

Abid Khan, MD
Resident
Rush University Medical Center
Chicago, Illinois

Muhammad Imran Khan, MD
Karachi, Pakistan

Omar Khan, MD, MHS, FAAFP[†]
Physician Leader of Primary Care &
    Community Medicine Service Line
Director of Global Health Residency
    Track in Family Medicine
Christiana Care Health System
Newark, Delaware

Rabeea Khan, MD
Resident Physician
Department of Ophthalmology
Kresge Eye Institute
Detroit, Michigan

Vikesh Khanijow, MD
Fellow
Gastroenterology
George Washington University Hospital
Washington, DC

Christopher R. Kieliszak, DO
Otolaryngology Resident Physician
Doctors Hospital
Columbus, Ohio

Luke D. Killpack, DO
Academic Primary Care Associates
Blacksburg, Virginia

Daniel Y. Kim, MD, FACS
Chairman
Department of Otolaryngology–Head &
    Neck Surgery
University of Massachusetts
Worcester, Massachusetts

Gemma Kim, MD
Assistant Professor and Program Director
    of Family Medicine
Department of Family Medicine
University of California, Riverside School
    of Medicine
Riverside, California

Tae K. Kim, MD
Assistant Professor and Regional Medical
    Director UCR Health
Department of Family Medicine
University of California, Riverside School
    of Medicine
Riverside, California

Walter M. Kim, MD, PhD[†]
Research/Clinical Fellow
Division of Gastroenterology
Brigham and Women's Hospital
Harvard Medical School
Boston, Massachusetts

Brian James Kimbrell, MD, FACS
Trauma Medical Director/Surgical Critical
    Care Director
Blake Medical Center
Bradenton, Florida
Assistant Clinical Professor
University of South Florida
Tampa, Florida

Ray S. King, MD, PhD
Department of Surgery
Medical College of Georgia
Georgia Regents University
Augusta, Georgia

Shawna King, DO
Resident
Bayfront Health St. Petersburg
St. Petersburg, Florida

Stella O. King, MD, MHA
Clinical Assistant Professor
Department of Family Medicine
University at Buffalo
Buffalo, New York

Cecilia M. Kipnis, MD[†]
Faculty
Department of Family Medicine
Naval Hospital Jacksonville
Jacksonville, Florida

Jeffrey T. Kirchner, DO, FAAFP, AAHIVS[†]
Medical Director
LGHP-Comprehensive Care for HIV
Lancaster General Health
Lancaster, Pennsylvania
Associate Clinical Professor
Department of Family and Community
  Medicine
Temple University School of Medicine
Philadelphia, Pennsylvania

Brandon Kirsch, MD
Department of Dermatology
Mayo Clinic
Jacksonville, Florida

Richard T. Klapchar, DO
Department of Otolaryngology–Head &
  Neck Surgery
Doctors Hospital
Columbus, Ohio

Gloria J. Klapstein, PhD
Associate Professor
Department of Basic Sciences
College of Osteopathic Medicine
Touro University California
Vallejo, California

Randolph J. Kline, MD[†]
Family Medicine Resident
David Grant Medical Center
Travis Air Force Base, California

Laura K. Klug, PharmD
Assistant Professor and Clinical
  Pharmacist
Department of Pharmacy Practice and
  Family Medicine
Creighton University School of Pharmacy
  and Health Professions
Omaha, Nebraska

Sandra L. Knaur, APRN, BC
Texas Pulmonary and Critical Care
  Consultants of Texas, PA
Fort Worth, Texas

Saranya Kodali, MD[†]
Internal Medicine Resident
Department of Internal Medicine
University of Massachusetts Medical
  School
Worcester, Massachusetts

Sharon L. Koehler, DO, FACS
Assistant Professor
Breast Surgical Oncology
Department of Medicine
Division of Surgery
New York Institute of Technology College
  of Osteopathic Medicine
Old Westbury, New York

Kimberly Kone, MD[†]
Resident in Family and Community
  Medicine
University of Texas Southwestern Medical
  Center
Dallas, Texas

Scott E. Kopec, MD
Associate Professor of Medicine
Director of Pulmonary and Critical Care
  Fellowship
Associate Director
Internal Medicine Residency
University of Massachusetts Medical
  School
Worcester, Massachusetts

Yash Kothari, MD[†]
Resident Physician
Internal Medicine Residency Program
University of Louisville
Louisville, Kentucky

Adam W. Kowalski, MD[†]
Family Medicine Residency
Carl R. Darnall Army Medical Center
Fort Hood, Texas

Rudolph M. Krafft, MD, FAAFP[†]
Clinical Professor
Department of Family and Community
  Medicine
Northeast Ohio University College of
  Medicine
Director of Family Medicine Residency
St. Elizabeth Mercy Health Center
Youngstown, Ohio

Sathya S. Krishnasamy, MD
Associate Professor of Medicine
Division of Endocrinology, Metabolism
  and Diabetes
University of Louisville
Louisville, Kentucky

Merrill Krolick, DO, FACC, FACP, FSCAI
Interventional Cardiology
The Heart Institute at Largo
Largo Medical Center
Largo, Florida

David C. Krulak, MD, MPH, MBA,
  FAAFP[†]
Physician
U.S. Navy
Aiea, Hawaii

David W. Kruse, MD
CAQ Primary Care Sports Medicine
Orthopaedic Specialty Institute
Orange, California

E. James Kruse, DO
Division Chief of Surgical Oncology
Department of Surgery
Georgia Regents University
Augusta, Georgia

Archana Kudrimoti, MD,–MBBS, MPH[†]
Assistant Professor
Clerkship Director
University Of Kentucky
Department of Family and Community
  Medicine
University of Kentucky Health Care at
  Turfland
Lexington, Kentucky

Karl A. Kuersteiner, MD[†]
Resident Physician
Department of Family Medicine
Naval Hospital Jacksonville
Jacksonville, Florida

Ajoy Kumar, MD, FAAFP
Chairman
Department of Family Medicine
Assistant Director
Bayfront Family Medicine Residency
Bayfront Health St. Petersburg
St. Petersburg, Florida

Barrett J. Kumar, DO, MSBA
Department of Internal Medicine
University Hospitals–Regional Hospitals
Cleveland, Ohio

Vineet Kumar, MD
Division of Cardiovascular Disease
University of Alabama at Birmingham
  School of Medicine
Birmingham, Alabama

Jason Kurland, MD
Assistant Professor of Medicine
Division of Renal Medicine
University of Massachusetts Medical School
Worcester, Massachusetts

Daniel B. Kurtz, PhD
Associate Professor and Chair of Biology
Utica College
Utica, New York

SreyRam Kuy, MD, MHS
Department of Surgery
Louisiana State University Health
  Sciences Center at Shreveport
Shreveport, Louisiana
Overton Brooks Veterans Affairs Medical
  Center
Washington, DC

Angela Kuznia, MD, MPH
Department of Family Medicine
Georgetown University Medical Center
Washington, DC

Melinda Y. Kwan, DO, MPH
Urgent Care/Family Medicine Physician
Urgent Care Department
Southwest Medical Associates
Las Vegas, Nevada

Nanette Lacuesta, MS, MD
Assistant Program Director
Riverside Methodist Hospital Family
    Medicine Residency Program
OhioHealth
Columbus, Ohio

John E. Laird, MD, FAAFP[†]
Staff Attending
Family Medicine Residency
Naval Hospital Camp Lejeune
Camp Lejeune, North Carolina

Nora E. Lamartine, MD
Resident
Department of Family Medicine and
    Community Health
University of Massachusetts Medical School
Worcester, Massachusetts

R. Aaron Lambert, MD[†]
Clinical Assistant Professor
Department of Family Medicine
Brody School of Medicine at East
    Carolina University
Greenville, North Carolina

Rahele Lameh, MD
Family Medicine Board Certified
Community Faculty
Family Medicine Department
The University of Texas Southwestern
    Dallas
Dallas, Texas

Stephen K. Lane, MD, FAAFP
Family Medicine
Scituate, Massachusetts

Jeffrey B. Lanier, MD, FAAFP[†]
Family Medicine Residency Program
Martin Army Community Hospital
Fort Benning, Georgia

Michael Lao, MD[†]
Resident in Urologic Surgery
Department of Urology
University of Connecticut Health Center
Farmington, Connecticut

Eduardo Lara-Torre, MD
Vice-Chairman for Academic Affairs
Residency Program Director
Carilion Clinic
Associate Professor
Departments of Obstetrics and
    Gynecology and Pediatrics
Virginia Tech Carilion School of
    Medicine
Roanoke, Virginia

Deborah A. Lardner, DO, DTM&H
Assistant Professor
Department of Family Medicine
Department of Emergency Medicine
New York Institute of Technology College
    of Osteopathic Medicine
New York Institute of Technology Center
    for Global Health
Old Westbury, New York

Richard A. Larson, MD
Professor of Medicine
Section of Hematology/Oncology
University of Chicago
Chicago, Illinois

Shane L. Larson, MD[†]
Staff Family Physician and Flight
    Surgeon
Department of Primary Care
Fort Carson, Colorado

Lakshmi Devi Nelson Lattimer, MD
Gastroenterology
George Washington University
Washington, DC

Justin P. Lavin, Jr., MD, FACOG
Chairman
Department of Obstetrics and
    Gynecology
Akron General Medical Center
Professor Emeritus of Obstetrics and
    Gynecology
Northeastern Ohio Medical University
Akron, Ohio

Ashik Lawrence, MD
Resident
East Jefferson General Hospital
Metairie, Louisiana

Miles C. Layton, DO[†]
Major, Medical Corps
Officer in Charge
Gastroenterology Clinic
Faculty of Family Medicine Residency
Martin Army Community Hospitals
Fort Benning, Georgia

Eleanor D. Lederer, MD, FASN
Kidney Disease Program
University of Louisville Hospital
Louisville, Kentucky

James J. Ledwith, Jr., MD, FAAFP
Residency Director
University of Massachusetts Fitchburg
    Family Medicine Residency Program
University of Massachusetts Medical
    School
Fitchburg, Massachusetts

Andrew G. Lee, MD
Professor of Ophthalmology, Neurology,
    and Neurosurgery
Weill Cornell Medical College
Chair of Ophthalmology
Houston Methodist Hospital
Adjunct Professor of Ophthalmology
Baylor College of Medicine
Clinical Professor of Ophthalmology
University of Texas Medical Branch–
    UTMB Galveston
University of Texas MD Anderson Cancer
    Center
Adjunct Professor of Ophthalmology
University of Iowa Hospitals and
    Clinics
Houston, Texas

Bianca Lee, DO, MS
Nassau University Medical Center
East Meadow, New York

Damon F. Lee, MD
Assistant Professor
Office of Medical Education
Assistant Clinical Professor
Department of Family Medicine and
    Community Health
John A. Burns School of Medicine
University of Hawaii
Honolulu, Hawaii

Daniel T. Lee, MD, MA
Clinical Professor of Family Medicine
David Geffen School of Medicine
University of California Los Angeles
Santa Monica, California

Ernestine Lee, MD
Assistant Professor
Department of Family Medicine
University of Texas at Austin
Austin, Texas

Ginny H. Lee, MD[†]
Department of Emergency Medicine
Summa Akron City Health System
Akron, Ohio

Hobart Lee, MD, FAAFP
Director and Assistant Professor
Family Medicine Residency Program
Loma Linda University School of Medicine
Loma Linda, California

Jennifer Lee, DO
Family Medicine Resident
Greenbrier Valley Medical Center
Lewisburg, West Virginia

F. Stuart Leeds, MD, MS
Assistant Professor of Family Medicine
Department of Family Medicine
Wright State University Boonshoft School
  of Medicine
Dayton, Ohio

Angelia Leipelt, BA, IBCLC, ICCE, CLE[†]
Lead Lactation Consultant
Dignity Health Methodist Hospital
Sacramento, California

Mark C. Lentner, DO
Department of Otolaryngology–Head &
  Neck Surgery
Philadelphia College of Osteopathic
  Medicine
Philadelphia, Pennsylvania

Maya Leventer-Roberts, MD, MPH
Pediatric Environmental Health Fellow
Department of Preventive Medicine
Icahn School of Medicine at Mount Sinai
New York, New York

Nikki A. Levin, MD, PhD
Associate Professor
Division of Dermatology and Department
  of Medicine
University of Massachusetts Medical
  School
Worcester, Massachusetts

Gary I. Levine, MD
Associate Professor
Department of Family Medicine
Brody School of Medicine at East
  Carolina University
Greenville, North Carolina

Douglas P. Lewis, MD, FAAFP
Associate Director
Via Christi Family Medicine Residency
Associate Director
Via Christi Adult Cystic Fibrosis Specialty
  Clinic
Clinical Assistant Professor
University of Kansas School of Medicine–
  Wichita
Wichita, Kansas

Anjie Li, MD[†]
Resident Physician
Department of Obstetrics and
  Gynecology
University of Massachusetts Medical
  School
Worcester, Massachusetts

Rung-chi Li, DO, PhD
Internal Medicine
The Christ Hospital
Cincinnati, Ohio

Jennifer Lin, DO
Family Medicine Resident
University of Massachusetts
Fitchburg, Massachusetts

Jonathan T. Lin, MD[†]
Housestaff of Internal Medicine
Department of Medicine
Icahn School of Medicine
New York, New York

Christopher Lin-Brande, MD[†]
Family Medicine Residency Program
David Grant Medical Center
Travis Air Force Base, Fairfield, California

Mary S. Lindholm, MD
Clinical Associate Professor and
  Clerkship Director
Department of Family Medicine and
  Community Health
University of Massachusetts Medical
  School
Worcester, Massachusetts

Melanie J. Lippmann, MD
Assistant Professor of Emergency
  Medicine
The Warren Alpert Medical School of
  Brown University
University Emergency Medicine
  Foundation
Rhode Island Hospital & The Miriam
  Hospital
Providence, Rhode Island

Katelin M. Lisenby, PharmD[†]
Assistant Clinical Professor
Department of Pharmacy Practice
Auburn University Harrison School of
  Pharmacy
Auburn, Alabama
Department of Family Medicine
University of Alabama College of
  Community Health Sciences
Tuscaloosa, Alabama

Kenneth Liu, PharmD
Adjunct Faculty, Massachusetts College
  of Pharmacy and Health Sciences
  University
Boston, Massachusetts

Kimberly E. Liu, MD, MSL, FRCSC
Assistant Professor
Centre for Fertility & Reproductive
  Health
Mount Sinai Hospital
Department of Obstetrics and
  Gynecology
University of Toronto
Toronto, Ontario, Canada

Jenifer R. Lloyd, DO, FAAD
Program Director
Dermatology
University Hospitals–Regional
  Hospitals
Richmond Heights, Ohio

Vincent Lo, MD, FAAFP
Senior Clinical Faculty
Mercy/Methodist Family Medicine
  Residency Program
Dignity Health Methodist Hospital of
  Sacramento
Sacramento, California
Associate Clinical Professor of Family
  Medicine
Department of Family and Community
  Medicine
University of California
Davis, California

Maria Lombardi, DO
Assistant Professor
Department of Pediatrics
New York Medical College
Valhalla, New York

Maria Cynthia S. Lopez, MD, FAAFP
Assistant Director of Family Medicine
  Residency
Bayfront Health St Petersburg
St. Petersburg, Florida

Gisela M. Lopez Payares, MD
Department of Family and Community
  Medicine
University of Texas Health Science
  Center at San Antonio
San Antonio, Texas

Bency K. Louidor-Paulynice, MD
Family Medicine
University of Massachusetts Medical School
Worcester, Massachusetts

Bruce L. Lovins, MD[†]
Hospitalist
Department of Medicine
Martin Army Community Hospital
Fort Benning, Georgia

Zhen Lu, MD
Chief Medical Director
Pacific Urgent Care & Family Medicine
Orange, California

Marie Luksch, DO
Obstetrics and Gynecology
Paoli Hospital
Paoli, Pennsylvania

John R. Luksch, DO
Chief Resident
Department of Family Medicine
Rowan University School of Osteopathic
    Medicine
Stratford, New Jersey

Alicia G. Lydecker, MD
Fellow in Medical Toxicology
Division of Medical Toxicology
Department of Emergency Medicine
University of Massachusetts Medical School
Worcester, Massachusetts

Ann M. Lynch, PharmD, RPh, AE-C
Associate Professor of Pharmacy
    Practice
Massachusetts College of Pharmacy and
    Health Sciences University
Worcester, Massachusetts

Paul Lyons, MD
Senior Associate Dean for Education
Chairman
Department of Family Medicine
Professor of Family Medicine
University of California, Riverside
Riverside, California

Theophile Lyotard, MD
Resident
Department of Family Medicine
Creighton University School of Medicine
Omaha, Nebraska

Jonathan MacClements, MD, FAAFP
Professor and Assistant Dean of
    Graduate Medical Education
Dell Medical School, University of Texas
    at Austin
Austin, Texas

Marina MacNamara, MD, MPH
Resident Physician
Family Medicine Residency Program
Mountain Area Health Education Center
Asheville, North Carolina

Douglas W. MacPherson, MD,
    MSc–CTM, FRCPC
Department of Pathology and Molecular
    Medicine
McMaster University
Hamilton, Ontario, Canada
Migration Health Consultants, Inc.
Qualicum Beach, British Columbia,
    Canada

Andrea Madrigrano, MD[†]
Assistant Professor
Department of Surgery
Rush University Medical Center
Chicago, Illinois

Michelle Magid, MD
Clinical Associate Professor
University of Texas Medical Branch
Clinical Assistant Professor
Texas A&M Health Science Center
Adjunct Faculty
Dell Medical School, University of Texas
    at Austin
Austin, Texas

Courtney Maiden, DO
Department of Family Medicine
Southeastern Regional Medical Center
Lumberton, North Carolina

Maricarmen Malagon-Rogers, MD
Pediatric Nephrologist
Associate Professor of Family Medicine
University of Tennessee, Graduate School
    of Medicine
Knoxville, Tennessee

Bryan Malave, MD[†]
Resident Physician
Department of Family Medicine
Martin Army Community Hospital
Fort Benning, Georgia

Uzma Malik, MD
Glen Cove, New York

Samir Malkani, MD, MRCP–UK
Associate Clinical Professor in Medicine
University of Massachusetts Medical
    School
Worcester, Massachusetts

Rubaiya Mallay, DO, FACOI, ACR
Division of Rheumatology
Suncoast Internal Medicine Consultants
Largo, Florida

Michael A. Malone, MD
Assistant Professor
Department of Family and Community
    Medicine
Penn State College of Medicine
Hershey, Pennsylvania

Mary Maloney, MD
Professor of Medicine and Director of
    Dermatologic Surgery
University of Massachusetts Medical
    School
Worcester, Massachusetts

Lee A. Mancini, MD, CSCS*D, CSN
Family Health Center
UMass Sports Medicine Center
Worcester, Massachusetts

Alison Mancuso, DO
Assistant Professor
Department of Family Medicine
Rowan University School of Osteopathic
    Medicine
Stratford, New Jersey

Krishna Manda, MD, MRCP
Renal Medicine
University of Massachusetts Memorial
    Health Care
Worcester, Massachusetts

Ninad T. Maniar, MBBS
Resident
Department of Internal Medicine
University of Louisville
Louisville, Kentucky

Mark J. Manning, DO, MsMEL
Chief
General Obstetrics and Gynecology
Assistant Professor
Department of Obstetrics and Gynecology
University of Massachusetts Medical School
Worcester, Massachusetts

Eric Ji-Yuan Mao, MD
Department of Medicine
Division of Gastroenterology
The Warren Alpert Medical School of
    Brown University
Providence, Rhode Island

Robert A. Marlow, MD, MA
Professor of Clinical Family Medicine
Department of Family, Community and
    Preventive Medicine
University of Arizona College of
    Medicine—Phoenix
Phoenix, Arizona
Associate Director/Director of Research
Family Medicine Residency Program
Scottsdale Healthcare
Scottsdale, Arizona

Wendy K. Marsh, MD, MSc
Associate Professor
Department of Psychiatry
University of Massachusetts Medical School
Worcester, Massachusetts

Cara Marshall, MD
Faculty
Lawrence Family Medicine Residency
Lawrence, Massachusetts
Assistant Professor
Department of Family Medicine and
    Community Health
University of Massachusetts Medical School
Worcester, Massachusetts

Michelle T. Martin, PharmD, BCPS,
    BCACP†
Clinical Pharmacist
University of Illinois Hospital and Health
    Sciences System
Clinical Assistant Professor
University of Illinois at Chicago College of
    Pharmacy
Chicago, Illinois

Stephen A. Martin, MD, EdM
Assistant Professor
Department of Family Medicine and
    Community Health
University of Massachusetts Medical School
Worcester, Massachusetts

Marni Martinez, APRN
Clinical Nurse Specialist
University of Texas at Austin
Austin, Texas

Carlos Martínez-Balzano, MD
Division of Lung, Allergy and Critical Care
    Medicine
University of Massachusetts Medical School
Worcester, Massachusetts

Mohamad Masoumy, MD, MS
Chief General Surgery Resident
Department of Surgery
Medical College of Georgia
Georgia Regents University
Augusta, Georgia

Jerin Mathew, MD
Nephrologist
Garfield Heights, Ohio

Donnah Mathews, MD, FACP†
Assistant Professor of Medicine
The Warren Alpert Medical School of
    Brown University
Medical Director of Clinical Management
Associate Medical Director, Home and
    Hospice Care of RI
Attending Physician
Department of General Medicine
Rhode Island Hospital
Providence, Rhode Island

Iryna Matkovska, DO
Resident Physician
Department of Emergency Medicine
Einstein Medical Center
Philadelphia, Pennsylvania

Douglas M. Maurer, DO, MPH, FAAFP†
Associate Professor of Family Medicine
Director of Faculty Development
    Fellowship
Madigan Army Medical Center
Tacoma, Washington

George H. Maxted, MD
Associate Program Director
Tufts University School of Medicine
Associate Program Director
Tufts University Family Medicine Program
    at Cambridge Health Alliance
Malden, Massachusetts

Beth Mazyck, MD
Associate Clinical Professor
Department of Family Medicine and
    Community Health
University of Massachusetts Medical
    School
Worcester, Massachusetts

Frank M. Mazzotta, DO
Clinical Instructor
Family and Community Medicine
Thomas Jefferson University Hospital
Philadelphia, Pennsylvania

Andrew J. McBride, MD
Resident
Department of Family Medicine and
    Community Health
Hospital of the University of Pennsylvania
Philadelphia, Pennsylvania

Casey McCann, MD†
Naval Hospital Pensacola
Pensacola, Florida

Kelly McCants, MD
Piedmont Heart Institute
Atlanta, Georgia

Margaret J. McCormick, MS, RN†
Clinical Associate Professor
Department of Nursing
Towson University
Towson, Maryland

Jonathan McDivitt, MD†
Cardiologist
United States Naval Ship Comfort—T-AH 20
Norfolk, Virginia

Kristina McGraw, DO
Assistant Professor
Family Medicine
West Virginia School of Osteopathic
    Medicine
Lewisburg, West Virginia

Jeannette M. McIntyre, MD†
Resident
Department of Family Medicine
Naval Hospital Jacksonville
Jacksonville, Florida

Elizabeth C. McKeen, MD†
Clinical Associate in Pediatrics
Boston Children's Hospital
Massachusetts General Hospital
Instructor in Pediatrics
Harvard Medical School
Boston, Massachusetts

Marc W. McKenna, MD†
Program Director of Family Medicine
Chestnut Hill Family Medicine
Chestnut Hill Hospital
Philadelphia, Pennsylvania

Donna-Marie McMahon, DO, FAAP†
Assistant Professor of Pediatrics
Director of the Doctor Patient Continuum
New York Institute of Technology College
    of Osteopathic Medicine
Old Westbury, New York

Vanessa W. McNair, MD, MPH†
Assistant Professor of Family Medicine
Jacksonville Family Medicine Residency
Naval Hospital Jacksonville
Jacksonville, Florida

Roger L. McRoberts, III, MD
Assistant Professor
Psychiatry
University of Texas Southwestern Austin
Austin, Texas

Colleen W. Meehan, MD, MPH[†]
Pediatric Resident
Department of Pediatrics
Children's National Medical Center
Washington, DC

Melissa K. Meghpara, DO
General Surgery Resident
Flushing Hospital Medical Center
Flushing, New York

Paavan Mehta, MD
University of Massachusetts Medical
    School
Worcester, Massachusetts

Donna I. Meltzer, MD
Clinical Associate Professor
Residency Director
Department of Family Medicine
SUNY Stony Brook
Stony Brook, New York

Daniel E. Melville, MD
Destination Health™
Southlake, Texas

Caleb J. Mentzer, DO
Resident
Department of General Surgery
Medical College of Georgia
Georgia Regents University
Augusta, Georgia

Brendan Merchant, MD
Cardiology Fellow
University of Massachusetts
Worcester, Massachusetts

Marcelle Meseeha, MD[†]
Chief Resident
Guthrie/Robert Packer Hospital Internal
    Medicine Residency Program
Sayre, Pennsylvania

Nessa S. Meshkaty, MD
Infectious Disease Department
Baystate Medical Center
Springfield, Massachusetts

Theo E. Meyer, MD, DPhil
Professor
Department of Cardiovascular Medicine
University of Massachusetts Medical
    School
Director, Cardiac Cath Lab
Department of Cardiology
UMass Memorial Medical Center
Worcester, Massachusetts

Christopher D. Meyering, DO[†]
Division Surgeon
1st Cavalry Division, U.S. Army
Fort Hood, Texas

Christina Mezzone, DO, MS
College of Osteopathic Medicine
New York Institute of Technology
Old Westbury, New York

Alyssa Miceli, DO[†]
Resident
University Hospitals–Regional Hospitals
Richmond Heights, Ohio

William E. Michael, MD[†]
Puget Sound Family Medicine
    Residency
Bremerton, Washington

Nicholas J. Michols, DO, ATC[†]
Resident Physician
Department of Family Medicine
Fort Belvoir Community Hospital
Fort Belvoir, Virginia

Tracy O. Middleton, DO
Clinical Professor and Chairman of
    Family Medicine
Midwestern University
Arizona College of Osteopathic
    Medicine
Glendale, Arizona

Mariya Milko, DO, MS[†]
Largo Medical Center
Largo, Florida

Heidi S. Millard, MD
Assistant Clinical Faculty
University of California, Riverside School
    of Medicine
Riverside, California

James P. Miller, MD[†]
Senior Pediatric Surgeon
Cook Children's Medical Center
Fort Worth, Texas

Jasmit S. Minhas, MD[†]
Resident Physician
Department of Internal Medicine
Lahey Hospital & Medical Center
Burlington, Massachusetts

Suzanne Minor, MD, FAAFP
Clerkship Director
Family Medicine
Assistant Professor
Division of Family Medicine
Department of Humanities, Health, and
    Society
Herbert Wertheim College of Medicine
Florida International University
Miami, Florida

Mark Minot, MD
Family Medicine Residency Program
Eisenhower Medical Center
Rancho Mirage, California

Tasaduq Mir, MD
Assistant Professor
Department of Family & Community
    Medicine
University of Texas Southwestern Medical
    Center
Dallas, Texas

Lauren C. Mitchell, DO[†]
Resident
Family Medicine
David Grant Medical Center
Travis Air Force Base, California

Sanjay Mohan, MD, MSCI
Assistant Professor of Medicine
Vanderbilt University School of Medicine
Nashville, Tennessee

Saadia Mohsin, MD
Resident Physician
Family Medicine
Summa Barberton Hospital
Barberton, Ohio

Tin Ming Timothy Mok, MD
House Staff Physician
Department of Family Medicine
Creighton University
Omaha, Nebraska

Maria Montanez, MD
School of Medicine
Family and Community Medicine
University of Texas Southwestern Austin
Austin, Texas

Mike Moore, PA, DO[†]
Madigan Army Medical Center
Tacoma, Washington

Tiffany A. Moore Simas, MD, MPH, MEd
Associate Professor of Obstetrics &
    Gynecology and Pediatrics
Department of Obstetrics & Gynecology
University of Massachusetts Medical
    School
Worcester, Massachusetts

Donald Morando, DO
Founding Program Director
Family Medicine Residency
Southeastern Regional Medical Center
Lumberton, North Carolina

M. Shawn Morehead, MD, MPH
Associate Director
St. Vincent's East Family Medicine
    Residency Program
Pinson, Alabama

Wynne S. Morgan, MD
Assistant Professor of Psychiatry &
    Pediatrics
Department of Psychiatry
Division of Child & Adolescent
    Psychiatry
University of Massachusetts Medical
    School
Worcester, Massachusetts

Jesse A. Morse, MD, MBA[†]
Family Medicine Resident
Department of Family Medicine
Creighton University Medical School
Omaha, Nebraska

Kelvin A. Moses, MD, PhD
Chief of Urology
Nashville General Hospital
Assistant Professor
Department of Urologic Surgery
Vanderbilt University Medical Center
Nashville, Tennessee

David A. Moss, MD[†]
Faculty
Nellis Air Force Base Family Medicine
    Residency
Las Vegas, Nevada

Timothy F. Mott, MD[†]
Assistant Professor
Family Medicine
Uniformed Services University of Health
    Sciences
Bethesda, Maryland

Josiah Moulton, DO
Resident
Scott Air Force Base
Saint Louis University
Belleville, Illinois

Mohammad Ansar Mughal, MD[†]
Community Medicine Associate
University Health System
San Antonio, Texas

Shani I. Muhammad, MD
Family Medicine Physician
Kaiser Permanente Fresno Medical
    Center
Fresno, California

S. Mimi Mukherjee, PharmD
Assistant Professor of Pharmacy Practice
Massachusetts College of Pharmacy and
    Health Sciences University
Worcester, Massachusetts
Clinical Pharmacist
Edward M. Kennedy Community Health
    Center
Framingham, Massachusetts

Joshua Mularella, DO
Assistant Professor
Department of Emergency Medicine
SUNY Upstate Medical University
Syracuse, New York

Sahil Mullick, MD
Family Medicine Residency Program
Department of Family Medicine
Creighton University
Omaha, Nebraska

Herbert L. Muncie, Jr., MD
Professor and Director of Student
    Education
Department of Family Medicine
Louisiana State University Health
    Sciences Center
New Orleans, Louisiana

Amanda B. Murchison, MD
Assistant Professor
Department of Obstetrics and Gynecology
Virginia Tech Carilion School of Medicine
Roanoke, Virginia

Erin A. Murphy, DO[†]
Family Medicine Resident
Family Medicine Residency
Naval Hospital Jacksonville
Jacksonville, Florida

Gregory Murphy, MD
Department of Urology
University of Connecticut Health Center
Farmington, Connecticut

Kathryn Myer, MD
Psychiatry Resident
University of Massachusetts Medical School
Worcester, Massachusetts

Catherine Mygatt, MD
Family Physician
Greater Lawrence Family Medicine
    Residency
Lawrence, Massachusetts

Aung S. Myint, DO
Internal Medicine Resident
Department of Medicine
George Washington University Hospital
Washington, DC

Jennifer Mytar, DO
Internal Medicine
The Christ Hospital
Cincinnati, Ohio

Adithi Naidu, MD
Resident
Department of Family Medicine and
    Community Health
University Hospitals Case Medical Center
Case Western Reserve University School
    of Medicine
Cleveland, Ohio

Urooj Najm, MBBS

Joshua E. Nash, DO
Surgical Critical Care/Trauma/Burn
    Fellow
Stroger Hospital of Cook County
Chicago, Illinois

Munima Nasir, MD
Assistant Professor
Department of Family and Community
    Medicine
Penn State Milton S. Hershey Medical
    Center
Hershey, Pennsylvania

Papia Nasiri, MD
Resident Physician
Department of Family and Community
    Medicine
Penn State Milton S. Hershey Medical
    Center
Hershey, Pennsylvania

Samah Nassereddine, MD
Internal Medicine Resident
George Washington University Hospital
Washington, DC

Eddie Needham, MD, FAAFP
Program Director and Academic
    Chairman
Florida Hospital Family Medicine
    Residency
Winter Park, Florida

Michael O. Needham, MD, CPT, MC, USA[†]
Staff Family Medicine Physician
United States Army Health Clinic
    Kaiserslautern
Kaiserslautern, Germany

Laurel A. Neff, DO[†]
Faculty Development Fellow
Department of Family Medicine
Madigan Army Medical Center
Tacoma, Washington

Holli K. Neiman-Hart, MD, FAAFP
Family Medicine Residency
West Virginia University
Morgantown, West Virginia

Clarice Nelson, MD
Department of Family Medicine
Prairie Star Health Center
Hutchinson, Kansas

Eric D. Nelson, MD
Pediatric Urologist
Assistant Professor of Urology
Connecticut Children's Medical Center
Hartford, Connecticut
University of Connecticut School of
    Medicine
Farmington, Connecticut

Nicole Nelson, DO[†]
Academic Chief Resident
Dwight D. Eisenhower Army Medical
    Center
Fort Gordon, Georgia

Vicki R. Nelson, MD, PhD
Department of Family Medicine and
    Community Health
University Hospitals Case Medical Center
Case Western Reserve University
Cleveland, Ohio

Brian E. Neubauer, MD[†]
Director and Assistant Professor of
    Cardiovascular-Pulmonary-Renal
    Module
Department of Medicine
F. Edward Hebert School of Medicine
Uniformed Services University of the
    Health Sciences
Bethesda, Maryland

Katie E. Neumayer, DO[†]
Department of Pediatrics
Madigan Army Medical Center
Tacoma, Washington

Jelaun Newsome, DO[†]
Department of Primary Care
U.S. Army Health Clinic Baumholder
Baumholder, Germany

Brigitte N. Ngo, DO[†]
Resident
University of Texas Austin DMS Family
    Medicine Residency Program
Austin, Texas

Alex Nguyen, MD[†]
Family Medicine Residency
Eglin Air Force Base
Valparaiso, Florida

Dana Nguyen, MD, FAAFP[†]
Assistant Professor
Department of Family Medicine
Uniformed Services University
Bethesda, Maryland

Nancy V. Nguyen, DO
Clinical faculty
Methodist Family Medicine Residency
    Program
Sacramento, California

Tam Nguyen, MD, FAAFP
Program Director
Family Medicine Residency Program
San Joaquin General Hospital
French Camp, California

Yummy Nguyen, MD[†]
Family Medicine Physician
Naval Hospital Pensacola
Pensacola, Florida

Stacey Nickoloff, DO
Program Director
Family Medicine Residency Program
Presence Resurrection Medical Center
Chicago, Illinois

Frederick W. Nielson, MD, Captain USAF[†]
Department of Family Medicine/Urgent
    Care
Osan Air Base, Republic of Korea

Maria De La Luz Nieto, MD[†]
Clinical Fellow and Instructor
Department of Obstetrics and Gynecology
Division of Urogynecology and
    Reconstructive Pelvic Surgery
University of North Carolina at Chapel Hill
Chapel Hill, North Carolina

Maria L. Nieves, MD[†]
Family Medicine Resident
Department of Family Medicine
Naval Hospital Jacksonville
Jacksonville, Florida

Elizabeth G. Nilson, MD, MPH, FACP
Program Director
Internal Medicine Residency
Assistant Professor
Tufts School of Medicine
General Internal Medicine
Lahey Hospital & Medical Center
Burlington, Massachusetts

G. Daud Noaz, MD, MSBME
Chief Resident
Louisiana State University Rural Family
    Medicine Residency Program
Bogalusa, Louisiana

Thomas Noh, MD
Resident
Department of Neurological Surgery
Henry Ford Hospital
Detroit, Michigan

David R. Norris, MD
Director and Associate Professor of
    Medical Student Programs
Department of Family Medicine
University of Mississippi Medical Center
Jackson, Mississippi

Bakr Nour, MD, PhD, FACS
Professor and Vice-Chairman
Department of Surgery
Weill Cornell Medical College, New York
    City
Senior Adviser to the Dean
Surgery Clerkship Director
Weill Cornell Medical College in Qatar
Al Rayyan, Qatar

Laura Novak, MD
Assistant Director Family Medicine
    Residency Program
Summa Barberton Family Medicine
    Residency
Barberton, Ohio

Rathna Nuti, MD[†]
Family Medicine Resident
Department of Family Medicine and
    Community
University of Texas Southwestern Medical
    Center
Dallas, Texas

Kamala Nyamathi, MD
Department of Family Medicine
Oregon Health & Science University
Portland, Oregon

Theodore X. O'Connell, MD
Residency Program Director
Family Medicine Residency Program
Kaiser Permanente Napa-Solano
Assistant Clinical Professor
Department of Family and Community
    Medicine
University of California San Francisco
San Francisco, California

John B. O'Donnell, MD, MS
Director
Preclinical Curriculum
College of Human Medicine
Michigan State University
Grand Rapids, Michigan

David T. O'Gurek, MD, FAAFP
Assistant Professor
Department of Family and Community
 Medicine
Temple University School of Medicine
Philadelphia, Pennsylvania

Elisa D. O'Hern, MD[†]
Pediatrician
Madigan Army Medical Center
Joint Base Lewis–McChord
Tacoma, Washington

Heather O'Mara, DO[†]
Staff
Family Medicine Residency Clinic
Womack Army Medical Center
Fort Bragg, North Carolina

Andrea Ochab, DO[†]
Naval Hospital Jacksonville
Jacksonville, Florida

Annie Oh, MD[†]
Assistant Professor
Division of Hematology/Oncology
University of Illinois at Chicago
Chicago, Illinois

Annie Lee Oh, MD
Assistant Professor of Clinical Medicine
Hematology/Oncology, Department of
 Medicine
The University of Illinois at Chicago
Chicago, Illinois

Jin Sol Oh, MD
General Surgery Resident
Department of General Surgery
Medical College of Georgia
Georgia Regents University
Augusta, Georgia

Arthur Ohannessian, MD
Health Sciences Clinical Assistant
 Professor
Residency Associate Program Director
Department of Family Medicine
David Geffen School of Medicine at
 UCLA
Los Angeles, California

Smriti Ohri, MD[†]
Assistant Professor
Department of Family Medicine
Oregon Health and Science University
Portland, Oregon

Amy Okpaku, DO[†]
Associate Program Director
University of Texas Austin DMS Family
 Medicine Residency
Austin, Texas

Erika Oleson, DO, MS
Assistant Professor
Division of Geriatric Medicine
Department of Family Medicine and
 Community Health
University of Massachusetts Medical
 School
Worcester, Massachusetts

Jacqueline L. Olin, MS, PharmD, BCPS,
 FASHP, FCCP
Professor of Pharmacy
Wingate University School of Pharmacy
Wingate, North Carolina

Karla A. Oliveros, MD
Department of Medicine
Universidad Catolica Santiago de
 Guayaquil
Guayaquil, Ecuador

Folashade Omole, MD, FAAFP
Professor and Vice-Chairman
Academic Affairs
Director of Integrative Medicine
Department of Family Medicine
Morehouse School of Medicine
Atlanta, Georgia

Jill SM Omori, MD
Associate Professor
Department of Family Medicine and
 Community Health
Office of Medical Education
John A. Burn School of Medicine
University of Hawaii
Honolulu, Hawaii

Imola K. Osapay, MD
Assistant Director
Family Practice - Barberton
Summa Health
Barberton, Ohio

Sean M. Oser, MD, MPH
Assistant Professor
Department of Family and Community
 Medicine
Pennsylvania State University College
 of Medicine
Hershey, Pennsylvania

Tamara K. Oser, MD
Assistant Professor
Department of Family and Community
 Medicine
Pennsylvania State University College
 of Medicine
Hershey, Pennsylvania

Chidinma Osineme, MD
Assistant Professor and Faculty
Department of Family and Community
 Medicine
Virginia Tech Carilion School of Medicine
 and Research Institute
Virginia Tech Carilion Family Medicine
 Residency Program
Roanoke, Virginia

Nilgun Ozturk, MD
UMass Memorial Medical Center
Worcester, Massachusetts

Soraira Pacheco, DO
Resident Physician
Department of Family Medicine
University of Texas Medical Branch
Galveston, Texas

Kelly Pagidas, MD
Women and Infants Hospital
Providence, Rhode Island

Rajandeep S. Paik, MD
Fellow-in-training
Department of Rheumatology
University of Massachusetts
Worcester, Massachusetts

Caitlin Pandolfo, MD
Residency Program
Department of Obstetrics &
 Gynecology
University of Massachusetts Medical
 School
Worcester, Massachusetts

Linda Paniagua, MD[†]
McGovern Medical Center
The University of Texas Health Sciences
 Center at Houston
Houston, Texas

Jon S. Parham, DO, MPH
Associate Professor and Associate
  Director of Predoctoral Education
Department of Family Medicine
University of Tennessee, Graduate School
  of Medicine
Knoxville, Tennessee

Douglas S. Parks, MD
Associate Professor
University of Wyoming Family Medicine
  Residency
University of Wyoming
Cheyenne, Wyoming

Naomi Parrella, MD[†]
Assistant Professor
Clinical Sciences Education Director,
  Family Medicine
Department of Family and Preventive
  Medicine
Chicago Medical School
Rosalind Franklin University of Medicine
  and Science
North Chicago, Illinois

David O. Parrish, MS, MD, FAAFP
Director of Family Medicine Residency
Bayfront Health St. Petersburg
St. Petersburg, Florida
Clinical Associate Professor
University of South Florida College of
  Medicine
Tampa, Florida

Sarah Parrott, DO
Assistant Professor
Division of Primary Care Medicine
Kansas City University of Medicine and
  Biosciences
Kansas City, Missouri

Aleta Paschal, MD
Medical College of Georgia
Augusta, University
Augusta, Georgia

Michael Passafaro, DO, DTM&H,
  FACEP, FACOEP[†]
Assistant Professor
Center for Global Health
Department of Clinical Specialties and
  Division of Emergency Medicine
New York Institute of Technology College
  of Osteopathic Medicine
Old Westbury, New York

Paul Pastor, MD
Catholic University of Santiago de
  Guayaquil
Guayaquil, Ecuador

Aniruddh Anil Patel, MD
Internal Medicine Residency Program
Department of Internal Medicine
University of Louisville School of
  Medicine
Louisville, Kentucky

Birju B. Patel, MD, FACP, AGSF[†]
Clinical Associate
Northeast Georgia Diagnostic Clinic
Atlanta Veterans Affairs Medical Center
Atlanta, Georgia

Chirag M. Patel, MD
Resident Physician
Internal Medicine Residency Program
University of Louisville
Louisville, Kentucky

Krunal Patel, MD
Resident, Internal Medicine
University of Massachusetts Medical
  School
Worcester, Massachusetts

Mahesh C. Patel, MD
Assistant Professor of Medicine
Division of Infectious Diseases,
  Immunology, and International
  Medicine
University of Illinois at Chicago College
  of Medicine
Chicago, Illinois

Manisha J. Patel, MD
Department of Internal Medicine
Lahey Hospital & Medical Center
Burlington, Massachusetts

Nihal K. Patel, MD
Gastroenterology Fellow
Dartmouth Hitchcock Medical Center
Lebanon, New Hampshire

Nupam A. Patel, MD
Resident
Pathology and Laboratory Medicine
University of Cincinnati College of
  Medicine
Cincinnati, Ohio

Palni Patel, PharmD
Adjunct Faculty
Massachusetts College of Pharmacy and
  Health Sciences University
Boston, Massachusetts

Ravin V. Patel, MD
Family Medicine
Department of Family Medicine
Saint Louis University/Belleville
  Campus
Belleville, Illinois

Jay R. Patibandla, MD[†]
Clinical Instructor of Obstetrics and
  Gynecology
Aultman Health Foundation Obstetrics
  and Gynecology Residency
Northeast Ohio Medical University
Canton, Ohio

Joseph E. Patruno, MD
Assistant Clinical Professor
University of South Florida College of
  Medicine
Lehigh Valley Health Network
Allentown, Pennsylvania

Jared M. Patton, MD, MS[†]
Resident Physician
Family Medicine Residency
Naval Hospital Camp Lejeune
Camp Lejeune, North Carolina

Candace Y. Pau, MD
Resident Physician
Family Medicine Residency Program
Kaiser Permanente Napa-Solano
Napa, California

Charles Pavia, PhD
Associate Professor of Microbiology
Departments of Medical Education and
  Biomedical Sciences
College of Osteopathic Medicine
New York Institute of Technology
Old Westbury, New York

Irina Pechenko, MD[†]
Family Medicine Residency Program
Martin Army Community Hospital
Fort Benning, Georgia

Maryse A. Pedoussaut, MD
Assistant Professor
Division of Medicine and Society
Department of Humanities, Health,
  and Society
Herbert Wertheim College of Medicine
Florida International University
Miami, Florida

Rebecca L. Peebles, DO[†]
Family Medicine Resident
David Grant Medical Center
Travis Air Force Base, California

Rod Pellenberg, MD
Nashville Pediatric Cardiology
Nashville, Tennessee

Randall Pellish, MD
Assistant Professor of Medicine
Department of Medicine
Program Director
Gastroenterology Fellowship
University of Massachusetts Medical
    School
Worcester, Massachusetts

Cinthya Pena Orbea, MD[†]
Internal Medicine
John H. Stroger Jr. Hospital of Cook
    Country
Chicago, Illinois

Brian P. Peppers, DO, PhD
Allergy and Immunology Fellow
University Hospitals–Regional Hospitals
Richmond Heights, Ohio

Ruben Peralta, MD, FACS
Director of Trauma and Critical Care
    Fellowship Program
Senior Consultant in Surgery, Emergency,
    Trauma and Critical Care Medicine
Vice-Chairman QPS Program
Department of Surgery
Associate Director of Trauma ICU
Department of Surgery
Hamad General Hospital
Department of Medical Education
Hamad Medical Corporation
Doha, Qatar

Luis Liu Perez, DO
Clinical Associate Professor of Family
    Medicine
Ohio University Heritage College of
    Osteopathic Medicine
Firelands Regional Medical Center
Sandusky, Ohio

T. Ray Perrine, MS, MD, FAAFP[†]
Attending Faculty
Family Medicine Residency Center
North Mississippi Medical Center
Tupelo, Mississippi

Christine S. Persaud, MD
Assistant Professor
Department of Orthopaedic Surgery and
    Rehabilitation Medicine
Medical Director
Division of Sports Medicine
SUNY Downstate Medical Center
Brooklyn, New York

Robert K. Persons, DO[†]
Staff Physician
Family Medicine Residency
Eglin Air Force Base
Valparaiso, Florida

Fahad Pervez, MD[†]
United States Air Force
Saint Louis University Family Medicine
    Residency Program
Belleville, Illinois

Bobby Peters, MD, FAAEM
Assistant Professor
Emergency Department
University of Iowa Hospitals
Iowa City, Iowa

Andrew H. Petersen, DO[†]
Department of Otolaryngology–Head &
    Neck Surgery
Doctors Hospital
Columbus, Ohio

Lindsay Petersen, MD
Clinical Lecturer and Surgical Breast
    Fellow
Department of Surgical Oncology
University of Michigan Health System
Ann Arbor, Michigan

Hugh R. Peterson, MD, FACP
Associate Professor of Medicine
Department of Internal Medicine
University of Louisville School of
    Medicine
Louisville, Kentucky

Kristopher S. Pfirman, DO
Chief Academic Resident
Department of Osteopathic Internal
    Medicine
Southeastern Regional Medical Center
Lumberton, North Carolina

David S. Pfoff, MD[†]
Chief of Ophthalmology
Ehrling Bergquist Clinic
Offutt Air Force Base, Nebraska

Ho Phong Pham, MD[†]
Family Medicine Residency Center
Carl R. Darnall Army Medical Center
Fort Hood, Texas

Karen S. Phelps, MD[†]
Dwight D. Eisenhower Army Medical
    Center
Fort Gordon, Georgia

Kelsey E. Phelps, MD
Assistant Clinical Faculty
Rural Family Medicine Residency
    Program
Louisiana State University
Bogalusa, Louisiana

Teny Anna Philip, MD
Department of Family and Community
    Medicine
University of Texas Health Science
    Center at San Antonio
San Antonio, Texas

Jeffrey Phillips, MD
Family Doctors, LLC
Tufts University School of Medicine
    Faculty
Tufts Residency at CHA Preceptor
UMass Medical School Preceptor
Swampscott, Massachusetts

Kantima Phisitkul, MD
Clinical Assistant Professor
Division of Nephrology
Department of Internal Medicine
University of Iowa Hospital and Clinics
Iowa City, Iowa

Jonathan Pickett, MD[†]
Madigan Army Medical Center
Tacoma, Washington

Gregory Piech, MD, MPH
Internal Medicine Resident
Department of Internal Medicine
George Washington University
Washington, DC

Deborah Pierce, DO
Associate Program Director and
    Osteopathic Director of Medical
    Education
Emergency Medicine Residency Program
Einstein Medical Center
Philadelphia, Pennsylvania

Jonathan Piercy, MD
Assistant Clinical Professor
Department of Family and Community
    Medicine
University of Kentucky College of
    Medicine
East Kentucky Family Medicine
    Residency Program
Hazard, Kentucky

Maria A. Pino, PhD, MS, RpH
Assistant Professor of Pharmacology
Department of Basic Biomedical Science
Touro College of Osteopathic Medicine
New York, New York

Walter L. Pipkin, MD
Associate Professor of Surgery and
    Pediatrics
Children's Hospital of Georgia
Georgia Regent's University
Augusta, Georgia

Jennifer M. Pisani, PharmD
Adjunct Assistant Professor
Massachusetts College of Pharmacy and
    Health Sciences University
Boston, Massachusetts

Maria M. Plummer, MD
Assistant Professor of Pathology
Department of Medical Education
New York Institute of Technology College
    of Osteopathic Medicine
Old Westbury, New York

Piotr Podlesny, MD[†]
Air Force Medicine
Family Medicine Residency Clinic
David Grant Medical Center
Travis Air Force Base, California

Anna C. Porter, MD
Assistant Professor of Medicine
Department of Medicine, Section of
    Nephrology
University of Illinois at Chicago
Chicago, Illinois

Jennifer Luo Powell, DO
Family Medicine Resident
Department of Family Medicine and
    Community Health
University of Massachusetts Medical
    School
Worcester, Massachusetts

James E. Powers, DO, FACEP, FAAEM
Associate Dean for Clinical Integration
Professor of Emergency Medicine
Campbell University School of
    Osteopathic Medicine
Lillington, North Carolina

Faruq Pradhan, MBBCh
Internal Medicine Resident
Lahey Hospital & Medical Center
Burlington, Massachusetts

Pia Prakash, MD
Department of Gastroenterology and
    Liver Diseases
George Washington University
Washington, DC

Tharani Vadivelu Prasad, MD
Resident
Department of Family and Community
    Medicine
University of Texas Health Science
    Center at San Antonio
San Antonio, Texas

Colleen M. Prinzivalli, PharmD, BCPS,
    CGP
Director of Clinical Pharmacy Services
Dovetail Health
Needham, Massachusetts

Barbara J. Provo, MSN, RN, FNP-BC,
    CWON
Nurse Practitioner and Clinical
    Coordinator
Wound and Ostomy Clinic
Froedtert Hospital & Medical College of
    Wisconsin
Milwaukee, Wisconsin

George G.A. Pujalte, MD, FACSM
Sports Medicine
Departments of Family Medicine, and
    Orthopedics
Mayo Clinic Health System
Waycross, Georgia

Margaret Pyle, MD
Resident
University of Massachusetts Medical
    School
Worcester, Massachusetts

Natasha J. Pyzocha, DO[†]
Resident Physician
Department of Family Medicine
Madigan Army Medical Center
Tacoma, Washington

Lina N. Qazi, DO
Family Medicine Resident
Southeastern Regional Medical Center
Lumberton, North Carolina

Sascha Qian, MD
Resident Physician
Department of Anesthesiology
New York-Presbyterian Hospital–
    Columbia
New York, New York

Juan Qiu, MD, PhD
Associate Professor
Department of Family and Community
    Medicine
Pennsylvania State University College of
    Medicine
Hershey, Pennsylvania

Jeffrey D. Quinlan, MD, FAAFP[†]
Associate Professor and Vice-Chairman
Department of Family Medicine
Uniformed Services University of the
    Health Sciences
Bethesda, Maryland

Patricia Martinez Quinones, MD
Surgery Resident
General Surgery Program
Augusta University
Augusta, Georgia

Jeremy Raab, MD[†]
National Capital Consortium Family
    Medicine Residency
Fort Belvoir Community Hospital
Fort Belvoir, Virginia

Naureen Bashir Rafiq, MBBS, MD
Creighton University Medical Center
Bellevue, Nebraska

Jyoti Ramakrishna, MD
Chief
Pediatric Gastroenterology and Nutrition
Floating Hospital for Children
Tufts Medical Center
Boston, Massachusetts

Kalyanakrishnan Ramakrishnan, MD
Professor
Department of Family and Preventive
    Medicine
University of Oklahoma Health Sciences
    Center
Oklahoma City, Oklahoma

Muthalagu Ramanathan, MD
Assistant Professor of Medicine
Associate Director of BMT Program
University of Massachusetts Medical
    School
Worcester, Massachusetts

Swathi A.N. Rao, MD[†]
Department of Endocrinology
Riverview Health
Noblesville, Indiana

Marina Rasnow-Hill, MD
Clinical Faculty
Department of Family Medicine/Obstetrics
Mercy/Methodist Family Medicine
    Residency Program
Sacramento, California

Wasiq Faraz Rawasia, MD
Cardiovascular Medicine Fellow
University of Louisville
Louisville, Kentucky

Sean Rea, DO
Southeastern Regional Medical Center
Lumberton, North Carolina

Donovan S. Reed, BS[†]
F. Edward Hebert School of Medicine
Uniformed Services University of the
    Health Sciences
Bethesda, Maryland

Grant M. Reed, DO
Resident Physician of Family Medicine
A.T. Still University
Medical College of Wisconsin
Waukesha, Wisconsin

Tyler R. Reese, MD[†]
Family Medicine Residency Program
Tripler Army Medical Center
Honolulu, Hawaii

Jennifer Reidy, MD, MS, FAAHPM
Co-Chief
Division of Palliative Care
University of Massachusetts Memorial
    Medical Center
Worcester, Massachusetts

Stephanie W. Reiser, DO[†]
Family Medicine Resident
Department of Family Medicine
Offutt Air Force Base/University of
    Nebraska Medical Center
Omaha, Nebraska

Caitlyn M. Rerucha, MD[†]
Adjunct Faculty, Medical Director
    Copperas Cove Medical Home
Department of Family Medicine and
    Community Health
Carl R. Darnall Army Medical Center
Fort Hood, Texas

Emily Reus, MD
Resident
UMass Memorial Medical Center
Worcester, Massachusetts

Jonathan D. Reves, DO
Internal Medicine Resident
Southeastern Regional Medical Center
Lumberton, North Carolina

Leigh G. Rexius, DO[†]
Resident
Womack Army Medical Center
Fort Bragg, North Carolina

Emmanuel Reyes-Ramos, MD
George Washington University
Washington, DC

Harlan G. Rich, MD, FACP, AGAF
Associate Professor of Medicine
The Warren Alpert Medical School of
    Brown University
University Medicine Foundation, Inc.
Director of Endoscopy
Rhode Island Hospital
Providence, Rhode Island

Andrew Richardson, MD
Family Medicine Resident
Texas A&M Family Medicine Residency
    Program
Bryan, Texas

John M. Richardson, MD[†]
Family Medicine Resident
Fort Belvoir Family Medicine Residency
Fort Belvoir, Virginia

Sean W. Richardson, DO[†]
Martin Army Community Hospital
Fort Benning, Georgia

Harry Richter, III, MD
Associate Professor
Rush University Medical Center
Chicago, Illinois

Matthew J. Richter, DO[†]
Family Medicine Resident
Department of Family Medicine
Naval Hospital Camp Lejeune
Camp Lejeune, North Carolina

Angela M. Riegel, DO[†]
Family Medicine Faculty
Offutt Air Force Family Medicine
    Residency
Offutt Air Force Base, Nebraska

Lyrad K. Riley, MD[†]
Director of Maternity Care Services
Eglin AFB Family Medicine Residency
    Program
Eglin Air Force Base
Valparaiso, Florida

Sonia Rivera-Martinez, DO, FACOFP
Assistant Professor
Department of Family Medicine
New York Institute of Technology College
    of Osteopathic Medicine
Old Westbury, New York

Anthony F. Rizzo, DO
Family Medicine Resident
Presence Resurrection Medical Center
Chicago, Illinois

Ramona Roach-Davis, DNP, FNP-BC[†]
Hoover Family Medicine
MedCenter Hoover
Hoover, Alabama

Michele Roberts, MD, PhD
Clinical Genetics
Anatomic and Clinical Pathology
Paxton, Massachusetts

Sean C. Robinson, MD
Clinical Instructor
Department of Family Medicine
Oregon Health and Science University
Portland, Oregon

Jack Rock, MD
Vice-Chairman of Education
Department of Neurosurgery
Director of Neurosurgery Residency
    Program
Co-Director
Surgical Neuro-Oncology Clinic and
    Metastatic Tumor—Brain Program
Director of Skullbase and Pituitary Tumor
    Program
Henry Ford Hospital
Detroit, Michigan

Patrick J. Rogers, DO
Emergency Medicine Resident
Department of Emergency Medicine
Rutgers-Robert Wood Johnson Medical
    School
New Brunswick, New Jersey

Theodore Rogers, DO[†]
Family Medicine Resident
Naval Hospital Camp LeJeune
Jacksonville, North Carolina

Tyler S. Rogers, MD[†]
Resident Physician
Department of Family and Community
    Medicine
Dwight D. Eisenhower Army Medical Center
Fort Gordon, Georgia

Andrew Romney, DO[†]
Family Medicine Resident
Nellis Air Force Base
Las Vegas, Nevada

Jose Rose, PA-C[†]
Physician Assistant
Fort Drum, New York

Noah M. Rosenberg, MD
Assistant Professor
Department of Family Medicine and
    Community Health
University of Massachusetts Medical School
Worcester, Massachusetts

Montiel T. Rosenthal, MD
Associate Professor and Director of
 Maternity Services
Department of Family and Community
 Medicine
University of Cincinnati College of
 Medicine
Cincinnati, Ohio

David A. Ross, MD
Resident Physician
Department of Family Medicine and
 Community Health
University of Pennsylvania
Philadelphia, Pennsylvania

Michael J. Ross, MD
Associate Professor of Medicine
Division of Nephrology
Icahn School of Medicine at Mount Sinai
New York, New York

Steven Rougas, MD, MS
Assistant Professor of Emergency Medicine
The Warren Alpert Medical School of
 Brown University
Providence, Rhode Island

Anna Rudnicki, MD†
Assistant Professor of Medicine
Division of Pulmonary, Allergy, and Critical
 Care Medicine
University of Massachusetts Medical School
Worcester, Massachusetts

Joshua J. Ruiz, DO
Internal Medicine Resident
Southeastern Health
Lumberton, North Carolina

Lloyd A. Runser, MD, MPH†
Associate Program Director
Scholarly Activity Coordinator
Family Medicine Residency
Department of Family Medicine
Womack Army Medical Center
Fort Bragg, North Carolina

Travis C. Russell, MD, FAWM†
Core Faculty
Nellis Family Medicine
Nellis Air Force Base
Las Vegas, Nevada

Emilio A. Russo, MD
Chief of Staff
Our Lady of the Angels Hospital
Program Director
Rural Family Medicine Residency Program
Louisiana State University
Bogalusa, Louisiana
Assistant Professor
Department of Family Medicine
Louisiana State University Health
 Sciences Center
New Orleans, Louisiana

Veronica J. Ruston, DO, Capt, USAF, MC†
Department of Family Health
Luke Air Force Base
Luke Air Force Base, Arizona

Anup K. Sabharwal, MD, MBA, FACE,
 CCD
Division of Endocrinology, Diabetes, and
 Metabolism
Herbert Wertheim College of Medicine
Florida International University
Miami, Florida

Komel Safdar, MBBS
Education
King Edward Medical College
Lahore, Pakistan

Daniel W. Saltzman, DO
Resident
Department of Emergency Medicine
Rutgers-Robert Wood Johnson Medical
 School
New Brunswick, New Jersey

Kathryn Samai, PharmD, BCPS
Assistant Professor of Pharmacy Practice
Lake Erie College of Osteopathic
 Medicine School of Pharmacy
Bradenton, Florida

Arthur B. Sanders, MD, MHA†
Professor
Department of Emergency Medicine
University of Arizona College of Medicine
Tucson, Arizona

Adam K. Saperstein, MD, FAAFP†
Assistant Professor
Department of Family Medicine
Uniformed Services University of the
 Health Sciences
Bethesda, Maryland

Yona Saperstein, MD
Department of Family Medicine
SUNY Downstate Medical Center
Brooklyn, New York

Steven B. Sapida, DO†
Naval Hospital Jacksonville
Jacksonville, Florida

John A. Saryan, MD
Allergy and Immunology, Asthma Center
Lahey Hospital & Medical Center
Burlington, Massachusetts
Lahey Medical Center, Peabody
Peabody, Massachusetts

Robert T. Sataloff, MD
Philadelphia Ear, Nose and Throat
 Associates—PENTA
Philadelphia, Pennsylvania

Thomas M. Savage, MD
Bayfront Health St. Petersburg
St. Petersburg, Florida

Paul A. Savel, MD†
Supervisory Physician
Department of Family Medicine
Madigan Army Medical Center
Tacoma, Washington

Shailendra K. Saxena, MD, PhD
Assistant Professor
Department of Family Medicine
Creighton University School of Medicine
Omaha, Nebraska

Durr-e-Shahwaar Sayed, DO
Faculty Physician
Department of Family Medicine
Inspira Health Network
Glassboro, New Jersey

Payam Sazegar, MD, CCFP
Clinical Assistant Professor
Department of Family Practice
University of British Columbia Faculty of
 Medicine
Vancouver, British Columbia, Canada

Catherine Scarbrough, MD
Assistant Professor
Department of Family Medicine
University of Alabama College of
 Community Health Sciences
Tuscaloosa, Alabama

Matthew J. Schear, DO, MS
Resident Ophthalmologist
Department of Osteopathic Manipulative
 Medicine
Hofstra North Shore—Long Island Jewish
 School of Medicine
Great Neck, New York

Jessica M. Schechtman, DO[†]
Clinical Instructor of Obstetrics and
   Gynecology
Aultman Health Foundation Obstetrics
   and Gynecology Residency
Northeast Ohio Medical University
Canton, Ohio

Edward Scheiner, DO
Advanced ENT
Sewell, New Jersey

Fred J. Schiffman, MD
Sigal Family Professor of Humanistic
   Medicine
The Warren Alpert Medical School of
   Brown University
Providence, Rhode Island

Jonathan Schimmel, MD
Resident
Department of Emergency Medicine
Rhode Island Hospital
Brown University
Providence, Rhode Island

Benjamin N. Schneider, MD
Assistant Dean for Student Affairs
Assistant Professor of Family Medicine
Oregon Health & Science University
Portland, Oregon

Brian J. Schneider, MD[†]
Sports Medicine Fellow
University of Colorado
Denver, Colorado

Sebastian Schnellbacher, DO[†]
Madigan Army Medical Center
Tacoma, Washington

Lisa M. Schroeder, MD
Assistant Director
Summa Barberton Family Practice
   Residency Program
Barberton, Ohio

Jennifer B. Schwartz, MD
Family and Sports Medicine Physician
Beth Israel Deaconess Medical Center
Boston, Massachusetts

Erik J. Schweitzer, MD MPH[†]
Assistant Professor of Family Medicine
Department of Family Medicine
Uniformed Services University of the
   Health Sciences
Bethesda, Maryland

Christopher J. Scola, MD
Assistant Clinical Professor of Medicine
University of Connecticut School of
   Medicine
Chief, Rheumatology Division
Hartford Hospital
Hartford, Connecticut

Ingrid U. Scott, MD, MPH
Professor of Ophthalmology and Public
   Health Sciences
Penn State Hershey Eye Center
Penn State College of Medicine
Hershey, Pennsylvania

Stephen Scott, MD, MPH
Associate Professor of Family Medicine
Associate Dean for Student Affairs
Weill Cornell Medical College in Qatar
Doha, Qatar

Gail Scully, MD, MPH
University of Massachusetts Memorial
   Medical Center
University of Massachusetts Medical
   School
Worcester, Massachusetts

Paul E. Seales, MD[†]
Resident
Department of Family Medicine
Naval Hospital Jacksonville
Jacksonville, Florida

Sajeewane M. Seales, MD
Department of Family Medicine
Naval Hospital Jacksonville
Jacksonville, Florida

David P. Sealy, MD
Professor of MUSC Greenwood AHEC
Program Director
Self Regional Healthcare Sports
   Medicine Fellowship
Greenwood, South Carolina

Margaret Seaver, MD, MPH
Palliative Medicine Service
Lahey Hospital & Medical Center
Burlington, Massachusetts

L. Michelle Seawright, DO[†]
Family Medicine Residency
Naval Hospital Camp Lejeune
Camp Lejeune, North Carolina

Sheila M. Seed, PharmD, MPH, RPh
Associate Professor of Pharmacy
   Practice
Vice-Chairman of Pharmacy Practice
Department of Pharmacy Practice
Massachusetts College of Pharmacy and
   Health Sciences University
Worcester, Massachusetts

Erin S. Seefeldt, MD[†]
Associate Program Director
Madigan Ophthalmology
Tacoma, Washington
Assistant Professor of Surgery
Uniformed Services University of the
   Health Sciences
Bethesda, Maryland

Amy Seery, MD
Assistant Professor
Department of Family and Community
   Medicine
University of Kansas School of Medicine–
   Wichita
Wichita, Kansas

Christopher R. Selinsky, DO[†]
Department of Otolaryngology–Head &
   Neck Surgery
Doctor's Hospital
Ohio University Heritage College of
   Osteopathic Medicine
Athens, Ohio

Peter J. Sell, DO, FAAP
Associate Professor
Department of Pediatrics
Critical Care Pediatrics and Child
   Protection Program
University of Massachusetts Medical School
Worcester, Massachusetts

Jessica T. Servey, MD, Col, USAF, MC[†]
Assistant Dean for Faculty Development
Associate Professor of Family Medicine
Uniformed Services University of the
   Health Sciences
Bethesda, Maryland

Tarsheen K. Sethi, MBBS
Clinical Fellow
Department of Medicine/Hematology-
   Oncology
Vanderbilt University Medical Center
Nashville, Tennessee

Patricia Seymour, MD, FAAFP, FHM
Assistant Professor
Department of Family Medicine and
    Community Health
University of Massachusetts Medical School
Worcester, Massachusetts

Chirag N. Shah, MD
Assistant Professor
Department of Emergency Medicine
Rutgers-Robert Wood Johnson Medical
    School
New Brunswick, New Jersey

Maulin Shah, DO
Family Medicine Resident
Department of Family Medicine
Firelands Regional Medical Center
Ohio University Heritage College of
    Osteopathic Medicine
Athens, Ohio

Meera Shah, MD, MS, AAHIVS[†]
HIV/AIDS and Transgender Care
    Provider
Callen-Lorde Community Health Center
New York, New York

Sachin P. Shah, MD
Lahey Hospital & Medical Center
Burlington, Massachusetts

Samir A. Shah, MD, FACG, FASGE,
    AGAF
Clinical Professor of Medicine
The Warren Alpert Medical School of
    Brown University
Chief of Gastroenterology
Department of Medicine
The Miriam Hospital
Providence, Rhode Island

S. David Shahbodaghi, MD, MPH[†]
Family Medicine Resident
Dwight D. Eisenhower Army Medical
    Center
Fort Gordon, Georgia

Kevin C. Shannon, MD, MPH, FAAFP
Associate Professor
Department of Family Medicine
Loma Linda University School of
    Medicine
Loma Linda, California

Musa A. Sharkawi, MBBCh, BAO
Resident Physician
Department of Internal Medicine
Lahey Hospital & Medical Center
Burlington, Massachusetts

Victoria R. Sharon, MD, DTMH
Assistant Professor of Dermatology &
    Mohs Surgery Director
Dermatology Inpatient Consultation
University of California, Davis
Davis, California

Cameron M. Shawver, DO[†]
Nellis Family Medicine Residency
Mike O'Callaghan Federal Medical
    Center
Nellis Air Force Base
Las Vegas, Nevada

Karen Sheflin, DO
Assistant Professor
Department of Family Medicine
College of Osteopathic Medicine
New York Institute of Technology
Old Westbury, New York

Paula A. Shelton, MD
Family Medicine
University of Texas Health Science
    Center at San Antonio
San Antonio, Texas

Nicole Shields, MD
Assistant Professor of Family Medicine
DeBusk College of Osteopathic
    Medicine
Lincoln Memorial University
Harrogate, Tennessee

Jeffrey Shih, MD
Assistant Professor of Medicine
Advanced Heart Failure and Cardiac
    Transplantation
Cardiovascular Medicine
University of Massachusetts
Worcester, Massachusetts

Naomi S. Shin, MD
Department of Internal Medicine
Mount Auburn Hospital
Cambridge, Massachusetts

Sonya Shipley, MD
Assistant Professor
Department of Family Medicine
University of Mississippi Medical Center
Jackson, Mississippi

Matthew W. Short, MD, FAAFP[†]
Director of Transitional Year Program
Associate Director of Medical Education
Madigan Army Medical Center
Tacoma, Washington
Associate Professor of Family Medicine
Uniformed Services University of the
    Health Sciences
Bethesda, Maryland

Sydney Short, MD
Cardiologist
Duke Cardiology and Cardiovascular
    Surgery of Lumberton
Lumberton, North Carolina

Suzanne Shurtz, MLIS, AHIP
Associate Professor
Instructional Services Librarian
Texas A&M University Medical Sciences
    Library
Joint Associate Professor
Department of Internal Medicine
Texas A&M Health Science Center
    College of Medicine
College Station, Texas

Aamir Siddiqi, MD[†]
Director of Clinical Services
Norris Health Center
University of Wisconsin—Milwaukee
Milwaukee, Wisconsin

Najm Hasan Siddiqui, MD
Hospitalist Physician
Parkview Medical Center
Pueblo, Colorado

Julia Siegel, MD
University of Massachusetts Medical School
Worcester, Massachusetts

Samuel N. Sigoloff, DO, CPT, MC[†]
Family Medicine Resident
Fort Benning, Georgia

Kimberly Sikule, MD
Resident
Family Medicine Residency
Barre Family Health Center
Worcester, Massachusetts

Hugh Silk, MD, MPH, FAAFP
Professor
Department of Family Medicine and
    Community Health
University of Massachusetts Medical
    School
Worcester, Massachusetts

Matthew A. Silva, PharmD, RPh, BCPS
Professor of Pharmacy Practice
Massachusetts College of Pharmacy and
    Health Sciences University
Worcester, Massachusetts

Lauren M. Simon, MD, MPH, FAAFP,
    FACSM
Associate Professor
Department of Family Medicine
Director of Primary Care Sports Medicine
Loma Linda University School of
    Medicine
Loma Linda, California

Marvin H. Sineath, Jr., MD, CAQSM[†]
Family Medicine Residency
Sports Medicine Director
Nellis Air Force Base, Nevada

Amy M. Singer, DO
Administrative Chief Resident
Department of Family Medicine
University of Texas Health Science
    Center at San Antonio
San Antonio, Texas

Nick Singh, MD[†]
Resident
Fort Hood, Texas

Nga Yan Siu, DO, MS
College of Osteopathic Medicine
New York Institute of Technology
Old Westbury, New York

Ana Lucia Siu Chang, MD
Resident Physician
Department of Family Medicine
University of Texas Medical Branch
Galveston, Texas

Maja Skikic, MD[†]
Department of Psychiatry
Vanderbilt University Medical Center
Nashville, Tennessee

Brian G. Skotko, MD, MPP
Co-Director
Down Syndrome Program
Division of Medical Genetics
Massachusetts General Hospital
Boston, Massachusetts

Dawn Sloan, MD
Faculty Development Fellow
Madigan Army Medical Center
Tacoma, Washington

Jennifer M. Slowik, DO, MS[†]
Family Medicine Physician
Department of Family Medicine
Martin Army Community Hospital
Fort Benning, Georgia

Jason C. Sluzevich, MD
Assistant Professor of Dermatology
Mayo Clinic
Jacksonville, Florida

Adam J.T. Smith, MD, PhD
Resident Physician
Department of Radiation Medicine
University of Kentucky
Lexington, Kentucky

Andrew Smith, MD
Greater Lawrence Family Health Center
Lawrence, Massachusetts

Dennis Smith, DO
Program Director
North Mississippi Medical Center Family
    Medicine Residency Program
Tupelo, Mississippi

Dustin K. Smith, DO[†]
Assistant Professor
Department of Family Medicine
Uniformed Services University of the
    Health Sciences
Faculty
Jacksonville Family Medicine Residency
    Program
Naval Hospital Jacksonville
Jacksonville, Florida

Elizabeth Smith, MD[†]
Eglin Air Force Base

Hedy Smith, MD, PhD[†]
Associate Professor and Director of
    Non-Malignant Hematology Services
Department of Hematology and
    Oncology
Tufts Medical Center
Boston, Massachusetts

Kayla J. Smith, MD
Georgia Regents University
Augusta, Georgia

Morgan Ashleigh Smith, DO[†]
General Surgery Resident
Department of Surgery
Georgia Regents University
Augusta, Georgia

Ruth Smith, MD[†]

Savannah W. Smith, MD[†], CPT, MC, USA
Family Medicine Resident
Martin Army Community Hospital
Fort Benning, Georgia

John C. Smulian, MD, MPH
Division of Maternal Fetal Medicine
Department of Obstetrics and
    Gynecology
Lehigh Valley Health Network
Allentown, Pennsylvania
University of South Florida-Morsani
    College of Medicine
Tampa, Florida

Matthew R. Snead, DO
Internal Medicine Resident Physician
Southeastern Health
Lumberton, North Carolina

Caroline K. Snowberger, DO
Resident
Department of Family Medicine
Christiana Care Hospital
Wilmington, Delaware

Christopher J. Snyder, MD[†]

Matthew J. Snyder, DO[†]
Associate Program Director
Saint Louis University Family Medicine
    Residency Program
Belleville, Illinois

Leah Soley, MD
Family Medicine
Pensacola, Florida

D'Ann Somerall, DNP, FNP-BC
Associate Professor
Assistant Master of Science in Nursing
    Program Director
Family Nurse Practitioner Specialty Track
    Coordinator
Family, Community, Health Systems
University of Alabama at Birmingham
Birmingham, Alabama

William E. Somerall, Jr., MD, MEd
Visiting Associate Professor School of
    Nursing
Adult/Acute Health, Chronic Care &
    Foundations
School of Nursing
University of Alabama at Birmingham
Birmingham, Alabama

Adam J. Sorscher, MD
Assistant Professor
Department of Family and Community
    Medicine
Geisel School of Medicine
Hanover, New Hampshire

Andres F. Sosa, MD
Assistant Professor of Medicine
Interventional Pulmonary
Division of Lung, Allergy and Critical Care
    Medicine
UMass Memorial Medical Center
Worcester, Massachusetts

Alison Southern, MD, MS, FACEP
Associate Program Director
Department of Emergency Medicine
Summa Akron City Hospital
Akron, Ohio

Charles M. Sow, MD
Associate Professor
Department of Family Medicine
Morehouse School of Medicine
Atlanta, Georgia

Thomas C. Spalla, MD
Director
ENT Facial Plastic Surgery at Cooper
    University Hospital
Assistant Professor
Cooper Medical School of Rowan
    University
Camden, New Jersey
Adjunct Professor
Department of Otolaryngology–Head &
    Neck Surgery
Drexel University College of Medicine
Philadelphia, Pennsylvania

Mikayla Spangler, PharmD[†]
Associate Professor
Departments of Pharmacy Practice and
    Family Medicine
Creighton University
Omaha, Nebraska

Kellie A. Sprague, MD
Director, Bone Marrow Transplant
    Program
Tufts Medical Center
Assistant Professor of Medicine
Tufts University School of Medicine
Boston, Massachusetts

Dana Sprute, MD, MPH, FAAFP[†]
Associate Professor of Medicine
Dell Medical School, University of Texas
    at Austin
Austin, Texas

Laura Steadman, EdD, CRNP, MSN,
    RN[†]
Assistant Professor
School of Nursing
University of Alabama at Birmingham
Birmingham, Alabama

Susan L. Steffans, DO
Assistant Professor
Department of Family & Community
    Medicine
A.T. Still University School of Osteopathic
    Medicine in Arizona
Mesa, Arizona

Daniel J. Stein, MD, MPH
Resident Physician
Department of Internal Medicine
University of Virginia Health System
Charlottesville, Virginia

Kim Michal Stein, MD
Resident Physician
University of Virginia Health System
Charlottesville, Virginia

Anne Steiner, MD
Director of Ocular Surface Center
North Shore LIJ Health System
Assistant Professor of Ophthalmology
Hofstra-NSLIJ School of Medicine
Great Neck, New York

Kyle Stephens, DO, MPH
Resident Physician
Mercy/Methodist Family Medicine
    Residency Program
Sacramento, California

Mark B. Stephens, MD, MS, FAAFP,
    CAPT, MC, USN[†]
Professor and Chairman
Department of Family Medicine
Uniformed Services University of the
    Health Sciences
Bethesda, Maryland

Nathaniel Stepp, DO, LCDR, USN[†]
Family Medicine Physician
Family Medicine Residency Staff
Naval Hospital Camp Lejeune
Camp Lejeune, North Carolina

William A. Stevens, MD[†]

J. Herbert Stevenson, MD[†]
Director of the Sports Medicine
    Fellowship Program
Associate Professor University of
    Massachusetts
Department of Family Medicine
Joint Appointment Department of
    Orthopedics
University of Massachusetts
Worcester, Massachusetts

Sheila O. Stille, DMD
Associate Professor and Assistant GPR
    Director
Department of Surgical Dentistry
University of Colorado School of Dental
    Medicine
Aurora, Colorado

Marcus F. Stoddard, MD
Professor of Medicine
Director
Non-invasive Cardiology Division
Cardiovascular Medicine
University of Louisville
Louisville, Kentucky

Helenka Stone, MD
Resident Physician
Department of Family Medicine
Creighton University
Omaha, Nebraska

Jeffrey G. Stovall, MD
Associate Professor
Department of Psychiatry
Vanderbilt University School of Medicine
Nashville, Tennessee

Celeste Straight, MD[†]
Resident Physician
Department of Obstetrics and
    Gynecology
University of Massachusetts Memorial
    Hospital
Worcester, Massachusetts

Melody L. Strattan, DO
Cardiology Fellow
Largo Medical Center
Largo, Florida

Adam Strosberg, DNP, ARNP-BC
Board Certified Family Nurse Practitioner
Broward Health and Florida Atlantic
    University
Fort Lauderdale, Florida

Sujit Suchindran, MD MPH
Senior Staff Physician
Department of Infectious Diseases
Lahey Hospital & Medical Center
Burlington, Massachusetts

Karyn M. Sullivan, PharmD, MPH
Associate Professor of Pharmacy
    Practice
Massachusetts College of Pharmacy and
    Health Sciences University
Worcester, Massachusetts

Heather Summe, MD, MS
Dermatology Resident
University of Massachusetts Medical
    School
Worcester, Massachusetts

Nina E. Suresh, MD, MS
Resident Physician
New York-Presbyterian Phyllis and David
  Komansky Center for Children's Health
Weill Cornell Medical Center
New York, New York

Shima Syed, MD[†]
Staff Physician
Department of Family and Community
  Medicine
Dwight D. Eisenhower Army Medical
  Center
Fort Gordon, Georgia

Michelle E. Szczepanik, MD[†]
Sports Medicine Director
Department of Family and Community
  Medicine
Carl R. Darnall Army Medical Center
Fort Hood, Texas

Alfonso Tafur, MD, MS, RPVI
Assistant Professor of Medicine
Department of Medicine—Cardiovascular
Oklahoma University Health Sciences
  Center
Oklahoma City, Oklahoma

Denisse V. Tafur, MD
Guayaquil, Ecuador

Timothy R. Takagi, MD
Faculty Physician
Associate Residency Director
Methodist Family Medicine Residency
  Program
Dignity Health Methodist Hospital of
  Sacramento
Sacramento, California

Amar Talati, DO
Resident Physician
Bayfront Health Family Medicine
  Residency
Bayfront Health St. Petersburg
St. Petersburg, Florida

Asif Talukder, MD
Resident Physician
Department of Surgery
Georgia Regents University
Augusta, Georgia

Krystal M. Tamura, MD
Faculty and Inpatient Medical Director
Department of Family Medicine
St. Anthony North Family Medicine
  Residency
Westminster, Colorado

Irene J. Tan, MD, FACR
Associate Professor of Clinical Medicine
Department of Medicine, Section of
  Rheumatology
Temple University School of Medicine
Philadelphia, Pennsylvania

Christopher L. Tangen, DO[†]
Medical Director of Sports Medicine
University Hospitals–Regional Hospitals
Richmond Campus
Richmond Heights, Ohio

Michael T. Tanoue, MD[†]
Resident, Internal Medicine
New York-Presbyterian Hospital
Weill Cornell Medical College
New York, New York

Craig Van Tassel, DO[†]
Naval Hospital Jacksonville
Jacksonville, Florida

Paul A. Tate, Jr., MD[†]
Womack Army Medical Center
Family Medicine Residency
Fort Bragg, North Carolina

Eugene M. Tay, MD, MS
Assistant Clinical Professor
Department of Family Medicine
Michigan State University
Grand Rapids, Michigan

Amber C. Taylor, MD[†]
Family Medicine Resident
Family Medicine Residency
Offutt Air Force Base
University of Nebraska Medical Center
Omaha, Nebraska

Danielle Taylor, DO, MS
Obstetrics and Gynecology Resident
Akron General Medical Center
Akron, Ohio

James L. Taylor, PharmD
Clinical Pharmacy Manager, Ambulatory
  Care
Family Medicine Residency Center
North Mississippi Medical Center
Tupelo, Mississippi

Timothy J. Taylor, DO[†]
Instructor
Campbell University College of
  Osteopathic Medicine
Lumberton, North Carolina

Bethany N. Teer, MD[†]
Family Medicine Residency Faculty
Department of Family and Community
  Medicine
Carl R. Darnall Army Medical Center
Fort Hood, Texas

Meaghan Tenney, MD
Assistant Professor
Section of Gynecologic Oncology
Department of Obstetrics and
  Gynecology
University of Chicago Medicine
Chicago, Illinois

Anna Cecilia S. Tenorio, MD
Academic Chief Resident
Department of Family and Community
  Medicine
University of Texas Health Science
  Center at San Antonio
San Antonio, Texas

Nimmy Thakolkaran, MD
Resident
Department of Family Medicine
Mount Sinai Hospital
Chicago, Illinois

Wesley M. Theurer, DO, MBA, MPH[†]
Womack Army Medical Center
Fort Bragg, North Carolina

Ian D. Thomas, MD
Pediatric Chief Resident
University of Arizona
Tucson, Arizona

Dena Thompson, DO
Resident
Southeastern Health
Lumberton, North Carolina

Margaret E. Thompson, MD, FAAP
Associate Professor of Family Medicine
Assistant Dean for the Clinical Curriculum
Michigan State University College of
  Human Medicine
Grand Rapids, Michigan

Matthew W. Thompson, MD[†]
Family Medicine Resident
Department of Family Medicine
Womack Army Medical Center
Fort Bragg, North Carolina

Matthew E. Tick, DO
Resident Physician
Department of Internal Medicine
George Washington University
Washington, DC

Robert J. Tiller, MD, FAAFP
Family Medicine Residency Program
    Director
Associate Professor of Family Medicine
Self Regional Healthcare
Greenwood, South Carolina

Bryan Tischenkel, MD
Columbia University Medical Center
New York-Presbyterian Hospital
New York, New York

Jonathan Tisdell, MD
Neurologist
Saint Vincent Hospital
Worcester, Massachusetts

Adam Z. Tobias, MD, MPH, FACEP
Assistant Professor of Emergency
    Medicine
University of Pittsburgh School of
    Medicine
Pittsburgh, Pennsylvania

Rachelle E. Toman, MD, PhD
Medical Director and Assistant Program
    Director
Georgetown University-Providence
    Hospital Family Medicine Residency
Washington, DC

Sebastian T. Tong, MD, MPH
Assistant Professor
Department of Family Medicine and
    Population Health
Virginia Commonwealth University
Richmond, Virginia

Tiffany Tonismae, MD
Virginia Tech Carilion
Roanoke, Virginia

Moshe S. Torem, MD, DLFAPA
Professor of Psychiatry
Northeast Ohio Medical University
Rootstown, Ohio
Chief of Integrative Medicine
Akron General Medical Center
Akron, Ohio

John R. Torro, MD
Faculty Attending Physician
Lawrence Family Medicine Residency
Lawrence, Massachusetts

Sunkaru Touray, MBChB, MSc[†]
Fellow in Pulmonary Diseases & Critical
    Care Medicine
Department of Pulmonary and Critical
    Care Medicine
University of Massachusetts Medical
    School
Worcester, Massachusetts

Huy Tan Tran, MD, LCDR, MC, USN[†]
Family Medicine Resident
Naval Hospital Camp Pendleton
Camp Pendleton, California

Vu D. Tran, MD[†]
Department of Family Medicine
Summa Barberton Hospital
Barberton, Ohio

Kashyap Trivedi, MD
Hertz and Associates in Gastroenterology
Los Alamitos, California

Rupal Trivedi, MD
Assistant Professor
Department of Family and Community
    Medicine
Saint Louis University School of Medicine
St. Louis, Missouri

Zoltan Trizna, MD, PhD
Dermatology and Dermatological Surgery
Austin, Texas

Katherine M. Tromp, PharmD[†]
Assistant Professor of Pharmacy Practice
Lake Erie College of Osteopathic
    Medicine School of Pharmacy
Bradenton, Florida

Caroline Tschibelu, MD[†]
House Staff
Department of Emergency Medicine
Robert Wood Johnson University Hospital
New Brunswick, New Jersey

Artsiom Tsyrkunou, MD, MPH
Primary Care Physician
Hillcrest Family Health Center
Berkshire Medical Center
Pittsfield, Massachusetts

Annie Marian Tubman, MD
Family Medicine Resident
Family Medicine of Southwest
Vancouver, Washington

Sarwada Tuladhar Jha, MBBS
Resident Physician
Department of Family Medicine
Creighton University Medical Center
Omaha, Nebraska

Bradley M. Turner, MD, MPH, MHA
Assistant Professor
University of Rochester
Rochester, New York

Auguste Turnier, MD
Internist/Gastroenterologist, Private
    Practice
Haddonfield, New Jersey

Cheryll Udani, MD
Resident
University of Texas Health Science
    Center at San Antonio
San Antonio, Texas

John K. Uffman, MD, MPH[†]
Pediatric Surgery
Cook Children's Medical Center
Fort Worth, Texas

Katherine S. Upchurch, MD
Clinical Professor of Medicine
University of Massachusetts Medical
    Group
Clinical Chief
Division of Rheumatology
University of Massachusetts Memorial
    Medical Group
Worcester, Massachusetts

Geraldine N. Urse, DO, FACOFP,
    MHPEd
Director of Medical Education/DIO
Doctors Hospital
Columbus, Ohio

Onameyore Utuama, MD, MPH
Morehouse School of Medicine Family
    Medicine Residency
Atlanta, Georgia

Nancy J. Vacca, MD
University of Texas Health Science
    Center at San Antonio
San Antonio, Texas

Santiago O. Valdes, MD, FAAP
Assistant Professor
Lillie Frank Abercrombie Section of
    Pediatric Cardiology
Texas Children's Hospital
Baylor College of Medicine
Houston, Texas

Anthony Valdini, MD, MS, FACP, FAAFP
Clinical Professor of Family Medicine and
    Community Health
University of Massachusetts School of
    Medicine
Lawrence, Massachusetts

Olga Valdman, MD
Assistant Professor
Department of Family Medicine
University of Massachusetts Medical School
Worcester, Massachusetts

Tricia Elaine VanWagner, MD[†]
Assistant Professor in Family Medicine
Uniformed Services University of the
    Health Sciences
Naval Hospital Sigonella
Sigonella, Italy

Kathleen M. Vazzana, DO
Pediatric Resident
Department of Pediatrics
University of Florida at Arnold Palmer
    Hospital for Children
Orlando, Florida

Nandhini Veeraraghavan, MD, CAQSM[†]
Associate Program Director
Department of Family Medicine
Sacred Heart Hospital
Allentown, Pennsylvania

Julian Vega, DO[†]
Family Medicine Resident
Martin Army Community Hospital
Fort Benning, Georgia

Suman Vellanki, MD
Family Medicine Resident
Summa Barberton Hospital
Barberton, Ohio

Sandhya Ventrapragada, MBBS, MD
Primary Care Physician
Department of Internal Medicine
Edward M. Kennedy Community Health
    Center
Framingham, Massachusetts

Conrad H. Vinalon, MD
Bayfront Health Family Medicine
    Residency
Bayfront Health St. Petersburg
St. Petersburg, Florida

Alicia Huff Vinyard, DO[†]
General Surgery Resident Physician
Department of General Surgery
Georgia Regents University
Augusta, Georgia

Siva Vithananthan, MD, FACS
Associate Professor of Surgery—Clinical
The Warren Alpert Medical School of
    Brown University
Providence, Rhode Island

Kirsten Vitrikas, MD[†]
Program Director
David Grant United States Air Force
    Family Medicine Residency
Travis Air Force Base, California

Theresa T. Vo, MD[†]
Department of Family Medicine
Dell Medical School, University of Texas
    at Austin
Austin, Texas

John T. Vogel, DO[†]
Family Medicine Faculty Physician
David Grant Medical Center
Travis Air Force Base, California

Yongkasem Vorasettakarnkij, MD, MSc
Faculty of Medicine
Department of Medicine
Chulalongkorn University
Cardiac Center
King Chulalongkorn Memorial Hospital
Thai Red Cross Society
Bangkok, Thailand

Gillian R. Wackowski, DO[†]
Resident
Jacksonville Family Medicine Residency
    Program
Navy Hospital Jacksonville
Jacksonville, Florida

Joseph R. Wagner, MD
Director of Robotic Surgery, Hartford
    Hospital
Minimally Invasive Surgery and Urologic
    Oncology
Hartford Healthcare Medical Group
Hartford, Connecticut

Cynthia M. Waickus, MD, PhD[†]
Associate Chair for Educational
    Programs
Department of Family Medicine
Rush Medical College
Chicago, Illinois

Jeffrey H. Walden, MD
Assistant Professor
University of North Carolina Department
    of Family Medicine
Cone Health Family Medicine Residency
Greensboro, North Carolina

Leslie A. Waldman, MD, FAAFP[†]
Associate Program Director
Puget Sound Family Medicine Residency
Bremerton, Washington

Shawn M. Wallace, MD
Family Medicine Residency
Bayfront Health St. Petersburg
St. Petersburg, Florida

Anne Walsh, MMSc, PA-C, DFAAPA
Instructor of Clinical Family Medicine
Department of Family Medicine
Keck School of Medicine
University of Southern California
Los Angeles, California

Nathaniel J. Walsh, MD
General Surgery Resident
Department of General Surgery
Medical College of Georgia
Georgia Regents University
Augusta, Georgia

Katrina E. Walters, MD, FAAFP, FM[†]
Director
Obstetrics Fellowship Program
Department of Family and Community
    Medicine
Carl R. Darnall Army Medical Center
Fort Hood, Texas

Kenneth C. Walters, MD
Medical Center at Augusta University
Augusta, Georgia

Hsin-Yi Janey Wang, MD
Family Medicine
University of Texas Health Science
    Center at San Antonio
San Antonio, Texas

Jeff Wang, MD, MPH[†]
Sports Medicine Fellow
University of Massachusetts Medical
    School
Worcester, Massachusetts

Ryan Wargo, PharmD, BCACP[†]
Assistant Professor and Director of
    Admissions
Lake Erie College of Osteopathic
    Medicine School of Pharmacy
Bradenton, Florida

Donald E. Watenpaugh, PhD
Adjunct Professor
Department of Integrative Physiology
University of North Texas Health Science
    Center
Fort Worth, Texas

Pamela Waters, MD
Resident
Eglin Air Force Base Hospital
Eglin Air Force Base
Valparaiso, Florida

Mohammed Abdalaziz Wazzan, MD,
    MBBS
George Washington University
Washington, DC

Christopher J. Weber, MD[†], LT, MC, USN
Family Medicine Resident
Department of Family Medicine
Naval Hospital Jacksonville
Jacksonville, Florida

Jill T. Wei, MD
Clinical Instructor
Department of Family Medicine
University of California Los Angeles,
 Santa Monica Bay Physicians
Santa Monica, California

Patrice M. Weiss, MD, FACOG
Executive Vice President and Chief
 Medical Officer
Professor
Department of Obstetrics and
 Gynecology
Virginia Tech Carilion School of Medicine
Carilion Clinic
Roanoke, Virginia

Frederick C. Weitendorf, RPH, RN
ICCU Clinical Pharmacist
Department of Pharmacy
Robley Rex VA Medical Center
Louisville, Kentucky

Mark Weitzel, DO
Otolaryngology Department
Philadelphia College of Osteopathic
 Medicine
Philadelphia, Pennsylvania

Jennifer J. Greene Welch, MD
Assistant Professor of Pediatrics
Pediatric Hematology/Oncology
The Warren Alpert Medical School of
 Brown University
Providence, Rhode Island

Jeremy B. Wells, MD
Primary Care Sports Medicine Physician
Department of Sports Medicine
Hattiesburg Clinic
Hattiesburg, Mississippi

Katie L. Westerfield, DO[†]
Family and Undergraduate Student
 Coordinator
Family Medicine Residency Program
Martin Army Community Hospital
Fort Benning, Georgia

Vernon Wheeler, MD, FAAFP[†]
Family Practice Physician
Fort Hood, Texas

Chris Wheelock, MD
PeaceHealth Southwest Washington
 Clinical Assistant Professor
Family Medicine
University of Washington
Vancouver, Washington

Ebony Whisenant, MD[†]
Assistant Professor of Family Medicine
Department of Medicine, Family Medicine
 and Community Health
Florida International University, Herbert
 Wertheim College of Medicine
Miami, Florida

Kimara Whisenant, MD
Bako Pathology
Atlanta, Georgia

Charles Whitaker, MD
Assistant Professor of Neurology
Neuromuscular Neurologist
Director of Muscular Dystrophy Clinic for
 Children
Hospital for Special Care
University of Connecticut School of
 Medicine
New Britain, Connecticut

Cassandra White, MD
Assistant Professor of Surgery
Medical College of Georgia
Georgia Regents University
Augusta, Georgia

Christopher White, MD, JD, MHA
Assistant Professor of Psychiatry &
 Family Medicine
University of Cincinnati College of
 Medicine
Cincinnati, Ohio

Jeremy S. White, MD
Internal Medicine Resident
University of Alabama at Birmingham
Birmingham, Alabama

Anne M. Valeri White, DO, FAAFP
Associate Director of Family Medicine
 Residency
Summa Akron City Hospital
Akron, Ohio
Clinical Assistant Professor of Family
 Medicine
Northeast Ohio Medical University
Rootstown, Ohio
Clinical Assistant Professor of Family
 Medicine
Ohio University Heritage College of
 Osteopathic Medicine
Athens, Ohio

Margaret Whitney, MD
Department of Obstetrics and
 Gynecology
Carilion Clinic
Roanoke, Virginia

Abbott Cotton Widdicombe, MD
Emergency Medicine Residency
Yale-New Haven Medical Center
New Haven, Connecticut

Susanne Wild, MD
Clinician Educator
Family Medicine Residency
Banner University Medical Center
 Phoenix
Clinical Assistant Professor
Department of Family and Community
 Medicine
University of Arizona College of
 Medicine–Phoenix
Phoenix, Arizona

Brittany L. Wiles, MD[†]
Department of Family Medicine
Naval Hospital Jacksonville
Jacksonville, Florida

Joanne Wilkinson, MD, MSc
Department of Family Medicine
Boston Medical Center
Boston, Massachusetts

Joshua Scott Will, DO[†]
Chief
Department of Women's Health and
 Newborn Care
Martin Army Community Hospital
Fort Benning, Georgia

Midhuna William, MD
Department of Family Medicine
Carilion Clinic
Virginia Tech School of Medicine
Roanoke, Virginia

Faren H. Williams, MD, MS[†]
Chief, Physical Medicine & Rehabilitation
Clinical Professor
Department of Orthopedics and Physical
 Rehabilitation
University of Massachusetts Medical
 School
Worcester, Massachusetts

Paul N. Williams, MD, FACP
Assistant Professor of Clinical Medicine
Primary Care Program Director
Temple University Hospital Internal
 Medicine Residency Program
Philadelphia, Pennsylvania

Alan J. Williamson, MD, Lr Col, USAF, MC[†]
Family Health Clinic Medical Director
Ehrling Bergquist Clinic
Offutt Air Force Base, Nebraska

Shenelle Wilson, MD
Urology Resident
Georgia Regents University
Augusta, Georgia

Amy B. Wilson-LaMothe, PharmD, BCPS
Assistant Professor of Pharmacy Practice
Massachusetts College of Pharmacy and Health Sciences University
Worcester, Massachusetts

Scott A. Wiltz, MD, MPH, FAAFP[†]
Associate Residency Director
Eglin Air Force Base Family Medicine Residency
Eglin Air Force Base
Valparaiso, Florida

Norton Winer, MD
Assistant Clinical
Professor of Neurology
Case Western Reserve University School of Medicine
Cleveland, Ohio

Robyn Wing, MD
Pediatric Emergency Medicine Fellow
Departments of Pediatrics & Emergency Medicine
Division of Pediatric Emergency Medicine
The Warren Alpert Medical School of Brown University
Providence, Rhode Island

Fawn Winkelman, DO
Board Certified Osteopathic Family Medicine
Boca Raton, Florida
Clinical Assistant Professor at the Department of Family Medicine
Nova Southeastern University College of Osteopathic Medicine
Fort Lauderdale, Florida

Kirsten A. Winnie, MD[†]
Family Medicine Resident
Offutt Air Force Base Family Medicine Residency Program
University of Nebraska Medical Center
Omaha, Nebraska

Christopher M. Wise, MD
W. Robert Irby Professor
Department of Medicine
Division of Rheumatology, Allergy, and Immunology
Medical College of Virginia
Virginia Commonwealth University
Richmond, Virginia

Sean R. Wise, MD[†]
Director of Sports Medicine
Family Medicine Residency
Womack Army Medical Center
Fort Bragg, North Carolina

Amy L. Wiser, MD
Assistant Professor
Assistant Residency Director of Education
Department of Family Medicine
Oregon Health & Science University
Portland, Oregon

Jeffrey D. Wolfrey, MD
Chair, Department of Family Medicine
Banner United Medical Center Phoenix
Clinical Professor
Department of Family and Community Medicine
University of Arizona College of Medicine—Phoenix
Phoenix, Arizona

Wendy Hin-Wing Wong, MD, MPH
Department of Emergency Medicine
The Warren Alpert Medical School of Brown University
Providence, Rhode Island

J. Andrew Woods, PharmD, BCPS
Associate Professor of Pharmacy
Wingate University School of Pharmacy
Charlotte, North Carolina

Dawna H. Woodyear, MD
Assistant Professor
University of Pittsburgh School of Medicine
Department of Family and Community Medicine
Medical Director
University of Pittsburgh Medical Center Matilda Theiss Health Center
Pittsburgh, Pennsylvania

Leah R. Evans Wong, MD, MEd
Pediatrics Resident
Department of Pediatrics
University of Massachusetts Medical School
Worcester, Massachusetts

Bart D. Worthington, DO, MS[†]
Family Medicine Resident
Saint Louis University Family Medicine Residency Program—Belleville
Belleville, Illinois

Frances Yung-tao Wu, MD
Assistant Director
Robert Wood Johnson Somerset Family Medicine Residency
Robert Wood Johnson Somerset
Somerville, New Jersey

Maria Harsha Wusu, MD, MSEd
Chief Resident
Department of Family Medicine
Boston Medical Center
Boston, Massachusetts

Kristen M. Wyrick, MD[†]
Assistant Professor of Family Medicine
Uniformed Service University of the Health Sciences
Bethesda, Maryland

Ewa M. Wysokinska, MD
Willmar Cancer Center
Willmar, Minnesota

Michael Y. Yang, MD[†]
Chestnut Hill Hospital
Philadelphia, Pennsylvania

Rebecca R. Yeager, MD
Family Medicine Resident
Department of Family Medicine
The Christ Hospital
University of Cincinnati
Cincinnati, Ohio

Dinesh Yogaratnam, PharmD
Assistant Professor of Pharmacy Practice
Massachusetts College of Pharmacy and Health Sciences University
Worcester, Massachusetts

James R. Yon, MD
Trauma, Burns, and Critical Care Fellow
John H. Stroger, Jr. Hospital of Cook County
Chicago, Illinois

Robert A. Yood, MD
Chief of Rheumatology
Reliant Medical Group
Clinical Professor of Medicine
University of Massachusetts Medical School
Worcester, Massachusetts

Kyung In Yoon, MD
Department of Emergency Medicine
Robert Wood Johnson University Hospital
New Brunswick, New Jersey

Daniel Young, MD
Residency Director
UHS Wilson Family Medicine Residency
UHS Hospitals
Johnson City, New York

Lester Young, MD
Trauma and Critical Care Surgery
Medical College of Georgia
Georgia Regents University
Augusta, Georgia

Edward L. Yourtee, MD, FACP
Chief Medical Officer
Parkland Medical Center
Derry, New Hampshire

Jacqueline L. Yurgil, DO[†]
Family Physician
Warner Robins, Georgia

Edlira Yzeiraj, DO, MS
Internal Medicine
Cleveland Clinic
Cleveland, Ohio

Christine C. Zacharia, MD
Clinician Educator
Department of Endocrinology
NorthShore University Health System
Evanston, Illinois

Isabel Zacharias, MD
Staff Physician
Department of Gastroenterology
UMass Memorial Medical Center
Worcester, Massachusetts

Amy M. Zack, MD, FAAFP
Family Medicine Physician
Associate Program Director, Family
    Medicine
Department of Family Medicine
MetroHealth Medical Center/Case
    Western Reserve University
Cleveland, Ohio

Matthew Zanghi, MD
University of Massachusetts Medical
    School
Worcester, Massachusetts

Steven M. Zeddun, MD[†]
Assistant Professor of Medicine
Division of Gastroenterology and Liver
    Diseases
George Washington University
Washington, DC

Youhua Zhang, MD, PhD
Assistant Professor
Department of Biomedical Sciences
College of Osteopathic Medicine
New York Institute of Technology
Old Westbury, New York

Ruslan Zhuravsky, DO
Otolaryngology and Facial Plastic Surgery
Rowan University School of Osteopathic
    Medicine
Stratford, New Jersey

Derek G. Zickgraf, DO[†]
Family Physician and Brigade Surgeon
8th Military Police Brigade
Schofield Barracks, Hawaii

Gennine M. Zinner, RNCS, ANP[†]
Nurse Practitioner
Boston Health Care for the Homeless
    Program
Clinical Faculty
Massachusetts General Hospital Institute
    of Health Professions
Boston, Massachusetts

Kimberly Zoberi, MD
Department of Family Medicine
St. Louis University School of Medicine
St. Louis, Missouri

Susan Zweizig, MD
Director
Division of Gynecologic Oncology
Department of Obstetrics and
    Gynecology
University of Massachusetts
Worcester, Massachusetts

Seth Zwillenberg, MD
Clinical Associate Professor of Pediatrics
    and Otolaryngology
Drexel University College of Medicine
Philadelphia, Pennsylvania

[†]*The views expressed are those of the authors and do not reflect the official policy of the Department of the Army, Department of the Navy, the Department of Defense, or the United States Government.*

CONTENTS

lxii • • • Contents

Topics

Contents

Diagnosis and Treatment: An Algorithmic Approach

This section contains flowcharts (or algorithms) to help the reader in the diagnosis of clinical signs and symptoms and treatment of a variety of clinical problems. They are organized by the presenting sign, symptom, or diagnosis.

These algorithms were designed to be used as a quick reference and adjunct to the reader's clinical knowledge and impression. They are not an exhaustive review of the management of a problem, nor are they meant to be a complete list of diseases.

ABDOMINAL PAIN, CHRONIC

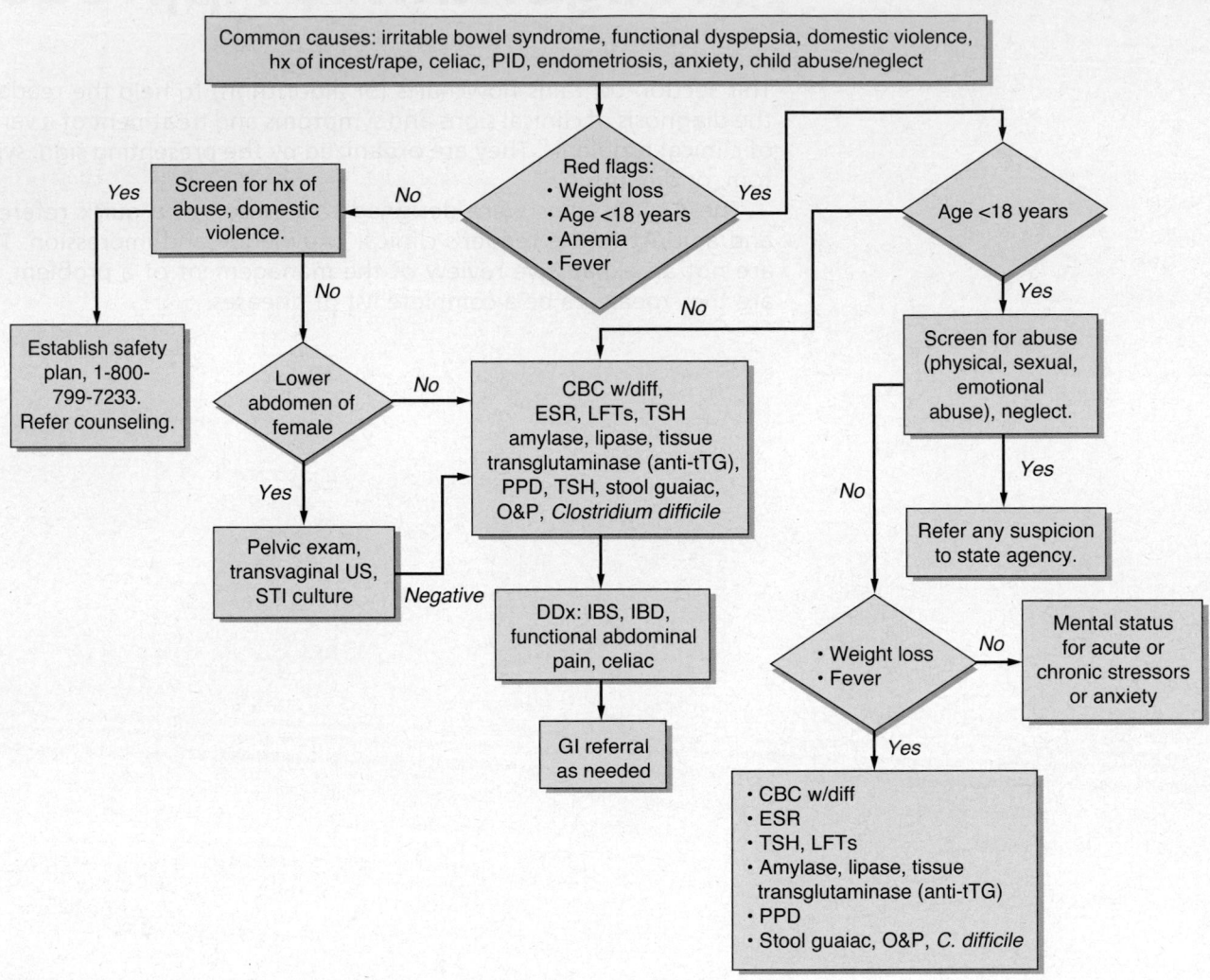

Common causes: irritable bowel syndrome, functional dyspepsia, domestic violence, hx of incest/rape, celiac, PID, endometriosis, anxiety, child abuse/neglect

Red flags:
• Weight loss
• Age <18 years
• Anemia
• Fever

No → Screen for hx of abuse, domestic violence. → *Yes* → Establish safety plan, 1-800-799-7233. Refer counseling.

No → Lower abdomen of female

No → CBC w/diff, ESR, LFTs, TSH amylase, lipase, tissue transglutaminase (anti-tTG), PPD, TSH, stool guaiac, O&P, *Clostridium difficile*

Yes → Pelvic exam, transvaginal US, STI culture → *Negative*

DDx: IBS, IBD, functional abdominal pain, celiac

GI referral as needed

Yes → Age <18 years

Yes → Screen for abuse (physical, sexual, emotional abuse), neglect.

Yes → Refer any suspicion to state agency.

No → • Weight loss • Fever → *No* → Mental status for acute or chronic stressors or anxiety

Yes →
• CBC w/diff
• ESR
• TSH, LFTs
• Amylase, lipase, tissue transglutaminase (anti-tTG)
• PPD
• Stool guaiac, O&P, *C. difficile*

Note: Only check for *Clostridium difficile* if the patient has concomitant diarrhea.

Shadi Hamdeh, MD and Adil Abdalla, MD

Camilleri M. Management of patients with chronic abdominal pain in clinical practice. *Neurogastroenterol Motil.* 2006;18(7):499–506.

ABDOMINAL PAIN, LOWER

Abdominal abscess, adenitis, aortic aneurysm, appendicitis, inflammatory bowel disease, diverticulitis, ectopic pregnancy, endometriosis, ischemic bowel, ovarian rupture or torsion, pancreatitis, PID, pyelonephritis, strangulated hernia

Duration of symptoms

Acute

Chronic

Physical exam indicating rebound tenderness, guarding, or other signs of a severe and acute disease process

Female patient of childbearing capacity

Yes

No

Yes

No

History of cyclic pain symptoms

Yes

No

Strangulated hernia, appendicitis, AAA, ovarian torsion, ruptured ovarian cyst, colitis, pancreatitis, mesenteric adenitis, ectopic pregnancy, ischemic bowel

Pyelonephritis, Crohn disease, ulcerative colitis, abdominal or retroperitoneal abscess

Endometriosis, IBS, ovarian cyst, mittelschmerz

IBS, PID, interstitial cystitis, ectopic pregnancy

Consider: KUB, CT abdomen/pelvis with contrast if creatinine ≤1.3, CBC, CMP, hCG, UA, lipase, stool guaiac, colonoscopy, surgical consult

Consider: hCG, CBC, UA with culture, pelvic ultrasound with transvaginal if needed

Diverticulitis, ischemic bowel, IBS. Consider: CBC, CMP, UA, lipase, CT abdomen/pelvis with contrast if creatinine ≤1.3, depression, domestic violence

Andrew G. Alexander, MD, Maegen Dupper, MD, and Heidi S. Millard, MD

Cartwright SL, Knudson MP. Diagnostic imaging of acute abdominal pain in adults. *Am Fam Physician*. 2015;91(7):452–459.

ABDOMINAL PAIN, UPPER

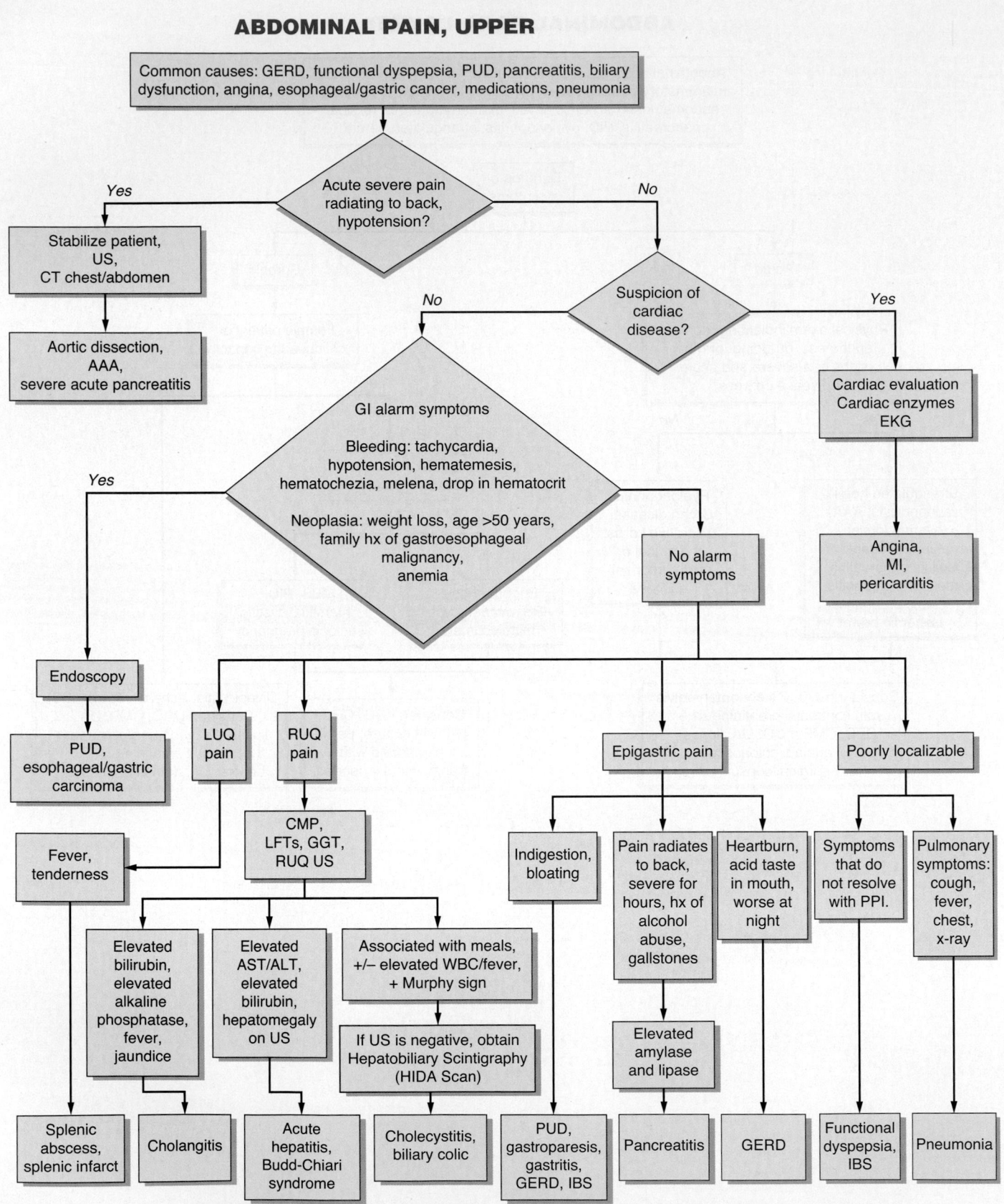

Matthew Chandler, MD and Marie L. Borum, MD, EdD, MPH

Yamamoto W, Kono H, Maekawa M, et al. The relationship between abdominal pain regions and specific diseases: an epidemiologic approach to clinical practice. *J Epidemiol.* 1997;7(1):27–32.

ACETAMINOPHEN POISONING, TREATMENT

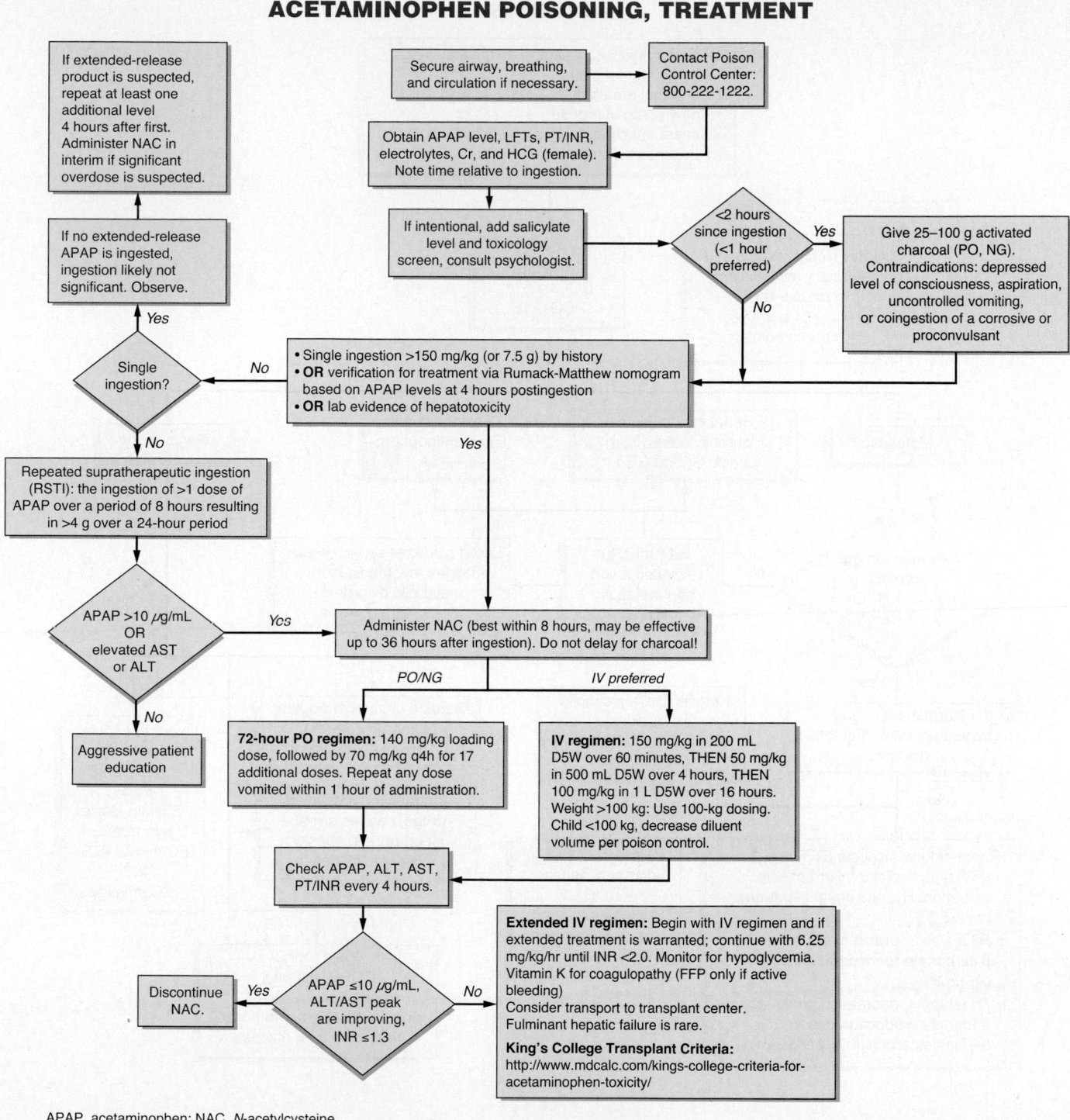

APAP, acetaminophen; NAC, N-acetylcysteine

Marissa T. Casagrande, PharmD, Ryan B. Feeney, PharmD, and Frank M. Mazzotta, DO

Hodgman MJ, Garrard AR. A review of acetaminophen poisoning. *Crit Care Clin.* 2012;28(4):499–516.

ACIDOSIS

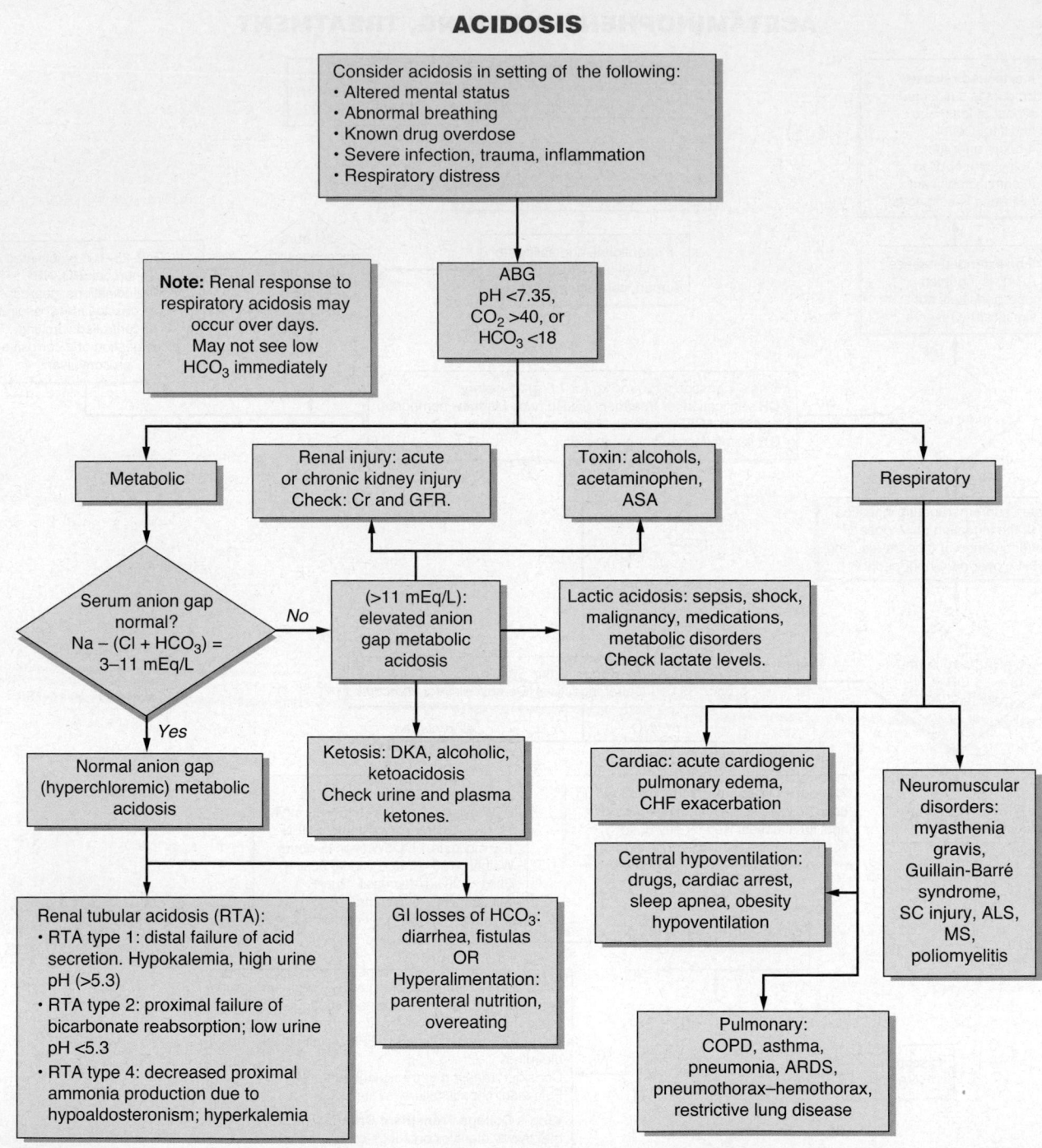

Consider acidosis in setting of the following:
- Altered mental status
- Abnormal breathing
- Known drug overdose
- Severe infection, trauma, inflammation
- Respiratory distress

Note: Renal response to respiratory acidosis may occur over days. May not see low HCO_3 immediately

ABG
pH <7.35,
CO_2 >40, or
HCO_3 <18

Metabolic

Renal injury: acute or chronic kidney injury Check: Cr and GFR.

Toxin: alcohols, acetaminophen, ASA

Respiratory

Serum anion gap normal?
$Na - (Cl + HCO_3) = 3-11$ mEq/L

No

(>11 mEq/L): elevated anion gap metabolic acidosis

Lactic acidosis: sepsis, shock, malignancy, medications, metabolic disorders Check lactate levels.

Yes

Normal anion gap (hyperchloremic) metabolic acidosis

Ketosis: DKA, alcoholic, ketoacidosis Check urine and plasma ketones.

Cardiac: acute cardiogenic pulmonary edema, CHF exacerbation

Neuromuscular disorders: myasthenia gravis, Guillain-Barré syndrome, SC injury, ALS, MS, poliomyelitis

Renal tubular acidosis (RTA):
- RTA type 1: distal failure of acid secretion. Hypokalemia, high urine pH (>5.3)
- RTA type 2: proximal failure of bicarbonate reabsorption; low urine pH <5.3
- RTA type 4: decreased proximal ammonia production due to hypoaldosteronism; hyperkalemia

GI losses of HCO_3: diarrhea, fistulas OR Hyperalimentation: parenteral nutrition, overeating

Central hypoventilation: drugs, cardiac arrest, sleep apnea, obesity hypoventilation

Pulmonary: COPD, asthma, pneumonia, ARDS, pneumothorax–hemothorax, restrictive lung disease

Katelin Engerer, MD and Robert J. Hyde, MD, MA, NRP, FACEP

Kaplan LJ, Frangos S. Clinical review: acid-base abnormalities in the intensive care unit—part II. *Crit Care*. 2005;9(2):198–203.

ACNE

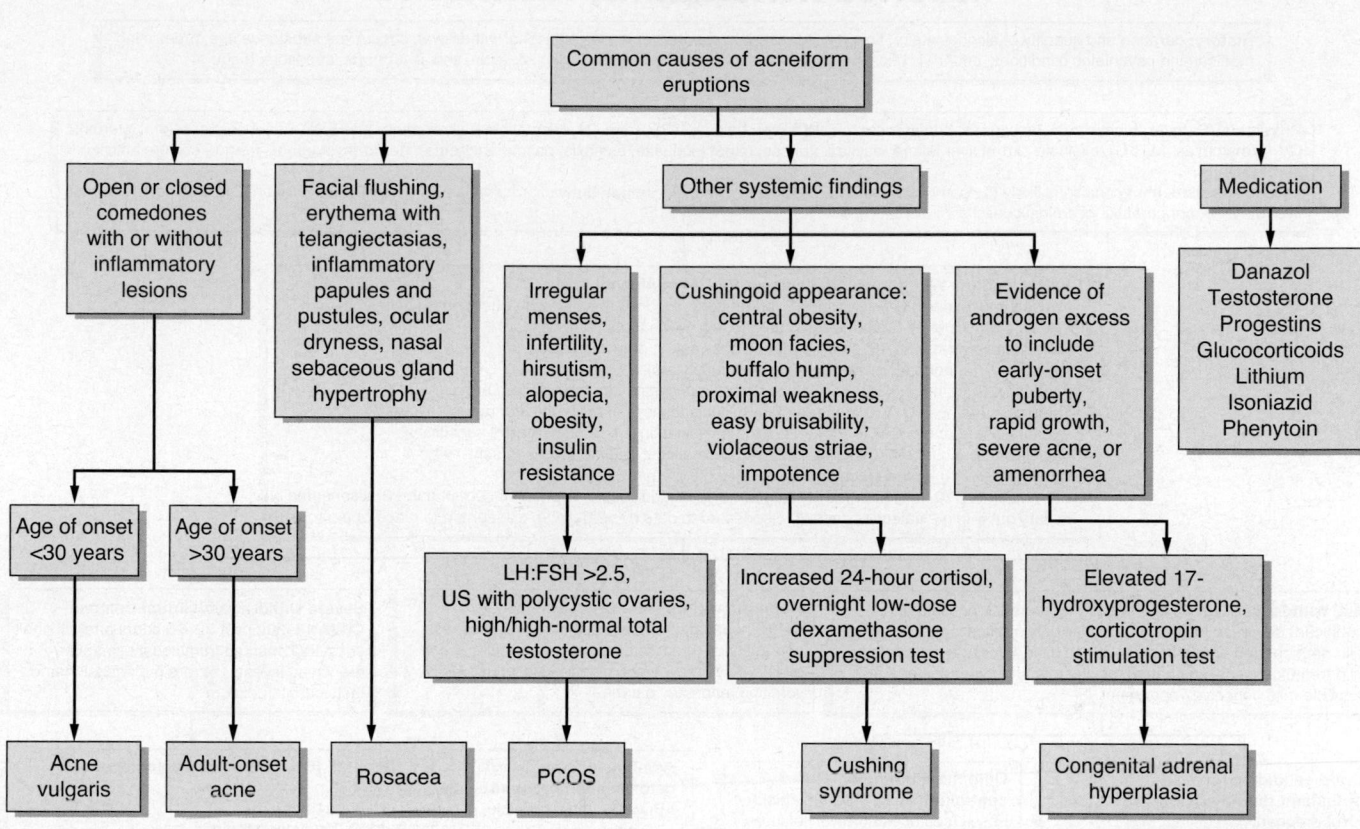

Jason N. Butler, DO, MS and Lloyd A. Runser, MD, MPH

Lolis MS, Bowe WP, Shalita AR. Acne and systemic disease. *Med Clin North Am.* 2009;93(6):1161–1181.

ALCOHOL WITHDRAWAL, TREATMENT

History: duration and quantity of alcohol intake, time since last drink, previous episodes of alcohol withdrawal, concurrent substance use, preexisting medical and psychiatric conditions, prior detoxification admissions, prior seizure activity, living situation, social supports, stressors, triggers

Physical: VS (fever, tachycardia, tachypnea, hypertension), **CIWA** (see below), MSE, (arousal, orientation, hallucinations), HEENT (diaphoresis, scleral icterus), CV (arrhythmias, M/R/G), evaluate s/sx of liver failure (ascites, varices, caput medusae, asterixis, palmar erythema), neuro (nystagmus, tremor, seizure activity).

Include assessment of conditions likely to *complicate*, *exacerbate*, or *precipitate* alcohol withdrawal: arrhythmias, CHF, CAD, dehydration, GI bleeding, infections, liver disease, pancreatitis, neurologic deficits.

Clinical Institute Withdrawal Assessment (CIWA) of Alcohol Scale
- Nausea and vomiting 0–7 (0, none; 4, intermittent; 7, constant nausea; frequent dry heaves/vomiting)
- Tremor 0–7 (0, none; 4, moderate; 7, severe; even with arms not extended)
- Paroxysmal sweats 0–7 (0, none; 4, beads of sweat; 7, drenching sweats)
- Anxiety 0–7 (0, none; 4, moderate; 7, acute panic state)
- Agitation 0–7 (0, none; 4, moderately restless; 7, constantly thrashing about or pacing)
- Tactile disturbances 0–7 (0, none; 4–7 for hallucinations; 1–3 for pruritus or paresthesias)
- Auditory disturbances 0–7 (0, none; 4–7 for hallucinations; 1–3 for increased sensitivity)
- Visual disturbances 0–7 (0, none; 4–7 for hallucinations; 1–3 for increased sensitivity)
- Headache 0–7 (0, no headache; 4, moderate; 7, extremely severe)
- Orientation 0–4 (0, fully oriented; 1, cannot do serial additions or is uncertain about date; 2, disoriented to date but within 2 calendar days; 3, disoriented to date by >2 days; 4, disoriented to place or person)

Mild withdrawal—CIWA 0–7 onset 5–8 hours after cessation or significant decrease in consumption: anxiety, restlessness, agitation, mild nausea, decreased appetite, sleep disturbance, facial sweating, mild tremulousness, fluctuating tachycardia and hypertension, possible mild cognitive impairment

Moderate withdrawal—CIWA 8–14 onset 24–72 hours after cessation: marked restlessness and agitation, moderate tremulousness with constant eye movement, diaphoresis, nausea, vomiting, anorexia, diarrhea

Severe withdrawal/delirium tremens—CIWA 15–30 onset 72–96 hours after alcohol cessation: marked tremulousness, fever, drenching sweats, severe hypertension and tachycardia, delirium

Good candidate for outpatient therapy:
- Not pregnant
- No comorbid illnesses requiring hospitalization
- No history of seizures
- Not a suicide risk
- Low risk of delirium tremens
- No history of unsuccessful outpatient detoxification
- Good access to follow-up medical care
- Tolerating oral medication
- Adequate social support available

Outpatient therapy contraindicated: pregnant, history of seizures or withdrawal seizures, chronic or acute comorbid illness requiring inpatient observation, lack of ability to follow-up

High risk of delirium tremens:
- Age >30 years
- Heavy drinking >8 years
- Drinking >100 g ethanol/day
- Random BAC >200 mg/dL
- Elevated MCV
- Cirrhosis

Admit to inpatient ward/detoxification program
- Private room if possible
- VS q4h
- CIWA q1–3h
- Institute seizure precautions
- Intravenous fluids

Admit to ICU for inpatient detoxification
- VS q30min
- CIWA q1h
- NPO, intravenous fluids
- Lateral decubitus position, restrain if necessary
- Glucose, sodium, potassium, phosphate, and magnesium replacement as needed

Treat as outpatient
- Thiamine 100 mg once daily for 5 days
- Folic acid 1 g once daily for 5 days
- Evaluate daily until symptoms decrease
- Assess blood pressure, heart rate, and CIWA-Ar score at each follow-up visit.
- Perform alcohol breath analysis randomly.
- Facilitate entry into a long-term outpatient therapy program (Alcoholics Anonymous).
- **If patient misses an appointment or resumes drinking, refer to addiction specialist or inpatient treatment facility.**

Labs:
- Toxicology screen/EtOH level to assess need for and timing of withdrawal regimen
- CBC, electrolytes, phosphate, magnesium; B_{12} and folate to be repleted regardless of blood levels
- Amylase/lipase if suspected pancreatitis
- PT, PTT if suspected liver failure

Imaging:
- Head CT if history of trauma, mental status changes greater than expected, or focal neurologic changes.
- Consider addition of EEG if focal neurologic signs or prolonged postictal state seizure.

Medications:
- Diazepam 5–20 mg IV q10min until calm, then q1h to maintain light somnolence for duration of delirium
If severe liver disease, severe asthma or respiratory failure, elderly, debilitated, or low serum albumin:
- Lorazepam 1–4mg IV q10min until calm, then q1h to maintain light somnolence for duration of delirium

Example outpatient regimen:
Fixed diazepam schedule
Day 1: 10 mg q6h
Day 2: 10 mg q8h
Day 3: 10 mg q12h
Day 4/5: 10 mg at bedtime

Symptom-triggered diazepam schedule:
Give dose if CIWA >8.
Day 1: 10 mg q4h PRN
Day 2: 10 mg q6h PRN
Day 3: 10 mg q6h PRN
Days 4/5: 10 mg twice a day PRN

Discharge planning:
- CIWA scores <8–10 for 24 hours
- Begin 1:1 or group therapy
- Discharge to treatment center, day program, home
- Facilitate entry into Alcoholics Anonymous.
- Evaluate for outpatient treatment with benzodiazepine.
- Nutrition/social work consultation

Medications:
Nutritional replacement
- Thiamine 100 mg IV/IM or PO once daily for 5 days
- Folic acid 1 g PO once daily for 5 days
Sympatholytic adjunctive therapy (no effect on prevention of withdrawal seizure and should be used with benzodiazepine therapy)
- Atenolol 50–100 mg once daily
- Clonidine 0.2 mg 3 times daily
For hallucinations associated with withdrawal:
- Haloperidol 2–5 mg IM/PO q1–4h max 5 mg/day
- Use only in conjunction with benzodiazepines and with extreme caution as haloperidol may lower seizure threshold.

Medications:
Long-acting benzodiazepines (diazepam) have rapid onset of action and provide smooth treatment course with fewer breakthrough symptoms.
- Diazepam 20 mg PO q1–2h until CIWA <8
OR
- Diazepam 2–5 mg IV/min—maximum 10–20 mg q1h

Short-acting benzodiazepines (lorazepam) may have lower risk when there is concern about prolonged sedation, for example, elderly patients or those with severe hepatic insufficiency.
- Lorazepam 1–2 mg PO q2–4h until CIWA <8

Paul A. Tate, Jr., MD and Paul A. Savel, MD

Muncie HL Jr, Yasinian Y, Oge' L. Outpatient management of alcohol withdrawal syndrome. *Am Fam Physician.* 2013;88(9):589–595.

ALKALINE PHOSPHATASE ELEVATION

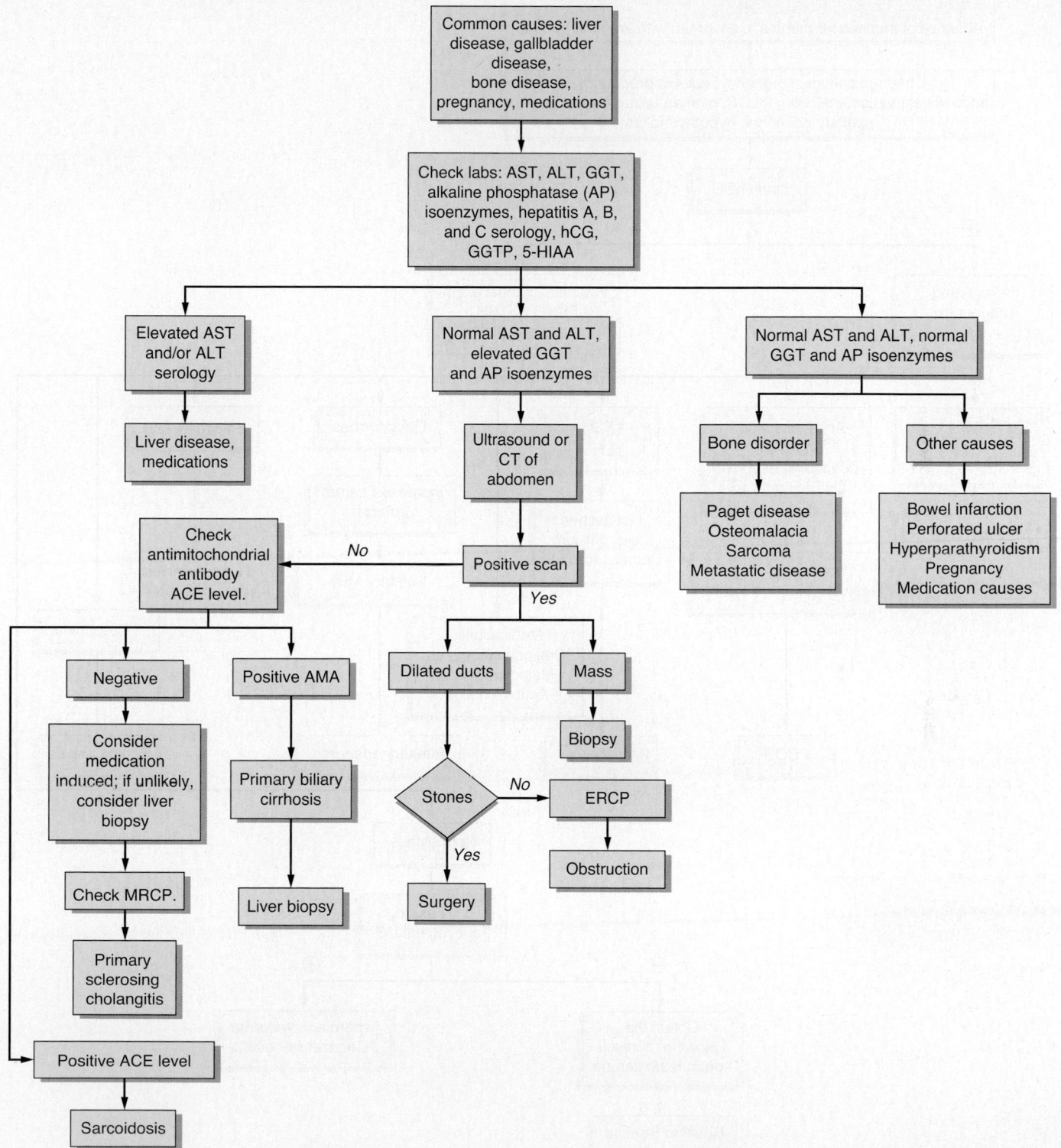

Reem Hadi, MD and Fozia Akhtar Ali, MD

Siddique A, Kowdley KV. Approach to a patient with elevated serum alkaline phosphatase. *Clin Liver Dis*. 2012;16(2):199–229.

AMENORRHEA, SECONDARY

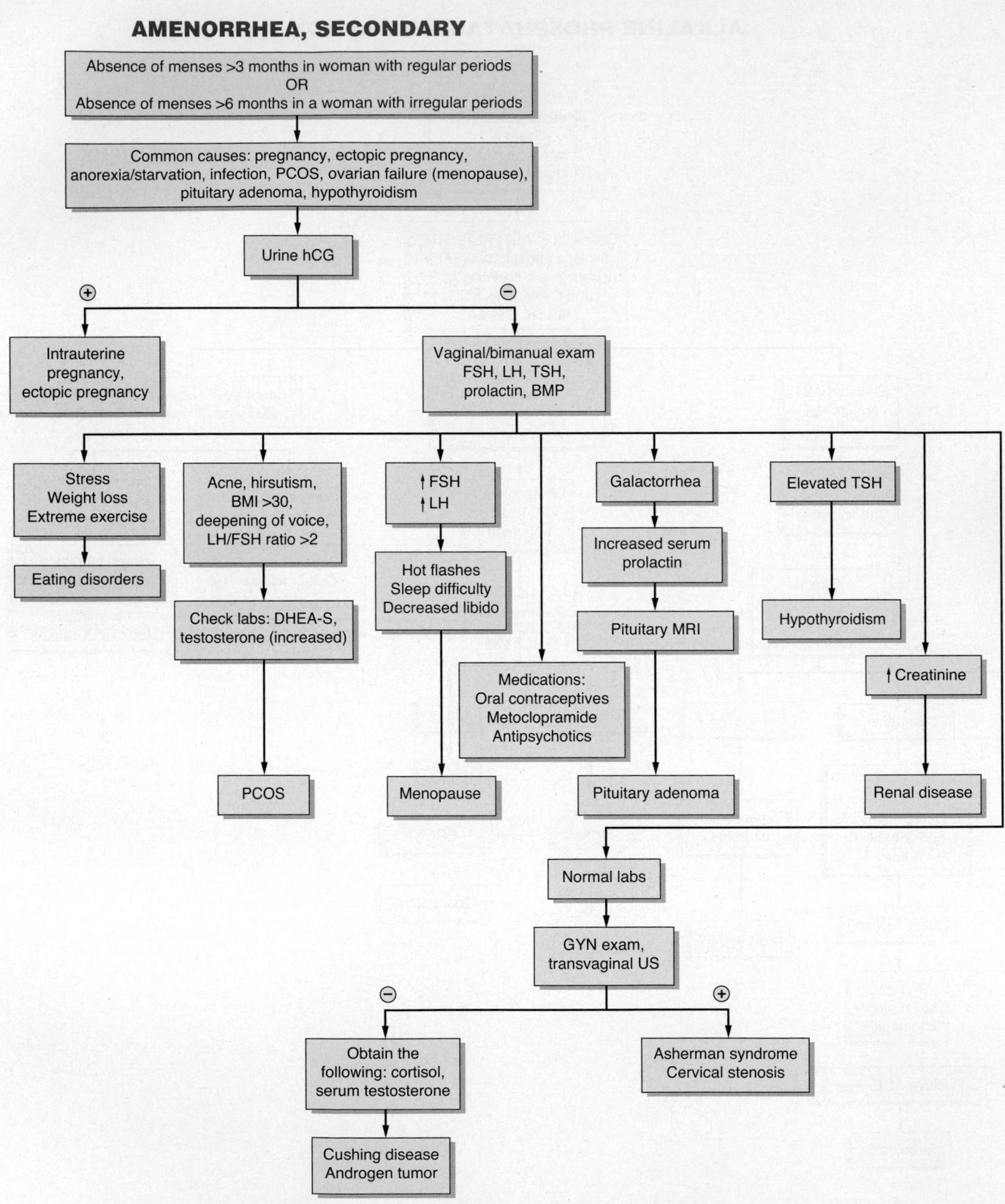

Absence of menses >3 months in woman with regular periods
OR
Absence of menses >6 months in a woman with irregular periods

Common causes: pregnancy, ectopic pregnancy, anorexia/starvation, infection, PCOS, ovarian failure (menopause), pituitary adenoma, hypothyroidism

Urine hCG

(+)
Intrauterine pregnancy, ectopic pregnancy

(−)
Vaginal/bimanual exam FSH, LH, TSH, prolactin, BMP

Stress
Weight loss
Extreme exercise
→ Eating disorders

Acne, hirsutism, BMI >30, deepening of voice, LH/FSH ratio >2
→ Check labs: DHEA-S, testosterone (increased)
→ PCOS

↑ FSH
↑ LH
→ Hot flashes
Sleep difficulty
Decreased libido
→ Menopause

Medications:
Oral contraceptives
Metoclopramide
Antipsychotics

Galactorrhea
→ Increased serum prolactin
→ Pituitary MRI
→ Pituitary adenoma

Elevated TSH
→ Hypothyroidism

↑ Creatinine
→ Renal disease

Normal labs
→ GYN exam, transvaginal US

(−)
Obtain the following: cortisol, serum testosterone
→ Cushing disease
Androgen tumor

(+)
Asherman syndrome
Cervical stenosis

Maria Montanez, MD and Fozia Akhtar Ali, MD

Master-Hunter T, Heiman DL. Amenorrhea: evaluation and treatment. *Am Fam Physician.* 2006;73(8):1374–1382.

ANEMIA

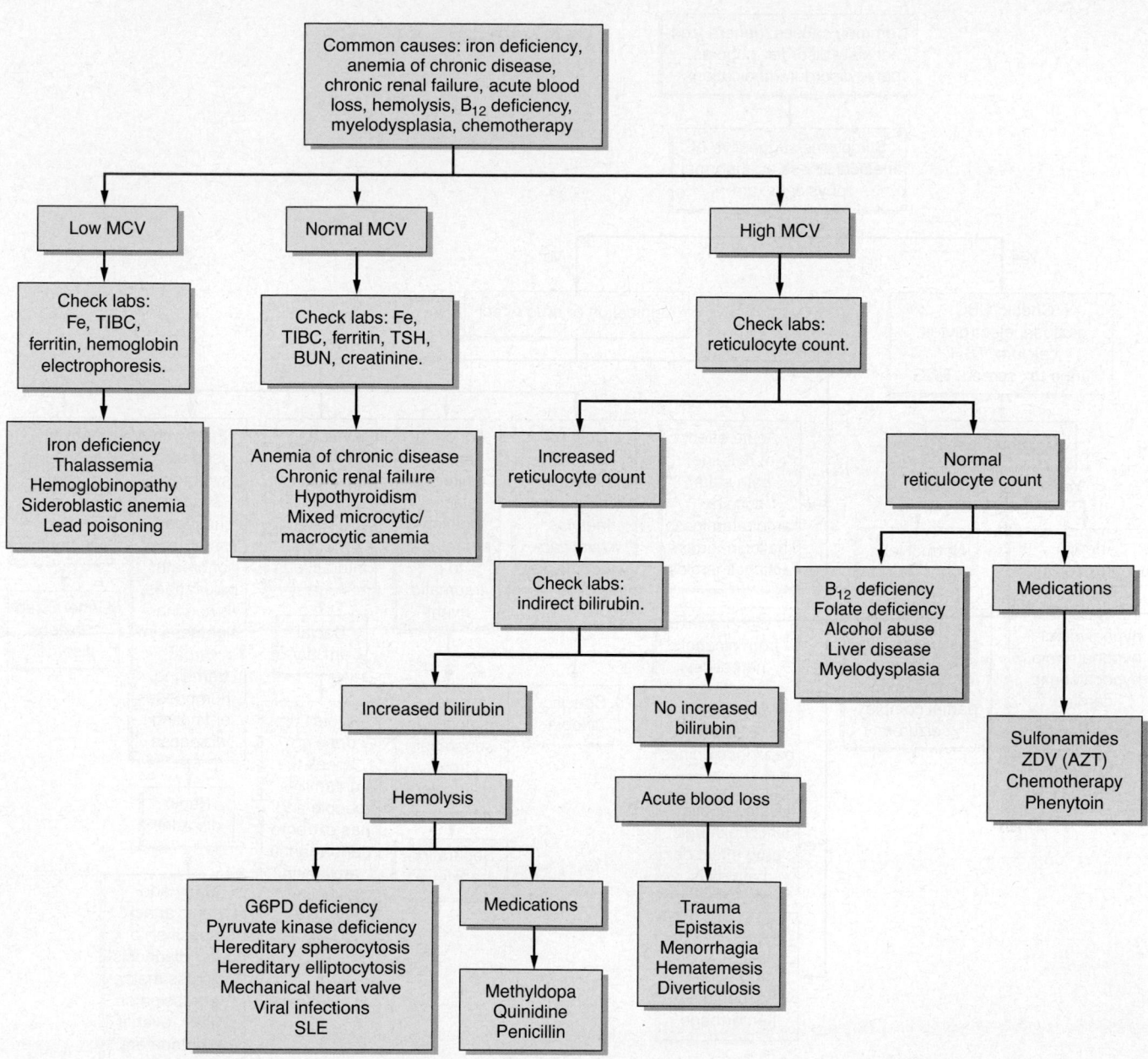

Robert A. Baldor, MD, FAAFP and Alan M. Ehrlich, MD

Smith DL. Anemia in the elderly. *Am Fam Physician*. 2000;62(7):1565–1572.

ANXIETY

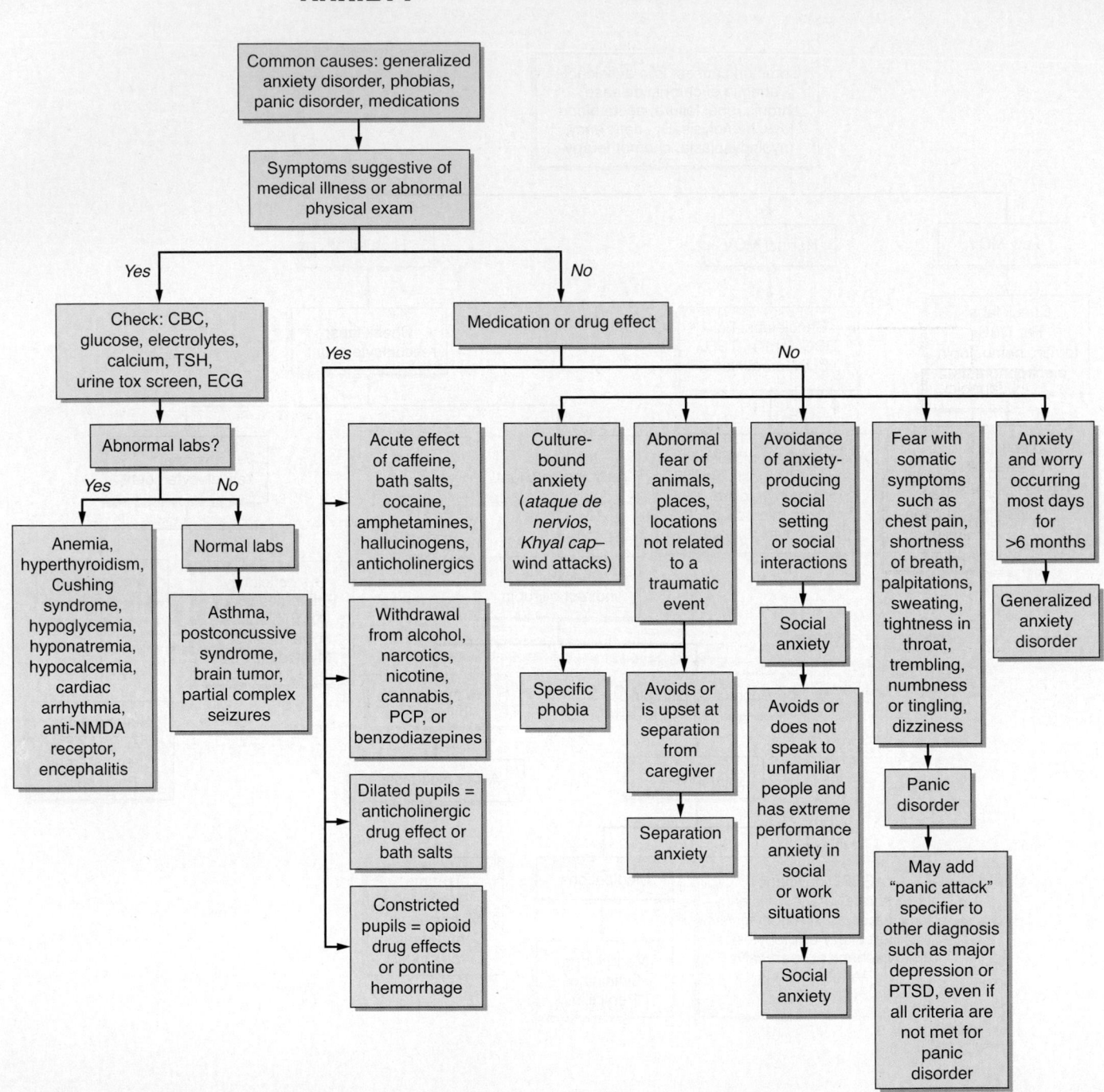

Bettina Bernstein, DO

Combs H, Markman J. Anxiety disorders in primary care. *Med Clin North Am.* 2014;98(5):1007–1023.

AST ELEVATION

Daniel J. Stein, MD, MPH and Stephen K. Lane, MD, FAAFP

Giboney PT. Mildly elevated liver transaminase levels in the asymptomatic patient. *Am Fam Physician.* 2005;71(6):1105–1110.

ASTHMA EXACERBATION, PEDIATRIC ACUTE

Initial evaluation: brief history of present illness, physical exam
Asthma history: emergency department visits, hospital and ICU admissions, home medications, frequency of oral steroid use, history of intubation, rapidly progressive episodes, food allergies
Physical exam: auscultation, use of accessory muscles, ability to speak, heart rate, oxygen saturation, PEF, or FEV_1

Severity	Respiratory rate (<6 years)	(>6 years)	Wheezing	Inspiration: expiratory ratio	Accessory muscle use	Oxygen saturation (room air)
Normal	30	20	None	2:1	None	99–100%
Mild	31–35	21–35	End expiration	1:1	+	96–98%
Moderate	46–60	36–50	Entire expiration	1:2	++	93–95%
Severe	>60	>50	Inspiration and expiration (may have silent chest)	1:3	+++	<93%

FEV_1 or PEF ≥40%
Mild exacerbation: inhaled β-agonist (nebulized or MDI with spacer q20–30min × 3 doses, consider systemic corticosteroids (PO/IM) if not immediate response or history of recent course of corticosteroids, check initial oxygen saturation level; no need for continue pulse-ox monitoring.
*Consider levalbuterol in place of albuterol if h/o ADR.

FEV_1 or PEF ≥40%
Moderate exacerbation: inhaled β-agonist in combination with ipratropium (nebulized) q20–30min × 3 doses, systemic corticosteroids (PO/IM), supplemental O_2 to achieve SaO_2 >90%
*Consider levalbuterol in place of albuterol if h/o ADR.

FEV_1 or PEF <40%
Severe exacerbation: inhaled β-agonist in combination with ipratropium (nebulized) q20–30min × 3 doses or continuous for 1 hour, systemic corticosteroids (PO/IM/IV), supplemental O_2 to achieve SaO_2 >90%, consider IM epinephrine if imminent respiratory failure.
*Consider levalbuterol in place of albuterol if h/o ADR.

Discharge criteria met?
In the first 2 hours:
• Decreased/absent wheezing and retractions
• Sustained SaO_2 >90% at least 60 minutes after last albuterol dose

Yes | *No*

FEV_1 or PEF <40%
Severe exacerbation: severe symptoms at rest, accessory muscle use, no improvement after initial treatment, nebulized β-agonist in combination with ipratropium q30–45min or continuous, consider magnesium sulfate IV; next then, consider terbutaline infusion if no response; consider heliox; consider endotracheal intubation for presumed or actual respiratory failure; make admit decision in <4 hours.

FEV_1 or PEF 40–69%
Moderate exacerbation:
Inhaled β-agonist q60min; continue treatment 1–3 hours, provided there is improvement; make admit decision in <4 hours; reassess after each treatment.

Improved FEV_1/PEF (lung function tests)
Discharge home
Patient education: Review home medications and inhaler/spacer technique.
Instructions for close follow-up within 1 week.
Continue treatment with inhaled β-agonist and PO corticosteroid.
Continue or consider initiation of inhaled corticosteroid.
Written asthma action plan
Prevention of acute exacerbation (trigger control/allergen avoidance)

Admission: ICU or closely monitored on floor

No

Improved FEV_1/PEF
Discharge criteria met?
In the first 2 hours:
• Decreased/absent wheezing and retractions
• Sustained SaO_2 >90% at least 60 minutes after last albuterol dose

Yes

Jasmit S. Minhas, MD and John A. Saryan, MD

National Asthma Education and Prevention Program. Expert Panel Report 3 (EPR-3): guidelines for the diagnosis and management of asthma—summary report 2007. *J Allergy Clin Immunol.* 2007;120(5)(Suppl):S94–S138.

ASTHMA, INITIAL TREATMENT

Management of chronic asthma
Classification of asthma severity in youth ≥12 years of age and adults

Components of severity	Intermittent	Mild persistent	Moderate persistent	Severe persistent
Daytime symptoms	≤2 days/week	>2 days/week but not every day	Daily	Throughout the day
Nighttime awakenings	≤2 times/month	3 or 4 times/month	>1 time weekly but not nightly	Often 7 times weekly
Short-acting β_2-agonist use for symptom control	≤2 days/week	>2 days/week but not daily and not >1 time on any day	Daily	Several times daily
Interference with normal activity	None	Minor limitation	Some limitation	Extremely limited
Lung function	• Normal FEV_1 between exacerbations • FEV_1 >80% predicted • FEV_1/FVC normal	• FEV_1 >80% predicted • FEV_1/FVC normal	• FEV_1 >60%, but <80% predicted • FEV_1/FVC reduced 5%	• FEV_1 <60% predicted • FEV_1/FVC reduced >5%
Asthma exacerbations requiring oral steroids	0–1/year	≥2/year	≥2/year	≥2/year

Recommended step for initiating treatment	Step 1	Step 2	Step 3	Step 4, 5, or 6
Preferred and alternative pharmacotherapy based on step	*Preferred:* Short-acting β_2-agonist as needed	*Preferred:* Low-dose ICS *Alternative:* Leukotriene modifier or theophylline	*Preferred:* Low-dose ICS + LABA or medium-dose ICS *Alternative:* Low-dose ICS + leukotriene modifier, theophylline, or zileuton	**Step 4** *Preferred:* Medium-dose ICS + LABA *Alternative:* Medium-dose ICS + leukotriene modifier, theophylline, or zileuton Identify triggers (cold air, dust, allergic exposures/pets), and control exposures. **Step 5** *Preferred:* High-dose ICS + LABA, and consider omalizumab for patients with allergies Identify triggers and control exposures. **Step 6** *Preferred:* High-dose ICS + LABA + oral corticosteroid, and consider omalizumab for patients with allergies Identify patients at risk for reactions to aspirin and NSAIDs, and avoid exposure.

At each step, discuss patient education, environmental control, and management of comorbidities.

Michael C. Barros, PharmD, BCPS, BCACP, Colleen M. Prinzivalli, PharmD, BCPS, CGP, and Alia Chisty, MD, MS FACP

Elward KS, Pollart SM. Medical therapy for asthma: updates from the NAEPP guidelines. *Am Fam Physician*. 2010;82(10):1242–1251.

ASTHMA, MAINTENANCE

Assessing control
Reevaluate patient in 2–6 weeks and adjust therapy based on components of control.

Well-controlled

Symptoms	≤2 days/week
Nighttime awakenings	≤2 times/month
Interference with normal activity	None
Short-acting β_2-agonist use for symptoms control	≤2 days/week
FEV$_1$ or peak flow	>80% predicted/ personal best
Exacerbations requiring oral steroids	0–1/year

Treatment:
- Maintain current step.
- Regular follow-up every 1–6 months.
- Consider step down if controlled for >3 months.

Not well-controlled

Symptoms	>2 days/week
Nighttime awakenings	1–3 times/week
Interference with normal activity	Some limitation
Short-acting β_2-agonist use for symptoms control	>2 days/week
FEV$_1$ or peak flow	60–80% predicted/ personal best
Exacerbations requiring oral steroids	≥2/year

Treatment:
- Step up 1 step.
- Reevaluate in 2–6 weeks.

Very poorly controlled

Symptoms	Throughout the day
Nighttime awakenings	≥4 times/week
Interference with normal activity	Extremely limited
Short-acting β_2-agonist use for symptoms control	Several times per day
FEV$_1$ or peak flow	<60% predicted/ personal best
Exacerbations requiring oral steroids	≥2/year

Treatment:
- Consider oral corticosteroids.
- Step up 1–2 steps.
- Reevaluate in 2 weeks.

FEV$_1$, forced expiratory volume in 1 second.

Michael C. Barros, PharmD, BCPS, BCACP, Colleen M. Prinzivalli, PharmD, BCPS, CGP, and Alia Chisty, MD, MS, FACP

Elward KS, Pollart SM. Medical therapy for asthma: updates from the NAEPP guidelines. *Am Fam Physician.* 2010;82(10):1242–1251.

ATAXIA

Acute (seconds–days)

- Obtain careful exposure history; consider infectious evaluation (CBC with diff, lumbar puncture), CT scan, or MRI.
- Toxins (alcohol, carbon monoxide, carbon tetrachloride, heavy metals, toluene, toxic exposure to solvents, methylmercury poisoning)
- Medications (antiepileptics, chemotherapy agents, aminoglycosides, anticholinergics, metronidazole [Flagyl]-induced cerebellar toxicity)
- Infectious (meningoencephalitis, postinfectious cerebellitis—varicella, measles, EBV)
- Ischemic/hemorrhagic stroke
- Head or neck trauma

Subacute (days–weeks)

- Obtain anti-TTG, TSH, CBC, RPR, LFTs, B_{12}, TSH, calcium, phosphorus, PTH.
- Atypical infectious process (PML, prion disease, Whipple disease)
- Autoimmune diseases (MS, celiac disease with enteropathy, Hashimoto encephalopathy, neurosarcoidosis)
- Benign tumors (vestibular schwannoma, meningioma)
- Primary malignant tumors (ependymoma, glioma, hemangioblastoma, medulloblastoma)
- Metastatic tumors (breast, colon, lung, melanoma, renal cell CA)
- Lymphoma
- Alcohol abuse and vitamin deficiencies (Wernicke encephalopathy; vitamin B_{12}, E, and zinc deficiencies)
- Systemic disorders (movement disorders—Parkinson, chorea; hypothyroid; hypoparathyroid)

Chronic (months–years)

- Congenital (Arnold-Chiari malformation, Dandy-Walker syndrome, hydrocephalus, Joubert syndrome, rhombencephalosynapsis)
- Autosomal dominant (spinocerebellar ataxias, episodic ataxias, adult-onset leukodystrophy)
- Autosomal recessive (Friedreich ataxia, ataxia telangiectasia, Wilson disease)
- X-linked (Fragile-X)

Other

- Obtain RPR, B_{12}, CT, or MRI.
- Normal pressure hydrocephalus
- Sensory ataxia (tabes dorsalis, B_{12} deficiency)
- Migraine HA with brainstem aura
- Labyrinthitis Ménière disease Acoustic neuroma
- Dementia

Fozia Akhtar Ali, MD and Teny Anna Philip, MD

Brunberg JA. Ataxia. *AJNR Am J Neuroradiol.* 2008;29(7):1420–1422.

CARDIAC ARRHYTHMIAS

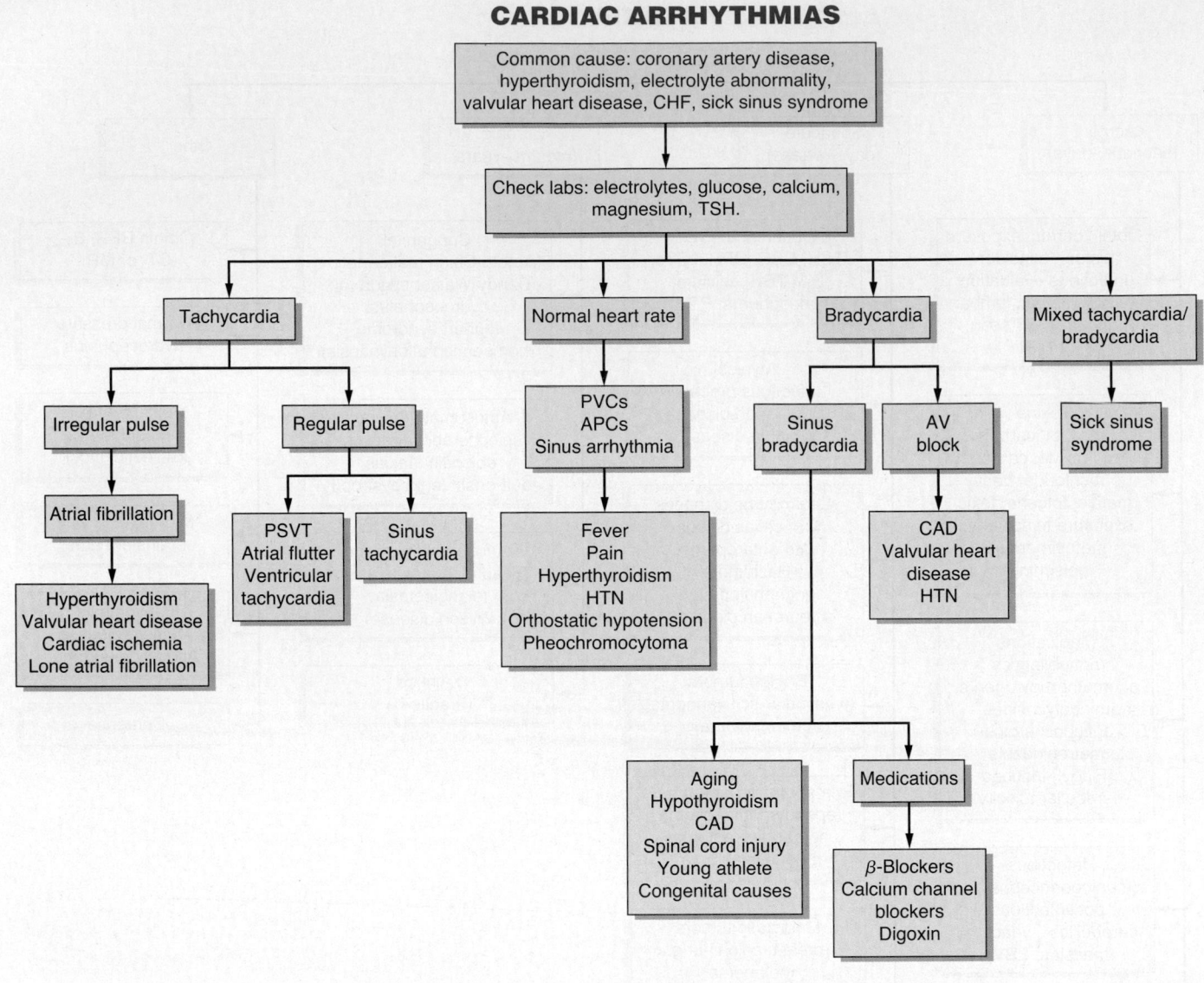

Common cause: coronary artery disease, hyperthyroidism, electrolyte abnormality, valvular heart disease, CHF, sick sinus syndrome

Check labs: electrolytes, glucose, calcium, magnesium, TSH.

Tachycardia

Normal heart rate

Bradycardia

Mixed tachycardia/bradycardia

Irregular pulse

Regular pulse

PVCs
APCs
Sinus arrhythmia

Sinus bradycardia

AV block

Sick sinus syndrome

Atrial fibrillation

PSVT
Atrial flutter
Ventricular tachycardia

Sinus tachycardia

Fever
Pain
Hyperthyroidism
HTN
Orthostatic hypotension
Pheochromocytoma

CAD
Valvular heart disease
HTN

Hyperthyroidism
Valvular heart disease
Cardiac ischemia
Lone atrial fibrillation

Aging
Hypothyroidism
CAD
Spinal cord injury
Young athlete
Congenital causes

Medications

β-Blockers
Calcium channel blockers
Digoxin

Amaninderapal S. Ghotra, MD, Suma Chennubhotla, MD, and Kelly McCants, MD

Link MS. Clinical practice. Evaluation and initial treatment of supraventricular tachycardia. *N Engl J Med.* 2012;367(15):1438–1448.

CERVICAL HYPEREXTENSION INJURY

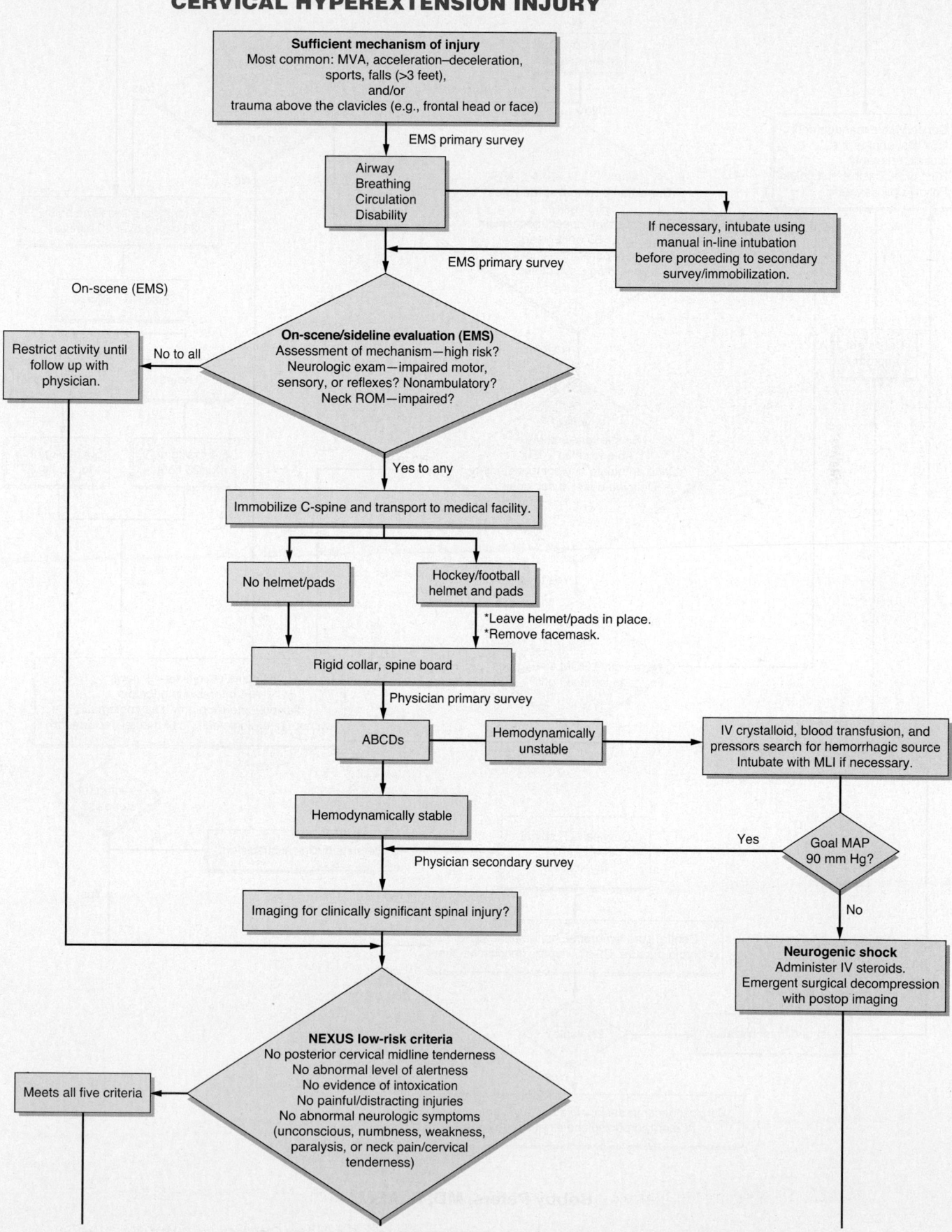

Sufficient mechanism of injury
Most common: MVA, acceleration–deceleration,
sports, falls (>3 feet),
and/or
trauma above the clavicles (e.g., frontal head or face)

EMS primary survey

Airway
Breathing
Circulation
Disability

If necessary, intubate using manual in-line intubation before proceeding to secondary survey/immobilization.

EMS primary survey

On-scene (EMS)

On-scene/sideline evaluation (EMS)
Assessment of mechanism—high risk?
Neurologic exam—impaired motor, sensory, or reflexes? Nonambulatory?
Neck ROM—impaired?

No to all → Restrict activity until follow up with physician.

Yes to any

Immobilize C-spine and transport to medical facility.

No helmet/pads

Hockey/football helmet and pads

*Leave helmet/pads in place.
*Remove facemask.

Rigid collar, spine board

Physician primary survey

ABCDs → Hemodynamically unstable → IV crystalloid, blood transfusion, and pressors search for hemorrhagic source Intubate with MLI if necessary.

Hemodynamically stable

Goal MAP 90 mm Hg?

Yes

No

Physician secondary survey

Imaging for clinically significant spinal injury?

Neurogenic shock
Administer IV steroids.
Emergent surgical decompression with postop imaging

NEXUS low-risk criteria
No posterior cervical midline tenderness
No abnormal level of alertness
No evidence of intoxication
No painful/distracting injuries
No abnormal neurologic symptoms
(unconscious, numbness, weakness, paralysis, or neck pain/cervical tenderness)

Meets all five criteria

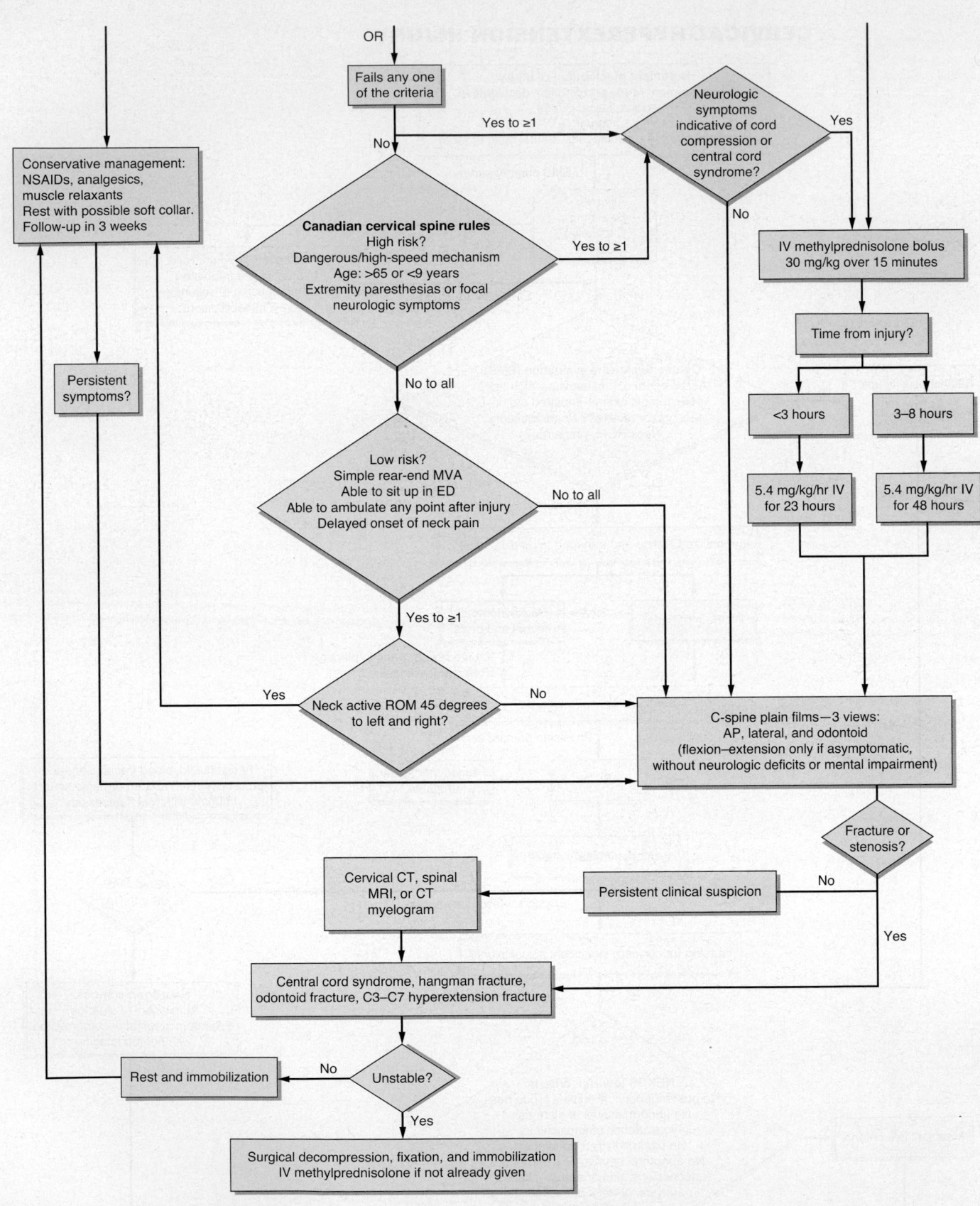

Bobby Peters, MD, FAAEM

Pimentel L, Diegelmann L. Evaluation and management of acute cervical spine trauma. *Emerg Med Clin North Am.* 2010;28(4):719–738.

CHEST PAIN/ACUTE CORONARY SYNDROME

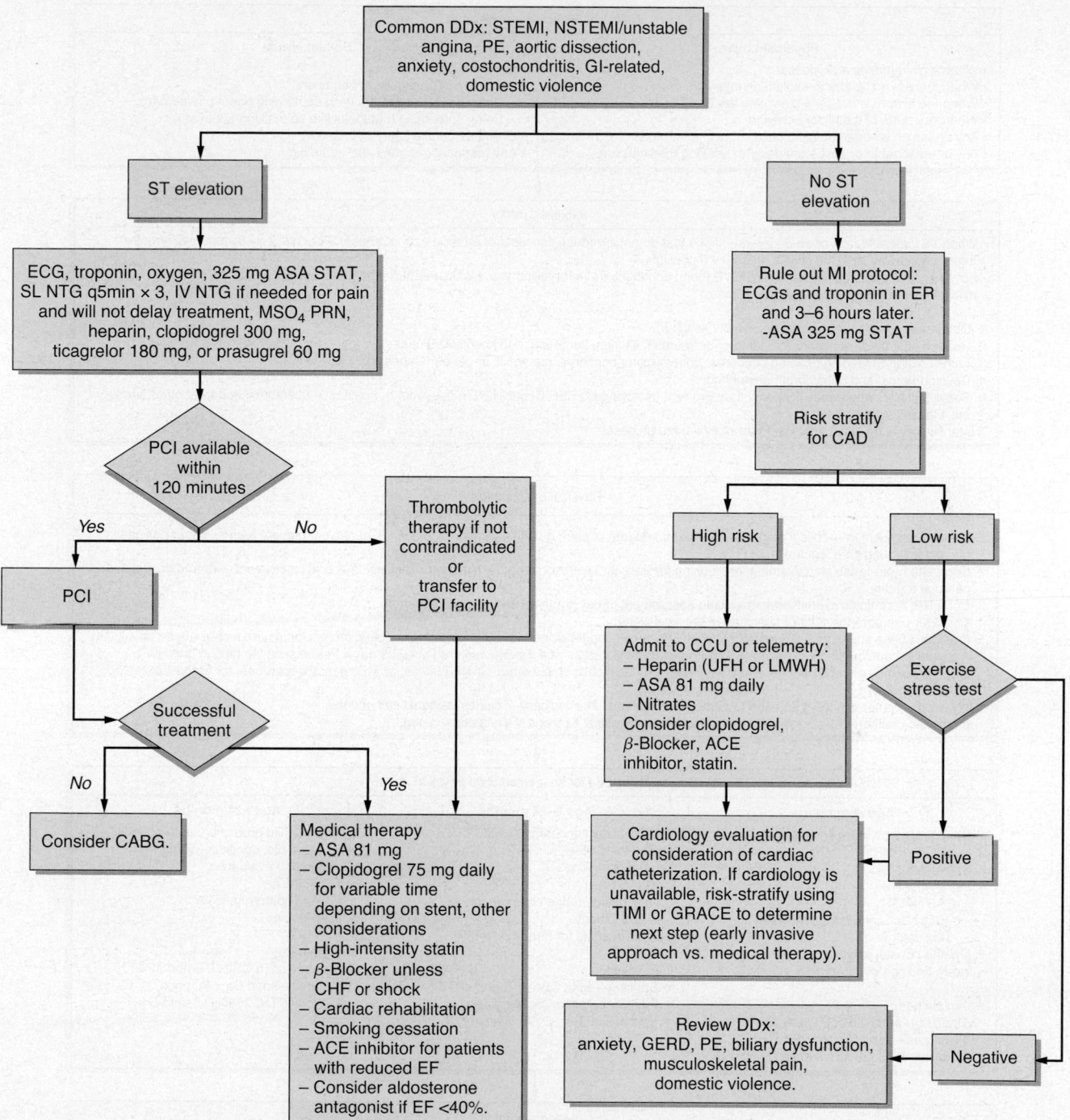

Jeremy Golding, MD, FAAFP

Amsterdam EA, Wenger NK, Brindis RG, et al. 2014 AHA/ACC guideline for the management of patients with non-ST-elevation acute coronary syndromes: executive summary: a report of the American College of Cardiology/American Heart Association Task Force on Practice Guidelines. *Circulation.* 2014;130(25):2354–2394.

CHILD ABUSE

When should you consider abuse?	
Physical abuse	**Sexual abuse**

• When a child makes a disclosure.
• When there is no history to explain an injury.
• When the history is not consistent with the injury seen.
• When key parts of the history change
• Any bruise on a nonambulating child
• Any unreasonable or persistent delay in seeking medical care
	• Child makes a disclosure.
	• Child displays sexualized behaviors.
	  – Doing something with/saying something about private parts
	  – Doing something that looks like sex/talking about sex.
	• Child has genital injury or infection.
	• Any pregnancy in child <16 years old

Medical history

• When >5 years old, ask open-ended questions that do not introduce concepts of abusive acts or abuser. For children <5 years old, acquire information away from the child's presence if possible.
• For all children: listen attentively, BELIEVE them, and thank them for telling you. Reassure them and avoid any anger, as the child may misinterpret this as you being angry at them.

1. Obtain a focused injury history (especially timeline).
2. Routine past medical history, including prior traumas, injuries, surgeries, and hospitalizations
3. Family history (bleeding/bruising concerns, bone/fracture concerns, metabolic or genetic issues)
4. Developmental and behavioral health history
5. Social history*: where they live, who they live with (including OTHER CHILDREN in household), substance use/abuse, job loss, other stressors, etc. Consult social worker if able.
*Note: History is the most important part of this entire process.

Physical examination

1. General assessment—child's alertness, demeanor, degree of pain, growth parameters, evidence of neglect (severe caries, diaper dermatitis, neglected wound care, cachexia, etc.)
2. Complete head-to-toe skin examination, looking for bruises, lacerations, burns, bites, etc. This includes oral cavity, ears, external genitalia, and perianal regions.
3. Complete neurologic examination (including assessment of development and behavioral health).
4. Consider photographs* and/or sketches of physical signs.
5. If sexual abuse suspected, a detailed genital examination should be performed by a trained medical professional (i.e., a child abuse physician). A sexual assault nursing evaluation (SANE) may be warranted as well if event occurred in last 5 days. Postassault lab testing and HIV prophylaxis may also be needed. Please contact your local child abuse team, SANE service, or emergency department for further assistance with management.
*Only secure cameras should be used to photograph patients. This typically excludes personal cell phones.
 If forensic photographs are needed, please contact local social services or child abuse team.

Diagnostic testing for suspected child physical abuse

Age ≤6 months	Age 6–24 months	Age >24 months

1. Child protection team consult
2. Head CT or MRI
3. Skeletal survey
4. Lab evaluation:
  a. AST/ALT
  b. Consider urine comprehensive toxicology.
5. Ophtho consult only if focal neuro exam findings or intracranial blood
 	
If unexplained:
• Bruising—send CBC, PT, and aPTT
• Fractures—send Ca, Mg, phos, alk phos, iPTH, 25-OH vitamin D
	1. Child protection team consult
	2. Skeletal survey
	3. Lab evaluation:
	  a. AST/ALT
	  b. Consider urine comprehensive toxicology.
	4. Low threshold for head CT or MRI
	
	If unexplained:
	• Bruising—send CBC, PT, and aPTT
	• Fractures—send Ca, Mg, phos, alk phos, iPTH, 25-OH vitamin D
		1. Consider child protection team consult.
		2. If >5 years old, consider history from child.
		3. Consider lab evaluation:
		  a. AST/ALT
		  b. Urine comprehensive toxicology
		
		If unexplained:
		• Bruising—send CBC, PT, and aPTT
		• Fractures—send Ca, Mg, phos, alk phos, iPTH, 25-OH vitamin D

Management

1. Referral to investigative agencies/child protection agencies according to state-specific mandated reporting laws. State reporting statutes and other resources available from Child Welfare Information Gateway (www.childwelfare.gov). Additional information on child abuse and neglect (SOCAN): www2.aap.org/sections/childabuseneglect/
2. Referral to appropriate medical providers (such as a pediatric trauma center)
3. Referral to appropriate behavioral health counselor for trauma symptom screening and education. Early mental health interventions (within the first 30 days following a traumatic event). Educational information under resources at the National Child Traumatic Stress Network webpage (http://www.nctsn.org/resources)
4. Medicolegal documentation
5. Safety plan in place prior to discharge with appropriate follow-up plan

Wynne S. Morgan, MD and Peter J. Sell, DO, FAAP

Campbell KA, Olson LM, Keenan HT. Critical elements in the medical evaluation of suspected child physical abuse. *Pediatrics.* 2015;136(1):35–43.

CHRONIC JOINT PAIN AND STIFFNESS

Kimberly Sikule, MD and J. Herbert Stevenson, MD

Pujalte GG, Albano-Aluquin SA. Differential diagnosis of polyarticular arthritis. *Am Fam Physician*. 2015;92(1):35–41.

CHRONIC OBSTRUCTIVE PULMONARY DISEASE (COPD), DIAGNOSIS AND TREATMENT

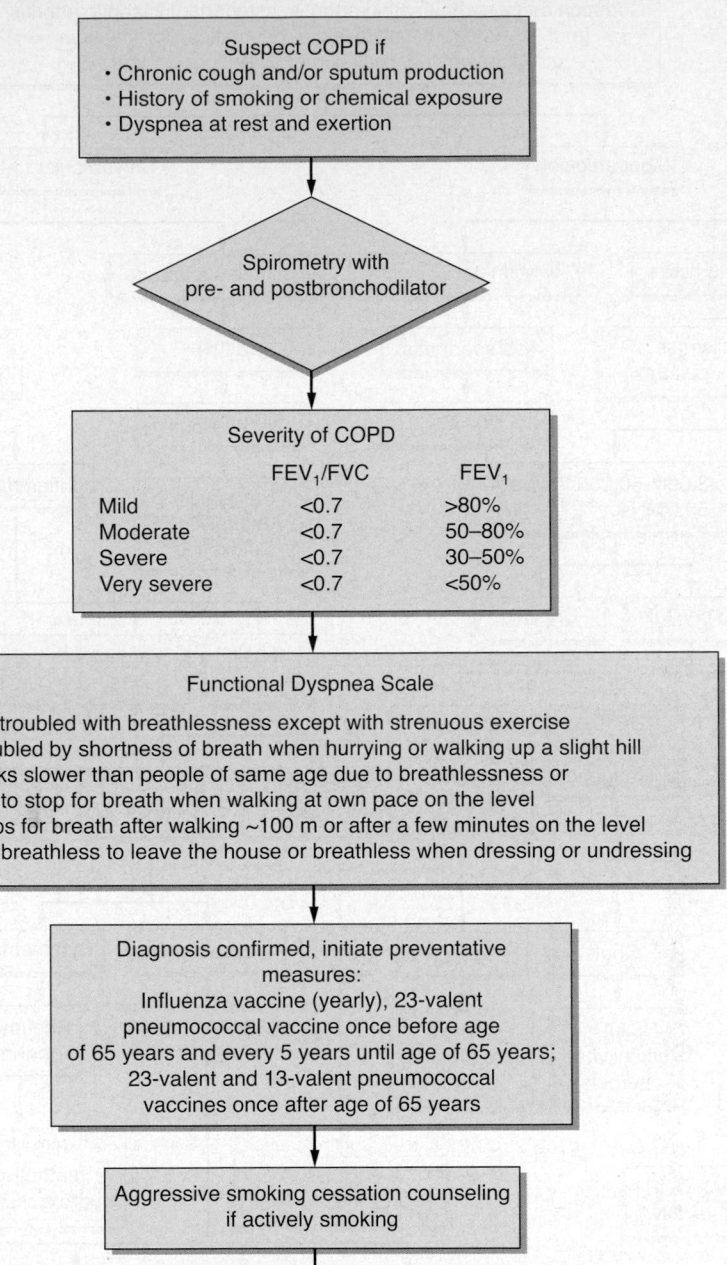

Suspect COPD if
- Chronic cough and/or sputum production
- History of smoking or chemical exposure
- Dyspnea at rest and exertion

↓

Spirometry with pre- and postbronchodilator

↓

Severity of COPD

	FEV$_1$/FVC	FEV$_1$
Mild	<0.7	>80%
Moderate	<0.7	50–80%
Severe	<0.7	30–50%
Very severe	<0.7	<50%

↓

Functional Dyspnea Scale

0 Not troubled with breathlessness except with strenuous exercise
1 Troubled by shortness of breath when hurrying or walking up a slight hill
2 Walks slower than people of same age due to breathlessness or has to stop for breath when walking at own pace on the level
3 Stops for breath after walking ~100 m or after a few minutes on the level
4 Too breathless to leave the house or breathless when dressing or undressing

↓

Diagnosis confirmed, initiate preventative measures:
Influenza vaccine (yearly), 23-valent pneumococcal vaccine once before age of 65 years and every 5 years until age of 65 years; 23-valent and 13-valent pneumococcal vaccines once after age of 65 years

↓

Aggressive smoking cessation counseling if actively smoking

↓

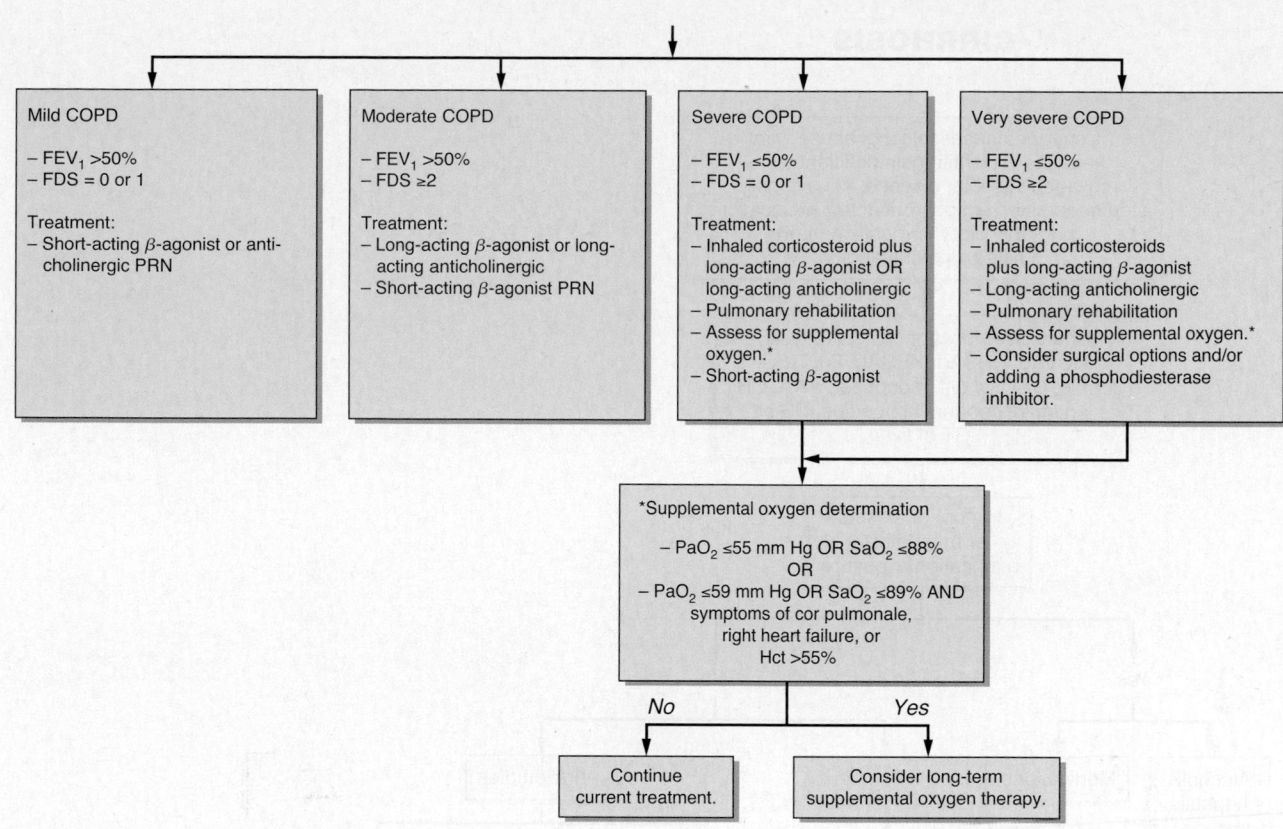

Mild COPD

– FEV_1 >50%
– FDS = 0 or 1

Treatment:
– Short-acting β-agonist or anti-cholinergic PRN

Moderate COPD

– FEV_1 >50%
– FDS ≥2

Treatment:
– Long-acting β-agonist or long-acting anticholinergic
– Short-acting β-agonist PRN

Severe COPD

– FEV_1 ≤50%
– FDS = 0 or 1

Treatment:
– Inhaled corticosteroid plus long-acting β-agonist OR long-acting anticholinergic
– Pulmonary rehabilitation
– Assess for supplemental oxygen.*
– Short-acting β-agonist

Very severe COPD

– FEV_1 ≤50%
– FDS ≥2

Treatment:
– Inhaled corticosteroids plus long-acting β-agonist
– Long-acting anticholinergic
– Pulmonary rehabilitation
– Assess for supplemental oxygen.*
– Consider surgical options and/or adding a phosphodiesterase inhibitor.

*Supplemental oxygen determination

– PaO_2 ≤55 mm Hg OR SaO_2 ≤88%
OR
– PaO_2 ≤59 mm Hg OR SaO_2 ≤89% AND symptoms of cor pulmonale, right heart failure, or Hct >55%

No

Yes

Continue current treatment.

Consider long-term supplemental oxygen therapy.

Scott E. Kopec, MD

Global Initiative for Chronic Obstructive Lung Disease. Global strategy for the diagnosis, management and prevention of chronic obstructive pulmonary disease. http://www.goldcopd.org/

CIRRHOSIS

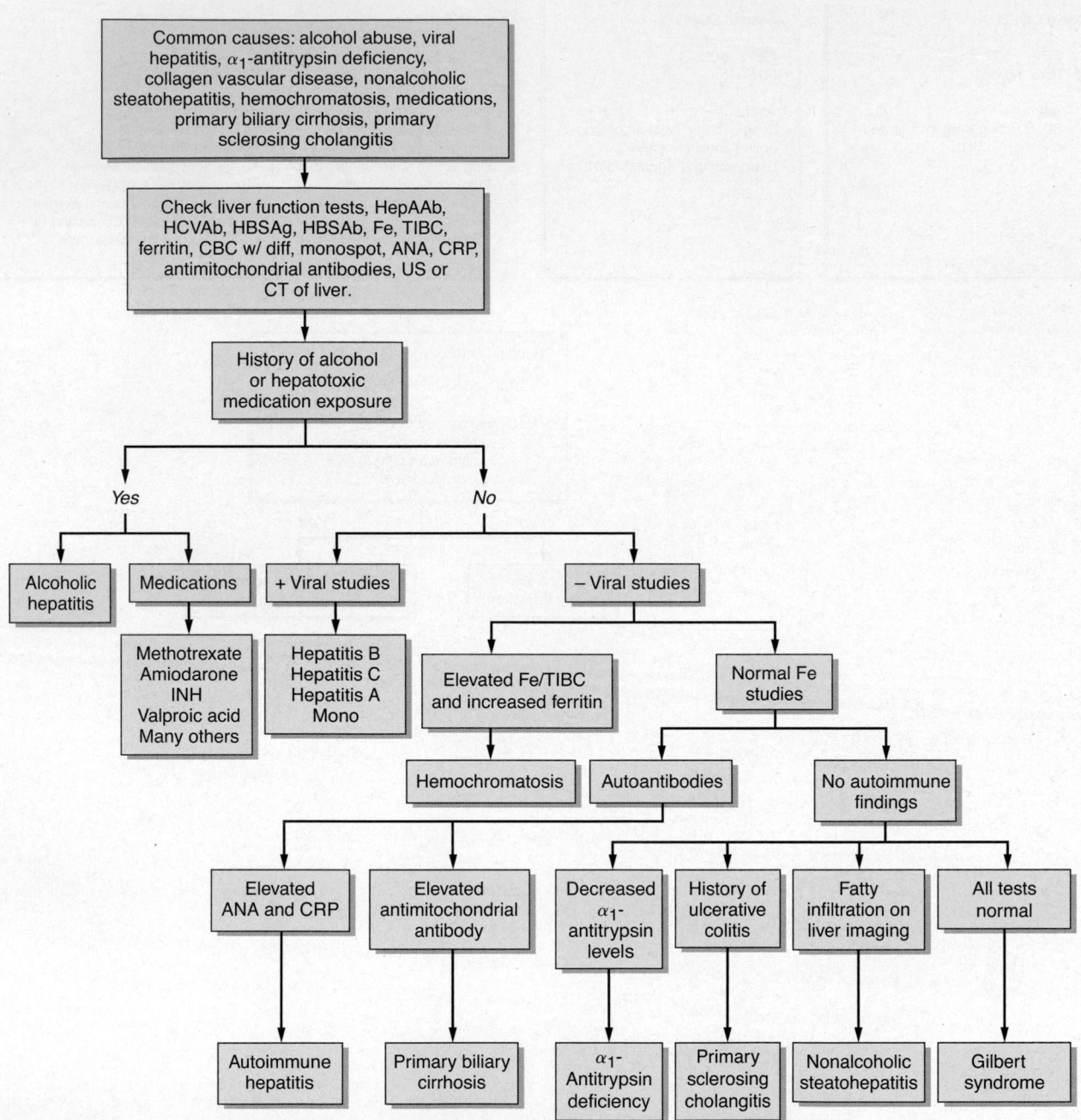

Common causes: alcohol abuse, viral hepatitis, α_1-antitrypsin deficiency, collagen vascular disease, nonalcoholic steatohepatitis, hemochromatosis, medications, primary biliary cirrhosis, primary sclerosing cholangitis

↓

Check liver function tests, HepAAb, HCVAb, HBSAg, HBSAb, Fe, TIBC, ferritin, CBC w/ diff, monospot, ANA, CRP, antimitochondrial antibodies, US or CT of liver.

↓

History of alcohol or hepatotoxic medication exposure

Yes →
- Alcoholic hepatitis
- Medications → Methotrexate, Amiodarone, INH, Valproic acid, Many others

No →
- + Viral studies → Hepatitis B, Hepatitis C, Hepatitis A, Mono
- − Viral studies →
  - Elevated Fe/TIBC and increased ferritin → Hemochromatosis
  - Normal Fe studies →
    - Autoantibodies →
      - Elevated ANA and CRP → Autoimmune hepatitis
      - Elevated antimitochondrial antibody → Primary biliary cirrhosis
    - No autoimmune findings →
      - Decreased α_1-antitrypsin levels → α_1-Antitrypsin deficiency
      - History of ulcerative colitis → Primary sclerosing cholangitis
      - Fatty infiltration on liver imaging → Nonalcoholic steatohepatitis
      - All tests normal → Gilbert syndrome

Robert A. Baldor, MD, FAAFP and Alan M. Ehrlich, MD

Porter ML, Dennis BL. Hyperbilirubinemia in the term newborn. *Am Fam Physician.* 2002;65(4):599–606.

CONCUSSION, SIDELINE EVALUATION
Stable, No C-spine injury

Concussion: traumatic event AND change in neurologic function OR one of the following signs/symptoms: **somatic** (HA, nausea/vomiting [N/V], dizziness, vertigo, visual problems, sensitivity to light or sound, numbness/tingling), **cognitive** (LOC, memory problems, feeling "foggy," slower reaction times, confusion), **emotional/behavioral** (i.e., irritability, sadness), **sleep** (i.e., drowsiness, difficulty falling asleep)

Evaluate ABCs and check for C-spine injury. Remove from play.

Stable and normal C-spine exam — *Unstable or C-spine injury possible*

Assess with standardized tool (SCAT3, SAC, Maddocks questions, BESS, etc.): vital signs, GCS, orientation, past and immediate memory, concentration, balance, coordination, delayed recall.
-SCAT3 available at http://physicians.cattonline.com/scat

Transfer to ED. Activate trauma team if needed. C-spine precautions if indicated. Continue to assess ABCs. Continue first aid.

Vital signs q5min: Do not leave patient alone.

Full history and PE (head and neck evaluation, complete neurologic exam)

Condition back to baseline — *Condition not back to baseline*

GCS ≤14, signs of altered mental status*, or signs of skull fracture

No — *Yes*

Continued monitoring at home and evaluation by medical professional within 24 hours

Occipital, parietal, or temporal scalp hematoma; LOC ≥5 seconds; severe mechanism of injury‡; or not acting normally per parent

Noncontrast head CT (or less commonly, MRI)

Abnormal — *Normal*

No — *Yes*

No imaging

Appropriate treatment (neurosurgical consult for bleeding or edema)

A. Follow up with medical professional in next 24 hours.
 • History and PE (including complete neurologic exam) using Sport Concussion Office Assessment Tool (SCOAT) available online www.sportsconcussion.co.za/Documents/SCOAT.pdf
Consider neuropsych testing.
 • If at neurologic baseline, review Return to Play protocol.
 • If not at neurologic baseline, consider ED evaluation or neuroimaging, close follow-up, and symptomatic treatment.
B. Consider neuropsych testing (paper-and-pencil, ImPACT, CogState, HeadMinder, ANAM, etc.).
 • The ideal timing, frequency, and type of neuropsych testing have not been determined.
 • Most concussions can be managed appropriately without the use of neuropsych testing.
 • Neuropsych testing may be most helpful for high-risk athletes, those with prior concussions, and those who may downplay symptoms in an effort to return to play sooner.
C. Return to Play protocol
No athlete may return to play the same day.
 • Once asymptomatic at a stage for 24 hours, may move on to next stage; if symptoms arise, must take a 24-hour period of complete rest before dropping back one stage and starting from there.
 • Most athletes should return no sooner than 6 days after concussion.
    o Stage 1: no activity (complete physical AND cognitive rest)
    o Stage 2: light aerobic exercise (walking, swimming, or stationary cycling at <70% max HR)
    o Stage 3: sport-specific exercise (sport-specific drills such as skating or running, no head impact activities)
    o Stage 4: noncontact training drills (progression to more complex training drills such as passing, may start progressive resistance training)
    o Stage 5: full contact practice
    o Stage 6: return to game play (should also be free of any medicines that could mask symptoms of concussion)
 • Please note initial cognitive rest, and a graded resumption of typical cognitive activity is also important. Patients may require accommodations such as a shortened school day, reduced academic workload, extended time for tests, and so on, when recovering from a concussion.
D. Symptom management: If concussive symptoms (typically HA, sleep, cognitive, and mood disturbances) are persistent and interfering with function, consider symptomatic treatment.
 • In the acute setting, ASA and NSAIDs should be used with caution due to increased risk of intracranial bleeding. Acetaminophen and physical modalities are OK.
 • If HA persists for a few days, consider typical abortive treatment. There is no established role for pharmacotherapy in the acute treatment of concussion-induced sleep, cognitive, or mood disturbances.
 • If symptoms persist beyond a few weeks, consider referral to specialist (neurology, sports medicine, etc.). Multidisciplinary approach is often needed.
 • If symptoms do not resolve despite appropriate evaluation and treatment, consider terminating athletic season or athletic career (no clear guidelines have been established; this decision should be made on a case-by-case basis).

*Signs of altered mental status: agitation, somnolence, repetitive questioning, or slow response to verbal communication
‡Severe mechanism of injury: motor vehicle crash with patient ejection, death of another passenger, or rollover; pedestrian or bicyclist without helmet struck by motorized vehicle; falls of >3 ft for patients <2 years old or >5 ft for patients ≥2 years old; or head struck by high-impact object

Caitlyn M. Rerucha, MD and Michelle E. Szczepanik, MD

Harmon KG, Drezner JA, Gammons M, et al. American Medical Society for Sports Medicine position statement: concussion in sport. *Br J Sports Med.* 2013;47(1):15–26.

CONGESTIVE HEART FAILURE: DIFFERENTIAL DIAGNOSIS

Common causes: CAD, MI, valvular disease, arrhythmia, idiopathic cardiomyopathy, pulmonary HTN, renal disease, medication noncompliance

Diagnosis made clinically

History: exercise intolerance, dyspnea on exertion or at rest, cough, orthopnea, paroxysmal nocturnal dyspnea, chest discomfort, fatigue, weight gain

Exam: elevated jugular venous pressure, rales, S_3/S_4 gallop, hepatojugular reflux, increased abdominal distention, pallor, lower, extremity edema

Testing: chest x-ray, EKG, troponin, echo, BNP, BMP, LFTs, TSH, UA, uric acid

Diagnosis of CHF: Framingham Diagnostic Criteria
Requires 2 major criteria or 1 major and 2 minor criteria

Major criteria
- Acute pulmonary edema
- Cardiomegaly
- Hepatojugular reflux
- Elevated jugular venous pressure
- Paroxysmal nocturnal dyspnea
- Rales
- S_3

Minor criteria
- Ankle edema
- Dyspnea on exertion
- Hepatomegaly
- Nocturnal cough
- Pleural effusion
- Tachycardia to >120 bpm

97% and 89% sensitive for systolic and diastolic heart failure, respectively

Not CHF | CHF

Alternative diagnosis:
- COPD
- Asthma
- Lung disease
- Pulmonary embolus

LVEF <50% (systolic HF)

LVEF >50% (diastolic HF)

Ischemic
- History of CAD/MI
- Positive stress test
- CAD on cardiac catheterization
- Troponin elevation

Evaluate for causes of CHF.
- Ischemic: CAD/MI
- Nonischemic: HTN, idiopathic CM, valvular disease, HOCM, arrhythmia, myocarditis/pericarditis, collagen vascular disease
- Due to volume: medication noncompliance, renal failure

Cardiac catheterization unless contraindicated

Nonischemic cardiomyopathy

Idiopathic cardiomyopathy

Other: HTN, thyrotoxicosis, alcoholism, chemotherapy-induced, cocaine, autoimmune, collagen vascular disease, infiltrative (amyloid, hemochromatosis), obstructive sleep apnea

Tachycardia-mediated (atrial fibrillation/flutter, SVT, frequent PVCs)

Valvular disease cardiomyopathy

Viral-mediated (coxsackievirus, adenovirus, HIV, EBV)

Michael T. Tanoue, MD, Parag Goyal, MD, and James M. Horowitz, MD, FACC

King M, Kingery J, Casey B. Diagnosis and evaluation of heart failure. *Am Fam Physician*. 2012;85(12):1161–1168.

CONSTIPATION, DIAGNOSIS AND TREATMENT (ADULT)

Rome III criteria
- Two of the following for 12 weeks in past 6 months:
  - <3 stools/week
  - For 25% of time, any of the following:
    - Hard stools
    - Straining
    - Manual assist
    - Sense of incomplete evacuation
    - Sense of anorectal blockade
- Rare loose stools without laxative use

Common causes: primary—functional, slow transit, pelvic floor dysfunction; secondary—IBS, diabetes mellitus, hypothyroidism, hypercalcemia, pregnancy, obstruction, medication side effect

History and physical: diet, fluid intake, exercise, Rome III criteria, digital rectal exam, abdominal exam, neurologic exam

Red flags: unintentional weight loss, hematochezia, family Hx IBD or colon cancer, positive fecal occult, anemia, new onset in age >50 years, change in stool size, neurologic findings

Yes → Colonoscopy

No

Medication Hx: anticholinergics, opiates, calcium channel blockers, antidepressants, antacids

Yes → Consider medication effect: Adjust and/or begin with empiric treatment.

No → Diagnostic testing: CBC, glucose, creatinine, calcium, TSH

Anemia

Hypothyroidism

Positive → Hypercalcemia

Diabetes mellitus

Negative

Empiric treatment: Increase exercise and water intake; trial of fiber of bulk-forming laxatives

Symptoms improved? No → Add polyethylene glycol and/or stimulant laxative.

Yes → Functional constipation

Symptoms improved? Yes → Functional constipation

No → Treatment failure → Diagnostic testing: colonic transit time (CTT) study, balloon expulsion test (BET), anorectal manometry (AM)

Abnormal CTT → Slow transit constipation → Treatments earlier, enemas, biofeedback

Normal CTT, abnormal BET, abnormal AM → Pelvic floor dysfunction → Treatments earlier, biofeedback, also Botox, surgery

Consider adjunctive agents such as lubiprostone and linaclotide.

Daniel J. Stein, MD, MPH and Stephen K. Lane, MD, FAAFP

Longstreth GF, Thompson WG, Chey WD, et al. Functional bowel disorders. *Gastroenterology.* 2006;130(5):1480–1491.

CONSTIPATION, TREATMENT (PEDIATRIC)

*Red flags:
Constipation <1 month
No meconium in 48 hours
Family history of Hirschsprung disease
Ribbon stools
Blood in the stools without anal fissures
Failure to thrive
Fever
Bilious vomiting
Abnormal thyroid gland
Severe abdominal distention
Perianal fistula
Abnormal position of anus
Absent anal or cremasteric reflex
Decreased lower extremity tone
Tuft of hair on spine
Sacral dimple
Gluteal cleft deviation
Extreme fear during anal inspection
Anal scars

Rome III Criteria (≥2 criteria):
≤2 defecations per week
At least one episode of incontinence per week after toilet training
History of excessive stool retention
History of painful/hard bowel movements
Presence of a large fecal mass
History of large diameter stools that may obstruct the toilet

Careful history and physical exam; digital rectal exam is not required for diagnosis.

Are red flags present?*

Yes → Obtain based on symptoms: CBC, glucose, TSH, calcium, glucose, creatinine, tissue transglutaminase (TTG), and endomysium antibody (EMA).

No → Functional constipation

Differential diagnosis:
Celiac disease
Hypothyroidism
Hypercalcemia
Hypokalemia
Diabetes mellitus
Drugs/toxins—opiates, anticholinergics, antidepressants, chemotherapy, heavy metals
Vitamin D intoxification
Botulism
Cystic fibrosis
Hirschsprung disease
Anal achalasia
Colonic inertia
Anal malformations
Pelvic mass
Spinal cord abnormalities
Abnormal abdominal musculature
Pseudoobstruction
Multiple endocrine neoplasia type 2B

Refer for specialty evaluation.

Fecal Impaction?

Yes → First line: polyethylene glycol 3350 1–1.5 g/kg/day for 3–6 days

Second line: enemas daily for 3–6 days

No → Maintenance therapy:
First line: PEG 0.4 g/kg/day adjusted for one to two soft bowel movements day

Lactulose is acceptable if PEG is not available.

Dietary changes/family education:
– High-fiber diet (1–5 years: 14 g/day; 5–13 years: 17–25 g/day; >13 years: 25–31 g/day). Increase fiber gradually to minimize flatulence.
– Limit caffeine and milk products (<16 oz/milk/day)
– If symptoms persist, add: <6 months—sorbitol-containing juices; >6 months—lactulose (1–3 mL/kg/day to max 60 mL/day) or polyethylene glycol 3350 (0.5–1 g/kg/day to max 17 g/day).

Bethany N. Teer, MD

Tabbers MM, DiLorenzo C, Berger MY, et al. Evaluation and treatment of functional constipation in infants and children: evidence-based recommendations from ESPGHAN and NASPGHAN. *J Pediatr Gastroenterol Nutr.* 2014;58(2):258–274.

CONTRACEPTION

Does she want short- or long-term contraception?

→ Short-term

Any contraindications against using estrogen?

Yes →

Condoms
Male condom: 82% effective
Female condom: 79% effective
– Both provide STD protection.

Other barrier methods:
– **Diaphragm**
– **Sponge**
– **Cervical cap**
– **± Spermicide**
– Efficacy 72.88%
– Less widely used
– Efficacy ↑ with dual contraceptive use for all barrier methods

Fertility awareness methods
– Less effective (76%)
– Nonhormonal, nonsurgical, natural methods
– Based on avoiding prime ovulation days during cycle
– **Ovulation**
– **Standard day**
– **2-day**
– **Symptothermal**

Yes →

Progestin only pill/mini pill
– Good efficacy (91%)
– Must be taken at same time every day
– Likely to cause breakthrough bleeding

No ↓

Can she reliably take medication daily?

Yes ↓

Breastfeeding <1 month

Yes →
No →

Combined oral contraceptive methods
– Good efficacy (91%)
– Many noncontraceptive benefits, ↓ dysmenorrhea, cycle control
– Continuous cycling/extended formulations available
– Daily dosing
– Estrogen-related AE, ↑ risk of VTE

No ↓

Transdermal method
– **Ortho Evra**
– Good efficacy (91%)
– Noncontraceptive benefits, ↓ dysmenorrhea, cycle control
– Once-weekly dosing
– 48-hour "window of forgiveness"
– Contraindicated in women >90 kg
– **Black box warning:** increased estrogen-related AE, especially VTE

Intravaginal method
– **NuvaRing**
– Good efficacy (91%)
– Lower hormone doses
– Simple to use
– Once a month dosing
– Many noncontraceptive benefits, ↓ dysmenorrhea, cycle control

→ Long-term

Does she want to have children in the future?

No ↓

Permanent methods

Sterilization methods
– Very effective (>99%)
– **Tubal ligation**—can be done laparoscopically or after a C-section
– **Vasectomy**—outpatient procedure

Yes ↓

Long-acting reversible methods

Injectable method
Depo-Provera
– Good efficacy (94%), good for 3 months
– High likelihood of unscheduled bleeding

Implantable methods
– **Implanon, Nexplanon**
– **Sino-implant**
– Very effective (>99%), good for 3–5 years
– Simple office procedure with no ongoing effort required
– High likelihood of unscheduled bleeding and/or prolonged amenorrhea

Intrauterine methods
– **Mirena IUD**
– **Skyla IUD**
– **Copper T 380A IUD**—nonhormonal
– Very effective (>99%), good for 5–10 years
– Outpatient office procedure with no ongoing effort required
– Prompt return to fertility
– Good when breastfeeding
– May cause irregular bleeding and cramping for first 3–6 months
– Option for adolescents and nulliparous women

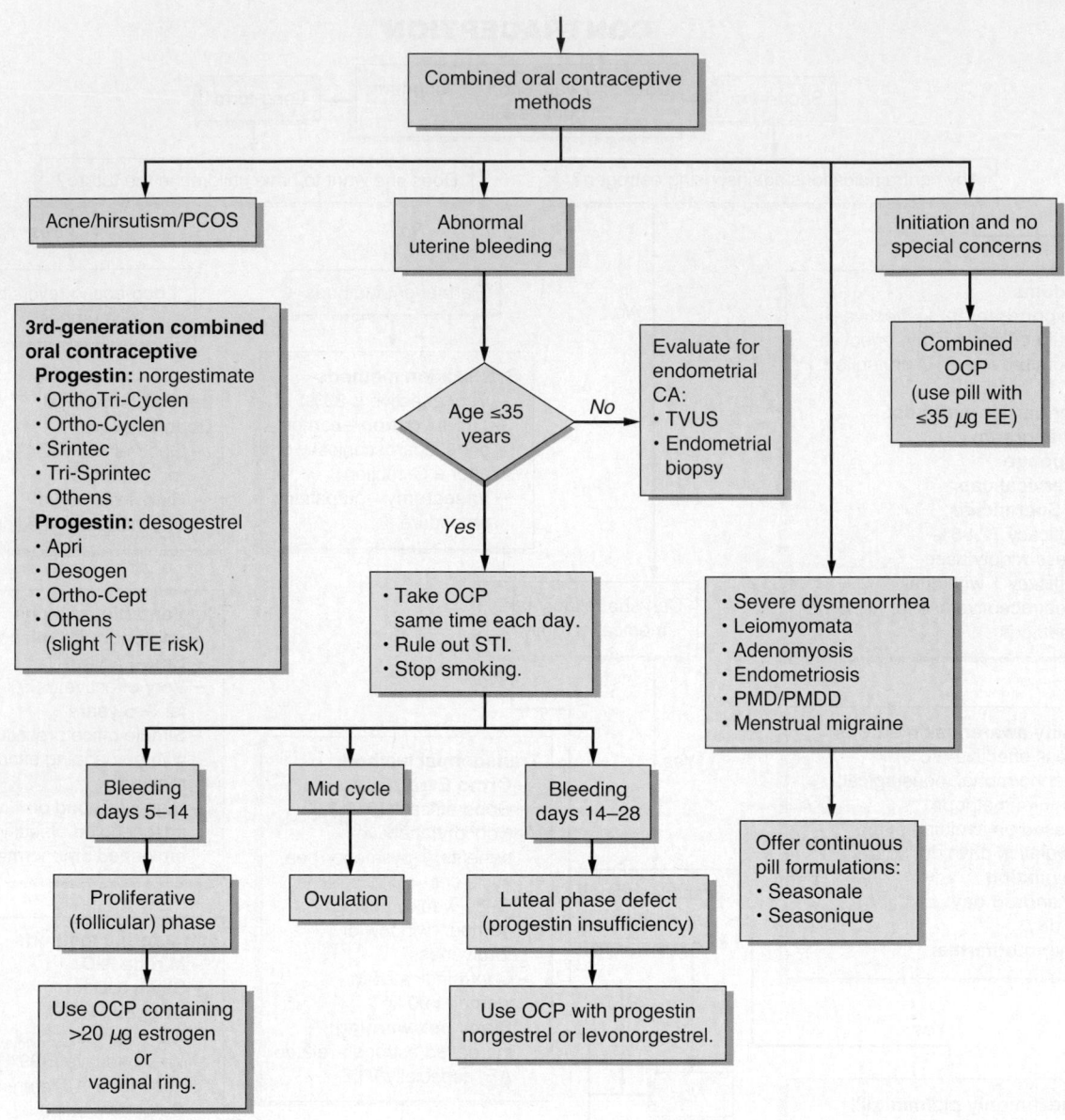

Combined oral contraceptive methods

Acne/hirsutism/PCOS

3rd-generation combined oral contraceptive
Progestin: norgestimate
- OrthoTri-Cyclen
- Ortho-Cyclen
- Srintec
- Tri-Sprintec
- Othens

Progestin: desogestrel
- Apri
- Desogen
- Ortho-Cept
- Othens
(slight ↑ VTE risk)

Abnormal uterine bleeding

Age ≤35 years → *No* → Evaluate for endometrial CA:
- TVUS
- Endometrial biopsy

Yes

- Take OCP same time each day.
- Rule out STI.
- Stop smoking.

Bleeding days 5–14 → Proliferative (follicular) phase → Use OCP containing >20 μg estrogen or vaginal ring.

Mid cycle → Ovulation

Bleeding days 14–28 → Luteal phase defect (progestin insufficiency) → Use OCP with progestin norgestrel or levonorgestrel.

Initiation and no special concerns → Combined OCP (use pill with ≤35 μg EE)

- Severe dysmenorrhea
- Leiomyomata
- Adenomyosis
- Endometriosis
- PMD/PMDD
- Menstrual migraine

Offer continuous pill formulations:
- Seasonale
- Seasonique

Amanda M. Carnes, MD

Division of Reproductive Health, National Center for Chronic Disease Prevention and Health Promotion, Centers for Disease Control and Prevention. U.S. Selected Practice Recommendations for Contraceptive Use, 2013: adapted from the World Health Organization selected practice recommendations for contraceptive use, 2nd edition. *MMWR Recomm Rep.* 2013;62(RR-05):1–60.

DEEP VENOUS THROMBOSIS, DIAGNOSIS AND TREATMENT

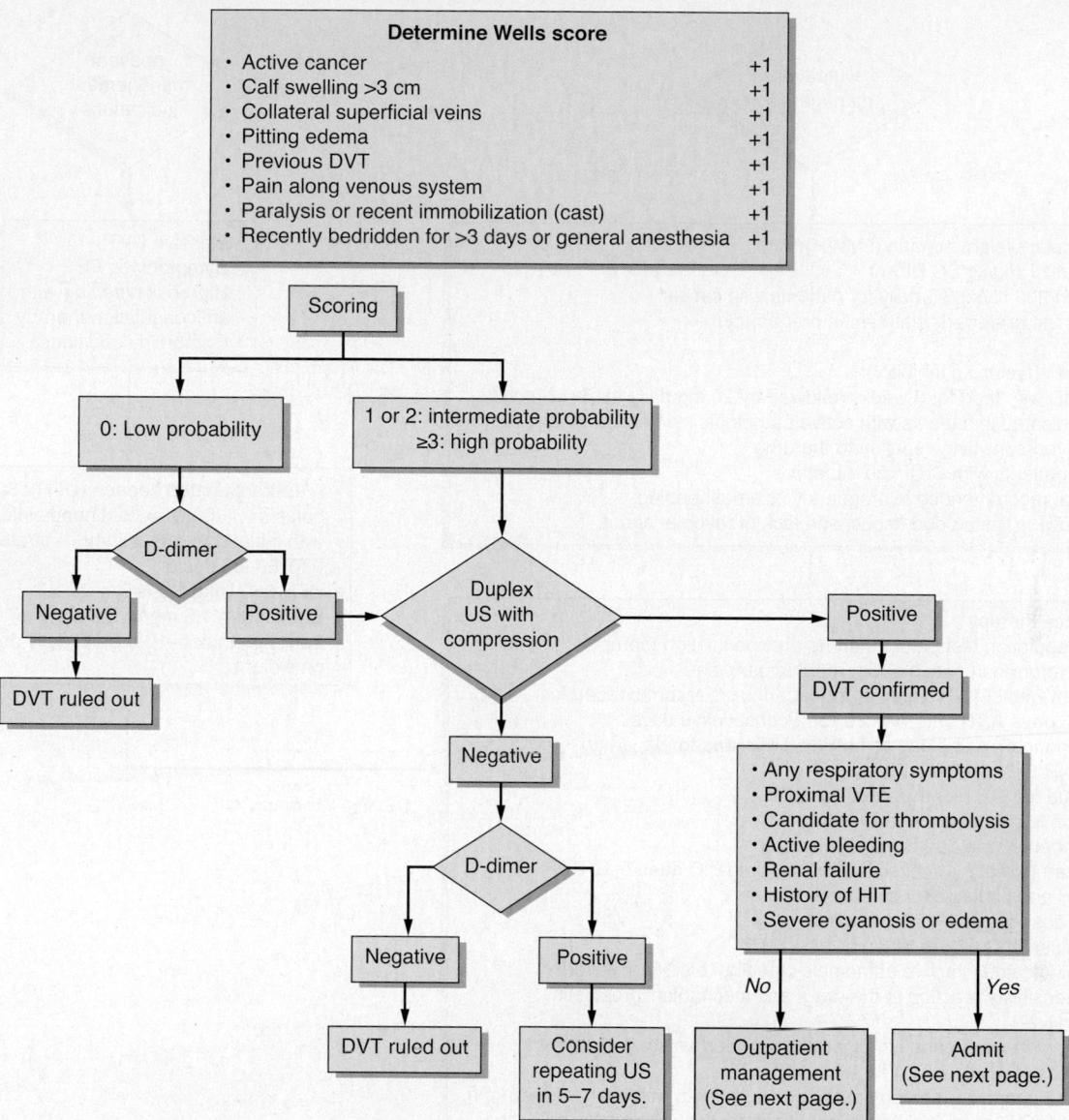

Determine Wells score

• Active cancer	+1
• Calf swelling >3 cm	+1
• Collateral superficial veins	+1
• Pitting edema	+1
• Previous DVT	+1
• Pain along venous system	+1
• Paralysis or recent immobilization (cast)	+1
• Recently bedridden for >3 days or general anesthesia	+1

Scoring

0: Low probability

1 or 2: intermediate probability
≥3: high probability

D-dimer

Negative → DVT ruled out

Positive

Duplex US with compression → Positive → DVT confirmed

Negative

D-dimer

Negative → DVT ruled out

Positive → Consider repeating US in 5–7 days.

• Any respiratory symptoms
• Proximal VTE
• Candidate for thrombolysis
• Active bleeding
• Renal failure
• History of HIT
• Severe cyanosis or edema

No → Outpatient management (See next page.)

Yes → Admit (See next page.)

Treatment

```
        ┌───────────────┐                              ┌───────────────┐
        │   Outpatient  │                              │   Inpatient   │
        │  management   │                              │  management   │
        └───────┬───────┘                              │  indications  │
                │                                      └───────┬───────┘
                ▼                                              ▼
```

Low-molecular-weight heparin (LMWH):
- Enoxaparin 1 mg/kg SC BID or
- Dalteparin 200 IU/kg SC daily for patients with cancer
- LMWH is the preferred treatment in pregnancy.

Rivaroxaban (factor Xa inhibitor):
- 15 mg BID with food for 3 weeks followed by 20 mg daily for 6–12 months
- Contraindicated in patients with active pathologic bleeding or history of severe hypersensitivity reaction to the drug
- Avoid in patients with CrCl <30 mL/min.
- Use is not recommended in pregnancy or breastfeeding.
- Current use is limited due to cost and lack of reversal agent.

- Massive DVT
- Symptomatic PE
- High-risk bleeding with anticoagulation therapy
- Comorbid conditions

- IV unfractionated heparin (UFH): 80 U/kg bolus or 5,000 U → continuous infusion with initial dose 18 U/kg/hr → titrate to goal PTT 60–85 sec or
- UFH 250 U/kg SC BID or
- Enoxaparin 1.5 mg/kg SC daily or
- Fondaparinux 5–10 mg SC daily depending on weight

Maintenance therapy
- Hypercoagulation test before starting anticoagulation therapy
- UFH is preferred in patients with renal impairment.
- Treatment with LMWH, UFH, or fondaparinux is recommended for at least 5 days **AND** until INR ≥ 2 for 2 consecutive days.
- Start warfarin on same day as LMWH, UFH, and fondaparinux
  - Goal INR 2–3
  - Continue for 3–6 months after first DVT.
  - Warfarin is contraindicated in pregnancy.
- Rivaroxaban 20 mg daily for 6–12 months
- Dabigatran (direct thrombin inhibitor): 150 mg BID after 7–10 days of LMWH and continue for at least 6 months
  - Adjust dose for CrCl <50 mL/min
  - Do not use in CrCl <15 mL/min
  - Contraindicated in active pathologic bleeding, history of severe hypersensitivity reaction to the drug, and mechanical prosthetic heart valve
  - Use is not recommended in bioprosthetic heart valve, pregnancy, and breastfeeding.
- LMWH or heparin SC can be continued for patients with allergy to warfarin.
- Consider IVC filter for individuals with contraindication to anticoagulation.

Bency K. Louidor-Paulynice, MD and Kimberly Bombaci, MD

Wells P, Forgie M, Rodger M. Treatment of venous thromboembolism. *JAMA*. 2014;311(7):717–728.

DEHYDRATION, PEDIATRIC

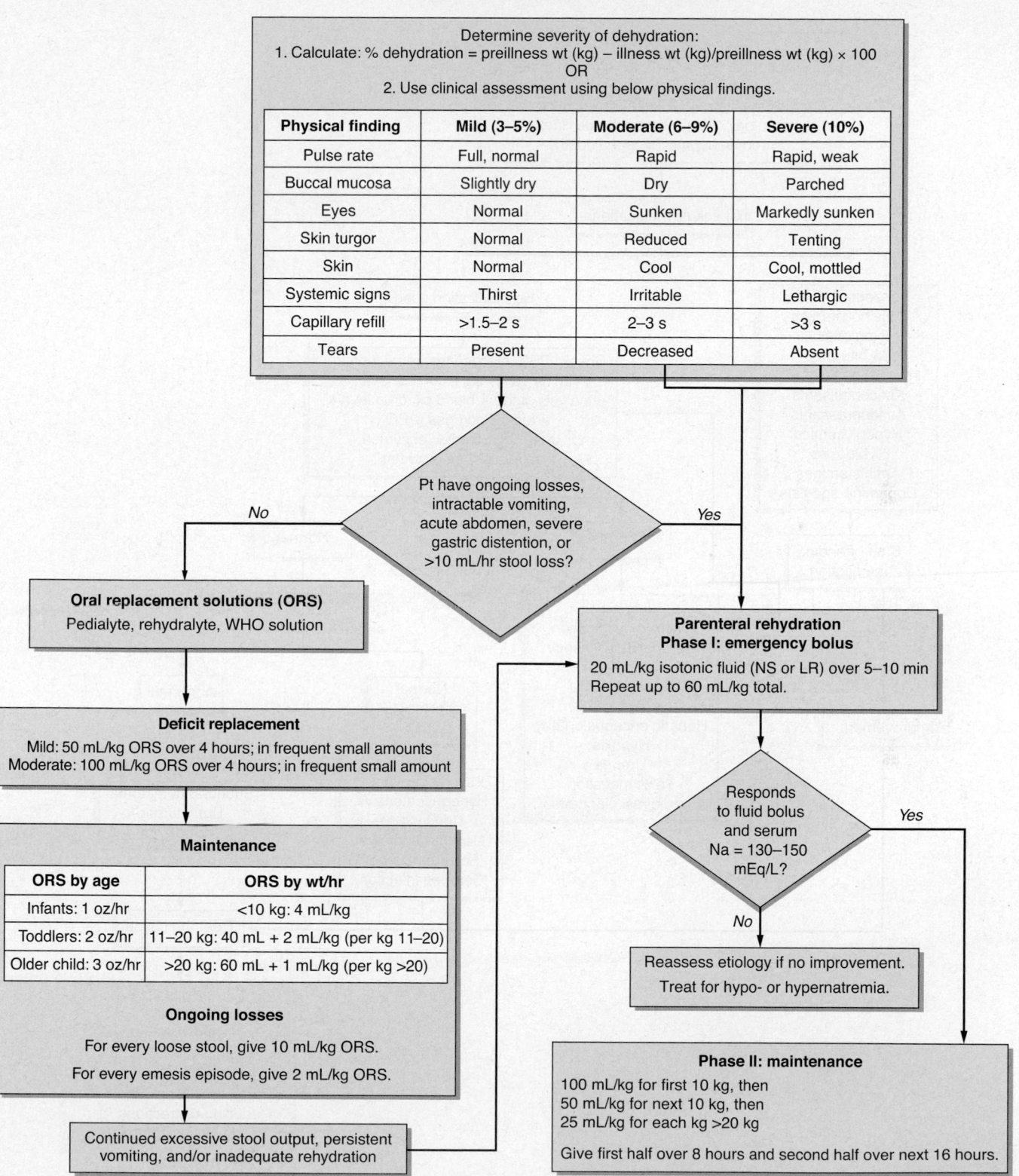

Determine severity of dehydration:
1. Calculate: % dehydration = preillness wt (kg) − illness wt (kg)/preillness wt (kg) × 100
OR
2. Use clinical assessment using below physical findings.

Physical finding	Mild (3–5%)	Moderate (6–9%)	Severe (10%)
Pulse rate	Full, normal	Rapid	Rapid, weak
Buccal mucosa	Slightly dry	Dry	Parched
Eyes	Normal	Sunken	Markedly sunken
Skin turgor	Normal	Reduced	Tenting
Skin	Normal	Cool	Cool, mottled
Systemic signs	Thirst	Irritable	Lethargic
Capillary refill	>1.5–2 s	2–3 s	>3 s
Tears	Present	Decreased	Absent

Pt have ongoing losses, intractable vomiting, acute abdomen, severe gastric distention, or >10 mL/hr stool loss?

No →

Oral replacement solutions (ORS)
Pedialyte, rehydralyte, WHO solution

Deficit replacement
Mild: 50 mL/kg ORS over 4 hours; in frequent small amounts
Moderate: 100 mL/kg ORS over 4 hours; in frequent small amount

Maintenance

ORS by age	ORS by wt/hr
Infants: 1 oz/hr	<10 kg: 4 mL/kg
Toddlers: 2 oz/hr	11–20 kg: 40 mL + 2 mL/kg (per kg 11–20)
Older child: 3 oz/hr	>20 kg: 60 mL + 1 mL/kg (per kg >20)

Ongoing losses

For every loose stool, give 10 mL/kg ORS.

For every emesis episode, give 2 mL/kg ORS.

Continued excessive stool output, persistent vomiting, and/or inadequate rehydration

Yes →

**Parenteral rehydration
Phase I: emergency bolus**
20 mL/kg isotonic fluid (NS or LR) over 5–10 min
Repeat up to 60 mL/kg total.

Responds to fluid bolus and serum Na = 130–150 mEq/L?

Yes →

No ↓

Reassess etiology if no improvement.
Treat for hypo- or hypernatremia.

Phase II: maintenance
100 mL/kg for first 10 kg, then
50 mL/kg for next 10 kg, then
25 mL/kg for each kg >20 kg

Give first half over 8 hours and second half over next 16 hours.

L. Michelle Seawright, DO and Nathaniel Stepp, DO, LCDR, USN

Tschudy M, Arcara K. *Harriet Lane Handbook*. 19th ed. Philadelphia, PA: Elsevier; 2012:271–291.

DELIRIUM

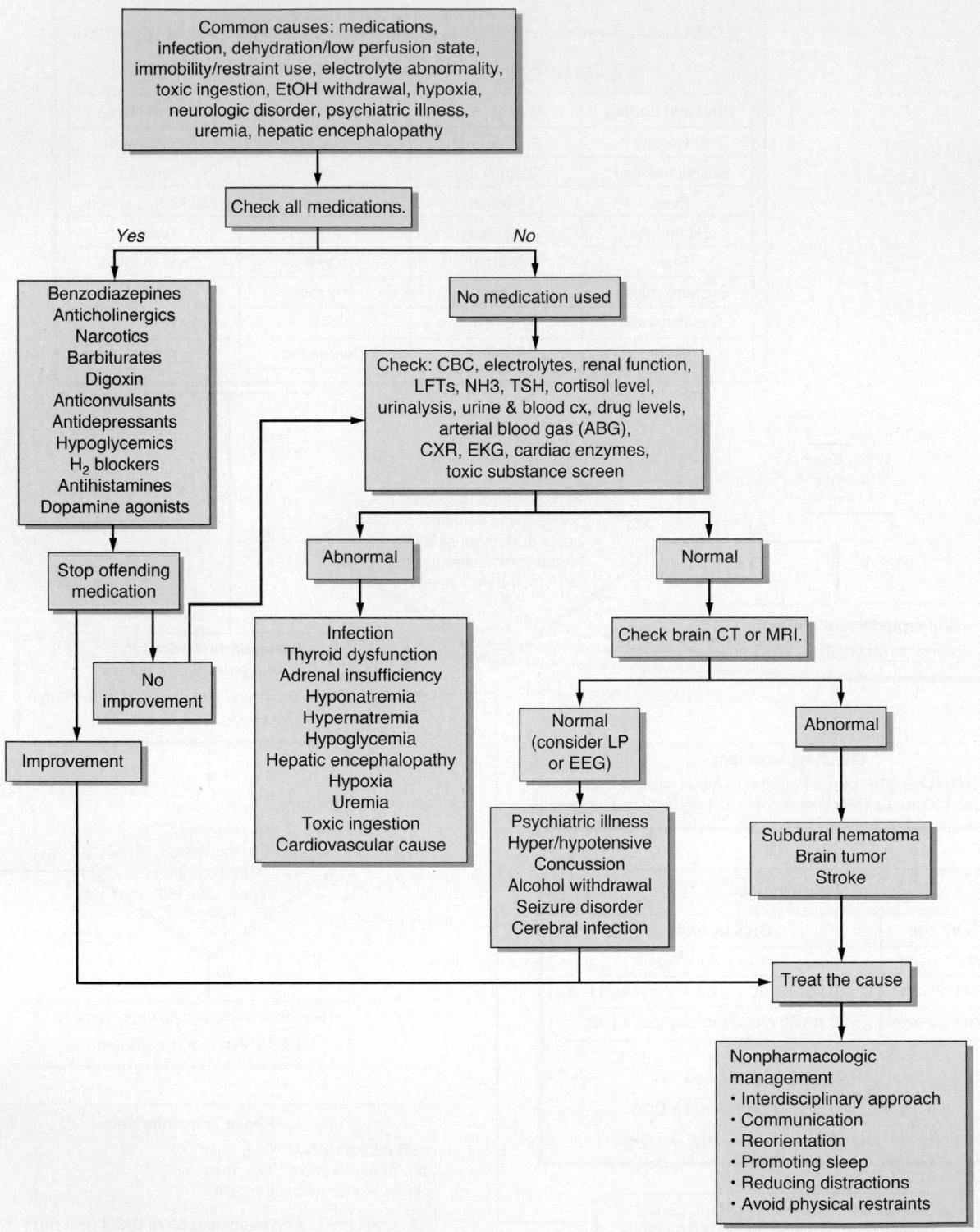

Michelle DiBetta, MD and Holly L. Baab, MD

Kalish VB, Gillham JE, Unwin BK. Delirium in older persons: evaluation and management. *Am Fam Physician*. 2014;90(3):150–158.

DEMENTIA

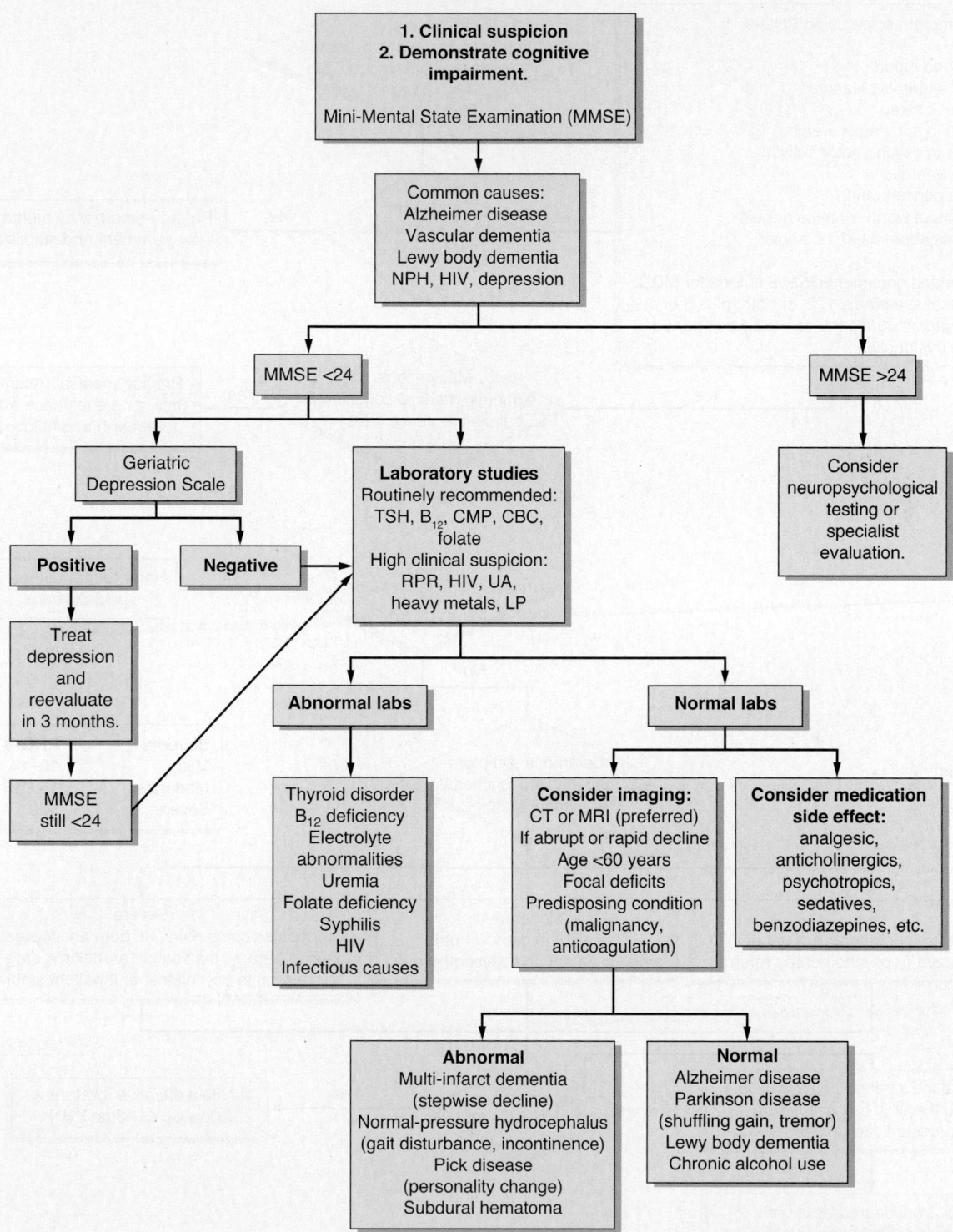

1. Clinical suspicion
2. Demonstrate cognitive impairment.

Mini-Mental State Examination (MMSE)

Common causes:
Alzheimer disease
Vascular dementia
Lewy body dementia
NPH, HIV, depression

MMSE <24

MMSE >24

Geriatric Depression Scale

Consider neuropsychological testing or specialist evaluation.

Positive

Negative

Treat depression and reevaluate in 3 months.

MMSE still <24

Laboratory studies
Routinely recommended:
TSH, B_{12}, CMP, CBC, folate
High clinical suspicion:
RPR, HIV, UA, heavy metals, LP

Abnormal labs

Normal labs

Thyroid disorder
B_{12} deficiency
Electrolyte abnormalities
Uremia
Folate deficiency
Syphilis
HIV
Infectious causes

Consider imaging:
CT or MRI (preferred)
If abrupt or rapid decline
Age <60 years
Focal deficits
Predisposing condition (malignancy, anticoagulation)

Consider medication side effect:
analgesic, anticholinergics, psychotropics, sedatives, benzodiazepines, etc.

Abnormal
Multi-infarct dementia (stepwise decline)
Normal-pressure hydrocephalus (gait disturbance, incontinence)
Pick disease (personality change)
Subdural hematoma

Normal
Alzheimer disease
Parkinson disease (shuffling gain, tremor)
Lewy body dementia
Chronic alcohol use

Kristin Grindstaff, DO and Casandra Cashman, MD, FAAFP

Simmons BB, Hartmann B, Dejoseph D. Evaluation of suspected dementia. *Am Fam Physician*. 2011;84(8):895–902.

DEPRESSIVE EPISODE, MAJOR

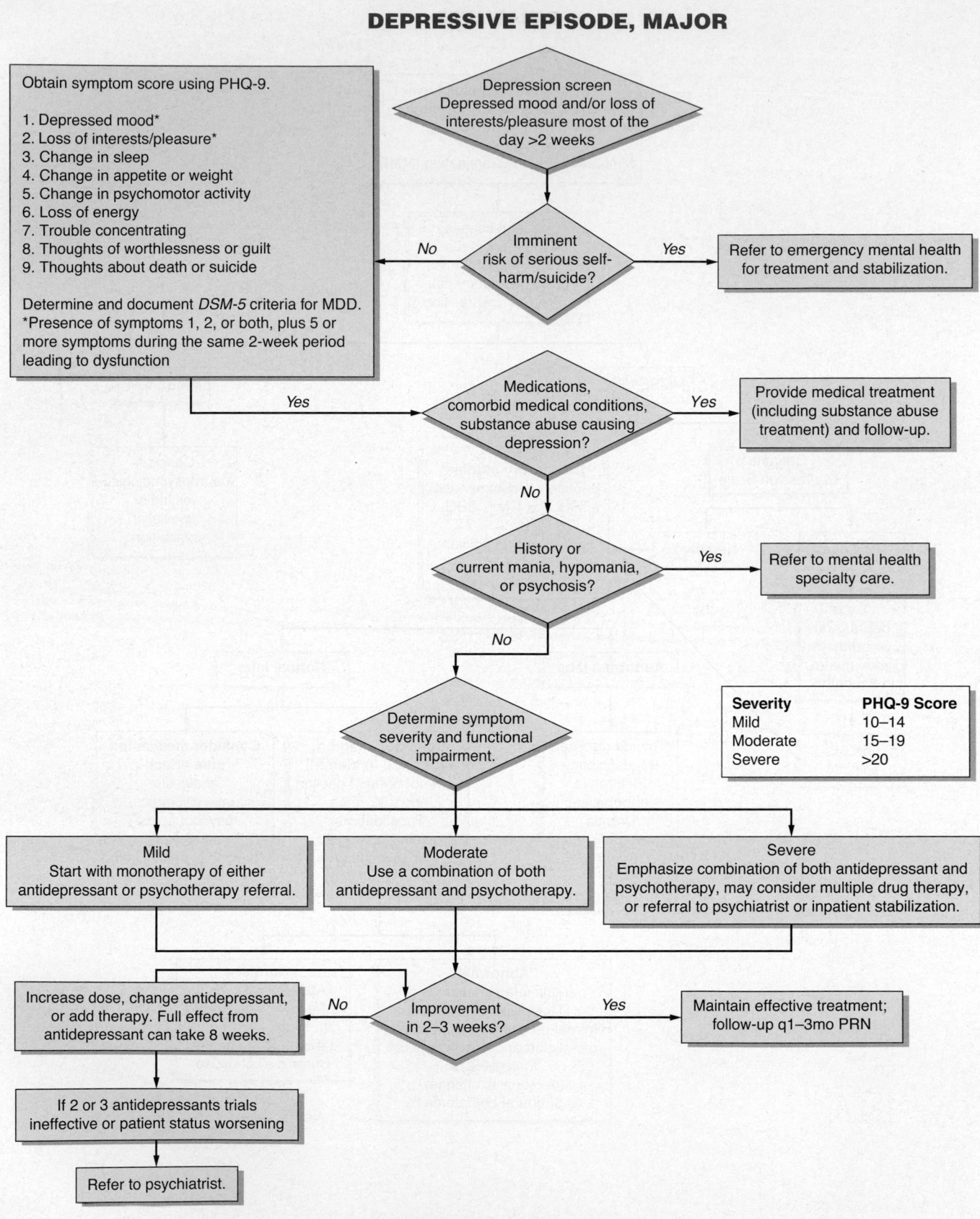

Wendy K. Marsh, MD, MSc

US Department of Veterans Affairs. *VA/DoD Clinical Practice Guideline for Management of Major Depressive Disorder.* Washington, DC: Department of Veteran Affairs; 2010.

DIABETIC KETOACIDOSIS (DKA), TREATMENT

DKA diagnostic criteria: serum glucose >250 mg/dL, arterial pH <7.3, serum bicarbonate <18 mEq/L, and moderate ketonuria/ketonemia
Complete initial evaluation. Check capillary glucose and serum/urine ketones to confirm hyperglycemia and ketonemia/ketonuria.

IV fluids

Start 1.0 L of 0.9% NaCl/hr.

Severe/ shock

Administer of 9% NaCl at 1–1.5 L over the 1st hour, then, if serum corrected Na is high or normal, give 0.45% NaCl at 250–500 mL/hr depending on hydration state.

Hemodynamic monitoring and pressors

Mild dehydration

Evaluate corrected serum
Corrected Na = measured Na + 0.016 × (glucose − 100)

Corrected serum Na ≥135 mEq/L → 0.45% NaCl (250–500 mL/hr)

Corrected serum Na <135 mEq/L → 0.9% NaCl (250–500 mL/hr)

Insulin

Regular insulin 0.1 U/kg IV bolus 1–2 hours after starting IV fluids

. . . then 0.1 U/kg/hr IV

Uncomplicated DKA

Initiate rapid-acting insulin bolus 0.3 U/kg SC then 0.2 U/kg SC 1 hour later.

Continue rapid acting insulin 0.2 U/kg SC q2h.

If serum glucose does not fall by 50–70 mg/dL in 1st hour, double IV dose or double SC bolus dose.

Potassium

Urine output >50 mL/hr

K^+ <3.3 mEq/L → Give 20–30 mEq K^+/hr and hold insulin until K^+ >3.3 mEq/L.

K^+ ≥5.3 mEq/L → Recheck every 2 hours.

K^+ ≥3.3 and <5.3 mEq/L → Add 20–30 mEq K^+ to each liter of IV fluid. Goal is K^+ between 4 and 5 mEq/L.

Assess need for bicarbonate.

pH <6.9

$NaHCO_3$ (100 mEq) in 400 mL H_2O with 20 mEq KCl. Give over 1 hour. Give at 200 mL/hr over 2 hours.

Repeat IV $NaHCO_3$ dose q2h until pH ≥6.9 and check serum K^+.

Laboratory evaluation

Initial: CBC, CMP, ABG, serum ketones, Mg, phosphate, UA, EKG, HbA1c; if indicated, CXR, BCx, UCx, amylase, lipase

Serial: in addition to clinical monitoring, glucose, electrolytes, venous blood gas, urine output

Calculated: effective osmolality, anion gap, corrected Na^+, urine output

Frequency: q1h initially, then q2–4h once stable until DKA resolution

---

Serum glucose <200 mg/dL

- 5% dextrose with 0.45% NaCl at 150–250 mL/hr
- Decrease insulin to 0.05–0.1 U/kg/hr IV.
- If using SC insulin instead of IV, decrease rapid acting SC bolus to 0.1 U/kg SC q2h.

Keep serum glucose between 150 and 200 mg/dL until resolution of DKA.

Resolution of DKA

Glucose <200 mg/dL, serum bicarbonate ≥18 mEq/L, and venous pH >7.3

Feed and change from IV to SC insulin regimen (0.5–0.8 U/kg/day for insulin naïve patients). Keep IV insulin running for 1–2 hours after SC doses. Look for causes of DKA.

Emily Bouley, MD and Frank J. Domino, MD

Westerberg DP. Diabetic ketoacidosis: evaluation and treatment. *Am Fam Physician.* 2013;87(5):337–346.

DIARRHEA, CHRONIC

Common causes: infectious (bacterial, viral, parasitic), inflammatory bowel disease, malignancy, irritable bowel syndrome, medications, thyroid dysfunction, food additives, malabsorption syndromes (celiac disease, pancreatic insufficiency)

History: bloody stools, medications, recent antibiotics, recent travel, family history, floating stools, relationship to food intake, surgical history (cholecystectomy, bowel resections), sexual history, recent hospitalization

Medications

Yes

No

Acid-reducing agents (PPIs, H$_2$ blockers), antacids (containing magnesium), antibiotics, NSAIDs, colchicine, herbal medications, vitamin and mineral supplements, antineoplastic agents, antiretroviral agents, sorbitol, fructose abuse, chronic laxative abuse

Labs: stool studies (culture, *Clostridium difficile*, ova + parasites), TSH, glucose, fecal fat, celiac serologies (TTG IgA), HIV

Abnormal

Stool positive for ova and parasites—parasitic infections (e.g., *Cryptosporidium*, *Giardia*, Microsporidium)

Positive *C. difficile* antigen/toxin or PCR—*C. difficile* infection

Positive fecal fat—see "Malabsorption" algorithm

Hyperthyroidism Diabetes

Normal

Positive celiac serologies (TTG, IgA, antiendomysial antibodies)

Colonoscopy

Abnormal exam and/or abnormal biopsies

Normal exam and biopsies

Positive stool cultures—bacterial infection (*Escherichia coli, Salmonella, Shigella, Campylobacter*)

Upper endoscopy to confirm diagnosis of celiac disease

Inflammatory bowel diseases, malignancy, ischemic colitis, infectious colitis, microscopic colitis

Irritable bowel syndrome

Lakshmi Devi Nelson Lattimer, MD and Marie L. Borum, MD, EdD, MPH

Schiller LR. Definitions, pathophysiology, and evaluation of chronic diarrhoea. *Best Pract Res Clin Gastroenterol.* 2012;25(5):551–562.

DISCHARGE, VAGINAL

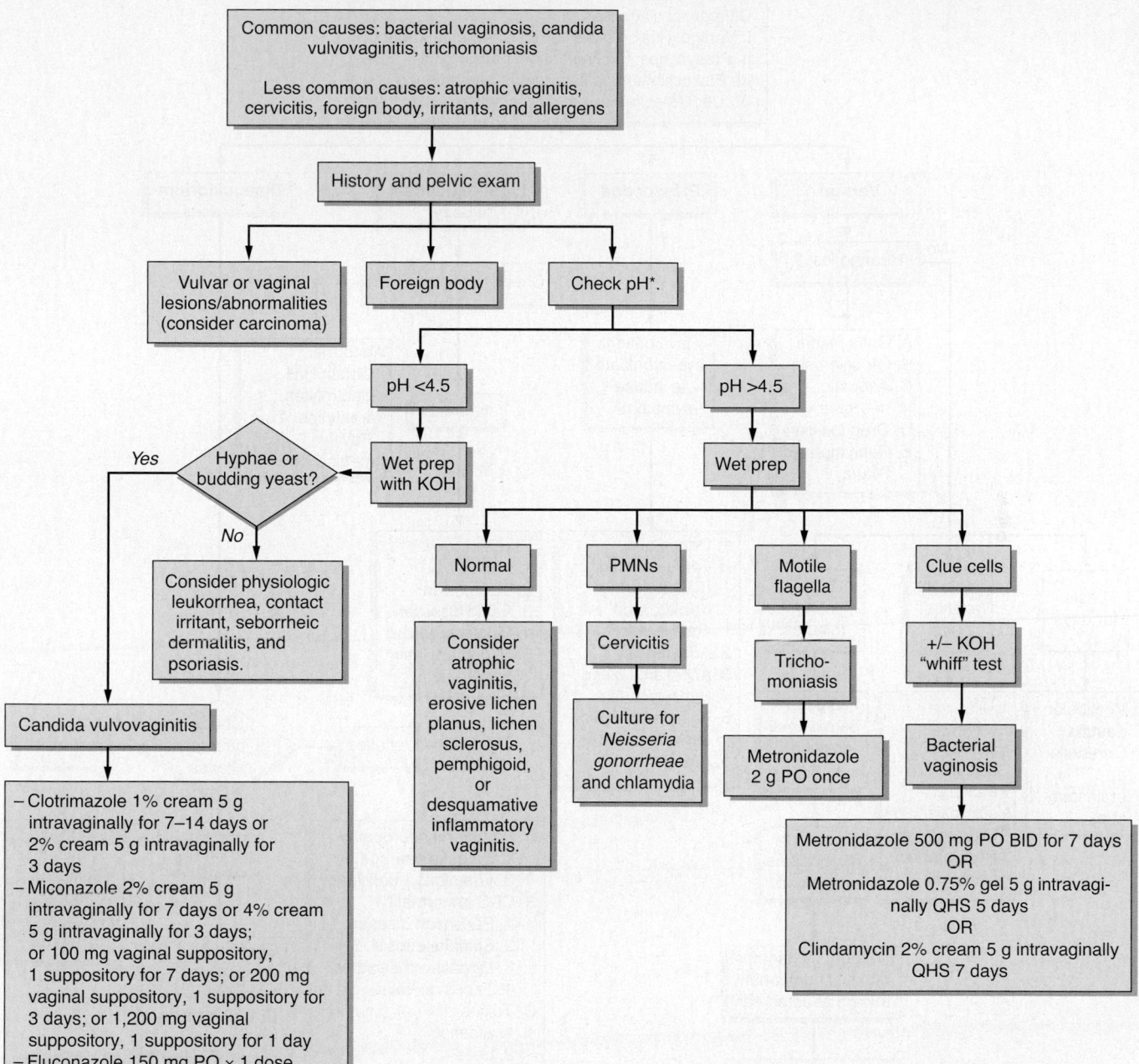

Common causes: bacterial vaginosis, candida vulvovaginitis, trichomoniasis

Less common causes: atrophic vaginitis, cervicitis, foreign body, irritants, and allergens

History and pelvic exam

- Vulvar or vaginal lesions/abnormalities (consider carcinoma)
- Foreign body
- Check pH*.

pH <4.5

pH >4.5

Hyphae or budding yeast?

Wet prep with KOH

Wet prep

Yes

No

Consider physiologic leukorrhea, contact irritant, seborrheic dermatitis, and psoriasis.

Normal

PMNs

Motile flagella

Clue cells

Consider atrophic vaginitis, erosive lichen planus, lichen sclerosus, pemphigoid, or desquamative inflammatory vaginitis.

Cervicitis

Tricho-moniasis

+/− KOH "whiff" test

Culture for *Neisseria gonorrheae* and chlamydia

Metronidazole 2 g PO once

Bacterial vaginosis

Candida vulvovaginitis

- Clotrimazole 1% cream 5 g intravaginally for 7–14 days or 2% cream 5 g intravaginally for 3 days
- Miconazole 2% cream 5 g intravaginally for 7 days or 4% cream 5 g intravaginally for 3 days; or 100 mg vaginal suppository, 1 suppository for 7 days; or 200 mg vaginal suppository, 1 suppository for 3 days; or 1,200 mg vaginal suppository, 1 suppository for 1 day
- Fluconazole 150 mg PO × 1 dose

Metronidazole 500 mg PO BID for 7 days
OR
Metronidazole 0.75% gel 5 g intravaginally QHS 5 days
OR
Clindamycin 2% cream 5 g intravaginally QHS 7 days

*pH is inaccurate if any blood is present and is less accurate at the extreme of ages.

Nicole Shields, MD

Hainer BL, Gibson MV. Vaginitis. *Am Fam Physician*. 2011;83(7):807–815.

DIZZINESS

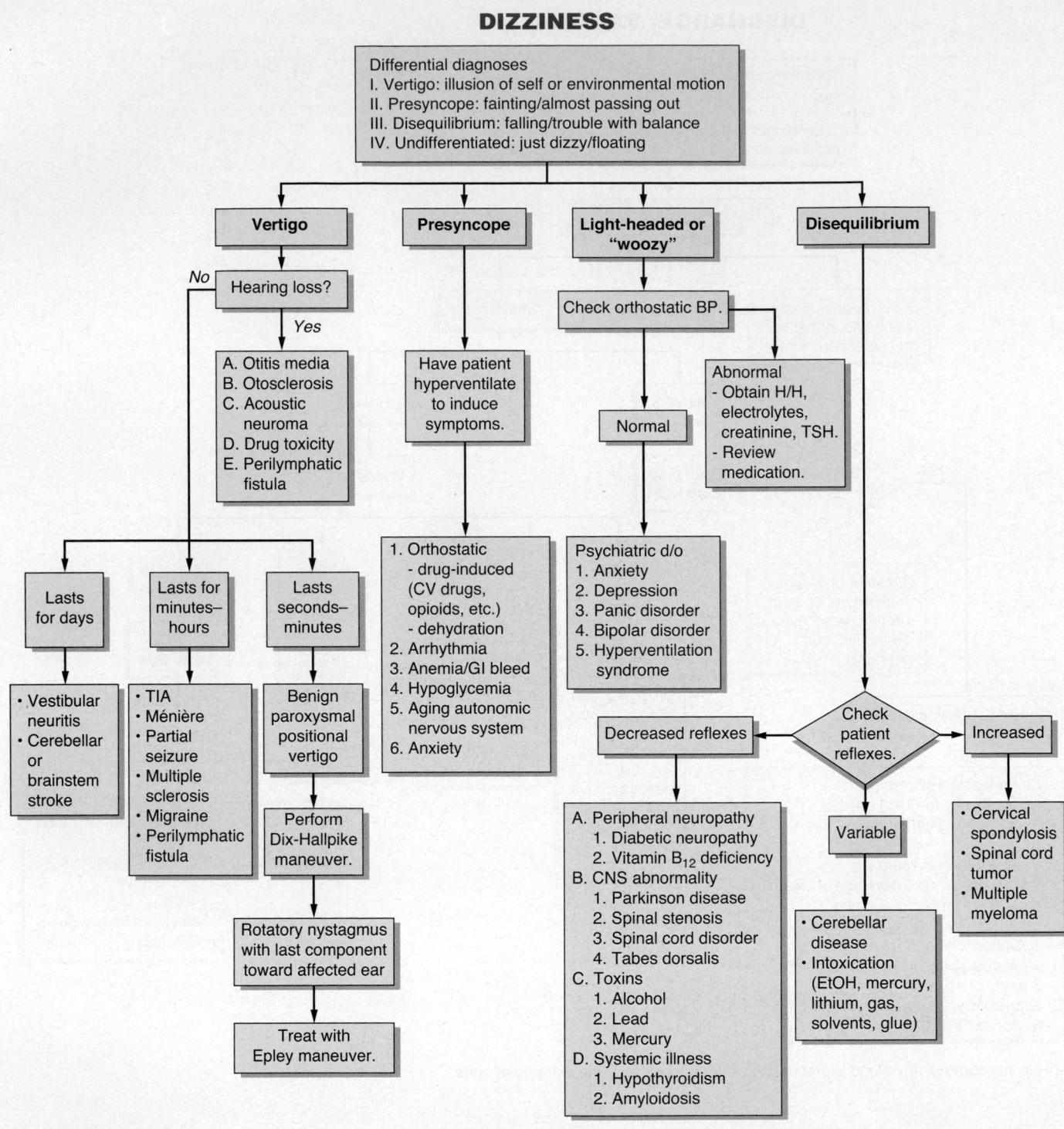

Differential diagnoses
I. Vertigo: illusion of self or environmental motion
II. Presyncope: fainting/almost passing out
III. Disequilibrium: falling/trouble with balance
IV. Undifferentiated: just dizzy/floating

Vertigo

No — **Hearing loss?**

Yes

A. Otitis media
B. Otosclerosis
C. Acoustic neuroma
D. Drug toxicity
E. Perilymphatic fistula

Lasts for days
- Vestibular neuritis
- Cerebellar or brainstem stroke

Lasts for minutes–hours
- TIA
- Ménière
- Partial seizure
- Multiple sclerosis
- Migraine
- Perilymphatic fistula

Lasts seconds–minutes
Benign paroxysmal positional vertigo

Perform Dix-Hallpike maneuver.

Rotatory nystagmus with last component toward affected ear

Treat with Epley maneuver.

Presyncope

Have patient hyperventilate to induce symptoms.

1. Orthostatic
   - drug-induced (CV drugs, opioids, etc.)
   - dehydration
2. Arrhythmia
3. Anemia/GI bleed
4. Hypoglycemia
5. Aging autonomic nervous system
6. Anxiety

Light-headed or "woozy"

Check orthostatic BP.

Normal

Abnormal
- Obtain H/H, electrolytes, creatinine, TSH.
- Review medication.

Psychiatric d/o
1. Anxiety
2. Depression
3. Panic disorder
4. Bipolar disorder
5. Hyperventilation syndrome

Disequilibrium

Check patient reflexes.

Decreased reflexes

A. Peripheral neuropathy
   1. Diabetic neuropathy
   2. Vitamin B_{12} deficiency
B. CNS abnormality
   1. Parkinson disease
   2. Spinal stenosis
   3. Spinal cord disorder
   4. Tabes dorsalis
C. Toxins
   1. Alcohol
   2. Lead
   3. Mercury
D. Systemic illness
   1. Hypothyroidism
   2. Amyloidosis

Variable
- Cerebellar disease
- Intoxication (EtOH, mercury, lithium, gas, solvents, glue)

Increased
- Cervical spondylosis
- Spinal cord tumor
- Multiple myeloma

Jamal Islam, MD, MS

Pigott DC, Rosko CI. The dizzy patient: an evidence-based diagnosis and treatment strategy. *Emerg Med Pract.* 2001;3(3):1–20.

DYSPEPSIA

Common causes: peptic ulcer (<10%), gastroesophageal cancer (<1%), gastroparesis, functional dyspepsia (>70%)

Main forms of functional dyspepsia: **epigastric pain syndrome** (intermittent pain/burning in epigastrium at least weekly) and **postprandial distress syndrome** (at least several episodes weekly of bothersome fullness after meals or early satiety). The two syndromes may both be present in the same patient.

GI red flags: onset at age 55 years or later (lower threshold in areas where gastric cancer is common, e.g., Southeast Asia); overt GI bleeding; dysphagia; persistent vomiting; unintentional weight loss; family hx gastric or esophageal cancer; palpable abdominal/epigastric mass; abnormal adenopathy; iron-deficiency anemia

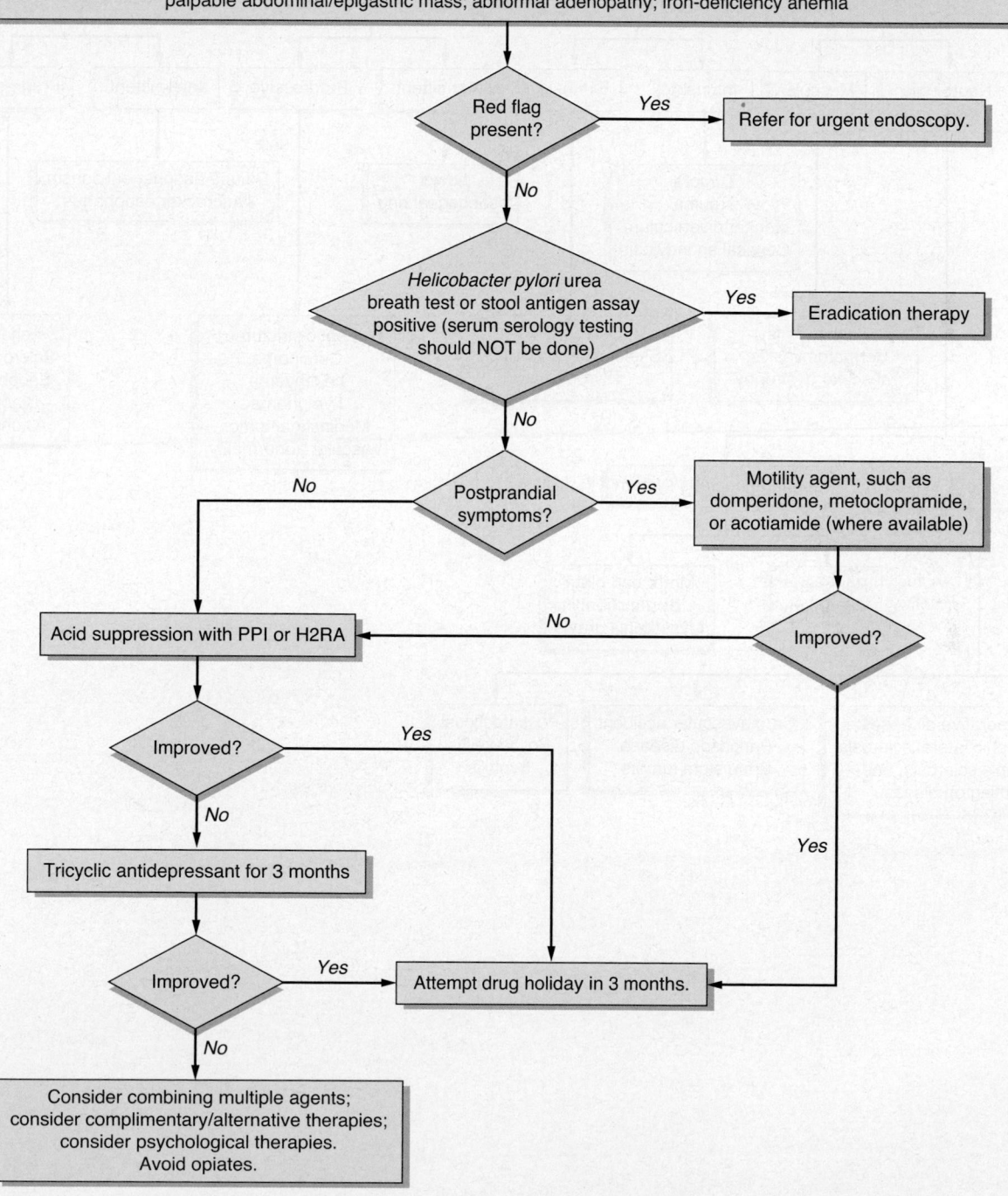

Jennifer L. Hamilton, MD, PhD, FAAFP

Talley NJ, Ford AC. Functional dyspepsia. *N Engl J Med.* 2015;373(19):1853–1863.

DYSPHAGIA

Shari Anthony, MD and Maria Cynthia S. Lopez, MD, FAAFP

Malagelada JR, Bazzoli F, Boeckxstaens G, et al. World gastroenterology organisation global guidelines: dysphagia—global guidelines and cascades update September 2014. *J Clin Gastroenterol*. 2015;49(5):370–378.

ERYTHROCYTOSIS

Common causes:
COPD, right-to-left cardiac shunt, obstructive sleep apnea, anabolic steroids/testosterone, renal cell CA, pheochromocytoma, uterine leiomyoma, high-affinity Hgb, polycythemia vera

↓

Definition:
Increase in red cell mass
Men with Hgb >18.5 or Hct >52%
Women with Hgb >16.5 or Hct >48%

↓

Oxygen saturation ≥92%

— No → **Workup of cardiopulmonary causes of erythrocytosis:** for example, COPD, right-to-left cardiac shunt, sleep apnea

Yes ↓

EPO level and JAK2 V617F PCR

EPO low and *JAK2* positive → **Polycythemia vera**

EPO low and *JAK2* negative → ***JAK2* exon 12: assessment**
⊕ → Polycythemia vera
⊖ → **Testing bone marrow biopsy, *BCR-ABL*, calreticulin PCR**

EPO elevated/normal and *JAK2* negative → **Secondary erythrocytosis**

↓

Causes and testing
Congenital
High oxygen affinity Hgb: P50 evaluation
Von Hippel-Lindau disease: genetic testing

Acquired
Renal cell carcinoma: CT scan
Pheochromocytoma: CT scan
Uterine leiomyoma: ultrasound
Use of androgen preparations: blood test

Manisha J. Patel, MD and Tarun Kewalramani, MD

Patnaik MM, Tefferi A. The complete evaluation of erythrocytosis: congenital and acquired. *Leukemia.* 2009;23(5):834–844.

FATIGUE

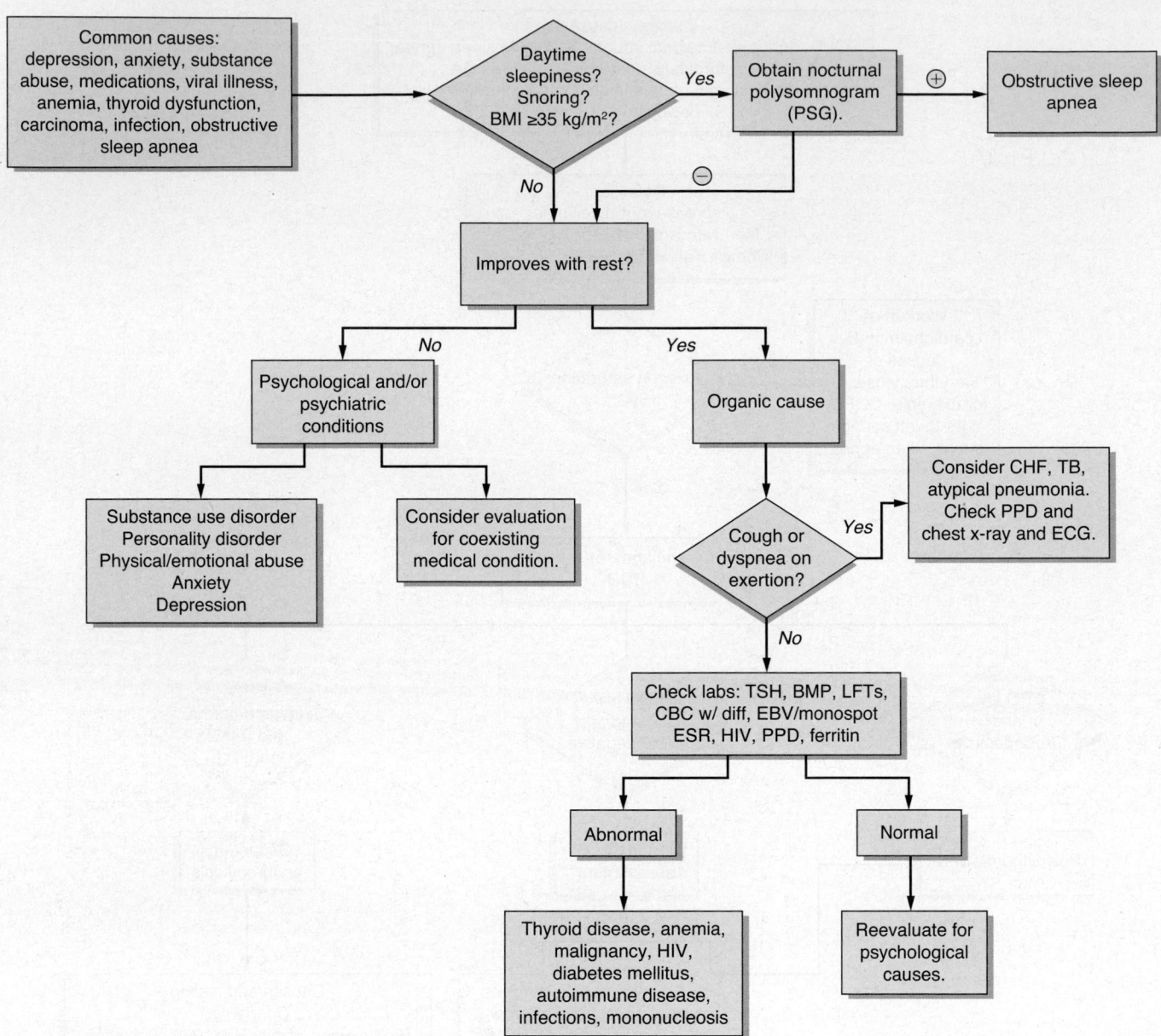

Paavan Mehta, MD and Frank J. Domino, MD

Rosenthal TC, Majeroni BA, Pretorius R, et al. Fatigue: an overview. *Am Fam Physician.* 2008;78(10):1173–1179.

FEVER IN THE FIRST 3 MONTHS OF LIFE

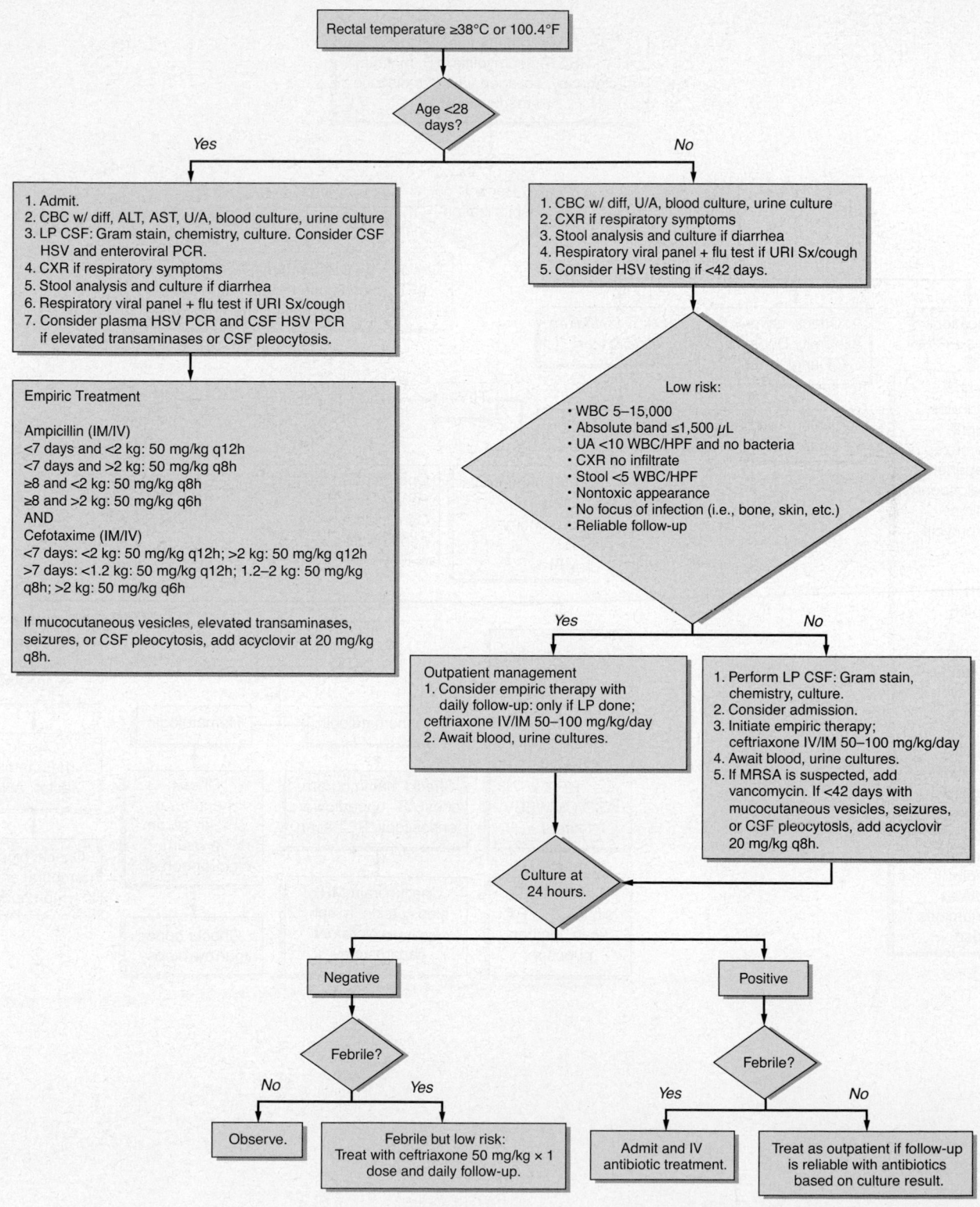

Rectal temperature ≥38°C or 100.4°F

Age <28 days?

Yes

1. Admit.
2. CBC w/ diff, ALT, AST, U/A, blood culture, urine culture
3. LP CSF: Gram stain, chemistry, culture. Consider CSF HSV and enteroviral PCR.
4. CXR if respiratory symptoms
5. Stool analysis and culture if diarrhea
6. Respiratory viral panel + flu test if URI Sx/cough
7. Consider plasma HSV PCR and CSF HSV PCR if elevated transaminases or CSF pleocytosis.

Empiric Treatment

Ampicillin (IM/IV)
<7 days and <2 kg: 50 mg/kg q12h
<7 days and >2 kg: 50 mg/kg q8h
≥8 and <2 kg: 50 mg/kg q8h
≥8 and >2 kg: 50 mg/kg q6h
AND
Cefotaxime (IM/IV)
<7 days: <2 kg: 50 mg/kg q12h; >2 kg: 50 mg/kg q12h
>7 days: <1.2 kg: 50 mg/kg q12h; 1.2–2 kg: 50 mg/kg q8h; >2 kg: 50 mg/kg q6h

If mucocutaneous vesicles, elevated transaminases, seizures, or CSF pleocytosis, add acyclovir at 20 mg/kg q8h.

No

1. CBC w/ diff, U/A, blood culture, urine culture
2. CXR if respiratory symptoms
3. Stool analysis and culture if diarrhea
4. Respiratory viral panel + flu test if URI Sx/cough
5. Consider HSV testing if <42 days.

Low risk:
- WBC 5–15,000
- Absolute band ≤1,500 μL
- UA <10 WBC/HPF and no bacteria
- CXR no infiltrate
- Stool <5 WBC/HPF
- Nontoxic appearance
- No focus of infection (i.e., bone, skin, etc.)
- Reliable follow-up

Yes

Outpatient management
1. Consider empiric therapy with daily follow-up: only if LP done; ceftriaxone IV/IM 50–100 mg/kg/day
2. Await blood, urine cultures.

No

1. Perform LP CSF: Gram stain, chemistry, culture.
2. Consider admission.
3. Initiate empiric therapy; ceftriaxone IV/IM 50–100 mg/kg/day
4. Await blood, urine cultures.
5. If MRSA is suspected, add vancomycin. If <42 days with mucocutaneous vesicles, seizures, or CSF pleocytosis, add acyclovir 20 mg/kg q8h.

Culture at 24 hours.

Negative

Febrile?

No → Observe.

Yes → Febrile but low risk: Treat with ceftriaxone 50 mg/kg × 1 dose and daily follow-up.

Positive

Febrile?

Yes → Admit and IV antibiotic treatment.

No → Treat as outpatient if follow-up is reliable with antibiotics based on culture result.

Robyn Wing, MD and William Jerry Durbin, MD

Byington CL, Reynolds CC, Korgenski K, et al. Costs and infant outcomes after implementation of a care process model for febrile infants. *Pediatrics.* 2012;130(1):e16–e24.

FEVER OF UNKNOWN ORIGIN

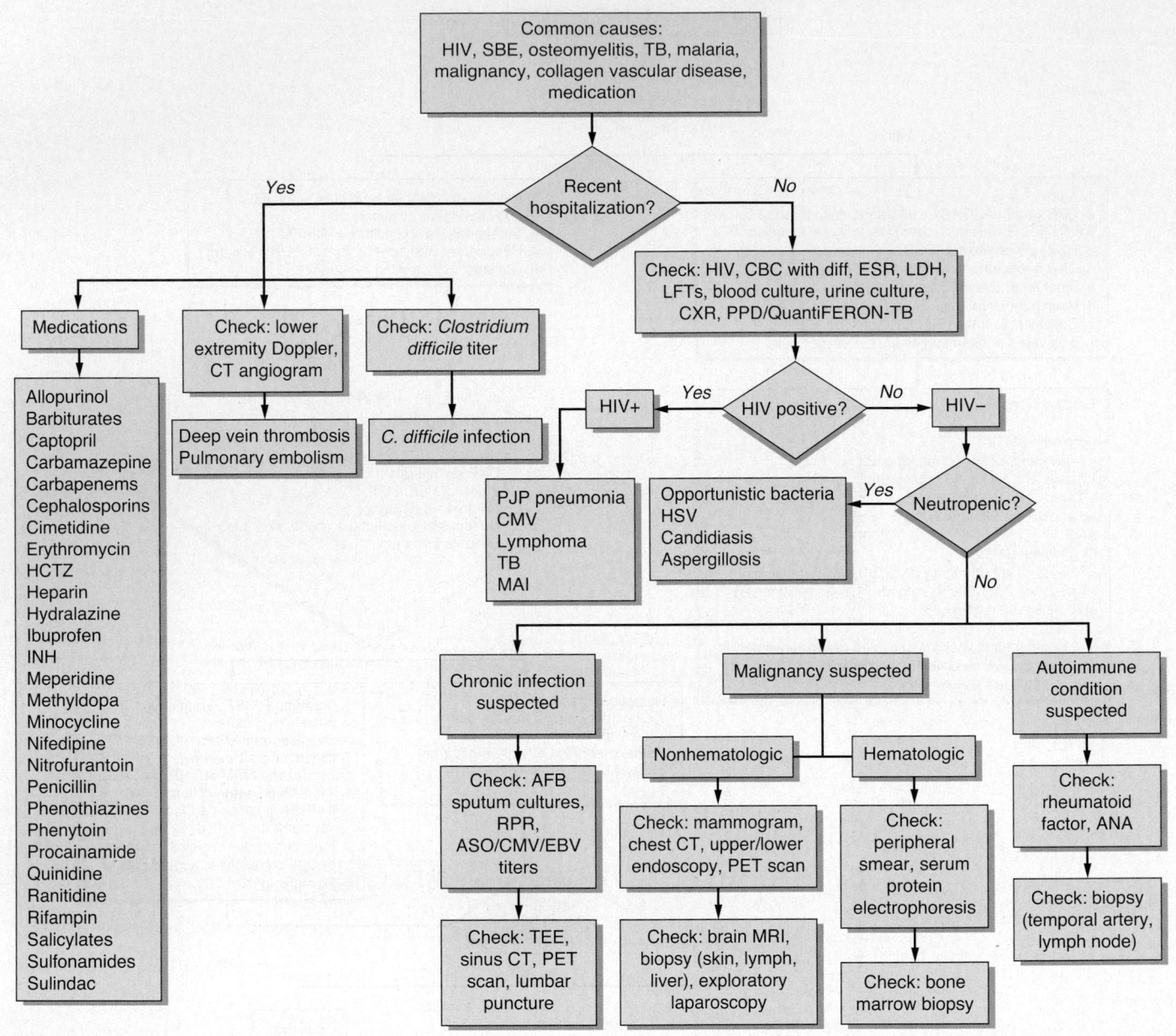

Rachelle E. Toman, MD, PhD, Megan Hollis, MD, and Angela Kuznia, MD, MPH

Hersch EC, Oh RC. Prolonged febrile illness and fever of unknown origin in adults. *Am Fam Physician.* 2014;90(2):91–96.

GAIT DISTURBANCE

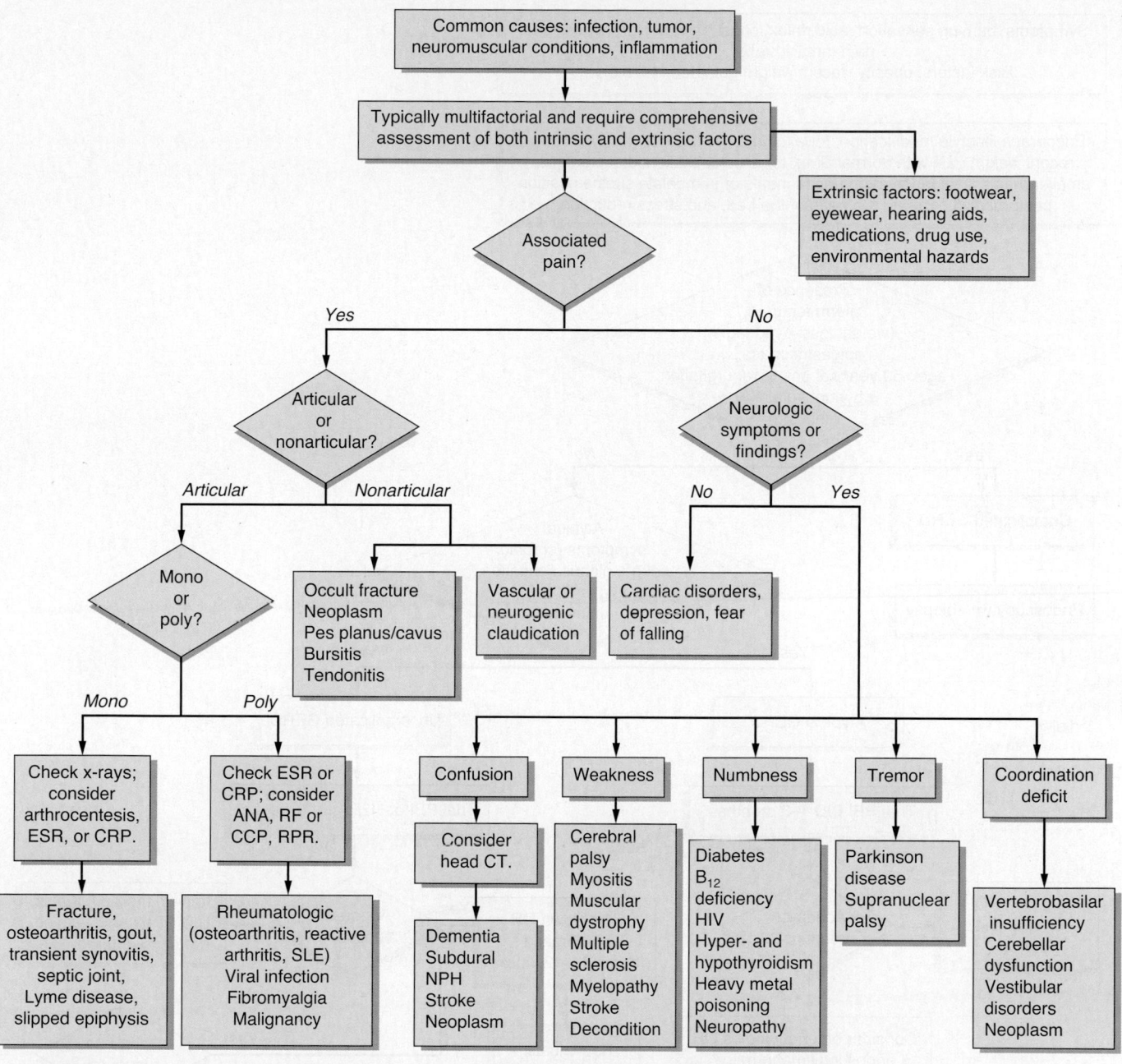

Common causes: infection, tumor, neuromuscular conditions, inflammation

Typically multifactorial and require comprehensive assessment of both intrinsic and extrinsic factors

Extrinsic factors: footwear, eyewear, hearing aids, medications, drug use, environmental hazards

Associated pain?

Yes

Articular or nonarticular?

Articular

Mono or poly?

Nonarticular

Occult fracture
Neoplasm
Pes planus/cavus
Bursitis
Tendonitis

Vascular or neurogenic claudication

No

Neurologic symptoms or findings?

No

Cardiac disorders, depression, fear of falling

Yes

Mono

Check x-rays; consider arthrocentesis, ESR, or CRP.

Poly

Check ESR or CRP; consider ANA, RF or CCP, RPR.

Confusion

Consider head CT.

Weakness

Numbness

Tremor

Coordination deficit

Fracture, osteoarthritis, gout, transient synovitis, septic joint, Lyme disease, slipped epiphysis

Rheumatologic (osteoarthritis, reactive arthritis, SLE)
Viral infection
Fibromyalgia
Malignancy

Dementia
Subdural
NPH
Stroke
Neoplasm

Cerebral palsy
Myositis
Muscular dystrophy
Multiple sclerosis
Myelopathy
Stroke
Decondition

Diabetes
B_{12} deficiency
HIV
Hyper- and hypothyroidism
Heavy metal poisoning
Neuropathy

Parkinson disease
Supranuclear palsy

Vertebrobasilar insufficiency
Cerebellar dysfunction
Vestibular disorders
Neoplasm

David T. O'Gurek, MD, FAAFP

Salzman B. Gait and balance disorders in older adults. *Am Fam Physician*. 2010;82(1):61–68.

GASTROESOPHAGEAL REFLUX DISEASE (GERD), DIAGNOSIS AND TREATMENT

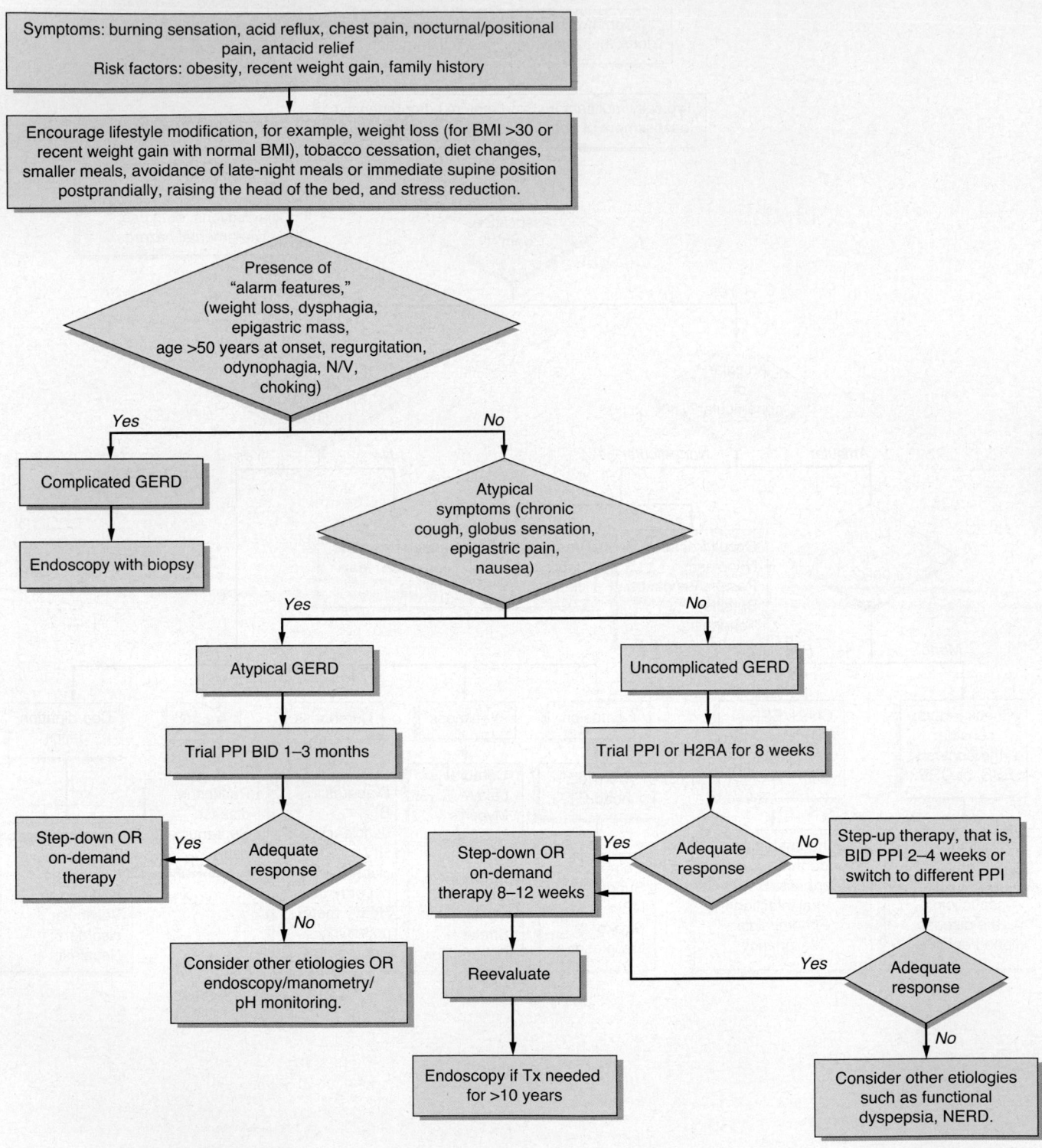

Aniruddh Anil Patel, MD and Thomas L. Abell, MD

Katz PO, Gerson LB, Vela MF. Guidelines for the diagnosis and management of gastroesophageal reflux disease. *Am J Gastroenterol.* 2013;108(3):308–328.

GENITAL ULCERS

Common causes: herpes simplex, syphilis, chancroid, granuloma inguinale

↓

Check labs: RPR, HIV, GC, and *Chlamydia* culture or DNA probe.

↓

Lesions painful?

Yes / **No**

Vesicles on erythematous base
↓
Unroof new vesicle to culture fluid.
↓
Herpes simplex

Tender papule erodes into a deep, painful ulcer with inguinal adenopathy, gray exudate with foul odor
↓
Gram stain shows gram-negative rods, "school of fish" appearance; culture difficult
↓
Chancroid

Evolves from pinpoint ulcer to a large sore, yellowish base; associated with recurrent oral ulcers
↓
Behçet disease

Indurated, smooth firm borders, usually singular unless HIV+
↓
RPR+, may confirm with FTA-ABS
↓
Syphilis

Starts as red nodule, spreads aggressively into an ulcer of rolled edges, resembling granulation
↓
Punch biopsy at ulcer edge
↓
Granuloma inguinale

Small, shallow genital or rectal papule or ulcer, no induration
↓
Chlamydia trachomatis L1, L2, or L3 culture
↓
Lymphogranuloma venereum

Chidinma Osineme, MD and Midhuna William, MD

Roett MA, Mayor MT, Uduhiri KA. Diagnosis and management of genital ulcers. *Am Fam Physician*. 2012:85(3):254–262.

GYNECOMASTIA

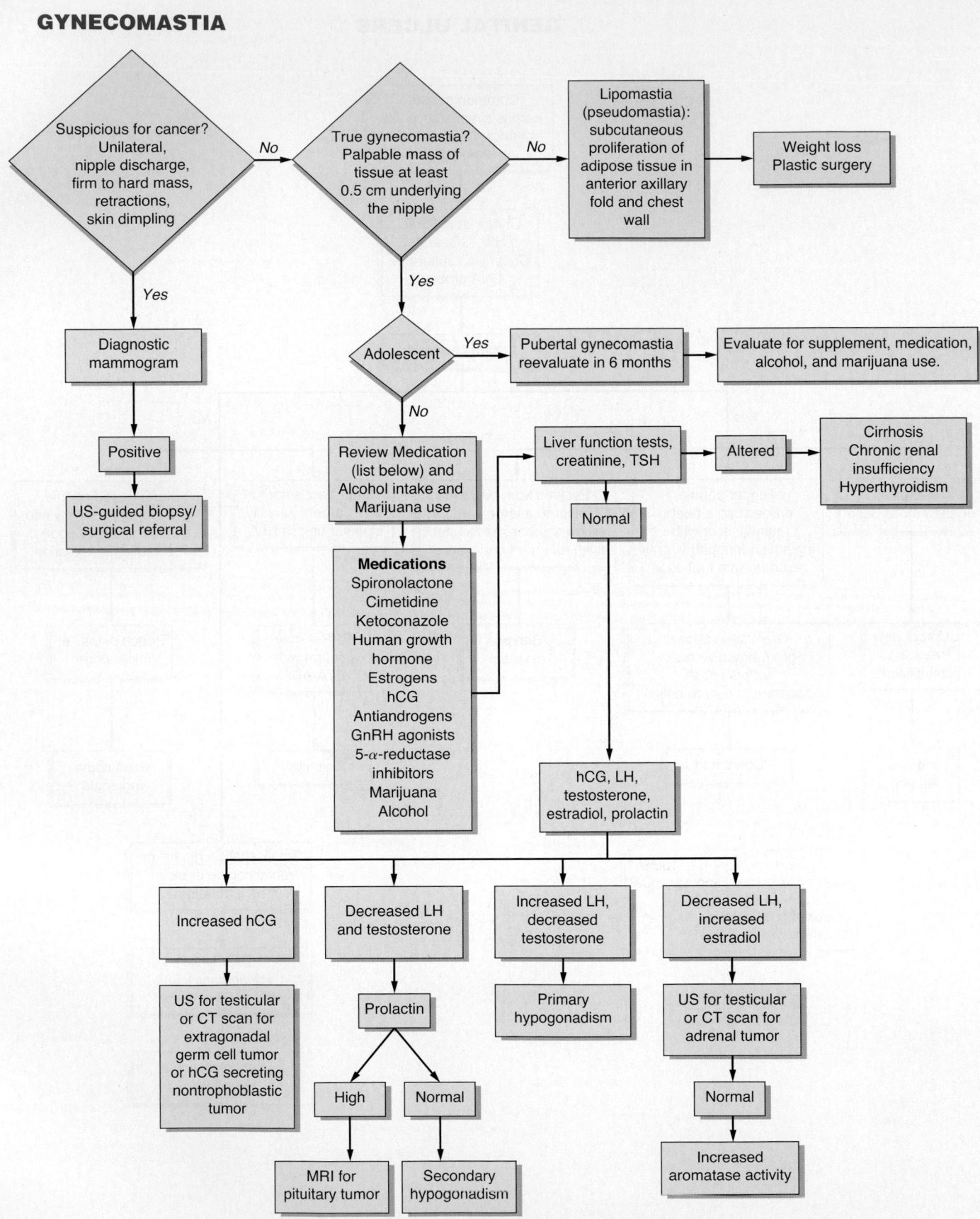

Katie L. Westerfield, DO and David C. Bury, DO

Narula HS, Carlson HE. Gynaecomastia—pathophysiology, diagnosis and treatment. *Nat Rev Endocrinol.* 2014;10(11):684–698.

HEADACHE, CHRONIC

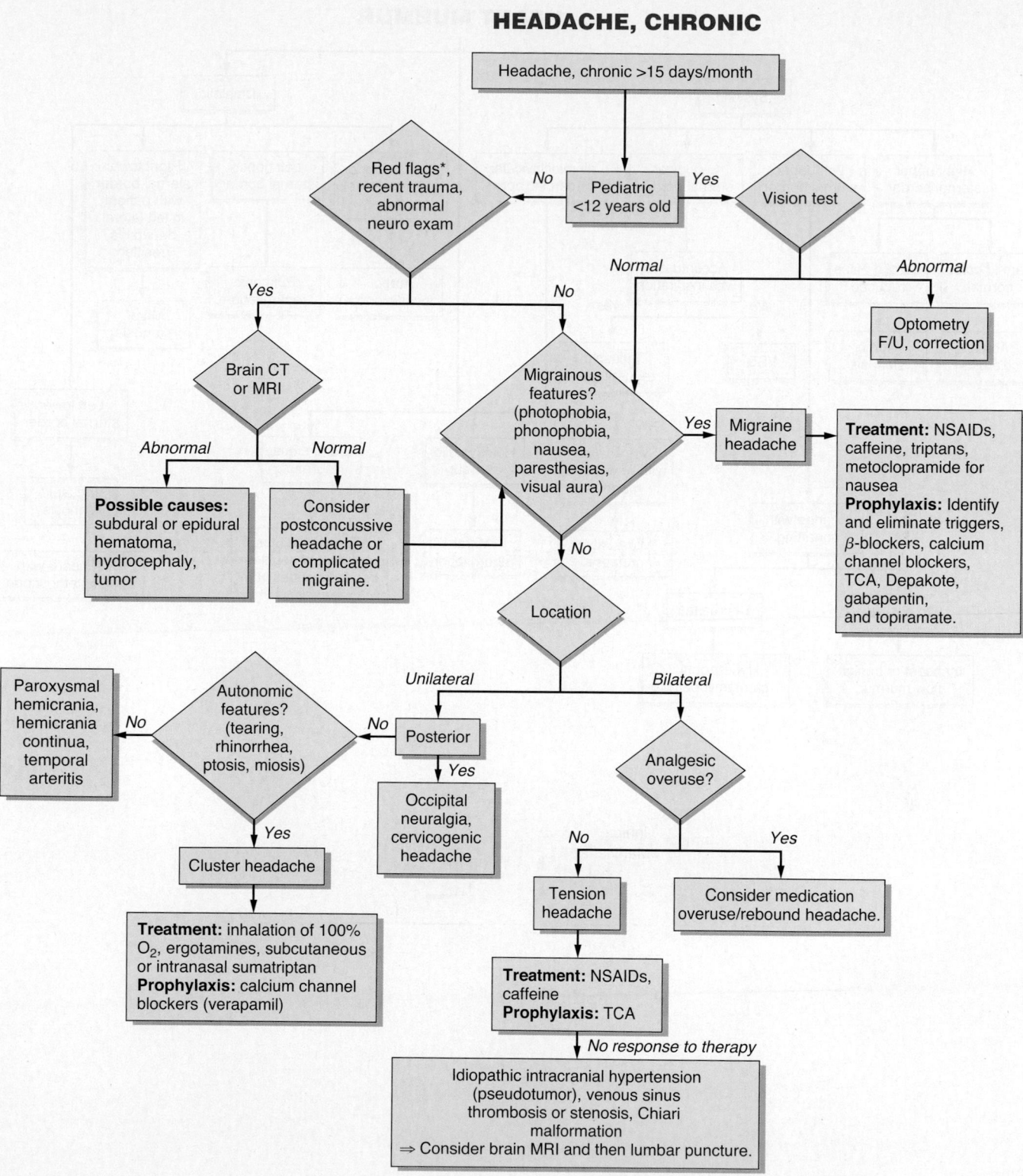

*Red flags include onset of headache after age 50 years, altered mental status (including confusion, personality changes), papilledema, report of "worst headache of my life," and focal neurologic deficits such as weakness or ataxia.

Amy Okpaku, DO

Yancey JR, Sheridan R, Koren KG. Chronic daily headache: diagnosis and management. *Am Fam Physician*. 2014;89(8):642–648.

HEART MURMUR

Michael Argyle, DO and Brett Johnson, DO

Bonow RO, Carabello BA, Chatterjee K, et al. 2008 Focused update incorporated into the ACC/AHA 2006 guidelines for the management of patients with valvular heart disease: a report of the American College of Cardiology/American Heart Association Task Force on Practice Guidelines (writing committee to revise the 1998 Guidelines for the Management of Patients With Valvular Heart Disease): endorsed by the Society of Cardiovascular Anesthesiologists, Society for Cardiovascular Angiography and Interventions, and Society of Thoracic Surgeons. *Circulation.* 2008;118(15):e523–e661.

HEEL PAIN

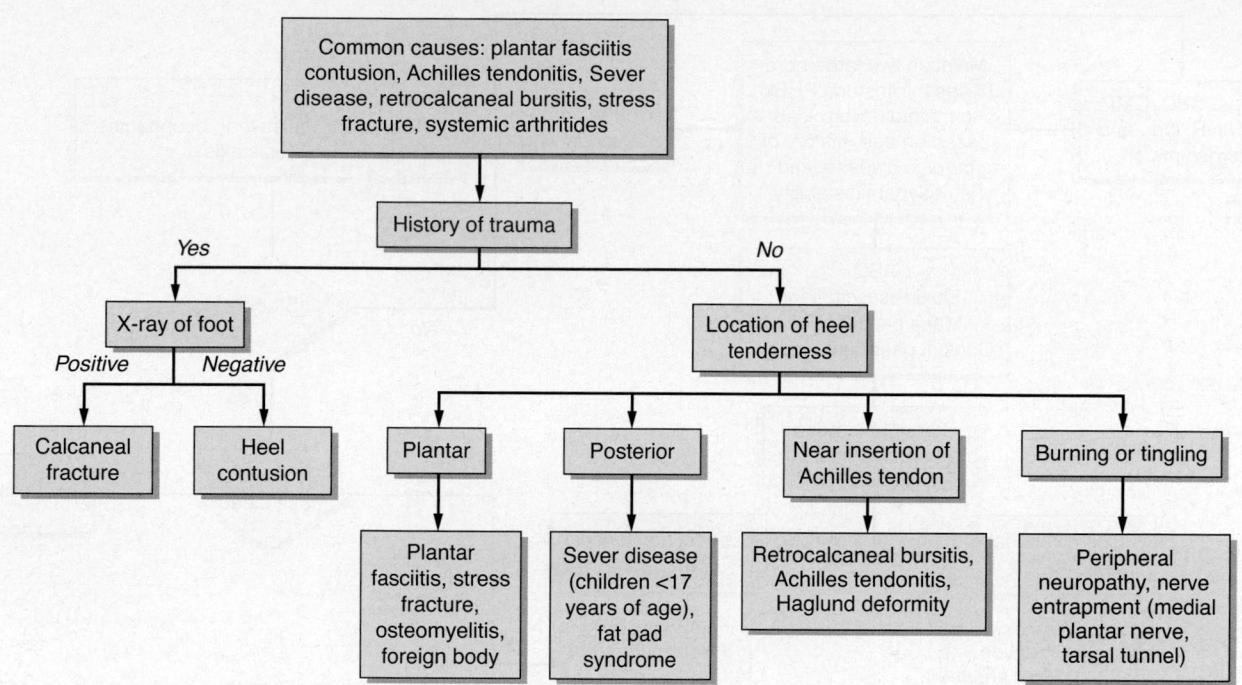

Common causes: plantar fasciitis contusion, Achilles tendonitis, Sever disease, retrocalcaneal bursitis, stress fracture, systemic arthritides

History of trauma

Yes — X-ray of foot
- *Positive* → Calcaneal fracture
- *Negative* → Heel contusion

No — Location of heel tenderness
- Plantar → Plantar fasciitis, stress fracture, osteomyelitis, foreign body
- Posterior → Sever disease (children <17 years of age), fat pad syndrome
- Near insertion of Achilles tendon → Retrocalcaneal bursitis, Achilles tendonitis, Haglund deformity
- Burning or tingling → Peripheral neuropathy, nerve entrapment (medial plantar nerve, tarsal tunnel)

Alec DeCastro, MD

Tu P, Bytomski JR. Diagnosis of heel pain. *Am Fam Physician.* 2011;84(8):909–916.

HEMATEMESIS (BLEEDING, UPPER GASTROINTESTINAL)

Labs: CBC, CMP, PT/INR, type and cross-match

Maintain two large bore IV lines; transfuse PRBC to maintain Hbg >7–8 based on age, history of cardiac disease, and hemodynamic stability.

Correct any coagulopathy.

Common causes: PUD, Mallory-Weiss tear, esophagitis, gastritis, varices, epistaxis

Stable — No / Yes

ABC
Fluid resuscitation
Make patient NPO
Consult gastroenterology

Start intravenous proton pump inhibitor.

Recent nose bleed — No / Yes → Epistaxis

Suspect variceal hemorrhage.

Suspect nonvariceal hemorrhage.

Start IV octreotide drip (3–5 days) and broad-spectrum antibiotics (5–7 days).

Perform upper endoscopy.

Perform urgent upper endoscopy with variceal ligation banding.

No source identified

Arteriovenous malformation, Mallory-Weiss tear, Dieulafoy ulcer

Erosive esophagitis

Peptic ulcer bleeding

Has the bleeding stopped?

Consider push enteroscopy, capsule endoscopy, colonoscopy, arteriography with embolization, induced bleed study, tagged red blood cell study.

Endoscopic therapy with epinephrine, thermocoagulation, or clipping

Continue proton pump inhibitor therapy.

Endoscopic therapy with epinephrine, thermocoagulation, or clips

Yes / No

Start prophylactic nonselective β-blocker.

Sengstaken-Blakemore tube

Has the bleeding stopped?

Yes / No

Repeat endoscopy in 1–2 weeks and reband as needed.

Emergent transjugular intrahepatic portosystemic shunt or surgery

Continue proton pump inhibitor therapy; eradicate *Helicobacter pylori* infection if present.

Reattempt upper endoscopy; otherwise, consider arteriography with embolization, or surgery.

Faruq Pradhan, MBBCh, Lisa N. Jarnagin, MBBCh, BAO, and Stephen C. Fabry, MD

Wilkins T, Khan N, Nabh A, et al. Diagnosis and management of upper gastrointestinal bleeding. *Am Fam Physician*. 2012;85(5):469–479.

HEMATURIA

Risk factors for urinary tract malignancy:
Age >35 years
Male sex
Analgesic abuse
Exposure to chemicals/dyes
Exposure to alkylating chemotherapeutic agents
Past or current smoking
Chronic UTI
Pelvic irradiation
Gross hematuria

Common causes: cystitis, urolithiasis, pyelonephritis, tumor, prostatitis

H&P Urinalysis Centrifuge → Supernatant red → Dipstick supernatant

Dipstick supernatant → Heme-negative → Beeturia Phenazopyridine Porphyria

Dipstick supernatant → Heme-positive → Plasma color → Clear → Myoglobinuria

Plasma color → Red → Hemoglobinuria

Sediment red → Hematuria → Microscopic urinalysis

Microscopic urinalysis → <3 RBC/HPF → Repeat UA 3 times at 6-week intervals.
Repeat UA 3 times at 6-week intervals → Negative → No further workup
Repeat UA 3 times at 6-week intervals → Positive → >3 RBC/HPF

Microscopic urinalysis → >3 RBC/HPF → Assess for UTI, vigorous exercise, menstruation, recent urologic procedure.

Repeat UA 6 weeks after Rx and discontinuation of contributing factor.
Repeat UA 6 weeks after Rx and discontinuation of contributing factor → Negative → No further workup
Repeat UA 6 weeks after Rx and discontinuation of contributing factor → Positive → Dysmorphic RBCs' proteinuria >200 mg/g

Dysmorphic RBCs' proteinuria >200 mg/g → Negative → Assess for risk factors for malignancy, renal insufficiency.
Dysmorphic RBCs' proteinuria >200 mg/g → Positive → Nephrology referral

Assess for risk factors for malignancy, renal insufficiency.
→ Low risk for malignancy, renal insufficiency
→ High risk for malignancy, normal renal functions

Low risk for malignancy, renal insufficiency → US/noncontrast CT and urology referral

High risk for malignancy, normal renal functions → CT with IV contrast and urology referral

US/noncontrast CT and urology referral → Cytoscopy ← CT with IV contrast and urology referral

Cytoscopy → Negative → Annual UA for 2 years
Cytoscopy → Positive → Treat

Annual UA for 2 years → Negative → Release from care.
Annual UA for 2 years → Positive → Repeat anatomic evaluation in 3–5 years.

Nephrology referral → Complements → Low
Nephrology referral → Complements → Normal

Complements → Low → Renal → Poststreptococcal GN MPGN
Complements → Low → Systemic diseases → SLE, cryoglobulinemia, bacterial endocarditis, shunt nephritis

Complements → Normal → Systemic diseases → PAN, GPA, HSP, GP, hypersensitivity vasculitis
Complements → Normal → Renal → IgA, idiopathic RPGN: anti-GBM, pauci-immune

Krishna Manda, MD, MRCP

Sharp VJ, Barnes KT, Erickson BA. Assessment of asymptomatic microscopic hematuria in adults. *Am Fam Physician*. 2013;88(11):747–754.

HEPATOMEGALY

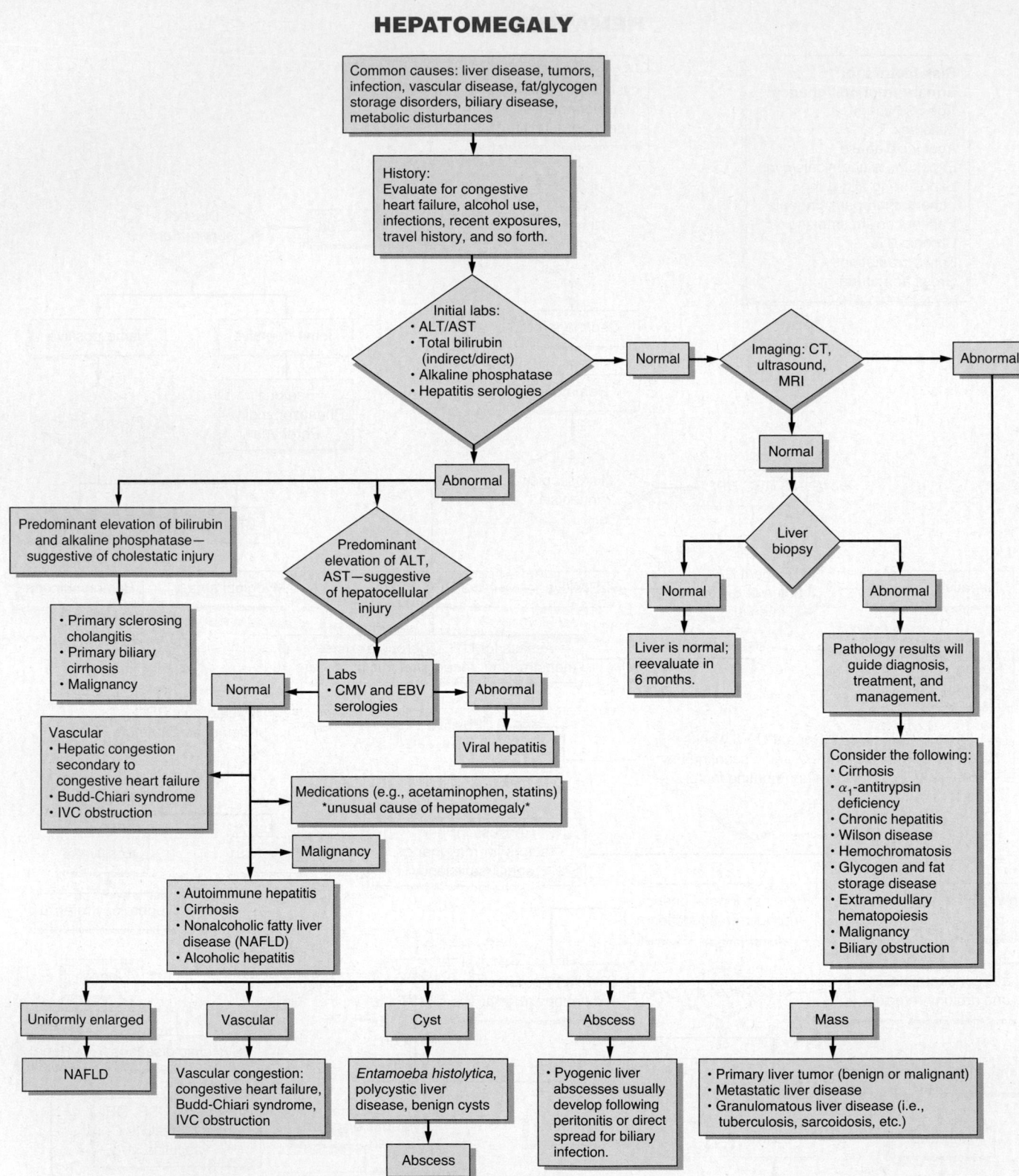

Common causes: liver disease, tumors, infection, vascular disease, fat/glycogen storage disorders, biliary disease, metabolic disturbances

History:
Evaluate for congestive heart failure, alcohol use, infections, recent exposures, travel history, and so forth.

Initial labs:
• ALT/AST
• Total bilirubin (indirect/direct)
• Alkaline phosphatase
• Hepatitis serologies

Normal → Imaging: CT, ultrasound, MRI → Abnormal

Normal → Liver biopsy → Abnormal

Normal → Liver is normal; reevaluate in 6 months.

Abnormal → Pathology results will guide diagnosis, treatment, and management.

Consider the following:
• Cirrhosis
• α_1-antitrypsin deficiency
• Chronic hepatitis
• Wilson disease
• Hemochromatosis
• Glycogen and fat storage disease
• Extramedullary hematopoiesis
• Malignancy
• Biliary obstruction

Abnormal

Predominant elevation of bilirubin and alkaline phosphatase—suggestive of cholestatic injury
• Primary sclerosing cholangitis
• Primary biliary cirrhosis
• Malignancy

Predominant elevation of ALT, AST—suggestive of hepatocellular injury

Labs
• CMV and EBV serologies

Normal / Abnormal → Viral hepatitis

Vascular
• Hepatic congestion secondary to congestive heart failure
• Budd-Chiari syndrome
• IVC obstruction

Medications (e.g., acetaminophen, statins) *unusual cause of hepatomegaly*

Malignancy

• Autoimmune hepatitis
• Cirrhosis
• Nonalcoholic fatty liver disease (NAFLD)
• Alcoholic hepatitis

Uniformly enlarged → NAFLD

Vascular → Vascular congestion: congestive heart failure, Budd-Chiari syndrome, IVC obstruction

Cyst → *Entamoeba histolytica*, polycystic liver disease, benign cysts → Abscess

Abscess → • Pyogenic liver abscesses usually develop following peritonitis or direct spread for biliary infection.

Mass → • Primary liver tumor (benign or malignant)
• Metastatic liver disease
• Granulomatous liver disease (i.e., tuberculosis, sarcoidosis, etc.)

Matthew Chandler, MD and Marie L. Borum, MD, EdD, MPH

Starr SP, Raines D. Cirrhosis: diagnosis, management, and prevention. *Am Fam Physician*. 2011;84(12):1353–1359.

HYPERCALCEMIA

Common causes: hyperparathyroidism, malignancy, hyperthyroidism, vitamin D toxicity, milk-alkali syndrome, medications

Obtain ionized calcium or total calcium: corrected Ca = total Ca + 0.8 × (4.5 − albumin level).

Clinical suspicion
Signs and symptoms of hypercalcemia:
GI: nausea, vomiting, anorexia, and constipation
Neurologic: lethargic, hypotonic, confused, or comatose
Renal: polyuria, nephrolithiasis, and dehydration
Cardiac: shortened heart rate–corrected QT intervals, broadened T waves, and 1st-degree atrioventricular block

Review medications:
increased calcium intake, vitamin A intoxication, vitamin D overdose, thiazides, milk-alkali syndrome, theophylline, lithium

Check parathyroid hormone.

Elevated PTH

Consider ectopic secretions of PTH (i.e., ovarian carcinoma).

Measure urinary calcium.

Elevated

Low

Consider primary hyperparathyroidism.

Consider surgery.

Consider familial hypocalciuric hypercalcemia (a decreased sensitivity of receptors requiring higher calcium levels to suppress PTH secretions).

Obtain detailed family hx.

Normal PTH or low

PTH-related protein (PTHrp) and 25-OH vitamin D and 1,25 OH vitamin D

Elevated PTHrp

Elevated 1,25 OH vitamin D

Normal or low 1,25 OH vitamin D

Consider malignancy: humoral hypercalcemia of malignancy (i.e., squamous cell carcinomas) OR local osteolytic hypercalcemia (i.e., multiple myeloma, bone metastases)

Consider endogenous production from granulomatous disease or lymphoproliferative disorders (i.e., TB and sarcoidosis).

Consider thyrotoxicosis, prolonged immobilization.

Elevated 25-OH vitamin D

Consider supplemental vitamin D overdose.

Review medications.

Deborah A. Lardner, DO, DTM&H and Michael Passafaro, DO, DTM&H, FACEP, FACOEP

Kacprowicz RF, Lloyd JD. Electrolyte complications of malignancy. *Emerg Med Clin North Am.* 2009;27(2):257–269.

HYPERKALEMIA

K >5.5 mEq/L

Common causes: renal failure, hyperglycemia, specimen delay and hemolysis, renal insufficiency, acidosis, rhabdomyolysis, insulin deficiency, adrenal insufficiency, medications, massive blood transfusions, tumor lysis, ischemic bowel

Weakness, nausea, paresthesias, palpitations, ileus, flaccid paralysis

ECG changes: peaked T waves, ↑ PR interval, ↑ QRS width, sine wave pattern, PEA

No

Repeat test.

Yes

Normal

Abnormal

Treat as acute hyperkalemia.

Pseudohyperkalemia: IVF with K, hemolyzed sample

Check medications.

No suspicious medications

ACEI, ARBs, β-blockers, NSAIDs, penicillin K, TMP-SMX, digitalis, K-sparing diuretics, heparin, cyclosporine, tacrolimus, pentamidine, succinylcholine

ABGs, GFR, Cr, BUN, glucose, electrolytes, digoxin levels, CPK, urine K+

Discontinue medication or adjust dose.

Urine K >30 mEq/L: transcellular shift

Urine K <30 mEq/L: impaired renal excretion

Acidosis
Rhabdomyolysis
Hyperglycemia
Burns

Renal insufficiency
Adrenal insufficiency
Hyporeninemic hypoaldosteronism

Matthew C. Kelly, MD and Michelle E. Szczepanik, MD

Kovesdy CP. Management of hyperkalemia: an update for the internist. *Am J Med.* 2015;128(12):1281–1287.

HYPERLIPIDEMIA

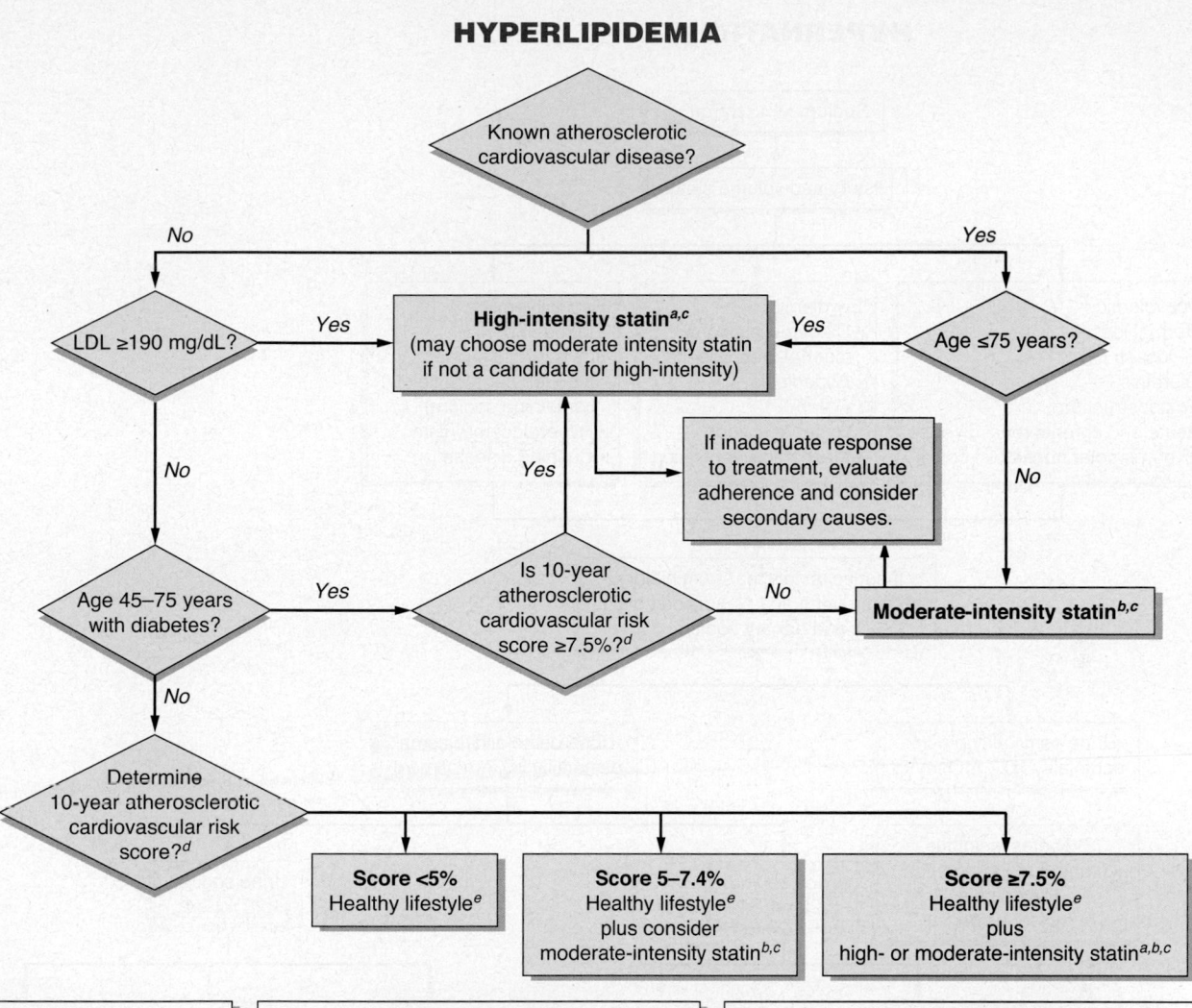

Known atherosclerotic cardiovascular disease?

No → **LDL ≥190 mg/dL?** — **Yes** → **High-intensity statin[a,c]** (may choose moderate intensity statin if not a candidate for high-intensity)

Yes → **Age ≤75 years?** — **Yes** → High-intensity statin[a,c]

If inadequate response to treatment, evaluate adherence and consider secondary causes.

Age ≤75 years? — **No** → **Moderate-intensity statin[b,c]**

LDL ≥190 mg/dL? — **No** → **Age 45–75 years with diabetes?** — **Yes** → **Is 10-year atherosclerotic cardiovascular risk score ≥7.5%?[d]** — **Yes** (to High-intensity statin) / **No** → **Moderate-intensity statin[b,c]**

Age 45–75 years with diabetes? — **No** → **Determine 10-year atherosclerotic cardiovascular risk score?[d]**

Score <5%
Healthy lifestyle[e]

Score 5–7.4%
Healthy lifestyle[e]
plus consider
moderate-intensity statin[b,c]

Score ≥7.5%
Healthy lifestyle[e]
plus
high- or moderate-intensity statin[a,b,c]

---

[a]High-intensity statin
Atorvastatin 40–80 mg/day
Rosuvastatin 20–40 mg/day

[b]Moderate-intensity statin
Atorvastatin 10–20 mg/day
Fluvastatin 40 mg twice daily
Fluvastatin XL 80 mg/day
Lovastatin 40 mg/day
Pitavastatin 2–4 mg/day
Pravastatin 40–80 mg/day
Rosuvastatin 5–10 mg/day
Simvastatin 20–40 mg/day

[c]Blood monitoring
Perform baseline ALT before starting therapy; monitor fasting lipid profile 4–12 weeks after starting or changing dose, every 3–12 months.

[d]Risk score calculators
Pooled cohort risk assessment equations:
http://my.americanheart.org/professional/StatementsGuidelines/PreventionGuidelines/Prevention-Guidelines_UCM_457698_SubHomePage.jsp;
http://www.acc.org/tools-and-practice-support/mobile-resources/features/2013-prevention-guidelines-ascvd-risk-estimator

[e]Healthy lifestyle
Diet of fruits, vegetables, fish, nuts, whole grains, and low in saturated fats. Thirty minutes of moderate-intensity aerobic **exercise** 5 days/week

Jason E. Cross, PharmD, Dinesh Yogaratnam, PharmD, and Sudeep K. Aulakh, MD, FACP, FRCPC

Stone NJ, Robinson JG, Lichtenstein AH, et al. 2013 ACC/AHA guideline on the treatment of blood cholesterol to reduce atherosclerotic cardiovascular risk in adults: a report of the American College of Cardiology/American Heart Association Task Force on Practice Guidelines. *Circulation.* 2014;129(25)(Suppl 2):S1–S45.

HYPERNATREMIA

Timothy J. Coker, MD

Braun MM, Barstow CH, Pyzocha NJ. Diagnosis and management of sodium disorders: hyponatremia and hypernatremia. *Am Fam Physician.* 2015;91(5):299–307.

HYPERTRIGLYCERIDEMIA

Steven W. Gale, MD and Timothy J. Coker, MD

Berglund L, Brunzell JD, Goldberg AC, et al. Evaluation and treatment of hypertriglyceridemia: an Endocrine Society clinical practice guideline. *J Clin Endocrinol Metab.* 2012;97(9):2969–2989.

HYPOALBUMINEMIA

Albumin <3.5 g/dL

History: edema, jaundice, alcoholism, hepatitis, foamy urine, muscle atrophy, ascitis, weight gain, loss of appetite, malnutrition, decreased PO intake, hyperlipidemia, diarrhea, vomiting, burns, inflammation

Decreased protein synthesis

Abnormal protein distribution

Protein loss

Cirrhosis, stigmas, ascites, spider angiomas

Hyperglycemia Low serum insulin

Physiologic stress (infection, surgery, trauma)

Hemodilutional states

Diabetes

↑ CRP and ESR

Peripheral edema, dyspnea, fatigue, ↑ BNP, crackles

Flank dullness, abdominal distension, fluid wave

Elevated β-hCG Amenorrhea

PLT <160,000/mm³

Elevated LFTs (esp. AST)

Positive hepatitis

INR ≥1.5

Elevated GGT

Alkaline phosphatase

Nodular liver on abdominal US

Acute and chronic inflammation

CHF

Ascites

Pregnancy

Diminished height
Poor weight gain
Deficit in lean body mass
Wasted
Stunted linear growth
Alopecia
Frequent infection
Vitamin deficiencies

Urine dipstick analysis

≥3–4 + protein

Liver cirrhosis

Decreased lymphocyte count, BUN, transferrin, prealbumin

Spot urine Random urine protein/Cr ratio ≥3–3.5

24-hour urine

If ≥3.5 g/24 hr

Malnutrition and starvation

Nephrotic syndrome

Enteral protein loss α₁-antitrypsin in stool

Skin burns and tissue damage

Upper GI endoscopy

Extensive skin burns

Protein-losing gastroenteropathy workup

Lawrence M. Gibbs, MD, MSEd

Gatta A, Verardo A, Bolognesi M. Hypoalbuminemia. *Intern Emerg Med.* 2012;7(Suppl 3):S193–S199.

HYPOCALCEMIA

Tiffany Burca, DO and Timothy J. Coker, MD

Michels TC, Kelly KM. Parathyroid disorders. *Am Fam Physician.* 2013;88(4):249–257.

HYPOGLYCEMIA

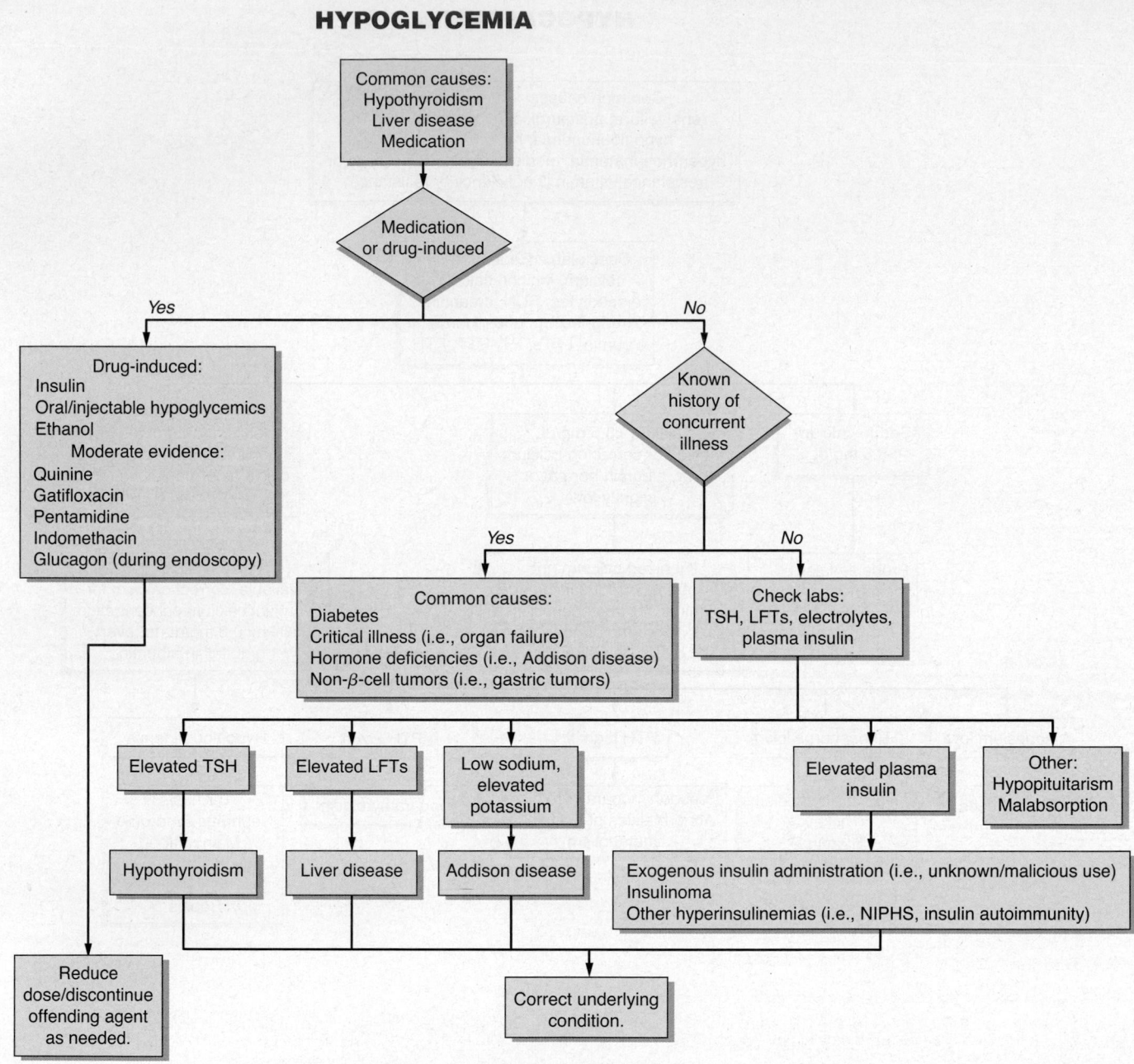

Aimee L. Dietle, PharmD and Stephanie J. Billings, MD

Martens P, Tits J. Approach to the patient with spontaneous hypoglycemia. *Eur J Intern Med.* 2014;25(5):415–421.

HYPOKALEMIA
Differential Diagnosis

GI losses

- Vomiting
- Diarrhea
- Nasogastric tube
- Laxative abuse
- Fistulas
- Villous adenoma
- Ureterosigmoidostomy
- Malabsorption
- Radiation enteropathy

Renal losses

Medications: diuretics (especially loop and thiazide), amphotericin B, aminoglycosides

Mineralocorticoid excess (hypertensive)
- Primary hyperaldosteronism
- Secondary hyperaldosteronism (CHF, cirrhosis, nephritic syndrome, renin-producing tumors)
- Bartter syndrome
- Gitelman syndrome
- Exogenous mineralocorticoids
- Liddle syndrome
- Vasculitis

Osmotic diuresis (e.g. poorly controlled diabetes)

Renal tubular acidosis (types I and II)

Poor dietary intake

- Alcoholism
- Tea and toast diet
- Anorexia nervosa

Intracellular shifts

- Metabolic alkalosis
- Insulin excess
- β-Adrenergic catecholamine excess (acute stress, B_2 agonists)
- Hypokalemic periodic paralysis
- Intoxications (theophylline, caffeine, barium, toluene)

Treatment of hypokalemia

Mild to moderate
K 2.5–3.4 mEq/L

Severe
K <2.5 mEq/L

PO replacement:
- KCl 40–120 mEq in divided doses

IV replacement only when PO repletion contraindicated

IV replacement:
- Peripheral line:
  o Up to 20 mEq/hr
  o Up to 60 mEq/L
- Central line (for concentrations >20 mEq/hr)

Nathaniel D. Cranney, DO and Bethany N. Teer, MD

Medford-Davis L, Rafique Z. Derangements of potassium. *Emerg Med Clin North Am.* 2014;32(2):329–347.

HYPONATREMIA

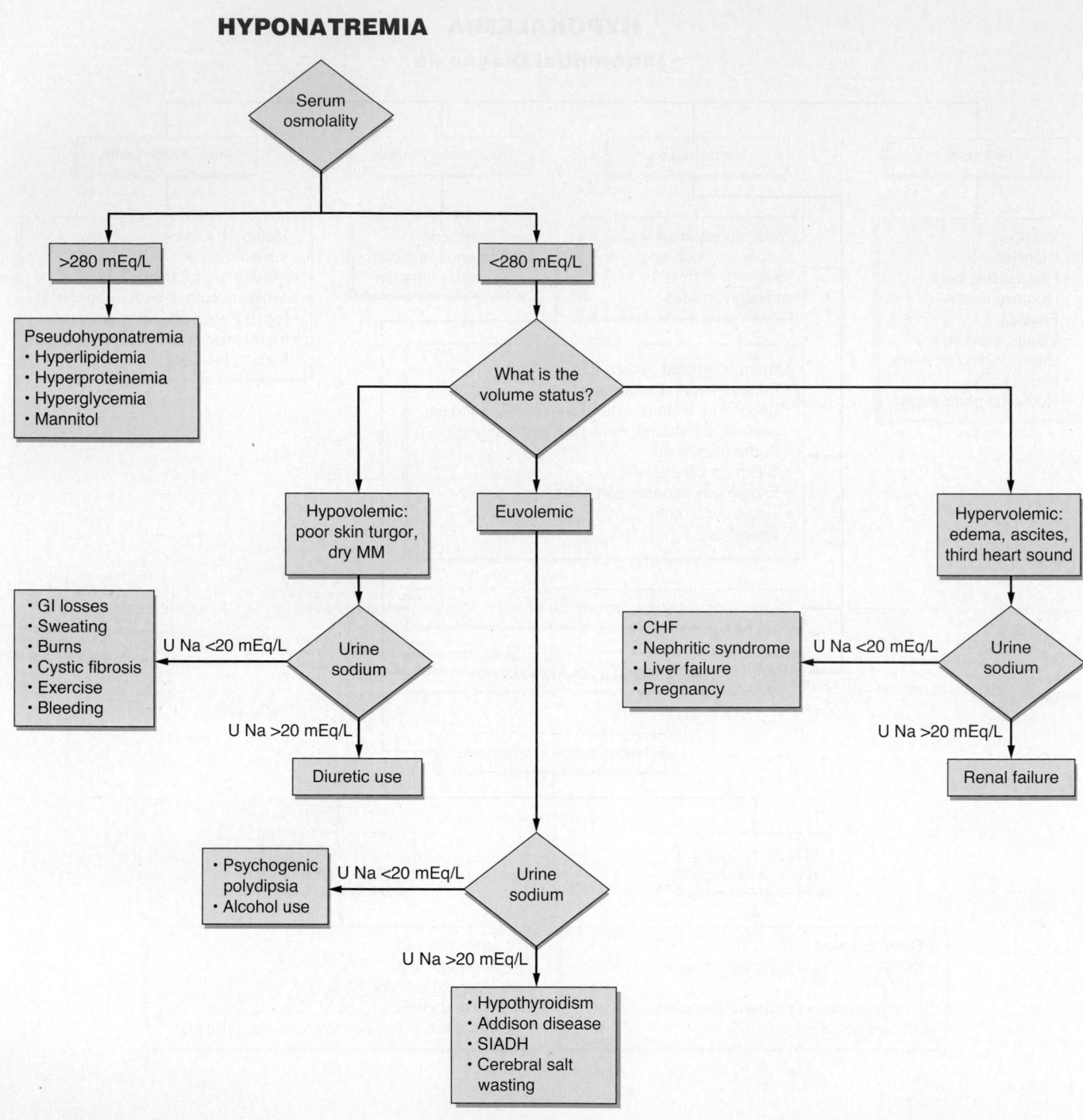

Sultan M. Babar, MD and R. Aaron Lambert, MD

Lien YH, Shapiro JI. Hyponatremia: clinical diagnosis and management. *Am J Med.* 2007;120(8):653–658.

HYPOTENSION

Resting SBP <90 mm Hg, MAP <60 mm Hg, or reduction in baseline BP (MAP) >30% or 40 mm Hg

Unstable

Stable

Organ hypoperfusion: abnormal mental status, clammy skin, thready rapid pulse, oliguria, metabolic acidosis, elevated lactate?

No →

Mild/moderate volume depletion
– Replete fluids and treat underlying cause.
– If more complex, check HCT, electrolytes, BUN, Cr.
– Monitor vital signs and orthostatics.
– Consider/anticipate early shock and treat as in algorithm below.

← Yes

Signs or history of potential volume loss: vomiting, diarrhea, fluid restriction, fever, intense physical activity?

Yes

No

Young healthy individual Normal SBP <90 mm Hg

Autonomic dysfunction
Medications
EtOH
Aging
Diabetes
Parkinson disease
Pregnancy
Prolonged bed rest
Recreational drug overdose

– Airway and breathing (intubation and mechanical ventilation if cannot protect airway, respiratory distress, hypoxemia or hypercarbia)
– Insert two large-bore IVs (or central venous catheter) and Foley catheter.
– Consider insertion of arterial line.
– Check EKG, CXR, CBC, electrolytes, renal function, PT/PTT.
– Closely monitor blood pressure while supine and upright, central venous pressure, intake/output.

Septic shock
Consider sources of bacteremia based on clinical symptoms and potential infectious entry sites.

Anaphylactic shock
Drug reactions
Insect bites
Transfusion reactions
Heavy metal poisoning

Neurogenic shock
Spinal cord injury
Severe head injury
Spinal anesthesia
Pharmacologic sympathetic blockade

Hypovolemic shock
Decreased JVP, CVP; history suggestive of hemorrhage, vomiting, diarrhea, burns, trauma; dry mucous membranes, decreased skin turgor

Increased JVP, CVP

Cardiogenic shock
Rales on physical exam
Myocardial infarction (most common cause)
Cardiomyopathy
Arrhythmia
Valvular heart disease

Obstructive shock
Pulmonary embolism
Clear lungs on physical exam
Tension pneumothorax (clinical diagnosis)
Pericardial tamponade
Severe constrictive pericarditis
Postintubation hypotension

– Blood cultures × 2
– Urinalysis
– Chest x-ray
– Further laboratory investigations and imaging based on suspected source of infection
– Consider ordering serum lactate levels based on severity of shock and trend following resuscitation.

– Intramuscular epinephrine immediately: Repeat doses q20min as needed.
– Antihistamines (both H1 and H2)
– Steroids (to prevent biphasic anaphylaxis)
– IV fluids

– IV fluids
– Supine or Trendelenburg position
– Maintain body temperature if febrile/hypothermic.

– Isotonic fluids
– Search for source of hemorrhage (internal or external) and control bleeding.
– PRBCs if large amount of blood loss
– Pressors* if patient remains hypotensive
– NGT if vomiting

– May require emergent bedside transthoracic echocardiogram
– Hemodynamic monitoring with Swan-Ganz catheter
  • Keep CO >4 L/min, CI >2.2.
– Patient may require inotropic support or vasopressors*.
– Avoid fluids if left ventricular filling pressure is elevated.
– Consider IABP.

– Specific therapy:
  • MI: standard medical therapy plus emergent revascularization
– Arrhythmia: urgent pharmacologic or electrical cardioversion if unstable
  • Valvular/structural defects: surgical repair
  • Tamponade: therapeutic pericardiocentesis
  • Pulmonary embolism: thrombolysis if persistent hypotension and no contraindications
  • Tension pneumothorax: chest tube
  • Pericarditis: pericardial stripping

– Early broad-spectrum antibiotics
– Early isotonic fluids—20–40 mL/kg (1–2 L) bolus. Crystalloid solution is equal to colloid in terms of outcome and significantly less expensive (Class I).
– May use pressors* if patient remains hypotensive after adequate fluid resuscitation
– Maintain MAP >65, urine output >0.5 mL/kg/hr, and CVP 8–12 mm Hg.
– Eradicate source (e.g., vascular access removal, abscess drainage).
– For refractory hypotension, consider stress dose steroids.
  • Dexamethasone is preferred to preserve later ACTH-stimulation test (Class IIb).
  • Vasopressin 0.04 U/min (range 0.01–0.04 U/min) may also be added to titrate down on other vasopressor agents (Class IIb).

*Vasopressors—goal to maintain MAP ≥65 mm Hg
If still hypotensive despite max dose of initial vasopressor agent, consider:
First-line agents: Add norepinephrine or dopamine (Class IIb), then add:
– Phenylephrine 100–180 μg/min then titrate to a maintenance dose of 40–60 μg/min (Class IIa); acts exclusively on α_1-receptors. Consider if severe tachycardia with other pressors.
– Epinephrine 1–4 μg/min (Class IIb). Epinephrine is the drug of choice in anaphylactic shock (Class I).
– Norepinephrine 8–12 μg/min starting dose (12 μg/min max) and titrate to desired BP. Titrate down to 2–4 μg/min when BP goal achieved (Class I). Vasopressor of choice for septic shock
– Dopamine 10–20 μg/kg/min and titrate up to 50 μg/kg/min max (Class I). Consider in those with reduced chronotropy and inotropy. Has increased β_1-receptor activity than norepinephrine. Renal dose no longer recommended.

Consider cardiac function: If reduced cardiac output or cardiac input on TTE or bedside echo, consider an agent that increases inotropy and peripheral vasodilator support to reduce afterload.
– Dobutamine 0.5–1.0 μg/kg/min, titrate to 40 μg/kg/min max. Maintenance dose is 2.5–50 μg/kg/min. Greatest arrhythmogenic potential as it is an adrenergic agent (Class IIa)
– Inamrinone (formerly amrinone) (Class IIb) 0.75 mg/kg bolus over 2–3 minutes. May repeat once then maintenance dose 5–15 μg/kg/min. Phosphodiesterase (PDE) inhibitor is theoretically less dysrhythmogenic.
– Milrinone 50 μg/kg bolus over 10 minutes then maintenance dose 0.375–0.75 μg/kg/min (Class IIb). Least risk of peripheral vasodilation. Newest PDE-inhibitor in the United States.

Amar Talati, DO and David O. Parrish, MS, MD, FAAFP

Mouncey PR, Osborn TM, Power GS, et al. Trial of early, goal-directed resuscitation for septic shock. *N Engl J Med.* 2015;372(14):1301–1311.

INFERLITY

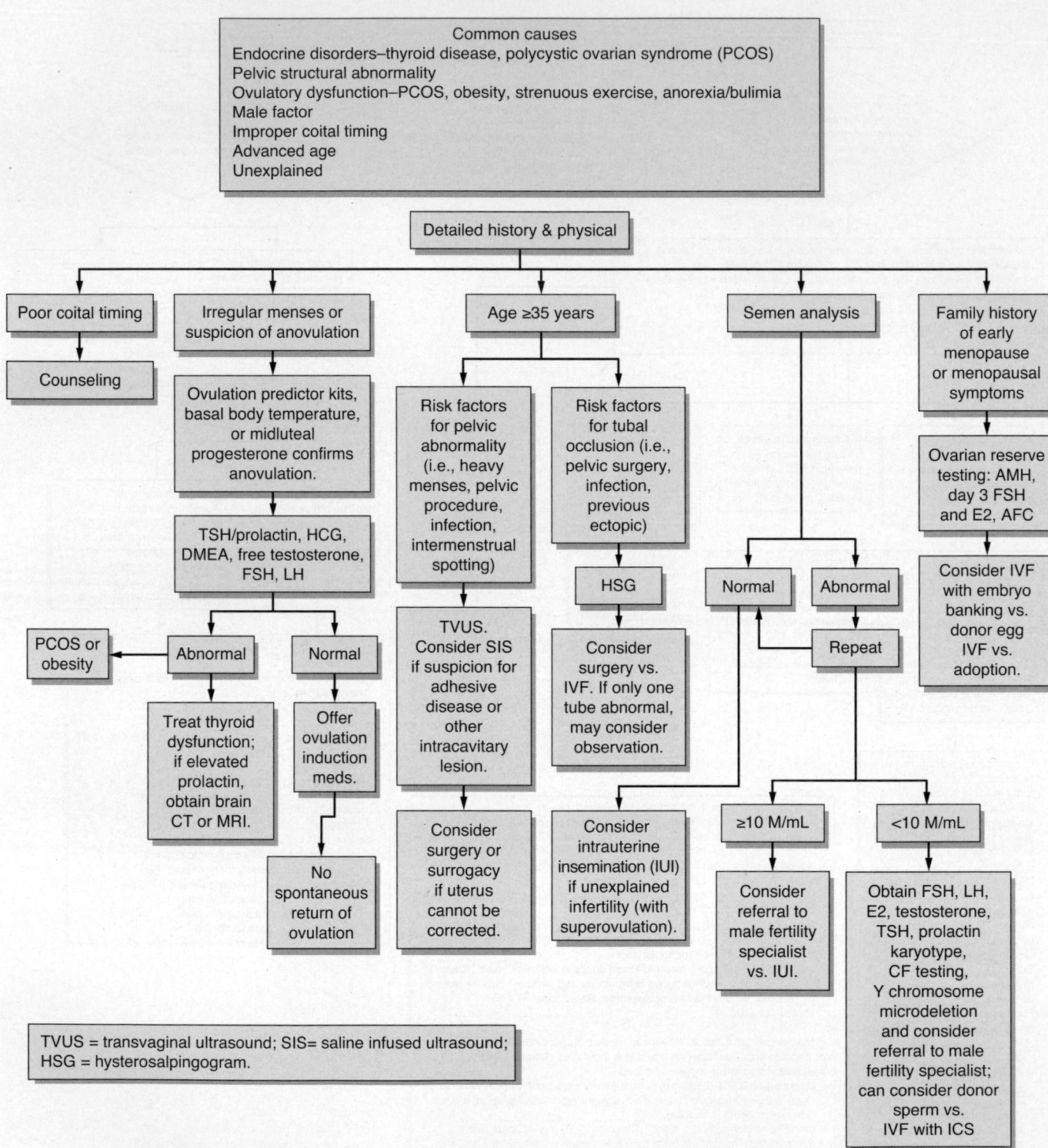

Common causes
Endocrine disorders–thyroid disease, polycystic ovarian syndrome (PCOS)
Pelvic structural abnormality
Ovulatory dysfunction–PCOS, obesity, strenuous exercise, anorexia/bulimia
Male factor
Improper coital timing
Advanced age
Unexplained

Detailed history & physical

Poor coital timing → Counseling

Irregular menses or suspicion of anovulation
→ Ovulation predictor kits, basal body temperature, or midluteal progesterone confirms anovulation.
→ TSH/prolactin, HCG, DMEA, free testosterone, FSH, LH
→ Abnormal → PCOS or obesity; Normal
Abnormal → Treat thyroid dysfunction; if elevated prolactin, obtain brain CT or MRI.
Normal → Offer ovulation induction meds. → No spontaneous return of ovulation

Age ≥35 years
Risk factors for pelvic abnormality (i.e., heavy menses, pelvic procedure, infection, intermenstrual spotting) → TVUS. Consider SIS if suspicion for adhesive disease or other intracavitary lesion. → Consider surgery or surrogacy if uterus cannot be corrected.
Risk factors for tubal occlusion (i.e., pelvic surgery, infection, previous ectopic) → HSG → Consider surgery vs. IVF. If only one tube abnormal, may consider observation. → Consider intrauterine insemination (IUI) if unexplained infertility (with superovulation).

Semen analysis
Normal / Abnormal
Abnormal → Repeat
≥10 M/mL → Consider referral to male fertility specialist vs. IUI.
<10 M/mL → Obtain FSH, LH, E2, testosterone, TSH, prolactin karyotype, CF testing, Y chromosome microdeletion and consider referral to male fertility specialist; can consider donor sperm vs. IVF with ICS

Family history of early menopause or menopausal symptoms
→ Ovarian reserve testing: AMH, day 3 FSH and E2, AFC
→ Consider IVF with embryo banking vs. donor egg IVF vs. adoption.

TVUS = transvaginal ultrasound; SIS= saline infused ultrasound; HSG = hysterosalpingogram.

Tiffany Tonismae, MD and Emily Evans-Hoeker, MD

Practice Committee of the American Society for Reproductive Medicine. Diagnostic evaluation of the infertile female: a committee opinion. *Fertil Steril.* 2015;103(6):e44–e50.

JAUNDICE

Jaundice: a yellow discoloration of skin, sclera, and mucous membranes by bilirubin, a bile pigment formed by the breakdown of heme rings; detected when the serum bilirubin level >3 mg/dL. Bilirubin is a product of hemoglobin breakdown in the spleen. Heme is converted to unconjugated bilirubin, bound to albumin, and then sent to the liver where it is then conjugated.

Common causes: Gilbert syndrome, hemolysis, hepatitis, and choledocholithiasis

CBC w/ diff, LFTs: ALT, AST, serum alkaline phosphatase (AP), total bilirubin (TB) and direct bilirubin (DB), haptoglobin, hepatitis serologies, amylase, lipase, hCG, urinalysis with urine bilirubin. US or CT

Unconjugated hyperbilirubinemia

No ← Direct bilirubin >0.3 mg/dL → Yes

Conjugated hyperbilirubinemia

Elevated AP — Yes → Intrahepatic ← No — Obstruction on imaging — Yes → Extrahepatic

No ↓

Prehepatic

- **Hemolytic anemia**
- **Reabsorption of large hematoma**

Labs: anemia, possible reticulocytosis, mild TB elevation (5 mg/dL), increased indirect bilirubin, normal DB levels, and negative urine bilirubin. All other LFTs are normal.

Unconjugated hyperbilirubinemia

- ○ **Gilbert syndrome:** mild defect in UDP glucuronosyltransferase (UGT, responsible for conjugation of bilirubin)
- ○ **Crigler-Najjar syndrome:** more severe defect in UGT, usually presents during infancy

Conjugated hyperbilirubinemia
- ○ **Dublin-Johnson syndrome:** defective secretion of conjugated bilirubin
- ○ **Rotor syndrome**

Both conjugated and unconjugated hepatocellular injury:

- ○ **Hepatitis:** viral, alcohol, or autoimmune insult leading to inflammation that impedes or prevents transport/secretion of conjugated bilirubin
- ○ **Medication/drug:** acetaminophen
- ○ **Cirrhosis**
- ○ **Congestive heart failure:** Hypoxia/anoxia of hepatocytes leads to cellular injury.

Intrahepatic cholestasis (No elevated LFTs, (primarily AP), US shows normal sized bile ducts)

Other:
- ○ **Medication/drug-induced**
- ○ **Total parenteral nutrition (TPN)**
- ○ **Sepsis**
- ○ **Sarcoidosis**
- ○ **Pregnancy**

Extrahepatic cholestasis (labs: elevated TB and DB, elevated AP, and positive urine bilirubin. US shows dilated bile duct[s].)

- **Choledocholithiasis**
- **Chronic pancreatitis:** alcohol
- **Cholangitis:** fever, pain and jaundice, altered mental status, sepsis
- **Biliary structure:** history of surgical/invasive procedure
- **Primary biliary cirrhosis**
- **Primary sclerosing cholangitis**
- **Biliary tract tumor/cholangiocarcinoma:** hepatomegaly, weight loss, abdominal pain
- **Pancreatic tumor:** painless jaundice, palpable gallbladder (rare)

Krunal Patel, MD and Isabel Zacharias, MD

Roche SP, Kobos R. Jaundice in the adult patient. *Am Fam Physician.* 2004;69(2):299–304.

KNEE PAIN

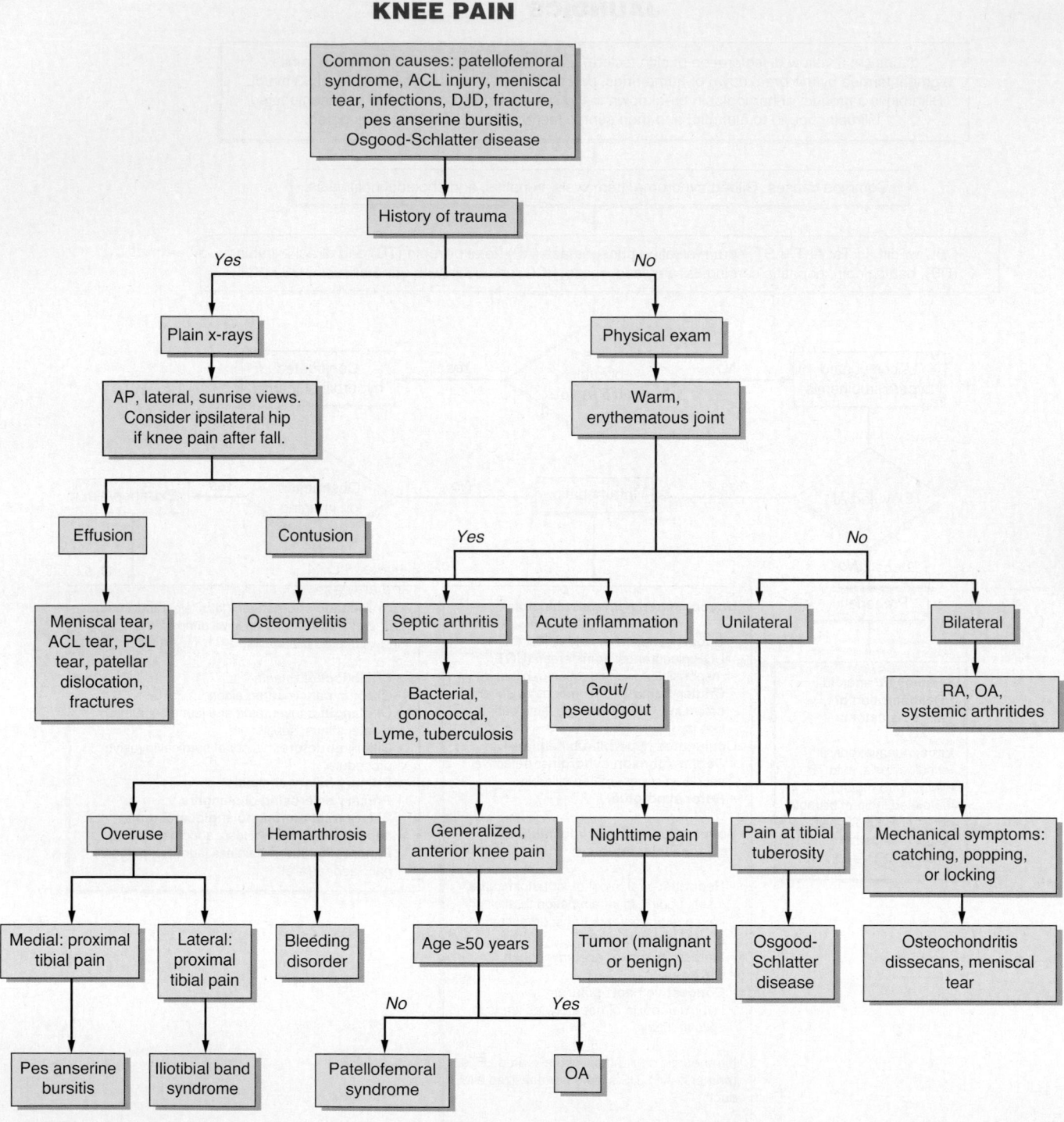

Alec DeCastro, MD

Calmbach WL, Hutchens M. Evaluation of patients presenting with knee pain: part I. History, physical examination, radiographs, and laboratory tests. *Am Fam Physician.* 2003;68(5):907–912.

LACTATE DEHYDROGENASE ELEVATION

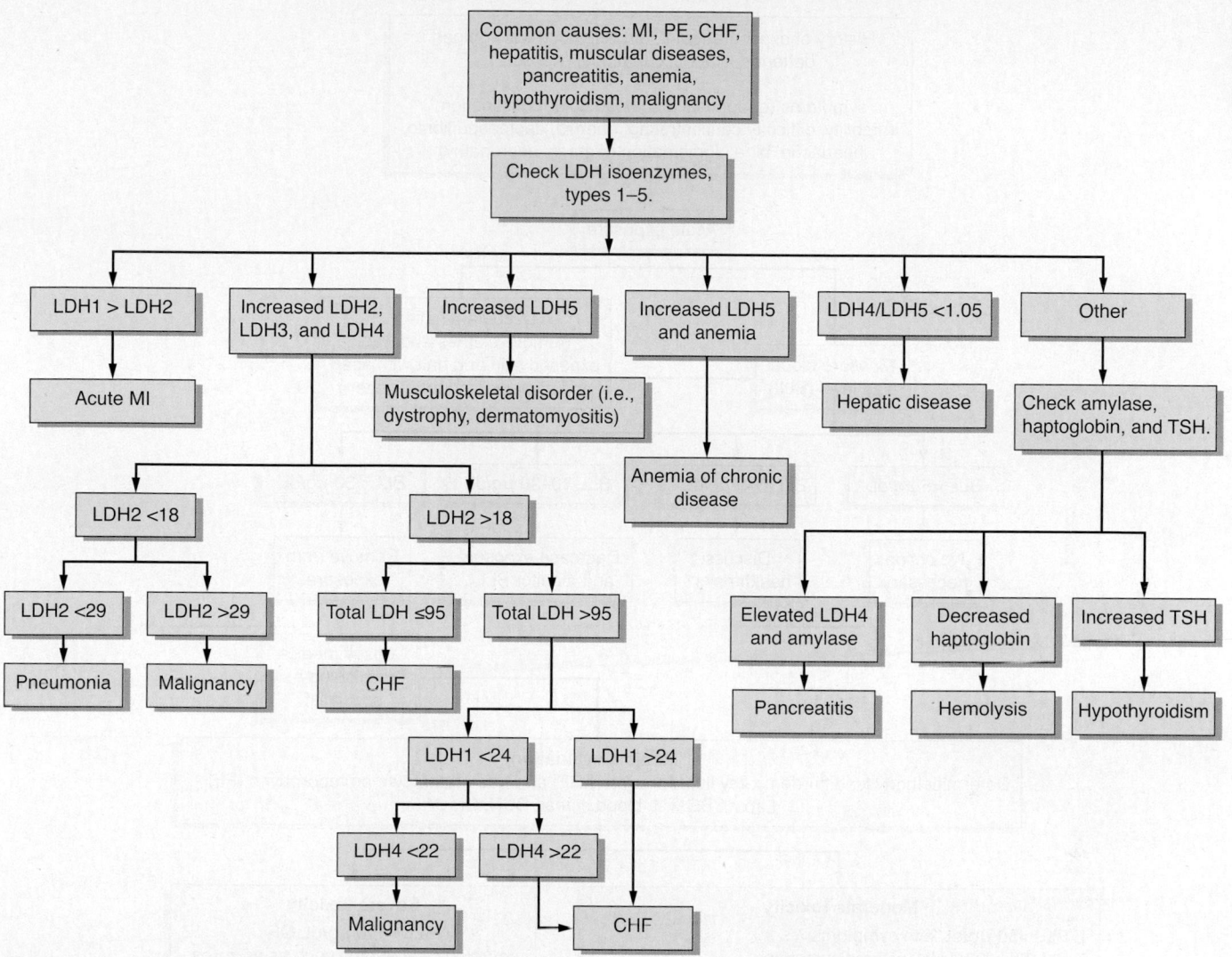

Curtis L. Galke, DO, FAAFP

Lossos IS, Breuer R, Intrator O, et al. Differential diagnosis of pleural effusion by lactate dehydrogenase isoenzyme analysis. *Chest*. 1997;111(3):648–651.

LEAD TOXICITY, DIAGNOSIS AND TREATMENT (ADULT)

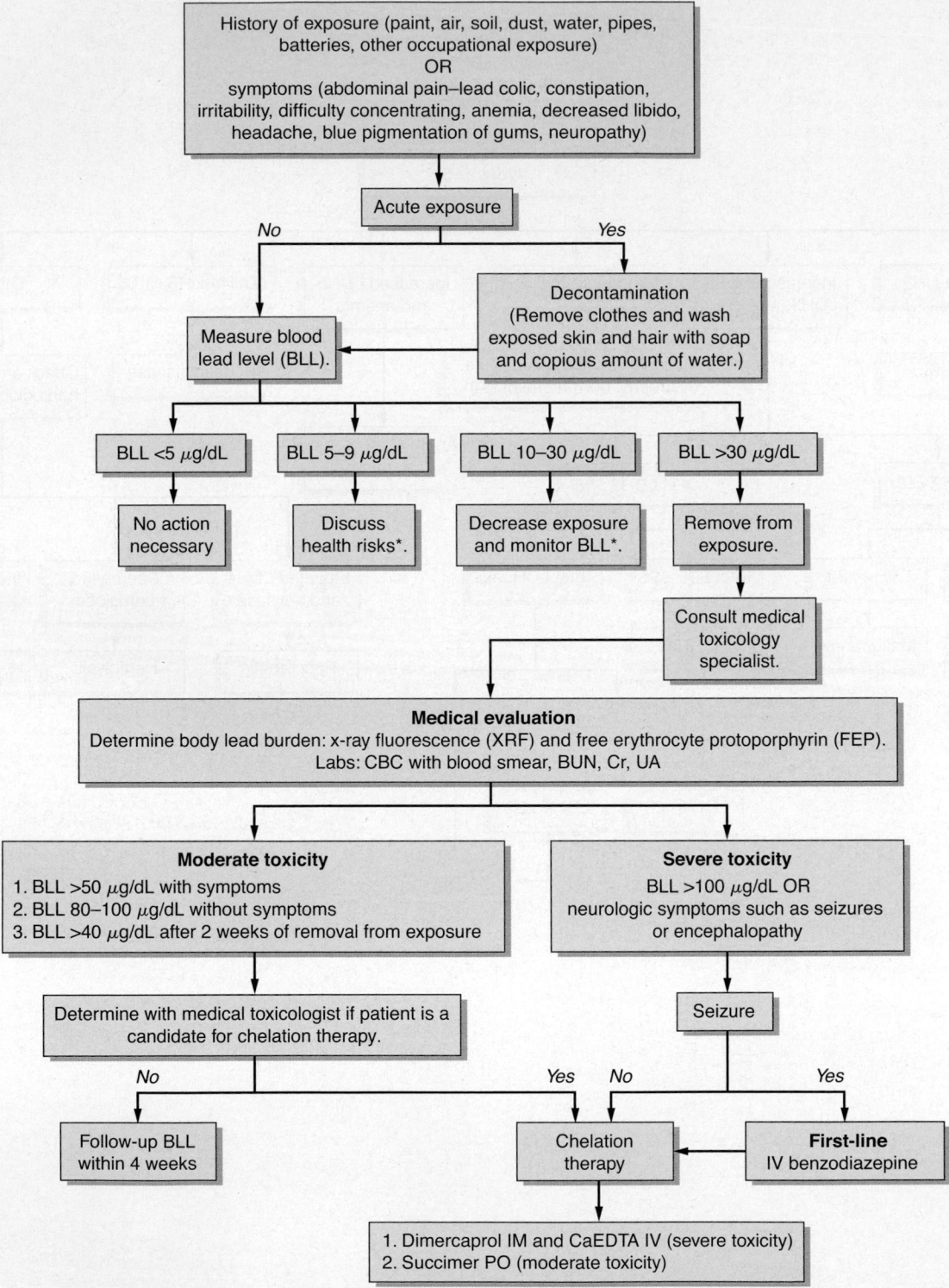

History of exposure (paint, air, soil, dust, water, pipes, batteries, other occupational exposure)
OR
symptoms (abdominal pain–lead colic, constipation, irritability, difficulty concentrating, anemia, decreased libido, headache, blue pigmentation of gums, neuropathy)

Acute exposure

No · Yes

Decontamination
(Remove clothes and wash exposed skin and hair with soap and copious amount of water.)

Measure blood lead level (BLL).

BLL <5 μg/dL → No action necessary

BLL 5–9 μg/dL → Discuss health risks*.

BLL 10–30 μg/dL → Decrease exposure and monitor BLL*.

BLL >30 μg/dL → Remove from exposure.

Consult medical toxicology specialist.

Medical evaluation
Determine body lead burden: x-ray fluorescence (XRF) and free erythrocyte protoporphyrin (FEP).
Labs: CBC with blood smear, BUN, Cr, UA

Moderate toxicity
1. BLL >50 μg/dL with symptoms
2. BLL 80–100 μg/dL without symptoms
3. BLL >40 μg/dL after 2 weeks of removal from exposure

Severe toxicity
BLL >100 μg/dL OR neurologic symptoms such as seizures or encephalopathy

Determine with medical toxicologist if patient is a candidate for chelation therapy.

Seizure

No · Yes · No · Yes

Follow-up BLL within 4 weeks

Chelation therapy

First-line IV benzodiazepine

1. Dimercaprol IM and CaEDTA IV (severe toxicity)
2. Succimer PO (moderate toxicity)

*If pregnant, reduce lead exposure for BLL 5–9 μg/dL and remove lead exposure for BLL >10 μg/dL.

Han Q. Bui, MD, MPH

Kosnett MJ, Wedeen RP, Rothenberg SJ, et al. Recommendations for medical management of adult lead exposure. *Environ Health Perspect.* 2007;115(3):463–471.

LOW BACK PAIN, CHRONIC

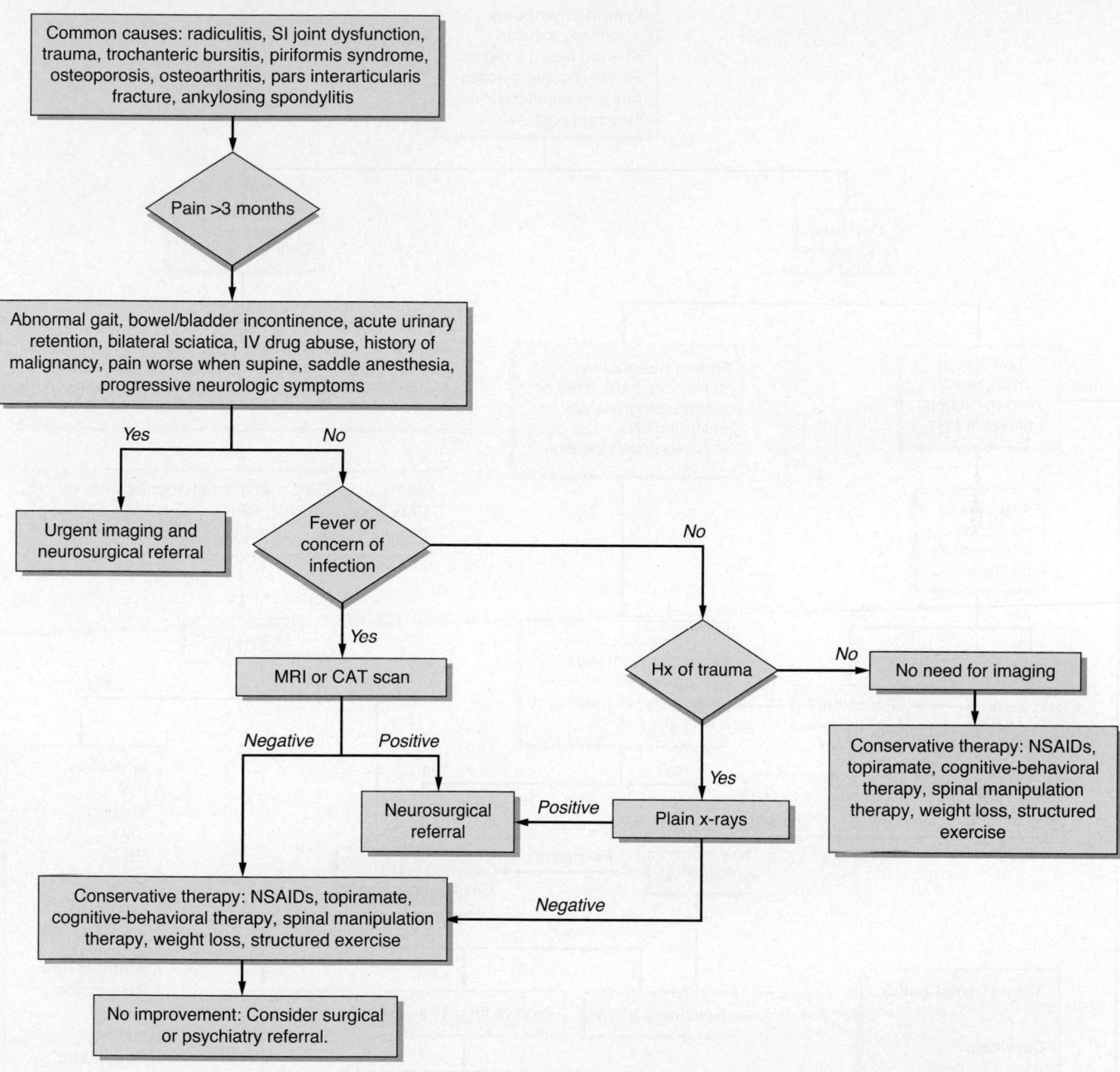

Common causes: radiculitis, SI joint dysfunction, trauma, trochanteric bursitis, piriformis syndrome, osteoporosis, osteoarthritis, pars interarticularis fracture, ankylosing spondylitis

Pain >3 months

Abnormal gait, bowel/bladder incontinence, acute urinary retention, bilateral sciatica, IV drug abuse, history of malignancy, pain worse when supine, saddle anesthesia, progressive neurologic symptoms

Yes — Urgent imaging and neurosurgical referral

No — Fever or concern of infection

No — Hx of trauma

Yes — MRI or CAT scan

Negative / *Positive*

Positive — Neurosurgical referral

No — No need for imaging

Plain x-rays

Negative — Conservative therapy: NSAIDs, topiramate, cognitive-behavioral therapy, spinal manipulation therapy, weight loss, structured exercise

Conservative therapy: NSAIDs, topiramate, cognitive-behavioral therapy, spinal manipulation therapy, weight loss, structured exercise

No improvement: Consider surgical or psychiatry referral.

Shawna King, DO and Holly L. Baab, MD

Herndon CM, Zoberi KS, Gardner BJ. Common questions about chronic low back pain. *Am Fam Physician.* 2015;91(10):708–714.

LYMPHADENOPATHY

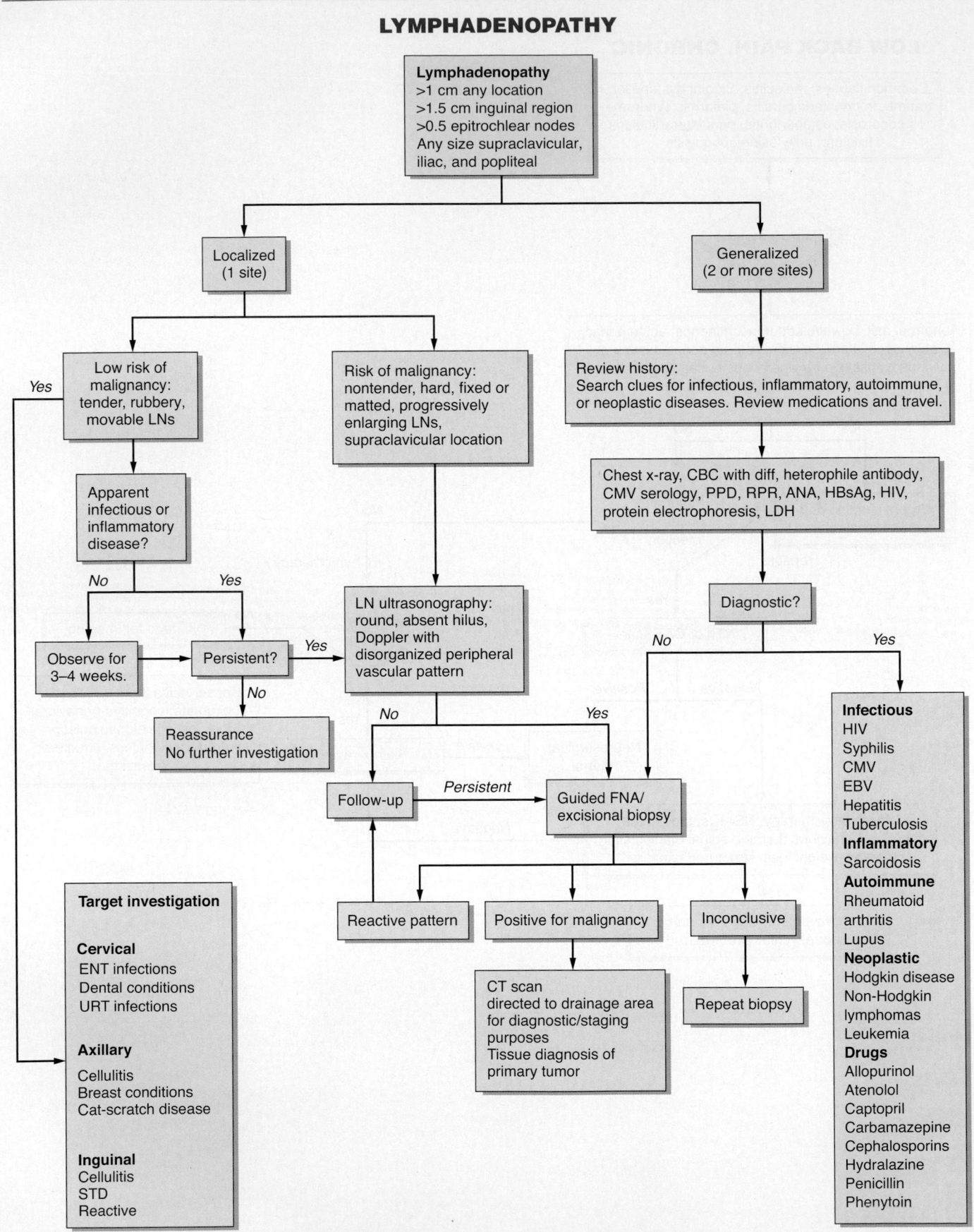

Lymphadenopathy
>1 cm any location
>1.5 cm inguinal region
>0.5 epitrochlear nodes
Any size supraclavicular, iliac, and popliteal

Localized (1 site)

Generalized (2 or more sites)

Low risk of malignancy: tender, rubbery, movable LNs

Risk of malignancy: nontender, hard, fixed or matted, progressively enlarging LNs, supraclavicular location

Review history:
Search clues for infectious, inflammatory, autoimmune, or neoplastic diseases. Review medications and travel.

Apparent infectious or inflammatory disease?

Chest x-ray, CBC with diff, heterophile antibody, CMV serology, PPD, RPR, ANA, HBsAg, HIV, protein electrophoresis, LDH

No *Yes*

Observe for 3–4 weeks.

Persistent?

Yes

LN ultrasonography: round, absent hilus, Doppler with disorganized peripheral vascular pattern

Diagnostic?

No   *Yes*

No

Reassurance
No further investigation

No   *Yes*

Follow-up —*Persistent*→ Guided FNA/excisional biopsy

Reactive pattern

Positive for malignancy

Inconclusive

CT scan
directed to drainage area for diagnostic/staging purposes
Tissue diagnosis of primary tumor

Repeat biopsy

Target investigation

Cervical
ENT infections
Dental conditions
URT infections

Axillary
Cellulitis
Breast conditions
Cat-scratch disease

Inguinal
Cellulitis
STD
Reactive

Infectious
HIV
Syphilis
CMV
EBV
Hepatitis
Tuberculosis
Inflammatory
Sarcoidosis
Autoimmune
Rheumatoid arthritis
Lupus
Neoplastic
Hodgkin disease
Non-Hodgkin lymphomas
Leukemia
Drugs
Allopurinol
Atenolol
Captopril
Carbamazepine
Cephalosporins
Hydralazine
Penicillin
Phenytoin

Pamela Waters, MD and Jonathan S. Bassett, MD

Mohseni S, Shojaiefard A, Khorgami Z, et al. Peripheral lymphadenopathy: approach and diagnostic tools. *Iran J Med Sci.* 2014;39(2)(Suppl):158–170.

LYMPHOPENIA

WBC <4,500/μL

Isolated neutropenia
ANC <1,500/μL

Isolated lymphopenia
ALC <1,500/μL

Concomitant anemia and/or
thrombocytopenia

Evaluate for neutropenia.

Evaluate for causes of pancytopenia.

Common causes
- **Infections** (including HIV, influenza, tuberculosis)
- **Medications** (especially prednisone and other immunosuppressives)
- **Nonpathologic lymphopenia** (especially in the elderly)

History of infection

Consider workup for the following:
- HIV
- Influenza
- Hepatitis
- Tuberculosis
- Malaria
- Histoplasmosis

History of suspicious medications
- Immunosuppressives
  - Prednisone, MTX, azathioprine, etc.
- Monoclonal antibody therapy
  - Rituximab
- Chemotherapy

Healthy elderly patient

In the absence of infection, weight loss, or other concerning history, no further investigation is neccssary.

Other
- Malnourishment
- Alcohol abuse
- Signs of underlying lymphoma or other malignancy
  - Weight loss, fever, night sweats
- Immune-mediated disease
  - RA, SLE, sarcoidosis, IBD
- Systemic, chronic disorders
  - CKD, CHF

Andrew Smith, MD and Erin Bassett-Novoa, MD

Brass D, Mckay P, Scott F. Investigating an incidental finding of lymphopenia. *BMJ.* 2014;348:g1721.

MENOPAUSE, EVALUATION AND MANAGEMENT

HRT
(use lowest effective dose for shortest duration possible.
Short-term use = 2–3 years; generally does not exceed 5 years)

Intact uterus?

Yes

No

Transdermal, oral, spray, gel, vaginal, or injectable estrogen + progesterone

Transdermal estrogen: Start 0.05 mg/day; max 0.10 mg/day

-OR-

Oral estrogen: 0.3, 0.45 mg, max 0.625 mg/day conjugated estrogens; 0.5–1 mg/day micronized estradiol

-OR-

Spray or gel: estradiol spray 0.021 mg delivered per spray; max 3 spray/day; 0.75 mg/day estradiol gel applied to large skin area

-OR-

Vaginal estrogen: 1 ring PV q3mo releases 50 or 100 μg/day estradiol.

-OR-

Injectable estrogen: 10–20 mg estradiol valerate IM q4wk

PLUS

Concomitant administration of one of the following:
1. **Medroxyprogesterone acetate (MPA)** 2.5 mg/day PO

-OR-

2. **Natural progesterone** 100–200 mg/day PO

Combined estrogen progesterone HRT

Combined estrogen and progesterone transdermal patches

Estradiol/levonorgestrel (delivers 0.045 mg/0.015 mg/day)

Estradiol/norethindrone acetate (delivers 0.05 mg/0.14 mg/day or = 0.05 mg/0.25 mg/day)

-OR-

Combined estrogen and progesterone pills

Estradiol 1 mg and drospirenone 0.5 mg

Ethinyl estradiol 2.5 or 5 μg and norethindrone acetate 0.5 or 1 mg

Conjugated estrogen 0.3, 0.45, or 0.625 mg and MPA 1.5, 2.5, or 5 mg

Estradiol 1 mg/norgestimate 0.9 mg

Topical estrogen therapy

Little or no estrogen is absorbed in bloodstream.
→ lower risk of side effects, but no effect on vasomotor symptoms. For use in patients with vaginal symptoms only.

Vaginal creams
0.01% estradiol cream PV daily equiv. to 0.1 mg

0.625 mg conjugated estrogen/g: 0.5 g PV daily × 21 days, then off for 7 days

Vaginal tablet:
Vaginal estradiol 10 μg tablet PV QD × 2 weeks, then 10 μg tablet PV twice weekly

Vaginal ring:
Vaginal estradiol that delivers 7.5 μg/day estradiol. Insert 1 ring PV q3mo.

Estrogen-only therapy
Transdermal
Oral
Spray/gel
Vaginal
Injectable

Do not use progesterone in women without a uterus.

Karen Browning, MD and Kelly Pagidas, MD

Huntzinger A. Practice guidelines: AHRQ releases evidence report on managing menopause-related symptoms. *Am Fam Physician.* 2005;72(4):709–710.

METABOLIC SYNDROME, TREATMENT

Identifiable risk factors:

1. Insulin resistance
2. Hypertension
3. Hyperlipidemia (elevated LDL, reduced HDL, and/or elevated triglycerides)
4. Abdominal obesity
5. Decreased physical inactivity
6. Aging
7. Hormonal imbalance
8. Microalbuminuria

Yes →

Assess:

1. Waist circumference
   • Men ≥40 inches (102 cm)
   • Women ≥35 inches (89 cm)
2. Serum triglyceride ≥150 mg/dL or on medication for the treatment of elevated triglyceride levels
3. HDL
   • Men <40 mg/dL
   • Women <50 mg/dL
4. Hypertension: ≥130/85 mm Hg or on medication for the treatment of hypertension
5. Glucose: fasting ≥100 mg/dL or on medication for the treatment of elevated fasting glucose levels

Does the patient meet 3 of the 5 criteria?

No → **Treat individual conditions.**

Yes → **Management:** First-line therapy treatment of any contributing risk factors

Treatment of inactivity:
30–60 minutes of continuous or intermittent moderate intensity activity

Treatment of elevated glucose:
Increased physical activity
Weight reduction
Oral hyperglycemic agents such as metformin to delay progression to DM

Treatment of abdominal obesity:
Weight reduction by 7–10% body weight through decrease in 500–1,000 calorie intake along with increased physical activity over 6–12 months
Maintenance of the weight reduction through consistent management/lifestyle changes through physical activity and reduced calorie intake

Treatment of hyperlipidemia:
Total fat 25–35% of total calories, saturated fat <7% of total calories
Medication therapy required with statin if any of the following:
1. +ASCVD and >21 years
2. LDL ≥190 mg/dL and 21 years
3. +DM age 40–75 years
4. ≥7.5% estimated 10-year ASCVD risk and age 40–75 years
5. Triglyceride ≥500 mg/dL

Treatment of hypertension:
JNC8 recommends therapy for BP >140/90 mm Hg for most patients. Lifestyle changes, moderation of alcohol consumption, sodium reduction, more of fresh fruits/vegetables, low-fat dairy products
Pharmacotherapy if necessary (first-line therapy: ACEI, ARB, CCB, or thiazide
Thiazides and CCBs are also considered first-line agents per JNC8.

Other clinical considerations:
– Treating sleep apnea with CPAP has shown significant improvement in metabolic profiles.
– New studies have shown treating patients with high-dose resveratrol for 16 weeks has significant improvements in formation and mineralization of new bone.
– Bariatric surgery has shown reductions in weight, insulin resistance, and inflammatory cytokines; however, currently, there are no accepted surgical interventions for metabolic syndrome.

Munawar Hayat, MD, Amber Durani, PA, and Tasaduq Mir, MD

Ginsberg HN. Treatment for patients with the metabolic syndrome. *Am J Cardiol*. 2003;91(7A):29E–39E.

MIGRAINE, TREATMENT

Suspected migraine headache
POUND:
Pulsatile quality
One-day duration (4–27 hours)
Unilateral location
Nausea or vomiting
Disabling intensity

With or without photophobia or phonophobia

Sudden onset | Age >55 years
Worst headache ever | Seizures
Increasing frequency | Fever, scalp tender
Worsening intensity | Systemic disease
Awakens from sleep | History trauma
Focal neurologic signs | Weight loss
Altered mental status | Myalgia
Precipitated by Valsalva | Exertion, bending

Yes → Consider alternate diagnosis and workup as directed by history and physical.

No → Meets criteria for migraine?
- **No** → Consider other headache syndrome.
- **Yes** → Classify as mild, moderate, or severe.

Mild → Acetaminophen (oral) → Resolved? **Yes** / **No**

Moderate → **NSAID (IV, oral)**
- Ibuprofen
- Diclofenac potassium
- Naproxen sodium
- Aspirin
→ Resolved? **Yes** / **No**

Simultaneous

Severe → ****Triptan**
- Sumatriptan (SC injection, nasal, oral)
- Zolmitriptan (nasal, oral, water)
- Rizatriptan (oral, water)
- Naratriptan (oral)
- Eletriptan (oral)
- Almotriptan (oral)
- Frovatriptan (oral)
→ Resolved? **Yes** / **No**

Rescue
- Ketorolac (IM)
- Indomethacin (oral or rectal)
- Prochlorperazine (oral or rectal)
- Chlorpromazine (oral)
- Dexamethasone or prednisone (IV)
- ***Opioid combination analgesic
→ Resolved? **Yes** / **No**

Aura?
- **Yes** → Magnesium sulfate (IV)
- **No**

Move to quiet, dark room
IV rehydration
Antiemetics PRN
- Hydroxyzine
- Metoclopramide
- Prochlorperazine
- Caffeine

- ***DHE (nasal, SC, IM self-injection)**
- Valproate (IV)
- Dexamethasone (IV)

Consider consultation with headache specialist.

Resolved? **Yes** / **No**

Ketorolac (IV) or opiates (IV, oral)

Resolved? **No** → Consult headache specialist. / **Yes**

• *****Butorphanol (IV, nasal spray)** Use in exceptional circumstances only.

Headache resolved

- Assess for hormone-related migraine.
- Consider prophylactic treatment as appropriate.

---

*Dihydroergotamine mesylate (DHE)
DHE must NOT be given to
- Pregnant or breastfeeding
- History of ischemic heart disease
- History of Prinzmetal angina
- Severe peripheral vascular disease
- Onset of chest pain after test dose
- Elevated blood pressure
- Within 24 hours of pain or ergot derivatives
- Basilar migraine with any three: diplopia, dysarthria, tinnitus, vertigo, temporary hearing loss, mental confusion
- Cerebrovascular disease

**5-HT (triptans)
- Avoid in patients with vascular disease, uncontrolled hypertension, and hemiplegic migraine.

***Opioids
- Avoid if at all possible due to medication headaches and dependency. This is especially true for butorphanol.

John M. Doan, DO and Robert K. Persons, DO

Worthington I, Pringsheim T, Gawel MJ, et al. Canadian Headache Society guideline: acute drug therapy for migraine headache. *Can J Neurol Sci.* 2013;40(5)(Suppl 3):S1–S80.

NAIL ABNORMALITIES

Dystrophic nails: Manicures/ pedicures Biting Rubbing

Nail fold

Nail line

Onycholysis: splitting nail plate from nail bed

Color change

Curving nails Longitudinal

Transverse

Erythema/ telangiectasias: SLE, Dermatomyositis, HIV/AIDS, Scleroderma, Rheumatoid arthritis, Hepatitis C

Red/tender swelling → Chronic?
- No → Infection, Herpetic whitlow
- Yes → Psoriasis, Reiter syndrome

Onychomycosis Psoriasis Trauma Vesicobullous disorders Squamous cell carcinoma

White: leukonychia → Chemotherapeutic drugs, Systemic disease

Green → *Pseudomonas aeruginosa*; pyocyanin production produces green color

Dark blue/red, black

Pincer nail: Medications, Psoriasis, Onychomycosis, SLE, Malignancy

Yellow → **Onychomycosis:** keratinaceous buildup under nail plate
- **Distal subungual onychomycosis** → Dermatophyte spread in palmar/plantar skin
- **Proximal subungual onychomycosis** → Fungus in deep nail plate; suspect immunosuppression

Clubbing: Cirrhosis, COPD, Celiac, Sprue

Koilonychia: iron deficiency anemia

Tiny linear discolorations?
- No → **Acute/painful/following trauma?**
  - No → Junctional nevus, Melanoma
  - Yes → Subungual hematoma
- Yes → **Splinter hemorrhages:** Bacterial endocarditis, Trauma, Psoriasis, Renal disease, Pulmonary disease, Endocrine disease

Horizontal
- **Migrates with nail growth: originates in nail plate** → Leukonychia (lines or spots related to random minor trauma to nail bed); Beau lines (any metabolic disease, trauma, Raynaud); Mees lines: heavy metal poisoning (arsenic); Renal failure
- **Does not migrate with nail growth: originates in nail bed** → Muehrcke lines (often in pairs): hypoalbuminemia

Longitudinal
- **Dark line: melanonychia**
  - **Single line** Nail matrix nevus, Melanoma, Normal variant in 90% black patients
  - **Multiple lines** HIV/AIDS, AZT, Hydroxychloroquine, Addison disease, Pregnancy, Trauma, Melanoma

Natasha J. Pyzocha, DO and Douglas M. Maurer, DO, MPH, FAAFP

Tully AS, Trayes KP, Studdiford JS. Evaluation of nail abnormalities. *Am Fam Physician.* 2012;85(8):779–787.

NEUTROPENIA

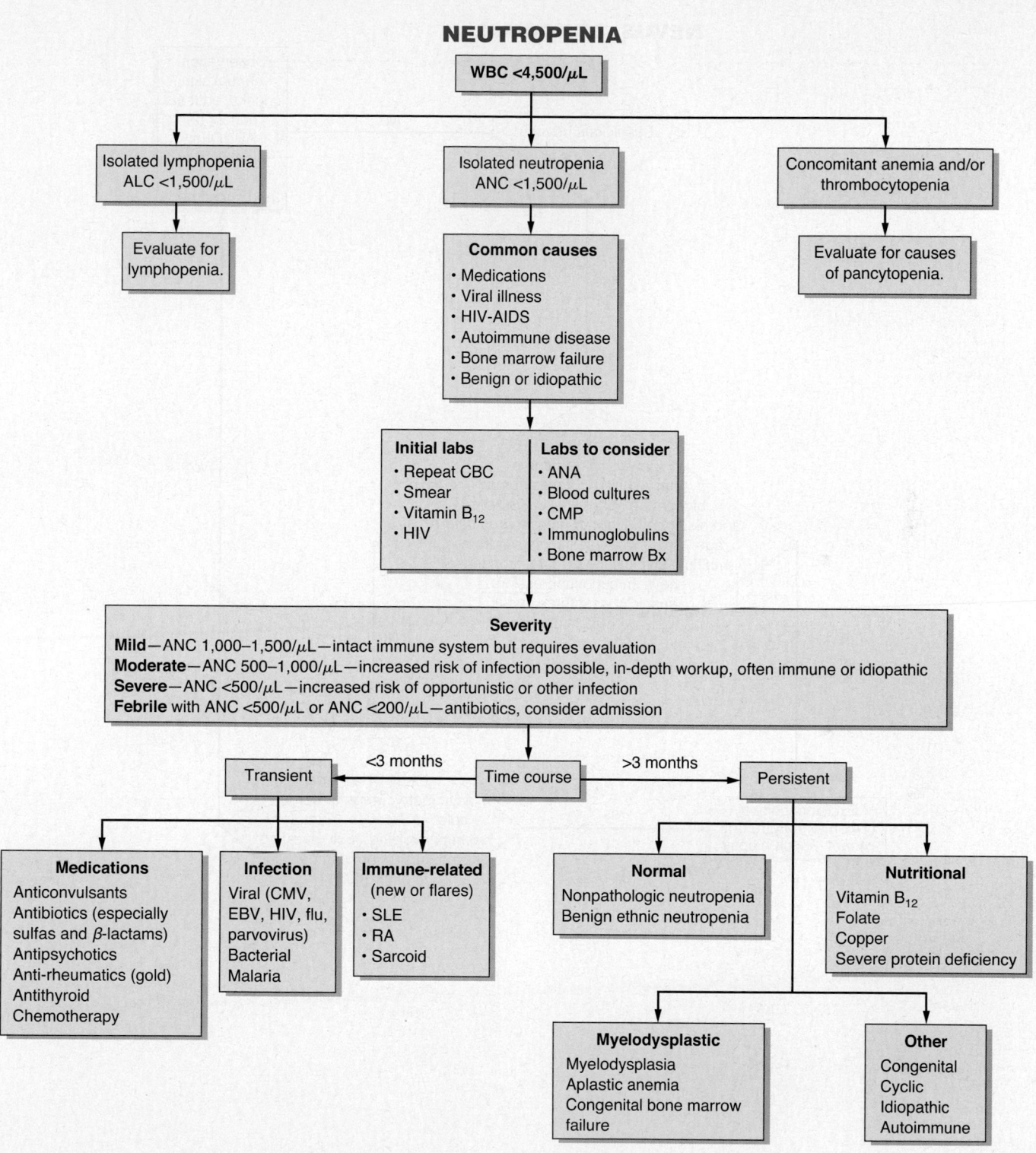

WBC <4,500/μL

Isolated lymphopenia
ALC <1,500/μL → Evaluate for lymphopenia.

Isolated neutropenia
ANC <1,500/μL

Concomitant anemia and/or thrombocytopenia → Evaluate for causes of pancytopenia.

Common causes
- Medications
- Viral illness
- HIV-AIDS
- Autoimmune disease
- Bone marrow failure
- Benign or idiopathic

Initial labs
- Repeat CBC
- Smear
- Vitamin B₁₂
- HIV

Labs to consider
- ANA
- Blood cultures
- CMP
- Immunoglobulins
- Bone marrow Bx

Severity
Mild—ANC 1,000–1,500/μL—intact immune system but requires evaluation
Moderate—ANC 500–1,000/μL—increased risk of infection possible, in-depth workup, often immune or idiopathic
Severe—ANC <500/μL—increased risk of opportunistic or other infection
Febrile with ANC <500/μL or ANC <200/μL—antibiotics, consider admission

Transient ← <3 months — Time course — >3 months → Persistent

Medications
Anticonvulsants
Antibiotics (especially sulfas and β-lactams)
Antipsychotics
Anti-rheumatics (gold)
Antithyroid
Chemotherapy

Infection
Viral (CMV, EBV, HIV, flu, parvovirus)
Bacterial
Malaria

Immune-related
(new or flares)
- SLE
- RA
- Sarcoid

Normal
Nonpathologic neutropenia
Benign ethnic neutropenia

Nutritional
Vitamin B₁₂
Folate
Copper
Severe protein deficiency

Myelodysplastic
Myelodysplasia
Aplastic anemia
Congenital bone marrow failure

Other
Congenital
Cyclic
Idiopathic
Autoimmune

Andrew Smith, MD and Erin Bassett-Novoa, MD

Newburger PE, Dale DC. Evaluation and management of patients with isolated neutropenia. *Semin Hematol.* 2013;50(3):198–206.

NEVUS, ABNORMAL

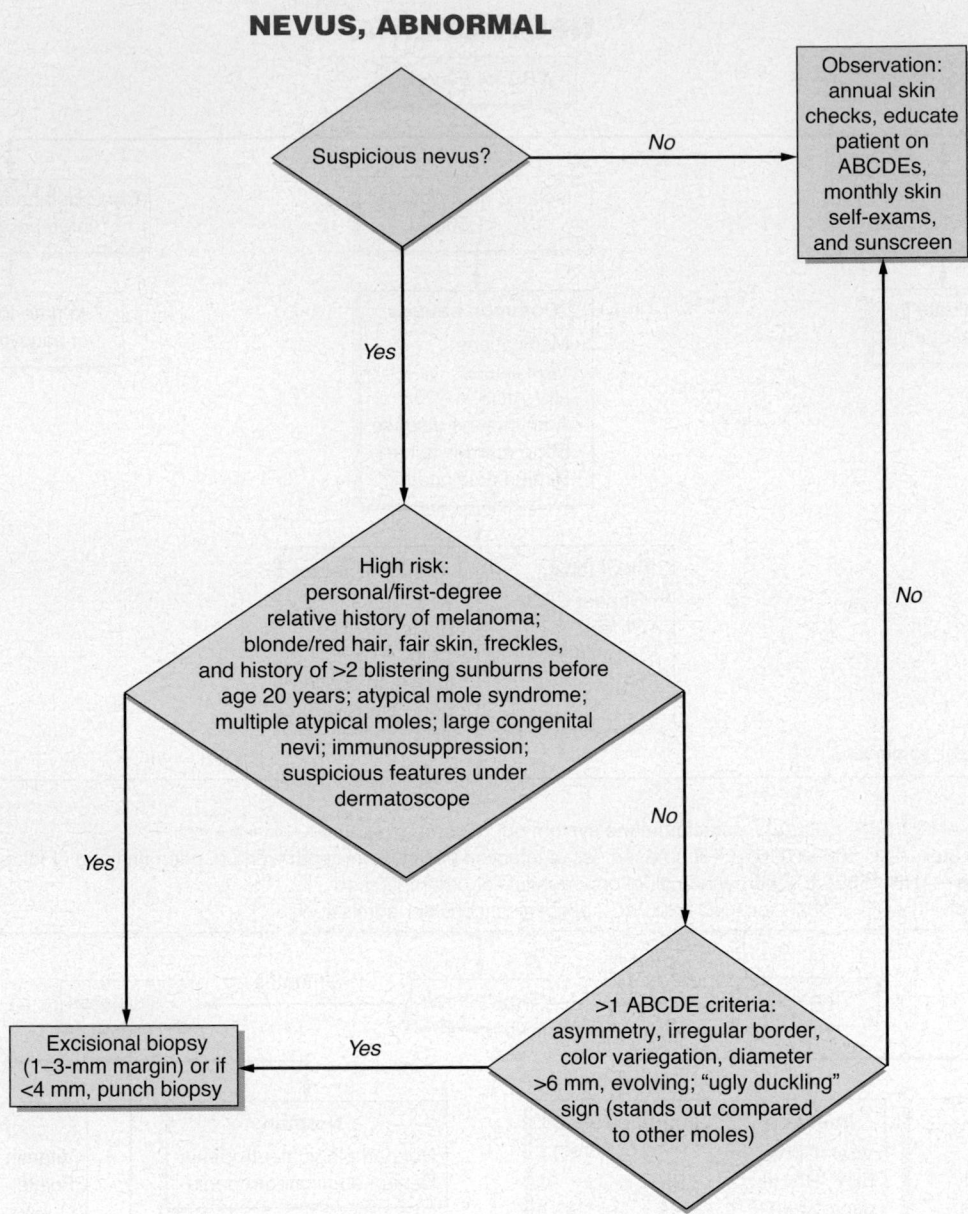

Amy Okpaku, DO

Perkins A, Duffy RL. Atypical moles: diagnosis and management. *Am Fam Physician*. 2015;91(11):762–767.

PAIN, CHRONIC

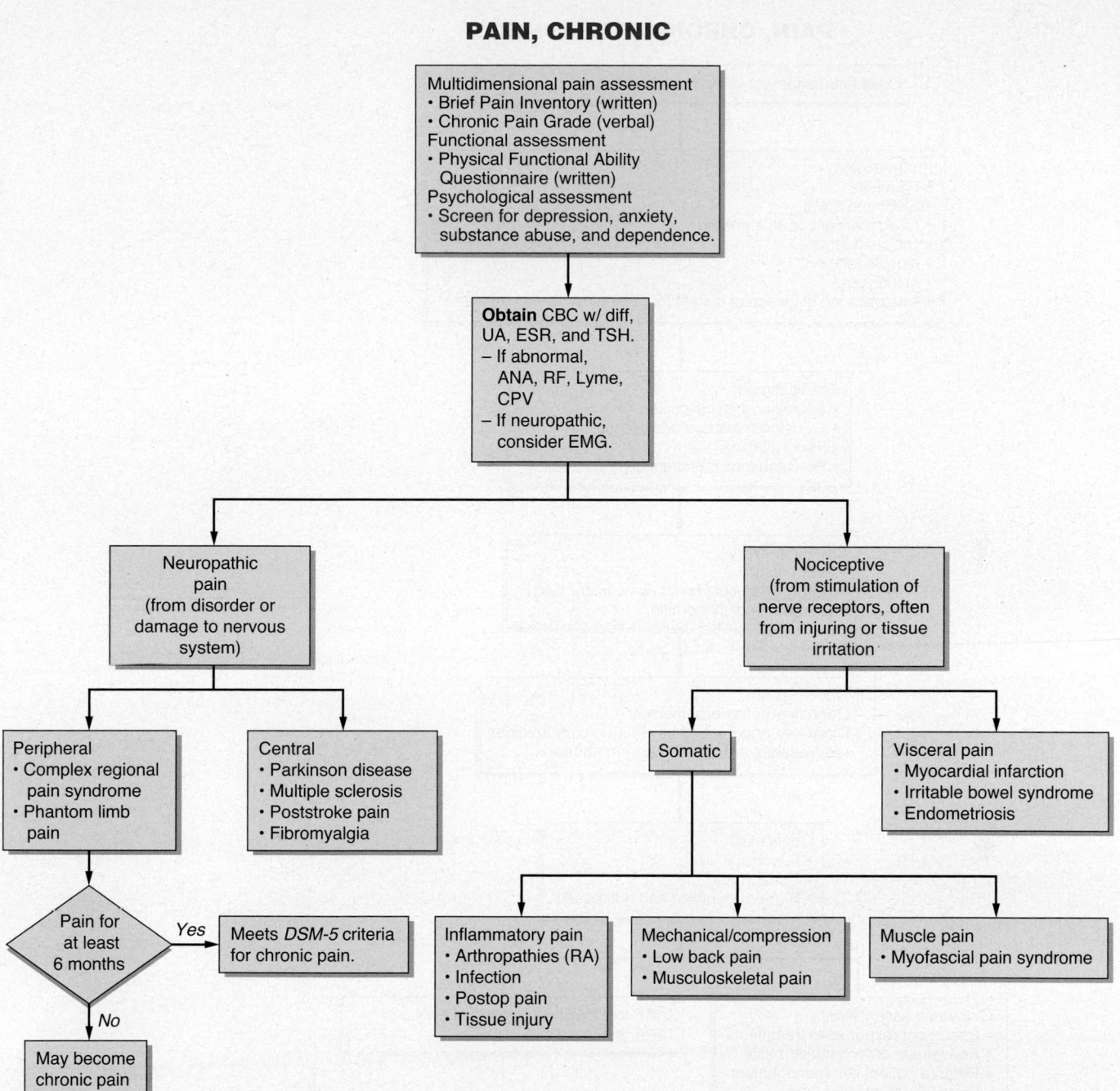

Multidimensional pain assessment
• Brief Pain Inventory (written)
• Chronic Pain Grade (verbal)
Functional assessment
• Physical Functional Ability Questionnaire (written)
Psychological assessment
• Screen for depression, anxiety, substance abuse, and dependence.

Obtain CBC w/ diff, UA, ESR, and TSH.
– If abnormal, ANA, RF, Lyme, CPV
– If neuropathic, consider EMG.

Neuropathic pain (from disorder or damage to nervous system)

Nociceptive (from stimulation of nerve receptors, often from injuring or tissue irritation

Peripheral
• Complex regional pain syndrome
• Phantom limb pain

Central
• Parkinson disease
• Multiple sclerosis
• Poststroke pain
• Fibromyalgia

Somatic

Visceral pain
• Myocardial infarction
• Irritable bowel syndrome
• Endometriosis

Pain for at least 6 months — *Yes* → Meets *DSM-5* criteria for chronic pain.

No

May become chronic pain

Inflammatory pain
• Arthropathies (RA)
• Infection
• Postop pain
• Tissue injury

Mechanical/compression
• Low back pain
• Musculoskeletal pain

Muscle pain
• Myofascial pain syndrome

Ashik Lawrence, MD, Anubhav Kaul, MD, and Margaret Seaver, MD, MPH

Institute for Clinical Systems Improvement. *Health Care Guideline: Assessment and Management of Chronic Pain.* 5th ed. Bloomington, MN: Institute of Clinical System Improvement; 2011.

PAIN, CHRONIC, TREATMENT

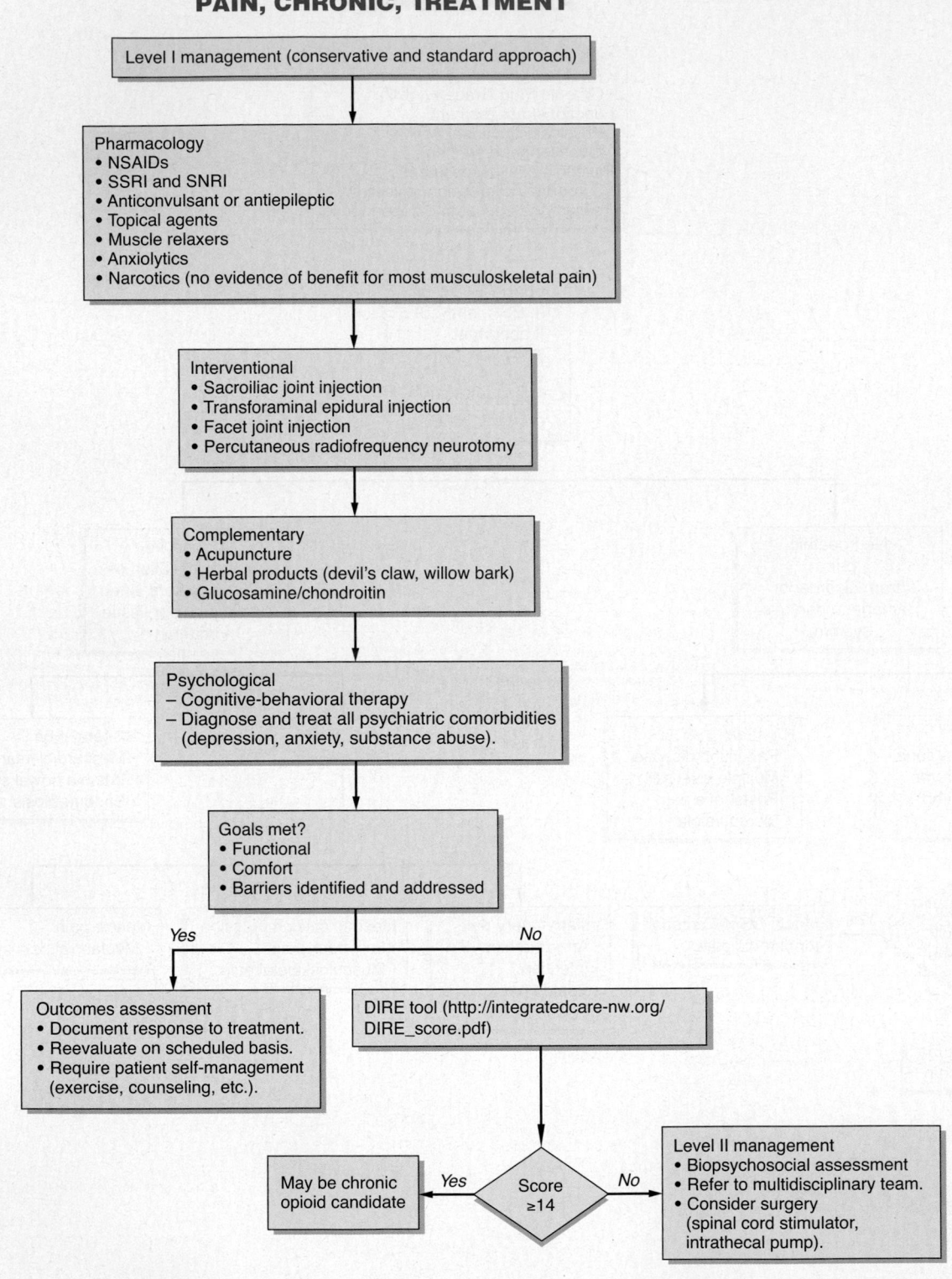

Ashik Lawrence, MD, Anubhav Kaul, MD, and Margaret Seaver, MD, MPH

Institute for Clinical Systems Improvement. *Health Care Guideline: Assessment and Management of Chronic Pain.* 5th ed. Bloomington, MN: Institute of Clinical System Improvement; 2011.

PALPABLE BREAST MASS

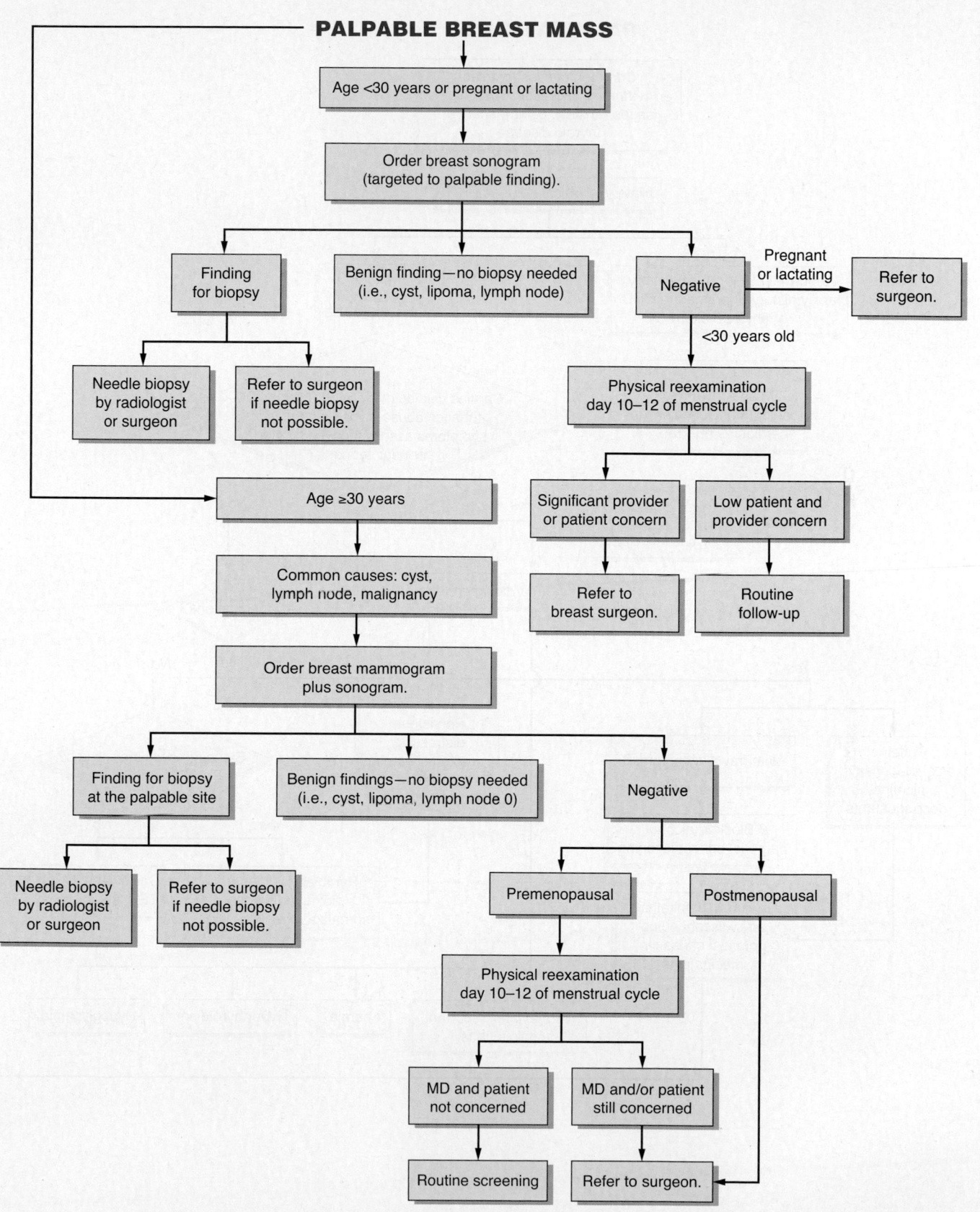

Lindsay Petersen, MD and Andrea Madrigrano, MD

Salzman B, Fleegle S, Tully AS. Common breast problems. *Am Fam Physician*. 2012;86(4):343–349.

PALPITATIONS

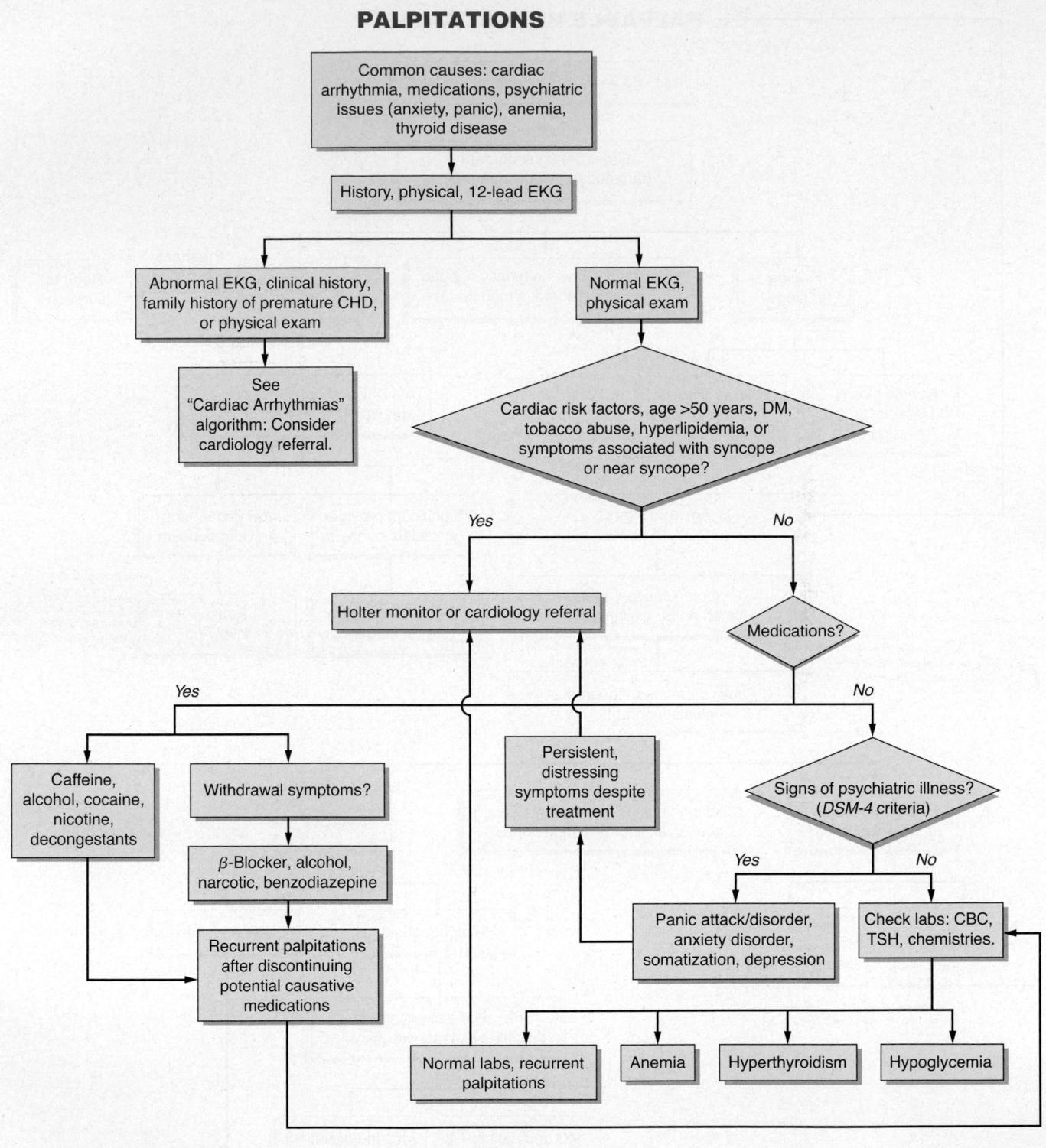

Common causes: cardiac arrhythmia, medications, psychiatric issues (anxiety, panic), anemia, thyroid disease

History, physical, 12-lead EKG

Abnormal EKG, clinical history, family history of premature CHD, or physical exam

See "Cardiac Arrhythmias" algorithm: Consider cardiology referral.

Normal EKG, physical exam

Cardiac risk factors, age >50 years, DM, tobacco abuse, hyperlipidemia, or symptoms associated with syncope or near syncope?

Yes   *No*

Holter monitor or cardiology referral

Medications?

Yes

No

Caffeine, alcohol, cocaine, nicotine, decongestants

Withdrawal symptoms?

β-Blocker, alcohol, narcotic, benzodiazepine

Recurrent palpitations after discontinuing potential causative medications

Persistent, distressing symptoms despite treatment

Signs of psychiatric illness? (*DSM-4* criteria)

Yes   *No*

Panic attack/disorder, anxiety disorder, somatization, depression

Check labs: CBC, TSH, chemistries.

Normal labs, recurrent palpitations

Anemia

Hyperthyroidism

Hypoglycemia

Abbott Cotton Widdicombe, MD and Frank J. Domino, MD

Wexler RK, Pleister A, Raman S. Outpatient approach to palpitations. *Am Fam Physician*. 2011;84(1):63–69.

PAP, NORMAL AND ABNORMAL IN NONPREGNANT WOMEN AGES 25 YEARS AND OLDER

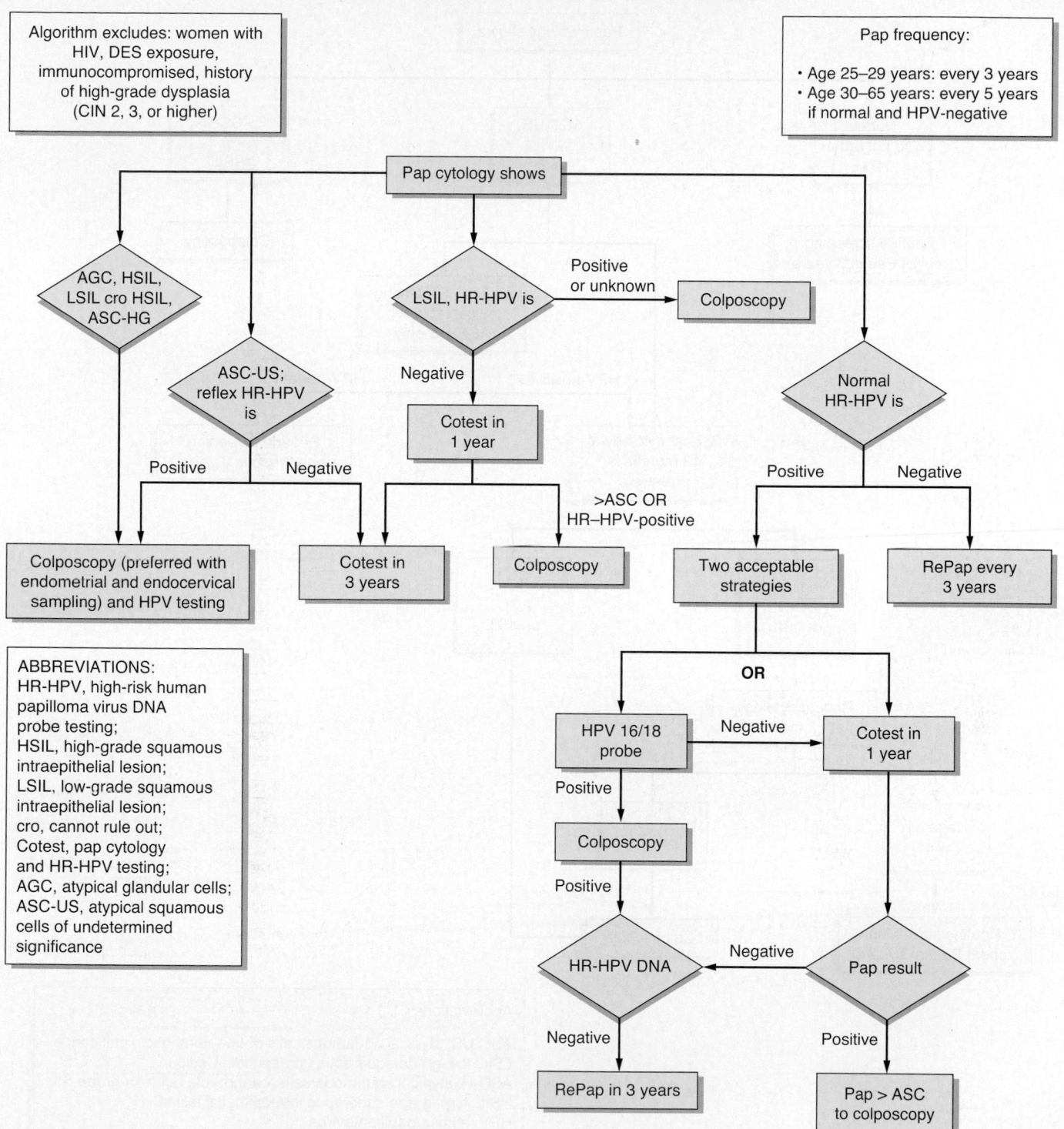

Algorithm excludes: women with HIV, DES exposure, immunocompromised, history of high-grade dysplasia (CIN 2, 3, or higher)

Pap frequency:
• Age 25–29 years: every 3 years
• Age 30–65 years: every 5 years if normal and HPV-negative

Pap cytology shows

AGC, HSIL, LSIL cro HSIL, ASC-HG

LSIL, HR-HPV is → Positive or unknown → Colposcopy

Negative

Normal HR-HPV is

ASC-US; reflex HR-HPV is

Cotest in 1 year

Positive   Negative

Positive   Negative

Colposcopy (preferred with endometrial and endocervical sampling) and HPV testing

Cotest in 3 years

Colposcopy

Two acceptable strategies

RePap every 3 years

>ASC OR HR–HPV-positive

ABBREVIATIONS:
HR-HPV, high-risk human papilloma virus DNA probe testing;
HSIL, high-grade squamous intraepithelial lesion;
LSIL, low-grade squamous intraepithelial lesion;
cro, cannot rule out;
Cotest, pap cytology and HR-HPV testing;
AGC, atypical glandular cells;
ASC-US, atypical squamous cells of undetermined significance

OR

HPV 16/18 probe → Negative → Cotest in 1 year

Positive

Colposcopy

Positive

HR-HPV DNA ← Negative ← Pap result

Negative

Positive

RePap in 3 years

Pap > ASC to colposcopy

Paul Pastor, MD

Adapted from American Society for Colposcopy and Cervical Pathology. Algorithms: updated consensus guidelines for managing abnormal cervical cancer screening tests and cancer precursors. http://www.asccp.org/Portals/9/docs/Algorithms%207.30.13.pdf. Accessed 2015.

PAP, NORMAL AND ABNORMAL IN WOMEN AGES 21–24 YEARS

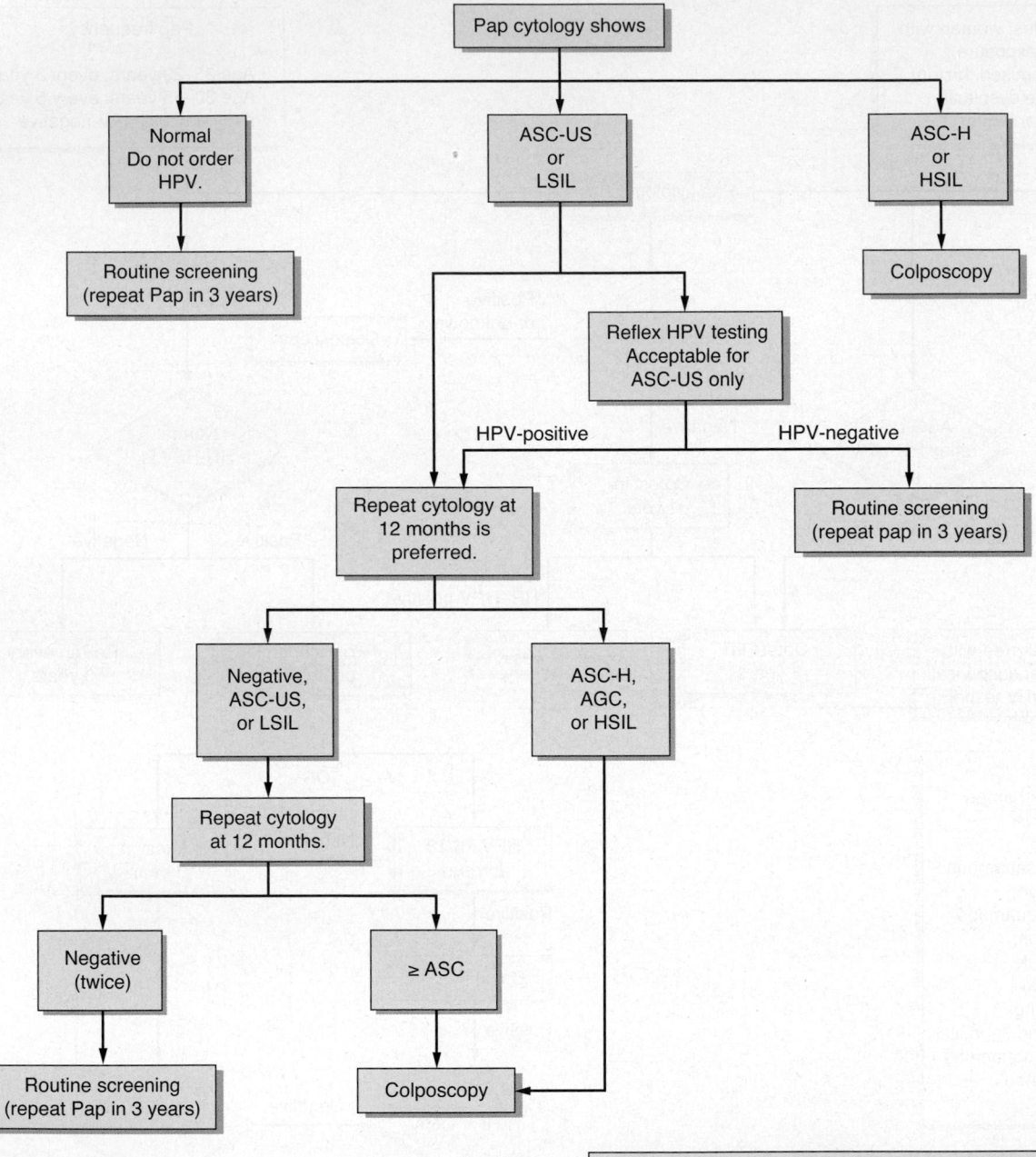

Susan L. Steffans, DO

American Society for Colposcopy and Cervical Pathology. Algorithms: updated consensus guidelines for management of abnormal cervical cancer screening tests and cancer precursors. http://www.asccp.org/Portals/9/docs/ASCCP%20Management%20Guidelines_August%202014.pdf. Accessed August 2015.

PARKINSON DISEASE, TREATMENT

Cardinal features
- Bradykinesia
- Resting tremor
- Rigidity
- Postural instability

Evaluate for underlying causes.

Drug-induced
- Antipsychotics
- Antidepressants (SSRI, TCA, MAOI)
- Levothyroxine
- Metoclopramide
- Diltiazem
- Medroxyprogesterone
- Valproate
- Lithium

Discontinue medication.

Parkinson disease

Alternative diagnosis
- Essential tremor
- Vascular parkinsonism
- Lewy body dementia
- Huntington disease
- Frontotemporal dementia with parkinsonism
- Progressive supranuclear palsy
- Spinocerebellar ataxia
- Multiple system atrophy
- Idiopathic basal ganglia calcification

Address underlying cause.

Goals of early management
- Symptom control
- Reduce functional disability.
- Slow disease progression.

- Encourage exercise, treat associated conditions.
- Offer physical therapy (gait, instability), speech therapy (speech volume), and occupational therapy (activities of daily living, safety, motor function).
- Initiate medications when symptoms significantly limit patient activities.

Motor symptoms

Nonmotor symptoms

Early disease
Dopamine agonist monotheraphy:
- Bromocriptine
- Pergolide
- Pramipexole
- Ropinirole

Late disease
Levodopa/carbidopa +/– dopamine agonist

Disease progression:
Dyskinesias
Motor fluctuations
Increased "off time"

Consider neurology referral.

Adjunct medication:
- MAO B inhibitors (rasagiline, selegiline)
- COMT inhibitors (entacapone)
- Apomorphine

Severe disease or unresponsive to medication:
Consider surgical referral for deep brain stimulation with use of implanted electrodes.

Sleep disturbance
- Sleep hygiene
- Change to levodopa/carbidopa (consider qHS).
- Add methylphenidate.
- Minimize dangerous activities (driving).

Autonomic dysfunction
- Erectile dysfunction: sildenafil
- Constipation: polyethylene glycol
- Drooling: Botox, glycopyrrolate

Psychiatric disorder
- Depression without cognitive impairment: TCA
- Psychosis: clozapine or quetiapine

Dementia
- Discontinue meds that contribute to cognitive impairment (dopaminergic or anticholinergic).
- Donezepil versus rivastigmine

Sarah Coles, MD and William Dabbs, MD

Gazewood JD, Richards DR, Clebak K. Parkinson disease: an update. *Am Fam Physician.* 2013;87(4):267–273.

PEDIATRIC EXANTHEMS, DIAGNOSTIC

URI symptoms present?

No

Roseola (sixth disease, exanthem subitum)
- Rash: erythematous maculopapular rash develops as fever resolves; starts on trunk and progresses to neck, extremities (rarely), face
- Prodrome: fever
- Enanthem: erythematous macules on soft palate
- Peak prevalence: 7–13 months

Yes

Enanthem (involvement of mucous membranes)?

No — **Vesicular?**

Yes — **Vesicular?**

No

Erythema infectiosum (fifth disease)
- Rash: intensely red malar rash "slapped cheek" followed in 1–2 days by reticular erythematous maculopapular rash on trunk, extremities, and buttocks; recrudescence can last up to months.
- Prodrome: generally mild, may have 1–4 days of headache, chills, URI symptoms
- Enanthem: none

Yes

Varicella (chickenpox)
- Rash: Macules form on trunk and spread to face and extremities; progress quickly in clusters to papules then tear-dropped shaped vesicles ("dew drops on a rose petal") that crust over or umbilicate
- Prodrome: 1–2 days of fever, malaise, anorexia
- Enanthem: Rarely, vesicles can lead to erosions of hard palate.

No

Yes

Coxsackie (hand-foot-mouth disease)
- Rash: Erythematous macules and papules ~2–3 mm found on palmar surface of hand, plantar surface of feet, and oral mucosa; progresses quickly through vesicular phase to form central gray ulcer
- Prodrome: 12–36 hours of cough, fever, malaise, anorexia, abdominal pain
- Enanthem: occurs with exanthem as painful ulcerative lesions commonly found on tongue, hard palate, and buccal mucosa

Koplik spots (white papules on buccal mucosa)?

No

Fast-spreading rash?

No

Rubella (third disease, German measles)
- Rash: erythematous maculopapular rash with downward progression from face
- Prodrome: 1–7 days of malaise, painful lymphadenopathy
- Enanthem: Forchheimer spots (petechia on soft palate)

Yes

Scarlet fever (second disease)
- Rash: rapidly progressing erythematous macules and pinpoint, blanchable papules ("goose pimples") with sandpaper texture, greatest intensity at skin folds occurring almost simultaneously with fever
- Prodrome: 1–2 days of fever, sore throat, vomiting, abdominal pain
- Enanthem: progression from white to red strawberry tongue
- Perform rapid strep testing, a throat culture, and initiate treatment.

Yes

Measles (first disease, rubeola)
- Rash: erythematous maculopapular rash (developing as fever progresses) with downward progression from face and brownish hue during resolution
- Prodrome: 3–4 days of conjunctivitis, coryza, fever, cough
- Enanthem: Koplik spots

Phillip Fournier, MD

Dyer JA. Childhood viral exanthems. *Pediatr Ann.* 2007;36(1):21–29.

PELVIC PAIN

Meredith Gray, MD and Isaiah Johnson, MD

Howard FM. Chronic pelvic pain. *Obstet Gynecol*. 2003;101(3):594–611.

POISON EXPOSURE AND TREATMENT
POISON EXPOSURE

Personal protective equipment; secure airway, breathing, circulation.
*Consider prolonged resuscitation effort (60 minutes) because intact neurologic survival is possible.

Check blood sugar (treat with 1 amp of D50); administer thiamine (100 mg IV/IM) and naloxone (0.4–2.0 mg q2–3min) if unresponsive.

Seizure control
1st-line benzodiazepines (BZD), 2nd-line barbiturates, avoid phenytoin.
Consider lorazepam 4 mg or diazepam 8 mg IV then phenobarbital 10–20 mg/kg IV or propofol 1 mg/kg IV.
*Pyridoxine up to 5 g IV if suspect isoniazid or mushroom poisoning

Correct hyperthermia (antipyretics ineffective).
Evaporative cooling, ice water immersion, ice packing, gastric lavage, peritoneal lavage

Collateral history from patient, family, or EMS; thorough physical exam

Contact Poison Control Center at 800-222-1222.

Initial workup: electrocardiogram, Tylenol level, ASA level, urinalysis with pH, hepatic function panel, comprehensive metabolic panel, pregnancy test (female), lactate, coagulation blood tests, salicylates, serum osmolality, serum ethanol level, blood gas (arterial or venous), chest x-ray, creatine kinase, carboxyhemoglobin, expanded urine drug screen

Consider drug immunoassay and drug levels for the following if indicated: digoxin, valproic acid, methotrexate, theophylline, carbamazepine, iron, lithium, phenobarbital, phenytoin, carbon monoxide, methemoglobin.

Bicarbonate for severe metabolic acidosis or widened QRS interval
*Instructions for drip below—titrate infusion to a target serum pH of 7.45–7.50.

GI decontamination only if supportive care not satisfactory and airway is secure. Consider activated charcoal 1 g/kg PO × 1 within an hour of ingestion or whole-bowel irrigation with polyethylene glycol at 1–2 L/hr via NGT.

Enhanced clearance with dialysis (aspirin, methanol, ethylene glycol, lithium, theophylline, isoniazid) or with urine alkalinization (urine pH >7.5)
*Instructions for drip below—titrate infusion to a target urine pH of >7.50.

Go to "Poison Treatment" algorithm.

POISON TREATMENT

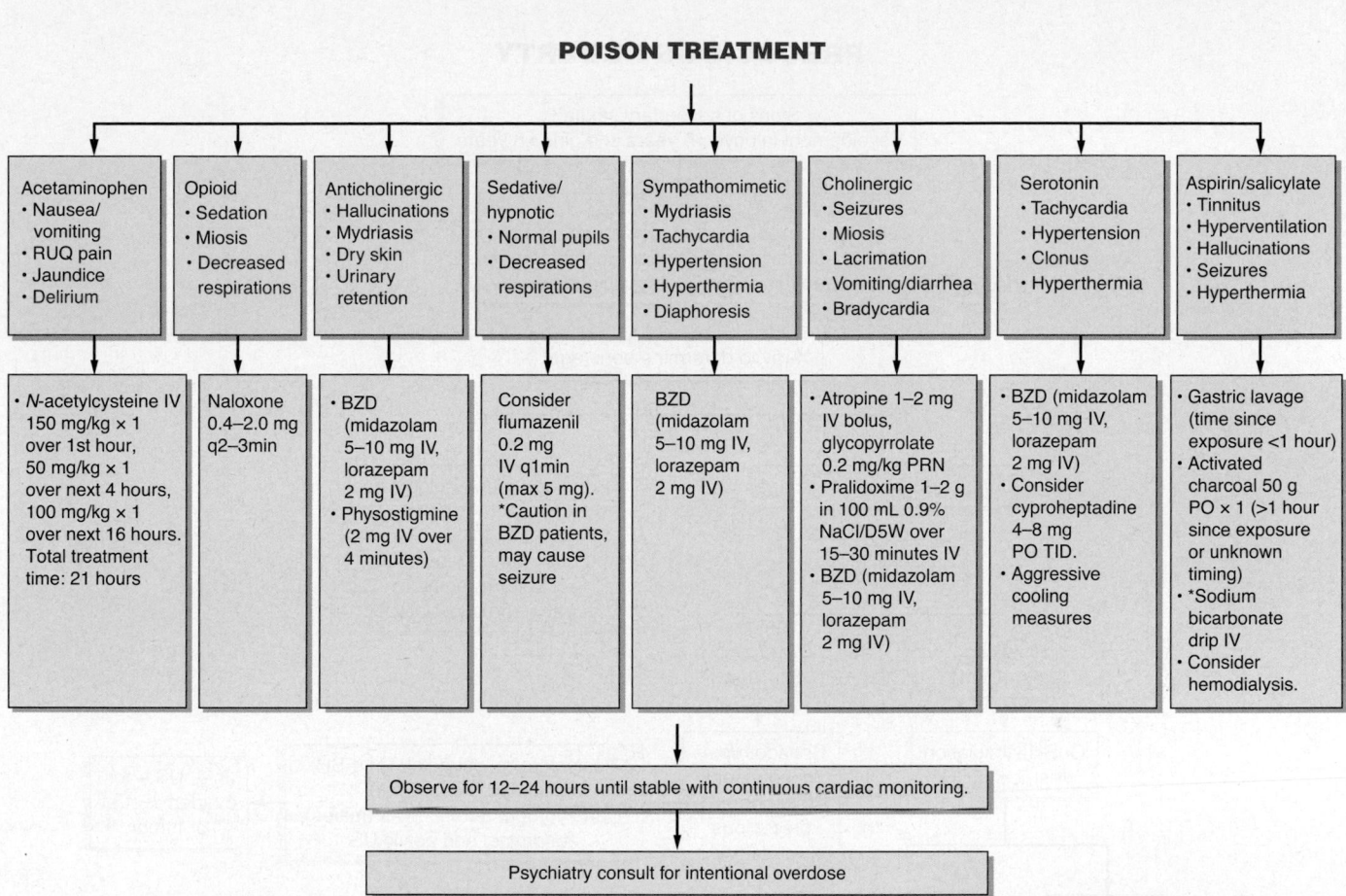

Acetaminophen
- Nausea/vomiting
- RUQ pain
- Jaundice
- Delirium

- *N*-acetylcysteine IV 150 mg/kg × 1 over 1st hour, 50 mg/kg × 1 over next 4 hours, 100 mg/kg × 1 over next 16 hours. Total treatment time: 21 hours

Opioid
- Sedation
- Miosis
- Decreased respirations

- Naloxone 0.4–2.0 mg q2–3min

Anticholinergic
- Hallucinations
- Mydriasis
- Dry skin
- Urinary retention

- BZD (midazolam 5–10 mg IV, lorazepam 2 mg IV)
- Physostigmine (2 mg IV over 4 minutes)

Sedative/hypnotic
- Normal pupils
- Decreased respirations

- Consider flumazenil 0.2 mg IV q1min (max 5 mg). *Caution in BZD patients, may cause seizure

Sympathomimetic
- Mydriasis
- Tachycardia
- Hypertension
- Hyperthermia
- Diaphoresis

- BZD (midazolam 5–10 mg IV, lorazepam 2 mg IV)

Cholinergic
- Seizures
- Miosis
- Lacrimation
- Vomiting/diarrhea
- Bradycardia

- Atropine 1–2 mg IV bolus, glycopyrrolate 0.2 mg/kg PRN
- Pralidoxime 1–2 g in 100 mL 0.9% NaCl/D5W over 15–30 minutes IV
- BZD (midazolam 5–10 mg IV, lorazepam 2 mg IV)

Serotonin
- Tachycardia
- Hypertension
- Clonus
- Hyperthermia

- BZD (midazolam 5–10 mg IV, lorazepam 2 mg IV)
- Consider cyproheptadine 4–8 mg PO TID.
- Aggressive cooling measures

Aspirin/salicylate
- Tinnitus
- Hyperventilation
- Hallucinations
- Seizures
- Hyperthermia

- Gastric lavage (time since exposure <1 hour)
- Activated charcoal 50 g PO × 1 (>1 hour since exposure or unknown timing)
- *Sodium bicarbonate drip IV
- Consider hemodialysis.

Observe for 12–24 hours until stable with continuous cardiac monitoring.

Psychiatry consult for intentional overdose

*To mix a bicarbonate drip: 150 mEq (3 amps) NaHCO$_3$ in 1 L of D5W, then start at a rate of 150–200 mL/hr.

Pediatric dosing (adult doses in algorithm)
- Activated charcoal (0.5–1.0 g/kg PO)
- Atropine (0.02 mg/kg IV)
- Bicarbonate (1–2 mEq/kg IV*)
- Chlorpromazine (not recommended)
- Cyproheptadine (0.25 mg/kg/day divided BID or TID)
- Dextrose (2.5 mL/kg of 10% or 1 mL/kg of 25% IV)
- Flumazenil (5 μg/kg IV)
- Glycopyrrolate (4 μg/kg IV)

- Lorazepam (0.05–0.1 mg/kg IV)
- Midazolam (0.1 mg/kg IV)
- Phenobarbital (10–20 mg/kg IV)
- Physostigmine (10–30 μg/kg IV)
- Polyethylene glycol (250–500 mL/hr PO/NG)
- Pralidoxime (20–40 mg/kg IV)
- Pyridoxine (same as adults)
- Naloxone (0.1 mg/kg IV q2–3min)
- Thiamine (not routinely given)

Andrew Romney, DO and Lee T. Church, MD

Frithsen IL, Simpson WM Jr. Recognition and management of acute medication poisoning. *Am Fam Physician*. 2010;81(3):316–323.

PRECOCIOUS PUBERTY

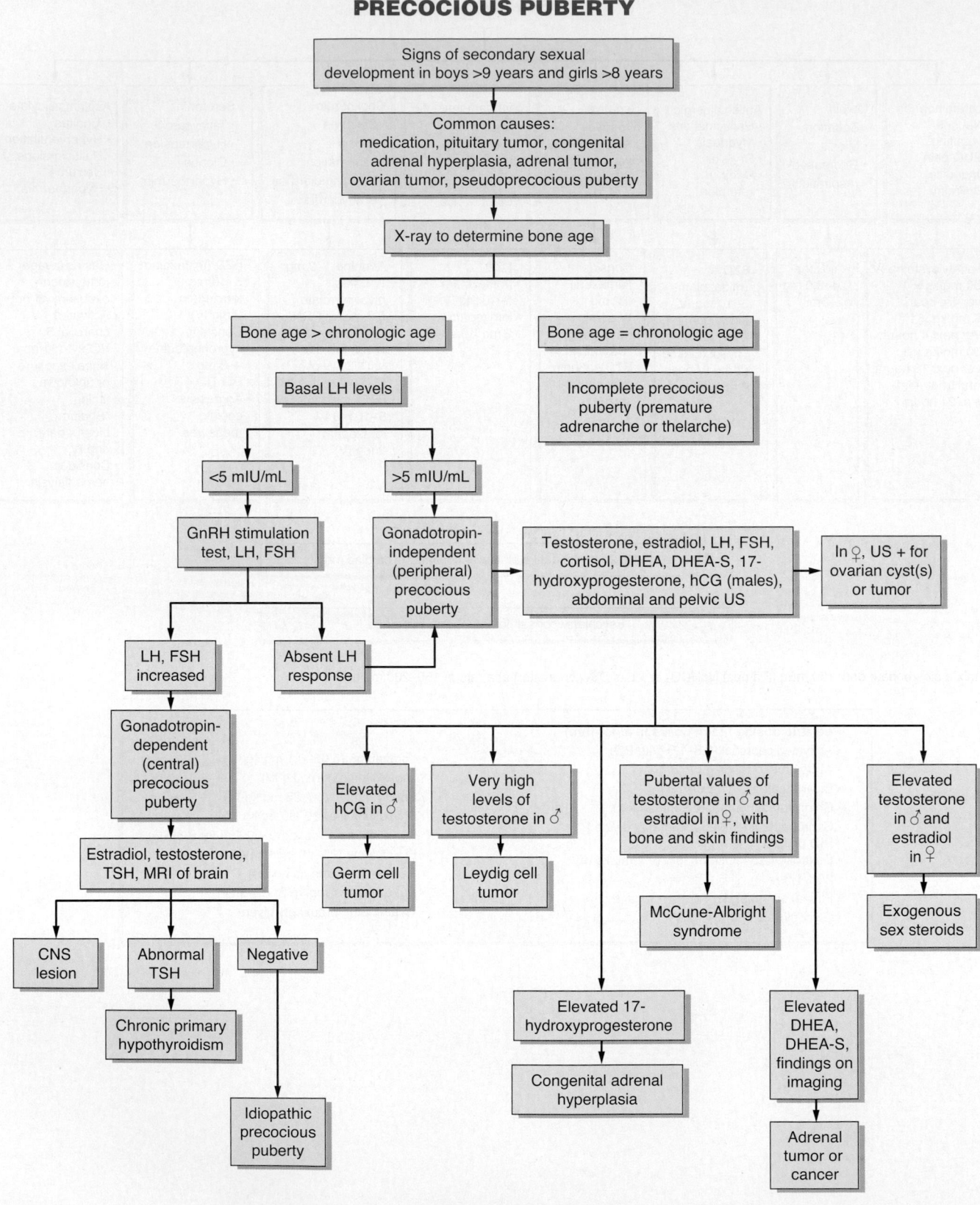

Nicole Shields, MD

Berberoğlu M. Precocious puberty and normal variant puberty: definiton, etiology, diagnosis and current management. *J Clin Res Pediatr Endocrinol.* 2009;1(4):164–174.

PREOPERATIVE EVALUATION OF NONCARDIAC SURGICAL PATIENT

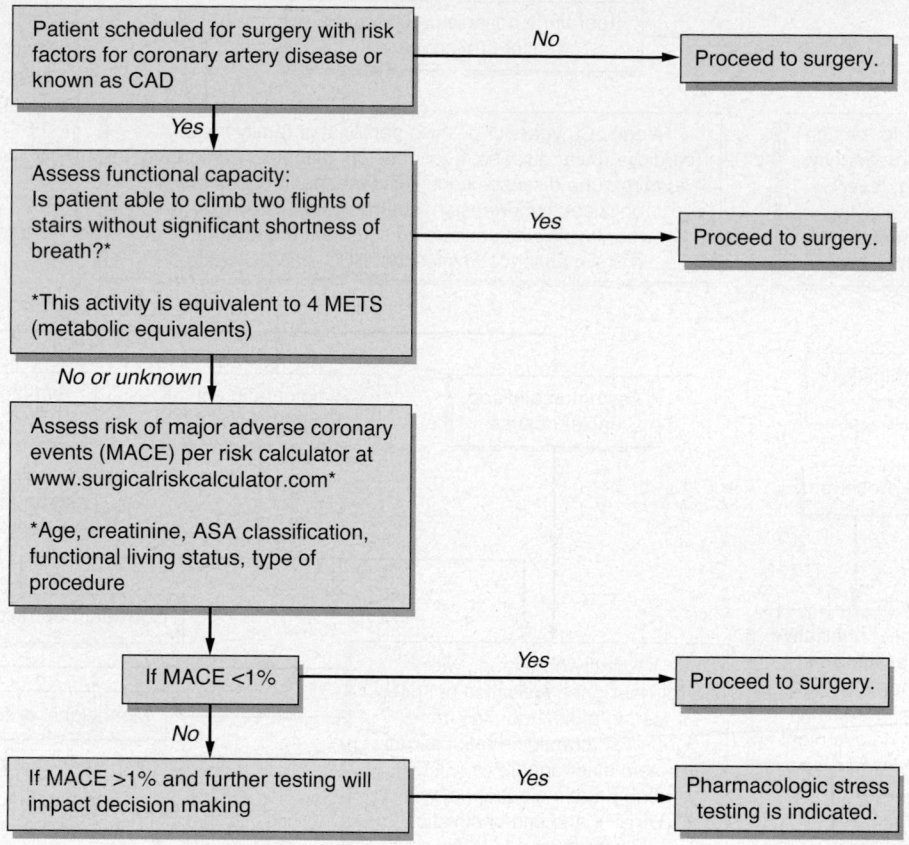

Andrew Grimes, MD and Stacy Jones, MD

Ghadimi K, Thompson A. Update on perioperative care of the cardiac patient for noncardiac surgery. *Curr Opin Anaesthesiol.* 2015;28(3):342–348.

PROTEINURIA

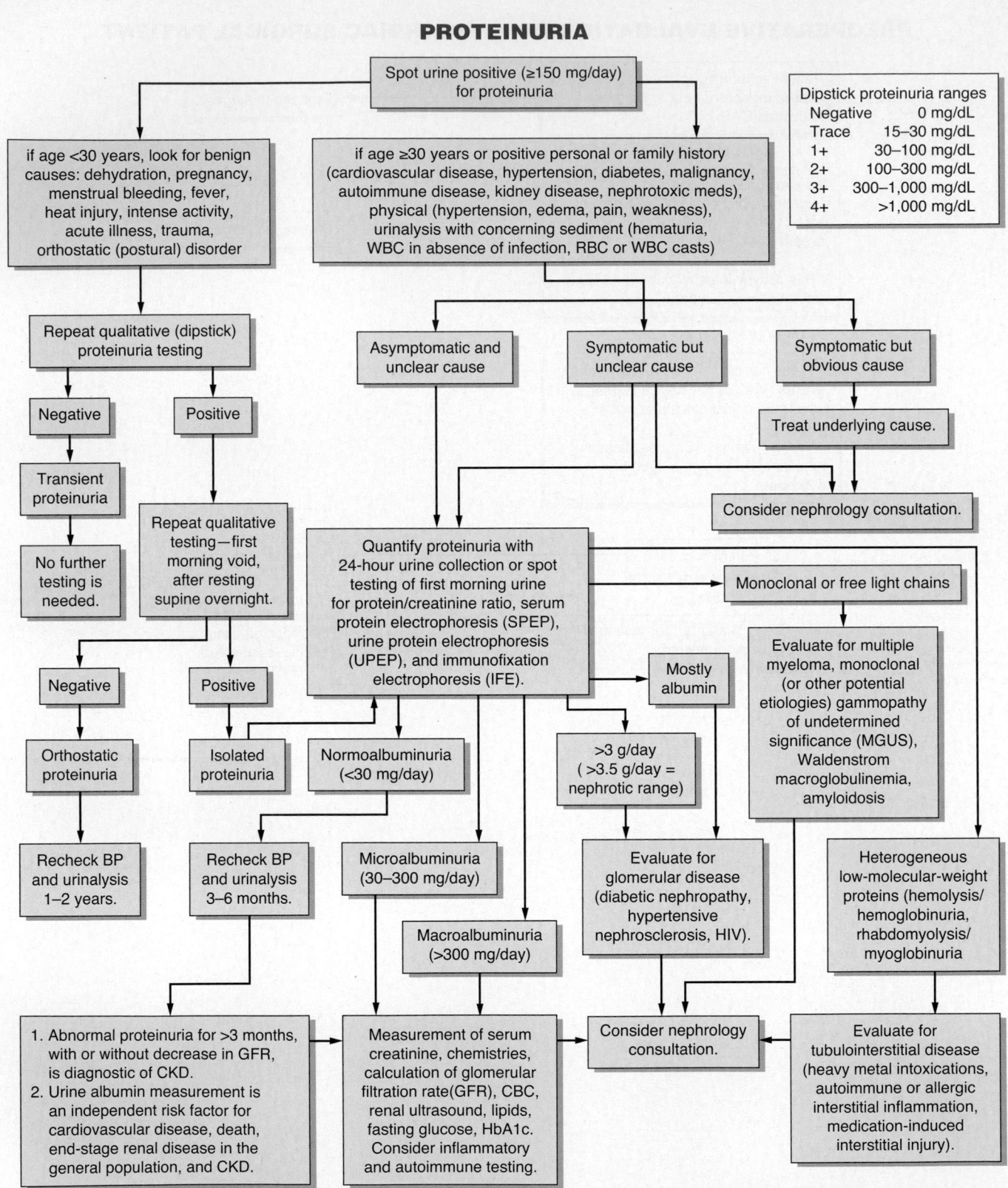

Spot urine positive (≥150 mg/day) for proteinuria

Dipstick proteinuria ranges
Negative   0 mg/dL
Trace   15–30 mg/dL
1+   30–100 mg/dL
2+   100–300 mg/dL
3+   300–1,000 mg/dL
4+   >1,000 mg/dL

if age <30 years, look for benign causes: dehydration, pregnancy, menstrual bleeding, fever, heat injury, intense activity, acute illness, trauma, orthostatic (postural) disorder

if age ≥30 years or positive personal or family history (cardiovascular disease, hypertension, diabetes, malignancy, autoimmune disease, kidney disease, nephrotoxic meds), physical (hypertension, edema, pain, weakness), urinalysis with concerning sediment (hematuria, WBC in absence of infection, RBC or WBC casts)

Repeat qualitative (dipstick) proteinuria testing

Asymptomatic and unclear cause

Symptomatic but unclear cause

Symptomatic but obvious cause

Negative

Positive

Treat underlying cause.

Transient proteinuria

Repeat qualitative testing—first morning void, after resting supine overnight.

Consider nephrology consultation.

No further testing is needed.

Quantify proteinuria with 24-hour urine collection or spot testing of first morning urine for protein/creatinine ratio, serum protein electrophoresis (SPEP), urine protein electrophoresis (UPEP), and immunofixation electrophoresis (IFE).

Monoclonal or free light chains

Negative

Positive

Mostly albumin

Evaluate for multiple myeloma, monoclonal (or other potential etiologies) gammopathy of undetermined significance (MGUS), Waldenstrom macroglobulinemia, amyloidosis

Orthostatic proteinuria

Isolated proteinuria

Normoalbuminuria (<30 mg/day)

>3 g/day (>3.5 g/day = nephrotic range)

Recheck BP and urinalysis 1–2 years.

Recheck BP and urinalysis 3–6 months.

Microalbuminuria (30–300 mg/day)

Evaluate for glomerular disease (diabetic nephropathy, hypertensive nephrosclerosis, HIV).

Heterogeneous low-molecular-weight proteins (hemolysis/ hemoglobinuria, rhabdomyolysis/ myoglobinuria

Macroalbuminuria (>300 mg/day)

1. Abnormal proteinuria for >3 months, with or without decrease in GFR, is diagnostic of CKD.
2. Urine albumin measurement is an independent risk factor for cardiovascular disease, death, end-stage renal disease in the general population, and CKD.

Measurement of serum creatinine, chemistries, calculation of glomerular filtration rate(GFR), CBC, renal ultrasound, lipids, fasting glucose, HbA1c. Consider inflammatory and autoimmune testing.

Consider nephrology consultation.

Evaluate for tubulointerstitial disease (heavy metal intoxications, autoimmune or allergic interstitial inflammation, medication-induced interstitial injury).

John M. Doan, DO and Robert K. Persons, DO

BMJ Best Practice. Assessment of proteinuria. http://us.bestpractice.bmj.com/best-practice/monograph/875.html Updated September 17, 2014. Accessed July 20, 2015.

PULMONARY EMBOLISM, DIAGNOSIS

Assess Pulmonary Embolism Rule Out Criteria (PERC)
If any of the following are true, then the patient is considered PERC-positive:
1. Patient is >49 years.
2. Patient's pulse >99 beats/min
3. Patient's pulse oximetry reading <95% on room air
4. Patient with hemoptysis
5. Patient taking exogenous estrogen
6. Patient had a previous VTE diagnosis.
7. Patient had surgery or trauma, which required intubation or hospitalization in the last 4 weeks.
8. Patient has unilateral leg swelling of the calves.

Assess the Clinical Pretest Probability of Pulmonary Embolism
Clinical pretest probability
(CPTP—modified Wells PE Score)
Clinical signs — 3
Alternative Dx unlikely — 3
Heart rate >100 — 1.5
Immobilization previous 4 days — 1.5
Previous DVT/PE — 1.5
Hemoptysis — 1
Malignancy — 1

PE less likely <4
PE likely >4

Anticoagulation:
Immediate treatment: at least 5 days of therapy regardless of INR
- Low-molecular-weight heparin
- Unfractionated heparin
- Fondaparinux
- Overlap with vitamin K antagonist for 2 days once INR is 2.0–3.0

Long-term treatment >3 months (based on risk factors and severity of PE):
- Vitamin K antagonist
- Extended treatment: indefinite (depends on risk factors and severity of PE)

Oral anticoagulation:
- Dabigatran (requires 5–10 days of parenteral anticoagulation before initiation)
- Rivaroxaban
- Apixaban

Low-risk patients consider outpatient treatment (troponin, BNP, and TTE can help with risk stratification).

Erynn E. Elleby, MD and Lawrence M. Gibbs, MD, MSEd

Dupras D, Bluhm J, Felty C, et al. Institute for clinical systems improvement. Venous thromboembolism diagnosis and treatment. https://www.icsi.org/_asset/sw0pgp/vte.pdf. Updated January 2013.

A-99

PULMONARY EMBOLISM, TREATMENT

Probability of pulmonary embolism above treatment threshold

Coagulation contraindicated?
• Prior intracranial bleed
• Ischemic stroke <3 months
• Suspected aortic dissection
• Active bleeding diathesis
• Recent brain or spinal surgery
• Closed head or facial trauma

IVC filter ←── Yes

No ↓

Massive pulmonary embolism? (SBP <90 mm Hg for >15 minutes) ── Yes → Thrombolysis contraindicated? ── Yes →

No ↓

Benefits of thrombolysis outweigh risks based on evidence of following clinical factors:
1. Hemodynamic instability
2. Worse respiratory insufficiency
3. Severe RV strain
4. Major myocardial necrosis?

── Yes

No

Embolectomy, per local expertise

Thrombolysis contraindicated? No ↓

Thrombolysis

Clinical improvement? ── No

Consider fondaparinux, lepirudin, or argatroban (Caution use of lepirudin in liver disease; caution use of argatroban in kidney disease.) and vitamin K antagonist with at least 5 days of concomitant therapy and INR ≥2 × 24 hours prior to discontinuing parenteral product with a goal INR of 2–3. Alternatively, consider using a new oral anticoagulant (dabigatran, apixaban, rivaroxaban, or edoxaban) without need for parenteral bridging.

Yes ←── History of heparin-induced thrombocytopenia? ←── Yes ── Clinical improvement?

Ryan B. Feeney, PharmD and Frank M. Mazzotta, DO

Jaff MR, McMurtry MS, Archer SL, et al. Management of massive and submassive pulmonary embolism, iliofemoral deep vein thrombosis, and chronic thromboembolic pulmonary hypertension: a scientific statement from the American Heart Association. *Circulation.* 2011;123(16):1788–1830.

RASH, FOCAL

7 classes of topical steroids based on ability to constrict capillaries. Class I, strongest; class VII, weakest						
Class I	**Class II**	**Class III**	**Class IV**	**Class V**	**Class VI**	**Class VII**
Clobetasol propionate ointment, cream, 0.05% (Temovate)	Fluocinonide ointment, cream, gel 0.05% (Lidex)	Triamcinolone acetonide ointment, 0.1% (Aristocort A)	Triamcinolone acetonide cream, 0.1% (Kenalog)	Fluocinolone acetonide cream, 0.025% (Synalar)	Desonide cream, 0.05% (DesOwen)	
Betamethasone dipropionate ointment, cream, 0.05% (Diprolene, Diprosone)	Amcinonide ointment, 0.1% (Cyclocort)	Betamethasone valerate ointment, 0.01% (Valisone)	Mometasone furoate cream, 0.1% (Elocon)	Fluticasone propionate cream, 0.05% (Cutivate)	Prednicarbate 0.1% cream (Dermatop)	Hydrocortisone, 0.5%, 1%, 2.5% (Hytone)
Halobetasol propionate ointment, cream, 0.05% (Ultravate)	Desoximetasone ointment, cream, 0.25%; gel, 0.05% (Topicort)	Fluticasone propionate ointment, 0.05% (Cutivate)	Hydrocortisone valerate ointment, 0.2% (Westcort)	Hydrocortisone valerate cream, 0.2% (Westcort)	Alclometasone dipropionate ointment, cream, 0.05% (Aclovate)	

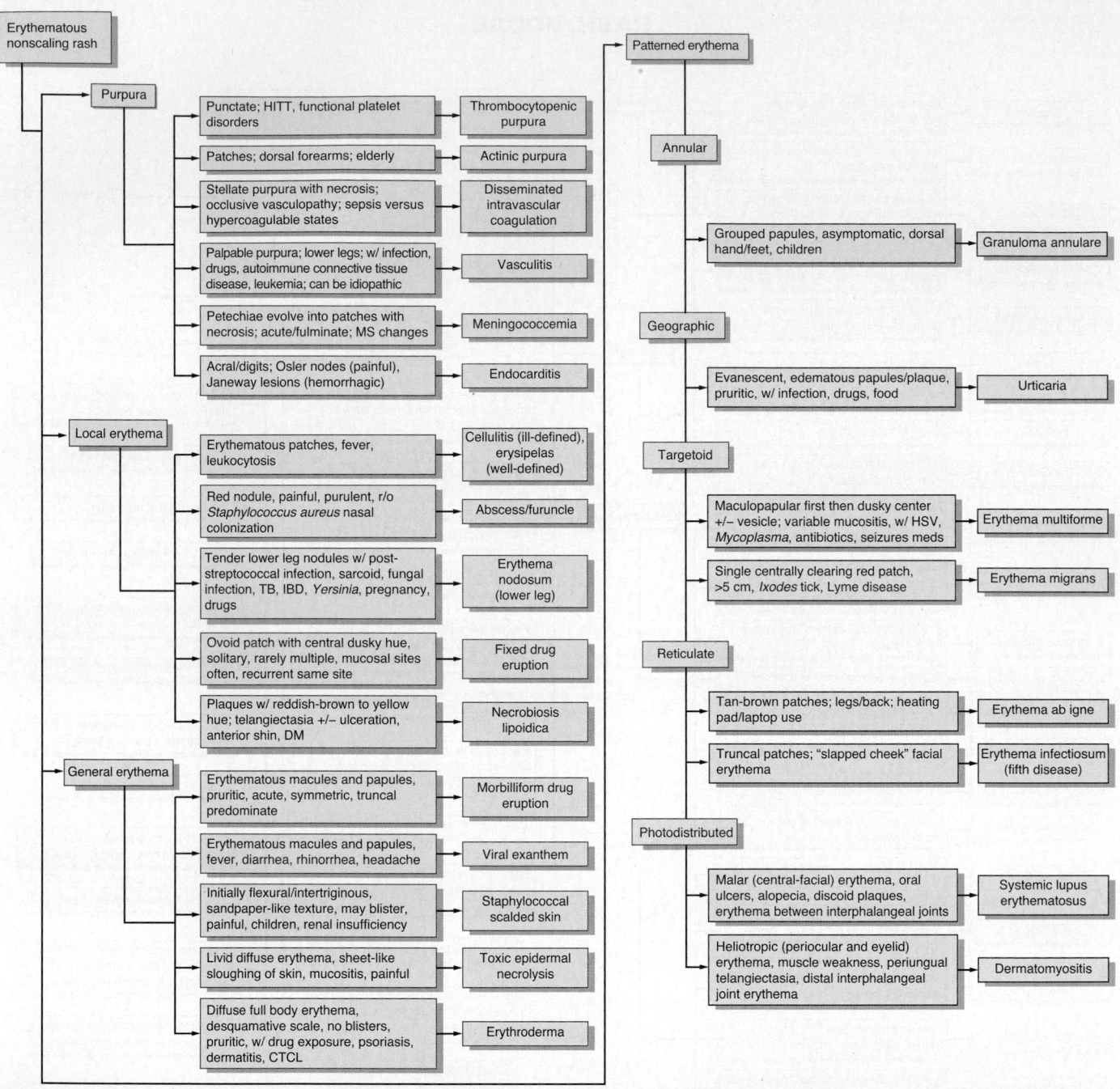

Erythematous nonscaling rash

Purpura
- Punctate; HITT, functional platelet disorders → Thrombocytopenic purpura
- Patches; dorsal forearms; elderly → Actinic purpura
- Stellate purpura with necrosis; occlusive vasculopathy; sepsis versus hypercoagulable states → Disseminated intravascular coagulation
- Palpable purpura; lower legs; w/ infection, drugs, autoimmune connective tissue disease, leukemia; can be idiopathic → Vasculitis
- Petechiae evolve into patches with necrosis; acute/fulminate; MS changes → Meningococcemia
- Acral/digits; Osler nodes (painful), Janeway lesions (hemorrhagic) → Endocarditis

Local erythema
- Erythematous patches, fever, leukocytosis → Cellulitis (ill-defined), erysipelas (well-defined)
- Red nodule, painful, purulent, r/o *Staphylococcus aureus* nasal colonization → Abscess/furuncle
- Tender lower leg nodules w/ post-streptococcal infection, sarcoid, fungal infection, TB, IBD, *Yersinia*, pregnancy, drugs → Erythema nodosum (lower leg)
- Ovoid patch with central dusky hue, solitary, rarely multiple, mucosal sites often, recurrent same site → Fixed drug eruption
- Plaques w/ reddish-brown to yellow hue; telangiectasia +/– ulceration, anterior shin, DM → Necrobiosis lipoidica

General erythema
- Erythematous macules and papules, pruritic, acute, symmetric, truncal predominate → Morbilliform drug eruption
- Erythematous macules and papules, fever, diarrhea, rhinorrhea, headache → Viral exanthem
- Initially flexural/intertriginous, sandpaper-like texture, may blister, painful, children, renal insufficiency → Staphylococcal scalded skin
- Livid diffuse erythema, sheet-like sloughing of skin, mucositis, painful → Toxic epidermal necrolysis
- Diffuse full body erythema, desquamative scale, no blisters, pruritic, w/ drug exposure, psoriasis, dermatitis, CTCL → Erythroderma

Patterned erythema

Annular
- Grouped papules, asymptomatic, dorsal hand/feet, children → Granuloma annulare

Geographic
- Evanescent, edematous papules/plaque, pruritic, w/ infection, drugs, food → Urticaria

Targetoid
- Maculopapular first then dusky center +/– vesicle; variable mucositis, w/ HSV, *Mycoplasma*, antibiotics, seizures meds → Erythema multiforme
- Single centrally clearing red patch, >5 cm, *Ixodes* tick, Lyme disease → Erythema migrans

Reticulate
- Tan-brown patches; legs/back; heating pad/laptop use → Erythema ab igne
- Truncal patches; "slapped cheek" facial erythema → Erythema infectiosum (fifth disease)

Photodistributed
- Malar (central-facial) erythema, oral ulcers, alopecia, discoid plaques, erythema between interphalangeal joints → Systemic lupus erythematosus
- Heliotropic (periocular and eyelid) erythema, muscle weakness, periungual telangiectasia, distal interphalangeal joint erythema → Dermatomyositis

7 classes of topical steroids based on ability to constrict capillaries. Class I, strongest; class VII, weakest						
Class I	**Class II**	**Class III**	**Class IV**	**Class V**	**Class VI**	**Class VII**
Clobetasol propionate ointment, cream, 0.05% (Temovate)	Fluocinonide ointment, cream, gel 0.05% (Lidex)	Triamcinolone acetonide ointment, 0.1% (Aristocort A)	Triamcinolone acetonide cream, 0.1% (Kenalog)	Fluocinolone acetonide cream, 0.025% (Synalar)	Desonide cream, 0.05% (Desowen)	
Betamethasone dipropionate ointment, cream, 0.05% (Diprolene, Diprosone)	Amcinonide ointment, 0.1% (Cyclocort)	Betamethasone valerate ointment, 0.01% (Valisone)	Mometasone furoate cream, 0.1% (Elocon)	Fluticasone propionate cream, 0.05% (Cutivate)	Prednicarbate 0.1% cream (Dermatop)	Hydrocortisone, 0.5%, 1%, 2.5% (Hytone)
Halobetasol propionate ointment, cream, 0.05% (Ultravate)	Desoximetasone ointment, cream, 0.25%; gel, 0.05% (Topicort)	Fluticasone propionate ointment, 0.05% (Cutivate)	Hydrocortisone valerate ointment, 0.2% (Westcort)	Hydrocortisone valerate cream, 0.2% (Westcort)	Alclometasone dipropionate ointment, cream, 0.05% (Aclovate)	

Brandon Kirsch, MD and Jason C. Sluzevich, MD

Ely JW, Seabury Stone M. The generalized rash: part I. Differential diagnosis. *Am Fam Physician*. 2010;81(6):726–734.

RECTAL BLEEDING AND HEMATOCHEZIA

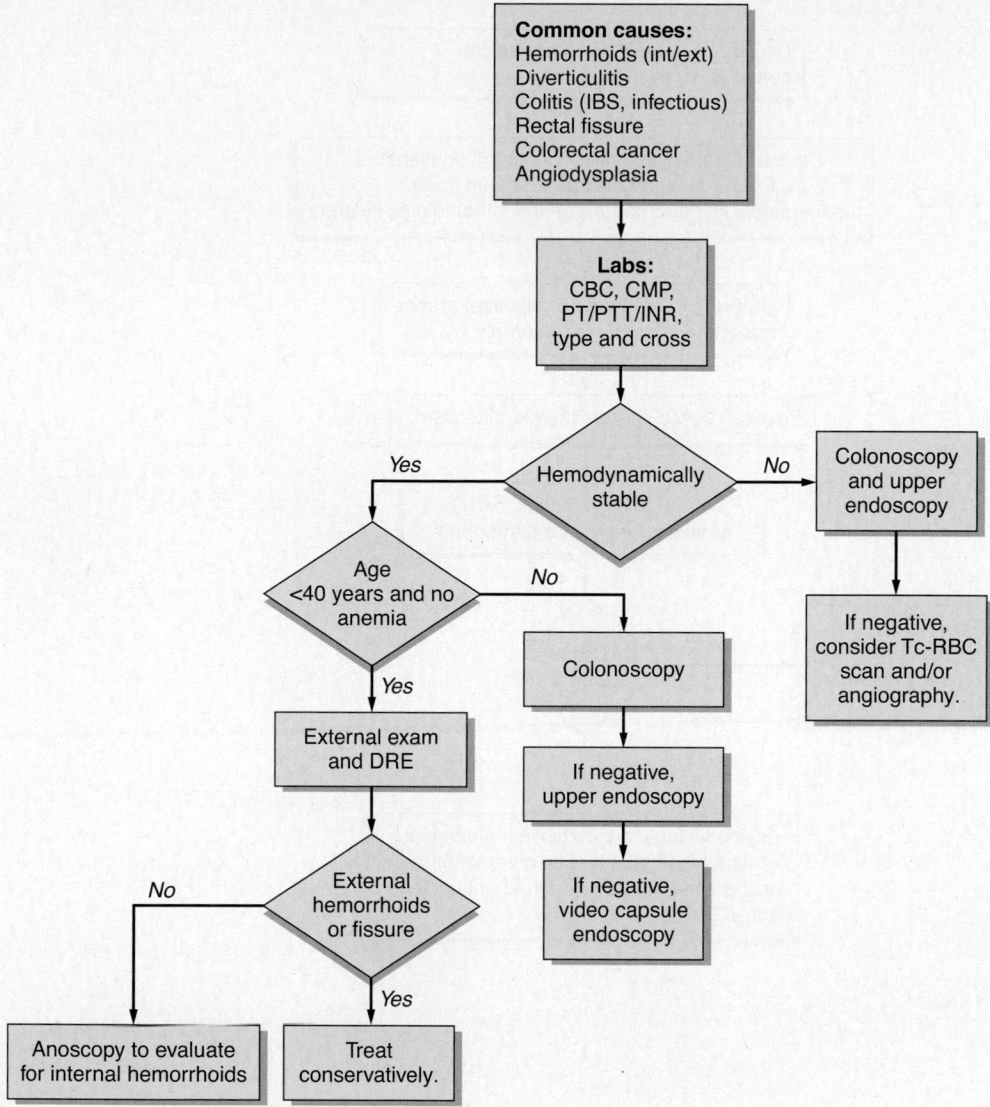

Common causes:
Hemorrhoids (int/ext)
Diverticulitis
Colitis (IBS, infectious)
Rectal fissure
Colorectal cancer
Angiodysplasia

Labs:
CBC, CMP,
PT/PTT/INR,
type and cross

Hemodynamically stable

Yes → Age <40 years and no anemia

No → Colonoscopy and upper endoscopy

Colonoscopy and upper endoscopy → If negative, consider Tc-RBC scan and/or angiography.

Age <40 years and no anemia — *No* → Colonoscopy

Age <40 years and no anemia — *Yes* → External exam and DRE

Colonoscopy → If negative, upper endoscopy → If negative, video capsule endoscopy

External exam and DRE → External hemorrhoids or fissure

External hemorrhoids or fissure — *No* → Anoscopy to evaluate for internal hemorrhoids

External hemorrhoids or fissure — *Yes* → Treat conservatively.

Mohammad Ansar Mughal, MD

Hoedema RE, Luchtefeld MA. The management of lower gastrointestinal hemorrhage. *Dis Colon Rectum*. 2005;48(11):2010–2024.

RECURRENT PREGNANCY LOSS

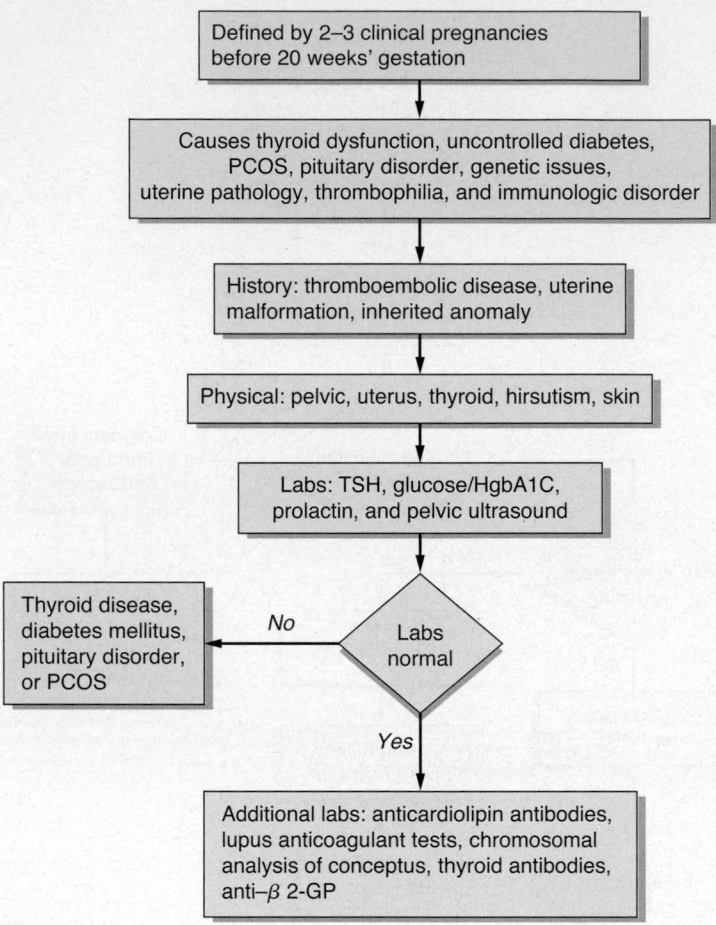

Defined by 2–3 clinical pregnancies before 20 weeks' gestation

↓

Causes thyroid dysfunction, uncontrolled diabetes, PCOS, pituitary disorder, genetic issues, uterine pathology, thrombophilia, and immunologic disorder

↓

History: thromboembolic disease, uterine malformation, inherited anomaly

↓

Physical: pelvic, uterus, thyroid, hirsutism, skin

↓

Labs: TSH, glucose/HgbA1C, prolactin, and pelvic ultrasound

↓

Labs normal

No → Thyroid disease, diabetes mellitus, pituitary disorder, or PCOS

Yes ↓

Additional labs: anticardiolipin antibodies, lupus anticoagulant tests, chromosomal analysis of conceptus, thyroid antibodies, anti–β 2-GP

Virginia Van Duyne, MD

Alijotas-Reig J, Garrido-Gimenez C. Current concepts and new trends in the diagnosis and management of recurrent miscarriage. *Obstet Gynecol Surv.* 2013;68(6):445–466.

RED EYE

Most common causes: conjunctivitis, episcleritis, scleritis, subconjunctival hemorrhage, uveitis, acute angle closure glaucoma, keratitis, corneal abrasion

Pain?

Yes

No

Blurred vision?

Yes

No/Maybe

Keratitis**
Photophobia, discharge
Fluorescein test positive
Blurry vision possible,
foreign body sensation

Corneal abrasion
Fluorescein test positive
Blepharospasm, blurry
vision possible

Scleritis*
Photophobia, no blurry
vision, no discharge or
foreign body sensation

Pupil

Constricted Sluggish

Middilated Nonreactive

Uveitis**
Photophobia with pain
worse with eye
movement and during
accommodation

**Acute angle-closure
glaucoma***
Photophobia, halos
around lights, nausea
and vomiting

Discharge?

Yes

No

Mucopurulent

Watery

**Subconjunctival
hemorrhage**
Asymptomatic,
self-limiting

Bacterial conjunctivitis
abrupt onset, morning
crusting

Allergic conjunctivitis
Very itchy associated
allergy symptoms,
accompanied foreign
body sensation

Viral conjunctivitis
Very contagious,
accompanied foreign
body sensation

Episcleritis
No photophobia,
no pain but foreign
body sensation or irritation,
rapid onset, self-limiting

*Urgent ophthalmology consultation
**Consultation within 24 hours

Drew-Anne Drapala, MD and Vincent Lo, MD, FAAFP

Cronau H, Kankanala RR, Mauger T. Diagnosis and management of red eye in primary care. *Am Fam Physician*. 2010;81(2):137–144.

SALICYLATE POISONING, ACUTE, TREATMENT

Assess airway, breathing, and circulation.
Provide appropriate ABC management. Avoid intubation unless patient is unable to protect airway. Intubation may increase acidosis and result in cardiovascular collapse.

Early toxicity: tachypnea, hyperpnea, nausea, vomiting, tinnitus, vertigo
Late toxicity: hyperthermia, hypotension, altered mental status

Does the patient exhibit signs of severe toxicity (altered mental status/coma, seizure, pulmonary edema, or need for endotracheal intubation and mechanical ventilation)?

No   *Yes*

History and physical
Obtain careful history of ingestion (time, reported ingestion, coingestants, etc.) and perform thorough physical exam for hemodynamic instability, alterations in respiratory pattern, and changes in mental status.

Initiate emergent hemodialysis
Begin volume resuscitation and alkalinization using 150 mEq (3 amps) $NaHCO_3$ + 40 mEq KCl in 1 L D5W unless prohibited by cerebral/pulmonary edema. Administer 25 g (1 amp) D50 for altered mental status. Do not delay treatment for diagnostic studies.

Note: Volume resuscitation and alkalinization are the mainstays of therapy and should be given to all symptomatic patients unless pulmonary or cerebral edema is present. Respiratory alkalosis (pH >7.5) is NOT a contraindication to therapy. Do not delay for charcoal or diagnostic studies.

Is the patient asymptomatic, stable, and known to have ingested <150 mg/kg?

No   *Yes*

Initial treatment
1. Early volume resuscitation with isotonic saline
2. Urinary alkalinization using 150 mEq (3 amps) $NaHCO_3$ + 40 mEq KCl mixed in 1 L D5W, infused at 2–3 mL/kg/hr.
3. Administer 1st-dose activated charcoal at 1 g/kg (max 50 g) ONLY if patient is alert, cooperative, and can tolerate. Consider additional doses of 25 g q3h if patient can tolerate and has bowel sounds on exam.

Evaluation/observation
Obtain first salicylate level, noting time since ingestion occurred.

ASA detectable?

No → Recheck if within 2 hours of presentation. Discharge after 6 hours observation if patient remains asymptomatic, and levels are nondetectable.

Yes → Recheck levels q2h until persistently within therapeutic range, trending down, or nondetectable. Routinely reassess for changes in clinical status, and initiate treatment if indicated.

Obtain diagnostic studies
Labs: salicylate level (note time since ingestion), ABG/VBG, basic electrolytes, BUN creatinine, LFTs, coags, UA. Obtain tox screen if polysubstance overdose suspected.
Imaging: chest radiograph (to evaluate for pulmonary edema). Consider head CT for altered mental status to evaluate for cerebral edema or alternative causes of mental status changes.

Presence of salicylate level >90 mg/dL, arterial pH <7.3, pulmonary or cerebral edema, renal failure, or has patient deteriorated?

No →

Maintenance therapy and evaluation
1. Continue bicarbonate infusion to maintain urine output of 1–2 mL/kg/hr.
2. Measure urine pH hourly and titrate infusion to goal pH of 7.5–8.0.
3. Measure serum K hourly and replete if <4.5 mEq/L.
4. Measure ABG or VBG hourly and decrease rate of bicarbonate drip if serum pH exceeds 7.6.
5. Measure serum salicylate level q2h until salicylate level begins to decline and acid–base status is normal.

Yes

Initiate hemodialysis.

Disposition
Treatment should be continued with frequent clinical assessment for improvement. Treatment and testing may be stopped ONLY when patient is asymptomatic, acid–base status is stable, AND salicylate level has fallen into therapeutic range (10–30 mg/dL).

Alicia G. Lydecker, MD, Matthew K. Griswold, MD, and Kavita Babu, MD

Chyka PA, Erdman AR, Christianson G, et al. Salicylate poisoning: an evidence-based consensus guideline for out-of-hospital management. *Clin Toxicol (Phila)*. 2007;45(2):95–131.

SEIZURE, NEW ONSET

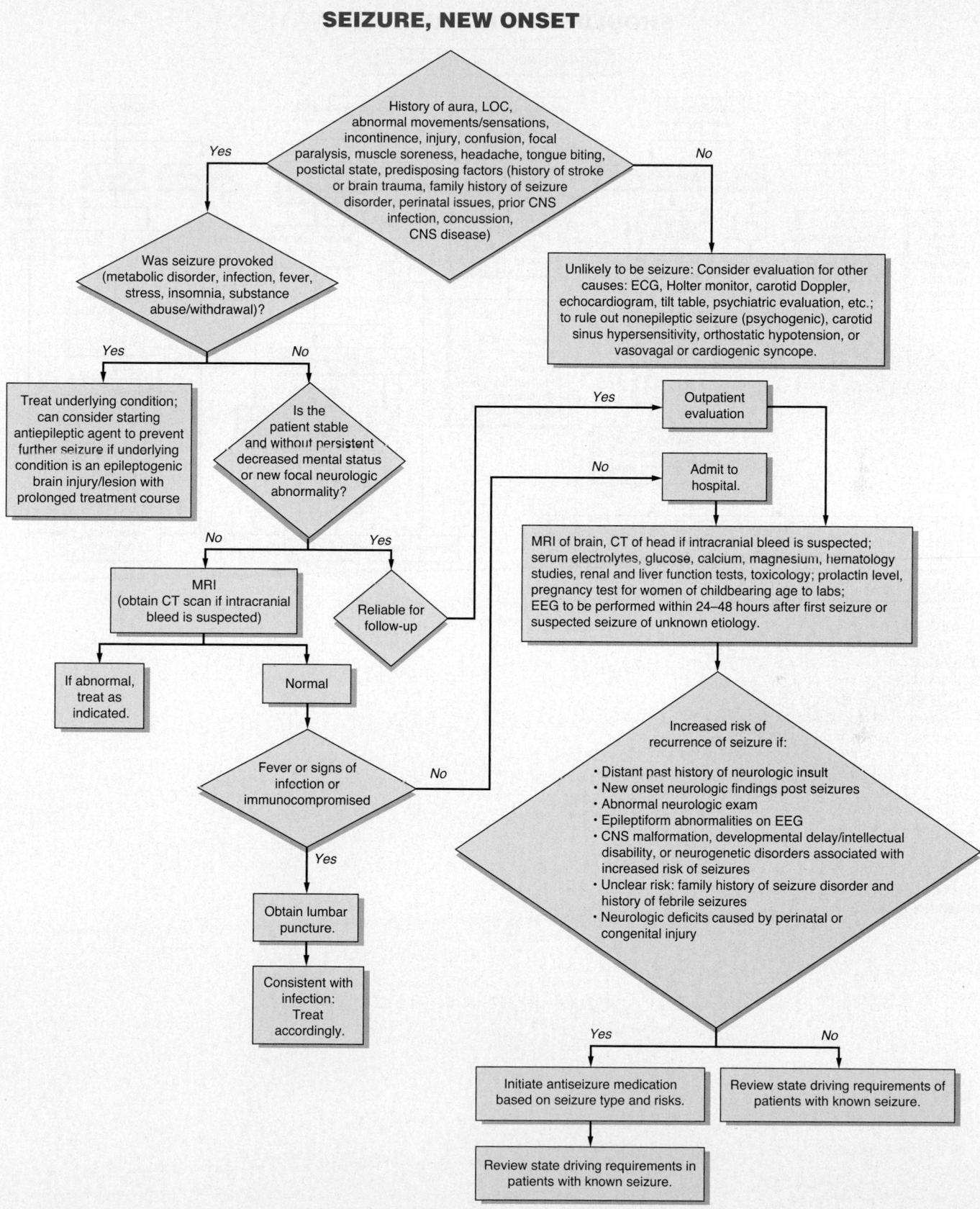

Andrew S. Hellenga, MD and Matthew J. Snyder, DO

Wilden JA, Cohen-Gadol AA. Evaluation of first nonfebrile seizures. *Am Fam Physician*. 2012;86(4):334–340.

SHOULDER PAIN, TREATMENT

Analgesics, NSAIDS, ice, activity modification

Myofascial or trigger point
→ PT
→ Dry needling TrP injection OMT Massage Myofascial release

Humeral Clavicle Scapula Fracture
→ Pain management Fracture management

Glenohumeral
→ OA
→ Anterior dislocation

OA → PT → IA CS → Surgical evaluation if refractory

Anterior dislocation → X-ray if first time and available → Reduce if negative fracture → PT → Surgical evaluation if recurrent or young and active

Adhesive capsulitis
→ Refer to PT. Consider IA CS injection.
→ Symptoms may take up to 1.5 years to resolve.
→ If not improving, consider:
• Repeat GH CS injection.
• Distention
• Manipulation under anesthesia
• Surgical release

Acromioclavicular
→ OA
→ Sprain/separation

OA → PT → IA CS

Sprain/separation → Immobilization for comfort → (2–3 days) → (4–6 weeks)

(2–3 days) → I
(4–6 weeks) → II → III → IV–VI

I, II, III → Conservative treatment → Surgical evaluation if refractory

IV–VI → Surgical repair

Rotator cuff
→ Tendinopathy
→ Tear
→ Labral tear

Tendinopathy → PT → SASD CS +/– GTN topical

Tear → Partial → Complete → PT and NSAIDs or SA CS injection → Surgical consult if:
• Not improving
• Disabling
• Young and acute traumatic tear
→ Surgical evaluation if refractory

Labral tear → PT → Surgical evaluation if refractory

Abbreviations
NSAIDS, nonsteroidal anti-inflammatory drugs; PT, physical therapy plus home exercise plan; OA, osteoarthritis; IA, intra-articular; TrP, trigger point; OMT, osteopathic manipulative therapy; CS, corticosteroid; GH, glenohumeral; SA, subacromial; GTN, glyceryl trinitrate

Shane L. Larson, MD and Derek G. Zickgraf, DO

Song A, Higgins LD, Newman J, et al. Glenohumeral corticosteroid injections in adhesive capsulitis: a systematic search and review. *PM R.* 2014;6(12):1143–1156.

SICKLE CELL ANEMIA, ACUTE, EVALUATION AND MANAGEMENT

This algorithm is meant to assist clinicians in the workup and management of common complications of sickle cell disease. It should not replace a physician's clinical judgment or be considered a standardized protocol for all patients.

Known Sickle Cell Patient (Part I of II)

Chief complaint
Joint/musculoskeletal pain

Chief complaint
Acute neurologic change or deficit

Chief complaint
Fever >101°F (38.3°C)

Possible causes
Vaso-occlusive crisis (VOC), infection

Possible causes
TIA, stroke, subarachnoid hemorrhage

Possible causes
Viral illness (respiratory, GI, or systemic viral infection, including parvovirus B19)
Pneumonia (esp. *Streptococcus pneumoniae* and atypicals)
Osteomyelitis (esp. *Salmonella, Escherichia coli, Staphylococcus aureus*)
Meningitis
UTI/pyelonephritis
Acute chest syndrome
Port/line infection
Other bacterial infections/sepsis (especially encapsulated bacterial organisms)

No specific physical findings
• Likely VOC

Warmth, swelling/effusion
over joint/skin
• In addition to VOC, consider infection (cellulitis, osteomyelitis, septic joint) or dactylitis If over hands/feet.
• Erythema may be seen with infection but is less likely with VOC.

Tests
• Full neurologic exam
• CBC w/ diff and retic
• Chem 10
• Type and crossmatch
• Noncontrast head CT to rule out bleeding ASAP
• MRI/MRA w/ diffusion-weighted images of brain to look for ischemia (may be deferred until after exchange transfusion)
• Consider LP after imaging if signs of infection.

Initial assessment
Must have rapid triage: exam, labs, and empiric antibiotics—goal within 1 hour of presentation

Localized hip pain or difficulty with ambulation
• Possible aseptic necrosis of femoral head

Treatment*
• Neurology and/or neurosurgery consults as indicated
• Hematology and transfusion medicine consults
• IV hydration[b] (maintenance or less if concern for increased ICP)
• Supplemental O_2 (adults); for peds, only if hypoxia is present
• Simple/exchange transfusion ASAP (do not wait for MRI or LP to be completed if stroke suspected)
• Abx if infectious cause suspected
• Admit (likely ICU)

Tests
• CBC w/ diff and retic (if H&H down and retic <0.5%, consider aplastic crisis)
• Blood cultures (draw off port or central line if present)
• UA C&S if GU Sx and all males <6 month/female <2 years
• Type and crossmatch
• CXR even if no respiratory Sx (acute chest may first present w/ fever)
• Throat cultures, viral panel, LP, stool studies if clinically indicated
• Imaging if osteomyelitis suspected

Tests
• CBC w/ diff & retic[a]
• Type and crossmatch
• Blood cultures if febrile or concern for osteomyelitis
• If bone infarct or aseptic necrosis suspected, consider MRI.
• Aspiration/analysis of joint fluid if effusion present
• If osteomyelitis suspected, consult radiology for MRI and/or bone marrow scan.

Treatment*
• Supplemental O_2 (adults); for peds, only if hypoxia is present
• IV hydration[b]
• Immediate empiric treatment w/ broad-spectrum Abx; consider additional coverage if port or line is present.
• May require simple/exchange transfusion for aplastic crisis
• Admit for severe bacterial infection, new chest infiltrate, or high-risk patient—hematology to determine risk based on age, appearance, exam, labs, and past medical Hx.
• Low-risk patient may be discharged home with follow-up per hematology's recommendations.

Treatment*
• Pain control **within 30 minutes of presentation**; start with PO meds, then IV.
• Supplemental O_2 (adults); for peds, only if hypoxia is present
• IV hydration[b]
• Abx if possible infectious cause (cover *Salmonella, E. coli,* staph/strep)
• May need simple/exchange transfusion
• Orthopedic consult for aseptic necrosis or osteomyelitis

Admit for treatment of any serious bacterial infection, if IV pain meds are needed to control pain, or if patient not tolerating oral hydration.

Mild/moderate pain
• Manage as outpatient or admit if other concerns.
• Acetaminophen, ibuprofen, or PO opioids
• Bowel regimen while on narcotics

Severe pain
• Admit for IV pain control—NSAIDs (ketorolac), opioids; consider patient-controlled analgesia (PCA).
• Bowel regimen while on narcotics

Sickle Cell Anemia, Acute, Evaluation and Management

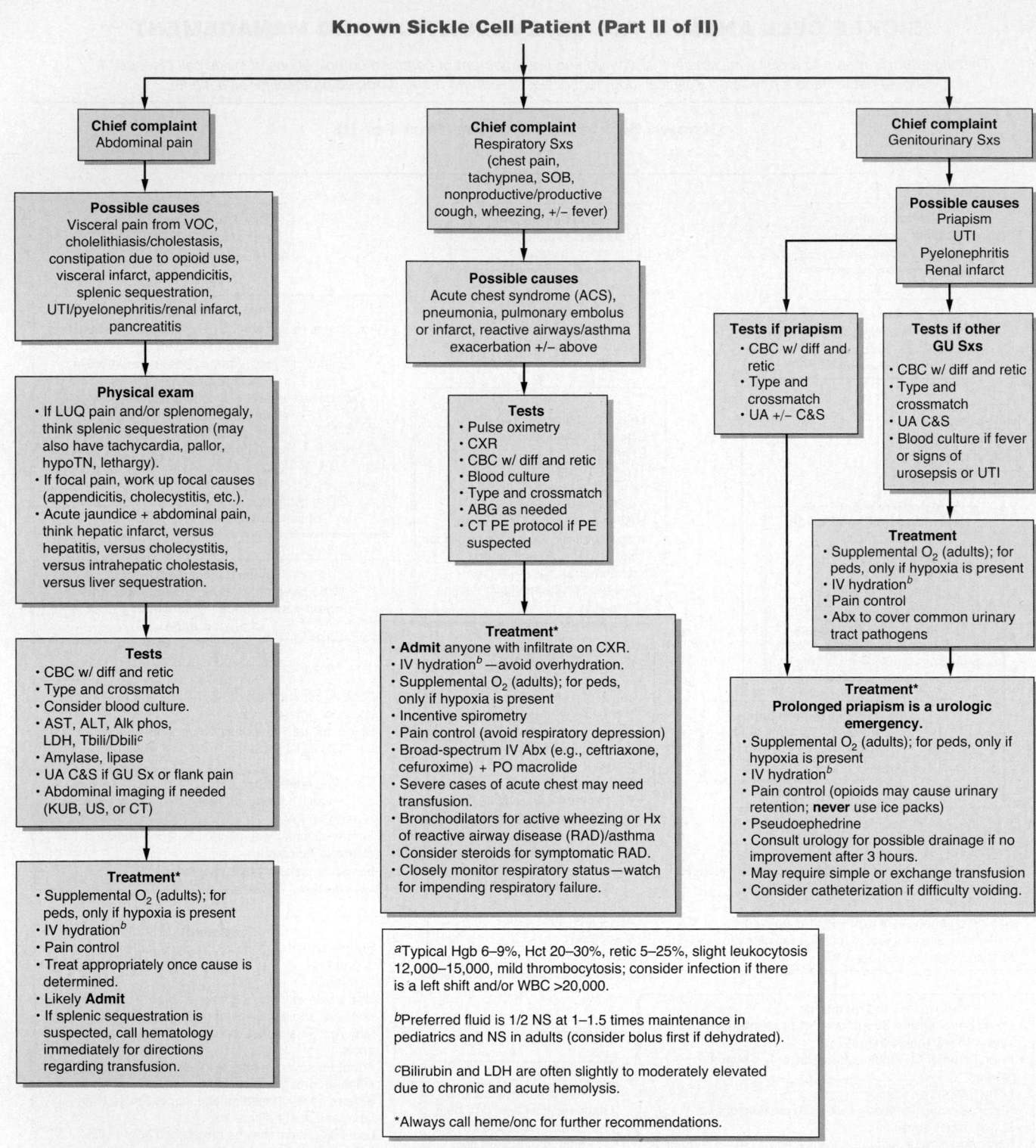

Known Sickle Cell Patient (Part II of II)

Chief complaint
Abdominal pain

Possible causes
Visceral pain from VOC, cholelithiasis/cholestasis, constipation due to opioid use, visceral infarct, appendicitis, splenic sequestration, UTI/pyelonephritis/renal infarct, pancreatitis

Physical exam
- If LUQ pain and/or splenomegaly, think splenic sequestration (may also have tachycardia, pallor, hypoTN, lethargy).
- If focal pain, work up focal causes (appendicitis, cholecystitis, etc.).
- Acute jaundice + abdominal pain, think hepatic infarct, versus hepatitis, versus cholecystitis, versus intrahepatic cholestasis, versus liver sequestration.

Tests
- CBC w/ diff and retic
- Type and crossmatch
- Consider blood culture.
- AST, ALT, Alk phos, LDH, Tbili/Dbili[c]
- Amylase, lipase
- UA C&S if GU Sx or flank pain
- Abdominal imaging if needed (KUB, US, or CT)

Treatment*
- Supplemental O_2 (adults); for peds, only if hypoxia is present
- IV hydration[b]
- Pain control
- Treat appropriately once cause is determined.
- Likely **Admit**
- If splenic sequestration is suspected, call hematology immediately for directions regarding transfusion.

Chief complaint
Respiratory Sxs (chest pain, tachypnea, SOB, nonproductive/productive cough, wheezing, +/– fever)

Possible causes
Acute chest syndrome (ACS), pneumonia, pulmonary embolus or infarct, reactive airways/asthma exacerbation +/– above

Tests
- Pulse oximetry
- CXR
- CBC w/ diff and retic
- Blood culture
- Type and crossmatch
- ABG as needed
- CT PE protocol if PE suspected

Treatment*
- **Admit** anyone with infiltrate on CXR.
- IV hydration[b] —avoid overhydration.
- Supplemental O_2 (adults); for peds, only if hypoxia is present
- Incentive spirometry
- Pain control (avoid respiratory depression)
- Broad-spectrum IV Abx (e.g., ceftriaxone, cefuroxime) + PO macrolide
- Severe cases of acute chest may need transfusion.
- Bronchodilators for active wheezing or Hx of reactive airway disease (RAD)/asthma
- Consider steroids for symptomatic RAD.
- Closely monitor respiratory status—watch for impending respiratory failure.

Chief complaint
Genitourinary Sxs

Possible causes
Priapism
UTI
Pyelonephritis
Renal infarct

Tests if priapism
- CBC w/ diff and retic
- Type and crossmatch
- UA +/– C&S

Tests if other GU Sxs
- CBC w/ diff and retic
- Type and crossmatch
- UA C&S
- Blood culture if fever or signs of urosepsis or UTI

Treatment
- Supplemental O_2 (adults); for peds, only if hypoxia is present
- IV hydration[b]
- Pain control
- Abx to cover common urinary tract pathogens

Treatment*
Prolonged priapism is a urologic emergency.
- Supplemental O_2 (adults); for peds, only if hypoxia is present
- IV hydration[b]
- Pain control (opioids may cause urinary retention; **never** use ice packs)
- Pseudoephedrine
- Consult urology for possible drainage if no improvement after 3 hours.
- May require simple or exchange transfusion
- Consider catheterization if difficulty voiding.

[a]Typical Hgb 6–9%, Hct 20–30%, retic 5–25%, slight leukocytosis 12,000–15,000, mild thrombocytosis; consider infection if there is a left shift and/or WBC >20,000.

[b]Preferred fluid is 1/2 NS at 1–1.5 times maintenance in pediatrics and NS in adults (consider bolus first if dehydrated).

[c]Bilirubin and LDH are often slightly to moderately elevated due to chronic and acute hemolysis.

*Always call heme/onc for further recommendations.

Andrew S. Hellenga, MD and Matthew J. Snyder, DO

New England Pediatric Sickle Cell Consortium. Clinical practice guidelines. http://www.nepscc.org/nepscc.html. Accessed 2015.

SUICIDE, EVALUATING RISK FOR

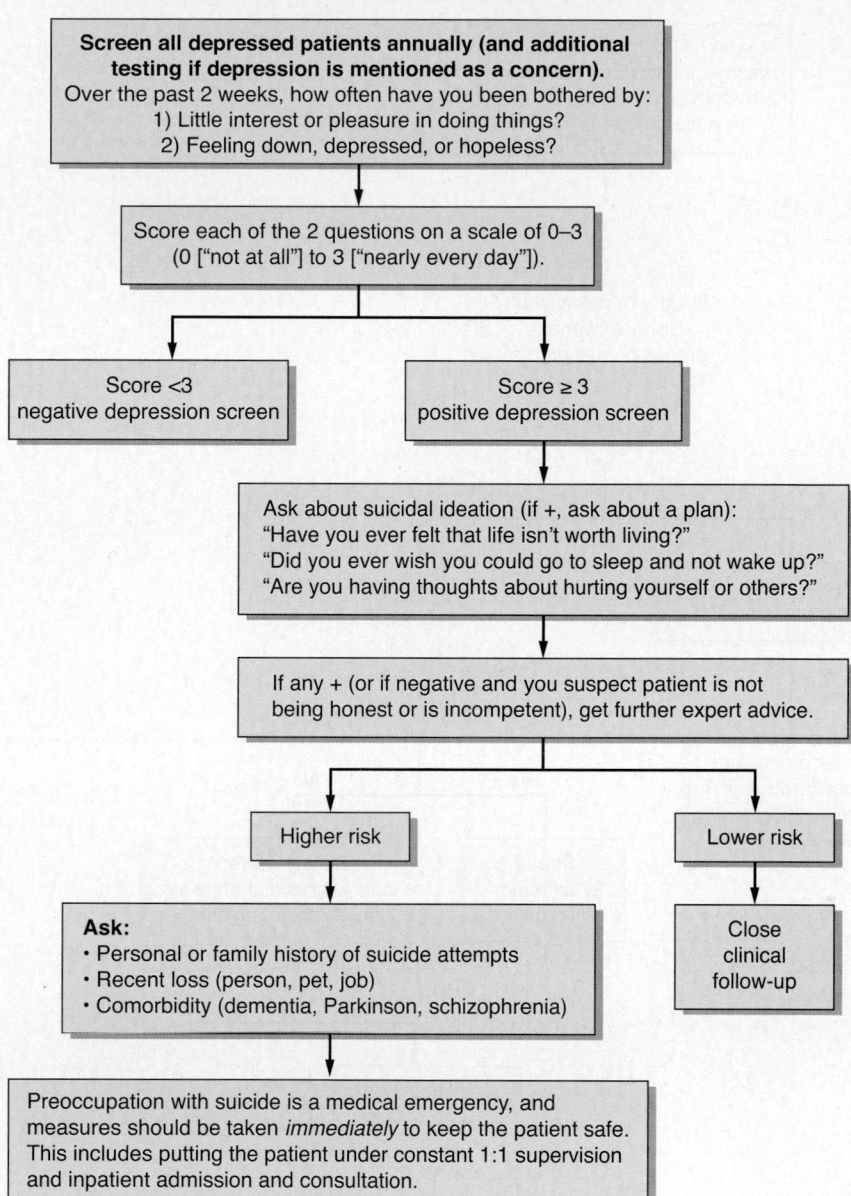

Screen all depressed patients annually (and additional testing if depression is mentioned as a concern).
Over the past 2 weeks, how often have you been bothered by:
1) Little interest or pleasure in doing things?
2) Feeling down, depressed, or hopeless?

Score each of the 2 questions on a scale of 0–3 (0 ["not at all"] to 3 ["nearly every day"]).

Score <3
negative depression screen

Score ≥ 3
positive depression screen

Ask about suicidal ideation (if +, ask about a plan):
"Have you ever felt that life isn't worth living?"
"Did you ever wish you could go to sleep and not wake up?"
"Are you having thoughts about hurting yourself or others?"

If any + (or if negative and you suspect patient is not being honest or is incompetent), get further expert advice.

Higher risk

Lower risk

Ask:
• Personal or family history of suicide attempts
• Recent loss (person, pet, job)
• Comorbidity (dementia, Parkinson, schizophrenia)

Close
clinical
follow-up

Preoccupation with suicide is a medical emergency, and measures should be taken *immediately* to keep the patient safe. This includes putting the patient under constant 1:1 supervision and inpatient admission and consultation.

Irene C. Coletsos, MD and Harold J. Bursztajn, MD

Posner K, Oquendo MA, Gould M, et al. Columbia Classification Algorithm of Suicide Assessment (C-CASA): classification of suicidal events in the FDA's pediatric suicidal risk analysis of antidepressants. *Am J Psychiatry.* 2007;164(7):1035–1043.

SYNCOPE

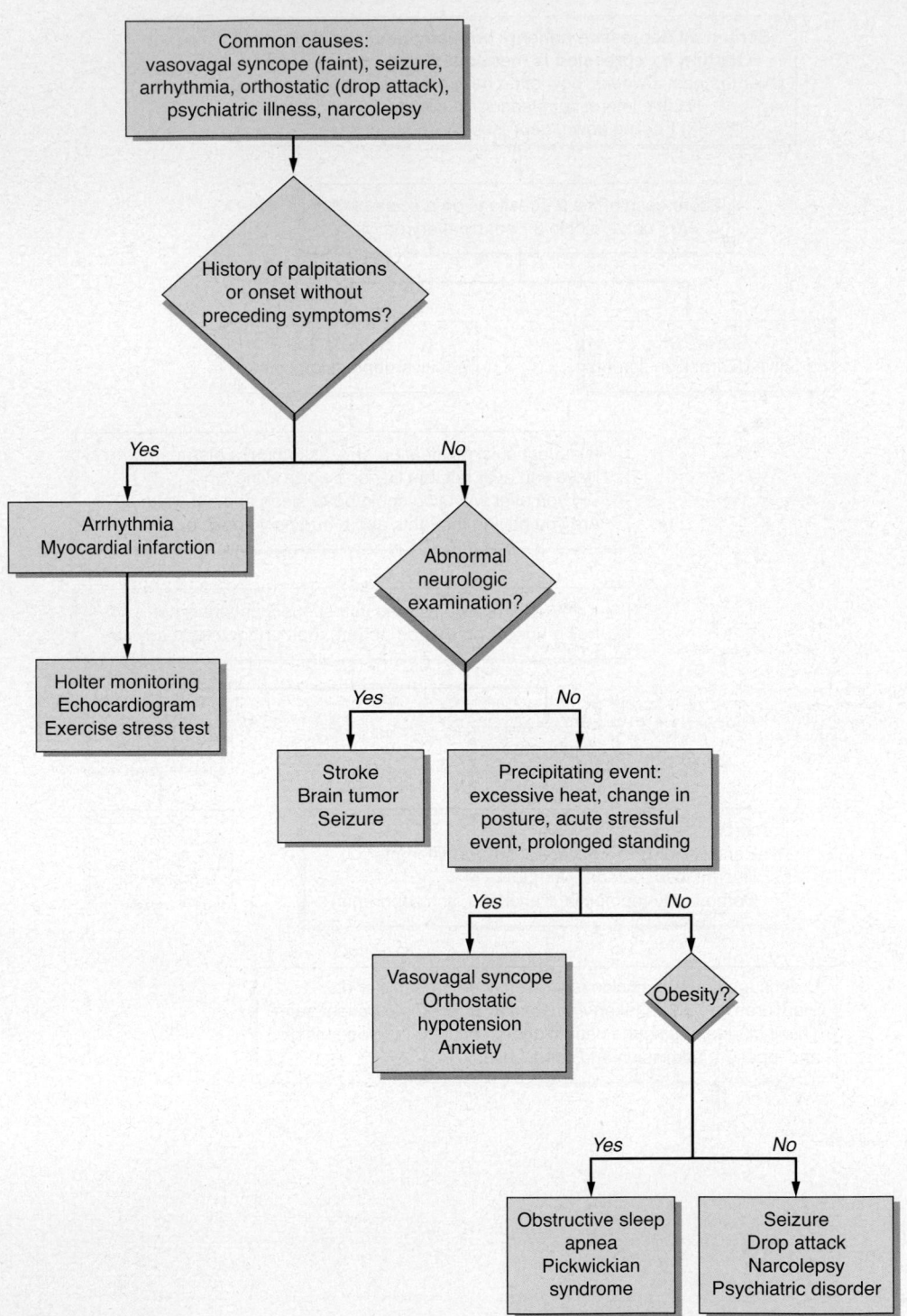

Common causes:
vasovagal syncope (faint), seizure, arrhythmia, orthostatic (drop attack), psychiatric illness, narcolepsy

History of palpitations or onset without preceding symptoms?

Yes

Arrhythmia
Myocardial infarction

Holter monitoring
Echocardiogram
Exercise stress test

No

Abnormal neurologic examination?

Yes

Stroke
Brain tumor
Seizure

No

Precipitating event: excessive heat, change in posture, acute stressful event, prolonged standing

Yes

Vasovagal syncope
Orthostatic hypotension
Anxiety

No

Obesity?

Yes

Obstructive sleep apnea
Pickwickian syndrome

No

Seizure
Drop attack
Narcolepsy
Psychiatric disorder

Tammy Donoway, DO, FAAFP

Gauer RL. Evaluation of syncope. *Am Fam Physician.* 2011;84(6):640–650.

THROMBOCYTOPENIA

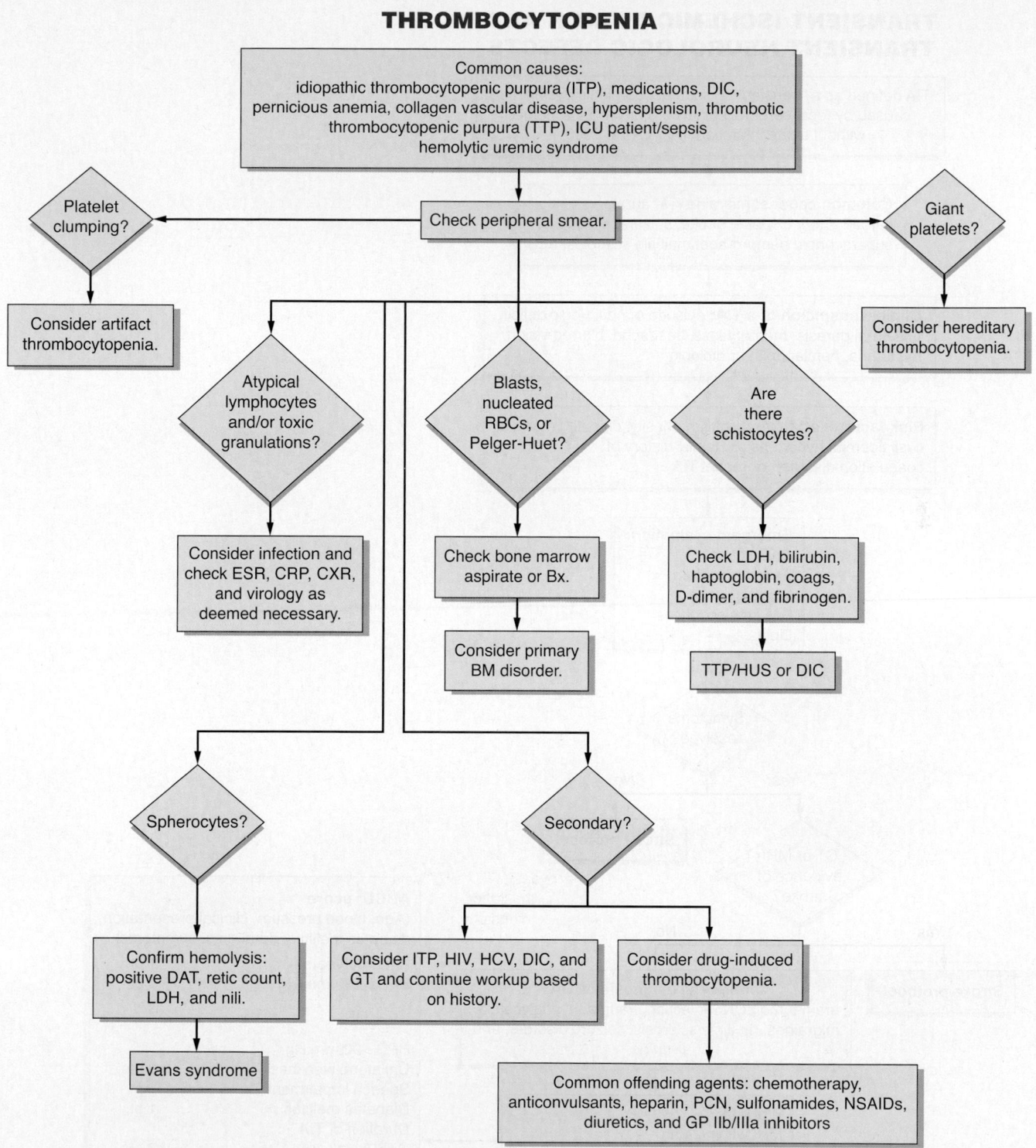

Common causes:
idiopathic thrombocytopenic purpura (ITP), medications, DIC, pernicious anemia, collagen vascular disease, hypersplenism, thrombotic thrombocytopenic purpura (TTP), ICU patient/sepsis hemolytic uremic syndrome

Check peripheral smear.

Platelet clumping? → Consider artifact thrombocytopenia.

Giant platelets? → Consider hereditary thrombocytopenia.

Atypical lymphocytes and/or toxic granulations? → Consider infection and check ESR, CRP, CXR, and virology as deemed necessary.

Blasts, nucleated RBCs, or Pelger-Huet? → Check bone marrow aspirate or Bx. → Consider primary BM disorder.

Are there schistocytes? → Check LDH, bilirubin, haptoglobin, coags, D-dimer, and fibrinogen. → TTP/HUS or DIC

Spherocytes? → Confirm hemolysis: positive DAT, retic count, LDH, and nili. → Evans syndrome

Secondary? → Consider ITP, HIV, HCV, DIC, and GT and continue workup based on history.

Consider drug-induced thrombocytopenia. → Common offending agents: chemotherapy, anticonvulsants, heparin, PCN, sulfonamides, NSAIDs, diuretics, and GP IIb/IIIa inhibitors

Nupam A. Patel, MD and Samuel B. Carli, MD

Reese JA, Li X, Hauben M, et al. Identifying drugs that cause acute thrombocytopenia: an analysis using 3 distinct methods. *Blood.* 2010;116(12):2127–2133.

TRANSIENT ISCHEMIC ATTACK AND TRANSIENT NEUROLOGIC DEFECTS

TIA defined as a "transient episode of neurologic dysfunction caused by focal cerebral spinal cord or retinal ischemia without acute infarction" (AHA/ASA, 2009).

Common causes: migraine (+/– aura), carotid artery disease, stroke, seizure, syncope, subarachnoid hemorrhage, multiple sclerosis, ALS

Clinical suspicion of a TIA: episode of neurologic deficit, unilateral paresis, memory loss, headache, blurred vision, dysarthria, hemianopia, or diplopia

Risk factors: cigarette smoking, obesity, diabetes mellitus, dyslipidemia, hypertension, family history of coagulation disorder, or recent TIA

Emergent evaluation:
EKG
Echocardiogram
Blood glucose
Serum electrolytes
Lipids

Symptoms resolved?

Yes   *No*

Stroke protocol

CT or MRI evidence of stroke?

Yes   No

Stroke protocol

Differential diagnosis of TIA: brain tumor, CNS infection, trauma, hypoglycemia, migraines, multiple sclerosis, seizure disorder, and vertigo

Workup:
MRI within 24 hr
Carotid studies
Consider ABCD² score for admission.

ABCD² score
(Age, blood pressure, clinical presentation, diabetes mellitus, duration of symptoms)

Age >60 years	1 pt.
BPS >140 mm Hg	1 pt.
OR	
BPD >90 mm Hg	
Unilateral weakness	2 pts.
Speech impairment	1 pt.
Diabetes mellitus	1 pt.
Duration of TIA	
>60 min	2 pts.
10–59 min	1 pt.

Admit patients with an ABCD² score >3 who present within 72 hr of symptom resolution, evidence of focal ischemia, or cannot complete outpatient workup.

Deborah A. Lardner, DO, DTM&H and Michael Passafaro, DO, DTM&H, FACEP, FACOEP

Simmons BB, Cirignano B, Gadegbeku AB. Transient ischemic attack: part I. Diagnosis and evaluation. *Am Fam Physician*. 2012;86(6):521–526.

TREMOR

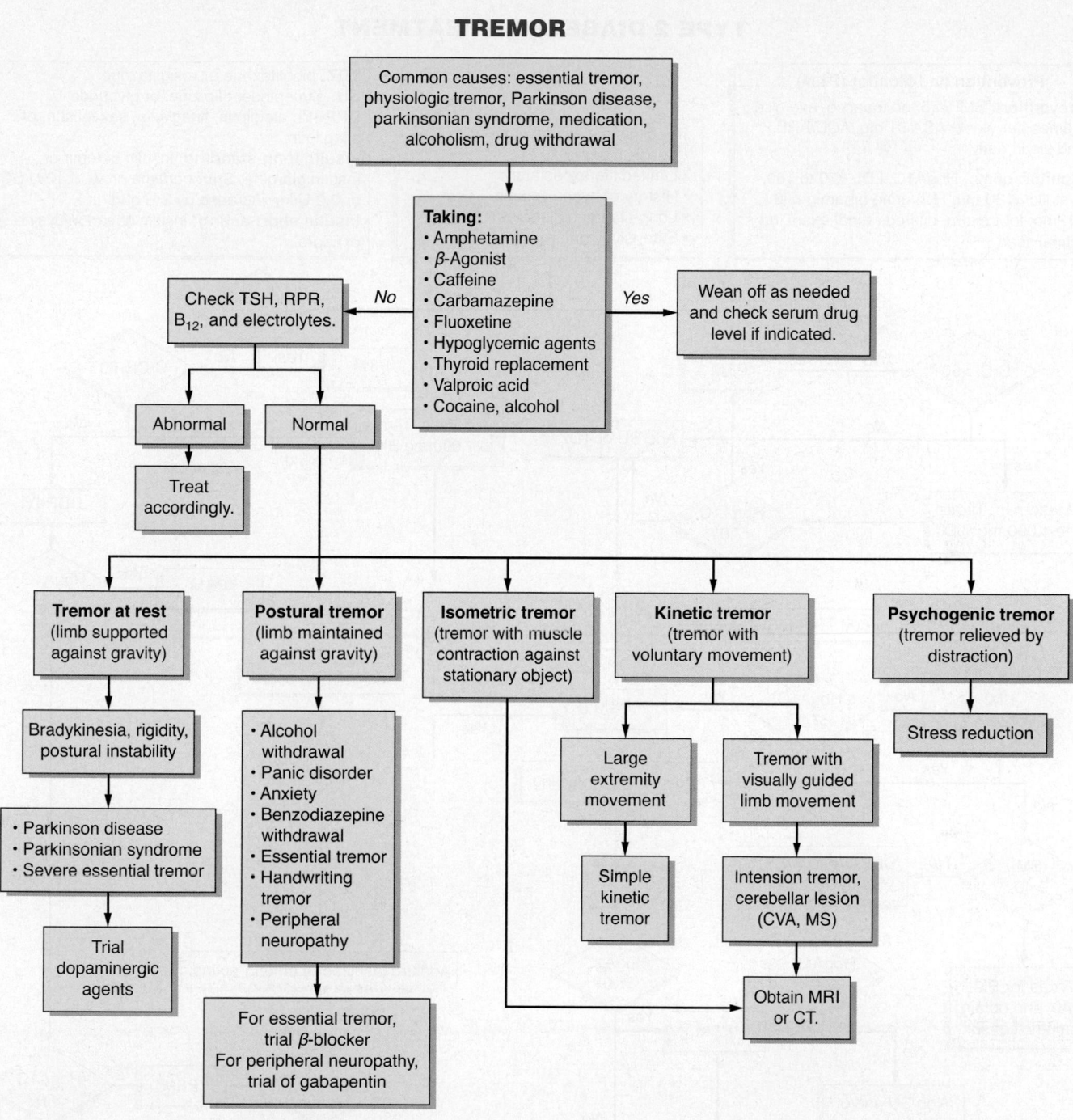

Kenneth Liu, PharmD, Steven J. Crosby, MA, BSP, RPh, FASCP, and Ildiko Halasz, MD

Crawford P, Zimmerman EE. Differentiation and diagnosis of tremor. *Am Fam Physician*. 2011;83(6):697–702.

TYPE 2 DIABETES, TREATMENT

*Prevention and Monitor (P&M)

Prevention: BMI <25, no tobacco, exercise 4 times per week, ASA 81 mg, ACE/ARB, and statin daily

Monitor: q6mo: HbgA1C, LDL <70 to 100, systolic <130 mm HG, urine albumin <30 q12mo: foot exam, dilated retinal exam, or retinal scan

Does this patient have the following?:
• Age >65 years
• Limited life expectancy
• History of hypoglycemia
• Long-standing diabetes
• Extensive comorbidities

TDZ: pioglitazone or rosiglitazone
SU: glimepiride, glipizide, or glyburide
DPP-IVi: alogliptin, linagliptin, saxagliptin, or sitagliptin
Insulin long-standing: insulin detemir or insulin glargine. Start bedtime or AM at 10 U SC or 0.2 U/kg; increase by 2 U q3d.
Insulin short-acting: insulin aspart, glulisine, or lispro

Andrew G. Alexander, MD

American Diabetes Association. Standards of medical care in diabetes—2015. *Diabetes Care*. 2015;38(1):S1–S94.

UREMIA

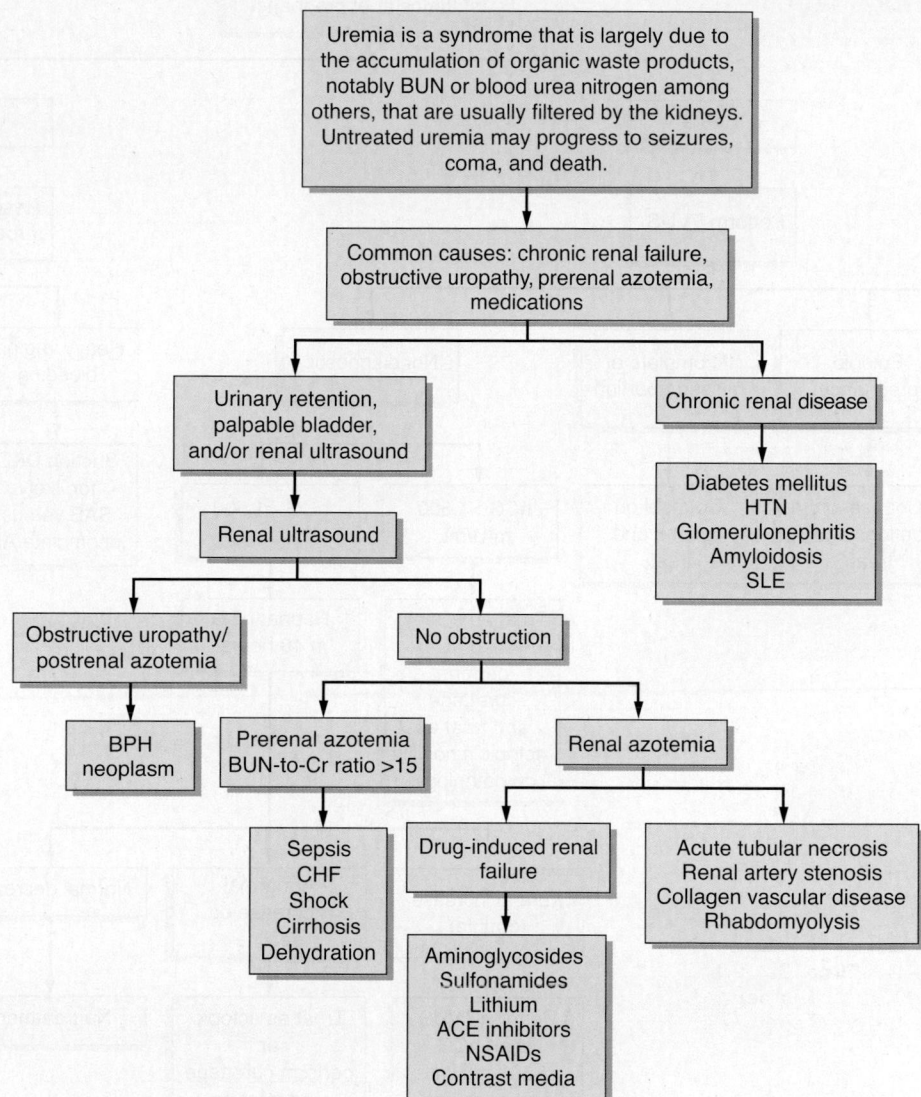

Uremia is a syndrome that is largely due to the accumulation of organic waste products, notably BUN or blood urea nitrogen among others, that are usually filtered by the kidneys. Untreated uremia may progress to seizures, coma, and death.

Common causes: chronic renal failure, obstructive uropathy, prerenal azotemia, medications

Urinary retention, palpable bladder, and/or renal ultrasound

Chronic renal disease

Diabetes mellitus
HTN
Glomerulonephritis
Amyloidosis
SLE

Renal ultrasound

Obstructive uropathy/ postrenal azotemia

No obstruction

BPH
neoplasm

Prerenal azotemia
BUN-to-Cr ratio >15

Renal azotemia

Sepsis
CHF
Shock
Cirrhosis
Dehydration

Drug-induced renal failure

Acute tubular necrosis
Renal artery stenosis
Collagen vascular disease
Rhabdomyolysis

Aminoglycosides
Sulfonamides
Lithium
ACE inhibitors
NSAIDs
Contrast media

Steven A. House, MD, FAAFP, FAAHPM, HMDC

Rahman M, Shad F, Smith MC. Acute kidney injury: a guide to diagnosis and management. *Am Fam Physician*. 2012;86(7):631–639.

VAGINAL BLEEDING DURING PREGNANCY

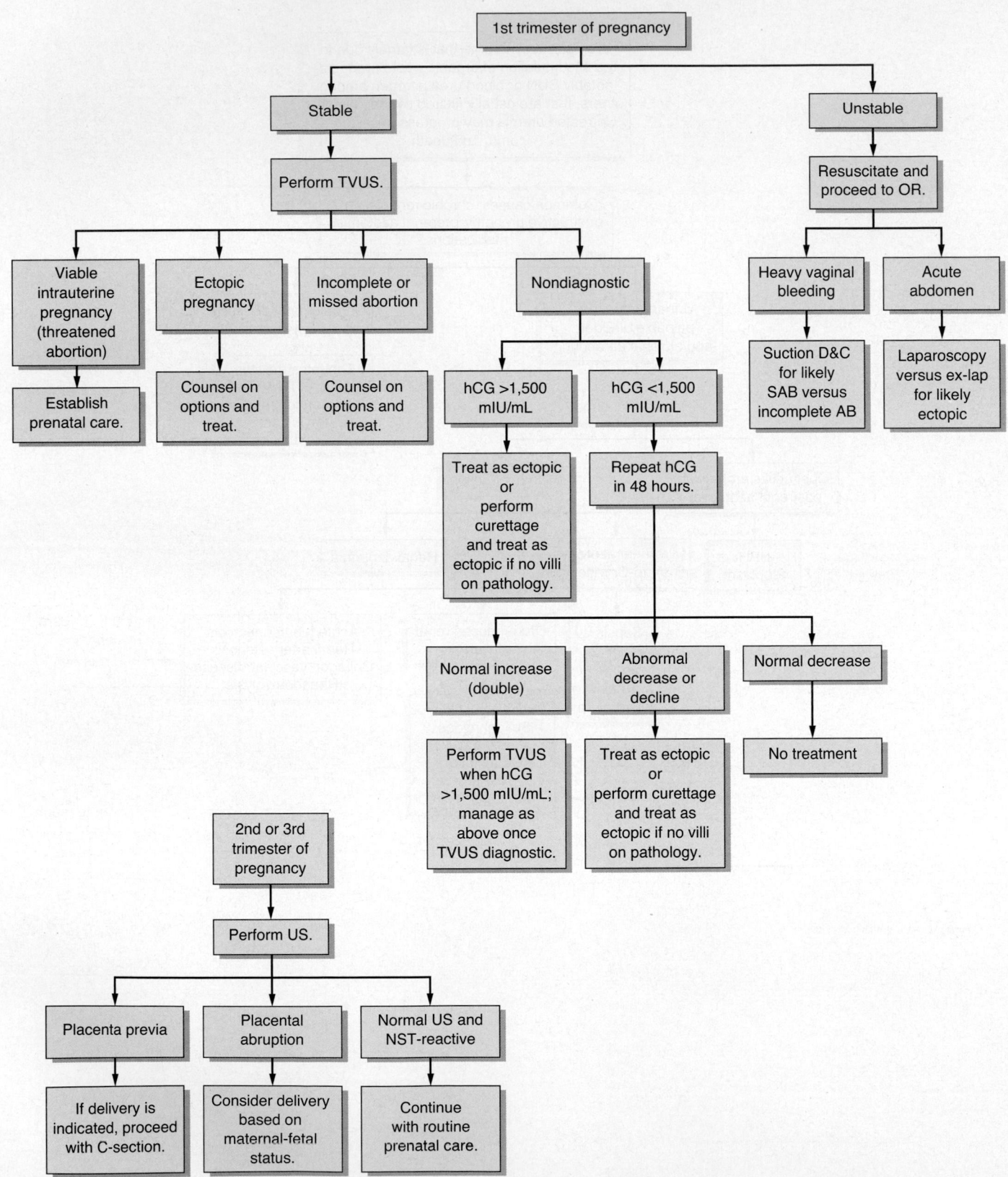

Emily Reus, MD and Mark J. Manning, DO, MsMEL

Gracia CR, Barnhart KT. Diagnosing ectopic pregnancy: decision analysis comparing six strategies. *Obstet Gynecol.* 2001;97(3):464–470.

VAGINAL BLEEDING, ABNORMAL

EMB, endometrial biopsy.

Tanya E. Anim, MD and Jennifer Tickal Keehbauch, MD

Sweet MG, Schmidt-Dalton TA, Weiss PM, et al. Evaluation and management of abnormal uterine bleeding in premenopausal women. *Am Fam Physician.* 2012;85(1):35–43.

VITAMIN D DEFICIENCY

Risk factors/common causes:

- Age >65 years
- Insufficient sunlight exposure (homebound, veiled)
- Renal disease
- Liver disease
- Depression

- Dark skin
- Insufficient dietary intake
- GI malabsorption
- Obesity (BMI >30)
- Immigrants to colder climates
- Chronic use of glucocorticoids
- Periosteal bone pain (e.g., sternum, tibia)

- GI malabsorption (celiac, cystic fibrosis, inflammatory bowel disease)
- Pregnancy
- Medications: anticonvulsants, antiretroviral, and glucocorticoids
- Gastrectomy or extensive bowel surgery

Significant risk factors?

→ **No** → Low suspicion for vitamin D deficiency

↓ **Yes**

Age <18 years?

← **Yes**

Requirements:
<1 year old: 400 IU/day
>1 year old: 600 IU/day
To reach levels >30 ng/mL, may require 1,000 IU/day.
Obese children: 2–3 times more vitamin D for their age group
Maintenance dose:
0–6 months: 1,000–2,000 IU/day
6 months–1 year: 1,500–2,000 IU/day
1–3 years: 2,500–4,000 IU/day
4–8 years: 3,000–4,000 IU/day
>8 years: 4,000 IU/day
Vitamin D deficiency:
0–1 year: 2,000 IU/day for 6 weeks or 50,000 IU weekly for 6 weeks followed by maintenance 400–1,000 IU/day
1–18 years: 2,000 IU/day for 6 weeks or 50,000 IU weekly for 6 weeks followed by maintenance 600–1,000 IU/day

→ **No** →

Lab: serum 25-hydroxyvitamin D concentration

Level <20 ng/mL (vitamin D deficiency)

Treatment

Start 50,000 IU (D_2 or D) once per week for 8 weeks, then 1,000–4,000 IU/day thereafter.

After 6 months, consider repeating serum 25-hydroxyvitamin D level.

Level <21–29 ng/mL (vitamin D insufficiency)

Treatment

600–2,000 IU/day

Level >30 ng/mL normal

Maintenance

In adults with adequate sun exposure; minimal intake:
19–50 years: 600 IU/day
50–70 years: 800 IU/day
(IOM states 600–4,000 IU/day safe)

Recheck serum 25-hydroxyvitamin D concentration.

Level <20 ng/mL?

→ **No** →

↓ **Yes**

Consult endocrinology if no malabsorptive disease.

Gisela M. Lopez Payares, MD and Fozia Akhtar Ali, MD

Holick MF, Binkley NC, Bischoff-Ferrari HA, et al. Evaluation, treatment, and prevention of vitamin D deficiency: an Endocrine Society clinical practice guideline. *J Clin Endocrinol Metab.* 2011;96(7):1911–1930.

WEIGHT LOSS, UNINTENTIONAL

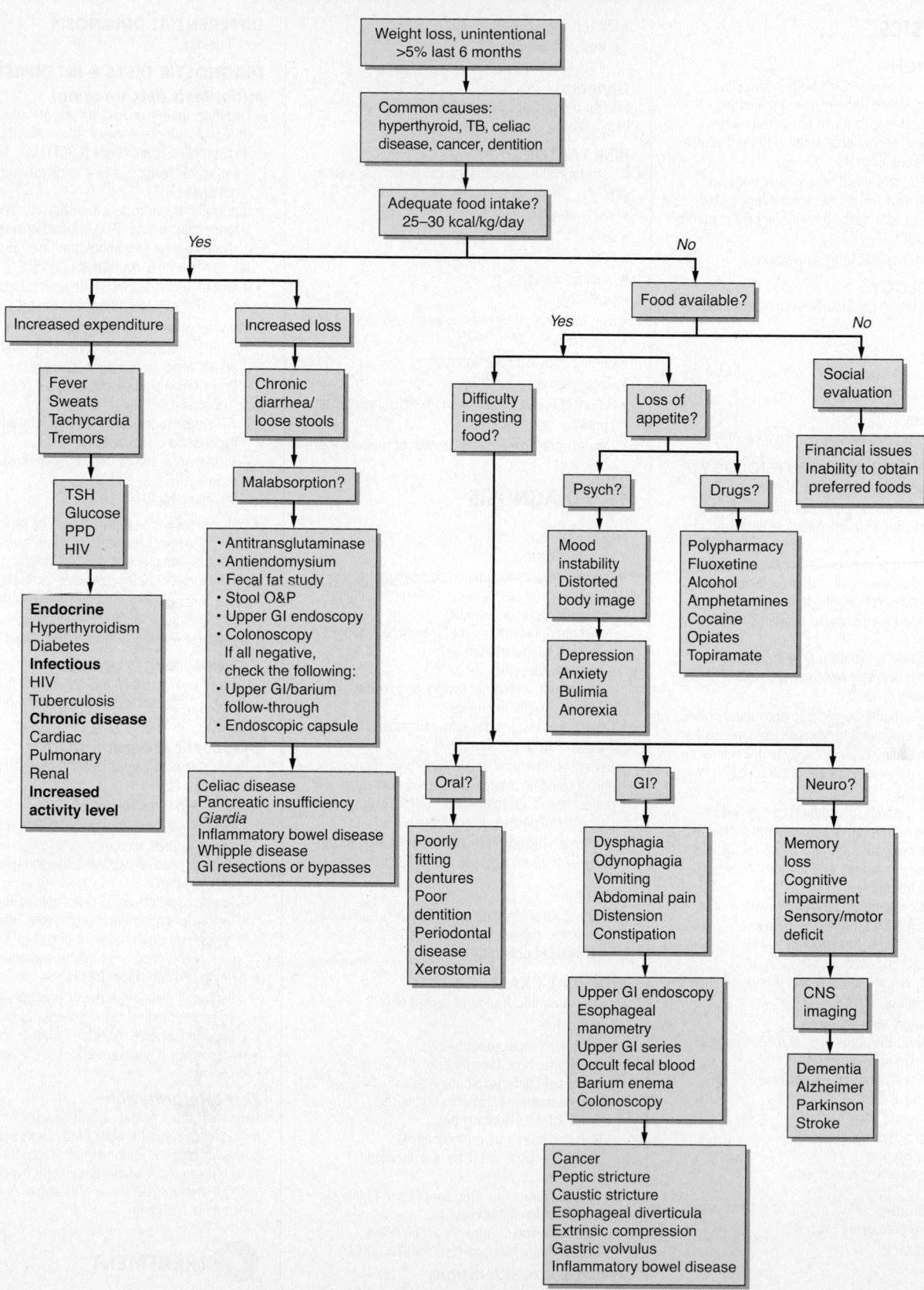

Weight loss, unintentional
>5% last 6 months

Common causes:
hyperthyroid, TB, celiac
disease, cancer, dentition

Adequate food intake?
25–30 kcal/kg/day

Yes

Increased expenditure

Fever
Sweats
Tachycardia
Tremors

TSH
Glucose
PPD
HIV

Endocrine
Hyperthyroidism
Diabetes
Infectious
HIV
Tuberculosis
Chronic disease
Cardiac
Pulmonary
Renal
**Increased
activity level**

Increased loss

Chronic
diarrhea/
loose stools

Malabsorption?

• Antitransglutaminase
• Antiendomysium
• Fecal fat study
• Stool O&P
• Upper GI endoscopy
• Colonoscopy
If all negative,
check the following:
• Upper GI/barium
follow-through
• Endoscopic capsule

Celiac disease
Pancreatic insufficiency
Giardia
Inflammatory bowel disease
Whipple disease
GI resections or bypasses

No

Food available?

Yes

Difficulty
ingesting
food?

Loss of
appetite?

Psych?

Mood
instability
Distorted
body image

Depression
Anxiety
Bulimia
Anorexia

Drugs?

Polypharmacy
Fluoxetine
Alcohol
Amphetamines
Cocaine
Opiates
Topiramate

No

Social
evaluation

Financial issues
Inability to obtain
preferred foods

Oral?

Poorly
fitting
dentures
Poor
dentition
Periodontal
disease
Xerostomia

GI?

Dysphagia
Odynophagia
Vomiting
Abdominal pain
Distension
Constipation

Upper GI endoscopy
Esophageal
manometry
Upper GI series
Occult fecal blood
Barium enema
Colonoscopy

Cancer
Peptic stricture
Caustic stricture
Esophageal diverticula
Extrinsic compression
Gastric volvulus
Inflammatory bowel disease

Neuro?

Memory
loss
Cognitive
impairment
Sensory/motor
deficit

CNS
imaging

Dementia
Alzheimer
Parkinson
Stroke

Crystal Amadi, MD and Fozia Akhtar Ali, MD

Gaddey HL, Holder K. Unintentional weight loss in older adults. *Am Fam Physician*. 2014;89(9):718–722.

ABNORMAL (DYSFUNCTIONAL) UTERINE BLEEDING

Stephen D. Cagle Jr., MD, Capt, USAF, MC • Matthew J. Snyder, DO

 BASICS

DESCRIPTION

- Abnormal uterine bleeding (AUB) is irregular menstrual bleeding (usually heavy, prolonged, or frequent); it is a diagnosis of exclusion after establishment of normal anatomy and the absence of other medical illnesses.
- The International Federation of Gynecology and Obstetrics (FIGO) revised the terminology system and now uses AUB rather than dysfunctional uterine bleeding (DUB).
- Commonly associated with anovulation

EPIDEMIOLOGY

Adolescent and perimenopausal women are affected most often.

Incidence

5% of reproductive age women will see a doctor in any given year for AUB.

Prevalence

10–30% of reproductive age women have AUB.

ETIOLOGY AND PATHOPHYSIOLOGY

- Anovulation accounts for 90% of AUB.
  - Loss of cyclic endometrial stimulation
  - Elevated estrogen levels stimulate endometrial growth.
  - No organized progesterone withdrawal bleeding
  - Endometrium eventually outgrows blood supply, breaks down, and sloughs from uterus.
  - 6–10% will have polycystic ovarian syndrome (PCOS).
- Adolescent AUB is usually due to an immature hypothalamic-pituitary-ovarian (HPO) axis that leads to anovulatory cycles.
- AUB can be broadly divided into anovulatory bleeding (usually irregular and unpredictable menses) or ovulatory bleeding (usually heavy regular menses) after pathologic causes of abnormal bleeding have been ruled out.
  - Pregnancy: ectopic pregnancy, threatened or incomplete abortion, or hydatidiform mole
  - Reproductive pathology and structural disorders
    ○ Uterus: leiomyomas, endometritis, hyperplasia, polyps, trauma
    ○ Adnexa: salpingitis, functional ovarian cysts
    ○ Cervix: cervicitis, polyps, STIs, trauma
    ○ Vagina: trauma, foreign body
    ○ Vulva: lichen sclerosus, STIs
- Malignancy of the vagina, cervix, uterus, and ovaries
- Systemic diseases
  - Inflammatory bowel disease
  - Hematologic disorders (e.g., von Willebrand disease, thrombocytopenia)
  - Advanced or fulminant liver disease
  - Chronic renal disease
- Diseases causing anovulation
  - Hyperthyroidism/hypothyroidism
  - Adrenal disorders
  - Pituitary disease (prolactinoma)
  - PCOS
  - Eating disorders
- Medications (iatrogenic causes)
  - Anticoagulants
  - Steroids
  - Tamoxifen
  - Hormonal medications: intrauterine devices (IUDs)
  - Selective serotonin reuptake inhibitors (SSRIs)
  - Antipsychotic medications

- Other causes of AUB
  - Excessive weight gain
  - Increased exercise

Genetics

Unclear but can include inherited disorders of hemostasis

RISK FACTORS

Risk factors for endometrial cancer (which can cause AUB)

- Age >40 years
- Obesity
- PCOS
- Diabetes mellitus
- Nulliparity
- Early menarche or late menopause (>55 years of age)
- Hypertension
- Chronic anovulation or infertility
- Unopposed estrogen therapy
- History of breast cancer or endometrial hyperplasia
- Tamoxifen use
- Family history: gynecologic, breast, or colon cancer

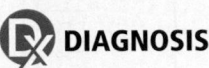 **DIAGNOSIS**

HISTORY

- Menstrual history
  - Onset, severity (quantified by pad/tampon use, presence and size of clots), timing of bleeding (unpredictable or episodic)
  - Menorrhagia with onset of menarche is suggestive of a coagulation disorder.
  - Menopausal status
  - Association with other factors (e.g., coitus, contraception, weight loss/gain)
- Gynecologic history: gravidity and parity, STI history, previous Pap smear results
- Review of systems (exclude symptoms of pregnancy and of bleeding disorders, bleeding from other orifices, stress, exercise, recent weight change, visual changes, headaches, galactorrhea)
- Medication history: Evaluate for use of aspirin, anticoagulants, hormones, and herbal supplements (1,2).

ALERT

Postmenopausal bleeding is any bleeding that occurs >1 year after the last menstrual period; cancer must always be ruled out (2)[C].

PHYSICAL EXAM

Discover anatomic or organic causes of AUB

- Evaluate for
  - Body mass index (obesity)
  - Pallor, vital signs (anemia)
  - Visual field defects (pituitary lesion)
  - Hirsutism or acne (hyperandrogenism)
  - Goiter (thyroid dysfunction)
  - Galactorrhea (hyperprolactinemia)
  - Purpura, ecchymosis (bleeding disorders)
- Pelvic exam
  - Evaluate for uterine irregularities and Tanner stage.
  - Check for foreign bodies.
  - Rule out rectal or urinary tract bleeding.
  - Include Pap smear and tests for STIs (2)[C].

Pediatric Considerations

Premenarchal children with vaginal bleeding should be evaluated for foreign bodies, physical/sexual abuse, possible infections, and signs of precocious puberty.

DIFFERENTIAL DIAGNOSIS

See "Etiology."

DIAGNOSTIC TESTS & INTERPRETATION

Initial Tests (lab, imaging)

- Everyone: urine human chorionic gonadotropin (hCG; rule out pregnancy and/or hydatidiform, mole) and complete blood count (CBC) (1)
  - For acute bleeding, a type and cross should be obtained (3)[C].
- If disorder of hemostasis is suspected, a partial thromboplastin time (PTT), prothrombin time (PT), activated partial thromboplastin time (aPTT), and fibrinogen level is appropriate (3)[C].
- If anovulation is suspected: thyroid stimulating hormone (TSH) level, prolactin level (1)
- Consider other tests based on differential diagnosis.
  - Follicle-stimulating hormone (FSH) level to evaluate for hypo- or hypergonadotropism
  - Coagulation studies and factors if coagulopathy is suspected (1)
  - 17-hydroxyprogesterone if congenital adrenal hyperplasia is suspected
  - Testosterone and/or dehydroepiandrosterone sulfate (DHEA-S) if PCOS
  - Screening for STI
- Endometrial biopsy (EMB) should be performed as part of the initial evaluation for postmenopausal uterine bleeding and in premenopausal women with risk factors for endometrial carcinoma (1)[A].
- TVUS, sonohysterography, and hysteroscopy may be similarly effective in detection of intrauterine pathology in premenopausal women with AUB (1)[A],(2)[C].
- If normal findings following imaging in patients without known risk factors for endometrial carcinoma, a biopsy should be performed if not done so previously (2)[C].

Diagnostic Procedures/Other

- Pap smear to screen for cervical cancer if age >21 years (2)[C]
- EMB should be performed in
  - Women age >35 years with AUB to rule out cancer or premalignancy
  - Postmenopausal women with endometrial thickness >5 mm
  - Women aged 18 to 35 years with AUB and risk factors for endometrial cancer (see "Risk Factors")
  - Perform on or after day 18 of cycle, if known; secretory endometrium confirms ovulation occurred.
- Dilation and curettage (D&C)
  - Perform if bleeding is heavy, uncontrolled, or if emergent medical management has failed.
  - Perform if unable to perform EMB in office (2)[C].
- Hysteroscopy if another intrauterine lesion is suspected

Test Interpretation

Pap smear could reveal carcinoma or inflammation indicative of cervicitis. Most EMBs show proliferative or dyssynchronous endometrium (suggesting anovulation) but can show simple or complex hyperplasia without atypia, hyperplasia with atypia, or endometrial adenocarcinoma.

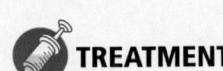 **TREATMENT**

Attempt to rule out other causes of bleeding prior to instituting therapy.

GENERAL MEASURES

NSAIDs (naproxen sodium 500 mg BID, mefenamic acid 500 mg TID, ibuprofen 600 to 1,200 mg/day) (1)[B]

- Decreases amount of blood loss compared with placebo, with no one clearly superior NSAID
- Diminishes pain

MEDICATION

First Line

- Acute, emergent, nonovulatory bleeding

  - Conjugated equine estrogen (Premarin): 25 mg IV q4h (max 6 doses) or 2.5 mg PO q6h should control bleeding in 12 to 24 hours (4)[A]
  - D&C if no response after two to four doses of Premarin or sooner if bleeding >1 pad/hr (2)[C]
  - Then change to oral contraceptive pill (OCP) or progestin for cycle regulation, that is, IUD (5)[A]

- Acute, nonemergent, nonovulatory bleeding
  - Combination OCP with ≥30 μg estrogen given as a taper. An example of a tapered dose: 4 pills/day for 4 days; 3 pills/day for 3 days; 2 pills/day for 2 days, daily for 3 weeks then 1 week off, then cycle on OCP for at least 3 months.

- Nonacute, nonovulatory bleeding (ranked in order as the best option based on efficacy, cost, side effects, and consumer acceptability) (5)[A]
  - Levonorgestrel IUD (Mirena) is the most effective form of progesterone delivery and is not inferior to surgical management.
  - Progestins: medroxyprogesterone acetate (Provera) 10 mg/day for 5 to 10 days each month. Daily progesterone for 21 days per cycle results in significantly less blood loss.
  - OCPs: 20 to 35 μg estrogen plus progesterone

- Do not use estrogen if contraindications, such as suspicion for endometrial hyperplasia or carcinoma, history of deep vein thrombosis (DVT), or the presence of smoking in women >35 years of age (relative contraindication), are present.
- Precautions
  - Failed medical treatment requires further workup.
  - Consider DVT prophylaxis when treating with high-dose estrogens (2)[C].

Second Line

- Leuprolide (varying doses and duration of action); gonadotropin-releasing hormone (GnRH) agonist
- Danazol (200 to 400 mg/day for a maximum of 9 months) is more effective than NSAIDs but is limited by androgenic side effects and cost. It has been essentially replaced by GnRH agonists.
- Antifibrinolytics such as tranexamic acid (Lysteda) 650 mg, 2 tablets TID (max 5 days during menstruation) (1)[A]
- Metformin or Clomid alone or in combination in women with PCOS who desire ovulation and pregnancy (6)[A]

ISSUES FOR REFERRAL

- If an obvious cause for vaginal bleeding is not found in a pediatric patient, refer to a pediatric endocrinologist or gynecologist (7).
- Patients with persistent bleeding despite medical treatment require reevaluation and referral to a gynecologist (7).

ADDITIONAL THERAPIES

- Antiemetics if treating with high-dose estrogen or progesterone (2)[C]
- Iron supplementation if anemia (usually iron deficiency) is identified

SURGERY/OTHER PROCEDURES

- Hysterectomy in cases of endometrial cancer or if medical therapy fails or if other uterine pathology is found

- Endometrial ablation is less expensive than hysterectomy and is associated with high patient satisfaction; failure of primary medical treatment is not necessary (1,4)[A].

  - This is a permanent procedure and should be avoided in patients who desire continued fertility.

INPATIENT CONSIDERATIONS

Admission Criteria/Initial Stabilization

Significant hemorrhage causing acute anemia with signs of hemodynamic instability; with acute bleeding, replace volume with crystalloid and blood, as necessary (1)[A].

Nursing

Pad counts and clot size can be helpful to determine and monitor amount of bleeding.

Discharge Criteria

- Hemodynamic stability
- Control of vaginal bleeding (2)[C]

 ONGOING CARE

FOLLOW-UP RECOMMENDATIONS

- Once stable from acute management, recommend follow-up evaluation in 4 to 6 months for further evaluation (5).
- Routine follow-up with a primary care or OB/GYN provider

Patient Monitoring

Women treated with estrogen or OCPs should keep a menstrual diary to document bleeding patterns and their relation to therapy.

DIET

No restrictions, although a 5% reduction in weight can induce ovulation in anovulation caused by PCOS (7)[C].

PATIENT EDUCATION

- Explain possible/likely etiologies.
- Answer all questions, especially those related to cancer and fertility.
- http://www.acog.org/Patients

PROGNOSIS

- Varies with pathophysiologic process
- Most anovulatory cycles can be treated with medical therapy and do not require surgical intervention.

COMPLICATIONS

- Iron deficiency anemia
- Uterine cancer in cases of prolonged unopposed estrogen stimulation

REFERENCES

1. Sweet MG, Schmidt-Dalton TA, Weiss PM, et al. Evaluation and management of abnormal uterine bleeding in premenopausal women. *Am Fam Physician*. 2012;85(1):35–43.
2. Committee on Practice Bulletins—Gynecology. Practice Bulletin No. 128: diagnosis of abnormal uterine bleeding in reproductive-aged woman. *Obstet Gynecol*. 2012;120(1):197–206.
3. American College of Obstetricians and Gynecologists. ACOG Committee Opinion No. 557: management of acute abnormal uterine bleeding in nonpregnant reproductive-aged women. *Obstet Gynecol*. 2013;121(4):891–896.
4. DeVore GR, Owens O, Kase N. Use of intravenous Premarin in the treatment of dysfunctional uterine bleeding—a double-blind randomized control study. *Obstet Gynecol*. 1982;59(3):285–291.
5. Marjoribanks J, Lethaby A, Farquhar C. Surgery versus medical therapy for heavy menstrual bleeding. *Cochrane Database Syst Rev*. 2006;(2):CD003855.
6. Schroeder BM. ACOG releases guidelines on diagnosis and management of polycystic ovary syndrome. *Am Fam Physician*. 2003;67(7):1619–1622.
7. Ely JW, Kennedy CM, Clark EC, et al. Abnormal uterine bleeding: a management algorithm. *J Am Board Fam Med*. 2006;19(6):590–602.

ADDITIONAL READING

- Farquhar C, Ekeroma A, Furness S, et al. A systematic review of transvaginal ultrasonography, sonohysterography and hysteroscopy for the investigation of abnormal uterine bleeding in premenopausal women. *Acta Obstet Gynecol Scand*. 2003;82(6):493–504.
- Kouides PA, Conard J, Peyvandi F, et al. Hemostasis and menstruation: appropriate investigation for underlying disorders of hemostasis in women with excessive menstrual bleeding. *Fertil Steril*. 2005;84(5):1345–1351.
- Lethaby AE, Cooke I, Rees M. Progesterone or progestogen-releasing intrauterine systems for heavy menstrual bleeding. *Cochrane Database Syst Rev*. 2005;(4):CD002126.
- Lethaby A, Farquhar C, Cooke I. Antifibrinolytics for heavy menstrual bleeding. *Cochrane Database Syst Rev*. 2000;(4):CD000249.
- Lethaby A, Irvine G, Cameron I. Cyclical progestogens for heavy menstrual bleeding. *Cochrane Database Syst Rev*. 2008;(1):CD001016.
- Lethaby A, Shepperd S, Cooke I, et al. Endometrial resection and ablation versus hysterectomy for heavy menstrual bleeding. *Cochrane Database Syst Rev*. 2000;(2):CD000329.

 SEE ALSO

- Dysmenorrhea; Menorrhagia (Heavy Menstrual Bleeding)
- Algorithm: Menorrhagia

 CODES

ICD10

- N93.9 Abnormal uterine and vaginal bleeding, unspecified
- N93.8 Other specified abnormal uterine and vaginal bleeding
- N91.2 Amenorrhea, unspecified

CLINICAL PEARLS

- AUB is irregular bleeding that occurs in the absence of pathology, making it a diagnosis of exclusion.
- Anovulation accounts for 90% of AUB.
- An EMB should be performed in all women >35 years of age with AUB to rule out cancer or premalignancy, and it should be considered in women aged 18 to 35 years with AUB and risk factors for endometrial cancer.
- It is appropriate to initiate medical therapy in females <35 years of age with no apparent risk of endometrial cancer prior to performing an EMB.

ABNORMAL PAP AND CERVICAL DYSPLASIA
Fozia Akhtar Ali, MD • Tharani Vadivelu Prasad, MD

BASICS

DESCRIPTION
- Cervical dysplasia: Premalignant cervical disease that is also called cervical intraepithelial neoplasia (CIN). Precancerous epithelial changes in the transformation zone of the uterine cervix almost always associated with human papillomavirus (HPV) infections.
- CIN encompasses a range of histologic diagnoses.
  - CIN I: mild dysplasia; low-grade lesion; cellular changes are limited to the lower 1/3 of the squamous epithelium.
  - CIN II: moderate dysplasia; high-grade lesion; cellular changes are limited to the lower 2/3 of the squamous epithelium.
  - CIN III or carcinoma in situ: severe dysplasia; high-grade lesion; cellular changes involve the full thickness of the squamous epithelium.
- System(s) affected: reproductive

ALERT
Incidence of cervical cancer has decreased by >50% in the last 30 years due to cervical cytology screening.

Pediatric Considerations
Cervical cancer is rare before age 21 years. Screening women younger than age 21 years (regardless of sexual history) does not reduce cervical cancer incidence and mortality compared with beginning screening at age 21 years. Screenings of adolescents lead to unnecessary evaluation and overtreatment of cervical lesions, which are highly likely to spontaneously regress (1)[A].

Geriatric Considerations
- Women age >65 years who have had adequate prior screening and no history of CIN II+ in the last 20 years should not be screened for cervical cancer. Adequate prior screening is defined as three consecutive, negative cytology results or two consecutive, negative HPV results within 10 years before cessation of screening (with the most recent test within the last 5 years).
- Routine screening should continue for at least 20 years after spontaneous regression or appropriate management of a high-grade precancerous lesion, even if this extends screening past the age 65 years.

Pregnancy Considerations
- Squamous intraepithelial lesions can progress during pregnancy but often regress postpartum.
- Colposcopy only to exclude the presence of invasive cancer in high-risk women
- Endocervical curettage is contraindicated during pregnancy (2).
- Unless cancer is identified or suspected, treatment of cervical intraepithelial neoplasia is contraindicated during pregnancy.

EPIDEMIOLOGY
- Cervical cancer is the 3rd most common cancer among women worldwide and ranks 14th for cancer deaths in women (3).
- Predominant age: can occur at any age, but incidence of CIN III peaks between ages 25 and 29; invasive disease peaks 15 years later. Cervical cancer most commonly occurs in women aged 35 to 55 years.

Incidence
The American Cancer Society estimates that, in 2014, 12,360 women will be diagnosed with invasive cervical cancer and 4,020 women will die from cervical cancer (4). Large declines in incidence rates over the past decades have begun to taper off. From 2006 to 2010, cervical cancer incidence rates have been stable in women younger than 50 years and decreasing by 3.1% per year in women 50 years and older.

Prevalence
- ~80% of sexually active women will have acquired a genital HPV infection by 50 years of age.
- Overall, 26.8% of women are HPV positive. Point prevalence of HPV positivity is highest in those 18 to 22 years of age (as high as 70%), falling off rapidly as women enter their 30s.

ETIOLOGY AND PATHOPHYSIOLOGY
HPV DNA is found in virtually all cervical carcinomas and precursor lesions worldwide.
- High-risk HPV types: 16, 18, 31, 33, 35, 45, 52, and 58 are common oncogenic virus types for cervical cancer.
- HPV 16 is the most carcinogenic HPV genotype and accounts for 55–60% of all cervical cancers.
- HPV 18 is the next most carcinogenic HPV genotype. HPV 18 causes a greater proportion of glandular cancers, adenocarcinoma, and adenosquamous carcinoma than squamous cell carcinoma.
- Most HPV infections are transient, becoming undetectable within 1 to 2 years. Persistent infections are what place women at significant risk for developing precancerous lesions.
- Low-risk types: HPV viral types 6, 11, 42, 43, and 44 are considered common low-risk types and may cause genital warts. HPV 6 and 11 (cause 90% of benign anogenital warts) can lead to low-grade squamous intraepithelial lesion (LSIL) and CIN I.

RISK FACTORS
- Previous or current HPV infection
- HIV infection and other immunosuppressive conditions
- In utero exposure to diethylstilbestrol
- Previous treatment of a high-grade precancerous lesion or cervical cancer
- Cigarette smoking
- Early age at first coitus (<20 years) and multiple sexual partners
- Some correlation with low socioeconomic status, high parity, oral contraceptive use, and poor nutrition

GENERAL PREVENTION
- Immunization: Immunization decreases high-risk HPV infections and cervical pathology for at least 5 to 7 years but has not yet been shown to decrease cervical cancer.
  - Ideally, HPV immunization of girls, boys, and women should be initiated prior to first intercourse.
    - Gardasil (quadrivalent: HPV 4):
      - Reduces dysplasia due to HPV types 16 and 18 (70% of cervical cancer) and types 6 and 11 (anogenital warts)
      - Three doses at 0, 2, and 6 months, approved for use in females ages 9 to 26 years. Only the quadrivalent vaccine is approved for males (ages 9 to 26 years) for prevention of anogenital warts.
    - Cervarix (bivalent: HPV 2): reduces dysplasia due to HPV 16 and 18 infection and CIN. Three doses at 0, 1, and 6 months, approved for use in females ages 10 to 25 years.
    - Gardasil 9: approved in December 2014 for use in females ages 9 to 26 and males ages 9 to 15; adds protection against five additional HPV types which cause approximately 25% of CIN II+ lesions
- Safe sex practices: condom use
- Screening
  - Pap smear is the main screening test for cervical cellular pathology.
  - Screening recommendations by age and source (see algorithm "Pap, Normal and Abnormal in Nonpregnant Women Ages 25 Years and Older" and separate algorithm "Pap, Normal and Abnormal in Women Ages 21–24 Years")
    - <21 years: Do not screen (5) (USPSTF/ASCCP/ACS/ASCP/ACOG).
  - Frequency of screening recommendation: USPSTF/ASCCP/ACS/ASCP generally agree by age and screen.
    - 21 to 29 years: Screen with cytology (Pap smear) every 3 years (5)[A]. Do not screen with HPV testing alone or combined with cytology (5).
    - 30 to 65 years: Screen with cytology every 3 years (acceptable) or cotesting (cytology/HPV testing) every 5 years (preferred).
    - >65 years (who have had adequate prior screening and are not high risk): Do not screen (5).
- Special circumstances: women after hysterectomy with removal of the cervix and with no history of CIN II+: Do not screen (6)[A].

DIAGNOSIS

HISTORY
Usually asymptomatic until there is invasive disease. Patients may present with vaginal discharge, abnormal vaginal bleeding, postcoital bleeding, pelvic pain, cervical mass, or bladder obstruction.

PHYSICAL EXAM
Pelvic exam occasionally reveals external HPV lesions. Examine for exophytic or ulcerative cervical lesions, with or without bleeding.

DIFFERENTIAL DIAGNOSIS
Acute or chronic cervicitis; cervical glandular hyperplasia; cervical polyp; cervical fibroid; HPV infection; invasive cervical malignancy; uterine malignancy

DIAGNOSTIC TESTS & INTERPRETATION
- Current evidence indicates no clinically important differences between conventional cytology and liquid-based cytology in detecting cervical cancer precursors (6)[A]. Conventional Pap smear involves a cervical sample plated on a microscope slide with fixative. Thin prep is a liquid-based collection and thin-layer preparation.
- Sensitivity of a single Pap smear for HSIL ~60–70%; specificity of ~90%. Pap smears done routinely at recommended intervals increase the sensitivity further.
- HPV viral typing: High-risk HPV subtype testing is more sensitive but less specific for identifying women with prevalent CIN III+.
- Cytology report component: specimen type (conventional Pap smear or liquid based), adequacy (presence of endocervical cells), and categorization (negative for intraepithelial lesion or malignancy or epithelial cell abnormality; i.e., squamous/glandular)

- Bethesda system (cytologic grading) epithelial cell abnormalities
  - Squamous cell
    - Atypical squamous cell (ASC) (of undetermined significance [ASC-US], cannot exclude high-grade squamous intraepithelial lesion [ASC-H])
    - HPV, mild dysplasia, CIN I
    - Moderate/severe dysplasia CIS, CIN II, and CIN III
  - Glandular cell
    - AGCs (atypical glandular cells)
      - AGCs: not otherwise specified
      - AGCs: favor neoplasia
    - AIS (adenocarcinoma in situ)
    - Adenocarcinoma

Diagnostic Procedures/Other
Algorithms differ for women age 21 to 24 years; see "ASCCP guidelines" (2) and algorithm "Pap, Normal and Abnormal in Women Ages 21–24 Years." Below recommendations for ages as noted.

- HPV positive, cytology negative (30 years of age and older)
  - Option 1: HPV DNA typing: if HPV 16 or 18 +, proceed to colposcopy; if negative, repeat cotesting at 1 year (6)[B].
  - Option 2: Repeat cotesting at 1 year: if ASC or HPV positive, proceed to colposcopy: if negative, repeat cotesting at 3 years.
- ASC-US: (>24 years of age)
  - Option 1: HPV testing (preferred)
    - If HPV positive, proceed to colposcopy (2)[B].
    - If HPV negative, repeat cotesting at 3 years (2)[B].
  - Option 2: Repeat cytology at 1 year (acceptable) (2)
    - If repeat cytology ASC or greater, proceed to colposcopy.
    - If repeat cytology is negative, proceed to routine screening in 3 years.
- ASC-H: Colposcopy is required.
- LSIL: (>24 years of age)
  - LSIL with negative HPV test: Repeat cotesting at 1 year (preferred).
    - If repeat cotesting is negative, repeat cotesting in 3 years.
    - If cotesting is positive, proceed to colposcopy.
  - LSIL with no HPV test or positive HPV test: Proceed to colposcopy.
  - LSIL in pregnancy: Colposcopy is preferred, but it is acceptable to defer colposcopy to postpartum (2).
- HSIL: loop electrosurgical excision procedure (LEEP) or colposcopy (2)[B]
- Atypical glandular cells: colposcopy with endocervical sampling and endometrial sampling (if 35 years or older or at risk for endometrial neoplasia) (2)[A]
- Atypical endometrial cells: endometrial and endo-cervical sampling
  - If negative, perform colposcopy.
- Women with no lesion on colposcopy or CIN I (preceded by "lesser abnormalities" such as ASC-US, LSIL, HPV 16+, HPV 18+, and persistent HPV)
  - Follow-up without treatment: cotesting at 12 months
  - If both HPV and cytology are negative, age-appropriate retesting 3 years later
  - If either positive, proceed to colposcopy. If persistent CIN I for at least 2 years, proceed to treatment with ablative or excisional methods.
- Ages 21 to 24: Management is slightly different than above; see "ASCCP guidelines" (2) or algorithm "Pap, Normal and Abnormal in Women Ages 21–24 Years."
- Age >30: If cytology is negative but HPV is positive, repeat cotesting at 1 year is acceptable.

Test Interpretation
Atypical squamous or columnar cells, coarse nuclear material, increased nuclear diameter, koilocytosis (HPV hallmark)

 TREATMENT

ASCCP guidelines: Evidence-based management algorithms guide Pap smear and postcolposcopic diagnostics and therapeutics and are available online at http://www.asccp.org/Guidelines (2).

GENERAL MEASURES
Office evaluation and observation; promote smoking cessation; promote protected intercourse; promote immunization.

MEDICATION
- Infective/reactive Pap smear: Treat trichomo-niasis, symptomatic candida, or shift in flora suggestive of bacterial vaginosis found on Pap smear results.
- Condyloma acuminatum: may be treated with cryotherapy or podophyllin topically q1–2wks or podofilox 0.5% applied BID × 3 days then off 4 days, repeated for 1 to 4 weeks, OR trichloroacetic acid applied topically by a physician and covered for 5 to 6 days, OR imiquimod cream 3 times per week at bedtime, up to 16 weeks

SURGERY/OTHER PROCEDURES
- Persistent CIN I, II, or III: ablative or excisional methods. If inadequate colposcopy for CIN II or III or recurrent CIN II or III, diagnostic excisional procedure is done. For adenocarcinoma in situ, hysterectomy is preferred.
- Cryotherapy, laser ablation, LEEP/large loop excision of transition zone, or cold-knife conization are all effective but require different training and with different side effects for patient. If cervical malignancy, see "Cervical Malignancy."

 ONGOING CARE

FOLLOW-UP RECOMMENDATIONS
After treatment (excision or ablation) of CIN II or III, women may reenter routine screening only after negative cotesting between 12 and 24 months. Screening should be continued for 20 years (6)[B].

DIET
Promote increased intake of antioxidant-rich foods.

PATIENT EDUCATION
HPV vaccination, smoking cessation, protected intercourse, regular screening with Pap smear per guidelines

PROGNOSIS
- Progression of CIN to invasive cervical cancer is slow, and the likelihood of regression is high: Up to 43% of CIN II and 32% of CIN III lesions may regress. CIN III has a 30% probability of becoming invasive cancer over a 30-year period, although only about 1% if treated.
- CIN III becomes invasive (7). Lesions discovered early are amenable to treatment with excellent results and few recurrences.
- One- and five-year relative survival rates for cervical cancer patients are 87% and 68%, respectively. The 5-year survival rate for patients diagnosed with localized disease is 91% (4).

COMPLICATIONS
Aggressive cervical surgery may be associated with cervical stenosis, cervical incompetence, and scarring affecting cervical dilatation in labor.

REFERENCES
1. Yang KY. Abnormal pap smear and cervical cancer in pregnancy. *Clin Obstet Gynecol*. 2012;55(3):838–848.
2. Massad S, Einstein MH, Huh WK, et al. 2012 updated consensus guidelines for the management of abnormal cervical cancer screening tests and cancer precursors. *J Low Genit Tract Dis*. 2013;17(5 Suppl 1):S1–S27.
3. American Cancer Society. Cancer facts & figures 2013. American Cancer Society Web site. http://www.cancer.org/acs/groups/content/@epidemiologysurveilance/documents/document/acspc-036845.pdf. Accessed July 7, 2015.
4. American Cancer Society. Cancer facts & figures 2014. American Cancer Society Web site. http://www.cancer.org/acs/groups/content/@research/documents/webcontent/acspc-042151.pdf. Accessed July 7, 2015.
5. U.S. Preventive Services Task Force. Cervical cancer: screening. U.S. Preventive Services Task Force Web site. http://www.uspreventiveservicestaskforce.org/Page/Document/UpdateSummaryFinal/cervical-cancer-screening. Accessed July 7, 2015.
6. American College of Obstetricians and Gynecologists. *ACOG Practice Bulletin No. 131: screening for cervical cancer*. Washington, DC: American College of Obstetricians and Gynecologists; 2012.
7. McCredie MR, Sharples KJ, Paul C, et al. Natural history of cervical neoplasia and risk of invasive cancer in women with cervical intraepithelial neoplasia 3: a retrospective cohort study. *Lancet Oncol*. 2008;9(5):425–434.

ADDITIONAL READING
American Society for Colposcopy and Cervical Pathology. Management guidelines. http://www.asccp.org/Guidelines-2/Management-Guidelines-2

 SEE ALSO

- Cervical Malignancy; Condylomata Acuminata; Trichomoniasis; Vulvovaginitis, Prepubescent
- Algorithm: Pap, Normal and Abnormal in Nonpregnant Women Ages 25 Years and Older; Pap, Normal and Abnormal in Women Ages 21-24 Years

CODES

ICD10
- R87.619 Unspecified abnormal cytological findings in specimens from cervix uteri
- N87.9 Dysplasia of cervix uteri, unspecified
- N87.1 Moderate cervical dysplasia

CLINICAL PEARLS
- HPV is present in virtually all cervical cancers (99.7%), but most HPV infections are transient.
- Vaccine should be offered prior to onset of any sexual activity for maximum effectiveness.
- Know and adhere to recognized screening guidelines to avoid the harms of overscreening.

ABORTION, SPONTANEOUS (MISCARRIAGE)

Clara M. Keegan, MD

 BASICS

DESCRIPTION

- Spontaneous abortion (SAb) (miscarriage) is the failure or loss of a pregnancy before 13 weeks' gestational age (WGA).
- Related terms
  - Anembryonic gestation: gestational sac on ultrasound (US) without visible embryo after 6 WGA
  - Complete abortion: entire contents of uterus expelled
  - Ectopic pregnancy: pregnancy outside the uterus
  - Embryonic or fetal demise: cervix closed; embryo or fetus present in the uterus without cardiac activity.
  - Incomplete abortion: abortion with retained products of conception, generally placental tissue
  - Induced or therapeutic abortion: evacuation of uterine contents or products of conception medically or surgically
  - Inevitable abortion: cervical dilatation or rupture of membranes in the presence of vaginal bleeding
  - Recurrent abortion: ≥3 consecutive pregnancy losses at <15 WGA
  - Threatened abortion: vaginal bleeding in the 1st trimester of pregnancy
  - Septic abortion: a spontaneous or therapeutic abortion complicated by pelvic infection; common complication of illegally performed induced abortions
- Synonym(s): miscarriage; early pregnancy loss
  - Missed abortion and blighted ovum are used less frequently in favor of terms representing the sonographic diagnosis.

EPIDEMIOLOGY

Predominant age: increases with advancing age, especially >35 years; at age 40 years, the loss rate is twice that of age 20 years.

Incidence

- Threatened abortion (1st-trimester bleeding) occurs in 20–25% of clinical pregnancies.
- Between 10% and 15% of all clinically recognized pregnancies end in SAb, with 80% of these occurring within 12 weeks after last menstrual period (LMP) (1).
- When both clinical and biochemical (β-hCG detected) pregnancies are considered, about 30% of pregnancies end in SAb.
- One in four women will have a SAb during her lifetime (1).

ETIOLOGY AND PATHOPHYSIOLOGY

- Chromosomal anomalies (50% of cases)
- Congenital anomalies
- Trauma
- Maternal factors: uterine abnormalities, infection (toxoplasma, other viruses, rubella, cytomegalovirus, herpesvirus), maternal endocrine disorders, hypercoagulable state

Genetics

Approximately 50% of 1st-trimester SAbs have significant chromosomal anomalies, with 50% of these being autosomal trisomies and the remainder being triploidy, tetraploidy, or 45X monosomies.

RISK FACTORS

Most cases of SAb occur in patients without identifiable risk factors; however, risk factors include the following:

- Chromosomal abnormalities
- Advancing maternal age

- Uterine abnormalities
- Maternal chronic disease (antiphospholipid antibodies, uncontrolled diabetes mellitus, polycystic ovarian syndrome, obesity, hypertension, thyroid disease, renal disease)
- Other possible contributing factors include smoking, alcohol, cocaine use, infection, and luteal phase defect.

GENERAL PREVENTION

- Insufficient evidence supports the use of aspirin and/or other anticoagulants, bed rest, hCG, immunotherapy, progestogens, uterine muscle relaxants, or vitamins for general prevention of SAb, before or after threatened abortion is diagnosed.
- By the time hemorrhage begins, 1/2 of pregnancies complicated by threatened abortion already have no fetal cardiac activity.

- Recurrent abortion: Women with a history of ≥3 prior SAbs may benefit from progestogens (OR 0.39, 95% CI 0.21–0.72) (2)[A].
- Antiphospholipid syndrome: The combination of unfractionated heparin and aspirin reduces risk of SAb in women with antiphospholipid antibodies and a history of recurrent abortion (RRR 46%, 95% CI 0.29–0.71) (3)[A].

DIAGNOSIS

HISTORY

- The possibility of pregnancy should be considered in a reproductive-age woman who presents with nonmenstrual vaginal bleeding.
- Vaginal bleeding
  - Characteristics (amount, color, consistency, associated symptoms), onset (abrupt or gradual), duration, intensity/quantity, and exacerbating/precipitating factors
  - Document LMP if known: allows calculation of estimated gestational age
- Abdominal pain/uterine cramping, as well as associated nausea/vomiting/syncope
- Rupture of membranes
- Passage of products of conception
- Prenatal course: toxic or infectious exposures, family or personal history of genetic abnormalities, past history of ectopic pregnancy or SAb, endocrine disease, autoimmune disorder, bleeding/clotting disorder

PHYSICAL EXAM

- Orthostatic vital signs to estimate hemodynamic stability
- Abdominal exam for tenderness, guarding, rebound, bowel sounds (peritoneal signs more likely with ectopic pregnancy)
- Speculum exam for visual assessment of cervical dilation, blood, and products of conception (confirms diagnosis of SAb)
- Bimanual exam to assess for uterine size–dates discrepancy and adnexal tenderness or mass

DIFFERENTIAL DIAGNOSIS

- Ectopic pregnancy: potentially life-threatening; must be considered in any woman of childbearing age with abdominal pain and vaginal bleeding
- Physiologic bleeding in normal pregnancy (implantation bleeding)
- Subchorionic bleeding
- Cervical polyps, neoplasia, and/or inflammatory conditions

- Hydatidiform mole pregnancy
- hCG-secreting ovarian tumor

DIAGNOSTIC TESTS & INTERPRETATION

Initial Tests (lab, imaging)

- Quantitative hCG
  - Particularly useful if intrauterine pregnancy (IUP) has not been documented by US.
  - Serial quantitative serum hCG measurements can assess viability of the pregnancy. Serum hCG should rise at least 53% every 48 hours through 7 weeks after LMP. An inappropriate rise, plateau, or decrease of hCG suggests abnormal IUP or possible ectopic pregnancy.
- Complete blood count (CBC) with differential
- Rh type
- Cultures: gonorrhea/chlamydia
- US exam to evaluate fetal viability and to rule out ectopic pregnancy (4)[A]

  - hCG >2,000 mIU/mL necessary to detect IUP via transvaginal US (TVUS), >5,500 mIU/mL for abdominal US
  - TVUS criteria for nonviable intrauterine gestation: 7-mm fetal pole without cardiac activity or 25-mm gestational sac without a fetal pole, IUP with no growth over 1 week, or previously seen IUP no longer visible
  - Structures and timing: with TVUS, gestational sac of 2 to 3 mm generally seen around 5 WGA; yolk sac by 5.5 WGA; fetal pole with cardiac activity by 6 WGA

Follow-Up Tests & Special Considerations

- In the case of vaginal bleeding with no documented IUP and hCG <2,000 mIU/mL, follow serum hCG levels weekly to zero.
- If levels plateau, consider ectopic pregnancy or retained products of conception. If levels are very high, consider gestational trophoblastic disease.
- If initial hCG level does not permit documentation of IUP by TVUS, follow serum hCG in 48 hours to document appropriate rise.
- Repeat US once hCG is at a level commensurate with visualization on US (see above).
- Provide patient with ectopic precautions in interim: worsening abdominal pain, dizziness/syncope, nausea/vomiting.
- In a pregnancy of unknown location with hCG rise <53% in 48 hours, offer methotrexate for treatment of presumed ectopic pregnancy.

Diagnostic Procedures/Other

- Fetal heart tones can be auscultated with Doppler starting between 10 and 12 WGA in a viable pregnancy.
- In threatened abortion, fetal cardiac activity at 7 to 11 WGA is 90–96% predictive of continued pregnancy.

 TREATMENT

GENERAL MEASURES

- Discuss contraception plan at the time of diagnosis of SAb, as ovulation can occur prior to resumption of normal menses.

- Expectant management ("watchful waiting") is 90% effective for incomplete abortion, although it may take several weeks for the process to be complete (1)[A]. This approach is only recommended in the 1st trimester and is more effective in women with symptoms of impending pregnancy loss (5)[C].

MEDICATION
- Long-term conception rate and pregnancy outcomes are similar for women who undergo expectant management, medical treatment, or surgical evacuation.
- Postinfection rates are lower with medical versus surgical management.

First Line
- Misoprostol: most common agent for inducing passage of tissue in missed or incomplete abortion
  - Off-label use; has not been submitted to the FDA for consideration for use in treatment of early pregnancy failure. Recognized by the World Health Organization (WHO) as a life-saving medication for this indication.
  - Efficacy: complete expulsion of products of conception in 71% by day 3, 84% by day 8
  - Efficacy depends on route of administration, gestational age of pregnancy, and dose.
  - Recommended dose is 800 μg vaginally; alternate regimens include the WHO regimen of 600 μg sublingually q3h for up to 3 doses; multidose regimens and oral dosing (including buccal and sublingual) may result in increased side effects.
- Common adverse effects include abdominal pain/cramping, nausea, and diarrhea. Pain increases at higher doses but is manageable with oral analgesia. There is no increase in nausea/diarrhea with a higher dose.
- Recommended for stable patients who decline surgery but do not want to wait for spontaneous passage of products of conception.

Second Line
- Rh-negative patients should be given Rh immunoglobulin (RhoGAM) 50 μg IM following a SAb.
- Women with evidence of anemia should receive iron supplementation.

ISSUES FOR REFERRAL
Patients should be monitored for up to 1 year for the development of pathologic grief. There is insufficient evidence to support counseling to prevent development of anxiety or depression related to grief following SAb.

SURGERY/OTHER PROCEDURES
- Uterine aspiration (suction dilation and curettage [D&C] or manual vacuum aspiration [MVA]) is the conventional treatment.
- Indications: septic abortion, heavy bleeding, hypotension, patient choice
- Risks (all rare): anesthesia (usually local), uterine perforation, intrauterine adhesions, cervical trauma, infection that may lead to infertility or increased risk of ectopic pregnancy
- When compared with expectant management, surgical intervention leads to fewer days of vaginal bleeding, with a lower risk of incomplete abortion and heavy bleeding but a higher risk of infection (6)[A].
- Vacuum aspiration (manual or electric) is considered preferable to sharp curettage, as aspiration is less painful, takes less time, involves less blood loss, and does not require general anesthesia. The WHO supports use of suction curettage over rigid metal curettage.
- Although data from induced abortions suggest that antibiotic prophylaxis with doxycycline 100 mg BID reduces the already rare risk of postprocedure infection, data are insufficient to support use of antibiotics after aspiration for SAb (7)[A].

COMPLEMENTARY & ALTERNATIVE MEDICINE
A systematic review of Chinese herbal medicine alone and in conjunction with Western medicine showed benefit over Western medicine alone in achieving continued viability at 28 weeks (number needed to treat [NNT] = 4.8 pregnancies with combined therapy). However, the available studies did not meet international standards for reporting quality (8)[C].

INPATIENT CONSIDERATIONS
Admission Criteria/Initial Stabilization
If the patient has orthostatic vital signs, initiate resuscitation with IV fluids and/or blood products, if needed.

IV Fluids
Hemodynamically unstable patients may require IV fluids and/or blood products to maintain BP.

 ONGOING CARE

FOLLOW-UP RECOMMENDATIONS
All patients should be offered follow-up in 2 to 6 weeks to monitor for resolution of bleeding, return of menses, and symptoms related to grief, as well as to review the contraception plan.

Patient Monitoring
- If SAb occurs in setting of previously documented IUP and abortion is completed with resumption of normal menses, it is not necessary to check or follow serum hCG to 0.
- After medical management, confirm complete expulsion with US or serial serum β-hCG (5)[C].
- If pregnancy is not immediately desired, offer effective contraception. Immediate insertion of an intrauterine device is both acceptable and safe.
- If pregnancy is desired, provide preconception counseling. There is no evidence that it is necessary to wait a certain number of cycles before attempting conception again.

DIET
NPO if patient is to undergo D&C under general anesthesia

PATIENT EDUCATION
- Pelvic rest for 1 week after D&C or MVA
- Advise patients to call with excessive bleeding (soaking two pads per hour for 2 hours), fever, pelvic pain, or malaise, which could indicate retained products of conception or endometritis.
- A patient fact sheet on miscarriage is available through the American Academy of Family Physicians at http://www.aafp.org/afp/2011/0701/p85.html.

PROGNOSIS
- Prognosis is excellent once bleeding is controlled.
- Recurrent abortion: Prognosis depends on etiology; up to 70% rate of success with subsequent pregnancy

COMPLICATIONS
- D&C or MVA: uterine perforation, bleeding, adhesions, cervical trauma, and infection that may lead to infertility or increased risk of ectopic pregnancy. Bleeding and adhesions more common with D&C than with MVA; all complications rare
- Retained products of conception

REFERENCES
1. Prine LW, MacNaughton H. Office management of early pregnancy loss. *Am Fam Physician.* 2011;84(1):75–82.
2. Haas DM, Ramsey PS. Progestogen for preventing miscarriage. *Cochrane Database Syst Rev.* 2013;(10):CD003511.
3. Empson M, Lassere M, Craig J, et al. Prevention of recurrent miscarriage for women with antiphospholipid antibody or lupus anticoagulant. *Cochrane Database Syst Rev.* 2005;(2):CD002859.
4. Doubilet PM, Benson CB, Bourne T, et al. Diagnostic criteria for nonviable pregnancy early in the first trimester. *N Engl J Med.* 2013;369(15):1443–1451.
5. Committee on Practice Bulletins—Gynecology. The American College of Obstetricians and Gynecologists Practice Bulletin No. 150. Early pregnancy loss. *Obstet Gynecol.* 2015;125(5):1258–1267.
6. Nanda K, Lopez LM, Grimes DA, et al. Expectant care versus surgical treatment for miscarriage. *Cochrane Database Syst Rev.* 2012;(3):CD003518.
7. May W, Gülmezoglu AM, Ba-Thike K. Antibiotics for incomplete abortion. *Cochrane Database Syst Rev.* 2007;(4):CD001779.
8. Li L, Dou L, Leung PC, et al. Chinese herbal medicines for threatened miscarriage. *Cochrane Database Syst Rev.* 2012;(5):CD008510.

ADDITIONAL READING
- Murphy FA, Lipp A, Powles DL. Follow-up for improving psychological well being for women after a miscarriage. *Cochrane Database Syst Rev.* 2012;(3):CD008679.
- Neilson JP, Gyte GM, Hickey M, et al. Medical treatments for incomplete miscarriage. *Cochrane Database Syst Rev.* 2013;(3):CD007223.
- Okusanya BO, Oduwole O, Effa EE. Immediate postabortal insertion of intrauterine devices. *Cochrane Database Syst Rev.* 2014;(7):CD001777.
- Tunçalp O, Gülmezoglu AM, Souza JP. Surgical procedures for evacuating incomplete miscarriage. *Cochrane Database Syst Rev.* 2010;(9):CD001993.

 SEE ALSO
- Ectopic Pregnancy
- Algorithm: Abortion, Recurrent

 CODES

ICD10
- O03.9 Complete or unspecified spontaneous abortion without complication
- O03.4 Incomplete spontaneous abortion without complication
- O02.1 Missed abortion

CLINICAL PEARLS
- Any pregnant woman with abdominal pain and/or vaginal bleeding must be evaluated to rule out ectopic pregnancy, which is potentially life threatening.
- As all options have similar long-term outcomes, patient preference should determine whether management is expectant, medical, or surgical.

ACETAMINOPHEN POISONING
Dawn Sloan, MD

 BASICS

DESCRIPTION
- A disorder characterized by hepatic necrosis following large ingestions of acetaminophen. Symptoms may vary from initial nausea, vomiting, diaphoresis, and malaise to jaundice, confusion, somnolence, coma, and death. The clinical hallmark is the onset of symptoms within 24 hours of ingestion of acetaminophen-only or combination products. Ideally, ingestion is treated before symptoms develop.
- Acetaminophen poisoning is most often encountered following large, single ingestions of acetaminophen-containing medications. Usual toxic doses are >10 g in adults and >200 mg/kg in children. However, poisoning also occurs after acute and chronic ingestions of lesser amounts in susceptible individuals, including those who regularly abuse alcohol, are chronically malnourished, or take medications that affect hepatic metabolism of acetaminophen.
- Therapeutic adult doses are 0.5 to 1 g q4–6h, up to a maximum of 4 g/day. Therapeutic pediatric doses are 10 to 15 mg/kg q4–6h, not to exceed 5 doses in 24 hours.
- System(s) affected: gastrointestinal, cardiovascular, renal/urologic
  – Multisystem organ failure can occur.
- Synonym(s): paracetamol poisoning

Geriatric Considerations
Hepatic damage may be increased if chronically taking hepatotoxic medications.

Pediatric Considerations
Hepatic damage at toxic acetaminophen levels is decreased in young children. This may be due to larger glutathione stores.

Pregnancy Considerations
- Increased incidence of spontaneous abortion, especially with overdose at early gestational age
- Incidence of spontaneous abortion or fetal death appears to be increased when *N*-acetylcysteine (NAC) treatment is delayed.
- IV NAC is generally preferred in pregnancy since it may offer greater bioavailability.

EPIDEMIOLOGY
- Predominant age: children and adults
- Predominant sex: no reported association

Incidence
>24,000 ED visits per year on average from 2004 to 2012 for acetaminophen-related overdoses in the United States

Prevalence
- >38,000 hospitalizations per year on average from 1998 to 2011 for acetaminophen-related poisonings in the United States
- <1% of hospitalizations in those <18 years old had coexistent liver toxicity.

ETIOLOGY AND PATHOPHYSIOLOGY
- Accidental or intentional ingestion of acetaminophen or combination medications containing acetaminophen
- 96% of ingested acetaminophen is metabolized in the liver, with only 2–4% excreted unchanged in the urine. When taken in therapeutic doses, 90–95% of hepatic metabolism occurs via glucuronidation and sulfation and results in the formation of benign metabolites. 5–10% of hepatic metabolism is by oxidation through the cytochrome P_{450} enzyme system (CYP 3A4 and CYP 2E1), which results in the formation of the toxic metabolite *N*-acetyl-*p*-benzoquinoneimine (NAPQI). NAPQI is rapidly conjugated with glutathione to form a nontoxic metabolite. The metabolites are excreted in the urine along with a small amount of unchanged drug. Hepatocellular damage typically occurs when toxic doses of acetaminophen result in saturation of the glucuronidation and sulfation pathways with subsequent production of excessive amounts of NAPQI. Available glutathione stores become depleted, NAPQI accumulates, and hepatocellular damage occurs.

RISK FACTORS
- Concurrent poisoning with other substances
- Psychiatric illness
- Previous toxic ingestions or suicide attempts
- Regular ingestion of large amounts of alcohol

GENERAL PREVENTION
Parent/caregiver education essential:
- Education during well-child exams regarding poisoning prevention
- Emergency telephone numbers

 DIAGNOSIS

- May present asymptomatic with history of ingestion in the last 8 hours, as signs and symptoms are related to liver toxicity and develop over the first 24 hours following large ingestions; may last as long as 8 days
- Symptoms may develop gradually following long-term ingestion of near-maximal therapeutic amounts of acetaminophen. Such patients may present in stages 1 to 3, without a history of ingestion of the usual toxic doses.
- Severe symptoms indicate large ingestions or coingestants:
  – Stage 1: first 24 hours after time of ingestion:
    ○ Nausea
    ○ Vomiting
    ○ Diaphoresis
  – Stage 2: 24 to 48 hours:
    ○ Right upper quadrant pain
    ○ Typically less nausea, vomiting, diaphoresis, and malaise than in stage 1
  – Stage 3: 72 to 96 hours:
    ○ Nausea, vomiting, and malaise reappear.
    ○ Severe poisonings may result in jaundice, confusion, somnolence, and coma.
  – Stage 4: 7 to 8 days:
    ○ Resolution of clinical signs in survivors
- Fulminant hepatic failure occurs in <1% of adults and is very rare in children <6 years of age.
- Patients with an unexplained rise in liver function tests (LFTs) with negative acetaminophen levels may be overdose patients presenting in stage 3.

HISTORY
Ingestion or suspected ingestion of acetaminophen-containing product

DIFFERENTIAL DIAGNOSIS
- Consider presence of coingestants, especially alcohol and aspirin.
- Other ingested toxins that produce severe acute hepatic injury, including the mushroom *Amanita phalloides* and products containing yellow phosphorus or carbon tetrachloride

DIAGNOSTIC TESTS & INTERPRETATION
Initial Tests (lab, imaging)
- Plasma acetaminophen levels should be drawn on all patients ≥4 hours after ingestion (levels prior to 4 hours not helpful).
- **ALT**, AST, PT/NR, bilirubin, lactate dehydrogenase (LDH)
- Electrolytes, glucose, BUN, creatinine
- Pregnancy screen in females (urine or serum)
- Urinalysis
- Consider arterial blood gas (ABG) if pH disturbance is suspected on clinical or lab grounds.
- Screens for suspected coingestants (aspirin, iron, etc.) may be positive (especially when suicide attempt is a possibility).
- With toxic ingestions, aspartate transaminase (AST; serum glutamic-oxaloacetic transaminase), alanine transaminase (ALT; serum glutamic-pyruvic transaminase), and bilirubin levels begin to rise in stage 2 and peak in stage 3.
- In severe poisonings, the prothrombin time (PT)/international normalized ratio (INR) will parallel these changes and should be monitored.
- Markedly elevated ALT levels are consistent with the diagnosis, and improvement in ALT is a good sign.
- Laboratory abnormalities usually resolve by stage 4.
- Renal function abnormalities are common in patients with hepatotoxicity.
- Evidence of damage to pancreas and heart may present following severe poisonings.
- Anion-gap metabolic acidosis due to accumulation of 5-oxoprolene may rarely be seen.
- Drugs that may alter lab results: none with clinically significant cross-reactivity with plasma acetaminophen assay
- Disorders that may alter lab results: diseases or toxic substances that damage the liver, particularly alcohol
- No specific imaging required

Follow-Up Tests & Special Considerations
ABG after hydration if pH is acidotic

Test Interpretation
Centrilobular hepatic necrosis

 TREATMENT

- Contact a regional/local poison control center for recommendations. In the United States: (800) 222-1222
- NAC should be given when plasma acetaminophen concentrations measured ≥4 hours after ingestion are in the "possible risk" or higher levels on the Rumack-Matthew nomogram. This corresponds to acetaminophen levels >150 µg/mL (993 µmol/L), >75 µg/mL (497 µmol/L), and >37 µg/mL (244 µmol/L) at 4, 8, and 12 hours after ingestion, respectively. See http://www.ars-informatica.ca/toxicity_nomogram.php?calc=acetamin or http://www.merckmanuals.com/professional/resources/clinical_calculators/name/calculator.html?WT.z_resource=Clinical Calculators.
- NAC should be started within 8 hours of ingestion for best chance of hepatic protection. Patients presenting near 8 hours should empirically receive NAC while waiting for labs.
- All patients with acetaminophen liver injury (even after 8 hours) should receive NAC.
- NAC therapy may be effective up to ≥36 hours after ingestion.

- Single-dose activated charcoal may be used if given within 1 hour of ingestion (especially in cases of coingestants) (1,2)[C],(3)[A], but not within 1 hour of administration of oral NAC. Never delay NAC for activated charcoal.
- Ipecac and gastric lavage are no longer recommended for routine use at home or in health care facilities (3)[C].

MEDICATION

First Line

- Acetylcysteine (NAC, Mucomyst) should be initiated within 8 hours of ingestion whenever possible; single-dose activated charcoal (1 g/kg PO) may be effective if given within 1 hour of ingestion. *Never delay oral NAC for activated charcoal.*
- Acetylcysteine may be given PO or IV, depending on situation and availability:
  - IV loading dose of Acetadote 150 mg/kg over 60 minutes followed by an infusion of 50 mg/kg over 4 hours (12.5 mg/kg/hr); this is followed by an infusion of 100 mg/kg over the next 16 hours (6.25 mg/kg/hr) (20-hour regimen)
  - Oral loading dose of 140 mg/kg, followed by 70 mg/kg q4h for 17 additional doses (72-hour regimen)
- Contraindications: medication allergies
- Precautions:
  - Oral NAC may cause significant nausea and vomiting due to its sulfur content; consider nasogastric tube.
  - Nausea can be treated with metoclopramide (Reglan), 1 to 2 mg/kg IV, or ondansetron (Zofran), 0.15 mg/kg IV (for age >4 years, usually 4 mg/dose).
  - IV NAC (Acetadote) may cause anaphylactoid reactions, including rash, bronchospasm, pruritus, angioedema, tachycardia, or hypotension (higher rates seen in asthmatics and those with atopy) (4,5)[C].
- Reactions usually occur with loading dose. Slow or temporarily stop the infusion; may concurrently treat with antihistamines
- Significant possible interactions: Activated charcoal given within 1 hour of oral NAC may adsorb NAC, limiting its effectiveness.

Second Line

Oral racemethionine (methionine)

ISSUES FOR REFERRAL

- Psychological evaluation in emergency room and close follow-up after intentional ingestions.
- Consider child abuse reporting if neglect led to overdose.

INPATIENT CONSIDERATIONS

Admission Criteria/Initial Stabilization

- Toxic and intentional ingestions
- Any reported ingestion with increased LFTs, acidosis on ABG, elevated creatinine, and so forth.
- Initiate aggressive age- and weight-appropriate IV hydration.

 ONGOING CARE

FOLLOW-UP RECOMMENDATIONS

- All patients should be evaluated at a health care facility.
- Patients with evidence of organ failure, increased LFTs, or coagulopathy should be evaluated for transfer to a site capable of liver transplant.
- Activity may be restricted if significant hepatic damage is present.
- Outpatient management of nontoxic accidental ingestions

Patient Monitoring

Ask about possible ingestion by others (i.e., suicide pacts).

DIET

No special diet, except with severe hepatic damage

PATIENT EDUCATION

- Patients should be counseled to avoid Tylenol if already using combination product(s) containing acetaminophen.
- Education of parents/caregivers during well-child visits
- Anticipatory guidance for caregivers, family, and cohabitants of potentially suicidal patients
- Education of patients taking long-term acetaminophen therapy

PROGNOSIS

- Complete recovery with early therapy
- <1% of adult patients develop hepatic failure. King criteria (pH <7.3, PT >100 s [INR >65], creatinine >3.4 mg/dL [>300 μmol/L]) is associated with a poor prognosis and possible need for liver transplant (6)[C]. Early referral increases the chance for transplant success (5)[A].
- Hepatic failure is very rare in children <6 years of age.

COMPLICATIONS

Rare following recovery from acute poisoning

REFERENCES

1. Brok J, Buckley N, Gluud C. Interventions for paracetamol (acetaminophen) overdose. *Cochrane Database Syst Rev.* 2006;(2):CD003328.
2. Gaudreault P. Activated charcoal revisited. *Clin Ped Emerg Med.* 2005;6:76–80.
3. Heard K. Gastrointestinal decontamination. *Med Clin North Am.* 2005;89(6):1067–1078.
4. Acetylcysteine (Acetadote) for acetaminophen overdosage. *Med Lett Drugs Ther.* 2005;47(1215–1216):70–71.
5. Culley CM, Krenzelok EP. A clinical and pharmacoeconomic justification for intravenous acetylcysteine: a US perspective. *Toxicol Rev.* 2005;24(2):131–143.
6. O'Grady JG, Alexander GJ, Hayllar KM, et al. Early indicators of prognosis in fulminant hepatic failure. *Gastroenterology.* 1989;97(2):439–445.

ADDITIONAL READING

- Ferner RE, Dear JW, Bateman DN. Management of paracetamol poisoning. *BMJ.* 2011;342:d2218.
- Larson AM, Polson J, Fontana RJ, et al. Acetaminophen-induced acute liver failure: results of a United States multicenter, prospective study. *Hepatology.* 2005;42(6):1364–1372.
- Major JM, Zhou EH, Wong HL, et al. Trends in rates of acetaminophen-related adverse events in the United States [published online ahead of print November 3, 2015]. *Pharmacoepidemiol Drug Saf.*
- Mund ME, Quarcoo D, Gyo C, et al. Paracetamol as a toxic substance for children: aspects of legislation in selected countries. *J Occup Med Toxicol.* 2005;10:43.

 SEE ALSO

Acetaminophen Poisoning, Treatment

 CODES

ICD

- T39.1X4A Poisoning by 4-Aminophenol derivatives, undetermined, init
- K71.10 Toxic liver disease with hepatic necrosis, without coma
- T39.1X1A Poisoning by 4-Aminophenol derivatives, accidental, init

CLINICAL PEARLS

- Contact a regional poison control center for management recommendations. In the United States: (800) 222-1222.
- NAC should be given when plasma acetaminophen concentrations measured ≥4 hours after ingestion are in the "possible risk" or higher levels on the Rumack-Matthew nomogram. This corresponds to acetaminophen levels >150 μg/mL (993 μmol/L), >75 μg/mL (497 μmol/L), and >40 μg/mL (265 μmol/L) at 4, 8, and 12 hours after ingestion, respectively.
- NAC should be started within 8 hours of ingestion for best chance of hepatic protection. Patients presenting near 8 hours should empirically receive NAC while waiting for labs.
- All patients with acetaminophen liver injury (even after 8 hours) should receive NAC.

ACL INJURY

Jeff Wang, MD, MPH • J. Herbert Stevenson, MD

 BASICS

DESCRIPTION

- The anterior cruciate ligament (ACL) is a primary knee stabilizer that serves to prevent excessive anterior translation and internal rotation of the tibia on the femur.
  - During dynamic movement, the ACL and posterior cruciate ligament (PCL) work together to stabilize the knee.
- ACL injuries are common and can occur through multiple mechanisms. >70% of ACL injuries are caused by noncontact forces.
- Although partial tears occur, complete ACL tears are more common.
- Due to differences in pelvic architecture and lower extremity alignment, female athletes are at 2 to 5 times higher at risk of ACL tear.
- ACL injury is associated with early onset of knee osteoarthritis.

EPIDEMIOLOGY

Incidence
- 250,000 ACL injuries annually in the United States
- Female incidence 2- to 5-fold > male (1)
- Greater incidence of noncontact ACL injuries in sports requiring cutting, pivoting, and rapid deceleration, such as basketball and soccer (1)

Prevalence
- Young athletes (15 to 25 years) sustain >50% of all ACL injuries (1)[B].
- >2/3 of patients with complete ACL tear have associated meniscal and/or articular cartilage injury.

Pediatric Considerations
- Rule out physeal injuries in skeletally immature patients.
- The incidence of ACL tears in patients with open physes has increased in recent years.
- ACL injury rates increase for both boys and girls after age 11 years.

ETIOLOGY AND PATHOPHYSIOLOGY

- Noncontact mechanisms: torsional or hyperextension forces creates anterior translation of the tibia relative to the femur. This creates excessive stress across the ACL with resultant rupture.
- Direct trauma: most often, a valgus blow to the knee with resultant trauma to ACL, medial collateral ligament, and lateral meniscus ("unhappy triad")

Genetics
A genetic predisposition has been identified. An association has been found between the genes encoding proteoglycans and the risk of ACL tears (7)[B].

RISK FACTORS

- Female athletes have increased risk.
  - Hormonal influence
    o Alterations in hormonal balance hypothesized to increase risk, but no conclusive evidence linking menstrual phase to ACL injury risk.

- Anatomic gender differences
  o Increased Q angle, increased genu valgum, narrower femoral notch size, smaller ACL
  o Neuromuscular imbalances (increased quadriceps activation, decreased hamstring activity during landings)
  - Movement patterns (sudden deceleration, change-of-direction cutting movements, landing from a jump in hyperextension)

GENERAL PREVENTION

- Neuromuscular training with proprioceptive, plyometric, and strength exercises significantly reduce noncontact ACL injuries in female athletes if performed several times a week for >6 weeks (2)[C].
- Prophylactic knee bracing does not prevent ACL injury.

COMMONLY ASSOCIATED CONDITIONS

- Meniscal tear
- Collateral ligament tear
- PCL tear
- Tibia or femur fractures
- Osteochondral injury
- Early-onset degenerative joint disease

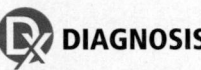 **DIAGNOSIS**

HISTORY
Describe mechanism
- Noncontact
  - Sudden deceleration
  - Cutting, sudden change in direction
  - Landing from a jump with the knee in extension
- Contact with player, object
- May recall sudden pop or snap
- Sudden pain and giving way
- Marked effusion/hemarthrosis within 4 to 12 hours
- "Pop" with deceleration or twisting movement associated with early effusion and inability to continue with participation are highly suggestive of ACL tear.

PHYSICAL EXAM
- Inspect for malalignment (fracture, dislocation).
- Palpate for effusion.
- Decreased range of motion (ROM)
  - Deficits may be secondary to pain, effusion, mechanical blocks (meniscal tear, loose body, torn ACL stump).
- Joint instability
- Difficulty bearing weight
- Evaluate integrity of extensor mechanism
- Special maneuvers (Lachman; anterior drawer; pivot shift) to assess ACL integrity
- Lachman test: most sensitive and highly specific diagnostic test for ACL injury in acute setting (3)[B]
  - Knee is placed in 20 to 30 degrees of flexion. Tibia is translated anteriorly with femur stabilized by the opposite hand. Increased anterior translation compared with uninjured knee indicates injury. Lack of a solid end point indicates rupture.

- Pivot shift test: less sensitive, but more than Lachman test: specific for ACL tear (3)[B]
  - Knee is placed in extension. Knee is flexed while valgus and internal rotation stress is applied. A positive test is anterior subluxation at 20 to 40 degrees of flexion.
- Anterior drawer test (3)[B]
  - Low sensitivity for ACL integrity, especially in acute setting
- Posterior drawer test assesses PCL integrity.
- McMurray test assesses for meniscal tears.
- Valgus/varus stress test for medial collateral ligament/lateral collateral (MCL/LCL) integrity

DIFFERENTIAL DIAGNOSIS
- Fracture
- Meniscal injury
- Patellar dislocation/subluxation
- Tendon disruption
- PCL injury
- Collateral ligament injury

DIAGNOSTIC TESTS & INTERPRETATION
Initial Tests (lab, imaging)
- Radiographs to rule out associated bony injury
- Anterior-posterior (AP), lateral, and tunnel views
  - Segond fracture: avulsion fracture of the lateral capsular margin of the tibia
  - Tibial eminence avulsion fracture
  - Fracture of proximal tibia or distal femur
  - Osteochondral injuries

Follow-Up Tests & Special Considerations
- MRI is the gold standard for imaging ligamentous and intra-articular structures. The sensitivity of MRI is 87–94%, specificity 88–93% (4).
- Secondary signs of ACL injury on MRI include contusion of the anterior femoral condyle and/or posterior tibial plateau, anterior translation of the tibia, an uncovered or displaced posterior horn of the lateral meniscus, PCL buckling, or a Segond fracture (an avulsion fracture of the lateral tibial condyle).
- Ultrasound is an emerging technique that is fast and noninvasive (5)[B].

Diagnostic Procedures/Other
Surgical management should be considered in the active population, young or old.

 TREATMENT

GENERAL MEASURES
- Acute injury: protection, relative rest, ice, compression, elevation, medications, modalities (PRICEMM) therapy
- Crutches may be useful until patient is able to ambulate without pain.
- Locked knee brace may be used initially for comfort. Use with caution and transition to a hinged knee brace as soon as possible to avoid quadriceps atrophy and stiffness.
- Aspiration of large effusion may alleviate pain and increase ROM.

MEDICATION

First Line
- Nonsteroidal anti-inflammatory drugs (NSAIDs)
  - Acute ligament sprains
    - Ibuprofen: 200 to 800 mg TID
    - Naproxen: 250 to 500 mg BID
- Acetaminophen: 3 g/day divided TID
- Opioids for severe pain (e.g., acetaminophen-hydrocodone)

ISSUES FOR REFERRAL
The decision to manage ACL tears surgically or nonsurgically ("conservatively") can be difficult. Consider surgical management in active patients or if the injury interferes with activities of daily living.

- Physical therapy is essential whether an athlete chooses nonsurgical or surgical treatment. Proper rehabilitation is time-consuming (6 to 12 months) and hard work. Physical therapy restores ROM, strength, and proprioception.
- Preoperative phase
  - Increase ROM and quadriceps strength, minimize inflammation.
- Early postoperative phase: weeks 2 to 4
  - ROM: Full extension is the primary goal. Rehabilitation begins immediately.
  - Progress to full weight bearing
- Intermediate postoperative phase: weeks 4 to 12
  - ROM: full flexion, hyperextension
  - Quadriceps and hamstring strengthening proprioceptive training, normalize gait
- Late postop phase: >3 months postop
  - Straight-line running
  - Increase speed, duration over 6 to 8 weeks
  - Progress to cutting and sport-specific drills
  - Strength and proprioceptive training

Geriatric Considerations
Management is based on anticipated activity level, associated injuries, coexisting medical conditions, and acute versus long-standing ACL deficiency.

SURGERY/OTHER PROCEDURES
- The decision for surgery depends on patient's activity level, age, associated injuries, and presence of osteoarthritis.
- There is an insufficient evidence to recommend surgery over conservative management in skeletally immature patients.
- No significant difference in patient-reported knee function or muscle strength between surgical and nonsurgical management (6)[B].
- In young, active adults with acute ACL tears, rehabilitation plus early ACL repair was not superior to a strategy of initial rehabilitation with delayed repair if rehabilitation alone failed. Rehabilitation alone results in an overall reduction of ACL reconstructions (6)[B].
- Reconstruction techniques
  - Bone-patella tendon-bone autograft
  - Hamstring autograft
  - Allograft tendon (from cadaver)

- No consistent significant differences in outcome between patellar tendon and hamstring tendon autografts
- In the hamstring autograft approach, double bundle is superior to the single bundle (7)[B].
- Concomitant meniscal tears are repaired at the time of ACL reconstruction.

INPATIENT CONSIDERATIONS
Admission Criteria/Initial Stabilization
Outpatient

 ONGOING CARE

FOLLOW-UP RECOMMENDATIONS
- ROM exercises to regain full flexion and extension
- Advance activity as tolerated

Patient Monitoring
Assess functional status, rehabilitative exercise compliance, and pain control at follow-up visit.

PROGNOSIS
- Athletes typically are out of competitive play for 6 to 9 months after injury for reconstructive surgery and rehabilitation.
- High prevalence of OA, even in those with early ACL reconstruction
- Delaying surgical repair of torn ACL increases risk of secondary meniscal injury.

COMPLICATIONS
- Instability
- Secondary meniscal and articular cartilage injury
- Early-onset degenerative arthritis
- Surgical risks
  - Infection, pulmonary embolism (PE), subsequent ACL graft rupture, laxity due to failure of graft remodeling

REFERENCES
1. Beynnon B, Vacek PM, Newell MK, et al. The effects of level of competition, sport, and sex on the incidence of first-time noncontact anterior cruciate ligament injury. Am J Sports Med. 2014;42(8):1806–1812.
2. Acevedo RJ, Rivera-Vega A, Miranda G, et al. Anterior cruciate ligament injury: identification of risk factors and prevention strategies. Curr Sports Med Rep. 2014;13(3):186–191.
3. Jain DK, Amaravati R, Sharma G. Evaluation of the clinical signs of anterior cruciate ligament and meniscal injuries. Indian J Orthop. 2009;43(4):375–378.
4. Grzelak P, Podgórski MT, Stefańczyk L, et al. Ultrasonographic test for complete anterior cruciate ligament injury. Indian J Orthop. 2015;49(2):143–149.
5. Grindem H, Eitzen I, Engbretsen L, et al. Nonsurgical or surgical treatment of ACL injuries: knee function, sports participation, and knee reinjury: the Delaware-Oslo ACL cohort study. J Bone and Joint Surg. 2014;96(15):1233–1241.
6. Koga H, Muneta T, Yagishita K, et al. Mid- to long-term results of single-bundle versus double-bundle anterior cruciate ligament reconstruction: randomized controlled trial. Arthroscopy. 2015;31(1):69–76.
7. Mannion S, Mtintsilana A, Posthumus M, et al. Genes encoding proteoglycans are associated with the risk of anterior cruciate ligament rupture. Br J Sports Med. 2014;48(22):1640–1646.

ADDITIONAL READING
- Christiansen BA, Anderson MJ, Lee CA, et al. Musculoskeletal changes following non-invasive knee injury using a novel mouse model of post-traumatic osteoarthritis. Osteoarthr Cartil. 2012;20(7):773–782.
- Frobell RB, Roos EM, Roos HP, et al. A randomized trial of treatment for acute anterior cruciate ligament tears. N Engl J Med. 2010;363(4):331–342.
- Hewett TE, Di Stasi SL, Myer GD. Current concepts for injury prevention in athletes after anterior cruciate ligament reconstruction. Am J Sports Med. 2013;41(1):216–224.
- Mohtadi NG, Chan DS, Dainty KN, et al. Patellar tendon versus hamstring tendon autograft for anterior cruciate ligament ruptures in adults. Cochrane Database Syst Rev. 2011;(9):CD005960.
- Silvers HJ, Mandelbaum BR. Prevention of anterior cruciate ligament injury in the female athlete. Br J Sports Med. 2007;(41 Suppl 1):i52–i59.
- White K, Di Stasi SL, Smith AH, et al. Anterior cruciate ligament- specialized post-operative return-to-sports (ACL-SPORTS) training: a randomized control trial. BMC Musculoskelet Disord. 2013;14:108.

 SEE ALSO

Algorithm: Knee pain

CODES

ICD10
- S83.519A Sprain of anterior cruciate ligament of unsp knee, init
- M23.619 Oth spon disrupt of anterior cruciate ligament of unsp knee
- S83.511A Sprain of anterior cruciate ligament of right knee, init

CLINICAL PEARLS
- Lachman test is the most sensitive and specific physical examination maneuver for diagnosing acute ACL injury.
- Bone contusion of the anterior femoral condyle and/or posterior tibial plateau on MRI is highly suggestive of ACL tear.
- 2/3 of complete ACL tears have associated meniscal or articular injuries.
- The decision for surgical repair is based on patient age, activity level, and associated symptoms.

ACNE ROSACEA

Daniel R. DiBlasi, DO • Shane L. Larson, MD

BASICS

DESCRIPTION
- Rosacea is a chronic condition characterized by recurrent episodes of facial flushing, erythema (due to dilatation of small blood vessels in the face), papules, pustules, and telangiectasia (due to increased reactivity of capillaries) in a symmetric, central facial distribution. Sometimes associated with ocular symptoms (ocular rosacea).
- Four subtypes:
  - Erythematotelangiectatic rosacea (ETR)
  - Papulopustular rosacea (PPR)
  - Phymatous rosacea
  - Ocular rosacea
- System(s) affected: skin/exocrine
- Synonym(s): rosacea

Geriatric Considerations
- Uncommon >60 years of age
- Effects of aging might increase the side effects associated with oral isotretinoin used for treatment (at present, data are insufficient due to lack of clinical studies in elderly patients ≥65 years).

EPIDEMIOLOGY
Prevalence
- Predominant age: 30 to 50 years
- Predominant sex: female > male. However, males are at greater risk for progression to later stages.

ETIOLOGY AND PATHOPHYSIOLOGY
- No proven cause
- Possibilities include the following:
  - Thyroid and sex hormone disturbance
  - Alcohol, coffee, tea, spiced food overindulgence (unproven)
  - Demodex follicular parasite (suspected)
  - Exposure to cold, heat
  - Emotional stress
  - Dysfunction of the GI tract

Genetics
People of Northern European and Celtic background commonly afflicted

RISK FACTORS
- Exposure to spicy foods, hot drinks
- Environmental factors: sun, wind, cold, heat

GENERAL PREVENTION
No preventive measures known

COMMONLY ASSOCIATED CONDITIONS
- Seborrheic dermatitis of scalp and eyelids
- Keratitis with photophobia, lacrimation, visual disturbance
- Corneal lesions
- Blepharitis
- Uveitis

DIAGNOSIS

HISTORY
- Usually have a history of episodic flushing with increases in skin temperature in response to heat stimulus in mouth (hot liquids), spicy foods, alcohol, sun exposure (solar elastosis)
- Acne may have preceded onset of rosacea by years; nevertheless, rosacea usually arises de novo without preceding history of acne or seborrhea.
- Excessive facial warmth and redness are the predominant presenting complaints. Itching is generally absent.

PHYSICAL EXAM
- Rosacea has typical stages of evolution:
  - The rosacea diathesis: episodic erythema, "flushing and blushing"
  - Stage I: persistent erythema with telangiectases
  - Stage II: persistent erythema, telangiectases, papules, tiny pustules
  - Stage III: persistent deep erythema, dense telangiectases, papules, pustules, nodules; rarely persistent "solid" edema of the central part of the face (phymatous)
- Facial erythema, particularly on cheeks, nose, and chin. At times, entire face may be involved.
- Inflammatory papules are prominent; pustules and telangiectasia may be present.
- Comedones are absent (unlike acne vulgaris).
- Women usually have lesions on the chin and cheeks, whereas the nose is commonly involved in men.
- Ocular findings (mild dryness and irritation with blepharitis, conjunctival injection, burning, stinging, tearing, eyelid inflammation, swelling, and redness) are present in 50% of patients.

DIFFERENTIAL DIAGNOSIS
- Drug eruptions (iodides and bromides)
- Granulomas of the skin
- Cutaneous lupus erythematosus
- Carcinoid syndrome
- Deep fungal infection
- Acne vulgaris
- Seborrheic dermatitis
- Steroid rosacea (abuse)
- Systemic lupus erythematosus
- Lupus pernio (sarcoidosis)

DIAGNOSTIC TESTS & INTERPRETATION
Diagnosis is based on physical exam findings.

Test Interpretation
- Inflammation around hypertrophied sebaceous glands, producing papules, pustules, and cysts
- Absence of comedones and blocked ducts
- Vascular dilatation and dermal lymphocytic infiltrate

TREATMENT

GENERAL MEASURES
- Proper skin care and photoprotection are important components of management plan (1)[B]. Use of mild, nondrying soap is recommended; local skin irritants should be avoided.
- Avoidance of triggers
- Reassurance that rosacea is completely unrelated to poor hygiene
- Treat psychological stress if present.
- Topical steroids should not be used, as they may aggravate rosacea.
- Avoid oil-based cosmetics:
  - Others are acceptable and may help women tolerate symptoms
- Electrodesiccation or chemical sclerosis of permanently dilated blood vessels
- Possible evolving laser therapy
- Support physical fitness.

MEDICATION

First Line

- Topical metronidazole preparations once (1% formulation) or twice (0.75% formulations) daily for 7 to 12 weeks was significantly more effective than placebo in patients with moderate to severe rosacea. A rosacea treatment system (cleanser, metronidazole 0.75% gel, hydrating complexion corrector, and sunscreen SPF 30) may offer superior efficacy and tolerability to metronidazole (2)[A].
- Azelaic acid (Finacea) is very effective as initial therapy; azelaic acid topical alone is effective for maintenance (3)[A].
- Topical ivermectin 1% cream (2)[A]
  - Recently found to be more effective than metronidazole for treatment of PPR
- Topical brimonidine tartrate 0.5% gel is effective in reducing erythema associated with ETR (4)[A].
  - α_2-Adrenergic receptor agonist; potent vasoconstrictor
- Doxycycline 40-mg dose is at least as effective as 100-mg dose and has a correspondingly lower risk of adverse effects but is much more expensive (5)[A].
- Precautions: Tetracyclines may cause photosensitivity; sunscreen is recommended.
- Significant possible interactions:
  - Tetracyclines: Avoid concurrent administration with antacids, dairy products, or iron.
  - Broad-spectrum antibiotics: may reduce the effectiveness of oral contraceptives; barrier method is recommended.

Second Line

- Topical erythromycin
- Topical clindamycin (lotion preferred)
  - Can be used in combination with benzoyl peroxide; commercial topical combinations are available
- Possible use of calcineurin inhibitors (tacrolimus 0.1%; pimecrolimus 1%). Pimecrolimus 1% is effective to treat mild to moderate inflammatory rosacea (6)[A].
- Permethrin 5% cream; similar efficacy compared to metronidazole (7)[B]. For severe cases, oral isotretinoin at 0.3 mg/kg for a minimum of 3 months.

Pediatric Considerations

Tetracyclines: not for use in children <8 years

Pregnancy Considerations

- Tetracyclines: not for use during pregnancy
- Isotretinoin: teratogenic; not for use during pregnancy or in women of reproductive age who are not using reliable contraception; requires registration with iPLEDGE program

ADDITIONAL THERAPIES

Cyclosporine 0.05% ophthalmic emulsion may be more effective than artificial tears for ocular rosacea.

SURGERY/OTHER PROCEDURES

Laser treatment is an option for progressive telangiectasias or rhinophyma.

 ## ONGOING CARE

FOLLOW-UP RECOMMENDATIONS

Outpatient treatment

Patient Monitoring

- Occasional and as needed
- Close follow-up and laboratory assessment for women using isotretinoin per prescribing instructions and iPLEDGE program guidance.

DIET

Avoid alcohol, excessive sun exposure, and hot drinks of any type.

PROGNOSIS

- Slowly progressive
- Subsides spontaneously (sometimes)

COMPLICATIONS

- Rhinophyma (dilated follicles and thickened bulbous skin on nose), especially in men
- Conjunctivitis
- Blepharitis
- Keratitis
- Visual deterioration

REFERENCES

1. Del Rosso JQ, Thiboutot D, Gallo R, et al. Consensus recommendations from the American Acne & Rosacea Society on the management of rosacea, part 3: a status report on systemic therapies. *Cutis.* 2014;93(1):18–28.
2. van Zuuren EJ, Fedorowicz Z, Carter BR, et al. Interventions for rosacea. *Cochrane Database Syst Rev.* 2015;(4):CD003262. doi:10.1002/14651858.CD003262.pub5.
3. Thiboutot DM, Fleischer AB, Del Rosso JQ, et al. A multicenter study of topical azelaic acid 15% gel in combination with oral doxycycline as initial therapy and azelaic acid 15% gel as maintenance monotherapy. *J Drugs Dermatol.* 2009;8(7):639–648.
4. Fowler J Jr, Jackson JM, Moore A, et al. Efficacy and safety of once-daily topical brimonidine tartrate gel 0.5% for the treatment of moderate to severe facial erythema of rosacea: results of two randomized, double-blind, and vehicle-controlled pivotal studies. *J Drugs Dermatol.* 2013;12(6):650–656.
5. Del Rosso JQ, Webster GF, Jackson M, et al. Two randomized phase III clinical trials evaluating anti-inflammatory dose doxycycline (40-mg doxycycline, USP capsules) administered once daily for treatment of rosacea. *J Am Acad Dermatol.* 2007;56(5):791–802.
6. Kim MB, Kim GW, Park HJ, et al. Pimecrolimus 1% cream for the treatment of rosacea. *J Dermatol.* 2011;38(12):1135–1139. doi:10.1111/j.1346-8138.2011.01223.x.
7. Koçak M, Yağli S, Vahapoğlu G, et al. Permethrin 5% cream versus metronidazole 0.75% gel for the treatment of papulopustular rosacea. A randomized double-blind placebo-controlled study. *Dermatology.* 2002;205(3):265–270.

ADDITIONAL READING

- Leyden JJ. Efficacy of a novel rosacea treatment system: an investigator-blind, randomized, parallel-group study. *J Drugs Dermatol.* 2011;10(10):1179–1185.
- Liu RH, Smith MK, Basta SA, et al. Azelaic acid in the treatment of papulopustular rosacea: a systematic review of randomized controlled trials. *Arch Dermatol.* 2006;142(8):1047–1052.

 ## SEE ALSO

- Acne Vulgaris; Blepharitis; Dermatitis, Seborrheic; Lupus Erythematosus, Discoid; Uveitis
- Algorithm: Acne

CODES

ICD10

- L71.9 Rosacea, unspecified
- L71.8 Other rosacea

CLINICAL PEARLS

- Rosacea usually arises de novo without any preceding history of acne or seborrhea.
- Rosacea may cause chronic eye symptoms, including blepharitis.
- Avoid alcohol, sun exposure, and hot drinks.
- Medication treatment resembles that of acne vulgaris, with oral and topical antibiotics.

ACNE VULGARIS

Gary I. Levine, MD

 BASICS

DESCRIPTION
- Acne vulgaris is a disorder of the pilosebaceous units. It is a chronic inflammatory dermatosis notable for open/closed comedones, papules, pustules, or nodules.
- Systems affected: skin/exocrine

Geriatric Considerations
Favre-Racouchot syndrome: comedones on face and head due to sun exposure

Pregnancy Considerations
- May result in a flare or remission of acne
- Erythromycin can be used in pregnancy; use topical agents when possible.
- Isotretinoin is teratogenic; pregnancy Category X
- Avoid topical tretinoin as it may cause retinoid embryopathy; class C (1).
- Contraindicated: isotretinoin, tazarotene, tetracycline, doxycycline, minocycline

Pediatric Considerations
- Neonatal acne (neonatal cephalic pustulosis) (2)
  – Newborn to 8 weeks; lesions limited to face; responds to topical ketoconazole 2% cream (3)
- Infantile acne
  – Newborn to 1 year; lesions on face, neck, back, and chest; no Rx required (3)
- Early–mid childhood acne
  – 1 to 7 years; rare; consider hyperandrogenism (3)
- Preadolescent acne
  – 7 to 11 years; common, 47% of children, usually due to adrenal awakening
- Do not use tetracycline in those <8 years of age (2,3); other therapies similar to adolescent acne

EPIDEMIOLOGY AND PATHOPHYSIOLOGY
- Predominant age: early to late puberty, may persist in 20–40% of affected individuals into 4th decade
- Predominant sex
  – Male > female (adolescence)
  – Female > male (adult)

Prevalence
- 80–95% of adolescents affected. A smaller percentage will seek medical advice.
- 8% of adults aged 25 to 34 years; 3% at 35 to 44 years
- African-Americans 37%, Caucasians 24%

ETIOLOGY AND PATHOPHYSIOLOGY
- Androgens (testosterone and dehydroepiandrosterone sulfate [DHEA-S]) stimulate sebum production and proliferation of keratinocytes in hair follicles (4).
- Keratin plug obstructs follicle os, causing sebum accumulation and follicular distention.
- *Propionibacterium acnes*, an anaerobe, colonizes and proliferates in the plugged follicle.
- *P. acnes* promote proinflammatory mediators, causing inflammation of follicle and dermis.

Genetics
- Familial association in 50%
- If a family history exists, the acne may be more severe and occur earlier.

RISK FACTORS
- Increased endogenous androgenic effect
- Oily cosmetics, cocoa butter
- Rubbing or occluding skin surface (e.g., sports equipment such as helmets and shoulder pads), telephone, or hands against the skin

- Polyvinyl chloride, chlorinated hydrocarbons, cutting oil, tars
- Numerous drugs, including androgenic steroids (e.g., steroid abuse, some birth control pills)
- Endocrine disorders: polycystic ovarian syndrome, Cushing syndrome, congenital adrenal hyperplasia, androgen-secreting tumors, acromegaly
- Stress
- High-glycemic load and possibly high-dairy diets may exacerbate acne (4,5).
- Severe acne may worsen with smoking.

COMMONLY ASSOCIATED CONDITIONS
- Acne fulminans, pyoderma faciale
- Acne conglobata, hidradenitis suppurativa
- Pomade acne
- SAPHO syndrome (synovitis, acne, pustulosis, hyperostosis, and osteitis)
- Pyogenic arthritis, pyoderma gangrenosum, and acne (PAPA) and seborrhea, acne, hirsutism, and alopecia (SAHA) syndromes
- Behçet syndrome, Apert syndrome
- Dark-skinned patients: 50% keloidal scarring and 50% acne hyperpigmented macules

 DIAGNOSIS

HISTORY
- Ask about duration, medications, cleansing products, stress, smoking, exposures, diet, and family history.
- Females may worsen 1 week prior to menses.

PHYSICAL EXAM
- Closed comedones (whiteheads)
- Open comedones (blackheads)
- Nodules or papules
- Pustules ("cysts")
- Scars: ice pick, rolling, boxcar, atrophic macules, hypertrophic, depressed, sinus tracts
- Grading system (American Academy of Dermatology, 1990) (4)
  – Mild: few papules/pustules; no nodules
  – Moderate: some papules/pustules; few nodules
  – Severe: numerous papules/pustules; many nodules
  – Very severe: acne conglobata, acne fulminans, acne inversa.
- Most common areas affected are face, chest, back, and upper arms (areas of greatest concentration of sebaceous glands) (4).

DIFFERENTIAL DIAGNOSIS
- Folliculitis: gram negative and gram positive
- Acne (rosacea, cosmetica, steroid-induced)
- Perioral dermatitis
- Chloracne
- Pseudofolliculitis barbae
- Drug eruption
- Verruca vulgaris and plana
- Keratosis pilaris
- Molluscum contagiosum
- Sarcoidosis
- Seborrheic dermatitis
- Miliaria

DIAGNOSTIC TESTS & INTERPRETATION
Initial Tests (lab, imaging)
Only indicated if additional signs of androgen excess; if so, test for free and total testosterone, DHEA-S, LH, and FSH (6)

 TREATMENT

- Comedonal (grade 1): keratolytic agent (7)[A] (see as follows for specific agents)
- Mild inflammatory acne (grade 2): benzoyl peroxide ± topical antibiotic + keratolytic agent
- Moderate inflammatory acne (grade 3): add systemic antibiotic to grade 2 regimen
- Severe inflammatory acne (grade 4): as in grade 3, or isotretinoin (7)[A]
- Topical retinoid plus a topical antimicrobial agent is 1st-line treatment for more than mild disease (8).
- Topical retinoid + antibiotic (topical or PO) is better than either alone for mild/moderate acne (7)[A].
- Topical retinoids are 1st-line agents for maintenance. Avoid long-term antibiotics for maintenance.
- Avoid topical antibiotics as monotherapy.
- Recommended vehicle type
  – Dry or sensitive skin: cream or ointment
  – Oily skin, humid weather: gel, solution, or wash
  – Hair-bearing areas: lotion, hydrogel, or foam
- Apply topical agents to entire affected area, not just visible lesions.
- Mild soap daily to control oiliness; avoid abrasives
- Avoid drying agents with keratolytic agents.
- Gentle cleanser and noncomedogenic moisturizer help decrease irritation.
- Oil-free, noncomedogenic sunscreens
- Stress management if acne flares with stress

MEDICATION

ALERT
Most prescription of topical medications are very expensive, costing from $100 to several hundred dollars per tube.

- Keratolytic agents (alpha-hydroxy acids, salicylic acid, azelaic acid) (side effects include dryness, erythema, and scaling; start with lower strength, increase as tolerated) (6,7)[A].

- Tretinoin (Retin-A, Retin A Micro, Avita, Atralin) varying strengths and formulations: apply at bedtime; wash skin, let skin dry 30 minutes before application
  – Retin-A Micro, Atralin, and Avita are less irritating, and stable with BP
  – May cause an initial flare of lesions; may be eased by 14-day course of oral antibiotics
  – Avoid in pregnant and lactating women.
- Adapalene (Differin): 0.1%, apply topically at night

  – Effective; less irritation than tretinoin or tazarotene (7)[A]

  – May be combined with benzoyl peroxide (Epiduo)—very effective in skin of color
- Tazarotene (Tazorac): apply at bedtime
  – Most effective and most irritating; teratogenic
- Azelaic acid (Azelex, Finevin): 20% topically, BID
  – Keratolytic, antibacterial, anti-inflammatory
  – Reduces postinflammatory hyperpigmentation in dark-skinned individuals
  – Side effects: erythema, dryness, scaling, hypopigmentation
  – Less effective in clinical use than in studies
  – Effective in postadolescent acne
- Salicylic acid: 2%, less effective and less irritating than tretinoin
- Alpha-hydroxy acids: available over-the-counter

- Topical antibiotics and anti-inflammatories
  - Topical benzoyl peroxide (6,7)[A]
    - 2.5% as effective as stronger preparations
    - Gel penetrates better into follicles
    - When used with tretinoin, apply benzoyl peroxide in morning and tretinoin at night
    - Side effects: irritation; may bleach clothes; photosensitivity
- Topical antibiotics (6,7)[A]
  - Erythromycin 2%
  - Clindamycin 1%
  - Metronidazole gel or cream: apply once daily
  - Azelaic acid (Azelex, Finevin): 20% cream: enhanced effect and decreased risk of resistance when used with zinc and benzoyl peroxide
  - Benzoyl peroxide-erythromycin (Benzamycin): especially effective with azelaic acid
  - Benzoyl peroxide-clindamycin (BenzaClin, DUAC, Clindoxyl)
  - Benzoyl peroxide-salicylic acid (Cleanse & Treat, Inova): similar in effectiveness to benzoyl peroxide-clindamycin
  - Sodium sulfacetamide (Sulfacet-R, Novacet, Klaron): useful in acne with seborrheic dermatitis or rosacea
  - Dapsone (Aczone) 5% gel: may cause yellow/orange skin discoloration when mixed with benzoyl peroxide
- Oral antibiotics: use for at least 6 to 8 weeks after initiation, discontinue after 12 to 18 weeks' duration; indicated when acne is more severe, trunk involvement, unresponsive to topical agents, or at greater risk for scarring (6,7,9)[A]
  - Tetracycline: 500 to 1,000 mg/day divided BID; high dose initially, taper in 6 months. Side effects: photosensitivity, esophagitis
  - Minocycline: 100 to 200 mg/day, divided daily—BID; side effects include photosensitivity, urticaria, gray-blue skin, vertigo, hepatitis
  - Doxycycline: 50 to 200 mg/day, divided daily—BID; side effects include photosensitivity
  - Erythromycin: 500 to 1,000 mg/day; divided BID–QID; decreasing effectiveness as a result of increasing *P. acnes* resistance
  - Trimethoprim-sulfamethoxazole (Bactrim DS, Septra DS): 1 daily or BID
  - Azithromycin (Zithromax): 500 mg 3 days/week × 1 month, then 250 mg every other day × 2 months
- Oral retinoids
  - Isotretinoin: 0.5 to 1 mg/kg/day divided BID to maximum 2 mg/kg/day divided BID for very severe disease; 60–90% cure rate; usually given for 12 to 20 weeks; maximum cumulative dose = 120 to 150 mg/kg; 20% of patients relapse and require retreatment (4,6,7)[A], 0.25 to 0.40 mg/kg/day in moderately severe acne
    - Side effects: teratogenic, pancreatitis, excessive drying of skin, hypertriglyceridemia, hepatitis, blood dyscrasias, hyperostosis, premature epiphyseal closure, night blindness, erythema multiforme, Stevens-Johnson syndrome, suicidal ideation, psychosis
    - Avoid tetracyclines or vitamin A preparations during isotretinoin therapy.
    - Monitor for pregnancy, psychiatric/mood changes, complete blood count (CBC), lipids, glucose, and liver function tests at baseline and every month.
    - Must be registered and adhere to manufacturer's iPLEDGE program (www.ipledgeprogram.com)

- Medications for women only
  - Oral contraceptives (4,6,7)[A],(10)
    - Norgestimate/ethinyl estradiol (OrthoTricyclen), norethindrone acetate/ethinyl estradiol (Estrostep), drospirenone/ethinyl estradiol (Yaz, Yasmin) are USFDA approved.
    - Levonorgestrel/ethinyl estradiol (Alesse) and most combined contraceptives effective
    - Spironolactone (Aldactone); 25 to 200 mg/day; antiandrogen; reduces sebum production

ISSUES FOR REFERRAL
Consider referral/consultation to dermatologist
- Refractory lesions despite appropriate therapy
- Consideration of isotretinoin therapy
- Management of acne scars

ADDITIONAL THERAPIES
- Acne hyperpigmented macules (11)
  - Topical hydroquinones (1.5–10%)
  - Azelaic acid (20%) topically
  - Topical retinoids
  - Corticosteroids: low dose, suppresses adrenal androgens (6)[B]
  - Dapsone 5% gel (Aczone): topical, anti-inflammatory; use in patients over 12 years
  - Sunscreen for prevention
- Light-based treatments
  - Ultraviolet A/ultraviolet B (UVA/UVB), blue or blue/red light; pulse dye, KTP, or infrared laser
  - Photodynamic therapy for 30 to 60 minutes with 5-aminolevulinic acid × 3 sessions is effective for inflammatory lesions.
    - Greatest use when used as adjunct to medications or if can't tolerate medications

SURGERY/OTHER PROCEDURES
- Comedo extraction after incising the layer of epithelium over closed comedo (6)[C]
- Inject large cystic lesions with 0.05 to 0.3 mL triamcinolone (Kenalog 2 to 5 mg/mL); use 30-gauge needle, inject through pore, slightly distend cyst (6)[C].
- Acne scar treatment: retinoids, steroid injections, cryosurgery, electrodessication, micro/dermabrasion, chemical peels, laser resurfacing

COMPLEMENTARY & ALTERNATIVE MEDICINE
Evidence suggests tea tree oil, seaweed extract, Kampo formulations, Ayurvedic formulations, rose extract, basil extract, epigallocatechin gallate, and tea extract may be useful (12).

ONGOING CARE

FOLLOW-UP RECOMMENDATIONS
Use oral or topical antibiotics for 3 months; taper as inflammatory lesions resolve. Do not use topical and oral antibiotic together.

DIET
Avoid high-glycemic index foods and milk (13)

PATIENT EDUCATION
- There may be a worsening of acne during first 2 weeks of treatment.
- Results are typically seen after a minimum of 4 weeks of treatment

PROGNOSIS
Gradual improvement over time (usually within 8 to 12 weeks after beginning therapy)

COMPLICATIONS
- Acne conglobata: severe confluent inflammatory acne with systemic symptoms
- Facial scarring and psychological distress, including anxiety, depression, and suicidal ideation (4)
- Postinflammatory hyperpigmentation, keloids, and scars are more common in skin of color

REFERENCES

1. Pugashetti R, Shinkai K. Treatment of acne vulgaris in pregnant patients. *Dermatol Ther*. 2013;26(4):302–311.
2. Friedlander SF, Baldwin HE, Mancini AJ, et al. The acne continuum: an age-based approach to therapy. *Semin Cutan Med Surg*. 2011;30(Suppl 3):S6–S11.
3. Admani S, Barrio VR. Evaluation and treatment of acne from infancy to preadolescence. *Dermatol Ther*. 2013;26(6):462–466.
4. Dawson AL, Dellavalle RP. Acne vulgaris. *BMJ*. 2013;346:f2634.
5. Burris J, Rietkerk W, Woolf K. Acne: the role of medical nutrition therapy. *J Acad Nutr Diet*. 2013;113(3):416–430.
6. Strauss JS, Krowchuk DP, Leyden JJ, et al. Guidelines of care for acne vulgaris management. *J Am Acad Dermatol*. 2007;56(4):651–663.
7. Feldman S, Careccia RE, Barham KL, et al. Diagnosis and treatment of acne. *Am Fam Physician*. 2004;69(9):2123–2130.
8. Thiboutot D, Gollnick H, Bettoli V, et al. New insights into the management of acne: an update from the Global Alliance to improve outcomes in Acne group. *J Am Acad Dermatol*. 2009;60(5 Suppl):S1–S50.
9. Del Rosso JQ, Kim G. Optimizing use of oral antibiotics in acne vulgaris. *Dermatol Clin*. 2009;27(1):33–42.
10. Heymann WR. Oral contraceptives for the treatment of acne vulgaris. *J Am Acad Dermatol*. 2007;56(6):1056–1057.
11. Woolery-Lloyd HC, Keri J, Doig S. Retinoids and azelaic acid to treat acne and hyperpigmentation in skin of color. *J Drugs Dermatol*. 2013;12(4):434–437.
12. Fisk WA, Lev-Tov HA, Sivamani RK. Botanical and phytochemical therapy of acne: a systematic review. *Phytother Res*. 2014;28(8):1137–1152.
13. Mahmood SN, Bowe WP. Diet and acne update: carbohydrates emerge as the main culprit. *J Drugs Dermatol*. 2014;13(4):428–435.

 SEE ALSO

- Acne Rosacea
- Algorithm: Acne

 CODES

ICD10
- L70.0 Acne vulgaris
- L70.4 Infantile acne
- L70.1 Acne conglobata

CLINICAL PEARLS
- Expect worsening for the first 2 weeks of treatment. Full results for changes in therapy take 8 to 12 weeks.
- Decrease topical frequency to every day or to every other day for irritation.
- Use BP every time a topical or oral antibiotic is used.

ACUTE CORONARY SYNDROMES: NSTE-ACS (UNSTABLE ANGINA AND NSTEMI)

Brendan Merchant, MD • Louis J. Berk, MD

 BASICS

DESCRIPTION
- Unstable angina (UA) and non–ST-segment eleva-tion myocardial infarction (NSTEMI) are acute coronary syndromes (ACS) without ST-segment elevation (NSTE-ACS).
- NSTEMI is defined by the rise and fall of cardiac biomarker values (preferably cardiac troponin) higher than the 99th percentile upper reference limit and accompanied by one of the following: symptoms of ischemia, new ST-segment T-wave changes, develop-ment of pathologic Q waves on ECG, or imaging evi-dence of new regional wall motion abnormality (1).
- UA, although clinically indistinguishable from NSTEMI (in an appropriate clinical setting, new-on-set anginal chest pain, or change in typical anginal pattern, or development of angina at rest, or change in typical anginal equivalent), can be differenti-ated from NSTEMI by a lack of elevation in cardiac biomarkers based on two or more samples collected at least 6 hours apart. Just as with NSTEMI, nonspe-cific ECG changes, such as ST-segment depressions or T-wave inversions, may be present (1).

EPIDEMIOLOGY
- Incidence of UA/NSTEMI increases with age (2).
- Presentation of coronary events in women is, on average, 10 years later than in men, with comparable rates of occurrence (2).

Incidence
Age-adjusted coronary heart disease (CHD) incidence rates (per 1,000 person-years): white men, 12.5; black men, 10.6; white women, 4.0; and black women, 5.1 (2)

Prevalence
For adults ≥20 years of age: 8.3% for men and 6.1% for women (2)

ETIOLOGY AND PATHOPHYSIOLOGY
- Platelet-rich thrombus forming on a disrupted plaque
- Dynamic obstruction triggered by intense spasm of a coronary artery, for example, Prinzmetal angina or coronary spasm induced by cocaine or methamphet-amine abuse
- Progressive mechanical limitation of coronary flow
- Coronary arterial inflammation
- Coronary dissection/rupture and thrombogenesis
- Myocardial oxygen demand exceeds supply
- UA/NSTEMI is usually caused by acute rupture of an atherosclerotic plaque, causing thrombosis and partial or total occlusion of a coronary artery (1).

RISK FACTORS
- Age
- Hypertension
- Tobacco use
- Diabetes mellitus
- Dyslipidemia
- Family history of early coronary artery disease (CAD)
- Sedentary lifestyle
- Overweight/obesity
- Psoriasis and other systemic inflammatory conditions

GENERAL PREVENTION
- Smoking cessation, healthy diet, weight control, physical activity
- If risk factors are present: BP control, lipid-lowering therapy, daily aspirin (in select patients)

COMMONLY ASSOCIATED CONDITIONS
- Cardiovascular disease (atherosclerotic, aneurysmal, autoimmune, peripheral)
- Other forms of heart disease (myocardial, valvular, high-output states)

 DIAGNOSIS

HISTORY
- Chest heaviness/tightness, with or without exertion, and increasing in frequency
- Pain or discomfort radiating to the neck, jaw, inter-scapular area, upper extremities, or epigastrium
- Associated symptoms of dyspnea, nausea, diaphore-sis, light-headedness, dysphoria
- History of myocardial ischemia (stable or unstable angina, MI, coronary bypass surgery, or percutane-ous coronary intervention [PCI])
- Family history of CAD or MI
- Risk factors for CAD and bleeding
- Use of phosphodiesterase-5 inhibitors (e.g., sildenafil) and concomitant nitrates
- Use of cocaine or amphetamines
- Medications and recent medication changes

PHYSICAL EXAM
- General: abnormal vital signs including tachycar-dia or bradycardia, hypertension or hypotension, widened pulse pressure, tachypnea, fever
- Neurologic: dizziness, syncope, fatigue, weakness, altered mental status
- Cardiovascular: dysrhythmia, jugular venous disten-tion (JVD), new murmur, rub or gallop, diminished peripheral pulses, carotid bruits
- Respiratory: tachypnea, increased work of breath-ing, crackles
- Musculoskeletal: Sharp pain reproducible with movement or palpation is unlikely to be cardiac.
- Skin: cool skin, pallor, diaphoresis, signs of dyslipid-emia (xanthomas, xanthelasma)

DIFFERENTIAL DIAGNOSIS
- Aortic dissection
- Pulmonary embolism
- Pleuropericarditis
- Perforating ulcer
- Gastroesophageal reflux disease (GERD) and spasm
- Esophageal perforation
- Biliary or pancreatic pain
- Dysrhythmia

Geriatric Considerations
Elderly patients, as well as women and those with diabetes, may have an atypical presentation without classic anginal symptoms.

DIAGNOSTIC TESTS & INTERPRETATION
Initial Tests (lab, imaging)
- 12-lead ECG (1)[A]: applies to both UA and NSTEMI
  - ST-segment depression and/or T-wave inversion:
    ○ ≥1-mm ST depression in ≥2 contiguous leads
    ○ T-wave inversions, other changes
    ○ ST depression and/or tall R wave in V_1/V_2 with upright T waves may indicate transmural STEMI of posterior wall.
    ○ If initial ECG is nondiagnostic but symptoms persist with suspicion for ACS, perform serial ECGs at 15- to 30-minute intervals.

- Serum biomarkers (negative by definition in UA)
  - NSTEMI is strictly defined as a rise and fall in serum biomarkers (usually troponin I or T, as they are more sensitive for detecting NSTEMI) exceed-ing the 99th percentile of a normal reference population. Troponin concentration rises 3 to 6 hours after onset of ischemic symptoms but can be delayed from 8 to 12 hours (troponin T is not specific in patients with renal dysfunction).
  - With contemporary troponin assays, CK-MB and myo-globin are not useful in the diagnosis of ACS (3)[A].
  - Patients with negative biomarkers within 6 hours of the onset of symptoms should have biomarkers remeasured 8 to 12 hours from onset of symptoms
- Chest x-ray
- Consider transthoracic echocardiography if not recently performed (1)[B].

Follow-Up Tests & Special Considerations
- Patients with ischemia are recommended to undergo an assessment of left ventricle (LV) func-tion to identify impaired function and/or need for appropriate medications such as ACE inhibitors, β-blockers, and aldosterone antagonists.
- Fasting lipid profile, preferably within 24 hours
- Complete blood count (CBC), basic metabolic panel, activated partial thromboplastin time (aPTT)
- Other laboratory tests:
  - Lactate dehydrogenase: increases within 24 hours, peaks 3 to 6 days, baseline 8 to 12 days (not routinely ordered)
  - Leukocytes: increase within several hours after MI, peak in 2 to 4 days
  - Brain natriuretic peptide (BNP): increases with MI, may not indicate heart failure

Pregnancy Considerations
Findings mimicking NSTEMI in pregnancy: ST depres-sion after anesthesia, increase in CK-MB after delivery, and mild increase in troponin in preeclampsia and gestational hypertension. Spontaneous coronary dis-section is a rare cause of ST elevation in pregnancy.

Diagnostic Procedures/Other
- Coronary angiography (discussed under "Treatment")
- If serial cardiac enzymes are negative and symptoms have resolved, consider stress testing, including either standard exercise treadmill test (ETT), stress echocardiography, or stress nuclear study (1)[B].
- Transesophageal echocardiography, contrast chest CT scan, or MRI generally are reserved for differ-entiating ACS and other causes of chest pain from aortic dissection.

Test Interpretation
- Subendocardial myocardial necrosis may be present.
- Atherosclerosis

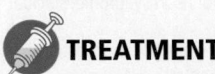 **TREATMENT**

GENERAL MEASURES
- Bed/chair rest with continuous ECG monitoring
- Antiarrhythmics as needed
- Anxiolytics as needed
- Deep vein thrombosis prophylaxis
- Continuation of aspirin, clopidogrel or prasugrel or ticagrelor, β-blockers, ACE inhibitors (or ARBs if ACE intolerant), lipid-lowering therapy

- Tight BP control
- Treatment for depression PRN (common post-MI)
- Cardiac rehabilitation and increased physical activity
- Smoking cessation
- Annual influenza vaccine

MEDICATION

First Line

- Aspirin, non–enteric-coated, initial dose of 162 to 325 mg PO or chewed to all patients (1)[A]
- P2Y12 Inhibitors
  - Clopidogrel, loading dose 300 to 600 mg followed by 75 mg/day (1)[B]; or ticagrelor, loading dose 180 mg followed by 90 mg BID (1)[B]. Clopidogrel is favored in patients with ≥2-degree heart block, hemoglobin <10 g/dL, platelet count <100,000 cell/mm^3, or liver disease.
  - Prasugrel is reserved for post-PCI patients treated with coronary stents, no history of stroke or TIA, <75 years, and weight >60 kg (1)[B].
  - Patients unable to take aspirin should receive a loading and maintenance dose of clopidogrel, ticagrelor, or prasugrel.
- Nitroglycerin (NTG) sublingual 0.4 mg every 5 minutes for total of three doses, then assess need for intravenous (IV) NTG (1)[C].
- Supplemental oxygen 2 to 4 L/min, maintaining arterial oxygen saturation >90% (1)[B]
- Morphine sulfate 2 to 4 mg IV (with increments of 2 to 8 mg IV repeated at 5- to 15-minute intervals) (1)[A]
- Oral β-blocker in patients without signs of heart failure, cardiogenic shock, or other contraindications (1)[B]. (IV β-blockers are potentially harmful when risk factors for shock are present.)
- In patients with concomitant ACS, stabilized heart failure, and reduced systolic function (LVEF <40%), the recommended β-blockers are metoprolol succinate, carvedilol, and bisoprolol (1)[C].
- Lipid-lowering therapy: initiate or continue high-intensity statin therapy (preferred due to nonlipid benefit on vascular function) (1)[A]; niacin or fibrate (1)[C] if statin use not possible
- Risk stratify using the TIMI or GRACE score to select use of early invasive approach (within 12 to 24 hours of admission) versus ischemia-guided therapy.
- Risks and benefits of the early invasive approach:
  - 33% relative risk reduction for both the end points of refractory angina and rehospitalization at 6 to 12 months (2)[A]
  - 27% and 22% relative risk reduction in rates of MI at 6 to 12 months and 3 to 5 years, respectively (2)[A]
  - Doubled risk of procedure-related MI and increased risk of minor periprocedural bleeding (1)[A]
- Invasive management
  - Benefits are more pronounced in higher risk patients, such as those with ECG changes or diabetes (2).
- Subsequent recommendations (1)[A]: For patients with elevated risk for clinical events or refractory angina or hemodynamic or electrical instability, initiate anticoagulant: enoxaparin or unfractionated heparin (UFH) or bivalirudin. Prior to angiography, add GP IIb/IIIa inhibitor (eptifibatide or tirofiban) or thienopyridine (clopidogrel or ticagrelor).

- Ischemia-guided therapy
  - For low-risk or selected intermediate-risk patients, based on patient or physician preference, or in chronic renal insufficiency stage IV: Initiate anticoagulant therapy: enoxaparin or UFH or fondaparinux; enoxaparin or fondaparinux preferable. Initiate clopidogrel or ticagrelor (1)[B].
- Contraindications: Prasugrel contraindicated in patients ≥75 years or those with history of CVA/TIA or increased bleeding risk. Ticagrelor contraindicated in ≥2-degree heart block.

Second Line

- ACE inhibitor in patients with pulmonary congestion or left ventricular ejection fraction (EF) ≤40%. Substitute ARB for ACE-intolerant patients (1)[A].
- Nondihydropyridine calcium channel blocker (CCB) (verapamil or diltiazem) to reduce myocardial oxygen demand when β-blockers are contraindicated if normal EF (1)[B]. Use oral long-acting CCB only after β-blockers and nitrates have been fully used (1)[C].
- Long-term nitrate therapy for recurrent angina/ischemia or heart failure (1)[C].
- Sublingual NTG at discharge (1)[C]

ISSUES FOR REFERRAL

Cardiology consultation is appropriate for likely UA/NSTEMI, particularly regarding the complexities of anticoagulation/antiplatelet therapy.

SURGERY/OTHER PROCEDURES

- Coronary reperfusion
  - PCI with stent placement
  - CABG surgery
- Intra-aortic balloon pump for severe ischemia, hypotension, refractory pain

INPATIENT CONSIDERATIONS

Admission Criteria/Initial Stabilization

- All patients with definite or suspected acute MI, ongoing pain, positive cardiac markers, ST deviations, hemodynamic abnormalities, probable or definite ACS
- Bed rest with continuous ECG monitoring, assess for reperfusion therapy, relieve ischemic pain, treat life-threatening complications, admit to coronary care unit.

ONGOING CARE

FOLLOW-UP RECOMMENDATIONS

- It is reasonable in patients with possible ACS who have normal serial ECGs and cardiac troponins to have a treadmill ECG, stress myocardial perfusion imaging, or stress echocardiography before discharge or within 72 hours after discharge (2)[A],(3)
- Follow up within 2 to 6 weeks (low risk) and 14 days (high risk).
- Refer to cardiac rehabilitation.

DIET

- Diet low in saturated fat, cholesterol, and sodium
- Request dietary consult.

PATIENT EDUCATION

- Education on new medications, diet, exercise, smoking cessation, lifestyle modification
- Resume exercise, sexual activity after outpatient reevaluation

PROGNOSIS

UA/NSTEMI patients have lower in-hospital mortality than those with STEMI but a similar or worse long-term outcome.

COMPLICATIONS

- Cardiogenic shock
- Heart failure
- Myocardial rupture
- Ventricular aneurysm
- Dysrhythmia
- Acute pulmonary embolism
- Acute thromboembolic stroke
- Pericarditis/Dressler syndrome
- Depression (increases mortality risk)
- Hyperglycemia

REFERENCES

1. Anderson JL, Adams CD, Antman EM, et al. 2012 ACCF/AHA focused update incorporated into the ACC/AHA 2007 guidelines for the management of patients with unstable angina/non-ST-elevation myocardial infarction: a report of the American College of Cardiology Foundation/American Heart Association Task Force on Practice Guidelines. *Circulation*. 2013;127(23):e663–e828.
2. Roger VL, Go AS, Lloyd-Jones DM, et al. Heart disease and stroke statistics—2012 update: a report from the American Heart Association. *Circulation*. 2012;125(1):e2–e220.
3. Amsterdam EA, Wenger NK, Brindis RG, et al. 2014 AHA/ACC guideline for the management of patients with non-ST-elevation acute coronary syndromes: a report of the American College of Cardiology/American Heart Association Task Force on Practice Guidelines. *J Am Coll Cardiol*. 2014;64(24): e139–e228. doi:10.1016/j.jacc.2014.09.017.

ADDITIONAL READING

- Cayla G, Silvain J, Collet JP, et al. Updates and current recommendations for the management of patients with non-ST-elevation acute coronary syndromes: what it means for clinical practice. *Am J Cardiol*. 2015;115(Suppl 5):10A–22A.
- Hoenig MR, Aroney CN, Scott IA. Early invasive versus conservative strategies for unstable angina and non-ST elevation myocardial infarction in the stent era. *Cochrane Database Syst Rev*. 2010;(3):CD004815.

CODES

ICD10

- I24.9 Acute ischemic heart disease, unspecified
- I20.0 Unstable angina
- I21.4 Non-ST elevation (NSTEMI) myocardial infarction

CLINICAL PEARLS

- Discontinue NSAIDs, nonselective or selective cyclooxygenase (COX)-2 agents, except for ASA, due to increased risks of mortality, reinfarction, hypertension, heart failure, and myocardial rupture.
- Discontinue clopidogrel or prasugrel or ticagrelor 5 to 7 days before elective CABG.
- Do not use nitrate products in patients who recently used a phosphodiesterase-5 inhibitor (24 hours of sildenafil or vardenafil, or 48 hours of tadalafil).
- Duration of antithrombotic therapy after NSTEMI depends on type of stent received and medications administered.
- Avoid β-blockers in cocaine or methamphetamine user.

ACUTE CORONARY SYNDROMES: STEMI

Kassie S. Johnson, MD • Fozia Akhtar Ali, MD

BASICS

DESCRIPTION
Acute myocardial infarction (AMI) is the rapid development of myocardial necrosis resulting from a sustained and complete absence of blood flow to a portion of the myocardium. ST-segment elevation myocardial infarction (STEMI) occurs when coronary blood flow ceases following thrombotic occlusion of a large coronary artery (usually) affected by atherosclerosis, causing transmural ischemia. This is accompanied by release of serum cardiac biomarkers and ST elevation (and likely a Q wave when infarction develops) on an ECG.

EPIDEMIOLOGY
Incidence
In the United States, estimated annual incidence of MI is 600,000 new and 320,000 recurrent attacks. In 2009, ~683,000 patients were discharged from United States hospitals diagnosed with acute coronary syndromes (ACS).

Prevalence
- Leading cause of morbidity and mortality in the United States
- ~7.5 million people in the United States are affected by MI.
- Prevalence increases with age and is higher in men (5.5%) than in women (2.9%).

ETIOLOGY AND PATHOPHYSIOLOGY
- Atherosclerotic coronary artery disease (CAD)
- Nonatherosclerotic
  - Emboli: for example, thrombi from left ventricle or atrium
  - Mechanical obstruction: chest trauma, dissection of aorta or coronary arteries
  - Increased vasomotor tone, variant angina
  - Arteritis, others: hematologic (disseminated intravascular coagulation [DIC]), aortic stenosis, cocaine, IV drug use, severe burns, prolonged hypotension
- Atherosclerotic lesions may be smooth and concentric or rough, eccentric, and fissured. Plaques that are rough and eccentric are more unstable, thrombogenic, and prone to rupture.

RISK FACTORS
Advancing age, hypertension, tobacco use, diabetes mellitus, dyslipidemia, family history of premature onset of CAD, sedentary lifestyle

GENERAL PREVENTION
Smoking cessation, healthy diet, weight control, regular physical activity, maintain goal blood pressure

COMMONLY ASSOCIATED CONDITIONS
Abdominal aortic aneurysm, extracranial cerebrovascular disease, atherosclerotic peripheral vascular disease

DIAGNOSIS

HISTORY
- Classically, sudden onset of chest heaviness/tightness, with or without exertion, lasting at least minutes
- Pain/discomfort radiating to neck, jaw, interscapular area, upper extremities, and epigastrium
- Previous history of myocardial ischemia (stable or unstable angina, MI, coronary bypass surgery, or percutaneous coronary intervention [PCI])

- Assess risk factors for CAD, history of bleeding, noncardiac surgery, family history of premature CAD.
- Medications: Ask if recent use of phosphodiesterase-5 inhibitors (if recent use, avoid concomitant nitrates).
- Alcohol and drug abuse (especially cocaine)

PHYSICAL EXAM
- General: restless, agitated, hypothermia, fever
- Neurologic: dizziness, syncope, fatigue, asthenia, disorientation (especially in the elderly)
- Cerebrovascular (CV): dysrhythmia, hypotension, widened pulse pressure, S_3 and S_4, jugular venous distention (JVD)
- Respiratory: dyspnea, tachypnea, crackles
- GI: abdominal pain, nausea, vomiting
- Musculoskeletal: pain in neck, back, shoulder, or upper limbs
- Skin: cool skin, pallor, diaphoresis

Geriatric Considerations
Elderly patients may have an atypical presentation, including silent or unrecognized MI, often with complaints of syncope, weakness, shortness of breath, unexplained nausea, epigastric pain, altered mental status, delirium. Patients with diabetes mellitus may have fewer and less dramatic chest symptoms.

DIFFERENTIAL DIAGNOSIS
Unstable angina, aortic dissection, pulmonary embolism (PE), perforating ulcer, pericarditis, dysrhythmias, gastroesophageal reflux disease (GERD) and spasm, biliary/pancreatic pain, hyperventilation syndrome

DIAGNOSTIC TESTS & INTERPRETATION

ALERT
The third universal definition for MI issued in 2012 by the American College of Cardiology, American Heart Association, European Society of Cardiology, and World Heart Federation revises older definitions of MI. It establishes the level of troponin necessary to diagnose MI in various clinical situations (e.g., after cardiac and noncardiac procedures). According to the definition, an MI diagnosis requires a cardiac troponin (I or T) level above the 99th percentile of a normal reference population, plus one or more of the following:
- Symptoms of ischemia
- New significant ST/T wave changes or left bundle branch block (LBBB)
- Pathologic Q waves on ECG
- New loss of viable myocardium or regional wall motion abnormality, as observed on imaging
- Intracoronary thrombus diagnosed by angiography or autopsy

Initial Tests (lab, imaging)
- Coronary angiography with measurement of fractional flow reserve (FFR)
- 12-lead ECG: ST-segment elevation in a regional pattern ≥1 mm ST elevation, with or without abnormal Q waves. ST depression ± tall R wave in V_1/V_2 may be STEMI of posterior wall. Absence of Q waves represents partial or transient occlusion or early infarction. New ST- or T-wave changes indicative of myocardial ischemia or injury. Consider right-sided and posterior chest leads if inferior MI pattern (examine V_3R, V_4R, V_7–V_9).

- ECG with continuous monitoring
  - 2D and M-mode echocardiography is useful in evaluating regional wall motion in MI and left ventricular function.
  - Portable echo can clarify diagnosis of STEMI if concomitant LBBB.
  - Useful in assessing mechanical complications and mural thrombus

Follow-Up Tests & Special Considerations
- Serum biomarkers
  - Troponin I and T (cTnI, cTnT) rise 3 to 6 hours after onset of ischemic symptoms.
  - Elevations in cTnI persist for 7 to 10 days, whereas those in cTnT persist for 10 to 14 days after MI.
  - Myoglobin fraction of creatine kinase (CK-MB): rises 3 to 4 hours after onset of myocardial injury; peaks at 12 to 24 hours and remains elevated for 2 to 3 days; CK-MB adds little diagnostic value in assessment of possible ACS to troponin testing.
  - Myoglobin: early marker for myocardial necrosis; rises 2 hours after onset of myocardial necrosis, reaches peak at 1 to 4 hours, and remains elevated for 24 hours; myoglobin adds little diagnostic value in assessment of possible ACS to troponin testing.
- Fasting lipid profile, CBC with platelets, electrolytes, magnesium, BUN, serum creatinine, and glucose; international normalized ratio (INR) if anticoagulation contemplated; brain natriuretic peptide (BNP) is elevated in acute MI; may or may not indicate heart failure

Pregnancy Considerations
Findings mimicking acute MI in pregnancy: ST-segment depression after anesthesia, increase in CK-MB after delivery, and mild increase in troponin I levels in preeclampsia and gestational hypertension

Diagnostic Procedures/Other
High-quality portable chest x-ray; transthoracic and/or transesophageal echocardiography, contrast chest CT scan, or MRI may occasionally be of value acutely. Coronary angiography is definitive test.

ALERT
Isosmolar contrast medium or low-molecular-weight contrast medium other than ioxaglate or iohexol is indicated in patients with chronic kidney disease undergoing angiography who are not having chronic dialysis.

Test Interpretation
Myocardial necrosis and atherosclerosis, if etiologic

TREATMENT

GENERAL MEASURES
- Admit to telemetry/coronary care unit (CCU) with continuous ECG monitoring and bed rest. Anxiolytics, if needed; stool softeners
- Antiarrhythmics, as needed, for unstable dysrhythmia; deep vein thrombosis (DVT) prophylaxis
- Continuation of aspirin 81 mg/day and clopidogrel 75 mg/day or prasugrel 10 mg/day or ticagrelor 90 mg twice daily, BB, ACE inhibitors (or ARB if ACE-intolerant), lipid-lowering therapy, tight BP control, progressively increased physical activity, smoking cessation, annual influenza vaccine

- Assess for depression, and treat with an SSRI or psychotherapy if present, as depression is present in 20% of patients post-MI and is a potent predictor for poor prognosis. Although it is unclear yet if treatment improves mortality, it does improve quality of life.

MEDICATION

Medication recommendations based on 2009 ACC/AHA (1) focused guideline updates [A] and [B] level recommendations and 2012 ESC STEMI guidelines (2)[A,B]

First Line

- Supplemental oxygen 2 to 4 L/min for patients with arterial oxygen saturation <90% or respiratory distress
- Nitroglycerin (NTG) sublingual 0.4 mg q5min for total of 3 doses, followed by nitroglycerin IV if ongoing pain and/or hypertension and/or management of pulmonary congestion if no contraindications exist (systolic <90 mm Hg or 30 mm Hg below baseline, right ventricle (RV) infarct, use of sildenafil within 24 hours or within 48 hours of tadalafil)
- Morphine sulfate 2 to 4 mg IV with increments of 2 to 8 mg IV repeated at 5- to 15-minute intervals to relieve pain or pulmonary congestion
- Antiplatelet agents
  - Aspirin (ASA), non–enteric-coated, initial dose 162 to 325 mg chewed (1)[A]
  - A loading dose of a thienopyridine is recommended for patients with STEMI for whom PCI is planned.
    - 600 mg of clopidogrel should be given as early as possible before or at the time of primary or nonprimary PCI.
    - Prasugrel 60 mg should be given as soon as possible for primary PCI. Do not use in patients likely to undergo coronary artery bypass graft (CABG) or with active bleeding, history of transient ischemic attack (TIA) or stroke, or additional risk factors for bleeding (body weight <60 kg or concomitant use of medications that increase risk of bleeding). (Generally, not recommended for patients age ≥75 years.)
    - Ticagrelor 180 mg loading dose
    - Duration of therapy with a thienopyridine varies. At least 12 months for patients receiving drug-eluting stent (DES) during PCI for ACS and up to 12 months for patients receiving bare-metal stent (BMS). Consider earlier discontinuation if risk of morbidity due to bleeding outweighs the benefits of therapy. Discontinue clopidogrel for at least 5 days or prasugrel at least 7 days prior to planned CABG. Management of patients on dual antiplatelet therapy (DAPT) who are referred for surgical procedures depends on the level of emergency and the thrombotic and bleeding risk of the individual patient.
  - For patients with STEMI undergoing nonprimary PCI
    - Continue clopidogrel in a patient who has received fibrinolytic therapy and has been given clopidogrel.
    - Administer loading dose of clopidogrel 600 mg if patient received a fibrinolytic without a thienopyridine or ticagrelor 180 mg or once the coronary anatomy is known and PCI is planned; administer a loading dose of prasugrel as soon as possible but not later than 1 hour after PCI. Administer loading dose of clopidogrel 300 mg in patients <75 years of age who received fibrinolytic therapy or who did not receive reperfusion therapy.
    - Clopidogrel 75 mg should be given with aspirin in patients with STEMI regardless of reperfusion therapy.

- β-blocker (BB) within 24 hours, if no contraindications exist (signs of congestive heart failure [CHF], low output state)
- Glycoprotein IIb/IIIa receptor antagonists at time of primary PCI in selected patients: abciximab, eptifibatide, or tirofiban
- ACE inhibitors should be initiated orally within 24 hours of STEMI in patients with anterior infarction, HF, or ejection fraction (EF ≤0.40) unless contraindicated.

PCI versus fibrinolysis: goal is to keep total ischemic time within 120 minutes. Door to needle time should be within 30 minutes or door to balloon time within 90 minutes.

- Coronary reperfusion therapy
  - Primary PCI (balloon angioplasty, coronary stents)
    - Symptom onset of ≤12 hours
    - Symptom onset of ≤12 hours and contraindication to fibrinolytic therapy irrespective of time delay
    - Cardiogenic shock or acute severe HF irrespective of time delay from onset of MI
    - Evidence of ongoing ischemia 12 to 24 hours after symptom onset
    - If substantial risk for intracranial hemorrhage (ICH)
    - Age <75 years with STEMI or LBBB who develop shock within 36 hours of AMI
  - Fibrinolysis
    - If EMS has fibrinolytic capability and the patient qualifies for therapy, prehospital fibrinolysis should be started within 30 minutes of FMS arrival on scene.
    - If presenting at a hospital without PCI capability and cannot be transferred to a PCI-capable facility to undergo PCI within 90 minutes of first medical contact
    - If no contraindications, administer within 12 hours, but not beyond 24 hours of onset of symptoms to patients with STEMI in ≥2 contiguous leads and/or new or presumably new LBBB.
      - Alteplase (rt-PA): 15-mg IV bolus, followed by 0.75 mg/kg (up to 50 mg) IV over 30 minutes, then 0.5 mg/kg (up to 35 mg) over 60 minutes; maximum 100 mg over 90 minutes
      - Reteplase (r-PA): 10 units IV bolus over 2 minutes, give 2nd bolus 30 minutes later.
      - Tenecteplase (TNK-tPA): 30 to 50 mg (based on weight) IV bolus over 5 to 10 seconds
    - Combination reperfusion with abciximab and half-dose r-PA or TNK-tPA
    - Use anticoagulants (unfractionated heparin [UFH], enoxaparin, or fondaparinux) as ancillary therapy to reperfusion therapy for minimum 48 hours and duration of admission (up to 8 days). Avoid UFH if >48 hours of anticoagulant required. Recommend supportive anticoagulant regimens in patients proceeding to primary PCI who have been treated with ASA and thienopyridine. Administer additional boluses of UFH as needed to maintain therapeutic clotting time levels in patients who received prior treatment with UFH. Bivalirudin recommended as a supportive measure for primary PCI in patients with or without prior treatment with UFH.

Second Line

- Long-acting nondihydropyridine calcium channel blocker (CCB) when BB is ineffective or contraindicated if EF is normal; do not use of immediate release nifedipine
- See chapter on "Heart Failure, Chronic" for additional medication management.

SURGERY/OTHER PROCEDURES

Intra-aortic balloon pump for cardiogenic shock; PCI of the left main coronary artery with stents as an alternative to CABG in patients with favorable anatomy and comorbid conditions that may increase risk of adverse surgical outcomes if CABG chosen

INPATIENT CONSIDERATIONS

Admission Criteria/Initial Stabilization

All patients with STEMI should be admitted to a CCU for evaluation and treatment. Transfer high-risk patients who receive fibrinolytic therapy as primary reperfusion therapy at a non–PCI-capable facility to a PCI-capable facility as soon as possible. Also admit suspected acute MI, ACS/positive cardiac markers or ST deviations, and hemodynamic abnormalities.

IV Fluids

Right ventricular infarction may need fluid resuscitation for hypotension.

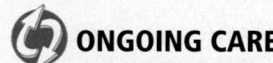 **ONGOING CARE**

FOLLOW-UP RECOMMENDATIONS

Follow up in 3 to 6 weeks of discharge. Identify high-risk patients for implantable cardioverter defibrillator (ICD) placement (especially those with EF <30%). Consider exercise-based cardiac rehabilitation program.

DIET

NPO for first 4 to 12 hours due to risk of emesis or aspiration

PATIENT EDUCATION

May resume sexual activity within 10 days, consistent with current exercise capacity. Driving can resume 1 week after discharge. Low-fat diet

COMPLICATIONS

Heart failure, myocardial rupture/left ventricular aneurysm, pericarditis, dysrhythmias, acute mitral regurgitation, severe depression (common)

REFERENCES

1. O'Gara PT, Kushner FG, Ascheim DD, et al. 2013 ACCF/AHA guideline for the management of ST-elevation myocardial infarction: executive summary: a report of the American College of Cardiology Foundation/American Heart Association Task Force on Practice Guidelines. *Circulation.* 2013;127(4):529–555.
2. Steg PG, James SK, Atar D, et al. ESC Guidelines for the management of acute myocardial infarction in patients presenting with ST-segment elevation. *Eur Heart J.* 2012;33(20):2569–2619.

 CODES

ICD10

- I24.9 Acute ischemic heart disease, unspecified
- I21.3 ST elevation (STEMI) myocardial infarction of unspecified site
- I25.10 Athscl heart disease of native coronary artery w/o ang pctrs

CLINICAL PEARLS

- Discontinue clopidogrel at least 5 to 7 days before elective CABG.
- For elective surgeries in patients on dual antiplatelet therapy (DAPT), it is recommended to wait until completion of mandatory regime and continue ASA perioperatively.

ACUTE KIDNEY INJURY

Jason Kurland, MD

 BASICS

DESCRIPTION
Abrupt loss of kidney function is defined as a rise in serum creatinine (SCr) of ≥0.3 mg/dL within 48 hours, or a 50% increase in SCr within 7 days, or oliguria of <0.5 mL/kg/hr for >6 hours, resulting in retention of nitrogenous waste as well as electrolyte, acid–base, and volume homeostasis abnormalities (1).

EPIDEMIOLOGY
Incidence
5% of hospital and 30% of ICU admissions have a diagnosis of acute kidney injury (AKI). 25% of patients develop AKI while in the hospital, and 50% of those cases are iatrogenic. Development of AKI in the inpatient setting is associated with a >4-fold increased risk of death (2).

ETIOLOGY AND PATHOPHYSIOLOGY
Can be divided into three categories: prerenal, intrarenal, and postrenal based on BUN/creatinine ratio
- Prerenal (BUN/creatinine ratio ≥20:1; ~55%)
  - Hypotension, volume depletion (GI losses, excessive sweating, diuretics, hemorrhage); renal artery stenosis/embolism; burns; heart failure; liver failure
  - Secondary to decreased renal perfusion (often due to hypovolemia) leading to a decrease in glomerular filtration rate (GFR); reversible if factors decreasing perfusion are corrected; otherwise, it can progress to an intrarenal pathology known as *ischemic acute tubular necrosis*.
- Intrarenal (BUN/creatinine <10:1; ~40%)
  - Acute tubular necrosis (ATN) (from prolonged prerenal state, radiographic contrast material, aminoglycosides, NSAIDs, or other nephrotoxic substances); glomerulonephritis (GN); acute interstitial nephritis (drug-induced); arteriolar insults; vasculitis; accelerated hypertension; cholesterol embolization (common after arterial procedures); intrarenal deposition/sludging (uric acid nephropathy and multiple myeloma [Bence-Jones proteins])
- Postrenal (BUN/creatinine 10 to 20:1; ~5%)
  - Extrinsic compression (e.g., benign prostatic hypertrophy [BPH], carcinoma, pregnancy); intrinsic obstruction (e.g., calculus, tumor, clot, stricture, sloughed papillae); decreased function (e.g., neurogenic bladder)
  - Secondary to extrinsic (e.g., BPH) or intrinsic (e.g., stones) obstruction of the urinary collection system

Genetics
No known genetic pattern

RISK FACTORS
- Chronic kidney disease (CKD)
- Comorbid conditions (e.g., diabetes, hypertension, heart failure, liver failure) (3)
- Advanced age
- Radiographic contrast material exposure
- Medications that impair autoregulation of GFR (NSAIDs, ACE-I/ARB, cyclosporine/tacrolimus)
- Nephrotoxic medications (e.g., aminoglycoside antibiotics, platinum-based chemotherapy)
- Volume depletion (e.g., diuretics, hemorrhage, GI losses)
- Sepsis (4)
- Surgery

- Rhabdomyolysis
- Solitary kidney (risk in nephrolithiasis)
- BPH
- Malignancy (e.g., multiple myeloma)

GENERAL PREVENTION
See "Treatment; General Measures."

COMMONLY ASSOCIATED CONDITIONS
Hyperkalemia, hyperphosphatemia, hypercalcemia, hyperuricemia, hydronephrosis, BPH, nephrolithiasis, congestive heart failure (CHF), uremic pericarditis, cirrhosis, CKD, malignant hypertension, vasculitis, drug reactions, sepsis, severe trauma, burns, transfusion reactions, recent chemotherapy, rhabdomyolysis, internal bleeding, dehydration

DIAGNOSIS

HISTORY
- General: PO intake, urine output, body weight, baseline creatinine (to assess magnitude of change), and medication use
- Prerenal: thirst, orthostatic dizziness
- Intrarenal: nephrotoxic medications, radiocontrast material, other toxins
  - Fever, arthralgias, and pruritic rash suggest allergic interstitial nephritis (AIN); although this triad is only present in 10% of cases.
  - Edema, hypertension, and oliguria with nephritic urine sediment (RBCs and RBC casts) point to glomerulonephritis or vasculitis
  - Livedo reticularis, SC nodules, and ischemic digits despite good pulses suggest atheroembolization.
  - Flank pain suggests occlusion of the renal artery or vein.
- Postrenal: Colicky flank pain that radiates to the groin suggests a ureteric obstruction such as a stone; nocturia, frequency, and hesitancy suggest prostatic disease; suprapubic and flank pain are usually secondary to distension of the bladder and collecting system; ask about anticholinergic drugs that could lead to neurogenic bladder.
- Uremic Sx: lethargy, nausea/vomiting, anorexia, pruritus, restless legs, sleep disturbance, hiccups

PHYSICAL EXAM
- Uremic signs: altered sensorium, seizures, asterixis, myoclonus, pericardial friction rub, peripheral neuropathies
- Prerenal signs: tachycardia, decreased jugular venous pressure (JVP), orthostatic hypotension, dry mucous membranes, decreased skin turgor; look for stigmata of associated comorbid conditions such as liver and heart failure, as well as sepsis.
- Intrinsic renal signs: pruritic rash, livedo reticularis, SC nodules, ischemic digits despite good pulses
- Postrenal signs: suprapubic distension, flank pain, enlarged prostate

DIFFERENTIAL DIAGNOSIS
See "Etiology."

DIAGNOSTIC TESTS & INTERPRETATION
Initial Tests (lab, imaging)
- Urinalysis: dipstick for blood and protein; microscopy for cells, casts, and crystals
- Casts: transparent hyaline casts—prerenal etiology; pigmented granular/muddy brown casts—ATN; WBC casts—acute interstitial nephritis; RBC casts—GN

- Urine eosinophils: ≥1% eosinophils by Hansel stain suggestive of acute interstitial nephritis (sensitivity, 67%; specificity, 83%)
- Urine electrolytes in an oliguric state
  - $FE_{Na} = [(U_{Na} \times P_{Cr})/(P_{Na} \times U_{Cr})] \times 100$, where U = urine, P = plasma, Na = sodium, Cr = creatinine; FE_{Na} <1%, likely prerenal; >2%, likely intrarenal
  - If patient is on diuretics, use FE_{urea} instead of FE_{Na}: $FE_{urea} = [(U_{urea} \times P_{Cr})/(P_{BUN} \times U_{Cr})] \times 100$; FE_{urea} <35% suggests prerenal etiology (5)[B].
- CBC, BUN, SCr, electrolytes (including Ca/Mg/P); consider arterial blood gases (ABGs).
- Common lab abnormalities in AKI
  - Increased: K^+, phosphate, Mg, uric acid
  - Decreased: Hct, Na, Ca
- Calculate creatinine clearance (CrCl) to ensure that medications are dosed appropriately.
  - Cockcroft-Gault equation for CrCl (mL/min) = $(140-age) \times$ (weight in kilograms) $\times$ (0.85 if female)/(72 × serum creatinine)
  - Note that estimating equations of CrCl/GFR are only valid when renal function (SCr) is at steady-state; anuria implies CrCl of 0.
  - Renal ultrasound (US): first-line; excludes postrenal causes if negative; identifies kidney size, hydronephrosis, and nephrolithiasis
  - Doppler-flow renal US: evaluates for renal artery stenosis/thrombosis; operator-dependent
  - Abdominal x-ray (kidney, ureter, bladder [KUB]): identifies calcification, renal calculi, kidney size
- Several novel biomarkers such as urinary IL-18, neutrophil gelatinase-associated lipocalin (NGAL), kidney injury molecule-1 (KIM-1), and plasma cystatin C, are currently being validated for their role in the initial evaluation and management of AKI (6)[C].

Follow-Up Tests & Special Considerations
- Consider CK (if suspect rhabdomyolysis) and immunologic testing (if suspect GN/vasculitis).
- More advanced imaging techniques should be considered if initial tests do not reveal etiology.
  - Prerenal: ultrasound as effective as CT for evaluating for obstruction
  - Noncontrast helical CT scan: considered most sensitive study for detecting nephrolithiasis
  - Radionucleotide renal scan: evaluates renal perfusion, function (GFR), and presence of obstructive uropathy and extravasation
  - MRI: Acute tubulointerstitial nephritis can show an increased T2-weighted signal. Gadolinium contrast is contraindicated if GFR <30 mL/min due to risk of nephrogenic systemic fibrosis.

Diagnostic Procedures/Other
Cystoscopy with retrograde pyelogram evaluates for bladder tumor, hydronephrosis, obstruction, and upper tract abnormalities without risk of contrast nephropathy.

Test Interpretation
Kidney biopsy: last resort if patient does not respond to therapy or other tests; do not reveal a diagnosis; most useful for evaluation of intrinsic AKI of unclear cause, such as AIN, GN, vasculitis, or renal transplant rejection

TREATMENT

GENERAL MEASURES
Identify and correct all prerenal and postrenal causes.

- Stop nephrotoxic drugs and renally dose others.
- Strictly record intake/output and daily weights.
- Optimize cardiac output to maintain renal perfusion.
- Follow nutrition suggestions and be aware of infections; treat aggressively if they occur.
- Avoid aspirin to reduce bleeding tendency.
- Indications for initiating hemodialysis in patients with AKI: volume overload, severe or progressive hyperkalemia, or severe metabolic acidosis refractory to medical management; advanced uremic complications (pericarditis, encephalopathy, bleeding diathesis)

MEDICATION
First Line
- Focus on treating the underlying cause and associated complications.
- Monitor and adjust fluids and electrolytes to prevent fluid overload, hyperkalemia, hyperphosphatemia, and hypermagnesemia.
  - If patient is oliguric and not volume overloaded, a fluid challenge may be appropriate with diligent monitoring for volume overload.
- Furosemide is ineffective in preventing and treating AKI (7)[A] but can judiciously be used to manage volume overload and/or hyperkalemia.
- Dopamine, natriuretic peptides, insulin-like growth factor, and thyroxine also have no benefit in the treatment of AKI.
- Fenoldopam, a dopamine agonist, has been equivocal in decreasing risk of RRT and mortality in setting of AKI; not currently recommended for use, large RCT in progress (1)[C]
- Hyperkalemia with ECG changes: Give IV calcium gluconate, isotonic sodium bicarbonate (only if acidemic, and avoid use of hypertonic "amps" of $NaHCO_3$), glucose with insulin, and/or high-dose nebulized albuterol (to drive K^+ into cells); Kayexalate and/or furosemide (to increase K^+ excretion); hemodialysis if severe/refractory
- Fluid restriction may be required for oliguric patients to prevent worsening hyponatremia.
- Metabolic acidosis (particularly pH <7.2): Sodium bicarbonate can be given; be aware of volume overload, hypocalcemia, hypokalemia.
- Effective strategies for AKI prevention: IV isotonic hydration, once-daily dosing of aminoglycosides (8)[A]; use of lipid formulations of amphotericin B, use of iso-osmolar nonionic contrast media
- Risk of contrast-induced AKI may be reduced by avoidance of hypovolemia: isotonic saline 1 mL/kg/hr morning of procedure and continued until next morning, or isotonic $NaHCO_3$ 3 mL/kg/hr × 1 hour before and 1 mL/kg/hr × 6 hours after contrast administration (9)[B]. N-acetylcysteine, although previously recommended, shown to have no benefit in recent large-scale RCT (10)[A].

Second Line
- Tamsulosin or other selective α-blockers for bladder outlet obstruction secondary to BPH
- Dihydropyridine calcium channel blockers may have a protective effect in posttransplant ATN.

ISSUES FOR REFERRAL
- Consider nephrology consultation.
- Urology consults for obstructive nephropathy

SURGERY/OTHER PROCEDURES
- Relief of obstruction with retrograde ureteral catheters/percutaneous nephrostomy
- Hemodialysis catheter placement

COMPLEMENTARY & ALTERNATIVE MEDICINE
Many herbal and dietary supplements can be nephrotoxic (aristolochic acid, licorice [*Glycyrrhiza glabra*], ephedra, star fruit [*Averrhoa carambola*], others).

INPATIENT CONSIDERATIONS
Admission Criteria/Initial Stabilization
Most patients with AKI will require admission; consider discharge in a stable patient with mild AKI and a clearly identified, reversible cause.

- Evaluate for and treat potentially life-threatening complications: hyperkalemia, metabolic acidosis, volume overload, advanced uremia
- If volume depleted, give isotonic IV fluids.
- Place a Foley catheter.

IV Fluids
Isotonic fluids should be used to treat hypovolemia.

Nursing
Place a Foley catheter; strict I/Os, daily weights

Discharge Criteria
- Stabilization of renal function and a concrete plan for continued treatment, if necessary
- Some patients may require dialysis until renal recovery.

 ONGOING CARE

FOLLOW-UP RECOMMENDATIONS
Nephrology follow-up if persistent renal impairment and/or proteinuria

DIET
- Total caloric intake should be 20 to 30 kcal/kg/day to avoid catabolism (1).
- Restrict Na^+ to 2 g/day (unless hypovolemic).
- Consider K^+ restriction (2 to 3 g/day) if hyperkalemic.
- If hyperphosphatemic, consider use of phosphate binders, although no evidence of benefit in AKI.
- Avoid magnesium- and aluminum-containing compounds.

PATIENT EDUCATION
Keep well-hydrated. Avoid nephrotoxic drugs, such as NSAIDs and aminoglycosides.

PROGNOSIS
- Depending on the cause, comorbid conditions, and age of patient, mortality ranges from 5% to 80%
- In cases of prerenal and postrenal failure, very good rates of recovery are positively correlated with shorter duration of AKI. Intrarenal etiologies usually take more time to recover. Overall, average recovery takes from days to months.
- Even with complete recovery from AKI, affected patients are at higher subsequent risk of developing CKD and ESRD (11).

COMPLICATIONS
Death, sepsis, infection, seizures, paralysis, peripheral edema, CHF, arrhythmias, uremic pericarditis, bleeding, hypotension, anemia, hyperkalemia, uremia

REFERENCES
1. International Society of Nephrology. Summary of recommendation statements. *Kidney Int Suppl.* 2012;2(1):8–12.
2. Wang HE, Muntner P, Chertow GM, et al. Acute kidney injury and mortality in hospitalized patients. *Am J Nephrol.* 2012;35(4):349–355.
3. Hilton R. Acute renal failure. *BMJ.* 2006;333(7572):786–790.
4. Lameire N. The pathophysiology of acute renal failure. *Crit Care Clin.* 2005;21(2):197–210.
5. Lameire N, Van Biesen W, Vanholder R. Acute renal failure. *Lancet.* 2005;365(9457):417–430.
6. McCullough PA, Kellum JA, Mehta RL, et al. ADQI consensus on AKI biomarkers and cardiorenal syndromes. *Contrib Nephrol.* 2013;182:45–64.
7. Ho KM, Sheridan DJ. Meta-analysis of frusemide to prevent or treat acute renal failure. *BMJ.* 2006;333(7565):420.
8. Venkataraman R, Kellum JA. Prevention of acute renal failure. *Chest.* 2007;131(1):300–308.
9. Merten GJ, Burgess WP, Gray LV, et al. Prevention of contrast-induced nephropathy with sodium bicarbonate: a randomized controlled trial. *JAMA.* 2004;291(19):2328–2334.
10. ACT Investigators. Acetylcysteine for prevention of renal outcomes in patients undergoing coronary and peripheral vascular angiography: main results from the randomized Acetylcysteine for Contrast-induced nephropathy Trial (ACT). *Circulation.* 2011;124(11):1250–1259.
11. Coca SG, Singanamala S, Parikh CR. Chronic kidney disease after acute kidney injury: a systematic review and meta-analysis. *Kidney Int.* 2012;81(5):442–448.

 SEE ALSO

- Glomerulonephritis, Acute; Hepatorenal Syndrome; Hyperkalemia; Prostatic Hyperplasia, Benign (BPH); Chronic Kidney Disease; Reye Syndrome; Rhabdomyolysis; Sepsis
- Algorithm: Anuria or Oliguria

CODES
ICD10
- N17.9 Acute kidney failure, unspecified
- N17.0 Acute kidney failure with tubular necrosis
- N00.9 Acute nephritic syndrome with unspecified morphologic changes

CLINICAL PEARLS
- Three categories of AKI: prerenal, intrarenal, and postrenal
  - Prerenal: decreased renal perfusion (often from hypovolemia) leading to a decrease in GFR; reversible if perfusion is restored
  - Intrarenal: intrinsic kidney damage; ATN is the most common cause via ischemic/nephrotoxic injury to the kidney.
  - Postrenal: secondary to extrinsic/intrinsic obstruction of the urinary collection system
- Recognize the need for emergent hemodialysis: severe hyperkalemia, metabolic acidosis, or volume overload refractory to conservative therapy; uremic pericarditis, encephalopathy, or neuropathy; and selected alcohol and drug intoxications

ADDISON DISEASE

Tya-Mae Y. Julien, MD

 BASICS

DESCRIPTION
- Primary adrenal gland insufficiency, which results from partial or complete destruction of the adrenal cells with inadequate secretion of glucocorticoids and mineralocorticoids
- ~80% of cases are caused by an autoimmune process, followed by tuberculosis (TB), AIDS, systemic fungal infections, and adrenoleukodystrophy
- Addison disease (primary adrenocortical insufficiency) can be differentiated from secondary (pituitary failure) and tertiary (hypothalamic failure) causes because mineralocorticoid function usually remains intact in secondary and tertiary causes.
- Addisonian (adrenal) crisis: acute complication of adrenal insufficiency (circulatory collapse, dehydration, hypotension, nausea, vomiting, hypoglycemia); usually precipitated by an acute physiologic stressor(s) such as surgery, illness, exacerbation of comorbid process, and/or acute withdrawal of long-term corticosteroid therapy
- System(s) affected: endocrine/metabolic
- Synonym(s): adrenocortical insufficiency; corticoadrenal insufficiency; primary adrenocortical insufficiency

EPIDEMIOLOGY
- Predominant age: all ages; typical age of presentation is 30 to 50 years
- Predominant sex: females > males (slight)
- No racial predilection

Incidence
0.6:100,000

Prevalence
4 to 6:100,000; possibly higher

ETIOLOGY AND PATHOPHYSIOLOGY
- Autoimmune adrenal insufficiency (~80% of cases in the United States)
- Infectious causes: TB (most common infectious cause worldwide), HIV (most common infectious cause in the United States, often with concomitant infections such as cytomegalovirus), Waterhouse-Friderichsen syndrome (most commonly meningococcus), fungal disease
- Bilateral adrenal hemorrhage and infarction (for patients on anticoagulants, 50% are in the therapeutic range)
- Antiphospholipid antibody syndrome
- Lymphoma, Kaposi sarcoma, metastasis (lung, breast, kidney, colon, melanoma); tumor must destroy 90% of gland to produce hypofunction
- Drugs (e.g., ketoconazole, fluconazole, etomidate)
- Surgical adrenalectomy, radiation therapy
- Sarcoidosis, hemochromatosis, amyloidosis
- Congenital enzyme defects (deficiency of 21-hydroxylase enzyme is most common), neonatal adrenal hypoplasia, congenital adrenal hyperplasia, familial glucocorticoid insufficiency, autoimmune polyglandular autoimmune syndromes 1 and 2, adrenoleukodystrophy
- Idiopathic
- Destruction of the adrenal cortex resulting in deficiencies in cortisol, aldosterone, and androgens

Genetics
- Autoimmune polyglandular syndrome (APS) type 2 genetics are complex and are associated with adrenal insufficiency, type 1 diabetes, and Hashimoto disease. APS type 2 is more common than APS type 1.
- APS type 1 is caused by mutations of the autoimmune regulator gene. Nearly all have the following triad: adrenal insufficiency, hypoparathyroidism, and mucocutaneous candidiasis before adulthood.
- Adrenoleukodystrophy is an X-linked recessive disorder resulting in toxic accumulation of unoxidized long-chain fatty acids.
- Increased risk with cytotoxic T-lymphocyte antigen 4 (CTLA-4)

RISK FACTORS
- 40% of patients have a 1st- or 2nd-degree relative with associated disorders.
- Chronic steroid use, then experiencing severe infection, trauma, or surgical procedures

GENERAL PREVENTION
- No preventive measures known for Addison disease; focus on prevention of complications
  - Anticipate adrenal crisis and treat before symptoms begin.
- Elective surgical procedures require upward adjustment in steroid dose.

COMMONLY ASSOCIATED CONDITIONS
- Diabetes mellitus
- Graves disease
- Hashimoto thyroiditis
- Hypoparathyroidism
- Hypercalcemia
- Ovarian failure
- Pernicious anemia
- Myasthenia gravis
- Vitiligo
- Chronic moniliasis
- Sarcoidosis
- Sjögren syndrome
- Chronic active hepatitis
- Schmidt syndrome

 DIAGNOSIS

HISTORY
- Weakness, fatigue
- Dizziness
- Anorexia, nausea, vomiting
- Abdominal pain
- Chronic diarrhea
- Depression (60–80% of patients)
- Decreased cold tolerance
- Salt craving

PHYSICAL EXAM
- Weight loss
- Low BP, orthostatic hypotension
- Increased pigmentation of high friction areas (extensor surfaces, plantar or palmar creases, dental-gingival margins, buccal and vaginal mucosae, lips, areolae, pressure points, scars, "tanning," freckles)
- Vitiligo
- Hair loss in females

DIFFERENTIAL DIAGNOSIS
- Secondary adrenocortical insufficiency (pituitary failure)
  - Withdrawal of long-term corticosteroid use
  - Sheehan syndrome (postpartum necrosis of pituitary)
  - Empty sella syndrome
  - Radiation to pituitary
  - Pituitary adenomas, craniopharyngiomas
  - Infiltrative disorders of pituitary (sarcoidosis, hemochromatosis, amyloidosis, histiocytosis X)
- Tertiary adrenocortical insufficiency (hypothalamic failure)
  - Pituitary stalk transection
  - Trauma
  - Disruption of production of corticotropic-releasing factor
  - Hypothalamic tumors
- Other
  - Myopathies
  - Syndrome of inappropriate antidiuretic hormone
  - Heavy metal ingestion
  - Severe nutritional deficiencies
  - Sprue syndrome
  - Hyperparathyroidism
  - Neurofibromatosis
  - Peutz-Jeghers syndrome
  - Porphyria cutanea tarda
  - Salt-losing nephritis
  - Bronchogenic carcinoma
  - Anorexia nervosa

DIAGNOSTIC TESTS & INTERPRETATION

Initial Tests (lab, imaging)
- Basal plasma cortisol and adrenocorticotropic hormone (ACTH) (low cortisol and high ACTH indicative of Addison disease) (1)[C]
- Standard ACTH stimulation test: Cosyntropin 0.25 mg IV; measure preinjection baseline and 60-minute postinjection cortisol levels (patients with Addison disease have low to normal values that do not rise).
- Insulin-induced hypoglycemia test
- Metapyrone test
- Autoantibody tests: 21-hydroxylase (most common and specific), 17-hydroxylase, 17-alpha-hydroxylase (may not be associated), and adrenomedullin
- Circulating very-long-chain fatty acid levels if boy or young man
- Low serum sodium
- Elevated serum potassium
- Elevated BUN, creatinine, calcium, thyroid-stimulating hormone (TSH)
- Low serum aldosterone
- Hypoglycemia when fasting
- Metabolic acidosis
- Moderate neutropenia
- Eosinophilia
- Relative lymphocytosis
- Anemia, normochromic, normocytic

Follow-Up Tests & Special Considerations
- Plasma ACTH levels do not correlate with treatment and should not be used for routine monitoring of replacement therapy.
- TSH: Repeat when condition has stabilized.
  - Thyroid hormone levels may normalize with the treatment of Addison disease.
- Drugs that may alter lab results: digitalis
- Disorders that may alter lab results: diabetes

Diagnostic Procedures/Other
- Abdominal CT scan: small adrenal glands in autoimmune adrenalitis; enlarged adrenal glands in infiltrative and hemorrhagic disorders
- Abdominal radiograph may show adrenal calcifications.
- Chest x-ray may show small heart size and/or calcification of cartilage.
- MRI of pituitary and hypothalamus if secondary or tertiary cause of adrenocortical insufficiency is suspected.
- CT-guided fine-needle biopsy of adrenal masses may identify diagnoses.

Test Interpretation
- Atrophic adrenals in autoimmune adrenalitis
- Infiltrative and hemorrhagic disorders produce enlargement with destruction of the entire gland.

TREATMENT

GENERAL MEASURES
Consider the 5 S's for the management of adrenal crisis:
- Salt, sugar, steroids, support, and search for a precipitating illness (usually infection, trauma, recent surgery, or not taking prescribed replacement therapy)

MEDICATION
First Line
- Chronic adrenal insufficiency
  - Glucocorticoid supplementation (2)[A]
    - Dosing: hydrocortisone 15 to 30 mg (or therapeutic equivalent) PO in 2 to 4 divided doses (to include morning rising and bedtime doses); dosage may vary and is usually lower in children and the elderly.
    - Precautions: hepatic disease, fluid disturbances, immunosuppression, peptic ulcer disease, pregnancy, osteoporosis
    - Adverse reactions: immunosuppression, osteoporosis, gastric ulcers, depression, hyperglycemia, weight gain, glaucoma
    - Drug interactions: concomitant use of rifampin, phenytoin, or barbiturates
  - Mineralocorticoid supplementation
    - Dosing: fludrocortisone 0.05 to 0.2 mg/day PO
  - May require salt supplementation
- Addisonian crisis
  - Hydrocortisone 100 mg IV followed by 10 mg/hr infusion or hydrocortisone 100 mg IV bolus q6–8h
  - IV glucose, saline, and plasma expanders
  - Fludrocortisone 0.05 mg/day PO (typically not required; high-dose hydrocortisone is an effective mineralocorticoid)

- Acute illnesses (fever, stress, minor trauma)
  - Double the patient's usual steroid dose, taper the dose gradually over a week or more, and monitor vital signs and serum sodium.
- Supplementation for surgical procedures
  - Administer hydrocortisone 25 to 150 mg or methylprednisolone 5 to 30 mg IV on the day of the procedure in addition to maintenance therapy; taper gradually to the usual dose over 1 to 2 days.

Second Line
- Addition of androgen therapy:
  - Dehydroepiandrosterone (DHEA) 25 to 50 mg PO once daily is sufficient to restore androgen levels to within normal range with minimal side effects and may improve well-being and sexuality in some women (3,4)[A].

INPATIENT CONSIDERATIONS
Admission Criteria/Initial Stabilization
- Presence of circulatory collapse, dehydration, hypotension, nausea, vomiting, hypoglycemia
- ICU admission for unstable cases
- Addisonian crisis:
  - Airway, breathing, and circulation management
  - Establish IV access; 5% dextrose and normal saline.
  - Administer hydrocortisone 100 mg IV bolus q6–8h; replacement with fludrocortisone is not necessary (high-dose hydrocortisone is an effective mineralocorticoid).
  - Correct electrolyte abnormalities.
  - BP support for hypotension
  - Antibiotics if infection suspected

IV Fluids
IV saline containing 5% dextrose and plasma expanders

ONGOING CARE

FOLLOW-UP RECOMMENDATIONS
- Verify adequacy of therapy: normal BP, serum electrolytes, plasma renin, and fasting blood glucose level
- Periodically assess for the development of long-term complications of corticosteroid use, including screening for osteoporosis, gastric ulcers, depression, and glaucoma.
- Lifelong medical supervision for signs of adequate therapy and avoidance of overdose
- Monitor for development of new autoimmune diseases.

DIET
Maintain water, sodium, and potassium balance.

PATIENT EDUCATION
- National Adrenal Diseases Foundation, Great Neck, NY 11021, (516) 487-4992 (http://www.nadf.us)
- Patient should wear or carry medical identification about the disease and the need for hydrocortisone or other replacement therapy.
- Instruct patient in self-administration of parenteral hydrocortisone for emergency situations.

PROGNOSIS
Requires lifetime treatment: Life expectancy approximates normal with adequate replacement therapy; without treatment, the disease is 100% lethal.

COMPLICATIONS
- Hyperpyrexia
- Psychotic reactions
- Complications from underlying disease
- Over- or underuse of steroid treatment
- Hyperkalemic paralysis (rare)
- Addisonian crisis

REFERENCES

1. Husebye ES, Allolio B, Arlt W, et al. Consensus statement on the diagnosis, treatment and follow-up of patients with primary adrenal insufficiency. *J Intern Med*. 2014;275(2):104–115.
2. Ekman B, Bachrach-Lindström M, Lindström T, et al. A randomized, double-blind, crossover study comparing two- and four-dose hydrocortisone regimen with regard to quality of life, cortisol and ACTH profiles in patients with primary adrenal insufficiency. *Clin Endocrinol (Oxf)*. 2012;77(1):18–25.
3. Gebre-Medhin G, Husebye ES, Mallmin H, et al. Oral dehydroepiandrosterone (DHEA) replacement therapy in women with Addison's disease. *Clin Endocrinol (Oxf)*. 2000;52(6):775–780.
4. McHenry CM, Bell PM, Hunter SJ, et al. Effects of dehydroepiandrosterone sulfate (DHEAS) replacement on insulin action and quality of life in hypopituitary females: a double-blind, placebo-controlled study. *Clin Endocrinol (Oxf)*. 2012;77(3):423–429.

 SEE ALSO

Algorithm: Adrenocortical Insufficiency

CODES

ICD10
- E27.1 Primary adrenocortical insufficiency
- A18.7 Tuberculosis of adrenal glands
- E27.2 Addisonian crisis

CLINICAL PEARLS

- 80% of cases are caused by an autoimmune process; the average age of diagnosis in adults is 40 years.
- Consider the 5 S's for the management of Addison disease: salt, sugar, steroids, support, and search for an underlying cause.
- The goal of steroid replacement therapy should be the lowest dose that alleviates patient symptoms while preventing adverse drug events.
- Plasma ACTH levels do not consistently correlate with treatment and should not be used alone for routine monitoring for efficacy of replacement therapy.
- Long-term use of steroids predisposes patients to the development of osteoporosis; screen accordingly and encourage calcium and vitamin D supplementation.

ADENOMYOSIS

Bradley M. Turner, MD, MPH, MHA • Amanda Martin Kelley, MD, MPH&TM

BASICS

DESCRIPTION
- Benign invasion of the endometrium into the myometrium, producing a diffusely enlarged uterus
- Microscopically, there are ectopic, nonneoplastic endometrial glands and stroma surrounded by hypertrophic and hyperplastic myometrium.
- Can be either diffuse or focal, depending on the extent of myometrial invasion
- In some cases, it may manifest as a circumscribed myometrial mass referred to as an adenomyoma.
- Most commonly affects the posterior wall of the uterus
- Typically associated with the uterus; however, the term "adenomyosis" can also be applied to benign hyperplastic changes in the bile ducts, gallbladder, and ampulla of Vater.

EPIDEMIOLOGY
- Most frequently presents in the 4th and 5th decades
- Wide variation among racial and ethnic groups and among different geographic regions

Incidence
- Variability in the criteria used for diagnosis make an accurate determination of true incidence difficult.
- Depending on the criteria used for diagnosis, the incidence has been estimated as between 5% and 50%.
- The incidence has been reported to be higher (35–50%) in women presenting with pelvic pain and infertility.

Prevalence
- As with incidence, an accurate determination of prevalence is difficult due to the variability in the criteria used for diagnosis.
- Depending on the criteria used for diagnosis, the prevalence has been reported to vary from 5% to 70%, with the mean frequency of adenomyosis at hysterectomy given as approximately 20–30%.

ETIOLOGY AND PATHOPHYSIOLOGY
- Adenomyosis has been described as an abnormal ingrowth and invagination of the basal endometrium into the inner layer of the myometrium (junctional zone [JZ]).
- The exact mechanism regarding how this occurs and is maintained is not clear and likely to be multifactorial.
- In women with adenomyosis, the JZ may represent a region of morphologic dysfunction and structural weakness, with varying susceptibility to invagination of endometrial stromal cells.
- Increased uterine pressure associated with pregnancy, leiomyomas, or other pathology may modulate the JZ environment, making it more susceptible to invagination of endometrial stromal cells.
- Other theories for pathogenesis include the following:
  - *Metaplasia theory*: metaplasia of myometrial smooth muscle cells
  - *Müllerian remnants theory*: de novo development from müllerian rests in the myometrium
  - *Tissue remodeling theory*: ectopic endometrial tissue arising secondary to tissue remodeling associated with uterine trauma either physiologic (e.g., during menstruation, childbirth, or spontaneous abortion) or iatrogenic (e.g., during uterine surgery)

- *Multipotential perivascular theory*: Multipotential perivascular stem cells may be associated with increased angiogenesis and pathophysiologic vascular remodeling, leading to vascular smooth muscle hypertrophy, proliferation, or migration.
- *Epithelial–mesenchymal transition theory*: Increased estrogen concentrations may enhance endometrial tissue growth, angiogenesis, and invagination into the JZ.
- *Hyperproliferation of uterine smooth muscle cell theory*: Activation of the MAPK/ERK pathway has been associated with hyperproliferative uterine smooth muscle cells in women with adenomyosis.
- *Mast cell activation theory*: Nerve growth factor, a mast cell–derived mediator, can be used as an indicator for the severity of adenomyosis. This and other mast cell–derived mediators may contribute to the differentiation and development of the myometrium and maintenance of adenomyosis.

Genetics
- DNA microarray and proteomics analysis have identified specific genes that are differentially expressed in adenomyosis and matched eutopic endometrium.
- Data suggest that genetic and epigenetic abnormalities contribute to the pathogenesis of adenomyosis.

RISK FACTORS
- Age >35 years, however, the disease may cause dysmenorrhea and chronic pelvic pain in women of younger age, including adolescents. Reports suggest that early-stage adenomyosis might present a different clinical phenotype compared to late-stage disease.
- Multiparity
- Tamoxifen treatment
- Other possible risk factors:
  - Previous uterine surgery (studies have been inconsistent)
  - Smoking (studies have been inconsistent)

COMMONLY ASSOCIATED CONDITIONS
- Leiomyomas (uterine fibroids)
- Endometriosis
- Endometrial polyps
- Urinary tract dysfunction

DIAGNOSIS

Pelvic pain, dysmenorrhea, and an enlarged uterus are the usual cues that prompt imaging by ultrasound or MRI; endometrial or uterine biopsies may be indicated in some cases.

HISTORY
- Presenting symptoms are nonspecific and the patient is often asymptomatic.
- Symptoms often include (1–4) the following:
  - Menorrhagia
  - Dysmenorrhea
  - Chronic pelvic pain
  - Abnormal uterine bleeding
- Urinary tract symptoms (e.g., stress urinary incontinence, urgency, daytime frequency, and urge urinary incontinence) have recently been associated with an increased incidence of adenomyosis; however, data are limited (5,6).

PHYSICAL EXAM
Uterus may be enlarged and tender (7).

DIFFERENTIAL DIAGNOSIS
- Pregnancy
- Benign uterine tumors
- Malignant uterine tumors
- Metastatic disease

DIAGNOSTIC TESTS & INTERPRETATION

Initial Tests (lab, imaging)
- Transvaginal ultrasound (TVUS) is the imaging method of choice for initial evaluation of suspected adenomyosis (2,4,7)[A].
- TVUS can be either two or three-dimensional (2)[A].
- Three-dimensional TVUS can provide JZ thickness.
- TVUS has a sensitivity of 72–82.5% and a specificity of 81–84.6% (4,7)[A].
- TVUS is less sensitive than MRI in differentiating adenomyosis from leiomyoma (2,7)[A].
- TVUS with power color flow Doppler can be used to differentiate adenomyosis from leiomyoma (2,4)[B], depending on the operator (2,7)[C].
- Although MRI is more sensitive (4,7)[A] than TVUS, the higher cost of the procedure limits its use as a first-line diagnostic tool.
- MRI has a sensitivity of 77–93% and a specificity of 67–99% (4,7)[A].
- Leiomyomas are associated with adenomyosis in 36–50% of cases, making MRI an ideal imaging method (4)[A].
- MRI should be considered when TVUS cannot provide a definitive diagnosis.

Diagnostic Procedures/Other
- Uterine biopsy with histologic interpretation
- Uterine-sparing operative treatment with histologic interpretation
- Hysterectomy with histologic interpretation

Test Interpretation
- The two-dimensional sonographic markers of adenomyosis include the following (2,4,7)[A]:

  - Uterine enlargement (with no visualized leiomyoma)
  - Cystic anechoic spaces or lakes in the myometrium
  - Uterine wall thickening
  - Subendometrial echogenic linear striations
  - Heterogeneous echo texture
  - Obscure endometrial/myometrial border
  - Thickening of the transition zone

- With three-dimensional TVUS, a JZ maximum (JZmax) ≥8 mm and a JZ maximum – JZ minimum (JZmin) ≥4 mm have been reported as significantly more associated with adenomyosis than two-dimensional features (2)[B].
- Features of adenomyosis on MRI include low-intensity widening of the JZ on T2-weighted images, which corresponds to smooth muscle hyperplasia and thickening of the JZ (2,4,7)[A].
- Three objective parameters have been identified for an MRI diagnosis of adenomyosis:

  - Thickening of the JZ to at least 8 to 12 mm (2)[B],(7)[A]
  - JZmax/total myometrium >40% (2,7)[B]
  - JZmax–JZmin >5 mm (2)[B]

- Histologic interpretation has traditionally been considered the most practicable way to establish a definitive diagnosis of adenomyosis (4,7)[C].

- Pathologic interpretation of uterine biopsy:
  - Presence of endometrial glands and stromal elements within the myometrium
  - Often difficult to definitively diagnose adenomyosis due to sampling bias and/or biopsy artifact (1)[A]
- Pathologic interpretation of uterine-sparing operative treatment and hysterectomy:
  - In morcellated specimens, diagnostic difficulty arises due to modification of the spatial arrangement of the tissue, leading to difficulty in referencing the surface. Sampling bias can also be an issue (1)[A].
  - Even in cases where the surface is accurately referenced, criteria vary among pathologists regarding the depth of invasion, which "definitively" defines adenomyosis (1,4,7,8)[A].

 TREATMENT

- The mainstay of treatment has been surgical therapy.
- Medical therapy shows promise in certain patients.

MEDICATION

- The levonorgestrel-releasing intrauterine system (Mirena) has been shown to result in a reduction of symptoms (6,9)[B].
- Gonadotropin-releasing hormone analogs have shown promise in several studies (9)[B].

ADDITIONAL THERAPIES

- Danazol has shown promise in several case series (8)[B].
- Immunomodulators of angiogenesis, and oral progestins (dienogest), may offer future options for medical treatment of adenomyosis (9,10)[B].

SURGERY/OTHER PROCEDURES

- Hysterectomy is curative.
- Uterine-sparing operative treatment (USOT) might be considered for women who wish to preserve fertility or do not wish to have a hysterectomy.
- USOT **excisional** techniques (1,8,11)[B]:
  - Complete excision (adenomyomectomy)
  - Cytoreduction (partial adenomyomectomy)
- USOT **nonexcisional** techniques (1,8,11–13)[B]:
  - Laparoscopic techniques including electrocoagulation, uterine artery ligation
  - Hysteroscopic techniques including endometrial ablation, endomyometrial resection
  - MRI or ultrasound-guided high-frequency ultrasound ablation (high-intensity focused ultrasound [HIFU])
  - Uterine artery embolization
  - Other reported techniques include the following: alcohol instillation (cystic adenomyosis), radiofrequency ablation (focal adenomyosis), microwave ablation, and thermoablation (diffuse adenomyosis)
- Of the nonexcisional techniques, HIFU and uterine artery embolization (UAE) seem to offer the most encouraging results (1)[C],(12,13)[B].

- Increasing percentages of necrosis after UAE may be an important factor associated with decreased recurrence of symptoms (14)[B].
- The impact of USOT on fertility outcomes are encouraging; however, data are lacking (11)[A].

 ONGOING CARE

PATIENT EDUCATION

Adenomyosis, PubMed health, at http://www.ncbi.nlm.nih.gov/pubmedhealth/PMHT0024411/

PROGNOSIS

- Adenomyosis is a benign proliferation of endometrial tissue.
- Symptoms usually resolve after menopause.
- Hysterectomy is curative.
- Additional studies are needed to determine the impact of untreated adenomyosis and USOT on fertility and reproductive outcomes.
- Additional studies are needed to clarify the role of medical treatment in women with adenomyosis.
- A consensus on the criterion for diagnosing adenomyosis needs to be reached.

COMPLICATIONS

- Anemia from blood loss associated with heavy periods
- Patients with adenomyosis have been reported to be at increased risk for malignant disease; however, to date, there has not been sufficient morphologic, genetic, or epigenetic evidence to substantiate the malignant transformation of adenomyosis.

REFERENCES

1. Taran FA, Stewart, EA, Brucker S. Adenomyosis: epidemiology, risk factors, clinical phenotype and surgical and interventional alternatives to hysterectomy. *Geburtshilfe Frauenheilkd*. 2013;73(9):924–931.
2. Exacoutos C, Manganaro L, Zupi E. Imaging for the evaluation of endometriosis and adenomyosis. *Best Pract Res Clin Obstet Gynaecol*. 2014;28(5):655–681.
3. Koike N, Tsunemi T, Uekuri C, et al. Pathogenesis and malignant transformation of adenomyosis (review). *Oncol Rep*. 2013;29(3):861–867.
4. Shwayder J, Sakhel K. Imaging for uterine myomas and adenomyosis. *J Minim Invasive Gynecol*. 2014;21(3):362–376.
5. Ekin M, Cengiz H, Öztürk E, et al. Genitourinary symptoms in patients with adenomyosis. *Int Urogynecol J*. 2013;24(3):509–512.
6. Ekin M, Cengiz H, Ayağ ME, et al. Effects of the levonorgestrel-releasing intrauterine system on urinary symptoms in patients with adenomyosis. *Eur J Obstet Gynecol Reprod Biol*. 2013;170(2):517–520.
7. Champaneria R, Abedin P, Daniels J, et al. Ultrasound scan and magnetic resonance imaging for the diagnosis of adenomyosis: systematic review comparing test accuracy. *Acta Obstet Gynecol Scand*. 2010;89(11):1374–1384.
8. Maheshwari A, Gurunath S, Fatima F, et al. Adenomyosis and subfertility: a systematic review of prevalence, diagnosis, treatment and fertility outcomes. *Hum Reprod Update*. 2012;18(4):374–392.
9. Benagiano G, Brosens I, Carrara S. Adenomyosis: new knowledge is generating new treatment strategies. *Womens Health (Lond Engl)*. 2009;5(3):297–311.
10. Hirata T, Izumi G, Takamura M, et al. Efficacy of dienogest in the treatment of symptomatic adenomyosis: a pilot study. *Gynecol Endocrinol*. 2014;30(10):726–729.
11. Grimbizis GF, Mikos T, Tarlatzis B. Uterus-sparing operative treatment for adenomyosis. *Fertil Steril*. 2014;101(2):472–487.
12. Dong X, Yang Z. High-intensity focused ultrasound ablation of uterine localized adenomyosis. *Curr Opin Obstet Gynecol*. 2010;22(4):326–330.
13. Popovic M, Puchner S, Berzaczy D, et al. Uterine artery embolization for the treatment of adenomyosis: a review. *J Vasc Interv Radiol*. 2011;22(7):901–909.
14. Bae SH, Kim MD, Kim GM, et al. Uterine artery embolization for adenomyosis: percentage of necrosis predicts midterm clinical recurrence. *J Vasc Interv Radiol*. 2015;26(9):1290.e2–1296.e2.

ADDITIONAL READING

- Benagiano G, Habiba M, Brosens I. The pathophysiology of uterine adenomyosis: an update. *Fertil Steril*. 2012;98(3):572–579.
- Fedele L, Bianchi S, Frontino G. Hormonal treatments for adenomyosis. *Best Pract Res Clin Obstet Gynaecol*. 2008;22(2):333–339.
- Streuli I, Santulli P, Chouzenoux S, et al. Activation of the MAPK/ERK cell-signaling pathway in uterine smooth muscle cells of women with adenomyosis *Reprod Sci*. 2015;22(12):1549–1560.
- Verit FF, Yucel O. Endometriosis, leiomyoma and adenomyosis: the risk of gynecologic malignancy. *Asian Pac J Cancer Prev*. 2013;14(10):5589–5597.
- Weiss G, Maseelall P, Schott LL, et al. Adenomyosis a variant, not a disease? Evidence from hysterectomized menopausal women in the Study of Women's Health Across the Nation (SWAN). *Fertil Steril*. 2009;91(1):201–206.

 CODES

ICD10

N80.0 Endometriosis of uterus

CLINICAL PEARLS

- Adenomyosis is often asymptomatic.
- Both TVUS and MRI are very accurate for the diagnosis of adenomyosis.
- MRI is more sensitive than TVUS, particularly in differentiating adenomyosis from leiomyoma. Differentiation of adenomyosis from leiomyoma is critical because the former is often treated with hysterectomy, whereas the latter is often treated with uterine conservation.
- Various medical and surgical therapeutic options, including uterine-sparing operative techniques, are available for adenomyosis.
- Hysterectomy is curative.

ADENOVIRUS INFECTIONS

Crystal Amadi, MD • Fozia Akhtar Ali, MD

 BASICS

DESCRIPTION
- Acute, typically self-limited, febrile illnesses characterized by inflammation of mucous membranes including the conjunctivae, and the respiratory and GI tracts.
- Adenovirus infections occur in epidemic and endemic situations:
  - Common types are as follows:
    - Acute febrile respiratory illness—affects primarily children
    - Acute respiratory disease—affects adults
    - Viral pneumonia—affects children and adults
    - Acute pharyngoconjunctival fever—affects children, particularly after summer swimming
    - Acute follicular conjunctivitis—affects all ages
    - Epidemic keratoconjunctivitis—affects adults
    - Intestinal infections leading to enteritis, mesenteric adenitis, and intussusception
  - Conjunctivitis
- System(s) affected: cardiovascular; GI; hematologic/lymphatic/immunologic; musculoskeletal; nervous; pulmonary; renal/urologic; ophthalmologic

Geriatric Considerations
Complications more likely in elderly populations

Pediatric Considerations
Viral pneumonia in infants and neonates (may be fatal)

EPIDEMIOLOGY
- Predominant age: <10 years, but epidemics in all ages
- Predominant sex: male = female
- Occurs worldwide and throughout the year but more frequently in warmer months

Incidence
- Common infection: 2–5% of all upper respiratory infections (URIs) and >10% of URIs in children
- Most individuals show evidence of prior adenovirus infection by age 10 years.
- Many adenovirus infections are subclinical or asymptomatic.
- 15–70% of conjunctivitis worldwide

ETIOLOGY AND PATHOPHYSIOLOGY
- DNA virus 60 to 90 nm in size, 6 species (A–F) with over 50 known serotypes
- Adenovirus can remain dormant in lymphoreticular tissue (adenoids and tonsils) after exposure and viral shedding may persist for months (1).
- Transmission
  - Aerosol droplets, fomites, fecal–oral
  - Virus can survive on skin and environmental surfaces.
  - Incubation period is 5 to 9 days (2).

- Most common known pathogens:
  - Types 1 to 5, 7, 14, and 21 cause upper respiratory illness and pneumonia.
  - Types 3, 7, and 21 cause pharyngoconjunctival fever.
  - Types 31, 40, and 41 cause gastroenteritis.
  - Types 8, 19, 37, 53, and 54 cause epidemic keratoconjunctivitis.
  - Types 5, 7, 14, and 21 cause more severe illness.

RISK FACTORS
- Large number of people gathered in a confined area (e.g., military recruits, college students, daycare centers, summer camps, community swimming pools)
- Immunocompromised are at risk for severe disease.

GENERAL PREVENTION
- Live, enteric-coated oral type 4 and type 7 adenovirus vaccine available for military recruits (or other personnel at high risk ages 17 to 50 years); reduces incidence of acute respiratory disease (3)
- Frequent hand washing
- Decontamination of environmental surfaces using chlorine, bleach, formaldehyde, or heat
- Universal precautions, particularly when examining patients with epidemic keratoconjunctivitis; droplet precautions if suspected adenoviral respiratory infection.
- Health care providers with suspected bilateral adenoviral conjunctivitis should avoid direct patient contact for 2 weeks after onset of symptoms in second eye.

COMMONLY ASSOCIATED CONDITIONS
- Otitis media
- Conjunctivitis
- Bronchiolitis
- Viral enteritis
- Less frequent syndromes (seen primarily in immunocompromised individuals): meningoencephalitis, hepatitis, myocarditis, pancreatitis, genital infections, intussusception and mesenteric adenitis hemorrhagic cystitis, and interstitial nephritis.

Dx DIAGNOSIS

HISTORY
Depends on type (see "Differential Diagnosis"). Common symptoms with most respiratory forms (4,5)
- Headache, malaise
- Sore throat
- Cough, coryza
- Fever (moderate to high)
- Vomiting, diarrhea, abdominal pain
- Ear pain
- Urinary symptoms/hematuria
- Eye redness and pain
- Irritative voiding symptoms (bladder involvement)

PHYSICAL EXAM
- Fever
- Tonsillar erythema/exudate
- Cervical lymphadenopathy
- Otitis media
- Conjunctivitis

DIFFERENTIAL DIAGNOSIS
- The following are the primary characteristics of the major adenovirus infections:
  - Acute respiratory illness
    - Mostly in children
    - Incubation period: 2 to 5 days
    - Malaise, fever, chills, headache, pharyngitis, hoarseness, dry cough
    - Fever lasting 2 to 4 days
    - Illness subsiding in 10 to 14 days
    - DDx: rhinovirus, influenza, parainfluenza, RSV
  - Viral pneumonia
    - Sudden onset of high fever, rapid infection of upper and lower respiratory tracts, skin rash, diarrhea
    - Occurs mostly in children aged a few days up to 3 years
    - DDx: bacterial pneumonia, RSV, influenza, parainfluenza
  - Acute pharyngoconjunctival fever
    - Spiking fever, headache, pharyngitis, conjunctivitis (typically unilateral), rhinitis, cervical adenitis
    - Subsides in 1 week
    - DDx: bacterial conjunctivitis, enterovirus, herpes simplex virus (HSV)
  - Epidemic keratoconjunctivitis
    - Usually unilateral onset of ocular redness and edema, periorbital edema, periorbital swelling, foreign body sensation
    - Lasts 3 to 4 weeks
    - DDx: bacterial conjunctivitis, enterovirus, HSV
  - Viral enteritis
    - Nausea/vomiting, diarrhea, abdominal pain
    - DDx: bacterial enteritis, bowel obstruction

DIAGNOSTIC TESTS & INTERPRETATION
Initial Tests (lab, imaging)
- Confirmation necessary only in severe cases and epidemics.
- Viral cultures from respiratory, ocular, or fecal sources
  - Pharyngeal isolate suggests recent infection.
- Adenovirus-specific ELISA; rapid but less sensitive than culture (6)[A]
- Adenovirus DNA via polymerase chain reaction (PCR)
- Rapid pathogen screening, Adeno Detector, is available for detecting adenoviral conjunctivitis (sensitivity, 89%; specificity, 94%); results in 10 minutes (7)[B]

- Antigen detection in stool for enteric serotypes
- Serologies (complement fixation) with a fourfold rise in serum antibody titer, identify recent adenoviral infection.
- Radiographs: bronchopneumonia in severe respiratory infections

Diagnostic Procedures/Other
Biopsy (lung or other) may be needed in severe or unusual cases; usually only in immunocompromised patients

Test Interpretation
- Varies with each virus
  - Severe pneumonia may show extensive intranuclear inclusions.
- *Bronchiolitis obliterans* may occur.

 TREATMENT

GENERAL MEASURES
- Treatment is supportive and symptomatic.
- Infections are usually benign and of short duration.

MEDICATION
First Line
- Acetaminophen 10 to 15 mg/kg PO for analgesia (avoid aspirin)
- Antivirals and immunotherapy for immunocompromised individuals and patients with severe disease are as follows:
  - No controlled trials showing benefit of any antiviral agents against human adenovirus infection; however, cidofovir (1 mg/kg every other day) is most commonly used.
  - For adenoviral conjunctivitis, topical ganciclovir 0.15% ophthalmic gel has been suggested for "off-label" use.

COMPLEMENTARY & ALTERNATIVE MEDICINE
Echinacea has not been shown to be better than placebo for treatment of viral URIs (8)[B].

INPATIENT CONSIDERATIONS
Admission Criteria/Initial Stabilization
Severely ill infants or immunocompromised patients with severe illness

Nursing
Hospitalized patients with adenoviral infections should be placed on contact precautions with droplet precautions added for those with respiratory illness.

 ONGOING CARE

FOLLOW-UP RECOMMENDATIONS
Rest during febrile phases

Patient Monitoring
For severe infantile pneumonia and conjunctivitis, daily physical exam until well.

DIET
No special diet

PATIENT EDUCATION
- Avoid aspirin in children.
- Give instructions for saline nasal spray, cough preparations, frequent hand washing, and surface cleaning.

PROGNOSIS
- Self-limited, usually without sequelae
- Severe illness and death in neonates and in immunocompromised hosts can occur; severe pneumonia in children <2 years can have a mortality rate as high as 16%.

COMPLICATIONS
Few, if any, recognizable long-term problems

REFERENCES

1. Wy Ip W, Qasim W. Management of adenovirus in children after allogeneic hematopoietic stem cell transplantation. *Adv Hematol.* 2013;2013:176418.
2. Lessler J, Reich NG, Brookmeyer R, et al. Incubation periods of acute respiratory viral infections: a systematic review. *Lancet Infect Dis.* 2009;9(5):291–300.
3. Lyons A, Longfield J, Kuschner R, et al. A double-blind, placebo-controlled study of the safety and immunogenicity of live, oral type 4 and type 7 adenovirus vaccines in adults. *Vaccine.* 2008;26(23):2890–2898.
4. Dominguez O, Rojo P, de Las Heras S, et al. Clinical presentation and characteristics of pharyngeal adenovirus infections. *Pediatr Infect Dis I.* 2005;24(8):733–734.
5. Centers for Disease Control and Prevention. Adenovirus symptoms. http://www.cdc.gov/adenovirus/about/symptoms.html.
6. Goto E. Meta-analysis of evaluating diagnostic accuracy of adenoclone (ELISA) for adenoviral infection among Japanese people. *Rinsho Byori.* 2010;58(2):148–155.
7. Kaufman HE. Adenovirus advances: new diagnostic and therapeutic options. *Curr Opin Ophthalmol.* 2011;22(4):290–293.
8. Barrett BP, Brown RL, Locken K, et al. Treatment of the common cold with unrefined echinacea. A randomized, double-blind, placebo-controlled trial. *Ann Intern Med.* 2002;137(12):939–946.

ADDITIONAL READING
- Houlihan C, Valappil M, Waugh S, et al. Severe adenovirus infection: an under-recognized disease with limited treatment options. *JICS.* 2012;13(4), October.
- Majeed A, Naeem Z, Khan DA, et al. Epidemic adenoviral conjunctivitis report of an outbreak in a military garrison and recommendations for its management and prevention. *J Pak Med Assoc.* 2005;55(7):273–275.
- Pihos AM. Epidemic keratoconjunctivitis: a review of current concepts in management. *J Optom.* 2013;6(2):69–74.

 SEE ALSO

Conjunctivitis, Acute; Intussusception; Pneumonia, Viral

 CODES

ICD10
- B34.0 Adenovirus infection, unspecified
- B30.1 Conjunctivitis due to adenovirus
- J12.0 Adenoviral pneumonia

CLINICAL PEARLS
- Adenovirus can mimic streptococcus pharyngitis with tonsillar exudates and cervical adenitis.
- Most common cause of strep-negative tonsillitis in young children
- Diagnosis only needs to be confirmed in severe cases and epidemics.
- Average incubation time is 5 to 6 days.
- Adenovirus conjunctivitis is highly contagious, handwashing and universal precautions help prevent spread.

ADHESIVE CAPSULITIS (FROZEN SHOULDER)

Brandon David Hecht, DO

 BASICS

DESCRIPTION
- Painful, gradual loss of both active and passive glenohumeral (GH) motion due to progressive fibrosis/contracture of the GH joint capsule
- The clinical course of adhesive capsulitis (AC) follows a predictable progression
  - Stage 1, freeze/pain: subacute onset of diffuse vague pain, lasting 2 to 9 months
  - Stage 2, frozen/adhesive: insidious onset of stiffness, lasting 4 to 12 months
  - Stage 3, thaw/recovery: gradual resolution over 5 to 24+ months. Resolution may be protracted (symptoms lasting >36 months) and incomplete but rarely results in a functional limitation.
- AC categorized as primary (idiopathic) and secondary (underlying or associated condition)
- System(s) affected: musculoskeletal
- Synonym(s): pericapsulitis; scapulohumeral periarthritis

EPIDEMIOLOGY
- Predominant age: 40 to 60 years
- Predominant sex: female > male

Prevalence
- General population: 2–5%
- Diabetics type 1 and type 2: 10–20%

ETIOLOGY AND PATHOPHYSIOLOGY
- Synovial inflammation and capsular fibrosis resulting in contracture of the rotator cuff, coracohumeral ligament, and anterior shoulder capsule restricting movement of the shoulder
- A poorly understood chronic inflammatory response with fibroblastic proliferation, possibly immunomodulated

Genetics
No known genetic predispositions

RISK FACTORS
- Sedentary vocation or lifestyle
- Age ≥40 years
- History of AC: 20–30% will develop the condition in contralateral shoulder.
- Minor injury: 20–30% of those with AC will report recent minor trauma to the shoulder.
- Systemic diseases: endocrinopathies, autoimmune disorders, atherosclerotic disease (see "Commonly Associated Conditions")

GENERAL PREVENTION
No current evidence regarding prevention

COMMONLY ASSOCIATED CONDITIONS
- Idiopathic AC associated with a history of Dupuytren contractures
- Secondary AC is associated with diabetes, thyroid disease, autoimmune diseases, rotator cuff injury or minor shoulder trauma, shoulder immobilization, history of stroke, or myocardial infarction.

 DIAGNOSIS

HISTORY
- Insidious onset of progressive, diffuse shoulder pain and stiffness
- Pain predominates early in the course of the disease:
  - Night pain often interrupts sleep.
  - Debilitating pain: achy at rest, sharper with movement, and poorly localized
  - Muscle spasm/pain in the neck, shoulder, acromioclavicular joint, and posterior thorax due to scapular overcompensation
- Stiffness predominates as pain begins to wane in later stages of disease:
  - Difficulties with activities of daily living (ADLs)
    - Inability to reach overhead or into back pocket
- Weakness
- Preceding injury, illness, or immobilization (secondary AC)

PHYSICAL EXAM
- Limited active and passive shoulder range of motion (ROM) in >1 plane of motion: Document ROM for forward flexion, abduction, and external and internal rotation at each visit.
- Diffuse shoulder tenderness with deep palpation
- Loss of natural arm swing with gait
- Normal strength (weakness may be present if pain inhibits effort, but objective strength testing typically reveals 5/5 strength in all planes)
- Special tests (Neer, Hawkins, etc.) are not diagnostic.
- No neurovascular deficits.

DIFFERENTIAL DIAGNOSIS
- Rotator cuff strain/tear/impingement syndrome
- GH or acromioclavicular joint osteoarthritis (OA)
- Cervical strain/radiculopathy/OA
- Myofascial pain syndrome
- Calcific tendonitis
- Fracture, dislocation
- Bony neoplasm/metastases

DIAGNOSTIC TESTS & INTERPRETATION
Initial Tests (lab, imaging)
No lab is diagnostic for primary (idiopathic) AC. Labs may help rule out underlying systemic diseases associated with secondary AC: Hbg A1C, TSH, and ESR.
- Plain radiograph (anteroposterior [AP], axillary, supraspinatus outlet views) to rule out OA, calcific tendinitis, avascular necrosis, osteomyelitis, fracture, dislocation, and tumor
- Radiographs are typically normal but may demonstrate disuse osteopenia of the proximal humerus in late AC.
- In secondary AC, MRI demonstrates characteristic thickening of the axillary pouch and helps to rule out other shoulder disorders.

Follow-up Tests & Special Considerations
- Serial exams in patients who present with non-specific shoulder pain and normal radiographs. At follow-up visits, the diagnosis of AC is supported if progressive motion restriction is identified in >1 plane of motion.
- Early in stage 1, pain is the predominant feature and restriction of motion may be difficult to identify. At 8-week follow-up, the patient may not complain of stiffness, but the loss of passive ROM may be easier to identify on exam.
- Early on, AC is difficult to distinguish from subacromial bursitis. The loss of passive external rotation may be the only finding that differentiates early AC from subacromial bursitis. The only other condition that may cause insidious loss of passive external rotation is GH arthritis.

Diagnostic Procedures/Other
Diagnostic subacromial anesthetic injection can help to differentiate AC from rotator cuff pathologies:
- Resolution of pain and restoration of ROM after subacromial injection suggests rotator cuff pathology or other cause of subacromial bursitis.
- Intact muscle strength with persistent active and passive ROM deficits and a firm mechanical end point are consistent with AC.

Test Interpretation
If performed, arthroscopy demonstrates capsular thickening and synovial inflammation with adhesions to the humerus.

TREATMENT

- Treatment is guided by the stage of AC at presentation. Conservative therapy is recommended initially (the first 4 to 6 months).
- Therapy includes combination of physical therapy, oral medications, and joint/bursal injections (1)[A].
- Structured physical therapy is superior to home exercises (2)[A].
- Patient education should include the following:
  - Expectations for a protracted recovery (months to years) characterized by resolution of pain prior to the return of function
  - Full ROM may never be recovered; however, functional limitations are uncommon.

GENERAL MEASURES
- Control pain, preserve mobility, and allow for restful sleep.
- Codman pendulum exercises: Lean forward onto table or chair with unaffected arm bending at the waist; let the affected arm dangle. Swing the affected arm slowly by moving the torso. Try smaller and then bigger circles (clockwise and counterclockwise).
- Climbing the wall: Put the hand flat on a wall in front of you; use the fingers to "climb" the wall; pause 30 seconds every few inches. Repeat the exercise after turning 90 degrees to wall (abduction).
- Heat and/or ice: may temporarily improve pain and secondary spasm
- Address underlying causes of secondary AC (see "Commonly Associated Conditions").
- Patient reassessment must be ongoing to reinforce expectations and determine patient's goals.

MEDICATION

First Line
- NSAIDs: widely used in the treatment of AC and thought to be most beneficial in stage 1 when pain is the predominant feature. If contraindicated, alternatives include acetaminophen or opioid analgesics. Concomitant use of NSAIDs with oral or injectable corticosteroids has no added benefit.
- Oral corticosteroids: rarely used in clinical practice, may have short-term improvement in pain and ROM (up to 6 weeks) early in the course of the disease (stage 1 and early stage 2)
  - Prednisolone: 30 mg/day for 3 weeks (alternatively 10 mg × 4 weeks, then 5 mg × 2 weeks)
- Subacromial (SA) corticosteroid injection: At any stage, SA injection in conjunction with physical therapy provides short-term (16 weeks) benefit in pain and ROM.
- Intra-articular (IA) corticosteroid injection short-term (16 weeks) improvement in pain and ROM if used in conjunction with physical therapy
  - No additional benefit with ultrasound guidance (3)[A]
  - Equal efficacy to scheduled NSAID therapy (4)[A]

Second Line
Tricyclic antidepressants (amitriptyline) have been used as neuromodulators. No evidence exists to support use in AC.

ISSUES FOR REFERRAL
- Some cases do not respond to nonoperative treatment.
- Orthopedic referral should be considered if patient has not responded adequately to conservative treatment within 4 to 6 months.

ADDITIONAL THERAPIES
- Physical therapy: additive effect when used in conjunction with other treatments (NSAIDs, injections, manipulation under anesthesia [MUA], surgical release), but there is no evidence to support the use of physical therapy alone in the treatment of AC (1,2)[A].
- Iontophoresis (electromotive drug administration) is generally not recommended in this condition.
- Although not commonly used, supervised neglect is a plausible treatment option for some patients as condition can resolve spontaneously over time.
- Capsular hydrodilation (arthrography distention): IA injection of large-volume saline with steroid or hyaluronic acid has demonstrated some short-term improvements (12 weeks) in pain and function (5)[A].
- IA hyaluronic acid: A systematic review showed no benefit when compared to IA corticosteroid when used in conjunction with physical therapy (6)[A].
- Suprascapular nerve block: may help with short-term pain relief
- Low-power laser therapy: superior to placebo (1)[A]
- Botox: Evidence suggests no benefit.

ALERT
Indications for more invasive options remain highly subjective and need to be individualized to each patient.

SURGERY/OTHER PROCEDURES
- Arthroscopic capsular release: most common surgical method for treating recalcitrant AC
  - Short-term benefits: improved pain and function
  - Long-term benefits: superior to conservative therapies in recalcitrant cases (5)[A]
- MUA: Outcomes are similar to those with conservative, noninvasive therapies; contraindicated in posttraumatic/postsurgical AC (5)[A]
- Transcatheter arterial embolization: Early evidence suggests benefit (7)[B].

COMPLEMENTARY & ALTERNATIVE MEDICINE
- Acupuncture: Insufficient evidence exists regarding the effectiveness of acupuncture for AC.
- Osteopathic manipulative technique: Evidence is equivocal.

INPATIENT CONSIDERATIONS
Admission Criteria/Initial Stabilization
Outpatient care

 ONGOING CARE

FOLLOW-UP RECOMMENDATIONS
Reinforce the natural course of the disease. Many patients are more likely to request invasive procedures (injections, capsular distension, MUA, surgery) when stiffness starts to affect ADLs.

Patient Monitoring
A multidisciplinary team approach helps reinforce the natural history of AC and provides patient encouragement.

DIET
No restrictions

PATIENT EDUCATION
Long-term course of treatment until resolution of symptoms; stretching and ROM exercises daily during and after improvement

PROGNOSIS
- Although AC is considered self-limiting, up to 50% of patients will have permanent restrictions of ROM (usually external rotation).
- Rare functional disability results

COMPLICATIONS
Surgical complications and complications due to MUA can be disabling but are uncommon.

REFERENCES

1. Jain TK, Sharma NK. The effectiveness of physiotherapeutic interventions in treatment of frozen shoulder/adhesive capsulitis: a systematic review. *J Back Musculoskelet Rehabil*. 2014;27(3):247–273.
2. Russel S, Jariwala A, Conlon R, et al. A blinded, randomized, controlled trial assessing conservative management strategies for frozen shoulder. *J Shoulder Elbow Surg*. 2014;23(4):500–507.
3. Prestgaard T, Wormgoor ME, Haugen S, et al. Ultrasound-guided intra-articular and rotator interval corticosteroid injections in adhesive capsulitis of the shoulder: a double-blind, sham-controlled randomized study. *Pain*. 2015;156(9):1683–1691.
4. Dehghan A, Pishgooei N, Salami MA, et al. Comparison between NSAID and intra-articular corticosteroid injection in frozen shoulder of diabetic patients; a randomized clinical trial. *Exp Clin Endocrinol Diabetes*. 2013;121(2):75–79.
5. Uppal HS, Evans JP, Smith C. Frozen shoulder: a systematic review of therapeutic options. *World J Orthop*. 2015;6(2):263–268.
6. Lee LC, Lieu FK, Lee HL, et al. Effectiveness of hyaluronic acid administration in treating adhesive capsulitis of the shoulder: a systematic review of randomized controlled trials. *Biomed Res Int*. 2015;2015:314120.
7. Okuno Y, Oguro S, Iwamoto W, et al. Short-term results of transcatheter arterial embolization of abnormal neovessels in patients with adhesive capsulitis: a pilot study. *J Shoulder Elbow Surg*. 2014;23(9):e199–e206.

ADDITIONAL READING

- Ewald A. Adhesive capsulitis: a review. *Am Fam Physician*. 2011;83(4):417–422.
- Maund E, Craig D, Suekarran S, et al. Management of frozen shoulder: a systematic review and cost-effectiveness analysis. *Health Technol Assess*. 2012;16(11):1–264.
- Rill BK, Fleckenstein CM, Levy MS, et al. Predictors of outcome after nonoperative and operative treatment of adhesive capsulitis. *Am J Sports Med*. 2011;39(3):567–574.
- Smith CD, Hamer P, Bunker TD. Arthroscopic capsular release for idiopathic frozen shoulder with intra-articular injection and a controlled manipulation. *Ann R Coll Surg Engl*. 2014;96(1):55–60.

CODES

ICD10
- M75.00 Adhesive capsulitis of unspecified shoulder
- M75.01 Adhesive capsulitis of right shoulder
- M75.02 Adhesive capsulitis of left shoulder

CLINICAL PEARLS
- Early-stage AC is difficult to distinguish from rotator cuff pathology. Restriction of external ROM suggests AC.
- Diagnostic subacromial bursa injection may help differentiate early AC from impingement syndrome. In AC, ROM deficits persist and strength is intact after injection.
- Normal radiographs in the setting of progressive restriction of motion in >1 plane confirms AC.
- Initial AC treatment is conservative.
- Invasive treatment options (capsular distention, MUA, and arthroscopy) can be considered after 4 to 6 months of conservative therapy. This is necessary in only about 10% of cases.

ADOPTION, INTERNATIONAL

Theodore R. Brown, DO, MPH, FAAFP

 BASICS

DESCRIPTION

Although international adoptions have decreased in the past 10 years, they still represent a significant portion of the roughly 135,000 yearly U.S. adoptions. The demographics of those children and their homelands have shifted significantly during that time. Diverse birth countries, disease exposures, and unknown health histories of these children make them a population that requires special attention. Although specialty clinics are becoming more prevalent, many adoptive parents will look to their primary care provider for their adoption health care needs.

EPIDEMIOLOGY

Incidence
- 7,092 children were adopted internationally in 2013.
- Approximately 5% of all U.S. adoptions are international, decreased from 17% in 2004.
- In 2013, the most common countries of origin for internationally adopted children were the following in descending order: China, Ethiopia, Ukraine, Haiti, Democratic Republic of Congo, Uganda, Russia, Nigeria, Philippines, and Bulgaria.
- In 2013, 8% of internationally adopted children were <1 year of age, 54% were ages 1 to 4 years, 29% were ages 5 to 12 years, and 9% were ≥13 years. 55% were girls.

RISK FACTORS
- Unknown birth, medical, and vaccination histories
- Possible exposure to toxins and/or inadequate nutrition in utero
- Exposures to infectious diseases are not commonly seen in the United States (1).
- Previous living conditions
  - Overcrowding
  - Institutionalization (orphanages)
- History of neglect, deprivation, or abuse
- For adoptive family, risks associated with required foreign travel (2)

GENERAL PREVENTION
- Required to be examined by a U.S. State Department physician in their native country before immigration to the United States; limited examination targeted at identifying diseases that would exclude qualifying for a visa
- Should be examined by a U.S. physician within 2 weeks of arrival or sooner if indicated (2)
- A follow-up visit 4 to 6 weeks after their postadoption appointment is recommended.
- All internationally adopted children should be screened for hearing, vision, growth, and developmental delays (3).
- Travel medicine visit for all family members traveling to adopted child's country (2)
- A preadoption visit between the adoptive family and physician can be helpful in clarifying medical diagnoses, reviewing available medical records, as well as photos and/or video that can help to confirm/refute specific diagnoses (1).

COMMONLY ASSOCIATED CONDITIONS
- 60% of international adoptees have a mild to moderate medical or developmental issue (4)
  - 20% have no issue; 20% have a severe problem.
- Infectious diseases, including the following:
  - Hepatitis A/B/C
  - Intestinal parasites

- Tuberculosis (TB), primarily latent
  - Syphilis, including inadequately treated
  - HIV
  - *Helicobacter pylori*
- Emotional or behavioral problems
- Developmental delay
- Fetal alcohol syndrome
- Feeding difficulties, malnutrition, rickets
- Anemia
- Congenital conditions (e.g., cleft lip/palate, orthopedic deformities)
- Prematurity or low birth weight
- Inadequate immunizations
- Lead poisoning
- Sensorineural and conductive hearing loss
- Strabismus, blindness

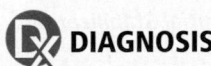 DIAGNOSIS

HISTORY
- Immunization records and titers (records that are "too perfect" should be reviewed carefully)
  - Some vaccinations are (e.g., *Haemophilus influenzae* type B [Hib], pneumococcal, varicella) not routine in other countries.
- Birth/prenatal history, including exposures
- Known family history of birth parents
- Prenatal and perinatal disease or toxin exposures
- Documented history of emotional or nutritional deprivation, or physical or sexual abuse
- Duration of time, if any, spent in orphanage
- Growth charts when available: The earliest sign of malnutrition is failure to gain weight; followed by slowed linear growth; and finally, lagging head circumference.
- Development, behavior, attachment, parent stress, and parent–child interactions should also be routinely monitored.

PHYSICAL EXAM
- Comprehensive unclothed physical exam, paced to child's comfort; particular attention to
  - Growth parameters
  - General appearance; presence of features suggestive of genetic disorder, syndromes, or congenital defects
  - Skin, for infection or signs of prior abuse (4)[C]
  - Genitalia, for signs of abuse or ritual cutting
  - Neurologic findings
  - May be child's first comprehensive exam; remain sensitive to child's cues and consider translator for older children.
- Evaluate for signs of dental decay, and refer for prompt treatment.
- Developmental assessment, especially for those with unknown date of birth (1)[C]

DIAGNOSTIC TESTS & INTERPRETATION
- Developmental screening: validated developmental screening tools at each visit to screen for potential developmental delay and to assess improvement, decline, and need for additional services
- Age-appropriate hearing and vision screening

Initial Tests (lab, imaging)
- Obtain: (1,5)[C],(2,6)[A]

  - Hepatitis A (Hep A IgM, Hep A IgG)
  - Hepatitis B (HBsAg, HBsAb, HBcAb)
  - Hepatitis C (enzyme immunoassay [EIA])

- HIV 1 and 2 antibody testing/ELISA
  - Syphilis: nontreponemal (RPR, VDRL, or ART) and treponemal (MHA-TP, FTA-ABS, or TPPA)
  - Tuberculin skin test (TST) in all ages or interferon-gamma release assay ages ≥5 years
  - Three stool specimens for ova and parasites, specific request for *Giardia intestinalis* and Cryptosporidium species testing of one sample
  - CBC with indices and differential
  - Blood lead concentration for ages ≤6 years
  - Thyroid-stimulating hormone (TSH)
  - Urinalysis
  - Hemoglobinopathy/blood disorder screen: sickle cell, thalassemia, glucose-6-phosphate dehydrogenase (G6PD) deficiency
- Consider based on clinical presentation:
  - Serologic testing for antibody titers depending on the availability/reliability of immunization records (see "MEDICATION") (7)[C]
  - Stool cultures for bacterial pathogens (for children with diarrhea) (1)[C]
  - *H. pylori* testing (for children with dyspepsia, abdominal pain, or anemia) (5)[C]
  - Ca^{++}, PO_4, alkaline phosphate, and 25 vitamin D level (if signs of rickets) (1)[C]
  - >12 months of age: for Chagas disease via *Trypanosoma cruzi*, serologic testing in adoptees from endemic countries (Mexico, Central and South America)
  - >24 months of age: for lymphatic filariasis in those with eosinophilia if from endemic countries (sub-Saharan Africa, Egypt, Southern Asia, Western Pacific Islands, the NE coast of Brazil, Guyana, Haiti, and the Dominican Republic) (6)[A]

Follow-Up Tests & Special Considerations

ALERT

If initially negative, repeat of HIV, Hep B, Hep C, and TB testing are recommended at 6 months; negative tests may represent a "window" period or be falsely negative due to malnutrition in the case of TST (5)[C].

- HIV: if antibody positive in children <18 months, confirm with DNA PCR (may represent maternal antibody) (2)[A].

- Hep C: confirm positive tests with recombinant immunoblot assay (RIBA) and/or HCV RNA PCR; an initial positive in children <18 months may be due to maternal antibody, repeat after 18 months of age.
- Positive TST (TB) must NOT be attributed to bacille Calmette-Guérin (BCG) vaccine and must be investigated; if not active disease, treat latent TB (5)[C].
- GI tract signs or symptoms occurring years after immigration: test for intestinal parasites.
- Eosinophilia >450 cells/mm³ with negative stool ova and parasites: serologic testing for *Schistosoma*; add *Strongyloides* for adoptees from sub-Saharan African, Latin American, and Southeast Asian countries (1)[C].
- Developmental screening: repeat at each visit and follow progress; 50–90% of internationally adopted children are delayed on adoption; however, most have normal cognition at long-term follow-up (3)[C].
- Social history screening: Behavioral concerns may first present during adolescence, even for children adopted in infancy.
- Serial evaluations to age 12 months for children with history of treated congenital syphilis: ophthalmologic, audiologic, neurologic, and developmental (5)[C]

TREATMENT

GENERAL MEASURES
- Regular diet for children who arrive malnourished
- Monitor linear growth.
- If developmental delay is diagnosed, consider early services (e.g., early intervention) or referral to developmental specialist.
- Recommend local support groups for parents.
- Attention to parental interactions: Postadoption depression may occur.

MEDICATION
- Immunizations/Catch-up per CDC schedule (http://www.cdc.gov/vaccines/schedules/)
  - No further Hep B vaccine needed if: HBsAg positive; HBsAb and HBcAb positive; or HBsAb positive and HB vaccine given appropriately
  - MMR should be used for vaccination for mumps and rubella, even in presence of measles antibodies (7)[C].
- Multiple approaches to children vaccinated outside the United States are acceptable (6)[A]:
  - Repeating questionable vaccinations negates the need to obtain serologic tests.
  - To minimize/avoid vaccine administration, check antibody titers.
- The following antibody titers can be measured:
  - Infants 6 to 12 months of age: polio, diphtheria, tetanus (latter two can serve as marker for DPT)
  - Children >12 months: Hep A, measles, mumps, rubella, varicella (7)[C]
- Adoptive parents, caretakers, and household members should be up to date on Tdap, Hep A, Hep B, and measles (2)[A],(4)[C].

ISSUES FOR REFERRAL
- Referrals are often necessary for diagnostic and treatment expertise; however, they should be minimized and planned carefully to ensure adjustment to the new home (1)[C].
  - Elective surgical procedures should likewise be deferred until the child has grown accustomed to his or her new home (3)[C].
- Individual or family counseling considered for all adoptive families for adjustment support
- Internationally adopted children may exhibit self-stimulating behaviors (e.g., rocking, head banging); may be related to prior sensory deprivation. These behaviors typically decrease with time, and no treatment is necessary if otherwise developing normally. If in doubt, refer to developmental pediatrics or occupational therapy.
  - If a child continues to have disruptive behaviors, or would rather self-soothe than seek nurturing human interaction, consider a thorough developmental evaluation.
  - Persistent behavioral issues in the parent–child interactions should be evaluated by a pediatric psychologist or psychiatrist (3)[C].
- Vision (strabismus in 10–25% of previously institutionalized adoptees): Refer to pediatric ophthalmology.
- Hearing (higher rates of conductive and sensorineural hearing loss): Refer to audiology and/or ENT for concerns, questionable screening results, or if slow to acquire language skills (3)[C].
- Pediatric dental evaluation by 12 months of age; sooner if signs of dental pathology are present (1)[C].

 ONGOING CARE

FOLLOW-UP RECOMMENDATIONS
Patient Monitoring
- Regular well-child visits, particularly within first months of entry into the United States
- Close monitoring of developmental milestones, behavior, and individual attachment

DIET
- Regular diet
- Up to 68% fall >2 standard deviations below the mean for one or more growth parameters; most begin to follow a curve <2 deviations from the mean within 9 to 12 months (3).

PATIENT EDUCATION
- Eating: Allow access to as much healthy food as the child wants so the child can learn self-regulatory behaviors of eating that may not have been learned in an institution (hunger, satiety) and can build trust with the parent(s) who feed him or her.
- Toileting: Some children may not be trained yet, others who were may regress and have accidents in their new home. Time, positive reinforcement, and avoiding punishment will resolve this issue as the child becomes comfortable with the new surroundings.
- Sleeping: Children must learn to trust their new home and parents, and thus, this is not a time for aggressive sleep rules. Parents should be present, physically and emotionally, just enough to let the child knows that he or she is safe; establishing and then gently reinforcing a bedtime ritual on arrival.
- Language: Adoptive family should learn key phrases in the child's native language prior to adoption. A translator should be available for school-aged children for the first few weeks; avoid the perception on the child's part that a translator's presence signifies potential return to his or her country.
- Adopted children may experience grieving of lost family, relationships, and culture, which is common, expected, and healthy behavior; encourage parents to acknowledge and work through this loss with their children, considering formal counseling, if needed (3).
- Children and families should be encouraged to learn about the culture of the birth country and the ethnic group of origin, including forming relationships with others of the same racial or ethnic group (4).

PROGNOSIS
- Degree of recovery of developmental delays is likely dependent on duration of time spent in an institution
  - Likelihood of long-term developmental, behavioral, or academic problems increases with adoption age.
  - Rate of recovery appears to exceed rate of normal development over a period of years and continues indefinitely (2).
- Some children may regress in previously acquired skills (1).
- When the child reaches adolescence, a desire to search for his or her biologic family is common (4).
- Adoption medicine is an evolving specialty, with an ever-increasing number of resources available, including the American Academy of Pediatrics' Council on Foster Care, Adoption, & Kinship Care (http://www2.aap.org/sections/adoption/index.html).

REFERENCES
1. Jones VF, High PC, Donoghue E, et al. Comprehensive health evaluation of the newly adopted child. *Pediatrics*. 2012;129(1):e214–e223.
2. Centers for Disease Control and Prevention. *CDC Health Information for International Travel 2014*. New York, NY: Oxford University Press; 2014.
3. Schulte EE, Springer SH. Health care in the first year after international adoption. *Pediatr Clin North Am*. 2005;52(5):1331–1349.
4. Barratt MS. International adoption. *Pediatr Rev*. 2013;34(3):145–146.
5. Miller LC. International adoption: infectious diseases issues. *Clin Infect Dis*. 2005;40(2):286–293.
6. American Academy of Pediatrics. Medical evaluation of internationally adopted children for infectious diseases. In: Pickering LK, ed. *Red Book: 2012 Report of the Committee on Infectious Diseases*. 29th ed. Elk Grove Village, IL: American Academy of Pediatrics; 2012.
7. Feja KN, Tolan RW Jr. Infections related to international travel and adoption. *Adv Pediatr*. 2013;60(1):107–139.

ADDITIONAL READING
- Dawood F, Serwint JR. International adoption. *Pediatr Rev*. 2008;29(8):292–294.
- Grogg SE, Grogg BC. Intercountry adoptions: medical aspects for the whole family. *J Am Osteopath Assoc*. 2007;107(11):481–489.
- Kroger AT, Sumaya CV, Pickering LK, et al. General recommendations on immunization: recommendations of the Advisory Committee on Immunization Practices (ACIP). *MMWR Recomm Rep*. 2011;60(RR02):1–60.
- U.S. Department of State, Bureau of Consular Affairs. The Hague Convention on Intercountry Adoption: a guide for prospective adoptive parents. http://travel.state.gov/content/dam/aa/pdfs/PAP_Guide_1.pdf.
- Weitzman C, Albers L. Long-term developmental, behavioral, and attachment outcomes after international adoption. *Pediatr Clin North Am*. 2005;52(5):1395–1419.

CODES

ICD10
- Z02.82 Encounter for adoption services
- Z62.821 Parent-adopted child conflict

CLINICAL PEARLS
- Initial labs: Hep B, Hep A, Hep C, HIV 1 and 2, syphilis, CBC, TSH, lead, G6PD deficiency, hemoglobin electrophoresis; PPD/TST (or IGRA ages ≥5 years), ova and parasites (three stool specimens, including single specimen for *Giardia* and *Cryptosporidium* antigens), urinalysis
- If initially negative, repeat of HIV, Hep B, Hep C, and TST testing are recommended at 6 months; negative tests may represent a "window" period or be falsely negative due to malnutrition in the case of TST.
- Immunizations per CDC schedule with catch-up (http://www.cdc.gov/vaccines/schedules/), as needed; ensure that adoptive family and caretakers are current on Tdap, Hep A, Hep B, measles.
- Internationally adopted children may exhibit self-stimulating behaviors (e.g., rocking, head banging), will typically decrease with time, and do not require treatment if otherwise developing normally; refer to developmental pediatrics or occupational therapy if there are concerns.
- Adoption medicine is an evolving specialty, with an ever-increasing number of resources available, including the American Academy of Pediatrics' Council on Foster Care, Adoption, & Kinship Care (http://www2.aap.org/sections/adoption/index.html).

ALCOHOL ABUSE AND DEPENDENCE

Gennine M. Zinner, RNCS, ANP

BASICS

DESCRIPTION
- Any pattern of alcohol use causing significant physical, mental, or social dysfunction; key features are tolerance, withdrawal, and persistent use despite problems.
- Alcohol abuse: maladaptive pattern of alcohol use manifested by ≥1 of:
  - Failure to fulfill obligations at work, school, or home
  - Recurrent use in hazardous situations
  - Recurrent alcohol-related legal problems
  - Continued use despite related social or interpersonal problems
- Alcohol dependence: maladaptive pattern of use manifested by ≥3 of the following:
  - Tolerance
  - Withdrawal
  - Using more than intended
  - Persistent desire or attempts to cut down/stop
  - Significant amount of time obtaining, using, or recovering from alcohol
  - Social, occupational, or recreational activities sacrificed for alcohol use
  - Continued use despite physical or psychological problems
- National Institute on Alcohol Abuse and Alcoholism criteria for "at-risk" drinking: men: >14 drinks a week or >4 per occasion; women: >7 drinks a week or >3 per occasion
- System(s) affected: nervous, gastrointestinal (GI)
- Synonym(s): alcoholism, alcohol abuse, alcohol dependence

Geriatric Considerations
- Common and underdiagnosed in elderly; less likely to report problem; may exacerbate normal age-related cognitive deficits and disabilities
- Multiple drug interactions
- Signs and symptoms may be different or attributed to chronic medical problem or dementia.
- Common assessment tools may be inappropriate.

Pediatric Considerations
- Children of alcoholics are at increased risk.
- In 2004, 28% of persons 12 to 20 years reported use in past month, one in five binge drink; binge drinkers are seven times more likely to report illicit drug use.
- Negative effect on maturation and development
- Early drinkers are four times more likely to develop a problem than those who begin >21 years.
- Depression, suicidal or disorderly behavior, family disruption, violence or destruction of property, poor school or work performance, sexual promiscuity, social immaturity, lack of interests, isolation, moodiness

Pregnancy Considerations
- Alcohol is teratogenic, especially during the 1st trimester; women should abstain during conception and throughout pregnancy.
- 10–50% of children born to women who are heavy drinkers will have fetal alcohol syndrome.
- Women experience harmful effects at lower levels and are less likely to report problems.

EPIDEMIOLOGY
- Predominant age: 18 to 25 years, but all ages affected
- Predominant sex: male > female (3:1)

Prevalence
- Lifetime prevalence: 13.6%
- 20% in primary care setting
- 48.2% of 21-year-olds in the United States reported binge drinking in 2004.

ETIOLOGY AND PATHOPHYSIOLOGY
- Multifactorial: genetic, environment, psychosocial
- Alcohol is a CNS depressant, facilitating γ-aminobutyric acid (GABA) inhibition and blocking N-methyl-D-aspartate receptors.

Genetics
50–60% of risk is genetic.

RISK FACTORS
- Family history
- Depression (40% with comorbid alcohol abuse)
- Anxiety
- Other substance abuse
- Tobacco
- Male gender
- Low socioeconomic status
- Unemployment
- Peer/social approval
- Family dysfunction or childhood trauma
- Posttraumatic stress disorder
- Antisocial personality disorder
- Bipolar disorder
- Eating disorders
- Criminal involvement

GENERAL PREVENTION
Counsel with family history and risk factors

COMMONLY ASSOCIATED CONDITIONS
- Cardiomyopathy, atrial fibrillation
- Hypertension
- Peptic ulcer disease/gastritis
- Cirrhosis, fatty liver, cholelithiasis
- Hepatitis
- Diabetes mellitus
- Pancreatitis
- Malnutrition
- Upper GI malignancies
- Peripheral neuropathy, seizures
- Abuse and violence
- Trauma (falls, motor vehicle accidents [MVAs])
- Severe psychiatric disorders (depression, bipolar, schizophrenia): >50% of patients with these disorders have a comorbid substance abuse problem.

DIAGNOSIS

HISTORY
- Behavioral issues
  - Anxiety, depression, insomnia
  - Psychological and social dysfunction, marital problems
  - Social isolation/withdrawal
  - Domestic violence
  - Alcohol-related legal problems
  - Repeated attempts to stop/reduce
  - Loss of interest in nondrinking activities
  - Employment problems (tardiness, absenteeism, decreased productivity, interpersonal problems, frequent job loss)
  - Blackouts
  - Complaints about alcohol-related behavior
  - Frequent trauma, MVAs, ED visits

- Physical symptoms
  - Anorexia
  - Nausea, vomiting, abdominal pain
  - Palpitations
  - Headache
  - Impotence
  - Menstrual irregularities
  - Infertility

PHYSICAL EXAM
- Physical exam may be completely normal.
- General: fever, agitation, diaphoresis
- Head/eyes/ears/nose/throat: plethoric face, rhinophyma, poor oral hygiene, oropharyngeal malignancies
- Cardiovascular: hypertension, dilated cardiomyopathy, tachycardia, arrhythmias
- Respiratory: aspiration pneumonia
- GI: stigmata of chronic liver disease, peptic ulcer disease, pancreatitis, esophageal malignancies, esophageal varices
- Genitourinary: testicular atrophy
- Musculoskeletal: poorly healed fractures, myopathy, osteopenia, osteoporosis, bone marrow suppression
- Neurologic: tremors, cognitive deficits (e.g., memory impairment), peripheral neuropathy, Wernicke-Korsakoff syndrome
- Endocrine/metabolic: hyperlipidemias, cushingoid appearance, gynecomastia
- Dermatologic: burns (e.g., cigarettes), bruises, poor hygiene, palmar erythema, spider telangiectasias, caput medusae, jaundice

DIFFERENTIAL DIAGNOSIS
- Other substance use disorders
- Depression
- Dementia
- Cerebellar ataxia
- Cerebrovascular accident (CVA)
- Benign essential tremor
- Seizure disorder
- Hypoglycemia
- Diabetic ketoacidosis
- Viral hepatitis

DIAGNOSTIC TESTS & INTERPRETATION
Screening:

- CAGE Questionnaire: (Cut down, Annoyed, Guilty, and Eye opener): >2 "yes" answers is 74–89% sensitive, 79–95% specific for alcohol use disorder; less sensitive for white women, college students, elderly. Not an appropriate tool for less severe forms of alcohol abuse (1)[A]

- Single question for unhealthy use: "How many times in the last year have you had X or more drinks in 1 day?" (X = 5 for men, 4 for women); 81.8% sensitive, 79% specific for alcohol use disorders (2)[C]

- Alcohol Use Disorders Identification Test (AUDIT): 10 items, if >4: 70–92% sensitive, better in populations with low incidence of alcoholism (3)[A]: http://www.nams.sg/addictions/Alcohol/Pages/Self-Assessment-Tool.aspx

Initial Tests (lab, imaging)
- CBC; liver function tests (LFTs); electrolytes; BUN/creatinine; lipid panel; thiamine; folate; hepatitis A, B, and C serology
- Amylase, lipase (if GI symptoms present)
- Serum levels increased in chronic abuse:
  - AST/ALT ratio >2.0
  - γ-glutamyl transferase (GGT)

- Carbohydrate-deficient transferrin
- Elevated mean corpuscular volume (MCV)
- ↑ Prothrombin time
- Uric acid
- ↑ Triglycerides and cholesterol (total)
- Often decreased
  - Calcium, magnesium, potassium, phosphorus
  - BUN
  - Hemoglobin, hematocrit
  - Platelet count
  - Serum protein, albumin
  - Thiamine, folate
- Blood alcohol concentration
  - >100 mg/dL in outpatient setting
  - >150 mg/dL without obvious signs of intoxication
  - >300 mg/dL at any time
- CAT scan or MRI of brain: cortical atrophy, lesions in thalamic nucleus, and basal forebrain
- Abdominal ultrasound (US): ascites, periportal fibrosis, fatty infiltration, inflammation

Test Interpretation
- Liver: inflammation or fatty infiltration (alcoholic hepatitis), periportal fibrosis (alcoholic cirrhosis occurs in only 10–20% of alcoholics)
- Gastric mucosa: inflammation, ulceration
- Pancreas: inflammation, liquefaction necrosis
- Heart: dilated cardiomyopathy
- Immune system: decreased granulocytes
- Endocrine organs: elevated cortisol levels, testicular atrophy, decreased female hormones
- Brain: cortical atrophy, enlarged ventricles

TREATMENT
- For management of acute withdrawal, please see "Alcohol Withdrawal."
- For outpatient withdrawal treatment, see "Alcohol Withdrawal, Treatment" or http://www.aafp.org/afp/2005/0201/p495.html

GENERAL MEASURES
- Brief interventions and counseling by clinicians have proven efficacy for problem drinking (4)[B].
- Treat comorbid problems (sleep, anxiety, etc.); but do not prescribe medications with cross tolerance to alcohol (benzodiazepine).
- Group programs and/or 12-step programs may have benefit in helping patients accept treatment.
- Research shows the benefit of referring patients with alcohol dependence to an addiction specialist or treatment program (3)[A].

MEDICATION
First Line
- Adjuncts to withdrawal regimens:
  - Naltrexone: 50 to 100 mg/day PO or 380 mg IM once every 4 weeks; opiate antagonist reduces craving and likelihood of relapse, decreases number of heavy drinking days in recalcitrant alcohol abusers (IM route may enhance compliance and thus efficacy) (3,5)[A].
  - Acamprosate (Campral): 666 mg PO TID beginning after completion of withdrawal; reduces relapse risk. If helpful, recommended to use for 1 year (6)[A].
  - Topiramate (Topamax): 25 to 300 mg/day PO or divided BID; enhances abstinence (3,5)[B] (not approved by FDA for use in alcohol dependence; off-label use)

- Supplements to all
  - Thiamine: 100 mg/day (1st dose IV prior to glucose to avoid Wernicke encephalopathy)
  - Folic acid: 1 mg/day
  - Multivitamin: daily
- Contraindications
  - Naltrexone: pregnancy, acute hepatitis, hepatic failure
  - Monitor LFTs.
- Precautions: organic pain, organic brain syndromes
- Significant possible interactions: alcohol, sedatives, hypnotics, naltrexone, and narcotics

ALERT
Treat acute symptoms if in alcohol withdrawal; give thiamine 100 mg/day with 1st dose prior to glucose.

Second Line
- Disulfiram: 250 to 500 mg/day PO; unproven efficacy; may provide psychological deterrent. Most effective if used with close supervision (5)[A]
- Selective serotonin reuptake inhibitors may be beneficial if comorbid depression exists (5)[A].

ISSUES FOR REFERRAL
Addiction specialist, 12-step or long-term program, psychiatrist

INPATIENT CONSIDERATIONS
Assess medical and psychiatric condition (CIWA >8).

Admission Criteria/Initial Stabilization
- Correct electrolyte imbalances, acidosis, hypovolemia (treat if in alcohol withdrawal).
- Thiamine: 100 mg IM, followed by 100 mg PO; folic acid: 1 mg/day
- Benzodiazepines used to lower risk of alcohol withdrawal, seizures

ONGOING CARE

FOLLOW-UP RECOMMENDATIONS
Patient Monitoring
- Outpatient detoxification: daily visits (not recommended for heavy alcohol abuse)
- Early outpatient rehabilitation: weekly visits
- Detoxification alone is not sufficient.

PATIENT EDUCATION
- American Council on Alcoholism: (800) 527-5344 or http://www.aca-usa.com/ (treatment facility locator, educational information)
- National Clearinghouse for Alcohol and Drug Information: (800) 729-6686 or http://www.health.org/
- Center for Substance Abuse Treatment: (800) 662-HELP or http://www.samhsa.gov/about-us/who-we-are/offices-centers/csat
- Alcoholics Anonymous: http://www.aa.org/
- Rational Recovery: https://rational.org/index.php?id=1
- Secular Organizations for Sobriety: http://www.centerforinquiry.net/sos
- http://www.alcoholanswers.org/: An evidence-based website for those seeking credible information on alcohol dependence and online support forums.

PROGNOSIS
- Chronic relapsing disease; mortality rate more than twice general population, death 10 to 15 years earlier
- Abstinence benefits survival, mental health, family, employment
- 12-step programs, cognitive behavior, and motivational therapies are often effective during 1st year following treatment.

COMPLICATIONS
- Cirrhosis (women sooner than men)
- GI malignancies
- Neuropathy, dementia, Wernicke-Korsakoff syndrome
- CVA
- Ketoacidosis
- Infection
- Adult respiratory distress syndrome
- Depression
- Suicide
- Trauma

REFERENCES
1. Dhalla S, Kopec JA. The CAGE questionnaire for alcohol misuse: a review of reliability and validity studies. *Clin Invest Med*. 2007;30(1):33–41.
2. Smith PC, Schmidt SM, Allensworth-Davies D, et al. Primary care validation of a single-question alcohol screening test. *J Gen Intern Med*. 2009;24(7):783–788.
3. Willenbring ML, Massey SH, Gardner MB. Helping patients who drink too much: an evidence-based guide for primary care clinicians. *Am Fam Physician*. 2009;80(1):44–50.
4. McQueen J, Howe TE, Allan L, et al. Brief interventions for heavy alcohol users admitted to general hospital wards. *Cochrane Database Syst Rev*. 2011;(8):CD005191.
5. Miller PM, Book SW, Stewart SH. Medical treatment of alcohol dependence: a systematic review. *Int J Psychiatry Med*. 2011;42(3):227–266.
6. Rösner S, Hackl-Herrwerth A, Leucht S, et al. Acamprosate for alcohol dependence. *Cochrane Database Syst Rev*. 2010;(9):CD004332.

ADDITIONAL READING
National Institute on Alcohol Abuse and Alcoholism. Helping patients who drink too much: a clinician's guide. http://www.niaaa.nih.gov/guide.

 SEE ALSO

Substance Use Disorders; Alcohol Withdrawal

CODES

ICD10
- F10.10 Alcohol abuse, uncomplicated
- F10.20 Alcohol dependence, uncomplicated
- F10.239 Alcohol dependence with withdrawal, unspecified

CLINICAL PEARLS
- CAGE Questionnaire: >2 "yes" answers is 74–89% sensitive, 79–95% specific for alcohol use disorder; less sensitive for white women, college students, elderly. Not an appropriate tool for less severe forms of alcohol abuse
- Single question for unhealthy use screening: "How many times in the last year have you had X or more drinks in 1 day?" (X = 5 for men, 4 for women); 81.8% sensitive, 79% specific for alcohol use disorders
- National Institute on Alcohol Abuse and Alcoholism criteria for "at-risk" drinking: men >14 drinks a week or >4 per occasion; women: >7 drinks a week or >3 per occasion

ALCOHOL WITHDRAWAL

Neela Bhajandas, PharmD • Matthew Hinton, PharmD • Paul N. Williams, MD, FACP

BASICS

DESCRIPTION
Alcohol withdrawal syndrome (AWS) is a spectrum of symptoms that results from abrupt cessation of alcohol in a dependent patient. Symptoms can begin within 5 hours of the last drink and persist for 5 to 10 days, ranging in severity.

EPIDEMIOLOGY
Each year, 8.2 million Americans meet diagnostic criteria for alcohol dependence. Data suggest that 2–9% of patients seen in a family physician's office have alcohol dependence. It is more prevalent among men, whites, Native Americans, younger and unmarried adults, and those with lower socioeconomic status; only 24% of those with dependence are ever treated. <5% of U.S. adults will experience withdrawal, but 8% of hospitalized patients exhibit signs and symptoms of withdrawal

ETIOLOGY AND PATHOPHYSIOLOGY
- Consumption of alcohol potentiates the effect of the inhibitory neurotransmitter γ-aminobutyric acid (GABA). With chronic alcohol ingestion, this repeated stimulation downregulates the inhibitory effects of GABA.
- Concurrently, alcohol ingestion inhibits the stimulatory effect of glutamate on the CNS, with chronic alcohol use upregulating excitatory NMDA glutamate receptors.
- When alcohol is abruptly stopped, the combined effect of a downregulated inhibitory neurotransmitter system (GABA-modulated) and upregulated excitatory neurotransmitter system (glutamate-modulated) results in brain hyperexcitability when no longer suppressed by alcohol; clinically seen as AWS.

Genetics
There is some evidence for a genetic basis of alcohol dependence.

RISK FACTORS
- High tolerance, prolonged use, high quantities
- Previous alcohol withdrawal episodes, detoxifications, alcohol withdrawal seizures, and delirium tremens (DTs)
- Serious medical problems
- Concomitant benzodiazepine (BZD) dependence

Geriatric Considerations
Elderly dependent on alcohol are more susceptible to withdrawal, and chronic comorbid conditions place them at higher risk of complications from withdrawal.

Pregnancy Considerations
Hospitalization or inpatient detoxification is usually required for treatment of acute alcohol withdrawal.

GENERAL PREVENTION
- Routinely screen all adults for alcohol misuse (1)[B].

- Screen with the **CAGE** or similar questionnaire
  - Feeling the need to **C**ut down
  - **A**nnoyed by criticism about alcohol use
  - **G**uilt about drinking/behaviors while intoxicated
  - "**E**ye opener" to quell withdrawal symptoms
  - Useful to detect problematic alcohol use, positive screen is ≥2 "yes" responses.
- 10-question AUDIT screening test is also useful to identify problem drinking.
- The "5 A's" is a screening tool used in primary care settings (Assess, Advise, Agree, Assist, Arrange).

COMMONLY ASSOCIATED CONDITIONS
- General: poor nutrition, electrolyte abnormalities (hyponatremia, hypomagnesemia, hypophosphatemia), thiamine deficiency, and dehydration
- GI: hepatitis, cirrhosis, varices, GI bleed
- Heme: splenomegaly, thrombocytopenia, macrocytic anemia
- Cardiovascular: cardiomyopathy, hypertension, atrial fibrillation, other arrhythmias
- CNS: trauma, seizure disorder, generalized atrophy, Wernicke-Korsakoff syndrome
- Peripheral nervous system: neuropathy, myopathy
- Pulmonary: aspiration pneumonitis or pneumonia; increased risk of anaerobic infections
- Psychiatric: depression, posttraumatic stress disorder, bipolar disease, polysubstance abuse

DIAGNOSIS

- *Diagnostic and Statistical Manual of Mental Disorders* AWS criteria are diagnosed when ≥2 of the following present within a few hours to several days after the cessation or reduction of heavy and prolonged alcohol ingestion (2)[C]:
  - Autonomic hyperactivity (sweating, tachycardia)
  - Increased hand tremor
  - Insomnia
  - Psychomotor agitation
  - Anxiety
  - Nausea
  - Vomiting
  - Grand mal seizures
  - Transient (visual, auditory, or tactile) hallucinations or illusions
- Criteria for DTs include ≥2 of the criteria for AWS and disturbances in orientation, memory, attention, awareness, visuospatial ability, or perception
- These should cause clinically significant distress or impair functioning and not be secondary to an underlying medical condition or mental disorder.
- There are three stages of AWS:
  - Stage 1 (minor withdrawal; onset 5 to 8 hours after cessation)
    - Mild anxiety, restlessness, and agitation
    - Mild nausea/GI upset and decreased appetite
    - Sleep disturbance
    - Sweating
    - Mild tremulousness
    - Fluctuating tachycardia and hypertension
  - Stage 2 (major withdrawal; onset 24 to 72 hours after cessation)
    - Marked restlessness and agitation
    - Moderate tremulousness with constant eye movements
    - Diaphoresis
    - Nightmares
    - Nausea, vomiting, diarrhea, anorexia
    - Marked tachycardia and hypertension
    - Alcoholic hallucinosis (auditory, tactile, or visual) may have mild confusion but can be reoriented.
  - Stage 3 (DTs; onset 72 to 96 hours after cessation)
    - Fever
    - Severe hypertension, tachycardia
    - Delirium
    - Drenching sweats
    - Marked tremors
    - Persistent hallucinations

- Alcohol withdrawal–associated seizures are often brief, generalized tonic–clonic seizures, and typically occur 6 to 48 hours after last drink.

HISTORY
Essential historical information should be as follows:
- Duration and quantity of alcohol intake, time since last drink
- Previous episodes/symptoms of alcohol withdrawal, prior detox admissions
- Concurrent substance use
- Preexisting medical and psychiatric conditions, prior seizure activity
- Social history: living situation, social support, stressors, triggers, and so forth

PHYSICAL EXAM
Should include assessment of conditions likely to complicate or that are exacerbated by AWS
- Cardiovascular: arrhythmias, heart failure, coronary artery disease
- GI: GI bleed, liver disease, pancreatitis
- Neuro: oculomotor dysfunction, gait ataxia, neuropathy
- Psych: orientation, memory (may be complicated by hepatic encephalopathy)
- General: hand tremor (6 to 8 cycles per second), infections

DIFFERENTIAL DIAGNOSIS
- Cocaine intoxication
- Opioid, marijuana, and methamphetamine withdrawal
- Anticholinergic drug toxicity
- Neuroleptic malignant syndrome
- ICU delirium
- Liver failure
- Sepsis, CNS infection, or hemorrhage
- Mania, psychosis
- Thyroid crisis (3)[C]

DIAGNOSTIC TESTS & INTERPRETATION
Initial Tests (lab, imaging)
- Blood alcohol level, urine drug screen
- CBC; comprehensive metabolic panel
- CNS imaging if acute mental status changes

TREATMENT

The goal is to prevent and treat withdrawal symptoms (e.g., seizures, DTs, cardiovascular events). This is done primarily with BZDs, which reduce the duration of symptoms and raise the seizure threshold.
- Exclude other medical and psychiatric causes.
- Provide a quiet, protective environment.
- The Clinical Institute Withdrawal Assessment for Alcohol Scale revised (CIWA-Ar) is useful for determining medication dosing and frequency of evaluation for AWS. Severity of symptoms are rated on a scale from 0 to 7, with 0 being without symptoms and 7 being the maximum score (except orientation and clouding of sensorium, scale 0 to 4)
  - Nausea and vomiting
  - Tremor
  - Paroxysmal sweats
  - Anxiety
  - Agitation
  - Tactile disturbances
  - Auditory disturbances

– Visual disturbances
– Headache or fullness in head
– Orientation and clouding of sensorium
- The maximum CIWA-Ar score achievable is 67.
  – Scores >8 are associated with mild withdrawal that will likely resolve without medication.
  – Scores between 8 and 15 are associated with moderate withdrawal which often require management with medication.
  – Scores >15 are considered severe withdrawal and are associated with the highest risk of seizures and development of DTs.
- Frequent reevaluation with CIWA-Ar score is crucial.

MEDICATION
First Line
- BZD monotherapy remains the treatment of choice (4)[A]; it is associated with fewer complications compared with neuroleptics (5)[A].

- BZD should be chosen by the following considerations:
  – Agents with rapid onset control agitation more quickly (e.g., IV diazepam [Valium]).
  – Long-acting BZDs (diazepam, chlordiazepoxide [Librium]) are more effective at preventing breakthrough seizures and delirium management.

  – Short-acting BZDs (lorazepam [Ativan], oxazepam [Serax]) are preferable when prolonged sedation is a concern (e.g., elderly patients or other serious concomitant medical illness) and preferable when severe hepatic insufficiency may impair metabolism (5)[A].
- BZD dosages will vary by patients. Given as symptom-triggered or fixed-schedule regimens. Symptom-triggered regimens have been found to require less BZD amounts and reduce hospitalization time (3)[A].

- Symptom-triggered regimen: Start with chlordiazepoxide 50 to 100 mg PO, repeat CIWA-Ar hourly and if score is ≥8, give additional dose of chlordiazepoxide 50 mg PO. Continue to reevaluate with CIWA-Ar hourly until adequate sedation achieved (score chlordiazepoxide with respective doses of diazepam, lorazepam, or oxazepam) (3)[C].

Second Line
- Thiamine: 100 mg daily IV or IM for at least 3 days (5)[C]
  – Note that IV glucose administered before treatment with thiamine may precipitate Wernicke encephalopathy and Korsakoff psychosis.
- β-Blockers (e.g., atenolol [Tenormin]) and α₂-agonists (e.g., clonidine [Catapres]) help to control hypertension and tachycardia and can be used with BZDs (3)[C]. Not used as monotherapy due to their inability to prevent DTs and seizures. May worsen underlying delirium.
- Carbamazepine: not recommended as first-line therapy; associated with reduced incidence of seizures but more studies are needed
- If the patient exhibits significant agitation and alcoholic hallucinosis, an antipsychotic (4,6)[C] (haloperidol [Haldol]) can be used, but this requires close observation, as it lowers the seizure threshold (3)[C].

- Neuroleptic agents are not recommended as monotherapy due to their association with increased mortality, longer duration of delirium, and complications when compared with sedative agents (7)[A].

ADDITIONAL THERAPIES
Peripheral neuropathy and cerebellar dysfunction merit physical therapy evaluation.

INPATIENT CONSIDERATIONS
Admission Criteria/Initial Stabilization
- CIWA-Ar score >15, or severe withdrawal
- Concurrent acute illness requiring in patient care
- Poor ability to follow up or no reliable social support
- Pregnancy
- Seizure disorder or history of severe alcohol-related seizures
- Suicide risk
- Concurrent BZD dependence
- Age >40 years old
- Prolonged heavy drinking >8 years
- Consumes >1 pint of alcohol or 12 beers per day
- Random blood alcohol level >200 mg/dL
- Elevated MCV, BUN
- Cirrhosis, liver failure

Discharge Criteria
CIWA-Ar scores of <10 on three consecutive determinations

 ONGOING CARE

FOLLOW-UP RECOMMENDATIONS
- Discharge arrangements include transfer to a treatment facility (e.g., sober house or residential program), outpatient substance abuse counseling, peer support groups (Alcoholics Anonymous), and the use of adjuvant treatment such as disulfiram (Antabuse), acamprosate (Campral), or naltrexone (ReVia, Vivitrol).
- Disulfiram: irreversibly inhibits aldehyde dehydrogenase, blocking alcohol metabolism, leading to an accumulation of acetaldehyde; therefore, it reinforces the individual's desires to stop drinking by providing a disincentive associated with increased acetaldehyde.
  – 250 to 500 mg/day PO for 1 to 2 weeks; maintenance 250 mg/day PO
  – Contraindications: concomitant use of metronidazole and ethanol-containing products, psychosis, severe myocardial disease, and coronary occlusion
- Acamprosate (666 mg PO TID): Glutamate and GABA modulator indicated to reduce cravings
  – Contraindications: renal impairment (CrCl <30 mL/min)
- Naltrexone (50 mg/day PO; 380 mg IM every 4 weeks): opiate receptor antagonist, theorized to attenuate pleasurable effects of alcohol and reduce craving. Initiate therapy after patient is opioid-free for at least 7 days.
  – Contraindications: acute hepatitis/liver failure, concomitant opioid therapy

Patient Monitoring
Frequent follow-up to monitor for relapse

PATIENT EDUCATION
- Alcoholics Anonymous: http://www.aa.org/
- SMART Recovery (Self-Management and Recovery Training): http://www.smartrecovery.org/ (not spiritually based)
- National Institute on Alcohol Abuse and Alcoholism: http://www.niaaa.nih.gov/guide/
- FamilyDoctor.Org: alcoholism (Spanish resources available)

PROGNOSIS
Mortality from severe withdrawal (DTs) is 1–5%.

COMPLICATIONS
Occurs more frequently in individuals who have prior episodes of withdrawal or concomitant illnesses.

REFERENCES
1. Moyer VA; U.S. Preventive Services Task Force. Screening and behavioral counseling interventions in primary care to reduce alcohol misuse: U.S. Preventive Services Task Force recommendation statement. *Ann Intern Med*. 2013;159(3):210–218.
2. American Psychiatric Association. *Diagnostic and Statistical Manual of Mental Disorders*. 5th ed. Arlington, VA: American Psychiatric Association; 2013.
3. Mayo-Smith MF. Pharmacological management of alcohol withdrawal. A meta-analysis and evidence-based practice guideline. American Society of Addiction Medicine Working Group on pharmacological management of alcohol withdrawal. *JAMA*. 1997;278(2): 144–151.
4. Amato L, Minozzi S, Vecchi S, et al. Benzodiazepines for alcohol withdrawal. *Cochrane Database Syst Rev*. 2010;(3):CD005063.
5. Amato L, Minozzi S, Davoli M. Efficacy and safety of pharmacological interventions for the treatment of the alcohol withdrawal syndrome. *Cochrane Database Syst Rev*. 2011;(6):CD008537.
6. Minozzi S, Amato L, Vecchi S, et al. Anticonvulsants for alcohol withdrawal. *Cochrane Database Syst Rev*. 2010;(3):CD005064.
7. Mayo-Smith MF, Beecher LH, Fischer TL, et al. Management of alcohol withdrawal delirium. An evidence-based practice guideline. *Arch Intern Med*. 2004;164(13):1405–1412.

ADDITIONAL READING
Sarff M, Gold JA. Alcohol withdrawal syndromes in the intensive care unit. *Crit Care Med*. 2010;38(9)(Suppl): S494–S501.

 SEE ALSO

Substance Use Disorders

 CODES

ICD10
- F10.239 Alcohol dependence with withdrawal, unspecified
- F10.230 Alcohol dependence with withdrawal, uncomplicated
- F10.231 Alcohol dependence with withdrawal delirium

CLINICAL PEARLS
- The kindling phenomenon has postulated that long-term exposure to alcohol affects neurons, resulting in increased alcohol craving and progressively worse withdrawal episodes (also known as allostasis).
- Any BZD dose should be patient-specific, sufficient to achieve and maintain a "light somnolence" (e.g., sleeping but easily arousable) and should be tapered off carefully even after AWS resolves to prevent BZD withdrawal.
- Administer thiamine before patient receives glucose, so as not to precipitate Wernicke encephalopathy.
- There should be frequent outpatient follow-up to monitor for relapse.
- Counsel patients taking disulfiram to avoid over-the-counter products that contain alcohol (i.e., mouthwashes).
- Avoid administering diazepam and lorazepam intramuscularly because of erratic absorption.

ALOPECIA

Amy M. Zack, MD, FAAFP

 BASICS

DESCRIPTION

- Alopecia: absence of hair from areas where it normally grows
  - Anagen phase: growing hairs, 90% scalp hair follicles at any time, lasts 2 to 6 years
  - Catagen phase: regression of follicle, <1% follicles, lasts 3 weeks
  - Telogen phase: Resting phase lasts 2 to 3 months, 50 to 150 telogen hairs shed per day.
- Classified as scarring (cicatricial), nonscarring, or structural
- Scarring (cicatricial) alopecia
  - Inflammatory disorders leading to permanent hair loss and follicle destruction
  - Includes lymphocytic, neutrophilic, and mixed subtypes
- Nonscarring alopecia
  - Lack of inflammation, no destruction of follicle
  - Includes focal, patterned, and diffuse hair loss such as androgenic alopecia, alopecia areata, telogen effluvium, anagen effluvium, syphilitic hair loss
- Structural hair disorders
  - Brittle or fragile hair from abnormal hair formation or external insult

EPIDEMIOLOGY

- Androgenic alopecia: onset in males between 20 and 25 years of age. Onset in females prior to 40 years of age, affecting as many as 70% of women >65 years of age
- Alopecia areata: onset usually prior to 30 years of age; men and women are equally affected. Well-documented genetic predisposition

Incidence

Incidence greatest in Caucasians, followed by Asians, African Americans, and Native Americans. In females, 13% premenopausal, with as many as 70% females >65 years of age

Prevalence

- Androgenic alopecia: in males, 30% Caucasian by 30 years of age, 50% by 50 years of age, and 80% by 70 years of age
- Alopecia areata: 1/1,000 with lifetime risk of 1–2%
- Scarring alopecia: rare, 3–7% of all hair disorder patients

ETIOLOGY AND PATHOPHYSIOLOGY

- Scarring (cicatricial) alopecia
  - Slick smooth scalp without follicles evident
  - Inflammatory disorders leading to permanent destruction of the follicle; it is not known what causes inflammation to develop.
  - Three major subtypes based on type of inflammation: lymphocytic, neutrophilic, and mixed.
  - Primary scarring includes discoid lupus, lichen planopilaris, dissecting cellulitis of scalp, primary fibrosing, among others.
  - Secondary scarring from infection, neoplasm, radiation, surgery, and other physical trauma, including tinea capitis
- Nonscarring alopecia
  - Focal alopecia
  - Alopecia areata
    - Patchy hair loss, usually autoimmune in etiology, T-cell–mediated inflammation resulting in premature transition to catagen then telogen phases

- May occur with hair loss in other areas of the body (alopecia totalis [entire scalp]), alopecia universalis (rapid loss of all body hair)
  - Nail disease frequently seen
  - High psychiatric comorbidity (1)
  - Alopecia syphilitica: "moth-eaten" appearance, secondary syphilis
  - Postoperative, pressure-induced alopecia: from long periods of pressure on one area of scalp
  - Temporal triangular alopecia: congenital patch of hair loss in temporal area, unilateral or bilateral
  - Traction alopecia: patchy, due to physical stressor of braids, ponytails, hair weaves
- Pattern hair loss
  - Androgenic alopecia: hair transitions from terminal to vellus hairs
  - Male pattern hair loss: androgen-mediated hair loss in specific distribution; bitemporal, vertex occurs where androgen sensitive hairs are located on scalp. This is a predominately-hereditary condition (2,3).
    - Increased androgen receptors, increased 5-alpha reductase leads to increased testosterone conversion in follicle to dihydrotestosterone (DHT). This leads to decreased follicle size and vellus hair (2,3).
    - Norwood Hamilton classification type I–VII
    - Female pattern hair loss: thinning on frontal and vertex areas (Ludwig classification, grade I–III). Females with low levels of aromatase have more testosterone available for conversion to DHT (4). This carries an unclear inheritance pattern (3).
    - Polycystic ovarian syndrome, adrenal hyperplasia, and pituitary hyperplasia all lead to androgen changes and can result in alopecia.
  - Drugs (testosterone, progesterone, danazol, adrenocorticosteroids, anabolic steroids)
- Trichotillomania: intentional pulling of hair from scalp. May present in variety of patterns
- Diffuse alopecia
  - Telogen effluvium: sudden shift of many follicles from anagen to telogen phase resulting in decreased hair density but not bald areas
    - May follow major stressors, including childbirth, injury, illness. Occurs 2 to 3 months after event.
    - Can be chronic with ongoing illness, including SLE, renal failure, IBS, HIV, thyroid disease, pituitary dysfunction.
    - Adding or changing medications (oral contraceptives, anticoagulants, anticonvulsants, SSRIs, retinoids, β-blockers, ACE inhibitors, colchicine, cholesterol-lowering medications, etc.)
    - Malnutrition from malabsorption, eating disorders; poor diet can contribute
  - Anagen effluvium
    - Interruption of the anagen phase without transition to telogen phase. Days to weeks after inciting event
    - Chemotherapy is most common trigger.
    - Radiation, poisoning, and medications can also trigger.
- Structural hair disorders
  - Multiple inherited hair disorders including Menkes disease, monilethrix, and so forth. These result in the formation of abnormal hairs that are weakened.
  - May also result from chemical or heat damaging from hair processing treatments

Genetics

- Family history of early patterned hair loss is common in androgenic alopecia, also in alopecia areata.
- Rare structural hair disorders may be inherited.

RISK FACTORS

- Genetic predisposition
- Chronic illness including autoimmune disease, infections, cancer
- Physiologic stress including pregnancy
- Poor nutrition
- Medication, chemotherapy, radiation
- Hair treatments, braids, weaves

GENERAL PREVENTION

Minimize risk factors where possible.

COMMONLY ASSOCIATED CONDITIONS

- See "Etiology and Pathophysiology."
- Vitiligo—4.1% patients with alopecia areata (AA), may be the result of similar autoimmune pathways (5).

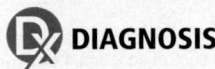 **DIAGNOSIS**

HISTORY

- Description of hair loss problem: rate of loss, duration, location, degree of hair loss, other symptoms including pruritus, infection, hair care, and treatments
- Medications
- Medical illness including chronic disease, recent illness, surgeries, pregnancy, thyroid disorder, iron deficiency, poisonings, exposures
- Psychological stress
- Dietary history and weight changes
- Family history of hair loss or autoimmune disorders

PHYSICAL EXAM

- Pattern of hair loss
  - Generalized, patterned, focal
  - Assess hair density, vellus versus terminal hairs, broken hair.
- Scalp scaling, inflammation, papules, pustules
- Presence of follicular ostia to determine class of alopecia
- Hair pull test
  - Pinch 25 to 50 hairs between thumb and forefinger and exert slow, gentle traction while sliding fingers up.
    - Normal: 1 to 2 dislodge
    - Abnormal: ≥6 hairs dislodged
    - Broken hairs (structural disorder)
    - Broken-off hair at the borders patch that are easily removable (in alopecia areata)
- Hair loss at other sites, nail disorders, skin changes
- Clinical signs of thyroid disease, lupus, or other diseases
- Clinical signs of virilization: acne, hirsutism, acanthosis nigricans, truncal obesity

DIFFERENTIAL DIAGNOSIS

Search for type of alopecia and then for reversible causes.

DIAGNOSTIC TESTS & INTERPRETATION

Initial Tests (lab, imaging)

- No testing may be indicated depending on clinical appearance.
- Nonandrogenic alopecia
  - TSH, CBC, ferritin
  - Consider: LFT, BMP, zinc, VDRL, ANA, prolactin all depending on clinical history and exam
- Androgenic alopecia: especially in females
  - Consider free testosterone and dehydroepiandrosterone sulfate

Diagnostic Procedures/Other

- Light hair-pull test: Pull on 25 to 50 hairs; ≥6 hairs dislodged is consistent with shedding (effluvium, alopecia areata).
- Direct microscopic exam of the hair shaft
  – Anagen hairs: elongated, distorted bulb with root sheath attached
  – Telogen hairs: rounded bulb, no root sheath
  – Exclamation point hairs: club-shaped root with thinner proximal shaft (alopecia areata)
  – Broken and distorted hairs may be associated with multiple hair dystrophies.
- Biopsy: most important in scarring alopecia
- Ultraviolet light fluorescence and potassium hydroxide prep (to rule out tinea capitis)

 TREATMENT

GENERAL MEASURES

- Consider potential harms and benefits to the patient prior to treatment. Many will gain an improved quality of life that is of benefit (3)[A].
- Stop any possible medication causes if possible; this will often resolve telogen effluvium (6)[C].
- Treat underlying medical causes (e.g., thyroid disorder, syphilis).
- Traction alopecia: Change hair care practices; education.
- Trichotillomania: often requires psychological intervention to induce behavior change

MEDICATION

- *Nonscarring*

Androgenic alopecia: Treatment must be continued indefinitely. Can use in combination

- Minoxidil (Rogaine): 2% topical solution (1 mL BID) for women, 5% topical solution (1 mL BID) or foam (daily) for men. Works in 60% of cases (2,4)[A]
  ○ Unclear mechanism of action; appears to prolong anagen phase (2)[A]
  ○ Adverse effects: skin irritation, hypertrichosis of face/hands, tachycardia. Category C in pregnancy (2,4)[A]
- Finasteride (Propecia): 1 mg/day for men and women (off label) (7,8)[A] 30–50% improvement in males, poor data in females (3)[A].
  ○ 5-alpha reductase inhibitor, reduces DHT in system, increases total and anagen hairs, slows transition of terminal to vellus hairs
  ○ Works best on vertex, least in anterior, temporal areas (2)[A]
  ○ Adverse effects: loss of libido, gynecomastia, depression. Caution in liver disease. Absolutely no use or contact during pregnancy, category X, reliable contraception required in female use (8)[A]
- Spironolactone (Aldactone): 100 to 200 mg/day (off-label) (4)[C]
  ○ Aldosterone antagonist, antiandrogen; blocks the effect of androgens, decreasing testosterone production
  ○ Adverse effects: dose-dependent, hyperkalemia, menstrual irregularity, fatigue; Category D in pregnancy
- Ketoconazole: decreases DHT levels at follicle, works best with minoxidil in female androgenic alopecia (8)[A]
- Combination: Finasteride + minoxidil has superior efficacy to monotherapy (3)[A].

Alopecia areata: no FDA-approved treatment; high rate of spontaneous remission in patchy AA. Treatments all focus on symptom management rather than etiology (9)[B].

- Intralesional steroids
  – Triamcinolone: 2.5 to 5 mg/mL (4)[C]
    ○ First line if <50% scalp involved
    ○ Inject 0.1 mL into deep dermal layer at 0.5 to 1 cm intervals with 1/2 in 30-gauge needle, every 4 to 6 weeks. Maximum 20 mg/session (1)[C]
    ○ Adverse effects: local burning, pruritus, skin atrophy
  – Topical steroids: very limited evidence for efficacy
  – Betamethasone: 0.1% foam shows limited hair regrowth (1)[C].
    ○ Adverse effects: folliculitis, high relapse rate after discontinuation

  – Systemic glucocorticoids: use in extensive, multifocal AA. May induce regrowth but requires long-term monthly treatment to maintain growth (1,9)[B].

    ○ Adverse effects: hyperglycemia, adrenal insufficiency, osteoporosis, cataracts, obesity
    ○ Psychiatric: SSRIs, psychiatric care, support groups

  – PUVA light therapy + prednisone: moderate effectiveness in diffuse AA (9)[B]

  – Tinea capitis: see "Tinea (Capitis, Corporis, Cruris)"

SURGERY/OTHER PROCEDURES

- Hair transplantation
- Wigs, hairpieces, extensions
- Surgical: graft transplantation, flap transplantation, or excision of the scarred area; used primarily in scarring alopecia

- Laser therapies to promote growth: lacks evidence (2)[A]

COMPLEMENTARY & ALTERNATIVE MEDICINE

- Many herbal medications are available; no clear evidence at this time.
- Volumizing shampoos can help remaining hair look fuller.

 ONGOING CARE

DIET

If nutritional deficit noted, supplementation may be necessary.

PATIENT EDUCATION

National Alopecia Areata Foundation: www.naaf.org

PROGNOSIS

- *Androgenic alopecia*: Prognosis depends on response to treatment.
- *Alopecia areata*: Often regrows within 1 year even without treatment. Recurrence common. 10% have severe, chronic form. Poor prognosis more likely with long duration, extensive hair loss, autoimmune disease, nail involvement, and young age
- *Telogen effluvium*: maximum shedding 3 months after the inciting event and recovery following correction of the cause. Usually subsides in 3 to 6 months but takes 12 to 18 months for cosmetically significant regrowth. Rarely, permanent hair loss, usually with long-term illness
- *Anagen effluvium*: Shedding begins days to a few weeks after the inciting event, with recovery following correction of the cause. Rarely, permanent hair loss
- *Traction alopecia*: Excellent prognosis with behavior modification

- *Cicatricial alopecia*: hair follicles permanently damaged; prognosis depends on type of alopecia and available treatments
- *Tinea capitis*: Excellent prognosis with treatment

REFERENCES

1. Alkhalifah A. Alopecia areata update. *Dermatol Clin*. 2013;31(1):93–108.
2. Banka N, Bunagan MJ, Shapiro J. Pattern hair loss in men: diagnosis and medical treatment. *Dermatol Clin*. 2013;31(1):129–140.
3. Blumeyer A, Tosti A, Messenger A, et al. Evidence-based (S3) guideline for the treatment of androgenetic alopecia in women and in men. *J Dtsch Dermatol Ges*. 2011;9(Suppl 6):S1–S57.
4. Rathnayake D, Sinclair R. Innovative use of spironolactone as an antiandrogen in the treatment of female pattern hair loss. *Dermatol Clin*. 2010;28(3):611–618.
5. Kumar S, Mittal J, Mahajan B. Colocalization of vitiligo and alopecia areata: coincidence or consequence? *Int J Trichology*. 2013;5(1):50–52.
6. Harrison S, Bergfeld W. Diffuse hair loss: its triggers and management. *Cleve Clin J Med*. 2009;76(6):361–367.
7. BMJ Best Practice. Epidemiology. http://bestpractice.bmj.com/best-practice/monograph/223/basics/epidemiology.html. Accessed 2013.
8. Atanaskova Mesinkovska N, Bergfeld WF. Hair: what is new in diagnosis and management? Female pattern hair loss update: diagnosis and treatment. *Dermatol Clin*. 2013;31(1):119–127.
9. Brzezińska-Wcisło L, Bergler-Czop B, Wcisło-Dziadecka D, et al. New aspects of the treatment of alopecia areata. *Postepy Dermatol Alergol*. 2014;31(4):262–265.

ADDITIONAL READING

Otberg N. Primary cicatricial alopecias. *Dermatol Clin*. 2013;31(1):155–166.

 SEE ALSO

- Tinea (Capitis, Corporis, Cruris); Syphilis; Lupus Erythematosus, Systemic (SLE); Polycystic Ovarian Syndrome (PCOS); Lichen Planus; Hyperthyroidism
- Algorithm: Alopecia

 CODES

ICD10

- L65.9 Nonscarring hair loss, unspecified
- L64.9 Androgenic alopecia, unspecified
- L63.9 Alopecia areata, unspecified

CLINICAL PEARLS

- History and physical are necessary in determining type of alopecia for appropriate treatment.
- Treatment of underlying medical condition or removal of triggering medication will often resolve hair loss.
- Educating the patient about the nature of the condition and expectations is key to care.
- Alopecia can affect the psychological condition of the patient, and it may be necessary to address this in any type of hair loss.

ALZHEIMER DISEASE

Jill Ann Grimes, MD

 BASICS

DESCRIPTION
- Alzheimer disease (AD) is the most common cause of dementia in the elderly.
- Degenerative neurologic disease with progressive impairment in ≥2:
  - Memory, executive function, attention, language, or visuospatial skills
  - With significant interference in ability to function in work, home, or social interactions
- *New diagnostic criteria* released in 2011 emphasize full spectrum of disease (1)[A]:
  - Preclinical AD (*research purposes only*: biomarkers present; subtle decline evident to patient but cognitive tests in "normal" range)
  - Mild cognitive impairment (MCI): Social, occupational, and functional skills are preserved despite significant decline in cognition.
  - Alzheimer dementia
- System(s) affected: nervous
- Synonym(s): presenile dementia; senile dementia of the Alzheimer type

Geriatric Considerations
Asymptomatic screening is not recommended.

EPIDEMIOLOGY
- Predominant age: >65 years
- 2/3 females, 1/3 males in United States

Incidence
1 in 8 Americans age >65 years (13%); nearly 50% once >85

Prevalence
>5.2 million in United States
- 200,000 younger onset (<65 years)

ETIOLOGY AND PATHOPHYSIOLOGY
- Unknown but involves amyloid beta accumulation initially, then synaptic dysfunction, neurodegeneration, and eventual neuronal loss
- Age, genetics, systemic disease, behaviors (smoking), and other host factors may influence the response to amyloid beta and/or the pace of progression toward the clinical manifestations of AD.

Genetics
- Positive family history in 50%, but 90% of AD is sporadic:
  - APOE4 increases risk but full unclear
- Familial/autosomal dominant AD accounts for <5% AD:
  - Amyloid precursor protein (APP), presenilin-1 (PS-1), and presenilin-2 (PS-2)

RISK FACTORS
- Aging, family history, APOE4, Down syndrome
- Cardiovascular and carotid artery disease
- Smoking (2- to 4-fold increase)
- Head trauma

GENERAL PREVENTION
- NSAIDs, estrogen, and vitamin E do NOT delay AD; insufficient evidence for statins (2)[A].
- Intellectual challenge (puzzles) and regular physical exercise may offer preventive benefit.
- Control vascular risk factors (e.g., hypertension); lowering cholesterol may retard pathogenesis of AD.

- Ginkgo biloba may be beneficial for cognition but not activities of daily living.
- Physical activities and omega-3 fatty acids may help to prevent or delay cognitive decline.
- Ultrasound (US) may help to identify asymptomatic patients at increased risk with chronic brain hypoperfusion secondary to cardiovascular or carotid artery pathology.

COMMONLY ASSOCIATED CONDITIONS
- Down syndrome
- Depression

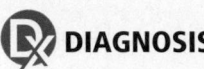 **DIAGNOSIS**

Degenerative neurologic disease with *progressive impairment in ≥2 areas*:
- Memory, executive function, attention, language, or visuospatial skills AND
- Significant interference in ability to function in work, home, or social interactions

HISTORY
- Include family members in interview (for accuracy and for behavioral assessment).
- Progressive and disruptive memory loss
- Depression, anhedonia, or apathy
- Intellectual decline, difficulty with calculations, multiple missed appointments
- Loss of interest, social withdrawal
- Date or time confusion
- Occupational dysfunction or personality change
- Restlessness and sleep disturbances

PHYSICAL EXAM
- Neurologic exam to rule out other causes
- Folstein Mini-Mental State Exam (MMSE): copyrighted but available (http://www.aafp.org/afp/20010215/703.html)
- Counting coins test: "If I gave you a nickel, quarter, dime, and penny, how much is that?"
- No focal neurologic signs
- Short-term memory loss
- Acalculia (e.g., cannot balance checkbook)
- Agnosia: inability to recognize objects
- Apraxia: inability to carry out movements
- Confabulation
- Delusions
- Impaired abstraction
- Decreased attention to hygiene
- Visuospatial distortion
- Late signs: psychotic features, mutism

DIFFERENTIAL DIAGNOSIS
- Depression
- Vascular dementia, multi-infarct dementia
- Lewy body disease
- Dementia associated with Parkinson disease
- Normal pressure hydrocephalus
- Creutzfeldt-Jakob disease
- End-stage multiple sclerosis
- Brain tumor: primary or metastatic
- Subdural hematoma
- Progressive multifocal leukoencephalopathy
- Metabolic dementia (hypothyroidism)
- Drug reactions, alcoholism, other addictions
- Dementia pugilistica

- Toxicity from liver and kidney failure
- Vitamin and other nutritional deficiencies
- Vasculitis
- Neurosyphilis

DIAGNOSTIC TESTS & INTERPRETATION
Neuropsychological testing: Order if clinical picture is confusing or to help determine level of independence for skills such as balancing checkbooks, driving, or managing medicines.

Initial Tests (lab, imaging)
- To help rule out other causes of dementia
  - CBC, ESR
  - Chemistry panel
  - Thyroid-stimulating hormone
  - Folate and B_{12} levels
  - Venereal disease reaction level (VDRL) or rapid plasma reagin (RPR)
  - HIV antibody (selected cases)
  - APOE4 or biomarker testing *is not routine*.
- **Imaging**: Controversy exists; may identify moderate cortical atrophy or ventricular enlargement.
  - Consider MRI or CT scan if
    ○ Cognitive decline is recent and rapid; age <60 years; history of stroke; gait disturbance or focal neurologic signs
    ○ Cancer, urinary incontinence, bleeding disorder, or current use of anticoagulants
  - Single-photon emission computed tomography (SPECT) and positron emission tomography (PET): only if diagnostic uncertainty after CT or MRI; *insufficient evidence to use alone*
  - Medicare pays for PET to distinguish AD from frontotemporal dementia under specific requirements; *this should not be routine*.

Follow-Up Tests & Special Considerations
Genetic testing for APOE4 or for familial AD types; discuss with genetic counselor

Test Interpretation
- Gross: diffuse cerebral atrophy in hippocampus, amygdala, and some subcortical nuclei
- Microscopic
  - Neuritic senile plaques
  - Neurofibrillary tangles
  - Pyramidal cell loss
  - Decreased cholinergic innervation (other neurotransmitters variably decreased)
  - Degeneration of locus ceruleus and basal forebrain nuclei of Meynert; amyloid angiopathy

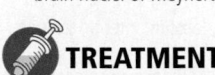 **TREATMENT**

GENERAL MEASURES
- Optimize treatment of associated comorbid conditions (including hearing and vision loss).
- Analyze environment for safety and security, and avoid sudden changes in environment.
- Assess spouse/caregiver burnout.
- Advance directives, living will, power of attorney

MEDICATION
First Line

2014 meta-analysis shows cholinesterase inhibitors (ChEIs) and memantine are "able to stabilize or slow decline in cognition, function, behavior, and global change" (3)[A].

- Debate continues regarding the clinical significance and cost-effectiveness of AD medication.

- ChEIs
  - Equally effective; all have potential for GI side effects; monitor for bradycardia/syncope; associated with abnormal dreams
  - When used for at least 6 months, provide mild benefit in cognition, ADL, and behavior. (No deterioration for 6 months is evidence of efficacy.)
  - Shown to reduce nursing home placement by 20% after 25 months of treatment
  - Best in mild to moderate disease (MMSE 10 to 24); *may* be effective in Lewy body dementia
  - Donepezil (Aricept): start at 5 mg/day PO; may increase to 10 mg/day after 1 month
  - Tablets disintegrating tablets; generic available
  - Caution with digoxin or beta-blockers (can cause 3rd-degree heart block)
  - Aricept 23-mg tablet approved in 2010
  - Rivastigmine (Exelon): start at 1.5 mg PO BID, increase by 1.5 mg BID every 2 weeks; maintenance 6 to 12 mg/day total
  - Capsule, solution, or patch (patch greatly reduces side effects)
  - Indicated for both AD and Parkinson dementia
  - Galantamine (Razadyne): start at 4 mg BID for 4 weeks, then increase by 4 mg BID every month with goal of 16 to 24 mg/day dose
  - Tablets, solution, extended-release (ER) capsule, and transdermal formulations (ER and transdermal have daily dosing)
- *N*-methyl-D-aspartate (NMDA) receptor antagonists (for moderate to severe AD; MMSE 5 to 14)
  - Monotherapy or in combination with acetylcholinesterase inhibitors
  - Memantine (Namenda): start 5 mg/day, with titrate to target dose of 10 mg BID after 4 weeks
  - Often improves behavioral issues
  - Beneficial for cognition and physician's global impression; increases risk of somnolence, weight gain, confusion, hypertension, nervous system disorders, and falling (4)[A]
- For depression (occurs in 1/3 of patients), SSRIs preferred first line.
- Insomnia
  - Trazodone 25 to 100 mg at bedtime, zolpidem (Ambien) 5 mg at bedtime, zaleplon (Sonata) 5 to 10 mg at bedtime, ramelteon (Rozerem) 8 mg at bedtime
  - Avoid diphenhydramine in elderly due to negative cognitive effects and risk of urinary retention (males).
- Moderate anxiety/restlessness: Consider low-dose, short-acting benzodiazepines, buspirone, or SSRIs (efficacy unproven).
- Severe aggressive agitation
  - Behavioral techniques and environmental modification help more than medications for wandering, restlessness, uncooperativeness, hoarding, and irritability:
    - Consider changing environment, rewards, behavioral redirection, hearing aids, and bright light therapy.
  - Memantine (Namenda): start at 5 mg/day, with starter pack titrating to target dose of 10 mg BID after 4 weeks
  - Antipsychotics (both conventional and atypical) are associated with increased mortality and acute care hospital admissions in elderly patients with dementia.
  - Antiepileptic agents (carbamazepine valproate, lamotrigine) have been used for their mood stabilizing properties.

- Precautions
  - Avoid anticholinergic drugs, such as tricyclic antidepressants and antihistamines.
  - Ginkgo biloba: Avoid anticoagulants and aspirin.
  - Benzodiazepines may produce paradoxical excitation or daytime drowsiness.
  - Triazolam (Halcion) can produce confusion, memory loss, and psychotic behavior.
  - Benzodiazepines may increase serum phenytoin concentration.
  - Cimetidine may increase benzodiazepine concentration.
  - Donepezil (Aricept): use with caution with anticholinergic medication, in sick sinus syndrome, or history of peptic ulcers
  - Paroxetine increases donepezil levels.

Second Line
Vitamin E, statins, estrogen, and NSAIDs should not be routinely recommended due to lack of evidence and safety concerns (1,2)[A].

ISSUES FOR REFERRAL
- Assess driving safety (vision, spatial relations, hearing, judgment):
  - http://www.nhtsa.gov/people/injury/olddrive/Driving%20Safely%20Aging%20Web/
- Support groups for patient and family: Alzheimer Association: http://www.alz.org/

ADDITIONAL THERAPIES
- Exercise to reduce restlessness
- Cognitive challenge; traditional and computerized training both effective
- Occupational, music, aroma, and pet therapy

COMPLEMENTARY & ALTERNATIVE MEDICINE
- Huperzine A 400 mg (herbal ChEIs) may improve cognition with minimal side effects (5)[A].
- Ginkgo biloba extracts (120 mg/day) show conflicting efficacy in treatment of AD but may be beneficial.
- Coenzyme Q10 is not effective.
- Acupuncture continues to be assessed and may enhance effectiveness of drugs in treating Alzheimer disease.

ONGOING CARE

FOLLOW-UP RECOMMENDATIONS
Patient Monitoring
- Schedule regular follow-up (3 months) to assess medical complications, provide support for family, and assess need for placement.
- Serial mental status testing is potentially helpful, but bedside tests (Folstein MMSE) offer wide variability and lack of sensitivity.

PATIENT EDUCATION
- Alzheimer Association: http://www.alz.org/
- Explain progressive nature of the disease and start advance directives planning as early as possible.

PROGNOSIS
Poor: Average survival from diagnosis is 4 to 8 years (diagnosis is often delayed).

COMPLICATIONS
- Behavioral: hostility, agitation, wandering, falls
- Metabolic: infection, dehydration, drug toxicity
- "Sundowning" (increase full-spectrum lights), depression (1/3 of patients), suicide

REFERENCES
1. McKhann GM, Knopman DS, Chertkow H, et al. The diagnosis of dementia due to Alzheimer's disease: recommendations from the National Institute on Aging-Alzheimer's Association workgroups on diagnostic guidelines for Alzheimer's disease. *Alzheimers Dement.* 2011;7(3):263–269.
2. McGuinness B, Craig D, Bullock R, et al. Statins for the treatment of dementia. *Cochrane Database Syst Rev.* 2014;8(7):CD007514.
3. Tan CC, Yu JT, Wang HF, et al. Efficacy and safety of donepezil, galantamine, rivastigmine, and memantine for the treatment of Alzheimer's disease: a systematic review and meta-analysis. *J Alzheimers Dis.* 2014;41(2):615–631.
4. Yang Z, Zhou X, Zhang Q. Effectiveness and safety of memantine treatment for Alzheimer's disease. *J Alzheimers Dis.* 2013;36(3):445–458.
5. Xing SH, Zhu CX, Zhang R, et al. Huperzine A in the treatment of Alzheimer's disease and vascular dementia: a meta-analysis. *Evid Based Complement Alternat Med.* 2014;2014:363985.

ADDITIONAL READING
- Birks JS, Grimley Evans J. Rivastigmine for Alzheimer's disease. *Cochrane Database Syst Rev.* 2015;(4):CD001191.
- Buckley JS, Salpeter SR. A risk-benefit assessment of dementia medications: systematic review of the evidence. *Drugs Aging.* 2015;32(6):453–467.
- Ehret MJ, Chamberlin KW. Current practices in the treatment of Alzheimer disease: where is the evidence after the phase III trials? *Clin Ther.* 2015;37(8):1604–1616.
- Zhou J, Peng W, Xu M, et al. The effectiveness and safety of acupuncture for patients with Alzheimer disease: a systematic review and meta-analysis of randomized controlled trials. *Medicine (Baltimore).* 2015;94(22):e933.

 ## SEE ALSO

Substance Use Disorders; Hypothyroidism, Adult; Depression

CODES

ICD10
- G30.9 Alzheimer's disease, unspecified
- G30.0 Alzheimer's disease with early onset
- G30.1 Alzheimer's disease with late onset

CLINICAL PEARLS
- Daily intellectual stimulation, such as puzzles, and moderate physical exercise may help prevent AD.
- Imaging studies have low yield in patients with a history typical of AD.
- Encourage families to join a chapter of the Alzheimer Association and to pursue advanced directive planning early in the course of the disease.
- Atypical antipsychotic medications increase mortality.

AMENORRHEA

Heidi L. Gaddey, MD • Stephanie W. Reiser, DO

BASICS

DESCRIPTION
- Primary amenorrhea
- Gonadal abnormalities
  – No menses by age 13 to 14 years with absence of secondary sexual characteristics OR
  – No menses by age 15 to 16 years with normal secondary characteristics
- Secondary amenorrhea: absence of menses for 3 months in a woman with previously normal menstruation or 6 months in a woman with a history of irregular cycles
- System(s) affected: endocrine/metabolic; reproductive

Pregnancy Considerations
Pregnancy is by far the most common cause of secondary amenorrhea.

EPIDEMIOLOGY
Prevalence
- Primary amenorrhea: <1% of female population
- Secondary amenorrhea: 3–5% of female population
- No evidence for race and ethnicity affecting prevalence

ETIOLOGY AND PATHOPHYSIOLOGY
- Primary amenorrhea
  – Hypothalamic–pituitary abnormalities
  – Constitutional delay of puberty
    ○ Eating disorder
    ○ Stress/exercise
    ○ Central lesions (tumors, hypophysitis, granulomas)
    ○ Pituitary dysfunction (hyperprolactinemia, abnormal secretion of follicle-stimulating hormone [FSH], luteinizing hormone [LH], or GnRH)
    ○ Thyroid dysfunction
  – Gonadal abnormalities
    ○ Chromosomal abnormalities (androgen insensitivity syndrome)
    ○ Euchromosomal gonadal agenesis or dysgenesis (Turner syndrome, Swyer syndrome, and pure gonadal dysgenesis)
    ○ Polycystic ovarian syndrome (PCOS)
    ○ Abnormal gonadotropin function
    ○ Autoimmune gonadal failure
    ○ Idiopathic gonadal failure
  – Anatomic abnormalities
    ○ Imperforate hymen
    ○ Transverse vaginal septum
    ○ Congenital absence of the cervix
    ○ Müllerian agenesis
- Secondary amenorrhea
  – Pregnancy
  – Thyroid disease
  – Functional hypothalamic amenorrhea (stress, weight loss, and/or excessive exercise)
  – Hyperprolactinemia (altered metabolism, ectopic production, breastfeeding/stimulation, hypothyroidism, medications, empty sella syndrome, pituitary adenoma)
  – If pregnancy, thyroid disease, and hyperprolactinemia are ruled out, consider the following:
    ○ Normogonadotropic amenorrhea: hyperandrogenic anovulation (acromegaly, androgen-secreting tumors, Cushing disease, exogenous androgens, nonclassical congenital adrenal hyperplasia, PCOS); outflow tract obstruction (Asherman syndrome, cervical stenosis, fibroids, polyps)

○ Hypergonadotropic hypogonadism: normal menopause; premature ovarian failure (autoimmune, chemotherapy, galactosemia, fragile X premutation and other genetic causes, 17-hydroxylase deficiency, idiopathic, mumps oophoritis, pelvic radiation)
○ Hypogonadotropic hypogonadism: eating disorders, CNS tumors, chronic illness, cranial radiation, excessive weight loss/exercise/malnutrition, hypothalamic or pituitary destruction, Sheehan syndrome
- Pathophysiology varies, depending on etiology.
- Primary amenorrhea should be evaluated in the context of presence or absence of secondary sexual characteristics.
- Can result from dysfunction in hypothalamic–pituitary–gonadal axis, anatomic abnormalities, or another endocrine gland disorder

Genetics
May occur with Turner syndrome or testicular feminization

RISK FACTORS
- Obesity
- Overtraining (prolonged, excessive exercise)
- Eating disorders
- Malnutrition
- Anovulatory disorders
- Psychosocial crisis
- Treatment with antipsychotic medications

GENERAL PREVENTION
Maintenance of proper body mass index (BMI) and healthy lifestyle with respect to food and exercise

COMMONLY ASSOCIATED CONDITIONS
- Premature ovarian failure may be associated with autoimmune abnormalities (autoimmune thyroiditis, type 1 diabetes).
- PCOS is associated with insulin resistance and obesity.
- Decreased exposure to estrogen may increase risk for osteopenia or osteoporosis.

DIAGNOSIS

HISTORY
- Review of systems including weight change, symptoms of pregnancy or menopause, virilizing changes, cyclic pelvic pain, galactorrhea, headaches, vision changes, fatigue, palpitations, polyuria/polydipsia
- Growth and pubertal development history, including age of breast development, pubertal growth spurt, and adrenarche
- History of chronic illness, trauma, surgery, medications, prior chemotherapy or radiation
- Psychiatric history
- Social history, including diet and exercise history, drug abuse, and sexual history
- Family history of delayed or absent puberty

PHYSICAL EXAM
- General appearance
- Vital signs, height, weight, growth percentile and BMI, hypotension, bradycardia, hypothermia (anorexia nervosa)
- HEENT exam: evidence of dental erosions, trauma to palate (bulimia), visual field defect, funduscopic changes, cranial nerve findings (prolactinoma), webbed neck (Turner syndrome), thyromegaly

- Skin exam: evidence of androgen excess (acne, hirsutism), acanthosis nigricans (PCOS), fine downy hair on body (anorexia nervosa), striae
- Breast: state of development, evidence of galactorrhea (prolactinoma), shield chest (Turner syndrome)
- Pelvic exam: presence or absence of pubic hair (if sparse: androgen insensitivity or deficiency); clitoromegaly (androgen excess); distention or bulging of external vagina (imperforate hymen); thin, pale vaginal mucosa without rugae (estrogen deficiency and ovarian failure); presence of cervical mucus (evidence for estrogen production); blind vaginal pouch (müllerian agenesis, androgen insensitivity syndrome); ovarian enlargement (tumors, PCOS, autoimmune oophoritis)

DIAGNOSTIC TESTS & INTERPRETATION
Initial Tests (lab, imaging)
- Primary amenorrhea
  – Serum prolactin (PRL) and thyroid-stimulating hormone (TSH)
  – If no secondary sexual characteristics, measure serum FSH and LH.
    ○ FSH/LH <5 IU/L suggests primary hypothalamic or pituitary etiology.
    ○ FSH >20 and LH >40 IU/L suggests gonadal failure, and karyotype analysis should be performed.
  – If secondary sexual characteristics are present, evaluate for anatomic abnormalities. If uterus is absent or abnormal, perform karyotype analysis, testosterone level, and dehydroepiandrosterone sulfate (DHEA-S).
- Secondary amenorrhea
  – Exclude pregnancy with hCG.
  – Serum TSH: Elevated in hypothyroidism, decreased in hyperthyroidism
  – Consider (low yield): serum chemistry, CBC, urinalysis to rule out underlying disease
  – PRL:
    ○ >100 ng/mL suggests empty sella syndrome or pituitary adenoma; perform MRI for evaluation.
    ○ <100 ng/mL: Evaluate for other etiologies, of which medications are most common.
- If PRL and TSH are normal, perform progestin challenge (see "Treatment").
  – If withdrawal bleed: normogonadotropic amenorrhea related to hyperandrogenic chronic anovulation, most commonly PCOS
  – If no withdrawal bleed: Follow up with estradiol priming (see "Diagnostic Procedures/Other" and "Treatment") and repeat progestin challenge:
    ○ If no bleed: Consider outflow tract obstruction.
    ○ If bleed occurs: Check FSH/LH: elevated in hypergonadotropic hypogonadism, decreased in pituitary tumors or hypogonadotropic hypogonadism
- If virilizing signs and significant acne are present, measure free testosterone, DHEA-S, and 17-OH progesterone levels. Initiate evaluation for androgen-secreting tumor if testosterone >200 ng/dL.
- Imaging is not generally indicated as a first approach.
- US may show ovarian cysts (PCOS), presence or absence of uterus, and endometrial thickness.
- An MRI of the pelvis can clarify any uterine or vaginal anomalies suggested by US or if pediatric patient is unable to tolerate transvaginal US probe.
- An MRI of the sella turcica if prolactinoma suspected (elevated PRL >100), and consider with functional hypothalamic amenorrhea (other adenomas)

Follow-Up Tests & Special Considerations

- Women <30 years with ovarian failure (see below) should have karyotype analysis and be investigated for premutations of FMR1 gene (fragile X syndrome) and for adrenal antibodies.
- If absence of uterus or foreshortened vagina, karyotype analysis should also be performed.
- Laparoscopy: diagnosis of streak ovaries (Turner syndrome) or polycystic ovaries
- Hysterosalpingogram: Rule out Asherman syndrome and other etiologies of outflow obstruction.

Diagnostic Procedures/Other

- If constitutional delay is suspected, obtain bone age.
- If hypothalamic amenorrhea from functional suppression is suspected, consider dual-energy x-ray absorptiometry (DEXA) scan to assess bone loss (1).

 TREATMENT

GENERAL MEASURES
Treatment depends on the underlying cause.

MEDICATION

- Progesterone challenge and replacement: medroxyprogesterone (Provera): 10 mg/day for 10 days will result in withdrawal bleed if hypothalamic–pituitary–gonadal axis is intact although experts disagree (2).
- Estrogen replacement: Cycling with a combination oral contraceptive (containing 35 or 50 μg of estrogen) or conjugated estrogen (Premarin) 0.625 mg for 25 days with progesterone added as above for the last 10 days will result in a withdrawal bleed if the uterus and lower genital tract are normal.
- Use of hormonal therapies will not correct the underlying problem. Other drugs might be required to treat specific conditions (e.g., bromocriptine for hyperprolactinemia).
- Use of hormonal replacement therapy is not recommended for long-term management of amenorrhea in older women.
  - May be safe for symptom management in young women
  - Give to maintain secondary sex characteristics and to prevent osteoporosis in adolescents and young women (3)[A].
- Combination estrogen/progesterone contraceptives (oral contraceptive pills [OCPs], patch, ring) replace estrogen and prevent pregnancy.
  - Have a positive effect on bone mineral density in oligo-/amenorrheic women but not in functional hypothalamic amenorrhea (4)[A]
  - Can decrease hirsutism in PCOS
- Calcium supplementation: 1,500 mg/day if cause is hypoestrogenism
- Because PCOS is related to insulin resistance, metformin (Glucophage) has been used (start at 500 mg BID) to correct metabolic abnormalities, improve ovulation, and restore normal menstrual patterns. Of note, treatment with metformin has shown an increase in clinical pregnancy rates but not in live birth rates (5)[A].
- Functional hypothalamic amenorrhea appears to improve with administration of exogenous leptin (still under investigation) (6)[C].

- Contraindications to estrogen administration
  - Pregnancy, thromboembolic disease, previous myocardial infarct or cerebrovascular accident, estrogen-dependent malignancy, severe hepatic impairment or disease
- Precautions
  - Patients with amenorrhea who desire pregnancy should not be given hormone replacement therapy but should receive treatment for infertility based on the specific cause.

ISSUES FOR REFERRAL
Many causes of amenorrhea require referral to specialists in ob/gyn, endocrine, surgery, and/or psychiatry.

SURGERY/OTHER PROCEDURES

- Hymenectomy for primary amenorrhea if due to imperforate hymen
- Lysis of adhesions in Asherman syndrome is often effective in restoring regular menses and fertility.
- If karyotype is XY, gonads must be removed due to increased risk of tumors.
- Patients with congenital short vagina can undergo surgery to create a functioning vagina.

 ONGOING CARE

FOLLOW-UP RECOMMENDATIONS
If overtraining is suspected, activity level should be reduced by 25–50%.

Patient Monitoring

- Depends on the cause and treatment chosen
- If hormonal replacement is used, discontinue after 6 months to assess spontaneous resumption of menses.

DIET

- Correct overweight or underweight by dietary management and behavior modification.
- If PCOS is the etiology, a weight-loss diet will help restore ovulation.

PATIENT EDUCATION

- Educate on the circumstances and complications of her condition and its underlying etiology.
- Specific educational resources are helpful (e.g., prenatal classes and menopause support groups).
- Discuss the expected duration of amenorrhea (temporary or permanent), effect on fertility, and the long-term sequelae of untreated amenorrhea (e.g., osteoporosis, vaginal dryness).
- Appropriate contraceptive advice should be given because fertility returns before menses.
- Additional support may be needed if the amenorrhea is associated with a reduction in, or loss of, fertility.

PROGNOSIS
Reflects the underlying cause. In functional hypothalamic amenorrhea, one study demonstrated 83% reversal rate in presence of obvious contributing factor.

COMPLICATIONS

- Estrogen-deficiency symptoms (e.g., hot flashes, vaginal dryness) and osteoporosis in prolonged hypoestrogenic amenorrhea
- Increased risk of endometrial cancer in patients whose amenorrhea is secondary to anovulation with estrogen excess (obesity, PCOS)
- Premature ovarian failure may increase cardiovascular risk.

REFERENCES

1. Gordon CM. Clinical practice. Functional hypothalamic amenorrhea. N Engl J Med. 2010;363(4):365–371.
2. Klein DA, Poth MA. Amenorrhea: an approach to diagnosis and management. Am Fam Physician. 2013;87(11):781–788.
3. Marjoribanks J, Farquhar C, Roberts H, et al. Long term hormone therapy for perimenopausal and postmenopausal women. Cochrane Database Syst Rev. 2012;(7):CD004143.
4. Liu SL, Lebrun CM. Effect of oral contraceptives and hormone replacement therapy on bone mineral density in premenopausal and perimenopausal women: a systematic review. Br J Sports Med. 2006;40(1):11–24.
5. Tang T, Lord JM, Norman RJ, et al. Insulin-sensitising drugs (metformin, rosiglitazone, pioglitazone, D-chiro-inositol) for women with polycystic ovary syndrome, oligo amenorrhoea and subfertility. Cochrane Database Syst Rev. 2012;(5):CD003053.
6. Chou SH, Chamberland JP, Liu X, et al. Leptin is an effective treatment for hypothalamic amenorrhea. Proc Natl Acad Sci U S A. 2011;108(16):6585–6590.

ADDITIONAL READING

- Practice Committee of American Society for Reproductive Medicine. Current evaluation of amenorrhea. Fertil Steril. 2008;90(Suppl 5):S219–S225.
- Santoro N. Update in hyper- and hypogonadotropic amenorrhea. J Clin Endocrinol Metab. 2011;96(11):3281–3288.

 SEE ALSO

- Osteoporosis; Hyperthyroidism; Hypothyroidism
- Algorithms: Amenorrhea, Primary; Amenorrhea, Secondary; Delayed Puberty

 CODES

ICD10

- N91.2 Amenorrhea, unspecified
- N91.0 Primary amenorrhea
- N91.1 Secondary amenorrhea

CLINICAL PEARLS

- First evaluate whether amenorrhea is primary or secondary and exclude pregnancy. TSH and PRL are usual first blood tests.
- Progestin challenge may cause withdrawal bleed in women with intact hypothalamic–pituitary–gonadal axis.

ANAL FISSURE

Anne Walsh, MMSc, PA-C, DFAAPA • Kashyap Trivedi, MD

 BASICS

DESCRIPTION
Anal fissure (fissure in ano): longitudinal tear in the lining of the anal canal distal to the dentate line, most commonly at the posterior midline; characterized by a knifelike tearing sensation on defecation, often associated with bright red blood per rectum. This very common benign anorectal condition is often confused with hemorrhoids. May be acute (<6 weeks) or chronic (>6 weeks) in duration

EPIDEMIOLOGY
- Affects all ages. Common in infants 6 to 24 months; not common in older children, suspect abuse, or trauma. Elderly is less common due to lower resting pressure in the anal canal.
- Sex: male = female; women are more likely to get anterior midline tears (25% vs. 8%).

Incidence
Exact incidence is unknown. Patients often treat with home remedies and do not seek medical care.

Prevalence
- 80% of infants, usually self-limited
- 20% of adults, most of whom do not seek medical advice

ALERT
- Lateral fissure: Rule out infectious disease.
- Atypical fissure: Rule out Crohn disease.

ETIOLOGY AND PATHOPHYSIOLOGY
High-resting pressure within the anal canal (usually as a result of constipation/straining) leads to ischemia of the anoderm, resulting in splitting of the anal mucosa during defecation and spasm of the exposed internal sphincter.

Genetics
None known

RISK FACTORS
- Constipation (25% of patients)
- Diarrhea (6% of patients)
- Passage of hard or large-caliber stool
- High-resting of internal anal sphincter (prolonged sitting, obesity)
- Trauma (sexual abuse, childbirth, mountain biking)
- Inflammatory bowel disease (Crohn disease)
- Infection (chlamydia, syphilis, herpes, tuberculosis)

GENERAL PREVENTION
All measures to prevent constipation; avoid straining and prolonged sitting on toilet.

COMMONLY ASSOCIATED CONDITIONS
Constipation, irritable bowel syndrome, Crohn disease, tuberculosis, leukemia, and HIV

 DIAGNOSIS

HISTORY
- Severe, sharp rectal pain, often with and following defecation but can be continuous; some patients will see bright red blood on the stool or when wiping.
- Occasionally, anal pruritus or perianal irritation

PHYSICAL EXAM
- Gentle spreading of the buttocks with close inspection of the anal verge will reveal a smooth-edged tear in the anodermal tissue, typically posterior midline, occasionally anterior midline, rarely eccentric to midline.
- Minimal edema, erythema, or bleeding may be seen.
- Chronic fissures may demonstrate rolled edges, hypertrophic papillae at proximal end, and a sentinel pile (tag) at distal end.

DIFFERENTIAL DIAGNOSIS
- Thrombosed external hemorrhoid: swollen, painful mass at anal verge
- Perirectal abscess: tender, warm erythematous induration or fluctuance
- Perianal fistula: abnormal communication between rectum and perianal epithelium with purulent drainage
- Pruritus ani: shallow excoriations rather than true fissure

DIAGNOSTIC TESTS & INTERPRETATION
Diagnostic Procedures/Other
- Avoid anoscopy/sigmoidoscopy initially unless necessary for other diagnoses.
- Rarely, due to pain, some patients may require exam under anesthesia in order to confirm the diagnosis.

 TREATMENT

The goal of treatment is to avoid repeated tearing of the anal mucosa with resultant spasm of the internal anal sphincter by decreasing the patient's high sphincter tone and addressing its underlying cause.

GENERAL MEASURES
- Wash area gently with warm water; consume high-fiber diet, increase fluids, add daily fiber supplement; avoid constipation, maintain healthy weight.
- Medical therapy for chronic fissures usually initiated in a stepwise manner: nitrates, calcium channel blockers, botulinum toxin (1)[B]

MEDICATION
First Line
Acute fissures—50% heal spontaneously with supportive measures:
- Stool softeners (docusate) daily
- Osmotic laxatives if needed (polyethylene glycol)
- Fiber supplements (e.g., psyllium, methylcellulose, inulin) and increased fluid intake
- Topical analgesics (2% lidocaine gel)
- Topical lubricants/emollients (Balneol cream)
- Sitz baths (sit in hot water bath for 10 to 20 minutes 2 to 3 times daily)

Second Line
Chronic fissures—require medical therapy (1,2)[A]:
- Chemical sphincterotomy
  - Topical nitroglycerin ointment 2% diluted to 0.2–0.4% applied QID; nitroglycerin 0.4% ointment available commercially (Rectiv): marginally but significantly better than placebo in healing (48.6% vs. 37%); late recurrence common (50%) (1)[A]; effect is to reduce resting anal pressure through the release of nitric oxide. Headache is a major side effect (20–30%).
  - Calcium channel blockers (e.g., nifedipine, diltiazem), oral or topical: no better than nitrates but with fewer side effects; effect is to relax the internal sphincter muscle, thereby reducing the resting anal pressure (3)[A].
  - Botulinum toxin 4 mL (20 units) injected into the internal sphincter muscle: no better than topical nitrates but with fewer side effects; effect is to inhibit the release of acetylcholine from nerve endings to inhibit muscle spasm (4)[B].

ISSUES FOR REFERRAL
- Late recurrence is common (50%) particularly if the underlying issue remains untreated (constipation, irritable bowel, etc.).
- Medical therapy usually is tried for 90 to 120 days prior to colorectal surgery referral.

ADDITIONAL THERAPIES
Anococcygeal support (modified toilet seat) may offer some advantage in chronic fissures to avoid surgery.

SURGERY/OTHER PROCEDURES
- Surgery reserved for failure of medical therapy; involves division of the internal sphincter muscle
- Lateral internal sphincterectomy is the surgical procedure of choice (90% healing) (5)[A].
  - Risk for fecal or flatus incontinence: 45% short term, 6–8% long term
- Botulinum toxin injections also first-line treatment; less effective (60–80% healing) than surgery but fewer complications (6)[C]
  - Risk for fecal or flatus incontinence: 18% short term, no long term
  - May be repeated as needed with same efficacy; higher doses are more effective.
- Controlled pneumatic balloon dilation may be used by gastroenterologists if surgical referral is not available; should not be used first line as benefits are not well documented. Uncontrolled manual dilation is no longer recommended (5,6)[C].

 ONGOING CARE

DIET
High fiber (>25 g/day; augment with daily fiber supplements); increase fluid intake.

PATIENT EDUCATION
- Avoid prolonged sitting or straining during bowel movements; drink plenty of fluids; avoid constipation; lose weight if obese.
- Avoid use of triple antibiotic ointment and long-term use of steroid creams to anal area.

PROGNOSIS
Most acute fissures heal within 6 weeks with conservative therapy. Medical therapy is less likely to be successful for chronic anal fissures; 40% failure rate.

COMPLICATIONS
Fecal and flatus incontinence, primarily associated with surgery (5–45% postop), which may become permanent (up to 8% long term, primarily to flatus)

REFERENCES

1. Altomare DF, Binda GA, Canuti S, et al. The management of patients with primary chronic anal fissure: a position paper. *Tech Coloproctol*. 2011;15(2):135–141.
2. Nelson RL, Thomas K, Morgan J, et al. Non surgical therapy for anal fissure. *Cochrane Database Syst Rev*. 2012;(2):CD003431.
3. Samim M, Twigt B, Stoker L, et al. Topical diltiazem cream versus botulinum toxin a for the treatment of chronic anal fissure: a double-blind randomized clinical trial. *Ann Surg*. 2012;255(1):18–22.
4. Madalinski MH. Identifying the best therapy for chronic anal fissure. *World J Gastrointest Pharmacol Ther*. 2011;2(2):9–16.
5. Nelson RL, Chattopadhyay A, Brooks W, et al. Operative procedures for fissure in ano. *Cochrane Database Syst Rev*. 2011;(11):CD002199.
6. Wald A, Bharucha AE, Cosman BC, et al. ACG clinical guideline: management of benign anorectal disorders. *Am J Gastroenterol*. 2014;109(8):1141–1157.

ADDITIONAL READING

- Fargo MV, Latimer KM. Evaluation and management of common anorectal conditions. *Am Fam Physician*. 2012;85(6):624–630.
- Gee T, Hisham RB, Jabar MF, et al. Ano-coccygeal support in the treatment of idiopathic chronic posterior anal fissure: a prospective non-randomised controlled pilot trial. *Tech Coloproctol*. 2013; 17(2):181–186.

- Sinha R, Kaiser AM. Efficacy of management algorithm for reducing need for sphincterotomy in chronic anal fissures. *Colorectal Dis*. 2012;14(6): 760–764.
- Sugerman DT. JAMA patient page. Anal fissure. *JAMA*. 2014;311(11):1171.
- Yiannakopoulou E. Botulinum toxin and anal fissure: efficacy and safety systematic review. *Int J Colorectal Dis*. 2012;27(1):1–9.

 CODES

ICD10
- K60.2 Anal fissure, unspecified
- K60.0 Acute anal fissure
- K60.1 Chronic anal fissure

CLINICAL PEARLS
- Avoid anoscopy or sigmoidoscopy initially unless necessary for other diagnoses.
- Best chance to prevent recurrence is to treat the underlying cause (e.g., chronic constipation).
- No medical therapy approaches the cure rate of surgery for chronic fissure.

ANEMIA, APLASTIC
Muthalagu Ramanathan, MD • Jan Cerny, MD, PhD

 BASICS

DESCRIPTION
- Pancytopenia due to hypocellular bone marrow without infiltrates or fibrosis. Classified as acquired (much more common) and congenital
- Acquired aplastic anemia: insidious onset; due to exogenous insult triggering an autoimmune reaction; often responsive to immunosuppression
- Congenital forms: rare, mostly present in childhood (exception is atypical presentation of Fanconi syndrome in adults; 30s for males and 40s for females)
- The occurrence of specific mutations in genes of the telomere complex in acquired aplastic anemia has blurred the distinction between the congenital and acquired forms.
- System(s) affected: heme/lymphatic/immunologic
- Synonym(s): hypoplastic anemia; panmyelophthisis; refractory anemia; aleukia hemorrhagica; toxic paralytic anemia

ALERT
- Early intervention for aplastic anemia greatly improves the chances of treatment success.
- Hematopoietic growth factors require close monitoring in newly diagnosed patients.

Geriatric Considerations
The elderly are often exposed to large numbers of drugs and therefore, may be more susceptible to acquired aplastic anemia.

Pediatric Considerations
- Congenital forms of aplastic anemia require different treatment regimens than acquired forms.
- Acquired aplastic anemia is seen in children exposed to ionizing radiation or treated with cytotoxic chemotherapeutic agents.

Pregnancy Considerations
- Pregnancy is a real but rare cause of aplastic anemia. Symptoms may resolve after delivery and with termination.
- Complications in pregnancy can occur from low platelet counts and paroxysmal nocturnal hemoglobinuria-associated aplastic anemia.

EPIDEMIOLOGY
- Predominant age: (1) biphasic 15 to 25 years (more common) and >60 years
- Predominant sex: male = female

Incidence
- 2 to 3 new cases per million per year in Europe and North America
- The incidence is 3-fold higher in Thailand and China versus the Western world.

ETIOLOGY AND PATHOPHYSIOLOGY
- Idiopathic (~70% of the cases)
- Drugs: phenylbutazone, chloramphenicol, sulfonamides, gold, cytotoxic drugs, antiepileptics (felbamate, carbamazepine, valproic acid, phenytoin)
- Viral: HIV, Epstein-Barr virus (EBV), nontypeable postinfectious hepatitis (not A, B, or C), parvovirus B19 (mostly in the immunocompromised), atypical mycobacterium
- Toxic exposure (benzene, pesticides, arsenic)
- Radiation exposure
- Immune disorders (systemic lupus erythematosus, eosinophilic fasciitis, graft vs. host disease)
- Pregnancy (rare)
- Congenital (Fanconi anemia, dyskeratosis congenita, Shwachman-Diamond syndrome, amegakaryocytic thrombocytopenia)
- The immune hypothesis: Activation of T cells with associated cytokine production leading to destruction or injury of hematopoietic stem cells. This leads to a hypocellular bone marrow without marrow fibrosis (2).
- The activation of T cells likely occurs because of both genetic and environmental factors. Exposure to specific environmental precipitants, diverse host, genetic risk factors, and individual differences in characteristics of immune response likely account for variations in its clinical manifestations and patterns of responsiveness to treatment.
- Telomerase deficiency leads to short telomeres. This leads to impaired regenerative capacity and hence, a reduction in marrow progenitors and qualitative deficiency in the repair capacity of hematopoietic tissue.
- Reduction of natural killer cells in the bone marrow

Genetics
- Telomerase mutations found in a small number of patients with acquired and congenital forms. These mutations render carriers more susceptible to environmental insults.
- Mutations in genes called TERC and TERT were found in pedigrees of adults with acquired aplastic anemia who lacked the physical abnormalities or a family history typical of inherited forms of bone marrow failure. These genes encode for the RNA component of telomerase.
- HLA-DR2 incidence in aplastic anemia is twice that in the normal population.

RISK FACTORS
- Treatment with high-dose radiation or chemotherapy
- Exposure to toxic chemicals
- Use of certain medications
- Certain blood diseases, autoimmune disorders, and serious infections
- Tumors of thymus (red cell aplasia)
- Pregnancy, rarely

GENERAL PREVENTION
- Avoid possible toxic industrial agents.
- Use safety measures when working with radiation.

 DIAGNOSIS

HISTORY
- Solvent and radiation history; family, environmental, travel, and infectious disease history
- Patients are often asymptomatic but may have frequent infections, fatigue, shortness of breath, headache, or bleeding/bruising.

PHYSICAL EXAM
- Mucosal hemorrhage, petechiae
- Pallor
- Fever
- Hemorrhage, menorrhagia, occult stool blood, melena, epistaxis
- Dyspnea
- Palpitations
- Progressive weakness
- Retinal flame hemorrhages
- Systolic ejection murmur
- Weight loss
- Signs of congenital aplastic anemia
  - Short stature
  - Microcephaly
  - Nail dystrophy
  - Abnormal thumbs
  - Oral leukoplakia
  - Hyperpigmentation (café au lait spots) or hypopigmentation

DIFFERENTIAL DIAGNOSIS
Includes other causes of bone marrow failure and pancytopenia
- Marrow replacement
  - Acute lymphoblastic leukemia
  - Lymphoma
  - Hairy cell leukemia (increased reticulin and infiltration of hairy cells)
  - Large granular lymphocyte leukemia
  - Fibrosis
- Megaloblastic hematopoiesis
  - Folate deficiency
  - Vitamin B_{12} deficiency
- Paroxysmal nocturnal hemoglobinuria, hemolytic anemia (dark urine), pancytopenia, and venous thrombosis (classically hepatic veins)
- Systemic lupus erythematosus
- Prolonged starvation or anorexia nervosa (bone marrow is gelatinous with loss of fat cells and increased ground substance)
- Transient erythroblastopenia of childhood
- Drug-induced agranulocytosis that may be reversible on withdrawal of drug
- Overwhelming infection
  - HIV with myelodysplasia
  - Viral hemophagocytic syndrome

DIAGNOSTIC TESTS & INTERPRETATION
Screening tests to exclude other etiologies
- CBC and absolute reticulocyte count
- Blood smear exam
- Cytogenetic studies of peripheral lymphocytes if <35 years of age to exclude Fanconi anemia
- Liver function test
- Viral serology: hepatitis A, B, C; EBV; cytomegalovirus (CMV); HIV
- Vitamin B_{12} and folate levels
- Autoantibody screening antinuclear antibody (ANA) and anti-DNA
- Flow cytometry looking for glycosylphosphatidylinositol (GPI), negative neutrophils and RBCs for detecting paroxysmal nocturnal hemoglobinuria
- Fetal hemoglobin in children
- Red cell adenosine deaminase (pure red cell aplasia)
- Cytogenetic analysis of bone marrow

Initial Tests (lab, imaging)
- CBC: pancytopenia, anemia (usually normocytic), leukopenia, neutropenia, thrombocytopenia
- Decreased absolute number of reticulocytes
- Increased serum iron secondary to transfusion
- Normal total iron-binding capacity (TIBC)
- High mean corpuscular volume (MCV) >104
- CD 34+ cells decreased in blood and marrow
- Urinalysis: hematuria
- Abnormal liver function tests (hepatitis)
- Increased fetal hemoglobin (Fanconi)
- Increased chromosomal breaks under specialized conditions (Fanconi)
- Molecular determination of abnormal gene (Fanconi)

- CT of thymus region if thymoma-associated RBC aplasia suspected
- Radiographs of radius and thumbs (if congenital anemia suspected)
- Renal ultrasound (to rule out congenital anemia or malignant hematologic disorder)
- Chest x-ray to exclude infections such as mycobacterial infection

Diagnostic Procedures/Other
Bone marrow aspiration and biopsy

Test Interpretation
- Normochromic RBC
- Bone marrow
  - Decreased cellularity (<10%): no fibrosis, no malignant cells seen
  - Decreased megakaryocytes
  - Decreased myeloid precursors
  - Decreased erythroid precursors
  - Prominent fat spaces and marrow stroma, polyclonal plasma cells

 TREATMENT

Early treatment increases the chance of success. Two major options: immunosuppressive therapy (1) and hematopoietic stem cell transplantation. Treatment decisions are based on age of the patient, severity of disease, and availability of a human leukocyte antigen (HLA)-matched sibling donor for transplantation.

GENERAL MEASURES
- Supportive measures: RBC and platelet transfusions. Use only irradiated leuko-reduced or CMV-negative blood initially if patient is a candidate for hematopoietic stem cell transplantation.
- Antibiotics, antifungals, antivirals when appropriate, especially if ANC <200 cells/μL
- Oxygen therapy for severe anemia
- Good oral hygiene
- Control menorrhagia with norethisterone or oral contraceptive pills.
- Avoid/discontinue causative agents/isolation if necessary.
- HLA testing on all patients and their immediate families
- Transfusion support (judiciously prescribed RBCs for severe anemia; platelets for severe thrombocytopenia)
  - Transfuse when
    ○ Hb <8 g/dL or if Hb <9 g/dL and symptomatic ± CHF (congestive heart failure)
    ○ Platelet count is <10 × 10^9 or if <20 × 10^9 with fever

MEDICATION
First Line
- Corticosteroids (methylprednisolone) are often given with immunosuppressive regimens.
- Immunosuppressive therapy (3)
  - A combination of antithymocyte globulin (ATG) plus cyclosporine. ATG eliminates lymphocytes, and cyclosporine blocks T-cell function.
- ATG
  - Horse serum containing polyclonal antibodies against human T cells
  - First choice treatment for patients >40 years of age and for younger patients without a compatible donor. Consider in patients 30 to 40 years of age.
  - May be used as a single agent but has better response in combination with cyclosporine

- Cyclosporine following initial ATG therapy for minimum of 6 months (4)
  - Monitor through blood levels. Normal values for assays vary.
  - Granulocyte-colony stimulating factor (G-CSF)
    ○ May be used in conjunction with ATG and cyclosporine
    ○ Shows faster neutrophil recovery but survival is not improved.
    ○ Treatment is costly and is disputed in two randomized trials.
  - Note: Relapses may occur after the initial response to the immunosuppressive therapy if cyclosporine is discontinued too early. Restarting cyclosporine can lead to a response in up to 25% of patients.
- Stem cell transplant: matched sibling allogeneic stem cell transplant for age <20 years and absolute neutrophil count (ANC) <500 or age 20 to 40 years and ANC <200

Second Line
- Rabbit ATG + cyclosporine
- Campath
- Androgen in a subset of patients who have anemia as a predominant feature
- Matched unrelated donor stem cell transplant
- Eltrombopag (5)
- Clinical trials: thrombopoietin (TPO) receptor agonists (6): http://patientrecruitment.nhlbi.nih.gov/AplasticAnemia.aspx

SURGERY/OTHER PROCEDURES
- First-line hematopoietic stem cell transplantation is recommended for patients with an HLA-identical donor and severe aplastic anemia when age <20 years and ANC <500 or age 20 to 40 years and ANC <200. Consider in patients 40 to 50 years of age in good general medical condition.
- Patients >40 years of age have higher rates of graft versus host disease and graft rejection.
- Unrelated donor transplants should be considered for patients age <40 years without HLA-matched sibling donor who failed first-line immunosuppressive therapy.
- Thymectomy for thymoma

INPATIENT CONSIDERATIONS
Nursing
If neutropenic, use antiseptic mouthwash such as chlorhexidine.

 ONGOING CARE

DIET
If neutropenic, avoid foods that can expose patient to bacteria, such as uncooked foods.

PATIENT EDUCATION
- Stay away from people who are sick; avoid large crowds.
- Wash your hands often.
- Brush and floss your teeth; get regular dental care to reduce risk of infections.
- Pneumonia vaccine and annual flu shot.
- Printed patient information available from Aplastic Anemia & MDS International Foundation, Inc., 800-747-2828. Web site: http://www.aamds.org/aplastic

PROGNOSIS
- Hematopoietic stem cell transplantation with HLA-matched sibling
  - Age <16 years, 91% at 5 years
  - Age >16 years, 70–80% at 5 years

- Immunosuppressive therapy using ATG and cyclosporine: overall survival of 75%; 90% among responders at 5 years

COMPLICATIONS
- Infection (fungal, sepsis)
- Graft versus host disease in bone marrow transplant recipients (acute 18%; chronic 26%)
- Side effects of immunosuppressant medications
- Hemorrhage
- Transfusion hemosiderosis
- Transfusion hepatitis
- Heart failure
- Development of secondary cancer: leukemia or myelodysplasia (15–19% risk at 6 to 10 years)
- Refractory pancytopenia

REFERENCES

1. Bacigalupo A, Passweg J. Diagnosis and treatment of acquired aplastic anemia. *Hematol Oncol Clin North Am*. 2009;23(2):159–170.
2. Townsley DM, Desmond R, Dunbar CE, et al. Pathophysiology and management of thrombocytopenia in bone marrow failure: possible clinical applications of TPO receptor agonists in aplastic anemia and myelodysplastic syndromes. *Int J Hematol*. 2013;98(1):48–55.
3. Brodsky RA, Jones RJ. Aplastic anaemia. *Lancet*. 2005;365(9471):1647–1656.
4. Bueno C, Roldan M, Anguita E, et al. Bone marrow mesenchymal stem cells from patients with aplastic anemia maintain functional and immune properties and do not contribute to the pathogenesis of the disease. *Haematologica*. 2014;99(7):1168–1175.
5. Desmond R, Townsley DM, Dunbar C, et al. Eltrombopag in aplastic anemia. *Semin Hematol*. 2015;52(1):31–37.
6. Scheinberg P, Young NS. How I treat acquired aplastic anemia. *Blood*. 2012;120(6):1185–1196.

 SEE ALSO

- Myelodysplastic Syndromes; Lupus Erythematosus, Systemic (SLE)
- Algorithm: Anemia

CODES

ICD10
- D61.9 Aplastic anemia, unspecified
- D61.89 Oth aplastic anemias and other bone marrow failure syndromes
- D61.01 Constitutional (pure) red blood cell aplasia

CLINICAL PEARLS
- Acquired aplastic anemia has an insidious onset, and is caused by an exogenous insult triggering an autoimmune reaction. This form is usually responsive to immunosuppressive therapy.
- Immunosuppressive therapy using ATG and cyclosporine: overall survival of 75%; 90% among responders at 5 years

ANEMIA, CHRONIC DISEASE
Christopher Lin-Brande, MD • Amy M. Davis, MD

BASICS

DESCRIPTION
- Otherwise known as anemia of chronic inflammation
- During chronic systemic infection, inflammation, or malignancy, the production of proinflammatory mediators causes inhibition of erythropoiesis as well as the imbalance in iron homeostasis (1).
- Anemia of chronic disease (ACD) is characterized as a normocytic, normochromic, hypoproliferative anemia and classically has low serum iron levels, elevated ferritin levels, and elevated total iron-binding capacity (TIBC) (1–3).
- Anemia is typically mild to moderate with hemoglobin rarely <8 g/dL.

EPIDEMIOLOGY
Prevalence
ACD is the second most common anemia after iron deficiency anemia (IDA) due to the aging population and the high prevalence of chronic infections and inflammatory disorders in the United States (4).

ETIOLOGY AND PATHOPHYSIOLOGY
- Production of red blood cells is decreased as a result of functional iron deficiency.
- In general, the severity of the anemia will correspond with the severity of the underlying disease (1).
- Proinflammatory cytokines such as interleukins (IL), tumor necrosis factor (TNF), bone morphogenic proteins (BMP), and interferons (IFN) create changes in iron homeostasis in several ways (1,4):
  - Dysregulating iron homeostasis
  - Diminishing proliferation as well as differentiation of red blood cell progenitor cells
  - Blunting the erythropoietic response
  - Increasing erythrocyte phagocytosis and apoptosis
- Iron overload and the proinflammatory cytokines IL-1, IL-6, and BMP6 increase the production of the iron-regulating hormone hepcidin in hepatocytes, macrophages, and enterocytes (1,4).
  - Hepcidin binds to ferroportin causing internalization and degradation, which prevents efflux of iron from stores in macrophages and hepatocytes (reticuloendothelial cell iron blockade) and prevents iron absorption by duodenal enterocytes.
    - This results in low serum iron levels and inhibited erythropoiesis known as iron-restricted erythropoiesis.
  - As a result, iron delivery to erythroid progenitor cells within bone marrow is reduced and erythropoiesis is diminished, causing anemia.
- Erythropoietin (EPO) production and the response to EPO by erythroid bone marrow is suppressed by proinflammatory cytokines such as IL-1,TNF-α, and IFN-γ (1).
- Inflammatory cytokines may also cause erythrophagocytosis and oxidative damage, reducing RBC survival.

COMMONLY ASSOCIATED CONDITIONS
- Chronic systemic diseases (2)
  - Rheumatoid arthritis (RA), systemic lupus erythematosus (SLE), sarcoidosis, temporal arteritis, inflammatory bowel disease (IBD), systemic inflammatory response syndrome (SIRS)
- Hepatic disease or failure
- Congestive heart failure or coronary artery disease
- Chronic kidney disease (CKD)

- Acute or chronic infections
  - Viral
    - HIV, HCV
  - Bacterial
    - Abscess, subacute bacterial endocarditis, tuberculosis, osteomyelitis
  - Fungal
  - Parasitic
- Malignancies
- Cytokine dysregulation (anemia of aging)
- Hypometabolic states
  - Protein malnutrition, thyroid disease, panhypopituitarism, diabetes mellitus, Addison disease

DIAGNOSIS

HISTORY
- ACD is often discovered incidentally on routine CBC with differential.
- ACD presents with the underlying causative infectious, inflammatory, or malignant process without any source of occult bleeding; often patients will have mild and vague anemia symptoms, such as fatigue, light-headedness, and palpitations (1).
- Those with a cardiovascular condition may experience symptoms of angina, shortness of breath, and reduced exercise capacity with even a moderate hemoglobin (Hgb) level (10 to 11 g/dL).

PHYSICAL EXAM
Physical exam findings are associated with the underlying condition.

DIFFERENTIAL DIAGNOSIS
- IDA
- Anemia of CKD
- Drug-induced marrow suppression or hemolysis
- Endocrine disorders
- Thalassemia
- Sideroblastic anemia
- Dilutional anemia

DIAGNOSTIC TESTS & INTERPRETATION
Initial Tests (lab, imaging)
- Hgb/Hct, MCV, reticulocyte count, ferritin, B_{12}/folate, serum iron, TIBC
- Hgb (1)
  - Typically, <13 g/dL in males or 12 g/dL in females
  - An Hgb of <8 g/dL typically suggests a concurrent secondary cause for the anemia.
- Mean corpuscular volume (MCV)
  - Usually normal (80 to 100 fL), but microcytosis may be present with concurrent iron deficiency or long-standing disease (<25% of cases)
- RBC morphology
  - Normocytic and normochromic
  - Increased protoporphyrin levels
- Serum ferritin
  - Nonspecific acute phase reactant
  - Normal or slightly elevated (30 to 200 μg/L)
  - In CKD, ferritin can reach 800 μg/L.
  - Serum ferritin levels <30 μg/L suggests coexisting iron deficiency.
- Serum iron levels
  - Low due to increased retention and decreased release from the RES
  - <50
- TIBC
  - Extremely low
  - <300

- Absolute reticulocyte count
  - Inappropriately low (reticulocyte index <20,000–25,000/μL) due to reduced erythropoiesis
- Serum B_{12} and folate
  - Diminished due decreased absorption or lacking in diet

	IDA	ACD	IDA+ACD
Iron	Low	Low	Low
Reticulocyte count	Low	Low	Low
Transferrin, TIBC	High	Low	Normal/high
Transferrin saturation	Low	Normal	Low
Ferritin	Low	Normal/high	Normal
sTfR index	High	Low	High
Hepcidin	Low	High	Normal
Inflammatory markers	Normal	High	High

Diagnostic Procedures/Other
- Traditional gold standard: bone marrow biopsy with Prussian blue stainable iron combined with anemia, hypoferremia, and low TSAT (1,2,4)
  - Staining is qualitative and may not be accurate.
- Reticulocyte Hgb concentration <28 pg (3)
- Soluble transferrin receptor (sTfR) and the sTfR/log ferritin index (5)[A]
  - Ratio reflects erythropoiesis within bone marrow and differentiates among ACD, IDA, and ACD + IDA.
    - However, sTfR alone may have greater clinical value than the sTfR index because transferrin is not affected by chronic disease/inflammation, unlike ferritin.
- Functional test: supplemental iron increase H/H in iron deficiency anemia and little effect on anemia of chronic disease
- Although a known cause of anemia may be present, iron, B_{12}, and folate deficiencies should be ruled out.

TREATMENT

GENERAL MEASURES
- Primary management should focus on the underlying cause of ACD (1,2,4).
  - Treatment of the primary disease will generally restore Hgb back to baseline.
- In cases where primary treatment is not possible (e.g. terminal cancer, end-stage renal disease), additional treatment can be considered.
  - The two main forms of treatment are erythropoietin stimulating agents (ESAs) and transfusions.
  - ACD is frequently responsive to ESAs (epoetin-α, darbepoetin) in pharmacologic doses (6).
  - Replete iron to maximize ESA effectiveness.
  - Transfusion should only be initiated in severe anemia or acute symptoms.
- Currently, no target Hgb exists but treatment to Hgb >13 g/dL is associated with adverse outcomes (1).
- Coexisting B_{12}, or folate deficiency should be considered and corrected in severe cases of anemia (7)[B].
  - Reduced dietary intake of nutrients is common among patients who are chronically ill.
  - Patients who regularly undergo hemodialysis will often lose these during treatment.

MEDICATION

- Erythropoietin-stimulating agents (ESAs)
  - Specifically approved for CKD, but there is evidence that they may also have applications in RA, IBD, HIV, and cancer
  - Indication for ESA therapy is an Hgb <10 g/dL (6)[C].
  - ESAs do not improve symptoms or outcomes in mild anemia of CHF (8)[A].
  - Do not use in certain cancers: breast, cervical, head and neck, lymphoid, and nonsmall cell lung cancers. Do not administer to patients with active malignancy not receiving curative therapy.
- Epoetin-α (1,6,9)
  - Indications
    ○ Hgb <10 g/dL
    ○ Fatigue or exertional intolerance
    ○ CKD (eGFR <60 mL/min)
    ○ Anemia due to IBD, RA, hepatitis C
    ○ Chemotherapy in patients with specific malignancies (palliative therapy)
  - Dosing and schedule
    ○ Lowest effective dose to maintain a Hgb level generally between 10 and 12 g/dL (1,6,9)
    ○ CKD associated: Start 50 to 100 U/kg SC/IV 3 times per week.
  - Patients with cancer who are undergoing chemotherapy: 150 U/kg SQ 3 times per week or 40,000 units once a week.
  - Adverse affects:
    ○ Increased risk of cardiovascular complications, mortality, and thromboembolism
    ○ Pure red cell aplasia (decrease in Hgb, low reticulocyte count, normal WBC and platelets)
    ○ Risk of tumor progression in certain cancer patients
- Darbepoetin-α
  - Long-acting, molecularly modified EPO preparation with a half-life 3 to 4 times longer than recombinant human EPO, reducing the frequency of injections to weekly or biweekly
  - Dosing and schedule
    ○ Administer SC/IV q1–2wk; hold if Hgb >12 g/dL; IV route is preferred in hemodialysis patients.
  - Adverse affects
    ○ Similar to EPO
- Epoetin-α or darbepoetin-α dose adjustments
  - Follow FDA-approved labeling.
  - Treatment beyond 6 to 8 weeks without appropriate rise of Hgb (>1 to 2 g/dL) is not recommended.

ADDITIONAL THERAPIES

- Iron (6)
  - Indications
    ○ Coexisting iron deficiency
    ○ Resistance to EPO
  - Forms
    ○ Oral: ferrous sulfate. Poorly tolerated (GI side effects), incomplete absorption (due to hepcidin)
    ○ Intravenous: ferric gluconate. iron sucrose, iron dextran (potential allergic and anaphylactoid reactions), ferumoxytol
  - Adverse affects
    ○ May stimulate hepcidin production and exacerbate iron restriction
  - Benefits
    ○ Relatively safe
    ○ Inexpensive
    ○ May decrease ESA requirements (DRIVE study)
- Transfusions
  - 1 to 2 U packed red blood cells (1)
  - Indications
    ○ Life-threatening/severe anemia: A "restrictive threshold" of Hgb 7 to 8 g/dL to guide transfusion in asymptomatic patients should be used (10)[A].

- Patients with underlying cardiac or pulmonary disease, active ACS, elderly patients, or patients with acute bleeding or hemorrhagic shock may require transfusion at Hgb of higher threshold (>10 g/dL).
  ○ Symptomatic anemia (chest pain, SOB, reduced exercise capacity), and/or EKG changes
  ○ Lack of response to medical therapy
  - Possible adverse affects
    ○ Infection (HIV, hepatitis)
    ○ Volume overload
    ○ Transfusion reaction
  - Specific benefits
    ○ Rapid correction of anemia
  - When an infection occurs during EPO therapy, it is best to cease EPO therapy and rely on transfusion therapy instead until the infection is properly treated.
- Future directions (1,4)
  - Antihepcidin antibodies, hepcidin-production inhibitors
  - Anti-BMP, anti–IL-6 antibodies
  - Ferroportin stabilizers
  - Vitamin D (lowers hepcidin)
  - Heparin (impairs hepcidin transcription)

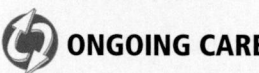 ## ONGOING CARE

FOLLOW-UP RECOMMENDATIONS
Referral to a hematologist is not always warranted.

Patient Monitoring
- Hgb should not be increased >11 to 12 g/dL because normalization of hemoglobin has been associated with higher mortality (9).
- Baseline and periodic monitoring of transferrin saturation, and ferritin levels every 3 months may be of value (6).

PATIENT EDUCATION
Patients receiving medical therapy should be advised about the following possible risks:

- Mortality, cardiovascular complications, thromboembolism, progression of cancer

PROGNOSIS
ACD does not typically progress.

COMPLICATIONS
- Adverse effects of ACD:
  - Mortality
  - Cardiovascular complications
  - Symptoms affecting daily life
- Adverse effects of ESAs:
  - Heightened risk of mortality and/or cardiovascular complications in CKD patients
  - Heightened risk of mortality and/or tumor progression in cancer patients
  - Elevated risk of thromboembolism

REFERENCES

1. Gangat N, Wolanskyj AP. Anemia of chronic disease. *Semin Hematol*. 2013;50(3):232–238.
2. Cullis JO. Diagnosis and management of anaemia of chronic disease: current status. *Br J Haematol*. 2011;154(3):289–300.
3. Thomas DW, Hinchliffe RF, Briggs C, et al. Guidelines for the laboratory diagnosis of functional iron deficiency. *Br J Haematol*. 2013;161(5):639–648.
4. Nemeth E, Ganz T. Anemia of inflammation. *Hematol Oncol Clin North Am*. 2014;28(4):671–681.
5. Infusino I, Braga F, Dolci A, et al. Soluble transferrin receptor (sTfR) and sTfR/log ferritin index for the diagnosis of iron-deficiency anemia. A meta-analysis. *Am J Clin Pathol*. 2012;138(5):642–649.

---

6. Kidney Disease: Improving Global Outcomes Anemia Work Group. KDIGO Clinical practice guideline for anemia in chronic kidney disease. *Kidney Inter Suppl*. 2012;2(4):279–335.
7. Macciò A, Madeddu C, Gramignano G, et al. The role of inflammation, iron, and nutritional status in cancer-related anemia: results of a large, prospective, observational study. *Haematologica*. 2015;100(1):124–132.
8. Kansagara D, Dyer E, Englander H, et al. Treatment of anemia in patients with heart disease: a systematic review. *Ann Intern Med*. 2014;159(11):746–757.
9. Babitt JL, Lin HY. Mechanisms of anemia in CKD. *J Am Soc Nephrol*. 2012;23(10):1631–1634.
10. Carson JL, Carless PA, Hebert PC. Transfusion thresholds and other strategies for guiding allogeneic red blood cell transfusion. *Cochrane Database Syst Rev*. 2012;(4):CD002042.

ADDITIONAL READING

- Besarab A, Bolton WK, Browne JK, et al. The effects of normal as compared with low hematocrit values in patients with cardiac disease who are receiving hemodialysis and epoetin. *N Engl J Med*. 1998;339(9):584–590.
- Fishbane S, Schiller B, Locatelli F, et al. Peginesatide in patients with anemia undergoing hemodialysis. *N Engl J Med*. 2013;368(4):307–319.
- Macdougall IC, Provenzano R, Sharma A, et al. Peginesatide for anemia in patients with chronic kidney disease not receiving dialysis. *N Engl J Med*. 2013;368(4):320–332.
- Pfeffer MA, Burdmann EA, Chen CY, et al. A trial of darbepoetin alfa in type 2 diabetes and chronic kidney disease. *N Engl J Med*. 2009;361(21):2019–2032.
- Singh AK, Szczech L, Tang KL, et al. Correction of anemia with epoetin alfa in chronic kidney disease. *N Engl J Med*. 2006;335(20):2085–2098.
- Swedberg K, Young JB, Anand IS, et al. Treatment of anemia with darbepoetin alfa in systolic heart failure. *N Engl J Med*. 2013;368(13):1210–1219.

 ## SEE ALSO

Iron Deficiency Anemia

 ## CODES

ICD10
- D63.8 Anemia in other chronic diseases classified elsewhere
- D63.0 Anemia in neoplastic disease
- D63.1 Anemia in chronic kidney disease

CLINICAL PEARLS

- ACD is the second most common anemia seen clinically.
- One of the most common diagnostic problems is making the distinction between ACD, IDA, and combined ACD + IDA.
  - Iron level is usually nondiagnostic.
  - Use markers such as transferrin/TIBC, TSAT, and ferritin to distinguish. New markers are under development (hepcidin, sTfR, sTfR index).
- IV iron should be given to all patients treated with ESAs.
- Hemoglobin should be kept in low to normal range.

ANEMIA, IRON DEFICIENCY
Deborah R. Erlich, MD, MMedEd

BASICS

DESCRIPTION
- Low serum iron associated with low hemoglobin (Hgb) or microcytic, hypochromic red blood cells (RBCs)
- Onset acute (rapid blood loss) or chronic (slow blood loss, deficient iron intake or absorption)
- Both low Hgb per RBC and fewer RBC in total lead to blood oxygen deficiency, which can have serious systemic consequences.
- System(s) affected: hematologic, lymphatic, immunologic, cardiac, gastrointestinal

Geriatric Considerations
Iron deficiency anemia is associated with increased hospitalization and mortality in older adults (1).

Pediatric Considerations
Infants who drink cow's milk or juice, live in poverty, are from developing countries or are of black or Native American descent are at high risk of iron deficiency anemia and should get iron supplements (2)[B].

Pregnancy Considerations
Iron supplements are recommended during pregnancy to improve maternal hematologic indexes, though significant clinical outcomes have not yet been proven (3)[A] other than neonatal birth weight (2)[B].

EPIDEMIOLOGY
- Iron deficiency is the most common nutritional deficiency in the world (4,5) and iron deficiency anemia (IDA) is the most common cause of anemia (50%) (4,6).
- Predominant age: all ages but especially toddlers and menstruating and pregnant women
- Predominant sex: female
- Predominant race: Mexican-American and black females (4)
- Common in both developing and developed countries

Incidence
- Adults: men 2%, women 15–20% annually
- Infants and toddlers: 3–5% annually
- Pregnant patients: maybe as high as 20% (2)

Prevalence
2 billion people worldwide (5)
- Infants and children age <12 years: 4–7%
- Men: 2–5%
- Menstruating women: 30% (5)

ETIOLOGY AND PATHOPHYSIOLOGY
Depletion of iron stores leads to decrease in both reticulocyte count and production of Hgb. Causes:
- Blood loss (menses, GI bleeding, trauma)
- Poor iron intake
- Poor iron absorption (e.g., atrophic gastritis, postgastrectomy, celiac disease)
- Increased demand for iron (e.g., infancy, adolescence, pregnancy, breastfeeding)

RISK FACTORS
- Premenopausal woman
- Frequent blood donor
- Pregnancy/lactation, young maternal age
- Strict vegan diet
- Use of NSAIDs

- Hospitalized with frequent blood draws
- Living in or visiting countries with endemic hookworm infection

GENERAL PREVENTION
- Screen asymptomatic pregnant women and high risk children at 1 year of age (6).
- Supplementation in asymptomatic children aged 6 to 12 months if at risk for IDA (e.g., malnutrition, abuse, cow's milk <12 months) (2,3)
- Iron- and vitamin C-rich diet for menstruating women
- Iron 30 mg/day for asymptomatic pregnant women (3)

COMMONLY ASSOCIATED CONDITIONS
- GI tract malignancy, peptic ulcer disease (PUD), Helicobacter pylori infection, irritable bowel disease
- Hookworm or other parasitic infestations
- Hypermetrorrhagia
- Pregnancy
- Obesity treated with gastric bypass surgery
- Malnutrition
- Medications such as NSAIDs or antacids

DIAGNOSIS

HISTORY
- Asymptomatic in most cases
- Weakness, fatigue, and/or malaise
- Exertional dyspnea
- Angina with coronary artery disease
- Headaches or inability to concentrate
- Melena
- Pica

PHYSICAL EXAM
- Pallor (skin, conjunctivae, sublingual)
- Tachycardia, tachypnea
- Cool extremities
- Brittle nails/hair
- Signs of heart failure

DIFFERENTIAL DIAGNOSIS
- GI bleeding (e.g., gastritis, PUD, carcinoma, varices, celiac disease)
- Chronic intravascular hemolysis (e.g., paroxysmal nocturnal hemoglobinuria, malfunctioning prosthetic valve)
- Defective iron usage (e.g., thalassemia trait, sideroblastosis, G6PD deficiency)
- Defective iron reutilization (e.g., infection, inflammation, cancer, hypothyroid, chronic diseases)
- Hypoproliferation (e.g., decreased erythropoietin from hypothyroidism, renal failure)
- Other anemias such as anemia of chronic disease, thalassemia, lead poisoning

DIAGNOSTIC TESTS & INTERPRETATION
Initial Tests (lab, imaging)
- Screen asymptomatic pregnant women and high risk children at 1 year of age (6).
- Test with signs and symptoms of anemia, and fully evaluate if iron deficiency is confirmed (2,5).
- Hgb (to define anemia):
  - <13 g in men and <12 g in women (WHO standards) (7)
  - Patients with comorbidities (e.g., chronic hypoxemia, smokers, high altitudes) may be anemic at higher Hgb levels.

- Mean corpuscular volume (MCV): <80 fL
  - MCV may be low normal in mild anemia, or hidden by large cells (reticulocytes, macrocytes).
- Ferritin is most sensitive and specific for diagnosing iron deficiency as cause of anemia (5):
  - <15 μg/L diagnoses IDA (<45 μg/L likely) (2)
  - >100 μg/L rules out iron deficiency
- Iron studies:
  - Decreased: ferritin, serum iron, transferrin saturation
  - Increased: total iron-binding capacity (TIBC), transferrin
- Red cell distribution width (RDW) increases with a mixed population of cells (e.g., mixed IDA and B_{12} deficiency).
- CBC with differential, peripheral smear, reticulocyte count, and index
  - Peripheral smear usually shows hypochromia and microcytosis, but may be normal, and reticulocyte production index is low (2).
- Consider testing for G6PD deficiency
- Evaluate for thalassemia
  - Very low MCV <80, elevated Hgb A2 or Hgb F, family history, and especially high or high normal RBC count
  - Microcytosis with ovalocytosis and unresponsive to iron suggests the thalassemia trait.
- IgA antiendomysial antibodies (IgA anti-EmA) and/or IgA antitissue transglutaminase (IgA- anti-TTG) for Celiac
- TSH for hypothyroidism
- An empiric trial of iron at 3 mg/kg/day may help diagnose decreased iron stores in children; reticulocytes become elevated in 7 to 10 days or Hgb increases >1 g/dL weekly, indicating iron deficiency.
- Drugs that may alter lab results:
  - Iron supplements or multivitamin–mineral preparations that contain iron
- Disorders that may alter lab results:
  - Elevated ferritin: acute or chronic liver disease, Hodgkin disease, acute leukemia, solid tumors, fever, acute inflammation, renal dialysis
  - Elevated Hgb: smoking, chronic hypoxemia, high altitude

Diagnostic Procedures/Other
- Stool guaiac
- Stool for ova and parasites if at risk
- Colonoscopy and endoscopy to evaluate for bleeding sites, and especially colorectal and gastric carcinoma for:
  - Premenopausal women with negative GYN workup and/or lack of response to iron
  - Men and postmenopausal women (6)[C]
- Bone marrow aspiration rarely performed

TREATMENT

GENERAL MEASURES
- Search for underlying cause and correct
- Avoid transfusions, except in rare cases.

MEDICATION
- Elemental iron 60 to 200 mg/day for adults (5,8)[C]
- Elemental iron 60 to 120 mg/day for pregnant women for treatment (8), 30 mg for prevention (3)[C]

- Elemental iron 15 mg/day for patients > age 80
- Elemental iron 3 to 6 mg/kg/day for children
- Ferrous sulfate 325 mg TID or ferrous gluconate 300 mg 1 to 3 tablets BID–TID, or ferrous fumarate 324 mg 1 tablet BID on an empty stomach 1 hour before meals (6)[C]
- Constipation will occur in ~1/4 of patients. Consider a stool softener along with iron.
  - Medications that reduce gastric acid secretion such as proton pump inhibitors and H_2 antagonists reduce iron absorption (6).
  - Special oral iron formulations (including enteric-coated iron) and compounds are expensive and reduce symptoms only to the degree that they reduce the delivery of iron.
- Liquid iron preparations (used for children) can also be used in adults when tablets are not absorbed or low tolerance requires a dose reduction.
  - Continued bleeding and untreated hypothyroidism are causes for "failure to respond" to iron.
  - Formula to determine elemental iron needed (7): Elemental iron (mg) = Dose (mL) = 0.0442 (Desired Hb − Observed Hb) × LBW + (0.26 × LBW)
    - Desired Hb = target Hgb in g/dL
    - Observed Hb = current Hgb in g/dL
    - LBW = lean body weight in kg
    - For males: LBW = 50 kg + 2.3 kg for each inch of height over 5 feet
    - For females: LBW = 45.5 kg + 2.3 kg for each inch of height over 5 feet
    - Normal Hgb (males and females)
      - >15 kg (33 lbs) . . . 14.8 g/dL
      - <15 kg (33 lbs) . . . 12.0 g/dL
- Consider parenteral iron for patients with an Hgb level <6 g/dL, malabsorption, chronic kidney disease, or failure to respond to higher oral doses with concomitant vitamin C (5).
- Issues for parenteral iron formulations:
  - Give test dose for iron dextran prior to first dose to avoid anaphylaxis; ferric gluconate or iron sucrose may be safer alternatives. Dimercaprol increases risk of nephrotoxicity.
  - Dosing is product dependent; refer to individual product for suggested dosing
- Blood transfusion for severe acute blood loss or severely symptomatic patients (e.g., demand ischemia due to anemia). Hgb threshold varies by risk factors and clinical scenario (5,9)[C].
- Relative contraindications (oral iron):
  - Tetracycline
  - Allopurinol
  - Antacids
  - Penicillamine
  - Fluoroquinolones
  - Vitamin E
- Precautions
  - Iron may cause dark stools and constipation.
  - Iron overdose is highly toxic; absorption is limited to 1 to 2 mg daily (5); keep tablets and liquids out of reach of small children.

ISSUES FOR REFERRAL
- Men and postmenopausal women with IDA (test for colon cancer)
- Pregnant women with Hgb level <9 g/dL
- Men or nonpregnant women with an Hgb level <6 g/dL
- Failure to respond to a 4- to 6-week trial of oral iron therapy

 ## ONGOING CARE

FOLLOW-UP RECOMMENDATIONS
Patient Monitoring
- Monitor patients every 3 to 12 months after Hgb normalizes (6)[C].
- Hgb increases 1 g/dL every 3 to 4 weeks.
- Iron stores may take up to 4 weeks to correct after Hgb normalizes.

DIET
- Iron-rich foods include red meat, poultry, and fish (all heme iron sources, best absorbed), and iron-fortified breads/cereals, lentils, beans, dark green vegetables, and raisins (all nonheme iron sources, less well absorbed) (10)
- Foods and beverages containing ascorbic acid (vitamin C) enhance iron absorption when taken simultaneously (7).
- Avoid milk or dairy products within 2 hours of iron tablet ingestion.
- Limit milk to 16 oz/day (adults).
- Limit tea, coffee, and caffeinated beverages.
- Increase fluid and dietary fiber to decrease likelihood of constipation.
- Limit foods with high levels of chemicals (phytates and polyphenols).

PATIENT EDUCATION
- http://familydoctor.org/familydoctor/en/diseases-conditions/anemia.html
- http://patient.info/pdf/4392.pdf

PROGNOSIS
- IDA can be resolved with iron therapy if the underlying cause is discovered and appropriately treated.
- Treat coexisting subclinical hypothyroidism and IDA together. Failure to treat hypothyroidism results in poor response to iron therapy.

COMPLICATIONS
- Hidden bleeding, particularly a bleeding malignancy
- Ischemic events or heart failure, especially in elderly
- Poor growth, failure to thrive, developmental delay in children (2,4)

REFERENCES
1. Culleton BF, Manns BJ, Zhang J, et al. Impact of anemia on hospitalization and mortality in older adults. *Blood*. 2006;107(10):3841–3846.
2. Killip S, Bennett JM, Chambers MD. Iron deficiency anemia. *Am Fam Physician*. 2007;75(5):671–678.
3. McDonagh M, Cantor A, Bougatsos C, et al. *Routine Iron Supplementation and Screening for Iron Deficiency Anemia in Pregnant Women: A Systematic Review to Update the U.S. Preventive Services Task Force Recommendation. Evidence Syntheses, No. 123*. Rockville, MD: Agency for Healthcare Research and Quality (US); 2015.
4. Centers for Disease Control and Prevention. Iron deficiency—United States, 1999–2000. *MMWR Morb Mortal Wkly Rep*. 2002;51(40):897–899.
5. Camaschella C. Iron-deficiency anemia. *N Engl J Med*. 2015;372(19):1832–1843.
6. Short MW, Domagalski JE. Iron deficiency anemia: evaluation and management. *Am Fam Physician*. 2013;87(2):98–104.
7. Johnson-Wimbley TD, Graham DY. Diagnosis and management of iron deficiency anemia in the 21st century. *Therap Adv Gastroenterol*. 2011;4(3):177–184.
8. Recommendations to prevent and control iron deficiency in the United States. Centers for Disease Control and Prevention. *MMWR Recomm Rep*. 1998;47(RR-3):1–29.
9. Murphy MF, Wallington TB, Kelsey P, et al. Guidelines for the clinical use of red cell transfusions. *Br J Haematol*. 2001;113(1):24–31.
10. National Institutes of Health Office of Dietary Supplements. Dietary Supplement Fact Sheet: Iron

ADDITIONAL READING
- Chertow GM, Mason PD, Vaage-Nilsen O, et al. On the relative safety of parenteral iron formulations. *Nephrol Dial Transplant*. 2004;19(6):1571–1575.
- de Benoist B, McLean E, Egli I, et al, eds. *Worldwide Prevalence of Anaemia 1993–2005. WHO Global Database on Anaemia*. Geneva, Switzerland: World Health Organization; 2008. http://whqlibdoc.who.int/publications/2008/9789241596657_eng.pdf
- Dubois RW, Goodnough LT, Ershler WB, et al. Identification, diagnosis, and management of anemia in adult ambulatory patients treated by primary care physicians: evidence-based and consensus recommendations. *Curr Med Res Opin*. 2006;22(2):385–395.
- Mabry-Hernandez IR. Screening for iron deficiency anemia—including iron supplementation for children and pregnant women. *Am Fam Physician*. 2009;79(10):897–898.
- Murray-Kolb LE, Beard JL. Iron deficiency and child and maternal health. *Am J Clin Nutr*. 2009;89(3):946S–950S.
- Tefferi A, Hanson CA, Inwards DJ. How to interpret and pursue an abnormal complete blood cell count in adults. *Mayo Clin Proc*. 2005;80(7):923–936.
- World Health Organization. *Guideline: Intermittent Iron and Folic Acid Supplementation in Menstruating Women*. Geneva, Switzerland: World Health Organization; 2011.

 ## SEE ALSO

Algorithm: Anemia

CODES

ICD10
- D50.9 Iron deficiency anemia, unspecified
- D62 Acute posthemorrhagic anemia
- D50.0 Iron deficiency anemia secondary to blood loss (chronic)

CLINICAL PEARLS
- IDA due to poor dietary iron intake is the most common anemia.
- Blood loss and reduced iron stores due to malabsorption or poor utilization are major risk factors for IDA.
- Premenopausal women and children are at the greatest risk for IDA.
- Cow's milk should not be given to any child age <12 months.
- Oral iron supplementation is the standard treatment for IDA.

ANEMIA, SICKLE CELL
Tipsuda Junsanto-Bahri, MD

 BASICS

DESCRIPTION
- Hereditary, hemoglobinopathy marked by chronic hemolytic anemia, periodic acute episodes of painful "crises," and increased susceptibility to infections
- The heterozygous condition (Hb A/S), sickle cell trait, is usually asymptomatic without anemia.
- Synonym(s): sickle cell disease (SCD); Hb SS disease

Pediatric Considerations
- Sequestration crises and hand–foot syndrome seen typically in infants/young children
- Strokes occur mainly in childhood.
- Adolescence/young adulthood
  - Frequency of complications and organ/tissue damage increases with age
  - Psychological complications: body image, interrupted schooling, restriction of activities, stigma of disease, low self-esteem

Pregnancy Considerations
- Complicated, especially during 3rd trimester and delivery
  - Fetal mortality 35–40%. Fetal survival is >90% if the fetus reaches the 3rd trimester.
  - High prevalence of small for gestational age (SGA) babies
- Increased risk of thrombosis, preterm delivery, pain, toxemia, infection, pulmonary infarction, phlebitis
- Partial exchange transfusion in 3rd trimester may reduce maternal morbidity and fetal mortality, but this is controversial.
- Chronic transfusions have been effective in diminishing pain episodes in pregnant women. However, this method should be used with caution due to risk of alloimmunization.

EPIDEMIOLOGY
Prevalence
- ~90,000 Americans have sickle cell anemia (SCA) and 3.5 million people in the United States have sickle cell trait.
- The condition affects mainly people of African descent. Hispanic, Middle-eastern, and Asian Indian ancestry may also be affected.

ETIOLOGY AND PATHOPHYSIOLOGY
- Hemoglobin S results from the substitution of the amino acid valine for glutamic acid at the sixth position of the β-globin chain
- HbS polymerizes in the RBC in the deoxygenated state resulting in RBC sickling.
- Sickle RBCs are inflexible, causes increased blood viscosity, stasis, obstruction of small arterioles and capillaries, and ischemia.
- Chronic anemia; crises
  - Vaso-occlusive crisis: tissue ischemia and necrosis; progressive organ failure/tissue damage from repeated episodes
  - Hand–foot syndrome: Vessel occlusion/ischemia affects small blood vessels in hands or feet.
  - Aplastic crisis: suppression of RBC production by severe infection (e.g., parvoviral and other viral infections)
  - Suppression of RBC production
  - Hyperhemolytic crisis: accelerated hemolysis with reticulocytosis; increased RBC fragility/shortened lifespan
  - Sequestration crisis: splenic sequestration of blood (only in young children as spleen is later lost to autoinfarction)

- Susceptibility to infection: impaired/absent splenic function leading to decreased ability to clear infection; defect in alternate pathway of complement activation.
- Increased RBC destruction causes decreased hemoglobin levels and results in anemia and fatigue.
- Sickle cells exhibit increased adhesion and decreased ability to maneuver through small vessels, leading to vaso-occlusion.

Genetics
- Autosomal recessive. Homozygous condition, Hb SS; heterozygous condition, Hb A/S
- The heterozygote condition can also be combined with other hemoglobinopathies: sickle-hemoglobin C disease (HbSC) and Sβ+ thalassemia are clinically similar to the heterozygous condition, whereas, Sβ thalassemia is clinically similar to the homozygous condition.

RISK FACTORS
- Vaso-occlusive crisis ("painful crisis"): hypoxia, dehydration, fever, infection, acidosis, cold, anesthesia, strenuous physical exercise, smoking
- Aplastic crisis (suppression of RBC production): severe infections, human parvovirus B19 infection, folic acid deficiency
- Hyperhemolytic crisis (accelerated hemolysis with reticulocytosis): acute bacterial infections, exposure to oxidant

GENERAL PREVENTION
- Prevention of crises
  - Avoid hypoxia, dehydration, cold, infection, fever, acidosis, and anesthesia.
  - Prompt management of fever, infections, pain
  - Hydration
  - Avoid alcohol and smoking.
  - Avoid high-altitude areas.
- Minimizing trauma: Aseptic technique is imperative.

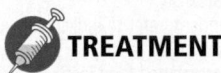 **DIAGNOSIS**

Diagnosis is often made by newborn screening programs.

HISTORY
- Often asymptomatic in early months of life due to presence of fetal hemoglobin
- In those >6 months of age, earliest symptoms are irritability and painful swelling of the hands and feet (hand–foot syndrome). May also see pneumococcal sepsis or meningitis, severe anemia and acute splenic enlargement (splenic sequestration), acute chest syndrome, pallor, jaundice, or splenomegaly.
- Manifestations in older children include anemia, severe or recurrent musculoskeletal or abdominal pain, aplastic crisis, acute chest syndrome, splenomegaly or splenic sequestration, and cholelithiasis.
- Painful crises in bones, joints, abdomen, back, and viscera account for 90% of all hospital admissions.
- Acute chest syndrome: tachycardia, fever, bilateral infiltrates caused by pulmonary infarctions

PHYSICAL EXAM
Fever, pale skin and nail beds, mild jaundice

DIFFERENTIAL DIAGNOSIS
Anemia: other hemoglobinopathies

DIAGNOSTIC TESTS & INTERPRETATION
Initial Tests (lab, imaging)
- Screening test: Sickledex test/Hb electrophoresis (diagnostic test of choice); SCA (FS pattern)
  - 80–100% Hb S, variable amounts of Hb F, and no Hb A1
  - Sickle cell trait (FS pattern): 30–45% Hb S, 50–70% Hb A1, minimal Hb F
- Hemoglobin ~5 to 10 g/dL; RBC indices: mean corpuscular volume (MCV) normal to increased; mean corpuscular hemoglobin concentration (MCHC) increased; reticulocytes 3–15%
- Leukocytosis; bands in absence of infection, platelets elevated; peripheral smear: sickled RBCs, nucleated RBCs, Howell-Jolly bodies
- Serum bilirubin mildly elevated (2 to 4 mg/dL); ferritin very elevated in multiply transfused patients; serum lactate dehydrogenase (LDH) elevated
- Fecal/urinary urobilinogen high
- Haptoglobin absent or very low
- Urine analysis: hemoglobinuria, hematuria (sickle cell trait may have painless hematuria), increased albuminuria (monitor for progressive kidney disease)
- Need for imaging depends on clinical circumstances
  - Bone scan to rule out osteomyelitis
  - CT/MRI to rule out CVA; high index of suspicion required for any acute neurologic symptoms other than mild headache.
  - Chest x-ray: may show enlarged heart; diffuse alveolar infiltrates in acute chest syndrome
  - Transcranial Doppler: start at age 2 years; repeat yearly. Transcranial Doppler ultrasound identifies children age 2 to 16 years at higher risk of stroke.
  - ECG to detect pulmonary hypertension and echocardiogram every other year from age 15 years and older.

Test Interpretation
Hyposplenism due to autosplenectomy is common; hypoxia/infarction in multiple organs

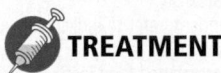 **TREATMENT**

GENERAL MEASURES
- Painful crises: hydration, analgesics; oxygen regardless of whether the patient is hypoxic (1)[A]
- Retinal evaluation starting at school age to detect proliferative sickle retinopathy (1,2)[A]

- Occupational therapy, cognitive and behavioral therapies, support groups
- All standard childhood vaccinations should be administered accordingly.
- Special immunizations
  - Influenza vaccine yearly
  - Conjugated pneumococcal vaccine (PCV13) at ages 2, 4, and 6 months; booster at 12 to 15 months.
  - Patients <5 years of age with incomplete vaccination history should receive catch-up doses accordingly.
  - Adults age ≥19 years who have functional asplenia and have not received pneumococcal vaccination should receive one dose PCV13, followed by administration of PPSV23 at least 8 weeks later (2)[A].

- Meningococcal vaccine:
  - 6 weeks old: Hib-MenCY at ages 2, 4, 6, and 12 months
  - 9 months old: two doses of MCV4 separated by 3 months
  - ≥2 years of age: two doses of MCV4-D-CRM separated by 2 months; boosters recommended every 5 years

MEDICATION

First Line

- Prophylactic penicillins indicated in infants and children starting at 2 months: A dose of 125 mg BID is recommended for children <5 years. A dose of 250 mg BID is recommended for children >5 years. Amoxicillin 20 mg/kg/day is an alternative to penicillin; if high risk remains, continue until puberty. Rising pneumococcal resistance to penicillin may change future recommendations (3)[A].
- Supplemental oxygen
- Painful crises (mild, outpatient)
  - Nonopioid analgesics (ibuprofen)
- Painful crises (severe, hospitalized)
  - Parenteral opioids (e.g., morphine on fixed schedule); patient-controlled analgesia (PCA) pump may be useful (2)[A].
- Hydroxyurea for prevention of painful acute chest syndrome, vaso-occlusive episodes, and very severe anemia. Increases fetal hemoglobin concentration. Adults: Start with 15 mg/kg/day single daily dose; Children: 20 mg/kg/day; titrate upward every 8 weeks (max dose of 35 mg/kg/day). Monitor blood counts satisfactory (avoid severe neutropenia, thrombocytopenia) (2)[A].
- Acute chest syndrome: may deteriorate quickly; monitor patients with vaso-occlusive crisis with incentive spirometry. Treat with aggressive management with oxygen, analgesics, antibiotics, simple or exchange transfusion (2)[A].
- Empiric antibiotics to cover *Mycoplasma pneumoniae*, and *Chlamydia pneumoniae* (cephalosporins or azithromycin) (1)[A]. If osteomyelitis, cover for *Staphylococcus aureus* and *Salmonella* (e.g., ciprofloxacin). Precautions: Avoid high-dose estrogen oral contraceptives; consider Depo-Provera. G-CSF use is contraindicated as it may lead to vaso-occlusive episodes and multiorgan failure.

Second Line

Folic acid: 0 to 6 months: 0.1 mg/day; 6 to 12 months: 0.25 mg/day; 1 to 2 years: 0.5 mg/day; >2 years of age: 1 mg/day

ADDITIONAL TREATMENT

Transfusions and additional therapies (4)[A]

- Transfusion for aplastic crises, severe complications (i.e., CVA), prophylactically before surgery, and treatment for acute chest syndrome; prophylactic transfusions for primary or secondary stroke prevention in children
- Preoperative transfusions have been shown to reduce the risk of perioperative complications.
- Avoid blood hyperviscosity.
- Consider chelation with deferasirox, an oral agent, if the patient is multiply transfused (after age 2 years). Red cell exchange transfusion minimizes risk of iron overload.

SURGERY/OTHER PROCEDURES

- Targeted fetal hemoglobin induction treatment (5)[A]
- Hematopoietic stem cell transplant (HSCT) (6)[A]: curative, but with significant morbidity and mortality; limited to individuals <16 years old.

INPATIENT CONSIDERATIONS

Admission Criteria/Initial Stabilization

Severe pain, suspected infection or sepsis, evidence of acute chest syndrome

IV Fluids

The preferred maintenance IV fluid is 1/2 NS, as NS may theoretically increase the risk of sickling.

 ONGOING CARE

FOLLOW-UP RECOMMENDATIONS

Patient Monitoring

- Treat infections early. Parents/patients: Any temperature of ≥101°F (38.3°C) requires immediate medical attention.
- For patients who receive chronic transfusions, monitor for hepatitis C and hemosiderosis.
- Periodic eye evaluations: starting age 10 years to detect proliferative sickle retinopathy; re-screen 1 to 2 year intervals (3)[A]
- Biannual examination for hepatic, renal, and pulmonary dysfunction
- Neuroimaging screening for risk of stroke: transcranial Doppler beginning at age 2 years and continuing up to age 16 years
- Baseline pulmonary evaluation at each visit to assess for wheezing, shortness of breath, or cough (indicators of disease severity and pulmonary hypertension). Echocardiography for symptomatic patients; right heart catheterization for diagnosis
- Consider venous thromboembolism (VTE) prophylaxis as there is an increased incidence of thromboembolism.

DIET

- Folic acid supplementation; avoid alcohol (leads to dehydration); maintain hydration
- Multivitamin without iron is recommended as there is high incidence of vitamin D deficiency and decreased bone marrow density in SCD patients.

PATIENT EDUCATION

- SickleCellKids.org—Education Web site for children with sickle cell anemia: http://www.sicklecelldisease.org
- American Sickle Cell Anemia Association: http://www.ascaa.org

PROGNOSIS

- Anemia occurs in infancy; sickle cell crises at 1 to 2 years of age; some children die in their first year.
- In adulthood, fewer crises, but more complications. Median age of death is 42 years for men and 48 years for women. Complications are mentioned below.

COMPLICATIONS

- Alloimmunization, bone infarct and osteomyelitis, aseptic necrosis of femoral head
- CVA (peak age 6 to 7 years), impaired mental development, even without history of stroke
- Cholelithiasis/abnormal liver function
- Chronic leg ulcers, poor wound healing
- Impotence, priapism, hematuria/hyposthenuria, renal complications (proteinuria)
- Retinopathy, splenic infarction (by age 10 years)
- Acute chest syndrome (infection/infarction) leading to chronic pulmonary disease
- Infections (pneumonia, osteomyelitis, meningitis, pyelonephritis); sepsis (leading cause of morbidity and mortality)
- Hemosiderosis (secondary to multiple transfusions)
- Substance abuse related to chronic opioid use

REFERENCES

1. Brousse V, Makani J, Rees DC. Management of sickle cell disease in the community. *BMJ*. 2014;348:g1765.
2. Yawn BP, Buchanan GR, Afenyi-Annan AN, et al. Management of sickle cell disease: summary of the 2014 evidence-based report by expert panel members. *JAMA*. 2014;312(10):1033–1048.
3. Cober MP, Phelps SJ. Penicillin prophylaxis in children with sickle cell disease. *J Pediatr Pharmacol Ther*. 2010;15(3):152–159.
4. Chou ST. Transfusion therapy for sickle cell disease: a balancing act. *Hematology Am Soc Hematol Educ Program*. 2013;2013:439–446.
5. Manwani D, Frenette PS. Vaso-occlusion in sickle cell disease: pathophysiology and novel targeted therapies. *Blood*. 2013;122(24):3892–3898.
6. Hsieh MM, Fitzhugh CD, Weitzel RP, et al. Non-myeloablative HLA-matched sibling allogeneic hematopoietic stem cell transplantation for severe sickle cell phenotype. *JAMA*. 2014;312(1):48–56.

ADDITIONAL READING

- Aragona E, Kelly MJ. Hyperhemolysis in sickle cell disease. *J Pediatr Hematol Oncol*. 2014;36(1):354–356. doi:10.1097/MPH.0b013e31828e529f.
- Costa VM, Viana MB, Aguiar RA. Pregnancy in patients with sickle cell disease: maternal and perinatal outcomes. *J Matern Fetal Neonatal Med*. 2015;28(6):685–689. doi:10.3109/14767058.2014.928855.
- Machado RF, Farber HW. Pulmonary hypertension associated with chronic hemolytic anemia and other blood disorders. *Clin Chest Med*. 2013;34(4):739–752.
- Naik RP, Streiff MB, Lanzkron S. Sickle cell disease and venous thromboembolism: what the anticoagulation expert needs to know. *J Thromb Thrombolysis*. 2013;35(3):352–358.

 SEE ALSO

Algorithm: Anemia

 CODES

ICD10

- D57.1 Sickle-cell disease without crisis
- D57.3 Sickle-cell trait
- D57.00 Hb-SS disease with crisis, unspecified

CLINICAL PEARLS

- Over 90,000 Americans have SCA (~1 in 375 African Americans). The preferred maintenance IV fluid is 1/2 NS, as NS may theoretically increase the risk of sickling.
- Painful crises in bones, joints, abdomen, back, and viscera account for 90% of all hospital admissions.
- Acute chest syndrome: tachycardia, fever, bilateral infiltrates caused by pulmonary infarctions

ANEURYSM OF THE ABDOMINAL AORTA

Michael J. Gray, MD, MA, MS, ATC

BASICS

DESCRIPTION
- An infrarenal aorta ≥3 cm in diameter is considered aneurysmal (1–5).
- Types
  - Fusiform aneurysm: involves the whole circumference or wall of the artery
  - Saccular aneurysm: does not involve the full circumference; often appears as an asymmetrical bleb or blister on side of aorta
- Clinical presentation relates to aneurysm location, size, type, and comorbid factors affecting patient. The majority are asymptomatic but may present with rupture, embolism, or thrombosis. Treatment and indications for surgical repair are dictated by risk of rupture, risk of surgical repair, and estimated patient life expectancy.
- Second most common disease to affect the aorta (5)
- System(s) affected: cardiovascular; neurologic; heme/lymphatic/immunologic
- Synonym(s): aortic aneurysms; AAA

Geriatric Considerations
Incidence of AAA, risk of rupture, and operative morbidity and mortality all rise with age.

Pediatric Considerations
Rare in children; may be associated with umbilical artery catheters, connective tissue diseases, arteritides, or congenital abnormalities

EPIDEMIOLOGY
- Frequency increases >50 years of age.
- Predominant sex: male > female (5:1) (1)

Incidence
- >15,000 deaths per year in United States
- 10th leading cause of death in men 65 to 75 years
- 3.9–7.2% males >50 years (3)
- 1.0–1.3% females >50 years (3)
- Females with 2 to 4 times increased risk of rupture (6)

Prevalence
- Depends on risk factors associated with AAA
- Prevalence of AAAs 2.9 to 4.9 cm in diameter ranges from 1.3% for men aged 45 to 54 years to 12.5% for men 75 to 84 years. Data for women are 0% and 5.2%, respectively; however, when detected, women presented at an older age and were more likely to present with a ruptured AAA. Female sex is an independent risk factor for *death* from AAA (2).

ETIOLOGY AND PATHOPHYSIOLOGY
- Vascular inflammatory degenerative disease, with major role of matrix metalloproteinases and inflammatory markers that result in aortic medial degeneration (4,6)
- Gradual and/or sporadic expansion of aneurysm and accumulation of mural thrombus (4)
- Mural thrombus can contribute to an area of localized hypoxia, thus, further weakening the aneurysm (4).
- Aneurysms tend to expand over time. (Laplace law: T [wall tension] = pressure × radius. Wall tension directly related to BP and radius of artery.) When wall tension exceeds wall tensile strength, rupture occurs (2,4).
- Average small AAA (<5.5 cm) grows at rate of 2.6 to 3.2 mm/year. Larger aneurysms grow faster rate as do aneurysms in current smokers; otherwise, no identifiable risk factors to assess which small AAAs will advance to require further intervention.
- Annual growth rate of 2.2 mm/year average for small aneurysms but increased in smokers; decreased in diabetics (4)

- 60–80% of AAAs between 40 and 49 mm will enlarge and require surgery in 5 years.
- Degenerative: atherosclerotic (80%); other causes: inflammatory diseases (5%), trauma, connective tissue disorders, infection (*Brucella, Salmonella, Staphylococcus*, tuberculosis)

Genetics
- Familial aggregations exist: Aneurysms may develop at an earlier age.
- 2 times risk of AAA if first-degree relative with AAA (1,2,6)
- 12–19% of patients with repair had first-degree relative with AAA (2).
- Marfan syndrome
- Ehlers-Danlos syndrome
- Polycystic kidney disease
- Tuberous sclerosis

RISK FACTORS
Older age, male, Northern European ethnicity, family history, smoking, hypertension (HTN), hyperlipidemia, peripheral vascular disease, peripheral aneurysms, chronic obstructive peripheral disease (COPD), obesity (2,4–6)

GENERAL PREVENTION
- Address cardiovascular disease risk factors.
- Follow screening guidelines: US screening for detection of AAA in male patients, 65 to 75 years, who have ever smoked.

COMMONLY ASSOCIATED CONDITIONS
- HTN, myocardial infarction (MI), heart failure, carotid artery, and/or lower extremity peripheral arterial disease
- Screening for thoracic aneurysm should also be considered.
- 20% of patients with AAA have concurrent thoracic aneurysm (5).

DIAGNOSIS

- Screening: recommended one-time US for AAA in men 65 to 75 years who have EVER smoked (3)[B], selective offer one-time US in men 65 to 75 years who have NEVER smoked (3)[C]
- U.S. Preventive Services Task Force recommends against routine screening for women who have NEVER smoked and states that there is insufficient evidence to make a recommendation for women 65 to 75 years old who have EVER smoked.
- Most often asymptomatic: discovered during exams for other complaints (1)
- Symptomatic: embolization, thrombosis, vague abdominal or back pain, syncope, lower extremity paralysis
- Rupture

ALERT
- The triad of shock, pulsatile mass, and abdominal pain always suggests rupture of AAA, and immediate surgical evaluation is recommended (2)[B].
  - Shock may be absent if rupture is contained.
  - Palpable pulsatile mass may be absent in up to 50% of patients with rupture.
  - Pain may radiate to the back, groin, flank (mimics urolithiasis), buttocks, or legs.
- Unusual presentations:
  - Primary aortoenteric fistula: erosion/rupture of AAA into duodenum
  - Aortocaval fistula: erosion/rupture of AAA into vena cava or left renal vein: 3–6%

- Inflammatory aneurysm: encasement by thick inflammatory rind; can cause chronic abdominal pain, weight loss, and elevated ESR. Surrounding viscera is densely adherent.

HISTORY
Abdominal or back pain; AAA risk factors

PHYSICAL EXAM
- Pulsatile supraumbilical mass
- Only 30–40% of AAA were detected by physical exam (6).
- Physical exam will only detect 76% of aneurysms >5 cm (6).
- 14% of AAA associated with femoral or popliteal aneurysms and 62–85% of patients with femoral or popliteal aneurysms will have an AAA (5,6); therefore, recommended AAA evaluation for all patients with known femoral or popliteal aneurysms (2)[B]
- Vague abdominal tenderness: may radiate to the back or flank
- Encroachment by aneurysm
  - Vertebral body erosion, gastric outlet obstruction, ureteral obstruction
  - Lower extremity ischemia secondary to embolization of mural thrombus
- Rupture leads to tachycardia, hypotension, evidence of shock and anemia, possible flank contusion (Grey-Turner sign) (6).

DIAGNOSTIC TESTS & INTERPRETATION
Initial Tests (lab, imaging)
- If rupturing AAA is considered: complete blood chemistry (chemistries, PT/INR, PTT, type and cross), ECG
- US: simplest and least expensive diagnostic procedure
- Multiple studies have demonstrated high sensitivity (94–100%) and specificity (98–100%) of US (3,6).
- Although effective in detecting AAA, US is a poor test to show leakage or rupture if bleeding is into the retroperitoneal space.
- Surveillance of asymptomatic aneurysm
  - 2.6 to 2.9 cm: Screen at 5-year intervals (6)[C].
  - 3.0 to 3.9 cm: Screen at 3-year intervals (2)[B],(6)[C].
  - 4.0 to 5.4 cm: Screen every 6 to 12 months (2)[A].
- CT scans are preferred preoperative study (caution with IV contrast in renal failure) (5).
- MRI/MRA can visualize AAA but is often not possible in emergent situations.
- Aortography does not define outer dimensions of aneurysm.
- Abdominal x-rays can be diagnostic if calcifications exist; not a diagnostic tool of choice (1,2)
- Ongoing research is exploring alternative diagnostic measurements, including measurement of total aortic volume versus single axial diameter measurement and measurement of total thrombus burden associated with AAA because this appears to have a greater risk association (2,4).

Follow-Up Tests & Special Considerations
- Evaluation for coronary artery disease is appropriate prior to elective AAA repair (i.e., cardiac clearance), including stress test, echocardiography, and ECG if appropriate (1).
- If AAA was discovered at any location, then full assessment of entire aorta including thoracic aorta and aortic valve is recommended (5)[C].
- Since AAA patients tend to have the same risk factor profile as coronary artery disease, general preventative cardiovascular disease measures should be initiated (5)[C].

Diagnostic Procedures/Other

ALERT
Use clinical judgment: Patients with known AAA having abdominal or back pain symptoms may be rupturing despite a negative CT scan.

DIFFERENTIAL DIAGNOSIS
• Other abdominal masses
• Other causes of abdominal or back pain (e.g., peptic ulcer disease, renal colic, diverticulitis, appendicitis, incarcerated hernia, bowel obstruction, GI hemorrhage, arthritis, metastatic disease, MI)

 TREATMENT

GENERAL MEASURES
• Treat atherosclerotic risk factors (2,5)[C].
• Medical optimization of cardiac, renal, and pulmonary conditions
• Smoking cessation (increased rate of expansion of 20–25% with continued smoking) and exercise (2)[B]
• Emergent treatment in unstable or symptomatic patients is immediate vascular surgery consultation, adequate IV access and resuscitation, type and cross for multiple units, and rapid bedside US.
• Less acute treatment of AAA/prevention of rupture is elective repair and risk factor modification.

MEDICATION
• β-Blockers should be used perioperatively in absence of contraindications (2,6)[A]; bronchodilators should be used for 2 weeks prior to repair for patients with COPD (6)[C].
• No medication has been proven to decrease the rate of growth or rupture (5).
• β-Blockers, statins, and aspirin may decrease risk of cardiovascular related mortality but no definitive decrease in AAA mortality (5).
• Doxycycline, previously theorized to decreased wall inflammation, has not been shown to have any effect on AAA (5).

SURGERY/OTHER PROCEDURES
Current recommendations
• Elective
  – 5.5-cm diameter is the threshold for repair in an "average" patient (2)[B].
  – Younger, low-risk patients with long life expectancy may prefer early repair.
  – Women or AAA with high risk of rupture: Consider elective repair at 4.5 to 5 cm.
  – Consider delayed repair in high-risk patients.
  – 5% perioperative mortality for open elective repair (2)
• High risk of rupture
  – Expansion >0.6 cm/year
  – Smoking/COPD severe/steroids
  – Family history; multiple relatives
  – Hypertension if poorly controlled
  – Shape is nonfusiform.
• High-risk patients for elective repair
  – Risk factors for open repair include age >70 years, COPD, chronic renal insufficiency (CRI), suprarenal clamp site, with 1-year mortality if no risk factors present of 1.2% and 67% for all four risk factors present.
  – Other poor prognostic factors include inactive/poor stamina, congestive heart failure, significant coronary artery disease, liver disease, family history of AAA.
  – Consider coronary revascularization prior to aneurysm repair if coronary artery disease (6)[B].

– Discontinue thienopyridine (clopidogrel and others); use 10 days prior to AAA repair, and restart immediately postoperatively (6)[C].
– Transfusion to hematocrit >28.0 if elective open repair was planned (6)[C]
• Emergent/symptomatic repair: traditionally, open repair; however, candidates with appropriate anatomy can have endovascular repair, with an estimated mortality of 32% for endovascular versus 44% open.
• Open repair versus endovascular repair (EVAR)
  – Open repair or EVAR in patients who are good or average surgical candidates (6)[B]
  – Open repair for patients who are unable to comply with the recommended periodic long-term surveillance (6)[B]
  – EVAR for patients at high surgical risk due to significant cardiac, pulmonary, or renal disease, but no significant mortality improvement compared with no therapy (6)[B]
  – EVAR tends to have improved procedural mortality (1.8% vs. 4.3%), but long-term mortality over 6 years is similar (7.5 deaths/patient-years for EVAR versus 7.7 deaths/patient-years for open repair), and EVAR patients require lifelong follow-up for monitoring (2,3).

INPATIENT CONSIDERATIONS
Risk of abdominal compartment syndrome after repair, 4–12%; usually associated with large fluid resuscitation

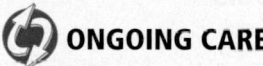 ONGOING CARE

FOLLOW-UP RECOMMENDATIONS
CT or MRI evaluation of the graft for EVAR surveillance at 1 month, 6 months, then annually (2)[B]

Patient Monitoring
BP and fasting lipid values: Control as for atherosclerotic disease (6)[C].

DIET
Low-fat, low-salt, and low-caffeine diet; nutrition optimized prior to elective repair; parenteral nutrition started within 7 days postoperatively if unable to have enteral feeds

PATIENT EDUCATION
Smoking cessation, aerobic exercise

PROGNOSIS
• Annual risk of rupture: (1)
  – <4-cm diameter: ~0% 4 to 4.9 cm: ~0.5–5%
  – 5 to 5.9 cm: ~3–15% 6 to 6.9 cm: ~10–20%
  – 7to 7.9 cm: ~20–40% >8 cm: 30–50%
• Patients with AAAs measuring ≥5.5 cm should undergo repair as should all patients with symptomatic AAA. Recommended routine surveillance at 1 year and every 5 years following repair (2).
• Only ~18% of patients with ruptured AAA survive.
• Despite a 5:1 ratio of AAA between males and females, women have higher AAA-associated mortality and morbidity, regardless of open or endovascular repair (2).
• 59–83% mortality if rupture occurs prior to hospitalization (3)

COMPLICATIONS
• Nonoperative: rupture, dissection, thromboembolization. Elective operative (conventional): death 2–8%, all cardiac 10–12% (MI 2–8%) (6)
• 5.1% of patients with EVAR repair required reintervention compared with 1.7 for open repair group.

• Pneumonia 5%, renal insufficiency 5–12%, bleeding 2–6%, DVT 5–8%, stroke 1–2%, rare <1% include graft thrombosis, graft infection, ureteral injury (6)

REFERENCES

1. Aggarwal S, Qamar A, Sharma V, et al. Abdominal aortic aneurysm: a comprehensive review. Exp Clin Cardiol. 2011;16(1):11–15.
2. Hirsch AT, Haskal ZJ, Hertzer NR, et al. ACC/AHA 2005 practice guidelines for the management of patients with peripheral arterial disease: a collaborative report. Circulation. 2006;113(1):e463–e654.
3. LeFevre ML. Screening for abdominal aortic aneurysm: U.S. Preventive Services Task Force recommendation statement. Ann Intern Med. 2014;161(4):281–290.
4. Moxon JV, Parr A, Emeto TI, et al. Diagnosis and monitoring of abdominal aortic aneurysm: current status and future prospects. Curr Probl Cardiol. 2010;35(10):512–548.
5. Erbel R, Aboyans V, Boileau C, et al. 2014 ESC Guidelines on the diagnosis and treatment of aortic diseases: document covering acute and chronic aortic diseases of the thoracic and abdominal aorta of the adult. The Task Force for the Diagnosis and Treatment of Aortic Diseases of the European Society of Cardiology (ESC). Eur Heart J. 2014;35(41):2873–2926.
6. Chaikof EL, Brewster DC, Dalman RL, et al. The care of patients with an abdominal aortic aneurysm: the Society for Vascular Surgery practice guidelines. J Vasc Surg. 2009;50(4 Suppl):S2–S49.

ADDITIONAL READING

• Rooke TW, Hirsch AT, Misra S, et al. 2011 ACCF/AHA focused update of the guideline for the management of patients with peripheral artery disease (updating the 2005 guideline): a report of the American College of Cardiology Foundation/American Heart Association Task Force on Practice Guidelines. J Am Coll Cardiol. 2011;58(19):2020–2045.
• Sweeting MJ, Thompson SG, Brown LC, et al. Meta-analysis of individual patient data to examine factors affecting growth and rupture of small abdominal aortic aneurysms. Br J Surg. 2012;99(5):655–665.

 SEE ALSO

Aortic Dissection; Ehlers-Danlos; Giant Cell Arteritis; Marfan Syndrome; Polyarteritis Nodosa; Turner Syndrome

 CODES

ICD10
• I71.4 Abdominal aortic aneurysm, without rupture
• I71.3 Abdominal aortic aneurysm, ruptured

CLINICAL PEARLS

• US is the procedure of choice for screening for AAA in any male >65 years with any history of tobacco use.
• Suspect AAA for any elderly patient with back, abdominal, or groin pain. Triad of hypotension/shock, pulsatile abdominal mass, and abdominal/back pain always suggests rupture, which requires emergent evaluation for surgery.
• 5.5 cm is the threshold diameter for elective surgical treatment (with some exceptions).

ANGIOEDEMA
Michelle T. Martin, PharmD, BCPS, BCACP • Jamie L. Berkes, MD

BASICS

DESCRIPTION
- Angioedema (AE) is an acute, localized swelling of skin, mucosa, and submucosa caused by extravasation of fluid into the affected tissues. It often resolves in hours to days, but it can be life-threatening if the upper airway is involved.
- Hereditary AE (HAE) and acquired AE (AAE) are diseases of the complement cascade that result in recurrent episodes of AE of the skin, upper airway, and GI tract.
- Synonym(s): angioneurotic edema; Quincke edema

EPIDEMIOLOGY
- Predominant age
  - Allergen, medication, or other triggers can affect all ages.
  - HAE: infancy to 2nd decade of life
  - AAE: Typically patients in 4th decade of life
- Predominant gender: male = female (except type III HAE, which affects more women than men)

Prevalence
- AE occurs in ~15% of the population over a lifetime.
- AE: 0.1–2.2% of patients receiving ACE inhibitors: African Americans have a four to five times greater risk of ACE inhibitor–induced AE than Caucasians.
- HAE: 1:10,000 to 50,000 population in the United States

ETIOLOGY AND PATHOPHYSIOLOGY
- Idiopathic
- Medication-induced
  - ACE inhibitors cause 10–25% of AE cases, mostly occurring within the 1st month of use. However, onset may be delayed by years.
  - Angiotensin-receptor blockers (ARBs) also can cause AE but more rarely than ACE inhibitors.
- Allergic triggers
  - Food allergens such as shellfish, nuts, eggs, milk, wheat, soy
  - Medications such as aspirin, NSAIDs, antibiotics, narcotics, and oral contraceptives
  - Latex, venom
- Physically induced: cold, heat, pressure, vibration, trauma, emotional stress, ultraviolet light
- Hereditary or acquired C1 INH deficiency
- Thyroid autoimmune disease–associated AE
- Type I hypersensitivity reaction
- Increase in vascular permeability secondary to IgE-mediated mast cell–stimulated histamine release or from activation of the complement system and an elevation in bradykinin (HAE)
- Attacks of HAE are triggered by prolonged mechanical pressure, cold, heat, trauma, emotional stress, menses, illness, and inflammation:
  - Type I HAE, the most common form, caused by decreased production of C1 esterase inhibitor (C1 INH), has autosomal dominant inheritance.
  - Type II HAE has functionally impaired C1 INH and autosomal dominant inheritance.
  - Type III (HAE-FXII) involves mutations in coagulation factor XII gene (occurs more frequently in women, often estrogen dependent, associated with estrogen administration); also, type III HAE-unknown exists.
- AAE is a rare condition:
  - Type I is associated with lymphoproliferative diseases or paraneoplastic diseases.
  - Type II is due to autoimmune disorders (anti-C1 INH antibody).
  - Affected patients have circulating antibodies directed either against specific immunoglobulins expressed on B cells (type I) or against C1 INH (type II).
  - AAE typically presents later in life (>40 years), and patients lack family history of AE.

Genetics
- HAE types I and II are autosomal dominant, whereas type III is dominant X-linked.
- HAE occurs in 25% of patients as a result of spontaneous genetic mutations.

RISK FACTORS
- Consuming medications and foods that can cause allergic reactions
- Preexisting diagnosis of HAE or AAE

GENERAL PREVENTION
- Avoid known triggers.
- Do not use ACE inhibitors in patients with C1 INH deficiency.

COMMONLY ASSOCIATED CONDITIONS
- Quincke disease (AE of the uvula)
- Urticaria

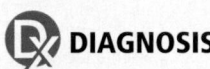

DIAGNOSIS

HISTORY
- Identify potential triggers, including medication history, recent exposure to allergens, physical elements, or trauma.
- In comparison with urticaria, AE typically is nonpruritic, but it can cause a burning sensation.
- Family history

PHYSICAL EXAM
- Acute onset of asymmetric localized swelling, usually of the face (eyelids, lips, ears, nose), tongue, larynx, and, less often, of the extremities or genitalia
- GI tract involvement may manifest as intermittent unexplained abdominal pain.

ALERT
10–35% of patients present with severe respiratory compromise requiring endotracheal intubation.

DIFFERENTIAL DIAGNOSIS
Urticaria (with AE in 40–50% of patients); allergic contact dermatitis; connective tissue disease: lupus, dermatomyositis; anaphylaxis; cellulitis; erysipelas; lymphedema; diffuse SC infiltrative process

DIAGNOSTIC TESTS & INTERPRETATION
Initial Tests (lab, imaging)
- If AE with urticaria and/or anaphylaxis, check for allergen-specific IgE to verify suspected trigger. Serum tryptase is elevated during acute AE (1)[C].
- Without a clear etiology and recurrence in AE and urticaria, check CBC and ESR:
  - Macrocytosis implies a pernicious anemia.
  - Eosinophilia may imply atopy or, rarely, a parasitic infection.
  - Elevated ESR may imply systemic disorders (1)[C].
- In recurrent AE without a clear etiology and without urticaria, consider ordering serum C4 level:
  - Low serum C4 is a sensitive but nonspecific screening test for hereditary and acquired C1 INH deficiency.
  - If C4 is normal, determine C1 INH level and function and recheck C4 during an acute attack.
  - If C4 level and C1 INH level and function are still normal, consider other causes (i.e., medications or HAE type III) for AE (2)[C].
  - If C4 level, C1 INH level, and C1 INH function are low, this indicates HAE type I.
  - HAE type II is characterized by low C4 and low C1 INH function, but C1 INH level can be normal or elevated (2)[C].
- C1q is decreased in ~75% of AAE but is usually normal in all types of HAE (2)[C].
- Abdominal radiographs and CT scan can demonstrate GI AE or ileus.
- C1 INH deficiency may occur in association with internal malignancy, so AE rarely can be a paraneoplastic disease. Imaging (CT scan, radiography, etc.) then would be done as part of a neoplastic workup for patients with AAE.

Follow-Up Tests & Special Considerations
If C4 and C1q are low (as in AAE), neoplastic and autoimmune workup is warranted. CBC, a peripheral smear, protein electrophoresis, immunophenotyping of lymphocytes, and imaging studies are often undertaken to rule out hematologic malignancies or cancer (1)[C].

Diagnostic Procedures/Other
Skin biopsy (may be nonspecific)

Test Interpretation
- Edema of deep dermis and SC tissue
- Variable perivascular and interstitial infiltrate

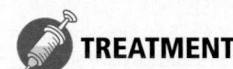

TREATMENT

GENERAL MEASURES
Intubation if airway is threatened

MEDICATION
First Line
- Acute allergic AE (with airway compromise)
  - Epinephrine 1:1,000; 0.3 mL IV or SC (1)[C]
  - Glucocorticoids (hydrocortisone 200 mg IV or Solu-Medrol 40 mg IV) (1)[C]
  - Diphenhydramine 50 mg IV
  - If medication induced, stop the causative agent.
- Idiopathic recurrent AE
  - 1st-generation antihistamines for acute AE (cause drowsiness)
  - Older children and adults: hydroxyzine (Vistaril) 5 mg/5 mL, 25-mg tablets 10 to 25 mg TID, or diphenhydramine (Benadryl) 25 to 50 mg q6h (3)[C]
  - Children <6 years of age: diphenhydramine 12.5 mg (elixir) q6–8h (5 mg/kg/day) (2)[C]
  - 2nd-generation H1 blockers: fexofenadine (Allegra) 180 mg/day BID, cetirizine (Zyrtec) 10 mg/day, desloratadine (Clarinex) 5 mg/day (3)[C]; use with caution in pregnancy and in the elderly.

- HAE chronic prophylaxis
  - A nanofiltered plasma-derived C1 INH (pdC1 INH) concentrate (Cinryze) dosed at 1,000 units/10 mL IV, rate of 1 mL/min (for 10 min) q3–4d. Administration setting options include clinic, home health care, and after proper training, home self-administration; risk of thromboembolic events (4)[C],(5)[B].
  - Attenuated androgens increase hepatic production of C1 INH: oral danazol 50 to 200 mg/day or oral stanozolol 2 mg/day; use lowest effective dose. Side effects include, but are not limited to, headache, weight gain, liver dysfunction, hirsutism, and menstrual disturbances. Monitor CBC, liver function tests, creatinine kinase, lactic dehydrogenase, fasting lipid profile, and urinalysis at baseline and q6mo. Abdominal US to be performed annually or q6mo if dose of danazol >200 mg/day. Danazol is not to be used in children, during the first 2 trimesters of pregnancy, during lactation, and in patients with hepatitis or cancer (2)[C].
- HAE short-term prophylaxis
  - Minor procedures (dental work): If C1 INH is available, no prophylaxis; otherwise, danazol 2.5 to 10 mg/kg/day (max 600 mg/day) and stanozolol 4 to 6 mg/day for 5 days prior to and 2 to 5 days after event (2)[C].
  - Major procedures (including intubation): C1 INH 1 (max 6) hour prior with additional dose on hand during procedure. If unavailable, danazol 2.5 to 10 mg/kg/day (max 600 mg/day) and solvent/detergent-treated plasma (SDP). If SDP unavailable, use fresh frozen plasma (FFP) 10 mL/kg; 2 to 4 units (400 to 800 mL) for an adult 1 to 6 hours prior
- Acute HAE treatment
  - C1 INH concentrate IV, dosed at 1,000 units if <50 kg; 1,500 units if 50 to 100 kg; 2,000 units if >100 kg (2)[C]
  - Recombinant human C1 INH isolated from the milk of transgenic rabbits (Ruconest—formerly Rhucin) was approved for acute HAE attacks. Trained patients may self-administer 50 IU/kg if <84 kg and 4,200 IU if ≥84 kg IV over 5 minutes. No more than two doses may be administered over 24 hours. Headache, nausea, and diarrhea may occur; and thromboembolic events or anaphylaxis are possible (6)[C].
  - Pasteurized human pdC1 INH (Berinert), dosed at 20 units/kg (available in 500 units/10 mL, max infusion rate of 4 mL/min IV via peripheral vein (4,7)[B]; DO NOT SHAKE (will denature the protein). Worsening of HAE pain was reported as the most severe adverse event.
  - Ecallantide (Kalbitor), a kallikrein inhibitor, is dosed in patients aged ≥16 years at 30 mg SC with three separate 10 mg/mL injections in the abdomen, thigh, or upper arm, and a second 30-mg dose may be repeated within 24 hours if needed (4,8)[B]. Injection-site rotation is not necessary but must be 2 inches away from attack site. A black box warning of anaphylaxis (potential adverse event) mandates administration in health care setting.
  - Icatibant (Firazyr), a bradykinin receptor-2 antagonist, is dosed at 30 mg SC over at least 30 seconds in the abdomen in patients aged ≥18 years and supplied in a prefilled 10 mg/mL

(3 mL) syringe for home administration. Subsequent doses of 30 mg may be repeated in 6-hour intervals (max 90 mg/24 hours) (4)[C],(9)[B].
  - Antihistamines and glucocorticoids typically do not benefit patients with HAE. Epinephrine can offer transient stabilization/improvement in laryngeal AE but is not sufficient for full treatment and does not alter the course of attack.
- Therapy under investigation for acute HAE treatment:
  - Cinryze has been studied for use during acute attacks (4)[C].
- Acute AAE treatment
  - C1 INH concentrate and FFP
  - Treatment of underlying lymphoproliferative disease is often curative in AAE type I.
  - Immunosuppressive therapy to suppress antibody production

Second Line
- HAE chronic prophylaxis: If pdC1 INH is unavailable and if patient cannot tolerate attenuated androgens, antifibrinolytic agents (plasmin inhibitors) such as tranexamic acid (not approved by the FDA in United States) 25 to 50 mg/kg/day divided BID or TID (3 to 6 g/day max) or ε-aminocaproic acid could be used. They are less effective than attenuated androgens and have many side effects. On rare occasions, they have been linked to (but not proven to cause) thrombophlebitis, embolism, or myositis (2)[C].
- Acute HAE: FFP if C1 INH concentrate is not available, but it can potentially worsen attack.
- Idiopathic AE: Oral doxepin (Sinequan) may be effective for AE (10 to 25 mg at bedtime).
- H2RA: Oral ranitidine (Zantac) 150 mg/day BID

SURGERY/OTHER PROCEDURES
Tracheostomy if progressive laryngeal edema prevents endotracheal intubation

INPATIENT CONSIDERATIONS
Admission Criteria
Ensure patent airway. If anaphylaxis, epinephrine (1:1,000) SC 0.3 to 0.5 mg q10–15min

IV Fluids
Given if needed to stabilize patient

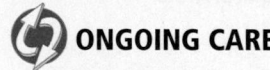 **ONGOING CARE**

FOLLOW-UP RECOMMENDATIONS
Patient Monitoring
- Diagnostic workup if symptoms are severe, persistent, or recurrent
- Protect airway if mouth, tongue, or throat is involved

DIET
Avoid known dietary allergens.

PATIENT EDUCATION
Educate on avoidance of triggers (i.e., food, medication, other physical stimuli), types of treatment, when to seek emergency care, and wearing Medic Alert bracelet.

PROGNOSIS
- AE symptoms often resolve in hours to 2 to 4 days. If airway is compromised, AE can be life-threatening.
- Patients with HAE have an average of 20 attacks/year; each may last 3 to 5 days. Prophylaxis can decrease the frequency of events and number of missed days of school or work.

COMPLICATIONS
Anaphylaxis

REFERENCES
1. Temiño VM, Peebles RS Jr. The spectrum and treatment of angioedema. *Am J Med*. 2008;121(4):282–286.
2. Zuraw BL, Bernstein JA, Lang DM, et al. A focused parameter update: hereditary angioedema, acquired C1 inhibitor deficiency, and angiotensin-converting enzyme inhibitor-associated angioedema. *J Allergy Clin Immunol*. 2013;131(6):1491–1493.
3. Frigas E, Park M. Idiopathic recurrent angioedema. *Immunol Allergy Clin North Am*. 2006;26(4):739–751.
4. Altman KA, Naimi DR. Hereditary angioedema: a brief review of new developments. *Curr Med Res Opin*. 2014;30(5):923–930.
5. Zuraw BL, Busse PJ, White M, et al. Nanofiltered C1 inhibitor concentrate for treatment of hereditary angioedema. *N Engl J Med*. 2010;363(6):513–522.
6. Riedl MA, Bernstein JA, Li H, et al. Recombinant human C1-esterase inhibitor relieves symptoms of hereditary angioedema attacks: phase 3, randomized, placebo-controlled trial. *Ann Allergy Asthma Immunol*. 2014;112(2):163.e1–169.e1.
7. Craig TJ, Levy RJ, Wasserman RL, et al. Efficacy of human C1 esterase inhibitor concentrate compared with placebo in acute hereditary angioedema attacks. *J Allergy Clin Immunol*. 2009;124(4):801–808.
8. Cicardi M, Levy RJ, McNeil DL, et al. Ecallantide for the treatment of acute attacks in hereditary angioedema. *N Engl J Med*. 2010;363(6):523–531.
9. Lumry WR, Li HH, Levy RJ, et al. Randomized placebo-controlled trial of the bradykinin B$_2$ receptor antagonist icatibant for the treatment of acute attacks of hereditary angioedema: the FAST-3 trial. *Ann Allergy Asthma Immunol*. 2011;107(6):529–537.

 SEE ALSO

Urticaria; Anaphylaxis

 CODES

ICD10
- T78.3XXA Angioneurotic edema, initial encounter
- D84.1 Defects in the complement system

CLINICAL PEARLS
- AE is an acute, localized swelling of skin, mucosa, and submucosa caused by extravasation of fluid into the affected tissues. It often resolves in hours to days, but it can be life-threatening if the upper airway is involved.
- HAE and AAE are diseases of the complement cascade that result in recurrent episodes of AE of the skin, upper airway, and GI tract.
- Trigger identification and avoidance are key in the prevention of AE.
- Patients with a history of allergies and AE should be prescribed an epinephrine autoinjector.

ANKLE FRACTURES

Wendy Hin-Wing Wong, MD, MPH • Jeffrey P. Feden, MD, FACEP

BASICS

- Bones: tibia, fibula, talus
- Mortise: tibial plafond, medial and lateral malleolus
- Ligaments: syndesmotic, lateral collateral, and medial collateral (deltoid) ligament

DESCRIPTION

- Two common classification systems help describe fractures (but do not always predict fracture stability)
  - Danis-Weber system: based on level of the fibular fracture in relationship to the syndesmosis
    - Type A: below syndesmosis (of tibiofibular joint). Usually stable (30% of ankle fractures)
    - Type B (most common): at syndesmosis. Can be stable or unstable (63%)
    - Type C: above syndesmosis. Usually unstable (7%)
  - Lauge-Hansen (LH): based on foot position and direction of applied force relative to the tibia
    - Supination-adduction (SA)
    - Supination-external rotation (SER): most common, 40–75% of fractures
    - Pronation-abduction (PA)
    - Pronation-external rotation (PER)
- Stability-based classification
  - Stable
    - Isolated lateral malleolar fractures (Weber A/B) without talar shift and with negative stress test
    - Isolated nondisplaced medial malleolar fractures
  - Unstable
    - Bi- or trimalleolar fractures
    - High fibular fractures (Weber C) or lateral malleolar fracture with medial injury and positive stress test
    - Lateral malleolar fracture with talar shift/tilt (bimalleolar equivalent)
    - Displaced medial malleolar fractures
- Pilon fracture: tibial plafond fracture due to axial loading (unstable)
- Maisonneuve: fracture of proximal 1/3 of fibula associated with ankle fracture (unstable); high risk of peroneal nerve injury

Pediatric Considerations

- Ankle fractures are more common than sprains in children compared to adults because ligaments are stronger than physis.
- Talar dome: osteochondral fracture of talar dome; suspect in child with nonhealing ankle "sprain" or recurrent effusions
- Tillaux: isolated Salter-Harris III of distal tibia with growth plate involvement
- Triplane fracture: Salter-Harris IV with fracture lines oriented in multiple planes: 2-, 3-, and 4-part variants

EPIDEMIOLOGY

- Ankle fractures are responsible for 9% of all adult and 5% of all pediatric fractures
- Peak incidence: females 45 to 64 years; males 8 to 15 years. Average is 46 years.

Incidence

- 107 to 184 per 100,000 people per year
- 3-fold increase in incidence predicted 2000 to 2030 in adults >60 years old

ETIOLOGY AND PATHOPHYSIOLOGY

- Most common: falls (38%), inversion injury (32%), sports-related (10%)
- Plantar flexion (joint less stable in this position)
- Axial loading: tibial plafond or pilon fracture

RISK FACTORS

- Age, fall, fracture history, polypharmacy, intoxication
- Obesity, sedentary lifestyle
- Sports, physical activity
- History of smoking or diabetes
- Alcohol or slippery surfaces

GENERAL PREVENTION

- Nonslip, flat, protective shoes
- Fall precautions in elderly

COMMONLY ASSOCIATED CONDITIONS

- Most ankle fractures are isolated injuries, but 5% have associated fractures, usually in ipsilateral lower limb.
- Ligamentous or cartilage injury (sprains)
- Ankle or subtalar dislocation
- Other axial loading or shearing injuries (i.e., vertebral compression or contralateral pelvic fractures)

DIAGNOSIS

HISTORY

- Location of pain, timing, and mechanism of injury (key historical element is exact mechanism)
- Weight-bearing status after injury
- History of ankle injury or surgery
- Tetanus status
- Assess for safety and fall risk (especially in elderly).

PHYSICAL EXAM

- Examine skin integrity (open vs. closed fracture).
- Assess point of maximal tenderness.
- Assess neurovascular status, pulses, motor/sensory exam, and ability to bear weight.
- Evaluate for compartment syndrome.
- Consider associated injuries (secondary survey).
- Assess ankle stability: anterior drawer test for the anterior talofibular ligament (ATFL), talar tilt test for lateral and medial ligaments, squeeze test and external rotation stress test for the tibiofibular syndesmosis

DIFFERENTIAL DIAGNOSIS

- Ankle sprain
- Other fractures: talus, 5th metatarsal, calcaneus

DIAGNOSTIC TESTS & INTERPRETATION

- Plain films: first line for suspected fractures (1)[A]
- Ottawa Ankle Rules (OAR): Overall sensitivity of 98% in adults, increases to 99.6% if applied within the first 48 hours after trauma (2)[A].

- OAR suggest films in patients aged 18 to 55 years if:
  - Tenderness at the posterior edge or tip of the medial malleolus, OR
  - Tenderness at the posterior edge or tip of the lateral malleolus, OR
  - Inability to bear weight both immediately and in the ED for four steps, OR
  - Tenderness at navicular or 5th metatarsal (Ottawa Foot Rules)
- If symptoms persist past 48 to 72 hours, obtain x-rays.
- In children >1 year old, OAR sensitivity is 98.5%.
- OAR not valid for intoxicated patients, those with multiple injuries, or sensory deficits (neuropathy)
- Three standard views
  - Anteroposterior (AP)
  - Lateral: talar dome/distal tibia incongruity indicate instability

- Mortise (15- to 25-degree internal rotation view): symmetry of mortise; space between the medial malleolus and talus should be ≤4 mm
- Additional stress view may demonstrate instability: increased medial clear space with manual external rotation

Pediatric Considerations

- Consider tenderness over distal fibula with normal films as Salter-Harris I.
- Stress views unnecessary in children and may cause physeal damage (3)[C].
- Salter-Harris V often missed, diagnosed when leg length discrepancy or angular deformity after Salter-Harris I; rare, 1% of fractures (3)[C]

Follow-Up Tests & Special Considerations

- CT recommended for operative planning in trimalleolar, Tillaux, triplane, pilon fractures, or fractures with intra-articular involvement (1)[A].

- MRI not routinely indicated; does not increase sensitivity for detecting complex ankle fractures (4)[C]
  - MRI useful for chronic instability, osteochondral lesions, occult fractures, and unexpected stiffness in children

Diagnostic Procedures/Other

- Ultrasound for soft tissue injury associated with displaced fractures (1)[A]

- Bone scan or MRI for stress fracture

TREATMENT

GENERAL MEASURES

- Immobilize in temporary cast/splint and protect with crutches/nonweight bearing
  - 1 to 2 weeks to allow decreased swelling, if not open or irreducible fracture (5)[C]

- Ice and elevate the extremity; pain due to swelling best controlled with elevation (6)[A]
  - Compression stockings offer no benefit for swelling (7)[A].

- Closed ankle fractures: stable versus unstable

  - Stable = nonoperative (1)[A]

  - Unstable = surgery
  - Lateral shift of talus ≥2 mm or displacement of either malleolus by 2 to 3 mm = surgery (5)[C]

  - In adults with displaced fractures: insufficient evidence if surgery or nonoperative management produces superior long-term outcomes (8)[A]

- Stable syndesmosis injury = nonoperative
- Fracture dislocations: urgent reduction
  - Do not wait for imaging if neurovascular compromise or obvious deformity.
  - Flex hip and knee 90 degrees for easier reduction.
  - Post reduction: neurovascular exam and x-rays

MEDICATION

First Line

- NSAIDs and/or acetaminophen for pain (1)[A]
- Initial IM pain injection (i.e., Ketorolac, ≥50 kg adult: 60 mg or 30 mg q6h, max 120 mg daily; children 2 to 16 years old, <50 kg or ≥ age 65 years: 1 mg/kg, 30 mg, or 15 mg q6h, max 60 mg daily) (6)[A]

- For suspected open fractures: tetanus booster, broad-spectrum cephalosporin and aminoglycoside within 3 hours post injury (5)[C]
- Intra-articular or hematoma block (1)[A]

Second Line
Opioid analgesics as adjunctive therapy (1)[A]

ISSUES FOR REFERRAL
- Consultation for neurovascular compromise, tenting of skin or open fracture, displaced or unstable fracture, compartment syndrome
- All other fractures: follow-up within 1 week and remain nonweight bearing. Consult orthopedics if not comfortable with routine fracture management.

ADDITIONAL THERAPIES
- Nonoperative = cast immobilization

  - No difference in type of immobilization (air-stirrup, cast, orthosis) (7)[A]
  - Initially nonweight bearing with crutches, then advance to 50% with crutches. Full weight bearing after 6 weeks post injury (6)[A]
  - If removable cast, gentle range of motion exercises at 4 weeks (6)[A]

- Open ankle fractures (2%)
  - Remove gross debris/contamination in ED.
  - Duration of optimal antibiotic therapy controversial
  - Surgical emergency, best if repaired within 24 hours

SURGERY/OTHER PROCEDURES
- Surgical options
  - Open reduction internal fixation (ORIF); preferred in athletes and unstable fractures
  - External fixation may be preferred in extreme tissue injury or comminuted fractures; may have more malunion compared to ORIF, but no difference in wound complications
- Timing of surgery
  - Immediately if neurovascular compromise, open fracture, unsuccessful reduction, tissue necrosis (5)[C]
  - Otherwise delay >5 days post injury because inflammation can affect wound healing (5)[C].
- Length of recovery: usually 6 to 8 weeks

Pediatric Considerations
- Salter-Harris I and II = nonoperative
  - Distal tibia: long leg cast for 4 to 6 weeks, then short leg cast for 2 to 3 weeks (4)[C]
  - Distal fibula: posterior splint or ankle brace 3 to 4 weeks, weight bearing. If displaced, then short leg cast 4 to 6 weeks, nonweight bearing (4)[C]
  - Limit reduction attempts because of potential injury to growth plate (3,4)[C].
  - Reduction not recommended if presenting ≥1 week post injury (4)[C]
  - Intra-articular displacement of ≥2 mm in child with >2 years growth remaining = ORIF (3)[C]
- Salter-Harris III and IV:
  - Distal tibia: if >2 mm displacement = ORIF (3)[C]
  - Distal fibula: rare, usually stable after tibial reduction (3)[C]
  - Tillaux and triplane: ORIF if displaced ≥2 mm (3,4)[C]

Geriatric Considerations
- Higher surgical risk due to age/comorbidities
- Osteoporosis increases risk of implant/fixation failure (8)[A].
- Risks from surgery/anesthesia: wound healing problems, pulmonary embolism, mortality, amputation, reoperation

INPATIENT CONSIDERATIONS
Admission Criteria/Initial Stabilization
Admit if:
- Emergency surgery required
- Patient nonadherent, lacks social support, unable to maintain non–weight-bearing status or has significant associated injuries
- Concerning mechanism of injury (i.e., syncope, myocardial infarction, head injury)

Nursing
Nonweight bearing, maintain splint/cast, apply ice, keep leg elevated, pain control, assist in ADLs

Discharge Criteria
- Ambulates with walker or crutches
- Medical workup (if needed) completed
- Orthopedic follow-up arranged

 ONGOING CARE

FOLLOW-UP RECOMMENDATIONS
Patient Monitoring
- Orthopedic follow-up: serial x-rays
  - In children, sclerotic lines on x-ray (Parker-Harris growth arrest lines) indicate growth disturbance (4)[C].
- Immobilize for 4 to 6 weeks, then progressive activity, weight bearing, with removable splint or boot (7)[A]
- Physical therapy referral: no difference in outcomes between stretching, manual therapy, exercise program (7)[A]

DIET
NPO if surgery is being considered.

PATIENT EDUCATION
- Ice and elevate for 2 to 3 weeks, use crutches/cane as instructed, splint/cast care (avoid getting wet, etc.)
- Notify physician if swelling increases, paresthesias, pain, or change in color of extremity

PROGNOSIS
- Good results can be achieved without surgery if fracture is stable.
  - Most return to activity within 3 to 4 months
- Most athletes return to preinjury activity levels.
- Increasing age, NOT injury severity, associated with worsening mobility after fracture (9)[B]

COMPLICATIONS
- Displaced fracture or instability
- Delayed union, malunion, or nonunion (0.9–1.9%)
- Postsurgical wound problems: loss of fixation, further surgery, amputation
- Deep venous thrombosis

- Complex regional pain syndrome, extensor retinaculum syndrome in children (4)[C]
- Infection (osteomyelitis)
- Posttraumatic arthritis, degenerative joint disease, growth arrest in children

REFERENCES

1. Ankle and foot disorders. In: Hegmann KT, ed. *Occupational Medicine Practice Guidelines. Evaluation and Management of Common Health Problems and Functional Recovery in Workers.* 3rd ed. Elk Grove Village, IL: American College of Occupational and Environmental Medicine; 2011:1–268. http://www.guideline.gov/content.aspx?id=36625&search=%22ankle+fractures%22. Accessed June 9, 2015.
2. Polzer H, Kanz KG, Prall WC, et al. Diagnosis and treatment of acute ankle injuries: development of an evidence-based algorithm. *Orthop Rev (Pavia).* 2012;4(1):e5.
3. Kay RM, Matthys GA. Pediatric ankle fractures: evaluation and treatment. *J Am Acad Orthop Surg.* 2001;9(4):268–278.
4. Parrino A, Lee MC. Ankle fractures in children. *Curr Orthop Pract.* 2013;24:617–624.
5. Mandi DM. Ankle fractures. *Clin Podiatr Med Surg.* 2012;29(2):155–186.
6. Work Loss Data Institute. *Ankle & Foot (Acute & Chronic).* Encinitas, CA: Work Loss Data Institute; 2013. http://www.guideline.gov/content.aspx?id=47571&search=ankle+fracture. Accessed June 18, 2015.
7. Lin CW, Donker NA, Refshauge KM, et al. Rehabilitation for ankle fractures in adults. *Cochrane Database Syst Rev.* 2012;(11):CD005595.
8. Donken CC, Al-Khateeb H, Verhofstad MH, et al. Surgical versus conservative interventions for treating ankle fractures in adults. *Cochrane Database Syst Rev.* 2012;(8):CD008470.
9. Keene D, James G, Lamb SE, et al. Factors associated with mobility outcomes in older people post-ankle fracture: an observational cohort study focusing on peripheral vessel function. *Injury.* 2013;44(7):987–993.

 CODES

ICD10
- S82.899A Oth fracture of unsp lower leg, init for clos fx
- S82.899B Oth fracture of unsp lower leg, init for opn fx type I/2
- S82.56XA Nondisp fx of medial malleolus of unsp tibia, init

CLINICAL PEARLS
- OAR are nearly 100% sensitive in determining the need for x-rays.
- Assess neurovascular status, ability to bear weight, associated injuries.
- Assess joint above (Maisonneuve).
- Normal x-rays with point tenderness indicate Salter-Harris type I fractures in children.

ANKYLOSING SPONDYLITIS

Damon F. Lee, MD

 BASICS

DESCRIPTION
- Ankylosing spondylitis (AS) is an axial inflammatory spondyloarthropathy (axSpA) characterized by radiologic evidence of sacroiliitis.
- System(s) affected: musculoskeletal; eyes; cardiac; neurologic; pulmonary
- Synonym(s): Marie–Strümpell disease; "bamboo spine"

EPIDEMIOLOGY
- Onset usually in early 20s; rarely occurs after age 40
- Male > female (approximately 2 to 3:1)

Incidence
Age- and gender-adjusted rate of 6.3 to 7.3/100,000 person-years

Prevalence
~0.55% for AS and ~1.4% for all axSpA in the United States (1)

ETIOLOGY AND PATHOPHYSIOLOGY
- Autoinflammation at sites of bacterial exposure (e.g., intestines) or mechanical stress in genetically susceptible individuals (2)
- Inflammation at the insertion of tendons, ligaments, and fasciae to bone (enthesopathy) causes erosion, remodeling, and new bone formation
- Inflammation-independent pathways of bony changes have also been hypothesized (2).

Genetics
- 80–90% of patients with AS are HLA-B27–positive.
- Other genetic associations include endoplasmic reticulum aminopeptidase 1 (ERAP1), interleukin 23 receptor (IL23R), and gene deserts on chromosome 2p15 and 21q22 (2).

RISK FACTORS
- HLA-B27
  - 1–8% of HLA-B27–positive adults have AS.
- Positive family history
  - HLA-B27–positive child of a parent with AS has a 10–30% risk of developing the disease.

COMMONLY ASSOCIATED CONDITIONS
- Uveitis/iritis (up to 40%)
- Enthesopathy: Achilles tendonitis, plantar fasciitis
- Dactylitis (sausage digit) from oligoarthritis
- Peripheral spondyloarthritis (SpA): psoriatic arthritis, reactive arthritis, inflammatory bowel disease (IBD)-related arthritis, juvenile idiopathic arthritis
- Aortitis and cardiac conduction defects

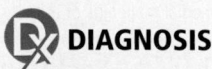 **DIAGNOSIS**

HISTORY
- Inflammatory back pain
  - Insidious onset
  - Duration >3 months
  - Morning stiffness in spine lasting >1 hour
  - Night time awakenings secondary to back pain
  - Pain and stiffness increase at rest and improve with activity
- Alternating buttock/hip pain is common.
- Constitutional symptoms (fatigue, weight loss, low-grade fever) are common.
- Inspirational chest pain due to enthesitis at costochondral junction and diminished chest wall expansion

- Other symptoms associated with enthesopathy (Achilles pain, plantar fascia pain); dactylitis (oligoarthritis); iritis (painful red eye, photophobia, vision changes)

PHYSICAL EXAM
- Sacroiliac joint tenderness, loss of lumbar lordosis, and cervical spine rotation
- Diminished range of motion in the lumbar spine in all three planes of motion
- Modified Wright-Schober test for lumbar spine flexion:
  - Mark patient's back over the L5 spinous process (or at dimples of Venus) and measure 10 cm above and 5 cm below this point. Normal is at least 5 cm of expansion between these two marks on maximal forward flexion.
- Thoracocervical kyphosis (usually after at least 10 years of symptoms)
- Occiput–wall distance increased (distance between occiput and wall when standing with back flat against a vertical surface; zero is normal)
- Respiratory excursion of chest wall
  - Normal is >5 cm of maximal respiratory excursion of chest wall measured at 4th intercostal space; <2.5 cm is consistent with AS.
- Tenderness of insertional sites—Achilles, plantar fascia
- Peripheral oligoarthritis/dactylitis seen mostly with peripheral SpA
- Cauda equina syndrome rarely occurs in late disease.
- Extra-articular manifestations: uveitis, psoriasis, IBD
- Aortic regurgitation murmur (1%)

DIFFERENTIAL DIAGNOSIS
- Nonradiographic axSpA (features AS without x-ray evidence of sacroiliitis; MRI detects changes earlier than plain films); other SpA
- Osteoarthritis of the axial spine
- Diffuse idiopathic skeletal hyperostosis (DISH)
- Osteitis condensans ilii: benign sclerotic changes in the iliac portion of the SI joint after pregnancy
- Infectious arthritis or discitis, unilateral sacroiliitis: tuberculosis, brucellosis, bacterial infection (particularly in IV drug users)

DIAGNOSTIC TESTS & INTERPRETATION
- Up to 10% of Caucasian population and 4% of African American population are HLA-B27–positive. Genetic testing is not necessary as part of initial evaluation, particularly with a consistent history and exam.
- ESR and C-reactive protein (CRP) may be mildly elevated or normal; if high, correlates with disease activity and prognosis.
- Absence of rheumatoid factor
- Mild normochromic anemia (15%)
- Synovial fluid: mild leukocytosis
- SI joints: Oblique projection is preferred.
  - X-ray changes may not be apparent for up to 10 years after disease onset. MRI is more sensitive; increased signal from the bone and bone marrow suggests osteitis and edema.
  - Sequential radiographic changes over time: widening of SI joint, erosions, sclerosis on both sides of joint not extending >1 cm from articular surface, and (lastly) ankyloses.

- Spine
  - Early plain radiograph changes: "shiny corners" due to osteitis and sclerosis at site of annulus fibrosus attachments to the corners of vertebral bodies with "squaring" due to erosion and remodeling of vertebral body; contrast-enhanced MRI is more sensitive for detecting early changes.
  - Late changes: ossification of annulus fibrosis resulting in bony bridging between vertebral bodies (syndesmophytes) giving classic "bamboo spine" appearance; ankylosis of apophyseal joints, ossification of spinal ligaments, and/or spondylo-discitis also occurs.
- Peripheral joints
  - Asymmetric pericapsular ossification, sclerosis, loss of joint space, and erosions may occur.

Diagnostic Procedures/Other
- ECG: conduction defects
- Echocardiogram: aortic valvular abnormalities
- Dual energy x-ray absorptiometry scan may reveal osteopenia/osteoporosis.

Test Interpretation
- Erosive changes and new bone formation at bony attachment of the tendons and ligaments result in ossification of periarticular soft tissues.
- Synovial hypertrophy and pannus formation, mononuclear cell infiltrate into subsynovium and subchondral bone marrow inflammation in the SI joint with erosions, followed by granulation tissue formation, and finally obliteration of joint space by fusion of joint and sclerosis of para-articular bone

 TREATMENT

GENERAL MEASURES
- Aggressive physical therapy is the most important nonpharmacologic management.
- Posture training and spinal range-of-motion exercises are essential.
- Firm bed; sleep in supine position without a pillow
- Breathing exercises 2 to 3 times per day
- Smoking cessation

MEDICATION
First Line
- Nonsteroidal anti-inflammatory drugs (NSAIDs) are first line for pain and stiffness in AS (3)[C].
- NSAIDs provide rapid and dramatic symptomatic relief, which may be diagnostic. No single NSAID preferred. Higher doses tend to be more efficacious.
- Continuous NSAID therapy may slow radiographic disease progression but may not be superior to intermittent therapy for symptom control (4)[A].
- Precautions
  - Consider CVD, GI, and renal risks of NSAIDs.
  - Consider GI prophylaxis (PPIs or misoprostol) while on NSAIDs in patients with hx of PUD, gastritis, or age >60 years
  - Use NSAIDS with caution in patients with a bleeding diathesis or patients receiving anticoagulants.
- Injection of intra-articular corticosteroids into SI joints and prostheses can provide transient relief, but systemic corticosteroids are usually ineffective.

Pregnancy Considerations

Infants exposed to NSAIDs in 1st trimester may have a higher incidence of cardiac malformations (5)[A].

Second Line

- Biologic agents: tumor necrosis factor (TNF)-α antagonists
  - Recommended for high disease activity or when a trial of two NSAIDs over 4 weeks have failed (3)[C]
  - FDA-approved agents for AS include etanercept (recombinant TNF receptor fusion protein), infliximab (chimeric monoclonal IgG1 antibody to TNF-α), adalimumab (fully humanized IgG1 monoclonal antibody to TNF-α), and golimumab (human IgG1 kappa monoclonal antibody to TNF-α).
  - Approved agents improve pain, function, and symptoms of AS as compared to placebo (6)[A].
  - No definitive evidence for TNF-α blockers with regards to disease remission, prevention of radiologic progression, or prevention of extra-articular manifestations (7).
  - Monoclonal TNF-α blockers are preferred when IBD is involved (3)[C].
  - Further investigation as to the effectiveness of TNF blocker therapy with NSAIDs is needed (8).
- Precautions with TNF-α blockers
  - Anti-TNFs increase the risk of serious bacterial, mycobacterial, fungal, opportunistic, and viral infections. Screen for tuberculosis and hepatitis B.
  - Monitor for reactivation of tuberculosis and invasive fungal infections, such as histoplasmosis, in all patients, especially those who travel to (or residents in) endemic areas.
  - Lymphomas, nonmelanoma skin cancers, and other malignancies have been reported in patients receiving anti-TNFs.
  - Immunizations (especially live vaccines) should be updated before initiating anti-TNFs; live vaccines are contraindicated once patients receive anti-TNFs.
- Disease-modifying antirheumatic drugs (DMARDs), such as methotrexate and sulfasalazine, are ineffective for axial disease; sulfasalazine may be effective for peripheral arthritis (3)[C].

ISSUES FOR REFERRAL

- Physical therapy can assist with treatment plan (including home regimens).
- Coordinate care with a rheumatologist for diagnosis, monitoring, and management (anti-TNF therapy).
- Management of aortic regurgitation, uveitis, spinal fractures, pulmonary fibrosis, hip joint involvement, renal amyloidosis, and cauda equina syndrome may require referral to appropriate specialty.

ADDITIONAL THERAPIES

- Bisphosphonate medications if osteopenia or osteoporosis is present
- Monitoring and management of CVD risk factors and comorbidities

SURGERY/OTHER PROCEDURES

- Evaluate for C-spine ankylosis/instability before intubation in patients with AS undergoing surgery.
- Total hip replacement if necessary to restore mobility and to control pain.
- Vertebral osteotomy can improve posture for patients with severe cervical or thoracolumbar flexion.

ONGOING CARE

FOLLOW-UP RECOMMENDATIONS
Patient Monitoring

- Symptom control and maintenance of mobility and function are primary treatment goals.
- Monitor posture and range of motion with 6- to 12-month visits; increase frequency if higher disease activity.
- Bath Ankylosing Spondylitis Disease Activity Index (BASDAI) or Ankylosing Spondylitis Disease Activity Score (ASDAS) can be used to measure disease activity.

PATIENT EDUCATION

- Maintain physical activity and posture.
- Swimming, tai chi, and walking are excellent activities.
- Avoid trauma/contact sports.
- Appropriate ergonomic modification of workplace
- Counsel about risk of spinal fracture.
- MedicAlert bracelet (helpful if intubation required)
- Arthritis Foundation: http://www.arthritis.org
- Spondylitis Association of America: http://www.spondylitis.org

PROGNOSIS

- Extent and rapidity of progression of ankylosis are highly variable.
- Progressive limitation of spinal mobility necessitates lifestyle modification.

COMPLICATIONS

- Spine
  - Spinal fusion causing kyphosis
  - Cervical spine fracture or subluxation carries high mortality rate; fracture can occur at any level of ankylosed spine.
  - Cauda equina syndrome (rare)
- Pulmonary: restrictive lung disease, upper lobe fibrosis (rare)
- Cardiac: conduction defects at atrioventricular (AV) node, aortic insufficiency, aortitis, pericarditis (extremely rare)
- Eye: uveitis and cataracts
- Renal: IgA nephropathy, amyloidosis ($<1\%$)
- GI: microscopic, subclinical ileal, and colonic mucosal ulcerations in up to 50% of patients, mostly asymptomatic

REFERENCES

1. Reveille JD, Weisman MH. The epidemiology of back pain, axial spondyloarthritis and HLA-B27 in the United States. *Am J Med Sci*. 2013;345(6):431–436.
2. Dougados M, Baeten D. Spondyloarthritis. *Lancet*. 2011;377(9783):2127–2137.
3. Braun J, van den Berg R, Baraliakos X, et al. 2010 update of the ASAS/EULAR recommendations for the management of ankylosing spondylitis. *Ann Rheum Dis*. 2011;70(6):896–904.
4. Guellec D, Nocturne G, Tatar Z, et al. Should non-steroidal anti-inflammatory drugs be used continuously in ankylosing spondylitis? *Joint Bone Spine*. 2014;81(4):308–312.
5. Adams K, Bombardier C, van der Heijde DM. Safety of pain therapy during pregnancy and lactation in patients with inflammatory arthritis: a systematic literature review. *J Rheumatol Suppl*. 2012;90:59–61.
6. Maxwell LJ, Zochling J, Boonen A, et al. TNF-alpha inhibitors for ankylosing spondylitis. *Cochrane Database of Syst Rev*. 2015;(4):CD005468. doi:10.1002/14651858.CD005468.pub2.
7. Gensler L, Inman R, Deodhar A. The "knowns" and "unknowns" of biologic therapy in ankylosing spondylitis. *Am J Med Sci*. 2012;343(5):360–363.
8. Sieper J. Treatment challenges in axial spondyloarthritis and future directions. *Curr Rheumatol Rep*. 2013;15(9):356. doi:10.1007/s11926-013-0356-9.

ADDITIONAL READING

- Baraliakos X, van den Berg R, Braun J, et al. Update of the literature review on treatment with biologics as a basis for the first update of the ASAS/EULAR management recommendations of ankylosing spondylitis. *Rheumatology (Oxford)*. 2012;51(8):1378–1387.
- Garg N, van den Bosch F, Deodhar A. The concept of spondyloarthritis: where are we now? *Best Pract Res Clin Rheumatol*. 2014;28(5):663–672.
- Sieper J. Developments in therapies for spondyloarthritis. *Nat Rev Rheumatol*. 2012;8(5):280–287.
- Sieper J, Rudwaleit M, Baraliakos X, et al. The Assessment of Spondyloarthritis International Society (ASAS) handbook: a guide to assess spondyloarthritis. *Ann Rheum Dis*. 2009;68(Suppl 2): ii1–ii44.
- van den Berg R, Baraliakos X, Braun J, et al. First update of the current evidence for the management of ankylosing spondylitis with non-pharmacological treatment and non-biologic drugs: a systematic literature review for the ASAS/EULAR management recommendations in ankylosing spondylitis. *Rheumatology (Oxford)*. 2012;51(8):1388–1396.

SEE ALSO

Arthritis, Psoriatic; Arthritis, Rheumatoid (RA); Crohn Disease; Reactive Arthritis (Reiter Syndrome); Ulcerative Colitis

CODES

ICD10

- M45.9 Ankylosing spondylitis of unspecified sites in spine
- M08.1 Juvenile ankylosing spondylitis
- M45.8 Ankylosing spondylitis sacral and sacrococcygeal region

CLINICAL PEARLS

- Diagnosis of AS is suggested by a history of inflammatory back pain, evidence of limited chest wall expansion, restricted spinal movements in all planes, radiographic evidence of sacroiliitis, and a therapeutic response to NSAIDs.
- HLA-B27 testing supports the diagnosis if clinical features are not definitive.
- MRI is more sensitive at detecting SI joint inflammation than plain radiography.
- Physical therapy is important in helping to maintain posture and mobility.
- NSAIDs and TNF-α blockers are the mainstays of pharmacologic treatment of AS.

ANORECTAL FISTULA

Nihal K. Patel, MD • David A. Greenwald, MD

 BASICS

DESCRIPTION

- An anorectal fistula is an open communication between an anal abscess and the perirectal skin.
- Anorectal fistulas typically form from an abscess of the anal crypt glands.
- The classification of fistulas grades severity and guides treatment. Five subtypes are described:
  - Submucosal or superficial: The fistula tracks beneath the submucosa and does not involve the sphincter mechanism (not classified under original Park classification).
  - Intersphincteric: The fistula travels along the intersphincteric plane (Park type 1).
  - Transsphincteric: The fistula traverses through the internal and external sphincter (type 2).
  - Suprasphincteric: The fistula originates at the dentate line and loops over the external sphincter, to the ischiorectal fossa (type 3).
  - Extrasphincteric (rare): high in the anal canal, (proximal to dentate line), does not involve sphincter complex (type 4)
- Fistulas can also be classified as low or high:
  - Low fistulas involve the distal 1/3 of the external sphincter muscle.
  - High fistulas involve more of the external sphincter.
- Fistulas may be simple or complex:
  - Simple fistulas are low and include superficial, intersphincteric, or low transsphincteric fistulas. They also involve only one communicating tract and are not associated with inflammatory bowel disease (IBD) or other organs (bladder).
  - Complex fistulas are higher along the gastrointestinal (GI) tract, have multiple tracts, involve other organs, are recurrent, or are associated with IBD or radiation.
  - System(s) affected: GI; skin/exocrine
  - Synonym(s): fistula-in-ano; anal fistula

EPIDEMIOLOGY

- The true prevalence is unknown because anorectal pain is commonly attributed to hemorrhoids.
- Mean age of presentation for anal abscess and fistula is 40 years (range 20 to 60).
- Predominant sex: Males are twice as likely to develop an abscess and/or fistula compared with females.
- Lifetime risk of developing fistula is 20–40% in Crohn disease patients.

ETIOLOGY AND PATHOPHYSIOLOGY

- Inspissated debris in an obstructed anal crypt gland results in suppuration and abscess formation along the path of least resistance in the perianal and perirectal spaces (cryptoglandular theory).

- Abscess rupture or drainage leads to an epithelialized track or fistula formation in ~1/3 of patients.
- Fistula formation also occurs in patients with IBD.
- Patients undergoing pelvic radiation are predisposed to fistula formation.
- Immunocompromised patients with primary perianal actinomycosis can (rarely) develop fistula-in-ano.
- Anorectal mucosal laceration due to rectal foreign bodies or trauma can cause abscess and fistula formation.

RISK FACTORS

- IBD (Crohn disease)
- Pelvic radiation
- Perianal trauma; previous anorectal abscess
- Pelvic carcinoma or lymphoma
- Ruptured anal hematoma
- Abscess formation due to acute appendicitis, salpingitis, or diverticulitis
- Tuberculosis (rare); syphilis; lymphogranuloma venereum
- Immunocompromised state (actinomycosis)

GENERAL PREVENTION

- Perianal hygiene
- Prevention or prompt treatment of anorectal abscess; management of commonly associated conditions or risk factors

COMMONLY ASSOCIATED CONDITIONS

- Anorectal abscess
- IBD (Crohn disease)
- Diabetes
- Chronic steroid treatment

DIAGNOSIS

HISTORY

- Perianal pain, pruritis, purulent (often malodorous) perianal drainage, and perirectal skin lesions
- Intermittent rectal pain is worse with defecation or sitting.
- Fever most common with abscesses, generally not common with fistulas

PHYSICAL EXAM

- Excoriations or inflammation of perianal skin
- Visible orifice; induration if opening is incomplete or blind
- Anorectal abscess palpated as an indurated or fluctuant tender perianal mass or small tender palpable lesion on rectal exam at level of anal crypt

- Anoscopy may reveal an internal orifice.
  - Goodsall rule can assist in determining course of the fistula tract (more predictive with posterior external anal openings):
    - If external opening is *anterior* to an imaginary line drawn transversely through the anal canal, fistula usually runs directly (radially) into the anal canal.
    - If external opening is within 3 cm of anal verge and *posterior* to line, fistula leads to a curved tract, with an internal opening in posterior commissure (except for a long anterior fistula).
    - In children, tract is usually straight.

DIFFERENTIAL DIAGNOSIS

- Pilonidal sinus; Hidradenitis suppurativa
- Hemorrhoids; Anal fissure, ulcer, or sores
- Infected inclusion cyst
- Urethroperineal fistulas
- Ischiorectal or high muscular abscess
- Rule out: Crohn disease, carcinoma, lymphoma, tuberculosis, chronic *Chlamydia trachomatis* infection, actinomycosis in immunocompromised, acute untreated pelvic inflammatory condition

DIAGNOSTIC TESTS & INTERPRETATION

Initial Tests (lab, imaging)

- Imaging helps define perianal anatomy.
- MRI and endoscopic ultrasound are preferred.
- MRI has ~80–90% overall concordance with surgical examination under anesthesia; accuracy improves with dedicated pelvic MRI to allow better resolution.
- Angulation of fistula from internal opening correlates with the type of fistula (acute angle likely high transsphincteric; obtuse angle likely lower fistula).
- Fistulography (insertion of catheter into external opening of fistula and injection of radiographic contrast material) is *not* preferred and generally not accurate when evaluating perianal disease. Fistulography is reserved for patients who may have a fistula between the rectum and another organ (such as bladder).
- CT is limited in evaluating perianal fistula tracts; more helpful for large perianal abscesses and inflammation
- Consider testing for syphilis for recurrent fistulas in sexually active patients.

Diagnostic Procedures/Other

- Anoscopy or sigmoidoscopy
- Colonoscopy and esophagogastroduodenoscopy if Crohn disease is suspected
- Probing into the tract may be done under anesthesia prior to surgery to determine course of fistula.
- Injection of dilute methylene blue or hydrogen peroxide intraoperatively may help identify internal opening.

TREATMENT

GENERAL MEASURES

- Surgical treatment is definitive (1)[A].

- Optimal surgical treatment based on correct fistula classification

- Goals of treatment include resolving the inflammatory process, maintaining continence, and preventing recurrence.

- Sitz baths 3 to 4 per day until definitive surgery

MEDICATION

- Medical management with antibiotics and immuno-suppressive agents plays a role in the treatment of fistulas due to Crohn disease, particularly if patients are minimally symptomatic.

- Studies have shown improvement (reduced pain, discharge, and induration) and healing in up to 80% of patients with 8 weeks of treatment using oral metronidazole in patients with Crohn disease.

- Use of infliximab has also been shown to be effective in healing perianal Crohn fistulas but has been associated with a high rate of recurrence.

- Antibiotics may be indicated if patients have signs of sepsis or an active infection with a concurrent anorectal abscess.

- Consider surgery in Crohn patients who fail long-term medical therapy.

SURGERY/OTHER PROCEDURES

- Choice of surgical procedure is a balance between achieving cure, avoiding recurrence, and maintaining fecal incontinence (2)[A].

- Low transsphincteric and simple intersphincteric fistulas can be treated with simple fistulotomy or fibrin sealant (fistula plug) (3)[A].

- Fistula plugs can be used as initial treatment for high transsphincteric fistulas. If the fistula recurs, then an advancement flap may be necessary.

- Complex fistulas should be treated with an endorectal advancement flap, which closes the internal opening of the fistula with a mobilized flap of healthy mucosal and submucosal tissue.

- Fistulotomy opens ("unroofs") the entire fistula tract (4)[B].

  - Fistula tract is cauterized or curetted and tract is marsupialized to promote healing.
  - Lower rates of recurrence compared to incision and drainage alone
  - Fistulotomy results in incontinence in about 12% of patients with simple fistulas, compared with almost 50% of patients with complex fistulas.

- A seton is a reactive suture or elastic that is used for drainage (noncutting seton) or to allow scarring of the tract (cutting seton). Cutting setons are tightened at regular intervals to allow slow cutting through the tract and causing scarring. Setons may be placed for complex fistulas treated with fistu-lotomy, for those that involve >30% of the external sphincter, are proximal to the dentate line, or are categorized as high transsphincteric fistulas.

- Postoperative: typically a same-day procedure; Sitz baths (Sit in warm bath for 20 minutes 3 to 4 times per day and after bowel movements.)

- Aggressive bowel regimen to prevent constipation

- Patients undergoing anal fistulotomy may benefit postoperatively from the use of topical application of sucralfate.

ONGOING CARE

FOLLOW-UP RECOMMENDATIONS

Resumption of activity as tolerated after surgery

Patient Monitoring

Anoscopy at 3 to 6 months following procedure; frequent follow-up to ensure complete healing and assess continence

DIET

High-fiber diet

PROGNOSIS

Postoperative healing:

- 4 to 5 weeks for perianal fistulas
- 12 to 16 weeks for deeper fistulas
- Postoperative healing may occur within 2 to 3 weeks in children.
- Healing may be delayed in Crohn disease.

COMPLICATIONS

- Fecal incontinence
- Constipation
- Rectovaginal fistula
- Delayed wound healing
- Low-grade carcinoma may develop in long-standing fistulas.
- Recurrent anorectal fistula if fistula is incompletely treated

REFERENCES

1. Whiteford MH, Kilkenny J III, Hyman N, et al. Practice parameters for the treatment of perianal abscess and fistula-in-ano (revised). *Dis Colon Rectum.* 2005;48(7):1337–1342.

2. Malik AI, Nelson RL. Surgical management of anal fistulae: a systematic review. *Colorectal Dis.* 2008;10(5):420–430.

3. Cirocchi R, Farinella E, La Mura F, et al. Fibrin glue in the treatment of anal fistula: a systematic review. *Ann Surg Innov Res.* 2009;3:12.

4. Rizzo JA, Naig AL, Johnson EK. Anorectal abscess and fistula-in-ano: evidence-based management. *Surg Clin North Am.* 2010;90(1):45–68.

ADDITIONAL READING

- A ba-bai-ke-re MM, Wen H, Huang HG, et al. Randomized controlled trial of minimally invasive surgery using acellular dermal matrix for complex anorectal fistula. *World J Gastroenterol.* 2010;16(26):3279–3286.

- Gupta PJ, Heda PS, Shrirao SA, et al. Topical sucralfate treatment of anal fistulotomy wounds: a randomized placebo-controlled trial. *Dis Colon Rectum.* 2011;54(6):699–704.

- Jacob TJ, Perakath B, Keighley MR. Surgical intervention for anorectal fistula. *Cochrane Database Syst Rev.* 2010;(5):CD006319.

- Lewis RT, Maron DJ. Anorectal Crohn's disease. *Surg Clin North Am.* 2010;90(1):83–97.

- Mishra A, Shah S, Nar AS, et al. The role of fibrin glue in the treatment of high and low fistulas in ano. *J Clin Diagn Res.* 2013;7(5):876–879.

- Niyogi A, Agarwal T, Broadhurst J, et al. Management of perianal abscess and fistula-in-ano in children. *Eur J Pediatr Surg.* 2010;20(1):35–39.

 SEE ALSO

Anorectal Abscess; Crohn Disease

CODES

ICD10

- K60.5 Anorectal fistula
- K60.3 Anal fistula
- K60.4 Rectal fistula

CLINICAL PEARLS

- Suspect anorectal fistula in patients with perianal pain, pruritis, purulent drainage, and perirectal skin lesions.

- Surgery is the traditional mainstay of treatment in patients who do not have Crohn disease.

- MRI or endoscopic ultrasound are the modalities of choice to define the anatomy of anorectal fistulas.

ANOREXIA NERVOSA
Umer Farooq, MD, MBBS • Wajiha Illyas, MD

 BASICS

DESCRIPTION
- Restriction of energy intake leading to significantly low weight in the context of age, sex, developmental trajectory, and physical health, with intense fear of weight gain and body image disturbance. Significantly low weight is defined as weight that is less than minimally normal/expected.
- *Diagnostic and Statistical Manual of Mental Disorders,* 5th edition (DSM-5), divides anorexia into two types:
  - Restricting type: not engaged in binge eating or purging behaviors for last 3 months
  - Binge eating/purging type: regularly engages in binge eating or purging behaviors (last 3 months)
- System(s) affected: cardiovascular, endocrine, metabolic, gastrointestinal, nervous, reproductive
- Severity of anorexia nervosa (AN) is based on BMI (per *DSM-5*):
  - Mild: BMI $\geq$ 17 kg/m^2
  - Moderate: BMI 16 to 16.99 kg/m^2
  - Severe: BMI 15 to 15.99 kg/m^2
  - Extreme: BMI < 15 kg/m^2

EPIDEMIOLOGY
- Predominant age: 13 to 20 years
- Predominant sex: female > male (10:1 female-to-male ratio)

Incidence
- 8 to 19 women/2 men per 100,000 per year

Prevalence
- 0.4% in women
- Less is known; however, an estimate suggests 0.3% in men (higher in gay and bisexual men).

ETIOLOGY AND PATHOPHYSIOLOGY
- Complex relationship among genetic, biologic, environmental, psychological, and social factors that result in the development of this disorder
- Subsequent malnutrition may lead to multiorgan damage.
- Serotonin, norepinephrine, and dopamine neuronal systems are implicated.

Genetics
- Underlying genetic vulnerability is likely but not well understood, some evidence of higher concordance rates in monozygotic twins than in dizygotic
- First-degree female relative with eating disorder increases risk 6- to 10-fold.

RISK FACTORS
- Female gender
- Adolescence
- Body dissatisfaction
- Perfectionism
- Negative self-evaluation
- Academic pressure
- Severe life stressors
- Participation in sports or artistic activities that emphasize leanness or involve subjective scoring: ballet, running, wrestling, figure skating, gymnastics, cheerleading, weight lifting
- Type 1 diabetes mellitus
- Family history of substance abuse, affective disorders, or eating disorder

GENERAL PREVENTION
Prevention programs can reduce risk factors and future onset of eating disorders (1)[A]:
- Target adolescents and young women 15 years of age or older.
- Encourage realistic and healthy weight management strategies and attitudes.
- Promote self-esteem.
- Reduce focus on thin as ideal.
- Decrease co-occurring anxiety/depressive symptoms and improve stress management.

COMMONLY ASSOCIATED CONDITIONS
- Mood disorder (major depression)
- Social phobia, obsessive-compulsive disorder
- Substance abuse disorder
- High rates of cluster C personality disorders

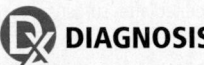 DIAGNOSIS

HISTORY
- Onset may be insidious or stress-related.
- Patient unlikely to self-identify problem (lack of insight into the illness); corroborate with parent/relative
- Restriction of energy intake relative to requirement, leading to significantly low body weight in the context of age, sex, developmental trajectory, and physical health
- Fear of weight gain and/or distorted body image
- Report feeling fat even when emaciated.
- Preoccupation with body size, weight control
- Elaborate food preparation and eating rituals.
- Other possible signs and symptoms:
  - Extensive exercise
  - Amenorrhea (primary or secondary)
  - Weakness, fatigue, cognitive impairment
  - Cold intolerance
  - Constipation, bloating, early satiety
  - Growth arrest, delayed puberty
  - History of fractures (decreased bone density)

PHYSICAL EXAM
- May be normal
- Abnormal vital signs: hypothermia, bradycardia, orthostatic hypotension
- Body weight <85% of expected
- Cardiac: dysrhythmias, midsystolic click of mitral valve prolapse
- Skin/extremities: dry skin; lanugo hair on extremities, face, and trunk; hair loss; edema
- Neurologic and abdominal exams: to rule out other causes of weight loss and vomiting

DIFFERENTIAL DIAGNOSIS
- Hyperthyroidism, adrenal insufficiency
- Inflammatory bowel disease, malabsorption
- Immunodeficiency, chronic infections
- Diabetes
- CNS lesion
- Bulimia, body dysmorphic disorder
- Depressive disorders with loss of appetite
- Anxiety disorder, food phobia
- Conversion disorder

DIAGNOSTIC TESTS & INTERPRETATION
- Psychological self-report screening tests may be helpful, but diagnosis is based on meeting the *DSM-5* criteria.

- Most findings are related directly to starvation and/or dehydration. All findings may be within normal limits.
- Screening tools:
  - SCOFF questionnaire (2)[B]
  - Eating Disorder Screen for Primary Care

Initial Tests (lab, imaging)
- CBC: anemia, leukopenia, thrombocytopenia
- Low serum luteinizing hormone, follicle-stimulating hormone; low serum testosterone in men
- Thyroid function tests: low thyroid-stimulating hormone with normal T$_3$/T$_4$
- Liver function tests: abnormal liver enzymes
- Chem 7: altered BUN, creatinine clearance; electrolyte disturbances
- Hypoglycemia, hypercholesterolemia, hypercortisolemia, hypophosphatemia
- Low sedimentation rate
- 12-Lead electrocardiogram to assess for prolonged QT interval
- Dual-energy x-ray absorptiometry of bone to assess for diminished bone density, only if underweight for >6 months

Test Interpretation
- Osteoporosis/osteopenia, pathologic fractures
- Sick euthyroid syndrome
- Cardiac impairment

ALERT
AN may exist concurrently with chronic medical disorders such as diabetes and cystic fibrosis.

 TREATMENT

GENERAL MEASURES
- Initial treatment goal geared to weight restoration; most managed as outpatients (OPs)
- OP treatment:
  - Interdisciplinary team (primary care physician, mental health provider, dietician)
  - Average weekly weight gain goal: 0.5 to 1.0 kg, with stepwise increase in calories
  - Cognitive-behavioral therapy (CBT), interpersonal psychotherapy, family-based therapy
  - Focus on health, not weight gain alone.
  - Build trust and a treatment alliance.
  - Involve the patient in establishing diet and exercise goals.
  - Challenge fear of uncontrolled weight gain; help the patient to recognize feelings that lead to disordered eating.
  - In chronic cases, goal may be to achieve a safe weight rather than a healthy weight.
- Inpatient treatment:
  - If possible, admit to a specialized eating disorders unit.
  - Assess risk for refeeding syndrome (metabolic shift from a catabolic to anabolic state).
  - Monitor vital signs, electrolytes, cardiac function, edema, and weight gain.
  - Initial supervised meals may be necessary.
  - Stepwise increase in activity
  - Tube feeding or total parenteral nutrition is used only as a last resort.
  - Supportive symptomatic care as needed

- Most patients should be treated as OPs using an interdisciplinary team.
- Behavioral therapies (e.g., cognitive-behavioral, interpersonal, or family therapy) should be offered (3–5)[A].
- CBT has demonstrated effectiveness as a means of improving treatment adherence and minimizing dropout among patients with AN (6)[A].

MEDICATION
First Line
- No medications are available that effectively treat patients with AN, but pharmacotherapy may be used as an adjuvant to CBTs (5,7)[A].
- If medications are used, start with low doses due to increased risk for adverse effects.
- SSRIs may:
  – Help to prevent relapse after weight gain
  – Treat comorbid depression or obsessive-compulsive disorder.
  – Use of atypical antipsychotics is being studied with mixed findings to date. Olanzapine is potentially beneficial as an adjuvant treatment of underweight individuals in the inpatient settings.
- Attend to black box warnings concerning antidepressants.

Second Line
- Management of osteopenia:
  – Primary treatment is weight gain.
  – Elemental calcium 1,200 to 1,500 mg/day plus vitamin D 800 IU/day
  – No indication for bisphosphonates in AN
  – Weak evidence for use of hormone-replacement therapy
- Psyllium (Metamucil) preparations to prevent constipation

ISSUES FOR REFERRAL
Patients with AN require an interdisciplinary team (primary care physician, mental health provider, nutritionist). An important step in management is to arrange OP mental health therapist.

INPATIENT CONSIDERATIONS
Admission Criteria/Initial Stabilization
- Suggested physiologic values: heart rate <40 beats/min, BP <90/60 mm Hg, symptomatic hypoglycemia, potassium <3 mmol/L, temperature <97.0°F (36.1°C), dehydration, other cardiovascular abnormalities, weight <75% of expected, rapid weight loss, lack of improvement while in OP therapy
- Suggested psychological indications: poor motivation/insight, lack of cooperation with OP treatment, inability to eat, need for nasogastric feeding, suicidal intent or plan, severe coexisting psychiatric disease, problematic family environment

Pediatric Considerations
- Children often present with nausea, abdominal pain, fullness, and inability to swallow.
- Additional indications for hospitalization: heart rate <50 beats/min, orthostatic BP, hypokalemia or hypophosphatemia, rapid weight loss even if weight not <75% below normal
- Children and adolescents should be offered family-based treatment.

Geriatric Considerations
Late-onset AN (>50 years of age) may be long-term disease or triggered by death of loved one, marital discord, or divorce.

Discharge Criteria
Discharge when medically stable. Arrange OP appointment with mental health provider and primary care provider.

 ONGOING CARE

FOLLOW-UP RECOMMENDATIONS
- Close follow-up until patient demonstrates forward progress in care plan
- Family and individual therapy is extremely important for the long-term benefits/outcomes.
- CBT is very helpful for the treatment of AN and may be helpful for the prevention of relapse.
- Emphasize importance of moderate activity for health, not thinness.

Patient Monitoring
- Level of exercise activity
- Weigh weekly until stable, then monthly
- Depression, suicidal ideation

DIET
- Dietary consultation while patient is hospitalized.
- Nutritional education programs

PATIENT EDUCATION
- Provide patients and families with information about the diagnosis and its natural history, health risks, and treatment strategies.
- http://www.mayoclinic.org/diseases-conditions/anorexia/home/ovc-20179508
- The National Alliance on Mental Illness: http://www.nami.org/Learn-More/Mental-Health-Conditions/Eating-Disorders

PROGNOSIS
- Prognosis: ~50% recover, 30% improve, 20% are chronically ill.
- Outcomes in men are likely better than in women.
- Mortality: 3%
- High risk of suicide in patients suffering from AN (8)[A]

COMPLICATIONS
- Refeeding syndrome
- Cardiac arrhythmia, cardiac arrest
- Cardiomyopathy, congestive heart failure
- Delayed gastric emptying, necrotizing colitis
- Seizures, Wernicke encephalopathy, peripheral neuropathy, cognitive deficits
- Osteopenia, osteoporosis

Pregnancy Considerations
- Fertility may be affected.
- Behaviors may persist, decrease, or recur during pregnancy and the postpartum interval.
- Increased risk for preterm labor, operative delivery, and infants with low birth weight; anemia, genitourinary infections, and labor induction should be managed as high risk.

REFERENCES
1. Stice E, Shaw H, Marti CN. A meta-analytic review of eating disorder prevention programs: encouraging findings. *Annu Rev Clin Psychol.* 2007;3:207–231.
2. Cotton MA, Ball C, Robinson P. Four simple questions can help screen for eating disorder. *J Gen Intern Med.* 2003;18(1):53–56.
3. Hay P, Bacaltchuk J, Claudino A, et al. Individual psychotherapy in the outpatient treatment of adults with anorexia nervosa. *Cochrane Database Syst Rev.* 2003;(4):CD003909.
4. Fisher CA, Hetrick SE, Rushford N. Family therapy for anorexia nervosa. *Cochrane Database Syst Rev.* 2010;(4):CD004780.
5. Bulik CM, Berkman ND, Brownley KA, et al. Anorexia nervosa treatment: a systematic review of randomized controlled trials. *Int J Eat Disord.* 2007;40(4):310–320.
6. Galsworthy-Francis L, Allan S. Cognitive behavioural therapy for anorexia nervosa: a systematic review. *Clin Psychol Rev.* 2014;34(1):54–72.
7. Claudino AM, Hay P, Lima MS, et al. Antidepressants for anorexia nervosa. *Cochrane Database Syst Rev.* 2006;(1):CD004365.
8. Zerwas S, Larsen JT, Petersen L, et al. The incidence of eating disorders in a Danish register study: associations with suicide risk and mortality. *J Psychiatr Res.* 2015;65:16–22.

ADDITIONAL READING
- American Psychiatric Association. *Practice Guideline for the Treatment of Patients with Eating Disorders.* 3rd ed. Arlington, VA: American Psychiatric Association; 2006
- Dalle Grave R. Eating disorders: progress and challenges. *Eur J Intern Med.* 2011;22(2):153–160.
- National Collaborating Centre for Mental Health. *Eating Disorders: Core Interventions in the Treatment and Management of Anorexia Nervosa, Bulimia Nervosa and Related Eating Disorders (NICE Guidelines).* Leicester, United Kingdom: British Psychological Society; 2004.

 SEE ALSO

- Amenorrhea; Osteoporosis; Bulimia Nervosa
- Algorithm: Weight Loss

 CODES

ICD10
- F50.00 Anorexia nervosa, unspecified
- F50.01 Anorexia nervosa, restricting type
- F50.02 Anorexia nervosa, binge eating/purging type

CLINICAL PEARLS
- "Are you satisfied with your eating patterns?" and/or "Do you worry that you have lost control over how you eat?" may help to screen those with an eating problem.
- Studies have shown patients with AN will not accept medications unless combined with psychotherapy.
- To care for a patient with AN, an interdisciplinary team that includes a medical provider, a dietician, and a behavioral health professional is the most accepted approach.
- Family analysis is necessary for the patients with AN to determine what kind of therapy would be most helpful.
- 3 months amenorrhea is no longer the criteria needed for the diagnosis of AN.

ANTIPHOSPHOLIPID ANTIBODY SYNDROME

Ho Phong Pham, MD • Dausen J. Harker, MD

BASICS

DESCRIPTION

Antiphospholipid antibody syndrome (APS) is an autoantibody-mediated thrombophilic disorder characterized by recurrent arterial or venous thrombosis and/or recurrent fetal loss in the presence of antiphospholipid antibodies (APAs). The APAs enhance clot formation by interacting with phospholipid-binding plasma proteins. The resulting APS can cause significant morbidity and mortality in both pregnant and nonpregnant individuals:

- Types of APS (based on clinical presentation)
  - Primary: occurs without associated underlying disease
  - Secondary: associated with autoimmune diseases (systemic lupus erythematosus [SLE] is most common); transient APAs linked to certain infections, drugs, and malignancies
  - Catastrophic APS (CAPS) a.k.a Asherson syndrome (<1%)
    ○ Most severe form of disease; characterized by thrombotic microangiopathy and associated with multiorgan failure
    ○ High mortality if treatment is delayed
    ○ Severe thrombocytopenia, hemolytic anemia, and DIC are additional features.
  - Associated clinical manifestations: livedo reticularis, cardiac valvular disease, thrombocytopenia, nephropathy, hemolytic anemia, coronary artery disease, and cognitive impairment

Pregnancy Considerations

- Complications include maternal thrombosis (stroke, venous thromboembolism [VTE]), fetal death, preeclampsia and placental insufficiency, fetal growth retardation, and preterm birth.
- Low-dose aspirin and low-molecular-weight heparin (LMWH) or unfractionated heparin are the drugs of choice in pregnancy.
- Prophylactic-dose heparin is recommended in the postpartum period (unless patient is on therapeutic anticoagulation) given high risk of thrombosis during this time. With adequate treatment, >70% of patients with APS deliver viable infants.

EPIDEMIOLOGY

- The prevalence of APAs increases with age but is not necessarily associated with a higher risk of thrombosis.
- For APS, female > male

Incidence

- In patients with positive APAs without prior risk of thrombosis, the annual incident risk of thrombosis is 0–3.8%. This risk is up to 5.3% in those with triple positivity (anticardiolipin antibodies, lupus anticoagulant (LAC), and anti–β2 glycoprotein-1 (GP1) antibodies positive).
- 10–15% of recurrent abortions are attributable to APS.

Prevalence

APAs are present in 1–5% of the general population and in ~40% of those with SLE. A higher prevalence is seen in those with VTE and stroke.

ETIOLOGY AND PATHOPHYSIOLOGY

- Anti–β2-GP1 antibodies play a central role in the pathogenesis of APS. The procoagulant effect is mediated by various possible mechanisms:
  - Endothelial effects: inhibition of prostacyclin production and loss of annexin V cellular shield
  - Platelet activation resulting in adhesion and aggregation
  - Interference of innate anticoagulant pathways (such as inhibition of protein C)
  - Complement activation
- Pregnancy-related complications are also a result of autoantibody-mediated effects:
  - Interference with expression of trophoblastic adhesion molecules resulting in abnormal placentation and placental thrombosis
- Proposed mechanisms: excess production of natural antibodies, molecular mimicry due to infections, exposure of phospholipid antigens during platelet activation, cardiolipin peroxidation, and genetic predisposition
- A "second hit" by environmental factors may be required to produce thrombosis.

Genetics

Most cases of APS are acquired. There are a few studies of familial occurrence of anticardiolipin antibodies and LAC. A valine 247/leucine polymorphism in β2-GP1 could be a genetic risk for the presence of anti–β2-GP1 antibodies and APS.

RISK FACTORS

- Age >55 years in males, >65 years in females
- Cardiovascular risk factors (hypertension, diabetes, obesity, smoking, combined oral contraceptive use)
- Underlying autoimmune disease (SLE, rheumatoid arthritis, collagen vascular disease, Sjögren syndrome, idiopathic thrombocytopenic purpura, Behçet syndrome)
- Surgery, immobilization, pregnancy

GENERAL PREVENTION

Risk factor modification: Control HTN and diabetes; smoking cessation; avoidance of oral contraceptives in high-risk patients; start thromboprophylaxis in established cases.

COMMONLY ASSOCIATED CONDITIONS

- Autoimmune diseases: SLE (most common), scleroderma, Sjögren syndrome, dermatomyositis, and rheumatoid arthritis
- Malignancy
- Infections: viral, bacterial, parasitic, and rickettsial
- Certain drugs associated with APA production without increased risk of thrombosis: phenothiazines, hydralazine, procainamide, and phenytoin
- Hemolysis, elevated liver enzymes, and low platelet count in association with pregnancy (HELLP) syndrome
- Sneddon syndrome (APS variant syndrome with livedo reticularis, HTN, and stroke)

DIAGNOSIS

Sapporo criteria, revised 2006:
- At least one of the following clinical criteria:
  - Vascular thrombosis
    ○ ≥1 clinical episodes of arterial, venous, or small vessel thrombosis, occurring within any tissue or organ and confirmed by unequivocal imaging studies or histopathology
    ○ Superficial venous thrombosis does not meet the criteria for APS.
  - Complications of pregnancy (any one of the following):
    ○ ≥3 consecutive spontaneous abortions before the 10th week of pregnancy, unexplained by maternal/paternal chromosomal abnormalities or maternal anatomic/hormonal causes
    ○ ≥1 unexplained deaths of morphologically normal fetuses (documented by ultrasonography or by direct examination) at ≥10th week of gestation
    ○ ≥1 premature births of morphologically normal newborn babies at ≤34th week of pregnancy due to severe preeclampsia, eclampsia, or placental insufficiency
- AND the presence of at least one of three laboratory findings (confirmed on ≥2 occasions at least 12 weeks apart):
  - LAC detected in blood
  - Anticardiolipin IgG and/or IgM antibodies present at moderate or high levels in the blood (>40 GPL or MPL or >99th percentile) via a standardized ELISA
  - Anti–β2-GP1 IgG and/or IgM antibodies in blood at a titer >99th percentile by standardized ELISA

HISTORY

- History of VTE or arterial thrombosis (stroke, MI)
- History of fetal loss or other obstetric complications
- Bleeding from thrombocytopenia if severe or acquired factor II deficiency
- Personal or family history of autoimmune disease

PHYSICAL EXAM

- Signs of venous thrombosis in extremities
- Skin manifestations, including a vasculitic rash in the form of palpable purpura or livedo reticularis or lower extremity ulcers
- Livedo reticularis
- Cardiac murmurs
- Focal neurologic or cognitive deficits

DIFFERENTIAL DIAGNOSIS

- Thrombophilic conditions
  - Inherited: deficiency of protein C, protein S, antithrombin III; mutation of factor V Leiden, prothrombin gene mutation
  - Acquired: neoplastic and myeloproliferative disorders, hyperviscosity syndromes, nephrotic syndrome
- Embolic disease secondary to atrial fibrillation, LV dysfunction, endocarditis, cholesterol emboli
- Heparin-induced thrombocytopenia
- Atherosclerosis
- CAPS: hemolytic-uremic syndrome, TTP, or malignant hypertension

DIAGNOSTIC TESTS & INTERPRETATION

- LAC assay and IgG and IGM anticardiolipin antibodies by ELISA, and anti–β2-GP1 IgG and IgM antibodies are diagnostic tests of choice.
- The LAC assay combines at least two out of three screening tests (prolongation of aPTT, dilute Russell viper venom time [dRVVT], and kaolin clotting) with two confirmatory tests.
- Anti–β2-GP1 antibodies are important in the pathogenesis of thrombosis. A positive LAC assay recognizes antibodies against β2-GP1 and prothrombin.
- The clinical significance of other autoantibodies (annexin V, phosphatidylserine, and phosphatidylinositol) remains unclear.

Initial Tests (lab, imaging)

- CBC, PT/INR, aPTT, LAC, anticardiolipin antibodies, anti–β2-GP1 antibodies (1)[B]

- Further testing for secondary causes such as SLE when clinically suspected
- Imaging is based on clinical picture, suspected sites of thrombosis, and organ involvement.

Follow-Up Tests & Special Considerations
- The results of LAC are difficult to interpret in patients treated with warfarin. Unfractionated heparin or LMWH and fondaparinux do not affect the LAC assay.
- Repeat testing at 12 weeks for persistence of APA.

Diagnostic Procedures/Other
Biopsy of the affected organ system may be necessary to distinguish from vasculitis.

Test Interpretation
Usual finding is thrombosis and minimal vascular or perivascular inflammation:
- Acute changes: capillary congestion and noninflammatory fibrin thrombi
- Chronic changes: ischemic hypoperfusion, atrophy, and fibrosis

 TREATMENT

MEDICATION
First Line
- Primary thromboprophylaxis: Low-dose aspirin is indicated in asymptomatic carriers of APAs with SLE and in pregnancy. It may be considered in other asymptomatic carriers. Hydroxychloroquine is recommended in all antiphospholipid-positive SLE patients.
- Secondary thromboprophylaxis: All symptomatic, nonpregnant patients with APS need indefinite anticoagulation. The target INR depends on the severity and type of thrombosis:
  – Venous thrombosis (first episode): warfarin with target INR of 2.0 to 3.0
  – Arterial thrombosis or recurrent venous thrombosis despite anticoagulation: warfarin with target INR 3.0 to 4.0
  – LMWH and fondaparinux are alternatives.
- New oral anticoagulants such as rivaroxaban, apixaban, and dabigatran; all have been approved for treatment of DVT/PE; studies in APS are lacking; a prospective randomized controlled trial of warfarin versus rivaroxaban in patients with thrombotic APS and with a target INR or 2.5 is underway.
  – Rituximab may be an option in severe cases, possibly in those with hematologic and microthrombotic/microangiopathic manifestations (2,3)[B].
- Danaparoid, fondaparinux, and argatroban can be considered in APS patients with heparin-induced thrombocytopenia.
- Newer oral anticoagulants (dabigatran, apixaban, and rivaroxaban) may be alternatives to warfarin with few drug interactions and no need for monitoring. The presence of APA interferes with hemostatic mechanisms and can interfere with anticoagulants. Ongoing phase III trials will help evaluate the role of new oral anticoagulants.
- Statins can decrease proinflammatory and prothrombotic state in APS. At this time, although they are not recommended in the absence of hyperlipidemia, APA-positive patients with recurrent thrombosis while adequately anticoagulated may benefit from statin therapy.
- B-cell inhibition may help in recalcitrant APS cases.
- Complement inhibition may be useful in cases refractory to anticoagulation, but further evaluation is needed.

- Peptide therapy may be a future treatment for APA-positive patients.
- Autologous hematopoietic stem cell transplantation may be an effective option for patients with concurrent complicated SLE and APS (4).
- Vitamin D deficiency/insufficiency should be corrected in all APA-positive patients, but its role in APS needs further study.
- Low-dose aspirin is superior to low-dose aspirin with low-dose warfarin due to decreased bleeding risk with no differences in number of thrombosis (5).
- CAPS: Anticoagulants and high-dose steroids may suffice in less severe cases. Aggressive treatment with either IVIG or plasmapheresis is often required in this life-threatening condition. These measures have improved survival to 66%.
- Treatment in pregnancy are as follows:
  – For women with no prior history of thrombosis and ≥2 early miscarriages, either 81 mg ASA alone or in combination with unfractionated heparin (5,000 to 10,000 units SC q12h) or LMWH (prophylactic dose). In those with a previous late pregnancy loss (>10 weeks' gestation) or preterm (<34 weeks) delivery due to severe preeclampsia, a combination of ASA and heparin is recommended.
  – In those with a history of thrombosis, low-dose ASA plus either therapeutic low-dose heparin (dosed every 8 to 12 hours to maintain mid-interval aPTT or factor Xa levels) or LMWH (therapeutic dose)
  – Refractory cases: Up to 30% of patients have recurrent pregnancy loss despite the use of ASA and heparin. There is no role for warfarin due to risk of teratogenicity (early pregnancy) and fetal bleeding (late pregnancy). Such cases are best managed in consultation with a maternal–fetal medicine specialist.

SURGERY/OTHER PROCEDURES
Patients with thrombosis may require thrombectomy or an IVC filter (depending on site) when anticoagulation is contraindicated.

 ONGOING CARE

FOLLOW-UP RECOMMENDATIONS
Patient Monitoring
- Standard guidelines for monitoring to maintain INR at goal with warfarin therapy
- Close monitoring is required during pregnancy.

DIET
Heart-healthy diet. Patients on warfarin should avoid foods rich in vitamin K (kale, spinach, sprouts, greens).

PATIENT EDUCATION
- Compliance with warfarin therapy to keep INR at goal
- Awareness of drug and diet interactions with warfarin
- Avoid oral hormonal contraceptives.

PROGNOSIS
- Pulmonary HTN, neurologic involvement, myocardial ischemia, nephropathy, gangrene of extremities, and catastrophic APS are associated with a worse prognosis.
- 30% risk of recurrent thrombosis in the absence of adequate anticoagulation

COMPLICATIONS
- Pregnancy complications and pulmonary HTN are associated with higher morbidity and mortality.
- Thrombotic complications are the most common cause of death.

REFERENCES
1. Giannakopoulos B, Passam F, Ioannou Y, et al. How we diagnose the antiphospholipid syndrome. *Blood*. 2009;113(5):985–994.
2. Arachchillage DJ, Cohen H. Use of new oral anticoagulants in antiphospholipid syndrome. *Curr Rheumatol Rep*. 2013;15(6):331.
3. Erkan D, Aguiar CL, Andrade D, et al. 14th International Congress on Antiphospholipid Antibodies: task force report on antiphospholipid syndrome treatment trends. *Autoimmun Rev*. 2014;13(6):685–696.
4. Statkute L, Traynor A, Oyama Y, et al. Antiphospholipid syndrome in patients with systemic lupus erythematosus treated by autologous hematopoietic stem cell transplantation. *Blood*. 2005;106:2700–2709.
5. Cuadrado MJ, Bertolaccini ML, Seed PT, et al. Low-dose aspirin vs low-dose aspirin plus low-intensity warfarin in thromboprophylaxis: a prospective, multicentre, randomized, open, controlled trial in patients positive for antiphospholipid antibodies (ALIWAPAS). *Rheumatology (Oxford)*. 2014;53(2):275–284.

ADDITIONAL READING
- Baker WF Jr, Bick RL, Fareed J. Controversies and unresolved issues in antiphospholipid syndrome pathogenesis and management. *Hematol Oncol Clin North Am*. 2008;22(1):155–174.
- Bramham K, Thomas M, Nelson-Piercy C, et al. First-trimester low-dose prednisolone in refractory antiphospholipid antibody-related pregnancy loss. *Blood*. 2011;117(25):6948–6951.
- Branch D, Holmgren C, Goldberg J. Practice bulletin no. 132: Antiphospholipid syndrome. *Obstet Gynecol*. 2012;120(6):1514–1521.
- Miyakis S, Lockshin MD, Atsumi T, et al. International consensus statement on an update of the classification criteria for definite antiphospholipid syndrome (APS). *J Thromb Haemost*. 2006;4(2):295–306.
- Ruiz-Irastorza G, Crowther M, Branch W, et al. Antiphospholipid syndrome. *Lancet*. 2010;376(9751):1498–1509.

CODES

ICD10
- D68.61 Antiphospholipid syndrome
- D68.69 Other thrombophilia
- D68.62 Lupus anticoagulant syndrome

CLINICAL PEARLS
- APS can be either primary, secondary, or present as a severe microvascular disease known as CAPS.
- Both clinical and laboratory criteria are required for diagnosis. The latter must be confirmed on two separate occasions at least 12 weeks apart.
- Thrombotic manifestations of APS can be either venous or arterial. Patients require lifelong anticoagulation.

ANTITHROMBIN DEFICIENCY

Ryan Wargo, PharmD, BCACP • Michelle I. Henne, MD • Holly L. Baab, MD

BASICS

DESCRIPTION
- Antithrombin is a glycoprotein that inhibits thrombin by forming an irreversible complex.
- There are two active sites: one that binds to heparin and one that binds to thrombin/target enzyme
- Antithrombin can also inhibit factors Xa, IXa, and XIa. This process is catalyzed by the presence of heparin.
- Patients deficient in antithrombin have an increased incidence of venous thrombosis, including deep vein thrombosis (DVT) of the lower extremity. Arterial thrombosis is much less common in patients deficient in antithrombin.
- System(s) affected: cardiovascular, nervous, pulmonary, reproductive, hematologic, lymphatic/immunologic hemic/lymphatic/immunologic
- Synonym(s): antithrombin III deficiency

EPIDEMIOLOGY
- Predominant age: Mean age of 1st thrombosis is in 2nd decade, usually after puberty.
- Predominant sex: male = female
- No racial or ethnic predisposition

Incidence
1/20 to 1/200 with thrombophilia (1)

Prevalence
1/2,000 to 1/5,000 of normal individuals (1)

ETIOLOGY AND PATHOPHYSIOLOGY
- Hereditary deficiency (2)
  - Type I deficiency is characterized by low levels of antigen (decreased synthesis). Plasma levels of antithrombin are often <50%.
  - Type II deficiency is found when the antithrombin molecule is dysfunctional (decreased function).
  - Type II deficiencies are due to mutations in either the active center of antithrombin that binds the target enzyme or the heparin-binding site.
  - No patients homozygous for defects in the active center have been described, suggesting that this is a lethal condition. Patients heterozygous for mutations in the heparin-binding site rarely have thrombotic episodes.
- Acquired deficiency (2)
  - Many clinical conditions are associated with antithrombin deficiency, such as those listed under "Follow-Up Tests & Special Considerations," but limited evidence suggests these deficiencies contribute to increased thrombosis.

Genetics
Autosomal dominant with variable clinical penetrance

RISK FACTORS
- Oral contraceptives, pregnancy, surgery, trauma, and the use of hormone replacement therapy (HRT) increase the risk of venous thrombosis in patients with antithrombin deficiency.
- Patients with antithrombin deficiency and another prothrombotic state, such as factor V Leiden or the prothrombin G20210A mutation, have increased rates of thrombosis.

Pregnancy Considerations
Increased thrombotic risk from 18% to 70% and specific complications may include preeclampsia, eclampsia, placental abruption, HELLP, premature birth, and recurrent pregnancy loss (3).

GENERAL PREVENTION
Patients with antithrombin deficiency without a history of thrombosis do not require prophylactic treatment.

COMMONLY ASSOCIATED CONDITIONS
Venous thromboembolism

DIAGNOSIS

HISTORY
- Previous thrombosis
- Family history of thrombosis
- Family history of antithrombin deficiency
- Recurrent pregnancy loss

PHYSICAL EXAM
Signs consistent with a deep or superficial venous thrombosis or pulmonary embolism

DIFFERENTIAL DIAGNOSIS
- Factor V Leiden
- Protein C deficiency
- Protein S deficiency
- Dysfibrinogenemia
- Dysplasminogenemia
- Homocystinemia
- Prothrombin G20210A mutation
- Elevated factor VIII levels

DIAGNOSTIC TESTS & INTERPRETATION
Initial Tests (lab, imaging)
- For evaluation of a new clot in a patient at risk: CBC with peripheral smear, PT/INR, aPTT, thrombin time, lupus anticoagulant, antiphospholipid antibodies, factor VIII, anticardiolipin antibody, anti-B2 glycoprotein antibody, activated protein C resistance, protein S antigen and resistance, antithrombin III assay, fibrinogen, factor V Leiden, prothrombin G20210A, homocysteine
- Testing should be done off heparin and at least 2 weeks after the 3 to 6 months course of oral anticoagulation.
- Another test to consider in the workup of antithrombin deficiency:
  - Antithrombin-heparin cofactor assay measures the ability of heparin to bind to antithrombin, which neutralizes the action of thrombin and factor Xa. This is an indirect measure of factor Xa and thrombin inhibition; the factor Xa inhibition activity being more specific. This assay will detect all currently recognized subtypes of hereditary antithrombin deficiency.
- Drugs that may alter lab results: heparin (increased clearance), estrogen, and L-asparaginase (decreased synthesis) can lower antithrombin levels.

Follow-Up Tests & Special Considerations
- The role of family screening for antithrombin deficiency is unclear because most patients with this mutation do not have thrombosis. Screening may be offered to pregnant women with a family history of factor protein S deficiency considering using oral contraceptives or pregnancy.
- Antithrombin levels are low in:
  - DIC
  - Sepsis
  - Burns
  - Severe trauma
  - Acute thrombosis
  - Pregnancy or postpartum
  - Liver disease
  - Nephrotic syndrome
  - Malignancy
  - Myeloproliferative disorders
- Antithrombin levels could be elevated by oral contraceptive pills.
- US to diagnose DVT if clinically indicated
- If DVT diagnosis in question, a negative D-dimer will help to rule out DVT.
- Spiral CT or V/Q scan to diagnose pulmonary embolism (PE) if clinically indicated
- V/Q scan may be difficult to interpret in patients with other lung disease.

Test Interpretation
Venous thrombosis

TREATMENT

GENERAL MEASURES
Routine anticoagulation for asymptomatic patients with antithrombin deficiency is not recommended (3,4)[C].

MEDICATION
First Line
- Patients with antithrombin deficiency and a first thrombosis should be anticoagulated initially with unfractionated heparin followed by oral anticoagulation with warfarin (5)[C].
- Heparin can be stopped after 5 total days of therapy provided the INR is 2 to 3 (5)[C].
- Oral anticoagulant should be started with the initial administration of heparin. Warfarin (Coumadin) 10 mg/day PO for the first 2 days, then adjusted to INR of 2 to 3. Patients should be maintained on warfarin for at least 6 months (5)[C].
- Recurrent thrombosis requires indefinite anticoagulation.
- Contraindications:
  - Active bleeding precludes anticoagulation; risk of bleeding is a relative contraindication to long-term anticoagulation.

- Precautions:
  - Observe patient for signs of embolization, further thrombosis, or bleeding.
  - Avoid IM injections.
  - Periodically check stool and urine for occult blood and monitor CBCs, including platelets.
  - Heparin-induced thrombocytopenia and/or paradoxical thrombosis with thrombocytopenia
- Significant possible interactions:
  - Agents that intensify the response to oral anticoagulants: Common anti-infective agents that potentially increase the effect of warfarin include ciprofloxacin, clarithromycin, erythromycin, metronidazole, trimethoprim-sulfamethoxazole, and azole antifungals. Additional interacting agents include alcohol, allopurinol, amiodarone, anabolic steroids, androgens, cimetidine, chloral hydrate, disulfiram, all NSAIDs, sulfinpyrazone, tamoxifen, thyroid hormone, vitamin E, ranitidine, salicylates, and acetaminophen
  - Agents that diminish the response to oral anticoagulants: aminoglutethimide, antacids, barbiturates, carbamazepine, cholestyramine, diuretics, griseofulvin, rifampin, oral contraceptives
  - See "Diet."

Second Line
- Argatroban: 0.4 to 0.5 μg/kg/min. Case reports describing the use of this direct thrombin inhibitor in patients with antithrombin deficiency have been published (5)[C].
- Antithrombin III (ATnativ, Thrombate III): 50 to 100 IU/min IV titrated to antithrombin level desired. Precise role in therapy remains unclear (5)[C].
- Low-molecular-weight heparin (LMWH) is difficult to manage in this population but is preferred during pregnancy (3,5)[C].

ISSUES FOR REFERRAL
- Recurrent thrombosis on anticoagulation
- Difficulty anticoagulating
- Genetic counseling

ADDITIONAL TREATMENT
- Patients with severe antithrombin deficiency may require plasma replacement of thrombin in order for heparin to be effective.
- Compression stockings for prevention

SURGERY/OTHER PROCEDURES
Thrombectomy may be indicated in complicated cases.

INPATIENT CONSIDERATIONS
Admission Criteria/Initial Stabilization
Complicated thrombosis, such as PE. Heparin initial bolus of 80 U/kg followed by infusion of 18 U/kg/hr. Frequent monitoring of the partial thromboplastin time (PTT) is important, as ~50% of patients deficient in antithrombin require >40,000 U of heparin daily to adequately prolong PTT.

Discharge Criteria
Stable on anticoagulation

 ONGOING CARE

FOLLOW-UP RECOMMENDATIONS
Patient Monitoring
Warfarin use requires periodic INR measurements (monthly after initial stabilization) with a goal of 2 to 3.

DIET
Foods high in vitamin K may interfere with anticoagulation on warfarin. Consider nutrition consultation.

PATIENT EDUCATION
- Patients should be educated about:
  - Use of oral anticoagulant therapy
  - Avoidance of NSAIDs while on warfarin
- The role of family screening is unclear, as most patients with this mutation do not have thrombosis. In a patient with a family history of factor V Leiden, consider screening during pregnancy or if considering oral contraceptive use.

PROGNOSIS
- The odds ratio of thrombosis in a patient with antithrombin deficiency is much higher than in patients with other thrombophilic conditions. The recurrence rate is similarly high.
- There is no difference in clinical severity between patients with type I defects and type II mutations.
- Overall, prognosis is good, if appropriately anticoagulated.

COMPLICATIONS
Recurrent thrombosis (requires indefinite anticoagulation)

REFERENCES

1. Lipe B, Ornstein DL. Deficiencies of natural anticoagulants, protein C, protein S, and antithrombin. *Circulation*. 2011;124(14):e365–e368.
2. Maclean PS, Tait RC. Hereditary and acquired antithrombin deficiency: epidemiology, pathogenesis and treatment options. *Drugs*. 2007;67(10):1429–1440.
3. James AH, Konkle BA, Bauer KA. Prevention and treatment of venous thromboembolism in pregnancy in patients with hereditary antithrombin deficiency. *Int J Womens Health*. 2013;5:233–241.
4. Rodgers GM. Role of antithrombin concentrate in treatment of hereditary antithrombin deficiency. An update. *Thromb Haemost*. 2009;101(5):806–812.
5. Guyatt GH, Akl EA, Crowther M, et al. Executive summary: Antithrombotic Therapy and Prevention of Thrombosis, 9th ed: American College of Chest Physicians Evidence-Based Clinical Practice Guidelines. *Chest*. 2012;141(2)(Suppl):7S–47S.

ADDITIONAL READING
De Stefano V, Rossi E. Testing for inherited thrombophilia and consequences for antithrombotic prophylaxis in patients with venous thromboembolism and their relatives. A review of the guidelines from Scientific Societies and Working Groups. *Thromb Haemost*. 2013;110(4):697–705.

 SEE ALSO

Deep Vein Thrombophlebitis

 CODES

ICD10
D68.59 Other primary thrombophilia

CLINICAL PEARLS
- Antithrombin levels will be low on heparin and during acute thrombosis.
- Diagnosis can be difficult. Conditions causing low levels of antithrombin III, such as pregnancy, liver disease, sepsis, and DIC, must be ruled out.
- Testing should be done off heparin and at least 2 weeks after the 3 to 6 months course of oral anticoagulation.
- For pregnant women with antithrombin deficiency but no prior history of VTE, antepartum and postpartum vigilance are recommended. Postpartum prophylaxis with prophylactic or intermediate-dose LMWH or vitamin K antagonists with target INR 2 to 3 for 6 weeks is only recommended if there is positive family history of VTE.

ANXIETY (GENERALIZED ANXIETY DISORDER)
Jay A. Brieler, MD • Clarice Nelson, MD

BASICS

DESCRIPTION
- Persistent, excessive, and difficult-to-control worry associated with significant symptoms of motor tension, autonomic hyperactivity, and/or disturbances of sleep or concentration.
- System(s) affected: nervous (resulting in increased sympathetic tone and increased catecholamine release); may have secondary effects on other symptoms such as cardiac (tachycardia) and GI (nausea, irregular bowels)

EPIDEMIOLOGY
Prevalence
- 12-month prevalence rate: 2–3%
- Lifetime prevalence rate: 5%
- Onset can occur any time in life but is typically during adulthood; median age of onset in the United States is 31 years.
- Predominant sex: female > male (2:1) (1)

ETIOLOGY AND PATHOPHYSIOLOGY
- May be mediated by abnormalities of neurotransmitter systems (i.e., serotonin, norepinephrine, and γ-aminobutyric acid [GABA])
- Associated with altered regional brain function (increased activity in the amygdala and prefrontal cortex) (2)

Genetics
- Strongly linked to depression in heritability studies
- A variant of the serotonin transporter gene (5HT1A) may contribute to both conditions; other genes (such as that for glutamic acid decarboxylase) also may play a role.

RISK FACTORS
- Caucasian race
- Adverse life events: stress, medical illness, disability, unemployment, and childhood physical and mental abuse
- Family history
- Lack of social support
- Obesity
- Comorbid psychiatric disorders (3)

GENERAL PREVENTION
- Regular exercise is associated with decreased anxiety and depression.
- CBT and parental intervention in children with social withdrawal or early anxiety may protect against the development of GAD (3).

COMMONLY ASSOCIATED CONDITIONS
- Major depressive disorder (>60%), dysthymia, bipolar disorder
- Alcohol/drug abuse
- Cigarette smoking in adolescence
- Panic disorder, agoraphobia, simple phobia, social anxiety disorder, anorexia nervosa

DIAGNOSIS

HISTORY
- Diagnosis is primarily made through history taking. Pathologic anxiety must be distinguished from normal anxiety reactions.

- *DSM-5* criteria are as follows:
  - Symptoms of excessive anxiety and worry must occur more often than not for at least 6 months.
  - Patient finds it difficult to control the worry.
  - At least three additional criteria are required for diagnosis of GAD in adults; only one is required in children.
    ◦ Restlessness or feeling keyed up or on edge
    ◦ Easily fatigued
    ◦ Difficulty concentrating or mind going blank
    ◦ Irritability
    ◦ Muscle tension
    ◦ Sleep disturbances (difficulty falling or staying asleep)
    ◦ Difficulty controlling worry
  - Persistent worry must cause significant distress or impairment in social, occupational, or other areas of functioning.
  - Focus of anxiety and worry is not consistent with or limited to the occurrence of other types of psychiatric disorders and is not directly related to posttraumatic stress disorder (PTSD).
  - Symptoms are not the result of a substance or other *DSM-5* diagnosis (4).

PHYSICAL EXAM
Useful for identifying other differential diagnosis (see below). No specific physical findings in GAD, but patient may exhibit irritability, bitten nails, tremor, or clammy hands.

DIFFERENTIAL DIAGNOSIS
- Cardiovascular: ischemic heart disease, valvular heart disease (mitral valve prolapse), cardiomyopathies, arrhythmias, congestive heart failure
- Respiratory: asthma, chronic obstructive pulmonary disease, pulmonary embolism
- CNS: stroke, seizures, dementia, migraine, vestibular dysfunction, neoplasms
- Metabolic and hormonal: hyper- or hypothyroidism, pheochromocytoma, adrenal insufficiency, Cushing syndrome, hypokalemia, hypoglycemia, hyperparathyroidism
- Nutritional: thiamine, pyridoxine, or folate deficiency; iron deficiency anemia
- Drug-induced anxiety: alcohol, sympathomimetics (cocaine, amphetamine, caffeine), corticosteroids, herbals (ginseng)
- Withdrawal: alcohol, sedative-hypnotics
- Psychiatric: other disorders (e.g., panic disorder, obsessive-compulsive disorder, PTSD, social phobia, adjustment disorder, and somatization disorder)

DIAGNOSTIC TESTS & INTERPRETATION
Initial Tests (lab, imaging)
- Laboratory tests are normal. Initial tests may include thyroid-stimulating hormone, CBC, basic metabolic panel, urine drug screen, and ECG.
- GAD-2: 2-question self-reporting scale (22% positive predictive value [PPV]/78% negative predictive value [NPV])
- PHQ-4 provides a very brief screen for both anxiety and depression (3).

Diagnostic Procedures/Other
Psychological testing
- GAD-7: 5 additional questions; provides more detailed information for treatment (29% PPV/71% NPV); also may be indicative of panic disorder (GAD-7: 29% PPV/71% NPV).

- Hamilton Anxiety Scale (HAM-A), Anxiety Disorders Interview Schedule (ADIS-IV)
- In pediatric populations: ADIS-IV Parent and Child Version, Multidimensional Anxiety Scale for Children (MASC), Screen for Child Anxiety Related Emotional Disorders (SCARED)

TREATMENT

GENERAL MEASURES
- Assess for suicidality given increased risk.
- Identify and treat coexisting substance abuse and other psychiatric conditions.

MEDICATION
Psychotherapeutic approaches

- Psychological treatments are effective in treating GAD: number needed to treat (NNT) = 2 (5)[A].
- Cognitive-behavioral therapy (CBT): Most well-studied psychological treatment; may improve comorbid conditions such as depression. Treatment of choice when available (3)[A]
- Relaxation/mindfulness training (3)[A]

- Psychodynamic psychotherapy: Treatment is focused on patient discovering and verbalizing unconscious conflicts (3)[C].

- Insufficient evidence to compare efficacy of the various treatment types at this time (5)[A]

First Line
- SSRI and SNRI antidepressants have demonstrated efficacy, are well-tolerated, do not cause abuse/dependence, and treat comorbid depression. Data to compare between agents are limited (6)[A].

- SSRIs
  - Paroxetine (Paxil): initially 10 to 20 mg/day; may titrate to a maximum of 50 mg/day (no added benefit more than 20 mg/day)
  - Escitalopram (Lexapro): initially 10 mg/day; may titrate to a maximum of 20 mg/day
  - Sertraline (Zoloft): initially 25 mg/day; may titrate to a maximum of 200 mg/day
  - Fluoxetine (Prozac) and citalopram (Celexa) likely have efficacy for GAD but do not have FDA indications

- SNRIs
  - Duloxetine (Cymbalta): initially 30 mg/day; may titrate to a maximum of 120 mg/day
  - Venlafaxine XR (Effexor XR): initially 37.5 to 75 mg/day; may titrate up by 75 mg every 4 days to a maximum of 225 mg/day

Second Line
- Benzodiazepines (efficacious in the short-term but less effective long-term), risk for dependence (5)[A]

  - Clonazepam (Klonopin): 0.25 mg BID; may increase to 4 mg/day divided BID
  - Diazepam (Valium): 2 to 5 mg BID–QID; may increase to a maximum of 40 mg/day
  - Lorazepam (Ativan): 0.5 mg BID–TID; may increase to 6 mg/day divided TID
  - Alprazolam (Xanax): 0.25mg TID; may increase to 4 mg/day

- Hydroxyzine (Vistaril, Atarax): CNS depressant, antihistamine, anticholinergic; decreased risk of dependence compared with benzodiazepines: usual dose: 50 to 100 mg PO QID; limit use in the elderly (3)[B]

- Azapirones: buspirone (BuSpar): less risk of dependence, although may be less effective. 15 mg/day divided BID–TID initially; maximum of 60 mg/day divided BID–TID (6)[A]
- Quetiapine (Seroquel): optimal dose 150 mg/day. Second-generation antipsychotic. Efficacious but less well-tolerated than SSRIs (6,7)[A].
- Pregabalin (Lyrica): has shown promise in decreasing anxiety scores and preventing relapse at 75 to 300 mg BID; may cause less sexual dysfunction and sleep disruption than SSRIs (6)[A]

- Tricyclic antidepressants (TCAs): imipramine (Tofranil): initially 25 to 50 mg/day; maximum of 300 mg/day, 100 mg/day in the elderly

Geriatric Considerations
- Avoid TCAs and long-acting benzodiazepines; benzodiazepines may cause delirium.
- Pregabalin may cause dizziness and somnolence.

Pediatric Considerations
- Black box warning (SSRIs): Antidepressants increase the risk of suicidal thinking and behavior in children, adolescents, and young adults.
- However, studies have also shown increase in suicide attempts in adolescents after SSRI discontinuation.
- Medications other than SSRIs have not been well-tested in pediatric populations.
- Anxiety and ADHD often co-occur.

Pregnancy Considerations
- Buspirone: Category B: secreted in breast milk; inadequate studies to assess risk
- Benzodiazepines: Category D: may cause lethargy and weight loss in nursing infants; avoid breastfeeding if the mother is taking chronically or in high doses
- SSRIs: if possible, taper and discontinue. After 20 weeks' gestation, there is increased risk of pulmonary hypertension; mild transient neonatal syndrome of CNS; and motor, respiratory, and GI signs. Studies regarding risk of autism show mixed results. Most are Category C:
  - Paroxetine: Category D: conflicting evidence regarding the risk of congenital cardiac defects and other congenital anomalies
  - Hydroxyzine: Category C: Case reports of neonatal withdrawal exist.

ALERT
Precautions

- Benzodiazepines: age >65 years, hepatic insufficiency, respiratory disease/sleep apnea, renal insufficiency, suicidal tendency, contraindicated with narrow-angle glaucoma, precaution with open-angle glaucoma; sudden discontinuation, especially of alprazolam, increases seizure risk. Long-term use has potential for tolerance and dependence; use with caution in patients with history of substance abuse.
- Buspirone: hepatic and/or renal dysfunction; monoamine oxidase inhibitor (MAOI) treatment
- TCAs: advanced age, glaucoma, benign prostatic hypertrophy, hyperthyroidism, cardiovascular disease, liver disease, urinary retention, MAOI treatment
- SSRIs: use caution in those with comorbid bipolar disorder; may trigger mania. Avoid with medications that may increase risk of serotonin syndrome.

ISSUES FOR REFERRAL
Concomitant depression or other comorbidities may warrant a psychiatric evaluation in light of increased suicide risk.

COMPLEMENTARY & ALTERNATIVE MEDICINE
- Patients frequently engage in complementary and alternative medicine (CAM); providers should be familiar with common therapies.

- Probable benefit but more study needed on several complementary therapies, including acupuncture, yoga, tai chi, and aromatherapy (8)[A].
- Kava: Some evidence for benefit over placebo in mild to moderate anxiety, but concern regarding potential hepatotoxicity persists. Safety is potentially affected by many factors, including manufacturing quality, plant part used, dose, and interactions with other substances (8)[A].
- Limited evidence to support other herbal medicines and St. John's wort likely not effective (8)[A]
- Strong evidence to support regular physical activity to relieve anxiety symptoms (8)[A]

INPATIENT CONSIDERATIONS
Patients at risk of suicide should be treated as inpatients; may be considered as well for patients with substantial interference in daily function.

 ## ONGOING CARE

FOLLOW-UP RECOMMENDATIONS
Patient Monitoring
- Follow up within 2 to 4 weeks from starting new medications.

- Medications should be continued past the initial period of response and probably for at least 6 months (6)[A].

- Monitor mental status on benzodiazepines and avoid drug dependence.
- Monitor BP, heart rate, and anticholinergic side effects of TCAs.
- Monitor all patients for suicidal ideation but especially those on SSRIs, SNRIs, and imipramine.

DIET
- Limit caffeine intake.
- Avoid alcohol (drug interactions, high rate of abuse, potential for increased anxiety).

PATIENT EDUCATION
- Regular exercise, especially yoga, may be beneficial for both anxiety and comorbid conditions.
- Psychoeducation regarding normal versus pathologic anxiety, the fight or flight response, and the physiology of anxiety can be extremely helpful.
- Moderate caffeine use; avoid alcohol and nicotine if possible.

PROGNOSIS
- Probability of recovery is approximately 40–60%, but relapse is common.
- Comorbid psychiatric disorders and poor relationships with spouse or family make relapse more likely (1).

REFERENCES

1. Weisberg RB. Overview of generalized anxiety disorder: epidemiology, presentation, and course. *J Clin Psychiatry*. 2009;70(Suppl 2):4–9.
2. Hilbert K, Leuken U, Beesdo-Baum K. Neural structures, functioning and connectivity in generalized anxiety disorder and interaction with neuroendocrine systems: a systematic review. *J Affect Disord*. 2014;158:114–126.
3. Patel G, Fancher TL. In the clinic. Generalized anxiety disorder. *Ann Intern Med*. 2013;159(11):ITC6-1–ITC6-11.
4. American Psychiatric Association. *Diagnostic and Statistical Manual of Mental Disorders*. 5th ed. Arlington, VA: American Psychiatric Association; 2013.
5. Cuijpers P, Sijbrandij M, Koole S, et al. Psychological treatment of generalized anxiety disorder: a meta-analysis. *Clin Psychol Rev*. 2014;34(2):130–140.
6. Baldwin DS, Waldman S, Allgulander C. Evidence-based pharmacological treatment of generalized anxiety disorder. *Int J Neuropsychopharmacol*. 2011;14(5):697–710.
7. Depping AM, Komossa K, Kissling W, et al. Second-generation antipsychotics for anxiety disorders. *Cochrane Database Syst Rev*. 2010;(12):CD008120.
8. Sarris J, Moylan S, Camfield DA, et al. Complementary medicine, exercise, meditation, diet, and lifestyle modification for anxiety disorders: a review of current evidence. *Evid Based Complement Alternat Med*. 2012;2012:809653.

 ## SEE ALSO

Algorithms: Depressive Episode, Major; Anxiety

 ## CODES

ICD10
- F41.9 Anxiety disorder, unspecified
- F41.1 Generalized anxiety disorder
- F41.8 Other specified anxiety disorders

CLINICAL PEARLS
- Psychiatric comorbidities, especially depression, are extremely common with GAD; patients are at increased risk for suicidality.
- CBT and SSRIs (possibly in combination) are the treatments of choice.
- Starting antidepressant medication at low doses, with careful titration to full therapeutic dosing, helps minimize side effects while maximizing efficacy.
- Benzodiazepines may be used initially but should be tapered and withdrawn if possible.
- CAM use is common, and certain therapies may be effective.

AORTIC VALVULAR STENOSIS

Michael T. Tanoue, MD • Parag Goyal, MD • James M. Horowitz, MD, FACC

 BASICS

DESCRIPTION

Aortic stenosis (AS) is a narrowing of the aortic valve area causing obstruction to left ventricular (LV) outflow. The disease has a long asymptomatic latency period, but development of severe obstruction or onset of symptoms such as syncope, angina, and congestive heart failure (CHF) are associated with a high mortality rate without surgical intervention.

EPIDEMIOLOGY

- Most common cause of LV outflow obstruction in both children and adults
- Predominant age
  - <30 years: congenital
  - 30 to 65 years: congenital or rheumatic fever
  - >65 years: degenerative calcification of aortic valve

Prevalence

- Affects 1.3% of population 65 to 74 years old, 2.4% 75 to 84 years old, 4% >84 years old (1)
- Bicuspid aortic valve: 1–2% of population. Bicuspid aortic valve predisposes to development of AS at an earlier age (1).

ETIOLOGY AND PATHOPHYSIOLOGY

- Progressive aortic leaflet thickening and calcification results in LV outflow obstruction. Obstruction causes increased afterload and over time, decreased cardiac output.
- Increase in LV systolic pressure is required to preserve cardiac output; this leads to development of concentric left ventricular hypertrophy (LVH). The compensatory LVH preserves ejection fraction but adversely affects heart functioning.
  - LVH impairs coronary blood flow during diastole by compression of coronary arteries and reduced capillary ingrowth into hypertrophied muscle.
  - LVH results in diastolic dysfunction by reducing ventricular compliance.
- Diastolic dysfunction necessitates stronger left atrial (LA) contraction to augment preload and maintain stroke volume. Loss of LA contraction by atrial fibrillation can induce acute deterioration.
- Diastolic dysfunction may persist after relief of aortic stenosis due to the presence of interstitial fibrosis.
- Angina: increased myocardial demand due to higher LV pressure. Myocardial supply is compromised due to LVH.
- Syncope (exertional): can be multifactorial from inability to augment cardiac output due to the fixed obstruction to LV outflow; arrhythmias; or most commonly, abnormal baroreceptor response resulting in failure to appropriately augment blood pressure
- Heart failure: Eventually, LVH cannot compensate for increasing afterload resulting in high LV pressure and volume, which are accompanied by an increase in LA and pulmonary pressures.
- Degenerative calcific changes to aortic valve (2)
  - Mechanism involves mechanical stress to valve leaflets as well as atherosclerotic changes to the valve tissue. Bicuspid valves are at higher risk for mechanical stress.
  - Early lesions: subendothelial accumulation of oxidized LDL and macrophages and T lymphocytes (inflammatory response)
  - Disease progression: fibroblasts undergo transformation into osteoblasts. Protein production of osteopontin, osteocalcin, and bone morphogenic protein-2 (BMP-2), which modulates calcification of leaflets.
- Congenital: unicuspid valve, bicuspid valve, tricuspid valve with fusion of commissures, hypoplastic annulus
- Rheumatic fever: chronic scarring with fusion of commissures

RISK FACTORS

- Congenital unicommissural valve or bicuspid valve (1)
  - Unicommissural valve: Most cases were detected during childhood.
  - Bicuspid valve: predisposes to the development of AS earlier in adulthood (4th to 5th decade) compared to tricuspid valve (6th to 8th decade)
- Rheumatic fever (1)
  - Prevalence of chronic rheumatic valvular disease has declined significantly in the United States.
  - Most cases are associated with mitral valve disease.
- Degenerative calcific changes
  - Most common cause of acquired AS in the United States
  - Risk factors are similar to that of coronary artery disease (CAD) and include the following: hypercholesterolemia, hypertension, smoking, male gender, age, and diabetes mellitus.

COMMONLY ASSOCIATED CONDITIONS

- CAD (50% of patients)
- Hypertension (40% of patients): results in "double-loaded" left ventricle (dual source of increased afterload as a result of obstruction from AS, and hypertension)
- Aortic insufficiency (common in calcified bicuspid valves and rheumatic disease)
- Mitral valve disease: 95% of patients with AS from rheumatic fever (RF) also have mitral valve disease
- LV dysfunction and CHF
- Acquired von Willebrand disease: Impaired platelet function and decreased vWF results in bleeding (ecchymosis and epistaxis) in 20% of AS patients. Severity of coagulopathy is directly related to severity of AS.
- Gastrointestinal arteriovenous malformations (AVMs)
- Cerebral or systemic embolic events due to calcium emboli

℞ DIAGNOSIS

HISTORY

- Primary symptoms: angina, syncope, and heart failure (3). Angina is the most frequent symptom. Syncope is often exertional. Heart failure symptoms include fatigue, exertional dyspnea, orthopnea, paroxysmal nocturnal dyspnea, and shortness of breath.
- Palpitations
- Neurologic events (transient ischemic attack or cerebrovascular accident) secondary to embolization
- Geriatric patients may have subtle symptoms such as fatigue and exertional dyspnea.
- Note: Symptoms do not always correlate with valve area (severity of AS) but most commonly occur when aortic valve area is <1 cm², jet velocity is > 4.0 m/s, or the mean transvalvular gradient is ≥ 40 mm Hg.

PHYSICAL EXAM

- Auscultation (3)
  - Harsh, systolic crescendo–decrescendo murmur is best heard at 2nd right sternal border and radiates into the carotid arteries. Peak of murmur correlates with severity of stenosis; later peaking murmur suggests greater severity.
  - High-pitched blowing diastolic murmur suggests associated aortic insufficiency.
  - Paradoxically split S2 or absent A2. Note: Normally split S2 reliably excludes severe AS.
  - S4 due to stiffening of the left ventricle
- Other associated signs (3) include *Pulsus parvus et tardus*: decreased and delayed carotid upstroke. LV heave. Findings of CHF: pulmonary and/or lower extremity edema

DIFFERENTIAL DIAGNOSIS

- Mitral regurgitation: high-frequency, pansystolic murmur, best heard at the apex, often radiates to the axilla
- Hypertrophic obstructive cardiomyopathy: also systolic crescendo–decrescendo murmur but best heard at left sternal border and may radiate into axilla. Murmur intensity increases by changing from squatting to standing and/or by Valsalva maneuver.
- Discrete fixed subaortic stenosis: 50–65% has associated cardiac deformity (patent ductus arteriosus [PDA], ventricular septal defect [VSD], aortic coarctation)
- Aortic supravalvular stenosis: Williams syndrome, homozygous familial hypercholesterolemia

DIAGNOSTIC TESTS & INTERPRETATION

Initial Tests (lab, imaging)

- Chest x-ray (CXR) (1)
  - May be normal in compensated, isolated valvular AS
  - Boot-shaped heart reflective of concentric hypertrophy
  - Poststenotic dilatation of ascending aorta and calcification of aortic valve (seen on lateral PA CXR)
- ECG: often normal ECG (ECG is nondiagnostic), or may show LVH, LA enlargement, and nonspecific ST- and T-wave abnormalities
- Echo indications
  - Initial workup
    - Doppler echocardiogram: primary test in the diagnosis and evaluation of AS
    - Assesses valve anatomy and severity of disease
    - Assesses LV wall thickness, size, and function, and pulmonary artery pressure
  - In known AS and changing signs/symptoms
  - In known AS and pregnancy due to hemodynamic changes of pregnancy
- Echo findings
  - Aortic valve thickening, calcification
  - Decreased aortic valve excursion
  - Reduced aortic valve area
  - Transvalvular gradient across aortic valve
  - LVH and diastolic dysfunction
  - LV ejection fraction
  - Wall-motion abnormalities suggesting CAD
  - Evaluate for concomitant aortic insufficiency or mitral valve disease.
- AS severity based on echo values (4)
  - Stage A (at risk): bicuspid aortic valve, sclerosis, or other congenital abnormality; mean pressure gradient: 0 mm Hg; jet vel. <2 m/s

- Stage B (progressive): bicuspid or trileaflet valve
  - Mild: mean pressure gradient: <20 mmHg; jet vel. 2.0 to 2.9 m/s
  - Moderate: mean pressure gradient: 20 to 40 mm Hg; jet vel. 3.0 to 3.9 m/s
- Stage C (asymptomatic severe AS):
  - C1 (without LV dysfunction): AVA ≤1.0 or AVAi ≤0.6 cm²/m²; mean pressure gradient: 40 to 60 mm Hg; jet vel. ≥4 to 5 m/s
  - C2 (with LV dysfunction): AVA ≤1.0 or AVAi ≤0.6 cm²/m²; mean pressure gradient: ≥40 mm Hg; jet vel. ≥4 m/s
- Stage D (symptomatic severe AS):
  - D1 (high-gradient): AVA ≤1.0 cm²; mean pressure gradient: >40 mm Hg; jet vel. >4 m/s
  - D2 (low-flow/low-gradient with reduced EF <50%): AVA ≤1.0 cm²; mean pressure gradient: <40 mm Hg; jet vel. <4 m/s
  - D3 (low-gradient, normal EF ≥50% or paradoxical low-flow severe AS): AVA ≤1.0 cm²; AVAi ≤0.6 cm²/m² and stroke volume index <35 mL/m²; mean pressure gradient: <40 mm Hg; jet vel. <4 m/s

Diagnostic Procedures/Other
- Exercise stress testing

  - Asymptomatic patients with severe AS (5)[B]: helpful to uncover subtle symptoms or changes, abnormal BP (increase <20 mm Hg), and ECG changes (ST depressions). 1/3 of patients develop symptoms with exercise testing; STOP testing at this point.
  - Symptomatic patients (5)[B]: DO NOT perform exercise stress testing, as it may induce hypotension or ventricular tachycardia.
  - CHF patients (5)[B]: Dobutamine stress echocardiography is reasonable to evaluate patients with low-flow/low-gradient AS and LV dysfunction.

- Cardiac catheterization

  - Perform prior to aortic valve replacement in patients with suspected CAD (5)[B]. Determines need for coronary artery bypass graft (CABG). If unambiguous diagnosis of AS, perform only coronary angiography.

  - Can also use if noninvasive testing is inconclusive or if there is discrepancy between severity of symptoms and findings on echo
  - Measures transvalvular flow and transvalvular pressure gradient, which facilitates calculation of effective valve area
  - Hemodynamic measurements with infusion of dobutamine can be useful for evaluation of patients with low-flow/low-gradient AS and LV dysfunction.

TEST INTERPRETATION
- Aortic valve: nodular calcification on valve cusps (initially at bases), cusp rigidity, cusp thickening, and fibrosis
- LVH, myocardial interstitial fibrosis
- 50% incidence of concomitant CAD

TREATMENT

MEDICATION
- No effective medical therapy for severe or symptomatic AS
- Prevention: currently no recommended medical therapy. Statins have been thought to slow progression if initiated during mild disease. However, this has not been supported by large, randomized controlled trials.

- Antibiotic prophylaxis against recurrent RF is indicated for patients with rheumatic AS (penicillin G 1,200,000 U IM q4wk; duration varies with age and history of carditis).
- Antibiotic prophylaxis is no longer indicated for prevention of infective endocarditis (5).
- Comorbidities: hypertension: angiotensin-converting enzyme (ACE) inhibitors, start with low dose and increase cautiously. Be cautious of vasodilators, which may cause hypotension.

SURGERY/OTHER PROCEDURES
- The only proven treatment for AS is valve replacement.
- Indications for aortic valve replacement (AVR) surgery:

  - Symptomatic and severe high-gradient AS by history or exercise testing (4)[B]
  - Asymptomatic, severe AS and LVEF < 50% (4)[B]
  - Severe AS (stage C or D) when undergoing other cardiac surgery (4)[B]

- AVR surgery is reasonable in patients who are:

  - Asymptomatic with severe AS (C1) with jet vel. ≥5 m/s and low surgical risk, decreased exercise tolerance, or have an exercise fall in blood pressure (4)[B]
  - Symptomatic stage D2, with a low-dose dobutamine stress with jet vel. ≥4.0 m/s or mean pressure gradient ≥40 mm Hg with ≤1.0 cm² at any dobutamine dose (4)[B]

  - Symptomatic stage D3 with LVEF >50% if clinical and hemodynamic data support valve obstruction as likely cause of symptoms (4)[C]
  - Stage B who are undergoing other cardiac surgery, or asymptomatic stage C1 with rapid disease progression and low surgical risk (4)[C]

ALERT
Note: If the aortic valve area is >1.5 cm² and the gradient is <15 mm Hg, there is no benefit from AVR.

- Transcatheter aortic valve replacement (TAVR) offers a less invasive option for some patients (6).
  - For those who are high at surgical risk and considered inoperable, TAVR has demonstrated superiority to medical therapy.
  - For those who are high at surgical risk, TAVR has demonstrated noninferiority to surgical AVR (6).
  - For those who are intermediate at surgical risk, TAVR may emerge as a reasonable alternative to surgical risk, though this indication has not yet been approved in the United States.
  - Valve-in-valve TAVR can be considered in high-risk patients with failed surgically implanted bioprosthetic valves.
- Percutaneous balloon valvuloplasty may have role in palliation or as a bridge to valve replacement in hemodynamically unstable or high-risk patients (5)[C] but is not recommended as an alternative to valve replacement.

ONGOING CARE

FOLLOW-UP RECOMMENDATIONS
- Advise patients to immediately report symptoms referable to AS.
- Asymptomatic patients: yearly history and physical (5)[C]

- Serial ECHO: yearly for severe AS, every 1 to 2 years for moderate AS, every 3 to 5 years for mild AS (5)[B]

PATIENT EDUCATION
Physical activity limitations
- Asymptomatic mild AS: no restrictions
- Asymptomatic moderate to severe AS: Avoid strenuous exercise. Consider exercise stress test prior to starting exercise program.

PROGNOSIS
- 25% mortality/year in symptomatic patients who do not undergo valve replacement; average survival is 2 to 3 years without AVR surgery.
- Median survival in symptomatic AS (3): heart failure: 2 years; syncope: 3 years; angina: 5 years
- Perisurgical mortality: AVR surgery has 4% mortality rate; AVR + CABG has 6.8% mortality rate
- Adverse postoperative prognostic factors: age, heart failure (HF) New York Heart Association (NYHA) class III/IV, cerebrovascular disease, renal dysfunction, CAD

REFERENCES
1. Carabello BA, Paulus WJ. Aortic stenosis. *Lancet*. 2009;373(9667):956–966.
2. Otto CM. Calcific aortic stenosis—time to look more closely at the valve. *N Engl J Med*. 2008;359(13):1395–1398.
3. Grimard BH, Larson JM. Aortic stenosis: diagnosis and treatment. *Am Fam Physician*. 2008;78(6):717–724.
4. Nishimura RA, Otto CM, Bonow RO, et al. 2014 AHA/ACC guideline for the management of patients with valvular heart disease: a report of the American College of Cardiology/American Heart Association Task Force on Practice Guidelines. *J Thorac Cardiovasc Surg*. 2014;148(1):e1–e132.
5. Bonow RO, Carabello BA, Kanu C, et al. ACC/AHA 2006 guidelines for the management of patients with valvular heart disease: a report of the American College of Cardiology/American Heart Association Task Force on Practice Guidelines (writing committee to revise the 1998 Guidelines for the Management of Patients With Valvular Heart Disease): developed in collaboration with the Society of Cardiovascular Anesthesiologists: endorsed by the Society for Cardiovascular Angiography and Interventions and the Society of Thoracic Surgeons. *Circulation*. 2006;114(5):e84–e231.
6. Smith CR, Leon MB, Mack MJ, et al. Transcatheter versus surgical aortic-valve replacement in high-risk patients. *N Engl J Med*. 2011;364(23):2187–2198.

CODES

ICD10
- I35.0 Nonrheumatic aortic (valve) stenosis
- I06.0 Rheumatic aortic stenosis
- Q23.0 Congenital stenosis of aortic valve

CLINICAL PEARLS
- AS is diagnosed on physical exam by a systolic crescendo–decrescendo murmur and delayed and diminished pulses.
- Symptomatic AS most commonly presents as angina, syncope, and heart failure.
- Symptomatic AS has a very poor prognosis, unless treated with surgical intervention.

APPENDICITIS, ACUTE

Anila Khaliq, MD • Komel Safdar, MBBS • Fariah Hanna, MBBS

BASICS

DESCRIPTION
- Acute inflammation of the vermiform appendix, first described by Reginald Fitz in 1886
- Arising from the base of the cecum in right lower quadrant (RLQ); can be localized anterior, posterior, medial, lateral to the cecum, as well as in the pelvis. Vascular supply by appendicular artery, a branch of the ileocolic artery. Nerve supply derived from the superior mesenteric plexus.
- Most common cause of acute surgical abdomen

EPIDEMIOLOGY
- Predominant age: 10 to 30 years: rare in infancy
- Predominant sex: slight male predominance:
  - Ages 10 to 30: male > female (3:2)
  - Age >30: male = female

Incidence
- 1 case per 1,000 people per year
- Lifetime incidence 1 in every 15 persons (7%)

Pregnancy Considerations
- Most common extrauterine surgical emergency
- No more common in pregnant versus nonpregnant women
- Higher rate of perforation; more likely to present with peritonitis

ETIOLOGY AND PATHOPHYSIOLOGY
The cause is thought to be obstruction of the appendiceal lumen. This leads to distention, ischemia, and bacterial overgrowth. Without intervention, most cases of appendicitis will lead to perforation and subsequently abscess formation or generalized peritonitis. Causes of obstruction:
- Fecaliths (most common)
- Lymphoid tissue hyperplasia (in children)
- Vegetable, fruit seeds, and other foreign bodies
- Intestinal worms (ascarids)
- Strictures, fibrosis, neoplasms

Genetics
First-degree relative with history of appendicitis increases risk, although no direct genetic link has been found.

RISK FACTORS
Adolescent males, familial tendency, intra-abdominal tumors

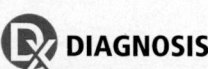

DIAGNOSIS

- Diagnosis of acute appendicitis relies on the history and physical examination with supporting laboratory studies and imaging.
- Scoring systems
  - Modified Alvarado Scoring System (MASS): The use of MASS in the diagnosis of acute appendicitis has been reported to improve the diagnostic accuracy and consequently reduces negative appendectomy and complication rates.
  - Use of MASS in for acute appendicitis in female patients should be supplemented by additional investigations like abdominal ultrasound or laparoscopy.
  - A MASS score above 7 should indicate appendectomy without the need for further imaging.

- A cutoff point of 6 for the MASS score will yield higher sensitivity and a better diagnosis of appendicitis but provides an increase in negative appendectomy.
- Pediatric Appendicitis Score—this has been developed to help predict the likelihood of acute appendicitis, although diagnosis is still considered a clinical decision.

HISTORY
- Classic history is vague periumbilical pain, followed by anorexia/nausea/vomiting. Over the next 4 to 48 hours, pain migrates to the RLQ.
- Only 50% of patients present with this classic history.
- Pain before vomiting (~100% sensitive), abdominal pain (~100%), pain migration (50%)
- Anorexia (~100%), nausea (90%), vomiting (75%), obstipation
- Atypical symptoms and pain associated with a retrocecal or pelvic appendix

PHYSICAL EXAM
- Fever; temperature >100.4°F (may be absent); tachycardia
- RLQ tenderness; maximal tenderness at McBurney point (1/3 the distance from the anterior superior iliac spine to the umbilicus)
- Voluntary and involuntary guarding
- Rovsing sign: RLQ pain with palpation of left lower quadrant
- Psoas sign: pain with right thigh extension (retrocecal appendix)
- Obturator sign: pain with internal rotation of flexed right thigh (pelvic appendix); local and suprapubic pain on rectal exam (pelvic appendix)
- Pelvic and rectal exams are necessary to rule out other causes of lower abdominal pain (e.g., pelvic inflammatory disease, prostatitis)
- Serial exams can be useful in indeterminate cases.

DIFFERENTIAL DIAGNOSIS
- GI:
  - Gastroenteritis, inflammatory bowel disease
  - Diverticulitis, ileitis
  - Cholecystitis, pancreatitis
  - Intussusception, volvulus
- Gynecologic:
  - Pelvic inflammatory disease, ectopic pregnancy
  - Ovarian cyst, ovarian torsion, tubo-ovarian abscess
  - Endometriosis
  - Ruptured Graafian follicle
- Urologic:
  - Testicular torsion, epididymitis
  - Kidney stones, prostatitis, cystitis, pyelonephritis
- Systemic:
  - Diabetic ketoacidosis
  - Henoch-Schönlein purpura
  - Sickle cell crisis
  - Porphyria
- Other:
  - Acute mesenteric lymphadenitis
  - No organic pathologic condition
  - Hernias
  - Psoas abscess

- Rectus sheath hematoma
- Epiploic appendagitis
- Pneumonia (basilar)

Pediatric Considerations
- Decreased diagnostic accuracy of history and physical exam
- Higher fever, more vomiting and diarrhea

Pregnancy Considerations
- Difficult diagnosis
- Normal response to infection/inflammation is suppressed.
- Appendix displaced out of pelvis by gravid uterus

Geriatric Considerations
Decreased diagnostic accuracy, more likely to be atypical presentation

DIAGNOSTIC TESTS & INTERPRETATION
Initial Tests (lab, imaging)
- Leukocytosis: WBC >10,000/mm³ (70%)
- Polymorphonuclear predominance or "left shift" (>90%)
- Human chorionic gonadotropin (hCG) (if negative, rule out ectopic pregnancy)
- Urinalysis: hematuria, pyuria (~30%)
- C-reactive protein: nonspecific inflammatory marker. When paired with an elevated WBC can increase the likelihood of appendicitis.
- Drugs may alter lab results: antibiotics, steroids.
- Imaging used in cases of suspected appendicitis when the diagnosis is not clear; is helpful to detect complications (abscess, perforation)
- Plain films: little utility, nonspecific findings, may visualize fecalith

- CT scan with contrast: sensitivity ~91–98%; specificity 95–99%; imaging modality of choice. However, growing concern regarding radiation dose, particularly in young patients (1)[A].
- Ultrasound: alternative in pregnant patients, children, and in women with suspected gynecologic pathology. Sensitivity and specificity vary by report and accuracy depends on the skill of the ultrasonographer. Can rule in appendicitis but cannot reliably exclude the diagnosis. Starting with an ultrasound and, if negative, obtaining a CT scan has been proposed as an effective workup strategy (2)[B].

- MRI: growing in popularity for diagnosing pregnant patients but also may be useful for patients with contrast allergies and/or patients with renal failure. Limitations include cost, availability, and time required to complete study.
- Radioisotope-labeled WBC scans: may be used in patients with indeterminate CT scans and suspected appendicitis as an alternative to observation or surgery. Limitations include availability and time required to complete study.

Diagnostic Procedures/Other
Exploratory laparotomy/laparoscopy: Acceptable nontherapeutic appendectomy rates vary based on age and gender and may be higher for females of childbearing age than males.

72

Test Interpretation

- Acute appendiceal inflammation, local vascular congestion, obstruction
- Gangrene, perforation with abscess (15–30%)
- Fecalith

 # TREATMENT

GENERAL MEASURES
Surgery (appendectomy) is the standard of care for acute, uncomplicated appendicitis.

MEDICATION
First Line
- Uncomplicated acute appendicitis: perioperative dose of antibiotic (3)[A]: single dose of cefoxitin or ampicillin/sulbactam (Unasyn) or cefazolin plus metronidazole

- Gangrenous or perforating appendicitis:
  – Broadened antibiotic coverage for aerobic and anaerobic enteric pathogens
  – Piperacillin and tazobactam (Zosyn) or ticarcillin and clavulanate (Timentin) or a 3rd-generation cephalosporin plus metronidazole are initial options.
  – Adjust dosage and choice of antibiotic based on intraoperative cultures.
  – Continue antibiotics for at least 7 days postoperatively or until patient becomes afebrile with normal WBC count.

Second Line
- Among patients with CT-proven, uncomplicated appendicitis, antibiotic treatment did not meet the prespecified criterion for noninferiority compared with appendectomy. Most patients randomized to antibiotic treatment for uncomplicated appendicitis did not require appendectomy during the 1-year follow-up period, and those who required appendectomy did not experience significant complications.

- In the case of acute appendicitis complicated by abscess formation or phlegmon in pediatric patients, some studies show initial conservative management with antibiotics alone to carry fewer risks and complications than emergent appendectomy (4)[A].

- Uncomplicated acute appendicitis: clindamycin plus one of the following: ciprofloxacin, levofloxacin, gentamicin, or aztreonam
- Gangrenous or perforated appendicitis: ciprofloxacin or levofloxacin plus metronidazole or monotherapy with a carbapenem (imipenem and cilastatin, meropenem, ertapenem)

ISSUES FOR REFERRAL
All cases of appendicitis require emergent surgical consultation.

SURGERY/OTHER PROCEDURES
- Inpatient surgery is indicated.
- Patients presenting within 72 hours of onset:
  – Immediate appendectomy; laparoscopic favored unless perforation (5)[A]
  – Drainage of abscess, if present
- Patients who present late (>4 to 5 days after symptom onset) may be treated initially with antibiotics, bowel rest, and drainage of any abscess. Later (4 to 10 weeks) appendectomy can then be performed in this subgroup only.

INPATIENT CONSIDERATIONS
Admission Criteria/Initial Stabilization
All patients with appendicitis should be admitted.

IV Fluids
Fluid resuscitation with normal saline (NS) or lactated Ringer (LR) solution. Correct fluid and electrolyte deficits.

Nursing
Preoperative preparation

Discharge Criteria
Tolerating PO; return of bowel function; afebrile; normal WBC

 # ONGOING CARE

FOLLOW-UP RECOMMENDATIONS
- Return to work is usually possible 1 to 2 weeks following most uncomplicated appendicitis.
- Restrict activity for 4 to 6 weeks after surgery: No heavy lifting (>10 lb) or strenuous physical activity.

PATIENT EDUCATION
Contact physician for postoperative development of:
- Anorexia, nausea, vomiting
- Abdominal pain, fever, chills
- Signs/symptoms of wound infection

PROGNOSIS
- Generally uncomplicated course in young adults with unruptured appendicitis
- Factors increasing morbidity and mortality: extremes of age, presence of appendiceal rupture
- Morbidity rates:
  – Nonperforated appendicitis: 3%
  – Perforated appendicitis: 47%
- Mortality rates:
  – Unruptured appendicitis: 0.1%
  – Ruptured appendicitis: 3%
  – Patients >60 years of age make up 50% of total deaths from appendicitis.
  – Older patients with ruptured appendix: 15%

Pediatric Considerations
- Rupture earlier
- Rupture rate: 15–60%

Pregnancy Considerations
- Rupture rate: 40%
- Fetal mortality rate: 2–8.5%

Geriatric Considerations
Rupture rate: 67–90%

COMPLICATIONS
- Wound infection, intra-abdominal abscess; lower rate with antibiotic prophylaxis (6)[A], intestinal fistulas
- Intestinal obstruction, paralytic ileus, incisional hernia
- Liver abscess (rare), pyelophlebitis

REFERENCES

1. Hlibczuk V, Dattaro JA, Jin Z, et al. Diagnostic accuracy of noncontrast computed tomography for appendicitis in adults: a systematic review. *Ann Emerg Med.* 2010;55(1):51.e1–59.e1.
2. Poortman P, Oostvogel HJ, Bosma E, et al. Improving diagnosis of acute appendicitis: results of a

diagnostic pathway with standard use of ultrasonography followed by selective use of CT. *J Am Coll Surg.* 2009;208(3):434–441.
3. Andersen BR, Kallehave FL, Andersen HK. Antibiotics versus placebo for prevention of postoperative infection after appendicectomy. *Cochrane Database Syst Rev.* 2005;(3):CD001439.
4. Simillis C, Symeonides P, Shorthouse AJ, et al. A meta-analysis comparing conservative treatment versus acute appendectomy for complicated appendicitis (abscess or phlegmon). *Surgery.* 2010;147(6):818–829.
5. Sauerland S, Lefering R, Neugebauer EA. Laparoscopic versus open surgery for suspected appendicitis. *Cochrane Database Syst Rev.* 2004;(4):CD001546.
6. Wilms IM, de Hoog DE, de Visser DC, et al. Appendectomy versus antibiotic treatment for acute appendicitis. *Cochrane Database Syst Rev.* 2011;(11):CD008359.

ADDITIONAL READING

- Kanumba ES, Mabula JB, Rambau P, et al. Modified Alvarado Scoring System as a diagnostic tool for acute appendicitis at Bugando Medical Centre, Mwanza, Tanzania. *BMC Surg.* 2011;11:4.
- Nasiri S, Mohebbi F, Sodagari N, et al. Diagnostic values of ultrasound and the Modified Alvarado Scoring System in acute appendicitis. *Int J Emerg Med.* 2012;5(1):26.
- Salminen P, Paajanen H, Rautio T, et al. Antibiotic therapy vs appendectomy for treatment of uncomplicated acute appendicitis: the APPAC randomized clinical trial. *JAMA.* 2015;313(23):2340–2348.

 ## SEE ALSO

Algorithm: Abdominal Rigidity

 ## CODES

ICD10
- K35.80 Unspecified acute appendicitis
- K35.2 Acute appendicitis with generalized peritonitis
- K35.3 Acute appendicitis with localized peritonitis

CLINICAL PEARLS
- Classic history of anorexia with periumbilical pain localizing to RLQ is the cornerstone of diagnosis for acute appendicitis.
- Diagnosis is much more challenging in children, pregnant patients, and the elderly due to varying symptoms and signs.
- In equivocal cases, CT of abdomen and pelvis is the diagnostic test of choice, although ultrasound and MRI are useful alternatives.
- Acute appendicitis is the most common surgical emergency during pregnancy.

ARTERITIS, TEMPORAL
Cynthia M. Waickus, MD, PhD

 BASICS

DESCRIPTION
- Technically termed giant cell arteritis (GCA)
- A chronic, generalized, cellular, and humoral immune-mediated vasculitis of large- and medium-sized vessels, predominantly affecting the cranial arteries originating from the aortic arch, although vascular involvement may be widespread. Inflammation of the aorta is observed in 50% of cases (1,2).
- Frequent features include fatigue, headaches, jaw claudication, loss of vision, scalp tenderness, polymyalgia rheumatica (PMR), and aortic arch syndrome (decreased or absent peripheral pulses, discrepancies of blood pressure, arterial bruits) (3).

EPIDEMIOLOGY
- The mean age of onset is approximately 75 years; rare <50 years.
- Women are affected about 2 times as often as men.
- Most common vasculitis in individuals of Northern European decent (Scandinavain countries)
- Rare in Asians and African Americans

Incidence
- Prevalence in individuals >50 years: 1 in 500 (1,4,5)
- Cyclic incidence: peaking every 5 to 7 years

ETIOLOGY AND PATHOPHYSIOLOGY
- The exact etiology of GCA remains unknown, although current theory suggests that advanced age, ethnicity, and specific genetic predisposition lead to a maladaptive response to endothelial injury, intimal hyperplasia, and ultimately vascular stenosis.
- Temporal arteritis (TA) is a chronic, systemic vasculitis primarily affecting the elastic lamina of medium- and large-sized arteries. Histopathology of affected arteries is marked by transmural inflammation of the intima, media, and adventitia, as well as patchy infiltration by lymphocytes, macrophages, and multinucleated giant cells. Mural hyperplasia can result in arterial luminal narrowing, resulting in subsequent distal ischemia (1,4,5).
- Current theory regarding the etiology of TA is that a maladaptive response to endothelial injury leads to an inappropriate activation of T cell–mediated immunity via immature antigen-presenting cells. The subsequent release of cytokines within the arterial vessel wall can attract macrophages and multinucleated giant cells, which form granulomatous infiltrates and give diseased vessels their characteristic histology. This also leads to an oligoclonal expansion of T cells directed against antigens in or near the elastic lamina. Ultimately, this cascade results in vessel wall damage, intimal hyperplasia, and eventual stenotic occlusion (5,6).
- In recent years, GCA and polymyalgia rheumatica (PMR) have increasingly been considered to be closely related conditions (3,4).

Genetics
The gene for HLA-DRB1–04 has been identified as a risk factor for TA, and polymorphisms of ICAM-1 have also been implicated (2).

RISK FACTORS
- Increasing age >70 years is the greatest risk factor.
- Genetic predisposition
- Environmental factors influence susceptibility (6–8).
- Heavy smoking and atherosclerotic disease are risk factors for females but not for males.

COMMONLY ASSOCIATED CONDITIONS
Polymyalgia rheumatica (PMR) may develop either before or after the arteritis (4,6).

 DIAGNOSIS

HISTORY
- Most common presenting symptom is headache (2/3 of patients) (1,3,7)[A].
- Constitutional symptoms (fever, fatigue, weight loss)
- Any visual disturbances (amaurosis fugax, diplopia)
- Vision loss (20% of patients)
- Jaw claudication (presence of symptom significantly increases likelihood of a positive biopsy)
- Scalp tenderness or sensitivity
- Claudication of upper extremities or tongue
- Symptoms of polymyalgia rheumatica (shoulder and hip girdle pain and stiffness)
- Distal extremity swelling/edema
- Upper respiratory symptoms

PHYSICAL EXAM
- Temporal artery abnormalities (beading, prominence, tenderness)
- Typically appear "ill"
- Decreased peripheral pulses in the presence of large vessel diseases
- Funduscopic exam shows pale and edema of the optic disk, scattered cotton wool patches, and small hemorrhages.
- Unlike other forms of vasculitis, GCA rarely involves the skin, kidneys, and lungs.

DIFFERENTIAL DIAGNOSIS
- *Classification criteria are as follows*:
  - Age >70 years
  - New localized headache
  - Temporal artery abnormality (tenderness to palpation, decreased or absent pulses)
  - ESR >50 mm/hr
  - Abnormal temporal artery biopsy showing vasculitis with predominance of mononuclear cell infiltration or granulomatous inflammation
- Three or more of the above symptoms: 95% sensitivity/91% specificity for GCA diagnosis (The American College of Rheumatology criteria for the classification of GCA)

DIAGNOSTIC TESTS & INTERPRETATION
Initial Tests (lab, imaging)
- ESR >50 mm/hr (86% sensitivity), although nonspecific (27%); infrequently, may be normal (3,7)[A]
- C-reactive protein (CRP) >2.45 mg/dL is a more sensitive marker of inflammation (97% sensitivity) and is associated with increased odds of a positive biopsy result.

- A normal ESR and/or CRP renders the diagnosis of GCA unlikely.
- Platelet count >400 × 10³
- Acute-phase reactants (fibrinogen, interleukin-6) are frequently elevated, but very nonspecific, and reserved for diagnostically difficult cases.
- Mild anemia: very nonspecific but may be associated with a lower rate of ischemic complications.
- Color Doppler US of the temporal artery may identify vascular occlusion, stenosis, or edema ("halo sign"); it is low cost and noninvasive but also very operator dependent and does not significantly improve on the clinical exam. It may aid in the diagnosis of larger vessel involvement (9).
- MRI and MRA allow for noninvasive evaluation of both the vessel lumen and the vessel wall and assess mural thickness (edema) and lumen diameter (occlusion). The information may aid in diagnosis, but results are affected by prior glucocorticoid treatment, perhaps indicating more value in assessing the disease course or relapse. Cost, logistics, and lack of validity data preclude its routine usefulness.
- Positron emission tomography (PET), like MRI/MRA and color Doppler, may be useful in diagnostically difficult cases to quantify the inflammatory burden and early in the course of disease, as the metabolic changes occur prior to structural vascular damage, but it also lacks studies to support its use (10).

Follow-Up Tests & Special Considerations
- Development of aortic aneurysms (late and potentially serious complication of GCA) can lead to aortic dissection.
- Due to the risk of irreversible vision loss, treatment with high-dose steroids should be started on strong clinical suspicion of temporal arteritis, prior to the temporal biopsy being done.

Diagnostic Procedures/Other
- Gold standard diagnostic study: histopalogic examination of the temporal artery biopsy specimen
- Overall sensitivity is 87%.
- The temporal artery is chosen because of its accessibility in the systemic disease, but any accessible cranial artery may be chosen.
- Length of biopsy specimen should be at least 2 cm to avoid false-negative results, as skip lesions may occur.
- Diagnostic yield of biopsy may be increased if procedure is coupled with imaging (high-resolution MRI or color Doppler US).
- Bilateral temporal artery biopsy should not be performed unless the initial histopathology is negative and the suspicion for GCA remains high.
- May be negative in up to 42% of patients, especially in large vessel disease
- Biopsy results are not affected by prior glucocorticoids, so treatment should not be delayed.

Test Interpretation
- Inflammation of the arterial wall, with fragmentation and disruption of the internal elastic lamina
- Multinucleated giant cells are found in <50% of cases and are not specific for the disease.
- Temporal arteritis occurs in three histologic patterns: classic, atypical, and healed.

TREATMENT

MEDICATION

First Line
Glucocorticoids:

- Prolonged treatment with glucocorticoids has been the mainstay of treatment and should be initiated immediately when the diagnostic suspicion for GCA is high (3)[A],(11)[B].
- Because of the risk of irreversible vision loss, treatment with high-dose steroids should be started on strong clinical suspicion of temporal arteritis, prior to the temporal biopsy being done.
- The typical dose of prednisone is 60 mg/day (or 1 mg/kg/day). Steroids should not be in the form of alternate day therapy, as this is more likely to lead to a relapse of vasculitis.
- The initial dose of steroids is continued for 2 to 4 weeks and slowly tapered over 9 to 12 months. Tapering may require ≥2 years.
- Oral steroids are at least as effective as IV steroids, except in the treatment of acute visual loss where IV steroids appear to offer significant benefit over oral steroids.
- It has been suggested that low-dose aspirin might be effective for patients with GCA (12)[B].
- Patients on corticosteroids should be placed on therapy to minimize osteoporosis unless there are contraindications.

Second Line
- Methotrexate as an adjunct to glucocorticoid therapy may have a modest effect in decreasing the relapse rate of temporal arteritis (13)[B],(14,15)[A].
- Therapies directed at TNF as adjunct to steroids have not shown significant benefit (15,16)[B]. Therapies directed at IL-6 blockade (tocilizumab – TCZ), and cyclophosphamide, have shown some benefit in patients who have not adequately responded to glucocorticoids (17,18)[A].

ONGOING CARE

FOLLOW-UP RECOMMENDATIONS
Sun avoidance and protection of the head and the face from photodamage may eventually prove to be important preventive measures for TA.

Patient Monitoring
- TA is typically self-limited and lasts several months or years.
- Overall, TA does not seem to decrease longevity. Nevertheless, it may lead to serious complications such as visual loss, which occurs in about 15–20% of patients.
- Another complication of GCA is the development of aortic aneurysms, usually affecting the ascending aorta. Yearly chest x-rays may be useful to identify this problem (19).
- About 50% of the patients with GCA will eventually develop polymyalgia rheumatica (stiffness of shoulder and hip girdle).

DIET
Calcium and vitamin D supplementation

PATIENT EDUCATION
- Consequences of discontinuing steroids abruptly (adrenal insufficiency, disease relapse)
- Risks of long-term steroid use (infection, hyperglycemia, weight gain, impaired wound healing, osteoporosis, hypertension)
- Possibility of relapse and importance of reporting new headaches and vision changes to provider immediately

PROGNOSIS
- Life expectancy is not affected by the disease unless severe aortitis is present.
- Once vision loss has occurred, it is unlikely to be recovered, but treatment resolves the other symptoms and prevents future vision loss and stroke.
- In most patients, glucocorticoid therapy can eventually be discontinued without complications. In a few patients, however, the disease is chronic and prednisone must be continued for years.
- Disease relapse is a distinct possibility.

COMPLICATIONS
- Vision loss with delayed diagnosis
- Glucocorticoid-related toxicity

REFERENCES

1. Ezeonyeji AN, Borg FA, Dasgupta B. Delays in recognition and management of giant cell arteritis: results from a retrospective audit. *Clin Rheumatol*. 2011;30(2):259–262.
2. Cantini F, Niccoli L, Storri L, et al. Are polymyalgia rheumatica and giant cell arteritis the same disease? *Semin Arthritis Rheum*. 2004;33(5):294–301.
3. Gonzalez-Gay MA, Vazquez-Rodriguez TR, Lopez-Diaz MJ, et al. Epidemiology of giant cell arteritis and polymyalgia rheumatica. *Arthritis Rheum*. 2009;61(10):1454–1461.
4. Robson JC, Kiran A, Maskell J, et al. The relative risk of aortic aneurysm in patients with giant cell arteritis compared with the general population of the UK. *Ann Rheum Dis*. 2015;(74)1:129–135.
5. Waldman CW, Waldman SD, Waldman RA. Giant cell arteritis. *Med Clin North Am*. 2013;97(2):329–335.
6. Weyand CM, Goronzy JJ. Immune mechanisms in medium and large-vessel vasculitis. *Nat Rev Rheumatol*. 2013;9(12):731–740.
7. Kermani TA, Warrington KJ. Recent advances in diagnostic strategies for giant cell arteritis. *Curr Neurol Neurosci Rep*. 2012;12(2):138–144.
8. Crowson CS, Matteson EL, Myasoedova E, et al. The lifetime risk of adult-onset rheumatoid arthritis and other inflammatory autoimmune diseases. *Arthritis Rheum*. 2011;63(3):633–639.
9. Arida A, Kyprianou M, Kanakis M, et al. The diagnostic value of ultrasonography-derived edema of the temporal artery wall in giant cell arteritis: a second meta-analysis. *BMC Musculoskelet Disord*. 2010;11:44.
10. Besson FL, Parienti JJ, Bienvenu B, et al. Diagnostic performance of ¹⁸F-fluorodeoxyglucose positron emission tomography in giant cell arteritis: a systematic review and meta-analysis. *Eur J Nucl Med Mol Imaging*. 2011;38(9):1764–1772.
11. Villa-Forte A. Giant cell arteritis: suspect it, treat it promptly. *Cleve Clin J Med*. 2011;78(4):265–270.
12. Lee MS, Smith SD, Galor A, et al. Antiplatelet and anticoagulant therapy in patients with giant cell arteritis. *Arthritis Rheum*. 2006;54(10):3306–3309.
13. Mahr AD, Jover JA, Spiera RF, et al. Adjunctive methotrexate for treatment of giant cell arteritis: an individual patient data meta-analysis. *Arthritis Rheum*. 2007;56(8):2789–2797.
14. Kötter I, Henes JC, Wagner AD, et al. Does glucocorticoid-resistant large-vessel vasculitis (giant cell arteritis and Takayasu arteritis) exist and how can remission be achieved? A critical review of the literature. *Clin Exp Rheumatol*. 2012;30(1 Suppl 70):S114–S129.
15. Borchers AT, Gershwin ME. Giant cell arteritis: a review of classification, pathophysiology, geo-epidemiology and treatment. *Autoimmun Rev*. 2012;11(6–7):A544–A554.
16. Yates M, Loke YK, Watts RA, et al. Prednisolone combined with adjunctive immunosuppression is not superior to prednisolone alone in terms of efficacy and safety in giant cell arteritis: meta-analysis. *Clin Rheumatol*. 2014;33(2):227–236.
17. Salvarani C, Magnani L, Catanoso M, et al. Tocilizumab: a novel therapy for patients with large-vessel vasculitis. *Rheumatology (Oxford)*. 2012;(51)1:151–156.
18. Quartuccio L, Masset M, De Maglio G, et al. Role of oral cyclophosphamide in the treatment of giant cell arteritis. *Rheumatology (Oxford)*. 2012;51(9):1677–1686.
19. Tomasson G, Peloquin C, Mohammad A, et al. Risk for cardiovascular disease early and late after a diagnosis of giant-cell arteritis: a cohort study. *Ann Intern Med*. 2014;160(2):73–80.

ADDITIONAL READING
Mukhtyar C, Guillevin L, Cid MC, et al. EULAR recommendations for the management of large vessel vasculitis. *Ann Rheum Dis*. 2009;68(3):318–323.

 SEE ALSO

Depression; Fibromyalgia; Headache, Cluster; Headache, Tension; Polymyalgia Rheumatica; Polymyositis/Dermatomyositis

 CODES

ICD10
- M31.6 Other giant cell arteritis
- M31.5 Giant cell arteritis with polymyalgia rheumatica

CLINICAL PEARLS
- Due to the risk of irreversible vision loss, treatment with high-dose steroids (prednisone 60 mg/day) should be started immediately in patients suspected of temporal arteritis.
- Temporal artery biopsy is the gold standard for diagnosis. Temporal artery biopsy is not likely to be affected by a few weeks of treatment.
- Treatment consists of a very slow steroid taper. Bone protection therapy and low-dose aspirin should be considered.
- Normal ESR level = value of age/2 for men and age + 10/2 for women

ARTHRITIS, JUVENILE IDIOPATHIC

Donna-Marie McMahon, DO, FAAP • Kathleen M. Vazzana, DO

BASICS

DESCRIPTION
- Juvenile idiopathic arthritis (JIA) is the most common chronic pediatric rheumatologic disease.
- JIA is associated with significant disability
  - Age of onset: <16 years
  - Joint swelling, restricted range of motion, warmth, redness, or pain are the most common symptoms.
  - ≥6 weeks of symptoms before diagnosis is common.
- Seven (International League of Associations for Rheumatology-ILAR) subtypes, determined by clinical characteristics in the first 6 months of illness (1):
  - Systemic (Still disease): 10%; preceded by febrile onset of ≥2 weeks with rash, serositis, hepatosplenomegaly, or lymphadenopathy (1)
  - Polyarticular rheumatoid factor (RF) (+): 5–10%; ≥5 joints involvement (1); large and small joints; RF positive on two tests ≥3 months apart (2)
  - Polyarticular RF (−): 10–30%; ≥5 (large and small) joints involved (1); RF negative (2)
  - Oligoarticular: 30–60%; involvement of 1 to 4 joints; risk for chronic uveitis in ANA (+) females (1) and axial skeletal involvement in older boys (2). Types: (i) monoarthritis (50%): knee, ankle, elbow; (ii) extended type: >4 joints after first 6 months
  - Psoriatic arthritis: 5%; arthritis with psoriasis or arthritis with >2 of the following: dactylitis, nail changes, psoriasis in a first-degree relative (1)
  - Enthesitis arthritis: 1–7%; oligo-polyarthritis in small or large joints and enthesis plus two of the following: sacroiliac or lumbosacral pain, Reiter syndrome family history or presence of acute anterior uveitis, HLA-B27 (+), ankylosing spondylitis, inflammatory bowel disease (1)[C]
  - Undifferentiated arthritis: arthritis that does not fulfill above categories or patients overlapping ≥2 categories (2)
- System(s) affected: musculoskeletal, hematologic, lymphatic, immunologic
- Synonyms: juvenile chronic arthritis; juvenile arthritis; juvenile rheumatoid arthritis (JRA); Still disease (2)

EPIDEMIOLOGY
- Male = female (1); onset: throughout childhood; 54% of cases occur in children 0 to 5 years (3).
- Polyarticular RF (+): female > male, 3:1 (2); onset: late childhood or adolescence (1)
- Polyarticular RF (−): female > male, 3:1; onset: early peak, 2 to 4 years; late peak, 6 to 12 years (2)
- Oligoarticular: female > male, 5:1; onset: 2 to 4 years (2)
- Psoriatic: female > male, 1:0.95 (2); onset: early peak, 2 to 3 years; late peak, 10 to 12 years (1)
- Enthesitis: female > male, 1:7; onset: early peak, 2 to 4 years; late peak, 6 to 12 years (2)
- Affected patients have an increased risk of developing cancer, although short-term risk is low (4).

Incidence
2 to 20/100,000 children <16 years in developed nations

Prevalence
16 to 150/100,000 children <16 years in developed nations (1)

ETIOLOGY AND PATHOPHYSIOLOGY
- Immunodysregulation of both humoral and cellular immunity. T lymphocytes play a key role.
- Genetic predisposition. IL2RA/CD25 and VTCN1 have been implicated as genetic loci.
- Environmental triggers, possibly infectious
  - Rubella or parvovirus B19 (5)
  - Heat shock proteins (5)
- Immunoglobulin or complement deficiency

Genetics
- Human leukocyte antigen (HLA) class I and II alleles
- HLA-A2 = early onset oligoarthritis in females
- HLA-DRB1*11 increases risk of systemic and oligo-JIA.
- HLA-B27 increases risk of enthesitis-related arthritis.
- HLA-DR4 is associated with polyarthritis RF (+) (5).

RISK FACTORS
Female gender 3:1

GENERAL PREVENTION
None identified.

COMMONLY ASSOCIATED CONDITIONS
Other autoimmune disorders, chronic anterior uveitis (iridocyclitis), nutritional impairment, growth issues (5)

DIAGNOSIS

Clinical criteria: age of onset <16 years and >6 weeks duration of objective arthritis (swelling or restricted range of motion of a joint accompanied by heat, pain, or tenderness with no other form of childhood arthritis) in ≥1 joints

HISTORY
- Arthralgias, fever, fatigue, malaise, myalgias, weight loss, morning stiffness, rash
- Limp, if lower extremity involvement
- Arthritis for ≥6 weeks

PHYSICAL EXAM
- Arthritis: swelling, effusion, limited range of motion, tenderness, pain with motion, warmth
- Rash, rheumatoid nodules, lymphadenopathy, hepato- or splenomegaly, enthesitis, dactylitis

DIFFERENTIAL DIAGNOSIS
- Legg-Calve-Perthes, toxic synovitis, growing pains, Perthes disease
- Septic arthritis, osteomyelitis, viral infection, mycoplasmal infection, Lyme disease
- Reactive arthritis: postinfectious, rheumatic fever, Reiter syndrome
- Inflammatory bowel disease: Crohn disease or ulcerative colitis
- Hemoglobinopathies, rickets
- Leukemia (particularly acute lymphocytic leukemia), bone tumors (osteoid osteoma), neuroblastoma
- Vasculitis, Henoch-Schönlein purpura, Kawasaki disease
- Systemic lupus erythematosus, dermatomyositis, mixed connective tissue disease, sarcoidosis, systemic sclerosis, collagen disorders
- Farber disease
- Accidental or nonaccidental trauma

DIAGNOSTIC TESTS & INTERPRETATION
Initial Tests (lab, imaging)
- CBC: leukocyte count is normal or markedly elevated (systemic), lymphopenia, reactive thrombocytosis, anemia. LFT (rule out hepatitis) and renal function studies (prior to therapy with potentially nephrotoxic drugs)
- Joint-fluid aspiration/analysis: Exclude infection.
- ESR and C-reactive protein are typically elevated. CRP often disproportionately elevated.
- Myeloid-related proteins (MRP 8/14) associated with flares
- Antinuclear antibodies (ANA)–positive patients have increased risk of uveitis. ANA positive in up to 70% with oligoarticular JIA
- RF (+): 2–10% (usually polyarticular); poor prognosis
- HLA-B27 positive: enthesitis-related arthritis
- Diagnostic radiography, MRI, US, and CT; no one modality has superior diagnostic value (6)[A].
- Radiograph of affected joint(s): **early** radiographic changes: soft tissue swelling, periosteal reaction, juxta-articular demineralization; **later** changes: joint space loss, articular surface erosions, subchondral cyst formation, sclerosis, joint fusion
- If orthopnea, obtain ECG to rule out pericarditis.
- Radionuclide scans: for infection/malignancy
- CT is best for bony abnormalities. MRI can assess synovial hypertrophy and cartilage degeneration. Also more sensitive to monitor clinical responsiveness to treatment in peripheral joints and disease activity

Follow-Up Tests & Special Considerations
- RF and ANA are present in mixed connective tissue disease (7)[B].
- When interpreting results of dual energy x-ray photon absorptiometry scans, it is important to use pediatric, not adult, controls as normative data.

Diagnostic Procedures/Other
Synovial biopsy: if synovial fluid cannot be aspirated or if infection is suspected in spite of negative synovial fluid culture

Test Interpretation
Synovial biopsy→ synovial cells hyperplasia, hyperemia, infiltration of small lymphocytes, and mononuclear cells

TREATMENT

GENERAL MEASURES
- Goal is to control active disease, extraarticular manifestations, and achieve clinical remission.
- All patients require regular (every 3 to 4 months for oligo-JIA and in ANA-positive patients) ophthalmic exams to uncover asymptomatic eye disease, particularly for 3 years following diagnosis.
- Moist heat or electric blanket for morning stiffness
- Splints for contractures
- Aerobic exercise: weight-bearing or aquatic therapy to improve functional capacity (8)

MEDICATION
First Line
- ≤4 joints
- NSAIDs: adequate in ~50%, symptoms often improve within days, full efficacy 2 to 3 months
- Drugs for children include the following:
  - Ibuprofen: 30 to 50 mg/kg/day, divided QID; max dose 2,400 mg/day
  - Naproxen: 10 mg/kg/day, divided BID; max dose 1,250 mg/day
  - Tolmetin sodium: 20 mg/kg/day, TID or QID; max dose 30 mg/kg/day
  - Diclofenac: 2 to 3 mg/kg, divided TID; max dose 50 mg TID

– Indomethacin: 1 to 2 mg/kg/day, divided BID to QID; max dose of 4 mg/kg/day
– NSAIDs are contraindicated if known allergy.
– Precautions: may worsen bleeding diatheses; use caution in renal insufficiency and hypovolemic states; take with food.
– Significant possible interactions: may lower serum levels of anticonvulsants and blunt the effect of loop diuretics. NSAIDs may increase serum methotrexate levels.
• Intra-articular long-acting corticosteroids: immediately effective. Improve synovitis, joint damage, and contractures and prevent leg length discrepancy (7)[B].
– Indication: patients with oligoarthritis who have failed a 2-month NSAID trial or with poor prognosis factors (9)[C]
– Example: triamcinolone hexacetonide
• ≥5 Joints
– If high disease activity or a failed 1 to 2 months NSAID trial→ methotrexate (9)[C]

Second Line
• 30–40% of patients require addition of disease-modifying antirheumatic drugs (DMARDs): methotrexate, sulfasalazine, leflunomide, and tumor necrosis factor (TNF) antagonists (etanercept, infliximab, adalimumab); newer biologic therapies, including IL-1 and IL-6 receptor antagonists, are currently under investigation
• Methotrexate: 10 mg/m^2/wk PO or SC (7)[B]
– Plateau of efficacy reached with 15 mg/m^2/wk; further increase in dosage is not associated with therapeutic benefit (10)[A].
• Sulfasalazine: oligoarticular and HLA-B27 spondyloarthritis (7)[B]
• Etanercept: 0.8 mg/kg (max of 50 mg/dose) given SC q1wk or 0.4 mg/kg SC twice a week (max of 25 mg/dose)
• Infliximab: 5 mg/kg q6–8wk
• Adalimumab: if weight 15 kg to <30 kg, 20 mg SC q2wk; if weight ≥30 kg, 40 mg SC q2wk
• Tocilizumab: IL-6 antibody demonstrating efficacy in phase III open label trials; ongoing studies to evaluate efficacy and appropriate dosing (7)[B]
• Anakinra: IL-1 receptor antibody under investigation with phase II and III clinical trials for systemic JIA (7)[B]
• Begin treatment with TNF-α inhibitors in children with a history of arthritis in ≤4 joints and significant active arthritis despite treatment with methotrexate or arthritis in ≥5 joints and any active arthritis following an adequate trial of methotrexate (9)[C].
• Begin treatment with anakinra in children with systemic arthritis and active fever whose treatment requires a second medication, in addition to systemic glucocorticoids (9)[C].
• Analgesics, including narcotics for pain control

ISSUES FOR REFERRAL
• Pediatric rheumatologist for management of JIA
• Orthopedics as needed for articular complicatoins
• Ophthalmology: for suspected uveitis
• Physical therapy to maintain range of motion, improve muscle strength and prevent deformities
• Occupational therapy to maintain and improve appropriate age-related functional activities
• Behavioral health if difficulty coping with disease

SURGERY/OTHER PROCEDURES
• Total hip and/or knee replacement for severe disease
• Soft tissue release if splinting/traction unsuccessful
• Correct limb length or angular deformities
• Synovectomy is rarely performed.

INPATIENT CONSIDERATIONS
Admission Criteria/Initial Stabilization
• Patient nonambulatory
• Signs/symptoms of pericarditis
• Persistent fever or diagnostic confusion to facilitate evaluation and workup
• Need for surgery

Discharge Criteria
Resolution of fever and swelling or serositis

 ## ONGOING CARE

FOLLOW-UP RECOMMENDATIONS
Patient Monitoring
Determined by medication and disease activity
• NSAIDs: periodic CBC, urinalysis, liver function tests (LFTs), renal function tests
• Aspirin and/or other salicylates: transaminase and salicylate levels, weekly for 1st month, then every 3 to 4 months
• Methotrexate: monthly LFTs, CBC, BUN, creatinine

DIET
Regular diet with special attention to adequate calcium, iron, protein, and caloric intake

PATIENT EDUCATION
• Ongoing education of patients and families with attention to psychosocial needs; school issues; educational needs; behavioral strategies for dealing with pain and noncompliance; use of health care resources; support groups
• Printed and audiovisual information available from local arthritis foundation

PROGNOSIS
• 50–60% ultimately remit, but functional ability depends on adequacy of long-term therapy (disease control, maintaining muscle and joint function).
• Poor prognosis is noted in patients with active disease at 6 months, polyarticular disease, extended pauciarticular disease course, female gender, RF (+), ANA (+), persistent morning stiffness, rapid appearance of erosions, hip involvement

COMPLICATIONS
• Blindness, band keratopathy, glaucoma, short stature, micrognathia if temporomandibular joint involvement, debilitating joint disease, disseminated intravascular coagulation, hemolytic anemia
• NSAIDs: peptic ulcer, GI hemorrhage, CNS reactions, renal disease, leukopenia
• DMARDs: bone marrow suppression, hepatitis, renal disease, dermatitis, mouth ulcers, retinal toxicity (antimalarials; rare)
• TNF antagonists: higher risk of infection
• Osteoporosis, avascular necrosis
• Methotrexate: Folate supplementation decreases hepatic/GI symptoms; may reduce stomatitis (11)[A].
• Macrophage activation syndrome: decreased blood cell precursors secondary to histiocyte degradation of marrow

REFERENCES
1. Restrepo R, Lee EY. Epidemiology, pathogenesis, and imaging of arthritis in children. *Orthop Clin North Am.* 2012;43(2):213–225.
2. Prince FH, Otten MH, van Suijlekom-Smit LW. Diagnosis and management of juvenile idiopathic arthritis. *BMJ.* 2010;341:c6434.
3. Behrens EM, Beukelman T, Gallo L, et al. Evaluation of the presentation of systemic onset juvenile rheumatoid arthritis: data from the Pennsylvania Systemic Onset Juvenile Arthritis Registry (PASOJAR). *J Rheumatol.* 2008;35(2):343–348.
4. Beukelman T, Haynes K, Curtis JR, et al. Rates of malignancy associated with juvenile idiopathic arthritis and its treatment. *Arthritis Rheum.* 2012;64(4):1263–1271.
5. Weiss JE, Ilowite NT. Juvenile idiopathic arthritis. *Rheum Dis Clin North Am.* 2007;33(3):441–470.
6. McKay GM, Cox LA, Long BW. Imaging juvenile idiopathic arthritis: assessing the modalities. *Radiol Technol.* 2010;81(4):318–327.
7. Kahn P. Juvenile idiopathic arthritis—current and future therapies. *Bull NYU Hosp Jt Dis.* 2009;67(3):291–302.
8. Klepper S. Making the case for exercise in children with juvenile idiopathic arthritis: what we know and where we go from here. *Arthritis Rheum.* 2007;57(6):887–890.
9. Beukelman T, Patkar NM, Saag KG, et al. 2011 American College of Rheumatology recommendations for the treatment of juvenile idiopathic arthritis: initiation and safety monitoring of therapeutic agents for the treatment of arthritis and systemic features. *Arthritis Care Res (Hoboken).* 2011;63(4):465–482.
10. Takken T, Van Der Net J, Helders PJ. Methotrexate for treating juvenile idiopathic arthritis. *Cochrane Database Syst Rev.* 2001;(4):CD003129.
11. Shea B, Swinden MV, Tanjong Ghogomu E, et al. Folic acid and folinic acid for reducing side effects in patients receiving methotrexate for rheumatoid arthritis. *Cochrane Database Syst Rev.* 2013;(5):CD000951.
12. Kemper AR, Van Mater HA, Coeytaux RR, et al. Systematic review of disease-modifying antirheumatic drugs for juvenile idiopathic arthritis. *BMC Pediatr.* 2012;12:29.

ADDITIONAL READING
Chang HJ, Burke AE, Glass RM. JAMA patient page. Juvenile idiopathic arthritis. *JAMA.* 2010;303(13):1328.

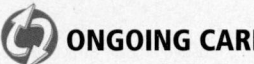 ## CODES

ICD10
• M08.90 Juvenile arthritis, unspecified, unspecified site
• M08.80 Other juvenile arthritis, unspecified site
• M08.00 Unsp juvenile rheumatoid arthritis of unspecified site

CLINICAL PEARLS
• JIA is the most common form of arthritis in children.
• JIA should be included in the differential diagnosis for a limping child.
• High-titer RF correlates with disease severity; positive RF titers confer poorer prognosis.
• DMARDs improve JIA-associated symptoms (12)[A].

ARTHRITIS, RHEUMATOID (RA)

Mariya Milko, DO, MS • Rubaiya Mallay, DO, FACOI, ACR

 BASICS

DESCRIPTION

- Chronic systemic autoimmune inflammatory disease with symmetric polyarthritis and synovitis
- Progressive chronic inflammation leads to large and small joint destruction, deformity, decline in functional status, and premature morbidity/mortality.
- System(s) affected: musculoskeletal, skin, hematologic, lymphatic, immunologic, muscular, renal, cardiovascular, neurologic, pulmonary

Geriatric Considerations
- Increased contribution of age-related comorbidities
- Decreased medication tolerance; increased incidence of hydroxychloroquine-associated maculopathy and sulfasalazine-induced nausea/vomiting, NSAID-induced gastric ulcers, and corticosteroid induced diabetes

Pregnancy Considerations
- Use effective contraception in patients taking disease-modifying antirheumatic drugs (DMARDs).
- Methotrexate and other DMARDS such as Arava, cyclophosphamide, and cyclosporine are teratogenic. Appropriate medication regimens for pregnant or breastfeeding patients is important.
- 50–80% of patients improve during pregnancy because of immunologic tolerance. Most relapse in 6 months. First episode may occur in pregnancy or postpartum.

EPIDEMIOLOGY

Incidence
- 25 to 30/100,000 cases for males
- 50 to 60/100,000 cases for females
- Peak age is 35 to 50 years.

Prevalence
General population: 0.3–1%

ETIOLOGY AND PATHOPHYSIOLOGY
- An insult (e.g., infection, smoking, trauma) precipitates an initial autoimmune reaction where antibody-complement complex activation ultimately results in endothelial activation, synovial hypertrophy, and joint inflammation. RA is a systemic disorder. Pathogenesis is mediated by abnormal B- and T-cell interactions and overproduction of cytokines such as TNF and IL-6.
- Multifactorial disease with genetic, host (hormonal, immunologic), and environmental (socioeconomic, smoking) factors

Genetics
- RA is 50% attributable to genetic causes. HLA-DR4 is a shared epitope in over 50% of cases.
- Monozygotic twin concordance 15–20%, suggesting that nongenetic roles also contribute to development of RA
- HLA DR4 and DRB1, STAT4, and CD40+ persons have increased relative risk.

RISK FACTORS
- Family history: First-degree relatives have 2- to 3-fold increased risk.
- Smokers have elevated relative risk of 1.4–2.2%
- Pregnancy and breastfeeding for 24 months lowers risk.
- Women affected 3:1, difference diminishes with age.

COMMONLY ASSOCIATED CONDITIONS
Accelerated atherosclerosis, pericarditis, amyloidosis, Felty syndrome (RA, splenomegaly, neutropenia), interstitial lung disease, pulmonary nodules, rheumatoid nodules, vasculitis, lymphomas, and carpal tunnel syndrome

 DIAGNOSIS

HISTORY
- Symmetric polyarthritis most commonly affecting the hands and feet

- Constitutional symptoms: fatigue, malaise, weight loss, low-grade fevers (1,2)[A],(3)[C]
- Articular symptoms: tender/swollen joints, early morning stiffness (at least 60 minutes), and difficulty with activities of daily living (ADL) (1,2)[A],(3)[C]
- Extra-articular involvement: skin, pulmonary, cardiovascular, and ocular symptoms; onset is typically insidious. Patients rarely present with abrupt onset of symptoms and extra-articular manifestations (1,2)[A],(3)[C].

PHYSICAL EXAM
- Evaluate for swollen, boggy, or tender joints:
  - Small joints: metacarpophalangeal (MCP), proximal intraphalangeal (PIP) leading to Boutonnière and swan-neck deformities, wrist, 2nd to 5th metatarsophalangeal (MTP), and thumb interphalangeal (IP) joints. Pain and decreased ROM; usually symmetric and affected first
  - Large joints: shoulders, elbows (rheumatoid nodules), hips, knees, and ankles will show evidence of effusions.
- Joint deformity, nodules, and fusion are late findings.
- Extra-articular findings associated with RA:
  - Splenomegaly, lymphadenopathy, subcutaneous nodules, peripheral neuropathy, and atlantoaxial joint instability. Axial migration of dens into foramen magnum may contribute to occipital headaches.
  - Cardiovascular mortality increased with RA— evaluate rhythm, presence of murmurs (valvular dysfunction), and for effusion
  - Pulmonary disease typically manifests as effusion and fibrosis (dullness, rales).

DIFFERENTIAL DIAGNOSIS
Sjögren syndrome, systemic lupus erythematosus (SLE), systemic sclerosis, adult Still disease, psoriatic arthritis, polymyalgia rheumatica (older), seronegative polyarthritis, erosive osteoarthritis, crystal arthropathy, septic arthritis, chronic Lyme disease, viral-induced arthritis (parvovirus B19, hepatitis C [with cryoglobulinemia]), occult malignancy, vasculitis (Behçet syndrome), inflammatory bowel disease, RS3PE hemochromatosis, sarcoidosis (3)[B]

DIAGNOSTIC TESTS & INTERPRETATION
Initial Tests (lab, imaging)
- CBC: Mild anemia and thrombocytosis are common and relate to disease activity (3)[C].

- ESR and C-reactive protein (CRP) are nonspecific markers used to assess disease activity (1)[A]
- Rheumatoid factor (RF): >1:80 in 70–80% of patients with RA (most commonly IgM Ab) (1)[A]
- Anticyclic citrullinated peptide antibodies (anti-CCP antibodies); specificity >90% (1)[A]

- Antinuclear antibody: present in 20–30%
- Electrolytes, creatinine, liver function, and urinalysis to assess comorbid states, establish baseline, and to assist with medication management (4)[C]
- Radiographic findings help establish diagnosis and monitor treatment (2)[C].
- MRI of hands and wrists looking for erosions, pannus, synovitis
- Diagnostic ultrasound: to assess for synovial thickening/erosions.
- Plain film radiographs are preferred for RA:
  - Initial radiographs of the hands, wrists, and feet
  - Hallmark is a lack of bony remodeling and symmetric joint space narrowing.
  - Earliest pattern of erosions is loss of cortical distinctness, followed by dot-dash pattern of cortical bone loss. Marginal erosions at cortical bone within joint capsule not covered by cartilage result in "mouse-ear" erosions.

Follow-Up Tests & Special Considerations
- 2010 American College of Rheumatology/European League Against Rheumatism (ACR/EULAR) criteria
- Patients with symptoms in at least one joint and definite clinical synovitis not explained by another disease
- A score of ≥6 is needed for to classify as definite RA
  - Joint score
    ○ 1 large joint: 0
    ○ 2 to 10 large joints: 1
    ○ 1 to 3 small joints (with or without large joints; distal interphalangeal [DIP], 1st MCP, and 1st MTP joints are excluded from assessment.): 2
    ○ 4 to 10 small joints (with/without large joints): 3
    ○ >10 joints (at least 1 small joint): 5
  - Serology score: At least one test is needed: negative RF (rheumatoid factor) and negative ACPA (anticitrullinated protein antibody): 0; low positive RF or low positive ACPA: 2; high positive RF or high positive ACPA: 3
  - Acute-phase reactants score: At least one result is needed. Normal CRP and normal ESR: 0; abnormal CRP or ESR: 1
  - Self-reported symptom duration score: <6 weeks: 0; ≥6 weeks: 1
- Patients with a score of <6/10 do not meet RA criteria, and reevaluation is likely necessary over time (3)[C].

Diagnostic Procedures/Other
- Joint aspiration can exclude crystal arthropathy and septic arthritis.
- Synovial fluid
  - Gram stain, cell count, culture, crystal analysis, and overall appearance
  - Yellowish-white, turbid, poor viscosity in RA
  - WBC increased (3,500 to 50,000 cells/mm^3)
  - Protein: ~4.2 g/dL (42 g/L)
  - Serum-synovial glucose difference ≥30 mg/dL (≥1.67 mmol/L)

 TREATMENT

Goals: Control disease activity and progression, relieve pain, maintain or improve function, and promote self-management to maximize activities of daily living.

GENERAL MEASURES

- Target treatment to achieve remission or minimize disease activity, prevent structural damage and disability (5)[A].
- Early, aggressive treatment prevents structural damage and disability (1)[A],(2–4)[C].
- Periodic evaluation of disease activity and extent of synovitis is important (1)[A].
- Arthritis self-management education (1)[A]

MEDICATION

- Early DMARD therapy to slow disease progression and induce remission is standard of care (1)[A].
- Symptomatic therapy in addition to DMARDs:
  - NSAIDs: naproxen (500 mg BID) or ibuprofen (800 mg TID) for symptomatic relief. If poor response to initial NSAID after 2 weeks, try alternative NSAID (1)[A].
  - If still poor response, prednisone (5 to 30 mg/day); taper off NSAID or prednisone as soon as effective control of disease activity with DMARD is achieved (1)[A].
- Notes on DMARD therapy

History of hepatitis, malignancy, and heart failure (HF) may alter first-line therapy (4)[C].

- Nonbiologic DMARDs
  - Should be started within 3 months of making the diagnosis of RA (1)[A]
  - Due to greater convenience, lower toxicity profiles and quicker onset of action, initial therapy is a nonbiologic DMARD: methotrexate, sulfasalazine, and leflunomide have comparable efficacy (1)[A].
  - Methotrexate is the first-line DMARD in patients with active RA; the optimal dosage should be reached within no more than 4 to 8 weeks (5)[A].
  - Methotrexate (MTX) (Rheumatrex): 7.5 to 25 mg/ week PO. DMARD with the most predictable benefit; many significant side effects, but the addition of folate reduces toxicity. Monitor CBC and renal and liver function every month × 3 months. Give with folic acid 1 mg PO daily. Contraindicated in renal and hepatic diseases, pregnancy, and breastfeeding (1)[A].
  - Sulfasalazine (SSZ): 500 mg/day, increase to 2 g/ day over 1 month; max: 2 to 3 g/day; 6-month trial. Monotherapy for low disease activity. Monitor CBC, liver enzymes every 2 weeks × 3 months, then every month × 3 months, then every 3 months. Screen for G6PD deficiency.
  - Leflunomide (Arava): loading dose 100 mg/day × 3 days, then 10 to 20 mg/day. GI side effects and potentially teratogenic; contraindicated in pregnancy. Monitor CBC, LFTs, and phosphate monthly for the first 6 months. Stop use if ALT >3× upper limit normal.
  - Antimalarials: hydroxychloroquine (HCQ) (Plaquenil) 400 mg QHS for 2 to 3 months, then 200 mg at bedtime; 6-month trial is usual. Usually used to treat milder forms or in combination with other DMARDs. Ophthalmologic exam every 6 to 12 months due to potential maculopathy. Adjust dose in renal insufficiency.
  - Minocycline (100 mg BID)
- Biologic DMARDs:
  - TNF inhibitors: IV infliximab (Remicade), SC adalimumab (Humira), and SC etanercept (Enbrel). No evidence that one is superior. Certolizumab pegol (Cimzia) and golimumab (Simponi), approved in moderate to severe disease.

- Janus kinase (JAK) inhibitor: Xeljanz, Interleukin-6 (IL-6) receptor antagonist: Actemra is approved to treat moderate to severe active rheumatoid arthritis in which methotrexate did not work well.
- Abatacept (Orencia) and Anakinra (Kineret) no longer considered cost-effective or efficacious treatment for RA (1)[A].
- Rituximab (Rituxan) is recommended with or without MTX for active moderate to severe RA with inadequate response to other DMARDs or failed anti-TNF agent (1)[A].
- All biologics are best used in combination with methotrexate (5)[A].
- Optimal dosage and duration of treatment unclear. Check purified protein derivative (PPD or QuantiF-ERON gold) prior to treatment and periodic CBC. Risk of lymphoma and CHF (1)[A].
- Ensure vaccinations are up-to-date prior to starting biologic agents. Recommended vaccinations: Pneumococcal, HPV, hepatitis B, influenza, varicella zoster (4)[C]
- Flare-ups
  - Intra-articular steroids: If disease is well-controlled after ruling out intra-articular infection (1)[A]. Can also use Acthar, a repository corticotropin injection. (5)[A].

ADDITIONAL THERAPIES

- Capsaicin cream: Apply 3 to 4 times per day. Best results are seen after 2 to 4 weeks of continuous use.
- Interdisciplinary care and management including physical therapy to minimize the consequences of loss of function, joint damage, maladaptive coping, and social isolation (1,4,6)[A]

SURGERY/OTHER PROCEDURES

- Surgical treatment including synovectomy, tendon reconstruction, joint fusion, and joint replacement may be considered to prevent disability in RA unresponsive to therapy or in advanced RA (1)[A].
- Important to get flexion/extension films of cervical spine prior to any surgery due to high risk of atlantoaxial joint instability and subluxation

 ONGOING CARE

The goals of comprehensive, interdisciplinary care are to inhibit the disease process, reduce pain, optimize symptom management (fatigue and stiffness), preserve joint integrity and joint function, maintain social and occupational roles, and maximize quality of life.

FOLLOW-UP RECOMMENDATIONS

- Encourage full activity as tolerated. Avoid heavy work or exercise during active (flare) phases. Emphasize exercise, mobility, and reduction of joint stress.
- Promote general health and psychosocial well-being.

Patient Monitoring

Address risk factors and evaluate for cardiovascular disease and osteoporosis. Disease Activity Score (DAS28) questionnaire for disease activity periodically and Health Assessment Questionnaire (HAQ) for functional status yearly.

DIET

Most beneficial diets for symptom control are gluten-free and vegetarian. Some benefits have been noted for "allergen-free," elemental, and Mediterranean diets.

PROGNOSIS

- Poor prognostic findings
  - Persistent moderate to severe disease; early or advanced age at disease onset
  - Many affected joints; swelling and pain in affected joints, positive MCP squeeze test, and PIP and MCP symmetric involvement
- 50% cannot function in their primary jobs within 10 years of onset.

REFERENCES

1. National Collaborating Centre for Chronic Conditions (UK). *Rheumatoid Arthritis: National Clinical Guideline for Management and Treatment in Adults* (NICE Clinical Guidelines, No. 79.). London, United Kingdom: Royal College of Physicians; 2009.
2. Aletaha D, Neogi T, Silman AJ, et al. 2010 rheumatoid arthritis classification criteria: an American College of Rheumatology/European League Against Rheumatism collaborative initiative. *Arthritis Rheum*. 2010;62(9):2569–2581.
3. Wasserman AM. Diagnosis and management of rheumatoid arthritis. *Am Fam Physician*. 2011;84(11):1245–1252.
4. Singh JA, Furst DE, Bharat A, et al. 2012 update of the 2008 American College of Rheumatology recommendations for the use of disease-modifying antirheumatic drugs and biologic agents in the treatment of rheumatoid arthritis. *Arthritis Care Res (Hoboken)*. 2012;64(5):625–639.
5. Gaujoux-Viala C, Gossec L, Cantagrel A, et al. Recommendations of the French Society for Rheumatology for managing rheumatoid arthritis. *Joint Bone Spine*. 2014;81(4):287–297.
6. Richards BL, Whittle SL, Buchbinder R. Neuromodulators for pain management in rheumatoid arthritis. *Cochrane Database Syst Rev*. 2012;(1):CD008921.

CODES

ICD10

- M06.9 Rheumatoid arthritis, unspecified
- M05.60 Rheu arthritis of unsp site w involv of organs and systems
- M05.30 Rheumatoid heart disease w rheumatoid arthritis of unsp site

CLINICAL PEARLS

- RA is an idiopathic, chronic, and systemic inflammatory disease characterized by symmetric polyarthritis and synovitis.
- Rheumatoid arthritis occurs in 1% of the U.S. population.
- Females have more articular disease; males have more systemic manifestations.
- Plain films are the imaging modality of choice in RA.
- Treatment with DMARDs within 3 months of diagnosis slows disease progression and improves chance for remission.
- Methotrexate is the first-line DMARD in patients with active RA.
- Atlantoaxial joint involvement leads to instability; avoid unnecessary manipulation of the cervical spine.

ARTHRITIS, SEPTIC
Jeffrey P. Feden, MD, FACEP

 BASICS

DESCRIPTION
- Infection due to bacterial invasion of the joint space
- Systems affected: musculoskeletal
- Synonyms: suppurative arthritis; infectious arthritis; pyarthrosis; pyogenic arthritis; bacterial arthritis

EPIDEMIOLOGY
- May occur at any age; higher incidence in very young and elderly
- Incidence:
  - 4 to 10/100,000 annual case rate (1)
- Prevalence: 27% of patients presenting with monoarticular arthritis have nongonococcal septic arthritis (2).
- Gender differences:
  - Gonococcal: female > male
  - Nongonococcal: male > female

ETIOLOGY AND PATHOPHYSIOLOGY
- Many different pathogenic organisms
- Nongonococcal:
  - *Staphylococcus aureus* (most common organism in adults)
    ○ MRSA risk increased in elderly, intravenous drug users (IVDU), postsurgical
  - *Streptococcus* spp. (second most common in adults)
  - Gram-negative rods (GNR): IVDU, trauma, extremes of age, immunosuppressed
- *Neisseria gonorrhea* (most common in young, sexually active adults)
- Other: rickettsial (e.g., Lyme), fungal, mycobacterial
- Risk by specific age (3):
  - <1 month: *Streptococcus aureus*, Group B strep (GBS), GNR
  - 1 month to 4 years: *Streptococcus aureus*, *Streptococcus pneumoniae*, *Neisseria meningitidis*
  - 16 to 40 years: *N. meningitidis*, *S. aureus*
  - >40 years: *S. aureus*
- Specific high-risk groups:
  - Rheumatoid arthritis: *S. aureus*
  - IVDU: *S. aureus*, GNR, opportunistic pathogens
  - Neonates: GBS
  - Immunocompromised: gram-negative bacilli, fungi
  - Trauma patients with open injuries: mixed flora
- Pathogenesis:
  - Hematogenous spread (most common)
  - Direct inoculation by microorganisms secondary to trauma or iatrogenesis (e.g., joint surgery)
  - Adjacent spread (e.g., osteomyelitis)
- Pathophysiology:
  - Microorganisms initially enter through synovial membrane and spread to the synovial fluid.
  - Resulting inflammatory response releases cytokines and destructive proteases leading to joint damage.
  - Microbial surface components recognizing adhesive matrix molecules (MSCRAMMs) on bacteria influence disease progression (4).

RISK FACTORS
- Age >80 years
- Low socioeconomic status; alcoholism
- Cellulitis and skin ulcers

- Prior violation of joint capsule
  - Prior orthopedic surgery
  - Intra-articular steroid injection
  - Trauma
- History of previous joint disease
  - Inflammatory arthritis (rheumatoid arthritis [RA]: 10-fold increased risk)
  - Osteoarthritis
  - Crystal arthritides
- Systemic illness
  - Diabetes mellitus, liver disease, HIV, malignancy, end-stage renal disease/hemodialysis, immunosuppression, sickle cell anemia
- Risks for hematogenous spread
  - IVDU, severe sepsis/systemic infection

GENERAL PREVENTION
- Prompt treatment of skin and soft tissue infections
- Control risk factors
- Immunization (*S. pneumoniae*; *N. meningitidis*)

 DIAGNOSIS

HISTORY
- Typical presentation includes a combination of joint pain, swelling, warmth, and decreased range of motion.
- Nongonococcal arthritis: predominantly monoarticular (80%)
  - Typically large joints (knee in 50% of cases)
  - Most patients report fever.
  - IV drug users may develop infection in axial joints (e.g., sternoclavicular joint).
  - Prosthetic joints may show minimal findings and present with draining sinus over the joint.
  - Patients on chronic immunosuppressive drugs and those receiving steroid joint injections may present atypically (no fever or joint pain).
- Pediatric considerations
  - Infants may present with refusal to move limb (can be mistaken as neurologic problem).
  - Hip joint pain may refer to the knee or thigh.
- Gonococcal arthritis
  - Bacteremic phase: migratory polyarthritis, tenosynovitis, high fever, chills, pustules (dermatitis-arthritis syndrome)
  - Localized phase: nonoarticular, low-grade fever

PHYSICAL EXAM
- Physical exam generally has poor sensitivity and specificity in the context of septic arthritis. Common findings include:
  - Limited range of motion
  - Joint effusion and tenderness
  - Erythema and warmth over affected joint
  - Pain with passive range of motion
- Septic arthritis of hip and shoulder involvement may reveal severe pain on range of motion and less obvious swelling on exam.
- Pediatric consideration: Infants with septic hip arthritis, keep the joint flexed and externally rotated.

DIFFERENTIAL DIAGNOSIS
- Crystal arthritis: gout, pseudogout, calcium oxalate, cholesterol
- Infectious arthritis: fungi, spirochetes, rheumatic fever, HIV, viral

- Inflammatory arthritis: RA, spondyloarthropathy, systemic lupus erythematosus, sarcoidosis
- Osteoarthritis
- Trauma: meniscal tear, fracture, hemarthrosis
- Other: bursitis, cellulitis, tendinitis

DIAGNOSTIC TESTS & INTERPRETATION
Initial Tests (lab, imaging)
- Synovial fluid analysis (gold standard):
  - Obtain prior to antibiotic therapy if possible
  - Include Gram stain, culture, cell count/differential, and crystal analysis.
  - Use blood culture bottles to increase yield.
  - Gram stain (positive in 50%) and culture (positive in 50–70%) should be sent with understanding of limitations.
  - >50,000 WBCs/HPF with >90% polymorphonuclear leukocytes is considered suggestive; however, *synovial WBC (sWBC) count alone is insufficient to rule in or rule out septic arthritis* (3)[A].
  - The presence of crystals (e.g., urate or calcium pyrophosphate) *does not exclude concurrent infectious arthritis* (5).
  - Prosthetic joint: WBC count is unreliable; a lower number of sWBCs may indicate infection.
- Serum tests:
  - WBC count alone is neither sensitive nor specific.
  - ESR with cutoff of >15 mm/hr has sensitivity up to 94% but poor specificity (6)[B].
  - CRP >20 mg/L has sensitivity of 92% (6)[B].
  - Serum procalcitonin >0.4 ng/mL has 85% sensitivity and 87% specificity (7)[B].
  - Synovial lactate is a potential biomarker (8,9)[C].
  - Blood cultures are positive in 50% of cases.
- Other tests:
  - Disseminated gonococcus: culture blood, cervix, urine, urethra, pharynx in addition to joint fluid
  - Suspected Lyme arthritis: send serum Lyme titers
- Pediatrics: No single lab test distinguishes septic arthritis from transient synovitis.
  - The combination of fever, non–weight bearing, and elevated ESR and CRP is suspicious, but synovial fluid should still be obtained.
- Imaging: helpful to identify effusion but does not differentiate septic from other forms of arthritis
  - Plain films:
    ○ Nondiagnostic for septic arthritis. Useful for other pathology such as trauma, soft tissue swelling, osteoarthritis, or osteopenia
    ○ May show nonspecific changes of inflammatory arthritis (i.e., erosions, joint destruction, joint space loss)
  - Ultrasound:
    ○ Identifies joint space to guide arthrocentesis
    ○ Recommended for aspiration of the hip
  - MRI:
    ○ Highly sensitive for effusion; increasing role to distinguish between transient synovitis and septic arthritis in children (10)[B]
  - Other imaging techniques:
    ○ CT is not routinely indicated.
    ○ Bone scans are not performed unless there is suspicion for osteomyelitis.

Diagnostic Procedures/Other

Arthrocentesis in all suspected cases (prior to initiation of antibiotics). Avoid contaminated tissue (e.g., overlying cellulitis) when performing arthrocentesis.

Test Interpretation

Synovial biopsy shows polymorphonuclear leukocytes and possibly the causative organism.

TREATMENT

GENERAL MEASURES

- Admit for parenteral antibiotics and monitoring. Antibiotics should begin immediately after arthrocentesis is performed and cultures requested.
- Removal of purulent material is *required* in these cases:
  - Pediatric: Surgical drainage and irrigation is recommended if hip involved due to high risk of avascular necrosis.
  - Prosthetic joint: Antibiotics and consult with orthopedics for consideration of replacement arthroplasty, resection arthroplasty, or débridement (11)[B].
- Treat for a total of 4 to 6 weeks in most cases.
  - Exception: gonococcal (2 to 3 weeks)
- Intra-articular antibiotics are not recommended.
- IV dexamethasone in conjunction with antibiotics may reduce long-term sequelae and improve recovery time in pediatric patients (12)[A].

MEDICATION

First Line

- Initial antibiotic choice is guided by Gram stain or most likely organism based on age and clinical history.
- Nongonococcal (13)[A]:
  - Gram-positive cocci:
    o Vancomycin 15 to 20 mg/kg 2 to 3 times daily or linezolid 600 mg twice daily
  - Gram-negative bacilli:
    o Cefepime 2 g twice daily or ceftriaxone 2 g daily or ceftazidime 2 g, 3 times daily or cefotaxime 2 g, 3 times daily
    o For cephalosporin allergy: Consider treatment with ciprofloxacin 400 mg, 3 times daily.
  - Negative Gram stain:
    o Vancomycin 15 to 20 mg/kg 2 to 3 times daily plus 3rd-generation cephalosporin until cultures and susceptibilities return
  - Duration of therapy: typically 2 weeks of IV and an additional 2 to 4 weeks PO while monitoring therapeutic response
- Gonococcal (14)[A]:
  - Ceftriaxone 1 g IV/IM daily for 7 to 14 days (and at least 24 to 48 hours after symptoms resolve)
  - May require concurrent drainage of affected joint
  - Concomitant treatment for *Chlamydia* (doxycycline 100 mg twice daily or azithromycin 1 g daily)
- Other considerations:
  - Narrow antibiotic therapy based on culture results
  - Consider *Salmonella* in pediatric patients with a history of sickle cell disease: 3rd-generation cephalosporin helpful in this instance.

  - Lyme arthritis: doxycycline 100 mg PO twice daily or amoxicillin 500 mg PO 3 times daily for 28 days if no neurologic involvement, otherwise ceftriaxone 2 g IV daily (15)[A]

ISSUES FOR REFERRAL

- Infectious disease and orthopedic consultations
- IVDU and immunosuppression warrant infectious disease consultation to guide therapy. Prosthetic joint infection is best managed with orthopedic consultation.

SURGERY/OTHER PROCEDURES

- Consider drainage in all cases, particularly shoulder, hip, and prosthetic joints.
- Other treatment options include repeat needle aspiration, arthroscopy, or arthrotomy.

ONGOING CARE

FOLLOW-UP RECOMMENDATIONS

Patient Monitoring

- Monitor synovial fluid to verify decreasing WBC and sterile fluid after initial treatment.
- If no improvement within 24 hours, reevaluate and consider arthroscopy.
- Follow-up at 1 week and 1 month after stopping antibiotics to ensure no relapse.

PROGNOSIS

- Early treatment improves functional outcome.
- Delayed recognition/treatment is associated with higher morbidity and mortality.
- Elderly, concurrent rheumatoid arthritis, *S. aureus* infections, and infection of hip and shoulder also increase risk of poor outcome.

COMPLICATIONS

- Mortality rate estimated at 11% (2)
- Limited joint range of motion, ankylosis
- Secondary osteoarthritis
- Flail, fused, or dislocated joint
- Sepsis, septic necrosis
- Sinus formation
- Osteomyelitis, postinfectious synovitis
- Limb length discrepancy (in children)

REFERENCES

1. Geirsson AJ, Statkevicius S, Vikingsson A. Septic arthritis in Iceland 1990–2002: increasing incidence due to iatrogenic infections. *Ann Rheum Dis*. 2008;67(5):638–643.
2. Mathews CJ, Weston VC, Jones A, et al. Bacterial septic arthritis in adults. *Lancet*. 2010;375(9717):846–855.
3. Margaretten ME, Kohlwes J, Moore D, et al. Does this adult patient have septic arthritis? *JAMA*. 2007;297(13):1478–1488.
4. Shirtliff ME, Mader JT. Acute septic arthritis. *Clin Microbiol Rev*. 2002;15(4):527–544.
5. Shah K, Spear J, Nathanson LA, et al. Does the presence of crystal arthritis rule out septic arthritis? *J Emerg Med*. 2007;32(1):23–26.
6. Hariharan P, Kabrhel C. Sensitivity of erythrocyte sedimentation rate and C-reactive protein for the exclusion of septic arthritis in emergency department patients. *J Emerg Med*. 2011;40(4):428–431.
7. Maharajan K, Patro DK, Menon J, et al. Serum Procalcitonin is a sensitive and specific marker in the diagnosis of septic arthritis and acute osteomyelitis. *J Orthop Surg Res*. 2013;8:19.
8. Lenski M, Scherer MA. The significance of interleukin-6 and lactate in the synovial fluid for diagnosing native septic arthritis. *Acta Orthop Belg*. 2014;80(1):18–25.
9. Carpenter CR, Schuur JD, Everett WW, et al. Evidence-based diagnostics: adult septic arthritis. *Acad Emerg Med*. 2011;18(8):781–796.
10. Yang WJ, Im SA, Lim GY, et al. MR imaging of transient synovitis: differentiation from septic arthritis. *Pediatr Radiol*. 2006;36(11):1154–1158.
11. Mittal Y, Fehring TK, Hanssen A, et al. Two-stage reimplantation for periprosthetic knee infection involving resistant organisms. *J Bone Joint Surg Am*. 2007;89(6):1227–1231.
12. Macchiaiolo M, Buonuomo PS, Mennini M, et al. Question 2: should steroids be used in the treatment of septic arthritis? *Arch Dis Child*. 2014;99(8):785–787.
13. Liu C, Bayer A, Cosgrove SE, et al. Clinical practice guidelines by the Infectious Diseases Society of America for the treatment of methicillin-resistant *Staphylococcus aureus* infections in adults and children. *Clin Infect Dis*. 2011;52(3):e18–e55.
14. Workowski KA, Berman S. Sexually transmitted diseases treatment guidelines, 2006. *MMWR Recomm Rep*. 2006;55(RR-11):1–94.
15. Wormser GP, Dattwyler RJ, Shapiro ED, et al. The clinical assessment, treatment, and prevention of lyme disease, human granulocytic anaplasmosis, and babesiosis: clinical practice guidelines by the Infectious Diseases Society of America. *Clin Infect Dis*. 2006;43(9):1089–1134.

CODES

ICD10

- M00.9 Pyogenic arthritis, unspecified
- M00.20 Other Streptococcal arthritis, unspecified joint
- M00.00 Staphylococcal arthritis, unspecified joint

CLINICAL PEARLS

- Because history, exam, and serum markers often confer little diagnostic benefit, arthrocentesis and synovial fluid analysis are mandatory in cases of suspected septic arthritis.
- Early IV antibiotics and drainage of infected joints are critical to successful management.
- Crystalline disease may coexist with septic arthritis.
- Initial antibiotic therapy is guided by results of aspiration (Gram stain), age, and patient-specific risk factors.

ARTHROPOD BITES AND STINGS

James E. Powers, DO, FACEP, FAAEM

BASICS

DESCRIPTION

Arthropods make up the largest division of the animal kingdom; two classes, insects and arachnids, have the greatest medical impact on humans. Arthropods affect humans by inoculating poison or irritative substances through a bite or sting, by invading tissue, or by contact allergy to their skin, hairs, or secretions. The greatest medical importance is transmission of infectious microorganisms that may occur during insect feeding. Sequelae to arthropod bites, stings, or contact may include the following:

- Local redness with itch, pain, and swelling: common, usually immediate and transient
- Large local reactions increasing over 24 to 48 hours
- Systemic reactions with anaphylaxis, neurotoxicity, organ damage, or other systemic toxin effects
- Tissue necrosis or secondary infection
- Infectious disease transmission: presentation may be delayed weeks to years

EPIDEMIOLOGY

Incidence

- Difficult to estimate, as most encounters unreported
- ~40 deaths per year in the United States from fatal anaphylactic reaction to insects but likely underreported (1)
- Unrecognized anaphylactic reactions to *Hymenoptera* stings may be cause of 1/4 of sudden and unexpected deaths outdoors (2).

Prevalence

Widespread, with regional and seasonal variations

ETIOLOGY AND PATHOPHYSIOLOGY

- Arthropods: four medically important classes
  - Insects: *Hymenoptera* (bees, wasps, hornets, fire ants), mosquitoes, bed bugs, flies, lice, fleas, beetles, caterpillars, and moths
  - Arachnids: spiders, scorpions, mites, and ticks
  - Chilopods (centipedes)
  - Diplopods (millipedes)
- Four general categories of pathophysiologic effects: toxic, allergic, infectious, and traumatic
  - Toxic effects of venom: local (tissue inflammation or destruction) versus systemic (neurotoxic or organ damage)
  - Allergic: Antigens in saliva may cause local inflammation. Exaggerated immune responses may result in anaphylaxis or serum sickness.
  - Trauma: Mechanical injury from biting or stinging causes pain, swelling, and portal of entry for bacteria and secondary infection. Retention of arthropod parts can cause a granulomatous reaction.
  - Infection: Arthropods are vectors and can transmit bacterial, viral, and protozoal diseases.

Genetics

Family history of atopy may be a factor in the development of more severe allergic reactions.

RISK FACTORS

- Previous sensitization is a key to most severe allergic reactions, but exposure history may not be recalled.
- Although most arthropod contact is inadvertent, certain activities, occupations, and travel increase risk.
- Greater risk for adverse outcome in young, elderly, immune compromised, or those with unstable cardiac or respiratory status
- Increased risk of anaphylaxis following insect sting in patients with mastocytosis (1)

GENERAL PREVENTION

- Avoidance of common arthropod habitats
- Insect repellents (not effective for bees, spiders, scorpions, caterpillars, bed bugs, fleas, ants)
  - N,N-diethyl-meta-toluamide (DEET)
    - Most effective broad-spectrum repellent against biting arthropods (3)
    - Formulations with higher concentrations (20–50%) are 1st-line choice when visiting areas of endemic arthropod-borne diseases (3).
    - Concentrations >30% give longer duration of effect
    - Safe for children >6 months of age and pregnant and lactating women (3)
  - Icaridin (formerly known as *picaridin*)
    - Use of concentrations <20% may require more frequent application to maintain effectiveness.
  - P-menthane-3,8-diol (PMD): component of lemon eucalyptus extract
    - Recommended alternative repellent to DEET at concentrations >20% (3)
    - May be used in children >6 months of age (3)
  - IR3535: less effective in most studies
  - Other botanical oils (citronella etc.): less effective than DEET; not for disease-endemic areas
- Barrier methods: clothing, bed nets
  - Use of light-colored pants, long-sleeved shirts, and hats may reduce arthropod impact.
  - Permethrin: Synthetic insecticide derived from chrysanthemum plant should not be applied to skin, but permethrin-impregnated clothing provides good protection against arthropods.
  - Mosquito nets: Insecticide-treated nets are advised for all travelers to disease-endemic areas at risk from biting arthropods (3).
  - WHO-recommended nets are Permanet 2.0 (Vestergaard), Olyset (Sumitomo), and Interceptor (BASF) (3).
- Desensitization 75–95% effective for *Hymenoptera*-specific venom
  - Skin tests are needed to determine sensitivity.
  - Refer to allergist/immunologist if candidate
- Fire ant control (but not elimination) possible
  - Baits; sprays, dusts, aerosols; biologic agents
- Risk of tick-borne diseases decreased by prompt removal of ticks within 24 hours of attachment.

DIAGNOSIS

HISTORY

- Sudden onset of pain or itching with visualization of arthropod
- Many cases unknown to patient or asymptomatic initially (bed bugs, lice, scabies, ticks). Consider in patients presenting with localized erythema, urticaria, wheals, papules, pruritus, or bullae.
- May identify insect by its habitat or by remnants brought by patient
- History of prior exposure useful but not always available or reliable
- Travel, occupational, social, and recreational history important

PHYSICAL EXAM

- If stinger is still present in skin, remove by flicking or scraping away from skin.
- Anaphylaxis is a clinical diagnosis. Essential to examine for signs and symptoms of anaphylaxis (4,5)
  - Erythema, urticaria, angioedema

- Itching/edema of lips, tongue, uvula; drooling
- Persistent vomiting
- Respiratory distress, wheeze, repetitive cough, stridor, dysphonia
- Hypotension, dysrhythmia, syncope, chest pain
- If anaphylaxis not present, exam focuses on the sting or bite itself. Common findings include local erythema, swelling, wheals, urticaria, papules, or bullae; excoriations from scratching.
- Thorough exam to look for arthropod infestation (lice, scabies) or attached ticks. Body lice usually found in seams of clothing. Skin scraping to identify scabies.
- Signs of secondary bacterial infection after 24 to 48 hours: increasing erythema, pain, fever, lymphangitis, or abscess
- Delayed manifestations of insect-borne diseases

DIFFERENTIAL DIAGNOSIS

- Urticaria and localized dermatologic manifestations:
  - Contact dermatitis, drug eruption, mastocytosis, bullous diseases, dermatitis herpetiformis, tinea, eczema, vasculitis, pityriasis, erythema multiforme, viral exanthem, cellulitis, abscess, impetigo, folliculitis, erysipelas, necrotizing fasciitis
- Anaphylactic-type reactions
  - Cardiac, hemorrhagic, or septic shock; acute respiratory failure, asthma; angioedema, urticarial vasculitis; flushing syndromes (catecholamines, vasoactive peptides); panic attacks, syncope
  - Differential diagnosis of the acute abdomen should include black widow spider bite.

DIAGNOSTIC TESTS & INTERPRETATION

Initial Tests (lab, imaging)

Seldom needed; basic lab parameters usually normal. Some findings may help confirm diagnosis of anaphylaxis:

- Plasma histamine levels elevated briefly after mast cell activation
- Serum tryptase within 15 minutes to 3 hours after onset of symptoms with second sample 24 hours later (5)

Follow-Up Tests & Special Considerations

- Severe envenomations may affect organ function and require monitoring of lab values (CBC, comprehensive metabolic panel, prothrombin time/international normalized ratio)
- Labs for arthropod-borne diseases, as indicated
  - Ticks: Lyme disease, Rocky Mountain spotted fever, relapsing fever, anaplasmosis, babesiosis, tularemia
  - Flies: tularemia, leishmaniasis, African trypanosomiasis, bartonellosis, loiasis
  - Fleas: plague, tularemia, murine typhus
  - Chigger mites: scrub typhus
  - Body lice: epidemic typhus, relapsing fever
  - Kissing bugs: Chagas disease
  - Mosquitoes: malaria, yellow fever, dengue fever, West Nile virus, equine encephalitis, chikungunya
- Refer to allergist for formal testing with history of anaphylaxis, significant systemic symptoms, progressively severe reactions (4,5)

Diagnostic Procedures/Other

Various skin tests and immunologic tests available to try to predict anaphylactic risk

TREATMENT

ALERT
- The more rapidly anaphylaxis develops, the more likely the reaction is to be severe and potentially life-threatening. Most deaths due to anaphylaxis occur within 30 to 60 minutes of sting.
- Epinephrine should be given as soon as diagnosis of anaphylaxis is suspected. Delay of epinephrine is associated with fatal anaphylaxis (4,5).
- Antihistamines and steroids do not replace epinephrine in anaphylaxis, and no direct outcome data regarding their effectiveness in anaphylaxis are available (4,5).
- Airway management critical if angioedema

GENERAL MEASURES
Local wound care, ice compress, elevation, analgesics

MEDICATION
First Line
- For arthropod bites/stings **with anaphylaxis**
  - There are no randomized controlled trials on treatments, so the following recommendations are all based on expert opinion consensus (5)[C].
  - Epinephrine: **most important:** IM injection in midanterolateral thigh (vastus lateralis muscle):
    ○ IM injection: epinephrine 1:1,000 (1 mg/mL): adult: 0.3 to 0.5 mg per dose; pediatric: give 0.01 mg/kg to a maximum dose of 0.5 mg per dose, can repeat every 5 to 15 minutes (5)
  - Positioning: supine with legs elevated
  - Oxygen 6 to 8 L/min up to 100%, as needed
  - IV fluids: Establish 1 to 2 large-bore IV lines. Normal saline rapid bolus 1 to 2 L IV; repeat as needed (pediatrics 20 to 30 mL/kg)
  - H_1 antihistamines: diphenhydramine 25 to 50 mg IV (pediatrics 1 to 2 mg/kg)
  - β_2 agonists: albuterol for bronchospasm nebulized 2.5 to 5 mg in 3 mL
  - Emergency treatment of refractory cases: consider epinephrine infusion, dopamine, glucagon, vasopressin, large-volume crystalloids (4,5)
- Arthropod bites/stings **without anaphylaxis**
  - Tetanus booster, as indicated
  - Oral antihistamines
    ○ Diphenhydramine
    ○ Cetirizine
    ○ H_2 blockers: ranitidine
  - Oral steroids: consider short course for severe pruritus; prednisone or prednisolone 1 to 2 mg/kg once daily
  - Topical intermediate-potency steroid cream or ointment × 3 to 5 days
    ○ Desoximetasone 0.05%
    ○ Triamcinolone 0.1%
    ○ Fluocinolone 0.025%
  - Wound care: antibiotics *only* if infection
  - Other specific therapies:
    ○ Scorpion stings: Treat excess catecholamine release (nitroprusside, prazosin, β-blockers). Diazepam for muscle spasms. Atropine for hypersalivation (6). Only one FDA-approved scorpion antivenom in United States and should be administered in conjunction with toxicologist. Black widow bites: Treat muscle spasms with diazepam and opioid analgesics PO or IV (6). Antivenom: available but should be administered in conjunction with toxicologist.
    ○ Poison control should be consulted for questions regarding management of envenomation. Poison Control hotline: 1-800-222-1222.
  - Fire ants: characteristically cause sterile pustules. Leave intact: Do not open or drain.

- Brown recluse spider: pain control, supportive treatment; surgical consult if débridement needed
- Ticks: early removal. Review guidelines for disease prophylaxis and treatment.
- Pediculosis: head, pubic, and body lice
  ○ First line: permethrin 1% (Nix) topical lotion. Apply to affected area, wash off in 10 minutes.
  ○ Alternatives: pyrethrin or malathion 0.5% lotion, ivermectin (not FDA approved for pediculosis) orally
  ○ Repeat above treatment in 7 to 10 days.
  ○ For eyelash infestation: Apply ophthalmic-grade petroleum jelly BID for 10 days.
- *Sarcoptes scabiei* scabies
  ○ Permethrin 5% cream: Apply to entire body. Wash off after 8 to 14 hours. Repeat in 1 week.
  ○ Ivermectin: 200 μg/kg PO once; repeat in 2 weeks (not FDA approved for this use)
  ○ Crotamiton 10% cream or lotion less efficacious; apply daily for 2 days after bathing.

Second Line
Second-line options for **anaphylaxis**:
- Ranitidine
- Methylprednisolone 1 mg/kg for 3 to 4 days or hydrocortisone 200 mg (5)

ISSUES FOR REFERRAL
Refer to allergist with history of anaphylaxis, severe systemic symptoms, or progressively severe reactions

SURGERY/OTHER PROCEDURES
Débridement and delayed skin grafting may be needed for brown recluse spider and other bites.

COMPLEMENTARY & ALTERNATIVE MEDICINE
- Some stings may be treated with a paste of 3 tsp of baking soda and 1 tsp water.
- None well tested

INPATIENT CONSIDERATIONS
Admission Criteria/Initial Stabilization
Anaphylaxis, vascular instability, neuromuscular events, pain, GI symptoms, renal damage/failure

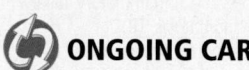

ONGOING CARE

FOLLOW-UP RECOMMENDATIONS
- Immunotherapy as recommended by allergist/consultant for anaphylaxis or serious reactions; venom immunotherapy cornerstone of treatment for *Hymenoptera*.
- Patient-administered epinephrine must be provided to patients with anaphylaxis. Consider "med-alert" identifiers (4,5).

Patient Monitoring
- Monitor for delayed effects, including infectious diseases from arthropod vectors.
- Serum sickness reactions, vasculitis (rare)

PATIENT EDUCATION
Avoidance and prevention

PROGNOSIS
- Excellent for local reactions
- For systemic reactions, best response with early intervention to prevent cardiorespiratory collapse

COMPLICATIONS
- Scarring
- Secondary bacterial infection
- Arthropod-associated diseases as mentioned earlier
- Psychological effects, phobias

REFERENCES
1. Tanskersley MS, Ledford DK. Stinging insect allergy: state of the art 2015. *J Allergy Clin Immunol Pract*. 2015;3(3):315–322.
2. Diaz JH. Recognition, management, and prevention of hymenopteran stings and allergic reactions in travelers. *J Travel Med*. 2009;16(5):357–364.
3. Moore SJ, Mordue Luntz AJ, Logan JG. Insect bite prevention. *Infect Dis Clin North Am*. 2012;26(3):655–673.
4. Simons FE, Ardusso LR, Bilò MB, et al. 2012 update: World Allergy Organization guidelines for the assessment and management of anaphylaxis. *Curr Opin Allergy Clin Immunol*. 2012;12(4):389–399.
5. De Bisschop MB, Bellou A. Anaphylaxis. *Curr Opin Crit Care*. 2012;18(4):308–317.
6. Quan D. North American poisonous bites and stings. *Crit Care Clin*. 2012;28(4):633–659.

ADDITIONAL READING
- Centers for Disease Control and Prevention. Protection against mosquitoes, ticks, & other insects & arthropods. http://wwwnc.cdc.gov/travel/yellowbook/2014/chapter-2-the-pre-travel-consultation/protection-against-mosquitoes-ticks-and-other-insects-and-arthropods. Accessed 2015.
- Centers for Disease and Prevention. FAQ. Insect repellent use & safety. http://www.cdc.gov/westnile/faq/repellent.html. Accessed 2015.
- Centers for Disease Control and Prevention. Tickborne diseases of the United States: a reference manual for health care providers. Third edition, 2015. Handbook available as a PDF at http://www.cdc.gov/ticks/
- Sicherer SH, Leung DY. Advances in allergic skin disease, anaphylaxis, and hypersensitivity reactions to foods, drugs, and insects in 2012. *J Allergy Clin Immunol*. 2013;131(1):55–66.
- Studdiford JS, Conniff KM, Trayes KP, et al. Bedbug infestation. *Am Fam Physician*. 2012;86(7):653–658.
- Swanson DL, Vetter RS. Bites of brown recluse spiders and suspected necrotic arachnidism. *N Engl J Med*. 2005;352(7):700–707.
- Warrell DA. Venomous bites, stings, and poisoning. *Infect Dis Clin North Am*. 2012;26(2):207–223.
- Juckett G. Arthropod bites. *Am Fam Physician*. 2013;88(12):841–847.

 # CODES

ICD10
- T63.481A Toxic effect of venom of arthropod, accidental, init
- T63.301A Toxic effect of unsp spider venom, accidental, init
- T63.484A Toxic effect of venom of oth arthropod, undetermined, init

CLINICAL PEARLS
- Urgent administration of epinephrine is a key to anaphylaxis treatment.
- Local treatment and symptom management are sufficient in most insect bites and stings.

ASCITES
Daniel J. Stein, MD, MPH • Stephen K. Lane, MD, FAAFP

 BASICS

DESCRIPTION
- Accumulation of fluid in the peritoneal cavity; may occur in conditions that cause generalized edema.
- Men generally have no fluid in peritoneal cavity; women may have up to 20 mL depending on menstrual phase.
- Ascites comes from Greek word *askos* (bag).

EPIDEMIOLOGY
- Children: nephrotic syndrome and malignancy most common
- Adults: cirrhosis (81%), cancer (10%), heart failure (3%), other (6%)

Incidence
~50–60% of patients with cirrhosis will develop ascites within 10 years (1).

Prevalence
10% of patients with liver cirrhosis have ascites.

ETIOLOGY AND PATHOPHYSIOLOGY
Portal hypertensive versus nonportal hypertensive etiologies
- Cannot reliably establish/confirm etiology without paracentesis
- Serum-ascites albumin gradient (SAAG), which is the (serum albumin level) − (ascites albumin level) differentiates causes

High portal pressure (SAAG ≥1.1)
- Cirrhosis
- Hepatitis (alcoholic, viral, autoimmune, medications)
- Acute liver failure
- Liver malignancy (primary or metastatic)
- Elevated right-sided filling pressures from heart failure or constrictive pericarditis
- Hepatic venous thrombosis (Budd-Chiari syndrome)
- Portal vein thrombosis

Normal portal pressure (SAAG <1.1)
- Peritoneal carcinomatosis
- Tuberculosis
- Severe hypoalbuminemia (nephrotic syndrome; severe enteropathy with protein loss)
- Meigs syndrome (ovarian cancer)
- Lymphatic leak (chylous ascites)
- Pancreatitis
- Inflammatory (vasculitis, lupus serositis, sarcoidosis)
- Other infections (parasitic, fungal)
- Hemoperitoneum from trauma or ectopic pregnancy

Pathophysiology of ascites is partially understood. It is best described for portal hypertensive (typically cirrhotic) ascites
- Most ascites is due to portal hypertension, with preferentially dilated splanchnic vasculature causing systemic hypotension.
- Reduced renal and carotid perfusion activates systemic vasoconstrictors and antinatriuretic mechanisms. This stimulates the sympathetic nervous system and renin-angiotensin-aldosterone system, culminating in sodium and water retention ascites and edema.

 DIAGNOSIS

HISTORY
- Progressive abdominal distention, which may be painless or painful.
- Weight gain, dyspnea/orthopnea, edema, early satiety, and nausea

- Patients with spontaneous bacterial peritonitis may present with fever, abdominal tenderness, and altered mentation.
- Individuals with underlying malignancy may present with weight loss.
- Address risk factors (e.g., EtOH use, TB exposure, prior malignancies, sexual partners, transfusion history)
- Obesity, hyperlipidemia and type 2 diabetes are associated with nonalcoholic steatohepatitis, which can progress to cirrhosis over time.

PHYSICAL EXAM
- Abdominal distention, flank dullness, shifting dullness, and puddle splash are most sensitive (83%) and specific (56%) exam findings (1).
- Edema (penile/scrotal, pedal), pleural effusion, rales
- Stigmata of cirrhosis (palmar erythema, spider angiomata, dilated abdominal wall collateral veins)
- Other signs of advanced liver disease: jaundice, muscle wasting, gynecomastia, leukonychia
- Signs of underlying malignancy: cachexia; umbilical (Virchow) node suggests upper abdominal malignancy.

DIAGNOSTIC TESTS & INTERPRETATION
Initial Tests (lab, imaging)
- Diagnostic paracentesis for fluid analysis should be obtained in all patients with ascites requiring hospital admission and in any new-onset or new-to-treatment patients with ascites (1)[C] to determine etiology and rule out infection.

  – Paracentesis has a complication rate of 1% (despite high prevalence of coexisting coagulation abnormalities). Routine attempts to correct platelet or coagulation defects are not needed (1)[B].

  – Ascitic fluid analysis should include (1)[C]:
    ○ Cell count and differential:
      ■ Polymorphonuclear leukocytes ≥250 cells/mm³ suggests infection.
    ○ Albumin level to calculate SAAG:
      ■ <1.1 g indicates a low portal pressure exudative process (i.e., inflammatory, biliary/pancreatic, carcinomatosis, TB)
      ■ ≥1.1 g indicates portal hypertensive/transudative process (cirrhosis, CHF, constrictive pericarditis, thrombosis)
    ○ Total protein (low in cirrhosis, nephrotic disease, and high in cardiac ascites. Cutoff approximately 25 g/L)
  – Other tests based on clinical scenario (1)[C]:
    ○ Bacterial gram stain/culture, if infection suspected (cirrhotic patients with ascites can fail to mount adequate fever or significant leukocytosis)
      ■ Fluid cultures are positive in 50–90% of cases of SBP.
      ■ Yield improved if inoculated to blood culture bottles at bedside and obtained before first dose of antibiotics.
    ○ Amylase (suspicion for bowel perforation, choledocholithiasis, or pancreatitis)
    ○ Triglyceride if fluid appears milky
    ○ Cytology if concern for malignancy (less sensitive in the absence of carcinomatosis)
    ○ Lactate dehydrogenase (LDH): An ascitic fluid–to–serum LDH ratio >1.0 can indicate infection, perforation, or tumor.
    ○ Carcinoembryonic antigen and alkaline phosphatase (elevated in viscous perforation)
- Myobacterial culture/TB complex PCR for suspicion of tuberculosis.

- Blood tests: BUN/creatinine, electrolytes (renal function)
  – Brain natriuretic peptide (heart failure)
  – Liver function tests and hepatitis serologies (hepatitis)
  – Albumin (needed for SAAG)
- Abdominal ultrasound can confirm ascites; highly sensitive, cost-effective, involves no radiation
- Portal Doppler can be obtained with ultrasound as first line to evaluate for thrombosis or cirrhosis.
- CT scan to rule out intra-abdominal pathology (e.g., malignancy)
- MRI preferred for evaluation of liver disease or confirmation of portal vein thrombosis

Diagnostic Procedures/Other
Laparoscopy: preferred if imaging and paracentesis are nondiagnostic
- Allows for direct visualization and biopsy of peritoneum, liver, and intra-abdominal lymph nodes
- Preferred for evaluating suspected peritoneal tuberculosis or malignancies

Test Interpretation
Cytology may reveal malignant cells: adenocarcinoma (ovary, breast, GI tract) or primary peritoneal carcinoma (most commonly associated with ascites)

 TREATMENT

For all patients:
- Daily weight
- Restrict dietary sodium to ≤2 g/day if the cause is due to portal hypertension (high SAAG) (1)[A].
- Water restriction (1 to 1.5 L/day) only necessary if serum sodium <120 to 125 mEq/L (1)[C]
- Creatinine >2.0 mg/dL: decrease diuretic doses, peritoneal paracentesis
- Avoid alcohol and ensure adequate nutrition if liver disease (1)[A].
- Baclofen may be used to reduce alcohol craving/consumption (1)[C].

MEDICATION

ALERT
Carefully approach diuresis; aggressive diuresis can induce prerenal acute kidney injury, encephalopathy, and hyponatremia. Monitor creatinine and electrolytes closely. Serum creatinine >2 mg/dL or serum sodium <120 mmol/L should prompt withdrawal of diuretics. NSAIDs may cause (or worsen) oliguria or azotemia and should be avoided. ACE inhibitors and angiotensin receptor blockers (ARBs) may be harmful in patients with cirrhosis/ascites due to an increased risk of hypotension and renal failure (1)[C]; ACE inhibitors and ARBs should be avoided in refractory ascites (1)[B]. Consider discontinuing β-blockers in patients with refractory ascites, worsening hypotension, or azotemia (1)[B].

First Line
- Sodium restriction and diuretics are the mainstay of treatment for patients with elevated portal pressures (1)[A]; other causes (e.g. carcinomatosis) are less likely to respond to medical therapy.
  – Spironolactone 100 to 400 mg daily PO; typical initial dose is 100 to 200 mg given in AM
    ○ Diuretic of choice due to its antialdosterone effects; can be used as single agent in patients with minimal ascites

– Furosemide 40 to 160 mg daily PO (avoid IV if possible); typical initial dose is 40 mg given in AM
  ○ Antinatriuretic effect helps to achieve negative sodium balance.
  ○ Not first-line as monotherapy but is an effective adjunct to potentiate the effect of spironolactone
– Most common (and preferred) regimen is spirono-lactone and furosemide together (maintaining a 100:40 ratio) for maximum efficacy and to maintain potassium homeostasis.
  ○ Titrate dose to desired result and monitor renal function regularly.
  ○ Follow daily weight.
• Diuretic-intractable ascites (10% of patients): persistent or worsening ascites despite maximum doses of spironolactone (400 mg/day) and furosemide (160 mg/day) and sodium restriction *or* progressive rise in creatinine to 2.0
  – *Ensure compliance with dietary sodium restriction using* 24-hour urine sodium excretion: in general, if <78 mEq/day, patient is compliant with 2-g dietary sodium restriction.
  – Therapeutic paracentesis or serial large-volume paracentesis (LVP) (see "Surgery/Other Procedures")

Second Line
• Midodrine 7.5 mg TID can be added to diuretic resistant or hypotensive patients and may improve survival (1)[B].

• Alternatives to spironolactone: amiloride up to 40 mg/day; triamterene up to 200 mg/day in divided doses (1)[C]

• Alternatives to furosemide: torsemide up to 100 mg/day; bumetanide up to 4 mg per day (1)[C]

• Vaptans may have a beneficial effect on hyponatre-mia and ascites, but routine use in ascites is not yet supported (2)[A].

ISSUES FOR REFERRAL
Consider referral for liver transplant in patients with decompensated liver disease, whether or not ascites is present/controlled. Liver transplant is the definitive treatment for portal hypertension (1)[B].

SURGERY/OTHER PROCEDURES
• Therapeutic paracentesis
  – Initial therapy if tense ascites is present (1)[C].

  – Serial (generally every 2 weeks) paracentesis can be used as second-line after diuretics in patients with elevated portal pressures (3)[B].

  – Complications: infection, hemodynamic collapse, acute renal failure

  – Similar complication rate as diuretics (3)[B]
  – Replace albumin when removing >5 L of ascites: 5.5 to 8 g albumin for each liter removed has been shown to decrease renal dysfunction, hypo-natremia post paracentesis, and overall morbidity (4)[A] for patients with portal hypertension; likely not needed for malignant ascites

  – Continue diuretics at 1/2 previous dose if transi-tioning to serial paracentesis in patients who fail diuretics alone.
• Transjugular intrahepatic portosystemic shunt (TIPS)
  – Used only in patients with elevated portal pressures

  – Fluoroscopically placed conduit from portal to hepatic vein for intractable ascites (5)[A]

    ○ At time of placement, portal pressure should drop ≥20 mm Hg or to <12 mm Hg, and asci-tes should be readily controlled with diuretics.

○ Yearly US to confirm shunt is functional.
○ 4 weeks after TIPS, urinary sodium and serum creatinine improve significantly and can normalize after 6 to 12 months in combination with diuretics (5). Dilation/replacement may be needed after 2 years.
○ Encephalopathy is a primary complication.

○ TIPS is superior to paracentesis for controlling ascites. No difference in mortality (5)[A].

• Peritoneovenous shunt (LeVeen or Denver shunt): drains ascites directly into the inferior vena cava
  – Clinical trials show poor long-term shunt patency, no survival advantage compared with medical therapy.
  – Complications include:
    ○ Bacteremia, bowel obstruction, and variceal bleed as a result of rapid volume overload from ascitic fluid into systemic circulation

    ○ Usually reserved for patients with refractory ascites who are not candidates for TIPS or liver transplant, and who have numerous abdominal adhesions, making repeated paracentesis unsafe (1)[A].

• Indwelling catheters with external drainage
  – Most useful in malignant ascites as a palliative measure
  – Overall low rate of infection
  – Can be drained at home
• Percutaneous endoscopic gastrostomy should be avoided in patients with ascites due to an associated high mortality rate following this procedure (1)[B].

COMPLEMENTARY & ALTERNATIVE MEDICINE
Caution advices with many herbal and other dietary supplements (risk drug interactions, hepatotoxicity, coagulopathy)

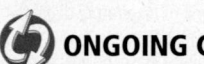 ONGOING CARE

PROGNOSIS
• Prognosis varies depending on underlying cause.
• Ascites in itself is rarely life threatening but can signify life-threatening disease (e.g., cancer, end-stage liver disease)

COMPLICATIONS
• Spontaneous bacterial peritonitis (SBP)
  – Ascitic fluid polymorphonuclear (PMN) leukocyte count ≥250 cells/mm³ or positive culture

    ○ Broad-spectrum antibiotics are as follows: Cefotaxime 2 g q8h or similar 3rd-generation cephalosporin is the treatment of choice for suspected SBP. Covers 95% of flora (including *Escherichia coli*, *Klebsiella*, pneumococci) (1)[A]
    ○ Lifetime antibiotic prophylaxis with norfloxacin or trimethoprim-sulfamethoxazole (TMP-SMX) is indicated in some patients who survive an epi-sode of SBP (1)[A]. Reduced incidence of SBP, delayed development of hepatorenal syndrome, and improved survival in cirrhosis (6)[C]

    ○ Suspect primary bacterial peritonitis (PBP) due to bowel perforations when ascitic fluid >250 cells/mm³ (often >5,000 cells/mm³), and any two of the following:
      ■ Ascitic fluid total protein >1 g/dL (often >3 g/dL)
      ■ Ascitic fluid glucose <50 mg/dL (or 2.8 mmol/L)
      ■ Ascitic fluid LDH that is 3-fold greater than serum LDH
• Hepatorenal syndrome: acute worsening of renal func-tion diagnosed when possible causes of acute renal failure are excluded, and at least 2 days of diuretic

withdrawal and maximal intravascular volume expan-sion with albumin (see "Hepatorenal Syndrome")
• Cellulitis is increasingly common in obese patients with brawny edema and should be treated with diuretics and appropriate antibiotics (1)[B].

REFERENCES
1. Runyon BA. Management of adult patients with ascites due to cirrhosis: update 2012. http://www.aasld.org/sites/default/files/guideline_documents/adultascitesenhanced.pdf. Accessed May 5, 2015.
2. Watson H, Jepsen P, Wong F, et al. Satavaptan treat-ment for ascites in patients with cirrhosis: a meta-analysis of effect on hepatic encephalopathy development. *Metab Brain Dis*. 2013;28(2):301–305.
3. Ginés P, Arroyo V, Quintero E, et al. Comparison of paracentesis and diuretics in the treatment of cir-rhotics with tense ascites. Results of a randomized study. *Gastroenterology*. 1987;93(2):234–241.
4. Bernardi M, Caraceni P, Navickis RJ, et al. Albumin infusion in patients undergoing large-volume paracentesis: a meta-analysis of randomized trials. *Hepatology*. 2012;55(4):1172–1181.
5. Rössle M, Gerbes AL. TIPS for the treatment of refractory ascites, hepatorenal syndrome and hepatic hydrothorax: a critical update. *Gut*. 2010;59(7):988–1000.
6. Fernández J, Navasa M, Planas R, et al. Primary prophylaxis of spontaneous bacterial peritonitis de-lays hepatorenal syndrome and improves survival in cirrhosis. *Gastroenterology*. 2007;133(3):818–824.

ADDITIONAL READING
• Becker G, Galandi D, Blum HE. Malignant ascites: systematic review and guideline for treatment. *Eur J Cancer*. 2006;42(5):589–597.
• Perumalswami PV, Schiano TD. The management of hospitalized patients with cirrhosis: the Mount Sinai experience and a guide for hospitalists. *Dig Dis Sci*. 2011;56(5):1266–1281.

 SEE ALSO

• Cirrhosis of the Liver; Hepatorenal Syndrome
• Algorithms: Congestive Heart Failure: Differential Diagnosis; Nephrotic Syndrome

 CODES

ICD10
• R18.8 Other ascites
• R18.0 Malignant ascites
• K70.31 Alcoholic cirrhosis of liver with ascites

CLINICAL PEARLS
• Cirrhosis remains the most common cause of ascites.
• Patients with new-onset ascites or hospitalized patients with ascites should have a diagnostic paracentesis.
• ACE inhibitors, ARBs, and β-blockers should be avoided in patients with ascites.
• Most common cause of "diuretic-intractable ascites" is noncompliance with dietary sodium restriction.
• First-line management of ascites is diuretics. Serial paracentesis or TIPS are second-line therapies.
• Ensure early referral of cirrhosis patients who are potential candidates for liver transplant.

ASTHMA
Urooj Najm, MBBS • Najm Hasan Siddiqui, MD

BASICS

DESCRIPTION
- Chronic, reversible inflammatory airway disease characterized by recurrent attacks of breathlessness and wheezing
- Four major classifications of asthma severity used primarily to initiate therapy (1,2):
  - Intermittent: symptoms ≤2 days/week, nighttime awakenings ≤2 times per month, short-acting β-agonist use ≤2 days/week, no interference with normal activity, and normal forced expiratory volume in 1 second (FEV_1) between exacerbations with FEV_1 (predicted) >80% and FEV_1/forced vital capacity (FVC) >80%
  - Mild persistent: symptoms >2 days/week but not daily, nighttime awakenings 3 to 4 times per month, short-acting β-agonist use >2 days/week but not daily, minor limitations in normal activity, and FEV_1 (predicted) >80% and FEV_1/FVC >80%
  - Moderate persistent: daily symptoms, nighttime awakenings ≥1 times per week but not nightly, daily use of short-acting β-agonist, some limitation in normal activity, and FEV_1 (predicted) 60–80% and FEV_1/FVC 75–80%
  - Severe persistent: symptoms throughout the day, nighttime awakenings often 7 times per week, short-acting β-agonist use several times a day, extremely limited normal activity, and FEV_1 (predicted) <60% and FEV_1/FVC <75%

EPIDEMIOLOGY
Prevalence
- Affects 5–10% of population
- One of the most common chronic diseases of childhood, affecting 7 million children
- In children, more common in boys than girls
- In adults, more common in women than men, African Americans than Caucasians

Pregnancy Considerations
In the United States, maternal asthma complicates approximately 4–8% of all pregnancies.

Geriatric Considerations
Prevalence of asthma in seniors (age ≥65 years) is 5.3%.

ETIOLOGY AND PATHOPHYSIOLOGY
- Airway inflammation begins with inflammatory cell infiltration, sub-basement fibrosis, mucus hypersecretion, epithelial injury, smooth muscle hypertrophy, angiogenesis that then leads to intermittent airflow obstruction, and bronchial hyperresponsiveness.
- Remodeling of airways may occur (1).

Genetics
- Inheritable component with complex genetics and environment interaction
- A gene-by-environment interaction occurs in which the susceptible host is exposed to environmental factors that are capable of generating immunoglobulin (Ig) E and sensitization occurs.

RISK FACTORS
- Host factors: genetic predisposition, gender, race, BMI
- Environmental: viral infections, animal and airborne allergens, tobacco smoke, and so on
- Exercise, obesity, and emotional stress
- Aspirin or NSAIDs hypersensitivity or β-blockers
- Food allergies and asthma → increased risk for fatal anaphylaxis from those foods

GENERAL PREVENTION
- Eliminate or modify exposure to asthma triggers (e.g., allergens, smoking, aspirin, NSAIDs).
- Consider allergen immunotherapy.
- Treat comorbidities such as allergic rhinitis.
- Annual influenza vaccine (inactivated influenza vaccine) for age <6 months
- Patients at risk for anaphylaxis should carry an EpiPen.

COMMONLY ASSOCIATED CONDITIONS
- Atopy: eczema, allergic conjunctivitis, allergic rhinitis
- Obesity (associated with higher asthma rates)
- Sinusitis
- Gastroesophageal reflux disease (GERD)
- Obstructive sleep apnea (OSA)
- Allergic bronchopulmonary aspergillosis (rare)
- Stress/depression

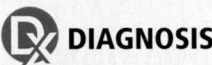

DIAGNOSIS

It is important to classify asthma severity.

HISTORY
- Question frequency of symptoms and rescue inhaler use.
- Symptoms include the following:
  - Cough (particularly if worse at night)
  - Wheeze
  - Chest tightness/difficulty breathing

PHYSICAL EXAM
- May be normal
- Focus on
  - General appearance: signs of respiratory distress such as use of accessory muscles
  - Upper respiratory tract: rhinitis, nasal polyps, swollen nasal turbinates
  - Lower respiratory tract: wheezing, prolonged expiratory phase
  - Skin: eczema

DIFFERENTIAL DIAGNOSIS
- In children
  - Upper airway diseases (allergic rhinitis or sinusitis)
  - Large airway obstruction (foreign body aspiration, vocal cord dysfunction, vascular ring or laryngeal web, laryngotracheomalacia, lymph nodes, or tumor)
  - Small airway obstruction (viral bronchiolitis, cystic fibrosis, bronchopulmonary dysplasia, heart disease)
  - Other causes (recurrent cough *not* due to asthma, aspiration/GERD)
- In adults
  - Chronic obstructive pulmonary disease, congestive heart failure, pulmonary embolism, benign or malignant tumor, pulmonary infiltration with eosinophilia, Churg-Strauss syndrome, drugs such as an ACE inhibitor, vocal cord dysfunction

DIAGNOSTIC TESTS & INTERPRETATION
Initial Tests (lab, imaging)
- Blood tests are not required but may find eosinophilia or elevated serum IgE levels.
- Spirometry: Normal test does not rule out asthma. It measures the FVC and the FEV_1. A reduced predicted ratio of FEV_1/FVC with reversibility (increase of 200 mL or 12% of FEV_1/FVC) after using a short-acting bronchodilator establishes the diagnosis.

- Bronchoprovocation (methacholine, histamine, cold air, or exercise) is used to simulate bronchoconstriction, which is very useful in atypical presentation/normal baseline spirometry. Abnormal test is not entirely specific for asthma, but normal test excludes asthma.
- Peak expiratory flow rates are inappropriate for diagnosis. Typically used for monitoring of symptoms in diagnosed asthma patients.
- Chest x-ray is used to exclude alternative diagnoses and to evaluate patients for complicating cardiopulmonary processes.

Follow-Up Tests & Special Considerations
Asthma action plan: Patients monitor their own symptoms and/or peak flow measurements.

Diagnostic Procedures/Other
- Allergy skin testing is not useful for diagnosis of asthma but may be considered to evaluate atopic triggers.
- Sweat testing in diagnosis of cystic fibrosis.
- Arterial blood gases are indicated for patients with respiratory distress and hypoxia.

Test Interpretation
Inflammatory cell infiltration, edema, goblet cell hyperplasia, smooth muscle hyperplasia, thickened basement membrane

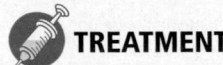

TREATMENT

GENERAL MEASURES
- Identify triggers and control exposures.
- Identify patients at risk for reactions to aspirin and NSAIDs and avoid exposure.
- All patients requiring inhaled agents should be prescribed with spacer (holding chamber) device.

MEDICATION
First Line
- Short-acting β-agonist (SABA) for quick relief of acute symptoms and to prevent exercise-induced bronchospasm (1)[A]

  - SABA include albuterol and levalbuterol (Xopenex) (3).
- Anticholinergic agent

  - Ipratropium bromide: used in combination with SABA for acute treatment, mainly in the ED (1)[A]
- Systemic corticosteroids can be used

  - In all patients with acute asthma exacerbations (4)[A]

  - In moderate to severe asthma as adjunct

  - Prednisolone 1 to 2 mg/kg/day or equivalent for up to 7 days in adults and for 3 days in children with no need for tapering (4)[A]

ALERT
- Use of holding chambers ("spacers") improves clinical benefit of inhaled agents and should be prescribed for all.
- HFA inhalers provide smaller particle size, better lung deposition, and less oropharyngeal deposition.
- All metered-dose inhalers (MDIs) need to be primed before use.
- Reserve nebulized delivery of medication for those unable to use spacer (e.g., infants, those intubated).
- All short-acting agents are pregnancy Category C.

Second Line

For long-term control

- Inhaled corticosteroids (ICS)

  – Most potent and effective long-term controller therapy for children and adults with persistent asthma and persistent asthma during pregnancy (1)[A]
  – Advice patients to rinse their mouth after inhalation to reduce adverse effects (1)[B].

  – Long-acting β_2-agonists (LABA)
    ○ Salmeterol or formoterol

    ○ Should not be used as monotherapy (1)[A]; doing so leads to an increased risk of severe outcomes, including death
  – Combination products, including LABA and ICS, are available and are indicated if ICS alone do not provide control; preferred in moderate and severe persistent disease (1,3)[A]. This is not recommended to treat acute symptoms or exacerbation (1)[D].
  – Leukotriene receptor agonists: alternative, not preferable for mild and moderate persistent asthma (1)[A]

    ○ Montelukast or zafirlukast (patients ≥5 years)
  – Lipoxygenase pathway inhibitor: alternative, not preferred for adjunctive treatment in adults (1)[D]: zileuton (patients ≥12 years)

  – Theophylline: not preferred as adjunctive therapy with inhaled corticosteroids (1)[A]. Monitoring of serum theophylline level is essential.
  – Cromolyn sodium and nedocromil are also alternatives; not preferred options for mild persistent asthma (1)[A]; can also be used before exercise and exposure to allergens for prevention of asthma

  – Immunomodulators

    ○ Omalizumab: adjunctive; not preferred therapy for patients ≥12 years with allergies and severe persistent asthma (1)[B]

ISSUES FOR REFERRAL

Referral to an asthma specialist (either a pulmonologist or an allergist) should be considered when

- Diagnosis unclear
- Additional asthma education needed
- Comorbidities: rhinitis, GERD, sinusitis, OSA
- Specialized testing (e.g., bronchoprovocation, skin testing)
- Specialized treatments (e.g., immunotherapy, anti-IgE therapy)
- Poorly controlled, moderate to severe persistent asthma in adults
- Moderate to persistent asthma in children
- Poorly controlled asthma: multiple emergency room visits for asthma

Pregnancy Considerations

- Poorly controlled asthma results in low birth weight, increased prematurity, and perinatal mortality.
- Albuterol is the preferred SABA, and budesonide is the preferred ICS due to excellent safety profile (1).
- Other ICS agents are pregnancy Category C, but no data indicate their unsafety in pregnancy (1). Montelukast and zafirlukast are Category B but are not studied extensively in pregnancy.

ADDITIONAL THERAPIES

- Allergen immunotherapy when clear relationship between symptoms and exposure to an unavoidable allergen
- Omalizumab (Xolair): anti-IgE therapy, approved for patients >12 years with moderate to severe asthma

INPATIENT CONSIDERATIONS

Admission Criteria/Initial Stabilization

No single measure is predictive.

- Dyspnea/hypoxia
- Poor or no response to SABA
- Peak expiratory flow (PEF) or FEV_1 <40%
- Decision for admission should be based on duration and severity of symptoms, severity of airflow obstruction, response to ED treatment, course and severity of prior exacerbations, access to medical care and medication, and adequacy of home condition (1).
- Supplemental oxygen to correct hypoxemia

- Repeated doses or continuous administration of SABA (1)[A]
- Ipratropium bromide may be used in the ED but is not for inpatient treatment (1)[B].
- Systemic corticosteroids for acute exacerbations (1)[A].
- Adjunctive therapy with $MgSO_4$ or helium–oxygen mixture (heliox) may be considered in severe cases (1)[B].

IV Fluids

- Avoid aggressive hydration in older children and adults.
- Monitor electrolytes.

Nursing

- Careful respiratory monitoring including vital signs, pulse oximetry, response and duration of response to SABA, and when possible, an objective measure of lung function such as PEF or FEV_1
- Asthma education

Discharge Criteria

- Minimal or absent asthma symptoms
- Hypoxia has resolved.
- FEV_1 or PEF ≥70% predicted or personal best
- Bronchodilator response sustained ≥60 minutes

 ONGOING CARE

FOLLOW-UP RECOMMENDATIONS

Smoking cessation counseling or elimination of secondhand smoke, if applicable

Patient Monitoring

- Quality-of-life measures: impact on activities, sleep, ED visits/hospitalizations, and so forth
- Pharmacotherapy: efficacy, compliance, side effects, technique
- Peak flow to evaluate if cough is due to exacerbation in those with known asthma.

DIET

Food allergies and sulfites (in food and wine) can precipitate symptoms for some patients.

PATIENT EDUCATION

- Patients' care plan and inhaled medication technique at every visit.
- American Academy of Allergy, Asthma & Immunology: 800-822-2762 or http://www.aaaai.org/
- American Lung Association: www.lungusa.org
- Asthma and Allergy Foundation of America: 800-727-8462 or http://www.aafa.org/
- Mattress and pillow covers DO NOT improve outcomes and should not be recommended.

PROGNOSIS

- Prognosis is good for male patients, nonsmokers, and children with mild disease.
- Asthma worsens in 1/3 of women during pregnancy and improves in another 1/3.

COMPLICATIONS

- Atelectasis
- Pneumonia
- Air leak syndromes: pneumomediastinum, pneumothorax
- Medication-specific side effects/adverse effects/interactions
- Respiratory failure
- Death: ~50% of asthma deaths occur in the elderly (age >65 years), and mortality is increasing in that population (5).

REFERENCES

1. National Heart, Lung, and Blood Institute. *National Asthma Education and Prevention Program Expert Panel Report 3: Guidelines for the Diagnosis and Management of Asthma*. Washington, DC: National Institutes of Health; 2007. NIH publication 08-5846.
2. Reddel HK, Taylor DR, Bateman ED, et al. An official American Thoracic Society/European Respiratory Society statement: asthma control and exacerbations: standardizing endpoints for clinical asthma trials and clinical practice. *Am J Respir Crit Care Med*. 2009;180(1):59–99.
3. Fanta CH. Asthma. *N Engl J Med*. 2009;360(10): 1002–1014.
4. Doherty S. Prescribe systemic corticosteroids in acute asthma. *BMJ*. 2009;338:b1234.
5. Stupka E, deShazo R. Asthma in seniors: part 1. Evidence for underdiagnosis, undertreatment, and increasing morbidity and mortality. *Am J Med*. 2009;122(1):6–11.

ADDITIONAL READING

Dombrowski MP, Schatz M. ACOG practice bulletin: clinical management guidelines for obstetrician-gynecologists number 90, February 2008: asthma in pregnancy. *Obstet Gynecol*. 2008;111(2, Pt 1): 457–464.

 SEE ALSO

Algorithm: Asthma Exacerbation, Pediatric Acute

CODES

ICD10

- J45.909 Unspecified asthma, uncomplicated
- J45.901 Unspecified asthma with (acute) exacerbation
- J45.20 Mild intermittent asthma, uncomplicated

CLINICAL PEARLS

- SABA is the most effective rescue therapy for acute asthma symptoms.
- Holding chambers should be used by all
- ICSs are the preferred long-term control therapy for patients of all ages.
- Peak flow is an inexpensive and easily available monitoring device once the diagnosis of asthma has been established.

ATELECTASIS

Bruce Jay Gardner, MD • Fahad Pervez, MD

BASICS

DESCRIPTION
- Incomplete expansion of lung tissue with resultant loss of lung volume and function, leading to impaired airway mucus clearance
- Broadly categorized as:
  - Obstructive: blockage within an airway
  - Nonobstructive: loss of contact between the parietal and visceral pleurae, replacement of lung tissue by scarring or infiltrative disease, surfactant dysfunction, and parenchymal compression
- Symptoms depends on the rapidity with which bronchial occlusion occurs, the size of the lung area affected, and the presence or absence of lung disease and comorbidities.
- Reduced respiratory gas exchange can lead to hypoxemia and other pulmonary complications.

EPIDEMIOLOGY
- Affects all ages; mean age is 60 years.
- Male = female. No racial predilection.

Incidence
- Round atelectasis (see "Initial Tests (lab, imaging)") is high in asbestos workers (65–70%).
- Incidence of lobar atelectasis depends on the collateral ventilation within each individual lung lobe.

Prevalence
Postoperative atelectasis is extremely common, affecting up to 90% of surgical patients, especially after major cardiac or GI procedures.

ETIOLOGY AND PATHOPHYSIOLOGY
- Obstructive (resorptive) atelectasis is more common and is caused by intrinsic respiratory blockage
  - Due to luminal blockage (foreign body, mucus plug, asthma, cystic fibrosis, trauma, tumor) or airway wall abnormality (congenital malformation, emphysema)
  - Distal to the obstruction, air is reabsorbed from the alveoli into the deoxygenated venous system, causing complete collapse of the alveolar tissue.
  - There are three collateral ventilation systems in each lobe: the pores of Kohn, canals of Lambert, and fenestrations of Boren. The patency and formation of the systems depends on multiple factors including age, lung disease, and FiO$_2$.
  - Age: Due to the late development of collaterals in children, atelectasis is frequently diagnosed after foreign body aspiration.
  - Emphysema: The fenestra of Boren in emphysematous patients often becomes enlarged; this enlargement can lead to a delay in atelectasis despite an obstructing lesion or mass.
  - FiO$_2$: Oxygen rapidly dissociates from alveoli to deoxygenated vessels in an obstructed airway. The 79% nitrogen in atmospheric air has a slower rate of dissociation from the alveoli, and thereby prevents collapse by maintaining positive pressure inside the alveoli. With increased FiO$_2$, the concentration of nitrogen is decreased predisposing patients to rapid development of atelectasis at the onset of obstruction.
- Nonobstructive atelectasis
  - Passive atelectasis: results from pleural membrane separation of the visceral and parietal layers
    - Pleural effusion, pneumothorax

- Compression atelectasis: alveoli compression leading to diminished resting volume (functional residual capacity [FRC]):
  - Space-occupying lesions, lymphadenopathy, cardiomegaly, abscess, chest wall pressure
- Adhesive atelectasis: surfactant dysfunction resulting in increased surface tension and alveoli collapse
  - Respiratory distress syndrome, acute respiratory distress syndrome (ARDS), radiation exposure, smoke inhalation, uremia
- Cicatrization: pleural or parenchymal scarring
  - Granulomatous disease, toxic inhalation, drug-induced fibrosis (e.g., amiodarone), radiation exposure
- Replacement atelectasis: diffuse tumor manifestation resulting in complete lobar collapse
  - Bronchioalveolar cell carcinoma
- Rounded atelectasis: distinct form of atelectasis following asbestos exposure
- Others
  - Hypoxemia due to pulmonary embolus
  - Muscular weakness (anesthesia, neuromuscular disease)

RISK FACTORS
- General anesthesia: positive fluid balance, ≥4 units blood transfusion, use of nasogastric tube, long-acting muscle relaxants, hypothermia, postoperative epidural anesthesia, ventilator settings with high tidal volume and plateau pressure
- Surgical procedures: cardiothoracic, upper GI, neurosurgery, oromaxillofacial, ENT, vascular
- Patient risk factors for developing postoperative atelectasis:
  - Age >60 and <6 years, chronic obstructive pulmonary disease (COPD), obstructive sleep apnea, CHF, alcohol abuse, pulmonary hypertension, albumin <3.5 g/dL, hemoglobin <10 g/dL, BMI >27 kg/m^2 (weak evidence), ASA class II+ functional dependence in activities of daily living (ADL), heart failure, smoking
- Intensive care and prolonged immobilization
- Brock syndrome: recurrent right middle lobe collapse secondary to airway disease, infection, or a combination thereof. The right middle lobe airway is long and thin and has the poorest drainage and clearance of the lobes, resulting in trapped mucus.

GENERAL PREVENTION
- Early mobilization, deep breathing exercises, coughing, and frequent changes in body position
- Preoperative physical therapy lowered rates of atelectasis, PNA, and LOS in elective cardiac surgery without improving other postoperative pulmonary complications or mortality (1)[A]. Further large RCTs are needed before conclusions can be made regarding the effect of chest physiotherapy and incentive spirometry.
- Mechanical ventilation settings with high tidal volumes (Vt >10 mL/kg), high plateau pressures (>30 cm H$_2$O), and without positive end-expiratory pressure (PEEP) are associated with postoperative pulmonary complications such as pneumonia and respiratory failure:
  - Ventilator-induced lung injury can be minimized by using low Vt and plateau pressures at sufficient PEEP while maintaining lower FiO$_2$ during anesthetic induction and intraoperatively.

- Application of continuous positive airway pressure (CPAP) during anesthesia induction and reversal of anesthesia-induced atelectasis after intubation by a recruitment maneuver may decrease postoperative pulmonary complications (2)[C].

COMMONLY ASSOCIATED CONDITIONS
- COPD and asthma
- Trauma
- ARDS, neonatal respiratory distress syndrome, pulmonary edema, pulmonary embolism
- Neuromuscular disorders (muscular dystrophy, spinal muscular atrophy, spinal cord injury), cystic fibrosis
- Respiratory syncytial virus (RSV), bronchiolitis
- Bronchial stenosis, pulmonic valve disease, pulmonary hypertension
- Pneumonia, pleural effusion, pneumothorax

DIAGNOSIS

HISTORY
- Frequently asymptomatic
- Tachypnea and sudden-onset dyspnea
- Nonproductive cough
- Pleuritic pain on affected side
- History of smoking, COPD, pulmonary insufficiency, exposure to radiation, asbestos, or other air pollutants

PHYSICAL EXAM
- Signs of hypoxia or cyanosis
- Tracheal or precordial impulse displacement toward the affected side; dullness to percussion
- Bronchial breathing if airway is patent
- Wheezing or absent breath sounds if airway is occluded
- Diminished chest expansion

DIFFERENTIAL DIAGNOSIS
See "Etiology and Pathophysiology."

DIAGNOSTIC TESTS & INTERPRETATION
Initial Tests (lab, imaging)
- CBC and sputum culture if infection suspected
- ABG: despite hypoxemia, the PaCO$_2$ level is usually normal or low
- Chest x-ray (CXR), PA and lateral
  - Raised diaphragm, flattened chest wall, movement of fissures and mediastinal structures toward the atelectatic region
  - Unaffected lung may show compensatory hyperinflation.
  - Wedge-shaped densities: obstructive atelectasis
  - Small, linear bands (Fleischner lines) often at lung bases: discoid (subsegmental or plate) atelectasis
  - Lobar collapse
    - Direct signs: displacement of fissures and opacification of the collapsed lobe. Right upper lobe collapse may display the inverted S sign of Golden, suggesting neoplastic shift of the minor fissure.
    - Indirect signs: displacement of the hilum, mediastinal shift toward the side of collapse, loss of volume of ipsilateral hemithorax, elevation of ipsilateral diaphragm, crowding of the ribs, compensatory hyperlucency of remaining lobes, and silhouetting of the diaphragm or heart border

- Air bronchograms: Evidence of pleural fluid or air may indicate compressive atelectasis.
- Adhesive atelectasis may present as a diffuse reticular granular pattern, progressing to a pulmonary edema pattern, and finally to bilateral opacification in severe cases.
- Pleural-based round density on CXR: round atelectasis
- Complete atelectasis of entire lung: opacification of the entire hemithorax and an ipsilateral shift of the mediastinum

Follow-Up Tests & Special Considerations
- Chest CT or MRI may be indicated to visualize airway and mediastinal structures and identify cause of atelectasis.
- Pulmonary function tests (PFTs) may detect restrictive disease, decreased respiratory muscle pressures, or airflow obstruction.
- Low serum albumin (<3.5 g/L) is a powerful marker of increased risk for postoperative pulmonary complications, including atelectasis.

Diagnostic Procedures/Other
Bronchoscopy can be considered in unexplained or refractory cases.

 TREATMENT

GENERAL MEASURES
- Prevention following surgery or general anesthesia using PEEP (2)[C]
- Treat the underlying cause.
- Ensure patient is lying on the unaffected side to promote drainage:
  - Maximize mobility and encourage frequent coughing and deep breathing.
- Incentive spirometry every hour while awake
  - Lack of evidence for incentive spirometry preventing postoperative pulmonary complications after coronary artery bypass graft (CABG) (3)[A]
- Initiate intubation and mechanical ventilation with PEEP in severe respiratory distress or hypoxemia:
  - Lower tidal volume (6 mL/kg) and lower end-inspiratory values (<30 mm Hg) are associated with reduced mortality.
  - PEEP 15 to 20 mL may be necessary to maintain arterial O_2 saturation in surfactant-impaired states.
- Postsurgical measures include positive airway pressure, continuous or intermittent.

MEDICATION
First Line
Pharmacotherapy should be tailored to address underlying cause:
- Antibiotics for infection
- Chemo/radiation therapy for tumor
- Steroids for asthma
- Effective analgesia to permit deep inspiration and coughing
- Mucolytics can be considered to promote airway clearance (NAC and saline most commonly studied).

Pediatric Considerations
- RhDNase may be effective clearing mucinous secretions in refractory mucous plugging in children.
- Chest physiotherapy (i.e., percussion, drainage, deep insufflation, and saline lavage) is a common treatment modality in the hospital setting. Caution must

be practiced when interpreting the possible positive effects as the number of patients studied is small, the results are not consistent across trials, data on safety are insufficient, and there may be limited applicability to current guidelines.

- Application of continuous distending pressure has some benefit in the treatment of preterm infants with respiratory distress syndrome and has the potential to reduce lung damage particularly if applied early (4)[A].

Second Line
Bronchofibroscopy in aspiration of inspissated secretions to improve airway clearance has been efficacious in several studies. However, debate continues regarding its efficacy in the treatment of atelectasis.

Pediatric Considerations
In obstructive atelectasis, bronchoscopy remains controversial. In the presence of a mucus plug or cast, bronchoscopy may be beneficial.

SURGERY/OTHER PROCEDURES
- Appropriate surgical resection for underlying disease (e.g., tumor, severe lymphadenopathy)
- Bronchoscopy

INPATIENT CONSIDERATIONS
Admission Criteria/Initial Stabilization
Ensure adequate oxygenation (may start with 100% FiO_2 then taper) and humidification

 ONGOING CARE

FOLLOW-UP RECOMMENDATIONS
Patient Monitoring
- Depends on underlying cause and comorbidities
- In uncomplicated cases of atelectasis associated with asthma or infection, outpatient monitoring is appropriate.

PATIENT EDUCATION
Maximize patient mobility and encourage frequent coughing and deep breathing.

PROGNOSIS
- For postoperative atelectasis, spontaneous resolution usually occurs within 24 hours but can persist for days after surgery.
- The prognosis of lobar atelectasis secondary to endobronchial obstruction depends on treatment of the underlying disease or malignancy.
- Surgical therapy is needed only for resectable causes or if chronic infection and bronchiectasis supervene.

COMPLICATIONS
- Pneumonia and pulmonary infections
- Acute atelectasis
  - Hypoxemia and respiratory failure
  - Postobstructive drowning of the lung
- Chronic atelectasis
  - Bronchiectasis
  - Pleural effusion and empyema

REFERENCES

1. Hulzebos EH, Smit Y, Helders PP, et al. Preoperative physical therapy for elective cardiac surgery patients. *Cochrane Database Syst Rev.* 2012;(11):CD010118.

2. Baltieri L, Santos LA, Rasera I Jr, et al. Use of Positive pressure in the bariatric surgery and effects on pulmonary function and prevalence of atelectasis: randomized and blinded clinical trial. *Arq Bras Cir Dig.* 2014;27(Suppl 1):26–30.

3. Freitas ER, Soares BG, Cardoso JR, et al. Incentive spirometry for preventing pulmonary complications after coronary artery bypass graft. *Cochrane Database Syst Rev.* 2012;(9):CD004466.

4. Ho JJ, Henderson-Smart DJ, Davis PG. Early versus delayed initiation of continuous distending pressure for respiratory distress syndrome in preterm infants. *Cochrane Database Syst Rev.* 2002;(2):CD002975.

ADDITIONAL READING

- Brower RG. Consequences of bed rest. *Crit Care Med.* 2009;37(10 Suppl):S422–S428.
- Ferreyra G, Long Y, Ranieri VM. Respiratory complications after major surgery. *Curr Opin Crit Care.* 2009;15(4):342–348.
- Guimarães MM, El Dib R, Smith AF, et al. Incentive spirometry for prevention of postoperative pulmonary complications in upper abdominal surgery. *Cochrane Database Syst Rev.* 2009;(3):CD006058.
- McCunn M, Sutcliffe AJ, Mauritz W, et al. Guidelines for management of mechanical ventilation in critically injured patients. *Trauma Care.* 2004;14(4):147–151.
- Mavros MN, Velmahos GC, Falagas ME. Atelectasis as a cause of postoperative fever: where is the clinical evidence? *Chest.* 2011;140(2):418–424.
- Qaseem A, Snow V, Fitterman N, et al. Risk assessment for and strategies to reduce perioperative pulmonary complications for patients undergoing noncardiothoracic surgery: a guideline from the American College of Physicians. *Ann Intern Med.* 2006;144(8):575–580.
- Tusman G, Böhm SH, Warner DO, et al. Atelectasis and perioperative pulmonary complications in high-risk patients. *Curr Opin Anaesthesiol.* 2012;25(1):1 10.
- Wu KH, Lin CF, Huang CJ, et al. Rigid ventilation bronchoscopy under general anesthesia for treatment of pediatric pulmonary atelectasis caused by pneumonia: a review of 33 cases. *Int Surg.* 2006;91(5):291–294.

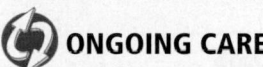 **CODES**

ICD10
J98.11 Atelectasis

CLINICAL PEARLS
- No strong clinical evidence supports atelectasis as an early cause of postoperative fever.
- Anesthesia-induced atelectasis occurs in almost all anesthetized patients.
- Bronchogenic carcinoma, which may present with atelectasis, must be excluded in all patients >35 years.
- In complete atelectasis of an entire lung, the mediastinal ipsilateral shift separates atelectasis from massive pleural effusion.
- Low serum albumin is a powerful predictor of postoperative pulmonary complications, including atelectasis.

ATRIAL FIBRILLATION AND ATRIAL FLUTTER

Youhua Zhang, MD, PhD • Bianca Lee, DO, MS

BASICS

This topic covers both atrial fibrillation (AFib) and atrial flutter (AFlut).

DESCRIPTION

- AFib: Paroxysmal or continuous supraventricular tachyarrhythmia characterized by rapid, uncoordinated atrial electrical activity and an irregularly irregular ventricular response. In most patients, the ventricular rate is rapid because the atrioventricular (AV) node is bombarded with very frequent atrial electrical impulses (400 to 600 bpm).
- AFlut: Paroxysmal or continuous supraventricular tachyarrhythmia with rapid but organized atrial electrical activity. The atrial rate is typically between 250 and 350 bpm and is often manifested as "saw-tooth" flutter (F) waves on the ECG, particularly in the inferior leads and V_1. AFlut commonly occurs with 2:1 or 3:1 AV block, so the ventricular response may be regular and typically at a rate of ∼150 bpm.
- AFib and AFlut are related arrhythmias, sometimes seen in the same patient. Distinguishing the two is important, as there may be implications for management.
- Clinical classifications:
  - Paroxysmal: self-terminating episodes, usually <7 days
  - Persistent: sustained >7 days, usually requiring pharmacologic or DC cardioversion to restore sinus rhythm
  - Permanent: Sinus rhythm cannot be restored or maintained. It is a shared decision between patient and clinician as to when to cease further attempts to restore and/or maintain sinus rhythm.
- Lone AFib occurs in patients <60 years (with possible genetic predisposition) who have no clinical or echocardiographic evidence of cardiovascular disease, including hypertension (HTN).

EPIDEMIOLOGY

- Incidence/prevalence increases significantly with age.
- Young patients with AFib, particularly lone AFib, are most commonly males.

Incidence

- AFib: from <0.1%/year <40 years to >1.5%/year >80 years
- Lifetime risk: 25% for those ≥40 years
- AFlut is less common.

Prevalence

- Estimated at 0.4–1% in general population, with 2.7 million patients in America
- Increase with age, up to 8% in those ≥80 years

ETIOLOGY AND PATHOPHYSIOLOGY

- Cardiac: HTN, ischemic heart disease, heart failure, valvular heart disease, cardiomyopathy, pericarditis, and infiltrative heart disease
- Pulmonary: pulmonary embolism (PE), chronic obstructive pulmonary disease (COPD), obstructive sleep apnea, pneumonia
- Ingestion: ethanol, caffeine
- Endocrine: hyperthyroidism, diabetes
- Obesity
- Postoperative: cardiac, pulmonary, or esophageal
- Idiopathic: lone AFib
- Patients with paroxysmal episodes are usually associated with premature atrial beats and/or bursts of tachycardia, originating in pulmonary vein ostia or other sites.

- Many patients with AFib are thought to have some degree of atrial fibrosis or scarring. This is often subclinical and usually not detectable with current cardiac imaging techniques but plays an important role in the pathogenesis of the arrhythmia.
- Autonomic (vagal and sympathetic) tone may play a role in triggering the arrhythmia.
- The presence of AFib is associated with electrical and structural remodeling processes that promote arrhythmia maintenance in the atria, termed "AFib begets AFib."

Genetics

Familial forms are rare but do exist. There are ongoing efforts to identify the genetic underpinnings of such cases.

RISK FACTORS

Age, HTN, and obesity are the most important risk factors for both AFib and AFlut.

GENERAL PREVENTION

Adequate control of HTN may prevent development of AFib due to hypertensive heart disease and is the most significant modifiable risk factor for AFib. Weight reduction may decrease the risk of AFib in obese patients. Ethanol consumption may trigger AFib in some.

COMMONLY ASSOCIATED CONDITIONS

HTN and other cardiac diseases

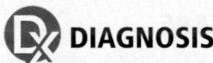

DIAGNOSIS

HISTORY

Symptoms vary from none to mild (palpitations, light-headedness, fatigue, poor exercise capacity) to severe (angina, dyspnea, syncope).

PHYSICAL EXAM

- AFib: irregularly irregular heart rate and pulse, frequently tachycardic, pulse deficit
- AFlut: similar to AFib but may have regular pulse

DIFFERENTIAL DIAGNOSIS

- Multifocal atrial tachycardia
- Sinus tachycardia with frequent atrial premature beats
- Paroxysmal supraventricular tachycardia (Wolff-Parkinson-White [WPW], atrioventricular nodal reentry tachycardia [AVNRT])

DIAGNOSTIC TESTS & INTERPRETATION

- AFib: The ECG is diagnostic, with findings of low-amplitude fibrillatory waves without discrete P waves and an irregularly irregular pattern of QRS complexes. There is often tachycardia in the absence of heart rate–controlling medications (1).
- AFlut: The ECG is again diagnostic. Saw-tooth flutter waves are the classic sign, generally best seen in the inferior leads, although ventricular rate may need to be slowed to see the waves. QRS complexes may be regular or irregular; there is usually tachycardia (1).
- Ambulatory rhythm monitoring (e.g., telemetry, Holter monitoring, event recorders) is helpful in diagnosing paroxysmal AFib or AFlut and monitoring for recurrence (1)[C].

Initial Tests (lab, imaging)

TSH, electrolytes, CBC, 2-D transthoracic echo-cardiogram, PT/INR (if anticoagulation is contemplated);digoxin level (if appropriate)

Follow-Up Tests & Special Considerations

- Occasional Holter monitoring and/or exercise stress testing to assess for adequacy of rate and/or rhythm control
- Chest x-ray (CXR) for cardiopulmonary disease
- ECG for signs of cardiac hypertrophy, ischemia, and/or other arrhythmias
- Transesophageal echocardiogram to detect left atrial appendage thrombus if cardioversion is planned
- Sleep study may be useful if sleep apnea is suspected.

Test Interpretation

- Atrial dilatation and fibrosis
- Atrial thrombus, especially in atrial appendage
- Valvular/rheumatic disease
- Cardiomyopathy

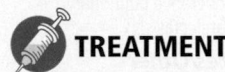

TREATMENT

MEDICATION

- Two primary issues in the management of AFib and/or AFlut:
  - Decisions on heart rate control (control ventricular rate while allowing AFib to continue) or rhythm control (terminate AFib and restore normal sinus rhythm)
  - Anticoagulation therapy to prevent thromboembolism (primarily stroke)
- Anticoagulation guidelines (the same for AFib and AFlut) (1,2)[C]:

- CHA_2DS_2VASc scoring (**C**HF [1 point], **H**TN [1 point], **A**ge ≥75 [2 points], **D**M [1 point], prior **S**troke or TIA [2 points]), **V**ascular disease (1 point), **A**ge 65 to 74 years (1 point), female **S**ex **c**ategory (1 point) (1–3). CHA_2DS_2VASc is the recommended stroke risk assessment for patients with nonvalvular AFib (1)[B].
  - In patients with nonvalvular AFib and a CHA_2DS_2VASc score of 0, antithrombotic therapy may be omitted, (1)[B].
  - In patients with nonvalvular AFib and a CHA_2DS_2VASc score of 1, no antithrombotic therapy or oral anticoagulant or aspirin is recommended (1)[C].

  - Unless contraindicated, patients with nonvalvular AFib with any high-risk factors for stroke (prior transient ischemic attack [TIA]/cerebrovascular accident [CVA]/thromboembolism) or a CHA_2DS_2VASc score ≥2 should receive oral anticoagulants. The following oral anticoagulants include warfarin maintaining an INR of 2.0 to 3.0 (1,3)[A], dabigatran (1)[B], rivaroxaban (1)[B], or apixaban (1)[B]. Patients with mechanical valves should maintain an INR of 2.0 to 3.0 or 2.5 to 3.5 dependent on the type and location of the prosthesis (1)[B]. For patients with AFib and mitral stenosis, a target INR range of 2.0 to 3.0 is recommended (2)[B].
  - Dabigatran (Pradaxa), a direct thrombin inhibitor, and apixaban (Eliquis) and rivaroxaban (Xarelto), factor Xa inhibitors, have recently been approved as alternatives to warfarin for the prevention of first and recurrent stroke in patients with nonvalvular AFib (1,3)[B]. The selection of an

antithrombotic should be individualized (1)[B]; consider the risks of each agent, cost, patient preference, and tolerability (1)[C].
  - ○ ALERT: Renal function should be evaluated prior to initiation of direct thrombin or factor Xa inhibitors (1)[B]. Dosing of such agents may in fact need individualized adjustment.
  - ○ ALERT: Direct thrombin inhibitor dabigatran should not be used in patients with AF and a mechanical heart valve (1)[B].
  - – Anticoagulation recommendations are independent of AFib pattern (paroxysmal, persistent, and permanent) (1,2)[B] although ongoing efforts to better understand who may be at greater and lesser risk of thromboembolism continue.
- Four classes of medications are available to achieve ventricular rate control: β-blockers (i.e., metoprolol), nondihydropyridine calcium channel blockers (i.e., verapamil, diltiazem), digoxin, and amiodarone. Optimal target for ventricular rate has not been firmly established, but there is evidence that aggressive control of the ventricular rate (<80 bpm) offers no benefit beyond more modest rate control (i.e., resting heart rate <110 bpm) (1,4)[B].

- Preventing rapid ventricular response (RVR) rates using AV nodal blocking medications is also often effective at controlling a patient's symptoms associated with AFib or AFlut. Patients in whom rate control cannot be achieved or who continue to have persistent symptoms despite reasonable heart rate control may require attempts at restoration of sinus rhythm.
- Of note, ventricular rate control can often be difficult to achieve in AFlut due to the more organized nature of the atrial electrical activity. For this reason, conversion to sinus rhythm is often the preferred strategy, and catheter ablation is also considered as a first-line treatment in recurrent AFlut (1).
- Restoration of sinus rhythm using electrical or pharmacologic cardioversion may significantly reduce the symptom burden of AFib or AFlut in many patients and may also be useful for controlling ventricular rate. Cardioversion does not impact the long-term risk/benefit ratio of anticoagulation:
  - – Cardioversion is most often performed electrically, but may also be achieved using antiarrhythmic drug therapy in some instances, by experienced clinicians (1)[A].
  - – If duration of AF is >48 hours or unknown, anticoagulate for ≥3 weeks before cardioversion to reduce the risk of stroke. Alternatively, once anticoagulation is established, a transesophageal echo may be performed to exclude the presence of left atrial thrombus, allowing cardioversion to proceed. After cardioversion, anticoagulation should be continued for ≥4 weeks in all patients in whom duration of AFib/AFlut is >48 hours, as the postcardioversion period is a time of increased stroke risk (1,2)[B].
- Randomized clinical trials (AFFIRM and RACE) comparing the outcomes of rate versus rhythm control found no difference in morbidity, mortality, and stroke rates in patients assigned to one therapy or the other (1).
- Chronic PO antiarrhythmic therapy to suppress AFib recurrence is available for appropriately selected patients. Expert consultation is recommended owing to the complexities of safe antiarrhythmic drug selection.

ISSUES FOR REFERRAL
Management of AFib or AFlut refractory to standard medical therapy (i.e., unable to achieve adequate rate control with medication or development of significant bradycardia with treatment) may require the use of

more aggressive treatments. These may include pacemaker implantation (to allow for more intensive pharmacologic blocking of the AV node) or an ablation procedure. AFlut in particular is often very amenable to ablation; thus, consideration should be given to early expert referral in appropriate patients. Antiarrhythmic drug therapy can often be very effective but should be prescribed by experienced practitioners.

SURGERY/OTHER PROCEDURES
- Electrophysiologic study and ablation may be considered for patients with either AFib or AFlut. In the case of AFlut, ablation is often a relatively straightforward procedure generally viewed as a first-line therapy due to its high rate of success in appropriate candidates. Ablation of AFib is a much more complex procedure with a more variable success rate; it continues to evolve. Thus, it is typically reserved for drug refractory patients.
- Cardiac surgery (e.g., the maze procedure, ligation of the left atrial appendage) may be considered in patients planning to undergo cardiac surgery for other reasons. Surgical therapy in isolation is rarely indicated for AFib or AFlut.

INPATIENT CONSIDERATIONS
Admission Criteria/Initial Stabilization
- Patients with significant symptoms, RVR, AFib/AFlut triggered by an acute process (e.g., MI, CHF, PE), or in whom antiarrhythmic therapy is being started likely require admission to the hospital for a period of stabilization.
- Outpatient management is reasonable for low-risk patients with controlled ventricular rates.
- Acute therapy for symptomatic or hemodynamically compromised patients with AFib or AFlut:
  - – IV β- or nondihydropyridine calcium channel blockers for control of ventricular rate. Once hemodynamically stable, oral medications may be administered (1)[B].
- Commonly used therapies in the acute setting include (1):
  - – Metoprolol tartrate: 2.5–5.0 mg IV bolus over 2 minutes; up to 3 doses
  - – Diltiazem: 0.25 mg/kg IV bolus over 2 minutes, then 5 to 15 mg/hr
  - – Some patients will be far more responsive to one class of agents than another. For this reason, if rate control is difficult to achieve, switching drug classes may be useful.
- Urgent cardioversion should be performed in hemodynamically unstable patients (1)[B]. It is somewhat unusual for AFib or AFlut alone to cause marked hemodynamic insult; thus, the possibility of a concurrent process should be considered in this setting.
- Consider the initiation of PO anticoagulation therapy. Inpatients may be "bridged" with IV or SC heparin or SQ low-molecular-weight heparin (LMWH) while waiting for warfarin to become effective (1)[C].

Discharge Criteria
Adequate rate or rhythm control without symptoms; long-term plan for anticoagulation established

ONGOING CARE
Many patients may benefit from elective expert consultation. In patients with no significant symptoms, if ventricular rate control or sinus rhythm is easily achieved and the choice of thromboembolic prevention is clear, management in a primary care setting may be appropriate.

FOLLOW-UP RECOMMENDATIONS
Patient Monitoring
Adequate anticoagulation levels (if warfarin is employed) should be determined at least weekly during initiation and monthly when stable (1)[A]. Ventricular rate control should be assessed on a regular basis.

DIET
Patients on warfarin should attempt to consume a stable amount of vitamin K.

PROGNOSIS
Anticoagulation reduces the annual embolic stroke rate from ~5–6% per year to 1–2% for most patients. AFib and AFlut may increase morbidity and mortality, but the overall prognosis is a function of underlying heart disease and adherence with therapy. Reported risk of anticoagulation varies but lies between 1% and 4% per year for major hemorrhage.

COMPLICATIONS
- Embolic stroke
- Peripheral arterial embolization
- Bleeding with anticoagulation
- Tachycardia-induced cardiomyopathy with prolonged periods of inadequate rate control

REFERENCES
1. January CT, Wann LS, Alpert JS, et al. 2014 AHA/ACC/HRS guideline for the management of patients with atrial fibrillation: a report of the American College of Cardiology/American Heart Association Task Force on Practice Guidelines and the Heart Rhythm Society. Circulation. 2014;130(23):2071–2104.
2. You JJ, Singer DE, Howard PA, et al. Antithrombotic therapy for atrial fibrillation: antithrombotic therapy and prevention of thrombosis, 9th ed: American College of Chest Physicians Evidence-Based Clinical Practice Guidelines. Chest. 2012;141(2 Suppl):e531S–e575S.
3. Furie KL, Goldstein LB, Albers GW, et al. Oral antithrombotic agents for the prevention of stroke in nonvalvular atrial fibrillation: a science advisory for healthcare professionals from the American Heart Association/American Stroke Association. Stroke. 2012;43(12):3442–3453.
4. Wann LS, Curtis AB, January CT, et al. 2011 ACCF/AHA/HRS focused update on the management of patients with atrial fibrillation (updating the 2006 guideline): a report of the American College of Cardiology Foundation/American Heart Association Task Force on Practice Guidelines. Circulation. 2011;123(1):104–123.

 CODES

ICD10
- I48.91 Unspecified atrial fibrillation
- I48.92 Unspecified atrial flutter
- I48.0 Paroxysmal atrial fibrillation

CLINICAL PEARLS
- Primary decision in persistent AFib is whether to strive for rate control or rhythm control. Younger patients often do better with a rhythm control strategy, whereas older patients often do well with rate control. Decision is complex.
- Anticoagulation recommendations are based on the risk of thromboembolism irrespective of the AFib pattern.

ATRIAL SEPTAL DEFECT
Edlira Yzeiraj, DO, MS • Edward A. Gotfried, DO, FACOS

 BASICS

DESCRIPTION
- Anatomy
  - Opening in the atrial septum allowing flow of blood between the two atria
  - Patent foramen ovale is also an open communication between the atria, but it is not considered an ASD because no septal tissue is missing.
- Types (by location in the interatrial septum) (1)
  - Classified based on their different anatomic location and abnormal embryogenesis: secundum ASD, primum ASD, sinus venosus ASD, coronary sinus ASD.
  - 70%: Ostium secundum defect occurs in the fossa ovalis region.
  - 15–20%: Ostium primum defect occurs in the inferior septum; often associated with cleft mitral valve and failure of endocardial cushion development.
  - 5–10%: Sinus venosus defect occurs in the superior-posterior septum near the orifice of the superior vena cava; usually associated with partial anomalous right upper pulmonary venous return.
  - Less than 1%: Coronary sinus defect: part of the entire common wall between the coronary sinus and the LA is absent.
- Hemodynamic effects
  - Left-to-right shunting in late ventricular systole and early diastole
  - Degree depends on size of the defect and relative pressures of the two ventricles.
  - Causes excessive blood flow through the right-sided circulation, ultimately leading to reactive pulmonary hypertension and heart failure
- Systems affected: cardiovascular; pulmonary

Pediatric Considerations
- Most cases of ASD are detected and corrected in the pediatric population.
- The smaller the defect and the younger the child, the greater the chance of spontaneous closure.

EPIDEMIOLOGY
Incidence
- Predominant age: present from birth, may be diagnosed at any age
- Slight female predominance (2)
- No race predilection
- 2/1,000 live births (3)

Prevalence
- ASDs account for 13% of congenital heart disorders (3)

ETIOLOGY AND PATHOPHYSIOLOGY
- Flow across ASD usually left-to-right shunt because of higher left-sided pressures:
  - Minimal right-to-left shunting in early ventricular systole, especially during inspiration
  - Increased right-sided pressure/pulmonary hypertension can cause reversal of shunt flow (Eisenmenger syndrome) with resulting cyanosis and clubbing.
- Symptoms typically occur due to right ventricular and pulmonary vascular volume overload and right-sided heart failure.

Genetics
- Most cases are spontaneous.
- 5% with chromosomal abnormalities; other rare mutations exist
- 25% prevalence in Down syndrome

RISK FACTORS
- Other congenital heart defects
- Family history (~7–10% recurrence)
- Thalidomide, alcohol exposure in utero, smoking, maternal age >35 years, and elevated blood glucose have been associated with increased risk (2).

COMMONLY ASSOCIATED CONDITIONS
- ASDs may occur as a component of other complex cardiac structural defects.
- Important to exclude anomalous pulmonary venous return
- Occasionally can indicate underlying genetic syndromes, for example: Holt-Oram (ASD present in 66%), Ellis-van Creveld, VACTERL syndrome, or Noonan syndrome.
- Overall, ~70% isolated (1)

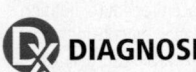 **DIAGNOSIS**

HISTORY
- Most ASDs are small and do not cause symptoms in infancy and childhood and are often found on routine physical examination when a cardiac murmur is detected incidentally.
- Infants with large ASDs may present with right-sided heart failure (more advanced, only 10% at diagnosis), recurrent respiratory infections, or failure to thrive.
- Should be considered in children with other congenital heart defects, Down syndrome
- In uncorrected defects, most people become symptomatic by age 40. Common symptoms in adults include atrial arrhythmias (the most frequent presenting symptom), exercise intolerance, dyspnea, and fatigue.

PHYSICAL EXAM
- Signs vary according to extent of shunting.
- Cardiac auscultation
  - *Fixed, widely split S_2 (key physical finding)*
  - May also have
    - Systolic ejection murmur (pulmonic flow murmur)
    - Low-pitched diastolic rumble (tricuspid flow murmur)
    - Diastolic murmur (pulmonic regurgitation)
    - Systolic murmur (mitral regurgitation)
- Right ventricular heave
- Palpable pulmonary artery pulse at left upper sternal border
- If heart failure has developed, may hear a 4th heart sound (right-sided)
- Signs of Eisenmenger syndrome:
  - Cyanosis and clubbing
  - Jugular venous distention and edema

DIFFERENTIAL DIAGNOSIS
- Other congenital heart disease
- Right bundle branch block (for widely split S_2)

DIAGNOSTIC TESTS & INTERPRETATION
Initial Tests (lab, imaging)
- Echocardiography is the test of choice (1)[C].
- Generally start with transthoracic Doppler imaging of the entire atrial septum (sensitivity is ~89% for secundum, ~100% for primum, and ~44% of sinus venosus ASDs), with progression to transesophageal echocardiography (TEE) if transthoracic echocardiography (TTE) is nondiagnostic.
- Patients with right ventricular overload by TTE but an otherwise negative study should have further testing.
- Oximetry: Cyanosis may suggest Eisenmenger syndrome (right-to-left shunting).

- ECG is not typically diagnostic, but findings include the following:
  - Right axis deviation
  - Right atrial enlargement (tall P in inferior leads)
  - Right ventricular conduction delay
  - Q wave in lead V_1
  - Right bundle branch block
  - Leftward axis, inverted P wave in lead III (sinus venosus)
  - Leftward axis (ostium primum)

Follow-Up Tests & Special Considerations
- Bubble contrast enhancement may be helpful.
- TEE may be required to define ASD morphology and to locate the pulmonary veins; often used prior to percutaneous closure. TEE has excellent sensitivity and specificity.

Diagnostic Procedures/Other
- Cardiac catheterization (1)[C]
  - Demonstrates right ventricle enlargement, location/fraction of the shunt, size of the ASD, any valvular disease, and overall anatomy
  - Used to assess pulmonary vascular resistance if pulmonary hypertension is suspected, particularly if surgery is planned
  - Generally not used in young patients for initial diagnosis, more often reserved for use when
    - Part of a planned interventional closure
    - Evaluating other disease simultaneously (e.g., coronary artery disease)
    - Visualization by other methods insufficient
- Cardiac magnetic resonance: a noninvasive follow-up to echo that allows viewing the defect/pulmonary veins and measurement of shunt fraction and right ventricular function—particularly useful for sinus venosus defects (2)
- Exercise testing: useful to quantify symptoms not consistent with clinical findings or to document change over time (1)[C]
- Chest x-ray: may demonstrate right ventricular and pulmonary artery enlargement, increased pulmonary vascular markings
- Cardiac CT scans can also define ASDs but with significant radiation exposure.

 TREATMENT

GENERAL MEASURES
- 75% of small secundum ASDs (<8 mm) will close spontaneously by 18 months of age; however, close follow-up is warranted (2).
- The likelihood of spontaneous closure is mainly determined by defect diameter: >10 mm at time of diagnosis is unlikely to spontaneously close (4).
- Primum and sinus venosus defects do not generally close and generally require surgical closure (2).

MEDICATION
First Line
- Treatment of secondary atrial fibrillation/supraventricular tachycardia with anticoagulation and cardioversion, followed by anticoagulation with maintenance of sinus rhythm if possible, or rate control if this fails (1)[A]
- Pulmonary vasodilator therapy may be considered for adults with progressive/severe pulmonary vascular disease (1)[B].

- Treatment of heart failure (diuretics, oxygen, digoxin, etc.)

Second Line
- Antibiotic prophylaxis is NOT recommended for unrepaired/isolated ASDs.

- The American Heart Association (AHA) recommends antibiotic prophylaxis against infective endocarditis during dental procedures for 6 months after the repair in patients whom a device or prosthetic material is used (5)[B].

  – In patients with repaired ASD who have a residual defect at or adjacent to the device, prophylaxis is recommended indefinitely.

  – If prophylaxis is indicated, for dental procedures, amoxicillin 2 g (adults) or 50 mg/kg (children). Other options include cephalosporins (e.g., ceftriaxone 1 g [adults] or 50 mg/kg [children] IM or IV) or clindamycin 600 mg PO (adults) or 20 mg/kg PO (children) or azithromycin 500 mg PO (adults) or 15 mg/kg (children) in patients who are penicillin-sensitive (5,6)[B].

- To prevent thrombus formation after device deployment, aspirin alone or a combination of aspirin and clopidogrel 75 mg for at least 6 months is recommended (7).

SURGERY/OTHER PROCEDURES
- The majority of small secundum defects, <6 mm, close spontaneously by 2 years of age, and some as late as 5 years. Closure is generally indicated in children with:
  – Defect >8 mm (unlikely to close) in children older than 2 years of age (to allow time for spontaneous closure, even though uncommon)
  – Defects of any size in a child older than 5 years with related symptoms
- Closure for secundum defects is not recommended in asymptomatic patients before 2 years of age given the possibility of spontaneous closure.
- In adults, secundum closure via percutaneous transcatheter device or surgery to reduce subsequent morbidity and mortality, if:
  – Right side heart enlargement regardless of symptoms (1)[B]
  – Pulmonary systemic flow ratio is 2:1 (or >1.5:1 and <21 years old according to the AHA)
  – Symptoms such as documented orthodeoxia/platypnea or paradoxical embolism (1)[C]
- Surgical repair is standard for a sinus venosus, coronary sinus, or primum ASD (1,2)[B]. These defects rarely close spontaneously and are not considered amenable to percutaneous closure.
- Percutaneous closure is considered the treatment of choice of secundum ASD in adults (8)[A]. It is a safe and effective with satisfactory long-term clinical follow up. In addition, the use of closure device does not significantly affect aortic or mitral valve function (8)[B].
- Secundum ASDs that are suitable for percutaneous closure should be ~35 mm in stretched balloon diameter and should have a sufficient rim of surrounding atrial tissue.
- Closure is not indicated for patients who have developed irreversible severe pulmonary hypertension without continued shunting or those who never develop symptoms and have an ASD <5 mm (1)[B].
- Overall, closing small asymptomatic secundum ASDs is controversial and not often done.
- Maze procedure may be considered before or after closure for patients with intermittent or chronic atrial tachyarrhythmias (1)[C].

FOLLOW-UP RECOMMENDATIONS
Echocardiography can be used to monitor both repaired and unrepaired ASDs.

Patient Monitoring
- In otherwise asymptomatic healthy children, follow up until defect has closed or become negligible in size.
- Appropriate evaluation and management for atrial tachyarrhythmias in patients with long-term follow-up (1)[C]
- If ASD repaired as an adult, periodic long-term follow-up is indicated (1)[C].
- ASDs repaired in childhood generally do not have late complications.
- In female patients with unrepaired ASD and Eisenmenger syndrome, pregnancy is not recommended due to increased risk of maternal and fetal mortality (1)[C].
- Pregnancy is well tolerated in patients with repaired ASD and small unrepaired ASDs (1)[A].
- Scuba diving and high-altitude travel must be approached with caution in patients with unrepaired ASDs; consultation is recommended.

PATIENT EDUCATION
For patient education materials on this topic, consult the following:
- American Heart Association: http://www.heart.org
- Mayo Clinic information: http://www.mayoclinic.com/health/atrial-septal-defect/DS00628

PROGNOSIS
- ASD closure in asymptomatic or minimally symptomatic adults reduces morbidity but not mortality (9).
- ASD closure before age 25 years in symptomatic adults reduces morbidity and likely also mortality.
- ASD repair deferred until after adolescence may not decrease long-term risk of future atrial arrhythmias.
- Up to 50% mortality by age 50 years in untreated symptomatic patients with large defects.

COMPLICATIONS
- Unrepaired: congestive heart failure, stroke, pulmonary hypertension/Eisenmenger syndrome, atrial arrhythmias, increased infection risk (pulmonary, cerebral abscess, infective endocarditis)
- Surgically repaired: late-onset arrhythmias 10 to 20 years after surgery (5%), perioperative atrial tachyarrhythmias in 10–13% of patients
- Device closure: device embolization (1%), cardiac perforation, thrombus formation, endocarditis, supraventricular arrhythmias, and device erosions

REFERENCES

1. Warnes CA, Williams RG, Bashore TM, et al. ACC/AHA 2008 guidelines for the management of adults with congenital heart disease: a report of the American College of Cardiology/American Heart Association Task Force on Practice Guidelines (Writing Committee to develop Guidelines on the Management of Adults with Congenital Heart Disease). Developed in collaboration with the American Society of Echocardiography, Heart Rhythm Society, International Society for Adult Congenital Heart Disease, Society for Cardiovascular Angiography and Interventions, and Society of Thoracic Surgeons. *J Am Coll Cardiol*. 2008;52(23):e143–e263.
2. Geva T, Martins JD, Wald RM. Atrial septal defects. *Lancet*. 2014;383(9932):1921–1932.
3. van der Linde D, Konings EE, Slager MA, et al. Birth prevalence of congenital heart disease worldwide: a systematic review and meta-analysis. *J Am Coll Cardiol*. 2011;58(21):2241–2247.
4. Hanslik A, Pospisil U, Salzer-Muhar U, et al. Predictors of spontaneous closure of isolated secundum atrial septal defect in children: a longitudinal study. *Pediatrics*. 2006;118(4):1560–1565.
5. Nishimura RA, Carabello BA, Faxon DP, et al. ACC/AHA 2008 guideline update on valvular heart disease: focused update on infective endocarditis: a report of the American College of Cardiology/American Heart Association Task Force on Practice Guidelines: endorsed by the Society of Cardiovascular Anesthesiologists, Society for Cardiovascular Angiography and Interventions, and Society of Thoracic Surgeons. *Circulation*. 2008;118(8):887–896.
6. Wilson W, Taubert KA, Gewitz M, et al. Prevention of infective endocarditis: guidelines from the American Heart Association: a guideline from the American Heart Association Rheumatic Fever, Endocarditis, and Kawasaki Disease Committee, Council on Cardiovascular Disease in the Young, and the Council on Clinical Cardiology, Council on Cardiovascular Surgery and Anesthesia, and the Quality of Care and Outcomes Research Interdisciplinary Working Group. *Circulation*. 2007;116(15):1736–1754.
7. Inglessis I, Landzberg MJ. Interventional catheterization in adult congenital heart disease. *Circulation*. 2007;115(12):1622–1633.
8. Scacciatella P, Marra S, Pullara A, et al. Percutaneous closure of atrial septal defect in adults: very long-term clinical outcome and effects on aortic and mitral valve function. *J Invasive Cardiol*. 2015;27(1):65–69.
9. Attie F, Rosas M, Granados N, et al. Surgical treatment for secundum atrial septal defects in patients >40 years old. A randomized clinical trial. *J Am Coll Cardiol*. 2001;38(7):2035–2042.

ADDITIONAL READING

Geva T, Martins JD, Wald RM. Atrial septal defects. *Lancet*. 2014;383(9932):1921–1932.

 SEE ALSO

Aortic Valvular Stenosis; Coarctation of the Aorta; Patent Ductus Arteriosus; Pulmonary Valve Stenosis; Tetralogy of Fallot; Ventricular Septal Defect

 CODES

ICD10
- Q21.1 Atrial septal defect
- Q21.2 Atrioventricular septal defect

CLINICAL PEARLS
- ASD is often missed due to subtle clinical presentation.
- Ideally, hemodynamically significant ASDs should be closed in early childhood, although some benefit from closure is present in older patients.
- Many ASDs can be treated by catheter-directed percutaneous closure rather than open-heart surgery.
- Routine endocarditis prophylaxis is not recommended for unrepaired ASDs.
- Generally, symptomatic and hemodynamically significant ASDs are repaired; management of asymptomatic small ASDs is debated.
- Patent foramen ovales, unlike large ASDs, are very common and generally require no treatment in asymptomatic individuals.

ATTENTION DEFICIT/HYPERACTIVITY DISORDER, ADULT

Yash Kothari, MD • Hugh R. Peterson, MD, FACP

BASICS

- Adult attention deficit hyperactivity disorder (adult ADHD) is a psychiatric condition resulting in inattention and/or hyperactivity or impulsivity. It is typically associated with a combination of low self-esteem, dysfunctional or unstable social relationships, and impaired academic/job performance.
- Adult ADHD has been shown to affect a significant portion of the adult population; >30% of patients diagnosed with ADHD as a child will continue to meet criteria as adults. Some others who no longer meet strict criteria still have significant residual ADHD traits (1).
- During transition from pediatric to adult care, poor control of high-risk behaviors during a hiatus of ADHD treatment can lead to increased morbidity.

DESCRIPTION

- Symptoms include difficulty concentrating, impulsivity, and hyperactivity/overactivity
- The three main types of ADHD are (i) hyperactivity-impulsivity predominant, (ii) inattentive predominant, and (iii) mixed.
- Cost to society in 2010 U.S. dollars estimated to be $105 to $194 billion from decreased productivity, lost income, and "spillover" costs ($33 to $43 billion) paid by families (1).

EPIDEMIOLOGY

Prevalence
General population prevalence for adult ADHD 2.5–4.4%, but population prevalence declines with age (2,3).

Genetics
ADHD patients often have first-degree relatives with ADHD. Some genes have been correlated with ADHD, although not necessary or sufficient for diagnosis (4).

RISK FACTORS

History of childhood and adolescent ADHD diagnosis, particularly symptoms of hyperactivity and/or impulsivity, persisting into adulthood. ADHD is more frequent in males than females (3).

COMMONLY ASSOCIATED CONDITIONS

- Substance use and substance abuse disorders
- Mood disorders
- Anxiety disorders
- Intellectual disabilities
- Obsessive-compulsive disorder (OCD)
- Tic disorders

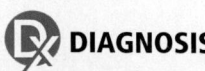

DIAGNOSIS

- Diagnosis is made from patient's history and detailing patient's current level of functioning in at least two different settings (e.g., work and home).

- It is particularly important to gather history of patient's childhood and school performance. ADHD symptoms should be present before age 12 years. If no diagnosis or concern for ADHD as a child, it is unlikely to be diagnosed as an adult.
- DSM-5 criteria are used for adults as well as children.

HISTORY

- History of childhood ADHD symptoms before age 12 years
- DSM-5 criteria include ≥5 hyperactivity/impulsivity symptoms and/or ≥5 inattentive symptoms. These symptoms must be present for ≥6 months.
- Symptoms must result in maladaptive behavior that impairs the patient's function.
- There must be clear evidence of impaired function due to inattention/hyperactivity in ≥2 settings (e.g., home and work).
- These symptoms must not be related to a psychotic episode, mood disorder, or an autistic spectrum disorder and must not be better explained by another DSM diagnosis.
- CAGE and substance abuse questions can help identify substance abuse issues but cannot determine whether substance abuse or adult is the primary disorder.
- Personal and family history of cardiac disease or sudden death should be documented.
- History of exposure to lead or other toxins
- History of thyroid disease

PHYSICAL EXAM

- Physical exam is key to ruling out other medical conditions.
- Focus on thyroid and neurologic examinations; look for findings suggestive of substance abuse.
- Record BP and baseline weight; monitor if starting medical treatment.

DIFFERENTIAL DIAGNOSIS

Hearing impairment; hyperthyroidism/hypothyroidism; sleep deprivation; sleep apnea; phenylketonuria; OCD; lead toxicity; substance abuse (5)[A]

DIAGNOSTIC TESTS & INTERPRETATION

- Adult ADHD screening tools: Retrospective scales include the Childhood Symptom Scale and the Wender Utah Rating Scale; current symptom scales include the Adult ADHD Rating Scale IV, Adult Self Report Scale Symptom Checklist, and the Connor Adult Rating Scale. These scales can take 5 to 20 minutes to complete.
- Provider/patient screening checklist
  – http://help4adhd.org/documents/AdultADHD SelfReportScale-ASRS-v1-1.pdf
  – http://webdoc.nyumc.org/nyumc_d6/files/psych_ adhd_screener.pdf
- ECG with concerns for cardiac disease in patient or family history
- Record baseline blood pressure, pulse, and BMI.

Initial Tests (lab, imaging)

- Thyroid-stimulating hormone (TSH)
- Liver function test monitoring (with atomoxetine)
- Rapid plasma reagin (RPR) or VDRL (Venereal Disease Research Laboratory) test
- Serum lead levels (pending history)

Follow-Up Tests & Special Considerations

- A history of childhood behaviors is helpful, but adult patients often don't accurately recall childhood symptomology.
- Seek the patient's permission to speak with family/friends/prior physicians and to seek school records and results of any psychological assessments.
- Inquire about family history of ADHD, family and personal substance abuse, and tic disorders to facilitate formulation of an accurate diagnosis and recognition of high-risk behaviors.
- Caution against stimulant use in pregnancy because of high risk of low fetal birth weight and preterm birth. Risks and benefits of treatment must be discussed in detail with patient and preferably with her spouse (6)[B].
- Caution against use of stimulants in adult patients with cardiac history.

ALERT

Mood disorders, generalized anxiety disorders, and substance abuse can also coexist with adult ADHD; treating both the ADHD and comorbid conditions will improve the patient's prognosis.

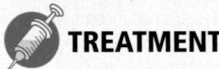

TREATMENT

- Most of the research and medication trials have been performed in children.
- There is increasing evidence that stimulants and nonstimulants used in children are also effective in adults (5)[A].

ALERT

Because stimulant medication may induce dependency, substance abuse, and diversion, it is necessary to do pill counts, screen urine for drugs, monitor behavior, and query prescription databases. Misuse of amphetamines may cause sudden death and serious cardiovascular adverse events.

GENERAL MEASURES

When prescribing stimulant medications for adults with ADHD, watch for misuse, abuse, and diversion of prescription medications. When substance abuse is not present, stimulants are first-line treatment for ADHD and highly efficacious. There are multiple formulations of stimulants, and patients may require trials of different dosages, formulations, and medications before an optimal response in symptoms and functions is achieved.

MEDICATION

- Psychotropic medications play a large part in the treatment of ADHD symptoms. Medications should be titrated slowly to effective dose to avoid side effects.
- Stimulants are more effective than antidepressants or nonstimulants, but up to 30% discontinue medications because of side effects.
- Stimulants can be divided into two different classes: Methylphenidate and amphetamine come in both short- and long-acting preparations.
- Antidepressants studied for ADHD include bupropion, which has been shown to have a medium effect compared with stimulants (6)[A].

First Line

- Stimulants: methylphenidate (Concerta, Ritalin), dexmethylphenidate (Focalin), dextroamphetamine/amphetamine (Adderall), dextroamphetamine (Dexedrine), lisdexamfetamine (Vyvanse)
  - Methylphenidate preparations are available in short-acting, intermediate-acting, long-acting, and patch formulations.
  - Ritalin LA may be used for patient's naive to stimulants. It can be started at 20 mg daily and dose titrated by 10 mg increments weekly to symptoms response. Maximum dose of 60 mg/day.
  - Concerta ER is another option in adults up to 65 years of age. Starting dose of 18 mg/day; adjust in increments of 18 mg weekly until symptoms improve. Maximum dose of 72 mg/day. Concerta also has an oral osmotic release to decrease abuse potential.
  - Amphetamines also come in immediate-release preparations and sustained-release preparations.
  - Dextroamphetamine is commonly used (half-life of 4 to 6 hours) with an initial dose of 5 mg twice daily; titrate up by 5 mg weekly to maximum of 20 mg twice daily.
    Caution: Immediate-release preparations have high abuse potential.
  - Dextroamphetamine/amphetamine (Adderall) is a 75%/25% mix that also comes in an extended-release form. Initial dosing can be started at 5 mg twice daily for short-acting or 20 mg once daily for long-acting, and increased by 5 mg/week for short-acting and 10 mg/week long-acting to a maximum of 40 to 60 mg total daily.
  - Lisdexamfetamine (Vyvanse) is an extended-release stimulant that is a prodrug requiring metabolization to active component, dextroamphetamine.
  - Dextroamphetamine can be initiated at 30 mg daily and titrated by 10 to 20 mg weekly to a maximum of 30 to 70 mg daily.

- Common side effects of stimulants include hypertension (HTN), tachycardia, insomnia, weight loss, stomach upset, increased anxiety/irritability, or worsening of tics (6)[A].
- Nonstimulants: Atomoxetine (Strattera) has been shown effective in adults with ADHD when compared to placebo (7)[B]. It may be given as a single dose or split dose and has low abuse potential, making it a better choice over a stimulant medication for patients with substance abuse history. Onset of effect may take up to 4 weeks. Atomoxetine may require dose adjustments with strong inhibitors of cytochrome P2D6 (e.g., Paxil or Prozac). Also, there are rare cases of liver damage associated with these medications. Monitor for increased suicidal thinking.

- Antidepressants: best used for those at high risk or with history of substance abuse disorder
  - Bupropion (Wellbutrin) is an antidepressant effective in adults with ADHD symptoms (6)[A].

ISSUES FOR REFERRAL

Patients with comorbid conditions may need referral for diagnosis and treatment. Consider cardiology consult for patients with known cardiac issues who may require stimulant treatment. Consider referral to obstetrician experienced in high-risk pregnancies when treating pregnant women with ADHD.

ADDITIONAL THERAPIES

Cognitive-behavioral therapy can be useful in conjunction with medication to help patient modify and cope with symptoms.

COMPLEMENTARY & ALTERNATIVE MEDICINE

Vitamin–mineral supplementation is an area of active research that holds promise for improved ADHD treatment (8)[A].

 ONGOING CARE

Transfer from pediatric to adult care must be closely coordinated to avoid hiatus in treatment.

FOLLOW-UP RECOMMENDATIONS

- Close follow-up of medication as dose is titrated.
- Continue to monitor for medication side effects.
- Repeat screening checklists to quantify benefit of interventions as needed.
- Reinforce behavioral change (e.g., self-initiated through cognitive-behavioral therapy), which is the essential goal of long-term management.

REFERENCES

1. Doshi JA, Hodgkins P, Kahle J, et al. Economic impact of childhood and adult attention-deficit/hyperactivity disorder in the United States. *J Am Acad Child Adolesc Psychiatry.* 2012;51(10): 990.e2–1002.e2.
2. Simon V, Czobor P, Bálint S, et al. Prevalence and correlates of adult attention-deficit hyperactivity disorder: meta-analysis. *Br J Psychiatry.* 2009;194(3):204–211.
3. Kessler RC, Adler L, Barkley R, et al. The prevalence and correlates of adult ADHD in the United States: results from the National Comorbidity Survey Replication. *Am J Psychiatry.* 2006;163(4):716–723.
4. Gatt JM, Burton KL, Williams LM, et al. Specific and common genes implicated across major mental disorders: a review of meta-analysis studies. *J Psychiatr Res.* 2015;60:1–13.
5. Castells X, Ramos-Quiroga JA, Bosch R, et al. Amphetamines for attention deficit hyperactivity disorder (ADHD) in adults. *Cochrane Database Syst Rev.* 2011;(6):CD007813.
6. Verbeeck W, Tuinier S, Bekkering GE. Antidepressants in the treatment of adult attention-deficit hyperactivity disorder: a systematic review. *Adv Ther.* 2009;26(2):170–184.
7. Asherson P, Bushe C, Saylor K, et al. Efficacy of atomoxetine in adults with attention deficit hyperactivity disorder: an integrated analysis of the complete database of multicenter placebo-controlled trials. *J Psychopharmacol.* 2014;28(9):837–846.
8. Rucklidge JJ, Frampton CM, Gorman B, et al. Vitamin-mineral treatment of attention-deficit hyperactivity disorder in adults: double-blind randomised placebo-controlled trial. *Br J Psychiatry.* 2014;204:306–315.

ADDITIONAL READING

- American Psychiatric Association. *Diagnostic and Statistical Manual of Mental Disorders.* 5th ed. Arlington, VA: American Psychiatric Association; 2013.
- Mongia M, Hechtman L. Cognitive behavior therapy for adults with attention-deficit/hyperactivity disorder: a review of recent randomized controlled trials. *Curr Psychiatry Rep.* 2012;14(5):561–567.
- Post RE, Kurlansik SL. Diagnosis and management of adult attention-deficit/hyperactivity disorder. *Am Fam Physician.* 2012;85(9):890–896.

 CODES

ICD10

- F90.9 Attention-deficit hyperactivity disorder, unspecified type
- F90.1 Attn-defct hyperactivity disorder, predom hyperactive type
- F90.0 Attn-defct hyperactivity disorder, predom inattentive type

CLINICAL PEARLS

- Adult ADHD results in inattention, easy distractibility, hyperactivity, and impulsive behavior; it is associated with low self-esteem, problematic interpersonal relationships, and difficulty meeting academic and job expectations.
- Psychotropic medications plus cognitive-behavioral treatments are the cornerstone of management.
- Substance abuse is a common comorbidity; recommend use of nonstimulant medication in those at high risk

ATTENTION DEFICIT/HYPERACTIVITY DISORDER, PEDIATRIC

Laura Novak, MD • Christina Emanuel, MD

 BASICS

DESCRIPTION
- Attention deficit hyperactivity disorder (ADHD) is a neurodevelopmental problem that manifests in early childhood characterized by distractibility, impulsivity, hyperactivity, and/or inattention.
- Three subsets: predominantly hyperactivity impulsive (ADHD-HI), predominantly inattentive (ADHD-I), or combined (ADHD-C)
- System(s) affected: nervous
- Synonym(s): attention deficit disorder; hyperactivity

EPIDEMIOLOGY
- Predominant age: onset <12 years; lasts into adolescence and adulthood; 50% meet diagnostic criteria by age 4 years
- Predominant sex: male > female (2:1); inattentive type (ADHD-I) may be more common in girls

Prevalence
11% of children 4 to 17 years old were diagnosed with ADHD as of 2011. Of those, 6.1% are receiving a medication for ADHD.

ETIOLOGY
Not definitive

Genetics
Familial pattern

RISK FACTORS
- Family history
- Medical causes (affecting brain development)
- Environmental causes (toxins such as lead, fetal alcohol, and nutritional deficiencies)

GENERAL PREVENTION
- Children are at risk for abuse, depression, and isolation.
- Parents need regular support and advice.

COMMONLY ASSOCIATED CONDITIONS
- Depression (in up to 1/3 of cases)
- Oppositional defiant disorder
- Conduct disorder
- Anxiety disorder
- Learning disabilities

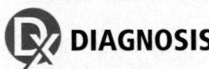 DIAGNOSIS

- American Academy of Pediatrics (AAP) guidelines recommend *DSM-5* criteria to establish diagnosis.
- *DSM-5* criteria for children <17 years: ≥6 inattention criteria and/or ≥6 hyperactivity/impulsivity criteria. Symptoms must occur often, be present before age of 12 years, for >6 months, be noticed in ≥2 settings (e.g., home, school), reduce quality of social or scholastic functioning, be excessive for development level of child, and are not better explained by or occur with another mental disorder (e.g., mood, anxiety, or personality disorder) (1)[A].

- Inattention
  - Careless mistakes in tasks; difficulty sustaining attention or in organizing tasks; does not seem to listen, follow through, or finish tasks; avoids tasks that require sustained mental effort; loses things; forgetful in daily activities

- Hyperactivity/impulsivity
  - Fidgets; difficulty remaining seated; runs/climbs excessively or inappropriately; difficulty playing quietly; acts as if "driven by a motor" or seeming to always be "on the go"; talks excessively; blurts out answers before question is complete; has difficulty waiting turn; interrupts others
- Children undergoing extreme stress (parent's divorce, illness, homelessness, abuse) may demonstrate ADHD behaviors secondary to stress (1). This can be assessed using the American Academy of Child and Adolescent Psychiatry (AACAP) screening tool.
- If diagnostic behaviors are noted in only one setting, explore the stressors in that setting.
- The diagnostic behaviors are more noticeable in tasks that require concentration or boredom tolerance than in free play or office situations.

HISTORY
- Birth and development history
- Psychosocial evaluation of home environment
- School performance history and school absences
- Psychiatric history or comorbid disorder(s)
- Cardiac history

PHYSICAL EXAM
- Baseline weight for future monitoring
- Note any soft neurologic signs, such as tics, clumsiness, mixed handedness
- Assess hearing and vision.

DIFFERENTIAL DIAGNOSIS
- Activity level appropriate for age
- Language or communication disorders
- Hearing/vision disorder
- Dysfunctional family situation
- Learning disability (e.g., dyslexia)
- Autism spectrum disorders
- Oppositional/defiant disorder or conduct disorder
- Tourette syndrome: motor and verbal tics
- Absence seizures (inattentive type ADHD only)
- Lead poisoning
- Sequelae of central nervous system infection/trauma
- Medication (decongestant, antihistamine, theophylline, phenobarbital)
- Sleep disorder (e.g., obstructive sleep apnea [OSA]) leading to daytime behavioral problems

DIAGNOSTIC TESTS & INTERPRETATION
- Behavior rating scales must be completed by parents, caregivers, and teachers prior to initiation of therapy and then repeated after therapy is started to gauge treatment efficacy.
- Forms are available from the ADHD toolkit at http://www.nichq.org/adhd.html (Vanderbilt Assessment Scales)
- Testing for learning disability (e.g., dyslexia) through the school may be needed.

Initial Tests (lab, imaging)
Lead level if high risk

Diagnostic Procedures/Other
- EEG if symptoms are highly suggestive of absence seizure disorder
- EKG if high risk

 TREATMENT

GENERAL MEASURES
- Parent/school/patient education
- Work closely with teacher.
- Behavioral therapy/environmental changes

MEDICATION
- 2011 AAP guideline recommends behavioral interventions for age 4 to 5, and behavioral interventions plus stimulant medications as first-line treatment for age 6 to 17 (2,3)[A].

- Stimulant choice should be based on cost, formulary, convenience, and duration. A second type of stimulant should be tried if the first treatment fails. All stimulant capsules can be opened and sprinkled (note Concerta is a pill)

First Line
Stimulant:
- Dexmethylphenidate
  - **Focalin:** initial: 2.5 mg BID; increase total daily by 2.5 to 5 mg weekly up to maximum dose of 20 mg/day
  - **Focalin XR:** initial: 5 mg in AM; increase daily dose by 5 mg weekly up to maximum dose of 30 mg/day
- Methylphenidate
  - SHORT-ACTING
    - Ritalin, Methylin: initial 5 mg BID before breakfast and lunch; increase by 5 to 10 mg weekly to maximum dose of 60 mg/day (2 or 3 divided doses)
  - INTERMEDIATE-ACTING
    - Ritalin SR: 20 mg once in AM; increase by 10 mg weekly up to 40 to 60 mg
    - Metadate ER: 10 mg BID; increase by 10 mg weekly to 40 to 60 mg
  - LONG-ACTING
    - Metadate CD: 20 mg in AM; increase by 10 to 20 mg weekly to 40 to 60 mg
    - Quillivant XR: 20 mg in AM; increase 10 to 20 mg weekly until 40 to 60 mg
    - Ritalin LA: 10 to 20 mg in AM; increase 10 mg weekly until 40 to 60 mg
    - Concerta: 18 to 36 mg in AM; increase by 18 mg weekly until 54 to 72 mg
    - Daytrana transdermal patch: 10 mg patch on (hip area) 2 hours before effect is needed; patch removed 9 hours after application; increase to next higher patch weekly until 30 mg patch if needed
- Dextroamphetamine
  - **Dexedrine spansule** (long-acting): 5 mg BID; increase by 5 mg weekly to maximum dose of 40 mg daily
- Dextroamphetamine and amphetamine
  - SHORT-ACTING
    - Adderall: 5 mg daily or BID; increase by 5 to 10 mg weekly to a maximum dose of 40 mg daily divided into 1 to 3 doses
  - LONG-ACTING
    - Adderall XR: 5 to 10 mg in AM; increase by 5 to 10 mg weekly until maximum dose of 30 mg/day
- Lisdexamfetamine
  - **Vyvanse:** 30 mg in AM; increase by 10 to 20 mg weekly up to a maximum of 70 mg/day

- Precautions:
  - If not responding, check compliance and consider another diagnosis.
  - Some children experience withdrawal (tearfulness, agitation) after a missed dose or when medication wears off. A small, short-acting dose at 4 PM may help to prevent this.
  - Stimulants are drugs of abuse and should be monitored carefully.
  - Drug holidays are not recommended.
- Common adverse effects:
  - Anorexia, insomnia, GI effects, and headache
- Significant possible interactions: may increase levels of anticonvulsants, SSRIs, tricyclics, and warfarin
- High caffeine energy drinks, albuterol inhalers and decongestants may increase side effects.
- The FDA reports permanent skin discoloration with Daytrana patches.

Pregnancy Considerations
Medications are Category C: caution in pregnancy

Second Line
Nonstimulant:
- **SNRI**
  - **Atomoxetine** (Strattera):
    - ≤70 kg: 0.5 mg/kg/day initial; increase after a minimum of 3 days to target dose of 1.2 mg/kg/day; maximum of 1.4 mg/kg/day
    - >70 kg: 40 mg daily; increase after minimum of 3 days to target dose of 80 mg/day; dose may be increased to maximum of 100 mg/day after additional 2 to 4 weeks
- **α^2-Agonist**
  - Modest efficacy, high side effects. Consider consultation before use.
    - **Clonidine XR (Kapvay):** 0.1 mg once daily at bedtime; increase by 0.1 mg weekly; doses should be taken twice daily with equal or higher split dosage given at HS; maximum of 0.4 mg/day; taper when discontinued
    - **Guanfacine XR (Intuniv):** 1 mg daily; increase by 1 mg weekly until 1 to 4 mg daily; taper when discontinued

ISSUES FOR REFERRAL
Should be considered for children <6 years old for psychological or medical complications, developmental disorder or intellectual disability, or poor response to medication

COMPLEMENTARY & ALTERNATIVE MEDICINE
- Surveys have shown that parents of children with ADHD use herbals and complementary treatments frequently (20–60%).
- Omega-3 fatty acids (found in fish oil and some supplements) showed improvement in rating scales in two double-blind, placebo-controlled studies of 116 and 130 patients (4).

 ONGOING CARE

FOLLOW-UP RECOMMENDATIONS
Patient Monitoring
- Parent/teacher rating scales
- Office visits to monitor side effects and efficacy: End points are improved grades, rating scales, family interactions, and peer interactions.
- Monitor growth (especially weight) and BP.

DIET
- "Insufficient evidence to suggest that dietary interventions reduce the symptoms of ADHD" (4).
- The AAP recommends that "For a child without a medical, emotional, or environmental etiology of ADHD behaviors, a trial of a preservative-free food coloring–free diet is a reasonable intervention" (4).

PATIENT EDUCATION
- Excellent reference: http://www.parentsmedguide.org
- Key points for parents:
  - Find things the child is good at and emphasize these; reinforce good behavior; give one task at a time; stop behavior with quiet discipline; coordinate homework with teachers; have external organization tools—charts, schedules, tokens
  - Develop an individualized education plan (IEP) with the school.
- Support groups:
  - Children and Adults with Attention Deficit Disorder (CHADD): http://www.chadd.org
  - Attention Deficit Disorder Warehouse: http://www.addwarehouse.com
  - National Information Center for Children and Youth with Disabilities: http://www.nichcy.org

PROGNOSIS
- May last into adulthood; plan for a transition at age 17 years
- Relative deficits in academic and social functioning may persist into late adolescence/adulthood.
- Encourage career choices that allow autonomy and mobility.

COMPLICATIONS
- Untreated ADHD can lead to failing in school, parental abuse, social isolation, and poor self-esteem.
- Possible withdrawal when medication wears off.
- Monitor growth with stimulant use. If appetite is poor, eat before the medication is given and after it wears off. Consider a shorter duration medication.
- Risk of substance abuse is controversial and seems to decrease with treatment of ADHD increased automobile accidents and injuries; decreases with medication

REFERENCES

1. American Psychiatric Association. *Diagnostic and Statistical Manual of Mental Disorders.* 5th ed. Washington, DC: American Psychiatric Association; 2013.
2. Rader R, McCauley L, Callen EC. Current strategies in the diagnosis and treatment of childhood attention-deficit/hyperactivity disorder. *Am Fam Physician.* 2009;79(8):657–665.
3. Wolraich M, Brown L, Brown RT, et al. ADHD: clinical practice guideline for the diagnosis, evaluation, and treatment of attention-deficit/hyperactivity disorder in children and adolescents. *Pediatrics.* 2011;128(5):1007–1022.
4. Sinn N. Nutritional and dietary influences on attention deficit hyperactivity disorder. *Nutr Rev.* 2008;66(10):558–568.

ADDITIONAL READING

- Laforett DR, Murray DW, Kollins SH. Psychosocial treatments for preschool-aged children with attention-deficit hyperactivity disorder. *Dev Disabil Res Rev.* 2008;14(4):300–310.
- Larson K, Russ SA, Kahn RS, et al. Patterns of comorbidity, functioning, and service use for US children with ADHD, 2007. *Pediatrics.* 2011;127(3):462–470.
- Millichap JG, Yee MM. The diet factor in attention-deficit/hyperactivity disorder. *Pediatrics.* 2012;129(2):330–337.

CODES

ICD10
- F90.9 Attention-deficit hyperactivity disorder, unspecified type
- F90.0 Attn-defct hyperactivity disorder, predom inattentive type
- F90.1 Attn-defct hyperactivity disorder, predom hyperactive type

CLINICAL PEARLS

- AAP recommends the use of stimulant medications as the first-line treatment.
- Children undergoing extreme stress (parent's divorce, illness, homelessness, abuse) may demonstrate ADHD behaviors secondary to stress.
- ADHD is 2 to 8 times more common in persons who have a first-degree relative with the condition.

ATYPICAL MOLE (DYSPLASTIC NEVUS) SYNDROME

Anne R. Atalig, MD, CPT • Mary DiGiulio, DO

BASICS

Atypical mole syndrome (AMS), also known as dysplastic nevi syndrome (DNS), B-K mole syndrome, or Clark nevi syndrome, is a condition characterized by a large number of pigmented nevi with architectural disorder, which arise sporadically or by inheritance, and are associated with an increased risk of melanoma.

DESCRIPTION
- There is no consensus on criteria for AMS.
- Elevated total body nevi count, including clinically atypical nevi, is usually >50 and often >100.
  - Larger number in hereditary AMS versus sporadic atypical nevi (as few as <10 in sporadic)
- Increased risk of melanoma (1,2)
  - Up to 90% occurrence by age 80 years in certain high-risk individuals
  - Earlier onset than sporadic melanoma cases
  - Most arise de novo than from an existing nevus
  - Higher risk for appearance at unusual sites (e.g., scalp)
- AMS terminology often used interchangeably with DNS, familial atypical multiple mole melanoma (FAMMM) syndrome, and B-K mole syndrome.
- Median age of diagnosis for melanoma in AMS is 10 to 20 years earlier than the general population, with documented cases of melanoma as early as in the 2nd and 3rd decades of life (3). Melanomas, in the setting of AMS, are most often superficial spreading or nodular type.

EPIDEMIOLOGY
Incidence
- Uncertain due to phenotype variability, limited data
- Up to 8% in Caucasian populations (4)
Prevalence
At least 32,000 cases in the United States per National Institutes of Health (NIH) (5)

ETIOLOGY AND PATHOPHYSIOLOGY
- Cyclin-dependent kinase inhibitor 2A (CDKN2A) mutations have been observed in familial DNS and multiple melanomas. The CDKN2A gene on 9p21 encodes for the proteins p16 and p14. p16 binds to CDK4/6 and is a negative cell-cycle regulator via inhibition of the CDK-cyclin D interaction needed for cell cycle progression from G1 to S. p14 functions by stabilizing the tumor-suppressor protein p53 in the G1 phase of the cell cycle.
- Familial cases of germline CDKN2A mutations are transmitted in an autosomal dominant fashion.
- No clear somatic mutation patterns in sporadic cases

Genetics
CDKN2A mutation observed in 25–40% of hereditary cases, with autosomal dominant inheritance but variable expressivity and incomplete penetrance

RISK FACTORS
Family history of melanoma or multiple nevi, sun exposure, neonatal blue-light phototherapy (6,7), history of painful sunburns

GENERAL PREVENTION
- No currently available prevention strategies
- Treatment is directed toward secondary prevention of melanoma complications with routine skin exams, biopsy of suspect lesions, and environmental risk mitigation (e.g., sun protection and sun avoidance).
- Experimental early detection protocols for pancreatic cancer is used with some high-risk individuals.

COMMONLY ASSOCIATED CONDITIONS
- Malignant melanoma, including ocular melanoma
- Ocular nevi
- Pancreatic cancer in CDKN2A mutation

DIAGNOSIS

AMS is a clinical diagnosis with various classifications schemes proposed. Although not widely accepted, diagnostic criteria, as defined by the NIH, require the three features of (i) malignant melanoma in ≥1 first- or second-degree relatives; (ii) numerous melanocytic nevi (frequently >50), some of which are clinically atypical; and (iii) nevi that have certain histologic features on pathologic examination (8).

HISTORY
- Changing lesions: bleeding, scaling, size, texture, nonhealing, hyper- or hypopigmentation
- Large number of nevi
- Congenital nevi
- Sun exposure habits
- Prior skin biopsies
- Prior melanoma
- Immunosuppression (e.g., AIDS, chemotherapy, pancreatic cancer)
- First- or second-degree relatives with:
  - AMS
  - Melanoma
  - Pancreatic cancer

PHYSICAL EXAM
- Full body skin exams
- Goal to distinguish melanoma from AMS
- ABCDE mnemonic for skins lesions concerning for melanoma: Asymmetry, Border irregularity, Color variegation, Diameter >6 mm, and Evolving lesion
  - Atypical mole (AM) is often defined as ≥5 mm + at least two other features.
  - Melanoma typically with several characteristics of ABCDEs, with increased specificity for melanoma using >6 mm for diameter
- "Ugly duckling sign" (9)[B]
  - Melanoma screening strategy of identifying malignant nevi straying from the predominant nevus pattern when numerous atypical nevi are present.
- Most common features of AM on dermoscopy magnification per the pattern analysis method include the following (10)[C]:
  - Atypical pigment network
  - Irregular/peripheral depigmentation areas
  - Irregular distribution of brown globules
  - Pigmentation with central heterogeneity and abrupt termination

- Some dermatoscopic features more suggestive of melanoma include the following (11)[C]:
  - Depigmented areas
  - Whitish veil
  - Homogenous areas distributed irregularly, in multiple areas, or >25% of total lesion
  - ≥4 colors

DIFFERENTIAL DIAGNOSIS
- Common nevus: acquired or congenital
- Melanoma
- Seborrheic keratosis
- Dermatofibroma
- Lentigo
- Pigmented actinic keratosis
- Pigmented basal cell carcinoma
- Blue rubber bleb nevus syndrome

DIAGNOSTIC TESTS & INTERPRETATION
Diagnosis is first suspected with history and physical exam, and then confirmed by biopsy and histopathology.

Initial Tests (lab, imaging)
- Dermoscopy can be used for more detailed exam to distinguish between benign and malignant lesions, and for further classification to 1 of 11 subtypes.
- Genetic testing is available for CDKN2A mutations, but it is not recommended outside of research studies as results cannot be adequately used for management or surveillance (11)[C].
- When the total nevus count is high and following each nevus is impractical, total body photography may aid in the evaluation of evolving nevi as well as in documenting new nevi (12)[C].

Diagnostic Procedures/Other
- Biopsy is recommended for any lesion where melanoma cannot be excluded.
- Biopsy entails full-thickness biopsy of the entire lesion with a narrow 1- to 3-mm margin of normal skin down to fat for adequate depth assessment (12)[C].
  - Excisional biopsy, elliptical or punch excision provides the most accurate diagnosis and should be performed when possible.
  - Scoop shave biopsy can also be used, but care must be taken to not transect the lesion.
- Reexcision of mild to moderately dysplastic nevi with positive margins may not change pathologic diagnosis, but for severely dysplastic nevi, consider reexcision, with surgical margins of 2 to 5 mm (13)[C].

Test Interpretation
"Dysplastic nevus" is a term more accurately reserved for histological findings. Features may include melanocyte proliferation in the dermoepidermal junction, bridging of rete ridges by melanocytic nests, dermal fibrosis, and interstitial lymphocytic inflammation.

TREATMENT

MEDICATION
No medications are available to treat AMS.

ISSUES FOR REFERRAL
- Consider referral to a dermatologist for routine skin exam in patients at high risk for melanoma.
- Ophthalmologic exams for ocular nevi/melanoma screening/papilledema
- Oncology or specialized genetics study group involvement if strong family predisposition to pancreatic cancer
- Cosmetic surgery consultation for cosmetically poor excision outcomes

ADDITIONAL THERAPIES
- Topical chemo- and immunotherapies have been unsuccessfully attempted to treat atypical moles.
- Laser treatment should be avoided because it is both unsafe and ineffective for melanocytic nevi.

SURGERY/OTHER PROCEDURES
Surgical excision of all atypical nevi is not recommended because most melanomas in AMS appear de novo on healthy skin and the procedure leads to both poor cosmetic outcomes and a false sense of security. Lesions suspicious for melanoma should be biopsied or removed surgically.

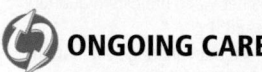 ONGOING CARE

FOLLOW-UP RECOMMENDATIONS
Close follow-up with a dermatologist or other experienced physician:
- Total body skin exam (including nails, scalp, genital area, and oral mucosa) every 6 months initially, starting at puberty; may be reduced to annually once nevi are stable
- Dermoscopic evaluation for suspect lesions
- Ocular exam for those with familial AMS
- Excision of suspect lesions
- Total body photography at baseline

Patient Monitoring
- Monthly self-exams of skin
- Sun avoidance and sun protection

PATIENT EDUCATION
For young adults aged 10 to 24 years with fair skin, counsel to minimize exposure to ultraviolet radiation to reduce risk of skin cancer (USPSTF Grade B)[A]. No evidence for adults >24 years (USPSTF Grade I)[A]

- Fair skin: light eye, hair, or skin color, freckles
- Educate on sun avoidance, proper application of sunscreen, use of protective clothing (e.g., hats), avoidance of tanning booths and sunburns.
- Teach "ABCDE" mnemonic + "ugly duckling sign" to assess nevi and identify potential melanomas.
- Provide instruction on skin self-exam techniques.
- A sample listing of patient-centric review sources on this topic are as follows:
  - American Academy of Dermatology (http://cancer.about.com/od/skincancermelanoma/p/abcdeskincancer.htm)
  - Skin Cancer Foundation (http://www.skincancer.org/skin-cancer-information/dysplastic-nevi)
  - Melanoma Research Foundation (http://www.melanoma.org/understand-melanoma/what-is-melanoma)

PROGNOSIS
- Most AM either regress or do not change.
- Multiple classification schemes have been developed over the years to delineate risk of melanoma in patients with AMS. Individuals with a family history of melanoma are at greatest risk. A classification system developed by Rigel (14) is simply and readily applied in the clinical setting. Points are assigned based on incidence of melanoma, with 1 point given for a personal history with melanoma and 2 points for each family member with melanoma (modified nuclear family consisting of first-degree relatives plus grandparents and uncles/aunts) and stratified as follows:
  - Score = 0, Rigel group 0, 6% 25-year accumulated risk for melanoma
  - Score = 1, Rigel group 1, 10% risk
  - Score = 2, Rigel group 2, 15% risk
  - Score ≥3, Rigel group 3, 50% risk
- The CDKN2A mutation has also been associated with a 60–90% risk of melanoma by age 80 years and a 17% risk for pancreatic cancer by age 75 years.

COMPLICATIONS
- Malignant melanoma
- Poor cosmetic outcomes from biopsy

REFERENCES
1. Newton JA, Bataille V, Griffiths K, et al. How common is the atypical mole syndrome phenotype in apparently sporadic melanoma? *J Am Acad Dermatol.* 1993;29(6):989–996.
2. Gandini S, Sera F, Cattaruzza MS, et al. Meta-analysis of risk factors for cutaneous melanoma: I. Common and atypical naevi. *Eur J Cancer.* 2005;41(1):28–44.
3. Silva JH, Sá BC, Avila AL, et al. Atypical mole syndrome and dysplastic nevi: identification of populations at risk for developing melanoma—review article. *Clinics (Sao Paulo).* 2011;66(3):493–499.
4. Naeyaert JM, Brochez L. Clinical practice. Dysplastic nevi. *N Engl J Med.* 2003;349(23):2233–2240.
5. Mize DE, Bishop M, Reese E, et al. Familial atypical multiple mole melanoma syndrome. In: Riegert-Johnson DL, Boardman LA, Hefferon T, et al, eds. *Cancer Syndromes.* Bethesda, MD: National Center for Biotechnology Information; 2009.
6. Csoma Z, Tóth-Molnár E, Balogh K, et al. Neonatal blue light phototherapy and melanocytic nevi: a twin study. *Pediatrics.* 2011;128(4):e856–e864.
7. Matichard E, Le Hénanff A, Sanders A, et al. Effect of neonatal phototherapy on melanocytic nevus count in children. *Arch Dermatol.* 2006;142(12):1599–1604.
8. Goldsmith LA, Askin FB, Chang AE, et al. NIH Consensus conference. Diagnosis and treatment of early melanoma. *JAMA.* 1992;268(10):1314–1319.
9. Scope A, Dusza SW, Halpern AC, et al. The "ugly duckling" sign: agreement between observers. *Arch Dermatol.* 2008;144(1):58–64.
10. Salopek TG, Kopf AW, Stefanato CM, et al. Differentiation of atypical moles (dysplastic nevi) from early melanomas by dermoscopy. *Dermatol Clin.* 2001;19(2):337–345.
11. Kefford R, Bishop JN, Tucker M, et al. Genetic testing for melanoma. *Lancet Oncol.* 2002;3(11):653–654.
12. Duffy K, Grossman D. The dysplastic nevus: from historical perspective to management in the modern era: part I. Historical, histologic, and clinical aspects. *J Am Acad Dermatol.* 2012;67(1):1.e1–1.e16.
13. Strazzula L, Vedak P, Hoang MP, et al. The utility of re-excising mildly and moderately dysplastic nevi: a retrospective analysis. *J Am Acad Dermatol.* 2014;71(6):1071–1076.
14. Rigel DS, Rivers JK, Friedman RJ, et al. Risk gradient for malignant melanoma in individuals with dysplastic naevi. *Lancet.* 1988;1(8581):352–353.

ADDITIONAL READING
- Czajkowski R, Placek W, Drewa G, et al. FAMMM syndrome: pathogenesis and management. *Dermatol Surg.* 2004;30(2, Pt 2):291–296.
- Farber MJ, Heilman ER, Friedman RJ. Dysplastic nevi. *Dermatol Clin.* 2012;30(3):389–404.
- Friedman RJ, Farber MJ, Warycha MA, et al. The "dysplastic" nevus. *Clin Dermatol.* 2009;27(1):103–115.
- Moloney FJ, Guitera P, Coates E, et al. Detection of primary melanoma in individuals at extreme high risk: a prospective 5-year follow-up study. *JAMA Dermatol.* 2014;150(8):819–827. doi: 10.1001/jamadermatol.2014.514.
- Robson ME, Storm CD, Weitzel J, et al. American Society of Clinical Oncology policy statement update: genetic and genomic testing for cancer susceptibility. *J Clin Oncol.* 2010;28(5):893–901.
- Slade J, Marghoob AA, Salopek TG, et al. Atypical mole syndrome: risk factor for cutaneous malignant melanoma and implications for management. *J Am Acad Dermatol.* 1995;32(3):479–494.

 CODES

ICD10
- D22.9 Melanocytic nevi, unspecified
- D22.4 Melanocytic nevi of scalp and neck
- D22.30 Melanocytic nevi of unspecified part of face

CLINICAL PEARLS
- Melanoma in AMS tends to arise from healthy skin despite a large number of atypical nevi.
- ~20% of individuals with familial AMS will develop pancreatic cancer by age 75 years.
- Patients with AMS tend to produce neoplasms in unusual sites such as the scalp, eyes, and sun-protected areas (e.g., gluteal folds).

AUTISM SPECTRUM DISORDERS

Macario C. Corpuz, MD, MBA, FAAFP • Jennifer Luo Powell, DO

BASICS

DESCRIPTION

- Group of neurodevelopmental disorders of early childhood: *DSM-5* has included autism spectrum disorders (ASDs) to include autistic disorder, childhood disintegrative disorder, Asperger disorder, pervasive developmental disorder not otherwise specified (PDD-NOS); and now, it also encompasses early infantile autism, childhood autism, Kanner autism, high-functioning autism, and atypical autism (1)[A].
- Two symptom clusters
- Social/communication
- Impairment of effective social skills and absent or impaired communication skills
- Fixed interests/repetitive behaviors
- Repetitive and/or stereotyped behaviors and interests, especially in inanimate objects (2)[A]
- Severity levels
  - Level 1: requiring support
  - Level 2: requiring substantial support
  - Level 3: requiring very substantial support
- Important to distinguish autism disorder from social (pragmatic) communication disorder. Separate *DSM-5* criteria for individuals with social communication deficits but do not meet autism-spectrum criteria.

EPIDEMIOLOGY

- Predominant age: onset in early childhood
- Predominant sex: male > female (5:1)

Pediatric Considerations

Symptom onset seen in children <3 years of age (except for childhood disintegrative disorder)

Prevalence

- According to the Centers for Disease Control and Prevention (CDC), an estimated 1/68 to 1/175 children, depending on the community
- Among 6 to 17 years–aged children within the United States, in 2011 to 2012, there is found to be a 2% (1 in 50) parent-reported prevalence compared to 1.16% (1 in 86) as reported in 2007.

ETIOLOGY AND PATHOPHYSIOLOGY

- No single cause has been identified.
- General consensus: A genetic abnormality leads to altered neurologic development.
- No scientific evidence relating vaccines, such as vaccines for measles, mumps, or rubella (MMR), or thimerosal causing ASDs (3)[C]
- Pathophysiology is incompletely understood.

Genetics

- High concordance in monozygotic twins
- Increased recurrence risk (2–18%) in subsequent siblings

RISK FACTORS

Siblings of affected children have a five times greater risk of developing autism. Prevalence ranging from 2% to 8%

GENERAL PREVENTION

- Early screening for early treatment means a better prognosis.
- Some ASDs are caused by genetic or chromosomal disorders.
- Economic costs
  - An additional $17,000 to $21,000 is an estimated cost for raising an ASD child.

- Medical costs for those with ASD in 2011 were estimated to be 4 to 6 times, ranging from $2,191 to $11,590 per child (4)[B].
- An estimated lifetime cost of services for an individual with ASD in 2011 is $3.8 million (5)[C].
- Due to caretaker burden, family earnings are found to be 28% less among families with ASD compared to children without health conditions (6)[C].

COMMONLY ASSOCIATED CONDITIONS

- Mental retardation, ADHD, anxiety, depression, or obsessive behavior
- Phenylketonuria (PKU), tuberous sclerosis, fragile X syndrome, Angelman syndrome, and fetal alcohol syndrome (rare)
- Seizures (increased risk if severe mental retardation)
- Maternal use of selective serotonin reuptake inhibitors (SSRIs) during pregnancy

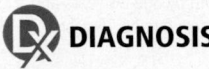

DIAGNOSIS

HISTORY

- Impairment in social interaction
  - Impairment in nonverbal behaviors such as eye-to-eye gaze, facial expression
  - Unable to develop peer relationships
  - Does not smile nor share emotions
  - Loss of social or emotional reciprocity
- Communication impairment
  - Delay or lack of development in language skills
  - Inability to initiate or sustain conversation
  - Stereotyped and repetitive use of language
  - Preoccupation with parts of toys or body parts
- Repetitive and stereotyped patterns of behavior
  - Excessively lines up toys or other objects
  - Unusually attached to one particular toy or object
  - Repetitive odd movements (toe walking, hand flapping)
  - Adherence to specific routines or rituals
- Prenatal, neonatal, and developmental history
- Seizure disorder
- Family history of autism, genetic disorders, learning disabilities, psychiatric illness, neurologic disorders, genetic disorders, or mental retardation
- Commonly associated with sleep disorders

PHYSICAL EXAM

- Macrocephaly in 25%; head circumference growth peaks at age 6 months and begins to decline by 1 year.
- Dysmorphic features consistent with genetic disorder (fragile X syndrome)
- Hypotonia occurs in autism but should prompt imaging.
- Wood lamp skin exam to rule out tuberous sclerosis

DIFFERENTIAL DIAGNOSIS

- Other mental and CNS disorders
- Obsessive-compulsive disorder
- Elective mutism
- Language disorder/hearing impairment
- Intellectual disability/global developmental delay
- Stereotyped movement disorder
- Severe early deprivation/reactive attachment disorder
- Anxiety disorder
- Social communication disorder
- Developmental language disorder

DIAGNOSTIC TESTS & INTERPRETATION

- Checklist for Autism in Toddlers (CHAT) to screen for ASDs at 18 months of age. (To order: http://www.autism.org.uk/working-with/health/screening-and-diagnosis/checklist-for-autism-in-toddlers-chat.aspx)

- The Pervasive Developmental Disorders Screening Test-II (PDDST-II) to screen for ASDs beginning at 18 months
- Modified Checklist for Autism in Toddlers (M-CHAT) to screen for ASDs at 16 to 30 months
- Social Communication Questionnaire (SCQ) (formerly Autism Screening Questionnaire)—used with children age 4+ years—the gold standard diagnostic interview used in research studies

Initial Tests (lab, imaging)

- Lead and PKU screening
- Karyotype and DNA analysis (fragile X, PKU, tuberous sclerosis, and others)
- Metabolic testing if signs of
  - Lethargy, limited endurance, unusual habits, hypotonia, recurrent vomiting and dehydration, developmental regression, or specific food intolerance
- MRI is useful only if focal neurologic symptoms.

Follow-Up Tests & Special Considerations

- Hearing tests: audiometry and brainstem auditory evoked response (BAERS)
- Comprehensive speech and language evaluation
- Evaluation by multidisciplinary team: includes a psychiatrist, neurologist, psychologist, speech therapist, and other autism specialists
- Intellectual level needs to be established and monitored, as it is one of the best measures of prognosis.
- Test used to follow autism are the following:
  - Autism Behavior Checklist (ABC)
  - Gilliam Autism Rating Scale (GARS)
  - Childhood Autism Rating Scale (CARS)
  - Autism Diagnosis Interview-Revised (ADI-R)
  - Autism Diagnostic Observation Schedule-Generic (ADOS-G) Imaging

Diagnostic Procedures/Other

EEG if history of seizures or spells

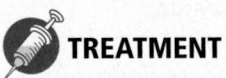

TREATMENT

GENERAL MEASURES

- Comprehensive structured educational programming of a sustained and intensive design, most commonly applied behavioral analysis therapy
- Core features of a successful education program
  - High staff–student ratio 1:2, or less
  - Individualized programming
  - Specialized teacher training with ongoing evaluation of teachers and programs
  - 25 hours a week minimum of specialized services
  - A structured routine environment that emphasizes attention, imitation, communication, socialization, and play interactions (7)[C]
  - Functional analysis of behavioral problems
  - Transition planning and involvement of the family
- Currently no cure for ASDs. Early diagnosis and initiation of multidisciplinary intervention help enhance functioning in later life.
- Early intensive behavioral intervention (EIBI) involving treatment for 20 to 40 hours per week is a well-established treatments for ASD.
- School-based special education for older children
- Some evidence indicates social skill groups can improve social competence for some children and adolescents with ASD.
- Find alternative methods of communication: sign language; picture exchange communication system

MEDICATION
- Autism behavior issues should be managed with maximal behavioral management prior to medication.
- Medication directed at managing symptoms

First Line
- No true first-line medical therapy; medications used to treat targeted symptoms
- Stimulants (such as methylphenidate): Efficacious in treating concomitant symptoms of ADHD such as impulsiveness, hyperactivity, and inattention; however, the magnitude of response is less than in typically developing children and adverse effects are more frequent.
- SSRIs have limited evidence for autism. It has shown help in reducing ritualistic behavior and improving mood and language skills. Initial choice for anxiety and depressive mood (8)[B]
- Risperidone has shown short-term efficacy for treatment for irritability, repetitious behaviors, and social withdrawal (9)[B]. Aripiprazole has shown efficacy for treating short-term irritability, hyperactivity, and repetitive movements (10)[B].
- Melatonin used for patients with concomitant sleep disorders

Second Line
- Vitamin B_6 and magnesium: inconclusive evidence in improving behavior, speech, and language of children with ASD (11)[C]
- Tricyclic antidepressants have limited and conflicting evidence of effect (12)[B].

ISSUES FOR REFERRAL
- Refer early to
  - Early learning for evaluation of behavior and language, genetic counseling, and audiology
- Consider referrals to psychiatry, ophthalmology, otolaryngology, neurology, and nutrition (13).
- Refer family members to parent support groups and respite programs.

COMPLEMENTARY & ALTERNATIVE MEDICINE
- Parent-mediated early intervention for young children with autism spectrum has sufficient evidence of benefit in child outcomes related to language understanding and severity of autism characteristics (14)[A].
- Music therapy has been shown to improve communication skills in autistic patients; however, more research is needed (15)[C].
- "Theory of mind," or related skills, can be taught to ASD patients, but further research is needed (16)[C].
- No evidence to support use of auditory integration therapy or other sound therapies as an effective treatment for ASD (17)[B].
- No evidence to support acupuncture for treatment of ASD (6)[C].
- IV secretin and pharmaceutical chelation has shown no evidence of efficacy and is not currently recommended as a treatment for ASD (18,19)[C].

 ONGOING CARE

FOLLOW-UP RECOMMENDATIONS
Patient Monitoring
- Constant monitoring by caregivers
- Reevaluation every 6 to 12 months by physician for seizures, sleep and nutritional problems, and prescribed medical management
- Intellectual and language testing every 2 years in childhood

DIET
- Gluten- and casein-free diets: Current evidence for efficacy is poor (20)[C].
- Omega-3 fatty acids supplementation has not been found to improve outcomes (21)[C].

PROGNOSIS
- Beginning treatment at a young age (2 to 4 years) results in better outcomes.
- Prognosis is closely related to initial intellectual abilities, with only 20% functioning above the mentally retarded level.
- Communicative language development before 5 years is also associated with a better outcome.
- The general expected course is for a lifelong need for supervised structured care.

COMPLICATIONS
- Increasing incidents of seizure disorders in up to 1 in 4 children
- Increased risk for physical and sexual abuse
- With pica, increased risk of lead poisoning
- Limited variety of food consumed due to dietary obsessions
- Increased risk for GI symptoms, including weight abnormalities and abnormal stool patterns

REFERENCES

1. Autism and Developmental Disabilities Monitoring Network Surveillance Year 2008 Principal Investigators; Centers for Disease Control and Prevention. Prevalence of autism spectrum disorders—Autism and Developmental Disabilities Monitoring Network, 14 sites, United States, 2008. *MMWR Surveill Summ.* 2012;61(3):1–19.
2. Blumberg SJ, Bramlett MD, Kogan MD, et al. Changes in prevalence of parent-reported autism spectrum disorder in school-aged U.S. children: 2007 to 2011–2012. *Natl Health Stat Report.* 2013;(65):1–11.
3. Demicheli V, Rivetti A, Debalini MG, et al. Vaccines for measles, mumps and rubella in children. *Cochrane Database Syst Rev.* 2012;(2):CD004407.
4. Lavelle TA, Weinstein MC, Newhouse JP, et al. Economic burden of childhood autism spectrum disorders. *Pediatrics.* 2014;133(3):e520–e529.
5. Ganz ML. The lifetime distribution of the incremental societal costs of autism. *Arch Pediatr Adolesc Med.* 2007;161(4):343–349.
6. Cidav Z, Marcus SC, Mandell DS. Implications of childhood autism for parental employment and earnings. *Pediatrics.* 2012;129(4):617–623.
7. Cheuk DK, Wong V, Chen WX. Acupuncture for autism spectrum disorders (ASD). *Cochrane Database Syst Rev.* 2011;(9):CD007849.
8. Williams K, Brignell A, Randall M, et al. Selective serotonin reuptake inhibitors (SSRIs) for autism spectrum disorders (ASD). *Cochrane Database Syst Rev.* 2013;(8):CD004677.
9. Jesner OS, Aref-Adib M, Coren E. Risperidone for autism spectrum disorder. *Cochrane Database Syst Rev.* 2007;(1):CD005040.
10. Ching H, Pringsheim T. Aripiprazole for autism spectrum disorders (ASD). *Cochrane Database Syst Rev.* 2012;(5):CD009043.
11. Nye C, Brice A. Combined vitamin B6-magnesium treatment in autism spectrum disorder. *Cochrane Database Syst Rev.* 2005;(4):CD003497.
12. Hurwitz R, Blackmore R, Hazell P, et al. Tricyclic antidepressants for autism spectrum disorders (ASD) in children and adolescents. *Cochrane Database Syst Rev.* 2012;(3):CD008372.
13. Reichow B, Steiner AM, Volkmar F. Social skills groups for people aged 6 to 21 with autism spectrum disorders (ASD). *Cochrane Database Syst Rev.* 2012;(7):CD008511.
14. Oono IP, Honey EJ, McConachie H. Parent-mediated early intervention for young children with autism spectrum disorders (ASD). *Cochrane Database Syst Rev.* 2013;(4):CD009774.
15. Geretsegger M, Elefant C, Mössler KA, et al. Music therapy for people with autism spectrum disorder. *Cochrane Database Syst Rev.* 2014;(6):CD004381.
16. Fletcher-Watson S, McConnell F, Manola E, et al. Interventions based on the Theory of Mind cognitive model for autism spectrum disorder (ASD). *Cochrane Database Syst Rev.* 2014;(3):CD008785.
17. Sinha Y, Silove N, Hayen A, et al. Auditory integration training and other sound therapies for autism spectrum disorders (ASD). *Cochrane Database Syst Rev.* 2011;(12):CD003681.
18. Williams K, Wray JA, Wheeler DM. Intravenous secretin for autism spectrum disorders (ASD). *Cochrane Database Syst Rev.* 2012;(4):CD003495.
19. James S, Stevenson SW, Silove N, et al. Chelation for autism spectrum disorder (ASD). *Cochrane Database of Syst Rev.* 2015;(5):CD010766.
20. Millward C, Ferriter M, Calver S, et al. Gluten- and casein-free diets for autistic spectrum disorder. *Cochrane Database Syst Rev.* 2008;(2):CD003498.
21. James S, Montgomery P, Williams K. Omega-3 fatty acids supplementation for autism spectrum disorders (ASD). *Cochrane Database Syst Rev.* 2011;(11):CD007992.

ADDITIONAL READING
- Reichow B, Barton EE, Boyd BA, et al. Early intensive behavioral intervention (EIBI) for young children with autism spectrum disorders (ASD). *Cochrane Database Syst Rev.* 2012;(10):CD009260.
- Vriend JL, Corkum PV, Moon EC, et al. Behavioral interventions for sleep problems in children with autism spectrum disorders: current findings and future directions. *J Pediatr Psychol.* 2011;36(9):1017–1029.

 SEE ALSO

Algorithm: Intellectual Disability

 CODES

ICD10
- F84.0 Autistic disorder
- F84.5 Asperger's syndrome
- F84.3 Other childhood disintegrative disorder

CLINICAL PEARLS
- ALARM mnemonic from the American Academy of Pediatrics (AAP)
- ASD is prevalent (screen ALL children between 18 and 24 months).
- Listen to parents when they feel something is wrong.
- Act early: Screen all children who fall behind in language and social developmental milestones (use early learning to help with evaluation).
- Refer to multidisciplinary teams (speech and language evaluation, genetic screening, social support groups).
- Monitor support for patient and families.

BABESIOSIS

Frederick W. Nielson, MD, Captain USAF • J. David Honeycutt, MD, FAAFP, FAWM

 BASICS

DESCRIPTION
- Rare tick-borne hemolytic disease caused by intraerythrocytic protozoan parasites of the genus *Babesia*
- Infrequently reported outside the United States
  - Sporadic cases have been reported from
    - France, Italy, the United Kingdom, Ireland, the former Soviet Union, Mexico (1)
    - China has reported a reemergence of cases.
  - In the United States, infections have been reported in many states, but most endemic areas are:
    - Islands off the coast of Massachusetts (including Nantucket and Martha's Vineyard)
    - New York (including Long Island, Shelter Island, and Fire Island)
    - Connecticut
    - In these areas, asymptomatic infection is common (1).
- Incubation period varies from 5 to 33 days:
  - Most patients do not recall specific tick exposure.
  - After transfusion of infected blood, the incubation period can be up to 9 weeks (1).
- System(s) affected: cardiovascular, gastrointestinal, hemic/lymphatic/immunologic, musculoskeletal, nervous, pulmonary, renal/urologic

Pediatric Considerations
Transplacental and perinatal transmission have been rarely reported (1,2).

Geriatric Considerations
- Morbidity and mortality are higher in patients >60 years.
- Cases occurring in patients >70 years are more common in those with medical comorbidities.

EPIDEMIOLOGY
Babesiosis affects patients of all ages. Most patients present in their 40s or 50s (1).

Incidence
- In 2012, there were 911 cases reported to the CDC.
- Prevalence is difficult to estimate due to lack of surveillance and asymptomatic infections.
- Transfusion-associated babesiosis and transplacental/perinatal transmission have been reported (1).
- A 1-year seroconversion study of patients in New York, at high risk for tick-borne diseases, showed antibodies to *Babesia microti* in 7 of 671 individuals (1%) (1).

ETIOLOGY AND PATHOPHYSIOLOGY
- *B. microti* (in the United States) and *Babesia divergens* and *Babesia bovis* (in Europe) cause most human infections (1). *B. divergens* and a new strain *Babesia ducani* appear to be more virulent. Other species have been identified in case reports. All share morphologic, antigenic, and genetic characteristics (1).

- Ixodid (hard-bodied) ticks, particularly *Ixodes dammini* (*Ixodes scapularis*: deer tick) and *Ixodes ricinus*, are the primary vectors. The white-footed mouse is the primary reservoir.
- Infection is passed to humans through the saliva of a nymphal-stage tick during a blood meal. Sporozoites introduced at the time of the bite enter red blood cells form merozoites through binary fission (classic morphology on blood smear). Humans are a dead-end host for *B. microti*.

RISK FACTORS
- Residing in endemic areas
- Asplenia
- Immunocompromised state

GENERAL PREVENTION
- Avoid endemic regions during the peak transmission months of May to September (1).
- Appropriate insect repellent is advised during outdoor activities, especially in wooded or grassy areas:
  - 10–35% N,N-diethyl-meta-toluamide (DEET) provides adequate protection (1).
- Early removal of ticks via daily skin checks; the tick must remain attached for at least 24 hours before the transmission of *B. microti* occurs (1).
- Examine pets for ticks.

COMMONLY ASSOCIATED CONDITIONS
- Coinfection with *Borrelia burgdorferi* and *B. microti*, particularly in endemic areas (1)
- Coinfection with *Ehrlichia* (1).

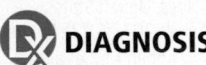 **DIAGNOSIS**

HISTORY
- Travel/exposure history
- Comorbidities (immunosuppression, chronic disease)
- Fever (68–89%), fatigue, (78–79%), chills (39–68%), sweats (41–56%), headache (32–75%), myalgia (32–37%), anorexia (24–25%), cough (17–23%), arthralgias (17–32%), nausea (9–22%). Other symptoms reported by case reports include abdominal pain, vomiting, diarrhea, and emotional lability.

PHYSICAL EXAM
- High fever (up to 40°C [104°F])
- Hemodynamic instability (shock in extremely ill)
- Hepatomegaly and splenomegaly (mild if noted)
- Rash (uncommon)
- CNS involvement includes headache, photophobia, neck and back stiffness, altered sensorium, and emotional lability.
- Jaundice and dark urine may develop later in course of illness.

DIFFERENTIAL DIAGNOSIS
- Bacterial sepsis
- Hepatitis
- Lyme disease
- Ehrlichiosis
- Leishmaniasis
- Malaria
- HIV
- EBV

DIAGNOSTIC TESTS & INTERPRETATION
Initial Tests (lab, imaging)
- Requires a high index of clinical suspicion. Nonspecific laboratory clues include evidence of mild to severe hemolytic anemia, normal to slightly depressed leukocyte count (1), elevated LDH or transaminase level, elevated BUN and Cr, proteinuria with hemoglobinuria (1,2).
- Definitive diagnosis is made by blood smear

  - A Wright- or Giemsa-stained peripheral blood smear demonstrates intraerythrocytic parasites (2)[B].

  - Dividing "cross-like" tetrads of merozoites (Maltese cross) are pathognomonic (2).
  - Serial blood smears may be required as low parasite load early in the illness may make identification difficult (2).
  - Can be confused with *Plasmodium falciparum* on peripheral smear
- If blood smears are negative but suspicion remains, IgM serologies through indirect immunofluorescent antibody testing (IFAT) for *B. microti* antigen are available:

  - The cutoff titer for a positive result varies by laboratory protocol. Titers of >1:64 or a 4-fold increase from baseline are consistent with *B. microti* infection (3). Titers may exceed >1:1,024 in acute infection (2)[B]. Titers often persists for 8 to 12 months and can last for years.

  - In New England, seroprevalence varies between 0.5% and 16% (3).

- Detection of *B. microti* by polymerase chain reaction (PCR) is more sensitive and equally specific in acute cases. PCR can also be used to monitor disease progression (2)[B]. Newer real-time PCR tests have a sensitivity and specificity approaching 100%.

- When lab tests are inconclusive and infection is strongly suspected, inoculation of laboratory animals with patient blood reveals *B. microti* organisms in the blood of the animal within 2 to 4 weeks (2).

Follow-Up Tests & Special Considerations
Monitoring intraerythrocytic parasitemia helps guide treatment (4)[C].

Diagnostic Procedures/Other
Based on blood smear, history, and epidemiologic information (2)

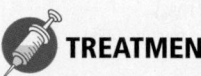 **TREATMENT**

GENERAL MEASURES
- In areas endemic for Lyme disease and ehrlichiosis, consider adding doxycycline (Vibramycin) 100 mg BID PO until serologic testing is completed (1)[C].
- Resistance to standard medications has emerged in severely immunocompromised patients (2).
- Consider treating asymptomatic patients if parasitemia persists for >3 months; otherwise, do not treat in absence of symptoms (1),(4)[C].

MEDICATION
First Line
- Mild to moderate infection with *B. microti*: 7 to 10 days of atovaquone 750 mg PO BID plus azithromycin 500 to 1,000 mg/day PO on day 1, followed by 250 mg/day afterward. Pediatrics: atovaquone 20 mg/kg (max 750 mg) BID and azithromycin 10 mg/kg (max 500 mg) on day 1, then 5 mg/kg (max 250 mg) (4)[B]. For severe *B. microti* infection: oral quinine 650 mg TID or QID plus oral clindamycin 600 mg TID for 7 to 10 days. Pediatrics: clindamycin 7 to 10 mg/kg (max 600 mg) TID or QID and quinine 8 mg/kg (max 650 mg) TID. IV formulations can be used (4)[C].
- Persistent or relapsing babesiosis: Treat for 6 weeks, including 2 weeks after *Babesia* is no longer detected on blood smear (5)[B].

Second Line
- Combination of quinine sulfate 650 mg PO TID and clindamycin 600 mg PO TID or 1.2 g parenterally BID for 7 to 10 days is the most commonly used treatment. Pediatric: quinine 8 mg/kg (max 650 mg) every 6 to 8 hours for 7 to 10 days and clindamycin 7 to 10 mg/kg (max 600 mg) PO q6–8h for 7 to 10 days. Some experts prefer this regimen for severe infections (4)[C].
- Other drugs including tetracycline, primaquine, sulfadiazine (Microsulfon), and sulfadoxine/pyrimethamine (Fansidar) have been evaluated. Results vary. Pentamidine (Pentam) is moderately effective in diminishing symptoms and decreasing parasitemia (1)[C].

ALERT
Clindamycin can lead to *Clostridium difficile*–associated diarrhea.

ISSUES FOR REFERRAL
Severe disease: Consider consultation with hematology and infectious disease for exchange transfusion in extremely ill patients (blood parasitemia >10%, massive hemolysis, and asplenia) (2)[C].

 ONGOING CARE

FOLLOW-UP RECOMMENDATIONS
- If left untreated, silent babesiosis may persist for months or years (2).
- 139 hospitalized cases in New York State between 1982 and 1993:
  - 9 patients (7%) died.
  - 25% of the patients were admitted to the ICU.
  - 25% hospitalized for >14 days.
- Alkaline phosphatase levels >125 U/L, WBC counts >5 × 10⁹/L, history of cardiac abnormality, history of splenectomy, presence of heart murmur, and parasitemia of 4% or higher are associated with disease severity (6)[B].

Patient Monitoring
The need for clinical and lab monitoring depends on disease severity. Severe infections: Follow hematocrit and parasitemia levels until clinical improvement and parasitemia is <5%. Mild to moderate: Expect clinical improvement within 48 hours and complete resolution within 3 months (4)[C].

COMPLICATIONS
While many remain asymptomatic, a case series noted the following complications in hospitalized patients: CHF (12%), DIC (18%), ARDS (21%), renal failure (6%), coma/lethargy (9%), death (9%). Other reported complications include neutropenia and myocardial infarction.

REFERENCES
1. Mylonakis E. When to suspect and how to monitor babesiosis. *Am Fam Physician.* 2001;63(10):1969–1974.
2. Vannier E, Krause PJ. Human babesiosis. *N Engl J Med.* 2012;366(25):2397–2407.
3. Vannier EG, Diuk-Wasser MA, Ben Mamoun C, et al. Babesiosis. *Infect Dis Clin North Am.* 2015;29(2):357–370.
4. Wormser GP, Dattwyler RJ, Shapiro ED, et al. The clinical assessment, treatment, and prevention of lyme disease, human granulocytic anaplasmosis, and babesiosis: clinical practice guidelines by the Infectious Diseases Society of America. *Clin Infect Dis.* 2006;43(9):1089–1134.
5. Krause PJ, Gewurz BE, Hill D, et al. Persistent and relapsing babesiosis in immunocompromised patients. *Clin Infect Dis.* 2008;46(3):370–376.
6. White DJ, Talarico J, Chang HG, et al. Human babesiosis in New York State: review of 139 hospitalized cases and analysis of prognostic factors. *Arch Intern Med.* 1998;158(19):2149–2154.

ADDITIONAL READING
- Deshpande A, Pasupuleti V, Thota P, et al. Community-associated *Clostridium difficile* infection and antibiotics: a meta-analysis. *J Antimicrob Chemother.* 2013;68(9):1951–1961.
- Florescu D, Sordillo PP, Glyptis A, et al. Splenic infarction in human babesiosis: two cases and discussion. *Clin Infect Dis.* 2008;46(1):e8–e11.
- Herwaldt BL, Linden JV, Bosserman E, et al. Transfusion-associated babesiosis in the United States: a description of cases. *Ann Intern Med.* 2011;155(8):509–519.
- Hilton E, DeVoti J, Benach JL, et al. Seroprevalence and seroconversion for tick-borne diseases in a high-risk population in the northeast United States. *Am J Med.* 1999;106(4):404–409.
- Joseph JT, Purtill K, Wong SJ, et al. Vertical transmission of *Babesia microti*, United States. *Emerg Infect Dis.* 2012;18(8):1318–1321.
- Kuwayama DP, Briones RJ. Spontaneous splenic rupture caused by *Babesia microti* infection. *Clin Infect Dis.* 2008;46(9):e92–e95.
- Martinot M, Zadeh MM, Hansmann Y, et al. Babesiosis in immunocompetent patients, Europe. *Emerg Infect Dis.* 2011;17(1):114–116.
- Mosqueda J, Olvera-Ramirez A, Aguilar-Tipacamu G, et al. Current advances in detection and treatment of babesiosis. *Curr Med Chem.* 2012;19(10):1504–1518.
- Teal AE, Habura A, Ennis J, et al. A new real-time PCR assay for improved detection of the parasite *Babesia microti.* *J Clin Microbiol.* 2012;50(3):903–908.

 CODES

ICD10
B60.0 Babesiosis

CLINICAL PEARLS
- If left untreated, silent babesial infection may persist for months or even years.
- Most patients do not recall tick exposure, and incubation can last up to a month.
- Ticks must remain in place for 24 hours to transmit infection—encourage daily "tick checks" if people are exposed in high-risk areas.
- First-line treatment for mild or moderate disease is atovaquone plus azithromycin.
- Patients with mild to moderate disease should show clinical improvement within 48 hours after starting therapy. Symptoms should fully resolve within 3 months.
- Coinfection with *B. burgdorferi* and *Ehrlichia* species is common in endemic areas. In areas endemic for Lyme disease and ehrlichiosis, consider adding doxycycline until serologic testing is completed.

BACK PAIN, LOW

Millicent King Channell, DO, MA, FAAO

BASICS

DESCRIPTION

- Low back pain (LBP) is extremely common and includes a wide range of symptoms involving the lumbosacral spine and pelvic girdle.
- LBP can be characterized by duration or associated symptoms.
- **Duration** (1)[A]
  - Acute (<6 weeks)
  - Subacute (>6 weeks but <3 months)
  - Chronic (>3 months)
- **Associated symptoms** (1)[A]
  - Localized/nonspecific "mechanical" LBP
  - Back pain with lower extremity symptoms
  - Systemic and visceral symptoms
- A specific cause is not found for most patients with LBP. Most cases resolve in 4 to 6 weeks.
- Rule out "red" flag symptoms indicating the need for immediate intervention.
- System(s) affected: musculoskeletal, neurologic
- Synonym(s): lumbago, lumbar sprain/strain, low back syndrome

EPIDEMIOLOGY

Incidence

- 1-year incidence: 6–15% (1)[A]
- LBP is one of the most common primary care complaints (1)[A].

Prevalence

- Lifetime prevalence: 84% (1)[A]
- Global point prevalence: 9% (1)[A]
- Predominant sex: male = female
- Age: The highest incidence is in the 3rd decade (20 to 29 years); overall prevalence increases with age until age 65 years and then declines (1)[A].

ETIOLOGY AND PATHOPHYSIOLOGY

A clear etiology is not found in most patients. Age-related degenerative changes of the lumbosacral spine, and atrophy of supporting musculature may contribute (2)[A].

RISK FACTORS

- Age (1)[A.]
- Activity (lifting, sudden twisting, bending) (1)[A]
- Obesity (1)[A]
- Sedentary lifestyle (1)[A]
- Physically strenuous work (1)[A]
- Psychosocial factors—anxiety, depression, stress (1)[A]
- Smoking (1)[A]

GENERAL PREVENTION

- Maintain normal weight (1)[A].
- Adequate physical fitness and activity (1)[A].
- Stress reduction (1)[A]
- Proper lifting technique and good posture
- Smoking cessation
- There is insufficient evidence to recommend for or against routine preventive measures in adults.

DIAGNOSIS

HISTORY

- Onset of pain (sudden or gradual) (1)[A]
- Pain from spinal structures (musculature, ligaments, facet joints, and disks) can refer to the thigh region but rarely below the knee (1)[A].
- Sacroiliac pain often refers to the thigh and can also radiate below the knee (1)[A].
- Irritation, impingement, or compression of lumbar nerve roots often results in more leg pain than back pain (1)[A].
- Pain from the L1–L3 nerve roots radiates to the hip and/or thigh, whereas pain from the L4–S1 nerve roots radiates below the knee.
- **Red flags**
  - Recent trauma
  - Neurologic deficits
    - Bowel/bladder incontinence or urinary retention
    - Saddle anesthesia
    - Weakness, falls
  - Night pain, sweats, fever, weight loss
  - Age >70 years with or without trauma
  - Age >50 years with minor trauma
  - History of cancer
  - Osteoporosis
  - Immunosuppression, prolonged glucocorticoid use
- **Yellow flags** predicting poor long-term prognosis
  - Lack of social support
  - Unsupportive work environment
  - Depression and/or anxiety
  - Abuse of alcohol or other substances
  - History of physical or sexual abuse
- Pain can be provoked with motion: flexion–extension, side-bending rotation, sitting, standing, and lifting. Pain often relieved with rest.
- Radicular pain may radiate to buttocks, thighs, and lower legs.

Pediatric Considerations

Back pain is not normal in children and must be carefully evaluated. Patients participating in gymnastics or other high impact sports (such as skateboarding and cheerleading) frequently land on their feet or buttocks. These can result in a vertebral fracture and/or damage to the intervertebral discs.

PHYSICAL EXAM

- Observe gait, position on examination table, and facial expressions.
- Test lumbar spine range of motion.
- Evaluate for point tenderness or muscle spasm.
  - Neurologic examination. Inspection: signs of muscle atrophy
  - Completely evaluate reflexes, strength, pulses, sensation
  - Straight leg test
  - FABER test (flexion, abduction, and external rotation)
  - Stork test: Stand on one leg with opposite hip held in flexion. Extend back. Pain in lumbosacral area is a positive test.

DIFFERENTIAL DIAGNOSIS

- Localized/nonspecific "mechanical" LBP (87%) (1)[A]

- Lumbar strain/sprain (70%)
  - Disc/facet degeneration (10%)
  - Osteoporotic compression fracture (4%)
  - Spondylolisthesis (2%)
  - Severe scoliosis, kyphosis
  - Asymmetric transitional vertebrae (<1%)
  - Traumatic fracture (<1%)
- Back pain with lower extremity symptoms (7%) (1)[A]
  - Disc herniation (4%)
  - Spinal stenosis (3%)
- Systemic and visceral symptoms (1)[A]
  - Neoplasia (0.7%)
    - Multiple myeloma; metastatic carcinoma
    - Lymphoma/leukemia
    - Spinal cord tumors, retroperitoneal tumors
  - Infection (0.01%)
    - Osteomyelitis
    - Septic discitis
    - Paraspinous abscess; epidural abscess
    - Shingles
  - Inflammatory disease (0.03%)
    - Ankylosing spondylitis, psoriatic spondylitis
    - Reactive arthritis
    - Inflammatory bowel disease
  - Visceral disease (0.05%)
    - Prostatitis
    - Endometriosis
    - Chronic pelvic inflammatory disease
    - Nephrolithiasis, pyelonephritis
    - Perinephric abscess
    - Aortic aneurysm
    - Pancreatitis; cholecystitis
    - Penetrating ulcer
  - Other
    - Osteochondrosis
    - Paget disease

DIAGNOSTIC TESTS & INTERPRETATION

Initial Tests (lab, imaging)

- Imaging studies are unnecessary during the first 6 weeks if no red flag signs or symptoms.
- X-ray of the lumbar spine (1,3,4)[A]
  - Not recommended for initial presentation or without red flags including trauma. Defer films for 6 weeks unless there is a high risk of disease.
  - Useful for bony etiology (e.g., fracture)
- MRI of the lumbar spine (1,3,4)[A] for patients presenting with neurologic deficits, failure to improve with 6 weeks of conservative treatment, or if there is a strong suspicion of cancer or cauda equina syndrome.
  - Useful for suspected herniated disc, nerve root compression, or metastatic disease
- CT scan of the lumbar spine (1,3,4)[A]
  - Appropriate alternative to MRI for patient with pacemaker, metallic hardware, or other contraindication to MRI
- Labs are unnecessary with initial presentation if no related red flags, signs, or symptoms present (1,3,4)[A]
- If infection or bone marrow neoplasm is suspected, consider (1,3,4)[A]
  - Complete blood count (CBC) with differential
  - Erythrocyte sedimentation rate (ESR)
  - C-reactive protein (CRP) level

Diagnostic Procedures/Other

Neurosurgical consult for acute neurologic deficits or suspected cauda equina syndrome (1,4)[A]

 TREATMENT

The primary goal is to provide supportive care and allow return to functional activity. Patients should be aware of alarm symptoms that prompt a return visit.

First Line

- Patient education (4)[A]

  - Reassure patients that pain is usually self-limited; treatment should relieve pain and improve function.
  - Encouraging activity as tolerated leads to quicker recovery.

- Medications (1,3,5)[A]

  - Acetaminophen 325 to 650 mg PO q4–6h PRN pain (max 4 g/day)
  - NSAIDs
    ○ Ibuprofen 400 to 600 mg PO 3 to 4 times daily (max 3,200 mg/day)
    ○ Naproxen 250 to 500 mg PO q12h (max 1,500 mg/day)

  - Manual medicine (4)[A], osteopathic manipulative treatments (OMT) (4)[A],(6)[B]: myofascial, counter-strain, bilateral ligamentous techniques, as well as muscle energy, if tolerated

- **Obstetric considerations** (6,7)[B]

  - Use medications cautiously in pregnancy—benefit must clearly outweigh risk.

- OMT and chiropractic care may be used in a multidisciplinary approach in the general population as well as the obstetric patient.

Second Line

- Second-line therapy for moderate to severe pain (1,3,5)[A]

  - Cyclobenzaprine 5 to 10 mg PO up to TID PRN (max 30 mg/day)
  - Tizanidine 2 mg PO up to TID PRN
  - Hydrocodone 2.5 to 10 mg PO q4–6h PRN pain; use of hydrocodone or other opioids for LBP is based on clinical judgment.

- Other treatments (1,3)[A]
  - Antidepressants (1,3,5)[A]

    ○ Tricyclic antidepressants (amitriptyline, nortriptyline, desipramine) have been shown in randomized trials to provide a small pain reduction in patients. No clear evidence that SSRIs are more effective than placebo in cases of chronic LBP.

- Injections (8)[A]

  - Facet: lumbar radiofrequency neurotomy, therapeutic facet joint nerve blocks in the lumbar spine, and lumbar intra-articular injections have all shown benefit

  - Epidural: provides short-term relief of persistent pain associated with documented radicular symptoms caused by herniated disc (1,3,4,8)[A]

Geriatric Considerations

- Older persons taking nonselective NSAIDs should use a proton pump inhibitor or misoprostol for gastrointestinal protection.
- Patients taking a COX-2 selective inhibitor with aspirin should use a proton pump inhibitor or misoprostol for gastrointestinal protection.
- Age-related decline in cytochrome P-450 function and polypharmacy (common in elderly patients) increases risk for adverse medication reactions.

COMPLEMENTARY & ALTERNATIVE MEDICINE

- Acupuncture is superior to no treatment, but evidence is mixed regarding the effectiveness of acupuncture over other treatment modalities (1,3,4)[A].
- Yoga can help with chronic LBP (1,3,4)[A].

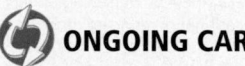 **ONGOING CARE**

FOLLOW-UP RECOMMENDATIONS

- Regular exercise (3,9)[A]
- Patient education regarding chronicity, recurrence, and red flags (3,9)[A]

Patient Monitoring

- Reassurance is key. Follow up within 2 to 4 weeks of initial presentation to monitor progress. Most patients spontaneously improve.
  - Assess severity and quality of pain as well as range of motion and other historical features (red flags).
- Reevaluate for possible underlying organic causes for pain if patients fail to improve.

COMPLICATIONS

- Regular NSAID use can increase risk of gastrointestinal toxicity and nephrotoxicity (1,4)[A].
- Acetaminophen has potential hepatotoxicity (1,4)[A].
- Centrally acting skeletal muscle relaxants and opioid agonists carry the risk for sedation, confusion, dependence, and abuse (1,4)[A].

REFERENCES

1. Golob AL, Wipf JE. Low back pain. *Med Clin North Am*. 2014;98(3):405–428.
2. Duffy RL. Low back pain: an approach to diagnosis and management. *Prim Care*. 2010;37(4):729–741.
3. Chaparro LE, Furlan AD, Deshpande A, et al. Opioids compared with placebo or other treatments for chronic low back pain: an update of the Cochrane Review. *Spine (Phila Pa 1976)*. 2014;39(7):556–563.
4. Casazza BA. Diagnosis and treatment of acute low back pain. *Am Fam Physician*. 2012;85(4):343–350.
5. Lee TJ. Pharmacologic treatment for low back pain: one component of pain care. *Phys Med Rehabil Clin N Am*. 2010;21(4):793–800.
6. Hensel KL, Buchanan S, Brown SK, et al. Pregnancy research on osteopathic manipulation optimizing treatment effects: the PROMOTE study. *Am J Obstet Gynecol*. 2015;212(1):108.e1–108.e9.
7. George JW, Skaggs CD, Thompson PA, et al. A randomized controlled trial comparing a multimodal intervention and standard obstetrics care for low back and pelvic pain in pregnancy. *Am J Obstet Gynecol*. 2013;208(4):295.e1–295.e7.
8. Manchikanti L, Kaye AD, Boswell MV, et al. A systematic review and best evidence synthesis of the effectiveness of therapeutic facet joint interventions in managing chronic spinal pain. *Pain Physician*. 2015;18(4):E535–E582.
9. Savigny P, Watson P, Underwood M; Guideline Development Group. Early management of persistent non-specific low back pain: summary of NICE guidance. *BMJ*. 2009;338:b1805.

ADDITIONAL READING

- de Leon-Casasola OA. Opioids for chronic pain: new evidence, new strategies, safe prescribing. *Am J Med*. 2013;126(3)(Suppl 1):S3–S11.
- Engers A, Jellema P, Wensing M, et al. Individual patient education for low back pain. *Cochrane Database Syst Rev*. 2008;(1):CD004057.
- Flynn TW, Smith B, Chou R. Appropriate use of diagnostic imaging in low back pain: a reminder that unnecessary imaging may do as much harm as good. *J Orthop Sports Phys Ther*. 2011;41(11):838–846.
- Henschke N, Ostelo RW, van Tulder MW, et al. Behavioural treatment for chronic low-back pain. *Cochrane Database Syst Rev*. 2010;(7):CD002014.
- Hutchinson AJ, Ball S, Andrews JC, et al. The effectiveness of acupuncture in treating chronic non-specific low back pain: a systematic review of the literature. *J Orthop Surg Res*. 2012;7:36.
- Kuijpers T, van Middelkoop M, Rubinstein SM, et al. A systematic review on the effectiveness of pharmacological interventions for chronic non-specific low-back pain. *Eur Spine J*. 2011;20(1):40–50.
- Urquhart DM, Hoving JL, Assendelft WW, et al. Antidepressants for non-specific low back pain. *Cochrane Database Syst Rev*. 2010;(1):CD001703.
- Walker BF, French SD, Grant W, et al. A Cochrane review of combined chiropractic interventions for low-back pain. *Spine (Phila Pa 1976)*. 2011;36(3):230–242.

 SEE ALSO

- Lumbar (Intervertebral) Disc Disorders
- Algorithm: Low Back Pain, Acute

 CODES

ICD10
- M54.5 Low back pain
- G89.29 Other chronic pain

CLINICAL PEARLS

- LBP is one of the most common complaints in primary care. Most patients do not have an identifiable cause of pain, and most cases resolve spontaneously within 4 to 12 weeks of onset.
- Assess for red flag symptoms in every patient.
- Labs and imaging studies are unnecessary for most cases of back pain if no red flag symptoms are present.
- In the absence of red flags, physical activity as tolerated speeds recovery.

BACTERIURIA, ASYMPTOMATIC

Mony Fraer, MD, FACP, FASN • Kantima Phisitkul, MD

 BASICS

DESCRIPTION
Asymptomatic bacteriuria (ASB) is diagnosed when significant bacteriuria is not accompanied by signs and symptoms attributable to urinary tract infection (UTI).

EPIDEMIOLOGY
Incidence
- General population: 3.5%
- Pregnancy: 7–10%
- Older women: 16–18%

Prevalence
- Variable, increased with age, female gender, sexual activity, and presence of genitourinary (GU) abnormalities
- Pregnancy: 2–10%
- Short- and long-term indwelling catheter 9–23% and 100%, respectively
- Long-term care residents in women 25–50% and men 15–40%

ETIOLOGY AND PATHOPHYSIOLOGY
- Microbiology is similar to that of other UTI, with bacteria originating from periurethral area, vagina, or gut.
- Organisms are less virulent in ASB than those causing UTI.
- The most common organism is *Escherichia coli*. Other common organisms are *Klebsiella pneumonia*, *Enterobacter*, *Proteus mirabilis*, *Staphylococcus aureus*, group B *Streptococcus* (GBS), and *Enterococcus*.

Genetics
Genetic variations that reduce toll-like receptor-4 function (TLR4) have been associated with ASB by lowering innate immune response and delaying bacterial clearance.

RISK FACTORS
- Older age
- Female gender
- Sexual activity, use of diaphragm with spermicide
- GU abnormalities: neurogenic bladder, urinary retention, urinary catheter use (indwelling, intermittent, or condom catheter)
- Institutionalized residents
- Diabetes mellitus
- Immunocompromised status
- Spinal cord injuries or functional impairment
- Hemodialysis
- Pregnancy (decreased peristalsis of the urinary tract)

COMMONLY ASSOCIATED CONDITIONS
Depends on the risk factors

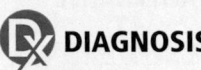 DIAGNOSIS

HISTORY
- Asymptomatic
- Lack of symptoms attributable to UTI such as fever, acute dysuria (<1 week), new or worsening urinary urgency/frequency/incontinence, or acute gross hematuria

PHYSICAL EXAM
- Afebrile
- No suprapubic and costovertebral angle tenderness

DIFFERENTIAL DIAGNOSIS
- UTI
- Contaminated urine specimen

DIAGNOSTIC TESTS & INTERPRETATION
Initial Tests (lab, imaging)
- Urinalysis (UA):
  - The presence of pyuria, leukocyte esterase, and nitrite in ASB is common.
- Urine culture
- Screening urine culture in asymptomatic patients is indicated in only two conditions:
  - Pregnancy: screening between 12 and 16 weeks' gestation or at first prenatal visit if later (1)[A]
  - Prior to transurethral resection of prostate (TURP) (1)[A] or any urologic interventions when mucosal bleeding is anticipated (1)[C].
- Screening for ASB in men and nonpregnant women is not recommended.

Follow-Up Tests & Special Considerations
- Noncontaminated urine specimen should be used for urine culture.
- In pregnancy, periodic screening urine culture should be done after ASB treatment (1)[A] but not required in GBS bacteriuria (2,3)[C].

Test Interpretation
- Patient with significant bacteriuria with or without pyuria and without symptoms referable to UTI should be diagnosed as ASB per Infectious Diseases Society of America.
  - Significant bacteriuria is defined based on type of urine specimen, sex, and the amount of bacteria.
  - By midstream, clean catch specimen
    - Male: >100,000 CFU/mL of single bacteria species
    - Female: the same criteria as male but needs two positive consecutive specimens
    - By catheterized specimen male and female: >100 CFU/mL of one bacterial species. Required one-time collection only
- The presence of pyuria or leukocyte esterase is common but not a marker of infection.
- Positive nitrite is an indicator of the presence of bacteriuria, but cannot differentiate UTI from ASB or poor collection technique.

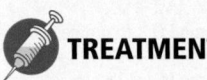 TREATMENT

GENERAL MEASURES

ALERT
- Antibiotic treatment of ASB is indicated in two conditions:
  - Pregnancy (1)[A]
    - Rationale: Treatment has been shown to significantly reduce the incidence of acute pyelonephritis and low birth weight.
  - Prior to urologic procedure particularly TURP (1)[A]
    - Rationale: Antibiotic treatment can effectively prevent postprocedure bacteremia and sepsis.
- Treatment of ASB in other conditions (nonpregnant women, diabetic women, indwelling catheter, patients with spinal cord injury, or the elderly living in the community) does not provide any known clinical benefit, does not reduce the risk of symptomatic infection nor improve morbidity or mortality. It increases health care cost, adverse drug side effects, development of resistant organisms, and reinfection rate (1,4).
- Inadequate evidence to guide management in nonurologic procedure and solid organ transplant (1,4)

MEDICATION

- Pregnancy
  - Intrapartum antibiotic prophylaxis with IV penicillin or clindamycin (penicillin allergy) is recommended for women with GBS bacteriuria occurring at any stage of pregnancy and of any colony count to prevent GBS disease in the newborn (2)[C].
  - No consensus on choice of antibiotics and duration of treatment in pregnancy; however, the cure rate is higher for the 4 to 7 days of treatment than one-day treatment (1)[A].
  - Choice of antibiotics should be guided by bacterial pathogen, local resistance rate, adverse effects, and comorbidities of patients (5).
  - Common oral antibiotics (FDA-B) that have been used
    - Nitrofurantoin 100 mg BID for 5 days (low level of resistance, may cause hemolysis in glucose-6-phosphate dehydrogenase deficiency)
    - Amoxicillin/clavulanate 500/125 BID for 5 to 7 days
    - Cefuroxime 250 mg BID for 5 days
    - Cephalexin 500 mg BID for 5 days
    - Fosfomycin 3 g for 1 single dose (not effective when glomerular filtration rate is less than 30 mL/min, may be used in highly resistant bacteria such as methicillin-resistant *Staphylococcus aureus* [MRSA], vancomycin-resistant enterococci [VRE], and extended-spectrum beta-lactamase [ESBL]-producing organism bacteria) (6)
  - Avoid trimethoprim in 1st trimester and near term. Avoid sulfa after 32 weeks' gestation.
  - Contraindicated: fluoroquinolones (FDA-C), tetracyclines (FDA-D)
- Prior to invasive urologic interventions
  - Initiate antibiotic the night before or immediately before the procedure (1)[A].
  - Antibiotic should be continued until the indwelling catheter is removed postprocedure (1)[B].

ONGOING CARE

FOLLOW-UP RECOMMENDATIONS

No consensus on screening frequency of ASB in pregnancy, but monthly screening of urine culture after ASB treatment is recommended except GBS (1,2).

Patient Monitoring

Development of any signs/symptoms of UTI should warrant antibiotic treatment.

DIET

Daily cranberry juice may reduce the frequency of ASB during pregnancy, but it has not been confirmed in large study (see "Additional Reading").

PATIENT EDUCATION

Patient should seek medical attention when UTI symptoms develop.

COMPLICATIONS

- Late pregnancy pyelonephritis occurs in 20–35% of women with untreated bacteriuria (20- to 30-fold higher than women with negative initial screening urine cultures or in whom bacteriuria was treated). Pyelonephritis is associated with premature delivery and worse fetal outcomes (infant with group B streptococcal infections, low-birth-weight infant). Antimicrobial treatment will decrease the risk of subsequent pyelonephritis from 20–35% to 1–4% and the risk of having a low-birth-weight baby from 15% to 5%.
- If bacteriuria remains untreated in patients who undergo traumatic urologic procedures, up to 60% develop bacteremia after the procedure and 5–10% progress to severe sepsis/septic shock.

REFERENCES

1. Nicolle LE, Bradley S, Colgan R, et al. Infectious Diseases Society of America guidelines for the diagnosis and treatment of asymptomatic bacteriuria in adults. *Clin Infect Dis*. 2005;40(5):643–654.
2. Zolotor AJ, Carlough MC. Update on prenatal care. *Am Fam Physician*. 2014;89(3):199–208.
3. Nicolle LE. Asymptomatic bacteriuria. *Curr Opin Infect Dis*. 2014;27(1):90–96.
4. Trautner BW, Grigoryan L. Approach to a positive urine culture in a patient without urinary symptoms. *Infect Dis Clin North Am*. 2014;28(1):15–31.
5. Mody L, Juthani-Mehta M. Urinary tract infections in older women: a clinical review. *JAMA*. 2014; 311(8):844–854.
6. Keating GM. Fosfomycin trometamol: a review of its use as a single-dose oral treatment for patients with acute lower urinary tract infections and pregnant women with asymptomatic bacteriuria. *Drugs*. 2013;73(17):1951–1966.

ADDITIONAL READING

- Ragnarsdóttir B, Svanborg C. Susceptibility to acute pyelonephritis or asymptomatic bacteriuria: host-pathogen interaction in urinary tract infections. *Pediatr Nephrol*. 2012;27(11):2017–2029.
- Wing DA, Rumney PJ, Preslicka CW, et al. Daily cranberry juice for the prevention of asymptomatic bacteriuria in pregnancy: a randomized, controlled pilot study. *J Urol*. 2008;180(4):1367–1372.

CODES

ICD10

- N39.0 Urinary tract infection, site not specified
- B96.20 Unsp Escherichia coli as the cause of diseases classd elswhr
- B96.1 Klebsiella pneumoniae as the cause of diseases classd elswhr

CLINICAL PEARLS

- ASB is a common and benign disorder for which treatment is not indicated in most patients.
- The presence of pyuria, leukocyte esterase, and nitrite is common in ASB and not an indication for antimicrobial treatment.
- Antibiotic treatment is indicated for ASB in pregnancy and patients who require urologic procedure in which mucosal bleeding is anticipated.
- Treatment of ASB in other conditions does not decrease the frequency of UTI or improve outcome.
- Overtreatment of ASB may result in negative consequences such as antimicrobial resistance, adverse drug reaction, and unnecessary cost.

BALANITIS, PHIMOSIS, AND PARAPHIMOSIS
James P. Miller, MD

BASICS

DESCRIPTION
- Balanitis:
  - An inflammation of the glans penis
  - Posthitis is an inflammation of the foreskin.
  - Balanitis xerotica obliterans (BXO) is lichen sclerosus of the glans penis (uncommon).
- Phimosis and paraphimosis:
  - Phimosis: tightness of the distal penile foreskin that prevents it from being drawn back from over the glans
  - Paraphimosis: constriction by foreskin of an uncircumcised penis, preventing the foreskin from returning to its position over the glans; occurs after the retracted foreskin becomes swollen and engorged; a urologic emergency
- System(s) affected: renal/urologic; reproductive; skin/exocrine

ALERT
- Recurrent infection and irritations (condom catheters) can lead to phimosis.
- Recurrent balanitis, either chemical or infectious, can lead to an acquired phimosis.
- Inappropriate forced reduction of a physiologic foreskin can lead to chronic scarring and acquired phimosis. Unfortunately, many times done due to instructions from health care providers.

EPIDEMIOLOGY
- Balanitis: predominant age: adult; predominant gender: male only
- Phimosis/paraphimosis: predominant age: infancy and adolescence; unusual in adults; risk returns in geriatrics; predominant sex: male only

Incidence
Balanitis: will affect 3–11% of males

Prevalence
Phimosis: in the United States: 8% of boys age 6 years and 1% of men >16 years of age (1)

ETIOLOGY AND PATHOPHYSIOLOGY
- Balanitis:
  - Allergic reaction (condom latex, contraceptive jelly)
  - Infections (*Candida albicans*, *Borrelia vincentii*, streptococci, *Trichomonas*, HPV)
  - Fixed-drug eruption (sulfa, tetracycline)
  - Plasma cell infiltration (Zoon balanitis)
  - Autodigestion by activated pancreatic transplant exocrine enzymes
- Phimosis:
  - Physiologic: present at birth; resolves spontaneously during the first 2 to 3 years of life through nocturnal erections, which slowly dilate the phimotic ring
  - Acquired: recurrent inflammation, trauma, or infections of the foreskin

- Paraphimosis:
  - Often iatrogenically or inadvertently induced by the foreskin not being pulled back over the glans after voiding, cleaning, cystoscopy, or catheter insertion

Geriatric Considerations
Condom catheters can predispose to balanitis.

Pediatric Considerations
Oral antibiotics predispose male infants to *Candida balanitis*. Inappropriate care of physiologic phimosis can lead to acquired phimosis by repeated forced reduction of the foreskin.

RISK FACTORS
- Balanitis:
  - Presence of foreskin
  - Morbid obesity
  - Poor hygiene
  - Diabetes; probably most common
  - Nursing home environment
  - Condom catheters
  - Chemical irritants
  - Edematous conditions: CHF, nephrosis
- Phimosis:
  - Poor hygiene
  - Diabetes by repeated balanitis
  - Frequent diaper rash in infants
  - Recurrent posthitis
- Paraphimosis:
  - Presence of foreskin
  - Inexperienced health care provider (leaving foreskin retracted after catheter placement)
  - Poor education about care of the foreskin

GENERAL PREVENTION
- Balanitis:
  - Proper hygiene and avoidance of allergens
  - Circumcision
- Phimosis/paraphimosis:
  - If the patient is uncircumcised, appropriate hygiene and care of the foreskin are necessary to prevent phimosis and paraphimosis.

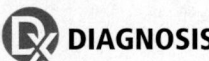

DIAGNOSIS

HISTORY
- Balanitis:
  - Pain
  - Drainage
  - Dysuria
  - Odor
  - Ballooning of foreskin with voiding
  - Redness
- Phimosis:
  - Painful erections
  - Recurrent balanitis
  - Foreskin balloons when voiding
  - Inability to retract foreskin at appropriate age

- Paraphimosis:
  - Uncircumcised
  - Pain
  - Drainage
  - Voiding difficulty

PHYSICAL EXAM
- Balanitis:
  - Erythema
  - Tenderness
  - Edema
  - Discharge
  - Ulceration
  - Plaque
- Phimosis:
  - Foreskin will not retract.
  - Secondary balanitis
  - Physiologic phimosis—preputial orifice appears normal and healthy
  - Pathologic phimosis—preputial orifice has fine white fibrous ring of scar
- Paraphimosis:
  - Edema of prepuce and glans
  - Drainage
  - Ulceration

DIFFERENTIAL DIAGNOSIS
- Balanitis:
  - Leukoplakia
  - Lichen planus
  - Psoriasis
  - Reiter syndrome
  - Lichen sclerosus et atrophicus
  - Erythroplasia of Queyrat
  - BXO: atrophic changes at end of foreskin; can form band that prevents retraction
- Phimosis/paraphimosis:
  - Penile lymphedema, which can be related to insect bites, trauma, or allergic reactions
  - Penile tourniquet syndrome: foreign body around penis, most commonly hair
  - Anasarca

DIAGNOSTIC TESTS & INTERPRETATION
Initial Tests (lab, imaging)
- Microbiology culture
- Wet mount
- Serology for syphilis
- Serum glucose; ESR (if concerns about Reiter syndrome)
- STD testing
- HIV testing
- Gram stain

Diagnostic Procedures/Other
Biopsy, if persistent

Pathologic Findings
Plasma cells infiltration with Zoon balanitis

TREATMENT

GENERAL MEASURES
- Consider circumcision for recurrent balanitis and paraphimosis.
- Warm compresses or sitz baths
- Local hygiene

MEDICATION
- Balanitis:
  - Antifungal:
    - Clotrimazole (Lotrimin) 1% BID
    - Nystatin (Mycostatin) BID–QID
    - Fluconazole: 150 mg PO single dose
- Antibacterial:
  - Bacitracin QID
  - Neomycin–polymyxin B–bacitracin (Neosporin) QID
  - If cellulitis, cephalosporin or sulfa drug PO or parenteral:
    - Dermatitis: topical steroids QID
    - Zoon balanitis: topical steroids QID
- Phimosis:
  - 0.05% fluticasone propionate daily for 4 to 8 weeks with gradual traction placed on foreskin (2)[B]
  - 1% pimecrolimus BID for 4 to 6 weeks. Not for use in children <2 years (3)[C].
- Paraphimosis:
  - Manual reduction, if possible (should be done with the patient sedated). Place the middle and index fingers of both hands on the engorged skin proximal to the glans. Place both thumbs on glans and, with gentle pressure, push on the glans and pull on the foreskin to attempt reduction. If unsuccessful, a dorsal slit will be necessary, with eventual circumcision after the edema resolves.
- Osmotic agents: granulated sugar placed on edematous tissue for several hours to reduce edema
- Puncture technique: Multiple punctures of foreskin with a 21-gauge needle will allow edematous fluid to escape and thus allow reduction.
- Dorsal slit; done by surgeon or urologist
- BXO:
  - 0.05% betamethasone BID
  - 0.1% tacrolimus BID

ISSUES FOR REFERRAL
Recurrent infections or development of meatal stenosis

SURGERY/OTHER PROCEDURES
- Balanitis and phimosis: Consider circumcision as preventive measure.
- For paraphimosis:
  - Represents a true surgical emergency to avoid necrosis of glans
  - Dorsal slit with delayed circumcision, if reduction is not possible
  - Operative exploration if the possibility of penile tourniquet syndrome cannot be eliminated. Hair removal cream can be applied if a hair is thought to be the cause of the tourniquet.

INPATIENT CONSIDERATIONS
Admission Criteria/Initial Stabilization
- Uncontrolled diabetes
- Sepsis

Nursing
Appropriate hygiene if condom catheters are used

Discharge Criteria
Resolution of problem

ONGOING CARE

FOLLOW-UP RECOMMENDATIONS
Patient Monitoring
Balanitis:
- Every 1 to 2 weeks until etiology has been established
- Persistent balanitis may require biopsy to rule out malignancy or BXO.
- Evaluation for resolution of phimosis

DIET
Weight reduction, if obese

PATIENT EDUCATION
- Need for appropriate hygiene
- Appropriate foreskin care
- Avoidance of known allergens
- No sexual activity for 2 to 3 weeks after circumcision

PROGNOSIS
Should resolve with appropriate treatment

COMPLICATIONS
- Meatal stenosis
- Premalignant changes from chronic irritation
- UTIs
- Acquired phimosis
- Unreducible paraphimosis can lead to gangrene
- Posthitis (inflammation of the prepuce)

REFERENCES
1. Oster J. Further fate of the foreskin. Incidence of preputial adhesions, phimosis, and smegma among Danish schoolboys. *Arch Dis Child*. 1968;43(228):200–203.
2. Zavras N, Christianakis E, Mpourikas D, et al. Conservative treatment of phimosis with fluticasone proprionate 0.05%: a clinical study in 1185 boys. *J Pediatr Urol*. 2009;5(3):181–185.
3. Georgala S, Gregoriou S, Georgala C, et al. Pimecrolimus 1% cream in non-specific inflammatory recurrent balanitis. *Dermatology*. 2007;215(3):209–212.

ADDITIONAL READING
- Kiss A, Csontai A, Pirót L, et al. The response of balanitis xerotica obliterans to local steroid application compared with placebo in children. *J Urol*. 2001;165(1):219–220.
- Palmer LS, Palmer JS. The efficacy of topical betamethasone for treating phimosis: a comparison of two treatment regimens. *Urology*. 2008;72(1):68–71.
- Pandher BS, Rustin MH, Kaisary AV. Treatment of balanitis xerotica obliterans with topical tacrolimus. *J Urol*. 2003;170(3):923.
- Stary A, Soeltz-Szoets J, Ziegler C, et al. Comparison of the efficacy and safety of oral fluconazole and topical clotrimazole in patients with candida balanitis. *Genitourin Med*. 1996;72(2):98–102.

 SEE ALSO

Reactive Arthritis (Reiter Syndrome)

CODES

ICD10
- N48.1 Balanitis
- N47.1 Phimosis
- N48.0 Leukoplakia of penis

CLINICAL PEARLS
- Balanitis is an inflammation of the glans penis. Posthitis is an inflammation of the foreskin. BXO is lichen sclerosus of the glans penis.
- With recurrent infections and a plaque, a biopsy should be done to rule out BXO or malignancy.
- If there is a true phimosis that interferes with appropriate hygiene, treat the phimosis with steroids or circumcision to help with hygiene.

BAROTRAUMA OF THE MIDDLE EAR, SINUSES, AND LUNG
Stephen L. Cook, MD • J. David Honeycutt, MD, FAAFP, FAWM

 BASICS

DESCRIPTION
- Barotrauma is tissue damage resulting from the direct effects of pressure changes or imbalances between ambient pressure and pressure within an enclosed body cavity.
- Body cavities at greatest risk for barotrauma
  - Middle ear (otic barotrauma)
  - Paranasal sinuses (sinus barotrauma)
  - Lungs (pulmonary barotrauma)
- Dental barotrauma
  - Dental work can create small pockets of air, which can damage teeth in scuba divers or aviators during ambient pressure changes.
- Synonym(s): dysbarism; aerotitis; otitic barotrauma; middle ear barotrauma; barotitis; barosinusitis

ALERT
- Dizziness and sensorineural hearing loss warrant immediate ENT referral for inner ear involvement.
- Valsalva maneuver can spread nasopharyngeal infection into the middle ear.

EPIDEMIOLOGY
Incidence
- Pulmonary barotrauma is second only to drowning as a leading cause of death among divers.
- Pulmonary barotrauma affects 2–3% of mechanically ventilated patients (1).
- Otic barotrauma is common in air travel, particularly among flight personnel (2).

Pediatric Considerations
- Children have difficulty opening the eustachian tube and commonly develop upper respiratory infections. This combination results in higher risk for otic and sinus barotraumas with smaller pressure changes than adults.
- Mechanical ventilation of neonates is associated with barotrauma and contributes to bronchopulmonary dysplasia.

Pregnancy Considerations
Increased nasal congestion in pregnancy increases the risk of barotitis media (barotrauma of the middle ear).

ETIOLOGY AND PATHOPHYSIOLOGY
- Boyle law relating volume and pressure of gases applies to all forms of barotrauma. When gas is trapped in a confined space, such as the middle ear, paranasal sinus, or lungs, a sudden decrease in ambient pressure causes expansion of the gas within the cavity.
- Otalgia (earache) and hearing loss occur as a result of stretching and deformation of the tympanic membrane.
- Sudden pressure differentials between middle and inner ear may lead to rupture of the round or oval window. This can create a labyrinthine fistula, which consequently can allow leakage of perilymph. Damage to inner ear may be permanent.
- When the transalveolar pressure disrupts the structural integrity of the alveolus, the alveolar wall can rupture, leading to interstitial emphysema, pneumothorax, or pneumomediastinum.
- Otic and sinus barotrauma:
  - Associated with rapid or extreme changes in ambient pressure: air travel, mountain climbing, scuba diving
    - Nasal congestion or eustachian tube dysfunction increases risk of damage.
  - Failure of eustachian tube to equilibrate pressure may distort the tympanic membrane, causing discomfort or rupture.
  - Rupture of round or oval membrane may cause inner ear barotrauma, vertigo, and sensorineural hearing loss.
- Pulmonary barotrauma
  - Iatrogenic complication of mechanical ventilation or hyperbaric oxygen treatment
  - Complication of rapid ascent or descent during scuba diving

RISK FACTORS
- Otic or sinus
  - Participation in high-risk activities without adequate pressure equilibration
    - Scuba diving, especially with rapid ascent or breath-holding
    - Airplane flight
    - Sky diving
    - High-altitude travel
    - High-impact sports: boxing, soccer, water skiing
  - Upper respiratory infections
  - Nasal congestion or allergic rhinitis
  - Eustachian tube dysfunction
  - Blast exposure
  - The most common complication of hyperbaric oxygen treatment is middle ear barotrauma, which can lead to permanent hearing loss and vertigo.
  - Pregnancy (associated nasal congestion)
  - Anatomic obstruction in the nasopharynx
    - Deviated nasal septum
    - Nasal polyps
    - Congenital anomalies, including cleft palate
  - Previous history of ear trauma
- Pulmonary
  - Iatrogenic:
    - Mechanical ventilation, especially in the presence of asthma, chronic interstitial lung disease, acute respiratory distress syndrome
    - Hyperbaric oxygen therapy
  - Scuba diving or other underwater activities
  - Air travel with preexisting pulmonary pathology

GENERAL PREVENTION
- Pulmonary barotrauma
  - Cautious use of mechanical ventilation, employing lung-protective vent settings (lower end-inspiratory airway pressures, lower tidal volumes of 6 mL/kg, higher positive end-expiratory pressures of 6 to 12 cm H_2O) (1)[A]
  - Cautious use of hyperbaric oxygen therapy
  - Avoid breath holding during ascent while scuba diving.
- Otic barotrauma
  - Avoid altitude changes or scuba diving with eustachian tube dysfunction.
  - Treat upper respiratory congestion.
- Equilibration of pressure: Valsalva maneuver, yawning, swallowing, drinking, or chewing gum

 DIAGNOSIS

HISTORY
- History of high-risk activity
- Otic (middle ear) barotrauma:
  - Otalgia, sensation of fullness or pressure in the ear
  - Hearing loss
  - Vertigo
  - Transient facial paralysis
  - Otorrhea
- All patients with middle ear barotrauma should be evaluated for inner ear barotrauma:
  - Hearing loss
  - Tinnitus
  - Vertigo
  - Disorientation
- Sinus barotrauma
  - Facial pain, sensation of fullness or pressure
- Pulmonary barotrauma: Ask about scuba diving, mechanical ventilation, air travel with preexisting lung disease:
  - Chest pain
  - Dyspnea
  - Shortness of breath
  - Hemoptysis

PHYSICAL EXAM
- Otic barotrauma
  - Otoscopic exam: otorrhea, pneumotoscopy
  - Assess balance and hearing.
  - Palpate eustachian tube for tenderness.
- Otic (middle ear) barotrauma
  - Conductive hearing loss with Weber and Rinne tests
  - Transient facial paralysis
- All patients with middle ear barotrauma should be evaluated for inner ear barotrauma:
  - Sensorineural hearing loss with Weber and Rinne tests
- Sinus barotrauma
  - Facial tenderness
- Pulmonary barotrauma
  - Hypoxia, hypotension
  - Auscultation, percussion
  - Assessment of respiratory distress

DIFFERENTIAL DIAGNOSIS
- Acute and chronic otitis media
- Otitis externa
- Temporomandibular joint syndrome
- Pulmonary: pulmonary embolism; complications of mechanical ventilation

DIAGNOSTIC TESTS & INTERPRETATION
Initial Tests (lab, imaging)
- Otic or sinus
  - CT to rule out underlying pathology, if suspected
    - Nasopharyngeal tumor (if enlarging facial/neck mass with or without nasal obstruction, recurrent epistaxis)
    - Chronic sinus disease (sinus pain, pressure, fullness, chronic posterior nasal drip/congestion)

- Pulmonary
  - Chest radiograph
  - Chest CT if unclear diagnosis by CXR
  - Arterial blood gases (ABG)
- Other: ultrasound

Diagnostic Procedures/Other
- Otic barotrauma
  - Tympanometry
  - Audiometry: conductive (middle ear) versus sensorineural (inner ear) hearing loss
  - Surgical exploration to rule out inner ear involvement, if suspected
- Pulmonary barotrauma: chest tube insertion, if clinically indicated, for pneumothorax

Test Interpretation
- Tympanic membrane (TM) retraction or bulging
  - Teed 0: no visible damage
  - Teed 1: congestion around umbo
  - Teed 2: congestion of entire TM
  - Teed 3: hemorrhage into middle ear
  - Teed 4: extensive middle ear hemorrhage; TM may rupture.
  - Teed 5: entire middle ear filled with deoxygenated blood
- Inner ear involvement with rupture of the round or oval windows, perilymphatic fistula, and leakage of perilymph into the middle ear
- Pulmonary barotrauma
  - Alveolar rupture may progress to interstitial emphysema, pneumoperitoneum, and pneumothorax.
- Petechial hemorrhages in area covered by diver's mask, as well as subconjunctival hemorrhages

 TREATMENT

GENERAL MEASURES
- Prevention/avoidance is best: Avoid flying or diving when risk factors are present.
- Autoinflate the eustachian tube during pressure changes (3)[B].
  - Valsalva during ascent and descent in air travel
  - Infants: breastfeeding, pacifier use, or bottle feed
  - ≥4 years: chewing gum
  - ≥8 years: blowing up a balloon
  - Adults: chewing gum, swallowing, or yawning
- The nasal balloon is effective for prevention (4)[B].
- Pressure-equalizing earplugs are not recommended in air travel and do not prevent ear barotrauma (5)[B].
- For inner ear barotrauma
  - Bed rest with head elevated to avoid leakage of perilymph
  - Tympanotomy and repair of round or oval window may be necessary.
  - Sudden or progressive sensorineural hearing loss accompanied by dizziness following barotrauma should prompt consideration of a perilymph fistula. Early surgical exploration is recommended to improve hearing and vestibular symptoms (6)[C].
- Lung protective settings during mechanical ventilation (1)[A]
  - Acute lung injury: NNT = 16
  - Lung injury: NNT = 11

- Treatment of pneumothorax
  - Removal of air from pleural space (chest tube; Heimlich valve)
- Correct iatrogenic cause (e.g., adjustment of mechanical ventilation).

MEDICATION
- Treat predisposing conditions (e.g., upper respiratory congestion prior to air travel):
  - Oral decongestants
  - Nasal decongestants
  - Antihistamines
- Antibiotics are not indicated for middle ear effusion secondary to barotrauma.
- Analgesics for pain control

ISSUES FOR REFERRAL
- Refer to otolaryngology if inner ear is exposed, perilymphatic fistula is present, or sensorineural hearing loss is experienced.
- Consult with a hyperbaric specialist if recompression is required.
- Chest tube placement

SURGERY/OTHER PROCEDURES
- If necessary, myringotomy or tympanoplasty
- Tympanotomy and repair of round or oval window may be necessary for inner ear barotrauma.
- Tube thoracostomy for persistent pneumothorax

INPATIENT CONSIDERATIONS
Admission Criteria/Initial Stabilization
- Patients with complicating emergencies (e.g., incapacitating pain requiring myringotomy, large tympanic perforation requiring tympanoplasty)
- Inner ear barotrauma with hearing loss
- Management of pneumothorax

 ONGOING CARE

FOLLOW-UP RECOMMENDATIONS
- No flying or diving until complete resolution of all signs and symptoms and Valsalva maneuver succeeds in equalizing pressure
- Complete bed rest for inner ear barotrauma
- No high-risk activities or air travel until pneumothorax is completely resolved

Patient Monitoring
- Repeat physical examination until symptoms are clear.
- Audiograms and tympanometry if tympanic rupture

PATIENT EDUCATION
- Demonstrate proper Valsalva maneuver.
- Appropriately treat sinus infections.
- American Academy of Pediatrics travel safety tips: https://www.aap.org/en-us/about-the-aap/aap-press-room/news-features-and-safety-tips/Pages/travel-safety-tips.aspx.
- Divers Alert Network of Duke University Medical Center information line: (919) 684-2948

PROGNOSIS
- Mild barotitis media may resolve spontaneously.
- Tympanic rupture takes weeks to months for healing.
- Hearing loss may be permanent in barotitis externa.
- Prognosis of pulmonary barotrauma depends on the extent of underlying pathology.

COMPLICATIONS
- Permanent hearing loss
- Ruptured tympanic membrane
- Chronic tinnitus, vertigo
- Fluid exudate in middle ear
- Perilymphatic fistula
- Sensorineural hearing loss

REFERENCES
1. Sutherasan Y, Vargas M, Pelosi P. Protective mechanical ventilation in the non-injured lung: review and meta-analysis. Crit Care. 2014;18(2):211.
2. Morgagni F, Autore A, Landolfi A, et al. Predictors of ear barotrauma in aircrews exposed to simulated high altitude. Aviat Space Environ Med. 2012;83(6):594–597.
3. Stangerup SE, Klokker M, Vesterhauge S, et al. Point prevalence of barotitis and its prevention and treatment with nasal balloon inflation: a prospective, controlled study. Otol Neurotol. 2004;25(2):89–94.
4. Landolfi A, Autore A, Torchia F, et al. Ear pain after breathing oxygen at altitude: prevalence and prevention of delayed barotrauma. Aviat Space Environ Med. 2010;81(2):130–132.
5. Klokker M, Vesterhauge S, Jansen EC. Pressure-equalizing earplugs do not prevent barotrauma on descent from 8000 ft cabin altitude. Aviat Space Environ Med. 2005;76(11):1079–1082.
6. Park GY, Byun H, Moon IJ, et al. Effects of early surgical exploration in suspected barotraumatic perilymph fistulas. Clin Exp Otorhinolaryngol. 2012;5(2):74–80.

 SEE ALSO

Algorithm: Ear Pain

 CODES

ICD10
- T70.0XXA Otitic barotrauma, initial encounter
- T70.1XXA Sinus barotrauma, initial encounter
- T70.29XA Other effects of high altitude, initial encounter

CLINICAL PEARLS
- Small children can equalize eustachian tube pressure by breastfeeding or sucking on bottles or pacifiers. Crying also serves as autoinflation.
- Pulmonary barotrauma is the second leading cause of death among divers.
- Otic barotrauma is common in air travel, especially among flight personnel.
- Pulmonary barotrauma is noted in 2–3% of mechanically ventilated patients.
- Sudden or progressive sensorineural hearing loss accompanied by dizziness following barotrauma suggests a perilymphatic fistula. Early surgical exploration is recommended to preserve hearing and vestibular functions.

BARRETT ESOPHAGUS

Eric Ji-Yuan Mao, MD • Harlan G. Rich, MD, FACP, AGAF

 BASICS

DESCRIPTION
- Metaplasia of the distal esophageal mucosa from native stratified squamous epithelium to abnormal columnar (intestinalized) epithelium, likely as a consequence of chronic GERD
- Predisposes to the development of adenocarcinoma of the esophagus

EPIDEMIOLOGY
- Predominant age: >50 years
- May occur in children (rare <5 years)

Incidence
- 10–15% of patients undergoing endoscopy for evaluation of reflux symptoms (1)
- Esophageal adenocarcinoma incidence is rising in the United States (1,2). From 1975 to 2001, there was nearly a 6-fold increase from 4 to 23 cases per million person-years.
- Attributed to changes in smoking and obesity rather than reclassification or overdiagnosis

Prevalence
- Difficult to ascertain because of different populations studied, varying definitions, and asymptomatic cases
- As many as 1.5 to 2.0 million adults in the United States (extrapolated from a 1.6% prevalence in Swedish general population) (1)

ETIOLOGY AND PATHOPHYSIOLOGY
- Chronic gastric reflux injures the esophageal mucosa, triggering columnar metaplasia. Refluxed bile acids likely induce differentiation in gastroesophageal junction (GEJ) cells.
- Columnar cells in the esophagus have higher malignant potential than squamous cells. Activation of *CDX2* gene and overexpression of HER2/neu (ERBB2) oncogene promotes carcinogenesis.
- Elevated levels of COX-2, a mediator of inflammation and regulator of epithelial cell growth, are associated with Barrett esophagus (2).
- Classic progression: normal epithelium → esophagitis → metaplasia (Barrett esophagus) → dysplasia (low- or high-grade) → adenocarcinoma

Genetics
- Familial predisposition to GERD and Barrett esophagus and multiple genetic markers have been identified.
- Acquired genetic changes lead to adenocarcinoma and are being investigated as biomarkers for risk stratification and early detection.

RISK FACTORS
- Chronic reflux (>5 years)
- Hiatal hernia
- Age >50
- Male gender
- White ethnicity—incidence in white males is much higher than white women and African American men
- Smoking history
- Intra-abdominal obesity
- Family history with at least one first-degree relative with Barrett esophagus or esophageal adenocarcinoma

GENERAL PREVENTION
Weight loss, smoking cessation, robust dietary intake of fruits and vegetables, and moderate wine consumption may decrease risk of Barrett esophagus and lower progression to esophageal cancer (3)[C].

COMMONLY ASSOCIATED CONDITIONS
GERD, obesity, hiatal hernia

 DIAGNOSIS

HISTORY
- Assess underlying risk factors.
- Common GERD symptoms: heartburn, regurgitation
- Less common symptoms include chest pain, odynophagia, chronic cough, water brash, globus sensation, laryngitis, or wheezing.
- Symptoms suggestive of complicated GERD or cancer include weight loss, anorexia, dysphagia, odynophagia, hematemesis, or melena.

ALERT
Up to 25% of patients with Barrett esophagus are asymptomatic (2).

PHYSICAL EXAM
No abnormal findings on physical exam are specific for Barrett esophagus. Perform a general physical examination including vital signs, oral examination, cardiopulmonary examination, abdominal examination, and lymph node examination.

DIFFERENTIAL DIAGNOSIS
- Erosive esophagitis
- GERD

DIAGNOSTIC TESTS & INTERPRETATION
Endoscopy with multiple biopsies for histologic examination are required to diagnose Barrett esophagus.
- Gastric fundic-type epithelium on pathology does not have clear malignant significance and may reflect sampling error.
- Specialized intestinal metaplasia at the GEJ: cancer risk difficult to assess with varying definitions of GEJ landmarks

ALERT
Screening for Barrett esophagus in the general population with GERD is **not** recommended. However, endoscopic screening for Barrett esophagus is suggested in men >60 years old with prolonged GERD symptoms (≥10 years) (4)[C].

Initial Tests (lab, imaging)
None:
- *Helicobacter pylori* testing is *not* indicated. Meta-analyses show an inverse relationship between *H. pylori* infections and Barrett esophagus, which may be related to decreased acid production (5)[C].
- No biomarkers are currently effective for diagnosis; many are under investigation for risk stratification (1),(3)[B].

Diagnostic Procedures/Other
- Endoscopy: visual identification of columnar epithelium (reddish, velvety appearance) replacing the squamous lining of the distal esophagus
- Disease extent: Long-segment (≥3 cm) versus short-segment (<3 cm)
- The Prague C (circumference) and M (maximum extent) criteria is a consensus-driven grading system used to describe Barrett esophagus using landmarks of the squamocolumnar junction, GEJ, extent of circumferential columnar lining, and extent of proximal extension of columnar mucosa.
  – White light endoscopy (preferably high resolution) is the standard for diagnosis.

- Advanced imaging techniques, such as narrow band imaging (NBI) and confocal laser endomicroscopy, may help identify dysplasia but are preliminary (1)[A].
- Systematic biopsies from endoscopy showing columnar epithelium confirm the diagnosis:
  – Seattle protocol: four-quadrant biopsies at regular intervals with additional biopsies of visible mucosal irregularities; more time-consuming but higher diagnostic yield than random biopsies (3)[A]
  – Capsule endoscopy is still developing and has lower sensitivity than conventional endoscopy (6)[B].

Test Interpretation
- Specialized intestinal metaplasia (also called specialized columnar epithelium) is diagnostic: Benign Barrett esophagus diagnosis is established by a single pathologist report (4)[C].
- Diagnosis of dysplasia (and grade) should be confirmed by two specialist gastrointestinal pathologists before treatment (4)[C].
- Cardia-type columnar epithelium may predispose to malignancy (unclear risk); International Consensus Group currently recommends defining Barrett esophagus by the presence of columnar mucosa in the esophagus with modifier of whether intestinal metaplasia is present. (4)[C].

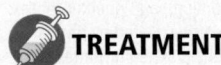 **TREATMENT**

ALERT
Neither suppression of gastric acid production via high-dose proton pump inhibitors (PPIs) nor reduction in esophageal acid exposure via antireflux surgery induces regression of Barrett esophagus. These therapies may, however, decrease cancer risk.

MEDICATION
- The goal of medical therapy is to control GERD to reduce esophagitis.
- Therapy usually does not result in reversal of Barrett esophagus but may decrease risk of progression to cancer (1,2)[A],(6,7)[B].

First Line
- Unlike the stepwise management of GERD without evidence of Barrett esophagus, patients with Barrett esophagus and GERD symptoms should be treated initially with a once-daily PPI.
- PPIs should be dosed 30 minutes before a meal (ideally, the first meal of the day).

ALERT
PPI therapy should be titrated to symptoms; pH monitoring is **not** recommended (1,2)[C].

- Chemoprevention of neoplastic progression is under active investigation.
- Case-controlled studies have shown that aspirin, and NSAIDs may prevent progression to esophageal cancer due to COX-2 inhibition:
  – COX-2 selective inhibitor celecoxib use not shown to affect progression of Barrett dysplasia to adenocarcinoma (2)[A].
  – Use of aspirin and a PPI for chemoprevention of esophageal cancer is under investigation (1–3).
  – Consider low-dose aspirin in patients with Barrett esophagus who also have risk factors for cardiovascular disease (2)[C].

- Statins, alone or in combination with aspirin or NSAIDs, appear to be effective in chemoprevention but are not yet routinely recommended (3)[B],(8)[A].

Second Line
If once-daily PPI does not control symptoms, move to twice-daily dosing (6)[A].

ISSUES FOR REFERRAL
- Initiate PPI therapy prior to endoscopy to reduce reactive esophagitis/atypia (6)[C].
- Refer patients considering esophagectomy to a high-volume institution.

ADDITIONAL THERAPIES
- Endoscopic eradication is any combination of endoscopic mucosal resection (EMR), photodynamic therapy (PDT), and radiofrequency ablation (RFA) to eliminate all Barrett epithelium.
- EMR: eradication rate 86–100%, excision to submucosa, allows staging, preferred for visible irregularities
- PDT: eradication rate 77–100% but strictures in 40%
- RFA: eradication rate 54–90%, comparable efficacy to PDT, fewer adverse effects

- Focal EMR combined with RFA of other areas is considered most effective eradication therapy (3)[B].

- Additional studies are still required before cryotherapy and other ablative procedures can be recommended.
- **Barrett esophagus with visible lesions:**
  – EMR with ablation if high-grade dysplasia or intramucosal cancer detected (4)[C]
- **Low-grade dysplasia:** Treatment is controversial.

  – Offer treatment such as RFA for low-grade dysplasia and high-risk features (multifocality, long segment length, persistence) (4)[C]. Endoscopic eradication may prevent progression to high-grade dysplasia or esophageal adenocarcinoma (3)[B],(9)[A].
- Endoscopic eradication therapy is recommended **for High-grade dysplasia**, without or with very limited submucosal invasion (stage T1SM1 or lower by endoscopic ultrasound) (1,2,6)[B].

ALERT
Endoscopic eradication is **not** recommended for Barrett esophagus without dysplasia. Surveillance should be continued in these patients.

SURGERY/OTHER PROCEDURES
Antireflux surgery such as fundoplication may control GERD symptoms but are not convincingly shown to reverse Barrett esophagus, decrease risk of cancer, or be superior to medical therapy (1,2)[A],(6)[B].

ALERT
Available data suggest that antireflux surgery does **not** decrease risk of esophageal cancer.
- Esophagectomy is definitive and should be offered as an alternative to endoscopic eradication therapy for high-grade dysplasia (1,3)[B]:

  – Preferred for patients with evidence of submucosal invasion (stage T1SM2 or higher)
  – Added benefit of lymph node removal
  – Mortality rate: <5% in patients with high-grade dysplasia who are otherwise healthy
  – Serious postoperative complications: 30–50%

  – Should ideally be performed by an experienced surgeon in a high-volume center (2,3)[A]

COMPLEMENTARY & ALTERNATIVE MEDICINE
A prospective study of 339 men and women with Barrett esophagus found those taking either a multivitamin, vitamin C, or vitamin E once a day were less likely to develop esophageal adenocarcinoma (10)[B].

Geriatric Considerations
Surveillance or no treatment may be preferable to endoscopic eradication therapy or esophagectomy in patients who are poor operative candidates.

 ## ONGOING CARE

FOLLOW-UP RECOMMENDATIONS
- Surveillance (to detect high-grade dysplasia or early carcinoma), while controversial, is recommended in patients with histologically confirmed Barrett-especially for those in high-risk groups.
- Surveillance intervals depend on the grade of dysplasia (3)[C].
- **No dysplasia**: 3 to 5 years
  – Discontinue surveillance if life expectancy is ≤5 years (4)[C].
- **Low-grade dysplasia**: 6 to 12 months
  – Routine surveillance if patients have confirmed absence of low-grade dysplasia after two consecutive endoscopies (4)[C]
- **Indefinite for dysplasia**: within 1 year
  – Increase acid suppression (4)[C].
- **High-grade dysplasia without eradication therapy**: 3 months

ALERT
- Adherence to recommended surveillance protocols may improve rates of dysplasia and cancer detection.
- Continue surveillance even if the patient has had endoscopic ablation therapy, antireflux surgery, or esophagectomy.

DIET
Avoid foods that can trigger reflux: caffeine, alcohol, chocolate, peppermint, carbonated drinks, garlic, onions, spicy foods, fatty foods, citrus, and tomato-based products.

PATIENT EDUCATION
- Lifestyle modifications: smoking cessation, weight loss, avoid supine position after meals, avoid tight-fitting clothes, elevate head of bed
- No evidence that treating GERD reverses Barrett esophagus or prevents esophageal cancer.

PROGNOSIS
Annual incidence of esophageal cancer in patients with Barrett esophagus is ≤0.33% per year (2,3)[B]:

- Low-grade dysplasia: may be transient; cancer risk 0.5–0.6% per year
- High-grade dysplasia: cancer risk 5–7% per year

COMPLICATIONS
Same as GERD: stricture, bleeding, ulceration

REFERENCES
1. Sharma P. Clinical practice. Barrett's esophagus. *N Engl J Med.* 2009;361(26):2548–2556.
2. Spechler SJ, Sharma P, Souza RF, et al. American Gastroenterological Association technical review on the management of Barrett's esophagus. *Gastroenterology.* 2011;140(3):e18–e52.
3. Spechler SJ, Sharma P, Souza RF, et al. American Gastroenterological Association medical position statement on the management of Barrett's esophagus. *Gastroenterology.* 2011;140(3):1084–1091.
4. Bennett C, Moayyedi P, Corley DA, et al. BOB CAT: a large-scale review and delphi consensus for management of Barrett's esophagus with no dysplasia, indefinite for, or low-grade dysplasia. *Am J Gastroenterol.* 2015;110(5):662–682.
5. Fischbach LA, Nordenstedt H, Kramer JR, et al. The association between Barrett's esophagus and *Helicobacter pylori* infection: a meta-analysis. *Helicobacter.* 2012;17(3):163–175.
6. Wang KK, Sampliner RE. Updated guidelines 2008 for the diagnosis, surveillance and therapy of Barrett's esophagus. *Am J Gastroenterol.* 2008;103(3):788–797.
7. Singh S, Garg SK, Singh PP, et al. Acid-suppressive medications and risk of oesophageal adenocarcinoma in patients with Barrett's oesophagus: a systematic review and meta-analysis. *Gut.* 2014;63(8):1229–1237.
8. Kastelein F, Spaander MC, Biermann K, et al. Nonsteroidal anti-inflammatory drugs and statins have chemopreventative effects in patients with Barrett's esophagus. *Gastroenterology.* 2011;141(6):2000–2008.
9. Phoa KN, van Vilsteren FG, Weusten BL, et al. Radiofrequency ablation vs endoscopic surveillance for patients with Barrett esophagus and low-grade dysplasia: a randomized clinical trial. *JAMA.* 2014;311(12):1209–1217.
10. Dong LM, Kristal AR, Peters U, et al. Dietary supplement use and risk of neoplastic progression in esophageal adenocarcinoma: a prospective study. *Nutr Cancer.* 2008;60(1):39–48.

ADDITIONAL READING
- Dunbar KB, Spechler SJ. Controversies in Barrett esophagus. *Mayo Clin Proc.* 2014;89(7):973–984.
- Zimmerman TG. Common questions about Barrett esophagus. *Am Fam Physician.* 2014;89(2):92–98.

 ## CODES

ICD10
- K22.70 Barrett's esophagus without dysplasia
- K22.719 Barrett's esophagus with dysplasia, unspecified
- K22.710 Barrett's esophagus with low grade dysplasia

CLINICAL PEARLS
- The incidence of esophageal carcinoma is rising faster than any other major malignancy. Barrett esophagus is a known precursor.
- Highest incidence is among white males >50 years.
- Endoscopic eradication therapy is preferred for high-grade dysplasia with or without submucosal invasion.
- Esophagectomy offers definitive therapy: Consider for all patients with high-grade dysplasia; preferred for patients with submucosal invasion.
- Promising areas for future research include the use of biomarkers for risk stratification, chemoprevention of neoplastic progression, capsule endoscopy for screening and the use of vitamins and antioxidants for prevention and treatment.

BASAL CELL CARCINOMA

William Farkas, DO, CPT, MC, USA • Sean R. Wise, MD

 BASICS

DESCRIPTION

Basal cell carcinoma (BCC) is the most common cancer, originating from the basal cell layer of the skin appendages.

- Rarely metastasizes but capable of local tissue destruction

Geriatric Considerations

Greater frequency in geriatric patients (ages 55 to 75 years have 100 times the incidence when compared with those aged <20 years)

Pediatric Considerations

- Rare in children, but childhood radiation treatment is contributory, as are frequent or severe sunburns.
- The Centers for Disease Control and Prevention recommend against using tanning beds and lamps in their guidelines for cancer prevention in school-age children.

EPIDEMIOLOGY

Worldwide, the most common form of cancer

Incidence

- Incidence in the United States: with squamous cell carcinoma, over 2 million cases each year. 4 to 5 times more common than squamous cell carcinoma.
- Predominant age: generally >40 years, although incidence increasing in younger populations
- Predominant sex: male > female (2:1 ratio)

ETIOLOGY AND PATHOPHYSIOLOGY

- UV-induced inflammation and cyclooxygenase activation in skin
- In chromosome 9q22, mutation of *PTCH1* (patched homolog 1), a tumor-suppressor gene that inhibits the hedgehog signaling pathway
- UV-induced mutations of the *TP53* (tumor protein 53), a tumor-suppressor gene
- Activation of *BCL2*, an antiapoptosis proto-oncogene

Genetics

- Several genetic conditions increase the risk of developing BCC:
  - Albinism (recessive alleles)
  - Xeroderma pigmentosum (autosomal recessive)
  - Bazex syndrome (rare, X-linked dominant)
  - Nevoid BCC syndrome/Gorlin syndrome (rare, autosomal dominant)
  - Cytochrome P-450 CYP2D6 and glutathione S-transferase detoxifying enzyme gene mutations (especially in truncal BCC, marked by clusters of BCCs and a younger age of onset)

RISK FACTORS

- Chronic sun exposure (UV radiation). Most common in the following phenotypes
  - Light complexion: skin type I (burns but does not tan) and skin type II (usually burns, sometimes tans)
  - Red or blond hair
  - Blue or green eyes
- Tendency to sunburn

- Male sex, although increasing risk in women due to lifestyle changes, such as tanning beds
- History of nonmelanoma skin cancer
  - After initial diagnosis of skin cancer, 35% risk of new nonmelanoma skin cancer at 3 years and 50% at 5 years
- Family history of skin cancer
- 3 to 4 decades after chronic arsenic exposure
- 2 decades after therapeutic radiation
- Chronic immunosuppression: transplant recipients (10 times higher incidence), patients with HIV or lymphomas

GENERAL PREVENTION

- Use broad-spectrum sunscreens of at least SPF 30 daily and reapply after swimming or sweating.
- Avoid overexposure to the sun by seeking shade between 10 AM and 4 PM, and wearing wide-brimmed hats and long-sleeved shirts.
- The American Cancer Society recommends cancer related checkups every 3 years in patients 20 to 40 years old, and yearly in patients older than 40 years.

COMMONLY ASSOCIATED CONDITIONS

- Cosmetic disfigurement because head and neck most often affected
- Loss of vision with orbital involvement
- Loss of nerve function due to perineural spread or extensive and deep invasion
- Ulcerating neoplasms are prone to infections.

 DIAGNOSIS

HISTORY

Exposure to risk factors, family history

PHYSICAL EXAM

- 80% on face and neck, 20% on trunk and lower limbs (mostly women)
- Nodular: most common (60%); presents as pinkish, pearly papule, plaque, or nodule, often with telangiectatic vessels, ulceration, and a rolled periphery usually on face (1)
  - Pigmented: presents as a translucent papule with "floating pigment"; more commonly seen in darker skin types; may give a blue, brown, or black appearance and be confused with melanoma (1)
- Superficial: 30%; light red, scaly plaque resembling eczema or psoriasis, but with raised, pearly white borders similar to the nodular subtype, usually on trunk or extremities; least invasive of BCC subtypes
- Morpheaform: 5–10%; resembles localized scleroderma; mass is ill-defined and often extends beyond visible lesion.

DIFFERENTIAL DIAGNOSIS

- Sebaceous hyperplasia
- Epidermal inclusion cyst
- Intradermal nevi (pigmented and nonpigmented)
- Molluscum contagiosum
- Squamous cell carcinoma (SCC)
- Nummular dermatitis

- Psoriasis
- Melanoma (pigmented lesions)
- Atypical fibroxanthoma
- Rare adnexal neoplasms

DIAGNOSTIC TESTS & INTERPRETATION

Diagnostic Procedures/Other

- Clinical diagnosis and histologic subtype are confirmed through skin biopsy and pathologic examination.
- Shave biopsy is typically sufficient; however, punch biopsy is more useful to assess depth of tumor and perineural invasion.
- If a genetic disorder is suspected, additional tests may be needed to confirm it.

Test Interpretation

- Nodular BCC
  - Extending from the epidermis are nodular aggregates of basaloid cells.
  - Tumor cells are uniform; rarely have mitotic figures; large, oval, hyperchromatic nuclei with little cytoplasm, surrounded by a peripheral palisade
  - Early lesions are usually connected to the epidermis, unlike late lesions.
  - Increased mucin in dermal stroma
    - Cleft formation (retraction artifact) common between BCC "nests" and stroma due to mucin shrinkage during fixation and staining
- Superficial BCC
  - Appear as buds of basaloid cells attached to undersurface of epidermis
  - Peripheral palisading
- Morpheaform BCC
  - Thin cords and strands of basaloid cells; embedded in dense, fibrous, scar-like stroma
  - Less peripheral palisading and retraction, greater subclinical involvement
- Infiltrating BCC
  - Like morpheaform BCC but no scar-like stroma and thicker, more spiky, irregular strands
  - Less peripheral palisading and retraction, greater subclinical involvement
- Micronodular BCC
  - Small, nodular aggregates of tumor cells
  - Less retraction artifact and higher subclinical involvement than nodular BCC

 TREATMENT

MEDICATION

- May be especially useful in those who cannot tolerate surgical procedures and in those who refuse to have surgery, as well as for low risk superficial and/or nodular BCC
- 5-fluorouracil cream inhibits thymidylate synthetase, interrupting DNA synthesis for superficial lesions in low-risk areas; primary treatment only; 5% applied BID for 3 to 10 weeks.

- Imiquimod (Aldara) cream approved for treatment of low-risk superficial BCC; daily dosing for 6 to 12 weeks; 90% histologic cure (1,2)[A]
- Neither imiquimod nor 5-FU is considered appropriate primary monotherapy for infiltrative or nodular BCC (1)[A].
- Topical treatment failure may yield skip lesions that yield false negative margins, making Mohs and excisional surgery potentially less effective (1)[A].

- Emerging therapies:
  - Vismodegib, a sonic hedgehog pathway inhibitor; for patients with advanced BCC when other options are exhausted; not considered appropriate therapy for low-risk tumors (1)[A].
  - Intralesional IFN-a-2B injection: some efficacy for small (<1 cm) nodular and superficial BCCs; relatively high cost, and frequent side effects (1,3)[A]

ADDITIONAL THERAPIES
- Radiation therapy
  - Useful for patients, typically older, who cannot or will not undergo surgery (1)[C]
  - Used following surgery, particularly if margins of tumor were not cleared
  - Cure rate is ~90%.
  - Tumors that recur in areas previously treated with radiation are harder to treat, and the area is more difficult to reconstruct.
  - Local treatment
  - Recurrence rates are 7–8%
- Photodynamic therapy (PDT)
  - 5-aminolevulinic acid, a photosensitizer, is activated by specific wavelengths of light, creating singlet oxygen radicals that destroy local tissue (no damage to surrounding or deep tissues).
  - Useful in areas where tissue preservation is cosmetically or functionally important; considered inferior to surgical excision in terms of efficacy (2)
  - When examining 5-year recurrence rates, may be equivalent to cryotherapy

SURGERY/OTHER PROCEDURES
- Surgical excision is first line treatment (3)[A]; specific treatment selection varies with extent and location of lesion as well as tumor border demarcation.

- High-risk areas
  - Inner canthus, nasolabial sulcus, philtrum, preauricular area, retroauricular sulcus, lip, temple, "mask areas" of the face (2)[C]
- Curettage and electrodesiccation
  - If nodular lesion <1 cm, in low-risk area, not deeply invasive
  - Avoid in the hair-bearing areas due to risk of the tumor extending down follicular structures.
  - 5-year cure rate of 92%; recurrence as high as 27% for high risk lesions
- Excision with postoperative margin assessment
  - Treatment of choice for low risk lesions <2 cm in diameter
  - Goal is 4 mm margin
  - 5-year cure rate of 98%

- Cryosurgery
  - Reserved for nodular and superficial BCC, not indicated for tumors with depth exceeding 3 mm
  - Typically for tumors with low risk of recurrence
  - May want pre- and posttreatment biopsies (2)[C]
  - 5-year cure rate of 99%
- Mohs surgery
  - Preferred microsurgically controlled surgical treatment for lesions in high-risk areas, recurrent lesions, and lesions exhibiting an aggressive growth pattern (1,2)[A]
  - Gold standard for maximizing tissue sparing for functional or cosmetic reasons (1)[A]
  - 5-year survival rate of 99%
  - Requires referral to appropriately trained dermatologic surgeon

INPATIENT CONSIDERATIONS
Outpatient, unless extensive lesion

 # ONGOING CARE

FOLLOW-UP RECOMMENDATIONS
- Avoid sun exposure.
- Oral retinoids may prevent the development of new BCCs in patients with Gorlin syndrome, renal transplant recipients, and patients with severe actinic damage.

Patient Monitoring
- Every 6 to 12 months for life
- Increased risk of other skin cancers
- Recurrence:
  - Local: follow NCCN 2015 guidelines for primary treatment
  - Regional: surgery and/or radiation therapy
  - Metastatic: multidisciplinary tumor board consultation

PATIENT EDUCATION
- Teach patient-appropriate sun-avoidance techniques, sunscreens, and so forth.
- Monthly skin self-exam
- Educate patients concerning adequate vitamin D intake.

PROGNOSIS
- Proper treatment yields 90–95% cure.
- Most recurrences happen within 5 years.
- Development of new BCCs: Some patients (36%) will develop a new lesion within 5 years.

COMPLICATIONS
- Local recurrence and spread
- Usually, recurrences will appear within 5 years.
- Metastasis: rare (<0.1%), but metastatic disease usually fatal within 8 months

REFERENCES
1. Firnhaber JM. Diagnosis and treatment of basal cell and squamous cell carcinoma. *Am Fam Physician*. 2012;86(2):161–168.
2. Clark CM, Furniss M, Mackay-Wiggan JM. Basal cell carcinoma: an evidence-based treatment update. *Am J Clin Dermatol*. 2014;15(3):197–216.
3. Bath-Hextall FJ, Perkins W, Bong J, et al. Interventions for basal carcinoma of the skin. *Cochrane Database Syst Rev*. 2007;(1):CD003412.

ADDITIONAL READING
- Kundu RV, Patterson S. Dermatologic conditions in skin of color: part I. Special considerations for common skin disorders. *Am Fam Physician*. 2013;87(12):850–856.
- Wong CS, Strange RC, Lear JT. Basal cell carcinoma. *BMJ*. 2003;327(7418):794–798.

CODES

ICD10
- C44.91 Basal cell carcinoma of skin, unspecified
- C44.31 Basal cell carcinoma of skin of other and unspecified parts of face
- C44.41 Basal cell carcinoma of skin of scalp and neck

CLINICAL PEARLS
- Nodular: pearly papule, plaque, or nodule often with telangiectatic vessels, ulceration, and a rolled periphery, usually on face
- Pigmented: presents as a translucent papule with "floating pigment"; more commonly seen in darker skin types
- Superficial: scaly papule or plaque with atrophic center, ringed by translucent micropapules, usually on trunk or extremities; more common in men
- Morpheaform: firm, smooth, flesh-colored, scar-like papule or plaque with ill-defined borders
- Use diagnostic keys above to differentiate between BCC and cutaneous SCC. SCC arises from actinic keratosis in 60% of cases and generally presents as an asymptomatic hyperkeratotic lesion. If unsure, biopsy or refer to a specialist.
- Some hyperpigmented BCCs may appear similar to melanoma. Remember the ABCDEs of melanoma recognition: **A**symmetry, **B**order irregularities, **C**olor variability, **D**iameter >6 mm, **E**nlargement. If unsure, refer to a specialist.
- The USPSTF concludes insufficient evidence and recommends for or against routine total body skin exams for melanoma, BCC, or SCC. Exams should be based on risk factors, including exposure and family and prior medical history. All patients should receive education about risks and self-exam.

BED BUGS

Fawn Winkelman, DO • Adam Strosberg, DNP, ARNP-BC

 BASICS

DESCRIPTION
- Nocturnal obligate blood parasites that take refuge on furniture and bedding
- 5 to 7 mm oval, reddish brown, flat, wingless

EPIDEMIOLOGY
Incidence
- According to the 2013 "Bugs Without Borders" survey, bed bug infestations are increasing and continue to remain the most difficult pest to treat, more difficult than cockroaches, termites, and ants (1)[B].
- Resurgence is due to the use of less toxic, less persistent insecticides as well as increased travel, use of secondhand furniture, and a high-turnover rate of residents in hotels.

Prevalence
- Infestations are increasing across the United States.
- Sharp increase in prevalence, as only 11% of survey respondents reported bed bug calls >10 years ago.
- Bed bug encounters have become more common in public places (schools, hospitals, hotels/motels, aircrafts) than in previous years, increasing by 10–30% (2)[B].

ETIOLOGY AND PATHOPHYSIOLOGY
- Insect family Cimicidae
- Three species that bite humans: *Cimex lectularius, Cimex hemipterus,* and *Leptocimex boueti* (2)[B]
- Most prevalent species are the *C. lectularius* (2)[B].
- Found in tropical or temperate climates
- Hide in crevices of mattresses, box springs, headboards, and baseboards
- Infestations occur in hotels/motels, hospitals, cinemas, transportation vehicles, aircrafts, and homes.

- Reactions range from an absent or minimal response to a more typical reaction presenting as pruritic, erythematous macules and papules or a less common urticarial and anaphylactic response.
- Skin reactions are due to host immunologic response to the parasite salivary proteins.
- Papular urticarial reactions are mediated via immunoglobulin (Ig) G antibody response to salivary proteins (3)[B].
- Bullous reactions are caused by an IgE-mediated hypersensitivity to nitrophorin, the substance that transports nitric oxide in bed bug saliva (3)[B].
- Bed bugs locate warmth and carbon dioxide production, which allows them to migrate to humans (4).

GENERAL PREVENTION
- Bed bug monitors and traps can be purchased, which contain carbon dioxide as well as heat to attract and trap the bugs but can be cost-prohibitive (5)[B].
- Avoidance of bed bugs: vacuum regularly, reduce clutter, seal cracks in walls, inspect luggage and clothing
- Launder all bedding and cloth items in 130°F (50°C) or hotter for 2 hours or 20°F (−5°C) or cooler for 5 days.
- If present in the home, eradication is essential via professional extermination. Some pest control companies have employed pest control canines to detect live bed bugs and eggs based on pheromones from the bed bugs but are expensive and generate false positives and negatives depending on the training of the dog (5)[B].

RISK FACTORS
- Immunologically weak or compromised
- Recent travel
- High turnover environment
- Secondhand furniture in home

 DIAGNOSIS

HISTORY
- Recent travel
- Blood specks on sheets
- Bed bug sighting
- New skin lesions in the morning
- Intense pruritus, pain, or burning

PHYSICAL EXAM
- Characteristic lesions are erythematous pruritic papules in an irregular linear pattern.
- Found on body surfaces exposed during sleeping such as face, neck, arms, legs, and shoulders
- May appear hours to days after being bitten
- Patients are usually asymptomatic but may be anaphylactic and present with papular urticaria, diffuse urticaria, and/or bullous lesions.

DIFFERENTIAL DIAGNOSIS
- Urticaria
- Insect or spider bite
- Scabies
- Dermatitis herpetiformis

DIAGNOSTIC TESTS & INTERPRETATION
Initial Tests (lab, imaging)
- Skin scraping with mineral oil preparation
- Skin biopsy

Test Interpretation
- Skin scraping is negative with mineral oil, which helps to exclude scabies.
- Skin biopsy shows nonspecific perivascular eosinophilic infiltrate consistent with arthropod bite reaction.

TREATMENT

GENERAL MEASURES
- Self-limited and resolves within 1 to 2 weeks
- Treat symptomatically
- Avoidance of the bed bugs by inspection
- Prevention by laundering bedding and cloth

MEDICATION
First Line
- Disease is self-limited; treat symptoms.
- Oral antihistamines (i.e., diphenhydramine, hydroxyzine)
- Topical antipruritics (i.e., pramoxine/calamine ointment or doxepin cream)
- Topical low to midpotency corticosteroids for 2 weeks (i.e., hydrocortisone, triamcinolone)
- Systemic corticosteroids (severe cases)

ADDITIONAL THERAPIES
- If secondarily infected, use topical or oral antibiotics against *Staphylococcus* and *Streptococcus* spp. (i.e., cephalexin, tetracycline, doxycycline, clindamycin, topical mupirocin).
- Epinephrine for anaphylaxis
- Professional extermination may be necessary.

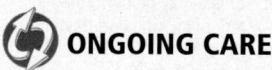 **ONGOING CARE**

FOLLOW-UP RECOMMENDATIONS
- Not necessary as disease is self-limited
- Recommended in extreme cases or if anaphylaxis ensues

PATIENT EDUCATION
- Avoid scratching to prevent superinfection.
- Inspect bedding, furniture, and luggage regularly.
- CDC: http://www.cdc.gov/parasites/bedbugs/
- EPA: http://www2.epa.gov/bedbugs

- MYTH 1: *Bed bugs are invisible.* They actually are nocturnal and hide during the daytime and adult bugs are about 1/4-inch long while eggs are the side of a pin head (6).
- MYTH 2: *Bed bugs reproduce rapidly.* Their life cycles are about 4 to 5 weeks (6), which is longer than the typical house fly.
- MYTH 3: *Bed bugs can live without feeding.* Bugs can only live about 3 to 5 months without a blood meal depending on climate (6).

COMPLICATIONS
- Bed bug dermatitis, allergic reactions, asthma exacerbations, anaphylaxis
- Significant psychological distress (insomnia, depression, anxiety, delusional parasitosis) (3)
- Secondary bacterial infections.
- Transmission of blood-borne diseases (rare)

REFERENCES
1. Studdiford JS, Conniff KM, Trayes KP, et al. Bedbug infestation. *Am Fam Physician.* 2012;86(7):653–658.
2. Kolb A, Needham GR, Neyman KM, et al. Bedbugs. *Dermatol Ther.* 2009;22(4):347–352.
3. Goddard J, deShazo R. Bedbugs (*Cimex lectularius*) and clinical consequences of their bites. *JAMA.* 2009;301(13):1358–1366.
4. Williams K, Willis MS. Bedbugs in the 21st century: the reemergence of an old foe. *Lab Medicine.* 2012;43:141–148.
5. Vaidyanathan R, Feldlaufer MF. Bed bug detection: current technologies and future directions. *Am J Trop Med Hyg.* 2013;88(4):619–625.
6. Ogg B. Bed bug myths—rely on research for facts. *The Nebline, University of Nebraska-Lincoln Extension.* 2012;347–348.

ADDITIONAL READING
- Lancaster Extension Education Center at http://lancaster.unl.edu/pest/bugs.shtml
- The National Pesticide Information Center (NPIC) 1-800-858-7378 or email at npic@ace.orst.edu.
- Thomas I, Kihiczak GG, Schwartz RA. Bedbug bites: a review. *Int J Dermatol.* 2004;43(6):430–433.

 CODES

ICD10
- S00.96XA Insect bite (nonvenomous) of unspecified part of head, initial encounter
- S10.96XA Insect bite of unspecified part of neck, initial encounter
- S40.269A Insect bite (nonvenomous) of unspecified shoulder, initial encounter

CLINICAL PEARLS
- 90% of infestations occur within 3 feet of beds.
- Wash bedding/clothing regularly in hot water.
- Vacuum carpet daily or steam clean daily.
- Inspect furniture, bedding, and luggage regularly.
- Use professional services if necessary.
- Patient education and vigilance is paramount for bed bug prevention and avoidance.
- Over-the-counter (OTC) products that contain pyrethroids are ineffective at killing bed bugs as they have become resistant over the years. These products can be identified with a suffix "-thrin" including permethrin, cyfluthirin, bifenthrin, and deltamethrin or fluvalinate and esfenvalerate (6).

BEHAVIORAL PROBLEMS, PEDIATRIC

William G. Elder, PhD

BASICS

DESCRIPTION
Behavior that disrupts at least one area of psycho-social functioning. Commonly reported behavioral problems are as follows:

- Noncompliance: active or passive refusal to do as requested by parent or other authority figure
- Temper tantrums: loss of internal control provoked by overtiredness, physical discomfort, or fear that leads to crying, whining, breath-holding, or in extreme cases, aggressive behavior
- Sleep problems: sleep patterns that are distressing to caregivers or child; difficulty going to sleep or staying asleep at night, nightmares, and night terrors
- Nocturnal enuresis: enuresis that occurs only at night in children >5 years of age with no medical problems
  - Primary: children who have never been dry at night
  - Secondary: children dry at night for at least 6 months
- Functional encopresis: repeated involuntary fecal soiling that is not caused by organic defect or illness
- Problem eating: "picky eating," difficult mealtime behaviors
- Normative sexual behaviors: developmentally appropriate behaviors in children in the absence of abuse
- Thumb-sucking: an innate reflex that is self-soothing; may be protective against sudden infant death. If persists, past eruption of primary teeth can affect teeth alignment and mouth shape.

EPIDEMIOLOGY
- Noncompliance: may manifest as children develop autonomy; males have a modestly greater likelihood of being noncompliant; decreases with age.
- Temper tantrums: 70% of 18- to 24-month-old children; 7% of 3- to 5-year-old children; in children with severe tantrums, 52% have other behavioral/emotional problems (1).
- Sleep problems
  - Night waking in 25–50% of infants 6 to 12 months; bedtime refusal in 10–30% of toddlers
  - Nightmares in 10–30% of preschoolers; peaks between ages 6 and 10 years
  - Night terrors in 1–6.5% early childhood; peaks between ages 4 and 12 years
  - Sleepwalking frequently in 3–5%; peaks between ages 5 and 8 years (2)
- Nocturnal enuresis
  - At least 20% of children in the 1st grade wet the bed occasionally; 4% wet ≥2 times per week.
  - At 10 years of age, 9% in boys, 3% in girls (3)
- Functional encopresis
  - Rare before age 3 years, most common in 5- to 10-year-olds; more common in boys (4)
- Problem eating
  - Prevalence peaks at 50% at 24 months of age; no relation to sex/ethnicity/income (5)
- Normative sexual behaviors
  - Rare in infancy, except hand to genital contact
  - Increased in 3- to 5-year-olds; less observed in >5-year-olds because more covert (6)
- Thumb-sucking: decreases with age; most children spontaneously stop between 2 and 4 years.

COMMONLY ASSOCIATED CONDITIONS
- Noncompliance: if exceeds what seems normative, rule out depression, compulsive patterns, adjustment disorder, inappropriate discipline
- Temper tantrums: difficult child temperament, stress

- Sleep problems: often with inconsistent bedtime routine or sleep schedule, stimulating bedtime environment; can be associated with hyperactive behavior, poor impulse control, and poor attention in young children (2). Acute or chronic anxiety is associated with insomnia.
- Enuresis: secondary often with medical problems, especially constipation, and frequent behavior problems, especially ADHD
- Functional encopresis: enuresis, UTIs, ADHD
- Normative sexual behaviors: family stressors such as separation or divorce (6)

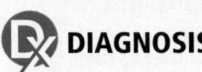

DIAGNOSIS

HISTORY
- Noncompliance: complete history from caregivers and teachers, if applicable; direct observation of child or child–caregiver interaction
  - Criteria is problematic for at least some adults, leading to difficult interactions for at least 6 months.
  - Reduces child's ability to take part in structured activities
  - Creates stressful relationships with compliant children
  - Disrupts academic progress; places child at risk for physical injury
- Temper tantrums: history, with focus on development, family functioning, or violence; may consist of stiffening limbs and arching back, dropping to the floor, shouting, screaming, crying, pushing/pulling, stamping, hitting, kicking, throwing, or running away (1)
- Sleep disorders: screening questions about sleep during well-child visit, such as the Bedtime problems, Excessive daytime sleepiness, Awakenings during the night, Regularity and duration of sleep, and Snoring (BEARS) screen; bedtime routine (2)[C]
- Nocturnal enuresis: severity, onset, and duration; daytime wetting or any associated genitourinary symptoms; family history of enuresis; medical and psychosocial history; constipation; child and caregiver's motivation for treatment (7)[C]
- Problem eating: review of child's diet, growth curves, nutritional needs, and caregiver's response to behavior (5)[C]
- Normative sexual behaviors: When was behavior first noticed? Any recent changes or stressors in family? Behavior solitary or with another; if with another, what age? Changes in frequency or nature of behaviors; occurs at home, daycare, school? Is behavior disruptive, intrusive, or coercive? (6) (See "Child Sexual Behavior Inventory" in the following discussion.)

PHYSICAL EXAM
- Nocturnal enuresis
  - Physical exam of abdomen for enlarged bladder, kidneys, or fecal masses; rectal exam if history of constipation; back for spinal dysraphism seen in dimpling or hair tufts
  - Neurologic exam: focus on lower extremities
  - Genitourinary exam
    - Males: meatal stenosis, hypospadias, epispadias, phimosis
    - Females: vulvitis, vaginitis, labial adhesions, ureterocele at introitus; wide vaginal orifice with scar or healed laceration may be evidence of abuse

- Functional encopresis
  - Height and weight; abdominal exam for masses or tenderness; rectal exam for tone, size of rectal vault, fecal impaction, masses, fissures, hemorrhoids; back for signs of spinal dysraphism seen in dimpling or hair tufts (4)

DIAGNOSTIC TESTS & INTERPRETATION
Initial Tests (lab, imaging)
- For nocturnal enuresis: urinalysis (dipstick test OK); if abnormal, consider urine culture.
  - For secondary enuresis: serum glucose, creatinine, thyrotropin (8)[C]
  - Urinary tract imaging and urodynamic studies if significant daytime symptoms with history or diagnosis of UTI or history of structural renal abnormalities (8)[C]
- For functional encopresis: tests for hypothyroidism or celiac disease if poor growth or family history; urinalysis and culture if enuresis or features of UTI (4)
  - Spine imaging if evidence of spinal dysraphism or if both encopresis and daytime enuresis; barium enema if suspect Hirschsprung disease

Follow-Up Tests & Special Considerations
Sleep disorders: Sleep studies may be performed in children if there is a history of snoring and daytime ADHD-type symptoms (2).

Diagnostic Procedures/Other
- Pediatric symptom checklist: https://brightfutures.org/mentalhealth/pdf/professionals/ped_sympton_chklst.pdf
- National Initiative for Children's Healthcare Quality (NICHQ) Vanderbilt Assessment (ADHD screen): http://www.myadhd.com/vanderbiltparent6175.html
- Child Sexual Behavior Inventory: Completed by female caregiver to assist with differentiation of normative versus abnormal behaviors particularly those related to sexual abuse: http://www.nctsnet.org/content/child-sexual-behavior-inventory-csbi

TREATMENT

- General: Educate caregiver about specific behavioral problem.
- Parent management training programs and techniques are effective for many child behavior problems (9)[A].
- Noncompliance: In the case of extreme child disobedience, consider parent training programs. Child may need to be formally screened for ADHD, obsessive-compulsive disorder (OCD), oppositional defiant disorder (ODD), or conduct disorder (CD).
- Temper tantrums: Remind caregiver this is a normal aspect of early childhood.
  - Educate caregiver that tantrums are not attention-seeking; although they may reveal that the child needs more attention from caregiver. This attention should be developmentally appropriate and not occur when the child is tantruming but at other times and prior to the tantrum.
  - If tantrum is set off by external factors, such as hunger or overtiredness, then correct.
  - Other methods for dealing with a tantrum include one of the following:
    - Ignore the tantrum; remove the child and place him or her in time-out (1 minute for each year of age); hold/restrain child until calmed down; provide child with clear, firm, and consistent instructions as well as enough time to obey.

- Sleep problems: Intervention consists largely of education of the caregiver who may need a roadmap for dealing with this difficult and distressing problem. Developmental stages; environmental factors and cues; caregiver emotions and reactions; and child fears, stress, and habits are all important factors in sleep onset and maintenance that should be explored and explained to the caregiver.
- Specific recommendations may also consist of other interventions including the following (2)[A]:
  - Graduated extinction: Caregiver ignores cries for specified period; can check at a fixed time or increasing intervals.
  - "Fading": gradual decrease in direct contact with the child as child falls asleep; goal is for the caregiver to exit the room and allow child to fall asleep independently.
  - Consider the "5S Intervention" for settling problems in toddlers (used to comfort infants in nurseries): swaddling, sucking, shushing, stomach/side position, and swinging.
  - If fearful, preferred routines or inert sprays or glitter spread by the child (while avoiding the eyes) may help the child feel more secure.
- Nocturnal enuresis
  - Bedwetting alarm: first-line therapy for caregivers who can overcome objection of having their sleep disturbed; about 2/3 of children respond while using the alarm; if enuresis recurs after use, it will often resolve with a second trial (7)[A].
  - Decrease fluids an hour before bedtime.
  - Little evidence from clinical trials but good empirical evidence for behavioral training, including positive reinforcement (small reward for each dry night) or responsibility training (if developmentally able, child is responsible for changing or washing sheets), encouraging daily bowel movements, and frequent bladder emptying during the day
- Functional encopresis
  - First disimpaction: PO with polyethylene glycol solution or mineral oil; if unsuccessful, manual mineral oil enemas
  - Maintenance therapy
    - Medical: osmotics, such as polyethylene glycol, fiber, lactulose; stimulants, such as senna or bisacodyl
    - Behavior modification: toileting after meals for 10 minutes 2 to 3 times a day, star charts, and rewards (4)[C]
- Problem eating
  - Avoid punishment, prodding, or rewards. Offer a variety of healthy foods at every meal; limit milk to 24 oz/day and decrease juice (5)[C].
- Normative sexual behavior: No treatment needed; caregivers may need encouragement not to punish or admonish child and to use gentle distraction to redirect behavior when in public setting.
- Thumb-sucking: Recommendations to caregivers include praising children when not sucking their thumb, offer alternatives that are soothing (e.g., stuffed toys), provide reminders or negative reinforcement in the form of a bandage around or bitters on the thumb (5)[C].

MEDICATION
Most pediatric behavioral issues respond well to nonpharmacologic therapy:
- Sleep disorders
  - For certain delayed sleep-onset disorders, after behavioral methods are exhausted, melatonin 0.5 to 10 mg PO can be tried while behavior modification is continued. Sleep latency is likely to be reduced. However, this is not approved by

the FDA for children. Expect rebound insomnia. Daytime exposure to bright or sunlight should be assured before treatment.
- Nocturnal enuresis
  - Desmopressin can decrease urine output to reduce enuresis episodes. Not before age 6 years; begin with 0.2 mg tablet nightly 1 hour before bedtime; titrate to 0.6 mg (8)[B]. However, use is questionable because its effects do not persist posttreatment (10)[A]. Intranasal formulations can cause severe hyponatremia, resulting in seizures and death in children. Behavioral interventions should be first-line treatment (7)[C].

ISSUES FOR REFERRAL
- A patient who exhibits self-injurious behaviors, slow recovery time from tantrums, more tantrums in the home than outside the home, or more aggressive behaviors toward others may require referral to a psychologist or psychiatrist.
- Children with chronic insomnia or anxiety that interferes with sleep should be referred to a psychologist or psychiatrist.
- A child with loud nightly snoring, with observed apnea spells, daytime excessive sleeping, and neurobehavioral signs such as mood changes, ADHD-like symptoms, or academic problems should be referred for sleep studies (2).
- With enuresis and obstructive sleep apnea symptoms, refer for sleep studies because surgical correction of airway obstruction often improves or cures enuresis and daytime wetting (8).
- Must distinguish sexual behavior problems: Developmentally inappropriate behaviors—greater frequency or much earlier age than expected—becomes a preoccupation, recurs after adult intervention/corrective efforts. If abuse is not suspected, consider referral to a child psychologist. If abuse is suspected, must report to child protective services (6).
- If disimpaction by either manual or medical methods is unsuccessful, consult gastroenterology or general surgery. Patients who show no improvement after 6 months of maintenance medical therapy should be referred to gastroenterology (4).
- Thumb-sucking resistant to behavioral intervention and threatening oral development may be evaluated by a pediatric dentist for use of habit-breaking dental appliances (5)[C].

 ## ONGOING CARE

DIET
Nutrition is very important in behavioral issues. Avoiding high-sugar foods and caffeine and providing balanced meals has been shown to decrease aggressive and noncompliant behaviors in children.

PATIENT EDUCATION
- Yale Parenting Center, Kazdin Method Sessions Webinars, $50.00 each. Cost http://yaleparentingcenter.yale.edu/kazdin-method-sessions
- See *Parent Training Programs: Insight for Practitioners* at: http://www.cdc.gov/violenceprevention/pdf/Parent_Training_Brief-a.pdf
- *The Happiest Baby Guide to Great Sleep: Simple Solutions for Kids from Birth to 5 Years.* Harvey Karp, MD New York, HarperCollins Publishers 2012, 384 pp.
- Products
  - Nytone Bed Wetting Alarms: by order to: http://www.nytone.com/products/nytone-enuresis-alarm?gclid=CM7Cm97i5rcCFSJ MgodW1wAgg

REFERENCES
1. Potegal M, Davidson RJ. Temper tantrums in young children: 1. Behavioral composition. *J Dev Behav Pediatr*. 2003;24(3):140–147.
2. Bhargava S. Diagnosis and management of common sleep problems in children. *Pediatr Rev*. 2011;32(3):91–98.
3. Robson WL. Clinical practice. Evaluation and management of enuresis. *N Engl J Med*. 2009;360(14):1429–1436.
4. Har AF, Croffie JM. Encopresis. *Pediatr Rev*. 2010;31(9):368–374.
5. Tseng AG, Biagioli FE. Counseling on early childhood concerns: sleep issues, thumb sucking, picky eating, and school readiness. *Am Fam Physician*. 2009;80(2):139–142.
6. Kellogg ND. Sexual behaviors in children: evaluation and management. *Am Fam Physician*. 2010;82(10):1233–1238.
7. Vande Walle J, Rittig S, Bauer S, et al. Practical consensus guidelines for the management of enuresis. *Eur J Pediatr*. 2012;171(6):971–983.
8. Ramakrishnan K. Evaluation and treatment of enuresis. *Am Fam Physician*. 2008;78(4):489–496.
9. Owen DJ, Slep AM, Heyman RE. The effect of praise, positive nonverbal response, reprimand, and negative nonverbal response on child compliance: a systematic review. *Clin Child Fam Psychol Rev*. 2012;15(4):364–385.
10. Glazener CM, Evans JH. Desmopressin for nocturnal enuresis in children. *Cochrane Database Syst Rev*. 2002;(3):CD002112.

ADDITIONAL READING
- Gringras P. When to use drugs to help sleep. *Arch Dis Child*. 2008;93(11):976–981.
- Gringras P, Gamble C, Jones AP, et al. Melatonin for sleep problems in children with neurodevelopmental disorders: randomised double masked placebo controlled trial. *BMJ*. 2012;345:e6664.
- Miller JW. Screening children for developmental behavioral problems: principles for the practitioner. *Prim Care*. 2007;34(2):177–201.
- Stein MT. Difficult behavior. In: Rudolph C, Rudolph A, Lister G, et al, eds., *Rudolph's Pediatrics*. 22nd ed. New York: McGraw-Hill, 2011:335–338.
- Strachan E, Staples B. Masturbation. *Pediatr Rev*. 2012;33(4):190–191.
- Zahrt DM, Melzer-Lange MD. Aggressive behavior in children and adolescents. *Pediatr Rev*. 2011;32(8):325–332.

CODES

ICD10
- F91.9 Conduct disorder, unspecified
- F91.1 Conduct disorder, childhood-onset type
- F91.2 Conduct disorder, adolescent-onset type

CLINICAL PEARLS
- Well-child visits provide opportunities for systematic screening for these common conditions.
- Parental education, including a review of age-appropriate discipline, is a key component of treatment.

BELL PALSY

Irina Pechenko, MD • Jeffrey B. Lanier, MD, FAAFP

 BASICS

DESCRIPTION

A peripheral lower motor neuron facial palsy, usually unilateral, which arises secondary to inflammation and subsequent swelling and compression of cranial nerve VII (facial) and the associated vasa nervorum

EPIDEMIOLOGY

- Affects 0.02% of the population annually
- Predominant sex: male = female
- Median age of onset is 40 years but affects all ages.
- Accounts for 60–75% of all cases of unilateral facial paralysis
- Occurs with equal frequency on the left and right sides of the face
- Most patients recover, but as many as 30% are left with facial disfigurement and pain.

Incidence

- 20 to 30 cases per 100,000 people in the United States per year
- Lowest in children ≤10 years of age; highest in adults ≥70 years of age
- Higher among pregnant women

Prevalence

Affects 40,000 Americans every year

ETIOLOGY AND PATHOPHYSIOLOGY

- Results from damage to the facial cranial nerve (VII)
- Inflammation of cranial nerve VII causes swelling and subsequent compression of both the nerve and the associated vasa nervorum.
- May arise secondary to reactivation of latent herpesvirus (herpes simplex virus [HSV] type 1 and herpes zoster virus) in cranial nerve ganglia or due to ischemia from arteriosclerosis associated with diabetes mellitus

Genetics

May be associated with a genetic predisposition, but it remains unclear which factors are inherited

RISK FACTORS

- Pregnancy, specially associated with severe preeclampsia (1)[A]
- Diabetes mellitus
- Age >30 years
- Exposure to cold temperatures
- Upper respiratory infection (e.g., coryza, influenza)
- Chronic HTN (1)[A]
- Obesity (1)[A]
- Migraine headache (2)[A]

COMMONLY ASSOCIATED CONDITIONS

- HSV
- Lyme disease
- Diabetes mellitus
- Hypertension
- Herpes zoster virus
- Ramsay-Hunt syndrome
- Sjögren syndrome
- Sarcoidosis
- Eclampsia
- Amyloidosis

 DIAGNOSIS

HISTORY

- Time course of the illness (rapid onset)
- Predisposing factors: recent viral infection, trauma, new medications, hypertension, diabetes mellitus
- Presence of hyperacusis or history of recurrent Bell palsy (both associated with poor prognosis)
- Any associated rash (suggestive of herpes zoster, Lyme disease, or sarcoid)
- Weakness on affected side of face, often sudden in onset
- Pain in or behind the ear in 50% of cases, which may precede the palsy in 25% of cases
- Subjective numbness on the ipsilateral side of the face
- Alteration of taste on the ipsilateral anterior 2/3 of the tongue (chorda tympani branch of the facial nerve)
- Hyperacusis (nerve to the stapedius muscle)
- Decreased tear production

PHYSICAL EXAM

- Neurologic
  - Determine if the weakness is caused by a problem in either the central or peripheral nervous systems.
  - Flaccid paralysis of muscles on the affected side, including the forehead
    ○ Impaired ability to raise the ipsilateral eyebrow
    ○ Impaired closure of the ipsilateral eye
    ○ Impaired ability to smile, grin, or purse the lips
    ○ Bell phenomenon: upward diversion of the eye with attempted closure of the lid
  - Patients may complain of numbness, but no deficit is present on sensory testing.
  - Examine for involvement of other cranial nerves.
- Head, ears, eyes, nose, and throat
  - Carefully examine to exclude a space-occupying lesion.
  - Perform pneumatic otoscopic exam.
- Skin: Examine for erythema migrans (Lyme disease) and vesicular rash (herpes zoster virus).

DIFFERENTIAL DIAGNOSIS

Etiologies include the following:

- Infectious
  - Acute or chronic otitis media
  - Malignant otitis externa
  - Osteomyelitis of the skull base
- Cerebrovascular
  - Brainstem stroke involving anteroinferior cerebellar artery
  - Aneurysm involving carotid, vertebral, or basilar arteries
- Neoplastic (Onset of palsy is usually slow and progressive and accompanied by additional cranial nerve deficits and/or headache.)
  - Tumors of the parotid gland
  - Cholesteatoma
  - Skull base tumor
  - Carcinomatous meningitis
  - Leukemic meningitis
- Traumatic
  - Temporal bone fracture
  - Mandibular bone fracture

- Other
  - Multiple sclerosis
  - Myasthenia gravis (should be considered in cases of recurrent or bilateral facial palsy)
  - Guillain-Barré syndrome (may also present with bilateral facial palsy)
  - Sjögren syndrome
  - Sarcoidosis
  - Amyloidosis
  - Melkersson-Rosenthal syndrome
  - Mononeuritis or polyneuritis

DIAGNOSTIC TESTS & INTERPRETATION

Initial Tests (lab, imaging)

- Blood glucose level (if diabetes a consideration)
- Lyme titer, ELISA, and Western blot for immunoglobulin (Ig) M, IgG for *Borrelia burgdorferi*
- ESR
- Consider CBC.
- Consider rapid plasma reagin test.
- Consider HIV test.
- In appropriate clinical circumstances, consider titers for varicella-zoster virus, cytomegalovirus, rubella, hepatitis A, hepatitis B, and hepatitis C.

Follow-Up Tests & Special Considerations

- CSF analysis
  - CSF protein is elevated in 1/3 of cases.
  - CSF cells show mild elevation in 10% of cases with a mononuclear cell predominance.
  - Not routinely indicated
- Salivary polymerase chain reaction for HSV1 or herpes zoster virus (largely reserved for research purposes)
- Facial radiographs
  - In the setting of trauma, evaluate for fracture.
- IV contrast–enhanced head CT
  - Evaluate for fracture.
  - Evaluate for stroke, if stroke is in the differential.
- IV contrast–enhanced brain MRI
  - Evaluate for central pontine, temporal bone, and parotid neoplasms.
  - Not routinely indicated

Diagnostic Procedures/Other

- Electromyograph: Nerve conduction on affected and nonaffected sides can be compared to determine the extent of nerve injury, especially if there is dense palsy or no recovery after several weeks.
- Electroneurography: Evoked potentials of affected and nonaffected sides can be compared.

Test Interpretation

Invasive diagnostic procedures are not indicated because biopsy could further damage cranial nerve XII.

TREATMENT

GENERAL MEASURES

- Artificial tears should be used to lubricate the cornea.
- The ipsilateral eye should be patched and taped shut at night to avoid drying and infection.

MEDICATION

- Corticosteroids decrease inflammation and limit nerve damage, thereby reducing the number of patients with residual facial weakness.

- Routine use of antiviral medication is not recommended. Antiviral agents targeting herpes simplex, when administered concurrently with corticosteroids, may further reduce the risk of unfavorable outcomes in patients with a dense Bell palsy (3)[A]:
  - Antivirals alone are less likely to produce full recovery than corticosteroids.
  - A combination of valacyclovir and steroids provides only minimal added benefit over steroid use alone (4)[B].
- Corticosteroids
  - Prednisolone: total of 500 mg over 10 days, 25 mg PO BID
    - Treatment with prednisolone within 48 hours of palsy onset has shown higher complete recovery rates and less synkinesis compared with no prednisolone (5)[B].
    - Antivirals in combination with corticosteroids
      - Valacyclovir: 1,000 mg TID for 7 days plus prednisolone 60 mg/day for 5 days; then tapered by 10 mg/day for total treatment length of 10 days (4)[B].
    - Steroids are recommended for all cases of Bell palsy.
    - Controversial whether antiviral treatment is necessary with steroids
      - American Academy of Otolaryngology–Head and Neck Surgery recommends antiviral treatment in all cases of Bell palsy cases (6)[A].
    - There is a strong recommendation to use corticosteroids for all patients with Bell palsy and strong recommendation against of antiviral treatment alone (6)[A].
- Contraindications
  - Documented hypersensitivity
  - Preexisting infections, including tuberculosis (TB) and systemic mycosis
- Precautions: Use with discretion in pregnant patients and those with peptic ulcer disease and diabetes.
- Significant possible interactions: measles-mumps-rubella, oral polio virus vaccine, and other live vaccines

Pregnancy Considerations
Steroids should be used cautiously during pregnancy; consult with an obstetrician.

ISSUES FOR REFERRAL
Patients may need to be referred to an ear, nose, and throat specialist or a neurologist.

ADDITIONAL THERAPIES
- Physical therapy: strong evidence that physical therapy combined with drug treatment has positive effect on grade and time of recovery compared with drug treatment only (7–9)[A].
- Electrostimulation and mirror biofeedback rehabilitation have limited evidence of effect (10)[C].
- Acupuncture with strong stimulation has shown some therapeutic promise.
- Routine use of eye-protective measures for patients with incomplete eye closure is recommended (6)[A].

SURGERY/OTHER PROCEDURES
- Surgical treatment of Bell palsy remains controversial and is reserved for intractable cases.

- There is an insufficient evidence to decide whether surgical intervention is beneficial or harmful in the management of Bell palsy (11)[B].
- In those cases where surgical intervention is performed, cranial nerve XII is surgically decompressed at the entrance to the meatal foramen where the labyrinthine segment and geniculate ganglion reside.
- Decompression surgery should not be performed >14 days after the onset of paralysis because severe degeneration of the facial nerve is likely irreversible after 2 to 3 weeks.
- A routine surgical decompression is not recommended (6)[B].

 ## ONGOING CARE

FOLLOW-UP RECOMMENDATIONS
Patient Monitoring
- Patients should start steroid treatment immediately and be followed for 12 months.
- Patients who do not recover complete facial nerve function should be referred to an ophthalmologist for tarsorrhaphy.

PATIENT EDUCATION
American Academy of Family Physicians: http://www.aafp.org/afp/2007/1001/p1004.html

PROGNOSIS
- Most patients achieve complete spontaneous recovery within 2 weeks. >80% recover within 3 months.
- 85% of untreated patients will experience the first signs of recovery within 3 weeks of onset.
- 16% are left with a partial palsy, motor synkinesis, and autonomic synkinesis.
- 5% experience severe sequelae, and a small number of patients experience permanent facial weakness and dysfunction.
- Poor prognostic factors include the following:
  - Age >60 years
  - Complete facial weakness
  - Hypertension
  - Ramsay-Hunt syndrome
- The Sunnybrook and House-Brackmann facial grading systems are clinical prognostic models that identify Bell palsy patients at risk for nonrecovery at 12 months.
- Treatment with prednisolone or no prednisolone and the Sunnybrook score are significant factors for predicting nonrecovery at 1 month (12)[C].
- Patients with no improvement or progression of symptoms should be referred to ENT (6)[A] and may require neuroimaging to rule out neoplasms (6)[A].

COMPLICATIONS
- Corneal abrasion or ulceration
- Steroid-induced psychological disturbances; avascular necrosis of the hips, knees, and/or shoulders
- Steroid use can unmask subclinical infection (e.g., TB).

REFERENCES
1. Katz A, Sergienko R, Dior U, et al. Bell's palsy during pregnancy: is it associated with adverse perinatal outcome? *Laryngoscope.* 2011;121(7): 1395–1398.
2. Peng KP, Chen YT, Fuh JL, et al. Increased risk of Bell palsy in patients with migraine: a nationwide cohort study. *Neurology.* 2015;84(2):116–124.
3. Thaera GM, Wellik KE, Barrs DM, et al. Are corticosteroid and antiviral treatments effective for bell palsy? A critically appraised topic. *Neurologist.* 2010;16(12):138–140.
4. Worster A, Keim SM, Sahsi R, et al. Do either corticosteroids or antiviral agents reduce the risk of long-term facial paresis in patients with new-onset Bell's palsy? *J Emerg Med.* 2010; 38(4):518–523.
5. Madhok V, Falk G, Fahey T, et al. Prescribe prednisolone alone for Bell's palsy diagnosed within 72 hours of symptom onset. *BMJ.* 2009;338:b255.
6. de Almeida JR, Guyatt GH, Sud S, et al. Management of Bell palsy: clinical practice guideline. *CMAJ.* 2014;186(12):917–922.
7. Teixeira LJ, Valbuza JS, Prado GF. Physical therapy for Bell's palsy (idiopathic facial paralysis). *Cochrane Database Syst Rev.* 2011;(12):CD006283.
8. Ferreira M, Marques EE, Duarte JA, et al. Physical therapy with drug treatment in Bell palsy: a focused review. *Am J Phys Med Rehabil.* 2015; 94(4):331–340.
9. Pourmomeny AA, Asadi S. Management of synkinesis and asymmetry in facial nerve palsy: a review article. *Iran J Otorhinolaryngol.* 2014; 26(77):251–256.
10. Alakram P, Puckree T. Effects of electrical stimulation on House-Brackmann scores in early Bell's palsy. *Physiother Theory Pract.* 2010;26(3): 160–166.
11. Axelsson S, Berg T, Jonsson L, et al. Prednisolone in Bell's palsy related to treatment start and age. *Otol Neurotol.* 2011;32(1):141–146.
12. Marsk E, Bylund N, Jonsson L, et al. Prediction of nonrecovery in Bell's palsy using Sunnybrook grading. *Laryngoscope.* 2012;122(4):901–906.

 ## SEE ALSO

Amyloidosis; Diabetes Mellitus, Type 1; Diabetes Mellitus, Type 2; Herpes Simplex; Herpes Zoster (Shingles); Lyme Disease; Sarcoidosis; Sjögren Syndrome

CODES

ICD10
G51.0 Bell's palsy

CLINICAL PEARLS

- Initiate steroids immediately following the onset of symptoms.
- Look closely at the voluntary movement on the upper part of the face on the affected side; in Bell palsy, all of the muscles are involved (weak or paralyzed); whereas in a stroke, the upper muscles are spared (because of bilateral innervation).
- Protect the affected eye with lubrication and taping.
- In areas with endemic Lyme disease, Bell palsy should be considered to be Lyme disease until proven otherwise.

BIPOLAR I DISORDER
Wendy K. Marsh, MD, MSc

 BASICS

DESCRIPTION
- Bipolar I (BP-I) is an episodic mood disorder of at least one manic or mixed (mania and depression) episode that causes marked impairment, psychosis, and/or hospitalization, major depressive, episodes are not required, but usually occur.
- Symptoms are not caused by a substance (e.g., drug), a general medical condition, or a medication.

Geriatric Considerations
New onset in older patients (>50 years of age) requires a workup for organic or chemically induced pathology.

Pediatric Considerations
Diagnosis less well defined, more rapid cycling, and mixed states. Depression often presents as irritable mood. There is an overlap with symptoms of attention deficit hyperactivity disorder (ADHD) and oppositional defiant disorder (ODD).

Pregnancy Considerations
- Potential teratogenic effects of commonly used medications (e.g., valproic acid)
- Postpartum caries risk of severe acute episode with psychosis and/or infanticidal ideation.

EPIDEMIOLOGY
- Onset usually between 15 and 30 years of age
- More common in separated/widowed/divorced persons

Prevalence
- 1.0–1.6% lifetime prevalence
- Equal among men and women (manic episodes more common in men; depressive episodes more common in women)
- Equal among races; however, clinicians tend to diagnose schizoaffective in African Americans with BP-I.

ETIOLOGY AND PATHOPHYSIOLOGY
Genetic predisposition and major life stressors can trigger initial and subsequent episodes:
- Dysregulation of biogenic amines or neurotransmitters (particularly serotonin, norepinephrine, and dopamine)
- MRI findings suggest abnormalities in prefrontal cortical areas, striatum, and amygdala that predate illness onset (1)[C].

Genetics
- Monozygotic twin concordance 40–70%
- Dizygotic twin concordance 5–25%
- 50% have at least one parent with a mood disorder
- First-degree relatives are 7 times more likely to develop BP-I than the general population.

RISK FACTORS
Genetics, major life stressors (especially loss of parent or spouse), or substance abuse

GENERAL PREVENTION
Treatment adherence and education can help to prevent relapses.

COMMONLY ASSOCIATED CONDITIONS
Substance abuse (60%), ADHD, anxiety disorders, and eating disorders

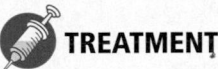 **DIAGNOSIS**

- The diagnosis of BP-I requires at least one manic or mixed episode (simultaneous mania and depression). Although a depressive episode is not necessary for the diagnosis, 80–90% of people with BP-I also experience depression.
- Manic episode, *DSM-5* criteria (2)
  – Distinct period of abnormally and persistently elevated, expansive, or irritable mood lasting plus increased activity or energy for at least 1 week (or any duration if hospitalization is necessary)
  – During the period of mood disturbance, three or more of the "DIG FAST" symptoms must persist (four if the mood is only irritable) and must be present to a significant degree.
    ○ Distractibility
    ○ Insomnia, decreased need for sleep
    ○ Grandiosity or inflated self-esteem
    ○ Flight of ideas or racing thoughts
    ○ Agitation or increase in goal-directed activity
    ○ Speech-pressured/more talkative than usual
    ○ Taking risks: excessive involvement in pleasurable activities that have a high potential for painful consequences (e.g., financial or sexual)
  – Mixed specifier: when three or more symptoms of opposite mood pole are present during primary mood episode, For example, mania with mixed features (of depression).

HISTORY
- Collateral information makes diagnostics more complete and is often necessary for a clear history.
- History: safety concerns (e.g., Suicidal/homicidal ideation? Safety plan? Psychosis present?), physical well-being (e.g., Number of hours of sleep? Appetite? Substance abuse?), personal history (e.g., Talkative? Speeding? Spending sprees or donations? Credit card debt? Promiscuous? Other risk-taking behavior? Legal trouble?)

PHYSICAL EXAM
- Mental status exam in acute mania
  – General appearance: bright clothing, excessive makeup, disorganized or discombobulated, psychomotor agitation
  – Speech: pressured, difficult to interrupt
  – Mood/affect: euphoria, irritability/expansive, labile
  – Thought process: flight of ideas (streams of thought occur to patient at rapid rate), easily distracted
  – Thought content: grandiosity, paranoia, hyperreligious
  – Perceptual abnormalities: 3/4 of manic patients experience delusions, grandiose, or paranoia.
  – Suicidal/homicidal ideation: Irritability or delusions may lead to aggression toward self or others; suicidal ideation is common with mixed episode.
  – Insight/judgment: poor/impaired
- See "Bipolar II Disorder" for an example of a mental status exam in depression.
- With mixed episodes, patients may exhibit a combination of manic and depressive mental states.

DIFFERENTIAL DIAGNOSIS
- Other psychiatric considerations: unipolar depression ± psychotic features, schizophrenia, schizoaffective disorder, personality disorders (particularly antisocial, borderline, histrionic, and narcissistic), ADD ± hyperactivity, substance-induced mood disorder
- Medical considerations: epilepsy (e.g., temporal lobe), brain tumor, infection (e.g., AIDS, syphilis), stroke, endocrine (e.g., thyroid) disease, multiple sclerosis
- In children, consider ADHD and ODD.

DIAGNOSTIC TESTS & INTERPRETATION
- BP-I is a clinical diagnosis.
- The Mood Disorder Questionnaire is a self-assessment screen for bipolar disorders (sensitivity 73%, specificity 90%) (3).
- Patient Health Questionnaire-9 helps to determine the presence and severity of a depressive episode.

Initial Tests (lab, imaging)
- TSH, CBC, BMP, LFTs, ANA, RPR, HIV, ESR
- Drug/alcohol screen with each presentation
- Dementia workup if new onset in seniors
- Consider brain imaging (CT, MRI) with initial onset of mania to rule out organic cause (e.g., tumor, infection, or stroke), especially with onset in elderly and if psychosis is present.

Diagnostic Procedures/Other
Consider EEG if presentation suggests temporal lobe epilepsy (hyperreligiosity, hypergraphia).

TREATMENT

- Ensure safety.
- Psychotherapy (e.g., cognitive-behavioral therapy, social rhythm therapy)
- Stress reduction
- Patient and family education

GENERAL MEASURES
- Psychotherapy for depression (e.g., cognitive-behavioral therapy, social rhythm, interpersonal) in conjunction with medications
- Regular daily schedule, exercise, a healthy diet, and sobriety

MEDICATION
First Line
- Treatment mood stabilizer(s) or other psychotropic medications. When combining, use different classes (e.g., an atypical antipsychotic and/or an antiseizure medication and/or lithium).
- Lithium (Lithobid, Eskalith, generic): dosing: 600 to 1,200 mg/day divided BID–QID; start 600 to 900 mg/day divided BID–TID, titrate based on blood levels. Warning: caution in kidney and heart disease; use can lead to diabetes insipidus or thyroid disease. Caution with diuretics or ACE inhibitors; dehydration can lead to toxicity (seizures, encephalopathy, arrhythmias). Pregnancy Category D (Ebstein anomaly). Monitor: Check ECG >40 years, TSH,

BUN, creatine, electrolytes at baseline and every 6 months; check level 5 to 7 days after initiation or dose change, then every 2 weeks × 3, then every 3 months (goal: 0.8 to 1.2 mmol/L).

- Antiseizure medications
  - Divalproex sodium, valproic acid (Depakote, Depakene, generic): dosing: start 250 to 500 mg BID–TID; maximum 60 mg/kg/day. Black box warnings: hepatotoxicity, pancreatitis, thrombocytopenia, pregnancy Category D. Monitor CBC and LFTs at baseline and every 6 months; check level 5 days after initiation and dose changes (goal: 50 to 125 μg/mL).
  - Carbamazepine (Equetro, Tegretol, generic): dosing: 800 to 1,200 mg/day PO divided BID–QID; start 100 to 200 mg PO BID and titrate to lowest effective dose. Warning: Do not use with TCA or within 14 days of an MAOI. Caution in kidney/heart disease; risk of aplastic anemia/agranulocytosis, enzyme inducer; pregnancy Category D. Monitor CBC and LFTs at baseline and every 3 to 6 months; check level 4 to 5 days after initiation and dose changes (goal: 4 to 12 μg/mL).
  - Lamotrigine (Lamictal, generic): dosing: 200 to 400 mg/day; start 25 mg/day for 2 weeks, then 50 mg/day for 2 weeks, then 100 mg/day for 1 week, then 150 mg/day. (Note: Use different dosing if adjunct to valproate). Warning: Titrate slowly (risk of Stevens-Johnson syndrome); caution with kidney/liver/heart disease; pregnancy Category C
  - Oxcarbazepine (Trileptal) dosing: 300 mg PO QD. Titrate to 1,800 to 2,400/day max.
- Atypical antipsychotics
  - Side effects: orthostatic hypotension, metabolic side effects (glucose and lipid dysregulation, weight gain), tardive dyskinesia, neuroleptic malignant syndrome (NMS), prolactinemia (except Abilify), increased risk of death in elderly with dementia-related psychosis, pregnancy Category C
  - Monitor LFTs, lipids, glucose at baseline, 3 months, and annually; check for extrapyramidal symptoms (EPS) with Abnormal Involuntary Movement Scale (AIMS) and assess weight (with abdominal circumference) at baseline, at 4, 8, and 12 weeks, and then every 3 to 6 months; monitor for orthostatic hypotension 3 to 5 days after starting or changing dose.
  - Risperidone (Risperdal, Risperdal Consta, generic): dosing: 1 to 6 mg/day divided QD–QID. IM preparation available (q2wk)
  - Olanzapine (Zyprexa, Zydis, generic): dosing: 5–20 mg/day; most likely to cause metabolic side effects (weight gain, diabetes)
  - Quetiapine (Seroquel, Seroquel XR, generic): dosing: in mania, 200 to 400 mg BID; in bipolar depression, 50 to 300 mg QHS. XR dosing 50 to 400 mg QHS
  - Aripiprazole (Abilify): dosing: 15 to 30 mg/day; less likely to cause metabolic side effects
  - Ziprasidone (Geodon): dosing: 40 to 80 mg BID; less likely to cause metabolic side effects. Caution: QTc prolongation (>500 ms) has been associated with use (0.06%). Consider ECG at baseline.
  - Asenapine: dosing: 5 to 10 mg sublingual BID
  - Lurasidone: dosing: 20 to 60 mg/day. FDA-approved for depression
  - Cariprazine:dosing: 1.5 to 6 mg/day. Start 1.5 mg

Second Line
- Antidepressants (in addition to mood stabilizers) have mixed evidence to support use.
- Benzodiazepines (for acute agitation with mania, associated anxiety)
- Sleep medications

ISSUES FOR REFERRAL
- Refer to psychiatry, depends on knowledge level of the doctor, stability of patient.
- Patients benefit from a multidisciplinary team, including a primary care physician, psychiatrist, and therapist.

ADDITIONAL THERAPIES
- Electroconvulsive therapy can be helpful in acute or treatment-resistant mania and depression.
- Modest evidence supports transcranial magnetic stimulation, vagus nerve stimulation, ketamine infusion, sleep deprivation, and hormone therapy (e.g., thyroid) in bipolar depression.

INPATIENT CONSIDERATIONS

Admission Criteria/Initial Stabilization
To admit involuntarily, the patient must have a psychiatric diagnosis (e.g., BP-I) and present a danger to self or others or the mental disease must be inhibiting the person from obtaining basic needs (e.g., food, clothing).

Nursing
Alert staff to potentially dangerous or agitated patients. Acute suicidal threats need continuous observation.

Discharge Criteria
Determined by safety

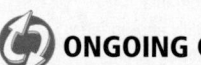 ONGOING CARE

FOLLOW-UP RECOMMENDATIONS
- Regularly scheduled visits support adherence with treatment.
- Frequent communication among primary care doctor, psychiatrist, and therapist

Patient Monitoring
Mood charts are helpful to monitor symptoms.

PATIENT EDUCATION
- National Alliance on Mental Illness (NAMI): http://www.nami.org/
- National Institutes of Mental Health (NIMH): http://www.nimh.nih.gov/index.shtml

PROGNOSIS
- Frequency and severity of episodes are related to medication adherence, consistency with therapy, quality of sleep, and support systems (4)[B].

- 40–50% of patients experience another manic episode within 2 years of first episode.
- 25–50% attempt suicide and 15% die by suicide.
- Substance abuse, unemployment, psychosis, depression, and male gender are associated with a worse prognosis.

REFERENCES
1. Fornito A, Yücel M, Wood SJ, et al. Anterior cingulate cortex abnormalities associated with a first psychotic episode in bipolar disorder. *Br J Psychiatry.* 2009;194(5):426–433.
2. American Psychiatric Association. *Diagnostic and Statistical Manual of Mental Disorders.* 5th ed. Arlington, VA: American Psychiatric Association; 2013.
3. Hirshfeld RM. Validation of the mood disorder questionnaire. *Bipolar Depression Bulletin.* 2004.
4. Depp CA, Moore DJ, Patterson TL, et al. Psycho-social interventions and medication adherence in bipolar disorder. *Dialogues Clin Neurosci.* 2008;10(2):239–250.

ADDITIONAL READING
- Agency for Healthcare Research and Quality. Antipsychotic medicines for treating schizophrenia and bipolar disorder: a review of the research for adults and caregivers. In: *Comparative Effectiveness Review Summary Guides for Consumers.* Rockville, MD: Agency for Healthcare Research and Quality; 2013.
- American Psychiatric Association. Practice guideline for the treatment of patients with bipolar disorder (revision). *Am J Psychiatry.* 2002;159(4)(Suppl):1–50.
- Licht RW. A new BALANCE in bipolar I disorder. *Lancet.* 2010;375(9712):350–352.
- Perlis RH, Brown E, Baker RW, et al. Clinical features of bipolar depression versus major depressive disorder in large multicenter trials. *Am J Psychiatry.* 2006;163(2):225–231.

 SEE ALSO

Algorithm: Depressive Episode, Major

 CODES

ICD10
- F31.9 Bipolar disorder, unspecified
- F31.10 Bipolar disorder, current episode manic without psychotic features, unspecified
- F31.30 Bipolar disord, crnt epsd depress, mild or mod severt, unsp

CLINICAL PEARLS
- BP-I is characterized by at least one manic or mixed episode that causes marked impairment, major depressive episodes usually occur, but are not necessary.
- 25–50% of BP-I patients attempt suicide and 15% die by suicide.
- There is no known way to prevent BP-I, but treatment adherence and education helps reduce further episodes.
- Goal of treatment is to decrease the intensity, length, and frequency of episodes as well as greater mood stability between episodes.

BIPOLAR II DISORDER

Wendy K. Marsh, MD, MSc

BASICS

DESCRIPTION
Bipolar II (BP-II) is a mood disorder characterized by at least one episode of major depression (with or without psychosis) and at least one episode of hypomania, a nonsevere mood elevation.

Geriatric Considerations
New onset in older patients (>50 years) requires a workup for organic or chemically induced pathology.

Pediatric Considerations
- Overlap with symptoms of attention deficit hyperactivity disorder (ADHD) and oppositional defiant disorder (ODD)
- Depression often presents as irritable mood.

Pregnancy Considerations
- Counsel women of childbearing age about potentially teratogenic effects of commonly used medications (e.g., valproic acid).
- Postpartum caries risk of severe acute episode with psychosis and /or infanticidal ideation.

EPIDEMIOLOGY
More common in women

Prevalence
0.5–1.1% lifetime prevalence

ETIOLOGY AND PATHOPHYSIOLOGY
- Dysregulation of biogenic amines or neurotransmitters (particularly serotonin, norepinephrine, and dopamine)
- Genetics
- Major life stressors increase risk of episode onset.

Genetics
Heritability estimate: >77%

GENERAL PREVENTION
No way to prevent the onset of BP-II, but treatment adherence and education can help to prevent further episodes.

COMMONLY ASSOCIATED CONDITIONS
Substance abuse or dependence, ADHD, anxiety disorders, and eating disorders

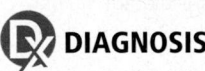 DIAGNOSIS

- *DSM-5* criteria: one hypomanic episode and at least one major depressive episode. The symptoms cause unequivocal change in functioning noticed by others but not severe enough to cause marked impairment (1)[C].
- Hypomania is a distinct period of persistently elevated, expansive, or irritable mood, different from usual euthymic mood, including increase in activity or energy lasting at least 4 days:
  – The episode must include at least three of the "DIG FAST" symptoms *plus increased energy* below (four if the mood is only irritable):
    ○ Distractibility
    ○ Insomnia, decreased need for sleep
    ○ Grandiosity or inflated self-esteem
    ○ Flight of ideas or racing thoughts

○ Agitation or increase in goal-directed activity (socially, at work or school, or sexually)
    ○ Speech-pressured/more talkative than usual
    ○ Taking risks: excessive involvement in pleasurable activities that have high potential for painful consequences (e.g., sexual or financial)
- Major depression
  – Depressed mood or diminished interest and four or more of the "SIG E CAPS" symptoms are present during the same 2-week period:
    ○ **S**leep disturbance (e.g., trouble falling asleep, early-morning awakening)
    ○ **I**nterest: loss or anhedonia
    ○ **G**uilt (or feelings of worthlessness)
    ○ **E**nergy, loss of
    ○ **C**oncentration, loss of
    ○ **A**ppetite changes, increase or decrease
    ○ **P**sychomotor changes (retardation or agitation)
    ○ **S**uicidal/homicidal thoughts
  – Rapid cycling is ≥4 mood episodes in 12 months (major depression or hypomania).
  – Mixed specifier: When three or more symptoms of opposite mood pole are present during primary mood episode, for example, hypomania with mixed features (of depression)
- Note: If symptoms have *ever* met criteria for a full manic episode or hospitalization was necessary secondary to manic/mixed symptoms or psychosis was present, then the diagnosis is BP-I.

HISTORY
Collateral information makes diagnostics more complete and is often necessary for a clear history.

PHYSICAL EXAM
- Mental status exam in hypomania
  – General appearance: usually appropriately dressed, with psychomotor agitation
  – Speech: may be pressured, talkative, difficult to interrupt
  – Mood/affect: euphoria, irritability/congruent, or expansive
  – Thought process: may be easily distracted, difficulty concentrating on one task
  – Thought content: usually positive, with "big" plans
  – Perceptual abnormalities: none
  – Suicidal/homicidal ideation: low incidence of homicidal or suicidal ideation
  – Insight/judgment: usually stable/may be impaired by their distractibility
- Mental status exam in acute depression
  – General appearance: unkempt, psychomotor retardation, poor eye contact
  – Speech: low, soft, monotone
  – Mood/affect: sad, depressed/congruent, flat
  – Thought process: ruminating thoughts, generalized slowing
  – Thought content: preoccupied with negative or nihilistic ideas
  – Perceptual abnormalities: 15% of depressed patients experience hallucinations or delusions.
  – Suicidal/homicidal ideation: Suicidal ideation is very common.
  – Insight/judgment: often impaired

DIFFERENTIAL DIAGNOSIS
- Other psychiatric considerations
  – BP-I disorder, unipolar depression, personality disorders (particularly borderline, antisocial, and narcissistic), ADD with hyperactivity, substance-induced mood disorder
- Medical considerations
  – Epilepsy (e.g., temporal lobe), brain tumor, infection (e.g., AIDS, syphilis), stroke, endocrine (e.g., thyroid disease), multiple sclerosis

DIAGNOSTIC TESTS & INTERPRETATION
- BP-II is a clinical diagnosis.
- Mood Disorder Questionnaire, self-assessment screen for BP, sensitivity 73%, specificity 90% (2)[B]
- Hypomania Checklist-32 distinguishes between BP-II and unipolar depression (sensitivity 80%, specificity 51%) (3)[B].
- Patient Health Questionnaire-9 helps to determine the presence and severity of depression.

Initial Tests (lab, imaging)
- Rule out organic causes of mood disorder during initial episode.
- Drug/alcohol screen is prudent with each presentation.
- Dementia workup if new onset in seniors
- With initial presentation: Consider CBC, chem 7, TSH, LFTs, ANA, RPR, HIV, and ESR.
- Consider brain imaging (CT, MRI) with initial onset of hypomania to rule out organic cause, especially with onset in the elderly.

TREATMENT

- Ensure safety.
- Medication management
- Psychotherapy (e.g., cognitive-behavioral therapy [CBT], social rhythm therapy, interpersonal therapy)
- Stress reduction
- Patient and family education
- Refer to psychiatrist.

GENERAL MEASURES
- Psychotherapy (e.g., CBT, social rhythm, interpersonal, family focused) in conjunction with medications
- Regular daily schedule, exercise, a healthy diet, and sobriety have been shown to help.

MEDICATION
- Less research has been conducted on the appropriate treatment of BP-II, but current consensus is to treat with the same medications as BP-I.
- Antidepressant medications must be used with caution during depressive episodes, because they may increase risk of hypomania or increase cycling (less common than with BP-I).

First Line

- When combining mood stabilizers, consider adding different classes (e.g., an atypical antipsychotic and/or an antiseizure medication and/or lithium).
- Lithium (Lithobid, Eskalith, generic): dosing 600 to 1,200 mg/day divided BID–QID, titrate based on blood levels:
  - Caution in kidney or heart disease; use can lead to diabetes insipidus, thyroid disease; caution in sodium-depleted patients (diuretics, ACE inhibitors); dehydration can lead to toxicity, which may cause seizures, encephalopathic syndrome, arrhythmias; pregnancy Category D (Ebstein anomaly with 1st-trimester use)
  - Monitor electrocardiogram in patients >40 years, TSH, BUN, creatinine, electrolytes at baseline and q6mo; check level 5 to 7 days after initiation or dose change, then q1–2wk × 3, then q3mo (goal: 0.8 to 1.2 mmol/L).
- Anticonvulsants
  - Valproic acid, divalproex sodium: dosing: Start 250 to 500 mg BID–TID, max 60 mg/kg/day. Warning: hepatotoxicity, pancreatitis, thrombocytopenia, pregnancy Category D (neural tube defects). Monitor CBC, LFTs at baseline and q6mo; check valproic acid level 5 days after initiation and dose changes (goal: 50 to 125 μm/mL).
  - Carbamazepine: dosing: 800 to 1,200 mg/day PO divided BID–QID, start 100 to 200 mg PO BID and titrate to lowest effective dose. Do not use with tricyclic antidepressants or within 14 days of monoamine oxidase inhibitor; caution with kidney or heart disease, may cause aplastic anemia/agranulocytosis. Monitor CBC, LFTs at baseline and q3–6mo; check level 4 to 5 days after initiation and dose changes (goal: 4 to 12 μm/mL).
  - Lamotrigine: treats depression only. Dosing: 200 mg/day start 25 mg for 2 weeks, then 50 mg for 2 weeks, then 100 mg for 1 week. (Note: different dosing if adjunct to valproate) Selected warnings: Titrate slowly (risk of Stevens-Johnson syndrome); caution with kidney, liver, or heart impairment. Monitor patient to monitor for rash.
- Atypical antipsychotics (AAs)
  - Side effects of AAs: orthostatic hypotension, negative metabolic side effects (effect glucose and lipid regulation, weight gain), tardive dyskinesia, neuroleptic malignant syndrome, prolactinemia increased risk of mortality in elderly with dementia-related psychosis, pregnancy Category C
  - Monitor LFTs, lipids, glucose at baseline, 3 months, and annually; check for extrapyramidal symptoms with Abnormal Involuntary Movement Scale (AIMS) and assess weight (with abdominal circumference) at baseline, then 4, 8, and 12 weeks, then q3–6mo; monitor for orthostatic hypotension 3 to 5 days after starting or changing dose.
  - Antimanic is a presumed class effect.
  - Aripiprazole: dosing: 15 mg/day, max 30 mg/day, less likely to cause metabolic side effects
  - Olanzapine: dosing: 5 to 20 mg/day, most likely AA to cause metabolic side effects (weight gain, diabetes mellitus)
  - Quetiapine: dosing: hypomania 200 to 400 mg BID; depression: 50 to 300 mg QHS
  - Risperidone: dosing: 1 to 6 mg/day QD–BID; generic and q2wk IM preparations available
  - Ziprasidone: dosing: 40 to 80 mg BID take with food. Less likely to cause metabolic side effects. Warning: QTc prolongation (>500 ms): consider baseline ECG.
  - Asenapine: dosing: 5 to 10 mg sublingual BID
  - Lurasidone: dosing: 20 to 60 mg/day. FDA-approved for depression.
  - Cariprazine: dosing:1.5 to 6 mg/day. Start 1.5 mg

Second Line

- Antidepressants (in addition to mood stabilizers) have better data in BP-II than BP-I.
- Sleep medications

ISSUES FOR REFERRAL

Patients benefit from care by a multidisciplinary team, including a primary care physician, therapist, and psychiatrist.

ADDITIONAL THERAPIES

- Electroconvulsive therapy for severe or treatment-resistant depression or mood elevation
- Modest evidence exists to support transcranial magnetic stimulation, vagal nerve stimulation, ketamine infusion, sleep deprivation, and hormone therapy (e.g., thyroid) in bipolar depression.

INPATIENT CONSIDERATIONS

If hospitalized for mood elevation symptoms, then diagnosis is mania and bipolar I. May be hospitalized for depression and be bipolar II

Admission Criteria/Initial Stabilization

To admit patients (>18 years) to a psychiatric unit involuntarily, they must have a psychiatric diagnosis and present a danger to themselves or others, or their mental disease must be inhibiting them from providing their basic needs (e.g., food, clothing, shelter).

Nursing

Acute suicidal threats require close observation.

Discharge Criteria

Determined by safety

ONGOING CARE

FOLLOW-UP RECOMMENDATIONS

- Regularly scheduled visits support treatment adherence.
- Frequent communication between primary care doctor, psychiatrist, and therapist ensures comprehensive care.

Patient Monitoring

Mood charts are helpful adjuncts to care.

PATIENT EDUCATION

- Support groups for patients and families are recommended.
- National Alliance on Mental Illness: http://www.nami.org/

PROGNOSIS

- Frequency and severity of problematic episodes are related to medication adherence, consistency with psychotherapy, sleep, support systems, regularity of daily activities, and social history.
- Substance abuse, unemployment, persistent depression, and male gender are associated with a worse prognosis.
- Although data are limited, evidence indicates that patients with BP-II may be at greater risk of both attempting and completing suicide than with BP-I and unipolar depression.

REFERENCES

1. American Psychiatric Association. *Diagnostic and Statistical Manual of Mental Disorders*. 5th ed. Arlington, VA: American Psychiatric Association; 2013.
2. Hirshfeld RM. Validation of the mood disorder questionnaire. *Bipolar Depression Bulletin*; 2004.
3. Angst J, Adolfsson R, Benazzi F, et al. The HCL-32: towards a self-assessment tool for hypomanic symptoms in outpatients. *J Affect Disord*. 2005;88(2):217–233.

ADDITIONAL READING

- American Psychiatric Association. Practice guideline for the treatment of patients with bipolar disorder (revision). *Am J Psychiatry*. 2002;159(4 Suppl):1–50.
- Benazzi F. A prediction rule for diagnosing hypomania. *Prog Neuropsychopharmacol Biol Psychiatry*. 2009;33(2):317–322.
- Benazzi F. Bipolar disorder—focus on bipolar II disorder and mixed depression. *Lancet*. 2007; 369(9565):935–945.
- Licht RW. A new BALANCE in bipolar I disorder. *Lancet*. 2010;375(9712):350–352.
- Perlis RH, Brown E, Baker RW, et al. Clinical features of bipolar depression versus major depressive disorder in large multicenter trials. *Am J Psychiatry*. 2006;163(2):225–231.

SEE ALSO

Algorithm: Depressive Episode, Major

CODES

ICD10
F31.81 Bipolar II disorder

CLINICAL PEARLS

- BP-II is characterized by at least one episode of major depression and one episode of hypomania.
- Patients may not recognize symptoms and or decline treatment during a hypomanic episode; they may enjoy the elevated mood and productivity.
- Patients with BP-II are at great risk of both attempting and completing suicide.

BITES, ANIMAL AND HUMAN

Kathryn Samai, PharmD, BCPS • Brian James Kimbrell, MD, FACS

 BASICS

DESCRIPTION
- Animal bites to humans from dogs (60–90%), cats (5–20%), rodents (2–3%), humans (2–3%), and rarely other animals, including snakes
- System(s) affected: potentially any

Pediatric Considerations
Young children are more likely to sustain bites and have bites that include the face, upper extremity, or trunk.

EPIDEMIOLOGY
- Predominant age: all ages but children > adults
- Predominant gender: dog bites, male > female; cat bites, female > male

Incidence
- 2 to 5 million animal bites per year in the United States
- Account for 1% of all emergency room visits
- 1–2% will require hospital admission, and 10 to 20 victims will die from bites annually (1).

ETIOLOGY AND PATHOPHYSIOLOGY
- Most dog bite wounds are from a domestic pet known to the victim.
- 89% of cat bites are provoked.
- Males, pit bull terriers, and German shepherds are most commonly associated with dog bites (2).
- Human bites are often the result of one person striking another in the mouth with a clenched fist.
- Bites can also occur incidentally in the case of paronychia due to nail biting, or thumb sucking, or "love nips" to the face, breasts, or genital areas.
- Animal bites can cause tears, punctures, scratches, avulsions, or crush injuries.
- Contamination of wound with flora from the mouth of the biting animal or from the broken skin of the victim can lead to infection.

RISK FACTORS
- Male dogs and older dogs are more likely to bite.
- Clenched-fist human bites are frequently associated with the use of alcohol.
- Patients presenting >8 hours following the bite are at greater risk of infection.

GENERAL PREVENTION
- Instruct children and adults about animal hazards and strongly enforce animal control laws.
- Educate dog owners.

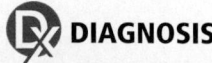 **DIAGNOSIS**

HISTORY
- Obtain detailed history of the incident (provoked or unprovoked).
- Type of animal
- Vaccine status
- Site of the bite
- Geographic setting

PHYSICAL EXAM
- Dog bites (60–90% of bites)
  - Hands and face most common site of injury in adults and children, respectively
  - More likely to have associated crush injury
- Cat bites (5–20% of bites)
  - Predominantly involve the hands, followed by lower extremities, face, and trunk

- Human bites (2–3% of bites)
  - Intentional bite: semicircular or oval area of erythema and bruising, with or without break in skin
  - Clenched-fist injury: small wounds over the metacarpophalangeal joints from striking the fist against another's teeth
- Signs of wound infection include fever, erythema, swelling, tenderness, purulent drainage, and lymphangitis.

ALERT
Cat bites (often puncture wounds) are twice as likely to cause infection as dog bites, with higher risks of osteomyelitis, tenosynovitis, and septic arthritis.

Pediatric Considerations
If human bite mark on child has intercanine distance >3 cm, bite probably came from an adult and should raise concerns about child abuse.

DIAGNOSTIC TESTS & INTERPRETATION
Initial Tests (lab, imaging)
- Drainage from infected wounds should be Gram-stained and cultured (3)[A].
  - If wound fails to heal, perform cultures for atypical pathogens (fungi, Nocardia, and mycobacteria) and ask lab to keep bacterial cultures for 7 to 10 days (some pathogens are slow-growing).
- 85% of bite wounds will yield a positive culture, with an average of five pathogens.
- Aerobic and anaerobic blood cultures should be obtained before starting antibiotics if bacteremia suspected (e.g., fever or chills).
- Previous antibiotic therapy may alter culture results.

ALERT
If bite wound is near a bone or joint, a plain radiograph is needed to check for bone injury and to use for comparison later if osteomyelitis is subsequently suspected (3)[B].

- Radiographs are needed to check for fractures in clenched-fist injuries.

Follow-Up Tests & Special Considerations
Subsequent suspicion of osteomyelitis warrants comparison of plain radiograph or MRI. Severe skull bites warrant a CT scan and ultrasound can be useful for detection of abscess.

Diagnostic Procedures/Other
Surgical exploration may be needed to ascertain extent of injuries or to drain deep infections (such as tendon sheath infections), especially in serious hand wounds.

Test Interpretation
- Dog bites (4,5)
  - Pasteurella species is present in 50% of bites.
  - Also found: viridans streptococci, Staphylococcus aureus, Staphylococcus intermedius, Bacteroides, Capnocytophaga canimorsus, Fusobacterium
- Cat bites (5)
  - Pasteurella species is present in 75% of bites.
  - Also found: Streptococcus spp. (including Streptococcus pyogenes), Staphylococcus spp. (including methicillin-resistant Staphylococcus aureus [MRSA]), Fusobacterium spp., Bacteroides spp., Porphyromonas spp., Moraxella spp.

- Human bites
  - Streptococcus spp., Staphylococcus aureus, Eikenella corrodens (29%), and various anaerobic bacteria (e.g., Fusobacterium, Peptostreptococcus, Prevotella, and Porphyromonas spp.)
  - Although rare, case reports have suggested transmission of viruses such as hepatitis, HIV, and herpes simplex.
- Reptile bites
  - If from a venomous snake, use antivenom. Bacteria: Pseudomonas aeruginosa, Proteus spp., Salmonella, Bacteroides fragilis, and Clostridium spp.
- Rodent bites
  - Streptobacillus moniliformis or Spirillum minor, which causes rat-bite fever
- Monkey bites
  - All monkey bites can transmit rabies, and bites of a macaque monkey may transmit herpes B virus, which is potentially fatal.

ALERT
Asplenic patients and those with underlying hepatic disease are at risk of bacteremia and fatal sepsis after dog bites infected with Capnocytophaga canimorsus (gram-negative rod).

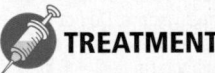 **TREATMENT**

GENERAL MEASURES
- Elevation of the injured extremity to prevent swelling
- Contact the local health department regarding the prevalence of rabies in the species of animal involved (highest in bats).
- Snake bite: If venomous, patient needs rapid transport to facility capable of definitive evaluation. If envenomation has occurred, patient should receive antivenom. Be sure patient is stable for transport; consider measuring and/or treating coagulation and renal status along with any anaphylactic reactions before transport.
- Monkey bite: Providers should contact CDC and administer an antiviral, such as valacyclovir, active against herpes B virus.

MEDICATION
- Consider need for antirabies therapy: rabies immunoglobulin and human diploid cell rabies vaccine for those bitten by wild animals (in the United States, primary vector is bat bite), rabid pets, unvaccinated pets, or if animal cannot be quarantined for 10 days.
- Tetanus toxoid (Td) for those previously immunized but >10 years since their last dose (3)[C]; tetanus, diphtheria, and pertussis (Tdap) is preferred over Td (3)
- A patient negative for anti-HBs and bitten by an HBsAg-positive individual should receive both hepatitis B immunoglobulin (HBIG) and hepatitis B vaccine.
- HIV postexposure prophylaxis is generally not recommended for human bites, given the extremely low risk for transmission, unless blood exposure to broken skin.
- Preemptive antibiotics are only recommended for human bites and high-risk wounds (deep puncture, crush injury, venous or lymphatic compromise, hands or near joint, face or genital area, immunocompromised hosts, requiring surgical repair, asplenic, advanced liver, edema).

- For preemptive and for empiric treatment of established infection, amoxicillin and clavulanate is first-line (3)[B],(6)
  - Adults: amoxicillin 875 mg/clavulanate 125 mg PO BID
  - Children: <3 months: 30 mg/kg/day PO q12h; ≥3 months and <40 kg: 45 mg/kg/day q12h; >40 kg, use adult dosing
    ○ Averse reaction: Amoxicillin and clavulanate should be given with food to decrease GI side effects.
    ○ Precautions: Dose antibiotics by body weight and renal function.
    ○ Significant possible interactions: Antibiotics may decrease efficacy of oral contraceptives.
  - Duration of therapy: preemptive, 3 to 5 days; treatment of cellulitis/skin abscess, 5 to 10 days; bacteremia, 10 to 14 days
  - Adults: clindamycin (300 mg PO TID) plus either
    ○ Trimethoprim-sulfamethoxazole (TMP-SMX; 1 DS tablet PO BID–TID) or
    ○ Ciprofloxacin (500 mg PO BID) for 7 to 21 days
    ○ Children: clindamycin (5 to 10 mg/kg IV [to a maximum of 600 mg] followed by 10 to 30 mg/kg/day in 3 to 4 divided doses to a maximum of 300 mg per dose) plus
    ○ TMP-SMX (8 to 10 mg/kg/day of trimethoprim) in 2 divided doses
- Avoid 1st-generation cephalosporins (e.g., cephalexin), penicillinase-resistant penicillins (e.g., dicloxacillin), macrolides (e.g., erythromycin), and clindamycin (when not administered with another agent) as they lack activity against *Pasteurella multocida* (dog/cat bites) and *E. corrodens* (human bites).

Pregnancy Considerations
- Penicillin-allergic pregnant women
  - Azithromycin 250 to 500 mg PO every day
- Observe closely and note potential increased risk of failure.

ALERT
Consider community acquired MRSA as possible pathogen (from human skin or colonized pet). If high suspicion, doxycycline or TMP-SMX provide good coverage (7).

ISSUES FOR REFERRAL
- Deep wounds to the hand and face should be referred to a hand surgeon or plastic surgeon, respectively.
- Bites from primates or unusual species of animals should be referred to infectious disease specialist.

SURGERY/OTHER PROCEDURES
- Copious irrigation of the wound with normal saline via a catheter tip is needed to reduce risk of infection.
- Devitalized tissue needs débridement.
- Débridement of puncture wounds is not advised.
- Primary closure can be considered if the wound is clean after irrigation and bite is <12 hours old and in bites to the face (cosmesis).
- Infected wounds and those at risk of infection (cat bites, human bites, bites to the hand, crush injuries, presentation >12 hours from injury) should be left open (8).

- Delayed primary closure in 3 to 5 days is an option for infected wounds.
- Splint hand if it is injured.
- Large, gaping wounds should be reapproximated with widely spaced sutures or Steri-Strips.

INPATIENT CONSIDERATIONS
Admission Criteria/Initial Stabilization
Patients with deep or severe wound infections, systemic infections requiring IV antibiotics, those requiring surgery, and the immunocompromised require ABCs for associated trauma or severe infection and IV antibiotic therapy
- Adults: ampicillin and sulbactam 1.5 to 3 g IV q6h *or* piperacillin and tazobactam 3.375 g IV q6h (3). Alternative: ciprofloxacin 400 mg IV q12h *or* levofloxacin 750 mg IV every day with metronidazole 500 mg IV q8h (3)
- Children: ampicillin and sulbactam 200 mg/kg/day IV given in 4 divided doses to a maximum of 3 g per dose

Discharge Criteria
Pending clinical improvement

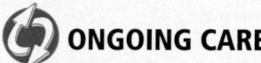

ONGOING CARE

FOLLOW-UP RECOMMENDATIONS
Patient Monitoring
- Patient should be rechecked in 24 to 48 hours if not infected at time of first encounter.
- Daily follow-up is warranted for infections.
- Subsequent revisions of empiric antibiotic therapy should be based on culture results and clinical response.

PATIENT EDUCATION
Educate parents at well-child checks about how to avoid animal bites.

PROGNOSIS
Wounds should steadily improve and close over by 7 to 10 days.

COMPLICATIONS
- Septic arthritis
- Osteomyelitis
- Extensive soft tissue injuries with scarring
- Hemorrhage
- Gas gangrene
- Sepsis
- Meningitis
- Endocarditis
- Posttraumatic stress disorder
- Death

REFERENCES

1. Goldstein EJ. New horizons in the bacteriology, antimicrobial susceptibility and therapy of animal bite wounds. *J Med Microbiol.* 1998;47(2):95–97.
2. Wiley JF II. Mammalian bites. Review of evaluation and management. *Clin Pediatr (Phila).* 1990;29(5):283–287.
3. Stevens DL, Bisno AL, Chambers HF, et al. Practice guidelines for the diagnosis and management of skin and soft tissue infections: 2014 update by the Infectious Disease Society of America. *Clin Infect Dis.* 2014;59(2):e10–e52.
4. Bini JK, Cohn SM, Acosta SM, et al. Mortality, mauling, and maiming by vicious dogs. *Ann Surg.* 2011;253(4):791–797.
5. Abrahamian FM, Goldstein EJ. Microbiology of animal bite wound infections. *Clin Microbiol Rev.* 2011;24(2):231–246.
6. Medeiros I, Saconato H. Antibiotic prophylaxis for mammalian bites. *Cochrane Database Syst Rev.* 2001;(2):CD001738.
7. Oehler RL, Velez AP, Mizrachi M, et al. Bite-related and septic syndromes caused by cats and dogs. *Lancet Infect Dis.* 2009;9(7):439–447.
8. Benson LS, Edwards SL, Schiff AP, et al. Dog and cat bites to the hand: treatment and cost assessment. *J Hand Surg Am.* 2006;31(3):468–473.

ADDITIONAL READING
- Okonkwo U, Changulani M, Moonot P. Animal bites: practical tips for effective management. *J Emerg Nurs.* 2008;34(3):225–226.
- Rittner AV, Fitzpatrick K, Corfield A. Best evidence topic report. Are antibiotics indicated following human bites? *Emerg Med J.* 2005;22(9):654.

 SEE ALSO

Cellulitis; Rabies; Snake Envenomation; *Bartonella* Infections

 CODES

ICD10
- S61.459A Open bite of unspecified hand, initial encounter
- S01.85XA Open bite of other part of head, initial encounter
- S20.97XA Other superficial bite of unspecified parts of thorax, initial encounter

CLINICAL PEARLS
- Wound cleansing, débridement, and culture are essential. Most wounds should be left open.
- Prophylaxis is recommended for human bites and high-risk wounds.
- Consider rabies and tetanus vaccination.
- Antibiotic and duration of therapy should be adjusted based on culture results and clinical improvement.
- Patients bitten by animals or humans require close follow-up to monitor for infection.

BLADDER CANCER
Margaret E. Thompson, MD, FAAP

BASICS

DESCRIPTION
- Primary malignant neoplasms arising in the urinary bladder
- Most common type is transitional cell carcinoma (90%).
- Other types include adenocarcinoma, small cell carcinoma, and squamous cell carcinoma.
- Rhabdomyosarcoma of the bladder may occur in children.

EPIDEMIOLOGY
Incidence
- Increases with age (median age at diagnosis is 73 years) (1)
- More common in Caucasians than in Asians or African Americans
- Male > female (4:1), but in smokers, risk is 1:1
- 35.8/100,000 men per year (1)
- 8.7/100,000 women per year (1)
- 20.5/100,000 men and women per year (1)

Prevalence
In 2012, 577,403 cases in the United States (1)

ETIOLOGY AND PATHOPHYSIOLOGY
Unknown, other than related to risk factors:
- 70–80% is nonmuscle invasive (in lamina propria or mucosa):
  - Usually highly differentiated with long survival
  - Initial event seems to be the activation of an oncogene on chromosome 9 in superficial cancers.
- 20% of tumors are muscle invasive (deeper than lamina propria) at presentation:
  - Tend to be high grade with worse prognosis
  - Associated with other chromosome deletions

Genetics
Hereditary transmission is unlikely, although transitional cell carcinoma pathophysiology is related to oncogenes.

RISK FACTORS
- Smoking is the single greatest risk factor (increases risk 4-fold) and increases risk equally for men and women (2).
- Use of pioglitazone for >1 year may be associated with an increased risk of bladder cancer. The risk seems to increase with duration of therapy and may also be present with other thiazolidinediones.
- Other risk factors:
  - Occupational carcinogens in dye, rubber, paint, plastics, metal, carbon black dust, and automotive exhaust
  - Schistosomiasis in Mediterranean (squamous cell) cancer
  - Arsenic in well water
  - History of pelvic irradiation
  - Chronic lower UTI
  - Chronic indwelling urinary catheter
  - Cyclophosphamide exposure
  - High-fat diet
  - Coffee consumption associated with reduced risk (RR 0.83; 95% CI, 0.73–0.94) (3)

ALERT
Any patient who smokes and presents with microscopic or gross hematuria or irritative voiding symptoms such as urgency and frequency not clearly due to UTI should be evaluated by cystoscopy for the presence of a bladder neoplasm.

GENERAL PREVENTION
- Avoid smoking and other risk factors.
- Counseling of individuals with occupational exposure
- The U.S. Preventive Services Task Force has concluded that there is an insufficient evidence to determine the balance between risk and harm of screening for bladder cancer (4)[B].

DIAGNOSIS

HISTORY
- Painless hematuria is the most common symptom.
- Urinary symptoms (frequency, urgency)
- Abdominal or pelvic pain in advanced disease
- Exposures (see "Risk Factors")

PHYSICAL EXAM
Normal in early cases, pelvic or abdominal mass in advanced disease, wasting in systemic disease

DIFFERENTIAL DIAGNOSIS
- Other urinary tract neoplasms
- UTI
- Prostatism
- Bladder instability
- Interstitial cystitis
- Urolithiasis
- Interstitial nephritis
- Papillary urothelial hyperplasia

DIAGNOSTIC TESTS & INTERPRETATION
Initial Tests (lab, imaging)
- Urinalysis is the initial test in patients presenting with gross hematuria or urinary symptoms such as frequency, urgency, and dysuria.
- Urine cytology (consult your local lab for volume needed and proper fixative/handling)
- Cystoscopy with biopsy is the gold standard for at-risk patients with painless hematuria.
- Macroscopic hematuria (55% sensitivity, positive predictive value [PPV] 0.22 for urologic cancer) (5)[C]

Follow-Up Tests & Special Considerations
- Urine cytology: 54% sensitivity overall (lower in less advanced tumors), 94% specific (6)[A]
- Other urine markers (of little clinical benefit):
  - Nuclear matrix protein-22 (NMP22): 67% sensitive, 78% specific (6)[A]
  - Bladder tumor–associated antigen stat: 70% sensitive, 75% specific, may be falsely positive in inflammatory conditions (6)[A]
  - Fluorescence in situ hybridization (FISH) assay: 69% sensitive, 78% specific (PPV 27.1, negative predictive value 95.3) for all tumors, more sensitive and specific for higher grade (7)[B]
  - *FGFR3* mutation has high specificity (99.9%) but low sensitivity (34.5%); PPV 95.2% (8)[A].
- *Bottom line: None of the urine markers is sensitive enough to rule out bladder cancer on its own.*
- Liver function tests, alkaline phosphatase if metastasis suspected
- Done for staging and to evaluate extent of disease but not for diagnosis itself:
  - CT urogram replacing IVP to image upper tracts if there is a suspicion of disease there
  - Diffusion-weighted MRI and multidimensional CT scan are undergoing study for use in diagnosis and staging of bladder tumors.

- For invasive disease, metastatic workup should include chest x-ray.
  - Bone scan should be performed if the patient has bone pain or if alkaline phosphatase is elevated.
- Urologic CT scan (abdomen, pelvis, with and without contrast) or MRI (40–98% accurate), with MRI slightly more accurate, is recommended if metastasis is suspected (9)[B].
- Regular cystoscopy (initiated at 3 months postprocedure) is indicated after transurethral resection of bladder tumor (TURBT) and intravesical chemotherapy for superficial bladder cancers.

Diagnostic Procedures/Other
- Cystoscopy with biopsy is the gold standard for diagnosis, but one study showed that 33% of patients had residual tumor after TURBT (9)[B].
- Using photodynamic diagnosis (PDD; employing a photosensitizing agent in the bladder that is taken up by tumor cells and visualized using a particular wavelength of light, which is changed to a different wavelength by the photosensitizing agent) has been shown to increase detection and identification of cancerous superficial tumors when compared with plain white light cystoscopy. A recent meta-analysis shows that this increases the likelihood of total resection (10)[A].

Test Interpretation
- Characterized as superficial (nonmuscle invasive) or invasive (muscle invasive)
- 70–80% present as superficial lesion.
- Superficial lesions
  - Carcinoma in situ: flat lesion, high grade
  - Ta: noninvasive papillary carcinoma
  - T1: extends into submucosa, lamina propria
- Invasive cancer
  - T2: invasion into muscle
    - pT2a: invasion into superficial muscle
    - pT2b: invasion into deep muscle
  - T3: invasion into perivesical fat
    - pT3a: microscopic
    - pT3b: macroscopic
  - T4: invasion into adjacent organs
    - aT4a: invades prostate, uterus, or vagina
    - aT4b: invades abdominal or pelvic wall
- N1–N3: invades lymph nodes
- M: metastasis to bone or soft tissue

TREATMENT

For nonmuscle-invasive bladder cancer, the treatment is generally removal via cystoscopic surgery (see earlier discussion re: PDD). For muscle-invasive cancer, a radical cystectomy with pelvic lymphadenectomy is preferred (11)[B].

MEDICATION
First Line
- A recent meta-analysis demonstrated neoadjuvant chemotherapy using platinum-based combination chemotherapy (with ≥1 of doxorubicin/epirubicin, methotrexate, or vinblastine), but not platinum alone, confers a significant survival advantage in patients with invasive bladder cancer, with an increase in survival at 5 years from 45% (without neoadjuvant treatment) to 50% (with treatment) (combined hazard ratio 0.86; 95% CI, 0.77–0.95) (12)[A].

- Intravesical bacillus Calmette-Guérin (BCG) after TURBT in high-grade lesions has been shown to decrease recurrence in Ta and T1 tumors (13)[A].

Second Line
- Chemotherapy is the first-line treatment for metastatic bladder cancer:
  - Methotrexate-vinblastine-doxorubicin-cisplatin (MVAC) is the preferred regimen.
- A recent review showed that gemcitabine plus cisplatin may be better tolerated and result in equivalent survival to MVAC, making it a possible first choice in metastatic bladder cancer.

ISSUES FOR REFERRAL
Patients with microscopic or gross hematuria not otherwise explained or resolving should be referred to a urologist for cystoscopy.

ADDITIONAL THERAPIES
Radiotherapy:
- In the United States, used for patients with muscle-invasive cancer who are not surgical candidates
- Preoperative (radical cystectomy) radiotherapy also an option
- Treatment of choice for muscle-invasive cancer in some European and Canadian centers:
  - 65 to 70 Gy over 6 to 7 weeks is standard.

SURGERY/OTHER PROCEDURES
- Surgery is definitive therapy for superficial and invasive cancer:
  - Superficial cancer: TURBT sometimes followed by intravesical therapy
- Invasive cancer
  - Radical cystectomy for invasive disease that is confined to the bladder is more effective than radical radiotherapy. There is insufficient evidence to recommend one form of urinary diversion over another (14).

INPATIENT CONSIDERATIONS
Admission Criteria/Initial Stabilization
Need for surgery or intensive therapy

 ONGOING CARE

FOLLOW-UP RECOMMENDATIONS
- Superficial cancers
  - Urine cytology alone has not been shown to be sufficient for follow-up.
  - Cystoscopy every 3 months for 18 to 24 months, every 6 months for the next 2 years, then annually
- Follow-up for invasive cancers depends on the approach to treatment.
- Patients treated with BCG require lifelong follow-up.

DIET
Continue adequate fluid intake.

PATIENT EDUCATION
Smoking cessation

PROGNOSIS
- 5-year relative survival rates (1)
  - Overall survival: 77.4%
    - In situ 95.9%
    - Localized: 69.9%
    - Regional metastasis: 34.0%
    - Distant metastasis: 5.4%
- Superficial bladder cancer
  - BCG treatment prevents recurrence versus TURBT alone; difference 30%, NNT 3.3
  - BCG prevents progression versus TURBT alone, difference 8%

- Invasive cancer
  - T2 disease: Radical cystectomy results in 60–75% 5-year survival.
  - T3 or T4 disease: Radical cystectomy results in 20–40% 5-year survival.
  - Neoadjuvant chemotherapy with cystectomy has led to varying degrees of increased survival.
  - Radiation with chemotherapy has led to varying degrees of increased survival.
- Metastatic cancer:
  - MVAC resulted in mean survival of 12.5 months.

COMPLICATIONS
- Superficial bladder cancer
  - Local symptoms
    - Dysuria, frequency, nocturia, pain, passing debris in urine
    - Bacterial cystitis
    - Perforation
  - General symptoms
    - Flulike symptoms
    - Systemic infection
- Invasive cancer
  - Symptoms related to definitive treatment, including incontinence, bleeding
  - Patients with neobladder at risk for azotemia and metabolic acidosis

REFERENCES

1. National Cancer Institute. SEER stat fact sheets: bladder cancer. http://seer.cancer.gov/statfacts/html/urinb.html. Accessed May 18, 2015.
2. Freedman ND, Silverman DT, Hollenbeck AR, et al. Association between smoking and risk of bladder cancer among men and women. *JAMA*. 2011;306(7):737–745.
3. Yu X, Bao Z, Zou J, et al. Coffee consumption and risk of cancers: a meta-analysis of cohort studies. *BMC Cancer*. 2011;11:96. doi: 10.1186/1471-2407-11-96.
4. Recommendation Summary. U.S. Preventive Services Task Force. http://www.uspreventiveservicestaskforce.org/Page/Topic/recommendation-summary/bladder-cancer-in-adults-screening. Accessed June 29, 2015.
5. Buntinx F, Wauters H. The diagnostic value of macroscopic haematuria in diagnosing urological cancers: a meta-analysis. *Fam Pract*. 1997;14(1):63–68.
6. Glas AS, Roos D, Deutekom M, et al. Tumor markers in the diagnosis of primary bladder cancer. A systematic review. *J Urol*. 2003;169(6):1975–1982.
7. Sarosdy MF, Kahn PR, Ziffer MD, et al. Use of a multitarget fluorescence in situ hybridization assay to diagnose bladder cancer in patients with hematuria. *J Urol*. 2006;176(1):44–47.
8. Karnes RJ, Fernandez CA, Shuber AP. A noninvasive mulitanalyte urine-based diagnostic assay for urothelial cancer of the bladder in the evaluation of hematuria. *Mayo Clin Proc*. 2012;87(9):835–342.
9. Kirkali Z, Chan T, Manoharan M, et al. Bladder cancer: epidemiology, staging and grading, and diagnosis. *Urology*. 2005;66(6 Suppl 1):4–34.
10. Mowatt G, N'Dow J, Vale L, et al. Photodynamic diagnosis of bladder cancer compared with white light cystoscopy: systematic review and meta-analysis. *Int J Technol Assess Health Care*. 2011;27(1):3–10.
11. Malkowicz SB, van Poppel H, Mickisch G, et al. Muscle-invasive urothelial carcinoma of the bladder. *Urology*. 2007;69(1 Suppl):3–16.
12. Advanced Bladder Cancer Overview Collaboration. Neoadjuvant chemotherapy for advanced bladder cancer. *Cochrane Database Syst Rev*. 2005;(2):CD005246
13. Shelley MD, Court JB, Kynaston H, et al. Intravesical bacillus Calmette-Guerin versus mitomycin C for Ta and T1 bladder cancer. *Cochrane Database Syst Rev*. 2003;(3):CD003231.
14. Cody JD, Nabi G, Dublin N, et al. Urinary diversion and bladder reconstruction/replacement using intestinal segments for intractable incontinence or following cystectomy. *Cochrane Database Syst Rev*. 2012;(2):CD003306.

ADDITIONAL READING
- Msaouel P, Koutsilieris M. Diagnostic value of circulating tumor cell detection in bladder and urothelial cancer: systematic review and meta-analysis. *BMC Cancer*. 2011;11:336.
- Sharma S, Ksheersagar P, Sharma P. Diagnosis and treatment of bladder cancer. *Am Fam Physician*. 2009;80(7):717–723.
- Zhu Z, Shen Z, Lu Y, et al. Increased risk of bladder cancer with pioglitazone therapy in patients with diabetes: a meta-analysis. *Diabetes Res Clin Pract*. 2012;98(1):159–163.

 SEE ALSO

- Hematuria
- Algorithm: Hematuria

 CODES

ICD10
- C67.9 Malignant neoplasm of bladder, unspecified
- C67.4 Malignant neoplasm of posterior wall of bladder
- C67.3 Malignant neoplasm of anterior wall of bladder

CLINICAL PEARLS
- Painless hematuria in smokers should be evaluated with cystoscopy.
- Be aware of potential link between pioglitazone treatment and risk for bladder cancer.
- The U.S. Preventive Services Task Force recommends against routine screening for bladder cancer.

BLEPHARITIS

Barton L. Blackorby, MD • Erin S. Seefeldt, MD

 BASICS

DESCRIPTION
- Common, usually chronic, inflammatory reaction of the eyelid margin
- Commonly presents as irritation, burning, redness, flaking, and crusting of the eyelids worse in morning
- Defined as anterior or posterior blepharitis with considerable overlap
  - Anterior blepharitis:
    ○ Staphylococcal
      ▪ Seborrheic
  - Posterior blepharitis:
    ○ Meibomian gland dysfunction (MGD)
- Areas affected: cornea, eyelid
- Can be primary or secondary to a systemic disease

EPIDEMIOLOGY
Incidence
- Very common
- All ethnic groups (Asians > Caucasians)
- Predominant age:
  - Nonstaphylococcal (average age: 50)
  - Staphylococcal (average age: <42)
- Predominant sex:
  - Nonstaphylococcal: male = female
  - Staphylococcal: male < female

RISK FACTORS
- Seborrheic dermatitis
- Contact dermatitis
- Herpes simplex dermatitis
- Varicella-zoster dermatitis
- Acne rosacea
- Immunocompromised state (e.g., AIDS, chemotherapy)
- Isotretinoin use
- Dry eye syndrome
- *Demodex folliculorum* infestation
- Giant papillary conjunctivitis

ETIOLOGY
- Seborrheic
  - Anterior eyelid inflammation secondary to increased and abnormal meibomian gland secretions
  - Eyelid erythema, crusting, and oily appearance
  - Can be associated with keratitis presenting as punctate epithelial erosions
  - Associated with acne rosacea
- Staphylococcal
  - Infection of the glands of the eyelid margin
  - Commonly caused by *Staphylococcus aureus* and coagulase-negative *Staphylococcus*, with occasional concomitant *Moraxella lacunata* infection
  - Crusting (golden) around eyelashes that is worse in the morning, collarette formation around lashes, scaling, crusting, and erythema
  - Severe cases are associated with keratitis and eyelid ulceration.

- Meibomian gland dysfunction: chronic obstruction and inflammation of the meibomian glands; associated with acne rosacea, acne vulgaris, and oral retinoid therapy
- Other types of blepharitis:
  - Contact dermatitis/blepharitis:
    ○ Develops from type IV hypersensitivity; common causes include ocular medications, topical anesthetics, antivirals, and cosmetics.
    ○ May occur with secondary *Staphylococcus* infection
  - Eczematoid blepharitis
    ○ Caused by type I hypersensitivity reaction to exotoxins and antigens from local flora
    ○ Strong association with eczema and asthma
    ○ Staphylococcal infection common
  - Parasitic blepharitis
    ○ Cylindrical sleeves along lashes
    ○ Found in 30% of chronic blepharitis

PATHOPHYSIOLOGY
- The exact etiopathogenesis is unknown.
- Suspected to be multifactorial
  - Chronic low-grade infections of the ocular surface with bacteria
  - Infestations with certain parasites such as the mite *Demodex*
  - Inflammatory skin conditions such as atopy and seborrhea

COMMONLY ASSOCIATED CONDITIONS
See "Risk Factors" and "Differential Diagnosis."

 DIAGNOSIS

HISTORY
- Duration of symptoms
- Unilateral or bilateral presentation
- Note any exacerbating conditions (e.g., smoke, allergens, wind, contact lenses).
- Pertinent past medical history: rosacea, herpetic zoster, autoimmune disease
- Current and recent medication use
- Recent exposure to infected individuals
- Frequently reported in all types of blepharitis
  - Burning
  - Itching
  - Eyelid erythema
  - Conjunctival infection (red eyes)
  - Lacrimation, tearing
  - Tear deficiency
  - Foreign body sensation
  - Photophobia (light sensitivity)
  - Impaired vision

PHYSICAL EXAM
- Test of visual acuity
- External exam (skin and eyelids)
  - Staphylococcal
    ○ Recurrent stye (external or internal hordeolum)
    ○ Missing, broken, or misdirected eyelashes (trichiasis)
    ○ Eyelid deposits: matted, hard scales; collarettes (ring-like formation around the lash shaft)
    ○ Ulcerations at base of eyelashes (rare)
    ○ Eyelid scarring may occur.
  - Seborrheic blepharitis
    ○ Eyelid deposits: dry flakes; oily or greasy secretions on lid margins and/or lashes
    ○ Associated dandruff of scalp and eyebrows
  - Meibomian gland dysfunction
    ○ Eyelash misdirection may occur with long-standing disease.
    ○ Eyelid deposits: fatty deposits; may be foamy
    ○ Eyelid margin thickening
    ○ Plugged meibomian gland orifices
      ▪ No expression of fluid upon gentle pressure of lid
    ○ Chalazion (sometimes multiple)
    ○ Eyelid scarring (notching) with long-term disease
    ○ Association with ocular rosacea
  - Mixed blepharitis: Signs and symptoms of >1 type of blepharitis may be present.

DIFFERENTIAL DIAGNOSIS
- Masquerade syndrome (1)
  - Persistent inflammation and thickening of eyelid margin may indicate squamous cell, basal cell, or sebaceous cell carcinoma masquerading as blepharitis. These carcinomas also may mimic styes or chalazia.
- Impetigo/erysipelas
- Herpetic zoster ophthalmicus
- Viral infections
- Contact or atopic dermatitis
- Medicamentosa

DIAGNOSTIC TESTS & INTERPRETATION
Follow-Up Tests & Special Considerations
- Consider masquerade syndrome in all cases of recurrent, persistent, or atypical chalazion; chronic unilateral unresponsive blepharoconjunctivitis; diffuse or nodular tumors of the eyelid; orbital mass developing after removal of an eyelid or caruncular tumor; and any tumor developing in a person with a history of ocular radiotherapy.
- Cultures in atypical blepharitis
- Biopsy in atypical cases for carcinoma
- Slit-lamp biomicroscopy
  - Examine tear film, eyelid margins, eyelashes, tarsal and bulbar conjunctiva, and cornea.
  - Fluorescein eye stain to evaluate for punctate epithelial keratitis
  - Inspect for loss of lashes (madarosis), whitening of the lashes (poliosis), trichiasis, crusting, eyelid margin ulcers, and lid irregularities.

TREATMENT

GENERAL MEASURES

- Promote proper eyelid hygiene (2,3)[C].
  - Apply warm compresses for several minutes at least once a day to soften adherent encrustations.
  - The eyelid margins then are scrubbed gently with eyelid cleanser or diluted baby shampoo twice a day to remove adherent material and clean the meibomian gland orifices (4)[C].
- Gentle vertical massage of the eyelids can help to express meibomian secretions in patients with meibomian gland dysfunction (2)[C].

- Discontinue soft contact lenses use during an acute case of blepharitis (3)[B].

MEDICATION

First Line

- According to Cochrane 2012, topical antibiotics provided some symptomatic relief and were effective in eradicating bacteria from the eyelid margin for anterior blepharitis. Lid hygiene may provide symptomatic relief for anterior and posterior blepharitis. The effectiveness of other treatments for blepharitis, such as topical steroids and PO antibiotics, was inconclusive (5)[A].
- No strong evidence supports any of the treatments in terms of curing chronic blepharitis (5)[A].

- Topical treatment to lid, if *Staphylococcus* likely:
  - Bacitracin ointment: 500 μg/g or (second choice)
  - Erythromycin: 0.5% ophthalmic ointment
    - The frequency and duration of treatment are guided by the severity (2)[C].
    - Topical corticosteroids (short term) should be used cautiously and briefly if at all and only for severe eyelid or ocular surface inflammation. The minimum effective dose and duration should be used; long-term use should be avoided if possible (6)[C].
- For patients with meibomian gland dysfunction inadequately controlled with eyelid hygiene, consider doxycycline 100 mg/day or tetracycline 1,000 mg/day in divided doses, tapered after clinical improvement (2 to 4 weeks) to doxycycline 50 mg/day or tetracycline 250 to 500 mg/day (2)[C].
- Oral azithromycin (500 mg/day for 3 days in three cycles with 7-day intervals) has been used successfully in the management of blepharitis associated with acne rosacea as an alternative to oral tetracyclines (2)[C].
- Because aqueous tear deficiency is common in blepharitis, use twice-daily artificial tears in addition to eyelid hygiene and medications.
- Contraindications: Allergy to medication; tetracyclines are not for use in pregnancy, nursing women, or children <8 years of age.
- Precautions
  - Tetracyclines can cause photosensitization, gastrointestinal upset, vaginitis, and rarely, azotemia. Tetracyclines have been implicated in cases of pseudotumor cerebri, and their metabolism may alter the effectiveness of certain medications (2).

- Corticosteroids may increase intraocular pressure and risk of cataract.
- Oral azithromycin can cause problems in patients with heart disease as it may cause irregular heart rhythms (2).

Second Line

Topical fluoroquinolones (e.g., gatifloxacin 0.3%, levofloxacin 0.5%, or moxifloxacin 0.5%) may be helpful for persistent or recurrent staphylococcal blepharitis or for those patients who prefer a solution.

ISSUES FOR REFERRAL

- Chronic recurrent blepharitis requires referral to an ophthalmologist for evaluation whether patient should continue soft lens use.
- A patient with chronic blepharitis that does not respond to therapy, particularly if associated with loss of eyelashes or corneal changes.

ADDITIONAL THERAPIES

Various commercial products are marketed to consumers and prescribed to patients; however, there is no substantial evidence of effectiveness (5)[A].

 ONGOING CARE

FOLLOW-UP RECOMMENDATIONS

Patient Monitoring

- Patients should schedule a return visit if their condition worsens despite treatment.
- Return visit intervals for patients with severe disease vary.
- If corticosteroid is prescribed, reevaluate within a few weeks to measure intraocular pressure and determine response to therapy.

PATIENT EDUCATION

- "Blepharitis Fact Sheet" from the American Academy of Ophthalmology
- Advise patient that blepharitis is a chronic condition likely to recur if eyelid hygiene is not maintained after antibiotic treatment is discontinued.

PROGNOSIS

Blepharitis cannot be permanently cured, and successful management is dependent on patient compliance with treatment regimen.

COMPLICATIONS

- Stye and chalazion
- Scarring of eyelid margin
- Corneal infection
- Superficial keratopathy
- Corneal neovascularization and ulceration
- Ectropion/entropion

REFERENCES

1. Tsai T, O'Brien JM. Masquerade syndromes: malignancies mimicking inflammation in the eye. *Int Ophthalmol Clin.* 2002;42(1):115–131.
2. American Academy of Ophthalmology Cornea/External Disease Panel. *Preferred Practice Pattern Guidelines: Blepharitis.* San Francisco, CA: American Academy of Ophthalmology; 2013.
3. Eyelid hygiene for blepharitis. *Insight.* 2011;36(1):24.
4. McCulley JP, Shine WE. Changing concepts in the diagnosis and management of blepharitis. *Cornea.* 2000;19(5):650–658.
5. Lindsley K, Matsumura S, Hatef E, et al. Interventions for chronic blepharitis. *Cochrane Database Syst Rev.* 2012;(5):CD005556.
6. Abelson MB, Cohane K, Fink K. Blepharitis: hiding in plain sight. *Rev Ophthalmol.* 2004;11(5):106–109.

 SEE ALSO

Lacrimal Disorders (Dry Eye Syndrome)

 CODES

ICD10

- H01.009 Unspecified blepharitis unspecified eye, unspecified eyelid
- H01.019 Ulcerative blepharitis unspecified eye, unspecified eyelid
- L21.8 Other seborrheic dermatitis

CLINICAL PEARLS

- Blepharitis is often a chronic condition; symptoms frequently can be lessened but rarely are eliminated.
- Promote proper eyelid hygiene.
- Bacitracin or erythromycin ophthalmic ointment is the first-line treatment if *Staphylococcus* is suspected.

BORDERLINE PERSONALITY DISORDER

Daniel E. Melville, MD • William G. Elder, PhD

 BASICS

DESCRIPTION

Beginning no later than adolescence or early adulthood, borderline personality disorder (BPD) is a consistent and pervasive pattern of labile affect and sense of self, impulsivity, and volatile interpersonal relationships (1):

- Common behaviors and variations:
  - Self-mutilation: pinching, scratching, cutting
  - Suicide: ideation, history of attempts, plans
  - Splitting: idealizing then devaluing others
  - Presentation of helplessness or victimization
  - High utilization of emergency department and resultant inpatient hospitalizations for psychiatric treatment
  - BPD patients are frequent users of primary care (2).
- High rate of associated mental disorders
- Typically display little insight into behavior

Geriatric Considerations
Illness (both acute and chronic) may exacerbate BPD and may lead to intense feelings of fear and helplessness.

Pediatric Considerations
Diagnosis is rarely made in children. Axis I disorders and general medical conditions are more probable.

Pregnancy Considerations
Physical, emotional, and social concerns may transiently mimic symptoms of BPD: Consider delay in diagnosis until pregnancy completed. Pregnancy may also induce stress or increased fears, resulting in escalation of borderline behaviors.

EPIDEMIOLOGY
Predominant age: Onset no later than adolescence or early adulthood (may go undiagnosed for years)

Prevalence
- General population: 0.5–5.9% of U.S. population (2)
- Estimated lifetime prevalence: 10–13% (2)
- 10% of all psychiatric outpatients and between 15% and 25% of patients in psychiatry inpatient settings have BPD (2).
- 20–30% of patients in primary care outpatient settings have a personality disorder.

ETIOLOGY AND PATHOPHYSIOLOGY
Undetermined, but generally accepted that psychiatric disorders are due to a combination of the following:

- Hereditary temperamental traits
- Environment (i.e., history of childhood sexual and/or physical abuse, history of childhood neglect, ongoing conflict in home)
- Stress is theorized to exert damaging effects on the brain, specifically the hippocampus (2,3).
- Neurobiologic research of BPD continues to increase the understanding of the etiology:
  - Abnormalities of the frontolimbic circuitry in relation to poor emotional stability (2)
  - Potential alterations in the sensitivity of opioid receptors and/or deficiencies with endogenous opioids (4)
  - Heightened activity in brain circuits involved in the experience of negative emotions and reduced activation that normally suppresses negative emotion once it is generated (5).

Genetics
First-degree relatives are at greater risk for this disorder (undetermined if due to genetic or psychosocial factors).

RISK FACTORS
- Genetic factors contribute; however, no specific genes have yet been identified as causative (2).
- Childhood sexual and/or physical abuse and neglect
- Disrupted family life
- Physical illness and external social factors may exacerbate borderline personality behaviors.

GENERAL PREVENTION
- Tends to be a multigenerational problem
- Children, caregivers, and significant others should have some time and activities away from the borderline individual, which may protect them.

COMMONLY ASSOCIATED CONDITIONS
Other psychiatric disorders, including:

- Co-occurring personality disorders, frequent
- Mood disorders, common
- Anxiety disorders, common
- Substance-related disorders, common
- Eating disorders, common
- Posttraumatic stress disorder, common
- BPD does not appear to be independently associated with increased risk of violence.

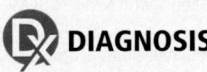 DIAGNOSIS

- The comprehensive evaluation should focus on (6)[B]:

  - Comorbid conditions
  - Functional impairments
  - Adaptive/maladaptive coping styles
  - Psychosocial stressors
  - Patient strengths; needs/goals

- Initial assessment should focus on determining treatment setting (6)[B]:

  - Establish treatment agreement with patient and outline treatment goals.
  - Assess suicide ideation and self-harm behavior.
  - Assess for psychosis.
  - Hospitalization is necessary if patient presents a threat of harm to self or others.

HISTORY
- Clinic visits for problems that do not have biologic findings
- Conflicts with medical staff members
- Idealizing or unexplained anger at physician
- History of unrealistic expectations of physician (e.g., "I know you can take care of me." "You're the best, unlike my last provider.")
- Obtain collateral information (i.e., from family, partner) about patient behaviors
- History of interpersonal difficulties, affective instability, and impulsivity
- History of self-injurious behavior, possibly with suicidal threats or attempts (7)

PHYSICAL EXAM
- BPD patients should have a thorough physical examination to help lower suspicion of organic disease (especially thyroid disease) (1,2).
- Often physical examination reveals no gross abnormalities, other than related to scarring from self-mutilation.

DIFFERENTIAL DIAGNOSIS
- Mood disorders:
  - Look at baseline behaviors when considering BPD versus mood disorder.
  - BPD symptoms increase the likelihood of misdiagnosing bipolar disorder.
  - In particular, disruptive mood dysregulation disorder, a new diagnosis appearing in DSM-5 and characterized by severe recurrent temper outbursts manifesting verbally or behaviorally and grossly out of proportion to the situation, may appear quite similar to the acting out and intense emotions seen in BPD. Look for other symptoms characteristic of BPD to differentiate (1).
- Psychotic disorder:
  - With BPD, typically only occurs under intense stress and is characterized as "micropsychotic."
- Other PD:
  - Thoughts, feelings, and behavior will differentiate BPD from other PDs.
- GMC:
  - Traits may emerge due to the effect of a GMC on the CNS.
- Substance use

DIAGNOSTIC TESTS & INTERPRETATION
- Consider age of onset. To meet criteria for BPD, borderline pattern will be present from adolescence or early adulthood.
- Formal psychological testing
- Rule out personality change due to a general medical condition (GMC) (1)[C]:
  - Traits may emerge due to the effect of a GMC on the CNS.
- Rule out symptoms related to substance use.
- If symptoms begin later than early adulthood or are related to trauma (e.g., after a head injury), a GMC, or substance use, then consider other diagnoses.

Diagnostic Procedures/Other
According to DSM-5 criteria, patient must meet at least five of the following criteria (1)[C]:

- Attempt to avoid abandonment
- Volatile interpersonal relationships
- Identity disturbance
- Impulsive behavior:
  - In ≥2 areas
  - Impulsive behavior is self-damaging.
- Suicidal or self-mutilating behavior
- Mood instability
- Feeling empty
- Is unable to control anger, or finds it difficult
- Paranoid or dissociative when under stress
- With advent of DSM-5, an alternative model is being promulgated that may come to define the diagnosis as impairments in personality functioning AND the presence of pathologic traits. Attention to these features may ultimately enhance provider understanding, diagnosis, and treatment of patients with personality dysfunction.
  - Criteria regarding personality functioning refer to impairments of self-functioning (i.e., identity or self-direction) AND interpersonal functioning (i.e., empathy or intimacy).
  - Pathologic personality traits refer to characteristics in the domains of negative affectivity (i.e., emotional liability, anxiousness, separation insecurity, depressivity); disinhibition (i.e., impulsivity, risk taking); OR antagonism (1).

TREATMENT

- Outpatient psychotherapy for BPD is the preferred treatment (2,6)[B]:
  - Dialectical behavior therapy (DBT) combines cognitive-behavioral techniques for emotional regulation and reality-testing with concepts of distress tolerance, acceptance, and self-awareness.
    - Following a dialectal process, therapists are tough-minded allies, who validate feelings and are unconditionally accepting, while also reminding patients to accept their dire level of emotional dysfunction and to apply better alternative behaviors.
    - DBT may be done individually and in groups.
- Consider transference-focused psychotherapy.
- Patient may need to be placed on suicide watch.
- Brief inpatient hospitalizations are ineffective in changing Axis II disorder behaviors:
  - Hospitalizations should be limited, and of short duration to adjust medications, implement psychotherapy for crisis intervention, and to stabilize patients from psychosocial stressors.
- Extended inpatient hospitalization should be considered for the following reasons (6)[B]:
  - Persistent/severe suicidal ideation or risk to others
  - Comorbid substance use and/or nonadherence to outpatient or partial hospitalization treatments
  - Comorbid Axis I disorders that may increase threat to life for the patient (i.e., eating disorders, mood disorders).

GENERAL MEASURES
Focus on patient management rather than on "fixing" behaviors:
- Schedule consistent appointment follow-ups to relieve patient anxiety.
- Meet with and rely on treatment team to avoid splitting of team by patient, and to provide opportunity to discuss patient issues.
- Treatment is usually most effective when both medications and psychotherapy are used simultaneously.

MEDICATION
- Although no specific medications are approved by the FDA to treat BPD, American Psychiatric Association (APA) guidelines recommend pharmacotherapy to manage symptoms (2)[A],(6)[B].
- Treat Axis I disorders (6)[B].
- Consider high rate of self-harm and suicidal behavior when prescribing (2)[A].
- APA guideline recommendations (6)[B]:
  - Affective dysregulation: mood stabilizers, SSRIs, and monoamine oxidase inhibitors (MAOIs)
  - Impulsive-behavioral control: SSRIs and mood stabilizers
  - Cognitive-perceptual symptoms: antipsychotics
- With more neurobiologic causes considered in relation to BPD, there is more emphasis on mood stabilizers and atypical antipsychotics, but research is uncertain and inconclusive (8)[B].
- Antipsychotics have short-lived benefit and offer no value other than transient treatment of cognitive perceptual symptoms (9)[B].

ISSUES FOR REFERRAL
- If hospitalized, consider for suicide risk, mood or anxiety disorders, or substance-related disorders.

- Urgency for scheduled follow-up depends on community resources (e.g., outpatient day programs for suicidal patients; substance abuse programs):
  - With increased risk for self-harm or self-defeating behaviors and low community resources, the patient can/will have increased need for frequent visits.

ADDITIONAL THERAPIES
Consider referring patient for specialized mental health behavioral services, including partial hospital therapy.

COMPLEMENTARY & ALTERNATIVE MEDICINE
Omega-3 fatty acid dietary supplementation has shown beneficial effects (2)[B].

INPATIENT CONSIDERATIONS
Admission Criteria/Initial Stabilization
Admit for inpatient services immediately in presence of psychosis or threat of injury to self or others; include police, as necessary, for safety measures.
- Assess suicidal ideation.
- Consider trial of antipsychotic medications for psychosis.

Nursing
Nurses can be instrumental in managing and calling patients, potentially relieving patient stress.

Discharge Criteria
- Patient should not present risk of harm to self or others and have a safety plan.
- Follow-up should be scheduled with a mental health specialist and primary care provider.

ONGOING CARE

FOLLOW-UP RECOMMENDATIONS
- Schedule visits that are short, more frequent, and focused to relieve patients' anxiety about relationships with their physician/provider and to help reduce risk of provider burnout.
- Maintain open lines of communication with mental health professionals providing psychological support.
- Emphasize importance of healthy lifestyle modifications (i.e., exercise, rest, diet).

Patient Monitoring
Monitor for suicidal or other self-harm behaviors.

PATIENT EDUCATION
Include patients in the diagnosis so they can make sense of their disease process and participate in the treatment strategy (6,9)[C].

PROGNOSIS
- Borderline behaviors may decrease with age and over time.
- Patients in treatment improve at a rate of seven times compared with following natural course (10).
- Treatment is complex and takes time.
- Medical focus includes patient management and caring for medical and Axis I disorders.

REFERENCES
1. American Psychiatric Association. *Diagnostic and Statistical Manual of Mental Disorders*. 5th ed. Arlington, VA: American Psychiatric Publishing; 2013.
2. Leichsenring F, Leibing E, Kruse J, et al. Borderline personality disorder. *Lancet*. 2011;377(9759):74–84.
3. Ruocco AC, Amirthavasagam S, Zakzanis KK. Amygdala and hippocampal volume reductions as candidate endophenotypes for borderline personality disorder: a meta-analysis of magnetic resonance imaging studies. *Psychiatry Res*. 2012;201(3):245–252.
4. Bandelow B, Schmahl C, Falkai P, et al. Borderline personality disorder: a dysregulation of the endogenous opioid system? *Psychol Rev*. 2010;117(2):623–636.
5. Ruocco A, Amirthavasagam S, Choi-Kain LW, et al. Neural correlates of negative emotionality in borderline personality disorder: an activation-likelihood-estimation meta-analysis. *Biol Psychiatry*. 2013;73(2):153–160.
6. Oldham JA. *Guideline Watch: Practice Guideline for the Treatment of Patients With Borderline Personality Disorder*. Arlington, VA: American Psychiatric Association; 2005.
7. Zanarini MC, Laudate CS, Frankenburg FR, et al. Reasons for self-mutilation reported by borderline patients over 16 years of prospective follow-up. *J Pers Disord*. 2013;27(6):783–794.
8. Feurino L III, Silk KR. State of the art in the pharmacologic treatment of borderline personality disorder. *Curr Psychiatry Rep*. 2011;13(1):69–75.
9. Sanislow CA, Marcus KL, Reagan EM. Long-term outcomes in borderline psychopathology: old assumptions, current findings, and new directions. *Curr Psychiatry Rep*. 2012;14(1):54–61.
10. Elder W, Walsh E. Personality disorders. In: South-Paul J, Matheny S, Lewis E, eds. *Current Diagnosis & Treatment in Family Medicine*. 3rd ed. New York, NY: McGraw-Hill; 2011.

CODES

ICD10
F60.3 Borderline personality disorder

CLINICAL PEARLS
- View BPD as a chronic condition with waxing and waning features. It is important to adjust medications/treatments as clinically appropriate when symptoms change.
- If there are problems with the patient disrespecting the physician or support staff, clear guidelines should be established with the treatment team and then with the patient.
- When considering terminating care, the patient may improve if empathetically confronted about certain behaviors and is given clear guidelines on how to behave in the clinic. It is the patient's job to follow the guidelines, and it is you and your team's job to enforce the guidelines. Designate a case management nurse or well-trained support staff person who can be the primary contact person for the patient.
- Have an agenda when you visit with BPD patients. Be cordial—they deserve the same professionalism any patient gets. Have and identify 1 to 2 issues to be discussed per clinic visit. Frequently scheduled visits can help with this.
- Regularly scheduled psychotherapy treatment helps physician performance by becoming the "home" for mental health treatment, leaving the physician to focus on the patient's immediate medical issues.

BRAIN INJURY, TRAUMATIC

Caleb J. Mentzer, DO • James R. Yon, MD

BASICS

DESCRIPTION
- Traumatic brain injury (TBI) is defined as an alteration in brain function, or other evidence of brain pathology, caused by an external force.
- System(s) affected: neurologic; psychiatric; cardiovascular; endocrine/metabolic; gastrointestinal
- Synonym(s): head injury, concussion

EPIDEMIOLOGY
Incidence
- 2.2 million ED visits and 280,000 hospitalizations/year
- 50,000 deaths/year; ~30% of all injury-related deaths
- Incidence in males twice that of females with 4-fold risk of fatal trauma

Prevalence
- Predominant age: 0 to 4 years, 15 to 19 years, and >65 years
- Predominant gender: male > female (2:1)

ETIOLOGY AND PATHOPHYSIOLOGY
- Falls (40%)
- Motor vehicle accidents (14%)
- Assault (10%)
- Child abuse (24% of TBI age 2 years and younger)
- Recreational activities (21% of pediatric TBI, peak seasons spring/summer; peak ages 10 to 14 years)
- Primary insult: direct mechanical damage
- Secondary insult: actuation of complex cellular and molecular cascades that promote cerebral edema, ischemia, and apoptotic cell death

RISK FACTORS
Alcohol and drug use, prior/recurrent head injury, contact sports, seizure disorder, ADHD, male sex, luteal phase of female menstrual cycle

Geriatric Considerations
Subdural hematomas are common after a fall or blow in elderly; symptoms may be subtle and not present until days after trauma. Many elderly patients are on antiplatelet or anticoagulation therapy.

GENERAL PREVENTION
- Safety education
- Seat belts; bicycle and motorcycle helmets
- Protective headgear for contact sports

Pediatric Considerations
Child abuse: Consider if dropped or fell <4 feet (e.g., off bed, couch), suspicious history, significant injury present, or any retinal hemorrhages.

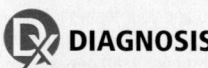

DIAGNOSIS

HISTORY
- Loss of consciousness (LOC), headache, vomiting, amnesia
- Epidural hemorrhage from blunt trauma: 30% with a "lucid interval" (initial LOC followed by recovery of consciousness, then LOC recurs and persists)

PHYSICAL EXAM
- Neurologic and cognitive testing is important.
- Repeat neurologic exams every 30 minutes until 2 hours after GCS reaches 15, then hourly for 4 hours, then every 2 hours.

- Evidence of increased intracranial pressure (ICP) (elevated BP, decreased pulse rate, or slow/irregular breathing [Cushing triad]—only 30% have all 3)
- Decorticate or decerebrate posturing
- Signs of basilar skull fracture: raccoon eyes, Battle sign, hemotympanum, CSF rhinorrhea or otorrhea)

DIFFERENTIAL DIAGNOSIS
Other causes of altered mental status (e.g., toxicologic, infectious, metabolic, vascular)

DIAGNOSTIC TESTS & INTERPRETATION
Initial Tests (lab, imaging)
- Mild TBI and concussions cognitive screening tests
  - Sports Concussion Assessment Tool V3 (SCAT3)
  - Child SCAT3
  - Concussion Recognition Tool (CRT)
  - Standardized Assessment of Concussion (SAC)
  - King-Devick Test
  - Balance Error Scoring System (BESS)
- Evaluate for coagulopathy.
- Type and screen for possible surgical intervention.
- Perform drug and alcohol screening.
- CT, noncontrast, is the study of choice to review bone windows, tissue windows, and subdural space.
- NEXUS II study demonstrated that if all eight clinical criteria are absent, there is a low likelihood of significant TBI:
  - Evidence of significant skull fracture (depressed, basilar, or diastatic)
  - Altered level of alertness
  - Neurologic deficit
  - Persistent vomiting
  - Presence of scalp hematoma
  - Abnormal behavior
  - Coagulopathy
  - Age >65 years

Follow-Up Tests & Special Considerations
Blast-related TBI: much higher rates of postconcussive syndrome, PTSD, depression, and chronic pain. Chronic impairment is strongly correlated with psychological factors. Return to battlefield guidelines similar to return to play in sports (see "General Measures") (1)[A]

Pediatric Considerations
Skull radiographs are not indicated unless abuse is suspected in which case they can detect fractures not seen under CT. No return to activity until they are asymptomatic, and return to school should precede return to sport/physical activity (2)[A].

Diagnostic Procedures/Other
- CSF rhinorrhea
  - Contains glucose; nasal mucus does not.
  - Check for the double-halo sign: If nasal discharge contains CSF and blood, two rings appear when placed on filter paper—a central ring followed by a paler ring.
- ICP monitors are associated with lower mortality, but use is not superior to nonuse (3)[A].

TREATMENT

GENERAL MEASURES
- Acute management depends on injury severity. Most patients need no interventions.
- Immediate goal: Determine who needs further therapy, imaging studies (CT), and hospitalization to prevent further injury.

- For the mildly injured patient
  - Early education is beneficial for recovery (4)[A].
  - **Return to play (RTP)**
    - Never RTP on same day.
    - Strict guidelines for graduated return to cognitive and physical activity when there are no evident signs or symptoms (physical, cognitive, emotional, or behavioral) on neuropsychological and clinical evaluation (2)[A]
- For the moderate to severely injured patient
  - Avoid hypotension or hypoxia. Head injury causes increased ICP secondary to edema, and cerebral perfusion pressure (CPP) should be maintained between 60 and 70 mm Hg (5)[A].
  - 30-degree head elevation decreases ICP and improves CPP.
  - Hyperventilation (hypocapnia)
    - Use should be limited to patients with impending herniation while preparing for definitive treatment or intraoperatively. Risk of worsening cerebral ischemia and organ damage (5–7)[A]
    - Addition of tromethamine can offset deleterious effects and lead to better outcomes (7)[A]
  - Mild systematic hypothermia lowers ICP but leads to increased rates of pneumonia. Selective brain cooling may also decrease ICP with improved outcomes at 2 years post injury (7)[A].
- Seizure prophylaxis
  - Does not change morbidity or mortality. Consider phenytoin or levetiracetam for 1 week post injury or longer for patients with early seizures, dural-penetrating injuries, multiple contusions, and/or subdural hematomas requiring evacuation (8)[A].

MEDICATION
First Line
- Pain
  - Morphine: 1 to 2 mg IV PRN, with caution, because it can depress mental status, further altering serial neurologic evaluations

ALERT
Bolus doses increase ICP and decrease CPP (9)[A].

- Increased ICP
  - Hypertonic saline: 2 mL/kg IV decreases ICP without adverse hemodynamic status; preferred agent (5,9)[A]
  - Mannitol: 0.25 to 2 g/kg (0.25 to 1 g/kg in children) given over 30 to 60 minutes in patients with adequate renal function. Prophylactic use is associated with worse outcomes (9)[A].
- Sedation
  - Propofol: preferred due to short duration of action. Avoid high doses to prevent propofol infusion syndrome. When combined with morphine, it can also effectively decrease ICP and decrease use of other meds (9)[A].
  - Midazolam: similar sedating effect to propofol but may cause hypotension (9)[A]
- Seizures
  - Phenytoin (Dilantin): 15 mg/kg IV (1 mg/kg/min IV, not to exceed 50 mg/min). Stop infusion if QT interval increases by >50%.

ALERT

Avoid corticosteroid use, as it increases mortality rates and risk of developing late seizures (9)[A]. Avoid barbiturates due to risk of hypotension (9)[A].

ISSUES FOR REFERRAL

Consult neurosurgery for:
- All penetrating head trauma
- All abnormal head CTs

ADDITIONAL THERAPIES

- Emerging therapies with limited but promising evidence: coma arousal therapy: amantadine, zolpidem, and levodopa/carbidopa; post coma therapy: bromocriptine
- Limited role for therapeutic hypothermia with defined physiologic parameters (10)[A]

SURGERY/OTHER PROCEDURES

- Early evacuation of trauma-related intracranial hematoma decreases mortality especially with GCS <6 and CT evidence of hematoma, cerebral swelling, or herniation (11)[A].
- Decompressive craniectomy reduces ICP especially when a large bone flap is removed. ONLY for adults and ONLY with GCS >6 (7)[A].
- Hyperbaric oxygen temporarily lowers ICP and improves mortality, but evidence is conflicting about outcomes at 6 to 12 months post injury (7)[A]. The combination of hyperbaric and normobaric hyperoxia reduces ICP and improves overall morbidity/mortality (12)[B].
- CSF drainage reduces ICP but has not been demonstrated to have long-term benefit (7)[A].
- CSF leakage often resolves in 24 hours with bed rest, but if not, may require surgical repair (5)[A].

COMPLEMENTARY & ALTERNATIVE MEDICINE

Music therapy in conjunction with multimodal stimulation improves awareness in comatose TBI patients (10)[B].

INPATIENT CONSIDERATIONS

Admission Criteria/Initial Stabilization

- Abnormal GCS or CT
- Clinical evidence of basilar skull fracture
- Persistent neurologic deficits (e.g., confusion, somnolence)
- Patient with no competent adult at home for observation
- Possibly admit: LOC, amnesia, patients on anticoagulants with negative CT
- ABCs take priority over head injury.
- C-spine immobilization should be considered in all head trauma.

IV Fluids

Use normal saline for resuscitation fluid.

Discharge Criteria

Normal CT with return to normal mental status and responsible adult to observe patient at home (see "Patient Monitoring")

 ONGOING CARE

FOLLOW-UP RECOMMENDATIONS

- Schedule regular follow-up within a week to determine return to activities.

- Rehabilitation indicated following a significant acute injury. Set realistic goals.
- For patients on anticoagulants, net benefit to restarting therapy after discharge despite increased bleeding risk.

Patient Monitoring

Patient should be discharged to the care of a competent adult with clear instructions on signs and symptoms that warrant immediate evaluation (e.g., changing mental status, worsening headache, focal findings, or any signs of distress). Patients should be monitored but not awakened from sleep.

DIET

As tolerated, monitor for signs of nausea.

PATIENT EDUCATION

Proper counseling, symptomatic management, and gradual return to normal activities are essential.

PROGNOSIS

- Gradual improvement may continue for years.
- 30–50% of severe head injuries may be fatal.
- Predicting outcome is difficult; many with even minor to moderate injuries have moderate to severe disability at 1 year, whereas prolonged coma may be followed by satisfactory outcome.
- Patients may have new-onset seizures over 2 years following trauma.
- Poor prognostic factors: low GCS on admission, nonreactive pupils, old age, comorbidity, midline shift

COMPLICATIONS

- Chronic subdural hematoma, which may follow even "mild" head injury, especially in the elderly; often presents with headache and decreased mentation
- Delayed hematomas and hydrocephalus
- Emotional disturbances and psychiatric disorders resulting from head injury may be refractory to treatment
- Seizures: seen in 50% of penetrating head injuries, 20% of severe closed head injuries, and <5% of head injuries overall. Hematomas increase risk of epilepsy.
- Postconcussion syndrome can follow mild head injury without LOC and includes headaches, dizziness, fatigue, and subtle cognitive or affective changes.
- Second-impact syndrome occurs when the CNS loses autoregulation. An individual with a minor head injury is returned to a contact sport and, following even minor trauma (e.g., whiplash), the patient loses consciousness and may quickly herniate, with a 50% mortality. A similar syndrome of malignant edema can occur in children with even a single injury.
- Increased risk for Alzheimer disease, Parkinson disease, and other brain disorders whose prevalence increases with age

REFERENCES

1. Rosenfeld JV, McFarlane AC, Bragge P, et al. Blast-related traumatic brain injury. *Lancet Neurol.* 2013;12(9):882–893.
2. McCrory P, Meeuwisse WH, Aubry M, et al. Consensus statement on concussion in sport: the 4th International Conference on Concussion in Sport held in Zurich, November 2012. *Br J Sports Med.* 2013;47(5):250–258.
3. Yuan Q, Wu X, Sun Y, et al. Impact of intracranial pressure monitoring on mortality in patients with traumatic brain injury: a systematic review and meta-analysis. *J Neurosurg.* 2015;122(3):574–587.
4. Nygren-de Boussard C, Holm LW, Cancelliere C, et al. Nonsurgical interventions after mild traumatic brain injury: a systematic review. Results of the International Collaboration on Mild Traumatic Brain Injury Prognosis. *Arch Phys Med Rehabil.* 2014;95(3)(Suppl):S257–S264.
5. Tsang KK, Whitfield PC. Traumatic brain injury: review of current management strategies. *Br J Oral Maxillofac Surg.* 2012;50(4):298–308.
6. Curley G, Kavanagh BP, Laffey JG. Hypocapnia and the injured brain: more harm than benefit. *Crit Care Med.* 2010;38(5):1348–1359.
7. Meyer MJ, Megyesi J, Meythaler J, et al. Acute management of acquired brain injury part I: an evidence-based review of non-pharmacological interventions. *Brain Inj.* 2010;24(5):694–705.
8. Agrawal A, Timothy J, Pandit L, et al. Post-traumatic epilepsy: an overview. *Clin Neurol Neurosurg.* 2006;108(5):433–439.
9. Meyer MJ, Megyesi J, Meythaler J, et al. Acute management of acquired brain injury part II: an evidence-based review of pharmacological interventions. *Brain Inj.* 2010;24(5):706–721.
10. Crossley S, Reid J, McLatchie R, et al. A systematic review of therapeutic hypothermia for adult patients following traumatic brain injury. *Crit Care.* 2014;18(2):R75.
11. Kim YJ. The impact of time to surgery on outcomes in patients with traumatic brain injury: a literature review. *Int Emerg Nurs.* 2014;22(4):214–219.
12. Rockswold SB, Rockswold GL, Zaun DA, et al. A prospective, randomized phase II clinical trial to evaluate the effect of combined hyperbaric and normobaric hyperoxia on cerebral metabolism, intracranial pressure, oxygen toxicity, and clinical outcome in severe traumatic brain injury. *J Neurosurg.* 2013;118(6):1317–1328.

 CODES

ICD10

- S06.9X0A Unsp intracranial injury w/o loss of consciousness, init
- S06.5X0A Traum subdr hem w/o loss of consciousness, init
- S06.6X0A Traum subrac hem w/o loss of consciousness, init

CLINICAL PEARLS

- TBI involves two distinct phases: the primary mechanical insult and secondary dysregulation of the cerebrovascular system with cerebral edema, ischemia, and cell-mediated death.
- Indications for imaging include evidence of skull fracture, altered consciousness, neurologic deficit, persistent vomiting, scalp hematoma, abnormal behavior, coagulopathy, age >65 years.
- Strict criteria exist for patients to return to normal sport activity following head injury to avoid the second-impact syndrome, which has 50% mortality.

BREAST ABSCESS

Lindsay Petersen, MD • Andrea Madrigrano, MD

 BASICS

DESCRIPTION
- Localized collection of pus within the breast parenchyma
- Can be associated with lactation or fistulous tracts secondary to squamous epithelial neoplasm or duct occlusion
- System(s) affected: skin/exocrine
- Synonym(s): mammary abscess; peripheral breast abscess; subareolar abscess; puerperal abscess

Pregnancy Considerations
Most commonly associated with postpartum lactation

EPIDEMIOLOGY
- Predominant age
  - Puerperal abscess: lactational
  - Subareolar abscess: postmenopausal
- Predominant sex: female
- Higher incidence in African American women

Incidence
- 0.1–0.5% of breastfeeding women
- Puerperal abscess rare after first 6 weeks of lactation

ETIOLOGY AND PATHOPHYSIOLOGY
- Delayed treatment of mastitis
- Puerperal abscesses: blocked lactiferous duct
- Subareolar abscess: squamous epithelial neoplasm with keratin plugs or ductal extension with associated inflammation
- Peripheral abscess: stasis within the duct leading to microbial accumulation and secondary abscess formation
- Microbiology
  - *Staphylococcus aureus* is most common cause.
  - Less common causes
    - *Streptococcus pyogenes; Escherichia coli; Bacteroides*
    - *Corynebacterium*
    - *Pseudomonas*
    - *Proteus*
- Methicillin-resistant *Staphylococcus aureus* (MRSA) is increasing. Risk factors for postpartum *S. aureus* (SA) breast abscess have not changed with rise in community-associated MRSA.

RISK FACTORS
- Puerperal mastitis
  - 5–11% progression to abscess:
    - Most often due to inadequate therapy
  - Risk factors (stasis):
    - Infrequent or missed feeds
    - Poor latch (1)
    - Damage or irritation of the nipple
    - Use of breast pump (2)
    - Illness in mother or baby
    - Rapid weaning
    - Blocked nipple or duct
- General factors
  - Smoking (3)
  - Diabetes (3)
  - Rheumatoid arthritis
  - Obesity (3)
- Medically induced factors
  - Steroids
  - Silicone/paraffin implant
  - Lumpectomy with radiation
  - Oral antibiotics during breastfeeding (mastitis) (2)
  - Topical antifungal medication during breastfeeding (mastitis) (2)
- Nipple retraction
- Nipple piercing (mastitis, subareolar abscess) (3)
- Higher recurrence rate if polymicrobial abscess

GENERAL PREVENTION
Early treatment of mastitis with milk expression, antibiotics, and compresses

COMMONLY ASSOCIATED CONDITIONS
Lactation

 DIAGNOSIS

HISTORY
- Tender breast lump, usually unilateral
- Breastfeeding
- Postmenopausal
- Systemic malaise (usually less than with mastitis)
- Localized erythema, edema, and pain
- Fever, nausea, vomiting, or spontaneous nipple drainage

PHYSICAL EXAM
- Fever, tachycardia
- Erythema of overlying skin
- Tenderness, fluctuance on palpation

- Draining pus or skin ulceration
- Local edema
- Nipple and skin retraction
- Regional lymphadenopathy

DIFFERENTIAL DIAGNOSIS
- Carcinoma (inflammatory or primary squamous cell)
- Engorgement
- Galactocele
- Tuberculosis (may be associated with HIV infection)
- Sarcoid; granulomatous mastitis
- Syphilis
- Foreign body reactions (e.g., to silicone and paraffin)
- Mammary duct ectasia

DIAGNOSTIC TESTS & INTERPRETATION
- CBC (leukocytosis)
- Elevated ESR
- Ultrasound (US) helps identify fluid collection within breast tissue.
- Culture and sensitivity of abscess fluid or expressed breast milk to identify pathogen (usually *Staphylococcus* or *Streptococcus*)
- MRSA is an increasingly important pathogen in both lactational and nonlactational abscesses.
- Other bacteria:
  - Nonlactational abscess and recurrent abscesses associated with anaerobic bacteria
    - *E. coli, Proteus*; mixed bacteria less common
- Mammogram to rule out carcinoma (generally not in acute phase)

Diagnostic Procedures/Other
Aspiration of abscess for culture (not accurate to exclude carcinoma)

Test Interpretation
- Squamous metaplasia of the ducts
- Intraductal hyperplasia
- Epithelial overgrowth
- Fat necrosis
- Duct ectasia

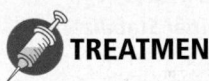 **TREATMENT**

GENERAL MEASURES
- Cold compresses for pain control
- Important to continue to breastfeed or express milk to drain the affected breast

136

MEDICATION

Combination of antibiotics and drainage for cure:

- Culture midstream sample of milk for mastitis.
- Culture abscess fluid for breast abscess.

- There is insufficient evidence regarding the effectiveness of antibiotic therapies for lactational mastitis alone (4)[A].

First Line

- NSAIDs for analgesia and/or antipyresis

- Dicloxacillin 500 mg QID for 10 to 14 days (5)[A]

- If no response in 24 to 48 hours, switch to cephalexin 500 mg QID for 10 to 14 days.
  – Or amoxicillin-clavulanate (Augmentin) 250 to 500 mg TID
- Clindamycin 300 mg QID if anaerobes are suspected
- If MRSA is a concern, TMP-SMZ DS 1 to 2 PO BID for 10 to 14 days. Clindamycin 300 mg PO QID as alternative
- *Contraindications*: antibiotic allergy
- In severe infections, vancomycin as an inpatient may be necessary.
  – Dose (30 mg/kg) IV in 2 divided doses every 24 hours may be necessary until culture results are available.
  – A 3rd-generation or a combination of a beta-lactam and beta-lactamase agent may need to be added as well.

SURGERY/OTHER PROCEDURES

- Aspiration with or without US guidance (6)[A]
- Consider US-guided percutaneous catheter placement if abscess >3 cm (6)[A].

- Serial aspirations under US may be necessary (q2–3d) if patients fail to respond (7)[C].

- Needle aspiration alone (without antibiotics) may be effective for small breast abscesses (8)[A].
- Consider incision and drainage if abscess is recurrent, chronic, or >5 cm (6)[A].

- Biopsy nonpuerperal abscesses to rule out carcinoma.
- Open all fistulous tracts, especially abscesses in nonlactating patients.

- US-guided aspiration with judicious use of antibiotics is superior to incision and drainage (9)[A].

COMPLEMENTARY & ALTERNATIVE MEDICINE

- Lecithin supplementation

- Acupuncture may help with breast engorgement, and prevention of breast abscess (10)[A].

INPATIENT CONSIDERATIONS

Admission Criteria/Initial Stabilization

Outpatient, unless systemically immunocompromised or septic

 ONGOING CARE

FOLLOW-UP RECOMMENDATIONS

Patient Monitoring

Ensure resolution to exclude carcinoma.

PATIENT EDUCATION

- Wound care
- Continue with breastfeeding or pumping (if breastfeeding is not possible due to location of abscess) to prevent engorgement.

PROGNOSIS

- Complete healing expected in 8 to 10 days
- Subareolar abscesses frequently recur, even after incision and drainage (I&D) and antibiotics; may require surgical removal of ducts

COMPLICATIONS

- Fistula: mammary duct or milk fistula
- Poor cosmetic outcome

REFERENCES

1. Branch-Elliman W, Golen TH, Gold HS, et al. Risk factors for *Staphylococcus aureus* postpartum breast abscess. *Clin Infect Dis*. 2012;54(1):71–77.
2. Mediano P, Fernández L, Rodríguez JM, et al. Case-control study of risk factors for infectious mastitis in Spanish breastfeeding women. *BMC Pregnancy Childbirth*. 2014;14:195.
3. Gollapalli V, Liao J, Dudakovic A, et al. Risk factors for development and recurrence of primary breast abscesses. *J Am Coll Surg*. 2010;211(1):41–48.
4. Jahanfar S, Ng CJ, Teng CL. Antibiotics for mastitis in breastfeeding women. *Cochrane Database Syst Rev*. 2013;(2):CD005458.
5. Cusack L, Brennan M. Lactational mastitis and breast abscess—diagnosis and management in general practice. *Aust Fam Physician*. 2011;40(12):976–979.
6. Lam E, Chan T, Wiseman SM. Breast abscess: evidence based management recommendations. *Expert Rev Anti Infect Ther*. 2014;12(7):753–762.
7. Elder EE, Brennan M. Nonsurgical management should be first-line therapy for breast abscess. *World J Surg*. 2010;34(9):2257–2258.
8. Thirumalaikumar S, Kommu S. Best evidence topic reports. Aspiration of breast abscesses. *Emerg Med J*. 2004;21(3):333–334.
9. Naeem M, Rahimnajjad MK, Rahimnajjad NA, et al. Comparison of incision and drainage against needle aspiration for the treatment of breast abscess. *Am Surg*. 2012;78(11):1224–1227.
10. Mangesi L, Dowswell T. Treatments for breast engorgement during lactation. *Cochrane Database Syst Rev*. 2010;(9):CD006946.

ADDITIONAL READING

- Berná-Serna JD, Berná-Mestre JD, Galindo PJ, et al. Use of urokinase in percutaneous drainage of large breast abscesses. *J Ultrasound Med*. 2009;28(4):449–454.
- Dabbas N, Chand M, Pallett A, et al. Have the organisms that cause breast abscess changed with time?—implications for appropriate antibiotic usage in primary and secondary care. *Breast J*. 2010;16(4):412–415.
- Rizzo M, Gabram S, Staley C, et al. Management of breast abscesses in nonlactating women. *Am Surg*. 2010;76(3):292–295.
- Trop I, Dugas A, David J, et al. Breast abscesses: evidence-based algorithms for diagnosis, management, and follow-up. *Radiographics*. 2011;31(6):1683–1699.

 CODES

ICD10

- N61 Inflammatory disorders of breast
- O91.13 Abscess of breast associated with lactation
- O91.12 Abscess of breast associated with the puerperium

CLINICAL PEARLS

- 5–11% of cases of puerperal mastitis go on to abscess (most often due to inadequate therapy for mastitis). Risk factors for mastitis are those that result in milk stasis (infrequent feeds, missing feeds).
- Abscesses not associated with lactation should be treated with antibiotics that cover anaerobic bacteria.
- The treatment of choice for most breast abscesses is the combination of antibiotics and aspiration.
- US-guided aspiration of breast abscess is preferred to incision and drainage in most cases.
- Continuing to empty the breast (feeding, pumping or expression of breast milk) is recommended during the presence of lactation-associated breast infection.

BREAST CANCER
Heather A. Dalton, MD • Amy M. Davis, MD

 BASICS

DESCRIPTION
- Malignant neoplasm of cells native to the breast—epithelial, glandular, or stroma
- Types: DCIS, infiltrating ductal carcinoma, infiltrating lobular carcinoma, Paget disease, phyllodes tumor, inflammatory breast cancer, angiosarcoma
- Molecular subtypes: luminal A (HR+/HER2−), triple negative (HR−/HER2−), luminal B (HR+/HER2+), HER2-enriched (HR−/HER2+)

EPIDEMIOLOGY
Incidence
- Estimated new female breast cancer (BC) cases for in situ 60,290; invasive 231,840 in 2015
- Estimated new male BC cases 2,350
- Estimated deaths in 2015 for females 40,290; males 440
- Second most common newly diagnosed cancer, leading cause of cancer death for U.S. women

Prevalence
Estimated 3.1 million of 162 million U.S. women (1.9%) as of January 1, 2014 (1)

ETIOLOGY AND PATHOPHYSIOLOGY
- Genes such as BRCA1 and BRCA2 function as tumor suppressor genes and mutation leads to cell cycle progression and limitations in DNA repair (2)
- Mutations in estrogen/progesterone induce cyclin D1 and c-myc expression, leading to cell cycle progression
- Additional tumors (33%) may cross-talk with estrogen receptors and epidermal growth factors receptors (EGFR), leading to similar abnormal cellular replication

Genetics
- Criteria for additional risk evaluation/gene testing in affected individual (2)[A]
  - BC at age ≤50 years
  - BC at any age and ≥1 family member with BC ≤50 years of age or ovarian/fallopian tube/primary peritoneal CA any age or ≥2 family members with BC or pancreatic CA any age or population at increased risk (e.g., Ashkenazi Jew with BC or ovarian CA at any age)
  - Triple-negative BC (ER−, PR−, HER2−)
  - Two BC primaries in single patient
  - Ovarian/fallopian tube/primary peritoneal CA
  - 1+ family member with BC and CA of thyroid, adrenal cortex, endometrium, pancreas, CNS, diffuse gastric, aggressive prostate (Gleason >7), leukemia, lymphoma, sarcoma, dermatologic manifestations, and/or macrocephaly, GI hamartomas
  - Male BC
  - Known BC susceptibility gene mutation in family
- Criteria for additional risk evaluation/gene testing in unaffected BC individual
  - First- or second-degree relative with BC ≤45 years of age
  - ≥2 breast primaries in one individual or ≥1 ovarian/fallopian tube/primary peritoneal CA from same side of family or ≥2 w/ breast primaries on same side of family
  - 1+ family member with BC and CA of thyroid, adrenal cortex, endometrium, pancreas, CNS, diffuse gastric, aggressive prostate (Gleason >7), leukemia, lymphoma, sarcoma, dermatologic manifestations, and/or macrocephaly, GI hamartomas

  - Ashkenazi Jewish with breast/ovary cancer at any age
  - Male BC
  - Known BC susceptibility gene mutation in family
- BRCA1 and BRCA2 account for 5–10% of female and 5–20% male cancers; 15–20% familial BCs
  - Mutations higher in Ashkenazi Jewish descent (2%)
  - Mutation in BRCA raises risk to 45–65% from 7% at age 70
- Other genes: ATM, BARD1, BRIP, CDH1, PTEN, STK11, CHEK2, p53, ERBB2, DIRAS3, NBN, RAD50, RAD51
- Cowden syndrome (PTEN): autosomal dominant, BC, hamartomas of skin, intestine, oral mucosa (trichilemmoma), microencephaly, endometrial CA, nonmedullary thyroid CA, benign thyroid lesions
- Li-Fraumeni syndrome (TP53): autosomal dominant, BC and CA in CNS, leukemia, sarcoma, osteosarcoma, adrenal cortex
- Ataxia-telangiectasia (ATM): autosomal recessive, ataxia, telangiectasia, lymphoma, leukemia, CA of breast, stomach, ovary
- Peutz-Jeghers (STK11): autosomal dominance; hamartomatous polyps of GI tract, mucocutaneous melanin in lips, buccal mucosa, fingers, toes; CA in GI, lung, breast, uterus, ovary

RISK FACTORS
- Risk Assessment Tool: http://www.cancer.gov/bcrisktool/
- >4.0 increase in relative risk: age >65, atypical hyperplasia, BRCA mutation, DCIS, LCIS, personal history <40, 2 or more first-degree relatives at early age
- 2.1 to 4.0 RR: post-menopausal, radiation history, dense breasts (>50%), single first-degree relative
- 1.1 to 2.0 RR: EtOH, Ashkenazi Jewish, DES exposure, early menarche, high socioeconomic status, first pregnancy >30, fibroadenoma, never breast fed, no full term pregnancies, obesity, personal history >40, personal history of endometrial, ovarian, colon cancer, HRT long term, recent OCP use
- 20–25% lifetime risk: BRCA mutation, first-degree relative with BRCA mutation, history of radiation age 10 to 30 years, Li-Fraumeni or Cowden syndrome or first-degree relative with the same
- 15–20% lifetime risk: personal history of BC, DCIS, LCIS, atypical ductal hyperplasia, atypical lobular hyperplasia, dense or unevenly dense breasts

GENERAL PREVENTION
- Maintain healthy weight—lean, avoid weight gain, limit high calorie foods, drinks
- Be physically active—150 minutes of moderate-intensity or 75 minutes vigorous activity weekly
- Eat healthy diet—limit processed/red meat, 2 1/2 cups of vegetables and fruits daily, limit refined-grain
- Limit EtOH to no more than 1 drink daily for women, 2 for men
- Clinical breast exam (CBE):
  - ACS: Does not recommend in average-risk
  - USPFTF: Insufficient evidence to assess clinical benefits and harms (3)[A]
- Mammography:
  - ACS: women 45 to 54 annually, >55 until <10 year life expectancy biennial; 40 to 44 optional
  - USPSTF: women biennial at age 50 to 74 (3)[B]

 DIAGNOSIS

HISTORY
- Painless lump in breast or axilla
- Breast pain, heaviness
- Swelling, thickening, redness of skin
- Nipple discharge (bloody), erosion, or retraction

PHYSICAL EXAM
- Visualize breasts with patient sitting for skin dimpling, peau d'orange, asymmetry
- Palpation of breast and regional lymph node exam: supraclavicular, infraclavicular, axillary

DIFFERENTIAL DIAGNOSIS
- Benign breast disease: fibrocystic disease, fibroadenoma, intraductal papilloma (bloody nipple discharge), duct ectasia, cyst, sclerosing adenosis, fat necrosis (s/p breast trauma)
- Infection: abscess, cellulitis, mastitis

DIAGNOSTIC TESTS & INTERPRETATION
Initial Tests (lab, imaging)
- Mammography BI-RADS: Breast Imaging–Reporting and Data System is a quality assurance (QA) method published by the American Radiology Society.
- BI-RADS interpretation: 0: incomplete (need additional imaging); 1: negative; 2: benign; 3: probably benign; 4: suspicious; 5: highly suggestive of malignancy; 6: known biopsy—proven malignancy
- All newly diagnosed BC: history and physical, CBC, LFTs, ALP, pathology review, ER/PR and HER2 status determination, genetic counseling if high risk, fertility counseling if indicated
- Palpable mass ≥30 years: Obtain mammogram.
  - If BI-RADS 1 to 3, then get ultrasound ± biopsy.
  - If BI-RADS 4 to 6, then get core needle biopsy ± surgical excision
- Palpable mass <30 years: Obtain ultrasound ± mammogram ± biopsy; if low clinical suspicion, observe for 1 to 2 menstrual cycles for resolution.
- Spontaneous, reproducible nipple discharge: Obtain mammogram, ± ultrasound.
  - If BI-RADS 1 to 3, then get ductogram or MRI.
  - If BI-RADS 4 to 5, then surgical excision
- Asymmetric thickening/nodularity ≥30 years: Obtain mammogram + ultrasound ± biopsy.
- Asymmetric thickening/nodularity <30 years: Obtain ultrasound ± mammogram ± biopsy.
- Skin changes, peau d'orange: Obtain mammogram ± ultrasound ± biopsy.

Follow-Up Tests & Special Considerations
- Early disease (clinical stage I and IIB)
- Consider additional studies only if signs and symptoms warrant.
- Advanced disease (stage IIIA or higher)
- Chest diagnostic CT, abdominal ± pelvis CT, FDG positron emission tomography (PET)/CT scan, bone scan or sodium fluoride PET/CT if FDG-PET/CT indeterminate
- Most common metastasis: lungs, liver, bone, brain
- Bone scan: localized pain, elevated alkaline phosphate
- Abdominal ± pelvis CT: abdominal symptoms, elevated alkaline phosphate, abnormal LFTs
- Chest imaging: pulmonary symptoms
- MRI: CNS/spinal cord symptoms

Diagnostic Procedures/Other

- Primary tumor: FNA, ultrasound-guided core needle biopsy, stereotactic-guided core needle biopsy ± wire localization, sentinel lymph node, surgical excision, sentinel lymph node biopsy; post biopsy may get inflammatory changes/hematoma.
- Genomic assay on formalin-fixed tissue for select +ER, −HER2, node negative tumor to assess chemotherapy responsiveness

Test Interpretation

- Ductal/lobular/other: tumor size, inflammatory component, invasive/noninvasive, margins, nodal involvement
- Nodal micrometastases: increased risk of disease recurrence
- ER, PR, HER2 assay

TREATMENT

MEDICATION

- Secondary prevention
  - ASA use at least once per week may be associated with as much as a 50% reduction in death from BC (see "Additional Reading")
  - Chemoprevention/hormone therapy for patients ages ≥35 years
  - Risk reduction for ER-positive tumors
- Hormone therapy for ER-positive tumors
  - Tamoxifen: premenopausal at diagnosis: 5-year treatment and consider for additional 5 years; avoid during lactation, pregnancy, or with history of deep venous thrombosis/pulmonary embolism; routine CYP2D6 testing not recommended; use strong CYP2D6-inhibiting medications with caution in conjunction
  - Aromatase inhibitors: postmenopausal women, 5-year treatment following tamoxifen for 4.5 to 6 years, or tamoxifen for up to 10 years
  - Ovarian ablation or suppression with luteinizing hormone–releasing hormone agonists: premenopausal women
  - Anti-HER2/neu antibody (e.g., trastuzumab) in select HER2/neu-positive patients
  - Monitor cardiac toxicity via ECG, especially with anthracycline.
- Neoadjuvant chemotherapy: Premenopausal women should be counseled on potential effect of chemotherapy on fertility, refer to fertility expert.
  - Locally advanced, inoperable advanced BC (stage III)
  - Early operable BC for breast conservation surgery
  - Triple negative BC
- Cytotoxic therapy: anthracyclines, taxanes, alkylating agents, antimetabolites
  - Higher risk patients with nonmetastatic operable tumors
  - Patients with high risk of recurrence after local treatment (serial/parallel [s/p] surgery ± radiation)
  - Online tool to estimate recurrence risk and benefits of adjuvant chemotherapy (http://www.adjuvantonline.com/online.jsp)
- Dose-dense chemotherapy demonstrates overall survival advantage in early BC (4)[A].
- Advanced disease
  - Hormone therapy
  - Cytotoxic therapy
  - Bisphosphonates to decrease skeletal complications
  - Antivascular endothelial growth factor antibody
  - Anti-HER2/neu antibody in select HER2/neu-positive patients

- Metastatic disease
  - Monitoring metastatic disease: system assessment, physical examination, performance status, weight, LFT/CBC, CT scan/chest/abdomen/pelvis, bone scan, PET/CT, tumor markers

SURGERY/OTHER PROCEDURES

Secondary prevention

- Risk-reducing mastectomy and bilateral salpingo-oophorectomy for breast and ovary CA syndromes
- Breast-conserving partial mastectomy/lumpectomy, if possible
- Negative margins; tumor usually <5 cm
- No prior breast radiation, relative contraindication: connective tissue disease (lupus, scleroderma)
- Modified radical mastectomy
- Large tumors; multicentric disease; young women with known *BRCA*; consider immediate or delayed reconstruction
- RT should be initiated without delay
- After breast-conserving therapy (BCT), stage I, IIA, IIB treatable with BCT + radiation
- Postmastectomy in select high-risk patients; palliation of metastatic disease; cord compression

Pregnancy Considerations

- TREATMENT varies on trimester
- Surgical: mastectomy or breast conservation: mastectomy preferred due to limitations of radiation during pregnancy.
- Sentinel lymph node biopsy: safe to use with lymphoscintigraphy
- Chemotherapy: appropriate in 2nd and 3rd trimesters, trastuzumab contraindicated
- RT: Avoid until after delivery.

INPATIENT CONSIDERATIONS

Discharge Criteria

Postmastectomy

- Complications: seroma, phantom breast syndrome, cellulitis, chest wall/axilla/arm pain, long thoracic nerve damage leading to winged scapula sign
- Lymphedema; avoid having BP taken on side of surgery

 ONGOING CARE

FOLLOW-UP RECOMMENDATIONS

- Every 4 to 6 months for 5 years, then annually
- No evidence to support the use of routine CBC, LFTs, "tumor markers", bone scan, CXR, liver ultrasound, CT scans, MRI, PET
- Mammogram/imaging 1 year after initial mammogram but 6 to 12 months postradiation, then annually
- Annual gynecologic exam for women on tamoxifen; bone mineral density at baseline and follow-up for women on aromatase inhibitors or with ovarian failure secondary to treatment

PROGNOSIS (5)

Stage	5-year Relative Survival Rate
0	100%
I	100%
II	93%
III	72%
IV	22%

COMPLICATIONS

- Hypercalcemia, metastatic disease, lymphedema
- Emotional issues (depression, body-image alteration)

REFERENCES

1. American Cancer Society. *Breast Cancer Facts & Figures 2015–2016*. Atlanta, GA: American Cancer Society; 2015. http://www.cancer.org.
2. National Comprehensive Cancer Network. NCCN Guidelines: Breast Cancer (Version 3.2015) © 2015. Breast Cancer National Comprehensive Cancer Network, Inc. http://www.nccn.org.
3. U.S. Preventive Services Task Force. Breast Cancer: Screening 2009. http://www.uspreventive servicestaskforce.org/Page/Document/Update SummaryFinal/breast-cancer-screening?ds=1&s= breast cancer.
4. Lyman GH, Barron RL, Natoli JL, et al. Systematic review of efficacy of dose-dense versus non-dose-dense chemotherapy in breast cancer, non-Hodgkin lymphoma, and non-small cell lung cancer. *Crit Rev Oncol Hematol*. 2012;81(3):296–308.
5. American Cancer Society. Breast Cancer Survival by stage. http://www.cancer.org.

ADDITIONAL READING

Rothwell PM, Wilson M, Price JF, et al. Effect of daily aspirin on risk of cancer metastasis: a study of incident cancers during randomised controlled trials. *Lancet*. 2012;379(9826):1591–1601.

 CODES

ICD10

- C50.919 Malignant neoplasm of unsp site of unspecified female breast
- D05.90 Unspecified type of carcinoma in situ of unspecified breast
- Z12.31 Encntr screen mammogram for malignant neoplasm of breast

CLINICAL PEARLS

- BC is most common CA death in U.S. women, lifetime risk of 1 in 8.
- High alcohol use, high body mass index (BMI), and physical inactivity are modifiable risk factors.
- Pursue/refer all abnormal breast physical examination/imaging findings.
- If patient ≥30 years of age with palpable mass, obtain mammogram, if <30 years of age obtain ultrasound.
- Normal mammography does not exclude possibility of CA with a palpable mass.

BREASTFEEDING

Angelia Leipelt, BA, IBCLC, ICCE, CLE • Ronald G. Chambers, Jr., MD, FAAFP

BASICS

- Breastfeeding is the natural process of feeding infant human milk directly from the breast.
- Breast milk is the preferred nutritional source and the normal and physiologic way to feed all newborns and infants.
- The American Academy of Pediatrics (AAP), the American Academy of Family Physicians (AAFP), WHO, and other medical organizations recommend exclusive breastfeeding for 6 months, with continuation of breastfeeding for ≥1 year as desired by the mother and infant (1)[A].

DESCRIPTION

- Maternal benefits (as compared with mothers who do not breastfeed) include the following (2):
  - Rapid involution/decreased postpartum bleeding (due to oxytocin release)
  - Association of decreased risk of postpartum depression and increased bonding
  - Associated postpartum weight loss
  - Decreased risk of breast cancer
  - Association of decreased risk of premenopausal ovarian cancer
  - Decreased risk of type 2 diabetes, hypertension, hyperlipidemia, rheumatoid arthritis and cardiovascular disease
  - Decreased risk of prematurity due to child spacing
  - Convenience and economic savings
- Infant benefits (as compared with children who are formula-fed) include the following (1,2):
  - Ideal food: easily digestible, nutrients well absorbed, less constipation
  - Lower rates of virtually all infections via maternal antibody protection
    - Fewer respiratory and GI infections
    - Decreased incidence of otitis media
    - Decreased risk of bacterial meningitis, pneumonia, and sepsis
    - Decreased incidence of necrotizing enterocolitis
  - Decreased incidence of obesity and type 1 and 2 diabetes
  - Decreased incidence of allergies, clinical asthma, and atopic dermatitis in childhood
  - Decreased risk of developing celiac disease and inflammatory bowel disease
  - Decreased risk of childhood leukemia
  - Decreased risk of sudden infant death syndrome (SIDS) and decreased mortality
  - Higher intelligence scores and better neurodevelopmental outcomes
  - Increased attachment between mother and baby
  - Decreased child abuse

EPIDEMIOLOGY

Incidence
- According to the most recent breastfeeding scorecard, United States breastfeeding rates are on the rise. Based on the CDC, in 2014: any breastfeeding: 79.2% (however, differs among different sociodemographic and culture) (3)
- Breastfeeding at 6 months: 49.4%
- Breastfeeding at 12 months: 26.7%
- Exclusive breastfeeding at 3 months: 40.7%
- Exclusive breastfeeding at 6 months: 18.8%

ETIOLOGY AND PATHOPHYSIOLOGY
The overarching mechanism of milk production is based on supply and demand.

- Stimulation of areola causes secretion of oxytocin.
- Oxytocin is responsible for let-down reflex when myoepithelial cells contract and milk is ejected into milk ducts (4).
- Sucking stimulates secretion of prolactin, which triggers milk production.
- Endocrine/metabolic: Cystic fibrosis, diabetes, galactosemia, phenylketonuria, and thyroid dysfunction may cause delayed lactation or decreased milk.

GENERAL PREVENTION

- Most vaccinations can be given to breastfeeding mothers. The CDC recommends that the diphtheria-tetanus-acellular pertussis, hepatitis B, inactivated influenza virus (as opposed to live attenuated), measles-mumps-rubella (MMR), and inactivated polio and varicella vaccines can be given. The CDC recommends avoiding the yellow fever or smallpox vaccine in breastfeeding mothers (5).
- The inactivated influenza virus is preferred to the live attenuated virus in women with infants' age 6 to 23 months, regardless of whether these infants are being breastfed (5).

DIAGNOSIS

PHYSICAL EXAM
Examine breasts, ideally during pregnancy, looking for scars, lumps, or inverted nipples. Confirm history of infertility, breast pathology, and previous breastfeeding problems.

ALERT
A breast lump should be followed to complete resolution or worked up if present and not just attributed to changes from lactation.

TREATMENT

GENERAL MEASURES
- Breastfeeding initiation

  - Initiate breastfeeding immediately after birth, ideally placing the infant on mother's chest, skin-to-skin, IN FIRST HOUR (1,6)[A].
  - Mother placed in a comfortable position, usually sitting or leaning back, with baby on chest allowing baby to move toward breast.
  - As baby opens wide, bring baby close, tucking baby in "belly to belly." Line baby's nose to nipple, baby tilts its head back with wide open mouth, bring baby close as baby latches to ensure baby's gum takes in more of the areola.
  - Baby's lips are flanged, rounded cheeks, no clicking or popping sounds and abscense of nipple pain when latched.
  - Feed baby on demand. Room-in and watch for hunger cues and cluster feeding.
  - Feed 2 to 8 times for first 24 hours and 8 to 15 times per 24 hours, feeding 10 or more minutes, emptying and alternating breasts.
  - Observation of a nursing session by an experienced physician, nurse, or lactation consultant
  - Avoid supplementation with formula or water unless medically indicated.

- Contraindications to breastfeeding are few (WHO) (1).
  - Maternal HIV (in industrialized world) or human T-cell leukemia virus (HTLV) infection
  - Active untreated tuberculosis
  - Active herpes simplex virus (HSV) lesions on the breast*
  - Substances of abuse without evaluation and review medications that will pass into human milk
  - Infants with galactosemia or maple syrup urine disease should not be fed with breast milk. Infants with phenylketonuria may be fed breast milk under close observation.
  - Mothers who develop varicella 5 days before through 2 days after delivery*
  - Mothers acutely infected with influenza H1N1 until afebrile*
  - Maternal hepatitis is NOT a contraindication.
  - *Expressed milk can be used.

ISSUES FOR REFERRAL
- Refer to trained physician, nurse, or IBCLC lactation consultant for inpatient and/or outpatient teaching.
- Frequent follow-up if having problems with latching, sore nipples, breast pain, or inadequate milk production.

COMPLEMENTARY & ALTERNATIVE MEDICINE
Galactagogues (7)[C]

- Metoclopramide, domperidone, oxytocin, fenugreek, goat's rue, and milk thistle have mixed results in improving milk production but efficacy and safety data are lacking in literature.

ONGOING CARE

FOLLOW-UP RECOMMENDATIONS
See mother and baby within a few days of hospital discharge, especially if first time breastfeeding.

- Risk factors for suboptimal initiation
  - Breast surgery, especially reduction surgery, prior to pregnancy may disrupt breast milk production in the future.
  - Severe postpartum hemorrhage may lead to Sheehan syndrome, which is associated with difficulty breastfeeding due to poor milk production.
  - Other factors: delivery mode, duration of labor, gestational age, maternal infection, parity, culture, mother–baby separation, maternal anxiety, artificial nipple, and nonbreast milk fluids.

Patient Monitoring
- Monitor infant's weight, behavior, and output closely.
- Supplementation with infant formula is recommended only if infant has lost ≥8–10% of birth weight or signs of dehydration such as decreased urine output.
- Supplementation without persistent breast stimulation with frequent feedings or breast pump use will decrease milk production and decrease breastfeeding success.

DIET
- For mothers:
  - Drink plenty of fluids: 8 glasses of liquid a day
  - Breastfeeding mothers require ~500 more calories a day than prepregnancy needs (1).
  - Gassy foods can cause baby to be fussy.

- Limit caffeine to 300 mg/day.
- Alcohol should be avoided. 1 to 2 drinks/week of alcohol may be okay, but mothers should avoid nursing 2 to 3 hours after a drink. <2% of alcohol is passed to baby via breast milk.
- Continue prenatal vitamin supplements.
- For infants:
  - In 2008, the AAP increased its recommended daily intake of vitamin D for infants from 200 to 400 IU. For exclusively breastfed babies, this will require taking a vitamin supplement, such as Poly-Vi-Sol or Vi-Daylin vitamin drops, 0.5 mL/day, beginning in the first few days of life (1).
  - In 2010, the AAP recommended adding supplementation for breastfed infants with oral iron 1 mg/kg/day beginning at age 4 months.
    - Preterm infants fed by human milk should receive an iron supplement of 2 mg/kg/day by 1 month of age, and this should be continued until the infant is weaned to iron-fortified formula or begins eating complementary foods that supply the 2 mg/kg of iron.
    - Fluoride supplement is unnecessary until 6 months of age (1).

PATIENT EDUCATION
- Primary care–initiated interventions and support measures to normalize breastfeeding have been shown to be successful with respect to child and maternal health outcomes (8).
  - U.S. Preventive Services Task Force (USPSTF) recommends structured breastfeeding education and behavioral counseling programs to promote breastfeeding.
    - Regular promotion of the advantages of breastfeeding/risks of not breastfeeding (6)[A]
    - Emphasize importance of exclusive breastfeeding for first 4 weeks of life to allow adequate buildup of sufficient milk supply.
- Milk usually transitions to mature milk about postpartum day 3 to 5.
- Frequent nursing (8–12 feedings per 24 hours by day 2)
- Baby should have 6 to 8 wet diapers/day and 3 to 4 bowel movements/day by day 6 to 8.
- Signs of adequate nursing
  - Baby feeding on demand.
  - Proper latching and positioning, nipples intact.
  - Hard breasts become soft after feeding.
  - Baby satisfied; appropriate weight gain (average 1 oz/day in first few months)
- Weaning
  - Solid food may be introduced at 6 months with continuation of breastfeeding.
  - Mothers returning to work/school should be introduced to alternative feeding methods 1 to 2 weeks prior. Initiate pumping to supply expressed breastmilk.
- Family planning
  - Lactational amenorrhea method (LAM): Breastfeeding may be used as effective birth control option if (i) infant is <6 months old, (ii) infant is exclusively breastfeeding, and (iii) mother is amenorrheic.
  - Other options include barrier methods, implants, Depo-Provera, PO contraception, and intrauterine devices (IUDs). ACOG recommends that progesterone-only pills be used 2 to 3 weeks postpartum, and that Depo-Provera, IUDs, combined OCPs, and Implanon can be used 6 weeks postpartum. However, ACOG recommends delaying use of combined OCPs until after 6 weeks postpartum when lactation is well established.

COMPLICATIONS
- Breast milk jaundice should be considered if jaundice persists for >1 week in an otherwise healthy, well-hydrated newborn. It peaks at 10 to 14 days.
- Plugged duct
  - Mother is well except for sore lump in one or both breasts and is without fever.
  - Use moist, hot packs on lump prior to, and during, nursing; more frequent nursing on affected side.
- Mastitis (see topic "Mastitis")
  - Sore lump in one or both breasts plus fever and/or redness on skin overlying lump
  - Use moist, hot packs on lump prior to, and during, nursing.
  - Antibiotics covering for *Staphylococcus aureus* (most common organism)
  - Other possible sources of fever should be ruled out, that is, endometritis and pyelonephritis.
  - Mother should get increased rest; use acetaminophen (Tylenol) PRN.
  - Fever should resolve within 48 hours or consider changing antibiotics. Lump should resolve. If it continues, an abscess may be present, requiring surgical drainage.
- Milk supply inadequate
  - Check infant weight gain.
  - Review signs of adequate supply; technique, frequency, and duration of nursing.
  - Check to see if mother has been supplementing with formula, thereby decreasing her own milk production.
- Sore nipples
  - Check technique and improve latch-on.
  - Baby should be taken off the breast by breaking the suction with a finger in the mouth.
  - Air-dry nipples after each nursing and/or coat with expressed breast milk.
  - Use lanolin cream to help in healing.
  - Do not wash nipples with soap and water.
  - Check for signs of thrush in baby and on mother's nipple. If affected, treat both.
  - Check for evidence of ankyloglossia (tongue tie) in the infant. Correction of ankyloglossia leads to decreased nipple soreness and improved breastfeeding.
  - Nipple bleb due to improper positioning. Moist heat and improve latching techniques.
- Flat or inverted nipples
  - When stimulated, inverted nipples will retract inward, flat nipples remain flat; check for this on initial prenatal physical.
  - Nipple shells, a doughnut-shaped insert, can be worn inside the bra during the last month of pregnancy to force the nipple gently through the center opening of the shell.
- Engorgement
  - Develops after milk first comes in (day 3 or 4 postpartum), resolves within a day or 2
  - Signs are warm, hard, sore breasts.
    - To resolve, offer baby more frequent nursing; breastfeed long enough to empty breasts.

REFERENCES
1. Johnston M, Landers S, Noble L, et al. Breastfeeding and the use of human milk. *Pediatrics*. 2012;129(3):e827–e841.
2. Ip S, Chung M, Raman G, et al. *Breastfeeding and Maternal and Infant Health Outcomes in Developed Countries*. Rockville, MD: Agency for Health Care Research and Quality; 2007.
3. Centers for Disease Control and Prevention. *Breastfeeding Report Card—United States, 2014*. Atlanta, GA: Centers for Disease Control and Prevention; 2014. http://www.cdc.gov/breastfeeding/pdf/2014breastfeedingreportcard.pdf. Accessed 2014.
4. Sinusas K, Gagliardi A. Initial management of breastfeeding. *Am Fam Physician*. 2001;64(6):981–988.
5. Centers for Disease Control and Prevention. *Breastfeeding Vaccinations*. Atlanta, GA: Centers for Disease Control and Prevention; 2010. http://www.cdc.gov/breastfeeding/recommendations/vaccinations.htm. Accessed 2014.
6. American College of Obstetricians and Gynecologists Women's Health Care Physicians; Committee on Health Care for Underserved Women. Committee Opinion No. 570: breastfeeding in underserved women: increasing initiation and continuation of breastfeeding. *Obstet Gynecol*. 2013;122(2, Pt 1):423–428.
7. Foranish AB, Yancey AM, Barnes KN, et al. The use of galactogogues in the breastfeeding mother. *Ann Pharmacother*. 2012;46(10):1392–1404.
8. Chantry CJ, Eglash A, Labbok M. Position on breastfeeding. *Breastfeed Med*. 2008;3(4):267–270.

ADDITIONAL READING
- American Academy of Pediatrics, American College of Obstetricians and Gynecologists. *Breastfeeding Handbook for Physicians*. Elk Grove Village, IL: American Academy of Pediatrics; 2006.
- Casey CF, Slawson DC, Neal LR. Vitamin D supplementation in infants, children, and adolescents. *Am Fam Physician*. 2010;81(6):745–748.
- Philipp BL, Bunik M, Chantry CJ, et al. ABM Clinical Protocol #7: Model Breastfeeding Policy (Revision 2010). *Breastfeed Med*. 2010;5(4):173–177.
- Wagner CL, Greer FR, Bhatia JJ, et al. Prevention of rickets and vitamin D deficiency in infants, children, and adolescents. *Pediatrics*. 2008;122(5):1142–1152.
- Websites/Books:
  - Baby Friendly USA at www.babyfriendly.org
  - La Leche League at www.llli.org
  - World Health Organization, United Nations Children's Fund. *Protecting, Promoting and Supporting Breastfeeding: The Special Role of Maternity Services. A Joint WHO/UNICEF Statement*. Geneva, Switzerland: World Health Organization; 1989. http://www.unicef.org/newsline/tenstps.htm.

 CODES

ICD10
Z39.1 Encounter for care and examination of lactating mother

CLINICAL PEARLS
- Women who do not receive support are at risk for shorter durations of breastfeeding (8).
- Breast milk is the optimal food for infants, with myriad health benefits for mothers and children.
- USPSTF recommends regular, structured education during pregnancy to promote breastfeeding.
- Vitamin D and iron supplementation should begin at birth and 4 months of age, respectively, for exclusively breastfed infants.

BRONCHIECTASIS

Sumera R. Ahmad, MD • Scott E. Kopec, MD

BASICS

DESCRIPTION
- Bronchiectasis is an irreversible dilatation of ≥1 airways accompanied by recurrent transmural bronchial infection/inflammation and chronic muco-purulent sputum production.
- Generally classified into cystic fibrosis (CF) and noncystic fibrosis (non-CF) bronchiectasis

EPIDEMIOLOGY
- Predominant age: most commonly presents in 6th decade of life
- Predominant sex: female > male

Incidence
Incidence has decreased in the United States for two reasons:
- Widespread childhood vaccination against pertussis
- Effective treatment of childhood respiratory infections with antibiotics

Prevalence
- Prevalence in adult U.S. population estimated to be >110,000 affected individuals.
- Internationally, prevalence increases with age from 4.2/100,000 persons aged 18 to 34 years to 271.8/100,000 among those aged 75 years and older (1).

ETIOLOGY AND PATHOPHYSIOLOGY
- CF bronchiectasis: bronchiectasis due to CF
- Non-CF bronchiectasis
  - Most cases are idiopathic.
  - Most commonly associated with non-CF bronchiectasis is childhood infection.
- Vicious circle hypothesis: Transmural infection, generally by bacterial organisms, causes inflammation and obstruction of airways. Damaged airways and dysfunctional cilia foster bacterial colonization, which leads to further inflammation and obstruction.

RISK FACTORS
- Nontuberculous mycobacterial infection is both a cause and a complication of non-CF bronchiectasis.
- Severe respiratory infection in childhood (measles, adenovirus, influenza, pertussis, or bronchiolitis)
- Systemic diseases (e.g., rheumatoid arthritis and inflammatory bowel disease)
- Chronic rhinosinusitis
- Recurrent pneumonia
- Aspirated foreign body
- Immunodeficiency
- Congenital abnormalities

GENERAL PREVENTION
- Routine immunizations against pertussis, measles, *Haemophilus influenza* type B, influenza, and pneumococcal pneumonia
- Genetic counseling if congenital condition is etiology
- Smoking cessation

COMMONLY ASSOCIATED CONDITIONS
- Mucociliary clearance defects
  - Primary ciliary dyskinesia
  - Young syndrome (secondary ciliary dyskinesia)
  - Kartagener syndrome
- Other congenital conditions
  - α1-antitrypsin deficiency
  - Marfan syndrome
  - Cartilage deficiency (Williams-Campbell syndrome)
- Chronic obstructive pulmonary disease

- Pulmonary fibrosis, causing traction bronchiectasis
- Postinfectious conditions
  - Bacteria (*H. influenzae* and *Pseudomonas aeruginosa*)
  - Mycobacterial infections (tuberculosis [TB] and *Mycobacterium avium* complex [MAC])
  - Whooping cough
  - Aspergillus species
  - Viral (HIV, adenovirus, measles, influenza virus)
- Immunodeficient conditions
  - Primary: hypogammaglobulinemia
  - Secondary: allergic bronchopulmonary aspergillosis (ABPA), posttransplantation
  - Sequelae of toxic inhalation or aspiration (e.g., chlorine, luminal foreign body)
- Rheumatic/chronic inflammatory conditions
  - Rheumatoid arthritis
  - Sjögren syndrome
  - Systemic lupus erythematosus
  - Inflammatory bowel disease
- Miscellaneous
  - Yellow nail syndrome

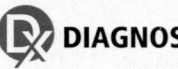

DIAGNOSIS

- Typical symptoms include chronic productive cough, wheezing, and dyspnea.
- Symptoms are often accompanied by repeated respiratory infections (2).
- Once diagnosed, investigate etiology.

HISTORY
- Any predisposing factors (congenital, infectious, and/or exposure-related)
- Immunization history

PHYSICAL EXAM
Symptoms are commonly present for many years and include the following:
- Chronic cough (90%)
- Sputum: may be copious and purulent (90%)
- Rhinosinusitis (60–70%)
- Fatigue: may be a dominant symptom (70%)
- Dyspnea (75%)
- Chest pain: may be pleuritic (20–30%)
- Hemoptysis (20–30%)
- Wheezing (20%)
- Bibasilar crackles (60%)
- Rhonchi (44%)
- Digital clubbing (3%)

DIFFERENTIAL DIAGNOSIS
- CF
- Chronic obstructive pulmonary disease
- Asthma
- Chronic bronchitis
- Pulmonary TB
- ABPA

DIAGNOSTIC TESTS & INTERPRETATION
- Spirometry
  - Moderate airflow obstruction and hyperresponsive airways
  - Forced expiratory volume in the 1st second of expiration (FEV_1): <80% predicted and FEV_1/FVC <0.7
- Special tests
  - Ciliary biopsy by electron microscopy
- Sputum culture
  - *H. influenzae*, nontypeable form (42%)

- *P. aeruginosa* (18%)
  - Cultures may also be positive for *Streptococcus pneumoniae*, *Moraxella catarrhalis*, MAC, and *Aspergillus*.
  - Of all isolates, 30–40% will show no growth.
- Special tests
  - Sweat test for CF
  - Purified protein derivative (PPD) test for TB
  - Skin test for *Aspergillus*
  - HIV
  - Serum immunoglobulins to test for humoral immunodeficiency
  - Protein electrophoresis to test for α1-antitrypsin deficiency
  - Barium swallow to look for abnormalities of deglutition, achalasia, esophageal hypomotility
  - pH probe to characterize reflux
  - Screening tests for rheumatologic diseases
- Chest radiograph
  - Nonspecific; increased lung markings or may appear normal
- Chest computed tomography (CT)
  - Noncontrast high-resolution chest CT is the most important diagnostic tool.
  - Bronchi are dilated and do not taper, resulting in "tram track sign"; parallel opacities seen on scan.
  - Varicose constrictions and balloon cysts may be seen.
  - For focal bronchiectasis, rule out endobronchial obstruction.
  - For exclusively upper lobe bronchiectasis, consider CF and ABPA.

Diagnostic Procedures/Other
- Bronchoscopy may be used to obtain cultures and evacuate sputum.
- Bronchoscopy for hemoptysis
- Bronchoscopy may be useful to rule out airway-obstructing lesions with focal bronchiectasis.

Test Interpretation
Bronchoscopy findings include the following:
- Dilatation of airways and purulent secretions
- Thickened bronchial walls with necrosis of bronchial mucosa
- Peribronchial scarring

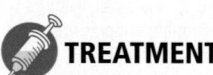

TREATMENT

- Treat underlying conditions.
- Recognize an acute exacerbation with 4 out of 9 criteria (3)
  - Change in sputum production
  - Increased dyspnea
  - Increased cough
  - Fever
  - Increased wheezing
  - Malaise, fatigue, lethargy
  - Reduced pulmonary function
  - Radiographic changes
  - Changes in chest sounds
- Non-CF bronchiectasis: determine cause of exacerbations; promote good bronchopulmonary hygiene via daily airway clearance.
- Consider surgical resection of damaged lung for focal disease that is refractory to medical management.
- Medical management: Reduce morbidity by controlling symptoms and preventing disease progression.
- Patients with non-CF bronchiectasis may not respond to CF treatment regimens in the same way as patients with CF do.

GENERAL MEASURES

- Maintain hydration (nebulized hypertonic saline, 3% or 7% may be used to help increase mucus clearance) (4)[A].
- Noninvasive positive-pressure ventilation

MEDICATION

- Insufficient evidence exists to support efficacy of short-course antibiotics in adults and children with bronchiectasis (5)[A].
- Frequent exacerbations may be treated with prolonged and aerosolized antibiotics (2)[A].
- Role of mucolytics, antiinflammatory agents, and bronchodilators is still unclear (2)[A].

First Line

- Antibiotics
  - Potentially useful in acute exacerbations
  - Chronic therapy decreases sputum volume and purulence, but it does not diminish the frequency of exacerbations (6)[A].
  - Patients may require twice the usual dose and longer treatment for 14 days (7)[C].
  - Sputum culture and sensitivity should direct therapy; antibiotic selection is complicated by a wide range of pathogens and resistant organisms.
  - Should be administered IV in cases of severe infection
    - Augmentin: 500 mg PO q8–12h. Pediatric: base dosing on amoxicillin content
    - Trimethoprim (TMP)/sulfamethoxazole (SMX) : 160 mg TMP/800 mg SMX PO q12h. Pediatric: ≥2 months, 8 mg/kg TMP and 40 mg/kg SMX PO/24 hours, administered in two divided doses q12h
    - Doxycycline and cefaclor given PO are also effective.
    - Nebulized aminoglycosides (tobramycin): 300 mg by aerosol BID (8)[B]
    - Ciprofloxacin: 750 mg PO q12h for adults for susceptible strain of *Pseudomonas*
    - Macrolides: appear to have immunomodulatory benefits
- Chronic use of azithromycin as an oral macrolide for 6 to 12 months in non-CF bronchiectasis has been shown to reduce exacerbations (9,10). Needs caution with respect to cardiovascular deaths, where it is a QTc-prolonging medication (9).
- Bronchodilators
  - Chronic use of β2-agonists (e.g., albuterol) reverses airflow obstruction.
- Inhaled corticosteroids
  - Insufficient evidence exists to recommend use of inhaled steroids with stable bronchiectasis (11)[A].
  - A therapeutic trial of inhaled steroids may be justified in adults with difficult-to-control symptoms (11)[A].
  - Decrease sputum and tend to improve lung function
    - Fluticasone propionate: 110 to 220 μg inhaled BID
  - Potential synergistic effect of long-acting β2-agonists with inhaled corticosteroids, allowing for lower steroid dose (12):
    - Budesonide 160 μg/Formoterol 4.5 μg 2 puffs inhaled BID

Second Line

Other broad-spectrum antimicrobials, including those with antipseudomonal coverage

ADDITIONAL THERAPIES

Sputum clearance techniques, including physiotherapy (percussion and postural drainage) and pulmonary rehabilitation (improves exercise tolerance)

SURGERY/OTHER PROCEDURES

- Surgery if area of bronchiectasis is localized and symptoms remain intolerable despite medical therapy or if disease is life-threatening (2)[A]
- Surgery effectively improves symptoms in 80% of these cases.

INPATIENT CONSIDERATIONS

Admission Criteria/Initial Stabilization

Bronchiectasis can present as a life-threatening massive hemoptysis. In this situation, in addition to airway protection and resuscitation, bronchial artery embolization or surgical intervention is necessary to control bleeding.

 ## ONGOING CARE

Long-term outpatient treatment recommendations for bronchiectasis in children (13)[B]:

- Children with CF and non–CF-related bronchiectasis should be treated by comprehensive interdisciplinary chronic disease management programs.
- Pathogen-directed aerosolized tobramycin treatment should be used long-term on a regular basis to improve the course of CF-related bronchiectasis.
- PO macrolide antibiotic use long term (up to 6 months) improves lung function among children with CF-related bronchiectasis.
- Long-term antibiotic use (PO or aerosolized) in children with non–CF-related bronchiectasis has not been studied enough to warrant routine use.
- Hypertonic saline administered by inhalation used long-term (48 weeks) improves lung function and is safer when used with pretreatment bronchodilator therapy among children who have CF.
- Nebulized dornase improves multiple pulmonary outcomes of children who have CF and is indicated for long-term use.
- Risks for long-term oral corticosteroid use outweigh pulmonary benefits in the treatment of CF-related bronchiectasis.
- High-dose ibuprofen therapy reduces the rate of decline among children with mild CF-related bronchiectasis and is indicated for long-term use.
- Mucolytic agents, airway-hydrating treatments, antiinflammatory therapy, chest physical therapy (CPT), and bronchodilator therapy have not been studied sufficiently long term in children with non–CF-related bronchiectasis to merit their routine use.

FOLLOW-UP RECOMMENDATIONS

Regular exercise is recommended.

Patient Monitoring

- Serial spirometry, every 2 to 5 years, to monitor the course of the disease
- Chest CTs to monitor progression of disease may be indicated with some conditions such as bronchiectasis with MAC infections.
- Routine microbiological sputum analysis

PATIENT EDUCATION

http://www.lungusa.org/

PROGNOSIS

- Mortality rate (death due directly to bronchiectasis) is 13%.
- *Pseudomonas* infection is associated with poorer prognosis.

COMPLICATIONS

- Hemoptysis
- Recurrent pulmonary infections
- Pulmonary hypertension
- Cor pulmonale
- Lung abscess

REFERENCES

1. Pappalettera M, Aliberti S, Castellotti P, et al. Bronchiectasis: an update. *Clin Respir J.* 2009;3(3):126–134.
2. ten Hacken NH, Wijkstra PJ, Kerstjens HA. Treatment of bronchiectasis in adults. *BMJ.* 2007;335(7629):1089–1093.
3. O'Donnell AE, Barker AF, Ilowite JS, et al. Treatment of idiopathic bronchiectasis with aerosolized recombinant human DNase I. rhDNase Study Group. *Chest.* 1998;113(5):1329–1334.
4. Kellett F, Robert NM. Nebulised 7% hypertonic saline improves lung function and quality of life in bronchiectasis. *Respir Med.* 2011;105(12):1831–1835.
5. Wurzel D, Marchant JM, Yerkovich ST, et al. Short courses of antibiotics for children and adults with bronchiectasis. *Cochrane Database Syst Rev.* 2011;(6):CD008695.
6. Evans DJ, Bara AI, Greenstone M. Prolonged antibiotics for purulent bronchiectasis in children and adults. *Cochrane Database Syst Rev.* 2007;(2):CD001392.
7. Pasteur MC, Bilton D, Hill AT. British Thoracic Society guideline for non-CF bronchiectasis. *Thorax.* 2010;65(Suppl 1):i1–i58.
8. Lobue PA. Inhaled tobramycin: not just for cystic fibrosis anymore? *Chest.* 2005;127(4):1098–1101.
9. Wong C, Jayaram L, Karalus N, et al. Azithromycin for prevention of exacerbations in non-cystic fibrosis bronchiectasis (EMBRACE): a randomised, double-blind, placebo-controlled trial. *Lancet.* 2012;380(9842):660–667.
10. Altenburg J, de Graaff CS, Stienstra Y, et al. Effect of azithromycin maintenance treatment on infectious exacerbations among patient with non-cystic fibrosis bronchiectasis: the BAT randomized controlled trial. *JAMA.* 2013;309(12):1251–1259.
11. Kapur N, Bell S, Kolbe J, et al. Inhaled steroids for bronchiectasis. *Cochrane Database Syst Rev.* 2009;(1):CD000996.
12. Martínez-García MÁ, Soler-Cataluña JJ, Catalán-Serra P, et al. Clinical efficacy and safety of budesonide-formoterol in non-cystic fibrosis bronchiectasis. *Chest.* 2012;141(2):461–468.
13. Redding GJ. Bronchiectasis in children. *Pediatr Clin North Am.* 2009;56(1):157–171.

 ## CODES

ICD10

- J47.9 Bronchiectasis, uncomplicated
- J47.1 Bronchiectasis with (acute) exacerbation
- J47.0 Bronchiectasis with acute lower respiratory infection

CLINICAL PEARLS

- Symptoms of bronchiectasis include chronic productive cough, wheezing, and dyspnea, often accompanied by repeated respiratory infections.
- A chest x-ray has poor sensitivity and specificity for the diagnosis; a noncontrast high-resolution chest CT is the most important diagnostic tool.
- Current practice guidelines recommend treating acute exacerbations with a 14-day course of antibiotics. Frequent exacerbations may be treated with prolonged and aerosolized antibiotics.

BRONCHIOLITIS

Dennis E. Hughes, DO, FACEP

 BASICS

DESCRIPTION
- Inflammation and obstruction of small airways and reactive airways generally affecting infants and young children—upper respiratory infection (URI) prodrome followed by increased respiratory effort and wheezing
- Usual course: insidious, acute, progressive
- Leading cause of hospitalizations in infants and children in most Western countries
- Predominant age: newborn–2 years (peak age <6 months). Neonates are not protected despite transfer of maternal antibody.
- Predominant sex: male > female

EPIDEMIOLOGY
Incidence
- 21% in North America
- May be seasonal (October–May in the Northern Hemisphere) and often occurs in epidemics
- 18.8% (90,000 annually) of all pediatric hospitalizations (excluding live births) in children <2 years
- Incidence increasing since 1980 (with concomitant increase in relative rate of hospitalization from 2002 to 2007).

ETIOLOGY AND PATHOPHYSIOLOGY
RSV accounts for 70–85% of all cases (children <12 months of age), but rhinovirus, parainfluenza virus, adenovirus, influenza virus, *Mycoplasma pneumoniae*, and *Chlamydophila pneumoniae* have all been implicated:
- Infection results in necrosis and lysis of epithelial cells and subsequent release of inflammatory mediators.
- Edema and mucus secretion, which combined with accumulating necrotic debris and loss of cilia clearance, results in airflow obstruction.
- Ventilation–perfusion mismatching resulting in hypoxia
- Air trapping is caused by dynamic airways narrowing during expiration, which increases work of breathing.
- Bronchospasm appears to play little or no role.

RISK FACTORS
- Secondhand cigarette smoke
- Low birth weight, premature birth
- Immunodeficiency
- Formula feeding (little or no breastfeeding)
- Contact with infected person (primary mode of spread)
- Children in daycare environment
- Congenital cardiopulmonary disease
- <12 weeks of age

GENERAL PREVENTION
- Handwashing or use of alcohol-based hand rubs (preferred)
- Contact isolation of infected babies
- Persons with colds should keep contact with infants to a minimum.
  - Breastfeeding of infants has been associated with reduced morbidity of disease.
- Palivizumab (Synagis), a monoclonal product, administered monthly, October–May, 15 mg/kg IM; used for RSV prevention ONLY in high-risk patients

Pediatric Considerations
Prior infection does not seem to confer subsequent immunity.

COMMONLY ASSOCIATED CONDITIONS
- Upper respiratory congestion
- Conjunctivitis
- Pharyngitis
- Otitis media
- Diarrhea

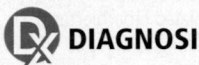 **DIAGNOSIS**

History and physical examination should be the basis for the diagnosis of bronchiolitis.

HISTORY
- Irritability
- Anorexia
- Fever
- Noisy breathing (due to rhinorrhea)
- Cough
- Grunting
- Cyanosis
- Apnea
- Vomiting

PHYSICAL EXAM
- Tachypnea
- Retractions (increased work of breathing)
- Rhinorrhea
- Wheezing
- Upper respiratory findings: pharyngitis, conjunctivitis, otitis

DIFFERENTIAL DIAGNOSIS
- Other pulmonary infections such as pertussis, croup, or bacterial pneumonia
- Aspiration
- Vascular ring
- Foreign body
- Asthma
- Heart failure
- Gastroesophageal reflux
- Cystic fibrosis

DIAGNOSTIC TESTS & INTERPRETATION
Laboratory and other ancillary testing (including chest x-ray) are not required if clinical diagnosis is bronchiolitis.

Initial Tests (lab, imaging)
- Arterial oxygen saturation by pulse oximetry. Results need to be interpreted in clinical context. Transient hypoxemia is a common phenomenon in healthy infants (1).
- Rapid respiratory viral antigen testing is not necessary during RSV season because the disease is managed symptomatically but may be useful for epidemiologic, hospital cohorting, or in the very young to reduce unnecessary other workup; also indicated in infants admitted while receiving palivizumab prophylaxis (if positive, prophylaxis may be discontinued).
- The American Association of Pediatrics (AAP) does not recommend routine RSV testing in infants and children with bronchiolitis.
- Chest x-ray findings are variable and may include atelectasis, peribronchial cuffing, hyperinflation, and perihilar infiltrates.

 TREATMENT

The cornerstone of therapy is supportive to include upper airway suctioning, prevention of significant and prolonged hypoxia, and dehydration. The other interventions noted have historically varying effect on the course of the illness despite numerous studies. Recent clinical practice guidelines do not support the routine use of corticosteroids, bronchodilators, or epinephrine. Parental education and support is vital (1)[A].

MEDICATION
First Line
- Humidified oxygen for hypoxia of <90% (pulse oximetry should be interpreted in context of clinical appearance of infant) (1)[C]

- Nebulized hypertonic saline (3%) can be effective in reducing LOS in hospitalized patients but not recommended use in the ED (1,2)[B].
- Antibiotics only if secondary bacterial infection present (rare). Not indicated for routine use (1)[B].

- Positive-pressure ventilation (PPV) in the form of continuous positive airway pressure (CPAP) can be used in cases of respiratory failure. There is limited clinical evidence other than observational studies (3)[C].
- High-flow nasal cannula oxygen widely used in various settings to improve oxygen saturation with resultant reduction in end-tidal CO_2 ($ETCO_2$) and respiratory rate, but overall effectiveness remains unproven to date (3)[C].

ADDITIONAL THERAPIES

- Ribavirin (palivizumab) for patients at high risk (for prophylaxis per CDC/AAP guidelines) (4)[A]
- Heliox therapy (70% helium and 30% oxygen) may be of benefit early in moderate to severe bronchiolitis to reduce degree of respiratory distress due to air flow restriction, but Cochrane review found little evidence of sustained benefit at 24 hours (5)[A].

- Although not routinely recommended, inhaled β-agonists (albuterol) can be effective in selected cases (particularly in patients with a history of bronchospasm).

INPATIENT CONSIDERATIONS

Bronchiolitis can be associated with apnea in children <6 weeks of age.

Admission Criteria/Initial Stabilization

- Respiratory rate >45 breaths/min with respiratory distress or apnea
- Hypoxia is common so clinical criteria are more helpful (pulse oximetry <94% used by many as cutoff).
- Ill or toxic appearance
- Underlying heart condition, respiratory condition, or immune suppression
- High risk for apnea (age <30 days, preterm birth [<37 weeks])
- Dehydrated or unable to feed
- Uncertain home care
- Use of Respiratory Distress Assessment Instrument may aid in determining admission. The five best predictors of admission, age, respiratory rate, heart rate, oxygen saturation, and duration of symptoms, were recently incorporated into a scoring instrument.
- Supplemental oxygen for pulse oximetry <94% on room air if clinically indicated. AAP recommends O_2 saturation >90% if infant otherwise well.

IV Fluids

Indicated only if tachypnea precludes oral feeding; weight-based maintenance rate plus insensible losses.

Discharge Criteria

Normal respiratory rate and no oxygen requirement: Recent small studies suggest that after a period of observation, children can be safely discharged on home oxygen with home health follow-up.

 ONGOING CARE

FOLLOW-UP RECOMMENDATIONS

Patient Monitoring

- Hospitalization is usually required only if oxygen is a requirement or unable to feed/drink.
- For a hospitalized patient, monitor as needed depending on the severity of the infection.
- If the patient is receiving home care, follow daily by telephone call for 2 to 4 days; the patient may need frequent office visits.

PATIENT EDUCATION

- American Academy of Pediatrics: http://www.aap.org
- American Academy of Family Physicians: http://www.familydoctor.org

PROGNOSIS

- Recovery time is variable. 40% can have symptoms at 14 days and 10% at 4 weeks.
- Mortality statistics differ but probably <1%.
- High-risk infants (bronchopulmonary dysplasia, congenital heart disease) may have a prolonged course.

COMPLICATIONS

- Bacterial superinfection
- Bronchiolitis obliterans
- Apnea
- Respiratory failure
- Death
- Increased incidence of development of reactive airway disease (asthma)

REFERENCES

1. Ralston SL, Lieberthal AS, Meissner HC, et al. Clinical practice guideline: the diagnosis, management, and prevention of bronchiolitis. *Pediatrics*. 2015;136(4):782.
2. Zhang L, Mendoza-Sassi RA, Wainwright C, et al. Nebulised hypertonic saline solution for acute bronchiolitis in infants. *Cochrane Database Syst Rev*. 2013;(7):CD006458.
3. Øymar K, Skjerven HO, Mikalsen IB. Acute bronchiolitis in infants, a review. *Scand J Trauma Resucs Emerg Med*. 2014;22:23.
4. Pickering LK, Kimberlin DW, Long SS, eds. *Red Book: 2012 Report of the Committee on Infectious Diseases*. 29th ed. Elk Grove Village, IL: American Academy of Pediatrics; 2012.
5. Liet JM, Ducruet T, Gupta V, et al. Heliox inhalation therapy for bronchiolitis in infants. *Cochrane Database Syst Rev*. 2015;(9):CD006915.

ADDITIONAL READING

- Beggs S, Wong ZH, Kaul S, et al. High-flow nasal cannula therapy for infants with bronchiolitis. *Cochrane Database Syst Rev*. 2014;(1):CD009609.
- Fernandes RM, Bialy LM, Vandermeer B, et al. Glucocorticoids for acute viral bronchiolitis in infants and young children. *Cochrane Database Syst Rev*. 2013;(6):CD004878.
- García CG, Bhore R, Soriano-Fallas A, et al. Risk factors in children hospitalized with RSV bronchiolitis versus non-RSV bronchiolitis. *Pediatrics*. 2010;126(6):e1453–e1460.

CODES

ICD10

- J21.9 Acute bronchiolitis, unspecified
- J21.0 Acute bronchiolitis due to respiratory syncytial virus
- J21.8 Acute bronchiolitis due to other specified organisms

CLINICAL PEARLS

- Bronchiolitis is the leading cause of hospitalizations in infants and children—especially <3 months of age.
- Diagnosis is a clinical one.
- Parental education and support is essential.
- Nasal and upper airway suctioning mainstay of treatment

BRONCHITIS, ACUTE

Alan Cropp, MD, FCCP • Ghazaleh Bigdeli, MD, FCCP

BASICS

DESCRIPTION
- Inflammation of trachea, bronchi, and bronchioles resulting from a respiratory tract infection or chemical irritant (1)
- Cough, the predominant symptom, may last as long as 3 weeks (2,3).
- Generally self-limited, with complete healing and full return of function (2)
- Most infections are viral if no underlying cardiopulmonary disease is present (2).
- Synonym(s): tracheobronchitis

Geriatric Considerations
Can be serious, particularly if part of influenza, with underlying COPD or CHF (3)

Pediatric Considerations
- Usually occurs in association with other conditions of upper and lower respiratory tract (trachea usually involved) (4)
- If repeated attacks occur, child should be evaluated for anomalies of the respiratory tract, immune deficiencies, or for chronic asthma.
- Acute bronchitis caused by RSV may be fatal.
- Antitussive medication not indicated in patients younger than age 6 years (2).

EPIDEMIOLOGY
- Predominant age: all ages
- Predominant gender: male = female

Incidence
- ~5% of adults per year (5)
- Common cause of infection in children (4)

Prevalence
Results in 10 to 12 million office visits per year

ETIOLOGY AND PATHOPHYSIOLOGY
- Viral infections such as adenovirus, influenza A and B, parainfluenza virus, coxsackie virus, RSV, rhinovirus, coronavirus (types 1 to 3), herpes simplex virus, metapneumonia virus (2)
- Bacterial infections, such as *Chlamydia pneumoniae* TWAR agent, *Mycoplasma*, *Bordetella pertussis*, *Haemophilus influenzae*, *Streptococcus pneumoniae*, *Moraxella catarrhalis*, and *Mycobacterium tuberculosis* (2)
- Secondary bacterial infection as part of an acute upper respiratory infection
- Possibly fungal infections
- Chemical irritants
- Acute bronchitis causes an injury to the epithelial surfaces, resulting in an increase in mucous production and thickening of the bronchiole wall (1).

Genetics
No known genetic pattern

RISK FACTORS
- Infants
- Elderly
- Air pollutants
- Smoking
- Secondhand smoke
- Environmental changes
- Chronic bronchopulmonary diseases
- Chronic sinusitis
- Tracheostomy or endobronchial intubation
- Bronchopulmonary allergy
- Hypertrophied tonsils and adenoids in children
- Immunosuppression
  - Immunoglobulin deficiency
  - HIV infection
  - Alcoholism
- Gastroesophageal reflux disease (GERD)

GENERAL PREVENTION
- Avoid smoking and secondhand smoke.
- Control underlying risk factors (i.e., asthma, sinusitis, and reflux).
- Avoid exposure, especially daycare.
- Pneumovax, influenza immunization

COMMONLY ASSOCIATED CONDITIONS
- Allergic rhinitis
- Sinusitis
- Pharyngitis
- Epiglottitis (rare but can be rapidly fatal)
- Coryza
- Croup
- Influenza
- Pneumonia
- Asthma
- COPD/emphysema
- GERD

DIAGNOSIS

HISTORY
- Sudden onset of cough and no evidence of pneumonia, asthma, exacerbation of COPD, or the common cold (3)
- Cough is initially dry and nonproductive, then productive; later, mucopurulent sputum, which may indicate secondary infection
- Cough lasts more than 5 days (1)
- Dyspnea, wheeze, and fatigue may occur.
- Possible contact with others who have respiratory infections (1)
- Fever is uncommon and may suggest pneumonia or influenza infection (1).

PHYSICAL EXAM
- Fever
- Tachypnea
- Pharynx injected
- Rales, rhonchi, wheezing
- No evidence of pulmonary consolidation

DIFFERENTIAL DIAGNOSIS
- Common cold
- Acute sinusitis
- Bronchopneumonia
- Influenza
- Bacterial tracheitis
- Bronchiectasis
- Asthma
- Reactive airways dysfunction syndrome (RADS)
- Allergy
- Eosinophilic pneumonitis
- Aspiration
- Retained foreign body
- Inhalation injury
- Cystic fibrosis
- Bronchogenic carcinoma
- Heart failure
- GERD
- Chronic cough

DIAGNOSTIC TESTS & INTERPRETATION
Initial Tests (lab, imaging)
- None normally needed; diagnosis is based on history and physical exam showing no postnasal drip or rales (1,3).
- For a complicated picture, consider the following:
  - WBC with differential
  - Sputum culture/sensitivity if CXR is abnormal (3)
  - Influenza titers (if appropriate for time of year) (1)
  - Viral panel
- No testing needed unless concerned about pneumonia
- CXR
  - Lungs normal, if uncomplicated
  - Helps to rule out other diseases (pneumonia) or complications

Follow-Up Tests & Special Consideration
- Arterial blood gases: hypoxemia (rarely)
- Pulmonary function tests (seldom needed during acute stages): increased residual volume, decreased maximal expiratory rate
- Procalcitonin level may influence use on antibiotics (6).
- Sputum culture in those patients intubated or with tracheostomy

TREATMENT

GENERAL MEASURES
- Outpatient treatment unless elderly or complicated by severe underlying disease
- Rest
- Stop smoking or avoid smoke.
- Steam inhalations
- Vaporizers
- Adequate hydration
- Antitussives
- Antibiotics are usually not recommended (1,3,7)[A].
- Treat associated illnesses (e.g., GERD).

MEDICATION

ALERT

Antibiotics are not recommended (1,3,6)[A] unless a treatable pathogen has been identified or significant comorbidities are present. This should be explained to patients who likely expect an antibiotic to be prescribed (3)[B].

First Line

- Supportive; increased fluids (cough results in increased fluid loss)
- Antipyretic analgesic such as aspirin, acetaminophen, or ibuprofen
- Decongestants if accompanied by sinus condition
- Cough suppressant for troublesome cough (not with COPD); honey, benzonatate (Tessalon), guaifenesin with codeine or dextromethorphan. Not indicated in children younger than age 6 years (2)[C]
- Mucolytic agents are not recommended (3)[B].
- Inhaled β-agonist (e.g., albuterol) or in combination with high-dose inhaled corticosteroids for cough with bronchospasm (2)[B]
- If influenza is highly suspected and symptom onset is <48 hours: oseltamivir (Tamiflu) or zanamivir (Relenza) (2)[B]
- Antibiotics ONLY if a treatable cause (i.e., pertussis) is identified (2)[A].
  - Clarithromycin (Biaxin): 500 mg q12h or azithromycin (Zithromax) Z-Pak for atypical or pertussis infection (1)[A]
  - In patients with acute bronchitis of a suspected bacterial cause, azithromycin tends to be more effective in terms of lower incidence of treatment failure and adverse events than amoxicillin or amoxicillin-clavulanic acid (8)[B].
    - Doxycycline: 100 mg/day × 10 days if *Moraxella*, *Chlamydia*, or *Mycoplasma* suspected
    - Quinolone for more serious infections or other antibiotic failure or in elderly or patients with multiple comorbidities
- Contraindication(s): Doxycycline and quinolones should not be used during pregnancy or in children.
- Precautions:
  - Multiple antibiotics have the potential to interfere with the effectiveness of PO contraceptives.
  - Antibiotic use can be associated with *Clostridium difficile* infections.
  - Cough and cold preparations should not be used in children <6 years (2)[B].

Second Line

Other antibiotics if indicated by sputum culture

ISSUES FOR REFERRAL

- Complications such as pneumonia or respiratory failure
- Comorbidities such as COPD
- Cough lasting >3 months

ADDITIONAL THERAPIES

- Antipyretic for fever (e.g., acetaminophen, aspirin, or ibuprofen)
- Inhaled β-agonist (e.g., albuterol) or in combination with high-dose inhaled corticosteroids for cough with bronchospasm (2)[B]
- Oral corticosteroids probably not indicated (2)[C]

COMPLEMENTARY & ALTERNATIVE MEDICINE

Throat lozenges for pharyngitis

INPATIENT CONSIDERATIONS

Admission Criteria/Initial Stabilization

- Hypoxia—may require supplemental oxygen
- Respiratory failure that may require CPAP/bilevel ventilation
- Severe bronchospasm
- Exacerbation of underlying disease
- Bronchodilators if patient is bronchospastic.

IV Fluids

May be helpful if patient is dehydrated

Nursing

- Ensure patient comfort and monitor for signs of deterioration, especially if underlying lung disease exists.
- May need to follow oxygen saturation in patients with underlying lung disease

Discharge Criteria

Improvement in symptoms and comorbidities

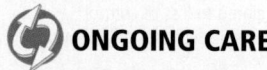 ## ONGOING CARE

FOLLOW-UP RECOMMENDATIONS

- Usually a self-limited disease not requiring follow-up
- Cough may linger for several weeks.
- In children, if recurrent, need to consider other diagnoses, such as asthma (7)

Patient Monitoring

- Oximetry until no longer hypoxemic
- Recheck for chronicity.

DIET

Increased fluids (3 to 4 L/day) while febrile

PATIENT EDUCATION

- For patient education materials favorably reviewed on this topic, contact the American Lung Association: 1740 Broadway, New York, NY 10019 (212) 315-8700; www.lungusa.org
- American Academy of Family Physicians: www.familydoctor.org

PROGNOSIS

- Usual: complete resolution
- Can be serious in the elderly or debilitated
- Cough may persist for several weeks after an initial improvement.
- Postbronchitic reactive airways disease (rare)
- Bronchiolitis obliterans and organizing pneumonia (rare)

COMPLICATIONS

- Superinfection such as bronchopneumonia
- Bronchiectasis
- Hemoptysis
- Acute respiratory failure
- Chronic cough

REFERENCES

1. Wenzel RP, Fowler AA III. Clinical practice. Acute bronchitis. *N Engl J Med*. 2006;355(20):2125–2130.
2. Albert RH. Diagnosis and treatment of acute bronchitis. *Am Fam Physician*. 2010;82(11):1345–1350.
3. Braman SS. Chronic cough due to acute bronchitis: ACCP evidence-based clinical practice guidelines. *Chest*. 2006;129(1)(Suppl):95S–103S.
4. Fleming DM, Elliot AJ. The management of acute bronchitis in children. *Expert Opin Pharmacother*. 2007;8(4):415–426.
5. Llor C, Moragas A, Bayona C, et al. Efficacy of anti-inflammatory or antibiotic treatment in patients with non-complicated acute bronchitis and discoloured sputum: randomised placebo controlled trial. *BMJ*. 2013;347:f5762.
6. Schuetz P, Amin DN, Greenwald JL. Role of procalcitonin in managing adult patients with respiratory tract infections. *Chest*. 2012;141(4):1063–1073.
7. Gonzales R, Anderer T, McCulloch CE, et al. A cluster randomized trial of decision support strategies for reducing antibiotic use in acute bronchitis. *JAMA Intern Med*. 2013;173(4):267–273.
8. Panpanich R, Lerttrakarnnon P, Laopaiboon M. Azithromycin for acute lower respiratory tract infections. *Cochrane Database Syst Rev*. 2008;(1):CD001954.

 ### SEE ALSO

- Asthma; Chronic Obstructive Pulmonary Disease and Emphysema
- Algorithm: Cough, Chronic

 ## CODES

ICD10

- J20.9 Acute bronchitis, unspecified
- J68.0 Bronchitis and pneumonitis due to chemicals, gases, fumes and vapors
- B97.0 Adenovirus as the cause of diseases classified elsewhere

CLINICAL PEARLS

- Acute bronchitis is a common and generally self-limited disease.
- It usually does not require treatment with antibiotics. This needs to be explained to patients who expect antibiotics to be prescribed.
- Cough may linger for several weeks.
- Recurrent or seasonal episodes may suggest another disease process, such as asthma.
- Fever is uncommon and should prompt investigation for pneumonia or influenza.

BULIMIA NERVOSA

Umer Farooq, MD, MBBS • Wajiha Illyas, MD

BASICS

DESCRIPTION
- A pattern of discrete periods of binge eating (within 2-hour period) along with lack of control over eating, followed by compensatory behaviors such as self induced vomiting, misuse of laxatives, and so forth.
- Both binge eating and compensatory behaviors happening at least once per week for 3 months
- *DSM-5* classifies bulimia nervosa as
  - Mild: 1 to 3 episodes of compensatory behaviors
  - Moderate: 4 to 7 episodes of compensatory behaviors
  - Severe: 8 to 13 episodes of compensatory behaviors
  - Extreme: 14 or more episodes of compensatory behaviors
- System(s) affected: oropharyngeal, endocrine/metabolic, gastrointestinal, dermatologic, cardiovascular, nervous

EPIDEMIOLOGY
- Predominant age: adolescents and young adults
- Mean age of onset: 18 to 21 years
- Predominant sex: female > male (10:1)

Incidence
28.8 women, 0.8 men per 100,000 per year

Prevalence
- More prevalent than anorexia nervosa
- 1–3% in women age 16 to 35 years
- 0.5% in young men (higher among gay and bisexual men)

ETIOLOGY AND PATHOPHYSIOLOGY
- Combination of biologic, psychological, environmental, and social factors. Unique contribution of any specific factor remains unclear.
- Strong evidence of serotonergic dysregulation in bulimia nervosa
- Substantial literature shows genetic evidence for bulimia nervosa (1)[B].

RISK FACTORS
- Female gender
- History of obesity and dieting
- Body dissatisfaction
- Critical comments about weight, body shape, or eating
- Severe life stressor
- Low self-esteem
- Perceived pressure to be thin
- Perfectionist or obsessive thinking
- Poor impulse control, substance abuse
- Environment stressing high achievement, physical fitness (e.g., armed forces, ballet, cheerleading, gymnastics, or modeling)
- Family history of substance abuse, affective disorders, eating disorder, or obesity
- Type 1 diabetes
- Sexual abuse is not causally related to bulimia.

GENERAL PREVENTION
- Prevention programs can reduce risk factors and future onset of eating disorders (2)[A].
- Target adolescents and young women ≥15 years

- Realistic and healthy weight management strategies and attitudes
- Decrease body dissatisfaction and promote self-esteem.
- Reduce focus on thin as ideal.
- Decrease anxiety/depressive symptoms and improve stress management.

COMMONLY ASSOCIATED CONDITIONS
- Major depression and dysthymia
- Anxiety disorders
- Substance use disorder
- Bipolar disorder
- Obsessive-compulsive disorder
- Borderline personality disorder

DIAGNOSIS

HISTORY
- Patients unlikely to self-identify binge eating or purging behaviors; corroborate with parent/relative
- Unhappiness and/or preoccupation with weight and diet attempts
- Pattern of binge eating and compensatory behaviors
  - Binge is context-specific (usually within 2-hour period, they will eat what would be an unusually large amount for most people)
  - Vomiting (often with little effort)
  - Vigorous aerobic exercise
  - Distress/shame-related to loss of control
- Depressed mood and self-depreciation following the binges
- Other possible signs and symptoms
  - Requesting weight loss help and mildly underweight to overweight
  - Diet pill, diuretic, laxative, ipecac, and thyroid medication use/abuse
  - Menstrual disturbance
  - Fatigue and lethargy
  - Abdominal pain, bloating, constipation, diarrhea, rectal prolapse
  - Sore throat
  - Thermal tooth sensitivity
  - Frequent fluctuations in weight
  - Omission/underdosing insulin in diabetes patients

PHYSICAL EXAM
- Often normal
- Bradycardia
- Eroded tooth enamel
- Perimylolysis
- Cheilosis
- Gingivitis
- Sialadenosis
- Asymptomatic, noninflammatory parotid gland enlargement
- Epigastric tenderness to palpation
- Calluses, abrasions, bruising on hand, thumb (Russell sign)
- Peripheral edema

DIFFERENTIAL DIAGNOSIS
- Anorexia, binge eating/purging type
- Major depressive disorder
- Addison disease
- Celiac disease

- Diabetes mellitus
- Hyperthyroidism, hypothyroidism
- Hyperpituitarism
- Hypothalamic brain tumor
- Kleine-Levin syndrome
- Body dysmorphic disorder
- Borderline personality disorder

DIAGNOSTIC TESTS & INTERPRETATION
All lab results may be within normal limits and are not necessary for diagnosis.

- Psychological self-report screening tests may be helpful, but diagnosis is based on meeting the *DSM-5* criteria:
  - SCOFF Questionnaire (3)[B]
  - Eating Disorder Screen for Primary Care

Initial Tests (lab, imaging)
- Blood work, CBC, and CMP
  - Hypokalemia, hypochloremia
  - Hypomagnesemia, hyponatremia, hypocalcemia, hypophosphatemia
  - Serum amylase levels
  - Alkalosis
  - Elevated BUN
  - Hypoglycemia
- Urinalysis
  - Increased urine specific gravity

Diagnostic Procedures/Other
- Electrocardiogram
- Bradycardia or arrhythmias
- Conduction defects
- Depressed ST segment due to hypokalemia

Test Interpretation
- Esophagitis
- Acute pancreatitis
- Cardiomyopathy and muscle weakness due to ipecac abuse
- Melanosis coli
- Cathartic colon syndrome
- Delayed or arrested skeletal growth
- Stress fracture
- Irreversible dental erosions
- Osteopenia/osteoporosis

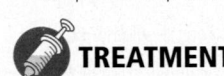

TREATMENT

- Cognitive-behavioral therapy (CBT) should be considered as first-line treatment (4,5)[A].
- Interpersonal therapies and group therapies have been found to be helpful.

GENERAL MEASURES
- Multidisciplinary team
  - Primary care physician, behavioral health provider, nutritionist
- Build trust; increase motivation for change.
- Assess psychological and nutritional status.
- Consider evidence-based self-help program.
- CBT for bulimia nervosa (4,5)[A]
  - Sixteen to twenty 50-minute appointments
  - Involve patient in establishing goals.

- Self-monitoring of food intake, frequency of binges/purges, related antecedents, consequences, thoughts, and emotions
- Self-monitoring of weight once per week
- Educate about ineffectiveness of purging for weight control and adverse outcomes.
- Establish prescribed eating plan to develop regular eating habits and realistic weight goal.
- Gradually introduce feared foods into diet.
- Problem-solve how to cope with triggers.
- Decrease ruminations about calories, weight, and purging.
- Challenge fear of loss of control.
- Establish relapse prevention plan.
- Gradual laxative withdrawal
- Interpersonal therapy
  - May act more slowly than CBT
- Transdiagnostic CBT
- Dialectical behavior therapy
- Family therapy for adolescents
- Nutritional education, relaxation techniques
- Educate patient to brush teeth and use baking soda to rinse mouth after vomiting.

MEDICATION
First Line
- Selective serotonin reuptake inhibitors (SSRIs) (6)[A], (7)[B], particularly fluoxetine (Prozac) titrated to 60 mg/day, are effective in reducing symptoms with relatively few side effects. Higher doses than standard doses for depression are often needed.

  - Combination of medication and CBT has been shown to have added benefit over medication or therapy alone.
- To prevent relapse, maintain antidepressant at full therapeutic dose for at least 1 year.
- Avoid bupropion: contraindicated due to its association with seizures in patients who purge
- Precautions
  - Serious toxicity following overdose is common.
  - Patients may vomit medications.

Second Line
- Select different SSRI.
- Ondansetron (Zofran) 4 to 8 mg TID between meals can help prevent vomiting.
- Psyllium (Metamucil) preparations, 1 tbs QHS with glass of water, can prevent constipation during laxative withdrawal.

ISSUES FOR REFERRAL
Patients with bulimia require a multidisciplinary team, including a primary care physician, behavioral health provider, and a nutritionist. Important part of treatment is to arrange mental health therapist for psychotherapy.

ADDITIONAL THERAPIES
Most patients can be treated as outpatients.

COMPLEMENTARY & ALTERNATIVE MEDICINE
Bright light therapy may help.

INPATIENT CONSIDERATIONS
- If possible, admit to a specialized eating disorders unit.
- Supervised meals and bathroom privileges
- Monitor weight and physical activity.
- Monitor electrolytes.
- Gradually shift control to patients as they demonstrate improvement.

Admission Criteria/Initial Stabilization
Hospitalize if severe malnutrition, dehydration, electrolyte disturbances, cardiac dysrhythmia, uncontrolled binging and purging, psychiatric emergency (threat to self/others), or if outpatient treatment failed

 ONGOING CARE

FOLLOW-UP RECOMMENDATIONS
Patient Monitoring
- Binge–purge activity, including antecedents and consequences
- Level of exercise activity
- Self-esteem, comfort with body and self
- Ruminations and depressive symptoms
- Repeat any abnormal lab values weekly or monthly until stable.

DIET
- Balanced diet, normal eating pattern
- Reintroduce feared foods.

PATIENT EDUCATION
- Astrachan-Fletcher E, Maslar M. *The Dialectical Behavior Therapy Skills Workbook for Bulimia: Using DBT to Break the Cycle and Regain Control of Your Life.* Oakland, CA: New Harbinger; 2009.
- http://www.nami.org/helpline/bulimia.htm

PROGNOSIS
- After effective CBT
  - In the short term, 50% of treated individuals do not meet criteria for diagnosis.
  - In the long term (2 to 10 years), 70% may be asymptomatic.
  - Symptomatic individuals may demonstrate remissions, relapses, subclinical, or other eating disorder–related behaviors.
- Untreated
  - Likely to remain chronic/relapsing problem
- Greater weight fluctuations, other impulsive behaviors, childhood obesity, low self-esteem, family history of alcohol abuse, psychiatric comorbidity, and personality disorder diagnoses (e.g., avoidant personality disorder) may predict poor prognosis.
- Mortality rate: 0.4%

COMPLICATIONS
- Substance use disorder
- Osteopenia/osteoporosis
- Stress fracture
- Gastric dilatation
- Boerhaave syndrome
- Mallory-Weiss tears
- Pseudo-Bartter syndrome
- Spontaneous pneumomediastinum
- Potassium depletion, cardiac arrhythmia, cardiac arrest
- Suicide

Pregnancy Considerations
Maternal and fetal problems if pregnant
- Binging/purging behaviors may persist, increase, or decrease with pregnancy.
- Increased risk for preterm delivery, operative delivery, and infants with low birth weight should be managed as high risk.

REFERENCES
1. Raevuori A. Genetic etiology of eating disorders. *Duodecim.* 2013;129(20):2126–2132.
2. Stice E, Shaw H, Marti CN. A meta-analytic review of eating disorder prevention programs: encouraging findings. *Annu Rev Clin Psychol.* 2007;3:207–231.
3. Cotton MA, Ball C, Robinson P. Four simple questions can help screen for eating disorders. *J Gen Intern Med.* 2003;18(1): 53–56.
4. Hay PP, Bacaltchuk J, Stefano S, et al. Psychological treatments for bulimia nervosa and binging. *Cochrane Database Syst Rev.* 2009;(4):CD000562.
5. Shapiro JR, Berkman ND, Brownley KA, et al. Bulimia nervosa treatment: a systematic review of randomized controlled trials. *Int J Eat Disord.* 2007;40(4):321–336.
6. Bacaltchuk J, Hay P, Trefiglio R. Antidepressants versus psychological treatments and their combination for bulimia nervosa. *Cochrane Database Syst Rev.* 2001;(4):CD003385.
7. Bellini M, Merli M. Current drug treatment of patients with bulimia nervosa and binge-eating disorder: selective serotonin reuptake inhibitors versus mood stabilizers. *Int J Psychiatry Clin Pract.* 2004;8(4):235–243.

ADDITIONAL READING
- American Psychiatric Association. *Practice Guideline for the Treatment of Patients with Eating Disorders.* 3rd ed. Washington, DC: American Psychiatric Association. http://www.psychiatry.org/
- National Institute for Clinical Excellence. *Eating Disorders: Core Interventions in the Treatment and Management of Anorexia Nervosa, Bulimia Nervosa and Related Eating Disorders (NICE Guidelines).* London, United Kingdom: National Institute for Clinical Excellence; 2004. http://www.nice.org.uk.

 SEE ALSO

- Anorexia Nervosa; Hyperkalemia; Laxative Abuse; Salivary Gland Tumors
- Algorithm: Weight Loss

CODES

ICD10
F50.2 Bulimia nervosa

CLINICAL PEARLS
- Asking "Are you satisfied with your eating patterns?" and/or "Do you worry that you have lost control over how much you eat?" may help to screen for an eating problem.
- Weight is not severely lowered as in anorexia nervosa.
- Consider using a stepped care approach. Start with a guided self-help program using instructional aids; next, begin CBT (e.g., 16 to 20 sessions over 4 to 5 months).
- SSRIs, particularly fluoxetine (60 mg daily), may be helpful as a first step or as an adjunctive treatment with CBT.

BUNION (HALLUX VALGUS)

Jennifer G. Chang, MD

BASICS

DESCRIPTION
- Lateral deviation of the great toe. Hallux valgus derives from the Latin for "big toe askew"; also commonly known as a bunion
- Lateral deviation of the great toe with medial deviation of the 1st metatarsal leads to a medial prominence of the 1st metatarsophalangeal (MTP) joint and a potentially painful and/or debilitating deformity.
- Progressive subluxation of the 1st MTP joint is common.
- System(s) affected: musculoskeletal/skin

EPIDEMIOLOGY
- Predominant age: more common in adults
  - Estimated 23% in adults aged 18 to 65 years
  - Estimated 35.7% in elderly >65 years
- Predominant sex: female > male by ~2:1

Prevalence
- Prevalence increases with age particularly in females.
- Juvenile hallux valgus
  - More common in girls (>80% of cases)
- Commonly bilateral
- Pain is not usually the presenting symptom.

ETIOLOGY AND PATHOPHYSIOLOGY
Multifactorial. Contributing factors include the following:
- Valgus deviation of the hallux promotes varus position of the 1st metatarsal.
- Medial MTP joint capsule stretches and attenuates while the lateral capsule contracts.
- Metatarsal head moves medially, shifting the sesamoid bones to a more lateral position.
- Extensor hallucis longus deviates laterally.
- Lateral and plantar migration of abductor hallucis moves the great toe into plantar flexion and lateral pronation.
- Medial collateral ligament stretches and eventually ruptures due to this deviation, decreasing stability and causing progressive subluxation of the 1st MTP joint.

RISK FACTORS
- Familial predisposition
- Abnormal biomechanics (i.e., flexible flat feet)
- Joint laxity; pronation of hindfoot; Achilles tendon contracture; pes planus (fallen arches)
- Metatarsus primus varus
- Amputation of second toe
- Inflammatory joint disease
- Neuromuscular disorders
- Improper footwear, narrow toe box

GENERAL PREVENTION
Proper footwear may decrease the progression of the disease.

COMMONLY ASSOCIATED CONDITIONS
- Medial bursitis of the 1st MTP joint (most common)
- Hammertoe deformity of the 2nd phalanx

- Plantar callus
- Metatarsalgia
- Degeneration of 1st metatarsal head cartilage
- Pronated feet; ankle equinus
- Onychocryptosis (ingrown toenail)
- Entrapment of the medial dorsal cutaneous nerve
- Synovitis of the MTP joint

DIAGNOSIS

- Based on clinical exam
- Radiographs are used for staging

HISTORY
- Painful MTP joint (most common symptom in adults)
- Abnormal position of great toe
- Enlargement of the MTP joint medially (patients complain of a "bump")
- Shoes don't fit properly
- Pain on ambulation
- Skin irritation, blistering, callus formation at 1st MTP

PHYSICAL EXAM
- Observe gait; may be antalgic due to pain
- Increased distal metatarsal articular angle (DMAA)
- Medial prominence at the MTP joint
- Medial inflammation and ulceration at the MTP joint
- Skin changes: inflammation, blistering, callus
- Great toe over- or underriding the second toe
- Examine the entire first ray for:
  - 1st MTP range of motion
  - 1st tarsometatarsal mobility
  - Neurovascular integrity
  - Degenerative osteoarthritis

DIFFERENTIAL DIAGNOSIS
- Trauma
  - Turf toe; sesamoiditis; stress fracture
- Infection
  - Osteomyelitis; septic arthritis
- Joint disorder
  - Osteoarthritis; rheumatoid arthritis; pseudogout; gout
- Tendon disorder
  - Tendinosis; tenosynovitis; tendon rupture
- Other
  - Bursitis; ganglia; foreign body granuloma

DIAGNOSTIC TESTS & INTERPRETATION
- Weight-bearing AP and lateral radiographs (sesamoid view optional) to assess:
  - Joint congruency and degenerative changes
  - Lateral sesamoid bone displacement (1)[A]
  - Rounded 1st MT head (1)[A]
  - Longer 1st metatarsal (1)[A]

- Radiographic parameters:
  - Hallux valgus angle (HA): Long axis of the 1st MT and proximal phalanx is normally <15 degrees.
  - Intermetatarsal angle (IM): Between long axis of 1st and 2nd MT is normally <9 degrees.
  - DMAA: Between 1st MT long axis and line through base of distal articular cap is normally <15 degrees.
  - Hallux valgus interphalangeus: Between long axis of distal phalanx and proximal phalanx is normally <10 degrees.

TREATMENT

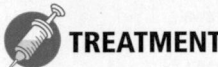

- Primary indication for treatment is pain.
- There are conservative and surgical approaches.
- Surgical treatment is generally more effective in improving pain but has attendant risks.

GENERAL MEASURES
Nonoperative treatment options may improve symptoms and delay the progression of hallux valgus deformity, although high-quality evidence is limited:
- Proper fitting footwear: low-heeled, wide-toe shoes to decrease stress on MTP joint (i.e., wide toe box)
- Orthoses to correct foot alignment (pes planus and overpronation). Improving gait may prevent bunion formation and reduce pressure on the MTP.
- Night splinting: In theory, splinting stabilizes and balances soft tissue structures around the MTP. Limited evidence shows improvement in degree of angulation in mild hallux valgus.
- Manual and manipulative therapy (MMT): stretches contracted soft tissue
- Foot exercises and stretching to improve intrinsic foot muscle strength and increase range of motion
- Pads/spacers: Pads decrease friction on the MTP joint. A toe spacer in the 1st interdigital space can straighten the hallux and may reduce pain (2)[C].

MEDICATION
- Topical and PO medications (NSAIDs) can be used to relieve pain and swelling. Other topical options include capsaicin cream.
- Corticosteroid injections improve pain.

ADDITIONAL THERAPIES
Custom orthoses are a safe intervention that may decrease pain at 6 and 12 months compared with no treatment; however, this improvement is less than that seen with surgical intervention (3)[B].

SURGERY/OTHER PROCEDURES

- Surgery is indicated if patient has severe pain, dysfunction, or persistent symptoms that do not abate with conservative therapy.
- Surgery is beneficial for patients with severe symptoms (3)[B]:
  - >150 different surgical techniques to treat hallux valgus; none has been proven to be superior, and no universally accepted standard exists for selecting a particular procedure over another.
  - Choice of surgical technique depends on the severity of disease, the HA and IM angles, congruency and subluxation of the MTP joint, patient-specific factors, and the pathologic element the surgeon determines needs correcting. Examples include the following:
    - ○ Arthrodesis: fusion of the 1st MTP joint; reserved for severe and/or recurrent hallux valgus
    - ○ Arthroplasty: removing the joint or replacing it with a prosthesis
    - ○ Exostectomy/bunionectomy: removing the medial bony prominence of the MTP joint
    - ○ Soft tissue realignment: alters the function of surrounding ligaments and tendons; used for minor, flexible deformities
    - ○ Osteotomy and realignment: can correct large deformities, but evidence of long-term outcome is lacking (4)[C]
    - ○ Mini-tight rope procedure: use of a Fiberwire to correct the misalignment of the deformity; reportedly allows for faster recovery and earlier weight bearing (5)[C] but may have high complication and failure rates (6)[C]
- Surgery can decrease pain and increase foot alignment. Some patients may have little to no improvement in symptoms despite interventions.
- Establish realistic expectations prior to surgery (7)[C].
- In pediatric patients, surgery should generally be delayed until skeletal maturity (8)[C].

COMPLEMENTARY & ALTERNATIVE MEDICINE

Marigold ointment may reduce pain and soft tissue swelling (9)[C].

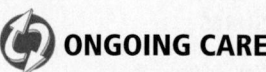 ONGOING CARE

FOLLOW-UP RECOMMENDATIONS

- Postoperative treatment includes physical therapy, physiotherapy, supportive footwear, continuous passive motion, or manual manipulation.
- Time until full weight bearing depends on the surgical procedure.

PROGNOSIS

Patient outcome varies depending on biomechanical factors, severity of the deformity, and treatment modality used. The radiologic HA angle predicts surgical outcomes. Patients with an HA angle <37 degrees have a higher chance of having the deformity successfully corrected with surgery compared with patients with an HA angle >37 degrees.

COMPLICATIONS

- Risks associated with surgery include infection, persistent pain, and poor cosmetic result.
- Additional risks vary with the surgical procedure.
- Other complications may include:
  - Early swelling
  - Hallux varus
  - Recurrence of bunion
  - Metatarsal fracture
  - Decreased sensation over the 1st metatarsal or phalanx

REFERENCES

1. Nix SE, Vicenzino BT, Collins NJ, et al. Characteristics of foot structure and footwear associated with hallux valgus: a systematic review. *Osteoarthritis Cartilage*. 2012;20(10):1059–1074.
2. Tehraninasr A, Saeedi H, Forogh B, et al. Effects of insole with toe-separator and night splint on patients with painful hallux valgus: a comparative study. *Prosthet Orthot Int*. 2008;32(1):78–83.
3. Torkki M, Malmivaara A, Seitsalo S, et al. Surgery vs orthosis vs watchful for hallux valgus: a randomized controlled trial. *JAMA*. 2001;285(19):2474–2480.
4. Choi JH, Zide JR, Coleman SC, et al. Prospective study of the treatment of adult primary hallux valgus with scarf osteotomy and soft tissue realignment. *Foot Ankle Int*. 2013;34(5):684–690.
5. Holmes GB Jr, Hsu AR. Correction of intermetatarsal angle in hallux valgus using small suture button device. *Foot Ankle Int*. 2013;34(4):543–549.
6. Dayton P, Sedberry S, Feilmeier M. Complications of metatarsal suture techniques for bunion correction: a systematic review of the literature. *J Foot Ankle Surg*. 2015;54(2):230–232.
7. Dux K, Smith N, Rottier FJ. Outcome after metatarsal osteotomy for hallux valgus: a study of postoperative foot function using revised foot function index short form. *J Foot Ankle Surg*. 2013;52(4):422–425.
8. Chell J, Dhar S. Pediatric hallux valgus. *Foot Ankle Clin*. 2014;19(2):235–243.
9. Deenik AR, de Visser E, Louwerens JW, et al. Hallux valgus angle as main predictor for correction of hallux valgus. *BMC Musculoskelet Disord*. 2008;9:70.

ADDITIONAL READING

- Maffulli N, Longo UG, Marinozzi A, et al. Hallux valgus: effectiveness and safety of minimally invasive surgery. A systematic review. *Br Med Bull*. 2011;97:149–167.
- Nix S, Smith M, Vicenzino B. Prevalence of hallux valgus in the general population: a systemic review and meta-analysis. *J Foot Ankle Res*. 2010;3:21.
- Perera AM, Mason L, Stephens MM. The pathogenesis of hallux valgus. *J Bone Joint Surg Am*. 2011;93(17):1650–1661.
- Smith SE, Landorf KB, Butterworth PA, et al. Scarf versus chevron osteotomy for the correction of 1–2 intermetatarsal angle in hallux valgus: a systematic review and meta-analysis. *J Foot Ankle Surg*. 2012;51(4):437–444.
- Trnka HJ, Krenn S, Schuh R. Minimally invasive hallux valgus surgery: a critical review of the evidence. *Int Orthop*. 2013;37(9):1731–1735.

CODES

ICD10

- M20.10 Hallux valgus (acquired), unspecified foot
- M20.11 Hallux valgus (acquired), right foot
- M20.12 Hallux valgus (acquired), left foot

CLINICAL PEARLS

- Avoid footwear with high heels, pointed toe boxes, or inadequate toe space to reduce development or progression of bunions.
- Surgery generally results in superior outcomes for pain relief in appropriately selected patients.
- No single surgical method has shown to be superior for long-term pain relief.
- Establish realistic expectations prior to surgery to improve patient satisfaction with surgical outcomes.

BURNS

Caleb J. Mentzer, DO • James R. Yon, MD

BASICS

DESCRIPTION
- Tissue injuries caused by application of heat, chemicals, electricity, or irradiation
- Extent of injury (depth of burn) is a result of intensity and duration of exposure.
  - 1st degree involves superficial layers of epidermis.
  - 2nd degree involves varying amounts of epidermis (with blister formation) and part of the dermis.
  - 3rd degree involves destruction of all skin elements (full thickness) with coagulation of subdermal plexus.
- System(s) affected: endocrine/metabolic, pulmonary, skin/exocrine

Geriatric Considerations
- Prognosis is worse for severe burns.
- Patients >60 years of age account for 11% all of burns.

Pediatric Considerations
Consider child abuse or neglect when dealing with hot water burns in children; abuse accounts for 15% of pediatric burns. Special concerns are sharply demarcated wounds, immersion injuries, and suspect stories. Involve child welfare services early.

EPIDEMIOLOGY
- Predominant age: 30 years; 13% infants; 11% >60 years of age
- Predominant gender: males account for 70%

Incidence
Per year in the United States
- 1.2 to 2 million burns; 700,000 emergency room visits; 45,000 to 50,000 hospitalizations; 3,900 deaths owing to burn-related complications
- In children: 250,000 burns; 15,000 hospitalizations; 1,100 deaths
- Estimated total cost of $2 billion annually for burn care
- House fires cause 75% of deaths.
- Burn deaths decreasing nationally due to improved prevention and treatment
- Increase in burns from the illegal production of methamphetamines. Patients can present with a combination of chemical burn, thermal burn, and explosion injury.

ETIOLOGY AND PATHOPHYSIOLOGY
- Open flame and hot liquid are the most common causes of burns (heat usually ≥45°C): Flame burns are more common in adults; scald burns are more common in children.
- Caustic chemicals or acids (may show little signs or symptoms for the first few days)
- Electricity (may have significant injury with very little damage to overlying skin)
- Excess sun exposure

RISK FACTORS
- Water heaters set too high
- Workplace exposure to chemicals, electricity, or irradiation
- Young children and older adults with thin skin are more susceptible to injury.
- Carelessness with burning cigarettes: related to 18% of fatal fires in 2006
- Inadequate or faulty electrical wiring

- Lack of smoke detectors: Lacking or nonfunctioning smoke alarms are implicated in 63% of residential fires.
- Arson: cause of 12.4% of fires that resulted in fatalities in 2012

GENERAL PREVENTION
Home safety education should be a key mechanism for injury prevention.
- Families educated on home safety were more likely to have safe hot water temperatures.
- Safety education results in more families having functioning smoke alarms and increased use of fireguards.

COMMONLY ASSOCIATED CONDITIONS
Smoke inhalation syndrome
- May involve thermal burn to respiratory mucosa (e.g., trachea, bronchi) as well as carbon monoxide inhalation
- Occurs within 72 hours of burn
- Should be suspected in all burns occurring in an enclosed space or exposure to explosions

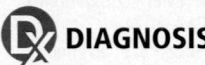

DIAGNOSIS

HISTORY
- History of source of burn
- In children or elderly: Check for consistency between the history and the burn's physical characteristics.

PHYSICAL EXAM
- 1st degree: Erythema of involved tissue, skin blanches with pressure, skin may be tender.
- 2nd degree: Skin is red and blistered, skin is very tender.
- 3rd degree: Burned skin is tough and leathery; skin is nontender.
- Rule of 9s (1)[C]
  - Each upper extremity: adult and child 9%
  - Each lower extremity: adult 18%; child 14%
  - Anterior trunk: adult and child 18%
  - Posterior trunk: adult and child 18%
  - Head and neck: adult 10%; child 18%
- Quick estimate: The surface area of the patient's hand (palmar surface plus fingers) is 1% of the body surface area (BSA).
- Careful documentation of extent of burn and the estimated depth of burn
- Check for any signs suggestive of potential airway involvement: singed nasal hair, facial burns, carbonaceous sputum, progressive hoarseness, inflamed oropharynx, circumferential burns around the neck, tachypnea

DIAGNOSTIC TESTS & INTERPRETATION
- Children: glucose (hypoglycemia may occur in children because of limited glycogen storage)
- Smoke inhalation: arterial blood gas, carboxyhemoglobin
- Electrical burns: ECG, urine myoglobin, creatine kinase isoenzymes

Initial Tests (lab, imaging)
- Labs: hematocrit; type and crossmatching; electrolytes, including BUN and creatinine; urinalysis
- Imaging: Chest radiograph; Xenon scan is useful in suspected smoke inhalation.

Diagnostic Procedures/Other
Bronchoscopy may be necessary in smoke inhalation to evaluate lower respiratory tract (2)[A].

TREATMENT

- Prehospital care (1)[C]
  - Remove the patient from the source of burn.
  - Extinguish and remove all burning clothing.
  - Room-temperature water may be poured onto burn but only in the first 15 minutes following burn exposure.
  - Wrap patient to prevent hypothermia.
  - All patients to receive 100% oxygen via face mask
- Hospitalization for all serious burns
  - 2nd-degree burns >10% of BSA
  - Any 3rd-degree burn
  - Burns of hands, feet, face, or perineum
  - Electrical or lightning burns
  - Inhalation injury
  - Chemical burns
  - Circumferential burn
- Transfer to burn center for (3)[C]
  - 2nd- and 3rd-degree burns >10% of BSA in patients <10 years and >50 years of age
  - 2nd-degree burns >20% of BSA and full-thickness burns >5% BSA in any age range
  - 3rd-degree burns in any age group
  - Burns of hands, feet, face, or perineum
  - Electrical or lightning burns
  - Inhalation injury
  - Chemical burns
  - Circumferential burn
  - Burns in patients with additional trauma (fractures, etc.) in which the burn is the more severe injury; otherwise, send to trauma center for stabilization.
  - Burn injuries in patients with preexisting medical conditions that could affect management, mortality, or recovery

GENERAL MEASURES
- Based on depth of burns and accurate estimate of total BSA involved (rule of 9s)
- Tetanus prophylaxis (if not current)
- Remove all rings, watches, and other items from injured extremities to avoid tourniquet effect.
- Remove clothing and cover all burned areas with dry sheets.
- Flush area of chemical burn (for ~2 hours).
- For all major burns, use 100% oxygen administration; consider early intubation.
- Do not apply ice to burn site.
- Nasogastric tube (high risk of paralytic ileus)
- Foley catheter
- Analgesia
- ECG monitoring in the first 24 hours following electrical burn
- Whirlpool hydrotherapy followed by silver sulfadiazine (Silvadene) occlusive dressings in severe burns
- Daily or BID cleansing with dressing changes
- Burn fluid resuscitation (1)[C]
  - Calculate fluid resuscitation from time of burn, not from time treatment begins.
  - 2 to 4 mL lactated Ringer × body weight (kg) × % BSA burn (1/2 given in first 8 hours, in second

8 hours, and in third 8 hours); in children, this is given in addition to maintenance fluids and is adjusted according to urine output and vital signs. Protocol-based resuscitation leads to superior outcomes.

– Colloid solutions are not recommended during the first 12 to 24 hours of resuscitation (1)[C],(4)[A].
– Other: Use of biologic membranes or skin substitutes may be indicated for burn coverage.
• Inhalation injury
– Intubation, ventilation with positive end-expiratory pressure assistance
– Hyperbaric oxygen treatment may be useful in patients with carbon monoxide levels >25%, patients with coma, focal neurologic deficit, ischemic ECG changes, and pregnant patients (1)[C].

MEDICATION

First Line

• IV morphine or hydromorphone (Dilaudid) for severe pain
• Oral analgesics, such as acetaminophen (Tylenol) with codeine, acetaminophen with oxycodone (Percocet), or acetaminophen with hydrocodone (Lortab) for moderate pain
• Silver sulfadiazine (Silvadene): Apply topically to burn site (can cause leukopenia). Do not use in sulfa-allergic patients, women who are pregnant/breastfeeding, or infants <2 months)
• Neosporin or bacitracin ointment: Apply to facial burns.
• Mupirocin: has potent inhibitory activity against methicillin-resistant Staphylococcus aureus (MRSA) (5)[B]
• Acticoat A.B. (a dressing consisting of two sheets of high-density polyethylene mesh coated with nano-crystalline silver) has a more controlled, prolonged release of silver, allowing less frequent dressing changes (5)[B].
• Electrical burn with myoglobinuria will require alkalinization of urine and mannitol.
• Consider H_2 blockers (e.g., famotidine) or proton pump inhibitors (e.g., lansoprazole, pantoprazole) for stress ulcer prophylaxis in severely burned patients.
• Tetanus toxoid/tetanus immunoglobulin
• There is no clear indication for prophylactic systemic antibiotics (5)[B].
• Use of negative pressure wound therapy may result in a low-protease environment with higher levels of angiogenic factor (vascular endothelial growth factor [VEGF]) during wound healing, leading to more chaotic, hyperkeratinized, thickened epidermis when compared with a standard hydrocolloid dressing (6)[C].

Second Line

• Mafenide (Sulfamylon) for full-thickness burn, best against Pseudomonas (Caution: metabolic acidosis, painful)
• Silver nitrate 0.5% (messy, leeches electrolytes from burn, causes water toxicity)
• Povidone–iodine (Betadine) may result in iodine absorption from burn and "tan eschar," makes débridement more difficult.
• Travase (enzymatic debridement)

SURGERY/OTHER PROCEDURES

• Escharotomy may be necessary in constricting circumferential burns of extremities or chest due to compartment syndrome.
• Tangential excision with split-thickness skin grafts: Early excision of burns results in a significant reduction in mortality (excluding patients with inhalational injury) and a significant decrease in hospital length of stay (7)[B].
• Various dressings (e.g., biosynthetic, biologic) are available to help reduce the number of dressing changes and promote healing.

 ## ONGOING CARE

FOLLOW-UP RECOMMENDATIONS
Early mobilization is the goal.

DIET
• High-protein, high-calorie diet when bowel function resumes
• Nasogastric tube feedings may be required in early postburn period.
• Total parenteral nutrition if NPO is expected for >5 days
• Early initiation of enteral nutrition in the first 24 hours of admission results in shorter intensive care unit (ICU) stay and lower wound infection rates

PATIENT EDUCATION
• Use of sunscreen: Skin grafts or newly epithelialized skin is highly sensitive to sun exposure and thermal extremes.
• Prevent access to electrical cords/outlets.
• Isolate household chemicals.
• Use low-temperature setting for water heater (<54°C).
• Household smoke detectors with special emphasis on maintenance
• Family/household evacuation plan
• Proper storage and use of flammable substances
• Burn management: http://www.aafp.org/afp/2000/1101/p2029.html
• Burn prevention: http://www.aafp.org/afp/2000/1101/p2032.html

PROGNOSIS
• 1st-degree burn: complete resolution
• 2nd-degree burn: epithelialization in 10 to 14 days (deep 2nd-degree burns probably will require skin graft)
• 3rd-degree burn: no potential for reepithelialization; skin graft is required.
• Baux score (sum of age and TBSA burned) and Denver 2 score (pulmonary score ranging 0 to 3, using PaO_2/FiO_2 cutoffs of 100, 175, and 250), renal score (0 to 3, using creatinine cutoffs of 1.8, 2.5, and 5.0 mg/dL), hepatic score (0 to 3, using bilirubin cutoffs of 2, 4, and 8 mg/dL), and cardiac score (0 to 3, based on number and dosage of inotropes) can be used to estimate mortality (8)[B].
• Length of hospital stay and need for ICU care depend on extent of burn, smoke inhalation, comorbidities, and age.
• Burn size is correlated to complications; >60% TBSA burned in children and >40% in adults are at increased risk for mortality and morbidity (8)[B].

• A 50% survival rate can be expected with a 62% burn in patients aged 0 to 14 years, 63% burn in patients aged 15 to 40 years, 38% burn in patients 40 to 65 years, and 25% burn in patients >65 years of age (1)[C].
• 90% of survivors can be expected to return to an occupation comparable to their preburn employment.

COMPLICATIONS
• Gastroduodenal ulceration (Curling ulcer)
• Marjolin ulcer: malignant squamous cell carcinoma developing in old burn site
• Signs of infection: discoloration, green fat, edema, eschar separation, and conversion of 2nd-degree to 3rd-degree wound
• Biopsy is the best way to diagnose wound infection.
• Burn wound sepsis: most commonly S. aureus (including MRSA), vancomycin-resistant enterococci, and gram-negative organisms (5)[B].
• Pneumonia
• Decreased mobility with possibility of future flexion contractures
• Hypertrophic scarring is common with burns.

REFERENCES

1. Teague H, Swencki SA, Tang A. The burned patient: assessment, diagnosis, and management in the ED. Trauma Reports. 2005;6(2):1–12.
2. Dries DJ, Endorf FW. Inhalation injury: epidemiology, pathology, treatment strategies. Scand J Trauma Resusc Emerg Med. 2013;21:31.
3. Bezuhly M, Fish JS. Acute burn care. Plast Reconstr Surg. 2012;130(2):349e–358e.
4. Perel P, Roberts I, Ker K. Colloids versus crystalloids for fluid resuscitation in critically ill patients. Cochrane Database Syst Rev. 2013;(2):CD000567.
5. Church D, Elsayed S, Reid O, et al. Burn wound infections. Clin Microbiol Rev. 2006;19(2):403–434.
6. Caulfield RH, Tyler MP, Austyn JM, et al. The relationship between protease/anti-protease profile, angiogenesis and re-epithelialisation in acute burn wounds. Burns. 2008;34(4):474–486.
7. Ong YS, Samuel M, Song C. Meta-analysis of early excision of burns. Burns. 2006;32(2):145–150.
8. Jeschke MG, Pinto R, Kraft R, et al. Morbidity and survival probability in burn patients in modern burn care. Crit Care Med. 2015;43(4):808–815.

CODES

ICD10
• T30.0 Burn of unspecified body region, unspecified degree
• T30.4 Corrosion of unspecified body region, unspecified degree

CLINICAL PEARLS
• 1st degree: erythema of involved tissue; skin blanches with pressure. Skin may be tender.
• 2nd degree: Skin is red and blistered. Skin is very tender.
• 3rd degree: Burned skin is tough and leathery. Skin is not tender.

BURSITIS, PES ANSERINE (PES ANSERINE SYNDROME)

Jennifer B. Schwartz, MD

BASICS

DESCRIPTION
- The pes anserinus ("goosefoot") is the combined insertion of the sartorius, gracilis, and semitendinosus ("SGT"-from medial to lateral) tendons on the anteromedial tibia.
- The pes anserine muscles help flex the knee and resist valgus stress
- The pes anserine bursa lies deep to the SGT tendons and superficial to the tibial attachment of the medial collateral ligament.
- *Pes anserine syndrome* is due to irritation of the bursa and/or tendons in this area

EPIDEMIOLOGY
Incidence
Inflammation of the pes anserine bursa is detected in up to 2.5% of MRI studies of patients with knee pain. The overall incidence is likely higher.

ETIOLOGY AND PATHOPHYSIOLOGY
Pes anserine bursitis occurs due to:
- Overuse injury
- Excessive valgus and rotary stresses
- Mechanical forces and degenerative changes
- Direct trauma

RISK FACTORS
- Obesity
- Age, female gender
- Pes planus; genu valgum
- Knee joint laxity/ligamentous injury
- Long distance running, hill running; change in mileage
- Swimming ("breaststroker's knee"); cycling
- Sports with side-to-side (cutting) activity (soccer, basketball, racquet sports)

COMMONLY ASSOCIATED CONDITIONS
- Osteoarthritis (OA)
  - Knee pain due to OA is often associated with pes anserine bursitis, both of which may need specific treatment.
  - Higher grades of OA associated with a thicker pes anserine bursa and larger area of bursitis (1,2)[C]
- Valgus knee deformity
- Obesity
- Diabetes mellitus (questionable association)

DIAGNOSIS

HISTORY
- Medial knee pain is the most common complaint.
- Changes in training regimen or mileage often accompany knee pain.
- Pain is located 4 to 6 cm distal to the medial joint line on the anteromedial aspect of the tibia.
- Pain exacerbated by knee flexion:
  - Going up or down stairs
  - Getting out of a chair

PHYSICAL EXAM
- Common findings include:
  - Tenderness to palpation at the pes anserine insertion
    ○ 30% of asymptomatic patients will have tenderness to deep palpation in this area.
  - Pain worsens with flexion of the knee against resistance.
  - Localized swelling of the pes anserine insertion
- Findings that suggest an alternative diagnosis: joint effusion, tenderness directly over the joint line, erythema or warmth, locking of the knee, systemic signs such as fever or pain with passive knee movement

DIFFERENTIAL DIAGNOSIS
- Medial collateral ligament injury
- Medial meniscal injury
- Medial plica syndrome
- Medial compartment OA
- Semimembranosus bursitis
- Popliteal/meniscal cyst
- Tibial stress fracture
- Septic arthritis

DIAGNOSTIC TESTS & INTERPRETATION
Initial Tests (lab, imaging)
- Primarily a clinical diagnosis
- Lab work not indicated. If infection is suspected: CBC, ESR, C-reactive protein, and joint fluid analysis are indicated.
- Imaging is not indicated unless there is concern for bony injury/fracture, ligamentous injury, or meniscal tear.

Follow-Up Tests & Special Considerations
- Ultrasound (US)
  - Can demonstrate focal edema within the pes anserine bursa but has poor correlation with clinical findings
  - Many patients with the clinical diagnosis of pes anserine bursitis have no morphologic changes of the pes anserine complex on US (3)[C].
- MRI: can demonstrate inflammation of the bursa, and delineate the pes anserine bursa from other structures. T2-weighted axial images are best on MRI (4)[C].
  - No large studies have evaluated the correlation between the clinical diagnosis of pes anserine bursitis and radiographic evidence of pes anserine pathology on MRI.
  - May see fluid in the pes bursa on MRI in 5% of asymptomatic patients (5)[C]

TREATMENT

Pes anserine bursitis is often self-limited. Conservative therapy is most common:
- Relative rest and activity modification to avoid offending movements (especially knee flexion)
- Ice to the affected area
- Physical therapy for knee strengthening and range of motion activities
- NSAIDs for pain control
- Corticosteroid injection for pain relief and as an antiinflammatory
- Weight loss to improve biomechanical forces at the knee

MEDICATION
First Line
NSAIDs, such as ibuprofen (800 mg PO TID) or naproxen (500 mg PO BID), are common 1st-line therapy.

Second Line
- Corticosteroid injection combined with local anesthetic provides relief in many patients (6)[C].
  - Inject at the point of maximal tenderness using standard aseptic technique
  - ~2 mL of anesthetic (i.e., 1% lidocaine) and 1 mL of steroid (i.e., 40 mg of methylprednisolone) is injected into the bursa using a small (e.g., 25-gauge, 1-inch) needle.

– Insert needle perpendicular to the skin until bone is felt and then withdraw slightly before injecting.
– Avoid injecting directly into the tendon (7)[C].
• US-guided injection is superior to blind injection (8)[C].
• Platelet-rich plasma injections also provide pain relief (9)[C].
• Injection of steroid and anesthetic provides pain relief, which allows for physical therapy and rehabilitative efforts.

ADDITIONAL THERAPIES
Physical therapy
• Hamstring and Achilles stretching
• Quadriceps strengthening—particularly of the vastus medialis (terminal 30 degrees of knee extension)
• Adductor strengthening

SURGERY/OTHER PROCEDURES
• No role for surgery in routine isolated cases
• Drainage or removal of bursa may be used in severe/refractory cases.

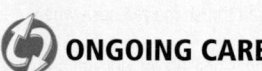 ONGOING CARE

Home exercise program focusing on flexibility and strengthening

DIET
Consider dietary changes as part of a comprehensive weight-loss program if obesity is a contributing factor.

PROGNOSIS
Most cases of pes anserine syndrome respond to conservative therapy. Recurrence is common, and multiple treatments may be required.

REFERENCES

1. Toktas H, Dundar U, Adar S, et al. Ultrasonographic assessment of pes anserinus tendon and pes anserinus tendinitis bursitis syndrome in patients with knee osteoarthritis. *Mod Rheumatol*. 2015;25(1):128–133.
2. Uysal F, Akbal A, Gökmen F, et al. Prevalence of pes anserine bursitis in symptomatic osteoarthritis patients: an ultrasonographic prospective study. *Clin Rheumatol*. 2015;34(3):529–533.
3. Helfenstein M Jr, Kuromoto J. Anserine syndrome [in English, Portuguese]. *Rev Bras Reumatol*. 2010;50(3):313–327.
4. Chatra PS. Bursae around the knee joints. *Indian J Radiol Imaging*. 2012;22(1):27–30.
5. Rennie WJ, Saifuddin A. Pes anserine bursitis: incidence in symptomatic knees and clinical presentation. *Skeletal Radiol*. 2005;34(7):395–398.
6. Yoon HS, Kim SE, Suh YR, et al. Correlation between ultrasonographic findings and the response to corticosteroid injection in pes anserine tendinobursitis syndrome in knee osteoarthritis patients. *J Korean Med Sci*. 2005;20(1):109–112.
7. Stephens MB, Beutler AI, O'Connor FG. Musculoskeletal injections: a review of the evidence. *Am Fam Physician*. 2008;78(8):971–976.
8. Finnoff JT, Nutz DJ, Henning PT, et al. Accuracy of ultrasound-guided versus unguided pes anserinus bursa injections. *PM R*. 2010;2(8):732–739.
9. Rowicki K, Płomiński J, Bachta A. Evaluation of the effectiveness of platelet rich plasma in treatment of chronic pes anserinus pain syndrome. *Ortop Traumatol Rehabil*. 2014;16(3):307–318.

ADDITIONAL READING
• Alvarez-Nemegyei J. Risk factors for pes anserinus tendinitis/bursitis syndrome: a case control study. *J Clin Rheumatol*. 2007;13(2):63–65.
• Wittich CM, Ficalora RD, Mason TG, et al. Musculoskeletal injection. *Mayo Clin Proc*. 2009;84(9):831–836; quiz 837.

CODES

ICD10
• M70.50 Other bursitis of knee, unspecified knee
• M70.51 Other bursitis of knee, right knee
• M70.52 Other bursitis of knee, left knee

CLINICAL PEARLS
• Consider pes anserine syndrome in patients presenting with medial knee pain.
• Pes anserine syndrome is relatively common in athletes and in older, obese patients with OA.
• Tenderness over the insertion of the pes anserine tendon on the medial aspect of the tibia 4 to 6 cm distal to the joint line is common in asymptomatic patients as well—correlation of the entire clinical picture is necessary for accurate diagnosis.
• Consider pes anserine syndrome in patients who have persistent symptoms associated with medial-sided OA
• Treatment is typically conservative. A local steroid/anesthetic injection may provide pain relief and enhance rehabilitation.

CANDIDIASIS, MUCOCUTANEOUS

Hugh Silk, MD, MPH, FAAFP • Sheila O. Stille, DMD • Azra Borogovac, MD

 BASICS

DESCRIPTION
- Heterogeneous mucocutaneous disorder caused by infection with *Candida* species
- Characterized by superficial infection of the skin, mucous membranes, and nails
- >20 *Candida* species cause infection in humans. *Candida albicans is most common.*
- Candidiasis affects:
  - Aerodigestive system
    - Oropharyngeal candidiasis (thrush): mouth, pharynx
    - Angular cheilitis: corner of the mouth
    - Esophageal candidiasis
    - Gastritis and/or ulcers, associated with thrush; alimental or perianal
  - Other systems
    - Candida vulvovaginitis: vaginal mucosa and/or vulvar skin
    - Candidal balanitis: glans of the penis
    - Candidal paronychia: nail bed or nail folds
    - Folliculitis
    - Interdigital candidiasis: webs of the digits
    - Candidal diaper dermatitis and intertrigo (within skin folds)
- Synonym(s): monilia; thrush; yeast; intertrigo

ALERT
Vaginal antifungal creams and suppositories can weaken condoms and diaphragms.

Pregnancy Considerations
- Vaginal candidiasis is common during pregnancy.
- Topical treatment during pregnancy should be extended by several days.
- Vaginal yeast infection at birth increases the risk of newborn thrush but is of no overall harm to baby.

EPIDEMIOLOGY
- Common in the United States; particularly with immunodeficiency and/or uncontrolled diabetes
- Age considerations
  - Infants and seniors: thrush and cutaneous infections (infant diaper rash)
  - Women of childbearing age: vaginitis
  - Prepubertal or postmenopausal: yeast vaginitis
  - Predominant sex: female > male

Incidence
Unknown—mucocutaneous candidiasis is common in immunocompetent patients. Complication rates are low.

Prevalence
Candida species are normal flora of oral cavity, pharynx, esophagus, and GI tract that are present in >70% of the U.S. population.

ETIOLOGY AND PATHOPHYSIOLOGY
C. albicans (responsible for 80–92% vulvovaginal and 70–80% oral isolates). Altered cell-mediated immunity against *Candida* species (either transient or chronic) increases susceptibility to infection.

Genetics
Chronic mucocutaneous candidiasis is a heterogeneous, genetic syndrome with infection of skin, nails, hair, and mucous membranes; typically presents in infancy.

RISK FACTORS
- Immunosuppression
- Antibacterial therapy (broad-spectrum antibiotics)
- Douches, chemical irritants, and concurrent vaginitides alter vaginal pH predisposing to candidal vaginitis.
- Denture wear
- Birth control pills; intrauterine devices
- Hyperglycemia; diabetes
- Uncircumcised men at higher risk for balanitis

GENERAL PREVENTION
- Use antibiotics and steroids judiciously; rinse mouth after inhaled steroid use (1)[A].
- Avoid douching. Treat other vaginal infections.
- Minimize perineal moisture (wear cotton underwear; frequent diaper changes).
- Clean dentures often; use well-fitting dentures, and remove during sleep.
- Optimize glycemic control in diabetics.
- Use preventive regimens during cancer treatments (2)[A].
- Treat with HAART in HIV-infected patients
- Antifungal prophylaxis against oral candidiasis is not recommended in HIV-infected adults unless patients have frequent or severe recurrences (3)[A].

COMMONLY ASSOCIATED CONDITIONS
- HIV
- Leukopenia
- Diabetes mellitus
- Cancer and other immunosuppressive conditions

 DIAGNOSIS

HISTORY
- Infants/children
  - Oral: adherent white patches on oral mucosae or on the tongue that do not wipe away easily
  - Perineal: erythematous rash with characteristic satellite lesions; painful if skin layer eroded. 40–75% of diaper rashes lasting >3 days are *C. albicans* (4,5)[A].
  - Angular cheilitis: painful fissures in corners of mouth
- Adults
  - Vulvovaginal lesions; whitish "curd-like" discharge; pruritus; burning
- Immunocompromised hosts
  - Oral: white, raised, painless, distinct patches; red, slightly raised patches
  - Esophagitis: dysphagia, odynophagia, retrosternal pain; usually concomitant thrush
  - GI symptoms: abdominal pain
  - Balanitis: erythema, erosions, scaling; dysuria
  - Folliculitis: follicular pustules
  - Interdigital: redness, itchiness at base and web-spaces of fingers and/or toes, possible maceration

PHYSICAL EXAM
- Infants/children
  - Oral: white, raised, distinct patches within the mouth; when wiped off reveals red base
  - Perineal: erythematous maculopapular rash with satellite pustules or papules
  - Angular cheilitis: tender fissures in mouth corners, often cracked and bleeding

- Adults
  - Vulvovaginal: thick, whitish, cottage cheese-like discharge; vagina or perineum erythema
- Immunocompromised hosts
  - Oral: white, raised, nontender, distinct patches; red, slightly raised patches; thick, dark-brownish coating; deep fissures
  - Esophagitis: often, oral thrush is visible.
  - Balanitis: erythema, linear erosions, scaling
  - Folliculitis: follicular pustules
  - Interdigital: redness, excoriations at base of fingers and/or toes, often maceration

DIFFERENTIAL DIAGNOSIS
- For oral candidiasis
  - Leukoplakia; lichen planus; geographic tongue
  - Herpes simplex; erythema multiforme
  - Pemphigus
- Baby formula or breast milk can mimic thrush—easier to remove than thrush (no red base when wiped away)
- Hairy leukoplakia: does not rub off; dorsum and lateral margins of tongue
- Angular cheilitis from vitamin B or iron deficiency, staphylococcal infection, or edentulous overclosure
- *Bacterial vaginosis* and *Trichomonas vaginalis* tend to have more odor, itch, and a different discharge.

DIAGNOSTIC TESTS & INTERPRETATION
Initial Tests (lab, imaging)
- 10% KOH slide preparation: mycelia (hyphae) or pseudo-mycelia (pseudohyphae) yeast forms; few WBC
- Associated with normal vaginal pH (<4.5)
- Barium swallow: cobblestone appearance, fistulas, or dilatation (denervation)

Diagnostic Procedures/Other
- If 1st-line treatment fails, obtain samples for culture
- Esophagitis may require endoscopy with biopsy (if suspicious for cancer).
- HIV seropositive patients with thrush and dysphagia relieved by antifungal have *Candida* esophagitis.

Test Interpretation
Biopsy: epithelial parakeratosis with polymorpho-nuclear leukocytes in superficial layers; periodic acid–Schiff staining reveals presence of candidal hyphae.

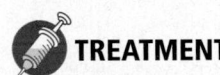 TREATMENT

GENERAL MEASURES
Screen for immunodeficiency.

MEDICATION
First Line
- Vaginal (choose 1)
  - Miconazole (Monistat) 2% cream: one applicator or 200 mg (one suppository), intravaginally qhs for 7 days
  - Clotrimazole (Gyne-Lotrimin, Mycelex): intravaginal tablets (100 mg qhs for 7 days; 200 mg qhs for 3 days; 500 mg daily for 1 day) or 2% cream (one applicator qhs for 3 days)
  - Fluconazole 150 mg PO single dose

- Oropharyngeal
  - Mild disease
    - Clotrimazole (Mycelex): oral 10 mg troche; 20 minutes 5 times daily for 7 to 14 days
    - Nystatin suspension: 100,000 U/mL swish and swallow 400,000 to 600,000 U 4 times per day
    - Nystatin pastilles: 200,000 U each, QID daily for 7 to 14 days (6)[B],(7)[A]
    - Denture wearers
      - Nystatin ointment: 100,000 U/g under denture and corners of mouth for 3 weeks
      - Remove dentures at night; clean 2× weekly with diluted (1:20) bleach.
  - Moderate to severe disease
    - Fluconazole: 200 mg load then 100 to 200 mg (>14 days of age: 6 mg/kg × 1 dose, then 3 mg/kg q24h × 7–14 days [max 100 mg/day])
- Esophagitis
  - Fluconazole: PO 400 mg load then 200 to 400 mg/day for 14 to 21 days or IV 400 mg (6 mg/kg) daily if oral therapy not tolerated

Pregnancy Considerations
2% miconazole cream, intravaginally, for 7 days in uncomplicated candidiasis. Systemic amphotericin B for invasive candidiasis in pregnancy.

Second Line
- Vaginal
  - Terconazole (Terazol): 0.4% cream (one applicator qhs for 7 days of induction therapy); 0.8% cream/80-mg suppositories (one applicator or one suppository qhs for 3 days)
  - For recurrent cases (≥4 symptomatic episodes in 1 year): induction therapy with 10 to 14 days of topical or oral azole, then, fluconazole, 150 mg once per week for 6 months (6)[A]
    - In HIV patients: Concerns with this regimen include emergence of drug resistance (8)[A].
- Oropharyngeal
  - Miconazole oral gel (20 mg/mL): QID, swish and swallow
  - Itraconazole (Sporanox) suspension: 200 mg (20 mL) daily; swish-swallow for 7 to 14 days
  - Posaconazole (Noxafil) oral suspension: 400 mg BID for 3 days, then 400 mg daily for up to 28 days
  - Amphotericin B (Fungizone) oral suspension (100 mg/mL): 1 mL QID daily, swish and swallow; use between meals
- Esophagitis
  - Amphotericin B (variable dosing) IV dose of 0.3 to 0.7 mg/kg daily; or an echinocandin should be used for patients who cannot tolerate oral therapy.
  - For refractory disease:
    - Itraconazole (Sporanox) oral solution: 200 mg daily
    - Posaconazole (Noxafil) oral suspension: 400 mg BID
    - Voriconazole (Vfend) 100 to 200 mg q12h PO or IV for 14 to 21 days (6)[A]
- Continue treatments for 2 days after infection gone:
  - Contraindications
    - Ketoconazole, itraconazole, or nystatin (if swallowed): severe hepatotoxicity
    - Amphotericin B: can cause nephrotoxicity
  - Precautions
    - Miconazole: can potentiate the effect of warfarin but drug of choice in pregnancy
    - Fluconazole: renal excretion: rare; hepatotoxicity: resistance frequent

- Itraconazole: Doubling the dosage results in ~3-fold increase in itraconazole plasma concentrations.
- Possible interactions (rarely seen with creams, lotions, or suppositories)
  - Fluconazole
    - Rifampin: decreased fluconazole concentrations
    - Tolbutamide: decreased concentrations
    - Warfarin, phenytoin, cyclosporine: altered metabolism; check levels.
  - Itraconazole: potent CYP 3A4 inhibitor. Carefully assess all coadministered medications.

ISSUES FOR REFERRAL
- Patients without obvious reasons for recurrent superficial candidal infections should be evaluated for concurrent immunodeficiency.
- GI candidiasis

ADDITIONAL THERAPIES
- For infants with thrush: Boil pacifiers and bottle nipples; assess mother's breasts/nipples for concurrent candida infection.
- For denture-related candidiasis: disinfect dentures (using soak solution of benzoic acid, 0.12% chlorhexidine gluconate, 1:20 NaOCl or alkalize proteases), and treat orally

COMPLEMENTARY & ALTERNATIVE MEDICINE
Probiotics: *Lactobacillus* and *Bifidobacterium* may inhibit *Candida* spp.

INPATIENT CONSIDERATIONS
Nursing
Proper oral hygiene. Protocols for brushing, denture care, and oral cavity moistening reduce oral candidiasis.

 ONGOING CARE

FOLLOW-UP RECOMMENDATIONS
Patient Monitoring
Immunocompromised persons benefit from regular evaluation and screening.

DIET
Active-culture yogurt or other live lactobacillus may decrease colonization; indeterminate evidence.

PATIENT EDUCATION
- Advise patients at risk for recurrence about overgrowth with antibacterial therapy.
- "Azole" medications are pregnancy Category C.

PROGNOSIS
- Benign prognosis in immunocompetent patients
- For immunosuppressed persons, *Candida* may become an AIDS-defining illness with significant morbidity.

COMPLICATIONS
In HIV patients, moderate immunosuppression (e.g., CD4 200 to 500 cells/mm^3) may be associated with chronic candidiasis. With more severe immunosuppression (e.g., CD4 <100 cells/mm^3), esophagitis or systemic infection are possible.

REFERENCES
1. Yang IA, Clarke MS, Sim EH, et al. Inhaled corticosteroids for stable chronic obstructive pulmonary disease. *Cochrane Database Syst Rev*. 2012;(7):CD002991.
2. Glenny AM, Gibson F, Auld E, et al. The development of evidence-based guidelines on mouth care

for children, teenagers and young adults treated for cancer. *Eur J Cancer*. 2010;46(8):1399–1412.
3. Panel on Opportunistic Infections in HIV-Infected Adults and Adolescents. Guidelines for the prevention and treatment of opportunistic infections in HIV-infected adults and adolescents: recommendations from the Centers for Disease Control and Prevention, the National Institutes of Health, and the HIV Medicine Association of the Infectious Diseases Society of America. Available at http://aidsinfo .nih.gov/contentfiles/lvguidelines/adult_oi.pdf. Accessed June 10, 2015.
4. Coughlin CC, Eichenfield LF, Frieden IJ. Diaper dermatitis: clinical characteristics and differential diagnosis. *Pediatr Dermatol*. 2014;31(Suppl 1):19–24.
5. Williams DW, Jordan RP, Wei XQ, et al. Interactions of *Candida albicans* with host epithelial surfaces. *J Oral Microbiol*. 2013;5.
6. Pappas PG, Kauffman CA, Andes D, et al. Clinical practice guidelines for the management of candidiasis: 2009 update by the Infectious Diseases Society of America. *Clin Infect Dis*. 2009;48(5):503–535.
7. Martins N, Ferreira IC, Barros L, et al. Candidasis: predisposing factors, prevention, diagnosis and alternative treatment. *Mycopathologia*. 2014;177(5–6):223–240.
8. Ray A, Ray S, George AT, et al. Interventions for prevention and treatment of vulvovaginal candidiasis in women with HIV infection. *Cochrane Database Syst Rev*. 2011;(8):CD008739.

ADDITIONAL READING
- Kumar S, Bansal A, Chakrabarti A, et al. Evaluation of efficacy of probiotics in prevention of candida colonization in a PICU—a randomized controlled trial. *Crit Care Med*. 2013; 41(2):565–572.
- Nyirjesy P, Sobel JD. Genital mycotic infections in patients with diabetes. *Postgrad Med*. 2013;125(3):33–46.
- Terai H, Shimahara M. Tongue pain: burning mouth syndrome vs Candida-associated lesion. *Oral Dis*. 2007;13(4):440–442.

 SEE ALSO

Candidiasis, Invasive; Candidiasis, Mucocutaneous; HIV/AIDS

 CODES

ICD10
- B37.9 Candidiasis, unspecified
- B37.0 Candidal stomatitis
- B37.49 Other urogenital candidiasis

CLINICAL PEARLS
- Candidiasis is generally a clinical diagnosis. KOH preparations are a simple confirmatory test in the office setting. Culture and biopsy are rarely needed to identify resistant strains.
- Person-to-person transmission is rare.
- If tongue pain continues after treatment, consider burning mouth syndrome. Obtain a biopsy if there is concern for oral cancer.
- Oral antifungal medications are hepatically metabolized and may have serious side effects.

CARBON MONOXIDE POISONING

Viren Kaul, MD • Faruq Pradhan, MBBCh • Anthony W. Gray, Jr., MD

 BASICS

DESCRIPTION

- Carbon monoxide (CO) is an odorless, tasteless, colorless gas that has the potential to cause sudden illness and even death if inhaled; it is a leading cause of poisoning death in the United States.
- CO is produced by combustion of carbon-containing compounds (wood, charcoal, oil, gas):
  - CO inhalation leads to displacement of oxygen from binding sites on hemoglobin.
  - Detrimental effects are related to tissue hypoxia from decreased oxygen content and a shift of the oxyhemoglobin dissociation curve to the left, further impairing oxygen unloading from hemoglobin.
- CO also binds to mitochondrial cytochrome oxidase, impairing adenosine triphosphate (ATP) production. It also binds to myoglobin thereby affecting muscle function.
- System(s) affected: cardiovascular, pulmonary, musculoskeletal, nervous

Pregnancy Consideration
Tissue hypoxia affects the fetal tissue. CO poisoning may cause significant fetal abnormalities, depending on the developmental stage. CO has a greater affinity for, and longer half-life when bound to fetal hemoglobin. Therefore, a pregnant mother potentially may be unaffected while the fetus is affected.

EPIDEMIOLOGY
Incidence
- ~50,000 emergency department visits annually (1)
- 235 CO exposure-related deaths were reported to U.S. poison centers between 2000 and 2009; however, this is likely an underestimation with closer 500 deaths occurring per year, on review of previous data. Unintentional poisoning is most common during winter months in cold climates, but can also occur in warm climates with use of generators, boats, and so forth.
- Intentional CO poisoning is ~10 times higher than unintentional poisonings.
- Likely markedly underdiagnosed because vague symptoms do not prompt individuals to seek medical attention

ETIOLOGY AND PATHOPHYSIOLOGY
- CO is rapidly absorbed in lungs.
- CO has ~240 times the affinity for hemoglobin compared to oxygen.
- CO binds to hemoglobin to form carboxyhemoglobin (COHb), resulting in impaired oxygen-carrying capacity, utilization, and delivery:
  - Leftward shift of the oxyhemoglobin dissociation curve occurs.
  - CO interferes with peripheral oxygen utilization by inactivating cytochrome oxidase.
- Delayed neurologic sequelae, related to lipid peroxidation by toxic oxygen species generated by xanthine oxidase
- The half-life of CO while the patient is breathing room air is ~320 minutes, while breathing 100% oxygen via a tight-fitting, nonrebreathing face mask is ~74 minutes, and with 100% hyperbaric oxygen is ~30 minutes.

- CO exposure also causes inflammation through separate pathways than those that cause cardiac and neurologic sequelae (2).
- Inhaled or ingested methylene chloride (from paint remover [dichloromethane]) is metabolized to CO by the liver, causing CO toxicity in the absence of ambient CO.

RISK FACTORS
- Alcohol use (3)
- Smoke inhalation
- Being in a closed or improperly ventilated space with a faulty furnace, stove, running engine, or any fuel-burning device
- Cigarette smoking
- Use of generators during power outages
- Extremes of age
- Predisposing cardiovascular disease, anemia, chronic respiratory conditions
- Exposure to exhaust (for example, riding in the back of enclosed pickup trucks or swimming near a motor boat) in precatalytic converter era automobiles.
- Employment in a coal mine, as an auto mechanic, paint stripper, or in the solvent industry
- Increased endogenous production in patients with hemolytic anemia

GENERAL PREVENTION
- Appropriate ventilation, especially where there are fuel-burning devices.
- Use of CO monitors
- Public education
- Determining the mechanism of exposure is critical in cases of accidental poisoning in order to limit future risk.
- Victims must not be discharged back to a contaminated environment.

COMMONLY ASSOCIATED CONDITIONS
- CO and cyanide poisoning can occur simultaneously following smoke inhalation (synergistic effect).
- Consider CO poisoning in a burn victim who has been in an enclosed space.

DIAGNOSIS

- Acute CO poisoning is suggested by history, physical exam, and an elevated COHb.
- Chronic CO intoxication is difficult to diagnose.
- The newest pulse CO-oximeters can screen for CO exposure using different wavelengths of light.
- Older pulse oximeters do not differentiate carboxyhemoglobin from oxyhemoglobin, causing normal pulse oximeter readings in hypoxic patients.
- A level >3% in a nonsmoker and >10% in a smoker confirms exposure, but the level does not correlate well with the severity of the acute illness or the long-term prognosis (2).

HISTORY
- No single symptom is sensitive or specific but may include the following:
  - Headaches: occurs in 84% patients
  - Dizziness

- Nausea, vomiting, diarrhea
- Weakness or fatigue
- Confusion or impaired judgment
- Seizures
- Chest pain
- Shortness of breath
- Loss of consciousness
- Visual disturbances

PHYSICAL EXAM
- "Cherry red" appearance of the lips and skin (<1% cases)
- Respiratory depression or tachypnea
- Cyanosis
- Visual-field defects, papilledema, or nystagmus
- CNS depression or coma, ataxia, seizure
- Tachycardia, hypotension, cardiac dysrhythmias, or even (cardiac) arrest

DIFFERENTIAL DIAGNOSIS
- Cyanide toxicity
- Viral syndromes
- Methylene chloride (dichloromethane) inhalation or ingestion
- Psychological disorders including major depressive disorder
- Other causes of mental status changes:
  - Infections such as meningitis or encephalitis
  - Metabolic causes such as hypoglycemia
  - Drugs: alcohol (EtOH) intoxication, opiates, acetylsalicylic acid (ASA) overdose
  - Trauma
  - CNS lesions

DIAGNOSTIC TESTS & INTERPRETATION
Initial Tests (lab, imaging)
- Measurement of COHb (may be low despite significant poisoning if patient had been treated with O_2 or has been breathing room air for a significant period of time before the level is drawn).
- ABG (looking for metabolic acidosis)
  - Blood PO_2 (PaO_2) tends to be normal as O_2 dissolved in blood is not affected by CO.
- Blood glucose
- Chemistries
- Anion gap = $([Na^+] + [K^+]) - ([Cl^-] + [HCO_3^-])$. HCO_3 decreased reflecting metabolic acidosis; anion gap >16
- Pregnancy test in all women of childbearing age
- Toxicology screen
- ECG in all patients
- Hemoglobin/hematocrit
- CK to evaluate rhabdomyolysis
- Cardiac enzymes in:
  - ≥65 years
  - Patient with cardiac risk factors or anemia
  - Patients with symptoms suggestive of cardiac ischemia
- Head CT/MRI scan is helpful to rule out other causes of neurologic decompensation. May also show infarction due to hypoxia/ischemia

Follow-Up Tests & Special Considerations
- Think of CO poisoning in younger patients with chest pain or symptoms suggestive of ischemia.
- Consider the diagnosis and inquire about exposure in afebrile patients with "flulike" symptoms, especially in the winter when flu and CO poisoning are both more common.
- Look for clusters of patients (coworkers, family members, school children) with similar symptoms.
- Patients with intentional poisoning require psychiatric evaluation when medically stable.

 TREATMENT

GENERAL MEASURES
- Prompt removal from the CO source
- Supportive care as necessary
- Intubation and mechanical ventilation may be necessary for severe intoxication, if patient is not able to protect airway, or has significant respiratory depression.
- Contact Poison Control Center at 800-222-1222 (United States only).

MEDICATION
Rapid reduction in tissue hypoxia with 100% oxygen via nonrebreathing reservoir face mask (4)[A] until COHb is normal (<3%) and patient is asymptomatic.

ADDITIONAL THERAPIES
- Hyperbaric oxygen has been somewhat controversial (4,5)[A]. Existing randomized trials do not establish whether the administration of hyperbaric oxygen to patients with CO poisoning reduces the incidence of adverse neurologic outcomes (5)[A].
- Despite this, hyperbaric oxygen recommended for levels >25–30%, evidence of cardiac involvement, severe acidosis, LOC, neurologic impairment, abnormal neuropsychiatric testing, age >36 years (6)[C].
- Hyperbaric oxygen has been shown to be safe in pregnant woman, but there have been no prospective studies of efficacy (4)[A]. International consensus favors it as part of a more aggressive role in treating pregnant women (6)[C].
- If no improvement occurs in cardiovascular or neurologic function within 4 hours, transport the patient to the nearest facility with hyperbaric oxygen, regardless of distance.

INPATIENT CONSIDERATIONS
Admission Criteria/Initial Stabilization
Patients whose symptoms do not improve after 4 to 5 hours of 100% O₂ should be transported to the nearest facility with hyperbaric oxygen. Those who demonstrate ECG or laboratory evidence of severe poisoning, who have evidence of end-organ damage, who require hyperbaric treatment, or who have another medical or social cause of concern should be hospitalized.

Discharge Criteria
Patients with mild symptoms from accidental poisoning can be managed in the ED and safely discharged.

 ONGOING CARE

FOLLOW-UP RECOMMENDATIONS
All patients treated for acute CO poisoning should be seen for clinical follow-up in 1 to 2 months after they are safely discharged (4). Patients should undergo neuropsychological testing if suspicion of cognitive impairment. Consider evaluation of family members or cohabitants.

Patient Monitoring
- Measurement of carboxyhemoglobin levels
- Arterial blood gases

PATIENT EDUCATION
- Professional installation and maintenance of combustion devices: 1-800-638-2772; Consumer Products Safety Commission hotline
- Some states require CO detector installation in homes, especially near bedrooms and potential sources.
- Annual furnace inspections (7)[B]

PROGNOSIS
Most survivors recover completely, with only a minority developing chronic neuropsychiatric impairment.

COMPLICATIONS
- Cardiac:
  - Myocardial infarction
  - Dysrhythmia
- Pulmonary:
  - Pulmonary edema
  - Pneumonia (aspiration)
- Neurologic:
  - Anoxic encephalopathy
  - Intellectual deterioration
  - Memory impairment
  - Parkinsonism
- Behavioral:
  - Irritability
  - Aggressiveness
  - Violence
  - Moodiness

Geriatric Considerations
Higher incidence of cardiovascular and neurologic disease, increasing complications

REFERENCES

1. Hampson NB, Weaver LK. Carbon monoxide poisoning: a new incidence for an old disease. *Undersea Hyperb Med*. 2007;34(3):163–168.
2. Weaver LK. Clinical practice. Carbon monoxide poisoning. *N Engl J Med*. 2009;360(12):1217–1225.
3. Yoon SS, Macdonald SC, Parrish RG. Deaths from unintentional carbon monoxide poisoning and potential for prevention with carbon monoxide detectors. *JAMA*.1998;279(9):685–687.
4. Hampson NB, Piantadosi CA, Thom SR, et al. Practice recommendations in the diagnosis, management, and prevention of carbon monoxide poisoning. *Am J Respir Crit Care Med*. 2012;186(11):1095–1101.
5. Buckley NA, Juurlink DN, Isbister G, et al. Hyperbaric oxygen for carbon monoxide poisoning. *Cochrane Database Syst Rev*. 2011;(4):CD002041. doi: 10.1002/14651858.CD002041.pub3.
6. Centers for Disease Control and Prevention. Carbon monoxide poisoning after a disaster. http://emergency.cdc.gov/disasters/carbonmonoxide.asp
7. Rupert DJ, Poehlman JA, Damon SA, et al. Risk and protective behaviours for residential carbon monoxide poisoning. *Inj Prev*. 2013;19(2):119–123.

ADDITIONAL READING
- Centers for Disease Control and Prevention. Unintentional, non-fire-related, carbon monoxide exposures—United States, 2001-2003. *MMWR Morb Mortal Wkly Rep*. 2005;54(2):36–39.
- Internet resources available at http://www.cpsc.gov, http://www.cdc.gov/co, and http://www.epa.gov/iaq/co.html.
- Iqbal S, Clower JH, Hernandez SA, et al. A review of disaster-related carbon monoxide poisoning: surveillance, epidemiology, and opportunities for prevention. *Am J Public Health*. 2012;102(10):1957–1963.
- Satran D, Henry CR, Adkinson C, et al. Cardiovascular manifestations of moderate to severe carbon monoxide poisoning. *J Am Coll Cardiol*. 2005;45(9):1513–1516.
- World Health Organization. World directory of poison centres. http://www.who.int/gho/phe/chemical_safety/poisons_centres/en/index.html.

 CODES

ICD10
- T58.91XA Toxic effect of carb monx from unsp source, acc, init
- T58.8X1A Toxic effect of carb monx from oth source, accidental, init
- T58.01XA Toxic effect of carb monx from mtr veh exhaust, acc, init

CLINICAL PEARLS
- The most appropriate intervention in the management of a CO-poisoned patient is a prompt removal from the source of CO and institution of 100% oxygen by high-flow face mask or endotracheal tube.
- A pregnant woman may appear normal while her fetus is severely affected.
- Consider CO poisoning in younger patients with chest pain or ischemia or in patients who present in clusters.
- COHb levels do not correlate well with symptoms, severity of illness, or outcome, so manage the patient, not the level.

CARDIOMYOPATHY

Timothy P. Fitzgibbons, MD, PhD • Theo E. Meyer, MD, DPhil

BASICS

DESCRIPTION
- Cardiomyopathy encompasses a large group of diseases of the myocardium that commonly result in mechanical pump dysfunction. The current classification scheme attempts to differentiate between myocardial diseases confined to the myocardium (primary) and those due to systemic disorders (secondary). Specific causes of myocardial dysfunction due to other cardiovascular disorders are considered a third, separate category (1).
- Classification of cardiomyopathy
  - Primary
    - Genetic
      - Hypertrophic cardiomyopathy (HCM)
      - Arrhythmogenic right ventricular cardiomyopathy/dysplasia (ARVC/D)
      - Left ventricular (LV) noncompaction (LVNC)
      - Glycogen storage (Danon type, PRKAG2)
      - Conduction defects
      - Mitochondrial myopathies
      - Ion channel disorders: long QT syndrome, Brugada, short QT syndrome, catecholaminergic ventricular tachycardia (CVPT), Asian SUNDS
    - Mixed
      - Dilated cardiomyopathy (DCM) (genetic or nongenetic)
      - Restrictive
    - Acquired
      - Myocarditis, stress cardiomyopathy, peripartum, tachycardia-induced, infants of type 1 diabetic mothers
  - Secondary (see list below)
    - Specific
      - Ischemic
      - Valvular
      - Hypertensive
      - Congenital heart disease
- Patients with end-stage cardiomyopathy have stage D heart failure or severe symptoms at rest refractory to standard medical therapy.
- System(s) affected: cardiovascular; renal

Pediatric Considerations
Etiology: idiopathic, viral, congenital heart disease, and familial

Pregnancy Considerations
May occur in women postpartum

EPIDEMIOLOGY
Predominant age: Ischemic cardiomyopathy is the most common etiology; predominantly in patients aged >50 years. Consider uncommon causes in young.

Incidence
- 60,000 patients <65 years old die each year from end-stage heart disease.
- 35,000 to 70,000 people might benefit from cardiac transplant or chronic support.

Prevalence
Most rapidly growing form of heart disease

ETIOLOGY AND PATHOPHYSIOLOGY
- Ischemic heart disease: most common etiology; up to 66% of patients
- Hypertension
- Valvular heart disease

- Primary genetic causes
- Congenital heart disease
- Peripartum/postpartum
- Endocrine
  - Diabetes mellitus
  - Hyperthyroidism
  - Hypothyroidism
  - Hyperparathyroidism
  - Pheochromocytoma
  - Acromegaly
- Nutritional deficiencies
  - Beriberi, pellagra, scurvy, selenium, carnitine, kwashiorkor
- Autoimmune/collagen
  - Systemic lupus erythematosus
  - Dermatomyositis
  - Rheumatoid arthritis
  - Scleroderma
  - Polyarteritis nodosa
- Infectious causes
  - Viral (e.g., HIV, coxsackievirus, adenovirus)
  - Bacterial and mycobacterial (e.g., diphtheria, rheumatic fever)
  - Parasitic (e.g., toxoplasmosis, *Trypanosoma cruzi*)
- Infiltrative (2)
  - Amyloidosis
  - Gaucher disease
  - Hurler disease
  - Hunter disease
  - Fabry disease
- Storage
  - Hemochromatosis
  - Fabry disease
  - Glycogen storage disease (type II, Pompe)
  - Niemann-Pick disease
- Neuromuscular/neurologic
  - Duchenne and Emery-Dreifuss muscular dystrophies
  - Friedreich ataxia
  - Myotonic dystrophy
  - Neurofibromatosis
  - Tuberous sclerosis
- Toxic
  - Alcohol
  - Drugs and chemotherapy: anthracyclines, cyclophosphamide, Herceptin
  - Radiation
  - Heavy metal, chemical agents
- Inflammatory (granulomatous):
  - Sarcoidosis
- Idiopathic
- Endomyocardial
  - Endomyocardial fibrosis
  - Hypereosinophilic syndrome (Loeffler endocarditis)

Genetics
Autosomal dominant HCM is the most common form of primary genetic cardiomyopathy (1/500 in the general population). Genetic causes of DCM are less common, accounting for 1/3 cases, with mostly autosomal dominant inheritance. LNC and ARVC are also inherited in an autosomal dominant fashion in addition to LQTS and other ion-channel disorders.

RISK FACTORS
- Hypertension
- Hyperlipidemia
- Obesity
- Coronary artery disease
- Diabetes mellitus

- Smoking
- Physical inactivity
- Excessive alcohol intake
- Dietary sodium
- Obstructive sleep apnea
- Chemotherapy

GENERAL PREVENTION
Reduce salt and water intake; home BP and daily weight measurement

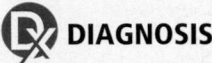

DIAGNOSIS

HISTORY
- Dyspnea at rest or with exertion
- Paroxysmal nocturnal dyspnea
- Orthopnea
- Postprandial dyspnea
- Right upper quadrant pain or bloating
- Midabdominal pain
- Fatigue
- Syncope
- Edema

PHYSICAL EXAM
- Tachypnea
- Cheyne-Stokes breathing
- Low pulse pressure
- Cool extremities
- Jugular venous distention
- Bibasilar rales
- Tachycardia
- Displaced point of maximal impulse (PMI)
- S_3 gallop
- Blowing systolic murmur
- Hepatosplenomegaly
- Ascites
- Edema

DIFFERENTIAL DIAGNOSIS
- Severe pulmonary disease
- Primary pulmonary hypertension
- Recurrent pulmonary embolism
- Constrictive pericarditis
- Some advanced forms of malignancy
- Anemia

DIAGNOSTIC TESTS & INTERPRETATION
- ECG: LV hypertrophy, interventricular conduction delay, atrial fibrillation, evidence of prior Q-wave infarction
- Hyponatremia
- Prerenal azotemia
- Anemia
- Mild elevation in troponin
- Elevated B-type natriuretic peptide (BNP) or pro-BNP
- Mild hyperbilirubinemia
- Elevated liver function tests
- Elevated uric acid

Initial Tests (lab, imaging)
- ECG
- Chest radiograph
  - Cardiomegaly
  - Increased vascular markings to the upper lobes
  - Pleural effusions may or may not be present.

- Echocardiography
  - In DCM, 4-chamber enlargement and global hypokinesis are present.
  - In HCM, severe LV hypertrophy is present.
  - Segmental contraction abnormalities of the LV are indicative of previous localized myocardial infarction.
- Cardiac MRI
  - May be useful to characterize certain nonischemic cardiomyopathies
- Stress myocardial perfusion imaging (MPI)
  - Recommended in those with new-onset LV dysfunction or when ischemia is suspected.

Diagnostic Procedures/Other
Cardiac catheterization

- Helpful to rule out ischemic heart disease
- Characterize hemodynamic severity
- Pulmonary artery catheters may be reasonable in patients with refractory heart failure to help guide management.

TREATMENT
See "Heart Failure, Chronic" for detailed treatment protocols.

GENERAL MEASURES
- Reduction of filling pressures
- Treatment of electrolyte disturbances

MEDICATION
First Line
- Systolic failure syndromes

  - ACE inhibitors: All considered equally effective; initiate at low doses and titrate as tolerated to target doses (3)[A].
  - ENTRESTO, a combination drug containing a neprilysin inhibitor and valsartan, was recently approved for the treatment of systolic HF (EF <40%) as an alternative to an ACE/ARB (4)[A].

  - Loop diuretics
    - May need to be given IV initially and then orally as patient stabilizes

  - Furosemide, 40 to 120 mg/day or TID (3)[A]

  - β-Blockers
    - Use with caution in acutely decompensated or low–cardiac output states.
    - Initiate with low doses and titrate as tolerated.

  - Metoprolol succinate, 12.5 to 200 mg/day; carvedilol, 3.125 to 25 mg BID; or bisoprolol, 1.25 to 10 mg/day (3)[A]
  - Patients with New York Heart Association (NYHA) II–IV heart failure, ejection fraction (EF) <35%, on standard therapy: aldosterone antagonists: spironolactone or eplerenone (3)[A]
  - Digoxin, 0.125 to 0.25 mg/day for symptomatic patients on standard therapy (3)[B]
  - Combination hydralazine/isosorbide dinitrate is first-line treatment in African American patients with class III–IV symptoms already on standard therapy and for all patients with reduced EF and symptoms incompletely responsive to ACE inhibitor and β-blocker (3)[A].

    - Contraindications

  - β-Blockers: low cardiac output, 2nd- or 3rd-degree heart block
  - Avoid use of diltiazem and verapamil in patients with systolic dysfunction.
  - Aldosterone antagonists: oliguria, anuria, renal dysfunction
  - Loop diuretics: hypokalemia, hypomagnesemia
  - ACE inhibitors: pregnancy, angioedema
- Precautions
  - In patients with chronic kidney disease, digoxin dosage should be ≤0.125 mg/day and drug levels followed carefully to avoid toxicity.
  - Closely monitor electrolytes.
  - ACE inhibitors: Initiate with care if BP is low. Begin with low-dose captopril, such as 6.25 mg TID.
  - β-Blockers: Avoid in patients with evidence of poor tissue perfusion; they may further depress systolic function.
  - Milrinone, dobutamine: long-term use associated with increased mortality
- Medications TO AVOID
  - NSAIDs
  - Glitazones
  - Cilostazol

Second Line
- Angiotensin receptor blockers as an alternative to ACE inhibitors

- Inotropic therapy (e.g., dobutamine or milrinone) for cardiogenic shock and support prior to surgery or cardiac transplantation (3)[B]
- Continuous inotrope infusion may be considered in stage D outpatients for symptom control in those who are not eligible for transplantation or mechanical circulatory support (3)[B].

ISSUES FOR REFERRAL
Management by a heart failure team improves outcomes and facilitates early transplant referral.

ADDITIONAL THERAPIES
- Prophylactic implantable cardioverter defibrillator (ICD) should be considered for patients with a left ventricular ejection fraction (LVEF) <35% and mild to moderate symptoms (3)[A].
- Cardiac resynchronization therapy (CRT) is recommended and should be considered for patients in sinus rhythm with a QRS >150 ms, LVEF <35%, in functional class (FC) I–III and ambulatory FC IV patients (3)[A].

- Patients with severe, refractory heart failure with no reasonable expectation of improvement should not be considered for an ICD.
- Consideration of an LV assist device as "permanent" or destination therapy or cardiac transplantation is reasonable in selected stage D patients.

ONGOING CARE

DIET
Low fat, low salt, fluid restriction

PROGNOSIS
~20–40% of patients in NYHA FC IV die within 1 year. With a transplant, 1-year survival is as high as 94%.

COMPLICATIONS
Worsening congestive heart failure syncope, renal failure, arrhythmias, or sudden death

REFERENCES
1. Maron BJ, Towbin JA, Thiene G, et al. Contemporary definitions and classification of the cardiomyopathies: an American Heart Association Scientific Statement from the Council on Clinical Cardiology, Heart Failure and Transplantation Committee; Quality of Care and Outcomes Research and Functional Genomics and Translational Biology Interdisciplinary Working Groups; and Council on Epidemiology and Prevention. *Circulation*. 2006;113(14):1807–1816.
2. Seward JB, Casaclang-Verzosa G. Infiltrative cardiovascular diseases: cardiomyopathies that look alike. *J Am Coll Cardiol*. 2010;55(27):1769–1779.
3. Yancy CW, Jessup M, Bozkurt B, et al. 2013 ACCF/AHA guideline for the management of heart failure: executive summary: a report of the American College of Cardiology Foundation/American Heart Association Task Force on Practice Guidelines. *Circulation*. 2013;128(16):1810–1852.
4. McMurray JJ, Packer M, Desai AS, et al. Angiotensin-neprilysin inhibition versus enalapril in heart failure. *N Engl J Med*. 2014; 371(11): 993–1004.

 SEE ALSO

- Alcohol Abuse and Dependence; Alcohol Withdrawal; Amyloidosis; Diabetes Mellitus, Type 1; Diabetes Mellitus, Type 2; Hypertension, Essential; Hypothyroidism, Adult; Hypertrophic Cardiomyopathy; Protein–Energy Malnutrition; Rheumatic Fever; Sarcoidosis
- Algorithm: Congestive Heart Failure: Differential Diagnosis

 CODES

ICD10
- I42.9 Cardiomyopathy, unspecified
- I42.0 Dilated cardiomyopathy
- I42.5 Other restrictive cardiomyopathy

CLINICAL PEARLS
- Cardiomyopathy represents the end-stage of a large number of disease processes involving the heart muscle.
- Ischemic, hypertensive, postviral, familial, alcoholic, and incessant tachycardia-induced are the most common cardiomyopathy varieties seen in the United States.
- Core therapy for heart failure applies salt restriction, diuretics, ACE inhibitors, β-blockers, digoxin, and electrical treatments, such as cardiac resynchronization and implantable defibrillators, as appropriate.

CAROTID STENOSIS

Edlira Yzeiraj, DO, MS • Maria M. Plummer, MD

 BASICS

Carotid stenosis may be caused by atherosclerosis, intimal fibroplasia, vasculitis, adventitial cysts, or vascular tumors; *atherosclerosis* is the most common etiology.

DESCRIPTION
- Narrowing of carotid artery lumen is typically due to atherosclerotic changes in the vessel wall. Atherosclerotic plaques are responsible for 90% of extracranial carotid lesions and up to 30% of all ischemic strokes.
- A "hemodynamically significant" carotid stenosis produces a drop in pressure, reduction in flow, or both and corresponds approximately to a 60% diameter-reducing stenosis (1).
- Carotid lesions are classified by the following:
  - Symptom status
    - Asymptomatic: tend to be homogenous and stable
    - Symptomatic (stroke, transient cerebral ischemic event): tend to be heterogeneous and unstable
  - Degree of stenosis
    - High grade: 80–99% stenosis
    - Moderate grade: 50–79% stenosis
    - Low grade: <50% stenosis

EPIDEMIOLOGY
More common in men and with increasing age (see "Risk Factors")

Incidence
Unclear (asymptomatic patients often go undiagnosed)

Prevalence
- Moderate stenosis (2)
  - Age <50 years: men 0.2%, women 0%
  - Age >80 years: men 7.5%, women 5%
- Severe stenosis (2)
  - Age <50 years: men 0.1%, women 0%
  - Age >80 years: men 3.1%, women 0.9%

ETIOLOGY AND PATHOPHYSIOLOGY
- Atherosclerosis begins during adolescence, consistently at carotid bifurcation. The carotid bulb has unique blood flow dynamics. Hemodynamic disturbances cause endothelial injury and dysfunction. Plaque formation in vessel wall results and stenosis then ensues.
- Initial cause not well understood, but certain risk factors are frequently present (see "Risk Factors"). Tensile stress on the vessel wall, turbulence, and arterial wall shear stress seem to be involved.

Genetics
- Increased incidence among family members
- Genetically linked factors
  - Diabetes mellitus (DM), race, hypertension (HTN), family history, obesity
  - In a recent single nucleotide polymorphism study, the following genes were strongly associated with worse carotid plaque: *TNFSF4, PPARA, TLR4, ITGA2,* and *HABP2.*

RISK FACTORS
- Nonmodifiable factors: advanced age, male sex, family history, cardiac disease, congenital arteriopathies (1)
- Modifiable factors: smoking, diet, dyslipidemia, physical inactivity, obesity, HTN, DM

GENERAL PREVENTION
- Antihypertensive treatment to maintain BP <140/90 mm Hg (systolic BP of 150 mm Hg is target in elderly) (3)[A]
- Smoking cessation to reduce the risk of atherosclerosis progression and stroke (3)
- Lipid control: regression of carotid atherosclerotic lesions seen with statin therapy (3)

COMMONLY ASSOCIATED CONDITIONS
- Transient ischemic attack (TIA)/stroke
- Coronary artery disease (CAD)/myocardial infarction (MI)
- Peripheral vascular disease (PVD)
- HTN
- DM
- Hyperlipidemia

 DIAGNOSIS

Screening for carotid stenosis is not recommended. However, in the setting of symptoms suggestive of stroke or TIA, workup for this condition may be indicated.

HISTORY
- Identification of modifiable and nonmodifiable comorbidities (see "Risk Factors")
- History of cerebral ischemic event
- Stroke, TIA, amaurosis fugax (monocular blindness), aphasia
- Coronary artery disease/MI
- Peripheral arterial disease
- Review of systems, with focus on risk factors for
  - Cardiovascular disease
  - Stroke (HTN and arrhythmia)

PHYSICAL EXAM
- Lateralizing neurologic deficits: contralateral motor and/or sensory deficit
- Amaurosis fugax: ipsilateral transient visual obscuration from retinal ischemia
- Visual field defect
- Dysarthria and in the case of dominant (usually left) hemisphere involvement, aphasia
- Carotid bruit (low sensitivity and specificity)

DIFFERENTIAL DIAGNOSIS
- Aortic valve stenosis
- Aortic arch atherosclerosis
- Arrhythmia with cardiogenic embolization
- Migraine
- Brain tumor
- Metabolic disturbances
- Functional/psychological deficit
- Seizure

DIAGNOSTIC TESTS & INTERPRETATION
Initial Tests (lab, imaging)
Workup for suspected TIA/stroke may include the following:
- CBC with differential
- Basic metabolic panel
- ESR (if temporal arteritis a consideration)
- Glucose/glycated hemoglobin (HbA1c)
- Fasting lipid profile
- Duplex ultrasonography is the recommended initial diagnostic test in asymptomatic patients with known or suspected carotid stenosis (3)[C].

- Duplex ultrasound (US) identifies ≥50% stenosis, with 98% sensitivity and 88% specificity.

Follow-Up Tests & Special Consideration
- Proceed to imaging if there is suggestion of stenosis from history or physical exam.
- Other noninvasive imaging techniques can add detail to duplex results:
  - CT angiography
    - 88% sensitivity and 100% specificity
    - Requires contrast load with risk for subsequent renal morbidity
  - MR angiography
    - 95% sensitivity and 90% specificity
    - Evaluates cerebral circulation (extracranial and intracranial) as well as aortic arch and common carotid artery
    - The presence of unstable plaque can be determined if the following characteristics are seen:
      - Presence of thin/ruptured fibrous cap
      - Presence of lipid-rich necrotic core
    - Tends to overestimate degree of stenosis

Diagnostic Procedures/Other
Cerebral (catheter) angiography is the traditional gold standard for diagnosis:
- Delineates anatomy pertaining to aortic arch and proximal vessels
- However, procedure is invasive and has multiple risks:
  - Contrast-induced renal dysfunction (1–5% complication rate)
  - Thromboembolic-related complications (1–2.6% complication rate) and neurologic complications
  - Should be used only when other tests are not conclusive

Test Interpretation
- Stenosis consistently occurs at carotid bifurcation, with plaque formation most often at proximal internal carotid artery:
  - Plaque is thickest at the carotid bifurcation.
  - Plaque occupies the intima and inner media and avoids outer media and adventitia.
- Plaque histology
  - Homogenous (stable) plaques seldom hemorrhage or ulcerate:
    - Fatty streak and fibrous tissue deposition
    - Diffuse intimal thickening
  - Heterogenous (unstable) plaques may hemorrhage or ulcerate:
    - Presence of lipid-laden macrophages, necrotic debris, cholesterol crystals
    - Ulcerated plaques
  - Soft and gelatinous clots with platelets, fibrin, and red and white blood cells

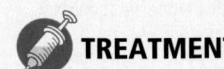 **TREATMENT**

Smoking cessation, BP control, use of antiplatelet medication, and statin medication are the primary treatments for both asymptomatic and symptomatic carotid stenosis.

GENERAL MEASURES
- Lifestyle modifications: dietary control and weight loss, exercise of 30 min/day at least 5 days/week.
- Patients should be advised to quit smoking and offered smoking cessation intervention to reduce the risk of atherosclerotic progression and stroke.

- Control of HTN with antihypertensive agents to maintain BP <140/90 mm Hg (3)[A]; <150/90 mm Hg in the elderly

MEDICATION

- Antihypertensive treatment (<140/90 mm Hg) (3)[A], <150/90 mm Hg in the elderly
- Diet, smoking cessation, and exercise are useful adjuncts to therapy.
- Statin initiation is recommended to reduce LDL cholesterol <100 mg/dL (3)[B]; choose moderate- to high-intensity statin therapy for anti-inflammatory benefit.
- In statin intolerance, LDL-lowering therapy with bile acid sequestrants and/or niacin is reasonable (3)[B].
- Aspirin: 75 to 325 mg/day (3)[A]
- If patient has sustained ischemic stroke or TIA, antiplatelet therapy with
  - Aspirin alone (75 to 325 mg/day) (3)[B] *or*
  - Clopidogrel alone (75 mg/day) (3)[B], *or*
  - Aspirin plus extended-release dipyridamole (25 and 200 mg BID, respectively) (3)[B]
  - A combination of clopidogrel plus aspirin is NOT recommended within 3 months post TIA or CVA (3)[B].

ISSUES FOR REFERRAL

- For acute symptomatic stroke, order imaging and contact neurology.
- For known carotid stenosis, some suggest duplex imaging every 6 months if stenosis is >50% and patient is a surgical candidate.

SURGERY/OTHER PROCEDURES

- Symptomatic carotid stenosis

  - Carotid endarterectomy (CEA) is recommended in symptomatic patients with a carotid stenosis of 70–99% without near-occlusion. Benefit in patients with carotid near-occlusion is uncertain in the long term (4)[A].
  - CEA is recommended for patients with a life expectancy of at least 5 years. The anticipated rate of perioperative stroke or mortality must be <6% (3)[A].
  - Treatment with aspirin (81 to 325 mg/day) is recommended for all patients who are having CEA. Aspirin should be started prior to surgery and continued for at least 3 months postsurgery but may be continued indefinitely (5)[B].
  - Carotid artery stenting (CAS) provides similar long-term outcomes as CEA (6)[A]. Age should be considered when planning a carotid intervention.
    - CAS has an increased risk of adverse cerebrovascular events in the elderly compared to the young but similar mortality risk. CEA is associated with similar neurologic outcomes in the elderly and young, at the expense of increased mortality (7)[A].
    - CAS is suggested in select patients with neck anatomy unfavorable for arterial surgery and those with comorbid conditions that greatly increase the risk of anesthesia and surgery (3)[A].
    - Dual antiplatelet therapy with aspirin (81 to 325 mg/day) plus clopidogrel (75 mg/day) is recommended for 30 days post CAS (3)[C].
- Asymptomatic patients

  - CEA is recommended by some for asymptomatic men who have 60–99% stenosis, have a life expectancy of at least 5 years, and the perioperative risk of stroke and death is <3% (6),(8)[B].
  - The advantage of surgical compared with medical therapy has decreased with contemporary medical management. It is not possible to make an evidence-based recommendation for or against surgical therapy with current literature (9)[A].

INPATIENT CONSIDERATIONS

Admission Criteria/Initial Stabilization

Any patient with presentation of acute symptomatic carotid stenosis should be hospitalized for further diagnostic workup and appropriate therapy.

Rapid evaluation for symptoms compatible with TIA should be obtained in the emergency department (ED) or inpatient setting.

Discharge Criteria

24 to 48 hours post CEA, if ambulating, taking adequate PO intake, and neurologically intact

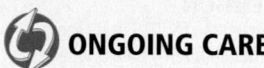 **ONGOING CARE**

FOLLOW-UP RECOMMENDATIONS

Patient Monitoring

- Duplex at 2 to 6 weeks postop
- Duplex every 6 to 12 months
- Reoperative CEA or CAS is reasonable, if there is rapidly progressive restenosis (3)[A].
- Patients with any of the following: renal failure, heart failure, diabetes, and age >80 years have a high-readmission rate following CEA; thus, intensive medical therapy and rigorous follow-up is recommended (10).

DIET

Low-fat, low-cholesterol, low-salt diet at discharge

PATIENT EDUCATION

For patient education materials on this topic, consult the following:

- American Heart Association: http://www.heart.org
- Mayo Clinic Information: http://www.mayoclinic.org/diseases-conditions/carotid-artery-disease/basics/definition/con-20030206

COMPLICATIONS

- Untreated: TIA/stroke (risk of ipsilateral stroke approximately 1.68% per year [10])
- Postoperative (s/p CEA)
  - Perioperative (within 30 days)
    - Stroke/death, cranial nerve injury, hemorrhage, hemodynamic instability, MI
  - Late (>30 days postop)
    - Recurrent stenosis, false aneurysm at surgical site

REFERENCES

1. Goldstein LB, Bushnell CD, Adams RJ, et al. Guidelines for the primary prevention of stroke: a guideline for healthcare professionals from the American Heart Association/American Stroke Association. *Stroke*. 2011;42(2):517–584.
2. de Weerd M, Greving JP, Hedblad B, et al. Prevalence of asymptomatic carotid artery stenosis in the general population: an individual participant data meta-analysis. *Stroke*. 2010;41(6):1294–1297.
3. Brott TG, Halperin JL, Abbara S, et al. 2011 ASA/ACCF/AHA/AANN/AANS/ACR/ASNR/CNS/SAIP/SCAI/SIR/SNIS/SVM/SVS guideline on the management of patients with extracranial carotid and vertebral artery disease: executive summary. *J Am Coll Cardiol*. 2011;57(8):1002–1044.
4. Rerkasem K, Rothwell PM. Carotid endarterectomy for symptomatic carotid stenosis. *Cochrane Database Syst Rev*. 2011;(4):CD001081.
5. Chaturvedi S, Bruno A, Feasby T. Carotid endarterectomy—an evidenced-based review: report of the Therapeutics and Technology Assessment Subcommittee of the American Academy of Neurology. *Neurology*. 2005;65(6):794–801.
6. Bonati LH, Lyrer P, Ederle J, et al. Percutaneous transluminal balloon angioplasty and stenting for carotid artery stenosis. *Cochrane Database Syst Rev*. 2012;(9):CD000515.
7. Antoniou GA, Georgiadis GS, Georgakarakos EI, et al. Meta-analysis and meta-regression analysis of outcomes of carotid endarterectomy and stenting in the elderly. *JAMA Surg*. 2013; 148(12):1140–1152.
8. Raman G, Moorthy D, Hadar N, et al. Management strategies for asymptomatic carotid stenosis: a systematic review and meta-analysis. *Ann Intern Med*. 2013;158(9):676–685.
9. Meschia JF, Bushnell C, Boden-Albala B, et al. Guidelines for the primary prevention of stroke: a statement for healthcare professionals from the American Heart Association/American Stroke Association. *Stroke*. 2014;45(12):3754–3832.
10. Fokkema M, Bensley RP, Lo RC, et al. In-hospital versus postdischarge adverse events following carotid endarterectomy. *J Vasc Surg*. 2013;57(6):1568–1575.

ADDITIONAL READING

- Go C, Avgerinos ED, Chaer RA, et al. Long-term clinical outcomes and cardiovascular events after carotid endarterectomy. *Ann Vasc Surg*. 2015;29(6):1265–1271.
- Jonas DE, Feltner C, Amick HR, et al. Screening for asymptomatic carotid artery stenosis: a systematic review and meta-analysis for the U.S. Preventive Services Task Force. *Ann Intern Med*. 2014;161(5):336–346.
- Paraskevas KI, Mikhailidis DP, Veith FJ. Comparison of the five 2011 guidelines treatment of carotid stenosis. *J Vasc Surg*. 2012;55(5):1504–1508.

 SEE ALSO

Algorithms: Transient Ischemic Attack and Transient Neurologic Defects; Stroke

 CODES

ICD10

- I65.29 Occlusion and stenosis of unspecified carotid artery
- I65.21 Occlusion and stenosis of right carotid artery
- I65.22 Occlusion and stenosis of left carotid artery

CLINICAL PEARLS

- Atherosclerosis is responsible for 90% of all cases of carotid artery stenosis.
- Duplex US is the best initial imaging modality.
- Antiplatelet therapy and aggressive treatment of vascular risk factors are the mainstays of medical therapy.
- Compared with CEA, CAS increases the risk of any stroke and decreases the risk of MI. For every 1,000 patients opting for stenting rather than endarterectomy, 19 more patients would have strokes and 10 fewer would have MIs.

CARPAL TUNNEL SYNDROME

Philip H. Aurigemma, MD • Marci D. Jones, MD

BASICS

DESCRIPTION
- Carpal tunnel syndrome (CTS) is a symptomatic compression neuropathy of the median nerve.
- Increased pressure within the carpal tunnel leads to compression of the median nerve and characteristic of motor-sensory findings.
- The dorsal element of the carpal tunnel is composed of the carpal bones. The transverse carpal ligament defines the palmar boundary:
  - The carpal tunnel contains nine flexor tendons in addition to the median nerve.
- Symptoms most commonly affect the dominant hand; >50% of patients will experience bilateral symptoms.
- System(s) affected: musculoskeletal, nervous

ALERT
Pregnancy: increased incidence during pregnancy (up to 20–45% of patients)

EPIDEMIOLOGY
- Predominant age: 40 to 60 years
- Predominant sex: female > male (3:1 to 10:1)

Incidence
- Two peaks: late 50s (women), late 70s (both genders)
- Incidence up to 276/100,000 has been reported.
- Incidence increases with age.

Prevalence
- 9% in women and 6% in men; 50 cases per 1,000 individuals per year in United States (1)[C]
- 14% in diabetics without neuropathy and 30% in patients with diabetic neuropathy
- Rising prevalence may be the result of increasing lifespan and increasing prevalence of diabetes.

ETIOLOGY AND PATHOPHYSIOLOGY
- Combination of mechanical trauma, inflammation, increased pressure, and ischemic injury to the median nerve within the carpal tunnel
- Acute CTS caused by rapid and sustained pressure in carpal tunnel, usually secondary to trauma, may require urgent surgical decompression.
- Chronic CTS divided into four categories (1)[C]:
  - Idiopathic: combination of edema and fibrous hypertrophy without inflammation
  - Anatomic: persistent median artery, ganglion cyst, infection, space-occupying lesion in carpal tunnel
  - Systemic: associated with conditions such as obesity, diabetes, hypothyroidism, rheumatoid arthritis, amyloidosis, scleroderma, renal failure, and drug toxicity
  - Exertional: repetitive use of hands and wrists, repeated palmar impact, use of vibratory tools. Repetitive use is an objective cause of CTS.

Genetics
Unknown; however, a familial type has been reported.

RISK FACTORS
- Prolonged postures in extremes of wrist flexion and extension; repetitive exposure to vibration
- Alterations of fluid balance: pregnancy, menopause, obesity, renal failure, hypothyroidism, congestive heart failure (CHF), and oral contraceptive use
- Neuropathic factors, such as diabetes, alcoholism, vitamin deficiency, or exposure to toxins, can elicit CTS symptoms.

GENERAL PREVENTION
There is no known prevention for CTS. It is recommended to take occasional (hourly) breaks when doing repetitive work involving hands.

COMMONLY ASSOCIATED CONDITIONS
- Diabetes, obesity; pregnancy; hypothyroidism
- Osteoarthritis of small joints of hand and wrist
- Hyperparathyroidism, hypocalcemia
- Miscellaneous associations include the following:
  - Acromegaly; lupus erythematosus; leukemia
  - Pyogenic infections; sarcoidosis
  - Primary amyloidosis; Paget disease
  - Hormone replacement therapy

DIAGNOSIS

HISTORY
- Patients report nocturnal pain, numbness, and tingling in the thumb, index, long, and radial portion of the ring fingers; patients may not localize and describe the entire hand as being affected.
- Hand weakness during tasks as opening jars is often noted early in the disorder.
- Atypical presentation involves paresthesias in radial digits, with pain radiating proximally along median nerve to elbow and sometimes the shoulder (1)[C].
- Symptoms characteristically are relieved by shaking or rubbing the hands.
- During waking hours, symptoms occur when driving, talking on the phone, and occasionally when using the hands for repetitive maneuvers.
- Presence of predisposing factors, such as diabetes, obesity, acromegaly, pregnancy

PHYSICAL EXAM
- Positive Tinel sign: Tapping over the palmar surface of the wrist proximal to the carpal tunnel may produce an electric sensation along the distribution of the median nerve (50% sensitivity; 77% specificity).
- Positive Phalen sign: Holding the wrist in fullly flexed position for 60 seconds precipitates paresthesias (68% sensitivity; 73% specificity).
- Durkan compression test: Direct compression of median nerve at carpal tunnel for 30 seconds elicits symptoms (87% sensitivity; 90% specificity) (1)[C].
- Wasting of thenar musculature is a late sign.
- Loss of 2-point discrimination
- Ulceration of tips of fingers is associated with loss of protective sensation.

DIFFERENTIAL DIAGNOSIS
- Cervical spondylosis (carpal tunnel may also occur with cervical spine disease; "double crush")
- Generalized peripheral neuropathy
- Brachial plexopathy, in particular upper trunk
- CNS disorders (multiple sclerosis, cerebral infarction)
- Thoracic outlet syndrome
- Pronator syndrome
- Anterior interosseous syndrome
- Musculoskeletal disorders of the wrist:
  - Trauma or distal radius fracture
  - Degenerative joint disease
  - Rheumatoid arthritis
  - Ganglion cyst
- Scleroderma

DIAGNOSTIC TESTS & INTERPRETATION
No laboratory test is diagnostic.

- Normal serum thyrotropin (thyroid-stimulating hormone [TSH]) and normal serum can exclude secondary conditions associated with CTS.

Initial Tests (lab, imaging)
- Special tests
  - Electrodiagnostic studies
    - Sensitivity 85%; specificity 95%
    - Nerve conduction studies compare latency and amplitude of median nerve across the carpal tunnel.
    - Prolonged distal latency of the median motor and/or sensory fibers may be seen. Axon loss is suggested with decreased amplitudes.
    - The most sensitive indicator is median sensory distal latency, which is prolonged in CTS. Sensory nerve action potentials may be reduced or unobtainable.
    - Electromyographic changes are indicative of long-standing or severe nerve dysfunction.
- Ulnar nerve stimulation should be performed to exclude generalized polyneuropathy.
- Standard radiographs of the wrist evaluate bony anatomy and degenerative joint disease.
- Special radiographic views of the carpal tunnel are of limited use.
- Magnetic resonance imaging and ultrasound are of limited benefit in diagnosis of CTS.

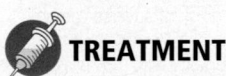

TREATMENT

GENERAL MEASURES
- Splinting of the wrist in a neutral position while sleeping may provide significant symptom relief:
  - Limited evidence indicates that splints worn at night are more effective than no treatment in the short term. Insufficient evidence to recommend a specific splint design or wearing regimen (2)[A].
- Splinting (sometimes prolonged) typically promotes symptom resolution.
- Corticosteroid injections are effective for up to 3 months compared with placebo (3)[A].
- Outcomes at 1 year show no benefit for local steroid injections compared to placebo (3)[A].

MEDICATION

First Line
NSAIDs, such as ibuprofen or naproxen sodium, are commonly used. There is insufficient evidence to determine their routine efficacy:

- Contraindications: GI intolerance
- Precautions: GI side effects of NSAIDs may preclude their use in selected patients.

Second Line
- Local steroid injection: Methylprednisolone injections are more effective than systemic steroids or placebo at 1 and 3 months and more effective than splinting at 6 months (4)[A].
- Response to injections can help confirm diagnosis of CTS and predict a better response to surgery.
- Side effects include reduction of collagen and proteoglycan synthesis, limiting tenocytes, and reducing mechanical strength of tendon, leading to further degeneration and risk for rupture.
- Oral steroids may provide a short-term improvement (2 to 8 weeks) in symptoms.
- The long-term risks of even a short course of steroids should be balanced with the limited potential benefit of symptom improvement.

ISSUES FOR REFERRAL
Preoperative electrodiagnostic studies are generally obtained prior to any surgical intervention.

SURGERY/OTHER PROCEDURES
- Completely dividing the transverse carpal ligament provides symptom relief in >95% of patients.
- Surgical decompression is an outpatient procedure performed under local or regional anesthesia.
- Healing of the incision generally takes 2 weeks; an additional 2 weeks may be required before using the affected hand for tasks requiring strength.
- Long-term results of open carpal tunnel release are excellent. Patients experience consistent pain relief for 10 to 15 years (5)[B].
- Recent randomized, controlled studies indicate that surgery leads to better functional improvements at 1 year compared with nonoperative management.
- Open versus endoscopic surgical procedures produce similar outcomes at 6 months. The approach should be based on surgeon and patient preference.
- Endoscopic carpal tunnel release allows a faster return to work.
- Risk of transient nerve injuries is higher with endoscopic release (6)[A].
- Therapeutic ultrasound, exercise, and mobilization techniques have limited benefit compared with other nonsurgical interventions. Poor quality evidence shows ultrasound may be more effective than placebo (7,8)[A].

COMPLEMENTARY & ALTERNATIVE MEDICINE
No trial data support the use of vitamin B_6 in the prevention or treatment of CTS.

INPATIENT CONSIDERATIONS

Admission Criteria/Initial Stabilization
Outpatient

 ## ONGOING CARE

FOLLOW-UP RECOMMENDATIONS

Patient Monitoring
- Patients treated nonoperatively (splinting, injections) require follow-up over 4 to 12 weeks to ensure adequate progress.
- There is only limited, low-quality evidence to suggest that rehabilitation exercises such as wrist immobilization, ice therapy, and multimodal hand rehabilitation are beneficial.
- 7–20% of patients treated surgically may experience recurrence.

PATIENT EDUCATION
- American Society for Surgery of the Hand: http://www.assh.org/Public/HandConditions/Pages/CarpalTunnelSyndrome.aspx
- For patient education materials, contact: American Academy of Family Physicians Foundation, P.O. Box 8418, Kansas City, MO 64114 (800) 274-2237, Ext. 4400.

PROGNOSIS
- Patients with severe CTS may not recover completely after surgical release. Paresthesias and weakness may persist, but night symptoms generally resolve.
- If untreated, more severe cases of CTS can lead to numbness and weakness in the hand, atrophy of the thenar muscles, and permanent loss of median nerve function.

COMPLICATIONS
- Postoperative infection (rare)
- Injury to the median nerve or its recurrent (motor) branch

REFERENCES

1. Cranford CS, Ho JY, Kalainov DM, et al. Carpal tunnel syndrome. J Am Acad Orthop Surg. 2007;15(9):537–548.
2. Page MJ, Massy-Westropp N, O'Connor D, et al. Splinting for carpal tunnel syndrome. Cochrane Database Syst Rev. 2012;(7):CD010003.
3. Atroshi I, Flondell M, Hofer M, et al. Methylprednisolone injections for the carpal tunnel syndrome: a randomized, placebo-controlled trial. Ann Intern Med. 2013;159(5):309–317.
4. Marshall S, Tardif G, Ashworth N. Local corticosteroid injection for carpal tunnel syndrome. Cochrane Database Syst Rev. 2007;(2):CD001554.
5. Louie DL, Earp BE, Collins JE, et al. Outcomes of open carpal tunnel release at a minimum of ten years. J Bone Joint Surg Am. 2013;95(12):1067–1073.
6. Sayegh ET, Strauch RJ. Open versus endoscopic carpal tunnel release: a meta-analysis of randomized controlled trials. Clin Orthop Relate Res. 2015;473(3):1120–1132.
7. Page MJ, O'Connor D, Pitt V, et al. Exercise and mobilisation interventions for carpal tunnel syndrome. Cochrane Database Syst Rev. 2012;(6):CD009899.
8. Page MJ, O'Connor D, Pitt V, et al. Therapeutic ultrasound for carpal tunnel syndrome. Cochrane Database Syst Rev. 2013;(3):CD009601.

ADDITIONAL READING

- Fowler JR, Gaughan JP, Ilyas AM. The sensitivity and specificity of ultrasound for the diagnosis of carpal tunnel syndrome: a meta-analysis. Clin Orthop Relat Res. 2011;469(4):1089–1094.
- Graham B. Nonsurgical treatment of carpal tunnel syndrome. J Hand Surg Am. 2009;34(3):531–534.
- Huisstede BM, Hoogvliet P, Randsdorp MS, et al. Carpal tunnel syndrome. Part I: effectiveness of nonsurgical treatments—a systematic review. Arch Phys Med Rehabil. 2010;91(7):981–1004.
- Middleton SD, Anakwe RE. Carpal tunnel syndrome. BMJ. 2014; 349: g6437.
- Peters S, Page MJ, Coppieters MW, et al. Rehabilitation following carpal tunnel release. Cochrane Database Syst Rev. 2013;(6):CD004158.
- Shi Q, MacDermid JC. Is surgical intervention more effective than non-surgical treatment for carpal tunnel syndrome? A systematic review. J Orthop Surg Res. 2011;6:17.
- Tai TW, Wu CY, Su FC, et al. Ultrasonography for diagnosing carpal tunnel syndrome: a meta-analysis of diagnostic test accuracy. Ultrasound Med Biol. 2012;38(7):1121–1128.
- Vasiliadis HS, Georgoulas P, Shrier I, et al. Endoscopic release for carpal tunnel syndrome. Cochrane Database Syst Rev. 2014;(1):CD008265.

 ## SEE ALSO

- Arthritis, Rheumatoid (RA); Hypoparathyroidism; Scleroderma; Lupus Erythematosus, Systemic (SLE)
- Algorithms: Carpal Tunnel Syndrome; Pain in Upper Extremity

 ## CODES

ICD10
- G56.00 Carpal tunnel syndrome, unspecified upper limb
- G56.01 Carpal tunnel syndrome, right upper limb
- G56.02 Carpal tunnel syndrome, left upper limb

CLINICAL PEARLS

- Paresthesias associated with CTS are characteristically confined to the thumb, index, long, and radial 1/2 of the ring fingers of the affected hand.
- Thenar atrophy is a late finding, indicating severe nerve damage.
- Durkan (carpal compression) test is superior to Tinel sign (tapping on median nerve over carpal tunnel) and Phalen maneuver (holding wrists in flexion) for the clinical diagnosis of CTS.
- Steroid injections offer short-term relief, but clinical outcomes at 1 year are no different than placebo.

CATARACT

Yasir Ahmed, MD • Ingrid U. Scott, MD, MPH

 BASICS

DESCRIPTION

- A cataract is any opacity or discoloration of the lens, localized or generalized; the term is usually reserved for changes that affect visual acuity (1,2).
- Etymology: from Latin *cataractes*, for "waterfall"; named after foamy appearance of opacity
- Leading cause of blindness worldwide, estimated 20 million people (1,2)
- Types include the following:
  - Age related: 90% of total
  - Metabolic (diabetes via accelerated sorbitol pathway, hypocalcemia, Wilson disease)
  - Congenital (1/250 newborns; 10–38% of childhood blindness)
  - Systemic disease associated (myotonic dystrophy, atopic dermatitis)
  - Secondary to associated eye disease, so-called complicated (e.g., uveitis associated with juvenile rheumatoid arthritis or sarcoid, tumor such as melanoma or retinoblastoma)
  - Traumatic (e.g., heat, electric shock, radiation, concussion, perforating eye injuries, intraocular foreign body)
  - Toxic/nutritional (e.g., corticosteroids)
- Morphologic classification:
  - Nuclear: exaggeration of normal aging changes of *central* lens nucleus, often associated with myopia due to increased refractive index of lens (some elderly patients consequently may be able to read again *without spectacles*, so-called second sight of the aged)
  - Cortical: outer portion of lens; may involve anterior, posterior, or equatorial cortex; radial, spoke-like opacities
  - Subcapsular: Posterior subcapsular cataract has more profound effect on vision than nuclear or cortical cataract; patients particularly troubled under conditions of miosis; near vision frequently impaired more than distance vision.
- System(s) affected: nervous

Geriatric Considerations
Some degree of cataract formation is expected in all people >70 years of age.

Pediatric Considerations
See "Congenital Cataract"; may present as leukocoria.

Pregnancy Considerations
See "Congenital Cataract" (i.e., medications, metabolic dysfunction, intrauterine infection, and malnutrition).

EPIDEMIOLOGY

Incidence
- ~48% of the 37 million cases of blindness worldwide result from cataracts (1,2).
- Leading cause of treatable blindness and vision loss in developing countries (1,2)
- Predominant age: depends on type of cataract
- Predominant sex: male > female

Prevalence
- Cataract type and prevalence are highly variable based on population demographic.
- An estimated 50% of people 65 to 74 years of age and 70% of people >75 years of age have age-related cataract.

ETIOLOGY AND PATHOPHYSIOLOGY
- Age-related cataract:
  - Continual addition of layers of lens fibers throughout life creates hard, dehydrated lens nucleus that impairs vision (nuclear cataract).
  - Aging alters biochemical and osmotic balance required for lens clarity; outer lens layers hydrate and become opaque, adversely affecting vision.
- Congenital:
  - Usually unknown etiology
  - Drugs (corticosteroids in 1st trimester, sulfonamides)
  - Metabolic (diabetes in mother, galactosemia in fetus)
  - Intrauterine infection during 1st trimester (e.g., rubella, herpes, mumps)
  - Maternal malnutrition
- Other cataract types:
  - Common feature is a biochemical/osmotic imbalance that disrupts lens clarity.
  - Local changes in lens protein distribution lead to light scattering (lens opacity).

Genetics
- Congenital (e.g., chromosomal disorders [Down syndrome])
- Genetics of age-related cataract are not yet established but likely multifactorial contribution.

RISK FACTORS
- Aging
- Cigarette smoking
- Ultraviolet (UV) sunlight exposure
- Diabetes
- Prolonged high-dose steroids
- Positive family history
- Alcohol

GENERAL PREVENTION
- Use of UV protective glasses
- Avoidance of tobacco products
- Effective control of diabetes
- Care with high-dose, long-term steroid use (systemic therapy > inhaled treatment)
- Protective methods using pharmaceutical intervention (e.g., antioxidants, acetylsalicylic acid [ASA], hormone replacement therapy [HRT]) show no proven benefit to date.

COMMONLY ASSOCIATED CONDITIONS
- Diabetes (especially with poor glucose control)
- Myotonic dystrophy (90% of patients develop visually innocuous change in 3rd decade; becomes disabling in 5th decade)
- Atopic dermatitis (AD) (10% of patients with severe AD develop cataracts in 2nd to 4th decades, often bilateral)
- Neurofibromatosis type 2

- Associated ocular disease or "secondary cataract" (e.g., chronic anterior uveitis, acute [or repetitive] angle-closure glaucoma or high myopia)
- Drug induced (e.g., steroids, chlorpromazine)
- Trauma

 DIAGNOSIS

HISTORY
- Age-related cataract:
  - Decreased visual acuity, blurred vision, distortion, or "ghosting" of images (1,2)
  - Problems with visual acuity in any lighting condition
  - Falls or accidents; injuries (e.g., hip fracture)
- Congenital: often asymptomatic, leukocoria, parents notice child's visual inattention or strabismus
- Other types of cataract:
  - May also present with decreased visual acuity
  - Appropriate clinical history or signs to help with diagnosis

PHYSICAL EXAM
- Visual acuity assessment for all cataracts
- Age-related cataract: lens opacity on eye examination
- Congenital:
  - Lens opacity present at birth or within 3 months of birth
  - Leukocoria (white pupil), strabismus, nystagmus, signs of associated syndrome (as with Down or rubella syndrome)
  - *Note:* must always rule out ocular tumor; early diagnosis and treatment of retinoblastoma may be lifesaving
- Other types of cataract: may present with decreased visual acuity associated with characteristic physical findings (e.g., metabolic, trauma)

DIFFERENTIAL DIAGNOSIS
- An opaque-appearing eye may be due to opacities of the cornea (e.g., scarring, edema, calcification), lens opacities, tumor, or retinal detachment. Biomicroscopic examination (slit lamp) or careful ophthalmoscopic exam should provide diagnosis.
- In the elderly, visual impairment is often due to multiple factors such as cataract and macular degeneration, both contributing to visual loss.
- Age-related cataract is significant if symptoms and ophthalmic exam support cataract as a major cause of vision impairment.
- Congenital lens opacity in the absence of other ocular pathology may cause severe amblyopia.
- *Note:* Cataract *does not* produce a relative afferent pupillary reaction defect. Abnormal pupillary reactions mandate further evaluation for other pathology.

DIAGNOSTIC TESTS & INTERPRETATION
- Visual quality assessment: Glare testing, contrast sensitivity is sometimes indicated.
- Retinal/macular function assessment: potential acuity meter testing
- Workup of underlying process

Test Interpretation

Consistent with lens changes found in the type of cataract; however, diagnosis is made by clinical examination.

 TREATMENT

- Outpatient (usually)
- ~1.64 million cataract extractions in the United States yearly (3,4)

GENERAL MEASURES

Eye protection from UV light

MEDICATION

There are currently no medications to prevent or slow the progression of cataracts.

ISSUES FOR REFERRAL

If patient has cataract and symptoms do not seem to support recommended surgery, a second opinion by another ophthalmologist may be indicated.

SURGERY/OTHER PROCEDURES

- Age-related cataract:
  - Surgical removal is indicated if visual impairment–producing symptoms are distressing to the patient, interfering with lifestyle or occupation, or posing a risk for fall or injury (3,4)[A].
  - Because significant cataract may develop gradually, the patient may not be aware of how it has changed his or her lifestyle. Physician may note a significant cataract, and patient reports "no problems." Thus, evaluation requires effective physician–patient exchange of information.
  - Surgical technique: Cataract extraction via small incisions, followed by implantation of a prosthetic intraocular lens; lenses have power calculated based on size of the eye and curvature of cornea usually to correct for distance vision; surgery performed on one (worse) eye, with contralateral surgery only after recovery and if deemed necessary; generally takes <1 hour depending on surgical technique
  - Anesthesia: usually regional injection or topical with sedation and monitoring of vital signs
  - Preoperative evaluation: by the primary care physician:
    - Patients on anticoagulants may need to be temporarily discontinued 1 to 2 weeks before surgery if possible (but not always necessary; thus, need to discuss with ophthalmologist).
    - Patients who have ever taken an α-blocker such as tamsulosin (Flomax) should alert their ophthalmologist (increased risk of intraoperative floppy iris syndrome [IFIS] even in patients who no longer use these drugs).

- Postoperative care: usually protective eye shield as directed, topical antibiotic, NSAIDs, and steroid ophthalmic medications; avoid lifting or bending over for a few weeks.
- Congenital cataract:
  - Treatment is surgical removal of cataract. Newborns may require surgery within days to reduce risk of severe amblyopia. Use of lens implants is controversial because the eyes are growing.
  - Postoperative care: long-term patching program for good eye to combat amblyopia; refractive correction of operative eye, with multiple repeat examinations; challenging for physician and parents

 ONGOING CARE

FOLLOW-UP RECOMMENDATIONS

Patient Monitoring

- As cataract progresses, an ophthalmologist may change spectacle correction to maintain vision. When this is no longer successful and interferes with patient's activities of daily living, surgery is indicated.
- Following surgery, spectacle correction may be required to maximize near and/or far visual acuity. Refraction is usually prescribed several weeks after surgery.

PATIENT EDUCATION

Medline Plus on cataracts at: https://www.nlm.nih.gov/medlineplus/cataract.html

PROGNOSIS

- Ocular prognosis is good after cataract removal if no prior or coexisting ocular disease: 94.3% of otherwise healthy eyes achieve best corrected visual acuity of 20/40 or better. Success rates are lower with comorbidities such as diabetes and glaucoma (5).
- In congenital cataracts, prognosis often is poorer because of the high risk of amblyopia.

COMPLICATIONS

- Vary widely from delay in visual recovery or protracted visual discomfort to blindness and loss of eye
- Nearly all reported complications occur rarely (<2% of eyes) except for posterior capsule opacification (14.7–42.7% of eyes, usually treated with Nd-YAG laser capsulotomy in office with a rate of 4–25.3%) (6,7)[B].
- Poor preoperative visual acuity is related to surgical complications (8).

REFERENCES

1. Asbell PA, Dualan I, Mindel J, et al. Age-related cataract. *Lancet*. 2005;365(9459):599–609.
2. Abraham AG, Condon NG, West Gower E. The new epidemiology of cataract. *Ophthalmol Clin North Am*. 2006;19(4):415–425.
3. Riaz Y, Mehta JS, Wormald R, et al. Surgical interventions for age-related cataract. *Cochrane Database Syst Rev*. 2006;(4):CD001323.
4. Fedorowicz Z, Lawrence D, Gutierrez P. Day care versus in-patient surgery for age-related cataract. *Cochrane Database Syst Rev*. 2005;(1):CD004242.
5. Biber JM, Sandoval HP, Trivedi RH, et al. Comparison of the incidence and visual significance of posterior capsule opacification between multifocal spherical, monofocal spherical, and monofocal aspheric intraocular lenses. *J Cataract Refract Surg*. 2009;35(7):1234–1238.
6. Findl O, Buehl W, Bauer P, et al. Interventions for preventing posterior capsule opacification. *Cochrane Database Syst Rev*. 2010;(2):CD003738.
7. Lundström M, Barry P, Henry Y, et al. Visual outcome of cataract surgery; study from the European Registry of Quality Outcomes for Cataract and Refractive Surgery. *J Cataract Refract Surg*. 2013;39(5):673–679.
8. Lundström M, Goh PP, Henry Y, et al. The changing pattern of cataract surgery indications: a 5-year study of 2 cataract surgery databases. *Ophthalmology*. 2015;122(1):31–38.

 SEE ALSO

- Algorithm: Cataracts
- Floppy Iris Syndrome

 CODES

ICD10

- H26.9 Unspecified cataract
- H25.9 Unspecified age-related cataract
- Q12.0 Congenital cataract

CLINICAL PEARLS

- Cataracts are the leading cause of blindness worldwide; 90% are age-related.
- Primary indication for cataract surgery is visual impairment leading to significant lifestyle changes for the patient.
- For congenital cataracts, must always rule out ocular tumor because early diagnosis and treatment of retinoblastoma may be lifesaving.
- Before prescribing an α-blocker for an older adult with hypertension or a prostate or urinary retention problem, consider whether the patient has cataracts (due to increased risk of IFIS).

CELIAC DISEASE
Jason E. Domagalski, MD, FAAFP • Matthew W. Short, MD, FAAFP

 BASICS

DESCRIPTION
- Autoimmune condition characterized by an immune-mediated reaction to dietary gluten (found in wheat, barley, rye) primarily affecting the small intestine in genetically predisposed individuals
- Presentations
  - Typical
    - Diarrheal illness characterized by villous atrophy with symptoms of malabsorption (steatorrhea, weight loss, vitamin deficiencies, anemia). Resolves with a gluten-free diet
    - <50% of adults present with GI symptoms.
  - Atypical
    - Minor GI symptoms, with a myriad of extraintestinal manifestations (e.g., anemia, dental enamel defects, neurologic symptoms, infertility)
  - Asymptomatic (silent) disease
    - Found when screening first-degree relatives
  - Latent
    - Positive laboratory tests and genetics, without signs/symptoms
- System(s) affected: gastrointestinal
- Synonym(s): celiac sprue; gluten enteropathy

EPIDEMIOLOGY
Incidence
- 1 to 13 per 100,000 worldwide (1)
- 6.5 per 100,000 in United States (2)
- Primarily impacts individuals of Northern European ancestry
- Predominant sex: female > male (3:2)

Prevalence
- 0.7% in United States; an estimated 3 million Americans have celiac disease (3).
- Prevalence is 8 to 204 per 100,000 worldwide and increasing (1).

ETIOLOGY AND PATHOPHYSIOLOGY
Sensitivity to gluten, specifically gliadin fraction. Tissue transglutaminase (tTG) modification of protein leads to immunologic cross-reactivity, inflammation, and tissue damage (villous atrophy) with subsequent malabsorption.

Genetics
Homogenicity for *HLA-DQ2* increases the risk of celiac disease and enteropathy-associated T-cell lymphoma.

RISK FACTORS
- First-degree relatives: 5–10% incidence (4)
- Monozygotic twins: 70% incidence
- 25% risk in family members with an autoimmune disease

Pediatric Considerations
No associations found with breastfeeding duration, age, concurrent infection, or gastroenteritis at time of gluten introduction.

GENERAL PREVENTION
Avoid gluten-containing products (wheat, barley, rye, and possibly oat products).

COMMONLY ASSOCIATED CONDITIONS
- *Dermatitis herpetiformis*: 85% of patients have celiac disease. All patients should follow gluten-free diet (4).
- Secondary lactase deficiency
- Osteopenia
- Thyroid disease: Hashimoto thyroiditis
- 3–10% of patients with type 1 diabetes also have celiac disease.
- Symptomatic iron deficiency, 10–15% have celiac disease
- Elevated AST and ALT (with no direct cause)
- Hyposplenism
- Irritable bowel syndrome (IBS)
- Restless leg syndrome
- Celiac disease is associated with increased risk for adenocarcinoma and lymphoma of the small bowel.
  - The risk of lymphoproliferative malignancies depends on small intestinal histopathology.
  - Little to no increased risk in latent celiac disease (seropositive but normal biopsy) (5)[A].
- Other autoimmune disorders

Pregnancy Considerations
- Prevalence of celiac disease: 2.5 to 3.5 times higher in women with unexplained infertility
- Up to 19% of men with celiac disease have androgen resistance. Semen quality and likelihood of pregnancy increase with gluten-free diet.
- Higher rates of low birth weight, spontaneous abortions, and stillbirths

Pediatric Considerations
Failure to thrive and delayed growth may be early manifestations. Some children may outgrow wheat intolerance after prolonged gluten-free diets but should watch for recurrence in middle age.

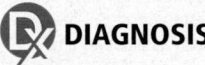 DIAGNOSIS

HISTORY
- Diarrhea, cramping, most common GI symptoms
- Steatorrhea (fatty stools)
- Muscle cramps
- Iron deficiency anemia
- Nervousness, depression
- Weight loss
- Failure to thrive (slowing velocity of weight gain)
- Weakness, fatigue
- Flatulence (can be explosive)
- Abdominal pain, nausea, vomiting
- Recurrent aphthous stomatitis
- Abdominal distention
- Delayed puberty
- Tingling numbness in hands, feet
- Bone or joint pain
- Migraines

PHYSICAL EXAM
Often normal but look for
- Oropharynx: aphthous stomatitis
- Skin: dermatitis herpetiformis (symmetric erythematous papules and blisters on elbows, knees, buttocks, and back)
- Abdomen: distention

DIFFERENTIAL DIAGNOSIS
- Short bowel syndrome
- Dyspepsia, gastroesophageal reflux disease (GERD)
- Pancreatic insufficiency
- Crohn disease; Whipple disease; tropical sprue
- Hypogammaglobulinemia
- Intestinal lymphoma
- HIV enteropathy
- Acute enteritis; radiation enteritis, eosinophilic gastroenteritis
- Giardiasis
- Pancreatic disease

DIAGNOSTIC TESTS & INTERPRETATION
Initial Tests (lab, imaging)
- Do not base diagnosis on serology alone. Patients with symptoms highly suggestive of celiac disease or those with positive serologies should undergo endoscopy for biopsy. Tissue biopsy is the gold standard for diagnosis.
- IgA antitissue transglutaminase (IgA-anti-tTG) is the preferred single serologic test in patients >2 (4)[C].
- Total serum IgA

ALERT
Positive IgA tTG has high sensitivity and specificity (sensitivity, 90–98%; specificity, 98%) if on normal (non-gluten-free) diet for at least 4 weeks.

- IgA-deficient patients have false-negative IgA anti-tTG antibodies.
- IgA deficiency is 10 to 15 times more prevalent in patients with celiac disease.
- The tTG antibody test is the preferred test (over the deamidated gliadin peptide [DGP] antibody) (6–8)[A].

Follow-Up Tests & Special Considerations
- If patient is IgA deficient OR if IgA anti-tTG are negative, follow up blood tests.
  - Anti-DGP IgA and IgG
    - Sensitivity, 94%; specificity, 99% (~anti-TTG)
- Do not use HLA DQ serotyping for initial diagnosis. Consider if discrepant serology–histology results in patients unable to test on gluten-free diet and children with Down syndrome (4)[C].
- Consider bone mineral density testing at diagnosis and after 1 year if osteopenia/osteoporosis on initial testing or 2 years if normal initially and patient still symptomatic or noncompliant.

Pediatric Considerations
- Antigliadin antibody (AgA–IgG and IgA) may be used for children age <2 years because tTG and endomysial (EMA) antibodies may be absent.
- Anti-DGP test is sensitive in children.
- IgA tTG >10 times normal with positive EMA testing and HLA-DQ2 has PPV of 97.4% and may not need confirmatory intestinal biopsies for diagnosis (4)[C].

Diagnostic Procedures/Other
- Endoscopy with a minimum of four biopsies of the distal duodenum and two of the duodenal bulb at time of initial evaluation correctly diagnosed 95% of children (4)[C].

- Video capsule endoscopy is a promising alternative with a sensitivity and specificity of 80% and 95%. Particularly helpful if antibody screening and clinical picture are consistent with celiac disease despite nondiagnostic duodenal biopsies (9)[A].

Test Interpretation
Small bowel biopsy

- Villous atrophy, hyperplasia and lengthening of crypts, infiltration of plasma cells, and intraepithelial lymphocytosis in lamina propria
- Villous atrophy also caused by Crohn disease, radiation enteritis, giardia and other food intolerances

 TREATMENT

GENERAL MEASURES
- Remove gluten from the diet.
  - Rice, corn, and soybean flour are safe and palatable substitutes (4)[C].
- Levels of IgA antigliadin normalize with gluten abstinence.
- LIFELONG abstinence is required; immune response to gluten will recur with resumption of gluten consumption.

MEDICATION
First Line
Usually no medications: Gluten-free diet is the treatment.

Second Line
- In refractory disease, consider
  - Steroids (prednisone, 40 to 60 mg/day PO in cases of refractory sprue)
  - Azathioprine (used with caution; use may lead to lymphoma)
  - Cyclosporine
  - Infliximab
  - Cladribine
- Patients may develop nutritional deficiencies depending on the severity of the disease.

Third Line
There are numerous clinical trials testing the efficacy of intraluminally acting agents such as *Lactobacilli* to gluten endopeptidases, inhibitors of transepithelial gliadin uptake, immunomodulation, and even vaccination (10). Findings are largely awaiting further validation.

ISSUES FOR REFERRAL
- Additional nutritional support
- Refractory disease

 ONGOING CARE

FOLLOW-UP RECOMMENDATIONS
- Consultation with registered dietitian
- Screen for osteoporosis and treat accordingly.

Patient Monitoring
- Repeat EGD if no clinical response to gluten-free diet or relapse in symptoms (4)[C].
- Follow anti-tTG IgA or deaminated antigliadin antibodies as a measure of response/compliance with diet (vs. antigliadin IgA or IgG).

DIET
- Remove gluten: wheat, rye, barley, and products with gluten additives.
- Dietary change is challenging (especially learning sources of "hidden" gluten) and should be coordinated with a skilled registered dietitian.

PATIENT EDUCATION
- Discuss how to recognize gluten in various products.
- Highlight potential complications and outcomes of failing to follow a gluten-free diet.

PROGNOSIS
- Good prognosis if adherent to gluten-free diet
- Patients should feel better within 7 days of dietary modification.
- Symptoms usually disappear in 4 to 6 weeks.
- It is unknown whether strict dietary adherence decreases cancer risk.

COMPLICATIONS
- Malignancy: <10% of patients (50% of whom develop small bowel lymphoma)
- Refractory disease (rare ~1–2% of all patients)
  - May respond to prednisone 40 to 60 mg/day PO
  - May need total parenteral nutrition
  - Two types: Type 2 has poor prognosis with 5-year survival of 44%.
- Chronic ulcerative jejunoileitis
  - Associated with multiple ulcers, intestinal bleeding, strictures, perforation, obstruction, and peritonitis.
  - 7% mortality
- Osteoporosis
- Dehydration
- Electrolyte depletion

REFERENCES

1. Kang JY, Kang AH, Green A, et al. Systematic review: worldwide variation in the frequency of coeliac disease and changes over time. *Aliment Pharmacol Ther*. 2013;38(3):226–245.
2. Riddle MS, Murray JA, Porter CK. The incidence and risk of celiac disease in a healthy US adult population. *Am J Gastroenterol*. 2012;107(8): 1248–1255.
3. Rubio-Tapia A, Ludvigsson JF, Brantner TL, et al. The prevalence of celiac disease in the United States. *Am J Gastroenterol*. 2012;107(10):1538–1544.
4. Rubio-Tapia A, Hill ID, Kelly CP, et al. ACG clinical guidelines: diagnosis and management of celiac disease. *Am J Gastroenterol*. 2013;108(5): 656–676.
5. Elfström P, Granath F, Ekström Smedby K, et al. Risk of lymphoproliferative malignancy in relation to small intestinal histopathology among patients with celiac disease. *J Natl Cancer Inst*. 2011;103(5):436–444.
6. Lewis NR, Scott BB. Meta-analysis: deamidated gliadin peptide antibody and tissue transglutaminase antibody compared as screening tests for coeliac disease. *Aliment Pharmacol Ther*. 2010;31(1):73–81.
7. Van der Windt DA, Jellema P, Mulder CJ, et al. Diagnostic testing for celiac disease among patients with abdominal symptoms: a systematic review. *JAMA*. 2010;303(17):1738–1746.
8. Sugai E, Vázquez H, Nachman F, et al. Accuracy of testing for antibodies to synthetic gliadin-related peptides in celiac disease. *Clin Gastroenterol Hepatol*. 2006;4(9):1112–1117.
9. Rokkas T, Niv Y. The role of video capsule endoscopy in the diagnosis of celiac disease: a meta-analysis. *Eur J Gastroenterol Hepatol*. 2012; 84(3):303–308.
10. Crowe S. Management of celiac disease: beyond the gluten-free diet. *Gastroenterology*. 2014; 146(7):1594–1596.

ADDITIONAL READING

- Bolotin D, Petronic-Rosic V. Dermatitis herpetiformis. Part II. Diagnosis, management, and prognosis. *J Am Acad Dermatol*. 2011;64(6):1027–1033.
- Celiac Disease Foundation: https://celiac.org/
- Celiac Disease Foundation. Quick start gluten-free diet guide for celiac disease and non-celiac gluten sensitivity. http://celiac.org/wp-content/uploads/2013 /12/quick-start-guide.pdf
- Celiac Sprue Association (CSA): http://www .csa.celiacs.org
- Giersiepen K, Lelgemann M, Stuhldreher N, et al. Accuracy of diagnostic antibody tests for coeliac disease in children: summary of an evidence report. *J Pediatr Gastroenterol Nutr*. 2012;54(2):229–241.
- Gluten Intolerance Group (GIG). https://www .gluten.org/
- Kagnoff MF. AGA Institute Medical Position Statement on the Diagnosis and Management of Celiac Disease. *Gastroenterology*. 2006;131(6):1977–1980.
- Rozenberg O, Lerner A, Pacht A, et al. A novel algorithm for the diagnosis of celiac disease and a comprehensive review of celiac disease diagnostics. *Clin Rev Allergy Immunol*. 2012;42(3):331–341.
- Welander A, Tjernberg AR, Montgomery SM, et al. Infectious disease and risk of later celiac disease in childhood. *Pediatrics*. 2010;125(3):e530–e536.

 SEE ALSO

Algorithms: Diarrhea, Chronic; Malabsorption Syndrome

 CODES

ICD10
K90.0 Celiac disease

CLINICAL PEARLS
- Test for celiac disease in patients with presumed IBS, dermatitis herpetiformis, or unexplained transaminitis.
- Test total IgA levels along with IgA anti-tTG antibodies in patients >2 years of age.
- Positive serology is not definitive; endoscopic biopsy is the gold standard for diagnosis.
- Standard of treatment is a gluten-free diet. Patient symptoms should improve within 7 days if fully compliant.

CELLULITIS
Jowhara Al-Qahtani, MD • Amer Homsi, MD • Bakr Nour, MD, PhD, FACS

 BASICS

DESCRIPTION
- An acute bacterial infection of the dermis and subcutaneous tissue
- Types and locations:
  - Periorbital cellulitis: bacterial infection of the eyelid and surrounding tissues (anterior compartment)
  - Orbital cellulitis: Infection of the eye posterior to the septum; sinusitis is the most common risk factor.
  - Facial cellulitis: preceded by upper respiratory infection or otitis media
  - Buccal cellulitis: infection of cheek in children associated with bacteremia (common before *Haemophilus influenzae* type B vaccine)
  - Peritonsillar cellulitis: common in children associated with fever, sore throat, and "hot potato" speech
  - Abdominal wall cellulitis: common in morbidly obese patients
  - Perianal cellulitis: sharply demarcated, bright, perianal erythema
  - Necrotizing cellulitis: gas-producing bacteria in the lower extremities; common in diabetics
- System(s) affected: skin/exocrine

EPIDEMIOLOGY
- Predominant sex: male = female (common in elderly and adults, except perianal cellulitis which is common in children)
- All-cause mortality for patient admitted with cellulitis is 7%. Recurrence rate of cellulitis is 8–20% (1)[A].

Incidence
200/100,000 patient/years

Prevalence
The exact prevalence is uncertain as cellulitis is common and not reportable. It affects all age groups and all races; however, certain types of cellulitis/microorganisms occur in certain populations. Community-acquired methicillin-resistant *Staphylococcus aureus* [CA-MRSA] has increased in athletes in contact sports (i.e., wrestling).

ETIOLOGY AND PATHOPHYSIOLOGY
Cellulitis is caused by bacterial penetration through a break in the skin. Hyaluronidase mediates subcutaneous (SC) spread.
- Microbiology
  - β-Hemolytic streptococci (groups A, B, C, G, and F), *S. aureus*, including MRSA and gram-negative aerobic bacilli, are the most common.
  - *S. aureus*: periorbital and orbital cellulitis and IV drug users
  - *Pseudomonas aeruginosa*: diabetics and other immunocompromised patients
  - *Aeromonas hydrophila* and *Vibrio vulnificus*: cellulitis caused by waterborne pathogens
  - *H. influenzae*: buccal cellulitis
  - Clostridia and non–spore-forming anaerobes: necrotizing cellulitis (crepitant/gangrenous)
  - *Streptococcus agalactiae*: cellulitis following lymph node dissection
  - *Pasteurella multocida* and *Capnocytophaga canimorsus*: cellulitis preceded by bites
  - *Streptococcus iniae*: immunocompromised hosts
  - Rare causes: *Mycobacterium*, fungal (mucormycosis, aspergillosis, syphilis)

Genetics
No genetic pattern

RISK FACTORS
- Disruption of skin barrier: trauma, infection, insect bites, injection drug use, body piercing
- Inflammation: eczema or radiation therapy
- Edema due to venous insufficiency. Lymphatic obstruction due to surgical procedures or congestive heart failure
- Elderly, diabetes, hypertension, obesity
- Recurrent cellulitis:

  - Cellulitis recurrence score (2)[A]
  - Recurrent cellulitis is seen in immunocompromised patients (HIV/AIDS, steroids and TNF-α inhibitor therapy, diabetes, hypertension, cancer, peripheral arterial or venous diseases, chronic kidney disease, dialysis, IV or SC drug use (2)[A].

GENERAL PREVENTION
- Good skin hygiene
- Support stockings to decrease edema
- Maintain tight glycemic control and proper foot care in diabetic patients

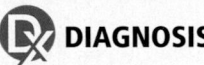 **DIAGNOSIS**

Primarily a clinical diagnosis

HISTORY
- Previous trauma, surgery, animal/human bites, dermatitis, fungal infection; all serve as a portal of entry for bacterial pathogens.
- Pain, itching, and/or burning
- Fever, chills, and malaise

PHYSICAL EXAM
- Localized pain and tenderness with erythema, induration, swelling, and warmth
- Peau d'orange appearance
- Regional lymphadenopathy
- Purulent drainage (from abscesses)
- Orbital cellulitis: proptosis, globe displacement, limitation of ocular movements, vision loss, diplopia
- Facial cellulitis: malaise, anorexia, vomiting, pruritus, burning, anterior neck swelling

DIFFERENTIAL DIAGNOSIS
Toxic shock syndrome, venous stasis dermatitis (commonly mistaken as cellulitis), bursitis, acute dermatitis or intertrigo, herpes zoster or herpetic whitlow, deep vein thrombosis or thrombophlebitis, acute gout or pseudogout, necrotizing fasciitis or myositis, gas gangrene, osteomyelitis, erythema chronicum migrans or malignancy, drug reaction, sunburn, or insect stings. Spider bites and MRSA cellulitis can present similarly.

DIAGNOSTIC TESTS & INTERPRETATION
Initial Tests (lab, imaging)
- If there are signs of systemic disease (fever, heart rate >100 bpm, or systolic blood pressure <90 mm Hg): blood cultures, CPK, CRP. Consider serum lactate levels.
- WBC has 84% specificity and 43% sensitivity; whereas CRP had a sensitivity of 67% and specificity of 95% (PPV 95% and NPV 68%).
- Aspirates from point of maximum inflammation yield 45% positive culture compared with 5% from leading edge
- Blood cultures: Pathogens are isolated in <5% of patients. Blood cultures in children are more likely to show a contaminant than true positive.
- Swab open cellulitis wounds for culture.
- Plain radiographs, CT, or MRI are useful if osteomyelitis, fracture, necrotizing fasciitis, or retained foreign body is suspected or underlying abscess.
- Gallium[67] scintillography helps detect cellulitis superimposed on chronic limb lymphedema.

Diagnostic Procedures/Other
Consider lumbar puncture in children with *H. influenzae* type B or if meningeal signs and facial cellulitis.

 TREATMENT

GENERAL MEASURES
- Immobilize and elevate the involved limb to reduce swelling.
- Sterile saline dressings or cool aluminum acetate compresses for pain relief
- Edema: compression stocking, pneumatic pumps. Diuretic therapy for CHF patients
- Mark the area of cellulitis to monitor progression.
- Tetanus immunization if needed, particularly if there is an open (traumatic) wound

MEDICATION
First Line
- Target treatment in the setting of known pathogens or certain exposure (animal bites)
- Antibiotic selection relies on clinical presentation:
  - Nonpurulent cellulitis
    - With nonpurulent drainage, target treatment toward β-hemolytic streptococci and MSSA.
    - Outpatient: treatment duration of 5 to 10 days
      - Oral: for mild cellulitis
        - Cephalexin 500 mg PO q6h; children: 25 to 50 mg/kg/day in 3 to 4 doses
        - Dicloxacillin 500 mg PO q6h; children: 25 to 50 mg/kg/day in 4 doses
        - Clindamycin 300 to 450 mg PO q6–8h; children: 20 to 30 mg/kg/day in 4 doses
      - IV: for rapidly progressing cellulitis
        - Cefazolin 1 to 2 g IV q8h; children: 100 mg/kg/day IV in 2 to 4 divided doses
        - Oxacillin 2 g IV q4h; children: 150 to 200 mg/kg/day IV in 4 to 6 doses
        - Nafcillin 2 g IV q4h; children: 150 to 200 mg/kg/day IV in 4 to 6 doses
        - Clindamycin 600 to 900 mg IV q8h; children: 25 to 40 mg/kg/day IV in 3 to 4 doses

- Purulent cellulitis (probable CA-MRSA)
  – Culture all purulent wounds and follow up in 48 hours.
  – Incise and drain abscess and start empiric antibiotic therapy. Modify based on culture results; tailor duration based on clinical response (3)[B]:
    ○ Oral
      ▪ Clindamycin 300 to 450 mg PO; children: 40 mg/kg/day in 3 to 4 doses
      ▪ Trimethoprim-sulfamethoxazole (TMP-SMZ) 1 DS tab PO BID; children: dose based on TMP at 8 to 12 mg/kg/day divided in 2 doses
      ▪ Doxycycline 100 mg PO BID; children >8 years of age: ≤45 kg: 4 mg/kg/day divided in 2 doses; >45 kg: 100 mg PO BID
      ▪ Minocycline 200 mg PO once, then 100 mg PO BID; children >8 years old: 4 mg/kg PO once, then 4 mg/kg PO BID
      ▪ Linezolid 600 mg PO BID; children <12 years: 10 mg/kg/dose (max 600 mg/dose) PO TID; ≥12 years: 600 mg PO BID
      ▪ Tedizolid 200 mg PO once daily; children: Dosing is not established.
    ○ IV
      ▪ Vancomycin 15 to 20 mg/kg/dose IV every 8 to 12 hours
      ▪ Daptomycin 4 mg/kg/dose IV once daily; if bacteremia is present or suspected: 6 mg/kg IV once daily
      ▪ Linezolid 600 mg IV BID
      ▪ Tedizolid 200 mg IV once daily
      ▪ Ceftaroline 600 mg IV q12h
      ▪ Tigecycline 100 mg IV once, thereafter 50 mg IV q12h
- Necrotizing cellulitis: requires broad-spectrum coverage to cover clostridial and anaerobic species: ampicillin-sulbactam 1.5 to 3.0 g q6–8h IV or piperacillin-tazobactam 3.37 g q6–8h IV plus ciprofloxacin 400 mg q12h IV plus clindamycin 600 to 900 mg q8h IV
- Freshwater exposure: penicillinase-resistant: penicillin plus gentamicin or fluoroquinolone; in salt water exposure: doxycycline 200 mg IV in 2 divided doses
- Bites: The combination of amoxicillin and clavulanic acid is recommended for human and dog bites. Ticarcillin and clavulanic acid or the combination of a 3rd-generation cephalosporin (i.e., ceftriaxone) plus metronidazole provides adequate parenteral therapy for animal or human bites. If allergic to penicillin, use fluoroquinolone plus metronidazole.
- Facial cellulitis in adults: ceftriaxone IV
- Diabetic foot infection: ampicillin/sulbactam or imipenem/cilastatin or meropenem; alternative: combinations of targeting anaerobes as well as gram-positive and gram-negative aerobes
- If severe infection, toxicity, immunocompromised patients, or worsening infection despite empirical therapy, admit for empiric antibiotic therapy covering MRSA.
- Recurrent streptococcal cellulitis: penicillin 250 mg BID, or if penicillin-allergic, use erythromycin 250 mg BID

Pediatric Considerations
- Avoid doxycycline in children ≥8 years old and during pregnancy.

Second Line
Mild infection
- Penicillin allergy: erythromycin 500 mg PO q6h
- Cephalexin remains a cost-effective therapy for outpatient management of cellulitis at current estimated MRSA levels.

SURGERY/OTHER PROCEDURES
- Débridement for gas and purulent matter
- Intubation or tracheotomy may be needed for cellulitis of the head or neck.

INPATIENT CONSIDERATIONS
Admission Criteria/Initial Stabilization
- Severe infection, suspicion of deeper or rapidly spreading infection, tissue necrosis, or severe pain
- Marked systemic toxicity or worsening symptoms that do not resolve after 24 to 48 hours of therapy
- Patients with underlying risk factors or severe comorbidities

 ONGOING CARE

FOLLOW-UP RECOMMENDATIONS
Patient Monitoring
- Repeat relevant labs (blood culture, CBC, potentially LP) if patient is toxic or not improving.
- Consider deep vein thrombosis prophylaxis.
- Cutaneous inflammation may worsen in the first 24 hours due to release of bacterial antigens. Symptomatic improvement usually occurs in 24 to 48 hours, but visible improvement may take 72 hours.

DIET
Glucose control in diabetics

PATIENT EDUCATION
Good skin hygiene.

PROGNOSIS
With adequate antibiotic treatment, prognosis is good.

- Low-dose penicillin prophylaxis in patients with recurrent cellulitis decreases recurrence (4)[A].

COMPLICATIONS
- Local abscess or bacteremia, sepsis
- Superinfection with gram-negative organisms
- Lymphangitis, especially if recurrent
- Thrombophlebitis or venous thrombosis
- Bacterial meningitis
- Gangrene

REFERENCES

1. Figtree M, Konecny P, Jennings Z, et al. Risk stratification and outcome of cellulitis admitted to hospital. *J Infect*. 2010;60(6):431–439.
2. Tay EY, Fook-Chong S, Oh CC, et al. Cellulitis recurrence score: a tool for predicting recurrence of lower limb cellulitis. *J Am Acad Dermatol*. 2015;72(1):140–145.
3. Champion AE, Goodwin TA, Brolinson PG, et al. Prevalence and characterization of methicillin-resistant *Staphylococcus aureus* isolates from healthy university student athletes. *Ann Clin Microbiol Antimicrob*. 2014;13(1):33.
4. Thomas KS, Crook AM, Nunn AJ, et al. Penicillin to prevent recurrent leg cellulitis. *N Engl J Med*. 2013;368(18):1695–1703.

ADDITIONAL READING

- Brook I. Management of human and animal bite wounds: an overview. *Adv Skin Wound Care*. 2005;18(4):197–203.
- Gunderson CG. Cellulitis: definition, etiology, and clinical features. *Am J Med*. 2011;124(12): 1113–1122.
- Kilburn SA, Featherstone P, Higgins B, et al. Interventions for cellulitis and erysipelas. *Cochrane Database Syst Rev*. 2010;(6):CD004299.
- Liu C, Bayer A, Cosgrove SE, et al. Clinical practice guidelines by the Infectious Diseases Society of America for the treatment of methicillin-resistant *Staphylococcus aureus* infections in adults and children. *Clin Infect Dis*. 2011;52(3):285–292.
- Oh CC, Ko HC, Lee HY, et al. Antibiotic prophylaxis for preventing recurrent cellulitis: a systematic review and meta-analysis. *J Infect*. 2014;69(1):26–34.
- Phoenix G, Das S, Joshi M. Diagnosis and management of cellulitis. *BMJ*. 2012;345:e4955.
- Quirke M, O'Sullivan R, McCabe A, et al. Are two penicillins better than one? A systematic review of oral flucloxacillin and penicillin V versus oral flucloxacillin alone for the emergency department treatment of cellulitis. *Eur J Emerg Med*. 2013;21(3):170–174.

 CODES

ICD10
- L03.90 Cellulitis, unspecified
- H05.019 Cellulitis of unspecified orbit
- L03.211 Cellulitis of face

CLINICAL PEARLS
- *S. aureus* and group A *Streptococcus* are the most common organisms that cause cellulitis.
- Consider MRSA if cellulitis is not responding to antibiotics in the first 48 hours.
- Rapid expansion of infected area with red/purple discoloration and severe pain may suggest necrotizing fasciitis, requiring urgent surgical evaluation.

CELLULITIS, ORBITAL
Robert Thomas Carlisle, MD, MPH

 BASICS

DESCRIPTION
- Acute, severe, vision-threatening infection of orbital contents posterior to orbital septum. Preseptal (previously referred to as periorbital) cellulitis is anterior to the septum. Distinguishing location determines the appropriate workup and treatment (1).
- Synonym(s): postseptal cellulitis

ALERT
- Differentiating orbital from preseptal cellulitis is the critical diagnostic step. Preseptal cellulitis can be identified at exam or, if needed, by CT scan.
- Diplopia, proptosis, vision loss, and fever suggest orbital involvement.
- Contrast CT is the imaging method of choice and should be done for suspicion of orbital cellulitis.
- Treat with immediate IV antibiotics; hospital admission and ophthalmology referral.
- Monitor frequently for vision loss, cavernous sinus thrombosis, abscess, and meningitis.
- Intraorbital foreign body (FB) may cause delayed orbital cellulitis.

EPIDEMIOLOGY
- No difference in frequency between genders in adults
- More common in children; mean age of surgical cases: 10.1 years; medical pediatric cases: 6.1 years
- Much less common than preseptal cellulitis

Incidence
Orbital cellulitis has declined since *Haemophilus influenzae* type b (Hib) vaccine was introduced in 1985. In 2000, incidence per 100,000 in California was 3.5 in whites, 6.1 in blacks, and 3.2 in Hispanics, compared to 6.5 in whites, 10.2 in blacks, and 5.5 in Hispanics in 1990.

ETIOLOGY AND PATHOPHYSIOLOGY
- Sinusitis is a major risk factor.
- The ethmoid sinus is separated from the orbit by the lamina papyracea ("layer of paper"), a thin bony separation, and is often the source of contiguous spread of infection to the orbit.
- The orbital septum is a connective tissue barrier that extends from the skull into the lid and separates the preseptal from the orbital space.
- Cellulitis in the closed bony orbit causes proptosis, globe displacement, orbital apex syndrome (mass effect on the cranial nerves), optic nerve compression, and vision loss.
- Orbital abscess (medial wall most common), meningitis, and cavernous sinus thrombosis may occur.
- Blood cultures are often negative.
- Cultures of surgical specimens in adults often grow multiple organisms, but >1/3 of cases have no pathogen recovered (2)[B].
- Most common organisms (3,4)[C]:
  - *Staphylococcus aureus*, *Streptococcus pneumoniae*, *Streptococcus anginosus*
- Less common organisms:
  - *Moraxella catarrhalis*, *H. influenzae*, group A β-hemolytic *Streptococcus*, *Pseudomonas aeruginosa*, anaerobes, phycomycosis (mucormycosis), aspergillosis, *Mycobacterium tuberculosis*, *Mycobacterium avium* complex, trichinosis, *Echinococcus*

- Hib was the most common organism prior to Hib vaccine, Since routine Hib vaccination in 1992, *Haemophilus* is no longer the leading cause of orbital cellulitis (3,4)[B].

Genetics
No known genetic predisposition

RISK FACTORS
- Sinusitis is present in 80–90% of cases (3)[C].
- Orbital trauma, retained orbital FB, ophthalmic surgery
- Dental, periorbital, skin, or intracranial infection; acute dacryocystitis and acute dacryoadenitis
- Immunosuppressed patients at increased of adverse outcomes

GENERAL PREVENTION
- Routine Hib vaccination
- Appropriate treatment of bacterial sinusitis
- Proper wound care and perioperative monitoring of orbital surgery and trauma
- Avoid trauma to the sinus passages.
- High index of suspicion in febrile patients presenting with eyelid and conjunctival pain, swelling, and erythema.

COMMONLY ASSOCIATED CONDITIONS
- >80% cases have contiguous sinusitis.
- Trauma and intraorbital FB
- Preseptal cellulitis
- Adverse outcomes of orbital apex syndrome, vision loss, ophthalmoplegia, abscess, meningitis, or cavernous sinus thrombosis

 DIAGNOSIS

HISTORY
- Complaints of acute onset red, swollen, tender eye or eyelid and pain with eye movements (5)[C]
- History of surgery, trauma, sinus or upper respiratory infection, dental infection
- Malaise, fever, stiff neck, mental status changes
- Specific signs of orbital cellulitis include:
  - Proptosis, double vision, ophthalmoplegia, vision loss (or decreased field of vision), pain with eye movement, decreased color vision (5)[C]

ALERT
- Severe septic appearance, mental status changes, contralateral cranial nerve palsy, or bilateral orbital cellulitis may indicate CNS involvement.
- MRSA orbital cellulitis may present without associated upper respiratory infection.

PHYSICAL EXAM
- Vital signs
  - Assess visual acuity (with glasses if required).
  - Lid exam and palpation of the orbit
  - Pupillary reflex for afferent pupillary defect
  - Extraocular movements; assess for pain with eye movement—if present, concerning for orbital cellulitis.
  - Red desaturation: Patient views red object with one eye and compares to the other; reduced red color may indicate optic nerve involvement.
  - Confrontation visual field testing

DIFFERENTIAL DIAGNOSIS
- Preseptal cellulitis
  - Eyelid erythema with or without conjunctival erythema, afebrile, no pain on eye movement, no diplopia, normal eye exam, vision intact (5)[C]
- Metastatic tumors and autoimmune inflammation may masquerade as orbital cellulitis in rare cases. Usually present with painless slow onset of symptoms
- Idiopathic orbital inflammatory disease (orbital pseudotumor) (3)[C]
  - Afebrile, normal WBCs; usually subacute, may have pain, responds to steroids
- Orbital FB
- Arteriovenous fistula (carotid-cavernous fistula)
  - Spontaneous or due to trauma; bruit may be present. Insidious, subacute onset
- Cavernous sinus thrombosis
  - Signs of orbital cellulitis with cranial nerves III, IV, V, and VI findings; often bilateral and acute
  - Severely ill
- Acute thyroid orbitopathy
  - Afebrile; possible signs of thyroid disease
  - Bilateral orbital involvement
- Orbital tumor
  - Acute rhabdomyosarcoma in children; acute lymphoblastic leukemia, or metastatic
  - Unilateral
  - Slow onset
- Trauma, insect bite, ruptured dermoid cyst (6)
- Clinical signs help distinguish preseptal from orbital cellulitis. Preseptal infection causes erythema, induration, and tenderness of the eyelid and/or periorbital tissues, and patients rarely show signs of systemic illness. Local skin trauma, lacerations, or bug bites can be seen. Extraocular movements and visual acuity are intact.
- Orbital cellulitis also presents with complaints of a red, swollen, painful eye or eyelid. It also results in proptosis, conjunctival edema, ophthalmoplegia (diminished ocular movement), or decreased visual acuity (7)[C].

- Staging in cases resulting from acute sinusitis (3)[A]
  - Stage I: no abscess
  - Stage IIa, b, c: small, large, or extending medial subperiosteal abscess
  - Stage III: orbital abscess
- Chandler staging: (6)[C]
  - Stage I: periorbital cellulitis (considered different entity)
  - Stage II: orbital lining edema, chemosis, proptosis, limitation of extraocular movement, fever
  - Stage III: includes stage II with subperiosteal abscess and occasional vision loss
  - Stage IV: orbital abscess, ophthalmoplegia with vision loss
  - Stage V: extension to cavernous sinus, subdural space, meninges, or brain (3,7)

DIAGNOSTIC TESTS & INTERPRETATION
- CBC with differential, C-reactive protein, ESR
- Cultures of eye secretions or nasopharyngeal aspirates are often contaminated by normal flora but may identify causative organism(s).
- Cultures from orbital and sinus abscesses more often yield positive results but should be limited

to cases where invasive procedures are indicated. Cultures from sinus aspirates and abscesses may grow multiple organisms.

- Blood cultures (often negative) should be obtained prior to initiation of antibiotic therapy.

Initial Tests (lab, imaging)

- CT scan of orbits and sinuses with axial and coronal views, with and without contrast, is the diagnostic modality of choice (8)[C]. US and MRI are alternatives (9)[B].

  – Thin section (2 mm) CT, coronal and axial views with bone windows to differentiate preseptal from orbital cellulitis, confirm extension into orbit, detect coexisting sinus disease, and identify orbital or subperiosteal abscesses that may require surgery.
  – Deviation of medial rectus indicates intraorbital involvement.
- MRI offers superior soft tissue resolution for identification of cavernous sinus thrombosis but is less effective for bone imaging.
- US is used to rule out orbital myositis, locate FBs or abscesses, and follow progression of drained abscess.

Follow-Up Tests & Special Considerations

- Consider a full-septic evaluation (including LP) before antibiotics in toxic patients or if meningitis is suspected (6)[C].
- Frequent eye exam and vital signs (q4h) are essential for timely treatment of associated conditions, such as meningitis or orbital abscess.

Diagnostic Procedures/Other

Consult ophthalmology for slit lamp and dilated funduscopic exam; exophthalmometry measurement for proptosis, color vision, automated visual field; and need for surgery.

TREATMENT

Admit patients with orbital cellulitis for monitoring of ocular status and treatment with broad-spectrum antibiotics (2).

MEDICATION

- Empiric antibiotic therapy to cover pathogens associated with acute sinusitis (*S. pneumoniae*, *H. influenzae*, *M. catarrhalis*, *Streptococcus pyogenes*), as well as for *S. aureus*, *S. anginosus*, and anaerobes
- Modify IV antibiotic treatment when sensitivities are available. Duration of IV therapy is usually a week, with additional PO therapy depending on response.
- PO antibiotic therapy for 2 to 3 weeks or longer (3 to 6 weeks) is recommended for patients with severe sinusitis and bony destruction.

First Line

- Ampicillin/sulbactam (Unasyn) or ceftriaxone plus metronidazole or clindamycin if anaerobic infection is suspected (2)
  – Ampicillin/sulbactam: 3 g IV q6h for adult; 200 to 300 mg/kg/day divided q6h for children
  – Ceftriaxone: 1 to 2 g IV q12h for adults or 100 mg/kg/day divided BID in children with max 4 g/day
  – Clindamycin: 600 mg IV q8h for adults; 20 to 40 mg/kg/day IV q6–8h for children (10)
  – Metronidazole: 500 mg IV q8 h for adult; 30 to 35 mg/kg/day divided q8h for children

- ALERT: In severe orbital cellulitis and in suspected or culture-proven MRSA infection, vancomycin remains the parenteral drug of choice. Use in conjunction with agents to cover gram-negative bacteria.
  – Vancomycin: 1 g IV q12h for adults; 40 mg/kg/day IV divided q8–12h, max daily dose 2 g for children (2)

ADDITIONAL THERAPIES

- Steroid use is controversial (3)[C].
- PO steroids as an adjunct to IV antibiotics for orbital cellulitis may speed resolution of inflammation (11)[C].
- Topical erythromycin or nonmedicated ophthalmic ointment protects the eye from exposure in cases with severe proptosis.
- PO antibiotics for ≥2 weeks are traditionally recommended following IV treatment.
- Children may be treated with amoxicillin/clavulanate 20 to 40 mg/kg/day divided TID or in adults 250 to 500 mg TID.

ISSUES FOR REFERRAL

Always admit to the hospital and consult with ophthalmology. Consider consultation with ID and ENT for orbital cellulitis; neurology/neurosurgery if intracranial spread is suspected

SURGERY/OTHER PROCEDURES

- IV antibiotic therapy is the initial therapy.
- Surgical intervention warranted for visual loss, complete ophthalmoplegia, or well-defined large abscess (>10 mm) on presentation or no clinical improvement after 24 to 48 hours of antibiotic therapy
- Trauma cases may need débridement or FB removal.
- Orbital abscess may need surgical drainage.
- Surgical drainage with 4 to 8 weeks of antibiotics is the treatment of choice for brain abscess.
- Surgical interventions may include external ethmoidectomy, endoscopic ethmoidectomy, uncinectomy, antrostomy, and subperiosteal drainage.

INPATIENT CONSIDERATIONS

Patients with orbital cellulitis should be admitted for IV antibiotics and serial eye exams to evaluate progression of infection or involvement of optic nerve.

- Follow temperature, WBC, visual acuity, pupillary reflex, ocular motility, and proptosis.
- Repeat CT scan, or surgical intervention, may be required for worsening orbital cellulitis cases.

ONGOING CARE

FOLLOW-UP RECOMMENDATIONS
Patient Monitoring
Serial visual acuity testing and slit lamp exams

ALERT
Bedside exam q4h is indicated, as complications can develop rapidly.

PATIENT EDUCATION

- Maintain proper hand washing and good skin hygiene.
- Avoid skin or lid trauma.

COMPLICATIONS

- Vision loss, CNS involvement, and death
- Permanent vision loss
  – Corneal exposure
  – Optic neuritis
  – Endophthalmitis

– Septic uveitis or retinitis
– Exudative retinal detachment
– Retinal artery or vein occlusions
– Globe rupture
– Orbital compartment syndrome
- CNS complications

– Intracranial abscess, meningitis, cavernous sinus thrombosis (4)[B]

REFERENCES

1. Pasternak A, Irish B. Ophthalmologic infections in primary care. *Clin Fam Pract.* 2004;6(1):19–33.
2. Seltz LB, Smith J, Durairaj VD, et al. Microbiology and antibiotic management of orbital cellulitis. *Pediatrics.* 2011;127(3):e566–e572.
3. Chadha NK. An evidence-based staging system for orbital infections from acute rhinosinusitis. *Laryngoscope.* 2012;122(Suppl 4):S95–S96.
4. Hauser A, Fogarasi S. Periorbital and orbital cellulitis. *Pediatr Rev.* 2010;31(6):242–249.
5. Carlisle RT, Digiovanni J. Differential diagnosis of the swollen red eyelid. *Am Fam Physician.* 2015;92(2):106–112.
6. Kloek CE, Rubin PA. Role of inflammation in orbital cellulitis. *Int Ophthalmol Clin.* 2006;46(2):57–68.
7. Distinguishing periorbital from orbital cellulitis. *Am Fam Physician.* 2003;67(6):1349–1353.
8. Mahalingam-Dhingra A, Lander L, Preciado DA, et al. Orbital and periorbital infections: a national perspective. *Arch Otolaryngol Head Neck Surg.* 2011;137(8):769–773.
9. Rudloe TF, Harper MB, Prabhu SP, et al. Acute periorbital infections: who needs emergent imaging? *Pediatrics.* 2010;125(4):e719–e726.
10. Bedwell J, Bauman NM. Management of pediatric orbital cellulitis and abscess. *Curr Opin Otolaryngol Head Neck Surg.* 2011;19(6):467–473.
11. Pushker N, Tejwani LK, Bajaj MS, et al. Role of oral corticosteroids in orbital cellulitis. *Am J Ophthalmol.* 2013;156(1):178.e1–183.e1.

CODES

ICD10

- H05.019 Cellulitis of unspecified orbit
- H05.011 Cellulitis of right orbit
- H05.012 Cellulitis of left orbit

CLINICAL PEARLS

- Most orbital cellulitis cases result from sinusitis.
- MRSA orbital cellulitis may present without associated upper respiratory infection.
- CT of orbits and sinuses with axial and coronal views with and without contrast is diagnostic modality of choice for suspected cases of orbital cellulitis.
- Patients with orbital cellulitis should be admitted for visual monitoring and IV antibiotic therapy.
- Older age (>10 years) and diplopia may predict need for surgical intervention in children.
- Ophthalmoplegia, mental status changes, contralateral cranial nerve palsy, or bilateral orbital cellulitis raise suspicion for intracranial involvement.

CELLULITIS, PERIORBITAL

Fozia Akhtar Ali, MD • Mohammad Ansar Mughal, MD

BASICS

DESCRIPTION
- An acute bacterial infection of the skin and subcutaneous tissue anterior to the orbital septum; not involving the orbital structures (globe, fat, and ocular muscles)
- Synonym(s): preseptal cellulitis

ALERT
It is essential to distinguish periorbital cellulitis from orbital cellulitis. Orbital cellulitis is a potentially life-threatening condition. *Orbital cellulitis is posterior to the orbital septum; symptoms include restricted eye movement, pain with eye movement, proptosis, and vision changes.*

EPIDEMIOLOGY
- Occurs more commonly in children; mean age 21 months
- 3 times more common than orbital cellulitis (1)[C]

Incidence
- Increased incidence in the winter months (due to increased cases of sinusitis) (1)[C]

ETIOLOGY AND PATHOPHYSIOLOGY
- The anatomy of the eyelid distinguishes periorbital (preseptal) from orbital cellulitis:
  - A connective tissue sheet (orbital septum) extends from the orbital bones to the margins of the upper and lower eyelids; it acts as a barrier to infection deep in the orbital structures.
  - Infection of tissues anterior to the orbital septum is periorbital (preseptal) cellulitis.
  - Infection deep to the orbital septum is orbital (postseptal) cellulitis.
- Periorbital cellulitis classically arises from a contiguous infection of soft tissues of the face.
  - Sinusitis (via lamina papyracea) extension
  - Local trauma; insect or animal bites
  - Foreign bodies
  - Dental abscess extension
  - Hematogenous seeding
- Common organisms (1)[C]
  - *Staphylococcus aureus*, typically MSSA (MRSA is increasing)
  - *Staphylococcus epidermidis*
  - *Streptococcus pyogenes*
- Atypical organisms
  - *Acinetobacter* sp.; *Nocardia brasiliensis*
  - *Bacillus anthracis*; *Pseudomonas aeruginosa*
  - *Neisseria gonorrhoeae*; *Proteus* sp.
  - *Pasteurella multocida*; *Mycobacterium tuberculosis*; *Trichophyton* sp. (ringworm)

- Since vaccine introduction, the incidence of *Haemophilus influenzae* has decreased. This organism should still be suspected in unimmunized or partially immunized patients.

Genetics
No known genetic predisposition.

RISK FACTORS
- Contiguous spread from upper respiratory infection
- Sinusitis
- Local skin trauma/puncture wound
- Insect bite
- Bacteremia

GENERAL PREVENTION
- Avoid dermatologic trauma around the eyes.
- Avoid swimming in fresh or salt water with facial skin abrasions.
- Routine vaccination: particularly *H. influenzae* type B and *Streptococcus pneumoniae*

DIAGNOSIS

HISTORY
- Induration, erythema, warmth, and/or tenderness of periorbital soft tissue, usually with normal vision and normal eye movements
- Chemosis (conjunctival swelling), proptosis; pain with extraocular eye movements can occur in severe cases of periorbital cellulitis, although these symptoms are more common with (and concerning for) orbital cellulitis.
- Fever (not always present)

ALERT
Pain with eye movement, fever, and conjunctival swelling raise the suspicion for orbital cellulitis.

PHYSICAL EXAM
- Vital signs and general appearance. (Patients with orbital cellulitis often appear systemically ill.)
- Thorough inspection of the eye and surrounding structures—lids, lashes, conjunctiva, and skin
- Erythema, swelling, and tenderness of lids without orbital congestion
  - Violaceous discoloration of eyelid is more commonly associated with *H. influenzae*.
- Evaluate for any skin break.
- Look for vesicles to rule out herpetic infection.
- Inspect nasal vaults and palpate sinuses for signs of acute sinusitis.
- Examine oral cavity for dental abscesses.
- Test ocular motility and visual acuity.

DIFFERENTIAL DIAGNOSIS
- Orbital cellulitis
  - Orbital cellulitis may have the same signs and symptoms as periorbital cellulitis, with more extensive proptosis, chemosis, ophthalmoplegia, decreased visual acuity, or fever.
- Abscess
- Dacryocystitis
- Hordeolum (stye)
- Allergic inflammation
- Orbital or periorbital trauma
- Idiopathic inflammation from orbital pseudotumor
- Orbital myositis
- Rapidly progressive tumors
  - Rhabdomyosarcoma
  - Retinoblastoma
  - Lymphoma
- Leukemia

DIAGNOSTIC TESTS & INTERPRETATION
Initial Tests (lab, imaging)
- CBC with differential
- Blood cultures (low yield) (2)[C]
- Wound culture of purulent drainage (if present)
- Imaging is indicated if there is suspicion for orbital cellulitis (marked eyelid swelling, fever, and leukocytosis or those who fail to improve on appropriate antibiotics in 24 to 48 hours).

- CT can evaluate the extent of infection and detect orbital inflammation or abscess (3)[B]:
  - The classic sign of orbital cellulitis on CT scan is bulging of the medial rectus.
  - CT should be performed with contrast, thin sections (2 mm); coronal and axial views with bone windows.

Follow-Up Tests & Special Considerations
- Children with periorbital or orbital cellulitis often have underlying sinusitis.
- If a child is febrile, <15 months old, and appears toxic, admit for blood cultures, antibiotic therapy, and consider lumbar puncture.

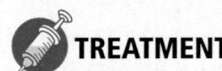

TREATMENT

MEDICATION
- Empiric antibiotic treatment to cover the most likely organisms (*Staphylococcus* and *Streptococcus*) (3)[C]
- Observe local prevalence of MRSA to determine need for coverage therapy.
- No evidence that IV antibiotics are more effective than PO in reducing recovery time or preventing secondary complications in the management of simple periorbital cellulitis (1)[C].
- No evidence for steroid use

First Line
- Uncomplicated posttraumatic
  - Usually due to skin flora, including *Staphylococcus* and *Streptococcus*
  - Cephalexin 500 mg PO q6h or dicloxacillin 500 mg PO q6h
  - Clindamycin 300 mg PO TID, doxycycline 100 mg PO BID, or trimethoprim-sulfamethoxazole (TMP-SMX) 1 to 2 DS tablets PO q12h if MRSA is suspected.
- Extension from sinusitis
  - Amoxicillin-clavulanate 875 mg PO BID
  - 3rd-generation cephalosporin (e.g., cefdinir 300 mg PO BID)
- Dental abscess
  - Amoxicillin-clavulanate 875 mg PO BID or clindamycin 300 mg PO TID
- Bacteremic cellulitis
  - May be associated with meningitis
  - Ceftriaxone 1 g IV q24h plus vancomycin 15 mg/kg/dose IV q8–12h or clindamycin 600 to 900 mg IV q8h to cover MRSA
- Duration of therapy should be 7 to 10 days
  - If symptoms do not improve within 24 hours, IV antibiotic therapy is indicated.

ISSUES FOR REFERRAL
Consult ENT and ophthalmology if there is concern of orbital cellulitis or when 1st-line treatment has failed (4).

SURGERY/OTHER PROCEDURES
- Usually not indicated in uncomplicated cases
- If there is an abscess or potential compromise of critical structures, orbital surgery is indicated.
- Diplopia is the strongest clinical predictor of surgery.

INPATIENT CONSIDERATIONS
Mild cases in adults and children >1 year of age can be managed on an outpatient basis, if the patient is stable and there are no systemic signs of toxicity.

Admission Criteria/Initial Stabilization
- Consider hospitalization and IV antibiotics:
  - If patient appears systemically ill
  - Children <1 year of age (4,5)[C]
  - Patients not immunized against *S. pneumoniae* or *H. influenzae*
  - If no signs of clinical improvement are apparent after 24 hours of antibiotic therapy
  - Cases with high suspicion of orbital cellulitis (eyelid swelling with reduced vision, diplopia, abnormal light reflexes, or proptosis)

Discharge Criteria
- No strict guidelines indicate when to switch from parenteral to PO therapy. In general, switch to PO therapy after the patient is afebrile and the skin findings have begun to resolve (typically 2 to 3 days).
- Continue therapy for 10 to 14 days for orbital cellulitis or complicated periorbital cellulitis.

 ONGOING CARE

FOLLOW-UP RECOMMENDATIONS
Patient Monitoring
Follow for signs of orbital involvement, including decreased visual acuity or painful/limited ocular motility.

PATIENT EDUCATION
- Maintain good skin hygiene.
- Avoid skin trauma.
- Report early skin changes (swelling, redness, and pain) if recurrent after a course of therapy.

PROGNOSIS
- With timely treatment, patients do well.
- A 10-day course of antibiotics is generally sufficient.
- Recurrent periorbital cellulitis occurs with ≥3 periorbital infections in 1 year with at least 1 month of in between episodes; must be differentiated from treatment failure due to antibiotic resistance (1)[C].

COMPLICATIONS
- Orbital cellulitis; orbital abscess formation
- Scarring
- Vision loss
- Cavernous sinus thrombosis
- Osteomyelitis

REFERENCES
1. Hauser A, Fogarasi S. Periorbital and orbital cellulitis. *Pediatr Rev.* 2010;31(6):242–249.
2. Baring DE, Hilmi OJ. An evidence based review of periorbital cellulitis. *Clin Otolaryngol.* 2011;36(1):57–64.
3. Beech T, Robinson A, McDermott AL, et al. Paediatric periorbital cellulitis and its management. *Rhinology.* 2007;45(1):47–49.
4. Upile NS, Munir N, Leong SC, et al. Who should manage acute periorbital cellulitis in children? *Int J Pediatr Otorhinolaryngol.* 2012;76(8):1073–1077.
5. Georgakopoulos CD, Eliopoulou MI, Stasinos S, et al. Periorbital and orbital cellulitis: a 10-year review of hospitalized children. *Eur J Ophthalmol.* 2010;20(6):1066–1072.

ADDITIONAL READING
- Chaudhry IA, Shamsi FA, Elzaridi E, et al. Inpatient preseptal cellulitis: experience from a tertiary eye care centre. *Br J Ophthalmol.* 2008;92(10):1337–1341. doi:10.1136/bjo.2007.128975.
- Goldstein SM, Shelsta HN. Community-acquired methicillin-resistant *Staphylococcus aureus* periorbital cellulitis: a problem here to stay. *Ophthal Plast Reconstr Surg.* 2009;25(1):77.
- Mahalingam-Dhingra A, Lander L, Preciado DA, et al. Orbital and periorbital infections: a national perspective. *Arch Otolaryngol Head Neck Surg.* 2011;137(8):769–773.
- Yeilding RH, O'Day DM, Li C, et al. Periorbital infections after Dermabond closure of traumatic lacerations in three children. *J AAPOS.* 2012;16(2):168–172.

 CODES

ICD10
L03.211 Cellulitis of face

CLINICAL PEARLS
- Periorbital (preseptal) and orbital (postseptal) cellulitis occur most commonly in children.
- It is critical to differentiate between periorbital cellulitis and orbital cellulitis; the latter is more dangerous and can be life threatening. Orbital cellulitis typically has fever, pain with eye movement, diplopia and/or proptosis. Prompt imaging is necessary if there is a concern for orbital cellulitis.
- CT scan of the patient's sinuses and orbits can be used to differentiate periorbital cellulitis from orbital cellulitis.
- The two most important predisposing factors for periorbital cellulitis are upper respiratory infections and eyelid trauma; sinusitis is more typically associated with orbital cellulitis (5)[C].

CEREBRAL PALSY

Christina Mezzone, DO, MS • Maria Lombardi, DO

BASICS

DESCRIPTION
Cerebral palsy (CP) is a group of clinical syndromes characterized by motor and postural dysfunction due to permanent and nonprogressive disruptions in the developing brain. Motor impairment resulting in activity limitation is necessary for this diagnosis. CP is classified by the nature of the movement disorder and its functional severity. Individuals with this disorder are affected with secondary musculoskeletal and neurologic problems (intellectual, sensory, speech and language impairment, and seizures).

EPIDEMIOLOGY
Incidence
- Overall, 1.5 to 2.5/1,000 live births
- Incidence increases as gestational age (GA) at birth decreases:
  - 146/1,000 for GA of 22 to 27 weeks
  - 62/1,000 for GA of 28 to 31 weeks
  - 7/1,000 for GA of 32 to 36 weeks
  - 1/1,000 for GA of 37+ weeks

Prevalence
3 to 4/1,000 of the population

ETIOLOGY AND PATHOPHYSIOLOGY
- Multifactorial; CP results from static injury or lesions in the developing brain, occurring prenatally, perinatally, or postnatally.
- Neuropathology linked to GA at time of brain insult
- Cytokines, free radicals, and inflammatory response are likely contributing factors.
- Etiology is most likely multifactorial and depends on timing of brain insult: prenatally, perinatally, or postnatally (see "Risk Factors").
- Spastic CP is most common, usually related to premature birth, with either periventricular leukomalacia or germinal matrix hemorrhage.
- Dystonic or athetotic CP, often resulting from kernicterus, is now rare due to improved management of hyperbilirubinemia.

Genetics
There are reports of associations between CP and polymorphisms of certain genes: thrombophilic, cytokines, and apolipoprotein E.

RISK FACTORS
- Prenatal: congenital anomalies, multiple gestation, in utero stroke, intrauterine infection (cytomegalovirus [CMV], varicella), intrauterine growth retardation (IUGR), clinical and histologic chorioamnionitis, antepartum bleeding, maternal factors (cognitive impairment, seizure disorders, hyperthyroidism), abnormal fetal position (e.g., breech)
- Perinatal: preterm birth, low birth weight, periventricular leukomalacia, perinatal hypoxia/asphyxia, intracranial hemorrhage/intraventricular hemorrhage, neonatal seizure or stroke, hyperbilirubinemia
- Postnatal: traumatic brain injury or stroke, sepsis, meningitis, encephalitis, asphyxia, and progressive hydrocephalus

GENERAL PREVENTION
- Treating mothers with magnesium sulfate during preterm delivery is neuroprotective for fetus and may reduce the risk of CP. Effect on term fetus is unknown.
- Improved management of hyperbilirubinemia with decrease in kernicterus has greatly reduced dyskinetic CP.
- Prevention or reduction of chorioamnionitis and premature births

COMMONLY ASSOCIATED CONDITIONS
- Seizure disorder (22–40%)
- Intellectual impairment (23–44%)
- Behavioral problems
- Speech and language impairment (42–81%)
  - May have an impact on expressive and/or receptive language
  - May be nonverbal
- Sensory impairments
  - Hearing deficits
  - Visual (62–71%): poor visual acuity, strabismus (50%), or hemianopsia
- Feeding impairment, swallowing dysfunction, and aspiration: when severe, may require gastrostomy feedings
- Poor dentition, excessive drooling
- GI conditions: constipation (59%), vomiting (22%), gastroesophageal reflux
- Decreased linear growth and weight abnormalities (under- and overweight)
- Osteopenia
- Bowel and bladder incontinence
- Orthopedic: contractures, hip subluxation/dislocation, scoliosis (60%)

DIAGNOSIS

- A clinical diagnosis including
  - Delayed motor milestones
  - Abnormal tone
  - Abnormal neurologic exam suggesting a cerebral etiology for motor dysfunction
  - Absence of regression (not losing function)
  - Absence of underlying syndromes or alternative explanation for etiology
- Although the pathologic lesion is static, clinical presentation may change as the infant grows and develops.
- Accurate early diagnosis remains difficult. Neurologic abnormalities observed in the first 1 to 2 years of life may resolve; be cautious of diagnosing CP before age 2 years.
- Serial exams are often required for a definitive diagnosis.

HISTORY
- Presentation: concerns over movements or delayed motor development
- Ask about
  - Prenatal, perinatal, and postnatal risk factors
  - Neurobehavioral signs
    ○ Poor feeding/frequent vomiting
    ○ Irritability
  - Timing of motor milestones: Delay in milestones is not sensitive or specific until after 6 months of age.
  - Abnormal spontaneous general movements
  - Asymmetry of movements such as early hand preference
- Regression of motor skills does not occur with CP.

PHYSICAL EXAM
- Assess for more than one type of neurologic impairment:
  - Spasticity: increased tone/reflexes/clonus
  - Dyskinesia: abnormal movements
  - Hypotonia: decreased tone
  - Ataxia: abnormal balance/coordination
- Areas of exam
  - Tone: may be increased or decreased
  - Trunk and head control: often poor but may be advanced due to high tone
  - Reduced strength and motor control
  - Persistence of primitive reflexes
  - Asymmetry of movement or reflexes
  - Decreased joint range of motion and contractures
  - Brisk deep tendon reflexes
  - Clonus
  - Delayed motor milestones: serial exams most effective
  - Gait abnormalities: scissoring, toe-walking
- CP is classified by the following:
  - Muscle tone or movement disorder
    ○ Spasticity
      ■ Unilateral: hemiplegic
      ■ Bilateral: diplegic (lower extremity [LE] > upper extremity [UE] involvement) or quadriplegic (UE ≥ LE involvement)
    ○ Dystonia: hypertonia and reduced movement
    ○ Choreoathetosis: irregular spasmodic involuntary movements of the limbs or facial muscles
    ○ Ataxia: loss of orderly muscular coordination
  - Motor function severity
    ○ The Gross Motor Function Classification System (GMFCS) scores I–IV
      ■ Score of I: ambulates without limitation
      ■ Score of II: ambulates without assistive devices but some limitation
      ■ Score of III: ambulates with assistive mobility devices
      ■ Score of IV: Self-mobility is limited, but technology can help.
      ■ Score of V: Self-mobility is severely limited, even with technology.
    ○ The Manual Ability Classification System (MACS) can be used to assess upper extremity and fine motor function.

DIFFERENTIAL DIAGNOSIS
Benign congenital hypotonia, brachial plexus injury, familial spastic paraplegia, dopa-responsive dystonia, transient toe-walking, muscular dystrophy, metabolic disorders (e.g., glutaric aciduria type 1), mitochondrial disorders, genetic disorders (e.g., Rett syndrome)

DIAGNOSTIC TESTS & INTERPRETATION
CP is a clinical diagnosis based on history, physical, and risk factors. Laboratory testing is not needed to make diagnosis but can help exclude other etiologies.
- Testing for metabolic and genetic syndromes (1)[C]
  - Not routinely obtained in the evaluation for CP.
  - Considered if no specific etiology is identified by neuroimaging or there are atypical features in clinical presentation.
  - Detection of certain brain malformations may warrant genetic or metabolic testing to identify syndromes.
- Screening for coagulopathies: Diagnostic testing for coagulopathies should be considered in children with hemiplegic CP with cerebral infarction identified on neuroimaging (1)[C].

Initial Tests (lab, imaging)
- Neuroimaging is not essential, but it is recommended in children with CP for whom the etiology has not been established (1)[C].
- MRI is preferred to CT if need to determine etiology and timing of a brain insult (1)[C].

- Abnormalities found in 80–90% of patients: brain malformation, cerebral infarction, intraventricular or other intracranial hemorrhage, periventricular leukomalacia, ventricular enlargement, or other CSF space abnormalities

Diagnostic Procedures/Other
- The Communication Function Classification System has recently been developed as another means of assessing verbal performance.
- International Classification of Functioning, Disability and Health for CP have been newly developed to standardize functional assessments.
- Screening for comorbid conditions: developmental delay/intellectual impairment, vision/hearing impairments, speech and language disorders, feeding/swallowing dysfunction, or seizures
- EEGs should only be obtained if there is a history of suspected seizures.

Test Interpretation
Perinatal brain injury may include the following:
- White matter damage
  - Most common in premature infants
  - Periventricular leukomalacia: gliosis with or without focal necrosis with resulting cysts and scarring; may be multiple lesions of various ages. Necrosis can lead to cysts/scarring.
  - Germinal matrix hemorrhage: may lead to intraventricular hemorrhage
- Gray matter damage: more common in term infants; cortical infarcts, focal neuronal damage, myelination abnormalities

 TREATMENT

Focuses on control of symptoms; treatments reduce spasticity to prevent painful contractures, manage comorbid conditions, and optimize functionality and quality of life.

GENERAL MEASURES
- Early intervention programs for preterm infants influences motor and cognitive outcomes (2)[A].
- Referral to early intervention for children ages 0 to 3 years is essential.
- Various therapy modalities enhance functioning:
  - Physical therapy to improve posture stability and gait, motor strength and control, and prevent contractures
  - Occupational therapy to increase functional activities of daily living and other fine motor skills
  - Speech therapy for verbal and nonverbal speech and to aid in feeding
- Equipment optimizes participation in activities:
  - Orthotic splinting (ankle–foot orthosis) maintains functional positioning and prevents contractures.
  - Spinal bracing (body jacket) may slow down scoliosis.
  - Augmentative communication with pictures, switches, or computer systems for nonverbal individuals
  - Therapeutic and functional electrical stimulation decreases activity limitation in gait.
  - Use of adaptive equipment such as crutches, walkers, gait trainers, and wheelchairs for mobility and standers for weight bearing

MEDICATION
First Line
- Diazepam (3)[A]
  - Short-term treatment for generalized spasticity; insufficient evidence on motor function
  - A γ-aminobutyric acid-A ($GABA_A$) agonist that facilitates CNS inhibition at spinal and supraspinal levels to reduce spasticity
  - Adverse effects: ataxia and drowsiness
  - Adult dose: 2 to 12 mg/dose PO q6–12h
  - Pediatric dose (<12 years and <15 kg): <8.5 kg: 0.5 to 1 mg HS; 8.5 to 15 kg: 1 to 2 mg HS; children 5 to 16 years of age and ≥15 kg: 1.25 mg TID
- Botulinum toxin type A (3)[A]
  - Acts at neuromuscular junction to inhibit the release of acetylcholine to reduce tone
  - Injected directly into muscles of interest for localized spasticity; insufficient evidence on motor function
  - Higher functional benefit when combined with occupational therapy
  - Lasts for 12 to 16 weeks following injection

Second Line
- Baclofen (3)[A]
  - $GABA_B$ agonist, facilitates presynaptic inhibition of mono- and polysynaptic reflexes
  - Adverse effects: drowsiness and sedation
  - Abrupt withdrawal symptoms: spasticity, hallucinations, seizures, confusion, hyperthermia
  - Adults: Initial dose is 5 mg TID; increase dosage every 3 days to an average maintenance dose of 20 mg TID 80 mg/day maximum
  - Pediatric dose (>2 years): initial 10 to 15 mg/day. Titrate to effective dose (maximum 40 mg/day). <8 years old: 60 mg/day maximum; >8 years old: 60 mg/day maximum
- Intrathecal baclofen (baclofen pump) (4)[A]
  - Continuous intrathecal route allows greater maximal response with smaller dosage to reduce spasticity.
  - May help ambulatory individuals with gait, but no improvement is seen in nonambulatory patients.
  - Adverse effects: infection, catheter malfunction, CSF leakage

ADDITIONAL THERAPIES
- Multidisciplinary care including ophthalmology; neurology; orthopedics; physiatry along with physical, occupational, and speech therapists
- A primary care "medical home" that coordinates medical and community services, provides support for the patient and the patient's family

SURGERY/OTHER PROCEDURES
- Dorsal root rhizotomy selectively cuts dorsal rootlets from L1–S2. Best for patients with normal intelligence with spastic diplegia. Decreases spasticity in lower limbs when done in conjunction with physiotherapy but associated with adverse effects. Evidence is lacking as to long-term outcomes.
- Surgical treatment of joint dislocations/subluxation, scoliosis management, tendon lengthening, gastrostomy

COMPLEMENTARY & ALTERNATIVE MEDICINE
- Hyperbaric oxygen is controversial and not recommended in those who do not suffer hypoxic ischemic encephalopathy (5)[A].
- Therapeutic horse riding or hippotherapy improves postural control and balance.
- Aquatherapy improves gross motor function in patients with various motor severities (6)[B].

 ONGOING CARE

PROGNOSIS
Reduced lifespan strongly associated with level of functional impairment and intellectual disability

REFERENCES
1. Ashwal S, Russman BS, Blasco PA, et al. Practice parameter: diagnostic assessment of the child with cerebral palsy: report of the Quality Standards Subcommittee of the American Academy of Neurology and the Practice Committee of the Child Neurology Society. *Neurology.* 2004;62(6):851–863.
2. Spittle A, Orton J, Anderson P, et al. Early developmental intervention programmes post-hospital discharge to prevent motor and cognitive impairments in preterm infants. *Cochrane Database Syst Rev.* 2012;(12):CD005495.
3. Delgado MR, Hirtz D, Aisen M, et al. Practice parameter: pharmacologic treatment of spasticity in children and adolescents with cerebral palsy (an evidence-based review): report of the Quality Standards Subcommittee of the American Academy of Neurology and the Practice Committee of the Child Neurology Society. *Neurology.* 2010;74(4):336–343.
4. Pin TW, McCartney L, Lewis J, et al. Use of intrathecal baclofen therapy in ambulant children and adolescents with spasticity and dystonia of cerebral origin: a systematic review. *Dev Med Child Neurol.* 2011;53(10):885–895.
5. Lacey DJ, Stolfi A, Pilati LE. Effects of hyperbaric oxygen on motor function in children with cerebral palsy. *Ann Neurol.* 2012;72(5):695–703.
6. Lai CJ, Liu WY, Yang TF, et al. Pediatric aquatic therapy on motor function and enjoyment in children diagnosed with cerebral palsy of various motor severities. *J Child Neurol.* 2015;30(2):200–208.

ADDITIONAL READING
- Himpens E, Van den Broeck C, Oostra A, et al. Prevalence, type, distribution, and severity of cerebral palsy in relation to gestational age: a meta-analytic review. *Dev Med Child Neurol.* 2008;50(5):334–340.
- Nguyen TM, Crowther CA, Wilkinson D, et al. Magnesium sulphate for women at term for neuroprotection of the fetus. *Cochrane Database Syst Rev.* 2013;(2):CD009395.
- O'Shea TM. Diagnosis, treatment, and prevention of cerebral palsy. *Clin Obstet Gynecol.* 2008;51(4):816–828.

 CODES

ICD10
- G80.9 Cerebral palsy, unspecified
- G80.1 Spastic diplegic cerebral palsy
- G80.2 Spastic hemiplegic cerebral palsy

CLINICAL PEARLS
- Management should focus on maximizing functioning and quality of life using multidisciplinary team approach.
- Regression of motor skills does not occur with CP.

CERVICAL HYPEREXTENSION INJURIES

Shane L. Larson, MD • Derek G. Zickgraf, DO

 BASICS

DESCRIPTION
- Class of neck injuries typically seen in rapid, forceful extension of the cervical spine (head extends posteriorly)
- Usually from motor vehicle accidents (MVA—whiplash), falls, or sports-related injuries (1)
- May involve
  - Injury to vertebral and paravertebral structures: fractures, dislocations, ligamentous tears, and disc disruption/subluxation
  - Spinal cord injury (SCI): traumatic central cord syndrome (CCS) secondary to cord compression or vascular insult, SCI without radiologic abnormality (see "SCIWORA")
  - Blunt cerebrovascular injury (BCVI): vertebral artery or carotid artery dissection
  - Soft tissue injury: cervical strain/sprain (i.e., whiplash), cervical stingers (see "Brachial Plexopathy")

EPIDEMIOLOGY
- Predominant age: Trauma and sports injuries are more common in young adults (average age 29.4 years); however, CCS mostly seen in older population (average age is 53 years)
- Predominant sex: male > female (1)

Incidence
In the United States
- Cervical fractures: 2 to 5/100 blunt trauma patients
- CCS: 3.6/100,000 people/year
- BCVI: estimated 1/1,000 of hospitalized trauma patients; incidence increased with cervical spine or thoracic injury
- Cervical strain: 3 to 4/1,000 people/year
- Whiplash is the most common injury in MVAs and accounts for 28% of all ED visits (2).
- Incidence of whiplash is 70 to 328/100,000 with rates peaking in 20- to 24-year-old females (3).
- 5% of trauma patients have spinal fractures and 20% of those have SCI.
- The incidence of traumatic SCI ranges from 2.3 to 83 cases per million population per year (2).

ETIOLOGY AND PATHOPHYSIOLOGY
Blunt trauma due to MVAs, sports injuries, falls, and assaults

RISK FACTORS
- Whiplash, initial injury: no seat belt use, female gender (3)[C]
- Chronic pain and/or disability: litigation, previous neck pain or injury, low education level (4,5)[C]
- Fractures: osteoporosis, conditions predisposing to spinal rigidity, such as ankylosing spondylitis or other spondyloarthropathies
- CCS: Preexisting spinal stenosis is present in >50% of cases, which may be
  - Acquired: prior trauma, spondylosis
  - Congenital: Klippel-Feil syndrome (congenital fusion of any 2 cervical vertebra)

GENERAL PREVENTION
Seat belts, use of proper safety equipment, rule changes, and technique-coaching emphasis in sports activities can potentially prevent or minimize injury.

COMMONLY ASSOCIATED CONDITIONS
Closed head injuries, whiplash-associated disorders (WAD), SCI, soft-tissue trauma

 DIAGNOSIS

HISTORY
Usually acute presentation with mechanism of cervical hyperextension (see "Etiology and Pathophysiology") and complaints of neck pain, stiffness, or headaches ± neurologic symptoms

PHYSICAL EXAM
- External signs of trauma on the head and neck such as abrasions, lacerations, or contusions are clues to mechanism and associated injuries.
- Presence, severity, and location of neck tenderness often helps localize involved structure(s):
  - Posterior midline, bony tenderness concerning for fracture
  - Paraspinal or lateral soft tissue tenderness suggests muscular/ligamentous injury.
  - Anterior tenderness concerning for vascular injury.
- Carotid bruit suggests carotid dissection.
- Neurologic exam: Paresthesias, weakness suggests SCI or stroke secondary to BCVI:
  - CCS often presents as
    - Distal > proximal symptom distribution, upper extremity > lower extremity
    - Extremity weakness/paralysis predominates.
    - Variable sensory changes below level of lesion (including paresthesias and dysesthesia)
    - Bladder/bowel incontinence may occur.

DIFFERENTIAL DIAGNOSIS
- Acute or chronic disc pathology (including herniation or internal disruption)
- Osteoarthritis
- Cervical radiculopathy
- For CCS
  - Bell cruciate palsy
  - Bilateral brachial plexus injuries
  - Carotid or vertebral artery dissection

DIAGNOSTIC TESTS & INTERPRETATION

Initial Tests (lab, imaging)
- Low-risk patients can be cleared clinically (without imaging) using either the Canadian C-spine Rule (CCR) or the National Emergency X-Ray Utilization Study (NEXUS) criteria (6)[B]:
  - CCR: Clinically clear a stable, adult patient with no history of cervical spine disease/surgery if all of the following conditions are met:
    - Glasgow Coma Scale (GCS) ≥15
    - Nonintoxicated patients without a distracting injury
    - No dangerous mechanism or extremity paresthesias
    - Age <65 years
    - At least 1 "low-risk factor" (i.e., simple rear-end MVA, ambulation at the accident scene, no midline cervical tenderness, delayed onset of neck pain, or sitting position at the time of exam)
  - NEXUS: Clinically clear if all of the following are met:
    - No alteration of mental status or intoxication
    - No focal/neurologic deficits
    - No distracting injury
    - No posterior, midline C-spine tenderness
  - Reported sensitivity/specificity: CCR (99.4%/45.1%), NEXUS (90.7%/36.8%)
- In patients with high-risk mechanism or any concerning historical/physical exam elements, imaging should strongly be considered. Choose from the

following options based on the suspected injury and level of clinical suspicion:
- Plain radiographs: recommended by some in patients who cannot be cleared clinically but still are in low-suspicion category: sensitivity for C-spine injury 39%:
  - Dynamic: flexion/extension; only if asymptomatic and no neurologic deficits or mental impairment, poor identification of ligamentous injury, limited diagnostic value (7)[A]
- CT: axial CT from occiput to T1 with coronal and sagittal reconstructions; has replaced plain radiography as the test of choice for cases with moderate to high clinical suspicion of C-spine injury, given high sensitivity (90–100%)
- MRI: test of choice in CCS with direct visualization of traumatic cord lesions (edema or hematomyelia), soft tissue compressing cord, and/or stenosis of canal. Detects ligamentous injury and abnormalities of intervertebral discs and soft tissues. MRI is poor with fractures due to false-positive results from nonspecific findings.
- CT angiography: visualization of cervical and cerebral vascular structures to detect BCVI, with reported sensitivity approaching 100% when a ≥16-slice CT scanner is used. MR angiography is an alternative modality, although accessibility and reported sensitivities of 47–50% limit its use settings.

Test Interpretation
- Vertebral fractures: See "General Measures."
- CCS: currently thought to be due to axonal disruption within the white matter of the lateral column, particularly the corticospinal tracts
- BCVI: intimal disruption, leading to thrombosis and embolization
- Acute cervical strain/sprain: Models based on animal, cadaver, and postmortem studies show myofascial tearing, edema, and inflammation.

Geriatric Considerations
- Degenerative changes of the C-spine may be confused with acute traumatic change, and osteopenia may limit fracture visualization on x-ray—CT more accurately makes this differentiation.
- Degenerative disease and osteopenia increases the risk of upper cervical spine injuries despite low-velocity trauma (3)[B].

Pediatric Considerations
Consider SCI without radiographic abnormality (SCIWORA): high incidence at <9 years and accounts for up to 50% of all pediatric cervical spine injuries. MRI may help detect the injury.

TREATMENT

GENERAL MEASURES
- Whiplash, WAD
  - Limited or no benefit to cervical collar; if needed, use for <72 hours (8)[C]
  - No advantage to engaging early multiprofessional intervention (e.g., pain management and psychology) (9)[C]
  - No evidence of different outcomes with physical therapy versus passive (immobilization, rest) treatment. Advance activity levels as tolerated.
  - Lack of clear effective treatments in current medical literature in absence of fracture (4)[B]

- Fractures
  - Stability determined by imaging; decompression, and stabilization are indicated in
    - Incomplete SCIs with spinal canal compromise
    - Clinical deterioration or failure to improve despite conservative management
  - Hangman fracture: traumatic spondylolisthesis of C2 with bilateral fractures through C2 pedicles, often with anterior subluxation of C2 over C3; can be unstable:
    - Managed with halo vest immobilization for 12 weeks until flexion/extension films normalize
  - Odontoid fractures: treated according to type:
    - I: through apex; usually stable; external immobilization with a cervical collar (less often halo vest) for up to 12 weeks
    - II: most common, at base of dens, usually unstable; nonunion rates of up to 67% with halo immobilization alone, especially with dens displacement >6 mm or age >50 years
    - III: through C2 body, usually stable; immobilization in halo or cervical collar for 12–20 weeks
  - Hyperextension teardrop fractures
    - If stable, rigid collar or cervicothoracic brace for 8 to 14 weeks
    - If unstable, halo brace for up to 3 months
- CCS: neck immobilization with cervical collar, physical therapy/occupational therapy (PT/OT)
- Cervical strain: No difference in outcomes with active (PT) versus passive (immobilization, rest) treatment; may use soft cervical collar for 10 days for symptomatic relief, then mobilize and increase activity as tolerated.
- Lack of clear effective treatments in current medical literature in absence of fracture (4)[B]

MEDICATION
- Fractures: pain control as needed with analgesics
- CCS: Within 8 hours of injury, consider methylprednisolone 30 mg/kg IV over 15 minutes, then continuous infusion 5.4 mg/kg/hr IV for 23 hours. Further improvement in motor function recovery may be seen if infusion is continued for 48 hours, especially if initial bolus administration is delayed by 3 to 8 hours after injury (10)[A].
- BCVI: Anticoagulation with IV heparin, followed by warfarin therapy for 3 to 6 months, then long-term antiplatelet therapy is a common practice. However, an antiplatelet agent is used as the sole initial therapy in patients with contraindications to anticoagulation. To date, no randomized controlled trials compare the efficacy of antiplatelet versus anticoagulant therapy, so evidence-based recommendations are unavailable.
- Cervical strain: muscle relaxants, acetaminophen/NSAIDs ± opiate analgesics are commonly used.

ISSUES FOR REFERRAL
- When cervical spine injury is suspected, the patient should be immobilized and sent to the ED.
- Emergent consultation from a spine surgeon for any concern for unstable fracture or SCI.

SURGERY/OTHER PROCEDURES
- Fractures
  - Hangman fracture: surgical fixation for excessive angulation or subluxation, disruption of intervertebral disc space, or failure to obtain alignment with external orthosis
  - Odontoid fractures
    - Type II: Early surgical stabilization is recommended in setting of age >50 years, dens displacement >5 mm, and specific fracture patterns.
    - Type III: Surgical intervention is often reserved for cases of nonunion/malunion after trial of external immobilization.

- CCS: Surgical decompression/fixation is indicated in setting of unstable injury, herniated disc, or when neurologic function deteriorates.
- BCVI: Surgical and/or angiographic intervention may be required if there is evidence of pseudoaneurysm, total occlusion, or transection of the vessel.

INPATIENT CONSIDERATIONS
Admission Criteria/Initial Stabilization
- Varies by injury; clinical judgment, imaging findings, concomitant injuries, and need for operative intervention
- Advanced Trauma Life Support protocol with backboard and collar

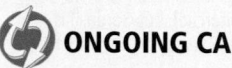 ONGOING CARE

FOLLOW-UP RECOMMENDATIONS
Patient Monitoring
Patients with known injuries will often be followed with serial imaging under the care of a specialist.

PATIENT EDUCATION
For patient instruction on prevention: ThinkFirst Foundation: http://www.thinkfirst.org

PROGNOSIS
- Presenting neurologic status is the most important.
- Fractures
  - Hangman fracture: 93–100% fusion rate after 8 to 14 weeks external immobilization
  - Odontoid fracture, fusion rate by type: type I ~100% with external immobilization alone; type II nonunion rates of up to 67% with halo immobilization alone, especially with dens displacement >6 mm or age >50 years; type III, 85% with external immobilization, 100% with surgical fixation
- BCVI: With early diagnosis and initiation of antithrombotic therapy, patients may have fewer neurologic sequelae.
- CCS
  - Spontaneous recovery of motor function in >50% of cases over several weeks, with younger patients more likely to regain function
  - Leg, bowel, and bladder functions return first, followed by upper extremities
- WAD: Prognostic factors for development of late whiplash syndrome (>6 months of symptoms affecting normal activity) include increased initial pain intensity, pain-related disability, and cold hyperalgesia (8).

COMPLICATIONS
- Fractures: instability or malunion/nonunion necessitating second operation, reactions, and infection related to orthosis
- BCVI: embolic ischemic events and pseudoaneurysm formation

REFERENCES
1. National Spinal Cord Injury Statistical Center. *Spinal Cord Injury: Facts and Figures at a Glance.* Birmingham, AL: National Spinal Cord Injury Statistical Center; 2015.
2. Oliver M, Inaba K, Tang A, et al. The changing epidemiology of spinal trauma: a 13-year review from a Level I trauma centre. *Injury.* 2012;43(8):1296–1300.
3. Quinlan KP, Annest JL, Myers B, et al. Neck strains and sprains among motor vehicle occupants—United States, 2000. *Accid Anal Prev.* 2004;36(1):21–27.
4. Wenzel HG, Mykletun A, Nilsen TI. Symptom profile of persons self-reporting whiplash: a Norwegian population-based study (HUNT 2). *Eur Spine J.* 2009;18(9):1363–1370.
5. Walton DM, Pretty J, MacDermid JC, et al. Risk factors for persistent problems following whiplash injury: results of a systematic review and meta-analysis. *J Orthop Sports Phys Ther.* 2009;39(5):334–350.
6. Stiell IG, Clement CM, McKnight RD, et al. The Canadian C-spine rule versus the NEXUS low-risk criteria in patients with trauma. *N Engl J Med.* 2003;349(26):2510–2518.
7. Sierink JC, van Lieshout WA, Beenen LF, et al. Systematic review of flexion/extension radiography of the cervical spine in trauma patients. *Eur J Radiol.* 2013;82(6):974–981.
8. Rasker JJ, Wolfe F. McLean et al.'s paper, "Incidence and predictors of neck and widespread pain after motor vehicle collision among U.S. litigants and nonlitigants". *Pain.* 2014;155(7):1416.
9. Jull G, Kenardy J, Hendrikz J, et al. Management of acute whiplash: a randomized controlled trial of multidisciplinary stratified treatments. *Pain.* 2013;154(9):1798–1806.
10. Bracken MB. Steroids for acute spinal cord injury. *Cochrane Database Syst Rev.* 2012;(1):CD001046.

ADDITIONAL READING
- Franz RW, Willette PA, Wood MJ, et al. A systematic review and meta-analysis of diagnostic screening criteria for blunt cerebrovascular injuries. *J Am Coll Surg.* 2012;214(3):313–327.
- Liu BC, Ivers R, Norton R, et al. Helmets for preventing injury in motorcycle riders. *Cochrane Database Syst Rev.* 2008;(1):CD004333.
- Shears E, Armitstead CP. Surgical versus conservative management for odontoid fractures. *Cochrane Database Syst Rev.* 2008;(4):CD005078.
- Watanabe M, Sakai D, Yamamoto Y, et al. Upper cervical spine injuries: age-specific clinical features. *J Orthop Sci.* 2010;15(4):485–492.

 SEE ALSO

Spine Injury: Cervical

 CODES

ICD10
- S13.4XXA Sprain of ligaments of cervical spine, initial encounter
- S13.101A Dislocation of unspecified cervical vertebrae, init encntr
- S14.109A Unsp injury at unsp level of cervical spinal cord, init

CLINICAL PEARLS
- Follow NEXUS or Canadian Cervical Spine rules on every patient with potential neck injury to determine imaging needs, but they do not supercede clinical judgment!
- Inquire about preexisting cervical spine conditions, especially in the elderly, as they may increase risk of injury or change radiographic interpretation.
- Suspect SCI until exam and imaging suggest otherwise.
- Consider BCVI when neurologic deficits are inconsistent with level of known injury or significant mechanism exists.

CERVICAL MALIGNANCY

Benjamin P. Brown, MD • Meaghan Tenney, MD

BASICS

DESCRIPTION
- Invasive cancer of the uterine cervix
- Commonly involves the vagina, parametria, and pelvic side walls
- Invasion of bladder, rectum, and other pelvic sites in advanced disease

EPIDEMIOLOGY

Incidence
- In the United States, cervical cancer is the third most common gynecologic malignancy.
- It is the second most common cancer among women in the developing world, with these patients representing >80% of reported cases.
- The disease has a bimodal distribution, with the highest risk among women aged 40 to 59 years and >70 years.

Prevalence
- In 2015, the American Cancer Society (ACS) estimated there were 12,900 new cases in the United States, with 4,100 deaths from the malignancy.
- African Americans and women in lower socioeconomic groups have the highest cervical cancer death rates.
- Hispanic and Latina women have the highest incidence of the malignancy.

ETIOLOGY AND PATHOPHYSIOLOGY
- Arises from preexisting dysplastic lesions, usually following persistent human papillomavirus (HPV) infection
- May be exophytic or endophytic
- Lymphatic spread
- Local tumor extension involving the bladder, ureters, rectum, and distant metastasis from hematogenous spread (Halstedian growth)
- Epidemiologic and experimental evidence supports HPV strains 16 and 18 as etiologic agents in ~70% of cervical cancers.
- Association with E6 and E7 oncogenic proteins responsible for malignant cell transformation by inactivation of p53 and Rb tumor suppressor genes
- Slow progression from dysplasia to invasive cancer allows time for screening and treatment of preinvasive disease.

Genetics
Not an inherited disease, except in very rare cases of Peutz-Jeghers syndrome

RISK FACTORS
- Causative agent in the majority of cases is persistent HPV infection.
- Other risk factors include the following:
  - Lack of regular Pap smears
  - Early coitarche
  - Multiple sexual partners
  - Unprotected sex
  - A history of sexually transmitted diseases (STDs)
  - Low socioeconomic status
  - High parity
  - Cigarette smoking
  - Immunosuppression
  - Diethylstilbestrol (DES) exposure in utero

GENERAL PREVENTION
- Patient education regarding safer sex
- Smoking cessation
- HPV vaccines
  - Gardasil vaccines: quadrivalent and 9-valent options; FDA approved in females and in males (for prevention of genital warts and anal cancer)
  - Cervarix vaccine: bivalent vaccine against oncogenic HPV strains 16 and 18
  - No vaccine yet conclusively shown to prevent cancer
  - Recommended age of vaccination is 11 to 12 years (prior to coitarche), but Gardasil is approved from 9 to 26 years and Cervarix from 10 to 25 years.
- Regular Pap smears and pelvic exams at appropriate intervals. In patients with no history of abnormal Paps, current guidelines from the American College of Obstetricians and Gynecologists (ACOG) are as follows:
  - Cytology alone every 3 years between 21 and 30 years
  - Cytology plus HPV testing every 5 years after 30 years (1)[C]
- The International Federation of Gynecology and Obstetrics (FIGO) recommends visual inspection with acetic acid (VIA) or Lugol's iodine (VILI) as alternatives to Pap smears in resource-poor settings (2)[C].
- Despite HPV vaccination, cervical cancer screening will remain the main preventive measure for both vaccinated and nonvaccinated women.

COMMONLY ASSOCIATED CONDITIONS
- Condyloma acuminata
- Preinvasive/invasive lesions of the vulva and vagina

DIAGNOSIS

HISTORY
- May be asymptomatic
- Most common symptom is vaginal bleeding, often postcoital.
- Other gynecologic symptoms include intermenstrual or postmenopausal bleeding and vaginal discharge.
- Other less common symptoms include low back pain with radiation down posterior leg, lower extremity edema, vesicovaginal and rectovaginal fistula, and urinary symptoms.

PHYSICAL EXAM
- Disease is staged clinically, not surgically.
- Thorough pelvic exam is essential:
  - Many patients have a normal exam, especially with microinvasive disease.
  - Lesions may be exophytic, endophytic, polypoid, papillary, ulcerative, or necrotic.
  - May have watery, purulent, or bloody discharge
- Bimanual and rectovaginal examination for uterine size, vaginal wall, rectovaginal septum, parametrial, uterosacral, and pelvic sidewall involvement
- Enlarged supraclavicular or inguinal lymphadenopathy, lower extremity edema, ascites, or decreased breath sounds with lung auscultation may indicate metastases or advanced stage disease.

DIFFERENTIAL DIAGNOSIS
- Marked cervicitis and erosion
- Glandular hyperplasia
- Sexually transmitted infection
- Cervical condyloma, leiomyoma, or polyp
- Metastasis from endometrial carcinoma or gestational trophoblastic neoplasia

DIAGNOSTIC TESTS & INTERPRETATION

Initial Tests (lab, imaging)
- Biopsy of gross lesions and colposcopically directed biopsies are the definitive means of diagnosis.
- CBC may show anemia.
- Urinalysis may show hematuria.
- In advanced disease, BUN, creatinine, and liver function tests (LFTs) may be helpful.
- CT scan of the chest, abdomen, and pelvis and/or a positron emission tomography (PET) scan
- Apart from chest x-ray (CXR) and intravenous pyelogram (IVP), imaging does not alter tumor stage.
- MRI may be helpful in evaluating parametrial involvement in patients who are surgical candidates or for radiation treatment planning.

Follow-Up Tests & Special Consideration
Prompt multidisciplinary plan of care

- Exam under anesthesia may help in determining clinical stage and disease extent and determine if patient is a surgical candidate.
- Endocervical curettage and cervical conization as indicated to determine depth of invasion and presence of lymphovascular involvement
- Cystoscopy to evaluate bladder invasion
- Proctoscopy for invasion into rectum

Test Interpretation
- Majority of cases (80%) are invasive squamous cell types usually arising from the ectocervix.
- Adenocarcinomas comprise 10–15% of cervical cancer arising from endocervical mucus-producing glandular cells. Often, no exophytic lesion but a "bulky" "barrel-shaped" cervix present on exam.
- Other cell types that may be present include rare mixed cell types, neuroendocrine tumors, sarcomas, lymphomas, and melanomas.

TREATMENT

GENERAL MEASURES
Improve nutritional state, correct any anemia, and treat any vaginal and/or pelvic infections.

MEDICATION
- Chemoradiation with cisplatin-containing regimen has superior survival rates over pelvic and extended-field radiation alone (3)[A].
- Neoadjuvant chemotherapy may improve survival for early and locally advanced tumors, but more data are needed (4)[A].

- Adjuvant chemotherapy after chemoradiation may improve progression-free survival in patients who receive primary chemoradiation for stages IIB–IVA tumors. The OUTBACK trial will further investigate these findings (http://www.clinicaltrials.gov).

- The addition of bevacizumab to standard combination chemotherapy (cisplatin/topotecan or cisplatin/paclitaxel) for recurrent, persistent, or metastatic disease has been shown to improve overall survival (5)[A].

ISSUES FOR REFERRAL
Multidisciplinary management of patients as needed and in a timely fashion

ADDITIONAL THERAPIES
- Chemoradiation (without surgery) is the first-line therapy for tumors stage IIB and higher (gross lesions with obvious parametrial involvement) and for most bulky stage IB2 tumors (6)[A].
- Combination of external beam pelvic radiation and brachytherapy is usually employed.
- If para-aortic lymph node metastases are suspected, extended-field radiation or lymph node dissection prior to radiation therapy may be performed.

SURGERY/OTHER PROCEDURES
- Surgical management is an option for patients with early-stage tumors.
- Removal of precursor lesions (cervical intraepithelial neoplasia [CIN]) by loop electrosurgical excision procedure (LEEP), cold knife conization, laser ablation, or cryotherapy
- Stage IA1 (lesions with <3-mm invasion from basement membrane) without lymphovascular space invasion: option of conization or simple extrafascial hysterectomy (6)[A]
- Stage IA2 (lesions with >3-mm but <5-mm invasion from basement membrane): option of radical hysterectomy with lymph node dissection or radiation, depending on clinical setting (6)[A]
- Stages IA2–IB1: Fertility-sparing radical trachelectomy may be considered in selected patients (6)[A].
- Stages IB1–IIA (gross lesions without obvious parametrial involvement): option of radical hysterectomy with lymph node sampling or primary chemoradiation with brachytherapy and teletherapy, depending on clinical setting (6)[A]
- Stage IVA (lesions limited to central metastasis to the bladder and/or rectum): Primary pelvic exenteration may be feasible (6)[A].
- Stage IVB disease is treated with goal of palliation. Early referral to palliative care should be made (6)[A],(7)[C].

Pregnancy Considerations
- Management is guided by consideration of stage of lesion, gestational age, and maternal assessment of risks and benefits from treatment.
- Abnormal cytology is best followed up by colposcopy with directed biopsies.
- CIN1 or less: postpartum follow-up
- CIN2–3: management per established guidelines
- Microinvasive carcinoma: conization or trachelectomy. If depth of invasion ≤3 mm, follow up at the 6-week postpartum visit
- Invasive carcinoma: definitive therapy, with timing determined by maternal preference, stage of disease, and gestational age

INPATIENT CONSIDERATIONS
Admission Criteria/Initial Stabilization
- Signs of active bleeding
- Urinary symptoms
- Dehydration

- Complications from surgery, chemotherapy, or radiation
- Active vaginal bleeding can be controlled with timely vaginal packing and radiation therapy.
- Recognition of ureteral blockage, hydronephrosis, urosepsis, and timely intervention

Discharge Criteria
Discharge criteria based on multidisciplinary assessment

 ONGOING CARE

FOLLOW-UP RECOMMENDATIONS
Patient Monitoring
- With completion of definitive therapy and based on individual risk factors, patients are evaluated with physical/pelvic examinations:
  - Every 3 to 6 months for 2 years
  - Every 6 to 12 months until the 5th year
  - Yearly thereafter (8)[C]
- Pap smears may be performed yearly but have a low sensitivity for detecting recurrence (8)[C].
- CT and PET scan are useful in locating metastases when recurrence is suspected (8)[C].
- Signs of recurrence include vaginal bleeding, unexplained weight loss, leg edema, and pelvic or thigh pain.

PATIENT EDUCATION
Patient education material available through the ACOG at http://www.acog.org, the Society of Gynecologic Oncology at http://www.sgo.org, the Foundation for Women's Cancer at http://www.foundationforwomenscancer.org, the American Cancer Society at http://www.cancer.org, and the National Cancer Institute at http://www.cancer.gov.

PROGNOSIS

Stage	5-y Survival (%)
1	76–98
2	66–73
3	40–42
4	9–22

COMPLICATIONS
- Loss of ovarian function from radiotherapy or indication for bilateral oophorectomy
- Hemorrhage
- Pelvic infection
- Genitourinary fistula
- Bladder dysfunction
- Sexual dysfunction
- Ureteral obstruction with renal failure
- Bowel obstruction
- Pulmonary embolism
- Lower extremity lymphedema

REFERENCES
1. Committee on Practice Bulletins—Gynecology. ACOG Practice Bulletin Number 131: screening for cervical cancer. *Obstet Gynecol.* 2012;120(5):1222–1238.
2. International Federation of Obstetrics and Gynecology. Global guidance for cervical cancer prevention and control. http://www.rho.org/files/FIGO_cervical_cancer_guidelines_2009.pdf.
3. Chemoradiotherapy for Cervical Cancer Meta-analysis Collaboration. Reducing uncertainties about the effects of chemoradiotherapy for cervical cancer: individual patient data meta-analysis. *Cochrane Database Syst Rev.* 2010;(1):CD008285.
4. Rydzewska L, Tierney J, Vale CL, et al. Neoadjuvant chemotherapy plus surgery versus surgery for cervical cancer. *Cochrane Database Syst Rev.* 2012;(12):CD007406.
5. Tewari KS, Sill MW, Long HJ III, et al. Improved survival with bevacizumab in advanced cervical cancer. *N Engl J Med.* 2014;370(8):734–743.
6. National Comprehensive Cancer Network. NCCN Clinical Practice Guidelines in Oncology: cervical cancer. http://www.nccn.org/professionals/physician_gls/pdf/cervical.pdf.
7. Smith TJ, Temin S, Alesi ER, et al. American Society of Clinical Oncology provisional clinical opinion: the integration of palliative care into standard oncology care. *J Clin Oncol.* 2012;30(8):880–887.
8. Salani R, Backes FJ, Fung MF, et al. Posttreatment surveillance and diagnosis of recurrence in women with gynecologic malignancies: Society of Gynecologic Oncologists recommendations. *Am J Obstet Gynecol.* 2011;204(6):466–478.

ADDITIONAL READING
- American Society for Colposcopy and Cervical Pathology. Algorithms: updated consensus guidelines for managing abnormal cervical cancer screening tests and cancer precursors. http://www.asccp.org/Portals/9/docs/ASCCP%20Management%20Guidelines_August%202014.pdf.
- Martin-Hirsch PP, Paraskevaidis E, Bryant A, et al. Surgery for cervical intraepithelial neoplasia. *Cochrane Database Syst Rev.* 2013;(12):CD001318.
- Scarinci IC, Garcia FA, Kobetz E, et al. Cervical cancer prevention: new tools and old barriers. *Cancer.* 2010;116(11):2531–2542.

 SEE ALSO

Abnormal Pap and Cervical Dysplasia

 CODES

ICD10
- C53.9 Malignant neoplasm of cervix uteri, unspecified
- C53.0 Malignant neoplasm of endocervix
- C53.1 Malignant neoplasm of exocervix

CLINICAL PEARLS
- Cervical cancer is the third most common gynecologic malignancy in the United States. Improving access to screening is likely to have the greatest impact in reduction of burden of disease.
- Women with cervical cancer may be asymptomatic and have a normal physical exam.
- Surgical management is an option for patients with early-stage tumors.
- Chemoradiation is the first-line therapy for higher stage tumors.

CERVICITIS, ECTROPION, AND TRUE EROSION

Cecilia M. Kipnis, MD • Gillian R. Wackowski, DO

BASICS

DESCRIPTION
- Cervicitis is an acute or chronic cervical inflammation; can be infectious or noninfectious.
- Ectropion is the eversion of the endocervix, exposing the columnar cells to the vaginal environment. This is more common in adolescents and pregnancy and can be confused for cervicitis.
- A true erosion occurs with the loss of overlying cervical epithelium due to trauma (e.g., forceful insertion of vaginal speculum in patient with atrophic mucosa).
- System(s) affected: reproductive

Geriatric Considerations
- Chronic cervicitis or a true erosion in postmenopausal women may be related to low levels of estrogen.
- Infectious cervicitis should not be overlooked in geriatric patients as many remain sexually active.

Pregnancy Considerations
All pregnant women should be screened for infectious cervicitis at the first prenatal visit by *screening for chlamydia*, and those with new or multiple sexual partners should also be screened for gonorrhea a (1).

Pediatric Considerations
Infectious cervicitis in children should lead to an investigation of possible sexual abuse.

EPIDEMIOLOGY
Incidence
- Cervicitis: most commonly due to infectious etiologies, including, but not limited to the following:
  - Chlamydia: 1,401,906 cases were reported to the CDC in 2013, 67% of reported cases occurring among 15- to 24-year-olds (2). Actual incidence is significantly higher.
  - Gonorrhea: second most commonly reported notifiable disease after chlamydia in the United States; 333,004 cases reported to the CDC in 2013 (2)
  - HSV and *Trichomonas*: these are not routinely reported to CDC but trend data show *Trichomonas* infections are up for a third year in a row (3).
  - *Mycoplasma genitalium*: increasingly recognized as a common sexually transmitted pathogen among high-risk, sexually active women (4)
- Ectropion: typically related to higher levels of estrogen; ectropion is common among adolescents, women using combined oral contraceptive pills (OCPs), and pregnant women.
  - Present in 14–37% of outpatients (5)
- True erosion: can be seen in women with cervical trauma

ETIOLOGY AND PATHOPHYSIOLOGY
- Cervicitis: Often, no specific etiology is identified.
  - Infectious: *Chlamydia trachomatis, Neisseria gonorrhoeae* are the most commonly identified pathogens; they affect the columnar epithelium of the endocervix. *Trichomonas vaginalis* and herpes simplex virus (HSV; especially primary infections of HSV-2) affect the squamous epithelium. Mycoplasmas (e.g., *M. genitalium*) are becoming increasingly recognized as causative organism.
  - Noninfectious: physical or chemical irritation (e.g., douching, latex exposure, contraceptive creams, or vaginal foreign bodies such as tampons, cervical caps), radiation therapy, inflammatory diseases, malignancy

- Ectropion
  - Hormonal changes with puberty, oral contraceptive use, or pregnancy
  - Resulting from cervical laceration during childbirth
- True erosion: injury to atrophic epithelium; estrogen-deficient states such as menopause

RISK FACTORS
- Infectious cervicitis (6)
  - Ages 15 to 25 is strongest predictor of risk
  - Multiple sexual partners
  - New sexual partner
  - Unprotected sex or sporadic use of condoms
  - History of sexually transmitted infection (STI)
  - Exchanging sex for money or drugs
  - Black and Hispanic race
  - Other reproductive tract infections: bacterial vaginitis, pelvic inflammatory disease (PID)
- Noninfectious cervicitis
  - Foreign objects: pessary, diaphragm, cervical cap, and so forth.
- Ectropion: adolescence, pregnancy, use of OCP
- True erosion: estrogen deficiency, trauma from foreign body

GENERAL PREVENTION
- STIs (chlamydia, gonorrhea, trichomoniasis)
- Advise use of condoms and safer sexual practices to prevent STIs.

Follow USPTF-recommended screening measures (6)[A]:

- Annual screening for *C. trachomatis* infection of all sexually active women ≤25 years and all older women at increased risk. Screen all pregnant women at the first prenatal visit.
- Annual screening for *N. gonorrhoeae* among sexually active women ≤25 years and all older women at increased risk (new or multiple partners, from communities with high prevalence). Screen among pregnant women at risk early in pregnancy (4).
- At least annual screening of trichomoniasis among HIV-positive women
- Treat sexual partners of infected women.
- Estrogen deficiency: estrogen replacement therapy

DIAGNOSIS

HISTORY
- Can be asymptomatic (4,6) or have increased or abnormal vaginal discharge
- Dyspareunia
- Lower abdominal pain/pelvic pain
- Postcoital or intermenstrual bleeding/spotting (4)

PHYSICAL EXAM
- Cervicitis: most evident is mucopurulent/purulent discharge from cervix and/or cervical friability (4)
- Other symptoms: erythema, ulceration (HSV), punctate hemorrhage ("strawberry" cervix appearance in trichomoniasis). Consider coexistence with PID with cervical motion tenderness on bimanual exam (6).
- Ectropion: Cervix appears red due to the color of the columnar epithelium.
- True erosion: vaginal bleeding, sharply defined ulcers of cervix

DIFFERENTIAL DIAGNOSIS
- Cervical dysplasia
- Cervical neoplasm
- Cervical polyp or fibroid
- Ruptured nabothian cyst

- Postcervical procedure (biopsy, LEEP, IUD insertion/ removal, aggressive pap smear)
- Bacterial vaginosis (discharge is noninflammatory)

DIAGNOSTIC TESTS & INTERPRETATION
- Nucleic acid amplification test (NAAT) is the recommended test by USPTF and CDC for *C. trachomatis*/*N. gonorrhoeae* detection (6)[A].

- Urine specimens are slightly less sensitive than clinical endocervical or self-collected vaginal swabs (4).
- NAAT is also the most sensitive test for *M. genitalium*, although testing for this is not widely available (4).
- Cultures may be used when evaluating a potential *N. gonorrhoeae* treatment failure (7).
- Vaginal wet mount for *T. vaginalis*
  - Culture, antigen assays, and NAAT should be considered when microscopy is unavailable or inconclusive. Sensitivity for microscopy is low (~50%).
  - Pap smears should not be used to diagnose trichomoniasis.
- If ulcerations are present, culture for HSV.

Diagnostic Procedures/Other
Colposcopy may be helpful in cases of chronic inflammation, with biopsy of suspicious areas.

TREATMENT

MEDICATION
First Line
- If infectious cervicitis suspected in high-risk patient, presumptive treatment is appropriate: ceftriaxone 250 mg single dose IM, followed by either azithromycin 1 g single dose or doxycycline 100 mg PO BID × 7 days. Option of ceftriaxone and azithromycin removes patient-compliance factor because they are 1-time doses and can be administered in office.
- Chlamydia: for nonpregnant women, azithromycin 1 g PO single dose or doxycycline 100 mg BID PO × 7 days; for pregnant women, azithromycin 1 g single dose or erythromycin base 500 mg QID PO × 7 days or erythromycin ethylsuccinate 800 mg QID × 7 days
- Gonorrhea: Due to increased resistance to antibiotics, the CDC currently recommends ceftriaxone 250 mg single dose IM, followed by either azithromycin 1 g PO single dose or doxycycline 100 mg PO BID × 7 days regardless of the chlamydial coinfection status.

- Trichomoniasis: metronidazole 2 g PO single dose or 500 mg PO BID × 7 days. A single oral dose of 2 g of tinidazole is also effective (6)[A].

- *M. genitalium*: azithromycin 1 g PO as a single dose or 500 mg PO once followed by 250 mg PO daily × 4 days
- Ectropion: none, unless patient is extremely symptomatic with copious discharge. In that case, acid-buffered vaginal jelly can be used to decrease discharge.
- True erosion: conjugated estrogen cream applied vaginally daily for 1 to 2 weeks, followed by maintenance dosing twice weekly or oral hormone replacement therapy (HRT)
- Contraindications:
  - Metronidazole: The manufacturer states that metronidazole is contraindicated in the 1st trimester in pregnancy but more recent meta-analyses suggest absence of teratogenicity.

– Doxycycline: do not use during pregnancy or lactation

– Estrogen: See extended list of contraindications to estrogen use in standard texts.

- Precautions:

  – Metronidazole and tinidazole: Avoid alcohol and breastfeeding during treatment and 12 to 24 hours after completion of treatment with metronidazole and 72 hours after completion of treatment with tinidazole (4)[A].

  – Doxycycline: possible fetal harm if used during pregnancy; staining of the infant's teeth if used during breastfeeding; allergy; photosensitization

  – Erythromycin: nausea or vomiting

  – Estrogens: history of estrogen-dependent neoplasms; history of thromboembolic diseases. See extended list of contraindications to estrogen therapy in standard texts.

- Significant possible interactions:

  – Metronidazole: ethanol

  – Doxycycline: dairy products, iron preparations, warfarin, and oral contraceptives (advise use of alternative contraceptive method)

  – Erythromycin: theophylline (elevated theophylline level)

  – Estrogen: N/A

Second Line

- Chlamydia

  – Levofloxacin 500 mg PO daily × 7 days

  – Ofloxacin 300 mg PO BID × 7 days (4)[A]

- Gonorrhea: If an injectable cephalosporin is not an option, oral cephalosporin therapy with azithromycin or doxycycline can be considered as 2nd-line therapy:

  – Cefixime: 400 mg PO single dose is an acceptable alternative to ceftriaxone, (however, necessitates that the patient return in 1 week for a test of cure) plus azithromycin 1 g single dose or doxycycline 100 mg PO BID × 7 days (8)[A].

  – In the case of a true penicillin allergy, alternative regimens include the following:

    ○ Azithromycin: 2 g PO as a single dose; however, due to evidence of increasing resistance to macrolides, use should be limited. Test of cure is recommended

    ○ CDC no longer recommends fluoroquinolones for treatment of gonorrhea due to emergence of fluoroquinolone-resistant *N. gonorrhoeae* in United States (8)[A].

    ○ *M. genitalium*: moxifloxacin 400 mg PO daily × 7 to 10 days (7)[C] in patients with persistent *M. genitalium* despite azithromycin treatment, although studies are limited

- Estrogen deficiency: A number of estrogen vaginal preparations are available commercially.

Pregnancy Considerations

Doxycycline and the quinolones are contraindicated in pregnancy.

SURGERY/OTHER PROCEDURES

- Ectropion: Symptomatic lesions can be treated with silver nitrate, or cryo and electrocautery (5).

- Chronic cervicitis with negative cultures and treatment failure may be treated with cryosurgery, electrocautery, or loop excision.

- Surgical management and cautery is generally considered overly invasive and should only be used in select patients with severe/significant symptoms who do not respond to other treatments.

Adverse effects can include continued or increased discharge, recurrence of lesion, and cervical stenosis which may affect fertility.

ONGOING CARE

FOLLOW-UP RECOMMENDATIONS

Patient Monitoring

- Test of cure for *C. trachomatis* is recommended in pregnant patients to document eradication of infection; perform at least 3 weeks following treatment.

- Reinfection with *Trichomonas*, gonorrhea, and chlamydia is common; repeat screening should be performed routinely for all patients 3 to 4 months following treatment (4)[A].

- Estrogen deficiency: Reexamine in 1 month to confirm healing.

ALERT

For *C. trachomatis*, the test of cure with nucleic acid amplification tests should not be done <3 weeks after treatment because of false-positive results due to dead organisms. For gonorrhea, however, the test of cure should be done at the infected anatomic site 1 week after treatment. The test of cure ideally should be performed with NAAT or culture.

PATIENT EDUCATION

If the etiology of cervicitis is a confirmed STI, the patient's sex partners within the preceding 60 days must be evaluated for *N. gonorrhoeae* or *C. trachomatis* and treated accordingly. Patient should abstain from sexual intercourse for 7 days after a single-dose regimen or after completion of a 7-day regimen to avoid reinfection.

PROGNOSIS

- Cervicitis: excellent after bacterial infection is eradicated

- Ectropion: spontaneous regression postpartum and with cessation of use of oral contraceptives

- True erosion: spontaneous healing

COMPLICATIONS

- Cervicitis due to *C. trachomatis* or *N. gonorrhoeae* carries an 8–10% risk of developing subsequent PID. Adolescents should be screened at least once yearly because they are a high-risk group for reinfection with sexually transmitted organisms.

- *M. genitalium* may be associated with PID.

- Women positive for HIV with cervicitis have an increased risk of viral shedding and transmission to sexual partners.

REFERENCES

1. Centers for Disease Control and Prevention; National Center for HIV/AIDS, Viral Hepatitis, STD, and TB Prevention (United States). Incidence, prevalence, and cost of sexually transmitted infections in the United States; CDC fact sheet. http://www.cdc.gov/std/stats/sti-estimates-fact-sheet-feb-2013.pdf.

2. Centers for Disease Control and Prevention. Reported STDs in the United States: 2013 national data for chlamydia, gonorrhea and syphilis; CDC fact sheet. http://www.cdc.gov/nchhstp/newsroom/docs/STD-Trends-508.pdf.

3. Centers for Disease Control and Prevention. 2013 sexually transmitted diseases surveillance Table 45. Selected STDs and complications—initial visits to physicians' offices, National Disease and Therapeutic Index, United States, 1966-2013. http://www.cdc.gov/std/stats13/tables/45.htm.

---

4. Workowski K, Bolan GA; Centers for Disease Control and Prevention. Sexually transmitted disease treatment guidelines, 2015. *MMWR Recomm Rep*. 2015;64(RR-03):1–137.

5. Wan YL, Edmondson RJ, Crosbie EJ. Intermenstrual and postcoital bleeding. *Obstet Gynaecol Reprod Med*. 2015;25(4):106–112.

6. U.S. Preventive Services Task Force. Final Recommendation Statement: Chlamydia and Gonorrhea: Screening. http://www.uspreventiveservicestaskforce.org/Page/Document/UpdateSummaryFinal/chlamydia-and-gonorrhea-screening?ds=1&s=chlamydia%20and%20gonorrhea%20screening. Accessed July 25, 2015

7. Manhart LE, Broad JM, Golden MR. *Mycoplasma genitalium*: should we treat and how? *Clin Infect Dis*. 2011;53(Suppl 3):S129–S142.

8. Centers for Disease Control and Prevention. Update to CDC's sexually transmitted diseases treatment guidelines, 2010: oral cephalosporins no longer a recommended treatment for gonococcal infections. *MMWR Morb Mortal Wkly Rep*. 2012;61(31):590–594.

ADDITIONAL READING

- Cazanave C, Manhart LE, Bébéar C. *Mycoplasma genitalium*, an emerging sexually transmitted pathogen. *Med Mal Infect*. 2012;42(9):381–392.

- Centers for Disease Control and Prevention. Recommendations for the laboratory-based detection of *Chlamydia trachomatis* and *Neisseria gonorrhoeae*—2014. *MMWR Recomm Rep*. 2014;63(RR-02):1–19.

- Cook RL, Hutchison SL, Østergaard L, et al. Systematic review: noninvasive testing for *Chlamydia trachomatis* and *Neisseria gonorrhoeae*. *Ann Intern Med*. 2005;142(11):914–925.

- Gülmezoglu AM, Azhar M. Interventions for trichomoniasis in pregnancy. *Cochrane Database Syst Rev*. 2011;(5):CD000220.

- Haggerty CL, Taylor BD. Mycoplasma genitalium: an emerging cause of pelvic inflammatory disease. *Infect Dis Obstet Gynecol*. 2011;2011:959816.

- Johnson LF, Lewis DA. The effect of genital tract infections on HIV-1 shedding in the genital tract: a systematic review and meta-analysis. *Sex Transm Dis*. 2008;35(11):946–959.

- Wilson JF. In the clinic. Vaginitis and cervicitis. *Ann Intern Med*. 2009;151(5):ITC3-1–ITC3-15.

 CODES

ICD10

- N72 Inflammatory disease of cervix uteri
- N86 Erosion and ectropion of cervix uteri

CLINICAL PEARLS

- If infectious cervicitis is suspected, treatment of choice is ceftriaxone 250 mg IM plus azithromycin 1 g PO × 1 dose. Do not wait for test results.

- Sexual partner(s) need to be treated.

- Positive results for *N. gonorrhoeae* or chlamydia should be reported to local or state health department.

CHICKENPOX (VARICELLA ZOSTER)
Kay A. Bauman, MD, MPH

 BASICS

DESCRIPTION
- Common, highly contagious generalized exanthem characterized by crops of pruritic vesicles on the skin and mucous membranes following exposure to varicella-zoster virus (VZV)
- VZV is spread by respiratory (airborne) droplets and direct contact with vesicles.
- VZV establishes latency in the dorsal root ganglia; reactivation results in zoster (shingles).
- Outbreaks tend to occur late winter through early spring in temperate climates.
- Usual incubation period is 14 to 16 days (range, 10 to 21). Patients are infectious from ~48 hours before appearance of vesicles until the final lesions have crusted. Historically, most people acquired chickenpox during childhood and developed lifelong immunity. Varicella is now part of recommended primary vaccination schedule.
- System(s) affected: nervous; skin/exocrine
- Synonym(s): varicella

EPIDEMIOLOGY
- Predominant age: peak incidence in preschoolers through 9 years but may occur at any age
- Predominant gender: male = female

Incidence
- Decreasing incidence since routine vaccination; estimated 3.5 million cases annually prior to vaccine, with an incidence of 8–9% in children age 1 to 9 years
- Reported U.S. varicella cases: 1991, 147,076; 2013, 11,359 cases (1,2)
- Prior to vaccine, ~100 deaths/year were reported in the United States; in 2013, there were 3 reported deaths (2).
- U.S. rates: 1994, prior to vaccine: 135.8/100,000 persons; 2012: 4.3/100,000 persons
- Rates of varicella in the United States dropped after vaccine introduction until mid-2000s when they plateaued; second dose of vaccine was recommended in 2006, and rates have again declined.
- In developing countries, varicella is still associated with a severe disease burden.
- Susceptible (immunologically naive) individuals exposed to varicella are at risk to develop disease and are also potentially infectious for 21 days.

ETIOLOGY AND PATHOPHYSIOLOGY
- Skin lesions are histologically identical to herpes simplex virus.
- In fatal cases, intranuclear inclusions are found in vascular endothelium and most organs.
- VZV is a double-stranded DNA virus of the α-Herpesviridae subfamily.
- Humans are primary disease reservoir.

RISK FACTORS
- No history of prior varicella infection or immunization
- Immunocompromised patients (especially children with leukemia/lymphoma in remission or receiving high-dose corticosteroids)
- Pregnancy

Geriatric Considerations
- Infection is more severe in adults than in children.
- Reactivation of latent infection causes zoster (shingles).

- Herpes zoster vaccine, a live attenuated vaccine licensed in 2006, is recommended as a single dose for all persons ≥60 years regardless of prior clinical history of shingles or chickenpox. It can be administered to persons ≥60 years who are receiving therapy to induce low-level immunosuppression but should not be given to highly immunocompromised patients. Giving the vaccine prior to starting chemotherapy significantly lowers risk of zoster (http://www.cdc.gov/vaccines/vpd-vac/shingles/hcp-vaccination.htm).
- Most common cause of death: primary viral pneumonia

Pediatric Considerations
- Neonates born to mothers who develop chickenpox from 5 days before to 2 days after delivery are at risk for serious disease and should receive varicella-zoster immune globulin (VZIG).
- Newborns are at highest risk for severe disease during the 1st month of life, especially if mother is seronegative.
- Delivery prior to 28 weeks increases risk.
- Varicella bullosa is seen mainly in children <2 years. Lesions appear as bullae instead of vesicles. The clinical course is similar.
- Most common cause of death: septic complications and encephalitis
- Avoid aspirin/acetylsalicylic acid in children because of link to Reye syndrome.

Pregnancy Considerations
- 25% risk of transplacental infection after maternal infection
- Congenital malformations are seen in 2% of patients when the fetus is infected during the 1st or 2nd trimesters, characterized by limb atrophy and scarring of the skin of the extremities and occasional CNS and eye manifestations.
- Morbidity (e.g., pneumonia) is increased in women infected during pregnancy.

GENERAL PREVENTION
- Isolate hospitalized patients.
- When indicated, passive immunization with IM VZIG should be given within 96 hours (but can be as long as up to 10 days) after exposure (3).
  - VZIG is recommended for people exposed to chickenpox or shingles who are immunocompromised, newborns of mothers with onset of chickenpox <5 days before delivery or <2 days after delivery, premature infants (<28 weeks) exposed in neonatal period either whose mothers are not immune, or babies who weigh <1,000 g regardless of maternal immunity (3).
- Active immunization after exposure prevents or reduces the severity of varicella if given within 72 hours postexposure.
- Active immunization: varicella virus vaccine (Varivax): live attenuated vaccine approved by FDA in 1995 for pediatric immunization and recommended by ACIP for immunization of healthy patients ≥12 months who have not had chickenpox
  - 12 months to 12 years: initial dose 0.5 mL SC at age 12 to 15 months; second dose at age 4 to 6 years. Prelicensure studies showed efficacy rates: 70–90% against any disease and 95% against severe disease 7 to 10 years after vaccination. Other studies showed 100% efficacy at 1 year and 98% at 2 years after vaccination.

Single dose is 85–94% effective in preventing severe disease. The two-dose regimen is 96–98% effective. Breakthrough disease generally has <50 lesions, shorter duration, and lower fever incidence (4)[A].
  - ≥13 years: two 0.5 mL SC doses 4 to 8 weeks apart, seroconversion rates 78–82% after one dose, 99% after two doses. Adult efficacy in lower end of this range
  - 2013 U.S. estimate: 91% one or more-dose vaccine coverage for children ages 19 to 35 months (5)
  - Vaccine side effects are pain and redness at the vaccine site. 1 in 10 develops fever. 1 in 25 will develop a mild varicella-like rash up to 1 month after vaccination.
  - Vaccine contraindications (6)
    - Severe allergic reaction (e.g., anaphylaxis) to a previous dose or vaccine component
    - Severe immunodeficiency (e.g., severely immunocompromised HIV patients, on chemotherapy, congenital immunodeficiency, or long-term immunosuppressive therapy)
    - Pregnancy
- MMRV vaccine, which combines the measles, mumps, and rubella vaccine with varicella, is equally effective. There are rare reports of an increased risk of febrile seizures 5 to 12 days after vaccination in 1/2,300 to 2,600 patients (7)[A].
- May be considered for a subset of HIV-positive children in CDC class I with CD4 >25%
  - Vaccine recipients who develop a rash should avoid contact with immunocompromised people, pregnant women who have never had chickenpox, and their newborns.
  - Children needing catch-up vaccination need at least 3 months between doses 1 and 2.

 DIAGNOSIS

HISTORY
- Prodromal symptoms: fever, malaise, anorexia, mild headache
- Malaise, muscle aches, arthralgias, and headache are more common in adults.
- Subclinical in ~4% of cases
- Characteristic rash

PHYSICAL EXAM
- Characteristic rash: crops of vesicles on erythematous bases ("dewdrops on a rose petal")
- Lesions erupt in successive crops.
- Progress from macule to papule to vesicle, then begin to crust
- Pruritic rash is present in various stages of development.
- Lesions may be present on mucous membranes, both oral and vaginal.

DIFFERENTIAL DIAGNOSIS
- Herpes simplex: herpes zoster
- Smallpox
- Impetigo
- Coxsackievirus infection
- Scabies
- Dermatitis herpetiformis
- Drug rash
- Rickettsial pox infection

DIAGNOSTIC TESTS & INTERPRETATION

The diagnosis of chickenpox is based primarily on clinical grounds. Other testing is generally used for complicated cases and epidemiologic studies.

Initial Tests (lab, imaging)

- Leukocyte count varies.
- Marked leukocytosis suggests secondary infection.
- Multinucleated giant cells on Tzanck smear from vesicle scrapings
- Isolate virus from human tissue culture.

Follow-Up Tests & Special Considerations

- Serologies can show response to acute infection (IgM) or prior infection (IgG).
- Visualization by electron microscopy, tissue culture (costly), and various methods of acute and convalescent sera collection: latex agglutination (most available), enzyme immunoassay, indirect immunofluorescence antibody, fluorescent antibody to membrane assay, or polymerase chain reaction (PCR) assay, which can detect wild from vaccine viral strains
- Vaccine-modified cases can be more difficult to diagnose; PCR testing of skin lesions (8)[B] is most sensitive and specific for diagnosing varicella, especially in vaccinated persons.

TREATMENT

Outpatient, except for complicated cases

GENERAL MEASURES

- Supportive/symptomatic treatment
- Antihistamines and/or oatmeal baths for itch
- Acetaminophen and/or ibuprofen for pain and fever
- Nail clipping in children can help prevent scarring or secondary infection from itching.

MEDICATION

First Line

- Supportive: antipyretics for fever; avoid aspirin in children.
- Local and/or systemic antipruritic agents for itching
- VZIG available for passive immunization for
  - Immunocompromised patients, newborn infants whose mothers have signs and symptoms of varicella around the time of delivery, premature infants born at 28 weeks or more whose mothers do not have evidence of immunity to varicella, and premature infants <28 weeks' gestation or who weigh <1,000 g regardless of mothers' evidence of immunity, VZIG should be given within 96 hours after exposure to be most beneficial (9).
- Acyclovir: decreases duration of fever and shortens time of viral shedding; recommended for adolescents, adults, and high-risk patients; most beneficial if initiated early in the disease (≤24 hours)
  - 2- to 16-year-old patients: 20 mg/kg/dose (max 800 mg/dose) QID for 5 days
  - Adults: 800 mg 5 times daily for 5 days

- Contraindication
  - Hypersensitivity to the drug
- Precautions
  - Renal insufficiency with acyclovir
  - Concurrent administration of probenecid increases half-life; increased effects with zidovudine (e.g., drowsiness, lethargy)

Second Line

- Famciclovir: 500 mg TID for 7 to 10 days (adults)
- Valacyclovir: 1 g TID for 7 to 10 days (adults)

ONGOING CARE

FOLLOW-UP RECOMMENDATIONS

Patient Monitoring

- Usually none is needed in mild cases. If complications occur, intensive supportive care may be required.
- Activity as tolerated. Children may return to school when lesions have completely scabbed.

DIET

No special diet

PATIENT EDUCATION

- In a healthy child, chickenpox is rarely serious and recovery is complete.
- Native chickenpox typically confers lifelong immunity.
- Second attack is rare, but subclinical infection can occur; happens occasionally after vaccination in children
- Infection becomes latent and may recur years later as herpes zoster in adults (and sometimes in children).
- Fatalities are rare.

COMPLICATIONS

- Although only 2% of cases are reported after 2nd decade, 35% of deaths occur in this age group.
- Secondary bacterial infection: cellulitis, abscess, erysipelas, sepsis, septic arthritis/osteomyelitis, or staphylococcal pyomyositis
- Pneumonia: 20–30% of adults with chickenpox have lung involvement; 1/400 is hospitalized.
- Encephalitis (the most common CNS complication)
- Meningitis
- Reye syndrome
- Purpura, thrombocytopenia
- Glomerulonephritis
- Arthritis
- Hepatitis

REFERENCES

1. Centers for Disease Control and Prevention. Summary of notifiable diseases: United States, 2009. *MMWR Morb Mortal Wkly Rep.* 2011;58(53): 1–100.
2. Notifiable Diseases and Mortality Tables. *MMWR Morb Mortal Wkly Rep.* 2014;63:715.
3. Centers for Disease Control and Prevention. FDA approval of an extended period for administering VariZIG for postexposure prophylaxis of varicella. *MMWR Morb Mortal Wkly Rep.* 2012;61(12):212.
4. Marin M, Güris D, Chaves SS, et al. Prevention of varicella: recommendations of the Advisory Committee on Immunization Practices (ACIP). *MMWR Recomm Rep.* 2007;56(RR04):1–40.
5. Elam-Evans LD, Yankey D, Singleton JA, et al. National, state, and selected local area vaccination coverage among children aged 19-35 months–United States, 2013. *MMWR Morb Mortal Wkly Rep.* 2014;63(34):741–748.
6. National Center for Immunization and Respiratory Diseases. General recommendations on immunization—recommendations of the Advisory Committee on Immunization Practices (ACIP). *MMWR Recomm Rep.* 2011;60(2):1–64.
7. Marin M, Broder KR, Temte JL, et al. Use of combination measles, mumps, rubella, and varicella vaccine: recommendations of the Advisory Committee on Immunization Practices (ACIP). *MMWR Recomm Rep.* 2010;59(RR03):1–12.
8. Leung J, Harpaz R, Baughman AL, et al. Evaluation of laboratory methods for diagnosis of varicella. *Clin Infect Dis.* 2010;51(1):23–32.
9. Centers for Disease Control and Prevention. Updated recommendations for use of VariZig—United States, 2013. *MMWR Morb Mortal Wkly Rep.* 2013;62(28):574–576.

ADDITIONAL READING

Galea SA, Sweet A, Beninger P, et al. The safety profile of varicella vaccine: a 10-year review. *J Infect Dis.* 2008;197(Suppl 2):S165–S169.

 SEE ALSO

Herpes Zoster

 CODES

ICD10

- B01.9 Varicella without complication
- B02.9 Zoster without complications
- P35.8 Other congenital viral diseases

CLINICAL PEARLS

- Varicella zoster infection is more likely to produce serious illness in adults than in children.
- Introduction of the varicella vaccine has reduced morbidity and mortality. Currently, two doses of vaccine are recommended.
- Herpes zoster vaccine is recommended for persons ≥60 years of age to prevent shingles.

CHILD ABUSE
Karen A. Hulbert, MD

 BASICS

DESCRIPTION
- Types of abuse: neglect (most common and highest mortality), physical abuse, emotional/psychological abuse, sexual abuse
- Neglect includes: physical (e.g., failure to provide necessary food or shelter or lack of appropriate supervision), medical (e.g., failure to provide necessary medical or mental health treatment), educational (e.g., failure to educate a child or attend to special education needs), and emotional (e.g., inattention to a child's emotional needs, failure to provide psychological care, or permitting the child to use alcohol or other drugs)
- System(s) affected: gastrointestinal (GI), endocrine/metabolic, musculoskeletal, nervous, renal, reproductive, skin/exocrine, psychiatric
- Synonym(s): suspected nonaccidental trauma; child maltreatment; child neglect

EPIDEMIOLOGY
Incidence
- The National Incidence Study (NIS) estimates the incidence of neglect in the United States using estimates from child protective services (CPS) statistics and other sources. Most recent *NIS-4* (published 2010) looked at data from 2004 to 2009.
- Using the stringent "harm standard" definition, >1.25 million children experience maltreatment (1 in 58).
- Using the "endangerment standard," 3 million children experienced maltreatment (1 child in 25) (1).

Prevalence
- In 2013, a nationally estimated 3 million referrals were made to CPS. Of those referrals, 677,997 were substantiated (60.9%). The number of child fatalities nationwide was 1,484 (2).
- The most common age of victims of abuse and neglect was <1 year old (2).
- The top three perpetrators (in order of prevalence) were parent, then "other relative," then unmarried partner (2).

RISK FACTORS
- All ages; male = female:
  - Risk of physical abuse increases with age.
  - Risk of fatal abuse is more common in those <2 years.
  - Physical abuse is 2.1 times higher among children with disabilities (2).
- Poverty, drug abuse, lower educational status, parental history of abuse, mentally ill parent/maternal depression, poor support network, and domestic violence:
  - Child abuse is 4.9 times more likely in family with spouse abuse (3).
  - Children in households with unrelated adults, 50 times more likely to die of inflicted injuries (3)
  - Adults who were abused as children are at higher risk of becoming abusers than those not abused.

GENERAL PREVENTION
- Know your patients and document their family situations; have increased suspicion to screen for risk factors at prenatal, postnatal, and pediatric visits.
- Physicians can educate parents on range of normal behaviors to expect in infants and children:
  - Anticipatory guidance on ways to handle crying infants; methods of discipline for toddlers

- Train first responders—teachers, childcare workers—to look for signs of abuse.
- Some studies suggest developing screening tools to identify high-risk families early and offer interventions such as early childhood home visitation programs.

COMMONLY ASSOCIATED CONDITIONS
- Failure to thrive
- Prematurity
- Developmental deficits
- Poor school performance
- Poor social skills
- Low self-esteem, depression

⊕ DIAGNOSIS

- Relatively minor injuries, frenulum tears, or bruising in precruising infants may be the first indications of child physical abuse; these minor, suspicious injuries have been termed "sentinel injuries" (4)[B].
- In a retrospective study of infants who were definitely abused, 27.5% had a sentinel injury (80% had a bruise), and in 41.9% of those cases, the parent reported that a medical provider was aware of the injury (4)[B].

- Documentation
  - The medical record is an important piece of evidence for investigation and litigation (5)[C].
  - Critical elements include the following (5)[C]:
    ○ Brief statement of child's disclosure or caregiver's explanation, including any alternate explanations offered
    ○ Time the incident occurred and date/time of disclosure
    ○ Whether witnesses were present
    ○ Developmental abilities of child
    ○ Objective medical findings
- DO NOT use terms such as "rule out," "R/O," and "alleged." They may cause ambiguity; clearly state physician opinion (5)[C].
- Documentation should include disposition of patient and record any report made to CPS (5)[C].

HISTORY

- History of a sentinel injury should prompt consideration of abuse; it may be the first and only abusive injury; there may be escalating and repeated violence instead of a single event of momentary loss of control (4)[B].

- Use nonjudgmental, open-ended questions (ask: who, what, when, and where; NEVER why).
- Use quotes whenever possible.
- Document past medical and developmental history, child's temperament, and interactions among family members.
- Suggestive of intentional trauma
  - No explanation or vague explanation (3)[C]
  - Important detail of explanation changes dramatically (3)[C].
  - Explanation is inconsistent with pattern, age, or severity (3)[C].
  - Explanation is inconsistent with child's physical or developmental abilities (3)[C].
  - Different witnesses provide markedly different history (3)[C].
  - Considerable delay in seeking treatment
- Nonspecific symptoms of abuse:
  - Behavior changes; self-destructive behavior
  - Anxiety and/or depression

- Sleep disturbances, night terrors
- School problems

PHYSICAL EXAM
- Explain what the exam will involve and why procedures are needed.
- Examine child in a comfortable setting.
- Allow child to choose who will be in the room.
- Use appropriate positions to examine the anal and genital areas of children.
- General assessment for signs of physical abuse, neglect, and self-injurious behaviors
- Thorough physical exam
  - Skin, head, eyes, ears, nose, and mouth
  - Chest/abdomen
  - Genital (consider exam under sedation) or refer to emergency department (ED)
  - Extremities, with focus on inner arms and legs
  - Growth data
- Maintain high index of suspicion for occult head, chest, and abdominal trauma.
- Physical abuse
  - Skin markings (e.g., lacerations, burns, ecchymoses, linear/shaped contusions, bites)
  - Immersion injuries with clearly distinguished outlines (e.g., from boiling water)
  - Oral trauma (e.g., torn frenulum, loose teeth)
  - Ear trauma (e.g., signs of ear pulling)
  - Eye trauma (e.g., hyphema, hemorrhage)
  - Head/abdominal blunt trauma
  - Fractures
- Sexual abuse
  - Unexplained penile, vaginal, hymenal, perianal, or anal injuries/bleeding/discharge
  - Pregnancy or STIs
  - Sperm is a definitive finding of child abuse.
- Neglect
  - Child may be low weight for height, unclean, or unkempt.
  - Rashes
  - Fearful or too trusting
  - Clinging to or avoiding caregiver
  - Flat or balding occiput
  - Abnormal development or growth parameters
- Measurements, photographs, and careful descriptions are critical for accurate diagnosis.
- Collaboration with specialist and child abuse assessment team (3)[C]

DIFFERENTIAL DIAGNOSIS
- Physical trauma
  - Accidental injury; toxic ingestion
  - Bleeding disorders (e.g., classic hemophilia)
  - Metabolic or congenital conditions
  - Conditions with skin manifestations (e.g., Mongolian spots, Henoch-Schönlein purpura, meningococcemia, erythema multiforme, hypersensitivity, car seat burns, staphylococcal scalded skin syndrome, chickenpox, impetigo)
  - Cultural practices (e.g., cupping, coining)
- Neglect
  - Endocrinopathies (e.g., diabetes mellitus)
  - Constitutional
  - GI (clefts, malabsorption, irritable bowel)
  - Seizure disorder
  - Sudden infant death syndrome (SIDS)
- Skeletal trauma
  - Obstetrical trauma
  - Nutritional (scurvy, rickets)
  - Infection (congenital syphilis, osteomyelitis)
  - Osteogenesis imperfecta

DIAGNOSTIC TESTS & INTERPRETATION
Initial Tests (lab, imaging)
- Directed by history and physical exam:
  - Urinalysis (e.g., abdominal/flank/back/genital trauma), urine DNA probe for STIs
  - Complete blood chemistry. Consideration of coagulation studies and platelet count (e.g., rule out bleeding disorder, abdominal trauma) as appropriate.
  - Electrolytes, creatinine, BUN, glucose
  - Liver and pancreatic function tests (e.g., abdominal trauma)
  - Guaiac stool (abdominal trauma)
- In cases of suspected neglect:
  - Stool exam, calorie count, purified protein derivative and anergy panel, sweat test, lead and zinc levels
- In cases of suspected sexual abuse:
  - STI testing: gonorrhea, chlamydia, *Trichomonas*; also consider HIV, herpes simplex virus (HSV), hepatitis panel, syphilis
  - Serum pregnancy test
- Skeletal survey is recommended for:
  - Infants <6 months with bruising, regardless of pattern (given rarity of accidental bruising in young nonmobile infants)
  - Children with bruising attributed to abuse or domestic violence
  - Children <12 months with bruising on the cheek, eye area, ear, neck, upper arm, upper leg, hand, foot, torso, buttocks, or genital area (6)[B]
  - All children with fractures and children with suspicious injuries <2 years:
    ○ Skeletal survey: X-rays include two views of each extremity; skull, anteroposterior (AP) and lateral; spine, AP and lateral; chest x-ray; and/or rib (posterior), abdomen, pelvis, hands, and feet.
    ○ Consider bone scan for acute rib fractures and subtle long bone fractures.
  - Intracranial and extracranial injury:
    ○ CT scan of head
    ○ Consider MRI of head/neck for better dating of injuries, looking at subtle findings, intercerebral edema, or hemorrhage.
  - Intra-abdominal injuries:
    ○ CT scan of abdomen

Follow-Up Tests & Special Considerations
- Bruising is a common presenting feature:
  - Bruising in babies who are not independently mobile is very uncommon (<1%).
- Patterns suggestive of abuse
  - Bruises seen away from bony prominences
  - Bruises to face, back, abdomen, arms, buttocks, ears, hands
  - Multiple bruises in clusters or uniform shape
  - Patterned injuries (such as bite marks or the imprint of an object like a belt or cord) should be considered inflicted until proven otherwise.
- Red flags (3)[B]
  - History that is inconsistent with the injury
  - No explanation offered for the injury or injury blamed on sibling or another child
  - History that is inconsistent with the child's developmental level
- Sexual abuse
  - Consider photocolposcopy.
  - <72 hours from time of abuse: Collect samples for the forensic laboratory (contact authorities for appropriate protocol).

Test Interpretation
- Spiral fractures in nonambulatory patients (children who are not walking or cruising should not have bruising or fractures from "falls")
- Chip or bucket-handle fractures
- Epiphyseal/metaphyseal rib fractures in infants
- Rupture of liver/spleen in abdominal blunt trauma
- Retinal hemorrhages in shaken baby syndrome
- Recent literature notes a greater risk of abuse with skull and femur fractures, unexplained injuries, and a delay in seeking care (7)[C].

 TREATMENT

GENERAL MEASURES
Test for STIs before treatment.

MEDICATION
First Line
Antibiotics as indicated for STIs

Second Line
Consider antidepressants if needed.

ALERT
Emergency contraception reduces rate of pregnancy after sexual assault:
- Levonorgestrel: single dose of 1.5 mg or two 0.75 mg doses taken together or 12 hours apart. Take as soon as possible; effective up to 72 hours (8)[A]
- Ulipristal (Ella): 30-mg single dose as soon as possible; effective up to 120 hours (8)[A]

ISSUES FOR REFERRAL
- Consider managing in ED to collect forensic specimens and maintain chain of evidence.
- Mandatory reporting to child protective authorities

INPATIENT CONSIDERATIONS
Admission Criteria/Initial Stabilization
- Moderate to severe injuries or unstable
- Acute psychological trauma
- If safety of child outside the hospital cannot be guaranteed

Discharge Criteria
- Child should be sent to another relative or into foster care if the suspected abuser lives with the child.
- Counseling for individual and family
- After initial evaluation, consider referral to sexual assault center.

 ONGOING CARE

FOLLOW-UP RECOMMENDATIONS
As clinically indicated
Patient Monitoring
- Refer to the state protective services.
- Monitor injury healing over time.
- Follow-up assessment for STIs that may not present acutely (e.g., HPV)

PROGNOSIS
Without intervention, child abuse is often a chronic and escalating phenomenon.

COMPLICATIONS
Growing evidence that sexual, physical, and emotional abuse in childhood are risk factors for poorer adult mental and physical health.

REFERENCES
1. Sedlak AJ, Mettenburg J, Basena M, et al. Fourth National Incidence Study of Child Abuse and Neglect (NIS-4): Report to Congress, Executive Summary. Washington, DC: U.S. Department of Health and Human Services, Administration for Children and Families; 2010.
2. U.S. Department of Health and Human Services, Administration for Children and Families, Administration on Children, Youth and Families, Children's Bureau. Child maltreatment 2013. http://www.acf.hhs.gov/programs/cb/resource/child-maltreatment-2013-data-tables. Accessed 2015.
3. Kellogg ND; American Academy of Pediatrics Committee on Child Abuse and Neglect. Evaluation of suspected child physical abuse. *Pediatrics*. 2007;119(6):1232–1241.
4. Sheets LK, Leach ME, Koszewski IJ, et al. Sentinel injuries in infants evaluated for child physical abuse. *Pediatrics*. 2013;131(4):701–707.
5. Jackson AM, Rucker A, Hinds T, et al. Let the record speak: medicolegal documentation in cases of child maltreatment. *Clin Ped Emerg Med*. 2006;7(3):181–185.
6. Wood JN, Fakeye O, Mondestin V, et al. development of hospital-based guidelines for skeletal survey in young children with bruises. *Pediatrics*. 2015;135 (2)e312–e320.
7. Preer G, Sorrentino D, Newton AW. Child abuse pediatrics: prevention, evaluation, and treatment. *Curr Opin Pediatr*. 2012;24(2):266–273.
8. Bosworth MC, Olusola PL, Low SB. An update on emergency contraception. *Am Fam Physician*. 2014;89(7):545–550.

ADDITIONAL READING
- Harris TS. Bruises in children: normal or child abuse? *J Pediatr Health Care*. 2010;24(4):216–221.
- van Rijn RR, Sieswerda-Hoogendoorn T. Educational paper: imaging child abuse: the bare bones. *Eur J Pediatr*. 2012;171(2):215–224.

CODES
ICD10
- T74.12XA Child physical abuse, confirmed, initial encounter
- T74.32XA Child psychological abuse, confirmed, initial encounter
- T74.22XA Child sexual abuse, confirmed, initial encounter

CLINICAL PEARLS
- When a bruise is present, it should be considered as potentially sentinel for physical abuse if no plausible explanation is given (4)[B].
- High index of suspicion is important for prevention and recognition of abuse.
- Neglect is the most common and lethal form of abuse and should be aggressively reported.
- Detailed exam with documentation is key.
- Mandated reporting is required for suspected child abuse and neglect; the physician does not have to prove abuse before reporting.
- Child Abuse Hotline https://www.childwelfare.gov/topics/responding/reporting/how/

CHLAMYDIA INFECTION (SEXUALLY TRANSMITTED)

Casandra Cashman, MD, FAAFP

 BASICS

DESCRIPTION
- *Chlamydia trachomatis* is an intracellular membrane-bound prokaryotic organism. Chlamydia derives from the Greek word for "cloak."
- Chlamydia is the most common bacterial sexually transmitted infection (STI) in the United States (1)[A].
- Transmitted through vaginal, anal, or oral sex; transmitted vertically during vaginal delivery
- Most cases are asymptomatic, especially in females. Untreated disease can lead to pelvic inflammatory disease (PID), ectopic pregnancy, and infertility.
- System(s) affected: reproductive

Pregnancy Considerations
Perinatal acquisition may result in neonatal pneumonia and/or conjunctivitis.

EPIDEMIOLOGY
Incidence
- Mandatory reporting started in 1985; there has generally been a steady increase in incidence since
- 1.4 million *reported* cases in 2013. Increasing incidence reflects broader screening, improved testing, and better reporting (as opposed to a large increase in disease burden). 2012 to 2013 is the first time since national reporting began that the rate of reported cases decreased.
- Swedish new variant chlamydia (nvCT) first reported in 2006; often produces false-negative tests; largely confined to Nordic countries.

Prevalence
- 446/100,000 people in the United States in 2012
- Populations most affected: young females, ethnic minorities
- Peak incidence: age 18 to 20 years
- Predominant sex: females > males. Females have >2.5 times higher reported incidence and prevalence than males. This likely reflects increased testing in females. Increasing use of urine screening may increase identification in males.
- Infection rates >7 times higher in blacks than whites. Rates are higher in larger urban areas.
- Highest male prevalence in heterosexual adolescents
- Estimated to affect ~2% of young sexually active individuals in the United States

ETIOLOGY AND PATHOPHYSIOLOGY
C. trachomatis serotypes D–K associated with genital tract infections. Chlamydia is an obligate intracellular organism. Chlamydia has biphasic life cycle. Exists extracellularly as elementary body (EB) that is metabolically inactive and infectious. Once taken up by host cell (typically columnar epithelium of the genital tract), the EB prevents lysosomal phagocytosis and transforms to reticulate body (RB) which requires energy from host cell to synthesize RNA, DNA, and proteins. After taking up host cell residence, EB are released and are capable of infecting neighboring cells or spreading the infection through sexual contact.

RISK FACTORS
Risk correlates with:
- Number of lifetime sexual partners and number of concurrent sexual partners
- No use of barrier contraception during intercourse
- Younger age (highest in females 15 to 19 years, males 20 to 24 years)
- Black/Hispanic/Native American and Alaskan Native ethnicity

GENERAL PREVENTION
- Screen populations with prevalence >5% at least annually (1)[A].
- Screening recommended if new or >1 sex partner in past 6 months; attending an adolescent clinic, family-planning clinic, STD or abortion clinic, or attending a jail or other detention center clinic. Screen if rectal pain, discharge or tenesmus, testicular pain; test all individuals with urethral or cervical discharge.
- All sexually active women ≤25 years of age should be screened at least yearly. Repeat testing in ~3 months is recommended for those who screen positive because reinfection rate is high regardless of whether the sexual partner is treated (2)[A].
- Consider screening sexually active men ≤25 years of age particularly in high-risk populations.
- Screen men who have sex with men annually.
- Nucleic acid amplification test (NAAT) is the preferred screening test in all circumstances except child sexual abuse involving boys or rectal/oropharyngeal testing in prepubescent girls. For these situations, culture and susceptibility testing is preferred (3)[A].
- Acceptable to screen women for chlamydia on same day as intrauterine device insertion—treat if positive (no need to remove IUD in this circumstance) (4)[B]

COMMONLY ASSOCIATED CONDITIONS
- Females
  - PID: ~10% develop PID within 12 months if untreated.
  - Infertility, ectopic pregnancy
  - Chronic pelvic pain
  - Urethral syndrome (dysuria, frequency, and pyuria in the absence of infection)
  - Arthritis (less common)
  - Spontaneous abortion
- Males
  - Epididymitis and nongonococcal urethritis
  - Reiter syndrome (HLA-B27)
  - Proctitis
- Neonates
  - Inclusion conjunctivitis (occurs in ~40% of exposed neonates)
  - Otitis media
  - Pneumonia
  - Pharyngitis
- Diseases caused by other chlamydial species
  - Lymphogranuloma venereum (LGV): *C. trachomatis* serotypes L1 to L3
  - Trachoma: *C. trachomatis* serotypes A–C

 DIAGNOSIS

Many patients are asymptomatic.

Pregnancy Considerations
- Test all patients at first prenatal visit.
- Test of cure 3 months after treatment for all pregnant patients
- Repeat test in 3rd trimester (2)[A].

HISTORY
- Complete sexual history, including number of sex partners (lifetime and past year), prior history of STIs, use of barrier protection, commercial sex work, oral or anal receptive intercourse, and partner fidelity
- In females, the most common symptoms are:
  - Mucopurulent vaginal discharge, dysuria (urethral syndrome), bartholinitis, abdominopelvic pain (endometritis, salpingitis/PID), right upper quadrant pain (Fitz-Hugh-Curtis syndrome)
- In males, the most common symptoms are:
  - Dysuria, urethral discharge (urethritis), scrotal pain (epididymitis), rectal pain or discharge (proctitis), acute arthritis (Reiter syndrome)

PHYSICAL EXAM
- Men and women: external genitalia (rash, lesions), urethral discharge, inguinal lymphadenopathy, pharyngeal exudate, and perianal lesions
- In addition, for women: cervix (discharge, motion tenderness), bimanual examination for cervical motion tenderness, uterine tenderness, ovarian or adnexal tenderness or mass
- LGV (*C. trachomatis* serovars L1, L2, or L3): Primary lesion is a small papule that may ulcerate at the site of transmission after an incubation period of 3 to 30 days. Unilateral tender lymphadenopathy. With rectal transmission, LGV causes an invasive proctocolitis.

DIFFERENTIAL DIAGNOSIS
- *Neisseria gonorrhoeae*: urethritis, proctitis, epididymitis, cervicitis, PID, Bartholin abscess
- *Mycoplasma* or *Ureaplasma urealyticum*: urethritis, epididymitis, Reiter disease, PID
- *C. trachomatis* (serotypes L1 to L3): LGV, proctitis
- Trichomoniasis

DIAGNOSTIC TESTS & INTERPRETATION
Initial Tests (lab, imaging)
- *Test of choice is NAAT*: sensitivity >95%; specificity >99%
- Urine is as sensitive as cervical swab.
- Patient self-collected vaginal swabs is also effective.
- Lab tests may remain positive for 3 weeks after successful treatment.
- Test for concurrent STIs, including gonorrhea, HIV, syphilis; perform cervical cancer (PAP) screening if clinically appropriate.

Follow-Up Tests & Special Considerations
See "Patient Monitoring."

TREATMENT

GENERAL MEASURES
- Offer patients concurrent testing for gonorrhea, HIV (after counseling and consent), and possibly syphilis. Also, ensure females are up to date with cervical cancer screening.
- Consider treating gonorrhea empirically.
- All partners (most recent partner and all partners within the past 60 days) should be tested and treated.

MEDICATION
First Line
- http://www.cdc.gov/std/treatment/2010/chlamydial-infections.htm
- Treatment of chlamydial urethritis, cervicitis (including sexual partners of infected persons)
- Azithromycin 1 g PO single dose *or*
- Doxycycline 100 mg PO BID for 7 days
- First-line PID treatment (outpatient)
  - Ceftriaxone 250 mg IM × 1 PLUS doxycycline 100 mg PO for 14 days with or without metronidazole 500 mg PO BID for 14 days *or*
  - Cefoxitin 2 g IM × 1 with probenecid 1 g PO × 1 *PLUS* doxycycline 100 mg PO for 14 days with or without metronidazole 500 mg PO BID for 14 days

- Azithromycin and ceftriaxone may be given simultaneously in the office to treat both chlamydia and gonorrhea. This reduces nonadherence (2)[A].
- Asymptomatic rectal chlamydia can be treated with doxycycline 100 mg BID for 7 days. Azithromycin 1 g for 1 day is slightly less effective but can also be used, especially if compliance or medication availability is an issue (5,6)[A].

ALERT
Use azithromycin with caution in patients with known QT prolongation, hypokalemia, hypomagnesemia, bradycardia, or who are currently treated with antiarrythmics.

Pregnancy Considerations
- Tetracyclines (doxycycline) and quinolones (ofloxacin, levofloxacin) are contraindicated in pregnant women.
- Consider the following:
  - Azithromycin 1 g PO *OR*
  - Amoxicillin 500 mg PO TID for 7 days (2)[A] OR
  - Erythromycin base 500 mg PO QID for 7 days

ALERT
Tetracyclines and quinolones are contraindicated in young children:

- <45 kg: erythromycin base or ethinyl succinate 500 mg/kg/day PO QID for 14 days
- >45 kg but <8 years: azithromycin 1 g PO for 1 day
- >8 years: adult regimen
- Rule out sexual abuse in children with chlamydial infections.

Second Line
For chlamydial urethritis/cervicitis

- Erythromycin base 500 mg PO QID for 7 days OR erythromycin ethylsuccinate 800 mg PO QID for 7 days
- Levofloxacin 500 mg PO daily for 7 days or orofloxacin 300 mg PO BID for 7 days

ADDITIONAL THERAPIES
Patient delivered partner therapy (PDPT) or expedited partner therapy (EPT): Provide medications or prescriptions to take to sexual partners of persons infected with STIs without clinical assessment.
- EPT reduces recurrence more effectively than traditional partner referral.
- http://www.cdc.gov/std/ept/legal/

INPATIENT CONSIDERATIONS
The following patients are recommended for inpatient treatment of PID: pregnancy, lack of response or intolerance to oral medicines, suspicion of poor compliance, severe clinical illness, pelvic abscess, and possible need for surgical intervention

Admission Criteria/Initial Stabilization
Outpatient treatment, unless moderately or severely ill

ONGOING CARE

FOLLOW-UP RECOMMENDATIONS
Patient and all partners should abstain from sexual contact until at least 7 days after completing treatment.

Patient Monitoring
- Test of cure: not routinely recommended, except in pregnancy
- Sexual partners should be treated.

PATIENT EDUCATION
- Counseling regarding safe sexual practices, use of barrier protection, and abstinence
- Patient and partner should complete antibiotic course.

PROGNOSIS
Prognosis is good following therapy.

COMPLICATIONS
- Both sexes: Chlamydial infection enhances transmission of and susceptibility to HIV.
- Females: tubal infertility (most common cause of acquired infertility), tubal (ectopic) pregnancy, chronic pelvic pain
  - Annual screening of sexually active women would prevent 61% of chlamydia-related PID.
- Males: transient oligospermia and postepididymitis urethral stricture (rare)

REFERENCES

1. Centers for Disease Control and Prevention. 2012 Sexually transmitted disease surveillance. http://www.cdc.gov/std/stats12/chlamydia.htm.
2. Workowski KA, Berman S, Bauer H, et al. Sexually transmitted diseases treatment guidelines, 2010. *MMWR Recomm Rep.* 2010;59(RR-12):1–110.
3. Centers for Disease Control and Prevention. Recommendations for the laboratory-based detection of *Chlamydia trachomatis* and *Neisseria gonorrhea*—2014. http://www.cdc.gov/mmwr/preview/mmwrhtml/rr6302a1.htm.
4. Sufrin CB, Postlethwaite D, Armstrong MA, et al. *Neisseria gonorrhea* and *Chlamydia trachomatis* screening at intrauterine device insertion and pelvic inflammatory disease. *Obstet Gynecol.* 2012;120(6):1314–1321.
5. Elgalib A, Alexander S, Tong CY, et al. Seven days of doxycycline is an effective treatment for asymptomatic rectal *Chlamydia trachomatis* infection. *Int J STD AIDS.* 2011;22(8):474–477.
6. Drummond F, Ryder N, Wand H, et al. Is azithromycin adequate treatment for asymptomatic rectal chlamydia? *Int J STD AIDS.* 2011;22(8):478–480.

ADDITIONAL READING

- Baud D, Goy G, Jaton K, et al. Role of *Chlamydia trachomatis* in miscarriage. *Emerg Infect Dis.* 2011;17(9):1630–1635.
- Price MJ, Ades AE, De Angelis D, et al. Risk of pelvic inflammatory disease following *Chlamydia trachomatis* infection: analysis of prospective studies with a multistate model. *Am J Epidemiol.* 2013;178(3):484–492.
- Ray WA, Murray KT, Hall K, et al. Azithromycin and the risk of cardiovascular death. *N Engl J Med.* 2012;366(20):1881–1890.
- Unemo M, Clarke IN. The Swedish new variant of Chlamydia trachomatis. *Curr Opin Infect Dis.* 2011;24(1):62–69.
- Won H, Ramachandran P, Steece R, et al. Is there evidence of the new variant *Chlamydia trachomatis* in the United States? *Sex Transm Dis.* 2013;40(5):352–353.

 SEE ALSO

Cervicitis, Ectropion, and True Erosion; Epididymitis; Gonococcal Infections; HIV/AIDS; Pelvic Inflammatory Disease (PID); Syphilis; Urethritis

CODES

ICD10
- A56.8 Sexually transmitted chlamydial infection of other sites
- A56.01 Chlamydial cystitis and urethritis
- A56.02 Chlamydial vulvovaginitis

CLINICAL PEARLS

- *C. trachomatis* is common in young sexually active individuals. Annual screening is recommended in sexually active women 25 years of age and younger.
- To prevent recurrence, treat patients and their partners concurrently.
- Test of cure is recommended for pregnant patients at 3 weeks. Pregnant women diagnosed in the 1st trimester should have a second test of cure 3 months after treatment.

CHLAMYDOPHILA PNEUMONIAE

Fozia Akhtar Ali, MD • Teny Anna Philip, MD

 BASICS

DESCRIPTION
- Chlamydophila pneumoniae (formerly known as Chlamydia pneumoniae) is an obligate intracellular gram-negative bacterium causing atypical pneumonia or bronchitis in adolescents and young adults (1).
- Associated with a more severe, persistent, latent infection in older adults
- Humans are the only known reservoir.

EPIDEMIOLOGY
- Responsible for 10–20% of community-acquired pneumonia (CAP) among adults, 2nd to mycoplasma in cases of atypical pneumonia (1)
- Epidemiologic studies suggest 4-year peaks.
- The incubation period is ~3 to 4 weeks.
- Most infected persons are asymptomatic.
- Typically presents as mild upper respiratory infection (URI). Bronchitis and pneumonia may follow in 1 to 4 weeks.
- Primary infection more common in ages 7 to 40 years; reinfection pneumonia more common in elderly
- Serologic evidence of previous infection is found in 50% of adults and 75% of elderly.
- Male > female (60–90%); possibly due to smoking

Incidence
- Outbreaks have occurred among military recruits, university students, and nursing home residents, with incidence highest in elderly.
- The overall incidence is unknown. Each year, an estimated 2 to 5 million cases of pneumonia (all causes) and 500,000 pneumonia-related hospitalizations occur in the United States (2).

Prevalence
10–20% of CAP cases among adults

ETIOLOGY AND PATHOPHYSIOLOGY
- The elementary body is the infectious form.
  - Rigid cell wall and relative metabolic inactivity allows the organism to survive outside of the host cell for a limited time.
- The elementary body infects the host cell by receptor-mediated endocytosis and becomes a reticulate body (3).
- Reticulate bodies divide intracellularly, forming intracytoplasmic inclusions that divide and release chlamydial antigens. This elicits a host immune response leading to mucus production in the nasal passages, sinuses, bronchial tree, and alveoli, along with nasopharyngeal and airway inflammation and bronchospasm.
- After 48 to 72 hours, the reticulate bodies become elementary bodies and are released by cell lysis.

RISK FACTORS
- Close quarters—classrooms, military barracks, shelters, and nursing homes.
- All ages at risk, but most common in school-age children. In the United States, 50% of adults have evidence of past infection by age 20. Reinfection throughout life appears to be common (2).

GENERAL PREVENTION
- Transmission is by respiratory droplets. Hand washing and avoiding exposure to infected persons are key preventive steps.
- Incidence high among military recruits during basic training; weekly azithromycin prophylaxis reduces case rate.

COMMONLY ASSOCIATED CONDITIONS
- Chronic obstructive pulmonary disease
- Asthma
- HIV infection
- Cystic fibrosis
- Diabetes mellitus

 DIAGNOSIS

HISTORY
- Illness varies in clinical severity from mild, self-limited URI to fulminant pneumonia.
- Onset is typically gradual.
- Sore throat and hoarseness may precede cough by a week or more, leading to biphasic constellation of symptoms (uncommon in *Legionella*, less common with *Mycoplasma, Streptococcus pneumoniae,* and *Haemophilus influenzae*).
- Dry cough
- Low-grade fever (usually early in illness); chills
- Rhinitis
- Headache, malaise, myalgias
- Sinus congestion
- Nausea
- Altered mental status; elderly patients are less likely to exhibit respiratory symptoms with pneumonia and may present with altered mental status or falls.

PHYSICAL EXAM
- General appearance usually nontoxic
- Fever
- Tachypnea
- Tachycardia
- Crackles or wheezing
- Bronchial breath sounds
- Percussion dullness and egophony less sensitive but more specific for pneumonia
- Pharyngeal erythema without exudate

DIFFERENTIAL DIAGNOSIS
- Other causes of atypical pneumonia, including *Mycoplasma pneumoniae* and *Legionella pneumophila*
- Other bacterial causes of pneumonia, including *S. pneumoniae, H. influenzae, Moraxella catarrhalis,* and *Staphylococcus aureus*
- Respiratory viruses: adenovirus, influenza A, influenza B, parainfluenza virus, and respiratory syncytial virus
- Endemic fungal pathogens: coccidioidomycosis, histoplasmosis
- Opportunistic fungal pathogens: *Candida* species, *Aspergillus* species, *Mucor* species, *Cryptococcus neoformans*
- Other: psittacosis, Q fever, TB, tularemia
- Conditions that mimic CAP: acute respiratory disease syndrome, idiopathic pulmonary fibrosis, neoplasm, pulmonary embolus, sarcoidosis, congestive heart failure

DIAGNOSTIC TESTS & INTERPRETATION
Initial Tests (lab, imaging)
- Microimmunofluorescence (MIF) test is most commonly used (and most practical) initial test.
  - Sensitivity of 50–90% if using paired sera
  - IgM 1:16 or higher
  - IgG 1:512 or higher
  - IgM may not be detectable early in the disease.
- Culture with oropharyngeal swab is the gold standard diagnostic method (not widely available).
  - Specificity 100%; sensitivity 50–70% (4)
  - Specimen should be kept cool and transported in specific media.
  - Most easily cultured using HL or HEp2 cells (5)
- PCR from pharyngeal swab or bronchioalveolar lavage specimen (30–95% sensitivity, >95% specificity) (4); during an outbreak, one study showed PCR was less sensitive (68% vs. 79%) but more specific (93% vs. 86%) than MIF IgM (6).
- White blood count is usually normal.
- Alkaline phosphatase levels may be elevated.
- Blood cultures are recommended if patient is toxic and requires ICU admission; otherwise less helpful.
- Complement fixation for *Chlamydia* is available but cannot distinguish *C. pneumoniae* from *Chlamydophila psittaci.*
- Chest x-ray (CXR) (7)[A] has no characteristic radiograph findings; CXR most commonly shows a single subsegmental infiltrate in the lower lobes.
- Pleural effusion seen in 20–25% of cases. ARDS is rare.
- Histologically, intra-alveolar inflammation with mild interstitial reaction is characteristic of chlamydial pneumonias. Alveolar lining cells contain intracytoplasmic inclusions.

Diagnostic Procedures/Other
Although serology is 95% specific, definitive diagnosis requires a positive culture or PCR testing.

TREATMENT

MEDICATION
Empiric coverage of atypical pathogens in patients with CAP has shown mortality benefit (8)[A].

First Line
Tetracyclines and macrolides are first choice (2).
- Doxycycline: 100 mg PO BID for 10 to 14 days (may use IV in inpatient setting) *OR*
- Azithromycin: 500 mg on day 1, then 250 mg on days 2 to 5 *OR*
- Clarithromycin: 500 mg q12h for 10 to 14 days *OR*
- Tetracycline: 500 mg PO QID for 10 to 14 days
  - Tetracyclines not for use during pregnancy or in children <8 years
  - Tetracyclines may cause photosensitivity; sunscreen is recommended.

Second Line
Alternative drugs
- Levofloxacin: 250 to 500 mg/day (PO or IV) or other respiratory fluoroquinolones have good bioavailability and the convenience of once-daily dosing but are recommended for use only when patients have failed treatment with a 1st-line drug, have had recent antibiotics, significant comorbidities, or have allergies to 1st-line medications.

Pregnancy Considerations
Avoid tetracyclines in pregnant women.

INPATIENT CONSIDERATIONS
- Usually outpatient care. Those with severe pneumonia or coexisting illness may require hospitalization.
- Pneumonia severity index can help predict morbidity and need for hospitalization (7).

Admission Criteria/Initial Stabilization
Infection in debilitated or hospitalized patients can be severe; ventilatory support for respiratory failure

Discharge Criteria
Reversal of respiratory distress, tolerating PO medications, otherwise stable medically, and clinically stable for discharge

ONGOING CARE

FOLLOW-UP RECOMMENDATIONS
Patient Monitoring
- Monitor patients weekly until well.
- Follow-up CXR can document resolution.
- Reinfection is possible.

PROGNOSIS
- Pneumonia is more likely to be life-threatening in older adults and patients with other underlying pulmonary disease (e.g., asthma, chronic obstructive pulmonary disease [COPD]) or the immune compromise (e.g., diabetes), with an overall 0.5–29% mortality rate.
- Death usually from secondary infection or underlying comorbidity

COMPLICATIONS
- Reactive airway disease
- Erythema nodosum
- Endocarditis
- Pericarditis or myocarditis
- Meningoencephalitis
- Possible association with atherosclerotic disease: *C. pneumoniae* has been cultured from atherosclerotic plaque in patients with coronary artery disease and stroke. Treatment for *C. pneumoniae* has not been shown to affect cardiovascular mortality.
- *C. pneumoniae* infection is associated with an increased risk for lung cancer (9).
- ARDS is rare.

REFERENCES

1. Blasi F, Tarsia P, Aliberti S. Chlamydophila pneumoniae. *Clin Microbiol Infect*. 2009;15(1):29–35.
2. Centers for Disease Control and Prevention. Chlamydophila pneumoniae infection. http://www.cdc.gov/pneumonia/atypical/chlamydophila.html. Accessed 2014.
3. Thibodeau KP, Viera AJ. Atypical pathogens and challenges in community-acquired pneumonia. *Am Fam Physician*. 2004;69(7):1699–1706.
4. Kumar S, Hammerschlag MR. Acute respiratory infection due to *Chlamydia pneumoniae*: current status of diagnostic methods. *Clin Infect Dis*. 2007;44(4):568–576.
5. Burillo A, Bouza E. Chlamydophila pneumoniae. *Infect Dis Clin North Am*. 2010;24(1):61–71.
6. Hvidsten D, Halvorsen DS, Berdal BP, et al. *Chlamydophila pneumoniae* diagnostics: importance of methodology in relation to timing of sampling. *Clin Microbiol Infect*. 2009;15(1):42–49.
7. Lutfiyya MN, Henley E, Chang LF, et al. Diagnosis and treatment of community-acquired pneumonia. *Am Fam Physician*. 2006;73(3):442–450.
8. Shefet D, Robenshtock E, Paul M, et al. Empiric antibiotic coverage of atypical pathogens for community acquired pneumonia in hospitalized adults. *Cochrane Database Syst Rev*. 2005;(2):CD004418.
9. Zhan P, Suo LJ, Qian Q, et al. Chlamydia pneumoniae infection and lung cancer risk: a meta-analysis. *Eur J Cancer*. 2011;47(5):742–747.

ADDITIONAL READING

Conklin L, Adjemian J, Loo J, et al. Investigation of a *Chlamydia pneumoniae* outbreak in a federal correctional facility in Texas. *Clin Infect Dis*. 2013; 57(5):639–647.

CODES

ICD10
J16.0 Chlamydial pneumonia

CLINICAL PEARLS

- Consider *C. pneumoniae* in well-appearing young patients presenting with CAP.
- Culture is the gold standard for diagnosis of *C. pneumoniae*. Serodiagnosis is used for acute infection.
- Tetracyclines or macrolides are initial drugs of choice.

CHOLELITHIASIS

Hongyi Cui, MD, PhD

BASICS

DESCRIPTION
- Cholelithiasis is the presence of cholesterol, pigment, or mixed stones (calculi) within the gallbladder.
- Synonym(s): gallstones

Pediatric Considerations
- Uncommon at <10 years
- Most gallstones in children are pigment stones associated with blood dyscrasias.

EPIDEMIOLOGY
Incidence
- Increased in Native Americans and Hispanics
- Increases with age by 1–3% per year; peaks at 7th decade; 2% of the U.S. population develops gallstones annually.

Prevalence
- Population: 8–10% of the United States; gallstones present in 20% >65 years of age
- Predominant sex: female > male (2 to 3:1)

ETIOLOGY AND PATHOPHYSIOLOGY
- Gallstone formation is a complex process mediated by genetic, metabolic, immune, and environmental factors. Gallbladder sludge (a mixture of cholesterol crystals, calcium bilirubinate granules, and mucin gel matrix) serves as the nidus for gallstone formation.
- Production of bile supersaturated with cholesterol (cholesterol stones) from excess cholesterol secretion precipitates as microcrystals that aggregate and expand. Stone formation is enhanced by biliary stasis or impaired gallbladder motility.
- Decrease in bile content of either phospholipid (lecithin) or decreased bile salt secretion
- Excess unconjugated bilirubin in patients with hemolytic diseases; passage of excess bile salt into the colon with subsequent absorption of excess unconjugated bilirubin in patients with inflammatory bowel disease (IBD) or after distal ileal resection (black or pigment stones)
- Hydrolysis of conjugated bilirubin or phospholipid by bacteria in patients with biliary tract infection or stricture (brown stones or primary bile duct stones; rare in the Western world and common in Asia)

RISK FACTORS
- Age (peak in 60s to 70s)
- Female gender, pregnancy, multiparity, obesity, and metabolic syndrome
- Caucasian, Hispanic, or Native American descent
- High-fat diet rich in cholesterol
- Cholestasis or impaired gallbladder motility in association with prolonged fasting, long-term total parenteral nutrition (TPN), and rapid weight loss
- Hereditary (p.D19H variant for the hepatic canalicular cholesterol transporter ABCG5/ABG8)
- Short gut syndrome, terminal ileal resection, inflammatory bowel disease
- Hemolytic disorders (hereditary spherocytosis, sickle cell anemia, etc.), cirrhosis (black/pigment stones)
- Medications (birth control pills, estrogen replacement therapy at high doses, and long-term corticosteroid or cytostatic therapy)
- Viral hepatitis, biliary tract infection and stricture (promotes intraductal formation of pigment stones)

GENERAL PREVENTION
- Ursodiol (Actigall) taken during rapid weight loss prevents gallstone formation.
- Regular exercise and dietary modification may reduce the incidence of gallstone formation.
- Lipid-lowering drugs (statins) may prevent cholesterol stone formation by reducing bile cholesterol saturation.

COMMONLY ASSOCIATED CONDITIONS
90% of people with gallbladder carcinoma have gallstones.

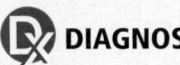

DIAGNOSIS

HISTORY
- Mostly asymptomatic (80%): 2% become symptomatic each year. Over their lifetime, <1/2 of patients with gallstones develop symptoms.
- Episodic right upper quadrant or epigastric pain lasting >15 minutes and sometimes radiating to the back (biliary colic), usually postprandially; pain sometimes awakens the patient from sleep; most patients develop recurrent symptoms after the first episode of biliary colic.
- Nausea, vomiting; indigestion or bloating sensation; fatty food intolerance

PHYSICAL EXAM
- Physical exam is *usually normal* in patients with cholelithiasis in the absence of an acute attack.
- Epigastric and/or right upper quadrant tenderness (Murphy sign) is the traditional physical finding—associated with cholecystitis.
- Charcot triad: fever, jaundice, right upper quadrant pain
- Reynold pentad: fever, jaundice, right upper quadrant pain, hemodynamic instability, mental status changes; classically associated with ascending cholangitis
- Flank and periumbilical ecchymoses (Cullen sign and Grey-Turner sign) in patients with acute hemorrhagic pancreatitis
- Courvoisier sign: palpable mass in the right upper quadrant in patient with obstructive jaundice most commonly due to tumors within the biliary tree or pancreas

DIFFERENTIAL DIAGNOSIS
- Peptic ulcer diseases and gastritis
- Hepatitis
- Pancreatitis
- Cholangitis
- Gallbladder cancer
- Gallbladder polyps
- Acalculous cholecystitis
- Biliary dyskinesia
- Choledocholithiasis

DIAGNOSTIC TESTS & INTERPRETATION
No lab study is specific for cholelithiasis.

Initial Tests (lab, imaging)
- Leukocytosis and elevated C-reactive protein level are associated with acute calculus cholecystitis.
- Ultrasound is the preferred imaging modality. US detects gallstones in 97–98% of patients.
- Thickening of the gallbladder wall (≥5 mm), pericholecystic fluid, and direct tenderness when the probe is pushed against the gallbladder (sonographic Murphy sign) are associated with acute cholecystitis.

- CT scan has no advantage over US except in detecting distal common bile duct stones.
- MR cholangiopancreatography (MRCP) is reserved for cases of suspected common bile duct stones. MRCP is recommended as a secondary imaging study if ultrasonography does not clearly demonstrate acute cholecystitis or gallstones (1)[C].
- Endoscopic US is as sensitive as endoscopic retrograde cholangiopancreatography (ERCP) for detection of common bile duct stones in patients with gallstone pancreatitis.
- Hepatobiliary iminodiacetic acid (HIDA) scan is useful in diagnosing acute cholecystitis secondary to cystic duct obstruction. It is also useful in differentiating acalculous cholecystitis from other causes of abdominal pain. False-positive results in fasting state, insufficient resistance of the sphincter of Oddi, and gallbladder agenesis.
- Cholecystokinin (CCK)-HIDA is specifically used to diagnose gallbladder dysmotility (biliary dyskinesia).
- 10–30% of gallstones are radiopaque calcium or pigment-containing gallstones and are more likely to be visible on plain x-ray. A "porcelain gallbladder" is a calcified gallbladder, visible by x-ray; associated with gallbladder cancer.

Test Interpretation
- Pure cholesterol stones are white or slightly yellow.
- Pigment stones may be black or brown. Black stones contain polymerized calcium bilirubinate, most often secondary to cirrhosis or hemolysis; these almost always form in the gallbladder.
- Brown stones are associated with biliary tract infection, caused by bile stasis, and as such may form either in the bile ducts or gallbladder.

TREATMENT

GENERAL MEASURES
- Treat symptomatic cholelithiasis.
- Conservative therapy is preferred during pregnancy. Surgery in the 2nd trimester if necessary.
- Prophylactic cholecystectomy for patients with calcified (porcelain) gallbladder (risk for gallbladder cancer), patients with large stones (>3 cm), patients with sickle cell disease, patients planning an organ transplant, and patients with recurrent pancreatitis due to microlithiasis
- In morbidly obese patients, simultaneous cholecystectomy may be performed in combination with bariatric procedures (2) to reduce subsequent stone-related comorbidities.

Geriatric Considerations
Gallstones are more common in the elderly. Age alone should not alter the therapeutic plan.

MEDICATION
First Line
- Analgesics for pain relief

  – NSAIDs are the first-choice treatment for pain control equivalent to opioid therapy (2)[A].

  – Opioids are an option for patients who cannot tolerate or fail to respond to NSAIDs.
- Antibiotics for patients with acute cholecystitis

- Prophylactic antibiotics in low-risk patients do not prevent infections during laparoscopic cholecystectomy (3,4)[A].

ISSUES FOR REFERRAL

Patients with retained or recurrent bile duct stones following cholecystectomy should be referred for ERCP.

SURGERY/OTHER PROCEDURES

- Surgery should be considered for patients who have symptomatic cholelithiasis or gallstone-related complications (cholecystitis) or in asymptomatic patients with immune suppression, calcified gallbladder, or family history of gallbladder cancer. Open or laparoscopic cholecystectomy (LC) has similar mortality and complication rates. LC offers less pain and quicker recovery. In well-selected patients, single-incision LC (SILC) and robotic LC are novel methods for the treatment of symptomatic cholelithiasis. SILC has not been shown to be superior to conventional multiport LC in terms of pain and risk of complications (5)[A]. Natural orifice transluminal endoscopic surgery (NOTES) is investigational. Surgery-related complications include common bile duct injury (0.5%), right hepatic duct/artery injury, retained stones, duct leak, biloma formation, and bile duct stricture.
  - Conversion to open procedure is based on clinical judgment. Male gender, previous upper abdominal surgery, thickened gallbladder wall, and acute cholecystitis increase the likelihood of need to convert to an open procedure.
  - In 10–15% of patients with symptomatic cholelithiasis, common bile duct (CBD) stones are detected by intraoperative cholangiogram (IOC). CBD stone(s) can be removed by laparoscopic CBD exploration or postoperative ERCP.
  - IOC helps delineate bile duct anatomy when dissection is difficult. Routine use of IOC is debatable but may be associated with decreased incidence of bile duct injury.
- Early LC (<24 hours after diagnosis of biliary colic) decreases hospital stay and operating time (6)[A].
- For patients with acute cholecystitis, early LC (<7 days of clinical presentation) seems safe and may shorten the total hospital stay versus delayed LC (>6 weeks after index admission with acute cholecystitis) (7)[A].
- Percutaneous cholecystostomy (PC) is used in high-risk patients with cholecystitis or gallbladder empyema. Interval cholecystectomy is advisable.
- Symptomatic patients who are not candidates for surgery or those who have small gallstones (5 mm or smaller) in a functioning gallbladder with a patent cystic duct are candidates for oral dissolution therapy (Actigall). However, the recurrence rate is >50% once the medication is discontinued.
- Extracorporeal shock wave lithotripsy is a noninvasive therapeutic alternative for symptomatic patients who are not candidates for surgery. It is useful for breaking down large bile duct stones before ERCP. Complications include biliary pancreatitis, hepatic hematoma, incomplete ductal stone clearance and recurrence, and so forth.

INPATIENT CONSIDERATIONS

For patients with symptomatic cholelithiasis, laparoscopic cholecystectomy is typically an outpatient procedure. For patients with complications (i.e., cholecystitis, cholangitis, pancreatitis), inpatient care is necessary.

Admission Criteria/Initial Stabilization

- Acute phase: NPO, IV fluids, and antibiotics
- Adequate pain control with narcotics and/or NSAIDs

 ONGOING CARE

FOLLOW-UP RECOMMENDATIONS
Patient Monitoring

- Follow for signs of symptomatic cholelithiasis
- Patients on oral dissolution agents should be followed with serial liver enzyme, serum cholesterol, and imaging studies.

DIET

A low-fat diet may be helpful.

PATIENT EDUCATION

- Change in lifestyle (e.g., regular exercise) and dietary modification (low-fat diet and reduction of total caloric intake) reduce gallstone-related hospitalizations.
- Patients with asymptomatic gallstones should be educated about the typical symptoms of biliary colic and gallstone-related complications.

PROGNOSIS

- <1/2 of patients with gallstones become symptomatic.
- Cholecystectomy: mortality <0.5% elective, 3–5% emergency; morbidity <10% elective, 30–40% emergency
- ~10–15% of the patients will have associated choledocholithiasis.
- After cholecystectomy, stones may recur within the biliary tree.

COMPLICATIONS

- Acute cholecystitis (90–95% secondary to gallstones)
- Gallstone pancreatitis
- Common bile duct stones with obstructive jaundice and acute cholangitis
- Biliary-enteric fistula and gallstone ileus; Bouveret syndrome is a variant of gallstone ileus where the gallstone lodges in the duodenum or pylorus causing a gastric outlet obstruction.
- Gallbladder cancer
- Mirizzi syndrome (extrinsic bile duct obstruction caused by gallstones lodged in gallbladder or cystic duct)

REFERENCES

1. American College of Radiology. ACR appropriateness criteria: right upper quadrant pain. http://www.acr.org/~/media/ACR/Documents/AppCriteria/Diagnostic/RightUpperQuadrantPain.pdf.
2. Colli A, Conte D, Valle SD, et al. Meta-analysis: nonsteroidal anti-inflammatory drugs in biliary colic. Aliment Pharmacol Ther. 2012;35(12):1370–1378.
3. Sanabria A, Dominguez LC, Valdivieso E, et al. Antibiotic prophylaxis for patients undergoing elective laparoscopic cholecystectomy. Cochrane Database Syst Rev. 2010;(12):CD005265.
4. Zhou H, Zhang J, Wang Q, et al. Meta-analysis: antibiotic prophylaxis in elective laparoscopic cholecystectomy. Aliment Pharmacol Ther. 2009;29(10):1086–1095.
5. Gurusamy KS, Vaughan J, Rossi M, et al. Fewer-than-four ports versus four ports for laparoscopic cholecystectomy. Cochrane Database Syst Rev. 2014;(2):CD007109.
6. Gurusamy KS, Koti R, Fusai G, et al. Early versus delayed laparoscopic cholecystectomy for uncomplicated biliary colic. Cochrane Database Syst Rev. 2013;(6):CD007196.
7. Gurusamy KS, Davidson C, Gluud C, et al. Early versus delayed laparoscopic cholecystectomy for people with acute cholecystitis. Cochrane Database Syst Rev. 2013;(6):CD005440.

ADDITIONAL READING

- Brown LM, Rogers SJ, Cello JP, et al. Cost-effective treatment of patients with symptomatic cholelithiasis and possible common bile duct stones. J Am Coll Surg. 2011;212(6):1049–1060.
- Gurusamy KS, Samraj K. Cholecystectomy versus no cholecystectomy in patients with silent gallstones. Cochrane Database Syst Rev. 2007;(1):CD006230.
- Keus F, Gooszen HG, van Laarhoven CJ. Open, small-incision, or laparoscopic cholecystectomy for patients with symptomatic cholecystolithiasis. An overview of Cochrane Hepato-Biliary Group reviews. Cochrane Database Syst Rev. 2010;(1):CD008318.
- Society for Surgery of the Alimentary Tract. SSAT patient care guidelines. Treatment of gallstone and gallbladder disease. J Gastrointest Surg. 2007;11(9):1222–1224.
- Uy MC, Talingdan-Te MC, Espinosa WZ, et al. Ursodeoxycholic acid in the prevention of gallstone formation after bariatric surgery: a meta-analysis. Obes Surg. 2008;18(12):1532–1538.
- Zehetner J, Pelipad D, Darehzereshki A, et al. Single-access laparoscopic cholecystectomy versus classic laparoscopic cholecystectomy: a systematic review and meta-analysis of randomized controlled trials. Surg Laparosc Endosc Percutan Tech. 2013;23(3):235–243.

 SEE ALSO

Cholangitis, Acute; Choledocholithiasis

 CODES

ICD10

- K80.20 Calculus of gallbladder w/o cholecystitis w/o obstruction
- K80.21 Calculus of gallbladder w/o cholecystitis with obstruction
- K80.01 Calculus of gallbladder w acute cholecystitis w obstruction

CLINICAL PEARLS

- Most patients with gallstones are asymptomatic.
- Transabdominal ultrasound is the preferred imaging modality for diagnosis of cholelithiasis (sensitivity, 97%; specificity, 95%).
- Laparoscopic cholecystectomy is the preferred procedure for symptomatic cholelithiasis; lithotripsy and oral dissolution therapy may be considered in rare circumstances.
- Acute acalculous cholecystitis is associated with bile stasis and gallbladder ischemia.
- Prophylactic cholecystectomy is not indicated in patients with asymptomatic gallstones.

CHRONIC COUGH

Jacqueline L. Olin, MS, PharmD, BCPS, FASHP, FCCP • Brian Hertz, MD • J. Andrew Woods, PharmD, BCPS

BASICS

DESCRIPTION
- Chronic cough is defined as a cough that persists for >8 weeks in adults.
- In children, chronic cough is often defined as a cough of >4 weeks in duration.
- Subacute cough describes a cough lasting 3 to 8 weeks.
- Patients present because of fear of the causative illness (e.g., cancer) as well as annoyance, self-consciousness, and hoarseness.
- System(s) affected: gastrointestinal (GI), pulmonary

EPIDEMIOLOGY
- Predominant age: all age groups
- Predominant sex: male = female, with females more likely to seek out medical attention

Incidence
Recurrent cough has been reported at 3–40% by various population estimates.

Prevalence
Chronic cough is one of the most common reasons for primary care visits.

ETIOLOGY AND PATHOPHYSIOLOGY
Varies with findings and disorders implicated
- Often multiple etiologies, but most are related to bronchial irritation. Most frequent etiologies (account for >90% of cases) in nonsmokers include the following:
  – Upper airway cough syndrome (UACS) (formerly referred to as *postnasal drip syndrome*) and other upper airway abnormalities, including allergic and vasomotor rhinitis syndromes
  – Asthma
  – Gastroesophageal reflux disease (GERD)
- Other causes:
  – ACE inhibitors
  – Chronic smoking or exposure to smoke or pollutants
  – Aspiration
  – Bronchiectasis
  – Infections (e.g., pertussis, tuberculosis)
  – Nonasthmatic eosinophilic bronchitis (NAEB)
  – Cystic fibrosis
  – Sleep apnea
  – Restrictive lung diseases (e.g., chronic interstitial lung disease)
  – Neoplasms: bronchogenic or laryngeal
  – Psychogenic (habit cough)
- Cough reflex hypersensitivity or cough hypersensitivity syndrome define a syndrome of cough with characteristic trigger symptoms not adequately explained by other medical conditions (1).

RISK FACTORS
Although various conditions may contribute to chronic cough, the main causes include smoking and pulmonary diseases.

COMMONLY ASSOCIATED CONDITIONS
Patients with UACS, asthma, and GERD may present with chronic cough as the only symptom and not the usual symptoms associated with the diagnoses.

DIAGNOSIS

HISTORY
- Patient age, associated signs/symptoms, medical history, medication history (i.e., ACE inhibitors), environmental and occupational exposures, potential for aspiration, and smoking history may make some causes more likely.
- The character of cough or description of sputum quality is rarely helpful in predicting the underlying cause.
- Cough diaries have not correlated well with objective measures.
- Hemoptysis or signs of systemic illness preclude empiric therapy.

PHYSICAL EXAM
- Signs and symptoms are variable and related to the underlying cause; usually, a nonproductive cough with no other signs or symptoms.
- Possible signs and symptoms of UACS, sinusitis, GERD, congestive heart failure, chronic stressors
- Absence of additional signs/symptoms of a particular condition not necessarily helpful
  – For example, 5% of patients with GERD have no other signs or symptoms and sometimes have poor response to empiric proton pump inhibitor (PPI) trials.

DIAGNOSTIC TESTS & INTERPRETATION
- Evaluation often starts with empiric therapy directed at likely underlying etiology and/or simple testing such as a chest x-ray (CXR).
- Extensive testing only if indicated by the history and physical

Pediatric Considerations
Children with chronic cough not responsive to an inhaled β-agonist and without overt stressors should undergo spirometry (if age-appropriate) and foreign body evaluation (CXR).

Initial Tests (lab, imaging)
- Evaluation will be dictated by findings in the comprehensive history and physical.
- Evaluation of peak flow may be indicated.
- If considering neoplasm, heart failure, or infectious etiologies, CXR or B-type natriuretic peptide (BNP) may be indicated.
- In cases of failure to respond to initial trial of empiric therapy, CXR may also be beneficial.

Follow-Up Tests & Special Considerations
- Examples:
  – If considering chronic obstructive pulmonary disease (COPD), asthma, or restrictive lung disease: spirometry
  – If suspicious of cystic fibrosis: sweat chloride testing
  – If suspicious of hypereosinophilic syndrome, tuberculosis, or malignancy: sputum for eosinophils and cytology
- If abnormal CXR, suspected neoplasm, or underlying pulmonary disorder, consider a chest CT.
- Consider pulmonary consultation.
- Refer to gastroenterologist for endoscopy.

Diagnostic Procedures/Other
If diagnosis suggested and inadequate response to initial measures, other procedures can be considered:
- Pulmonary function testing
- Purified protein derivative (PPD) skin testing
- Allergen testing

- 24-hour esophageal pH monitor
- Bronchoscopy, if history of hemoptysis or smoking with normal CXR
- Endoscopic or video fluoroscopic swallow evaluation or barium esophagram
- Sinus CT
- Ambulatory cough monitoring and cough challenge with citric acid, capsaicin, or other bronchodilator (at specialized cough clinic)
- Echocardiogram

Test Interpretation
Specific to underlying cause

TREATMENT

- With chronic cough, empiric treatment should be directed at the most common causes as clinically indicated (UACS, asthma, GERD) (2)[C].
- Oral antihistamine/decongestant therapy with a 1st-generation antihistamine or nasal steroid spray can be used as initial empiric treatment (2)[C].
- In patients with cough associated with the common cold, nonsedating antihistamines were not found to be effective in reducing cough (2)[C].
- In stable patients with chronic bronchitis, therapy with ipratropium bromide may reduce chronic cough (3)[C].
- Centrally acting antitussive drugs (dextromethorphan, hydrocodone) may be used for short-term symptomatic relief of coughing in patients with chronic bronchitis but have limited efficacy in cough due to upper respiratory infections (3)[C].
- For cough associated with lung cancer, narcotic cough suppressants are recommended (3)[C].
- The American Academy of Pediatrics does not recommend central cough suppressants for treating any kind of cough (2)[B].
- In children <14 years, when pediatric recommendations are not available, adult recommendations should be used with caution (2)[C].
- Some children with recurrent cough and no evidence of airway obstruction may benefit from an inhaled β-agonist (4)[C].
- In infants and children with nonspecific chronic cough, trials of empiric PPI therapy were not effective (5)[C].

GENERAL MEASURES
- In patients with chronic cough, considerations for potential etiology should include asthma (2)[B] or UACS (2)[C].
- With concomitant complaints of heartburn and regurgitation, GERD should be considered as a potential etiology (2)[C].
- 90% of patients will have resolution of cough after smoking cessation (2)[A].
- When indicated, ACE inhibitor therapy should be switched in patients in whom intolerable cough occurs (3)[A]. It may take several days or weeks for cough to resolve after stopping ACE inhibitor therapy.
- Empirically treat postnasal drip and GERD.
- Consider nonpharmacologic options, such as warm fluids, hard candy, or nasal drops. In infants and children, try clearing secretions with a bulb syringe.
- Attempt maximal therapy for single most likely cause for several weeks, then search for coexistent etiologies.

MEDICATION

- Treatments (nasal steroids, classic antihistamines, antacids, bronchodilators, inhaled corticosteroids, PPIs, antibiotics) should be directed at the specific cause of cough.
- If history and physical exam suggest GERD, may want to trial H₂ blocker or PPI therapy prior to further diagnostic testing.
- A comparative effectiveness review of 49 studies with common opioid and nonanesthetic antitussives stated there is some efficiency for treating cough in adults, but evidence is limited (6)[C].
- The FDA issued a public health advisory stating that OTC cough and cold medicines, including antitussives, expectorants, nasal decongestants, antihistamines, or combinations, should not be given to children <2 years. Subsequently, manufacturers have changed labeling to state "do not use" in children <4 years. National estimates have shown a decline in emergency department visits in children <2 years related to adverse events from cough and cold medicine ingestion (7).
- Routine empiric treatment of children with chronic cough with leukotriene receptor antagonists lacks evidence and cannot be recommended (8)[C]. A small pilot study with montelukast in adults demonstrated some symptom relief after 2 weeks of treatment (9)[A].

First Line

- In adults, oral antihistamine/decongestant therapy can be empiric treatment. Multiple formulations are available OTC in combination with other ingredients. Advise patients to review labels carefully or consult pharmacist:
  - Chlorpheniramine 2 mg/phenylephrine 5 mg/acetaminophen 325 mg (Tylenol Allergy Multi-Symptom) 2 caplets or gel caps PO q4h (maximum 12 caplets or gel caps in 24 hours; for patients >12 years)
  - Nasal steroids: fluticasone, budesonide, others, 1 spray BID
- Central cough suppressants for short-term symptomatic relief of nonproductive cough
  - Dextromethorphan 10 to 20 mg PO q4h for patients >12 years; use 5 to 10 mg PO q4h for patients 6 to 12 years
    - Concomitant use of dextromethorphan and agents with serotonergic activity (e.g., SSRIs) should be avoided due to risk of serotonin syndrome.
  - Narcotics: codeine 15 to 30 mg PO q6h; hydrocodone/acetaminophen (Vicodin) 5 mg PO q6h; hydrocodone/chlorpheniramine (Tussionex Pennkinetic) 10 mg (5 mL) PO q12h for patients ≥12 years (no benefit in children; no good efficacy data in adults)

Second Line

- A peripherally acting antitussive agent has been used:
  - In patients >10 years, benzonatate (Tessalon Perles) 100 to 200 mg PO TID as needed (maximum 600 mg/day)
- Results from a small randomized placebo-controlled trial (n = 27) demonstrated subjective cough score improvement in patients using slow-release morphine sulfate. Patients had failed with other antitussive therapies. Side effects included constipation and drowsiness, and there were no discontinuations due to adverse events (10)[A].
  - Morphine was administered 5 to 10 mg PO BID.

- An analysis of studies evaluating inhaled corticosteroid use in chronic cough for patients without additional indication such as asthma did not show consistent benefits (11)[C].

ISSUES FOR REFERRAL
Patients with chronic cough may benefit from evaluation by pulmonary, gastroenterology, ear-nose-and-throat (ENT), and/or allergy specialists.

SURGERY/OTHER PROCEDURES
Fundoplication may be effective for cough secondary to refractory GERD.

 ONGOING CARE

FOLLOW-UP RECOMMENDATIONS
Consider stepwise withdrawal of medications after resolution of cough.

Patient Monitoring
Frequent follow-up is necessary to assess the effectiveness of treatment

DIET
Dietary modification: Patients with GERD may benefit by avoiding ethanol, caffeine, nicotine, citrus, tomatoes, chocolate, and fatty foods.

PATIENT EDUCATION
- Reassure patient that most cases of chronic cough are not life-threatening and that the condition can usually be managed effectively.
- Counsel that several weeks to a month may be needed for significant reduction or elimination of cough
- Prepare the patient for the possibility of multiple diagnostic tests and therapeutic regimens because the treatment is very often empiric.

PROGNOSIS
- >80% of patients can be effectively diagnosed and treated using a systematic approach.
- Cough from any cause may take weeks to months until resolution, and resolution depends greatly on efficacy of treatment directed at underlying etiology.

COMPLICATIONS
- Cardiovascular: arrhythmias, syncope
- Stress urinary incontinence
- Abdominal and intercostal muscle strain
- GI: emesis, hemorrhage, herniation
- Neurologic: dizziness, headache, seizures
- Respiratory: pneumothorax, laryngeal, or tracheobronchial trauma
- Skin: petechiae, purpura, disruption of surgical wounds
- Medication side effects
- Other: negative impact on quality of life

REFERENCES

1. Morice AH, Millqvist E, Belvisi MG, et al. Expert opinion on the cough hypersensitivity syndrome in respiratory medicine. *Eur Respir J*. 2014;44(5):1132–1148.
2. Irwin RS, Baumann MH, Bolser DC, et al. Diagnosis and management of cough executive summary: ACCP evidence-based clinical practice guidelines. *Chest*. 2006;129(1)(Suppl):1S–23S.
3. Bolser DC. Cough suppressant and pharmacologic protussive therapy: ACCP evidence-based clinical practice guidelines. *Chest*. 2006;129(1)(Suppl):238S–249S.
4. Gupta A, McKean M, Chang AB. Management of chronic non-specific cough in childhood: an evidence-based review. *Arch Dis Child Educ Pract Ed*. 2007;92(2):33–39.
5. Chang AB, Lasserson TJ, Gaffney J, et al. Gastro-oesophageal reflux treatment for prolonged non-specific cough in children and adults. *Cochrane Database Syst Rev*. 2011;(1):CD004823.
6. Yancy WS Jr, McCrory DC, Coeytaux RR, et al. Efficacy and tolerability of treatments for chronic cough: a systematic review and meta-analysis. *Chest*. 2013;144(6):1827–1838.
7. Hampton LM, Nguyen DB, Edwards JR, et al. Cough and cold medication adverse events after market withdrawal and labeling revision. *Pediatrics*. 2013;132(6):1047–1054.
8. Chang AB, Winter D, Acworth JP. Leukotriene receptor antagonist for prolonged non-specific cough in children. *Cochrane Database Syst Rev*. 2006;(2):CD005602.
9. Mincheva RK, Kralimarkova TZ, Rasheva M, et al. A real-life observational pilot study to evaluate the effects of two-week treatment with montelukast in patients with chronic cough. *Cough*. 2014;10(1):2.
10. Morice AH, Menon MS, Mulrennan SA, et al. Opiate therapy in chronic cough. *Am J Respir Crit Care Med*. 2007;175(4):312–315.
11. Johnstone KJ, Chang AB, Fong KM, et al. Inhaled corticosteroids for subacute and chronic cough in adults. *Cochrane Database Syst Rev*. 2013;(3):CD009305.

ADDITIONAL READING
Dicpinigaitis PV, Morice AH, Birring SS, et al. Antitussive drugs—past, present, and future. *Pharmacol Rev*. 2014;66(2):468–512.

 SEE ALSO

- Asthma; Bronchiectasis; Congestive Heart Failure; Eosinophilic Pneumonias; Gastroesophageal Reflux Disease; Laryngeal Cancer; Lung, Primary Malignancies; Pertussis; Pulmonary Edema; Rhinitis, Allergic; Sinusitis; Tuberculosis
- Algorithm: Cough, Chronic

CODES

ICD10
- R05 Cough
- J44.9 Chronic obstructive pulmonary disease, unspecified
- J41.0 Simple chronic bronchitis

CLINICAL PEARLS
- Chronic cough is defined as a cough that persists for >8 weeks in adults.
- In patients with chronic cough, most frequent etiologies include a history of smoking, asthma, UACS, and GERD.
- The FDA issued a public health advisory stating that OTC cough and cold medicines should not be given to children <2 years. OTC cough expectorant and suppressant product labels state "do not use" in children <4 years.

CHRONIC FATIGUE SYNDROME

Anthony Valdini, MD, MS, FACP, FAAFP

 BASICS

DESCRIPTION

- A condition characterized by profound mental and physical exhaustion, with at least 6 months presence of multiple systemic and neuropsychiatric symptoms, and at least four of eight associated conditions are required per CDC definition:
  - Impaired memory
  - Sore throat
  - Tender lymph nodes
  - Persistent muscle or joint pain
  - New headaches
  - Nonrefreshing sleep
  - Postexertional malaise >24 hours
- Must have a new or definite onset (not lifelong)
- Fatigue is not relieved by rest and results in >50% reduction in previous activities (occupational, educational, social, and personal). Other potential medical causes must be ruled out (1).
- Exclusions: See "History."

EPIDEMIOLOGY

- Predominant age: 20 to 50 years
- Predominant sex: male < female
- All socioeconomic groups
- Associations between ethnicity and incidence have been reported. Higher rates found in ethnic minorities (Native Americans and African Americans) compared with white populations based on population studies. Service-based studies (tertiary care) have reported higher rates among whites or no association between incidence and ethnicity (2).

Prevalence

Estimates vary widely and depend on case definition and population studied, but a reasonable estimate using a strict case definition is 100 cases per 100,000 population. Community-based studies have reported prevalence rates of 0.23 and 0.42%.

ETIOLOGY AND PATHOPHYSIOLOGY

- Unknown and likely multifactorial
  - Possible interaction between genetic predisposition, environmental factors, an initiating stressor, and perpetuating factors
- A recent theory attributes possible neuroendocrine immunologic and biochemical effects in CFS to dysbiosis of the gut microbiome.
- Physiologic or environmental stressor could be precipitant.
- Many patients with chronic fatigue recall significant stressors (e.g., major medical procedure, loss of a loved one, loss of employment) in months before symptoms began.
- Systems hypothesized to contribute to altered physiology include the following:
  - Neuroendocrine (e.g., diminished cortisol response to increased corticotropin concentrations)
  - Immune (e.g., increased C-reactive protein and β-2 microglobulin)
  - Neuromuscular (e.g., dysfunction of oxidative metabolism)
  - Autonomic (Orthostatic hypotension is reported in a proportion of chronic fatigue syndrome [CFS] sufferers.)
  - Serotonergic (e.g., hyperserotonergic mechanisms or upregulation of serotonin receptors)

Genetics

Higher concordance among monozygotic twins compared with dizygotic twins

RISK FACTORS

Possible predisposing factors include the following: (3)

- Personality characteristics (neuroticism and introversion)
- Lifestyle
  - Childhood inactivity or overactivity
  - Inactivity in adulthood after infectious mononucleosis
  - Familial predisposition
  - Comorbid mood disorders of depression and anxiety
- Long-standing medical conditions in childhood
- Childhood trauma (emotional, physical, sexual abuse) (4)
- Prolonged idiopathic chronic fatigue
- Postinfectious fatigue and CFS have followed: mononucleosis, Ross River virus, *Coxiella burnetii*, herpes zoster, Q fever, and *Guardia lamblia*
- Because of concern for a possible "as yet undiscovered" infectious etiology, CFS patients were excluded from donating blood by the American Red Cross in 2010.

COMMONLY ASSOCIATED CONDITIONS

Common comorbidities include the following:

- Fibromyalgia (more common in women)
- Irritable bowel syndrome
- Gynecologic conditions (pelvic pain, endometriosis) and GYN surgeries (hysterectomy, oophorectomy) (5)
- Anxiety disorders
- Major depression
- Posttraumatic stress disorder (including physical and/or past sexual abuse)
- Domestic violence
- Attention deficit hyperactivity disorder (ADHD)
- Postural orthostatic tachycardia syndrome (POTS)
- Sleep disorders, including OSA
- Reduced left ventricular size and mass

DIAGNOSIS

HISTORY

- Discrete onset
- Profound mental and physical exhaustion
- At least 6 months presence of multiple systemic and neuropsychiatric symptoms
- Significantly interferes with daily activities/work
- At least four of eight associated conditions per CDC definition:
  - Impaired memory, sore throat, tender lymph nodes, persistent muscle or joint pain, new headaches, nonrefreshing sleep, postexertional malaise
- Exclusion criteria
  - <2 years after recovery of substance/alcohol abuse
  - Any past or current dx of anorexia nervosa or bulimia, dementia, schizophrenia, or bipolar disease
  - BMI ≥40
  - Malignancy
  - Previously diagnosed medical condition, unresolved clinically (e.g., hepatitis B or C)

PHYSICAL EXAM

Complete physical exam to rule out other medical causes for symptoms. Note: Tender adenopathy is one of the defining criteria.

ALERT

Detailed mental status examination (or referral to psychiatrist) to rule out other primary etiologies or comorbidities

DIFFERENTIAL DIAGNOSIS

- Idiopathic chronic fatigue (i.e., fatigue of unknown cause for >6 months without meeting criteria for CFS)
- Psychiatric disorders
  - Major depression
  - Somatization disorder
- Physiologic fatigue (inadequate or disrupted sleep, menopause)
- Pregnancy until 3 months postpartum
- Insomnia: primary (no clear etiology) versus secondary (e.g., due to anxiety, depression, environmental factors, poor sleep hygiene)
- Other known or defined systemic disease
- Endocrine disorder (hypothyroidism, Addison disease, Cushing syndrome, diabetes mellitus)
- Localized infection (e.g., occult abscess)
- Chronic or subacute bacterial disease (e.g., endocarditis)
- Lyme disease
- Fungal disease (e.g., histoplasmosis, coccidioidomycosis)
- Parasitic disease (e.g., amebiasis, giardiasis, helminth infestation)
- HIV or related disease
- Iatrogenic (e.g., medication side effects)
- Toxic agent exposure
- Obesity
- Malignancy
- Autoimmune disease
- Chronic inflammatory disease (sarcoidosis, Wegener granulomatosis)
- Neuromuscular disease (multiple sclerosis, myasthenia gravis)

DIAGNOSTIC TESTS & INTERPRETATION

No single diagnostic test available and finding an abnormal result is not always the same as discovering the cause of fatigue. Be prepared to renew the search for the cause if the problem is treated and the patient remains fatigued.

Initial Tests (lab, imaging)

- Standard laboratory tests are recommended to rule out other causes for symptoms:
  - Chemistry panel
  - CBC
  - Urinalysis
  - Thyroid-stimulating hormone (TSH)
  - ESR or C-reactive protein
  - Liver function
  - Screen for drugs of abuse
  - Age/gender-appropriate cancer screening
- Additional studies, if clinical findings are suggestive or patient at risk:
  - Antinuclear antibodies and rheumatoid factor (if elevated ESR)
  - Creatine kinase
  - Tuberculin skin test
  - Serum cortisol
  - HIV
  - Venereal Disease Research Laboratory or rapid plasma reagin
  - Lyme serology
  - IgA tissue transglutaminase
- No applicable imaging tests available; however, EEG and/or MRI may be useful if patient has CNS symptoms; polysomnography, if patient is sleepy (4).

Follow-Up Tests & Special Considerations

- Assess for comorbid psychiatric disorders.
- Assess for personality and psychosocial factors and maladaptive coping styles.

- In patients with sleep disturbance, polysomnography may reveal a treatable comorbid disease.

 TREATMENT

Focus on changes in lifestyle and insight, with a goal to avoid complicating treatments (e.g., addicting medications, invasive testing) or interventions that support secondary gain.

GENERAL MEASURES

ALERT
Treatment cornerstones include both cognitive-behavioral therapy (CBT) and graded exercise therapy. Medication is of little value. Two treatments have been shown effective, often used in combination (6)[A]:

- Individual CBT: Challenge fatigue-related cognition; plan social and occupational rehabilitation.
- Graded exercise therapy (GET): Track amount of exercise patient can do without exacerbating symptoms and gradually increase intensity and duration. Both involve a careful balance between activity and rest (7)[A]. Fear of movement and avoidance of physical activity are common in CFS.
- Patients learn how to gradually increase activity in a way that will not exacerbate their illness. Vigorous exercise can trigger relapse, perhaps related to immune dysregulation.
- Improves functional capacity and diminishes sense of fatigue
- GET is more effective with educational interventions using telephone reminders.
- Duration of illness does not predict treatment outcome; aggressive combined care is indicated for all.

MEDICATION
- No established pharmacologic treatment recommendations
- Studies have been conducted with antivirals, antidepressants, immunoglobulins, hydrocortisone, and modafinil. None has shown clear benefit.
- Agomelatine, an antidepressant with agonist activity at melatonin receptors, is promising in early studies (8)[C].
- If insomnia is present, use of nonaddicting sleep aids (hydroxyzine, trazodone, doxepin, etc.) may improve outcomes.

ISSUES FOR REFERRAL
- Psychiatrist to assist in managing comorbid disorders if needed
- Rehabilitative medicine

COMPLEMENTARY & ALTERNATIVE MEDICINE
- Insufficient to recommend any complementary and alternative medicine option for all (9)
- Social support groups have not proven to be effective.

 ONGOING CARE

FOLLOW-UP RECOMMENDATIONS
- Gradual increase in physical exercise with scheduled rest periods
- Avoid extended periods of rest.

Patient Monitoring
Although no consensus exists, periodic reevaluation is appropriate for support, relief of symptoms, and assessment for other possible causes of symptoms.

DIET
- No diet has been shown to be effective for treatment of CFS.
- Whether weight loss improves symptoms in obese CFS patients has yet to be tested.

PATIENT EDUCATION
- Patient education is an important part of treatment of CFS, such as education on the benefits of cognitive therapies, lifestyle changes, and pharmacologic therapy directed at specific-associated symptoms.
- Chronic Fatigue and Immune Dysfunction Syndrome Association of America: http://solvecfs.org/
- CDC, Chronic Fatigue Syndrome: http://www.cdc.gov/cfs/

PROGNOSIS
- Fluctuating course is common.
- Generally, improvement is slow, with a course of months to years.
- An estimated 5% fully recover.
- Patients with poor social adjustment, a strong belief in an organic etiology, financial secondary gain, or age >50 years are less likely to improve (10).

COMPLICATIONS
- CFS patients may reduce physical activity out of fear that it may worsen symptoms.
- Depression
- Unemployment: Although studies document improvement with treatment, <1/3 of patients in trials return to work.
- The U.S. Social Security Administration lists CFS as a bona fide form of disability.
- Receipt of government payments (secondary gain) has been associated with treatment nonresponse.
- Polypharmacy
- Chronic immune activation or an infection associated with CFS may play a role in an increased risk for non-Hodgkin lymphoma in elderly (>80 years) CFS patients.

REFERENCES
1. Baker R, Shaw EJ. Diagnosis and management of chronic fatigue syndrome or myalgic encephalomyelitis (or encephalopathy): summary of NICE guidance. *BMJ*. 2007;335(7617):446–448.
2. Dinos S, Khoshaba B, Ashby D, et al. A systematic review of chronic fatigue, its syndromes and ethnicity: prevalence, severity, co-morbidity and coping. *Int J Epidemiol*. 2009;38(6):1554–1570.
3. Lievesley K, Rimes KA, Chalder T. A review of the predisposing, precipitating and perpetuating factors in chronic fatigue syndrome in children and adolescents. *Clin Psychol Rev*. 2014;34(3):233–248.
4. Duffy FH, McAnulty GB, McCreary MC, et al. EEG spectral coherence data distinguish chronic fatigue syndrome patients from healthy controls and depressed patients—a case control study. *BMC Neurol*. 2011;11:82.
5. Boneva RS, Maloney EM, Lin JM, et al. Gynecological history in chronic fatigue syndrome: a population-based case-control study. *J Womens Health (Larchmt)*. 2011;20(1):21–28.
6. White PD, Goldsmith KA, Johnson AL, et al. Comparison of adaptive pacing therapy, cognitive behaviour therapy, graded exercise therapy, and specialist medical care for chronic fatigue syndrome (PACE): a randomised trial. *Lancet*. 2011;377(9768):823–836.

7. Nijs J, Paul L, Wallman K. Chronic fatigue syndrome: an approach combining self-management with graded exercise to avoid exacerbations. *J Rehabil Med*. 2008;40(4):241–247.
8. Pardini M, Cordano C, Benassi F, et al. Agomelatine but not melatonin improves fatigue perception: a longitudinal proof-of-concept study. *Eur Neuropsychopharmacol*. 2014;24(6):939–944.
9. Adams D, Wu T, Yang X, et al. Traditional Chinese medicinal herbs for the treatment of idiopathic chronic fatigue and chronic fatigue syndrome. *Cochrane Database Syst Rev*. 2009;(4):CD006348.
10. Cairns R, Hotopf M. A systematic review describing the prognosis of chronic fatigue syndrome. *Occup Med (Lond)*. 2005;55(1):20–31.

ADDITIONAL READING
- Carruthers BM, van de Sande MI, De Meirleir KL, et al. Myalgic encephalomyelitis: international consensus criteria. *J Intern Med*. 2011;270(4):327–328.
- Centers for Disease Control and Prevention. Diagnosis and management of chronic fatigue syndrome, CDC course for clinicians. http://www.cdc.gov/cfs/education/diagnosis/course.html.
- Freeman R, Wieling W, Axelrod FB, et al. Consensus statement on the definition of orthostatic hypotension, neurally mediated syncope and the postural tachycardia syndrome. *Clin Auton Res*. 2011;21(2):69–72.
- Social Security Administration. Providing medical evidence to the social security administration for individuals with chronic fatigue syndrome fact sheet. https://www.socialsecurity.gov/disability/professionals/cfs-pub063.htm.
- The IOM convened an expert panel at the request of several US government agencies. In the report submitted to HHS, they suggest changing name from CFS to "Systemic Exertion Intolerance Disease," and redefining diagnostic criteria. http://www.ncbi.nlm.nih.gov/pubmed/25695122.

 SEE ALSO

Algorithm: Fatigue

 CODES

ICD10
R53.82 Chronic fatigue, unspecified

CLINICAL PEARLS
- CFS and depression can be comorbid. However, to differentiate between the two, sore throat, tender lymph nodes, and postexercise fatigue are much more characteristic of CFS.
- No universal pharmacologic agents (e.g., antidepressants, immune modulators) have been shown to be consistently effective.
- ~70% of patients show improvement with CBT, compared to 55% with GET; in many cases, these two treatments can be undertaken in combination.
- There are many more patients with idiopathic chronic fatigue than true CFS. To diagnose CFS, CDC criteria need to be met; standardized instruments (SF-36, symptom index and Multidimensional Fatigue Inventory [MFI]) have been shown to be of use in the empirical diagnosis of CFS and may be helpful for following patients' progress.

CHRONIC KIDNEY DISEASE

Urooj Najm, MBBS • Najm Hasan Siddiqui, MD

BASICS

Chronic kidney disease (CKD) is defined as structural or functional abnormalities of the kidney for ≥3 months, as determined by either pathologic abnormalities or markers of damage—including abnormalities in blood or urine tests, histology, imaging studies, or history of kidney transplant—*or a* GFR <60 mL/min/1.73 m² for ≥3 months.

DESCRIPTION
- In 2012, Kidney Disease Improving Global Outcome (KDIGO) classified CKD in six categories by GFR estimation:
  - G1: kidney damage with normal or increased GFR ≥90 mL/min/1.73 m²
  - G2: mild ↓ GFR 60 to 89 mL/min/1.73 m²
  - G3a: mild to moderate ↓ GFR 45 to 59 mL/min/1.73 m²
  - G3b: moderate to severe ↓ GFR 30 to 44 mL/min/1.73 m²
  - G4: severe ↓ GFR 15 to 29 mL/min/1.73 m²
  - G5: kidney failure: GFR <15 mL/min/1.73 m² or dialysis
- CKD per albumin-to-creatinine ratio (ACR) category:
  - A1: normal to mildly increased: <30 mg/g or <3 mg/mmol
  - A2: moderately increased: 30 to 300 mg/g or 3 to 30 mg/mmol (formerly called microalbuminuria)
  - A3: severely increased: >300 mg/g or >30 mg/mmol (formerly called macroalbuminuria)
- System(s) affected: renal/urinary, cardiovascular, skeletal, endocrine, metabolic, hematologic, lymphatic, immune, neurologic
- Synonym(s): chronic renal failure; chronic renal insufficiency

Geriatric Considerations
GFR normally decreases with age, despite normal creatinine (Cr). Adjust renally cleared drugs for GFR in the elderly.

Pediatric Considerations
CKD definition is not applicable for children <2 years because of lower GFR even when corrected for body surface area. Calculated GFR based on serum Cr is used in this age group.

Pregnancy Considerations
- Renal function in CKD may deteriorate during pregnancy. Cr >1.5 and hypertension (HTN) are major risk factors for worsening renal function.
- Increased risk of premature labor, preeclampsia, and/or fetal loss
- ACE inhibitors and angiotensin receptor blockers (ARBs) are contraindicated due to teratogenicity. Use diuretics with caution.

EPIDEMIOLOGY
- Majority of people with CKD in stages 1 to 3
- African Americans are 3.6 times more likely to develop CKD than Caucasians.
- Predominant sex: Similar in both sexes; however, incidence rate of end-stage renal disease (ESRD) is 1.6 times higher in males than females.

Incidence
Estimated annual incidence of 1,700/1 million population

Prevalence
Overall prevalence of CKD is 14.2%. Unadjusted prevalence/incidence rates of ESRD (stage 5) are 1,752 and 362.4/1 million, respectively. Numbers do not reflect the burden of earlier stages of CKD (stages 1 to 4), which are estimated to affect 13.1% of the population nationwide or 26.3 million in the United States.

ETIOLOGY AND PATHOPHYSIOLOGY
Progressive destruction of kidney nephrons; GFR will drop gradually, and plasma Cr values will approximately double, with 50% reduction in GFR and 75% loss of functioning nephrons mass. Hyperkalemia usually develops when GFR falls to <20 to 25 mL/min. Anemia develops from decreased renal synthesis of erythropoietin.
- Renal parenchymal/glomerular
  - Nephritic: hematuria, RBC casts, HTN, variable proteinuria
    - Focal proliferative: IgA nephropathy, systemic lupus erythematosus (SLE), Henoch-Schönlein purpura, Alport syndrome, proliferative glomerulonephritis, crescentic glomerulonephritis
    - Diffuse proliferative: membranoproliferative glomerulonephritis, SLE, cryoglobulinemia, rapidly progressive glomerulonephritis (RPGN), Goodpasture syndrome
  - Nephrotic: proteinuria (>3.5 g/day), hypoalbuminemia, hyperlipidemia, and edema
    - Minimal change disease, membranous nephropathy, focal segmental glomerulosclerosis
    - Amyloidosis, diabetic nephropathy
- Vascular: HTN, thrombotic microangiopathies, vasculitis (Wegener), scleroderma
- Interstitial-tubular: infections, obstruction, toxins, allergic interstitial nephritis, multiple myeloma, connective tissue disease, cystic disease
- Postrenal: obstruction (benign prostatic hyperplasia), neoplasm, neurogenic bladder

Genetics
- Alport syndrome, Fabry disease, sickle cell anemia, SLE, and autosomal dominant polycystic kidney disease can lead to CKD.
- Polymorphisms in gene that encodes for podocyte nonmuscle myosin IIA are more common in African Americans than Caucasians and appear to increase risk for nondiabetic ESRD.

RISK FACTORS
- Type 1 or 2 diabetes mellitus (DM); most common
- Age >60 years
- Cardiovascular disease (e.g., HTN [common], renal artery stenosis, atheroemboli)
- Previous kidney transplant
- Urinary tract obstruction (e.g., benign prostatic hyperplasia)
- Autoimmune disease, vasculitis/connective tissue disorder
- Family history of CKD
- Nephrotoxic drugs (lithium, salicylate, high-dose or chronic NSAIDs, sulfa)
- Congenital anomalies, obstructive uropathy, renal aplasia/hypoplasia/dysplasia, reflux nephropathy
- Hyperlipidemia
- Low income/education/ethnic minority status
- Obesity/smoking/heroin use
- Chronic infection (hepatitis B, hepatitis C, HIV)

GENERAL PREVENTION
- Treat reversible causes: hypovolemia, infections, diuretics, drugs (NSAIDs, aminoglycosides, IV contrast).
- Treat risk factors: DM, HTN, hyperlipidemia, smoking, and obesity; adjust medication doses to prevent renal toxicity.

COMMONLY ASSOCIATED CONDITIONS
HTN, DM, cardiovascular disease

DIAGNOSIS

HISTORY
Patients with CKD stages 1 to 3 are usually asymptomatic; can present with
- Oliguria, nocturia, polyuria, hematuria, change in urinary frequency
- Bone disease
- Edema, HTN, dyspnea
- Fatigue, depression, weakness
- Pruritus, ecchymosis
- Metallic taste in mouth, anorexia, nausea, vomiting
- Hyperlipidemia, claudication, restless legs
- Erectile dysfunction, decrease libido, amenorrhea

PHYSICAL EXAM
- Volume status (pallor, BP/orthostatic; edema; jugular venous distention; weight)
- Skin: sallow complexion, uremic frost
- Ammonia-like odor (uremic fetor)
- Cardiovascular: Assess for murmurs, bruits, pericarditis.
- Chest: pleural effusion
- Rectal: enlarged prostate
- CNS: asterixis, confusion, seizures, coma, peripheral neuropathy

DIAGNOSTIC TESTS & INTERPRETATION
Initial Tests (lab, imaging)
- GFR can be estimated by multiple equations (freely available in medical calculators), including MDRD equation:
  - GFR (mL/min/1.73 m²) = 175 × [(serum Cr μmol/1/88.4)$^{-1.154}$] × [age (years)$^{-0.203}$] × 0.742 for females *or* 1.21 for African American
  - Often used as estimate in electronic health records
- Cr clearance (CrCl) can be calculated using Cockcroft-Gault formula
  - CrCl (male) = ([140 − age] × weight (kg)/(serum Cr × 72)]
  - CrCl (female) = CrCl (male) × 0.85
  - Formula used for determining cut points for renally adjusted medications
- Urine analysis
  - Urine microscopy: WBC casts in pyelonephritis, RBC casts in glomerulonephritis/vasculitis, dysmorphic RBCs
  - Urine electrolytes: sodium, Cr, urea (if on loop diuretics)
  - Proteinuria/albuminuria
    - 24-hour urine collection: >30 to 300 mg/24 hr (20 to 200 μg/min) is microalbuminuria and >300 mg/24 hr (>200 μg/min) is macroalbuminuria.
    - Albumin/Cr ratio (ACR): See "Description."

- Hematology: normochromic, normocytic anemia; increased bleeding time
- Chemistry
  - Elevated BUN, Cr, hyperkalemia, metabolic acidosis
  - Increased parathyroid hormone, decreased 25-(OH) vitamin D, hypocalcemia, hyperphosphatemia
  - Hyperlipidemia, decreased albumin

ALERT
Drugs that may alter lab result:

- Cimetidine: inhibits Cr tubular secretion
- Trimethoprim: inhibits Cr and K^+ secretion and may cause/worsen hyperkalemia
- Cefoxitin and flucytosine: increases serum Cr
- Diltiazem and verapamil (like ACE/ARBs) have significant antiproteinuric effects in patients with CKD.
- Ultrasound (initial test of choice): Small, echogenic kidneys; may see obstruction (e.g., hydronephrosis); cysts; kidneys may be enlarged with HIV and diabetic nephropathy.
- Doppler ultrasound to assess for renovascular disease, thrombosis
- Noncontrast CT scan: obstruction, calculi, cysts, neoplasm, renal artery stenosis
- MRI/MRA: Avoid gadolinium because of the risk of nephrogenic systemic fibrosis.
- Renal arteriogram for renal artery stenosis can be therapeutic (angioplasty or stenting).
- Renal scan to screen for differential function between kidneys
- Retrograde pyelogram: if strong suspicion for obstruction despite negative finding on ultrasound

Follow-Up Tests & Special Considerations
- Serology: antinuclear antibody (ANA); double-stranded DNA, antineutrophil cytoplasmic antibody; complements (C3, C4, CH50); anti-glomerular basement membrane (GBM) antibodies; hepatitis B, C; and HIV screening
- Serum and urine immunoelectrophoresis

Diagnostic Procedures/Other
Biopsy: hematuria, proteinuria, acute/progressive renal failure, nephritic or nephrotic syndrome

TREATMENT

GENERAL MEASURES
- Lowering salt intake to <2 g/day of sodium in adults, unless contraindicated (1)[C]
- Minimize radiocontrast exposure; prehydrate; N-acetylcysteine use is controversial. Avoid nephrotoxins (NSAIDs, aminoglycosides, etc.).
- Renal replacement: Prepare for dialysis or transplant when GFR <30 mL/min/1.73 m².
- Vaccines: pneumococcal, influenza
- Encourage smoking cessation, encourage weight loss (if applicable), and limit alcohol consumption.

MEDICATION
- HTN: Goal is BP <130/80 mm Hg (in nonhemodialysis patients) and <140/90 mm Hg (in patients on hemodialysis) in the nephrology literature, but more recent analysis based on outcomes suggests a universal BP target of <140/90 mm Hg (2).
- Antihypertensive agents should be selected based on the type of CKD and presence of cardiovascular disease.

- Long-acting (once daily) agents should be prescribed preferentially and given at bedtime.
- ACE inhibitors (drugs of choice) or ARBs for BP control and antiproteinuric effect
  - Potential for hyperkalemia
  - Can tolerate up to 30% rise in serum Cr unless hyperkalemia develops
  - If goal is not reached, add diuretic; thiazides are recommended for GFR ≥30 mL/min/1.73 m²; loop diuretics are recommended for GFR <30 mL/min/1.73 m²), followed by diltiazem or verapamil or a β-blocker.
- Secondary hyperparathyroidism
  - Cinacalcet, paricalcitol (decrease PTH levels)
- Recommended serum phosphate maintenance levels for CKD patients:

Stage	mg/day	mmol/L
Normal range (may vary by institution)	2.5–4.5	0.81–1.45
Stages 3 and 4 CKD (not on dialysis)	2.7–4.6	0.87–1.49
Stage 5 and ALL stages on dialysis	3.5–5.5	1.13–1.78

- Stages 3 to 5 CKD (not on dialysis): Restrict dietary phosphate to 800 to 1,000 mg/day.
  - Calcium-containing phosphate binders (with meals): calcium carbonate, calcium acetate (risk of hypercalcemia)
  - Noncalcium phosphate binders (with meals): sevelamer, lanthanum
  - Vitamin D: inactive vitamin D 25 (ergocalciferol or cholecalciferol), calcitriol (active vitamin D 1,25 [OH]): Vitamin D may increase absorption of phosphate by intestines and should not be started until serum phosphate concentration is controlled.
- Anemia: ferrous sulfate, erythropoietin-stimulating agents (ESAs): Before starting ESAs, nonrenal causes of anemia/iron stores should be checked. Start when Hgb <10 g/dL; goal range 10 to 11 g/dL, not to exceed 11.5 g/dL
- Hyperlipidemia: Statins with low-density lipoprotein (LDL) goal is similar to coronary heart disease patients (LDL <70 to 100).
- Glycemic control: Target HbA1c 7.0%, but it should be individualized based on life expectancy of patient, risk for adverse events related to glucose control, and patient preference (1). Tighter control may slow progression of microalbuminuria but may not reduce progression to ESRD and death in patients with type 2 diabetes. Use of metformin is not advised with serum Cr ≥1.5 mg/dL in males and ≥1.4 mg/dL in females because of possible risk of lactic acidosis.
- Metabolic acidosis: Start treatment when bicarb <20 mEq/L; goal 23 to 29 mEq/L
  - Sodium bicarbonate: daily dose of 0.5 to 1 mEq/kg/day or sodium citrate (should be avoided in patients taking aluminum-containing antacid)

ISSUES FOR REFERRAL
- Nephrology consult: GFR <15: immediate
- GFR 15 to 29: urgent
- GFR 30 to 59: nonurgent referral
- GFR 60 to 89: not required unless with comorbidities

SURGERY/OTHER PROCEDURES
Placement of dialysis access or transplantation

INPATIENT CONSIDERATIONS
Admission Criteria/Initial Stabilization
Uremia: nausea/vomiting, fluid overload, pericarditis, uremic encephalopathy, resistant HTN, hyperkalemia, metabolic acidosis, hyperphosphatemia

 ## ONGOING CARE

DIET
Nutrition consult for CKD diet: Protein restriction in early CKD is controversial but may be beneficial in ESRD; restricted intake of phosphates; sodium and water restriction to avoid volume overload; potassium restriction if hyperkalemic

PATIENT EDUCATION
National Kidney Federation patient Web site at: http://www.kidney.org/patients

PROGNOSIS
Patients with CKD gradually progress to ESRD, with bad prognoses. 5-year survival rate for U.S. patients on dialysis is ~35%.

COMPLICATIONS
HTN, anemia, secondary hyperparathyroidism, renal osteodystrophy, sleep disturbances, infections, malnutrition, electrolyte imbalances, platelet dysfunction/bleeding, pseudogout, gout, metabolic calcification, sexual dysfunction

REFERENCES
1. Mancia G, Fagard R, Narkiewicz K, et al. 2013 ESH/ESC guidelines for the management of arterial hypertension: the Task Force for the Management of Arterial Hypertension of the European Society of Hypertension (ESH) and of the European Society of Cardiology (ESC). J Hypertens. 2013;31(7):1281–1357.
2. Kidney Disease: Improving Global Outcomes (KDIGO) CKD Work Group. KDIGO 2012 clinical practice guideline for the evaluation and management of chronic kidney disease. Kidney Inter Suppl. 2013;3:1–150. www.kdigo.org/clinical_practice_guidelines/pdf/CKD/KDIGO_2012_CKD_GL.pdf

 ## SEE ALSO

- Hydronephrosis; Nephrotic Syndrome; Polycystic Kidney Disease; Proteinuria
- Algorithm: Anuria or Oliguria

 ## CODES

ICD10
- N18.9 Chronic kidney disease, unspecified
- Q63.9 Congenital malformation of kidney, unspecified
- N18.3 Chronic kidney disease, stage 3 (moderate)

CLINICAL PEARLS
- Maintaining BP <140/90 mm Hg is imperative (in patients not on dialysis).
- Avoid nephrotoxins including ACE/ARB in acute kidney injury (AKI) with or without CKD.
- CKD is a CHD risk equivalent.

CHRONIC OBSTRUCTIVE PULMONARY DISEASE AND EMPHYSEMA

Alan Cropp, MD, FCCP • Michael Apostolis, MD

BASICS

DESCRIPTION
- Chronic obstructive pulmonary disease (COPD) usually describes a mixture of chronic bronchitis and emphysema. It is characterized by airflow limitation that is not fully reversible, inflammation, and is progressive (1,2).
- Chronic bronchitis is defined clinically by increased mucus production and recurrent cough present on most days for at least 3 months per year during at least two consecutive years without another cause.
- Emphysema, the destruction of interalveolar septa, occurs in the distal or terminal airways and involves both airways and lung parenchyma.

EPIDEMIOLOGY
Incidence
Affects more than 5% of adults in the United States and is the 12th leading cause of morbidity (1)

Prevalence
- Third leading cause of death in the United States (1)
- Projected to be the third leading cause of death globally by 2020 (2)

ETIOLOGY AND PATHOPHYSIOLOGY
Cigarette and/or cannabis smoking, air pollution (including indoor), antiprotease deficiency (α_1-antitrypsin), occupational exposure (firefighters), infection (viral), occupational pollutants (cadmium, silica)
- Impaired gas (carbon dioxide and oxygen) exchange
- Chronic bronchitis: airway obstruction (3)
- Emphysema: destruction of lung parenchyma

Genetics
- Chronic bronchitis is not a genetic disorder.
- Antiprotease deficiency (due to α_1-antitrypsin deficiency) is an inherited, rare disorder due to two autosomal codominant alleles.

RISK FACTORS
- Smoking: passive smoking, especially adults whose parents smoked; cannabis use (one joint is equivalent to 2.5 to 5 cigarettes) (1–3)
- Severe pneumonia early in life including viral (4)
- Aging
- Lower level of education and poverty (4)
- Airway hyperactivity
- Indoor pollution (open fire for cooking or heating) (4)
- Occupational organic or inorganic dusts (4)

GENERAL PREVENTION
- Avoidance of smoking is the most important preventive measure.
- Early detection through pulmonary function tests (PFTs) in high-risk patients may be useful in preserving remaining lung function.

COMMONLY ASSOCIATED CONDITIONS
- Pulmonary: lung cancer, chronic respiratory failure, acute bronchitis, sleep apnea, pulmonary hypertension, asthma
- Cardiac: coronary artery disease, arrhythmia
- Ear, nose, and throat (ENT): chronic sinusitis, laryngeal carcinoma
- Miscellaneous: malnutrition, osteoporosis, muscle dysfunction, depression

DIAGNOSIS

HISTORY
- Discuss patient's use of tobacco and cannabis.
- Consider indoor pollution (coal furnace) (4).

- Review possible causes of exacerbation (e.g., recent infection) and history of cough, sputum, dyspnea
- Chronic bronchitis: cough, sputum production, frequent infections, intermittent dyspnea, wheeze, hemoptysis, morning headache, pedal edema
- Emphysema: minimal cough, scant sputum, dyspnea, weight loss, occasional infections

PHYSICAL EXAM
- Rarely diagnostic for COPD (2)
- Chronic bronchitis: cyanosis, wheezing, weight gain, diminished breath sounds, distant heart sounds
- Emphysema: barrel chest, minimal wheezing, accessory muscle use, pursed lip breathing, cyanosis slight or absent, breath sounds diminished

DIFFERENTIAL DIAGNOSIS
- Asthma (including occupational)
- Bronchiectasis
- Lung cancer
- Acute bronchitis
- Normal aging of lungs
- Chronic pulmonary embolism
- Sleep apnea
- Primary alveolar hypoventilation
- Chronic sinusitis
- Reactive airways dysfunction syndrome (RADS)
- Congestive heart failure (CHF)
- Bronchiolitis obliterans
- Gastroesophageal reflux disease
- Cystic fibrosis

DIAGNOSTIC TESTS & INTERPRETATION
Spirometry (the most reliable/objective measurement of airflow obstruction) (1–3)[A]

Initial Tests (lab, imaging)
- Spirometry (1–3) (see "Diagnostic Procedures")
- Chronic bronchitis
  - Arterial blood gases (ABGs) may show hypercapnia and hypoxia.
  - Hemoglobin may be increased.
- Emphysema
  - Normal serum hemoglobin or polycythemia
  - Normal $PaCO_2$ on ABGs unless forced expiratory volume in 1 second (FEV_1) <1 L, in which case it can be elevated
  - Mild hypoxia
- Chronic bronchitis CXR: increased bronchovascular markings and cardiomegaly
- Emphysema CXR: small heart, hyperinflation, flat diaphragms, and possibly bullous changes

Follow-Up Tests & Special Considerations
- Check continuous overnight oximetry in selected patients.
- α_1-Antitrypsin screening for those with COPD age <45 years, have a blood relative with this disease, or spirometry out of proportion to tobacco use
- Chest CT may show diffuse bullous changes or upper lobe predominance. Also, small lung nodules may be identified (5).

Diagnostic Procedures/Other
- PFTs (1,2)[A]

  - Not indicated during acute exacerbation (3)
  - Decreased FEV_1 and resulting reduction in FEV_1:FVC (forced vital capacity) ratio
  - Poor or absent reversibility to bronchodilator
  - Normal or reduced FVC
  - Normal or increased total lung capacity

- Increased residual volume and functional residual capacity
- Diffusing capacity is normal or reduced.
- Staging: Global Initiative for Obstructive Lung Disease (GOLD) criteria (3)
  - Mild COPD: FEV_1 ≥80% predicted
  - Moderate COPD: FEV_1 50–80% predicted
  - Severe COPD: FEV_1 30–50% predicted
  - Very severe COPD: FEV_1 <30% predicted or FEV_1 <50% predicted plus chronic respiratory failure

Test Interpretation
- Chronic bronchitis: bronchial mucous gland enlargement, increased number of secretory cells in surface epithelium, thickened small airways from edema and inflammation, smooth muscle hyperplasia, mucus plugging, bacterial colonization of airways
- Emphysema: entire lung affected, bronchi usually clear of secretions, anthracotic pigment, alveoli enlarged with loss of septa, cartilage atrophy, bullae

TREATMENT

GENERAL MEASURES
- Smoking cessation: This is the most important intervention to decrease risk (1,2)[A].
- Aggressive treatment of infections (3)[B]
- Treat any reversible bronchospasm.
- Home oxygen: may improve survival; should be initiated partial pressure of arterial oxygen (PaO_2) ≤55 mm Hg or pulse oximetry trends ≤88% (1)[A]
- Influenza and pneumococcal immunizations (2)[B]
- Tiotropium (Spiriva) may slow disease progression (6)[B].

MEDICATION
Medications help reduce symptoms and exacerbations (1).

First Line
- All patients should have a short-acting β-agonist (albuterol) to use as a rescue drug (1).
- Anticholinergics (2)[A]
  - Ipratropium (Atrovent), tiotropium (Spiriva), aclidinium bromide (Tudorza) AND/OR
- Long-acting β-agonists
  - Salmeterol (Serevent), formoterol (Foradil), one inhalation q12h; or arformoterol (Brovana), formoterol (Perforomist), nebulized q12h (1,2)[A]

ALERT
Acute exacerbation: Use oxygen, inhaled β-agonists, inhaled anticholinergic agents, and oral or IV corticosteroids prednisone (up to 1 mg/kg/day commonly 40 mg/day for 5 days) (7)[A]. Antibiotics should be given for those with moderate/severe exacerbations showing clinical signs of bacterial infection (increased sputum volume, increased sputum purulence); optimal antibiotic therapy has not been determined (3)[B].

Second Line
- Trial of inhaled corticosteroids for moderate or severe disease (2)[A]
  - May initiate earlier if suggestion of asthmatic component to disease
  - Systemic corticosteroids: Prednisone (Deltasone) can be given orally 7.5 to 15 mg/day in selected patients.

– Long-term monotherapy with steroids (oral or inhaled) is not recommended (2,3)[A].

– Inhaled corticosteroids are associated with an increased risk of pneumonia (3).

- Continuous home oxygen: may improve survival; should be initiated for severe resting hypoxemia ($PaO_2 \leq 55$ mm Hg or oxygen saturation $\leq 88\%$) or PaO_2 56 to 59 mm Hg with evidence of hypoxia (i.e., polycythemia or pulmonary hypertension) or pulse oximetry trends $\leq 88\%$ (1)[A]

- Theophylline if other long-term treatment is unavailable or unaffordable: 400 mg/day; increase by 100 to 200 mg in 1 to 2 weeks, if necessary (4)[B]

– Reduce dosage in patients with impaired renal or liver function, age >55 years, or CHF

– Monitor serum level. Therapeutic range is 8 to 13 μg/mL.

– Low-dose theophylline may help inflammatory component (4)[B].

- Combination of inhaled corticosteroid, long-acting β-agonist, and anticholinergic indicated for severe disease. Several combination medications are now available (2)[A].

- Mucolytic agents may improve secretions but do not improve outcomes.

- Phosphodiesterase-4 inhibitor (PDE4) inhibitor (roflumilast) in severe chronic bronchitis may reduce exacerbations (2)[B].

- α_1-Antitrypsin, if deficient: 60 mg/kg/week to maintain level >80 mg/dL

- Precautions
  – Sympathomimetics: excessive use may be dangerous. May need to reduce dosage or use levalbuterol (Xopenex) in patients with cardiovascular disease, hypertension (HTN), hyperthyroidism, diabetes, or seizures. Anticholinergics: narrow-angle glaucoma, benign prostatic hyperplasia, bladder neck obstruction
  – Corticosteroids: weight gain, diabetes, adrenal suppression, osteoporosis, infection (pneumonia)

- Sympathomimetics may be aerosolized.

- Anticholinergics: Ipratropium (Atrovent) may be aerosolized or combined with albuterol (Combivent Respimat).

ISSUES FOR REFERRAL
Severe exacerbation, frequent hospitalizations, age <40 years, rapid progression, weight loss, severe disease, or surgical evaluation

ADDITIONAL THERAPIES
- Adequate hydration and pulmonary hygiene
- Consider postural drainage, flutter valve, or other devices to assist mucus clearance.
- Pulmonary rehabilitation (1–3)[A]
- Intermittent, noninvasive ventilation may help in severe chronic respiratory failure.
- Short course of antibiotics (5 to 10 days) for acute exacerbations (2)[B]
- Immunizations
- Supplemental oxygen if indicated

SURGERY/OTHER PROCEDURES
- Lung reduction surgery (selected cases)
- Lung transplantation (selected cases)

INPATIENT CONSIDERATIONS
Admission Criteria/Initial Stabilization
- Outpatient treatment is usually adequate.
- Exacerbation with acute decompensation (hypoxemia, hypercarbia)

- Serious comorbidities (i.e., decompensated CHF)
- Systemic steroids reduce recovery time and improve hypoxia (2,7)[A]
- Supplemental oxygen and short-acting bronchodilators should be given (3).

ALERT
If not already in place, have patient delineate an advance directive.

- www.agingwithdignity.org, www.putitinwriting.org
- Progressive nature of disease and severity of treatment methods (ventilation, etc.) make revisiting patient preferences beneficial.

- Acute respiratory failure may require ICU and invasive or noninvasive ventilation (NIV) (2)[A].
- Systemic steroids (prednisone 40 mg/day for 5 days or equivalent) have been shown to reduce recovery time and improve hypoxia (7)[A].

Nursing
Teach proper inhaler use.

Discharge Criteria
- Ability to ambulate (3)

- Hypoxia can be treated with home oxygen (may only be temporary) (2)[A].

- Inhaled short-acting β-agonist therapy no more frequently than q4h (3)

- Ability to eat and sleep without interruption caused by dyspnea (3)

 ## ONGOING CARE

FOLLOW-UP RECOMMENDATIONS
- May taper or stop oral steroids as outpatient
- If pneumonia caused exacerbation, need to follow CXR or chest CT until clear or stable

- Pulmonary rehabilitation for exertional dyspnea (1)[A]

Patient Monitoring
- Severe or unstable patients should be seen monthly. When stable, see every 6 months.
- Check theophylline level with dose adjustment, then check every 6 to 12 months.
- With use of home oxygen, check ABGs yearly or with change in condition. Frequently monitor saturation (pulse oximetry). Some patients only desaturate at night, thus only need nocturnal oxygen.
- Yearly spirometry
- Travel at high altitude with supplemental oxygen if necessary.

- Baseline chest CT for patients aged 55 to 74 years with a 30 pack/year smoking history to look for lung nodules (5)[B]

- Discuss advance directive and health care proxy.

DIET
A high-protein low-carbohydrate diet may benefit those with hypercarbia.

PATIENT EDUCATION
American Lung Association: www.lung.org/lung-disease/copd/

PROGNOSIS
- Patient's age and postbronchodilator FEV_1 are the most important predictors of prognosis.

- Supplemental O_2, when indicated, is shown to increase survival (may only need at night) (1)[A].

- Smoking cessation improves prognosis—consider E-cigarettes (2).
- Malnutrition, cor pulmonale, hypercapnia, and pulse >100 indicate a poor prognosis.

COMPLICATIONS
- Malnutrition, poor sleep quality, infections, secondary polycythemia
- Acute or chronic respiratory failure, bullous lung disease, pneumothorax
- Arrhythmias, cor pulmonale, pulmonary HTN

REFERENCES
1. Qaseem A, Wilt TJ, Weinberger SE, et al. Diagnosis and management of stable chronic obstructive pulmonary disease: a clinical practice guideline update from the American College of Physicians, American College of Chest Physicians, American Thoracic Society, and European Respiratory Society. *Ann Intern Med*. 2011;155(3):179–191.
2. Vestbo J, Hurd SS, Agustí AG, et al. Global strategy for the diagnosis, management, and prevention of chronic obstructive pulmonary disease: GOLD executive summary. *Am J Respir Crit Care Med*. 2013;187(4):347–365.
3. Global Initiative for Chronic Obstructive Lung Disease. Global strategy for the diagnosis, management, and prevention of COPD. Revised 2013. http://www.goldcopd.org/guidelines-global-strategy-for-diagnosis-management.html
4. Lamprecht B, McBurnie MA, Vollmer WM, et al. COPD in never smokers: results from the population-based burden of obstructive lung disease study. *Chest*. 2011;139(4):752–763.
5. Detterbeck FC, Mazzone PJ, Naidich DP, et al. Screening for lung cancer: diagnosis and management of lung cancer, 3rd ed: American College of Chest Physicians evidence-based clinical practice guidelines. *Chest*. 2013;143(5)(Suppl):e78S–e92S.
6. Csikesz NG, Gartman EJ. New developments in the assessment of COPD: early diagnosis is key. *Int J Chron Obstruct Pulmon Dis*. 2014;9:277–286.
7. Leuppi JD, Schuetz P, Bingisser R, et al. Short-term vs conventional glucocorticoid therapy in acute exacerbations of chronic obstructive pulmonary disease: the REDUCE randomized clinical trial. *JAMA*. 2013;309(21):2223–2231.

 ## SEE ALSO

Bronchitis, Acute

 ## CODES

ICD10
- J44.9 Chronic obstructive pulmonary disease, unspecified
- J43.9 Emphysema, unspecified
- J42 Unspecified chronic bronchitis

CLINICAL PEARLS
- Consider screening PFTs on any high-risk patient.
- Overnight oximetry if daytime SaO_2 is borderline.
- Influenza/pneumococcal vaccines should be current.
- Advance directive before patient is seriously ill.
- Consider chest CT for patients age 55 to 74 years with a 30 pack/year smoking history for lung cancer screening.

CHRONIC PAIN MANAGEMENT: AN EVIDENCE-BASED APPROACH

Jennifer Reidy, MD, MS, FAAHPM

 BASICS

- Chronic pain is pain persisting beyond the time of normal tissue healing, usually >3 months.
- Over time, neuroplastic changes in the CNS transform pain into a chronic disease itself. Pain levels can exceed observed pathology on exam or imaging.
- Pain experience is inherently related to emotional, psychological, and cognitive factors.
- An epidemic of undertreated pain coexists with an epidemic of prescription drug abuse in the United States.
- Use a system-based practice to safely and effectively prescribe opioids when indicated for chronic nonmalignant pain.

EPIDEMIOLOGY

Incidence
Incidence is rising, but exact rate is unclear. The annual economic cost of chronic pain in the United States is estimated at $560 to $635 billion (1)[B].

Prevalence
In the United States, an estimated 100 million adults live with chronic pain—more than the total affected by heart disease, cancer, and diabetes combined (1)[B].
Chronic pain accounts for 20% of outpatient visits and 12% of all prescriptions (2)[B].

ETIOLOGY AND PATHOPHYSIOLOGY
- With intense, repeated, or prolonged stimulation of damaged or inflamed tissues, the threshold for activating primary afferent pain fibers is lowered, the frequency of firing is higher, and there is increased response to noxious and/or normal stimuli (peripheral and central sensitization). The amygdala, prefrontal cortex, and cortex are thought to relay emotions and thoughts that create the pain experience, and these areas may undergo structural and functional changes with chronic pain.
- Many patients have an identifiable etiology (most commonly musculoskeletal problems or headache), but pain levels can be worse than observable tissue injury. A significant percentage of patients have no obvious cause of chronic pain.

Genetics
Current research suggests genetic polymorphism in opioid receptors, which may affect patient's response and/or side effects to individual opioids.

RISK FACTORS
- Traumatic: motor vehicle accidents, repetitive motion injuries, sports injuries, work-related injuries, and falls
- Postsurgical: any surgery but especially back surgeries, amputations, and thoracotomies
- Medical conditions: See "Commonly Associated Conditions" later.
- Psychiatric comorbidities: substance abuse, depression, posttraumatic stress disorder (PTSD), personality disorders
- Aging: increased incidence with age but should not be considered a "normal" part of aging

GENERAL PREVENTION
- Avoidance of work-related injuries through the use of ergonomically correct workplace design
- Exercise and physical therapy to help prevent work-related low back pain

- Varicella vaccine and rapid treatment of shingles to lower risk of postherpetic neuralgia
- Tight glycemic control for diabetic patients, alcohol cessation for alcoholics, smoking cessation

COMMONLY ASSOCIATED CONDITIONS
Any chronic disease and/or its treatment can cause chronic pain, including diabetes, cardiovascular disease, HIV, progressive neurologic conditions, lung disease, cirrhosis, autoimmune disease, cancer, renal failure, depression, and mental illness.

 DIAGNOSIS

Chronic pain can be divided into two general categories:
- Nociceptive pain (two types)
  - Somatic: skin, bone, soft tissue disease; described as well-localized, sharp, stabbing, aching
  - Visceral: visceral inflammation/injury; described as poorly localized, dull, aching; may refer to sites remote from lesion
- Neuropathic pain: damaged peripheral or central nerves; described as burning, tingling, and/or numbness
  - Sympathetically mediated pain: Peripheral nerve injury can cause severe burning pain, swelling of the affected limb, and focal changes in sweat production and skin appearance. Example: complex regional pain syndrome

HISTORY
- Obtain pain history: location, onset, intensity, duration, quality, temporal pattern, exacerbating agents, alleviators, prior treatments
- Assess and document how pain affects patient's functioning and quality of life and what they expect from treatment.
- Screen for personal or family history of substance abuse (including tobacco addiction), mental health conditions, domestic violence, or sexual abuse.
- Use standardized tools: pain severity—Brief Pain Inventory (short form); mood—Patient Health Questionnaire-9 (PHQ-9); substance abuse—Screener and Opioid Assessment for Patients with Pain (SOAPP), multiple versions
- Use screening to risk stratify patients for risks of chronic opioid therapy and increased monitoring; a positive screen does not automatically exclude patients from opioid therapy.

PHYSICAL EXAM
Exam is guided by history and must include functional and mental assessments.

DIFFERENTIAL DIAGNOSIS
- The causes of pain are numerous, and clinic presentations are protean, depending on the individual patient.
- There is a spectrum of aberrant drug-taking behaviors, and differential diagnosis includes
  - Inadequate analgesia ("pseudoaddiction"), disease progression, opioid-resistant pain, opioid-induced hyperalgesia, addiction, opioid tolerance, self-medication of nonpain symptoms, criminal intent (diversion)

DIAGNOSTIC TESTS & INTERPRETATION
Testing is based on differential diagnosis of pain syndrome to elucidate etiology.

Initial Tests (lab, imaging)
- Urine drug screen: Order qualitative analysis for drugs of abuse and quantitative analysis for the drug you are prescribing.
- Most tests are immunoassays, which usually detect morphine and heroin but often not other opioids. Laboratory-based chromatography/spectrometry can identify specific drugs. Clinicians should be aware of uses and limitations of local laboratory testing (http://www.aafp.org/afp/2010/0301/p635.html).

Follow-Up Tests & Special Considerations
If patient is taking chronic opioid therapy, order random urine drug screens as part of the "universal precautions" approach (see "Ongoing Care").

Diagnostic Procedures/Other
- Consider interventional pain clinic for complicated joint injections and nerve root blocks, which can be diagnostic.
- If complex regional pain syndrome is suspected, a sympathetic block can be diagnostic and possibly prevent chronic pain.

TREATMENT

- Goals of treatment are restoring function and a decrease in pain while balancing risks and benefits of therapies.
- Intradisciplinary teams offer most effective approach to chronic pain, including its physical, emotional, and psychological aspects. These teams may include the patient, family, primary care doctor, nurse, pain management specialist, pharmacist, psychologist, psychiatrist, physical and occupational therapists, physiatrist, complementary medicine practitioners, social worker, and (if needed) addiction medicine specialist (3)[B].
- Treatment should always include nonpharmacologic therapies such as exercise, cognitive-behavioral therapy (CBT), patient and family education, yoga, massage, relaxation techniques, support groups, meditation, and acupuncture.

GENERAL MEASURES
Keep a pain and function diary to record pain and activity level and how much medication is taken.

MEDICATION
- Always begin with exercise, physical therapy, CBT, and self-management skills before or with pain medications. Use sequential time-limited trials of medications, starting at low doses, and gradually increasing until either effect or dose-limiting side effects are reached. Rational polypharmacy may be indicated (such as an opioid + neuropathic agent).
- For mild to moderate chronic pain
  - Acetaminophen: daily dose not to exceed total 4 g in healthy adults and 2 g in the elderly or those with hepatic disease or active or past history of alcohol use
  - NSAIDs: COX-2 selective inhibitors should be used with caution because of cardiac risks but may have less gastric risk. If high cardiac risk consider nonselective COX inhibitor (such as naproxen) with or without gastric prophylaxis (depending on ulcer risk).

- "Weak" opioids, including tramadol. Caution: Opioid analgesic combinations can lead to serious acetaminophen or NSAID toxicities if patients exceed safely prescribed doses.
- Topical agents: NSAIDs, lidocaine (gel is less expensive than patch), ketamine, capsaicin
- For neuropathic pain
  - Classes of medications include (i) tricyclic antidepressants (desipramine and nortriptyline have fewer side effects); (ii) serotonin-norepinephrine reuptake inhibitor (SNRI) antidepressants (duloxetine); (iii) anticonvulsants (alpha 2-delta ligands, gabapentin, and pregabalin); (iv) opioids, including tramadol. Example: combination of nortriptyline + gabapentin
  - See "Neuropathic Pain."
- For moderate to severe chronic pain
  - Strong opioids, including morphine, oxycodone, hydromorphone, oxymorphone, fentanyl. Check opioid equianalgesic tables for dosing by route of administration.
  - No evidence supports any of these strong opioids as superior or having improved side effect profile.
  - In patients with chronic back pain, opioids may be efficacious for short-term use, but long-term benefits and side effects are unclear; in addition, aberrant medication-taking behaviors range from 5% to 24%.
    ○ Morphine should be avoided in patients with significant renal insufficiency.
    ○ Methadone should only be prescribed by experienced providers. The only opioid that also acts as N-methyl-D-aspartate receptor antagonist, methadone has many drug interactions and can contribute to potentially fatal cardiac arrhythmias.
  - Once stable dose of opioids is established, change to sustained-release formulations if pain is constant or very frequent. Short-acting formulations are only for breakthrough or episodic pain.
  - Common side effects: constipation: Senna should be prescribed at time opioids are started; also nausea, sedation, mental status changes, and pruritus

ALERT
Patients on chronic opioid therapy must agree to monitoring. Clinicians should use universal precautions and systems-based practice, including written agreements, random urine drug screens, pill/patch counts, and other measures (see "Ongoing Care") (4,5)[B].

SURGERY/OTHER PROCEDURES
Consider interventional procedures, including joint injections, nerve blocks, spinal cord stimulation, and intrathecal medication among others, as needed.

COMPLEMENTARY & ALTERNATIVE MEDICINE
- Acupuncture: efficacy in chronic neck and back pain and fibromyalgia
- Exercise: efficacy in low back pain and fibromyalgia
- Improved mood and coping skills, decreased disability with CBT
- Mind–body interventions: yoga, tai chi, hypnosis, progressive muscle relaxation, meditation

 ONGOING CARE

FOLLOW-UP RECOMMENDATIONS
Patient Monitoring
- It can be difficult to identify appropriate pain relief–seeking behavior from inappropriate drug-seeking, but consistent patient–clinician relationships over time can often discern the difference.
- Always maintain a risk–benefit stance and avoid judging a patient.
- Assess and document benefits, pain levels, functioning, and quality of life. In general, patients successfully taking opioids for pain become more engaged (better relationships and productive work).
- At each visit, assess and document harm, using universal precautions approach. This system-based practice includes the following:
  - Informed consent for opioid therapy
  - Written or electronic agreement between patient and clinician
  - One prescribing clinician (or designee) and one pharmacy
  - No after-hours prescriptions or early refills
  - Mandatory police reports for medication thefts
  - Random urine drug tests, pill/patch counts
  - Requirements for patient to continue with physical therapy, counseling, psychiatric medications, or other necessary treatments
  - Participate in state's prescription drug monitoring program: See www.pmpalliance.org.
  - Taper and discontinue medications (10% dose reduction per week) if patient does not benefit, if side effects outweigh benefits, or if medications are abused or diverted. If addiction is suspected, always offer treatment for substance abuse (4,5)[B].

PATIENT EDUCATION
American Chronic Pain Association: http://theacpa.org/

COMPLICATIONS
- Rate of addiction in chronic pain patients is unclear (3–19% in published literature), but it may reflect rate in the general population.
- Definitions
  - Addiction: chronic biopsychologic disease characterized by impaired control over drug use, compulsive use, and continued use despite harm
  - Physical dependence: withdrawal syndrome produced by abrupt cessation or rapid dose reduction; is not addiction but a physiologic phenomenon
  - Tolerance: state of adaptation when a drug induces changes that diminish its effects over time
  - Diversion: selling drugs or giving them to persons other than for whom they are prescribed

ALERT
Caution: From 1999 to 2007, the rate of unintentional overdose death increased by 124%, largely due to prescription opioid overdoses (especially methadone). In 2011, prescription narcotic overdose was the leading cause of accidental death in the United States (http://www.cdc.gov/drugoverdose/index.html) (6)[B].

REFERENCES
1. Institute of Medicine, Committee on Advancing Pain Research, Care, and Education. *Relieving Pain in America: A Blueprint for Transforming Prevention, Care, Education and Research*. Washington, DC: The National Academies Press; 2011.
2. Alford DP, Krebs EE, Chen IA, et al. Update in pain medicine. *J Gen Intern Med*. 2010;25(11): 1222–1226.
3. Dobscha SK, Corson K, Perrin NA, et al. Collaborative care for chronic pain in primary care: a cluster randomized trial. *JAMA*. 2009;301(12): 1242–1252.
4. American Society of Anesthesiologists Task Force on Chronic Pain Management. Practice guidelines for chronic pain management: an updated report by the American Society of Anesthesiologists Task Force on Chronic Pain Management and the American Society of Regional Anesthesia and Pain Medicine. *Anesthesiology*. 2010;112(4):810–833.
5. Manchikanti L, Abdi S, Atluri S, et al. American Society of Interventional Pain Physicians (ASIPP) guidelines for responsible opiod prescribing in chronic non-cancer pain: Part 2—guidance. *Pain Physician*. 2012;15(3 Suppl):S67–S116.
6. Bohnert AS, Valenstein M, Bair MJ, et al. Association between opioid prescribing patterns and opioid overdose-related deaths. *JAMA*. 2011;305(13):1315–1321.

ADDITIONAL READING
- Federation of State Medical Boards of the United States, Inc. Model policy for the use of controlled substances for the treatment of pain www.painpolicy.wisc.edu/sites/www.painpolicy.wisc.edu/files/model04.pdf.
- Washington State Agency Medical Director's Group. Interagency guideline on opioid dosing for chronic non-cancer pain: an educational aid to improve care and safety with opioid therapy. www.agencymeddirectors.wa.gov.

 CODES

ICD10
- G89.29 Other chronic pain
- G89.21 Chronic pain due to trauma
- G89.28 Other chronic postprocedural pain

CLINICAL PEARLS
- Start with the presumption that the patient's pain is *real*, even if pathophysiologic evidence for it cannot be found.
- Emphasize that being pain-free may not be possible but that better function and quality of life can be shared goals.
- Use a multidisciplinary approach with nonpharmacologic therapies, exercise, patient self-management strategies and thoughtful medication use with clear goals, expectations, and documentation of care plan.
- Use universal precautions and systems-based practice to safely and effectively prescribe opioids for chronic pain.

CIRRHOSIS OF THE LIVER
Kathleen M. Donahue, DO

 BASICS

DESCRIPTION
A chronic hepatocellular disease involving inflammation, necrosis, and fibrosis potentially leading to liver failure and/or cancer

EPIDEMIOLOGY
- Predominant age: 40 to 50 years old
- Predominant sex: male > female; more women get cirrhosis from alcohol abuse.
- Ninth leading cause of death among U.S. adults

ETIOLOGY AND PATHOPHYSIOLOGY
- Chronic hepatitis C (26%)
- Alcohol abuse (21%)
- Hepatitis C with alcoholic liver disease (15%)
- Nonalcoholic steatohepatitis/obesity (~10%)
- Hepatitis B plus hepatitis D infection (15%)
- Other: hemochromatosis, autoimmune hepatitis, primary biliary cirrhosis, secondary biliary cirrhosis, primary sclerosing cholangitis, Wilson disease, α_1-antitrypsin deficiency, granulomatous disease (e.g., sarcoidosis); drug-induced liver disease (e.g., methotrexate, α-methyldopa, amiodarone); venous outflow obstruction (e.g., Budd-Chiari syndrome, veno-occlusive disease); chronic right-sided heart failure; tricuspid regurgitation; and rare genetic, metabolic, and infectious causes

Genetics
Hemochromatosis, Wilson disease, and α_1-antitrypsin deficiency in adults are associated with cirrhosis.

RISK FACTORS
Alcohol abuse, intravenous drug abuse, obesity, blood transfusion

GENERAL PREVENTION
- Mitigate risk factors (e.g., alcohol abuse): *>80% of chronic liver disease is preventable*.
- Limit alcohol consumption and advise weight loss in overweight or obese patients.
  - Elevated BMI and alcohol have an additive effect on liver disease (1).

COMMONLY ASSOCIATED CONDITIONS
Diabetes, alcoholism, drug abuse, depression, obesity

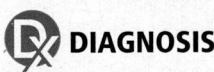 **DIAGNOSIS**

HISTORY
- Review risk factors (alcohol abuse, viral hepatitis, family history of primary liver cancer, other liver disease, or autoimmune disease)
- Symptoms
  - Fatigue, malaise, weakness
  - Anorexia, weight loss (weight gain if ascites/edema)
  - Right upper abdominal pain
  - Absent/irregular menses, chronic anovulation
  - Diminished libido, erectile dysfunction
  - Tea-colored urine, clay-colored stools
  - Edema, abdominal swelling/bloating
  - Bruising, bleeding, hematemesis, hematochezia, melena, pruritus
  - Night blindness

PHYSICAL EXAM
Physical exam may be normal until end-stage disease.
- Skin changes: spider angiomas, palmar erythema, jaundice, scleral icterus, ecchymoses, caput medusa, hyperpigmentation

- Hepatomegaly (small, fibrotic liver in end-stage disease)
- Splenomegaly (if portal hypertension)
- Central obesity
- Abdominal fluid wave, shifting dullness (ascites)
- Gynecomastia
- Dupuytren contractures
- Pretibial, presacral pitting edema and clubbing (especially in hepatopulmonary syndrome)
- Asterixis, mental status changes
- Muscle wasting, weakness
- Fetor hepaticus with severe portal-systemic shunting

DIFFERENTIAL DIAGNOSIS
Steatohepatitis, other causes of portal hypertension (e.g., portal vein thrombosis, lymphoma); metastatic or multifocal cancer in the liver; vascular congestion (e.g., cardiac cirrhosis); acute alcoholic hepatitis

DIAGNOSTIC TEST & INTERPRETATION
Initial Test (lab, imaging)
- Aspartate aminotransferase/alanine aminotransferase (AST/ALT): mildly elevated, typically AST > ALT; enzymes normalize as cirrhosis progresses.
- Elevated alkaline phosphatase (ALP), gamma-glutamyl transpeptidase (GGT), and total/direct bilirubin
- Anemia from hemolysis, folate deficiency, and/or splenomegaly
- Decreased platelet count
- Impaired synthetic liver function
  - Low albumin and cholesterol
  - Prolonged prothrombin (PT), international normalized ratio (INR), partial thromboplastin time (PTT). Vitamin K–dependent clotting factors (II, VII, IX, X)
- Progressive cirrhosis
  - Elevated ammonia level, BUN, sodium, and potassium
- α-Fetoprotein level to screen for hepatocellular carcinoma
- Abdominal ultrasound q6–12mo to screen for hepatocellular carcinoma
- Doppler ultrasound to assess liver parenchyma and hepatic/portal veins
- MRI best follow-up test for HCC if α-fetoprotein elevated and/or liver mass found on ultrasound
- Noninvasive modalities, such as elastography, are being researched as an alternative to liver biopsy (2).

Follow-Up Tests & Special Considerations
Consider the following:
- Hepatitis serologies (particularly B and C)
- Serum ethanol and GGT if alcohol abuse suspected
- Antimitochondrial antibody to screen for primary biliary cirrhosis
- Anti-smooth muscle and antinuclear antibodies to screen for chronic active (autoimmune) hepatitis
- Iron saturation (>50%) and ferritin (markedly increased) to screen for hemochromatosis; if abnormal, check hemochromatosis (HFE) genetics/mutation analysis.
- α_1-antitrypsin phenotype screen
- Ceruloplasmin level to screen for Wilson disease; if low, check copper excretion (serum copper plus 24-hour urine copper).

Diagnostic Procedures/Other
- Liver biopsy: required for definitive diagnosis, percutaneous if INR <1.5 and no ascites; otherwise, transjugular. Serologic testing gaining use as a surrogate for biopsy.

- Ultrasound-based elastography: noninvasive alternative to liver biopsy, not widely available; relies on increased "stiffness" of abnormal tissue to evaluate for fibrosis
- Endoscopy if portal hypertension to rule out esophageal varices/portal hypertensive gastropathy (3)[C]

Test Interpretation
- Fibrous bands and regenerative nodules are classic biopsy features of cirrhosis.
- Other histologic findings vary with etiology
  - Alcoholic liver disease: steatosis, polymorphonuclear (PMN) leukocyte infiltrate, ballooning degeneration of hepatocytes, Mallory bodies, giant mitochondria
  - Chronic hepatitis B and C: periportal lymphocytic inflammation
  - Nonalcoholic steatohepatitis (NASH): identical to alcoholic liver disease; steatosis may be absent in advanced disease ("burned-out NASH").
  - Biliary cirrhosis: PMN infiltrate in wall of bile ducts, inflammation increased in portal spaces, progressive loss of bile ducts in portal spaces.
  - Hemochromatosis: intrahepatic iron stores increased (iron stain or weighted biopsy tissue)
  - α_1-antitrypsin deficiency: positive periodic acid–Schiff (PAS) bodies in hepatocytes

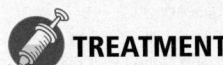 **TREATMENT**

Outpatient care except for major GI bleeding, altered mental status, sepsis/infection, rapid hepatic decompensation and renal failure.

GENERAL MEASURES
- Abstain from alcohol, drugs, hepatotoxic medications, and hepatotoxic herbs.
- Pneumococcal, hepatitis A/B, and influenza vaccines
- NASH: weight reduction, exercise, optimal control of lipids/glucose

MEDICATION
First Line
Treat the underlying cause first (*note prescribing precautions in decompensated cirrhosis*).
- Hepatitis C: Goal of treatment is to eradicate hepatitis C virus (HCV) RNA in serum. Combination therapy of pegylated interferon (PEG-IFN) with ribavirin is the standard of care for most genotypes.
- Hepatitis B: Goal of treatment is to achieve HBeAg seroconversion. Adefovir 10 mg PO daily, entecavir 0.5 to 1.0 mg PO daily, telbivudine 600 mg PO daily, or lamivudine 100 mg PO daily for minimum of 1 year, or continue for at least 6 months after HBeAg seroconversion; alternatively, PEG-IFN α-2a 180 μg SC weekly for 48 weeks. Lamivudine is no longer recommended as first-line agent due to high rates of resistance.
- Alcoholic hepatitis: Treat withdrawal; discriminant function >32 may benefit from prednisolone, 40 mg/day for 28 day with 2 to 4 weeks taper, to reduce mortality. Pentoxifylline for patients unable to tolerate steroids
- Biliary cirrhosis: ursodeoxycholic acid (ursodiol) 13 to 15 mg/kg PO divided BID–QID with food (4)[A]; bile acid sequestrants (BAS) are first-line therapy for pruritus: cholestyramine 4 to 8 g PO BID; antihistamines; rifampicin 150 to 300 mg PO BID; or opiate antagonists such as naltrexone 50 mg/day can be used for pruritus if ursodiol is ineffective.

- Wilson disease: initial treatment with penicillamine 1,000 to 1,500 mg/day PO BID–QID or trientine 750 to 1,500 mg/day PO BID–TID on empty stomach. Trientine (Syprine) is better tolerated. After 1 year, zinc acetate 150 mg/day PO BID–TID for maintenance. Zinc for presymptomatic, pregnant, and pediatric populations.
- Autoimmune (chronic active) hepatitis: prednisone 30 to 60 mg/day initially, maintenance 5 to 20 mg/day with or without azathioprine (Imuran) 0.5 to 1.0 mg/kg; adjust to keep transaminase levels normal. The combination is preferred. Discontinue maintenance after at least 24 months of treatment if AST and ALT are normal.
- Esophageal varices: propranolol 40 to 160 mg or nadolol 40 mg daily to lower portal pressure by 20 mm Hg, systolic pressure from 90 to 100 mm Hg, and pulse rate by 25% (3)[A].
- Ascites/edema: low-sodium (<2 g/day) diet and spironolactone 100 to 400 mg/day with or without furosemide 40 to 160 mg/day PO; torsemide may substitute for furosemide.
- Encephalopathy: lactulose 15 to 45 mL BID, titrate to induce three loose bowel movements daily. Combination therapy with rifaximin (550 mg PO BID) is recommended regimen to prevent recurrent hepatic encephalopathy (5)[B].
- Pruritus: ursodiol, cholestyramine, or antihistamines (e.g., hydroxyzine)
- Renal insufficiency: Stop diuretics and nephrotoxic drugs, normalize electrolytes, and hospitalize for plasma expansion or dialysis.
- Prophylactic antibiotics for invasive procedures, GI bleeding, or history of spontaneous bacterial peritonitis (3)[A]
- Proton pump inhibitor for esophageal varices requiring banding or portal hypertensive gastropathy (6)[A]

ISSUES FOR REFERRAL
Evaluate for liver transplant at onset of complications (ascites, variceal bleeding, encephalopathy), jaundice, or liver lesion suggestive of hepatocellular carcinoma and/or when evidence of hepatic dysfunction develops (Child-Turcotte-Pugh >7 and Model for End-stage Liver Disease [MELD] >10).

SURGERY/OTHER PROCEDURES
- Varices: endoscopic ligation, typically 4 to 6 treatments (if acute bleed, use pre-esophagogastroduodenoscopy [EGD] octreotide as vasoconstrictor); transjugular intrahepatic shunt (TIPS) second-line or salvage therapy for acute bleed (3)
- Ascites: if tense, therapeutic paracentesis every 2 weeks PRN; caution if pedal edema absent
- Fulminant hepatic failure: liver transplantation
- Hepatocellular carcinoma: curable if small with radiofrequency ablation or resection and transplant

COMPLEMENTARY & ALTERNATIVE MEDICINE
- Zinc sulfate 220 mg BID may improve dysgeusia and appetite; adjunct for hepatic encephalopathy
- Milk thistle (silymarin) may lower transaminases and improve symptoms.
- Danshen and huang qi injections may promote improvement; further studies needed (7)[B].
- Hepatotoxicity and drug interactions are common with many herbal medications (8).

INPATIENT CONSIDERATIONS
Admission Criteria/Initial Stabilization
Major GI bleeding, altered mental status, sepsis/infection, rapidly progressing hepatic decompensation, renal failure

 ONGOING CARE

FOLLOW-UP RECOMMENDATIONS
Regular physical conditioning may help with fatigue.
Patient Monitoring
- Once stable, monitor liver enzymes, platelets, and PT q6–12mo.
- Patients over 55 years with chronic hepatitis B or C, elevated INR, or low platelets are at highest risk for HCC. Serial α-fetoprotein and liver ultrasound screening q6–12mo in patients with cirrhosis (9)[C].
- Endoscopy at diagnosis and every 3 years (compensated) and every 1 year (decompensated) to screen for varices (3)[C]

DIET
- Protein (1.0 to 1.5 g/kg body weight), high fiber, daily multivitamin (without iron), and sodium (<2 g/day, essential if ascites/edema)
- Protein restriction is no longer recommended (10).
- Coffee consumption has a graded and inverse association with liver cancer (11)[A].

PATIENT EDUCATION
- Educate about when to seek emergency care (e.g., hematemesis, altered mental status).
- Maintain sobriety and smoking cessation (no cannabis).
- Update required immunizations; hepatitis C transmission precautions

PROGNOSIS
- At diagnosis of cirrhosis, expect 5 to 20 years of asymptomatic disease.
- After onset of complications, death typically within 5 years without transplant
  - 5% per year develop HCC.
  - 50% of cirrhotics develop ascites over 10 years; 50% 5-year survival once ascites develops
  - Acute variceal bleeding is the most common fatal complication; 30% mortality
  - Median survival after complications (ascites, variceal bleeding, encephalopathy) develop is 1.5 years (7).
  - With transplant, 85% survive 1 year; after transplant, ~5% annual mortality
- <25% of eligible patients receive a transplant because of donor organ shortage.

COMPLICATIONS
Ascites, edema, infections, encephalopathy, GI bleeding, esophageal varices, gastropathy, colopathy, hepatorenal syndrome, hepatopulmonary syndrome, hepatocellular carcinoma, fulminant hepatic failure, complications after transplant (e.g., surgical, rejection, infections)

REFERENCES
1. Hart CL, Morrison DS, Batty GD, et al. Effect of body mass index and alcohol consumption on liver disease: analysis of data from two prospective cohort studies. *BMJ*. 2010;340:c1240.
2. Tsochatzis EA, Gurusamy KS, Ntaoula S, et al. Elastography for the diagnosis of severity of fibrosis in chronic liver disease: a meta-analysis of diagnostic accuracy. *J Hepatol*. 2011;54(4):650–659.
3. Garcia-Tsao G, Sanyal AJ, Grace ND, et al. Prevention and management of gastroesophageal varices and variceal hemorrhage in cirrhosis. *Hepatology*. 2007;46(3):922–938.
4. Lindor KD, Gershwin ME, Poupon R, et al. Primary biliary cirrhosis. *Hepatology*. 2009;50(1):291–308.
5. Sharma BC, Sharma P, Lunia MK, et al. A randomized, double-blind, controlled trial comparing rifaximin plus lactulose with lactulose alone in treatment of overt hepatic encephalopathy. *Am J Gastroenterol*. 2013;108(9):1458–1463.
6. Leontiadis GI, Sharma VK, Howden CW. Proton pump inhibitor therapy for peptic ulcer bleeding: Cochrane collaboration meta-analysis of randomized controlled trials. *Mayo Clin Proc*. 2007;82(3):286–296.
7. Zhu C, Cao H, Zhou X, et al. Meta-analysis of the clinical value of danshen injection and huangqi injection in liver cirrhosis. *Evid Based Complement Alternat Med*. 2013;2013:842824.
8. Verma S, Thuluvath PJ. Complementary and alternative medicine in hepatology: review of the evidence of efficacy. *Clin Gastroenterol Hepatol*. 2007;5(4):408–416.
9. Yang JD, Roberts LR. Hepatocellular carcinoma: a global view. *Nat Rev Gastroenterol Hepatol*. 2010;7(8):448–458.
10. Tsiaousi ET, Hatzitolios AI, Trygonis SK, et al. Malnutrition in end stage liver disease: recommendations and nutritional support. *J Gastroenterol Hepatol*. 2008;23(4):527–533.
11. Bravi F, Bosetti C, Tavani A, et al. Coffee reduces risk for hepatocellular carcinoma: an updated meta-analysis. *Clin Gastroenterol Hepatol*. 2013;11(11):1413–1421.

ADDITIONAL READING
- Chou R, Wasson N. Blood tests to diagnose fibrosis or cirrhosis in patients with chronic hepatitis C virus infection: a systematic review. *Ann Intern Med*. 2013;158(11):807–820.
- Nierhoff J, Chávez Ortiz AA, Herrmann E, et al. The efficiency of acoustic radiation force impulse imaging for the staging of liver fibrosis: a meta-analysis. *Eur Radiol*. 2013;23(11):3040–3053.

 SEE ALSO

Algorithm: Cirrhosis

 CODES

ICD10
- K74.60 Unspecified cirrhosis of liver
- K70.30 Alcoholic cirrhosis of liver without ascites
- K74.69 Other cirrhosis of liver

CLINICAL PEARLS
- 80% of chronic liver disease that leads to cirrhosis is preventable (primarily alcohol abuse).
- Check abdominal ultrasound every 6 months for early detection of hepatocellular carcinoma.
- Update necessary immunizations and treat underlying cause (hepatitis C, alcohol abuse, etc.).

CLOSTRIDIUM DIFFICILE INFECTION

Darren S. Bryan, MD • James R. Yon, MD

 BASICS

DESCRIPTION
- *Clostridium difficile* is a gram-positive, spore-forming anaerobic bacillus that releases toxins to produce clinical disease.
- Infection caused by *C. difficile* is frequently associated with antibiotic use, hospitalization, and age.
- Severity of infection can range from diarrhea to pancolitis, perforation, and death.
- System(s) affected: gastrointestinal
- Synonyms(s): *C. difficile*-associated disease or diarrhea (CDAD); *C. difficile* colitis; *C. difficile*

EPIDEMIOLOGY
Incidence
- *C. difficile* infection is among the most common causes of hospital-acquired infection. The incidence appears to be rising (1).
- There are approximately 15 new cases per 1,000 clinical discharges. Higher with increased age (2)
- Rates of complications associated with *C. difficile* such as treatment failure and recurrence are also increasing (1).

Prevalence
- *C. difficile* causes ~25% of all cases of antibiotic-associated diarrhea
- Prevalence of community-acquired *C. difficile* infection is increasing. Up to 40% of patients will require hospitalization (2).
- *C. difficile* is present as a commensurate organism in 2–5% of the adult U.S. population.

ETIOLOGY AND PATHOPHYSIOLOGY
- *C. difficile* are motile bacteria existing in vegetative and spore forms. Spores can survive for months in harsh conditions and outside of the body.
- Spread by fecal–oral contact. Acid-resistant spores pass through stomach, and reside predominantly in the colon.
- Colonic colonization causes disruptions in barrier functions of the normal microbiome (2).
- *C. difficile* is noninvasive. Toxins are produced that mediate disease:
  - Toxins A (enterotoxin) and B (cytotoxin) attract neutrophils and monocytes, degrading colonic epithelial cells, and causing clinical disease.
- BI/NAP1/027 strain of *C. difficile* has been shown to produce a much more virulent form of disease, with increased endotoxin concentrations. It is associated with increased rates of colectomy and death.

Genetics
No known genetic factors

RISK FACTORS
- Host risk factors
  - Age >65 years
  - Hospitalization or stay in long-term health care facility. The length of stay is directly correlated with the risk for *C. difficile* infection.
  - Comorbidities, including inflammatory bowel disease, immunosuppression, tube feeding, chronic liver disease, and end-stage renal disease
  - Previous *C. difficile* infection

- Factors that disrupt normal colonic microbiota:
  - Exposure to almost all antibiotics (including perioperative prophylaxis) is associated with an increased risk for *C. difficile* infection.
  - Most commonly implicated antibiotics include: ampicillin, amoxicillin, clindamycin, cephalosporins, and fluoroquinolones
- Recurrence from prior infection
  - Recurrence rates approximately 20% after initial episode. More likely to have recurrence with each additional episode (2)
- Patients who have had colectomy for *C. difficile* infection can have colonization of the ileum. Community-acquired *C. difficile* infections (no overnight admission in >12 weeks) are more frequent in patients without other risk factors (younger, no recent antibiotic exposure).

Geriatric Considerations
C. difficile is the most common cause of acute diarrheal illness in long-term care facilities. Elderly patients also commonly have multiple other risk factors (comorbid disease, antibiotic exposure, medication use).

Pediatric Considerations
- Neonates have a higher rate of *C. difficile* colonization (25–80%) but are generally less symptomatic than adults (possibly due to immature toxin receptors)
- Frequently serve as carrier for symptomatic infection in adults

GENERAL PREVENTION
- A comprehensive infection control program decreases the incidence of *C. difficile* infection.
- 2010 Society for Healthcare Epidemiology of America (SHEA)/Infectious Diseases Society of America (IDS) guidelines:
  - For health care workers, patients, and visitors:
    - Contact precautions, including gloves and gowns, on entry to room
    - Alcohol-based hand sanitizers not effective. Hand hygiene with soap and water before and after patient interaction
    - Accommodate patients with *C. difficile* infection in private rooms, if possible.
  - Environmental cleaning and disinfection
    - Disinfection with hypochlorite solution or other spore-killing solutions
    - Identification and reduction of environmental sources of *C. difficile*, including the use of nondisposable rectal thermometers
  - Antimicrobial use restrictions
    - Minimize the frequency and duration of antibiotic therapy.

COMMONLY ASSOCIATED CONDITIONS
Pseudomembranous colitis, toxic megacolon, sepsis, colonic perforation

Rx DIAGNOSIS

HISTORY
- Age and underlying comorbidities
- Recent antibiotic use
- Diarrhea (defined as >3 stools in 24 hours) that is watery, foul-smelling, and sometimes bloody (1)
- Fever (<10%), anorexia, nausea
- Recent hospitalization or stay at nursing facility

PHYSICAL EXAM
Physical exam findings range from mild abdominal pain to peritoneal findings and shock:
- Mild or moderate disease: mild lower abdominal pain, often cramping pain
- Severe disease: fever, nausea/vomiting, dehydration
- Severe, complicated disease: shock, peritonitis, ileus

DIFFERENTIAL DIAGNOSIS
- Antibiotic-associated diarrhea
- Inflammatory bowel disease
- Enteric infections
- Food poisoning

DIAGNOSTIC TESTS & INTERPRETATION
- SHEA/IDSA guidelines (2)
  - Mild or moderate disease: leukocytosis with white blood cell (WBC) count <15,000 cells/μL and a serum creatinine level <1.5× the premorbid level
  - Severe, uncomplicated disease: leukocytosis with WBC count >15,000 cells/μL or a serum creatinine level >1.5× the premorbid level
  - Severe, complicated disease: markers of severe infection include hypotension, sepsis, markedly elevated WBC count, and bandemia
    - Other signs seen on imaging include obstruction, perforation, toxic megacolon, and colonic wall thickening

Initial Tests (lab, imaging)
- Polymerase chain reaction (PCR)-based testing is preferred for *C. difficile*. Rapid, highly sensitive, and hightly specific (2)[B]

- Alternative to PCR: screening and confirmatory testing. *C. difficile* common antigen tests: Tests for glutamate dehydrogenase (GDH), found in both toxic and nontoxic strains of *C. difficile* (sensitivity, 85–95%; specificity, 89–99%).
- Confirmatory: enzyme immunoassay for toxins (A/B or A); rapid results, inexpensive, easy to use (sensitivity 63–94%)
- Stool culture is the most sensitive test; however, non–toxin-producing strains also detected.

- Repeat testing during the same episode of diarrhea is not recommended. Stool carriage persists for 3 to 6 weeks after successful treatment (2)[A].

Diagnostic Procedures/Other
- Endoscopy can be used to evaluate for pseudomembranes and exclude other conditions
  - While not all patients with *C. difficile* infection have pseudomembranes, their presence is pathognomonic for *C. difficile*.
- Flexible sigmoidoscopy may miss 15–20% of pseudomembranes present in the proximal colon.
- Colonoscopy evaluates the entire colon: used when diagnosis is in doubt or severity demands rapid diagnosis
- Plain films may show thumbprinting and colonic distension.
- CT may show mucosal wall thickening, thickened colonic wall, and pericolonic inflammation.

Test Interpretation
Pseudomembranes consist of inflammatory and cellular debris that forms visible exudates that can obscure the underlying mucosa. These exudates have a yellow to grayish color.

TREATMENT

GENERAL MEASURES
- Avoid antimotility agents and opiates.
- Avoid indiscriminate use of antibiotics.
- Proton pump inhibitors associated with recurrent infection, however have not shown to be causal
- Discontinue offending antibiotic, if possible.

MEDICATION

First Line
- Mild or moderate infection (3)[A]
  - Oral metronidazole is the drug of choice for mild to moderate *C. difficile* infection:
    - 500 mg PO TID for 10 to 14 days
    - If patient is unable to take oral medications, then intravenous (IV) metronidazole or intraluminal vancomycin can be used.
- Severe infection (3)[A]
  - Enteral vancomycin is 1st-line therapy in patients with severe or fulminant *C. difficile* infection:
    - 125 mg PO QID for 10 to 14 days
    - Vancomycin retention enema if unable to take PO, or if there is evidence of poor gastrointestinal motility
- Severe, complicated infection—consider surgical and critical care consultation (3)[A]
  - Vancomycin: 500 mg PO QID and metronidazole 500 mg PO TID
- 1st recurrence
  - Treat the same as 1st episode
- 2nd recurrence
  - Vancomycin taper and/or pulse: vancomycin 125 mg PO QID for 10 to 14 days, then 125 mg PO BID for 7 days, then 125 mg PO once daily for 7 days, then 125 mg PO every 2 to 3 days for 2 to 8 weeks:
    - Pulse dosing every 2 to 3 days allows spores to germinate and then be killed.

ALERT
When using vancomycin for treatment of *C. difficile* infection, oral or rectal formulations must be used. IV formulations are not excreted into the colonic lumen.

Second Line
- Vancomycin: indicated for patients who cannot tolerate or have failed metronidazole therapy and for those who are pregnant
- Fidaxomicin is another option 200 mg PO BID. Similar cure rates to vancomycin and lower recurrence rates, however can be cost prohibitive.
- Fidaxomicin rapidly kills *C. difficile* whereas vancomycin inhibits growth. Fidaxomicin has a narrow antimicrobial spectrum and helps preserve normal anaerobic flora.
- Fecal transplant: stool from healthy, screened donor. Administered via either rectal or oral route. Highly effective treatment for recurrent infections (>90% cure rate) when offending antibiotic stopped. Recipient gut flora have been transformed in as few as 3 days following fecal transplantation (4)[A].

SURGERY/OTHER PROCEDURES
- Most patients improve with conservative management and oral antibiotics.
- Patients with severe fulminant colitis develop paralytic ileus, leading to distention (megacolon), and potential perforation.
- Severe lower quadrant abdominal pain or signs of hemodynamic instability in the setting of known infection should prompt surgical and critical care consultation.

ALERT
BI/NAP1/027 strain associated with fulminant colitis, often requiring surgical intervention. More common in younger patients with severe disease.

COMPLEMENTARY & ALTERNATIVE MEDICINE
- Adjunctive therapy with intravenous immunoglobulin (IVIG) has shown initial promise, but more data are required before routine clinical use.
- Probiotics have an (strain-specific) inhibitory effect on *C. difficile* and may play a role in prevention.
- Other investigational treatment options:
  - New antibiotics (Rifalazil, Tolevamer, and Ramoplanin)
  - Monoclonal antibodies to directly modulate the effects of toxins
  - Vaccine form of *C. difficile* antitoxin antibody

INPATIENT CONSIDERATIONS

Admission Criteria/Initial Stabilization
- Hypovolemia
- Inability to keep up with enteric losses
- Hematochezia
- Electrolyte disturbances

IV Fluids
To maintain volume status

Discharge Criteria
- Decreased diarrhea severity and frequency
- Tolerating oral diet and medications
- Do not repeat testing for toxins, as they may shed for weeks following an acute infection.

ONGOING CARE

FOLLOW-UP RECOMMENDATIONS
Many patients can be treated as outpatients.

Patient Monitoring
- Relapses of colitis occur in 15–30%
- Relapses typically occur 2 to 10 days after discontinuing antibiotics.

DIET
Regular diet or NPO if severe and surgical evaluation required

PATIENT EDUCATION
Educate patients about *C. difficile* transmission, the importance of hand washing, and the appropriate use of antibiotics.

ALERT
Alcohol-based hand sanitizers are not effective against *C. difficile*. Wash with soap and water.

PROGNOSIS
- Most patients improve with conservative management and oral antibiotics.
- 1–3% of patients develop severe/fulminant colitis requiring emergency colectomy.

REFERENCES
1. Khanna S, Pardi DS. *Clostridium difficile* infection: management strategies for a difficult disease. *Therap Adv Gastroenterol*. 2014;7(2):72–86.
2. Leffler DA, Lamont JT. *Clostridium difficile* infection. *N Engl J Med*. 2015;372(16):1539–1548.
3. Debast SB, Bauer MP, Kuijper EJ; European Society of Clinical Microbiology and Infectious Diseases: update of the treatment guidance document for *Clostridium difficile* infection. *Clin Microbiol Infect*. 2014;20(Suppl 2):1–26.
4. Shankar V, Hamilton MJ, Khoruts A, et al. Species and genus level resolution analysis of gut microbiota in *Clostridium difficile* patients following fecal microbiota transplantation. *Microbiome*. 2014;2:13.

ADDITIONAL READING
- Cohen SH, Gerding DN, Johnson S, et al. Clinical practice guidelines for *Clostridium difficile* infection in adults: 2010 update by the Society for Healthcare Epidemiology of America (SHEA) and the Infectious Diseases Society of America (IDSA). *Infect Control Hosp Epidemiol*. 2010;31(5):431–455.
- Kassam Z, Lee CH, Yuan Y, et al. Fecal microbiota transplantation for *Clostridium difficile* infection: systematic review and meta-analysis. *Am J Gastroenterol*. 2013;108(4):500–508.
- McCollum DL, Rodriguez JM. Detection, treatment, and prevention of *Clostridium difficile* infection. *Clin Gastroenterol Hepatol*. 2012;10(6):581–592.

CODES

ICD10
A04.7 Enterocolitis due to Clostridium difficile

CLINICAL PEARLS
- *C. difficile* is spread by fecal–oral contact.
- Alcohol-based hand sanitizers are ineffective against *C. difficile*. Wash hands with soap and water.
- Testing and treatment of asymptomatic patients is not recommended.
- PCR is the preferred initial test.
- Patients may shed organism or toxin for weeks after treatment. Repeat toxin assays following treatment are not helpful.
- Metronidazole remains the drug of choice for mild to moderate disease.

COLIC, INFANTILE
Daniel T. Lee, MD, MA • Arthur Ohannessian, MD

BASICS

DESCRIPTION
- Colic is defined as excessive crying in an otherwise healthy baby.
- A commonly used criteria is the Wessel criteria or the Rule of Three: crying lasts for:
  - >3 hr/day
  - >3 days/week
  - Persists >3 weeks
- Many clinicians no longer use the criterion of persistence for >3 weeks because few parents or clinicians will wait that long before evaluation or intervention.
- Some clinicians feel that colic represents the extreme end of the spectrum of normal crying, whereas most feel that colic is a distinct clinical entity.

EPIDEMIOLOGY
Incidence
- Predominant age: between 2 weeks and 4 months of age
- Predominant sex: male = female

Prevalence
- Probably between 10% and 25% of infants
- Range is somewhere between 8% and 40% of infants.

Pediatric Considerations
This is a problem during infancy.

ETIOLOGY AND PATHOPHYSIOLOGY
The cause is unknown. Factors that may play a role include the following:
- Infant gastroesophageal reflux disease
- Allergy to cow's milk, soy milk, or breast milk protein
- Fruit juice intolerance
- Swallowing air during the process of crying, feeding, or sucking
- Overfeeding or feeding too quickly; underfeeding also has been proposed.
- Inadequate burping after feeding
- Family tension
- Parental anxiety, depression, and/or fatigue
- Parent–infant interaction mismatch
- Baby's inability to console him- or herself when dealing with stimuli
- Increased gut hormone motilin, causing hyperperistalsis
- Functional lactose overload (i.e., breast milk that has a lower lipid content can have faster transit time in the intestine, leading to more lactose fermentation in the gut and hence gas and distension) (1)[C]
- Tobacco smoke exposure

RISK FACTORS
- Physiologic predisposition in infant but no definitive risk factors have been established. However, emerging data suggest maternal smoking or exposure to nicotine replacement therapy during pregnancy is associated with higher incidence of infantile colic (2)[B].
- Infants with a maternal history of migraine headaches are twice as likely to have colic (3)[B].

GENERAL PREVENTION
Colic is generally not preventable.

DIAGNOSIS

HISTORY
- Evaluation for Wessel criteria: crying lasts for >3 hr/day, >3 days/week, and persists >3 weeks.
- The colicky episodes may have a clear beginning and end.
- The crying is generally spontaneous, without preceding events triggering the episodes.
- The crying is typically different from normal crying. Colicky crying may be louder, more turbulent, variable in pitch, and appear more like screaming.
- The infant may be difficult to soothe or console regardless of how the parents try to help.
- The infant acts normally when not colicky.
- Assess the support system of caregivers and families, including coping skills.

PHYSICAL EXAM
- A comprehensive physical exam is normal.
- Because excessive crying may be a risk factor for shaken baby syndrome or other forms of child abuse (4)[B], be sure to examine the child carefully for signs of shaken baby syndrome or other types of child abuse.

DIFFERENTIAL DIAGNOSIS
Any organic cause for excessive or qualitatively different crying in infants such as:
- Infections (e.g., meningitis, sepsis, otitis media, or UTI)
- GI issues such as gastroesophageal reflux disease, intussusception, lactose intolerance, constipation, anal fissure, or strangulated hernia
- Trauma, which includes foreign bodies, corneal abrasion, occult fracture, digit or penile hair tourniquet syndrome, or child abuse

DIAGNOSTIC TESTS & INTERPRETATION
Initial Tests (lab, imaging)
Clinical diagnosis; no testing is done unless clinical symptoms imply other cause (UTI, weight loss, etc.).

Diagnostic Procedures/Other
A thorough history and physical exam should be performed to rule out other causes. Otherwise, no diagnostic procedures or imaging is indicated.

TREATMENT

GENERAL MEASURES
- Soothe by holding and rocking the baby.
- Use a pacifier.
- Use of gentle rhythmic motion (e.g., strollers, infant swings, car rides).
- Place near white noise (e.g., vacuum cleaner, clothes dryer, white noise machine).
- Crib vibrators or car ride simulators have not proven to be helpful (5)[B].
- Increased carrying or use of infant carrier has not been shown to improve colic (5)[B].
- Burping does not significantly lower colic events and can cause significant increase in regurgitation episodes (6)[B].
- Employ the 5 Ss (need to be done concurrently):
  - Swaddling: tight wrapping with blanket; may be especially beneficial in infants <8 weeks old (7)[B]
  - Side: laying baby on side
  - Shushing: loud white noise
  - Swinging: rhythmic, jiggly motion
  - Sucking: sucking on anything (e.g., nipple, finger, pacifier)

MEDICATION
- None as no medication found to be beneficial and safe. Probiotics are safe and effective (see Complementary and Alternative Medicine).
- Dicyclomine (Bentyl) has been proven beneficial, but the potential serious adverse effects (apnea, seizures, and syncope) have precluded its use. Furthermore, the manufacturer has made the medication contraindicated for infants <6 months (8)[B].
- Simethicone has not been shown to be beneficial (8)[B].
- Omeprazole has not been shown to be beneficial (9)[B].

ISSUES FOR REFERRAL
Excessive vomiting, poor weight gain, recurrent respiratory diseases, or bloody stools should prompt referral to a specialist.

COMPLEMENTARY & ALTERNATIVE MEDICINE
- Recent data from a large randomized controlled study involving nine neonatal units in Italy found that prophylactic use of *Lactobacillus reuteri* was beneficial. At 3 months of age, the mean duration of crying time (38 vs. 71 minutes; $p < .01$), the mean number of regurgitations per day (2.9 vs. 4.6; $p < .01$), and the mean number of evacuations per day (4.2 vs. 3.6; $p < .01$) for the *L. reuteri* DSM 17938 and placebo groups, respectively, were significantly different (10)[A].
- However, the effect of *L. reuteri* has not been as robust in infants already diagnosed with colic. A placebo-controlled study of 50 infants given *L. reuteri* had significantly reduced median daily crying times throughout the study (370 to 35 min/day vs. 300 to 90 min/day in placebo group). However, weight gain, stooling frequency, and incidence of regurgitation were similar in both groups (11)[B].
- *L. reuteri* is available as over-the-counter drops, but it is not regulated by the FDA.
  - A 2013 systematic review found probiotics effective for breastfed infants but not formula-fed infants. Infant massage and crib vibrator were found to reduce colic symptoms by 50% in a small RCT (12)[B].
- Anecdotal evidence that car rides, both real and simulated via podcast (https://www.youtube.com/watch?v=8KAXmIe-T_4), or running a vacuum cleaner near the baby may be effective.
- Herbal teas and supplements may help but are not recommended because of limited, inconclusive evidence. Examples:
  - One study concluded that herbal teas containing mixtures of chamomile, vervain, licorice, fennel, and balm-mint used up to TID may be beneficial (4)[C]. However, the study used high dosages, raising clinical concerns that this therapy may impair needed milk consumption in infants and be impractical to administer. In addition, preparations used in the study may not be commercially available in the United States.

– A second double-blind, randomized trial of 0.1% fennel seed oil emulsion versus placebo demonstrated a decrease in colic symptoms according to the Wessel criteria. However, this preparation of fennel seed oil is not commercially available in the United States, and the long-term health effects are unknown (13)[B].

• A home-based intervention focusing on reducing infant stimulation and synchronizing infant sleep–wake cycles with the environment, as well as parental support, has been shown to be effective (14)[B].

• Use of music may help (15,16)[C].
• Chiropractic treatment has shown no benefit over placebo.
• Infant massage has not been shown to be helpful.

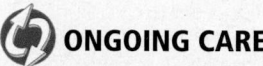 ONGOING CARE

FOLLOW-UP RECOMMENDATIONS
Frequent outpatient visits as needed for parental reassurance, education, and monitoring and to ensure the health of the infant and parents

Patient Monitoring
Follow for proper feeding, growth, and development.

DIET
• If breastfeeding:
  – Continue breastfeeding. Switching to formula probably will not help.
  – Possible therapeutic benefit from eliminating milk products, eggs, wheat, and/or nuts from the diet of breastfeeding mothers (5)[B]
  – Along with eliminating the preceding foods from the maternal diet, removing soy, nuts, and fish may be beneficial.
• If formula feeding:
  – Feeding the infant in a vertical position using a curved bottle or bottle with collapsible bag may help to reduce air swallowing.
  – If no intervention or dietary change has improved the situation, consider a 1-week trial of hypoallergenic formulas such as whey hydrolysate (e.g., Good Start) or casein hydrolysate (e.g., Alimentum, Nutramigen, Pregestimil) (5)[B],(8)[C].
  – The American Academy of Pediatrics concluded that there is no proven role for soy formula in the treatment of colic (17)[C].
  – Adding fiber to formula also has not been shown to be helpful (5,15)[B].
• Supplementing with sucrose solution may be helpful, but the effect may be short-lived (<1 hour) (5,8)[B].
• Despite the proposed mechanism of functional lactose overload, use of lactase enzymes in formula or breast milk or given directly to the infant has no therapeutic benefit (5)[B].

PATIENT EDUCATION
• Reassure parents that colic is not the result of bad parenting, and advise parents about having proper rest breaks, adequate sleep, and help in caring for the infant.
• Explain the spectrum of crying behavior.
• Avoid over- or underfeeding.

• Instruct in better feeding techniques such as improved bottles (low air, curved) and sufficient burping after feeding.
• Colic information at American Family Physician: www.aafp.org/afp/2004/0815/p741.html

PROGNOSIS
• Usually subsides by 3 to 6 months of age, often on its own
• Despite apparent abdominal pain, colicky infants eat well and gain weight normally.
• A handful of studies indicate temper tantrums may be more common among formerly colicky infants as studied in toddlers up to 4 years old (18,19)[C].
• Colic has no bearing on the baby's intelligence or future development.

COMPLICATIONS
• Colic is self-limiting and does not result in lasting effects to infant or maternal mental health (20)[C].
• However, case-control studies have shown an increased incidence of diagnosing childhood migraine headaches in patients with a history of colic during infancy (21)[B].

REFERENCES

1. Douglas P, Hill P. Managing infants who cry excessively in the first few months of life. *BMJ*. 2011;343:d7772.
2. Milidou I, Henriksen TB, Jensen MS, et al. Nicotine replacement therapy during pregnancy and infantile colic in the offspring. *Pediatrics*. 2012;129(3):e652–e658.
3. Romanello S, Spiri D, Marcuzzi E, et al. Association between childhood migraine and history of infantile colic. *JAMA*. 2013;309(15):1607–1612.
4. Reijneveld SA, van der Wal MF, Brugman E, et al. Infant crying and abuse. *Lancet*. 2004;364(9442): 1340–1342.
5. Garrison MM, Christakis DA. A systematic review of treatments for infant colic. *Pediatrics*. 2000;106(1, Pt 2):184–190.
6. Kaur R, Bharti B, Saini SK. A randomized controlled trial of burping for the prevention of colic and regurgitation in healthy infants. *Child Care Health Dev*. 2015;41(1):52–56.
7. van Sleuwen BE, L'hoir MP, Engelberts AC, et al. Comparison of behavior modification with and without swaddling as interventions for excessive crying. *J Pediatr*. 2006;149(4):512–517.
8. Wade S, Kilgour T. Extracts from "clinical evidence": infantile colic. *BMJ*. 2001;323(7310): 437–440.
9. Moore DJ, Tao BS, Lines DR, et al. Double-blind placebo-controlled trial of omeprazole in irritable infants with gastroesophageal reflux. *J Pediatr*. 2003;143(2):219–223.
10. Indrio F, Di Mauro A, Riezzo G, et al. Prophylactic use of a probiotic in the prevention of colic, regurgitation, and functional constipation: a randomized clinical trial. *JAMA Pediatr*. 2014;168(3):228–233.
11. Savino F, Cordisco L, Tarasco V, et al. *Lactobacillus reuteri* DSM 17938 in infantile colic: a randomized, double-blind, placebo-controlled trial. *Pediatrics*. 2010;126(3):e526–e533.

12. Huhtala V, Lehtonen L, Heinonen R, et al. Infant massage compared with crib vibrator in the treatment of colicky infants. *Pediatrics*. 2000;105(6):E84.
13. Alexandrovich I, Rakovitskaya O, Kolmo E, et al. The effect of fennel (*Foeniculum vulgare*) seed oil emulsion in infantile colic: a randomized, placebo-controlled study. *Altern Ther Health Med*. 2003;9(4):58–61.
14. Keefe MR, Lobo ML, Froese-Fretz A, et al. Effectiveness of an intervention for colic. *Clin Pediatr (Phila)*. 2006;45(2):123–133.
15. Clemons RM. Issues in newborn care. *Prim Care*. 2000;27(1):251–267.
16. McCollough M, Sharieff GQ. Common complaints in the first 30 days of life. *Emerg Med Clin North Am*. 2002;20(1):27–48.
17. O'Connor NR. Infant formula. *Am Fam Physician*. 2009;79(7):565–570.
18. Canivet C, Jakobsson I, Hagander B. Infantile colic. Follow-up at four years of age: still more "emotional." *Acta Paediatr*. 2000;89(1):13–17.
19. Rautava P, Lehtonen L, Helenius H, et al. Infantile colic: child and family three years later. *Pediatrics*. 1995;96(1, Pt 1):43–47.
20. Clifford TJ, Campbell MK, Speechley KN, et al. Sequelae of infant colic: evidence of transient infant distress and absence of lasting effects on maternal mental health. *Arch Pediatr Adolesc Med*. 2002;156(12):1183–1188.
21. Gelfand AA, Thomas KC, Goadsby PJ. Before the headache: infant colic as an early life expression of migraine. *Neurology*. 2012;79(13):1392–1396.

ADDITIONAL READING
• Anabrees J, Indrio F, Paes B, et al. Probiotics for infantile colic: a systematic review. *BMC Pediatr*. 2013;13:186.
• Johnson JD, Cocker K, Chang E. Infantile colic: recognition and treatment. *Am Fam Physician*. 2015;92(7):577–582.
• Savino F, Pelle E, Palumeri E, et al. *Lactobacillus reuteri* (American Type Culture Collection Strain 55730) versus simethicone in the treatment of infantile colic: a prospective randomized study. *Pediatrics*. 2007;119(1):e124–e130.

 CODES

ICD10
R10.83 Colic

CLINICAL PEARLS
• Colic is defined as excessive crying in an otherwise healthy baby.
• Excessive crying may be a risk factor for shaken baby syndrome or other forms of child abuse.
• Usually subsides spontaneously by 3 to 6 months of age
• Provide advice, support, and reassurance to parents.
• Prevent caregiver burnout by advising parents to get proper rest breaks, sleep, and help in caring for the infant.

COLITIS, ISCHEMIC

Pia Prakash, MD • Mohammed Abdalaziz Wazzan, MD, MBBS • Marie L. Borum, MD, EdD, MPH

BASICS

Ischemic colitis (IC) results from decreased blood flow to the colon with resultant inflammation and tissue damage.

DESCRIPTION
- More common in the elderly but can affect patients of all ages
- Patients present in several ways:
  - *Nonacute IC* from a chronic process with irreversible ischemic injury
  - *Acute process* with self-limited transient mucosal ischemia
- IC is self-limited and reversible in 80% of patients:
  - 20% of patients progress to full-thickness necrosis requiring surgical intervention.
- Most commonly, ischemia is related to a nonocclusive reduction in blood flow:
  - Occlusive events are less common.
- Presentation varies, but patients with acute IC typically present with localized abdominal pain and tenderness. Frequent loose, bloody stools may be seen within 12 to 24 hours of onset.
- Laboratory and radiographic findings are nonspecific and must be correlated with clinical presentation.
- Colonoscopy is the gold standard for diagnosis of IC.
- In the absence of complications, most patients recover with supportive care including IV fluids, bowel rest, and clinical monitoring.

EPIDEMIOLOGY
- Men and women are at equal risk.
- Patients with inflammatory bowel disease or COPD have an increased risk.
- Evidence of IC seen in 1 of every 100 endoscopies

Geriatric Considerations
Rare in patients <60 years old. 70 years is the average age at diagnosis.

Incidence
- 4.5 to 44 cases per 100,000 in the general population
- 1 of every 2,000 hospital admissions
- True incidence may be underestimated due to nonspecific clinical manifestations.

Prevalence
19 cases per 100,000 in the general population

ETIOLOGY AND PATHOPHYSIOLOGY
- Reduced blood flow to the colon, compromises the ability to meet metabolic demands
- Most commonly, an acute, self-limited process
- The colon is perfused by both the superior and inferior mesenteric arteries (SMAs and IMAs) and branches of the internal iliac arteries. Occlusion of branches of the SMA or IMA rarely leads to ischemic consequences due to extensive collateral circulation.
- Watershed areas of the colon (splenic flexure and rectosigmoid junction) are most susceptible to ischemic damage. Blood is carried by narrow branches of the SMA and IMA to these areas, putting them at increased risk for ischemia. The splenic flexure is supplied by the terminal branches of the SMA, and the rectosigmoid junction is supplied by the terminal branches of the IMA.
- Left colon is more commonly affected than the right.

- The rectum is often spared because of additional blood supply from the internal iliac arteries.
- Poor perfusion may result from systemic disease, local vascular compromise, and anatomic or functional changes in the colon itself. An occlusion of large vessels is usually not identified.
  - Hypoperfusion from shock, trauma
  - Embolic occlusion of mesenteric vessels
  - Hypercoagulable states, vasculitis
  - Sickle cell disease
  - Arterial thrombosis; venous thrombosis
  - Mechanical colonic obstruction (e.g., tumor, adhesions, hernia, volvulus, prolapse, diverticulitis)
  - Surgical complications (e.g., related to abdominal aortic aneurysm repair)
  - Medications (intestinally active vasoconstrictive substances, medications that induce hypotension and thus, hypoperfusion)
  - Cocaine abuse
  - Aortic dissection
  - Strenuous physical activity (e.g., long-distance running)
- Acute IC is largely self-limited and often resolves without long-term complications.
- Repeated episodes of ischemia and inflammation may result in chronic colonic ischemia, possible stricture formation, recurrent bacteremia, and sepsis. These patients may have unresolving areas of colitis and require segmental colonic resection.

RISK FACTORS
- Age >60 years (90% of patients)
- Smoking (most common cause of recurrent IC) (1)
- Hypertension, diabetes mellitus
- Rheumatologic disorders/vasculitis
- Cerebrovascular disease, ischemic heart disease
- Recent abdominal surgery
- Constipation-inducing medications
- History of vascular surgery
- Hypoalbuminemia; hemodialysis
- Smoking, hypercoagulability, oral contraceptive (2)
- AAA repair (IMA ligation) (2)
- IBS-C (related to treatment with serotonin antagonist) (2)

DIAGNOSIS

- Diagnosis is based on history, risk factors, and physical examination (3)[A].
- Laboratory values and radiographic findings are usually nonspecific (3)[A].
- Colonoscopy is diagnostic (3)[A].

HISTORY
- Abdominal pain is the most common symptom (4).
- Symptoms vary depending on severity (5)[A].
- Sudden-onset, mild to moderate abdominal pain with tenderness over the affected segment of bowel (3)[A]
- Sudden urge to defecate followed by passage of either bright red or maroon stool (5)[A]
- Lower GI bleeding is rarely heavy (3)[A].
- Loose, bloody bowel movements may occur, typically within 12 to 24 hours of abdominal pain onset (5)[A].

PHYSICAL EXAM
- Individual signs and symptoms are poorly predictive of IC (6)[A].
- Vital signs: hypotension; tachycardia
- Tenderness to palpation over the involved segment of bowel (5)[A]
- Abdominal distention with vomiting due to an associated ileus (3)[A]
- In the uncommon setting of transmural ischemia, patients may develop peritoneal signs such as rebound and guarding (7)[A].

DIFFERENTIAL DIAGNOSIS
- Infectious colitis (7)[A]
- Inflammatory bowel disease (ulcerative colitis, Crohn disease) (7)[A]
- Colon cancer (7)[A]; diverticulitis (7)[A]
- Pseudomembranous colitis (6)[A]

DIAGNOSTIC TESTS & INTERPRETATION
- Depends on the clinical presentation, extent of colonic involvement, transmural involvement, and acuity (3)[A].
- CT scan is the initial diagnostic test for patients with nonspecific abdominal pain (6)[A].
- Colonoscopy is the most sensitive diagnostic test (3)[A].
- Radiographic tests and laboratory values are nonspecific (6)[A].

Initial Tests (lab, imaging)
- The following lab markers of ischemia are not specific to IC and are more common in severe ischemia (6)[A]:
  - CBC (leukocytosis) (6)[A]
  - BMP, ABG (signs of metabolic acidosis) (6)[A]
  - Lactate (6)[A], CPK (6)[A]
  - Alkaline phosphatase (6)[A]
  - Lactate dehydrogenase (LDH) (6)[A], amylase (6)[A]

  - Procalcitonin (8)
  - Hypoxia inducible factor 1-alpha (9)
  - Abdominal plain film should be obtained:

    ○ 20% of patient show signs of IC such as thumbprinting and mural thickening (7)[A].
    ○ Necessary to rule out bowel perforation and pneumoperitoneum (7)[A]
- No role for routine mesenteric angiography (3)[A], but it can help detect the cause of IC (10).
- Abdominal CT scan with contrast should be obtained in suspected IC (3)[A]:

  - The most common CT findings are moderate continuous circumferential thickening of colonic wall and pericolonic fat stranding (10).
  - Other common CT findings include hyperdense mucosa, submucosal edema, and mesenteric inflammation (3)[A].
  - Pneumatosis, pneumoperitoneum, and free peritoneal fluid suggest advanced ischemia (3)[A].

Follow-Up Tests & Special Considerations

- Stool cultures, fecal leukocytes, stool ova, and parasites to rule out infection (6)[A]
- Patients undergoing aortic surgery may need post-operative colonoscopy within 2 to 3 days to look for signs of IC (5)[A].
- Cardiac workup including electrocardiogram, Holter monitoring, or transthoracic echocardiogram to exclude cardiogenic embolism as indicated (6)[A].

Diagnostic Procedures/Other

- Colonoscopy is gold standard; sigmoidoscopy also used (3)[A]
- Cyanotic hemorrhagic tissue and edematous mucosa suggests ischemia (5)[A].
  - Segmental distribution (watershed), hemorrhagic nodules, and rectal sparing (5)[A]
  - "Colon single-stripe sign" is a single line of erythema, with a 75% histopathologic yield (5)[A].
  - Routine biopsy is no longer advised, as results are typically nonspecific (3)[A].
- In cases of isolated right colon ischemia, noninvasive vascular imaging studies are recommended to evaluate acute SMA occlusion (5)[A].

Test Interpretation

- Fulminant gangrenous IC seen in 15% of cases requires surgical intervention (3)[A].
- Acute transient IC seen in 85% of cases requires clinical evaluation for further workup (3)[A].
- Biopsied specimens reveal mucosal infarction and ghost cells, which show normal cellular outlines but lack intracellular contents (3)[A].

 TREATMENT

- Treatment depends on disease severity (3)[A].
- Continuous clinical monitoring, including vital signs and serial abdominal exams (7)[A]
- In the absence of colonic necrosis or perforation, most patients respond to supportive care (5)[A]: Bowel rest (5)[A]
  - IV fluids to maintain hemodynamic stability (5)[A]
  - Broad-spectrum antibiotics to cover aerobic and anaerobic bacteria to avoid bacterial translocation secondary to colonic mucosal damage (5)[A]
    - ○ Ciprofloxacin 400 mg IV BID or 500 mg PO BID
    - ○ Metronidazole 500 mg PO/IV TID
  - Avoid intestinally active vasoconstrictive medications (5)[A].
  - Avoid systemic corticosteroids, which may worsen ischemic damage and increase risk of perforation (3)[A].
  - If ileus is present, place nasogastric tube (3)[A].
- If radiographic abnormalities are present, serial abdominal x-rays help follow improvement (5)[A].
- If signs of clinical deterioration are present despite supportive care, including increased abdominal pain, peritoneal signs, persistent diarrhea, bleeding, or sepsis, consider surgery (3)[A].

MEDICATION

- Broad-spectrum antibiotics (i.e., metronidazole, ciprofloxacin) (5)[A]
- If cardiac workup reveals CHF or cardiac arrhythmias, initiate appropriate medical treatment (5)[A].

ADDITIONAL THERAPIES

Stem cell implantation in ischemic colonic wall in a rat model enhanced tissue healing by promoting angiogenesis (11)[B].

SURGERY/OTHER PROCEDURES

- 20% of patients require surgical intervention (12)[A].
- Evidence of pneumatosis intestinalis, portal vein air, or free peritoneal air are indications for immediate surgery (3)[A].
- Surgery may be indicated for the following:
  - Peritoneal signs, increased abdominal tenderness, new-onset shock, lactic acidosis, or acute renal failure (3)[A]
  - Diarrhea, lower GI bleeding, or exudative colitis persisting past 14 days (3)[A]
- Most common surgical intervention is colectomy with end ileostomy (6)[A].
  - Cholecystectomy may prevent resuscitation-related acute acalculous cholecystitis (3)[A].

 ONGOING CARE

DIET

- Bowel rest until symptoms resolve
- Parenteral nutrition for patients needing prolonged bowel rest who have contraindications to surgery.

PROGNOSIS

- In most patients, IC symptoms resolve in 24 to 48 hours.
- Radiographic or endoscopic resolution within 2 weeks.
- Right-sided IC appears to be the most significant predictor of outcome. Patients with right-sided IC have a 2-fold increase in mortality and a 5-fold increase in morbidity.
- Secondary cardiovascular prevention minimizes recurrence.
- Male gender, low hemoglobin, low serum albumin, high BUN, and presence of metabolic acidosis are poor prognostic factors (2)
- Chronic kidney disease, COPD, long-term care facilities increase mortality in IC (2,13)

COMPLICATIONS

20–30% of patients develop chronic IC, with persistent diarrhea or stricture formation requiring surgical intervention.

REFERENCES

1. Sherid M, Sifuentes H, Samo S, et al. Risk factors of recurrent ischemic colitis: a multicenter retrospective study. Korean J Gastroenterol. 2014;63(5):283–291.
2. Brandt LJ, Feuerstadt P, Longstreth GF, et al. ACG clinical guideline: epidemiology, risk factors, patterns of presentation, diagnosis, and management of colon ischemia (CI). Am J Gastroenterol. 2015;110(1):18–44.
3. Moszkowicz D, Mariani A, Trésallet C, et al. Ischemic colitis: the ABCs of diagnosis and surgical management. J Visc Surg. 2013;150(1):19–28.
4. Yadav S, Dave M, Edakkanambeth Varayil J, et al. A population-based study of incidence, risk factors, clinical spectrum, and outcomes of ischemic colitis. Clin Gastroenterol Hepatol. 2015;13(4):731–738.e6.
5. Feuerstadt P, Brandt LJ. Colon ischemia: recent insights and advances. Curr Gastroenterol Rep. 2010;12(5):383–390.
6. Theodoropoulou A, Koutroubakis IE. Ischemic colitis: clinical practice in diagnosis and treatment. World J Gastroenterol. 2008;14(48):7302–7308.
7. Sun MY, Maykel JA. Ischemic colitis. Clin Colon Rectal Surg. 2007;20(1):5–12.
8. Cosse C, Sabbagh C, Browet F, et al. Serum value of procalcitonin as a marker of intestinal damages: type, extension, and prognosis. Surg Endosc. 2015;29(11):3132–3139.
9. Harki J, Sana A, van Noord D, et al. Hypoxia-inducible factor 1-α in chronic gastrointestinal ischemia. Virchows Arch. 2015;466(2):125–132.
10. Sherid M, Samo S, Sulaiman S, et al. Is CT angiogram of the abdominal vessels needed following the diagnosis of ischemic colitis? A multicenter community study. ISRN Gastroenterol. 2014;2014:756926.
11. Joo HH, Jo HJ, Jung TD, et al. Adipose-derived stem cells on the healing of ischemic colitis: a therapeutic effect by angiogenesis. Int J Colorectal Dis. 2012;27(11):1437–1443.
12. Tortora A, Purchiaroni F, Scarpellini E, et al. Colitides. Eur Rev Med Pharmacol Sci. 2012;16(13):1795–1805.
13. Yoon SY, Jung SA, Na SK, et al. What's the clinical features of colitis in elderly people in long-term care facilities? Intest Res. 2015;13(2):128–134.

ADDITIONAL READING

- Iacobellis F, Berritto D, Somma F, et al. Magnetic resonance imaging: a new tool for diagnosis of acute ischemic colitis? World J Gastroenterol. 2012;18(13):1496–1501.
- O'Neill S, Yalamarthi S. Systematic review of the management of ischaemic colitis. Colorectal Dis. 2012;14(11):e751–e763. doi:10.1111/j.1463-1318.2012.03171.x.
- Paterno F, McGillicuddy EA, Schuster KM, et al. Ischemic colitis: risk factors for eventual surgery. Am J Surg. 2010;200(5):646–650.

CODES

ICD10

- K55.9 Vascular disorder of intestine, unspecified
- K55.0 Acute vascular disorders of intestine
- K55.1 Chronic vascular disorders of intestine

CLINICAL PEARLS

- Suspect IC in patients with multiple risk factors who present with abdominal pain and loose bloody stools.
- Colonoscopy is the diagnostic gold standard.
- Most often, IC is self-limited, responding well to conservative management with IV fluids, bowel rest, and empiric broad-spectrum antibiotics.
- Peritoneal signs or lack of clinical improvement suggests more extensive ischemia and require surgical intervention.
- Right-sided IC is associated with higher morbidity and mortality.

COLONIC POLYPS

Marcelle Meseeha, MD • Maximos Attia, MD

 BASICS

DESCRIPTION
- Intraluminal colonic protrusions; most commonly sporadic, or part of polyposis syndromes.
- Classified according to size:
  – Diminutive ≤5 mm, small 6 to 9 mm, large ≥10 mm (1)
- Morphologic classification:
  – Depressed, flat, sessile, or pedunculated
- Clinical significance:
  – >95% of colon adenocarcinoma arise from polyps.

EPIDEMIOLOGY
Colorectal polyps are more common in:
- Western countries
- Men
- Non-Caucasian (2)

Incidence
Incidence increases with age.

Prevalence
- 15–20% of all adults
- 30% of U.S. population >50 years
- 6% of children (2)
- 12% of children with lower GI bleed (2)

ETIOLOGY AND PATHOPHYSIOLOGY
Divided into:
- Mucosal
  – Neoplastic
    ○ Adenomatous polyps (tubular >80%, villous 5–15%, tubulovillous 5–15%)
    ○ Serrated polyps
      ■ Sessile serrated polyps are common, more in proximal colon, with low malignant potential if with no dysplasia, and significant malignant potential if dysplastic.
      ■ Traditional serrated adenoma is uncommon, more often noted in distal colon, with significant malignant potential (1).
  – Non-neoplastic polyps (hyperplastic, juvenile polyps, hamartomas, inflammatory pseudopolyps)
    ○ Hyperplastic polyps are very common, more in distal colon, with very low malignant potential (1).
    ○ Juvenile polyps are common in childhood, benign hamartomas, more in rectosigmoid, and not premalignant (2).
- **Submucosal** (lipomas, lymphoid aggregates, carcinoids)

Genetics
- Inactivation of tumor suppressor genes as adenomatous polyposis coli (APC) or mismatch repair genes (*MLH1*) causes polyps to grow into cancer.
- Familial adenomatous polyposis (FAP) is autosomal dominant. By age 40, almost all patients develop colorectal cancer (CRC).
- MUTYH-associated polyposis (MAP) is autosomal recessive caused by biallelic mutations in MUTYH gene.
- Juvenile polyposis syndrome (JPS) is autosomal dominant. 50–60% of patients have a mutation in the *SMAD4* or *BMPR1A* gene. By age 35, 20% of patients develop CRC (2).

RISK FACTORS
- Family history of intestinal polyposis, polyps, or CRC
- Advancing age
- Male
- High-fat, low-fiber diet
- Tobacco use
- Excessive alcohol intake: >8 drinks a week
- Inflammatory bowel disease is associated with a decreased prevalence of colon polyps (IBD associated with higher risk of colon cancer).

GENERAL PREVENTION
- Low-fat, high-fiber diet
- Avoid smoking.
- Decrease alcohol intake.
- Use of NSAIDs and calcium is associated with decreased incidence and recurrence of polyps (3)[A].
- No lower rates of CRC with azathioprine, 6-mercaptopurine, folate, calcium, multivitamins, or statins

COMMONLY ASSOCIATED CONDITIONS
Hereditary polyposis syndromes:
- Adenomatous
  – Familial adenomatous polyposis (FAP)
    ○ Classic (CFAP)
    ○ Attenuated (AFAP)
  – MUTYH-associated polyposis (MAP)
  – FAP variants:
    ○ Gardner syndrome
    ○ Turcot syndrome
- Hamartomatous
  – Peutz-Jeghers syndrome (PJS)
  – Juvenile polyposis syndrome (JPS)
  – Familial juvenile polyposis
  – Cowden syndrome

ALERT
JPS impose a higher risk of CRC, although juvenile polyps are not premalignant.

 DIAGNOSIS

HISTORY
- Usually normal
- Generally asymptomatic
- Painless rectal bleeding, bright or dark red, mixed with stools, dripping, or on wiping
- Diarrhea or mucous stool
- Abdominal pain
- Constipation
- Chronic bleeding resulting in iron deficiency anemia
- McKittrick-Wheelock syndrome; large hypersecretory rectosigmoid villous adenoma, resulting in persistent severe diarrhea, electrolyte disorder, dehydration, and prerenal acute renal failure
- Social and family history

PHYSICAL EXAM
- Usually normal
- Rectal polyps noted as prolapsed or palpated on DRE
- FOBT by DRE is less effective than FOBT by stool passed spontaneously.

DIAGNOSTIC TESTS & INTERPRETATION

Initial Tests (lab, imaging)
- CBC; anemia with chronic bleeding
- Basic metabolic panel; electrolyte disorder with hypersecretory adenomas
- Fecal occult blood test (FOBT), an insensitive screening test, as small polyps don't usually bleed, includes:
  – Guaiac (gFOBT)—uses a chemical indicator with color change in presence of blood
  – Immunochemical (iFOBT or fecal immunochemical test [FIT])—uses antibodies against human hemoglobin
- Stool DNA test is more sensitive and less specific than fecal immunochemical test (FIT).

Diagnostic Procedures/Other
- Colonoscopy is the gold standard test for detection of polyps and polypectomy. Not a perfect screening test, with increased miss rate with right-sided colon polyps, smaller polyp size, low quality of colon prep, less endoscopist experience
- Computed tomographic colonography (CTC) is less sensitive with flat polyps and requires excellent bowel preparation.
- Double-contrast barium enema
- Colon capsule endoscopy
- Enhanced optical technologies can potentially differentiate between neoplastic and non-neoplastic colonic lesions (4)[A].
- Enhanced optical technologies include:
  – Narrowed spectrum endoscopy (narrow-band imaging [NBI])
  – Image-enhanced endoscopy (i-scan)
  – Fujinon intelligent chromoendoscopy (FICE)
  – Confocal laser endomicroscopy (CLE)
- Patients with >10 colorectal adenomas should get genetic testing for APC and MUTYH (5)[C].

Test Interpretation
- Tubular adenoma
  – Gross: tend to be polypoid
  – Micro: dysplastic epithelium with a tubular architecture
- Villous adenoma
  – Gross: tend to be sessile
  – Micro: dysplastic epithelium with fine finger-like projections
- Tubulovillous adenomas have a combination of tubular and villous architecture.
- Hyperplastic polyps are composed of hyperplastic colonic mucosa.
- Hamartomatous polyps include muscularis mucosa.
- Juvenile polyp
  – Gross: pedunculated, smooth, red mass, 1 to 3 cm (2).

 TREATMENT

SURGERY/OTHER PROCEDURES
- Colonic polypectomy; diagnostic, therapeutic
- Techniques are as follows:
  – Snare polypectomy with electrocautery for pedunculated polyps
  – Endoscopic mucosal resection for sessile polyps
  – Endoscopic submucosal dissection

- Colorectal surgery; prophylactic in FAP and MAP and when there are numerous polyps or persistent bleeding (2,5)[C]:
  – Total colectomy ileorectal anastomosis
  – Proctocolectomy ileal pouch anal anatomosis
- Chemoprevention: NSAIDs and calcium may reduce incidence and recurrence of polyps in patients with FAP and MAP (3)[A].

 ONGOING CARE

FOLLOW-UP RECOMMENDATIONS
Follow-up colonoscopy in:

- 10 years if no polyps or distal small hyperplastic polyps (<10 mm) (1)[B]
- 5 to 10 years if 1 to 2 small tubular adenomas (<10 mm) (1)[B]
- 3 years if 3 to 10 adenomas if any polyp ≥6 mm (1)[B] or if all polyps <6 mm (1)[C]
- <3 years if >10 adenomas (1)[B]
- 3 years if one or more adenomas ≥10 mm (1)[A]
- 3 years if one or more adenomas with villous features of any size or with HGD (1)[B]
- 5 years if sessile serrated polyp(s) <10 mm with no dysplasia (1)[C]
- 3 years if sessile serrated polyp(s) ≥10 mm or with dysplasia or traditional serrated adenoma (1)[C]
- 1 year if serrated polyposis syndrome (1)[B]

Patient Monitoring
- Colonoscopy for CRC screening starts at age 50 years and earlier for at-risk patients.
- Stop screening if life expectancy is <10 years.
- In CFAP and AFAP, screen for extracolonic manifestations: thyroid cancer, desmoid tumors, and gastroduodenal polyposis (every 6 months to 5 years) (5)[C]
- In families, lifetime screening is indicated in mutation carriers (5)[C]:
  – In CFAP: with sigmoidoscopy or colonoscopy every 1 to 2 years starting at age of 10 to 11 years
  – In AFAP and MAP: with colonoscopy every 1 to 2 years starting at age of 18 to 20 years
- After colorectal surgery, surveillance of the rectum (every 6 to 12 months) or pouch (every 6 months to 5 years) is indicated (5)[C].
- First-degree relatives of patients with JPS require screening by colonoscopy and upper endoscopy after age 12 (2)[C].

DIET
Low-fat, high-fiber diet has been recommended but with insufficient evidence.

PATIENT EDUCATION
Importance of colonoscopy as a screening tool for reduction of incidence of colorectal cancer

PROGNOSIS
- Regression or no change in size, more with small hyperplastic polyps and with patients on NSAIDs
- Recurrence: Juvenile polyps recur in 45% of children with multiple polyps and 17% of children with solitary polyps (2).
- Increase in size, more with large adenomas
- Progression to cancer
- Risk factors for colon cancer (6)[A]:
  – Polyp pathology
    ○ Adenomatous
    ○ Serrated
    ○ With high-grade dysplasia
    ○ With >25% villous histology
    ○ Polyp size >1 cm in diameter
    ○ Polyps located in proximal colon
    ○ More than three polyps
- Recurrence rates <10% postpolypectomy

COMPLICATIONS
- Polyps: progression to cancer
- Polypectomy: bleeding 2–11%, perforation 0–1%, higher with endoscopic submucosal dissection
- Colonoscopy: complications related to anesthesia and procedure itself

REFERENCES
1. Lieberman DA, Rex DK, Winawer SJ, et al. Guidelines for colonoscopy surveillance after screening and polypectomy: a consensus update by the US Multi-Society Task Force on Colorectal Cancer. *Gastroenterology*. 2012;143(3):844–857.
2. Thakkar K, Fishman DS, Gilger MA. Colorectal polyps in childhood. *Curr Opin Pediatr*. 2012;24(5):632–637.
3. Johnson CC, Hayes RB, Schoen RE, et al. Nonsteroidal anti-inflammatory drug use and colorectal polyps in the prostate, lung, colorectal, and ovarian cancer screening trial. *Am J Gastroenterol*. 2010;105(12):2646–2655.
4. Wanders LK, East JE, Uitentuis SE, et al. Diagnostic performance of narrowed spectrum endoscopy, autofluorescence imaging, and confocal laser endomicroscopy for optical diagnosis of colonic polyps: a meta-analysis. *Lancet Oncol*. 2013;14(13):1337–1347.
5. Stoffel EM, Mangu PB, Limburg PJ. Hereditary colorectal cancer syndromes: American Society of Clinical Oncology clinical practice guideline endorsement of the familial risk-colorectal cancer: European Society for Medical Oncology clinical practice guidelines. *J Oncol Pract*. 2015;11(3): e437–e441.
6. Gao Q, Tsoi KK, Hirai HW, et al. Serrated polyps and the risk of synchronous colorectal advanced neoplasia: a systematic review and meta-analysis. *Am J Gastroenterol*. 2015;110(4):501–509.

ADDITIONAL READING
- Ashraf I, Paracha SR, Arif M, et al. Digital rectal examination versus spontaneous passage of stool for fecal occult blood testing. *South Med J*. 2012;105(7):357–361.
- Brenner H, Hoffmeister M, Arndt V, et al. Protection from right- and left-sided colorectal neoplasms after colonoscopy: population-based study. *J Natl Cancer Inst*. 2010;102(2):89–95.
- Cooper K, Squires H, Carroll C, et al. Chemoprevention of colorectal cancer: systematic review and economic evaluation. *Health Technol Assess*. 2010;14(32):1–206.
- Farraye FA, Odze RD, Eaden J, et al. AGA medical position statement on the diagnosis and management of colorectal neoplasia in inflammatory bowel disease. *Gastroenterology*. 2010;138(2):738–745.
- Imperiale TF, Ransohoff DF, Itzkowitz SH, et al. Multitarget stool DNA testing for colorectal-cancer screening. *N Engl J Med*. 2014;370(14):1287–1297.
- Lee BG, Shin SH, Lee YA, et al. Juvenile polyp and colonoscopic polypectomy in childhood. *Pediatr Gastroenterol Hepatol Nutr*. 2012;15(4):250–255.
- Sonnenberg A, Genta RM. Low prevalence of colon polyps in chronic inflammatory conditions of the colon. *Am J Gastroenterol*. 2015;110(7):1056–1061.
- Summers RM. Polyp size measurement at CT colonography: what do we know and what do we need to know? *Radiology*. 2010;255(3):707–720.

 SEE ALSO

Colorectal Cancer

 CODES

ICD10
- K63.5 Polyp of colon
- D12.6 Benign neoplasm of colon, unspecified
- K51.40 Inflammatory polyps of colon without complications

CLINICAL PEARLS
- Progression from normal mucosa to polyp to carcinoma is a sequence that takes years to develop.
- Colonoscopy is the gold standard tool for diagnosis of polyps and reduction of CRC incidence.
- Small hyperplastic polyps should be biopsied to differentiate adenomatous and serrated polyps.
- Use of NSAIDs and calcium is associated with decreased incidence and recurrence of polyps.

COLORECTAL CANCER
Stephen Scott, MD, MPH

BASICS

DESCRIPTION
- Colorectal cancer (CRC) denotes a neoplasm that develops in the colon or rectum.
- CRC is the second leading cause of cancer deaths and is the third most common cancer in men and women in the United States.
- Screening for CRC reduces the incidence of and mortality from CRC.

EPIDEMIOLOGY
Incidence
93,090 new cases of colon cancer; 39,610 new cases of rectal cancer; and 49,700 deaths from colon and rectal cancer combined were estimated in the United States in 2015 (1).

Prevalence
- The lifetime risk for developing CRC in the United States is about 1 in 21 (4.8%).
- Incidence and death rates have been declining due to improved screening, prevention, and treatment.

ETIOLOGY AND PATHOPHYSIOLOGY
- Progression from the first abnormal cells to the appearance of CRC usually occurs over 10 to 15 years; a disease characteristic that contributes to the effectiveness of prevention.
- High-risk polyp findings include multiple polyps, villous polyps, and larger polyps.
- Hyperplastic polyps are less likely to evolve into CRC.
- Multiple genetic and environmental factors have been linked to the development of CRC.

Genetics
- There does not seem to be a single genetic pathway to CRC.
- <10% of CRC cases are linked to an inherited gene
  - APC, a tumor suppressor gene, is altered in familial adenomatous polyposis (FAP).
  - Genes encoding DNA mismatch repair (MMR) enzymes are implicated in hereditary nonpolyposis colon cancer (HNPCC): MLH1, MSH2, MSH6, PMS1, PMS2, and others.
  - STK11, a tumor suppressor gene, is altered in Peutz-Jeghers syndrome.
- Sporadic cases of CRC have been linked to oncogenes: Kras, c-Myc, c-Src, HER-2/neu, and others.

RISK FACTORS
- Age: >90% of people diagnosed with CRC are >50 years of age.
- Personal history of colorectal polyps
  - Risks increase with multiple polyps, villous polyps, and larger polyps.
- Personal history of cancer
  - Rectal cancer has higher incidence of local recurrence than proximal cancers (20–30% vs. 2–4%).
- History of inflammatory bowel disease
  - Prevalence of CRC in ulcerative colitis and Crohn disease is ~3%, with a cumulative risk of CRC of 2% at 10 years, 8% at 20 years, and 18% at 30 years.

- Family history of CRC
  - Having a single first-degree relative with a history of CRC increases risk 1.7-fold.
  - Risk is more than double for those who have a history of CRC or polyps in:
    - Any first-degree relative <60 years of age
    - ≥2 first-degree relatives, regardless of age
- Inherited syndromes
  - HNPCC also called Lynch syndrome.
    - Often develops at younger age (Average age at diagnosis of CRC is 44 years.)
    - Lifetime risk of CRC is 52–69%.
    - Accounts for ~2% of all CRCs
  - FAP
    - Affected individuals develop hundreds to thousands of polyps in colon and rectum.
    - CRC usually present by age 40 years.
    - Accounts for <1% of CRCs
  - Peutz-Jeghers syndrome
    - Individuals may have freckles (mouth, hands, feet) and large polyps in GI tract.
    - Greatly increased risk for CRC and cancers
- Race and ethnicity
  - African Americans have the highest CRC incidence and mortality rates in the United States.
  - Several different gene mutations have been identified among Ashkenazi Jews.
- Miscellaneous
  - Patients with obesity, diabetes, acromegaly, smoking, and alcohol use are at increased risk.

GENERAL PREVENTION
- Diets high in fruits and vegetables have been linked with decreased risk; those high in red and processed meats may increase CRC risk.
- Some studies suggest that vitamin D, calcium, folate, and fiber may lower CRC risk; more research is needed to understand how diet affects risks of CRC.
- People who are physically inactive are at higher risk for CRC.
- Long-term smokers are more likely than nonsmokers to develop and die from CRC.
- CRC has been linked to heavy alcohol consumption; may be related to low folate intake or absorption
- NSAIDs may reduce risk in some groups; experts do not recommend NSAID use as a cancer prevention strategy in people at average risk for CRC.
- Colon cancer screening is one of the most powerful tools in preventing colon cancer.

ALERT
The U.S. Preventive Services Task Force (USPSTF) strongly recommends that clinicians screen men and women between the ages of 50 and 75 years for CRC using fecal occult blood testing, sigmoidoscopy, or colonoscopy.

- American Cancer Society recommendations for screening include the following (2):
  - Fecal occult blood testing annually
  - Fecal immunochemical test (FIT) annually
  - Flexible sigmoidoscopy every 5 years
  - Colonoscopy every 10 years
  - CT colonography every 5 years (colonoscopy completed if positive)*
  - Double-contrast barium enema every 5 years*
  - Stool DNA test (sDNA) every 3 years*

  - *The USPSTF does not recommend barium enema as a screening test and concludes the evidence is insufficient to assess the benefits and harms of CT colonography and stool DNA testing as screening modalities for CRC.
- Screening in high-risk groups
  - People with a personal history of polyps need more frequent colonoscopy screening, depending on risk (i.e., 1 or 2 <1-cm polyps with low-grade dysplasia is deemed low-risk and may warrant repeat colonoscopy in 5 to 10 years; decision is influenced by family history, age, quality of initial colonoscopy, and patient comorbidities).
  - People who have a family history of CRC or adenomatous polyps before age 60 years should begin colonoscopy at age 40 or 10 years younger than the age of relative at cancer diagnosis, whichever is earlier.
  - People with inflammatory bowel disease should have regular surveillance colonoscopy with biopsies to detect dysplasia; guidelines for timing and location vary by professional society but generally indicate starting surveillance by ~8 years of onset of disease followed by surveillance every 1 to 2 years.
  - Genetic testing may be appropriate for individuals with a strong family history of CRC or polyps:
    - Family members of a person affected by HNPCC should start colonoscopy surveillance as early as age 20 years.
    - Individuals with suspected FAP should have yearly flexible sigmoidoscopy beginning at age 10 to 12 years; those who test positive for the gene linked to FAP may consider colectomy.

DIAGNOSIS

HISTORY
- Many patients with CRC are asymptomatic.
- Common presenting symptoms and signs in symptomatic patients include the following:
  - Abdominal pain or cramping
  - Change in bowel habits (constipation, diarrhea, narrowing of stool)
  - Rectal bleeding, dark stools, or blood in stool
  - Weakness or fatigue
  - Anemia
  - Weight loss
- Other presentations may include symptoms due to the presence of metastatic lesions (lymph nodes, liver, lung, peritoneum), fever of unknown origin, and *Streptococcus bovis* or *Clostridium septicum* sepsis.

PHYSICAL EXAM
- Weight loss
- Signs of anemia (i.e., conjunctival pallor)
- Palpable abdominal mass

DIFFERENTIAL DIAGNOSIS
- >95% of CRCs are adenocarcinomas.
- Other colonic tumors include carcinoid tumors, lymphomas, and Kaposi sarcoma in HIV.
- Many conditions can mimic CRC, including other cancers, hemorrhoids, inflammatory bowel disease, infection, and extrinsic masses (i.e., cysts, abscesses).

DIAGNOSTIC TESTS & INTERPRETATION
Initial Tests (lab, imaging)
- CBC (to evaluate anemia)
- Liver function (CRC may spread to the liver)
- Colonoscopy
- CT colography if colonoscopy incomplete

Follow-Up Tests & Special Considerations
- Carcinoembryonic antigen (CEA) should be obtained preoperatively to assist with follow-up screening.
- CT to evaluate presence of metastatic disease
- Chest x-ray to evaluate presence of chest metastases
- Endoscopic ultrasound (EUS) may be used to evaluate the extent of rectal cancers; endorectal MRI may also provide further detail.
- Intraoperative US may be used to evaluate solid organs (e.g., the liver) after tumor resection.
- Positron emission tomography (PET) may be used in some cases to detect metastatic disease.

Diagnostic Procedures/Other
- Biopsy is usually performed (most often during colonoscopy) if CRC is suspected.
- CT needle-guided biopsy may be needed to evaluate a suspected tumor or metastasis.

Test Interpretation
The American Joint Committee on Cancer (AJCC) TNM staging is preferred
- Stage 0: limited to the mucosa (carcinoma in situ or intramucosal carcinoma (Tis, N0, M0)
- Stage I: invades mucosa (T1) or muscularis propria (T2); no invasion of lymph nodes or distant sites (T1, N0, M0 or T2, N0, M0)
- Stage IIA: invades pericolorectal tissues; no lymph nodes or distant sites (T3, N0, M0)
- Stage IIB: penetrates to surface of visceral peritoneum; no lymph nodes or distant sites (T4a, N0, M0)
- Stage IIC: directly invades or adherent to other organs or structures (T4b, N0, M0)
- Stage IIIA: invades submucosa or muscularis propria with spread to 1 to 3 lymph nodes; no distant sites (T1, N1, M0 or T2, N1, M0)
- Stage IIIB: invades pericolorectal tissues or surface of visceral peritoneum + spread to 1 to 3 lymph nodes; no distant sites (T3, N1, M0, or T4a, N1, M0)
- Stage IIIC: invades pericolorectal tissues or peritoneum or other organs and to ≥4 nearby lymph nodes; no distant sites (any T3 or T4, N2, M0)
- Stage IVA: any level of invasion with spread to one organ or site (any T, any N, M1a)
- Stage IVB: any level of invasion with spread to more than one organ or site or peritoneum (any T, any N, M1b)

TREATMENT
MEDICATION
Surgical resection is the primary treatment for CRC, as noted in the following texts. Adjuvant chemotherapy is most clearly beneficial for stage III (node-positive) disease, in which improvements of ~30% may be achieved in both disease recurrence and overall survival, compared with nontreated controls. Chemotherapeutic regimens for metastatic disease may extend overall survival from 6 months to ~2 years (3)[B].

First Line
Combination chemotherapy is common and may include oxaliplatin, irinotecan, fluorouracil, leucovorin, and capecitabine.

Geriatric Considerations
Elderly patients tend to tolerate CRC chemotherapy and should be considered for treatment.

Second Line
Targeted therapies may be used alongside first-line agents or alone if first-line agents are ineffective
- Bevacizumab (Avastin) is a monoclonal antibody that targets vascular endothelial growth factor (VEGF); inhibits angiogenesis
- Cetuximab (Erbitux) and panitumumab (Vectibix) are monoclonal antibodies that target epidermal growth factor receptor (EGFR).
- Aflibercept and regorafenib are newer agents with actions on VEGF.

SURGERY/OTHER PROCEDURES
- Surgery is the primary treatment for localized CRC
  - May involve segmental resection, hemicolectomy, or colectomy, as well as resection of nodes, depending on size and invasion
  - Laparoscopic-assisted colectomy is an emerging option for earlier stage tumors.
  - Surgery for rectal cancer may include local transanal, low anterior, or abdominoperineal resection or pelvic exenteration.
- Radiation therapy is most often used for peritoneal or rectal cancers; it may also be used to relieve symptoms.

COMPLEMENTARY & ALTERNATIVE MEDICINE
- May serve as an adjunct to treatment for CRC
- 70–75% of cancer survivors report using at least one type of complementary and alternative medicine (CAM), and almost all report that the alternative therapy improved well-being.

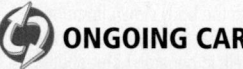 ONGOING CARE

FOLLOW-UP RECOMMENDATIONS
Patient Monitoring
- People with a personal history of proximal cancer (nonrectal) should have follow-up colonoscopy in 1 year and, if normal, in 3 and 5 years subsequently.
- CEA and/or CA 19-9 are used to detect recurrence in people treated for CRC. (Note: CEA levels may be elevated in ulcerative colitis, nonmalignant GI tumors, liver disease, lung disease, and in smokers.)

PATIENT EDUCATION
- NIH: Colorectal cancer: http://www.nlm.nih.gov/medlineplus/colorectalcancer.html
- NCI: Colorectal cancer: http://www.cancer.gov/types/colorectal
- AAFP: Colorectal Cancer: http://www.aafp.org/afp/2015/0115/p93-s1.html

PROGNOSIS
5-year relative survival rate is determined by stage (adjusted for patients dying of other diseases): stage I: 93%; stage II: 72–85%; stage III: 44–83%; stage IV: 8%.

COMPLICATIONS
- Colorectal surgery: pain, deep vein thrombosis, anastomotic leaks, infection, scarring, bowel obstruction
- Chemotherapy: hair loss, nausea, vomiting, bruising, fatigue, increased risk for infections
- Radiation therapy: skin irritation, nausea, rectal pain, incontinence, bladder irritation, fatigue, and sexual problems

REFERENCES
1. Siegel RL, Miller KD, Jemal A. Cancer statistics, 2015. *CA Cancer J Clin.* 2015;65(1), 5–29.
2. American Cancer Society. Guidelines for the early detection of cancer. http://www.cancer.orghealthy/findcancerearly/cancerscreeningguidelinesamerican cancer-society-guidelines-for-the-earlydetection-of-cancer. Accessed 2015.
3. Brenner H, Kloor M, Pox CP. Colorectal cancer. *Lancet.* 2014;383(9927):1490–1502.

ADDITIONAL READING
- Benson AB III, Venook AP, Bekaii-Saab T, et al. Colon cancer, version 3.2014. *J Natl Compr Canc Netw.* 2014;12(7):1028–1059.
- National Institutes of Health, National Cancer Institute. Colorectal cancer—for patients. http://www.cancer.gov/types/colorectal/. Accessed 2015.

 CODES

ICD10
- C19 Malignant neoplasm of rectosigmoid junction
- C18.9 Malignant neoplasm of colon, unspecified
- C20 Malignant neoplasm of rectum

CLINICAL PEARLS
- The USPSTF recommends screening beginning at age 50 years and notes that evidence supports fecal occult blood testing (yearly), sigmoidoscopy, or colonoscopy (every 10 years).
- High-risk polyp findings include multiple polyps, villous polyps, and larger polyps; hyperplastic polyps are less likely to become cancerous.
- 10% of cases of CRC occur in people <50 years of age. People who have a family history of CRC without other risks (i.e., polyposis syndrome) should begin colonoscopy at age 40 years or 10 years younger than the age of relative at cancer diagnosis, whichever is earlier.
- Iron deficiency anemia in the elderly should prompt a search for CRC and should not be attributed to normal aging.

COMPLEMENTARY AND ALTERNATIVE MEDICINE

Paul Crawford, MD

 BASICS

- Complementary and alternative medicine (CAM) are medical and health care systems, practices, and products not presently considered part of conventional medicine.
- The National Center for Health Statistics (NCHS) 2012 survey (1) reports nonvitamin, nonmineral dietary supplements, chiropractic or osteopathic manipulation, yoga, and massage therapy were the most common complementary health approaches used.
- Medical professionals who incorporate CAM into their medical practice will often refer to their health care model as "integrative medicine."

DESCRIPTION

- Definitions and additional terms
  - *Complementary medicine* is used with conventional medicine to address a health concern. For example, massage plus physical therapy to address low back pain or medication plus osteopathic manipulation to address recurrent headaches.
  - *Alternative medicine* is used in place of conventional medicine to promote healing of conditions that cannot be explained by the conventional biomedical model or for which the effectiveness of therapy is not yet established by clinical research.
  - *Integrative medicine* is the combination of allopathic medicine with CAM and may be provided to the patient by a single licensed medical professional trained in CAM or by a group of diverse health care providers.
  - *Holistic* is a descriptive term for a practitioner's approach to patient care. A holistic practitioner assesses the emotional, spiritual, mental, and physical state of wellness of the client, then works to provide comprehensive care. A holistic practice may include practitioners of different disciplines to best address all aspects of wellness or illness.
- *Biologically based therapies*: diets, herbals, vitamins, supplements, flower essences
- Manipulative and body-based methods
  - Massage therapy is the manipulation of the body's soft tissues, whereby the licensed practitioner uses knowledge of anatomy and physiology to restore function, promote relaxation, and relieve pain. There are several different types of massage.
  - Osteopathic manipulative medicine focuses on the musculoskeletal system. It includes indirect techniques (e.g., muscle energy, myofascial release, osteopathy in the cranial field, and strain–counterstrain approach), as well as direct action techniques (high-velocity thrusts).
  - Craniosacral therapy is a gentle manual treatment focusing on the release of bony and fascial restrictions in the craniosacral system (cranium, sacrum, spinal cord, meninges, CSF).
  - Chiropractic therapy focuses on the musculoskeletal and nervous systems and how imbalances in these systems can affect general health. It is used to treat back, neck, and joint pain. Doctors of Chiropractic (DCs) complete 4 to 5 years of intensive training in anatomy, physiology, and manipulation.

- Mind–body medicine
  - Meditation is a practice of detachment in which a person sits quietly, generally focusing on the breath, while releasing all thoughts from the mind with the intention to center the self, restore balance, and enhance well-being. Mindfulness meditation involves making oneself aware of the most immediate of activities in order to gain control over actions and anxiety.
  - Spiritual practices; for example, prayer
  - Yoga is an exercise of mindfulness, meditation, strength, and balance. It is composed of *asanas* (postures) and *pranayamas* (focused breathing).
  - Aromatherapy uses highly concentrated plant extracts to stimulate healing processes. These aromatic oils are rubbed on the skin, aerosolized, or used in compresses.
  - Relaxation techniques include breathing exercises, progressive muscle relaxation, and guided imagery.
  - *Tai chi* and *qi gong* are Chinese exercise systems that combine meditation, regulated breathing, and flowing dance-like movements to enhance and balance *chi* (*qi*), or life force energy.
- Alternative medical systems
  - Traditional Chinese medicine incorporates Chinese herbs and acupuncture. Acupuncture is the practice of regulating *chi* by inserting hair-thin needles at specific points along meridian pathways of the body. *Chi* movement is responsible for animating and protecting the body; relieving pain; and regulating blood, oxygen, and nourishment to every cell.
  - Ayurvedic medicine originated in India and is one of the world's oldest medical systems. It uses healing modalities and herbs to integrate and balance the body, mind, and spirit.
  - Homeopathy is a system of therapy based on the concept that very dilute quantities of an offending agent can stimulate the body's own immune system to produce a reaction against this offense, thereby healing itself. In general, homeopathic remedies are considered safe and unlikely to cause serious adverse reactions. Only three states license homeopaths.
  - Naturopathy is based on providing natural and minimally invasive options for prevention and treatment of disease. Treatment regimens can include herbs, vitamins, supplements, dietary counseling, homeopathic remedies, manipulative therapies, acupuncture, and hydrotherapy. Four-year doctoral training programs are available; however, only 20 states/territories have licensing laws for naturopathic practitioners.
- Energy therapies
  - *Reiki*, which means "source energy," is a healing practice from Japan. Laying hands lightly on the patient or holding the hands just above the body, the *reiki* practitioner facilitates spiritual and physical healing by stimulating a patient's life force energy.
- Common reasons patients choose CAM
  - Additive therapy to address aspects not provided for in conventional medical treatment
  - Conventional medicine has been unsuccessful in fully addressing ailment.

  - Preventive health care
  - Desire for a holistic and natural approach to well-being
  - Preference for noninvasive treatment options
  - Concern about side effects of medication
  - Desire for spiritual support to be incorporated into healing practice
  - Cultural or familial belief system may be more aligned with "natural" solutions not provided for or supported by the standard allopathic model of health care.

EPIDEMIOLOGY

- All ages use CAM, but it is most prevalent among adults aged 30 to 69 years.
- Gender ratio: female > male
- College graduates and residents from western states are more likely to use CAM.
- Cancer survivors are more likely than the general population to use CAM.
- Six most used CAM therapies based on the NCHS 2012 survey. These CAM therapies were used by the indicated percentage of survey participants:
  - Nonvitamin, nonmineral dietary supplements (17.9%)
  - Chiropractic and osteopathic manipulation (8.5%)
  - Yoga (8.4%)
  - Massage (6.8%)
  - Meditation (4.1%)
  - Special diets (3.0%)

 TREATMENT

- Variable evidence supports safety and efficacy of
  - Meditation for lowering BP (2)[C]
  - Acupuncture for chronic low back pain (3)[B]
  - Acupuncture to improve fertility (4)[C]
  - Spinal manipulative therapy for prophylactic treatment of headaches
  - Ginger for nausea, including that associated with chemotherapy
  - Manipulation, massage, and mobilization for acute low back and posterior neck pain
  - Massage therapy to promote weight gain in preterm infants
  - Massage (30 minutes × 3) during labor shortens the second stage and reduces pain (5)[A].
  - Acupuncture for chemotherapy-induced nausea and vomiting
  - Tai chi for improving balance and decreasing the risk of and fear of falling in elderly
  - Mind–body techniques for migraines, chronic pain, and insomnia
  - Homeopathic remedy for the treatment of chemotherapy-induced stomatitis in children
  - Riboflavin for migraine prophylaxis
  - Horse chestnut seed extract to improve lower leg venous tone, pain, and edema
  - Glucosamine for osteoarthritis and knee pain
  - Yoga and meditation appear to improve endothelial function in patients with CAD and can have potential beneficial effects on depressive disorders.
  - Yoga throughout pregnancy shortens labor by 140 to 190 minutes

- Exercise in both preconception and early pregnancy reduces chance of gestational diabetes mellitus (6)[A].
- Breast stimulation in late pregnancy increases successful induction of labor (NNT 3.2) and reduces postpartum hemorrhage (NNT 19) (7)[A].
- Oral probiotics in preterm infants to decrease necrotizing enterocolitis and reduce mortality (8)[A].
- Oral probiotics to prevent URIs in children and influenza in the elderly (9,10)[A]
- Oral probiotics to shorten the duration of acute and antibiotic-associated diarrhea and as prophylaxis for traveler's diarrhea (10),(11)[A],(12,13)
- Vitamin D 800 IU/day may reduce falls and fractures in the elderly (14)[A].

- *Acupuncture* for recurrent headache
- Evidence supports safety, but evidence regarding efficacy is inconclusive:
  - *Homeopathy* for induction and augmentation of labor
  - Chondroitin sulfate is ineffective for osteoarthritis.
  - *Sterile water injections* do not reduce pain in labor.
  - Omega-3 fatty acids may reduce inflammation and anxiety in young healthy adults.
  - *Dietary fat reduction* for certain types of cancer
  - *Mind–body techniques* for metastatic cancer
  - *Copper and magnetic bracelets* for pain
  - *Vitamin D levels* >30 ng/mL correlate with lower risk of some cancers. Adequate vitamin D intake may decrease atopy and asthma symptoms.
- Evidence supports efficacy, but evidence regarding safety is inconclusive:
  - St. John's wort extract for short-term treatment of depression in adults
  - Licorice for gastritis
- Evidence indicates serious risk:
  - Black cohosh, blue cohosh, and evening primrose oil are unsafe to induce labor.
  - Delay in seeking medical care or replacement of curative conventional treatment
  - Use of toxic herbs or substances
  - Known herb–drug interactions

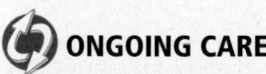 ONGOING CARE

PATIENT EDUCATION
The National Center for Complementary and Integrative Health (https://nccih.nih.gov/)

COMPLICATIONS

ALERT
Ginkgo and St. John's wort account for most herb–drug interactions described in the medical literature.

- Herbs with possible adverse effects
  - Serious adverse events from herbal remedies remain uncommon.
  - Some ethnic medicines, as those prescribed by practitioners of Ayurveda or traditional Chinese medicine, may intentionally contain heavy metals or other toxic substances. These are usually listed by their pharmacopeial names, for example, Qian Dan = lead oxide.

- Bitter orange (*Citrus sinensis*): sympathomimetic; increases heart rate (HR), BP
- California poppy (*Eschscholzia californica*): may cause respiratory depression, drowsiness; contains opioids
- Cascara sagrada (*Frangula purshiana*): depletes serum potassium
- Chaparral (*Larrea tridentata*): hepatotoxic
- Ephedra (*Ephedra* spp.): sympathomimetic; increases HR, BP; insomnia, gastric distress
- Ginkgo (*Ginkgo biloba*): extravasation, increased bleeding time
- Guarana (*Paullinia cupana*): tachycardia, hypertension; contains caffeine
- Kava (*Piper methysticum*): decreases use of niacin; possibly hepatotoxic
- Licorice (*Glycyrrhiza* spp.): Long-term use depletes serum potassium
- Lily of the valley (*Convallaria majalis*): contains cardiac glycosides
- Poke root (*Phytolacca species*): strong gastric irritant, may cause sedation
- Senna (*Cassia senna*): depletes serum potassium
- Snakeroot (*Aristolochia* spp.): nephrotoxic
- St. John's wort (*Hypericum perforatum*): numerous drug interactions; induces CYP(3a4) pathway, speeding metabolism of many drugs
- Wormwood (*Artemisia absinthium*): elevates serotonin level, may raise BP
- Yohimbe (*Pausinystalia yohimbe*): elevates BP

Geriatric Considerations
Gingko biloba commonly interacts with Coumadin.

Pediatric Considerations

ALERT
Iron is a leading cause of accidental poisoning in children <6 years of age. Minerals (i.e., potassium, calcium, magnesium, zinc, copper, and selenium) may cause toxicity.

- Vitamin A is most common cause of hypervitaminosis.
- Beta-carotene may have a limited potential for overdose.

REFERENCES

1. Peregoy JA, Clarke TC, Jones LI, et al. *Regional variation in use of complementary health approaches by U.S. adults. NCHS data brief, no 146.* Hyattsville, MD: National Center for Health Statistics; 2014.
2. Anderson JW, Liu C, Kryscio RJ. Blood pressure response to transcendental meditation: a meta-analysis. *Am J Hypertens.* 2008;21(3):310–316.
3. Manheimer E, White A, Berman B, et al. Meta-analysis: acupuncture for low back pain. *Ann Intern Med.* 2005;142(8):651–663.
4. Park JJ, Kang M, Shin S, et al. Unexplained infertility treated with acupuncture and herbal medicine in Korea. *J Altern Complement Med.* 2010;16(2):193–198.
5. Mortazavi SH, Khaki S, Moradi R, et al. Effects of massage therapy and presence of attendant on pain, anxiety and satisfaction during labor. *Arch Gynecol Obstet.* 2012;286(1):19–23.
6. Tobias DK, Zhang C, van Dam RM, et al. Physical activity before and during pregnancy and risk of gestational diabetes mellitus: a meta-analysis. *Diabetes Care.* 2011;34(1):223–229.
7. Kavanagh J, Kelly AJ, Thomas J. Breast stimulation for cervical ripening and induction of labour. *Cochrane Database Syst Rev.* 2005;(3):CD003392.
8. AlFaleh K, Anabrees J, Bassler D, et al. Probiotics for prevention of necrotizing enterocolitis in preterm infants. *Cochrane Database Syst Rev.* 2011;(3):CD005496.
9. Guillemard E, Tondu F, Lacoin F, et al. Consumption of a fermented dairy product containing the probiotic Lactobacillus casei DN-114001 reduces the duration of respiratory infections in the elderly in a randomised controlled trial. *Br J Nutr.* 2010;103(1):58–68.
10. Hojsak I, Snovak N, Abdović S, et al. Lactobacillus GG in the prevention of gastrointestinal and respiratory tract infections in children who attend day care centers: a randomized, double-blind, placebo-controlled trial. *Clin Nutr.* 2010;29(3):312–316.
11. Johnston BC, Supina AL, Ospina M, et al. Probiotics for the prevention of pediatric antibiotic-associated diarrhea. *Cochrane Database Syst Rev.* 2007;(2):CD004827.
12. Hickson M, D'Souza AL, Muthu N, et al. Use of probiotic Lactobacillus preparation to prevent diarrhoea associated with antibiotics: randomised double blind placebo controlled trial. *BMJ.* 2007;335(7610):80.
13. McFarland LV. Meta-analysis of probiotics for the prevention of traveler's diarrhea. *Travel Med Infect Dis.* 2007;5(2):97–105.
14. Makariou S, Liberopoulos EN, Elisaf M, et al. Novel roles of vitamin D in disease: what is new in 2011? *Eur J Intern Med.* 2011;22(4):355–362.

CODES

Z76.89 Persons encountering health services in other specified circumstances

CLINICAL PEARLS

- Oral probiotics reduce respiratory and diarrheal infections and reduce mortality in preterm infants.
- Acupuncture is effective for back pain, headaches, and infertility.
- Yoga and breast stimulation shorten labor.
- Ginkgo and St. John's wort account for most herb–drug interactions described in the medical literature.

COMPLEX REGIONAL PAIN SYNDROME

Dennis E. Hughes, DO, FACEP

 BASICS

DESCRIPTION

- Complex regional pain syndrome (CRPS) is a pain syndrome that is seemingly disproportionate in time or degree to any known trauma or lesion.
  - Type I: no nerve injury (reflex sympathetic dystrophy [RSD])
  - Type II: associated with a demonstrable nerve injury (causalgia)
- Synonym(s): traumatic erythromelalgia; Weir Mitchell causalgia; causalgia; reflex sympathetic dystrophy; posttraumatic neuralgia; sympathetically maintained pain

EPIDEMIOLOGY

- Incidence of 5.46/100,000 and prevalence of 20.57/1,000,000 in United States
- Peak age 50 to 70 years
- Predominant gender: female > male (3:1, 60–81%); favoring postmenopausal
- Recent studies found 3.8% occurrence after wrist fracture and 7% occurrence after intra-articular ankle fracture—both independent high risk for CPRS (1)[B].
- More prevalent in patients that report higher than usual expected pain in early phases of trauma (1)[B].

ETIOLOGY AND PATHOPHYSIOLOGY

- Poorly understood activation of abnormal sympathetic reflex that lowers pain threshold.
  - Increased excitability of nociceptive neurons in the spinal cord; "central sensitization"
  - Exaggerated responses to normally nonpainful stimuli (hyperalgesia, allodynia)
- Other than known nerve injury (type II or causalgia), no known definitive pathogenesis

Genetics

No known genetic pattern

RISK FACTORS

- Minor or severe trauma (upper extremity fracture noted in 44%)
- Surgery (particularly carpal tunnel release)
- Lacerations
- Burns
- Frostbite
- Casting/immobilization after extremity injury
- Penetrating injury
- Polymyalgia rheumatica
- Myocardial infarction (MI)
- Cerebral vascular accident

GENERAL PREVENTION

- Early mobilization after fracture, stroke, and MI has proven benefit in reducing incidence of CRPS.

- One study of wrist fractures found that addition of 500 mg/day of vitamin C lowered rates of CRPS.
- There is evidence that limiting use of tourniquets, liberal regional anesthetic use, and ensuring adequate perioperative analgesia can reduce the incidence of CRPS-I.

COMMONLY ASSOCIATED CONDITIONS

- Serious injury to bone and soft tissue
- Herpes zoster
- Postherpetic neuralgia results from partial or complete damage to afferent nerve pathways.
- Pain occurs in dermatomes as a sequela of herpes zoster.

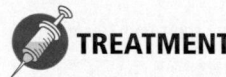 **DIAGNOSIS**

Unprovoked pain is the hallmark of the condition, and the diagnosis of CRPS is excluded by the existence of conditions that would otherwise account for the degree of symptoms. Clinical diagnostic criteria (2):

HISTORY

- Continuing pain which is disproportionate to any inciting event.
- One reported symptom in 3 of the 4 following categories:
  - Sensory: hyperalgesia and/or allodynia
  - Vasomotor: skin, temperature, color asymmetry
  - Sudomotor/edema: edema, sweating changes, or sweating asymmetry
  - Motor/trophic: decreased range of motion or motor dysfunction and/or trophic changes (hair, nail, skin) (1)

PHYSICAL EXAM

At least one sign at evaluation in 2 of the following:

- Sensory: hyperalgesia (to pinprick) or allodynia (to light touch, pressure, or joint movement)
- Vasomotor: evidence of temperature, skin, color asymmetry
- Sudomotor/edema: evidence of edema or sweating changes or asymmetry
- Motor/trophic: decreased range of motion, motor dysfunction, or trophic changes in hair, nails, skin (1)

DIFFERENTIAL DIAGNOSIS

- Infection
- Hypertrophic scar
- Bone fragments
- Neuroma
- CNS tumor or syrinx
- Deep vein thrombosis or thrombophlebitis
- Thoracic outlet syndrome

DIAGNOSTIC TESTS & INTERPRETATION

Initial Tests (lab, imaging)

- CBC
- Erythrocyte sedimentation rate (ESR)
- Plain radiographs may show patchy demineralization within 3 to 6 weeks of onset of CRPS that are more pronounced than would be see from disuse alone.
- 3-phase bone scanning has varying sensitivity but is most accurate for support of the diagnosis when there is diffuse activity (especially on phase 3).
- Bone density

Diagnostic Procedures/Other

- Electromyelography (EMG) shows nerve injury with type II CRPS.
- Sudomotor function testing (resting sweat testing, resting skin temperature, quantitative sudomotor axon reflex testing—all related to increased autonomic activity of the affected limb)

Test Interpretation

- Partial or complete damage to afferent nerve pathways and probably reorganized central pain pathways
- Nerves most commonly involved are median and sciatic.
- Atrophy in affected muscles
- Incomplete nerve plexus lesion

TREATMENT

GENERAL MEASURES

Discourage maladaptive behaviors (pain medication seeking, secondary gain). Principle of functional restoration is a stepwise and multidisciplinary approach.

MEDICATION

First Line

- NSAIDS recommended early in course but mixed support in literature
- The following have literature support of either limited or suggestive benefit in treatment of CRPS-I:
  - Corticosteroids (prednisone 30 mg/day for 2 to 12 weeks with taper) are the only class of drugs that have direct clinical trial support early in the course.
  - Gabapentin 600 to 1,800 mg/day for 8 weeks following diagnosis
  - 50% DMSO cream applied to affected extremity up to 5 times daily
  - N-acetylcysteine 600 mg TID
  - Bisphosphonates (alendronate) at 40 mg/day (however, optimal dose uncertain)
  - Nifedipine 20 mg/day showed benefit early in the course of the condition.

- Although many have advocated the use of tricyclic antidepressants in the treatment of CRPS, there is no credible evidence of improvement of pain. They may be helpful in controlling depressive symptoms that develop with disease progression (2).

ISSUES FOR REFERRAL
- After 2 months of the illness, psychological evaluation is generally indicated to identify and treat any comorbid conditions.
- Identifying local resources and early referral for expert management give increased likelihood of long-term success in controlling condition.

ADDITIONAL THERAPIES
Type I
- Physical and occupational therapy (beneficial to the overall prognosis for recovery)
  - Should be started early
    - "Mirror therapy" has shown good results.
- Transcutaneous nerve stimulation
- Psychotherapy
- Use of subdissociative (0.2 to 0.5 mg/kg) infusions of ketamine has shown some promise but effects seem to be time limited (3)[B].

SURGERY/OTHER PROCEDURES
- Type II responds more favorably to nerve-directed treatment
  - Sympathetic blocks
  - Cervicothoracic or lumbar sympathectomies have little data to support their use and should be used judiciously after all other therapies have failed (4)[A].
- Anesthetic blockade (chemical or surgical) of sympathetic nerve function
  - Transient relief suggests that chemical or surgical sympathectomy will be helpful.
  - Little in the way of quality clinical trials exist to support local sympathetic blockage as the gold standard of therapy.
- IV regional sympathetic block with guanethidine or reserpine by pain specialist or anesthetist
- Transcutaneous electric nerve stimulation (controversial)
- Inject myofascial painful trigger points

- Spinal cord stimulation (quality of life improved only with implanted system)
- Intrathecal analgesia
- Amputation as a last resort in severe cases, with patients reporting improved quality of life

COMPLEMENTARY & ALTERNATIVE MEDICINE
- Vitamin C (500 mg/day) may help to prevent CRPS in those with wrist fracture.
- Briskly rub the affected part several times per day
- Acupuncture
- Hypnosis can be suggested.
- Relaxation training (alternate muscle relaxing and contracting)
- Biofeedback
- Whirlpool baths

INPATIENT CONSIDERATIONS
Admission Criteria/Initial Stabilization
Only for proposed surgical therapy

 ONGOING CARE

FOLLOW-UP RECOMMENDATIONS
Weekly, to monitor progress and initiate additional modalities as needed

PATIENT EDUCATION
- Stress need to remain active physically
- Instruct carefully about any prescribed medications.
- Reflex Sympathetic Dystrophy Syndrome Association, http://rsds.org/, 203-877-3790
- American RSD Hope Group, www.rsdhope.org, 207-583-4589

PROGNOSIS
Most improve with early treatment, but symptoms may be lifelong if there is limited response to initial treatments.

COMPLICATIONS
- Depression
- Disability
- Opioid dependence

REFERENCES
1. Pons T, Shipton EA, Williman J, et al. Potential risk factors for the onset of complex regional pain syndrome type 1: a systematic literature review. *Anesthesiol Res Pract.* 2015;2015:956539.
2. Harden RN, Oaklander AL, Burton AW, et al. Complex regional pain syndrome: practical diagnostic and treatment guidelines, 4th edition. *Pain Med.* 2013;14(2):180–229.
3. Azari P, Lindsay DR, Briones D, et al. Efficacy and safety of ketamine in patients with complex regional pain syndrome: a systematic review. *CNS Drugs.* 2012;26(3):215–228.
4. Straube S, Derry S, Moore RA, et al. Cervicothoracic or lumbar sympathectomy for neuropathic pain and complex regional pain syndrome. *Cochrane Database Syst Rev.* 2013;(9):CD002918.

ADDITIONAL READING
- Goebel A. Complex regional pain syndrome in adults. *Rheumatology (Oxford).* 2011;50(10):1739–1750.
- Perez RS, Zollinger PE, Dijkstra PU, et al. Evidence based guidelines for complex regional pain syndrome type 1. *BMC Neurol.* 2010;10:20.

CODES

ICD10
- G90.50 Complex regional pain syndrome I, unspecified
- G90.519 Complex regional pain syndrome I of unspecified upper limb
- G90.529 Complex regional pain syndrome I of unspecified lower limb

CLINICAL PEARLS
- A pain syndrome disproportioned to injury
- Pain control and early mobility are the key to recovery.
- Avoid use of opiate analgesics.
- Use a multidisciplinary approach.

CONDYLOMATA ACUMINATA

Morgan Ashleigh Smith, DO • Tayseer Husain Chowdhry, MD, MA • E. James Kruse, DO

 BASICS

DESCRIPTION
- Condylomata acuminata are soft, skin-colored, fleshy lesions (commonly called genital warts) that are caused by human papillomavirus (HPV):
  - Warts appear singly or in groups (a single wart is a "condyloma"; multiple warts are "condylomas" or "condylomata"); small or large; typically appear on the anogenital skin (penis, scrotum, introitus, vulva, perianal area); and may occur in the anogenital tract (vagina, cervix, rectum, urethra, anus); also conjunctival, nasal, oral, and laryngeal warts
- System(s) affected: skin/exocrine, reproductive, occasionally respiratory
- HIV considerations:
  - Treatment of external genital warts should not be different for HIV-infected persons (1).
  - Lesions may be larger or more numerous (1)
  - May not respond as well to therapy as immunocompetent persons (1)

Pediatric Considerations
- Consider sexual abuse if seen in children, although children can be infected by other means (e.g., transfer from wart on another child's hand or prolonged latency period) (2).
- American Academy of Pediatrics recommends all school-aged children who present with lesions be evaluated for abuse and screened for other STDs (2).

Pregnancy Considerations
- Warts often grow larger during pregnancy and regress spontaneously after delivery.
- Virus does not cross the placenta. Treatment during pregnancy is somewhat controversial. Cesarean section is not absolutely indicated for maternal condylomata (3)[A].
- Cervical infection has been found to be a risk factor for preterm birth (3)[A].
- Few documented cases of laryngeal papillomas due to HPV transmission at the time of delivery. Although rare, the condition is life-threatening (4).
- HPV vaccination is contraindicated in pregnancy.
- The safety of imiquimod, sinecatechins, podophyllin, and podofilox during pregnancy has not been established (3)[C].

EPIDEMIOLOGY
- HPV types 6 and 11 associated with 90% of condylomata acuminata. Types 16, 18, 31, 33, and 35 may be found in warts and may be associated with high-grade intraepithelial dysplasia in immunocompromised states such as HIV.
- Highly contagious; incubation period may be from 1 to 8 months. Initial infections may very well go unrecognized, so a "new" outbreak may be a relapse of an infection acquired years prior.
- Predominant age: 15 to 30 years
- Predominant sex: 1:1 male to female
- Most infections are transient and clear spontaneously within 2 years.

Incidence
One study population demonstrated that from 2007 to 2010, with the introduction of HPV vaccines, the incidence of genital warts decreased 35% (from 0.94% per year to 0.61% per year) in females <21 years, and decreased 19% in males <21.

Prevalence
- Most common viral sexually transmitted infection (STI) in the United States. Most sexually active men and women will have acquired a genital HPV infection, usually asymptomatic, at some time.
- Peak prevalence in ages 17 to 33 years
- 10–20% of sexually active women may be actively infected with HPV. Studies in men suggest a similar prevalence.
- Pregnancy and immunosuppression favor recurrence and increased growth of lesions.

ETIOLOGY AND PATHOPHYSIOLOGY
HPV is a circular, double-stranded DNA molecule. There are >120 HPV subtypes. HPV types that cause genital warts do not cause anogenital cancers.

RISK FACTORS
- Usually acquired by sexual activity
  - Young adults and adolescents
  - Multiple sexual partners; short interval between meeting new sex partner and first intercourse
  - Not using protective barriers
  - Young age of commencing sexual activity
  - History of other STI
- Immunosuppression (particularly HIV)

GENERAL PREVENTION
- Sexual abstinence or monogamy
- Quadrivalent HPV vaccine available against genital warts and cervical cancer. This vaccine is targeted to adolescents before the period of their greatest risk for exposure to HPV. The vaccine does not treat previous infections:
  - Immunity has been documented to last at least 5 years after HPV vaccination.
  - The HPV quadrivalent vaccine (Gardasil) protects against the two most common HPV serotypes (types 6 and 11, which cause most anogenital warts) and the two most cancer-promoting types (16 and 18) (5).
  - Quadrivalent vaccine is indicated for females and males ages 9 to 26 years: Vaccine is administered IM; 3 doses at 0, 2, and 6 months to achieve optimal seroconversion (6).
  - Vaccine efficacy for preventing external genital warts is related to age of administration of 1st dose: 76% if aged <20 years, 93% if <14 years.
- Bivalent HPV vaccine is available but does not cover the HPV types that cause most condyloma lesions (Cervarix) (5).
- Quadrivalent vaccine has been proven effective in prevention of external lesions in males 16 to 26 years of age (5).
- Use of condoms is partially effective, although warts may be easily spread by lesions not covered by a condom (e.g., 40% of infected men have scrotal warts).
- Abstinence until treatment completed

COMMONLY ASSOCIATED CONDITIONS
- >90% of cervical cancer associated with HPV types 16, 18, 31, 33, and 35
- 60% of oropharyngeal and anogenital squamous cell carcinomas are associated with HPV
- STIs (e.g., gonorrhea, syphilis, chlamydia), AIDS

 DIAGNOSIS

HISTORY
- Explore sexual history, contraception use, and other lifestyle topics.
- Most warts are asymptomatic but symptoms include
  - Pruritus, burning, redness, pain, bleeding
  - Vaginal discharge
  - Large warts may cause obstructive symptoms in the anus (with defecation) or vaginal canal (with intercourse or childbirth)

PHYSICAL EXAM
- Lesions often have a typical rough, warty appearance with multiple fingerlike projections but may be soft, sessile, and smooth.
- Large lesions are cauliflower-like and may grow to >10 cm.
- Most common sites: penis, vaginal introitus, and perianal region
- May be seen anywhere on the anogenital epithelium or in the anogenital tract
- Warts often occur in clusters.
- Bleeding or irritation of the lesions may be noted.

DIFFERENTIAL DIAGNOSIS
- Condylomata lata (flat warts of syphilis)
- Lichen planus
- Normal sebaceous glands
- Seborrheic keratosis
- Molluscum contagiosum
- Keratomas, micropapillomatosis
- Scabies
- Crohn disease
- Skin tags
- Melanocytic nevi
- Vulvar intraepithelial neoplasia
- Squamous cell carcinoma

DIAGNOSTIC TESTS & INTERPRETATION
- Diagnosis is usually clinical, made by unaided visual examination of the lesions.
- Biopsy
- Acetowhitening test: Subclinical lesions can be visualized by wrapping the penis with gauze soaked with 5% acetic acid (vinegar) for 5 minutes. Using a 10× hand lens or colposcope, warts appear as tiny white papules. A shiny white appearance of the skin represents foci of epithelial hyperplasia (subclinical infection), but because of low specificity, the CDC recommends against routine use of this test to screen for HPV mucosal infection.

Initial Tests (lab, imaging)
- Usually not required for diagnosis
- Serologic tests for syphilis may be helpful to rule out condylomata lata.
- Other testing for STIs
- Pap smear may be indicated.

Follow-Up Tests & Special Considerations
Because squamous cell carcinoma may resemble or coexist with condylomata, biopsy may be considered for lesions refractory to therapy.

Diagnostic Procedures/Other
- Biopsy with highly specialized identification techniques, such as HPV DNA detected through polymerase chain reaction, is rarely useful.

- Colposcopy, antroscopy, anoscopy, and urethroscopy may be required to detect anogenital tract lesions.
- Screening men who have sex with men (MSM) with anal Pap smears is controversial.

 TREATMENT

GENERAL MEASURES
- May resolve spontaneously
- Change therapy if no improvement after 3 treatments, not complete clearance after 6 treatments, or therapy's duration or dosage exceeds manufacturer's recommendations.
- Appropriate screening/counseling of partners

MEDICATION
First Line
- No single therapy for genital warts is ideal for all patients or clearly superior to other therapies.
- Recommendations for external genital warts, patient-applied:

  – Podofilox (Condylox): antimitotic action; apply 0.5% solution or gel to warts twice daily (allowing to dry) for 3 consecutive days at home followed by 4 days of no therapy; may repeat up to 4 total cycles; maximum of 0.5 mL/day or area less than 10 cm^2 (3)[A],(7)
  – Imiquimod (Aldara): immune enhancer; self-treatment with a 5% cream applied once daily at bedtime 3 times weekly until warts resolve for up to 16 weeks. Wash off with soap and water 6 to 10 hours after application. Imiquimod has been noted to weaken condoms and diaphragms; therefore, patients should refrain from sexual contact while the cream is on the skin (3)[A],(8).
  – Sinecatechins (Veregen): immune enhancer and antioxidant, extract from green tea; apply a 0.5-cm strand of ointment 3 times daily for up to 16 weeks. Do not wash off after use (3)[A].

- Recommendations for external genital warts, provider-applied:

  – Cryotherapy: liquid nitrogen applied to warts for two 10-second bursts with thawing in between; usually requires 2 to 3 weekly sessions (3)[A]
  – Podophyllin 10–25% in tincture of benzoin. Apply directly to warts, air-dry in office before coming into contact with clothes. Wash off in 1 to 4 hours. Repeat every 7 days in office until gone (3)[A],(7).
  – Trichloroacetic acid (TCA): 80% solution. Apply only to warts; powder/talc to remove unreacted acid. Repeat in office at weekly intervals; ideal for isolated lesions in pregnancy (3)[A].
- Recommendations for exophytic cervical warts: biopsy to exclude high-grade squamous intraepithelial lesion (SIL) (3)[A]
- Recommendations for vaginal warts: cryotherapy or TCA or bichloracetic acid (BCA) 80–90% (3)[A]
- Recommendations for urethral meatus warts: cryotherapy or podophyllin 10–25% in compound tincture of benzoin (3)[A]
- Recommendations for anal warts: cryotherapy, TCA or BCA 80–90%, or surgery; specialty consultation for intra-anal warts (3)[A]

Pregnancy Considerations
Cryotherapy, surgery, or TCA. Medications contraindicated in pregnancy: podophyllin, podophyllotoxin, sinecatechins, interferon, and imiquimod (3)[C]

Second Line
Intralesional interferon, photodynamic therapy, topical cidofovir (3)[A]

SURGERY/OTHER PROCEDURES
- Larger warts may require surgical excision, laser treatment, or electrocoagulation (including infrared therapy):

  – Precaution: Laser treatment may create smoke plumes that contain HPV. CDC recommendation is for the use of a smoke evacuator no less than 2 inches from the surgical site. Masks are recommended; N95 the most efficacious (9)[A].

- Intraurethral, external (penile and perianal), anal, and oral lesions can be treated with fulgurating CO$_2$ laser. Oral or external penile/perianal lesions can also be treated with electrocautery or surgery.

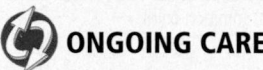 **ONGOING CARE**

FOLLOW-UP RECOMMENDATIONS
No restrictions, except for sexual contact

Patient Monitoring
- Patients should be seen every 1 to 2 weeks until lesions resolve.
- Patients should follow up 3 months after completion of treatment.
- Persistent warts require biopsy.
- Sexual partners require monitoring.

PATIENT EDUCATION
- Provide information on HPV, STI prevention, and condom use.
- Explain to patients that it is difficult to know how or when a person acquired an HPV infection; a diagnosis in one partner does not prove sexual infidelity in the other partner.
- Emphasize the need for women to follow recommendations for regular Pap smears.

PROGNOSIS
- Asymptomatic infection persists indefinitely.
- Treatment has not clearly been shown to decrease transmissible infectivity.
- Warts may clear with treatment or resolve spontaneously. However, recurrences are frequent, particularly in the first 3 months, and may necessitate repeated treatments.

COMPLICATIONS
- Cervical dysplasia (probably does not occur with type 6 or 11, which cause most warts)
- Malignant change: Progression of condylomata to cancer rarely, if ever, occurs, although squamous cell carcinoma may coexist in larger warts.
- Urethral, vaginal, or anal obstruction from treatment
- The prevalence of high-grade dysplasia and cancer in anal canal is higher in HIV-positive than in HIV-negative patients, probably because of increased HPV activity.

REFERENCES
1. Gormley RH, Kovarik CL. Human papillomavirus-related genital disease in the immunocompromised host: part II. *J Am Acad Dermatol.* 2012;66(6):883. e1–883.e17; quiz 899–900.
2. Unger ER, Fajman NN, Maloney EM, et al. Anogenital human papillomavirus in sexually abused and nonabused children: a multicenter study. *Pediatrics.* 2011;128(3):e658–e665.
3. Workowski KA, Bolan GA; Centers for Disease Control and Prevention. Sexually transmitted diseases treatment guidelines, 2015. *MMWR Recomm Rep.* 2015;64(RR-03):1–137.
4. Gerein V, Schmandt S, Babkina N, et al. Human papilloma virus (HPV)-associated gynecological alteration in mothers of children with recurrent respiratory papillomatosis during long-term observation. *Cancer Detect Prev.* 2007;31(4):276–281.
5. Centers for Disease Control and Prevention. FDA licensure of bivalent human papillomavivaccine (HPV2, Cervarix) for use in females and updated HPV vaccination recommendations from the Advisory Committee on Immunization Practices (ACIP). *MMWR Morb Mortal Wkly Rep* 2010;59(20):626–629.
6. Centers for Disease Control and Prevention. Recommendations on the use of quadrivalent human papillomavirus vaccine in males—Advisory Committee on Immunization Practices (ACIP), 2011. *MMWR Morb Mortal Wkly Rep.* 2011;60(50):1705–1708.
7. Stockfleth E, Beti H, Orasan R, et al. Topical Polyphenon E in the treatment of external genital and perianal warts: a randomized controlled trial. *Br J Dermatol.* 2008;158(6):1329–1338.
8. Gotovtseva EP, Kapadia AS, Smolensky MH, et al. Optimal frequency of imiquimod (aldara) 5% cream for the treatment of external genital warts in immunocompetent adults: a meta-analysis. *Sex Transm Dis.* 2008;35(4):346–351.
9. NIOSH Health Hazard Evaluation and Technical Assistance Reports, HETA 85-126-1932 (1988) and HETA 88-101-2008 (1990)

ADDITIONAL READING
- Bauer HM, Wright G, Chow J. Evidence of human papillomavirus vaccine effectiveness in reducing genital warts: an analysis of California public family planning administrative claims data, 2007–2010. *Am J Public Health.* 2012;102(5):833–835.
- Giuliano AR, Palefsky JM, Goldstone S, et al. Efficacy of quadrivalent HPV vaccine against HPV infection and disease in males. *N Engl J Med.* 2011;364(5):401–411.
- Gormley RH, Kovarik CL. Human papillomavirus-related genital disease in the immunocompromised host: part I. *J Am Acad Dermatol.* 2012;66(6):867. e1–867.e14; quiz 881–882.

 CODES

ICD10
A63.0 Anogenital (venereal) warts

CLINICAL PEARLS
- Condylomata acuminata are soft, skin-colored, fleshy lesions caused by HPV subtypes 6, 11, 16, 18, 31, 33, and 35.
- Quadrivalent HPV vaccine addresses the two most common HPV serotypes to be contracted in warts types 6 and 11 and the two most cancer-promoting types 16 and 18 (Gardasil).
- Vaccine: 0.5 mL IM first dose and at months 2 and 6
- The majority of sexually active men and women will have acquired a genital HPV infection, usually asymptomatic, at some time.
- No single therapy for genital warts is ideal for all patients or clearly superior to other therapies.
- Quadrivalent HPV vaccine is effective in preventing HPV infection, particularly if administered prior to the onset of engaging in sexual activity. Gardasil is approved and recommended for use in males and females aged 9 to 26 years.

CONJUNCTIVITIS, ACUTE
Frances Yung-tao Wu, MD

BASICS

DESCRIPTION
- Inflammation of the bulbar and/or palpebral conjunctiva of <4 weeks' duration
- System(s) affected: nervous, skin/exocrine
- Synonym(s): pink eye

Geriatric Considerations
- Suspect autoimmune, systemic, or irritative conditions.
- If purulent, risk of bacterial cause increases with age, the combo of age >65 years and bilateral lid adherence = risk >70% (1)[B].

Pediatric Considerations
- Neonatal conjunctivitis may be gonococcal, chlamydial, irritative, or related to dacryocystitis.
- Pediatric ER study; 78% positive bacterial culture, mostly *Haemophilus influenzae*; 13% no growth; other studies showed >50% adenovirus.
- Children <5 years were 7 times more likely to be bacterial than were older children or adults.
- Daycare regulations sometimes require any child with presumed conjunctivitis to be treated with a topical antibiotic, despite lack of evidence (2)[A].

EPIDEMIOLOGY
- Predominant age
  – Pediatric: viral, bacterial
  – Adult: viral, bacterial, allergic
- Predominant sex: male = female

Incidence
In the United States: variable, but accounts for 1–2% of all ambulatory office visits

ETIOLOGY AND PATHOPHYSIOLOGY
- Viral
  – Adenovirus (common cold), coxsackievirus (implicated in recent hemorrhagic conjunctivitis epidemics in Asia and Middle East)
  – Enterovirus (acute hemorrhagic conjunctivitis)
  – Herpes simplex
  – Herpes zoster or varicella
  – Measles, mumps, or influenza
- Bacterial
  – *Staphylococcus aureus* or *epidermidis*
  – *Streptococcus pneumoniae*
  – *H. influenzae* (children)
  – *Pseudomonas* spp. or anaerobes (in contact lens users)
  – *Acanthamoeba* from contaminated contact lens solution may cause keratitis.
  – *Neisseria gonorrhoeae* and *meningitidis*
  – *Chlamydia trachomatis*: gradual onset >4 weeks
- Allergic
  – Hay fever, seasonal allergies, atopy
- Nonspecific
  – Irritative: topical medications, wind, dry eye, UV light exposure, smoke
  – Autoimmune: Sjögren syndrome, pemphigoid, Wegener granulomatosis
  – Rare: Rickettsia, fungal, parasitic, tuberculosis, syphilis, Kawasaki disease, chikungunya, Graves, gout, carcinoid, sarcoid, psoriasis, Stevens-Johnson, Reiter syndrome

RISK FACTORS
- History of contact with infected persons
- Sexually trasmitted disease (STD) contact: gonococcal, chlamydial, syphilis, or herpes
- Contact lenses: pseudomonal or acanthamoeba keratitis
- Epidemic bacterial (streptococcal) conjunctivitis reported in school settings

GENERAL PREVENTION
- Wash hands frequently.
- Demonstrate eyedropper technique: While eye is closed and head back, several drops over nasal canthus; then open eyes to allow liquid to enter. Never touch tip of dropper to skin or eye.

COMMONLY ASSOCIATED CONDITIONS
- Viral infection (e.g., common cold)
- Possible STD

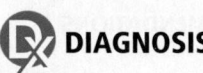

DIAGNOSIS

HISTORY

ALERT
Red flag: Any decrease in visual acuity is not consistent with conjunctivitis alone; must document normal vision for diagnosis of isolated conjunctivitis.

- Viral: contact or travel
  – May start with one eye, then both
  – If herpetic, recurrences or vesicles on skin
- Bacterial: difficult to distinguish from viral, unless contact lens user. Assume bacterial in contact lens wearer unless cultures are negative. If recent STD, suspect chlamydia or gonococcus.
- Allergic: itching, atopy, seasonal, dander
- Irritative: Feels dry, exposure to wind, tear film deficit may persist 30 days after acute conjunctivitis, chemicals, or drug: atropine, aminoglycosides, iodide, phenylephrine, antivirals, bisphosphonates, retinoids, topiramate, chamomile, COX-2 inhibitors.
- Foreign body: Redness may persist 24 hours after removal.

PHYSICAL EXAM
- General: common to all types of conjunctivitis
  – Red eye, conjunctival injection
  – Foreign body sensation
  – Eyelid sticking or crusting, discharge
  – Normal visual acuity and pupillary reactivity
- Viral
  – Palpable preauricular lymphadenopathy may be present.
  – Hemorrhagic coxsackievirus-related epidemics were reported.
  – Severe viral: herpes simplex or zoster:
    ○ Burning sensation, rarely itching
    ○ Unilateral, herpetic skin vesicles in herpes zoster
    ○ Palpable preauricular node
- Bacterial (non-STD): may be epidemic
  – Mild pruritus, discharge mild to heavy
  – Conjunctival chemosis/edema
  – If contact lens user, must rule out pseudomonal (or other bacterial) keratitis.
- Bacterial: gonococcal (or meningococcal) hyperacute infection
  – Rapid onset 12 to 24 hours
  – Severe purulent discharge
  – Chemosis/conjunctival/eyelid edema
  – Rapid growth of superior corneal ulceration
  – Preauricular adenopathy
  – Signs of STDs (chlamydia, GC, HIV, etc.)
- Allergic
  – Itching predominant
  – Seasonal or dander allergies
  – Chemosis/conjunctival/eyelid edema
- Nonspecific irritative
  – Dry eyes, intermittent redness, chemical/drug exposure
  – Foreign body: may have redness and discharge 24 hours after removal
- Must document normal visual acuity.
- Cornea should be clear and without fluorescein uptake. Cloudy or ulcerated signifies keratitis; consult ophthalmologist.
- Recommend fluorescein exam: Evert lid to inspect for foreign bodies.
- Skin: Look for herpetic vesicles, nits on lashes (lice), scaliness (seborrhea), or styes.
- Limbal flush at corneal margin if uveitis
- If pupil is irregular (i.e., penetrating foreign body), emergent referral is warranted.
- Discharge but no conjunctival injection: blepharitis

DIFFERENTIAL DIAGNOSIS
- Uveitis (iritis, iridocyclitis, choroiditis): limbal flush (red band at corneal margin), hazy anterior chamber, and decreased visual acuity
- Penetrating ocular trauma: emergently hospitalize
- Acute glaucoma (emergency): headache, corneal clouding, poor visual acuity
- Corneal ulcer(s) or foreign body: lesions on fluorescein exam
- Dacryocystitis: tenderness and swelling over tear sac (below medial canthus)
- Scleritis and episcleritis: red injected vessels radially oriented, sectoral (pie wedge), nodularity of sclera
- Pingueculitis: inflammation of a yellow nodular or wedge-like area of chronic conjunctival degeneration (pinguecula)
- Ophthalmia neonatorum: neonates in the first 2 days of life (gonococcal; 5 to 12 days of life): chlamydial, HSV, very rare *N. meningitidis*. Consider specialty consultation for required systemic therapy.
- Blepharitis: Lid margins are inflamed producing itching, scale, or discharge, but no conjunctival injection.

DIAGNOSTIC TESTS & INTERPRETATION
- Usually not needed initially for the most common causes
- Culture swab if STD is suspected, very severe symptoms, or patient is a contact lens user
- Viral swab for detection of adenovirus is not yet in common use.

Diagnostic Procedures/Other
- Fluorescein exam for ulcer or abrasion on cornea
- Small superficial foreign bodies may be removed with irrigation or moistened swab.

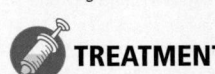

TREATMENT

GENERAL MEASURES
- Infectious conjunctivitis rarely needs antibiotics and resolve on their own.
- Clean eyelid with wet cloth up to QID.
- Stop use of contact lenses while red.
- Patching of eye is not beneficial.

MEDICATION

First Line
- Viral (nonherpetic)
  - Artificial tears for symptomatic relief
  - Vasoconstrictor/antihistamine (e.g., naphazoline/pheniramine) QID for severe itching
  - May consider topical antibiotic (see bacterial below) if return to daycare requires treatment
- Viral (herpetic) (by ophthalmologist)
  - Ganciclovir gel: 0.15%, 5 times per day for 7 days (3)[B]
  - Acyclovir: PO 400 mg 5 times per day for herpes simplex virus (HSV); 800 mg for zoster for 7 days
- Bacterial (non-STI): 3 days cool compress before starting any antibiotic showed no adverse consequences and decreased unnecessary Rx (4)[A].
  - After 3 days, consider topical antibiotics (NNT 7 at day 6) as a reasonable option for delayed treatment: Polymyxin B–Bacitracin ophthalmic ointment: Apply 4 times per day for 5 to 7 days.
  - Polymyxin B-trimethoprim solution 1 gtt 4 times per day for 5 days
  - Erythromycin ophthalmic ointment: 1/2 inch BID–QID for 5 days
  - Sodium sulfacetamide (10% solution) (Bleph-10): 2 drops q4h (while awake) for 5 days
  - Tobramycin or gentamicin: 0.3% ophthalmic drops/ointment q4h (drops) to q8h (ointment) for 7 days
- Bacterial (gonococcal)
  - Neonates: Hospitalize for IV therapy.
  - Adults: ceftriaxone: 1 g IM as single dose and topical bacitracin ophthalmic ointment 1/2 inch QID. Neonates 25 to 50 mg/kg IV or IM, not to exceed 125 mg, as a single dose. Chlamydia in neonates requires oral erythromycin ethylsuccinate: 50 mg/kg/day divided q6h PO for 14 days, max 3 g/day.
- Allergic and atopic (listed by approximate, increasing cost, from lowest to highest): All are efficacious, but evidence favoring one over another is inconclusive (5)[A].
  - Ketotifen (Zaditor, Alaway, and other generics over-the-counter [OTC]): 0.25% 1 drop BID
  - Cromolyn (Opticrom): 4% QID
  - Azelastine: 0.05% 1 gtt BID
  - Pemirolast (Alamast): 0.1% 1 gtt QID
  - Alcaftadine (Lastacaft): 0.25% 1 gtt QD
  - Emedastine: 0.05% 1 drop QID
  - Epinastine (Elestat): 0.05% BID
  - Ketorolac (Acular): 0.1% 1 drop QID
  - Olopatadine (Pataday, Patanol): 0.1% 1 drop BID or 0.2% 1 drop daily
  - Bepotastine (Bepreve): 1.5% 1 gtt BID
  - Lodoxamide tromethamine (Alomide): 0.1% 1 gtt QID
  - Nedocromil (Alocril): 2% 1 gtt BID
  - Oral nonsedating antihistamines (cetirizine [Zyrtec] 10 mg/day, fexofenadine [Allegra] 60 mg BID, etc.) may treat nasal symptoms but cause ocular drying. Oral antihistamine (e.g., diphenhydramine 25 mg TID) in severe cases of itching
- Contraindications: Avoid topical steroids unless able to monitor intraocular pressure. Also, case report of HSV keratitis presenting without distinguishing findings from viral conjunctivitis would discourage initial use of steroids. Steroids were not beneficial in treatment of bacterial keratitis (6)[A]. Topical immune modulators (tacrolimus, cyclosporine) should be reserved for specialist use only in the most difficult cases.

- Precautions
  - Do not allow dropper to touch the eye.
  - Case reports of eye irritation from gentamicin in infants, moxifloxacin in adults, sulfacetamide in allergic individuals
  - Vasoconstrictor/antihistamine: rebound vasodilation after prolonged use

Second Line
- Viral and allergic: numerous OTC products
- Bacterial: second line (quinolones used as postop or known resistant organisms)
  - Ofloxacin: 0.3% 1 gtt 4 times per day for 7 days
  - Ciprofloxacin: 0.3% 1 gtt 4 times per day for 7 days
  - Levofloxacin: 0.3% 1 gtt 4 times per day for 7 days
  - Gatifloxacin: 0.3% 1 gtt 3 times per day for 7 days
  - Moxifloxacin: 0.5% 1 gtt 3 times per day for 7 days
  - Besifloxacin: 0.6% 1 gtt 3 times per day for 7 days
  - Azithromycin: 1.5% 2 times per day for 3 days

ISSUES FOR REFERRAL
Any significantly decreased visual acuity, herpetic keratitis, or contact lens–related bacterial conjunctivitis warrants ophthalmologic consultation.

COMPLEMENTARY & ALTERNATIVE MEDICINE
As condition is usually benign and self-limited, saline flushes, cool compresses, and similar treatments help.

INPATIENT CONSIDERATIONS
Acute gonococcal conjunctivitis (or very rare case of meningococcal conjunctivitis) requires inpatient treatment with ceftriaxone 50 mg/kg IV everyday (pediatric), 1 g IM for 1 (adult) along with ophthalmologic consultation.

Admission Criteria/Initial Stabilization
Penetrating ocular trauma, gonococcal conjunctivitis

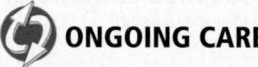 ## ONGOING CARE

FOLLOW-UP RECOMMENDATIONS
- If not resolved within 5 to 7 days, alternate diagnoses should be considered or consultation obtained, although some epidemic keratoconjunctivitis and other adenoviral conjunctivitis typically last 1 to 2 weeks.
- Children may be excluded from school until eye is no longer red, if viral or bacterial, depending on school policy. Allergic conjunctivitis should be able to return to school with doctor's note.

PATIENT EDUCATION
- Patients should not wear contacts until their eyes are fully healed (typically 1 week).
- Patients should discard current pair of contacts.
- Patients should discard any eye makeup that they have been using, especially mascara.
- Cool, moist compress can ease irritation and itch.

PROGNOSIS
- Viral: 5 to 10 days for pharyngitis with conjunctivitis, 2 weeks with adenovirus
- Herpes simplex: 2 to 3 weeks
- Most common bacterial-H flu, staph, strep: self–limited; 74–80% resolution within 7 days, whether treated or not

COMPLICATIONS
- Corneal scars with herpes simplex
- Lid scars or entropion with varicella zoster and chlamydia
- Corneal ulcers or perforation, very rapid with gonococcal

- Hypopyon: pus in anterior chamber
- Chlamydial neonatal (ophthalmic): could have concomitant pneumonia
- Otitis media may follow *H. influenzae* conjunctivitis.
- The very rare *N. meningitidis* conjunctivitis may be followed by meningitis.

REFERENCES
1. van Weert HC, Tellegen E, Ter Riet G. A new diagnostic index for bacterial conjunctivitis in primary care. A re-derivation study. *Eur J Gen Pract*. 2014; 20(3):202–208.
2. Steeples L, Mercieca K. Acute conjunctivitis in primary care: antibiotics and placebo associated with small increase in proportion cured by 7 days compared with no treatment. *Evid Based Med*. 2012;17(6):177–178.
3. Wilhelmus KR. Antiviral treatment and other therapeutic interventions for herpes simples virus epithelial keratitis. *Cochrane Database Syst Rev*. 2015;(1):CD002898.
4. Sheikh A, Hurwitz B, van Schayck CP, et al. Antibiotics versus placebo for acute bacterial conjunctivitis. *Cochrane Database Syst Rev*. 2012;(9):CD001211.
5. Castillo M, Scott NW, Mustafa MZ, et al. Topical antihistamines and mast cell stabilisers for treating seasonal and perennial allergic conjunctivitis. *Cochrane Database Syst Rev*. 2015;(6):CD009566.
6. Herretes S, Wang X, Reyes JM. Topical corticosteroids as adjunctive therapy for bacterial keratitis. *Cochrane Database Syst Rev*. 2014;(10):CD005430.

ADDITIONAL READING
Narayana S, McGee S. Bedside diagnosis of the "red eye" a systematic review. *Am J Med*. 2015;28(11):1220.e1–1224.e1.

 ### SEE ALSO
- Rhinitis, Allergic
- Algorithm: Eye Pain

 ### CODES

ICD10
- H10.30 Unspecified acute conjunctivitis, unspecified eye
- H10.33 Unspecified acute conjunctivitis, bilateral
- H10.32 Unspecified acute conjunctivitis, left eye

CLINICAL PEARLS
- Conjunctivitis does *not* alter visual acuity; decreased acuity or photophobia should prompt consideration of more serious ophthalmic disorders.
- Culture discharge in all *contact lens wearers*, consider referral, and remind patient to throw away current contacts and avoid contacts until eyes are fully healed.
- Antibiotic therapy is of no value in viral conjunctivitis (most cases of infectious conjunctivitis) and does not significantly alter the course of most types of bacterial conjunctivitis (therefore, it is optional in these cases).

CONSTIPATION

S. Mimi Mukherjee, PharmD • Sandhya Ventrapragada, MBBS, MD

BASICS

Unsatisfactory defecation characterized by infrequent stools, difficult stool passage, or both. Characteristics include <3 bowel movements a week, hard stools, excessive straining, prolonged time spent on the toilet, a sense of incomplete evacuation, and abdominal discomfort/bloating.

DESCRIPTION
• System(s) affected: gastrointestinal (GI)
• Synonym(s): obstipation

Geriatric Considerations
Colorectal neoplasms may be associated with constipation; new-onset constipation after age 50 years is a "red flag." Use warm water enemas for impaction instead of sodium phosphate enema in geriatric patients. Sodium phosphate enemas have been associated with fatalities and severe electrolyte disturbances (1)[B].

Pediatric Considerations
Consider Hirschsprung disease (absence of colonic ganglion cells): 25% of all newborn intestinal obstructions, milder cases diagnosed in older children with chronic constipation, abdominal distension, decreased growth; 5:1 male-to-female ratio; associated with inherited conditions such as Down syndrome

Pregnancy Considerations
Avoid misoprostol. Other agents consider risks versus benefits.

EPIDEMIOLOGY
• More pronounced in children and elderly
• Predominant sex: female > male (2:1)
• Nonwhites > whites

Incidence
• 5 million office visits annually
• 100,000 hospitalizations

Prevalence
~15% of population affected

ETIOLOGY AND PATHOPHYSIOLOGY
• As food leaves the stomach, the ileocecal valve relaxes (gastroileal reflex) and chyme enters the colon (1 to 2 L/day) from the small intestine. In the colon, sodium is actively absorbed in exchange for potassium and bicarbonate. Water follows the osmotic gradient. Peristaltic contractions move chyme through the colon into the rectum. Chyme is converted into feces (200 to 250 mL).
• Normal transit time is 4 hours to reach the cecum and 12 hours to reach the distal colon.
• Defecation reflexively follows once stool reaches the rectal vault. This reflex can be inhibited by voluntarily contracting the external sphincter or facilitated by straining to contract the abdominal muscles while voluntarily relaxing the anal sphincter. Rectal distention initiates the defecation reflex. The urge to defecate occurs as rectal pressures increase. Distention of the stomach by food also initiates rectal contractions and a desire to defecate (gastrocolic reflex).

• Primary constipation
  – Slow colonic transit time (13%)
  – Pelvic floor/anal sphincter dysfunction (25%)
  – Functional: normal transit time and sphincter function, subjective symptoms (bloating, abdominal discomfort, perceived difficulty defecating, presence of hard stools) (69%)
• Secondary constipation
  – Irritable bowel syndrome (IBS)
  – Endocrine dysfunction (diabetes mellitus, hypothyroid)
  – Metabolic disorder (increased calcium, decreased potassium)
  – Mechanical (obstruction, rectocele)
  – Pregnancy
  – Neurologic disorders (Hirschsprung, multiple sclerosis, spinal cord injuries)
• Medication effect
  – Anticholinergic effects (antidepressants, narcotics, antipsychotics)
  – Antacids (calcium, aluminum)
  – Nondihydropyridine calcium channel blockers, especially verapamil

Genetics
Unknown but may be familial

RISK FACTORS
• Extremes of life (very young and very old)
• Polypharmacy
• Sedentary lifestyle or condition
• Improper diet and inadequate fluid intake

GENERAL PREVENTION
High-fiber diet, adequate fluids, exercise, and training to "obey the urge" to defecate

COMMONLY ASSOCIATED CONDITIONS
• General debilitation (disease or aging)
• Dehydration
• Hypothyroidism
• Hypokalemia
• Hypercalcemia

DIAGNOSIS

ALERT
Red flags:

• New onset after age of 50 years
• Hematochezia/melena
• Unintentional weight loss
• Anemia
• Neurologic defects

HISTORY
Rome III criteria (2)[C]:
• At least two of the following for 12 weeks in the previous 6 months:
  – <3 stools/week
  – Straining at least 1/4 of the time
  – Hard stools at least 1/4 of time
  – Need for manual assist at least 1/4 of time
  – Sense of incomplete evacuation at least 1/4 of time
  – Sense of anorectal blockade at least 1/4 of time
• Loose stools rarely seen without use of laxatives.

PHYSICAL EXAM
• Vital signs, height, weight
• Digital rectal exam (masses, pain, stool, fissures, hemorrhoids, anal tone)
• Abdominal/gynecologic exam (masses, pain)
• Neurologic exam

DIFFERENTIAL DIAGNOSIS
Congenital
• Hirschsprung disease/syndrome
• Hypoganglionosis
• Congenital dilation of the colon
• Small left colon syndrome

DIAGNOSTIC TESTS & INTERPRETATION
Primarily a clinical diagnosis

Initial Tests (lab, imaging)
CBC, glucose, TSH, calcium, and creatinine routinely and sigmoid/colonoscopy if red flags are present

Follow-Up Tests & Special Considerations
• If condition is refractory, pursue further testing:
  – Colonoscopy
  – Barium enema to look for obstruction and/or megarectum, megacolon, or Hirschsprung disease
• Additional testing
  – Measure colonic transit time by ingesting radiopaque (Sitz-Mark) markers.
  – Plain abdominal film obtained 5 days later (120 hours): Retention of >20% markers indicates slow transit.
  – Markers seen exclusively in distal colon/rectum suggests defecatory disorder.

Diagnostic Procedures/Other
Consider referral in refractory cases:
• Balloon expulsion
• Defecography using a barium paste
• Anorectal manometry with a rectal catheter

Test Interpretation
• Most cases are functional.
• Paucity or absence of intramural enteric ganglia in certain cases of congenital or acquired megacolon
• Neuromuscular abnormalities in certain cases of pseudo-obstruction

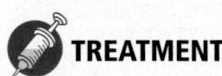

TREATMENT

Address immediate concerns:
• Bloating/discomfort/straining: osmotic agents
• Postoperative, after childbirth, hemorrhoids, fissures: stool softener to aid defecation
• If impacted: manual disimpaction, then treat the chronic underlying condition

GENERAL MEASURES
• Attempt to eliminate medications that may cause or worsen constipation.
• Increase fluid intake.
• Increase fiber in diet.
• Enemas if other methods fail

MEDICATION

In patients with no known secondary causes of constipation, conservative nonpharmacologic treatment is recommended.

- Regular exercise
- Increased fluid intake
- Bowel habit training

First Line

Bulking agents (must be accompanied by adequate amounts of liquid to be useful):

- Hydrophilic colloids (bulk-forming agents)
  - Psyllium (Konsyl, Metamucil, Perdiem Fiber): 1 tbsp in 8-oz liquid PO daily up to TID
  - Methylcellulose (Citrucel): 1 tbsp in 8-oz liquid PO daily up to TID
  - Polycarbophil (Mitrolan, FiberCon): 2 caplets with 8-oz liquid PO up to QID
- Stool softeners
  - Docusate sodium (Colace): 100 mg PO TID
- Osmotic laxatives
  - Polyethylene glycol (PEG) (MiraLax) 17 g/day PO dissolved in 4 to 8 oz of beverage (current evidence shows PEG to be superior to lactulose) (3)[B]
  - Lactulose (Chronulac) 15 to 60 mL PO QHS (flatulence, bloating, cramping)
  - Sorbitol: 15 to 60 mL PO QHS (as effective as lactulose)
  - Magnesium salts (milk of magnesia) 15 to 30 mL PO once daily; avoid in renal insufficiency

Second Line

- Stimulants (irritate bowel, causing muscle contraction; usually combined with a softener; work in 8 to 12 hours)
  - Senna/docusate (Senokot-S, Ex-lax, Peri-Colace): 1 to 2 tablets or 15 to 30 mL PO at bedtime
  - Bisacodyl (Dulcolax, Correctol): 1 to 3 tablets PO daily
- Lubricants (soften stool and facilitate passage of the feces by its lubricating oily effects)
  - Mineral oil (15 to 45 mL/day)
  - Short-term use only. Can bind fat-soluble vitamins, with the potential for deficiencies; may similarly decrease absorption of some drugs
  - Avoid in those at risk for aspiration (lipoid pneumonia)
- Suppositories
  - Osmotic: sodium phosphate
  - Lubricant: glycerin
  - Stimulatory: Bisacodyl
  - Enemas: saline (Fleet enema)
- Lubiprostone (Amitiza): a selective chloride channel activator; 24 μg PO BID
- Linaclotide (Linzess): guanylate cyclase-C agonist; dose: 145 μg PO once daily; adult use only
  - Avoid in children <6 years.
  - Peripherally acting μ-opioid receptor antagonists, indicated for opioid-induced constipation
  - Methylnaltrexone (Relistor): dose: 38 to <62 kg: 8 mg; 62 to 114 kg: 12 mg SC every other day PRN
  - Naloxegol (Movantik): dose: 12.5 to 25.0 mg PO daily, discontinue other laxatives for 3 days when initiating naloxegol, avoid in patients on strong Cyp3A4 inhibitors due to increased naloxegol levels and risk of opioid withdrawal

- Prokinetic agents (partial 5-HT4 agonists) have been withdrawn due to cardiac side effects; only available via IND protocols: tegaserod (Zelnorm), cisapride (Propulsid)
- Other agents not approved by the FDA:
  - Misoprostol (Cytotec): a prostaglandin that increases colonic motility
  - Colchicine: neurogenic stimulation to increase colonic motility

ADDITIONAL THERAPIES

Other nonpharmacologic therapies include the following:

- Biofeedback therapy
- Behavior therapy
- Probiotics
- Electric stimulation

SURGERY/OTHER PROCEDURES

Surgery rarely indicated

INPATIENT CONSIDERATIONS

Toxic megacolon

Nursing

Manual disimpaction occasionally required in chronic refractory cases

 ONGOING CARE

FOLLOW-UP RECOMMENDATIONS

Encourage exercise and physical activity.

Patient Monitoring

If functional constipation persists, consider organic cause.

DIET

Increase fiber (bloating and gas can be problematic):

- Gradually increase intake to 25 g/day over a 6-week period.
- Bran (hard outer layer of cereal grains)
- Vegetables and fruits
- Whole grain foods
- Encourage liberal intake of fluids.

PATIENT EDUCATION

- Occasional mild constipation is normal.
- Bowel training: the best time to move bowels is in the morning, after eating breakfast, when the normal bowel transit and defecation reflexes are functioning.

PROGNOSIS

- Occasional constipation responsive to simple measures is harmless.
- Habitual constipation can be a lifelong nuisance.
- Patients with neurologic compromise can suffer from ill effects such as obstipation, impaction, and toxic megacolon.
- No evidence for laxative dependence
- No evidence for harm from stimulant use; melanosis coli may develop, but it is a benign condition.

COMPLICATIONS

- Volvulus
- Toxic megacolon
- Acquired megacolon in severe, long-standing cases
- Fluid and electrolyte depletion: laxative abuse

- Rectal ulceration (stercoral ulcer) related to recurrent fecal impaction
- Anal fissures

REFERENCES

1. Ori Y, Rozen-Zvi B, Chagnac A, et al. Fatalities and severe metabolic disorders associated with the use of sodium phosphate enemas: a single center's experience. *Arch Intern Med*. 2012;172(3):263–265.
2. Bharucha AE, Pemberton JH, Locke GR III. American Gastroenterological Association technical review on constipation. *Gastroenterology*. 2013;144(1):218–238.
3. Lee-Robichaud H, Thomas K, Morgan J, et al. Lactulose versus polyethylene glycol for chronic constipation. *Cochrane Database Syst Rev*. 2010;(7):CD007570.

ADDITIONAL READING

- Basilisco G, Coletta M. Chronic constipation: a critical review. *Dig Liver Dis*. 2013;45(11):886–893.
- Bove A, Pucciani F, Bellini M, et al. Consensus statement AIGO/SICCR: diagnosis and treatment of chronic constipation and obstructed defecation (part I: diagnosis). *World J Gastroenterol*. 2012; 18(14):1555–1564.
- Dimidi E, Christodoulides S, Fragkos KC, et al. The effect of probiotics on functional constipation in adults: a systematic review and meta-analysis of randomized controlled trials. *Am J Clin Nutr*. 2014;100(4):1075–1084.
- Ford AC, Moayyedi P, Lacy BE, et al. American College of Gastroenterology monograph on the management of irritable bowel syndrome and chronic idiopathic constipation. *Am J Gastroenterol*. 2014;109(Suppl 1):S2–S26.
- van Dijk M, Benninga MA, Grootenhuis MA, et al. Chronic childhood constipation: a review of the literature and the introduction of a protocolized behavioral intervention program. *Patient Educ Couns*. 2007;67(1–2):63–77.

CODES

ICD10

- K59.00 Constipation, unspecified
- K59.01 Slow transit constipation
- K59.09 Other constipation

CLINICAL PEARLS

- Constipation is unsatisfactory defecation with infrequent stools, difficult stool passage, or both for 3 months.
- Functional constipation (normal transit time and sphincter function) is most common.
- Workup red flags: onset >50 years, hematochezia/melena, unintentional weight loss, anemia, neurologic defects
- Osmotic agents (PEG) have the most evidence supporting clinical effectiveness.

CONTRACEPTION

Kim Michal Stein, MD • Melissa J. Fullerton, MD

BASICS

DESCRIPTION
- Medications or procedures that control timing of pregnancies and prevent unintended pregnancies
- Contraception options are divided into two major categories: hormonal and nonhormonal.
- The most effective methods of contraception are vasectomy, female sterilization, and the long-acting reversible contraceptives (LARCs).

EPIDEMIOLOGY
Incidence
- The estimated prevalence of contraception use among reproductive age women is 63% worldwide and 77% in the United States (1).
- 49% of all pregnancies in the United States are unintended, and half occur in women using a form of reversible contraception.
- 43% of all unintended pregnancies in the United States result in termination.
- The most frequently used forms of contraception in the United States (in order of prevalence) are oral contraceptive pills (OCPs), female sterilization, male condom, male sterilization, and depot injectables.
- Although LARCs are one of the most effective forms of contraception, they are among the least used methods in the United States.

RISK FACTORS
- Unintended pregnancy: higher rates among women ages 18 to 24 and >40 years, unmarried/cohabitating women, women with less than a college education, and minority women
- Contraception discontinuation or nonuse: patient or partner dissatisfaction with prior methods of contraception or intolerable side effects

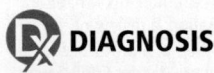

DIAGNOSIS

HISTORY
- Review past medical history, family history, social history, as well as sexual and pregnancy history, and prior experience with contraceptives and prior STDs.
- Important history/contraindications
  - Estrogen-progestin contraceptives
    - Absolute: age ≥35 years and smoking ≥15 cigarettes per day, SBP ≥160 mm Hg or DBP ≥100 mm Hg, multiple CAD risk factors, prior venous thromboembolism (or known hypercoagulability), ischemic heart disease, stroke, complicated valvular disease, systemic lupus, migraine with aura, breast cancer, cirrhosis, or hepatocellular adenoma or malignant hepatoma
    - Relative: age ≥35 years and smoking <15 cigarettes per day, breastfeeding, HTN 140 to 159 mm Hg or diastolic 90 to 99 mm Hg (or well-controlled on medications), migraines without aura but ≥35 years, or breast cancer history in remission >5 years
  - Progestin-only pill/Depo/Implant
    - No absolute
    - Relative: bariatric surgery, ischemic heart disease, history of stroke, lupus, migraine with aura, breast cancer, severe cirrhosis, hepatocellular adenoma, or malignant hepatoma
  - IUD—Mirena
    - Absolute: postseptic abortion, postpartum sepsis, cervical cancer, gestational trophoblastic disease, endometrial cancer, unexplained

vaginal bleeding, symptomatic PID, distorted uterine cavity, current purulent cervicitis or known chlamydia/gonorrhea
    - Relative: ischemic heart disease, lupus, severe cirrhosis, hepatocellular adenoma or malignant hepatoma, increased risk of STDs, solid organ transplant
  - IUD—ParaGard
    - Absolute: same as Mirena
    - Relative: severe thrombocytopenia, increased risk of STDs, solid organ transplant

DIAGNOSTIC TESTS & INTERPRETATION
- A negative pregnancy test (urine or serum) is advised prior to initiating contraception.
- Testing for gonorrhea and chlamydia should be considered but is not required prior to IUD insertion, although need to rule out symptomatic infections.
- Pap smear if otherwise indicated
- Screen for hypertension [A].
- In family history of thrombophilia, testing can be considered before initiation of estrogen-containing contraception, especially if specific defect is known.

TREATMENT

GENERAL MEASURES
- Methods should be selected based on patient preference, effectiveness, desire for sexually transmitted disease (STD) prevention, side effects, and contraindications.
- General categories included hormonal and nonhormonal methods.
  - Nonhormonal methods include condoms, diaphragm, cervical cap, copper IUD, vasectomy, female sterilization, fertility awareness, sponge, spermicides, and abstinence.
  - Hormonal methods include combined oral contraceptives (COCs), patch, ring, injectables, intrauterine devices (IUDs), and implants.

MEDICATION
- Estrogen-progestin contraceptives
  - Mechanism of action: Work by suppression of ovulation, thickening cervical mucus, and endometrial changes that interfere with transport of sperm to egg and with implantation
  - Efficacy: failure rate of about 4.8% at 1 year
  - Side effects: nausea, bloating, headaches, mastalgia, depression, acne, and hirsutism
  - Side effect management: Breakthrough bleeding is usually self-limiting after 3 months; if persists, change pill. Amenorrhea: rule out pregnancy
  - Combined oral contraception (COCs): Pill
    - All COCs contain the same type of estrogen (ethinyl estradiol) but differ in the level of estrogen (range of 10 to 50 μg) and the type of progestin
    - Newer progestins (such as norgestimate and desogestrel) are less androgenic but may have increased rate of venous thromboembolism (VTE).
    - Start with a pill that is inexpensive (generic); contains an average amount of estrogen (30 to 35 μg).
    - Dosing: Most pills have a 21/7 regimen (21 active days and 7 placebo). Alternatively, can take active pills continuously with four yearly scheduled withdrawal bleeds.
    - Initiation: first day start (begin the pill on the first day of menses), quick start (begin pill on day medication is obtained), or Sunday start (begin pill on first Sunday)

  - Weekly hormonal patch (Ortho Evra): releases 20 μg/day ethinyl estradiol and 150 μg/day norelgestromin
    - Applied transdermally and changed weekly
    - Produces higher serum estrogen levels than oral 20 μg pill and may be associated with a slightly increased risk of blood clot
    - Patch may cause local skin irritation; not as reliable in women >90 kg.
  - Vaginal contraceptive ring (NuvaRing):
    - Flexible polymer ring with 15 μg/day of ethinyl estradiol and 120 μg/day of etonogestrel absorbed via vaginal wall
    - Inserted into vagina for 3 weeks/cycle or use continuous cycling for 4 weeks then replace immediately with a fresh ring (off label)
    - Though systemic exposure to estrogen is about 50% of exposure with COCs, the risk of blood clots is about the same.
- Progestin-only birth control
  - Mechanism of action: thickening cervical mucus and thinning endometrial lining
  - Progestin-only pill (Micronor)
    - Efficacy: failure rate of about 0.3% with perfect use, 9% with typical use at 1 year
    - Can be used in women with contraindication for estrogen, including breastfeeding women after 6 weeks postpartum.
    - Dosing: 1 pill taken daily, no placebo days; needs to be taken at the same time daily
    - Side effects: irregular bleeding
  - Injectable contraceptive (medroxyprogesterone)
    - Efficacy: failure rate of 0.2% with perfect use, 6% with typical use at 1 year
    - Dosing: Depo-Provera 150 mg IM or Depo-SubQ Provera 104 mg SQ, both are given every 3 months. Contraceptive levels of hormone persist for up to 4 months (2- to 4-week margin of safety).
    - Side effects include irregular bleeding, weight gain (average of 5 lb/year of use), and amenorrhea.
- LARCs: IUDs and implantable devices [A]
  - Mirena (levonorgestrel IUD):
    - Mechanism of action: sterile inflammatory reaction due to foreign body that is toxic to sperm and ova, thickens cervical mucus, endometrial decidualization and glandular atrophy, inhibiting sperm-egg binding, partial inhibition of ovarian follicular development and ovulation
    - Efficacy: failure rate of 0.2% with both perfect and typical use at 1 year
    - Dosing: IUD releases 20 μg/day of levonorgestrel (very low serum levels).
    - Approved for use up to 5 years; has been used off label for up to 7 years
    - Safe in nulliparous women/teenagers
    - Can be inserted immediately postpartum or immediately following dilation and curettage for miscarriage or abortion, but these are associated with higher rates of expulsion compared to delayed placement (6 to 10 weeks)
    - Side effects: irregular menstrual spotting for the first 3 to 6 months that usually resolves after 6 months of use; may see absence of menses after 1 year
    - Side effect management: Consider trial of COCs or estrogen alone for spotting and cramps.
    - Can reduce heavy bleeding in women with menorrhagia
  - Skyla (levonorgestrel-releasing intrauterine system):
    - Similar to Mirena but releases lower hormone dose (14 μg/day initially, down to 5 μg/day

of levonorgestrel), slightly smaller, and lasts 3 years. Smaller insertion tube might make this an easier IUD for nulliparous women. More bleeding days than Mirena
- ParaGard (Copper IUD):
  ○ Mechanism of action: In addition to sterile inflammatory reaction due to foreign body, free copper and copper salts enhance the cytotoxic inflammatory reaction—toxic to sperm and ova.
  ○ Efficacy: failure rate of 0.6% with perfect use, 0.8% with typical use at 1 year
  ○ Approved for up to 10 years
  ○ Same insertion timing as Mirena
  ○ Side effects: blood loss and cramping
- Nexplanon (etonogestrel implant):
  ○ Mechanism of action: same as progestin-only pill or medroxyprogesterone
  ○ Efficacy: failure rate of 0.05% with perfect use, 0.3% with typical use at 1 year
  ○ Dosing: 40 mm × 2 mm semi-rigid plastic rod containing 68 mg of etonogestrel. Initially releases 60 to 70 μg/day, down to 25 to 30 μg/day at the end of the third year
  ○ Effective for up to 3 years
  ○ Must be inserted only by certified providers
  ○ Side effects: menstrual irregularities (common first 6 to 12 months), amenorrhea after 1 year
• Emergency contraception: should be initiated as soon as possible post-unprotected intercourse. Copper IUD is the most effective, followed by levonorgestrel, ulipristal and Yuzpe method (least effective) (2)[A]
- Copper-bearing IUD (ParaGard): Insert up to 5 days after intercourse; failure rate of 0.04–0.19%.
- Levonorgestrel: 1.5 mg taken as two 0.75-mg tablets (Plan B) or one 1.5-mg tablet (Plan B 1-Step). 1.1–2.4% failure rate. Less nausea than "Yuzpe regimen." Available over the counter; may be less expensive if prescribed. Most effective within 72 hours, efficacy declines with time
- Ulipristal acetate (Ella): 30 mg × 1 dose; Selective progesterone modulator, effective up to 5 days after unprotected intercourse with minimal decline in efficacy. About 2% failure rate
- Estradiol/levonorgestrel (Preven, Lo Ovral, Ogestrel): "Yuzpe regimen" 50 μg/0.25 mg, 2 tablets q12h (4 tablets total). Any OC may be used as long as the dose of estrogen component ≥100 μg/dose. About 3.2% failure rate. *Note:* Antiemetic should be given 1 to 2 hours before each dose.

ADDITIONAL THERAPIES
• Condoms: failure rate of 2% with perfect use, 18% with typical use at 1 year
• Spermicides: All contain nonoxynol-9; may alter vaginal flora and mucosal barrier. 28% failure at 1 year with typical use
• Sponge (Today Sponge): Soft foam disk contains nonoxynol-9. Moisten with water before use; effective for 24 hours; must leave in for 6 hours after use; less effective in parous women. 12–24% failure at 1 year with typical use
• Diaphragm: dome-shaped device made of latex or silicone with flexible spring-activated rim, works by preventing sperm from entering cervix; used with spermicides. 12–16% failure at 1 year with typical use

SURGERY/OTHER PROCEDURES
Permanent sterilization
• Female: tubal ligation or Essure (micro-insert system placed hysteroscopically). Essure requires confirmation of tubal occlusion with hysterosalpingogram 3 months postprocedure. 0.5% failure at 1 year

• Male: vasectomy. Less complicated than female. 0.15% failure at 1 year

COMPLEMENTARY & ALTERNATIVE MEDICINE
• Fertility awareness methods: calendar method, cervical mucus method, temperature method. Low cost but generally not as effective as other methods. 24% failure at 1 year with typical use
• Withdrawal method: Male partner withdraws from vagina before ejaculation. Failure if not timed accurately. 22% failure at 1 year with typical use
• Lactational amenorrhea method: Breastfeeding is effective contraception only if (i) the infant is <6 months old, (ii) the infant is exclusively breastfeeding, and (iii) the mother has not resumed regular menses. 7% failure at 1 year with typical use

Pediatric Considerations
• AAP and ACOG recommend LARCs as the most effective in sexually active adolescents.
• Contraception counseling should include anticipated adverse effects, need to use condoms for STD prevention, and indications for emergency contraception (including options and how to obtain).

 ## ONGOING CARE

FOLLOW-UP RECOMMENDATIONS
Patient Monitoring
• Pelvic exam, Pap smear, and STI testing per guidelines and routine follow-up 2 to 3 months postinitiation of all methods to assess tolerance
• Check for IUD strings 1 month after insertion; spontaneous expulsion rate highest in the first month.
• BP check within 3 months of initiation in patients on estrogen containing methods

DIET
St. John's wort may alter estrogen levels, reducing efficacy or causing breakthrough bleeding.

PATIENT EDUCATION
• Diaphragm: device inspected prior to each use, 1 tablespoon of spermicide in hollow of the dome, diaphragm is inserted into the vagina, additional applicator of spermicide placed in vagina. If placed >6 hours prior to intercourse need additional applicator of spermicide. Position needs to be checked post intercourse, and additional spermicide applied prior to each new episode of intercourse. Diaphragm should remain in place for at least 6 hours after the last episode of intercourse to maximize effectiveness.
• Male condoms: New condom is placed on the penis before genital contact, remains intact until the penis is withdrawn, new condom needs to be used with every act of intercourse.
• IUD: Patient should monitor presence of the string monthly following menses.
• OCP: Pill should be taken at approximately the same time each day. Back up birth control method is needed for the first 7 days with quick start and Sunday start methods.

COMPLICATIONS
• Estrogen-progestin contraceptives:
  - Serious (requires discontinuation): stroke, thromboembolism, hypertension, myocardial infarction, and cholestatic jaundice

  - Overall 5-fold increased risk of venous thrombosis compared to nonusers, comparable to the 4-fold increased risk of venous thrombosis during pregnancy (3)[B]
• Injectable contraceptive:
  - Potential for decreased bone mineral density (BMD) if used for ≥2 years. Mostly recovers after discontinuation. Consider calcium/vitamin D supplementation if prolonged use.
• Nexplanon: insertion site reaction including pain, bleeding, paresthesias, and infection
• IUDs:
  - Pelvic inflammatory disease (PID): Treat without removal unless serious infection or failure to respond to therapy.
  - Uterine perforation
  - Absolute risk of ectopic pregnancy is reduced with IUD, but if pregnancy does occur, there is a higher risk that it will be ectopic.
• Sponge and diaphragm: rarely associated with toxic shock syndrome

REFERENCES
1. Alkema L, Kantorova V, Menozzi C, et al. National, regional, and global rates and trends in contraceptive prevalence and unmet need for family planning between 1990 and 2015: a systematic and comprehensive analysis. *Lancet.* 2013;381(9878):1642–1652.
2. Cheng L, Gülmezoglu AM, Piaggio G, et al. Interventions for emergency contraception. *Cochrane Database Syst Rev.* 2008;(2):CD001324.
3. van Hylckama Vlieg A, Helmerhorst FM, Vandenbroucke JP, et al. The venous thrombotic risk of oral contraceptives, effects of oestrogen dose and progestogen type: results of the MEGA case-control study. *BMJ.* 2009;339:b2921.

ADDITIONAL READING
• CDC Medical Eligibility Criteria for Contraceptive Use, 2010. Available as chart, app for smartphone ("CDC Contraception")
• Chart comparing contraceptive methods: ARHP Method Match at http://www.arhp.org/methodmatch/

 ## CODES

ICD10
• Z30.9 Encounter for contraceptive management, unspecified
• Z30.41 Encounter for surveillance of contraceptive pills
• Z30.431 Encounter for routine checking of intrauterine contracep dev

CLINICAL PEARLS
• Hormonal and IUD contraceptives may be initiated immediately if the likelihood of pre-existing pregnancy is low.
• Contraception method should be chosen based on individual patient needs.
• LARC methods provide high efficacy and convenience for patients.
• All patients should be counseled on emergency contraception options.

COR PULMONALE

Parag Goyal, MD • Sergey G. Gurevich, MD • James M. Horowitz, MD, FACC

BASICS

DESCRIPTION
- Enlargement and subsequent dysfunction and failure of the right ventricle (RV) in the presence of pulmonary hypertension secondary to abnormalities of the pulmonary system, including disorders of the lung parenchyma, pulmonary circulation, chest wall, and ventilatory mechanisms.
- For the purposes of this review, pulmonary arterial hypertension (WHO Group I) will not be considered as a cause of cor pulmonale.
- May occur in acute or chronic setting
  - Acute: rapid increase of pulmonary arterial pressure resulting in RV overload, dysfunction, and potential cardiovascular collapse
  - Chronic: progressive hypertrophy and dilation of the RV over months to years, leading to dysfunction, and potentially failure

EPIDEMIOLOGY
- ~6–7% of all types of adult heart disease in United States
- Estimated 10–30% of heart failure admissions in the United States are the result of cor pulmonale, most commonly related to chronic obstructive pulmonary disease (COPD).

Incidence
Difficult to assess: Best estimate is 1/10,000 to 3/10,000/year.

Prevalence
Difficult to assess: Best estimate is 2/1,000 to 6/1,000.

ETIOLOGY AND PATHOPHYSIOLOGY
- Acute: A sudden event, such as large pulmonary embolism (PE), increases resistance to blood flow in the pulmonary vasculature, causing a quick and significant increase of pressure proximally. The RV is unable to overcome this pressure, leading to low RV cardiac output, which ultimately leads to low left ventricle (LV) cardiac output. Increased RV pressures in conjunction with a low cardiac output may cause coronary ischemia, further impairing cardiac output and potentially causing complete cardiovascular collapse.
- Chronic: A disorder of the pulmonary system causing chronic hypoxia leads to vasoconstriction of the pulmonary vasculature. Over time, the pulmonary vasculature hypertrophies and the intrinsic vasodilatory mechanisms (mediated by nitric oxide) become dysregulated, leading to increases in pulmonary vasculature resistance. The resulting pulmonary hypertension (WHO Group III) transmits increased pressures and volumes to the thin-walled, low-pressure RV, causing maladaptive remodeling (concentric hypertrophy, followed by eccentric dilation frequently with associated tricuspid regurgitation) and subsequent impairment in RV systolic and diastolic function.
- Pulmonary disorders
  - Lung parenchymal disease: COPD (most common), interstitial lung disease (ILD)
  - Pulmonary circulation: thromboembolic disease (associated with pulmonary hypertension WHO Group IV)
  - Chest wall: severe obesity, kyphoscoliosis
  - Ventilation: obstructive sleep apnea (OSA) and obesity hypoventilatory syndrome, neuromuscular diseases such as Guillain-Barré syndrome, muscular dystrophy, myasthenia gravis, spinal cord injuries
- LV failure is not considered a cause of cor pulmonale.

RISK FACTORS
- Acute cor pulmonale (most commonly caused by PE)
  - Risk factors associated with PE:
    - Vessel injury
    - Stasis
    - Hypercoagulable states
- Chronic cor pulmonale (most commonly caused by underlying pulmonary disorder)
  - Risk factors associated with pulmonary disorders
    - Tobacco use (COPD)
    - Occupational exposures (ILD)
    - Hypercoagulable state (chronic thromboembolic disease)
    - Obesity, age (chest wall abnormalities)

GENERAL PREVENTION
Management of underlying pulmonary disorder, including aggressive correction of hypoxia and acidosis, which may contribute to worsening pulmonary hypertension.

COMMONLY ASSOCIATED CONDITIONS
Pulmonary hypertension, defined as the presence of a resting mean pulmonary artery pressure (PAP) >25 mm Hg

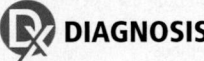

DIAGNOSIS

HISTORY
- Dyspnea is the most common symptom, although nonspecific; may be present at rest, with exertion, or occur as paroxysmal nocturnal dyspnea
- Other pulmonary symptoms: pleuritic chest pain, cough, hemoptysis
- General heart failure symptoms: fatigue, lethargy, syncope; exertional angina less likely
- Right-sided heart failure symptoms: anorexia, early satiety, right upper quadrant discomfort from hepatic congestion, lower extremity edema
- Hoarseness secondary to compression of the left recurrent laryngeal nerve by enlarged pulmonary vessels
- Cardiovascular collapse, shock, and/or cardiac arrest may occur in acute or advanced chronic setting.

PHYSICAL EXAM
- Peripheral edema is the most common sign of right-sided heart failure, although it is nonspecific.
- General: pallor, diaphoresis, cyanosis, tachypnea
- Neck: jugular venous distension, with prominent *a*-wave
- Lungs: tachypnea, wheezing
- Heart
  - Increased intensity of pulmonic component of second heart sound (P_2)
  - Splitting of S_2 over the cardiac apex with inspiration
  - Audible right-sided S_3 or S_4
  - Jugular venous pressure (JVP), with prominent v-wave
  - RV heave
  - Pansystolic murmur heard best at right midsternal border increasing with inspiration, consistent with tricuspid regurgitation (typically a late sign)
  - Early diastolic murmur heard best at left upper sternal border, consistent with pulmonary regurgitation
- Abdomen: hepatomegaly
- Extremities: clubbing, bilateral lower extremity edema, also signs of deep vein thrombosis (DVT) such as tenderness or unilateral swelling

DIFFERENTIAL DIAGNOSIS
Other causes of right-sided failure:
- Left-sided heart failure (WHO Group II)
- WHO Groups I and V pulmonary hypertension
- Right-sided intrinsic cardiomyopathy

DIAGNOSIS TESTS & INTERPRETATION
- 2D echocardiogram (1)[C]
  - Initial diagnostic test of choice
  - Elevated PAP
  - Right ventricular hypertrophy
  - Bulging of the interventricular septum into the LV with systole
  - Flattening of the interventricular or interatrial septum
  - Dilation and hypokinesis of the RV
  - Tricuspid regurgitation
  - Dilation of the right atrium
  - Acute thromboembolic pulmonary disease as evidenced by right ventricular hypokinesis with sparing of the apex (McConnell sign)
  - Echocardiography can over- or underestimate the PAP depending on image quality or operator. PAP should therefore be verified by catheter.
- MRI
  - If echocardiography is inconclusive or as a substitute
  - Most accurate modality for diagnosing emphysema and ILD
  - Can assess pressures, size, function, myocardial mass, and viability
  - Despite being superior to echocardiogram, diagnosis of cor pulmonale still requires assessment via catheterization.
- Right heart catheterization (1)[C]
  - Gold standard for diagnosis of pulmonary hypertension, and therefore critical for diagnosis of cor pulmonale
  - Elevated central venous pressure (CVP)
  - Mean PAP >25 mm Hg at rest
  - Absence of left heart failure (pulmonary capillary wedge pressure <15 mm Hg)

Initial Tests (lab, imaging)
- CBC may show signs of polycythemia due to chronic hypoxia.
- Basic metabolic panel (BMP) may demonstrate elevated creatinine secondary to poor cardiac output.
- Liver function tests (LFTs) may be abnormal due to hepatic congestion or poor cardiac output secondary to RV failure.

- Brain natriuretic peptide (BNP) and cardiac troponin can be elevated secondary to right ventricular strain.
- D-dimer may be positive as evidence of underlying thromboembolic pulmonary disease.
- Arterial blood gas may show hypercapnia due to COPD.
- ECG often shows signs of right-sided enlargement.
  – Right axis deviation
  – An R/S wave ratio >1 in V_1
  – Right ventricular hypertrophy (R wave in V_1 and V_2 with S waves in V_5 and V_6)
  – Right atrial enlargement as evidenced by P pulmonale (increased amplitude of P wave in lead II)
  – Incomplete or complete right bundle branch block
  – $S_1S_2S_3$ pattern or $S_1Q_3T_3$ inverted pattern
- Chest x-ray
  – Cardiomegaly
  – Enlargement of the central pulmonary arteries and reduced size of peripheral vessels (oligemia)
  – Reduced retrosternal space due to right ventricular enlargement on lateral views
  – Enlargement of the right atrium resulting in prominence of the right heart border
  – Evidence of COPD, ILD, and structural disease (i.e., kyphosis)
  – Evidence of PE (Westermark sign and Hampton hump)
- Spiral CT scan of chest
  – Diagnosis of acute PE
  – Diagnosis of COPD and ILD
- Ventilation/perfusion scan (V/Q)
  – High specificity and sensitivity for acute and chronic thromboembolic disease
  – May be used for diagnosis of acute thromboembolic disease if contraindication to chest spiral CT
  – May be preferred to chest spiral CT for diagnosis of chronic thromboembolic pulmonary disease, given higher sensitivity (can detect peripheral pulmonary emboli otherwise missed by spiral CT)
  – Diagnosis of chronic thromboembolic disease may warrant confirmation by pulmonary angiography.
- Pulmonary angiography
  – Gold standard in diagnosis of chronic thromboembolic pulmonary disease
- Polysomnography
  – Gold standard for diagnosis of OSA
- Pulmonary function tests (PFTs)
  – Impaired diffusion capacity
  – Obstructive or restrictive ventilatory defects (ILD, structural abnormalities, and COPD)

 TREATMENT

Reduce symptoms and improve quality of life and survival. Reduce disease burden via oxygenation, preservation of cardiac function, and attenuation of pulmonary hypertension.

GENERAL MEASURES
- Treat underlying disease (2)[A].

  – For underlying pulmonary disease, bronchodilators and/or steroids may be beneficial.
  – For underlying chronic thromboembolic disease, anticoagulation may be indicated.

- Supportive therapy as necessary
  – Continuous positive airway pressure/bilevel positive airway pressure may be used for hypoxia/sleep disorders.
  – Ventilation using positive-pressure masks, negative-pressure body suits, or mechanical ventilation is suggested for patients with neuromuscular disease.
  – Phlebotomy may be indicated for severe polycythemia (hematocrit >55%).

MEDICATION

- Oxygen (3)[A]

  – Long-term continuous oxygen therapy improves the survival of hypoxemic patients with COPD and cor pulmonale.
  – All patients with pulmonary hypertension whose PaO_2 is consistently <55 mm Hg or saturation ≤88% at rest, during sleep, or with ambulation should be prescribed oxygen to keep O_2 >92 mm Hg.

- Preservation of cardiac function (4)[B]

  – Inotropes: Dobutamine and milrinone may improve cardiac output; should be reserved for hemodynamically unstable patients
  – Diuretics: decrease RV filling pressures; also reduces peripheral edema secondary to RHF
    ○ Excessive volume depletion should be avoided.
    ○ Monitor closely for metabolic alkalosis, as this may suppress ventilatory drive and contribute to hypoxia.
- Ameliorate pulmonary hypertension (1,4)[C]
  – Treatment of underlying disease is hallmark of management.
  – When refractory to traditional medical treatment, advanced therapies may be beneficial, although evidence is lacking.
  – For chronic thromboembolic associated pulmonary hypertension (WHO Group IV), riociguat and macitentan may be used.

ISSUES FOR REFERRAL
Patients with cor pulmonale should be referred to a specialized center for expert consultation.

SURGERY/OTHER PROCEDURES
- Endarterectomy for chronic thromboembolic disease (WHO Group IV)
- Moderate to severe disease refractory to medication may require lung and/or heart transplantation.

 ONGOING CARE

DIET
Salt and fluid restriction

PATIENT EDUCATION
- Smoking cessation and avoidance of exposure to secondary smoke is strongly recommended.
- Level of physical activity should be discussed with physician.
- Pregnancy should be avoided.

PROGNOSIS
- Patients with cor pulmonale resulting from COPD have a greater likelihood of dying than do similar patients with COPD alone.
- Pulmonary arterial pressure is a reliable indicator of prognosis; higher pressure is associated with a worse prognosis.
- In patients with COPD and mild disease (PAP 20 to 35 mm Hg), 5-year survival is 50%.

REFERENCES
1. Galiè N, Hoeper MM, Humbert M, et al. Guidelines for the diagnosis and treatment of pulmonary hypertension: the Task Force for the Diagnosis and Treatment of Pulmonary Hypertension of the European Society of Cardiology (ESC) and the European Respiratory Society (ERS), endorsed by the International Society of Heart and Lung Transplantation (ISHLT). *Eur Heart J.* 2009:30(20):2493–2537.
2. McLaughlin VV, Archer SL, Badesch DB, et al. ACCF/AHA 2009 expert consensus document on pulmonary hypertension a report of the American College of Cardiology Foundation Task Force on Expert Consensus Documents and the American Heart Association developed in collaboration with the American College of Chest Physicians; American Thoracic Society, Inc.; and the Pulmonary Hypertension Association. *J Am Coll Cardiol.* 2009;53(17):1573–1619.
3. Naeije R. Pulmonary hypertension and right heart failure in chronic obstructive pulmonary disease. *Proc Am Thorac Soc.* 2005;2(1):20–22.
4. Price LC, Wort SJ, Finney SJ, et al. Pulmonary vascular and right ventricular dysfunction in adult critical care: current and emerging options for management: a systematic literature review. *Crit Care.* 2010;14(5):R169.

 SEE ALSO

Chronic Obstructive Pulmonary Disease and Emphysema; Congestive Heart Failure: Differential Diagnosis; Pulmonary Arterial Hypertension; Pulmonary Embolism

CODES

ICD10
- I27.81 Cor pulmonale (chronic)
- I26.09 Other pulmonary embolism with acute cor pulmonale

CLINICAL PEARLS
- Treatment of cor pulmonale requires treatment of the underlying disease.
- Continuous, long-term oxygen therapy improves life expectancy and quality of life in cor pulmonale.
- Referral of patients with cor pulmonale to a specialized center is strongly recommended.

CORNEAL ABRASION AND ULCERATION
Caroline A. Coicou, MD • Christine S. Persaud, MD

 BASICS

DESCRIPTION
- Corneal abrasions result from scratching, denuding, abrading, or cutting of the epithelial layer of the cornea. They are usually traumatic and accidental but can occur spontaneously as well.
- Corneal ulcers usually represent an infection deeper in the cornea by bacteria, viruses, or fungi as a result of breakdown in the protective epithelial barrier.
- Both corneal abrasions and ulcerations can result in scarring, which may impair vision.
- Both lesions can occur centrally or marginally.

EPIDEMIOLOGY
Incidence
- Corneal abrasion is the most common ophthalmologic visit to the emergency department and is a commonly seen problem in urgent care:
  - 64% of cases are caused by direct minor trauma to eye.
  - 12% of cases are due to contact lens–related problems.
- Ulceration is also common in the United States.

ETIOLOGY AND PATHOPHYSIOLOGY
- Corneal abrasions most commonly result from accidental trauma (e.g., fingernail scratch, makeup brush):
  - Dirt, sand, sawdust, or other foreign body gets caught under eyelid.
- Corneal ulcers result from presence of an entryway to the external eye through dry eye; burns; abrasion; contact lenses; inappropriate use of topical anesthetics, antibiotics, or antiviral drops; immunosuppressant drugs; diabetes; or immunodeficiency. Causes of ulcerations include the following:
  - Infection with gram-positive organisms ~29–53% (*Staphylococcus aureus* and coagulase-negative *Streptococcus* are common ones)
  - Infection with gram-negative organisms ~47–50% (*Pseudomonas* being most common, followed by *Serratia marcescens*, *Proteus mirabilis*, and gram-negative enteric bacilli)

ALERT
Patients with contact lenses may have colonization of the cornea with *Pseudomonas* and other gram-negative bacteria and should be treated with ophthalmic quinolones or aminoglycosides to prevent corneal ulceration and infection (1)[A].

- Viral infections, especially herpes
- Fungal infections (*Candida, Aspergillus, Fusarium, Acanthamoeba*) in agricultural workers or associated with ocular corticosteroid use
- Autoimmune disorders, such as rheumatoid arthritis (RA), systemic lupus erythematosus (SLE), and scleroderma, are the usual cause of peripheral ulcerative keratitis.
- Vitamin A deficiency may cause corneal necrosis or keratomalacia.

RISK FACTORS
- Any abrasive injury
- Foreign body in eye
- Contact lenses (especially soft lenses and extended-wear lenses)
- Blepharitis
- Dry eye syndrome
- Entropion (with lashes scratching cornea)
- Chronic topical steroid use
- Abuse of topical anesthetics
- Autoimmune disorders
- Vitamin A deficiency
- Chronic corneal exposure (e.g., Bell palsy, exophthalmos)
- Recent eye surgery: Trendelenburg position is newly identified as a risk factor for corneal abrasion (2).
- Immunosuppression and trigeminal nerve abnormalities
- Flash burn (welding burn or prolonged gazing directly at bright sunlight; symptoms often begin several hours after exposure)

GENERAL PREVENTION
- Eye protection to avoid injury during work, crafts, and sports
- Proper contact lens handling
  - Do not sleep while wearing contact lens.
- Artificial tears for those with inability to blink or known dry eyes
- Lenses to block UV rays (e.g., welding helmets)

COMMONLY ASSOCIATED CONDITIONS
- Chronic ulcerations may be associated with neurotrophic keratitis due to lack of 5th nerve innervation of the cornea. Individuals with thyroid disease, diabetes, or immunosuppressive conditions are particularly at risk.
- Any cause of fat malabsorption may be associated with vitamin A deficiency.

 DIAGNOSIS

HISTORY
- Sudden onset of eye pain, photophobia, tearing, foreign body sensation, blurring of vision, and/or conjunctival injection
- Abrasions and ulcerations are usually unilateral.
- History remarkable for contact lens use, dry eyes, rubbing eye, history of trauma from foreign body, or chemical burn
- History of connective tissue disorder

PHYSICAL EXAM
- Visual acuity may be decreased if abrasion or ulcer is centrally located.
- Conjunctival injection
- Increased lacrimation on affected side
- Photophobia
- Blepharospasm

- Lesion seen on slit-lamp exam and area of damage shows fluorescein uptake; staining seen using Wood lamp or cobalt blue slit lamp:
  - "Dendritic" staining pattern with fluorescein indicative of viral keratitis
- Examine for foreign body under eyelids or in cornea ("rust ring")

DIFFERENTIAL DIAGNOSIS
- Foreign body in eye
- Unilateral iritis
- Acute or chronic glaucoma
- Keratitis
- Scleritis with corneal melting
- Herpes simplex or zoster
- Bilateral or true idiopathic lesions may suggest basement membrane dystrophy.

DIAGNOSTIC TESTS & INTERPRETATION
Initial Tests (lab, imaging)
- Culture ulcer and contact lens, if applicable.
- Pretreatment with topical antibiotics may alter culture results.

Diagnostic Procedures/Other
Scrapings of the corneal ulcer for culture and sensitivity ideally should be obtained before beginning local antibiotics. The sample should be plated directly onto the culture medium.

Test Interpretation
Scrapings for Gram and Giemsa stain may demonstrate bacteria, yeast, or intranuclear inclusions that may aid in the diagnosis.

TREATMENT

GENERAL MEASURES
- Simple corneal abrasions can be managed by primary care physicians, but consider referral for lesions larger than 4 mm. See indications for referral in the following text.
- All patients with corneal ulceration should be referred immediately to an ophthalmologist. Corneal cultures should be obtained before starting antibiotics. If immediate referral is not possible, it is reasonable to start antibiotics without delay.
- Flash burns from welding or prolonged exposure to sunlight may be treated like corneal abrasions (3)[C].
- Topical ophthalmic steroids should be avoided: may delay healing of corneal abrasions (4)[C]. Use of topical anesthetics outside of clinical settings should be avoided: may develop corneal toxicity with prolonged use (5)[A]

MEDICATION
First Line
- Eye patching does not reduce pain or speed the healing process (6)[A].
- Topical NSAIDs have been proven to reduce eye pain (6)[A].

  – Ophthalmic NSAIDs: Diclofenac 0.1% QID helps relieve moderate pain:
    ○ Alternatives include ketorolac 0.5% and bromfenac 0.09%
    ○ Caution: Ophthalmic NSAIDs may rarely cause corneal melting and perforation.
- Ophthalmic antibiotics may help prevent further infection and ulceration of corneal abrasions (3)[C].
- Some ophthalmic antibiotics include ciprofloxacin 0.3%, ofloxacin 0.3%, gentamicin 0.3%, erythromycin 0.5%, polymyxin B/trimethoprim (Polytrim), and tobramycin 0.3%:
  – Ointment preparations may be more soothing to the eye than solutions.
  – Topical antibiotics should be continued until eye pain is resolved.
  – Chloramphenicol should be avoided due to high risk of toxicity and Stevens-Johnson syndrome.
- Large corneal abrasions (>4 mm) or very painful abrasions should be treated with a combination of topical antibiotic and topical NSAID.
- Reevaluate in 24 hours. If improving, no need for further follow-up (3)[C].
- Fungal keratitis is treated with a protracted course of topical antifungal agents (by ophthalmologist).
- A combination of cryotherapy and antifungal agents for treatment of fungal corneal ulcer could help facilitate the practice of fungal keratitis treatment in the future (7).
- Herpetic keratitis should be referred promptly to ophthalmologist and treated initially with trifluridine:
  – Vidarabine and acyclovir are alternatives.

Second Line
- Oral analgesic medication (hydrocodone and other opioids) if topical analgesia not adequate
- Supplemental topical cycloplegics (i.e., homatropine 5% and cyclopentolate 1%) have not been found to be beneficial in relieving pain in corneal abrasion (8)[B].
- Topical 0.3% HA provided a promising treatment for superficial corneal abrasion caused by mechanical damage (9).
- Sodium hyaluronate reduces reepithelialization time when used after mechanical abrasions of the cornea (10).
- In the management of traumatic corneal abrasions, the administration of an eye gel containing sodium hyaluronate and xanthan gum is able to reduce the length of occlusive patching (11).

ISSUES FOR REFERRAL
- Consultation with an ophthalmologist is recommended for all ulcers to help determine appropriate therapy. Moreover, ulcers need corneal cultures to be taken directly onto culture media.
- Also refer to ophthalmologist if there is history of the following:
  – Significant ocular trauma
  – Corneal infection is suspected (including viral keratitis).
  – Recurrent or nonhealing abrasion is encountered despite standard treatment.
  – Severe ocular pain not explained by apparent pathology (e.g., traumatic iritis)

 ONGOING CARE

FOLLOW-UP RECOMMENDATIONS
Patient Monitoring
- Contact lens wearer should be monitored daily with slit lamp for signs of secondary infection.
- Minor abrasion should be reevaluated only if it becomes more painful (3)[C].
- Large abrasion (>4 mm) should be reevaluated in 24 hours, and if improving, no need to follow further unless symptoms worsen again (3)[C].

PATIENT EDUCATION
- Prevention of abrasions and proper handling of contact lenses can prevent recurrence of corneal ulcers.

PROGNOSIS
- Corneal abrasions and ulcerations should improve daily and heal with appropriate therapy.
- If healing does not occur within 24 to 48 hours or the lesion extends, obtain an ophthalmology consultation.

COMPLICATIONS
- Recurrence
- Scarring of the cornea
- Loss of vision
- Corneal perforation

REFERENCES
1. Dargin JM, Lowenstein RA. The painful eye. *Emerg Med Clin North Am*. 2008;26(1):199–216, viii.
2. Segal KL, Fleischut PM, Kim C, et al . Evaluation and treatment of perioperative corneal abrasions. *J Ophthalmol*. 2014;2014:901901.
3. Fraser S. Corneal abrasion. *Clin Ophthalmol*. 2010;4:387–390.
4. Tomas-Barberan S, Fagerholm P. Influence of topical treatment on epithelial wound healing and pain in the early postoperative period following photorefractive keratectomy. *Acta Ophthalmol Scand*. 1999;77(2):135–138.
5. Duffin RM, Olson RJ. Tetracaine toxicity. *Ann Ophthalmol*. 1984;16(9):836, 838.
6. Turner A, Rabiu M. Patching for corneal abrasion. *Cochrane Database Syst Rev*. 2006;(2):CD004764.
7. Chen Y, Yang W, Gao M, et al. Experimental study on cryotherapy for fungal corneal ulcer. *BMC Ophthalmol*. 2015;15:29.
8. Carley F, Carley S. Towards evidence based emergency medicine: best BETs from the Manchester Royal Infirmary. Mydriatics in corneal abrasion. *Emerg Med J*. 2001;18(4):273.
9. Lin T, Gong L. Sodium hyaluronate eye drops treatment for superficial corneal abrasion caused by mechanical damage: a randomized clinical trial in the People's Republic of China. *Drug Des Devel Ther*. 2015;9:687–694.
10. Moreira LB, Scalco R, Hara S. Corneal reepithelialization time with instillation of eye drops containing sodium hyaluronate and carboxymethylcellulose [in Portuguese]. *Arq Bras Oftalmol*. 2013;76(5):292–295.
11. Faraldi F, Papa V, Santoro D, et al. A new eye gel containing sodium hyaluronate and xanthan gum for the management of post-traumatic corneal abrasions. *Clin Ophthalmol*. 2012;6:727–731.

ADDITIONAL READING
- Ehlers JP, Shah CP, Fenton GL. *The Wills Eye Manual: Office and Emergency Room Diagnosis and Treatment of Eye Disease*. Baltimore, MA: Lippincott Williams & Wilkins; 2008.
- Watson SL, Barker NH. Interventions for recurrent corneal erosions. *Cochrane Database Syst Rev*. 2007;(4):CD001861, revised in *Cochrane Database Syst Rev*. 2012;(9):CD001861.
- Wilhelmus KR. Therapeutic interventions for herpes simplex virus epithelial keratitis. *Cochrane Database Syst Rev*. 2008;(1):CD002898.
- Wipperman JL, Dorsch JN. Evaluation and management of corneal abrasions. *Am Fam Physician*. 2013;87(2):114–120.

 CODES

ICD10
- S05.00XA Inj conjunctiva and corneal abrasion w/o fb, unsp eye, init
- H16.009 Unspecified corneal ulcer, unspecified eye
- H16.049 Marginal corneal ulcer, unspecified eye

CLINICAL PEARLS
- Contact lens use should be discontinued until corneal abrasion or ulcer is healed and pain is fully resolved.
- Eye patching is not recommended.
- Prescribe topical and/or oral analgesic medication for symptom relief and consider ophthalmic antibiotics.
- Prompt referral to an ophthalmologist should be made with suspicion of an ulcer, recurrence of abrasion, retained foreign body, viral keratitis, significant visual loss, or lack of improvement despite therapy.

CORNS AND CALLUSES

Neil J. Feldman, DPM, FACFAS

BASICS

DESCRIPTION
- A callus (tyloma) is a diffuse area of hyperkeratosis, usually without a distinct border.
  - Typically, the result of exposure to repetitive forces, including friction and mechanical pressure; tend to occur on the palms of hands and soles of feet (1).
- A corn (heloma) is a circumscribed hyperkeratotic lesion with a central conical core of keratin that causes pain and inflammation. The conical core in a corn is a thickening of the stratum corneum.
- Hard corn or heloma durum (more common): more often on toe surfaces, especially 5th toe (proximal interphalangeal [PIP] joint)
- Soft corn (heloma molle): commonly in the interdigital space (1)
- Digital corns are also known as clavi.
- Intractable plantar keratosis is usually located under a metatarsal head (1st and 5th most common), is typically more difficult to resolve, and often is resistant to usual conservative treatments.

EPIDEMIOLOGY
Corns and calluses have the largest prevalence of all foot disorders.

Incidence
Incidence of corns and calluses increases with age. Less common in pediatric patients. Women affected more often than men. Blacks report corns and calluses 30% more often than whites.

Prevalence
- 9.2 million Americans
- ~38/1,000 people affected

ETIOLOGY AND PATHOPHYSIOLOGY
Increased activity of keratinocytes in superficial layer of skin leading to hyperkeratosis. This is a normal response to excess friction, pressure, or stress.
- Calluses typically arise from repetitive friction, motion, or pressure to skin.
- Soft corns arise from increased moisture from perspiration leading to skin maceration, along with mechanical irritation, especially between toes.
- Hard corns are an extreme form of callus with a keratin-based core. Often found on the digital surfaces and commonly linked to bony protrusions, causing skin to rub against shoe surfaces.

Genetics
No true genetic basis was identified because most corns and calluses are due to mechanical stressors on the foot/hands.

RISK FACTORS
- Extrinsic factors producing pressure, friction, and local stress
  - Ill-fitting shoes
  - Not using socks, gloves
  - Manual labor
  - Walking barefoot
  - Activities that increase stress applied to skin of hands or feet (running, walking, sports)
- Intrinsic factors
  - Bony prominences: bunions, hammertoes
- Enlarged bursa or abnormal foot function/structure: hammertoe, claw toe, or mallet toe deformity

GENERAL PREVENTION
External irritation is by far the most common cause of calluses and corns. General measures to reduce friction on the skin are recommended to reduce incidence of callus formation. Examples include wearing shoes that fit well and using socks and gloves.

Geriatric Considerations
In elderly patients, especially those with neurologic or vascular compromise, skin breakdown from calluses/corns may lead to increased risk of infection/ulceration. 30% of foot ulcers in the elderly arise from eroded hyperkeratosis. Regular foot exams are emphasized for these patients as well as diabetic patients (2).

COMMONLY ASSOCIATED CONDITIONS
- Foot ulcers, especially in diabetic patients or patients with neuropathy or vascular compromise
- Infection: look for warning signs of:
  - Increasing size or redness
  - Puslike drainage
  - Increased pain/swelling
  - Fever
  - Change in color of fingers or toes
- Signs of gangrene

DIAGNOSIS

- Most commonly a clinical diagnosis based on visualization of the lesion
- Examination of footwear may also provide clues.

HISTORY
- Careful history can usually pinpoint cause.
- Ask about neurologic and vascular history and diabetes. These may be risk factors for progression of corns/calluses to frank ulcerations and infection.

PHYSICAL EXAM
- Calluses
  - Thickening of skin without distinct borders
  - Often on feet, hands; especially over palms of hands, soles of feet
  - Colors from white to gray-yellow, brown, red
  - May be painless or tender
  - May throb or burn
- Corns
  - Hard corns: commonly on dorsum of toes or dorsum of 5th PIP joint
    - Varied texture: dry, waxy, and transparent to a hornlike mass
    - Distinct borders
    - More common on feet
    - Often painful
  - Soft corns
    - Often between toes, especially between 4th and 5th digits at the base of the webspace
    - Often yellowed, macerated appearance
    - Often extremely painful

DIFFERENTIAL DIAGNOSIS

- Plantar warts (typically a loss of skin lines within the wart), which are viral in nature
- Porokeratoses (blocked sweat gland)
- Underlying ulceration of skin, with or without infection (rule out especially with diabetic patients)

DIAGNOSTIC TESTS & INTERPRETATION

Initial Tests (lab, imaging)
- Radiographs may be warranted if no external cause is found. Look for abnormalities in foot structure, bone spurs.
- Use of metallic radiographic marker and weight-bearing films often highlight the relationship between the callus and bony prominence.

Diagnostic Procedures/Other
Biopsy with microscopic evaluation in rare cases

Test Interpretation
Abnormal accumulation of keratin in epidermis, stratum corneum

 TREATMENT

GENERAL MEASURES

- Débridement of affected tissue and use of protective padding
- Low-heeled shoes; soft upper with deep and wide toebox
- Extra-width shoes for 5th-toe corns
- Avoidance of activities that contribute to painful lesions
- Prefabricated or custom orthotics

MEDICATION

- Most therapy for corns and calluses can be done as self-care in the home (1).
- Use bandages, soft foam padding, or silicone sleeve over the affected area to decrease friction on the skin and promote healing with digital clavi.
- Use socks or gloves regularly.
- Use lotion/moisturizers for dry calluses and corns.
- Keratolytic agents, such as urea or ammonium lactate, can be applied safely.
- Use sandpaper discs or pumice stones over hard, thickened areas of skin.

Geriatric Considerations
Use of salicylic acid corn plasters can cause skin breakdown and ulceration in patients with thin, atrophic skin; diabetes; and those with vascular compromise. The skin surrounding the callus will often turn white and can become quite painful. Aggressive use of pumice stones can also lead to skin breakdown, especially surrounding the callus.

ISSUES FOR REFERRAL

- May benefit from referral to podiatrist if use of topical agents and shoe changes are ineffective
- Abnormalities in foot structure may require surgical treatment.
- Diabetic, vascular, and neuropathic patients may benefit from referral to podiatrist for regular foot exams to prevent infection or ulceration.

SURGERY/OTHER PROCEDURES

- Surgical treatment to areas of protruding bone where corns and calluses form
- Rebalancing of foot pressure through functional foot orthotics
- Shaving or cutting off hardened area of skin using a chisel or 15-blade scalpel. For corns, remove keratin core and place pad over area during healing.

COMPLEMENTARY & ALTERNATIVE MEDICINE

- Many over-the-counter topical creams, ointments, and lotions are available for calluses (Kera brand, CalleX, Urea, Lac-Hydrin). Do not use on broken skin.
- Warm water/Epsom salt soaks.

INPATIENT CONSIDERATIONS

Admission Criteria/Initial Stabilization
- Admission usually not necessary, unless progression to ulcerated lesion with signs of severe infection, gangrene
- May require aggressive débridement in operating room should an abscess or deep space infection be suspected. Deep-space infections can develop where an abscess can penetrate into tendon sheaths and/or deep compartments within the foot or hand, potentially leading to rapid sepsis. Vascular status must be assessed and vascular referral considered.

Nursing
Wound care, dressing changes for infected lesions

 ONGOING CARE

PATIENT EDUCATION

- General information: http://www.mayoclinic.org/diseases-conditions/corns-and-calluses/basics/definition/con-20014462
- American Podiatric Medical Association: http://www.apma.org

PROGNOSIS

Complete cure is possible once factors causing pressure or injury are eliminated.

COMPLICATIONS

Ulceration, infection

REFERENCES

1. Freeman DB. Corns and calluses resulting from mechanical hyperkeratosis. *Am Fam Physician*. 2002;65(11):2277–2280.
2. Pinzur MS, Slovenkai MP, Trepman E, et al. Guidelines for diabetic foot care: recommendations endorsed by the Diabetes Committee of the American Orthopaedic Foot and Ankle Society. *Foot Ankle Int*. 2005;26(1):113–119.

ADDITIONAL READING

Theodosat A. Skin diseases of the lower extremities in the elderly. *Dermatol Clin*. 2004;22(1):13–21.

 CODES

ICD10
L84 Corns and callosities

CLINICAL PEARLS

Most therapy for corns and calluses can be done as self-care in the home using padding over the affected area to decrease friction or pressure. However, if simple home care is not helpful, then removal of the lesions is often immediately curative.

CORONARY ARTERY DISEASE AND STABLE ANGINA

Melody L. Strattan, DO • Merrill Krolick, DO, FACC, FACP, FSCAI

 BASICS

DESCRIPTION
- Coronary artery disease (CAD) refers to the atherosclerotic narrowing of the epicardial coronary arteries. It may manifest insidiously as angina pectoris or as an acute coronary syndrome (ACS).
- Stable angina is a chest discomfort due to myocardial ischemia that occurs predictably at a certain level of exertion or emotional stress.
- The spectrum of ACS includes unstable angina (UA), non–ST segment elevation myocardial infarction (NSTEMI), and ST elevation myocardial infarction (STEMI). See separate chapters on these ACS.
- Definitions
  - Typical angina: exhibits three classical characteristics: (i) substernal chest tightness, pressure, or heaviness that frequently radiates to the jaw, back, or arms and generally lasts from 2 to 15 minutes; (ii) occurs in a consistent pattern at a certain level of myocardial oxygen demand from exertion, emotional stress, or increased sympathetic tone; and (iii) relieved with rest or sublingual nitroglycerin.
  - Atypical angina: exhibits two of the above typical characteristics
  - Noncardiac chest pain: exhibits ≤1 of the above typical characteristics
  - Anginal equivalent: Patients may present without chest discomfort but with nonspecific symptoms such as dyspnea, diaphoresis, fatigue, belching, nausea, light-headedness, or indigestion that occur with exertion or stress.
  - Unstable angina: anginal symptoms that are new or changed in character to become more frequent, more severe, or both; it is considered an ACS but does not present with cardiac biomarker elevation.
  - NSTEMI: Presents with cardiac biomarker elevation. Ischemic ECG changes may be present, but there is no ST segment elevation.
  - STEMI: defined by ST elevations on ECG and elevated cardiac biomarkers; generally caused by acute plaque rupture and complete obstruction of the culprit vessel
- Canadian Cardiovascular Society grading scale:
  - Class I: Angina does not limit ordinary physical activity, occurring only with strenuous or prolonged exertion (7 to 8 METs).
  - Class II: Angina causes slight limitation of ordinary activity. It occurs when walking rapidly, uphill, or >2 blocks; climbing >1 flight of stairs; or with emotional stress (5 to 6 METs).
  - Class III: Angina causes marked limitation of ordinary physical activity. It occurs when walking one to two blocks or climbing one flight of stairs (3 to 4 METs).
  - Class IV: Angina occurs with any physical activity and may occur at rest (1 to 2 METs).

Geriatric Considerations
- Elderly may present with atypical symptoms.
- Other physical limitations may delay recognition of angina until it occurs with minimal exertion or at rest.
- Maintain a high degree of suspicion during evaluation of dyspnea and other nonspecific complaints.
- Geriatric patients may be very sensitive to the side effects of medications used to treat angina.

EPIDEMIOLOGY
- CAD is the leading cause of death for adults both in the United States and worldwide.
- CAD is responsible for about 30% of all deaths, averaging 1 death every 40 seconds in the United States alone.
- Global cost of CAD in 2010 $863 billion
- ~80% of CAD is preventable with healthy lifestyle.

Incidence
In the United States, the lifetime risk of a 40-year-old developing CAD is 49% for men and 32% for women.

Prevalence
In the United States, 17.6 million people carry a diagnosis of CAD, 10.2 million with angina pectoris (1).

ETIOLOGY AND PATHOPHYSIOLOGY
- Anginal symptoms occur during times of myocardial ischemia caused by a mismatch between coronary perfusion and myocardial oxygen demand.
- Atherosclerotic narrowing of the coronary arteries is the most common etiology of angina, but it may also occur in those with significant aortic stenosis, pulmonary hypertension, hypertrophic cardiomyopathy, coronary spasm, or volume overload.
- Sensory nerves from the heart enter the spinal cord at levels C7–T4, causing diffuse referred pain/discomfort in the associated dermatomes.

RISK FACTORS
- Traditional risk factors: hypertension, ↓HDL, smoking, diabetes, premature CAD in 1st-degree relatives (men <55 years old; women <65 years old), age (>45 for men, >55 for women)
- Nontraditional risk factors: obesity, sedentary lifestyle, abnormal ankle-brachial indices, renal disease

GENERAL PREVENTION
- Smoking cessation
- Regular aerobic exercise program
- Weight loss for obese patients (goal BMI <25 kg/m^2)
- BP control (goal <140/90 mm Hg; <150/90 mm Hg for those ≥60 years old) (2)
- Diabetes management
- Lipid-lowering therapy (statins) for those with diabetes, known CAD, and for 10-year risk ≥7.5%
- Low-dose aspirin may be considered in those with 10-year risk ≥10%.

COMMONLY ASSOCIATED CONDITIONS
Hyperlipidemia, peripheral vascular disease, cerebrovascular disease, hypertension, obesity, diabetes

DIAGNOSIS

HISTORY
- Careful history is important to elicit symptoms.
- Pain may be described with a clenched fist over the center of the chest (Levine sign).
- Discomfort is usually not affected by position or deep inspiration.
- Episodes of angina are generally of the same character and in the same location.
- Recent decrease in level of physical activity may be due to worsening anginal symptoms.
- Dyspnea on exertion may present as the only symptom. Atypical symptoms are more likely in women, the elderly, and diabetic patients.
- May present with symptoms similar to gastric reflux or GI upset (indigestion, nausea, diaphoresis)
- Ascertain whether symptoms are similar to those with previously diagnosed heart disease.

PHYSICAL EXAM
- Normal physical exam does not exclude the diagnosis of angina or CAD.
- Cardiac exam may reveal dysrhythmias, heart murmurs indicative of valvular disease, gallops, or signs of congestive heart failure.
- Evidence of peripheral vascular disease (diminished pulses, bruits, abdominal aortic aneurysm [AAA])

DIFFERENTIAL DIAGNOSIS
- Vascular: aortic dissection, pericarditis, myocarditis, myocardial infarction
- Pulmonary: pleuritis, pulmonary embolism, pneumothorax
- Gastroesophageal: gastric reflux, esophageal spasm, peptic ulcer
- Musculoskeletal: costochondritis, arthritis, muscle strain, rib fracture
- Other: anxiety, psychosomatic, cocaine abuse

DIAGNOSTIC TESTS & INTERPRETATION

Initial Tests (lab, imaging)
- Serial cardiac troponin to rule out myocardial infarction (MI)
- CBC to evaluate for anemia, infectious cause (1)[C]
- Fasting lipid profile (1)[C]
- Fasting glucose or hemoglobin A1C (1)[C]
- Basic metabolic panel to rule out electrolyte abnormalities and assess renal function.
- ECG
  - Should be routinely obtained unless there is a noncardiac cause of the chest pain (1)[C]
  - Frequently unremarkable between angina episodes; may show signs of myocardial ischemia during symptomatic episodes, evidence of old MI
  - Left bundle branch block or ventricular pacing makes interpretation unreliable.
- Chest x-ray may exclude other causes of pain (1)[C].

Follow-Up Tests & Special Considerations
- Goal is to detect possible high-risk coronary lesions, where intervention would improve long-term mortality or alleviate anginal symptoms.
- Stress testing is most helpful for patients at intermediate risk of heart disease.
  - Exercise testing for those who can physically exercise (≥5 metabolic equivalents [METS]) (1)[A]
    - Standard exercise ECG for those with normal baseline ECG
    - Exercise stress testing with echo or perfusion imaging for those with abnormal baseline ECG or in premenopausal women
  - In patients who cannot tolerate exercise, consider pharmacologic stress testing (1)[A].
- Echocardiogram should be obtained in patients with a new or loud (≥III/VI) murmur, evidence of myocardial infarction, symptoms of heart failure, concern for hypertrophic cardiomyopathy or pericardial effusion, and in those with new arrhythmias (1)[A].
- Echocardiogram can be considered in patients with hypertension or diabetes and abnormal ECG (1)[A].
- CT coronary angiography or MRI angiography can be alternative to stress testing in patients with continued symptoms despite negative or inconclusive stress testing for anatomic definition of disease.

Diagnostic Procedures/Other

- Cardiac catheterization with coronary angiography is the gold standard for confirmation and delineation of coronary disease and direction of interventional therapy or surgery.
- Significant CAD is defined as ≥50% stenosis of the left main coronary artery or ≥70% stenosis of other major coronary arteries by angiography.
- Borderline lesions may be assessed with a pressure wire. Fractional flow reserve (FFR) of ≤0.8 demonstrates a hemodynamically significant lesion.

 TREATMENT

GENERAL MEASURES

- BP control goal: <140/90 mm Hg for most, except in elderly (2)[A]

- Smoking cessation goal: complete cessation, no exposure to secondhand smoke or E-cigarettes
- Physical activity goal: 30 to 60 minutes of moderate aerobic activity, at least 5 (preferably 7) days/week
- Weight management goal: BMI 18.5 to 24.9 kg/m²; waist circumference <35 inches (women) or <40 inches (men)
- Glycemic control in diabetics: Goal is strict glucose control while avoiding hypoglycemic episodes.

MEDICATION

First Line

- β-Blockers: decrease myocardial oxygen demand by lowering heart rate, BP, and contractility.

  - Improve mortality in patients with MI or heart failure; use as initial therapy (1)[A]

  - Can improve symptoms of angina
  - Metoprolol (25 to 400 mg daily [succinate] or divided BID [tartrate]) or carvedilol (3.125 to 25 mg BID). Adjust doses according to clinical response. Maintain resting heart rate 50 to 60 bpm.
  - Side effects bradycardia, fatigue, sexual dysfunction

- Calcium channel blockers (CCBs): cause arterial vasodilation, decreased myocardial oxygen demand, and improved coronary blood flow. Similar effectiveness to β-blockers; may be used instead of, or in addition to β-blockers (1)[A]. Only long-acting CCBs should be used:

  - Dihydropyridine CCBs: nifedipine (30 to 90 mg/day), amlodipine (5 to 10 mg/day), or felodipine (2.5 to 10 mg/day): vasodilators
  - Nondihydropyridine CCBs such as diltiazem (120 to 480 mg/day) or verapamil (120 to 480 mg/day) also have negative inotropic effects; should not be used in those with EF <40%. Side effects include constipation and peripheral edema. The nondihydropyridine CCBs may also cause bradycardia or precipitate heart failure in those with severe systolic dysfunction (ejection fraction <40%).

- Nitrates: Dilate systemic veins and arteries (including coronary vessels) and cause decreased preload. At higher doses, they decrease BP and thus, afterload, increasing myocardial flow.

  - Sublingual nitroglycerin 0.4 mg every 5 minutes for 2 to 3 doses may be used for acute anginal episodes (1)[A].

  - Long-acting nitrates such as isosorbide mononitrate (30 to 240 mg daily [extended release]) can be used for angina prophylaxis.
  - Side effects include headache and hypotension, but tend to improve with continued usage.

- Lipid-lowering agents:

  - High-intensity statin therapy is indicated for all patients with CAD regardless of lipid levels (3)[A].

  - Statin therapy should also be encouraged for those with high CAD risk.
  - Atorvastatin (10 to 80 mg/day) and rosuvastatin (5 to 40 mg/day) are high-intensity statins.
  - Statins reduce risk of MI & revascularization need.
  - Side effects include myalgias, transaminitis, rhabdomyolysis (rare), impaired glucose tolerance.
- Aspirin: Decreases risk of thrombosis by inhibiting cyclo-oxygenase and thromboxane.

  - Aspirin (75 to 162 mg/day) decreases risk of first MI and reduces adverse cardiovascular events in those with stable angina (1)[A].
  - Clopidogrel (75 mg/day) may be used in patients with contraindications to aspirin (1)[A].

  - Dual antiplatelet therapy with aspirin + clopidogrel, prasugrel, or ticagrelor is indicated after percutaneous coronary intervention.
- Angiotensin-converting enzyme inhibitors (ACEIs): act on the renin-angiotensin-aldosterone system to reduce BP and afterload. They also have effects on cardiac remodeling after MI.

  - ACEIs such as lisinopril (5 to 40 mg/day) and enalapril (2.5 to 20 mg BID) have been shown to reduce both cardiovascular death and MI in patients with CAD and left ventricular systolic dysfunction (1)[A].

  - Angiotensin receptor blockers such as candesartan (4 to 32 mg daily) may be used in patients intolerant to ACEIs.
  - Side effects include cough (ACEIs only), hyperkalemia, and angioedema.

Second Line

Ranolazine (500 to 1000 mg BID) decreases calcium overload in myocytes, acting as an antianginal/anti-ischemic agent.

- Does not affect heart rate or BP
- Use as adjunctive therapy when symptoms persist despite optimal doses of other antianginals
- Side effects can include nausea, constipation, dizziness, QT prolongation, and headache.

SURGERY/OTHER PROCEDURES

- Revascularization should be considered when noninvasive testing suggests a high-risk lesion. It can also be performed if optimal medical therapy is inadequate to control symptoms.
- Percutaneous coronary intervention (PCI) with balloon angioplasty and/or stent placement (with drug-eluting or bare-metal stent) is performed for significant lesions. Additional techniques include laser therapy and atherectomy.
- PCI does not decrease mortality or risk of MI vs. with medical management with stable angina.
- Coronary artery bypass graft (CABG) is preferred over PCI for those with severe left main coronary stenosis, significant lesions in ≥3 major coronary arteries, and for lesions not amenable to PCI.

COMPLEMENTARY & ALTERNATIVE MEDICINE

Relaxation/stress reduction therapy for angina

INPATIENT CONSIDERATIONS

Admission Criteria/Initial Stabilization

Inpatient evaluation of patients with changes in anginal symptoms representing unstable angina (an ACS)

Discharge Criteria

Without myonecrosis, discharge after appropriate risk stratification.

 ONGOING CARE

FOLLOW-UP RECOMMENDATIONS

- Lifestyle modifications should be aggressively stressed at every visit.
- Patients should be followed clinically; routine stress testing is not necessary for asymptomatic patients.

Patient Monitoring

Frequent follow-up after initial event: every 4 to 6 months in 1st year, then 1 to 2 times per year

DIET

- Reduced intake of trans-fatty acids (1)[C]
- Adherence to dietary modification for comorbid conditions (diabetes, heart failure, hypertension)

PROGNOSIS

Variable; depends on severity of symptoms, extent of CAD, and left ventricular function

COMPLICATIONS

ACS, arrhythmia, cardiac arrest, heart failure

REFERENCES

1. Fihn SD, Gardin JM, Abrams J, et al. 2012 ACCF/AHA/ACP/AATS/PCNA/SCAI/STS guideline for the diagnosis and management of patients with stable ischemic heart disease. *J Am Coll Cardiol*. 2012;60(24):e44–e164.
2. James PA, Oparil S, Carter BL, et al. 2014 Evidence-based guideline for the management of high blood pressure in adults: report from the panel members appointed to the Eighth Joint National Committee (JNC 8). *JAMA*. 2014;311(5):507–520.
3. Stone NJ, Robinson JG, Lichtenstein AH, et al. 2013 ACC/AHA guideline on the treatment of blood cholesterol to reduce atherosclerotic cardiovascular risk in adults. *Circulation*. 2014;129(25 Suppl 2): S1–S45.

 SEE ALSO

Algorithm: Chest Pain/Acute Coronary Syndrome

 CODES

ICD10

- I25.119 Athscl heart disease of native cor art w unsp ang pctrs
- I25.118 Athscl heart disease of native cor art w oth ang pctrs
- I20.9 Angina pectoris, unspecified

CLINICAL PEARLS

- Maximize antianginal therapy: Combine β-blockers, CCBs, and nitrates as tolerated.
- Lifestyle changes and optimal medical therapy must be emphasized to prevent progression of atherosclerosis and to control contributing risk factors.

COSTOCHONDRITIS

Smriti Ohri, MD

 BASICS

DESCRIPTION
- Anterior chest wall pain associated with pain and tenderness of the costochondral and costosternal regions
- System(s) affected: musculoskeletal
- Synonym(s): costosternal syndrome; parasternal chondrodynia; anterior chest wall syndrome (1)

EPIDEMIOLOGY
- Predominant age: 20 to 40 years
- Predominant gender: female

Incidence
- 30% of chest pain visits in emergency room (2)
- 20% of chest pain visits in primary care office were due to musculoskeletal causes with 13% because of costochondritis (3).

ETIOLOGY AND PATHOPHYSIOLOGY
Not fully understood

RISK FACTORS
- Unusual physical activity or overuse that stresses the upper extremity
- Recent trauma (including motor vehicle accident, domestic violence) or new activity
- Recent upper respiratory infection (URI) with coughing

 DIAGNOSIS

- Pain is usually sharp, achy, or pressure-like
- Pain involves multiple and mostly unilateral 2nd to 5th costal cartilages.
- Exacerbated by upper body movements and exertional activities
- Reproduced by palpation of the affected cartilage segments
- Chest tightness is often associated with the pain.

HISTORY
- A complete and thorough history is mandatory for the diagnosis, with special emphasis on cardiac risk factor evaluation.
- Social history: careful screening and evaluation for domestic violence and substance abuse

PHYSICAL EXAM
- A physical exam to exclude more serious conditions that may present with chest pain is necessary for the diagnosis.
- Tenderness elicited over the costochondral junctions is necessary to establish the diagnosis but does not completely exclude other causes of chest pain.
- If swelling or redness of costal cartilage is present, this may be termed as Tietze syndrome.
- Movement of upper extremity of the same side may reproduce the pain (1).
- Palpation of epigastric region to evaluate for gastroesophageal reflux disease (GERD) and deep palpation in right upper quadrant of abdomen to evaluate gallbladder

Pediatric Considerations
- Consider psychogenic chest pain in children who perceive family discord.
- Consider slipping rib syndrome in children with chronic chest and abdominal pain (4).

Geriatric Considerations
- Presents with multiple problems capable of causing chest pain, making a thorough history and physical exam imperative
- Consider herpes zoster in elderly patients with nonspecific musculoskeletal chest pain.

DIFFERENTIAL DIAGNOSIS
- Cardiac
  - Coronary artery disease (CAD)
  - Cardiac contusion from trauma
  - Aortic aneurysm
  - Pericarditis
  - Myocarditis
- Gastrointestinal
  - Gastroesophageal reflux
  - Peptic esophagitis
  - Esophageal spasm
  - Cholecystitis
- Musculoskeletal (4)
  - Fibromyalgia
  - Slipping rib syndrome
  - Costovertebral arthritis
  - Painful xiphoid syndrome
  - Rib trauma
  - Ankylosing spondylitis
  - Precordial catch syndrome
- Psychogenic
  - Anxiety disorder
  - Panic attacks
  - Hyperventilation
- Respiratory
  - Asthma
  - Pulmonary embolism
  - Pneumonia
  - Chronic cough
  - Pneumothorax
- Other
  - Domestic violence and abuse
  - Herpes zoster
  - Spinal tumor
  - Metastatic cancer
  - Substance abuse (cocaine)

DIAGNOSTIC TESTS & INTERPRETATION
- The diagnosis of costochondritis is primarily based on a thorough history and physical exam.
- Laboratory exams should be used to exclude other differential diagnosis.
- ESR is inconsistently elevated.

Initial Tests (lab, imaging)
No imaging is indicated for the diagnosis of costochondritis; chest x-ray and rib films are often normal.

Diagnostic Procedures/Other
- None indicated for the diagnosis of costochondritis.
- Consider ECG in patients age >35 years, those with history or risk of CAD (5)[C].
- Consider chest x-ray in patients with cardiopulmonary symptoms (5)[C].
- Consider spiral CT for pulmonary embolism and D-dimer if history or risk factors are present.

Test Interpretation
Costochondral joint inflammation

TREATMENT

Reassurance of benign nature of condition and potential for long, slow recovery from pain

GENERAL MEASURES
- Rest and heat (or ice massage, whichever makes the patient feel better) (6,7)[C]
- Stretching exercises
- Minimizing activities that provoke the symptoms (e.g., reducing the frequency or intensity of exercise or work activities) (6,7)[C]

MEDICATION
- Pain relief with NSAIDs (ibuprofen, naproxen, or diclofenac); acetaminophen or other analgesics may be considered in noninflammatory disorders (6,7)[C].
- Use of skeletal muscle relaxants may be beneficial if associated with muscle spasm.

ISSUES FOR REFERRAL
Consider referral to physical therapy or osteopathy. Refractory cases of costochondritis can be treated with local injections of combined lidocaine (Xylocaine)/corticosteroid into costochondral areas if severe; however, this is rarely necessary (8)[C].

COMPLEMENTARY & ALTERNATIVE MEDICINE
Limited data on use of manipulation or ice massage but may be safely tried if patient is interested.

INPATIENT CONSIDERATIONS
Admission Criteria/Initial Stabilization
Only indicated if differential diagnosis is unclear and cardiac or other more serious etiology of chest pain is being considered

 ONGOING CARE

FOLLOW-UP RECOMMENDATIONS
Follow up within 1 week if diagnosis is unclear or symptoms do not abate with conservative treatment.

PATIENT EDUCATION
- Educate the patient in regard to the self-limited (although potentially recurrent) nature of the illness.
- Instruct patient on proper physical activity regimens to avoid overuse syndromes.
- Stress importance of avoiding sudden, significant changes in activity.

PROGNOSIS
- Self-limited illness lasts for weeks to months but usually abates by 1 year, although sometimes chronic especially in adolescents.
- Often recurs

COMPLICATIONS
Incomplete attention to differential diagnosis or overly aggressive interventions to ensure a more life-threatening diagnosis is not missed.

REFERENCES

1. Proulx AM, Zryd TW. Costochondritis: diagnosis and treatment. *Am Fam Physician*. 2009;80(6):617–620.
2. Disla E, Rhim HR, Reddy A, et al. Costochondritis. A prospective analysis in an emergency department setting. *Arch Intern Med*. 1994;154(21):2466–2469.
3. Klinkman MS, Stevens D, Gorenflo DW. Episodes of care for chest pain: a preliminary report from MIRNET. Michigan Research Network. *J Fam Pract*. 1994;38(4):345–352.
4. Ayloo A, Cvengros T, Marella S. Evaluation and treatment of musculoskeletal chest pain. *Prim Care*. 2013;40(4):863–887. doi:10.1016/j.pop.2013.08.007.
5. Miller CD, Lindsell CJ, Khandelwal S, et al. Is the initial diagnostic impression of "noncardiac chest pain" adequate to exclude cardiac disease? *Ann Emerg Med*. 2004;44(6):565–574.
6. How J, Volz G, Doe S, et al. The causes of musculoskeletal chest pain in patients admitted to hospital with suspected myocardial infarction. *Eur J Intern Med*. 2005;16(6):432–436.
7. Spalding L, Reay E, Kelly C. Cause and outcome of atypical chest pain in patients admitted to hospital. *J R Soc Med*. 2003;96(3):122–125.
8. Aspegren D, Hyde T, Miller M. Conservative treatment of a female collegiate volleyball player with costochondritis. *J Manipulative Physiol Ther*. 2007;30(4):321–325.

ADDITIONAL READING
- Cayley WE Jr. Diagnosing the cause of chest pain. *Am Fam Physician*. 2005;72(10):2012–2021.
- Freeston J, Karim Z, Lindsay K, et al. Can early diagnosis and management of costochondritis reduce acute chest pain admissions? *J Rheumatol*. 2004;31(11):2269–2271.
- Verdon F, Herzig L, Burnand B, et al. Chest pain in daily practice: occurrence, causes and management. *Swiss Med Wkly*. 2008;138(23–24):340–347.

 CODES

ICD10
M94.0 Chondrocostal junction syndrome [Tietze]

CLINICAL PEARLS
- A very common disorder, accounting for perhaps 30% of all cases of chest pain
- Diagnosis is based primarily on history and physical with lab and other testing done to exclude various differentials based on thorough history and risk factors.
- Educate the patient in regard to the self-limited (although potentially recurrent) nature of the illness. Instruct patient on proper physical activity regimens to avoid overuse syndromes.

COUNSELING TYPES
William T. Garrison, PhD

BASICS

DESCRIPTION

- Psychotherapeutic and counseling interventions play an important role in the management of chronic and acute-onset diseases and disorders. They are typically the primary initial mode of evaluation and/or treatment for most mild to moderate psychiatric disorders that reach criteria using the *DSM-5* (1) or *ICD-10* (2) diagnostic classification systems. It should be noted that the *DSM* system has recently been revised with significant changes in several disorder categories and their criteria. Treatment and successful control of either medical or psychological conditions require some form of professional counseling experience. Best outcomes occur when they are employed by a skilled practitioner. However, psychotherapy differs from generic counseling, which can take many forms and is delivered commonly in nonmedical settings, with mixed results.
- Counseling approaches are usually tailored to the specific presenting problem or issue and serve educational and emotional support functions. Typically, such counseling in medical settings will be time-limited and problem-focused and often not intended to lead to major medical symptom relief or major behavioral changes.
- The goals of psychotherapy range from increasing individual psychological insight and motivation for change to reduction of interpersonal conflict in the marriage or family, reduction of chronic or acute emotional suffering, and reversal of dysfunctional or habitual behaviors. There are several general types of psychotherapy, starting with individual, marital, or family approaches. In addition, a number of psychological theories guide various methods and treatment philosophies. The following is a brief overview of commonly used psychotherapeutic and counseling methods.
- Psychodynamic therapy: Unconscious conflict manifests as patient's symptoms/problem behaviors:
  - Short-term (4 to 6 months) and long-term (≥1 year)
  - Focus is on increasing insight of underlying conflict or processes to initiate symptomatic change.
  - Therapist actively helps patient identify patterns of behavior stemming from existence of an unconscious conflict or motivations that may not be accurately perceived.
- Cognitive-behavioral therapy (CBT): Patterns of thoughts and behaviors can lead to development and/or maintenance of symptoms. Thought patterns may not accurately reflect reality and may lead to psychological distress:
  - Therapy aims at modifying thought patterns by increasing cognitive flexibility and changing dysfunctional behavioral patterns.
  - Encourages patient self-monitoring of symptoms and the precursors or results of maladaptive behavior

- Uses therapist-assisted challenges to patient's basic beliefs/assumptions
- May use *exposure*, a procedure derived from basic learning theories, which encourages gradual steps toward change.
- Can be offered in group or individual formats
- Therapist's role is suggestive and supportive.
- Dialectical behavior therapy (DBT): Techniques such as social skills training, mindfulness, and problem solving are used to modulate impulse control and affect management:
  - Derivative of CBT
  - Originally used in treatment of patients with self-destructive behaviors (e.g., cutting, suicide attempts)
  - Seeks to change rigid patterns of cognitions and behaviors that have been maladaptive
  - Uses both individual and group treatment modalities
  - Therapist takes an active role in interpretation and support.
- Interpersonal psychotherapy: Interpersonal relationships in a patient's life are linked to symptoms. Therapy seeks to alleviate symptoms and improve social adjustment through exploration of patient's relationships and experiences. Focus is on one of four potential problem areas:
  - Grief
  - Interpersonal role disputes
  - Role transitions
  - Interpersonal deficits: Therapist works with the patient in resolving the problematic interpersonal issues to facilitate change in symptoms.
- Family therapy: focuses on the family as a unit of intervention
  - Uses psychoeducation to increase patient's and family's insight
  - Teaches communication and problem-solving skills
- Motivational interviewing: focuses on motivation as a key to successful change process
  - Short-term and problem-focused
  - Focuses on identifying discrepancies between goals and behavior
  - "5 A's" model is a brief counseling framework developed specifically for physicians to effect behavioral change in patients:
    ○ Assess for a problem.
    ○ Advise making a change.
    ○ Agree on action to be taken.
    ○ Assist with self-care support to make the change.
    ○ Arrange follow-up to support the change.
- Counseling (heterogeneous treatment)
  - Often focuses on situational factors maintaining symptoms
  - Often encourages the use of community resources
- Behavioral therapy: relatively nontheoretical approach to behavioral change or symptom reduction/eradication through application of principles of stimulus and response

Pediatric Considerations

- Important distinctions are made between psychotherapy and counseling for children/teens compared to adults/couples.
- The focus of evaluation must include attention to parent and family processes and factors. Interventions typically include interactions and sessions with parents as well as collateral work with teachers and other school personnel.
- Younger children will often be evaluated and diagnosed through behavioral descriptions provided by parents and other adults who know them well as well as through direct observation and/or play techniques. Children of all ages should be screened using behavioral checklists that are norm-referenced for age.
- Any child or teenager who requests counseling should be interviewed initially by the primary care provider and referred appropriately. Most referrals will be in response to parental request, however.
- Psychotherapeutic interventions with the strongest empirical basis with children include behavior therapy/modification, CBT, and family/parenting therapy. Play therapy has the least empirical support, and insight-oriented therapies appear to be more effective with older children (>11 years).
- There is controversy regarding the efficacy of psychopharmacologic treatment in preadolescents, although clear benefits have been demonstrated in some studies. Treatment guidelines for mild to moderate depressed mood and/or anxiety disorders typically recommend pediatric CBT initially, and studies have typically supported this approach in preteen and milder cases.

EPIDEMIOLOGY

- ~18.8 million adults suffer from clinical depression, and 20 million suffer from a diagnosable anxiety disorder.
- One in four Americans report seeking some form of mental health treatment in their adult life. This includes generic counseling in nonmedical settings such as work, clergy, or school settings and also includes visits to primary care providers. It is estimated that between 3.5% and 5% of adults in the United States actually participate in formal mental health psychotherapy annually.
- Public health experts report that the majority of those adults with diagnosable psychiatric disorders, however, do not receive professional mental health services. This is due to multiple factors, including failure to identify, noncompliance with psychiatric referral, regional shortages of providers, economic barriers, and excessive time duration from referral to available service.
- A large study conducted between 1987 and 1997 concluded that the percentage of adults in psychotherapy remained relatively stable over that decade, the use of psychopharmacology doubled, and older adults (aged 55 to 64 years) increasingly sought psychotherapy services. In that same study, it was found that psychotherapy duration (number of sessions) decreased substantially and about 1/3 of psychotherapy patients only attended one or two sessions.

RISK FACTORS

The need for psychotherapy or counseling services is directly and indirectly associated with a host of socioeconomic and biogenetic factors, including the general effects of poverty, family or marital dysfunction; life stressors; medical diseases or conditions; and individual biologic predisposition to mental health disorders.

GENERAL PREVENTION

It is generally assumed that early identification and intervention of child and adolescent psychopathology increases the likelihood of reducing the risk for adult psychopathology, but this has not been sufficiently validated in all categories of psychological disorders. Data support such claims in disorders such as childhood ADHD, anxiety disorders, and habit disorders of childhood, however.

 TREATMENT

GENERAL MEASURES

There is evidence of a "dose effect" in psychotherapy outcomes research, with some investigators suggesting that 6 to 8 sessions are necessary to yield positive initial effects and upward of 15 to 20 sessions for longer term, sustainable therapeutic effects. This dose effect may not be applicable to counseling services with primarily informational or emotional/supportive functions. Also, long-term therapy should be evaluated at 6- to 12-month intervals to determine efficacy.

MEDICATION

- Psychotherapy is most likely to be accompanied by use of pharmaceutical adjuncts in moderate to severe cases of psychological dysfunction that do not respond to other therapies or in cases of extremely poor quality of life or high risk. The most common examples are in cases of clinical depression or anxiety that clearly incapacitates the patient or significantly reduces his or her quality of life. Patients at risk for suicide or who represent a danger to others are also candidates for acute psychopharmacotherapy. Studies suggest that verbal and behaviorally oriented therapies can add efficacy to medication treatment in both depression and anxiety.
- There is controversy in the research field regarding the efficacy of medication alone versus psychotherapy alone versus combined treatments. The most recent consensus has been that combined treatments in moderate to severe psychological dysfunction are most likely to render positive short-term results and increase the likelihood that such effects can be sustained over time.

ADDITIONAL THERAPIES

- Anxiety disorders
  - Panic disorder with and without agoraphobia: CBT, psychodynamic therapy
  - Generalized anxiety disorder: CBT
  - Obsessive-compulsive disorder: CBT
  - Posttraumatic stress disorder: CBT
  - Specific phobia: CBT
  - Social phobia: CBT
- Mood disorders
  - Unipolar depression: CBT, interpersonal therapy, psychodynamic therapy
  - Bipolar disorder: family therapy, interpersonal therapy, CBT
  - Schizophrenia: psychodynamic therapy, family therapy, CBT
- Eating disorders
  - Binge eating disorder: CBT, interpersonal therapy
  - Bulimia nervosa: CBT, interpersonal therapy
- Personality disorders
  - Borderline: DBT, CBT
- Substance-use disorders
  - Alcohol: counseling, CBT, motivational interviewing
  - Cocaine: CBT, counseling
  - Heroin: CBT, counseling
  - Smoking: 5 A's
- Somatoform disorders:
  - Hypochondriasis: CBT
  - Body dysmorphic disorder: CBT

COMPLEMENTARY & ALTERNATIVE MEDICINE

A host of nonempirically based psychological and nutritional therapies can be found outside of mainstream medicine and psychological science. Very little or no evidence exists to support such experimental therapies, but all have the considerable power of the placebo effect fueling their anecdotal supports or claims. Placebo effects are also thought to be powerfully enhanced by the use of ingested or applied substances that create real physiologic, although not therapeutic, changes in the patient. If it makes them feel different, they are more likely to believe it helps.

 ONGOING CARE

FOLLOW-UP RECOMMENDATIONS

Patient Monitoring

There is evidence of a "dose effect" in psychotherapy outcomes research, with some investigators suggesting that 6 to 8 sessions are necessary to yield positive initial effects and upward of 15 to 20 sessions for longer term, sustainable therapeutic effects. This dose effect may not be applicable to counseling services with primarily informational or emotional/supportive functions. Because many patients cease attendance to psychotherapy sessions after one or a few sessions, most interventions of this type cannot be accurately evaluated by the referring provider. Long-term therapy should also be evaluated for effectiveness at regular periods.

REFERENCES

1. American Psychiatric Association. *Diagnostic and Statistical Manual of Mental Disorders*. 5th ed. Arlington, VA: American Psychiatric Association; 2013.
2. World Health Organization. *The ICD-10 Classification of Mental and Behavioural Disorders: Clinical Descriptions and Diagnostic Guidelines*. Geneva, Switzerland: World Health Organization; 1992.

ADDITIONAL READING

- Bortolotti B, Menchetti M, Bellini F, et al. Psychological interventions for major depression in primary care: a meta-analytic review of randomized controlled trials. *Gen Hosp Psychiatry*. 2008;30(4): 293–302.
- Eddy KT, Dutra L, Bradley R, et al. A multidimensional meta-analysis of psychotherapy and pharmacotherapy for obsessive-compulsive disorder. *Clin Psychol Rev*. 2004;24(8):1011–1030.
- Furukawa TA, Watanabe N, Churchill R. Combined psychotherapy plus antidepressants for panic disorder with or without agoraphobia. *Cochrane Database Syst Rev*. 2007;(1):CD004364.
- Hunot V, Churchill R, Silva de Lima M, et al. Psychological therapies for generalised anxiety disorder. *Cochrane Database Syst Rev*. 2007;(1):CD001848.

 CODES

ICD10

- Z71.9 Counseling, unspecified
- Z71.89 Other specified counseling
- Z63.9 Problem related to primary support group, unspecified

CLINICAL PEARLS

- Combined medication and psychotherapeutic treatments in moderate to severe psychological dysfunction are most likely to render positive short-term results and increase the likelihood such effects can be sustained over time.
- Relapse is common over time and/or as treatments are discontinued.
- Children <10 years may benefit significantly from counseling or psychotherapy alone for symptom relief.
- Older children and those with more severe symptoms typically require psychopharmacologic options in concert with counseling or verbal therapy approaches.

CROHN DISEASE

Eric Ji-Yuan Mao, MD • Samir A. Shah, MD, FACG, FASGE, AGAF

 BASICS

DESCRIPTION

A chronic, relapsing inflammatory GI tract disorder, most commonly involving the terminal ileum (80%)

- Hallmark features
  - Transmural inflammation which can result in fibrosis, stricture formation, and fissures leading to sinus tracts, abscesses, or fistulas.
  - Noncaseating granulomas (30%), crypt abscesses
  - Skip lesions: patchy, segmental distribution of disease; lesions may affect multiple bowel segments, interspersed with areas of normal mucosa; disease can also be continuous, potentially mimicking ulcerative colitis (UC).
  - Diverse presentations: ileocolitis (50%); isolated colitis (20%) are most common. In cases of isolated colitis, 10% involve the rectum and 33% involve the anorectal area.
- Early disease
  - Ulcerations: focal lesions with surrounding edema, resembling aphthous ulcers
  - Perianal disease (pain, anal fissures, perirectal abscess) may precede intestinal disease.
  - May present as wasting illness or anorexia
- Developed disease
  - Mucosal cobblestoning; luminal stenosis; creeping fat; fissures between mucosal folds result in strictures/adhesions and/or fistulae

EPIDEMIOLOGY

Incidence

- In North America, 8 to 15 cases/100,000 adults; incidence is rising in North America and Western Europe.
- Bimodal age distribution: Predominant age is 15 to 25 years, with a second smaller peak at 50 to 70 years.
- Women slightly more affected than men; increased incidence in northern climates
- Increased risk in whites versus non-whites: 2 to 5 times
- Increased risk in Ashkenazi Jews: 3 to 5 times

Prevalence

U.S. adults: 100 to 200 cases/100,000

ETIOLOGY AND PATHOPHYSIOLOGY

- General: Clinical manifestations result from activation of inflammatory cells, whose by-products produce nonspecific tissue injury.
- Mechanism of diarrhea: excess fluid secretion and impaired fluid absorption; bile salt malabsorption in inflamed ileum, with steatorrhea, bacterial overgrowth
- Multifactorial: Genetic, environmental triggers, and immunologic abnormalities result in inflammation and tissue injury in genetically predisposed individuals.

Genetics

Of CD patients, 15% have a first-degree relative with inflammatory bowel disease (IBD); first-degree relative of an IBD patient has 3 to 30 times increased risk of developing IBD by age 28 years. At least 163 different genes associated with IBD.

- Mutations in susceptibility loci
  - Ileal CD: IBD1 gene (chromosome 16)
  - Early-onset CD (age ≤15 years): mutations in 5q31-33 (IBD5), 21q22, and 20q13
  - North American white men with CD: 30% have HLA-DR7 and DQ4.

- Extraintestinal manifestations of CD: mutations in HLA-A2, HLA-DR1, HLA-DQw5
- Others: IL-10, IL-23 receptors; ATG16L1; IRGM
- Genetic syndromes associated with IBD: Turner and Hermansky-Pudlak syndromes, glycogen storage disease type 1b

RISK FACTORS

- Environmental factors
  - Cigarette smoking doubles the risk of developing CD; tobacco cessation may reduce frequency of flares and reduce relapses after surgery.
  - Dietary factors: higher incidence if diet high in refined sugars, animal fat, protein (meat, fish)
  - *Salmonella* or *Campylobacter* increase risk of developing IBD
  - *Clostridium difficile* infection may trigger flare of IBD and make treatment more difficult.
- Immunologic abnormalities: an aggressive immune response against commensal enteric bacteria
  - Tumor necrosis factor (TNF): upregulation of inflammatory Th1 cytokines
  - Tissue inflammation may result from increased secretion of cytokine IL-17 by Th17 subset of CD4+ T cells.

COMMONLY ASSOCIATED CONDITIONS

- Extraintestinal manifestations
  - Arthritis (20%): seronegative, primarily involving large joints; axial arthritis or ankylosing spondylitis (AS), and sacroiliitis (SI).
  - Skin disorders (10%): erythema nodosum, pyoderma gangrenosum, psoriasis
  - Ocular disease (5%): uveitis, iritis, episcleritis
  - Kidney stones: calcium oxalate stones (from steatorrhea and diarrhea) or uric acid stones (from dehydration and metabolic acidosis)
  - Fat-soluble vitamin deficiency (A, D, E, K), B_{12}
  - Osteopenia and osteoporosis; hypocalcemia
  - Hypercoagulability: venous thromboembolism prophylaxis essential in hospitalized patients
  - Gallstones: cholesterol stones resulting from impaired bile acid reabsorption
  - Primary sclerosing cholangitis (5%): more common in men with UC; asymptomatic, elevated alkaline phosphatase as marker
  - Autoimmune hemolytic anemia
- Conditions correlated with increased disease activity
  - Peripheral arthropathy (but not SI and AS)
  - Episcleritis (but not uveitis)
  - Oral aphthous ulcers and erythema nodosum
  - SI, AS, and uveitis are associated with HLA-B27.
- Other significant complications: GI bleed, toxic megacolon, bowel perforation/peritonitis, malignancy, sclerosing cholangitis, rectovaginal fistula

 DIAGNOSIS

HISTORY

Hallmarks: fatigue, fever, weight loss, prolonged diarrhea, perianal disease, crampy abdominal pain, with or without gross bleeding. Children may present with failure to thrive.

- Factors exacerbating CD: concurrent infection, smoking, NSAIDs, and possibly stress

PHYSICAL EXAM

Presentation varies with location of disease.

- General: signs of sepsis/disease activity (fever, tachycardia, hypotension) or wasting/malnutrition
- Abdominal: focal or diffuse tenderness, distension, rebound/guarding; rectal bleeding

- Perianal: fistulae, fissures
- Skin: erythema nodosum; psoriasis

DIFFERENTIAL DIAGNOSIS

- Acute, severe abdominal pain: perforated viscus, pancreatitis, appendicitis, diverticulitis, bowel obstruction, kidney stones, ovarian torsion
- Chronic diarrhea with crampy pain (colitis-like): UC, radiation colitis, infection, drugs, ischemia, microscopic colitis, IBD, celiac disease, malignancy (lymphoma, carcinoma), carcinoid
- Wasting illness: malabsorption, malignancy, psychiatric illness

DIAGNOSTIC TESTS & INTERPRETATION

Initial Tests (lab, imaging)

- CBC, chem 10, LFTs, erythrocyte sedimentation rate, C-reactive protein, serum iron, vitamin B_{12}, vitamin D-25 OH
- If diarrhea, stool specimen for routine culture, fecal leukocytes, *C. difficile*, and ova and parasites
- In hospitalized patients with severe flare-ups, KUB to rule out toxic megacolon
- Colonoscopy with ileoscopy provides the greatest diagnostic sensitivity and specificity for colonic disease.
- Small bowel: sensitivity of CT or magnetic resonance enterography (MRE) better than small bowel follow through. MRE has no radiation exposure (important in younger patients). Capsule endoscopy allows small bowel visualization but no biopsy (1)[A].

  - Signs of small bowel disease: narrowed lumen with nodularity and/or string sign; cobblestone appearance, fistula and abscess formation, bowel loop separation (transmural inflammation)
- Gastroduodenal: upper GI endoscopy
  - Signs of gastroduodenal disease: antral narrowing and segmental duodenal stricturing; inflammatory mucosal disease on endoscopy
- Perirectal complications: combination of endoscopic ultrasound (EUS) or MRI with exam under anesthesia
- Contraindications to endoscopy: perforated viscus, recent myocardial infarction, severe diverticulitis, toxic megacolon, or inability to undergo appropriate bowel preparation. In most cases, unprepared limited sigmoidoscopy allows adequate visualization to assess severity, extent, and aspirate stool for *C. difficile*, obtain biopsies to assess histologic severity, and exclude other disorders (e.g., cytomegalovirus).

Follow-Up Tests & Special Considerations

Evidence of complications

- Stricture: obstructive signs such as nausea, vomiting, pain, weight loss, diarrhea, or inability to pass gas/feces
- Abscess/phlegmon: localized abdominal peritonitis with fever and abdominal pain; diffuse peritonitis suggests intestinal perforation or abscess rupture (may be masked by steroids, opiates).
- Fistulae (33–50% of patients, after 10 to 20 years of disease, respectively)
  - Enteroenteric: asymptomatic or a palpable, commonly indolent abdominal mass
  - Enterovesical: pneumaturia, recurrent polymicrobial UTI
  - Retroperitoneal: psoas abscess, ureteral obstruction
  - Enterovaginal: vaginal passage of gas or feces; clear, nonfeculent drainage from ileal fistula may be misdiagnosed as primary vaginal infection.

Diagnostic Procedures/Other
How to distinguish CD from UC
- CD: small bowel disease, rectal sparing; skip lesions; granulomas, perianal disease, and/or fistulae; no gross bleeding: RLQ pain is common.
  - Commercially available antibody tests (overall 70% sensitive): anti-Saccharomyces cerevisiae antibody (ASCA), Cbir-1, OmpC, I2
- UC: diffuse, continuous involving the rectum; loss of vascularity, friable tissue; perinuclear antineutrophil cytoplasmic antibody (pANCA); LLQ pain; typically only affects colon; rectal bleeding common

ALERT
CD can mimic UC with continuous bowel involvement; 10–15% of cases are difficult to differentiate; diagnosed as IBD unclassified (IBD-U).

 # TREATMENT

- Disease severity: Crohn Disease Activity Index (CDAI)
  - Asymptomatic: spontaneously, after medical/surgical intervention, or while on steroids (CDAI <150)
  - Mild to moderate CD: ambulatory patients able to tolerate PO intake without dehydration, obstruction, or >10% weight loss. No abdominal tenderness, toxicity, or mass (CDAI 150 to 220)
  - Moderate to severe CD: Patients who have failed initial treatment or who continue to have mild symptoms such as fever, weight loss, and abdominal pain (CDAI 220 to 450).
  - Severe: persistent symptoms despite outpatient therapy with glucocorticoids and/or biologics, or fulminant disease (peritonitis, cachexia, intestinal obstruction, abscess) (CDAI >450)
- General strategies
  - Step-up approach: Begin treatment with milder therapy (5-ASA, antibiotics) followed by more aggressive agents (steroids, immunomodulators, anti-TNF agents), as needed.
  - Top-down approach: Early management with immunomodulators and/or anti-TNF agents before patients receive steroids, become steroid-dependent, or require surgery.

GENERAL MEASURES
Additional therapies depend on location of disease.
- Oral lesions: triamcinolone acetonide in benzocaine and carboxymethyl cellulose or topical sucralfate for aphthous ulcers, cheilitis, and/or granulomatous sialadenitis
- Gastroduodenal CD: no clinical trials, although slow-release mesalamine may be beneficial, as it is partially released in proximal small bowel. Case reports note success of anti-TNF therapies. Symptomatic relief possible from proton pump inhibitors, H_2-receptor blockers, and/or sucralfate.
- Ileitis: supplementation of fat-soluble vitamins, iron, B_{12}, folate, and calcium to prevent bone loss
- Treatment toxicity: pancreatitis, bone marrow toxicity, lymphoma, nonmelanoma skin cancer, infections (TB, histoplasmosis, others), malignancy

MEDICATION
First Line
- Asymptomatic patients: observation alone
- Mild CD
  - 5-Aminosalicylates have minimal role in CD management. They can be used for colonic CD without deep ulcerations or penetration/fibrostenosing disease (2)[C].

- Antibiotics use is controversial. Controlled trials have not consistently demonstrated efficacy (2)[C].
- Glucocorticoid therapy: controlled ileal release budesonide (9 mg/day for 8 to 16 weeks, then discontinued over 2- to 4-week taper) for distal ileum and/or right colon involvement (2,3)[A]
- Consider adjunctive therapy: antidiarrheals (loperamide); bile acid-binding resin (cholestyramine 4 to 12 g/day); probiotics (either alone or in combination may prevent recurrent inflammation and reduce symptoms in acute CD).
- Induction/maintenance: 5-ASA is not recommended (3)[C]. Controlled ileal release budesonide, 9 mg/day, is effective for maintenance for up to 6 months (2)[A].
- Moderate to severe CD
  - Induction: prednisone 40 to 60 mg/day (2)[A] or controlled-release budesonide (for isolated, moderate ileitis) or anti-TNF agents as initial induction agent or for lack of response to corticosteroid or immunomodulator (2,3)[A]
  - Maintenance: no role for mesalamine. If steroids required for induction, use immunomodulator (2,3)[B] or biologic (anti-TNF agent) (2)[A],(3)[B] for maintenance.
  - Except for budesonide, do not use steroids for maintenance (1)[A].
- Severe disease: immunomodulators, anti-TNF agents ± steroids
  - Azathioprine or 6-mercaptopurine: thiopurine methyltransferase (TPMT) and LFTs prior to initiation. Check CBC/LFTs q2–3mo.
  - Methotrexate: effective for steroid-dependent and steroid-refractory CD (2)[B]
    ○ Folic acid 1 mg/day; follow LFTs
  - Anti-TNF therapies: active disease, fistulae, steroid sparing, some extraintestinal disease. Infliximab, adalimumab, certolizumab pegol
    ○ Check for evidence of TB and HBV infection prior to initiation of anti-TNF therapy.
    ○ Avoid live vaccines.
    ○ Monitoring: Consider anti-drug Ab levels to assess for immunogenicity. Serum concentrations of anti-TNF agents may also correlate with disease activity.
- Combination therapy
  - Azathioprine + infliximab is more effective than either alone if no previously treatment with either.
  - Rare complication: hepatosplenic T-cell lymphoma (fatal, mostly seen in young males)
- Anti-adhesion molecules: prevent inflammatory cells from entering GI tract
  - Vedolizumab: gut-specific, can be used in anti-TNF failures or anti-TNF naive patients as induction and maintenance; given IV, no risk of progressive multifocal leukoencephalopathy (PML); FDA approved May 2014
  - Natalizumab: non–gut-specific, PML risk (1/1,000). Can minimize risk by testing for John Cunningham (JC) virus antibody. However, can avoid risk of PML now with vedolizumab.

ADDITIONAL THERAPIES
Complications
- Peritonitis: bowel rest and antibiotic therapy (7 to 10 days parenteral antibiotics, followed by 2- to 4-week course of PO ciprofloxacin and metronidazole); surgery, as indicated
  - Consider holding steroids which mask sepsis.

- Abscess: antibiotics, percutaneous drainage, or surgery with resection of affected segments
- Small bowel obstruction: IV hydration, nasogastric (NG) suction, total parenteral nutrition (TPN) for malnutrition, resolution typically in 24 to 48 hours. Surgery for nonresponders

 ## ONGOING CARE

FOLLOW-UP RECOMMENDATIONS
Patient Monitoring
Vaccinations in CD
- Check titers; avoid live vaccines (MMR, varicella, zoster) in patients on immunosuppressive therapy (steroids, 6MP, AZA, MTX, or anti-TNF).
- Regardless of immunosuppression: HPV, influenza, pneumococcal, meningococcal, hepatitis A, B; Tdap

PATIENT EDUCATION
Crohn and Colitis Foundation of America (800) 343-3637; www.ccfa.org

REFERENCES
1. Baumgart DC, Sandborn WJ. Crohn's disease. *Lancet*. 2012;380(9853):1590–1605.
2. Lichtenstein GR, Hanauer SB, Sandborn WJ, et al. Management of Crohn's disease in adults. *Am J Gastroenterol*. 2009;104(2):465–483.
3. Talley NJ, Abreu MT, Achkar JP, et al. An evidence-based systematic review on medical therapies for inflammatory bowel disease. *Am J Gastroenterol*. 2011;106(Suppl 1):S2–S25.

ADDITIONAL READING
Bernstein CN. Treatment of IBD: where we are and where we are going. *Am J Gastroenterol*. 2015; 110(1):114–126.

CODES

ICD10
- K50.919 Crohn's disease, unspecified, with unspecified complications
- K50.00 Crohn's disease of small intestine without complications
- K50.10 Crohn's disease of large intestine without complications

CLINICAL PEARLS
- The incidence of CD has risen over the past 4 decades.
- MRE allows assessment of luminal and extraluminal CD without radiation exposure.
- Assess for TB and HBV infection prior to initiating anti-TNF therapy.
- Cigarette smoking doubles the risk of developing CD; tobacco cessation may reduce frequency of flares and need for surgery.
- Test for *C. difficile* infection when evaluating diarrhea in all CD patients.
- Hospitalized CD patients require deep vein thrombosis prophylaxis.

CROUP (LARYNGOTRACHEOBRONCHITIS)

Garreth C. Debiegun, MD, FACEP, FAWM

 BASICS

DESCRIPTION

- Croup is a subacute viral illness characterized by upper airway symptoms such as barking cough, stridor, and fever. "Croup" is used to refer to viral laryngotracheitis or laryngotracheobronchitis (LTB), although it is sometimes used for LTB with pneumonitis, bacterial tracheitis, or spasmodic croup.
- Most common cause of upper airway obstruction or stridor in children
- Spasmodic croup: noninfectious form with sudden resolution
  - No fever or radiographic changes
  - Initially treated as croup
  - Usually self-limiting and resolves with mist therapy at home
  - Often recurs on same night or in 2 to 3 nights
- System(s) affected: pulmonary, respiratory
- Synonym(s): infectious croup; viral croup

EPIDEMIOLOGY

- Predominant age
  - Common among children 7 months to 3 years
  - Most common during the 2nd year of life
  - Rare among those >6 years
- Predominant sex: male > female (1.5:1)
- Timing
  - Possible during any time of year but is most common in autumn and winter (with parainfluenza 1 and respiratory syncytial virus [RSV])

Incidence

- Six cases per year per 100 children <6 years old
- 1.5–6% of cases require hospitalization.
- 2–6% of those require intubation.
- Decreasing incidence in the United States and Canada

ETIOLOGY AND PATHOPHYSIOLOGY

- Subglottic region/larynx is entirely encircled by the cricoid cartilage.
- Inflammatory edema and subglottic mucus production decrease airway radius.
- Small children have small airways with more compliant walls.
- Negative-pressure inspiration pulls airway walls closer together.
- Small decrease in airway radius causes significant increase in resistance (Poiseuille law: resistance proportional to $1/radius^4$).
- Usually viruses that initially infect oropharyngeal mucosa and then migrate inferiorly
- Parainfluenza virus
  - Most common pathogen: 75% of cases
  - Type 1 is the most common, causing 18% of all cases of croup.
  - Types 2, 3, and 4 are also common.
  - Type 3 may cause a particularly severe illness.
- Other viruses: RSV, paramyxovirus, influenza virus type A or B, adenovirus, rhinovirus, enteroviruses (coxsackie and echo), reovirus, measles virus where vaccination not common, and metapneumovirus
- *Haemophilus influenzae* type B now rare with routine immunization
- May have bacterial cause: *Mycoplasma pneumoniae* has been reported.

RISK FACTORS

- History of croup
- Recurrent upper respiratory infections
- Atopic disease increases the risk of spasmodic croup.

COMMONLY ASSOCIATED CONDITIONS

- If recurrent (>2 episodes in a year) or during first 90 days of life, consider host factors.
- Underlying anatomic abnormality (e.g., subglottic stenosis)
  - In one study, found to be present in 59% children with recurrent croup
- Paradoxical vocal cord dysfunction
- Gastroesophageal reflux disease
- Neonatal intubation

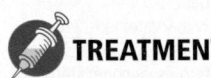 **DIAGNOSIS**

- Most children who present with acute onset of barky cough, stridor, and chest wall indrawing have croup.
- Croup is a clinical diagnosis; lab tests and imaging serve only ancillary purposes.
- Classic "seal-like" barking, spasmodic cough
- May have biphasic stridor
- Low- to moderate-grade fever
- Upper respiratory infection prodrome lasting 1 to 7 days
- Severity usually is determined by clinical observation for signs of respiratory effort: nasal flaring, retractions, tripoding, sniffing position, abdominal breathing, and tachypnea. Later symptoms: hypoxia/cyanosis or fatigue
- Westley croup score (≤2 mild; 3 to 7 moderate; ≥8 severe), most useful for research purposes
  - Level of consciousness: normal, including sleep, 0; disoriented, 5
  - Cyanosis: none, 0; with agitation, 4; at rest, 5
  - Stridor: none, 0; with agitation, 1; at rest, 2
  - Air entry: normal, 0; decreased, 1; markedly decreased, 2
  - Retractions: none, 0; mild, 1; moderate, 2; severe, 2
- No change in stridor with positioning
- Nontender larynx
- Inflamed subglottic region with normal-appearing supraglottic region
- Differentiate from epiglottitis: non-toxic-appearing, normal voice, no drooling, is coughing (1).

HISTORY

- 2 to 3 days of nonspecific prodromal syndrome with low-grade fever, coryza, and rhinorrhea
- Onset and recurrence at night when child is sleeping
- Symptoms often resolve en route to the hospital, as the child is exposed to cool night air.
- Lack of prodrome indicates spasmodic croup.

PHYSICAL EXAM

- Pulse oximetry often is normal because there is no disturbance of alveolar gas exchange.
- Overall appearance: Is the child comfortable or struggling?
- Work of breathing: labored or comfortable?
- Sound of breathing and voice: hoarse, stridor, inspiratory wheezing, short sentences?
- Observed/subjective tidal volume: sufficient for child's size?

DIFFERENTIAL DIAGNOSIS

- Epiglottitis: currently rare
- Foreign body aspiration
- Subglottic stenosis (congenital or acquired)
- Bacterial tracheitis
- Simple upper respiratory infection
- Retropharyngeal or peritonsillar abscess
- Trauma
- Allergic reaction (acute angioneurotic edema)
- Airway anomalies (e.g., tracheo-/laryngomalacia)
- Other anatomic obstructions: subglottic hemangioma, subglottic cyst

DIAGNOSTIC TESTS & INTERPRETATION

- No laboratory abnormality is diagnostic.
- WBCs may be low, normal, or elevated.
- Lymphocytosis is expected but not required.
- Rapid antigen or viral culture tests are available in some centers.
  - Guide isolation precautions, not management.

Initial Tests (lab, imaging)

- Posteroanterior and lateral neck films show funnel-shaped subglottic region with normal epiglottis: "steeple," "hourglass," or "pencil point" sign (present in 40–60% of children with LTB).
- CT may be more sensitive for defining obstruction in a confusing clinical picture.
- Patient should be monitored during imaging; airway obstruction may occur rapidly.

Test Interpretation

- Inflammatory reaction of respiratory mucosa
- Loss of epithelial cells
- Thick mucoid secretions

TREATMENT

GENERAL MEASURES

- Minimize lab tests, imaging, and procedures that upset the child; agitation worsens tachypnea and can be more detrimental than accepting a clinical diagnosis.
- ECG monitoring and pulse oximetry
  - Frequent checks are more sensitive to worsening disease than is pulse oximetry.

MEDICATION

First Line

- Well established in the literature; cornerstones of treatment are immediate nebulized epinephrine and dexamethasone.
- Racemic or L-epinephrine (Equal efficacy and side effect profiles; L-epinephrine is used for most other hospital purposes and is less expensive.) (2)[A]
  - Reserved for more severe cases with stridor at rest
  - Racemic epinephrine: 0.05 mL/kg/dose (max 0.5 mL) of 2.25% solution nebulized in normal saline to total volume of 3 mL
  - L-epinephrine: 0.5 mL/kg/dose (max 5 mL) of a 1:1,000 dilution nebulized

- Onset in 1 to 5 minutes, duration of 2 hours
- Repeat as necessary if side effects are tolerated.
- Observe child for 2 hours to ensure no recurrence after epinephrine wears off.
- Corticosteroids
  - Dexamethasone (least expensive, easiest), 0.15–0.6 mg/kg; higher doses have been traditional care, but studies have shown 0.15 mg/kg has equal efficacy (3)[B]. Single dose; IV/IM/PO has proven equal efficacy.
  - Randomized controlled trials show this begins to improve symptoms within 30 minutes (4)[A]; full effect by 4 hours
  - Other steroids (betamethasone, budesonide (5)[A], prednisolone) are beneficial; there may be minimal superiority of dexamethasone; also, dexamethasone carries benefit of single-dose administration (6,7)[A].
- Heliox: a helium–oxygen mixture
  - Smaller, lower mass helium molecule (compared with nitrogen) theoretically maintains laminar flow in narrower airways and serves as bridge therapy to steroids.
  - Minimum of 60% helium must be used; 70% is preferable; 79% if patient has no oxygen requirement.
  - Limited data; a Cochrane review found no benefit in mild cases but likely benefit in moderate to severe croup as a bridge to steroid effect (8)[A].
- Antibiotics are not indicated in this viral illness.
  - Antecedent or subsequent bacterial infection is possible but uncommon.
- Oxygen as needed
- Humidified air shows no clinical benefit.

Second Line
Oseltamivir for influenza A

SURGERY
- Intubation rarely is required; tube 0.5 to 1 mm smaller than normal.
  - After trial of medical management, intubation is for fatigue caused by work of breathing or beginning total obstruction; not secondary to low oxygen saturation
  - Extubate in 3 to 5 days when there is an appropriate air leak around the endotracheal tube.
- Tracheotomy: rarely; maintenance 3 to 7 days

COMPLEMENTARY & ALTERNATIVE MEDICINE
- Although proven no benefit in hospital, may be helpful at home. Do not use high-temperature misters (e.g., teakettles) because of a risk of burns. A hot shower running in a bathroom is a good steam generator.
- Some children respond well to cold, dry air.
- Probiotics may decrease the incidence of upper respiratory tract infections (9)[A].

INPATIENT CONSIDERATIONS
Admission Criteria/Initial Stabilization
- Minor cases need no visit to a hospital or primary care physician (PCP).
- Outpatient care in mild cases
- Admit patients who do not respond to therapy or have recurrent stridor at rest after epinephrine wears off. Also admit those who have oxygen requirement, pneumonia, or congestive heart failure.
- In most cases, observation in the ED after medical management is sufficient.

Discharge Criteria
- >2 hours since last epinephrine
- No stridor at rest, no difficulty breathing
- Child able to tolerate liquids PO
- No underlying medical condition
- Caretakers able to assess changes to clinical picture and reaccess medical care

 ## ONGOING CARE

FOLLOW-UP RECOMMENDATIONS
Patient Monitoring
Most patients will be seen in an ED or PCP office setting.

DIET
- NPO and IV fluids for severe cases
- Frequent small feedings with increased fluids for mild cases

PATIENT EDUCATION
- Must keep the patient quiet; crying may exacerbate symptoms.
- Educate parents about when to seek emergency care if mild cases progress.
- Provide emotional support and reassurance for the patient.

PROGNOSIS
- Up to 1/3 of patients will have a recurrence.
- Recovery is usually full and without lasting effects.
- If multiple recurrences, consider referral to ENT specialist to evaluate for possible anatomic etiology.

COMPLICATIONS
- Rare
- Subglottic stenosis in intubated patients
- Bacterial tracheitis
- Cardiopulmonary arrest
- Pneumonia

REFERENCES

1. Tibballs J, Watson T. Symptoms and signs differentiating croup and epiglottitis. *J Paediatr Child Health*. 2011;47(3):77–82.
2. Bjornson C, Russell KF, Vandermeer B, et al. Nebulized epinephrine for croup in children. *Cochrane Database Syst Rev*. 2013;10:CD006619.
3. Dobrovoljac M, Geelhoed GC. 27 years of croup: an update highlighting the effectiveness of 0.15 mg/kg of dexamethasone. *Emerg Med Australas*. 2009;21(4):309–314.
4. Dobrovoljac, Geelhoed GC. How fast does oral dexamethasone work in mild to moderately severe croup? A randomized double-blinded clinical trial. *Emerg Med Australas*. 2012;24(1):79–85.
5. Cetinkaya F, Tüfekçi BS, Kutluk G. A comparison of nebulized budesonide, and intramuscular, and oral dexamethasone for treatment of croup. *Int J Pediatr Otorhinolaryngol*. 2004;68(4):453–456.
6. Russell KF, Liang Y, O'Gorman K, et al. Glucocorticoids for croup. *Cochrane Database Syst Rev*. 2011;(1):CD001955.
7. Garbutt JM, Conlon B, Sterkel R, et al. The comparative effectiveness of prednisolone and dexamethasone for children with croup: a community-based randomized trial. *Clin Pediatr (Phila)*. 2013;52(11):1014–1021.
8. Moraa I, Sturman N, McGuire T, et al. Heliox for croup in children. *Cochrane Database Syst Rev*. 2013;(12):CD006822.
9. Hao Q, Lu Z, Dong BR, et al. Probiotics for preventing acute upper respiratory tract infections. *Cochrane Database Syst Rev*. 2011;(9):CD006895.

ADDITIONAL READING
- Bjornson CL, Johnson DW. Croup. *Lancet*. 2008;371(9609):329–339.
- Cherry JD. Clinical practice. Croup. *N Engl J Med*. 2008;358(4):384–391.

 ## SEE ALSO

Bronchiolitis; Epiglottitis; Tracheitis, Bacterial

 ## CODES

ICD10
- J05.0 Acute obstructive laryngitis [croup]
- J20.9 Acute bronchitis, unspecified
- J38.5 Laryngeal spasm

CLINICAL PEARLS
- Parainfluenza virus is the most common pathogen but caused by many viruses.
- Nebulized epinephrine only for stridor at rest
- Dexamethasone 0.6 mg/kg PO × 1
- Lateral neck films show funnel-shaped subglottic region with normal epiglottis: "steeple," "hourglass," or "pencil point" sign (present in 40–60% of children with LTB).

C

CRYPTOGENIC ORGANIZING PNEUMONIA

Roselyn Jan Wuthrich Clemente-Fuentes, MD • Merima Bucaj, DO

 BASICS

DESCRIPTION

- Cryptogenic organizing pneumonia or COP (previously known as bronchiolitis obliterans organizing pneumonia or BOOP) is a primary (cryptogenic) or secondary process of the lungs characterized by granulation-like tissue involving the distal airways and alveoli.
- COP is a restrictive problem that is completely reversible.
- A specific reaction of lung tissue to a variety of injuries, but exact pathogenesis is unknown
- It may occur as patchy infiltrates, or it may be nodular or secondary to another lung disease.
- May also appear to be a migrating process
- May have a gradual or sudden onset.
- Lungs show a pattern of multiple patchy pneumonia, which are seen on the chest x-ray (CXR) as patchy alveolar or ground glass opacifications, with or without interstitial infiltrates; there may be air bronchograms as well.
- Most cases will respond to corticosteroids, which may have to be given for a year or more.
- Synonym(s): bronchiolitis obliterans organizing pneumonia; intraluminal fibrosis of distal airways; idiopathic BOOP; obliterative bronchiolitis

Geriatric Considerations
More common than originally thought and may be sudden and very severe

Pediatric Considerations
Rare but has been reported after viral pneumonia

EPIDEMIOLOGY
- Incidence/prevalence in the United States: estimated at 0.01% but may be underdiagnosed
- Predominant age: reported cases range age 0 to 70 years; most commonly seen in age 40s to 60s

Prevalence
Unknown

ETIOLOGY AND PATHPHYSIOLOGY
Idiopathic: a complex response to a variety of injuries such as toxic inhalation, postmycoplasma, viral and bacterial infection, aspiration, immunologic factors, drugs

Genetics
No known genetic component

RISK FACTORS
- Immunocompromised patients, including transplant recipients and AIDS patients
- Other autoimmune conditions
- Reported frequency of tobacco use in diagnosed cases 25–50%, making smoking unlikely to be a precipitating factor

GENERAL PREVENTION
Except for prevention of relapse, none known

ASSOCIATED CONDITIONS
- Drug-induced pneumonitis
  - Paraquat poisoning
  - Amiodarone toxicity
  - Acebutolol toxicity
  - Amphotericin B
- β-Blockers
  - Bleomycin
  - Carbamazepine
  - Cephalosporins
  - Gold
  - Minocycline
  - Nitrofurantoin
  - Phenytoin
  - Sulfamethoxypyridazine
  - Sulfasalazine
  - Ticlopidine
- Antineoplastic agents
  - Freebase cocaine pulmonary toxicity
  - Overdose of L-tryptophan
- Infections
  - Chronic infectious pneumonia
  - Malaria
  - Chlamydia
  - Legionella
  - Mycoplasma
  - Pneumocystis
  - Cryptococcus
- Immunocompromised (AIDS or bone marrow, lung, renal transplantation)
- Malignancy: colon, breast, lymphoma
- Bronchial obstruction (lack of mucociliary clearance), which is lung cancer
- Connective tissue diseases
  - COP itself is an autoimmune connective tissue disorder, so autoimmune connective tissue disorders confer a higher risk of acquiring the disease.
  - Rheumatoid arthritis
  - Sjögren syndrome
  - Polymyositis
  - Scleroderma
  - Essential mixed cryoglobulinemia
  - Wegener granulomatosis
- Miscellaneous
  - Cystic fibrosis
  - Bronchopulmonary dysplasia
  - Renal failure
  - Congestive heart failure (CHF)
  - Adult respiratory distress syndrome (ARDS)
- Idiopathic pulmonary fibrosis
  - Chronic eosinophilic pneumonia
  - Hypersensitivity pneumonitis
  - Histiocytosis X
  - Sarcoidosis
  - Pneumoconioses
- Radiation pneumonitis

DIAGNOSIS

Consider differential in patients presenting with

- Flulike illness that lasts 4 to 10 weeks or longer. Most have been treated with empiric antibiotics without success.
- Fatigue, fever, and weight loss >10 lbs
- Persistent nonproductive cough
- Dyspnea may be severe.
- Bilateral crackles

HISTORY
- Fatigue/malaise
- Fever/chills
- Weight loss
- Dry cough
- Dyspnea
- No improvement after multiple courses of antibiotics
- Other symptoms suggestive of connective tissue disease such as joint pain, dry eyes/mucus membranes, etc.
- A history of exposure to new medication, radiation, and other environmental exposures that may predispose

PHYSICAL EXAM
- Hypoxia
- Cyanosis
- Respiratory distress
- Bilateral crackles
- Wheezing
- Dry cough
- Shortness of breath
- Rarely: hemoptysis, respiratory distress

DIFFERENTIAL DIAGNOSIS
- Usual interstitial pneumonitis
- Noninfectious diseases
- Tuberculosis
- Sarcoidosis
- Histoplasmosis
- Berylliosis
- Goodpasture syndrome
- Neoplasm
- Polyarteritis nodosa
- Systemic lupus erythematosus
- Wegener granulomatosis
- Sjögren syndrome
- Chronic eosinophilic pneumonia
- Cryptogenic bronchiolitis

DIAGNOSTIC TESTS & INTERPRETATION
- May have normal or nonspecific laboratory findings
- Leukocytosis with a normal differential
- Elevated ESR/CRP
- Eosinophilia
- If secondary to autoimmune process, it may have elevated levels of antinuclear antibodies (ANA), rheumatoid factor (RF), anti-SSA/Ro, anti-SSB/La, anti-Jo, etc.
- Check HIV status.
- Negative cultures
- Negative serology for Mycoplasma, Coxiella, Legionella, psittacosis, and fungus
- Negative viral studies
- CXR: often appears more normal than the physical examination
  - CXR may show bilateral patchy alveolar opacities (typical pattern), often in the middle or upper lung area, a ground glass pattern that may have air bronchograms.
  - CXR can also reveal a solitary focal nodule or mass known as a focal pattern (1)[B].
- Throughout the disease, new infiltrates may appear or may seem to migrate.
- Effusions and cavitary lesions are rare on x-ray.
- Patients with linear opacities at lung bases may have a poorer prognosis.
- CT scans more accurately define the distribution and extent of the patchy alveolar opacities with areas of hyperlucency. Findings are commonly described as a "reversed halo sign" or "atoll sign," a focal round area of ground glass attenuation; however, this is a nonspecific finding (2,3)[A].
- Up to 90% of CT scans may show airspace consolidation with air bronchograms.
- Pulmonary function shows a restrictive/obstructive pattern.

- Flow-volume loop shows terminal airway obstruction.
- The involved area may seem to migrate.
- Ventilation–perfusion ratio scan: matched patchy defects

Diagnostic Procedures/Other
- In one study, open lung biopsy established the correct diagnosis in 1/3 of patients (4)[B].
- Transbronchial biopsy has yielded a correct diagnosis in 2/3 of cases (4,5)[B].

- Consider steroids for a diagnostic trial. If a diagnostic trial is successful, be prepared to treat the patient for at least 1 year. Relapses are common after stopping treatment.
- Bronchoalveolar lavage (BAL) fluid in patients with COP have shown larger amounts of natural killer cells, natural killer T-like cells, Fas and tumor necrosis factor receptor expression indicating cytotoxicity and local inflammation (5,6)[C]. In one specific study, the most frequent BAL profile was mixed alveolitis with lymphocytic predominance, a CD4/CD8 index of 0.4, and foamy macrophages, which was shown to be specific (88.8%) but not sensitive (4)[C].

Test Interpretation
- Intraluminal fibrosis of distal airspaces is the major pathologic feature.
- Fibroblasts and plugs of inflammatory cells and loose connective tissue fill these distal airways, known as Masson bodies.
  - Characteristic "butterfly" pattern of intraluminal granulation tissue plugs extending from alveoli to bronchioles
- Inflammatory cells are mainly lymphocytes and plasma cells.
- Interstitial fibrosis is present.
- Plugs of edematous granulation tissue in the terminal and respiratory bronchioles and alveolar ducts do not cause permanent damage.

TREATMENT

- Observation for patients with minimal symptoms and absent/mild PFT abnormalities as may spontaneously resolve. Reassess at 8 to 12 week intervals (8)[C].
- Inpatient care may be required for rapidly progressive disease or respiratory failure for high dose IV steroids and supportive care

GENERAL MEASURES
- Monitor blood gases or pulse oximetry.
- Oxygen, as necessary

MEDICATION
First Line
Prednisone

- 1 mg/kg (up to 60 mg/day) for 1 to 3 months, then 40 mg/day for 3 months, then 10 to 20 mg/day for up to 1 year (1)[A]

- May consider a 6-month-only taper or alternate day dosing for 1 year to limit steroid exposure
- Increase length of taper for patients on long-term therapy to avoid precipitating Addisonian crisis.
- Treatment may be needed for ≥1 year.

- In one study, the best response to corticosteroid therapy was seen in individuals <35 years of age, nonsmokers, and with morphologic features (large bronchial plugs, mild inflammatory reaction) and immunohistochemical markers (presence of collagen IV, absence of collagen III, CD-68-positive cells and positive VEGF) (7)[B].

- Precautions: Be aware of the patient's TB status and history of peptic ulcer disease. Long-term steroid treatment is associated with significant adverse effects, including adrenal suppression, infection, Cushing syndrome, fluid retention, osteoporosis, hyperkalemia, and poor wound healing.

Pediatric Considerations
Prednisone: 1 mg/kg q24h for 1 month, followed by weaning over several months

Second Line
- Steroids other than prednisone may be used.
- Prescribe antimicrobials if the original infection is persistent. The proper choice depends on the pathogen.
- Anecdotal use of inhaled triamcinolone and cyclophosphamide has been reported.
- Macrolide antibiotics have also been used for their anti-inflammatory properties; however, not employed in most cases (4)[C].
- If unresponsive to systemic glucocorticoids, can consider second immunosuppressive such as azathioprine or cyclophosphamide (9,10)[C]

ISSUES FOR REFERRAL
Patients should be followed by a pulmonologist.

ONGOING CARE

FOLLOW-UP RECOMMENDATIONS
Patient Monitoring
- Frequent visits, weekly at first
- Prednisone must be continued because of the chance of relapse.
- Monitor the lung disease and the side effects of prednisone therapy.
  - Annual TB screening
  - Monthly CBC
  - Funduscopic examination every 3 to 6 months
  - Serial dual energy x-ray absorptiometry (DEXA) scans for osteoporosis

DIET
No special diet

PATIENT EDUCATION
- Compliance: Emphasize the need to continue prednisone because of the chance of a relapse.
- Recurrence in up to 1/3 who do not complete full steroid treatment (1)

PROGNOSIS
Typically complete recovery, but individual case management is mandatory.

COMPLICATIONS
- Bronchiectasis
- Most people recover completely without permanent sequelae if full course of steroids completed.
- Death occurs in up to 7% but usually in individuals who are elderly or have preexisting comorbid conditions.

REFERENCES

1. Cottin V, Cordier JF. Cryptogenic organizing pneumonia. *Semin Respir Crit Care Med*. 2012;33(5):462–475.
2. Marchiori E, Zanetti G, Hochhegger B, et al. Reversed halo sign on computed tomography: state-of-the-art review. *Lung*. 2012;190(4):389–394.
3. Marchiori E, Irion KL, Zanetti G, et al. Atoll sign or reversed halo sign? Which term should be used? *Thorax*. 2011;66(11):1009–1010.
4. Drakopanagiotakis F, Paschalaki K, Abu-Hijleh M, et al. Cryptogenic and secondary organizing pneumonia: clinical presentation, radiographic findings, treatment response, and prognosis. *Chest*. 2011;139(4):893–900.
5. Jara-Palomares L, Gomez-Izquierdo L, Gonzalez-Vergara D, et al. Utility of high-resolution computed tomography and BAL in cryptogenic organizing pneumonia. *Respir Med*. 2010;104(11):1706–1711.
6. Papakosta D, Manika K, Gounari E, et al. Bronchoalveolar lavage fluid and blood natural killer and natural killer T-like cells in cryptogenic organizing pneumonia. *Respirology*. 2014;19(5):748–754.
7. Ye Q, Dai H, Sarria R, et al. Increased expression of tumor necrosis factor receptors in cryptogenic organizing pneumonia. *Respir Med*. 2011;105(2):292–297.
8. Bradley B, Branley HM, Egan JJ, et al. Interstitial lung disease guideline: the British Thoracic Society in collaboration with the Thoracic Society of Australia and New Zealand and the Irish Thoracic Society. *Thorax*. 2008;63(Suppl 5):v1–v58.
9. Purcell IF, Bourke SJ, Marshall SM. Cyclophosphamide in severe steroid-resistant bronchiolitis obliterans organizing pneumonia. *Respir Med*. 1997;91(3):175–177.
10. Vaz AP, Morais A, Melo N, et al. Azithromycin as an adjuvant therapy in cryptogenic organizing pneumonia [in Portuguese]. *Rev Port Pneumol*. 2011;17(4):186–189.

 SEE-ALSO

Sjögren syndrome

 CODES

ICD10
J84.116 Cryptogenic organizing pneumonia

CLINICAL PEARLS
- COP is a restrictive problem that is completely reversible.
- Major risk factors for COP include immunosuppression. No known association with smoking.
- Consider COP in prolonged respiratory illness with fatigue, nonproductive cough, and weight loss unresponsive to multiple antibiotics.
- When diagnosing COP, one should perform an autoimmune workup.
- The classic CT finding of COP is the "reversed halo sign" also known as "atoll sign."
- The histopathology characteristic of excessive proliferation of granulation tissue that may extend into the "butterfly" pattern
- COP treatment is a prolonged course of corticosteroids.

CRYPTORCHIDISM

Pamela Ellsworth, MD

 BASICS

DESCRIPTION
- Incomplete or improper descent of one or both testicles; also called *undescended testes* (1)
- Normally, descent is in the 7th to 8th month of gestation. The cryptorchid testis may be palpable or nonpalpable.
- Types of cryptorchidism
  - Abdominal: located inside the internal ring
  - Canalicular: located between the internal and external rings
  - Ectopic: located outside the normal path of testicular descent from abdominal cavity to scrotum; may be ectopic to perineum, femoral canal, superficial inguinal pouch (most common), suprapubic area, or opposite hemiscrotum
  - Retractile: fully descended testis that moves freely between the scrotum and the groin
  - Iatrogenic: Previously descended testis becomes undescended secondary to scar tissue after inguinal surgery, such as an inguinal hernia repair or hydrocelectomy.
  - Also may be referred to as palpable versus nonpalpable (1)
- System(s) affected: reproductive
- Synonym(s): undescended testes (UDT)

EPIDEMIOLOGY
Incidence
- Predominant age: premature newborns
- Predominant sex: male only

Prevalence
- In the United States, cryptorchidism occurs in 1–3% of full-term and 15–30% of premature newborn males (2).
- Spontaneous testicular descent occurs by age 1 to 3 months in 50–70% of full-term males with cryptorchidism.
- Descent at 6 to 9 months of age is rare (3).

ETIOLOGY AND PATHOPHYSIOLOGY
- Not fully known
- May involve alterations in
  - Mechanical factors (gubernaculum, length of vas deferens and testicular vessels, groin anatomy, epididymis, cremasteric muscles, and abdominal pressure), hormonal factors (gonadotropin, testosterone, dihydrotestosterone, and müllerian-inhibiting substance[MIS]), and neural factors (ilioinguinal nerve and genitofemoral nerve)
  - Major regulators of testicular descent from intra-abdominal location into the bottom of the scrotum are the Leydig cell–derived hormones, testosterone, and insulin-like growth factor 3 (IGF-3).
  - Mutations in the gene for IGF-3 and in the androgen receptor gene have been evaluated as possible causes of cryptorchidism as well as chromosomal alterations (1).
  - Environmental factors acting as endocrine disruptors of testicular descent also may contribute to the etiology of cryptorchidism (4).
- Risk of ascent may be as high as 32% in retractile testis (5).

Genetics
Occurrence of UDT in siblings, as well as fathers, suggests a genetic etiology.

RISK FACTORS
- Family history of cryptorchidism: highest risk if brother had UDT, followed by uncle, then father (6)
- Low birth weight, prematurity, and small for gestational age are associated with a substantial increase in incidence of cryptorchidism (1). Retractile testes are at increased risk for ascent (5).

COMMONLY ASSOCIATED CONDITIONS
- Inguinal hernia/hydrocele
- Abnormalities of vas deferens and epididymis
- Intersex abnormalities
- Hypogonadotropic hypogonadism
- Germinal cell aplasia
- Prune-belly syndrome
- Meningomyelocele
- Hypospadias
- Wilms' tumor
- Prader-Willi syndrome
- Kallmann syndrome
- Cystic fibrosis

 DIAGNOSIS

HISTORY
- ≥1 testicles in a site other than the scrotum
- May be an isolated defect or associated with other congenital anomalies

PHYSICAL EXAM
- Performed with warm hands, with child in sitting, standing, and squatting position
- A Valsalva maneuver and applied pressure to lower abdomen may help to identify the testes, especially a gliding testis.
- Failure to palpate a testis after repeated exams suggests an intra-abdominal or atrophic testis.
- An enlarged contralateral testis in the presence of a nonpalpable testis suggests testicular atrophy/absence.
- Testes should be palpated for quality and position at each recommended well-child visit (1)[B].

DIFFERENTIAL DIAGNOSIS
- Retractile testis (hypermobile testis) a normally descended testis that ascends into the inguinal canal because of an active cremasteric reflex (more common in males 4 to 6 years of age)
- Atrophic testis: may occur as a result of neonatal torsion
- Vanished testis may be the result of a lack of development or in utero torsion.

DIAGNOSTIC TESTS & INTERPRETATION
Initial Tests (lab, imaging)
- In phenotypic male newborn with bilateral, nonpalpable UDTs, hormone levels are helpful to determine whether the testes are present and should be evaluated for possible disorder of sexual development (1)[A].
  - Luteinizing hormone (LH)
  - Follicle-stimulating hormone (FSH)
  - MIS
  - Testosterone
  - Serum electrolytes
  - Karyotype

- If bilateral nonpalpable testes and presenting >3 months of age, a human chorionic gonadotropin (hCG) stimulation test to determine presence or absence of testicular tissue (hCG 2,000 IU/day for 3 days, and check testosterone before and after stimulation) as well as gonadotropins—to say testes are absent—need negative stimulation test and elevated gonadotropins (7).
- Ultrasound or other imaging modalities should not be performed in the evaluation of boys with cryptorchidism prior to referral to a specialist, as they are rarely needed in decision making (1)[B].

Follow-Up Tests & Special Considerations
- In newborns and children <6 months of age, periodic examination to determine if testis is palpable and descended prior to considering further intervention (1)
- In the absence of spontaneous testicular descent by 6 months of age (gestational age adjusted), infant should be referred to appropriate specialist and should perform surgery within 1 year (1,8)[B].
- In children with retractile testes, examination should be performed at least yearly to rule out subsequent ascent (1)[B].
- Best accuracy in predicting monarchism in boys 11 to 30 months of age with unilateral nonpalpable UDT if unilateral nonpalpable undescended testis and contralateral descended testis is 19 to 20 mm or greater in length measured by caliper (9)[B].

Diagnostic Procedures/Other
Laparoscopy is useful in a child with nonpalpable cryptorchidism to confirm testicular absence or presence accurately and to determine the feasibility of performing a standard orchidopexy.

Test Interpretation
- Higher incidence of carcinoma in UDT and alterations in spermatogenesis (10)
- Histologic changes occur by 1.5 years of age and include smaller seminiferous tubules, fewer spermatogonia, and more peritubular tissue (10,11).

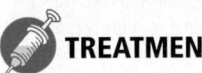 TREATMENT

GENERAL MEASURES
- Rule out retractile testis.
- Appropriate health care: outpatient until surgery is performed
- Administration of chorionic gonadotropin may cause testicular descent in some boys. Reports of efficacy are inconsistent. American Urological Association (AUA) guidelines on cryptorchidism do not recommend use of hormonal therapy to induce testicular descent due to low response rate and lack of evidence for long-term efficacy (1).

MEDICATION
Medical therapy is not indicated in the United States per the AUA guidelines on cryptorchidism 2014 (1).

ISSUES FOR REFERRAL
- ≥1 testes not descended by 6 months age (1)[B]
- Bilateral nonpalpable UDTs (1)
- Newly diagnosed cryptorchidism after 6 months of age (1)[B]

SURGERY/OTHER PROCEDURES

- Reasons to consider: avoids torsion, averts trauma, decreases but does not eliminate risk of malignancy, and prevents further alterations in spermatogenesis
- In the absence of spontaneous testicular descent by 6 months of age (gestational age-adjusted), surgery should be performed within 1 year (1)[B].
- Prepubertal orchiopexy decreases risk of testicular cancer and results in 2- to 6-fold reduction in relative risk compared to postpubertal orchiopexy (1,12–14).
- Laparoscopy/abdominal exploration is performed first if testis is nonpalpable (15).
- If palpable, an inguinal approach is usually performed. If low-lying, a single incision scrotal approach can also be considered but may increase the risk of hernia (16,17).

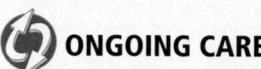 **ONGOING CARE**

FOLLOW-UP RECOMMENDATIONS

- Initial follow-up within 1 month of surgery and periodically thereafter to assess testicular size/growth.
- Patients with retractile testes should be examined at least annually to monitor for secondary ascent until testis is no longer retractile (1)[B].

Patient Monitoring

- Patients should be followed after surgery to evaluate testicular growth.
- Testicular tumors occur mainly during or after puberty; thus, these children should be taught self-examination when they are older.

DIET

No restrictions

PATIENT EDUCATION

Discuss with parents about causes, available treatments and possible effects on patient's reproductive potential and also increased risk for testicular cancer and need for regular self-examination.

PROGNOSIS

- Disorder is usually corrected with medical or surgical therapy; however, there are possible lifelong consequences.
- If testicle is absent or orchiectomy is required, may consider placement of testicular prosthesis
- Early orchiopexy may decrease risk of testicular damage and risk of malignancy.

COMPLICATIONS

- Progressive failure of spermatogenesis, if left untreated; even with orchiopexy, the fertility rate is still reduced, especially with bilateral UDTs.
- Spermatogenesis is related to the duration of cryptorchidism and the location of the testis (18).
- Formerly, bilaterally cryptorchid men had a greater decrease in fertility compared with unilateral cryptorchid male and the general male population (1,19–23).
- Abnormalities also have been identified in the contralateral descended testis, although less severe.

REFERENCES

1. Kolon TF, Herndon CDA, Baker LA, et al. Evaluation and treatment of cryptorchidism: AUA guideline. https://www.auanet.org/education/guidelines/cryptorchidism.cfm
2. Sijstermans K, Hack WW, Meijer RW, et al. The frequency of undescended testis from birth to adulthood: a review. *Int J Androl*. 2008;31(1):1–11.
3. Berkowitz GS, Lapinski RH, Dolgin SE, et al. Prevalence and natural history of cryptorchidism. *Pediatrics*. 1993;92(1):44–49.
4. Main KM, Skakkebaek NE, Toppari J. Cryptorchidism as part of the testicular dysgenesis syndrome: the environmental connection. *Endocr Dev*. 2009;14:167–173.
5. Agarwal PK, Diaz M, Elder JS. Retractile testis—is it really a normal variant? *J Urol*. 2006;175(4):1496–1499.
6. Elert A, Jahn K, Heidenreich A, et al. Population-based investigation of familial undescended testis and its association with other urogenital anomalies. *J Pediatr Urol*. 2005;1(6):403–407.
7. Docimo SG, Silver RI, Cromie W. The undescended testicle: diagnosis and management. *Am Fam Physician*. 2000;62(9):2037–2044.
8. Klein MD. Referral to pediatric surgical specialists. *Pediatrics*. 2014;133(2):350–356.
9. Braga LH, Kim S, Farrokhyar F, et al. Is there an optimal contralateral cut-off size that predicts monarchism in boys with nonpalpable testes? *J Pediatr Urol*. 2014;10(4): 693–698.
10. Cortes D, Thorup JM, Visfeldt J. Cryptorchidism: aspects of fertility and neoplasms. A study including data of 1,335 consecutive boys who underwent testicular biopsy simultaneously with surgery for cryptorchidism. *Horm Res*. 2001; 55(1):21–27.
11. Park KH, Lee JH, Han JJ, et al. Histological evidences suggest recommending orchiopexy within the first year of life for children with unilateral inguinal cryptorchid testis. *Int J Urol*. 2007;14(7): 616–621.
12. Wood HM, Elder JS. Cryptorchidism and testicular cancer: separating fact from fiction. *J Urol*. 2009; 181(2):452–461.
13. Walsh TJ, Dall'Era MA, Croughan MS, et al. Prepubertal orchiopexy for cryptorchidism may be associated with lower risk of testicular cancer. *J Urol*. 2007;178(4 Pt 1):1440–1446.
14. Pettersson A, Richiardi L, Nordenskjold A, et al. Age at surgery for undescended testis and risk of testicular cancer. *N Engl J Med*. 2007;356(18): 1835–1841.
15. Patil KK, Green JS, Duffy PG. Laparoscopy for impalpable testes. *BJU Int*. 2005;95(5):704–708.
16. Al-Mandil M, Khoury AE, El-Hout Y, et al. Potential complications with the prescrotal approach for the palpable undescended testis? A comparison of single prescrotal incision to the traditional inguinal approach. *J Urol*. 2008;180(2):686–689.
17. Na SW, Kim SO, Hwang EC, et al. Single scrotal incision orchiopexy for children with palpable low-lying undescended testis: early outcome of a prospective randomized controlled study. *Korean J Urol*. 2011;52(9):637–641.
18. Wilkerson ML, Bartone FF, Fox L, et al. Fertility potential: a comparison of intra-abdominal and intracanalicular testes by age groups in children. *Horm Res*. 2001;55(1):18–20.
19. Bremholm Rasmussen T, Ingerslev HJ, Høstrup H. Bilateral spontaneous descent of the testis after the age of 10: subsequent effects on fertility. *Br J Surg*. 1988;75(8):820–823.
20. Gilhooly PE, Meyers F, Lattimer JK. Fertility prospects for children with cryptorchidism. *Am J Dis Child*. 1984;138(10):940–943.
21. Fallon B, Kennedy TJ. Long-term follow-up of fertility in cryptorchid patients. *Urology*. 1985; 25(5):502–504.
22. Gracia J, Sánchez Zalabardo J, Sánchez García J, et al. Clinical, physical, sperm and hormonal data in 251 adults operated on for cryptorchidism in childhood. *BJU Int*. 2000;85(9):1100–1103.
23. Trsinar B, Muravec UR. Fertility potential after unilateral and bilateral orchiopexy for cryptorchidism. *World J Urol*. 2009;27(4):513–519.

ADDITIONAL READING

- Barthold JS. Undescended testis: current theories of etiology. *Curr Opin Urol*. 2008;18(4):395–400.
- Barthold JS, González R. The epidemiology of congenital cryptorchidism, testicular ascent and orchiopexy. *J Urol*. 2003;170(6 Pt 1):2396–2401.
- Cortes D. Cryptorchidism—aspects of pathogenesis, histology and treatment. *Scand J Urol Nephrol Suppl*. 1998;196:1–54.
- Fantasia J, Aidlen J, Lathrop W, et al. Undescended testes: a clinical and surgical review. *Urol Nurs*. 2015;35(3):117–126.
- Foresta C, Zuccarello D, Garolla A, et al. Role of hormones, genes, and environment in human cryptorchidism. *Endocr Rev*. 2008;29(5):560–580.
- Hutson JM, Balic A, Nation T, et al. Cryptorchidism. *Semin Pediatr Surg*. 2010;19(3):215–224.
- Kollin C, Hesser U, Ritzén EM, et al. Testicular growth from birth to two years of age, and the effect of orchidopexy at age nine months: a randomized, controlled study. *Acta Paediatr*. 2006; 95(3):318–324.
- Lee PA. Fertility after cryptorchidism: epidemiology and other outcome studies. *Urology*. 2005;66(2): 427–431.

 CODES

ICD10

- Q53.9 Undescended testicle, unspecified
- Q53.10 Unspecified undescended testicle, unilateral
- Q53.20 Undescended testicle, unspecified, bilateral

CLINICAL PEARLS

- If testicular descent does not occur by 6 months of age, it is unlikely to occur. Therefore, refer patients to a specialist if a testis has not descended by 6 months of age.
- Children with bilateral, nonpalpable UDTs require laboratory evaluation to determine if viable testicular tissue is present and to rule out disorder of sexual differentiation.
- Radiologic imaging has no role in the initial evaluation of cryptorchidism.
- The risk of infertility is increased with bilateral UDTs.

CUSHING DISEASE AND CUSHING SYNDROME

Linda Paniagua, MD • Geetha Gopalakrishnan, MD

BASICS

DESCRIPTION
- Clinical abnormalities associated with chronic exposure to excessive amounts of cortisol (the major adrenocorticoid)
- Cushing syndrome is defined as excessive corticosteroid exposure from exogenous sources (medications) or endogenous sources (pituitary, adrenal, pulmonary, etc.) or tumor. Exogenous intake of steroids is the primary cause of Cushing syndrome.
- Cushing disease is defined as glucocorticoid excess due to excessive adrenocorticotropic hormone (ACTH) secretion from a pituitary tumor, the most common cause of primary Cushing syndrome.
- System(s) affected: endocrine/metabolic, musculoskeletal, skin/exocrine, cardiovascular; neuropsychiatric

Pediatric Considerations
- Rare in infancy and childhood
- Cushing disease accounts for approximately 75% of all cases of Cushing syndrome in children >7 years.
- In children <7 years, adrenal causes of Cushing syndrome (adenoma, carcinoma, or bilateral hyperplasia) are more common.
- Most common presenting symptom is lack of growth consistent with the weight gain.

Pregnancy Considerations
- Pregnancy may exacerbate disease.
- Cortisol levels increase in normal pregnancy states.

EPIDEMIOLOGY
Incidence
Uncommon: 0.7 to 2.4/1 million per year (1)

Prevalence
2–5% prevalence reported in difficult-to-control diabetics with obesity and hypertension (HTN)

ETIOLOGY AND PATHOPHYSIOLOGY
- Syndrome: excessive corticosteroid exposure from exogenous sources (medications) or endogenous sources (pituitary, adrenal, pulmonary, etc.) or tumor
- Disease: pituitary tumor causing excess ACTH (corticotropin)
- General population
  - Exogenous glucocorticoids
  - Endogenous ACTH–dependent hypercortisolism: 80–85%
    ○ ACTH-secreting pituitary tumor: 75%
    ○ Ectopic ACTH production (e.g., small cell carcinoma of lung, bronchial carcinoid): 20%
  - Endogenous ACTH–independent hypercortisolism: 15–20%
    ○ Adrenal adenoma
    ○ Adrenal carcinoma
    ○ Macronodular or micronodular hyperplasia
- Pediatric/adolescent (1)
  - Adrenal hyperplasia secondary to McCune-Albright: mean age 1.2 years
  - Adrenocortical tumors: mean age 4.5 years
  - Ectopic ACTH syndrome: mean age 10.1 years
  - Primary pigmented nodular adrenocortical disease: mean age 13.0 years
  - Cushing disease: mean age 14.1 years
- Pregnancy (2)
  - Pituitary-dependent Cushing syndrome: 33%
  - Adrenal causes: 40–50%
  - ACTH-independent adrenal hyperplasia: 3%

Genetics
- Multiple endocrine neoplasia
- Carney complex (an inherited multiple neoplasia syndrome)
- McCune-Albright syndrome (mutation of GNAS1 gene)
- Familial isolated pituitary adenomas (mutations in the aryl hydrocarbon receptor–interacting protein gene)

RISK FACTORS
- Prevalent sex: female > male (3:1) (3)
- Most often occurs between the ages of 25 and 40 years
- Prolonged use of corticosteroids

GENERAL PREVENTION
Avoid corticosteroid exposure, when possible.

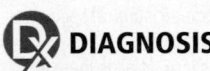

DIAGNOSIS

HISTORY
- Weight gain: 95%
- Decreased libido: 90%
- Menstrual irregularity: 80%
- Depression/emotional lability: 50–80%
- Easy bruising: 65%
- Diabetes or glucose intolerance: 60%

PHYSICAL EXAM
- Obesity (usually central): 95%
- Facial plethora: 90%
- Moon face (facial adiposity): 90%
- Thin skin: 85%
- Hypertension: 75%
- Skeletal growth retardation in children (epiphyseal plates remain open): 70–80%
- Hirsutism: 75%
- Proximal muscle weakness: 60%
- Purple striae on the skin
- Increased adipose tissue in neck and trunk
- Acne

DIFFERENTIAL DIAGNOSIS
- Obesity
- Diabetes mellitus
- HTN
- Metabolic syndrome X
- Polycystic ovarian disease
- Pseudo-Cushing (e.g., alcoholism, physical stress, severe major depression)

DIAGNOSTIC TESTS & INTERPRETATION
Initial Tests (lab, imaging)
- Recent guidelines (4)[C]
  - The 2008 Endocrine Society guidelines recommend against widespread testing for Cushing syndrome except in patients with the following:
    ○ Adrenal incidentaloma
    ○ Multiple progressive features suggestive of Cushing syndrome
    ○ Unusual features for their age such as osteoporosis and HTN
    ○ Abnormal growth (children)
- Late-night salivary cortisol, 24-hour urinary free cortisol, or low-dose dexamethasone suppression testing

- Elevated late-night salivary cortisol: Obtain at least two measurements. Cortisol secretion is highest in the morning and lowest between 11 PM and midnight. The nadir of serum cortisol is maintained in pseudo-Cushing (e.g., obesity, alcoholism, depression) but not in Cushing syndrome. Sensitivity and specificity are >90–95% (5,6)[B].
- 24-hour urinary free cortisol level: Obtain ≥2 samples to rule out intermittent hypercortisolism if results are normal and suspicion is high. Also measure 24-hour urinary creatinine excretion to verify adequacy of collection. Results may be falsely low if glomerular filtration rate <30 mL/min. Overall sensitivity and specificity varies, 90–97% and 85–96%, respectively (5)[B]. Avoid drinking excessive amounts of water due to risk of false-positive values. False-positive values can be seen in the presence of pseudo-Cushing states.

- Low-dose dexamethasone suppression testing: Dexamethasone 1 mg is given between 11 PM and midnight, and fasting plasma cortisol is measured between 8 and 9 AM the following morning. A serum cortisol level below 1.89 μg/dL excludes Cushing syndrome, but specificity is limited. The presence of pseudo-Cushing states (depression, obesity, etc.), hepatic or renal disease, or any drug that induces cytochrome P-450 enzymes may cause a false result.
- High-dose dexamethasone suppression test may be useful when baseline ACTH levels are indeterminate:

- 8 mg overnight dexamethasone suppression test: 8 mg of oral dexamethasone is given at 11 PM, with measurement of an 8-AM cortisol level the next day. A baseline 8-AM cortisol measurement is also obtained the morning prior to ingesting dexamethasone. Suppression of serum cortisol level to <50% of baseline is suggestive of a pituitary source of ACTH rather than ectopic ACTH or primary adrenal disease. Sensitivity and specificity are 95% and 100%, respectively (7)[B].

- If the initial results are positive or if clinical suspicion is high, perform additional studies to confirm diagnosis. Other tests to consider include the following:

- Awake midnight plasma cortisol: Obtain samples on three consecutive nights. A late-evening serum cortisol >7.5 μg/dL has a sensitivity of 96% and specificity of 100% (8)[B]. Persistently elevated serum cortisol implies Cushing syndrome; nadir of serum cortisol is maintained in obese patients but not in Cushing.
- Corticotropin-releasing hormone (CRH) after dexamethasone: used to distinguish Cushing syndrome from pseudo-Cushing syndrome. Dexamethasone 0.5 mg is given q6h for 48 hours starting at noon. CRH (1 μg/kg) is given 2 hours after the last dose of dexamethasone. Plasma cortisol is >1.4 μg/dL 15 minutes after CRH in patients with Cushing syndrome but not in those with pseudo-Cushing (9)[B].

- Pituitary MRI scan if pituitary tumor is suspected
- Abdominal CT scan if adrenal disease is suspected
- Chest CT scan if ectopic ACTH secretion is suspected
- Octreotide scintigraphy to look for occult ACTH-secreting tumor
- Dual energy x-ray absorptiometry to evaluate for osteoporosis

ALERT
- Antiepileptic drugs, progesterone, oral contraceptives (withdraw estrogen-containing drugs 6 weeks before testing), rifampin, and spironolactone may cause a false-positive dexamethasone suppression test.
- Pregnancy (4)[C]: Urine-free cortisol is recommended instead of dexamethasone testing in the initial evaluation of pregnant women. Only urine free cortisol in the 2nd or 3rd trimester >3 times the upper limit of normal can be taken to indicate Cushing syndrome.
- Epilepsy (4)[C]: best to use measured cortisol from saliva and urine instead of serum cortisol after dexamethasone. No data to guide length of time needed after withdrawal of such medication to allow dexamethasone metabolism to return to normal; such medication change may not be clinically possible.

Follow-Up Tests & Special Considerations
- Once the diagnosis of Cushing syndrome is confirmed, localization is the next step:
  – ACTH level: elevated in ACTH-dependent Cushing syndrome (e.g., pituitary and ectopic tumor) and low in ACTH-independent Cushing syndrome (e.g., adrenal tumors and exogenous glucocorticoids)
  – High-dose dexamethasone suppression testing: used to distinguish between an ACTH-secreting pituitary tumor and ectopic ACTH-secreting tumors. 0.5 mg dexamethasone is given q6h for 8 doses, with serum cortisol measured at 2 and 6 hours after last dose (sensitivity 79%, specificity 74%) (7)[B].
- Diagnosis of Cushing syndrome is complicated by the nonspecificity and high prevalence of clinical symptoms in patients without the disorder and involves a variety of tests of variable sensitivity and specificity. Efficient screening and confirmatory procedures are essential before considering therapy.

Diagnostic Procedures/Other
Diagnostic procedure depends on clinical judgment. Inferior petrosal sinus sampling with CRH stimulation can be considered if ACTH-dependent tumor is suspected but not localized.

Test Interpretation
- Thyroid function suppressed
- HTN
- Dyslipidemia
- Polycystic ovarian syndrome/hyperandrogenism
- Oligomenorrhea/hypogonadism
- Myopathy/cutaneous wasting
- Neuropsychiatric problems
- Ipsilateral adrenal gland hyperplasia and contralateral adrenal gland atrophy
- Hypercoagulable state
- Osteoporosis
- Nephrolithiasis
- Growth hormone reduced

 TREATMENT

MEDICATION
- Drugs usually not effective for primary long-term treatment; used in preparation for surgery or as adjunctive treatment after surgery, pituitary radiotherapy, or both.
- Metyrapone, ketoconazole, and mitotane all lower cortisol by directly inhibiting synthesis and secretion in the adrenal gland. Replacement glucocorticoid therapy is often required. As initial treatment, remission rates up to 85% (10,11)[C].
- Mifepristone is a potent glucocorticoid receptor antagonist. It is FDA approved to control hyperglycemia in adults with endogenous Cushing syndrome who

have type 2 diabetes or glucose intolerance secondary to hypercortisolism that has not responded to (or who are not candidates for) surgery.
- Pasireotide is a somatostatin receptor ligand with affinity for somatostatin receptor 5. It has been approved for adult Cushing disease treatment by the FDA.

SURGERY/OTHER PROCEDURES
- Transsphenoidal surgery
  – Primary treatment for Cushing disease due to remission range of 65–90% (12)[C]
  – Resection of the ACTH-producing ectopic tumor
- Adrenal surgery
  – For unilateral adrenal adenomas, laparoscopic surgery is the treatment of choice.
  – For nodular hyperplasia, bilateral adrenalectomy is usually recommended.
  – For patients with Cushing disease, bilateral laparoscopic adrenalectomy can be considered if the patient has persistent disease even after pituitary surgery and radiotherapy.
- RADIOTHERAPY and stereotactic radiosurgery (SRS) can be used to treat persistent hypercortisolism after transsphenoidal surgery in Cushing disease.
- Fractionated radiotherapy
  – Rates of remission range from 56% to 84% [B].
  – Its related complications of hypopituitarism has limited its usefulness [A].
- Stereotactic radiosurgery
- Rates of remission range from 17% to 83% [A].
- Can be used as primary treatment without resection in patients with cavernous sinus tumors

 ONGOING CARE

PATIENT EDUCATION
- Teaching regarding diet and monitoring daily weight, early treatment of infections, emotional lability
- National Adrenal Disease Foundation. Great Neck, NY 11021; 516-407-4992

PROGNOSIS
- Guardedly favorable prognosis with surgery for Cushing disease; generally chronic course with cyclic exacerbations and rare remissions
- Better prognosis following surgery for benign adrenal tumors; long-term recurrence rate is 20%.
- Poor with small cell carcinoma of the lung producing ectopic hormone; neuroendocrine tumors (bronchial carcinoid) have much better prognosis.

COMPLICATIONS
- Osteoporosis
- Increased susceptibility to infections
- Metastases of malignant tumors
- Increased cardiovascular risk even after treatment
- Lifelong glucocorticoid dependence following treatment with bilateral adrenalectomy
- Nelson syndrome (pituitary tumor) after treatment with bilateral adrenalectomy (can occur in 8–38% of patients)

REFERENCES
1. Storr HL, Chan LF, Grossman AB, et al. Pediatric Cushing's syndrome: epidemiology, investigation and therapeutic advances. *Trends Endocrinol Metab*. 2007;18(4):167–174.
2. Lindsay JR, Nieman LK. Adrenal disorders in pregnancy. *Endocrinol Metab Clin North Am*. 2006;35(1):1–20.
3. Newell-Price J, Bertagna X, Grossman AB, et al. Cushing's syndrome. *Lancet*. 2006;367(9522): 1605–1617.
4. Nieman LK, Biller BM, Findling JW, et al. The diagnosis of Cushing's syndrome: an Endocrine Society clinical practice guideline. *J Clin Endocrinol Metab*. 2008;93(5):1526–1540.
5. Putignano P, Toja P, Dubini A, et al. Midnight salivary cortisol versus urinary free and midnight serum cortisol as screening tests for Cushing's syndrome. *J Clin Endocrinol Metabol*. 2003;88(9):4153–4157.
6. Yaneva M, Mosnier-Pudar H, Dugué MA, et al. Midnight salivary cortisol for the initial diagnosis of Cushing's syndrome of various causes. *J Clin Endocrinol Metab*. 2004;89(7):3345–3351.
7. Aytug S, Laws ER Jr, Vance ML. Assessment of the utility of the high-dose dexamethasone suppression test in confirming the diagnosis of Cushing disease. *Endocr Pract*. 2012;18(2):152–157.
8. Isidori AM, Kaltsas GA, Pozza C, et al. The ectopic adrenocorticotropin syndrome: clinical features, diagnosis, management, and long-term follow-up. *J Clin Endocrinol Metabol*. 2006;91(2):371–377.
9. Yanovski JA, Cutler GB Jr, Chrousos GP, et al. Corticotropin-releasing hormone stimulation following low-dose dexamethasone administration. A new test to distinguish Cushing's syndrome from pseudo-Cushing's states. *JAMA*. 1993;269(17):2232–2238.
10. Findling JW, Raff H. Cushing's syndrome: important issues in diagnosis and management. *J Clin Endocrinol Metab*. 2006;91(10):3746–3753.
11. Nieman LK, Ilias I. Evaluation and treatment of Cushing's syndrome. *Am J Med*. 2005;118(12):1340–1346.
12. Biller BM, Grossman AB, Stewart PM, et al. Treatment of adrenocorticotropin-dependent Cushing's syndrome: a consensus statement. *J Clin Endocrinol Metab*. 2008;93(7):2454–2462.

 SEE ALSO

Algorithm: Cushing Syndrome

CODES

ICD10
- E24.9 Cushing's syndrome, unspecified
- E24.0 Pituitary-dependent Cushing's disease
- E24.2 Drug-induced Cushing's syndrome

CLINICAL PEARLS
- Cushing disease is due to excessive ACTH secretion from a pituitary tumor, resulting in corticosteroid excess.
- Cushing syndrome is due to excessive corticosteroid exposure from exogenous sources (medications) or endogenous sources (pituitary, adrenal, pulmonary, etc.) or tumor.
- Depression, alcoholism, medications, eating disorders, and other conditions can cause mild clinical and laboratory findings similar to those in Cushing syndrome (pseudo-Cushing syndrome).

CUTANEOUS DRUG REACTIONS
Mary Iaculli, DO • Joanne Wilkinson, MD, MSc

 BASICS

DESCRIPTION
- An adverse cutaneous reaction in response to administration of a drug. Rashes are the most common adverse drug reactions.
- Severity can range from mild eruptions that resolve within 48 hours after the removal of the inciting agent to severe skin damage with multiorgan involvement.
- Morbilliform/simple exanthem (75–95%) and urticarial (5–6%) eruptions are most common, but multiple morphologic types may occur.
- System(s) affected: skin/mucosa/exocrine, hematologic/lymphatic/immunologic

EPIDEMIOLOGY
- All ages affected
- Predominant sex: female > male
- No correlation between development of adverse reaction and patient's age, diagnosis, or survival.
- Special consideration in the geriatric population who are on multiple medications: increased likelihood of severe cutaneous and systemic reactions; also consider in the pediatric group: difficult to distinguish from viral exanthems

Incidence
In the United States, prevalence of 2–3% in hospitalized patients; estimated 1/1,000 hospitalized patients has had a severe cutaneous reaction.

ETIOLOGY AND PATHOPHYSIOLOGY
- Predictable adverse reactions are due to overdose, side effect, or drug interaction.
- Unpredictable reactions include intolerance, drug idiosyncrasy secondary to abnormality in metabolism, or immune reaction. >700 drugs are known to cause a dermatologic reaction:
  - Immunologically mediated reaction: immunoglobulin (Ig) E–mediated reaction (type I hypersensitivity), cytotoxic/IgG/IgM induced (type II), immune complex reactions (type III), and delayed-type hypersensitivity (type IV) with T cells, eosinophils, neutrophils, and monocytes
  - Acneiform: OCPs, corticosteroids, iodinated compounds, hydantoins, lithium
  - Erythema multiforme/Stevens-Johnson syndrome (SJS)/toxic epidermal necrolysis (TEN): >100 drugs reported. Most common include sulfonamides, cephalosporins NSAIDs, barbiturates, hydantoins, anticonvulsants tetracycline, terbinafine.
  - Fixed drug eruptions: NSAIDS, sulfonamides, tetracycline, barbiturates, salicylates, OCPs
  - Lichenoid: thiazides, NSAIDs, gold, ACE inhibitors, proton pump inhibitors, antimalarials, sildenafil
  - Photosensitivity: doxycycline, thiazides, sulfonylureas, quinolones, sulfonamides, NSAIDs
  - Hypersensitivity vasculitis: hydralazine, penicillins, cephalosporins, thiazides, gold, sulfonamides, NSAIDs, propylthiouracil
  - Drug rash with eosinophilia and systemic symptoms (DRESS) syndrome: anticonvulsants, sulfonamides, dapsone, minocycline, allopurinol
  - Acute generalized exanthematous pustulosis (AGEP): penicillins, cephalosporins, macrolides, calcium channel blockers, antimalarials, carbamazepine, acetaminophen, terbinafine, nystatin, vancomycin
  - Sweet syndrome (acute febrile neutrophilic dermatosis): sulfa drugs, granulocyte colony-stimulating factor (G-CSF), granulocyte-macrophage colony-stimulating factor (GM-CSF), diazepam, minocycline, nitrofurantoin, captopril, penicillamine
  - Serum sickness-like reaction: cephalosporins, penicillins, TMP-SMX, propranolol, bupropion, minocycline
  - Morbilliform/urticarial/exfoliative erythroderma: numerous medications, including penicillins, cephalosporins, sulfonamides, tetracyclines, ibuprofen, naproxen, allopurinol, acetylsalicylic acid, radiocontrast media (1)[A]

Genetics
Genetics may play a role, as certain HLA antigens have been associated with increased predisposition to specific drug eruptions:
- HLA-B*5801, HLA-B*5701, and HLA-B*1502 have been linked to allopurinol-induced and carbamazepine-induced SJS/TEN, respectively.
- HLA class I antigens, such as HLA-A2, HLA-B12, and HLA-B22, have been linked to TEN and fixed drug eruptions, respectively.

RISK FACTORS
Previous drug reaction, multiple medications, concurrent infections, immunocompromised, disorders of metabolism, and certain genetic HLA haplotypes

GENERAL PREVENTION
Always ask patients about prior adverse drug events. Be aware of medications with higher incidence of reactions as well as drug cross-reactions.

 DIAGNOSIS

HISTORY
- New medications within the preceding 6 weeks, most commonly within preceding 2 weeks: all oral, parenteral, and topical agents, including over the counter drugs, vitamins, and herbal remedies
- Consider other etiologies: bacterial infections, viral exanthems, or underlying skin disease including cutaneous lymphoma

PHYSICAL EXAM
May present as a number of different eruption types, including, but not limited to the following:
- Morbilliform eruptions (exanthems)
  - Most frequent cutaneous reaction (75–95%); difficult to distinguish from viral exanthem; often secondary to antibiotic
  - Starts on trunk as pruritic red macules and papules and extends to extremities in confluent fashion, sparing face, palms, soles, and mucous membranes
  - Onset 7 to 21 days after drug initiation (2)[C].
- Urticaria
  - Pruritic erythematous wheals distributed anywhere on the body, including mucous membranes; may progress to angioedema, appears as nonpitting edema without erythema or margins
  - Individual lesions fade within 24 hours, but new lesions may develop (2).
- Acneiform eruptions
  - Folliculocentric, monomorphous pustules typically involving the face, chest, and back distinguished from acne vulgaris by absence of gross and/or microscopic comedones
  - Often may become secondarily infected (2)[C]
- Fixed drug eruptions
  - Single/multiple, round, sharply demarcated, violaceous plaques with gray center that may leave postinflammatory hyperpigmentation; occur on skin or mucous membrane
  - Appear shortly after drug exposure and recur in identical location after reexposure; some patients have a refractory period during which the drug fails to activate lesions.
  - Onset usually is 48 hours after ingestion of drug (2).
- AGEP
  - Multiple nonfollicular sterile pustules on erythematous background with desquamation after 7 to 10 days
  - Involves intertriginous areas but can be generalized and involve the face
  - Appears similar to pustular psoriasis, but AGEP has fever and marked leukocytosis with neutrophilia and/or eosinophilia (2)[C]
- DRESS syndrome
  - Classic triad of fever, exanthem, and internal organ involvement with possible pharyngitis and lymphadenopathy
  - Can lead to exfoliative dermatitis, often accompanied by facial edema
  - Internal organ involvement: 80% hepatic, 40% renal, 33% pulmonary, and cardiac lab tests show elevated liver transaminases and eosinophilia.
  - Onset 2 to 8 weeks after drug exposure; may develop 3 months or later into therapy (3)[B].
- Erythema multiforme
  - Relatively common, acute, often recurrent
  - Most commonly associated with herpes simplex virus and other viral/bacterial etiologies (i.e., mycoplasma); less likely secondary to drug exposure. 50% with unknown etiology
  - Three-zone target lesions and raised atypical two-zone targets with localized erythema
  - Lesions predominant on distal extremities including on acral surface with limited mucosal involvement; <10% epidermal detachment (4)[B]
- SJS/TEN
  - Classification and distinction between SJS and TEN determined by affected body surface area (BSA)
    - SJS: <10% BSA; SJS-TEN overlap: 10–30% BSA; TEN: >30% BSA
  - Unlike erythema multiforme, strong association with preceding drug exposure as opposed to infection except in children where infection is more common (e.g., mycoplasma)
  - Onset is 1 to 3 weeks after starting offending agent: Flat atypical two-zone target lesions and erythematous macules that are truncal and generalized with mucosal involvement
  - May develop confluent areas of bullae, erosions, and necrosis; significant risk for infection and sepsis
  - SJS: 5–15% mortality; TEN: 30% mortality (5)[C],(6)[A]
- Lichenoid eruptions
  - Flat-topped, violaceous, pruritic papules on extensor surfaces and involving oral mucosa
  - Reticular pattern: Lesions heal with hyperpigmentation.
  - Chronic lesions persist for weeks/months after the drug discontinued (2)
- Photosensitivity reaction
  - Phototoxic reactions: occur within 24 hours of light exposure with exaggerated sunburn reaction; confined to sun-exposed areas
  - Photoallergic reactions: caused by UVA exposure; more pruritic than painful; can involve non–sun-exposed areas

- Hypersensitivity vasculitis
  - Petechiae/palpable purpura and/or maculopapular rash concentrated on lower extremities and dependent areas
  - Biopsy shows neutrophils around an arteriole or venule.
  - Possible renal, joint, and CNS involvement with fever, myalgias, arthritis, and abdominal pain (2)
- Sweet syndrome
  - Fever, neutrophilia, tender edematous violaceous papules, plaques, or nodules, with or without pustules/vesicles that spontaneously resolve
  - May have oral ulcers or ocular manifestations, such as conjunctivitis
  - Classically seen in young women after a mild respiratory illness or GI infection, but 7–56% associated with malignancy and pregnancy
- Serum sickness–like reaction
  - Fever, nonspecific cutaneous eruption with possible bullous lesions, arthralgias
  - Onset 7 to 14 days
- Exfoliative dermatitis/erythroderma
  - Generalized erythema with exfoliation and/or fine desquamation over 90% of body surface
  - Difficult to distinguish between drug, primary cutaneous lymphoma, or inflammatory etiology
  - Lymphadenopathy, hepatosplenomegaly, leukocytosis, eosinophilia, or anemia may be present.
  - Increased risk of secondary infection and insensible fluid and temperature loss with hemodynamic instability

DIFFERENTIAL DIAGNOSIS
- Viral exanthem: Presence of fever, lymphocytosis, and other systemic findings may help in narrowing differential.
- Primary dermatosis: Correlation of drug withdrawal to rash resolution may clarify diagnosis; skin biopsy is helpful.
- Bacterial infection: Cultures of pustules may distinguish primary infection from AGEP and acneiform eruptions.

DIAGNOSTIC TESTS & INTERPRETATION
Initial Tests (lab, imaging)
A minimum number of tests are useful in evaluating for internal organ involvement. CBC with differential; significant eosinophilia may be seen in DRESS and other drug-induced allergic reactions. LFT, urinalysis, and serum creatinine; chest x-ray if suspected vasculitis

Diagnostic Procedures/Other
- Special tests depend on suspected mechanism:
  - Type I: skin/intradermal testing, radioallergosorbent (RAST)
  - Type II: direct/indirect Coombs test
  - Type III: ESR, C-reactive protein, ANA, antihistone antibody, tissue biopsy for immunofluorescence studies
  - Type IV: patch testing, lymphocyte proliferation assay (investigational)
  - Anaphylaxis/nonimmunologic mast and basophil cell reaction: serum tryptase levels
- Cultures useful in excluding infectious etiology; skin biopsy is nonspecific but useful in characterizing an eruption and excluding primary skin pathologies.
- Develop a timeline documenting the onset and duration of all drugs, dosages, and onset of cutaneous eruption (1)[A].

Test Interpretation
- Nonspecific histologic findings are superficial epidermal and dermal infiltrates composed variably of lymphocytes, neutrophils, and eosinophils.

- SJS/TEN: partial or full-thickness necrosis of the epidermis necrotic keratinocytes, vacuolization leading to subepidermal blister at basal membrane zone

TREATMENT

GENERAL MEASURES
- Monitor for signs of impending cardiovascular collapse: Anaphylactic reactions, DRESS, SJS/TEN, extensive bullous reactions, and generalized erythroderma may require inpatient treatment.
- Do not rechallenge with drugs causing urticaria, bullae, angioedema, DRESS, anaphylaxis, or erythema multiforme.

MEDICATION
- Withdrawal of offending drug. Depending on the type of eruption, symptomatic treatment may be useful, but most require no additional therapy except cessation of offending agent.
- Anaphylaxis or widespread urticaria: epinephrine 0.1 to 0.5 mg (1:1,000 [1 mg/mL] solution) SC every 5 to 15 min; prednisone may be given to prevent recurrence.
- Acute urticaria (<6 weeks) and chronic urticaria (>6 weeks): 2nd-generation antihistamines (preferred, less sedating): cetirizine 10 to 20 mg daily, loratadine 10 to 20 mg daily, fexofenadine 180 mg daily, levocetirizine 5 to 10 mg daily. 1st-generation antihistamines: diphenhydramine 10 to 25 mg QHS, hydroxyzine 10 to 25 mg TID, doxepin 10 to 50 mg QHS H_2 antagonists: cimetidine 400 mg BID, ranitidine 150 mg BID
- Anaphylaxis, severe urticaria: prednisone PO 1 mg/kg in tapering doses
- Erythema multiforme
  - Treatment is generally supportive with management of suspected underlying infection.
  - Herpes simplex virus (HSV)–associated: prophylaxis with acyclovir 400 mg BID, valacyclovir 500 to 1,000 mg/day, or famciclovir 250 mg BID
  - "Magic mouthwash" BID or TID is helpful for mucosal erosions. Consider ophthalmology consult for severe ocular involvement (4)[B].
- SJS/TEN: Treatment is supportive. Consult with a dermatologist and ophthalmologist. Systemic corticosteroid use remains controversial. Consider IVIG 2 to 3 g/kg for severe disease. In pediatric TEN patients, low-dose IVIG (0.05 to 0.1 g/kg/day) was effective. Varied success rates reported with use of anti–tumor necrosis factor-α agents, cyclosporine, cyclophosphamide, and plasmapheresis (5)[C],(6)[A].
- DRESS: prompt removal of offending drug and supportive measures; high-potency topical steroids for rash; systemic steroids with severe organ involvement; prednisone 0.5 to 2 mg/kg/day with prolonged taper 8 to 12 weeks (3)[B].

ONGOING CARE

FOLLOW-UP RECOMMENDATIONS
Patient Monitoring
- For urticarial, bullous, DRESS, or erythema multiforme spectrum lesions, close follow-up is needed.
- Patients with anaphylaxis/angioedema should be given EpiPen for secondary prevention and a Med-Alert bracelet; label the patient's medical record with the agent and reaction.
- If the patient needs to take the inciting drug (e.g., antibiotic) in the future, induction of drug tolerance or graded challenge procedures may be necessary.

PROGNOSIS
- Eruptions generally begin fading within days after removing offending agent. With morbilliform eruptions, eruption may spread distally even when agent is removed, resolving over time.
- Anaphylaxis, angioedema, DRESS, SJS/TEN, and bullous reactions are potentially fatal.

COMPLICATIONS
Anaphylaxis, bone marrow suppression, hepatitis (dapsone, hydantoin), renal failure, and pulmonary and thyroid toxicity

REFERENCES

1. Joint Task Force on Practice Parameters, American Academy of Allergy, Asthma and Immunology, American College of Allergy, Asthma and Immunology, et al. Drug allergy: an updated practice parameter. *Ann Allergy Asthma Immunol*. 2010;105(4):259–273.
2. Ahmed AM, Pritchard S, Reichenberg J. A review of cutaneous drug eruptions. *Clin Geriatr Med*. 2013;29(2):527–545.
3. Chen YC, Chiu HC, Chu CY. Drug reaction with eosinophilia and systemic symptoms: a retrospective study of 60 cases. *Arch Dermatol*. 2010;146(12):1373–1379.
4. Wetter DA, Davis MD. Recurrent erythema multiforme: clinical characteristics, etiologic associations, and treatment in a series of 48 patients at Mayo Clinic, 2000 to 2007. *J Am Acad Dermatol*. 2010;62(1):45–53.
5. Mockenhaupt M. Stevens-Johnson syndrome and toxic epidermal necrolysis: clinical patterns, diagnostic considerations, etiology, and therapeutic management. *Semin Cutan Med Surg*. 2014;33(1):10–16.
6. Schneck J, Fagot JP, Sekula P, et al. Effects of treatments on the mortality of Stevens-Johnson syndrome and toxic epidermal necrolysis: a retrospective study on patients included in the prospective EuroSCAR study. *J Am Acad Dermatol*. 2008;58(1):33–40.

CODES

ICD10
- L27.1 Loc skin eruption due to drugs and meds taken internally
- L50.0 Allergic urticaria
- R21 Rash and other nonspecific skin eruption

CLINICAL PEARLS
- Virtually, any drug can cause a rash; antibiotics are the most common culprits that cause cutaneous drug reactions.
- Focus on drug history with new suspicious skin eruptions.
- Usually self-limited after withdrawal of offending agent
- Symptoms such as tongue swelling/angioedema, skin necrosis, blisters, high fever, dyspnea, and mucous membrane erosions signify more severe drug reactions.
- Useful resources: Drug Eruption Reference Manual by Jerome Litt; www.drugeruptiondata.com; www.druginteractions.com

CYSTIC FIBROSIS

Brandon W. Bonds, MD • Tatiana P. Ivan, MD

BASICS

DESCRIPTION
- Cystic fibrosis (CF) is an autosomal recessive genetic mutation (CFTR gene) that most prominently affects the pulmonary and pancreatic systems.
- The GI, endocrine, and reproductive systems as well as the liver, sinuses, and skin can all be involved.
- Initially a pediatric disease, CF has become a chronic pediatric and adult medical condition as improvements in medical care have led to a dramatic increase in long-term survival.

EPIDEMIOLOGY
CF is the most common lethal inherited disease in Caucasians and is found in every racial group.

Incidence
Number of infants born with CF in relation to the total number of live births in the United States
- 1 in 3,000 Caucasians
- 1 in 4,000 to 10,000 Latin Americans
- 1 in 15,000 to 20,000 African Americans
- 1 in 30,000 Asian Americans

Prevalence
- 30,000 patients with CF living in the United States
- ~1,000 new diagnoses are made annually.

ETIOLOGY AND PATHOPHYSIOLOGY
- Abnormal CFTR function leads to abnormally viscous secretions that alter organ function.
- The lungs: obstruction, infection, and inflammation negatively affect lung growth, structure, and function
  - Decreased mucociliary clearance
  - Infection is accompanied by an intense neutrophilic response.
  - Degradation of supporting tissues causes bronchiectasis and eventual failure.

Genetics
CFTR gene (cystic fibrosis transmembrane conductance regulator): >1,500 mutations exist that can cause varying severity of phenotypic CF, all of which are recessively inherited. Most common is loss of the phenylalanine residue at 508th position (deltaF508), which accounts for 8.7% of affected alleles in the CF population in the United States. *G551D* mutation accounts for 4.3% of affected alleles.

RISK FACTORS
CF is a single-gene disorder. The severity of the phenotype can be affected by the specific CFTR mutation (most predictive of pancreatic disease), other modifier genes (CFTM1 for meconium ileus), gastroesophageal reflux disease (GERD), severe respiratory virus infection, and environmental factors such as tobacco smoke exposure.

GENERAL PREVENTION
Preconception counseling
- American Congress of Obstetricians and Gynecologists (ACOG) recommends preconception or early (1st/2nd trimester) genetic analysis for all North American couples planning a pregnancy, with appropriate counseling to identified carriers and genetic analysis of siblings of known CF patients.
- Universal newborn screening (NBS) has been integral in early diagnosis (62% of new CF diagnosis in 2013 were found by NBS)
- Patients diagnosed prior to onset of symptoms have better lung function, nutritional outcomes, and should receive referral and early intervention services by an accredited regional CF center.

Pregnancy Considerations
- Pulmonary disease may worsen during pregnancy.
- CF may cause increased incidence of preterm delivery, IUGR, and cesarean section (1)[A].
- Advances in fertility treatments now allow men with CF to father children (2)[A].

DIAGNOSIS

HISTORY
- Suspect with failure to thrive, steatorrhea, and recurrent respiratory problems
  - Chronic/recurrent respiratory symptoms, including airway obstruction and infections**
  - Persistent infiltrates on chest x-rays (CXRs)
  - Hypochloremic metabolic acidosis
- Hx during neonatal period
  - Meconium ileus (20%) (generally considered pathopneumonic for CF)
  - Prolonged jaundice
- Hx during infancy
  - Failure to thrive
  - Chronic diarrhea
  - Anasarca/hypoproteinemia
  - Pseudotumor cerebri (vitamin A deficiency)
  - Hemolytic anemia (vitamin E deficiency)
- Hx during childhood
  - Recurrent endobronchial infection
  - Bronchiectasis
  - Chronic pansinusitis
  - Steatorrhea
  - Poor growth
  - DIOS
  - Allergic bronchopulmonary aspergillosis
- Hx for adolescence and adulthood (7% diagnosed >18 years old) (3)[A]
  - Recurrent endobronchial infection
  - Bronchiectasis
  - Allergic bronchopulmonary aspergillosis
  - Chronic sinusitis
  - Hemoptysis
  - Pancreatitis
  - Portal hypertension
  - Azoospermia
  - Delayed puberty

PHYSICAL EXAM
- Respiratory
  - Rhonchi and/or crackles
  - Hyperresonance on percussion
  - Nasal polyps
- GI: Hepatosplenomegaly when cirrhosis is present.
- Other: digital clubbing, growth retardation, and pubertal delay

COMMONLY ASSOCIATED CONDITIONS
- CF-related diabetes (CFRD)
  - May present as steady decline in weight, lung function, or increased frequency of exacerbation
  - Leading comorbid complication (20.3%)
  - Result of progressive insulin deficiency
  - Early screening and treatment may improve reduced survival found in CFRD (4)[A].
- Upper respiratory
  - Rhinosinusitis is seen in up to 100% of patients with CF.
  - Nasal polyps are seen in up to 86% of patients.

- The GI tract
  - Pancreatic exocrine insufficiency (85–90%) (1)[A]
  - Malabsorption of fat, protein, and fat-soluble vitamins (A, D, E, and K)
  - Hepatobiliary disease (10.8%)
  - Focal biliary cirrhosis
  - Cholelithiasis
  - Meconium ileus at birth (10–15%) (5)[A]
  - Distal intestinal obstruction syndrome (DIOS): intestinal blockage that typically occurs in older children and adults (5.1%) (2)[A]
  - GERD (31.3%) (2)[A]
- Endocrine
  - Bone mineral disease (14.8%) (2)[A]
  - Joint disease (2.9%) (2)[A]
  - Hypogonadism
  - Frequent low testosterone levels in men
  - Menstrual irregularities are common.
- Reproductive organs
  - Congenital bilateral absence of the vas deferens: obstructive azoospermia in 98% of males
- Depression (12%) (2)[A]

DIFFERENTIAL DIAGNOSIS
- Immunologic
  - Severe Combined Immunodeficiency
- Pulmonary
  - Difficult-to-manage asthma
  - COPD
  - Recurrent pneumonia
  - Chronic/recurrent sinusitis
  - Primary ciliary dyskinesia
- Gastrointestinal
  - Celiac disease
  - Protein-losing enteropathy
  - Pancreatitis of unknown etiology
  - Shwachman-Diamond syndrome

DIAGNOSTIC TESTS & INTERPRETATION
Initial Tests (lab, imaging)
- NBS tests blood levels of immunoreactive trypsin (IRT) (2)[A].
- Patients must have clinical symptoms of CF involving at least one organ system
- Sweat test (gold standard)
  - Sweat chloride
    - >60 mmol/L (on 2 occasions) is (+) for CF.
    - <40 mmol/L is normal.
  - CFTR mutation analysis
  - Limited panel testing: Allele-specific polymerase chain reaction (PCR) identifies >90% of mutations; finite chance of false-negative finding. Full-sequence testing is more costly and time-consuming.
  - Nasal potential difference (when sweat test and DNA testing inconclusive)
  - CXR

Follow-Up Tests & Special Considerations
To further investigate the presence of CF-related complications, these tests are generally ordered:
- Sputum culture (common CF organisms)
- Pulmonary function tests (PFTs)
- 72-hour fecal fat, stool elastase
- Oral glucose tolerance test (OGTT) annually after age 10 years

- Head CT: Abnormal sinus CT findings are nearly universal in CF and may include mucosal thickening, intraluminal sinus polyps, and sinus effusions.
- Chest CT (not routine): useful when unusual findings noted on CXR

Diagnostic Procedures/Other
- Flexible bronchoscopy
- Bronchoalveolar lavage

TREATMENT

GENERAL MEASURES
- CF Foundation Guidelines call for yearly evaluation:
  - 4 office visits, 4 respiratory cultures, PFTs q6mo, and at least 1 evaluation by a multidisciplinary team including dietician, GI, and social worker
  - PFT goals: >75% predicted for adults, >100% predicted for children <18 years old
  - Annual screening for ABPA for patients >6 years old with total serum IgE concentration
  - Annual influenza vaccination for all CF patients age >6 months and all other age appropriate recommended vaccines
  - Screen all adults for osteoporosis with a DXA scan.
  - Annual measurement of fat soluble vitamins to rule out vitamin deficiencies
  - Annual LFTs
  - Decrease exposure to tobacco smoke
  - All patients should be followed in a CF center (accredited sites are listed at www.cff.org).
- Infant care:
  - Monthly visits for first 6 months of life and then every 2 months until 1 year of life
  - Fecal elastase testing and salt supplementation after diagnosis
  - Consider palivizumab for RSV prophylaxis in infants with CF <2 years (6)[A].
  - Avoidance of smoke

MEDICATION
- Pulmonary infections:
  - Antibiotics, oral
    - *Staphylococcus aureus*: Bactrim (MRSA), doxycycline (MRSA) or cephalexin
    - *Pseudomonas aeruginosa*: fluoroquinolones
  - Antibiotics, inhaled
    - TOBI (tobramycin): for *P. aeruginosa*, nebulizer twice daily for 28 days; stop for 28 days, then resume use (7)[A]
    - Colistin (more commonly used in Europe)
    - Cayston (aerosolized aztreonam) (7)[A]
  - Antibiotics, IV
    - *S. aureus*: Cefazolin or nafcillin
    - Methicillin-resistant *S. aureus* (MRSA): vancomycin or linezolid
    - *P. aeruginosa*: Zosyn or ceftazidime plus aminoglycoside (tobramycin)
    - Dual therapy synergistic
- Medications recommended for chronic use in pulmonary disease:
  - Recombinant human DNAse (Dornase alpha) (7)[A]
  - Hypertonic saline
  - High-dose ibuprofen in patients 6 to 17 years old with FEV_1 ≤60 PPV
  - Inhaled tobramycin or aztreonam in *P. aeruginosa* positive patients

- Azithromycin in *P. aeruginosa* positive patients
- Ivacaftor (VX770): A small-molecule CFTR potentiator shown to improve lung function and improve risk of pulmonary exacerbations in patients 6 years and older with at least one copy of *G551D* mutation (7)[A].
- Inhaled steroids are not recommended for chronic use in the absence of asthma or ABPA.
- Insufficient evidence to recommend for or against chonic use: inhaled β-agonist, inhaled anticholinergics, leukotriene modifiers, inhaled colistin
  - Pancreatic enzymes (87.3%) (2)[A]
    - Often combined with H_2 blocker or PPI to increase effectiveness
  - Fat-soluble vitamin supplementation (A, D, E, and K)
  - Liver disease (cholestasis)
    - Ursodeoxycholic acid has not been proven effective.

ADDITIONAL THERAPIES
- High frequency chest wall oscillation vest is the most widely used airway clearance technique.
- Aerobic exercise is used as an adjunct therapy for airway clearance (8)[A].
  - CF-related bone disease: Consider bisphosphonate therapy.

SURGERY/OTHER PROCEDURES
- Timing for lung transplantation (bilateral) is polyfactorial (9)[A].
- 5-year posttransplant survival is up to 62%.
- Liver transplantation is reserved for progressive liver failure ± portal hypertension with GI bleeding.
- Nasal polypectomy in 4.5% of CF patients (2)[A]

INPATIENT CONSIDERATIONS
Admission Criteria/Initial Stabilization
- CF exacerbations should always be admitted on contact precautions and private rooms.
- Pulmonary exacerbation (most common reason for admission)
- Bowel obstruction (due to DIOS, previously known as meconium ileus equivalent [MIE])
- Pancreatitis (in pancreatic-sufficient patients)
- Nasal cannula oxygen when SaO_2 <90%

IV Fluids
- Increased salt loss increases risk of hyponatremic hypochloremic dehydration.
- Cautious use of IV fluids

ONGOING CARE

FOLLOW-UP RECOMMENDATIONS
- Upon discharge for a pulmonary exacerbation, follow-up with CF provider within 2 to 4 weeks
- Routine clinic visits every 3 months, with airway cultures and pulmonary function testing
- Annual comprehensive nutritional evaluation (5)[A]

DIET
High-calorie, high-fat diet titrated to specific BMI goals established by the CF Foundation nutrition guidelines. If not meeting nutritional goals, dietician, pancreatize enzyme, and oral or tube supplemental feeding should be considered if indicated (8)[A].

PATIENT EDUCATION
Cystic Fibrosis Foundation: www.cff.org

PROGNOSIS
- Median survival is 40.7 years.
- Progression of lung disease usually determines length of survival.

REFERENCES
1. Grigoriadis C, Tympa A, Theodoraki K. Cystic fibrosis and pregnancy: counseling, obstetrical management and perinatal outcome. *Invest Clin*. 2015;56(1):66–73.
2. Cystic Fibrosis Foundation Patient Registry. *Annual Data Report*. Bethesda, MD: Cystic Fibrosis Foundation; 2013.
3. Gilljam M, Ellis L, Corey M, et al. Clinical manifestations of cystic fibrosis among patients with diagnosis in adulthood. *Chest*. 2004;126(4): 1215–1224.
4. Moran A, Brunzell C, Cohen RC, et al. Clinical care guidelines for cystic fibrosis-related diabetes: a position statement of the American Diabetes Association and a clinical practice guideline of the Cystic Fibrosis Foundation, endorsed by the Pediatric Endocrine Society. *Diabetes Care*. 2010;33(12):2697–2708.
5. O'Sullivan BP, Freedman SD. Cystic fibrosis. *Lancet*. 2009;373(9678):1891–1904.
6. Borowitz D, Robinson KA, Rosenfeld M, et al. Cystic Fibrosis Foundation evidence-based guidelines for management of infants with cystic fibrosis. *J Pediatr*. 2009;155(6)(Suppl):S73–S93.
7. Mogayzel PJ Jr, Naureckas ET, Robinson KA, et al. Cystic fibrosis pulmonary guidelines. Chronic medications for maintenance of lung health. *Am J Respir Crit Care Med*. 2013;187(7):680–689.
8. Flume PA, Robinson KA, O'Sullivan BP, et al. Cystic fibrosis pulmonary guidelines: airway clearance therapies. *Respir Care*. 2009;54(4):522–537.
9. Weill D, Benden C, Corris PA, et al. A consensus document for the selection of lung transplant candidates: 2014—an update from the Pulmonary Transplantation Council of the International Society for Heart and Lung Transplantation. *J Heart Lung Transplant*. 2015;34(1):1–15.

CODES

ICD10
- E84.9 Cystic fibrosis, unspecified
- E84.11 Meconium ileus in cystic fibrosis
- E84.0 Cystic fibrosis with pulmonary manifestations

CLINICAL PEARLS
- Meconium ileus is virtually pathognomonic for CF.
- When sweat test is equivocal, CFTR genetic testing is diagnostic.
- CF must be considered in *any* child with chronic diarrhea, especially if associated with poor growth or failure to thrive.
- All children with nasal polyps, digital clubbing, or bronchiectasis should be evaluated.
- A rapid decline in pulmonary function suggests the acquisition of resistant organisms (e.g., *Burkholderia cepacia*), CFRD, allergic bronchopulmonary aspergillosis (ABPA), or GERD.

DE QUERVAIN TENOSYNOVITIS

Jeff Wang, MD, MPH • J. Herbert Stevenson, MD

 BASICS

DESCRIPTION
- First identified in 1895, de Quervain tenosynovitis is a painful condition due to stenosis of the tendon sheath in the first dorsal compartment of the radial aspect of the wrist.
- Caused by repetitive motion of the extensor pollicis brevis (EPB) and abductor pollicis longus (APL) over the radial styloid with resultant irritation of the surrounding tendon sheath

EPIDEMIOLOGY
- The predominant age range is 30 to 50 years.
- Women are affected more commonly than men (1).

Incidence
- The overall incidence of de Quervain tenosynovitis is 0.9/1,000 person-years (1).
- For patients age >40 years, the incidence is 1.4/1,000 person-years compared with 0.6/1,000 person-years for those younger than 20 years.
- Women have an incidence rate ratio of 2.8/1,000 person-years compared with 0.6/1,000 person-years in men.
- The incidence ratio rate of de Quervain tenosynovitis is 1.3/1,000 person-years in blacks and 0.8/1,000 person-years in whites.

ETIOLOGY AND PATHOPHYSIOLOGY
- Repetitive motions of the wrist and/or thumb result in microtrauma and thickening of the tendons (EPB, APL) and surrounding tendon sheath
- EPB and APL movement is resisted as they glide over the radial styloid causing pain with movements of the thumb and wrist.

RISK FACTORS
- Women age 30 to 50 years
- Pregnancy (primarily 3rd trimester and postpartum)
- African American
- Systemic diseases (e.g., rheumatoid arthritis)
- Participation in activities that include repetitive motion or forceful grasping with thumb and wrist deviation such as golf, fly fishing, racquet sports, rowing, or bicycling
- Repetitive movements with the hand/thumb requiring forceful grasping with wrist involving ulnar/radial deviation; dental hygienists, musicians, carpenters, assembly workers, and machine operators

GENERAL PREVENTION
Avoid overuse or repetitive movements of the wrist and/or thumb associated with forceful grasping and ulnar/radial deviation.

 DIAGNOSIS

HISTORY
- Repetitive motion activity; overuse of wrist or thumb
- Gradually worsening pain along the radial aspect of the thumb and wrist with certain movements, particularly ulnar deviation of the wrist
- Pregnancy
- Sports, leisure, and occupational history
- Trauma (rare)

PHYSICAL EXAM
- Pain over the radial styloid exacerbated when patients move the thumb or make a fist.
- Crepitus with movement of the thumb
- Swelling over the radial styloid and base of the thumb
- Decreased range of motion of the thumb
- Pain over the 1st dorsal compartment on resisted thumb abduction or extension
- Tenderness may extend proximally or distally along the tendons with palpation or stress.
- Finkelstein test: The examiner grasps the affected thumb and deviates the hand sharply in the ulnar direction. A positive test occurs when there is pain along the distal radius.
- Eickhoff test: Patient grasps a flexed thumb and the examiner deviates the wrist in an ulnar direction.
- Finkelstein test is more sensitive for determining tenosynovitis of the APL and EPB tendons (2)[A].

DIFFERENTIAL DIAGNOSIS
- Scaphoid fracture
- Scapholunate ligament tear
- Dorsal wrist ganglion
- Osteoarthritis of the 1st carpometacarpal joint
- Flexor carpi radialis tendonitis
- Infectious tenosynovitis
- Tendonitis of the wrist extensors
- Intersection syndrome
- Trigger thumb

DIAGNOSTIC TESTS & INTERPRETATION
Initial Tests (lab, imaging)
- Primarily a clinical diagnosis. Radiographs of the wrist to rule out other pathology, such as carpometacarpal (CMC) arthritis, if the diagnosis is in question.
- MRI is the imaging test of choice to rule out coexisting soft tissue injury or wrist joint pathology.

Follow-Up Tests & Special Considerations
Ultrasound can help to detect anatomic variations in the 1st dorsal extensor compartment of the wrist and target corticosteroid injections (3),(4)[C],(5)[B].

Test Interpretation
Inflamed and thickened retinacular sheath of the tendon

TREATMENT

- Most cases of de Quervain syndrome are self-limited.
- Rest and NSAIDs (2)[A]
- Ice (15 to 20 minutes 5 to 6 times a day)
- Immobilization with a thumb spica splint (2)[A]
- Occupational therapy (6)[A]
- Corticosteroid injection (ultrasound guided) (7)[A]
- Consider surgery if conservative measures fail >6 months.

GENERAL MEASURES
- If full relief is not achieved, a corticosteroid injection of the tendon sheath can improve symptoms.
- Anatomic variation, including two tendon sheaths in the 1st compartment or the EPB tendon traveling in a separate compartment may complicate treatment. Ultrasound can distinguish these variants and improve anatomic accuracy of injections (3),(8)[B],(9,10).
- Surgical release may be indicated after 3 to 6 months of conservative treatment if symptoms persist. Surgery is highly effective and has a relatively low rate of complications.

MEDICATION
First Line
Splinting, rest, and NSAIDs

Second Line
- Corticosteroid injection of the tendon sheath has shown significant cure rates. An 83% success rate after single injection has been reported. Additional injections are sometimes required (7)[A].
- Corticosteroid injection plus immobilization is more effective than immobilization alone (5)[B].
- Addition of hyaluronic acid to the corticosteroid injection improves outcome and reduces recurrence (11)[B].
- A 4-point injection technique may be preferred to 1- and 2-point injection techniques in high-resistance training athletes (12)[B].

- Percutaneous tenotomy and/or injection of platelet-rich plasma are newer techniques that show promise for treatment of de Quervain tenosynovitis.

ISSUES FOR REFERRAL
Referral to a hand surgeon is indicated if there is no improvement with conservative therapy.

ADDITIONAL THERAPIES
- Hand therapy, along with iontophoresis/phonophoresis, may help improve outcomes in persistent cases.
- Patients may use thumb-stretching exercises as part of their rehabilitation.

SURGERY/OTHER PROCEDURES
- Indicated for patients who have failed conservative treatment
- Endoscopic release may provide earlier relief, fewer superficial radial nerve complications, and greater patient satisfaction with resultant scar compared to open release (5)[B].

INPATIENT CONSIDERATIONS
Admission Criteria/Initial Stabilization
Hospitalization for care associated with surgical treatment

 ONGOING CARE

FOLLOW-UP RECOMMENDATIONS
- Additional corticosteroid injection may be performed at 4 to 6 weeks if symptoms persist. Caution with repeat steroid injections.
- Avoid repetitive motions and activities that cause pain.

DIET
As tolerated

PATIENT EDUCATION
Activity modification: Avoid repetitive movement of the wrist/thumb and forceful grasping.

PROGNOSIS
Extremely good with conservative treatment. Complete resolution can take up to 1 year. 95% success rates have been shown with conservative therapy over 1 year. Up to 1/3 of patients will have recurrence (7)[A].

COMPLICATIONS
- Most complications are secondary to treatment. This includes GI, renal, and hepatic injury secondary to NSAID use.

- Nerve damage may occur during surgery (13)[B].
- Hypopigmentation, fat atrophy, bleeding, infection, and tendon rupture have been reported as potential adverse events from corticosteroid injection. Ultrasound guidance reduces the rate of complications (14)[B].
- If not appropriately treated, thumb flexibility may be lost due to fibrosis.

REFERENCES

1. Wolf JM, Sturdivant RX, Owens BD. Incidence of de Quervain's tenosynovitis in a young, active population. *J Hand Surg Am*. 2009;34(1):112–115.
2. Huisstede BM, Coert JH, Fridén J, et al. Consensus on a multidisciplinary treatment guideline for de Quervain disease: results from the European HANDGUIDE study. *Phys Ther*. 2014;94(8):1095–1110.
3. Lee KH, Kang CN, Lee BG, et al. Ultrasonographic evaluation of the first extensor compartment of the wrist in de Quervain's disease. *J Orthop Sci*. 2014;19(1):49–54.
4. Di Sante L, Martino M, Manganiello I, et al. Ultrasound-guided corticosteroid injection for the treatment of de Quervain's tenosynovitis. *Am J Phys Med Rehabil*. 2013;92(7):637–638.
5. Kang HJ, Koh IH, Jang JW, et al. Endoscopic versus open release in patients with de Quervain's tenosynovitis: a randomised trial. *Bone Joint J*. 2013;95-B(7):947–951.
6. Goel R, Abzug JM. de Quervain's tenosynovitis: a review of the rehabilitative options. *Hand (N Y)*. 2015;10(1):1–5.
7. Ashraf MO, Devadoss VG. Systematic review and meta-analysis on steroid injection therapy for de Quervain's tenosynovitis in adults. *Eur J Orthop Surg Traumatol*. 2014;24(2):149–157.
8. Kume K, Amano K, Yamada S, et al. In de Quervain's with a separate EPB compartment, ultrasound-guided steroid injection is more effective than a clinical injection technique: a prospective open-label study. *J Hand Surg Eur Vol*. 2012;37(6):523–527.
9. Kwon BC, Choi SJ, Koh SH, et al. Sonographic identification of the intracompartmental septum in de Quervain's disease. *Clin Orthop Relat Res*. 2010;468(8):2129–2134.
10. Rousset P, Vuillemin-Bodaghi V, Laredo JD, et al. Anatomic variations in the first extensor compartment of the wrist: accuracy of US. *Radiology*. 2010;257(2):427–433.
11. Orlandi D, Corazza A, Fabbro E, et al. Ultrasound-guided percutaneous injection to treat de Quervain's disease using three different techniques: a randomized controlled trial. *Eur Radiol*. 2015;25(5):1512–1519.
12. Pagonis T, Ditsios K, Toli P, et al. Improved corticosteroid treatment of recalcitrant de Quervain tenosynovitis with a novel 4-point injection technique. *Am J Sports Med*. 2011;39(2):398–403.
13. Scheller A, Schuh R, Hönle W, et al. Long-term results of surgical release of de Quervain's stenosing tenosynovitis. *Int Orthop*. 2009;33(5):1301–1303.
14. Jeyapalan K, Choudhary S. Ultrasound-guided injection of triamcinolone and bupivacaine in the management of de Quervain's disease. *Skeletal Radiol*. 2009;38(11):1099–1103.

ADDITIONAL READING
- Choi SJ, Ahn JH, Lee YJ, et al. De Quervain disease: US identification of anatomic variations in the first extensor compartment with an emphasis on sub-compartmentalization. *Radiology*. 2011;260(2):480–486.
- Peters-Veluthamaningal C, van der Windt DA, Winters JC, et al. Corticosteroid injection for de Quervain's tenosynovitis. *Cochrane Database Syst Rev*. 2009;(3):CD005616.

 SEE ALSO

Algorithm: Pain in Upper Extremity

 CODES

ICD10
M65.4 Radial styloid tenosynovitis [de Quervain]

CLINICAL PEARLS
- Repetitive movements of the wrist and thumb, and activities that require forceful grasping are the most common causes of de Quervain tenosynovitis.
- Initial treatment is typically conservative.
- Corticosteroid injections are helpful and have lower complication rates if done under ultrasound guidance.
- Surgery is helpful for recalcitrant cases.

D

DEEP VEIN THROMBOPHLEBITIS

Denisse V. Tafur, MD • Alfonso Tafur, MD, MS, RPVI

BASICS

DESCRIPTION
- Development of blood clot within the deep veins, usually accompanied by inflammation of the vessel wall
- Major clinical consequences are embolization (usually to the lung) and postphlebitic syndrome.
- System(s) affected: cardiovascular

EPIDEMIOLOGY
- Age and gender adjusted incidence of venous thromboembolism (VTE) is 100 times higher in the hospital than in the community. Almost half of all VTEs occur either during or soon after discharge from a hospital stay or surgery.
- Of patients with VTE, 1/3 die within 30 days, 20% will have sudden death due to pulmonary embolism (PE). The 28-day DVT fatality rate is 9%.

Incidence
- In the United States, VTE occurs for the first time in 100/100,000 persons/year.
- ~2/3 of the new VTE cases are DVT alone.
- Higher incidence among Caucasians and African Americans relative to Hispanics and Asians
- Complicates ~1/1,000 pregnancies

Prevalence
Variable; depends on medical condition or procedure
- 22–52% of the patients with PE have DVT.
- 25% of patients with superficial venous thrombosis (1)[B]
- Present in 11% of patients with acquired brain injury entering to neurorehabilitation

ETIOLOGY AND PATHOPHYSIOLOGY
Factors involved may include venous stasis, endothelial injury, and abnormalities of coagulation.

Genetics
- Factor V Leiden is found in 5% of the population and in 20% of all VTE events. It is the most common thrombophilia. Homozygosity is found in 1/5,000 persons. It increases the risk of VTE 3- to 8-fold in heterozygous carriers and 50- to 80-fold in homozygous.
- Prothrombin 20210A is found in 3% of Caucasians. Increases the risk of thrombosis ~3-fold.

RISK FACTORS
- Acquired: age, previous thrombosis, immobilization, major surgery, orthopedic surgery, malignancy, oral contraceptives, hormonal replacement therapy, antiphospholipid syndrome, polycythemia vera, paroxysmal nocturnal hemoglobinuria, pregnancy/puerperium, diabetes who developed VTE
- Inherited: antithrombin deficiency, protein C deficiency, protein S deficiency, factor V Leiden R506Q, prothrombin G20210A, dysfibrinogenemia
- Mixed/unknown: hyperhomocysteinemia, high levels of factor VIII, high levels of thrombin activatable fibrinolysis inhibitor (TAFI), high levels of factor XI

GENERAL PREVENTION
- Mechanical thromboprophylaxis is recommended in patients with high bleeding risk and as adjunct to anticoagulant-based thromboprophylaxis.
- Compression stockings have conflicting data on postthrombotic syndrome prevention (2)[B].

- Risk stratification of hospitalized patients using standardized scores is recommended (i.e., Caprini score).
- For acutely ill and for critically ill hospitalized patients at increased risk of thrombosis, low-molecular-weight heparin [LMWH], low-dose unfractionated heparin [LDUH], or fondaparinux are recommended (3)[C].
- Rivaroxaban and apixaban are approved in United States for surgical DVT prevention.
- For most patients, prolonged secondary prophylaxis is not recommended.

DIAGNOSIS

Modified Wells criteria
- Active cancer +1 point. Calf swelling >3 +1 point. Collateral superficial veins +1 point. Pitting edema +1 point. Previous documented DVT +1 point. Swelling of entire leg +1 point. Localized pain along distribution of deep venous system +1 point. Paralysis, paresis, or recent cast immobilization of lower extremities +1 point. Recently bedridden >3 days or major surgery requiring regional or general anesthetic in past 4 weeks +1 point. Alternative diagnosis at least as likely −2 points
  - Interpretation: Score 0 to 1 DVT unlikely. Score ≥2: moderate to high probability.

HISTORY
- Establish pretest probability based on Wells criteria.
- Classify as "provoked" or "idiopathic" based on underlying risk factors, that is, surgery, cancer, pregnancy, trauma.
- Clinical assessment of bleeding risk: bleeding with previous history of anticoagulation, history of liver disease, recent interventions, history of GI bleed

PHYSICAL EXAM
- Physical exam is only 30% accurate for DVT.
- Resistance to dorsiflexion of the foot (Homan sign) is unreliable.
- Swelling of collateral veins. Massive edema with cyanosis is a medical emergency (phlegmasia cerulea dolens, rare).
- Thoracic outlet maneuvers in upper extremity DVT
- Attention to signs of possible malignancy

DIFFERENTIAL DIAGNOSIS
Cellulitis, fracture, ruptured synovial cyst (Baker cyst), lymphedema, muscle strain/tear, extrinsic compression of vein (e.g., by tumor/enlarged lymph nodes), compartment syndrome, localized allergic reaction

DIAGNOSTIC TESTS & INTERPRETATION
Initial Tests (lab, imaging)
- D-dimer (sensitive but not specific; has a high negative predictive value [NPV])
- Patients with a prior DVT and those with malignancy have a high rate of VTE, which decreases the NPV of Wells prediction rule (4).
- CBC, platelet count, activated partial thromboplastin time (aPTT), prothrombin time (PT)/INR
- In young patients with idiopathic/recurrent VTE, consider thrombophilia testing.
- Compression ultrasound (CUS): noninvasive; sensitive and specific for popliteal, femoral thrombi but has poor ability to detect calf vein thrombi
- Contrast venography: gold standard, is technically difficult, risk of morbidity

- Impedance plethysmography: as accurate as duplex US, less operator dependent but poor at detecting calf vein thrombi; not widely available
- MR venography: as accurate as contrast venography; may be useful for patients with contraindications to IV contrast
- ^{125}I-fibrinogen scan: detects only active clot formation; very good at detecting ongoing calf thrombi; takes 4 hours for results
- In patients with suspected DVT, the choice of diagnostic test process should be guided by the assessment of the pretest probability.
  - Low pretest probability: D-dimer, proximal CUS
  - Moderate pretest probability: D-dimer, proximal CUS, whole leg US
  - High pretest probability: proximal CUS, whole leg US
  - If negative, no further testing is recommended.
  - If positive
    o Low pretest probability, then CUS
    o Moderate pretest probability, then proximal CUS/whole leg US
    o CUS: if positive, treat DVT; if negative
  - Low pretest probability, no further testing
  - Moderate pretest probability, repeat proximal CUS in 1 week

Follow-Up Tests & Special Considerations
Risk of an underlying malignancy is more likely if recurrent VTE, risk 3.2 (95% CI 2.0–4.8). Unprovoked VTE, 4.6 times higher (vs. secondary); upper extremity DVT, not catheter associated; odds ratio (OR) 1.8, abdominal DVT; OR 2.2, (5) bilateral lower extremity DVT, OR 2.1 (5)

TREATMENT

MEDICATION
All proximal DVTs should receive treatment. Consider starting therapy even before confirmation in patients with high pretest probability.

First Line
- Unfractionated heparin (UFH)
  - IV drip: initial dose of 80 U/kg or 5,000 U followed by continuous infusion of 18 U/kg/hr. Target an aPTT ratio >1.5. The aPTT prolongation should correspond to a 0.3 to 0.7 anti-Xa level.
  - SC UFH: monitored: 17,500 U or 250 U/kg BID with aPTT adjustment to an equivalent to 0.3 to 0.7 anti-Xa. Alternatively, fixed dose: 333 U/kg followed by BID dose 250 U/kg.
- Enoxaparin (Lovenox): 1 mg/kg/dose SC q12h or 1.5 mg/kg/dose OD
- Dalteparin (Fragmin): 200 U/kg SC q24h
- Fondaparinux (Arixtra): 5 mg (body weight <50 kg), 7.5 mg (body weight = 50 to 100 kg), or 10 mg (body weight >100 kg) SC once daily
- Rivaroxaban (Xarelto): 15 mg PO twice daily with food for the first 3 weeks.
- Apixaban (Eliquis): 10 mg PO twice daily for 1 week followed by 2.5 to 5 mg PO twice daily
- 2016 CHEST guidelines recommend using dabigatran, rivaroxaban, apixaban, or edoxaban instead of vitamin K antagonists for the first 3 months' treatment. Evidence to support these recommendations remains mixed. Because of cost and insurance coverage, implementation of these recommendations will be variable (http://journal.publications .chestnet.org/article.aspx?articleid=2479255).

- Maintenance therapy
  - Warfarin (Coumadin): 5 mg/day for 3 days, then adjust to a target INR of 2 to 3; overlap with injectable anticoagulant for minimum of 5 days and two consecutive therapeutic INRs
  - Rivaroxaban (Xarelto): 20 mg PO once daily with food after the first 3 weeks
  - Apixaban (Eliquis): 2.5 to 5 mg PO twice daily after the first 1 week
  - Dabigatran (Pradaxa): 150 mg PO twice daily (CrCl >30 mL/min) after 5 to 10 days of parenteral anticoagulant
  - Edoxaban (Savaysa): 60 mg PO once daily following 5 to 10 days of initial therapy with a parenteral anticoagulant (30 mg If CrCl 15 to 50 mL/min or ≤60 kg)
- Adverse effects
  - Heparin or LMWH: bleeding, edema, injection site irritation, skin eruptions, hematoma, thrombocytopenia
  - Fondaparinux: bleeding, injection site irritation, rash, fever, anemia
  - Warfarin: bleeding, skin necrosis, teratogenicity
  - Rivaroxaban: bleeding, anemia, rash, increase in transaminases
  - Dabigatran: bleeding, rash, edema
  - Edoxaban: bleeding, rash, anemia
- Contraindications
  - Heparin or LMWH: bleeding, heparin hypersensitivity, heparin-induced thrombocytopenia (HIT), idiopathic thrombocytopenic purpura (ITP)
  - Fondaparinux: bleeding, thrombocytopenia
  - Warfarin: current bleeding, alcoholism, preeclampsia, pregnancy, surgery

Second Line
Heparin can be given by intermittent SC self-injection.

Pregnancy Considerations
- Warfarin (Coumadin) is a teratogen; treat with full-dose heparin initially, followed by SC heparin starting at 15,000 U q12h.
- Warfarin is safe with breastfeeding.
- LMWH, dalteparin, fondaparinux, apixaban are pregnancy Category B.
- Dabigatran, Edoxaban are pregnancy Category C.

ADDITIONAL THERAPIES
Edoxaban (recently FDA approved) after initial treatment with heparin is as effective as warfarin in preventing recurrences in patients with acute VTE and has less bleeding complications (6)[B].

SURGERY/OTHER PROCEDURES
- In selected patients with proximal DVT (iliofemoral DVT, <2 weeks of symptoms, good functional status, >1 year of life expectancy), consider catheter-directed thrombolysis/open thrombectomy.
- When anticoagulants have failed or are contraindicated, filtering devices are recommended in the acute setting.

INPATIENT CONSIDERATIONS
Admission Criteria/Initial Stabilization
Admission for respiratory distress, proximal VTE, candidate for thrombolysis, active bleeding, renal failure, phlegmasia cerulea dolens, history of HIT

Nursing
Limb elevation and multilayered compression.

Discharge Criteria
Medically stable and properly anticoagulated; overlap of anticoagulation and warfarin monitoring may be done as an outpatient.

 ## ONGOING CARE

FOLLOW-UP RECOMMENDATIONS
- Gradual resumption of normal activity, with avoidance of prolonged immobility
- Duration of warfarin treatment after DVT
  - 3 months for treatment of a DVT secondary to a reversible risk factor
  - Patients with unprovoked DVT can be considered for prolonged secondary prophylaxis
    - In patients who have completed 3 months of anticoagulation after an unprovoked VTE, a positive D-dimer 1 month after discontinuation of therapy correlates with the risk of VTE recurrence (7)[A].

Patient Monitoring
- Monitor platelet count while on heparin, LMWH, fondaparinux.
- An anti-Xa activity level may help guide LMWH titration of therapy, but it is not usually needed.
- Investigate significant bleeding (e.g., hematuria or GI hemorrhage) because anticoagulant therapy may unmask a preexisting lesion (e.g., cancer, peptic ulcer disease, or arteriovenous malformation).

PATIENT EDUCATION
- Patients should wear compression stockings post-DVT.
- Dietary habits should be discussed when warfarin is initiated to ensure that intake of vitamin K–rich foods is monitored.

PROGNOSIS
- 20% of untreated proximal (e.g., above the calf) DVTs progress to pulmonary emboli, and 10–20% of those are fatal; with anticoagulant therapy, mortality is decreased 5- to 10-fold.
- DVT confined to the infrapopliteal veins has a small risk of embolization but can propagate into the proximal system.

COMPLICATIONS
PE (fatal in 10–20%), arterial embolism (paradoxical embolization) with arteriovenous (AV) shunting, chronic venous insufficiency, postphlebitic syndrome (pain and swelling in affected limb without new clot formation), treatment-induced hemorrhage, soft tissue ischemia associated with massive clot and high venous pressures; phlegmasia cerulea dolens (rare but a surgical emergency)

REFERENCES
1. Decousus H, Quéré I, Presles E, et al. Superficial venous thrombosis and venous thromboembolism: a large, prospective epidemiologic study. Ann Intern Med. 2010;152(4):218–224.
2. Kahn S, Shapiro S, Wells P, et al. Compression stockings to prevent post-thrombotic syndrome: a randomised placebo-controlled trial. Lancet. 2014;383(9920):880–888.
3. Holbrook A, Schulman S, Witt DM, et al. Evidence-based management of anticoagulant therapy: Antithrombotic Therapy and Prevention of Thrombosis, 9th ed: American College of Chest Physicians evidence-based clinical practice guidelines. Chest. 2012;141(2 Suppl):e152S–e184S.
4. Geersing GJ, Zuithoff NP, Kearon C, et al. Exclusion of deep vein thrombosis using the Wells rule in clinically important subgroups: individual patient data meta-analysis. BMJ. 2014;348:g1340.
5. Tafur AJ, Kalsi H, Wysokinski WE, et al. The association of active cancer with venous thromboembolism location: a population-based study. Mayo Clin Proc. 2011;86(1):25–30.
6. Büller HR, Décousus H, Grosso MA, et al. Edoxaban versus warfarin for the treatment of symptomatic venous thromboembolism. N Engl J Med. 2013;369(15):1406–1415.
7. Palareti G, Cosmi B, Legnani C, et al. D-dimer testing to determine the duration of anticoagulation therapy. N Engl J Med. 2006;355(17):1780–1789.

ADDITIONAL READING
- Agnelli G, Büller HR, Cohen A, et al. Oral apixaban for the treatment of acute venous thromboembolism. N Eng J Med. 2013;369(9):799–808.
- Bauersachs R, Berkowitz SD, Brenner B, et al. Oral rivaroxaban for symptomatic venous thromboembolism. N Eng J Med. 2010;363(26):2499–2510.
- Kyrle PA, Rosendaal FR, Eichinger S. Risk assessment for recurrent venous thrombosis. Lancet. 2010;376(9757):2032–2039.
- Lyman GH, Khorana A, Kuderer N, et al. Venous thromboembolism prophylaxis and treatment in patients with cancer: American Society of Clinical Oncology clinical practice guideline update. J Clin Oncol. 2013;31(17):2189–2204.
- Prins MH, Lensing AW, Bauersachs R, et al. Oral rivaroxaban versus standard therapy for the treatment of symptomatic venous thromboembolism: a pooled analysis of the EINSTEIN-DVT and PE randomized studies. Thromb J. 2013;11(1):21.
- Schulman S, Kearon C, Kakkar AK, et al. Dabigatran versus warfarin in the treatment of acute venous thromboembolism. N Engl J Med. 2009;361(24):2342–2352.

 ### SEE ALSO

Antithrombin Deficiency; Factor V Leiden; Protein C Deficiency; Protein S Deficiency; Prothrombin 20210 (Mutation); Pulmonary Embolism

 ### CODES

ICD10
- I80.209 Phlbts and thombophlb of unsp deep vessels of unsp low extrm
- I80.299 Phlebitis and thombophlb of deep vessels of unsp low extrm
- I80.10 Phlebitis and thrombophlebitis of unspecified femoral vein

CLINICAL PEARLS
- Many cases are asymptomatic and are diagnosed after embolization.
- Of the patients with superficial thrombophlebitis, 25% will have DVT at presentation.
- Heparin and warfarin should overlap for a minimum of 5 days to achieve target INR.
- The current American Society of Clinical Oncology guidelines acknowledge the value of primary prophylaxis in selected patients with active cancer receiving outpatient chemotherapy.

DEHYDRATION

Jerin Mathew, MD • Mony Fraer, MD, FACP, FASN

BASICS

DESCRIPTION
- Dehydration is a state of negative fluid balance; strictly defined as free water deficiency
- The two types of dehydration:
  – Water loss
  – Salt and water loss (combination of dehydration and hypovolemia)

EPIDEMIOLOGY
- Cause of 10% of all pediatric hospitalizations in the United States
- Gastroenteritis, one of its leading causes, accounts to 13/1,000 children <5 years of age annually in the United States.

Incidence
- More than half a million hospital admissions annually in the United States for dehydration
- Of hospitalized older persons, 7.8% have the diagnosis of dehydration (1).
- Worldwide, ~3 to 5 billion cases of acute gastroenteritis occur each year in children <5 years of age, resulting in nearly 2 million deaths.

ETIOLOGY AND PATHOPHYSIOLOGY
- Negative fluid balance occurs when ongoing fluid losses exceed fluid intake.
- Fluid losses can be insensible (sweat, respiration), obligate (urine, stool), or abnormal (diarrhea, vomiting, osmotic diuresis in diabetic ketoacidosis).
- Negative fluid balance can ultimately lead to severe intravascular volume depletion (hypovolemia) and ultimately end-organ damage from inadequate perfusion.
- The elderly are at increased risk as kidney function, urine concentration, thirst sensation, aldosterone secretion, release of vasopressin, and renin activity are all significantly lowered with age.
- Decreased intake
- Increased output: vomiting, diarrheal illnesses, sweating, frequent urination
- Third spacing of fluids: effusions, ascites, capillary leaks from burns, or sepsis

Genetics
Some underlying causes of dehydration have a genetic component (diabetes), whereas others do not (gastroenteritis).

RISK FACTORS
- Children <5 years of age at highest risk
- Elderly
- Decreased cognition
- Lack of access to water such as in critically sick intubated patients

GENERAL PREVENTION
- Patient/parent education on the early signs of dehydration
- Observing universal precautions (including hand hygiene)

Geriatric Considerations
A systematic approach in assessing risk factors is necessary for early prevention and management of dehydration in the elderly, especially those in long-term care facilities.

COMMONLY ASSOCIATED CONDITIONS
- Hypo-/hypernatremia
- Hypokalemia
- Hypovolemic shock
- Renal failure

DIAGNOSIS

Calculate % dehydration = (preillness weight – illness weight)/preillness weight × 100. Supplement this along with the ongoing fluid loss.

Clinical Finding (2)	Mild	Moderate	Severe
Dehydration: children	5–10%	10–15%	>15%
Dehydration: adults	3–5%	5–10%	>10%
General condition: infants	Thirsty, alert, restless	Lethargic/drowsy	Limp, cold, cyanotic extremities, may be comatose
General condition: older children	Thirsty, alert, restless	Alert, postural dizziness	Apprehensive, cold, cyanotic extremities, muscle cramps
Quality of radial pulse	Normal	Thready/weak	Feeble or impalpable
Quality of respiration	Normal	Deep	Deep and rapid/tachypnea
BP	Normal	Normal to low	Low (shock)
Skin turgor	Normal skin turgor	Reduced skin turgor, cool skin	Skin tenting, cool, mottled, acrocyanotic skin
Eyes	Normal	Sunken	Very Sunken
Tears	Present	Absent	Absent
Mucous membranes	Moist	Dry	Very dry
Urine output	Normal	Reduced	None passed in many hours
Anterior fontanelle	Normal	Sunken	Markedly sunken

HISTORY
- Fever
- Intake (including description and amount)
- Diarrhea (including duration, frequency, consistency, ± mucus/blood)
- Vomiting (including duration, frequency, consistency, ± bilious/nonbilious)
- Urination pattern
- Sick contacts
- Medication history (e.g., diuretics, laxatives)

PHYSICAL EXAM
- The most useful individual signs for identifying dehydration in children are prolonged capillary refill time, abnormal skin turgor, and abnormal respiratory pattern (3).
- Vitals: pulse, BP, temperature
- Orthostatic vital signs: Take BP and heart rate (HR) while supine, sitting, and standing.
  – Systolic BP decrease by 20, diastolic BP decrease by 10, or HR increase by 20 highly suggestive of hypovolemia (4)
- Weight loss: <5%, 10%, or >15%
- Mental status
- Head: sunken anterior fontanelle (for infants)
- Eyes: sunken, ± tear production
- Mucous membranes: tacky, dry, or parched
- Capillary refill: ranges from brisk to >3 seconds

DIFFERENTIAL DIAGNOSIS
- Decreased intake: ineffective breastfeeding, inadequate thirst response, anorexia, malabsorption, metabolic disorder, obtunded state
- Excessive losses: gastroenteritis, diarrhea, febrile illness, diabetic ketoacidosis, hyperglycemia, hyperosmolar hyperglycemic state, diabetes insipidus, intestinal obstruction, sepsis

DIAGNOSTIC TESTS & INTERPRETATION
Initial Tests (lab, imaging)
- For mild dehydration: generally not necessary
- For moderate to severe dehydration
  – Blood work, including electrolytes, BUN, creatinine, and glucose
  – Urinalysis (specific gravity, hematuria, glucosuria)
- Imaging does not play a role in the diagnosis of dehydration, unless diagnosis of the specific medical condition causing the dehydration requires imaging.
- In adults, there is evidence to support the use of inferior vena cava collapsibility as a surrogate marker for volume status.

Pediatric Considerations
Infants and the elderly may not concentrate urine maximally, so a nonelevated specific gravity should not be reassuring.

TREATMENT

MEDICATION

First Line
- Oral rehydration is the first-line treatment in dehydrated children. If this is unsuccessful, use IV rehydration. If IV unobtainable, nasogastric (NG) rehydration can be considered (5).
- Oral rehydration is the first-line treatment in dehydrated adults as long as they can tolerate fluids. Have a lower threshold for IV rehydration if needed.
- If the patient is experiencing excessive vomiting, consider using an antiemetic.
- Ondansetron (PO/IV) may be effective in decreasing the rate of vomiting, improving the success rate of oral hydration, preventing the need for IV hydration, and preventing the need for hospital admission (6,7).
- Other antiemetics can be used.

Second Line
- Loperamide may reduce the duration of diarrhea compared with placebo in children with mild to moderate dehydration (two randomized controlled trials [RCTs] yes, one RCT no).
- In children ages 3 to 12 years with mild diarrhea and minimal dehydration, loperamide decreases diarrhea duration and frequency when used with oral rehydration.

Pediatric Considerations
Given a higher risk for serious adverse events, loperamide is not indicated for children <3 years of age with acute diarrhea.

ISSUES FOR REFERRAL
- For severe dehydration, critical care referral and ICU-level care may be warranted.
- Surgical consultation for acute abdominal issues

SURGERY/OTHER PROCEDURES
For specific underlying causes of dehydration, such as intestinal obstruction or appendicitis

INPATIENT CONSIDERATIONS

Admission Criteria/Initial Stabilization
- Intractable vomiting/diarrhea
- Electrolyte abnormalities
- Hemodynamic instability
- Inability to tolerate oral rehydration therapy (ORT)
- Stabilize ABCs.
- If mild dehydration, try ORT.
- If excessive vomiting/severe dehydration with shock, start IV access and IV fluids immediately.

IV Fluids
- Stage I
  - For moderate to severe dehydration in children: isotonic saline or Ringer lactate solution bolus of 10 to 20 mL/kg; may repeat up to 60 mL/kg; if still hemodynamically unstable, consider colloid replacement (blood, albumin, fresh frozen plasma) and address other causes for shock.
  - For moderate to severe hypovolemia in adults: isotonic saline or Ringer lactate 20 mL/kg/hr until normal state of consciousness returns/vital signs stabilize. Also consider colloid replacement if continued fluids required beyond 3 L.
- Stage II: Replace fluid deficit along with maintenance over 48 hours. Fluid deficit = preillness weight − illness weight.

- An alternative IV treatment option for moderate (10%) dehydration in children
  - Bolus with NS/LR at 20 mL/kg for 1 hour
  - Replete fluid deficit with D5 1/2 NS + 20 mEq KCl/L at 10 mL/kg for 8 hours (hours 2 to 9).
  - Replete 1.5 for maintenance fluids with D5 1/4 NS + 20 mEq/L of KCl for 16 hours (hours 10 to 24).
- An alternative to IV fluids is hypodermoclysis, the SC infusion of fluids into the body.
  - Indications: hydration of patients with mild to moderate dehydration who do not tolerate oral intake because of cognitive impairment, severe dysphagia, advanced terminal illness, or intractable vomiting. It is also indicated to prevent dehydration, especially in frail elderly residents living in long-term care settings who reject the oral route for any reason; useful technique for patients with difficult IV access
  - Contraindications: severe dehydration or shock, patients with coagulopathy or receiving full anticoagulation, patients with severe generalized edema (anasarca) or congestive heart failure, and those with fluid overload (8)

Nursing
Strict inputs and outputs: oral and IV input and output of urine and stool, which may include weighing wet diapers

Discharge Criteria
- Input > output
- Underlying etiology treated and improving

 ONGOING CARE

FOLLOW-UP RECOMMENDATIONS
Activity as tolerated
- If mild to moderate dehydration, the patient may be mobile without restrictions, although watch for orthostasis/falls.
- If moderate to severe dehydration, bed rest.

Patient Monitoring
Ongoing surveillance for recurrence

DIET
- Bland food such as bananas, rice, apples, toast (BRAT) diet
- If diarrhea, avoid dairy for 48 hours after symptoms resolve. One review of weak RCTs and three of five subsequent RCTs found that lactose-free feeds reduced the duration of diarrhea in children with mild to severe dehydration, compared with lactose-containing feeds. However, two subsequent RCTs found no difference between lactose-free and lactose-containing feeds in duration of diarrhea.
- Small frequent sips of room temperature liquids
- For children, Pedialyte (liquid or popsicles)
- Continue breastfeeding ad lib.

PATIENT EDUCATION
- Patients should go to the nearest emergency facility or call 911 if they or their child feels faint or dizzy when rising from a sitting or lying position, becomes lethargic and/or confused, or complains of a rapid heart rate.
- Patients should call their physician if they are unable to keep down any fluids, vomiting has been going on >24 hours in an adult or >12 hours in a child, diarrhea has lasted >2 days in an adult/child, or an infant/child is much less active than usual or is very irritable.

- Patient information on dehydration: http://www.mayoclinic.org/diseases-conditions/dehydration/basics/definition/con-20030056

PROGNOSIS
Self-limited if treated early; potentially fatal

COMPLICATIONS
- Seizures
- Renal failure
- Cardiovascular arrest

REFERENCES

1. Thomas DR, Cote TR, Lawhorne L, et al. Understanding clinical dehydration and its treatment. *J Am Med Dir Assoc.* 2008;9(5):292–301.
2. Gorelick MH, Shaw KN, Murphy KO. Validity and reliability of clinical signs in the diagnosis of dehydration in children. *Pediatrics.* 1997;99(5):E6.
3. Steiner MJ, DeWalt DA, Byerley JS. Is this child dehydrated? *JAMA.* 2004;291(22):2746–2754.
4. Lanier JB, Mote MB, Clay EC. Evaluation and management of orthostatic hypotension. *Am Fam Physician.* 2011;84(5):527–536.
5. Rouhani S, Meloney L, Ahn R, et al. Alternative rehydration methods: a systematic review and lessons for resource-limited care. *Pediatrics.* 2011;127(3):e748–e757.
6. Colletti JE, Brown KM, Sharieff GQ, et al. The management of children with gastroenteritis and dehydration in the emergency department. *J Emerg Med.* 2010;38(5):686–698.
7. Carter B, Fedorowicz Z. Antiemetic treatment for acute gastroenteritis in children: an updated Cochrane systematic review with meta-analysis and mixed treatment comparison in a Bayesian framework. *BMJ Open.* 2012;2(4):e000622.
8. Lopez JH, Reyes-Ortiz CA. Subcutaneous hydration by hypodermoclysis. *Rev Clin Gerontol.* 2010;20(2):105–113.

 SEE ALSO

Oral Rehydration

 CODES

ICD10
- E86.0 Dehydration
- E87.1 Hypo-osmolality and hyponatremia
- E86.1 Hypovolemia

CLINICAL PEARLS
- Dehydration is the result of a negative fluid balance and is a common cause of hospitalization in both children and the elderly.
- Begin by assessing the level of dehydration and determining the underlying cause.
- Treatment is directed at restoring fluid balance via oral rehydration (first-line) therapy or IV fluids and treating underlying causes.

DELAYED SLEEP-WAKE PHASE DISORDER (DSWPD)

Adam J. Sorscher, MD

BASICS

DESCRIPTION
- Circadian rhythm sleep disorders (CRSDs) are a family of conditions that occur when an individual's preferred timing of sleep is not synchronized to commitments to job, school, family, or social engagements. In CRSDs, intrinsic sleep is normal (i.e., there is no sleep fragmenting condition such as obstructive sleep apnea or periodic limb movement disorder). However, when forced by obligations to attempt sleep at nonpreferred times, individuals with CRSDs may complain of both sleep-initiation insomnia and excessive sleepiness in their wake time. These symptoms resolve entirely if the individual is allowed to sleep at his or her preferred time.
- Delayed sleep-wake phase disorder (DSWPD) is marked by a stable but persistent inability to initiate sleep at a desired time. Individuals are typically unable to initiate sleep until 2 to 6 hours later than societal norms (typically after 2 AM), and this frequently results in insufficient sleep/sleepiness in the day that follows.

EPIDEMIOLOGY
DSWPD is the most common circadian rhythm disorder seen by referral in sleep medicine clinics.

Prevalence
DSWPD has an estimated prevalence of 0.1–0.2% in the general population. It is most common in adolescents, with a prevalence of 7–16%.

ETIOLOGY AND PATHOPHYSIOLOGY
In all mammals, an oscillating signal from the suprachiasmatic nucleus (SCN) in the anterior hypothalamus establishes circadian rhythms, including the propensity to be awake or asleep. The average period of this signal in humans is 24.2 hours, slightly longer than the environmental day. Certain factors, most significantly morning light, shift the timing of the circadian rhythm and thereby synchronize it to the shorter environmental cycle day by day. DSWPD occurs when the circadian rhythm is not adequately synchronized to the shorter 24-hour environmental cycle, creating a mismatch between them. Some theories to account for inadequate synchronization are that it occurs in individuals who have an abnormally long circadian period (>25 hours) or whose circadian clock does not properly respond to synchronizing agents such as light (1).
- Release of melatonin from the pineal gland in the evening initiates a cascade of events that usually triggers sleep behavior several hours later. Studies suggest that the timing of melatonin release within the circadian cycle is delayed by 40 to 120 minutes in late adolescence compared with prepuberty. This suggests that the tendency for teenagers to delay sleep onset is largely a genetically programmed developmental phenomenon.

- DSWPD is the result of biologic, behavioral, and psychosocial factors. The relative contributions of genetically predetermined endogenous factors (the shifting of the circadian phase just described) versus voluntary behaviors that delay bedtime are not fully delineated.

Genetics
Emerging evidence indicates a genetic component to DSWPD—a positive family history is reported in approximately 40% of individuals. In one familial case report, DSWPD was shown to occur in an autosomal dominant inheritance pattern. Polymorphisms in circadian rhythm genes such as *hPer3* and *clock* among individuals with DSWPD constitute evidence of a genetic component to the disorder (2).

RISK FACTORS
DSWPD primarily affects adolescents and young adults—a cohort who have a biologic tendency to delay the onset of sleep yet often need to be up early for school/work responsibilities. Children with autism spectrum disorders also frequently have disturbed circadian rhythm cycles.

GENERAL PREVENTION
In DSWPD (and all CRSDs), careful attention to sleep hygiene is necessary to establish and maintain a desired sleep schedule. The most important behavioral practices needed to prevent an undesirably late fall-asleep time are as follows:
- Maintain a regular sleep/wake schedule 7 days/week.
- Avoid daytime napping.
- Minimize caffeine and stimulants.
- Avoid stimulating activities in the late evening, such as computer, TV, and social interactions. A 30-minute "wind-down" time prior to bedtime in which homework, socializing, and electronic devices are off-limits is helpful.
- If computer screens are to be used in the evening, consider "apps" that filter out blue and green wavelengths because these frequencies are especially potent at further delaying the onset of sleep.
- Attempt to arise at a similar time on weekends as on school/work mornings—adolescents who sleep *ad lib* on the weekends (sometimes into the afternoon) often find that they have especially great difficulty initiating sleep on Sunday night and, thus, get the week off to a bad start.

DIAGNOSIS

HISTORY
- People with DSWPD report both sleep initiation insomnia and excessive sleepiness in the daytime. They do not initiate sleep until 2 to 6 hours later than normative sleep times and they struggle to awaken for school/work in the morning.
- Careful questioning should explore for competing/comorbid causes of insomnia (poor sleep hygiene, significant mental health disorders, restless legs syndrome, medical conditions/medication side effects, and substance abuse disorders) and for competing/comorbid causes of hypersomnolence (symptoms of

narcolepsy and obstructive sleep apnea, voluntary insufficient sleep, medical conditions/medication side effects, and substance abuse disorders).
- In contrast to DSWPD, individuals with psychophysiologic insomnia (psychologically conditioned arousal when attempting to initiate sleep) do not usually experience genuine hypersomnolence in the daytime despite short sleep times overnight, but instead complain of fatigue.
- People with DSWPD will have no complaint about sleep/wakefulness and their sleep will be of normal duration when they are able to sleep at their preferred time (e.g., their sleep/wakefulness complaints resolve when on summer vacation from school, when they can choose their own preferred sleep-wake schedule).

PHYSICAL EXAM
Explore for features of sleep apnea, a competing cause of hypersomnolence: obesity/large neck circumference; hypertension; crowded oropharynx

DIFFERENTIAL DIAGNOSIS
DSWPD and other CRSDs are unique in that they are often marked by the twin complaints of insomnia when attempting to sleep *and* hypersomnolence in the wake period. Other sleep disorders usually cause either insomnia or hypersomnolence but not both. DSWPD and other CRSDs resolve entirely if the individual is allowed to sleep at his or her preferred time.

DIAGNOSTIC TESTS & INTERPRETATION
- Diagnosis of DSWPD is made primarily by thorough history taking.
- Sleep logs completed over 3 weeks time graphically reveal fall-asleep times that are consistently 2 to 6 hours later than societal norms and much later wake-up times (not infrequently in the afternoon) on days off from school/work (3)[B].
- Wrist actigraphy (using a wristwatch-like device with an accelerometer), undertaken for 3 weeks, also provides an accurate display of sleep and wake timing but is usually not reimbursable by insurance and is not needed if the individual can complete sleep logs (3)[B].
- Testing in the sleep lab is not indicated unless a suspicion exists of comorbid intrinsic disorders of sleep, such as sleep apnea, narcolepsy, or parasomnias (unusual behaviors arising out of sleep) (3)[A].

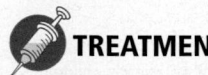

TREATMENT

- The goal of treatment in DSWPD is to help the individual consistently initiate sleep at an earlier time. The principal therapies that advance sleep onset are light and melatonin (factors that shift the circadian rhythm are called zeitgebers). Comparatively, light is much more potent than melatonin in its phase-shifting ability. The phase-shifting effects of light and melatonin depend on the timing at which they are provided as depicted in the phase-response curve (see online version). Key points: Light will advance sleep onset to an earlier time if provided after the body's temperature nadir that occurs ~2/3 through the habitual sleep phase and for several hours thereafter. Proper timing is critical because exposure to light in the evening or *before* the temperature nadir (i.e., in the initial 2/3 of the sleep period) will have the opposite effect—it will further delay sleep onset. For melatonin, the most potent phase-advancing effect occurs if it is provided in the evening, 4 to 6 hours before an individual's usual sleep onset time.

- Use the following rules to guide prescribing of light in order to advance sleep phase (3)[B]:

  – No single rule exists for intensity, duration, or wavelength for light therapy. Most protocols employ a 2,500 to 10,000 lux full-spectrum light box, set 2 to 3 feet from the individual for 30 to 120 minutes. A common prescription is 10,000 lux box for 30 minutes upon awakening in the morning. Retailers of full-spectrum light boxes abound on the Internet. Sunlight, when present in the morning in warm-weather seasons, is equally effective.
  – Prescribe exposure to full-spectrum light immediately upon awakening. (Note: Although the phase-advancing effect of light is actually greatest if it is provided *immediately* after the body temperature nadir that occurs ~2/3 through the sleep period, the strategy of waiting until the habitual waking time is preferred for these reasons: [i] it acknowledges that it is onerous for the individual to wake up artificially early for light therapy and [ii] it minimizes the risk of unintentionally providing light *before* the temperature nadir, which further delays the sleep phase.)
  – Light exposure in the evening has the effect of delaying sleep phase and worsening DSWPD. Instruct individuals to limit light exposure in the evening (consider using sunglasses or curtailing outdoor activities in warm-weather months).
  – Contraindications to phototherapy include retinopathy, photosensitivity, and bipolar disorder.

MEDICATION

- Prescribe melatonin to be taken 4 to 6 hours before the habitual (usual) fall-asleep time, *not* at bedtime. Melatonin in minute doses is as effective as higher doses in producing phase-shift; therefore, use the lowest dose available—usually 1 or 3 mg (3)[B].
- Once earlier sleep onset and wake-up occurs, adjust the timing of therapies every 3 to 5 days—continue to use light directly upon awakening; provide melatonin earlier and earlier in the evening corresponding to 4 to 6 hours before the newly observed fall-asleep time.

ALERT

Melatonin has a weak sedating effect, and individuals should be counseled not to drive/operate dangerous machines after taking the medication. Other side effects include headache and unusual taste in mouth.

ISSUES FOR REFERRAL

- Referral for evaluation and testing at a sleep clinic is not necessary in most cases of DSWPD. The chief indications for referral are suspicion of the following comorbid disorders:
  – Obstructive sleep apnea: indicated by loud snoring, obesity/large neck, witnessed apneas, and history of hypertension
  – Narcolepsy: indicated by severe levels of daytime sleepiness, despite adequate sleep quantity, and sometimes accompanied by cataplexy (bouts of sudden muscular weakness triggered by strong emotions)
  – Parasomnias: undesirable experiential/behavioral phenomena that arise out of sleep, such as dangerous sleepwalking or dream-enactment behavior
- In addition, many individuals with the complaint of insomnia/sleepiness have comorbid mental health disorders, primarily depression and possibly substance abuse. Referral for mental health disorders/substance abuse treatment is indicated if these are present.

ADDITIONAL THERAPIES

- Chronotherapy is an older strategy in which the individual is instructed to delay sleep and wake times by 2 to 3 hours every 2 to 3 days, shifting the sleep cycle across the 24-hour day, until the individual reaches a desired bedtime. Carried out over several weeks, this protocol is extremely disruptive to daytime schedules and also has not been demonstrated to be effective. It is seldom used (4).

- Some early reports suggest that vitamin B_{12} has circadian phase-shifting properties. This finding has not been confirmed in subsequent investigations, and presently, no evidence seen of benefit to the use of this supplement in CRSDs (3)[B].

- Use of sedative-hypnotic medications to treat the insomnia component and stimulant medications to treat daytime sleepiness has not been shown to be effective in the context of DSWPD (3)[C].

 ## ONGOING CARE

Remind patients to practice healthy sleep behaviors (see "General Prevention") if they wish to maintain an earlier sleep/wake pattern.

PATIENT EDUCATION

http://www.aafp.org/afp/1999/0401/p1918.html

REFERENCES

1. Wyatt JK, Stepanski EJ, Kirkby J. Circadian phase in delayed sleep phase syndrome: predictors and temporal stability across multiple assessments. *Sleep.* 2006;29(8):1075–1080.
2. Ebisawa T, Uchiyama M, Kajimura N, et al. Association of structural polymorphisms in the human *period3* gene with delayed sleep phase syndrome. *EMBO Rep.* 2001;2(4):342–346.
3. Morgenthaler TI, Lee-Chiong T, Alessi C, et al. Practice parameters for the clinical evaluation and treatment of circadian rhythm sleep disorders. An American Academy of Sleep Medicine report. *Sleep.* 2007;30(11):1445–1459.
4. Sack RL, Auckley D, Auger RR, et al. Circadian rhythm sleep disorders: part II, advanced sleep phase disorder, delayed sleep phase disorder, free-running disorder, and irregular sleep-wake rhythm. An American Academy of Sleep Medicine review. *Sleep.* 2007;30(11):1484–1501.

ADDITIONAL READING

- Barion A, Zee PC. A clinical approach to circadian rhythm sleep disorders. *Sleep Med.* 2007;8(6):566–577.
- Kanathur N, Harrington J, Lee-Chiong T Jr. Circadian rhythm sleep disorders. *Clin Chest Med.* 2010;31(2):319–325.
- Kripke DF, Rex KM, Ancoli-Israel S, et al. Delayed sleep phase cases and controls. *J Circadian Rhythms.* 2008;6:6.
- Wilson SJ, Nutt DJ, Alford C, et al. British Association for Psychopharmacology consensus statement on evidence-based treatment of insomnia, parasomnias and circadian rhythm disorders. *J Psychopharmacol.* 2010;24(11):1577–1601.

CODES

ICD10
G47.21 Circadian rhythm sleep disorder, delayed sleep phase type

CLINICAL PEARLS

- The tendency to become "night-owlish" with adolescence is, to a large extent, a biologically programmed phenomenon, not strictly a behavioral choice. Enlightened public policy would recognize this and allow for later start times for high schools.
- DSWPD can be diagnosed with careful history taking and sleep logs; referral for formal sleep studies is usually not indicated.
- Use of light and melatonin can shift habitual sleep onset and offset time by their action on the human circadian rhythm.
- To maintain a desirable sleep phase, individuals with DSWPD usually need to maintain meticulous attention to sleep hygiene, including a regular sleep/wake schedule 7 days/week, to avoid lapsing into a delayed phase pattern.

DELIRIUM

Whitney A. Gray, CRNP • Katrina A. Booth, MD

BASICS

DESCRIPTION
- A neurologic complication of illness and/or medication(s), especially common in older patients, manifested by new confusion and impaired attention
- A medical emergency requiring immediate evaluation to decrease morbidity and mortality
- System(s) affected: nervous
- Synonym(s): acute confusional state, altered mental status, organic brain syndrome, acute mental status change

EPIDEMIOLOGY
- Predominant age: older persons
- Predominant sex: male = female

Incidence
- >50% in older ICU patients
- 11–51% in postoperative patients
- 10–40% in hospitalized older patients

Prevalence
- 8–17% in older ED patients
- 14% in older postacute care patients

ETIOLOGY AND PATHOPHYSIOLOGY
- Multifactorial: believed to result from a decline in physiologic reserves with aging, resulting in a vulnerability to new stressors
- Neuropathophysiology is not clearly defined; cholinergic deficiency, dopamine excess, and neuroinflammation are the leading hypotheses.
- Often interaction between predisposing and precipitating risk factors
- With more predisposing factors (i.e., frail patients), fewer precipitating factors are needed to cause delirium.
- If few predisposing factors (e.g., very robust patients), more precipitating factors are needed to cause delirium.
- Multicomponent approach addressing contributing factors can reduce incidence and complications.

RISK FACTORS
- Predisposing risk factors (1)
  - Advanced age, >70 years
  - Preexisting cognitive impairment
  - Functional impairment
  - Dehydration; high BUN:creatinine ratio
  - History of alcohol abuse
  - Malnutrition
  - Hearing or vision impairment
- Precipitating risk factors
  - Severe illness in any organ system(s)
  - Environmental irritants (urinary catheter, restraints)
  - Polypharmacy (≥5 medications)
  - Specific medications, especially benzodiazepines, opioids (meperidine), and anticholinergics (diphenhydramine)
  - Pain
  - Any iatrogenic event
  - Surgery
  - Sleep deprivation

GENERAL PREVENTION
Follow treatment approach.

COMMONLY ASSOCIATED CONDITIONS
Multiple but most common are the following:
- New medicine or medicine changes
- Infections (especially lung, urine, and blood stream, but consider meningitis as well)
- Toxic-metabolic (especially low sodium, elevated calcium, renal failure, and hepatic failure)

- Heart attack or stroke
- Alcohol or drug withdrawal
- Preexisting cognitive impairment increases risk

DIAGNOSIS

Diagnosis is made using a careful history, behavioral observation, and cognitive assessment.

- *DSM-5* is the current standard; diagnostic criteria include (2):
  - Disturbance in attention and awareness
  - Change in cognition not due to dementia
  - Onset over short (hours to days) period and fluctuates during course of day
  - Evidence from history, exam, or lab that disturbance is caused by physiologic consequence of medical condition, intoxicating substance, medication use, or more than one cause
- The confusion assessment method (CAM) is the most well-validated and tested clinical tool and has been adapted for ICU setting in adults (CAM-ICU) and children (pediatric CAM-ICU [pCAM-ICU]) (3)[B].

ALERT
- Key diagnostic features of the CAM
  - Acute change in mental status that fluctuates
  - Abnormal attention and either disorganized thinking or altered level of consciousness
- Several nondiagnostic symptoms may be present:
  - Short- and long-term memory problems
  - Sleep–wake cycle disturbances
  - Hallucinations and/or delusions
  - Emotional lability
  - Tremors and asterixis
- Subtypes based on level of consciousness
  - Hyperactive delirium (15%): Patients are loud, agitated, and disruptive.
  - Hypoactive delirium (20%): quietly confused; sleepy, may sit and not eat, drink, or move
  - Mixed delirium (50%): features of both hyperactive and hypoactive delirium
  - Normal consciousness delirium (15%): still displays disorganized thinking, along with acute onset, inattention, and fluctuation

HISTORY
- Time course of mental status changes
- Recent medication changes
- Symptoms of infection
- New neurologic signs
- Abrupt change in functional ability

PHYSICAL EXAM
- Comprehensive cardiorespiratory exam is essential.
- Focal neurologic signs are usually absent.
- Mini-mental state exam (MMSE) is the most well-known and studied cognitive screen, but it may not be the most appropriate in an acute care setting; shorter cognitive screens have been studied in delirious patients (i.e., short blessed test [SBT], Brief Alzheimer's Screen [BAS], and Ottawa 3DY) and may be helpful if performed serially over time. Most patients will perform poorly if delirium is present; dementia cannot be diagnosed during delirium.
- GI/GU exam for constipation/urinary retention

DIFFERENTIAL DIAGNOSIS
- Depression (slow onset, disturbance of mood, normal level of consciousness, fluctuates weeks to months)

- Dementia (insidious onset, memory problems, normal level of consciousness, fluctuates days to weeks)
- Psychosis (rarely sudden onset in older adults)

DIAGNOSTIC TESTS & INTERPRETATION

Initial Tests (lab, imaging)
- Guided by history and physical exam
  - CBC with differential
  - Comprehensive metabolic panel (CMP)
  - Urinalysis, urine culture, blood culture
  - Medication levels (digoxin, theophylline, antiepileptics where applicable)
- Chest radiograph for most
- ECG as necessary
- Others, if indicated by history and exam

Follow-Up Tests & Special Considerations
- If lab tests listed above do not indicate a precipitator of delirium, consider
  - Arterial blood gases
  - Troponin
  - Toxicology screen
  - Ammonia
  - Thyroid-stimulating hormone
- Noncontrast-enhanced head CT scan if
  - Unclear diagnosis
  - Recent fall
  - Receiving anticoagulants
  - New focal neurologic signs
  - Need to rule out intracranial mass before lumbar puncture

Diagnostic Procedures/Other
- Lumbar puncture (rarely necessary)
  - Perform if clinical suspicion of a CNS bleed or infection is high.
- EEG (rarely necessary)
  - Consider after above evaluation if cause remains unclear or suspicion of seizure activity.

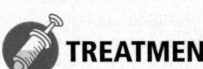

TREATMENT

- The best treatment is prevention (4)[A].
- Addressing six risk factors (i.e., cognitive impairment, sleep deprivation, dehydration, immobility, vision impairment, and hearing impairment) in at-risk hospitalized patients can reduce the incidence of delirium by 33%.
- Principles: Maintain safety, identify causes, and manage symptoms.
- Stabilize vital signs and ensure immediate evaluation.

GENERAL MEASURES
- Postoperative patients should be monitored and treated for
  - Myocardial infarction/ischemia
  - Infection (i.e., pneumonia, UTI)
  - Pulmonary embolism
  - Urinary or stool retention (attempt catheter removal by postoperative day 2)
- Anesthesia route (general vs. epidural) does not affect the risk of delirium.

- ICU sedation-avoidance of benzodiazepines may reduce risk (5)[B].

- Multifactorial treatment: Identify contributing factors and provide preemptive care to avoid iatrogenic problems, with special attention to
  - CNS oxygen delivery (attempt to attain):
    - $SaO_2 > 90\%$ with goal of $SaO_2 > 95\%$
    - Systolic BP <2/3 of baseline or >90 mm Hg
    - Hematocrit >30%

D

- Fluid/electrolyte balance
  - Sodium, potassium, and glucose normal (glucose <300 mg/dL in diabetics)
  - Treat fluid overload or dehydration.
- Treat pain
  - Schedule acetaminophen (650 mg QID) if daily pain
  - Opioids alone (morphine) or in combination (oxycodone, hydrocodone) may be used for breakthrough pain.

ALERT
- Avoid meperidine (Demerol).
- Eliminate unnecessary medications.
  - Investigate new symptoms as potential medication side effects (i.e., Beers medications).
- Regulate bowel/bladder function.
  - Bowel movement at least every 48 hours
  - Screen for urinary retention
- Prevent major hospital-acquired problems.
  - 6-inch thick foam mattress overlay or a pressure-reducing mattress
  - Avoid urinary catheter.
  - Incentive spirometry
  - Venous thromboembolism (VTE) prophylaxis if bed-fast
  - Early mobilization
  - Environmental stimulation
    - Glasses and hearing aids
    - Clock and calendar
    - Soft lighting
    - Music and television, if desired
  - Sleep
    - Quiet environment
    - Soft music
    - Therapeutic massage
- Restraints increase risk of falls/injury
  - Use only in the most difficult-to-manage patients, as briefly as possible

MEDICATION
- Nonpharmacologic approaches are preferred for initial treatment, but medication may be needed for agitation management, especially in the ICU setting (6)[C].
- Medications treat only the symptoms and do not address the underlying cause.
- No medication is FDA approved for delirium.
- Medications should not be used prophylactically.

First Line
- Antipsychotics
  - Haloperidol (Haldol): initially, 0.25 to 0.5 mg PO/IM; reevaluate and potentially redose hourly. Critical care guidelines do not support use of antipsychotics for prevention of ICU delirium (5).
  - Quetiapine (Seroquel) 12.5 to 25 mg PO BID
  - Risperidone (Risperdal) 0.25 to 0.5 mg/day PO
- Benzodiazepines should be avoided except in alcohol withdrawal or if patient taking at baseline because delirium could be a sign of withdrawal.
- Lorazepam (Ativan): initially, 0.25 to 0.5 mg PO/IM/IV q6–8h; may need to adjust to effect (caution in patients with impaired liver function)
- Contraindications: Avoid typical antipsychotics in patients with Parkinsonism or Parkinson disease.
- Precautions: Typical antipsychotics may cause extrapyramidal effects; benzodiazepines may cause delirium. Both increase fall risk. Antipsychotics may prolong the QT interval.

Second Line
- Olanzapine (Zyprexa) 2.5 to 5.0 mg/day PO
- Multiple trials demonstrate adverse events with cholinesterase inhibitors in the management of delirium; evidence does not support their use.

ISSUES FOR REFERRAL
Geriatric, psychiatric, or neurologic consultation is helpful if delirium is not easily explainable or resolving after full evaluation. Interprofessional team approach is best.

ADDITIONAL THERAPIES
Early mobilization critical
- Out of bed several hours daily starting on hospital day 2 (or postoperative day 1) if no contraindications
- Daily therapy if not ambulating or functioning independently

INPATIENT CONSIDERATIONS
General measures described earlier are also applicable to delirium prevention.

Admission Criteria/Initial Stabilization
New delirium is a medical emergency and requires admission, except in the setting of palliative home care.

IV Fluids
As needed for dehydration

Nursing
- Screen for development of delirium.
- Assessment of precipitants/contributing factors (pain, constipation, urinary retention)
- Reorient; maintain day/night orientation.
- Institute skin care program and turning regimen for immobile patients.
- Maintain and encourage mobility.
- Encourage family presence and participation.

Discharge Criteria
- Resolution of precipitating factor(s)
- Safe discharge site if delirium is slow to resolve

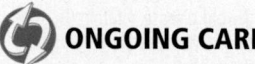 ## ONGOING CARE

FOLLOW-UP RECOMMENDATIONS
- If delirium at discharge, often needs postacute facility and ongoing assessment for resolution
- If no delirium at discharge and going home, follow-up with primary care physician in 1 to 2 weeks

Patient Monitoring
- Evaluate and assess mental status daily.
- Continued evaluation for precipitating cause(s)

DIET
- Liberalize diet to increase oral intake
- Nutritional supplements (1 to 3 cans/day) if intake poor
- Consider temporary nasogastric tube if unable to eat and bowels working.

PROGNOSIS
- May take weeks/months to fully resolve
- Usually improves with treatment of underlying condition(s); can lead to chronic cognitive impairment
- Delirium significantly increases a person's chance of dying even up to 1 year later.

COMPLICATIONS
- Falls
- Pressure ulcers
- Malnutrition
- Functional decline
- Future cognitive dysfunction
- Higher risk for institutionalization
- Death

REFERENCES
1. Inouye SK, Westendorp RG, Saczynski JS. Delirium in elderly people. *Lancet.* 2014;383(9920):911–922.
2. American Psychiatric Association. *Diagnostic and Statistical Manual of Mental Disorders.* 5th ed. Arlington, VA: American Psychiatric Association; 2013.
3. van Eijk MM, van Marum RJ, Klijn IA, et al. Comparison of delirium assessment tools in a mixed intensive care unit. *Crit Care Med.* 2009;37(6):1881–1885.
4. Reston JT, Schoelles KM. In-facility delirium prevention programs as a patient safety strategy: a systematic review. *Ann Intern Med.* 2013;158 (5 Pt 2):375–380.
5. Kalabalik J, Brunetti L, El-Srougy R. Intensive care unit delirium: a review of the literature. *J Pharm Pract.* 2014;27(2):195–207.
6. Barr J, Fraser GL, Puntillo K, et al. Clinical practice guidelines for the management of pain, agitation, and delirium in adult patients in the intensive care unit. *Crit Care Med.* 2013;41(1):263–306.

ADDITIONAL READING
- Inouye SK, Robinson T, Blaum C, et al. Amercian Geriatrics Society abstracted clinical practice guideline for postoperative delirium in older adults. *J Am Geriatr Soc.* 2015;63(1):142–150.
- National Clinical Guideline Centre. *Delirium: Diagnosis, Prevention, and Management.* London, United Kingdom: National Clinical Guideline Centre; 2010.
- Quinlan N, Marcantonio ER, Inouye SK, et al. Vulnerability: the crossroads of frailty and delirium. *J Am Geriatr Soc.* 2011;59(Suppl 2):S262–S268.

 ## SEE ALSO
- Dementia; Depression; Substance Use Disorders
- Algorithm: Delirium

 ## CODES

ICD10
- R41.0 Disorientation, unspecified
- F19.931 Oth psychoactive substance use, unsp w withdrawal delirium
- F10.231 Alcohol dependence with withdrawal delirium

CLINICAL PEARLS
- The CAM criteria for delirium are acute onset of fluctuating mental status, inattention, and either disorganized thinking or altered level of consciousness.
- Hypoactive subtype of delirium can easily be missed.
- Addressing six risk factors (i.e., cognitive impairment, sleep deprivation, dehydration, immobility, vision impairment, and hearing impairment) in hospitalized patients can reduce the incidence of delirium by 33%.
- Delirium may not resolve as soon as the treatable contributors resolve; may take weeks or months
- Avoid diphenhydramine and benzodiazepines in older patients. Nonpharmacologic measures are preferable as a sleep aid.

DEMENTIA
Umer Farooq, MD, MBBS • Wajiha Illyas, MD

 BASICS

DESCRIPTION
- *DSM-5* classifies dementias under neurocognitive disorders (major and mild).
- Evidence of cognitive decline from previous level of performance in one of cognitive domains (attention, executive function, learning, and memory). The cognitive deficits interfere significantly with ADLs (for major only) and do not occur exclusively in the context of delirium or any other mental disorder.
- *DSM-5* specifies the cause of neurocognitive decline secondary to the following:
  - Alzheimer dementia (AD)
    - Progressive cognitive decline; most common in age > 65 years
  - Vascular dementia (VaD)
    - Usually correlated with a cerebrovascular event and/or cerebrovascular disease
    - Stepwise deterioration with periods of clinical plateaus
  - Lewy body dementia
    - Fluctuating cognition associated with parkinsonism, hallucinations and delusions, gait difficulties, and falls
  - Frontotemporal dementia
    - Language difficulties, personality changes, and behavioral disturbances
  - Creutzfeldt-Jakob disease (CJD)
    - Very rare; rapid onset
  - HIV dementia
  - Substance-/medication induced neurocognitive disorder

EPIDEMIOLOGY
Prevalence
- In patients age ≥71 years
  - AD: 5–10% up to 25% after 7th decade of life
  - VaD: 17%
  - Other: 13%
- Estimated 5.4 million Americans had AD in 2010.
  - 5 million >65 years of age; 200,000 <65 years
  - Prevalence expected to double by 2030

ETIOLOGY AND PATHOPHYSIOLOGY
- AD: involves β-amyloid protein accumulation and/or neurofibrillary tangles (NFTs), synaptic dysfunction, neurodegeneration, and eventual neuronal loss
- Age, genetics, systemic disease, smoking, and other host factors may influence the β-amyloid accumulation and/or the pace of progression toward the clinical manifestations of AD.
- VaD: cerebral atherosclerosis/emboli with clinical/subclinical infarcts

Genetics
- AD: Positive family history in 50%, but 90% AD is sporadic: *APOE4* increases risk but full role unclear.
- Familial/autosomal dominant AD accounts for <5% AD: amyloid precursor protein (APP), presenilin-1 (PSEN-1), and presenilin-2 (PSEN-2)

RISK FACTORS
- Age; sex: female > male
- Genetic predisposition
- Hypertension: AD; VaD
- Hypercholesterolemia: AD; VaD
- Diabetes: VaD
- Cigarette smoking: VaD

- Endocrine/metabolic abnormalities: hypothyroidism, Cushing syndrome, thiamine and vitamin B_{12} deficiency
- Chronic alcoholism, other drugs
- Lower educational status
- Head injury early in life
- Sedentary lifestyle

GENERAL PREVENTION
- Treat reversible causes of dementia, such as drug-induced, alcohol-induced, and vitamin deficiencies.
- Treat hypertension, hypercholesterolemia, and diabetes.
- No evidence for statins (or any other specific medication) to prevent onset of dementia (1)[A]
- BP control and low-dose aspirin may prevent or lessen cognitive decline in VaD.

COMMONLY ASSOCIATED CONDITIONS
- Anxiety and major depression
- Psychosis (delusions; delusions of persecution are common)
- Delirium
- Behavioral disturbances (agitation, aggression)
- Sleep disturbances

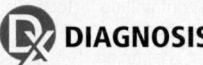 **DIAGNOSIS**

HISTORY
Probable diagnosis AD (2)[B]:
- Age between 40 and 90 years (usually >65 years)
- Progressive cognitive decline of insidious onset
- No disturbances of consciousness
- Deficits in areas of cognition
- No other explainable cause of symptoms
- Specifically rule out thyroid disease, vitamin (B_{12}) deficiency, grief reaction, and depression
- Supportive factors: family history of dementia

PHYSICAL EXAM
- Often normal physical
- No disturbances of consciousness
- Cognitive decline demonstrated by standardized instruments, including the following:
  - Mini-mental state exam
  - Montreal Cognitive Assessment (MoCA) Test
  - ADAS-Cog
  - Clock draw test
  - Use caution in relying solely on cognition scores, especially in those with learning difficulty, language barriers, or similar limitations.

DIFFERENTIAL DIAGNOSIS
- Major depression
- Medication side effect
- Chronic alcohol use
- Delirium
- Subdural hematoma
- Normal pressure hydrocephalus
- Brain tumor
- Thyroid disease
- Parkinson disease
- Vitamin B_{12} deficiency
- Toxins (aromatic hydrocarbons, solvents, heavy metals, marijuana, opiates, sedative-hypnotics)

DIAGNOSTIC TESTS & INTERPRETATION
Initial Tests (lab, imaging)
- Used to rule out causes
  - CBC, CMP
  - Thyroid-stimulating hormone
  - Vitamin B_{12} level
- Select patients
  - HIV, rapid plasma regain (RPR)
  - Erythrocyte sedimentation rate (ESR)
  - Folate
  - Heavy metal and toxicology screen
- Research studies with cerebrospinal fluid (CSF) biomarkers in patient with confirmed AD have shown decreased A β (1 to 42) and increased tau and p-tau levels, which are specific features of AD, and CSF tau proteins are increased in CJD (3)[A].
- Neuroimaging (CT/MRI of brain): cerebral atrophy
  - Early age of onset (<65 years), rapid progression, focal neurologic deficits, cerebrovascular disease risk, or atypical symptoms: neuroimaging (MRI/CT) to rule out other causes
  - Important findings
    - AD: diffuse cerebral atrophy starting in association areas, hippocampus, amygdala
    - VaD: old infarcts, including lacunar

Diagnostic Procedures/Other
PET scan is not routinely recommended; has been approved to differentiate between Alzheimer disease and frontotemporal dementia

Test Interpretation
AD
- Neurofibrillary tangles: abnormally phosphorylated tau protein
- Senile plaques: amyloid precursor protein derivatives
- Microvascular amyloid

 TREATMENT

GENERAL MEASURES
- Daily schedules and written directions
- Emphasis on nutrition, personal hygiene, accident-proofing the home, safety issues, sleep hygiene, and supervision
- Socialization (adult daycare)
- Sensory stimulation (display of clocks and calendars) in the early to middle stages
- Discussion with the family concerning support and advance directives

MEDICATION
- Cognitive dysfunction
- Medications for AD show a small, statistically significant improvement in some cognitive measures, but it remains unclear if the improvement is clinically significant (4)[A].
- Cognitive dysfunction, mild
  - Cholinesterase inhibitors: donepezil (Aricept), 5 to 10 mg/day; rivastigmine (Exelon), 1.5 to 6 mg BID, transdermal system 4.6 mg/24 hr and 9.5 mg/24 hr; galantamine (Razadyne), 4 to 12 mg BID, extended release 8 to 24 mg/day
    - Adverse events: nausea, vomiting, diarrhea, anorexia, nightmares, bradycardia/syncope

○ Galantamine warning: associated with mortality in patients with mild cognitive impairment in clinical trial

○ Start drug with lowest acquisition cost; also consider adverse event profile, adherence, medical comorbidity, drug interactions, and dosing profiles.

• Cognitive dysfunction, moderate to severe
  − Cholinesterase inhibitors OR
  − Memantine (Namenda), 5 to 20 mg/day
    ○ Adverse events: dizziness, confusion, headache, constipation
    ○ OR combination cholinesterase inhibitor and memantine

• Commonly associated conditions
  − Psychosis and agitation/aggressive behavior
    ○ Look for precipitating factors (infection, pain, depression, medications).
    ○ Nonpharmacologic therapies (behavioral interventions, music therapy, etc.) are preferred as first-line treatment.
    ○ Mood stabilizers (valproic acid, carbamazepine) have been used, although evidence is lacking.
    ○ For moderate/severe symptoms; antipsychotics: Initiate low doses, risperidone 0.25 to 1 mg/day; olanzapine 1.25 to 5 mg/day; quetiapine 12.5 to 50 mg/day; aripiprazole 5 mg/day; ziprasidone 20 mg/day
    ○ Atypical antipsychotics associated with a better side effect profile: Quetiapine and aripiprazole are often first-line due to decreased extrapyramidal side effect.

ALERT
Black box warning on antipsychotics due to increased mortality in elderly with dementia

• Depression and insomnia
  − Depression
    ○ Selective serotonin reuptake inhibitors (SSRIs): Initiate low doses, citalopram (Celexa) 10 mg/day, escitalopram (Lexapro) 5 mg/day, sertraline (Zoloft) 25 mg/day.
    ○ Adverse events: nausea, vomiting, agitation, parkinsonian effects, sexual dysfunction, hyponatremia
    ○ Venlafaxine, mirtazapine, and bupropion are also useful.
  − Sleep disturbances
    ○ Low-dose antidepressants (e.g., Remeron) have significant sedative properties at 7.5 or 15 mg.
    ○ Trazodone 25 to 100 mg is frequently used because of better side effect profile.
  − Psychosis and agitation/aggressive behavior
    ○ Some data for SSRIs
    ○ Benzodiazepines if agitation with anxiety; in elderly, use PRN.

Geriatric Considerations
Initiate pharmacotherapy at low doses and titrate slowly up if necessary.

• Benzodiazepine are potentially inappropriate for older adults; yet, their use persists.

ALERT
Benzodiazepine use is associated with increased fall risk (5)[B].

• Watch decreased renal function and hepatic metabolism.

ISSUES FOR REFERRAL
Neuropsychiatric evaluation particularly helpful in early stages or mild cognitive impairment

ADDITIONAL THERAPIES
Behavioral modification

• Socialization, such as adult daycare, to prevent isolation and depression
• Sleep hygiene program as alternative to pharmaceuticals for sleep disturbance
• Scheduled toileting to prevent incontinence

COMPLEMENTARY & ALTERNATIVE MEDICINE
• Vitamin E is no longer recommended due to lack of evidence.
• Ginkgo biloba is not recommended due to lack of evidence.
• NSAIDs, selegiline, and estrogen lack efficacy and safety data.

INPATIENT CONSIDERATIONS
Admission Criteria/Initial Stabilization
• Worsening physical health issues
• Psychiatry admission may be required because of safety concerns (self-harm/harm to others), self-neglect, aggressive behaviors, or other behavioral issues.

 ONGOING CARE

FOLLOW-UP RECOMMENDATIONS
Patient Monitoring
• Progression of cognitive impairment by use of standardized tool (e.g., MMSE, ADAS-Cog)
• Development of behavioral problems: sleep, depression, psychosis
• Adverse events of pharmacotherapy
• Nutritional status
• Caregiver evaluation of stress
• Evaluate issues that may affect quality of life.

PATIENT EDUCATION
• Safety concerns
• Long-term issues: management of finances, medical decision making, possible placement when appropriate; legal guardianship, if necessary, to avoid capacity and competency issues
• Advance directives
• National Institute on Aging. About Alzheimer's disease: other dementias. http://www.nia.nih.gov/alzheimers/topics/other-dementias

PROGNOSIS
• AD: usually steady progression leading to profound cognitive impairment
  − Average survival of AD is about 8 years.
• VaD: incrementally worsening dementia, but cognitive improvement is unlikely
• Secondary dementias: Treatment of the underlying condition may lead to improvement. Commonly seen with normal pressure hydrocephalus, hypothyroidism, and brain tumors.

COMPLICATIONS
• Wandering
• Delirium
• Sundown syndrome: It is frequently common in older people (who are sedated) and also in people who have dementia (adverse reaction to small dose of psychoactive substances).
• Falls with injury
  − Hip fracture
  − Head trauma/hematomas
• Neglect and abuse
• Caregiver burnout

REFERENCES
1. McGuinness B, Craig D, Bullock R, et al. Statins for the prevention of dementia. *Cochrane Database Syst Rev.* 2009;(2):CD003160.
2. Blass DM, Rabins PV. In the clinic. Dementia. *Ann Intern Med.* 2008;148(7):ITC4-1–ITC4-16.
3. van Harten AC, Kester MI, Visser PJ, et al. Tau and p-tau as CSF biomarkers in dementia: a meta-analysis. *Clin Chem Lab Med.* 2011;49(3):353–366.
4. Birks J. Cholinesterase inhibitors for Alzheimer's disease. *Cochrane Database Syst Rev.* 2006;(1):CD005593.
5. Softic A, Beganlic A, Pranjic N, et al. The influence of the use of benzodiazepines in the frequency falls in the elderly. *Med Arch.* 2013;67(4):256–259.

ADDITIONAL READING
• Lyketsos CG, Colenda CC, Beck C, et al. Position statement of the American Association for Geriatric Psychiatry regarding principles of care for patients with dementia resulting from Alzheimer dementia. *Am J Geriatr Psychiatry.* 2006;14(7):561–572.
• National Collaborating Centre for Mental Health. *Dementia: The NICE-SCIE Guideline on Supporting People with Dementia and Their Carers in Health and Social Care.* London, United Kingdom: British Psychological Society, Royal College of Psychiatrists; 2007. http://www.nice.org.uk/nicemedia/live/10998/30320/30320.pdf
• Rabins PV, Blacker D, Rovner BW, et al. American Psychiatric Association practice guideline for the treatment of patients with Alzheimer's disease and other dementias. Second edition. *Am J Psychiatry.* 2007;164(12)(Suppl):5–56.

 SEE ALSO

Algorithm: Dementia

 CODES

ICD10
• F03 Unspecified dementia
• G30.9 Alzheimer's disease, unspecified
• F01.50 Vascular dementia without behavioral disturbance

CLINICAL PEARLS
• Medications for AD show a small, statistically significant improvement in some cognitive measures, but it remains unclear if the improvement is clinically significant.
• Do not forget the role of adult protective services in case of elderly abuse.
• A particular concern in nursing homes relates to the use of physical restraints and antipsychotic medication, which are regulated in the United States by the Omnibus Reconciliation Act of 1987.

DEMENTIA, VASCULAR

Birju B. Patel, MD, FACP, AGSF • N. Wilson Holland, MD, FACP, AGSF

BASICS

Vascular dementia is a heterogeneous disorder caused by the sequel of cerebrovascular disease that manifests in cognitive impairment affecting memory, thinking, language, behavior, and judgment.

DESCRIPTION
- Vascular dementia (previously known as multi-infarct dementia) was first mentioned by Thomas Willis in 1672. Later, it was further described in the late 19th century by Binswanger and Alzheimer as a separate entity from dementia paralytica caused by neurosyphilis. This concept has evolved tremendously since the advent of neuroimaging modalities.
- Synonym(s): vascular cognitive impairment (VCI); vascular cognitive disorder (VCD); arteriosclerotic dementia; poststroke dementia; senile dementia due to hardening of the arteries; Binswanger disease. *Diagnostic and Statistical Manual of Mental Disorders (DSM-5)* categorizes vascular dementia as mild or major VCD.

EPIDEMIOLOGY
Second most common cause of dementia after Alzheimer dementia in the elderly

Incidence
About 6 to 12 cases/1,000/person age >70 years

Prevalence
- ~1.2–4.2% in those age >65 years
- 14–32% prevalence of dementia after a stroke

ETIOLOGY AND PATHOPHYSIOLOGY
Upon autopsy of those with dementia, many have significant vascular pathology are present, but this is not necessarily correlated clinically with vascular dementia. No set pathologic criteria exist for the diagnosis of vascular dementia such as those that exist for Alzheimer dementia. Pathology includes the following:
- Large vessel disease: cognitive impairment that follows a stroke
- Small vessel disease: includes white matter changes (leukoaraiosis), subcortical infarcts, and incomplete infarction. This is usually the most common cause of multi-infarct dementia.
- Subcortical ischemic vascular disease: due to small vessel involvement within cerebral white matter, brain stem, and basal ganglia. Lacunar infarcts and deep white matter changes are typically included in this category.
- Noninfarct ischemic changes and atrophy
- Transient ischemic attack (TIA)/stroke
- Vascular, demographic, genetic factors
- Vascular disease (i.e., hypertension [HTN], peripheral vascular disease [PVD], atrial fibrillation, hyperlipidemia, diabetes)

Genetics
- Cerebral autosomal dominant arteriopathy with subcortical infarcts (CADASIL) is caused by a mutation in the *NOTCH3* gene on chromosome 19 that results in leukoencephalopathy and subcortical infarcts. This is clinically manifested in recurrent strokes and associated cognitive decline.

- Apolipoprotein E gene type: Those with ApoE4 subtypes are at higher risk of developing both vascular and Alzheimer dementia.
- Amyloid precursor protein (APP) gene: leads to a form of vascular dementia called heritable cerebral hemorrhage with amyloidosis (1)

RISK FACTORS
- Age
- Previous stroke
- Smoking
- Diabetes (especially with frequent hypoglycemia)
- HTN
- Atrial fibrillation
- PVD
- Hyperlipidemia
- Metabolic syndrome
- Coronary atherosclerotic heart disease (2)

GENERAL PREVENTION
- Optimization and aggressive treatment of vascular risk factors, such as HTN, diabetes, and hyperlipidemia (3)[C]
- HTN is the single most modifiable risk factor and treatment for it must be optimized.
- Smoking is associated with white matter changes on imaging which may be associated with small vessel disease and vascular dementia progression (4)[B].
- Lifestyle modification: weight loss, physical activity, smoking cessation
- Medication management for vascular risk reduction: aspirin usage, statin therapy for hyperlipidemia, antihypertensive therapy (5)[B]

COMMONLY ASSOCIATED CONDITIONS
- CADASIL
- Cerebral amyloid angiopathy (CAA): accumulation of amyloid in cerebral vasculature resulting in infarctions and hemorrhages

DIAGNOSIS

Differentiation between Alzheimer dementia and vascular dementia can be difficult, and significant overlap is seen in the clinical presentation of these two dementias. The diagnosis of vascular dementia is a clinical diagnosis.

HISTORY
- Gradual, stepwise progression is typical.
- Ask about onset and progression of cognitive impairment and the specific cognitive domains involved.
- Ask about vascular risk factors and previous attempts to control these risk factors.
- Ask about medication compliance.
- Ask about urinary incontinence and gait disturbances. Abnormal gait and falls are strong predictors of development of vascular dementia, particularly unsteady, frontal, and hemiparetic types of gait.

- Look for early symptoms, including difficulty performing cognitive tasks, memory, mood, and assessment of instrumental activities of daily living (IADLs).
- Past history may include TIAs, cerebrovascular accidents (CVAs), coronary atherosclerotic heart disease, atrial fibrillation, hyperlipidemia, and/or PVD.

PHYSICAL EXAM
- Screen for HTN. Average daily BP and not office BP is associated with progression of cerebrovascular disease and cognitive decline in the elderly.
- Focal neurologic deficits may be present.
- Gait assessment is important, especially looking at gait initiation, gait speed, and balance (6)[C],(7)[B].
- Check for carotid bruits as well as abdominal bruits and assess for presence of PVD.
- Check body mass index and waist circumference.
- Do a thorough cardiac evaluation that includes looking for arrhythmias (i.e., atrial fibrillation).

DIFFERENTIAL DIAGNOSIS
- Alzheimer dementia
- Depression
- Drug intoxication
- CNS tumors
- Hypothyroidism
- Vitamin B_{12} deficiency

DIAGNOSTIC TESTS & INTERPRETATION
- Cognitive testing, such as Mini-Mental Status Exam (MMSE), Saint Louis University Mental Status (SLUMS), and Montreal Cognitive Assessment (MOCA), provides more definitive information in terms of cognitive deficits, especially executive function, which may be lost earlier in vascular dementia.
- Neuropsychological testing may also be beneficial, especially in evaluating multiple cognitive domains and their specific involvements and deficits.

Initial Tests (lab, imaging)
As appropriate, consider CBC, comprehensive metabolic profile, lipid panel, thyroid function, hemoglobin A1C, and vitamin B_{12}.
- Imaging is used in conjunction with history and physical examination to support a clinical diagnosis of vascular dementia.
- Cognitive deficits observed clinically do not always have to correlate with findings found on neuroimaging studies.
- MRI is best in terms of evaluation of subtle subcortical deficits.
- White matter changes and specific location of these changes can be associated with executive dysfunction and episodic memory impairment (8)[C].

TREATMENT

Prevention is the real key to treatment:
- Control of risk factors, including HTN, hyperlipidemia, and diabetes
- Avoidance of tobacco and smoking cessation
- Healthy, low-cholesterol diet

MEDICATION

- Acetylcholinesterase inhibitors may be used but are of limited benefit in vascular dementia (9)[A].
- Clinical evidence for use of memantine is limited with the clinical benefit likely modest.
- Controlling BP with any antihypertensive medications, treatment of dyslipidemia (e.g., statins), and treatment of diabetes are very important.
- Nicardipine has been studied and has been found to have some neuroprotective effects for vascular dementia (10)[B].
- Selective serotonin receptor inhibitors (SSRIs) may be of benefit for agitation and psychosis in vascular dementia (11)[A].

ADDITIONAL THERAPIES

- Limit alcohol drink intake to ≤1/day in women and 2/day in men.
- Heavy sustained alcohol use contributes to HTN.
- Aspirin and/or clopidogrel may be useful in some cases.

SURGERY

Carotid endarterectomy/stenting should be considered if evidence of significant internal carotid artery stenosis (i.e., >70–80%).

COMPLEMENTARY & ALTERNATIVE MEDICINE

Ginkgo biloba should be avoided due to increased risk of bleeding, especially in CAA.

INPATIENT CONSIDERATIONS

- Remain sensitive to functional assessment and avoidance of pressure ulcers after CVAs.
- Avoid Foley catheter usage unless absolutely necessary due to increased risk of infection.

Nursing

- Nonpharmacologic approaches to behavior management should be attempted prior to medication usage.
- Providing optimal sensory input to patients with cognitive impairment is important during hospitalizations to avoid delirium and confusion. Patients should be given frequent cues to keep them oriented to place and time. They should be informed of any changes in the daily schedule of activities and evaluations. Family and caregivers should be encouraged to be with patients with dementia as much as possible to further help them from becoming confused during hospitalization. Recreational, physical, occupational, and music therapy can be beneficial during hospitalization in avoiding delirium and preventing functional decline.
- Particular emphasis has to be placed on screening for, and optimizing, the mood of the patient. Depression is very common in older patients, especially those who have had strokes and have become hospitalized. Depression in itself can present as "pseudodementia" with worsening confusion during hospitalization and is a treatable condition.

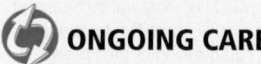 ONGOING CARE

Vascular dementia is a condition that should be followed with multiple visits in the office setting with goals of optimizing cardiovascular risk profiles for patients. Future planning and advanced directives should be addressed early. Family and caregiver evaluation and burden should also be evaluated.

FOLLOW-UP RECOMMENDATIONS

Perform regular follow-up with a primary care provider or geriatrician for risk factor modification and education on importance of regular physical and mental exercises as tolerated.

Patient Monitoring

Appropriate evaluation and diagnosis of this condition, need for future planning, optimizing vascular risk factors, lifestyle modification counseling, therapeutic interventions

DIET

- The American Heart Association diet and dietary approaches to stop hypertension (DASH) diet is recommended for optimal BP and cardiovascular risk factor control.
- Low-fat, decreased concentrated sweets and carbohydrates, especially in those with metabolic syndrome

PATIENT EDUCATION

- Lifestyle modification is important in vascular risk reduction (smoking cessation, exercise counseling, dietary counseling, weight-loss counseling).
- Optimizing vascular risk factors via medications (i.e., HTN, diabetes, atrial fibrillation, PVD, heart disease)
- Avoiding smoking, including secondhand smoke
- Home BP monitoring and glucometer testing of blood sugars if HTN, impaired glucose tolerance and/or diabetes is present.

PROGNOSIS

- Lost cognitive abilities that persist after initial recovery of deficits from stroke do not usually return. Some individuals can have intermittent periods of self-reported improvement in cognitive function.
- Risk factors for progression of cognitive and functional impairment poststroke include age, pre-stroke cognitive abilities, depression, polypharmacy, and decreased cerebral perfusion during acute stroke.

COMPLICATIONS

- Physical disability from stroke
- Severe cognitive impairment
- Death

REFERENCES

1. Russell MB. Genetics of dementia. *Acta Neurol Scand Suppl*. 2010;(190):58–61.
2. Gorelick PB, Scuteri A, Black SE, et al. Vascular contributions to cognitive impairment and dementia: a statement for healthcare professionals from the American Heart Association/American Stroke Association. *Stroke*. 2011;42(9):2672–2713.
3. Hasnain M, Vieweg WV. Possible role of vascular risk factors in Alzheimer's disease and vascular dementia. *Curr Pharm Des*. 2014;20(38):6007–6013.
4. Power MC, Deal JA, Sharrett AR, et al. Smoking and white matter hyperintensity progression: the ARIC-MRI Study. *Neurology*. 2015;84(8):841–848.
5. White WB, Wolfson L, Wakefield DB, et al. Average daily blood pressure, not office blood pressure, is associated with progression of cerebrovascular disease and cognitive decline in older people. *Circulation*. 2011;124(21):2312–2319.
6. Montero-Odasso M, Verghese J, Beauchet O, et al. Gait and cognition: a complementary approach to understanding brain function and the risk of falling. *J Am Geriatr Soc*. 2012;60(11):2127–2136.
7. Verghese J, Lipton RB, Hall CB, et al. Abnormality of gait as a predictor of non-Alzheimer's dementia. *N Engl J Med*. 2002;347(22):1761–1768.
8. Smith EE, Salat DH, Jeng J, et al. Correlations between MRI white matter lesion location and executive function and episodic memory. *Neurology*. 2011;76(17):1492–1499.
9. Kavirajan H, Schneider LS. Efficacy and adverse effects of cholinesterase inhibitors and memantine in vascular dementia: a meta-analysis of randomised controlled trials. *Lancet Neurol*. 2007;6(9):782–792.
10. Amenta F, Lanari A, Mignini F, et al. Nicardipine use in cerebrovascular disease: a review of controlled clinical studies. *J Neurol Sci*. 2009;283(1–2):219–223.
11. Seitz DP, Adunuri N, Gill SS, et al. Antidepressants for agitation and psychosis in dementia. *Cochrane Database Syst Rev*. 2011;(2):CD008191.

 SEE ALSO

Alzheimer Disease; Depression; Mild Cognitive Impairment

 CODES

ICD10

- F01.50 Vascular dementia without behavioral disturbance
- F01.51 Vascular dementia with behavioral disturbance

CLINICAL PEARLS

- Executive dysfunction and gait abnormalities are often seen early and are more pronounced in vascular dementia as opposed to Alzheimer dementia.
- Memory is relatively preserved in vascular dementia when compared with Alzheimer dementia in the early stages of this disease.
- Stepwise progression, as opposed to progressive decline in Alzheimer dementia, is typical.
- Considerable overlap exists between vascular dementia and Alzheimer dementia in clinical practice and classification into one of these categories is often difficult.

DENTAL INFECTION

Hugh Silk, MD, MPH, FAAFP • Sheila O. Stille, DMD • Nina E. Suresh, MD, MS

 BASICS

DESCRIPTION
- Very painful area ± swelling in the head and neck region arising from the teeth and supporting structures; if left untreated, can lead to serious and potentially life-threatening illnesses
- Assume any head and neck infection or swelling to be odontogenic in origin until proven otherwise.

EPIDEMIOLOGY
Incidence
- Caries (a.k.a. tooth decay or cavity) is a contagious bacterial infection that causes demineralization and destruction of the hard tissues of the teeth (enamel, dentin, and cementum).
- Transmitted vertically from caregivers
- Completely preventable disease with good oral hygiene and diet
- The introduction of fluoride has dramatically decreased dental caries.

Prevalence
- 23% of 2- to 5-year-olds have caries (1)[A].
- Rates are higher in Hispanic and black children (1)[A].
- Percentage of children 6 to 19 years with untreated dental caries: 19.1% (2011 to 2012) (2)[A]
- 92% of adults 20 to 64 years have had dental caries; 23% have untreated dental caries (2005 to 2008) (2)[A]
- 25% of children 5 to 17 years account for 80% of caries in the United States.
- 5% of adults age 20 to 64 years has no teeth.

ETIOLOGY AND PATHOPHYSIOLOGY
Caries or trauma can lead to pulpal death, which in turn leads to infection of pulp and/or abscess of adjacent tissues via direct or hematogenous bacterial colonization.
- *Streptococcus mutans* vertically transmitted to newly dentate infants from caregivers
- Acidic secretions from *S. mutans* are implicated in early caries.
- Often polymicrobial mix of strict anaerobes and facultative anaerobes in dental abscess
- Anaerobes, including *peptostreptococci, Bacteroides, Prevotella,* and *Fusobacterium,* have been implicated. *Lactobacilli* not seen in healthy subjects but seen in those with rampant caries (3)[B].

RISK FACTORS
- Low socioeconomic status
- Parent and/or sibling with history of caries or existing untreated dental caries
- Previous caries
- Poor access to dental and health care
- Fear of dentist
- Poor oral hygiene
- Poor nutrition, including diet containing high level of sugary foods and drinks
- Trauma to the teeth or jaws
- Inadequate access to and use of fluoride
- Gingival recession (increased risk of root caries)
- Physical and mental disabilities

- Decreased salivary flow (e.g., use of anticholinergic medications, immunologic diseases, radiation therapy to head and neck)

GENERAL PREVENTION
- Prevent caries and contagious bacterial infection (*S. mutans*).
- Majority of dental problems can be avoided through flossing; brushing with fluoride toothpaste, systemic fluoride (fluoridated bottled water; fluoride supplements for high-risk patients in nonfluoridated areas), and fluoride varnish for moderate- to high-risk pediatric patients; and regular dental cleanings (4)[B].
- Consider prevention of transmission of *S. mutans* from mother to infant by improving mother's dentition and decreasing mother's bacterial load through proper dental care, chlorhexidine gluconate rinses, and use of xylitol products. Avoid smoking, which is linked to severe periodontal disease (5)[A].
- Good control of systemic diseases (e.g., diabetes)
- Fluoride varnish provided by dental or medical primary care providers twice per year (4)[B]

COMMONLY ASSOCIATED CONDITIONS
- Rampant caries throughout dentition, faulty restorations, extractions, crowding, and multiple missing teeth
- Periapical abscesses associated with necrotic teeth
- Periodontal abscesses
- Soft tissue cellulitis
- Periodontitis (deep inflammation ± infection of gingiva, alveolar bone support, and ligaments)

 DIAGNOSIS

HISTORY
- Pain at infected site or referred pain to ears, jaw, cheek, neck, or sinuses. Unexplained headaches.
- Sensitivity to hot or cold stimuli
- Unprovoked, intermittent, or constant throb along nerve pathway
- Pain on biting or chewing
- Trismus (inability to open mouth)
- Bleeding or purulent drainage from gingival tissues
- When severe infection (systemic)
  - Fever
  - Difficulty breathing or swallowing
  - Mental status changes
- Children <4 years with stiff neck, sore throat, and dysphagia should be worked up for retropharyngeal abscess secondary to primary molar infection

PHYSICAL EXAM
- Gingival edema and erythema
- Cheek (extraoral swelling) or intraoral swelling
- Presence of fluctuant mass
- Suppuration of gingival margin or from tooth
- Submandibular or cervical lymphadenopathy on side of complaint
- Severe (systemic) infection may present with dysphagia, fever, and signs of airway compromise.

DIFFERENTIAL DIAGNOSIS
- Bacterial or viral throat infection
- Pericoronitis (inflammation ± infection of gum flap over mandibular last molar, typically third molars)
- Otitis media
- Sinusitis
- Viral (HSV1, herpangina, hand-foot-mouth disease) or aphthous stomatitis
- Temporomandibular joint (TMJ) dysfunction (myofascial pain, +/− internal derangement of TMJ)
- Parotitis
- Cyst
- Jaw pain can be anginal equivalent, especially in women, and especially lower left side of the jaw.

DIAGNOSTIC TESTS & INTERPRETATION
Initial Tests (lab, imaging)
- No initial labs needed, unless patient looks acutely ill
- If acutely ill
  - Consider CBC with differential.
  - Culture and sensitivity; if abscess present, aspirate pus and culture for aerobes and anaerobes (3)[A].
  - Polymicrobial infections, most likely anaerobic gram-negative rods and anaerobic gram-positive cocci (4)[B]
- Individual dental films of suspected teeth, including root apices; test with palpation, percussion, and cold sensitivity to diagnose correct tooth
- Panoramic film of the teeth and jaw for evaluation of the extent of infection

Follow-Up Tests & Special Considerations
- Panoramic radiograph on patients with trismus
- In large facial swellings extending below inferior border of mandible or into infraorbital space (eye closing), CT scan can be used to determine the extent and density of the swelling, locating the abscess within the soft tissue and bone, and airway involvement. This aids in determining treatment course and planning need for and location of external drainage by oral and maxillofacial surgeon or ENT.

TREATMENT
- Place patient on appropriate antibiotic, if indicated (if systemic). Pain without swelling or systemic signs of infection does not warrant antibiotic use.
- If localized infection, incision and drainage may be warranted.
- Appropriate pain control: Anti-inflammatory agents are 1st line; short-course opioids in some cases (6)[A].
- Refer to dentist as soon as possible for definitive treatment: root canal or extraction or gum therapy (7)[B].
- If infection is severe (systemic symptoms), consider hospitalization with IV antibiotics until stabilized. Patient may need intraoral or extraoral incision and drainage of abscess as well. Definitive treatment necessary to prevent progression or recurrence.

GENERAL MEASURES
- Ibuprofen 600 to 800 mg (peds: 10 mg/kg) q6h or acetaminophen 650 to 1,000 mg (peds: 10 to 15 mg/kg) q4–6h PRN for pain
- For more severe pain, consider acetaminophen or ibuprofen + short course of opioids.
- Can consider local anesthetic nerve block with long-acting anesthetic (bupivacaine) as adjunct; avoid penetrating infection with needle to avoid tracking infection.

MEDICATION
First Line
- Amoxicillin: 500 mg TID for 7 to 10 days; in children, 40 to 60 mg/kg/day divided TID
- If penicillin-allergic, use clindamycin 300 mg PO TID for 7 days.

Second Line
If long-standing infection or previously antibiotic-treated infection that does not respond to 1st-line treatment
- Clindamycin: 300 mg PO TID for 7 to 10 days
- Amoxicillin/clavulanic acid (500 mg/125 mg), 1 tablet PO TID for 7 days
- If severe infection, consider IV antibiotics (ampicillin-sulbactam, cefoxitin, cefotetan)
- Consider double coverage with metronidazole 500 mg PO TID for 7 days for better bone penetration and good anaerobic coverage. Do not use metronidazole alone. Will increase development of resistant strains; can be used with amoxicillin or clindamycin

ISSUES FOR REFERRAL
A dentist should be consulted and follow-up definitive care appointment should be secured prior to discharge from medical office, emergency room, or hospital unit.

SURGERY/OTHER PROCEDURES
- Incision and drainage of abscess should be performed if abscess is large and fluctuant.
- Root canal or extraction should be performed as definitive treatment.

INPATIENT CONSIDERATIONS
Admission Criteria/Initial Stabilization
Criteria for hospital admission include swelling involving deep spaces of the neck, floor of the mouth, or infraorbital region; deviation of the airway; unstable vital signs; fever; chills; raspy voice; confusion or delirium; or evidence of invasive infection or cellulitis.
- Secure airway, if compromised, with either endotracheal intubation or tracheotomy.
- IV fluid resuscitation with normal saline may be indicated in acutely ill patients.

Nursing
- Ensure good oral hygiene.
- Rinse or swab mouth with chlorhexidine gluconate BID.
- Use warm saltwater rinses several times per day to encourage drainage, especially after incision and drainage. In conjunction, use ice packs on outside of face to decrease swelling and help encourage drainage into mouth.

Discharge Criteria
Discharge patient if
- Airway not compromised
- Abscess and sepsis eliminated
- Able to take PO intake and ambulate.

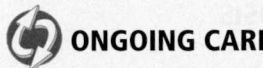 ONGOING CARE

Educate patient in need for proper oral hygiene, need for follow-up dental care, and need for routine dental care and stress medical complications that can and have occurred due to lack of dental care.

FOLLOW-UP RECOMMENDATIONS
- Follow up with dentist within 24 hours.
- Ensure adequate PO intake, including protein.

DIET
- Maintain a healthful diet; bacteria thrive on refined sugar and starch.
- Avoid sugary foods that stick between the teeth.
- Avoid continuous sugary/carbonated drinks throughout day; encourage water as beverage of choice between meals.

Pediatric Considerations
In children, limit the frequency of sugary drinks and advise against sleeping with a bottle to decrease the chance of dental caries.

PATIENT EDUCATION
- Manage dental disease, comprehensively—caries and periodontal disease need to be controlled.
- Minimally, biannual dental visits after disease control
- Nutritional education
  - Limit the frequency of sugar/carbonated drinks and sugary or sticky foods.
- In young children, avoid sleeping with a bottle to decrease the chance of dental caries.
- Brush twice daily and floss daily
- Caretakers should tend to their personal oral hygiene ± chlorhexidine gluconate rinses in first 3 years of the child's life to decrease the risk of transmission of the caries-causing microorganisms.

PROGNOSIS
Prognosis is excellent with proper treatment.

COMPLICATIONS
- Ludwig angina
- Retropharyngeal and mediastinal infection
- Osteomyelitis
- Endocarditis
- Submental infection
- Submandibular infection
- Can cause unstable diabetes in diabetics/worsen preexisting heart disease
- Brain abscess/death

REFERENCES
1. Dye BA, Thornton-Evans G, Li X, et al. Dental caries and sealant prevalence in children and adolescents in the United States, 2011–2012. NCHS data brief, no 191. Hyattsville, MD: National Center for Health Statistics; 2015. http://www.cdc.gov/nchs/data/databriefs/db191.htm. Accessed 2015.
2. National Center for Health Statistics. Health, United States, 2011: with special feature on socioeconomic status and health. Table 76. Hyattsville, MD: National Center for Health Statistics; 2012. http://www.cdc.gov/nchs/data/hus/hus11.pdf/. Accessed 2014.
3. Robertson D, Smith AJ. The microbiology of the acute dental abscess. J Med Microbiol. 2009;58(Pt 2):155–162.
4. Marinho VC, Higgins JP, Logan S, et al. Topical fluoride (toothpastes, mouth rinses, gels or varnishes) for preventing dental caries in children and adolescents. Cochrane Database Syst Rev. 2003;(4):CD002782.
5. Mickenautsch S, Yengopal V. Anticariogenic effect of xylitol versus fluoride—a quantitative systematic review of clinical trials. Int Dent J. 2012;62(1):6–20.
6. Ong CK, Seymour RA. An evidence-based update of the use of analgesics in dentistry. Periodontol 2000. 2008;46:143–164.
7. Douglass AB, Douglass JM. Common dental emergencies. Am Fam Physician. 2003;67(3):511–516.

ADDITIONAL READING
- Clark MB, Douglass AB, Maier R, et al. Smiles for Life: A National Oral Health Curriculum. 3rd ed. Leawood, KS: Society of Teachers of Family Medicine; 2010. http://www.smilesforlifeoralhealth.com/buildcontent.aspx?tut=555&pagekey=62948&cbreceipt=0. Accessed 2014.
- Douglas JM, Clark MB. Integrating oral health into overall health care to prevent early childhood caries: need, evidence, and solutions. Pediatr Dent. 2015;37(3):266–274.
- Dye BA, Li X, Beltrán-Aguilar ED. Selected oral health indicators in the United States, 2005-2008. NCHS data brief, no 96. Hyattsville, MD: National Center for Health Statistics; 2012.
- Flynn TR. What are the antibiotics of choice for odontogenic infections, and how long should the treatment course last? Oral Maxillofac Surg Clin North Am. 2011;23(4):519–536.
- Lockhart PB, ed. Oral Medicine and Medically Complex Patients. 6th ed. New York, NY: Elsevier; 2013.
- U.S. Preventive Services Task Force. Dental caries in children from birth through age 5 years: screening. AHRQ Publication No. 12-05170-EF-2. http://www.uspreventiveservicestaskforce.org/Page/Topic/recommendation-summary/dental-caries-in-children-from-birth-through-age-5-years-screening. Accessed 2014.

 CODES

ICD10
- K02.9 Dental caries, unspecified
- K04.7 Periapical abscess without sinus
- K12.2 Cellulitis and abscess of mouth

CLINICAL PEARLS
- Do not ignore toothache pain.
- Treat patients with facial swelling aggressively, as infections can spread quickly, leading to significant morbidity or death.
- Promote prevention (oral hygiene, fluoride, dental visits) to avoid infections.

DEPRESSION

Rachel Bramson, MD • Michael L. Brown, MD • Suzanne Shurtz, MLIS, AHIP

BASICS

DESCRIPTION
- A primary mood disorder characterized by a sustained depressed mood and/or decreased interest in things that used to give pleasure (anhedonia), which represents a change from previous functioning.
- Variants: (1) major depressive disorder (MDD), (2) dysthymic disorder, and (3) depressive disorder not otherwise specified (NOS). (Last two disorders have slightly different diagnostic criteria but are still treated as below.)

EPIDEMIOLOGY
Incidence
In United States, 6.9% of 18 years of age or older in the past year

Prevalence
- 16.2% lifetime risk of having MDD
- Patients can relapse; risk decreases with longer remission period but increases in patients with severe episodes, episodes at a younger age, and multiple episodes.
- Predominant age
  - Low risk before early teens but highest prevalence in teens and young adults
- Predominant gender
  - Females > males (2:1)

ETIOLOGY AND PATHOPHYSIOLOGY
Complex etiology with two major models in the literature
- *Monoamine-deficiency hypothesis*: symptoms related to decreased levels of norepinephrine (dullness and lethargy) and serotonin (irritability, hostility, and suicidal ideation) in multiple regions of the brain; other neurotransmitters involved include dopamine, acetylcholine, γ-aminobutyric acid (GABA), glutamate
- *Stress/hypothalamic–pituitary–adrenal axis*: Abnormalities in cortisol response lead to depression; elevated cortisol levels can be associated with depression, but cortisol tests are not indicated for diagnosis.
- Other areas of research interest: inflammatory processes and abnormal circadian rhythms; impaired synthesis/metabolism of neurotransmitters
- Environmental factors and learned behavior may affect neurotransmitters and/or have an independent influence on depression.

Genetics
Multiple gene loci place a person at increased risk when faced with environmental stressor; twin studies suggest 37% concordance (1).

RISK FACTORS
- Female > male (2:1)
- Severity of 1st episode
- Persistent sleep disturbances
- Presence of chronic disease(s), recent myocardial infarction (MI), cardiovascular accident (CVA)
- Strong family history (depression, bipolar, suicide, substance abuse), spouse with depression
- Substance abuse and dependence, domestic abuse/violence
- Losses, stressors, unemployment
- Single, divorced, or unhappily married

COMMONLY ASSOCIATED CONDITIONS
- Bipolar disorder, cyclothymic disorder, grief reaction, anxiety disorders, somatoform disorders, schizophrenia/schizoaffective disorders

- Medical comorbidity
- Substance abuse

DIAGNOSIS

HISTORY
DSM-5 requires all of the following criteria for MDD:
- Criterion A: ≥5 of the following symptoms present nearly every day during the same 2-week period, with at least one of the five being either depressed mood or loss of interest or pleasure:
  - Depressed mood most of the day by subjective report or observation from other people
  - Diminished interest or pleasure in all activities most of the day by subjective report or observation from other people
  - Decreased or increased appetite or significant weight loss without dieting
  - Insomnia or hypersomnia
  - Fatigue or energy loss
  - Restlessness, irritability, or withdrawal observable by others
  - Worthlessness, excessive/inappropriate guilty feelings
  - Diminished thinking/concentration, poor memory, indecisiveness
  - Recurrent thoughts of death, suicidal ideations, and may or may not have a specific plan
- Criterion B: symptoms cause significant social, occupational, or functional distress or impairment
- Criterion C: symptoms not attributable to substance effects or other medical conditions

Geriatric Considerations
- Difficult to diagnose due to medical comorbidity
- Can present with memory difficulties as chief complaint; treatment reverses memory difficulty
- Can be the initial presentation of irreversible dementia
- Geriatric Depression Scale (GDS 15) improves rate of diagnosis in primary care setting (2,3)[A].

Pediatric Considerations
- Can present as irritable or angry rather than sad or dejected
- Failure to make expected weight gains can substitute weight loss symptom above
- A sudden and remarkable drop in grades can indicate difficulty concentrating.
- Can present with separation anxiety

PHYSICAL EXAM
Complete physical with focus on endocrine, cardiac, neurologic, and psychiatric (affect, attention, cognition, memory); look for evidence of contributing medical or neurologic disorder

DIFFERENTIAL DIAGNOSIS
- Psychiatric: depressed phase of bipolar disorder—inquire if prior mania, family or personal history of bipolar disorder, prior agitation or excitement with antidepressant medication. If positive, monitor carefully for mood elevation or destabilization, adjustment disorder, and bereavement.
- Neurologic or degenerative CNS diseases, dementias
- Medical comorbidity: adrenal disease, thyroid disorders, diabetes, metabolic abnormalities (hypercalcemia), liver/renal failure, malignancy, chronic fatigue syndrome, fibromyalgia, lupus
- Nutritional: pernicious anemia, pellagra
- Medications/substances: abuse, side effects, overdose, intoxication, dependence, withdrawal

DIAGNOSTIC TESTS & INTERPRETATION
- A clinical diagnosis made by eliciting personal, family, social, and psychosocial factors
- The Patient Health Questionnaire-9 (PHQ-9) is a brief screening test valid for diagnosis of MDD in primary care settings (3)[A].
- Other validated standard rating scales include the following: Beck Depression Inventory, Zung, GDS 15, and so forth. Rating scales are also useful to track response to treatment over time (3)[A].
- Rule out hypothyroidism, anemia, and metabolic disorders with TSH, CBC, and comprehensive metabolic panel (CMP)
- Order urine drug screen if symptoms suggest intoxication.

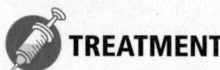

TREATMENT

American Psychiatric Association (APA) 2010 guidelines recommend phasic approach: acute phase (first 3 months), continuation phase (4 to 9 months), and maintenance (9 months until discontinuation) (4)[A].

- Acute phase
  - Full evaluation, including risk to self and others, with selection of appropriate treatment setting (hospitalization for those at risk of harm to self or others, or so incapacitated as to be unable to take care of themselves and/or who have no support system to assist with treatment)
  - Goal should be symptom remission, with intervention based on clinical picture, including patient's preference, availability of services
  - For mild to moderate depression, psychotherapies (individual, interpersonal, or cognitive-behavioral therapy [CBT]) and/or medication are recommended.
  - For refractory/severe depression, medication is indicated.
  - For patients not responding to medication alone, CBT should be initiated.
  - Continue to increase dosage q3–4wk until symptoms in remission. Full medication effect is complete in 4 to 6 weeks. Augmentation with 2nd medication may be necessary.
  - See within 2 to 4 weeks of starting medication and q2wk until improvement, then monthly to monitor medication changes.
  - ≥6 visits recommended for monitoring (younger patients; those at high suicide risk, see within 1st week, and follow frequently)
- Continuation/maintenance phase
  - Regular visits to monitor for signs of relapse, q3–6mo if stable; depression rating scales should be used.
  - Once remission achieved, dosage should be continued for at least 6 to 9 months to reduce relapse; CBT is also effective in reducing relapse (visits typically q2wk).
  - If/when drug discontinuation is considered, medications should be tapered gradually (weeks to months).

ISSUES FOR REFERRAL
- Refer immediately for active suicidal ideations, psychosis, severe agitation, severe self-neglect, and significant risk of self-harm.
- Refer to psychiatry for failed response to medication trials, suspected bipolar disorder, more persistent suicidal thoughts, and self-neglect.

MEDICATION

- Effectiveness of medications is comparable between/within classes; selection should be based on provider familiarity and patient characteristics/preferences (5)[A].

- Selective serotonin reuptake inhibitors (SSRIs) and tricyclic antidepressants (TCAs) are effective, but TCAs are second line due to side effects and lethality in overdose. Tolerability is much poorer than newer antidepressants.

- First-line SSRIs* (starting dose; usual dose)
  – Fluoxetine (Prozac): 20 mg/day; 20 to 60 mg/day
  – Sertraline (Zoloft): 50 mg/day; 50 to 200 mg/day
  – Paroxetine (Paxil): 10 mg/day; 20 to 50 mg/day
  – Paroxetine CR (Paxil CR): 12.5 mg/day; 25 to 62.5 mg/day
  – Citalopram (Celexa): 20 mg/day; 20 to 40 mg/day (higher doses not advised; EKG monitoring for doses >40 mg/day due to increased risk of QTc prolongation)
  – Escitalopram (Lexapro): 10 mg/day; 10 to 20 mg/day
  – Precautions: abrupt discontinuation may result in withdrawal symptoms (i.e., dizziness, nausea, headache, paresthesia)
  – Fluoxetine, paroxetine may raise serum levels of other drugs; escitalopram, sertraline have minimal to no drug interactions.
  – Common side effects: sexual dysfunction (20%), nausea, GI upset, dizziness, insomnia, headache; typically resolve in the 1st week
  – Less common side effects: drowsiness, weight gain, emotional blunting, dry mouth
  – *Lower starting doses for elderly, adolescents, those with comorbid conditions, panic disorder, significant anxiety, or hepatic conditions

- Others (starting dose; usual dose)
  – Venlafaxine (Effexor, Effexor XR): 37.5 mg/day; 300 mg/day
  – Bupropion XL (Wellbutrin XL): 150 mg/day; 300 to 450 mg/day (precautions: powers seizure threshold at doses >450 mg/day)
  – Duloxetine (Cymbalta): 30 mg/day; 60 to 120 mg/day
  – Desvenlafaxine (Pristiq): 50 to 100 mg/day
  – Vilazodone: start 10 mg/day; usual target 40 mg/day
  – Vortioxetine: start 5 mg/day; target dose 20 mg/day
  – Levomilnacipran: start 20 mg/day; target dose 40 to 120 mg/day

Second Line

- TCAs (starting dose; usual dose)
  – Amitriptyline (Elavil): 25 to 50 mg/day; 100 to 300 mg/day
  – Nortriptyline (Pamelor): 25 mg/day; 50 to 150 mg/day
  – Doxepin (Sinequan): 25 to 50 mg/day; 100 to 300 mg/day
  – Imipramine (Tofranil, Tofranil-PM): 25 to 50 mg/day; 100 to 300 mg/day
  – Desipramine (Norpramin): 25 to 50 mg/day; 100 to 300 mg/day
  – Precautions: advanced age, glaucoma, benign prostate hyperplasia, hyperthyroidism, cardiovascular disease, liver disease, monamine oxidase inhibitor (MAOI) treatment, potential for fatal overdose, arrhythmia, worsening glycemic control; *SSRIs recommended for patients with diabetes (4)[A]
  – Common side effects: dry mouth, blurred vision, constipation, urinary retention, tachycardia, confusion/delirium; elderly particularly susceptible

- α_2-Antagonists (sedating) (starting dose; usual dose)
  – Mirtazapine (Remeron): 15 mg/day; 15 to 45 mg/day

- Atypical antipsychotics
  – Adjunctive treatment: aripiprazole or quetiapine
  – Treatment-resistant depression (TRD): olanzapine
  – Significant side effects: dyslipidemia, hypertriglyceridemia, glucose dysregulation, diabetes mellitus, hyperprolactinemia, tardive dyskinesia, neuroleptic malignant syndrome, QTc prolongation (6)[A]
  – Recommended for depression with psychotic features; consult with psychiatry and consider carefully before starting (4)[A].

- Significant potential interactions
  – TCAs: amphetamines, barbiturates, clonidine, epinephrine, ethanol, norepinephrine
  – ALL ANTIDEPRESSANTS: allow 14-day washout period before starting MAOIs
  – MAOIs: not recommended in primary care. Significant drug and food interactions limit use.

ALERT

- Black box warning: increased risk of suicidality in children, adolescents, and young adults up to age 25 years who are treated with antidepressants. Although this has not been extended to adults, suicide risk assessments are warranted for all patients.
- Serotonin syndrome—a rare but potentially lethal complication from rapid increase in dose or new addition of medication with serotonergic effects
- Caution with personal or family history of bipolar disorder: Antidepressants can precipitate mania.

Pregnancy Considerations
SSRIs: Fluoxetine, sertraline, and bupropion considered safe in pregnancy (paroxetine, Category D; other SSRIs, Category C).

ADDITIONAL THERAPIES

- Electroconvulsive therapy (ECT) for refractory cases
- Repetitive transcranial magnetic stimulation (rTMS) may be helpful for TRD (6)[A].

COMPLEMENTARY & ALTERNATIVE MEDICINE

Used in mild depression but *not* regulated by FDA nor recommended by APA

- Hypericum perforatum (St. John's wort): multiple drug interactions; not safe in pregnancy
- Data do not support S-adenosyl methionine (SAM-e) or acupuncture.

INPATIENT CONSIDERATIONS

Admission Criteria/Initial Stabilization
Inpatient care is indicated for severe depression, patients at risk of suicide/homicide, and for comorbid conditions.

Discharge Criteria
Depressive symptoms abating, no longer suicidal, appropriate outpatient follow-up in place

 ONGOING CARE

PATIENT EDUCATION

- Depression is a common medical illness, not a character defect.
- Emphasize the need for long-term treatment and follow-up, which includes lifestyle changes.
- Exercise, good sleep hygiene, good nutrition, and decreased use of tobacco and alcohol are recommended. The optimal regimen is one the patient prefers and will adhere to.

PROGNOSIS

- 70% show significant improvement
- Of patients with a single depressive episode, 50% will relapse over their lifetime.

COMPLICATIONS

- Suicide
- Lower quality of life

REFERENCES

1. Flint J, Kendler KS. The genetics of major depression. *Neuron.* 2014;81(3):484–503.
2. Mitchell AJ, Bird V, Rizzo M, et al. Diagnostic validity and added value of the Geriatric Depression Scale for depression in primary care: a meta-analysis of GDS30 and GDS15. *J Affect Disord.* 2010;125(1–3):10–17.
3. Deneke DE, Schultz H, Fluent TE. Screening for depression in the primary care population. *Prim Care.* 2014;41(2):399–420.
4. American Psychiatric Association. Practice guidelines for the treatment of patients with major depressive disorder. http://www.psychiatryonline.com/pracGuide/pracGuideTopic_7.aspx. Accessed 2015.
5. Arroll B, Elley CR, Fishman T, et al. Antidepressants versus placebo for depression in primary care. *Cochrane Database Syst Rev.* 2009;(3):CD007954.
6. McIntyre RS, Filteau MJ, Martin L, et al. Treatment-resistant depression: definitions, review of the evidence, and algorithmic approach. *J Affect Disord.* 2014;156:1–7.

ADDITIONAL READING

- American Psychiatric Association. *Diagnostic and Statistical Manual of Mental Disorders.* 5th ed. Arlington, VA: American Psychiatric Association; 2013.
- Patient Health Questionnaire (PHQ) Screeners: http://www.phqscreeners.com/overview.aspx?Screener=03_GAD-7

 SEE ALSO

Algorithms: Depressed Mood Associated with Medical Illness; Depressive Episode, Major

CODES

ICD10

- F32.9 Major depressive disorder, single episode, unspecified
- F33.9 Major depressive disorder, recurrent, unspecified
- F34.1 Dysthymic disorder

CLINICAL PEARLS

- Therapeutic alliance is important to treatment success.
- Given the high recurrence rates, long-term treatment is often necessary.

DEPRESSION, ADOLESCENT

Nanette Lacuesta, MS, MD • Joseph Gladwell, MD

 BASICS

DESCRIPTION
- *DSM-5* depressive disorders include disruptive mood dysregulations disorder (DMDD), major depressive disorder (MDD), dysthymia, premenstrual dysphoric disorder, substance-/medication-induced depressive disorder, and other nonspecific depression. This chapter focuses on MDD.
- MDD is a primary mood disorder characterized by sadness and/or irritable mood with impairment of functioning; abnormal psychological development; and a loss of self-worth, energy, and interest in typically pleasurable activities.
- DMDD is characterized by a chronic, severe persistent irritability with frequent temper outbursts in response to frustration.
- Dysthymic disorder is differentiated from major depression by less intense symptoms that are more persistent, lasting at least 1 year.
- Adolescents with depression are likely to suffer broad functional impairment across social, academic, family, and occupational domains, along with a high incidence of relapse and a high risk for substance abuse and other psychiatric comorbidity.

EPIDEMIOLOGY
Incidence
During adolescence, the cumulative probability of depression ranges from 5% to 20% (1,2).

Prevalence
- MDD: 6–12% of adolescents; twice as common in females (1)
- DMDD: 2–5%; more prominent in males (3)

ETIOLOGY AND PATHOPHYSIOLOGY
- Unclear; low levels of neurotransmitters (serotonin, norepinephrine) may produce symptoms; decreased functioning of the dopamine system also contributes.
- External factors may affect neurotransmitters independently.

Genetics
- Offspring of parents with depression have three to four times increased rates of depression compared with offspring of parents without mood disorder (2).
- Family studies indicate that anxiety in childhood tends to precede adolescent depression (2).

RISK FACTORS
- Increased three to six times if first-degree relative has a major affective disorder; three to four times in offspring of parents with depression
- Prior depressive episodes
- History of low self-esteem, anxiety disorders, attention deficit hyperactivity disorder (ADHD), and/or learning disabilities
- Hormonal changes during puberty
- Female gender
- Low socioeconomic status
- General stressors: adverse life events, difficulties with peers, loss of a loved one, academic difficulties, abuse, chronic illness, and tobacco abuse

GENERAL PREVENTION
Insufficient evidence for universal depression prevention programs (psychological and social) (4)[B]
- Some evidence indicates that child and adolescent mental health can be improved by successfully treating maternal depression (2,4)[A].

- Agency for Healthcare Research and Quality (AHRQ) recommends the screening of adolescents (12 to 18 years of age) for major depressive disorder when systems are in place to ensure accurate diagnosis, psychotherapy (cognitive-behavioral or interpersonal), and follow-up (5)[C].

COMMONLY ASSOCIATED CONDITIONS
- 2/3 of adolescents with depression have at least one comorbid psychiatric disorder.
- 20% meet the criteria for generalized anxiety disorder.
- Also associated with behavioral disorders, substance abuse, eating disorders

 DIAGNOSIS

HISTORY
- Adolescents may present with medically unexplained somatic complaints (fatigue, irritability, headache).
- Based on *DSM-5* criteria, ≥5 of the following symptoms have been present during the same 2-week period and represent a change from previous functioning: At least one of the symptoms is either depressed mood or loss of interest or pleasure (3):
  – Criterion A
    ○ Depressed mood most of the day, nearly every day by either subjective report or observation by others (feelings of sadness, emptiness, hopelessness; in children, can be irritability)
    ○ Markedly diminished interest or pleasure in all activities most of the day, nearly every day
    ○ Significant weight loss when not dieting or weight gain (>5% body weight in 1 month)
    ○ Insomnia or hypersomnia
    ○ Psychomotor agitation or retardation nearly every day
    ○ Fatigue or loss of energy
    ○ Feelings of worthlessness or excessive or inappropriate feelings of guilt nearly every day
    ○ Diminished ability to think or concentrate, or indecisiveness, nearly every day
    ○ Recurrent thoughts of death, recurrent suicidal ideation, or attempt
  – Criterion B. Symptoms cause clinically significant distress or impairment in social, occupational, or other important areas of functioning.
  – Criterion C. Episode is not attributable to substances' effects or other medical conditions.
  – Criterion D. Episode is not better explained by a schizoaffective, schizophreniform, or delusional disorder.
  – Criterion E. There has never been a manic or hypomanic episode.

PHYSICAL EXAM
- Psychomotor retardation/agitation may be present.
- Clinicians should carefully assess patients for signs of self-injury (wrist lacerations) or abuse.

DIFFERENTIAL DIAGNOSIS
- Normal bereavement
- Substance-induced mood disorder
- Bipolar disorder
- Mood disorder secondary to a medical condition (thyroid, anemia, vitamin deficiency, diabetes)
- Organic CNS diseases
- Malignancy
- Infectious mononucleosis or other viral diseases
- ADHD, posttraumatic stress disorder (PTSD), eating disorders, and anxiety disorders
- Sleep disorder

DIAGNOSTIC TESTS & INTERPRETATION
Initial Tests (lab, imaging)
May be used to rule out other diagnoses (i.e., CBC, TSH, glucose, mono spot, and urine drug)

Follow-Up Tests & Special Considerations
None with sufficient sensitivity/specificity for diagnosis

Diagnostic Procedures/Other
- Depression is primarily diagnosed after a formal interview, with supporting information from caregivers and teachers.
- Standardized tests are useful as screening tools and to monitor response to treatment but should not be used as the sole basis for diagnosis:
  – Beck Depression Inventory (BDI): ages 12 to 18 years (2)[A]
  – Child Depression Inventory (CDI): ages 7 to 17 years
  – Reynolds Adolescent Depression Scale (RADS): teenagers in grades 7 to 12
  – Mood and Feelings Questionnaire (MFQ) (6)[A]
  – Patient Health Questionnaire-9 (PHQ-9): ages 13 to 17 years with ideal cut point of 11 or higher (instead of 10 used for adults) (7)[B]
- The USPSTF concludes that the current evidence is insufficient to assess the balance of benefits and harms of screening for suicide risk in adolescents in a primary care setting (8)[C].

TREATMENT

GENERAL MEASURES
- Active support and monitoring with short validated scales should be used in mild cases for 6 to 8 weeks.
- Psychotherapy and/or medication should be considered if active support and monitoring do to improve symptoms (9)[A].
- Treatment should include psychoeducation, supportive management, and family and school involvement (10)[C].
- Initial management should include treatment planning and ensuring that the patient and family is comfortable with the plan (11)[C].
- A Cochrane review showed that there was no significant difference between remission rates for adolescents treated with cognitive behavioral therapy (CBT) versus medication or combination therapy immediately postintervention (12)[A].
- A multitreatment meta-analysis showed that combined fluoxetine/CBT had higher efficacy than monotherapies, but other SSRIs such as sertraline and escitalopram were better tolerated (9)[A].

MEDICATION
First Line

- Fluoxetine: for depression in age >8 years. Starting dose of 10 mg/day; effective dose of 10 to 60 mg/day The most studied SSRI and with the most favorable effectiveness and safety data has the longest half-life of the SSRIs and is not generally associated with withdrawal symptoms between doses or upon discontinuation (13)[A].
- Escitalopram: for depression in age >12 years. Starting dose of 5 mg/day; effective dose of 10 to 20 mg/day (13)[A].
- Citalopram: for depression in age >12 years. Starting dose of 10 mg/day; effective dose of 10 to 40 mg/day (13)[A].
- Sertraline: for depression in age >12 years. Starting dose of 25 mg/day; effective dose of 50 to 200 mg/day (13)[A]
- Can titrate dose every 1 to 2 weeks if no significant adverse effects emerge (headaches, GI upset, insomnia, agitation, behavior activation, suicidal thoughts) (13)[A]
- SSRI black box warning to monitor for worsening condition, behavior changes, and suicidal thoughts (13)[A]
- Antidepressant treatment should be continued for 6 to 12 months after the resolution of symptoms at the same dosage (10)[C].
- Given their rates of increased drug metabolism, adolescents may be at higher risk for withdrawal symptoms from SSRIs than adults; if these are present, twice-daily dosing may be considered (9)[A].
- All other SSRIs except fluoxetine should be slowly tapered when discontinued (9)[A].

Pediatric Considerations

- Tricyclic antidepressants (TCAs) have not been proven to be effective in adolescents and should not be used (9)[A].
- Paroxetine (SSRI): Avoid use due to short half-life, associated withdrawal symptoms, and higher association with suicidal ideation.

ISSUES FOR REFERRAL

- Collaborative care interventions between mental health and primary care have a greater improvement in depressive symptoms after 12 months (14)[B].
- Primary care providers should provide initial treatment of pediatric depression. Refer to a child psychiatrist for severe, recurrent, or treatment-resistant depression or if the patient has comorbidities (13)[A].

COMPLEMENTARY & ALTERNATIVE MEDICINE

- Physical exercise and light therapy may have a mild to moderate effect (15)[B].
- St. John's wort, acupuncture, S-adenosylmethionine, and 5-hydroxytryptophan have not been shown to have an effect or have inadequate studies to support use in adolescent depression (15)[B].

INPATIENT CONSIDERATIONS
Admission Criteria/Initial Stabilization
If severely depressed, psychotic, suicidal, or homicidal, one-on-one supervision may be needed.

 ONGOING CARE

Patient Monitoring

- Systematic and regular tracking of goals and outcomes from treatment should be performed, including assessment of depressive symptoms and functioning in home, school, and peer settings (13)[A].
- Diagnosis and initial treatment should be reassessed if no improvement is noted after 6 to 8 weeks of treatment (13)[A].
- The goal of treatment should be no symptoms or a significant reduction of depressive symptoms for 2 weeks (10)[C].
- Educate patients and family members about the causes, symptoms, course and treatments of depression, risks of treatments, and risk of no treatment.

PROGNOSIS
- 60–90% of episodes remit within 1 year.
- 50–70% of remissions develop subsequent depressive episodes within 5 years.

- Depression in adolescence predicts mental health disorders in adult life, psychosocial difficulties, and ill health (2)[A].
- Baseline symptom severity and comorbid anxiety may impact treatment response (16)[A].
- Parental depression at baseline significantly affects intervention effects (4)[A].

COMPLICATIONS
- Treatment-induced mania, aggression, or lack of improvement in symptoms
- School failure/refusal
- Suicide

REFERENCES

1. Clark MS, Jansen KL, Cloy JA. Treatment of childhood and adolescent depression. *Am Fam Physician*. 2012;86(5):442–448.
2. Thapar A, Collishaw S, Pine DS, et al. Depression in adolescence. *Lancet*. 2012;379(9820):1056–1067.
3. American Psychiatric Association. *Diagnostic and Statistical Manual of Mental Disorders*. 5th ed. Arlington, VA: American Psychiatric Association; 2013.
4. Beardslee WR, Brent DA, Weersing VR, et al. Prevention of depression in at-risk adolescents: longer-term effects. *JAMA Psychiatry*. 2013;70(11):1161–1170.
5. U.S. Preventive Services Task Force. Screening and treatment for major depressive disorder in children and adolescents: US Preventive Services Task Force Recommendation Statement. *Pediatrics*. 2009;123(4):1223–1228.
6. Thapar A, Collishaw S, Potter R, et al. Managing and preventing depression in adolescents. *BMJ*. 2010;340:c209.
7. Larun L, Nordheim LV, Ekeland E, et al. Exercise in prevention and treatment of anxiety and depression among children and young people. *Cochrane Database Syst Rev*. 2006;(3):CD004691.
8. Richardson LP, McCauley E, Grossman DC, et al. Evaluation of the Patient Health Questionnaire-9 item for detecting major depression among adolescents. *Pediatrics*. 2010;126(6):1117–1123.
9. Ma D, Zhang Z, Zhang X, et al. Comparative efficacy, acceptability, and safety of medicinal, cognitive-behavioral therapy, and placebo treatments for acute major depressive disorder in children and adolescents: a multiple-treatments meta-analysis. *Curr Med Res Opin*. 2014;30(6):971–995.
10. Birmaher B, Brent D. Practice parameter for the assessment and treatment of children and adolescents with depressive disorders. *J Am Acad Child Adolesc Psychiatry*. 2007;46(11):1503–1526.
11. Cheung AH, Zuckerbrot RA, Jensen PS, et al. Guidelines for Adolescent Depression in Primary Care (GLAD-PC): II. Treatment and ongoing management. *Pediatrics*. 2007;120(5):e1313–e1326.
12. Cox GR, Callahan P, Churchill R, et al. Psychological therapies versus antidepressant medication, alone and in combination for depression in children and adolescents. *Cochrane Database Syst Rev*. 2014;(11):CD008324.
13. Cheung AH, Kozloff N, Sacks D. Pediatric depression: an evidence-based update on treatment interventions. *Curr Psychiatry Rep*. 2013;15(8):381.
14. Reeves GM, Riddle MA. A practical and effective primary care intervention for treating adolescent depression. *JAMA*. 2014;312(8):797–798.
15. Popper CW. Mood disorders in youth: exercise, light therapy, and pharmacologic complementary and integrative approaches. *Child Adolesc Psychiatr Clin N Am*. 2013;22(3):403–441.
16. Nilsen TS, Eisemann M, Kvernmo S. Predictors and moderators of outcome in child and adolescent anxiety and depression: a systematic review of psychological treatment studies. *Eur Child Adolesc Psychiatry*. 2013;22(2):69–87.

ADDITIONAL READING

- Emslie GJ, Mayes T, Porta G, et al. Treatment of resistant depression in adolescents (TORDIA): week 24 outcomes. *Am J Psychiatry*. 2010;167(7):782–791.
- LeFevre ML. Screening for suicide risk in adolescents, adults, and older adults in primary care: U.S. Preventive Services Task Force recommendation statement. *Ann Intern Med*. 2014;160(10):719-726.

 CODES

ICD10
- F32.9 Major depressive disorder, single episode, unspecified
- F33.9 Major depressive disorder, recurrent, unspecified
- F33.8 Other recurrent depressive disorders

CLINICAL PEARLS

- Adolescent depression is underdiagnosed and often presents with irritability and anhedonia.
- Fluoxetine is the most studied FDA approved for treatment of adolescent depression.
- Escitalopram, citalopram, and sertraline are also FDA-approved antidepressants.
- CBT combined with fluoxetine is efficacious for adolescents with major depression.
- Paroxetine and TCAs should not be used to treat adolescent depression.
- Referral to a child psychiatrist is appropriate for complex cases or treatment-resistant depression.
- Monitor all adolescents with depression for suicidality, especially during the 1st month of treatment with an antidepressant.

DEPRESSION, GERIATRIC

Jennifer M. Slowik, DO, MS • Rachel M. Jones, DO • Jeffrey B. Lanier, MD, FAAFP

BASICS

DESCRIPTION
- Depression is a primary mood disorder characterized by a depressed mood and/or a markedly decreased interest or pleasure in normally enjoyable activities most of the day, almost every day for at least 2 weeks, and causing significant distress or impairment in daily functioning with at least four other symptoms of depression.
- It is not considered a part of normal aging.

EPIDEMIOLOGY
Prevalence rates among the elderly vary largely depending on the specific diagnostic instruments used and their current health and/or home environment:
- 5% of community-dwelling elderly
- 5–10% seen in primary care clinics
- 10–37% of hospitalized elderly patients
- 12–27% of nursing home residents

ETIOLOGY AND PATHOPHYSIOLOGY
- Significant gaps exist in the understanding of the underlying pathophysiology
- Ongoing research has identified several possible mechanisms, including the following:
  - Monoamine transmission and associated transcriptional and translational activity
- Epigenetic mechanisms and resilience factors
- Neurotrophins, neurogenesis, neuroimmune systems, and neuroendocrine systems
- Depression appears to be a complex interaction between heritable and environmental factors.

RISK FACTORS
- General
  - Female sex
  - Lower socioeconomic status
  - Chronic physical health condition(s)
  - History of mental health problems
  - Family history of depression
  - Death of a loved one
  - Caregiving
  - Social isolation
  - Lack/loss of social support
  - Significant loss of independence
  - Uncontrolled or chronic pain
  - Insomnia/sleep disturbance
- Prevalence of depression in medical illness
  - Stroke (22–50%)
  - Cancer (18–50%)
  - Myocardial infarction (15–45%)
  - Parkinson disease (10–39%)
  - Rheumatoid arthritis (13%)
  - Diabetes mellitus (5–11%)
  - Alzheimer dementia (5–15%)
- Suicide
  - Suicide is the 11th leading cause of death in the United States for all ages.
  - Suicide rates are higher for Americans age >65 years compared with the general population (~15/100,000 people)
  - Suicide rates are highest for males aged >75 years (rate 38.5/100,000).

DIAGNOSIS

HISTORY
- Depressed mood most of the day, nearly every day, and/or loss of interest/pleasure in life for at least 2 weeks

- Other common symptoms include the following:
  - Feeling hopeless, helpless, or worthless
  - Insomnia and loss of appetite/weight (alternatively, hypersomnia with increased appetite/weight in atypical depression)
  - Fatigue and loss of energy
  - Somatic symptoms (headaches, chronic pain)
  - Neglect of personal responsibility or care
  - Psychomotor retardation or agitation
  - Diminished concentration, indecisiveness
  - Thoughts of death or suicide
- Screening with "SIGECAPS"
  - **S**leep: changes in sleep habits from baseline, including excessive sleep, early waking, or inability to fall asleep
  - **I**nterest: loss of interest in previously enjoyable activities (anhedonia)
  - **G**uilt: excessive or inappropriate guilt that may or may not focus on a specific problem or circumstance
  - **E**nergy: perceived lack of energy
  - **C**oncentration: inability to concentrate on specific tasks
  - **A**ppetite: increase/decrease in appetite
  - **P**sychomotor: restlessness and agitation or the perception that everyday activities are too strenuous to manage
  - **S**uicidality: desire to end life or hurt oneself, harmful thoughts directed internally, recurrent thoughts of death or thoughts of homicidality

PHYSICAL EXAM
Mental status exam, thorough neurologic exam, and general physical exam to rule out other conditions

DIFFERENTIAL DIAGNOSIS
Concurrent medical conditions, cognitive disorders, and medications may cause symptoms that mimic depression:
- Medical conditions: hypothyroidism, vitamin B_{12} or folate deficiency, liver or renal failure, cancers, stroke, sleep disorders, electrolyte imbalances, Cushing disease, chronic fatigue syndrome
- Dementia and neurodegenerative disorders
- Delirium
- Medication-induced: interferon-α, β_2-blockers, isotretinoin, benzodiazepines, glucocorticoids, levodopa, clonidine, H_2 blockers, baclofen, varenicline, metoclopramide, reserpine
- Psychiatric disorders: adjustment disorder with depressed mood, grief reaction, bipolar disorder, dysthymic disorder, anxiety disorders, substance abuse–related mood disorders, psychotic disorders

DIAGNOSTIC TESTS & INTERPRETATION
Initial Tests (lab, imaging)
Initial laboratory evaluation is done primarily to rule out potential medical factors that could be causing symptoms.
- Thyroid-stimulating hormone (hypothyroidism)
- CBC with differential (anemia, infection)
- Vitamin B_{12}, folic acid (deficiencies)
- Urinalysis (urinary tract infection, glucosuria)
- Comprehensive metabolic panel (uremia, hypo- or hyperglycemia, hypo- or hypernatremia, hypercalcemia, liver failure)
- Urine drug screen
- 24-hour urine free cortisol (Cushing disease)

Follow-Up Tests & Special Considerations
Additional testing for possible confounding medical and cognitive disorders, as warranted. May consider a sleep study for patients with decreased energy, sleep disturbances, changes in concentration or psychomotor activity.

Diagnostic Procedures/Other
Validated screening tools and rating scales:
- Geriatric Depression Scale: 15- or 30-point scales
- Patient Health Questionnaire (PHQ-2 or PHQ-9)
- Hamilton Depression Rating Scale
- Beck Depression Inventory
- Cornell Scale for Depression in Dementia (1)[A]

TREATMENT

Although response alone, usually interpreted as a 50% reduction in symptoms, can be clinically meaningful, the goal is to treat patients to the point of remission (i.e., essentially the absence of depressive symptoms).

GENERAL MEASURES
- Lifestyle modifications:
  - Increase physical activity
  - Improve nutrition
  - Encourage social interactions
  - Exercise: may be beneficial for depression in the elderly population (2)[A]
- Psychotherapy: Studies do show some benefit in depressed elderly patients (3)[B]:
  - Cognitive-behavioral therapy
  - Problem-solving therapy
  - Interpersonal therapy
  - Psychodynamic psychotherapy

MEDICATION
- Typically more conservative initial dosing and titration of antidepressants in the elderly, starting with 1/2 of the usual initiation dose and increasing within 2 to 4 weeks, as tolerated
- Continue titrating dose every 2 to 4 weeks, as appropriate to reach an adequate treatment dose.

First Line
- SSRIs have been found to be effective in treating depression in the elderly (4)[A].
- No single SSRI clearly outperforms others in the class; choice of medication often reflects side effect profile or practitioner familiarity (5)[A]:
  - Citalopram: Start at 10 mg/day. Treatment range 10 to 20 mg/day.
  - Sertraline: Start at 25 to 50 mg/day. Treatment range 50 to 200 mg/day.
  - Escitalopram: Start at 10 mg/day. Treatment range 10 to 20 mg/day.
  - Fluoxetine: Start at 10 mg/day. Treatment range 20 to 60 mg/day
  - Paroxetine: Start at 10 mg/day. Treatment range 20 to 40 mg/day.
- SSRIs should not be used concomitantly with monoamine oxidase inhibitors (MAOIs)
- Common side effects—increased risk of falls, nausea, diarrhea, sexual dysfunction

Second Line
- Atypical antidepressants: more effective than placebo in treatment of depression in the elderly, although additional studies are needed to better delineate patient factors that determine response:
  - Bupropion (sustained/twice a day and extended/once daily available): start at 150 mg/day. Increase dose in 3 to 4 days. Treatment range 300 to 450 mg/day. Avoid in patients with elevated seizure risk, tremors, or anxiety (5)[B].

– Venlafaxine (immediate- and extended-release available): start at 37.5 mg/day extended-release and titrate weekly. Treatment range 150 to 225 mg/day. May be associated with elevated BP at higher doses (5)[C].

– Duloxetine: start at 20 to 30 mg/day. Treatment range 60 to 120 mg/day. Also may be associated with elevated BP (5)[A].

– Mirtazapine: start at 7.5 to 15 mg nightly. Treatment range 30 to 45 mg/day; can produce problems with dry mouth, weight gain, sedation, and cognitive dysfunction (5)[B].

– Desvenlafaxine: 50 mg/day in AM; higher doses do not confer additional benefit; 50 mg every other day if CrCl <30 mL/min (6)[A].

ISSUES FOR REFERRAL
Depression with suicidal ideation, psychotic depression, bipolar disorder, comorbid substance abuse issues, polypharmacy, severe or refractory illness

ADDITIONAL THERAPIES
• For patients who have not responded to initial SSRI trial:

– Switch to a different SSRI medication, switch to an atypical antidepressant, or augment initial antidepressant with bupropion (7)[A]

• Second generation antipsychotic agents (5)[C]:
– Aripiprazole: 2 to 5 mg/day. Treatment range 5 to 15 mg/day; can produce sedation, weight gain, increased cholesterol levels
– Should only be used for augmentation in conjunction with other antidepressant medications
• Tricyclic antidepressants (TCAs):
– Nortriptyline: 25 to 50 mg nightly. Treatment range 75 to 150 mg nightly; can produce anticholinergic effects, weight gain, increase risk of falls (5)[C]

– TCAs have been shown to be effective in treating depression in the elderly. However, they are difficult for elderly patients to tolerate due to side effect profile and are potentially lethal in overdose, limiting their use as initial treatment agents (4)[A].

• MAOIs also appear more effective than placebo in the treatment of depression in the elderly. They are not used frequently in clinical practice due to potential side effects and necessary dietary restrictions (4)[A].

• Although not FDA approved—buspirone, lithium, or triiodothyronine are sometimes used off-label to augment a primary antidepressant (7)[B].

• Evidence for benefit of antidepressants in the treatment of depression in patients with dementia is equivocal. Consideration should be made for a limited trial with close monitoring for symptom improvement or side effects and used only in patients with severe symptoms (8)[A].

• Electroconvulsive therapy (ECT): has been shown to produce remission of depressive symptoms in the elderly. It should be considered as an initial option for patients with severe or psychotic depression (9)[B].

COMPLEMENTARY & ALTERNATIVE MEDICINE
• Acupuncture: equally beneficial as counseling (10)[B]
• St. John's wort may have minimal benefit and has numerous drug interactions (11)[A].

• Tryptophan and hydroxytryptophan: 150 to 300 mg/day; possible efficacy, additional investigation required (12)[B]

INPATIENT CONSIDERATIONS
Inpatient care is indicated in cases of imminent safety risk (e.g., acutely suicidal patients) or for those patients unable to care adequately for themselves due to depression.

 ONGOING CARE

FOLLOW-UP RECOMMENDATIONS
Due to the delay of benefit following initiation of antidepressant therapy, it is necessary to ensure open communication with the patient to prevent premature discontinuation of therapy. An adequate explanation of potential side effects with instructions to call the office before discontinuing therapy is imperative.

Patient Monitoring
• A patient with severe depression who exhibits suicidality may require admission to an appropriate facility.
• Monitor for worsening anxiety symptoms or increase in suicidality especially in the week following initiation of antidepressants.

DIET
No dietary restrictions are necessary, except for patients taking MAOIs, which necessitates dietary restriction of foods high in tyramine.

PATIENT EDUCATION
• Depression is a treatable illness.
• Medications may need to be taken for at least 2 to 4 weeks before any beneficial effect is noted and may take 6 to 8 weeks to reach maximum efficacy.
• Depression is often a recurring illness.
• National Suicide Prevention Lifeline at 1-800-273-TALK (8255) is a free, 24-hour hotline available to anyone in suicidal crisis or emotional distress. Calls will be routed to the nearest crisis center.

PROGNOSIS
• Treatment outcomes in the elderly may be worse than in the general population, possibly mediated by physical comorbidities and other factors.
• Depending on the population studied and specific clinical measures used, estimates vary for initial clinical response and remission (between 30% and 70%).

COMPLICATIONS
• Impairment in social, occupational, or interpersonal functioning
• Difficulty performing activities of daily living and self-care
• Increase in medical services utilization and increased costs of care
• Suicide

REFERENCES
1. Wongpakaran N, Wongpakaran T. Cornell scale for depression in dementia: study of residents in a northern thai long-term care home. *Psychiatry Investig.* 2013;10(4):359–364. doi:10.4306/pi.2013.10.4.359.
2. Blake H, Mo P, Malik S, et al. How effective are physical activity interventions for alleviating depressive symptoms in older people? A systematic review. *Clin Rehabil.* 2009;23(10):873–887.
3. Wilson KC, Mottram PG, Vassilas CA. Psychotherapeutic treatments for older depressed people. *Cochrane Database Syst Rev.* 2008;(1):CD004853.
4. Wilson K, Mottram P, Sivanranthan A, et al. Antidepressant versus placebo for depressed elderly. *Cochrane Database Syst Rev.* 2001;(2):CD000561.
5. Taylor WD. Clinical practice. Depression in the elderly. *N Engl J Med.* 2014;371(13):1229–1236.
6. Nelson JC, Delucchi K, Schneider LS. Efficacy of second generation antidepressants in late-life depression: a meta-analysis of the evidence. *Am J Geriatr Psychiatry.* 2008;16(7):558–567.
7. Ruhé HG, Huyser J, Swinkels JA, et al. Switching antidepressants after a first selective serotonin reuptake inhibitor in major depressive disorder: a systematic review. *J Clin Psychiatry.* 2006;67(12):1836–1855.
8. Nelson JC, Devanand DP. A systematic review and meta-analysis of placebo-controlled antidepressant studies in people with depression and dementia. *J Am Geriatr Soc.* 2011;59(4):577–585.
9. Van der Wurff FB, Stek ML, Hoogendijk WL, et al. Electroconvulsive therapy for the depressed elderly. *Cochrane Database Syst Rev.* 2003;(2):CD003593.
10. MacPherson H, Richmond S, Bland M, et al. Acupuncture and counselling for depression in primary care: a randomised controlled trial. *PLoS Med.* 2013;10(9):e1001518.
11. Linde K, Mulrow CD, Berner M, et al. St John's wort for depression. *Cochrane Database Syst Rev.* 2005;(2):CD000448.
12. Shaw K, Turner J, Del Mar C. Tryptophan and 5-hydroxytryptophan for depression. *Cochrane Database Syst Rev.* 2002;(1):CD003198.

 SEE ALSO

Algorithms: Depressed Mood Associated with Medical Illness; Depressive Episode, Major

 CODES

ICD10
• F32.9 Major depressive disorder, single episode, unspecified
• F03 Unspecified dementia
• F43.21 Adjustment disorder with depressed mood

CLINICAL PEARLS
• Depression is not a normal part of aging.
• Depression in the elderly may be difficult to diagnose precisely due to medical and cognitive comorbidities.
• Depression may present primarily with cognitive dysfunction and this may improve with treatment of the depression.
• A multidisciplinary approach to the treatment of depression is often the most efficacious.
• SSRIs are considered 1st-line therapy for safety and tolerability. A full remission may take upward of 12 weeks of treatment. Long-term treatment may be needed to prevent recurrence.

DEPRESSION, POSTPARTUM
Kathryn Myer, MD • Nancy Byatt, DO, MBA, FAPM

 BASICS

DESCRIPTION
- Major depressive disorder (MDD) that recurs or has its onset in the postpartum period
- May also occur in mothers adopting a baby or in fathers
- Postpartum depression (PPD) is similar to non-pregnancy depression (sleep disorders, anhedonia, psychomotor changes, etc.); it most often has its onset within the first 12 weeks postpartum yet can occur within 1 year after delivery.
- Different than postpartum "blues" (sadness and emotional lability), which is experienced by 30–70% of women and has an onset and resolution within first 10 days postpartum.

EPIDEMIOLOGY
Incidence
14.5% of women have a new episode of major or minor depression during postpartum period (1).

Prevalence
- More than 50% of women with postpartum depression enter pregnancy depressed or have an onset during pregnancy (2).
- As many as 19.2% women suffer from depression within 3 months in the postpartum period (3).

ETIOLOGY AND PATHOPHYSIOLOGY
- May be related to sensitivity in hormonal fluctuations, including estrogen; progesterone; and other gonadal hormones as well as neuroactive steroids; cytokines; hypothalamic–pituitary–adrenal (HPA) axis hormones; altered fatty acid, oxytocin, and arginine vasopressin levels; and genetic and epigenetic factors
- Multifactorial including biologic–genetic predisposition in terms of neurobiologic deficit, destabilizing effects of hormone withdrawal at birth, inflammation, and psychosocial stressors

RISK FACTORS
- Previous episodes of PPD
- History of MDD
- MDD during pregnancy
- Anxiety during pregnancy
- History of premenstrual dysphoria
- Family history of depression
- Unwanted pregnancy
- Socioeconomic stress
- Low self-esteem
- Young maternal age
- Alcohol abuse
- Marital conflict
- Multiple births
- African Americans and Hispanics may have higher rates of PPD.
- Preterm and low birth weight baby
- Postpartum pain, sleep disturbance, and fatigue
- Recent immigrant status
- Increased stressful life events
- History of childhood sexual abuse
- Decision to decrease antidepressants during pregnancy
- Intimate partner violence (4)

GENERAL PREVENTION
- Universal screening during pregnancy to allow for detection and treatment
- Screen using Edinburgh Postnatal Depression Scale during pregnancy and the postpartum year: http://www.testandcalc.com/etc/tests/edin.asp
- Postnatal visits, psychotherapy, and/or psychoeducation for high-risk women
- For women with depression during pregnancy, psychotherapy or treatment with antidepressants during pregnancy may prevent PPD.
- Depression care manager who provides education, routine telephone contact, and follow-up to engage women in treatment

COMMONLY ASSOCIATED CONDITIONS
- Bipolar mood disorder
- Depressive disorder not otherwise specified
- Dysthymic disorder
- Cyclothymic disorder
- MDD

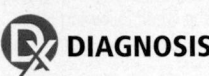 **DIAGNOSIS**

HISTORY
- Increased/decreased sleep
- Decreased interest in formerly compelling or pleasurable activities
- Guilt, low self-esteem
- Decreased energy
- Decreased concentration
- Increased/decreased appetite
- Psychomotor agitation or retardation
- Suicidal ideation

DIFFERENTIAL DIAGNOSIS
- Baby blues: not a psychiatric disorder; mood lability resolves within days
- Postpartum psychosis: a psychiatric emergency
- Postpartum anxiety/panic disorder
- Postpartum obsessive-compulsive disorder
- Hypothyroidism
- Postpartum thyroiditis: can occur in up to 5.7% of patients in the United States and can present as depression (5)

DIAGNOSTIC TESTS & INTERPRETATION
Initial Tests (lab, imaging)
Thyroid-stimulating hormone (TSH), B_{12}, folate and Vitamin D

Diagnostic Procedures/Other
- Edinburgh Postnatal Depression Scale is a validated screening tool.
- The Patient Health Questionnare-9 (PHQ-9) is a validated commonly used screening tool.
- Edinburgh Postnatal Depression Scale (Partner Version): to be completed by mother's partner to obtain his or her view of mother's depression

 TREATMENT

GENERAL MEASURES
- Outpatient individual psychotherapy in combination with pharmacotherapy
- Interpersonal psychotherapy and cognitive behavioral therapy

- Strongly consider pharmacotherapy when symptoms are moderate or severe.
- Assess suicidal ideation.
- Assess homicidal ideation and thoughts of harming the baby.
- Thoughts of harming the baby require immediate hospitalization.
- Visiting nurse services can provide direct observations of the mother regarding safety concerns and mother–child bonding.

MEDICATION
First Line
- For nonbreastfeeding women, selection of antidepressants is similar to nonpostpartum patients.
- Selective serotonin reuptake inhibitors (SSRIs) are generally effective and safe:
  – Fluoxetine (Prozac): 20 to 80 mg/day PO (most activating of all SSRIs)
  – Sertraline (Zoloft): 50 to 200 mg/day PO (mildly sedating)
  – Paroxetine (Paxil): 20 to 60 mg/day PO (sedating)
  – Citalopram (Celexa): 20 to 40 mg/day PO (FDA recommendation)
  – Escitalopram (Lexapro): 10 to 20 mg/day PO
- Tricyclic antidepressants (TCAs) are effective and less expensive yet also are lethal in overdose and have unfavorable side effects:
  – Avoid TCAs in mothers with a history of suicidal ideation.
- Bupropion (Wellbutrin): 150 to 450 mg/day PO in patients with depression plus psychomotor retardation and hypersomnia and with weight gain. Bupropion is less likely to cause weight gain or sexual dysfunction and is highly activating.
- Mirtazapine (Remeron): 15 to 45 mg/day PO at bedtime; may assist with sleep restoration and weight gain; no sexual dysfunction
- Serotonin–norepinephrine reuptake inhibitors (SNRIs)
  – Venlafaxine (Effexor XR): a dual-action antidepressant that blocks the reuptake of serotonin in doses of up to 150 mg/day and then blocks the reuptake of norepinephrine in doses of 150 to 450 mg/day PO
  – Duloxetine (Cymbalta): more balanced serotonin/norepinephrine reuptake throughout dosing; 40 to 60 mg/day PO (doses >60 mg have not been demonstrated to be more effective)
  – Desvenlafaxine (Pristiq): 50 mg/day PO
- Bipolar disorder requires treatment with mood stabilizer.
- Among breastfeeding mothers
  – Breastfeeding should generally not preclude treatment with antidepressants.
  – SSRIs and some other antidepressants are considered a reasonable option during breastfeeding.
  – All antidepressants are excreted in breast milk but are generally compatible with lactation.
  – Paroxetine and sertraline have lower translactal passage.
  – SSRIs and nortriptyline have a better safety profile.
  – Translactal passage is greater with fluoxetine and citalopram (4)[B].
  – Start with low doses and increase slowly. Monitor infant for adverse side effects.
  – Continuing an efficacious medication is preferred over switching antidepressants to avoid exposing the mother and infant to the risks of untreated PPD (4)[B].

– Breastfeeding women need additional education and support regarding the risks and benefits of use of antidepressants during breastfeeding.
– Consider negative effects of untreated PPD on infant and child development.

– Discussions of the treatment options with the patient and her partner when possible. Take into account the patient's personal psychiatric history and previous response to treatment, the risks of no treatment or undertreatment, available data about the safety of medications during breastfeeding, and her individual expectations and treatment preferences (6)[B].

– For further information: http://toxnet.nlm.nih.gov/

Second Line
Consider switching to a different antidepressant or augmentation if patient has a lack of response. Electroconvulsive therapy (ECT) is an option for depressed postpartum women who do not respond to antidepressant medications, have severe or psychotic symptoms, cannot tolerate antidepressant medications, are actively engaged in suicidal self-destructive behaviors, or have a previous history of response to ECT (7)[B].

ISSUES FOR REFERRAL
• Obtain psychiatric consultation for patients with psychotic symptoms.
• Strongly consider immediate hospitalization if delusions or hallucinations are present.
• Hospitalization is indicated if mother's ability to care for self and/or infant is significantly compromised.

ADDITIONAL THERAPIES
• Psychoeducation, including providing reading material for the patient and family
• Psychotherapy: Interpersonal psychotherapy, cognitive behavioral therapy, and psychodynamic psychotherapy have shown to be effective (5)[B].

COMPLEMENTARY & ALTERNATIVE MEDICINE
• Breastfeeding has been associated with reduced stress and improved maternal mood.
• Infant massage, infant sleep intervention, exercise, and bright light therapy may be beneficial (7)[B].

INPATIENT CONSIDERATIONS

ALERT
Obtain psychiatric consultation for patients with psychotic symptoms. If delusions or hallucinations are present, strongly consider immediate hospitalization. The psychotic mother should *not* be left alone with the baby.

Admission Criteria/Initial Stabilization
Presence of suicidal or homicidal ideation and/or psychotic symptoms and/or thoughts of harming baby and/or inability to care for self or infant, severe weight loss

Discharge Criteria
• Absence of suicidal or homicidal ideation and/or psychotic symptoms and/or thoughts of harming the baby
• Mother must be able to care for self and infant.

 ONGOING CARE

FOLLOW-UP RECOMMENDATIONS
Patient Monitoring
• Collaborative care approach, including primary care visits and case manager follow-ups
• Consultation with the infant's doctor, particularly if the mother is breastfeeding while taking psychotropic medications

DIET
• Good nutrition and hydration, especially when breastfeeding
• Mixed evidence to support the addition of multivitamin with minerals and omega-3 fatty acids

PATIENT EDUCATION
• *This Isn't What I Expected: Overcoming Postpartum Depression*, by Karen R. Kleinman and Valerie Davis Raskin
• *Down Came the Rain: My Journey Through Postpartum Depression*, by Brooke Shields, 2005
• *Behind the Smile: My Journey Out of Postpartum Depression*, by Marie Osmond, Marcia Wilkie, and Judith Moore, 2001
• Web resources
– Postpartum Support International: http://www.postpartum.net/
– La Leche League: http://www.llli.org/
– http://toxnet.nlm.nih.gov/
– http://www.mededppd.org/
– http://www.womensmentalhealth.org/
– http://www.motherrisk.org/
– http://www.step-ppd.com/

PROGNOSIS
• Treatment of maternal depression to remission has been shown to have a positive impact on children's mental health.
• Some patients, particularly those with undertreated or undiagnosed depression, may develop chronic depression requiring long-term treatment.
• Untreated maternal depression is linked to impaired mother–infant bonding and cognitive and language development delay in infants and children (8).
• Postpartum psychosis is associated with tragic outcomes such as maternal suicide and infanticide.

COMPLICATIONS
• Suicide
• Self-injurious behavior
• Psychosis
• Neglect of baby
• Harm to the baby

REFERENCES
1. Stuart-Parrigon K, Stuart S. Perinatal depression: an update and overview. *Curr Psychiatry Rep.* 2014;16(9):468.
2. Wisner KL, Sit DK, McShea MC, et al. Onset timing, thoughts of self-harm, and diagnoses in postpartum women with screen-positive depression findings. *JAMA Psychiatry.* 2013;70(5):490–498.
3. Bobo WV, Yawn PB. Concise review for physicians and other clinicians: postpartum depression. *Mayo Clin Proc.* 2014;89(6):835–844.
4. Gavin NI, Gaynes BN, Lohr KN, et al. Perinatal depression: a systematic review of prevalence and incidence. *Obstet Gynecol.* 2005;106(5 Pt 1): 1071–1083.
5. Cerulli C, Talbot NL, Tang W, et al. Co-occurring intimate partner violence and mental health

diagnoses in perinatal women. *J Womens Health (Larchmt).* 2011;20(12):1797–1803.
6. Nicholson WK, Robinson KA, Smallridge RC, et al. Prevalence of postpartum thyroid dysfunction: a quantitative review. *Thyroid.* 2006;16(6):573–582.
7. Pearlstein T, Howard M, Salisbury A, et al. Postpartum depression. *Am J Obstet Gynecol.* 2009;200(4):357–364.
8. Fitelson E, Kim S, Baker AS, et al. Treatment of postpartum depression: clinical, psychological and pharmacological options. *Int J Womens Health.* 2010;3:1–14.

ADDITIONAL READING
• Edinburgh Postnatal Depression Scale. http://www.fresno.ucsf.edu/pediatrics/downloads/edinburghscale.pdf.
• Gjerdingen D, Katon W, Rich DE. Stepped care treatment of postpartum depression: a primary care-based management model. *Womens Health Issues.* 2008;18(1):44–52.
• Harrington AR, Greene-Harrington CC. Healthy Start screens for depression among urban pregnant, postpartum and interconceptional women. *J Natl Med Assoc.* 2007;99(3):226–231.
• Hirst KP, Moutier CY. Postpartum major depression. *Am Fam Physician.* 2010;82(8):926–933.
• Howard LM, Boath E, Henshaw C. Antidepressant prevention of postnatal depression. *PLoS Med.* 2006;3(10):e389.
• Kendall-Tackett K. A new paradigm for depression in new mothers: the central role of inflammation and how breastfeeding and anti-inflammatory treatments protect maternal mental health. *Int Breastfeed J.* 2007;2:6.
• Musters C, McDonald E, Jones I. Management of postnatal depression. *BMJ.* 2008;337:a736.
• Ng RC, Hirata CK, Yeung W, et al. Pharmacologic treatment for postpartum depression: a systematic review. *Pharmacotherapy.* 2010;30(9):928–941.
• Sit DK, Wisner KL. Identification of postpartum depression. *Clin Obstet Gynecol.* 2009;52(3):456–468.
• Tammentie T, Tarkka MT, Astedt-Kurki P, et al. Family dynamics and postnatal depression. *J Psychiatr Ment Health Nurs.* 2004;11(2):141–149.

 CODES

ICD10
• F53 Puerperal psychosis
• O90.6 Postpartum mood disturbance

CLINICAL PEARLS
• PPD is a common, debilitating medical condition that impairs a mother's ability to function and interact with her infant and family.
• Universal screening for depression is recommended during the 1st and 3rd trimester and at regular intervals during the postpartum period.
• Early diagnosis and treatment are vital, as untreated PPD can lead to developmental difficulties for the infant and prolonged disability and suffering for the mother.
• Breastfeeding is recommended for maternal and child health. Several medication options for treating depression in mothers are safe for breastfeeding infants.
• Treatment with antidepressants should be individualized for breastfeeding mothers (4)[B].

DEPRESSION, TREATMENT RESISTANT

Michelle Magid, MD • Roger L. McRoberts, III, MD

 BASICS

DESCRIPTION
- Major depressive disorder (MDD) that has failed to respond to ≥2 adequate trials of antidepressant therapy in ≥2 different classes (1).
- Antidepressant therapy must be given for 6 weeks at standard doses before being considered a failure.

EPIDEMIOLOGY
- Depression affects >18 million people in the United States and >340 million people worldwide.
- 16% lifetime risk of MDD (2,3)
- Approximately 1/3 of patients with MDD will develop treatment-resistant depression (3,4).

ETIOLOGY AND PATHOPHYSIOLOGY
- Unclear. Low levels of neurotransmitters (serotonin, norepinephrine, dopamine) have been indicated.
- Serotonin has been linked to irritability, hostility, and suicidal ideation.
- Norepinephrine has been linked to low energy.
- Dopamine may play a role in low motivation and depression with psychotic features.
- Environmental stressors such as abuse and neglect may affect neurotransmission.
- Inflammation and oxidative stress in the brain can contribute to treatment-resistant depression (5).

Genetics
A genetic abnormality in the serotonin transporter gene (5-HTTLPR) may increase risk for treatment-resistant depression.

RISK FACTORS
- Severity of disease
- Mislabeling patients with depression who are bipolar
- Comorbid medical disease (including chronic pain)
- Comorbid personality disorder
- Comorbid anxiety disorder
- Comorbid substance abuse
- Familial predisposition to poor response to antidepressants

GENERAL PREVENTION
- Medication adherence in combination with psychotherapy
- Maintenance electroconvulsive therapy (ECT) may prevent relapse.

COMMONLY ASSOCIATED CONDITIONS
- Suicide
- Bipolar disorder
- Substance use disorders
- Anxiety disorders
- Dysthymia
- Eating disorders
- Somatic symptom disorders

 DIAGNOSIS

HISTORY
- Symptoms are the same as in MDD. However, patients do not respond to standard form of treatment. Severity and duration are extreme.
- Especially important to screen for suicidality in treatment-resistant depression
- Screening with SIGECAPS
  - Sleep: too much or too little
  - Interest: failure to enjoy activities
  - Guilt: excessive and uncontrollable
  - Energy: poor energy
  - Concentration: inability to focus on tasks
  - Appetite: too much or too little
  - Psychomotor changes: restlessness/agitation or slowing/lethargy
  - Suicidality: desire to end life

PHYSICAL EXAM
Mental status exam may reveal poor hygiene, poor eye contact, blunted affect, tearfulness, weight loss or gain, psychomotor retardation, or agitation.

DIFFERENTIAL DIAGNOSIS
- Bipolar disorder
- Dysthymia
- Dementia
- Early-stage Parkinson disease
- Personality disorder
- Medical illness such as malignancy, thyroid disease, HIV
- Substance use disorders

DIAGNOSTIC TESTS & INTERPRETATION
Initial Tests (lab, imaging)
- Used to rule out medical factors that could be causing/contributing to treatment resistance
  - CBC
  - Complete metabolic profile, including liver tests, calcium, and glucose
  - Urine drug screen
  - Thyroid-stimulating hormone (TSH)
  - Vitamin D level (25-OH vitamin D)
  - Testosterone, if applicable
- CT or MRI of the brain if neurologic disease, tumor, or dementia is suspected.

Follow-Up Tests & Special Considerations
Delirium and dementia may often look like depression.

Diagnostic Procedures/Other
- Depression is a clinical diagnosis.
- Validated depression rating scales to assist
  - Beck Depression Inventory
  - Hamilton Rating Scale for Depression
  - Patient Health Questionnaire 9 (PHQ-9)

 TREATMENT

MEDICATION
First Line
- Please see "Depression" topic. When those fail, augmentation and combination strategies are as follows:
  - Antidepressants in combination
    - Citalopram (Start 20 mg/day. Max dose 40 mg/day) + bupropion (start 100 mg BID; max dose 450 mg total) (4,6)[B]
    - Tricyclic antidepressants (TCAs) and selective serotonin reuptake inhibitors (SSRIs) may be used in combination. Proceed with caution due to risk of serotonin syndrome. Citalopram (start 20 mg/day; max dose 40 mg/day) + nortriptyline (start 50 mg at bedtime; max dose 150 mg at bedtime)
  - Antidepressants + antipsychotics
    - Citalopram (start 20 mg/day; max dose 40 mg/day) + aripiprazole (2 to 5 mg/day, different mechanism of action at higher doses) OR + risperidone (start 0.5 to 1 mg at bedtime; max dose 6 mg/day) OR + quetiapine (start 25 mg at bedtime; titrate to 100 to 300 mg at bedtime. Max dose 600 mg/day) (7,8)[A]
  - Antidepressant + lithium
    - TCA: nortriptyline (start 50 mg at bedtime; max dose 150 mg at bedtime) + lithium (start 300 mg at bedtime; max dose 900 mg BID) (1,7,9)[A]
    - SSRI: citalopram (start 20 mg/day; max dose 40 mg QD) + lithium (start 300 mg at bedtime; max dose 900 mg BID) (1,4,7)[B]
  - Antidepressant + thyroid supplementation
    - Citalopram (start 20 mg/day; max dose 40 mg/day) + triiodothyronine (T3) (12.5 to 50 μg/day) (4,10)[B]
- In all above combinations, citalopram (Celexa) can be replaced with other SSRIs such as fluoxetine (Prozac) 20 to 80 mg/day, sertraline (Zoloft) 50 to 200 mg/day, and escitalopram (Lexapro) 10 to 20 mg/day or with serotonin–norepinephrine reuptake inhibitors (SNRIs) duloxetine (Cymbalta) 30 to 120 mg/day, venlafaxine XR (Effexor XR) 75 to 225 mg/day, or desvenlafaxine (Pristiq) 50 to 100 mg/day.
- Maximum doses for medication in treatment-resistant cases may be higher than in treatment-responsive cases.

Second Line
Monamine oxidase inhibitor (MAOI)
- Tranylcypromine (Parnate): start 10 mg BID, increase 10 mg/day every 1 to 3 weeks; max dose 60 mg/day
- Selegiline transdermal (Emsam patch): Apply 6-mg patch daily, increase 3 mg/day; max dose 12 mg/day

- Side-effect profile (e.g., hypertensive crisis), drug–drug interactions, and dietary restrictions make MAOIs less appealing. Patch version does not require dietary restrictions at lower doses.
- High risk of serotonin syndrome, if combined with another antidepressant; 2-week washout period is advised.

ISSUES FOR REFERRAL
Treatment-resistant depression should be managed in consultation with a psychiatrist.

ADDITIONAL THERAPIES
- First line
  - ECT: safe and effective treatment for treatment-resistant and life-threatening depression, with a 60–90% success rate (11,12)[A]:
    - Known to rapidly relieve suicidality, psychotic depression, and catatonia
    - Controversy due to cognitive side effects during the treatment
    - 3 types of lead placements
      - Bitemporal: rapid and effective. Usually need 6 to 10 treatments at 1.5× seizure threshold
      - Right unilateral: may be slightly less rapid but fewer cognitive side effects. Usually need 8 to 12 treatments at 6× seizure threshold
      - Bifrontal: newer technique that may offer similar speed to bitemporal, with slightly improved side-effect profile
- Second line
  - Deep brain stimulation (DBS): Surgical implantation of intracranial electrodes, connected to an impulse generator implanted in the chest wall (13,14)[C]:
    - Reserved for those who have failed medications, psychotherapy, and ECT
    - Preliminary data are promising, showing 40–70% response rate and 35% remission rate, but further trials are warranted.
  - Transcranial magnetic stimulation (TCMS): Noninvasive brain stimulation technique that is generally safe. A few case reports on efficacy in treatment-resistant depression but thus far is only FDA approved for less severe forms of the illness (9,14)[C].
  - Vagus nerve stimulation (VNS): Surgical implantation of electrodes onto left vagus nerve. Its use in treatment-resistant depression has become limited in recent years (13)[C].
  - Ketamine—not FDA approved, but evidence of rapid improvement in mood and suicidal thinking, although the literature is limited. In addition, the effects of ketamine appear temporary, disappearing after days to weeks (9,15)[C].

INPATIENT CONSIDERATIONS
Admission Criteria/Initial Stabilization
Inpatient care is indicated for severely depressed, psychotic, catatonic, or suicidal patients.

Discharge Criteria
Symptoms improving, no longer suicidal, psychosocial stressors addressed

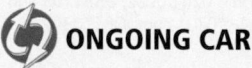# ONGOING CARE

FOLLOW-UP RECOMMENDATIONS
- Frequent visits (i.e., every month)
- During follow-up, evaluate side effects, dosage, and effectiveness of medication as well as need for referral to ECT.
- Patients who have responded to ECT may need maintenance treatments (q3–12wk) to prevent relapse.
- Combination of lithium/nortriptyline after ECT appears to be as effective as maintenance ECT in reducing relapse.

DIET
Patients on MAOIs need dietary restriction.

PATIENT EDUCATION
Educate patients that depression is a medical illness, not a character defect.
- Review signs and symptoms of worsening depression and when patient needs to come in for further evaluation.
- Discuss safety plan to address suicidal thoughts.

PROGNOSIS
With medication adherence, close follow-up, improved social support, and psychotherapy, prognosis improves.

COMPLICATIONS
- Suicide
- Disability
- Poor quality of life

REFERENCES
1. Keller MB. Issues in treatment-resistant depression. *J Clin Psychiatry*. 2005;66(Suppl 8):5–12.
2. Kessler RC, Berglund P, Demler O, et al. The epidemiology of major depressive disorder: results from the National Comorbidity Survey Replication (NCS-R). *JAMA*. 2003;289(23):3095–3105.
3. Olchanski N, McInnis Myers M, Halseth M, et al. The economic burden of treatment-resistant depression. *Clin Ther*. 2013;35(4):512–522.
4. Rush AJ, Trivedi MH, Wisniewski SR, et al. Acute and longer-term outcomes in depressed outpatients requiring one or several treatment steps: a STAR*D report. *Am J Psychiatry*. 2006;163(11):1905–1917.
5. Bakunina N, Pariante CM, Zunszain PA. Immune mechanisms linked to depression via oxidative stress and neuroprogression [published online ahead of print January 10, 2015]. *Immunology*. 2015;144;365–373. doi: 10.1111/imm.12443.
6. Trivedi MH, Fava M, Wisniewski SR, et al. Medication augmentation after the failure of SSRIs for depression. *N Engl J Med*. 2006;354(12):1243–1252.
7. Hicks P, Hicks XP, Meyer H, et al. How best to manage treatment-resistant depression? *J Fam Pract*. 2010;59(9):490–497.
8. Maglione M, Maher AR, Hu JH, et al. *Off-Label Use of Atypical Antipsychotics: An Update*. Rockville, MD: Agency for Healthcare Research and Quality; 2011. Report No. 11-EHC087-EF. AHRQ Comparative Effectiveness Reviews.
9. Holtzheimer PE. Advances in the management of treatment-resistant depression. *Focus (Am Psychiatr Publ)*. 2010;8(4):488–500.
10. Nierenberg AA, Fava M, Trivedi MH, et al. A comparison of lithium and T(3) augmentation following two failed medication treatments for depression: a STAR*D report. *Am J Psychiatry*. 2006;163(9):1519–1530.
11. American Psychiatric Association. Practice guideline for the treatment of patients with major depressive disorder, third edition. *Am J Psychiatry*. 2010;167(10):1–118. http://psychiatryonline.org/data/Books/prac/PG_Depression3rdEd.pdf
12. Weiner RD. *The Practice of Electroconvulsive Therapy: Recommendations for Treatment, Training, and Privileging: A Task Force Report of the American Psychiatric Association*. 2nd ed. Washington, DC: American Psychiatric Association; 2001:5–25.
13. Morishita T, Fayad SM, Higuchi MA, et al. Deep brain stimulation for treatment-resistant depression: systematic review of clinical outcomes. *Neurotherapeutics*. 2014;11(3):475–484.
14. Holtzheimer PE III, Mayberg HS. Deep brain stimulation for treatment-resistant depression. *Am J Psychiatry*. 2010;167(12):1437–1444.
15. Caddy C, Giaroli G, White TP, et al. Ketamine as the prototype glutamatergic antidepressant: pharmacodynamic actions, and a systematic review and meta-analysis of efficacy. *Ther Adv Psychopharmacol*. 2014;4(2):75–99.

CODES

ICD10
- F32.9 Major depressive disorder, single episode, unspecified
- F33.9 Major depressive disorder, recurrent, unspecified

CLINICAL PEARLS
- Treatment-resistant depression is common, affecting 1/3 of those with MDD.
- Combination and augmentation strategies with antidepressants, antipsychotics, and mood stabilizers can be helpful.
- ECT should be considered in severe and life-threatening cases.

DERMATITIS HERPETIFORMIS

Geoffrey Strider Farnsworth, MD

 BASICS

DESCRIPTION
- Dermatitis herpetiformis (DH) presents as a chronic, relapsing, polymorphous, intensely pruritic, erythematous papulovesicular eruption with symmetrical distribution primarily involving extensor skin surfaces of the elbows, knees, buttocks, back, and scalp.
- DH is an autoimmune disease associated with gluten sensitivity with genetic, environmental, and immunologic influences.
- DH is distinguished from other bullous diseases by characteristic histologic and immunologic findings, as well as associated gluten-sensitive enteropathy (GSE).
- System(s) affected: skin
- Synonym(s): Duhring disease, Duhring-Brocq disease

EPIDEMIOLOGY
- Occurs most frequently in those of Northern European origin
- Rare in persons of Asian or African American origin
- Predominant age: most common in 4th and 5th decades but may present at any age
- Childhood DH is rare in most countries, although an Italian study showed 27% of patients were younger than the age of 10 and 36% younger than the age of 20.
- Predominant gender: Adults: male > female (1.5:1 in the United States, 2:1 worldwide) Children: female > male

Incidence
1/100,000 persons per year in the United States

Prevalence
11/100,000 persons in the U.S. population; as high as 39/100,000 persons worldwide

ETIOLOGY AND PATHOPHYSIOLOGY
- Evidence suggests that epidermal transglutaminase (eTG) 3, a keratinocyte enzyme involved in cell envelope formation and maintenance, is the autoantigen in DH.
- eTG is highly homologous with tissue transglutaminase (tTG), which is the antigenic target in celiac disease and GSE.
- The initiating event for DH is presumed to be the interaction of wheat peptides with tTGs, which results in the formation of an autoantigen with high affinity for particular class II major histocompatibility complex (MHC) molecules.
- Presentation of the autoantigen leads to activation of T cells and the humoral immune system.
- IgA antibodies against tTG cross-react with eTG and result in IgA-eTG immune complexes that are deposited in the papillary dermis. Subsequent activation of complement and recruitment of neutrophils to the area result in inflammation and microabscesses.
- Skin eruption may be delayed up to 5 to 6 weeks after exposure to gluten.
- Gluten applied directly to the skin does not result in the eruption, whereas gluten taken by mouth or rectum does. This implies necessary processing by the GI system.
- Thought to be immune complex–mediated disease

Genetics
- High association with human leukocyte antigen DQ2 (95%), with remaining patients being positive for DQ8, DR4, or DR3
- Strong association with combination of alleles DQA1*0501 and DQB1*0201/0202, DRB1*03 and DRB1*05/07, *or* DQA1*0301 and DQB1*0302

RISK FACTORS
- GSE: >90% of those with DH will have GSE, which may be asymptomatic.
- Family history of DH or celiac disease

GENERAL PREVENTION
Gluten-free diet (GFD) results in improvement of DH and reduces dependence on medical therapy. GFD also may reduce the risk of lymphomas associated with DH.

COMMONLY ASSOCIATED CONDITIONS
- Hypothyroidism is the most common autoimmune condition associated with DH.
- GSE, gluten ataxia
- Gastric atrophy, hypochlorhydria, pernicious anemia
- GI lymphoma, non-Hodgkin lymphoma
- Hyperthyroidism, thyroid nodules, thyroid cancer
- IgA nephropathy
- Autoimmune disorders, including systemic lupus erythematosus, dermatomyositis, Sjögren syndrome, rheumatoid arthritis, sarcoidosis, Raynaud phenomenon, insulin-dependent diabetes mellitus, myasthenia gravis, Addison disease, vitiligo, alopecia areata, primary biliary cirrhosis, and psoriasis

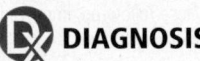 **DIAGNOSIS**

Diagnosis of DH involves a clinicopathologic correlation among clinical presentation, histologic and direct immunofluorescence evaluation, serology, and response to therapy or dietary restriction.

HISTORY
- Waxing and waning, intensely pruritic eruption with papules and tiny vesicles
- Eruption may worsen with gluten intake.
- GI symptoms may be absent or may not be reported until prompted.

PHYSICAL EXAM
- Classic lesions described as symmetric, grouped, erythematous papules and vesicles
- More commonly presents with erosions, excoriations, lichenification, hypopigmentation, and/or hyperpigmentation secondary to scratching and healing of old lesions
- Areas involved include extensor surfaces of elbows (90%), knees (30%), shoulders, buttocks, and sacrum. The scalp is also frequently affected. Oral lesions are rare.
- In children, purpura may be visible on digits and palmoplantar surfaces.
- Adults with associated enteropathy are most often asymptomatic, with about 20% experiencing steatorrhea and <10% with findings of bloating, diarrhea, or malabsorption.
- Children with associated enteropathy may present with abdominal pain, diarrhea, iron deficiency, and reduced growth rate.

DIFFERENTIAL DIAGNOSIS
- In adults
  - Bullous pemphigoid: linear deposition of C3 and IgG at the basement membrane zone
  - Linear IgA disease: homogeneous and linear deposition of IgA at the basement membrane zone, absence of GSE
  - Prurigo nodularis
  - Urticaria: wheals, angioedema, dermal edema
  - Erythema multiforme
- In children
  - Atopic dermatitis: face and flexural areas
  - Scabies: interdigital areas, axillae, genital region
  - Papular urticaria: dermal edema
  - Impetigo

DIAGNOSTIC TESTS & INTERPRETATION
Initial Tests (lab, imaging)
- Serum IgA tTG antibodies: Detection of tTG antibodies was noted to be up to 95% sensitive and >90% specific for DH in patients on unrestricted diets (1,2)[A].
- Serum IgA eTG antibodies: Antibodies to eTG, the primary autoantigen in DH, were shown to be more sensitive than antibodies to tTG in the diagnosis of patients with DH on unrestricted diets (95% vs. 79%) but is not widely available in all labs (1,2)[A].
- Serum IgA endomysial antibodies: have a sensitivity between 50% and 100% and a specificity close to 100% in patients on unrestricted diets but is more expensive, time-consuming, and operator-dependent than tTG (2)

Follow-Up Tests & Special Considerations
Serologic assessment of anti-tTG and anti-eTG correlate with intestinal involvement of disease and in conjunction with antiendomysial antibodies (EMA) may be useful in monitoring major deviations from GFD (1,2).

Diagnostic Procedures/Other
The "gold standard" for diagnosing DH is a skin biopsy of perilesional skin evaluated via direct immunofluorescence, which demonstrates granular IgA deposited in dermal papillae and/or basement membrane (1,2)[A],(3)[C].

Test Interpretation
- Direct immunofluorescence of perilesional skin reveals a granular pattern of IgA deposition in the dermal papillae (1,2).
- Histopathology of lesion with routine staining reveals neutrophilic microabscesses in the tips of the dermal papillae and may show subepidermal blistering (1,2).

 TREATMENT

GENERAL MEASURES
- GFD is the mainstay of treatment and can lead to complete resolution of symptoms (1,2)[A].
- Typically requires 18 to 24 months of strict adherence to GFD prior to resolution of skin lesions without other treatment.
- Lesions can recur within 12 weeks of reintroduction of gluten.

MEDICATION
Medication is useful for immediate symptom management but should be used as an adjunct to dietary modification (2).

First Line
- Dapsone is approved by the FDA for use in DH and is the most widely used medication (2,4)[A]. Initial dosing of 50 mg/day typically results in improvement of symptoms within 24 to 48 hours; can increase dose to 200 mg to obtain control (1)[C]. Use minimum effective dose with slow titration based on patient response and tolerability. Average maintenance dose is 1 mg/kg/day (50 to 150 mg/day). Minor outbreaks on the face and scalp are common even with treatment. Not ideal for long-term use in DH.

- Dapsone works by inhibiting neutrophil recruitment and IL-8 release, inhibiting the respiratory burst of neutrophils, and protecting cells from neutrophil-mediated injury, thereby suppressing the skin reaction. It has no role in preventing IgA deposition or mitigating the immune reaction in the gut (2,4).
- Precautions
  – Common side effects include nausea, vomiting, headache, dizziness, weakness, and hemolysis.
  – A drop in hemoglobin of 1 to 2 g is characteristic with dapsone 100 mg/day.
  – G6PD deficiency increases severity of hemolytic stress. Dapsone should be avoided, if possible, in those who are G6PD-deficient.
  – Dose-related methemoglobinemia may occur with doses >100 mg/day. Cimetidine may reduce the severity of this side effect.
  – Risk of distal motor neuropathy

ALERT
- Monitor for potentially fatal dapsone-induced sulfone syndrome: fever, jaundice and hepatic necrosis, exfoliative dermatitis, lymphadenopathy, methemoglobinemia, and hemolytic anemia.
- Can occur 48 hours or 6 months after treatment, most often 5 weeks after initiation

Pediatric Considerations
- <2 years: Dosing is not established.
- >2 years: 0.5 to 1.0 mg/kg/day

Pregnancy Considerations
- Category C: Safety during pregnancy is not established.
- Secreted in breast milk and will produce hemolytic anemia in infants
- Adherence to a strict GFD 6 to 12 months before conception should be considered with the hope of eliminating need for dapsone during pregnancy.

Second Line
- High-potency topical steroids can be used acutely to control symptoms until dapsone becomes effective (1)[C].
- Sulfapyridine (1 to 2 g/day) is FDA approved for use in DH and is thought to be the active metabolite in sulfasalazine (2 to 4 g/day) (2,5)[B]. Common side effects include nausea, vomiting, and anorexia. Enteric-coated form may reduce side effects. Other side effects include agranulocytosis, hypersensitivity reactions, hemolytic anemia, proteinuria, and crystalluria (2,5).

ISSUES FOR REFERRAL
Over time, interdisciplinary treatment may involve a dermatologist, gastroenterologist, and registered dietician. Genetic counseling and testing should be considered on diagnosis (1,2).

ADDITIONAL THERAPIES
A single case report describes topical dapsone therapy as potential alternative treatment or as an adjunct to oral dapsone to decrease systemic exposure and risk of severe side effects. However, it has not been studied extensively (6)[C].

ONGOING CARE

FOLLOW-UP RECOMMENDATIONS
Patient Monitoring
- Every 6 to 12 months by physician and dietician to evaluate GFD adherence and recurrence of symptoms
- Adherence to GFD can be monitored with serologic levels of anti-tTG, anti eTG, and EMA levels (1).

- Patients on dapsone require lab monitoring weekly for the 1st month, biweekly for 2 months, then every 3 months for the duration of medication use (1,4).

DIET
GFD
- Grains that should be avoided: wheat (includes spelt, kamut, semolina, and triticale), rye, and barley (including malt)
- Safe grains (gluten-free): rice, amaranth, buckwheat, corn, millet, quinoa, sorghum, teff (an Ethiopian cereal grain), and oats
- Care should be taken to avoid gluten-free grains that are contaminated with sources of gluten during processing such as oats.
- Sources of gluten-free starches that can be used as flour alternatives
  – Cereal grains: amaranth, buckwheat, corn, millet, quinoa, sorghum, teff, rice (white, brown, wild, basmati, jasmine), and montina
  – Tubers: arrowroot, jicama, taro, potato, and tapioca
  – Legumes: chickpeas, lentils, kidney beans, navy beans, pea beans, peanuts, and soybeans
  – Nuts: almonds, walnuts, chestnuts, hazelnuts, and cashews
  – Seeds: sunflower, flax, and pumpkin

PATIENT EDUCATION
- Patients on dapsone should be made aware of potential hemolytic anemia and the signs associated with methemoglobinemia.
- American Academy of Dermatology, 930 N. Meacham Road, P.O. Box 4014, Schaumberg, IL 60168-4014; (708) 330-0230
- The University of Chicago Celiac Disease Center, 5841 S. Maryland Ave., Mail Code 4069, Chicago, IL 60637; (773) 702-7593; www.celiacdisease.net or http://www.cureceliacdisease.org/
- Gluten Intolerance Group of North America, 31214-124 Ave. SE, Auburn, WA 98092; (206) 246-6652; fax (206) 246-6531; https://www.gluten.org/
- The Celiac Disease Foundation, 13251 Ventura Blvd., #1, Studio City, CA 9160; (818) 990-2354; fax (818) 990-2379

PROGNOSIS
- Lifelong disease with favorable prognosis
- 10- to 15-year survival rates do not seem to differ from general population.
- Remission in 10–15%
- Skin disease responds readily to dapsone. Occasional new lesions (2 to 3 per week) are to be expected and are not an indication for altering daily dosage.
- Strict adherence to a GFD improves clinical symptoms and decreases dapsone requirement. GFD is the only sustainable method of eliminating cutaneous and GI disease.
- Risk of lymphoma may be decreased in those who maintain a GFD.

COMPLICATIONS
- Majority of complications are associated with GSE.
- Malnutrition, weight loss, nutritional deficiencies (folate, B_{12}, iron)
- Abdominal pain, dyspepsia
- Osteoporosis, dental abnormalities
- Autoimmune diseases
- Lymphomas

REFERENCES
1. Antiga E, Caproni M. The diagnosis and treatment of dermatitis herpetiformis. *Clin Cosmet Investig Dermatol*. 2015;8:257–265.
2. Bolotin D, Petronic-Rosic V. Dermatitis herpetiformis. Part II. Diagnosis, management, and prognosis. *J Am Acad Dermatol*. 2011;64(6):1027–1033.
3. Junkins-Hopkins JM. Dermatitis herpetiformis: pearls and pitfalls in diagnosis and management. *J Am Acad Dermatol*. 2010;63(3):526–528.
4. Wozel G, Blasum C. Dapsone in dermatology and beyond. *Arch Dermatol Res*. 2014;306(2):103–124.
5. Willsteed E, Lee M, Wong LC, et al. Sulfasalazine and dermatitis herpetiformis. *Australas J Dermatol*. 2005;46(2):101–103.
6. Handler MZ, Chacon AH, Shiman MI, et al. Letter to the editor: application of dapsone 5% gel in a patient with dermatitis herpetiformis. *J Dermatol Case Rep*. 2012;6(4):132–133.

ADDITIONAL READING
- Bolotin D, Petronic-Rosic V. Dermatitis herpetiformis. Part I. Epidemiology, pathogenesis, and clinical presentation. *J Am Acad Dermatol*. 2011;64(6):1017–1024.
- Cardones AR, Hall RP III. Management of dermatitis herpetiformis. *Immunol Allergy Clin North Am*. 2012;32(2):275–281.
- Cardones AR, Hall RP III. Pathophysiology of dermatitis herpetiformis: a model for cutaneous manifestations of gastrointestinal inflammation. *Immunol Allergy Clin North Am*. 2012;32(2):263–274.
- Kárpáti S. An exception within the group of autoimmune blistering diseases: dermatitis herpetiformis, the gluten-sensitive dermopathy. *Immunol Allergy Clin North Am*. 2012;32(2):255–262.
- Paek SY, Steinberg SM, Katz SI. Remission in dermatitis herpetiformis: a cohort study. *Arch Dermatol*. 2011;147(3):301–305.

 See Also

- Celiac Disease
- Algorithm: Rash, Focal

 CODES

ICD10
L13.0 Dermatitis herpetiformis

CLINICAL PEARLS
- DH is a chronic, relapsing, intensely pruritic rash that often presents with erosions, excoriations, lichenification, and pigmentary changes secondary to scratching and healing of old papulovesicular lesions.
- Strong association with gluten-sensitive enteropathy
- Diagnosis established with perilesional skin biopsy showing direct immunofluorescence demonstrating granular IgA deposits in the dermal papillae.
- Serologic levels of IgA transglutaminase aid in diagnosis and monitoring of deviations from GFD.
- Mainstay of treatment is a GFD with dapsone used primarily for short-term symptom relief.

DERMATITIS, ATOPIC
Dennis E. Hughes, DO, FACEP

 BASICS

DESCRIPTION
- A chronic, relapsing, pruritic eczematous condition affecting characteristic sites
- Early onset cases have coexisting allergen sensitization more often than late onset.
- Clinical phenotypical presentation is highly variable, suggesting multifactorial pathophysiology.
- May have significant effect on quality of life for patient and family

EPIDEMIOLOGY
- 45% of all cases begin in the first 6 months of life with 95% onset prior to age 5 years.
- 70% of affected children will have a spontaneous remission before adolescence.
- Incidence on the rise for the past 3 decades in industrialized countries; overall, affects ~15% of children at some time (United States)
- Also, may have late-onset dermatitis in adults or relapse of childhood condition—primarily hand eczema
- Asians and blacks are affected more often than whites.
- 60% if one parent is affected; rises to 80% if both parents are affected

ETIOLOGY
- Two main hypothesis: immunologic with unbalanced immune response and/or skin barrier dysfunction (1)
- Alteration in stratum corneum results in transepidermal water loss and defect in barrier function.
- Epidermal adhesion is reduced either as a result of (i) genetic mutation resulting in altered epidermal proteins or (ii) defect in immune regulation causing an altered inflammatory response.
- Interleukin-31 (IL-31) upregulation is thought to be a major factor in pruritus mediated by cytokines and neuropeptides rather than histamine excess.

Genetics
- Recent discovery of association between atopic dermatitis (AD) and mutation in the filaggrin gene (on chromosome 1), which codes for a skin barrier protein (2)
- Both epidermal and immune coding likely involved

RISK FACTORS
- "Itch–scratch cycle" (stimulates histamine release)
- Skin infections
- Emotional stress
- Irritating clothes and chemicals
- Excessively hot or cold climate
- Food allergy in children (in some cases)

- Exposure to tobacco smoke
- Family history of atopy
  - Asthma
  - Allergic rhinitis

COMMONLY ASSOCIATED CONDITIONS
- Food sensitivity/allergy in many cases
- Asthma
- Allergic rhinitis
- Hyper-IgE syndrome (Job syndrome)
  - AD
  - Elevated IgE
  - Recurrent pyodermas
  - Decreased chemotaxis of mononuclear cells

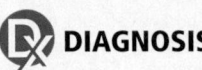 **DIAGNOSIS**

HISTORY
Presence of major symptoms, including relapsing of condition, family history, typical distribution, and morphology necessary to make diagnosis of AD

PHYSICAL EXAM
Primarily skin manifestations
- Distribution of lesions
  - Infants: trunk, face, and flexural surfaces; diaper-sparing
  - Children: antecubital and popliteal fossae
  - Adults: hands, feet, face, neck, upper chest, and genital areas
- Morphology of lesions
  - Infants: erythema and papules; may develop oozing, crusting vesicles
  - Children and adults: Lichenification and scaling are typical with chronic eczema as a result of persistent scratching and rubbing (lichenification rare in infants).
- Associated signs
  - Facial erythema, mild to moderate
  - Perioral pallor
  - Infraorbital fold (Dennie sign/Morgan line)-atopic pleat
  - Dry skin progressing to ichthyosis
  - Increased palmar linear markings
  - Pityriasis alba (hypopigmented asymptomatic areas on face and shoulders)
  - Keratosis pilaris

DIFFERENTIAL DIAGNOSIS
- Photosensitivity rashes
- Contact dermatitis (especially if only the face is involved)
- Scabies
- Seborrheic dermatitis (especially in infants)

- Psoriasis or lichen simplex chronicus if only localized disease is present in adults
- Rare conditions of infancy
  - Histiocytosis X
  - Wiskott-Aldrich syndrome
  - Ataxia-telangiectasia syndrome
- Ichthyosis vulgaris

DIAGNOSTIC TESTS & INTERPRETATION
Initial Tests (lab, imaging)
- No test is diagnostic.
- Serum IgE levels are elevated in as many as 80% of affected individuals, but test is not routinely ordered.
- Eosinophilia tends to correlate with disease severity.
- Scoring atopic dermatitis (SCORAD) is scoring system for AD comprising scores for area, intensity, and subjective symptoms.

 TREATMENT

GENERAL MEASURES
- Minimize flare-ups and control the duration and intensity of flare-up.
- Avoid agents that may cause irritation (e.g., wool, perfumes).
- Minimize sweating.
- Lukewarm (not hot) bathing
- Minimize use of soap (superfatted soaps best).
- Sun exposure may be helpful.
- Humidify the house.
- Avoid excessive contact with water.
- Avoid lotions that contain alcohol.
- If very resistant to treatment, search for a coexisting contact dermatitis.

Pediatric Considerations
Chronic potent fluorinated corticosteroid use may cause striae, hypopigmentation, or atrophy, especially in children.

MEDICATION
First Line
- Frequent systemic lubrication with thick emollient creams (e.g., Eucerin, Vaseline) over moist skin is the mainstay of treatment before any other intervention is considered (1)[A].
- Infants and children: 0.5–1% topical hydrocortisone creams or ointments (use the "fingertip unit [FTU]" dosing) (1)[C]

- Adults: higher potency topical corticosteroids in areas other than face and skin folds
- Short-course, higher potency corticosteroids for flares; then return to the lowest potency (creams preferred) that will control dermatitis.
- Antihistamines for pruritus (e.g., hydroxyzine 10 to 25 mg at bedtime and as needed)

Second Line
- Topical immunomodulators (tacrolimus or pimecrolimus) for episodic use for children >2 years. There is a black box warning from the FDA regarding potential cancer risk.
- Plastic occlusion in combination with topical medication to promote absorption
- For severe AD, consider systemic steroids for 1 to 2 weeks (e.g., prednisone 2 mg/kg/day PO [max 80 mg/day] initially, tapered over 7 to 14 days).
- Topical tricyclic doxepin, as a 5% cream, may decrease pruritus.
- Modified Goeckerman regimen (tar and ultraviolet light)
- Low-dose methotrexate was established as effective treatment in adults, and recent review suggests it is safe for children and adolescents (3)[B].

ISSUES FOR REFERRAL
- Ophthalmology evaluation for persistent vernal conjunctivitis
- If using topical steroids around eyes for extended periods, ophthalmology follow-up for cataract evaluation

ADDITIONAL THERAPIES
- Methods to reduce house mite allergens (micropore filters on heating, ventilation, and air-conditioning systems; impermeable mattress covers)
- Behavioral relaxation therapy to reduce scratching
- Bleach baths may reduce staph colonization, but definitive evidence for benefit in the condition is lacking. Recommend 1/2 cup of standard 6% household bleach for a full tub of water and soak for 5 to 10 minutes, blotting skin dry upon leaving the bath.

COMPLEMENTARY & ALTERNATIVE MEDICINE
- Evening primrose oil (includes high content of fatty acids)
  - May decrease prostaglandin synthesis
  - May promote conversion of linoleic acid to omega-6 fatty acid
- Probiotics may reduce the severity of the condition, thus reducing medication use.

 ONGOING CARE

FOLLOW-UP RECOMMENDATIONS
Patient Monitoring
Evaluate to ensure that secondary bacterial or fungal infection does not develop as a result of disruption of the skin barrier. Most patients with AD are colonized by *Staphylococcus*. There is a little evidence for the routine use of antimicrobial interventions to reduce skin bacteria, but treatment of clinical infection with coverage for *Staphylococcus* is recommended.

DIET
- Trials of elimination may find certain "triggers" in some patients.
- Breastfeeding in conjunction with maternal hypoallergenic diets may decrease the severity in some infants.

PATIENT EDUCATION
- http://www.aad.org/skin-conditions/dermatology-a-to-z/atopic-dermatitis
- National Eczema Association: www.nationaleczema.org

PROGNOSIS
- Chronic disease
- Declines with increasing age
- 90% of patients have spontaneous resolution by puberty.
- Localized eczema (e.g., chronic hand or foot dermatitis, eyelid dermatitis, or lichen simplex chronicus) may continue in some adults.

COMPLICATIONS
- Cataracts are more common in patients with AD.
- Skin infections (usually *Staphylococcus aureus*); sometimes subclinical
- Eczema herpeticum
  - Generalized vesiculopustular eruption caused by infection with herpes simplex or vaccinia virus
  - Causes acute illness requiring hospitalization
- Atrophy and/or striae if fluorinated corticosteroids are used on face or skin folds
- Systemic absorption may occur if large areas of skin are treated, particularly if high-potency medications and occlusion are combined.

REFERENCES
1. Thomsen SF. Atopic dermatitis: natural history, diagnosis, and treatment. *ISRN Allergy.* 2014;2014:354250.
2. Wollenberg A, Seba A, Antal AS. Immunological and molecular targets of atopic dermatitis treatment. *Br J Dermatol.* 2014;170(Suppl 1):7–11.
3. Deo M, Yung A, Hill S, et al. Methotrexate for treatment of atopic dermatitis in children and adolescents. *Int J Dermatol.* 2014;53(8):1037–1041.

ADDITIONAL READING
- Boguniewicz M, Leung DY. Recent insights into atopic dermatitis and implications for management of infectious complications. *J Allergy Clin Immunol.* 2010;125(1):4–13.
- Catherine Mack Correa M, Nebus J. Management of patients with atopic dermatitis: the role of emollient therapy. *Dermatol Res Pract.* 2012;2012:836931.
- Lifschitz C. The impact of atopic dermatitis on quality of life. *Ann Nutr Metab.* 2015;66(Suppl 1): 34–40.

 SEE ALSO

Algorithm: Rash, Focal

 CODES

ICD10
- L20.9 Atopic dermatitis, unspecified
- L20.89 Other atopic dermatitis
- L20.83 Infantile (acute) (chronic) eczema

CLINICAL PEARLS
- Institute early and proactive treatment to reduce inflammation. Use the lowest potency topical steroid that controls symptoms.
- Monitor for secondary bacterial infection.
- Frequent systemic lubrication with thick emollient creams (e.g., Eucerin, Vaseline) over moist skin is the mainstay of treatment before any other intervention is considered.

D

DERMATITIS, CONTACT

Aamir Siddiqi, MD

BASICS

DESCRIPTION
- A cutaneous reaction to an external substance
- Primary irritant dermatitis is due to direct injury of the skin. It affects individuals exposed to specific irritants and generally produces discomfort immediately after exposure (1).
- Allergic contact dermatitis (ACD) affects only individuals previously sensitized to a substance. It represents a delayed hypersensitivity reaction, requiring several hours for the cascade of cellular immunity to be completed to manifest itself (2).
- System(s) affected: skin/exocrine
- Synonym(s): dermatitis venenata

EPIDEMIOLOGY
Common

Incidence
Occupational contact dermatitis: 20.5/100,000 workers/year in one Australian study

Prevalence
- Contact dermatitis represents >90% of all occupational skin disorders.
- Predominant sex: male = female
  - Variations due to differences in exposure to offending agents, as well as normal cutaneous variations between males and females (eccrine and sebaceous gland function and hair distribution)

Geriatric Considerations
Increased incidence of irritant dermatitis secondary to skin dryness

Pediatric Considerations
Increased incidence of positive patch testing due to better delayed hypersensitivity reactions (3)

ETIOLOGY AND PATHOPHYSIOLOGY
Hypersensitivity reaction to a substance generating cellular immunity response (4)
- Plants
  - Urushiol (allergen): poison ivy, poison oak, poison sumac
  - Primary contact: plant (roots/stems/leaves)
  - Secondary contact: clothes/fingernails (not blister fluid)
- Chemicals
  - Nickel: jewelry, zippers, hooks, and watches (5)
  - Potassium dichromate: tanning agent in leather
  - Paraphenylenediamine: hair dyes, fur dyes, and industrial chemicals
  - Turpentine: cleaning agents, polishes, and waxes
  - Soaps and detergents

- Topical medicines
  - Neomycin: topical antibiotics
  - Thimerosal (Merthiolate): preservative in topical medications
  - Anesthetics: benzocaine
  - Parabens: preservative in topical medications
  - Formalin: cosmetics, shampoos, and nail enamel

Genetics
Increased frequency of ACD in families with allergies

RISK FACTORS
- Occupation
- Hobbies
- Travel
- Cosmetics
- Jewelry

GENERAL PREVENTION
- Avoid causative agents.
- Use of protective gloves (with cotton lining) may be helpful.

DIAGNOSIS

HISTORY
- Itchy rash
- Assess for prior exposure to irritating substance.

PHYSICAL EXAM
- Acute
  - Papules, vesicles, bullae with surrounding erythema
  - Crusting and oozing
  - Pruritus
- Chronic
  - Erythematous base
  - Thickening with lichenification
  - Scaling
  - Fissuring
- Distribution
  - Where epidermis is thinner (eyelids, genitalia)
  - Areas of contact with offending agent (e.g., nail polish)
  - Palms and soles relatively more resistant, although hand dermatitis is common.
  - Deeper skin folds spared
  - Linear arrays of lesions
  - Lesions with sharp borders and sharp angles are pathognomonic.
- Well-demarcated area with a papulovesicular rash

DIFFERENTIAL DIAGNOSIS
- Based on clinical impression
  - Appearance, periodicity, and localization
- Groups of vesicles
  - Herpes simplex
- Diffuse bullous or vesicular lesions
  - Bullous pemphigoid
- Photodistribution
  - Phototoxic/allergic reaction to systemic allergen
- Eyelids
  - Seborrheic dermatitis
- Scaly eczematous lesions
  - Atopic dermatitis
  - Nummular eczema
  - Lichen simplex chronicus
  - Stasis dermatitis
  - Xerosis

DIAGNOSTIC TESTS & INTERPRETATION

Diagnostic Procedures/Other
Consider patch tests for suspected allergic trigger (systemic corticosteroids or recent, aggressive use of topical steroids may alter results).

Test Interpretation
- Intercellular edema
- Bullae

TREATMENT

GENERAL MEASURES
- Remove offending agent:
  - Avoidance
  - Work modification
  - Protective clothing
  - Barrier creams, especially high-lipid content moisturizing creams (e.g., Keri lotion, petrolatum, coconut oil)
- Topical soaks with cool tap water, Burow solution (1:40 dilution), saline (1 tsp/pt water), or silver nitrate solution
- Lukewarm water baths
- Aveeno oatmeal baths
- Emollients (white petrolatum, Eucerin)

MEDICATION

First Line

- Topical medications (6)[A]
  - Lotion of zinc oxide, talc, menthol 0.15% (Gold Bond), phenol 0.5%
  - Corticosteroids for ACD as well as irritant dermatitis
    - High-potency steroids: fluocinonide (Lidex) 0.05% gel, cream, or ointment TID–QID
    - Use high-potency steroids only for a short time, then switch to low- or medium-potency steroid cream or ointment
    - Caution regarding face/skin folds: use lower potency steroids, and avoid prolonged usage. Switch to lower potency topical steroid once the acute phase is resolved.
- Calamine lotion for symptomatic relief
- Topical antibiotics for secondary infection (bacitracin, erythromycin)
- Systemic
  - Antihistamine
    - Hydroxyzine: 25 to 50 mg PO QID, especially useful for itching
    - Diphenhydramine: 25 to 50 mg PO QID
    - Cetirizine 10 mg PO BID–TID
- Corticosteroids
  - Prednisone: taper starting at 60 to 80 mg/day PO, over 10 to 14 days
  - Used for moderate to severe cases
  - May use burst dose of steroids for up to 5 days
- Antibiotics for secondary skin infections
  - Dicloxacillin: 250 to 500 mg PO QID for 7 to 10 days
  - Amoxicillin-clavulanate (Augmentin): 500 mg PO BID for 7 to 10 days
  - Erythromycin: 250 mg PO QID in penicillin-allergic patients
  - Trimethoprim-sulfamethoxazole (Bactrim DS): 160 mg/800 mg (1 tablet) PO BID for 7 to 10 days (suspected resistant *Staphylococcus aureus*)
- Precautions
  - Antihistamines may cause drowsiness.
  - Prolonged use of potent topical steroids may cause local skin effects (atrophy, stria, telangiectasia).
  - Use tapering dose of oral steroids if using >5 days.

Second Line

Other topical or systemic antibiotics, depending on organisms and sensitivity

Pregnancy Considerations

Usual caution with medications.

ISSUES FOR REFERRAL

May need referral to a dermatologist or allergist if refractory to conventional treatment

COMPLEMENTARY & ALTERNATIVE MEDICINE

The use of complementary and alternative treatment is a supplement and not an alternative to conventional treatment.

Admission Criteria/Initial Stabilization

Rarely needs hospital admission

ONGOING CARE

FOLLOW-UP RECOMMENDATIONS

Stay active, but avoid overheating.

Patient Monitoring

- As necessary for recurrence
- Patch testing for etiology after resolved

DIET

No special diet

PATIENT EDUCATION

- Avoidance of irritating substance
- Cleaning of secondary sources (nails, clothes)
- Fallacy of blister fluid spreading disease

PROGNOSIS

- Self-limited
- Benign

COMPLICATIONS

- Generalized eruption secondary to autosensitization
- Secondary bacterial infection

REFERENCES

1. Ale IS, Maibacht HA. Diagnostic approach in allergic and irritant contact dermatitis. *Expert Rev Clin Immunol*. 2010;6(2):291–310.
2. Tan CH, Rasool S, Johnston GA. Contact dermatitis: allergic and irritant. *Clin Dermatol*. 2014;32(1):116–124.
3. Admani S, Jacob SE. Allergic contact dermatitis in children: review of the past decade. *Curr Allergy Asthma Rep*. 2014;14(4):421.
4. Martin SF. Contact dermatitis: from pathomechanisms to immunotoxicology. *Exp Dermatol*. 2012;21(5):382–389.
5. Tuchman M, Silverberg JI, Jacob SE, et al. Nickel contact dermatitis in children. *Clin Dermatol*. 2015;33(3):320–326.
6. Usatine RP, Riojas M. Diagnosis and management of contact dermatitis. *Am Fam Physician*. 2010;82(3):249–255.

See Also

Algorithm: Rash, Focal

CODES

ICD10

- L25.9 Unspecified contact dermatitis, unspecified cause
- L23.9 Allergic contact dermatitis, unspecified cause
- L25.5 Unspecified contact dermatitis due to plants, except food

CLINICAL PEARLS

- Anyone exposed to irritants or allergic substances is predisposed to contact dermatitis, especially in occupations that have high exposure to chemicals.
- The most common allergens causing contact dermatitis are plants of the *Toxicodendron* genus (poison ivy, poison oak, poison sumac).
- Poison-ivy dermatitis typically requires 10 to 14 days of topical or oral steroid therapy to prevent recurrent eruption.
- The usual treatment for contact dermatitis is avoidance of the allergen or irritating substance and temporary use of topical steroids.
- A contact dermatitis eruption presents in a nondermatomal geographic fashion due to the skin being in contact with an external source.

DERMATITIS, DIAPER

Dennis E. Hughes, DO, FACEP

 BASICS

DESCRIPTION
- Diaper dermatitis is a rash occurring under the covered area of a diaper. It is usually initially a contact dermatitis.
- System(s) affected: skin/exocrine
- Synonym(s): diaper rash; nappy rash; napkin dermatitis

Geriatric Considerations
Incontinence is a significant cofactor.

EPIDEMIOLOGY
Incidence
- The most common dermatitis found in infancy
- Peak incidence: 7 to 12 months of age, then decreases
- Lower incidence reported in breastfed babies due to lower pH, urease, protease, and lipase activity.

Prevalence
Prevalence has been variably reported from 4–35% in the first 2 years of life.

ETIOLOGY AND PATHOPHYSIOLOGY
- Immature infant skin with histologic, biochemical, functional differences compared to mature skin (1)
- Wet skin is central in the development of diaper dermatitis, as prolonged contact with urine or feces results in susceptibility to chemical, enzymatic, and physical injury; wet skin is also penetrated more easily.
- Fecal proteases and lipases are irritants.
- Superhydrase urease enzyme found in the stratum corneum liberates ammonia from cutaneous bacteria.
- Fecal lipase and protease activity is increased by acceleration of GI transit; thus, a higher incidence of irritant diaper dermatitis is observed in babies who have had diarrhea in the previous 48 hours.
- Once the skin is compromised, secondary infection by *Candida albicans* is common. 40–75% of diaper rashes that last >3 days are colonized with *C. albicans*.

- Bacteria may play a role in diaper dermatitis through reduction of fecal pH and resulting activation of enzymes.
- Allergy is exceedingly rare as a cause in infants.

RISK FACTORS
- Infrequent diaper changes
- Improper laundering (cloth diapers)
- Family history of dermatitis
- Hot, humid weather
- Recent treatment with oral antibiotics
- Diarrhea (>3 stools per day increases risk)
- Dye allergy
- Eczema may increase risk.

GENERAL PREVENTION
Attention to hygiene during bouts of diarrhea

COMMONLY ASSOCIATED CONDITIONS
- Contact (allergic or irritant) dermatitis
- Seborrheic dermatitis
- Psoriasis
- Candidiasis
- Atopic dermatitis

 DIAGNOSIS

HISTORY
- Onset, duration, and change in the nature of the rash
- Presence of rashes outside the diaper area
- Associated scratching or crying
- Contact with infants with a similar rash
- Recent illness, diarrhea, or antibiotic use
- Fever
- Pustular drainage
- Lymphangitis

PHYSICAL EXAM
- Mild forms consist of shiny erythema ± scale.
- Margins are not always evident.
- Moderate cases have areas of papules, vesicles, and small superficial erosions.

- It can progress to well-demarcated ulcerated nodules that measure ≥1 cm in diameter.
- It is found on the prominent parts of the buttocks, medial thighs, mons pubis, and scrotum.
- Skin folds are spared or involved last.
- *Tidemark dermatitis* refers to the bandlike form of erythema of irritated diaper margins.
- Diaper dermatitis can cause an id reaction (autoeczematous) outside the diaper area.

DIFFERENTIAL DIAGNOSIS
- Contact dermatitis
- Seborrheic dermatitis
- Candidiasis
- Atopic dermatitis
- Scabies
- Acrodermatitis enteropathica
- Letterer-Siwe disease
- Congenital syphilis
- Child abuse
- Streptococcal infection
- Kawasaki disease
- Biotin deficiency
- Psoriasis
- HIV infection

DIAGNOSTIC TESTS & INTERPRETATION
Initial Tests (lab, imaging)
Rarely needed

Follow-Up Tests & Special Considerations
- Consider a culture of lesions or a potassium hydroxide (KOH) preparation.
- The finding of anemia in association with hepatosplenomegaly and the appropriate rash may suggest a diagnosis of Langerhans cell histiocytosis or congenital syphilis.
- Finding mites, ova, or feces on a mineral oil preparation of a burrow scraping can confirm the diagnosis of scabies.

Test Interpretation
- Biopsy is rare.
- Histology may reveal acute, subacute, or chronic spongiotic dermatitis.

TREATMENT

Prevention is the key to treatment of this condition.

GENERAL MEASURES
- Expose the buttocks to air as much as possible.
- Use mild, slightly acidic cleanser with water; no rubbing and pat dry.
- Avoid impermeable waterproof pants during treatment (day or night); they keep the skin wet and subject to rash or infection.
- Change diapers frequently, even at night, if the rash is extensive.
- Superabsorbable diapers are beneficial, as they wick urine away from skin and still allow air to permeate (2)[C].
- Discontinue using baby lotion, powder, ointment, or baby oil (except zinc oxide).
- Use of appropriately formulated baby wipes (fragrance-free) is safe and as effective as water (3)[B].
- Apply zinc oxide ointment or other barrier cream to the rash at the earliest sign and BID or TID (e.g., Desitin or Balmex). Thereafter, apply to clean, thoroughly dried skin (4)[C].
- Cornstarch can reduce friction. Talc powders that do not enhance the growth of yeast can provide protection against frictional injury in diaper dermatitis, but do not form a continuous lipid barrier layer over the skin and obstruct the skin pores. These treatments are not recommended.

MEDICATION
First Line
- For a pure contact dermatitis, a low-potency topical steroid (hydrocortisone 0.5–1% TID for 3 to 5 days) and removal of the offending agent (urine, feces) should suffice.
- If candidiasis is suspected or diaper rash persists, use an antifungal such as miconazole nitrate 2% cream, miconazole powder, econazole (Spectazole), clotrimazole (Lotrimin), or ketoconazole (Nizoral) cream at each diaper change.
- If inflammation is prominent, consider a very low-potency steroid cream such as hydrocortisone 0.5–1% TID along with an antifungal cream ± a combination product such as clioquinol–hydrocortisone (Vioform–Hydrocortisone) cream.

- If a secondary bacterial infection is suspected, use an antistaphylococcal oral antibiotic or mupirocin (Bactroban) ointment topically.
- Precautions: Avoid high- or moderate-potency steroids often found in combination of steroid antifungal mixtures—these should never be used in the diaper area.

Second Line
Sucralfate paste for resistant cases

ISSUES FOR REFERRAL
Consider if a systemic disease such as Langerhans cell histiocytosis, acrodermatitis enteropathica, or HIV infection is suspected

INPATIENT CONSIDERATIONS
Admission Criteria/Initial Stabilization
- Febrile neonates
- Recalcitrant rash suggestive of immunodeficiency
- Toxic-appearing infants
Nursing
Assist first-time parents with hygiene education.

 ONGOING CARE

FOLLOW-UP RECOMMENDATIONS
Patient Monitoring
Recheck weekly until clear; then at times of recurrence.

PATIENT EDUCATION
Patient education is vital to the treatment and prevention of recurrent cases.

PROGNOSIS
- Quick, complete clearing with appropriate treatment
- Secondary candidal infections may last a few weeks after treatment has begun.

COMPLICATIONS
- Secondary bacterial infection (consider community-acquired methicillin-resistant *Staphylococcus aureus* [MRSA] in pustular dermatitis that does not respond to normal therapy)
- Rare complication is inoculation with group A β-hemolytic *Streptococcus* resulting in necrotizing fasciitis.
- Secondary yeast infection

REFERENCES
1. Stamatas GN, Tierney NK. Diaper dermatitis: etiology, manifestations, prevention, and management. *Pediatr Dermatol*. 2014;31(1):1–7.
2. Erasala GN, Romain C, Merlay I. Diaper area and disposable diapers. *Curr Probl Dermatol*. 2011;40:83–89.
3. Lavender T, Furber C, Campbell M, et al. Effect on skin hydration of using baby wipes to clean the napkin area of newborn babies: assessor-blinded randomised controlled equivalence trial. *BMC Pediatr*. 2012;12:59.
4. Humphrey S, Bergman JN, Au S. Practical management strategies for diaper dermatitis. *Skin Therapy Lett*. 2006;11(7):1–6.

ADDITIONAL READING
Serdaroğlu S, Üstünbaş TK. Diaper dermatitis (napkin dermatitis, nappy rash). *J Turk Acad Dermatol*. 2010;4(4):04401r.

 SEE ALSO

Algorithm: Rash, Focal

 CODES

ICD10
- L22 Diaper dermatitis
- B37.2 Candidiasis of skin and nail

CLINICAL PEARLS
- Hygiene is the main preventative measure.
- Look for secondary infection in persistent cases.

DERMATITIS, SEBORRHEIC

Juan Qiu, MD, PhD

 BASICS

DESCRIPTION
Chronic, superficial, recurrent inflammatory rash affecting sebum-rich, hairy regions of the body, especially the scalp, eyebrows, and face

EPIDEMIOLOGY
Incidence
- Predominant age: infancy, adolescence, and adulthood
- Predominant sex: male > female

Prevalence
Seborrheic dermatitis: 3–5%

ETIOLOGY AND PATHOPHYSIOLOGY
- Skin surface yeasts *Malassezia* (formerly *Plasmodium ovale*) may be a contributing factor (1,2).
- The mite *Demodex folliculorum* may have a direct/indirect role (3).
- Genetic and environmental factors: Flares are common with stress/illness.
- Parallels increased sebaceous gland activity in infancy and adolescence or as a result of some acnegenic drugs.
- Seborrheic dermatitis is more common in immunosuppressed patients, suggesting that immune mechanisms are implicated in the pathogenesis of the disease, although the mechanisms are not well defined (1).

Genetics
Positive family history; no genetic marker is identified to date.

RISK FACTORS
- Parkinson disease
- AIDS (disease severity correlated with progression of immune deficiency)
- Emotional stress
- Medications may flare/induce seborrheic dermatitis: auranofin, aurothioglucose, buspirone, chlorpromazine, cimetidine, ethionamide, gold, griseofulvin, haloperidol, interferon-α, lithium, methoxsalen, methyldopa, phenothiazine, psoralen, stanozolol, thiothixene, trioxsalen (2)

GENERAL PREVENTION
Seborrheic skin should be washed more often than usual.

COMMONLY ASSOCIATED CONDITIONS
- Parkinson disease
- AIDS

 DIAGNOSIS

Diagnosis of seborrheic dermatitis usually can be made by history and physical exam.

HISTORY
- Intermittent active phases manifest with burning, scaling, and itching, alternating with inactive periods; activity is increased in winter and early spring, with remissions commonly occurring in summer.
- Infants
  - Cradle cap: greasy scaling of scalp, sometimes with associated mild erythema
  - Diaper and/or axillary rash
  - Age at onset typically ~1 month
  - Usually resolves by 8 to 12 months
- Adults
  - Red, greasy, scaling rash in most locations consisting of patches and plaques with indistinct margins
  - Red, smooth, glazed appearance in skin folds
  - Minimal pruritus
  - Chronic waxing and waning course
  - Bilateral and symmetric
  - Most commonly located in hairy skin areas: scalp and scalp margins, eyebrows and eyelid margins, nasolabial folds, ears and retroauricular folds, presternal area, middle to upper back, buttock crease, inguinal area, genitals, and armpits

PHYSICAL EXAM
- Scalp appearance varies from mild, patchy scaling to widespread, thick, adherent crusts. Plaques are rare.
- Seborrheic dermatitis can spread onto the forehead, the posterior part of the neck, and the postauricular skin, as in psoriasis.
- Skin lesions manifest as brawny or greasy scaling over red, inflamed skin.
- Hypopigmentation is seen in African Americans.
- Infectious eczematoid dermatitis, with oozing and crusting, suggests secondary infection.
- Seborrheic blepharitis may occur independently.

DIFFERENTIAL DIAGNOSIS
- Atopic dermatitis: Distinction may be difficult in infants.
- Psoriasis
  - Usually knees, elbows, and nails are involved.
  - Scalp psoriasis will be more sharply demarcated than seborrhea, with crusted, infiltrated plaques rather than mild scaling and erythema.
- Candida
- Tinea cruris/capitis: Suspect these when usual medications fail/hair loss occurs.
- Eczema of auricle/otitis externa
- Rosacea
- Discoid lupus erythematosus: Skin biopsy will be beneficial.
- Histiocytosis X: may appear as seborrheic-type eruption
- Dandruff: scalp only, noninflammatory

DIAGNOSTIC TESTS & INTERPRETATION
Diagnostic Procedures/Other
Consider biopsy if
- Usual therapies fail
- Petechiae is noted.
- Histiocytosis X is suspected.
- Fungal cultures in refractory cases or when pustules and alopecia are present.

Test Interpretation
Nonspecific changes
- Hyperkeratosis, acanthosis, accentuated rete ridges, focal spongiosis, and parakeratosis are characteristic.
- Parakeratotic scale around hair follicles and mild superficial inflammatory lymphocytic infiltrate

 TREATMENT

GENERAL MEASURES
- Increase frequency of shampooing.
- Sunlight in moderate doses may be helpful.
- Cradle cap
  - Frequent shampooing with a mild, nonmedicated shampoo
  - Remove thick scale by applying warm mineral oil, then wash off 1 hour later with a mild soap and a soft-bristle toothbrush or terrycloth washcloth.
- Adults: Wash all affected areas with antiseborrheic shampoos. Start with over-the-counter products (selenium sulfide) and increase to more potent preparations (containing coal tar, sulfur, or salicylic acid) if no improvement is noted.
- For dense scalp scaling, 10% liquor carbonic detergens in Nivea oil may be used at bedtime, covering the head with a shower cap. This should be done nightly for 1 to 3 weeks.

MEDICATION

First Line

- Cradle cap: Use a coal tar shampoo or ketoconazole (Nizoral) shampoo if the nonmedicated shampoo is ineffective.
- Adults
  - Topical antifungal agents
    - Ketoconazole or miconazole 2% shampoo twice a week for clearance, then once a week or every other week for maintenance (1,4–6)[A]
    - Ketoconazole (Nizoral) and sertaconazole 2% cream may be used to clear scales in other areas (1,4–6)[A].
    - Ciclopirox 1% shampoo twice weekly (1)[A]
  - Topical corticosteroids
    - Begin with 1% hydrocortisone and advance to more potent (fluorinated) steroid preparations, as needed (1,4–6)[A].
      - Avoid continuous use of the more potent steroids to reduce the risk of skin atrophy, hypopigmentation, or systemic absorption (especially in infants and children).
      - Precautions: Fluorinated corticosteroids and higher concentrations of hydrocortisone (e.g., 2.5%) may cause atrophy or striae if used on the face or on skin folds.
  - Other topical agents
    - Coal tar 1% shampoo twice a week
    - Selenium sulfide 2.5% shampoo twice a week (1,4–6)[A]
    - Zinc pyrithione shampoo twice a week
    - Lithium succinate ointment twice a week
- Once controlled, washing with zinc soaps or selenium lotion with periodic use of steroid cream may help to maintain remission.

Second Line

- Calcineurin inhibitors
  - Pimecrolimus 1% cream BID (7)[B]
  - Tacrolimus 0.1% ointment BID (1,4–6)[A]
- Systemic antifungal therapy
  - Data are limited.
  - For moderate to severe seborrheic dermatitis
    - Ketoconazole: 200 mg/day (8)[A]
    - Itraconazole: 200 mg/day (8)[A]
    - Daily regimen for 1 to 2 months followed by twice-weekly dosing for chronic treatment
    - Monitor potential hepatotoxic effects.
- Low-molecular-weight hyaluronic acid
  - Hyaluronic acid sodium salt gel 0.2% BID (9)[B]

ISSUES FOR REFERRAL

No response to first-line therapy and concerns regarding systemic illness (e.g., HIV)

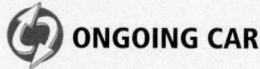

ONGOING CARE

FOLLOW-UP RECOMMENDATIONS

Patient Monitoring

Every 2 to 12 weeks, as necessary, depending on disease severity and degree of patient sophistication

PATIENT EDUCATION

http://familydoctor.org/familydoctor/en/diseases-conditions/seborrheic-dermatitis.html

PROGNOSIS

- In infants, seborrheic dermatitis usually remits after 6 to 8 months.
- In adults, seborrheic dermatitis is usually chronic and unpredictable, with exacerbations and remissions. Disease is usually easily controlled with shampoos and topical steroids.

COMPLICATIONS

- Skin atrophy/striae is possible from fluorinated corticosteroids, especially if used on the face.
- Glaucoma can result from use of fluorinated steroids around the eyes.
- Photosensitivity is caused occasionally by tars.
- Herpes keratitis is a rare complication of herpes simplex: Instruct patient to stop eyelid steroids if herpes simplex develops.

REFERENCES

1. Dessinioti C, Katsambas A. Seborrheic dermatitis: etiology, risk factors, and treatment: facts and controversies. *Clin Dermatol*. 2013:31(4):343–351.
2. Hay RJ. Malassezia, dandruff and seborrhoeic dermatitis: an overview. *Br J Dermatol*. 2011;165(Suppl 2):2–8.
3. Karincaoglu Y, Tepe B, Kalayci B, et al. Is *Demodex folliculorum* an aetiological factor in seborrhoeic dermatitis? *Clin Exp Dermatol*. 2009;34(8): e516–e520.
4. Clark GW, Pope SM, Jaboori KA. Diagnosis and treatment of seborrheic dermatitis. *Am Fam Physician*. 2015;91(3):185–190.
5. Stefanaki I, Katsambas A. Therapeutic update on seborrheic dermatitis. *Skin Therapy Lett*. 2010;15(5):1–4.
6. Kastarinen H, Oksanen T, Okokon EO, et al. Topical anti-inflammatory agents for seborrheic dermatitis of the face or scalp. *Cochrane Database Syst Rev*. 2014;(5):CD009446.
7. Kim GK, Rosso JD. Topical pimecrolimus 1% cream in the treatment of seborrheic dermatitis. *J Clin Aesthet Dermatol*. 2013;6(2):29–35.
8. Gupta AK, Richarson M, Paquet M. Systematic review of oral treatments for seborrheic dermatitis. *J Eur Acad Dermatol Venereol*. 2014:28(1):16–26.
9. Schlesinger T, Rowland Powell C. Efficacy and safety of a low molecular weight hyaluronic acid topical gel in the treatment of facial seborrheic dermatitis final report. *J Clin Aesthet Dermatol*. 2014:7(5):15–18.

ADDITIONAL READING

- Bikowski J. Facial seborrheic dermatitis: a report on current status and therapeutic horizons. *J Drugs Dermatol*. 2009;8(2):125–133.
- Darabi K, Hostetler SG, Bechtel MA, et al. The role of Malassezia in atopic dermatitis affecting the head and neck of adults. *J Am Acad Dermatol*. 2009;60(1):125–136.
- Johnson BA, Nunley JR. Treatment of seborrheic dermatitis. *Am Fam Physician*. 2000;61(9):2703–2710, 2713–2714.
- Naldi L, Rebora A. Clinical practice. Seborrheic dermatitis. *N Engl J Med*. 2009;360(4):387–396.
- Shemer A, Kaplan B, Nathansohn N, et al. Treatment of moderate to severe facial seborrheic dermatitis with itraconazole: an open non-comparative study. *Isr Med Assoc J*. 2008;10(6):417–418.

 SEE ALSO

Algorithm: Rash, Focal

 CODES

ICD10

- L21.9 Seborrheic dermatitis, unspecified
- L21.1 Seborrheic infantile dermatitis
- L21.0 Seborrhea capitis

CLINICAL PEARLS

- Search for an underlying systemic disease in a patient who is unresponsive to usual therapy.
- In adults, seborrheic dermatitis is usually chronic and unpredictable, with exacerbations and remissions. Disease is usually easily controlled with shampoos and topical steroids.

D

DERMATITIS, STASIS
Joseph A. Florence, MD • Fereshteh Gerayli, MD, FAAFP

BASICS

DESCRIPTION
- Chronic, eczematous, erythema, scaling, and noninflammatory edema of the lower extremities accompanied by cycle of scratching, excoriations, weeping, crusting, and inflammation in patients with chronic venous insufficiency, due to impaired circulation and other factors (nutritional edema)
- Clinical skin manifestation of chronic venous insufficiency usually appears late in the disease.
- May present as a solitary lesion
- System(s) affected: skin/exocrine
- Synonym(s): gravitational eczema; varicose eczema; venous dermatitis

EPIDEMIOLOGY
Incidence
In the United States: common in patients age >50 years; annual incidence of varicose vein 2–2.6%

Prevalence
- Prevalence of varicose vein is 7% (5–30%) and symptomatic chronic venous insufficiency is 0.86%
- Predominant age: adult, geriatric
- Predominant sex: female > male

Geriatric Considerations
Prevalence
- Common in this age group:
  - Estimated to affect 15 to 20 million patients age >50 years in the United States

ETIOLOGY AND PATHOPHYSIOLOGY
- Incompetence of perforating veins causing blood to backflow to the superficial venous system leading to venous hypertension (HTN) and cutaneous inflammation
- Deposition of fibrin around capillaries
- Microvascular abnormalities
- Ischemia
- Continuous presence of edema in ankles, usually present because of venous valve incompetency (varicose veins)
- Weakness of venous walls in lower extremities
- Trauma to edematous, ischemic skin
- Itch may be caused by inflammatory mediators (from mast cells, monocytes, macrophages, or neutrophils) liberated in the microcirculation and endothelium.
- Abnormal leukocyte–endothelium interaction is proposed to be a major factor.
- A cascade of biochemical events leads to ulceration.

Genetics
Familial link probable

RISK FACTORS
- Previous deep venous thrombosis
- Chronic edema (due to CHF, pulmonary HTN, obstructive sleep apnea; cirrhosis, nephrotic syndrome, or medication)
- Previous pregnancy
- Obesity
- Atopy
- Superimposed itch scratch cycle
- Trauma
- Genetic propensity
- Prolonged medical illness
- Secondary infection
- Low-protein diet
- Old age
- Tight garments that constrict the thigh
- Vein stripping
- Vein harvesting for coronary artery bypass graft surgery
- Previous cellulitis

GENERAL PREVENTION
- Use compression stockings to avoid recurrence of edema and to mobilize the interstitial lymphatic fluid from the region of stasis dermatitis and also following DVT.
- Topical lubricants twice a day to prevent fissuring and itching

COMMONLY ASSOCIATED CONDITIONS
- Varicose veins
- Venous insufficiency
- Other eczematous disease
- Hyperhomocysteinemia
- Venous HTN
- Most diseases that worsen peripheral edema (e.g. CHF, diastolic dysfunction)

DIAGNOSIS

HISTORY
- Older than 50 years with exception of acquired venous insufficiency due to surgery, trauma, or thrombosis (1)
- Pruritus, pain, and burning may precede skin signs, which are aggravated during evening hours.
- Insidious onset (2)
- Usually bilateral (3)
- Reddish-brown skin discoloration (3)
- Edema—initially develops around the ankle (3)
- Trauma is more indicative of cellulitis (3).

PHYSICAL EXAM
- Evaluation of the lower extremities characteristically reveals:
  - Bilateral, pitting edema (4,5)
  - Typically with erythema, hyperpigmentation—more common in the lower 1/3 of the extremity and medially (4,5)
- Violaceous (sometimes brown), erythematous-colored lesions due to deoxygenation of venous blood (postinflammatory hyperpigmentation and hemosiderin deposition within the cutaneous tissue)
  - Serous drainage, weeping, crusting, inflammation of the skin
  - Superficial desquamation (4)
  - May present as a solitary lesion mimicking a neoplasm (6)

DIFFERENTIAL DIAGNOSIS
- Cellulitis or erysipelas
- Trauma-related inflammation
- Deep vein thrombosis
- Nonspecific dermatitis
- Thrombophlebitis
- Contact dermatitis
- Vasculitis
- Basal cell or squamous cell carcinoma
- Lipodermatosclerosis
- Lymphedema
- Eosinophilic cellulitis
- Other eczematous diseases

DIAGNOSTIC TESTS & INTERPRETATION
Initial Tests (lab, imaging)
- Blood tests usually not indicated unless cellulitis and/or sepsis are suspected. Leukocytosis is more likely with true cellulitis (3).
- If stasis dermatitis is secondary to venous thrombosis, a thorough hematologic workup may be indicated to rule out hypercoagulability states.
- Duplex ultrasound imaging may diagnose deep venous thrombosis or severe valve damage secondary to past thrombosis.
- Potentially more accurate gold standards (e.g., skin biopsy) would introduce considerable risk to study patients and would not be acceptable from an ethical standpoint (3)

Diagnostic Procedures/Other
- Rule out arterial insufficiency (check peripheral pulses); ankle brachial pressure index (ABPI or ABI).
- Check for diabetes.

Test Interpretation
- ABPI <0.8 is suggestive of arterial insufficiency.
- ABPI can be falsely elevated in diabetic patients and others with distal small vessel calcifications.
- Arterial duplex ultrasound and angiography are the gold standards.

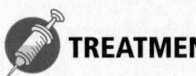

TREATMENT

GENERAL MEASURES
- Primary role of treatment is to reverse effects of venous HTN.
- Typically outpatient:
  - Reduce edema:
    - Leg elevation: heels higher than knees; knees higher than hips
    - Compression therapy: elastic bandage wraps: ace bandages or Unna paste boot (zinc gelatin) or compression stockings (Jobst or nonfitted type) (7)[A]
    - Graduated elastic compression of 30 to 40 mm Hg at the ankle improves ulcer healing rate and may prevent ulcer recurrence (7)[A]
    - No specific type of topical dressing (hydrocolloid versus simple nonadherent dressing) superior to another when used with compression therapy to maintain moist wound environment. Multilayer or bilayer compression bandages—more effective than nonelastic or short stretch bandages for severe cases (7)[A].
    - High compression is contraindicated in arterial insufficiency; pneumatic compression devices (7)[A].
  - Treat infection: Debride the ulcer base of necrotic tissue.
- Activity:
  - Avoid standing still.
  - Stay active and exercise regularly.
  - Elevate foot of bed unless contraindicated.
- Inpatient, for endovascular radiofrequency ablation, vein stripping, sclerotherapy, or skin grafts; treatment of advanced cellulitis or venous ulcers
  - Venous ulcer treatment includes autolytic, biologic, chemical, mechanical, and surgical.

MEDICATION
First Line
- Topical moisturizers, emollients, and barrier creams (e.g., white petroleum, lanolin, etc.) aid with

antipruritic treatment via reducing transepidermal water loss (8)[B].

- No evidence for routine use of systemic or topical antibiotics unless clear evidence of infection (9)[A].
- Uncomplicated stasis dermatitis can be treated with short courses of topical steroids (8,10[B]. (Topical triamcinolone 0.1% cream/ointment TID or betamethasone valerate 0.1% cream/ointment/solution TID) (10)[B].
- Topical antipruritic: pramoxine, camphor, menthol, and doxepin 5% cream (8)[B]
- Antipruritic medications (e.g., diphenhydramine, cetirizine hydrochloride, desloratadine) (8)[B]
- Pentoxifylline (400 mg TID) is effective in treating venous leg ulcer and may be effective in the absence of compression (11)[A].
- Enteric-coated aspirin (at least 300 mg) daily improves venous ulcer healing (12)[B].
- In light of increasing bacterial resistance to antibiotics, current guidelines recommend the use of antibacterial preparations only for clinical infection (cellulitis, increased pain, warmth, malodorous exudate) not for bacterial colonization (9)[A].
- Current evidence does not support the routine use of honey or silver-based products (9)[A].
- There is no reliable evidence in the effectiveness of topical preparations such as povidone-iodine, peroxide based preparations, mupirocin, chlorhexidine (9)[A].
- Insufficient evidence exists to either support or refute the routine use of silver sulfadiazine (SSD) for ambulatory patients with either partial-thickness burns or stasis dermatitis ulcers to decrease mortality, prevent infection, or augment wound healing (9)[A].
- If secondary infection, treat with PO antibiotics for *Staphylococcus* or *Streptococcus* organisms (e.g., dicloxacillin 250 mg QID, levofloxacin 500 mg QID, clindamycin 300 mg QID, or trimethoprim-sulfamethoxazole DS BID (3)[B].

Second Line
Consider antibiotics on basis of culture results of exudate from infected ulcer craters.

ISSUES FOR REFERRAL
- Consider referral for nonhealing ulcer.
- Arterial insufficiency
- Uncertain diagnosis
- Rheumatoid arthritis
- Patch testing to evaluate for contact dermatitis
- Associated disease (e.g., symptomatic varicose veins)

ADDITIONAL THERAPIES
If the patient is on amlodipine therapy, consider discontinuing amlodipine (13)[B].

SURGERY/OTHER PROCEDURES
Sclerotherapy and surgery may be required for associated disease.

ONGOING CARE

FOLLOW-UP RECOMMENDATIONS
Patient Monitoring
- If Unna boot compression is used: Cut off and reapply boot once a week. Unna boots reduce edema by compression and prevent scratching.
- Regular use of high compression stockings reduces chance of recurrent venous ulcer (14)[A].

DIET
lose weight, if overweight.

PATIENT EDUCATION
- Encourage staying active to keep circulation and leg muscles in good condition. Walking is ideal.
- Keep legs elevated while sitting or lying.
- Do not wear girdles, garters, or pantyhose with tight elastic tops.
- Do not scratch.
- Avoid leg injury.
- Elevate foot of bed with 2- to 4-inch blocks.
- Apply compression stockings prior to getting out of bed when less edema is present. Regular use of high compression stockings may prevent recurrence of venous ulcers.

PROGNOSIS
- Chronic course with intermittent exacerbations and remissions
- The healing process for ulceration is often prolonged and may take months.

COMPLICATIONS
- Sensations of itching, pain, and burning have negative impact on the quality of life (2)[B].
- Secondary bacterial infection
- DVT
- Bleeding at dermatitis sites
- Squamous cell carcinoma in edges of long-standing stasis ulcers
- Scarring, which in turn leads to further compromise to blood flow and increased likelihood of minor trauma

REFERENCES

1. Beauregard S, Gilchrest BA. A survey of skin problems and skin care regimens in the elderly. *Arch Dermatol.* 1987;123(12):1638–1643.
2. Duque M, Yosipovitch G, Chan YH, et al. Itch, pain, and burning sensation are common symptoms in mild to moderate chronic venous insufficiency with an impact on quality of life. *J Am Acad Dermatol.* 2005;53(3):504–508.
3. David CV, Chira S, Eells SJ, et al. Diagnostic accuracy in patients admitted to hospitals with cellulitis. *Dermatol Online J.* 2011;17(3):1.
4. Bailey E, Kroshinsky D. Cellulitis: diagnosis and management. *Dermatol Ther.* 2011; 24(2):229–239.
5. Farage MA, Miller KW, Berardesca E, et al. Clinical implications of aging skin: cutaneous disorders in the elderly. *Am J Clin Dermatol.* 2009;10(2):73–86.
6. Weaver J, Billings SD. Initial presentation of stasis dermatitis mimicking solitary lesions: a previously unrecognized clinical scenario. *J Am Acad Dermatol.* 2009;61(6):1028-1032.
7. O'Meara S, Cullum N, Nelson EA, et al. Compression for venous leg ulcers. *Cochrane Database Syst Rev.* 2012;(11):CD000265.
8. Patel T, Yosipovitch G. Therapy of pruritus. *Expert Opin Pharmacother.* 2010;11(10):1673–1682.
9. O'Meara S, Al-Kurdi D, Ologun Y, et al. Antibiotics and antiseptics for venous leg ulcers. *Cochrane Database Syst Rev.* 2014;(1):CD003557.
10. Weiss SC, Nguyen J, Chon S, et al. A randomized controlled clinical trial assessing the effect of betamethasone valerate 0.12% foam on the short-term treatment of stasis dermatitis. *J Drugs Dermatol.* 2005;4(3):339–345.
11. Jull A, Arroll B, Paraq V, et al. Pentoxifylline for treating venous leg ulcers. *Cochrane Database Syst Rev.* 2007;(3):CD001733.
12. Layton AM, Ibbotson SH, Davies JA, et al. Randomised trial of oral aspirin for chronic venous leg ulcers. *Lancet.* 1994;344(8916):164–165.
13. Gosnell AL, Nedorost ST. Stasis dermatitis as a complication of amlodipine therapy. *J Drugs Dermatol.* 2009;8(2):135–137.
14. Nelson EA, Bell-Syer SE, Cullum NA. Compression for preventing recurrence of venous ulcers. *Cochrane Database Syst Rev.* 2000;(4):CD002303.

ADDITIONAL READING
- Collins L, Seraj S. Diagnosis and treatment of venous ulcers. *Am Fam Physician.* 2010;81(8):989–996.
- Partsch H, Flour M, Smith PC; International Compression Club. Indications for compression therapy in venous and lymphatic disease consensus based on experimental data and scientific evidence. Under the auspices of the IUP. *Int Angiol.* 2008;27(3):193–219.
- Sippel K, Mayer D, Ballmer B, et al. Evidence that venous hypertension causes stasis dermatitis. *Phlebology.* 2011;26(8):361–365.

 SEE ALSO
- Varicose Veins
- Algorithm: Rash, Focal

 CODES

ICD10
- I83.10 Varicose veins of unsp lower extremity with inflammation
- I83.11 Varicose veins of right lower extremity with inflammation
- I83.12 Varicose veins of left lower extremity with inflammation

CLINICAL PEARLS
- Treatment of edema associated with stasis dermatitis via elevation and/or compression stockings is essential for optimal results.
- Pentoxifylline 1,200 mg daily and aspirin 300 mg daily improve venous ulcer healing.
- No difference in healing rate of venous stasis ulcers by use of hydrocolloid dressing versus simple non-adherent dressing when used beneath compression. Decision about the dressing should be based on local cost and patient or physician's preferences (7)[A].
- Mild topical corticosteroids reduce inflammation and itching; however, these may potentiate infection; high-potency topical corticosteroids should be avoided due to increased risk of atrophy and ulceration.

DIABETES MELLITUS, TYPE 1
Matthew C. Brown, MD • Courtney Dawley, DO

 BASICS

DESCRIPTION
- Type 1 diabetes mellitus (T1DM) is a chronic disease caused by pancreatic insufficiency (deficiency) of insulin production.
- Results in hyperglycemia and end-organ complications (e.g., accelerated atherosclerosis, neuropathy, nephropathy, and retinopathy)
- Features include the following:
  - Patients are insulinopenic and require insulin.
  - Polyphagia, polydipsia, and polyuria
  - Ketosis
  - Usually rapid onset
  - Body habitus: normal or thin physique
- System(s) affected: endocrine/metabolic

Pregnancy Considerations
- Hyperglycemia increases the incidence of congenital malformations. Tight control of blood sugar prior to conception (goal A1C <7%) is important (1).
- Women with microalbuminuria during the 1st trimester are at increased risk for preeclampsia and preterm delivery.
- A safe pregnancy is possible with vaginal delivery of a term baby. Close monitoring of blood sugar during labor is important.
- Many drugs used to treat diabetic complications are relatively/absolutely contraindicated in pregnancy.

EPIDEMIOLOGY
- Age of onset peaks between 5 and 7 years of age and again around puberty; rapid decline in incidence after adolescence.
- Slightly more common in males than females
- Overall incidence is increasing worldwide.
- More cases are diagnosed in the autumn and winter than in spring and summer.

Incidence
- 18/100,000 per year in the United States (0 to 60/100,000 worldwide) (2)
- Average lifetime prevalence risk of T1DM in the general population is 0.4%.
- Racial predilection for whites
- African Americans have lowest overall incidence.

Pediatric Considerations
- Although onset is usually before the age of 19 years, T1DM can occur for the first time in patients who are well into their 30s.
- Young children are more likely to present in diabetic ketoacidosis (DKA) due to atypical presentation and because they may not express thirst or obtain fluids as readily as older children or adults.

ETIOLOGY AND PATHOPHYSIOLOGY
- Genetic predisposition is thought to exist.
- Alteration in immunologic integrity, placing the β-cell at special risk for inflammatory damage
- Autoantibodies present in >90% of patients at presentation: glutamic acid decarboxylase (GAD), insulinoma-associated autoantigen 2 (IA2A), zinc transporter 8 (ZnT8A), and insulin (IAA) (2)

- Associated environmental triggers (none have been verified):
  - Vitamin D deficiency
  - Infant feeding practices (short-term breastfeeding, early exposure to complex proteins)
  - Viruses (e.g., enteroviruses, retroviruses)
  - Environmental toxins
- Various epigenetic modifications of gene expression (DNA methylation, histone modifications, and micro-RNA dysregulation) have been noted, further suggesting a role between genetics and environment in the development of T1DM (3).

Genetics
- T1DM is a polygenic disorder with 40+ loci known to affect susceptibility to the disease (2).
- Genes located on major histocompatibility complex (MHC) on chromosome 6 provide about half of the genetic susceptibility leading to T1DM risk (2).
- HLA class II shows the strongest association with T1DM risk, but class I MHCs also affect risk (2).

RISK FACTORS
- Certain human leukocyte antigen (HLA) types, MHC classes, and autoantibodies (2)
- Increased susceptibility to T1DM is inheritable (3):
  - Only 10–15% of newly diagnosed T1DM patients have a positive family history of T1DM.
  - Among autoimmune conditions, T1DM has the highest concordance rates in monozygotic twins.
  - Average prevalence risk of T1DM in children of patients with T1DM is ~6%.
  - Relative risk for siblings of patients with T1DM is about 15%.
- See environmental triggers above (2).

COMMONLY ASSOCIATED CONDITIONS
- Autoimmune diseases, such as celiac disease, vitamin B$_{12}$ deficiency, and hypothyroidism
- T1DM can also be seen as part of autoimmune polyendocrine syndromes.

 DIAGNOSIS

DIFFERENTIAL DIAGNOSIS
- Benign renal glycosuria
- Glucose intolerance
- Type 2 diabetes
- Consider monogenic diabetes if
  - Diabetes is diagnosed before 6 months of age.
  - Strong family history of diabetes without classic features of type 2 diabetes
  - Mild fasting hyperglycemia
  - Nonobese diabetic child with negative autoantibodies
- Secondary diabetes
  - Pancreatic disease (chronic pancreatitis, cystic fibrosis, hereditary hemochromatosis)
  - Endocrine-associated diabetes: acromegaly, Cushing syndrome, pheochromocytoma, glucagonoma, neuroendocrine tumors
  - Drug- or chemical-induced glucose intolerance: glucocorticosteroids, HIV protease inhibitors, atypical antipsychotics, tacrolimus, cyclosporine
- Acute poisonings (salicylate poisoning can cause hyperglycemia and glycosuria and may mimic DKA)

DIAGNOSTIC TESTS & INTERPRETATION
Initial Tests (lab, imaging)
- *Criteria for the diagnosis of diabetes (1)[C]:
  - Fasting glucose ≥126 mg/dL (7.0 mmol/L)
  - Random of ≥200 mg/dL (11.1 mmol/L) in a patient with classic symptoms of hyperglycemia
  - Oral glucose tolerance test; plasma glucose ≥200 mg/dL 2 hours after a glucose load of 1.75 g/kg (max dose 75 g)
  - Glycated hemoglobin (HbA1c) level ≥6.5%
  - *In the absence of unequivocal hyperglycemia, results should be confirmed by repeat testing.
- Other tests to consider:
  - Serum electrolytes, especially in sicker patients who may have ketoacidosis
  - Urinalysis for glucose, ketones, and microalbuminuria
  - Pancreatic autoantibodies
    ○ Islet cell, IAA, GAD, IA2A, and ZnT8A
  - CBC (WBC count and hemoglobin may be elevated)
- C-peptide insulin level if needed to differentiate from type 2 diabetes

Test Interpretation
Inflammatory changes, lymphocytic infiltration around the islets of Langerhans, or islet cell loss

HISTORY
- Polyuria and polydipsia (4)[C]
  - Polyuria may present as nocturia, bedwetting, or incontinence in a previously continent child.
  - Polyuria may be difficult to appreciate in diaper-clad children.
- Weight loss 10–30%
  - Often almost devoid of body fat at diagnosis due to hypovolemia and increased catabolism
- Prolonged or recurrent candidal infection, usually in the diaper area
- Increased fatigue, lethargy, muscle cramps
- Abdominal discomfort, nausea
- Vision changes, such as blurriness
- Altered school or work performance

 TREATMENT

GENERAL MEASURES
- Overall control of carbohydrate metabolism for all pediatric age ranges (1)[C]
  - Before meals, strive for blood glucose levels in range of 90 to 1,300 mg/dL (5.0 to 7.2 mmol/L)
  - Bedtime/overnight: 90 to 150 mg/dL (5.0 to 8.3 mmol/L)
  - A1c goal: <7.5% across all pediatric age groups
  - A1c <7.0% is reasonable if achieved without excessive hypoglycemia.
- Very tight control might be dangerous in young children due to risk of repeated hypoglycemia.
- Adult A1c goal: <7.0% (1)[B]
  - A1c <6.5% is reasonable in select individuals (1)[C].
  - Less stringent A1c goals (such as <8%) may be appropriate for others (1)[B].

- Normal growth and development and overall good health (asymptomatic) (4)[C]:
  - Reach optimal height for genetic potential.
  - Appropriate and timely pubertal maturation
  - Coping psychosocial development: normal school or work attendance and performance; normal goals/career plans. Screen children ≥10 years of age annually for depression.
- Prevent acute complications, including the following:
  - Hypoglycemic insulin reactions
  - Ketoacidosis
- Delay or prevent chronic end-organ complications

MEDICATION

- Most type 1 diabetes patients will require some form of insulin supplementation, either multiple-dose insulin injections or continuous subcutaneous insulin infusion (1)[A].

- Types of insulin (1)[C]:
  - Long-acting insulin analogues: insulin glargine (Lantus) and insulin detemir (Levemir). These should not be mixed with other insulins in the same syringe.
  - Intermediate-acting insulin (NPH)—Humulin N or Novolin N—can be mixed with other insulins
  - Short-acting (regular) insulin: Novolin R or Humulin R
  - Very rapid-acting insulin analogues: insulin lispro (Humalog), insulin aspart (Novolog), and insulin glulisine (Apidra)

First Line

- Flexible intensive insulin therapy is the gold standard.

- Multiple dose insulin (MDI) or continuous subcutaneous insulin infusion (CSII) have equal efficacy (1)[B].

- Total initial dose is 0.2 to 0.4 U/kg/day for insulin-naïve patients (will often need 0.6 to 0.7 U/kg/day).
- 40–60% of total dose given as basal insulin, with the rest as bolus insulin

- MDI regimen (1)[A],(5)[C]:

  - Basal, long-acting insulin once or twice a day
  - Prandial, short-acting insulin based on number of carbohydrate portions (e.g., 1:10, meaning 1 U of insulin for every 10 g of carbohydrate to be eaten)
  - Correctional short-acting mealtime insulin based on premeal blood glucose level (subtract target blood glucose level and divided by sensitivity factor)
  - Administration of the mealtime insulin before a meal may be more efficacious than during or after the meal.
- CSII regimen:
  - May use regular insulin or rapid-acting insulin analogues
  - Basal insulin is infused continuously at a preset rate, and bolus doses are given with meals as above.

Second Line

- Twice-daily injections with NPH along with regular or rapid-acting insulin
- Not physiologic, but lower cost and fewer injections may improve adherence in the less-motivated patient.

- Premixed insulin available as NPH/regular (Novolin or Humulin 70/30) or NPH/rapid-acting insulin (e.g., Novolog 75/25 Mix or Humulin 75/25 Mix) (5)[C]
- Pancreatic transplantation is usually reserved for patients with end-stage renal failure, who may receive kidney-pancreatic transplants at the same time.
- Oral hypoglycemics not indicated in type 1 diabetes (except in obese patients, who may have a combination of type 1 and type 2): Metformin (Glucophage)

INPATIENT CONSIDERATIONS

Newly diagnosed type 1 diabetics may require hospitalization during initiation of insulin therapy.

 ONGOING CARE

FOLLOW-UP RECOMMENDATIONS

- Normal; full participation in sports activities
- Regular aerobic exercise is recommended.

Patient Monitoring

- BP monitoring at every office visit. If elevated, consider an ACE inhibitor or an angiotensin receptor blocker; avoid in pregnancy (1)[C].
- Monitor height, weight, and sexual maturation (in children) (5)[C].
- Daily home blood glucose monitoring with home blood glucose meter: Blood tests should be done at least 4 to 6 times daily (more frequently in pump patients) for optimal monitoring.
- Quarterly measurement of HbA1c
- Annual screenings (1)[C]:
  - Microalbuminuria for earliest signs of possible nephropathy
  - Ophthalmology exam (after 3 to 5 years of diabetes, also depending on glycemic control); annually thereafter
  - Annual lipid profile, thyroid levels, blood chemistries, CBC
  - Annual influenza vaccine in patients ≥6 months of age
  - Pneumococcal polysaccharide vaccine to all patients ≥2 years
  - Hepatitis B vaccination to unvaccinated adults aged 19 to 59 years

DIET

- American Diabetic Association diet: http://www.diabetes.org/food-and-fitness/food/
- Carbohydrate counting using insulin-to-carbohydrate ratio with all meals and snacks; allows patient flexibility in eating and ability to eat almost anything

PROGNOSIS

- Initial remission or honeymoon phase with decreased insulin needs and easier control, usually 3 to 6 months
- Current prognosis for reduced life expectancy:
  - Increasing longevity and quality of life with careful blood glucose monitoring, improvement in insulin delivery regimens, and appropriate glycemic control

COMPLICATIONS

- Microvascular disease (retinopathy, nephropathy, neuropathy)
- Hyperlipidemia
- Macrovascular disease (coronary and cerebral artery disease)
- Chronic foot ulcers/amputations

- Hypoglycemia
- DKA
- Excessive weight gain
- Increased risk for preeclampsia and preterm delivery
- Driving mishaps
- Psychological problems of chronic disease

REFERENCES

1. American Diabetes Association. Standards of medical care in diabetes. *Diabetes Care*. 2015;38(Suppl 1): S77–S79.
2. Atkinson MA, Eisenbarth GS, Michels AW. Type 1 diabetes. *Lancet*. 2014;383(9911):69–82.
3. Stankov K, Benc D, Draskovic D. Genetic and epigenetic factors in etiology of diabetes mellitus type 1. *Pediatrics*. 2013;132(6):1112–1122.
4. Silverstein J, Klingensmith G, Copeland K, et al. Care of children and adolescents with type 1 diabetes: a statement of the American Diabetes Association. *Diabetes Care*. 2005;28(1):186–212.
5. Mooradian AD, Bernbaum M, Albert SG. Narrative review: a rational approach to starting insulin therapy. *Ann Intern Med*. 2006;145(2):125–134.

ADDITIONAL READING

- Cox DJ, Ford D, Gonder-Frederick L, et al. Driving mishaps among individuals with type 1 diabetes: a prospective study. *Diabetes Care*. 2009;32(12): 2177–2180.
- Gillett MJ. International Expert Committee report on the role of the A1c assay in the diagnosis of diabetes: Diabetes Care 2009;32(7):1327–1334. *Clin Biochem Rev*. 2009;30(4):197–200.
- Husebye ES, Anderson MS. Autoimmune polyendocrine syndromes: clues to type 1 diabetes pathogenesis. *Immunity*. 2010;32(4):479–487.

 SEE ALSO

Diabetes Mellitus, Type 2; Diabetic Ketoacidosis

 CODES

ICD10

- E10.9 Type 1 diabetes mellitus without complications
- E10.8 Type 1 diabetes mellitus with unspecified complications
- E10.69 Type 1 diabetes mellitus with other specified complication

CLINICAL PEARLS

- Polyuria may present as nocturia, bedwetting, or incontinence in a previously continent child.
- Young children are more likely to present in DKA because they may not express thirst or obtain fluids as readily as older children or adults.
- Onset usually before the age of 19 years, but type 1 diabetes can present in patients who are well into their 30s.

DIABETES MELLITUS, TYPE 2
Swathi A.N. Rao, MD • Sathya S. Krishnasamy, MD

 BASICS

DESCRIPTION
- Can manifest as nonketotic hyperglycemia and is due to a progressive insulin secretory defect in the setting of insulin resistance
- Significant contributing factor to blindness, renal failure, and lower limb amputations

Geriatric Considerations
Monitor elderly for hypoglycemia; adjust doses for renal/hepatic dysfunction and cognitive function.

Pediatric Considerations
Incidence is increasing and parallels weight gain.

Pregnancy Considerations
First-line drug is insulin (class B), but metformin and glyburide are alternatives that do not cause adverse effects in some females (1,2)[A].

EPIDEMIOLOGY
Incidence
1.7 million new diagnoses/year in 2012

Prevalence
- In 2012, 29.1 million Americans or 9.3% of the population had DM; men and women equally affected
- 7.6% of non-Hispanic Caucasians, 12.8% of Hispanics, 13.2% of non-Hispanic African Americans, 9% of Asian Americans, and 15.9% of Native Americans

ETIOLOGY AND PATHOPHYSIOLOGY
- Peripheral insulin resistance, defective insulin secretion, increased gluconeogenesis, altered gut microbiome. Genetic factors: monogenic (e.g., *PPARγ* and insulin gene mutations) and polygenic
- Obesity, hemochromatosis
- Drug- or chemical-induced (e.g., glucocorticoids, highly active antiretroviral therapy [HAART], atypical antipsychotics, posttransplant immunosuppressants)

Genetics
50% concordance in monozygotic twins

RISK FACTORS
- Family hx of DM in first-degree relative, genetic factors, ethnicity (African American, Latino, Native American, Asian, and Pacific Islander)
- Gestational diabetes or history of baby with birth weight ≥4 kg (9 lb), PCOS, obesity (BMI ≥25 kg/m²) and visceral adiposity, hypertriglyceridemia or low high-density lipoprotein, sedentary lifestyle, impaired fasting glucose (IFG)/impaired glucose tolerance (IGT)/metabolic syndrome (1)[A]

GENERAL PREVENTION
Weight loss of 5–10% body weight, exercise 150 minutes/week, decrease in fat and caloric intake. Follow USDA dietary recommendation of 14 g fiber/1,000 kcal; metformin, acarbose, or TZDs in high-risk prediabetics with cardiovascular risk factors (1)[A]

COMMONLY ASSOCIATED CONDITIONS
Hypertension, hyperlipidemia, metabolic syndrome, fatty liver disease, infertility, PCOS, acanthosis nigricans (1)[A]

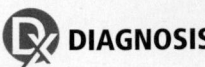 **DIAGNOSIS**

HISTORY
Polyuria, polydipsia, polyphagia, weight loss, weakness, fatigue, blurry vision, and frequent infections

PHYSICAL EXAM
BMI, funduscopic exam, oral exam, cardiopulmonary exam, abdominal exam for hepatomegaly, focused neurologic exam, and diabetic foot exam

DIFFERENTIAL DIAGNOSIS
- Type 1 DM
- Cushing syndrome, acromegaly, and glucagonoma

DIAGNOSTIC TESTS & INTERPRETATION
Initial Tests (lab, imaging)
Criteria for diagnosis
- HbA1c ≥6.5% is diagnostic.
- Hyperglycemic crisis + random plasma glucose ≥200 mg/dL (11.1 mmol/L) *or*
- Fasting plasma glucose (FPG) ≥126 mg/dL (7.0 mmol/L) *or*
- 2-hour postprandial plasma glucose ≥200 mg/dL (11.1 mmol/L) after a 75-g glucose load after overnight fast of at least 8 hours

- If equivocal, repeat testing (1,3)[A].

Follow-Up Tests & Special Considerations
Screen patients with history of gestational diabetes for persistent diabetes/prediabetes 6 to 12 weeks postpartum with OGTT, 1 year postpartum, and at least every 3 years thereafter (2,3)[A].

 TREATMENT

- Use an individualized, patient-centered approach with attention to cost, comorbidities, and compliance.
- A1C targets
  - A1C ≤6.5%: for nonpregnant adults with long life expectancy, no cardiovascular disease, DM for a short duration, and no hx of hypoglycemia. If not achievable safely, <7.0% (1,3)[A].
  - For those with a limited life expectancy, advanced micro- or macrovascular complications, extensive comorbidities, and history of hypoglycemia or long-standing DM goal A1C of 7–8% per AACE, <8% per ADA (1,3)[A]
  - Individualized goals for high glycators/variation in hemoglobin glycation index (4)[A]
- FPG goal is <110 mg/dL (5.5 mmol/L) and 2-hour postprandial goal is <140 mg/dL (1)[A]. Per ADA, recommended 2-hour postprandial goal: 80 to 130 mg/dL and peak postprandial glucose <180 mg/dL (1)[A]

- General approach
  - Individualized medical nutrition therapy by certified nutritionist and individualized exercise regimen with at least 150 minutes of moderate-intensity exercise per week
  - If A1C is <7.5%, oral monotherapy in the form of biguanides, GLP-1 receptor agonist, DPP-4 inhibitor, SGLT2 inhibitor, or α–glucosidase inhibitor. Consider TZD, glinide, or sulfonylureas but with caution due to side effects.
  - If 7.5% < A1C <9.0%, metformin plus second medication, ideally weight-neutral or weight loss-promoting with low risk of hypoglycemia
  - If A1C ≥9.0%, initiate insulin alone or in combination with oral agents (1)[A].

GENERAL MEASURES
- Comprehensive diabetic foot exam annually (3)[A].
- Nephropathy: annual urine microalbumin to creatinine ratio and eGFR or albumin excretion rate (1,3)[A]

- Retinopathy: dilated fundoscopic exam by ophthalmologist at diagnosis and every 2 years if normal, otherwise annually (3)[A]
- If 40 to 75 years old, begin a statin—moderate intensity for low-risk and high-intensity statin if ≥7.5% ASCVD risk (3,5)[A].
- Low-dose aspirin for all adults with CVD risk unless contraindicated.
- Hypertension: goal BP <130/80 mm Hg (SBP <120 mm Hg preferred if tolerated). ACE inhibitor/ARB first-line antihypertensives (3)[A]
- Vaccination: Follow CDC recommendations (1,3)[A]. Limit protein intake to 0.8 to 1 g/kg body weight/day for diabetics with early stages of CKD and to 1 g/kg body weight/day for those with advanced CKD (1,3)[A].

PATIENT EDUCATION
Diabetes self-management education and support by certified diabetes educator (1,3)[A].

MEDICATIONS
First Line
- Biguanides
  - Metformin (Glucophage, Fortamet, Riomet, Glumetza): preferred first medication. Promotes weight loss and improves insulin resistance. Dosage: 500 to 2,000 mg in divided doses or ER 1,000 to 2,000 mg every evening. Maximum effective dose 2,000 mg/day
  - Avoid metformin and combination drugs containing metformin in renal insufficiency, prior to radiocontrast agent use, surgery, and severe acute illnesses (e.g., liver disease, cardiogenic shock, pancreatitis, hypoxia) due to increased risk of lactic acidosis.
  - Caution with acute heart failure, alcohol abuse, elderly (can merge with previous bullet)
  - Associated with GI side effects, vitamin B_{12} deficiency (3)[A].
- Dipeptidyl peptidase-4 inhibitors
  - Weight neutral with minimal risk for hypoglycemia; dose adjustments in renal function decline with exception of linagliptin
  - Sitagliptin (Januvia): 100 mg/day
  - Saxagliptin (Onglyza): 2.5 mg/day, maximum 5 mg/day
  - Linagliptin (Tradjenta): 5 mg/day
  - Alogliptin (Nesina) 25 mg/day. Significant interactions with metformin (3)[A]
  - Linagliptin/metformin (Jentadueto): 2.5/500 mg PO BID, maximum 2.5/1,000 mg PO BID (3)[A]
- Sulfonylureas
  - Caution with renal or liver disease, sulfa allergy, creatinine clearance <50 mL/min, elderly, pregnancy
  - Glipizide (Glucotrol): 2.5 to 40 mg/day. Dosage >10 mg/day given BID 30 minutes before meals
  - Glipizide extended-release: 5 to 20 mg/day
  - Glyburide (DiaBeta, Glynase, Micronase): 1.25 to 20 mg/day, Glynase 0.75 to 12 mg/day
  - Glimepiride (Amaryl): 1 to 8 mg/day (3)[A]
  - Drugs that may potentiate effects of sulfonylureas: salicylates, clofibrate, warfarin (Coumadin), ethanol, and ACE inhibitors
- Thiazolidinediones
  - Obtain baseline liver function tests: if abnormal, use with caution. Contraindicated in patients with NYHA Class III or IV heart failure.
  - Pioglitazone (Actos): 15 to 45 mg/day

– Cumulative use of pioglitazone or rosiglitazone was not associated with the incidence of bladder cancer in a large, pooled multipopulation analysis (6)[A].

– Duetact (pioglitazone hydrochloride and glimepiride): 30/2 mg PO daily with meal
– Rosiglitazone (Avandia): 4 to 8 mg/day

Second Line

- Insulin: rapid (aspart, lispro, glulisine); short (regular insulin); intermediate (neutral protamine hagedorn); long-acting (glargine, detemir); premixed (several types)
  – May be used in combination with certain oral agents. Combination basal/bolus insulin may be used (0.5 to 2 U/kg/day) after failure of oral agents.
  – Long-acting insulins have lower risk of hypoglycemia than short-acting insulin.
  – Insulin detemir (Levemir) or insulin glargine (Lantus): 10 units (or 0.1 to 0.2 units/kg) once daily in the evening or 2 divided doses (already mentioned). Onset of action 1 hour. No peak. Duration of action is 16 to 23 hours.

  – Human insulin inhalation powder (Afrezza): given as a single inhalation before a meal, in combination with long-acting insulin; contraindicated in chronic lung disease; can cause edema when given with TZDs (3)[B]
  – Concentrated human regular insulin (U-500) Eli Lilly: used for extreme insulin resistance (7)[B]
  – Toujeo Solostar pen (glargine U300) Sanofi-Aventis: used for insulin resistant patients. Improvement in nocturnal hypoglycemia compared to U100 glargine (8)[A]. Consider insulin pump therapy and V-Go in select patients (3)[A].

- Amylinomimetic
  – Pramlintide (Symlin): 60 to 120 μg SC before every major meal
  – Prandial insulins (short-acting/rapid-acting) should be reduced by 50% if pramlintide is initiated to avoid hypoglycemia.

  – Avoid anticholinergics that slow intestinal absorption of nutrients (3)[A].

- GLP-1 (glucagonlike peptide-1) receptor agonist (incretins)
  – Exenatide (Byetta): 5 to 10 μg SC BID within 60 minutes before meals and at least 6 hours apart. Extended-release formulation (Bydureon): 2 mg SC weekly
  – Liraglutide (Victoza): 0.6 mg/day SC for 1 week, then increase to 1.2, maximum 1.8 mg/day. Less expensive and better tolerated than exenatide; contraindicated in patients with personal or family history of medullary thyroid cancer or (MEN) type 2 (black box warning).
  – Liraglutide (Saxenda): 3 mg SC daily approved for treatment of obesity.
  – Albiglutide (Tanzeum): 30 to 50 mg SC qwk in a single-dose pen
  – Dulaglutide (Trulicity) 0.75 to 1.5 mg weekly: 2 mg/wk

  – Associated increased risk of acute pancreatitis with GLP-1 agonists and DPP4 inhibitors and caution with use in CKD ≥ stage 4. GLP-1 analogs and Symlin require insulin adjustment and may exacerbate gastroparesis (3,9)[A].

- α-Glucosidase inhibitors
  – Acarbose (Precose): 25 to 100 mg TID
  – Miglitol (Glyset): 25 to 100 mg TID
  – Take at beginning of meals to decrease postprandial hyperglycemia.
  – Avoid in renal insufficiency and bowel diseases.

  – Drug binders, such as cholestyramine resin, should be taken at least 2 hours apart from α-glucosidase inhibitors (3)[A].

- Meglitinides
  – Repaglinide (Prandin): 0.5 to 4 mg before meals; may be useful in patients with sulfa allergy or renal impairment
- Diphenylalanine derivatives
  – Nateglinide (Starlix): 60 to 120 mg before meals TID (3)[A]
- Bile acid sequestrants
  – Colesevelam: 3.75 g/day or 1.875 g BID (3)[A]
- Dopamine-2 agonists
  – Bromocriptine mesylate immediate release (Cycloset): 0.8 to 1.6 mg/day within 2 hours of awakening

  – Alters hypothalamic regulation of metabolism and reduces hepatic gluconeogenesis (10)[A].
  – May cause dizziness, nausea, fatigue, rhinitis (3)[A]
- SGLT2 inhibitors
  – Inhibits glucose reabsorption by sodium glucose cotransporter-2 inhibition
  – Canagliflozin (Invokana):100 to 300 mg single dose before breakfast; adjust dose with renal function decline
  – Dapagliflozin (Farxiga): 5 to 10 mg daily; avoid use if eGFR <60
  – Empagliflozin (Jardiance): 10 to 25 mg daily; avoid use if eGFR <45
  – Xigduo (dapagliflozin-metformin): 5/100, 10/1,000 mg PO daily

  – May cause hypotension, genital mycotic infections, UTI, impairment of renal function, electrolyte abnormalities, elevated LDL, and DKA and increased fracture risk (canagliflozin) (3)[A]

- Drug interactions: Thiazides cause IGT and fluoroquinolones can cause hyper- and hypoglycemia.

SURGERY/OTHER PROCEDURES

For patients with BMI >35 m^2/kg, consider bariatric surgery (11)[B].

COMPLEMENTARY & ALTERNATIVE MEDICINE

Cinnamon may improve glycemic control, with improvements in A1C and FBG (12)[B].

 ONGOING CARE

FOLLOW-UP RECOMMENDATIONS

Patient Monitoring

- Office visit frequency per physician discretion, use telemedicine/mobile communications and home BG monitoring.
- Monitor glucose, HbA1c, BP, body weight, lipid profile, and renal and liver function.
- A1c twice a year for patients with well-controlled blood glucose and quarterly for patients with hyperglycemia or recent changes in therapy
- Consider CGM as clinically indicated.

PROGNOSIS

There is evidence that intensive glycemic control in newly diagnosed diabetics may reduce long-term CVD rates.

COMPLICATIONS

- Emergencies: hyperosmolar coma, DKA, hypoglycemia
- CVD: CAD, PVD, stroke; microvascular: peripheral neuropathy, proliferative retinopathy, nephropathy, erectile dysfunction, and CKD; ophthalmic: blindness, cataracts, glaucoma, retinopathy; GI: NAFLD, gastroparesis, diarrhea; neurologic: autonomic dysfunction; foot ulcers and soft tissue infections

REFERENCES

1. Handelsman Y, Bloomgarden ZT, Grunberger G, et al. American association of clinical endocrinologists and american college of endocrinology: clinical practice guidelines for developing a diabetes mellitus comprehensive care plan—2015. *Endocr Pract*. 2015;21(Suppl 1):1–87.
2. Metzger BE, Buchanan TA, Coustan DR, et al. Summary and recommendations of the Fifth International Workshop-Conference on Gestational Diabetes Mellitus. *Diabetes Care*. 2007;30 (Suppl 2):S251–S260.
3. Standards of medical care in diabetes—2015: summary of revisions. *Diabetes Care*. 2015;38(Suppl):S4.
4. Hempe JM, Liu S, Myers L, et al. The hemoglobin glycation index identifies subpopulations with harms or benefits from intensive treatment in the ACCORD trial. *Diabetes Care*. 2015;38(6):1067–1074.
5. Stone NJ, Robinson JG, Lichtenstein AH, et al. 2013 ACC/AHA guideline on the treatment of blood cholesterol to reduce atherosclerotic cardiovascular risk in adults: a report of the American College of Cardiology/American Heart Association Task Force on Practice Guidelines. *Circulation*. 2014;129(25)(Suppl 2):S1–S45.
6. Levin D, Bell S, Sund R, et al. Pioglitazone and bladder cancer risk: a multipopulation pooled, cumulative exposure analysis. *Diabetologia*. 2015;58(3):493–504.
7. Boldo A, Comi RJ. Clinical experience with U500 insulin: risks and benefits. *Endocr Pract*. 2012;18(1):56–61.
8. Ritzel R, Roussel R, Bolli GB, et al. Patient-level meta-analysis of the EDITION 1, 2 and 3: glycaemic control and hypoglycaemia with new insulin glargine 300 U/ml versus glargine 100 U/ml in people with type 2 diabetes. *Diabetes Obes Metab*. 2015;17(9):859–867.
9. Fakhoury WK, Lereun C, Wright D. A meta-analysis of placebo-controlled clinical trials assessing the efficacy and safety of incretin-based medications in patients with type 2 diabetes. *Pharmacology*. 2010;86(1):44–57.
10. Defronzo RA. Bromocriptine: a sympatholytic, d2-dopamine agonist for the treatment of type 2 diabetes. *Diabetes Care*. 2011;34(4):789–794.
11. Schauer PR, Kashyap SR, Wolski K, et al. Bariatric surgery versus intensive medical therapy in obese patients with diabetes. *N Engl J Med*. 2012;366(17):1567–1576.
12. Akilen R, Tsiami A, Devendra D, et al. Cinnamon in glycaemic control: systematic review and meta analysis. *Clin Nutr*. 2012;31(5):609–615.

 SEE ALSO

- Diabetes Mellitus, Type 1; Diabetic Ketoacidosis; Hypertension, Essential
- Algorithm: Type 2 Diabetes, Treatment

CODES

ICD10

- E11.9 Type 2 diabetes mellitus without complications
- E11.319 Type 2 diabetes mellitus with unspecified diabetic retinopathy without macular edema
- E11.21 Type 2 diabetes mellitus with diabetic nephropathy

CLINICAL PEARLS

Individualized, patient-centered approach to management.

DIABETIC KETOACIDOSIS

Melanie J. Lippmann, MD

 BASICS

DESCRIPTION
- A life-threatening medical emergency in diabetics secondary to severe insulin deficiency and characterized by hyperglycemia, ketosis, and metabolic acidosis
- System(s) affected: endocrine/metabolic

EPIDEMIOLOGY
Incidence
- In the United States: 46 episodes/10,000 diabetics; 2/100 patient-years of type 1 diabetes mellitus (DM) (1)
- Predominant age: 19 to 44 years (56%) and 45 to 65 years (24%); only 18% are <20 years.

ETIOLOGY AND PATHOPHYSIOLOGY
A deficiency of insulin, exacerbated by an increase in counterregulatory hormones (e.g., catecholamines, cortisol, glucagon, and growth hormone) leading to a hyperglycemic crisis, osmotic diuresis, ketosis with metabolic acidosis, and frequently accompanied by electrolyte disturbances
- Noncompliance/insufficient insulin: 25%
- Infection: 30–40%
- First presentation of DM: 10–25%
- Myocardial infarction (MI): 5–7%
- No cause identified: 10–30%
- Cerebrovascular accident (CVA)
- Medications (corticosteroids, sympathomimetics, atypical antipsychotics)
- Illicit drugs (cocaine)
- Trauma
- Surgery
- Emotional stress
- Pregnancy

RISK FACTORS
- Type 1 > type 2 DM
- Younger patients at higher risk

GENERAL PREVENTION
- Close monitoring of glucose during periods of stress, infection, and trauma
- Careful insulin control and regular monitoring of blood glucose levels
- "Sick day" management instructions

COMMONLY ASSOCIATED CONDITIONS
Complications of chronic (and poorly controlled) DM such as nephropathy, neuropathy, and retinopathy

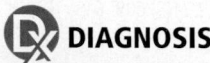 **DIAGNOSIS**

HISTORY
- Recent illness, injury, or surgery
- Changes in diet or medications
- Missed insulin doses/noncompliance or failure of insulin pump
- Weight loss in patients recently diagnosed with type 1 DM
- Polyuria, nocturia
- Polydipsia, polyphagia
- Generalized weakness
- Malaise, fatigue, lethargy
- Anorexia or increased appetite
- Nausea, vomiting
- Abdominal pain
- Decreased perspiration
- Fever

PHYSICAL EXAM
- Hypotension
- Tachycardia
- Hypothermia or fever
- Tachypnea, Kussmaul respirations
- Fruity odor of ketotic breath (acetone smell)
- Decreased reflexes
- Abdominal tenderness, decreased bowel sounds
- Dry mucous membranes, poor skin turgor
- Decreased perspiration
- Altered mental status
- Coma

DIFFERENTIAL DIAGNOSIS
- Hyperosmolar hyperglycemic crisis
- Alcoholic ketoacidosis
- Starvation ketosis
- Toxic ingestions (e.g., salicylates, methanol)
- Lactic acidosis
- Uremia/chronic renal failure
- Sepsis
- Acute pancreatitis

DIAGNOSTIC TESTS & INTERPRETATION
- ECG
  - Usually shows sinus tachycardia
  - Changes consistent with electrolyte abnormalities
  - Ischemia/MI as a precipitating factor
- Urine and blood cultures
- Consider lumbar puncture (meningitis).
- Chest x-ray to rule out possible infectious etiology

Initial Tests (lab, imaging)

ALERT
- Diagnostic criteria (1)[C]:
  - Hyperglycemia (glucose usually 250 to 800 mg/dL)
  - Low HCO_3 (usually ≤18 mEq/L)
  - Metabolic acidosis on arterial blood gases (pH <7.3)
  - Anion gap = serum sodium − (serum chloride + bicarbonate), >10 mmol
- Other important labs:
  - Serum ketosis: Check β-hydroxybutyrate (β-HB) instead of ketones to evaluate ketosis (2)[B]. β-HB is the predominant ketone produced and is preferred over serum ketones. β-HB >3 mg/dL is abnormal and should be decreased to <1.5 mg/dL within 12 to 24 hours (3)[B].
  - Urine ketosis (urinalysis [UA]) may only identify acetoacetate and not β-HB.
  - Glycosuria
  - Hyperamylasemia, hyperlipasemia
  - Hypertriglyceridemia/hypercholesterolemia
  - Increased creatinine and BUN: Markedly increased serum ketones may cross-react and cause a falsely high serum creatinine.
  - Pseudohyponatremia: Hyperglycemia or hypertriglyceridemia may cause an artificially low sodium concentration. The measured sodium is suppressed by 1.6 mg/dL for every 100 mg/dL of glucose over 100 mg/dL.
  - Decreased calculated total body K⁺: Severe acidosis gives an artificially high K⁺ level.
  - Increased serum osmolality (mOsm/kg) = [2 × serum Na (mEq/L) + glucose (mg/dL)/18 + BUN (mg/dL)/2.8]; if calculated osmolality <320 mOsm/kg, consider etiologies other than diabetic ketoacidosis (DKA)
  - Elevated base deficit
  - A1C helps determine history of diabetic control.

- CBC, electrolytes, BUN, creatinine
- Serum β-HB or ketones
- Arterial blood gases (ABGs); venous blood gases (VBGs) may also be used (VBG pH correlates with 0.03 lower than ABG pH).
- Chest x-ray to rule out pulmonary infection
- Head CT scan if suspected CVA or cerebral edema
- If necessary, cardiac enzymes and blood cultures

Diagnostic Procedures/Other
Only if surgical problem is the underlying precipitant (e.g., appendicitis, cholecystitis)

 TREATMENT

- Oxygen and airway management, as needed
- Establish IV access.
- Cardiac monitoring
- Start isotonic crystalloid solution (0.9% saline).
- Fingerstick glucose testing

GENERAL MEASURES
- All but mild cases require inpatient management.
- Severe DKA requires an ICU setting.
- Goals
  - Fluid resuscitation
  - Insulin therapy to normalize serum glucose
  - Resolution of anion gap acidosis
  - Correction of electrolytes
- Identify and treat the precipitating cause (e.g., infection, MI)
- Laboratory testing during management:
  - Serum glucose q1–2h until stable
  - Electrolytes, phosphorus, and venous pH q2–6h as needed

MEDICATION
First Line
- Insulin (1)[C]
  - Bolus 0.1 U/kg IV then continuous infusion at 0.1 U/kg/hr (do not use initial insulin bolus in children)
  - If without bolus, 0.14 U/kg/hr continuous infusion (4)
  - Aim for rate of serum glucose decline of 100 mg/dL/hr
  - When glucose 200 mg/dL, reduce infusion to 0.02 to 0.05 U/kg/hr IV or give rapid-acting insulin at 0.1 U/kg SC q2h; goal glucose is 150 to 200 mg/dL.
  - Overlap and continue IV insulin infusion for 1 to 2 hours after SC insulin is initiated.
- IV fluids to correct dehydration: Start with 0.9% NaCl bolus, calculate corrected sodium; if serum Na⁺ is high, consider 0.45% NaCl to replace free fluid loss or when adding potassium replacement.
  - When glucose is 200 mg/dL, change to 5% dextrose with 0.45% NaCl at 150 to 250 mL/hr.
- Potassium: falsely elevated due to acidosis; when K⁺ ≤5.2 mg/dL and if urine output is adequate, start replacement with 20 to 30 mEq/L of K⁺ in 1 L IV fluids (1).
  - Hold insulin if K⁺ ≤3.3 mg/dL; give IV potassium 20 to 30 mEq/hr with fluids until >3.3 mg/dL to prevent cardiac arrhythmia (class III).
  - For each 0.1 unit of pH, serum K⁺ will change by ~0.6 mEq in opposite direction.

- Phosphorus: Routine replacement may lead to hypocalcemia; if very low (<1.0), give 20 to 30 mEq/L of K-Phos in fluids.

- Sodium bicarbonate: no demonstrable benefit with a pH >7.0 (2,5)[B]; rehydration usually leads to resolution of acidosis. Guidelines recommend its use with pH <6.9 or in patients with life-threatening hyperkalemia; however, there is evidence that it may increase cerebral edema, especially in children (6)[A].

- Magnesium: If Mg ≤1.8 mg/dL and the patient is symptomatic, consider replacement.
- Precautions
  - If the patient is on an insulin pump, it should be stopped.
  - If glucose does not fall by 10% in 1st hour, give regular insulin 0.14 U/kg IV bolus, then continuous infusion at previous rate.
  - If using bicarbonate, add 100 mmol or 2 ampules of sodium bicarbonate to 400 mL isotonic solution with 20 mEq KCL over 200 mL/hr for 2 hours until venous pH is >7.0, then stop infusion (1).

Second Line
Insulin, SC or IM: Load with 0.3 U/kg SC, followed by 0.1 U/kg/hr; space dosing to q2h once glucose <250 mg/dL; in uncomplicated DKA, may be safe and cost effective (7)[B]

Pediatric Considerations
- Children with moderate to severe DKA should be transferred to the nearest pediatric critical care hospital.
- Cerebral edema is a rare complication (~ 1%) but has a mortality of 20–50%:
  - Diagnostic criteria exist for diagnosis; CT may rule out alternative diagnoses (8).
  - Treat with IV bolus of mannitol 1 g/kg in 20% solution, reduce IV fluid rate, and consider hypertonic 3% saline (9).

Geriatric Considerations
Must be careful with impaired renal function or congestive heart failure when correcting fluid and electrolyte abnormalities

Pregnancy Considerations
- Pregnancy itself is diabetogenic and also results in a compensated respiratory alkalosis (HCO_3 19 to 20 mEq/L) with theoretically reduced buffering capacity
- Pregnant women are more susceptible to DKA.
- Euglycemic DKA
- Increased risk of preeclampsia and fetal death
- β-Tocolytics and corticosteroids can trigger DKA.
- Perinatal death: 9–35%

INPATIENT CONSIDERATIONS
Admission Criteria/Initial Stabilization
ADA admission guidelines: blood glucose >250 mg/dL; pH <7.3; HCO_3 ≤15 mEq/L; ketones in urine; ICU setting for severe DKA (10)

IV Fluids
- 1 to 1.5 L over the 1st hour, then, if serum corrected Na is high or normal, give 0.45% NaCl at 250 to 500 mL/hr depending on hydration state.
- Switch to 5% dextrose in 0.45% saline at maintenance rate when serum glucose <200 mg/dL; maintain blood glucose between 150 and 250 mg/dL.

- Overly rapid correction of fluid balance may precipitate cerebral edema (2)[C]; if the blood glucose level is falling too rapidly, consider using a 10% dextrose solution instead.

Pediatric Considerations
Bolus 10 to 20 mL/kg initially; 4-hour fluid total should be <50 mL/kg to reduce chance of cerebral edema.

Discharge Criteria
- Discharge when DKA has resolved: anion gap <12, glucose <200 mg/dL; pH >7.3; bicarbonate >18 mEq/L; additionally, patients must be tolerating PO intake and able to resume home medication regimen.
- Underlying precipitant (e.g., infection) must be identified and treated.

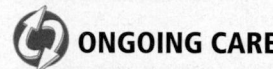

ONGOING CARE

FOLLOW-UP RECOMMENDATIONS
Patient Monitoring
- Monitor mental status, vital signs, and urine output q30–60min until improved, then q2–4h.
- Monitor blood sugar q1h until <200 mg/dL, then q2–6h.
- Monitor electrolytes, BUN, venous pH, and creatinine q2–4h.

DIET
- NPO initially
- Advance to preketotic diet when nausea and vomiting are controlled.
- Avoid foods with high glycemic index (e.g., soft drinks, fruit juice, white bread, etc.).

PROGNOSIS
- 16% of all diabetes-related fatalities
- Overall DKA mortality of 0.5–2%..
- In children <10 years of age, DKA causes 70% of diabetes-related fatalities.

COMPLICATIONS
- Cerebral edema (most common cause of death in children with DKA)
- Pulmonary edema
- Vascular thrombosis
- Hypokalemia
- Hypophosphatemia
- Cardiac dysrhythmia (secondary to hypokalemia or acidosis)
- MI, myocardial injury
- Acute gastric dilatation
- Late hypoglycemia (secondary to treatment)
- Erosive gastritis
- Infection, mucormycosis
- Respiratory distress

REFERENCES

1. Kitabchi AE, Umpierrez GE, Miles JM, et al. Hyperglycemic crises in adult patients with diabetes. *Diabetes Care.* 2009;32(7):1335–1343.
2. Agus MS, Wolfsdorf JI. Diabetic ketoacidosis in children. *Pediatr Clin North Am.* 2005;52(4):1147–1163.

---

3. Trachtenbarg DE. Diabetic ketoacidosis. *Am Fam Physician.* 2005;71(9):1705–1714.
4. Kitabchi AE, Murphy MB, Spencer J, et al. Is a priming dose of insulin necessary in a low-dose insulin protocol for the treatment of diabetic ketoacidosis? *Diabetes Care.* 2008;31(11):2081–2085.
5. Kitabchi AE, Umpierrez GE, Murphy MB, et al. Hyperglycemic crises in diabetes. *Diabetes Care.* 2004;27(Suppl 1):S94–S102.
6. Chua HR, Schneider A, Bellomo R. Bicarbonate in diabetic ketoacidosis—a systematic review. *Ann Intensive Care.* 2011;1(1):23.
7. Umpierrez GE, Latif K, Stoever J, et al. Efficacy of subcutaneous insulin lispro versus continuous intravenous regular insulin for the treatment of patients with diabetic ketoacidosis. *Am J Med.* 2004;117(5):291–296.
8. Watts W, Edge JA. How can cerebral edema during treatment of diabetic ketoacidosis be avoided? *Pediatr Diabetes.* 2014;15(4):271–276.
9. Brown TB. Cerebral oedema in childhood diabetic ketoacidosis: is treatment a factor? *Emerg Med J.* 2004;21(2):141–144.
10. American Diabetes Association. Hospital admission guidelines for diabetes. *Diabetes Care.* 2004;27(Suppl 1):S103.

ADDITIONAL READING
- American Diabetes Association. Standards of medical care in diabetes—2013. *Diabetes Care.* 2013;36(Suppl 1):S11–S66.
- Sheikh-Ali M, Karon BS, Basu A, et al. Can serum beta-hydroxybutyrate be used to diagnose diabetic ketoacidosis? *Diabetes Care.* 2008;31(4):643–647.

 SEE ALSO

Diabetes Mellitus, Type 1

 CODES

ICD10 .
- E10.10 Type 1 diabetes mellitus with ketoacidosis without coma
- E13.10 Oth diabetes mellitus with ketoacidosis without coma
- E10.11 Type 1 diabetes mellitus with ketoacidosis with coma

CLINICAL PEARLS
- Admit if blood glucose >250 mg/dL, pH <7.3, HCO_3 ≤15 mEq/L, and ketones in urine.
- Potassium is falsely elevated due to acidosis; start replacement when K^+ ≤5.2 mg/dL and urine output is adequate.

DIABETIC POLYNEUROPATHY

Samir Malkani, MD, MRCP–UK

 BASICS

DESCRIPTION
Peripheral nerve dysfunction seen in diabetes; several patterns described (1):
- Symmetric polyneuropathy
  - Distal sensory or sensorimotor
  - Proximal lower extremity polyneuropathy
- Focal and multifocal neuropathy
  - Cranial neuropathy
  - Focal limb or truncal neuropathy
  - Radiculoplexus neuropathy (diabetic amyotrophy)
- Acute painful small fiber neuropathy
- Autonomic neuropathies
- Chronic inflammatory demyelinating polyneuropathy (CIDP)

EPIDEMIOLOGY
Prevalence
- Generalized polyneuropathy
  - 10% at diabetes diagnosis
  - 50% at 25 years
  - Cross-sectional prevalence: 15% by symptoms; 50% by nerve conduction
- Autonomic neuropathy: 16.7% in a United Kingdom study

ETIOLOGY AND PATHOPHYSIOLOGY
- Metabolic derangement due to hyperglycemia
  - Aldose reductase converts excess glucose to sorbitol, which causes nerve damage.
  - Nonenzymatic glycation of neural proteins and lipids forms damaging advanced glycosylation end products.
  - Protein kinase C activation causes vascular endothelial changes.
  - Oxidative stress from excessive production of reactive oxygen species
  - Cyclo-oxygenase 2 and poly (ADP ribose) polymerase activation
- Vasculopathy causing nerve ischemia: predominant factor in mononeuropathies

RISK FACTORS
- Poor glycemic control
- Duration of diabetes
- Hypertension
- Hyperlipidemia
- Alcohol consumption

GENERAL PREVENTION
Maintenance of normal blood sugar

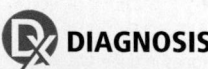 **DIAGNOSIS**

HISTORY
- Most common form (typical): symmetric distal sensory or sensorimotor polyneuropathy
  - Distressing numbness, tingling, pain of legs/feet, usually worse at night; allodynia; hyperalgesia
  - Sometimes silent sensory loss, patient unaware
  - Ataxia due to proprioceptive loss
  - Neuropathic foot ulcers due to analgesia and repetitive injury
  - Neuropathic degeneration of foot joints
  - Hands involved late
  - Distal muscle involvement, usually mild
- Symmetric proximal polyneuropathy
  - Proximal leg weakness and wasting
  - Muscles of shoulder girdle rarely involved
  - Pain and sensory changes less prominent
- Focal cranial or limb mononeuropathy
  - May involve 3rd, 4th, 6th, or 7th cranial nerve
  - Femoral, sciatic, or peroneal neuropathy: weakness or pain in nerve distribution
  - Any major peripheral nerve can be involved.
- Truncal neuropathies: painful radiculopathy over dermatomes
- Lumbar radiculoplexus neuropathy (diabetic amyotrophy)
  - Unilateral hip, thigh pain
  - Pelvic girdle and thigh weakness with atrophy
  - Recovery over months
- Diabetic autonomic neuropathy
  - GI: nocturnal diarrhea, sometimes alternating with constipation; gastroparesis with postprandial fullness; nausea and vomiting
  - Cardiovascular: postural dizziness, exercise intolerance
  - Urogenital: urinary hesitancy, overflow incontinence; erectile dysfunction; vaginal dryness; sexual dysfunction
  - Sudomotor: anhidrosis or hyperhidrosis; gustatory sweating of head and upper body
- CIDP: progressive, severe motor loss
- Diabetic cachexia: painful small fiber neuropathy with prominent weight loss and depression

PHYSICAL EXAM
- Symmetric distal polyneuropathy
  - "Stocking-and-glove" distal sensory loss
  - Large-fiber neuropathy: loss of perception of vibration and light touch (10-G monofilament)
  - Small-fiber involvement: loss of temperature and pinprick
  - Absent ankle reflexes
  - Wasting, weakness of small muscles in foot; changes to arch of foot or clawing of toes
  - With small-fiber involvement, there may be lack of objective sensory deficit despite pain.
- Symmetric proximal polyneuropathy
  - Proximal leg, arm wasting, and weakness
  - Loss of patellar reflexes
- Focal cranial or limb mononeuropathy
  - 3rd cranial nerve palsy: painful ophthalmoplegia and ptosis; preserved pupillary reflexes (in contrast to compressive palsies)
  - 6th cranial nerve: lateral gaze palsy
  - Femoral neuropathy: weakness of lower leg extension, hip flexion, quadriceps wasting, absent patellar reflex, sensory loss in anterior thigh
  - Sciatic neuropathy: pain or sensory loss in back of thigh and leg; weakness of hamstrings, lower leg muscles
  - Peroneal neuropathy: foot drop
- Truncal neuropathies: sensory loss along dermatome
- Lumbar radiculoplexopathy (amyotrophy)
  - Weakness and wasting pelvic girdle and thigh
  - Sensory loss in L2–L3
  - Absent patellar reflex
- Autonomic neuropathy
  - Cardiovascular: resting tachycardia; orthostatic hypotension
  - Gastroparesis: postprandial distension; gastric splash
- CIDP: motor weakness

DIFFERENTIAL DIAGNOSIS
- Uremic polyneuropathy
- Drug induced
  - Antineoplastic drugs: cisplatin, vincristine
  - Isoniazid
  - Amiodarone
- Toxic
  - Chronic arsenic poisoning
  - *n*-Hexane, methyl-*n*-butyl ketone
- Nutritional deficiency
  - Usually associated with alcoholism
- Paraneoplastic polyneuropathy
- Hypothyroidism

DIAGNOSTIC TESTS & INTERPRETATION
Initial Tests (lab, imaging)
- Fasting plasma glucose, 2-hour glucose tolerance test or hemoglobin A1c for diagnosis and to assess glycemic control
- Serum B_{12}
- Thyroid function
- Creatinine and BUN
- Syphilis testing
- Serum protein electrophoresis
- Vitamin D
- In mononeuropathy/mononeuritis multiplex, test for vasculitis, paraproteinemia, and sarcoid.
- In radiculopathy or mononeuropathy, imaging studies to exclude compressive lesions

Diagnostic Procedures/Other
- Bedside testing of vibration perception with 128-Hz tuning fork, monofilament perception of 10G filament
- Quantitative sensory testing for vibratory and thermal thresholds
  - Standardized measures for assessing severity and risk of foot ulceration
- Electromyogram nerve conduction velocity
  - Useful to confirm mononeuropathy and entrapment syndromes
  - Sensitive but nonspecific index of presence and severity of diabetic polyneuropathy
  - In small unmyelinated fiber painful neuropathy, test may be normal.
- Lumbar puncture
  - In CIDP, elevation of spinal fluid protein
- Skin biopsy with epidermal nerve fiber density
  - Enables direct study of small nerve fibers that are difficult to assess electrophysiologically
- Corneal confocal microscopy
  - Noninvasive approach based on examination of corneal innervation

Test Interpretation
- In nerve biopsy of peripheral nerve, Wallerian degeneration, focal axonal swellings containing neurofilaments, axonal atrophy, and demyelination are seen.
- Thick neural capillary basement membrane and endothelial proliferation
- Obliterative microvascular lesions and perivascular inflammation

TREATMENT

GENERAL MEASURES

- Maintain blood glucose close to normal.
- Provide appropriate footwear to prevent pressure damage to insensate feet.

MEDICATION

First Line

- Management of pain and sensory neuropathy
  - Tricyclic antidepressants (TCA) (2),(3)[A] (off-label)
- Analgesia may be related to effects on sodium channels. NNT ~1.5 to 5.5, NNH ~3 to 16
- Amitriptyline 25 to 150 mg at bedtime
- Nortriptyline (25 to 150 mg); desipramine (25 to 200 mg) is less sedating than amitriptyline but limited trial data.
- Anticholinergic side effects may occur.
  - Calcium channel modulators: gabapentin (2),(3)[A] (off-label)
- Binds Ca^{2+} channel-associated protein α_2-δ, inhibits neurotransmitter release
- Dose range from 300 to 1,200 mg TID, NNT ~4 to 12
- Reduce dose in renal insufficiency.
- Adverse effects: dizziness, fatigue, edema
- Fewer side effects than TCA
  - Calcium channel modulators: pregabalin (2),(3)[A]
- Binds same calcium channel as gabapentin
- Linear pharmacokinetics, unlike gabapentin
- Usual dose: 150 to 300 mg/day, NNT ~3 to 6
- Adverse effects are dizziness and edema.
  - Duloxetine (2),(3)[A]
- Selective serotonin and norepinephrine reuptake inhibitor
- Usual dose is 60 mg/day. NNT ~3 to 6
- Adverse effects are nausea and dizziness.
- Management of autonomic neuropathy
  - Orthostatic hypotension
    - Fludrocortisone (off-label)
    - Midodrine (off-label)
  - Gastroparesis
    - Metoclopramide or domperidone
    - Erythromycin (off-label)
  - Diabetic diarrhea
    - Loperamide
    - Clonidine (off-label)
    - Octreotide (off-label)
    - Antibiotics for bacterial overgrowth
  - Hyperhidrosis
    - Propantheline (off-label)

Geriatric Considerations

Anticholinergic effects of TCAs may cause urinary retention and arrhythmias.

Second Line

- Antidepressants
  - Venlafaxine (2),(3)[B] (75 to 225 mg daily) (off-label)
    - Serotonin-norepinephrine reuptake inhibitor

- Anticonvulsants
  - Carbamazepine (3)[C] (off-label)
    - Blocks sodium channels
    - Dose 100 to 800 mg/day
- Topical therapies
  - Capsaicin 0.075% cream applied TID
    - Depletes C fibers in skin of substance P
  - Lidocaine 5% (700 mg) patches applied daily to feet (off-label):
    - Causes sodium channel blockade
- Opiate analgesia
  - Tramadol (3)[B] (off-label) : 100 to 400 mg/day, NNT 3 to 8
    - Binds opiate receptors; also inhibits reuptake of norepinephrine and serotonin; fewer opiate side effects
  - Tapentadol (3)[B]
    - Binds to μ-opiate receptor and inhibits norepinephrine uptake
- α-lipoic acid (3)[C]
  - Antioxidant properties may limit free radical–mediated damage.
  - 600 mg/day PO dose showed benefit in small studies; intravenous more effective.

ISSUES FOR REFERRAL

If CIDP is suspected, refer to neurologist for investigation and treatment.

ADDITIONAL THERAPIES

- Transcutaneous electrical nerve stimulation
- Percutaneous nerve stimulation
- Electrical spinal cord stimulation
- Actovegin, dextromethorphan with quinidine
- C-peptide

COMPLEMENTARY & ALTERNATIVE MEDICINE

Acupuncture, Reiki, electromagnetic field treatment: no convincing trial data

SURGERY/OTHER PROCEDURES

Electrical spinal cord stimulation

ONGOING CARE

PROGNOSIS

- Generalized symmetric polyneuropathies
  - Usually slow, chronic progression
  - Insensitive but painless foot as pain lessens
- Focal neuropathies
  - Recovery over months to years

COMPLICATIONS

- Claw foot deformity
- Neurotropic ulceration
  - Painless ulcers on weight-bearing area
  - Callus formation is a precursor to ulceration.
- Neuropathic arthropathy
  - Results in complete disorganization of joint structure in foot, Charcot joint

REFERENCES

1. Albers JW, Pop-Busui R. Diabetic neuropathy: mechanisms, emerging treatments, and subtypes. *Curr Neurol Neurosci Rep.* 2014;14(8):473.
2. Griebeler ML, Morey-Vargas OL, Brito JP, et al. Pharmacologic interventions for painful diabetic neuropathy: an umbrella systematic review and comparative effectiveness network meta-analysis. *Ann Intern Med.* 2014;161(9):639–649.
3. Kaku M, Vinik A, Simpson DM. Pathways in the diagnosis and management of diabetic polyneuropathy. *Curr Diab Rep.* 2015;15(6):609.

ADDITIONAL READING

- Bril V, England J, Franklin GM, et al. Evidence-based guideline: treatment of painful diabetic neuropathy: report of the American Academy of Neurology, the American Association of Neuromuscular and Electrodiagnostic Medicine, and the American Academy of Physical Medicine and Rehabilitation. *Neurology.* 2011;76(20):1758–1765.
- Javed S, Petropoulos IN, Alam U, et al. Treatment of painful diabetic neuropathy. *Ther Adv Chronic Dis.* 2015;6(1):15–28.
- Saarto T, Wiffen PJ. Antidepressants for neuropathic pain: a Cochrane review. *J Neurol Neurosurg Psychiatry.* 2010;81(12):1372–1373.
- Tesfaye S, Boulton AJ, Dickenson AH. Mechanisms and management of diabetic painful distal symmetrical polyneuropathy. *Diabetes Care.* 2013;36(9):2456–2465.

SEE ALSO

Diabetes Mellitus, Type 1; Diabetes Mellitus, Type 2

CODES

ICD10

- E10.42 Type 1 diabetes mellitus with diabetic polyneuropathy
- E11.42 Type 2 diabetes mellitus with diabetic polyneuropathy
- E13.42 Oth diabetes mellitus with diabetic polyneuropathy

CLINICAL PEARLS

- Occasionally, when glycemic control improves dramatically, as can occur when treatment for diabetes is initiated, there may be a worsening of neuropathy symptoms. Symptoms usually stabilize and gradually improve as glycemic control is maintained.
- It is common to combine agents with different mechanisms of action in the management of neuropathic pain. Topical therapies can be combined with systemic therapies. There is limited evidence-based data to support combination therapy.

DIARRHEA, ACUTE

Pia Prakash, MD • Bedoor Alabbas, MD • Marie L. Borum, MD, EdD, MPH

 BASICS

DESCRIPTION
- Acute diarrhea is an abnormal increase in stool water content, volume, or frequency (≥3 in 24 hours) for <14 days duration.
- Acute viral diarrhea (50–70%)
  - Most common; usually occurs for 1 to 3 days and is typically self-limited
- Bacterial diarrhea (15–20%)
  - Develops 6 to 24 hours after ingestion of contaminated food
  - Suspect when concurrent illness in others who have shared potentially contaminated food
  - Suspect *Clostridium difficile* in patients with recent antibiotic use or hospitalization.
- Protozoal infections (10–15%)
  - Prolonged, watery diarrhea in areas with contaminated water supply
  - Consider if diarrhea lasts >7 days.
- Traveler's diarrhea typically begins 3 to 7 days after arrival in foreign location; rapid onset

EPIDEMIOLOGY
- In developing countries, acute diarrhea is more common in children. No age predilection in developed countries
- Acute diarrhea accounts for >128,000 U.S. hospital admissions and approximately 1.5 million worldwide deaths annually (1).

Prevalence
- 7th leading cause of death worldwide (1)
- Affects 11% of the general population
- In developing countries, acute diarrhea is most common in children aged >5 years.
- Rotavirus and adenovirus common in children >2 years
- In developing world, acute diarrhea is largely due to contaminated food and water.

ETIOLOGY AND PATHOPHYSIOLOGY
- Bacterial
  - *Escherichia coli*
  - *Salmonella*
  - *Shigella*
  - *Campylobacter jejuni*
  - *Vibrio parahaemolyticus*
  - *Vibrio cholerae*
  - *Yersinia enterocolitica*
  - *C. difficile*
  - *Staphylococcus aureus*
  - *Bacillus cereus*
  - *Clostridium perfringens*
  - *Listeria monocytogenes*
- Viral
  - Rotavirus and norovirus (most common)
  - Adenovirus
  - Astrovirus
  - Cytomegalovirus (in immunocompromised)
- Protozoal
  - *Giardia lamblia*
  - *Entamoeba histolytica*
  - *Cryptosporidium*
  - *Isospora belli*
  - *Cyclospora*
  - *Microspora*

- Pathophysiology (2)
  - Noninflammatory: increased intestinal secretions without disruption of intestinal mucosa
  - Inflammatory: disrupts intestinal mucosal integrity, with subsequent tissue invasion/damage
- Viral diarrhea: changes in small intestine cell morphology that include villous shortening, increased number of crypt cells, and increased cellularity of the lamina propria
- Bacterial diarrhea: Bacterial invasion of colonic wall leads to mucosal hyperemia, edema, and leukocytic infiltration.

RISK FACTORS
- Travel to developing countries
- Failure to observe food/water precautions
- Immunocompromised host
- Antibiotic use
- Proton pump inhibitor (PPI) use (3)
- Daycare attendance
- Nursing home residence
- Pregnancy (12-fold increase for listeriosis) (2)

GENERAL PREVENTION
- Frequent hand washing
- Proper food and water precautions, particularly during foreign travel—"boil it, peel it, cook it, or forget it"
- Avoid undercooked meats, raw fish, unpasteurized milk.
- Rotavirus vaccine (for infants) (4)
- Typhoid fever and cholera vaccine (for travel to endemic areas) (5,6)
- Probiotics have not been shown to prevent traveler's diarrhea (7).

COMMONLY ASSOCIATED CONDITIONS
- Inflammatory bowel disease
- Immunocompromise (HIV, malignancy, chemotherapy)

 DIAGNOSIS

HISTORY
- Duration of symptoms <14 days
- Historical clues for dehydration: orthostatic hypotension, dizziness, increased thirst, decreased urinary output, or altered mental status
- Description of stool—characteristics and output
  - Frequency
  - Quantity
  - Character: presence of mucus, blood, or fat
  - Consistency
  - Floating (8)[A]
- *Giardia* associated with pale, greasy stools
- Weight loss
- Associated symptoms: change in appetite, abdominal pain or bloating, nausea/vomiting, or fever
- Recent hospitalization or antibiotic use
- Travel history
- Ingestion of raw or undercooked meat; raw seafood; unpasteurized milk
- Sick contacts (8)[A]

- Immunocompromised state
- Pregnancy
- Daycare attendance
- Nursing home residence

PHYSICAL EXAM
- General: fever, volume status—pulse; blood pressure
- Cardiovascular: tachycardia, orthostatic hypotension
- Abdominal: bowel sounds, abdominal distention, abdominal tenderness, masses, hepatomegaly
- Rectal: stool with blood or mucus, tenderness
- Skin: turgor and capillary refill

Geriatric Considerations
Watery diarrhea with chronic constipation may be caused by fecal impaction or obstructing neoplasm.

DIFFERENTIAL DIAGNOSIS
- Inflammatory bowel disease
- Malabsorption
- Medications (cholinergic agents, magnesium-containing antacids, chemotherapy, antibiotics)
- *C. difficile* colitis secondary to antibiotic use
- Diverticulitis; ischemic colitis
- Spastic (irritable) colon
- Fecal impaction
- Endocrinopathies: thyroid disease
- Neoplasia

DIAGNOSTIC TESTS & INTERPRETATION
Initial Tests (lab, imaging)
- CBC
  - Leukocytosis, anemia from blood loss, eosinophilia (parasite infection)
- Serum electrolytes
- BUN and creatinine may elevate with volume depletion.
- Nonanion gap metabolic acidosis
- Stool sample
  - Occult blood present in inflammatory bowel disease, bowel ischemia, and certain bacterial infections
  - Fecal leukocytes
  - Stool ova and parasites
  - Stool culture
    ○ For bloody diarrhea, consider *Salmonella, Shigella, Campylobacter, E. coli* 0157:H7, *Y. enterocolitica, E. histolytica.*
  - *C. difficile* toxin (especially with recent hospitalization or antibiotic use) (8)[B]
  - *Giardia* ELISA >90% sensitive in at-risk population
  - Abdominal radiographs (flat plate and upright) if severe abdominal pain or concern for obstruction
  - Abdominal CT scan is preferred to evaluate intra-abdominal and intestinal disease.

Diagnostic Procedures/Other
- Consider sigmoidoscopy or colonoscopy in patients with persistent diarrhea, when there is no clear diagnosis after routine blood and stool tests, and if empiric or supportive therapy is ineffective.
- Consider colonoscopy in immunocompromised patients to evaluate for CMV colitis.
- Colonoscopy helps to distinguish infectious diarrhea from inflammatory bowel disease.

TREATMENT

GENERAL MEASURES

- Oral rehydration and electrolyte management are key elements in successful treatment (9)[A].

- Diet, as tolerated—"if the gut works, use it"
- IV fluids if patient cannot tolerate oral rehydration or presents with severe dehydration

MEDICATION

First Line

- Consider empiric antibiotics (fluoroquinolones or macrolides) in patients with signs and symptoms of systemic infection and severe cases of traveler's diarrhea (10).
  - Fever
  - Bloody diarrhea
  - Presence of fecal leukocytes
  - Immunocompromised host
  - Signs of volume depletion
  - Symptoms >1 week
- Tailor antibiotics to stool culture results (11)
  - *Giardia*: metronidazole, tinidazole
  - *E. histolytica*: metronidazole
  - *Shigella*: ciprofloxacin or azithromycin
  - *Campylobacter*: azithromycin or erythromycin
  - *C. difficile*: metronidazole, PO vancomycin, or fidaxomicin
  - Traveler's diarrhea: patients without fever or dysentery: rifaximin 200 mg PO TID or ciprofloxacin 500 mg PO BID. Patients with fever or dysentery: azithromycin 500 mg PO × 1 on day 1 followed by 250 mg PO for 4 days
- General considerations
  - Antibiotics are not recommended in *Salmonella* infections unless caused by *Salmonella typhosa*, or if the patient is febrile or immunocompromised.
  - Avoid antibiotics in patients with *E. coli* 0157:H7 due to risk for hemolytic-uremic syndrome.
  - Antibiotics are not indicated for foodborne toxigenic diarrhea.
  - Avoid antimotility agents (e.g., loperamide) when possible in patients suspected of having infectious diarrhea (especially, *E. coli* 0157:H7) or antibiotic-associated colitis.
  - Antimotility agents, when used in combination with antibiotics, may speed recovery from traveler's diarrhea (12)[A].
- Significant medication interactions
  - Salicylate absorption from bismuth subsalicylate can cause toxicity in patients already taking aspirin-containing compounds and may alter anticoagulation control in patients taking warfarin.
  - Avoid alcoholic beverages with metronidazole due to the possibility of a disulfiram reaction.

COMPLEMENTARY & ALTERNATIVE MEDICINE

- Probiotic use above 10^{10}/g may help in patients with antibiotic-associated diarrhea (3)[A].
- The use of probiotics is controversial in the treatment of acute diarrhea. Probiotics should be avoided in immunocompromised patients (3,13)[A].
- Probiotics shorten the duration of symptoms in pediatric (14).
- Zinc supplementation can decrease diarrhea-related morbidity and mortality (15)[A].

INPATIENT CONSIDERATIONS

Admission Criteria/Initial Stabilization

Outpatient management, except for patients who are severely ill with signs of volume depletion

 ONGOING CARE

DIET

- Early refeeding is encouraged. Regular diets are as effective as restricted diets.
- The traditional bananas, rice, applesauce, toast (BRAT) diet has little evidence-based support, despite heavy clinical use, and may result in suboptimal nutrition.
- During periods of active diarrhea, coffee, alcohol, dairy products, fruits, vegetables, red meats, and heavily seasoned foods may exacerbate symptoms.

PATIENT EDUCATION

See guidelines in "General Prevention" section.

PROGNOSIS

Acute diarrhea is rarely life-threatening if adequate hydration is maintained.

COMPLICATIONS

- Volume depletion, shock
- Sepsis
- Anemia
- Hemolytic uremic syndrome with *E. coli* 0157:H7
- Guillain-Barré syndrome with *C. jejuni*
- Reactive arthritis with *Salmonella, Shigella,* and *Yersinia*
- Functional bowel disorders (e.g., postinfectious irritable bowel syndrome [PI-IBS]) (16)

REFERENCES

1. World Health Organization. The top 10 causes of death in the world, 2000 and 2012 fact sheet. http://www.who.int/mediacentre/factsheets/fs310/en/
2. Barr W, Smith A. Acute diarrhea. *Am Fam Physician*. 2014;89(3):180–189.
3. Janarthanan S, Ditah I, Adler DG, et al. *Clostridium difficile*-associated diarrhea and proton pump inhibitor therapy: a meta-analysis. *Am J Gastroenterol*. 2012;107(7):1001–1010.
4. Soares-Weiser K, Maclehose H, Bergman H, et al. Vaccines for preventing rotavirus diarrhoea: vaccines in use. *Cochrane Database Syst Rev*. 2012;(11):CD008521.
5. Anwar E, Goldberg E, Fraser A, et al. Vaccines for preventing typhoid fever. *Cochrane Database Syst Rev*. 2014;(1):CD001261.
6. Sinclair D, Abba K, Zaman K, et al. Oral vaccines for preventing cholera. *Cochrane Database Syst Rev*. 2011;(3):CD008603.
7. Ritchie ML, Romanuk TN. A meta-analysis of probiotic efficacy for gastrointestinal diseases. *PLoS One*. 2012;7(4):e34938.
8. Pawlowski SW, Warren CA, Guerrant R. Diagnosis and treatment of acute or persistent diarrhea. *Gastroenterology*. 2009;136(6):1874–1886.
9. DuPont HL. Clinical practice. Bacterial diarrhea. *N Engl J Med*. 2009;361(16):1560–1569.
10. Dryden MS, Gabb RJ, Wright SK. Empirical treatment of severe acute community-acquired gastroenteritis with ciprofloxacin. *Clin Infect Dis*. 1996;22(6):1019–1025.
11. DuPont HL. Acute infectious diarrhea in immunocompetent adults. *N Engl J Med*. 2014;370(16):1532–1540.
12. Riddle MS, Arnold S, Tribble DR. Effect of adjunctive loperamide in combination with antibiotics on treatment outcomes in traveler's diarrhea: a systematic review and meta-analysis. *Clin Infect Dis*. 2008;47(8):1007–1014.
13. Goldenberg JZ, Ma SS, Saxton JD, et al. Probiotics for the prevention of *Clostridium difficile*-associated diarrhea in adults and children. *Cochrane Database Syst Rev*. 2013;(5):CD006095.
14. Corrêa NB, Penna FJ, Lima FM, et al. Treatment of acute diarrhea with *Saccharomyces boulardii* in infants. *J Pediatr Gastroenterol Nutr*. 2011;53(5):497–501.
15. Walker CL, Black RE. Zinc for the treatment of diarrhoea: effect on diarrhoea morbidity, mortality and incidence of future episodes. *Int J Epidemiol*. 2010;39(Suppl 1):i63–i69.
16. Schwille-Kiuntke J, Mazurak N, Enck P. Systematic review with meta-analysis: post-infectious irritable bowel syndrome after travellers' diarrhoea. *Aliment Pharmacol Ther*. 2015;41(11):1029–1037.

ADDITIONAL READING

- Chen CC, Kong MS, Lai MW, et al. Probiotics have clinical, microbiologic, and immunologic efficacy in acute infectious diarrhea. *Pediatr Infect Dis J*. 2010;29(2):135–138.
- DuPont HL. Systematic review: the epidemiology and clinical features of travellers' diarrhoea. *Aliment Pharmacol Ther*. 2009;30(3):187–196.
- Johnston BC, Ma SS, Goldenberg JZ, et al. Probiotics for the prevention of *Clostridium difficile*-associated diarrhea: a systematic review and meta-analysis. *Ann Intern Med*. 2012;157(12):878–888.
- Koo HL, DuPont HL. Rifaximin: a unique gastrointestinal-selective antibiotic for enteric diseases. *Curr Opin Gastroenterol*. 2010;26(1):17–25.
- McFarland LV. Evidence-based review of probiotics for antibiotic-associated diarrhea and *Clostridium difficile* infections. *Anaerobe*. 2009;15(6):274–280.

 SEE ALSO

Botulism; Cholera; Food Poisoning, Bacterial

 CODES

ICD10

- R19.7 Diarrhea, unspecified
- A09 Infectious gastroenteritis and colitis, unspecified
- A08.4 Viral intestinal infection, unspecified

CLINICAL PEARLS

- Viruses are the most common causes of acute diarrheal illness in the United States.
- Oral rehydration is the most important step in treating acute diarrhea.
- Routine stool culture is not recommended, unless the patient presents with bloody diarrhea, fever >38.5°C, severe dehydration, signs of inflammatory disease, persistent symptoms >3 to 7 days, or immunosuppression.
- Start empiric antibiotics in patients who are severely ill or immunocompromised.

DIARRHEA, CHRONIC

Aung S. Myint, DO • Matthew Chandler, MD • Marie L. Borum, MD, EdD, MPH

 BASICS

DESCRIPTION

- An increase in frequency of defecation or decrease in stool consistency (typically >3 loose stools per day) for >4 weeks (1–3):
  - Etiologies include osmotic, secretory, malabsorptive, inflammatory, and hypermotility.
  - Infectious etiologies are less common in chronic diarrhea.
- System(s) affected: gastrointestinal (GI)

EPIDEMIOLOGY

Prevalence
Variable depending on etiology, but overall ~3–5% of the U.S. population is affected (3)

ETIOLOGY AND PATHOPHYSIOLOGY
In most cases, chronic diarrhea is the result of disturbances in the intestinal luminal water and electrolyte balance. This varies depending on etiology.

- Osmotic (fecal osmotic gap >125 mOsm/kg) (2,3)
  - Carbohydrate malabsorption
    ○ Disaccharides including lactose
    ○ Monosaccharides including fructose
    ○ Polyols including sorbitol, xylitol, sucralose, and saccharin (common sugar substitutes)
    ○ These substances cannot be metabolized, thus creating an osmotic gradient.
  - Substances including magnesium, phosphate, and sulfate
- Secretory (fecal osmotic gap <50 mOsm/kg) (2,3)
  - Stimulant laxative ingestion
  - Postcholecystectomy
    ○ Excessive bile salts in intestinal lumen cause cholerheic diarrhea; often resolves in 6 to 12 months
  - Ileal bile acid malabsorption
    ○ Ileal resection of <100 cm leads to cholerheic diarrhea due to excessive colonic bile salts.
  - Disordered motility
    ○ Postvagotomy
    ○ Diabetic autonomic neuropathy
    ○ Hyperthyroidism
  - Neuroendocrine tumors
    ○ VIPoma
    ○ Gastrinoma
    ○ Somatostatinoma
    ○ Carcinoid syndrome
  - Metastatic medullary carcinoma of the thyroid
  - Systemic mastocytosis
  - Protein-losing enteropathy
- Malabsorption (2,3)
  - Whipple disease
  - Giardiasis
  - Celiac disease
  - Short bowel syndrome
    ○ Ileal resection of >100 cm leads to insufficient bile salt concentrations in the duodenum for optimal fat absorption, leading to fat and fat-soluble vitamin malabsorption.
  - Small intestinal bacterial overgrowth
  - Pancreatic exocrine insufficiency (CF, chronic pancreatitis)
  - Inadequate bile acid production/secretion
- Inflammatory (2,3)
  - Ulcerative colitis
  - Crohn disease
  - Microscopic colitis (lymphocytic or collagenous)
  - Vasculitis
  - Radiation enterocolitis
  - Eosinophilic enterocolitis

- Hypermotility (normal fecal osmotic gap) (1–3)
  - Irritable bowel syndrome (IBS)
  - Functional diarrhea
- Drugs: NSAIDs, colchicine, metformin, digoxin, SSRIs (3)
- Herbal products: St. John's wort, echinacea, garlic, saw palmetto, ginseng, cranberry extract, *aloe vera*
- Infectious (2,3)
  - Bacterial: *Clostridium difficile, Mycobacterium avium intracellulare*
  - Viral: cytomegalovirus
  - Parasitic: *Giardia lamblia, Cryptosporidium, Isospora*
  - Helminthic: *Strongyloides*

Genetics
- Celiac disease is associated with HLA-DQ2 and HLA-DQ8 haplotypes on major histocompatibility complex (MHC) class II antigen-presenting cells (4).
- IBD is polygenic (5).
- Cystic fibrosis (CF) is caused by a mutation in the CF transmembrane conductance regulator (CFTR), resulting in abnormal exocrine gland secretions.
- Familial diarrhea syndrome is linked to a missense mutation in GUCY2C resulting in hyperactivation of CFTR (6).

RISK FACTORS
- Osmotic
  - Excessive ingestion of nonabsorbable carbohydrates
  - Lactose intolerance
  - Celiac disease
- Secretory
  - Extensive small bowel resection/ileal surgery
  - History of neuroendocrine disease
  - History of stimulant laxative abuse
  - Dysmotility syndromes
- Malabsorptive
  - CF
  - Chronic alcohol abuse
  - Chronic pancreatitis/pancreatic insufficiency
  - Celiac disease
  - Medications (e.g., orlistat, acarbose)
- Inflammatory
  - Inflammatory bowel disease (IBD)
  - NSAID use
  - Thoracoabdominal radiation
  - HIV/AIDS
  - Antibiotic use
  - Immunosuppressant therapy
- Hypermotility
  - Psychosocial stress
  - Preceding infection
- Genetic predisposition

ALERT
Diabetes mellitus and/or prior cholecystectomy both cause secretory and osmotic diarrhea.

GENERAL PREVENTION
- Variable depending on etiology of the diarrhea
- Treat the underlying disorder.

COMMONLY ASSOCIATED CONDITIONS
- Extraintestinal manifestations of IBD include arthralgias, aphthous stomatitis, uveitis/episcleritis, erythema nodosum, pyoderma gangrenosum, perianal fistulas, rectal fissures, ankylosing spondylitis, and primary sclerosing cholangitis.
- Celiac disease is associated with dermatitis herpetiformis.
- A significant number of patients with IBS have psychiatric comorbidities.

Dx DIAGNOSIS

HISTORY
- Detailed history of symptoms, including the following (1–3):
  - Onset, pattern, and frequency
  - Stool volume and quality (including presence of blood or mucus)
  - Presence of nocturnal symptoms
  - Travel history
  - Antibiotic exposure
  - Dietary habits
  - Current medications
  - Family history
- Determine aggravating or alleviating factors, including changes with oral intake or improvement with selective food avoidance (e.g., dairy products).
- Evaluate for recent unintentional weight loss.
- Complete review of systems, including rashes, arthritis, ocular problems, heat intolerance, polyuria/polydipsia, headache, fever, flushing, alcohol intake
- IBS or functional diarrhea by Rome III criteria (3):
  - IBS: recurrent abdominal pain or discomfort at least 3 days/month in last 3 months. ≥2 of the following criteria must be met:
    ○ Improvement with defecation
    ○ Onset associated with change in frequency of stool
    ○ Onset associated with change in form of stool
  - Functional diarrhea: loose or watery stools ≥75% of the time without pain for >3 months (symptoms >6 months)

PHYSICAL EXAM
- General: Assess for volume depletion, nutritional status, recent weight loss (2,3).
- Skin: flushing (carcinoid), erythema nodosum (IBD), pyoderma gangrenosum (IBD), ecchymoses (vitamin K deficiency), dermatitis herpetiformis (celiac disease) (1–3)
- HEENT: iritis/uveitis (IBD)
- Neck: goiter (hyperthyroid), lymphadenopathy (Whipple disease)
- Cardiovascular: tachycardia (hyperthyroid)
- Pulmonary: wheezing (carcinoid)
- Abdomen: hyperactive bowel sounds (IBD), abdominal distention (IBD/IBS), diffuse tenderness (IBD/IBS)
- Anorectal: anorectal fistulas (IBD), anal fissures (IBD)
- Extremities: arthritis (IBD)
- Neurologic: tremor (hyperthyroid)

DIFFERENTIAL DIAGNOSIS
See above.

DIAGNOSTIC TESTS & INTERPRETATION
Initial Tests (lab, imaging)
- Blood: CBC with differential, electrolytes (Mg, P, Ca), total protein, albumin, thyroid-stimulating hormone (TSH), free T4, erythrocyte sedimentation rate, iron studies (2,3)
- Stool: WBCs, culture, ova and parasites, *Giardia* stool antigen, *C. difficile* toxin, stool electrolytes (fecal osmotic gap), fecal occult blood, qualitative fecal fat (Sudan stain) (2,3).
- Plain film of the abdomen to evaluate for obstruction, toxic megacolon, bowel ischemia (1)
- CT to rule out chronic pancreatitis if abnormal pancreatic enzymes or evidence of malabsorption (1,2)

Follow-Up Tests & Special Considerations

- Celiac disease: antiendomysial antibody IgA, antitissue transglutaminase (TTG) IgA, antigliadin (AGA) IgA, serum IgA (10% of celiac patients have IgA deficiency that may result in false-negative results) (4)[A]
- Chronic pancreatic insufficiency: fecal elastase (2)[A]
- Protein-losing enteropathy: fecal α_1 antitrypsin (2)[A]
- Carbohydrate malabsorption: fecal pH (3)[A]

- Small bowel overgrowth: hydrogen breath test

- Prior history of hospitalization or antibiotics: C. difficile toxin (3)[A]
- HIV ELISA, special stains for Isospora and Cryptosporidium (2)[A]

- Allergy testing (2)[C]
- Neuroendocrine tumor
  - Serum: chromogranin A, VIP, gastrin (1,3)
  - Urine: 5-HIAA, histamine (1,3)

Diagnostic Procedures/Other

- Ileocolonoscopy with biopsies: to diagnose IBD, microscopic colitis, CMV colitis, and colorectal neoplasia (7)[A]
- Flexible sigmoidoscopy: especially if pregnant, with comorbidities, or if left-sided symptoms predominate (tenesmus and urgency) (7)[A]

- Esophagogastroduodenoscopy (EGD) with small bowel biopsies if malabsorption is suspected:
  - Celiac, Giardia infection, Crohn disease, eosinophilic gastroenteropathy, Whipple disease, intestinal amyloid, pancreatic insufficiency (7)[A]

- Capsule endoscopy if further evaluation of small bowel is needed (7)[C]
- Upper GI series with small bowel follow-through
- CT or magnetic resonance (MR) enterography (1,2)

Test Interpretation

- Celiac disease: Marsh classification:
  - Intraepithelial lymphocytosis, crypt hyperplasia, villous atrophy (4)
- Crohn disease: cobblestoning, linear ulcerations, skip lesions, noncaseating granulomas
- Ulcerative colitis: crypt abscesses, superficial inflammation
- Lymphocytic colitis: increased intraepithelial infiltration of lymphocytes, increased inflammatory cells within the lamina propria, normal mucosal architecture (8)
- Melanosis coli suggests laxative abuse (2).

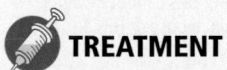

TREATMENT

GENERAL MEASURES

- Volume resuscitation if necessary (2)[A]
- Electrolyte replacement if indicated (2)[A]

- If stable, treatment is generally outpatient.

MEDICATION

First Line

- Based on underlying cause:
  - Lactose intolerance: lactose-free diet (9)[A]
  - Cholecystectomy or ileal resection: cholestyramine or colestipol 2 to 16 g/day PO divided (10)[A]

  - Diabetes: aggressive diabetes management and glucose control
  - Hyperthyroidism: methimazole 5 to 20 mg/day PO, propylthiouracil (PTU) 100 to 150 mg/day PO divided; thyroid ablation

  - C. difficile: vancomycin 125 mg PO q6h or metronidazole (Flagyl) 500 mg PO q8h or fidaxomicin 200 mg PO BID

  - G. lamblia: metronidazole 250 mg PO Q8H, nitazoxanide 500 mg PO q12h (2)[A]
  - Whipple disease: ceftriaxone 2 g IV for 14 days then Bactrim DS 160/800 mg PO BID for 1 to 2 years (11)[A]
  - Small intestinal bacterial overgrowth: rifaximin 550 mg PO BID, fluoroquinolones 250 to 750 mg PO BID, metronidazole 500 mg PO q6–8h, penicillins (12)[A]
  - Pancreatic insufficiency: pancreatic enzyme replacement (1)[A]

  - HIV/AIDS: antiretroviral therapy

  - Microscopic colitis: budesonide 9 mg/day PO, mesalamine 800 mg PO TID, Pepto-Bismol 786 mg PO TID (8)[A]
  - IBD: 5-aminosalicylic acid (5-ASA), corticosteroids (short-term only), antibiotics (short-term only), immunomodulators (6-mercaptopurine [6-MP], azathioprine, methotrexate), anti-TNF therapy (infliximab, adalimumab, certolizumab) (5)[A]
  - Neuroendocrine tumor: octreotide 100 to 600 μg/day SC (2,13)[A]
  - Celiac disease: gluten-free diet (wheat/barley/rye avoidance) (4)[A]
  - IBS diarrhea predominant: rifaximin 550 mg PO BID, alosetron 0.5 to 1 mg PO BID, peppermint oil (14)[A]

- Symptom relief:
  - Loperamide (Imodium) 4 to 8 mg/day PO divided
  - Diphenoxylate-atropine (Lomotil) 1 to 2 tabs PO BID–QID (2)[A]

SURGERY/OTHER PROCEDURES

- Resection of neuroendocrine tumors (13)[A]

- Intestinal resection for medically refractory IBD

- Fecal transplant for recurrent C. difficile infection (14)[A]

COMPLEMENTARY & ALTERNATIVE MEDICINE

Many homeopathic and naturopathic formulations are available; most have not been evaluated by the FDA.

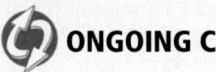 ONGOING CARE

DIET

Abstain from gluten-containing foods, nonabsorbable carbohydrates, lactose-containing products, and food allergens depending of etiology of diarrhea.

PATIENT EDUCATION

- Reassure patient of wide variation in what is accepted as "normal" bowel habits.
- Restrict colon stimulants.
- Specific education and dietary changes based on underlying etiology.

PROGNOSIS

Depends on etiology

COMPLICATIONS

- Fluid and electrolyte abnormalities (1,3)
- Malnutrition (1); anemia (1,3)
- Malignancy (colon cancer in IBD, small bowel cancer in celiac disease and Crohn disease, lymphoma with IBD therapies) (5)
- Infection with immunomodulator, biologic, and corticosteroid therapies for IBD (5)

REFERENCES

1. Schiller LR. Definitions, pathophysiology, and evaluation of chronic diarrhoea. Best Pract Res Clin Gastroenterol. 2012;26(5):551–562.
2. Fine KD, Schiller LR. AGA technical review on the evaluation and management of chronic diarrhea. Gastroenterology. 1999;116(6):1464–1486.
3. Juckett G, Trivedi R. Evaluation of chronic diarrhea. Am Fam Physician. 2011;84(10):1119–1126.
4. Rubio-Tapia A, Hill ID, Kelly CP, et al. ACG clinical guidelines: diagnosis and management of celiac disease. Am J Gastroenterol. 2013;108(5): 656–676.
5. Talley NJ, Abreu MT, Achkar JP, et al. An evidence-based systematic review on medical therapies for inflammatory bowel disease. Am J Gastroenterol. 2011;106(Suppl 1):S2–S25.
6. Fiskerstrand T, Arshad N, Haukanes BI, et al. Familial diarrhea syndrome caused by an activating GUCY2C mutation. N Engl J Med. 2012;366(17):1586–1595.
7. Shen B, Khan K, Ikenberry SO, et al. The role of endoscopy in the management of patients with diarrhea. Gastrointest Endosc. 2010;71(6): 887–892.
8. Temmerman F, Baert F. Collagenous and lymphocytic colitis: systematic review and update of the literature. Dig Dis. 2009;27(Suppl 1):137–145.
9. Shaukat A, Levitt MD, Taylor BC, et al. Systematic review: effective management strategies for lactose intolerance. Ann Intern Med. 2010;152(12): 797–803.
10. Wilcox C, Turner J, Green J. Systematic review: the management of chronic diarrhoea due to bile acid malabsorption. Aliment Pharmacol Ther. 2014;39(9):923–939.

ADDITIONAL READING

van Nood E, Vrieze A, Nieuwdorp M, et al. Duodenal infusion of donor feces for recurrent Clostridium difficile. N Engl J Med. 2013;368(5):407–415.

 SEE ALSO

Algorithm: Diarrhea, Chronic

 CODES

ICD10

K52.9 Noninfective gastroenteritis and colitis, unspecified

CLINICAL PEARLS

- Consider IBS, IBD, malabsorption syndromes (such as lactose intolerance), celiac disease, over-the-counter medications, and herbal products and chronic infections (particularly in patients who are immunocompromised).
- The appropriate workup is based on a comprehensive medical history.

DIFFUSE INTERSTITIAL LUNG DISEASE

Jacqueline L. Olin, MS, PharmD, BCPS, FASHP, FCCP • J. Andrew Woods, PharmD, BCPS • Brian Hertz, MD

 BASICS

DESCRIPTION

- Interstitial lung diseases (ILDs) represent a diverse group of chronic progressive lung diseases associated with alveolar inflammation and/or potentially irreversible pulmonary fibrosis.
- >200 individual diseases may present with similar characteristics, making ILD difficult to classify.
- A classification scheme proposed by the American Thoracic Society and European Respiratory Society includes these subtypes:
  - Known causes (environmental, occupational, or drug-associated disease)
  - Systemic disorders (e.g., sarcoidosis, Wegener granulomatosis, collagen vascular disease)
  - Rare lung diseases (e.g., pulmonary histiocytosis, lymphangioleiomyomatosis)
  - Idiopathic interstitial pneumonias (IIPs)
- Based on clinical, radiologic, and histologic features, IIPs are further subclassified into the following diagnoses (1):
  - Major IIPs, including idiopathic pulmonary fibrosis (IPF), nonspecific interstitial pneumonia (NSIP), respiratory bronchiolitis-associated ILD (cryptogenic organizing pneumonia [COP], etc.)
  - Rare IIPs
  - Unclassifiable IIPs
- Classification of IIPs and relationships between the subtypes are difficult to classify due to mixed patterns of injury (1).

Pediatric Considerations

ILD in infants and children represents a heterogeneous group of respiratory disorders. Diseases result from a variety of processes involving genetic factors and inflammatory or fibrotic responses, and processes are distinct from those that cause ILD in adults (2). Some diseases result from developmental disorders and growth abnormalities in infancy (2,3). After common causes are excluded, referral of infants to a subspecialist is recommended (2).

EPIDEMIOLOGY

Incidence

- Exact incidence and prevalence are difficult to determine because of differences in case definitions and procedures used in diagnosis.
- Cited incidence of IPF in the United States: 16.3 to 17.4/100,000 (4) and pediatric ILD of 1.32/1,000,000 (3)

Prevalence

Cited prevalence of IPF in the United States: 42.7 to 63 cases/100,000 in the general population (4) and pediatric ILD of 3.6/1 million (3)

ETIOLOGY AND PATHOPHYSIOLOGY

- Alveolar inflammation may progress into irreversible fibrosis.
- Varying degrees of ventilatory dysfunction occur among the ILD subtypes.
- ILD associated with collagen vascular disease and systemic connective disorders can manifest involvement of skin, joints, muscular, and ocular systems.
- Some types of ILD associated with specific exposures:
  - Medications (amiodarone, antibiotics [especially nitrofurantoin], chemotherapy agents, gold, illicit drugs)
  - Inorganic dusts (silicates, asbestos, talc, mica, coal dust, graphite)
  - Organic dusts (moldy hay, inhalation of fungi, bacteria, animal proteins)
  - Metals (tin, aluminum, cobalt, iron, barium)
  - Gases, fumes, vapors, aerosols

Genetics

Some subtypes of ILD may be associated with specific predisposing genes and environmental exposures; however, the role of genetic factors is unknown.

RISK FACTORS

- Environmental or occupational exposure to inorganic or organic dusts
- 66–75% of patients with ILD have a history of smoking.
- Due to diversity of diseases, age is not a reliable predictor of pathology:
  - Most patients with connective tissue disease-related pathology and inherited subtypes present between ages 20 and 40 years.
  - Median age of patients with IPF is 66 years. Studies of clinical predictors of survival including age, ethnicity, and smoking status have been inconsistent (5).

GENERAL PREVENTION

Avoiding environmental/occupational exposure to organic or inorganic dust and smoking cessation may reduce incidence or improve clinical course in patients with established ILD.

COMMONLY ASSOCIATED CONDITIONS

Many systemic disorders and primary diseases are associated with ILD. A partial list includes the following:

- Collagen vascular disease
- Sarcoidosis
- Amyloidosis
- Goodpasture syndrome
- Churg-Strauss syndrome
- Wegener granulomatosis

DIAGNOSIS

- Accurate diagnosis is imperative, as treatment choices and prognosis can vary with pathogenesis.
- Diagnosis of IPF requires exclusion of other known ILD causes, the presence of a UIP pattern on high-resolution computed tomography (HRCT), and/or surgical lung biopsy pattern (6).

HISTORY

- Symptoms may include progressive exertional dyspnea and nonproductive cough.
- Patients may also present with hemoptysis or fatigue.
- Obtaining a history of illness duration (acute vs. chronic), potential environmental/occupational exposures, travel, medical conditions (including systemic diseases), and medication reconciliation is important in assessing the cause of the ILD.
- Some cases of lung disease may occur weeks to years after discontinuation of an offending agent (e.g., carmustine).

PHYSICAL EXAM

Physical findings are usually nonspecific. Some common features includes the following:

- Crackles (typically present on auscultation of lung bases on posterior axillary line)
- Rales
- Inspiratory "squeaks"
- Clubbing of the digits and cyanosis in advanced disease

DIFFERENTIAL DIAGNOSIS

- Acute pulmonary edema
- Diffuse hemorrhage
- Atypical pneumonia
- Diffuse bronchoalveolar cell carcinoma or lymphatic spread of tumor

DIAGNOSTIC TESTS & INTERPRETATION

Initial Tests (lab, imaging)

- O_2 saturation
- Peak expiratory flow rate
- CBC with differential, comprehensive metabolic profile
- CRP or sedimentation rate
- Chest x-ray (CXR): most commonly reticular pattern, less commonly nodular or mixed patterns

Follow-Up Tests & Special Considerations

HRCT of the chest is the most useful tool for distinguishing among ILD subclasses, especially if normal CXRs:

- If indicated, arterial blood gas (ABG), hypersensitivity pneumonitis panel, plasma ACE inhibitor concentration (sarcoidosis)
- If a systemic disorder is suspected, consider antinuclear antibody (ANA), rheumatoid factor (RF), erythrocyte sedimentation rate (ESR), and antineutrophil cytoplasmic antibodies (ANCA).

Diagnostic Procedures/Other

- Pulmonary function testing (PFT; spirometry, lung volumes, carbon monoxide diffusing capacity)
  - Commonly demonstrates a restrictive defect (decreased vital capacity and total lung capacity)
  - Forced vital capacity (FVC) has been shown to decline 100 to 200 mL/year in the placebo arm of IPF patients in clinical trials (5).
- Bronchoscopy
  - Bronchoalveolar lavage (BAL) cellular analysis studies may be useful in distinguishing subtypes (including sarcoidosis, hypersensitivity pneumonitis, cancer). If performed, the BAL target site should be chosen based on the HRCT finding (7).
  - Bronchoscopic transbronchial lung biopsy may help diagnose sarcoidosis and, on occasion, is sufficiently supportive of other ILD diagnoses.
- Thoracoscopic surgery for lung biopsy has the greatest diagnostic specificity for ILDs but is less frequently used given improved specificity of HRCT. May be indicated if a diagnosis cannot be determined from transbronchial biopsy or HRCT

Test Interpretation

- Diagnostic classifications of IIPs are based on histopathologic patterns seen on lung biopsy.
- Major histologies include an inflammation and fibrotic and granulomatous changes.
- Characteristic changes on HRCT may help to distinguish between the following subtypes:
  - Reticulonodular, ground glass opacities, and, in later stages, honeycombing may be seen.
  - Associated hilar and mediastinal adenopathy are characteristic of stage I and II sarcoidosis.
- No specific test is the gold standard, which emphasizes the importance of a multidisciplinary consensus for diagnosis with clinical, radiologic, and pathologic findings.

TREATMENT

- Evidence does not support the routine use of any specific therapy for ILD in general, and especially IPF (6).
- No survival benefit of home oxygen use in ILD (8)[A].
- Corticosteroids have a role in some ILD subtypes (9)[A].
- Current evidence does not clearly support routine use of noncorticosteroid anti-inflammatory agents for IPF, including cyclosporine, azathioprine, colchicines, cyclophosphamide, cytokines, bosentan, etanercept, methotrexate, N-acetylcysteine, or interferon.
- Clinical trials have indicated that anticoagulation (warfarin) and endothelin receptor antagonists (ambrisentan, bosentan) are ineffective, potentially harmful, and therefore not recommended in the treatment of IPF.
- Lung transplant among selected IPF patients has demonstrated median survival of 4.5 years (10)[A].

GENERAL MEASURES
- Avoid/minimize offending environmental/occupational exposures/medications.
- Smoking cessation
- Supplemental oxygen, if indicated

MEDICATION
First Line
- Corticosteroids are most effective for certain ILDs, especially exacerbations of sarcoidosis, NSIP, COP, and hypersensitivity pneumonitis. However, response rates have been variable across and within subtypes. The optimal dose and duration of therapy are unknown.
- Common starting dose of prednisone is 0.5 to 1 mg/kg/day for 4 to 12 weeks, with potential up-titration to 0.5 mg/kg based on patient response.

Second Line
- Two antifibrotic agents were approved in 2014 for IPF, which have demonstrated modest slowing of FVC decline over 52 weeks compared to placebo. Both medications decreased all-cause mortality rates. Longer term studies are not yet available. It is not clear if FVC is the most conclusive meaningful efficacy variable for IPF.
  - Pirfenidone (Esbriet), an orally active antifibroblast agent has demonstrated a favorable risk-to-benefit profile in three randomized, placebo-controlled trials of IPF patients with mild-to-moderate impairment of lung function. The ASCEND trial demonstrated that pirfenidone led to a significant reduction in rate of decline in FVC compared with placebo. Notable secondary endpoints include the following: significant improvement in progression-free survival; in pooled analysis that included patients from other phase 3 trials, there was a significant reduction in all-cause death as well as death from IPF. Adverse effects from the ASCEND trial were GI related (nausea, vomiting, anorexia, weight loss, GERD, and dyspepsia), rash, insomnia, dizziness, fatigue, and aminotransferase elevation. Most were mild to moderate in nature and did not result in pirfenidone discontinuation. Pirfenidone is not recommended for patients with severe liver impairment or ESRD (requiring dialysis) (11)[A].
  - Pirfenidone is titrated over 2 weeks to 801 mg orally 3 times daily with food.
  - Nintedanib (Ofev), a tyrosine kinase inhibitor, reduced the annual rate of decline in FVC and fewer acute exacerbations occurred compared to placebo. The most common adverse effects are GI upset (nausea, vomiting, diarrhea, abdominal pain),

anorexia, aminotransferase elevation, and hypertension. It is not recommended in moderate to severe liver impairment and can cause birth defects (12)[A].
  - Nintedanib is given at 150 mg orally twice daily with food.
- The addition of tacrolimus to corticosteroids (with cyclosporine, cyclophosphamide, or no additional therapy) demonstrated improved event-free survival in patients with ILD complicated with polymyositis or dermatomyositis (13)[A].
- Several second-line agents have been used in Wegener granulomatosis:
  - Cyclophosphamide is commonly used in treatment of Wegener granulomatosis. It is given 1.5 to 2 mg/kg/day PO for 3 to 6 months.
  - Methotrexate has been used in treatment of mild Wegener granulomatosis in combination with corticosteroids. A studied dosing regimen consisted of an initial methotrexate dose of 0.3 mg/kg (maximum dose of 15 mg) once weekly, with 2.5 mg titration each week (maximum dose of 25 mg/week).
  - Other second-line agents that have been studied include mycophenolate, mofetil, and rituximab.

SURGERY/OTHER PROCEDURES
Single- or double-lung transplantation may be a treatment of last resort. Some ILDs associated with systemic disease may recur in the recipient lung.

ONGOING CARE

FOLLOW-UP RECOMMENDATIONS
Follow-up testing should include PFTs, cardiopulmonary stress test, pulse oximetry, and CXR.

PATIENT EDUCATION
National Heart, Lung, and Blood Institute: http://www.nhlbi.nih.gov/health/health-topics/topics/ipf/

PROGNOSIS
IPF confers the worst prognosis (median survival of 2.5 to 3 years) (5). A clinical prediction model to estimate the risk of death from ILD has been described (14). Other subtypes, including hypersensitivity pneumonitis, nonspecific interstitial pneumonia, and cryptogenic organizing pneumonia, have a good prognosis.

COMPLICATIONS
- Cor pulmonale
- Pneumothorax
- Progressive respiratory failure

REFERENCES

1. Travis WD, Costabel U, Hansell DM, et al. An official American Thoracic Society/European Respiratory Society statement: update of the international multidisciplinary classification of the idiopathic interstitial pneumonias. Am J Respir Crit Care Med. 2013;188(6):733–748.
2. Kurland G, Deterding RR, Hagood JS, et al. An official American Thoracic Society clinical practice guideline: classification, evaluation, and management of childhood interstitial lung disease in infancy. Am J Respir Crit Care Med. 2013;188(3):376–394.
3. Cazzato S, di Palmo E, Ragazzo V, et al. Interstitial lung disease in children. Early Hum Dev. 2013; 89(Suppl 3):S39–S43.
4. Nalysnyk L, Cid-Ruzafa J, Rotella P, et al. Incidence and prevalence of idiopathic pulmonary fibrosis: review of the literature. Eur Respir Rev. 2012;21(126):355–361.
5. Ley B, Collard HR, King TE Jr. Clinical course and prediction of survival in idiopathic pulmonary fibrosis. Am J Respir Crit Care Med. 2011;183(4):431–440.
6. Raghu G, Collard HR, Egan JJ, et al. An official ATS/ERS/JRS/ALAT statement: idiopathic pulmonary fibrosis: evidence-based guidelines for diagnosis and management. Am J Respir Crit Care Med. 2011;183(6):788–824.
7. Meyer KC, Raghu G, Baughman RP, et al. An official American Thoracic Society clinical practice guideline: the clinical utility of bronchoalveolar lavage cellular analysis in interstitial lung disease. Am J Respir Crit Care Med. 2012;185(9):1004–1014.
8. Crockett A, Cranston JM, Antic N. Domiciliary oxygen for interstitial lung disease. Cochrane Database Syst Rev. 2010;(3):CD002883.
9. Richeldi L, Davies HR, Ferrara G, et al. Corticosteroids for idiopathic pulmonary fibrosis. Cochrane Database Syst Rev. 2009;(3):CD002880.
10. Kistler KD, Nalysnyk L, Rotella P, et al. Lung transplantation in idiopathic pulmonary fibrosis: a systematic review of the literature. BMC Pulm Med. 2014;14:139.
11. King TE Jr, Bradford WZ, Castro-Bernardini S, et al. A phase 3 trial of pirfenidone in patients with idiopathic pulmonary fibrosis. N Engl J Med. 2014;370(22):2083–2092.
12. Richeldi L, du Bois RM, Raghu G, et al. Efficacy and safety of nintedanib in idiopathic pulmonary fibrosis. N Engl J Med. 2014;370(22): 2071–2082.
13. Kurita T, Yasuda S, Oba K, et al. The efficacy of tacrolimus in patients with interstitial lung diseases complicated with polymyositis or dermatomyositis. Rheumatology (Oxford). 2015;54(8):1536.
14. Ryerson CJ, Vittinghoff E, Ley B, et al. Predicting survival across chronic interstitial lung disease: the ILD-GAP model. Chest. 2014;145(4):723–728.

ADDITIONAL READING

- Martinez FJ, de Andrade JA, Anstrom KJ, et al. Randomized trial of acetylcysteine in idiopathic pulmonary fibrosis. N Engl J Med. 2014;370(22): 2093–2101.
- Noth I, Anstrom KJ, Calvert SB, et al. A placebo-controlled randomized trial of warfarin in idiopathic pulmonary fibrosis. Am J Respir Crit Care Med. 2012;186(1):88–95.
- Spagnolo P, Del Giovane C, Luppi F, et al. Non-steroid agents for idiopathic pulmonary fibrosis. Cochrane Database Syst Rev. 2010;(9):CD003134.

CODES

ICD10
- J84.9 Interstitial pulmonary disease, unspecified
- J84.10 Pulmonary fibrosis, unspecified
- J84.111 Idiopathic interstitial pneumonia, not otherwise specified

CLINICAL PEARLS
- ILD differs from chronic obstructive pulmonary disease (COPD); anatomically, ILD involves the lung parenchyma (i.e., alveoli) and COPD involves both airways and alveoli.
- In some cases, avoiding or minimizing offending environmental/occupational exposures, medications, and smoking may alter disease severity.

D

DIVERTICULAR DISEASE
Jin Sol Oh, MD • David Hardy, MD, RPVI • Steven B. Holsten, Jr., MD, FACS

BASICS

DESCRIPTION
Diverticular disease includes asymptomatic diverticulosis, symptomatic uncomplicated diverticular disease, uncomplicated diverticulitis, complicated diverticulitis, and diverticular bleeding.
- Diverticulum (single) or diverticula (multiple) are outpouchings of colonic mucosa and submucosa through weakened muscle layers in the colonic wall.
  - Less common in vegetarians and more common in cultures with low-fiber diets
  - Most diverticula occur on the left side of the colon; Asian populations have more right-sided diverticula.
  - Prevalence of diverticulosis and the number of diverticula increase with age.
- Symptomatic uncomplicated diverticular disease: recurrent abdominal pain attributed to diverticula in the absence of macroscopically overt colitis or diverticulitis (1)
- Uncomplicated diverticulitis: diverticular inflammation and/or infection without systemic sequelae
- Complicated diverticulitis inflammation/infection with secondary abscess formation, bowel obstruction or perforation, peritonitis, fistula, or stricture formation
- Diverticular bleeding occurs in 3–5% of patients with diverticular disease.
  - Accounts for >40% of lower GI bleeds and 30% of cases of hematochezia in general
  - Bleeding more common with right-sided diverticula
- System(s) affected: entire GI tract except the rectum

EPIDEMIOLOGY
Incidence
- Diverticulosis affects 60% of the population above the age of 60, and 70% by age of 80.
- 1–2% of the general population is affected by diverticulitis over the course of a lifetime (1).
- Traditionally, 15–25% of patients with diverticulosis were thought to develop diverticulitis in their lifetime. The true incidence of diverticulitis is likely <5%.
- Yearly mortality rate: 2.5/100,000

Prevalence
- Increased from 62 to 75/100,000 persons from 1998 to 2005; large increase in incidence for patients <45 years of age due to changes in diet
- Male = female overall. More common in men <65 years of age and more common in women >65 years

ETIOLOGY AND PATHOPHYSIOLOGY
Diverticula form where intestinal blood flow (vasa recta) penetrates the colonic mucosa. This results in decreased resistance to intraluminal pressure. Diverticulitis occurs when there is diverticular inflammation, infection, and/or perforation.
- Age-related degeneration of mucosal wall, increased intraluminal pressure from dense, fiber-depleted stools, and abnormal colonic motility contribute to diverticular disease.
- Thinning of the vasa recta over the neck of the diverticula increases susceptibility to bleeding.
- Diverticulitis occurs when local inflammation and infection contribute to tissue necrosis with risk for mucosal micro- or macroperforation.
- Most right-sided diverticula are true diverticula (all layers of the colonic wall).
- Most left-sided diverticula are pseudodiverticula (outpouchings of the mucosa and submucosa only).

- Surgical and autopsy studies show mycosis, a constellation of thickened circular muscle (pseudo-hypertrophy due to increased elastin in the taeniae), short taeniae, and luminal narrowing.
- Diverticulitis: inflammation with lymphocytic infiltrate, ulceration, mucin depletion necrosis, Paneth cell metaplasia, and cryptitis
- Alterations in intestinal microbiota contribute to chronic inflammation (1,2).
- Diverticular disease and irritable bowel syndrome (IBS) may be on the same disease continuum.

Genetics
- No known genetic pattern
- Asian and African populations have lower overall prevalence but develop diverticular disease with adoption of a Western lifestyle.

RISK FACTORS
- Age >40 years
- Low-fiber diet
- Sedentary lifestyle, obesity
- Previous diverticulitis. Risk rises with the number of diverticula
- Smoking increases the risk of perforation (1).
- NSAIDs, steroids, and opiate analgesics increase risk for diverticular bleeding. Calcium channel blockers and statins appear to protect against diverticular bleeding.

GENERAL PREVENTION
High-fiber diet or nonabsorbable fiber (psyllium) (>30 g/day of fiber)

COMMONLY ASSOCIATED CONDITIONS
Connective tissue diseases, colon cancer, and inflammatory bowel disease

DIAGNOSIS

HISTORY
- Diverticulosis
  - 80–85% of patients are asymptomatic. Of the 15–20% with symptoms, 1–2% will need hospitalization and 0.5% will need surgery.
  - Abdominal pain is most common symptom: dull, colicky, primarily left lower quadrant (LLQ). Pain can be exacerbated by eating and by bowel movement or passage of flatus.
  - Diarrhea or constipation
- Diverticulitis: uncomplicated (75%) and complicated (25%)
  - Abdominal pain: acute onset, typically in LLQ
  - Fever and/or chills
  - Anorexia, nausea (20–62%), or vomiting
  - Constipation (50%) or diarrhea (25–35%)
  - Dysuria and urinary frequency suggest bladder or ureteral irritation.
  - Pneumaturia and fecaluria can occur if colovesical fistula develops.
- Diverticular bleeding
  - Melena, hematochezia
  - Painless rectal bleeding
- Immunocompromised patients may not present with fever or leukocytosis but are at higher risk for perforation and abscess formation (2).

PHYSICAL EXAM
- Diverticulosis
  - Exam may be completely normal.
  - May have intermittent distension or tympany
  - No signs of peritoneal inflammation
  - May have heme + stools

- Diverticulitis
  - Abdominal tenderness usually localized to the LLQ.
  - Rebound tenderness, involuntary guarding, or rigidity (suggests peritoneal inflammation or potential bowel perforation)
  - Palpable mass in LLQ (20%) that is tender, firm, or fixed.
  - Abdominal distension and tympany
  - Bowel sounds hypoactive or could be high-pitched and intermittent if obstruction ensues
  - Rectal exam may reveal tenderness or mass.
  - Colovaginal, colovesical, and perirectal fistulae may be the initial manifestation (rarely).

DIFFERENTIAL DIAGNOSIS
IBS, lactose intolerance, carcinoma, inflammatory bowel disease, fecal impaction, incarcerated hernia, gallbladder disease, angiodysplasia, colitis, acute appendicitis, ectopic pregnancy

DIAGNOSTIC TESTS & INTERPRETATION
Initial Tests (lab, imaging)
- WBC is normal in diverticulosis and up to 45% of cases of diverticulitis. As diverticulitis worsens, WBC typically elevated with left shift.
- Hemoglobin normal (unless bleeding)
- ESR elevated in diverticulitis
- Urinalysis (UA) may show microscopic pyuria or hematuria.
- Urine culture: usually normal. Persistent infection suspicious for colovesical fistula
- Blood cultures positive in systemic cases of diverticulitis
- Diverticulosis
  - Asymptomatic diverticulosis is a common incidental finding on routine colonoscopy.
- Diverticulitis
  - Plain films of the abdomen (acute abdominal series—supine and upright) to assess for air under the diaphragm (bowel perforation) and signs of bowel obstruction (dilated loops of bowel)
  - CT scan with IV, oral, and rectal contrast to stage disease and map treatment plan (3)[A]
  - Ultrasound and magnetic resonance imaging are useful alternative.
  - Barium enema is not recommended due to risk of peritoneal extravasation.
- Diverticular bleeding/hematochezia
  - Endoscopy is the test of choice to evaluate GI bleeding (4,5).
  - Angiography if bleeding obscures endoscopy or when endoscopy cannot visualize a source (4,5)

Diagnostic Procedures/Other
- For evaluation of suspected diverticular bleeding
  - Place NG tube for lavage to exclude upper GI bleeding (4).
  - 99mTc-pertechnetate–labeled RBC scan (more sensitive) with follow-up angiography to localize bleeding (not studied in a comparison trial) (4,5)
- For diverticulitis, gallium- or indium-labeled leukocytes to localize abscess (rarely used)

TREATMENT

GENERAL MEASURES
- Diverticulosis: Outpatient therapy with fiber supplementation and/or bulking agents (psyllium) is recommended (preferably >20 to 30 g/day) (3)[A].
- Uncomplicated diverticulitis: pain, tenderness, leukocytosis, but no toxicity or peritoneal signs;

use oral antibiotics. 1–2% of subjects require hospitalization for toxicity, septicemia, peritonitis, or failure of symptoms to resolve. Up to 30% of patients may require surgery at first episode of diverticulitis. Recurrent bouts of diverticulitis increase need for surgical intervention.

- Complicated diverticulitis: Hinchey classification to describe severity:
  - Stage I: diverticulitis + confined paracolic abscess or phlegmon
  - Stage II: diverticulitis + distant abscess
  - Stage III: diverticulitis + purulent peritonitis
  - Stage IV: diverticulitis + fecal peritonitis
- Patients who are septic or hemodynamically unstable require hospitalization, bowel rest, and broad-spectrum antibiotic therapy until symptoms improve.
- Symptomatic improvement is expected within 2 to 3 days. Antibiotics should be continued for 7 to 10 days.
- 80% of diverticular bleeding resolves spontaneously (4).

MEDICATION

First Line

- Symptomatic uncomplicated diverticular disease: cyclical rifaximin 400 mg PO BID for 7 days every month or continuous mesalamine 800 mg PO BID (3)[B]

- Diverticulitis
  - Outpatient: PO antibiotics: cover for anaerobes and gram-negatives with:
    - A fluoroquinolone (ciprofloxacin 750 mg BID or levofloxacin 750 QD) plus metronidazole 500 mg TID (may use clindamycin if metronidazole intolerant) or
    - Trimethoprim/sulfamethoxazole DS BID plus metronidazole 500 TID
    - Treat for 7 to 10 days

  - The routine use of antibiotics in uncomplicated diverticulitis is controversial (6)[A].

  - Inpatient: Use IV antibiotics.
    - Monotherapy with a β-lactam/β-lactamase inhibitor: piperacillin/tazobactam (3,375 g IV QID) or ampicillin/sulbactam 3 g IV q6h or ertapenem (1 g IV QD)
    - Penicillin-allergic patient: quinolone (levofloxacin 750 mg IV QD plus metronidazole 500 mg IV TID)
    - Unresponsive or severe disease: imipenem or meropenem

  - Recurrences of acute diverticulitis may be decreased by using mesalamine ± rifaximin (7) [A] or probiotics.

- Diverticular bleeding
  - Consider vasopressin 0.2 to 0.3 units/min through selective intra-arterial catheter.
- Precautions
  - Avoid morphine and other opiates that may increase intraluminal pressure or promote ileus.
  - Increased fiber intake is not recommended in the acute management of diverticulitis.

Second Line

- Outpatient: amoxicillin/clavulanate monotherapy (875/125 mg BID) (contraindicated in patients with clearance <30 mL/min) or moxifloxacin (400 mg PO QD) plus metronidazole (500 mg PO TID)
- Severely ill inpatients: ampicillin (500 mg IV q6h) + metronidazole (500 mg IV TID) + a quinolone or ampicillin + metronidazole + an aminoglycoside

ISSUES FOR REFERRAL

- After resolution of diverticulitis, (typically 6 to 8 weeks), perform colonoscopy to exclude malignancy, fistula, strictures, or inflammatory bowel disease (3).
- Patients with complicated diverticulitis (hemodynamic instability or failure to respond to initial IV antibiotic therapy) should have appropriate surgical and critical care/infectious disease consultations.

SURGERY/OTHER PROCEDURES

- Indication for emergent surgery: peritonitis, uncontrolled sepsis, perforated viscus, colonic obstruction, or acute deterioration

- Elective resection in nonemergent or recurrent cases of diverticulitis is a case-by-case decision (3)[B]:

  - After first episode of diverticulitis, there is a 33% chance of recurrence. After a second episode, there is a 66% chance of further recurrence.
  - Most complications occur during first bout of diverticulitis.
  - Emergent surgery carries a much higher risk of morbidity/mortality.
  - Recommendations for elective surgery are based on severity of complications (not solely on number of recurrences).

  - Elective resection is typically advised after recovery from a complicated diverticulitis treated nonoperatively (3)[B].

  - Younger patients are more likely to have recurrence.
  - Immunocompromised patients are more likely to present with acute complicated diverticulitis, fail medical management, and have complications from elective surgery.
- Large abscesses (>4 cm) can be drained using radiographic guidance and managed nonoperatively (3).
- Diverticular bleeding
  - Endoscopy and hemostasis by epinephrine injection, electrocautery, or clipping can be achieved (5).
  - Angiography can identify bleeding source and embolize the feeding artery (5).
  - Patient with massive bleeding and recurrent bleeding requires limited or subtotal colonic resection.

COMPLEMENTARY & ALTERNATIVE MEDICINE

Probiotics such as Lactobacillus casei and Escherichia coli Nissle 1917 have been used with mixed success to prevent recurrence.

INPATIENT CONSIDERATIONS

Admission Criteria/Initial Stabilization

- Admit for toxicity, sepsis, and/or peritonitis.
- Admit patients who cannot tolerate oral intake or who need IV fluids, analgesics, antibiotics, bowel rest, and NG suction.

ONGOING CARE

DIET

- NPO during acute diverticulitis; advance diet as tolerated as bowel function returns
- Patients with known diverticulosis or a history of diverticulitis should consume a high-fiber diet (>30 g/day) to prevent recurrence (8).

PROGNOSIS

- Typically good with early detection and prompt treatment
- Risk for recurrence increases with each subsequent bout of diverticulitis.

- Rebleeding occurs in up to 6%.
- Diverticulitis recurs more often in younger patients, but severity is similar to elderly.

COMPLICATIONS

Hemorrhage, perforation, peritonitis, obstruction, abscess, or fistula

REFERENCES

1. Strate LL, Modi R, Cohen E, et al. Diverticular disease as a chronic illness: evolving epidemiologic and clinical insights. Am J Gastroenterol. 2012;107(10):1486–1493.
2. Sheth AA, Longo W, Floch MH. Diverticular disease and diverticulitis. Am J Gastroenterol. 2008;103(6):1550–1556.
3. Rafferty J, Shellito P, Hyman NH, et al. Practice parameters for sigmoid diverticulitis. Dis Colon Rectum. 2006;49(7):939–944.
4. Zuccaro G Jr. Management of the adult patient with acute lower gastrointestinal bleeding. American College of Gastroenterology. Practice Parameters Committee. Am J Gastroenterol. 1998;93(8):1202–1208.
5. Ghassemi KA, Jensen DM. Lower GI bleeding: epidemiology and management. Curr Gastroenterol Rep. 2013;15(7):333.
6. Shabanzadeh DM, Wille-Jørgensen P. Antibiotics for uncomplicated diverticulitis. Cochrane Database Syst Rev. 2012;(11):CD009092.
7. Gatta L, Vakil N, Vaira D, et al. Efficacy of 5-ASA in the treatment of colonic diverticular disease. J Clin Gastroenterol. 2010;44(2):113–119.
8. Ravikoff JE, Korzenik JR. Presentations the role of fiber in diverticular disease. J Clin Gastroenterol. 2011;45:S7–S11.

ADDITIONAL READING

- Boynton W, Floch M. New strategies for the management of diverticular disease: insights for the clinician. Therap Adv Gastroenterol. 2013;6(3):205–213.
- Katz LH, Guy DD, Lahat A, et al. Diverticulitis in the young is not more aggressive than in the elderly, but it tends to recur more often: systematic review and meta-analysis. J Gastroenterol Hepatol. 2013;28(8):1274–1281.
- Templeton AW, Strate LL. Updates in diverticular disease. Curr Gastroenterol Rep. 2013;15(8):339.

 CODES

ICD10

- K57.90 Dvrtclos of intest, part unsp, w/o perf or abscess w/o bleed
- K57.30 Dvrtclos of lg int w/o perforation or abscess w/o bleeding
- K57.92 Diverticulitis of intestine, part unspecified, without perforation or abscess without bleeding

CLINICAL PEARLS

- Diverticular disease is age-related and more common in Western cultures due to diet and lifestyle.
- Patients with known diverticular disease should consume a high-fiber diet (>30g/day).
- Decision for elective surgery in diverticulitis is made on a case-by-case basis.

DOMESTIC VIOLENCE

Rhonda A. Faulkner, PhD • Luis T. Garcia, MD

 BASICS

DESCRIPTION
- Domestic violence (DV) is the behavior in any relationship that is used to gain or maintain power and control over an intimate partner.
- May include physical, sexual, and/or emotional abuse; economic or psychological actions; or threats of actions that influence another person
- Although women are at greater risk of experiencing DV, it occurs among patients of any race, age, sexual orientation, religion, gender, socioeconomic background, and education level.
- Synonym(s): intimate partner violence (IPV); spousal abuse; family violence

EPIDEMIOLOGY
Incidence
8% in the United States; women are more likely to report partner violence than men.

Prevalence
- DV occurs in 1 of 4 American families. Nearly 5.3 million incidents of DV occur each year among U.S. women aged ≥18 and 3.2 million incidents among men.
- DV results in nearly 2 million injuries and up to 4,000 deaths annually in the United States.
- 30% of women and 22% of men have experienced physical, sexual, or psychological IPV during their lifetime in the United States.
- 14–35% of adult female patients in emergency departments report experiencing DV within the past year.
- Costs of DV are estimated to exceed $5.8 billion annually, of which $4.1 billion are for direct medical and mental health services.
- DV survivors have a 1.6- to 2.3-fold increase in health care use compared with the nonabused population.

Geriatric Considerations
- 4–6% of elderly are abused, with ~2 million elderly persons experiencing abuse and/or neglect each year. In 90% of cases, the perpetrator is a family member.
- Elder abuse is any form of mistreatment that results in harm or loss to an older person; may include physical, sexual, emotional, financial abuse, and/or neglect.

Pediatric Considerations
- >3 million children aged 3 to 17 years are at risk of witnessing acts of DV.
- ~1 million abused children are identified in the United States each year.
- Children living in violent homes are at increased risk of physical, sexual, and/or emotional abuse; anxiety and depression; decreased self-esteem; emotional, behavioral, social, and/or physical disturbances; and lifelong poor health.

Pregnancy Considerations
DV occurs during 7–20% of pregnancies. Women with unintended pregnancy are at 3 times greater risk of DV. 25% of abused women report exacerbation of abuse during pregnancy. There is a positive correlation between DV and postpartum depression.

RISK FACTORS
- Patient/victim risk factors
  - Substance abuse
  - Poverty/financial stressors/unemployment
  - Recent loss of social support
  - Family disruption and life cycle changes
  - History of abusive relationships or witness to abuse as child
  - Mental or physical disability in family
  - Social isolation
  - Pregnancy
  - Attempting to leave the relationship
- Abuser risk factors
  - Substance abuse (e.g., PCP, cocaine, amphetamines, alcohol)
  - Young age
  - Unemployment
  - Low academic achievement
  - Witnessing or experiencing violence as child
  - Depression
  - Personality disorders
  - Threatening to self or others
  - Violence to children or violence outside the home
- Relational risk factors
  - Marital conflict
  - Marital instability
  - Economic stress
  - Traditional gender role norms
  - Poor family functioning
  - Obsessive, controlling relationship

Geriatric Considerations
Factors associated with the abuse of older adults include increasing age, nonwhite race, low-income status, functional impairment, cognitive disability, substance use, poor emotional state, low self-esteem, cohabitation, and lack of social support.

Pediatric Considerations
Factors associated with child abuse or neglect include low-income status, low maternal education, nonwhite race, large family size, young maternal age, single-parent household, parental psychiatric disturbances, and presence of a stepfather.

DIAGNOSIS

- DV is often underdiagnosed, with only 10–12% of physicians conducting routine screening.
- Although prevalence of DV in primary care settings is 7–50%, <15% are screened.
- Pregnancy increases risk.
- Barriers to screening: time constraints, discomfort with the subject, fear of offending the patient, and lack of perceived skills and resources to manage DV
- Abused patients may refuse to disclose abuse for many reasons, which includes the following:
  - Not feeling emotionally ready to admit the reality of the situation
  - Shame and self-blame
  - Feelings of failure if abuse is admitted
  - Fear of rejection by the physician
  - Fear of retribution from abuser
  - Belief that abuse will not happen again
  - Belief that no alternatives or available resources exist

HISTORY
- Physicians should introduce the subject of DV in a general way (i.e., "I routinely ask all patients about domestic violence. Have you ever been in a relationship where you were afraid?").
- How to screen
  - Screen patient alone, without partner or others present.
  - Ask screening questions in patient's primary language; do not use children or other family members as interpreters.
- Partner violence screen (sensitivity 35–71%; specificity 80–94%)
  - "Have you ever been hit, kicked, punched, or otherwise, hurt by someone within the past year? If so, by whom?"
  - "Do you feel safe in your current relationship?"
  - "Is there a partner from a previous relationship who is making you feel unsafe now?"
- CDC-recommended RADAR system
  - **R:** Routinely screen every patient; make screening a part of everyday practice in prenatal, postnatal, routine gynecologic visits, and annual health screenings.
  - **A:** Ask questions directly, kindly, and be nonjudgmental.
  - **D:** Document findings in the patient's chart using the patient's own words, with details. Use body maps and photographs as necessary.
  - **A:** Assess the patient's safety and see if the patient has a safety plan.
  - **R:** Review options for dealing with DV with the patient and provide referrals.
- SAFE questions
  - **S**tress/safety: "Do you feel safe in your relationship?"
  - **A**fraid/abused: "Have you ever been in a relationship where you were threatened, hurt, or afraid?"
  - **F**riends/family: "Are your friends or family aware that you have been hurt? Could you tell them, and would they be able to give you support?"
  - **E**mergency plan: "Do you have a safe place to go and the resources you need in an emergency?"
- "How often does your partner: physically hurt you? insult or talk down to you? threaten you with harm? scream or curse at you?"
- Assess pregnancy difficulties such as poor/late prenatal care, low–birth-weight babies, and perinatal deaths.
- Pelvic and abdominal pain, chronic without demonstrable pathology
- Headaches, back pain
- Gynecologic disorders
- Sexually transmitted infections (STIs) including HIV/AIDS
- Depression, suicidal ideation, anxiety, fatigue
- Substance abuse
- Eating disorders
- Overuse of health services/frequent emergency room visits
- Noncompliance

PHYSICAL EXAM
- Clinical presentation/psychological signs and symptoms
  - Delay in seeking treatment
  - Inconsistent explanation of injuries
  - Reluctance to undress
  - Signs of battered woman syndrome and/or post-traumatic stress disorder (PTSD) (flat affect/avoidance of eye contact, evasiveness, heightened startle response, sleep disturbance, traumatic flashbacks)
  - Depression, anxiety, chronic fatigue, substance abuse
  - Suspicious partner accompaniment at appointment; overly solicitous partner and/or refusal to leave exam room
- Physical signs and symptoms
  - Tympanic membrane rupture
  - Rectal or genital injury (centrally located injuries with bathing-suit pattern of distribution—concealable by clothing)

– Head and neck injuries (site of 50% of abusive injuries)
– Facial scrapes, loose or broken tooth, bruises, cuts, or fractures to face or body
– Knife wounds, cigarette burns, bite marks, welts with outline of weapon (such as belt buckle)
– Broken bones
– Defensive posture injuries
– Injuries inconsistent with the explanation given
– Injuries in various stages of healing

DIAGNOSTIC TESTS & INTERPRETATION

- The U.S. Preventive Services Task Force (USPSTF) in 2013 issued guidelines recommending that clinicians screen all women of childbearing age (14 to 46 years old) for DV and provide or refer women to intervention services when appropriate (1)[B].

- Other recommendations
  – American College of Physicians (ACP) recommends routine screening for DV for all women in primary care settings at periodic intervals and when women present for emergency care with traumatic injuries.
  – The American Medical Association (AMA) recommends that all patients be routinely screened for DV with inquiry into history of family violence.
  – The World Health Organization (WHO) recommends against DV screening or routine inquiry about exposure to DV; however, they recommend asking about exposure to DV when assessing conditions that may be caused or complicated by abuse (2)[B].
  – U.S. Surgeon General and American Association of Family Practitioners recommend that physicians consider the possibility of DV as a cause of illness and injury.
  – The Partner Violence Screen is a 3-question screening tool with a high specificity.
  – There is no evidence of harm in screening for DV.

Pediatric Considerations
American Academy of Pediatrics (AAP) and AMA recommend that physicians remain alert for signs and symptoms of child physical and sexual abuse in the routine exam.

Pregnancy Considerations
American Congress of Obstetrics and Gynecologists (ACOG) and AMA guidelines on DV recommend that physicians routinely assess all pregnant women for DV. ACOG recommends periodic screening throughout obstetric care (at the first prenatal visit, at least once per trimester, at the postpartum checkup).

Initial Tests (lab, imaging)
Liver function tests (LFTs), amylase, lipase if abdominal trauma is suspected

 TREATMENT

- Treatment includes initial diagnosis; ongoing medical care; emotional support, counseling, and patient education regarding the DV cycle; referrals to community and supportive services as needed.
- On diagnosis, use the SOS-DoC intervention:
- **S:** Offer *S*upport and assess *S*afety
  – Support: "You are not to blame. I am sorry this is happening to you. There is no excuse for DV."
  – Remind patient of your commitment to confidential communication.
  – Safety: Listen and respond to safety issues for the patient: "Do you feel safe going home?"; "Are your children safe?"

- **O:** Discuss *O*ptions, including safety planning and follow-up.
  – Provide information about DV and help when needed. Make referrals to local resources:
    ○ "Do you need or want to access a safety shelter or DV service agency?"
    ○ "Do you want police intervention and if so, would you like me to call the police so they can make a report with you?"
    ○ Offer numbers to local resources and National DV Hotline: 1-800-799-SAFE (open 24/7; can provide physicians in every state with information on local resources).
- **S:** Validate patient's *S*trengths:
  – "It took courage for you to talk with me today. You have shown great strength in very difficult circumstances."
- **Do:** *Do*cument observations, assessment, and plans:
  – Use patient's own words regarding injury and abuse.
  – Legibly document injuries: Use a body map.
  – If possible, take instant photographs of patient's injuries if given patient consent.
  – Make patient safety plan. Prepare patient to get away in an emergency:
    ○ Encourage patient to keep the following items in a safe place: keys (house and car); important papers (Social Security card, birth certificates, photo ID/driver's license, passport, green card); cash, food stamps, credit cards; medication for self and children; children's immunization records; important phone numbers/addresses (friends, family, local shelters); personal care items (e.g., extra glasses).
    ○ Encourage patient to arrange a signal with someone to let that person know when she or he needs help.
- **C:** Offer *C*ontinuity:
  – Offer a follow-up appointment and assess barriers to access.

GENERAL MEASURES
- Reporting child and elder abuse to protective services is mandatory in most states. Several states have laws requiring mandatory reporting of IPV.
- Contact the local DV program to find out about laws and community resources before they are needed.
- Display resource materials (National DV Hotline: 1-800-799-SAFE) in the office, all exam rooms, and restrooms.

ADDITIONAL THERAPIES
- National DV Hotline: 1-800-799-SAFE (7233)
- Post in all exam rooms posters in both English and Spanish; available at http://www.thehotline.org/resources/download-materials/

 ONGOING CARE

FOLLOW-UP RECOMMENDATIONS
- Schedule prompt follow-up appointment.
- Inquire about what has happened since last visit.
- Review medical records and ask about past episodes to convey concern for the patient and a willingness to address this health issue openly.
- DV often requires multiple interventions over time before it is resolved.

PATIENT EDUCATION
- Counsel patients about nonviolent ways to resolve conflict.
- Educate patients about the cycle of violence.
- Counsel parents about developmentally appropriate ways to discipline their children.
- Educate parents about the negative consequences of arguments on children and each other.
- National Coalition Against Domestic Violence: http://www.ncadv.org/
- CDC: http://www.cdc.gov/violenceprevention/

PROGNOSIS
Most DV perpetrators do not voluntarily seek therapy unless pressured by partners or upon legal mandate. Current evidence is insufficient on effectiveness of therapy for perpetrators.

REFERENCES
1. U.S. Preventive Services Task Force. *Screening for Intimate Partner Violence and Abuse of Elderly and Vulnerable Adults*. Rockville, MD: Agency for Healthcare Research and Quality; 2013.
2. Feder G, Wathen CN, MacMillan HL. An evidence-based response to intimate partner violence: WHO guidelines. *JAMA*. 2013;310(5):479–480.

ADDITIONAL READING
- Cronholm PF, Fogarty CT, Ambuel B, et al. Intimate partner violence. *Am Fam Physician*. 2011;83(10): 1165–1172.
- Hegarty K, O'Doherty L, Taft A, et al. Screening and counselling in the primary care setting for women who have experienced intimate partner violence (WEAVE): a cluster randomised controlled trial. *Lancet*. 2013;382(9888):249–258.
- Wu Q, Chen HL, Xu XJ. Violence as a risk factor for postpartum depression in mothers: a meta-analysis. *Arch Womens Ment Health*. 2012;15(2):107–114.

CODES

ICD10
- T74.91XA Unspecified adult maltreatment, confirmed, initial encounter
- T74.11XA Adult physical abuse, confirmed, initial encounter
- T74.31XA Adult psychological abuse, confirmed, initial encounter

CLINICAL PEARLS
- Display resource materials in the office (e.g., posting abuse awareness posters/National DV Hotline, 1-800-799-SAFE, in both English and Spanish, in all exam rooms and restrooms).
- Given the high prevalence of DV and the lack of harm and potential benefits of screening, routine screening is recommended.
- For those who screened positive, offer resources, reassure confidentiality, and provide close follow-up.

DOWN SYNDROME
Michele Roberts, MD, PhD • Brian G. Skotko, MD, MPP

 BASICS

DESCRIPTION
- Down syndrome (DS) is a congenital condition associated with intellectual disability and an increased risk of multisystem medical problems.
- System(s) affected: neurologic (100%), cardiac (40–50%), GI (8–12%)
- Synonym(s): trisomy 21

Pediatric Considerations
Murmur may not be present at birth. Delay in recognition of heart condition may lead to irreversible pulmonary hypertension.

Geriatric Considerations
- Life expectancy has increased to ~60 years
- Age-related health issues occur at earlier age than in the general population.
- Communication difficulties may interfere with prompt recognition of some medical issues.

Pregnancy Considerations
- American Congress of Obstetricians and Gynecologists (ACOG) recommends all pregnant women be offered traditional prenatal screening and diagnostic testing for DS.
  - Maternal prenatal screening may be performed in the 1st or 2nd trimester.
  - Prenatal diagnostic tests include chorionic villus sampling or amniocentesis.
- ACOG and the Society for Maternal-Fetal Medicine (SMFM) acknowledge that any women may choose noninvasive prenatal screening (NIPS), although conventional screening tests remain most appropriate for most women. Amercian College of Medical Genetics and Genomics (ACMG) recommends all women be offered NIPS.
- Most, but not all, men with DS are believed to be infertile.
- Most women with DS are subfertile but can conceive children with and without DS.

EPIDEMIOLOGY
Incidence
In the United States, 1 per 792 live births, ~5,300 births/year (1)

Prevalence
~250,000 persons in the United States (2)

ETIOLOGY AND PATHOPHYSIOLOGY
- Etiology: presence of all or part of an extra chromosome 21
- Trisomy 21: 95% of DS, an extra chromosome 21 is found in all cells due to nondisjunction, usually in maternal meiosis.
- Translocation DS: 3–4% of DS, extra chromosome 21q material is translocated to another chromosome (usually 13, 14, or 21); ~25% have parental origin.
- Mosaic trisomy 21: 1–2% of DS, manifestations may be milder.

Genetics
- Online Mendelian Inheritance in Man (OMIM) 190685
- Inheritance: most commonly sporadic nondisjunction resulting in trisomy 21

- Chance of having another child with DS is
  - 1% (or age risk, whichever is greater) after conceiving a pregnancy with nondisjunction trisomy 21
  - 10–15% for mothers/sisters and 3–5% for fathers/brothers who carry balanced translocation with chromosome 21
  - 100% if the parental balanced translocation is 21:21 (45,t[21:21])
  - Unclear after child with mosaic DS but ~1%

RISK FACTORS
- DS believed to occur in all races with equal frequency.
- Chance of having an infant with DS increases with mother's age.
- Relatively more infants with DS are born to younger mothers because younger women are more likely to become pregnant.
- Prenatal diagnosis of DS is more common in older women, and a high percentage of such pregnancies are electively terminated.

GENERAL PREVENTION
- No prevention for nondisjunction trisomy 21
- Preimplantation diagnosis with in vitro fertilization (IVF), prenatal diagnosis and termination, and adoption are current options for expectant parents who do not wish to raise a child with DS.

COMMONLY ASSOCIATED CONDITIONS
- Cardiac
  - Congenital heart defects (40–50%)
- GI/growth
  - Feeding problems are common in infancy.
  - Structural defects (~12%)
  - Gastroesophageal reflux
  - Constipation
  - Celiac disease (~5%)
- Pulmonary
  - Tracheal stenosis/tracheoesophageal fistula
  - Pulmonary hypertension
  - Obstructive sleep apnea (50–75%)
- Genitourinary
  - Cryptorchidism, hypospadias
- Hematologic/neoplastic
  - Transient myeloproliferative disorder (~10%): generally resolves spontaneously; can be preleukemic (acute megakaryoblastic leukemia [AMKL]) in 20–30%
  - Leukemia (AMKL or acute lymphoblastic leukemia [ALL]) in 0.5–1%
  - Decreased risk of most solid tumors; increased risk of germ cell tumors
- Endocrine
  - Hypothyroidism: congenital or acquired (13–63%) (3)
  - Diabetes
- Skeletal
  - Atlantoaxial instability (15%): ~2% symptomatic
  - Short stature is common.
  - Scoliosis (some cases have adult onset)
  - Hip problems (1–4%)
- Immune/rheumatologic
  - Abnormal immune function with increased rate of respiratory infections
  - Increased risk of autoimmune disorders, including Hashimoto thyroiditis, celiac disease, and alopecia

- Neurologic
  - Intellectual ability ranging from mild to severe disability. Average is moderate intellectual disability.
  - Autism spectrum disorder (<18%); autism (<6%)
  - Seizures: (8%), typically occurring <1 year of age or >30 years of age
  - Alzheimer disease: at least 40% at age 40 years develop signs of dementia; percentage increases with age
- Psychiatric
  - Attention deficit hyperactivity disorder (ADHD), obsessive-compulsive disorder (OCD), oppositional-defiant disorder (ODD), and autism spectrum disorder increased frequency in children.
  - Generalized depression and anxiety with increased frequency in young adults/adults
- Sensory
  - Hearing loss (75%): mostly conductive due to high frequency of asymptomatic middle ear effusion; otitis media (50–70%)
  - Visual impairment (60%): mostly strabismus (refractive errors, 15%), nystagmus, cataracts (15%)
- Dermatologic
  - Xerosis, eczema, palmoplantar hyperkeratosis, atopic or seborrheic dermatitis, onychomycosis, syringomas, furunculosis/folliculitis

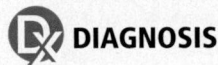 DIAGNOSIS

HISTORY
~85% of mothers of infants with DS learn of the diagnosis postnatally, although this is changing with the availability of NIPS.

PHYSICAL EXAM
- Typical growth curves should be used (4).
- Infants and children
  - Brachycephaly (100%)
  - Hypotonia (80%)
  - Small ears, often low set and simplified
  - Upslanting palpebral fissure (90%)
  - Epicanthic folds (90%)
  - Brushfield spots
  - Depressed nasal bridge
  - Short neck, often with increased nuchal folds
  - Single palmar crease, single flexion crease on fifth finger
  - Increased space between toes 1 and 2, fifth finger clinodactyly, brachydactyly

DIAGNOSTIC TESTS & INTERPRETATION
Initial Tests (lab, imaging)
- Maternal prenatal screening includes the following:
  - 1st trimester: combined screen (maternal age, β-human chorionic gonadotropin [β-hCG], pregnancy-associated plasma protein A [PAPP-A], and nuchal translucency)
  - 2nd trimester: quad screen (α-fetoprotein, β-hCG, estriol, inhibin-A)
  - Sequential screen (combined screen in 1st trimester, if abnormal, obtain amniocentesis *or* await 2nd trimester quad screening)
  - Integrated screen (combined screening in 1st trimester plus quad screen in 2nd trimester)
  - NIPS with cell-free DNA (beginning at 10 weeks' gestation)

- Prenatal diagnosis includes the following:
  – Chorionic villus sampling: 1st trimester, ~99% accurate, ~1% miscarriage
  – Amniocentesis: 2nd trimester, ~99% accurate, ~0.25% miscarriage rate
- Postnatal diagnosis
  – Fluorescence in situ hybridization (FISH) can be performed at time of clinical suspicion, but karyotype should always be done to differentiate type of DS.
  – Parental (and adult-aged sibling) karyotype is indicated only if translocation DS found in child.
- Labs for newborns
  – Echo, with or without murmur (4)
  – CBC with differential (to look for transient myeloproliferative disorder) (4)
  – Thyroid-stimulating hormone (TSH) (4)
  – Audiogram (4)
  – Ophthalmologic exam (look for red reflex) (4)
  – Swallowing study for those with feeding difficulties (4)

Follow-Up Tests & Special Considerations
- After delivering a prenatal diagnosis, the physician should offer "Understanding a Down Syndrome Diagnosis" (www.lettercase.org) (5).
- If the diagnosis is postnatal, the mother and her partner should be informed of the diagnosis promptly by a physician (preferably the obstetrician and pediatrician or family physician), on the basis of clinical observations and before the karyotype is available, but with consideration of extenuating circumstances (e.g., mother's medical condition). The spouse/partner and infant should be present unless this would cause undue delay. The meeting should be private. Refer to the baby by name (6).
- In the postnatal setting, the physician should be knowledgeable on the subject of DS and should conduct a discussion with content that is current, respectful, balanced, informative, and realistic, but not overly pessimistic, concentrating on what is relevant to the first year of life (6,7).
- Cardiac follow-up, as indicated (4).

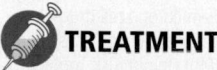 TREATMENT

GENERAL MEASURES
Genetic evaluation and counseling

ISSUES FOR REFERRAL
- Infant stimulation programs (early intervention) (8)[A]
- Lactation consultant
- Physical/occupational/speech therapy (8)[A]
- Educational inclusion often successful.
- Pediatric cardiologist, if indicated.
- DS specialty clinics can improve medical outcomes (9)[B].

SURGERY/OTHER PROCEDURES
Repair of congenital anomalies is appropriate. Plastic surgery for facial features is not recommended.

COMPLEMENTARY & ALTERNATIVE MEDICINE
- There is no evidence to support the use of antioxidant or folinic acid supplements in children with DS.
- Craniosacral manipulation is dangerous due to potential atlantoaxial instability.

- Sicca is illegal in United States, potentially dangerous, and without any evidence of benefit.
- Piracetam is much publicized, without scientific evidence of benefit.

INPATIENT CONSIDERATIONS
Admission Criteria/Initial Stabilization
If the social situation indicates adoption, consider the National Down Syndrome Adoption Network (NDSAN) (www.ndsan.org), national registry of families seeking to adopt a child with DS.

 ONGOING CARE

FOLLOW-UP RECOMMENDATIONS
Patient Monitoring
The American Academy of Pediatrics recommends ongoing assessment and review, at least annually, the following surveillance (4)[C]:
- Vision: Assess for strabismus, cataracts, and nystagmus by ophthalmologist by 6 months, annually between ages 1 and 5 years; every 2 years ages 5 to 13 years; every 3 years ages 13 to 21 years.
- Hearing: neonatal screen with auditory brainstem response (ABR) or otoacoustic emissions (OAE), then audiogram every 6 months until age 3 years, then annually
- Thyroid: initial newborn screen. Repeat TSH at 6 months, 12 months, and then annually (4)[C]
- Screening for celiac disease (total IgA and tissue transglutaminase [TTG]-IgA) annually, if symptomatic
- Three-view cervical spine films if patient symptomatic, beginning at 3 to 5 years of age
- Hemoglobin annually to screen for iron deficiency anemia
- Repeat echocardiogram in teens if with murmur or fatigue

DIET
- No special diet, but caloric needs are lower in adolescents/adults with DS than their peers.
- Obesity is prevalent at all ages.
- No scientific evidence supports megavitamin therapy or dietary supplements.

PATIENT EDUCATION
- National Down Syndrome Congress 800-232-NDSC; www.ndsccenter.org
- National Down Syndrome Society 800-221-4602; www.ndss.org
- The LuMind Down Syndrome Research Foundation provides information on the latest research for people with DS: www.lumindfoundation.org
- www.lettercase.org provides peer-reviewed booklet for parents who have received a prenatal diagnosis of DS and have not yet made a decision about their pregnancy.
- downsyndromepregnancy.org provides a free downloadable book for expectant mothers who have decided to continue their pregnancies after a prenatal diagnosis of DS.
- www.downsyndromediagnosis.org

PROGNOSIS
- Associated congenital anomalies are the immediate concern during the newborn period.
- 99% of young adults/adults with DS report being happy with their lives (10).
- Life expectancy ~60 years

REFERENCES
1. de Graaf G, Buckley F, Skotko BG. Estimates of the live births, natural losses, and elective terminations with Down syndrome in the United States. *Am J Med Genet A.* 2015;167A(4):756–767.
2. Parker SE, Mai CT, Canfield MA, et al. Updated national birth prevalence estimates for selected birth defects in the United States, 2004–2006. *Birth Defects Res A Clin Mol Teratol.* 2010;88(12):1008–1016.
3. Purdy IB, Singh N, Brown WL, et al. Revisiting early hypothyroidism screening in infants with Down syndrome. *J Perinatol.* 2014;34(12):936–940.
4. Bull MJ, Saal HM, Braddock SR, et al. Health supervision for children with Down syndrome. *Pediatrics.* 2011;128(2):393–406.
5. Skotko BG, Kishnani PS, Capone GT, et al. Prenatal diagnosis of Down syndrome: how best to deliver the news. *Am J Med Genet A.* 2009;149A(11):2361–2367.
6. Sheets KB, Crissman BG, Feist CD, et al. Practice guidelines for communicating a prenatal or postnatal diagnosis of Down syndrome: recommendations of the national society of genetic counselors. *J Genet Couns.* 2011;20(5):432–441.
7. Skotko BG, Capone GT, Kishnani PS, et al. Postnatal diagnosis of Down syndrome: synthesis of the evidence on how best to deliver the news. *Pediatrics.* 2009;124(4):e751–e758.
8. Blauw-Hospers CH, Hadders-Algra M. A systematic review of the effects of early intervention on motor development. *Dev Med Child Neurol.* 2005;47(6):421–432.
9. Skotko BG, Davidson EJ, Weintraub GS. Contributions of a specialty clinic for children and adolescents with Down syndrome. *Am J Med Genet A.* 2013;161A(3):430–437.
10. Skotko BG, Levine SP, Goldstein R. Self-perceptions from people with Down syndrome. *Am J Med Genet A.* 2011;155A(10):2360–2369.

ADDITIONAL READING
University of Kentucky's Human Development Institute. *National Center for Prenatal and Postnatal Down Syndrome Resources.* Lexington, KY: University of Kentucky's Human Development Institute; 2012. www.downsyndromediagnosis.org

 SEE ALSO

Algorithm: Intellectual Disability

 CODES

ICD10
- Q90.9 Down syndrome, unspecified
- Q90.1 Trisomy 21, mosaicism (mitotic nondisjunction)
- Q90.0 Trisomy 21, nonmosaicism (meiotic nondisjunction)

CLINICAL PEARLS
- 99% of young adults/adults with DS report being happy with their lives.
- DS specialty clinics can improve medical outcomes.

DRUG ABUSE, PRESCRIPTION

Carolyn Cammarano, PharmD, RPh • Matthew A. Silva, PharmD, RPh, BCPS • Jeffrey Baxter, MD

BASICS

DESCRIPTION
- Prescription drug abuse behaviors exist on a continuum and may include the following:
  - Use of medication for nonmedical reasons such as to get high or enhance performance
  - Use of medication for medical reasons other than what the prescriber intended
  - Use of medication for any reason by someone other than the person for whom the medication was originally prescribed
- Commonly abused prescription medications include opioid analgesics (morphine, oxycodone, hydrocodone, oxymorphone, hydromorphone, fentanyl, methadone, buprenorphine), stimulants (amphetamine, methylphenidate), benzodiazepines (alprazolam, clonazepam), and barbiturates (secobarbital, amobarbital).
- *Diversion* is a term used to describe the rerouting of medications from prescriptions or other legitimate supplies for recreational use or criminal activity, such as selling prescription medication for personal profit.

EPIDEMIOLOGY
- In 2011, 56% of the 2.5 million drug-related ED visits attributed to drug misuse and abuse were due to pharmaceuticals (1.4 million) (1).
- Prescription opioids are the second most commonly used class to initiate illicit drug use (1.9 million) (2).

Incidence
- Predominant sex: males > females (2)
- Predominant age: highest among adults 18 to 25 years, then adolescents and teens 12 to 17 years, followed by adults ≥26 years (2)
- >20% of the 3.1 million persons who were first-time substance abusers in 2011 used prescription medications nonmedically (2).
- The average age of persons with the first reported instance of nonmedical prescription drug use is 22.4 years (2).

Prevalence
- The number of persons with nonmedical opioid dependence increased from 936,000 in 2002 to 1.4 million in 2011 (2).
- Lifetime prevalence of prescription drug abuse is highest for opioids, benzodiazepines, and stimulants.

ETIOLOGY AND PATHOPHYSIOLOGY
- Prescription medications are now perceived by young adults to be more socially acceptable than other illicit drugs.
- Pharmacokinetics, compound purity, government approval, and extensive media advertising, along with personal or family experiences with prescription medication, contribute to perceived advantages of prescription drug misuse over street drugs and other illicit substances.

Genetics
Variant alleles affecting the expression and function of opioid, dopamine, acetylcholine, serotonin, and GABA may explain susceptibility to all forms of prescription and nonprescription drug abuse behaviors.

RISK FACTORS
- Sociodemographic, psychosocial, pain- and drug-related factors
- Genetics and environment; family history

GENERAL PREVENTION
- Educate and raise awareness about the dangers of misuse and abuse of prescription drugs. Focus on individuals, then families, then communities.
- Educate and reinforce safe practices in evaluating patients and prescribing medications. Use office-based peer-to-peer education and follow-up with pharmacies when abuse behaviors are suspected.
- Develop or adopt a standard practice agreement for prescribing and monitoring controlled substances with abuse potential (3–5)
- Prescription monitoring programs (PMP) show fair evidence in reducing doctor shopping but have not reliably shown reductions in ED visits for drug overdose and prescription drug abuse–related deaths (3).
- Avoid prescribing benzodiazepines and hypnotics to elderly (6).
- Avoid using benzodiazepines >2 to 4 weeks.
- Minimize controlled substances when patients have a personal or family history of substance abuse or psychiatric disorders (7).
- Limit or avoid prescribing controlled medications on first visit and until a relationship can be established.
- Take a thorough history, contact family members and past prescribers, and perform observed urine drug screens. Stop prescribing prescription analgesics for chronic pain when they are not working, if a patient is unable to take medications as prescribed or if there are problems related to opioid and nonopioid analgesics. Identify and treat underlying substance abuse problems, and involve behavioral health providers when possible.
- Effective intranasal naloxone education and distribution to opioid users, family, friends, and social service agency staff contacts in communities with >1 enrollment/100,000 people and 5 or more opioid-related overdose fatalities reduce new opioid overdose deaths (8)[B].
- Consider providing spouse/family members and/or caretakers access to and education on intranasal naloxone use in the event of a suspected opioid overdose (8)[B].

COMMONLY ASSOCIATED CONDITIONS
- Benzodiazepines: withdrawal syndromes/delirium, psychosis, anxiety, sleep driving, blackout states, cognitive impairment, impaired driving while awake; increased fall risk and mortality in elderly patients
- Amphetamines: hypertension, tachyarrhythmias, myocardial ischemia, seizures, hypothermia, psychosis, hallucinations, paranoia, anxiety
- Opioids: respiratory depression and death with overdose, low testosterone, and sexual dysfunction with chronic abuse. Methadone is associated with QT prolongation, which increases risk for torsades de pointes.

DIAGNOSIS

Screening: "How many times in the past year have you used an illegal drug or used a prescription medication for nonmedical reasons?"; primary care setting sensitivity of 100% and specificity of ~75% (9)[C]

HISTORY
Consider aberrant behaviors found when taking a history. Patient may ask for dose escalations and early refills ("spilled the bottle . . .", "pharmacist shorted me . . .", etc.), has strong preference for one drug, targets appointments at end of day and after hours, and shows hostile/threatening behavior or overly flattering behavior.

DIAGNOSTIC TESTS & INTERPRETATION
- Urine drug screens are recommended to identify patients who are noncompliant or abusing prescription drugs despite limited evidence of reliability and accuracy (3,10)[C].
- Urine drug screen (UDS): Order an expanded panel to detect commonly used opioids (ask specifically for semisynthetics [hydrocodone, hydromorphone, oxycodone] and synthetics [methadone, fentanyl, propoxyphene, meperidine]) along with tramadol and buprenorphine.
- Clonazepam and lorazepam rarely show up as benzodiazepines in routine UDS and should be ordered specifically.

Initial Tests (lab, imaging)
- Interpretation: Results are positive if drugs that are not prescribed are present; positive in presence of illicit drugs (marijuana, cocaine); suspect diversion if negative for prescribed drug.
- Be suspicious if patient refuses test.
- OxyContin will only be positive for oxycodone.
- Hydrocodone will be positive for hydrocodone and hydromorphone.
- Codeine will be positive for codeine plus morphine.
- Heroin will be positive for morphine.
- Thus, if UDS is positive for morphine, it could mean that a patient took morphine, codeine, heroin, or hydrocodone.

Diagnostic Procedures/Other
Cut down, Anger at being questioned about use, Guilt about prior use, Eye-opener use early in day (CAGE) or Alcohol use disorders identification test (AUDIT) to assess current alcohol use. Drug abuse screening test (DAST) helps determine patient's involvement with drugs over the past year. Details: http://counsellingresource.com/lib/quizzes/drug-testing/drug-abuse/. Screener and Opioid Assessment for Patients with Pain (SOAPP); Opioid Risk Tool (ORT); and Diagnosis, Intractability, Risk, Efficacy (DIRE) are tools used to assess risk of opioid misuse (11)[C].

Test Interpretation
See "History."

TREATMENT

- Whenever there is evidence of prescription opioid abuse, the controlled substance should be tapered to begin discontinuing drug therapy (3)[C].
- Benzodiazepines cannot be stopped abruptly for risk of seizures and death. A Cochrane Review supported a gradual benzodiazepine withdrawal over 10 weeks (12)[A].
- Amphetamines can be stopped abruptly without risk of severe withdrawal or death.
- The general approach to treatment includes inpatient, residential, or outpatient detoxification as required; counseling and intensive counseling as needed; and ongoing medication-assisted treatment.

GENERAL MEASURES

Alcoholics Anonymous/Narcotics Anonymous is helpful, as are Al-Anon/Alateen for family members. Nonjudgmental interactions and cognitive-behavioral therapy focused on motivational interviewing, goal-setting, and brief interventions help manage anxiety, insomnia, and denial and improve willingness to change.

MEDICATION

- Opioid detoxification programs use clonidine (13)[A], buprenorphine (13,14)[A], or methadone (15)[A] under the direction of an addiction specialist. Buprenorphine is as effective as methadone but safer (16)[A]. Both buprenorphine and methadone are more effective than clonidine for detoxification.

- Buprenorphine and methadone have been found to be similarly effective when used in long-term opioid maintenance therapy. Long-term therapy supervised by an addiction specialist is preferable to short-term detoxification.

- Subutex (buprenorphine) lacks naloxone and is prone to diversion and abuse because patients can crush, snort, or shoot to get high. Suboxone (buprenorphine and naloxone) discourages abuse and diversion because naloxone displaces buprenorphine binding to opioid receptors. Newer Suboxone sublingual film is preferred as the dosage form is difficult to adulterate.

- There is neither support for using or converting to long half-life benzodiazepines before beginning a slow, gradual 10-week benzodiazepine taper, although diazepam is often preferred, nor are there any benefits shown using propranolol, buspirone, progesterone, hydroxyzine, or dothiepin to manage withdrawal symptoms. Carbamazepine may be useful in patients who were dependent on ≥20 mg diazepam equivalents daily, and antidepressants may be helpful for depression and anxiety linked to benzodiazepine withdrawal.

- Atomoxetine and bupropion SR can also be helpful in managing ADHD symptoms in select patients.

ISSUES FOR REFERRAL

Refer to chemical dependency groups/addiction specialists/pain management and psychiatry/psychology when patients have polysubstance abuse and to treat underlying mood and anxiety disorders, PTSD, and ADHD.

COMPLEMENTARY & ALTERNATIVE MEDICINE

Acupuncture, yoga, meditation, or martial arts may aid in anxiety management and stress reduction.

INPATIENT CONSIDERATIONS

Admission Criteria/Initial Stabilization

Indications for inpatient detoxification are concomitant alcohol and benzodiazepine dependence (increased risk of seizures), mental confusion/delirium, history of seizures, psychosis, active suicidal ideation, serious comorbid medical issues, and absence of social support.

 ONGOING CARE

PATIENT EDUCATION

- Advise patients receiving controlled medication to keep them hidden and inaccessible to others. Inform patients that giving their medication to others may result in legal charges. Warn about potential addiction when starting controlled substances and about withdrawal symptoms when a medication is stopped abruptly. Warn of the dangers of respiratory depression and death when opioids are mixed with benzodiazepines. Advise patients on controlled substances; avoid all alcohol and any illicit drugs.

- Tell patient to come to you if he or she begins to need medication in increasing amounts, uses it to feel high or overcome stress, or spends a lot of time craving it and thinking about the next dose. Emphasize that you will create a mutual plan to stop the medication and try something new. Inform spouse/family members when family dynamics are an important behavioral component.

REFERENCES

1. U.S. Department of Health and Human Services, Substance Abuse and Mental Health Services Administration. Drug Abuse Warning Network, 2011: National Estimates of Drug-Related Emergency Department Visits. Rockville, MD: Center for Behavioral Health Statistics and Quality, 2013.
2. Substance Abuse and Mental Health Services Administration. *Results from the 2011 National Survey on Drug Use and Health: Summary of National Findings*. Rockville, MD: Substance Abuse and Mental Health Services Administration; 2012. HHS Publication No. (SMA) 12–4713.
3. Manchikanti L, Abdi S, Atluri S, et al. American Society of Interventional Pain Physicians (ASIPP) guidelines for responsible opioid prescribing in chronic non-cancer pain: part I–evidence assessment. *Pain Physician*. 2012;15(3 Suppl):S1–S65.
4. Hariharan J, Lamb GC, Neuner JM. Long-term opioid contract use for chronic pain management in primary care practice. A five year experience. *J Gen Intern Med*. 2007;22(4):485–490.
5. Starrels JL, Becker WC, Alford DP, et al. Systematic review: treatment agreements and urine drug testing to reduce opioid misuse in patients with chronic pain. *Ann Intern Med*. 2010;152(11):712–720.
6. American Geriatrics Society 2012 Beers Criteria Update Expert Panel. American Geriatrics Society updated Beers Criteria for potentially inappropriate medication use in older adults. *J Am Geriatr Soc*. 2012;60(4):616–631.
7. Miotto K, Kaufman A, Kong A, et al. Managing co-occurring substance use and pain disorders. *Psychiatr Clin North Am*. 2012;35(2):393–409.
8. Walley AY, Xuan Z, Hackman HH, et al. Opioid overdose rates and implementation of overdose education and nasal naloxone distribution in Massachusetts: interrupted time series analysis. *BMJ*. 2013;346:f174.
9. Smith PC, Schmidt SM, Allensworth-Davies D, et al. A single-question screening test for drug use in primary care. *Arch Intern Med*. 2010;170(13):1155–1160.
10. Manchikanti L, Abdi S, Atluri S, et al. American Society of Interventional Pain Physicians (ASIPP) guidelines for responsible opioid prescribing in chronic non-cancer pain: part 2–guidance. *Pain Physician*. 2012;15(3 Suppl):S67–S116.
11. Chou R, Fanciullo GJ, Fine PG, et al. Clinical guidelines for the use of chronic opioid therapy in chronic noncancer pain. *J Pain*. 2009;10(2):113–130.
12. Denis C, Fatséas M, Lavie E, et al. Pharmacological interventions for benzodiazepine mono-dependence management in outpatient settings. *Cochrane Database Syst Rev*. 2006;(3):CD005194.
13. Gowing L, Ali R, White JM. Buprenorphine for the management of opioid withdrawal. *Cochrane Database Syst Rev*. 2009;(3):CD002025.
14. Maremmani I, Gerra G. Buprenorphine-based regimens and methadone for the medical management of opioid dependence: selecting the appropriate drug for treatment. *Am J Addict*. 2010;19(6):557–568.
15. Mattick RP, Breen C, Kimber J, et al. Methadone maintenance therapy versus no opioid replacement therapy for opioid dependence. *Cochrane Database Syst Rev*. 2009;(3):CD002209.
16. Mattick RP, Breen C, Kimber J, et al. Buprenorphine maintenance versus placebo or methadone maintenance for opioid dependence. *Cochrane Database Syst Rev*. 2014;(2):CD002207.

 CODES

ICD10

- F19.10 Other psychoactive substance abuse, uncomplicated
- F11.10 Opioid abuse, uncomplicated
- F15.10 Other stimulant abuse, uncomplicated

CLINICAL PEARLS

- Education and prescription monitoring programs are important for preventing prescription drug abuse.
- Use a standardized office practice agreement when prescribing controlled substances.
- Screening: "How many times in the past year have you used an illegal drug or prescription medication for nonmedical reasons?"
- Avoid prescribing controlled substances and nonbenzodiazepine hypnotics to patients at risk for substance abuse or with an Axis 1 or Axis 2 diagnosis.
- Discontinue prescription opioid analgesics if pain or functionality does not improve and if there's evidence of prescription or illicit drug abuse (i.e., positive UDS, driving while intoxicated [DWI], accidental or intentional overdose, early refills).
- Limit benzodiazepine use to 2 to 4 weeks.
- Conduct frequent, observed Urine screen.
- Addiction is a potentially fatal disease.

DUCTAL CARCINOMA IN SITU

Bradley M. Turner, MD, MPH, MHA • David G. Hicks, MD

 BASICS

DESCRIPTION

- Ductal carcinoma in situ (DCIS) is a heterogeneous group of lesions that have in common the presence of a clonal proliferation of neoplastic epithelial cells confined to ducts and lobules.
- Considered a premalignant lesion—the neoplastic cells are not invasive (pure DCIS).
- Classified as low, intermediate, or high-grade
- Mortality from DCIS with subsequent progression to invasive breast carcinoma (IBC) is low, regardless of histologic type or type of treatment.

EPIDEMIOLOGY

Incidence
- Estimated 58,168 new diagnoses of DCIS in 2014.
- DCIS accounts for approximately 80–85% of in situ breast carcinomas (lobular carcinoma in situ [LCIS] accounts for approximately 15–20%).
- Stable incidence in women ≥50 years of age over the last several years.
- Increasing incidence in women <50 years of age over the last several years.
- Represents ~26% of all new IBC—an estimated 60,290 new cases in 2015.
- Incidence rate of DCIS is comparable among women of different ethnicities.

ETIOLOGY AND PATHOPHYSIOLOGY
- A non-obligate precursor to IBC
- Presumed to be the final step prior to invasive breast cancer, part of a poorly understood spectrum of polyclonal and clonal epithelial proliferative lesions.
- Either low- or high-grade DCIS has the potential for subsequent invasion into the surrounding stroma; however, the changes necessary for transition to IBC are poorly understood.
- Molecular evidence suggests that low- and high-grade DCIS are genetically distinct lesions, with high-grade DCIS associated with more aggressive disease.

Genetics
- Low-grade DCIS typically shows diffuse and strong expression of estrogen receptor (ER) and progesterone receptor (PR), without HER2 protein overexpression or amplification.
- High-grade DCIS not consistently ER+ or PR+; frequent HER2 protein overexpression and amplification; commonly associated with p53 gene mutations.
- HER2 overexpression is even more frequent in high-grade DCIS compared to IBC.
- *BRCA1* and *BRCA2* associations observed
- If patients are high risk, consider genetic counseling after diagnosis of DCIS.

RISK FACTORS
- Similar to IBC, although not as strongly associated
- Female gender, older age, nulliparity, late age at first birth, late age at menopause, family history of a first-degree relative with breast cancer, prior breast biopsies, long-term use of postmenopausal hormone replacement therapy, elevated body mass index in postmenopausal women not taking hormone replacement, high mammographic breast density
- Association with smoking, lactation, early menarche, increased alcohol consumption, and oral contraceptive use are less clear.

GENERAL PREVENTION
- Screening may result in overdiagnosis with little or no reduction in the incidence of advanced cancers.
- General screening guidelines have been suggested for asymptomatic women with an average risk of breast carcinoma.
- Women with increased risk should have more aggressive screening (risk assessment tool available at http://www.cancer.gov/bcrisktool/Default.aspx).
- General screening guidelines—U.S. Preventive Services Task Force (USPSTF)
  – Biennial mammography for women aged 50 to 74 years.
  – Avoid routine screening mammography in women aged 40 to 49 years of age. The decision to start biennial mammographic screening before age 50 years should be individualized based on the patient's values regarding specific benefits or harms.
  – Discourage teaching of breast self-exam (BSE).
  – Insufficient evidence to assess the value of clinical breast exam (CBE) in women after age 40 years. If this service is offered, the patient should understand this uncertainty.
  – Insufficient evidence to assess the benefit or harm of digital mammography or MRI over film mammography. If this service is offered, the patient should understand this uncertainty.
- General screening guidelines—National Comprehensive Cancer Network (NCCN)
  – NCCN recommends that women should be familiar with their breast, promptly report changes to their health care provider, and that periodic, consistent BSE may facilitate breast self-awareness.
  – Ages 25 to 39 years: breast awareness, CBE every 1 to 3 years
  – Age 40 years and older: breast awareness, annual CBE, annual screening mammography
- Clinicians should use judgment when applying screening guidelines.
- Mammography screening should be individualized.
- If no intervention would occur based on screening findings, patient should not undergo screening.
- Risk reduction
  – Assess for familial/genetic and other elements that contribute to an increased risk of breast cancer.
  – Lifestyle modifications: Limit alcohol intake to <1 drink/day, exercise, maintain healthy diet, and weight control.
  – Risk reduction surgery supported for carefully selected women at high risk of breast cancer who desire this intervention.
  – Risk reduction agents (i.e., tamoxifen) are recommended in certain high-risk women ≥35 years of age.

 DIAGNOSIS

HISTORY
- Most DCIS is now diagnosed by screening mammography (presence of microcalcifications in approximately 72%); patients may be asymptomatic with nonpalpable mass (12%) (1,2)[A].
- More advanced lesions may present with a palpable mass, spontaneous nipple discharge, or Paget disease (1,3)[A].

PHYSICAL EXAM
- CBE with inspection of breasts with patient in upright and supine position, evaluating for asymmetry, spontaneous discharge, skin changes (peau d'orange, erythema, scaling), nipple retraction/excoriation (Paget disease).
- Palpation of all breast quadrants with patient in upright and supine position, including lymph node examination (axillary, supraclavicular, and internal mammary nodes).
- Positive clinical findings: Refer for consideration of diagnostic imaging and/or surgical evaluation, unless <30 years of age with a low clinical suspicion (observe 1 to 2 menstrual cycles; if positive clinical findings persist, refer for imaging) (3)[A].

DIFFERENTIAL DIAGNOSIS

Usual ductal hyperplasia, flat epithelial atypia, atypical ductal hyperplasia (ADH), LCIS, microinvasive carcinoma (1)[A]

DIAGNOSTIC TESTS & INTERPRETATION

Initial Tests (lab, imaging)
- Mammography Breast Imaging Reporting and Data System (BI-RADS) developed by the American College of Radiology is used for uniform reporting of mammography results.
- BI-RADS interpretation: **Categories (0 to 6) 0:** incomplete and needs additional imaging; **1:** negative; **2:** benign finding; **3:** probably benign finding; **4:** suspicious abnormality; **5:** highly suggestive of malignancy; **6:** known biopsy-proven malignancy
- Similar BI-RADS interpretations for diagnostic ultrasound (US).
- Screening BI-RADS category 0: diagnostic workup with consideration for diagnostic imaging
- Screening BI-RADS categories 1 and 2: screening recommendations.
- Screening BI-RADS category 3: diagnostic imaging at 6 months, then every 6 to 12 months for 2 to 3 years; consider biopsy if patient anxious or follow-up uncertain.
- Screening BI-RADS categories 4 and 5: diagnostic imaging with follow-up
- Screening BI-RADS category 6: technically not a "screening" category other than to assess a known cancer that might need additional evaluation. NCCN guidelines for breast cancer should be followed.
- DCIS is commonly seen on imaging as clustered microcalcifications (2)[A].
- Diagnostic imaging will result in consideration for tissue biopsy.

Follow-Up Tests & Special Considerations
- US is not recommended for screening (3)[A].
- The sensitivity of breast MRI screening is higher than mammography but has lower specificity resulting in a greater number of false positives (2,3)[A].
- Screening with MRI is only recommended in certain women: *BRCA* mutation, first-degree relative of *BRCA* carrier, ≥20% lifetime risk of breast cancer, radiation to chest between the ages of 10 and 30 years, presence of Li-Fraumeni, Cowden, or Bannayan-Riley-Ruvalcaba syndrome in patient or first-degree relative (3)[A].
- Screening with MRI is not recommended in women with <15% lifetime risk of breast cancer.

- MRI can also complement mammography in the diagnostic setting, particularly in patients with skin changes (3)[A].
- Although MRI and US are complementary diagnostic methods to mammography, US is less sensitive in detecting most microcalcifications and MRI does not typically detect microcalcifications at all (2,3)[A].
- Pathology
  - Tissue is necessary for diagnosis: typically core needle (CN) or vacuum-assisted (VA) biopsy (mammographic/stereotactic, US, or MRI guided). Open surgical biopsy can be performed in patients not amenable to CN or VA biopsy.
  - Fine-needle aspiration (FNA) is not adequate for specific diagnosis of DCIS; however, it can suggest the presence of neoplastic cells.
  - Histologic classification
    - Classification is subjective; however, traditionally classified as either low, intermediate, or high-grade based on architectural patterns (comedo, solid, cribiform, clinging, papillary, and micropapillary), nuclear grade (I, II, or III), and the absence or presence of necrosis (1,2).
    - Ductal intraepithelial neoplasia (DIN) is an alternative histologic classification incoporating size as a discriminating factor (2,4)[C].
    - Grade is more important for prognosis, risk for progression, and local recurrence.
    - Comedo-type necrosis (necrosis filling central portion of involved duct), is typically seen in high-grade DCIS, with varying degrees of necrosis in other types of DCIS.
  - Determination of ER and PR status (1)[A].
  - Studies show unclear or weak evidence of HER2 status as a prognostic indicator in DCIS (5)[A].

TREATMENT

SURGERY/OTHER PROCEDURES

- Surgery is the primary treatment option. Options for surgery are based on risk of recurrence, anatomic location, extent of disease, and the ability to achieve "negative" margins (5)[A].
- Positive margins are considered "ink on tumor" (6)[A].
- Negative margins controversial with DCIS (5)[C]
- Margins <1 mm considered inadequate (1,5)[A]
- Totality of evidence may not support distinguishing between margins of "no ink on tumor" and margins of <1 mm (6)[C].
- Margins <1 mm at the breast fibroglandular boundary (chest wall or skin) do not mandate surgical excision but may be an indication for higher boost dose radiation in patients opting for breast conservation (5)[A].
- Surgical options include the following:
  - **Breast conservation (lumpectomy) without lymph node procedure, with or without whole breast radiation therapy** (5)[A]
  - A sentinel lymph node biopsy should strongly be considered if the lumpectomy is in an anatomic location compromising the performance of a future sentinel lymph node procedure (5)[C].
  - Radiation decreases recurrence rates by about 50% (2,7,8)[A].
  - ~50% of recurrences are pure DCIS; ~50% are IBC (1,5)[A].

- Recurrence generally requires mastectomy with consideration for systemic treatment (2)[C].
- Patients not amenable to margin-free lumpectomy should have total mastectomy (5)[C].
- **Mastectomy with or without sentinel node biopsy ± breast reconstruction** (5)[A]
- Mastectomy provides maximum local control.
- Rates of recurrence for DCIS and IBC are similar to lumpectomy.
- Recurrence should be treated with wide local excision, chest wall radiation, and consideration for systemic treatment (5)[A].
- Long-term cause-specific survival seems to be equivalent to lumpectomy with whole breast radiation (5)[A].
- Secondary chemoprevention following breast-conserving surgery for ER + DCIS
- Tamoxifen for 5 years (5)[A]
- Considered in lumpectomy patients with or without whole breast radiation (5)[A]
- Benefit of tamoxifen and trastuzumab in patients with ER-negative/HER2-positive disease is unclear (1,9,10)[C].

ONGOING CARE

FOLLOW-UP RECOMMENDATIONS

- History and physical exam every 6 months for first 5 years, then annually
- Mammography 6 to 12 months after whole breast radiation, then every 12 months
- If treated with tamoxifen, monitor per NCCN guidelines for breast cancer risk reduction (5,10).

PROGNOSIS

- Good prognosis: 10-year breast cancer-specific survival rates of >95%; overall mortality after diagnosis of treated pure DCIS generally >98%
- Risk of local recurrence after mastectomy generally reported as 1–2% (higher in some studies).
- Higher risk of local recurrences after breast-conserving therapy in younger age (particularly before age 40 years), larger tumor size, high nuclear grade, comedo-type necrosis, and close/positive margin status (related to DCIS volume)
- ER+ tumors are associated with lower risk for recurrence.
- The Oncotype Dx DCIS score, a multigene assay including seven DCIS related genes, offers hope for quantifying the risk of local recurrence of DCIS or the development of IBC in certain patient populations (tumors ≤ 2.5 cm, negative margins) (11,12)[B].

REFERENCES

1. Siziopikou KP. Ductal carcinoma in situ of the breast: current concepts and future directions. *Arch Pathol Lab Med.* 2013;137(4):462–466.
2. Lee RJ, Vallow LA, McLaughlin SA, et al. Ductal carcinoma in situ of the breast. *Int J Surg Oncol.* 2012;2012:123549.
3. NCCN clinical practice guidelines in oncology: breast cancer screening and diagnosis (Version 1.2014) 2014. National Comprehensive Cancer Network Web site. http://www.nccn.org. Accessed June 3, 2015.
4. Tavassoli FA. Breast pathology: rationale for adopting the ductal intraepithelial neoplasia (DIN) classification. *Nat Clin Pract Oncol.* 2005;2(3):116–117.
5. NCCN clinical practice guidelines in oncology: breast cancer (Version 2.2015) 2015. National Comprehensive Cancer Network Web site. http://www.nccn.org. Accessed June 3, 2015.
6. Moran MS, Schnitt SJ, Giuliano AE, et al. Society of Surgical Oncology-American Society for Radiation Oncology concensus guideline on margins for breast-conserving surgery with whole-breast irradiation in stages I and II invasive breast cancer. *Ann Surg Oncol.* 2014;21(3):704–716.
7. Donker M, Litiére S, Werutsky G, et al. Breast-conserving treatment with or without radiotherapy in ductal carcinoma in situ: 15-year recurrence rates and outcome after a recurrence, from the EORTC 10853 randomized phase III trial. *J Clin Oncol.* 2013;31(32):4054–4059.
8. Goodwin A, Parker S, Ghersi D, et al. Post-operative radiotherapy for ductal carcinoma in situ of the breast. *Cochrane Database Syst Rev.* 2013;(11):CD000563.
9. Carraro DM, Elias EV, Andrade VP. Ductal carcinoma in situ of the breast: morphological and molecular features implicated in progression [published ahead of print November 21, 2013]. *Biosci Rep.*
10. NCCN clinical practice guidelines in oncology: breast cancer (Version 1.2015) 2015. National Comprehensive Cancer Network Web site. http://www.nccn.org. Accessed June 3, 2015.
11. Solin LJ, Gray R, Baehner FL, et al. A multigene expression assay to predict local recurrence risk for ductal carcinoma in situ of the breast. *J Natl Cancer Inst.* 2013;105(10):701–710.
12. Alvarado M, Carter DL, Guenther JM, et al. The impact of genomic testing on the recommendation for radiation therapy in patients with ductal carcinoma in situ: a prospective clinical utility assessment of the 12-gene DCIS score result. *J Surg Oncol.* 2015;111(8):935–940.

 SEE ALSO

Breast Cancer

 CODES

ICD10
- D05.10 Intraductal carcinoma in situ of unspecified breast
- D05.11 Intraductal carcinoma in situ of right breast
- D05.12 Intraductal carcinoma in situ of left breast

CLINICAL PEARLS

- DCIS is a heterogeneous group of noninvasive neoplastic lesions arising from the breast ductal epithelial cells.
- The incidence of DCIS has continued to increase in women <50 years of age, with a more stable incidence in women ≥50 years of age.
- The goal of DCIS treatment is to prevent recurrence and progression to IBC.
- The Oncotype DX DCIS score may be useful in identifying patients at higher risk for recurrence or progession to IBC.
- Current standard of care is breast-conserving therapy with consideration for postoperative whole breast radiation therapy and/or postsurgical tamoxifen therapy, unless otherwise contraindicated.
- With appropriate therapy, the overall prognosis of pure DCIS is good.

DUPUYTREN CONTRACTURE

Joshua L. Eaton, MD, FAWM • Alex Nguyen, MD

BASICS

DESCRIPTION
- Palmar fibromatosis; caused by progressive fibrous proliferation and tightening of the fascia of the palms, resulting in flexion deformities and loss of function
- Not the same as "trigger finger," which is caused by thickening of the distal flexor tendon
- Similar change rarely occurs in plantar fascia, usually appearing simultaneously.
- System(s) affected: musculoskeletal
- Synonyms: morbus Dupuytren; Dupuytren disease; "Celtic hand"

EPIDEMIOLOGY
Prevalence
- Increases with age; mean prevalence in western countries: 12%, 21%, and 29% at ages 55, 65, and 75 years, respectively. Norway: 30% of males >60 years; Spain: 19% of males >60 years
- More common in Caucasians of Scandinavian or Northern European ancestry

ETIOLOGY AND PATHOPHYSIOLOGY
Unknown; possibly a T-cell–mediated autoimmune disorder. Occurs in three stages:
- Proliferative phase: proliferation of myofibroblasts with nodule development on palmar surface
- Involutional stage: spread along palmar fascia to fingers with cord development
- Residual phase: spread into fingers with cord tightening and contracture formation

Genetics
- Autosomal dominant with incomplete penetrance:
  – Siblings with 3-fold risk
- 68% of male relatives of affected patients develop disease at some time.

RISK FACTORS
- Smoking (mean: 16 pack-years; odds ratio: 2.8)
- Increasing age
- Male/Caucasian; male > female (1.7:1)
- Workers exposed to vibration—risk doubles if regular (weekly) exposure
- Diabetes mellitus (increases with duration of DM, usually mild; middle and ring finger involved)
- Epilepsy
- Chronic illness (e.g., pulmonary tuberculosis, liver disease, HIV)
- Hypercholesterolemia
- Alcohol consumption

GENERAL PREVENTION
Avoid risk factors, especially if a strong family history.

COMMONLY ASSOCIATED CONDITIONS
- Alcoholism
- Epilepsy
- Diabetes mellitus
- Chronic lung disease
- Occupational hand trauma (vibration)
- Hypercholesterolemia
- Carpal tunnel syndrome
- Peyronie disease

DIAGNOSIS

HISTORY
- Caucasian male aged 50 to 60 years
- Family history
- Mild pain early:
  – Begins in palm and spreads to digits
- Unilateral or bilateral (50%)
- Right hand more frequent
- Ring finger more frequent
- Ulnar digits are more affected than radial digits
- Flexion contracture of metacarpophalangeal (MCP) before proximal interphalangeal (PIP) joint

PHYSICAL EXAM
- Painless plaques or nodules in palmar fascia
- Cordlike band in the palmar fascia
- Skin adheres to fascia and becomes puckered.
- Palpable subcutaneous nodules
- Reduced flexibility of MCP and PIP joints
- No sign of inflammation
- Web space contractures
- Ectopic Dupuytren can involve plantar (Ledderhose—10%) and penile (Peyronie—2%) fascia.
  – Knuckle pads over PIP:
    ○ Garrod nodes associated with severe disease
  – Disease stages:
    ○ Early: skin pits (can also be seen in nevoid basal cell cancer and palmar keratosis)
    ○ Intermediate: nodules and cords. Nerves and vessels can be entwined in cords.
    ○ Late: contractures

DIFFERENTIAL DIAGNOSIS
- Tendon abnormalities
- Camptodactyly: early teens; tight fascial bands on ulnar side of small finger
- Diabetic cheiroarthropathy: all four fingers
- Volkmann ischemic contracture

DIAGNOSTIC TESTS & INTERPRETATION
Diagnostic Procedures/Other
MRI can assess cellularity of lesions that correlate with recurrence after surgery.

Test Interpretation
- Myofibroblasts predominate
- Nodules: lumps fixed to skin hypercellular masses
- Cords: organized collagen type III arranged parallel and hypocellular
- First stage (proliferative): increased myofibroblasts
- Second stage (residual): dense fibroblast network
- Third stage (involutional): Myofibroblasts disappear.

TREATMENT

GENERAL MEASURES
- Physiotherapy alone is ineffective:
  – Intermittent splinting is unlikely to be effective.
  – Continuous splinting may help pre- and postop.
- Follow isolated involvement of palmar fascia conservatively.
- MCP joint involvement can be followed conservatively if flexion contracture is <30 degrees.

MEDICATION
First Line
- Clostridial collagenase injections (FDA-approved in 2010):
  – Degrades collagen to allow manual rupture of diseased cord
  – Best for isolated cord of MCP joint
  – 5-year recurrence rate of 47%; comparable with surgical recurrence rates (1)[B]
  – More rapid recovery of hand function compared to limited fasciectomy with fewer serious adverse events (2)[B]
  – Complications: injection site reaction, skin tear
  – Can do two cords concurrently
  – Can be effective for postsurgical recurrence
- Steroid injection:
  – Can treat acute nodules or painful knuckle pads
  – Serial triamcinolone injections improved long-term outcomes when combined with needle aponeurotomy (3)[B].

Second Line
Surgery for contracture >30%

ISSUES-FOR-REFERRAL
- Any involvement of PIP joints
- MCP joints contracted >30 degrees
- Positive Hueston tabletop test: When the palm is placed on a flat surface, the digits cannot be simultaneously placed fully on the same surface as the palm because of flexion contractures.

ADDITIONAL THERAPIES
- Percutaneous and needle fasciotomy:
  - Best for MCP joint; improvement of 93% versus 57% for PIP joint (4)[B]
  - Recurrence common; 50%
  - Shown to be effective for recurrent disease (4)[B]
  - Better for MCP joints in patients with comorbid conditions; lower complication rate, but higher recurrence (5)[C]
- Continuous elongation (atraumatic elongation using an external device, typically on 4th and 5th digits prepares a severely contracted joint for surgery (6)[B].

SURGERY/OTHER PROCEDURES
- Dermofasciectomy/limited fasciectomy/segmental aponeurectomy:
  - Greater initial correction over nonincisional treatment; higher complication rates (5)[C]
  - Night extension orthosis in combination with standard hand therapy no different maintaining finger extension than hand therapy alone in the 3 months following surgical release (6)[B].
- Indications:
  - Any involvement of the PIP joints
  - MCP joints contracted at least 30 degrees
  - Positive Hueston tabletop test
- May require skin grafts for wound closure with severe cutaneous shrinkage
- 80% have full range of movement with early surgery.
- Amputation of 5th digit if severe and deforming
- MCP joints respond better to surgery than PIP joints, especially if contracted >45 degrees.

ONGOING CARE

FOLLOW-UP RECOMMENDATIONS
Patient Monitoring
Regular follow-up every 6 months to 1 year

PATIENT EDUCATION
- Avoid risk factors (alcohol, vibratory exposure, etc.), especially if strong family history.
- Mild disease: Passively stretch digits twice a day and avoid recurrent gripping of tools.

PROGNOSIS
- Unpredictable but usually slowly progressive
- 10% may regress spontaneously.
- Dupuytren diathesis predicts aggressive course. Features include ethnicity (Nordic), family history, bilateral lesions outside of palm, age <50 years—all factors with 71% risk of recurrence compared to baseline 23% without any risk factors.
- Prognosis is better for MCP versus PIP joint after surgery and collagenase injection.

COMPLICATIONS
- Reflex sympathetic dystrophy postsurgery
- Operative nerve injury
- Postoperative recurrence in 46–80%
- Postoperative hand edema and skin necrosis
- Digital infarction

REFERENCES
1. Peimer CA, Blazar P, Coleman S, et al. Dupuytren contracture recurrence following treatment with collagenase *Clostridium histolyticum* (CORDLESS [Collagenase Option for Reduction of Dupuytren Long-Term Evaluation of Safety Study]): 5-year data. *J Hand Surg Am.* 2015;40(8):1597–1605.
2. Zhou C, Hovius SE, Slijper HP, et al. Collagenase *Clostridium histolyticum* versus limited fasciectomy for Dupuytren's contracture: outcomes from a multicenter propensity score matched study. *Plast Reconstr Surg.* 2015;136(1):87–97.
3. McMillan C, Binhammer P. Steroid injection and needle aponeurotomy for Dupuytren disease: long-term follow-up of a randomized controlled trial. *J Hand Surg Am.* 2014;39(10):1942–1947.
4. van Rijssen AL, Werker PM. Percutaneous needle fasciotomy for recurrent Dupuytren disease. *J Hand Surg Am.* 2012;37(9):1820–1823.
5. Henry M. Dupuytren's disease: current state of the art. *Hand (N Y).* 2014;9(1):1–8.
6. Collis J, Collocott S, Hing W, et al. The effect of night extension orthoses following surgical release of Dupuytren contracture: a single-center, randomized, controlled trial. *J Hand Surg Am.* 2013;38(7):1285.e2–1294.e2.

ADDITIONAL READING
- Ball C, Pratt AL, Nanchahal J. Optimal functional outcome measures for assessing treatment for Dupuytren's disease: a systematic review and recommendations for future practice. *BMC Musculoskelet Disord.* 2013;14:131.
- Eaton C. Evidence-based medicine: Dupuytren contracture. *Plast Reconstr Surg.* 2014;133(5): 1241–1251.
- Lanting R, Broekstra DC, Werker PM, et al. A systematic review and meta-analysis on the prevalence of Dupuytren disease in the general population of Western countries. *Plast Reconstr Surg.* 2014;133(3): 593–603.
- Michou L, Lermusiaux JL, Teyssedou JP, et al. Genetics of Dupuytren's disease. *Joint Bone Spine.* 2012;79(1):7–12.
- Sweet S, Blackmore S. Surgical and therapy update on the management of Dupuytren's disease. *J Hand Ther.* 2014;27(2):77–84.

 CODES

ICD10
M72.0 Palmar fascial fibromatosis [Dupuytren]

CLINICAL PEARLS
- Dupuytren contracture is a fixed flexion deformity of (most commonly) the 4th and 5th digits due to palmar fibrosis. 90% of cases are progressive.
- Refer patients with involvement of the PIP joints or MCP involvement with contractures of >30 degrees.
- Both surgical and enzymatic fasciotomy have high rate of recurrence.

D

DYSHIDROSIS
Cara Marshall, MD

 BASICS

DESCRIPTION
- A skin rash (dermatitis) within the "dyshidrosis" family. Literature supports the presence of several different classes within the family dyshidrosis but no general agreement about a strict definition of these classes.
- Dyshidrotic eczema
  - Common, chronic, or recurrent; nonerythematous; symmetric vesicular eruption primarily of the palms, soles, and interdigital areas
  - Associated with burning, itching, and pain
- Pompholyx (from Greek "bubble")
  - Rare condition characterized by abrupt onset of large bullae.
  - Sometimes used interchangeably with dyshidrotic eczema (small vesicles). Some believe these to be discrete entities.
- Lamellar dyshidrosis
  - Fine, spreading exfoliation of the superficial epidermis in the same distribution as described above.
- System(s) affected: dermatologic, exocrine, immunologic
- Synonym(s): cheiropompholyx, keratolysis exfoliativa, vesicular palmoplantar eczema, desquamation of interdigital spaces, palmar pompholyx reaction, acute and recurrent hand dermatitis (1)

EPIDEMIOLOGY
Incidence
- Mean age of onset is 40 years and younger
- Male = female
- Comprises 5–20% of hand eczema cases

Prevalence
20 cases/100,000 populations

ETIOLOGY AND PATHOPHYSIOLOGY
- Exact mechanism unknown; thought to be multifactorial
- Dermatopathology: spongiosis with intraepidermal vesicles
- Despite the name, sweat glands are not altered/affected (2)
- Vesicles remain intact due to thickness of stratum corneum of palmar/plantar skin (1).
- Exact cause not known.
- Aggravating factors (debated)
  - Hyperhidrosis (in 40% of patients with the condition)
  - Climate: hot/cold weather; humidity
  - Contact sensitivity (in 30–67% of patients with the condition) (2)
  - Nickel, cobalt, and chromate sensitivity (may include implanted orthopedic or orthodontic metals) (1)
  - Irritating compounds and solutions
  - Stress
  - Dermatophyte infection (present in 10% of patients with the condition) (2)
  - Prolonged wear of occlusive gloves
  - IV immunoglobulin therapy
  - Smoking

Genetics
- Atopy: 50% of patients with dyshidrotic eczema have atopic dermatitis (1)
- Rare autosomal dominant form of pompholyx found in Chinese population maps to chromosome 18q22.1–18q22.3 (2).

RISK FACTORS
- Many risk factors are disputed in the literature, with none being consistently associated.
- Atopy
- Other dermatologic conditions
  - Atopic dermatitis (early in life)
  - Contact dermatitis (later in life)
  - Dermatophytosis
- Sensitivity to
  - Foods
  - Drugs: neomycin, quinolones, acetaminophen, and oral contraceptives
  - Contact and dietary: nickel (more common in young women), chromate (more common in men), and cobalt (1)
  - Smoking in males

GENERAL PREVENTION
- Control emotional stress.
- Avoid excessive sweating.
- Avoid exposure to irritants.
- Avoid diet high in metal salts (chromium, cobalt, nickel).
- Avoid smoking.

COMMONLY ASSOCIATED CONDITIONS
- Atopic dermatitis
- Allergic contact dermatitis
- Parkinson disease
- HIV (2)

 DIAGNOSIS

HISTORY
- Episodes of pruritic rash
- Recent emotional stress
- Familial or personal history of atopy
- Exposure to allergens or irritants (3)
  - Occupational, dietary, or household
  - Cosmetic and personal hygiene products
  - Vesicular eruption typically occurs 24 hours after allergen challenge (1).
- Costume jewelry use
- IV immunoglobulin therapy
- HIV
- Smoking

PHYSICAL EXAM
- Symmetric distribution on the palms and soles; also may affect the dorsal aspects of hands and feet
- Lesions may not heal completely between flares (1).
- Early findings
  - 1 to 2 mm, clear, nonerythematous, deep-seated vesicles

- Late findings
  - Unroofed vesicles with inflamed bases
  - Desquamation
  - Peeling, rings of scale, or lichenification common

DIFFERENTIAL DIAGNOSIS
- Vesicular tinea pedis/manuum
- Vesicular id reaction
- Contact dermatitis (allergic or irritant)
- Scabies
- Chronic vesicular hand dermatitis
- Drug reaction
- Dermatophytid
- Bullous disorders: dyshidrosiform bullous pemphigoid, pemphigus, bullous impetigo, epidermolysis bullosa
- Pustular psoriasis
- Acrodermatitis continua
- Erythema multiforme
- Herpes infection
- Pityriasis rubra pilaris
- Vesicular mycosis fungoides

DIAGNOSTIC TESTS & INTERPRETATION
Follow-Up Tests & Special Considerations
- Skin culture in suspected secondary infection (most commonly, *Staphylococcus aureus*) (4)
- Consider antibiotics based on culture results and severity of symptoms.

Diagnostic Procedures/Other
- Diagnosis is based on clinical exam.
- Potassium hydroxide (KOH) wet mount (if concerned about dermatophyte infection)
- Patch test (if suspecting allergic cause)

Test Interpretation
- Fine, 1- to 2-mm spongiotic intraepidermal vesicles with little to no inflammatory change
- No eccrine glandular involvement
- Thickened stratum corneum

TREATMENT

GENERAL MEASURES
- Avoid possible causative factors: stress, direct skin contact with irritants, nickel, occlusive gloves, household cleaning products, smoking, sweating
- Use moisturizers/emollients for symptomatic relief and to maintain effective skin barrier.
- Skin care
  - Wear shoes with leather rather than rubber soles (e.g., sneakers).
  - Wear socks and gloves made of cotton and change frequently.
  - Wash infrequently, carefully dry, then apply emollient.
  - Avoid direct contact with fresh fruit (5)[C].

MEDICATION

First Line

- Mild cases: topical steroids (high potency) (2)[B]
  - Considered cornerstone of therapy but limited published evidence
- Moderate to severe cases
  - Ultrahigh-potency topical steroids with occlusion over treated area (4)[B]
  - Prednisone 40 to 100 mg/day tapered after blister formation ceases (2)[B]
  - Psoralens plus ultraviolet (UV)-A therapy (PUVA), either systemic/topical or immersion in psoralens (2)[B]
- Recurrent cases (4)[B]
  - Systemic steroids at onset of itching prodrome
  - Prednisone 60 mg PO for 3 to 4 days

Second Line

- Topical calcineurin inhibitors (mitigate the long-term risks of topical steroid use)
  - Topical tacrolimus (6)[B]
  - Topical pimecrolimus (6)[B]
  - May not be as effective on plantar surface
- Other therapies (typically with dermatology consultation)
  - Oral cyclosporine (4)[B]
  - Injections of botulinum toxin type A (BTXA) (6)[B]
    - Newer topical forms of BTXA currently being developed show promise
    - Painful, requires nerve block
  - Systemic alitretinoin (teratogenic) (5)[B]
  - Topical bexarotene (a teratogenic retinoid X receptor agonist approved for use in cutaneous T-cell lymphoma) (6)[B]
  - Methotrexate (6)[C]
  - Azathioprine (1)[C]
  - Disulfiram or sodium cromoglycate in nickel-allergic patients (1)[C]
  - Mycophenolate mofetil (2)[C]
  - Tap water iontophoresis (2)[C]

ISSUES FOR REFERRAL

- Allergist (if allergen testing required)
- Psychologist (if stress modification needed)

ADDITIONAL TREATMENT

- Radiation therapy (1)[C]
- UV-free phototherapy (5)[C]
- Treat underlying dermatophytosis (1).

COMPLEMENTARY & ALTERNATIVE MEDICINE

- Topical treatments to minimize pruritus (not curative) (4)[C]: Burow solution (aluminum acetate) or vinegar compresses
- Exposure to sunlight as maintenance therapy, 12 minutes every other day, 10 to 15 exposures (5)[C]
- Dandelion juice (avoid in atopic patients) (6)[C]

ONGOING CARE

FOLLOW-UP RECOMMENDATIONS

Patient Monitoring

- Dyshidrotic Eczema Area and Severity Index (DASI) (1)
- Parameters used in the DASI score
  - Number of vesicles per square centimeter
  - Erythema
  - Desquamation
  - Severity of itching
  - Surface area affected
- Grading: mild (0 to 15), moderate (16 to 30), severe (31 to 60)
- Monitor BP and glucose in patients receiving systemic corticosteroids.
- Monitor for adverse effects of medications.

DIET

- Consider diet low in metal salts if there is history of nickel sensitivity (4)[B].
- Updated recommendations for low-cobalt diet are available (1).

PATIENT EDUCATION

- Instructions on self-care, complications, and avoidance of triggers/aggravating factors
- PubMed Health: Dyshidrotic Eczema at: http://www.ncbi.nlm.nih.gov/pubmedhealth/PMH0001835/

PROGNOSIS

- Condition is benign.
- Usually heals without scarring.
- Lesions may spontaneously resolve.
- Recurrence is common.

COMPLICATIONS

- Secondary bacterial infections (S. aureus most common)
- Dystrophic nail changes
- Fissures
- Skin tightening/discomfort
- Psychological distress

REFERENCES

1. Veien NK. Acute and recurrent vesicular hand dermatitis. Dermatol Clin. 2009;27(3):337–353.
2. Wollina U. Pompholyx: a review of clinical features, differential diagnosis, and management. Am J Clin Dermatol. 2010;11(5):305–314.
3. Guillet MH, Wierzbicka E, Guillet S, et al. A 3-year causative study of pompholyx in 120 patients. Arch Dermatol. 2007;143(12):1504–1508.
4. Lofgren SM, Warshaw EM. Dyshidrosis: epidemiology, clinical characteristics, and therapy. Dermatitis. 2006;17(4):165–181.
5. Letić M. Use of sunlight to treat dyshidrotic eczema. JAMA Dermatol. 2013;149(5):634–635.
6. Wollina U. Pompholyx: what's new? Expert Opin Investig Drugs. 2008;17(6):897–904.

ADDITIONAL READING

- Chen JJ, Liang YH, Zhou FS, et al. The gene for a rare autosomal dominant form of pompholyx maps to chromosome 18q22.1–18q22.3. J Invest Dermatol. 2006;126(2):300–304.
- Molin S, Diepgen TL, Ruzicka T, et al. Diagnosing chronic hand eczema by an algorithm: a tool for classification in clinical practice. Clin Exp Dermatol. 2011;36(6):595–601.
- Schuttelaar ML, Coenraads PJ, Huizinga J, et al. Increase in vesicular hand eczema after house dust mite inhalation provocation: a double-blind, placebo-controlled, cross-over study. Contact Dermatitis. 2013;68(2):76–85.
- Soler DC, Bai X, Ortega L, et al. The key role of aquaporin 3 and aquaporin 10 in the pathogenesis of pompholyx. Med Hypotheses. 2015;84(5):498–503.
- Stuckert J, Nedorost S. Low-cobalt diet for dyshidrotic eczema patients. Contact Dermatitis. 2008;59(6):361–365.
- Sumila M, Notter M, Itin P, et al. Long-term results of radiotherapy in patients with chronic palmoplantar eczema or psoriasis. Strahlenther Onkol. 2008;184(4):218–223.
- Tzaneva S, Kittler H, Thallinger C, et al. Oral vs. bath PUVA using 8-methoxypsoralen for chronic palmoplantar eczema. Photodermatol Photoimmunol Photomed. 2009;25(2):101–105.

SEE ALSO

Algorithm: Rash, Focal

CODES

ICD10

L30.1 Dyshidrosis [pompholyx]

CLINICAL PEARLS

- Dyshidrosis is a transient, recurrent vesicular eruption most commonly of the palms, soles, and interdigital areas.
- Etiology and pathophysiology are unknown but are most likely related to a combination of genetic and environmental factors.
- Best prevention is effective skin care and limiting exposure to irritating agents.
- Treatments are based on disease severity; preferred treatments include topical steroids, oral steroids, and calcineurin inhibitors.
- Condition is benign and usually heals spontaneously and without scarring. Medical treatment decreases healing time and risk for progression to secondary bacterial infection.

DYSMENORRHEA

Taiwona Elliott, DO

BASICS

DESCRIPTION
- Pelvic pain occurring at/around time of menses; a leading cause of absenteeism for women <30 years old
- Primary dysmenorrhea: pelvic pain without pathologic physical findings
- Secondary dysmenorrhea: often more severe, results from specific pelvic pathology. Severity based on activity impairment
  - Mild: painful, rarely limits daily function, or requires analgesics
  - Moderate: daily activity affected, rare absenteeism, and requires analgesics
  - Severe: daily activity affected, likelihood absenteeism, limited benefit from analgesics
- System affected: reproductive
- Synonym(s): menstrual cramps

EPIDEMIOLOGY
- Predominant age
  - Primary: onset 6 to 12 months after the start of menarche, teens to early 20s
  - Secondary: 20s to 30s
- Predominant sex: women only

Prevalence
- Up to 90% of menstruating females have experienced primary dysmenorrhea.
- Up to 42% lose days of school/work monthly due to dysmenorrhea.
- Up to 20% reported impairment in daily activities.

ETIOLOGY AND PATHOPHYSIOLOGY
- Primary: Elevated prostaglandin (PGF2α) production through indirect hormonal control (stimulation of production by estrogen) causes nonrhythmic hypercontractility and increased uterine muscle tone with vasoconstriction and resultant uterine ischemia. Ischemia results in hypersensitization of type C pain nerve fibers. Intensity of cramps directly proportional to amount of PGF2α released.
- Secondary
  - Endometriosis (most common cause)
  - Congenital abnormalities of uterine/vaginal anatomy
  - Cervical stenosis
  - Pelvic inflammatory disease
  - Adenomyosis
  - Ovarian cysts
  - Pelvic tumors, especially leiomyomata (fibroids) and uterine polyps

Genetics
Not well studied

RISK FACTORS
- Primary (1)
  - Cigarette smoking
  - Alcohol use
  - Early menarche (age <12 years)
  - Age <30 years
  - Irregular/heavy menstrual flow
  - Nonuse of oral contraceptives
  - Sexual abuse
  - Psychological symptoms (depression, anxiety, increased stress, etc.)
  - Nulliparity
- Secondary (10%)
  - Pelvic infection
  - Use of intrauterine device (IUD)

- Structural pelvic malformations
- Family history of endometriosis in first-degree relative

GENERAL PREVENTION
- Primary: Choose a diet low in animal fats.
- Secondary: Reduce risk of sexually transmitted infections (STIs).

Pediatric Considerations
Onset with first menses raises probability of genital tract anatomic abnormality (i.e., transverse vaginal septum, imperforate or minimally perforated hymen, uterine anomalies).

COMMONLY ASSOCIATED CONDITIONS
- Irregular/heavy menstrual periods
- Longer menstrual cycle length/duration of bleeding
- Endometriosis

DIAGNOSIS

Based on characteristic history of suprapubic/low back cramping/pain occurring at or near menstrual flow onset lasting for 8 to 72 hours (2).

HISTORY
- Primary: Onset once ovulatory cycles are established in adolescents; 6 to 12 months after menarche on average
- Patients may have associated nausea, vomiting, diarrhea, headache, fatigue, or pain radiating into the inner thighs.
- Recurrence at or just before the onset of the menstrual flow
  - Pelvic pain occurring between menstrual periods is not likely to be dysmenorrhea.
  - Present with most menstrual periods (cyclic)
- Relief associated with the following:
  - Continued bleeding for the usual duration
  - Use of analgesics, especially NSAIDs
  - Orgasm
  - Local heat application
- Response to NSAIDs helps confirm diagnosis.
- Secondary: associated with chronic pelvic pain, mid-cycle pain, dyspareunia, and abnormal uterine bleeding

PHYSICAL EXAM
- Primary: Physical exam typically is normal. Examine to rule out secondary dysmenorrhea. Pelvic exam is recommended if sexually active to rule out infection.
- Secondary: Evaluate for cervical discharge, uterine enlargement, tenderness, irregularity, or fixation.

DIFFERENTIAL DIAGNOSIS
- Primary: History is characteristic.
- Secondary
  - Pelvic/genital infection
  - Complication of pregnancy
  - Missed/incomplete abortion
  - Ectopic pregnancy
  - Uterine/ovarian neoplasm
  - Endometriosis
  - UTI
  - Complication with IUD use

DIAGNOSTIC TESTS & INTERPRETATION
Initial Tests (lab, imaging)
- Pregnancy test
- Urine testing for infection
- Gonorrhea/chlamydia cervical testing, especially in women age <25 years and in high-prevalence areas.

- Primary: Consider pelvic ultrasound to rule out secondary abnormalities if history is not characteristic or suspected abnormality on exam.
- Secondary: Ultrasound/laparoscopy to define anatomy for severe/refractory cases. MRI may be useful as second-line noninvasive imaging if ultrasound is nondiagnostic and torsion, deep endometriosis, or adenomyosis suspected.

Follow-Up Tests & Special Considerations
Counsel regarding appropriate preventive measures for STI and pregnancy.

Diagnostic Procedures/Other
Laparoscopy is rarely needed.

Test Interpretation
- Primary: none
- Secondary: Specific anatomic abnormalities may be noted (see "Differential Diagnosis").

Pregnancy Considerations
Consider ectopic pregnancy when pelvic pain occurs with vaginal bleeding.

TREATMENT

- Reassure the patient that treatment success is very likely with adherence to recommendations.
- Relief may require the use of several treatment modalities at the same time.

GENERAL MEASURES
- Exercise and local heat are noninvasive general measures to relieve pain.
- High-frequency transcutaneous electrical nerve stimulation (TENS) has been found to be beneficial. There is conflicting evidence for low-frequency TENS.
- Secondary dysmenorrhea: Treatment of infections; suppression of endometrium if endometriosis suspected; remove IUD if contributing factor.

MEDICATION
First Line
- NSAIDs: No NSAID has been found to be superior to others. Medication should be taken on scheduled dosing 1 to 2 days *prior* to onset of menses and continued for 2 to 3 days (2,3)[A]. If one NSAID preparation does not work, another NSAID preparation should be tried.

  - Ibuprofen 400 mg q8h
  - Naproxen sodium 500 mg BID
  - Celecoxib 400 mg × 1, then 200 mg q12h
  - Mefenamic acid 500 mg × 1, then 250 mg q6h

- Hormonal contraceptives: recommended for primary dysmenorrhea in women desiring contraception (2)[B]. Directly limits endometrial growth resulting in reduced prostaglandin production and intrauterine pressure. Continuous rather than cyclic dosing may initially be more effective at reducing pain, however, may have similar benefit after 6 months (4)[B]. Estrogen-containing contraceptives are recommended as first-line for secondary dysmenorrhea due to endometriosis, although progestin-only methods have also been shown to be beneficial (2)[B].
- Levonorgestrel IUDs can decrease primary dysmenorrhea (5)[B].

- Potential contraindications to NSAIDs and combined oral contraceptives (COCs)
  - Platelet disorders
  - Gastric ulceration or gastritis

- Thromboembolic disorders
- Vascular disease
- Migraine with aura
- Precautions
  - GI irritation
  - Lactation
  - Coagulation disorders
  - Impaired renal function
  - Heart failure
  - Liver dysfunction
- Significant possible interactions
  - Coumadin-type anticoagulants
  - Aspirin with other NSAIDs

Second Line

- Local heat can help relieve pain and may be as effective as NSAIDs (2)[B].
- Exercise may have beneficial effects in relieving pain (6)[B].
- β_2-adrenoceptor agonists have not definitively been shown to relieve pain in dysmenorrhea (7)[B].
- Behavioral interventions, such as relaxation exercises, may help alleviate pain in primary dysmenorrhea.

SURGERY/OTHER PROCEDURES
Laparoscopic uterosacral nerve ablation has been shown to relieve pain at >12 months postoperatively.

COMPLEMENTARY & ALTERNATIVE MEDICINE

- Spinal manipulation has not been shown to be effective in treating pain (8)[A].
- Chinese herbal medicine shows promising evidence of decreasing pain, but more evidence is needed.
- Acupuncture treatments have been shown to decrease pain in dysmenorrhea, but further randomized, well-designed studies are needed (2,9)[B].
- Acupoint stimulation, particularly noninvasive stimulation (acupressure), can relieve pain (10)[B].
- Aromatherapy abdominal massage performed daily for 10 minutes, 7 days prior to onset of menses can decrease primary dysmenorrhea (11)[B].
- Further research needed to determine benefit and safety for use of oral fennel, extracorporeal magnetic innervation, vitamin K_1 injection into the spleen-6 acupuncture point, use of high-frequency vibratory stimulation tampon, and vaginal sildenafil.

INPATIENT CONSIDERATIONS
Both primary and secondary dysmenorrhea are usually managed in the outpatient setting.

Admission Criteria/Initial Stabilization
- Primary: outpatient care
- Secondary: usually outpatient care

 ONGOING CARE

FOLLOW-UP RECOMMENDATIONS
Normal

DIET
- Vitamin B_1 100 mg daily, omega-3 fatty acid, and fish oil supplementation may be beneficial (12)[B].
- Magnesium has been shown to be useful, but the correct dosage has not been determined.
- Insufficient evidence to show usefulness of zinc and vitamin E at this time
- Low-fat vegetarian diet can be helpful in some patients (12).

PATIENT EDUCATION
Reassure the patient that primary dysmenorrhea is treatable with the use of NSAIDs, COCs, IUD, or local heat; and that it will usually abate with age and parity.

PROGNOSIS
- Primary: reduced with age and parity
- Secondary: likely to require therapy based on underlying cause

COMPLICATIONS
- Primary: anxiety and/or depression
- Secondary: infertility from underlying pathology

REFERENCES

1. Ju H, Jones M, Mishra G. The prevalence and risk factors of dysmenorrhea. *Epidemiol Rev.* 2014;36:104–113.
2. Osayande AS, Mehulic S. Diagnosis and initial management of dysmenorrhea. *Am Fam Physician.* 2014;89(5):341–346.
3. Lethaby A, Duckitt K, Farquhar C. Non-steroidal anti-inflammatory drugs for heavy menstrual bleeding. *Cochrane Database Syst Rev.* 2013;(1):CD000400.
4. Dmitrovic R, Kunselman AR, Legro RS. Continuous compared with cyclic oral contraceptives for the treatment of primary dysmenorrhea: a randomized controlled trial. *Obstet Gynecol.* 2012;119(6):1143–1150.
5. Lindh I, Milsom I. The influence of intrauterine contraception on the prevalence and severity of dysmenorrhea: a longitudinal population study. *Hum Reprod.* 2013;28(7):1953–1960.
6. Brown J, Brown S. Exercise for dysmenorrhoea. *Cochrane Database Syst Rev.* 2010;(2):CD004142.
7. Fedorowicz Z, Nasser M, Jagannath VA, et al. Beta2-adrenoceptor agonists for dysmenorrhoea. *Cochrane Database Syst Rev.* 2012;(5):CD008585.
8. Kannan P, Claydon LS. Some physiotherapy treatments may relieve menstrual pain in women with primary dysmenorrhea: a systematic review. *J Physiother.* 2014;60(1):13–21.
9. Reyes-Campos MD, Díaz-Toral LG, Verdín-Terán SL, et al. Acupuncture as an adjunct treatment for primary dysmenorrhea: a comparative study. *Med Acupunct.* 2013;25(4):291–294.
10. Chen MN, Chien LW, Liu CF. Acupuncture or acupressure at the Sanyinjiao (SP6) Acupoint for the treatment of primary dysmenorrhea: a meta-analysis. *Evid Based Complement Alternat Med.* 2013;2013:493038.
11. Marzouk TM, El-Nemer AM, Baraka HN. The effect of aromatherapy abdominal massage on alleviating menstrual pain in nursing students: a prospective randomized cross-over study. *Evid Based Complement Alternat Med.* 2013;2013:742421.
12. Hansen SO, Knudsen UB. Endometriosis, dysmenorrhoea and diet. *Eur J Obstet Gynecol Reprod Biol.* 2013;169(2):162–171.

ADDITIONAL READING

- Akin MD, Weingand KW, Hengehold DA, et al. Continuous low-level topical heat in the treatment of dysmenorrhea. *Obstet Gynecol.* 2001;97(3):343–349.
- Allen LM, Lam AC. Premenstrual syndrome and dysmenorrhea in adolescents. *Adolesc Med State Art Rev.* 2012;23(1):139–163.
- Altunyurt S, Göl M, Altunyurt S, et al. Primary dysmenorrhea and uterine blood flow: a color Doppler study. *J Reprod Med.* 2005;50(4):251–255.
- Bayer LL, Hillard PJ. Use of levonorgestrel intrauterine system for medical indications in adolescents. *J Adolesc Health.* 2013;52(4 Suppl):S54–S58.
- Cho SH, Hwang EW. Acupuncture for primary dysmenorrhoea: a systematic review. *BJOG.* 2010;117(5):509–521.
- Dawood MY. Primary dysmenorrhea: advances in pathogenesis and management. *Obstet Gynecol.* 2006;108(2):428–441.
- Eby GA. Zinc treatment prevents dysmenorrhea. *Med Hypotheses.* 2007;69(2):297–301.
- Kannan P, Claydon LS, Miller D, et al. Vigorous exercises in the management of primary dysmenorrhea: a feasibility study. *Disabil Rehabil.* 2015:37(15):1334–1339.
- Khan KS, Champaneria R, Latthe PM. How effective are non-drug, non-surgical treatments for primary dysmenorrhoea? *BMJ.* 2012;344:e3011.
- Latthe P, Mignini L, Gray R, et al. Factors predisposing women to chronic pelvic pain: systematic review. *BMJ.* 2006;332(7544):749–755.
- Polat A, Celik H, Gurates B, et al. Prevalence of primary dysmenorrhea in young adult female university students. *Arch Gynecol Obstet.* 2009;279(4):527–532.
- Proctor M, Farquhar C. Diagnosis and management of dysmenorrhea. *BMJ.* 2006;332(7550):1134–1138.
- Zahradnik HP, Hanjalic-Beck A, Groth K. Non-steroidal anti-inflammatory drugs and hormonal contraceptives for pain relief from dysmenorrhea: a review. *Contraception.* 2010;81(3):185–196.
- Zannoni L, Giorgi M, Spagnolo E, et al. Dysmenorrhea, absenteeism from school, and symptoms suspicious for endometriosis in adolescents. *J Pediatr Adolesc Gynecol.* 2014;27(5):258–265.
- Zhu X, Proctor M, Bensoussan A, et al. Chinese herbal medicine for primary dysmenorrhea. *Cochrane Database Syst Rev.* 2008;(2):CD005288.

 SEE ALSO

- Endometriosis
- Dyspareunia
- Menorrhagia
- Premenstrual Syndrome (PMS) and Premenstrual Dysphoric Disorder (PMDD)
- Algorithm: Pelvic Pain

 CODES

ICD10
- N94.6 Dysmenorrhea, unspecified
- N94.4 Primary dysmenorrhea
- N94.5 Secondary dysmenorrhea

CLINICAL PEARLS

- Dysmenorrhea is a leading cause of absenteeism for women age <30 years.
- In women who desire contraception, hormonal contraceptives are the preferred treatment.
- All NSAIDs studied have been found to be equally effective in the relief of dysmenorrhea and should be initiated 1 to 2 days prior to onset of menses with scheduled dosing.

DYSPAREUNIA

Scott T. Henderson, MD

 BASICS

DESCRIPTION

- Recurrent and persistent genital pain associated with sexual activity, which is not exclusively due to lack of lubrication or vaginismus.
- May be the result of organic, emotional, or psychogenic causes
  - Primary: present throughout one's sexual history
  - Secondary: arising from some specific event or condition (e.g., menopause, drugs)
  - Superficial: pain at, or near, the introitus or vaginal barrel associated with penetration
  - Deep: pain after penetration located at the cervix or lower abdominal area
  - Complete: present under all circumstances
  - Situational: occurring selectively with specific situations
- System(s) affected: reproductive

EPIDEMIOLOGY

- Predominant age: all ages
- Predominant sex: female > male

Incidence

>50% of all sexually active women will report dyspareunia at some time.

Geriatric Considerations

Incidence increases dramatically in postmenopausal women primarily because of vaginal atrophy.

Prevalence

- Most sexually active women will experience dyspareunia at some time in their lives.
  - ~15% (4–40%) of adult women will have dyspareunia on a few occasions during a year.
  - ~1–2% of women will have painful intercourse on a more-than-occasional basis.
  - Male prevalence is ~1%.

ETIOLOGY AND PATHOPHYSIOLOGY

- Disorders of vaginal outlet
  - Adhesions
  - Condyloma
  - Clitoral irritation
  - Episiotomy scars
  - Fissures
  - Hymeneal ring abnormalities
  - Inadequate lubrication
  - Infections
  - Lichen planus
  - Lichen sclerosus
  - Postmenopausal atrophy
  - Psoriasis
  - Trauma
  - Vulvar papillomatosis
  - Vulvar vestibulitis/vulvodynia
- Disorders of vagina
  - Abnormality of vault owing to surgery or radiation
  - Congenital malformations
  - Inadequate lubrication
  - Infections
  - Inflammatory or allergic response to foreign substance
  - Masses or tumors
  - Pelvic relaxation resulting in rectocele, uterine prolapse, or cystocele

- Disorders of pelvic structures
  - Endometriosis
  - Levator ani myalgia/spasm
  - Malignant or benign tumors of the uterus
  - Ovarian pathology
  - Pelvic adhesions
  - Pelvic inflammatory disease (PID)
  - Pelvic venous congestion
  - Prior pelvic fracture
  - Uterine fibroids
- Disorders of the GI tract
  - Constipation
  - Crohn disease
  - Diverticular disease
  - Fistulas
  - Hemorrhoids
  - Inflammatory bowel disease
- Disorders of the urinary tract
  - Interstitial cystitis
  - Ureteral or vesical lesions
  - Urethritis
- Chronic disease
  - Behçet syndrome
  - Diabetes
  - Sjögren syndrome
- Male
  - Cancer of penis
  - Genital muscle spasm
  - Infection or irritation of penile skin
  - Infection of seminal vesicles
  - Lichen sclerosus
  - Musculoskeletal disorders of pelvis and lower back
  - Penile anatomy disorders
  - Phimosis
  - Prostate infections and enlargement
  - Testicular disease
  - Torsion of spermatic cord
  - Urethritis
- Psychological disorders
  - Anxiety
  - Conversion reactions
  - Depression
  - Fear
  - Hostility toward partner
  - Phobic reactions
  - Psychological trauma

RISK FACTORS

- Fatigue
- Stress
- Depression
- Diabetes
- Estrogen deficiency
  - Menopause
  - Lactation
- Previous PID
- Vaginal surgery
- Alcohol/marijuana consumption
- Medication side effects (antihistamines, tamoxifen, bromocriptine, low-estrogen oral contraceptives, SSRIs, depo-medroxyprogesterone, desipramine)

Pregnancy Considerations

Pregnancy is a potent influence on sexuality; dyspareunia is common. Women who experience delivery interventions including episiotomy are at greater risk than women who deliver over an intact perineum or have an unsutured tear.

COMMONLY ASSOCIATED CONDITIONS

Vaginismus

Pregnancy Considerations

Episiotomies do not have a protective effect (1)[A].

 DIAGNOSIS

HISTORY

- Identify pain characteristics
  - Onset
  - Duration
  - Location: entry versus deep, single versus multiple sites; positional
  - Intensity/quality: varying degrees of pelvic/genital pressure, aching, tearing, and/or burning
  - Pattern (precipitating or aggravating factors): when pain occurs (at entry, during, or after intercourse)
  - Relief measures: Avoid intercourse, change positions, and have intercourse only at certain times of the month.
- Include menstrual, obstetric, reproductive, sexual, domestic violence, and rape histories with medical, surgical, and psychosocial history

PHYSICAL EXAM

- A complete exam, including a focused pelvic exam, to identify pathology and provide patient education.
- Because examination often reproduces the pain, examiner should be cautious and sensitive to patient's anxiety. Exam must include inspection and palpation of vulva and vaginal areas, palpation of the uterine and adnexal structures, and a rectovaginal exam. Sensory mapping with a cotton-tipped applicator to identify sensitive and painful areas.
- Inspect and palpate urethra and base of the bladder.

DIFFERENTIAL DIAGNOSIS

Vaginismus

DIAGNOSTIC TESTS & INTERPRETATION

Initial Tests (lab, imaging)

Based on history and exam findings

- Wet mount
- Gonorrhea and chlamydia cultures
- Herpes culture
- Urinalysis and urine culture
- Pap smear

Follow-Up Tests & Special Considerations

- Serum estradiol if vulvodynia or atrophic vaginitis
- Voiding cystourethrogram if urinary tract involvement
- GI contrast studies if GI symptoms
- Ultrasound and CT scan are of limited value; perform if clinically indicated.

Diagnostic Procedures/Other
Based on history and exam findings
- Colposcopy and biopsy if vaginal/vulvar lesions
- Laparoscopy if complex deep-penetration pain
- Cystoscopy if urinary tract involvement
- Endoscopy if GI involvement

Test Interpretation
Depends on etiology

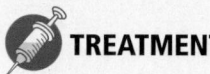 TREATMENT

- Potential relationships exists between primary dyspareunia and vaginismus, low libido, and arousal disorders.
- Endocrine factors, such as primary amenorrhea, might reduce the biologic basis of sexual response.
- If pain prevents penetration, severe vaginismus may be present.

GENERAL MEASURES
- Educate the patient and partner regarding the nature of the problem. Reassure both that there are solutions to the problem.
- Initiate specific treatment when initial evaluation identifies an organic cause.
- Once organic causes are ruled out, treatment is a multidimensional and multidisciplinary approach (2)[C].
  - Individual behavioral therapy
    - Indicated to help the patient deal with intrapersonal issues and assess the role of the partner
  - Couple behavioral therapy
    - Indicated to help resolve interpersonal problems
    - May involve short-term structured intervention or sexual counseling
    - Designed to desensitize systemically uncomfortable sexual responses and intercourse through a series of interventions over a period of weeks
    - Interventions range from muscle relaxation and mutual body massage to sexual fantasies and erotic massage.

MEDICATION
First Line
Depends on the etiology
- Antibiotics, antifungals, or antivirals, as indicated, for infection
- Vaginal moisturizers and lubricants for dryness
- Analgesics and topical anesthetics for pain
- Topical estrogen for vaginal and vulvar atrophy
- Neuropathic pain associated with vulvar vestibulitis/vulvodynia may respond to tricyclic antidepressants (amitriptyline or nortriptyline) or gabapentin.

Second Line
Ospemifene for moderate to severe symptoms due to menopause-related vulvar and vaginal atrophy (3)[B]

ISSUES FOR REFERRAL
Referral for long-term therapy may be necessary.

ADDITIONAL THERAPIES
Physical therapy for pelvic floor muscle pain

SURGERY/OTHER PROCEDURES
- Laparoscopic excision of endometriotic lesions has shown benefit (4)[C].
- Surgical vestibulectomy can be considered if medical measures fail with vulvar vestibulitis (5)[B].

COMPLEMENTARY & ALTERNATIVE MEDICINE
- Sitz baths may relieve painful inflammation.
- Perineal massage
- Antioxidants may improve symptoms associated with endometriosis.

 ONGOING CARE

FOLLOW-UP RECOMMENDATIONS
Patient Monitoring
- Outpatient follow-up depends on therapy.
- Every 6 to 12 months once resolved

DIET
A high-fiber diet may help if constipation is a contributing cause.

PATIENT EDUCATION
- Boston Women's Health Book Collective. *Our Bodies, Ourselves: A New Edition for a New Era.* New York, NY: Simon & Schuster; 2005.
- Kegel exercise information
- Provide couples with information about sexual arousal techniques.

PROGNOSIS
Depends on underlying cause but most patients will respond to treatment.

REFERENCES
1. Carroli G, Mignini L. Episiotomy for vaginal birth. *Cochrane Database Syst Rev.* 2009;(1):CD000081.
2. Crowley T, Richardson D, Goldmeier D. Recommendations for the management of vaginismus: BASHH Special Interest Group for Sexual Dysfunction. *Int J STD AIDS.* 2006;17(1):14–18.
3. Portman DJ, Bachmann GA, Simon JA, et al. Ospemifene, a novel selective estrogen receptor modulator for treating dyspareunia associated with postmenopausal vular and vaginal atrophy. *Menopause.* 2013; 20(6):623–630.
4. Ferrero S, Abbamonte LH, Giordano M, et al. Deep dyspareunia and sex life after laparoscopic excision of endometriosis. *Hum Reprod.* 2007;22(4):1142–1148.
5. Steege JF, Zolnoun DA. Evaluation and treatment of dyspareunia. *Obstet Gynecol.* 2009;113(5):1124–1136.

ADDITIONAL READING
- Boardman LA, Stockdale CK. Sexual pain. *Clin Obstet Gynecol.* 2009;52(4):682–690.
- Frank JE, Mistretta P, Will J. Diagnosis and treatment of female sexual dysfunction. *Am Fam Physician.* 2008;77(5):635–642.
- Sung SC, Jeng CJ, Lin YC. Sexual health care for women with dyspareunia. *Taiwan J Obstet Gynecol.* 2011;50(3):268–274.

 SEE ALSO

- Balanitis; Endometriosis; Pelvic Inflammatory Disease (PID); Sexual Dysfunction in Women; Genito-Pelvic Pain/Penetration Disorder (Vaginismus); Vulvovaginitis, Estrogen Deficient; Vulvovaginitis, Prepubescent
- Algorithms: Dyspareunia; Discharge, Vaginal

 CODES

ICD10
- N94.1 Dyspareunia
- F52.6 Dyspareunia not due to a substance or known physiol cond

CLINICAL PEARLS
- Careful history to determine if patient feels pain before, during, or after intercourse will help identify cause.
  - Pain before intercourse suggests a phobic attitude toward penetration and/or the presence of vestibulitis.
  - Pain during intercourse combined with the location of the pain is most predictive of the causes of pain.
  - Introital pain after intercourse suggests vestibulitis in women of childbearing age, hypertonic pelvic floor, or vulvovaginal dystrophia.
- Potential relationship exists between primary dyspareunia and vaginismus, low libido, and arousal disorders.
- Episiotomy does not offer any benefit in the prevention of dyspareunia; an episiotomy in fact may cause more future discomfort.

DYSPEPSIA, FUNCTIONAL

Kristina Burgers, MD, FAAFP • Matthew W. Short, MD, FAAFP

 BASICS

DESCRIPTION

- The presence of bothersome postprandial fullness, early satiety, or epigastric pain/burning in the absence of causative structural disease (to include normal upper endoscopy) for the preceding 3 months with initial symptom onset at least 6 months prior to diagnosis (Rome III criteria)
- Rome III criteria divide patients into two subtypes:
  - Postprandial distress syndrome
  - Epigastric pain syndrome
- System(s) affected: GI
- Synonym(s): idiopathic dyspepsia; nonulcer dyspepsia; nonorganic dyspepsia; postprandial distress syndrome; and epigastric pain syndrome

EPIDEMIOLOGY

Incidence
Unknown, accounts for 70% of patients with dyspepsia, and ~5% of primary care visits

Prevalence
- 15–30% prevalence in developed countries (3–10% when strict Rome III criteria are used)
- Predominant age: adults but can be seen in children
- Predominant gender: female > male

ETIOLOGY AND PATHOPHYSIOLOGY
Unknown, but proposed mechanisms or associations include gastric motility disorders, visceral pain hypersensitivity, *Helicobacter pylori* infection, alteration in upper GI microbiome, medications, anxiety, and depression

Genetics
Possible link to G-protein *β*-3 subunit 825 CC genotype and serotonin transport genes

Pediatric Considerations
Be alert for family system dysfunction.

Pregnancy Considerations
Pregnancy may exacerbate symptoms.

Geriatric Considerations
Patients >50 years with new-onset dyspepsia should have an upper endoscopy.

RISK FACTORS
- Other functional disorders
- Anxiety/depression psychosocial factors: divorce, unemployment
- Smoking

GENERAL PREVENTION
Avoid foods and habits known to exacerbate symptoms.

COMMONLY ASSOCIATED CONDITIONS
Other functional bowel disorders

 DIAGNOSIS

HISTORY
- Postprandial fullness (1)[B]
- Early satiety (1)[B]
- Epigastric pain (1)[B]
- Epigastric burning (1)[B]

- Symptoms for 3 months (1)[C]
- Warning signs that necessitate endoscopy include (2,3)[C]:
  - Unintended weight loss
  - Progressive dysphagia
  - Persistent vomiting
  - GI bleeding
  - Family history of cancer
  - Age >55 years

PHYSICAL EXAM
- Document weight status and vital signs.
- Examine for signs of systemic illness.
  - Murphy sign for cholelithiasis
  - Rebound and guarding for ulcer perforation
  - Palpation during muscle contraction for abdominal wall pain
  - Jaundice
  - Thyromegaly

DIFFERENTIAL DIAGNOSIS
- Peptic ulcer disease; gastroesophageal reflux disease
- Cholecystitis
- Gastric or esophageal cancer; esophageal spasm
- Malabsorption syndromes; celiac disease
- Pancreatic cancer; pancreatitis
- Inflammatory bowel disease; carbohydrate malabsorption; gastroparesis
- Ischemic bowel disease
- Intestinal parasites
- Irritable bowel syndrome
- Ischemic heart disease
- Diabetes mellitus; thyroid disease
- Connective tissue disorders
- Conversion disorder
- Medication effects

DIAGNOSTIC TESTS & INTERPRETATION

Initial Tests (lab, imaging)
- Functional dyspepsia is a diagnosis of exclusion. Order labs are based on clinical suspicion (3)[C].
- CBC (if anemia or infection are suspected)
- LFT (if hepatobiliary disease is suspected)

- Test for *H. pylori* (stool antigen or urea breath test) in areas of high *H. pylori* prevalence (3,4)[A].

- Upper endoscopy for patients >55 years or those with alarm symptoms (weight loss, signs of blood loss, dysphagia, concern for cancer) (3)[C]
- Perform upper endoscopy if patient does not respond to gastric acid suppression trial (3)[C].
- A self-report questionnaire can help assess and track symptoms (3)[C].

Diagnostic Procedures/Other
Esophageal manometry or gastric accommodation studies are rarely needed (3)[C].

Test Interpretation
None (by definition this a functional disorder)

 TREATMENT

GENERAL MEASURES
- Few effective treatment options are available (5).
- Reassurance and physician support are helpful (3)[C].
- Treatment is based on presumed etiologies.
- Discontinue offending medications (3)[C].

MEDICATION

First Line

- Treat *H. pylori* if confirmed on testing (3,4)[A].
- Trial of once daily proton pump inhibitor (PPI) medication (e.g., omeprazole 20 mg PO QD) or H2RA (e.g., ranitidine 150 mg BID) for up to 8 weeks in patients without alarm symptoms (3,5)[A]

Second Line

- Trial of low-dose tricyclic antidepressant (TCA) medication is helpful in epigastric pain syndrome but not postprandial distress syndrome (amitriptyline 10 mg at bedtime); consider doubling dose after a few days (2,5)[A],(6)[B]; caution in elderly.
- Trazodone 25 mg at bedtime is an alternative (2,5) [A]. Consider a 1-month trial of prokinetic medication (metoclopramide) or buspirone if no response to TCA (2,5)[B]. Caution with metoclopramide in elderly due to side effects of tardive dyskinesia and parkinsonian symptoms.

ADDITIONAL THERAPIES

- Stress reduction (2,5)[A]
  - Relaxation techniques
  - Physical exercise
  - Reflux precautions where applicable
- Psychotherapy effective in some patients (2)[A],(3)[B]

COMPLEMENTARY & ALTERNATIVE MEDICINE

Alternative approaches need further study.

- Peppermint oil +/− caraway oil
- Probiotics have theoretical benefit but few controlled trials (5)[B].
- Hypnotherapy may help (3)[B].
- Transcutaneous electroacupuncture may help (3)[B].

 ONGOING CARE

FOLLOW-UP RECOMMENDATIONS

Patient Monitoring

- Provide ongoing support and reassurance.
- Upper endoscopy if persistent symptoms
- Change medications if no change after 4 weeks (3)[C].
- Discontinue drug therapy after symptom resolution (3)[C].

DIET

- Limited data to support dietary modification
- Consider limiting fatty foods (2,5)[C].
- Avoid foods that exacerbate symptoms: wheat and cow milk proteins, peppers or spices, coffee, tea, and alcohol (2,5)[C].

PATIENT EDUCATION

Reassurance and stress reduction techniques

PROGNOSIS

Long-term/chronic symptoms with symptom-free periods

COMPLICATIONS

Iatrogenic, from evaluation to rule out serious pathology

REFERENCES

1. Tack J, Talley NJ. Functional dyspepsia—symptoms, definitions and validity of the Rome III criteria. *Nat Rev Gastroenterol Hepatol*. 2013;10(3):134–141.
2. Vanheel H, Tack J. Therapeutic options for functional dyspepsia. *Dig Dis*. 2014;32(3):230–234. doi:10.1159/000358111.
3. Miwa H, Kusano M, Arisawa T, et al. Evidence-based clinical practice guidelines for functional dyspepsia. *J Gastroenterol*. 2015;50(2):125–139. doi:10.1007/s00535-104-1022-3.
4. Zhao B, Zhao J, Cheng WF, et al. Efficacy of *Helicobacter pylori* eradication therapy on functional dyspepsia: a meta-analysis of randomized controlled studies with 12-month follow-up. *J Clin Gastroenterol*. 2014;48(3):241–247.
5. Stein B, Everhart KK, Lacy BE. Treatment of functional dyspepsia and gastroparesis. *Curr Treat Options Gastroenterol*. 2014;12(4):385–397. doi:10.1007/s11938-014-0028-5.
6. Talley NJ, Locke GR, Saito Y, et al. Effect of amitriptyline and escitalopram on functional dyspepsia: a multicenter, randomized controlled study. *Gastroenterology*. 2015;149(2):340.e2–349.e2. doi:10.1053/j.gastro.2015.04.020.

ADDITIONAL READING

- Amini M, Ghamar Chehreh ME, Khedmat H, et al. Famotidine in the treatment of functional dyspepsia: a randomized double-blind, placebo-controlled trial. *J Egypt Public Health Assoc*. 2012;87(1–2):29–33.
- Ford AC, Moayyedi P. Dyspepsia. *Curr Opin Gastroenterol*. 2013;29(6):662–668. doi:10.1097/MOG.0b013e328365d45d.

- Ganesh M, Nurko S. Functional dyspepsia in children. *Pediatr Ann*. 2014;43(4):e101–e105. doi:10.3928/00904481-20140325-12.
- Graham D, Rugge M. Clinical practice: diagnosis and evaluation of dyspepsia. *J Clin Gastroenterol*. 2010;44(3):167–172.
- Kaminski A, Kamper A, Thaler K, et al. Antidepressants for the treatment of abdominal pain-related functional gastrointestinal disorders in children and adolescents. *Cochrane Database Syst Rev*. 2011;(7):CD008013.
- Lacy BE, Talley NJ, Locke GR III, et al. Review article: current treatment options and management of functional dyspepsia. *Aliment Pharmacol Ther*. 2012;36(1):3–15.
- Lan L, Zeng F, Liu GJ, et al. Acupuncture for functional dyspepsia. *Cochrane Database Syst Rev*. 2014;(10):CD008487.
- Loyd RA, McClellan DA. Update on the evaluation and management of functional dyspepsia. *Am Fam Physician*. 2011;83(5):547–552.
- Oustamanolakis P, Tack J. Dyspepsia: organic versus functional. *J Clin Gastroenterol*. 2012;46(3):175–190.
- Overland MK. Dyspepsia. *Med Clin North Am*. 2014;98(3):549–564.
- Tack J, Masaoka T, Janssen P. Functional dyspepsia. *Curr Opin Gastroenterol*. 2011;27(6):549–557.

 SEE ALSO

- Irritable Bowel Syndrome
- Algorithms: Dyspepsia

 CODES

ICD10

K30 Functional dyspepsia

CLINICAL PEARLS

- Dyspepsia without underlying organic disease is termed functional or idiopathic.
- Consider empiric treatment with acid suppression as first-line therapy for functional dyspepsia.
- Extensive diagnostic testing is not recommended unless alarm symptoms are present.

D

DYSPHAGIA

Felix B. Chang, MD, DABMA, FAAMA

 BASICS

Difficulty transmitting the alimentary bolus from the mouth to stomach

DESCRIPTION

- Oropharyngeal dysphagia: difficulty transferring food bolus from oropharynx to proximal esophagus
- Esophageal dysphagia: difficulty moving food bolus through the body of the esophagus to the pylorus

EPIDEMIOLOGY

10% of individuals >50 years of age

Prevalence

- Common primary care complaint
- Rates of impaired swallowing in nursing home residents range from 29% to 32%.

ETIOLOGY AND PATHOPHYSIOLOGY

- Oropharyngeal (transfer dysphagia):
  - Mechanical causes: pharyngeal and laryngeal cancer, acute epiglottitis, carotid body tumor, pharyngitis, tonsillitis, strep throat, lymphoid hyperplasia of lingual tonsil, lateral pharyngeal pouch, hypopharyngeal diverticulum
- Esophageal:
  - Esophageal mechanical lesions: carcinomas, esophageal diverticula, esophageal webs, Schatzki ring, structures (peptic, chemical, trauma, radiation), foreign body
  - Extrinsic mechanical lesions: peritonsillar abscess, thyroid disorders, tumors, mediastinal compression, vascular compression (enlarged left atrium, aberrant subclavius, aortic aneurysm), osteoarthritis cervical spine, adenopathy, esophageal duplication cyst
- Neuromuscular: achalasia, diffuse esophageal spasm, hypertonic lower esophageal sphincter, scleroderma, nutcracker esophagus, CVA, Alzheimer disease, Huntington chorea, Parkinson disease, multiple sclerosis, skeletal muscle disease (polymyositis, dermatomyositis), neuromuscular junction disease (myasthenia gravis, Lambert-Eaton syndrome, botulism), hyper- and hypothyroidism, Guillain-Barré syndrome, systemic lupus erythematous, acute lymphoblastic leukemia, amyloidosis, diabetic neuropathy, brainstem tumors, Chagas disease
- Infection: diphtheria, chronic meningitis, tertiary syphilis, Lyme disease, rabies, poliomyelitis, CMV, esophagitis (*Candida*, herpetic)
- Globus phenomenon

RISK FACTORS

- Children: hereditary and/or congenital malformations
- Adults: age >50 years. Elderly: GERD, stroke, COPD, chronic pain
- Smoking, excess alcohol intake, obesity
- Medications: quinine, potassium chloride, vitamin C, tetracycline, Bactrim, clindamycin, NSAIDs, procainamide, anticholinergics, bisphosphates
- Neurologic events or diseases: CVA, myasthenia gravis, multiple sclerosis, Parkinson disease, amyotrophic lateral sclerosis (ALS), Huntington chorea
- HIV patients with CD4 cell count <100 cells/mm^3
- Trauma or irradiation of head, neck, and chest; mechanical lesions

- Extrinsic mechanical lesions: lung, thyroid tumors, lymphoma, metastasis
- Iron deficiency
- Anterior cervical spine surgery (up to 71% in the first 2 weeks postop; 12–14% at 1 year postop)
- Dysphagia lusoria (vascular abnormalities causing dysphagia): complete vascular ring, double aortic arch, right aortic arch with retroesophageal left subclavian artery and left ligamentum arteriosum, and right aortic arch with mirrow-image branching and left ligamentum arteriousum

GENERAL PREVENTION

- Correct poorly fitting dentures in older patients.
- Educate patients on prolonged chewing and drinking large volumes of water to accompany meals.
- Liquid and soft food diet in appropriate patients
- Avoid alcohol with meals.
- Prophylactic swallowing exercises in patients with head and neck cancer undergoing chemoradiation

COMMONLY ASSOCIATED CONDITIONS

Peptic structure, esophageal webs and rings, carcinoma; history of stroke, dementia, pneumonia

 DIAGNOSIS

HISTORY

- Dysphagia to both solids and liquids from the onset of deglutition is likely an esophageal motility disorder.
- Oropharyngeal dysphagia presents as difficulty in initiating the swallowing process.
- Dysphagia for solids that later progresses to involve liquids more likely reflects mechanical obstruction.
- Progressive dysphagia is usually caused by cancer or a peptic stricture. Intermittent dysphagia is most often related to a lower esophageal ring.
- Inquire about heartburn, weight loss, hematemesis, coffee ground emesis, anemia, regurgitation of undigested food particles, and respiratory symptoms.
- Inquire about regurgitation, aspiration, or drooling immediately after swallowing.
  - May represent oropharyngeal dysphagia
- Does the food bolus feel stuck?
  - Upper sternum or back of throat may represent oropharyngeal dysphagia, whereas sensation over the lower sternum is typical of esophageal dysphagia.
- Is odynophagia present?
  - May represent inflammation, achalasia, diffuse esophageal spasm, esophagitis, pharyngitis, pill-induced esophagitis, cancer
- Globus sensation ("lump in the throat")?
  - Indicates cricopharyngeal or laryngeal disorders.
- History of sour taste in the back of the throat or history of chronic heartburn suggests GERD.
- Inquire about alcohol and/or tobacco use.
- Are there associated symptoms such as weight loss or chest pain?
  - Double aortic arch, right aortic arch with retroesophageal left subclavian artery and left ligamentum arteriosum
  - Anticholinergics, antihistamines, and some antihypertensives can decrease salivary production.

- Halitosis: Rule out diverticulitis.
- Prior history of a connective tissue disorder
- Changes in speech, hoarseness, weak cough, dysphonia? Rule out neuromuscular dysfunction.

PHYSICAL EXAM

- General: vital signs
- Skin:
  - Telangiectasia, sclerodactyly, calcinosis (r/o autoimmune disease); Reynaud phenomenon, sclerodactyly may be found in CREST syndrome or systemic scleroderma; stigmata of alcohol abuse (palmar erythema; telangiectasia)
- Head, eye, ear, nose, throat (HEENT):
  - Oropharyngeal:
    ○ Pharyngeal erythema/edema, tonsillitis, pharyngeal ulcers or thrush, odynophagia (bacterial, viral, fungal infections)
    ○ Tongue fasciculations (ALS)
  - Neck:
    ○ Neck masses, lymphadenopathy, neck tenderness, goiter
    ○ Neck tenderness: acute thyroiditis
- Neurologic:
  - Cranial nerve exam:
    ○ Sensory: cranial nerves V, IX, and X
    ○ Motor: cranial nerves V, VII, X, XI, and XII
  - CNS, mental status exam, strength testing, Horner syndrome, ataxia, cogwheel rigidity (CVA, dementia, Parkinson disease, Alzheimer disease)
    ○ Eye position, extraocular motility
  - Informal bedside swallowing evaluation:
    ○ Observe level of consciousness, postural control-upright position, oral hygiene, mobilization of oral secretions.

DIFFERENTIAL DIAGNOSIS

See "Etiology and Pathophysiology."

DIAGNOSTIC TESTS & INTERPRETATION

Adults: (1)[C]

- Barium swallow
- Fiberoptic endoscopic examination of swallowing (FEES)
- Gastroesophageal endoscopy
- Barium cine/video esophagogram
- Ambulatory 24-hour pH testing
- Esophageal manometry
- Videofluoroscopic swallowing study (VFSS): oropharyngeal dysphagia

Initial Tests (lab, imaging)

- Guided by diagnostic considerations (2)[C]
  - CBC (infection and inflammation)
  - Serum protein and albumin levels for nutritional assessment
  - Thyroid function studies to detect dysphagia associated with hypothyroidism or hyperthyroidism, cobalamin levels
  - Antiacetylcholine antibodies (myasthenia)
- Barium swallow: detects strictures or stenosis

Follow-Up Tests & Special Considerations

- CT scan of chest
- MRI of brain and cervical spine

- Videofluoroscopic swallowing function study (VSFS) (lips, tongue, palate, pharynx, larynx, proximal esophagus)
- Fiberoptic endoscopy and videofluoroscopy are similar in terms of diagnostic sensitivity (3)[C].

Diagnostic Procedures/Other
Endoscopy with biopsy; esophageal manometry; esophageal pH monitoring

Test Interpretation
- Squamous cell or adenocarcinoma
- Barrett metaplasia
- Fibrous tissue of a ring, web, or stricture
- Loss of smooth muscle (scleroderma)

 TREATMENT

GENERAL MEASURES
Exclude cardiac disease. Ensure airway patency and adequate pulmonary function. Assess nutritional status. Speech therapy evaluation is helpful.

MEDICATION
First Line
- For esophageal spasms: calcium channel blockers: nifedipine 10 to 30 mg TID; imipramine 50 mg at bedtime; sildenafil 50 mg/day PRN
- For esophagitis:
  - Antacids: Tums, Mylanta, Maalox
  - H_2 blockers:
    - Cimetidine: up to 1,600 mg orally per day in 2 or 4 divided doses for 12 weeks
    - Ranitidine: initial 150 mg orally 4 times daily and maintenance 150 mg orally twice daily
    - Nizatidine: 150 mg orally twice daily for 12 weeks
    - Famotidine: 20 to 40 mg orally twice daily for 12 weeks
  - Proton pump inhibitors:
    - Omeprazole: 20 mg once daily for 4 to 8 weeks
    - Lansoprazole: 30 mg once daily for up to 8 weeks
    - Rabeprazole: 20 mg orally once daily for 4 to 8 weeks
    - Esomeprazole: 20 to 40 mg orally once daily for 4 to 8 weeks
    - Pantoprazole: 40 mg orally once daily for up to 8 weeks
  - Prokinetic agents: rarely used
  - Precautions: may need to use liquid forms of medications because patients might have difficulty swallowing pills

ISSUES FOR REFERRAL
- Gastroenterology: endoscopy, refractory symptoms
- Surgery: dilation, esophageal myotomy, biopsy

ADDITIONAL THERAPIES
Speech therapy to assess swallowing; nutritional evaluation for dietary and positioning recommendations; physical therapy for muscle-strengthening exercise; no eating at bedtime; remaining upright after eating
- Self-expanded metal stent is safe, effective, and quicker in palliating dysphagia compared to other modalities.

SURGERY/OTHER PROCEDURES
- Esophageal dilatation (pneumatic or bougie)
- Esophageal stent; laser for cancer palliation (4)[A]
- Treatment for underlying problem (e.g., thyroid goiter, vascular ring, esophageal atresia)
- Nd:YAG laser incision of lower esophageal rings refractory to dilation
- Photodynamic therapy (cancer) (4)[C]
- Cricopharyngeal myotomy (oropharyngeal dysphagia)
- Surgery for Zenker diverticulum, refractory strictures, or myotomy (for achalasia)
- Percutaneous endoscopic gastrostomy (PEG) decreases risk of dysphagia when compared with nasogastric tube.

COMPLEMENTARY & ALTERNATIVE MEDICINE
- Acupuncture has been used for neurogenic dysphagia.
- Electroacupuncture combined with dilating granule has been used in the treatment of GERD.
- Insufficient evidence for routine use of botulinum toxin

INPATIENT CONSIDERATIONS
Admission Criteria/Initial Stabilization
- Complete or partial esophageal obstruction with malnutrition or hypovolemia/dehydration
- Comorbid conditions complicating dysphagia
- Need for enteral feeding
- Outpatient for conditions where patient is able to maintain nutrition and has little risk of complications.
- Hospitalization may be required for adults when dysphagia is associated with total or near-total obstruction of esophageal lumen.
- Hospitalization may be needed for endoscopy and/or esophageal dilation and is generally indicated for diagnostic or therapeutic surgical procedures.

IV Fluids
For dehydrated, hypovolemic patients, and patients with impaired consciousness

Discharge Criteria
Tolerating adequate diet without nausea/pain

 ONGOING CARE

DIET
See "General Prevention."

PATIENT EDUCATION
Dietary modification; no eating at bedtime; remaining upright after eating; smoking cessation

PROGNOSIS
Vary with specific diagnosis.

COMPLICATIONS
- Oropharyngeal: pneumonia, lung abscess, aspiration, airway obstruction
- Malnutrition and dehydration

REFERENCES
1. American College of Radiology. ACR appropriateness criteria for dysphagia. National Guideline Clearinghouse. https://www.guidelinecentral.com/summaries/acr-appropriateness-criteria-dysphagia/. Accessed 2014.
2. Al-Hussaini A, Latif EH, Singh V. 12-minute consultation: an evidence-based approach to the management of dysphagia. *Clin Otolaryngol*. 2013; 38(3):237–243.
3. ASGE Standards of Practice Committee, Pasha SF, Acosta RD, et al. The role of endoscopy in the evaluation and management of dysphagia. *Gastrointest Endosc*. 2014;79(2):191–201.
4. Dai Y, Li C, Xie Y, et al. Interventions for dysphagia in oesophageal cancer. *Cochrane Database Syst Rev*. 2014;(10):CD005048.

ADDITIONAL READING
- Anderson U, Beck A, Kjaersgaard A, et al. Systematic review and evidence based recommendations on texture modified foods and thickened fluids for adults (≥18 years) with oropharyngeal dysphagia. *e-SPEN Journal*. 2013;8(4):e127–e134.
- Cho SK, Lu Y, Lee DH. Dysphagia following anterior cervical spinal surgery: a systematic review. *Bone Joint J*. 2013;95-B(7):868–873.
- Geeganage C, Beavan J, Ellender S, et al. Interventions for dysphagia and nutritional support in acute and subacute stroke. *Cochrane Database Syst Rev*. 2012;(10):CD000323.
- Regan J, Murphy A, Chiang M, et al. Botulinum toxin for upper oesophageal sphincter dysfunction in neurological swallowing disorders. *Cochrane Database Syst Rev*. 2014;(5):CD009968.

CODES

ICD10
- R13.10 Dysphagia, unspecified
- R13.12 Dysphagia, oropharyngeal phase
- R13.14 Dysphagia, pharyngoesophageal phase

CLINICAL PEARLS
- Preventing aspiration is a priority.
- Swallow therapy is recommended in patients with oropharyngeal dysphagia following a stroke, head or neck trauma, surgery, or degenerative neurologic diseases.
- Patients with oropharyngeal dysphagia usually report feeling an obstruction in the neck and point to this area when asked to identify the site of their symptoms.
- Weight loss is usually associated with malignancy or achalasia.
- Most patients with Sjögren syndrome have associated dysphagia.

ECTOPIC PREGNANCY
Ryan J. Callery, MD

 BASICS

DESCRIPTION
Ectopic: pregnancy implanted outside the confines of the uterine cavity. Subtypes include:
- Tubal: pregnancy implanted in any portion of the fallopian tube
- Abdominal: pregnancy implanted intra-abdominally, most commonly after tubal abortion or rupture of tubal ectopic pregnancy
- Heterotopic: pregnancy implanted intrauterine and a separate pregnancy implanted outside uterine cavity
- Ovarian: implantation of pregnancy in ovarian tissue
- Cervical: implantation of pregnancy in cervix
- Intraligamentary: implantation of pregnancy within the broad ligament

EPIDEMIOLOGY
Incidence
- 108,800 cases in 1992 in the United States, according to CDC census (most recent data available) meaning that 1.5–2.0% of all pregnancies were ectopic. The true incidence is difficult to estimate because many patients are treated in the outpatient setting.
- In the United States, ectopic pregnancy is the leading cause of 1st-trimester maternal deaths and accounts for 6% of all pregnancy-related deaths.
- Heterotopic pregnancy, although rare (1:30,000), occurs with greater frequency in women undergoing in vitro fertilization (IVF) (1/1,000).

Prevalence
~33% recurrence rate if prior ectopic pregnancy

ETIOLOGY AND PATHOPHYSIOLOGY
- 97% of ectopic pregnancies occur in the fallopian tube, of which, 55% in the ampullary portion of the tube, 25% in the isthmus, and 17% in the fimbria.
- Of the remaining 3%, most are ovarian, cervical, abdominal pregnancies, or heterotopic.
- For a tubal pregnancy, impaired movement of the fertilized ovum to the uterine cavity due to dysfunction of the tubal cilia, scarring, or narrowing of the tubal lumen
- Other locations are rare but may occur from reimplantation of an aborted tubal pregnancy or from uterine structural abnormalities (mainly cervical pregnancy).

RISK FACTORS
- History of pelvic inflammatory disease (PID), endometritis, or current gonorrhea/chlamydia infection
- Previous ectopic pregnancy
- History of tubal surgery (~33% of pregnancies after tubal ligation will be ectopic)
- Pelvic adhesive disease (infection or prior surgery)
- Use of an intrauterine device (IUD): Overall chance of pregnancy of any type with an IUD is low; however, there is an increased likelihood of ectopic location if pregnancy occurs. IUDs reduce absolute risk of ectopic pregnancy.
- Use of assisted reproductive technologies
- Diethylstilbestrol exposure in utero (DES was last used in 1972)
- Tobacco use
- Patients with disorders that affect ciliary motility may be at increased risk (e.g., endometriosis, Kartagener).

GENERAL PREVENTION
- Reliable contraception or abstinence
- Screening and treatment of STIs (i.e., gonorrhea, chlamydia) that can cause PID and tubal scarring

 DIAGNOSIS

HISTORY
In >50% of presenting cases, patients have sudden-onset abdominal pain coupled with cessation of/or irregular menses. Other common symptoms include nausea and/or vomiting, vaginal bleeding, and pain referred to the shoulder (from hemoperitoneum).

PHYSICAL EXAM
- Abdominal tenderness ± rebound tenderness
- Vaginal bleeding
- Palpable mass on pelvic exam (adnexal or cul-de-sac fullness)
- Cervical motion tenderness
- In cervical cases, an hourglass-shaped cervix might be noted.
- In cases of rupture and significant intraperitoneal bleeding, signs of shock such as pallor, tachycardia, and hypotension may be present.

DIFFERENTIAL DIAGNOSIS
- Missed, threatened, inevitable, or completed abortion
- Gestational trophoblastic neoplasia ("molar pregnancy")
- Appendicitis
- Salpingitis, PID
- Ruptured corpus luteum or hemorrhagic cyst
- Ovarian tumor, benign or malignant
- Ovarian torsion
- Cervical polyp, cancer, trauma, or cervicitis

DIAGNOSTIC TESTS & INTERPRETATION
Initial Tests (lab, imaging)
- Human chorionic gonadotropin (hCG): Serial quantitative serum levels normally increase by at least 53% every 48 hours: Abnormal rise should prompt workup for gestational abnormalities. Clinical impression of acute abdomen/intraperitoneal bleeding concurrent with a positive hCG level is indicative of ectopic pregnancy until proven otherwise (1).
- CBC and ABO type and antibody screen
- Serum progesterone level (>20 mg/mL associated with lower risk of ectopic pregnancy). In women with pain and/or bleeding who have an inconclusive US, serum progesterone level <3.2 ng/mL ruled out a viable pregnancy in 99.2% of women (2).
- Under investigation: evaluation of serum progesterone levels in conjunction with vascular endothelial growth factor, inhibin A, and activin A using an algorithm. This diagnosed patients with ectopic pregnancy with 99% accuracy (3).
- Transvaginal US (TVUS) is the gold standard for diagnosis:
  - Failure to visualize a normal intrauterine gestational sac when serum hCG is above the discriminatory level (>1,500 to 2,000 IU/L) suggests an abnormal pregnancy (4).
  - Recent studies show an hCG level of 3,500 IU/L to be associated with a 99% probability of detecting a normal intrauterine gestational sac in clinical practice (5).
  - These values are not valid for multiple gestations
- MRI is also useful but costly and rarely used if TVUS is available.

Diagnostic Procedures/Other
- In the setting of an undesired pregnancy, sampling of the uterine cavity with endometrial biopsy or D&C can identify the presence/absence of intrauterine chorionic villi. When an intrauterine pregnancy (IUP) has been evacuated by curettage, hCG levels should drop by 15% the next day (6).
- Historically, culdocentesis was performed to confirm suspected hemoperitoneum prior to surgical management. Currently, TVUS quantification of pelvic fluid is sufficient.

Test Interpretation
Products of conception (POC; especially chorionic villi) outside the uterine cavity

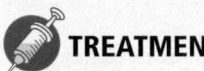 **TREATMENT**

MEDICATION
- Methotrexate (MTX): treatment for unruptured tubal pregnancy or for remaining POCs after laparoscopic salpingostomy. MTX inhibits DNA synthesis via folic acid antagonism by inactivating dihydrofolate reductase. Most effective when pregnancy is <3 cm diameter, hCG <5,000 mIU/mL, and no fetal heart movement is seen. Success rate is 88% if hCG <1,000 mIU/mL, 71% if hCG <2,000 mIU/mL:
  - Dosage:
    - Single: IM methotrexate: 50 mg/m² of body surface area; may repeat once (preferred method) if <15% decline in hCG by day 7
    - Double dose: methotrexate 50 mg/m² of body surface area once and then repeated on day 4; if <15% decline in hCG on day 7, may repeat dose on days 7 and 11
    - Multidose: methotrexate 1 mg/kg IM/IV every other day, with leucovorin 0.1 mg/kg IM in between. Maximum 4 doses; course may be repeated 7 days after last dose if necessary.
  - Contraindications
    - Hemodynamic instability or any evidence of rupture
    - Moderate to severe anemia
    - Severe hepatic or renal dysfunction
    - Immunodeficiency
  - Relative contraindications
    - Fetal heart rate seen
    - Large gestational sac
    - Noncompliance or limited access to hospital or transportation
    - High hCG count >5,000 mIU/mL
- Precautions: immunologic, hematologic, renal, GI, hepatic, and pulmonary disease, or interacting medications
- Pretreatment testing: serum hCG, CBC, liver and renal function tests, blood type, and screen
- Patient counseling: During therapy, refrain from use of alcohol, aspirin, NSAIDs, and folate supplements (decreases efficacy of MTX); avoid excessive sun exposure.
  - Adherence to scheduled follow-up appointments is critical.
  - Increased abdominal pain may occur during treatment; however, severe pain, nausea, vomiting, bleeding, dizziness, or light-headedness may indicate treatment failure and require urgent evaluation.
- Rupture of ectopic pregnancy during MTX treatment ranges from 7% to 14%.
- Side effects include stomatitis, conjunctivitis, abdominal cramping, and rarely neutropenia, pneumonitis, or alopecia (7–9).

ISSUES FOR REFERRAL
- Consider gynecologic consultation if not experienced in medical management.
- Refer to a gynecologist for surgical care.

ADDITIONAL THERAPIES
- Physician or patient may elect for surgical treatment as primary method, then postop hCG should guide need for MTX.
- After evidence of medical failure or tubal rupture, surgery is necessary.
- Surgery may either be salpingostomy (with preservation of tube) or salpingectomy (tubal removal). Abdominal entry is typically laparoscopic.
- Treatment of cervical, ovarian, abdominal, or other ectopic pregnancy is complicated and requires immediate specialist referral.
- Follow all patients treated medically to an hCG of 0 to ensure that there is no need for surgical intervention.
- Offer anti-D Rh prophylaxis at a dose of 50 μg to all Rh-negative women who have a surgical procedure to manage an ectopic pregnancy.
- Expectant management to allow for spontaneous resolution of ectopic pregnancy is acceptable in asymptomatic patients with no evidence of rupture or hemodynamic instability coupled with an appropriately low hCG (<200 mIU/mL) and no extrauterine mass suggestive of ectopic. Ruptured tubal pregnancies may occur even with extremely low hCG levels (<100 mIU/mL) (10).

SURGERY/OTHER PROCEDURES
- Indications include ruptured ectopic pregnancy, inability to comply with medical follow-up, previous tubal ligation, known tubal disease, current heterotopic pregnancy, desire for permanent sterilization at time of diagnosis.
- Laparoscopy is the first-line surgical management.
- Salpingostomy is preferred in patients who wish to maintain fertility particularly if contralateral tube is damaged/absent:
  - No difference in recurrence rate compared to salpingectomy (11).
  - Persistent trophoblastic tissue with salpingostomy remains in the fallopian tube in 4–15% of cases.
- Salpingectomy is indicated for uncontrolled bleeding, recurrent ectopic pregnancy, severely damaged tube, large gestational sac, or patient desire for sterilization.

INPATIENT CONSIDERATIONS
Admission Criteria/Initial Stabilization
- Fails criteria for methotrexate management, suspicion of rupture, orthostatic, shock, and severe abdominal pain requiring IV narcotics
- Inpatient observation in the setting of an uncertain diagnosis, particularly with an unreliable patient, may be appropriate.
- Surgical emergency
  - Two IV access lines should be placed immediately if suspicion of rupture; aggressive resuscitation as needed
  - Blood product transfusion if necessary en route to OR
  - In cases of shock, pressors and cardiac support may be necessary.

IV Fluids
- Unnecessary for a stable ectopic pregnancy being medically treated
- Critical for a surgical patient who is bleeding

Nursing
Strict input/output, hourly vitals, orthostatics if mobile, frequent abdominal exams, serial hematocrit, pad counts if heavy vaginal bleeding

Discharge Criteria
Afebrile, abdominal pain resolving or resolved, diagnosis established, surgical treatment, and recovery is complete

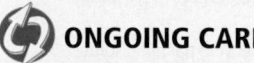 ONGOING CARE

FOLLOW-UP RECOMMENDATIONS
Patient Monitoring
- Serial serum quantitative hCG until level drops to zero:
  - After methotrexate administration, a strict monitoring protocol should be followed (8).
  - Following salpingostomy, weekly levels are appropriate.
  - Following salpingectomy, further follow-up may be unnecessary.
- Pelvic US for persistent or recurrent masses
- Pain control: brief course of narcotics usually necessary
- Liver and renal function tests following methotrexate administration if repeat dosing is required
- Delay of subsequent pregnancy for at least 3 months after treatment with methotrexate due to teratogenicity (folate deficiency)

DIET
- During treatment, avoid foods and vitamins high in folate (leafy greens, liver, edamame) due to interaction with methotrexate efficacy.
- Maintain excellent hydration.

PATIENT EDUCATION
- Signs and symptoms of ectopic pregnancy should be reviewed.
- Patients should be encouraged to plan subsequent pregnancies and seek early medical care on discovery of future pregnancies.

PROGNOSIS
- Chronic ectopic pregnancies are rare and treated with surgical removal of the fallopian tube.
- Future fertility depends on fertility prior to ectopic pregnancy and degree of tubal compromise.
- ~66% of women with a history of ectopic pregnancy will have a future IUP if they are able to conceive.
- If infertility persists beyond 12 months, the fallopian tubes should be evaluated.

COMPLICATIONS
- Hemorrhage and hypovolemic shock
- Persistent trophoblastic tissue after medical or surgical management
- Infection
- Infertility
- Blood transfusions with associated infections/transfusion reaction
- Disseminated intravascular coagulation in the setting of massive hemorrhage

REFERENCES

1. Barnhart KT, Sammel MD, Rinaudo PF, et al. Symptomatic patients with an early viable intrauterine pregnancy: HCG curves redefined. *Obstet Gynecol*. 2004;104(1):50–55.
2. Verhaegen J, Gallos ID, van Mello NM, et al. Accuracy of single progesterone test to predict early pregnancy outcome in women with pain or bleeding: meta-analysis of cohort studies. *BMJ*. 2012;345:e6077.
3. Rausch ME, Sammel MD, Takacs P, et al. Development of a multiple marker test for ectopic pregnancy. *Obstet Gynecol*. 2011;117(3):573–582.
4. Barnhart K, Mennuti MT, Benjamin I, et al. Prompt diagnosis of ectopic pregnancy in an emergency department setting. *Obstet Gynecol*. 1994;84(6):1010–1015.
5. Connolly A, Ryan DH, Stuebe AM, et al. Reevaluation of discriminatory and threshold levels for serum β-hCG in early pregnancy. *Obstet Gynecol*. 2013;121(1):65–70.
6. Seeber BE, Barnhart KT. Suspected ectopic pregnancy. *Obstet Gynecol*. 2006;107(2 Pt 1):399–413.
7. Bachman EA, Barnhart K. Medical management of ectopic pregnancy: a comparison of regimens. *Clin Obstet Gynecol*. 2012;55(2):440–447.
8. Practice Committee of the American Society for Reproductive Medicine. Medical treatment of ectopic pregnancy. *Fertil Steril*. 2006;86(5 Suppl 1):S96–S102.
9. Menon S, Colins J, Barnhart KT. Establishing a human chorionic gonadotropin cutoff to guide methotrexate treatment of ectopic pregnancy: a systematic review. *Fertil Steril*. 2007;87(3):481–484.
10. American College of Obstetricians and Gynecologists. ACOG Practice Bulletin No. 94: medical management of ectopic pregnancy. *Obstet Gynecol*. 2008;111(6):1479–1485.
11. Mol F, van Mello NM, Strandell A, et al. Salpingotomy versus salpingectomy in women with tubal pregnancy (ESEP study): an open-label, multicentre, randomised controlled trial. *Lancet*. 2014;383(9927):1483–1489.

ADDITIONAL READING
- Barnhart KT. Clinical practice. Ectopic pregnancy. *N Engl J Med*. 2009;361(4):379–387.
- Hajenius PJ, Mol F, Mol BW, et al. Interventions for tubal ectopic pregnancy. *Cochrane Database Syst Rev*. 2007;(1):CD000324.
- National Institute for Clinical Excellence. Ectopic Pregnancy and Miscarriage: *Diagnosis and Initial Management in Early Pregnancy of Ectopic Pregnancy and Miscarriage*. London, United Kingdom: National Institute for Clinical Excellence; 2012.
- Sagiv R, Debby A, Feit H, et al. The optimal cutoff level of human chorionic gonadotropin for efficacy of methotrexate treatment in women with extrauterine pregnancy. *Int J Gynaecol Obstet*. 2012:116(2):101–104.

 CODES

ICD10
- O00.9 Ectopic pregnancy, unspecified
- O00.1 Tubal pregnancy
- O00.0 Abdominal pregnancy

CLINICAL PEARLS
- Ectopic pregnancy is the leading cause of 1st-trimester maternal death and accounts for 6% of U.S. pregnancy deaths.
- 97% of ectopic pregnancies occur in the fallopian tube.
- Diagnosis requires high clinical suspicion in the setting of abdominal pain and a positive pregnancy test.

EJACULATORY DISORDERS

Payam Sazegar, MD, CCFP

BASICS

DESCRIPTION

- Premature ejaculation (PE): inability to control ejaculatory reflex resulting in ejaculation sooner than desired; most common type of sexual dysfunction affecting all age groups:
  - Defined (ISSM 2007) as an ejaculation that always or nearly always occurs prior to or within 1 minute of penetration; an inability to ejaculate on all or nearly all penetrations and with negative personal consequences (1,2).
  - Natural biologic response is to ejaculate within 2 to 5 minutes after vaginal penetration.
  - Ejaculatory control is an acquired behavior that increases with experience.
- Delayed ejaculation (DE): prolonged time to ejaculate (>30 minutes) despite desire, stimulation, and erection
- Aspermia (lack of sperm in the ejaculate):
  - Anejaculation (AE): lack of emission or contractions of bulbospongiosus muscle
  - Retrograde ejaculation (RE): partial or complete ejaculation of semen into the bladder
  - Obstruction: ejaculatory duct obstruction or urethral obstruction
- Painful ejaculation: genital or perineal pain during or after ejaculation
- Ejaculatory anhedonia: normal ejaculation lacking orgasm or pleasure
- Hematospermia: presence of blood in the ejaculate
- Ejaculatory duct obstruction
- Synonym(s): rapid ejaculation; retarded ejaculation; inhibited orgasm in males; ejaculatory dysfunction

EPIDEMIOLOGY

Prevalence

- PE is common. Reported prevalence in U.S. males ranges from 20–30% depending definition.
- DE is reported in 5–8% of men age 18 to 59 years, but <3% experience the problem for >6 months.
- Predominant age: all sexually mature age groups
- Predominant sex: male only

ETIOLOGY AND PATHOPHYSIOLOGY

Male sexual response:

- Erection mediated by parasympathetic nervous system
- Normal ejaculation consists of three phases:
  - Emission phase: Semen is deposited into urethra by contraction of prostate, seminal vesicles, and vas deferens; under autonomic sympathetic control.
  - Ejaculation phase: Semen is forcibly propelled out of urethra by rhythmic contractions of bulbospongiosus and ischiocavernosus muscles. This is mediated by the somatic nervous system on the motor branches of the pudendal nerve. Bladder neck contracture induced by α-adrenergic receptors ensures antero-grade ejaculation.
  - Orgasm: the pleasurable sensation associated with ejaculation (cerebral cortex); smooth muscle contraction of accessory sexual organs; release of pressure in posterior urethra
- PE has many theoretical causes:
  - Penile hypersensitivity
  - 5-hydroxytryptamine (5-HT) receptor sensitivity
  - Sexual inexperience
  - High level of sexual arousal and/or long interval since last ejaculation
  - Fear of sexual transmitted infections (STIs)
  - Anxiety or guilty feelings about sex
  - Lack of privacy
  - Interpersonal maladaptation (e.g., marital problems, unresponsiveness of partner)
- DE:
  - Rarely due to underlying painful disorder (e.g., prostatitis, seminal vesiculitis)
  - Psychogenic
  - Sexual performance anxiety and other psychosocial factors
  - Medications may impair ejaculation (e.g., MAOIs, SSRIs, α- and β-blockers, thiazides, antipsychotics, tricyclic and quadricyclic antidepressants, NSAIDs, opiates, alcohol).
- Never any ejaculate:
  - Congenital structural disorder (Müllerian duct cyst, Wolffian abnormality)
  - Acquired (radical prostatectomy, postinfectious, posttraumatic, T10–T12 neuropathy)
- AE:
  - Retroperitoneal lymph node (LN) dissection
  - Spinal cord injury or other (traumatic) sympathetic nerve injury
  - Medications (α- and β-blockers, benzodiazepines, SSRIs, MAOIs, TCAs, antipsychotics, aminocaproic acid
  - Diabetes mellitus (DM) (neuropathy)
  - Radical prostatectomy
- RE:
  - Transurethral resection of the prostate (25%) or other prostate resection procedures
  - Surgery on the neck of the bladder
  - Extensive pelvic surgery
  - Retroperitoneal LN dissection for testicular cancer (also may produce failure of emission)
  - Neurologic disorders (MS, DM)
  - Medications (α-blockers, in particular tamsulosin, ganglion blockers, antipsychotics)
  - Urethral stricture (may be posttraumatic)
- Painful ejaculation:
  - Infection or inflammation (orchitis, epididymitis, prostatitis, urethritis)
  - Ejaculatory duct obstruction
  - Seminal vesicle calculi
  - Obstruction of the vas deferens
  - Psychological/functional
- Ejaculatory anhedonia:
  - Medications
  - Psychological
  - Hormonal imbalances
  - Decreased libido
- Hematospermia (often unable to find cause):
  - Inflammation/infection
  - Calculi: bladder, seminal vesicle, prostate, urethra
  - Trauma to genital area (cycling, constipation)
  - Obstruction
  - Cyst
  - Tumor (prostate cancer [1–3% present with hematospermia])
  - Arteriovenous malformations
  - Iatrogenic
  - Hypertension

COMMONLY ASSOCIATED CONDITIONS

- Neurologic disorders (e.g., multiple sclerosis [MS])
- DM
- Prostatitis
- Ejaculatory duct obstruction
- Urethral stricture
- Psychological disorders
- Endocrinopathies
- Relationship/interpersonal difficulties

DIAGNOSIS

- Ejaculation occurs before individual wishes (PE).
- Ejaculation does not occur following normal stimulation (including masturbation).

HISTORY

- Detailed sexual history, including:
  - Time frame of the problem
  - Quality of patient's sexual response
  - Sense of ejaculatory control and sexual distress
  - Overall assessment of the relationship
  - Ask specific questions as patients often reluctant to discuss openly
- Detailed history of recent and current medications
- History of past trauma or recent infections
- Past surgical history with particular attention to genitourinary (GU) surgeries
- Supplements and alternative therapies tried
- Many men do not distinguish initially between problems related to erection and ejaculation.
- Some men have unrealistic expectations of ejaculatory response and frequency.
- Include the sexual partner in the interview, especially if the patient expresses a belief that he is not meeting his partner's needs.
- In review of systems, elicit any evidence of testosterone deficiency or prolactin excess especially if anhedonia present.

PHYSICAL EXAM

- Check vitals. Look for focal neurologic signs (MS, spinal cord injury) and psychiatric disorders.
- Thorough GU exam, including:
  - Size and texture of testes and epididymis
  - Verification of the presence of the vas deferens
  - Location and patency of urethral meatus
  - Digital rectal examination to evaluate prostate consistency and size and possible midline lesions

DIAGNOSTIC TESTS & INTERPRETATION

- Laboratory test results may be normal.
- Fasting glucose or HgbA1c to rule out diabetes
- Postorgasmic urinalysis will confirm RE. Semen fructose level, sperm count, and viscosity can be measured. Patient may complain of cloudy urine.
- AE will have fructose negative, sperm negative, nonviscous postorgasmic urinalysis
- In painful ejaculation, urinalysis and urine culture
- If prostate cancer is considered, check prostate-specific antigen (PSA).
- In anhedonia, consider checking testosterone, prolactin, glucose, and thyroid levels.
- In hematospermia, painful ejaculation, or if ejaculatory duct obstruction is considered, transrectal ultrasound (TRUS) may be helpful.
- TRUS-guided seminal vesicle aspiration; if ejaculatory duct obstruction is present, then the aspirate will contain sperm.
- If suspicious of anatomic abnormality, can get scrotal US and/or MRI

TREATMENT

GENERAL MEASURES

- Identifying any medical cause (even if not reversible) helps patient accept condition.
- Improve partner communication.
- Psychological counseling for patient and partner

- Reduce performance pressure through reassurance
- Use of a variety of resources may be necessary (e.g., psychiatrist, psychologist, sex therapist, vascular surgeon, urologist, endocrinologist, neurologist).
- PE:
  - Use sensate focus therapy (gradual progression of nonsexual contact to sexual contact).
  - Quiet vagina: female partner stops moving just prior to ejaculation
  - Techniques to learn ejaculatory control (e.g., coronal squeeze technique [squeezing the glans penis until ejaculatory urge ceases] or start-and-stop technique [cessation of penile stimulation when ejaculation approaches and resumption of stimulation when ejaculatory feeling ends]) (3)[B]
- DE:
  - Change to antidepressant less likely to cause DE (citalopram, fluvoxamine, nefazodone).
- AE/RE:
  - Discontinue offending medication(s).
  - Diabetic control
  - If urethral obstruction present, refer to urologist
  - RE may be helped if intercourse occurs when bladder is full.
  - Consider penile vibratory stimulation (effective in spinal cord injuries >T10) or electroejaculation (place on monitor if lesions above T6 because autonomic dysreflexia may result) to collect sperm in AE cases.
- Painful ejaculation:
  - Counseling may be beneficial.
  - If seminal vesicle stones are possible, refer to urologist
- Hematospermia:
  - Often resolves spontaneously, without known cause
  - May try empiric antibiotic, but little evidence to support
  - If persistent or high degree of suspicion for abnormality, refer to urologist.

MEDICATION
- PE:
  - Treating underlying erectile dysfunction (if identified) with PDE5 inhibitors
- First line:
  - Topical anesthetic gel applied (2.5% prilocaine ± 2.5% lidocaine [EMLA]) 2.5 g under a condom for 30 minutes prior to intercourse (4,5)[A]
  - Daily dosing of clomipramine 20 to 50 mg, sertraline 25 to 200 mg, fluoxetine 5 to 20 mg, or paroxetine 10 to 40 mg can delay ejaculation within 1 to 3 weeks of starting medication (4)[A].
  - Dapoxetine, a short-acting SSRI, used "on demand" 30 to 60 mg 1 to 2 hours prior to sex (2,4)[A].
  - Tramadol 5 to 50 mg used "on demand" 2 hours before sex. Effective in many studies (6)[A].
  - Some other "'on-demand" options include: clomipramine 20 to 40 mg 4 to 24 hours before intercourse, sertraline 50 mg 4 to 8 hours before intercourse, and paroxetine 20 mg 3 to 4 hours before intercourse (2)[A]
  - Consider switching antidepressants to bupropion, nefazodone, or mirtazapine.
  - Second line: behavioral/sex therapy, pelvic floor muscle therapy (3)[B]

- DE (limited options):
  - Patients who must continue SSRIs may respond to bupropion, buspirone (1)[B], or yohimbine (1)[C] before intercourse.
  - Sex therapy, self-stimulation therapies (1)[B]
  - Some evidence that amantadine or cyproheptadine may be helpful (2)[B]
- AE/RE:
  - α-Agonists and antihistamines can be helpful but are not approved by the FDA.
  - First line:
    - Pseudoephedrine 60 mg po daily to QID (7)[A]
    - Imipramine 25 to 75 mg po BID (7)[A]
  - Second line: For RE, can try postejaculation bladder harvest of sperm (if fertility desired). For AE, can try midodrine, penile vibratory stimulation, or electroejaculation (7)[B].
- Painful ejaculation:
  - Treat underlying infection/inflammatory process
  - α-Blockers may have some benefit.

ISSUES FOR REFERRAL
The following conditions, when suspected, should be referred to a urologist:
- Ejaculatory duct obstruction
- Seminal vesicle or prostatic stones
- Urethral obstruction
- Vas deferens obstruction
- Calculi
- Persistent or severe hematospermia

SURGERY/OTHER PROCEDURES
Surgical treatment of ejaculatory duct obstruction:
- Transurethral resection of the ejaculatory ducts

 ONGOING CARE

PATIENT EDUCATION
See "General Measures."

PROGNOSIS
Often improves with therapy and counseling

COMPLICATIONS
Psychological impact on some males: signs of severe inadequacy, self-doubt, additional anxiety, and guilt

REFERENCES
1. Rowland D, McMahon CG, Abdo C, et al. Disorders of orgasm and ejaculation in men. *J Sex Med*. 2010;7(4 Pt 2):1668–1686.
2. McMahon CG, Jannini E, Waldinger M, et al. Standard operating procedures in the disorders of orgasm and ejaculation. *J Sex Med*. 2013;10(1):204–229.
3. Melnik T, Althof S, Atallah AN, et al. Psychosocial interventions for premature ejaculation. *Cochrane Database Syst Rev*. 2011;(8):CD008195.
4. Porst H. An overview of pharmacotherapy in premature ejaculation. *J Sex Med*. 2011;8(Suppl 4): 335–341.
5. Wyllie MG, Powell JA. The role of local anaesthetics in premature ejaculation. *BJU Int*. 2012;110(11 Pt C): E943–E948.
6. Kirby EW, Carson CC, Coward RM. Tramadol for the management of premature ejaculation: a timely systematic review. *Int J Impot Res*. 2015;27(4):121–127.
7. Barazani Y, Stahl PJ, Nagler HM, et al. Management of ejaculatory disorders in infertile men. *Asian J Androl*. 2012;14(4):525–529.

ADDITIONAL READING
- Gur S, Sikka SC. The characterization, current medications, and promising therapeutics targets for premature ejaculation. *Andrology*. 2015;3(3):424–442.
- Jefferys A, Siassakos D, Wardle P. The management of retrograde ejaculation: a systematic review and update. *Fertil Steril*. 2012;97(2):306–312.
- Siegel AL. Pelvic floor muscle training in males: practical applications. *Urology*. 2014;84(1):1–7.

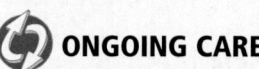 CODES

ICD10
- F52.4 Premature ejaculation
- N53.11 Retarded ejaculation
- N53.14 Retrograde ejaculation

CLINICAL PEARLS
- If erectile dysfunction is contributing to ejaculatory difficulty, management of erectile dysfunction should precede attempted management of ejaculatory disorders.
- Medications should always be thoroughly reviewed because they may be the primary cause of ejaculatory disorders.
- PE and DE generally have both psychogenic and physical causes, whereas AE and RE are due to organic neurogenic/autonomic dysfunction.
- A multidisciplinary approach, including the primary care physician, urologists, psychologists, and other appropriate health care professionals, is essential to the proper treatment of ejaculatory disorders.

ELDER ABUSE

Nitin Budhwar, MD • Kimberly Kone, MD

BASICS

DESCRIPTION

- The National Center of Elder Abuse divides abuse into three categories (older than age 60) (1)[A]:
  - **Domestic:** Abuse from someone who has a special relationship with the elderly individual (spouse, child, friend, or in-home caregiver) that occurs in the home of the elderly or caregiver.
  - **Institutional:** Occurs in the setting of a facility that is responsible for caring for the elderly, such as a nursing home or long-term care facility.
  - **Self-neglect:** The behavior of the elderly individual leads to harm.
- Types of abuse in estimated order of occurrence:
  - Self-neglect (estimated 50%). The most common form of abuse (2)[C].
  - Financial
  - Neglect
  - Emotional
  - Physical
  - Sexual
  - Taken advantage of: Misinformation and unregulated online pharmaceutical, financial companies, and so forth, that specifically target the elderly leading to deleterious outcomes (3)[C].

EPIDEMIOLOGY

Incidence
Estimate is that as many as 1:10 have been victims of abuse, placing a conservative number at 50,000 cases per year. Majority of whom are believed to be women (4)[A].

Prevalence
A recent national survey measuring prevalence of abuse in individuals of at least 60 years and older found that 11.9% of the surveyed population suffered some form of abuse:
- 5.2% encountered financial mistreatment by family members
- 5.1% suffered potential neglect
- 4.6% encountered emotional mistreatment, mostly by humiliation or verbal abuse
- 1.6% encountered physical mistreatment, mostly through battery
- 0.6% sexually mistreated, mostly through forced intercourse

ETIOLOGY AND PATHOPHYSIOLOGY
The etiology of elder abuse is a complex biopsychosocial combination of increased dependence on the caregiver by the victim in a suboptimal environment with poor behavioral coping methods, which is compounded by increased stress.

Genetics
Not contributory

RISK FACTORS
- The victim:
  - Advanced age
  - Exploitable resources
  - Prior history of abuse in life
  - Dementia or other cognitive impairment
  - Female gender
  - Disability in caring for him/herself
  - Depression
  - Social isolation
  - Stress: health, financial, or situational

- The abuser:
  - Mental illness
  - Financial dependency
  - Substance abuse
  - History of violence
  - Other antisocial behavior (5)[C]

GENERAL PREVENTION
- Improve patient social contact and support.
- Identify and correct potential risk factors for elder abuse:
  - Home visit to identify for potential risks of fall hazards and barriers to ambulation that could lead to fractures and functional decline that could leave the individual vulnerable to abuse
  - Evaluate for assistive devices that help the patient independently complete his/her ADLs and prevent caregiver dependence.
  - Screen for depression using validated tools like the Geriatric Depression Scale.
  - Early identification and treatment of cognitive impairment
- Identify caregiver stress and burden; refer to community programs that aid with emotional assistance.
- Advance life directives planning, including identifying possible caregivers, choosing a medical power of attorney (MPOA), estate, and will planning, and so forth.

COMMONLY ASSOCIATED CONDITIONS
Most common associated conditions with elder abuse are also identified as risk factors: social isolation, increased dependence for ADL/IADLs, depression, cognitive impairment, and aggressive behavior (5) [C],(6)[B].

DIAGNOSIS

A high index of suspicion when risk factors are present is important; types of abuse should be kept in mind as some types might not be obvious. It can be difficult to diagnose elder abuse in a single clinic visit, so it is important to get social services involved and to consider doing home visits, when abuse is suspected (5)[C].

HISTORY
It is important to take a detailed history with focus on the living arrangements, degree of functionality, who the caregivers are, and other risk factors listed above. Pay attention to clues such as withdrawal from normal activities or a sudden change in finances or abrupt changes to a will.

PHYSICAL EXAM
- It is important objectively to document positive and negative findings in your physical exam and to be very detailed because it can be admissible in court if abuse is suspected.
- Vital signs: Check weight and assess for progressive loss in weight; BP and pulse rate can be an indicator of dehydration that could be secondary to neglect.
- General overall appearance:
  - Wasting or cachexia
  - Poor hygiene, unkempt clothing
  - If the patient is bedbound, it is important to assess the integrity of the mattress and sheets. Look for excessive skin flakes, hair, or urine-soiled mattresses.
- Oral exam:
  - Assess for poor dentition, oral ulcers, or abscesses.

- Skin exam:
  - Most bruises from elder abuse are large (>5 cm) and located on the face, lateral arm, or back.
  - Bite or burn marks
  - It is important to check for pressure ulcers on the bony prominences of the patient: elbows, sacrum, heels, and scapula
- Mental/psychiatric:
  - Withdrawn, anxious, fearful, blunted
- Genital/rectal exam if sexual abuse is suspected (4)[A].

DIFFERENTIAL DIAGNOSIS
- Advanced dementia can present with individuals appearing withdrawn and they are often malnourished.
- Elderly with advanced dementia of Alzheimer type or Lewy body dementia can present with delusions of persecution and aggression that can be confused for elder abuse.
- Patients with Parkinson disease often fall and may exhibit fractures and bruises on a frequent basis that may mimic recurrent physical abuse.
- Coagulopathy seen in patients in advanced malignancy with bone marrow suppression or invasion, and those on chronic antiplatelet therapy can appear with bruising that can be easily confused with elder abuse.
- Wasting from malignancy, infections, chronic disease
- Thyroid disorder can present with altered mental status (AMS), depression, or anxiety.
- Chronic lung disease can present with decreased weight.
- Delirium from acute electrolyte disturbances, infectious etiology, or cardiovascular compromise can all present similar to elder abuse.
- Impaired financial status can also be confused with self-neglect.

DIAGNOSTIC TESTS & INTERPRETATION
The following workup is recommended:
- Nutritional assessment: iron, vitamin B_{12}, folate, thiamine, albumin, prealbumin, CBC, LFTs, electrolytes
- Malignancy workup, as per current guidelines
- If bruising is noted, check for coagulopathies (e.g., platelets, bleeding times, PT/INR, and PTT)
- If cognitive impairment is observed, check thyroid-stimulating hormone, vitamin B_{12} level; consider syphilis and HIV testing if indicated.
- Assessment of infection: may include urinalysis and culture, chest radiograph, blood count, and cultures
- Radiographic imaging of areas below soft tissue injury is indicated if there is evidence of infection (osteomyelitis) at a pressure ulcer site or bruising of a limb (fracture).
- If physical abuse is suspected and cognitive impairment present, then cranial imaging to look for hemorrhage (e.g., subdural) is indicated using CT scan or MRI.

Diagnostic Procedures/Other
- Pulse test: Check BP and pulse in presence and absence of suspected abuser. Elevation of either in the presence of the suspected abuser should raise suspicion. Useful in patients with dementia or other condition that makes history-taking difficult.
- Folstein Mini-Mental State Examination (MMSE), Montreal Cognitive Assessment (MOCA), or other validated tools to assess for cognitive impairment if suspected

- Geriatric Depression Scale if suspected
- Documentation: Practitioners may make statements of "suspected mistreatment," but should avoid making definitive diagnosis of abuse in their initial assessment, unless it is very obvious.

TREATMENT

Most states require all health care providers to report suspected elder abuse to a local agency such as the Adult Protective Services (http://www.nccafv.org/state_elder_abuse_hotlines.htm).

MEDICATION
None

INPATIENT CONSIDERATIONS
Admission Criteria/Initial Stabilization
- Victims of elder abuse should be admitted to the hospital if there are no safe discharge alternatives.
- Management of uncontrolled chronic conditions due to neglect (i.e., wound care from ulcers or infections)
- Cases of suspected abuse *must be reported* to the state's Adult Protective Services agency or a designated alternative (e.g., if patient resides in nursing home, then report to that state's regulatory entity). Social services may help. If physical harm has occurred, consider reporting to local law enforcement for investigation.
- Hospital security may need to be notified if restricted visitor access to a patient is required, and the patient's name may be hidden from the public hospital census.
- If the patient is a victim of elder abuse, he/she must be relocated to a safer alternative and may need admission for sequelae caused by the abuse.

Discharge Criteria
Victims should not be discharged to a potentially abusive environment. Alternatives to discharge to the unsafe environment may include:
- Friend or family member
- Nursing home
- Personal care home
- Assisted living facility
- Local victims' rescue or sheltering program if available

ONGOING CARE

FOLLOW-UP RECOMMENDATIONS
Victims of abuse should not be discharged without adequate follow-up, including:
- Primary care physician visit within 1 week
- Follow-up with Adult Protective Services or other agency; a home visit should be scheduled prior to discharge if the patient is going back home.

- Home Health Agency for assessment of safety (physical therapy)
- Follow-up with appropriate mental health care

Patient Monitoring
The patient should have frequent visits and be followed through the appropriate agencies to reduce continuation of abuse and to identify recurring abuse.

PATIENT EDUCATION
- For Elder Abuse Resources in your state, you can go to the National Center of Elder Abuse at www.ncea.aoa.gov
- Or your local representative by calling 1-800-677-1166

PROGNOSIS
Elder abuse and self-neglect are associated with an overall increased risk in mortality (7)[B].

COMPLICATIONS
Complications of elder abuse can lead to worsening depression, increased mortality, and overall poor quality of life.

REFERENCES

1. National Center on Elder Abuse. *Elder Abuse Prevalence and Incidence.* Washington, DC: National Center on Elder Abuse; 2005.
2. Mosqueda L, Dong X. Elder abuse and self-neglect: "I don't care anything about going to the doctor, to be honest. . ." *JAMA.* 2011;306(5):532–540.
3. Liang BA, Lovett KM, Mackey TK. Elder abuse. *J Am Geriatr Soc.* 2012;60(2):398–400.
4. Committee opinion no. 568: elder abuse and women's health. *Obstet Gynecol.* 2013;122(1):187–191.
5. Halphen JM, Varas GM, Sadowsky JM. Recognizing and reporting elder abuse and neglect. *Geriatrics.* 2009;64(7):13–18.
6. Acierno R, Hernandez MA, Amstadter AB, et al. Prevalence and correlates of emotional, physical, sexual, and financial abuse and potential neglect in the United States: the National Elder Mistreatment Study. *Am J Public Health.* 2010;100(2):292–297.
7. Dong X, Simon M, Mendes de Leon C, et al. Elder self-neglect and abuse and mortality risk in a community-dwelling population. *JAMA.* 2009;302(5):517–526.

ADDITIONAL READING

- Burnett J, Dyer CB, Halphen JM, et al. Four subtypes of self-neglect in older adults: results of a latent class analysis. *J Am Geriatr Soc.* 2014;62(6):1127–1132.
- Cooper C, Katona C, Finne-Soveri H, et al. Indicators of elder abuse: a crossnational comparison of psychiatric morbidity and other determinants

in the ad-hoc study. *Am J Geriatr Psychiatry.* 2006;14(6):489–497.
- Lachs MS, Pillemer K. Elder abuse. *Lancet.* 2004;364(9441):1263–1272.
- Lachs MS, Williams CS, O'Brien S, et al. Adult protective service use and nursing home placement. *Gerontologist.* 2002;42(6):734–739.
- Lachs MS, Williams CS, O'Brien S, et al. The mortality of elder mistreatment. *JAMA.* 1998;280(5):428–432.
- Widera E, Steenpass V, Marson D, et al. Finances in the older patient with cognitive impairment: "He didn't want me to take over". *JAMA.* 2011;305(7):698–706.
- Wiglesworth A, Austin R, Corona M, et al. Bruising as a marker of physical elder abuse. *J Am Geriatr Soc.* 2009;57(7):1191–1196.
- Wiglesworth A, Mosqueda L, Mulnard R, et al. Screening for abuse and neglect of people with dementia. *J Am Geriatr Soc.* 2010;58(3):493–500.

 # CODES

ICD10
- T74.11XA Adult physical abuse, confirmed, initial encounter
- T74.21XA Adult sexual abuse, confirmed, initial encounter
- T74.01XA Adult neglect or abandonment, confirmed, initial encounter

CLINICAL PEARLS
- Elder abuse, or elder mistreatment, is a condition in which the physical, psychological, or financial well-being of an older adult is infringed upon through intentional acts or lack of action, even if harm is not intended.
- It is important to identify vulnerable individuals through proper evaluation of potential risk factors for abuse (social isolation, depression, cognitive impairment, disability requiring assistance, and financial dependence by the caregiver).
- Correction of risk factors is important to reduce the incidence of elder abuse (strengthen the patients' social support, treat depression, provide the patient with assistive devices, screen for cognitive impairment with a trial of medication if possible, and identify caregiver burn out).
- Clearly document your physical exam with only specific objective findings.
- Contact APS or your local resources if elder abuse is suspected; it is unlawful not to report suspected elder abuse.

ENCOPRESIS

Jay Fong, MD • William T. Garrison, PhD

 BASICS

DESCRIPTION

- Voluntary or involuntary fecal soilage in a (typically) previously toilet-trained child
  - Age may be chronologic or developmental.
  - No underlying organic disease
  - At least one event per month for 3 months
  - Classified into functional constipation (retentive encopresis) and functional nonretentive fecal incontinence (FNRFI); both cause fecal incontinence. There is no constipation in FNRFI. *Functional constipation is more common.*
- System(s) affected: GI; psychological
- Synonym(s): fecal incontinence, soiling

EPIDEMIOLOGY

Incidence
Predominant sex: male > female (4 to 6:1). Constipation accounts for 3% of general pediatric referrals; up to 84% of constipated children have fecal incontinence at some point.

Prevalence
Occurs in 1–3% of children 4 years of age

ETIOLOGY AND PATHOPHYSIOLOGY

- In 90% of cases, encopresis develops as a consequence of chronic constipation, with resulting overflow incontinence (*retentive encopresis*). The other 10% are caused by specific organic etiologies.
- Chronic constipation with irregular and incomplete evacuation results in progressive rectal distension and stretching of the internal/external anal sphincters.
- As a child habituates to chronic rectal distension, they may no longer sense the normal urge to defecate. Eventually, soft or liquid stool leaks around the retained fecal mass.
- Many children voluntarily withhold stool in response to the urge to defecate for fear of pain or a preoccupation with not interrupting social activities.
- Psychological
  - Stool withholding, fear, anxiety
  - Difficulty with toilet training, including unusual anxiety or conflict with parent
  - Resistance to using public toilet facilities, such as school bathrooms or outdoor toilets
  - Known association with sexual abuse in boys; likely similar association in girls
  - Developmental delay
- Anatomic
  - Rectal distension and desensitization
  - Anal fissure or painful defecation
  - Muscle hypotonia
  - Slow intestinal motility
  - Hirschsprung disease
  - Cystic fibrosis
  - Spinal cord defects (e.g., spina bifida)
  - Congenital anorectal malformations
  - Anal stenosis
  - Anterior displacement of the anus
  - Postoperative stricture of anus or rectum
  - Pelvic mass
  - Neurofibromatosis

- Dietary or metabolic
  - Inadequate dietary fiber
  - Excessive protein or milk intake
  - Inadequate water intake
  - Hypothyroidism
  - Hypercalcemia
  - Hypokalemia
  - Diabetes insipidus; diabetes mellitus
  - Food allergy
  - Gluten enteropathy
- Medication side effects

Genetics
None known; although incidence may be higher in children with family history of constipation.

RISK FACTORS
- Male gender
- Constipation
- Very low birth weight
- Painful defecation
- Difficulty with bowel training, including social pressure related to early daycare placement
- Organic/anatomic causes
- Anxiety and depression
- Insufficient fluid or fiber intake
- Refusal to use public restrooms
- Attention deficit

GENERAL PREVENTION
Family education: toilet training when ready, optimize fluid and fiber intake

COMMONLY ASSOCIATED CONDITIONS
- Constipation, Hirschsprung disease
- Cerebral palsy, cystic fibrosis
- Developmental and behavioral diagnoses, urinary incontinence

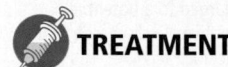 **DIAGNOSIS**

HISTORY
- Signs/symptoms of constipation:
  - Hard, large-caliber stools
  - <3 defecations/week
  - Pain or discomfort with stool passage, withholding of stool
  - Blood on stool or in diaper/toilet bowl
  - Decreased appetite
  - Abdominal pain that improves with stool passage.
  - Hiding while defecating before child is toilet-trained; avoiding use of the toilet
  - Diet low in fiber or fluids, high in dairy products
  - No stool passage in the first 48 hours of life
  - Pasty stool on underclothes
  - Recurrent UTIs
- Abrupt onset after age 5 years more likely to be associated with psychological trauma.
- Overlap with attention deficit disorder (ADD) common in children >5 years
- Medication use: opiates, phenobarbital, and tricyclic antidepressants (TCAs)
- Family history of constipation

PHYSICAL EXAM
- Neurologic exam of lower extremities and perineal area, with attention to S1–S4 distribution, perineal sensation, cremasteric reflex, and anal sphincter tone
- Genital examination and digital rectal exam: Assess for anal fissures, sphincter tone, rectal distension/impaction, occult or visible blood.
- Abdominal exam: bowel sounds, percussion note (tympany), abdominal distension; palpate for stool (most common in left lower quadrant).

DIAGNOSTIC TESTS & INTERPRETATION
Most cases of encopresis can be diagnosed by history and physical.

Initial Tests (lab, imaging)
- Only to rule out organic causes
- UA/urine culture: UTI/glucosuria
- Thyroid function tests: hypothyroidism
- Electrolyte panel, including calcium: hypokalemia, hypercalcemia, or hyperglycemia
- Abdominal plain films if impaction is suspected and not detected by abdominal or rectal exam.

Follow-Up Tests & Special Considerations
- Failure to pass meconium within 48 hours of birth, failure to thrive, bloody diarrhea, or bilious vomiting in a neonate should be promptly evaluated to exclude aganglionic megacolon.
- Constipation and diarrhea, rash, failure to thrive, or recurrent pneumonia should prompt evaluation for cystic fibrosis. Patients with abdominal distension or ileus should be evaluated for possible obstruction.

Diagnostic Procedures/Other
Manometric studies may be useful in patients who have constipation that does not respond to treatment.

TREATMENT

GENERAL MEASURES
- Anticipatory guidance relative to toilet training including advice about when children should reduce reliance on diapers or use pull-ups during the daytime hours (average age for toilet training in girls is 29 months; 31 months for boys).
- Eliminate impaction prior to maintenance therapy.
- Avoid frequent and repeated rectal exams, enemas, and suppositories, especially in infants.
- Once stools are regular in frequency, child should sit on toilet BID at the same time each day for 10 to 15 minutes and for 10 to 15 minutes after meals. Incorporate positive reinforcement for successful bowel movements.

MEDICATION
- Remove impaction and start maintenance treatment.
- No randomized, controlled studies have compared methods of disimpaction: can use oral agents, enemas, and rectal suppositories; oral agents are least traumatic. Glycerin suppositories are best option for infants.

First Line
- Disimpaction with polyethylene glycol (PEG)
  – Give 17 g (240 mL) water or juice: 1 to 1.5 g/kg/day for 3 days for disimpaction
  – 0.4 to 0.8 g/kg/day for maintenance
- Disimpaction with mineral oil for child >1 year; give 15 to 30 mL/year of age to max 240 mL.
  – Maintenance: 1 to 3 mL/kg/day or divided BID
  – May mix with orange juice to make palatable; avoid in infants to avoid aspiration pneumonia.
- Other maintenance regimens include the following:
  – Milk of magnesia (MOM) 400 mg (5 mL): 1 to 2 mL/kg/day BID
  – Lactulose 10 g (15 mL): 1 to 3 mL/kg/day divided BID
  – Senna syrup 8.8 g sennoside (5 mL): age 2 to 6 years: 2.5 to 7.5 mL/day divided BID; age 6 to 12 years: 5 to 15 mL/day divided BID
  – Bisacodyl suppository 10 mg: 0.5 to 1 suppository once or twice per day

ISSUES FOR REFERRAL
If symptoms do not improve after 6 months of good compliance with a multifactorial treatment model, refer to pediatric gastroenterologist for recommendations and further evaluation.

ADDITIONAL THERAPIES
Behavioral treatment and counseling

SURGERY/OTHER PROCEDURES
If ongoing constipation is refractory to a combination of medical and behavioral therapy, consider anorectal manometry to evaluate for internal anal sphincter achalasia (or ultrashort-segment Hirschsprung disease). If present, this condition can be treated successfully in most patients with an internal sphincter myectomy.

COMPLEMENTARY & ALTERNATIVE MEDICINE
- Children with volitional stool holding who receive behavioral treatment in addition to medications are more likely to have resolution of encopresis at 3 and 6 months than children receiving medication alone (1)[A].
- No evidence that biofeedback training adds benefit to conventional treatment for functional fecal incontinence in children (2)[A]
- Behavioral interventions combined with laxative therapy (rather than laxative therapy alone) improve continence in children with functional fecal incontinence associated with constipation (1)[B].

INPATIENT CONSIDERATIONS
Admission Criteria/Initial Stabilization
- Continued soiling and recurrent impaction on outpatient medical therapy, whether from lack of medication efficacy or patient nonadherence
- Decreased intake leading to malnutrition or dehydration
- Recalcitrant vomiting or concern for obstruction
- Involve appropriate agencies if concern for abuse
- Hospital admission and abdominal films may be necessary to ensure complete removal of impaction. This may include direct gastric administration of balanced electrolyte–PEG solutions if the patient cannot tolerate by mouth. Serial abdominal films and observation of the rectal effluent can help to determine treatment adequacy.

IV Fluids
IV fluids if the patient is dehydrated and having difficulty tolerating oral hydration

Nursing
Nursing to document stool output and character

Discharge Criteria
- Stools that are looser in consistency and clearer in appearance are a successful inpatient end point.
- Abdominal radiographs showing less fecal loading (compared with a pretreatment radiograph) with improving serial abdominal exams

 ONGOING CARE

FOLLOW-UP RECOMMENDATIONS
Patient Monitoring
- Continue maintenance treatment for 6 months to 2 years with visits every 4 to 10 weeks for support and to ensure compliance; more frequent visits with oppositional or anxious children
- Telephone or virtual visits can be used to adjust doses and to provide ongoing encouragement.
- Treat recurrences of impaction promptly.
- Emphasize compliance with medication and self-initiation of regular bathroom visits.
- Children who do not progress using a well-designed behavior plan should be referred for more in-depth mental health evaluation and counseling.

DIET
Adequate fluid and fiber intake (2)[A]. Reduce cow's milk products. Avoid excessive consumption of bananas, rice, apples, and gelatin.

PATIENT EDUCATION
- Demystify defecation.
- Carefully explain the treatment plan including medications and dietary changes.
- Avoid punishment for inadvertent soiling.
- In children >4 years of age, explain to parents how overreliance on diapers and pull-ups (while convenient) can prolong the problem.
- Always attempt to use positive reinforcement for successful toilet sits and medication compliance.
- If positive approach is unsuccessful, consider removing desired privileges (e.g., TV, video games) for noncompliance with behavioral plan. Some children respond well to a token economy (earned privileges) to promote desired behavior.

PROGNOSIS
- Many children exhibit a good response and relapse due to noncompliance by parents and/or child.
- From 30% to 50% of children may still have encopresis after 5 years of treatment.
- Children with psychosocial or emotional problems preceding the encopresis are more recalcitrant to treatment.

COMPLICATIONS
- Colitis due to excessive enema/suppository
- Perianal dermatitis
- Anal fissure

REFERENCES
1. Brazzelli M, Griffiths PV, Cody JD, et al. Behavioural and cognitive interventions with or without other treatments for the management of faecal incontinence in children. *Cochrane Database Syst Rev.* 2011;(12):CD002240.
2. Tabbers MM, DiLorenzo C, Berger MY, et al. Evaluation and treatment of functional constipation in infants and children: evidence-based recommendations from ESPGHAN and NASPGHAN. *J Pediatr Gastroenterol Nutr.* 2014;58(2):258–274.

ADDITIONAL READING
- Borowitz SM, Cox DJ, Tam A, et al. Precipitants of constipation during early childhood. *J Am Board Fam Pract.* 2003;16(3):213–218.
- Constipation Guideline Committee of the North American Society for Pediatric Gastroenterology, Hepatology and Nutrition. Evaluation and treatment of constipation in infants and children: recommendations of the North American Society for Pediatric Gastroenterology, Hepatology and Nutrition. *J Pediatr Gastroenterol Nutr.* 2006;43(3):e1–e13.
- Levitt M, Peña A. Update on pediatric faecal incontinence. *Eur J Pediatr Surg.* 2009;19(1):1–9.
- Loening-Baucke V, Pashankar DS. A randomized, prospective, comparison study of polyethylene glycol 3350 without electrolytes and milk of magnesia for children with constipation and fecal incontinence. *Pediatrics.* 2006;118(2):528–535.

CODES

ICD10
- R15.9 Full incontinence of feces
- R15.1 Fecal smearing
- F98.1 Encopresis not due to a substance or known physiol condition

CLINICAL PEARLS
- 90% of encopresis results from chronic constipation.
- Address toddler constipation early by decreasing excessive milk intake, increasing fruits/vegetables intake, and ensuring adequate fluid and fiber intake.
- Eliminate fecal impaction before initiating maintenance therapy.

E

ENDOCARDITIS, INFECTIVE

Danielle DeFoe, MS, DO • Theodore B. Flaum, DO, FACOFP

 BASICS

DESCRIPTION

- An infection of the valvular (primarily) and mural (rarely) endocardium
- System(s) affected: cardiovascular, endocrine/metabolic, hematologic/lymphatic, immunologic, pulmonary, renal/urologic, skin/exocrine, neurologic
- Synonym(s): bacterial endocarditis; subacute bacterial endocarditis (SBE); acute bacterial endocarditis (ABE)

EPIDEMIOLOGY

Incidence

- Increase in incidence in United States from 11 per 100,000 to 15 per 100,00 between 2000 and 2011
- 1.5–3.0% incidence 1 year after prosthetic valve replacement; at 5 years, the incidence is 3–6%.
- Increasing incidence of cardiovascular device-related infections, due to higher frequency of implantable devices, especially in the elderly

ETIOLOGY AND PATHOPHYSIOLOGY

- ABE: *Staphylococcus aureus*; *Streptococcus* groups A, B, C, G; *Streptococcus pneumoniae*; *Staphylococcus lugdunensis*; *Enterococcus* spp. (gram-positive); *Haemophilus influenzae* or *parainfluenzae*; *Neisseria gonorrhoeae* (gram-negative)
- SBE: α-Hemolytic streptococci (viridans group strep), *Streptococcus bovis*, *Enterococcus* spp., *Staphylococcus aureus*, *Staphylococcus epidermidis* (gram-positive); HACEK organisms: *Haemophilus aphrophilus* or *paraphrophilus*, *Actinobacillus* (*Aggregatibacter*) *actinomycetemcomitans*, *Cardiobacterium hominis*, *Eikenella corrodens*, *Kingella kingae*
- Endocarditis in IV drug abusers (tricuspid valve): *Staphylococcus aureus*, *Enterococcus* spp. (gram-positive); *Pseudomonas aeruginosa*, *Burkholderia cepacia*, other bacilli (gram-negative); *Candida* spp.
- Early prosthetic-valve endocarditis (<60 days after valve implantation): *Staphylococcus aureus*, *Staphylococcus epidermidis* (gram-positive); gram-negative bacilli; fungi: *Candida* spp., *Aspergillus* spp.
- Late prosthetic valve endocarditis (>60 days after valve implantation): α-Hemolytic streptococci, *Enterococcus* spp., *S. epidermidis* (gram-positive); *Candida* spp., *Aspergillus* spp.
- Culture-negative endocarditis: 10% of cases; *Bartonella quintana* (homeless); *Brucella* spp., fungi, *Coxiella burnetii* (Q fever), *Chlamydia trachomatis*, *Chlamydophila psittaci*, HACEK organisms; Abiotrophia (formerly B$_6$-deficient streptococci); use of antibiotics prior to blood cultures
- Device-related endocarditis: coagulase-negative staphylococci or *S. aureus*

RISK FACTORS

- Injection drug use, IV catheterization, certain malignancies (colon cancer), poor dentition, chronic hemodialysis
- High-risk conditions
  - Prosthetic cardiac valve, implantable devices (pacemaker, automatic implantable cardioverter defibrillator [AICD]), total parenteral nutrition
  - Previous infective endocarditis (IE)
  - Congenital heart disease (CHD): unrepaired cyanotic CHD, including palliative shunts and conduits; repaired CHD with prosthetic device during the first 6 months; repaired CHD with residual defects at or near prosthetic site; cardiac transplant with valvulopathy (1)[B]

GENERAL PREVENTION

- Maintain good oral hygiene.
- Antibiotic prophylaxis is only recommended for high-risk cardiac conditions (1)[B]—prosthetic heart valve, history of endocarditis, transplant with abnormal valvular function, CHD (see "Risk Factors").
- *Procedures requiring prophylaxis*
  - Oral/upper respiratory tract: any manipulation of gingival tissue or periapical region of teeth or perforation of the oral mucosa (1)[B], invasive respiratory procedures involving incision, or biopsy of the respiratory mucosa merit prophylaxis; amoxicillin 2 g PO (if penicillin allergic, clindamycin 600 mg PO) 30 to 60 minutes before procedure or ampicillin 2 g IV/IM are first-line prophylactic choices. For penicillin-allergic patients, use clindamycin 600 mg IV, or cephalexin 2 g PO, or azithromycin/clarithromycin 500 mg PO, or cefazolin/ceftriaxone 1 g IV/IM 30 minutes before procedure. Pediatric doses are amoxicillin 50 mg/kg PO (max 2 g), cephalexin 50 mg/kg PO (max 2 g), clindamycin 20 mg/kg PO (max 600 mg), and ampicillin or ceftriaxone 50 mg/kg (maximum 1 g) IM/IV.
  - GI/GU: Only consider coverage for enterococcus (with penicillin, ampicillin, piperacillin, or vancomycin) for patients with an established infection undergoing procedures (1)[B].
  - Cardiac valvular surgery or placement of prosthetic intracardiac/intravascular materials: perioperative cefazolin 1 to 2 g IV 30 minutes preop, or vancomycin 15 mg/kg (maximum 1 g) (penicillin-allergic patients) 60 minutes preop (1)[B]
  - Skin: incision and drainage of infected tissue; use agents active against skin pathogens (e.g., cefazolin 1 to 2 g IV q8h or vancomycin 15 mg/kg q12h; max 1 g) if penicillin-allergic or if methicillin-resistant *Staphylococcus aureus* (MRSA) suspected.

DIAGNOSIS

- Modified Duke Criteria for Diagnosis of IE (2)[B] (definite: 2 major criteria, or 1 major and 3 minor criteria, or 5 minor criteria; possible: 1 major and 1 minor criteria, or 3 minor criteria)
- Major clinical criteria
  - Positive blood culture: isolation of typical microorganism for IE from two separate blood cultures or persistently positive blood culture
  - Single positive blood culture for *C. burnetii* or anti–phase-1 IgG antibody titer >1:800
  - Positive echocardiogram: presence of vegetation, abscess, or new partial dehiscence of prosthetic valve; must be performed rapidly if IE is suspected
  - New valvular regurgitation (change in preexisting murmur not sufficient)
- Minor criteria
  - Predisposing heart condition or IV drug use
  - Fever ≥38.0°C (100.4°F)
  - Vascular phenomena: major arterial emboli, septic pulmonary infarcts, mycotic aneurysm, intracranial hemorrhage, conjunctival hemorrhage, Janeway lesions
  - Immunologic phenomena: glomerulonephritis, Osler nodes, Roth spots, rheumatoid factor (RF)
  - Microbiologic evidence: positive blood culture but not a major criterion (excluding single positive

cultures for coagulase-negative staphylococci and organisms that do not cause endocarditis) or serologic evidence of infection likely to cause IE

HISTORY

- Fever (>38°C), chills, cough, dyspnea, orthopnea; especially in subacute endocarditis: night sweats, weight loss, fatigue
- Predisposition to IE (see "Risk Factors")
- Symptoms of transient ischemic attack, cerebrovascular accident (CVA), or myocardial infarction (MI) on presentation

PHYSICAL EXAM

- Most patients with IE have new murmur or change in existing murmur. Signs of heart failure (rales, edema) if valve function is compromised.
- Peripheral stigmata of IE: splinter hemorrhages in fingernail beds, Osler nodes on fleshy portions of extremities, "Roth spot" retinal hemorrhages, Janeway lesions (cutaneous evidence of septic emboli), palatal or conjunctival petechiae, splenomegaly, hematuria (due to emboli or glomerulonephritis)
- Neurologic findings consistent with CVA, such as visual loss, motors weakness, and aphasia

DIFFERENTIAL DIAGNOSIS

Fever of unknown origin, infected central venous catheter, marantic endocarditis, connective tissue diseases, intra-abdominal infections, rheumatic fever, salmonellosis, brucellosis, malignancy, tuberculosis, atrial myxoma, septic thrombophlebitis

DIAGNOSTIC TESTS & INTERPRETATION

- When patient is not critically ill; three sets of blood cultures drawn >2 hours apart from different sites *before administration* of *antibiotics*.
- In acutely ill patients, draw three sets of blood cultures over a 1-hour period *prior to empiric antibiotic therapy.*
- Leukocytosis common in acute endocarditis
- Anemia, decreased C3, C4, CH50, and RF in subacute endocarditis
- ESR, C-reactive protein (CRP)
- Hematuria, microscopic or macroscopic
- Consider serologies for *Chlamydia*, Q fever, *Legionella*, and *Bartonella* in "culture-negative" endocarditis.
- Transthoracic or transesophageal echocardiogram (TTE/TEE) should be performed as soon as IE is suspected.
- Baseline ECG may provide clues to extension of infection.
- CT scan may help locate embolic abscesses (e.g., splenic abscess).
- Vegetations are composed of platelets, fibrin, and colonies of microorganisms. Destruction of valvular endocardium, perforation of valve leaflets, rupture of chordae tendineae, abscesses of myocardium, rupture of sinus of Valsalva, and pericarditis may occur.
- Emboli, abscesses, and/or infarction may occur in any organ system.
- Immune-complex glomerulonephritis

TREATMENT

MEDICATION

First Line

- Initial empirical treatment should be started after three sets of blood cultures have been drawn while waiting for a causative organism to be identified.
  - Native valves: Ampicillin-sulbactam 12 g/day IV divided into 4 doses with gentamicin 3 mg/kg/day

IV/IM in 2 or 3 doses. If penicillin allergic, use vancomycin 30 mg/kg/day IV in 2 doses with gentamicin 3 mg/kg/day IV/IM in 2 or 3 doses and with ciprofloxacin 1,000 mg/day PO or 800 mg/day IV, both in 2 doses (3)[A].
  – Prosthetic valves: Vancomycin 30 mg/kg/day IV in 2 doses with gentamicin 3 mg/kg/day IV/IM in 2 doses and rifampin 1,200 mg/day PO in 2 doses, if <12 months postsurgery. If >12 months, use native valve regimen (3)[A].

- Penicillin-susceptible viridans group streptococci or *S. bovis*

  – Native valve: penicillin G 12 to 18 million U/day IV continuously or in 4 to 6 doses or ceftriaxone 2 g/day IV/IM in 1 dose, both for 4 weeks (2)[B]
  – Prosthetic valve: penicillin G 24 million U/day IV continuously or 4 to 6 doses for 6 weeks or ceftriaxone 2 g/day IV/IM in 1 dose ± gentamicin 3 mg/kg IV/IM q24h for 2 weeks (peak gentamicin level 3 μg/mL and trough <1 μg/mL) (2)[B]

- Penicillin-resistant viridans group streptococci or *S. bovis*

  – Native valve: penicillin G 24 million U/day IV, either continuously or in 6 equally divided doses or ceftriaxone 2 g/day IV/IM in 1 dose for 4 weeks + gentamicin 3 mg/kg IV/IM q24h for 2 weeks (peak gentamicin level 3 μg/mL and trough <1 μg/mL) (2)[B]
  – Prosthetic valve: Regimen is equivalent, but length of therapy is 6 weeks for all antibiotics.

- *Staphylococcus*

  – Native valve: oxacillin or nafcillin 12 g IV every day for 4 to 6 weeks. The use of gentamicin is optional (e.g., patients with severe sepsis) and at most limited to 3 days. According to BSAC and IDSA guidelines, for MRSA bacteremia, the use of gentamicin is no longer recommended for staphylococcal native valve IE. For oxacillin-resistant strains, use vancomycin 15 mg/kg/day IV q12h for 6 weeks for goal trough of 15 to 20 μg/mL (2)[B].
  – Prosthetic valve: oxacillin or nafcillin 12 g/day IV in 4 to 6 doses + rifampin 300 mg IV/PO q8h, for 6 weeks, + gentamicin 3 mg/kg/day IV for first 2 weeks (peak gentamicin level 3 μg/mL and trough <1 μg/mL). For oxacillin-resistant strains, use vancomycin 15 mg/kg/day IV q12h, + rifampin 300 mg IV/PO q8h, both for 6 weeks, + gentamicin 3 mg/kg/day IV/IM in 2 to 3 doses for the first 2 weeks (peak gentamicin level 3 μg/mL and trough <1 μg/mL) (2)[B].

- Penicillin-sensitive *Enterococcus*, native or prosthetic valve: ampicillin 12 g IV divided q4h *or* penicillin G 18 to 30 million U/day IV continuously or in 6 doses plus gentamicin 3 mg/kg IV q8h for 4 to 6 weeks (peak gentamicin level 3 μg/mL and trough <1 μg/mL) (2)[B]. Consider expert consultation for penicillin-resistant enterococci.

- *HACEK* organisms: ceftriaxone 2 g IM or IV q24h for 4 weeks (2)[B] *or* ampicillin-sulbactam 12 g IV divided q4h for 4 weeks *or* ciprofloxacin 1 g/day PO or 800 mg/day IV in 2 equally divided doses for 4 weeks
  – Cardiac device-related endocarditis: Whole device removal is recommended for all patients with lead infection, followed by antibiotic therapy based on organism susceptibility (4)[B].

- Precautions: In patients with renal impairment, dosage adjustment should be made for penicillin G, gentamicin, cefazolin, ampicillin, ampicillin/sulbactam, ciprofloxacin, and vancomycin.

Rapid infusion of vancomycin <1 hour may cause "red man syndrome" due to histamine release, not an allergic reaction. Treat with antihistamines and decrease infusion rate.
- Interactions: Vancomycin + gentamicin increases renal toxicity. Rifampin increases the requirement for Coumadin and oral hypoglycemic agents.

Second Line
For patients allergic to penicillin:

- Penicillin-susceptible or resistant viridans group streptococci or *S. bovis*: vancomycin 30 mg/kg (not to exceed 2 g/day) IV for 4 weeks (6 weeks for prosthetic valve endocarditis) for goal trough of 15 to 20 μg/mL (2)[B]
- *Enterococcus*, native or prosthetic valve: Desensitization to penicillin should be considered. Vancomycin 15 mg/kg (usual dose, 1 g) IV q12h, + gentamicin or streptomycin (peak gentamicin level 3 μg/mL and trough <1 μg/mL) for 4 to 6 weeks (6 weeks for prosthetic valve endocarditis) (2)[B]
- *Staphylococcus* of native valve: cefazolin 2 g IV q8h (not to be used in patients with immediate-type hypersensitivity to penicillin) for 4 to 6 weeks *or* vancomycin 30 mg/kg (usual dose, 1 g) IV q12h for a goal trough of 15 to 20 μg/mL, for 6 weeks (2)[B]

SURGERY/OTHER PROCEDURES
Surgery is required in 50% of IE cases. Indications include (3)[A]:

- Heart failure due to of aortic or mitral valve disease Prevention of embolism: aortic or mitral valve vegetations >10 mm with prior embolic episodes; isolated very large vegetation >15 mm; in patients with major ischemic stroke, surgery is delayed for at least 4 weeks, if possible (5)[C].
- Uncontrolled infection: persistent fever and positive cultures >7 to 10 days; infection caused by fungi or resistant organism; presence of abscess, fistula, false aneurysm, or enlarging vegetations
- Early prosthetic valve IE

ONGOING CARE

FOLLOW-UP RECOMMENDATIONS
Patient Monitoring
- Check gentamicin peak (~3 μg/mL) and trough (<1 μg/mL) levels if used for >5 days and with renal dysfunction. Perform twice-weekly BUN and serum creatinine while on gentamicin. Consider audiometry baseline and follow-up during long-term aminoglycoside therapy.
- Check vancomycin trough (15 to 20 μg/mL) levels in all patients (typically prior to 4th dose) (3)[B].
- Baseline ECG; monitor ECG for conduction disturbances/MI in initial weeks of therapy.
- TTE at the conclusion of therapy
- Blood cultures q48h until negative

PROGNOSIS
Late complications contribute to the poor prognosis of IE. The main complications are heart failure, reinfection, and cerebral emboli. 10-year survival is 60–90% (6)[A].

COMPLICATIONS
- Cerebral complications are the most frequent and severe, occurring in 15–20% of patients (1)[A].

- Emboli: arterial (e.g., MI, mesenteric, splenic, cerebral infarction), infectious (e.g., abscesses of heart, lung, brain, meninges, bone, pericardium)
  – Neurologic events are the most frequent complications in patients with IE requiring ICU admission. Ischemic stroke is the presenting symptom of IE in 20% of cases (6)[A].
- Inflammatory/immune disorders (e.g., arthritis, myositis, glomerulonephritis)
- Other complications: congestive heart failure (CHF), ruptured valve cusp, sinus of Valsalva aneurysm, arrhythmia, and mycotic aneurysms

REFERENCES
1. Wilson W, Taubert KA, Gewitz M, et al. Prevention of infective endocarditis: guidelines from the American Heart Association: a guideline from the American Heart Association Rheumatic Fever, Endocarditis, and Kawasaki Disease Committee, Council on Cardiovascular Disease in the Young, and the Council on Clinical Cardiology, Council on Cardiovascular Surgery and Anesthesia, and the Quality of Care and Outcomes Research Interdisciplinary Working Group. *Circulation*. 2007;116(15):1736–1754.
2. Baddour LM, Wilson WR, Bayer AS, et al. Infective endocarditis: diagnosis, antimicrobial therapy, and management of complications: a statement for healthcare professionals from the Committee on Rheumatic Fever, Endocarditis, and Kawasaki Disease, Council on Cardiovascular Disease in the Young, and the Councils on Clinical Cardiology, Stroke, and Cardiovascular Surgery and Anesthesia, American Heart Association: endorsed by the Infectious Diseases Society of America. *Circulation*. 2005;111(23):e394–e434.
3. Hoen B, Duval X. Clinical practice. Infective endocarditis. *N Engl J Med*. 2013;368(15):1425–1433.
4. Baddour LM, Epstein AE, Erickson CC, et al. Update on cardiovascular implantable electronic device infections and their management: a scientific statement from the American Heart Association. *Circulation*. 2010;121(3):458–477.
5. Byrne JG, Rezai K, Sanchez JA, et al. Surgical management of endocarditis: the society of thoracic surgeons clinical practice guideline. *Ann Thorac Surg*. 2011;91(6):2012–2019.
6. Sonneville R, Mirabel M, Hajage D, et al. Neurologic complications and outcomes of infective endocarditis in critically ill patients: the ENDOcardite en REAnimation prospective multicenter study. *Crit Care Med*. 2011;39(6):1474–1481.

CODES

ICD10
- I33.0 Acute and subacute infective endocarditis
- I39 Endocarditis and heart valve disord in dis classd elswhr
- A54.83 Gonococcal heart infection

CLINICAL PEARLS
- Antibiotic prophylaxis is recommended for patients with artificial heart valves, history of IE, CHDs, and cardiac transplants with valvulopathy.
- TEE/TTE and blood cultures are the mainstays for the diagnosis of IE.
- Most common organisms involved in IE are viridians *Streptococcus* spp. and *Staphylococcus*.

ENDOMETRIAL CANCER AND UTERINE SARCOMA

Jay R. Patibandla, MD • Michael P. Hopkins, MD, MEd

 BASICS

DESCRIPTION

- Endometrial cancer: malignancy of the endometrial lining of the uterus
  - Two types
    - Type I: estrogen dependent, grade 1 or grade 2, better prognosis, endometrioid histology
    - Type II: estrogen independent, higher grade, more aggressive, include grade 3 endometrioid and nonendometrioid: serous, clear cell, mucinous, poor prognosis (1)[A]
- Cell types: adenocarcinoma, adenosquamous (malignant squamous elements), clear cell, and papillary serous
- Sarcomas: malignancy of the uterine mesenchyme and mixed tumors
  - Mixed müllerian sarcoma (carcinosarcoma): Heterologous sarcoma elements are not native to the müllerian system (e.g., cartilage or bone); homologous sarcoma elements are native to the müllerian system (40–50% prevalence of all sarcomas).
  - Leiomyosarcoma develops in the myometrium, characterized by cellular atypic mitoses and coagulative necrosis (30% prevalence of all sarcomas).
  - Endometrial stromal sarcoma develops from the stromal component of the endometrium (15% prevalence of all sarcomas).
  - Poorer prognosis (2)[C]
- Predominant age
  - Endometrial cancer: Most patients are postmenopausal:
    - Average age of diagnosis: 63 years old
  - Sarcomas: occurs in both pre- and postmenopausal:
    - Average age of diagnosis: 40 to 69 years old (2)[C]
- 70% of endometrial cancer is stage I at the time of diagnosis.
- System(s) affected: reproductive
- Synonym(s): uterine cancer; endometrial cancer; corpus cancer

Pregnancy Considerations
This malignancy is not associated with pregnancy.

EPIDEMIOLOGY

Incidence
- Endometrial cancer is the most common gynecologic malignancy; fourth most common cancer in women and eighth leading cause of cancer-related death in women worldwide.
- In the United States, it is estimated that endometrial cancer will account for 54,870 new cases and 10,170 deaths in 2015 (2)[C].

Prevalence
500,000 women in the United States

ETIOLOGY AND PATHOPHYSIOLOGY
Continuous estrogen stimulation unopposed by progesterone
- Endometrial: unopposed estrogen
  - Estrogen replacement therapy without concomitant progesterone increases the risk. Addition of progesterone decreases risk to that of general population.
- Sarcomas: etiology unknown

Genetics
- Endometrial: Lynch syndrome (hereditary nonpolyposis colorectal cancer)
- Sarcoma: African American, higher incidence of leiomyosarcoma, childhood retinoblastoma survivors

RISK FACTORS
- Early menarche/late menopause
- Nulliparity
- Personal or family history of colon or reproductive system cancer
- Obesity
- Diabetes mellitus
- Hypertension
- Polycystic ovarian syndrome
- Estrogen-secreting tumor
- Endometrial hyperplasia
- Unopposed estrogens
- Tamoxifen use
- Increasing age

GENERAL PREVENTION
- In young women who are obese or anovulatory, the risk of endometrial cancer can be reduced by taking oral contraceptive pills, permanently losing weight, or taking cyclic progesterone to prevent unopposed estrogen's effects on the uterus (3)[A].
- Estrogen replacement therapy should always include progesterone unless the woman has had a hysterectomy (3)[A].
- Cigarette smoking has been associated with a lower risk of type I endometrial cancer; however, it is not recommended secondary to its many health risks and increase risk of type II endometrial cancer.

COMMONLY ASSOCIATED CONDITIONS
- Endometrial hyperplasia: 1–25% will progress to endometrial adenocarcinoma:
  - Simple without atypia
  - Complex without atypia
  - Simple with atypia
  - Complex with atypia
    - 43% with complex hyperplasia with atypia have concurrent endometrial cancer.
- Endometrial cancer patients should be screened regularly for breast and colon cancer because of an increased risk of these cancers.
- Patients who have breast or colon cancer are at increased risk for endometrial cancer.
- Granulosa cell tumors of the ovary produce estrogen; these patients will have an increased risk of endometrial cancer.

DIAGNOSIS

HISTORY
- Endometrial cancer
  - Postmenopausal bleeding is the most frequent sign. Any spotting or abnormal discharge mandates evaluation.
  - Premenopausal patients with history of anovulation and heavy, irregular, or prolonged periods that fail multiple medical managements mandate evaluation.
- Sarcoma
  - Mixed müllerian sarcoma: bleeding and prolapsing tissue, pain (2)[C]
  - Leiomyosarcoma: pelvic pain, pressure, uterine mass, abnormal bleeding

PHYSICAL EXAM
Pelvic exam: enlarged, fixed

DIFFERENTIAL DIAGNOSIS
- Atypical complex hyperplasia: a premalignant lesion of the endometrium
- Cervical cancer
- Ovarian cancer invading the uterus
- Endometriosis
- Adenomyosis
- Leiomyoma

DIAGNOSTIC TESTS & INTERPRETATION

Initial Tests (lab, imaging)
- Liver and renal function tests
- Transvaginal ultrasound usually shows increased endometrial thickness (>4 mm in postmenopausal patients or in patients with irregular or heavy periods if >35 years of age) (1)[A].
- Levels of cancer antigen 125 (CA-125) may be elevated when intra-abdominal disease is present (1)[A].
- Chest x-ray (CXR): Most common site of metastases is the lungs.
- Mammogram and colonoscopy: Endometrial cancer is associated with breast and colon cancer.

Follow-Up Tests & Special Considerations
- Endometrial cancer is mostly localized to the uterus, therefore preop evaluation for metastasis is not needed unless metastasis is already suspected (2)[A].
- CT scan, PET/CT, MRI, CA-125: not part of the routine evaluation but may be needed if metastasis is suspected; patient is a poor operative candidate or pathology returns high grade (G3 endometroid, papillary serous, clear cell, carcinosarcoma) (2)
- MRI has been reported to show the depth of myometrial penetration accurately but is not always cost-effective (4)[A].

Diagnostic Procedures/Other
- Office endometrial biopsy (90% accurate): If negative with high suspicion for cancer or patient continues to have bleeding, a dilation and curettage (D&C) is necessary (2)[B]. Endometrial stromal sarcoma and leiomyosarcoma rarely are diagnosed preoperatively. Any patient with history of irregular, heavy, or prolonged periods should undergo endometrial biopsy prior to endometrial ablation procedures.
- Fractional D&C is 99% accurate except in cases of sarcoma.
- If surgical approach is favored, D&C with hysteroscopic guidance is recommended over D&C alone, due to its ability to pick up discrete lesions (2)[A].

Test Interpretation
- Federation of Gynecology and Obstetrics Staging System: revised 2009
  - Stage I (confined to corpus uteri)
    - A: no or <1/2 myometrial invasion
    - B: invasion ≥1/2 the myometrium
  - Stage II: Tumor invades cervical stroma but does not extend beyond the uterus.
  - Stage III: local and/or regional spread
    - A: uterine serosal and/or adnexal invasion
    - B: vaginal and/or parametrial involvement
    - C: metastases to pelvic and/or para-aortic lymph nodes

○ IIIC1: +pelvic nodes
○ IIIC2: +para-aortic lymph nodes positive pelvic lymph nodes
– Stage IV: Tumor invades bladder and/or bowel mucosa and/or distant metastases:
○ A: Tumor invades bladder and/or bowel mucosa.
○ B: distant metastases, including intra-abdominal metastases and/or inguinal lymph nodes (1)[A]
• Uterine sarcoma criteria for diagnosis: mitotic index, cellular atypia, and areas of coagulative necrosis separated from tumor (5)[C]

 TREATMENT

GENERAL MEASURES
• Main treatment for uterine cancer is surgery.
• Radiation is used to prevent tumor recurrence at the vaginal cuff.

MEDICATION
First Line
• Endometrial
– Chemotherapy for advanced or recurrent disease incurable with surgery and radiation
○ Paclitaxel + carboplatin (2)[B]
○ Doxorubicin + cisplatin + paclitaxel
• Hormonal therapy
– Medroxyprogesterone acetate: for recurrence or metastases
– Megestrol (Megace) 160 mg/day for at least 2 months for women with premalignant lesions, atypical complex hyperplasia, or well-differentiated endometrial cancer in patients desiring fertility. Follow with D&C to determine cancer resolution.
– Levonorgestrel-containing intrauterine device: as mentioned earlier for patients who desire future fertility (3,6,7)[A]
• Sarcoma
– Chemotherapy
○ Doxorubicin as single agent or in combination (5)[A]
• Hormonal
– Tamoxifen or aromatase inhibitors; not fully studied
– Progesterones (3)[A]

ADDITIONAL THERAPIES
Radiation therapy
• Nonoperative candidates: radiation therapy alone
• Low risk: no adjuvant radiation therapy
• Intermediate risk: Consider adjuvant vaginal brachytherapy; reduces local recurrences but has no effect on overall survival
• High risk: chemotherapy and radiation therapy in some cases (4,8)[A]

SURGERY/OTHER PROCEDURES
Surgical staging
• Extrafascial hysterectomy and bilateral salpingo-oophorectomy
• Cytologic washings
• Pelvic and para-aortic lymph node dissection
• Omental sampling, as indicated
• Optimal tumor debulking (1)[A]

Geriatric Considerations
Older (and obese) patients may be at high risk for surgery. Alternative radiation therapy can be considered.

INPATIENT CONSIDERATIONS
Admission-Criteria/Initial Stabilization
• Excessive vaginal bleeding
• Preoperative stabilization
Nursing
Routine; ensure postoperative pain is controlled.
Discharge Criteria
Postsurgical criteria: pain controlled, tolerating diet, ambulating, and voiding

 ONGOING CARE

FOLLOW-UP RECOMMENDATIONS
Follow-up visit for speculum and rectovaginal exam every 3 to 6 months for 2 years, then every 6 months for 3 years, and then annually for life (2)[C]

PATIENT MONITORING
• Annual CXR is no longer recommended.
• CT scan or PET/CT scan of the chest, abdomen, and pelvis should be used only to investigate suspicion of recurrent disease, not routinely

DIET
As tolerated and according to comorbidities

PATIENT EDUCATION
After surgery:
• No intercourse for ~6 weeks
• No lifting >10 to 15 lb
• No driving until pain-free
• Do not expect resumption of full activity for 6 weeks.

PROGNOSIS
5-year survival rates
• Uterine adenocarcinoma

Stage	Survival (%)
IA	88
IB	75
II	69
IIIA	58
IIIB	50
IIIC	47
IVA	17
IVB	15

• Uterine carcinosarcoma

Stage	Survival (%)
I	70
II	45
III	30
IV	15

(3,4)[A]

COMPLICATIONS
• Surgical: excessive bleeding, wound infection, lymphedema, deep vein thrombosis (DVT), and damage to the urinary or intestinal systems
• Radiation: diarrhea, ileus, bowel obstruction or fistula, radiation cystitis, proctitis, vaginal stenosis, DVT
• Chemotherapy: per the drug given

REFERENCES
1. Creasman W. Revised FIGO staging for carcinoma of the endometrium. *Int J Gynaecol Obstet*. 2009;105(2):109.
2. American College of Obstetricians and Gynecologists. ACOG practice bulletin, clinical management guidelines for obstetrician-gynecologists, number 149, April 2015: endometrial cancer. *Obstet Gynecol*. 2015;125(4):1006–1026.
3. Polyzos NP, Pavlidis N, Paraskevaidis E, et al. Randomized evidence on chemotherapy and hormonal therapy regimens for advanced endometrial cancer: an overview of survival data. *Eur J Cancer*. 2006;42(3):319–326.
4. Humber C, Tierney J, Symonds P, et al. Chemotherapy for advanced, recurrent or metastatic endometrial carcinoma. *Cochrane Database Syst Rev*. 2005;(4):CD003915.
5. Gadducci A, Cosio S, Romanini A, et al. The management of patients with uterine sarcoma: a debated clinical challenge. *Crit Rev Oncol Hematol*. 2008;65(2):129–142.
6. Bramwell VH, Anderson D, Charette ML. Doxorubicin-based chemotherapy for the palliative treatment of adult patients with locally advanced or metastatic soft tissue sarcoma. *Cochrane Database Syst Rev*. 2003;(3):CD003293.
7. Fleming GF, Brunetto VL, Cella D, et al. Phase III trial of doxorubicin plus cisplatin with or without paclitaxel plus filgrastim in advanced endometrial carcinoma: a Gynecologic Oncology Group study. *J Clin Oncol*. 2004;22(11):2159–2166.
8. Einhorn N, Tropé C, Ridderheim M, et al. A systematic overview of radiation therapy effects in uterine cancer (corpus uteri). *Acta Oncol*. 2003;42(5–6):557–561.

 SEE ALSO

• Cervical Malignancy
• Algorithm: Pelvic Pain

 CODES

ICD10
• C54.1 Malignant neoplasm of endometrium
• C55 Malignant neoplasm of uterus, part unspecified
• C54.2 Malignant neoplasm of myometrium

CLINICAL PEARLS
• Most common presenting symptom is abnormal uterine bleeding.
• Any patient with history of irregular, heavy, or prolonged periods should undergo endometrial biopsy.
• Primary cause is unopposed estrogen.
• Endometrial thickness on transvaginal ultrasound of <5 mm makes endometrial cancer very unlikely.
• Primary treatment is with surgery, with possible chemotherapy ± radiation.

ENDOMETRIOSIS

Andrew G. Alexander, MD • Maegen Dupper, MD • Heidi S. Millard, MD

 BASICS

DESCRIPTION

- Endometriosis is a common but potentially painful and debilitating estrogen-dependent gynecologic condition affecting women of predominately reproductive age (1)[A].
- Symptoms and signs generally consists of pelvic pain and decreased fertility.
- Due to estrogen-dependent implants of endometrial tissue found outside the uterus. Although endometriomas have been recorded in liver, bowel, umbilicus, lung, and other tissue, the most common pathologic sites are:
  - Peritoneum(bladder, cul-de-sac, pelvic walls, ligaments, and fallopian tubes)
  - Ovaries
  - Rectovaginal septum
- Ectopic endometrial implants proliferate and slough with the menstrual cycle
- Stage I (minimal) to IV (severe). Staging is useful in therapeutic planning but does not correlate with pain severity.

EPIDEMIOLOGY

Prevalence

- Female only
- Affects 11% of fertile women (2)
- Found in 30–50% of infertile women
- Found in 50–60% of women and adolescent women with pelvic pain

Pediatric Considerations

Endometriosis may begin with puberty as endometrial implants are dependent on ovarian hormones. This can lead to debilitating pelvic pain and severe dysmenorrhea associated with missed school, social, and family activities.

Pregnancy Considerations

The presence of endometriosis decreases fecundability from 15–20% per month to 2–10% per month. 25–50% of infertile women have endometriosis. However, pelvic endometriosis generally improves during pregnancy.

Geriatric Considerations

Although menopause often results in a resolution of symptoms, pelvic endometriosis may extend into menopause and is exacerbated by hormone replacement therapy (HRT).

ETIOLOGY AND PATHOPHYSIOLOGY

- Not fully understood, several factors are believed to play a role, including immunologic changes and genetic predisposition in the presence of abnormal proliferating endometrial tissue implants causing chronic peritoneal inflammation.
- Theories include:
  - **Sampson theory:** Retrograde menstruation results in peritoneal implantation and disease
  - **Halban theory:** Distant disease is probably caused by hematogenous/lymphatic dissemination or metaplastic transformation.
  - **Coelomic metaplasia:** Coelomic epithelium remains undifferentiated in the peritoneal cavity and differentiates to form functioning endometrium.

- Endometrial-associated infertility is multifactorial:
  - Pelvic inflammation
  - Anatomic disruption of pelvic structures (involvement of the fallopian tube may cause isthmic tubal obstruction)
  - Proliferation and activation of peritoneal macrophages (may predispose to gamete phagocytosis)
  - Alteration in eutopic endometrium

Genetics

Odds ratio of symptomatic endometriosis with a first degree affected relative is 7.2. Those with affected first-degree relatives have a 26% chance of severe manifestations, versus 12% if no first degree affected relatives.

RISK FACTORS

- Family history
- Menstruation and ovulation
- Delayed childbirth

GENERAL PREVENTION

- Suppression of heavy menstruation and ovulation with oral contraceptives during adolescence may delay sequelae.
- Some factors are considered protective:
  - Fruits, green vegetables, n-3 long-chain fatty acids
  - Aerobic exercise may decrease pelvic pain.
- Early diagnosis and treatment might help prevent sequelae.

COMMONLY ASSOCIATED CONDITIONS

Associated with increased risks for cancer of the ovary, breast, endometrium; increased risk for cutaneous melanoma, non-Hodgkin lymphoma, autoimmune diseases, asthma, and cardiovascular disease

 DIAGNOSIS

- History: dysmenorrhea (50–90% of cases) due to deep infiltrating endometrial implants
- Dyspareunia due to lesions of the cul-de-sac, uterosacral ligaments, and posterior vaginal fornix
- Dyschezia due to involvement of the rectosigmoid colon and rectovaginal regions
- Chronic pelvic pain (≥6 months) that worsens with time and begins 1 to 2 days prior to menstrual cycles
- Hematochezia
- Cyclic nausea, abdominal distention
- Infertility (late finding)
- History of pelvic pain, infertility, and hysterectomy in first- or second-degree relative

PHYSICAL EXAM

- Focal pain/tenderness on pelvic exam is associated with endometriosis in 66% of patients.
- Pelvic mass may be present.
- Immobile pelvic organs (frozen pelvis)
- Rectovaginal exam revealing uterosacral nodules, beading, or tenderness
- An exquisitely tender "barb" stabbing pain in the region of the uterosacral ligament is found in severe cases.

DIFFERENTIAL DIAGNOSIS

Differential diagnosis of pelvic pain includes all causes of acute abdomen and

- Complications of intrauterine/ectopic pregnancy
- Pelvic adhesions
- Acute salpingitis/pelvic inflammatory disease
- Ruptured ovarian cyst
- Uterine leiomyomas
- Adenomyosis
- Irritable bowel syndrome
- Inflammatory bowel disease
- Pelvic malignancy
- Cystitis
- Depression
- History of sexual abuse
- Chronic pain syndrome

DIAGNOSTIC TESTS & INTERPRETATION

Initial Tests (lab, imaging)

- Labs are only useful to rule out other diagnoses; there are no useful labs to rule in endometriosis.
- CA-125 levels are not recommended (3)[C] due to low sensitivity.
- If history and physical exam reveal adnexal pain or tenderness with/without fullness on pelvic exam
  - Transvaginal ultrasound (US) and MRI are equally effective in detecting ovarian endometriomas: sensitivity, 80–90%; specificity, 60–98% for both
  - US is preferred (less costly).
  - Both modalities are poor in detecting peritoneal implants and adhesions.

Diagnostic Procedures/Other

Definitive diagnosis is made by the gross and microscopic characteristics of tissue visualized and biopsied during laparoscopy or laparotomy.

Test Interpretation

- Laparoscopically visualized red and blue-black lesions described as "powder-burns," adhesions, and "chocolate cysts" on the ovarian and peritoneal surfaces.
- Histologically described endometrial glands and stroma on analysis of biopsied lesions

TREATMENT

GENERAL MEASURES

Management is dependent on multiple factors:

- Age and reproductive desires of the patient
- The certainty of the diagnosis
- The degree of degradation on quality of life due to pain and infertility
- The threat to other organ systems: GI tract, bladder

MEDICATION

Medications are used to improve the patient's quality of life through symptom relief, and to prevent progression of the disease and its potential to cause organ dysfunction.

First Line
Women found to have endometriomas during incidental surgery or studies may not need any treatment. Others with minimal symptoms may find sufficient relief with NSAID medications. Increased exercise, especially aerobic, may help others.

- NSAIDs initiated at the beginning or just before menses. Evidence is inconclusive on effectiveness (4)[B].
- Cyclic combined oral contraceptive pills (OCPs) suppress ovulation.

Second Line
- Low-dose OCPs or low-dose progestins with recommendations to switch from cyclic to continuous contraception for 3 to 6 months if symptoms persist or if there is chronic, noncyclic pelvic pain
  - Levonorgestrel intrauterine device (IUD) (Mirena) found to decrease recurrence of painful menstruation (although not FDA approved for this indication).
- Medroxyprogesterone acetate 150 mg IM 3 months. Prolonged use may lead to loss of bone mineral density of uncertain clinical significance. Gonadotropin-releasing hormone (GnRH) agonists: Inhibit pituitary gonadotropin synthesis and induce a hypoestrogenic state.
- Norethindrone acetate 5 mg PO once daily plus conjugated equine estrogen 0.625 mg PO once daily

Third Line
If symptoms and signs continue, physicians should be experienced in the use and side effects of gonadotropin-releasing hormone analogues prior to their use (symptoms return in as many as 70% of treated patients):

- Leuprolide acetate (Depo-Lupron) 3.75 mg IM each month or 11.25 mg IM every 3 months (gluteal)
- Nafarelin (Synarel) intranasal one spray (200 μg) in one nostril each morning and the other nostril each evening (start between days 2 and 4 of menstrual cycle)
- Goserelin (Zoladex) implant 3.6 mg SC in upper abdominal wall every 28 days
- Danazol: also effective, with side effects similar to GnRH analogs
- Aromatase inhibitors (anastrozole and letrozole) prolong the remission induced by gonadotropin-releasing hormone medications.

ALERT
Calcium (1,000 to 1,500 mg/day) with vitamin D 1,000 to 2,000 IU daily or low-dose estrogen with progestogen (5)[B] is recommended when using GnRH agonists to prevent calcium loss.

ISSUES FOR REFERRAL
- Refer early to a physician with expertise in medical and surgical treatment of endometriosis, especially if the patient desires to conceive in the future.
- Indications for referral to a properly experienced gynecologist include the following:
  - Need for definitive diagnosis
  - Failure to respond to a conservative or first-line therapy
  - Chronic pelvic pain
  - Delayed fertility

ADDITIONAL THERAPIES
Regular exercise and counseling for pain-management strategies. Narcotics are contraindicated for chronic pain.

SURGERY/OTHER PROCEDURES
Surgery (laparoscopy or laparotomy) is both diagnostic and therapeutic (first line or when conservative measures fail):

- Peritoneal endometriosis: laser ablation/excision/fulguration
- Ovarian endometriosis (endometriomas) >3 to 4 cm: ablation, excision, drainage
- Lysis of adhesions (LOA)
- Hysterectomy with bilateral salpingo-oophorectomy for debilitating symptoms refractory to other medical or surgical treatments:
  - Relieves pain in 80–90%, but pain recurs in 10% within 1 to 2 years after surgery
  - Postoperative HRT should include estrogen and progestogen or progesterone
- Interruption of nerve pathways: laparoscopic ablations and presacral neurectomy improve dysmenorrhea
- Fertility procedures: Ablation or excision of lesions with LOA is recommended to treat infertility in stages I–II disease:
  - Spontaneous conception should be attempted for 1 year prior to assisted reproduction techniques.
  - Disease does not endanger in vitro fertilization (IVF) pregnancies.

ALERT
Surgery for endometriomas may decrease ovarian reserve in advanced disease

COMPLEMENTARY & ALTERNATIVE MEDICINE
- Osteopathic manipulative therapy found to improve quality of life (3)[C].
- Postsurgical use of Chinese herbal medicine has been found to be effective.

- Acupuncture may be more effective than Danazol to decrease pain, irregular menstruation, and perineal swelling (6)[B].

- Osteopathic manipulation

ONGOING CARE

FOLLOW-UP RECOMMENDATIONS
Routine gynecologic care

Patient Monitoring
Symptomatic and asymptomatic pelvic masses
http://www.acog.org/

PROGNOSIS
- Excellent, especially if diagnosis and treatment plans are initiated early in disease course
- Poor for recovery of fertility if the disease has progressed to stage III/IV
- Symptoms and signs improve after bilateral oophorectomy.

COMPLICATIONS
Sequelae include chronic pelvic pain, reduced quality of life, repetitive surgical intervention, depression, infertility, medication side effects and costs, and infertility.

REFERENCES
1. Brown J, Farquhar C. Endometriosis: an overview of Cochrane Reviews. *Cochrane Database Syst Rev*. 2014;(3):CD009590.
2. Buck Louis GM, Hediger ML, Peterson CM, et al. Incidence of endometriosis by study population and diagnostic method: the ENDO study. *Fertil Steril*. 2011;96(2):360–365.
3. Daraï C, Deboute O, Zacharopoulou C, et al. Impact of osteopathic manipulative therapy on quality of life of patients with deep infiltrating endometriosis with colorectal involvement: results of a pilot study. *Eur J Obstet Gynecol Reprod Biol*. 2015;188:70–73.
4. Allen C, Hopewell S, Prentice A, et al. Nonsteroidal anti-inflammatory drugs for pain in women with endometriosis. *Cochrane Database Syst Rev*. 2009;(2):CD004753.
5. Giudice LC. Clinical practice. Endometriosis. *N Engl J Med*. 2010;362(25):2389–2398.
6. Zhu X, Hamilton KD, McNicol ED. Acupuncture for pain in endometriosis. *Cochrane Database Syst Rev*. 2011;(9):CD007864.

ADDITIONAL READING
- Davis L, Kennedy SS, Moore J, et al. Modern combined oral contraceptives for pain associated with endometriosis. *Cochrane Database Syst Rev*. 2007;(3):CD001019.
- de Ziegler D, Borghese B, Chapron C. Endometriosis and infertility: pathophysiology and management. *Lancet*. 2010;376(9742):730–738.
- Fujii S. MR Imaging of endometriosis. In: Harada T, ed. *Endometriosis: Pathogenesis and Treatment*. Tottori, Japan: Springer; 2014.
- Hughes E, Brown J, Collins JJ, et al. Ovulation suppression for endometriosis. *Cochrane Database Syst Rev*. 2007;(3):CD000155.
- Jacobson TZ, Duffy JM, Barlow D, et al. Laparoscopic surgery for pelvic pain associated with endometriosis. *Cochrane Database Syst Rev*. 2009;(4):CD001300.
- Koga K, Yoshino O, Hirota Y, et al. Infertility treatment of endometriosis patients. In: Harada T, ed. *Endometriosis: Pathogenesis and Treatment*. Tottori, Japan: Springer; 2014.
- Practice Committee of American Society for Reproductive Medicine. Treatment of pelvic pain associated with endometriosis. *Fertil Steril*. 2008;90(5 Suppl):S260–S269.

CODES

ICD10
- N80.9 Endometriosis, unspecified
- N80.3 Endometriosis of pelvic peritoneum
- N80.2 Endometriosis of fallopian tube

CLINICAL PEARLS
- Severe dysmenorrhea and dyspareunia are never normal. Failure to respond to NSAIDs and/or OCPs warrants further investigation.
- A rectovaginal exam can be useful in patients suspected of having endometriosis.

ENDOMETRITIS AND OTHER POSTPARTUM INFECTIONS

Justin P. Lavin, Jr., MD, FACOG • Ayesha Hasan, MD • Danielle Taylor, DO, MS

 BASICS

DESCRIPTION
- Endometritis (infection of the endometrium) is the most common postpartum infection.
- Bacterial infection of genital tract, usually within the 1st week after delivery, can occur as late as 1 to 6 weeks postpartum.
- Less common are postpartum infections of the myometrium and parametrial tissues. Vaginal and cervical infections, perineal cellulitis, pelvic cellulitis, septic pelvic vein thrombophlebitis, and parametrial phlegmon are other less-common postpartum infections of the pelvic region.
- System(s) affected: reproductive
- Synonym(s): postpartum infection; endometritis; endoparametritis; endomyometritis; myometritis; endomyoparametritis; metritis; metritis with pelvic cellulitis

EPIDEMIOLOGY
Incidence
Predominant age and gender: women of childbearing years

Prevalence
- Occurs after 1–3% of all births
- Infection is 10 times more likely after cesarean section
  - 2–15% of infections occur prior to labor
  - 30–35% occur after labor in absence of appropriate antibiotic prophylaxis; 2–15% occur after labor with appropriate prophylaxis
  - Fifth leading cause of maternal mortality, accounting for 11% of maternal deaths

ETIOLOGY AND PATHOPHYSIOLOGY
- Endometritis is more common in labors complicated by chorioamnionitis.
- Other infections follow trauma to the perineum, vagina, cervix, and uterus.
- Postpartum infections are typically polymicrobial, involving organisms ascending from the lower genital tract:
  - Aerobic isolates (70%): *Streptococcus faecalis, Streptococcus agalactiae, Streptococcus viridans, Staphylococcus aureus, Escherichia coli*
  - Anaerobic isolates (80%): *Peptococcus* sp., *Peptostreptococcus* sp., *Clostridium* sp., *Bacteroides bivius, Bacteroides fragilis, Fusobacterium* sp.
- Other genital mycoplasmata
- Consider herpes simplex virus and cytomegalovirus, particularly in immunocompromised patients failing to improve on appropriate antibiotics.
- Thrombosis of any pelvic vein, including vena cava
- Phlegmon on leaves of the broad ligament

RISK FACTORS
- Cesarean delivery is the primary risk factor.
- Chorioamnionitis
- Bacterial vaginosis
- Group B streptococcal colonization of genital tract
- HIV infection
- Prolonged labor
- Prolonged rupture of membranes
- Multiple vaginal examinations
- Internal fetal monitoring during labor
- Operative vaginal delivery
- Manual extraction of the placenta
- Low socioeconomic status
- Obesity
- Anemia
- Care in a teaching hospital

GENERAL PREVENTION
- Vaginal delivery
  - Avoid unnecessary vaginal examinations.
  - Treat chorioamnionitis during labor.
  - Avoid manual placental extraction and retained placental products.
  - Consider antibiotic prophylaxis for third- and fourth-degree laceration (1)[B].
  - Use aseptic technique for operative vaginal delivery.
  - Antibiotic prophylaxis for operative vaginal delivery is not necessary (2)[A].
- Cesarean delivery
  - Preoperative preparation using a paint and scrub technique with a 10% povidone iodine scrub and topical solution decreases puerperal infection by up to 38% (3)[B].
  - Prophylactic antibiotics before both emergency and scheduled cesarean deliveries prior to skin incision reduces the prevalence of postpartum infection (4)[A],(5,6)[B].
    - Antibiotics should be administered within 1 hour of the surgery start time (6)[B].
    - Appropriate administration of antibiotics results in a 40% reduction in postpartum maternal infections without any increase in neonatal infectious outcomes (6)[B].
  - Extending the spectrum of coverage to include both a cephalosporin and a macrolide may further decrease infection risk (7)[A],(8)[B].
  - Vaginal preparation with povidone iodine solution immediately before cesarean delivery reduces the risk of postoperative endometritis (9)[A].
  - Weight-based antibiotic dosage helps ensure appropriate tissue concentrations prior to skin incision (10).

COMMONLY ASSOCIATED CONDITIONS
- Chorioamnionitis
- Wound infection

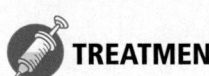 **DIAGNOSIS**

HISTORY
- History of cesarean delivery or chorioamnionitis
- Fever and chills
- Malaise
- Headache
- Anorexia
- Abdominal pain
- Heavy vaginal bleeding or foul smelling lochia

PHYSICAL EXAM
- Oral temperature >38°C (100.4°F)
- Tachycardia
- Uterine tenderness on exam
- Other localized abdominopelvic tenderness on exam
- Purulent or malodorous lochia
- Heavy vaginal bleeding
- Ileus
- Group A or B streptococcal bacteremia may have no localizing signs.

DIFFERENTIAL DIAGNOSIS
- "5 Ws": Wind (pneumonia); Water (UTI); Wound infection; Wow (mastitis); Wonder drug (medication-related fever)
- Viral syndrome; dehydration
- Thrombophlebitis
- Thyroid storm
- Appendicitis

DIAGNOSTIC TESTS & INTERPRETATION
Initial Tests (lab, imaging)
- CBC: Interpret with care (*Physiologic leukocytosis may be as high as 20,000 WBCs.*).
- Two sets of blood cultures (especially with suspected sepsis)
- Note: Diagnosis often made on clinical grounds. Potential testing includes:
  - Genital tract cultures and rapid test for group B streptococci (may be done during labor)
  - Amniotic fluid Gram stain: usually polymicrobial
  - Uterine tissue cultures: Prep the cervix with Betadine and use a shielded specimen collector or Pipelle; difficult to obtain without contamination
- If patient is not responsive to antibiotics in 24 to 48 hours:
  - Ultrasound for retained products of conception, pelvic abscess, or mass
  - CT or MRI looking for pelvic vein thrombophlebitis, abscess, or deep-seated wound infection

Diagnostic Procedures/Other
Paracentesis/culdocentesis with culture rarely necessary

Test Interpretation
- Superficial layer of infected necrotic tissue in microscopic sections of uterine lining
- >5 NEUTROPHILS per high-power field in superficial endometrium; ≥1 plasma cell in endometrial stroma

TREATMENT

MEDICATION
First Line
- Clindamycin 900 mg IV q8h + gentamicin 5 mg/kg IV q24h (11)[A]
- Potential side effects include nephrotoxicity, ototoxicity, pseudomembranous colitis, or diarrhea (in up to 6%).

Second Line
- Ampicillin-sulbactam 3 g IV q6h
- Metronidazole 500 mg q8–12h + penicillin 5,000,000 U q6h, or
- Ampicillin 2 g q6h + gentamicin 5 mg/kg q24h (11)[A]
- Cefoxitin 2 g IV q6h. Add ampicillin 2 g IV q6h, if clinical failure after 48 hours
- Cefotetan 2 g IV q12h. Add ampicillin 2 g IV q6h, if clinical failure after 48 hours (11)[A]

- Note: Base therapy on cultures, sensitivities, and clinical response.
- Contraindications
  – Drug allergy
  – Renal failure (aminoglycosides)
  – Avoid sulfa, tetracyclines, and fluoroquinolones before delivery and if breastfeeding. Metronidazole is relatively contraindicated if breastfeeding.
- Precautions:
  – Clindamycin and other antibiotics occasionally cause pseudomembranous colitis.
  – Antibiotic-associated diarrhea (*Clostridium difficile*)
- Note: Consider adding a macrolide antibiotic (for chlamydia coverage) for infections occurring after 48 hours.
- Note: Heparin typically indicated for septic pelvic vein thrombophlebitis; requires 10 days of full anticoagulation

SURGERY/OTHER PROCEDURES
- Curettage for retained products of conception
- Surgery to drain abscess
- Surgery to decompress the bowel
- Surgical drainage of a phlegmon is not advised unless it is suppurative. Surgical removal of other inflamed tissue is usually not required.

INPATIENT CONSIDERATIONS
Admission Criteria/Initial Stabilization
- Inpatient care is recommended for postpartum infections.
- Many infections occur after hospital discharge.
- IV antibiotics and close observation for severe infections
- Open and drain infected wounds.
- Optimize fluid status.

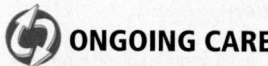 ## ONGOING CARE

FOLLOW-UP RECOMMENDATIONS
Patient Monitoring
- Individualize according to severity
- IV antibiotics can be stopped when the patient is afebrile for 24 to 48 hours.
- Oral antibiotics on discharge are not necessary, unless patient was bacteremic; then continue oral antibiotics to complete a 7-day course.

DIET
As tolerated, although may be limited by ileus

PATIENT EDUCATION
- Advise patient to contact physician with fever >38°C (100.4°F) postpartum, heavy vaginal bleeding, foul-smelling lochia, or other symptoms of infection.
- Information available at http://www.healthline.com/health/pregnancy/complications-postpartum-endometritis

PROGNOSIS
With supportive therapy and appropriate antibiotics, most patients improve quickly and recover without complication.

COMPLICATIONS
- Resistant organisms; peritonitis; pelvic abscess
- Septic pelvic thrombophlebitis
- Ovarian vein thrombosis
- Sepsis; death

REFERENCES
1. Duggal N, Mercado C, Daniels K, et al. Antibiotic prophylaxis for prevention of postpartum perineal wound complications: a randomized controlled trial. *Obstet Gynecol*. 2008;111(6):1268–1273.
2. Liabsuetrakul T, Choobun T, Peeyananjarassri K, et al. Antibiotic prophylaxis for operative vaginal delivery. *Cochrane Database Syst Rev*. 2014;(10):CD004455.
3. Weed S, Bastek JA, Sammel MD, et al. Comparing postcesarean infectious complication rates using two different skin preparations. *Obstet Gynecol*. 2011;117(5):1123–1129.
4. Smaill FM, Grivell GM. Antibiotic prophylaxis versus no prophylaxis for preventing infection after cesarean section. *Cochrane Database Sys Rev*. 2014;(10):CD007482.
5. Dinsmoor MJ, Gilbert S, Landon MB, et al. Perioperative antibiotic prophylaxis for non-laboring cesarean delivery. *Obstet Gynecol*. 2009;114(4):752–756.
6. American College of Obstetricians and Gynecologist. ACOG practice bulletin No. 120: use of prophylactic antibiotics in labor and delivery. *Obstet Gynecol*. 2011;117(6):1472–1483.
7. Costantine MM, Rahman M, Ghulmiyah L, et al. Timing of perioperative antibiotics for cesarean delivery: a metaanalysis. *Am J Obstet Gynecol*. 2008;199(3):301.e1–301.e6.
8. Tita AT, Owen J, Stamm AM, et al. Impact of extended-spectrum antibiotic prophylaxis on incidence of postcesarean surgical wound infection. *Am J Obstet Gynecol*. 2008;199(3):303.e1–303.e3.
9. Haas DM, Morgan S, Contreras K. Vaginal preparation with antiseptic solution before cesarean section for preventing postoperative infections. *Cochrane Database Syst Rev*. 2014;(12):CD007892.
10. Pevzner L, Swank M, Krepel C, et al. Effects of maternal obesity on tissue concentrations of prophylactic cefazolin during cesarean delivery. *Obstet Gynecol*. 2011;117(4):877–882.
11. French LM, Smaill FM. Antibiotic regimens for endometritis after delivery. *Cochrane Database Syst Rev*. 2015;(2):CD001067.

ADDITIONAL READING
- Baaqeel H, Baaqeel R. Timing of administration of prophylactic antibiotics for caesarean section: a systematic review and meta-analysis. *BJOG*. 2013;120(6):661–669.
- Bianco A, Roccia S, Nobile CG, et al. Postdischarge surveillance following delivery: the incidence of infections and associated factors. *Am J Infect Control*. 2013;41(6):549–553.
- Maharaj D. Puerperal pyrexia: a review. Part I. *Obstet Gynecol Surv*. 2007;62(6):393–399.
- Maharaj D. Puerperal pyrexia: a review. Part II. *Obstet Gynecol Surv*. 2007;62(6):400–406.
- Srinivas SK, Fager C, Lorch SA. Variations in postdelivery infection and thrombosis by hospital teaching status. *Am J Obstet Gynecol*. 2013;209(6):567.e1–567.e7.
- Sun J, Ding M, Liu J, et al. Prophylactic administration of cefazolin prior to skin incision versus antibiotics at cord clamping in preventing postcesarean infectious morbidity: a systematic review and meta-analysis of randomized controlled trials. *Gynecol Obstet Invest*. 2013;75(3):175–178.

 ## SEE ALSO

Algorithm: Pelvic Pain

 ## CODES

ICD10
- O86.12 Endometritis following delivery
- O86.4 Pyrexia of unknown origin following delivery
- O86.13 Vaginitis following delivery

CLINICAL PEARLS
- Postpartum endometritis follows 1–3% of all births.
- Infections are typically polymicrobial and involve organisms ascending from the lower genital tract.
- Evidence supports antibiotic prophylaxis prior to skin incision for all cesarean deliveries but not for operative vaginal deliveries.
- clindamycin 900 mg IV q8h and gentamicin 5 mg/kg q24h are recommended as first-line therapy for endometritis. Treat until the patient is afebrile for 24 to 48 hours, at which point antibiotics can be stopped completely (except in cases of documented bacteremia, which require a 7-day course of therapy).
- If no improvement occurs on antibiotics, consider retained placental products, abscess, wound infection, hematoma, cellulitis, phlegmon, or septic pelvic vein thrombosis.

ENURESIS

Cody B. Godfrey, DO • Swati Avashia, MD, FAAP

BASICS

DESCRIPTION
- Classification
  - Primary nocturnal enuresis (NE): 80% of all cases; child/adult who has never established urinary continence on consecutive nights for a period of ≥6 months
  - Secondary NE: 20% of cases; resumption of enuresis after at least 6 months of urinary continence
- NE: intermittent nocturnal incontinence after the anticipated age of bladder control (age 5 years)
  - Primary monosymptomatic NE (PMNE): bed wetting with no history of bladder dysfunction or other lower urinary tract (LUT) symptoms
  - Nonmonosymptomatic NE (NMNE): bed wetting with LUT symptoms such as frequency, urgency, daytime wetting, hesitancy, straining, weak or intermittent stream, posturination dribbling, lower abdominal or genital discomfort, or sensation of incomplete emptying

ALERT
Adult-onset NE with absent daytime incontinence is a serious symptom; complete urologic evaluation and therapy are warranted.

- System(s) affected: nervous, renal/urologic
- Synonym(s): bed wetting; sleep enuresis; nocturnal incontinence; primary NE

EPIDEMIOLOGY
Incidence
- Depends on family history
- Spontaneous resolution: 15% per year, 99% of children are dry by age 15 years.

Prevalence
- Very common. 5 to 7 million children in the U.S.
- 40% of 3-year-olds; 10% of 6-year-olds; 3% of 12-year-olds; 1% of adults
- Male > female (3:1)
- Nocturnal > day (3:1)

Geriatric Considerations
Infrequent; often associated with daytime incontinence (formerly referred to as diurnal enuresis)

ETIOLOGY AND PATHOPHYSIOLOGY
- A disorder of sleep arousal, a low nocturnal bladder capacity, and nocturnal polyuria are the three factors that interrelate to cause NE.
- Both functional and organic causes (below); many theories, none absolutely confirmed
- Detrusor instability
- Deficiency of arginine vasopressin (AVP); decreased nocturnal AVP or decreased AVP stimulation secondary to an empty bladder (bladder distension stimulates AVP)
- Maturational delay of CNS
- Severe NE with some evidence of interaction between bladder overactivity and brain arousability: association with children with severe NE and frequent cortical arousals in sleep
- Organic urologic causes in 1–4% of enuresis in children: UTI, occult spina bifida, ectopic ureter, lazy bladder syndrome, irritable bladder with wide bladder neck, posterior urethral valves, neurologic bladder dysfunction
- Organic nonurologic causes: epilepsy, diabetes mellitus, food allergies, obstructive sleep apnea, chronic renal failure, hyperthyroidism, pinworm infection, sickle cell disease
- NE occurs in all stages of sleep.

Genetics
Most commonly, NE is an autosomal-dominant inheritance pattern with high penetrance (90%).
- 1/3 of all cases are sporadic.
- 75% of children with enuresis have a first-degree relative with the condition.
- Higher rates in monozygotic versus dizygotic twins (68% vs. 36%)
- If both parents had NE, risk in child is 77%; 44% if one parent is affected. Parental age of resolution often predicts when child's enuresis should resolve.

RISK FACTORS
- Family history
- Stressors (emotional, environmental) common in secondary enuresis (e.g., divorce, death)
- Constipation
- Encopresis
- Organic disease: 1% of monosymptomatic NE (e.g., urologic and nonurologic causes)
- Psychological disorders
  - Comorbid disorders are highest with secondary NE: depression, anxiety, social phobias, conduct disorder, hyperkinetic syndrome, internalizing disorders
  - Association with ADHD; more pronounced in ages 9 to 12 years
- Altered mental status or impaired mobility

GENERAL PREVENTION
No known measures

COMMONLY ASSOCIATED CONDITIONS
- Obstructive sleep apnea syndrome: atrial natriuretic factor inhibits renin-angiotensin-aldosterone pathway leading to diuresis
- Constipation (1/3 of patients with NE)
- Behavioral problems (specifically ADHD)

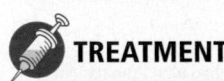

DIAGNOSIS

HISTORY
- Age of onset, duration, severity
- LUT tract symptoms
- Constipation and encopresis (15% with comorbid encopresis)
- Daily intake patterns
- Voiding and elimination patterns (voiding diary)
- Psychosocial history
- Family history of enuresis
- Investigation and previous treatment history

PHYSICAL EXAM
- ENT: evaluation for adenotonsillar hypertrophy
- Abdomen: enlarged bladder, kidneys, fecal masses, or impaction
- Back: Look for dimpling or tufts of hair on sacrum.
- Genital urinary exam
  - Males: meatal stenosis, hypospadias, epispadias, phimosis
  - Females: vulvitis, vaginitis, labial adhesions, ureterocele at introitus; evidence of abuse
- Rectal exam: tone and constipation
- Neurologic exam, especially lower extremities

DIFFERENTIAL DIAGNOSIS
- Primary NE
  - Delayed physiologic urinary control
  - UTI (both)
  - Spina bifida occulta

- Obstructive sleep apnea (both)
- Idiopathic detrusor instability
- Previously unrecognized myelopathy or neuropathy (e.g., multiple sclerosis, tethered cord, epilepsy)
- Anatomic urinary tract abnormality (e.g., ectopic ureter)
- Secondary NE
  - Bladder outlet obstruction
  - Neurologic disease, neurogenic bladder (e.g., spinal cord injury)

DIAGNOSTIC TESTS & INTERPRETATION
Initial Tests (lab, imaging)
- Only obligatory test in children is urinalysis.
- Urinalysis and urine culture: UTI, pyuria, hematuria, proteinuria, glycosuria, and poor concentrating ability (low specific gravity) may suggest organic etiology, especially in adults.
- Urinary tract imaging is usually not necessary.
- If abnormal clinical findings or adult onset: renal and bladder US
- IV pyelogram, voiding cystourethrogram (VCUG), or retrograde pyelogram as indicated
- Spine radiographs for spina bifida occulta

Follow-Up Tests & Special Considerations
- Secondary enuresis: serum glucose, BUN, creatinine, thyroid-stimulating hormone (TSH), urine culture
- In children, imaging and urodynamic studies are helpful for significant daytime symptoms, history of UTIs, suspected structural abnormalities, and in refractory cases.

Diagnostic Procedures/Other
Urodynamic studies may be beneficial in adults and nonmonosymptomatic NE.

Test Interpretation
- Dysfunctional voiding
- Detrusor instability and/or reduced bladder capacity most common findings

TREATMENT

GENERAL MEASURES
- Use nonpharmacologic approaches as first line before prescribing medications (1)[A].
- Simple behavioral interventions (e.g., scheduled wakening, positive reinforcement, bladder training, diet changes) are effective though less so than alarms or medications (2)[B].

  - Explain the three pathophysiologic factors.
  - Encourage normal drinking patterns during daytime hours and reduction of intake in the hours prior to sleep.
  - Emphasize regular bedtime with full night's sleep.
  - Scheduled voiding before bed
  - Nightlights to light the way to the bathroom
  - Reward system for dry nights
  - Use pull up over regular underwear or cloth underwear with built in waterproof barrier.
- Do not shame or punish bedwetting but have the child participate in removing and laundering soiled bedding and garments.

- If behavioral interventions alone have no success, combined therapy (e.g., enuresis alarm, bladder training, motivational therapy, and pelvic floor muscle training) is more effective than each component alone or than pharmacotherapy (1)[A].

- Enuresis alarms (bells or buzzers)
  - 66–70% success rate; must be used nightly for 3 to 4 months; offers cure; significant parental involvement; disruption of sleep for entire family
  - In children, number needed to treat (NNT) = 2 (3)[A].
  - If successful, it should be used until 14 consecutive dry nights achieved (4)[B].
- See "Patient Education" for options.

MEDICATION
First Line
- Desmopressin (DDAVP): synthetic analogue of vasopressin that decreases nocturnal urine output (5)[A]
  - Adults only: 20 mg (2 sprays) intranasally at bedtime
  - FDA recommends against use in children due to reports of severe hyponatremia resulting in seizures and deaths in children using intranasal formulations of desmopressin.
  - Oral DDAVP: dose-dependent: begin at 0.2 mg tablet taken at bedtime on empty stomach; may titrate to 0.6 mg
    - Maximally effective in 1 hour; cleared within 9 hours
    - Trial nightly for 6 months, then stop for 2 weeks for test of dryness
    - Suspend dose in children who experience acute condition affecting fluid/electrolyte balances (fever, vomiting, diarrhea, vigorous exercise).
  - 10–70% success; safe even when used for >12 months; high relapse rate after discontinuation without a structured withdrawal program
  - In children, NNT = 6 (6)[A].
- Anticholinergics
  - Oxybutynin (Ditropan, Ditropan XL, Oxytrol patch): anticholinergic; smooth muscle relaxant, antispasmodic; may increase functional bladder capacity and aids in timed voiding (6)[B]
    - Ditropan: adults and children >5 years of age: 5 mg PO TID to QID; children 1 to 5 years of age: 0.02 mg/kg/dose BID to QID (syrup 5 mg/5 mL)
    - Ditropan XL: adults: 5 mg/day PO; increase to 30 mg/day PO (5-, 10-mg tabs)
    - Oxytrol patch: 1 patch every 3 to 4 days (3.9 mg/patch) (periodic trials off the medication, that is, weekends or weeks at a time, will help determine efficacy and resolution of primary disturbance)
    - Ditropan: 5 to 10 mg at night; 30–50% success; 50% relapse after stopped
  - Tolterodine (Detrol, Detrol LA): anticholinergic; fewer side effects than Ditropan (7)[B]
    - Detrol: 1 to 2 mg PO BID
    - Detrol LA: 2 to 4 mg/day

Pediatric Considerations
FDA recommends against using intranasal formulations of desmopressin in children due to reports of severe hyponatremia resulting in seizures and deaths (8)[A].

Second Line
- Imipramine (Tofranil): tricyclic antidepressant, anticholinergic effects; increases bladder capacity, antispasmodic properties
  - Primarily in adults; use in children is reserved for resistant cases.
  - Dose: adults, 25 to 75 mg and children >6 years, 10 to 25 mg PO at bedtime; increase by 10 to 25 mg at 1- to 2-week intervals; treat for 2 to 3 months; then taper

- 25–30% success when used <3 months.
- Pretreatment ECG recommended identifying underlying rhythm disorders.
- Precautions
  - Oxybutynin: glaucoma, myasthenia gravis, GI or genitourinary obstruction, ulcerative colitis, megacolon; use a decreased dose in the elderly.
  - Tolterodine: urinary retention, gastric retention, or uncontrolled narrow-angle glaucoma; significant drug interactions with CYP2D6, CYP3A3/4 substrates
  - DDAVP: Avoid in patients at risk for electrolyte changes or fluid retention (congestive heart failure [CHF], renal insufficiency). Stop during gastroenteritis or other acute illness with risk of dehydration.
  - Imipramine: Do not use with monoamine oxidase inhibitors (MAOIs), hypotension, and arrhythmias; low-toxic therapeutic ratio
- Combination therapy with DDAVP and oxybutynin has better results than individual use (7)[B].
- Prostaglandin inhibitors (e.g., indomethacin) have been studied; may increase bladder capacity, not as effective as DDAVP, and increase adverse effects (7)[B]

ALERT
Imipramine: cardiotoxicity and death with overdose

ISSUES FOR REFERRAL
- Primary NE: persistent enuresis despite nonpharmacologic and pharmacologic therapies
- Diurnal incontinence or nonmonosymptomatic enuresis with voiding dysfunction or underlying medical condition

ADDITIONAL THERAPIES
Individual and family psychotherapy, crisis intervention

SURGERY/OTHER PROCEDURES
Only for surgically correctable causes (e.g., tethered cord, ectopic ureter, benign prostatic hypertrophy, obstructive sleep apnea)

COMPLEMENTARY & ALTERNATIVE MEDICINE
Acupuncture and hypnosis are other treatments offered; small amounts of supportive data (9,10)[B]

 ONGOING CARE

FOLLOW-UP RECOMMENDATIONS
Patient Monitoring
DIET
- Limit fluid and caffeine intake 2 hours before sleep.
- Limit dairy products 4 hours before sleep (decrease osmotic diuresis).

PATIENT EDUCATION
Web resources for hypnosis scripts, alarms, and supplies
- http://www.hypnoticworld.com/hypnosis-scripts/habits-disorders/enuresis
- www.bedwettingstore.com/index.htm; www.drisleeper.com; www.enurad.com; www.nitetrain-r.com; www.sleepydryalarm.com; www.wetstop.com; www.pottypager.com/

PROGNOSIS
In children, NE is usually self-limiting; 1% will persist as adult; evaluate for organic causes.

COMPLICATIONS
UTI, perineal excoriation, psychological disturbance (especially in children)

REFERENCES
1. Robson WL. Clinical practice. Evaluation and management of enuresis. *N Engl J Med.* 2009;360(14):1429–1436.
2. Caldwell PH, Nankivell G, Sureshkumar P. Simple behavioural interventions for nocturnal enuresis in children. *Cochrane Database Syst Rev.* 2013;(7):CD003637.
3. Glazener CM, Evans JH, Peto RE. Alarm interventions for nocturnal enuresis in children. *Cochrane Database Syst Rev.* 2005;(2):CD002911.
4. Bayne AP, Skoog SJ. Nocturnal enuresis: an approach to assessment and treatment. *Pediatr Rev.* 2014;35(8):327–335.
5. Vande Walle J, Stockner M, Raes A, et al. Desmopressin 30 years in clinical use: a safety review. *Curr Drug Saf.* 2007;2(3):232–238.
6. Glazener CM, Evans JH. Desmopressin for nocturnal enuresis in children. *Cochrane Database Syst Rev.* 2002;(3):CD002112.
7. Deshpande AV, Caldwell PH, Sureshkumar P. Drugs for nocturnal enuresis in children (other than desmopressin and tricyclics). *Cochrane Database Syst Rev.* 2012;(12):CD002238.
8. Graham KM, Levy JB. Enuresis. *Pediatr Rev.* 2009;30(5):165–172.
9. Neveus T, Eggert P, Evans J, et al. Evaluation and treatment for monosymptomatic enuresis: a standardization document from the International Children's Continence Society. *J Urol.* 2010;183(2):441–447.
10. Bower WF, Diao M. Acupuncture as a treatment for nocturnal enuresis. *Auton Neurosci.* 2010;157(1–2):63–67.

ADDITIONAL READING
Vande Walle J, Rittig S, Bauer S, et al. Practical consensus guidelines for the management of enuresis. *Eur J Pediatr.* 2012;171(6):971–983.

 SEE ALSO
- Incontinence, Urinary Adult Female; Incontinence, Urinary Adult Male
- Algorithm: Enuresis

CODES
ICD10
- N39.44 Nocturnal enuresis
- R32 Unspecified urinary incontinence
- F98.0 Enuresis not due to a substance or known physiol condition

CLINICAL PEARLS
- Initial evaluation is history, exam, and urinalysis.
- For PMNE in children, if the condition is not distressing to child and caretakers, treatment is unnecessary.
- Behavioral and lifestyle interventions are the first-line treatment for PMNE, alarms and desmopressin are the most effective treatments.
- Dryness is possible for most children.

EOSINOPHILIC ESOPHAGITIS

Peter I. Chung, MD • Benjamin Hyatt, MD

 BASICS

Eosinophilic esophagitis (EoE) is a chronic, immune-mediated, inflammatory esophageal disease characterized clinically in adults by dysphagia, food impaction, and heartburn and in children with non-specific abdominal complaints, abdominal pain, and failure to thrive. Histologically, EoE is characterized by eosinophilic predominate inflammation (1)[A].

EPIDEMIOLOGY
All ages, most common in 20s to 30s; male > female, 3:1

Incidence
Incidence in general population is approximately 1 case in 10,000 persons per year (2)[A].

Prevalence
Gradually increasing, perhaps due to better case finding, understanding of EoE in multiple clinical guises; 45 to 55/100,000

- Increased prevalence in those with celiac disease.

ETIOLOGY AND PATHOPHYSIOLOGY
- Believed to be an atopic inflammatory disease, whose pathogenesis is an aberrant immune response to antigenic stimulation
- Like eczema and asthma, T-helper 2 (T_H2) lymphocytes play a role, as do mixed IgE and non–IgE-mediated allergic responses to food and environmental allergens.
- Although not well-understood, the pathophysiology of EoE is postulated to be due to increased recruitment and activation of eosinophils in the esophagus. Eosinophil chemoattractants include eotaxin-3, IL-5, and IL-13.

Genetics
- EoE susceptibility may be caused by polymorphisms in thymic stromal lymphopoietin protein (TSLP) (3)[A].
- Potential new subphenotype of EoE (may also overlap with GERD): proton pump inhibitor (PPI)–responsive esophageal eosinophilia, where PPIs may act to decrease the inflammatory response in EoE (3)[A]

RISK FACTORS
- EoE is commonly associated with atopy/allergic disorders, such as asthma, hay fever, or eczema (1,4)[A].
- High rate of associated food antigen allergies/anaphylaxis

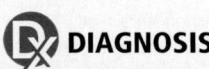 **DIAGNOSIS**

There are no pathognomonic findings for EoE. A definitive diagnosis is made by esophageal endoscopy and biopsy.

HISTORY
- Solid food dysphagia and food impaction are the most common symptoms and are usually present for 3 to 4 years prior to the diagnosis.
- Patients may also have reflux symptoms. Often, the diagnosis is entertained after patients fail a trial of antireflux medications. Other common complaints include nausea or vomiting, regurgitation, chest pain, upper abdominal pain, or decreased appetite.
- Patients may also have a history of food or environmental allergies, as well as asthma or atopic conditions (e.g., dermatitis).

PHYSICAL EXAM
No specific physical exam findings are associated with the diagnosis. However, signs and symptoms of allergies or asthma with symptoms of ongoing dysphagia or GERD-like symptoms should raise suspicion; some patients will have signs indicating weight loss or malnutrition.

DIFFERENTIAL DIAGNOSIS
- GERD
  - Associated with EoE; diseases may coexist in individual patients.
- PPI-responsive esophageal eosinophilia (PPI-REE)
  - Characteristics of PPI-REE
    - Shows classic EoE symptoms
    - Diagnosis of GERD has been excluded.
    - Responds to PPIs clinically and histologically
- Secondary causes of esophageal eosinophilia including celiac disease, Crohn esophagitis, infection, vasculitis, PPIs, achalasia, connective tissue disease, eosinophilic gastrointestinal diseases
- Functional dyspepsia
- Congenital rings
- Esophageal carcinoma
- Esophageal motility disorders

DIAGNOSTIC TESTS & INTERPRETATION
- To exclude PPI-REE, patients with suspected EoE should be given a 2-month course of PPI followed by endoscopy with biopsies.
- Solid food dysphagia is an indication for esophago-gastroduodenoscopy (EGD), as are other concerning or "red-flag" symptoms, many of which occur in patients with EoE; they include the following:
  - Odynophagia
  - Weight loss
  - Early satiety or vomiting
  - Aspiration/wheezing or cough
  - GI bleeding
  - Unexplained iron deficiency anemia
  - Male >45 years with long-standing symptoms
- GERD patients who show no symptomatic improvement after 8 to 12 weeks of a PPI should also be considered for EGD and biopsy.
- Serum IgE levels are elevated in 70% of patients.
- Peripheral eosinophilia occurs in 10–50% of patients.

Follow-Up Tests & Special Considerations
Testing for asthma and IgE-mediated food/inhalant allergies, if clinically relevant, can help manage coexisting atopic conditions:

- Serum IgE, skin prick test, or atopy patch test

Diagnostic Procedures/Other
EGD: 17% of biopsy-proven cases of EoE had an endoscopically normal exam (5)[A].

- Endoscopic findings: esophageal rings (trachealization), strictures, white plaques or exudates, linear furrows, narrow-caliber esophagus, and pallor or decreased vasculature
  - Esophageal biopsies are required for diagnosis; two to four biopsies from both proximal and distal esophagus. At initial diagnosis, biopsies should be obtained from antrum and/or duodenum to rule out other causes of esophageal eosinophilia in all children and adults with gastric or small intestinal symptoms or endoscopic abnormalities (1)[A].
    - Biopsy specimen: Pathologic findings may include surface layering of eosinophils, eosinophilic microabscesses, subepithelial lamina propria fibrosis, or basal cell hyperplasia.
- Barium contrast radiography
  - Can help to identify anatomic abnormalities in EoE but has a low sensitivity for diagnosis
  - May be an alternative to repeated endoscopies in previously treated patients who have changing symptoms
- pH monitoring: may be helpful in differentiating EoE from GERD
- Consensus American Gastroenterological Association guidelines for diagnosis of EoE (1)[A]
  - Clinical symptoms of esophageal dysfunction
  - ≥15 eosinophils in one high-power field on biopsy
  - Mucosal eosinophilia is isolated to esophagus and persists after PPI use.
  - Secondary causes of esophageal eosinophilia are excluded.

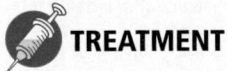 **TREATMENT**

End points of therapy of EoE include improvements in clinical symptoms and reducing esophageal eosinophilic inflammation. Defining evidence-based end points in EoE is still an area of active research (1)[A].

MEDICATION
First Line
- Corticosteroids
  - Topical steroids (swallowed, not inhaled) are the first-line pharmacologic treatment.
    - Initial dosing for treatment of EoE: Swallowed fluticasone dose in adults is 880 to 1,760 μg/day in a divided dose and in children is determined based on age or weight.

Swallowed budesonide dose in adults is 2 mg/day, typically in divided doses; in children determined based on age or weight. Initial duration of treatment is 8 weeks. Medication should be discontinued if patient develops side effects or other intolerances. Patients have relapsed after withdrawal of the medication. Inhaled topical steroid trials are ongoing.

- Systemic steroids: Prednisone can be helpful if topical steroids are not effective or for patients who require a more rapid improvement to symptoms, such as those with refractory dysphagia and in patients who are hospitalized. Long-term toxicity limits use (1)[A].

- Diet
  - Dietary elimination is considered initial therapy in both children and adults.
  - Three dietary regimens have been shown to be effective in treatment of EoE: (i) elemental amino acid–based diet; (ii) elimination diet based on various food allergy tests; and (iii) six-food elimination diet of the most common food groups known to trigger EoE: wheat, soy, cow's milk, eggs, nuts, and seafood. All three methods have been shown to be effective in children for both clinical and histologic improvement, with the elemental diet being most effective:

    ○ In children, success rates of 77–98% have been reported for clinical and histologic remission using an elemental amino acid formula. A retrospective chart review comparing the three diets showed that the elemental diet was superior, with 96% remission (6)[B]. Yet, this treatment has not gained popularity because of its high cost, impaired quality of life, and overall practicality.
  - In adults, food allergy plays an important role in EoE, and six-food elimination diet (SFED) is an effective therapy (7)[B]:

    ○ Gonsalves et al. evaluated SFED in adult patients with EoE and demonstrated clinical, endoscopic, and histologic improvement. Symptoms improved in 94% of patients. Reintroduction of eliminated food caused reactivation of EoE with wheat (60%) and cow's milk (50%) as the leading causative agents. Skin-prick allergy testing was only 13% predictive in identifying food triggers.

Second Line
- Endoscopic esophageal dilation

  - May be used effectively in symptomatic patients with strictures that are resistant to medical or dietary treatments and initially in patients with severe and symptomatic esophageal stenosis (1)[A]
  - A systematic review showed that 92% of patients treated with dilation had improvement in dysphagia symptoms for up to 1 to 2 years.
  - Patients should be informed of the risks of esophageal dilation. The most common risk is postprocedure chest pain, which occurs in 75% of patients. The perforation rate for dilation is 0.3%, contrary to early reports which showed higher rates of perforation. Bleeding requiring endoscopic intervention or blood products is very rare, with only one occurrence reported to date (1,4)[A].

ISSUES FOR REFERRAL
Refer to an allergist and/or nutritionist to help identify/manage allergic disorders and diet regimens.

ADDITIONAL THERAPIES
Other pharmacologic therapies

- Montelukast, mepolizumab (IL-5 monoclonal antibody), acid suppression therapy, purine analogues, anti-TNF therapy. Biologic agents have been well-tolerated with low adverse effects (AEs); yet, no studies have shown prolonged symptomatic relief (1)[A].

- Antihistamines: Case studies showed no benefit.

ONGOING CARE

FOLLOW-UP RECOMMENDATIONS

- EoE is a chronic disease with symptom recurrence after discontinuing treatment the rule rather than the exception. Prevention of progression of esophageal dysfunction is primary. Maintenance therapy with swallowed topical corticosteroid therapy and/or dietary restriction should be considered in all patients after clinicopathologic remission indefinitely or PRN (1)[A]. This is not yet standardized; only one RCT maintenance study has been done using low-dose budesonide (0.25 mg BID) versus placebo after remission for 50 weeks. Those maintained on budesonide had modest reduction in eosinophilia and fewer symptom recurrences, but there was still significant recurrence (8)[A]. As such, ongoing therapy needs to be tailored to individual patient cases.

- Patient should be counseled on the high likelihood of symptom recurrence after discontinuing treatment.

Patient Monitoring
- No guidelines yet established. It is reasonable to order periodic endoscopy based on symptoms or after completing a recent therapeutic regimen.
- There is no evidence to date of esophageal malignancy or hypereosinophilic syndromes associated with EoE.
- Esophageal candidiasis is a common side effect of chronic corticosteroid therapy.

PROGNOSIS
EoE does not seem to affect life expectancy. Quality of life is affected to some extent due to the chronic nature of the disease, difficulty in adhering to a restrictive diet, and so forth. Nutritional status can be maintained with appropriate care and diligence.

COMPLICATIONS
- Food impaction
- Esophageal stricture/ring/narrowing
- Nutritional deficiencies
- Subglottic stenosis or laryngeal edema is very rare.

REFERENCES

1. Dellon ES, Gonsalves N, Hirano I, et al. ACG clinical guidelines: evidenced based approach to diagnosis and management of esophageal eosinophilia and eosinophilic esophagitis (EoE). *Am J Gastroenterol.* 2013;108(5):679–692.
2. Dellon ES. Epidemiology of eosinophilic esophagitis. *Gastroenterol Clin North Am.* 2014;43(2):201–218.
3. Liacouras CA, Furuta GT, Hirano I, et al. Eosinophilic esophagitis: updated consensus recommendations for children and adults. *J Allergy Clin Immunol.* 2011;128(1):3.e6–20.e6.
4. Bohm ME, Richter JE. Review article: oesophageal dilation in adults with eosinophilic oesophagitis. *Aliment Pharmacol Ther.* 2011;33(7):748–757.
5. Kim HP, Vance RB, Shaheen NJ, et al. The prevalence and diagnostic utility of endoscopic features of eosinophilic esophagitis: a meta-analysis. *Clin Gastroenterol Hepatol.* 2012;10(9):988.e5–996.e5.
6. Henderson CJ, Abonia JP, King EC, et al. Comparative dietary therapy effectiveness in remission of pediatric eosinophilic esophagitis. *J Allergy Clin Immunol.* 2012;129(6):1570–1578.
7. Gonsalves N, Yang GY, Doerfler B, et al. Elimination diet effectively treats eosinophilic esophagitis in adults; food reintroduction identifies causative factors. *Gastroenterology.* 2012;142(7):1451. e1–1459.e1.
8. Straumann A, Conus S, Degen L, et al. Long-term budesonide maintenance treatment is partially effective for patients with eosinophilic esophagitis. *Clin Gastroenterol Hepatol.* 2011;9(5):400. e1–409.e1.

ADDITIONAL READING

- Dellon ES, Jensen ET, Martin CF, et al. Prevalence of eosinophilic esophagitis in the United States. *Clin Gastroenterol Hepatol.* 2014;12(4):589.e1–596.e1.
- Stewart MJ, Shaffer E, Urbanski SJ, et al. The association between celiac disease and eosinophilic esophagitis in children and adults. *BMC Gastroenterol.* 2013;13:96.

CODES

ICD10
K20.0 Eosinophilic esophagitis

CLINICAL PEARLS

- Food impaction or recurrent solid food dysphagia in a young, adult male: Think EoE.
- EoE commonly mimics disorders like GERD and PPI-REE.
- A PPI trial is now required prior to the diagnosis of EoE.
- Remember "red flags" in patients with GERD: dysphagia, odynophagia, weight loss, early satiety or vomiting, aspiration/wheezing/cough, GI bleeding, unexplained iron deficiency anemia, age >50 years. Each "red flag" justifies EGD.

EPICONDYLITIS

Kevin Heaton, DO

 BASICS

DESCRIPTION
- Tendinopathy of the elbow characterized by pain and tenderness at the origins of the wrist flexors/extensors at the humeral epicondyles
- May be acute (traumatic) or chronic (overuse)
- Two types
  - Medial epicondylitis ("golfer's elbow")
    - Involves the wrist flexors and pronators, which originate at the medial epicondyle
  - Lateral epicondylitis ("tennis elbow")
    - Involves the wrist extensors and supinators, which originate at the lateral epicondyle
- May be caused by many different athletic or occupational activities
- Common in carpenters, plumbers, gardeners, and athletes
- Usually involves the dominant arm
- Lateral epicondylitis is more common.

EPIDEMIOLOGY
- Predominant age: >40 years
- Predominant sex: male = female

Incidence
- Common overuse injury
- Lateral > medial
- Estimated between 1% and 3%

Prevalence
- Lateral epicondylitis: 1.3%
- Medial epicondylitis: 0.4%

ETIOLOGY AND PATHOPHYSIOLOGY
- Acute (tendonitis)
  - Inflammatory response to injury
- Chronic (tendinosis)
  - Overuse injury
  - Tendon degeneration, fibroblast proliferation, microvascular proliferation, lack of inflammatory response
- Repetitive wrist flexion or extension places strain across enthesis of flexor/extensor group
- Tool/racquet gripping
- Shaking hands
- Sudden maximal muscle contraction
- Direct blow

RISK FACTORS
- Repetitive wrist motions
  - Flexion/pronation: medial
  - Extension/supination: lateral
- Smoking
- Obesity
- Upper extremity forceful activities

GENERAL PREVENTION
- Limit overuse of the wrist flexors, extensors, pronators, and supinators.
- Use proper techniques when working with hand tools or playing racquet sports.
- Use lighter tools and smaller grips.

 DIAGNOSIS

HISTORY
- Pain typically localized to lateral or medial elbow.
- Occupational activities
- Sports participation
- Direct trauma
- Duration and location of symptoms
- Prior treatments or medication use
- Pain with gripping
- Sensation of mild forearm weakness

PHYSICAL EXAM
- Localized pain just distal to the affected epicondyle
- Increased pain with wrist flexion/pronation (medial)
- Increased pain with wrist extension/supination (lateral)
- Medial epicondylitis
  - Tenderness at origin of wrist flexor tendons
  - Increased pain with resisted wrist flexion and pronation
  - Normal elbow range of motion
  - Increased pain with gripping
- Lateral epicondylitis
  - Tenderness at origin of wrist extensors
  - Increased pain with resisted wrist extension/supination
  - Normal elbow range of motion
  - Increased pain with gripping

DIFFERENTIAL DIAGNOSIS
- Elbow osteoarthritis
- Epicondylar fractures
- Posterior interosseous nerve entrapment (lateral)
- Ulnar neuropathy (medial)
- Synovitis
- Medial collateral ligament injury
- Referred pain from shoulder or neck

DIAGNOSTIC TESTS & INTERPRETATION
Initial Tests (lab, imaging)
No imaging is required for initial evaluation and treatment of a classic overuse injury.

Follow-Up Tests & Special Considerations
- Anterior-posterior/lateral radiographs if decreased range of motion, trauma, or no improvement with initial conservative therapy. Assess for fractures or signs of arthritis.
- For recalcitrant cases
  - Musculoskeletal ultrasound (US) reveals abnormal tendon appearance (e.g., tendon thickening, partial tear at tendon origin, calcifications). US can also guide injections of steroid and/or anesthetic.
  - MRI can show intermediate or high T2 signal intensity within the common flexor or extensor tendon or the presence of peritendinous soft tissue edema.

Diagnostic Procedures/Other
Infiltration of local anesthetic with subsequent resolution of symptoms supports the diagnosis if clinically in doubt.

TREATMENT

GENERAL MEASURES
Initial treatment consists of activity modification, counterforce bracing, oral or topical NSAIDs, ice, and physical therapy:
- Observation: If left untreated, symptoms typically last between 6 months and 2 years. For patients with good function and minimal pain, consider conservative management using a "wait and see" approach based on patient preference.
- Modify activity, encourage relative rest, and correct faulty biomechanics
- Counterforce bracing with a forearm strap is easy and inexpensive. Systematic reviews are inconclusive about overall efficacy, but initial bracing may improve the ability to perform daily activities in the first 6 weeks.
- Consider nighttime wrist splinting for repetitive daily activities if counterforce bracing fails.
- Ice frequently after activities
- Physical therapy
  - Begin once acute pain is resolved. Infiltration of local anesthetic can reduce pain and allow for physical therapy
  - Eccentric strength training and stretching program
  - US therapy
  - Corticosteroid iontophoresis
  - Dry needling

MEDICATION
First Line
- Topical NSAIDs: Low-quality evidence suggests topical NSAIDS are significantly more effective than placebo with respect to pain and number needed to treat to benefit (NNT = 7) in the short term (up to 4 weeks) with minimal adverse effects (1)[A].
- Oral NSAIDs: Unclear efficacy with respect to pain and function, but may offer short-term pain relief. Associated with adverse GI effects (1)[A].

Second Line
Corticosteroid injections: Short-term (≤8 weeks) reduction in pain. No benefits found for intermediate or long-term outcomes (2)[A].

ISSUES FOR REFERRAL
Failure of conservative therapy

ADDITIONAL THERAPIES

- Platelet-rich plasma (PRP) injections
  - Injection of concentrated autologous PRP leads to a local inflammatory response. Platelets degranulate, release growth factors, and stimulate the physiologic healing cascade
  - PRP treatment of chronic lateral epicondylitis significantly reduces pain and increases function. The benefit exceeds that of corticosteroid injection even after a follow-up of 2 years (3)[B].
- Autologous blood injections
  - Stimulates the inflammatory cascade within the degenerated tendon by providing cellular and humoral mediators for regeneration.
  - More effective at 3 months then corticosteroid injection for improving pain, function and grip strength (4)[B]
- US-guided percutaneous needle tenotomy
  - Injection of a local anesthetic followed by US-guided tendon fenestration, aspiration, and abrasion of the underlying bone. Thought to break apart scar tissue and stimulate inflammation and healing.
- Prolotherapy
  - Injection of a dextrose solution into and around the tendon attachment stimulates a localized inflammatory response, leading to increased blood flow to stimulate healing.
- Glyceryl trinitrate (GTN) transdermal patch
  - Nitric oxide (NO) is a small free radical generated by nitric oxide synthases. NO is expressed by fibroblasts and is postulated to aid in collagen synthesis. Topical application of GTN theoretically improves healing by this mechanism. 1/4 of a 5-mg/24-hour GTN transdermal patch is applied once daily for up to 24 weeks.
  - Significant decrease in pain are seen at 3 weeks and 6 months compared to placebo patch (5)[B].
- Botulinum toxin A for chronic lateral epicondylitis
  - Injections into the forearm extensor muscles (60 units) can be performed in the outpatient setting.

SURGERY/OTHER PROCEDURES

- Elbow surgery may be indicated in refractory cases:
  - Fair evidence for treatment (6)[B]
  - Involves débridement and tendon release
  - Can be performed open or arthroscopically

- Denervation of the lateral humeral epicondyle
  - Transection of the posterior cutaneous nerve of the forearm with implantation into the triceps may help with chronic symptoms and pain.

COMPLEMENTARY & ALTERNATIVE MEDICINE

Acupuncture: effective for short-term pain relief for lateral epicondyle pain

 ONGOING CARE

PROGNOSIS

Good: Majority resolve with conservative care.

REFERENCES

1. Pattanittum P, Turner T, Green S, et al. Non-steroidal anti-inflammatory drugs (NSAIDs) for treating lateral elbow pain in adults. *Cochrane Database Syst Rev.* 2013;(5):CD003686.
2. Krogh TP, Bartels EM, Ellingsen T, et al. Comparative effectiveness of injection therapies in lateral epicondylitis: a systematic review and network meta-analysis of randomized controlled trials. *Am J Sports Med.* 2013;41(6):1435–1446.
3. Gosens T, Peerbooms JC, van Laar W, et al. Ongoing positive effect of platelet-rich plasma versus corticosteroid injection in lateral epicondylitis: a double-blind randomized controlled trial with 2-year follow-up. *Am J Sports Med.* 2011;39(6):1200–1208.
4. Arik HO, Kose O, Guler F, et al. Injection of autologous blood versus corticosteroid for lateral epicondylitis: a randomised controlled study. *J Orthop Surg (Hong Kong).* 2014;22(3):333–337.
5. Ozden R, Uruç V, Doğramaci Y, et al. Management of tennis elbow with topical glyceryl trinitrate. *Acta Orthop Traumatol Turc.* 2014;48(2):175–180.
6. Yeoh KM, King GJ, Faber KJ, et al. Evidence-based indications for elbow arthroscopy. *Arthroscopy.* 2012;28(2):272–282.

ADDITIONAL READING

- Cullinane FL, Boocock MG, Trevelyan FC. Is eccentric exercise an effective treatment for lateral epicondylitis? A systematic review. *Clin Rehabil.* 2014;28(1):3–19.

- Dingemanse R, Randsdorp M, Koes BW, et al. Evidence for the effectiveness of electrophysical modalities for treatment of medial and lateral epicondylitis: a systematic review. *Br J Sports Med.* 2014;48(12):957–965.
- Green S, Buchbinder R, Barnsley L, et al. Acupuncture for lateral elbow pain. *Cochrane Database Syst Rev.* 2002;(1):CD003527.
- Kalichman L, Bannuru RR, Severin M, et al. Injection of botulinum toxin for treatment of chronic lateral epicondylitis: systematic review and meta-analysis. *Semin Arthritis Rheum.* 2011;40(6):532–538.
- McShane JM, Shah VN, Nazarian LN. Sonographically guided percutaneous needle tenotomy for treatment of common extensor tendinosis in the elbow: is a corticosteroid necessary? *J Ultrasound Med.* 2008;27(8):1137–1144.
- Rose NE, Forman SK, Dellon AL. Denervation of the lateral humeral epicondyle for treatment of chronic lateral epicondylitis. *J Hand Surg Am.* 2013;38(2):344–349.

 SEE ALSO

Algorithm: Pain in Upper Extremity

CODES

ICD10

- M77.00 Medial epicondylitis, unspecified elbow
- M77.10 Lateral epicondylitis, unspecified elbow
- M77.01 Medial epicondylitis, right elbow

CLINICAL PEARLS

- Medial epicondylitis (golfer's elbow) is characterized by pain and tenderness at the tendinous origins of the wrist flexors at the medial epicondyle.
- Lateral epicondylitis (tennis elbow) is characterized by pain and tenderness at the tendinous origins of the wrist extensors at the lateral epicondyle.
- Left untreated, symptoms typically last between 6 months and 2 years.
- Most patients improve using conservative treatment with bracing, activity modification, and physical therapy.

E

EPIDIDYMITIS

Thomas M. Savage, MD • Holly L. Baab, MD

BASICS

- Acute epididymitis: pain for <6 weeks
- Chronic epididymitis: pain for ≥3 months

DESCRIPTION

- Inflammation (infectious or noninfectious) of epididymis resulting in scrotal pain and swelling, induration of the posterior epididymis, and eventual scrotal wall edema, involvement of the adjacent testicle, and hydrocele formation.
- Epididymitis with involvement of testis is named epididymo-orchitis
- Classification: infectious (bacterial, viral, fungal, parasitic) versus sterile (chemical, traumatic, autoimmune, idiopathic, industrial, noninfectious, vasoepididymal reflux syndrome, vasal reflux syndrome); chronic versus acute
- System(s) affected: reproductive

EPIDEMIOLOGY

- Predominant age: usually younger, sexually active men or older men with UTIs; in older men, usually secondary to bladder outlet obstruction
- Predominant sex: male only

Pediatric Considerations

In prepubertal boys: Epididymitis is found to be the most common cause of acute scrotum—more common than testicular torsion.

Incidence

- Common (600,000 cases annually in the United States) (1)
- 1 in 1,000 males per year

Prevalence

Common

ETIOLOGY AND PATHOPHYSIOLOGY

- Infectious epididymitis
  - Retrograde passage of urine or urinary bacteria from the prostate or urethra to the epididymis via the ejaculatory ducts and the vas deferens; rarely, hematogenous spread
  - Causative organism is identified in 80% of patients and varies according to patient age.
- Sterile epididymitis
  - Chemical epididymitis occurs when sterile urine flows backward from the urethra to the epididymis
  - Can develop as a sequelae of strenuous exercise with a full bladder when urine is pushed through internal urethral sphincter (located at proximal end of prostatic urethra)
  - Reflux of urine through orifice of ejaculatory ducts at verumontanum may occur with history of urethritis/prostatitis, as inflammation may produce rigidity in musculature surrounding orifice to ejaculatory ducts, holding them open.
  - Exposure of epididymis to foreign fluid may produce inflammatory reaction within 24 hours.
- <35 years and sexually active
  - Usually *Chlamydia trachomatis* or *Neisseria gonorrhoeae*
  - Look for serous urethral discharge (chlamydia) or purulent discharge (gonorrhea)
  - With anal intercourse, likely *Escherichia coli* or *Haemophilus influenzae*
- >35 years
  - Coliform bacteria usually, but sometimes *Staphylococcus aureus* or *Staphylococcus epidermidis*
  - In elderly men, often with distal urinary tract obstruction, benign prostatic hyperplasia (BPH), UTI, or catheterization

- Tuberculosis (TB), if sterile pyuria, nodularity of vas deferens (hematogenous spread), and recent infection. TB is the most common granulomatous disease affecting the epididymitis (2).
  - Sterile urine reflux after transurethral prostatectomy
  - Granulomatous reaction following BCG intravesical therapy for bladder cancer
- Prepubertal boys
  - Usually coliform bacteria
  - Evaluate for underlying congenital abnormalities, such as vesicoureteral reflux, ectopic ureter, or anorectal malformation (rectourethral fistula).
- Amiodarone may cause noninfectious epididymitis; resolves with decreasing drug dosage.
- Syphilis, blastomycosis, coccidioidomycosis, and cryptococcosis are rare causes, but brucellosis can be a common cause in endemic areas.

RISK FACTORS

- UTI
- Prostatitis
- Indwelling urethral catheter
- Urethral instrumentation or transurethral surgery
- Urethral or meatal stricture
- Transrectal prostate biopsy
- Prostate brachytherapy (seeds) for prostate cancer
- Anal intercourse
- High-risk sexual activity
- Strenuous physical activity
- Prolonged sedentary periods
- Bladder obstruction (benign prostatic hyperplasia, prostate cancer)
- HIV-immunosuppressed patient
- Severe Behçet disease
- Presence of foreskin
- Constipation
- Sterile epididymitis
  - Increased intra-abdominal pressure (due to frequent physical strain)
    ○ Military recruits, especially who begin physically unprepared.
    ○ Laborers; restaurant kitchen workers
    ○ Full bladder during intense physical exertion

GENERAL PREVENTION

- Vasectomy or vasoligation during transurethral surgery
- Safer sexual practices
- Mumps vaccination
- Antibiotic prophylaxis for urethral manipulation
- Early treatment of prostatitis/BPH
- Avoid vigorous rectal exam with acute prostatitis.
- Emptying the bladder prior to physical exertion
- Physically conditioning the body prior to engaging in regular intense physical exertion
- Treat constipation.

COMMONLY ASSOCIATED CONDITIONS

- Prostatitis/urethritis/orchitis
- Hemospermia
- Constipation
- UTI

DIAGNOSIS

- Scrotal pain, sometimes radiating to the groin region, may begin acutely over several hours.
- Urethral discharge or symptoms of UTI, such as frequency of urination, dysuria, cloudy urine, or hematuria

- Initially, only the posterior-lying epididymis, usually the lowermost tail section, is very tender and indurated; will eventually progress to involvement of body and head of epididymis
- Elevation of the testes/epididymis reduces the discomfort (Prehn sign).
- Entire hemiscrotum becomes swollen and red; the testis becomes indistinguishable from the epididymis; the scrotal wall becomes thick and indurated; and reactive hydrocele may occur.
- Sterile epididymitis
  - Unilateral scrotal pain and swelling preceded by several hours of intense physical exertion. Patient may recall full bladder prior to exertion.
  - No symptoms of infection

Pediatric Considerations

- In prepubertal patients, may be postinfectious inflammatory condition; treat with anti-inflammatories, analgesics.
- Antibiotic therapy can be reserved for young infants and those with pyuria or positive urine cultures (3).
- Bacteremia from *H. influenzae* infection may produce acute epididymitis.
- In adolescent males, particularly age >13 years, must rule out testicular torsion.
- History not helpful in distinguishing epididymitis from testicular torsion

Geriatric Considerations

Diabetics with sensory neuropathy may have no pain despite severe infection/abscess.

PHYSICAL EXAM

- The tail of the epididymis is larger in comparison with the contralateral side.
- Epididymis is markedly tender to palpation.
- Absence of a cremasteric reflex should raise suspicion for testicular torsion.

DIFFERENTIAL DIAGNOSIS

- Epididymal congestion following vasectomy
- Testicular torsion
- Torsion of testicular appendages
- Orchitis
- Testicular malignancy
- Testicular trauma
- Epididymal cyst
- Inguinal hernia
- Urethritis
- Spermatocele
- Hydrocele
- Hematocele
- Varicocele
- Epididymal adenomatoid tumor
- Epididymal rhabdomyosarcoma
- Vasculitis (Henoch-Schönlein purpura)

DIAGNOSTIC TESTS & INTERPRETATION

Initial Tests (lab, imaging)

- All suspected cases should be evaluated for objective evidence of inflammation by one of the following:
  - Urinalysis preferably on first-void urine to evaluate for positive leukocyte esterase
  - Gram stain urethral discharge. ≥2 WBC per oil immersion field. Also for evaluation of presence or absence of gonococcal infection
  - Microscopic examination of sediment from a spun first-void urine with ≥10 WBC per high power field.

- Urine culture, preferably first-void
- Urine GC/chlamydia testing by NAAT for all suspected cases (2)[A].
- CRP >24 mg/L suggestive of epididymitis (4)[C]
- Urinalysis clear and culture-negative suggest sterile epididymitis.
- If testicular torsion cannot be excluded (especially in children), Doppler ultrasound is test of choice (1).
- In adult men, Doppler ultrasound: sensitivity and specificity of 100% in evaluation of acute scrotum (5)

Pediatric Considerations
Further radiographic imaging in children should be done to rule out anatomic abnormalities.

Diagnostic Procedures/Other
This is a clinical diagnosis.

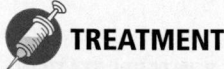 TREATMENT

GENERAL MEASURES
- Bed rest or restriction on activity
- Athletic scrotal supporter
- Scrotal elevation
- Ice pack wrapped in towel
- Avoid constipation.
- Spermatic cord block with local anesthesia in severe cases
- If chemical epididymitis
  - No strenuous physical activity and avoidance of any Valsalva maneuvers for several weeks.
  - Empty bladder prior to strenuous exercises

MEDICATION
First Line
- <35 years, or suspected STD etiology: doxycycline 100 mg PO BID for 10 days (C. trachomatis coverage) PLUS ceftriaxone 250 mg IM for 1 (N. gonorrhoeae coverage). Refer sexual partner(s) for evaluation and treatment if contact within 60 days of the onset of symptoms (2)[A].
- ≥35 years, not suspecting STD etiology with suspected enteric organism (i.e., bacteriuria due to bladder outlet obstruction, prostate biopsy, urinary instrumentation, systemic disease, and/or immunosuppression)
  - Levofloxacin (Levaquin) 500 mg/day PO for 10 days OR
  - Ofloxacin 300 mg PO BID for 10 days (2)[A]
- Men who are at risk for both STD and enteric organism (i.e., men who have sex with men who report insertive anal intercourse): ceftriaxone 250 mg IM for 1 plus fluoroquinolone as above (2)[A].
- Analgesia (infectious and chemical epididymitis)
  - NSAIDs (e.g., naproxen or ibuprofen) for mild to moderate pain
  - Consider corticosteroid if patient cannot tolerate NSAID.
  - Acetaminophen-codeine or acetaminophen-oxycodone for moderate to severe pain
- Septic or toxic patient
  - 3rd-generation cephalosporin or aminoglycoside
- For Behçet, sarcoid, Henoch-Schönlein purpura
  - Corticosteroids, such as methylprednisolone, 40 mg/day recommended

Second Line
- Trimethoprim-sulfamethoxazole (Bactrim, Septra) double-strength PO BID for 10 to 14 days; increasing bacterial resistance may limit effectiveness.
- Add rifampin (rifampicin) or vancomycin, as required.

ISSUES FOR REFERRAL
- If suspicion is high for testicular torsion or cancer, consult a urologist.
- Epididymitis in prepubertal boys requires a urology referral due to high incidence of associated urogenital abnormalities.
- If medical management fails, should be referred to urologist to rule out anatomic abnormality or chemical epididymitis.

SURGERY/OTHER PROCEDURES
- Vasostomy to drain infected material if severe or refractory case
- Scrotal exploration if unable clinically to distinguish between epididymitis and testicular torsion
- Drainage of abscesses, epididymectomy (acute suppurative), or epididymo-orchiectomy in severe cases refractory to antibiotics
- Surgery to correct underlying anatomic abnormality or obstruction

INPATIENT CONSIDERATIONS
Admission Criteria/Initial Stabilization
- Intractable pain
- Sepsis
- Abscess
- Persistent vomiting
- Scheduled surgery
- Purulent drainage
- Most cases can be managed with outpatient care

 ONGOING CARE

FOLLOW-UP RECOMMENDATIONS
Patient Monitoring
- Return to office if symptoms fail to improve within 72 hours of treatment for reevaluation of diagnosis and therapy (2).
- In chemical epididymitis, follow up in 4 weeks to assess efficacy of NSAIDs and lifestyle changes.

DIET
If constipation is contributing to pain or chemical epididymitis, then consider constipation prevention and/or treatment.

PATIENT EDUCATION
- Stress completing course of antibiotics, even when asymptomatic
- Early recognition and treatment of UTI or prostatitis
- Safer sexual practices
- If chemical epididymitis, then educate on noninfectious etiology and proper lifestyle changes.

PROGNOSIS
- Pain improves within 1 to 3 days, but induration may take several weeks/months to completely resolve.
- If bilateral involvement, sterility may result.
- In chemical epididymitis, symptoms usually resolve in <1 week.

COMPLICATIONS
- Recurrent epididymitis
- Infertility
- Oligospermia
- Testicular necrosis or atrophy
- Secondary abscess formation
- Fournier gangrene (necrotizing synergistic infection)

REFERENCES
1. Trojian TH, Lishnak TS, Heiman D. Epididymitis and orchitis: an overview. Am Fam Physician. 2009;79(7):583–587.
2. Workowski KA, Bolan GA; Centers for Disease Control and Prevention. Sexually transmitted diseases treatment guidelines, 2015. MMWR Recomm Rep. 2015;64(RR-03):1–137.
3. Santillanes G, Gausche-Hill M, Lewis RJ. Are antibiotics necessary for pediatric epididymitis? Pediatr Emerg Care. 2011;27(3):174–178.
4. Crawford P, Crop JA. Evaluation of scrotal masses. Am Fam Physician. 2014;89(9):723–727.
5. Rizvi SA, Ahmad I, Siddiqui MA, et al. Role of color Doppler ultrasonography in evaluation of scrotal swellings: pattern of disease in 120 patients with review of literature. Urol J. 2011;8(1):60–65.

ADDITIONAL READING
- Akinci E, Bodur H, Cevik MA, et al. A complication of brucellosis: epididymoorchitis. Int J Infect Dis. 2006;10(2):171–177.
- Bennett RT, Gill B, Kogan SJ. Epididymitis in children: the circumcision factor? J Urol. 1998;160(5):1842–1844.
- Somekh E, Gorenstein A, Serour F. Acute epididymitis in boys: evidence of a post-infectious etiology. J Urol. 2004;171(1):391–394.
- Tracy CR, Steers WD, Costabile R. Diagnosis and management of epididymitis. Urol Clin North Am. 2008;35(1):101–108; vii.
- Wolin LH. On the etiology of epididymitis. J Urol. 1971;105(4):531–533.

CODES

ICD10
- N45.1 Epididymitis
- N45.3 Epididymo-orchitis
- N45.4 Abscess of epididymis or testis

CLINICAL PEARLS
- With epididymitis, the pain is gradual in onset and the tenderness is mostly posterior to the testis. With testicular torsion, the symptoms are quite rapid in onset, the testis will be higher in the scrotum and may have a transverse lie, and the cremasteric reflex will be absent. The absence of leukocytes on urine analysis and decreased blood flow on scrotal ultrasound with Doppler will suggest torsion.
- Prostatic massage is contraindicated in epididymitis because of the risk for worsening local infection and the potential for sepsis are increased with acute prostatitis.
- Chemical epididymitis is a clinical diagnosis of exclusion, and infectious causes are much more common; but certain occupations, such as soldiers and laborers, must be considered.

EPISCLERITIS

Sean M. Oser, MD, MPH • Tamara K. Oser, MD

BASICS

- Episcleritis is the localized inflammation of the vascular connective tissue superficial to the sclera.
- Usually a self-limited condition, typically resolving within 3 weeks
- Most cases resolve without treatment.
- Topical lubricants and/or topical corticosteroid treatment may relieve symptoms while awaiting spontaneous resolution.

DESCRIPTION
- Edema and injection confined to the episcleral tissue
- Two types
  - Simple (diffuse scleral involvement—more common)
  - Nodular (focal area[s] of involvement—less common)

EPIDEMIOLOGY
Slight female predominance (~60–65%)

Incidence
- May occur at any age
- Peak incidence in 40s to 50s
- Community incidence not well-known (~20 to 50 cases/100,000 person-years)

Prevalence
Not historically well-known; a recent community study found a prevalence of 53 cases/100,000 persons.

ETIOLOGY AND PATHOPHYSIOLOGY
Etiology: Usually idiopathic, but other causes may be found (either nonimmune or immune).

Pathophysiology
- Nonimmune (e.g., dry eye syndrome, with histology showing widespread vasodilation, edema, lymphocytic infiltration)
- Immune (systemic vasculitis or rheumatologic disease)

COMMONLY ASSOCIATED CONDITIONS
- Usually not associated with another condition
- Less commonly associated conditions include the following:
  - Rheumatoid arthritis
  - Vasculitis
  - Inflammatory bowel disease
  - Ankylosing spondylitis
  - Systemic lupus erythematosus
  - Gout
  - Herpes zoster
  - Hypersensitivity disorders
    - Rosacea
    - Contact dermatitis
    - Penicillin sensitivity
    - Erythema multiforme

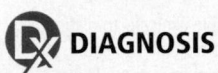

DIAGNOSIS

Episcleritis is a clinical diagnosis (1,2)[C].

HISTORY
- History should elicit potential causative factors, recurrence, or associated systemic disease (2)[C].
- Pain is often absent; when present, it is usually mild and localized to the eye (1–3)[C].
- Mild tearing may be present (2)[C].

PHYSICAL EXAM
- Check visual acuity; decreased vision is very unusual with episcleritis, and its presence should raise suspicion for another condition such as scleritis (1–3)[C].
- Focal hyperemia (2,4)[C]
- Pupils equal and reactive (2)[C]
- Superficial episcleral vascular dilation (1,2)[C]
- Episcleral edema (1,2)[C]
  - Diffuse in simple episcleritis
  - Focal in nodular episcleritis

- Tenderness over involved area may be present (2)[C] but is usually absent (3,4)[C].
- Superficial episcleral vascular hyperemia blanches with topical phenylephrine (1,4)[C].

ALERT
Recurrent episodes, difficulty confirming the diagnosis, or worsening symptoms require prompt ophthalmology referral (2)[C].

DIFFERENTIAL DIAGNOSIS
- Scleritis
- Bacterial conjunctivitis
- Viral conjunctivitis
- Herpes (ulcerative) keratitis
- Superficial keratitis
- Increased intraocular pressure (ocular hypertension)

DIAGNOSTIC TESTS & INTERPRETATION
Most patients with episcleritis do not require any further lab work or diagnostic studies (5)[C].

TREATMENT

MEDICATION
Treatment for episcleritis typically consist of symptomatic relief. The goal is to suppress the inflammation, which will, in turn, relieve the discomfort or pain. In most cases, treatment is not needed.

First Line
Topical lubricants such as artificial tears are typically used for initial management of symptomatic episcleritis (2)[C].

Second Line
- Topical corticosteroids are useful when discomfort is not sufficiently controlled by conservative measures (2,5,6)[C].
  - Fluorometholone 0.1% drops 4 times daily; if not effective, may increase frequency
  - Prednisolone 0.5–1% eye drops
- Refractory episcleritis may be treated with oral NSAIDs, typically indomethacin 25 mg 3 or 4 times daily (5)[C].

ISSUES FOR REFERRAL

Recurrent episodes, uncertain diagnosis, and/or worsening symptoms should prompt ophthalmology referral. Rarely, episcleritis may progress to scleritis in which case ophthalmology referral is also recommended.

ADDITIONAL THERAPIES

- Topical NSAIDs have not been shown to have a significant benefit over artificial tears (7)[B].
- When episcleritis results from viral infection, appropriate antiviral therapy is indicated (6)[C].

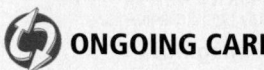 ONGOING CARE

FOLLOW-UP RECOMMENDATIONS

Episcleritis is usually self-limited (up to 21 days) and does not typically require follow-up.

PROGNOSIS

- Most patients have no ocular complications.
- Prognosis for episcleritis is excellent, with most patients making a full recovery.

COMPLICATIONS

Associated complications are rare, even at tertiary care referral centers, where referral bias likely overestimates their community incidence. When complications do occur, they tend not to be severe.

- Anterior uveitis may occur in 4–16% of cases (1,5,6)[C].
- Decreased vision may occur in 0–4% of cases (1,5,6)[C].
- Ocular hypertension has been reported in 0–3.5% of cases (1,5,6)[C].

REFERENCES

1. Sainz de la Maza M, Molina N, Gonzalez-Gonzalez LA, et al. Clinical characteristics of a large cohort of patients with scleritis and episcleritis. *Ophthalmology*. 2012;119(1):43–50.
2. Cronau H, Kankanala RR, Mauger T. Diagnosis and management of red eye in primary care. *Am Fam Physician*. 2010;81(2):137–144.
3. Garrity JA. Ocular manifestations of small-vessel vasculitis. *Cleve Clin J Med*. 2012;79(Suppl 3):S31–S33.
4. Galor A, Thorne JE. Scleritis and peripheral ulcerative keratitis. *Rheum Dis Clin North Am*. 2007;33(4):835–854.
5. Jabs DA, Mudun A, Dunn JP, et al. Episcleritis and scleritis: clinical features and treatment results. *Am J Ophthalmol*. 2000;130(4):469–476.
6. Berchicci L, Miserocchi E, Di Nicola M, et al. Clinical features of patients with episcleritis and scleritis in an Italian tertiary care referral center. *Eur J Ophthalmol*. 2014;24(3):293–298.
7. Williams CP, Browning AC, Sleep TJ, et al. A randomised, double-blind trial of topical ketorolac vs artificial tears for the treatment of episcleritis. *Eye (Lond)*. 2005;19(7):739–742.

ADDITIONAL READING

- Homayounfar G, Borkar DS, Tham VM, et al. Clinical characteristics of scleritis and episcleritis: results from the Pacific Ocular Inflammation Study. *Ocul Immunol Inflamm*. 2014;22(5):403–404.

- Homayounfar G, Nardone N, Borkar DS, et al. Incidence of scleritis and episcleritis: results from the Pacific Ocular Inflammation Study. *Am J Ophthalmol*. 2013;156(4):752–758.
- Honik G, Wong IG, Gritz DC. Incidence and prevalence of episcleritis and scleritis in Northern California. *Cornea*. 2013;32(12):1562–1566.

 CODES

ICD10

- H15.109 Unspecified episcleritis, unspecified eye
- H15.129 Nodular episcleritis, unspecified eye
- H15.102 Unspecified episcleritis, left eye

CLINICAL PEARLS

- Episcleritis typically is a benign, self-limited disorder.
- Is often not painful and presents without decrease in visual acuity
- Although treatment is often not needed, when employed, the goal is symptomatic relief while awaiting spontaneous resolution.
- Topical lubricants and/or topical corticosteroid treatment may relieve symptoms.
- Associated complications are uncommon and not severe but may include anterior uveitis, decreased vision, and ocular hypertension.
- Episcleritis can be an early presentation of scleritis, which is more severe. Accurate diagnosis of episcleritis is important.

E

EPISTAXIS

Brian E. Neubauer, MD

 BASICS

DESCRIPTION
- Hemorrhage from the nose involving either the anterior or posterior mucosal surfaces
- Synonym(s): nosebleed
- Intractable or refractory epistaxis: recurrent or persistent despite appropriate packing or multiple episodes during a short period, each requiring medical attention

EPIDEMIOLOGY
Incidence
- In the United States: common
- Estimated lifetime prevalence: ~60%
- Bimodal, with peaks in children up to 15 years and in adults >50 years, particularly ages 70 to 79 years
- Most common in males <49 years.
- Rare in children <2 years.
- ~6% of patients require medical or surgical intervention; accounts for ~1 in 200 ER visits

ETIOLOGY AND PATHOPHYSIOLOGY
- Local versus systemic disease. Most are due to local causes.
- Anterior: 90–95% of all cases (Kiesselbach plexus)
- Posterior: 5–10% of cases. Usually branches of sphenopalatine arteries: may be asymptomatic or may present with other symptoms (hematemesis, hemoptysis)
- Idiopathic
- Local inflammation/irritation
  - Infection (viral URI, sinusitis, TB, syphilis)
  - Irritant inhalation (smoking, rhinitis)
  - Topical steroid or antihistamine use
  - Septal deviation (more air movement on one side)
  - Low humidity, nasal oxygen use, CPAP
  - Tumors: benign, malignant
  - Vascular malformations
- Trauma
  - Epistaxis digitorum (nose picking)
  - Foreign bodies
  - Septal perforation
  - Nasal fracture
  - Nasal surgery
- Systemic
  - Thrombocytopenia
  - Congenital or acquired coagulopathies
  - Liver or renal disease
  - Chronic alcohol abuse
  - Leukemia
  - Anticoagulant drug use
  - CHF
  - Hereditary hemorrhagic telangiectasia (HHT)
  - Collagen abnormalities

- Mitral valve stenosis
- Multiple myeloma
- Polycythemia vera

RISK FACTORS
- Local irritation from multiple causes (see "Etiology and Pathophysiology")
- Medications/supplements including aspirin, clopidogrel, ginseng, garlic, ginkgo biloba, warfarin, and other anticoagulants

GENERAL PREVENTION
- Humidification at night
- Cut fingernails to minimize picking.
- For topical-nasal medication users, direct spray laterally away from septum. Use opposite hand to spray (i.e., right hand to spray in left nostril).
- Petroleum jelly to prevent anterior mucosal drying

COMMONLY ASSOCIATED CONDITIONS
- Vascular malformation/telangiectasia (HHT)
- Neoplasm (rare, but consider in persistent unilateral cases)
- Systemic
  - Coagulopathy: primary or iatrogenic
  - Thrombocytopenia
  - Cirrhosis
  - Renal failure
  - Alcoholism
- No proven association with hypertension (HTN) but may make control of bleeding more difficult.

 DIAGNOSIS

HISTORY
- Assess patency or airway and cardiovascular stability first.
- Initial presentation, including detail on which side bleeding began, anterior or posterior, duration.
- Trauma includes nose picking, other precipitating events.
- Previous episodes
- Comorbid conditions (cardiovascular compromise symptoms)
- Current medications including over-the-counter and supplements

PHYSICAL EXAM
- Blood loss through one or both nostrils in most cases is due to anterior nasal septal bleeding and can often be directly visualized.
- Focus on localizing site of bleeding to anterior versus posterior nasal cavity.
- Patient is seated, head forward, to avoid blood going down the posterior pharynx.
- Use of nasal speculum improves visualization.

DIFFERENTIAL DIAGNOSIS
- Diagnosis usually apparent; the differential for the etiology is key.
- Posterior bleeding must be included in the differential for any chronic blood loss.

DIAGNOSTIC TESTS & INTERPRETATION
- Indicated only in complicated cases and/or profuse blood loss
- Lab testing is not indicated in most uncomplicated cases in which bleeding is reasonably easily controlled and is not truly hemorrhagic.

Initial Tests (lab, imaging)
- Mild cases, responsive to pressure: no labs
- For recurrent or intractable cases
  - CBC, PT/PTT, BMP
- PT/PTT if on warfarin or other medications affecting coagulation.
- Cross-match when appropriate.
- Toxicology screen when nasal use of illicit drugs is suspected
- For most cases, imaging is not indicated.

Follow-Up Tests & Special Considerations
If recurrent unilateral epistaxis, especially if not responding to treatment measures, consider evaluation for neoplasm.

Diagnostic Procedures/Other
Nasal endoscopy

Pediatric Considerations
More likely anterior, idiopathic, and recurrent

Geriatric Considerations
More likely to be posterior bleed

 TREATMENT

- Most cases are managed as outpatient (1)[B].

- Home use—Nosebleed QR: a nonprescription powder of hydrophilic polymer with potassium salt; induces scab formation
- Patient applies direct pressure by pinching the lower part of the nose (nasal ala) for 5 to 20 minutes without a break. This will stop active bleeding in most patients.
- An ice pack placed over the dorsum of the nose may help with hemostasis.
- Inspect the nasal septum for the bleeding site.

GENERAL MEASURES
Resuscitation, as indicated. Use universal "ABC" approach.

MEDICATION

First Line

- If general measures fail, affected naris may be sprayed with topical vasoconstrictor, such as:
  - Phenylephrine: 0.5–1%
  - Oxymetazoline: 0.05%
  - Epinephrine: 1:1,000
  - Cocaine: 4%

Second Line

- Chemical (silver nitrate) or electrical cautery
- Nasal packing: ribbon gauze, nasal tampons, nasal balloon catheter
- For intractable/refractory: Consider surgical ligation, endoscopic ligation/cautery, endovascular embolization.

ISSUES FOR REFERRAL

- Posterior bleeding frequently requires an otolaryngology consultation.
- Anterior bleeding that fails conservative measures, packing, and cauterization
- Recurrent episodes
- Patients with HHT should establish care with ENT early.

ADDITIONAL THERAPIES

- Nasal packing: either with ribbon gauze or preformed nasal tampons. Systemic prophylactic antibiotics are unnecessary in the majority of patients with nasal packs; topical antibiotics may be as effective and cheaper (2)[B].
- FloSeal: A biodegradable hemostatic sealant (a thrombin-type gel) in one study is more effective and better tolerated than packing (3)[B].

- If an actively bleeding anterior septal site is visualized, this may be treated with gentle and specific silver nitrate cautery for ~10 seconds for definitive treatment. 75% silver nitrate is preferred. Apply in a spiral fashion, starting around the bleeding vessel, moving inward.
- Limit cautery (silver nitrate) to one side of septum, or wait 4 to 6 weeks in between treatments to reduce risk of perforation.
- Posterior: posterior packing or tamponade with balloon devices (Foley catheter has been used). Inpatient monitoring is generally required.

- Recurrent epistaxis: Cochrane review in children shows no difference in effectiveness between antiseptic nasal cream, petroleum jelly, silver nitrate cautery, or no treatment (4)[A].
  - Silver nitrate cautery followed by 4 weeks of antiseptic cream may be better than antiseptic cream alone (5)[B].

SURGERY/OTHER PROCEDURES

- Packing
  - Layering of Vaseline ribbon gauze (1/2 inch)
    - For gauze packing, be certain that both ends of the ribbon gauze protrude from the nostril.

- Packing is layered from the floor upward.
  - Secure packing with gauze across the outside of the nostril.
  - Nasal tampon may be used after lubricating the tip with KY Jelly or antibiotic cream or ointment.
  - Additional saline may be needed to expand the tampon if the bleeding has slowed.
  - Merocel and Rapid Rhino packs are easier to use than gauze packing and are usually well tolerated.
- Posterior bleed
  - In the emergent setting, this may be attempted utilizing a Foley catheter or a specific posterior packing balloon.
  - With both methods, the tubing is introduced through the nose similar to the passage of a nasogastric tube. Once it reaches the posterior oral pharynx, the balloon is inflated and the tubing is pulled back outward to tamponade the posterior bleeding source.
    - If using a Foley catheter (10 to 14F catheter), the balloon can be inflated with 10 mL of saline.
    - Traction is maintained with an umbilical cord clamp with adequate padding between the clip and the nose to avoid injury.

INPATIENT CONSIDERATIONS

Consider hospitalization for elderly or for patients with posterior bleeding or coagulopathy. May also consider if significant comorbidities

Admission Criteria/Initial Stabilization

- Posterior bleed
- Hemodynamic changes
- Clotting dysfunction
- Universal "airway/breathing/circulation" (ABC) approach. Stop blood loss.

 ## ONGOING CARE

FOLLOW-UP RECOMMENDATIONS

Patient Monitoring

- When significant blood loss, hemodynamic monitoring
- 24-Hour minimum of packing in place; some authors recommend 3 to 5 days. The latter recommendation carries the risk of mucosal injury and toxic shock syndrome. The former has the risk of rebleed, which usually occurs between 24 and 48 hours.

PATIENT EDUCATION

- Demonstrate proper pinching pressure techniques.
- Avoidance of trauma or irritants is key.
- Management of systemic illness and proper use of medication

PROGNOSIS

- Most are self-limited.
- Good results with proper treatment

COMPLICATIONS

- Septal perforation
- Pressure-induced tissue necrosis of the nasal mucosa
- Toxic shock syndrome with packing
- Arrhythmias triggered by packing (particularly posterior)

REFERENCES

1. Melia L, McGarry GW. Epistaxis: update on management. *Curr Opin Otolaryngol Head Neck Surg.* 2011;19(1):30–35.
2. Biggs TC, Nightingale K, Patel NN, et al. Should prophylactic antibiotics be used routinely in epistaxis patients with nasal packs? *Ann R Coll Surg Engl.* 2013;95(1):40–42.
3. Mathiasen RA, Cruz RM. Prospective, randomized, controlled clinical trial of a novel matrix hemostatic sealant in patients with acute anterior epistaxis. *Laryngoscope.* 2005;115(2):899–902.
4. Qureshi A, Burton MJ. Interventions for recurrent idiopathic epistaxis (nosebleeds) in children. *Cochrane Database Syst Rev.* 2012;(9):CD004461.
5. Calder N, Kang S, Fraser L, et al. A double-blind randomized controlled trial of management of recurrent nosebleeds in children. *Otolaryngol Head Neck Surg.* 2009;140(5):670–674.

ADDITIONAL READING

- Manes RP. Evaluating and managing the patient with nosebleeds. *Med Clin North Am.* 2010;94(5): 903–912.
- Schlosser RJ. Clinical practice. Epistaxis. *N Engl J Med.* 2009;360(8):784–789.

 ## CODES

ICD10

R04.0 Epistaxis

CLINICAL PEARLS

- Most episodes are anterior in etiology and respond to timed pressure over the anterior nares for 5 to 20 minutes.
- Most are idiopathic or as a result of nose picking.
- Posterior nosebleeds can be asymptomatic or present with nausea, hematemesis, or heme-positive stool.
- Consider evaluation for neoplasm if recurrent unilateral episodes.

ERECTILE DYSFUNCTION

Michael C. Barros, PharmD, BCPS, BCACP • Neela Bhajandas, PharmD • Paul N. Williams, MD, FACP

 BASICS

DESCRIPTION
- Erectile dysfunction (ED): the consistent or recurrent inability to acquire or sustain an erection of sufficient rigidity and duration for sexual intercourse
- In the past, ED was assumed to be a symptom of the aging process in men, but it can result from concurrent medical conditions of the patient or from medications that patients may be taking to treat those conditions.
- Sexual problems are frequent among older men and have a detrimental effect on their quality of life but are infrequently discussed with their physicians (1).
- Synonym(s): impotence

ALERT
When ED occurs in a younger man, it is associated with a significantly increased risk of future cardiac events (2).

EPIDEMIOLOGY
Incidence
It is estimated that >600,000 new cases of ED will be diagnosed annually in the United States, although this may be an underestimation of the true incidence, as ED is vastly underreported.

Prevalence
Overall prevalence for ED:
- 52% in men age 40 to 70 years
- Age-related increase ranging from 12.4% in men age 40 to 49 years up to 46.6% in men age 50 to 69 years

ETIOLOGY AND PATHOPHYSIOLOGY
- ED is a neurovascular event.
  - With stimulation, there is release of nitrous oxide, which increases production of guanosine 3',5'-cyclic monophosphate (cGMP).
  - This leads to relaxation of cavernous smooth muscle, leading to increased blood flow to penis.
  - As cavernosal sinusoids distend with blood, there is passive compression of subtunical veins, which decreases venous outflow, and this leads to an erection.
- Alterations in any of these events leads to ED.
- ED may result from problems with systems required for normal penile erection.
  - Vascular: diseases that compromise blood flow
    - Peripheral vascular disease, arteriosclerosis, essential hypertension
  - Neurologic: diseases that impair nerve conduction to brain or penile vasculature
    - Spinal cord injury, stroke, diabetes
  - Endocrine: diseases associated with changes in testosterone, luteinizing hormone, prolactin levels
  - Structural: phimosis, lichen sclerosis, congenital curvature
  - Psychological: patients suffering from malaise, depression, performance anxiety
- Social habits such as smoking or excessive alcohol intake
- Medications may cause ED.
- Structural injury or trauma (bicycling accident)

Genetics
Rarely related to chromosomal disorders

RISK FACTORS
- Advancing age
- Cardiovascular disease
- Diabetes mellitus
- Metabolic syndrome
- Sedentary lifestyle
- Cigarette smoking
- Urologic surgery, radiation, trauma/injury to pelvic area or spinal cord
- Medications that induce ED
  - SSRIs, β-blockers, clonidine, digoxin, spironolactone, antiandrogens, corticosteroids, H_2 blockers
- Central neurologic and endocrinologic conditions
- Substance abuse
- Psychological conditions: stress, anxiety, or depression

GENERAL PREVENTION
The two best ways to prevent ED are by the following:
- Making healthy lifestyle choices by exercising regularly, eating well-balanced meals, limiting alcohol, and avoiding smoking
- Treating existing health problems and working with your patients to manage diabetes, heart disease, and other chronic problems

ALERT
Aging alone is not a cause.

COMMONLY ASSOCIATED CONDITIONS
- Cardiovascular disease:
  - Men with ED have a greater likelihood of having angina, myocardial infarction, stroke, transient ischemic attack, congestive heart failure, or cardiac arrhythmia compared to men without ED (3).
- Diabetes
- Psychiatric disorders

 DIAGNOSIS

Inability to achieve or maintain erection satisfactory for intercourse

HISTORY
- Identify concurrent medical illnesses or surgical procedures, history of trauma, and a list of current medications (e.g., antihypertensive meds).
- Psychosocial history: smoking, ethanol intake, recreational drug use, anxiety and depression, satisfaction with current relationship
- Presence or absence of morning erections
- Speed of onset and duration of symptoms
- Relationship of symptoms to libido
- Detailed sexual history important to rule out premature ejaculation, as this is frequently confused with ED

PHYSICAL EXAM
- Signs and symptoms of hypogonadism: gynecomastia, small testicles, decreased body hair
- Penile plaques (Peyronie disease)
- Detailed examination of the cardiovascular, neurologic, and genitourinary systems
  - Blood pressure
  - Check femoral and lower extremity pulses to assess vascular supply to genitals.
  - Check anal sphincter tone and genital reflexes, including cremasterics and bulbocavernosus.

DIFFERENTIAL DIAGNOSIS
- Premature ejaculation
- Decreased libido
- Anorgasmia
- Sudden versus chronic ED

DIAGNOSTIC TESTS & INTERPRETATION
Vascular and/or neurologic assessment, and monitoring of nocturnal erections may be indicated in selected patients but not for routine workup (4)[C].

Initial Tests (lab, imaging)
- Hgb A1c, lipid panel, TSH, and morning total testosterone level (3)[C]
- Doppler, angiogram, and cavernosogram are available radiologic modalities but not recommended in routine practice for the diagnosis of ED (4)[C].

Follow-Up Tests & Special Considerations
Other hormonal tests, such as prolactin, should only be ordered when there is suspicion for a specific endocrinopathy.

Diagnostic Procedures/Other
Questionnaires can be offered to assess the severity of ED, including the International Index of Erectile Function (IEFF) and its validated and more easily administered abridged version, the Sexual Health Inventory for Men (SHIM) (4)[C].

TREATMENT
- Lifestyle modifications and managing medications contributing to ED is first-line therapy for ED (5)[C]. Use least invasive therapy first; reserve more invasive therapies for nonresponders.
- Phosphodiesterase type 5 (PDE-5) inhibitor choice should be based on patient's preference (cost, ease of use, and adverse effects).

GENERAL MEASURES
- Psychotherapy alone or in combination with psychoactive drugs may be helpful in men whose ED is related to depression or anxiety.
- Weight loss and increased physical activity for obese men with ED

MEDICATION
First Line
PDE-5 inhibitors are effective in the treatment of ED in many men, including those with diabetes mellitus and spinal cord injury and sexual dysfunction associated with antidepressants (3)[A]. There is insufficient evidence to support the superiority of one agent over the others (5)[A]:

- Sildenafil (Viagra): usual daily dose: 50 to 100 mg within at least 60 minutes of sexual intercourse
- Vardenafil (Levitra): usual daily dose 5 to 20 mg within at least 60 minutes of sexual intercourse

- Vardenafil (Staxyn): ODT: usual dose 10 mg within 60 minutes of sexual intercourse
- Tadalafil (Cialis): usual daily dose 5 to 20 mg within at least 30 minutes of sexual intercourse or 2.5 mg once daily without regard to sexual activity
- Avanafil (Stendra): usual daily dose: 50 to 200 mg within at least 15 to 30 minutes of sexual intercourse
  - Adverse effects of PDE-5 inhibitors: headache, facial flushing, dyspepsia, nasal congestion, dizziness, hypotension, increased sensitivity to light (sildenafil and vardenafil), vision changes, lower back pain (tadalafil), and priapism (with excessive doses)
  - Sildenafil and vardenafil should be taken on an empty stomach for maximum effectiveness.

Geriatric Considerations
Use doses at the lower end of the dosing range for elderly patients.
- Sildenafil 25 mg daily
- Vardenafil 5 mg daily

Second Line
Intraurethral and intracavernosal injectables are second-line therapies shown to be effective and should be administered based on patient preference (3)[B]. Intraurethral suppositories are a less invasive treatment option than intracavernosal injections; however, they are not as effective (5)[C]. Alprostadil, also known as prostaglandin E1, causes smooth muscle relaxation of the arterial blood vessels and sinusoidal tissues in the corpora:

- Intraurethral alprostadil (Muse):
  - Urethral suppository: 125-, 250-, 500-, and 1,000-μg pellets. Administer 5 to 50 minutes before intercourse. No more than 2 doses in 24 hours are recommended.
- Intracavernosal alprostadil (available in 2 formulations):
  - Alprostadil (Caverject): usual dose: 10 to 20 μg, with max dose of 60 μg. Injection should be made at right angles into one of the lateral surfaces of the proximal third of the penis using a 0.5-inch, 27- or 30-gauge needle. Do not use >3 times a week or more than once in 24 hours.
  - Alprostadil may also be combined with papaverine (Bimix) plus phentolamine (Tri-Mix).

ALERT
- Initial trial dose of second-line agents should be administered under supervision of a specialist or primary care physician with expertise in these therapies.
- Patient should notify physician if erection lasts >4 hours for immediate attention.
- Vacuum pump devices are a noninvasive second-line option and are available over the counter. Do not use vacuum devices in men with sickle cell anemia or blood dyscrasias.
- Testosterone supplementation in men with hypogonadism improves ED and libido (3)[B]. Available formulations include injectable depots, transdermal patches and gels, SC pellets, and oral therapy.
- Contraindications:
  - Nitroglycerin (or other nitrates) and phosphodiesterase inhibitors: potential for severe, fatal hypotension

- Precautions/side effects:
  - Testosterone: precautions: Exogenous testosterone reduces sperm count and thus do not use in patients wishing to keep fertility; side effects: acne, sodium retention
  - Intraurethral suppository: local penile pain, urethral bleeding, dizziness, and dysuria
  - Intracavernosal injection: penile pain, edema and hematoma, palpable nodules or plaques, and priapism
  - Sildenafil: hypotension (caution for patients on nitrates)
  - PDE-5 inhibitors: Use caution with congenital prolonged QT syndrome, class Ia or II antiarrhythmics, nitroglycerin, α-blockers (e.g., terazosin, tamsulosin), retinal disease, unstable cardiac disease, liver and renal failure.
  - Significant possible interactions
  - PDE-5 inhibitor concentration is affected by CYP3A4 inhibitors (e.g., erythromycin, indinavir, ketoconazole, ritonavir, amiodarone, cimetidine, clarithromycin, delavirdine, diltiazem, fluoxetine, fluvoxamine, grapefruit juice, itraconazole, nefazodone, nevirapine, saquinavir, and verapamil). Serum concentrations and/or toxicity may be increased. Lower starting doses should be used in these patients.
  - PDE-5 inhibitor concentration may be reduced by rifampin and phenytoin.

ADDITIONAL THERAPIES

Behavioral therapy: Couples therapy aimed at improving relationship difficulties found that men who received this therapy plus sildenafil had more successful intercourse than those who received only sildenafil (6)[A].

SURGERY/OTHER PROCEDURES
Penile prosthesis should be reserved for patients who have failed or are ineligible first- or second-line therapies.

COMPLEMENTARY & ALTERNATIVE MEDICINE
Trazodone, yohimbine, and herbal therapies are not recommended for the treatment of ED, as they have not proven to be efficacious.

ONGOING CARE

FOLLOW-UP RECOMMENDATIONS
Patient Monitoring
Treatment should be assessed at baseline and after the patient has completed at least 1 to 3 weeks of a specific treatment: Monitor the quality and quantity of penile erections, and monitor the level of satisfaction patient achieves.

DIET
Diet and exercise recommended to achieve a normal body mass index; limit alcohol

PROGNOSIS
- All commercially available PDE-5 inhibitors are equally effective. In the presence of sexual stimulation, they are 55–80% effective.
  - Lower success rates with diabetes mellitus and radical prostatectomy patients who suffer from ED.
- Overall effectiveness is 70–90% for intracavernosal alprostadil and 43–60% for intraurethral alprostadil (4)[B].
- Penile prostheses are associated with an 85–90% patient satisfaction rate (4)[C].

REFERENCES

1. Lindau ST, Schumm LP, Laumann EO, et al. A study of sexuality and health among older adults in the United States. N Engl J Med. 2007;357(8): 762–774.
2. Inman BA, Sauver JL, Jacobson DJ, et al. A population-based, longitudinal study of erectile dysfunction and future coronary artery disease. Mayo Clin Proc. 2009;84(2):108–113.
3. Heidelbaugh JJ. Management of erectile dysfunction. Am Fam Physician. 2010;81(3):305–312.
4. McVary KT. Clinical practice. Erectile dysfunction. N Engl J Med. 2007;357(24):2472–2481.
5. The American Urological Association. Guideline on the management of erectile dysfunction: diagnosis and treatment recommendations. Reviewed and Validity Confirmed in 2011. http://www.auanet.org/education/guidelines/erectile-dysfunction.cfm. Accessed 2015.
6. Melnik T, Soares BG, Nasselo AG. Psychosocial interventions for erectile dysfunction. Cochrane Database Syst Rev. 2007;(3):CD004825.

CODES

ICD10
- N52.9 Male erectile dysfunction, unspecified
- N52.1 Erectile dysfunction due to diseases classified elsewhere
- F52.21 Male erectile disorder

CLINICAL PEARLS

- Nitrates should be withheld for 24 hours after sildenafil or vardenafil administration and for 48 hours after use of tadalafil. PDE-5 inhibitors are contraindicated in patients taking concurrent nitrates of any form (regular or intermittent nitrate therapy), as it can lead to severe hypotension and syncope.
- Reserve surgical treatment for patients who do not respond to drug treatment.
- The use of PDE-5 inhibitors with α-adrenergic antagonists may increase the risk of hypotension. Tamsulosin is the least likely to cause orthostatic hypotension.
- Avanafil should not be used with strong CYP3A4 inhibitors and max dose should be 50 mg with moderate CYP3A4 inhibitors.
- ED serves as a predictor for future cardiovascular events; thus, these patients should be followed vigilantly.

ERYSIPELAS

Fozia Akhtar Ali, MD • Mary Anne de la Cruz Estacio, DO

BASICS

DESCRIPTION
- Distinct form of cellulitis notable for acute, well-demarcated, superficial bacterial skin infection with lymphatic involvement almost always caused by *Streptococcus pyogenes*
- Usually acute, but a chronic recurrent form also exists (1)
- Nonpurulent
- System(s) affected: skin, exocrine
- Synonym(s): St. Anthony's Fire

EPIDEMIOLOGY
- Predominant age: infants, children, and adults >40 years
- Greatest in elderly (>75 years)
- No gender/racial predilection
- Affects all races

Incidence
- Erysipelas occurs in ~1/1,000 persons/year (2).
- Incidence on the rise since the 1980s (3)

Prevalence
Unknown

ETIOLOGY AND PATHOPHYSIOLOGY
- Group A streptococci induce inflammation and activation of the contact system, a proinflammatory pathway with antithrombotic activity, releasing proteinases and proinflammatory cytokines.
- The generation of antibacterial peptides and the release of bradykinin, a proinflammatory peptide, increase vascular permeability and induce fever and pain.
- The M proteins from the group A streptococcal cell wall interact with neutrophils, leading to the secretion of heparin-binding protein, an inflammatory mediator that also induces vascular leakage.
- This cascade of reactions leads to the symptoms seen in erysipelas: fever, pain, erythema, and edema.
- Group A β-hemolytic streptococci primarily; commonly *S. pyogenes*, occasionally, other *Streptococcus* groups C/G
- Rarely, group B streptococci/*Staphylococcus aureus* may be involved.

RISK FACTORS
- Disruption in the skin barrier (surgical incisions, insect bites, eczematous lesions, local trauma, abrasions, dermatophytic infections, intravenous drug user [IVDU])
- Chronic diseases (diabetes, malnutrition, nephrotic syndrome, heart failure)
- Immunocompromised (HIV)/debilitated
- Fissured skin (especially at the nose and ears)
- Toe-web intertrigo and lymphedema (2)
- Leg ulcers/stasis dermatitis
- Venous/Lymphatic insufficiency (saphenectomy, varicose veins of leg, phlebitis, radiotherapy, mastectomy, lymphadenectomy)
- Alcohol abuse
- Morbid obesity
- Recent streptococcal pharyngitis
- Varicella

GENERAL PREVENTION
- Good skin hygiene
- It is recommended that predisposing medical conditions, such as tinea pedis and stasis dermatitis, be appropriately managed first.
- Men who shave within 5 days of facial erysipelas are more likely to have a recurrence.
- With recurrences, search for other possible sources of streptococcal infection (e.g., tonsils, sinuses).
- Compression stockings should be encouraged for patients with lower extremity edema.
- Consider suppressive prophylactic antibiotic therapy, such as penicillin, in patients with >2 episodes in a 12-month period.

Pediatric Considerations
Group B *Streptococcus* may be a cause of erysipelas in neonates/infants.

DIAGNOSIS

Prodromal symptoms before the skin eruption of erysipelas may include:
- Moderate- to high-grade fever
- Chills
- Headache
- Malaise
- Anorexia, usually in the first 48 hours (4)[B]
- Vomiting
- Arthralgias

ALERT
It is important to differentiate erysipelas from a methicillin-resistant *S. aureus* (MRSA) infection, which usually presents with an indurated center, significant pain, and later evidence of abscess formation.

PHYSICAL EXAM
- Vital signs: moderate- to high-grade fever with resultant tachycardia. Hypotension may occur.
- The presence of a fever in erysipelas can be considered a differentiating factor from other skin infections.
- Headache and vomiting may be prominent.
- Acute onset of intense erythema; well-demarcated painful plaque (5)
- Peau d'orange appearance
- Milian's ear sign (erythema involves skin of ear as well as face implies erysipelas)
- Vesicles and bullae may form but are not uniformly present.
- Desquamation may occur later.
- Lymphangitis
- Location
  - Lower extremity 70–80% of cases
  - Face involvement is less common (5–20%), especially nose and ears.
  - Chronic form usually recurs at site of the previous infection and may recur years after initial episode.
- Patients on systemic steroids may be more difficult to diagnose because signs and symptoms of the infection may be masked by anti-inflammatory action of the steroids.

- Systemic toxicity resolves rapidly with treatment; skin lesions desquamate on days 5 to 10 but usually heal without scarring.
- In geriatric patients, facial involvement presents in a butterfly pattern. Pustules characteristically absent and regional lymphadenopathy with lymphangitic streaking is seen.

Pediatric Considerations
- Abdominal involvement is more common in infants, especially around umbilical stump.
- Face, scalp, and leg involvement are common in older children due to the excoriations of anterior rhinitis sicca allowing an easy port of entry.

Geriatric Considerations
- Fever may not be as prominent.
- Face and lower extremity are the most common areas.
- High-output cardiac failure may occur in debilitated patients with underlying cardiac disease.
- More susceptible to complications

DIFFERENTIAL DIAGNOSIS
- Cellulitis (margins are less clear and does not involve ear)
- Necrotizing fasciitis (systemic illness and more pain)
- Skin abscess (feel for area of fluctuance)
- DVT (need to rule out if clinically suspected)
- Acute gout (check patient history)
- Insect bite (check patient history)
- Dermatophytes
- Impetigo (blistered/crusted appearance; superficial)
- Ecthyma (ulcerative impetigo)
- Herpes zoster (dermatomal distribution)
- Erythema annulare centrifugum (raised pink-red ring/bull's-eye marks)
- Contact dermatitis (no fever, pruritic, not painful)
- Giant cell urticaria (transient, wheal-appearance, severe itching)
- Angioneurotic edema (no fever)
- Scarlet fever (widespread rash with indistinct borders and without edema; rash is most common early in skin folds; develops generalized "sandpaper" feeling as it progresses)
- Toxic shock syndrome (diffuse erythema with evidence of multiorgan involvement)
- Lupus (of the face; less fever, positive antinuclear antibodies)
- Polychondritis (common site is the ear)
- Other bacterial infections to consider:
  - Meat, shellfish, fish, and poultry workers: *Erysipelothrix rhusiopathiae* (known as erysipeloid)
  - Human bite: *Eikenella corrodens*
  - Cat/dog bite: *Pasteurella multocida/Capnocytophaga canimorsus*
  - Salt water exposure: *Vibrio vulnificus*
  - Fresh/brackish water exposure: *Aeromonas hydrophilia*

DIAGNOSTIC TESTS & INTERPRETATION
Reserve diagnostic tests for severely ill, toxic patients, or those who are immunosuppressed.

Initial Tests (lab, imaging)
- Leukocytosis
- Blood culture (<5% positive)
- Elevated erythrocyte sedimentation rate (ESR) and C-reactive protein (CRP)
- Streptococci may be cultured from exudate/noninvolved sites.

Test Interpretation
Biopsy is not needed. However, skin findings would show
- Dermal and epidermal edema, extending into the SC tissues
- Peau d'orange appearance caused by edema in the superficial tissue surrounding the hair follicles
- Vasodilation and enlarged lymphatics
- Mixed interstitial infiltrate mainly consisting of neutrophils and mononuclear cells
- Endothelial cell swelling
- Gram-positive cocci in lymphatics and tissue with rare invasion of local blood vessels
- Fibrotic thickening of lymphatic vessel walls with possible luminal occlusion may be seen in recurrent erysipelas.

 TREATMENT

GENERAL MEASURES
- Symptomatic treatment of myalgias and fever
- Adequate fluid intake
- Local treatment with cold compresses
- Elevation of affected extremity
- Appropriate therapy for any underlying predisposing condition

MEDICATION
- Antibiotics cure 50–100% of infections, but which regimen is most successful is unclear
- Antibiotics may be as effective when given orally versus intravenously.
- A 5-day course of antibiotics may be as effective as a 10-day course at curing (6)[A].

First Line
- Adults
  - Extremities, nondiabetic
    - Primary
      - Penicillin G: 1 to 2 million U IV q6h *or* cefazolin 1 g IV q8h
    - Alternative (if penicillin-allergic)
      - Vancomycin 15 mg/kg IV q12h
      - When afebrile **Pen VK** 500 mg PO QID AC and HS
  - Total 10 days, diabetics
    - Early-mild:
      - Trimethoprim-sulfamethoxazole (TMP-SMX)-DS: 1 to 2 tabs PO BID and penicillin VK 500 mg PO QID *or* cephalexin 500 mg PO QID
  - Severe disease
    - IMP or MER or ERTA IV and linezolid 600 mg IV/PO BID. *or* vancomycin IV or daptomycin 4 mg/kg IV q24h
  - Facial
    - Primary
      - Vancomycin: 15 mg/kg (actual weight) IV q8–12h with target trough 15 to 20
    - Alternative
      - Daptomycin 4 mg/kg IV q24h or linezolid: 600 mg IV q12h
- Children
  - Penicillin G
    - 0 to 7 days, <2,000 g: 50,000 U/kg q12h
    - 8 to 28 days, <2,000 g: 75,000 U/kg q8h
    - 0 to 7 days, >2,000 g = 50,000 U/kg q8h
    - 8 to 28 days, >2,000 g = 50,000 U/kg q6h
    - >28 days to 50,000 U/kg per day

  - Cefazolin
    - 0 to 7 days, <2,000 g: 25 mg/kg q12h
    - 8 to 28 days, <2,000 g: 25 mg/kg q12h
    - 0 to 7 days, >2,000 g = 25 mg/kg q12h
    - 8 to 28 day, >2,000 g = 25 mg/kg q8h
    - >28 days to 25 mg/kg q8h
- No reported group A streptococci resistance to β-lactam antibiotics
- In chronic recurrent infections, prophylactic treatment after the acute infection resolves:
  - Penicillin G benzathine: 1.2 million U IM q4wks *or* penicillin VK 500 mg PO BID *or* azithromycin 250 mg PO QD
- If staphylococcal infection is suspected or if patient is acutely ill, consider a β–lactamase-stable antibiotic.
- Consider community-acquired MRSA, and depending on regional sensitivity, may treat MRSA with TMP-SMX DS 1 tab PO BID or vancomycin 1 g IV q12h or doxycycline 100 mg PO BID

ISSUES FOR REFERRAL
Recurrent infection, treatment failure

ADDITIONAL THERAPIES
Some patients may notice a deepening of erythema after initiating antimicrobial therapy. This may be due to the destruction of pathogens that release enzymes, increasing local inflammation. In this case, treatment with corticosteroids, in addition to antimicrobials, can mildly reduce healing time and antibiotic duration in patients with erysipelas. Consider prednisolone 30 mg/day with taper over 8 days (7).

INPATIENT CONSIDERATIONS
Admission Criteria/Initial Stabilization
- Patient with systemic toxicity
- Patient with high-risk factors (e.g., elderly, lymphedema, postsplenectomy, diabetes)
- Failed outpatient care

IV Fluids
IV therapy if systemic toxicity/unable to tolerate PO

Discharge Criteria
No evidence of systemic toxicity with resolution of erythema and swelling

 ONGOING CARE

FOLLOW-UP RECOMMENDATIONS
Bed rest with elevation of extremity during acute infection, then activity as tolerated

Patient Monitoring
Patients should be treated until all symptoms and skin manifestations have resolved.

PATIENT EDUCATION
Stress importance of completing prescribed medication regimen

PROGNOSIS
- Patients should recover fully if adequately treated.
- May experience deepening of erythema after initiation of antibiotics
- Most respond to therapy after 24 to 48 hours.
- Mortality is <1% in patients receiving appropriate treatment.
- Bullae formation suggests longer disease course, and often indicates a concomitant *S. aureus* infection that may require antibiotic coverage for MRSA.

- Chronic edema/scarring may result from chronic recurrent cases.
- Rarely, obstructive lymphadenitis may result from chronic recurrent cases.

COMPLICATIONS
- Recurrent infection
- Abscess (suggests staphylococcal infection)
- Necrotizing fasciitis
- Lymphedema (most prominent risk factor for recurrence) (8)
- Bacteremia, which may lead to sepsis
- Pneumonia (due to sepsis/toxin-producing organism)
- Meningitis (due to sepsis/toxin-producing organism)
- Embolism
- Gangrene
- Bursitis, septic arthritis, tendinitis, or osteitis

REFERENCES
1. Gabillot-Carré M, Roujeau JC. Acute bacterial skin infections and cellulitis. *Curr Opin Infect Dis.* 2007;20(2):118–123.
2. Bernard P. Management of common bacterial infections of the skin. *Curr Opin Infect Dis.* 2008;21(2):122–128.
3. Celestin R, Brown J, Kihiczak G, et al. Erysipelas: a common potentially dangerous infection. *Acta Dermatovenerol Alp Pannonica Adriat.* 2007;16(3):123–127.
4. Stevens DL, Bisno AL, Chambers HF, et al. Practice guidelines for the diagnosis and management of skin and soft-tissue infections. *Clin Infect Dis.* 2005;41(10):1373–1406.
5. Breen JO. Skin and soft tissue infections in immunocompetent patients. *Am Fam Physician.* 2010;81(7): 893–899.
6. Morris AD. Cellulitis and erysipelas. *BMJ Clin Evid.* 2008;2008:1708.
7. Bergkvist PI, Sjöbeck K. Antibiotic and prednisolone therapy of erysipelas: a randomized, double blind, placebo-controlled study. *Scand J Infect Dis.* 1997;29(4):377–382.
8. Inghammar M, Rasmussen M, Linder A. Recurrent erysipelas—risk factors and clinical presentation. *BMC Infect Dis.* 2014;14:270.

ADDITIONAL READING
Gilbert D, Chambers HF, Eliopoulos GM, et al, eds. *The Sanford Guide to Antimicrobial Therapy.* 44th ed. Sperryville, VA: Sanford Guides; 2014.

 CODES

ICD10
A46 Erysipelas

CLINICAL PEARLS
- Athlete's foot is the most common portal of entry.
- Erysipelas is distinguished from cellulitis by its sharp, shiny, fiery-red, raised border.
- In recurrent cases, search for other possible source of streptococcal infection (e.g., tonsils, sinuses, intertrigo).
- Most erysipelas infections now occur on the legs, rather than the face.

ERYTHEMA MULTIFORME

Tyler S. Rogers, MD • John Scott Earwood, MD

 BASICS

- Erythema multiforme (EM) is relatively common, acute, reccurent, self-limiting inflammatory disease.
  - Mostly (~90% of cases) triggered by infectious agents (up to 50% by herpes simplex virus [HSV]-1 or -2), or less commonly, by drugs and vaccinations (1,2)
  - Skin lesions include acrally distributed, distinct targetoid lesions with concentric color variation, sometimes accompanied by oral, genital, or ocular mucosal lesions (1,3).
  - Flat, atypical lesions and macules with or without blisters are more suggestive of Stevens-Johnson syndrome (SJS) or toxic epidermal necrolysis (TEN) (4,5,6).
- There is no universal diagnostic criteria, but clinical history, clinical examination, skin biopsy, laboratory studies, and special consideration of persistent EM are all included in making a diagnosis.

DESCRIPTION
- Two subtypes, erythema multiforme minor (EMm) and erythema multiforme major (EMM), with the former involving none or one mucous membrane, and the latter involving at least two mucous membrane sites. EMM is now separate from SJS and TEN (4).
- Recurrent EM is defined as >3 attacks but has a mean number of 6 attacks (range 2 to 24) per year and a mean duration of 6 to 9.5 years (range 2 to 36) (1).

EPIDEMIOLOGY
Incidence
Annual U.S. incidence is estimated at 0.01–1% (1).
Prevalence
- Peak incidence in 20s and 40s; rare <3 years and >50 years of age (4)
- Male > female (3:2 to 2:1)

ETIOLOGY AND PATHOPHYSIOLOGY
- The exact pathophysiology of EM is incompletely understood but appears to be the result of a TH1-mediated immune reponse to an inciting event such as infection or drug exposure.
- Genetic susceptibility can be a predisposing factor in some patients with EM. Different HLA alleles have been found to be consistent in patients with EM.
- HSV containing a certain *HSV pol*, a polymerase associated with the HSV-triggered EM seems to involve autoimmune activation (1)
- With electron microscopy, there is evidence of lichenoid inflammatory infiltrate and epidermal necrosis including circulating immune complexes, deposition of C3, IgM, and fibrin around the upper dermal blood vessels.
- SJS and TEN have an increased granulysin and perforin expression within T cells than in EM (5,6).
- Previous viral infections, particularly; also Epstein-Barr, coxsackie, echovirus, varicella, mumps, poliovirus, hepatitis C, cytomegalovirus, HIV, molluscum contagiosum virus (1)
- Bacterial infections, particularly *M. pneumoniae;* other reported bacterial infections include *Treponema pallidum* and *Gardnerella vaginalis* (1)

- Medications, including NSAIDs, antibiotics, sulfonamides, and antiepileptics (1,3)
- Vaccines: stronger association with HPV, MMR, and small pox vaccines, but also associated with hepatitis B, meningococcal, pneumococcal, varicella, influenza, diphtheria-pertussis-tetanus, and *H. influenzae* (2,7)
- Occupational exposures: herbicides (alachlor and butachlor), iodoacetonitrile
- Radiation therapy
- Premenstrual hormone changes (3)
- Malignancy (3)

Genetics
Strong association with HLA-DQB10301, particularly in herpes-related cases (1); possible association in recurrent cases with HLA-B35, -B62, -DR53

RISK FACTORS
Previous history of EM

GENERAL PREVENTION
- Known or suspected etiologic agents should be avoided.
- Acyclovir or valacyclovir may help prevent herpes-related recurrent EM.

COMMONLY ASSOCIATED CONDITIONS
See "Etiology and Pathophysiology" earlier.

 DIAGNOSIS

Clinical

HISTORY
- Absent or mild prodromal symptoms
- Acute, self-limiting, episodic course
- History of new medication
- Preceding HSV infection 10 to 15 days before the skin eruptions
- Rash involving the skin and sometimes the mucous membrane, most commonly the mouth.
- Symptoms of any of the infections associated with EM, most commonly HSV and *Mycoplasma pneumoniae*

PHYSICAL EXAM
- Acral extremities
- Symmetric cutaneous eruptions composed of targetoid lesions with concentric color variation.
- Mucosal involvement
  - Oral involvement manifest as erythema, erosions, bullae, and ulcerations on both nonkeratinized and keratinized mucosal surfaces and on the vermilion of the lips. Minimal involvement in EMm, if present, most commonly involves the mouth.
  - Can include any mucosal tissue including genital, ocular, oral, and so forth
  - At least two mucosal sites involved in EMM, including eyes (conjunctivitis, keratitis); mouth (stomatitis, cheilitis, characteristic blood-stained crusted erosions on lips); and probable trachea, bronchi, GI tract, or genital tract (balanitis and vulvitis) (6)

DIFFERENTIAL DIAGNOSIS
- SJS
  - Generalized distribution of lesions; concentrated on the trunk
  - Macular atypical targetoid lesions
  - Flat target lesions or macules with coalescence of lesions
  - Blisters and skin detachment <10% of the total body surface area (6)
  - 1–5% mortality (4)
  - Presence of constitutional symptoms with presence of high fever (>38.5°C) more likely with SJS than EM
  - More likely to have mucosal involvement at ≥2 sites, lymphadenopathy, high C-reactive protein levels (>10 mg/dL), and hepatic dysfunction, and >90% have severe mucosal involvement at least at one site (1)
- TEN
  - Similar to SJS but has full-thickness skin necrosis and skin detachment >30% of the total body surface area (6,8)
  - 34–40% mortality rate (4)
- Urticaria
- Fixed drug eruption
- Bullous pemphigoid
- Paraneoplastic pemphigoid
- Sweet syndrome
- Rowell syndrome
- Polymorphus light eruption
- Cutaneous small-vessel vasculitis
- Mucocutaneous lymph node syndrome
- Erythema annulare centrifugum
- Acute hemorrhagic edema of infancy
- Subacute cutaneous lupus erythematosus
- Contact dermatitis
- Pityriasis rosea
- HSV
- Secondary syphilis
- Tinea corporis
- Dermatitis herpetiformis
- Herpes gestationis
- Septicemia
- Serum sickness
- Viral exanthem
- Rocky Mountain spotted fever
- Meningococcemia
- Lichen planus
- Behçet syndrome
- Recurrent aphthous ulcers
- Herpetic gingivostomatitis
- Granuloma annulare

DIAGNOSTIC TESTS & INTERPRETATION
- No lab test is indicated to make the diagnosis of EM (1,4,9).
- Skin biopsy of lesional and perilesional tissue in equivocal conditions
- Direct and indirect immunofluorescence (DIF and IIF) to differentiate EM from other vesiculobullous diseases. DIF is detected on a biopsy of perilesional skin, and IIF is detected from a blood sample (1).
- HSV tests in recurrent EM (serologic tests, swab culture, or tests using skin biopsy sample to check HSV antigens or DNA in keratinocytes by DIF or direct fluorescent antibody [DFA] or polymerase chain reaction [PCR])
- Antibody staining to IFN-γ and TNF-α to differentiate HSV from drug-associated EM
- As the second most common cause of EM, *M. pneumoniae* should be worked up with CXR, swabs, and serologic test.
- In persistent EM, check complement levels (1).

Initial Tests (lab, imaging)
No imaging studies are indicated in most cases unless there is suspicion for *M. pneumoniae*.

Follow-Up Tests & Special Considerations
Chest x-ray may be necessary if an underlying pulmonary infection (*M. pneumoniae*) is suspected.

Test Interpretation
- Vacuolar interface dermatitis with CD4+ T lymphocytes and histiocytes in papillary dermis and the dermal–epidermal junction
- Superficial perivascular lymphocytic inflammation
- Satellite cell necrosis
- Necrotic keratinocytes mainly in the basal layer
- Papillary dermal edema

 TREATMENT

GENERAL MEASURES
- Step 1 DISCONTINUE OR TREAT INCITING FACTOR (1,4,9)
- Wound care for severe cases with epidermal detachment.
- Oral lesions should be addressed to insure maintenance of PO intake. This can include oral anesthetic solutions and antiseptic rinses.

MEDICATION
- Acute EM
  - Discontinuation of inciting factors and treatment of underlying disease (1,4,9)[B]
  - Symptomatic treatment with oral antihistamines and topical (1)[B]
  - HSV-induced EM: Most recent sources report no proven effect on the course of EM using antivirals with acute mild EM (1,9)[B]
  - *M. pneumoniae*-associated EM may require antibiotics.
- Mucosal membrane EM
  - Consider high-potency topical corticosteroid gel, oral antiseptic, and oral anesthetic solutions if mild.
  - If more severe, consider prednisone 40 to 60 mg/day with dosage tapered over 2 to 4 weeks (1)[B].
  - Ophthalmology consultation is imperative for ocular involvement (4)[A].

- Recurrent EM
  - First-line treatment for HSV-associated and idiopathic recurrent EM is antiviral prophylaxis; 12 to 24 months of prophylaxis is most effective (1,10)[B].
  - Therapy includes acyclovir 400 mg BID, valacyclovir 500 mg BID, famciclovir 250 mg BID (1)[B]
  - Second-line therapy includes dapsone (100 to 150 mg/day), azathioprine (Imuran, 100 to 150 mg/day), thalidomide (100 to 200 mg/day), tacrolimus (0.1% ointment daily), mycophenolate mofetil (CellCept 1,000 to 1,500 mg BID), hydroxychloroquine (400 mg/day) (1)[B]

INPATIENT CONSIDERATIONS
Admission Criteria/Initial Stabilization
- Care at home
- Hospitalization needed for fluid and electrolyte management in patient with severe mucous membrane involvement, impaired oral intake, and dehydration
- IV antibiotics if secondary infection develops

 ONGOING CARE

FOLLOW-UP RECOMMENDATIONS
Patient Monitoring
- The disease is self-limiting.
- Complications are rare, with no mortality.

DIET
As tolerated, with increased fluid intake

PATIENT EDUCATION
- The disease is self-limiting. However, the recurrence risk may be 30%.
- Avoid any identified etiologic agents.

PROGNOSIS
- Rash evolves over 1 to 2 weeks and subsequently resolves within 2 to 6 weeks, generally without scarring or sequelae.
- Following resolution, there may be some postinflammatory hyper- or hypopigmentation.

COMPLICATIONS
Secondary infection

REFERENCES

1. Sokumbi O, Wetter DA. Clinical features, diagnosis, and treatment of erythema multiforme: a review for the practicing dermatologist. *Int J Dermatol*. 2012;51(8):889–902.
2. Rosenblatt AE, Stein SL. Cutaneous reactions to vaccinations. *Clinical Dermatology*. 2015;33(3):327–332.
3. Levin J, Hofstra T. Recurrent erythema multiforme. *JAMA*. 2014;312(4):426–427.
4. Habif TP. Erythema multiforme. *Clinical Dermatology*. 5th ed. St. Louis, MO: Mosby-Elsevier; 2010:710–714.
5. Iwai S, Sueki H, Watanabe H, et al. Distinguishing between erythema multiforme major and Stevens-Johnson syndrome/toxic epidermal necrolysis immunopathologically. *J Dermatol*. 2012;39(9):781–786.
6. Scwartz RA, McDonough PH, Lee BW. Toxic epidermal necrolysis: part I. Introduction, history, classification, clinical features, systemic manifestations, etiology, and immunopathogenesis. *J Am Acad Dermatol*. 2013;69(2):173.e1–173.e13.
7. Storie EB, Perry A. Erythema multiforme following smallpox vaccination. *Mil Med*. 2014;179(1):e113–e115.
8. Scwartz RA, McDonough PH, Lee BW. Toxic epidermal necrolysis: part II. Prognosis, sequelae, diagnosis, differential diagnosis, prevention, and treatment. *J Am Acad Dermatol*. 2013;69(2):187.e1–187.e16.
9. Sola CA, Beute TC. Erythema multiforme. *J Spec Oper Med*. 2014;14(3):90–92.
10. Wetter DA, Davis MD. Recurrent erythema multiforme: clinical characteristics, etiologic associations, and treatment in a series of 48 patients at Mayo Clinic, 2000 to 2007. *J Am Acad Dermatol*. 2010;62(1):45–53.

 SEE ALSO

Cutaneous Drug Reactions; Dermatitis Herpetiformis; Pemphigoid Gestationis; Stevens-Johnson Syndrome; Toxic Epidermal Necrolysis; Urticaria

 CODES

ICD10
- L51.9 Erythema multiforme, unspecified
- L51.8 Other erythema multiforme
- L51.0 Nonbullous erythema multiforme

CLINICAL PEARLS
- EM is diagnosed clinically by careful review of the history, thorough detailed physical exam, and by excluding other similar disorders. No lab tests are required for the diagnosis.
- Typical lesions are characteristic targetoid or "iris" lesions but can include raised targetoids.
- Lesions are symmetrically distributed on palms, soles, dorsum of the hands, and extensor surfaces of extremities and face. The oral mucosa is the most affected mucosal region in EM.
- Management of EM involves determining the etiology when possible. The first step is to treat the suspected infection or discontinue the causative drug.
- Complications are rare. Most cases are self-limited. However, the recurrence risk may be as high as 30%.
- Recurrent cases often are secondary to HSV infection. Antiviral therapy may be beneficial.

ERYTHEMA NODOSUM

Faruq Pradhan, MBBCh • Fredric D. Gordon, MD, AGAF

 BASICS

DESCRIPTION
- A delayed-type hypersensitivity reaction to various antigens, or an autoimmune reaction presenting as a panniculitis that affects subcutaneous fat
- Clinical pattern of multiple, bilateral, erythematous, tender nodules in a typically pretibial distribution that undergo a characteristic pattern of color changes, similar to that seen in bruises. Unlike erythema induratum, the lesions of erythema nodosum (EN) do not typically ulcerate.
- Occurs most commonly on the shins; less commonly on the thighs, forearms, trunk, head, or neck
- Often associated with nonspecific prodrome including fever, weight loss, and arthralgia
- Often idiopathic but may be associated with a number of clinical entities
- Usually remits spontaneously in weeks to months without scarring, atrophy, or ulceration
- Uncommon to have recurrences after initial presentation

Pregnancy Considerations
May have repeat outbreaks during pregnancy

Pediatric Considerations
Rare pediatric variant has lesions only on palms or soles, often unilateral. Typically has a shorter duration in children than adults.

EPIDEMIOLOGY
Incidence
- 1 to 5/100,000/year
- Predominant age: 20 to 30 years
- Predominant sex: female > male (6:1) in adults

Prevalence
Varies geographically depending on the prevalence of disorders associated with EN

ETIOLOGY AND PATHOPHYSIOLOGY
- Idiopathic: up to 55%
- Infectious: 44%. Streptococcal pharyngitis (most common), mycobacteria, mycoplasma, chlamydia, mycoplasma, coccidiodomycosis, rarely can be caused by *Campylobacter* spp., ricketssiae, *Salmonella* spp., psittacosis, syphilis
- Sarcoidosis: 11–25%
- Drugs: 3–10%. Sulfonamides, amoxicillin, oral contraceptives, bromides, azathioprine, vemurafenib

- Pregnancy: 2–5%,
- Enteropathies: 1–4%. Ulcerative colitis, Crohn disease, Behçet disease, celiac disease, diverticulitis
- Rare causes: <1% (1)
  - Fungal: dermatophytes, coccidioidomycosis, histoplasmosis, blastomycosis
  - Viral/chlamydial: infectious mononucleosis, lymphogranuloma venereum, paravaccinia, HIV
  - Malignancies: lymphoma/leukemia, sarcoma, myelodysplastic syndrome
  - Sweet syndrome

RISK FACTORS
See "Etiology and Pathophysiology."

COMMONLY ASSOCIATED CONDITIONS
See "Etiology and Pathophysiology."

 DIAGNOSIS

HISTORY
- Often a prodrome 1 to 3 weeks prior to onset of lesions; can consist of malaise, fever, weight loss, cough, and arthralgia
- Increasingly tender nodules on the legs, usually over the shins
- Fever, malaise, chills, fatigue
- Headache
- Can precede systemic process by weeks

PHYSICAL EXAM
- Lesions initially present as warm, tender, erythematous firm nodules and become fluctuant, gradually fading to resemble a bruise over 1 to 2 months (erythema contusiformis).
- Typically pretibial, although can extend proximally to involve thighs or trunk (atypically can involve extensor surface of forearms)
- Diameter varies from 1 to 10 cm with poor demarcation.

DIFFERENTIAL DIAGNOSIS
- Nodular vasculitis or erythema induratum (warm ulcerating calf nodules)
- Superficial thrombophlebitis
- Cellulitis
- Weber-Christian disease (violaceous, scarring nodules)
- Lupus panniculitis
- Cutaneous polyarteritis nodosa

- Sarcoidal granulomas
- Cutaneous T-cell lymphoma
- EN leprosum (clinically similar to EN but shows vasculitis on histopathology)
- Subcutaneous infection (including staphylococcus, *Sporothrix schenckii*, *Nocardia brasiliensis*, *Mycobacterium marinum*, *Leishmania braziliensis*)

DIAGNOSTIC TESTS & INTERPRETATION
Diagnosis is made clinically, with support of testing
- ESR or C-reactive protein (CRP): often elevated, but can be normal in up to 40% (2)[C]
- CBC: mild leukocytosis (2)[C]
- Urine pregnancy test (2)[C]
- Throat culture, antistreptolysin O titer (2)[C]
- Blood and/or stool culture, stool ova and parasites (O&P)
- Tuberculin skin testing (2)[C]
- Seronegative rheumatoid factor

Initial Tests (lab, imaging)
CXR for hilar adenopathy or infiltrates related to sarcoidosis or tuberculosis (2)[C]

Diagnostic Procedures/Other
Deep-incisional or excisional skin biopsy including subcutaneous tissue; rarely necessary except in atypical cases with ulceration, duration >12 weeks, or absence of nodules overlying lower limbs (3)[C]

Test Interpretation
- Septal panniculitis without vasculitis
- Neutrophilic infiltrate in septa of fat tissue early in course
- Actinic radial (Miescher) granulomas, consisting of collections of histocytes around a central stellate cleft, may be seen.
- Fibrosis, paraseptal granulation tissue, lymphocytes, and multinucleated giant cells predominate late in course (4).

 TREATMENT

- Condition usually self-limited within 1 to 2 months
- All medications listed as treatment for EN are off-label uses of the medications. There are no specific FDA-approved medications.

GENERAL MEASURES
- Mild compression bandages and leg elevation may reduce pain. (Wet dressings, hot soaks, and topical medications are not useful.)
- Discontinue potentially causative drugs.
- Treat underlying disease.
- Indication for treatment is poorly defined in literature; hence, therapy specifically for EN is directed towards symptom management.

MEDICATION

First Line
- NSAIDs:
  - Ibuprofen 400 mg PO q4–6h (not to exceed 3,200 mg/day)
  - Indomethacin 25 to 50 mg PO TID
  - Naproxen 250 to 500 mg PO BID
- Precautions
  - GI upset/bleeding (avoid in Crohn or ulcerative colitis)
  - Fluid retention
  - Renal insufficiency
  - Dose reduction in elderly, especially those with renal disease, diabetes, or heart failure
  - May mask fever
  - NSAIDs can increase cardiovascular (CV) risk.
- Significant possible interactions
  - May blunt antihypertensive effects of diuretics and β-blockers
  - NSAIDs can elevate plasma lithium levels.
  - NSAIDs can cause significant elevation and prolongation of methotrexate levels.

Second Line
- Potassium iodide 400 to 900 mg/day divided BID or TID for 3 to 4 weeks (for persistent lesions); need to monitor for hyperthyroidism with prolonged use; pregnancy class D (5)[B]

- Corticosteroids for severe, refractory, or recurrent cases in which an infectious workup is negative. Prednisone 1 mg/kg/day for 1 to 2 weeks is the recommended dose/duration. Potential side effects include hyperglycemia, hypertension, weight gain, worsening gastroesophageal reflux disease, mood changes, bone loss, osteonecrosis, and proximal myopathy (1)

- For EN related to Behçet disease, one can also consider colchicine 0.6 to 1.2 mg BID. Potential side effects include GI upset and diarrhea (6)[B].

INPATIENT CONSIDERATIONS

Admission Criteria/Initial Stabilization
Occasionally, admission may be needed for the antecedent illness (e.g., tuberculosis).

ONGOING CARE

FOLLOW-UP RECOMMENDATIONS
- Keep legs elevated
- Elastic wraps or support stockings may be helpful when patients are ambulating.

Patient Monitoring
Monthly follow-up or as dictated by underlying disorder

DIET
No restrictions

PATIENT EDUCATION
- Lesions will resolve over a few weeks to months
- Scarring is unlikely.
- Joint aches and pains may persist.
- <20% recur

PROGNOSIS
- Individual lesions resolve generally within 2 weeks.
- Total time course of 6 to 12 weeks but may vary with underlying disease.
- Joint aches and pains may persist for years.
- Lesions do not scar.
- Recurrences: occurs over variable periods, averaging several years; seen most often in sarcoid, streptococcal infection, pregnancy, and oral contraceptive use. If medication induced, avoid recurrent exposure.

COMPLICATIONS
- Vary according to underlying disease
- None expected from lesions of EN

REFERENCES
1. Schwartz RA, Nervi SJ. Erythema nodosum: a sign of systemic disease. *Am Fam Physician*. 2007;75(5):695–700.
2. Cribier B, Caille A, Heid E, et al. Erythema nodosum and associated diseases. A study of 129 cases. *Int J Dermatol*. 1998;37(9):667–672.
3. Requena L, Yus ES. Erythema nodosum. *Dermatol Clin*. 2008;26(4):425–438.
4. Sánchez Yus E, Sanz Vico MD, de Diego V. Miescher's radial granuloma. A characteristic marker of erythema nodosum. *Am J Dermatopathol*. 1989;11(5):434–442.
5. Horio T, Imamura S, Danno K, et al. Potassium iodide in the treatment of erythema nodosum and nodular vasculitis. *Arch Dermatol*. 1981;117(1):29–31.
6. Yurdakul S, Mat C, Tüzün Y, et al. A double-blind trial of colchicine in Behçet's syndrome. *Arthritis Rheum*. 2001;44(11):2686–2692.

ADDITIONAL READING
- Bartyik K, Várkonyi A, Kirschner A, et al. Erythema nodosum in association with celiac disease. *Pediatr Dermatol*. 2004;21(3):227–230.
- Chong TA, Hansra NK, Ruben BS, et al. Diverticulitis: an inciting factor in erythema nodosum. *J Am Acad Dermatol*. 2012;67(1):e60–e62.
- Harris T, Henderson MC. Concurrent Sweet's syndrome and erythema nodosum. *J Gen Intern Med*. 2011;26(2):214–215.
- Jeon HC, Choi M, Paik SH, et al. A case of assisted reproductive therapy-induced erythema nodosum. *Ann Dermatol*. 2011;23(3):362–364.
- Schwartz RA, Nervi SJ. Erythema nodosum: a sign of systemic disease. *Am Fam Physician*. 2007;75(5):695–700.
- Then C, Langer A, Adam C, et al. Erythema nodosum associated with myelodysplastic syndrome: a case report. *Onkologie*. 2011;34(3):126–128.

CODES

ICD10
- L52 Erythema nodosum
- A18.4 Tuberculosis of skin and subcutaneous tissue

CLINICAL PEARLS
- Lesions of EN appear to be erythematous patches, but when palpated, their underlying nodularity is appreciated.
- Evaluation for a concerning underlying etiology is necessary in EN, but most cases are idiopathic.
- EN in the setting of hilar adenopathy may be seen with multiple etiologies and does not exclusively indicate sarcoidosis.
- In patients with a history of Hodgkin lymphoma, EN may be an early sign of recurrence.

ESOPHAGEAL VARICES
Edward Feller, MD, FACP, FACG

 BASICS

DESCRIPTION
- Dilated distal esophageal veins connecting the portal and systemic circulations
- Results from portal hypertension (most commonly due to liver cirrhosis), resistance to portal blood flow, and increased portal venous blood inflow
- Superficial location of distal esophageal veins makes them susceptible to rupture.
- Esophageal variceal rupture: Most common fatal complication of cirrhosis; severity of liver disease correlates with presence of varices and risk of bleeding.

EPIDEMIOLOGY
Incidence
- At diagnosis, 30% of cirrhotic patients have varices; increases to 90% at 10 years (1).
- 1-year rate of first variceal bleeding is 5% for small varices, 15% for large varices.

Pediatric Considerations
Portal hypertension is common in chronic liver disease in children. No clear guidelines for screening; pharmacologic or endoscopic treatment are equivalent (2)[A].

Prevalence
- 50% of patients with esophageal varices will experience bleeding at some point.
- Variceal bleeding: 15–20% mortality in the following 6 weeks after the episode
- Gender: male > female

ETIOLOGY AND PATHOPHYSIOLOGY
- Fibrous tissue and regenerative nodules in cirrhosis lead to splanchnic arteriolar vasodilatation, increased portal inflow, and increased resistance to outflow resulting in portal hypertension. Increased production of endothelin-1 and decreased production of nitrous oxide causes intrahepatic vasoconstriction, with further reduction in flow (1).
- Portal hypertension: pressure gradient >10 mm Hg between the portal vein and inferior vena cava. Collateral vessels (varices) form to decompress portal circulation.
- Cirrhotic portal hypertension
  - >90% of cases due to alcohol and HCV
  - Less common: hemochromatosis, hepatitis B, nonalcoholic fatty liver disease, primary biliary cirrhosis and autoimmune cirrhosis
- Noncirrhotic portal hypertension
  - Extrahepatic portal or splenic vein thrombosis, trauma, chronic pancreatitis, thrombotic disease, polycythemia
  - Metastasis to liver sinusoids/portal vein: lymphoma, leukemia, hepatoma, or other carcinomas
  - Metabolic disease altering liver sinusoids: amyloidosis, Gaucher disease, Budd-Chiari syndrome, veno-occlusive disease

Genetics
Cirrhosis is rarely hereditary.

RISK FACTORS
- Cirrhosis due to any cause
- In cirrhotic patients, thrombocytopenia and splenomegaly, correlated with portal hypertension, are independent predictors of esophageal varices.
- Noncirrhotic portal hypertension

- Increased bleeding risk in known varices include varix size and endoscopic signs (red wale marks, cherry-red spots); vessel wall thickness; abrupt increase in variceal pressure (i.e., Valsalva maneuver)
- MELD/Child-Pugh score; presence of portal vein thrombosis; high hepatic venous pressure gradient [HVPG]

GENERAL PREVENTION
- Prevent underlying causes: alcoholism, hepatitis B vaccine, needle hygiene, detox in IV drug use (IVDU) to avoid HCV exposure; specific screening and therapy for hepatitis B and C, hemochromatosis (1)
- See "Treatment" for prevention of first and second bleeds.

COMMONLY ASSOCIATED CONDITIONS
- Portal hypertensive gastropathy; varices in stomach, duodenum, colon, rectum (causes massive bleeding, unlike hemorrhoids); rarely at umbilicus (caput medusa) or ostomy sites
- Isolated gastric varices can occur due to splenic vein thrombosis/stenosis from hypercoagulability/contiguous inflammation (most commonly, chronic pancreatitis). Tumors can compress/infiltrate the splenic vein leading to pressure increase in short gastric veins. Signs of portal hypertension or esophageal varices may be absent (3).
- Other complications of cirrhosis: hepatic encephalopathy, ascites, hepatorenal syndrome, spontaneous bacterial peritonitis, hepatocellular carcinoma

DIAGNOSIS

- First indication of varices often associated with GI bleeding episode: painless hematemesis, hematochezia, and/or melena
- Occult bleeding (anemia): uncommon

HISTORY
- Underlying history of cirrhosis/liver disease. Variceal bleed can be initial presentation of previously undiagnosed cirrhosis.
- Alcoholism, exposure to blood-borne viruses
- Hematemesis, melena, or hematochezia
- Rapid upper GI bleed can present as rectal bleeding.

PHYSICAL EXAM
- Assess hemodynamic stability: hypotension, tachycardia (active bleeding).
- Assess airway integrity.
- Abdominal exam—liver palpation/percussion (often small and firm with cirrhosis)
- Splenomegaly, ascites (shifting dullness; puddle splash)
- Visible abdominal periumbilical collateral circulation (caput medusae)
- Peripheral stigmata of alcoholism: spider angiomata on chest/back, palmar erythema, testicular atrophy, gynecomastia
- Anal varices (which collapse with digital pressure, whereas hemorrhoids do not)
- Hepatic encephalopathy; asterixis
- Blood on rectal exam

DIFFERENTIAL DIAGNOSIS
- Upper GI bleeding: 10–30% are due to varices.
  - In patients with known varices, as many as 50% bleed from nonvariceal sources.
  - Peptic ulcer; gastritis
  - Gastric/esophageal malignancy
  - Congestive gastropathy of portal hypertension
  - Arteriovenous malformation
  - Mallory-Weiss tears
  - Aortoenteric fistula
  - Hemoptysis; nosebleed
- Lower GI bleeding
  - Rectal varices; hemorrhoids
  - Colonic neoplasia
  - Diverticulosis/arteriovenous malformation
  - Rapidly bleeding upper GI site
- Continued/recurrent bleeding risk: actively bleeding/large varix, high Childs-Pugh severity score, infection, renal failure

DIAGNOSTIC TESTS & INTERPRETATION
Initial Tests (lab, imaging)
- Anemia: Hemoglobin may be normal in active bleeding; may require 6 to 24 hours to equilibrate; other causes of anemia are common in cirrhotics.
- Thrombocytopenia: most sensitive and specific lab parameter, correlates with portal hypertension, large esophageal varices
- Abnormal aspartate aminotransferase (AST), alanine aminotransferase (ALT), alkaline phosphatase, bilirubin; prolonged PT, low albumin suggest cirrhosis (4).
- BUN, creatinine (BUN often elevated in GI bleed)
- Esophagogastroduodenoscopy (3)[A]

  - Can identify actively bleeding varices as well as large varices and stigmata of recent bleeding
  - Can treat bleeding with esophageal band ligation (preferred to sclerotherapy); prevent rebleeding; detect gastric varices, portal hypertensive gastropathy; diagnose alternative bleeding sites
  - Can identify and treat nonbleeding varices appearing as protruding submucosal veins in the distal third of the esophagus

Diagnostic Procedures/Other
- HVPG >10 mm Hg: significant portal hypertension (normal: 1 to 5 mm Hg) (3)[A]

- Video capsule endoscopy screening: may be an alternative for those unwilling to undergo screening endoscopy
- Doppler sonography (second line): demonstrates patency, diameter, and flow in portal and splenic veins, and collaterals; very sensitive for gastric varices; documents patency after ligation or transjugular intrahepatic portosystemic shunt (TIPS).
- MRI (second line, not routine): demonstrates large vascular channels in abdomen, mediastinum; demonstrates patency of intrahepatic portal and splenic vein
  - Venous-phase celiac arteriography: demonstrates portal vein and collaterals; diagnoses hepatic vein occlusion
  - Portal pressure measurement using retrograde catheter in hepatic vein

TREATMENT

GENERAL MEASURES
- Treat underlying comorbidities related to cirrhosis.
- Variceal bleeding is often complicated by hepatic encephalopathy and infection.

- Active bleeding (5)[A]
  - IV access, hemodynamic resuscitation
  - Type and crossmatch packed RBCs. Overtransfusion increases portal pressure and increases rebleeding risk.
  - Treat coagulopathy as necessary. Fresh frozen plasma may increase blood volume and increase rebleeding risk.
  - Avoid sedation, monitor mental status, and avoid nephrotoxic drugs and β-blockers acutely.
  - Thiamine replacement as indicated, monitor blood glucose, risk for alcohol withdrawal, and delirium tremens
  - IV octreotide to lower portal venous pressure as adjuvant to endoscopic management. IV bolus of 50 μg followed by drip of 50 μg/hr.
  - Terlipressin (alternative): 2 mg q4h IV for 24 to 48 hours, then 1 mg q4h
  - Urgent upper GI endoscopy for diagnosis and treatment
    - Variceal band ligation preferred to sclerotherapy for bleeding varices. Also for nonbleeding medium-to-large varices to decrease bleeding risk
    - Ligation: lower rates of rebleeding, fewer complications, more rapid cessation of bleeding, higher rate of variceal eradication
- Repeat ligation/sclerosant for rebleeding.
- If endoscopic treatment fails to stop bleeding, consider per oral placement of Sengstaken-Blakemore-type tube to stabilize patient for TIPS.
- As many as 2/3 of patients with variceal bleeding develop an infection, most commonly spontaneous bacterial peritonitis, UTI, or pneumonia. Antibiotic prophylaxis with oral norfloxacin 400 mg or IV ceftriaxone 1 g q12h for up to a week.
- In active bleeding, avoid β-blockers, which decrease BP and blunt the physiologic increase in heart rate during acute hemorrhage.
- Prevent recurrence of acute bleeding
  - Vasoconstrictors: terlipressin, octreotide (reduce portal pressure)
  - Endoscopic band ligation (EBL): if bleeding recurs/portal pressure measurement shows portal pressure remains >12 mm Hg
  - TIPS: Second-line therapy if above methods fail; TIPS decreases portal pressure by creating communication between hepatic vein and an intrahepatic portal vein branch.

MEDICATION
Primary prevention of variceal bleeding (6)[A]

- Endoscopy: assesses variceal size, presence of red wale sign (longitudinal variceal reddish streak that suggests either a recent bleed or a pending bleed) to determine risk stratification
  - Endoscopy every 2 to 3 years if cirrhosis but no varices; every 1 to 2 years if small varices and not receiving β-blockers

First Line
- (Not actively bleeding). Nonselective β-blockers reduce portal pressure and decrease risk of first bleed from 25% to 15% in primary prophylaxis.

Used in cirrhosis with small varices and increased hemorrhage risk, as well as cirrhosis + medium-to-large varices (6)[A]

- Propranolol: 20 mg BID increase until heart rate decreased by 25% from baseline
- Nadolol 80 mg daily; increase as above
- Contraindications: severe asthma

- Chronic prevention of rebleeding (secondary prevention): Nonselective β-blockers and EBL reduce rate of rebleeding to a similar extent, but β-blockers reduce mortality, whereas ligation does not (7)[A].

Second Line
Obliteration of varices with esophageal banding for those intolerant of medication prophylaxis

- During ligation: proton pump inhibitors, such as lansoprazole 30 mg/day, until varices obliterated

ISSUES FOR REFERRAL
Referral considerations include endoscopy, liver transplantation, and interventional radiology for TIPS.

ADDITIONAL THERAPIES
Patients should receive pneumococcal vaccine and hepatitis A/B virus (HAV/HBV) vaccine.

SURGERY/OTHER PROCEDURES
- Esophageal transection: in rare cases of uncontrollable, exsanguinating bleeding
- Liver transplantation

INPATIENT CONSIDERATIONS
Admission Criteria/Initial Stabilization
Inpatient for acute bleeding and hemodynamic stabilization, therapeutic endoscopy. ICU care is the most appropriate initially.

Discharge Criteria
Bleeding cessation; hemodynamic stability and appropriate treatment plan for comorbidities

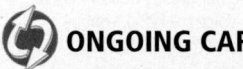 ONGOING CARE

FOLLOW-UP RECOMMENDATIONS
Patient Monitoring
- Close monitoring of vital signs.
- Endoscopic variceal ligation, repeated every 1 to 4 weeks until varices eradicated
- If TIPS, repeat endoscopy for rebleeding.
- Endoscopic screening in patients with known cirrhosis every 2 to 3 years; yearly in patients with decompensated cirrhosis

PATIENT EDUCATION
National Digestive Information Clearinghouse, (http://www.niddk.nih.gov/health-information/health-topics/digestive-diseases/Pages/default.aspx) or American Liver Foundation, (http://www.liverfoundation.org/)

PROGNOSIS
- Depends on underlying comorbidities
- In cirrhosis, 1-year survival is 50% for those surviving 2 weeks following a variceal bleed.
- In-hospital mortality remains high related to severity of underlying cirrhosis, ranging from 0% in Child A to 32% in Child C disease (5).
- Prognosis in noncirrhotic portal fibrosis is better than for cirrhotics.

COMPLICATIONS
- Formation of gastric varices or varices in other uncommon locations may occur after eradication of esophageal varices.

- Esophageal varices can recur.
- Hepatic encephalopathy, renal dysfunction, hepatorenal syndrome
- Infections are common after banding/ligation of varices.

REFERENCES
1. Asrani SK, Kamath PS. Natural history of cirrhosis. *Curr Gastroenterol Rep.* 2013;15(2):308.
2. Pinto RB, Schneider AC, da Silveira TR. Cirrhosis in children and adolescents: an overview. *World J Hepatol.* 2015;7(3):392–405.
3. de Franchis R, Dell'Era A. Invasive and noninvasive methods to diagnose portal hypertension and esophageal varices. *Clin Liver Dis.* 2014;18(2):293–302.
4. Woreta TA, Alqahtani SA. Evaluation of abnormal liver tests. *Med Clin North Am.* 2014;98(1):1–16.
5. Herrera JL. Management of acute variceal bleeding. *Clin Liver Dis.* 2014;18(2):347–357.
6. Simonetto DA, Shah VH, Kamath PS. Primary prophylaxis of variceal bleeding. *Clin Liver Dis.* 2014;18(2):335–345.
7. Albillos A, Tejedor M. Secondary prophylaxis for esophageal variceal bleeding. *Clin Liver Dis.* 2014;18(2):359–370.

ADDITIONAL READING
- Kochhar GS, Navaneethan U, Hartman J, et al. Comparative study of endoscopy vs. transjugular intrahepatic portosystemic shunt in management of gastric variceal bleeding. *Gastroenterol Rep (Oxf).* 2015;3(1):75–82.
- Zanetto A, Senzolo M, Ferrarese A, et al. Assessment of bleeding risk in patients with cirrhosis. *Curr Hepatol Rep.* 2015;14(1):9–18.

 SEE ALSO

Cirrhosis of the Liver; Portal Hypertension

 CODES

ICD10
- I85.00 Esophageal varices without bleeding
- I85.01 Esophageal varices with bleeding
- I85.10 Secondary esophageal varices without bleeding

CLINICAL PEARLS
- Cirrhosis is the most common underlying cause of esophageal variceal bleeding.
- In acute bleeding, avoid β-blockers, which decrease BP and blunt the physiologic increase in heart rate.
- In acute bleeding, overtransfusion can elevate portal pressure and increases bleeding risk.
- Thrombocytopenia is the most sensitive marker of increased portal pressure, large esophageal varices.
- During bleeding, consider antibiotic prophylaxis for spontaneous peritonitis and other infections with IV ciprofloxacin or oral norfloxacin for 7 to 10 days.

E

ESSENTIAL TREMOR SYNDROME

Jonathon M. Firnhaber, MD

 BASICS

DESCRIPTION
- A postural (occurring with voluntary maintenance of a position against gravity) or kinetic (occurring during voluntary movement) flexion–extension tremor that is slow and rhythmic and primarily affects the hands and forearms, head, and voice with a frequency of 4 to 12 Hz
- Older patients tend to have lower frequency tremors, whereas younger patients exhibit frequencies in the higher range.
- May be familial, sporadic, or associated with other movement disorders
- Can begin at any age but the incidence and prevalence increase with age
- The tremor can be exacerbated by emotional or physical stresses, fatigue, and caffeine.
- System(s) affected: neurologic, musculoskeletal, ear/nose/throat (ENT) (voice)

EPIDEMIOLOGY
Essential tremor is the most common pathologic tremor in humans.

Incidence
- Can occur at any age but bimodal peaks exist in the 2nd and 6th decades
- Incidence rises significantly after age 49 years.

Prevalence
The overall prevalence for essential tremor has been estimated between 0.4% and 0.9% but is increased in older (65 years) patients to 4.6% and in advanced age (95 years) up to 22% (1)[B].

ETIOLOGY AND PATHOPHYSIOLOGY
- Suspected to originate from an abnormal oscillation within thalamocortical and cerebello-olivary loops, as lesions in these areas tend to reduce essential tremor
- Essential tremor is not a homogenous disorder; many patients have other motor manifestations and nonmotor features, including cognitive and psychiatric symptoms.

Genetics
- Positive family history in 50–70% of patients; autosomal dominant inheritance is demonstrated in many families, but twin studies suggest that environmental factors are also involved.
- A link to genetic loci exists on chromosomes 2p22–2p25, 3q13, and 6p23. In addition, a Ser9Gly variant in the dopamine D_3 receptor gene on 3q13 has been suggested as a risk factor.

COMMONLY ASSOCIATED CONDITIONS
- Can be present in 10% of patients with Parkinson disease (PD); characteristics of PD that distinguish it from essential tremor include 3- to 5-Hz resting tremor; accompanying rigidity, bradykinesia, or postural instability; and no change with alcohol consumption.
- Patients with essential tremor have a 4% risk of developing PD. Although action tremors may precede PD, they will be diagnosed as essential tremor as long as the bradykinesia and rigidity of PD are not yet present (1)[B].
- Resting tremor, typically of the arm, may be seen in up to 20–30% of patients with essential tremor. Although action tremor is the hallmark feature of essential tremor, it is commonly found in patients with PD as well.

 DIAGNOSIS

HISTORY
- Core criteria for diagnosis
  - Bilateral (less likely unilateral) action (postural or kinetic) tremor of the hands and forearms that is most commonly asymmetric
  - Absence of other neurologic signs, with the exception of cogwheel phenomenon
  - May have isolated head tremor with no signs of dystonia
- Secondary criteria include long duration (>3 years), positive family history, and beneficial response to alcohol (2)[C].

PHYSICAL EXAM
- Tremor can affect upper limbs (~95% of patients).
- Less commonly, the tremor affects head (~34%), lower limbs (~30%), voice (~12%), tongue (~7%), face (~5%), and trunk (~5%).

DIFFERENTIAL DIAGNOSIS
- PD
- Wilson disease
- Hyperthyroidism
- Multiple sclerosis
- Dystonic tremor
- Cerebellar tremor
- Asterixis
- Psychogenic tremor
- Orthostatic tremor
- Drug-induced or enhanced physiologic tremor (amiodarone, cimetidine, lamotrigine, itraconazole, valproic acid, SSRIs, steroids, lithium, cyclosporine, β-adrenergic agonists, ephedrine, theophylline, tricyclic antidepressants [TCAs], antipsychotics) (3)[B].

DIAGNOSTIC TESTS & INTERPRETATION
Initial Tests (lab, imaging)
- No specific biologic marker or diagnostic test is available.
- Ceruloplasmin and serum copper to rule out Wilson disease
- Thyroid-stimulating hormone to rule out thyroid dysfunction
- Serum electrolytes, BUN, creatinine
- Brain MRI usually is not necessary or indicated unless Wilson disease is found or exam findings imply central lesion.

Diagnostic Procedures/Other
- Accelerometry evaluates tremor frequency and amplitude; >95% of PD cases exhibit frequencies in the 4- to 6-Hz range, and 95% of essential tremor cases exhibit frequencies in the 5- to 8-Hz range.
- Surface electromyography is less helpful in distinguishing essential tremor from PD.

Test Interpretation
Posture-related tremor

TREATMENT

MEDICATION
Pharmacologic treatment should be considered when tremor interferes with activities of daily living (ADLs) or causes psychological distress.

First Line
- Propranolol 60 to 320 mg/day in divided doses or in long-acting formulation reduces limb tremor magnitude by ~50%, and almost 70% of patients experience improvement in clinical rating scales. There is insufficient evidence to recommend propranolol for vocal tremor. Single doses of propranolol, taken before social situations that are likely to exacerbate tremor, are useful for some patients.
- Primidone 25 mg at bedtime, gradually titrated to 150 to 300 mg at bedtime, improves tremor amplitude by 40–50%. Maximum dose is 750 mg/day, with doses >250 mg/day typically divided to BID or TID. Low-dose therapy (<250 mg/day) is just as effective as high-dose (750 mg/day) therapy.
- Propranolol and primidone have similar efficacy when used as initial therapy for limb tremor; both carry a level A recommendation (4)[A].
- 30–50% of patients will not respond to either propranolol or primidone.

Second Line

- Topiramate at a mean dose of 292 mg/day demonstrated significantly greater reduction in tremor rating scale (TRS) compared with placebo (7.70 vs. 0.08; p <.005; baseline TRS = 37.0) in a small study combining results of three double-blind, randomized, controlled trials following a common protocol. Use is limited by dropout rates as high as 40% due to appetite suppression, weight loss, paresthesias, and concentration difficulties (5)[B].
- Gabapentin up to 400 mg TID
- Sotalol, nadolol, and atenolol are alternative β-blockers; each has less evidence than propranolol to support use.
- Clonazepam and alprazolam should be used with caution because of abuse potential.
- Clozapine has shown efficacy at doses of 6 to 75 mg/day but is recommended only for refractory cases of limb tremor because of a 1% risk of agranulocytosis. The American Academy of Neurology (AAN) indicates that insufficient evidence exists to support or refute the efficacy of clozapine for chronic use (4)[A].
- Memantine, in a pilot study using doses up to 40 mg/day, showed significant benefit in a small subset of the study group. Adverse events at this dose included dizziness, somnolence, and poor energy (6)[B].
- Pramipexole, at a dose of 2.1 mg/day, demonstrated moderate efficacy in reducing severity of tremor in a pilot study of 29 patients. Immediate- and extended-release formulations were equally effective (7)[B].
- Levetiracetam and 3,4-diaminopyridine are probably ineffective at reducing limb tremor and should not be considered according to the AAN (4)[A].
- Other medications that have been evaluated for treatment of essential tremor, with limited data to support their use, include acetazolamide, clonidine, flunarizine, methazolamide, nimodipine, olanzapine, phenobarbital, pregabalin, quetiapine, sodium oxybate, and zonisamide (4)[A].

- Alcohol may provide transient improvement in symptoms, but its brief duration of action, subsequent rebound, and associated risk of developing alcohol addiction make it a less attractive option for longer term treatment. Alcohol may be an appropriate option for short-term, situation-specific improvement in symptoms.

- Botulinum toxin A injections should be offered as a treatment option for cervical dystonia (level A recommendation from AAN) and may be offered for blepharospasm, focal upper extremity dystonia, adductor laryngeal dystonia, and upper extremity essential tremor. Limited data support its use for head and voice tremor (8)[B].

ISSUES FOR REFERRAL
Referral to a neurologist can help to differentiate those with dystonia, neuropathic tremor, PD, or drug-induced tremor.

SURGERY/OTHER PROCEDURES

- Deep brain stimulation provides a magnitude of benefit that is superior to all available medications and may be used to treat medically refractory limb tremor; it has fewer adverse effects than thalamotomy (9)[B].

- Bilateral thalamic stimulation is effective in reducing tremor and functional disability; however, dysarthria is a possible complication.
- Unilateral thalamotomy may be used to treat limb tremor that is refractory to medical management.
- Bilateral thalamotomy is not recommended because of adverse side effects.

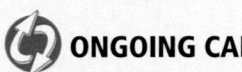 ONGOING CARE

DIET
Avoid caffeine.

PROGNOSIS
Tremor tends to worsen with age, increasing in amplitude.

REFERENCES

1. Elias WJ, Shah BB. Tremor. *JAMA*. 2014;311(9): 948–954.
2. Bain P, Brin M, Deuschl G, et al. Criteria for the diagnosis of essential tremor. *Neurology*. 2000;54 (11 Suppl 4):S7.
3. Zeuner KE, Deuschl G. An update on tremors. *Curr Opin Neurol*. 2012;25(4):475–482.
4. Zesiewicz TA, Elble RJ, Louis ED, et al. Evidence-based guideline update: treatment of essential tremor: report of the Quality Standards Subcommittee of the American Academy of Neurology. *Neurology*. 2011;77(19):1752–1755.
5. Connor GS, Edwards K, Tarsy D. Topiramate in essential tremor: findings from double-blind, placebo-controlled, crossover trials. *Clin Neuropharmacol*. 2008;31(2):97–103.
6. Handforth A, Bordelon Y, Frucht SJ, et al. A pilot efficacy and tolerability trial of memantine for essential tremor. *Clin Neuropharmacol*. 2010;33(5):223–226.
7. Herceg M, Nagy F, Pál E, et al. Pramipexole may be an effective treatment option in essential tremor. *Clin Neuropharmacol*. 2012;35(2):73–76.
8. Simpson DM, Blitzer A, Brashear A, et al. Assessment: botulinum neurotoxin for the treatment of movement disorders (an evidence-based review): report of the Therapeutics and Technology Assessment Subcommittee of the American Academy of Neurology. *Neurology*. 2008;70(19):1699–1706.
9. Flora ED, Perera CL, Cameron AL, et al. Deep brain stimulation for essential tremor: a systematic review. *Mov Disord*. 2010;25(11):1550–1559.

ADDITIONAL READING

- Buijink AW, Contarino MF, Koelman JH, et al. How to tackle tremor—systematic review of the literature and diagnostic work-up. *Front Neurol*. 2012;3:146.
- Deuschl G, Raethjen J, Hellriegel H, et al. Treatment of patients with essential tremor. *Lancet Neurol*. 2011;10(2):148–161.
- Sullivan KL, Hauser RA, Zesiewicz TA. Essential tremor. Epidemiology, diagnosis, and treatment. *Neurologist*. 2004;10(5):250–258.
- Thenganatt MA, Louis ED. Distinguishing essential tremor from Parkinson's disease: bedside tests and laboratory evaluations. *Expert Rev Neurother*. 2012;12(6):687–696.

 CODES

ICD10
G25.0 Essential tremor

CLINICAL PEARLS

- Core criteria for diagnosis of essential tremor include bilateral action (intention) tremor of the hands, forearm, and/or head without resting component.
- Beneficial response to alcohol and positive family history help to differentiate essential tremor from PD (PD is characterized by tremor at rest, bradykinesia, and rigidity, and it does not improve with alcohol use).
- 10% of patients with PD will have both resting tremors of PD and essential (intention) tremors.
- Wilson disease, thyroid disease, and medication effect should be ruled out.
- Brain MRI is usually not necessary or indicated.
- First-line treatments include propranolol and primidone.

EUSTACHIAN TUBE DYSFUNCTION
Adam W. Kowalski, MD • Vernon Wheeler, MD, FAAFP

 BASICS

DESCRIPTION
- Eustachian tube dysfunction (ETD) represents a spectrum of disorders involving an impairment in the functional valve of the eustachian tube of the middle ear.
- ETD can be classified as *patulous dysfunction*, in which the eustachian tube is excessively open, or *dilatory dysfunction*, in which there is failure of the tubes to dilate (i.e., open) appropriately.
- Pathophysiology is thought to be related to pressure dysregulation, impaired protection secondary to reflux of irritating material into the middle ear, or impaired clearance by the mucociliary system.
- May occur in the setting of pressure changes (e.g., scuba diving or air travel) or acute upper airway inflammation (e.g., allergic or infectious rhinosinusitis, acute otitis media)
- Chronic ETD may lead to a retracted tympanic membrane, recurrent serous effusion, recurrent otitis media (OM), adhesive OM, chronic mastoiditis, or cholesteatoma.
- System(s) affected: auditory
- Synonym(s): auditory tube dysfunction; eustachian tube disorder; blocked eustachian tube; patulous eustachian tube

ALERT
- Sudden sensorineural hearing loss (SSNHL) can be misdiagnosed as ETD.
- A simple 512-Hz tuning fork test lateralizes to the opposite ear in SSNHL and to the affected ear in ETD with conductive hearing loss.
- Any SSNHL is a medical emergency and should be referred to an otolaryngologist immediately.

EPIDEMIOLOGY
- Limited quality studies on epidemiology of ETD
- Most common in children <5 years of age, thought to be related to anatomical differences (see "Etiology and Pathophysiology" section)
- Usually decreases with age

Incidence
70% of children by age 7 years have experienced ETD.

Prevalence
- 1% of the adult population
- Males > females
- Highest prevalence among Native Americans, Inuits, Australian Aborigines, Hispanics, Africans

ETIOLOGY AND PATHOPHYSIOLOGY
- Under normal circumstances, the eustachian tube (ET) is closed but can open to release a small amount of air to equalize pressure between the middle ear and the surrounding atmosphere.
- ETD is failure of the ET, palate, nasal cavities, and nasopharynx to regulate middle ear and mastoid pressure.
- ET functions
  - Ventilation/regulation of middle ear pressure
  - Protection from nasopharyngeal secretions
  - Drainage of middle ear fluid
  - ET is closed at rest and opens with yawning, swallowing, and chewing.
- Cycle of dysfunction: Structural or functional obstruction of the ET compromises three functions
  - Negative pressure develops in middle ear.
  - Serous exudate is drawn from the middle ear by negative pressure or refluxed into the middle ear if the ET opens momentarily.

- Infection of static fluid causes edema and release of inflammatory mediators, which exacerbates cycle of inflammation and obstruction.
- In children, a horizontal and shorter ET predisposes to difficulties with ventilation and drainage.
- Adenoid hypertrophy can block the torus tubarius (proximal opening of the ET).
- In adults, paradoxical closing with swallowing has been noted in a majority of affected patients.
- Tumors that impair/occlude the ET proximally or distally, or that invade the tensor veli palatini and impair normal swallow regulation, can also lead to dysfunction.

Genetics
Twin studies show a genetic component. Specific genetic cause is still undefined.

RISK FACTORS
- Adult and pediatric
  - Allergic rhinitis, tobacco exposure, GERD, chronic sinusitis, adenoid hypertrophy or nasopharyngeal mass, neuromuscular disease, altered immunity
- Pediatric
  - In addition to the earlier mentioned, prematurity and low birth weight, young age, daycare, crowded living conditions, low socioeconomic status, prone sleeping position, prolonged bottle use, craniofacial abnormalities (e.g., cleft palate, Down syndrome)

Pregnancy Considerations
ETD may be exacerbated by rhinitis of pregnancy; symptoms resolve postpartum.

GENERAL PREVENTION
- Control sources of upper airway inflammation: allergies, infectious rhinosinusitis, GERD
- Autoinsufflation of middle ear (i.e., blow gently against pinched nostril and closed mouth)
- Avoid atmospheric pressure changes (e.g., plane flight, scuba diving) in the setting of acute allergy exacerbation or URI.
- Avoid exposure to environmental irritants: tobacco smoke and pollutants.

COMMONLY ASSOCIATED CONDITIONS
- Hearing loss
- OM: acute, chronic, and serous
- Chronic mastoiditis
- Cholesteatoma
- Allergic rhinitis
- Chronic sinusitis/URI
- Adenoid hypertrophy
- GERD
- Cleft palate
- Down syndrome
- Obesity
- Nasopharyngeal carcinoma or other tumor

 DIAGNOSIS

HISTORY
- Symptoms of ear pain, fullness, "plugging," hearing loss, tinnitus, popping or snapping noises, and vertigo are commonly seen with ETD.
- Other historical elements
  - Unilateral or bilateral. Adults presenting with persistent unilateral symptoms should be evaluated for nasopharyngeal process (tumor).

- History of previous ear infections, surgeries, head trauma, recent flying or diving
- Voice change (hypo- or hypernasal voice, consider NP mass or palatal dysfunction)
- Differentiate patulous dysfunction, in which patient's own voice and breath sounds are amplified (autophony), from dilatory dysfunction, in which patient complains more of ear pain, "plugged" ear, hearing loss, and tinnitus.

- ETDQ-7 is a new questionnaire to attempt to quantify ETD in adult patients. Based on presence and intensity of symptoms in past 1 month, severity is rated on 1 to 7 scale, with 1 indicating no problem and 7 indicating severe problems. A total score cutoff >14.5 categorizes patient as having diagnosis of ETD (1,2)[B]. Data is limited but promising. Questions:
  - Pressure in ears in past 1 month?
  - Pain in ears in past 1 month?
  - A feeling that ears are clogged or "under water"?
  - Ear symptoms when you have cold or sinusitis?
  - Crackling or popping sounds in the ears?
  - Ringing in ears?
  - A feeling that your hearing is muffled?

PHYSICAL EXAM
- Pneumatic otoscopy: retracted tympanic membrane, effusion, decreased drum movement
- Toynbee maneuver: view changes of the drum while patient autoinsufflates against closed lips and pinched nostrils; may show various degrees of retraction
  - Entire drum may be retracted and "lateralize" with insufflation.
  - Posterosuperior quadrant (pars flaccida) may form a retraction pocket.
- Tuning fork tests: 512-Hz fork placed on the forehead lateralizes to affected ear (Weber test); the fork will be louder behind the ear on the mastoid than in front of the ear (bone conduction > air conduction, Rinne test) in conductive hearing loss.
- Nasopharyngoscopy: adenoid hypertrophy or nasopharyngeal mass
- Anterior rhinoscopy: deviated nasal septum, polyps, mucosal hypertrophy, turbinate hypertrophy

DIFFERENTIAL DIAGNOSIS
- SSNHL (a medical emergency)
- Tympanic membrane perforation
- Barotrauma
- Temporomandibular joint disorder
- Ménière disease
- Superior semicircular canal dehiscence

DIAGNOSTIC TESTS & INTERPRETATION
Initial Tests (lab, imaging)
- Radiologic studies are not performed routinely if clinical signs/symptoms suggest ETD.
- CT scan (not necessary) may show changes related to OM or middle ear/mastoid opacification.
- Functional MRI might determine cause of ETD (in recalcitrant cases), as the ET opening can be visualized during Valsalva.

Diagnostic Procedures/Other
- Audiogram may show conductive hearing loss.
- Tympanometry: type B or C tympanograms indicate fluid or retraction, respectively. Negative middle ear peak pressures seen even with normal (type A) tympanograms.

TREATMENT

- Due to limited high-quality evidence, it is difficult to recommend any one treatment option/intervention as superior (3)[C].
- Use of a "nasal balloon" shown effective for clearing OM with effusion; unclear of benefit for ETD
- Generally, principle of treatment is to remove or fix the underlying cause (e.g., infection, tumor, perforation of TM, restore tensor palitini muscle, etc.) and hopefully end or at least reduce cycle of infection/inflammation.
- Although no evidence exists, some consider antibiotics for AOM; decongestants, nasal steroids, antihistamines (if allergic rhinitis is present), and surgery/procedures for recalcitrant cases
- Tympanostomy tubes ± adenoidectomy when indicated for recurrent ear infections or severe progressive retractions

MEDICATION

- Only when infection such as AOM is suspected as driving cause of ETD should antibiotics be given; large study giving antibiotics to children with OM with effusion showed no benefit (4)[A].
- Few data support pharmacologic treatments such as decongestants, nasal steroids, or antihistamines for ETD.
- Medication options are for treatment of comorbid conditions.
- Decongestants, topical, oral
  - Avoid prolonged use (>3 days); can cause rhinitis medicamentosa.
  - Decongestants are most useful for acute ETD related to a resolving URI.
  - Decongestants are not typically used for relief of chronic ETD in children.
    - Phenylephrine: adults and children ≥12 years of age, 1 tablet (10 mg) q4h PRN; children 6 to 11 years of age, 5 mg q4h PRN; children 4 to 5 years of age, 2.5 mg q4h PRN
    - Pseudoephedrine: adults, 60 mg q4–6h PRN; children 6 to 12 years of age, 30 mg q4–6h PRN; children 4 to 5 years of age, 15 mg q4–6h PRN
    - Oxymetazoline: adults and children ≥6 years of age, 1 to 2 sprays each nostril q12h PRN. Limit use to ≤3 days.
    - Phenylephrine: adults, 1 to 2 sprays each nostril q4h PRN. Limit use to ≤3 days.
- Nasal steroids (may be beneficial for those with allergic rhinitis) (5)[A]
  - Beclomethasone (Beconase, Vancenase): adults and children ≥12 years of age, 1 to 2 sprays each nostril BID; children 6 to 11 years of age, 1 spray each nostril BID. Not recommended for children <6 years of age
  - Budesonide (Rhinocort): adults and children ≥6 years of age, 1 spray each nostril daily
  - Ciclesonide (Omnaris) (a prodrug activated on nasal mucosa): adults and children ≥6 years of age, 2 sprays each nostril daily
  - Flunisolide (Nasarel, Nasalide): adults and children ≥6 years of age, 2 sprays each nostril BID
  - Fluticasone furoate (Veramyst): adults and children ≥12 years of age, 2 sprays each nostril daily; children 2 to 11 years of age, 1 spray each nostril daily
  - Fluticasone propionate (Flonase): adults 1 to 2 sprays each nostril daily; children ≥4 years of age, 1 spray each nostril daily
  - Mometasone (Nasonex): adults and children ≥12 years of age, 2 sprays each nostril daily; children 2 to 12 years of age, 1 spray each nostril daily
  - Triamcinolone (Nasacort): adults and children ≥6 years of age, 1 to 2 sprays each nostril daily; children 2 to 5 years of age, 1 spray each nostril daily
- 2nd-generation H_1 antihistamines (may be beneficial for those with ETD and chronic rhinitis)
  - Cetirizine (Zyrtec) (tablets, chewable tablets, liquid): adults and children ≥6 years of age, 5 to 10 mg/day PO; children 12 months to 5 years of age: 2.5 mg/day PO, may increase to BID; children 6 to <12 months of age: 2.5 mg/day PO
  - Desloratadine (Clarinex) (tablets, Reditabs, liquid): adults and children ≥12 years of age, 5 mg/day PO; children 6 to 11 years of age, 2.5 mg/day PO; children 12 months to 5 years of age, 1.25 mg/day PO; children 6 to 11 months of age, 1 mg/day PO
  - Fexofenadine (Allegra) (tablets, Reditabs, liquid): adults and children ≥12 years of age, 60 mg PO BID or 180 mg/day PO; children 2 to 11 years of age, 30 mg PO BID
  - Levocetirizine (Xyzal) (tablets, liquid): adults and children ≥12 years of age, 2.5 to 5 mg PO every evening; children 6 to 11 years of age, 2.5 mg PO every evening; children 6 months to 5 years of age, 1.25 mg PO every evening
- Antihistamine nasal sprays (may be beneficial for those with ETD and chronic rhinitis)
  - Azelastine (Astepro or Astelin): adults and children ≥12 years of age, 1 to 2 sprays each nostril BID; children 6 to 11 years of age, 1 spray each nostril BID
  - Olopatadine (Patanase): adults and children ≥12 years of age, 2 sprays each nostril BID; children 6 to 11 years of age, 1 spray each nostril BID

SURGERY/OTHER PROCEDURES

- Myringotomy and pressure equalization tube placement to ventilate middle ear, relieve pressure, and prevent sequelae of chronically retracted drum
- Patients with ETD during pressure changes may benefit from minimally invasive laser eustachian tuboplasty.
- New studies are emerging regarding balloon tuboplasty, but to date are very limited in terms of efficacy, safety, and long-term outcomes (6)[B].
- Adenoidectomy if hypertrophied tissue is present.
  - In children, first set of tubes are typically placed alone. Adenoidectomy is performed with second set of tubes if problems recur.
  - Some advocate adenoidectomy even in absence of excess tissue; reduces frequency and number of subsequent tubes

 ONGOING CARE

FOLLOW-UP RECOMMENDATIONS

- Monitor pressure equalization tubes every 6 to 8 months in children and every 6 to 12 months in adults.
- Monitor tympanic membrane retraction pocket for progression every 6 to 12 months to allow for early intervention for progression in hearing loss, obvious ossicular erosion, or cholesteatoma.

DIET

Breastfeeding is associated with lower incidence of ETD and OM.

PROGNOSIS

If symptoms of ETD persist beyond age 7 years, patient is more likely to have long-term problems and require regular monitoring.

COMPLICATIONS

Morbidity related to hearing compromise or associated sequela of chronic ear infections

REFERENCES

1. McCoul ED, Anand VK, Christos PJ. Validating the clinical assessment of eustachian tube dysfunction: the Eustachian Tube Dysfunction Questionnaire (ETDQ-7). *Laryngoscope.* 2012;122(5):1137–1141.
2. Van Roeyen S, Van de Heyning P, Van Rompaey V. Value and discriminative power of the seven-item Eustachian tube dysfunction questionnaire. *Laryngoscope.* 2015;125(11):2553–2556.
3. Norman G, Llewellyn A, Harden M, et al. Systematic review of the limited evidence base for treatments of Eustachian tube dysfunction: a healthy technology assessment. *Clin Otolaryngol.* 2014;39(1):6–21.
4. van Zon A, van der Heijden GJ, van Dongen TM, et al. Antibiotics for otitis media with effusion in children. *Cochrane Database Syst Rev.* 2012;(9): CD009163.
5. Simpson SA, Lewis R, van der Voort J, et al. Oral or topical nasal steroids for hearing loss associated with otitis media with effusion in children. *Cochrane Database Syst Rev.* 2011;(5):CD001935.
6. Gürtler N, Husner A, Flurin H. Balloon dilation of the eustachian tube: early outcome analysis. *Otol Neurotol.* 2015;36(3):437–443.

ADDITIONAL READING

- Bluestone CD. Studies in otitis media: Children's Hospital of Pittsburgh-University of Pittsburgh progress report—2004. *Laryngoscope.* 2004;114(11, Pt 3 Suppl 105):1–26.
- Gluth MB, McDonald DR, Weaver AL, et al. Management of Eustachian tube dysfunction with nasal steroid spray: a prospective, randomized, placebo-controlled trial. *Arch Otolaryngol Head Neck Surg.* 2011;137(5):449–455.
- Seibert JW, Danner CJ. Eustachian tube function and the middle ear. *Otolaryngol Clin North Am.* 2006;39(6):1221–1235.
- Williamson I, Vennik J, Harnden A, et al. Effect of nasal balloon autoinflation in children with otitis media with effusion in primary care: an open randomized controlled trial. *CMAJ.* 2015;187(13): 961–969.

 SEE ALSO

Algorithm: Ear Pain

CODES

ICD10

- H69.90 Unspecified Eustachian tube disorder, unspecified ear
- H69.00 Patulous Eustachian tube, unspecified ear
- H68.109 Unspecified obstruction of Eustachian tube, unspecified ear

CLINICAL PEARLS

- ETD can be acute or chronic. Treatment is based on the underlying etiology.
- Weber test: 512-Hz fork placed on the forehead lateralizes to affected ear in ETD and opposite ear in SSNHL
- SSNHL (medical emergency) can be misdiagnosed as ETD and should always be ruled out, especially in patients with unilateral symptoms.

FACTOR V LEIDEN

Marina Rasnow-Hill, MD

 BASICS

DESCRIPTION

- Factor V Leiden is a genetic mutation at the activated protein C (APC) cleavage site on the factor V and Va molecule leading to the most common form of inherited thrombophilia.
- System(s) affected: cardiovascular, gastrointestinal, hemo-/lymphatic/immunologic, nervous, pulmonary, reproductive
- Synonym(s): factor V Leiden thrombophilia; factor V Leiden mutation; hereditary APC resistance

Pediatric Considerations
Potential for increased thrombosis risk in patients with factor V Leiden and concomitant risks

Pregnancy Considerations
- Recurrent late pregnancy loss is a possible complication.
- Increased thrombotic risk in pregnancy and postpartum (additive) especially in homozygous state
- Possible increased risk of IUGR, preeclampsia, placental abruption, evidence mixed (1)

EPIDEMIOLOGY

Prevalence
Studies estimate ~5–8% occurrence of heterozygosity in Caucasians, Hispanic Americans ~2%, African Americans ~1%, and Asian Americans ~0.45%.

ETIOLOGY AND PATHOPHYSIOLOGY

- Factor V circulates in the plasma. When exposed to tissue factor from endothelial activation, factor V amplifies the production of thrombin which in turn further promotes clotting by activating factor V into procoagulant factor Va.
- For balance, thrombin also promotes APC production which will cleave and inactivate factor V, Va, and VIII, thereby keeping the clotting cascade in check (negative feedback loop).
- In factor V leiden, a point mutation at the binding site of APC (Arg506Glu) renders it less able to cleave factor V or Va. This, in turn, reduces the anticoagulant role of factor V as a cofactor to APC, and increases the *procoagulant* role of activated factor V, as there is now 20-fold slower degradation of factor Va Leiden.

RISK FACTORS

- Risk for venous thromboembolism (VTE) is ~7-fold in heterozygous and ~80-fold in homozygous factor V Leiden individuals, compared with individuals without the mutation (2). This risk is compounded/increased by the presence of the following:
  - Having non-O blood type (A, B, or AB) (increased risk 2- to 4-fold)
  - Oral contraceptives: homozygotes up to 100-fold; heterozygotes, 35-fold. The increased risk is halved when the patient uses desogestrel-containing oral contraceptives.

- Hormone replacement therapy (HRT) and selective estrogen receptor modulators (SERMs) both increase the risk of thrombosis; in patients with factor V Leiden, that risk is compounded.
- Pregnancy and *homozygous* factor V Leiden increase the risk of thrombosis 7- to 16-fold during pregnancy and the puerperium.
- Data are conflicting with regard to risk for recurrent VTE for patients with factor V Leiden but trend toward an increased risk (1,3).

GENERAL PREVENTION

ALERT
Patients with factor V Leiden without thrombosis do not require prophylactic anticoagulation.

COMMONLY ASSOCIATED CONDITIONS
Venous thrombosis

 DIAGNOSIS

HISTORY
- Previous thrombosis
- Family history of thrombosis

PHYSICAL EXAM
- Family history of factor V Leiden mutation
- Findings suggestive of VTE in any form (DVT, PE, cerebral vein thrombosis); 10–26% of patients with VTE are carriers of the factor V Leiden mutation.
- Thrombosis in unusual locations, such as the sagittal sinus, or mesentery and portal systems, although these are less common in patients with factor V Leiden than in patients with deficiency of protein C or S.
- There is a weak, however significant, association between procoagulant states (including factor V Leiden) and coronary events in younger patients (4).

DIFFERENTIAL DIAGNOSIS
- Protein C deficiency
- Protein S deficiency
- Antithrombin deficiency
- Other causes of APC resistance (e.g., antiphospholipid antibodies)
- Dysfibrinogenemia
- Dysplasminogenemia
- Homocystinemia
- Prothrombin 20210 mutation
- Elevated factor VIII levels

DIAGNOSTIC TESTS & INTERPRETATION

Initial Tests (lab, imaging)
- For evaluation of a new clot in patient at risk: CBC with peripheral smear, PT/INR, aPTT, thrombin time, lupus anticoagulant, antiphospholipid antibodies, factor VIII, anticardiolipin antibody, anti-$\beta(2)$GP-I antibodies, APC resistance, protein S antigen and resistance, antithrombin III assay, fibrinogen, factor V Leiden, prothrombin G20210A

- Genetic test: DNA-based test for factor V mutation; will be unaffected by anticoagulation and other drugs
- Functional test: plasma-based coagulation assay using factor V–deficient plasma to which patient plasma is added along with purified APC. The relative prolongation of the activated partial thromboplastin time (aPTT) is used to assay for the defect. Heparin, direct thrombin inhibitors, and factor Xa inhibitor may cause false-negative results. In the absence of exposure to anticoagulants, functional testing is preferred to genomic for cost and time to diagnosis (5)[A].
- Extremity US for DVT
- V/Q scan or spiral CT for PE

Follow-Up Tests & Special Considerations
- US may not show DVT acutely; repeat in 5 to 7 days if strong suspicion.
- V/Q scan for evaluation of PE may be difficult to interpret in smokers or those with underlying lung disease.

Diagnostic Procedures/Other
Magnetic resonance angiography (MRA), venography, or arteriography to detect thrombosis

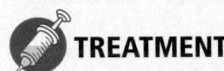 **TREATMENT**

Only indicated if thrombotic event

GENERAL MEASURES

- Like general VTE treatment, patients with factor V Leiden and a first thrombosis should be anticoagulated initially with heparin or LMWH and warfarin for at least 3 months.
- Treatment with low-molecular-weight heparin (LMWH) is recommended over unfractionated heparin, unless the patient has severe renal failure (6)[A].
- Treat as outpatient, if possible (6)[A]
- Initiate warfarin with LMWH on the first treatment day and discontinue LMWH after minimum of 5 days and when INR >2 for two consecutive days (6)[A].
- Patients should be maintained on warfarin with an INR of 2 to 3 for at least 3 months (6)[A].
- For those patients with recurrence, the risks and benefits of indefinite anticoagulation need to be assessed.

MEDICATION

First Line
- LMWH:
  - Enoxaparin (Lovenox): 1 mg/kg SC BID, start warfarin simultaneously, continue enoxaparin for minimum of 5 days and until INR is >2 for two consecutive days, at which time enoxaparin can be stopped.
  - Fondaparinux (Arixtra): 5 mg (body weight <50 kg), 7.5 mg (body weight 50 to 100 kg), or 10 mg (body weight >100 kg) SC daily

- Tinzaparin (Innohep): 175 anti-Xa IU/kg SC daily for minimum of 5 days and patient is adequately anticoagulated with warfarin (INR of at least 2 for two consecutive days)
- Dalteparin (Fragmin): 200 IU/kg SC daily
- Oral anticoagulant
  - Warfarin (Coumadin) PO with dose adjusted to an INR of 2 to 3 (3)[A].
- Contraindications
  - Active bleeding precludes anticoagulation
  - Risk of bleeding is a relative contraindication to long-term anticoagulation.
  - Warfarin is contraindicated in patients with history of warfarin skin necrosis (6)[A].
  - Warfarin is contraindicated in pregnancy.
- Precautions
  - Observe patient for signs of embolization, further thrombosis, or bleeding
  - Avoid IM injections. Periodically check stool and urine for occult blood; monitor CBCs, including platelets.
  - Heparin: thrombocytopenia and/or paradoxic thrombosis with thrombocytopenia
  - Warfarin: necrotic skin lesions (typically breasts, thighs, or buttocks)
  - LMWH: adjust dosage in renal insufficiency. May also need dose adjustment in pregnancy
- Significant possible interactions
  - Agents that intensify the response to oral anticoagulants: alcohol, allopurinol, amiodarone, anabolic steroids, androgens, many antimicrobials, cimetidine, chloral hydrate, disulfiram, all NSAIDs, sulfinpyrazone, tamoxifen, thyroid hormone, vitamin E, ranitidine, salicylates, acetaminophen
  - Agents that diminish the response to anticoagulants: aminoglutethimide, antacids, barbiturates, carbamazepine, cholestyramine, diuretics, griseofulvin, rifampin, oral contraceptives

Second Line
- Heparin 80 mg/kg IV bolus followed by 18 g/kg/hr continuous infusion
- Adjust dose depending on aPTT.
- In patients requiring large daily doses of heparin, measure an anti-Xa level for dose guidance.
- Alternatively, for outpatients, weight-adjusted subcutaneous unfractionated heparin with 333 U/kg first, then 250 U/kg, without monitoring (6)[A]
- Consider deficiency of antithrombin as a comutation in patients with significant elevated heparin requirements.

ISSUES FOR REFERRAL
- Recurrent thrombosis on anticoagulation
- Difficulty anticoagulating
- Genetic counseling
- Homozygous state in pregnancy

SURGERY/OTHER PROCEDURES
- Anticoagulation must be held for surgical interventions.
- For most patients with DVT, recommendations are against routine use of vena cava filter in addition to anticoagulation except when there is contraindication for anticoagulation (6)[A].
- Thrombectomy may be necessary in some cases.

INPATIENT CONSIDERATIONS
Admission Criteria/Initial Stabilization
Complicated thrombosis, such as PE

Nursing
- Teach LMWH and warfarin use.
- See above for drug interactions.

Discharge Criteria
Stable on anticoagulation

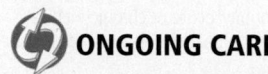 ONGOING CARE

FOLLOW-UP RECOMMENDATIONS
Patient Monitoring
Warfarin use requires periodic (~monthly after initial stabilization) INR measurements, with a goal of 2 to 3 (6)[A].

DIET
- No restrictions
- Large amounts of foods rich in vitamin K may interfere with anticoagulation with warfarin.

PATIENT EDUCATION
- Patients should be educated about the following:
  - Use of oral anticoagulant therapy
  - Avoidance of NSAIDs while on warfarin
- The role of family screening is unclear, as most patients with this mutation do not have thrombosis. In a patient with a family history of factor V Leiden, consider screening during pregnancy or if considering oral contraceptive use.

PROGNOSIS
- Most patients heterozygous for factor V Leiden do not have thrombosis.
- Homozygotes have about a 50% lifetime incidence of thrombosis.
- Recurrence rates after a first thrombosis are not clear, with some investigators finding rates as high as 5% and others finding rates similar to the general population.
- Despite the increased risk for thrombosis, factor V Leiden does not increase overall mortality.

COMPLICATIONS
- Recurrent thrombosis
- Bleeding on anticoagulation

REFERENCES
1. Lijfering WM, Middeldorp S, Veeger NJ, et al. Risk of recurrent venous thrombosis in homozygous carriers and double heterozygous carriers of factor V Leiden and prothrombin G20210A. *Circulation.* 2010;121(15):1706–1712.
2. Rosendaal FR, Koster T, Vandenbroucke JP, et al. High risk of thrombosis in patients homozygous for factor V Leiden (activated protein C resistance). *Blood.* 1995;85(6):1504–1508.
3. Eichinger S, Weltermann A, Mannhalter C, et al. The risk of recurrent venous thromboembolism in heterozygous carriers of factor V Leiden and a first spontaneous venous thromboembolism. *Arch Intern Med.* 2002;162(20):2357–2360.
4. Ye Z, Liu EH, Higgins JP, et al. Seven haemostatic gene polymorphisms in coronary disease: meta-analysis of 66,155 cases and 91,307 controls. *Lancet.* 2006;367(9511):651–658.
5. Prüller F, Weiss EC, Raggam RB, et al. Activated protein C resistance assay and factor V Leiden. *N Engl J Med.* 2014;371(7):685–686.
6. Guyatt GH, Akl EA, Crowther M, et al. Executive summary: antithrombotic therapy and prevention of thrombosis, 9th ed: American College of Chest Physicians evidence-based clinical practice guidelines. *Chest.* 2012;141(2)(Suppl):7S–47S.

ADDITIONAL READING
Seligsohn U, Lubetsky A. Genetic susceptibility to venous thrombosis. *N Engl J Med.* 2001;344(16):1222–1231.

 SEE ALSO

Deep Vein Thrombophlebitis

 CODES

ICD10
D68.51 Activated protein C resistance

CLINICAL PEARLS
- Extremely rare in Asian and African populations
- Asymptomatic patients with factor V Leiden do not need anticoagulation.
- For pregnant women homozygous for factor V Leiden but no prior history of VTE, postpartum prophylaxis with prophylactic or intermediate-dose LMWH or vitamin K antagonists with target INR 2 to 3 for 6 weeks is recommended. Antepartum prophylaxis is added if there is positive family of VTE.

FAILURE TO THRIVE
Durr-e-Shahwaar Sayed, DO

BASICS

DESCRIPTION
- Failure to thrive (FTT) is not a diagnosis but a sign of inadequate nutrition in young children manifested by a failure of physical growth, usually affecting weight. In severe cases, decreased length and/or head circumference may develop.
- Various parameters are used to define FTT, but in clinical practice, it is commonly defined as either weight for age that falls below the 5th percentile on more than one occasion or weight that drops two or more major percentile lines on standard growth charts.
- A combination of anthropometric criteria rather than one criterion should be used to identify children at risk of FTT (1)[C].

Pediatric Considerations
- Children with genetic syndromes, intrauterine growth restriction (IUGR), or prematurity follow different growth curves.
- 25% of children will decrease their weight or height crossing ≥2 major percentile lines in the first 2 years of life. These children are failing to reach their genetic potential or demonstrating constitutional growth delay (slow growth with a bone age < chronologic age). After shifting down, these infants grow at a normal rate along their new percentile and do not have FTT.

EPIDEMIOLOGY
Incidence
- Predominant age: 6 to 12 months; 80% <18 months
- Predominant sex: male = female

Prevalence
- As many as 10% of children seen in primary care have signs of growth failure.
- 1–5% of pediatric inpatient admissions are for FTT.
- Occurs more frequently in children living in poverty (1)

ETIOLOGY AND PATHOPHYSIOLOGY
- Mismatch between caloric intake and caloric expenditure
- Often grouped into four major categories:
  - Inadequate caloric intake (most frequent)
  - Inadequate caloric absorption
  - Excessive caloric expenditure
  - Defective utilization
- Traditionally, FTT was classified as organic or nonorganic, but most cases are multifactorial.
- FTT often begins with a specific event and may lead to persistent difficulties.
- Causes of FTT can be grouped by pathophysiology (including examples):
  - Inadequate intake: breastfeeding difficulty, incorrect formula preparation, poor transition to food (6 to 12 months), poor feeding habits (e.g., excessive juice, restrictive diets), mechanical problems (e.g., oromotor dysfunction, congenital anomalies, GERD, CNS or PNS anomalies), oral aversion, poverty, neglect, poor parent–child interaction
  - Inadequate absorption: necrotizing enterocolitis, short gut syndrome, biliary atresia, liver disease, cystic fibrosis, celiac disease, milk protein allergy, vitamin/mineral deficiency
  - Increased expenditure: hyperthyroidism, congenital/chronic cardiopulmonary disease, HIV, immunodeficiencies, malignancy, renal disease
  - Defective utilization: metabolic disorders, congenital infections (TORCH: toxoplasmosis, other agents, rubella, cytomegalovirus, herpes simplex)

Genetics
Multiple genetic disorders can cause FTT.

RISK FACTORS
- Psychosocial risks
  - Poverty, parent(s) with mental health disorder or cognitive impairment, poor parenting skills or hypervigilant parents, families with unique health/nutritional beliefs, physical or emotional abuse, substance abuse, and social isolation
- Medical risks
  - Intrauterine exposures, history of IUGR (symmetric or asymmetric), congenital abnormalities, oromotor dysfunction, premature or sick newborn, infant with physical deformity, acute or chronic medical conditions, developmental delay, lead poisoning, anemia

Pregnancy Considerations
FTT is linked to intrauterine exposures, IUGR, and prematurity.

GENERAL PREVENTION
- Educate parents on normal feeding and parenting skills.
- Access to supplemental feeding programs (women, infants, and children [WIC])

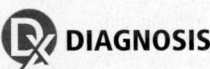
DIAGNOSIS

HISTORY
- Prenatal and developmental history
- Past medical history: acute/chronic disease affecting caloric intake, digestion, absorption, or causing increased energy need or defective utilization
- Medication history, including complementary and alternative medications
- Family history: stature of parents and growth trajectories of siblings, chronic diseases, genetic disorders, developmental delay
- Diet history from birth: breastfeeding or formula feeding; timing and introduction of solids; who feeds the child, when, and how often; placement of child during feeds; amounts consumed/caloric intake; beverages consumed; snacking; vomiting or stooling associated with feeds; oral aversions or unusual behaviors during feeding
- Social history: family composition, socioeconomic status, child-rearing beliefs, stressors, parental depression, parental substance abuse, caretaker personal history of abuse/neglect
- Review of systems: anorexia, activity level, mental status, fevers, dysphagia, vomiting, gastroesophageal reflux, stooling pattern/consistency, dysuria, urinary frequency

PHYSICAL EXAM
- A combination of anthropometric criteria, rather than one criterion should be used (1)[C].
- Accurate measurement of height, weight, and head circumference on National Center for Health Statistics (NCHS) growth charts (www.cdc.gov/growthcharts) (2).
- The World Health Organization (WHO) growth charts may be more appropriate for breastfed infants (www.who.int/childgrowth/standards/en/).
- Growth charts exist for many other syndromes/conditions such as Down syndrome, Turner syndrome, and the premature infant.
- Exam should assess for the following:
  - Signs of dehydration or severe malnutrition are as follows:
    - Severity of malnutrition estimated via Gomez classification: Compare current weight for age with expected weight for age (50th percentile): severe, <60% of expected; moderate, 61–75%; mild, 76–90%.
  - Underlying medical disease
  - Dysmorphic features
  - Mental status (alert, responsive to stimuli)
  - Any signs of physical abuse and/or neglect
- Observe interaction with caregivers and feeding techniques, specifically bonding and social/psychological cues.

DIFFERENTIAL DIAGNOSIS
Differentiate based on growth patterns
- FTT classically presents as low weight for age, normal linear growth, normocephalic or low weight for age, followed by decreased linear growth or low weight for age, leading to decreased linear growth and decreased head circumference (without neurologic signs).
  - In this situation, consider differential diagnosis as outlined in "Etiology and Pathophysiology."
- If low linear growth with normal weight for length or low linear growth and proportionately low weight and decreased head circumference:
  - Consider genetic potential (constitutional short stature or growth delay), genetic syndromes, teratogens, endocrine disorders
- If microcephaly with prominent neurologic signs, with poor growth secondary to presumed neurologic disorder:
  - Consider TORCH infections, genetic syndromes, teratogens, brain injury (i.e., hypoxic/ischemic)

DIAGNOSTIC TESTS & INTERPRETATION
- Labs useful only in ~1% of cases and are generally not recommended (1)[C].
- A period of addressing nutritional causes is preferable prior to extensive labs and other workup.

Initial Tests (lab, imaging)
Labs should be ordered based on history and physical exam findings and the age of the patient.
- Tests often considered in initial evaluation:
  - CBC, ESR
  - Electrolytes, BUN/creatinine, liver function tests
  - Urinalysis and urine culture
  - Lead level
- Other tests as dictated by the history and exam:
  - TSH, amylase/lipase, serum zinc level, iron studies, karyotype, genetic testing, sweat chloride test, stool for ova and parasite or fat/reducing substances, guaiac, α-1-antitrypsin and elastase, radioallergosorbent test for IgE food allergies, tissue transglutaminase and total IgA (celiac sprue), P-ANCA and anti–*Saccharomyces cerevisiae* antibodies (for inflammatory bowel disease [IBD]), TB test, HIV, ELISA, hepatitis A and B, other infections

Follow-Up Tests & Special Considerations
- Prospective 3-day food diary for accurate record of caloric intake should be obtained.
- Home visit by a clinician to observe infant feeding, interaction of caretakers, and home environment (3)
- Observe breastfeeding and/or formula preparation to ensure adequacy and offer instruction.

- Additional indicated evaluations may be performed by dietitians, occupational, physical and speech therapists, social workers, developmental specialists, psychiatrists, psychologists, visiting nurses, lactation consultants, and/or child protection services.
- Can consider
  – Skeletal survey if suspicion of physical abuse
  – Bone age if possible endocrine disorder
  – Swallowing studies, small bowel follow-through if possible oromotor dysfunction, GERD, structural abnormalities
  – Brain imaging if microcephalic and/or neurologic findings on examination

 TREATMENT

GENERAL MEASURES
- Treat underlying conditions.
- Caregiver and infant interaction should be evaluated in infants and children with FTT.
- Age appropriate nutritional counseling should be provided (1)[C].
  – The goal is to improve nutrition to allow catch-up growth (weight gain 2 to 3 times > average for age).
- Calculate energy needs based on recommended energy intake for age, increased by 50%.
  – Recommended energy intake (use expected, not actual weight, to calculate needs)
    ○ 0 to 1 month: 120 kcal/kg/day
    ○ 1 to 2 months: 115 kcal/kg/day
    ○ 2 to 3 months: 105 kcal/kg/day
    ○ 3 to 6 months: 95 kcal/kg/day
    ○ 6 months to 3 years: 90 kcal/kg/day (4)[C]
- Alternatively, may calculate caloric requirements for infants to achieve catch-up growth
  – kcal/kg/day required = RDA for age (kcal/kg) × ideal weight for height/actual weight, where ideal weight for height is the median weight for the patient's height
- Try various strategies to increase caloric intake, such as the following:
  – Optimize breastfeeding support, consider supplementation.
    Higher calorie formulas
  – Addition of rice cereal or fats to current foods
  – Limit intake of milk to 24 to 32 oz/day.
  – Avoid juice and soda.
  – Vitamin and/or nutritional supplements
  – Assist with social and family problems (WIC, food stamps, and other transitional assistance).
- Rapid high-calorie intake can cause diarrhea, malabsorption, hypokalemia, and hypophosphatemia. Therefore, increasing formulas more than 24 kcal/oz is not recommended.
- The target energy intake should be slowly increased to goal over 5 to 7 days.
- Catch-up growth should be seen in 2 to 7 days.
- Accelerated growth should be continued for 4 to 9 months to restore weight and height.

MEDICATION
Use only for identified underlying conditions.

ISSUES FOR REFERRAL
- Refer as indicated for underlying conditions.
- Multidisciplinary care is beneficial (1)[A]. Specialized multidisciplinary clinics may be of benefit for children with complicated situations, failure to respond to initial treatment, or when the PCP does not have access to specialized services such as nutrition, psychology, PT/OT, and speech therapy (2).

ADDITIONAL THERAPIES
In severe cases, nasogastric tube feedings or gastrostomy may be considered.

INPATIENT CONSIDERATIONS
Most cases of FTT can be managed as outpatients.

Admission Criteria/Initial Stabilization
Hospitalization should be considered if (1)[C]:
- Outpatient management fails.
- There is evidence of severe dehydration or malnutrition.
- There are signs of abuse or neglect.
- There are concerns that the psychosocial situation presents harm to child.
- During catch-up growth, some children will develop nutritional recovery syndrome:
  – Symptoms include sweating, increased body temperature, hepatomegaly (increased glycogen deposits), widening of cranial sutures (brain growth > bone growth), increased periods of sleep, fidgetiness, and mild hyperactivity.
- There may also be an initial period of malabsorption with resultant diarrhea.

Discharge Criteria
Catch-up growth should be seen in 2 to 7 days. If this is not seen, reevaluation of causes is needed.

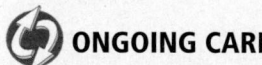 ONGOING CARE

FOLLOW-UP RECOMMENDATIONS
- If specific disease is identified, follow-up as indicated.
- Close long-term follow-up with frequent visits is important to create and maintain a healthy, supportive environment (3).
- Children with history of FTT are at increased risk of recurrent FTT, and growth should be monitored closely (1,4).
- If the family fails to comply, child protection authorities must be notified.

DIET
Nutritional requirements for a "normal" child:
- Infant
  – 120 kcal/kg/day, decreased to 95 kcal/kg/day at 6 months; if breastfed, ensure appropriate frequency and duration of feeding.
  – Between 6 and 12 months, continue breast milk and/or formula, but pureed foods should be consumed several times a day during this period.
- Toddler
  – Three meals plus two nutritional snacks, 16 to 32 oz of milk/day; avoid juice and soda, and feed in a social environment.
  – Do not restrict fat and cholesterol in children <2 years.
- Rate of weight gain expected for age:
  – 0 to 3 months: 26 to 31 g/day
  – 3 to 6 months: 17 to 18 g/day
  – 6 to 9 months: 12 to 13 g/day
  – 9 to 12 months: 9 g/day
  – 1 to 3 years: 7 to 9 g/day

PATIENT EDUCATION
- Counsel parents regarding the need to avoid "food battles," which worsen the problem.
- Educate parents regarding infant social and physiologic cues, formula/food preparation, proper feeding techniques, and importance of relaxed and social mealtimes.
- When environmental deprivation is identified, educating in a nonpunitive way is essential.
- "Failure to thrive: What this means for your child," available from AAFP at: www.aafp.org/afp/2011/0401/p837.html
- WIC provides grants to states for supplemental foods, health care referrals, and nutrition education for low-income pregnant, breastfeeding, and nonbreastfeeding postpartum women and to infants and children up to age 5 years at nutritional risk: www.fns.usda.gov/wic/

PROGNOSIS
- Many children with FTT show adequate improvement in dietary intake with intervention.
- Some studies looking at children with FTT have demonstrated an association with later problems with cognitive development, behavioral issues, and growth, but there is no consensus on these long-term outcomes or their clinical significance (1).
- Children with FTT are at increased risk for future undernutrition, overnutrition, and eating disorders.

REFERENCES
1. Cole SZ, Lanham JS. Failure to thrive: an update. *Am Fam Physician*. 2011;83(7):829–834.
2. Grissom M. Disorders of childhood growth and development: failure to thrive versus short stature. *FP Essent*. 2013;410:11–19.
3. Shields B, Wacogne I, Wright CM. Weight faltering and failure to thrive in infancy and early childhood. *BMJ*. 2012;345:e5931.
4. Krugman SD, Dubowitz H. Failure to thrive. *Am Fam Physician*. 2003;68(5):879–884.

ADDITIONAL READING
- Atalay A, McCord M. Characteristics of failure to thrive in a referral population: implications for treatment. *Clin Pediatr (Phila)*. 2012;51(3):219–225.
- Jaffe AC. Failure to thrive: current clinical concepts. *Pediatr Rev*. 2011;32(3):100–107.
- Kerzner B, Milano K, MacLean WC Jr, et al. A practical approach to classifying and managing feeding difficulties. *Pediatrics*. 2015;135(2):344–353.

 CODES

ICD10
- R62.51 Failure to thrive (child)
- P92.6 Failure to thrive in newborn

CLINICAL PEARLS
- FTT is a sign of inadequate nutrition.
- Underlying medical and/or social issues are generally suggested by history and physical exam, and extensive laboratory or imaging tests are rarely needed.
- A multidisciplinary team approach to diagnosis and treatment is critical to help children with FTT and their families.
- Prompt diagnosis and intervention is important to decrease the risk of adverse effects.

FEMALE ATHLETE TRIAD

Andrew J. McBride, MD • Rahul Kapur, MD, CAQSM

 BASICS

Syndrome of three interrelated clinical entities: low energy availability (EA) (with or without disordered eating [DE]), menstrual dysfunction (MD), and low bone mineral density (BMD) (1).

DESCRIPTION

- Female athlete triad was first described in 1992: Patients may meet criteria for only one or two parts of the triad.
- Prevention and early intervention are essential to prevent progression to serious clinical end points of eating disorders, amenorrhea, and osteoporosis.
- 2014 Female Athlete Triad Coalition Consensus Statement and the 2007 American College of Sports Medicine (ACSM) Position Stand suggest (1):
  - Each component of the triad represents a spectrum ranging from health to dysfunction.
  - Energy availability is fundamental to the propagation of the triad.
  - Full recovery is not possible without correction of low energy availability.
- Energy availability (EA)
  - Dietary energy intake minus exercise energy expenditure. The core element of the triad.
  - Represents the amount of dietary energy remaining for bodily functions after correcting for exercise training
  - Low EA results in reduced capacity for cellular maintenance, thermoregulation, and growth.
  - Low EA serves a causal role in the induction of exercise-associated menstrual disturbances.
  - Low EA occurs either intentionally or inadvertently. Examples include increasing training disproportionately to energy intake; DE; and reducing energy intake by restricting, fasting, binging, and purging or use of diet pills, laxatives, diuretics, or enemas. Not all athletes meet diagnostic criteria from *Diagnostic and Statistical Manual of Mental Disorders* 5th edition (*DSM-5*) for eating disorders.
- Menstrual dysfunction (MD)
  - Low EA alters the hypothalamic-pituitary axis, resulting in decreased estrogen levels.
  - MD ranges from eumenorrhea to amenorrhea.
  - MD includes athletes who have low estrogen levels but still experience menstruation.
  - Energy deficit results in menstrual dysfunction at ~30 kcal/kg lean body mass per day.
  - MD includes luteal suppression (shortened luteal phase, prolonged follicular phase, and decreased estradiol level), anovulation, oligomenorrhea (menstrual cycle >35 days), and primary and secondary hypothalamic amenorrhea.
  - Primary amenorrhea, although less common, can occur in young athletes. Secondary amenorrhea is defined as the absence of menstrual cycles for >3 months after menarche established.
  - Although hypothalamic suppression is the most common cause of secondary amenorrhea in these athletes, other causes must be ruled out.
- BMD
  - Ranges from optimal bone health to osteoporosis
  - Bone health encompasses bone strength as well as bone quality. The current practice standard (dual-energy x-ray absorptiometry) measures bone density not bone quality. However, newer research using peripheral quantitative CT scans have shown that amenorrheic female athletes have a lower proportion of cortical bone, which is

thought to be related to deficient mineralization and may be responsible for the increased fracture risk (2). This research may help providers better understand why two athletes with the same BMD may have very different bone fracture histories.
  - ○ ACSM Position Stand recommends using the International Society of Clinical Densitometry (ISCD) guidelines for BMD Z-scores <−2.0.
  - ○ Because most athletes have a higher BMD than nonathletes, ACSM recommends further workup for any athlete with a Z-score <−1, even in the absence of fracture.
  - Endothelial dysfunction
  - ○ Emerging evidence suggests that the female athlete triad is associated with endothelial dysfunction. Reduced levels of estrogen alter vasodilation. Athletic amenorrhea is associated with reduced brachial artery flow-mediated dilation, which has a 95% positive predictive value for coronary endothelial dysfunction. Consequences include decreased blood flow to muscles during exercise and accelerated atherosclerosis. In the future, this clinical syndrome may be considered a tetrad (3).

EPIDEMIOLOGY

Prevalence

- Overall prevalence: 0–16% of female athletes (4). Prevalence of two criteria varies: MD + BMD 0–8% (n = 460), MD + LE 18% (n = 80), and BMD + LE 4% (n = 80) (4)
- DE higher than general population (4)
- Menstrual dysfunction: Prevalence of secondary amenorrhea is as high as 60% in female athletes compared to 2–5% in the general population (4).
- Bone health: Using the World Health Organization (WHO) criteria for low BMD, prevalence of osteopenia (T-score between −1 and −2) ranges from 0% to 40% in female athletes, as compared to ~12% in the general population (4).

ETIOLOGY AND PATHOPHYSIOLOGY

- Low EA disrupts the hypothalamic-pituitary-ovarian axis, decreasing pulsatile gonadotropin-releasing hormone (GnRH) release (5).
- Low GnRH levels decrease luteinizing hormone (LH) and follicle-stimulating hormone (FSH) levels, decreasing estrogen production with resultant menstrual dysfunction.
- Estrogen deficiency negatively affects bone density. A chronic state of malnutrition reduces the rate of bone formation and increases the rate of bone resorption. Changes in bone metabolism occur within 5 days of reductions in EA.

RISK FACTORS

- History of menstrual irregularities and amenorrhea; history of stress fractures and recurrent or nonhealing injuries; history of critical comments about eating or weight from parent or coach; history of depression; history of dieting; personality factors including perfectionism and/or obsessiveness, overtraining, and inappropriate coaching behaviors (1)
- Lean physique, sports with an aesthetic component (ballet, figure skating, gymnastics, distance running, diving, and swimming), or sports with weight classifications (martial arts and wrestling). Frequent weigh-ins, consequences for weight gain, and win-at-all-cost attitude all increase risk (6).
- A lack of family or social support; intense training hours; social isolation or entering a new

environment (boarding school or college); an athlete with comorbid psychological conditions (anxiety, depression, and/or obsessive-compulsive disorder)

GENERAL PREVENTION

- Education of athletes (middle school through college), coaches, trainers, parents, and physicians. Young athletes are extremely impressionable and may turn negative comments and unhealthy advice into maladaptive eating and exercising habits.
- General screening during preparticipation exam (PPE) and annual physicals is endorsed by AAP, AAFP, ACSM, AAOSM, and AMSSM (6).
- Female Athlete Triad Coalition has 11-question screening to use during PPE (1).
- Screen athletes presenting with "red flag" conditions such as fractures, weight changes, fatigue, amenorrhea, bradycardia, orthostatic hypotension, syncope, arrhythmias, electrolyte abnormalities, or depression.

COMMONLY ASSOCIATED CONDITIONS

- Anorexia nervosa, bulimia nervosa, avoidant or restrictive food intake disorder, and other psychological disorders, including low self-esteem, depression, and anxiety (5)
- Low BMD predisposes athletes to stress fractures and may not be fully reversible. This may lead to a higher rate of fractures after menopause.

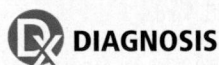 **DIAGNOSIS**

The female athlete triad is a clinical diagnosis based primarily on patient history. Screening for the female athlete triad at annual sports physicals or during routine exams and acute visits if there are concerns (1,5)[A]. There are several screening tools that have been validated for use in female athletes, including Athletic Milieu Direct Questionnaire (AMDQ), Brief Eating Disorders in Athletes Questionnaire (BEDA-Q), and Female Athlete Screening Tool (FAST) (7). However, there is no current consensus on which tool to use in practice (7).

HISTORY

Assess menstrual history (including oral contraceptive use), fracture history, and symptoms of depression. Assess dietary practices, eating behaviors, and history of weight changes. Dietary intake logs and a nutritional assessment by a sports dietitian can help. Assess body image; fear of weight gain; fluctuations in weight; history of DE; and use of laxatives, diet pills, or enemas.

PHYSICAL EXAM

- Height, weight, body mass index (BMI) <17.5% kg/m² or <85% of expected body weight in adolescents (1)[A]
- Common findings include bradycardia, orthostatic hypotension, hypothermia, cold or cyanotic extremities, lanugo, parotid gland enlargement or tenderness, epigastric tenderness, eroded tooth enamel, and knuckle or hand calluses (Russell sign).
- Patients with amenorrhea should undergo a pelvic exam to verify the presence of a uterus and evaluate for outflow tract abnormalities. Vaginal atrophy may be present if the patient is hypoestrogenic.

DIFFERENTIAL DIAGNOSIS

Screen for anorexia nervosa, bulimia nervosa, avoidant/restrictive food intake disorder, and

rumination disorder using the *DSM-5* criteria. Rule out the following in amenorrheic patients:
- Pregnancy
- Endocrine abnormalities: thyroid dysfunction, Cushing syndrome
- Hypothalamic dysfunction: psychological stress-induced amenorrhea, medication-induced amenorrhea, Kallmann syndrome
- Pituitary dysfunction: prolactinoma, Sheehan syndrome, sarcoidosis, empty sella syndrome
- Ovarian dysfunction: polycystic ovarian syndrome, premature ovarian failure, menopause, gonadal dysgenesis, Turner syndrome, ovarian neoplasm, autoimmune disease
- Uterine dysfunction: Asherman syndrome, absence of uterus

DIAGNOSTIC TESTS & INTERPRETATION
Initial Tests (lab, imaging)
- Basic metabolic panel, magnesium, phosphorus, albumin, CBC with differential, ESR, thyroid-stimulating hormone (TSH), calcium, 25-OH vitamin D, and urinalysis (1,6)
- Evaluation for secondary amenorrhea includes urine hCG, FSH, LH, prolactin, and TSH.
- Pelvic ultrasound in patients with hyperandrogenism to exclude polycystic ovaries or virilizing ovarian tumors
- ECG to rule out prolonged QT interval

Follow-Up Tests & Special Considerations
- BMD testing by dual-energy x-ray absorptiometry (DEXA) is based on a risk stratification model (1). Risk factors include DE, eating disorders >6 months, hypoestrogenism, amenorrhea, oligomenorrhea, and/or in patients with a history of stress fractures or fractures from minimal impact.
- If components of the triad persist, ISCD 2013 guidelines suggest reevaluation by the same DEXA machine every 1 to 2 years.

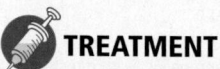 ## TREATMENT

- The goal is to optimize nutritional status and treat maladaptive behavioral disorders (1,4)[A].
- A multidisciplinary team includes a physician, registered dietitian, and behavioral health provider. Build open lines of communication with coaches, trainers, and family.
- A positive EA of >30 kcal/kg of fat-free muscle mass/day is sufficient to restore menses (5)[A].
- Physically active females should strive for an EA of >45 kcal/kg of fat-free muscle mass/day (1)[A].

MEDICATION
First Line
- Increasing EA through appropriate nutrition is the best strategy for normalizing gonadotropin pulsatility and release. The use of combination oral contraceptive pills (cOCPs), hormone replacement therapy (HRT), and/or bisphosphonates has not been clearly shown to increase BMD or aid in the restoration of normal menstrual cycling. cOCPs or transdermal estradiol with cyclic progesterone can be considered in patients with particularly low BMD Z-scores and fracture histories who do not respond to 1 year of nonpharmacologic management.

- cOCP or transdermal estradiol can also be given to minimize further bone loss in patients >16 years and <21 years who, despite adequate nutrition and body weight gain, continue to have decreasing BMD and functional hypothalamic amenorrhea.
- Provide calcium and vitamin D supplementation to maintain serum levels within 32 to 50 mg/mL (1)[A].

INPATIENT CONSIDERATIONS
Evaluate patients with eating disorders for potentially life-threatening conditions requiring hospital admission, including bradycardia, severe orthostatic hypotension, significant electrolyte imbalances, hypothermia, arrhythmias, or prolonged QT interval.

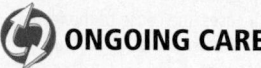 ## ONGOING CARE

- Patients should have regular follow-up with a multidisciplinary treatment team (6)[A].
- Cognitive-behavioral therapy (CBT) is effective for exercising women with ED and may be more beneficial than nutritional counseling alone in women with DE behavior.
- "Clearance and Return to Play (RTP) Guidelines by Medical Risk Stratification" help determine when to allow an athlete to return to competition. More research is needed to validate this model (1)[A].
- To continue training and competing, athletes with eating disorders must agree to the following stipulations as part of a behavioral contract: to comply with all treatment strategies; to be closely monitored by health care providers; to place treatment goals over training goals; and to modify the type, duration, and intensity of training or competition as necessary.

PATIENT EDUCATION
All young female patients should be counseled on the importance of proper nutrition, calcium, and vitamin D intake and the benefits of regular weight-bearing exercise. Patients presenting with ≥1 components of the triad should be educated about the short- and long-term effects of low BMD (1,4)[A].

PROGNOSIS
- The short- and long-term prognosis for patients with female athlete triad depends on time to diagnosis and response to treatment.
- It is estimated that amenorrheic women will lose 2–3% of bone mass per year without intervention.
- With early diagnosis and treatment using a multidisciplinary team, the prognosis for patients with the female athlete triad is good. Patients regain normal menstrual cycling and increase BMD.
- Because the triad often occurs within the age window of optimal bone strengthening, patients with a prolonged disease course may suffer from complications of decreased BMD throughout their adolescent and adult life.
- Patients with DE behaviors often require long-term therapy to manage their disease.

REFERENCES
1. De Souza MJ, Nattiv A, Joy E, et al. 2014 Female Athlete Triad Coalition consensus statement on treatment and return to play of the female athlete triad: 1st International Conference held in San Francisco, CA, May 2012, and 2nd International Conference held in Indianapolis, IN, May 2013. *Clin J Sport Med.* 2014;24(2):96–119.
2. Mallinson RJ, De Souza MJ. Current perspectives on the etiology and manifestation of the "silent" component of the female athlete triad. *Int J Womens Health.* 2014;6:451–467.
3. Lanser EM, Zach KN, Hoch AZ. The female athlete triad and endothelial dysfunction. *PM R.* 2011;3(5):458–465.
4. Barrack MT, Ackerman KE, Gibbs JC. Update on the female athlete triad. *Curr Rev Musculoskeletal Med.* 2013;6(2):195–204.
5. Temme KE, Hoch AZ. Recognition and rehabilitation of the female athlete triad/tetrad: a multidisciplinary approach. *Curr Sports Med Rep.* 2013;12(3):190–199.
6. Deimel JF, Dunlap BJ. The female athlete triad. *Clin Sports Med.* 2012;31(2):247–254.
7. Knapp J, Aerni G, Anderson J. Eating disorders in female athletes: use of screening tools. *Curr Sports Med Rep.* 2014;13(4):214–218.

ADDITIONAL READING
Nattiv A, Loucks AB, Manore MM, et al. American College of Sports Medicine position stand. The female athlete triad. *Med Sci Sports Exerc.* 2007;39(10):1867–1882.

 ### SEE ALSO

Algorithms: Amenorrhea, Primary (Absence of Menarche by Age 16); Amenorrhea, Secondary; Weight Loss, Unintentional

 ### CODES

ICD10
- F50.9 Eating disorder, unspecified
- N91.2 Amenorrhea, unspecified
- R53.83 Other fatigue

CLINICAL PEARLS
- The female athlete triad consists of: low EA (with or without DE), MD, and low BMD. Athletes may exhibit varying degrees of dysfunction in any of these three areas.
- Screen at-risk women to allow for early diagnosis and intervention.
- Early intervention by a multidisciplinary team, including physicians, registered dietitians, mental health professionals, coaches, trainers, and parents, is the most successful strategy to minimize further bone loss, recover BMD, and regain normal menstrual function.
- Current guidelines recommend screening for abnormal BMD using DEXA studies for patients with DE, eating disorders >6 months, hypoestrogenism, amenorrhea, oligomenorrhea, and/or in patients with a history of stress fractures or fractures from minimal impact.

F

FEVER OF UNKNOWN ORIGIN (FUO)

Scott T. Henderson, MD

BASICS

DESCRIPTION
- Classic definition
  - Repeated fever >38.3°C
  - Fever duration at least 3 weeks
  - Uncertain diagnosis after 1 week of study in the hospital
- The FUO definition has evolved over time and should be based on characteristics and patient subtypes. In-hospital evaluation has been eliminated in previously healthy people.
- Some expand the definition to include nosocomial, neutropenic, and shorter duration HIV-associated fevers.

EPIDEMIOLOGY
Incidence
Incidence unclear

ETIOLOGY AND PATHOPHYSIOLOGY
- >200 causes; each with prevalence of ≤5%
- Most commonly, FUO is an atypical presentation of a common condition.
- Spectrum of causes varies by geography
- Infection
  - Abdominal or pelvic abscesses
  - Amebic hepatitis
  - Catheter infections
  - Cytomegalovirus
  - Dental abscesses
  - Endocarditis/pericarditis
  - HIV (advanced stage)
  - Mycobacterial infection (often with advanced HIV)
  - Osteomyelitis
  - Renal
  - Sinusitis
  - Wound infections
  - Other miscellaneous infections
- Neoplasms
  - Atrial myxoma
  - Colorectal cancer
  - Hepatoma
  - Lymphoma
  - Leukemia
  - Solid tumors (renal cell carcinoma)
- Noninfectious inflammatory disease
  - Connective tissue diseases
    o Adult Still disease
    o Rheumatoid arthritis
    o Systemic lupus erythematosus
  - Granulomatous disease
    o Crohn disease
    o Sarcoidosis
  - Vasculitis syndromes
    o Giant cell arteritis
    o Polymyalgia rheumatica
- Other causes
  - Alcoholic hepatitis
  - Cerebrovascular accident
  - Cirrhosis

- Medications
  o Allopurinol, captopril, carbamazepine, cephalosporins, cimetidine, clofibrate, erythromycin, heparin, hydralazine, hydrochlorothiazide, isoniazid, meperidine, methyldopa, nifedipine, nitrofurantoin, penicillin, phenytoin, procainamide, quinidine, sulfonamides
- Endocrine disease
- Factitious/fraudulent fever
- Occupational causes
- Periodic fever
- Pulmonary emboli/deep vein thrombosis
- Thermoregulatory disorders
- In up to 20–30% of cases, the cause of the fever will not be identified despite thorough workup.

RISK FACTORS
- Recent travel
- Exposure to biologic or chemical agents
- HIV-infection (particularly in advanced stages)
- Elderly
- Drug abuse
- Immigrants
- Young female health care workers (consider factitious fever)

Geriatric Considerations
Noninfectious inflammatory diseases are the most frequent causes in high-income countries. This most commonly includes temporal arteritis, polymyalgia rheumatica, or rheumatoid arthritis. In elderly patients with infections, common causes include intra-abdominal abscess, complicated urinary tract infection, tuberculosis, and endocarditis. Other common causes of FUO in patients >65 years include malignancies, particularly hematologic malignancies and drug-induced fever.

Pediatric Considerations
- ~50% of FUO in published pediatric case series are infectious. Collagen vascular disease, malignancy are also common (1)[A].
- Inflammatory bowel is a common cause in older children and adolescents.

DIAGNOSIS

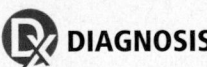

HISTORY
- Common constitutional symptoms
  - Chills, night sweats, myalgias, weight loss with an intact appetite (infectious)
  - Arthralgias, myalgias, fatigue (inflammatory)
  - Fatigue, night sweats, weight loss with loss of appetite (neoplasms)
- Past medical history: chronic infections, abdominal diseases, transfusion history, malignancy, psychiatric illness, and recent hospitalization
- Past surgical history: type of surgery performed, postoperative complications, and any indwelling foreign material
- Obtain a comprehensive list of all medications, including over-the-counter and herbal remedies.
- Family history, such as periodic fever syndromes and recent febrile illnesses in family members to which the patient may have been exposed

ALERT
Obtain a thorough travel, psychosocial, occupational, sexual, and drug use history.

PHYSICAL EXAM
- Physical findings with high diagnostic yield
  - Funduscopic exam for choroid tubercles or Roth spots
  - Temporal artery tenderness
  - Oral-mucosal lesions
  - Auscultation for bruits and murmurs
  - Abdominal palpation for organomegaly
  - Rectal examination
  - Testicular examination
  - Lymph node examination
  - Skin and nail bed exam for clubbing, nodules, lesions, and erosions
  - Focal neurologic signs
  - Bony tenderness or joint effusion
  - Serial exams are often helpful for evolving physical signs associated with FUO (e.g., lesions associated with endocarditis).

DIFFERENTIAL DIAGNOSIS
See "Etiology and Pathophysiology."

DIAGNOSTIC TESTS & INTERPRETATION
Initial Tests (lab, imaging)
- CBC
- Peripheral blood smear
- Electrolytes, BUN and creatinine
- Lactate dehydrogenase
- Calcium
- LFTs
- C-reactive protein, ESR
- HIV testing
- Blood cultures (not to exceed six sets)
- Urinalysis and urine culture
- Chest x-ray
- CT or MRI of abdomen and pelvis (with directed biopsy, if indicated) (2)[C]

Follow-Up Tests & Special Considerations
- Rheumatoid factor and antinuclear antibody test
- Serologic tests: Epstein-Barr, hepatitis, syphilis, Lyme disease, Q fever, cytomegalovirus, amebiasis, coccidioidomycosis
- Serum ferritin
- Serum protein electrophoresis
- Sputum and urine cultures for TB
- Thyroid function tests
- Tuberculin skin test
  - May not be helpful if anergic or acute infection
  - If test negative, repeat in 2 weeks
  - If indicated, consider an interferon gamma release assay (IGRA) test.
- Technetium-based scan, if infectious process or tumor suspected (2)[B]
- FDG-PET/CT scan if infectious process, inflammatory process, or tumor suspected; PET scans have a high negative predictive value and good sensitivity (but may have false positives) (3)[A].

- Ultrasound of abdomen and pelvis (plus directed biopsy, if indicated) if renal obstruction or gallbladder/biliary tree pathology suspected
- Echocardiogram if cardiac valve lesions (endocarditis), atrial myxomas, or pericardial effusion is suspected
- Lower-extremity Doppler if deep vein thrombosis/pulmonary embolism suspected
- CT scan of chest if pulmonary emboli suspected
- Indium-labeled leukocyte scanning if inflammatory process or occult abscess suspected
- Bone scan if osteomyelitis or metastatic disease suspected

Diagnostic Procedures/Other
- Liver biopsy if granulomatous disease suspected (2)[C]
- Temporal artery biopsy, particularly in the elderly
- Lymph node, muscle, or skin biopsy, if clinically indicated
- Bone marrow aspiration biopsy with smear, culture, histologic examination, and flow cytometry
- Spinal tap, if clinically indicated

Test Interpretation
Depends on etiology

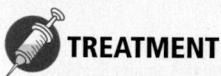

TREATMENT

GENERAL MEASURES
- Treatment depends on the specific etiology.
- Therapeutic trials are a last resort and should be as specific as possible based on available clinical evidence. Such "shotgun" approaches are discouraged because they obscure the clinical picture, have untoward effects, and do not provide a diagnostic solution (2)[C].

MEDICATION
First Line
- First-line drugs depend on the diagnosis.
- Evidence does not support isolated treatment of fever (4)[C].

Second Line
Only if the patient has localizing symptoms associated with the fever or continues to decline, consider a therapeutic trial—consultation with appropriate specialists (infectious disease, rheumatology) is recommended in this case.
- Antibiotic trial based on patient's history and suspected culture negative endocarditis
- Antituberculous therapy if there is a high risk for TB pending definitive culture results
- Corticosteroid trial based on patient's history (once occult malignancy is ruled out) if temporal arteritis is suspected

ALERT
If a steroid trial is initiated, patient may have a relapse after treatment or if certain conditions (e.g., TB) have been undiagnosed.

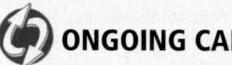

ADDITIONAL THERAPIES
Febrile patients have increased caloric and fluid demands.

SURGERY/OTHER PROCEDURES
The need for exploratory laparotomy has been largely eliminated with the advent of more sophisticated tests and imaging modalities.

INPATIENT CONSIDERATIONS
Admission Criteria/Initial Stabilization
- Reserved for the ill and debilitated
- Consider if factitious fever has been ruled out or an invasive procedure is indicated

 ## ONGOING CARE

FOLLOW-UP RECOMMENDATIONS
Patient Monitoring
If the etiology of the fever remains unknown, repeat the history, physical exam, and screening lab studies.

DIET
No specific dietary recommendations have been shown to ameliorate undiagnosed fever.

PATIENT EDUCATION
Maintain an open line of communication between physician and patient/family as the workup progresses:
- The extended time required in establishing a diagnosis can be frustrating.

PROGNOSIS
- Depends on etiology and age
  - Patients with HIV have the highest mortality.
- 1-year survival rates (reflecting deaths due to all causes)

Age	Survival
<35 years	91%
35–64 years	82%
>64 years	67%

COMPLICATIONS
Depends on etiology

Pregnancy Considerations
Fever increases the risk of neural tube defects in pregnancy and can also trigger preterm labor.

REFERENCES

1. Chow A, Robinson JL. Fever of unknown origin in children: a systematic review. *World J Pediatr*. 2011;7(1):5–10.
2. Mourad O, Palda V, Detsky AS. A comprehensive evidence-based approach to fever of unknown origin. *Arch Intern Med*. 2003;163(5):545–551.
3. Hao R, Yuan L, Kan Y, et al. Diagnostic performance of 18F-FDG PET/CT in patients with fever of unknown origin: a meta-analysis. *Nucl Med Commun*. 2013;34(7):682–688.
4. Hersch EC, Oh RC. Prolonged febrile illness and fever of unknown origin in adults. *Am Fam Physician*. 2014;90(2):91–96.

ADDITIONAL READING

- Ben-Baruch S, Canaani J, Braunstein R, et al. Predictive parameters for a diagnostic bone marrow biopsy specimen in the work-up of fever of unknown origin. *Mayo Clin Proc*. 2012;87(2):136–142.
- Hayakawa K, Ramasamy B, Chandrasekar PH. Fever of unknown origin: an evidence-based review. *Am J Med Sci*. 2012;344(4):307–316.
- Varghese GM, Trowbridge P, Doherty T. Investigating and managing pyrexia of unknown origin in adults. *BMJ*. 2010;341:C5470.

 ### SEE ALSO

- Arthritis, Juvenile Idiopathic; Colorectal Cancer; Cytomegalovirus (CMV) Inclusion Disease; Endocarditis, Infective; Hepatoma; HIV/AIDS; Lupus Erythematosus, Discoid; Osteomyelitis; Polyarteritis Nodosa; Polymyalgia Rheumatica; Pulmonary Embolism; Rheumatic Fever; Sinusitis; Stroke, Acute; Arteritis, Temporal
- Algorithms: Fever in the First 3 Months of Life; Fever of Unknown Origin

CODES

ICD10
R50.9 Fever, unspecified

CLINICAL PEARLS

- A sequential approach to FUO based on a careful history, physical examination, and targeted testing/imaging typically leads to a rational diagnosis in most cases.
- Use empiric therapy only in carefully defined circumstances.
- FUO cases that defy precise diagnosis after intensive investigation and prolonged observation generally carry a favorable prognosis.
- FUO in older persons may represent an atypical presentations of a common disease.
- The most common causes of FUO in high-income countries are noninfectious inflammatory diseases and cases that remain idiopathic.

F

FIBROCYSTIC CHANGES OF THE BREAST

Alain Michael P. Abellada, MD

 BASICS

DESCRIPTION

- Fibrocystic changes (FCC) is not a disease but refers to a constellation of benign histologic findings. It is the most frequent female benign clinical breast finding.
- The most common symptoms are cyclic pain and tenderness, swelling, and fullness.
- The breast tissue may feel dense with areas of thicker tissue having an irregular, nodular, or ridge-like surface.
- Women may experience sensitivity to touch with a burning sensation. For some women, the pain is so severe that it limits exercise or the ability to lie prone.
- Usually affects both breasts, most often in the upper outer quadrant where most of the milk-producing glands are located.
- Histologically, in addition to macrocysts and microcysts, FCC may contain solid elements including adenosis, sclerosis, apocrine metaplasia, stromal fibrosis, and epithelial metaplasia and hyperplasia.
  - Depending on the presence of epithelial hyperplasia, fibrocystic change is classified as nonproliferative, proliferative without atypia, or proliferative with atypia.
- System(s) affected: endocrine/metabolic, reproductive
- Synonym(s): diffuse cystic mastopathy; fibrocystic disease; chronic cystic mastitis; or mammary dysplasia

EPIDEMIOLOGY

FCC occurs with great frequency in the general population. It affects women between the ages of 25 and 50 years and it is rare below the age of 20.

Incidence

Unknown but very frequent

Prevalence

Up to 1/3 of women aged 30 to 50 years have cysts in their breasts. It most commonly presents in the 3rd decade, peaks in the 4th decade when hormonal function is at its peak, and sharply diminishes after menopause.

- With hormone replacement therapy, FCC may extend into menopause
- Less common in East Asian races

ETIOLOGY AND PATHOPHYSIOLOGY

- FCC originates from an exaggerated response of breast stroma and epithelium to a variety of circulating and locally produced hormones (mainly estrogen and progesterone) and growth factors.
- Cysts may form due to dilatation of the lobular acini possibly due to imbalance of fluid secretion and resorption, or due to obstruction of the duct leading to the lobule.

RISK FACTORS

- In many women, methylxanthine-containing substances (e.g., coffee, tea, cola, and chocolate) can potentiate symptoms of FCC, though a direct causality has not been established.
- Diet high in saturated fats may increase risk of FCC.

COMMONLY ASSOCIATED CONDITIONS

FCC categorized as proliferative with atypia confers a higher risk of breast cancer.

 DIAGNOSIS

HISTORY

- Obtain personal history of breast biopsy and family history of breast disease (benign or malignant). It is important to ascertain if the patient has a known family history of *BRCA1* or *BRCA2*-related cancer.
- Inquire regarding pertinent signs/symptoms, such as breast pain, engorgement, nipple discharge, palpable lumps, tenderness.
  - Symptomatically, the condition is manifested as premenstrual cyclic mastalgia, with pain and tenderness to touch.

PHYSICAL EXAM

- The patient should be examined in the following positions while disrobed down to the waist (1):
  - With the patient standing with arms at sides, observe for elevation of the level of a nipple, dimpling, bulging, and peau d'orange.
  - With the patient's arms raised above her head, observe for dimpling and elevation of the nipple (may accentuate a mass fixed to the pectoral fascia). If so, have the patient push her hands down against her hips to flex and tense the pectoralis major muscles, move the mass to determine fixation to the underlying fascia.
  - If the patient has large and pendulous breasts, ask her to lean forward, so that her breasts hang free from the chest wall (retraction and masses may become more evident).
  - With the patient lying supine, palpate with the pads of the three middle fingers (with varying pressures from light, to medium, to deep), rotating the fingers in small circular motions and moving in vertical overlapping passes from rostral to caudal and then back caudal to rostral in the next pass. The lateral half of the breast is best palpated with the patient rolled onto the contralateral hip and the medial half with the patient supine, both with the ipsilateral hand behind the head. The entire breast from the second to sixth rib and from the left sternal border to the midaxillary line must be palpated against the chest wall.
- Be certain to examine the creases under and between the breasts. If the patient has noted a lump, ask her to point it out; always palpate the opposite breast first.
- Patients with fibrocystic changes have clinical breast findings that range from mild alterations in texture to dense, firm breast tissue with palpable masses.

DIFFERENTIAL DIAGNOSIS

- Pain
  - Mastitis
  - Costochondritis
  - Pectoralis muscle strain
  - Neuralgia
  - Breast cancer
  - Angina pectoris
  - Gastroesophageal reflux (GERD)
  - Superficial phlebitis of the thoracoepigastric vein (Mondor disease)
- Masses
  - Breast cancer
  - Sebaceous cyst
  - Fibroadenoma
  - Lipoma
  - Fat necrosis
- Skin changes
  - Breast cancer (peau d'orange: thickened skin similar to peel of an orange)
  - Eczema

DIAGNOSTIC TESTS & INTERPRETATION

- Evaluation should focus on excluding breast cancer.
- Testing may be conducted based on a level of clinical suspicion.
- FCC can be evaluated with mammogram, though dense breast tissue may appear normal in women <35 years of age.
- Ultrasound is the most important method in assessing a cyst.

Initial Tests (lab, imaging)

- On mammogram, FCC appears as nodular densities of breast tissue; solitary cysts can appear as round or ovoid or well-circumscribed masses, usually with low to intermediate density. FCC may also contain calcifications.
- On ultrasound, if a simple cyst is demonstrated as an anechoic structure with imperceptible wall and posterior acoustic enhancement, benign diagnosis is confirmed and no further imaging or intervention is indicated. However, if the cyst appears to be thick-walled and/or contains internal echoes, differential diagnosis should include a complicated cyst, an abscess, a galactocele, or a focal duct ectasia in the appropriate clinical contexts.
- MRI is indicated in patients with *BRCA1* or *BRCA2* mutation or in any woman with ≥25% lifetime risk for breast cancer.
- On MRI, cystic changes are well-circumscribed lesions of high-signal intensity on T2-weighted sequences and of low-signal intensity on T1-weighted images.

Diagnostic Procedures/Other

- Fine-needle aspiration (FNA) and biopsy:
  - Allows differentiation of cystic and solid lesions
  - Aspirate may be straw-colored, dark brown, or green.
  - Cells sent for cytology can reveal cancer with high accuracy.
  - Low morbidity
- If mass disappears, no further evaluation is necessary (including cytologic evaluation of aspirated fluid).

- On the basis of the presence and degree of epithelial hyperplasia, FCC is comprised of nonproliferative, (approximately 65% of the total), proliferative without, (approximately 30% of the total), and proliferative with atypia, (approximately 5% to 8% of the total) (2).

Test Interpretation

Certain histologic changes in the setting of fibrocystic change confer an increased risk for breast cancer:

- Nonproliferative changes: relative risk of 1.2 to 1.4
- Proliferative disease (PD) without atypia: relative risk of 1.7 to 2.1
- PD with atypia: relative risk ≥4 (3)[B]

 TREATMENT

- After ruling out malignancy by means of examination and/or imaging and diagnostic procedures, FCC may not require treatment and often resolves with time.
- Cool compresses, avoiding trauma, and around-the-clock wearing of a well-fitting, supportive brassiere may be useful for symptom relief.

MEDICATION

First Line

For cyclic pain and swelling: NSAIDs:

- Ibuprofen 400 mg QID/PRN
- Naproxen 500 mg BID/PRN

Second Line

- Oral contraceptives may be useful in modulating symptoms or in preventing the development of new changes.
- For severe pain, consider the following (4,5)[B]:
  - Danazol (Danocrine) 100 to 400 mg/day divided in 2 doses for 4 to 6 months
  - Bromocriptine 1.25 to 2.5 mg BID for 3 months
  - Tamoxifen 10 mg/day for 3 to 6 months
  - These medications are not without serious side effects and thorough counseling is required. Consultation with a breast specialist may be considered.
- Bromocriptine, danazol, and tamoxifen all significantly reduced pain. Tamoxifen was found to have the fewest adverse effects (4)[A].

ISSUES FOR REFERRAL

- If discrete palpable lesion in a woman ≥35 years: US, then refer to a surgeon.
- If discrete palpable lesion in a woman >35 years: Diagnostic mammography ± US, then refer to surgeon.

SURGERY

- Breast cyst aspiration can be both diagnostic and therapeutic.
- Core-needle biopsies performed under stereotactic guidance with vacuum assistance has similar accuracy in distinguishing between malignant and benign lesions compared to open surgical biopsy (6)[A].

COMPLEMENTARY & ALTERNATIVE MEDICINE

- The use of vitamin E has shown effectiveness in treating breast pain due to FCC (3)[B].
- Evening primrose oil and pyridoxine have not been shown to reduce mastalgia (4)[A],(7)[B].

 ONGOING CARE

FOLLOW-UP RECOMMENDATIONS

Condition is benign, chronic, and recurrent.

Patient Monitoring

- Follow-up times are variable, depending on the clinical situation and pertinent family history.
- US is useful to differentiate cysts from solid lesions and in evaluating women <35 years of age for FCC but is not useful for screening.
- Screening mammograms should be obtained after age 40 to 50 years. Refer to the USPSTF, ACOG, or ACS recommendations for screening schedules.

DIET

The role of caffeine consumption in the development and treatment of FCC has never been proven; however, some patients report relief of symptoms after abstinence from coffee, tea, and chocolate.

PATIENT EDUCATION

- Patient information on fibrocystic breasts from the Mayo Foundation for Medical Education and Research: http://www.mayoclinic.org/diseases-conditions/fibrocystic-breasts/basics/definition/con-20034681
- Information on breast cancer prevention from the National Cancer Institute: http://www.cancer.gov/
- Information on fibrocystic breasts from the American Cancer Society: http://www.cancer.org/healthy/findcancerearly/womenshealth/non-cancerousbreastconditions/non-cancerous-breast-conditions-finding-benign-br-cond

REFERENCES

1. Barton MB, Harris R, Fletcher SW. The rational clinical examination. Does this patient have breast cancer? The screening clinical breast examination: should it be done? How? *JAMA*. 1999;282(13):1270–1280.
2. Hartmann LC, Sellers TA, Frost MH, et al. Benign breast disease and the risk of breast cancer. *N Engl J Med*. 2005;353(3):229-237.
3. Parsay S, Olfati F, Nahidi S. Therapeutic effects of vitamin E on cyclic mastalgia. *Breast J*. 2009;15(5):510-514.
4. Srivastava A, Mansel RE, Arvind N, et al. Evidence-based management of mastalgia: a meta-analysis of randomised trials. *Breast*. 2007;16(5):503–512.
5. Mousavi SR, Mousavi SM, Samsami M, et al. Comparison of tamoxifen with danazol in the management of fibrocystic disease. *Int J Med Sci*. 2011;2:329–331.
6. Bruening W, Fontanarosa J, Tipton K, et al. Systematic review: comparative effectiveness of core-needle and open surgical biopsy to diagnose breast lesions. *Ann Intern Med*. 2010;152(4):238–246.
7. Horner NK, Lampe JW. Potential mechanisms of diet therapy for fibrocystic breast conditions show inadequate evidence of effectiveness. *J Am Diet Assoc*. 2000;100(11):1368–1380.

ADDITIONAL READING

- Amin AL, Purdy AC, Mattingly JD, et al. Benign breast disease. *Surg Clin North Am*. 2013;93(2):299–308.
- Griffin JL, Pearlman MD. Breast cancer screening in women at average risk and high risk. *Obstet Gynecol*. 2010;116(6):1410–1421.
- Jatoi I. Screening clinical breast examination. *Surg Clin North Am*. 2003;83(4):789–801.
- Klein S. Evaluation of palpable breast masses. *Am Fam Physician*. 2005;71(9):1731–1738.
- Meisner AL, Fekrazad MH, Royce ME. Breast disease: benign and malignant. *Med Clin North Am*. 2008;92(5):1115–1141.
- Morris EA. Diagnostic breast MR imaging: current status and future directions. *Magn Reson Imaging Clin N Am*. 2010;18(1):57–74.
- Rinaldi P, Ierardi C, Costantini M, et al. Cystic breast lesions: sonographic findings and clinical management. *J Ultrasound Med*. 2010;29(11):1617–1626.
- Santen RJ, Mansel R. Benign breast disorders. *N Engl J Med*. 2005;353(3):275–285.
- Saslow D, Boetes C, Burke W, et al. American Cancer Society guidelines for breast screening with MRI as an adjunct to mammography. *CA Cancer J Clin*. 2007;57(2):75–89.

CODES

ICD10

- N60.19 Diffuse cystic mastopathy of unspecified breast
- N60.09 Solitary cyst of unspecified breast
- N60.29 Fibroadenosis of unspecified breast

CLINICAL PEARLS

- FCC of the breast comprise a spectrum of histopathologic changes are a common finding in reproductive-aged women. The former term of fibrocystic disease is a misnomer.
- Atypia, as demonstrated histopathologically, confers an increased cancer risk.
- NSAIDs are the first-line treatment. OCPs, Danazol, Bromocripine, and Tamoxifen are second-line treatments, though not without considerable adverse effects. Caution should be used and consultation with a breast specialist is recommended.

FIBROMYALGIA

F. Stuart Leeds, MD, MS

BASICS

DESCRIPTION
- Chronic, widespread noninflammatory musculoskeletal pain syndrome with multisystem manifestations. Although the specific pathophysiology has not been elucidated, it is generally thought to be a disorder of altered central pain regulation.
- Synonym(s): FMS; fibrositis, fibromyositis (misnomers); "psychogenic rheumatism" (archaic and inaccurate)

EPIDEMIOLOGY
Incidence
- Predominant sex: female > male (70–90% are females) (1)
- Predominant age range: 20 to 65 years

Prevalence
2–5% of adult U.S. population (2); 8% of primary care patients

ETIOLOGY AND PATHOPHYSIOLOGY
- Idiopathic, but appears to be a primary disorder of central pain processing, termed central sensitization (3). Afferent augmentation of peripheral nociceptive stimuli
- Alterations in neuroendocrine, neuromodulation, neurotransmitter, neurotransporter, biochemical, and neuroreceptor function/physiology
- Sleep abnormalities—α-wave intrusion (4)
- Inflammation is not a feature of fibromyalgia.

Genetics
- Genetics
  - High familial aggregation
  - Inheritance is unknown but likely polygenic.
  - Odds ratio may be as high as 8.5 for a first-degree relative of a familial proband (5).
- Environmental—several triggers have been described:
  - Physical trauma or severe illness
  - Stressors (e.g., work, family, life events, and physical/sexual abuse)
  - Viral and bacterial infections

RISK FACTORS
- Female gender
- Poor functional status
- Negative/stressful life events
- Low socioeconomic status

GENERAL PREVENTION
No known strategies for prevention.

COMMONLY ASSOCIATED CONDITIONS
- Often a comorbid condition with other rheumatologic or neurologic disorders
- Obesity is frequently present and is associated with increased severity of symptoms (6).

DIAGNOSIS

- Original 1990 ACR criteria, still widely used: (i) pain in all four quadrants, (ii) axial (neck/spine) involvement, (iii) tender points (TPs) ≥11, (iv) no other explanation for symptoms (2)
- Per the 2010 revised ACR criteria (2)
  - Based on Widespread Pain Index (WPI) and Symptom Score (SS)
    - Must have (WPI ≥7 + SS ≥5) or (WPI ≥3 and SS ≥9); and
    - Symptoms for >3 months; and
    - No other explanation for these symptoms

- A questionnaire tool to facilitate WPI/SS patient scoring and diagnosis may be found at: www.fmnetnews.com/docs/NewFibroCriteriaSurvey.pdf
- This tool assesses the following:
  - WPI counts the number of sites of regional pain occurring over past week (**score 0 to 19 sites**)
  - The SS scale score is the sum of two parts.
    - Part 1 grades the three key symptoms: **fatigue**, **waking unrefreshed**, and **cognitive symptoms**
    - Part 2 counts 40+ associated symptoms, ranking them from "none" to "many"
    - The parts are added together to give a total SS of **0 to 12**.
- The Visual Analogue Scale Fibromyalgia Impact Questionnaire (VASFIQ) (7) is recommended for initial and serial assessment of patient's functional status. It may be found at: http://www.ncbi.nlm.nih.gov/pmc/articles/PMC3383533/figure/fig1-1759720X11416863/
- Enhancements to the 2010 criteria, termed **2011modCr** and **2013altCr** (8) have been proposed, but are not yet widely accepted.

HISTORY
- Universal symptoms include
  - Chronic widespread pain ≥3 months: bilateral limbs and in the axial skeleton
  - Fatigue and sleep disturbances
- Often present:
  - Mood disorders, including depression, anxiety, and panic symptoms
  - Cognitive impairment: qualitatively different from that seen in isolated mood disorders ("fibro fog") (9)
  - Headaches: typically, tension and migraine types
  - Other regional pain syndromes, such as irritable bowel syndrome, chronic pelvic pain, vulvodynia, and interstitial cystitis
  - Paresthesias, often "nonanatomic"
  - Exercise intolerance, dyspnea, and palpitations
  - Sexual dysfunction
  - Ocular dryness
  - "Multiple chemical sensitivity" and an increased tendency to report drug reactions
  - Impaired social/occupational functioning
  - Symptoms can wax and wane on a day-to-day basis, varying in quality, intensity, and location.

PHYSICAL EXAM
- Classic fibromyalgia TPs: 9 symmetric pairs (5 anterior, 4 posterior) located at anterior sternocleidomastoids, upper mid-trapezius, medial 2nd intercostal spaces, lateral epicondyles, medial fat pad of knees, and posteriorly, at occipital insertions, upper medial scapular insertions, upper outer quadrants of gluteals, and posterior greater trochanters. The presence of ≥11 TPs carries a sensitivity of 88.4% and specificity 81.1% for the disease (2). These are distinct from the "trigger points" found in myofascial pain syndrome.
- Joints examined for swelling, tenderness, erythema, decreased range of motion, crepitus, and cystic or mass lesions—all typically absent in isolated fibromyalgia.
- Document absence of inflammatory musculoskeletal disease features (e.g., no synovitis, enthesopathy, dermatologic/ocular findings)
- Neurologic exam: may demonstrate generalized or "nonanatomic" dysesthesia, hyper- or hypesthesia

DIFFERENTIAL DIAGNOSIS
- RA, SLE, sarcoidosis, and other inflammatory connective tissue disorders
- Diffuse/advanced OA

- Seronegative spondyloarthropathies (AS, psoriatic arthritis, etc.)
- Polymyalgia rheumatica
- Inherited myopathies
- Drug-induced and endocrine myopathies
- Viral/postviral polyarthralgia
- Anemia and iron deficiency
- Electrolyte disturbances: Mg, Na, K, Ca
- Obstructive sleep apnea
- Osteomalacia/vitamin D deficiency
- Opioid-induced hyperalgesia
- Hypothyroidism
- Multiple sclerosis
- Lyme disease
- Hepatitis B and C (chronic)
- Inclusion-body myositis
- Spinal stenosis/neuropathies
- Peripheral vascular disease
- Somatoform disorder
- Overlap syndromes
  - Chronic fatigue syndrome/chronic fatigue immune dysfunction syndrome (CFIDS)
  - Myofascial pain syndrome (more anatomically localized than fibromyalgia, but they may co-occur)

DIAGNOSTIC TESTS & INTERPRETATION
Initial Tests (lab, imaging)
- CBC with differential, ESR or CRP, CPK, TSH, comprehensive metabolic profile; consider 25-OH vitamin D, Mg, B_{12}, folate, and urine drug screen
- ANA, RF, and other rheumatologic labs unnecessary, unless there is evidence of an inflammatory connective tissue disorder.
- Imaging is not indicated, except to exclude other diagnoses.

Diagnostic Procedures/Other
- Sleep studies may be indicated to rule out obstructive sleep apnea or narcolepsy.
- Consider psychiatric or neuropsychiatric evaluation for mood disorders and cognitive disturbances.

TREATMENT

According to the HHS National Guideline Summary (10) and other sources, evidence-based interventions include the following:
- Nonpharmacologic treatment critical to successful outcomes
- Nonpharmacologic

  - Educate the patient about the diagnosis, signs, symptoms, and treatment options (10)[A].

  - Provide Internet education resources.
    - www.fmaware.org
    - www.nfra.net
    - www.fmnetnews.com

  - Use the VASFIQ for initial assessment and interval evaluation during treatment (10)[A].
  - Cognitive-behavioral therapy improves mood, energy, pain, and functional status (10)[A].
  - Aerobic exercise: moderately intense, with gradual progression to avoid symptom exacerbation (11)[A]

  - Weight loss may augment the benefits of exercise.

  - Strength/resistance training—mild to moderate (11)[A]
  - Aquatic exercise training (12)[A]

  - Sleep hygiene

- Pharmacologic
  - The three FDA-approved drugs are duloxetine, milnacipran, and pregabalin; others are used off-label.

MEDICATION

First Line

- Amitriptyline: 10 to 50 mg PO at bedtime to treat pain, fatigue, and sleep disturbances (13)[A]
- Duloxetine: initially 30 mg/day for 1 week, then increase to 60 mg/day as tolerated. Taper if discontinued (13)[A].
- Milnacipran: day 1: 12.5 mg/day; days 2 to 3, begin dividing doses: 12.5 mg BID; days 4 to 7: 25 mg BID; after day 7: 50 mg BID; max dose 100 to 200 mg BID. Taper if discontinued (13)[A].
- Pregabalin: Start with 75 mg BID, titrate over 1 week to 150 mg BID; max dose 450 mg/day divided BID–TID (14)[A].
- Cyclobenzaprine 5 mg HS; titrate up to 10 mg BID–TID (10)[B].

Second Line

- Gabapentin start at 300 mg HS, titrate to 1,200 to 2,400 mg/day divided BID–TID (10)[B].
- Fluoxetine 10 to 80 mg/day PO (higher doses may be more effective). Taper if discontinued (10)[B].
- Paroxetine CR 12.5 to 62.5 mg/day. Taper if discontinued (10)[B].

- Tramadol 50 to 100 mg q6h; likely more effective in combination with acetaminophen (10)[C]
- Several investigational agents show some promise of benefit, including pramipexole (15), naltrexone, quetiapine, sodium oxybate (4), nabilone, and pirlindole (16)
- Cholecalciferol may be beneficial in patients with low 25-OH vitamin D levels (17).

- Medications likely to be ineffective (10)[C] include NSAIDs, opioids, benzodiazepines, magnesium, guaifenesin, thyroxine, corticosteroids, DHEA, melatonin, calcitonin; also antiepileptic agents (other than pregabalin and gabapentin) (18)[A].

- *Note that, given the frequent co-presentation of fibromyalgia with other pain syndromes, it may be reasonable to treat the latter with NSAIDs, corticosteroids, opioids, and other such agents in conjunction with evidence-based fibromyalgia therapies.*

ISSUES FOR REFERRAL

In the case of unclear diagnosis or poor response to therapy, may refer to rheumatology, neurology, and/or pain management.

COMPLEMENTARY & ALTERNATIVE MEDICINE

- Acupuncture (especially electroacupuncture), biofeedback, hypnotherapy (10,19)[B]
- Balneotherapy (mineral-rich baths) (10)[B]

- Yoga, tai chi, and qi gong—improve sleep, fatigue, and quality of life but may not decrease pain (20).
- Limited double-blind trials have shown effectiveness of supplementation with S-adenosyl methionine, and acetyl-L-carnitine.
- Transcranial direct current or magnetic stimulation and repetitive transcranial magnetic stimulation (21,22)

- Likely to be ineffective: chiropractic treatment, massage, electrotherapy, ultrasound, trigger point injections (10)[A]

 ## ONGOING CARE

FOLLOW-UP RECOMMENDATIONS
Patient Monitoring
- For efficacy of therapy at 2- to 4-week intervals
- Advance exercise gradually to maintain tolerability

DIET
No proven efficacy of any specific diet. Caloric or carbohydrate restriction may be helpful in obese patients.

PROGNOSIS
- 50% partial remission after 2 to 3 years of therapy (23)
- Typically has fluctuating, chronic course
- Poorer outcome tied to greater duration/severity of symptoms, depression, advanced age, lack of social support

REFERENCES

1. Jones GT, Atzeni F, Beasley M, et al. The prevalence of fibromyalgia in the general population: a comparison of the American College of Rheumatology 1990, 2010, and modified 2010 classification criteria. *Arthritis Rheumatol*. 2015;67(2):568–575.
2. Wolfe F, Häuser W. Fibromyalgia diagnosis and diagnostic criteria. *Ann Med*. 2011;43(7):495–502.
3. Smith HS, Harris R, Clauw D. Fibromyalgia: an afferent processing disorder leading to a complex pain generalized syndrome. *Pain Physician*. 2011;14(2):E217–E245.
4. Russell IJ, Holman AJ, Swick TJ, et al. Sodium oxybate reduces pain, fatigue, and sleep disturbance and improves functionality in fibromyalgia: results from a 14-week, randomized, double-blind, placebo-controlled study. *Pain*. 2011;152(5):1007–1017.
5. Arnold LM, Hudson JI, Hess EV, et al. Family study of fibromyalgia. *Arthritis Rheum*. 2004;50(3):944–952.
6. Okifuji A, Donaldson GW, Barck L, et al. Relationship between fibromyalgia and obesity in pain, function, mood, and sleep. *J Pain*. 2010;11(12):1329–1337.
7. Boomershine CS, Emir B, Wang Y, et al. Simplifying fibromyalgia assessment: the VASFIQ Brief Symptom Scale. *Ther Adv Musculoskelet Dis*. 2011;3(5):215–226.
8. Bennett RM, Friend R, Marcus D, et al. Criteria for the diagnosis of fibromyalgia: validation of the modified 2010 preliminary American College of Rheumatology criteria and the development of alternative criteria. *Arthritis Care Res (Hoboken)*. 2014;66(9):1364–1373.
9. Glass JM. Cognitive dysfunction in fibromyalgia and chronic fatigue syndrome: new trends and future directions. *Curr Rheumatol Rep*. 2006;8(6):425–429.
10. National Guideline Clearinghouse. Guideline summary NGC-7367: management of fibromyalgia syndrome in adults. http://f.i-md.com/medinfo/material/8d0/4eb2854244ae46d1d13648d0/4eb2855d44ae46d1d13648d3.pdf. Accessed 2014.
11. Häuser W, Klose P, Langhorst J, et al. Efficacy of different types of aerobic exercise in fibromyalgia syndrome: a systematic review and meta-analysis of randomised controlled trials. *Arthritis Res Ther*. 2010;12(3):R79.
12. Bidonde J, Busch AJ, Webber SC, et al. Aquatic exercise training for fibromyalgia. *Cochrane Database Syst Rev*. 2014;(10):CD011336.
13. Häuser W, Petzke F, Üçeyler N, et al. Comparative efficacy and acceptability of amitriptyline, duloxetine and milnacipran in fibromyalgia syndrome: a systematic review with meta-analysis. *Rheumatology (Oxford)*. 2011;50(3):532–543.
14. Häuser W, Walitt B, Fitzcharles MA, et al. Review of pharmacological therapies in fibromyalgia syndrome. *Arthritis Res Ther*. 2014;16(1):201.
15. Holman AJ, Myers RR. A randomized, double-blind, placebo-controlled trial of pramipexole, a dopamine agonist, in patients with fibromyalgia receiving concomitant medications. *Arthritis Rheum*. 2005;52(8):2495–2505.
16. Tort S, Urrútia G, Nishishinya MB, et al. Monoamine oxidase inhibitors (MAOIs) for fibromyalgia syndrome. *Cochrane Database Syst Rev*. 2012;(4):CD009807.
17. Wepner F, Scheuer R, Schuetz-Wieser B, et al. Effects of vitamin D on patients with fibromyalgia syndrome: a randomized placebo-controlled trial. *Pain*. 2014;155(2):261–268.
18. Wiffen PJ, Derry S, Moore RA, et al. Antiepileptic drugs for neuropathic pain and fibromyalgia—an overview of Cochrane reviews. *Cochrane Database Syst Rev*. 2013;(11):CD010567.
19. Deare JC, Zheng Z, Xue CC, et al. Acupuncture for treating fibromyalgia. *Cochrane Database Syst Rev*. 2013;(5):CD007070.
20. Langhorst J, Klose P, Dobos GJ, et al. Efficacy and safety of meditative movement therapies in fibromyalgia syndrome: a systematic review and meta-analysis of randomized controlled trials. *Rheumatol Int*. 2013;33(1):193–207.
21. Marlow NM, Bonilha HS, Short EB. Efficacy of transcranial direct current stimulation and repetitive transcranial magnetic stimulation for treating fibromyalgia syndrome: a systematic review. *Pain Pract*. 2013;13(2):131–145.
22. Castillo-Saavedra L, Gebodh N, Bikson M, et al. Clinically effective treatment of fibromyalgia pain with high-definition transcranial direct current stimulation: phase II open-label dose optimization [published online ahead of print October 9, 2015]. *J Pain*.
23. Forseth KO, Førre O, Gran JT. A 5.5 year prospective study of self-reported musculoskeletal pain and of fibromyalgia in a female population: significance and natural history. *Clin Rheumatol*. 1999;18(2):114–121.

ADDITIONAL READING

Theadom A, Cropley M, Smith HE, et al. Mind and body therapy for fibromyalgia. *Cochrane Database Syst Rev*. 2015;(4):CD001980.

 ## SEE ALSO

Algorithm: Fatigue

 ## CODES

ICD10
M79.7 Fibromyalgia

CLINICAL PEARLS

- Use rigorous ACR criteria to make the diagnosis.
- Fibromyalgia is not a somatoform disorder and is not merely a manifestation of depression or anxiety, although as with all chronic pain syndromes, it is frequently associated with mood disturbances.
- Best outcomes occur in patients who understand their illness and are willing to actively engage in a multimodal treatment plan, including exercise, medication, CBT, and lifestyle modifications.

F

FOLLICULITIS

David L. Anderson, MD • Thomas P. Garigan, MD, MA

 BASICS

DESCRIPTION

- Superficial inflammation of a follicle, usually a hair follicle, caused by infection, local trauma, or chemical irritation (1)
- Can occur anywhere on the body that hair is found
- Most frequent symptom is pruritus.
- Painless or tender pustules, vesicles, or pink/red papulopustules up to 5 mm in size.
- Most commonly infectious in etiology:
  - *Staphylococcus aureus* bacteria (most common)
  - *Pseudomonas aeruginosa* infects areas of the body exposed to poorly chlorinated hot tubs, pools, or contaminated water.
  - *Aeromonas hydrophila* with recreational water exposure
  - Fungal (dermatophytic, *Pityrosporum*, *Candida*)
  - Viral (VZV, herpes simplex virus [HSV])
  - Parasitic (*Demodex* spp. mites, schistosomes)
- Noninfectious types
  - Acneiform folliculitis
  - Actinic superficial folliculitis
  - Acne vulgaris
  - Keloidal folliculitis
  - Folliculitis decalvans
  - Perioral dermatitis
  - Rosacea
  - Fox-Fordyce disease
  - Pruritus folliculitis of pregnancy
  - Eosinophilic pustular folliculitis (three variants: Ofuji disease in patients of Asian descent, HIV-positive/immunocompromised, infantile)
  - Toxic erythema of the newborn
  - Eosinophilic folliculitis (seen in HIV-positive/immunocompromised)
  - Follicular mucinosis
- Skin disorders may produce a follicular eruption that includes the following:
  - Pseudofolliculitis: similar in appearance; occurs after shaving; affects the face, scalp, pubis, and legs. Pseudofolliculitis barbae, or razor bumps, occurs frequently in black men.
  - Atopic dermatitis
  - Follicular psoriasis

EPIDEMIOLOGY
Affects persons of all ages, gender, and race

ETIOLOGY AND PATHOPHYSIOLOGY
Predisposing factors to folliculitis
- Chronic staphylococcal carrier
- Diabetes mellitus
- Malnutrition
- Pruritic skin disease (e.g., scabies, eczema, etc.)
- Exposure to poorly chlorinated swimming pools/hot tubs or water contaminated with *P. aeruginosa*, *A. hydrophila*, or schistosomes
- Occlusive corticosteroid use (for multiple hours)
- Bacteria
  - Superficial or deep
  - Most frequently due to *S. aureus* (increasing number of MRSA cases)
  - Also due to *Streptococcus* species, *Pseudomonas* (following exposure to water contaminated with the species), or *Proteus*.
  - May progress to furunculosis (painful pustular nodule with central necrosis that leaves a permanent scar after healing)

- Fungal
  - Dermatophytic (tinea capitis, corporis, pedis)
  - Pityrosporum (Pityrosporum orbiculare) commonly affecting teenagers and men, predominantly on upper chest and back
  - *Candida albicans*, although rare, has been reported with broad spectrum antibiotic use, glucocorticoid use, immunosuppression, and in those who abuse heroin, resulting in candidemia that leads to pustules and nodules in hair-bearing areas.
- Viral
  - HSV
  - May be due to molluscum contagiosum, usually a sign of immunosuppression
- Parasitic
  - *Demodex* spp. mites (most commonly *Demodex folliculorum*)
  - Schistosomes (swimmer's itch)
- Acneiform type commonly drug-induced (systemic and topical corticosteroids, lithium, isoniazid, rifampin), EGFR inhibitors
- Severe vitamin C deficiency
- Actinic superficial type occurs within 24 to 48 hours of exposure to the sun, resulting in multiple follicular pustules on the shoulders, trunk, and arms.
- Acne vulgaris
- Keloidal folliculitis is a chronic condition affecting mostly black patients; involves the neck and occipital scalp, resulting in hypertrophic scars and hair loss; usually secondary to folliculitis barbae from shaving
- Folliculitis decalvans is a chronic folliculitis that leads to progressive scarring and alopecia of the scalp.
- Rosacea consists of papules, pustules, and/or telangiectasias of the face; individuals are genetically predisposed. *Helicobacter pylori* and *D. folliculorum* have also been implicated.
- Perioral dermatitis seen most commonly in children and young women; restricted to the perioral region as well as the lower eyelids. May be due to cosmetics, hyperandrogenemia, or use of fluorinated topical corticosteroids
  - Typically spares vermillion border
- Fox-Fordyce disease affects the skin containing apocrine sweat glands (i.e., axillae), resulting in chronic pruritic, annular, follicular papules.
- Eosinophilic pustular folliculitis (EPF) has three variants: classic (Ofuji disease), associated with HIV infection, and infantile
- Toxic erythema of the newborn is a self-limiting pustular eruption usually appearing during the first 3 to 4 days of life and subsequently fading in the following 2 weeks.
- Malassezia infections in adult males with lesions on trunk (2)

RISK FACTORS
- Hair removal (shaving, plucking, waxing, epilating agents)
- Other pruritic skin conditions: eczema, scabies
- Occlusive dressing or clothing
- Personal carrier or contact with methicillin-resistant *S. aureus* (MRSA)–infected persons
- Diabetes mellitus
- Immunosuppression (medications, chemotherapy, HIV)
- Use of hot tubs or saunas
- Use of EGFR inhibitors
- Chronic antibiotic use (gram-negative folliculitis)

GENERAL PREVENTION
- Good hygiene practices
  - Wash hands frequently.
  - Antimicrobial soap
  - Wash towels, clothes, and linens frequently with hot water to avoid reinfection.
- Good hair removal practices
  - Exfoliate beforehand.
  - Use witch hazel, alcohol, or Tend Skin afterward.
  - Shave in direction of hair growth; use moisturizer/warm water.
  - Decrease frequency of shaving
  - Use clippers primarily or single-blade razors if straight shaving is desired.

COMMONLY ASSOCIATED CONDITIONS
- Impetigo
- Furunculosis
- Scabies
- Acne
- Follicular psoriasis
- Eczema

 DIAGNOSIS

HISTORY
- Recent use of hot tubs, swimming pools, topical corticosteroids, certain hair styling and shaving practices, antibiotics or systemic steroids
- HIV status
- History of STDs (specifically syphilis)
- MRSA exposures/carrier status
- Ask about home and work environment (risk/exposure potential)
- Pityrosporum folliculitis occurs more often in warm, moist climates.
- Inquire about the timeline in which the lesions have occurred, including previous similar episodes.

PHYSICAL EXAM
- Characteristic lesions are 1- to 5-mm–wide vesicles, pustules, or papulopustules with surrounding erythema.
- Rash occurs on hair-bearing skin, especially the face (beard), proximal limbs, scalp, and pubis.
- Pseudomonal folliculitis appears as a widespread rash, mainly on the trunk and limbs.
- In pseudofolliculitis, the growing hair curls around and penetrates the skin at shaved areas.

DIFFERENTIAL DIAGNOSIS
- Acne vulgaris/acneiform eruptions
- Arthropod bite
- Contact dermatitis
- Cutaneous candidiasis
- Milia
- Atopic dermatitis
- Follicular psoriasis
- Hidradenitis suppurativa

DIAGNOSTIC TESTS & INTERPRETATION
Initial Tests (lab, imaging)
- Diagnosis is usually made clinically, taking risk factors, history, and location of lesion into account.
- Culture and Gram stain of the pustule by scraping the pustule with a no. 15 blade and not directly swabbing the skin to identify infectious agent and sensitivities to antibiotics

- KOH preparation as well as Wood lamp fluorescence to identify *Candida* or yeast
- Tzanck smear where suspicion of herpetic simplex viral folliculitis is high

Follow-Up Tests & Special Considerations
- If risk factors or clinical suspicion exist, consider serologies for HIV or syphilis.
- If recurrent, consider HIV testing and A1C/fasting blood sugar testing to evaluate for diabetes.
- Punch biopsy may be considered if lesions persist despite treatment (3)[C].

Test Interpretation
- Treat positive bacterial culture according to sensitivities.
- Positive HIV serology: Follow up with CD4 count and punch biopsy to rule out eosinophilic folliculitis.
- Eosinophilic folliculitis: Collect eosinophils within superficial follicle (4).

 TREATMENT

GENERAL MEASURES
- Lesions usually resolve spontaneously.
- Avoid shaving and waxing affected areas (5)[C].
- Warm compresses may be applied TID.
- Systemic antibiotics are typically unnecessary.
- Topical mupirocin may be used in presumed *S. aureus* infection.
- Topical antifungals for fungal folliculitis (2)[B]
- Preventive measures are keys to avoidance of recurrence:
  - Antibacterial soaps (Dial soap, chlorhexidine, or benzyl peroxide wash when showering/bathing)
  - Bleach baths (1/2 cup of 6% bleach per standard bathtub, and soak for 5 to 15 minutes followed by water rinse 1 to 2 times a week)
  - Keep skin intact; daily skin care with noncomedogenic moisturizers; avoid scratching.
  - Clean shaving instruments daily or use disposable razor, disposing after 1 use.
  - Change washcloths, towels, and sheets daily.

MEDICATION
Antiseptic and supportive care is usually enough. Systemic antibiotics may be used with questionable efficacy.

First Line
- Staphylococcal folliculitis
  - Mupirocin ointment applied TID for 10 days
  - Cephalosporin (cephalexin): 250 to 500 mg PO QID for 7 to 10 days
  - Dicloxacillin: 250 to 500 mg PO QID for 7 to 10 days
- For MRSA
  - Bactrim DS: 1 to 2 tablets (160 mg/800 mg) BID PO for 5 to 10 days
  - Clindamycin: 300 mg PO TID for 10 to 14 days
  - Minocycline: 200 mg PO initially then 100 mg BID for 5 to 10 days
  - Doxycycline: 50 to 100 mg PO BID for 5 to 10 days
- Pseudomonal folliculitis
  - Topical dilute acetic acid baths
  - Ciprofloxacin: 500 to 750 mg PO BID for 7 to 14 days only if patient is immunocompromised or lesions are persistent
- Eosinophilic folliculitis/eosinophilic pustular folliculitis
  - HAART treatment for HIV-positive–related causes
  - Topical corticosteroids: betamethasone 0.1% BID for 3 to 24 weeks *or*
  - Antihistamines (hydroxyzine, cetirizine) *or*
  - Tacrolimus topically BID for 3 to 24 weeks *or*

- Isotretinoin 0.5 mg/kg/day PO for 4 to 8 weeks *or*
  - Itraconazole or metronidazole
- Fungal folliculitis
  - Topical antifungals: ketoconazole 2% cream or shampoo or selenium sulfide shampoo daily *or*
  - Econazole cream applied to affected area BID for 2 to 3 weeks
    - Systemic antifungals for relapses fluconazole (100 to 200 mg/day for 3 weeks) *or* itraconazole (200 mg/day for 1 to 3 weeks)
    - Griseofulvin (tinea capitis in children; 10 to 20 mg/kg/day for 6 weeks minimum)
- Parasitic folliculitis
  - 5% permethrin: Apply to affected area, leave on for 8 hours, and wash off.
  - Ivermectin: 200 μg/kg × 1 followed by topical permethrin
- Herpetic folliculitis
  - Valacyclovir: 500 mg PO TID for 5 to 10 days or
  - Famciclovir: 500 mg PO TID for 5 to 10 days or
  - Acyclovir: 200 mg PO 5 times daily for 5 to 10 days

ISSUES FOR REFERRAL
Unusual or persistent cases should be biopsied and then referred to dermatology.

ADDITIONAL THERAPIES
Public Health Measures
- Outbreaks of culture-positive *Pseudomonas* hot tub folliculitis should be reported so that source identification can be determined and superchlorination (14 parts/million) can occur.

SURGERY/OTHER PROCEDURES
Incision and drainage is unlikely to be necessary and typically not preferred due to potential for scar formation.

 ONGOING CARE

FOLLOW-UP RECOMMENDATIONS
Patient Monitoring
- Resistant cases should be followed every 2 weeks until cleared.
- One return visit in 2 weeks if symptoms abate

DIET
For obese patients, weight reduction will decrease skin-on-skin friction.

PATIENT EDUCATION
Avoid shaving in involved areas.

PROGNOSIS
- Usually resolves with treatment; however, *S. aureus* carriers may experience recurrences.
- Mupirocin nasal treatment for carrier status and for family/household members might be helpful.
- Resistant or severe cases may warrant testing for diabetes mellitus or immunodeficiency (HIV) (3)[C].

COMPLICATIONS
- Primary complication is recurrent folliculitis.
- Extensive scarring with hyperpigmentation
- Progression to furunculosis or abscesses

REFERENCES
1. Breitkopf T, Leung G, Yu M, et al. The basic science of hair biology: what are the causal mechanisms for the disordered hair follicle? *Dermatol Clin*. 2013;31(1):1–19.
2. Song HS, Kim SK, Kim YC. Comparison between *Malassezia* folliculitis and non-*Malassezia* folliculitis. *Ann Dermatol*. 2014;26(5):598–602.
3. Tilley DH, Satter EK, Kakimoto CV, et al. Disseminated verrucous varicella zoster with exclusive follicular involvement. *Arch Dermatol*. 2012;148(3):405–407.
4. Annam V, Yelikar BR, Inamadar AC, et al. Clinico-patholigical study of itchy folliculitis in HIV-infected patients. *Indian J Dermatol Venereol Leprol*. 2010;76(3):259–262.
5. Khanna N, Chandramohan K, Khaitan BK, et al. Post waxing folliculitis: a clinicopathological evaluation. *Int J Dermatol*. 2014;53(7):849–854.

ADDITIONAL READING
- Bachet JB, Peuvrel L, Bachmeyer C, et al. Folliculitis induced by EGFR inhibitors, preventive and curative efficacy of tetracyclines in the management and incidence rates according to the type of EGFR inhibitor administered: a systematic literature review. *Oncologist*. 2012;17(4):555–568.
- Böer A, Herder N, Winter K, et al. Herpes folliculitis: clinical, histopathological, and molecular pathologic observations. *Br J Dermatol*. 2006;154(4):743–746.
- Brooke RCC, Griffiths CEM. Folliculitis decalvans. *Clin Exp Dermatol*. 2001;26(1):120–122.
- Ellis E, Scheinfeld N. Eosinophilic pustular folliculitis: a comprehensive review of treatment options. *Am J Clin Dermatol*. 2004;5(3):189–197.
- Fiorillo L, Zucker M, Sawyer D, et al. The *Pseudomonas* hot-foot syndrome. *N Engl J Med*. 2001;345(5):335–338.
- Fridkin SK, Hageman JC, Morrison M, et al. Methicillin-resistant *Staphylococcus aureus* disease in three communities. *N Engl J Med*. 2005;352(14):1436–1444.
- James WD. Clinical practice. Acne. *N Engl J Med*. 2005;352(14):1463–1472.
- Luelmo-Aguilar J, Santandreu MS. Folliculitis: recognition and management. *Am J Clin Dermatol*. 2004;5(5):301–310.
- Nervi SJ, Schwartz RA, Dmochowski M. Eosinophilic pustular folliculitis: a 40 year retrospect. *J Am Acad Dermatol*. 2006;55(2):285–289.

 SEE ALSO

Algorithm: Rash, Focal

 CODES

ICD10
- L73.9 Follicular disorder, unspecified
- L66.2 Folliculitis decalvans
- L73.8 Other specified follicular disorders

CLINICAL PEARLS
- Folliculitis lesions are typically 1 to 5 mm clusters of pruritic erythematous papules and pustules.
- Most commonly due to *S. aureus*. If community has increased incidence of MRSA, consider anti-MRSA treatment.
  - It is extremely important to educate patients on proper hygiene and skin care techniques in order to prevent chronic or recurrent cases.

FOOD ALLERGY

Stanley Fineman, MD

 BASICS

DESCRIPTION
- Hypersensitivity reaction caused by certain foods
- System(s) affected: gastrointestinal, hemic/lymphatic/immunologic, pulmonary, skin/exocrine
- Synonym(s): allergic bowel disease; dietary protein sensitivity syndrome

EPIDEMIOLOGY
- Predominant age: all ages but more common in infants and children
- Predominant sex: male > female (2:1)

Incidence
Prospective studies indicate ~2.5% of infants experience hypersensitivity reactions to cow's milk in their 1st year of life (1)[B].

Prevalence
- The true prevalence of IgE-mediated food allergy when assessed by double-blind, placebo-controlled food challenge is 3% (2)[B].
- The self-reported prevalence of food allergy is 12% in children and 13% in adults (2)[B].
- In young children, the most common food allergies are cow's milk (2.5%), egg (1.3%), peanut (0.8%), and wheat (0.4%) (3)[B].
- Adults tend to have allergies to shellfish (2%), peanut (0.6%), tree nuts (0.5%), and fish (0.4%).
- In general, only 3–4% of children >4 years of age have persisting food allergy; food allergy is frequently a transient phenomenon (4)[B].
- 20% of children with peanut protein allergy may outgrow their sensitivity by school age.

ETIOLOGY AND PATHOPHYSIOLOGY
Allergic response triggered by immunologic mechanisms, such as the classic IgE-allergic response or nonimmunologic-mediated mechanisms
- Any food or ingested substance can cause allergic reactions:
  - Most commonly implicated foods include cow's milk, egg whites, wheat, soy, peanuts, fish, tree nuts (walnut and pecan), and shellfish.
- Several food dyes and additives may elicit non–IgE-mediated allergic-like reactions.

Genetics
In family members with a history of food hypersensitivity, the probability of food allergy in subsequent siblings may be as high as 50%.

RISK FACTORS
- Persons with allergic or atopic predisposition have increased risk of hypersensitivity reaction to food.
- Family history of food hypersensitivity

GENERAL PREVENTION
- Avoidance of offending food
- In patients at risk for anaphylaxis, epinephrine autoinjectors should be readily available.

DIAGNOSIS

PHYSICAL EXAM
- GI (system usually affected)
  - More common: nausea, vomiting, diarrhea, abdominal pain, occult bleeding, flatulence, and bloating
  - Less common: malabsorption, protein-losing enteropathy, eosinophilic-enteritis, colitis
- Dermatologic
  - More common: urticaria/angioedema, atopic dermatitis, pallor, or flushing
  - Less common: contact rashes
- Respiratory
  - More common: allergic rhinitis, asthma and bronchospasm, cough, serous otitis media
  - Less common: pulmonary infiltrates (Heiner syndrome), pulmonary hemosiderosis
- Neurologic
  - Less common: migraine headaches
- Other symptoms
  - Systemic anaphylaxis, vasculitis

DIFFERENTIAL DIAGNOSIS
- A careful history is necessary to document a temporal relationship with the manifestations of suspected food hypersensitivity.
- True food allergy or hypersensitivity should be differentiated from food intolerance which may present with similar symptoms.
- GI (irritable bowel syndrome, celiac sprue, dumping syndrome, inflammatory bowel diseases, etc.), dermatologic, respiratory, neurologic, psychiatric (generalized anxiety disorder, personality disorders, etc.), or other systemic manifestations may mimic a variety of clinical entities.

DIAGNOSTIC TESTS & INTERPRETATION
Initial Tests (lab, imaging)
- CBC with differential: Eosinophilia in blood or tissue suggests atopy.
- Serum IgA antitissue transglutaminase (IgA-anti-TTG)
- Epicutaneous (prick or puncture) allergy skin tests are used to document IgE-mediated immunologic hypersensitivity and can be done using commercially available extracts (variable sensitivities) or fresh-food skin testing.
- Skin testing using the suspect food is helpful. If positive on skin test, an oral challenge may aid in diagnosis. The overall correlation between commercially available allergy skin testing and oral food challenge is 60% but increases to 90% when fresh food skin testing is done (i.e., a positive skin test correlates with a positive challenge to a particular food)
  - Skin testing has a high sensitivity (low false-negative rate) *but* a low specificity (high false-positive rate) so *only* skin test against antigens found on history (5)[C].
- Food-specific IgE assays (radioallergosorbent [RAST] and fluorescent enzyme immunoassay [FEI]) detect specific IgE antibodies to offending foods and are less sensitive to skin testing.
  - In certain laboratories, the ImmunoCap food-specific IgE was almost as accurate as a skin test in predicting positive oral challenges.

- Using a serum assay alone to diagnose food allergy has been shown to result in misdiagnosis of true clinical food allergic sensitivity, particularly in children with atopic dermatitis. Do not test using a panel but rather for specific IgE to foods based on patient history.
- Periodic monitoring of the peanut-specific IgE levels every 2 years may be helpful. If the level of peanut-specific IgE falls to <0.5 kU/L, then a cautious oral challenge under the supervision of an allergist may be considered. A fresh food skin test with peanut protein should be considered prior to the oral challenge (6)[B].
- Patch testing for foods for determining delayed-sensitivity immunologic reactions, in patients with eosinophilic esophagitis and atopic dermatitis, is considered of marginal benefit (7)[B].
- Widespread allergy skin testing or serum IgE tests are *not* recommended because of their poor predictive value without a clinical correlating history (3)[B].
- Leukocyte histamine release and assays for circulating immune complexes are predominantly research procedures and are of limited use in clinical practices:
  - Assays for IgG and IgG 4 subclass antibodies are commercially available.
  - No convincing data suggest that these tests are reliable for the diagnosis of food allergy (4)[B].
- The provocative injection and sublingual provocative tests are highly controversial and have been proven useless for diagnosis of food allergy.
- The leukocytotoxic assay is an unproven diagnostic procedure and is not useful for the diagnosis of allergy (7)[B].
- Other unproven diagnostic procedures that are not recommended include provocative neutralization, lymphocyte stimulation, hair analysis, and applied kinesiology (3)[B].

Diagnostic Procedures/Other
Elimination and challenge test is the best procedure for confirming food allergy:
- The suspected food is eliminated from the diet for 1 to 2 weeks.
- The patient's symptoms are monitored. If they disappear or substantially improve, an oral challenge with the suspected food should be performed under medical supervision.
- Optimally, this challenge should be performed in a double-blind, placebo-controlled manner.
- Patients with history of anaphylaxis should not have an oral challenge unless lack of IgE sensitivity can be documented.
- Most allergic reactions will occur within 30 minutes to 2 hours after challenge, although late reactions have also been described that may occur from 12 to 24 hours.
- Consider referral to gastroenterology for endoscopy and/or psychiatry if history and testing are inconclusive.

Test Interpretation
Pathologic findings are not common in food allergies; however, inflammatory changes can sometimes be seen in the GI tract. The diagnosis of eosinophilic esophagitis is defined by the finding of >15 to 20 eosinophils per high-power field on esophageal biopsy (8)[C].

TREATMENT

GENERAL MEASURES
- Avoiding the offending food is the most effective mode of treatment for patients with food allergies.
- Those patients with exquisite and severe allergy hypersensitivity to a food should be more cautious in their avoidance of that food. They should carry epinephrine for self-administration in the event that the offending food is ingested unknowingly and a subsequent immediate reaction develops.
- Immunotherapy or hyposensitization with food extracts by various routes, including SC immunotherapy or sublingual neutralization, are not recommended. Research studies are in progress, but immunotherapy is considered experimental at this time.

MEDICATION
- Patients with significant type 1, IgE-mediated hypersensitivity should have epinephrine for autoinjection available in case of accidental ingestion and resulting severe anaphylactic reaction.
- After receiving epinephrine for a systemic anaphylactic reaction to a food, the patient should be monitored in a medical facility because 15–25% of patients may require >1 dose of epinephrine.
- Symptomatic treatment for milder reactions (e.g., antihistamine)
- The use of cromolyn has been suggested but is not recommended for use in most patients with food allergy.

COMPLEMENTARY & ALTERNATIVE MEDICINE
There are reports of benefit using various Chinese herbal medicines in laboratory animals with induced food allergy. Benefits have not been reported in humans at this time.

ONGOING CARE

FOLLOW-UP RECOMMENDATIONS
Patient Monitoring
As needed

DIET
- As determined by tests and clinical evaluation
- Strict avoidance of offending food

PATIENT EDUCATION
- Patients should be counseled by a dietitian to maintain a nutritionally sound diet despite avoiding those foods to which the patient is sensitive.
- Patient support: Food Allergy Research & Education, Inc.: 7925 Jones Branch Drive Suite 1100 McLean, VA 22102 Toll-Free: 800-929-4040; Web site www.foodallergy.org
- Other information available at: www.allergyasthmanetwork.org, www.acaai.org, and www.aaaai.org

PROGNOSIS
- Most infants will outgrow their food hypersensitivity by 2 to 4 years:
  - It may be possible to reintroduce the offending food cautiously into the diet (particularly helpful when the food is one that is difficult to avoid). It is critical that a specific IgE to the offending food is checked, optimally by fresh food allergy skin test, and is negative prior to an oral challenge.
  - 20% of young children with peanut allergy experience resolution by the age of 5 years.
  - 42% of children with egg allergy and 48% of children with milk allergy develop clinical tolerance and lose their sensitivity over time (1)[C].
- Adults with food hypersensitivity (particularly to milk, fish, shellfish, or nuts) tend to maintain their allergy for many years (3)[B].

COMPLICATIONS
- Anaphylaxis
- Angioedema
- Bronchial asthma
- Enterocolitis
- Eosinophilic esophagitis
- Eczematoid lesions

REFERENCES

1. Sicherer SH, Sampson HA. Food allergy: epidemiology, pathogenesis, diagnosis, and treatment. *J Allergy Clin Immunol.* 2014;133(2):291–307.
2. Rona RI, Keil T, Summers C, et al. The prevalence of food allergy: a meta-analysis. *J Allergy Clin Immunol.* 2007;120(3):638–646.
3. Boyce JA, Assa'ad A, Burks AW, et al. Guidelines for the diagnosis and management of food allergy in the United States: summary of the NIAID-sponsored expert panel report. *J Allergy Clin Immunol.* 2010;126(6):1105–1118.
4. Burks AW, Tang M, Sicherer S, et al. ICON: food allergy. *J Allergy Clin Immunol.* 2012;129(4):906–920.
5. Sicherer SH, Wood RA. Advances in diagnosing peanut allergy. *J Allergy Clin Immunol Pract.* 2013;1(1):1–13.
6. Fleischer DM, Bock SA, Spears GC, et al. Oral food challenges in children with a diagnosis of food allergy. *J Pediatr.* 2011;158(4):578.e1–583.e1.
7. Spergel JM, Brown-Whitehorn T, Beausoleil JL, et al. Predictive values for skin prick test and atopy patch test for eosinophilic esophagitis. *J Allergy Clin Immunol.* 2007;119(2):509–511.
8. Spergel JM, Brown-Whitehorn TF, Cianferoni A, et al. Identification of causative foods in children with eosinophilic esophagitis treated with an elimination diet. *J Allergy Clin Immunol.* 2012;130(2):461.e5–467.e5.
9. Greer FR, Sicherer SH, Burks AW, et al. Effects of early nutritional interventions on the development of atopic disease in infants and children: the role of maternal dietary restriction, breastfeeding, timing of introduction of complementary foods, and hydrolyzed formulas. *Pediatrics.* 2008;121(1):183–191.
10. Du Toit G, Roberts G, Sayre PH, et al. Randomized trial of peanut consumption in infants at risk for peanut allergy. *N Engl J Med.* 2015;372(9):803–813.

ADDITIONAL READING
- American College of Allergy, Asthma, & Immunology. Food allergy: a practice parameter. *Ann Allergy Asthma Immunol.* 2006;96(3)(Suppl 2):S1–S68.
- Høst A, Halken S. A prospective study of cow milk allergy in Danish infants during the first 3 years of life. Clinical course in relation to clinical and immunological type of hypersensitivity reaction. *Allergy.* 1990;45(8):587–596.
- Maloney JM, Rudengren M, Ahlstedt S, et al. The use of serum-specific IgE measurements for the diagnosis of peanut, tree nut, and seed allergy. *J Allergy Clin Immunol.* 2008;122(1):145–151.

 SEE ALSO

Anaphylaxis; Celiac Disease; Irritable Bowel Syndrome

 CODES

ICD10
- T78.1XXA Oth adverse food reactions, not elsewhere classified, init
- T78.00XA Anaphylactic reaction due to unspecified food, init encntr
- L27.2 Dermatitis due to ingested food

CLINICAL PEARLS
- Recent studies suggest that up to 20% of children with peanut allergy may outgrow their sensitivity:
  - Periodic monitoring of the peanut-specific IgE levels every 2 years may be helpful. If the level of peanut-specific IgE falls to <0.5 kU/L, then a cautious oral challenge under the supervision of an allergist may be considered. A FRESH FOOD skin test with peanut protein should be considered prior to the oral challenge (1)[B].
- Oral itching following ingestion of fresh fruit may be a warning of risk for anaphylaxis but may also represent oral allergy syndrome.
  - This syndrome is the result of cross-reacting proteins in pollens (e.g., patients sensitive to birch tree pollen frequently have cross-reactivity to fresh apples and pears. Cooked fruits are usually tolerated) (1)[B].
- Current evidence does not support a major role for maternal dietary restrictions during pregnancy or lactation in the prevention of atopic disease in infants. It is generally recommended to exclusively breastfeed for the first 6 months of life, particularly when there is a family history of atopy and food allergy. Although solid foods should not be introduced before 4 to 6 months of age, there is no convincing evidence that delaying their introduction beyond this period has a significant protective effect on the development of allergies (9)[C].
- There is a recent evidence suggesting that children 4 to 11 months of age who have eczema or other food allergy may benefit from early introduction of peanut protein. Allergy skin testing should be a consideration prior to introducing peanut protein (10).

F

FOOD POISONING, BACTERIAL
Jewell P. Carr, MD • Daniel J. Fisher, MD

BASICS

DESCRIPTION
- Food poisoning (also known as foodborne illness) is a state resulting from the consumption of contaminated food (1).
- The illness may be caused by bacterial, parasitic, or viral infection or by toxins produced by bacteria (2).

EPIDEMIOLOGY
Incidence
- The Centers for Disease Control and Prevention (CDC) estimates that roughly 1 in 6 Americans (48 million people) get sick, 128,000 are hospitalized, and 3,000 die of foodborne diseases annually (3).
- Contaminated produce is the most common source of diarrhea due to foodborne infection (1).
- No pathogen is identified in 80% of cases of foodborne illness (3).
- Noroviruses are responsible for >50% of cases of foodborne illness (1).
- According to CDC data, the bacterial pathogens most commonly contributing to foodborne illness are *Salmonella* (nontyphoidal) *Campylobacter*, *Clostridium perfringens*, and *Staphylococcus aureus* (3).

ETIOLOGY AND PATHOPHYSIOLOGY
- Short incubation period (1 to 6 hours): likely preformed toxin–induced
  - *Bacillus cereus*
    - Food sources: improperly cooked rice/fried rice and red meats
    - Causes sudden onset of severe nausea and vomiting. Diarrhea may be present.
  - *S. aureus*
    - Food sources: nonrefrigerated or improperly refrigerated meats and potato and egg salads
    - Causes sudden onset of severe nausea and vomiting. Abdominal cramps and fever may be present.
- Medium incubation period (8 to 16 hours)
  - *Bacillus cereus* (toxin)
    - Food sources: meat, stew gravy, vanilla sauce
    - Causes watery diarrhea, abdominal cramps, nausea
  - *C. perfringens*
    - Food sources: dry/precooked meats and poultry
    - Causes watery diarrhea, nausea, abdominal cramps
- Long incubation period (>16 hours)
  - Toxin-producing organisms:
    - *Clostridium botulinum*: Source is commercially canned or improperly home-canned foods. Causes vomiting, diarrhea, slurred speech, diplopia, dysphagia, and descending muscle weakness/flaccid paralysis
    - Enterohemorrhagic *Escherichia coli* (e.g., 0157:H7): Food sources are undercooked beef, especially hamburger, unpasteurized milk, raw fruits and vegetables, and contaminated water. Causes severe diarrhea that often becomes bloody, abdominal pain, vomiting. More common in children <4 years of age
    - Enterotoxigenic *E. coli*: Food sources are foods or water contaminated by human feces. Causes watery diarrhea, abdominal cramps, and vomiting
    - *Vibrio cholerae*: Food sources are contaminated water, fish, and shellfish, especially food sold by street vendors. Causes profuse watery

diarrhea and vomiting, which can lead to severe dehydration and death within hours
  - Invasive organisms: often bloody stool and fever
    - *Salmonella*: Food sources are contaminated eggs, poultry, unpasteurized milk or juice, cheese, contaminated raw fruits and vegetables, and contaminated peanut butter. Causes watery diarrhea, fever, abdominal cramps, vomiting
    - *Campylobacter jejuni*: Food sources are raw and undercooked poultry, unpasteurized milk, and contaminated meats. Causes diarrhea (may be bloody), cramps, vomiting, fever
    - *Shigella*: Food sources are food or water contaminated by human fecal material. Causes abdominal cramps, fever, diarrhea
    - *Vibrio parahaemolyticus*: Food source is raw shellfish. Causes nausea, vomiting, diarrhea, abdominal pain
    - *Vibrio vulnificus*: Food source is undercooked and raw seafood; wounds exposed to sea water. Causes vomiting, diarrhea, abdominal pain, bacteremia, wound infections; can be fatal in patients with liver disease or those who are immunocompromised
    - *Yersinia enterocolitica* and *Y. pseudotuberculosis*: Food sources are undercooked pork, unpasteurized milk, tofu, contaminated water. Causes appendicitis-like symptoms: abdominal pain, fever, diarrhea, vomiting; occurs primarily in older children and younger adults
    - *Listeria*: Sources include unpasteurized/contaminated milk, soft cheese, and processed/delicatessen meats. Causes nausea, vomiting, fever, watery diarrhea

RISK FACTORS
- Recent travel to a developing country (1)
- Food handlers, daycare attendees, nursing home residents, and recently hospitalized patients (2)
- Altered immunity due to underlying disease or medications (1); patients taking antacids, H2 blockers, and proton pump inhibitors (1)
- Cross-contamination and subsequent ingestion of improperly prepared and stored foods

GENERAL PREVENTION
- When preparing food at home:
  - Wash hands, cutting boards, and surfaces before food preparation and after preparing each food item.
  - Wash fresh produce thoroughly before eating.
  - Keep raw meat, poultry, fish, and their juices away from other food that will not be cooked (e.g., salad).
  - Do not put cooked protein or washed produce back into containers or on surfaces where unwashed or raw food was stored.
  - Thoroughly cook meat to the following internal temperature:
    - Fresh beef, veal, pork, and lamb: 145°F
    - Ground meats and egg dishes: 160°F
    - Poultry: 165°F
    - Cook chicken eggs thoroughly until the yolk is firm.
  - Refrigerate leftovers within 2 to 3 hours in clean, shallow, and covered containers. If the temperature is >90°F, refrigerate within 1 hour.
- When traveling to underdeveloped countries:
  - Eat only freshly prepared foods.
  - Avoid beverages and foods prepared with non-potable water.

  - Other risky foods include raw or undercooked meat and seafood, unpeeled raw fruits, and vegetables.
  - Bottled, carbonated, and boiled beverages are generally safe to drink.
- Concerning prevention, improved hygiene and sanitation reduces the risk of traveler's diarrhea, but the prevention strategy "Boil it, Cook it, Peel it, or Forget it" has inconsistent and limited evidence (4,5)[C].
- Chemoprophylaxis for traveler's diarrhea (trips <14 days):
  - Bismuth subsalicylate 525 mg QID (4)[A]
  - Ciprofloxacin 500 mg daily or BID (4)[A]
  - Rifaximin 200 mg daily or BID (4)[A]

DIAGNOSIS

HISTORY
- Onset, duration, frequency, severity, and character (i.e., watery, bloody, mucus-filled, etc.) of diarrhea should be noted (2).
- The definition of diarrhea is >3 or more unformed stools daily or the passage of >250 g of unformed stool per day (1).
- Suspect bacterial food poisoning when multiple persons have rapid onset of symptoms after eating the same meal; have high fever, blood, or mucus in stool; severe abdominal pain; signs of dehydration; or recent travel to a foreign country (1,2).
- Any of the following should prompt further evaluation and possible supportive treatment: high fever (≥101.3°F), ≥6 stools/day, blood in the stools, elevated white blood cell count, signs of dehydration, and diarrheal illness that lasts >2 to 3 days (1).
- Suspect *Clostridium difficile* colitis if with recent prolonged antibiotic use or recurrent *C. difficile* infection in repeated episodes (1,6).

PHYSICAL EXAM
- Focus on signs of dehydration: delayed capillary refills, increased skin turgor, dry mucous membranes, and orthostatic changes (2).
- Fever may be suggestive of a more invasive or toxin producing bacteria (2).
- Abdominal exam: important to assess for pain and to differentiate between other acute abdominal processes (2)
- Rectal exam may be useful to assess for blood, rectal pain or consistency of stool (2).

DIFFERENTIAL DIAGNOSIS
- Infectious gastrointestinal illness of any kind (i.e., viral or parasitic)
- *C. difficile* colitis
- Inflammatory bowel disease
- Appendicitis and other acute abdominal surgical processes
- Hepatitis
- Malabsorption

DIAGNOSTIC TESTS & INTERPRETATION
Initial Tests (lab, imaging)
- Culture of stool and sensitivity, fecal leukocytes, and Hemoccult testing; consider ova and parasites if dehydration, history of foreign travel, or symptoms lasting >2 weeks (1)[C].
- CBC, BMP for severe cases with dehydration, inpatient, and nursing home exposure (1)[C]

- Flexible sigmoidoscopy and colonoscopy are reserved for severe cases or when pathogen is suspected in setting of negative stool cultures (1).
- Abdominal CT may be helpful when intra-abdominal pathology or bowel disease are in the differential (1).

Follow-Up Tests & Special Considerations
Epidemiologic investigation may be warranted.

 TREATMENT

Most cases of food poisoning are self-limiting and do not require medication.

MEDICATION
First Line
- Children, the elderly, and pregnant patients with signs of mild diarrhea should be started on oral rehydration solution to prevent dehydration (2)[C].
- Oral rehydration options can be purchased or mixed simply from common home ingredients: 6 tsp sugar and 1/2 tsp salt in 1 L of clean, potable water (2)[B].
- Travelers may consider empiric treatment for diarrhea with a single dose of ciprofloxacin 750 mg together with loperamide (2)[A].
- Empiric antibiotic therapy for traveler's diarrhea should be considered in cases of moderate to severe disease (4)[A].

Second Line
For severe cases of food poisoning (up to 8% have bacteremia) or if the patient has a prosthetic valve, the following medications are recommended.
- *B. cereus* (2)
  - Supportive care only
- *Campylobacter jejuni* (1,2,5)
  - Mild: supportive care only—antibiotics may induce resistance (5)
  - Severe: azithromycin 500 mg/day for 3 to 5 days or ciprofloxacin 500mg BID to QID for 5 to 7 days
- *C. botulinum*
  - Supportive care. Antitoxin can be helpful if administered early in the course of the illness.
- *C. perfringens*
  - Supportive care only
- *C. difficile* (1,2,6)
  - Mild disease: metronidazole 500 mg TID for 10 days (6)[A]
  - Moderate disease: vancomycin 125 mg PO QID for 14 days (6)[A]
  - Severe disease: vancomycin 500 mg PO QID plus metronidazole 500 mg IV every 8 hours (6)[A]; or fidaxomicin 200 mg BID for 10 days
  - Discontinue offending antibiotic if applicable.
- Enterohemorrhagic *E. coli* (e.g., 0157:H7) (1)
  - Supportive care only. Closely monitor renal function, hemoglobin, and platelets. Infection associated with hemolytic uremic syndrome (HUS). Antibiotics may increase this risk.
- Enterotoxigenic *E. coli* (common cause of traveler's diarrhea) (1,2,4,5)
  - Generally self-limited. Antibiotics shorten course of illness (4,5)[A]
  - Ciprofloxacin 500 mg BID or 750 mg daily for 1 to 3 days; azithromycin 1 g × single dose or daily for 3 days; or rifaximin 200 mg TID for 3 days
- *Salmonella*, nontyphoidal (1,2,4,5)
  - No therapy in mild disease—increases duration of shedding without reducing disease duration (5)

  - Moderate: ciprofloxacin 500 mg BID for 5 to 7 days, levofloxacin 500 mg daily for 7 to 10 days or TMP/SMX DS 160/800 mg twice per day for 5 to 7 days
  - Severe diarrhea, immunocompromised, systemic signs, positive blood cultures: IV ceftriaxone 1 to 2 g daily for 7 to 10 days
- *Shigella* (1,2)
  - Ciprofloxacin 500 mg BID or 750 mg daily for 3 days, or 2-g single dose; alternative options: azithromycin 500 mg twice per day for 3 days, TMP/SMX DS 160/800 mg twice per day for 5 days, or ceftriaxone 2 to 4 g single dose
- *S. aureus* (1)
  - Supportive care only
- Noncholeraic *Vibrio* (1)
  - Ciprofloxacin 750 mg daily for 3 days or azithromycin 500 mg daily for 3 days
- *Vibrio cholerae* (1)
  - Doxycycline 300 mg 1-time dose in most cases or tetracycline 500 mg QID for 3 days or erythromycin 250 mg TID for 3 days or azithromycin 500 mg/day for 3 days
- *Yersinia* (2)
  - Usually supportive care only
  - Severe: doxycycline combine with aminoglycoside; TMP/SMX DS 160/800 mg BID for 5 days; or ciprofloxacin 500 mg BID for 7 to 10 days

ADDITIONAL THERAPIES
- For severe nausea and vomiting, promethazine is effective in adults. Ondansetron is effective in children (4).
- Loperamide 4 mg initially, then 2 mg after each loose stool to a maximum of 8 mg in a 24-hour period may be used *unless* high fever, bloody diarrhea, and/or severe abdominal pain present (signs of enteroinvasion) (4)[A]
- Bismuth subsalicylate (Pepto-Bismol) 525 mg QID is moderately effective in traveler's diarrhea (4)[A].
- Probiotics (i.e., *Lactobacillus* sp.) have been shown to reduce severity and sometimes duration by 24 hours. May also decrease likelihood of antibiotic-associated diarrhea (1,2). However, the evidence for their use is inconsistent (4)[C].
- Diligent hand washing during course will decrease spread (2)[A].

 ONGOING CARE

DIET
- Avoid food while nausea is present, but drink plenty of fluids in frequent sips.
- As the nausea subsides, drink adequate fluids; add in bland, low-fat meals; and rest. Avoid alcohol, coffee, nicotine, and spicy foods.
- Nursing infants should continue to be breastfed on demand, and infants and older children should be offered their usual food.
- For diarrhea, consider a bland diet (BRAT: Bananas, Rice, Apples, Toast-dry).
- Limiting dairy till 24 hours after last diarrhea episode may assist in symptom reduction.

PROGNOSIS
Most infections are self-limited and will resolve over the course of 4 to 5 days. If antibiotics are given in moderate to severe traveler's diarrhea, the duration may shorten to a day and a half (Steffen).

COMPLICATIONS
- Dehydration (2)
- Hemolytic uremic syndrome (HUS following *E. coli* 0157:H7 infection) (5)
- Guillain-Barré syndrome after *Campylobacter* enteritis (1)
- Reactive arthritis after salmonella, shigella, or yersinia infections (1)
- *Clostridium difficile* colitis after antibiotic use (6)
- Postinfectious irritable bowel (1)

REFERENCES
1. DuPont HL. Acute infectious diarrhea in immunocompetent adults. *N Engl J Med.* 2014;370(16):1532–1540.
2. Barr W, Smith A. Acute diarrhea in Adults. *Am Fam Physician.* 2014;89(3):180–189.
3. Centers for Disease Control and Prevention. *Trends in Foodborne Illness in the United States, 2013.* Atlanta, GA: Centers for Disease Control and Prevention; 2014. http://www.cdc.gov/foodborneburden/trends-in-foodborne-illness.html.
4. Steffen R, Hill DR, Dupont HL. Traveler's diarrhea: a clinical review. *JAMA.* 2015;313(1):71–80.
5. Zollner-Schwetz I, Krause R. Therapy of acute gastroenteritis: role of antibiotics. *Clin Microbiol Infect.* 2015;21(8):744–749. http://dx.doi.org/10.1016/j.cmi.2015.03.002.
6. Leffler DA, Lamont JT. Clostridium difficile infection. *N Engl J Med.* 2015;372(16):1539–1548.

ADDITIONAL READING
- Allen SJ, Martinez EG, Gregorio GV, et al. Probiotics for treating acute infectious diarrhoea. *Cochrane Database Syst Rev.* 2010;(11):CD003048.
- Kalyoussef S, Feja KN. Foodborne illnesses. *Adv Pediatr.* 2014;61(1):287–312.

 SEE ALSO

Appendicitis, Acute; Botulism; Brucellosis; Dehydration; Diarrhea, Acute; Guillain-Barré Syndrome; Hypokalemia; Intestinal Parasites; Salmonella Infection; Typhoid Fever

CODES
ICD10
- A05.9 Bacterial foodborne intoxication, unspecified
- A02.0 Salmonella enteritis
- A04.5 Campylobacter enteritis

CLINICAL PEARLS
- Consider bacterial food poisoning when multiple people present after ingesting the same food with fevers and blood/mucus in stool or have recently returned from a developing nation.
- Consider culture and antibiotics in a prolonged febrile state with blood/mucus in stool, septicemic states, and traveler's diarrhea.
- With signs of enteroinvasion (high prolonged fever, bloody diarrhea, severe pain, septicemia), consider withholding antispasmodics (e.g., loperamide).

FROSTBITE

Donald Morando, DO • Lina N. Qazi, DO • Courtney Maiden, DO

 BASICS

DESCRIPTION
- A localized complication of exposure to cold, causing tissue to freeze, resulting in diminished blood flow to the affected part (especially hands, face, or feet).
- System(s) affected: endocrine/metabolic, skin/exocrine
- Synonym(s): dermatitis congelationis; frostnip; environmental injuries

EPIDEMIOLOGY
- Predominant age: all ages
- Predominant sex: male = female

ETIOLOGY AND PATHOPHYSIOLOGY
- Prolonged exposure to cold
- Refreezing thawed extremities
- Ice crystals form intracellularly, damaging capillaries
- Vasoconstriction reduces blood flow and microclotting leads to ischemia.
- Cellular dehydration, abnormal electrolyte concentrations due to the above and ultimately cell death
- In severe cases, deep tissue freezing may occur with damage to underlying blood vessels, muscles, and nerve tissue.
- With rewarming, the ice crystals melt and injured endothelium promotes edema resulting in the formation of epidermal blisters.
- Inflammatory mediators, prostaglandins, and thromboxane A2 induce vasoconstriction and platelet aggregation, worsening ischemia.

RISK FACTORS
- Environmental: lack of proper clothing or shelter resulting in prolonged exposure to below freezing temperatures
- Substance abuse, especially alcohol
- Age: infants and elderly
- Previous cold-related injury
- Decreased caloric intake (<1,500 calories/day)
- Dehydration or hypovolemia
- Underlying psychiatric disturbance
- Smoker
- Lean body mass
- Raynaud phenomenon
- Peripheral vascular disease
- Diabetes

GENERAL PREVENTION
- Dress in layers with appropriate cold weather gear, avoid clothing that is too constricting.
- Cover exposed areas and extremities appropriately.
- Prepare properly for trips to cold climates.
- Minimize wind exposure.
- Stay dry.

- Avoid alcohol.
- Ensure adequate hydration and caloric intake.
- Supplemental oxygen at very high altitudes (>7,500 meters)

COMMONLY ASSOCIATED CONDITIONS
- Alcohol and/or drug abuse
- Hypothermia

 DIAGNOSIS

HISTORY
- Throbbing pain
- Paresthesia
- Excessive sweating
- Joint pain
- Determine duration and severity of cold exposure.

PHYSICAL EXAM
- Feet, hands, and face are the most commonly affected.
- Classified as superficial or deep injuries
- Superficial: Only the skin and subcutaneous tissues are involved. Tissue is pliable. White mottled appearance with minimal capillary refill. Erythematous and edematous on rewarming, blisters are usually clear and neurovascular compromise is reversible.
- Deep: Injury extends into the bone. Tissue remains mottled and pulseless after rewarming, loss of sensation persists. Infrequent hemorrhagic blister formation. Tissue loss is common. High risk of infection

DIFFERENTIAL DIAGNOSIS
- Frostnip: a superficial cold injury that does not cause permanent damage
- Chilblains (pernio): an inflammatory reaction to short-term cold, wet exposure without tissue freezing
- Immersion syndrome (trench foot): inflammatory reaction to prolonged cold, wet exposure, typically socks or footwear

DIAGNOSTIC TESTS & INTERPRETATION
ECG in hypothermia may show bradycardia, atrial fibrillation, atrial flutter, ventricular fibrillation, diffuse T-wave inversion, Osborn waves (upward-going "hump" following S wave in the RST segment).

Initial Tests (lab, imaging)
- Baseline labs: CBC, CMP, UA for myoglobinuria, culture wound if suspected infection
- Triple-phase bone scan can identify tissue viability at early stage and facilitate early débridement.
- Other imaging techniques sometimes used include MRI/MRA, infrared thermography, angiography, digital plethysmography, and laser Doppler studies.

Test Interpretation
- Ice crystallization in the intravascular extracellular space
- Atrophy
- Fibroblastic proliferation
- Skin necrosis

 TREATMENT

Geriatric Considerations
- Associated disease states increase mortality.
- Periarticular osteoporosis complicates
- More prone to hypothermia

Pediatric Considerations
Loss of epithelial growth centers

ALERT
Acidosis

GENERAL MEASURES
- Admit patient to a burn center for deep injuries.
- Increase patient's body temperature to 34°C.
- Only warm areas of injury if possibility of refreezing can be excluded. Warm affected parts of body in 37–39°C water with antiseptics (iodine, polyhexanide) for 15 to 60 minutes or until skin color changes to red/violet (1)[C].
- Apply topical aloe vera gel before dressing.
- Débride open blisters only, débridement of tense, cloudy, or clear blisters at discretion of provider
- Splint and elevate affected extremity.
- Tetanus prophylaxis
- Analgesia and hydration, oral hydration if patient is alert and has no GI symptoms, otherwise IV hydration with warm normal saline in small boluses.
- Ibuprofen 400 mg BID
- Daily bathing in warm water containing antiseptics with active and passive mobilization
- Dry, loose bulky dressings, including in between fingers/toes (2)[C]
- Prohibit smoking
- Regular monitoring for reperfusion, consider experimental vasodilatation, thrombolytics, or sympathectomy for failed reperfusion (1)[C].

MEDICATION
First Line
- tPA administered within 24 hours of injury may prevent damage from thrombosis and may reduce amputation rate (3),(4)[B].

- Low-molecular-weight dextran to decrease blood viscosity should be considered in patients not given other systemic treatments (e.g., thrombolysis) (2)[C].

- Aspirin 250 mg plus buflomedil 400 mg IV followed by 8 days of iloprost 0.5 to 2 mg/kg/min for 6 hr/day may prevent amputation in patients with frostbite extending to the proximal phalanx (5)[B].

- Tetanus toxoid
- Ibuprofen 400 mg q12h to inhibit prostaglandins (6)[C]
- NSAIDs for mild to moderate pain; for severe pain, narcotic analgesia
- Systemic antibiotics should be used for proven infection, trauma, or cellulitis. Prophylactic antibiotics are not recommended (7)[C].
- **Precautions:** tPA should not be used with history of recent bleeding, stroke, ulcer, and so forth.

Second Line
Pentoxifylline has been tried with some success (6)[C].

ADDITIONAL THERAPIES
- Heated oxygen
- Warm IV fluids via central venous pressure line
- Avoid rubbing the affected area, as this can lead to further tissue destruction and worse outcomes.

SURGERY/OTHER PROCEDURES
- Urgent surgery is rarely needed, except fasciotomy for compartment syndrome.
- Suspect compartment syndrome if tissue swollen and compartment pressures >37 to 40 mm Hg.
- Fasciotomy is indicated if elevated compartment pressures (2)[B]
- Surgical débridement, as needed, to remove necrotic tissue
- Amputation should not be considered until tissues are definitively dead: may take ~3 weeks to know whether the tissue is permanently injured.
- Imaging with 99 mTc bone scan and/or MRA should be considered in severe cases to help determine extent of injury and assess viability of surrounding tissue. Imaging can help determine need for surgery (8).

INPATIENT CONSIDERATIONS
Admission Criteria/Initial Stabilization
Hospitalization is generally recommended unless no blisters are present after rewarming (4,8).
- Institute emergency measures for hypothermic patient without pulse or respiration. Such measures may include CPR and internal warming with warm IV fluids and warm oxygen (see topic "Hypothermia").
- Prevent refreezing.
- It may be necessary to keep the frostbitten part frozen until the patient can be transported to a care facility. Prolonged freezing is preferable to warming and refreezing (9)[C].
- Remove nonadherent wet clothing and shoes.
- Treat for hypothermia.
- Treat for pain.
  - NSAIDs and/or narcotics, if needed.
- Do not rub areas to warm them; increased tissue damage may occur (3)[C].
- Avoid pressure on frostbitten body parts except when the life of the patient or rescuer is in danger (10)[C].

IV Fluids
If patient cannot tolerate oral fluids or has altered mental status, give warmed normal saline in small boluses (2)[C].

 ONGOING CARE

FOLLOW-UP RECOMMENDATIONS
Outpatient or inpatient, depending on severity
- As tolerated; protect injured body parts.
- Initiate physical therapy once healing progresses sufficiently.
- Avoid nicotine.

- Avoid recurrent cold exposure.
- Properly fitting attire; consider custom footwear if feet were affected (7).

Patient Monitoring
- Preferably, electronic probe for temperature monitoring (rectal or vascular)
- Follow-up for physical therapy progress, infection, other complications

DIET
- As tolerated
- Warm oral fluids

PATIENT EDUCATION
- Refer to local library for information.
- Provide education on
  - Exposure protection
  - Risk factors for frostbite injuries
  - Early signs and symptoms of frostbite

PROGNOSIS
- Anesthesia and bullae may occur.
- The affected areas will heal or mummify without surgery; the process may take 6 to 12 months for healing.
- Patient may be sensitive to cold and experience burning and tingling.
- Cyanotic nonblanching skin and blisters with dark fluid suggest worse prognosis (9)[C].
- Loss of sensation after rewarming indicates poor prognosis.

COMPLICATIONS
- Hyperglycemia
- Acidosis
- Refractory arrhythmias
- Tissue loss: Distal parts of an extremity may undergo spontaneous amputation.
- Gangrene
- Hyperhidrosis due to nerve injury
- Decreased hair and nail growth
- Raynaud phenomenon
- Chronic regional pain
- Localized osteoporosis
- Death

REFERENCES
1. Sachs C, Lehnhardt M, Daigeler A, et al. The triaging and treatment of cold-induced injuries. *Dtsch Arztebl Int*. 2015;112(44):741–747.
2. McIntosh SE, Hamonko M, Freer L, et al. Wilderness Medical Society practice guidelines for the prevention and treatment of frostbite. *Wilderness Environ Med*. 2011;22(2):156–166.
3. Bruen KJ, Ballard JR, Morris SE, et al. Reduction of the incidence of amputation in frostbite injury with thrombolytic therapy. *Arch Surg*. 2007;142(6):546–551.
4. Jurkovich GJ. Environmental cold-induced injury. *Surg Clin North Am*. 2007;87:247–267.
5. Cauchy E, Cheguillaume B, Chetaille E. A controlled trial of a prostacyclin and rt-PA in the treatment of severe frostbite. *N Engl J Med*. 2011;364(2):189–190.

6. Imray C, Grieve A, Dhillon S. Cold damage to the extremities: frostbite and non-freezing cold injuries. *Postgrad Med J*. 2009;85(1007):481–488.
7. Handford C, Buxton P, Russell K, et al. Frostbite: a practical approach to hospital management. *Extrem Physiol Med*. 2014;3:7.
8. Ingram BJ, Raymond TJ. Recognition and treatment of freezing and nonfreezing cold injuries. *Curr Sports Med Rep*. 2013;12(2):125–130.
9. Biem J, Koehncke N, Classen D, et al. Out of the cold: management of hypothermia and frostbite. *CMAJ*. 2003;168(3):305–311.
10. State of Alaska Department of Health and Social Services. Cold injuries guidelines: Alaska Multilevel 2003 version. http://www.hypothermia.org/Hypothermia_Ed_pdf/Alaska-Cold-Injuries.pdf.

ADDITIONAL READING
- Cappaert TA, Stone JA, Castellani JW, et al. National Athletic Trainers' Association position statement: environmental cold injuries. *J Athl Train*. 2008;43(6):640–658.
- Murphy JV, Banwell PE, Roberts AH, et al. Frostbite: pathogenesis and treatment. *J Trauma*. 2000;48(1):171–178.
- Twomey JA, Peltier GL, Zera RT. An open-label study to evaluate the safety and efficacy of tissue plasminogen activator in treatment of severe frostbite. *J Trauma*. 2005;59(6):1350–1354.

 SEE ALSO
- Hypothermia
- Algorithm: Hypothermia

 CODES

ICD10
- T33.90XA Superficial frostbite of unspecified sites, init encntr
- T34.90XA Frostbite with tissue necrosis of unsp sites, init encntr
- T33.829A Superficial frostbite of unspecified foot, initial encounter

CLINICAL PEARLS
- Frostbite is considered a tetanus-prone injury. Treat as any injury involving tissue destruction.
- Avoid rewarming en route to the hospital if there is a chance of refreezing. Avoid burns to affected areas, which may be numb and insensitive to heat.
- It is difficult to assess degree of tissue involvement early on. Delay surgery until definite tissue destruction is present.

F

FURUNCULOSIS

Zoltan Trizna, MD, PhD

BASICS

DESCRIPTION
- Acute bacterial abscess of a hair follicle (often *Staphylococcus aureus*)
- System(s) affected: skin/exocrine
- Synonym(s): boils

EPIDEMIOLOGY
Incidence
- Predominant age
  - Adolescents and young adults
  - Clusters have been reported in teenagers living in crowded quarters, within families, or in high school athletes.
- Predominant sex: male = female

Prevalence
Exact data are not available.

ETIOLOGY AND PATHOPHYSIOLOGY
- Infection spreads away from hair follicle into surrounding dermis.
- Pathogenic strain of *S. aureus* (usually); most cases in United States are now due to community-acquired methicillin-resistant *S. aureus* (CA-MRSA) whereas methicillin-sensitive *S. aureus* (MSSA) is most common elsewhere (1).

Genetics
Unknown

RISK FACTORS
- Carriage of pathogenic strain of *Staphylococcus* sp. in nares, skin, axilla, and perineum
- Rarely, polymorphonuclear leukocyte defect or hyperimmunoglobulin E–*Staphylococcus* sp. abscess syndrome
- Diabetes mellitus, malnutrition, alcoholism, obesity, atopic dermatitis
- Primary immunodeficiency disease and AIDS (common variable immunodeficiency, chronic granulomatous disease, Chediak-Higashi syndrome, C3 deficiency, C3 hypercatabolism, transient hypogammaglobulinemia of infancy, immunodeficiency with thymoma, Wiskott-Aldrich syndrome)
- Secondary immunodeficiency (e.g., leukemia, leukopenia, neutropenia, therapeutic immunosuppression)
- Medication impairing neutrophil function (e.g., omeprazole)
- The most important independent predictor of recurrence is a positive family history.

GENERAL PREVENTION
Patient education regarding self-care (see "General Measures"); treatment and prevention are interrelated.

COMMONLY ASSOCIATED CONDITIONS
- Usually normal immune system
- Diabetes mellitus
- Polymorphonuclear leukocyte defect (rare)
- Hyperimmunoglobulin E–*Staphylococcus* sp. abscess syndrome (rare)
- See "Risk Factors."

DIAGNOSIS

HISTORY
- Located on hair-bearing sites, especially areas prone to friction or repeated minor traumas (e.g., underneath belt, anterior aspects of thighs, nape, buttocks)
- No initial fever or systemic symptoms
- The folliculocentric nodule may enlarge, become painful, and develop into an abscess (frequently with spontaneous drainage).

PHYSICAL EXAM
- Painful erythematous papules/nodules (1 to 5 cm) with central pustules
- Tender, red, perifollicular swelling, terminating in discharge of pus and necrotic plug
- Lesions may be solitary or clustered.

DIFFERENTIAL DIAGNOSIS
- Folliculitis
- Pseudofolliculitis
- Carbuncles
- Ruptured epidermal cyst
- Myiasis (larva of botfly/tumbu fly)
- Hidradenitis suppurativa
- Atypical bacterial or fungal infections

DIAGNOSTIC TESTS & INTERPRETATION
Initial Tests (lab, imaging)
Obtain culture if with multiple abscesses marked by surrounding inflammation, cellulitis, systemic symptoms such as fever, or if immunocompromised.

Follow-Up Tests & Special Considerations
- Immunoglobulin levels in rare (e.g., recurrent or otherwise inexplicable) cases
- If culture grows gram-negative bacteria or fungus, consider polymorphonuclear neutrophil leukocyte functional defect.

Test Interpretation
Histopathology (although a biopsy is rarely needed)
- Perifollicular necrosis containing fibrinoid material and neutrophils
- At deep end of necrotic plug, in SC tissue, is a large abscess with a Gram stain positive for small collections of *S. aureus*.

TREATMENT

GENERAL MEASURES
- Moist, warm compresses (provide comfort, encourage localization/pointing/drainage) 30 minutes QID
- If pointing or large, incise and drain: consider packing if large or incompletely drained.
- Routine culture is not necessary for localized abscess in nondiabetic patients with normal immune system.
- Sanitary practices: Change towels, washcloths, and sheets daily; clean shaving instruments; avoid nose picking; change wound dressings frequently; do not share items of personal hygiene (2)[B].

MEDICATION
First Line
- Systemic antibiotics usually *unnecessary*, unless extensive surrounding cellulitis or fever
- If suspecting MRSA, see "Second Line."

- If multiple abscesses, lesions with marked surrounding inflammation, cellulitis, systemic symptoms such as fever, or if immunocompromised: place on antibiotics therapy directed at *S. aureus* for 10 to 14 days.
  – Dicloxacillin (Dynapen, Pathocil) 500 mg PO QID *or* cephalexin 500 mg PO QID *or* clindamycin 300 mg TID, if penicillin-allergic

Second Line
- Resistant strains of *S. aureus* (MRSA): clindamycin 300 mg q6h or doxycycline 100 mg q12h or trimethoprim-sulfamethoxazole (TMP-SMX DS) 1 tab q8–12h or minocycline 100 mg q12h
- If known or suspected impaired neutrophil function (e.g., impaired chemotaxis, phagocytosis, superoxide generation), add vitamin C 1,000 mg/day for 4 to 6 weeks (prevents oxidation of neutrophils).
- If antibiotic regimens fail:
  – May try PO pentoxifylline 400 mg TID for 2 to 6 months
  – Contraindications: recent cerebral and/or retinal hemorrhage; intolerance to methylxanthines (e.g., caffeine, theophylline); allergy to the particular drug selected
  – Precautions: prolonged prothrombin time (PT) and/or bleeding; if on warfarin, frequent monitoring of PT

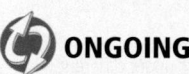 ONGOING CARE

FOLLOW-UP RECOMMENDATIONS
Patient Monitoring
Instruct patient to see physician if compresses are unsuccessful.

DIET
Unrestricted

PROGNOSIS
- Self-limited: usually drains pus spontaneously and will heal with or without scarring within several days.
- Recurrent/chronic: may last for months or years

- If recurrent, usually related to chronic skin carriage of staphylococci (nares or on skin). Treatment goals are to decrease or eliminate pathogenic strain *or* suppress pathogenic strain.
  – Culture nares, skin, axilla, and perineum (culture nares of family members).
  – Mupirocin 2%: Apply to both nares BID for 5 days each month.
  – Culture anterior nares every 3 months; if failure, retreat with mupirocin or consider clindamycin 150 mg/day for 3 months.
- Especially in recurrent cases, wash entire body and fingernails (with nailbrush) daily for 1 to 3 weeks with povidone-iodine (Betadine), chlorhexidine (Hibiclens), or hexachlorophene (pHisoHex soap), although all can cause dry skin.

COMPLICATIONS
- Scarring
- Bacteremia
- Seeding (e.g., septal/valve defect, arthritic joint)

REFERENCES
1. Demos M, McLeod MP, Nouri K. Recurrent furunculosis: a review of the literature. *Br J Dermatol*. 2012;167(4):725–732.
2. Fritz SA, Camins BC, Eisenstein KA, et al. Effectiveness of measures to eradicate *Staphylococcus aureus* carriage in patients with community-associated skin and soft-tissue infections: a randomized trial. *Infect Control Hosp Epidemiol*. 2011;32(9):872–880.

ADDITIONAL READING
- El-Gilany AH, Fathy H. Risk factors of recurrent furunculosis. *Dermatol Online J*. 2009;15(1):16.
- Ibler KS, Kromann CB. Recurrent furunculosis—challenges and management: a review. *Clin Cosmet Investig Dermatol*. 2014;7:59–64.
- McConeghy KW, Mikolich DJ, LaPlante KL. Agents for the decolonization of methicillin-resistant *Staphylococcus aureus*. *Pharmacotherapy*. 2009;29(3):263–280.
- Rivera AM, Boucher HW. Current concepts in antimicrobial therapy against select gram-positive organisms: methicillin-resistant *Staphylococcus aureus*, penicillin-resistant pneumococci, and vancomycin-resistant enterococci. *Mayo Clin Proc*. 2011;86(12):1230–1243.

- Wahba-Yahav AV. Intractable chronic furunculosis: prevention of recurrences with pentoxifylline. *Acta Derm Venereol*. 1992;72(6):461–462.
- Winthrop KL, Abrams M, Yakrus M, et al. An outbreak of mycobacterial furunculosis associated with footbaths at a nail salon. *N Engl J Med*. 2002;346(18):1366–1371.

 SEE ALSO

Folliculitis; Hidradenitis Suppurativa

 CODES

ICD10
- L02.92 Furuncle, unspecified
- L02.12 Furuncle of neck
- L02.429 Furuncle of limb, unspecified

CLINICAL PEARLS
- Pathogens may be different in different localities. Keep up-to-date with the locality-specific epidemiology.
- If few, furuncles/furunculosis do not need antibiotic treatment. If systemic symptoms (e.g., fever), cellulitis, or multiple lesions occur, oral antibiotic therapy is used.
- Other treatments for MRSA include linezolid PO or IV and IV vancomycin.
- Folliculitis, furunculosis, and carbuncles are parts of a spectrum of pyodermas.
- Other causative organisms include aerobic (e.g., *Escherichia coli, Pseudomonas aeruginosa,* and *Streptococcus faecalis*), anaerobic (e.g., *Bacteroides, Lactobacillus, Peptobacillius,* and *Peptostreptococcus*), and *Mycobacteria*.
- Decolonization (treatment of the nares with topical antibiotic) is only recommended if the colonization was confirmed by cultures because resistance is common and treatment is of uncertain efficacy.

F

GALACTORRHEA

Nicole Nelson, DO • David Bode, MD

 BASICS

DESCRIPTION
- Milky nipple discharge not associated with gestation or present >1 year after weaning. Galactorrhea does not include serous, purulent, or bloody nipple discharge.
- System(s) affected: endocrine/metabolic, nervous, reproductive
- Synonym(s): disordered lactation; nipple discharge

Pregnancy Considerations
Most cases of galactorrhea during pregnancy are physiologic.

EPIDEMIOLOGY
- Predominant age: 15 to 50 years (reproductive age)
- Predominant sex: female > male (rare, e.g., in patients with multiple endocrine neoplasia type 1 [MEN1], the most common anterior pituitary tumors are prolactinomas)

Incidence
Common

Prevalence
6.8% of women referred to physicians with a breast complaint have nipple discharge.

ETIOLOGY AND PATHOPHYSIOLOGY
Disorders of lactation are associated with elevated prolactin levels, either from overproduction or loss of inhibitory regulation by dopamine.
- Nipple stimulation
- Pituitary gland overproduction
  - Prolactinoma
- Loss of dopamine via hypothalamic dysregulation
  - Craniopharyngiomas
  - Meningiomas or other tumors
  - Sarcoid
  - Irradiation
  - Vascular insult
  - Stalk disruption
  - Traumatic injury
- Medications that suppress dopamine (1):
  - Typical and atypical antipsychotics
  - SSRIs
  - Tricyclic antidepressants
  - Cimetidine
  - Ranitidine
  - Reserpine
  - α-Methyldopa
  - Verapamil
  - Estrogens
  - Isoniazid
  - Opioids
  - Stimulants
  - Neuroleptics
  - Metoclopramide
  - Domperidone
  - Protease inhibitors

- Chest wall injury
  - Zoster, surgical, or other trauma
- Postoperative condition, especially oophorectomy
- Renal failure
- Other causes
  - Primary hypothyroidism
  - Cirrhosis
  - Cushing disease
  - Ectopic prolactin secretion
  - Renal failure
  - Sarcoid
  - Lupus
  - Multiple sclerosis
  - Polycystic ovary syndrome
- Idiopathic
  - Normal prolactin levels

GENERAL PREVENTION
- Frequent nipple stimulation can cause galactorrhea.
- Avoid medications that can suppress dopamine.

COMMONLY ASSOCIATED CONDITIONS
See "Etiology and Pathophysiology."

 DIAGNOSIS

- Findings vary with causes
- Look for signs/symptoms of associated conditions:
  - Adrenal insufficiency
  - Acromegaly
  - Hypothyroidism
  - Chest wall conditions

HISTORY
- Usually bilateral milky nipple discharge; may be spontaneous or induced by stimulation
- Determine possibility of pregnancy or recent discontinuation of lactation
- Signs of hypogonadism from hyperprolactinemia
  - Oligomenorrhea, amenorrhea
  - Inadequate luteal phase, anovulation, infertility
  - Decreased libido (especially in affected males)
- Mass effects from pituitary enlargement
  - Headache, cranial neuropathies
  - Bitemporal hemianopsia, amaurosis, scotomata

PHYSICAL EXAM
Breast examination should be performed with attention to the presence of spontaneous or induced nipple discharge.

DIFFERENTIAL DIAGNOSIS
- Pregnancy-induced lactation or recent weaning
- Nonmilky nipple discharge
  - Intraductal papilloma
  - Fibrocystic disease
- Purulent breast discharge
  - Mastitis
  - Breast abscess
  - Impetigo
  - Eczema
- Bloody breast discharge: Consider malignancy (Paget disease, breast cancer).

DIAGNOSTIC TESTS & INTERPRETATION
Perform formal visual field testing if pituitary adenoma suspected.

Initial Tests (lab, imaging)
- Prolactin level, thyroid-stimulating hormone, pregnancy test, liver, and renal functions
- Drugs that may alter lab results: medications that can cause hyperprolactinemia
- Situations that may alter lab results:
  - Lab evaluation of prolactin may be falsely elevated by a recent breast examination.
  - Vigorous exercise
  - Sexual activity
  - High-carbohydrate diet
  - Consider repeating the test under different circumstances if the value is borderline (30 to 40) elevated.
- Prolactin levels may fluctuate. Elevated prolactin levels should be confirmed with at least one additional level drawn in a fasting, nonexercised state, with no breast stimulation (2)[C].
- Prolactin levels >250 ng/mL are highly suggestive of a pituitary adenoma (3)[C].
- If a breast mass is palpated in the setting of nipple discharge, evaluation of that mass is indicated with mammogram and/or ultrasound.
- Pituitary MRI with gadolinium enhancement if the serum prolactin level is significantly elevated (>200 ng/mL) or if a pituitary tumor is otherwise suspected.

Follow-Up Tests & Special Considerations
- Consider evaluation of follicle-stimulating hormone and luteinizing hormone if amenorrheic.
- Consider evaluation of growth hormone levels if acromegaly suspected.
- Measure adrenal steroids if signs of Cushing disease present.

Diagnostic Procedures/Other
If diagnosis is in question, confirm by microscopic evaluation that nipple secretions are lipoid.

Test Interpretation
None, unless pituitary resection required

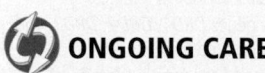 TREATMENT

- Avoid excess nipple stimulation.
- Idiopathic galactorrhea (normal prolactin levels) does not require treatment.
- Discontinue causative medications, if possible.
- Treat to manage symptoms, reduce patient anxiety, and restore fertility.
- Treat tumors >10 mm (even if asymptomatic) to reduce pituitary tumor size or prevent progression to avoid neurologic sequelae.
- If microadenoma, watchful waiting can be appropriate because 95% do not enlarge.

MEDICATION

- Dopamine agonists work to reduce prolactin levels and shrink tumor size. Therapy is suppressive, not curative (4)[C].
- Treatment is discontinued when tumor size has reduced or regressed completely or after pregnancy has been achieved.
- Cabergoline (Dostinex)
  - Start at 0.25 mg PO twice weekly and increase by 0.25 mg monthly until prolactin levels normalize. Usual dose ranges from 0.25 to 1 mg PO once or twice weekly.
  - More effective and better tolerated than bromocriptine (5)[A]
  - Convenient dosing
- Although cabergoline has been associated with valvular heart disease in patients treated for Parkinson disease, the lower doses used in treatment of prolactinomas have not been adequately studied (6)[C].
- Bromocriptine
  - Start at 1.25 mg/day PO with food and increase weekly by 1.25 mg/day until therapeutic response achieved (usually 2.5 to 15 mg/day, divided once daily/TID).
  - More expensive and more frequent dosing; however, most providers have experience with this effective drug.
  - Long-term treatment can cause woody fibrosis of the pituitary gland.
- Contraindications are similar for all and include the following:
  - Uncontrolled hypertension
  - Sensitivity to ergot alkaloids
- Precautions
  - Nausea, vomiting, and drowsiness are common.
  - Orthostasis, light-headedness, or syncope
  - Hypertension, seizures, acute psychosis, and digital vasospasm are rare.
- Significant possible interactions
  - Phenothiazines, butyrophenones; other drugs listed under "Etiology and Pathophysiology"

SURGERY/OTHER PROCEDURES

- Surgery
  - Macroadenomas need surgery if (a) medical management does not halt growth, (b) neurologic symptoms persist, (c) size >10 mm, or (d) patient cannot tolerate medications. Also considered in young patients with microadenomas to avoid long-term medical therapy.
  - Transsphenoidal pituitary resection
  - 50% recurrence after surgery
- Radiotherapy
  - Radiation is an alternative tumor therapy for macroprolactinomas not responsive to other modes of treatment:
    ○ 20–30% success rate
    ○ 50% risk of panhypopituitarism after radiation
    ○ Risk of optic nerve damage, hypopituitarism, neurologic dysfunction, and increased risk for stroke and secondary brain tumors

ONGOING CARE

FOLLOW-UP RECOMMENDATIONS

- Outpatient care unless pituitary resection required
- Bromocriptine patients need adequate hydration
- Dopamine agonist therapy should be discontinued in pregnancy.

Patient Monitoring

- Varies with cause
- Check prolactin levels every 6 weeks until normalized, then every 6 to 12 months.
- Monitor visual fields and/or MRI at least yearly until stable.

DIET

No restrictions

PATIENT EDUCATION

- Warn about symptoms of mass enlargement in pituitary.
- Discuss treatment rationale, risks of treating, and expectant management.
- Patient education material available from American Family Physician: www.aafp.org/afp/20040801/553ph.html

PROGNOSIS

- Depends on underlying cause
- Symptoms can recur after discontinuation of a dopamine agonist.
- Surgery can have 50% recurrence.
- Prolactinomas <10 mm can resolve spontaneously.

COMPLICATIONS

- If enlarging pituitary adenoma, risk of permanent visual field loss
- Panhypopituitarism can complicate radiation or surgical therapy.
- Osteoporosis if amenorrhea persists without estrogen replacement.

REFERENCES

1. Molitch ME. Drugs and prolactin. *Pituitary*. 2008;11(2):209–218.
2. Huang W, Molitch ME. Evaluation and management of galactorrhea. *Am Fam Physician*. 2012;85(11):1073–1080.
3. Melmed S, Casanueva FF, Hoffman AR, et al. Diagnosis and treatment of hyperprolactinemia: an Endocrine Society clinical practice guideline. *J Clin Endocrinol Metab*. 2011;96(2):273–288.
4. Majumdar A, Mangal NS. Hyperprolactinemia. *J Hum Reprod Sci*. 2013;6(3):168–175.
5. Wang AT, Mullan RJ, Lane MA, et al. Treatment of hyperprolactinemia: a systematic review and meta-analysis. *Syst Rev*. 2012;1:33.
6. Córdoba-Soriano JG, Lamas-Oliveira C, Hidalgo-Olivares VM, et al. Valvular heart disease in hyperprolactinemic patients treated with low doses of cabergoline. *Rev Esp Cardiol*. 2013;66(5):410–412.

ADDITIONAL READING

- Mancini T, Casanueva FF, Giustina A. Hyperprolactinemia and prolactinomas. *Endocrinol Metab Clin North Am*. 2008;37(1):67–99.
- Patel BK, Falcon S, Drukteinis J. Management of nipple discharge and the associated imaging findings. *Am J Med*. 2015;128(4): 353–360.

SEE ALSO

Hyperprolactinemia

CODES

ICD10

- N64.3 Galactorrhea not associated with childbirth
- N64.52 Nipple discharge

CLINICAL PEARLS

- Galactorrhea is a common disorder, affecting up to 50% of reproductive-age women.
- Common causes include idiopathic, from excess nipple stimulation, dopamine-suppressing medications, or pituitary prolactinoma
- Most cases may be adequately evaluated by thyroid-stimulating hormone, prolactin, and human chorionic gonadotropin measurement, with additional testing as suggested by the presence of other symptoms or signs.
- Lab evaluation of prolactin may be falsely elevated due to recent sexual activity, breast examination, exercise, or a high-carbohydrate diet. Repeat any borderline elevation before continuing evaluation or initiating treatment.
- Evaluate prolactin >200 ng/mL (or suspicion of pituitary macroadenoma) with a gadolinium-enhanced MRI.

G

GAMBLING ADDICTION

Rebecca Collins, DO, MPH, FAAFP

 BASICS

DESCRIPTION

Gambling is the act of placing something of value at risk in the hopes of gaining something of greater value. Pathologic gambling (PG) and problem gambling affect up to 15 million Americans with the number of those affected increasing, especially in young people. The essential feature of gambling disorder is persistent and recurrent maladaptive gambling behavior that disrupts personal, family, and/or vocational pursuits. Individuals with gambling disorder have high rates of comorbidity with other mental disorders (substance use, depression, anxiety, and personality disorders). There is a debate as to whether gambling addiction is an impulse-control disorder or a non-substance abuse–related disorder.

EPIDEMIOLOGY

- Predominant sex: male > female, though gap narrowing
- Rates of pathologic and problem gambling are higher in adolescents and middle-age persons than older adults.
- The younger a person starts gambling, the more likely he or she is to become a pathologic gambler.
- Economics: $0.5 trillion wagered in United States annually.

Prevalence

- Lifetime gambling disorder prevalence is 0.4–1% in the U.S. adults.
  - Males 0.6%, females 0.2%
  - African American 0.9%, Caucasian 0.4%, Hispanic 0.3%
- Living in closer proximity to a casino increases prevalence.

GENERAL PREVENTION

- Focus on treatment; patient education; awareness of risk factors, associated conditions, and warning signs of pathologic or problematic gambling behaviors.
- Primary prevention using educational programs that target at-risk youth and adults
- Public health interventions: Decrease available gambling locations and lottery venues, ban advertising for gambling activities, keep lottery tickets out of sight, add warning label of risk of problem gambling to packaging of gambling products, enforce legal age of gambling, moratorium on building new casinos (1).

ETIOLOGY AND PATHOPHYSIOLOGY

- *DSM-5* characterizes gambling disorder as a non-substance related and addictive disorder; however, there is a debate whether it is an impulse-control disorder or possibly both.
- Impulse control: changes in serotonin metabolites in pathologic gamblers and patients with impulse-control disorders
- Substance abuse: similarities found between PG and substance use (tolerance, withdrawal, anticipatory craving, relapses)
- The brains of pathologic gamblers may have some predisposition to illness. Functional MRI studies indicate that the ventromedial prefrontal cortex is less activated when gambling stimuli are presented to pathologic gamblers.

- Abnormalities in the neurotransmitters serotonin, norepinephrine, dopamine, and glutamate may be implicated in PG.
  - Norepinephrine: Low levels seem to help a patient avoid gambling, whereas high levels may lead to poor decision making.
  - Serotonin: involved in impulse control by helping a patient weigh the risks of gambling
  - Dopamine: High levels in the nucleus accumbens while gambling lead to a pleasurable rush may induce reversible PG in Parkinson patients who take dopamine agonists.
- Medicine classes for each category have been used to treat.

Genetics

- *SLC6A4* serotonin transporter gene has been associated with PG in males but not in females.
- Dopamine receptor genes *DRD1*, *DRD2*, *DRD3*, and *DRD4* have been correlated with PG.
- More prevalent among first-degree relatives of alcoholics than among general population.

RISK FACTORS

- Some types of gambling present a greater risk to cause PG than other types: pull tabs, casino gambling, bingo, and card games outside a casino
- Being involved with several gaming modalities is related to PG and suggests that the gambler is very captivated with risking money for excitement as opposed to risking money for social pleasure or for an interest in sports.
- Lower socioeconomic status
- Adults in mental health treatment
- Substance abuse (nicotine, alcohol, inhalants, marijuana)
- Positive family history
- Antisocial personality disorder, depressive and bipolar disorders, other substance abuse disorders (especially alcohol)

COMMONLY ASSOCIATED CONDITIONS

- Poor nutrition
- Stress-related medical conditions (e.g., peptic ulcer disease [PUD], hypertension, migraine, palpitations)
- Suicidal ideation and attempts
- Substance abuse disorder (especially alcohol)
- Attention deficit hyperactivity disorder
- Bipolar disorder and other mood disorders
- Impulse-control disorders
- Personality disorders
- Incarceration
- Financial problems (e.g., previous bankruptcy)

 DIAGNOSIS

DSM-5 criteria for gambling disorder (2):

- Persistent and recurrent gambling behavior leading to significant impairment or distress as indicated by ≤4 of the following in a 12-month period, AND gambling behavior is not better explained by a manic episode:
  - Often preoccupied with gambling
  - Need to gamble with increasing amounts of money to achieve the desired excitement

  - Repeated unsuccessful efforts to control, cut back, or stop gambling
  - Restless or irritable when attempting to cut down or stop gambling
  - Often gambles when feeling distressed (e.g., helpless, guilty, anxious, depressed)
  - After losing money gambling, often returns another day to get even ("chasing" one's loses)
  - Lies to conceal the extent of involvement with gambling
  - Has jeopardized or lost a significant relationship, job, or educational or career opportunity because of gambling
  - Relies on others to provide money to relieve a desperate financial situation caused by gambling ("bailout" behavior)
- Specifiers:
  - Episodic: meets diagnostic criteria at >1 time point with symptoms subsiding for at least several months
  - Persistent: continuous symptoms for multiple years
  - Early remission: After criteria met previously, none met for ≥3 months but <12 months.
  - Sustained remission: After criteria met previously, no criteria met for ≥12 months.
  - Current severity: mild (4 to 5 criteria), moderate (6 to 7 criteria), or severe (8 to 9 criteria)

HISTORY

- Preoccupation with gambling and chasing losses are most frequently endorsed criteria.
- Those with moderate to severe forms of disorder are usually the individuals who present for treatment.
- May have distortions in thinking (e.g., denial, superstitions, sense of power and control over outcome of chance events)
- Preoccupation with money; belief that money is the cause and solution to their problems
- Personality characteristics: impulsivity, competitive, energetic, restless OR depressed, lonely, helpless, guilty
- 50% of patients in treatment for PG have suicidal ideation, 17% have suicide attempts.
- Symptoms can develop anytime from adolescence through older adulthood.
- Amounts of money wagered is not in themselves indicative of gambling disorder (some individuals can wager thousands of dollars per month and not have a problem, some may wager much smaller amounts but experience substantial gambling-related difficulties).
- Loss of important relationships with family or friends
- Absenteeism or poor work/school performance
- Poor general health; high use of medical services
- Unexplained new financial problems
- New participation in illegal or dishonest money-making endeavors or activities
- Disruptions in personal life or career
- Patient may ask his or her family and friends to pay off his or her debts ("bailing them out").

DIFFERENTIAL DIAGNOSIS
- Social gambling
- Professional gambling
- Bipolar disorder, manic episode
- Personality disorder
- Other medical conditions (patients on dopaminergic medications, e.g., Parkinson)

DIAGNOSTIC TESTS & INTERPRETATION
- South Oaks Gambling Screen (SOGS):
  - Most extensively used and validated screening tool
  - 20-question screen for PG
  - Score of 3 to 4 suggests problem gambling.
  - Score of ≥5 indicates probable PG.
  - Criticized as having high false-positive rate and being too lengthy to administer
- Gamblers Anonymous 20 questions:
  - Easily obtainable from Gamblers Anonymous Web site
  - Scores of >7 are indicative of problem/PG.
- Lie/Bet method: "Have you ever had to lie to people important to you about how much you gambled?" "Have you ever felt a need to bet more money?":
  - A patient who answers at least one question with a "Yes" suggests further investigation needed to see if criteria are met for PG.
  - This test has been shown to have >85% specificity and >95% sensitivity.

Initial Tests (lab, imaging)
None usually indicated

TREATMENT

To treat PG, treat comorbidities first. The usual comorbid disorders are substance abuse, bipolar disorder, ADHD, and other impulse-control disorders. Nonpharmacologic therapies are more effective than pharmacologic therapies. Some data suggest that gambling abstinence is not necessary for treatment; patients can still exhibit controlled gambling.

GENERAL MEASURES
- Get a sense of the patient's readiness for change.
- Provide intervention/patient education. Although there are no FDA-approved drug treatments for PG, make clinically based medication recommendations.
- Screen for and treat comorbid conditions.
- Provide referrals:
  - Addiction psychiatrist/counselor
  - Gamblers Anonymous
  - Consumer credit organizations
  - Bankruptcy lawyers
  - Gam-Anon for family members

MEDICATION
- There are no FDA-approved medicines for gambling addiction; pharmacotherapy is most effective when directed toward patient's comorbid psychiatric condition (3)[A].
- SSRIs:
  - Currently seen as beneficial for treating comorbid impulse-control disorders, although their efficacy has been under question for PG
  - All studies with SSRIs limited due to small size, short follow-up, conflicting outcomes, and in some cases study design; confirmation for some positive findings need larger randomized controlled trials with extended follow-up before recommendations for use can be made

- Opiate antagonists have the ability to decrease dopamine release in the dopamine reward pathway. Naltrexone and nalmefene have been reported to cause improvements on gambling symptom assessment scores (4,5)[B].

ADDITIONAL THERAPIES
- Cognitive-behavioral therapy (CBT):
  - The main effective interventions for PG are psychoeducation, cognitive restructuring, problem solving, social skills training, and relapse prevention. Studies indicated that CBT resulted in significant improvement as short-term therapy.
  - CBT may be done in several formats: individual, group, brief group, and dual diagnosis. All these formats have been shown to be effective. Group therapy is favored because patients are often extroverted. Couple or family therapy also may be used.
- Gamblers Anonymous:
  - A 12-step program similar to Alcoholics Anonymous for a person suffering from a gambling addiction.
  - Dropout rate is high if this is the only means of therapy.
  - Patients may deny need to attend in the first place, and for that reason, Gamblers Anonymous may not be appropriate for patients who are in the precontemplation stage.
- Motivational enhancement therapy (MET):
  - Provides nonargumentative exploration of patient's stage of change
  - Patient receives positive reinforcement from clinician.
  - Motivational enhancement strategies support self-efficacy.
  - Improves patient rapport; aids in removing barriers to treatment
  - In one study, MET alone did not show any improvement, but MET and CBT together improved outcome measures.
- Because of increased suicide rates, patients may need to be hospitalized acutely for safety and to prevent gambling.
- Because patients are at increased risk from mental and physical illness, they benefit from relaxation exercises to reduce stress, identify triggers, substitute gambling with other activities and a complete physical and lab work with nutrition evaluation.

ONGOING CARE

FOLLOW-UP RECOMMENDATIONS
Patients seeking treatment for gambling addiction should be followed routinely to monitor the response to treatment, tolerance to medications, and relapse.

PATIENT EDUCATION
- Gamblers Anonymous:
  - http://www.gamblersanonymous.org/ga/
  - National hotline 1-888-GA-HELPS (888-424-3577)
- Gam-Anon: support group for spouses, family, or close friends: http://www.gam-anon.org/
- Responsible Gambling Council: http://www.responsiblegambling.org/
- Humphrey H. This Must Be Hell: A Look at Pathological Gambling. Bloomington, IN: iUniverse; 2000.
- Lee B. Born To Lose: Memoirs of a Compulsive Gambler. Center City, MN: Hazelden; 2005.

PROGNOSIS
- Patients with gambling addiction can be treated but many relapse.
- 36–39% of patients did not experience any gambling-related problems according to one study, and only 7–12% sought formal treatment or Gamblers Anonymous meetings.
- Roughly 1/3 of patients who have a gambling addiction recover without any intervention.

REFERENCES
1. Poulin C. Gambling. *CMAJ*. 2006;175(10):1208.
2. American Psychiatric Association. *Diagnostic and Statistical Manual of Mental Disorders*. 5th ed. Arlington, VA: American Psychiatric Association; 2013:585–589.
3. Dell'Osso B, Allen A, Hollander E. Comorbidity issues in the pharmacological treatment of pathological gambling: a critical review. *Clin Pract Epidemiol Ment Health*. 2005;1:21.
4. Kim SW, Grant JE, Adson DE, et al. Double-blind naltrexone and placebo comparison study in the treatment of pathological gambling. *Biol Psychiatry*. 2001;49(11):914–921.
5. Grant JE, Potenza MN, Hollander E, et al. Multicenter investigation of the opioid antagonist nalmefene in the treatment of pathological gambling. *Am J Psychiatry*. 2006;163(2):303–312.

ADDITIONAL READING
- Chou KL, Afifi TO. Disordered (pathologic or problem) gambling and axis I psychiatric disorders: results from the National Epidemiologic Survey on Alcohol and Related Conditions. *Am J Epidemiol*. 2011;173(11):1289–1297.
- Leung KS, Cottler LB. Treatment of pathological gambling. *Curr Opin Psychiatry*. 2009;22(1):69–74.
- Nussbaum D, Honarmand K, Govoni R, et al. An eight component decision-making model for problem gambling: a systems approach to stimulate integrative research. *J Gambl Stud*. 2011;27(4):523–563.
- Okuda M, Balán I, Petry NM, et al. Cognitive-behavioral therapy for pathological gambling: cultural considerations. *Am J Psychiatry*. 2009;166(12):1325–1330.

CODES

ICD10
- F63.0 Pathological gambling
- Z72.6 Gambling and betting

CLINICAL PEARLS
- Several brief screening strategies can be used to identify PG, including the SOGS, the Gamblers Anonymous 20 questions, and the Lie/Bet method.
- To treat PG, first treat comorbidities such as substance abuse, bipolar disorder, ADHD, and other mental health/substance abuse disorders.
- Nonpharmacologic therapies are more effective than pharmacologic therapies. There is no FDA-approved therapy for PG.
- Patients seeking treatment for gambling addiction should be followed routinely by physicians and counselors to monitor the response to treatment, tolerance to medications, and possibility of relapse.

GANGLION CYST

Matthew W. Thompson, MD • William Fiden, MD

BASICS

- Ganglion cysts are common benign tumors that are not related to nerve tissue (as implied incorrectly by the name).
- Can be located anywhere throughout the body but usually adjacent to or within joints and tendons, with the most common locations being the wrist, foot, and ankle
- Not a true cyst as microscopic examination does not show an epithelial lining
- Most are asymptomatic except for changing size. Local nerve compression can result in pain or activity limitation.
- Synonym(s): synovial cyst; myxoid cyst; Gideon disease; Bible bump.

EPIDEMIOLOGY
- Can affect all age groups. Unusual in children
- Most common in ages 20 to 40 years and twice as common in women
- Common in dorsal wrist, radial wrist, and dorsum of the distal interphalangeal (DIP) joint (referred to as a mucous cyst)
- Mucous cysts are usually seen in older patients.
- 60–70% of hand and wrist ganglion cysts are on the dorsal wrist; 15–20% are on the volar wrist.

Prevalence
- Prevalence of wrist ganglia in patients presenting with wrist pain is as high as 19%.
- Prevalence of ganglia in patients with a palpable mass in the wrist is as high as 27%.
- Reported prevalence in ankles is 5.6%.

ETIOLOGY AND PATHOPHYSIOLOGY
Pathogenesis is unclear. Cysts are filled with mucin and communicate with the adjacent joint space, tendon and/or tendon sheath via a stalk. Several theories about their orgin include:
- Herniation of synovial lining creates a one-way valve. Although this is supported by dye studies, the lack of a synovial (epithelial) lining in the cyst wall makes this less likely.
- Mucoid degeneration of connective tissue results in formation of hyaluronic acid, leading to cystic space formation. Studies haven't confirmed this hypothesis.

- Joint stress leads to a tear in the joint capsule or tendon sheath allowing synovial fluid to leak into surrounding tissues. Local irritation leads to production of fluid and a pseudocapsule forms (explaining the lack of an epithelial lining).
- Recurrent stress may stimulate mucin production by nearby mesenchymal cells (seen on electron microscopy) resulting in cyst formation.

Genetics
No specific genetic links have been found.

RISK FACTORS
- Female > male
- Osteoarthritis for mucoid cysts
- Joint trauma (possible but not proven)

COMMONLY ASSOCIATED CONDITIONS
Mucous cysts are usually associated with osteoarthritis at the DIP joint.

DIAGNOSIS

Usually made on basis of history and physical examination

HISTORY
- Patients presents with an asymptomatic mass that has been present for months or years (most common) or when the cyst become painful, causes weakness, increases in size or interfers with activities.
- Pain is typically annoying as opposed to debilitating.
- Variable in size and location
- May increase in size and pain with activity and recede with rest

PHYSICAL EXAM
- Mass
  - Rubbery
  - Subcutaneous
  - May transilluminate
  - Fixed to the tendon sheath and only slightly mobile
  - No overlying skin changes

- Palpation may cause pain due to nerve compression.
- Small ganglions may only be palpable in full wrist flexion or extension.
- Occult ganglions are not palpable but can be quite painful.

DIFFERENTIAL DIAGNOSIS
- Carpal bossing: a small, immovable mass of bone on the back of the wrist
- Giant cell tumor, lipoma, sarcoma, hamartoma, interosseous neuroma
- Epidermal inclusion cyst
- True synovial cyst
- Anomalous musculature
- Tenosynovitis

DIAGNOSTIC TESTS & INTERPRETATION
Unless diagnosis is unclear, imaging is not necessary.

Initial Tests (lab, imaging)
- Most are apparent clinically and do not need imaging
- Plain films can exclude bony pathology but rarely alter the course of treatment.
- Other options to exclude occult ganglions:
  - Ultrasound; MRI
  - Arthroscopy
- US and MRI have similar rates of sensitivity and specificity. US is less expensive than MRI but more operator-dependent.
- Arthroscopy is used for both diagnostic and therapeutic purposes and can be considered when initial workup is nondiagnostic and conservative treatment is not effective.

Test Interpretation
- Gross pathologic evaluation shows that cysts are often multilobulated.
- Microscopic exam reveals a relatively acellular outer wall with several layers of randomly oriented collagen fibers and mesenchymal cells in the collagen fibers.
- Cyst fluid is highly viscous and contains glucosamine, albumin, globulin, and hyaluronic acid.
- Histopathologically identical regardless of anatomic location

TREATMENT

Four primary treatment options include:

- Reassurance and observation: Ganglia are not likely to be malignant or to cause damage. May treat with splinting and NSAIDs if desired for comfort
  - Multiple studies suggest spontaneous cyst resolution in half of patients over 5 years (1,2)[A].
- Closed rupture: historically done by hitting cyst with a book ("King James Bible treatment")
  - Results in initial treatment decreased clinical symptoms by 22–66%, recurrence is common.
  - Typically a home remedy.
- Aspiration: can be done in the office under local anesthesia with a 16-gauge needle at base of the cyst. Studies demonstrate mixed results on aspirations with 30–85% success with multiple aspirations (1,2)[A]. Volar wrist ganglia should not be aspirated without US guidance due to risk of damage to neurovascular structures. Mucous cysts can be aspirated, but recurrence is >50% and pain may not resolve if due to underlying osteoarthritis.
  - Concurrent injection of steroids or hyaluronidase have mixed results and are not clearly more effective than aspiration alone. Steroids have the additional risk of fat atrophy and skin depigmentation.
  - Multiple cyst punctures are not more effective than simple aspiration.
  - Sclerotherapy or injections that increase inflammation and cause fibrosis to reduce recurrence are less common due to concerns for joint damage.
- Surgical excision

MEDICATION

First Line
- NSAIDs for pain relief
- No other medications have been shown to be effective.

SURGERY/OTHER PROCEDURES
- Recurrence rates vary among studies but have been as low as 0–28%. Results better at high-volume centers and actual recurrence rates are likely higher.
  - Arthroscopic excision is as good as open excision with better cosmetic outcomes and a faster return to normal function (3)[A].

- A 6-year study comparing blind aspiration, surgery, and watchful waiting showed:
  - Recurrence rates of 58% after aspiration, 39% after surgery, and 58% in untreated patients.
  - Patient satisfaction was 81% with aspiration, 83% with surgery, and 53% with reassurance.
  - There was no significant difference in pain, weakness, or stiffness between groups.
  - Pain was reduced significantly in all groups.
  - Time away from work is greater with excision compared to aspiration and reassurance.
  - Neither aspiration nor surgical excision provides a clear long-term benefit over simple observation. The primary benefit of surgery is early cosmetic resolution (4)[B].
- Bottom line
  - Surgery appears to provide the lowest rates of cyst recurrence but does not provide significantly higher pain reduction or patient satisfaction.
  - Determine the patient's reasons for seeking medical attention. Education alone can provide adequate treatment.

 ONGOING CARE

May require supervised hand therapy after surgical repair to improve stiffness and function

FOLLOW-UP RECOMMENDATIONS
- Hand/occupational therapy may be helpful if ganglion symptoms persist despite rest.
- Manage expectations about recurrence.

PROGNOSIS
- Generally very good
- Up to 50% will resolve with watchful waiting.
- Higher rate of resolution in children

COMPLICATIONS
- Risk of recurrence is present regardless of treatment; no specific recommendations to minimize this risk.
- Risks of surgical excision include the following:
  - Residual pain
  - Poor cosmesis
  - Neuropathy
  - Stiffness and instability of the wrist, especially scapholunate ligament instability
  - Open excision if arthroscopic treatment fails to resolve symptoms

REFERENCES

1. Suen M, Fung B, Lung CP. Treatment of ganglion cysts. *ISRN Orthop*. 2013;2013:940615.
2. Meena S, Gupta A. Dorsal wrist ganglion: current review of literature. *J Clin Orthop Trauma*. 2014;5(2):59–64.
3. Bontempo NA, Weiss AP. Arthroscopic excision of gangion cysts. *Hand Clin*. 2014;30(1):71–75.
4. Dias JJ, Dhukaram V, Kumar P. The natural history of untreated dorsal wrist ganglia and patient reported outcome 6 years after intervention. *J Hand Surg Eur Vol*. 2007;32(5):502–508.

ADDITIONAL READING

Gant J, Ruff M, Janz BA. Wrist ganglions. *J Hand Surg Am*. 2011;36(3):510–512.

 SEE ALSO

Algorithm: Pain in Upper Extremity

CODES

ICD10
- M67.40 Ganglion, unspecified site
- M67.48 Ganglion, other site
- M67.439 Ganglion, unspecified wrist

CLINICAL PEARLS

- Ganglion cysts (technically not true cysts) are the most common wrist masses.
- Diagnosis is based on history and physical examination.
- Treatment options include observation, aspiration, and excision. Long-term outcomes are generally similar with all three approaches.
- Volar wrist ganglia should not be aspirated without ultrasound guidance due to the risk of damage to neurovascular structures from blind aspiration.

GASTRITIS
Miles C. Layton, DO • Matthew W. Short, MD, FAAFP

 BASICS

DESCRIPTION
- Inflammation of the gastric mucosa with a spectrum of clinical findings
- Patchy erythema of gastric mucosa
  - Common on endoscopy; usually insignificant
- Erosive gastritis or reactive gastropathy
  - A reaction to mucosal injury by a noxious agent (especially NSAIDs or alcohol)
- Reflux gastritis
  - A reaction to protracted reflux exposure to biliary and pancreatic fluid, usually associated with a pyloric defect
  - Typically limited to the prepyloric antrum
- Hemorrhagic gastritis (stress ulceration)
  - A reaction to hemodynamic disorder (e.g., hypovolemia or hypoxia [as in shock])
  - Common in ICU patients, particularly after severe burns and trauma
  - Seen rarely with dabigatran (oral thrombin inhibitor)
- Infectious gastritis
  - Commonly associated with *Helicobacter pylori*, colonizing organism in much of world's population
  - Viral infection, usually as a component of systemic infection, is common.
  - Significant infection by other microbes is rare.
- Atrophic gastritis
  - Frequent in the elderly
  - Primarily from long-standing *H. pylori* infections
  - May be caused by prolonged PPI use
  - Major risk factor for gastric cancer
  - Associated with primary (pernicious) anemia
  - Autoimmune disease
- Synonym(s): erosive gastritis; reflux gastritis; hemorrhagic gastritis; acute gastritis

Geriatric Considerations
Persons age >60 years often harbor *H. pylori* infection.

Pediatric Considerations
Gastritis rarely occurs in infants or children.

EPIDEMIOLOGY
- Predominant age: all ages
- Predominant sex: male = female

ETIOLOGY AND PATHOPHYSIOLOGY
- Noxious agents cause a breakdown in the gastric mucosal barrier, leaving the epithelial cells unprotected.
- Infection: *H. pylori* (most common cause), *Staphylococcus aureus* exotoxins, and viral infection
- Alcohol
- Aspirin and other NSAIDs
- Bile reflux
- Pancreatic enzyme reflux
- Portal hypertensive (HTN) gastropathy
- Emotional stress

Genetics
Unknown, but observational studies show that 10% of a given population is never colonized with *H. pylori*, regardless of exposure. Genetic variations in *TLR1* may help explain some of this observed variation in individual risk for *H. pylori* infection.

RISK FACTORS
- Age >60 years
- Exposure to potentially noxious drugs or chemicals (e.g., alcohol or NSAIDs)
- Hypovolemia, hypoxia (shock), burns, head injury, complicated postoperative course
- Autoimmune diseases (thyroid disease and diabetes)
- Family history of *H. pylori* and/or gastric cancer
- Stress (hypovolemia or hypoxia)
- Tobacco use
- Radiation
- Ischemia
- Pernicious anemia
- Gastric mucosal atrophy

GENERAL PREVENTION
- Avoid injurious drugs or chemical agents.
- Patients with hypovolemia or hypoxia (especially patients confined to an intensive care ward) should receive prophylactic antacid therapy.
- In ICU patients (particularly burn and trauma), H_2 receptor antagonists, prostaglandins, or sucralfate commonly used for gastric mucosal protection
- Consider testing for *H. pylori* (and eradicating if present) in patients on long-term NSAID therapy.

COMMONLY ASSOCIATED CONDITIONS
- Gastric or duodenal peptic ulcer
- Primary (pernicious) anemia—atrophic gastritis
- Portal HTN, hepatic failure
- Gastric lymphoma linked to lymphoid follicles

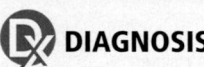 **DIAGNOSIS**

HISTORY
- Nondescript epigastric distress, often aggravated by eating and often severe.
- Burning epigastric pain
- Anorexia
- Nausea, with or without vomiting
- Significant bleeding is unusual except in hemorrhagic gastritis.
- Hiccups
- Bloating or abdominal fullness

PHYSICAL EXAM
- Assess vital signs. Abdominal exam often normal
- Mild epigastric tenderness
- May have heme-positive stool
- Stool may be black in color.
- Examine for stigmata of chronic alcohol abuse.

DIFFERENTIAL DIAGNOSIS
- Functional abdominal pain (dyspepsia)
- Peptic ulcer disease
- Viral gastroenteritis
- Pancreatic disease
- Gastric cancer (elderly)
- Cholecystitis
- Pancreatic disease (inflammation vs. tumor)

DIAGNOSTIC TESTS & INTERPRETATION
Initial Tests (lab, imaging)
- Usually normal
- CBC to evaluate for blood loss/anemia
- ^{13}C-urea breath test for *H. pylori*
  - 95% specifity and sensitivity

- *H. pylori*, serology serum IgG
  - Inexpensive
  - 85% sensitivity, 79% specifity
  - Positive in history of colonization or prior infections, therefore, cannot be used to assess eradication
- Stool analysis for fecal *H. pylori* antigen
  - 95% specifity and sensitivity
- Gastric acid analysis may be abnormal but is not a reliable indicator of gastritis.
- Low serum pepsinogen I (PG I) relative to PG II is associated with fundal intestinal metaplasia.
- Drugs that may alter lab results: Antibiotics or PPIs may affect urea breath test for *H. pylori*.
  - Hold PPIs for 2 weeks, H_2 receptor antagonists for 24 hours, and antibiotics for 4 weeks prior to stool or breath tests (1,2)[C].

Follow-Up Tests & Special Considerations
Endoscopy for *H. pylori*
- Culture; polymerase chain reaction (PCR); histology; rapid urease testing

Diagnostic Procedures/Other
- Gastroscopy with biopsy allows for a precise diagnosis and is a first-line diagnostic tool in:
  - Age >55 years with new-onset signs and symptoms
  - Weight loss, persistent vomiting, or GI bleed (1)[C]
- Biopsies (multiple) in both body and antrum recommended if there is a poor response to the initial treatment (3)[C],(4)[B]. *Patient must discontinue PPIs for 2 weeks prior to endoscopy to improve accuracy of result.*

Test Interpretation
Acute or chronic inflammatory infiltrate in gastric mucosa, often with distortion or erosion of adjacent epithelium. Presence of *H. pylori* often confirmed

 TREATMENT

GENERAL MEASURES
- Treatment of *H. pylori* is required to relieve symptoms.
- Parenteral fluid and electrolyte supplements if oral intake is compromised.
- Consider discontinuing NSAIDs.
- Encourage alcohol and smoking cessation.
- Endoscopy indicated for patients not responsive to treatment

MEDICATION
First Line
- Antacids: best given in liquid form, 30 mL 1 hour after meals and at bedtime; useful mainly as an emollient
- H_2 receptor antagonists (e.g., cimetidine [Tagamet]): oral cimetidine 300 mg q6h (or ranitidine [Zantac] 150 mg BID or famotidine [Pepcid] 20 mg BID or nizatidine [Axid]150 mg BID not shown to be clearly superior to antacids
- Sucralfate (Carafate): 1 g q4–6h on an empty stomach; rationale uncertain but empirically helpful
- Prostaglandins (misoprostol [Cytotec]): can help allay gastric mucosal injury; suggested dosage 100 to 200 μg QID

- PPIs can be used if there is no response to antacids or H₂ receptor blockers (e.g. omeprazole 20 mg daily or BID or esomeprazole 20 mg daily or BID)
- *H. pylori* eradication
  – Clarithromycin triple therapy (CTT)
    ○ A short-course therapy (10 to 14 days) of amoxicillin 1 g BID, standard dose PPI BID (omeprazole 20 mg BID, etc.), and clarithromycin 500 mg BID (1,2,5)[A]
    ○ 70–85% eradication
    ○ Optimal treatment still undefined.
    ○ IF PCN ALLERGIC: Substitute amoxicillin with metronidazole 500 mg BID.
  – Bismuth quadruple therapy (BQT)
    ○ PPI (omeprazole 20 mg) BID plus bismuth (Pepto-Bismol) 30 mL liquid or 2 tablets QID plus metronidazole 250 mg QID plus tetracycline 500 mg QID for 10 to 14 days (1,2,5,6)[A]
    ○ 75–90% eradication
    ○ Use as initial therapy in areas of high clarithromycin resistance (>15%).
    ○ Consider in penicillin-allergic patients.
- *H. pylori* alternative treatment: Consider sequential antibiotic therapy with standard dose PPI (i.e., omeprazole 20 mg) and amoxicillin 1 g BID for 5 days followed by clarithromycin 500 mg and tinidazole 500 mg BID with standard dose PPI (omeprazole 20 mg) BID for 5 days. Some studies show it works just as well or better than triple therapy (1,2)[B],(5)[A].
- *H. pylori* treatment failure: use a different regimen, avoiding clarithromycin (unless resistance testing confirms susceptibility):
  – BQT for 7 to 14 days (1,2,5)[A]
  – Consider levofloxacin 250 mg BID, amoxicillin 1 g BID, and standard dose PPI BID for 14 days in those who fail two attempts (1,2,5)[A].
- Consider probiotics in known symptomatic *H. pylori*, to decrease the density of *H. pylori* in the gastric antrum and body, decrease severity of gastritis, peptic ulcers, and possibly slow the progression toward atrophic gastritis and gastric adenocarcinoma (7)[A],(8)[C],(9)[A].
  – Probiotics alone likely do not eradicate *H. pylori*.
- Contraindications: hypersensitivity
- Precautions:
  – If bismuth is prescribed, warn the patient about the side effect of stool becoming black.
  – Refer to the manufacturer's profile of each drug.
- Significant possible interactions: Refer to the manufacturer's profile of each drug.

INPATIENT CONSIDERATIONS
Gastritis may occur in ICU patients.

Admission Criteria/Initial Stabilization
Outpatient, except for severe hemorrhagic gastritis

ONGOING CARE

FOLLOW-UP RECOMMENDATIONS
Usually no restrictions

- Confirm *H. pylori* eradication in patients with:
  – Gastric ulcer
  – Persistent dyspepsia despite treatment
  – *H. pylori* associated mucosa-associated lymphoid tissue (MALT) lymphoma
  – History of resection of gastric cancer

Patient Monitoring
- Repeat gastroscopy after 6 weeks if gastritis was severe or if patient has a poor treatment response.
- Surveillance gastroscopy every 3 to 5 years in patients with atrophic gastritis in both the antrum and body; within 1 year for patients with low-grade dysplasia, (with extensive biopsy sampling); 6 and 12 months in patients with high-grade dysplasia (4)[B]

DIET
Restrictions, if any, depend on symptom severity (e.g., bland, light, soft foods); avoid caffeine and spicy foods and alcohol.

PATIENT EDUCATION
- Smoking cessation; limit alcohol
- Dietary changes
- Relaxation therapy
- Avoid NSAIDs as possible

PROGNOSIS
- Most cases clear spontaneously when the cause has been identified and treated.
- Recurrence of *H. pylori* infection requires a repeated course of treatment.

COMPLICATIONS
- Bleeding from extensive mucosal erosion or ulceration
- Clearing *H. pylori* before chronic gastritis develops may prevent development of gastric cancer.

REFERENCES

1. McColl KE. Clinical practice. Helicobacter pylori infection. *N Engl J Med*. 2010;362(17):1597–1604.
2. Chey WD, Wong BC; Practice Parameters Committee of the American College of Gastroenterology. American College of Gastroenterology guideline on the management of *Helicobacter pylori* infection. *Am J Gastroenterol*. 2007;102(8):1808–1825.
3. Hirota WK, Zuckerman MJ, Adler DG, et al. ASGE guideline: the role of endoscopy in the surveillance of premalignant conditions of the upper GI tract. *Gastrointest Endosc*. 2006;63(4):570–580.
4. Dinis-Ribeiro M, Areia M, de Vries AC, et al. Management of precancerous conditions and lesions in the stomach (MAPS): guideline from the European Society of Gastrointestinal Endoscopy (ESGE), European Helicobacter Study Group (EHSG), European Society of Pathology (ESP), and the Sociedade Portuguesa de Endoscopia Digestiva (SPED). *Endoscopy*. 2012;44(1):74–94.
5. Malfertheiner P, Megraud F, O'Morain CA, et al. Management of Helicobacter pylori infection—the Maastricht IV/Florence Consensus report. *Gut*. 2012;61(5):646–664.
6. Venerito M, Krieger T, Ecker T, et al. Meta-analysis of bismuth quadruple therapy versus clarithromycin triple therapy for empiric primary treatment of *Helicobacter pylori* infection. *Digestion*. 2013;88(1):33–45.
7. Patel A, Shah N, Prajapati JB. Clinical application of probiotics in the treatment of *Helicobacter pylori* infection—a brief review. *J Microbiol Immunol Infect*. 2014;47(5):429–437.
8. Emara MH, Elhawari SA, Yousef S, et al. Emerging role of probiotics in the management of *Helicobacter pylori* infection: histopathologic perspectives [published online ahead of print May 22, 2015]. *Helicobacter*. 2015:1–8.
9. Ruggiero P. Use of probiotics in the fight against *Helicobacter pylori*. *World J Gastrointest Pathophysiol*. 2014;5(4):384–391.

ADDITIONAL READING

- El-Zimaity H, Serra S, Szentgyorgyi E, et al. Gastric biopsies: the gap between evidence-based medicine and daily practice in the management of gastric *Helicobacter pylori* infection. *Can J Gastroenterol*. 2013;27(10):e25–e30.
- Eslami L, Nasseri-Moghaddam S. Meta-analyses: does long-term PPI use increase the risk of gastric premalignant lesions? *Arch Iran Med*. 2013;16(8):449–458.
- Graham DY, Rimbara E. Understanding and appreciating sequential therapy for *Helicobacter pylori* eradication. *J Clin Gastroenterol*. 2011;45(4):309–313.
- Lanza FL, Chan FK, Quigley EM, et al. Guidelines for prevention of NSAID-related ulcer complications. *Am J Gastroenterol*. 2009;104(3):728–738.

CODES

ICD10
- K29.70 Gastritis, unspecified, without bleeding
- K29.71 Gastritis, unspecified, with bleeding
- K29.00 Acute gastritis without bleeding

CLINICAL PEARLS

- *H. pylori* is the most common cause of gastritis.
- >50% of adult patients are colonized with *H. pylori*.
- *H. pylori* antibodies decline in the year after treatment and should not be used to determine eradication. *H. pylori* antibody titers rise significantly with reinfection.
- *H. pylori* stool antigen tests can be used before and after therapy to assess for eradication and reinfection.
- Several courses of rescue therapy may be necessary to eradicate *H. pylori*.
- Discontinue PPIs 2 weeks prior to endoscopy to improve diagnostic accuracy in cases of suspected gastritis.
- Consider probiotics as adjunct treatment in symptomatic *H. pylori* gastritis.

G

GASTROESOPHAGEAL REFLUX DISEASE

Anna Cecilia S. Tenorio, MD • Fozia Akhtar Ali, MD

 BASICS

DESCRIPTION
Backward flow of stomach acid or contents into the mouth or esophagus that occurs for twice a week for several weeks, causing symptoms of discomfort often described as heartburn, acid indigestion, and acid reflux

EPIDEMIOLOGY
Incidence
Incidence: 5 per 1,000 person-years

Prevalence
- Prevalence of gastroesophageal reflux disease (GERD) is about 10–20% in the United States and United Kingdom, and in Asia is about 5%.
- 40% of adults in the United States have symptoms of reflux.
- 50–85% of GERD patients have nonerosive reflux disease
- Chronic GERD is a risk factor for Barrett esophagus.
- 10% of patients with chronic GERD have Barrett esophagus.
- Risk of adenocarcinoma without Barrett esophagus and no dysplasia: 0.1–0.5% per patient year
- Risk of adenocarcinoma with Barrett esophagus and high–grade dysplasia: 6–19% per patient-year
- Pediatric population: Regurgitation occurs at least once a day in 67% of 4-month-old infants. Prevalence decreased to 21% at age 6 to 7 months, and down to 5% at age 10 to 12 months.

ETIOLOGY AND PATHOPHYSIOLOGY
- The pattern and mechanism of reflux varies depends on the severity of disease.
- GERD begins with contact of acidic stomach contents with the squamous mucosal lining of the esophagus, at the esophagogastric junction (EGJ).
- Usually affected by inappropriate transient lower esophageal sphincter relaxation. Foods that are spicy, acidic and high in fat, caffeine, alcohol, tobacco, anticholinergic medications, nitrates, smooth muscle relaxants affect LES relaxation.
- Most people with severe GERD have some evidence of hiatal hernia, which affects GERD by (1):
  - Trapping acid in the hernia sac
  - Impaired acid emptying
  - Increasing retrograde acid flow rate
  - Reducing the EGJ sphincter pressure
  - Increased frequency of transient lower esophageal sphincter relaxations

Genetics
Genetic heterogeneity has been associated with GERD.

RISK FACTORS
- Obesity
- Hiatal hernia
- Scleroderma
- Alcohol use
- Tobacco use
- Pregnancy

GENERAL PREVENTION
- Decrease consumption of food and beverage triggers such as spicy, fatty foods, alcohol and caffeine
- Weight loss
- Avoid lying down soon after eating a meal.
- Tobacco and alcohol cessation
- Elevated head of bed when sleeping at night
- Avoid having meals close to bedtime.

- Infants: Use car seat for 2 to 3 hours after meals; thickened feedings

COMMONLY ASSOCIATED CONDITIONS
- Nonerosive esophagitis
- Erosive esophagitis
- Irritable bowel syndrome
- Peptic ulcer disease
- Extraesophageal reflux: aspiration, chronic cough, laryngitis, vocal cord granuloma, sinusitis, otitis media
- Halitosis
- Hiatal hernia: acid pocket (zone of high acidity in the proximal stomach after a meal) above the diaphragm in patients with hiatal hernia is a risk factor (2)[B]
- Peptic stricture: 10% of patients with GERD
- Barrett esophagus
- Esophageal adenocarcinoma

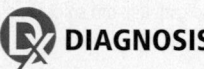 **DIAGNOSIS**

- Typical symptoms: acid regurgitation, heartburn, dysphagia (mostly post prandial)
- Atypical symptoms: epigastric fullness/pressure/pain, dyspepsia, nausea, bloating, belching, chest pain, lump in throat
- Extraesophageal signs and symptoms: chronic cough, bronchospasm, wheezing, hoarseness, sore throat, asthma, laryngitis, dental erosions

HISTORY
- Heartburn: retrosternal burning sensation
- Regurgitation; sour or acid taste in mouth ("water brash")
- Symptoms worse with bending or recumbency
- Extraesophageal symptoms (cough; wheezing; hoarseness)
- Diet, alcohol and tobacco use
- Diagnosis often solely based on history and clinical symptoms

PHYSICAL EXAM
Typically unremarkable
- BMI
- Rare epigastric tenderness or palpable epigastric mass
- Look for stigmata of chronic systemic disease or alcohol use.

DIFFERENTIAL DIAGNOSIS
- Infectious esophagitis (*Candida*, herpes, HIV, cytomegalovirus)
- Chemical esophagitis
- Pill-induced esophagitis
- Eosinophilic esophagitis
- Nonulcer dyspepsia
- Biliary tract disease
- Radiation injury
- Crohn disease
- Angina/coronary artery disease
- Esophageal stricture or anatomic defect (ring, sling)
- Esophageal adenocarcinoma
- Achalasia
- Scleroderma
- Peptic ulcer disease

DIAGNOSTIC TESTS & INTERPRETATION
Patients with typical symptoms of GERD and without alarm symptoms (dysphagia odynophagia, weight loss, early satiety, anemia, new onset, male >50 years)

should be initially treated empirically with antisecretory agents without any further diagnostic testing.

Initial Tests (lab, imaging)
- Indication for blood work depends on clinical presentation. Check for anemia (history of bleeding; or possible poor B_{12} absorption due to chronic proton pump inhibitor [PPI] use).
- Patients with GERD presenting with noncardiac chest pain should undergo evaluation first before the onset of treatment.

Diagnostic Procedures/Other
- Upper endoscopy
  - First-line diagnostic test for those with alarm signs and uncontrolled symptoms (2)[B]
  - Indications for UGI endoscopy
    - Alarm symptoms such as dysphagia, bleeding, anemia, weight loss, recurrent vomiting
    - Persistent typical GERD symptoms despite empiric treatment of twice-daily PPI for 4 to 8 weeks
    - Men >50 years old with chronic GERD (>5 years) and other risk factors: hiatal hernia, high BMI, tobacco use, high abdominal fat distribution
    - History of severed erosive esophagitis to assess healing and check for Barrett esophagus and other UGI pathology
    - Surveillance in patients with history of Barrett's esophagus
  - ~50–70% of patients with heartburn have negative endoscopy findings
- Savary-Miller classification
  - Grades esophagitis based on endoscopy
    - Grade I: ≥1 nonconfluent reddish spots, with or without exudate
    - Grade II: erosive and exudative lesions in the distal esophagus; may be confluent but not circumferential
    - Grade III: circumferential erosions in the distal esophagus
    - Grade IV: chronic complications such as deep ulcers, stenosis, or scarring with Barrett metaplasia
- Esophageal manometry
  - Not recommended for primary GERD diagnosis; a second option for those with GERD and normal endoscopy (2)[B]
  - Diagnose motility disorders: functional heartburn, achalasia, and distal esophageal spasm.
  - Used to evaluate peristaltic function preoperatively and to record LES pressure
- Ambulatory reflux (ph) monitoring
  - Used to evaluate possible excessive esophageal acid exposure to those with GERD, normal endoscopy and no PPI response (2)[B]
  - Used also to document frequency of reflux
  - Need to discontinue PPI use for 7 days prior to procedure
- Barium swallow: not used for GERD diagnosis. Used to evaluate complaints of dysphagia to outline anatomic abnormalities (hiatal hernia)

Test Interpretation
- Acute inflammation (especially eosinophils)
- Epithelial basal zone hyperplasia seen in 85%
- Barrett epithelial change: Gastric columnar epithelium replaces squamous epithelium in distal esophagus (metaplasia).

TREATMENT

GENERAL MEASURES
Lifestyle changes are first-line intervention:

- Elevate head of bed (2)[B].
- Avoid meals 2 to 3 hours before bedtime (2)[B].
- Avoid stooping, bending and tight-fitting garments.
- Avoid medications that relax LES (anticholinergic drugs; calcium channel blockers).
- Weight loss (2)[B]
- Tobacco cessation and alcohol avoidance
- Limit consumption of patient-specific food triggers (global elimination of all reflux-causing foods is not necessary or beneficial).
- Stepped therapy
  - Phase I: lifestyle and diet modifications, antacids plus H$_2$ blockers or PPIs
  - Phase II: If symptoms persist, consider endoscopic evaluation.
  - Phase III: If symptoms still persist, consider surgical options.

MEDICATION
First Line
- H$_2$ blockers in equipotent oral doses (e.g., cimetidine 800 mg BID or 400 mg QID, ranitidine 150 mg BID, famotidine 20 mg BID, or nizatidine 150 mg BID)
  - Renally dosed
- PPIs: Irreversibly bind proton pump (H$^+$/K$^+$ ATPase), effective onset within 4 days. Omeprazole 20 to 40 mg/day, lansoprazole 15 to 30 mg/day, dexlansoprazole 30 mg/day, pantoprazole 40 mg/day, rabeprazole 20 mg/day, esomeprazole 40 mg/day
  - No major differences in efficacy among PPIs (3)[A]
  - Dose 30 to 60 minutes before meals with the exception of dexlansoprazole (2)[A].
  - PPIs may increase risk of hypomagnesemia, hip fracture, *Clostridium difficile* infection, vitamin B$_{12}$ deficiency, and community acquired pneumonia.
- PPI is more effective than H$_2$ blocker and prokinetics for healing erosive esophagitis and nonerosive esophagitis (4)[A].
- Erosive esophagitis: 8 weeks of PPI effective in 90%

Pediatric Considerations
Antacids or liquid H$_2$ blockers and PPIs are available. Prokinetics have a minimal role due to safety concerns and limited efficacy.

Second Line
- Antacids or barrier agents (sucralfate 1 g PO QID 1 hour before meals and at bedtime for 4 to 8 weeks) may relieve breakthrough symptoms.
- Prokinetics: metoclopramide 5 to 10 mg before meals
- Baclofen as add-on therapy with a PPI
- Precautions
  - Blood dyscrasias and anemia with PPIs and H$_2$ blockers
  - Metoclopramide is a dopamine blocker; risk of dystonia and tardive dyskinesia
  - Tachyphylaxis may occur with H$_2$ blockers.
- Significant possible interactions
  - PPIs and H$_2$ blockers: multiple cytochrome P450 drug interactions; that is, warfarin, phenytoin, antifungals, digoxin

SURGERY/OTHER PROCEDURES
- Laparoscopic fundoplication (wrapping gastric fundus around distal esophagus) increases pressure gradient between stomach and esophagus.

- Bariatric surgery
  - Surgery indicated if : Patient desires to discontinue medical therapy, has side effects with medical therapy, large hiatal hernia, esophagitis refractory to medical therapy, or refractory symptoms (4)[A].
  - Pre-op ambulatory pH monitor is mandatory in patients without evidence of erosive esophagitis (4)[A].
  - Rule out esophageal dysmotility prior to surgery by manometry to rule out achalasia or scleroderma like esophagus (4)[A].
  - Best surgical response is seen in patients with typical symptoms who respond well to PPI therapy.
  - If it is estimated that a patient will require >10 years of PPI treatment, surgery may be more cost-effective.
  - Bariatric surgery can be considered for patients with comorbid obesity. Gastric bypass is preferred (4)[A].

Pediatric Considerations
Surgery for severe symptoms (apnea, choking, persistent vomiting)

ONGOING CARE

FOLLOW-UP RECOMMENDATIONS
Patient Monitoring
- Monitor and follow symptoms over time.
- Repeat endoscopy at 4 to 8 weeks if there is a poor symptomatic response to medical therapy, especially in older patients.
- Endoscopic surveillance every 2 to 3 years in patients with Barrett esophagus to screen for malignant transformation (in patients who would opt for treatment if cancer is detected)

DIET
Avoid foods that can trigger or make symptoms worse.

PATIENT EDUCATION
Lifestyle and dietary modifications: Eat small meals; avoid lying down soon after meals; elevate head of bed; weight loss; smoking cessation; avoid alcohol and caffeine.

PROGNOSIS
- Symptoms and esophageal inflammation often return promptly when treatment is withdrawn. To prevent relapse of symptoms, continue antisecretory therapy (in addition to lifestyle and dietary modifications).
  - PPI maintenance therapy likely improves quality of life better than H$_2$ blocker maintenance.
  - Full-dose PPIs are more effective than half-dose for maintenance (4)[A].
  - In erosive esophagitis, daily maintenance therapy with PPI prevents relapse; intermittent PPI therapy not as effective (2)[A]
- Medical and surgical therapy are equally effective for symptom reduction (4)[A].
- Antireflux surgery
  - 90–94% symptom response. Patients with persistent symptoms should have repeat anatomic evaluation (endoscopy or esophagram).
  - Some surgically treated patients eventually require medical therapy.
- Regression of Barrett epithelium does not routinely occur despite aggressive medical or surgical therapy.

COMPLICATIONS
- Peptic stricture: 10–15%
- Barrett esophagus: 10%
  - Adenocarcinoma cancer develops at an annual rate of 0.5%.

- Primary treatment for Barrett esophagus with high-grade dysplasia is endoscopic radiofrequency ablation.
- Extraesophageal symptoms: hoarseness, aspiration (including pneumonia)
- Bleeding due to mucosal injury
- Noncardiac chest pain

Geriatric Considerations
Complications more likely (e.g., aspiration pneumonia)

REFERENCES

1. Lee YY, McColl KE. Pathophysiology of gastroesophageal reflux disease. *Best Pract Res Clin Gastroenterol*. 2013;27(3):339–351.
2. Kahrilas PJ, Shaheen NJ, Vaezi MF, et al. American Gastroenterological Association medical position statement on the management of gastroesophageal reflux disease. *Gastroenterology*. 2008;135(4):1383. e5–1391.e5.
3. Agency for Healthcare Research and Quality. Comparing effectiveness of management strategies for gastroesophageal reflux disease. An update to the 2005 report. http://effectivehealthcare.ahrq.gov/index.cfm/search-for-guides-reviews-and-reports/?productid=781&pageaction=displayproduct/. Accessed 2015.
4. Katz PO, Gerson LB, Vela MF. Guidelines for the diagnosis and management of gastroesophageal reflux disease. *Am J Gastroenterol*. 2013;108(10):308–328.

ADDITIONAL READING

- Anderson WD III, Strayer SM, Mull SR. Common questions about the management of gastroesophageal reflux disease. *Am Fam Physician*. 2015;91(10):692–697.
- Campanozzi A, Boccia G, Pensabene L, et al. Prevalence and natural history of gastroesophageal reflux: a pediatric prospective survey. *Pediatrics*. 2009;123(3):779–783.
- El-Serag HB, Sweet S, Winchester CC, et al. Update on the epidemiology of gastro-oesophageal reflux disease: a systematic review. *Gut*. 2014;63(6):871–880.

SEE ALSO

Algorithms: Abdominal Pain, Upper; Dyspepsia

CODES

ICD10
- K21.9 Gastro-esophageal reflux disease without esophagitis
- K21.0 Gastro-esophageal reflux disease with esophagitis

CLINICAL PEARLS

- GERD is primarily diagnosed by history.
- GERD should be considered in nonsmokers who have chronic cough (>3 weeks).
- PPI treatment does not appear to inhibit neoplastic progression in Barrett esophagus.
- No evidence to support that patients with GERD should routinely be tested for *Helicobacter pylori*.
- Empiric treatment with H$_2$ blockers or PPI leads to symptomatic relief in most cases. Persistent symptoms should be evaluated with endoscopy.

G

GENITO-PELVIC PAIN/PENETRATION DISORDER (VAGINISMUS)

Jeffrey D. Quinlan, MD, FAAFP

 BASICS

Genito-pelvic pain/penetration disorder is the name of the conditions formally known as vaginismus and dyspareunia. Vaginismus results from involuntary contraction of the vaginal musculature. Primary vaginismus occurs in women who have never been able to have penetrative intercourse. Women with secondary vaginismus were previously able to have penetrative intercourse but are no longer able to do so.

DESCRIPTION
- Persistent or recurrent difficulties for 6 months or more with at least one of the following:
  - Inability to have vaginal intercourse/penetration on at least 50% of attempts
  - Marked genito-pelvic pain during at least 50% of vaginal intercourse/penetration attempts
  - Marked fear of vaginal intercourse/penetration or of genito-pelvic pain during intercourse/penetration on at least 50% of vaginal intercourse/penetration attempts
  - Marked tensing or tightening of the pelvic floor muscles during attempted vaginal intercourse/penetration on at least 50% of occasions
- The disturbance causes marked distress or interpersonal difficulty.
- Dysfunction is not as a result of:
  - Nonsexual mental disorder
  - Severe relationship stress
  - Other significant stress
  - Substance or medication effect
- Specify if with a general medical condition (e.g., lichen sclerosis, endometriosis) (1).

Pregnancy Considerations
- May first present during evaluation for infertility
- Pregnancy can occur in patients with genito-pelvic pain/penetration disorder when ejaculation occurs on the perineum.
- Vaginismus may be an independent risk factor for cesarean delivery.

EPIDEMIOLOGY
Incidence
The incidence of vaginismus is thought to be about 1–17% per year worldwide. In North America, 12–21% of women have genito-pelvic pain of varying etiologies (2).

Prevalence
- True prevalence is unknown due to limited data/reporting.
- Population-based studies report prevalence rates of 0.5–30%.
- Affects women in all age groups.
- Approximately 15% of women in North America report recurrent pain during intercourse.

ETIOLOGY AND PATHOPHYSIOLOGY
Most often multifactorial in both primary and secondary vaginismus
- Primary
  - Psychological and psychosocial issues
    - Negative messages about sex and sexual relations in upbringing may cause phobic reaction.
    - Poor body image and limited understanding of genital area
    - History of sexual trauma
  - Abnormalities of the hymen
  - History of difficult gynecologic examination
- Secondary
  - Often situational
  - Often associated with dyspareunia secondary to:
    - Vaginal infection
    - Inflammatory dermatitis
    - Surgical or postdelivery scarring
    - Endometriosis
    - Inadequate vaginal lubrication
    - Pelvic radiation
    - Estrogen deficiency
  - Conditioned response to pain from physical issues previously listed

RISK FACTORS
- Most often idiopathic
- Although the exact role in the condition is unclear, many women report a history of abuse or sexual trauma.
- Often associated with other sexual dysfunctions

COMMONLY ASSOCIATED CONDITIONS
- Marital stress, family dysfunction
- Anxiety
- Vulvodynia/vestibulodynia

 DIAGNOSIS

DSM-5 has combined vaginismus and dyspareunia in a condition called genito-pelvic pain/penetration disorder.

HISTORY
- Complete medical history
- Full psychosocial and sexual history, including the following:
  - Onset of symptoms (primary or secondary)
  - If secondary, precipitating events, if any
  - Relationship difficulty/partner violence
  - Inability to allow vaginal entry for different purposes
    - Sexual (penis, digit, object)
    - Hygiene (tampon use)
    - Health care (pelvic examination)
  - Infertility
  - Traumatic experiences (exam, sexual, etc.)
  - Religious beliefs
  - Views on sexuality

PHYSICAL EXAM
- Pelvic examination is necessary to exclude structural abnormalities or organic pathology.
- Educating the patient about the examination and giving her control over the progression of the examination is essential, as genital/pelvic examination may induce varying degrees of anxiety in patients.
- Referral to a gynecologist, family physician, or other provider specializing in the treatment of sexual disorders may be appropriate.
- Contraction of pelvic floor musculature in anticipation of examination may be seen.
- Lamont classification system aids in the assessment of severity
  - First degree: Perineal and levator spasm relieved with reassurance.
  - Second degree: Perineal spasm maintained throughout the pelvic exam.
  - Third degree: levator spasm and elevation of buttocks
  - Fourth degree: levator and perineal spasm and elevation with adduction and retreat

DIFFERENTIAL DIAGNOSIS
- Vaginal infection
- Vulvodynia/vestibulodynia
- Vulvovaginal atrophy
- Urogenital structural abnormalities
- Interstitial cystitis
- Endometriosis

DIAGNOSTIC TESTS & INTERPRETATION
No laboratory tests indicated unless signs of vaginal infection are noted on examination. When diagnosing of this disorder has been conducted, five factors should be considered.
- Partner factors
- Relationship factors
- Individual vulnerability factors
- Cultural/religious factors
- Medical factors

Test Interpretation
Not available; may be needed to check for secondary causes

 TREATMENT

- Genito-pelvic pain penetration disorder may be successfully treated (2)[B].
- Outpatient care is appropriate.
- Treatment of physical conditions, if present, is first line (see "Secondary" under "Etiology and Pathophysiology").
- Role for pelvic floor physical therapy and myofascial release

- Some evidence suggests that cognitive-behavioral therapy may be effective, including desensitization techniques, such as gradual exposure, aimed at decreasing avoidance behavior and fear of vaginal penetration (3)[A].
- Based on a Cochrane review, a clinically relevant effect of systematic desensitization cannot be ruled out (4)[A].
- Evidence suggests that Masters and Johnson sex therapy may be effective (5)[B].
  - Involves Kegel exercises to increase control over perineal muscles
  - Stepwise vaginal desensitization exercises
    ○ With vaginal dilators that the patient inserts and controls
    ○ With woman's own finger(s) to promote sexual self-awareness
    ○ Advancement to partner's fingers with patient's control
    ○ Coitus after achieving largest vaginal dilator or three fingers; important to begin with sensate-focused exercises/sensual caressing without necessarily a demand for coitus
    ○ Female superior at first; passive (nonthrusting); female-directed
    ○ Later, thrusting may be allowed.
- Topical anesthetic or anxiolytic with desensitization exercises may be considered.
- Patient education is an essential component of treatment (see "Patient Education" section).

MEDICATION

- Antidepressants and anticonvulsants have been used with limited success. Low-dose tricyclic antidepressant (amitriptyline 10 mg) may be initiated and titrated as tolerated (6)[B].
- Topical anesthetics or anxiolytics may be utilized in combination with either cognitive-behavioral therapy or desensitization exercises as noted above (4)[B].
- Botulinum neurotoxin type A injections may improve vaginismus in patients who do not respond to standard cognitive-behavioral and medical treatment for vaginismus.
  - Dosage: 20, 50, and 100 to 400 U of botulinum toxin type A injected in the levator ani muscle have been shown to improve vaginismus (4)[B].
- Intravaginal botulinum neurotoxin type A injection (100 to 150 U) followed by bupivacaine 0.25% with epinephrine 1:400,000 intravaginal injection (20 to 30 mL) while the patient is anesthetized may facilitate progressive placement of dilators and ultimately resolution of symptoms (7)[B].

ISSUES FOR REFERRAL
For diagnosis and treatment recommendations, the following resources may be consulted:
- Obstetrics/gynecology
- Pelvic floor physical therapy
- Psychiatry
- Sex therapy
- Hypnotherapy

SURGERY/OTHER PROCEDURES
Contraindicated

COMPLEMENTARY & ALTERNATIVE MEDICINE
- Biofeedback
- Functional electrical stimulation

 ONGOING CARE

FOLLOW-UP RECOMMENDATIONS
Desensitization techniques of gentle, progressive, patient-controlled vaginal dilation

Patient Monitoring
General preventive health care

DIET
No special diet

PATIENT EDUCATION
- Education about pelvic anatomy, nature of vaginal spasms, normal adult sexual function
- Handheld mirror can help the woman to learn visually to tighten and loosen perineal muscles.
- Important to teach the partner that spasms are not under conscious control and are not a reflection on the relationship or a woman's feelings about her partner
- Instruction in techniques for vaginal dilation
- Resources
  - American College of Obstetricians & Gynecologists (ACOG), 409 12th St., SW, Washington, DC 20024-2188; 800-762-ACOG. http://www.acog.org/
  - Valins L. When a Woman's Body Says No to Sex: Understanding and Overcoming Vaginismus. New York, NY: Penguin; 1992.

PROGNOSIS
Favorable, with early recognition of the condition and initiation of treatment

REFERENCES
1. American Psychiatric Association. *Diagnostic Statistical Manual of Mental Disorders*. 5th ed. Arlington, VA: American Psychiatric Association; 2013.
2. Landry T, Bergeron S. How young does vulvo-vaginal pain begin? Prevalence and characteristics of dyspareunia in adolescents. *J Sex Med*. 2009;6(4):927–935.
3. ter Kuile MM, Both S, van Lankveld JJ. Cognitive behavioral therapy for sexual dysfunctions in women. *Psychiatr Clin North Am*. 2010;33(3):595–610.
4. Melnik T, Hawton K, McGuire H. Interventions for vaginismus. *Cochrane Database Syst Rev*. 2012;(12):CD001760.
5. Pereira VM, Arias-Carrión O, Machado S, et al. Sex therapy for female sex dysfunction. *Int Arc Med*. 2013;6(1):37.
6. Crowley T, Goldmeier D, Hiller J. Diagnosing and managing vaginismus. *BMJ*. 2009;338:b2284.
7. Pacik PT. Vaginismus: review of current concepts and treatment using botox injections, bupivacaine injections, and progressive dilation with the patient under anesthesia. *Aesthetic Plast Surg*. 2011;35(6):1160–1164.

ADDITIONAL READING
- Basson R, Wierman ME, van Lankveld J, et al. Summary of the recommendations on sexual dysfunctions in women. *J Sex Med*. 2010;7(1, Pt 2):314–326.
- Jeng CJ, Wang LR, Chou CS, et al. Management and outcome of primary vaginismus. *J Sex Marital Ther*. 2006;32(5):379–387.
- Pacik PT. Understanding and treating vaginismus: a multimodal approach. *Int Urogynecol J*. 2014;25(12):1613–1620.
- Reissing ED, Binik YM, Khalifé S, et al. Etiological correlates of vaginismus: sexual and physical abuse, sexual knowledge, sexual self-schema, and relationship adjustment. *J Sex Marital Ther*. 2003;29(1):47–59.
- Simons JS, Carey MP. Prevalence of sexual dysfunctions: results from a decade of research. *Arch Sex Behav*. 2001;30(2):177–219.
- ter Kuile MM, van Lankveld JJ, de Groot E, et al. Cognitive-behavioral therapy for women with lifelong vaginismus: process and prognostic factors. *Behav Res Ther*. 2007;45(2):359–373.

 SEE ALSO

Dyspareunia; Sexual Dysfunction in Women

 CODES

ICD10
- N94.2 Vaginismus
- N94.1 Dyspareunia

CLINICAL PEARLS
- In a patient with suspected genito-pelvic pain penetration disorder, a complete medical history, including a comprehensive psychosocial and sexual history and a patient-centric, patient-controlled educational pelvic exam should be conducted.
- This condition can be treated effectively.
- Cognitive-behavioral therapy may be effective for the treatment of this condition.
- Botox injection therapy is in the experimental stages but looks promising for the treatment of vaginismus. Bupivacaine and dilation under general anesthesia has also been tried as a treatment for vaginismus.

G

GIARDIASIS

Iryna Matkovska, DO • Deborah Pierce, DO • Merle A. Carter, MD, FACEP

BASICS

DESCRIPTION
- Intestinal infection caused by the protozoan parasite *Giardia lamblia*:
  - *G. lamblia* is also called *Giardia duodenalis* and *Giardia intestinalis*.
- Infection results from ingestion of cysts, which transform into trophozoites:
  - Trophozoites colonize the small intestine and cause symptoms.
  - Cycle is continued when the trophozoites encyst in the small intestine and are subsequently transmitted through water, food, or hands contaminated by feces of infected person.
- Most infections result from fecal–oral transmission or ingestion of contaminated water (e.g., swimming).
- Less commonly, giardiasis is the result of contaminated food.

EPIDEMIOLOGY
- Predominant age:
  - All ages but most common in early childhood ages 1 to 9 years and adults 35 to 44 years
- Predominant gender:
  - Male > female (slightly)
- Minimal seasonal variability; slight increase in summer

Pediatric Considerations
Most common in early childhood

Prevalence
- 5% of patients with stools submitted for ova and parasite exams
- >19,000 cases/year in reportable U.S. states:
  - *Giardia* is not reportable in Indiana, Kentucky, Mississippi, North Carolina, and Texas.

ETIOLOGY AND PATHOPHYSIOLOGY
Giardia trophozoites colonize the surface of the proximal small intestine: The mechanism of diarrhea is unknown.

Genetics
No known genetic risk factors

RISK FACTORS
- Daycare centers
- Anal intercourse
- Wilderness camping
- Travel to developing countries
- Children adopted from developing countries
- Public swimming pools
- Pets with Gardia infection/diarrhea

GENERAL PREVENTION
- Hand hygiene
- Water purification when camping and when traveling to developing countries
- Properly cook all foods.

COMMONLY ASSOCIATED CONDITIONS
Hypogammaglobulinemia and possibly IgA deficiency: diarrhea more severe and prolonged in these patients

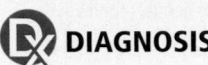

DIAGNOSIS

HISTORY
- 25–50% of infected persons are symptomatic.
- Symptoms usually appear 1 to 2 weeks after exposure.
- Chronic diarrhea (can last for weeks)
- Abdominal bloating
- Flatulence
- Loose, greasy, foul-smelling stools that tend to float
- Weight loss
- Nausea
- Lactose intolerance

PHYSICAL EXAM
- Typically normal vital signs
- Nonspecific; abdominal exam; may have bloating tenderness or increased bowel sounds

DIFFERENTIAL DIAGNOSIS
- Cryptosporidiosis, isosporiasis, cyclosporiasis
- Other causes of malabsorption include celiac sprue, tropical sprue, bacterial overgrowth syndromes, and Crohn ileitis.
- Irritable bowel (diarrhea without weight loss)

DIAGNOSTIC TESTS & INTERPRETATION
Initial Tests (lab, imaging)
- Stool for ova and parasites:
  - Repeat 3 times on separate days
  - Cysts in fixed or fresh stools, and occasionally, trophozoites are found in fresh diarrheal stools.
- Limitations: experienced operator, intermittent shedding of ova may not be present in stool sample, labor intensive

  - ELISA: sensitivity and specificity of 100% and 91.5% respectively (compared to 50–70% sensitivity using microscopy) (1)[B].

- Polymerase chain reaction (PCR) techniques are more sensitive than microscopy but have not been widely adopted due to high cost.

- Rapid detection tests have been studied showing high detection rates not widely available (2)[B].

Follow-Up Tests & Special Considerations
String test (Entero-test):
- A gelatin capsule on a string is swallowed and left in the duodenum for several hours or overnight. The string is removed and visualized microscopically.

Diagnostic Procedures/Other
Esophagogastroduodenoscopy (EGD) with biopsy and sample of small intestinal fluid

Test Interpretation
Intestinal biopsy shows flattened, mild lymphocytic infiltration and trophozoites on the surface.

TREATMENT

Outpatient for mild cases; inpatient if symptoms are severe enough to cause dehydration warranting parenteral fluid replacement

GENERAL MEASURES
- Medical therapy for all infected individuals
- Fluid replacement if dehydrated

MEDICATION
First Line
- Metronidazole (Flagyl): 250 mg PO TID for 5 to 7 days (2)[B]
- Tinidazole: 2 g PO single dose (50 mg/kg up to 2 g for children)
- Albendazole: 400 mg/day PO for 5 days:
  - Albendazole has comparable effectiveness to metronidazole with fewer side effects and lower cost.
- Precautions:
  - Theoretical risk of carcinogenesis with metronidazole
- Significant possible interactions: occasional disulfiram reaction with metronidazole or tinidazole

Pregnancy Considerations
Medications to treat giardiasis are relatively contraindicated during pregnancy; consider appropriate consultation with infectious disease or maternal–fetal medicine specialist.

Pediatric Considerations
In one study, administration of vitamin A reduced prevalence of *G. lamblia* (3)[A].

Second Line

- Furazolidone: 8 mg/kg/day TID for 10 days (slightly less effective but commonly used in pediatrics because it is well tolerated); not available in United States
- Paromomycin (Humatin): a nonabsorbable aminoglycoside that is probably less effective but commonly recommended in pregnancy because of lower risk of teratogenicity
- Quinacrine: 100 mg TID for 5 to 7 days; withdrawn from the U.S. market
- Nitazoxanide suspension was approved by the FDA in 2003 for treatment of giardiasis in children 1 to 11 years. Children aged 1 to 4 years receive 100 mg BID and age 5 to 11 years receive 200 mg BID for 3 days.
- Two other nitroimidazole antibiotics, ornidazole and secnidazole, are effective against *Giardia* but are not available in the United States.

ADDITIONAL THERAPIES

- There have been anecdotal reports of herbal products containing *Mentha crispa* being effective in the treatment of *Giardia*. When studied, it was much less effective than secnidazole (a metronidazole analog).
- A recent study showed tetrahydrolipstatin (Orlistat) had activity against *Giardia* (may be a potential treatment option in the future for patients who are resistant to metronidazole) (4)[C].
- In mouse studies, auranofin, miltefosine, disulfiram, and omeprazole have all shown effective activity against *G. lamblia*. Research is still needed in humans (5–8)[C].

 ONGOING CARE

FOLLOW-UP RECOMMENDATIONS
Patient Monitoring
Symptoms, weight, stool exams if patients fail to improve

DIET
Low lactose, low fat, monitor for dehydration

PATIENT EDUCATION

- Hand washing may be more important than water purification to prevent transmission in outdoor enthusiasts.
- Lactose intolerance may follow *Giardia* infection and cause of persistent diarrhea posttreatment. Consider low-lactose diet.
- CDC Facts about *Giardia* and Swimming Pools: http://www.cdc.gov/healthywater/pdf/swimming/resources/giardia-factsheet.pdf
  – Don't swim if you have diarrhea.
  – Wash hands with soap after changing diapers before returning to the pool.

  – Do not ingest pool, lake, or river water.
  – Use chlorine to kill *Gardia* in water used for recreational activities.

PROGNOSIS
- Untreated giardiasis lasts for weeks.
- Most (90%) patients respond to treatment within a few days:
  – Most nonresponders or relapses respond to a second course with the same or a different agent.

COMPLICATIONS
Malabsorption, reactive arthritis, and weight loss, lactose intolerance

ALERT
Notifiable disease

REFERENCES

1. Jahan N, Khatoon R, Ahmad S. A comparison of microscopy and enzyme linked immunosorbent assay for diagnosis of *Giardia lamblia* in human faecal specimens. *J Clin Diagn Res*. 2014;8(11): DC04–DC06.
2. Van den Bossche D, Cnops L, Verschueren J, et al. Comparison of four rapid diagnostic tests, ELISA, microscopy and PCR for the detection of *Giardia lamblia*, *Cryptosporidium* spp. and *Entamoeba histolytica* in feces. *J Microbiol Methods*. 2015; 110:78–84.
3. Lima AA, Soares AM, Lima NL, et al. Effects of vitamin A supplementation on intestinal barrier function, growth, total parasitic, and specific *Giardia* spp infections in Brazilian children: a prospective randomized, double-blind, placebo-controlled trial. *J Pediatr Gastroenterol Nutr*. 2010;50(3):309–315.
4. Hahn J, Seeber F, Kolodziej H, et al. High sensitivity of *Giardia duodenalis* to tetrahydolipstatin (orlistat) in vitro. *PLoS One*. 2013;8(8):e71597.
5. Tejman-Yarden N, Miyamoto Y, Leitsch D, et al. A reprofiled drug, auranofin, is effective against metronidazole-resistant *Giardia lamblia*. *Antimicrob Agents Chemother*. 2013;57(5):2029–2035.
6. Eissa MM, Amer EI. *Giardia lamblia*: a new target for miltefosine. *Int J Parasitol*. 2012;42(5):443–452.
7. Galkin A, Kulakova L, Lim K, et al. Structural basis for inactivation of *Giardia lamblia* carbamate kinase by disulfiram. *J Biol Chem*. 2014;289(15): 10502–10509.
8. Reyes-Vivas H, de la Mora-de la Mora I, Castillo-Villanueva A, et al. Giardial triosephosphate isomerase as possible target of the cytotoxic effect of omeprazole in *Giardia lamblia*. *Antimicrob Agents Chemother*. 2014;58(12):7072–7082.

ADDITIONAL READING

- Almirall P, Escobedo AA, Ayala I, et al. Mebendazole compared with secnidazole in the treatment of adult giardiasis: a randomised, no-inferiority, open clinical trial. *J Parasitol Res*. 2011;2011:636857.
- Cañete R, Rodríguez P, Mesa L, et al. Albendazole versus metronidazole in the treatment of adult giardiasis: a randomized, double-blind, clinical trial. *Curr Med Res Opin*. 2012;28(1):149–154.
- Lal A, Hales S, French N, et al. Seasonality in human zoonotic enteric diseases: a systematic review. *PLoS One*. 2012;7(4):e31883.
- Solaymani-Mohammadi S, Genkinger JM, Loffredo CA, et al. A meta-analysis of the effectiveness of albendazole compared with metronidazole as treatments for infections with *Giardia duodenalis*. *PLoS Negl Trop Dis*. 2010;4(5):e682.
- Teles NS, Fechine FV, Viana FA, et al. Evaluation of the therapeutic efficacy of *Mentha crispa* in the treatment of giardiasis. *Contemp Clin Trials*. 2011; 32(6):809–813.
- Yoder JS, Harral C, Beach MJ. Giardiasis surveillance— United States, 2006–2008. *MMWR Surveill Summ*. 2010;59(6):15–25.

 SEE ALSO

Algorithm: Diarrhea, Chronic

 CODES

ICD10
A07.1 Giardiasis [lambliasis]

CLINICAL PEARLS

- Daycare facilities and public swimming pools are common sources of *Giardia* (don't assume camping or travel is required).
- Metronidazole has high cure rates (but is often poorly tolerated).
- Most treatment failures respond to a second course of antibiotics (with same or other drugs).
- A single FA or ELISA is as sensitive as three stool samples for ova and parasites for detecting *Giardia*.

G

GILBERT DISEASE
Robert A. Marlow, MD, MA

 BASICS

DESCRIPTION
Mild, chronic, or intermittent unconjugated hyperbilirubinemia (not due to hemolysis) with otherwise normal liver function (1)

Pediatric Considerations
Rare for the disorder to be diagnosed before puberty (2)

Pregnancy Considerations
The relative fasting that may occur with morning sickness can elevate bilirubin level.

EPIDEMIOLOGY
- Predominant age: present from birth but most often presents in the 2nd or 3rd decade of life; heterozygous for single abnormal gene (3)
- Predominant sex: male > female (2 to 7:1)

Prevalence
Prevalence in the United States: ~7% of the population (4); ~1 in 3 of those affected are not aware that they have the disorder.

ETIOLOGY AND PATHOPHYSIOLOGY
The hyperbilirubinemia results from impaired hepatic bilirubin clearance (~30% of normal). Hepatic bilirubin conjugation (glucuronidation) is reduced, although this is likely not the only defect (3).

Genetics
A gene defect resulting in reduced bilirubin uridine diphosphate–glucuronosyltransferase-1 appears to be necessary but not sufficient for Gilbert syndrome (5).

RISK FACTORS
Male gender

COMMONLY ASSOCIATED CONDITIONS
Gilbert disease may be part of a spectrum of hereditary disorders that includes types I and II Crigler-Najjar syndrome.

 DIAGNOSIS

HISTORY
No significant symptoms, although a variety of nonspecific symptoms have been described. An episode of nonpruritic jaundice can be triggered by stressors such as fasting, dehydration, infections, physical exertion, lack of sleep, and surgery. Some medications may also trigger episodes of jaundice, such as drugs that inhibit glucuronyl transferase, such as gemfibrozil and the protease inhibitors atazanavir and indinavir. Any symptoms present during an episode of jaundice, including fatigue, are caused by the triggering factor and are not directly a result of the Gilbert disease (6).

PHYSICAL EXAM
No abnormal physical findings other than occasional mild jaundice that can be precipitated by the above-mentioned triggers (fasting, dehydration, infections, physical exertion, lack of sleep, and surgery).

DIFFERENTIAL DIAGNOSIS
- Hemolysis
- Ineffective erythropoiesis (megaloblastic anemias, certain porphyrias, thalassemia major, sideroblastic anemia, severe lead poisoning, congenital dyserythropoietic anemias)
- Cirrhosis
- Chronic persistent hepatitis
- Pancreatitis
- Biliary tract disease

DIAGNOSTIC TESTS & INTERPRETATION
Initial Tests (lab, imaging)
- Bilirubin: Elevated but <6 mg/dL (103 μmol/L) and usually <3 mg/dL (51 μmol/L), virtually all unconjugated (indirect), with conjugated bilirubin within the normal range and/or <20% of the total bilirubin (6).
- CBC with peripheral smear is normal.
- Reticulocyte count is normal.
- Liver function tests (LFTs) (aspartate aminotransferase [AST], alanine transaminase [ALT], alkaline phosphatase, and gamma-glutamyl transpeptidase [GGT]) are normal.
- Fasting and postprandial serum bile acids are normal.
- Up to 60% of patients have clinically insignificant mild hemolysis that frequently can only be detected with sophisticated red cell survival studies.
- Drugs that may alter lab results: Bilirubin level may be raised by nicotinic acid and lowered by phenobarbital.
- Disorders that may alter lab results: Bilirubin levels increase during fasting and may increase during a febrile illness.

Follow-Up Tests & Special Considerations
If history, physical exam, and laboratory tests are normal, see the patient on two to three further occasions during the ensuing 12 to 18 months. If the patient develops no symptoms, reticulocytosis, or new liver function abnormalities, make the diagnosis of Gilbert disease.

Diagnostic Procedures/Other

ALERT
A liver biopsy is not usually needed to exclude other diagnoses (4).

- Some clinicians recommend confirming the diagnosis by reducing daily caloric intake to 400 kcal for 48 hours, which results in a 2- to 3-fold increase in unconjugated bilirubin, but other clinicians consider this impractical and nonspecific for Gilbert disease.
- After 12 hours of fasting, an increase of total bilirubin to >1.9 mg/dL 2 hours after an oral dose of rifampin 900 mg distinguishes patients with Gilbert disease with a sensitivity of 100% and a specificity of 100% (7).

TREATMENT

- Outpatient
- The most important treatment is to make a positive diagnosis of Gilbert disease to reassure the patient and prevent further unnecessary procedures.

 ONGOING CARE

FOLLOW-UP RECOMMENDATIONS
Patient Monitoring
If history, physical exam, and laboratory tests are normal, see the patient on two to three further occasions during the ensuing 12 to 18 months. If the patient develops no symptoms, reticulocytosis, or new liver function abnormalities, make the diagnosis of Gilbert disease.

PATIENT EDUCATION
Reassure the patient that the condition is benign with no known sequelae.

PROGNOSIS
- The disorder is benign with an excellent prognosis.
- There is some preliminary evidence that patients with Gilbert disease may have a lower incidence of cardiovascular disease (8,9). Elevated levels of bilirubin may exert an antioxidation effect (9).
- Patients with Gilbert syndrome are able to serve as donors for right lobe of liver for transplantation (10).

COMPLICATIONS
No known complications

REFERENCES

1. Bosma PJ. Inherited disorders of bilirubin metabolism. *J Hepatol*. 2003;38(1):107–117.
2. Fretzayas A, Moustaki M, Liapi O, et al. Gilbert syndrome. *Eur J Pediatr*. 2012;171(1):11–15.
3. Strassburg CP. Pharmacogenetics of Gilbert's syndrome. *Pharmacogenomics*. 2008;9(6):703–715.
4. Radu P, Atsmon J. Gilbert's syndrome—clinical and pharmacological implications. *Isr Med Assoc J*. 2001;3(8):593–598.
5. Bosma PJ, Chowdhury JR, Bakker C, et al. The genetic basis of the reduced expression of bilirubin UDP-glucuronosyltransferase 1 in Gilbert's syndrome. *N Engl J Med*. 1995;333(18):1171–1175.
6. Claridge LC, Armstrong MJ, Booth C, et al. Gilbert's syndrome. *BMJ*. 2011;342:d2293.
7. Murthy GD, Byron D, Shoemaker D, et al. The utility of rifampin in diagnosing Gilbert's syndrome. *Am J Gastroenterol*. 2001;96(4):1150–1154.
8. Inoguchi T, Sasaki S, Kobayashi K, et al. Relationship between Gilbert syndrome and prevalence of vascular complications in patients with diabetes. *JAMA*. 2007;298(12):1398–1400.
9. Bulmer AC, Blanchfield JT, Toth I, et al. Improved resistance to serum oxidation in Gilbert's syndrome: a mechanism for cardiovascular protection. *Atherosclerosis*. 2008;199(2):390–396.
10. Demirbas T, Piskin T, Dayangac M, et al. Right-lobe liver transplant from donors with Gilbert syndrome. *Exp Clin Transplant*. 2012;10(1):39–42.

 CODES

ICD10
- E80.4 Gilbert syndrome
- E80.6 Other disorders of bilirubin metabolism

CLINICAL PEARLS

- Gilbert disease: a mild chronic or intermittent unconjugated hyperbilirubinemia (not due to hemolysis) with otherwise normal liver function
- The hyperbilirubinemia results from impaired hepatic bilirubin clearance (30% of normal). Hepatic bilirubin conjugation (glucuronidation) is reduced, although this is likely not the only defect.
- The most important reason to make the diagnosis of Gilbert disease is to reassure the patient that this is a benign condition with no known sequelae and to prevent unnecessary procedures.
- To diagnose Gilbert disease: History, physical exam, and laboratory tests (LFTs, reticulocytosis, etc.) are normal on visits every 6 months over 18 months.
- A liver biopsy is not usually needed to rule out other liver diseases. The diagnosis can be confirmed by otherwise normal LFTs, no evidence of hemolysis, and the response to fasting or a dose of rifampin.
- The etiology of Gilbert disease can result when the patient has a gene defect resulting in reduced conjugation of bilirubin. The gene defect is necessary but not sufficient to produce Gilbert disease.

G

GINGIVITIS

Hugh Silk, MD, MPH, FAAFP • Sheila O. Stille, DMD • Nerissa P. Duchin, MD

 BASICS

DESCRIPTION
Gingivitis is a reversible form of inflammation of the gingiva. It is a mild form of periodontal disease. Classification includes the following:
- Plaque-induced
- Not plaque-induced (bacterial, viral, or fungal; e.g., acute necrotizing gingivitis, Vincent disease ["trench mouth"], denture-related)
- Modified by systemic factors (e.g., pregnancy, puberty, HIV, diabetes, smoking, leukemia)
- Modified by medications (calcium channel blockers, antipsychotics, antiepileptics, antirejection medications, hormones)
- Modified by malnutrition (vitamin deficiencies)
- System(s) affected: gastrointestinal; ears, nose, throat; dental
- Synonym(s): mild periodontal disease; gum disease

Geriatric Considerations
More frequent in this age group (due more to additive effects than to increased susceptibility)

Pediatric Considerations
Mild cases common in children (most common form of pediatric periodontal disease) and usually require no specific interventions other than improved oral hygiene

Pregnancy Considerations
- Very common in pregnant women; hormonal effect
- Self-limited

EPIDEMIOLOGY
- Predominant age: children, teenagers, and young adults. Predominant sex: slightly more males than female
- Prevalence ~50% of children
- ~90% of adolescents and adult population
- ~30–75% of pregnant women

ETIOLOGY AND PATHOPHYSIOLOGY
Inflammation of gingiva. This can progress to deeper, destructive inflammation. If involving supporting bone, will be classified as periodontitis, not gingivitis.
- Usually noncontagious
- Inadequate plaque removal
- Blood dyscrasias (pregnancy)
- Oral contraceptives
- Allergic reactions
- Nutritional deficiencies
- Vasoconstriction (nicotine, methamphetamine)
- Endocrine/hormonal variations
  - Pregnancy
  - Menses
  - Menarche
- Chronic debilitating disease
- Vincent disease
  - Synergistic infection with fusiform bacillus (*Fusobacterium* spp.) and spirochete (*Borrelia vincentii*)
- Pathology
  - Acute or chronic inflammation
  - Hyperemic capillaries
  - Polymorphonuclear infiltration
  - Papillary projections in subepithelial tissue
  - Fibroblasts

Genetics
Possible genetic link (up to 30% of population); rare condition called hereditary gingival fibromatosis associated with hirsutism

RISK FACTORS
- Poor dental hygiene/plaque formation
- Pregnancy
- Uncontrolled diabetes mellitus
- Malocclusion or dental crowding
- Smoking
- Mouth breathing
- Xerostomia
- Faulty dental restoration
- HIV-positive; AIDS
- Stress
- Hospitalization (1)[A]
- Vitamin C deficiency; coenzyme Q10 deficiency
- Dental appliances (dentures, braces)
- Eruption of primary or secondary teeth
- Necrotizing ulcerative gingivitis
  - Stress
  - Lack of sleep
  - Malnutrition
  - Viral illness
  - Typically teens and young adults
- Bronchial asthma and other respiratory diseases (2,3)[B]
- Rheumatoid arthritis (4)[B]

GENERAL PREVENTION
- Good oral hygiene
  - Adults
    - Regular twice-daily brushing with fluoride toothpaste and increased benefit of using circular oscillating electric brush rather than regular brush or sonic/vibration (5,6)[A]
    - Daily "high-quality" flossing (studies show that flossing only helps when it is done correctly) (7)[A]
    - Chlorhexidine with oral hygiene better than other oral rinse agents (8,9)[A]
      - Use in acute phase sparingly (10)[B]
  - Pediatrics
    - Regular twice-daily brushing with fluoride toothpaste under parental supervision until full manual dexterity (~8 years of age)
    - Regular flossing if no spaces between teeth
- Cleaning by a dentist or hygienist every 6 months or more frequently, if indicated
- Mouth rinse with essential oils (menthol, thymol, eucalyptol; e.g., Listerine) combined with brushing (11)[B]
  - Caution: Long-term use of alcohol-based mouth rinse may be associated with an increased risk of oral cancer (12)[B].

COMMONLY ASSOCIATED CONDITIONS
- Periodontitis
- Glossitis
- Pedunculated growths (pyogenic granulomata)

 DIAGNOSIS

HISTORY
- Gum erythema, swelling, and edema
- Gums are tender when touched but otherwise painless.
- Bleeding of gums when brushing, flossing, or eating
- Inquire about HIV risk, pregnancy, nutritional deficiencies, diabetes, and other risk factors as indicated (see "Risk Factors").
- Smoking history
- Oral hygiene, dental visit history

PHYSICAL EXAM
- Normal gums should appear pink, firm, stippled, and scalloped.
- Gingivitis—marginal gum swelling and edema (usually painless, except to touch)
- Gum erythema: bright red or red-purple appearance
- Bleeding with manipulation of gums
- Change of normal gum contours
- Plaque (soft) and calculus (not easily removed)
- Edema of interdental papillae
- HIV gingivitis
  - Also called linear gingival erythema
  - Narrow band of bright red inflamed gum surrounding neck of tooth
  - Painful
  - Bleeds easily
  - Rapid destruction of gingival tissue and can progress to periodontitis with destruction of underlying support tissues (periodontal ligament, supporting alveolar bone)
- Vincent disease
  - Ulcers
  - Fever
  - Malaise
  - Regional lymphadenopathy
  - Pain
  - Mouth odor

DIFFERENTIAL DIAGNOSIS
- Periodontitis (deeper inflammation, causing destruction to connective tissue, ligaments, and alveolar bone)
- Glossitis
- Desquamative gingivitis (painful, persistent, usually middle-aged women)
- Pericoronitis (gum flap traps food and plaque over partially erupted third molar), common in adolescence
- Gingival ulcers (aphthous, herpetic, malignancy, TB, syphilis)
- Specific forms of gingivitis: See "Description," including acute necrotizing ulcerative gingivitis (Vincent disease) and HIV gingivitis (linear gingival erythema).

DIAGNOSTIC TESTS & INTERPRETATION
Initial Tests (lab, imaging)
- No tests usually needed
- Possible smear or culture to identify causative agent (HIV gingivitis includes gram-negative anaerobes, enteric strains, and *Candida*)
- Labs for contributing conditions (HIV, pregnancy, diabetes, nutritional deficiencies)

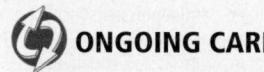

TREATMENT

GENERAL MEASURES
- Stop any contributing medications.
- Remove irritating factors (plaque, calculus, faulty dental restorations, or partial dentures).
- Good oral hygiene (see "General Prevention")
- Regular dental checkups (for scaling and polishing if plaque and/or tartar are present)
- Smoking cessation
- Warm saline rinses BID
- Special care needs patients: use of tray-applied 10% carbamide peroxide gels (13)[C]

MEDICATION
First Line
- Chlorhexidine rinses or varnishes may be used (14)[B].
- Mouth rinses with essential oils (EOMW) may be equally effective to chlorhexidine for reduction of gingival inflammation (while EOMW is not as effective for plaque control) (15)[A].
- Both chlorhexidine and EOMW rinses are as clinically effective as oral prophylaxis and oral hygiene instruction at 6-month recall (16)[B].

- Antibiotics indicated only for acute necrotizing ulcerative gingivitis (Vincent disease)
- Antibiotics
  - Penicillin V: pediatric dose, 25 to 50 mg/kg/day divided q6h; adult dose, 250 to 500 mg q6h, OR
  - Metronidazole: pediatric dose, 30 mg/kg/day PO/IV divided q6h; maximum 4 g/day; adult dose, 500 mg BID or TID for 10 days OR
  - Amoxicillin/clavulanic acid: pediatric dose, 30 mg/kg/day PO divided q12h; info: use 125 mg/31.25 mg/5 mL susp; adult dose, 875 mg/ 125 mg PO BID for 10 days
  - Erythromycin: pediatric dose 30 to 40 mg/kg/day divided q6h; adult dose, 250 mg q6h
  - Doxycycline: adult dose, 100 mg BID 1st day, then QD for 10 days
- Topical corticosteroids
  - Triamcinolone 0.1% in Orabase (spray or ointment), applied locally TID, QID
    ∘ Contraindications
      ▪ Allergy to specific medication
- Precautions
  - Erythromycin frequently causes GI issues.

Second Line
- Acetaminophen or ibuprofen for any pain (rare)
- Other antibiotics or antifungal rinses or systemic according to culture or smear
- Decapinol oral rinse (surfactant that acts as a physical barrier, making it harder for bacteria to stick to tooth and mucosal surfaces) to reduce bacteria (not recommended for pregnant women or children <12 years); should be used in conjunction with other oral hygiene practices when those practices alone are not enough

ISSUES FOR REFERRAL
- Dental referral for cleanings and further treatment, as needed
- If gingivitis becomes periodontitis, deep root scaling, planing, and antibiotics may be indicated.

SURGERY/OTHER PROCEDURES
- Débridement for acute necrotizing gingivitis
- Minor surgery may be necessary to correct tissue overgrowth for gingivitis caused by medicines.

COMPLEMENTARY & ALTERNATIVE MEDICINE
- Bilberry: potentially helpful in reducing inflammation and stabilizing collagen tissue
- Coenzyme Q10: topically, to restore coenzyme Q10 deficiency
- Replace any other deficiencies (e.g., vitamin C).

ONGOING CARE

FOLLOW-UP RECOMMENDATIONS
- Outpatient
- No restrictions

Patient Monitoring
Until clear; dental follow-up for continued cleanings and secondary prevention

DIET
- Well-balanced diet that includes fruits, vegetables, vitamin C; avoid sugary snacks and drinks, which contribute to plaque formation.
- Soft foods during flare, if significant inflammation/bleeding

PATIENT EDUCATION
- Good oral hygiene, including twice-daily brushing with circular oscillating electric brush, fluoridated toothpaste, and daily flossing; regular dental visits
- Printable and viewable patient information available under "gum diseases" from the American Dental Association at http://www.mouthhealthy.org/en/ and the American Academy of Periodontology under "patient resources" at http://www.perio.org/

PROGNOSIS
- Usual course: acute, relapsing, intermittent; chronic
- Prognosis: generally favorable, responds well to appropriate treatment
- Left untreated, may progress to periodontitis (controversial), which is a major cause of tooth loss

COMPLICATIONS
Severe periodontal disease (which is associated with heart disease, diabetes, and preterm birth)

REFERENCES

1. Terezakis E, Needleman I, Kumar N, et al. The impact of hospitalization on oral health: a systematic review. J Clin Periodontol. 2011;38(7):628–636.
2. Stensson M, Wendt LK, Koch G, et al. Oral health in pre-school children with asthma—followed from 3 to 6 years. Int J Paediatr Dent. 2010;20(3):165–172.
3. Widmer RP. Oral health of children with respiratory diseases. Paediatr Respir Rev. 2010;11(4):226–232.
4. Keles ZP, Keles GC, Avci B, et al. Analysis of YKL-40 acute-phase protein and interleukin-6 levels in periodontal disease. J Periodontol. 2014;85(9):1240–1246.
5. Yaacob M, Worthington HV, Deacon SA, et al. Powered versus manual toothbrushing for oral health. Cochrane Database Syst Rev. 2014;(6):CD002281.
6. Klukowska M, Grender JM, Conde E, et al. A 12-week clinical comparison of an oscillating-rotating power brush versus a marketed sonic brush with self-adjusting technology in reducing plaque and gingivitis. J Clin Dent. 2013;24(2):55–61.
7. Sambunjak D, Nickerson JW, Poklepovic T, et al. Flossing for the management of periodontal diseases and dental caries in adults. Cochrane Database Syst Rev. 2011;(12):CD008829.
8. Van Strydonck DA, Slot DE, Van der Velden U, et al. Effect of a chlorhexidine mouthrinse on plaque, gingival inflammation and staining in gingivitis patients: a systematic review. J Clin Periodontol. 2012;39(11):1042–1055.
9. Babu JP, Garcia-Godoy F. In vitro comparison of commercial oral rinses on bacterial adhesion and their detachment from biofilm formed on hydroxyapatite disks. Oral Health Prev Dent. 2014;12(4):365–371.
10. Eliot MN, Michaud DS, Langevin SM, et al. Periodontal disease and mouthwash use are risk factors for head and neck squamous cell carcinoma. Cancer Causes Control. 2013;24(7):1315–1322.
11. Cortelli SC, Cortelli JR, Shang H, et al. Gingival health benefits of essential-oil and cetylpyridinium chloride mouthrinses: a 6-month randomized clinical study. Am J Dent. 2014 Jun;27(3):119–126.
12. McCullough M, Farah CS. The role of alcohol in oral carcinogenesis with particular reference to alcohol-containing mouthwashes. Aust Dent J. 2008;53(4):302–305.
13. Lazarchik DA, Haywood VB. Use of tray-applied 10 percent carbamide peroxide gels for improving oral health in patients with special-care needs. J Am Dent Assoc. 2010;141(6):639–646.
14. Puig Silla M, Montiel Company JM, Almerich Silla JM. Use of chlorhexidine varnishes in preventing and treating periodontal disease. A review of the literature. Med Oral Patol Oral Cir Bucal. 2008;13(4):E257–E260.
15. Van Leeuwen MP, Slot DE, Van der Weijden GA. Essential oils compared to chlorhexidine with respect to plaque and parameters of gingival inflammation: a systematic review. J Periodontol. 2011;82(2):174–194.
16. Osso D, Kanani N. Antiseptic mouth rinses: an update on comparative effectiveness, risks and recommendations. J Dent Hyg. 2013;87(1):10–18.

SEE ALSO

- Dental Infection; Glossitis
- Algorithm: Bleeding Gums

CODES

ICD10
- K05.10 Chronic gingivitis, plaque induced
- K05.11 Chronic gingivitis, non-plaque induced
- K05.00 Acute gingivitis, plaque induced

CLINICAL PEARLS
- Gingivitis may be prevented and treated with regular dental cleanings, good oral hygiene, and use of certain mouth rinses including chlorhexidine.
- Untreated, gingivitis may progress to periodontitis, a possible contributor to systemic inflammation and its consequences (e.g., coronary artery disease and uncontrolled diabetes).
- New-onset or difficult-to-treat gingivitis, consider differential of etiology: pregnancy, HIV, diabetes, medications, and vitamin deficiencies.

G

GLAUCOMA, PRIMARY CLOSED-ANGLE

H. Anh Hinshaw, MD • David S. Pfoff, MD

BASICS

DESCRIPTION
- Primary angle closure suspect (PACS): eye has narrow or occludable anterior chamber angle, but no other abnormalities (1)
- Primary angle closure (PAC): signs of trabecular meshwork obstruction appear, such as increased intraocular pressure (IOP) or synechiae formation (1)
  - Acute angle closure: sudden block of meshwork by iris (2)
  - Subacute (intermittent) angle closure: periodic acute episodes with normal IOP between (2)
  - Chronic angle closure: most common, refers to an eye with permanent closure of areas of the anterior chamber angle by peripheral anterior synechiae (1)[C]
- Primary angle closure glaucoma (PACG): glaucomatous optic neuropathy and visual field loss are present (1)[C].

Geriatric Considerations
Increased risk with age and prior history of cataract, hyperopia, and/or uveitis

Pregnancy Considerations
Medications used may cross the placenta and be excreted into breast milk.

EPIDEMIOLOGY
- Age >40 years
- Female > male
- Inuit and Asian > African and European

Prevalence
- Estimated that over 23 million (in 2020) and 32 million (in 2040) people worldwide will have PACG with the majority in Asia (3)
- PACG is not as common in the United States, accounts for 10% of all glaucoma (2).

ETIOLOGY AND PATHOPHYSIOLOGY
- Iridotrabecular contact (ITC): instigating factor; peripheral iris apposition to the posterior trabecular meshwork (1)
- ITC causes obstruction of aqueous humor outflow through the trabecular meshwork, which causes elevation in IOP. Prolonged ITC can cause scarring to form, degradation of trabecular meshwork, and loss of vision (1).
- Most common underlying mechanism of PAC is anterior lens displacement, leading to pupillary block in which aqueous humor egress through the pupil is limited. This causes pressure to build posterior in the peripheral iris, leading to anterior bowing of the iris and closing of the angle (1,2).
- Other mechanisms include predisposing ocular anatomy, such as plateau iris (2)

Genetics
First-degree relatives have a 1–12% increased risk in whites, 6 times greater risk in Chinese patients with positive family history.

RISK FACTORS
- Hyperopia
- Age >40 years
- Shallow anterior chamber
- Female gender
- Family history of angle closure
- Asian or Inuit descent
- Short axial length
- Thick crystalline lens

- Anterior positioned lens
- Plateau iris
- Drugs that can induce angle-closure:

  - Adrenergic agonists (albuterol, phenylephrine), anticholinergics (oxybutynin, atropine, botulinum toxin A), antihistamines, antidepressants including selective serotonin reuptake inhibitors (SSRIs) and tricyclic antidepressants (TCAs), cholinergic agents, sulfa-based drugs, topiramate, cocaine, ecstasy (4)[A]

GENERAL PREVENTION
- Routine eye exam with gonioscopy for high-risk populations
- U.S. Preventive Services Task Force: insufficient evidence to recommend for or against screening adults for open-angle glaucoma (5)[A]
- Prophylactic laser iridotomy for PACS patients has been found to be effective in preventing PACG.
- Prophylactic laser iridotomy in contralateral eye of patients that have had unilateral acute PAC has been effective in preventing acute attacks in the contralateral eye (2)[C].

COMMONLY ASSOCIATED CONDITIONS
- Cataract
- Hyperopia
- Microphthalmos
- Systemic hypertension

DIAGNOSIS

HISTORY
- Patient's previous medical and ophthalmologic history
- Family history of glaucoma
- Obtain history of prescription, over-the-counter, and herbal medications
- Precipitating factors (dim light, medicines)
- Review of symptoms
- Acute (6)[C]
  - Severe eye pain
  - Blurred vision
  - Eye redness
  - Halos around lights/objects
  - Frontal headache
  - Nausea and vomiting, which may lead to erroneous abdominal exploration
- Chronic (2)[C]
  - May have subacute symptoms (intermittent subacute attacks)
  - Compromised peripheral, then central vision
  - Usually asymptomatic until advanced vision loss has occurred.

PHYSICAL EXAM
- Includes, but is not limited to, the following in the undilated eye (1)[C]
  - Visual acuity
  - Visual field testing and ocular motility
  - Pupil size and reactivity (mid-dilated, minimally reactive)
  - External examination
  - Undilated fundus exam (congestion, cupping, atrophy of optic nerve)
  - Slit-lamp exam (anterior segments)
  - Tonometry (determination of IOP)
  - Gonioscopy (visualization of the angle)

- Acute (6)[C]
  - Elevated IOP (>21 mm Hg)
  - Corneal microcystic edema (haze)
  - Hyperemic conjunctiva
  - Mid-dilated, nonreactive, or irregular pupil
  - Shallow anterior chamber, often with inflammatory reaction (cell and flare in anterior chamber)
  - Pain with eye movement
  - Closed angle by gonioscopy or anterior segment optical coherence tomography (AS-OCT)
- Chronic (6)[C]
  - Multiple peripheral anterior synechiae
  - Normal or elevated IOP
  - Increased cup-to-disc ratio or excavation of disc
  - Glaucoma flecks (lens) and iris atrophy (previous acute attacks)

DIFFERENTIAL DIAGNOSIS
- Acute orbital compartment syndrome
- Traumatic hyphema
- Conjunctivitis, episcleritis
- Corneal abrasion
- Glaucoma, malignant or neovascular
- Herpes zoster ophthalmicus
- Iritis and uveitis
- Orbital/periorbital infection
- Vitreous or subconjunctival hemorrhage
- Tight necktie, causing increased IOP
- Lens-induced angle closure

DIAGNOSTIC TESTS & INTERPRETATION
Initial Tests (lab, imaging)
Ultrasound (US) biomicroscopy AS-OCT (1)[C]

Diagnostic Procedures/Other
Careful ophthalmic examination, including gonioscopy and tonometry (1)[C]

Test Interpretation
- Narrow or closed anterior angle
- Corneal stromal and epithelial edema
- Endothelial cell loss (guttata)
- Iris stromal necrosis
- Anterior subcapsular cataract (*glaukomflecken*)
- Optic disc congestion, cupping, excavation
- Optic nerve atrophy

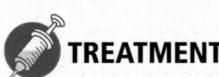

TREATMENT

Goals of treatment (1)[C]:
- Reverse or prevent angle-closure process
- Control IOP
- Prevent damage to the optic nerve

GENERAL MEASURES
- For acute attack: ocular emergency
  - Manage nausea and pain
  - Immediate ophthalmology consultation
  - Goals of therapy through medical and surgical treatment: reduce IOP to <35 mm Hg or by >25% of presenting IOP (7)[B]

MEDICATION
- During acute attack, therapy can be initiated with 2% pilocarpine, 0.5% timolol maleate, and 1% apraclonidine drops 1 minute apart, and acetazolamide 500 mg PO, glycerin (Osmoglen) (50%) 6 oz PO, and IV mannitol 20% 1.5 to 2g/kg infused over 30 to 60 minutes for a rapid decrease in IOP; after the cornea clears, a peripheral iridotomy is done (8)[C].

- Additionally, medical therapy to decrease IOP and clear the cornea prior to surgery can also be accomplished using some or all of the following (1,9)[C]:
  - Carbonic anhydrase inhibitors (CAIs):
    - Contraindications/precautions: sulfa allergy, hepatic insufficiency
    - Systemic:
      - Acetazolamide (Diamox): 500 mg IV/PO; may repeat with 250 mg in 4 hours to a maximum of 1 g/day
      - Methazolamide (Neptazane): 50 to 100 mg PO BID–TID
    - Topical:
      - Dorzolamide (Trusopt) 2% eyedrops: 1 drop in affected eye(s) TID
      - Brinzolamide (Azopt) 1% suspension: 1 drop in affected eye(s) TID
  - β-Blockers:
    - Contraindications/precautions: decompensated heart failure, sinus bradycardia, heart block, severe COPD/asthma
      - Timolol (Timoptic) 0.25–0.5% solution: 1 drop in affected eye(s) BID
      - Timolol (Timolol GFS, Timoptic-XE) 0.25–0.5% gel-forming solution: 1 drop daily
      - Levobunolol (Betagan) 0.5% solution: 1 drop in affected eye(s) 1 to 2 times daily
      - Betaxolol (Betoptic) 0.5% solution: 1 to 2 drops in affected eye(s) BID
      - Carteolol (Ocupress)1% solution: 1 drop in affected eye(s) BID
      - Metipranolol (Optipranolol) 0.3% solution: 1 drop in affected eye(s) BID
  - α_2-Agonists: (used as adjunct therapy)
    - Contraindications/precautions: MAO inhibitor therapy
      - Brimonidine (Alphagan P) 0.15%, 0.2% solution: 1 drop in affected eye(s) TID
      - Apraclonidine (Iopidine) 0.5% solution: 1 to 2 drops in affected eye(s) TID
  - Prostaglandin analogs:
    - Precautions: changes to iris, eyelid, and eyelash pigmentation, eyelash growth, irritation, redness; can cause corneal epithelium herpes to recur
      - Latanoprost (Xalatan) 0.005% solution: 1 drop in affected eye(s) daily
      - Travoprost (Travatan Z) 0.004% solution: 1 drop in affected eye(s) daily
      - Bimatoprost (Lumigan) 0.01% solution: 1 drop in affected eye(s) daily
      - Tafluprost (Zioptan) 0.0015% solution: 1 drop in affected eye(s) nightly
      - Unoprostone (Rescula) 0.15% solution: 1 drop in affected eye(s) BID
  - Direct cholinergic agonists:
    - Precautions: may worsen the condition due to anterior rotation of the lens–iris diaphragm, impaired night vision, color vision changes
      - Pilocarpine (Isopto Carpine) (1%, 2%, 4% solution): 1 drop up to 6 times daily to reduce IOP; for acute attack, 1 drop of 1–2% in affected eye(s) every 10 minutes up to 3 doses
  - Cholinesterase inhibitor:
    - Precautions: may worsen the condition due to anterior rotation of the lens–iris diaphragm, impaired night vision
      - Echothiophate iodide (Phospholine Iodide) 0.125% solution: 1 drop BID
    - Combination products:
      - Timolol-Dorzolamide (Cosopt) 0.5%/2% solution: 1 drop in affected eye(s) BID
      - Timolol-Brimonidine (Combigan) 0.5%/0.2% solution: 1 drop in affected eye(s) BID
      - Brinzolamide-Brimonidine (Simbrinza) 1%/0.2% solution: 1 drop in affected eye(s) TID

ADDITIONAL THERAPIES
Keep patient supine.

SURGERY/OTHER PROCEDURES
- Acute (1)[C],(6)[B]
  - Laser peripheral iridotomy is preferred surgical treatment, but surgical iridectomy can be used if laser is not available.
- Subacute and chronic (1,5,10)[B]
  - Laser iridectomy for pupillary block
  - Goniosynechialysis to separate synechiae
  - Phacoemulsification to remove cataract

INPATIENT CONSIDERATIONS
Admission Criteria/Initial Stabilization
- Patient requires metabolic ± electrolyte and volume status monitoring (with osmotic agents).
- Facilitate close ophthalmology monitoring.

 ONGOING CARE

FOLLOW-UP RECOMMENDATIONS
Schedule an immediate ophthalmologic follow-up.

Patient Monitoring
- Postsurgical follow-up
- Evaluation of the contralateral eye
- Routine monitoring after acute attack per ophthalmologist recommendations

PATIENT EDUCATION
- Advise patient to seek emergency medical attention if experiencing a change in visual acuity, blurred vision, eye pain, or headache.
- If narrow angles, but no peripheral iridotomy performed: Avoid decongestants, motion sickness medications, adrenergic agents, antipsychotics, antidepressants, and anticholinergic agents.
- Correct eyedrop administration technique, including the following:
  - Remove contact lenses before administration and wait 15 minutes before reinserting.
  - Allow at least 5 minutes between administration of multiple ophthalmic products.
- Patients with significant visual impairment should be referred to vision rehab and social services.
- Patient education materials:
  - Glaucoma Research Foundation: http://www.glaucoma.org
  - National Eye Institute: http://www.nei.nih.gov

PROGNOSIS
- With timely treatment, most patients do not have permanent vision loss.
- Prognosis depends on ethnicity, underlying eye disease, and time-to-treatment.

COMPLICATIONS
- Chronic corneal edema
- Corneal fibrosis and vascularization
- Iris atrophy
- Cataract
- Optic atrophy
- Malignant glaucoma
- Central retinal artery/vein occlusion
- Permanent decrease in visual acuity
- Repeat episode
- Fellow (contralateral) eye attack

REFERENCES

1. American Academy of Ophthalmology. *Primary Angle Closure Preferred Practice Pattern*. San Francisco, CA: American Academy of Ophthalmology; 2010. http://www.aao.org.
2. Patel K, Patel S. Angle-closure glaucoma. *Dis Mon*. 2014;60(6):254–262.
3. Tham YC, Li X, Wong TY, et al. Global prevalence of glaucoma and projections of glaucoma burden through 2040: a systematic review and meta-analysis. *Ophthalmology*. 2014;121(11): 2081–2090.
4. Subak-Sharpe I, Low S, Nolan W, et al. Pharmacological and environmental factors in primary angle-closure glaucoma. *Br Med Bull*. 2010;93: 125–143.
5. Moyer VA. Screening for glaucoma: U.S. Preventive Services Task Force Recommendation Statement. *Ann Intern Med*. 2013;159(7): 484–489.
6. Saw SM, Gazzard G, Friedman DS. Interventions for angle-closure glaucoma: an evidence-based update. *Ophthalmology*. 2003;110(10): 1869–1878.
7. Choong YF, Irfan S, Menage MJ. Acute angle closure glaucoma: an evaluation of a protocol for acute treatment. *Eye (Lond)*. 1999;13(Pt 5): 613–616.
8. Pokhrel PK, Loftus SA. Ocular emergencies. *Am Fam Physician*. 2007;76(6):829–836.
9. Kolko M. Present and new treatment strategies in the management of glaucoma. *Open Ophthalmol J*. 2015;9:89–100.
10. Qing G, Wang N, Mu D. Efficacy of goniosynechialysis for advanced chronic angle-closure glaucoma. *Clin Ophthalmol*. 2012;6:1723–1729.

 SEE ALSO

Glaucoma, Primary Open-Angle

 CODES

ICD10
- H40.20X0 Unsp primary angle-closure glaucoma, stage unspecified
- H40.219 Acute angle-closure glaucoma, unspecified eye
- H40.2290 Chronic angle-closure glaucoma, unsp eye, stage unspecified

CLINICAL PEARLS
- Examiner can determine if patient is hyperopic by observing the magnification of the patient's face through his or her glasses (myopic lenses minify).
- A careful history may reveal similar episodes of angle closure that resolved spontaneously.
- Miotics, such as pilocarpine, can be effective during mild attacks, but in the setting of high IOP (due to iris sphincter ischemia), other agents such as CAIs, prostaglandin analogs, α_2-agonists, and β-blockers are necessary.

G

GLAUCOMA, PRIMARY OPEN-ANGLE

Richard W. Allinson, MD

 BASICS

DESCRIPTION
- Primary open-angle glaucoma (POAG) is an optic neuropathy resulting in visual field loss frequently associated with increased intraocular pressure (IOP).
- Normal IOP is 10 to 22 mm Hg. However, glaucomatous optic nerve damage also can occur with normal IOP and as a secondary manifestation of other disorders such as corticosteroid-induced glaucoma.
- System(s) affected: nervous
- Synonym(s): chronic open-angle glaucoma

Pregnancy Considerations
Prostaglandins should be avoided during pregnancy in the treatment of POAG.

EPIDEMIOLOGY
Incidence
- Predominant age: usually >40 years
- Increases with age
- Predominant gender: male = female

Prevalence
Prevalence in persons >40 years of age is ~1.8%.

Geriatric Considerations
Increasing prevalence with increasing age

ETIOLOGY AND PATHOPHYSIOLOGY
- Abnormal aqueous outflow resulting in increased IOP
- Normally, aqueous is produced by the ciliary epithelium of the ciliary body and is secreted into the posterior chamber of the eye.
- Aqueous then flows through the pupil and enters the anterior chamber to be drained by the trabecular meshwork in the iridocorneal angle of the eye into the Schlemm canal and into the venous system of the episclera.
- 5–10% of the total aqueous outflow leaves via the uveoscleral pathway.
- Impaired aqueous outflow through the trabecular meshwork
  - Increased resistance within the aqueous drainage system

Genetics
A family history of glaucoma increases the risk for developing glaucoma.

RISK FACTORS
- Increased IOP
- Myopia
- Diabetes mellitus (DM)
- African American
- Elderly
- Hypothyroidism
- Positive family history
- Central corneal thickness <550 μm
- Larger vertical cup-to-disc ratio (CDR)
- Larger horizontal CDR
- CDR asymmetry
- Disc hemorrhage
- Prolonged use of topical, periocular, inhaled, or systemic corticosteroids
- Obstructive sleep apnea
- Hypertension (1)[B]
- Corneal hysteresis (CH) (2)[B]
  - A measure of the viscoelastic damping of the cornea
  - Lower CH associated with faster rates of visual field loss

GENERAL PREVENTION
Possible reduced risk of open-angle glaucoma with long-term use of oral statins among persons with hyperlipidemia

COMMONLY ASSOCIATED CONDITIONS
DM

 DIAGNOSIS

HISTORY
Painless, slowly progressive visual loss; patients are generally unaware of the visual loss until late in the disease. Central visual acuity remains unaffected until late in the disease.

PHYSICAL EXAM
- Visual acuity and visual field assessment
- Ophthalmoscopy to assess optic nerve for glaucomatous damage
- Increased IOP
- CDR >0.5: Normal eyes show a characteristic configuration for disc rim thickness of inferior ≥ superior ≥ nasal ≥ temporal (ISNT rule).
- Earliest visual field defects are paracentral scotomas and peripheral nasal steps.

DIFFERENTIAL DIAGNOSIS
- Normal-tension glaucoma
- Optic nerve pits
- Anterior ischemic optic neuropathy
- Compressive lesions of the optic nerve or chiasm
- Posthemorrhagic (shock optic neuropathy)

DIAGNOSTIC TESTS & INTERPRETATION
Initial Tests (lab, imaging)
Optical coherence tomography can be useful in the detection of glaucoma by measuring the thickness of the retinal nerve fiber layer (RNFL).
- RNFL is thinner in patients with glaucoma.
- RNFL tends to be thinner with older age, in Caucasians, greater axial length, and smaller optic disc area.

Diagnostic Procedures/Other
- Visual field testing: perimetry
  - A multifocal intraocular lens may reduce visual sensitivity on standard automated perimetry.
- Tonometry to measure IOP

Test Interpretation
- Atrophy and cupping of optic nerve
- Loss of retinal ganglion cells (RGCs) and their axons produces defects and thinning in the RNFL.
- Significant RGC loss may occur at specific location before corresponding visual field loss is detected (3)[B].

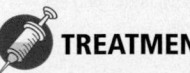 **TREATMENT**

GENERAL MEASURES
- Early Manifest Glaucoma Trial
  - Early treatment delays progression.
  - The magnitude of initial IOP reduction influences disease progression (4)[A].
- Ocular Hypertension Treatment Study
  - Patients who only had increased IOP in the range of 24 to 32 mm Hg were treated with topical ocular hypotensive medication.
  - Treatment produced ~20% reduction in IOP

- At 5 years, treatment reduced the incidence of POAG by >50%: 9.5% in the observation group versus 4.4% in the medication-treated group (5)[A].
- The Advanced Glaucoma Intervention Study
  - Eyes were randomized to laser trabeculoplasty or filtering surgery when medical therapy failed.
  - In follow-up, if IOP was always <18 mm Hg, visual fields tended to stabilize. When IOP was >17 mm Hg, >1/2 the time, patients tended to have worsening of visual fields (6)[A].
  - Whites did better with trabeculectomy first whereas African Americans did better with argon laser trabeculoplasty as the initial procedure.
- Collaborative Initial Glaucoma Treatment Study
  - Both initial medical and surgical (trabeculectomy) treatment achieved significant IOP reduction, and both had little visual field loss over time (7)[A].
  - There was a 5-year risk of endophthalmitis of 1.1% after trabeculectomy (8)[A].

MEDICATION
- >1 medication, with different mechanisms of action, may be needed.
- When ≥3 medications are required, compliance is difficult, and surgery may be needed. Ocular hypotensive agent categories
  - β-Adrenergic antagonists (nonselective and selective): decrease aqueous formation; best when used as an add-on therapy: timolol 0.25% (initial) to 0.5% one drop in affected eye q12h; gel-forming solution (0.35% or 0.5%) one drop in affected eye once daily; betaxolol 0.5% one drop in affected eye twice daily
  - Parasympathomimetics (miotic), including cholinergic (direct-acting) and anticholinesterase agents (indirect-acting parasympathomimetic): increase aqueous outflow
    - Pilocarpine 1–4%: one drop in affected eye BID to QID (cholinergic)
- Carbonic anhydrase inhibitors (oral, topical): decrease aqueous formation
  - Acetazolamide: 250 mg PO 1 to 4 times per day
  - Dorzolamide 2%: one drop TID
  - Brinzolamide 1%: one drop TID
- Adrenergic agonists (nonselective and selective α_2-adrenergic agonists)
  - Epinephrine 0.5–2%: One drop BID and Propine (dipivefrin) 0.1% one drop BID are both nonselective agents that increase aqueous outflow through the trabecular meshwork and increase uveoscleral outflow.
  - Brimonidine tartrate 0.1%: One drop TID (α_2-adrenergic agonist) decreases aqueous formation and increases uveoscleral outflow.
- Prostaglandin analogues: enhance uveoscleral outflow and increase aqueous outflow through the trabecular meshwork: latanoprost 0.005% one drop at bedtime; travoprost 0.004% one drop at bedtime
- Hyperosmotic agents: increase blood osmolality, drawing water from the vitreous cavity
  - Mannitol 20% solution: administered IV at 2 g/kg of body weight
  - Glycerin 50% solution: administered PO; dosage is usually 4 to 7 oz.
- Contraindications/precautions
  - Nonselective β-adrenergic antagonists: Avoid in asthma, chronic obstructive pulmonary disease (COPD), 2nd- and 3rd-degree atrioventricular (A-V) block, and decompensated heart failure.

Betaxolol is a selective β-adrenergic antagonist and is safer in pulmonary disease.
– Parasympathomimetics (miotic): Indirect-acting parasympathomimetic agents increase risk of ocular and systemic side effects and are used rarely.
– Carbonic anhydrase inhibitors
  ○ Do not use with sulfa drug allergies.
  ○ Do not use with cirrhosis because of the risk of hepatic encephalopathy.
- Adrenergic agonists: Caution is recommended when using brimonidine and monoamine oxidase (MAO) inhibitor or tricyclic antidepressant (TCA) and in patients with vascular insufficiency. Brimonidine can cause excessive sleepiness and lethargy in children.
- Prostaglandin analogues: caution with uveitis and avoided during pregnancy
- Hyperosmotic agents
  – Glycerin can produce hyperglycemia or ketoacidosis in diabetic patients.
  – Can cause congestive heart failure
  – Do not use in patients with anuria.
- Precautions
  – β-Adrenergic antagonists: caution with obstructive pulmonary disease, heart failure, and DM
  – Parasympathomimetics (miotic): cause pupillary constriction and may cause decreased vision in patients with a cataract; may cause eye pain or myopia due to increased accommodation. All miotics break down the blood–aqueous barrier and may induce chronic iridocyclitis.
  – Adrenergic agonists (e.g., brimonidine): caution with vascular insufficiency
  – Contact lens wearers: Many products contain benzalkonium chloride; remove contact lens prior to administration and wait 15 minutes before reinsertion.
  – Prostaglandin analogues may cause increased pigmentation of the iris and periorbital tissue (eyelid).
    ○ Increased pigmentation and growth of eyelashes
    ○ Should be used with caution in active intraocular inflammation (iritis/uveitis)
    ○ Caution is also advised in eyes with risk factors for herpes simplex, iritis, and cystoid macular edema.
    ○ Macular edema may be a complication associated with treatment.
- Hyperosmotic agents: caution in diabetics; dehydrated patients; and those with cardiac, renal, and hepatic disease
- Significant possible interactions: β-adrenergic antagonists: caution in patients taking calcium antagonists because of possible A-V conduction disturbances, left ventricular failure, or hypotension
- Parasympathomimetics (miotic): Indirect-acting parasympathomimetic agents, anticholinesterase eye drops, can reduce serum pseudocholinesterase levels. If succinylcholine is used for induction of general anesthesia, prolonged apnea may result.

SURGERY/OTHER PROCEDURES
- Argon laser trabeculoplasty (ALT)
  – Can be applied up to 180 degrees of the trabecular meshwork
  – Improves aqueous outflow
  – The Glaucoma Laser Trial Research Group showed in newly diagnosed, previously untreated patients with POAG that ALT was as effective as topical glaucoma medication within the first 2 years of follow-up.
  – Usually reserved for patients needing better IOP control while taking topical glaucoma drops
- Selective laser trabeculoplasty (SLT)
  – 532-nm Nd:YAG laser
  – Appears to be as effective as ALT in lowering IOP

- Trabeculectomy (glaucoma filtering surgery)
  – Usually reserved for patients needing better IOP control after maximal medical therapy and who may have previously undergone an ALT
  – Mitomycin C can be applied at the time of surgery to increase the chances of a surgical success.
  – Subconjunctival bevacizumab may be a beneficial adjunctive therapy for reducing late surgical failure after trabeculectomy.
- Shunt (tube) surgery
  – For example, Molteno and Ahmed devices
  – Generally reserved for difficult glaucoma cases in which conventional filtering surgery has failed or is likely to fail
- Tube Versus Trabeculectomy (TVT) Study
  – After 5 years of follow-up, both procedures were associated with similar IOP reduction and the number of glaucoma medications needed (9)[A].
- Ciliary body ablation: indicated to lower IOP in patients with poor visual potential or those who are poor candidates for filtering or shunt procedures
- Canaloplasty can control IOP in patients with POAG. Canaloplasty involves the placement of a microcatheter circumferentially through Schlemm canal, vasodilation of the canal, and placement of a nylon tensioning suture.
- Cataract extraction can decrease IOP in patients with ocular hypertension (10)[A].

 ONGOING CARE

FOLLOW-UP RECOMMENDATIONS
Patient Monitoring
- Monitor vision and IOP every 3 to 6 months.
- Visual field testing every 6 to 18 months
- Optic nerve evaluation every 3 to 18 months, depending on POAG control
- A worsening of the mean deviation by 2 dB on the Humphrey field analyzer and confirmed by a single test after 6 months had a 72% probability of progression.
- The IOP response to ocular hypotensive agents tends to be reduced in persons with thicker corneas.

PATIENT EDUCATION
POAG is a silent robber of vision, and patients may not appreciate the significance of their disease until much of their visual field is lost.

PROGNOSIS
- With standard glaucoma therapy, the rate of visual field loss in POAG is slow.
- Patients still may lose vision and develop blindness, even when treated appropriately.
- The rate of legal blindness from POAG over a follow-up of 22 years is 19%.
- The rate of progression of visual field loss increases with older age.

COMPLICATIONS
Blindness

REFERENCES
1. Zhao D, Cho J, Kim MH, et al. The association of blood pressure and primary open-angle glaucoma: a meta-analysis. *Am J Ophthalmol*. 2014;158(3):615.e9–627.e9.
2. Medeiros FA, Meira-Freitas D, Lisboa R, et al. Corneal hysteresis as a risk factor for glaucoma

progression: a prospective longitudinal study. *Ophthalmology*. 2013;120(8):1533–1540.
3. Alasil T, Wang K, Yu F, et al. Correlation of retinal nerve fiber layer thickness and visual fields in glaucoma: a broken stick model. *Am J Ophthalmol*. 2014;157(5):953–959.
4. Heijl A, Leske MC, Bengtsson B, et al. Reduction of intraocular pressure and glaucoma progression: results from the Early Manifest Glaucoma Trial. *Arch Ophthalmol*. 2002;120(10):1268–1279.
5. Kass MA, Heuer DK, Higginbotham EJ, et al. The Ocular Hypertension Treatment Study: a randomized trial determines that topical ocular hypotensive medication delays or prevents the onset of primary open-angle glaucoma. *Arch Ophthalmol*. 2002;120(6):701–713.
6. The Advanced Glaucoma Intervention Study (AGIS): 7. The relationship between control of intraocular pressure and visual field deterioration. *Am J Ophthalmol*. 2000;130(4):429–440.
7. Lichter PR, Musch DC, Gillespie BW, et al. Interim clinical outcomes in the Collaborative Initial Glaucoma Treatment Study comparing initial treatment randomized to medications or surgery. *Ophthalmology*. 2001;108(11):1943–1953.
8. Zahid S, Musch DC, Nizol LM, et al. Risk of endophthalmitis and other long-term complications of trabeculectomy in the Collaborative Initial Glaucoma Treatment Study (CIGTS). *Am J Ophthalmol*. 2013;155(4):674–680, 680.e1.
9. Gedde SJ, Schiffman JC, Feuer WI, et al. Treatment outcomes in the Tube Versus Trabeculectomy (TVT) Study after five years of follow-up. *Am J Ophthalmol*. 2012;153(5):789.e2–803.e2.
10. Mansberger SL, Gordon MO, Jampel H, et al. Reduction in intraocular pressure after cataract extraction: the Ocular Hypertension Treatment Study. *Ophthalmology*. 2012;119(9):1826–1831.

ADDITIONAL READING
- Aychoua N, Junoy Montolio FG, Jansonius NM. Influence of multifocal intraocular lenses on standard automated perimetry test results. *JAMA Ophthalmol*. 2013;131(4):481–485.
- Lin CC, Hu CC, Ho JD, et al. Obstructive sleep apnea and increased risk of glaucoma: a population-based matched-cohort study. *Ophthalmology*. 2013;120(8):1559–1564.

CODES

ICD10
- H40.11X0 Primary open-angle glaucoma, stage unspecified
- H40.11X1 Primary open-angle glaucoma, mild stage
- H40.11X2 Primary open-angle glaucoma, moderate stage

CLINICAL PEARLS
- Topical or systemic steroids can cause the IOP to increase.
- Pain is not a frequent symptom of POAG.
- Painless, slowly progressive visual loss; patients generally are unaware of the visual loss until late in the disease. Central visual acuity remains unaffected until late in the disease.
- Patients still may lose vision and develop blindness, even when treated appropriately.

G

GLOMERULONEPHRITIS, ACUTE

Jonathan T. Lin, MD • Michael J. Ross, MD

 BASICS

DESCRIPTION
- Acute glomerulonephritis (GN) is an inflammatory process involving the glomerulus of the kidney, resulting in a clinical syndrome consisting of hematuria, proteinuria, and renal insufficiency, often in association with hypertension and edema.
- Acute GN may be caused by primary glomerular disease or secondary to systemic disease:
  - Postinfectious GN
  - IgA nephropathy/Henoch-Schönlein purpura (HSP)
  - Antiglomerular basement membrane disease (anti-GBM disease)
  - Antineutrophil cytoplasmic antibody (ANCA)–associated GN
  - Membranoproliferative GN (MPGN)
  - Lupus nephritis
  - Cryoglobulin-associated GN
- Clinical severity ranges from asymptomatic microscopic or gross hematuria to a rapid loss of kidney function over days to weeks, termed rapidly progressive GN (RPGN).

ALERT
Urgent investigation and treatment are required to avoid irreversible loss of kidney function.

EPIDEMIOLOGY
- Postinfectious GN
  - Most commonly follows group A β-hemolytic *Streptococcus* infection but can occur as a result of other bacterial infections or less commonly in the setting of viral or parasitic infections
  - Accounts for 80% of acute GN in children
  - May also occur in the setting of infective endocarditis
- IgA nephropathy
  - Most common form of primary acute GN
  - Occurs mainly in the 2nd and 3rd decades
  - Male > female (2:1)
  - Incidence differs geographically: Asia > United States
  - HSP typically childhood illness, usually <10 years old
- Anti-GBM disease
  - A notable cause of the pulmonary–renal syndrome known as Goodpasture disease
  - Peak distribution in 3rd and 6th decades
- ANCA-associated GN
  - Often has a relapsing and remitting course
  - Four disease presentations:
    - Granulomatosis with polyangiitis (GPA) formerly Wegener granulomatosis
    - Microscopic polyangiitis (MPA)
    - Isolated Pauci-immune GN—when isolated to kidneys
    - Eosinophilic granulomatosis with polyangiitis (EGPA), formerly Churg-Strauss disease—GN relatively common but renal involvement rarely severe
  - Older patients are more commonly affected, although this GN can affect any age group.
- MPGN
  - May be primary or secondary
  - May present in the setting of a systemic viral (hepatitis B or hepatitis C) or rheumatologic illness
  - Classification by immunofluorescence: immune complex mediated or complement

mediated (dense deposit disease [DDD] and C3 glomerulonephritis [C3GN])
  - Classification by electron microscopy: MPGN types I–III
- Lupus nephritis
  - 30–70% of systemic lupus patients will have renal involvement.
  - Several histologic variants but diffuse proliferative GN most severe and requires urgent treatment
- Cryoglobulin-associated vasculitis
  - 80% of cases are associated with hepatitis C infection.

ETIOLOGY AND PATHOPHYSIOLOGY
- In general, an immunologic mechanism triggers inflammation and proliferation of glomerular tissue.
- Postinfectious GN: immune complex disease with host immune reaction to nephritogenic strains of streptococci as a trigger
- IgA nephropathy: relates to an abnormal glycosylation of IgA
- Anti-GBM disease: caused by autoantibodies that target type IV collagen of basement membranes
- ANCA-associated GN: Autoantibodies against neutrophil granules are involved in the pathogenesis.
- MPGN: An immune or genetic etiology is presumed, which triggers glomerular deposits and inflammation.
- Lupus nephritis: an immune complex–mediated glomerular disease
- Cryoglobulin-associated GN: An immune etiology is presumed but not clearly defined.

Genetics
Genetic factors are likely to play a role in susceptibility to many of the acute GNs, although these have not been sufficiently defined to be clinically useful in most circumstances.

RISK FACTORS
- Epidemics of nephritogenic strains of streptococci are triggers for postinfectious GN.
- Hepatic cirrhosis, celiac disease, and HIV infection place patients at risk for IgA nephropathy.
- Anti-GBM disease has been associated with influenza A infection and inhaled hydrocarbon solvent exposure.
- ANCA-associated GN is increased in settings where there is increased silica exposure (i.e., earthquakes and farming).
- Infection with hepatitis B or C is known to be associated with MPGN.
- Infection with hepatitis C is a risk factor for developing cryoglobulinemic GN.
- Mutations in alternate complement pathway genes are associated with complement-mediated MPGN.

GENERAL PREVENTION
Early detection is paramount.

 DIAGNOSIS

HISTORY
- Patients may report cola- or tea-colored urine and decreased urine volume.
- Edema occurs in many patients, typically in face and lower extremities.
- Shortness of breath may occur with significant fluid overload.

- Generalized malaise
- Timing
  - Postinfectious GN typically occurs 1 to 3 weeks after pharyngitis or 2 to 6 weeks after skin infection.
  - IgA nephropathy may present within several days after an acute infection.
- Patients may also present with complaints more specific to the associated disease:
  - Joint pain or rash in lupus nephritis
  - Hemoptysis in pulmonary–renal syndromes (see "Physical Exam")
  - Sinusitis, pulmonary infiltrates, arthralgias in ANCA-associated GN
  - Abdominal or joint pain and purpura in IgA–HSP
  - Purpura and skin vasculitis in cryoglobulinemia-associated GN

PHYSICAL EXAM
- A complete physical exam may discover clues to systemic disease as a potential cause.
- Sinus disease: ANCA-associated GN, most commonly GPA
- Pharyngitis or impetigo: postinfectious GN or IgA nephropathy
- Pulmonary hemorrhage (pulmonary–renal syndrome): anti-GBM disease/Goodpasture, ANCA-associated GN, or lupus nephritis
- Hepatomegaly or liver tenderness could point to cryoglobulinemia-associated GN or IgA nephropathy.
- Purpura may point to ANCA-associated GN or HSP/IgA nephropathy.

DIFFERENTIAL DIAGNOSIS
Nonglomerular hematuria: trauma, prostate diseases, urologic cancer, cystitis, nephrolithiasis, renal cysts

DIAGNOSTIC TESTS & INTERPRETATION
Initial Tests (lab, imaging)
- Urinalysis with examination of sediment
  - Dysmorphic RBCs or RBC casts on urine microscopy indicate glomerular hematuria and strongly suggest the diagnosis of an acute GN.
  - Pyuria and white blood cell casts may also be present.
- Electrolytes, BUN, creatinine, CBC
- Antistreptolysin O titer, streptozyme: often positive in poststreptococcal GN
- Complement levels (C3, C4)
  - C3 complement levels are low in postinfectious GN.
  - C3 and C4 are abnormal in lupus nephritis and MPGN.
  - C4 can be low in cryoglobulinemia.
- Proteinuria: 24-hour collection or random urine protein/creatinine ratio
  - Typically mild to moderate proteinuria, sometimes nephrotic range
- Antinuclear antibody (ANA) to rule out lupus nephritis
- ANCA antibody screen: MPO and PR3 antibodies
- Anti-GBM antibody
- Hepatitis B surface antigen and antibody
- Hepatitis C antibody
- HIV testing
- A chest x-ray may be useful in the setting of hemoptysis or a suspected infiltrate on exam.

Test Interpretation
- Renal biopsy
- If clinical picture is consistent with postinfectious GN in a child, a biopsy may not be required.
- If there is clinical suspicion for other causes of acute GN, renal biopsy should be done.
- Light microscopy
  - Diffuse hypercellularity suggests a proliferative disease such as IgA nephropathy, lupus nephritis, or postinfectious GN.
  - Presence of glomerular crescents correlates with RPGN and disease severity.
- Immunofluorescence
  - Isolated mesangial IgA staining is pathognomonic for IgA nephropathy, with the absence of immune complex staining suggesting ANCA-associated GN.
  - Pattern of IgG, IgM, C3, and C4 staining may also aid in characterizing the GN.
  - Lupus nephritis typically positive for all immunoglobulins and complements ("full house")
- Electron microscopy: The location of immunoglobulin deposits is useful in pointing to a particular diagnosis.

 TREATMENT

Supportive in postinfectious GN

MEDICATION
First Line
- Hypertension
  - Diuretics are useful for management of salt retention and edema.
  - Calcium channel blockers
  - Avoid angiotensin-converting enzyme inhibitors (ACE-I) or angiotensin receptor blockers (ARBs) if acute renal dysfunction is present.
- Peripheral edema: Loop diuretics are often required due to the degree of edema.
- Pulmonary edema: oxygen and diuretics

Second Line
- Each of the glomerular diseases often requires a specific treatment plan based on renal biopsy results; therefore, a nephrologist is often the guiding care at this point.
- Empiric pulse methylprednisolone prior to kidney biopsy may be indicated in cases of RPGN (1)[C].
- Crescents on renal biopsy may be an indication for steroids in postinfectious GN and in other cases, are often an indication for potent immunosuppressive medications in addition to steroids (2)[C].
- Steroids plus either cyclophosphamide, rituximab, or mycophenolate may be used to treat ANCA-associated renal disease and proliferative forms of lupus nephritis (2–6)[A].
- Plasmapheresis may also be considered in some cases for RPGN or anti-GBM disease or ANCA-associated renal disease with diffuse pulmonary hemorrhage (2)[C],(4,7)[A].
- Dialysis may be needed for uremia, hyperkalemia refractory to medical management, intractable acidosis, and diuretic-resistant pulmonary edema.
- IgA nephropathy: ACE-Is or ARBs recommended for patients with proteinuria (1,2)[C], selected patients may benefit from immunosuppression.

ISSUES FOR REFERRAL
Consultation with a nephrologist is usually required to assist with renal biopsy to confirm diagnosis and assist with management.

INPATIENT CONSIDERATIONS
Admission Criteria/Initial Stabilization
Consider admission for patients with no urine output, rapidly deteriorating renal function, significant hypertension, and suspicion of pulmonary hemorrhage or fluid overload that is compromising heart or respiratory function.

Discharge Criteria
Hemodynamically stable patients without complications may be managed as outpatients.

 ONGOING CARE

FOLLOW-UP RECOMMENDATIONS
Patient Monitoring
- Depends on type of GN
- Regular BP checks and urinalysis to detect recurrence, assessment of renal function to detect acute or follow chronic renal disease as a result of the primary event, and regular clinical assessment to detect suspicious symptoms that may herald a recurrence (i.e., rash, joint complaint, hemoptysis)
- Periodic reassessment of serology tests to detect asymptomatic individuals

DIET
- No-added-salt diet and fluid restriction until edema and hypertension clear
- Avoid high-potassium foods if significant renal dysfunction is present.

PATIENT EDUCATION
- National Kidney Foundation, https://www.kidney.org/atoz/content/glomerul

PROGNOSIS
- In general, the prognosis depends on the cause of the GN.
- The GN may be self-limited (as often is the case in postinfectious GN) or part of a chronic disease that makes the possibility of recurrence of acute disease likely, with the potential for progressive loss of renal function over time.
- Some forms of acute GN (including ANCA associated and severe lupus) require long-term immunosuppression to prevent recurrence.

COMPLICATIONS
- Hypertensive retinopathy and encephalopathy
- RPGN
- Microscopic hematuria may persist for years.
- Chronic kidney disease
- Nephrotic syndrome (~10%)

REFERENCES
1. Chadban SJ, Atkins RC. Glomerulonephritis. *Lancet.* 2005;365(9473):1797–1806.
2. Beck L, Bomback AS, Choi MJ, et al. KDOQI US commentary on the 2012 KDIGO clinical practice guideline for glomerulonephritis. *Am J Kidney Dis.* 2013;62(3):403–441. doi:10.1053/j.ajkd.2013.06.002.
3. Hahn BH, McMahon MA, Wilkinson A, et al. American College of Rheumatology guidelines for screening, treatment, and management of lupus nephritis. *Arthritis Care Res (Hoboken).* 2012;64(6):797–808. doi:10.1002/acr.21664.
4. Walters G, Willis NS, Craig JC. Interventions for renal vasculitis in adults. *Cochrane Database Syst Rev.* 2008;(3):CD003232. doi:10.1002/14651858.CD003232.pub2.
5. Stone JH, Merkel PA, Spiera R, et al. Rituximab versus cyclophosphamide for ANCA-associated vasculitis. *N Engl J Med.* 2010;363(3):221–232. doi:10.1056/NEJMoa0909905.
6. Bomback AS, Appel GB. Updates on the treatment of lupus nephritis. *J Am Soc Nephrol.* 2010;21(12):2028–2035. doi:10.1681/ASN.2010050472.
7. Jayne DR, Gaskin G, Rasmussen N, et al. Randomized trial of plasma exchange or high-dosage methylprednisolone as adjunctive therapy for severe renal vasculitis. *J Am Soc Nephrol.* 2007;18(7):2180–2188.

 SEE ALSO

- Acute Kidney Injury (Acute Renal Failure); Glomerulonephritis, Postinfectious; Henoch-Schönlein Purpura; Hyperkalemia; Hypertensive Emergencies; IgA Nephropathy; Nephrotic Syndrome; Vasculitis
- Algorithm: Hematuria

 CODES

ICD10
- N00.9 Acute nephritic syndrome with unsp morphologic changes
- N00.2 Acute nephritic syndrome w diffuse membranous glomrlneph
- N00.8 Acute nephritic syndrome with other morphologic changes

CLINICAL PEARLS
- Dysmorphic RBCs and RBC casts are a key component of the urinalysis in GN.
- Postinfectious GN in children is typically a self-limited disease.
- Searching for other organ involvement is useful in establishing a definitive diagnosis.
- With the discovery of a GN, monitor the initial renal function labs frequently to identify a RPGN.

G

GLOMERULONEPHRITIS, POSTINFECTIOUS

Rebecca S. Domalski, DO • Theodore B. Flaum, DO, FACOFP

 BASICS

DESCRIPTION
Postinfectious glomerulonephritis (PIGN) is an immune complex disease preceded by nonrenal infection with certain strains of bacteria, most commonly *Streptococcus* and *Staphylococcus*. The most common form of PIGN, poststreptococcal glomerulonephritis (PSGN), predominantly affects children. The clinical presentation varies from asymptomatic to the acute nephritic syndrome, characterized by gross hematuria, proteinuria, edema, hypertension (HTN), and acute kidney injury.

EPIDEMIOLOGY
A global decline in incidence, especially in developed countries is attributed to better hygiene and a decreased incidence of streptococcal skin infections: Of cases, 97% occur in developing countries. PSGN is primarily a pediatric disease, but a recent increase has been seen in nonstreptococcal GN in adults.

Incidence
- Pediatrics: 24.3 cases/100,000 persons per year in developing countries; 6 cases/100,000 persons per year in developed countries
- Adults: 2 cases/100,000 persons per year in developing countries; 0.3 cases/100,000 persons per year in developed countries
- Worldwide, 34% of cases are now seen in adults with a global burden of 68,000 cases per year.
- Male > female (2:1) (1)

ETIOLOGY AND PATHOPHYSIOLOGY
- Glomerular immune complex disease induced by specific nephritogenic strains of bacteria:
  - Group A β-hemolytic *Streptococcus* (GAS)
  - Staphylococcus (predominantly *Staphylococcus aureus*; more commonly methicillin-resistant *S. aureus* [MRSA], occasionally coagulase-negative *Staphylococcus*)
  - Gram-negative bacteria including *Escherichia coli*, *Yersinia*, *Pseudomonas*, and *Haemophilus* (1)
- Proposed mechanisms for the glomerular injury (2):
  - Deposition of circulating immune complexes with streptococcal or staphylococcal antigens—these complexes can be detected in patients with streptococcal- or staphylococcal-related GN but do not correlate to disease activity (3).
  - In situ immune complex formation from deposition of antigens within the glomerular basement membrane (GBM) and subsequent antibody binding
  - In situ glomerular immune complex formation promoted by antibodies to streptococcal or staphylococcal antigens
  - Alteration of normal renal antigen leading to molecular mimicry that elicits an autoimmune response
- Glomerular immune complex causing complement activation and inflammation:
  - Nephritis-associated plasmin receptor (NAPlr): activates plasmin, contributes to activation of the alternative complement pathway

- Streptococcal pyrogenic exotoxin B (SPE B): binds plasmin and acts as a protease; promotes the release of inflammatory mediators
- Activation of the alternative complement pathway causes initial glomerular injury as evidenced by C3 deposition and decreased levels of serum C3. The lectin pathway of complement activation has also been recently implicated in glomerular injury (4).

RISK FACTORS
- Children 5 to 12 years of age
- Older patients (>65 years of age) (1):
  - Patients with immunocompromising comorbid conditions
  - Diabetes
  - Alcohol abuse

GENERAL PREVENTION
- Early antibiotic treatment for streptococcal and staphylococcal infections, when indicated, although efficacy in preventing GN is uncertain
- Improved hygiene
- Prophylactic penicillin treatment to be used in closed communities and household contacts of index cases in areas where PIGN is prevalent

COMMONLY ASSOCIATED CONDITIONS
Streptococcal infection, staphylococcal infection

 DIAGNOSIS

HISTORY
- Patients present with acute nephritic syndrome, characterized by sudden onset of hematuria associated with edema and HTN 1 to 2 weeks after an infection
- A triad of edema, hematuria, and HTN is classic.
- Urine described as "tea-colored" or "cola-colored."
- PIGN in children usually follows GAS skin/throat infection.
- The latent period between GAS infection and PIGN depends on the site of infection: 1 to 3 weeks following GAS pharyngitis and 3 to 6 weeks following GAS skin infection.

- Adult PIGN most commonly follows staphylococcal infections (3 times more common than streptococcal infections) of the upper respiratory tract, skin, heart, lung, bone, or urinary tract. Studies show 7–16% of cases of adult PIGN have no preceding evidence of infection and, in 24–59% the offending microorganism cannot be identified (5)[A].

PHYSICAL EXAM
- Edema: present in ~2 of 3 adult patients due to sodium and water retention; less common in pediatric patients
- Gross hematuria: present in 25–60% of patients
- HTN: present in 80–90% of patients and varies from mild to severe; secondary to fluid retention Hypertensive encephalopathy is an uncommon but serious complication
- Microscopic hematuria: subclinical cases of PIGN
- Respiratory distress: due to pulmonary edema (rare)

DIFFERENTIAL DIAGNOSIS
The diagnosis of PIGN is generally by history once the diagnosis of acute nephritis is made, with documentation of a recent infection and nephritis beginning to resolve 1 to 2 weeks after presentation. However, with progressive disease >2 weeks, persistent hematuria/HTN >4 to 6 weeks, or no adequate documentation of a GAS or other infection, the differential diagnosis of GN needs to be considered and renal biopsy ordered:

- Membranoproliferative glomerulonephritis (MPGN): The presentation of MPGN may be indistinguishable initially with hematuria, HTN, proteinuria, and hypocomplementemia after an upper respiratory infection. However, patients with MPGN continue to have persistent nephritis and hypocomplementemia beyond 4 to 6 weeks and possibly also have a further elevation in serum creatinine. Patients with PIGN tend to have resolution of their disease and a return of normal C3 and CH50 levels within 2 to 4 weeks.
- Secondary causes of GN: Lupus nephritis and Henoch-Schönlein purpura nephritis have features similar to PIGN. Extrarenal manifestations and laboratory tests for these underlying systemic diseases help differentiate them from PIGN. Hypocomplementemia is not characteristic of Henoch-Schönlein purpura and the hypocomplementemia that occurs in lupus nephritis is with reductions in both C3 and C4, whereas C4 levels are normal in PIGN.
- IgA nephropathy often presents after an upper respiratory infection. It can be distinguished from PIGN based on a shorter time frame between the upper respiratory illness and hematuria, as well as history of gross hematuria, as PIGN recurrence is rare. IgA nephropathy is a chronic illness and will recur. Patients with IgA nephropathy have normal C3/C4 levels.
  - Note: IgA-dominant PIGN is a newly recognized form of PIGN occurring in poststaphylococcal GN. This differs from primary IgA nephropathy in that these patients do not have a history of renal disease (1)[A].
- Pauci-immune crescentic GN: In elderly patients with severe renal failure and active urine sediment, this is much more common, so antineutrophil cytoplasmic antibody (ANCA) testing should be done (1)[A].

DIAGNOSTIC TESTS & INTERPRETATION
Initial Tests (labs, imaging)
Urinalysis shows hematuria; can be with/without RBC casts and pyuria. Proteinuria is present, but nephrotic range proteinuria is uncommon in children (more likely in adults).

Follow-Up Tests & Special Considerations
- Culture: PSGN usually presents weeks after a GAS infection; only ~25% of patients will have either a positive throat or skin culture.
- Complement: 90% of pediatric patients (slightly fewer adult patients) will have depressed C3 and CH50 levels in the first 2 weeks of the disease, whereas C2 and C4 levels remain normal. C3 and CH50 levels return to normal within 4 to 8 weeks after presentation.

- Creatinine: elevated to the point of renal insufficiency in 25–83% of cases, more commonly in adults (83%) (4)[A].
- Serology: Elevated titers of antibodies support evidence of a recent GAS infection. Streptozyme test measuring antistreptolysin O (ASO), antihyaluronidase (AHase), antistreptokinase (ASKase), anti–nicotinamide-adenine dinucleotidase (anti-NAD), and anti-DNAse B antibodies: positive in >95% of patients with PSGN due to pharyngitis and 80% with skin infections. In pharyngeal infection, ASO, anti-DNAse B, anti-NAD, and AHase titers are elevated. In skin infections, only the anti-DNAse and AHase titers are typically elevated.

Diagnostic Procedures/Other
Renal biopsy is rarely done in children; recommended in most adults to confirm the diagnosis and rule out other glomerulopathies with similar clinical presentations that require immunosuppressive treatment.

Test Interpretation
- Light microscopy: diffuse proliferative glomerulonephritis with prominent endocapillary proliferation and numerous neutrophils within the capillary lumen. Deposits may also be found in the mesangium ("starry sky"). Severity of involvement varies and correlates with clinical findings. Crescent formation is uncommon and is associated with a poor prognosis.
- Immunofluorescence microscopy: Deposits of C3 and IgG distributed in a diffuse granular pattern.
- Electron microscopy: dome-shaped subepithelial electron-dense deposits that are referred to as "humps." These deposits are immune complexes, and they correspond to the deposits of IgG and C3 found on immunofluorescence. Rate of clearance of these deposits affects recovery time.
- Renal biopsy: usually not performed in most patients to confirm the diagnosis of PIGN as clinical history is highly suggestive and resolution of PIGN typically begins within 1 week of presentation. A biopsy is done when other glomerular disorders are being considered, such as in the case of persistently low C3 levels beyond 6 weeks for possible diagnosis of MPGN, recurrent episodes of hematuria suggestive of IgA nephropathy, or a progressive increase in serum creatinine not characteristic of PIGN.

TREATMENT

MEDICATION
- No specific therapy exists for PIGN, and no randomized controlled trials indicate that aggressive immunosuppressive therapy has a beneficial effect in patients with rapidly progressive crescentic disease. Despite this, patients with >30% crescents on renal biopsy are often treated with steroids (4)[A].

- Older patients often require hospitalization to prevent and treat complications of heart failure (HF) from volume overload (1).
- Management is supportive, with focus on treating the clinical manifestations of PIGN. These include HTN and pulmonary edema:
  - General measures include salt and water restriction and loop diuretics.
  - Calcium channel blockers/angiotensin-converting enzyme (ACE) inhibitors may be used in cases of severe HTN (4)[A].
- Patients with evidence of persistent bacterial infection should be given a course of antibiotic therapy.

SURGERY/OTHER PROCEDURES
Acute dialysis is required in approximately 50% of elderly patients (1).

ONGOING CARE

FOLLOW-UP RECOMMENDATIONS
Patient Monitoring
- Repeat urinalysis to check for clearance of hematuria and/or proteinuria.
- Consider other diagnosis if no improvement within 2 weeks.
- Recurrence is rare.

DIET
Renal diet if requiring instances of dialysis

PROGNOSIS
- Most children with PIGN have an excellent outcome, with >90% of cases achieving full recovery of renal function.
- Elderly patients, especially adults, develop HTN, recurrent proteinuria, and renal insufficiency long after the initial illness. Adults with multiple comorbid factors have the worst prognosis and highest incidence of chronic renal injury following PIGN (1).
- Complete remission in adult PIGN is only 26–56%. This has declined since the 1990s, suggesting prognosis is worsening (5).
- The presence of diabetes, higher creatinine levels, and more severe glomerular disease (e.g., crescents) on biopsy are all risk factors for developing end-stage renal disease (1).

REFERENCES
1. Nasr SH, Radhakrishnan J, D'Agati VD. Bacterial infection-related glomerulonephritis in adults. *Kidney Int*. 2013;83(5):792–803.
2. Nadasdy T, Hebert LA. Infection-related glomerulonephritis: understanding mechanisms. *Semin Nephrol*. 2011;31(4):369–375.
3. Uchida T, Oda T, Watanabe A, et al. Clinical and histologic resolution of poststreptococcal glomerulonephritis with large subendothelial deposits and kidney failure. *Am J Kidney Dis*. 2011;58(1):113–117.
4. Ramdani B, Zamd M, Hachim K, et al. Acute postinfectious glomerulonephritis. *Nephrol Ther*. 2012;8(4):247–258.
5. Wen YK. Clinicopathological study of infection-associated glomerulonephritis in adults. *Int Urol Nephrol*. 2010;42(2):477–485.

ADDITIONAL READING
- Eison TM, Ault BH, Jones DP, et al. Post-streptococcal acute glomerulonephritis in children: clinical features and pathogenesis. *Pediatr Nephrol*. 2011;26(2):165–180.
- Nasr SH, Fidler ME, Valeri AM, et al. Postinfectious glomerulonephritis in the elderly. *J Am Soc Nephrol*. 2011;22(1):187–195.
- Nast CC. Infection-related glomerulonephritis: changing demographics and outcomes. *Adv Chronic Kidney Dis*. 2012;19(2):68–75.
- Rodriguez-Iturbe B, Musser JM. The current state of poststreptococcal glomerulonephritis. *J Am Soc Nephrol*. 2008;19(10):1855–1864.
- Singh GR. Glomerulonephritis and managing the risks of chronic renal disease. *Pediatr Clin North Am*. 2009;56(6):1363–1382.

CODES

ICD10
- N05.9 Unsp nephritic syndrome with unspecified morphologic changes
- N00.9 Acute nephritic syndrome with unsp morphologic changes

CLINICAL PEARLS
- PIGN is an immune complex disease occurring after infection with certain strains of bacteria, most commonly group A *Streptococcus pyogenes*.
- The clinical presentation varies from asymptomatic to the acute nephritic syndrome, characterized by gross hematuria, proteinuria, edema, HTN, and acute kidney injury.
- Treatment is primarily supportive and includes treating HTN and edema, along with antibiotics for any ongoing bacterial infection.
- Persistent nephritis and low C3 levels for >2 weeks should prompt evaluation for other causes of GN, such as MPGN or systemic lupus erythematosus nephritis.

G

GLUCOSE INTOLERANCE

Kristina McGraw, DO • Jennifer Lee, DO • Robert A. Baldor, MD, FAAFP

 BASICS

DESCRIPTION
- Glucose intolerance is a chronic condition defined as blood glucose higher than considered normal, yet does not meet criteria levels for diabetes.
- Individuals with impaired fasting glucose (IFG) and/or impaired glucose intolerance (IGT) have been referred to as having prediabetes:
  – IFG: 100 to 125 mg/dL
  – IGT: 140 to 199 mg/dL 2 hours after ingestion of 75 g oral glucose load
  – Hemoglobin A1c as a screening test 5.7–6.4% (1)

EPIDEMIOLOGY
- As of 2010, it is estimated that one of every three U.S. adults ≥20 years of age have prediabetes (2).
- An estimated 86 million people in the United States are living with prediabetes.
- Only 11% of people with prediabetes are aware of their condition (3).
- Prediabetes has a 37% prevalence among adults >20 years old and 51% of adults ≤65 years in the United States (4).

Incidence
- 15–30% of people with prediabetes will develop type 2 diabetes within 5 years.
- Prospective studies indicate that A1c range of 5.5–6.0% have a 5-year cumulative incidence from 9% to 25% for developing diabetes (2).
- Highest incidence in American Indians/Alaska Natives, non-Hispanic blacks, and Hispanics (2)

ETIOLOGY AND PATHOPHYSIOLOGY
Insulin resistance and progressive insulin secretory defect (5)

RISK FACTORS
- Body mass index (BMI) ≥25: overweight
- Obesity and metabolic syndrome
- 10-fold risk increase for future diabetes in A1c ranges 5.7–6.4%
- History of gestational diabetes (GDM)
- Sedentary lifestyle
- Glucocorticoids and antipsychotic use

GENERAL PREVENTION
- Lifestyle modification with weight reduction and increased physical activity
- A decrease in excess body fat provides the greatest risk reduction.
- Medical therapy: weight loss medications
  – Phentermine
  – Orlistat
  – Lorcaserin
  – Phentermine topiramate ER
- Surgical therapy (BMI ≥35)
  – Lap band
  – Gastric sleeve
  – Gastric bypass
- Patients with other cardiovascular risk factors (e.g., dyslipidemia, hypertension, obesity, tobacco use) should receive appropriate counseling to modify diet and exercise.

Pregnancy Considerations
- Screening for diabetes in pregnancy is based on risk factor analysis:
  – High risk: first prenatal visit
  – Average risk: 24 to 28 weeks' gestation
- Women with GDM should be screened for diabetes 6 to 12 weeks' postpartum (6).

COMMONLY ASSOCIATED CONDITIONS
- Obesity (abdominal and visceral obesity)
- Dyslipidemia with high triglycerides (TG)
- Metabolic syndrome
- PCOS
- GDM
- Low HDL
- HTN
- Congenital diseases (Down, Turner, Klinefelter, and Wolfram syndromes)

 DIAGNOSIS

Who to screen
- BMI ≥25
- Age >45 years
- First-degree relative with diabetes
- Low HDL <35 mg/dL
- High TG >250 mg/dL
- HTN: BP >140/90 mm Hg or on treatment
- Hx of GDM
- Physical inactivity
- Hx of cardiovascular disease
- Ethnic group at increased risk (non-Hispanic black, Native American, Hispanics, Asian American, Pacific Islander)
- HgbA1c ≥5.7%, IGT, or IFG on previous testing
- PCOS
- Conditions associated with insulin resistance such as severe obesity or acanthosis nigricans

HISTORY
- No clear symptoms
- Polyuria
- Polydipsia
- Weight loss
- Blurred vision
- Polyphagia

PHYSICAL EXAM
- General physical exam
- BMI assessment

DIFFERENTIAL DIAGNOSIS
- Type A insulin resistance
- Leprechaunism
- Rabson-Mendenhall syndrome
- Lipoatrophic diabetes
- Pancreatitis
- Cystic fibrosis
- Hemochromatosis
- Acromegaly

- Cushing syndrome
- Glucagonoma
- Pheochromocytoma
- Hyperthyroidism
- Somatostatinoma
- Aldosteronoma
- Drug-induced hyperglycemia
  – Thiazide diuretics (high doses)
  – β-blockers
  – Corticosteroids (including inhaled corticosteroids)
  – Thyroid hormone
  – α-Interferon
  – Pentamidine
  – Protease inhibitors
  – Atypical antipsychotics

DIAGNOSTIC TESTS & INTERPRETATION
Initial Tests (lab, imaging)
- Fasting glucose
- 2-Hour OGTT
- HbA1c
- Repeat screen at least at 3-year intervals with normal results or sooner depending on risk status (5).

Follow-Up Tests & Special Considerations
- Fasting lipid profile
- Creatinine and GFR
- Urinalysis
- Microalbumin-to-creatinine ratio
- Thyroid-stimulating hormone with free T$_4$

 TREATMENT

- Lifestyle aimed at increasing physical activity and weight loss prevents or delays the development of diabetes in people with IGT and IFG (6)[C].

- Exercise and lifestyle:
  – At least 150 minute/week of moderate-intensity aerobic exercise and/or at least 90 minute/week of vigorous aerobic exercise
  – Resistance exercise improves insulin sensitivity to the same extent as aerobic exercise; resistance training 3 times per week is recommended for those with type 2 diabetes
  – Smoking cessation
- Follow-up counseling (6)[B]
- Diabetes prevention programs are cost effective (6)[B].

  – Diabetes prevention program (participants <60 years of age, BMI ≥35 kg/m^2, women with a history of gestational diabetes) showed that loss of weight through diet and exercise reduces risk of developing diabetes by 58% and demonstrated that lifestyle modification decreases risk of diabetes more than metformin.

- Because of its effectiveness, low cost, and long-term safety, the ADA recommends consideration of metformin for prevention of diabetes in individuals with IGT [A], IFG [C], or an A1c 5.7–6.4% [C], especially for those with BMI >35kg/m^2, aged <60 years, and women with history of GDM [A].

- Dietary recommendations:
  - Either low-carbohydrate, low-fat calorie-restricted, or Mediterranean diets may be effective.
  - Diets high in fiber-rich foods, such as vegetables, fruits, whole grains, seeds, and nuts plus white meat sources are protective against type 2 diabetes (7).
  - Restrict beverages containing simple sugars, as they increase risk of diabetes (7).
  - Intake of polyunsaturated fatty acid (PUFA) may improve glycemic control; however, data is inconsistent regarding PUFA and other types of fatty acids (7).
  - Individuals who have prediabetes or diabetes should receive individualized medical nutrition therapy (MNT) as needed to achieve treatment goals, preferably provided by a registered dietitian familiar with the components of diabetes MNT (6).

MEDICATION

First Line
Metformin (drug of choice) 500 mg BID or 850 mg daily may reduce incidence of new-onset diabetes and BMI (level 2); contraindicated with Cr >1.5 in males and >1.4 in females increases risk of lactic acidosis (6).

Second Line
Acarbose: started as 50 mg PO once daily and titrated to 100 mg PO TID, may reduce incidence of diabetes; GI upset is common (7).

ISSUES FOR REFERRAL
- Nutritionist
- Diabetes educator/registered dietitian upon diagnosis
- Exercise physiologist
- Lifestyle coaching

ADDITIONAL THERAPIES
- Weight loss of 5–10% improves glycemic control, increases insulin sensitivity, improves lipids, and lowers BP.
- Alternative/botanical therapy:
  - Fenugreek, bitter melon, and cinnamon have reduced hyperglycemia and improved insulin sensitivity in studies by Deng (8) and Graf et al. (9).

ONGOING CARE

FOLLOW-UP RECOMMENDATIONS
Patient Monitoring
- Consider self-monitoring of blood glucose.
- At least annual monitoring for development of diabetes with HbA1c, 2-hour OGTT, or fasting glucose
- BP should be routinely measured.
- Annual testing for lipid abnormalities and microalbuminuria (for detection and therapy modification of incipient diabetic nephropathy)

DIET
- Monitor carbohydrate intake.
- Macronutrient distribution should be based on individual assessment of eating patterns, preferences, and metabolic goals.
- Consider Mediterranean diet.

- Maximize low glycemic index foods.
- Low-fat (<25%) intake: Saturated fat intake should be <7% of total calories.
- Minimize *trans* fat intake.
- Low-sodium intake <2,300 mg/day
- High-fiber (~50 g/day; 14 g/1,000 kcal) and whole-grain intake
- Drink ample quantities of water, minimum of 64 oz of water daily, and strictly avoid sugar-sweetened beverages.
- Moderate alcohol intake: 1 drink/day for women; 2 drinks/day for men

PROGNOSIS
- Individuals with IFG and/or IGT have high risk for the future development of diabetes.
- Prediabetes increases the risk of developing type 2 diabetes, heart disease, and stroke.
- The potential impact of interventions to reduce mortality or the incidence of cardiovascular disease has not been demonstrated to date.
- 20–70% of individuals with prediabetes who do not lose weight, change their dietary habits, and/or engage in moderate physical activity will progress to type 2 diabetes within 3 to 6 years (7).
- HbA1c >6.5% at age 12 to 39 years associated with increased risk of death before age 55 years compared with HbA1c <5.7%

COMPLICATIONS
- Cardiovascular disease
- PAD
- Stroke: 2 to 4 times higher risk
- Ketoacidosis
- Sexual dysfunction
- Gastroparesis
- Nephropathy and potential for renal failure
- Retinopathy and potential for loss of vision
- Peripheral and autonomic neuropathy

REFERENCES

1. Nathan DM, Davidson MB, DeFronzo RA, et al. Impaired fasting glucose and impaired glucose tolerance: implications for care. *Diabetes Care*. 2007;30(3):753–759.
2. Centers for Disease Control and Prevention. *National Diabetes Statistics Report: Estimates of Diabetes and Its Burden in the United States*, 2014. Atlanta, GA: U.S. Department of Health and Human Services; 2014.
3. Centers for Disease Control and Prevention. Awareness of prediabetes—United States, 2005–2010. *MMWR Morb Mortal Weekly Rep*. 2013:62(11):209–212.
4. Centers for Disease Control and Prevention. Prediabetes facts. http://www.cdc.gov/diabetes/basics/prediabetes.html. Accessed 2014.
5. American Diabetes Association. Diagnosis and classification of diabetes mellitus. *Diabetes Care*. 2014;37(Suppl 1):S81–S90.
6. American Diabetes Association. Standards of medical care in diabetes—2014. *Diabetes Care*. 2014;37(Suppl 1):S14–S80.
7. Stull AJ. Lifestyle approaches and glucose intolerance [published online ahead of print October 14, 2014]. *Am J Lifestyle Med*. doi: 10.1177/1559827614554186.
8. Deng R. A review of the hypoglycemia effects of five commonly used herbal food supplements. *Recent Pat Food Nutr Agric*. 2012;4(1):50–60.
9. Graf BL, Raskin I, Cefalu WT, et al. Plant-derived therapeutics for the treatment of metabolic syndrome. *Curr Opin Investig Drugs*. 2010;11(10):1107–1115.

ADDITIONAL READING
- Maruthur NM, Ma Y, Delahanty LM, et al. Early response to preventive strategies in the Diabetes Prevention Program. *J Gen Intern Med*. 2013;28(12):1629–1636.
- Ramachandran A, Riddle MC, Kabali C, et al. Relationship between A1C and fasting plasma glucose in dysglycemia or type 2 diabetes: an analysis of baseline data from the ORIGIN trial. *Diabetes Care*. 2012;35(4):749–753.

CODES

ICD10
- E74.39 Other disorders of intestinal carbohydrate absorption
- R73.09 Other abnormal glucose
- R73.01 Impaired fasting glucose

CLINICAL PEARLS
- Lifestyle optimization is essential for all patients with prediabetes.
- Research shows that you can lower your risk for type 2 diabetes by 58% by losing 7% of your body weight (or 15 lb if you weigh 200 lb).
- Exercising moderately (such as brisk walking) 30 minutes/day, 5 days a week
- Consider concurrent cardiovascular risks and further workup as indicated clinically.
- Patient education and lifestyle reinforcement should be emphasized in all clinical encounters.

G

GONOCOCCAL INFECTIONS

Paul Lyons, MD

 BASICS

DESCRIPTION
A sexually or vertically transmitted bacterial infection caused by *Neisseria gonorrhoeae*:

- *N. gonorrhoeae* is a fastidious gram-negative intracellular diplococcus (1)[A].
- Presents as conjunctival, pharyngeal, urogenital or anorectal infections. Urogenital infections are most common (1)[A].
- Hematogenous dissemination also occurs leading to fever, skin lesions, arthralgias, purulent or sterile arthritis, tenosynovitis, endocarditis, or (rarely) meningitis (1)[A].
- Asymptomatic carrier state can occur in both sexes.
- In newborns, gonococcal ophthalmia neonatorum, a purulent conjunctivitis, may occur after vaginal delivery by an infected mother, potentially leading to blindness if not treated promptly (1,2)[A].
- System(s) affected: cardiovascular, musculoskeletal, nervous, reproductive, skin/exocrine
- Synonym(s): gonococcal infection (GC); clap

EPIDEMIOLOGY
- Predominant age: 15 to 24 years (1,2)[A]
- Predominant sex: women 105/100,000; men 92/100,000 (2)[A]

Incidence
CDC 2012: 334,826 reported cases (107.5/100,000 U.S. population) (2)[A]

Prevalence
Incidence and prevalence of are approximately equal. The true prevalence is higher due to the asymptomatic nature of the disease (2)[A]:

- Rates peaked in mid-1970s and fell 74% over the next 20 years with national control program (2)[A].
- Highest rate: women aged 20 to 24 years (578/100,000) followed by women aged 15 to 19 years (521/100,000) (2)[A]
- Blacks (462/100,000) have higher reported rates of infections than whites (31/100,000) (2)[A].
- The southern regions of the United States have higher reported rates. Highest reported state rate is Mississippi (231/100,000) (2)[A].

ETIOLOGY AND PATHOPHYSIOLOGY
Infection requires four steps: (i) mucosal attachment. Bacterial proteins bind to receptors on host cells; (ii) local penetration/invasion; (iii) local proliferation; (iv) inflammatory response or dissemination *N. gonorrhoeae* (gonococcus). *N. gonorrhoeae* spreads most commonly during sexual relations.

Genetics
Congenital deficiency of late components of complement cascade (C7 to C9) are prone to develop dissemination of local gonococcal infections.

RISK FACTORS
- History of previous gonorrhea infection or other STIs
- Sexual exposure to an infected individual without barrier protection (condom)
- New/multiple sexual partners
- Inconsistent condom use
- Commercial sex work or drug use
- Infants: infected mother

- Children: sexual abuse by infected individual
- Autoinoculation (finger to eye)

GENERAL PREVENTION
- Condoms offer partial protection. They must be used appropriately for protection during oral, anal, and vaginal intercourse.
- Treat sexual contacts; consider expedited partner therapy (EPT) (2,3)[A].

COMMONLY ASSOCIATED CONDITIONS
Other STIs: *Chlamydia*, syphilis, HIV, hepatitis B, herpes (2–4)[A]

 DIAGNOSIS

HISTORY
- Sexual history
  - Number of partners and age of onset of sexual activity; STI history
  - New/recent change in sexual partner
  - Contact with commercial sex workers
  - Condom use
  - Menses and possibility of pregnancy
- *10% males and 20–40% of women are asymptomatic* (2)[A].
- If symptomatic, explore the onset, context, duration, timing, severity, and associated symptoms:
  - Symptoms typically appear within 1 to 14 days after exposure (when present) (1)[A].
- Ocular symptoms: discharge, itch, redness (1)[A]
- Pharyngeal symptoms: asymptomatic infection (98%), sore throat (1)[A]
- GI symptoms: acute diarrhea (1)[A]
- Urinary symptoms: urinary frequency, urgency, dysuria (1)[A]
- Urethral symptoms: copious urethral discharge (1,2)[A]
  - Males: scant to copious purulent urethral discharge (82%), dysuria (53%), testicular pain (1%), asymptomatic infection (10%), proctitis
  - Females: asymptomatic cervical infection (20%), endocervical discharge (96%), vaginal discharge, Bartholin gland swelling, dysmenorrhea, menometrorrhagia, abdominal pain/tenderness, dyspareunia, cervical motion tenderness, rebound, infertility, chronic pelvic pain
- Either sex, for receptive anal intercourse: rectal discharge, tenesmus, rectal burning; can be asymptomatic.
- Disseminated syndromes (1,2)[A]
  - Fever, chills, malaise, skin rash, arthralgia
  - Endocarditis: high fevers
  - Meningitis: meningeal signs, headache, skin lesions, fever, altered mental status

PHYSICAL EXAM
- General: fever, chills (1)[A]
- Ocular: purulent discharge, conjunctivitis, chemosis, eyelid edema, corneal ulceration (1)[A]
- Pharyngeal infection: exudative pharyngitis (<1%) (1)[A]
- GI: acute diarrhea, hyperactive bowel sounds (1)[A]
- Genitourinary (GU) (1)[A]
  - Males: urethral discharge, testicular tenderness (1%)
  - Females: endocervical discharge, Bartholin gland abscess, abdominal pain/tenderness, cervical motion tenderness, rebound tenderness

- Either sex, for receptive anal intercourse: Rectal discharge; rectal exam may be normal (1)[A].
- Disseminated syndromes (1)[A]:
  - Fever, chills, malaise, tenosynovitis, maculopapular-pustular rash, polyarthralgia—typically large joints (knee, wrist, ankle), purulent arthritis
  - Endocarditis: rapid cardiac valve destruction, heart murmurs, high fevers
  - Meningitis: meningeal signs, headache, skin lesions, fever, altered mental status

DIFFERENTIAL DIAGNOSIS
Chlamydia trachomatis, UTIs, other vaginitis, or urethritis (bacterial, viral, or parasitic)

DIAGNOSTIC TESTS & INTERPRETATION
Initial Tests (lab, imaging)
- Nucleic acid amplification (NAAT) is the most sensitive and specific test for *N. gonorrhoeae* (2)[A]. Other options include:
  - Genital culture
  - Add pharyngeal culture in adolescents
  - Gram stain (recommended for urethritis)
  - Urethral smear, sensitivity in symptomatic male: ≥95%; sensitivity of endocervical smear in infected woman: 40–60%; specificity: 100%
- DNA probes and polymerase chain reaction (PCR) sensitivity: 92–99% dependent on population; specificity: >97%; can replace culture
- Blood culture is 50% sensitive in disseminated disease. Joint fluid culture is 50% sensitive in septic arthritis. Screen for additional STIs, especially chlamydia, syphilis, and HIV.
- Imaging is not generally recommended.

Follow-Up Tests & Special Considerations
- Test of cure is not generally recommended (1–3)[A].
- Follow-up testing may be considered in cases of recurrent infection, when oral cephalosporin treatment is used and/or in areas where significant antibiotic resistance exists (2,3)[A].
- Pelvic ultrasound or CT scan may demonstrate thick, dilated fallopian tubes or abscess formation.

Diagnostic Procedures/Other
Culdocentesis may demonstrate free purulent exudate and provide material for Gram staining and culture. Gram-staining material from unroofed skin lesions may show typical organisms.

Test Interpretation
- Gram-negative intracellular diplococci
- Nonpathologic gram-negative diplococci may be found in extragenital locations. For this reason, Gram stain of pharyngeal or rectal swabs is not recommended.

TREATMENT
GENERAL MEASURES
- STI counseling and condom use
- In children and adolescents, suspect sexual abuse.

MEDICATION
- *N. gonorrhoeae* multidrug antimicrobial resistance continues to increase: *CDC recommends dual therapy for all uncomplicated GC infections in U.S. adults and adolescents* (both to treat for concomitant chlamydia and to increase efficacy against drug-resistant strains) (2–4)[A].

- Quinolones are not recommended (2–4)[A].
- *If treatment fails, check culture and sensitivities, and report to CDC through local health authorities (2–4)[A].*
- Treat with regimen that is also effective against uncomplicated genital chlamydial infection (2–4)[A].

First Line

- Uncomplicated urogenital, anorectal, and pharyngeal gonorrheal infection (2,3)[A]
  - Ceftriaxone 250 mg IM in a single dose
  - *PLUS* treatment for chlamydia (azithromycin 1 g PO single dose or doxycycline 100 mg PO BID for 7 days)
- Pharyngitis: ceftriaxone 250 mg IM once PLUS treatment for chlamydia (azithromycin 1 g PO single dose or doxycycline 100 mg PO BID for 7 days) (1–3)[A]
- Conjunctivitis: ceftriaxone, 1 g IM single dose (1–3)[A]
- Pelvic inflammatory disease (PID): Parenteral and oral treatments are equivalent for mild to moderate severity PID. If using IV therapy, switch to PO within 24 to 48 hours of clinical improvement (1–3)[A].
  - Cefotetan 2 g IV q12 OR cefoxitin 2 g IV q6h + doxycycline 100 mg PO or IV q12h
  - Clindamycin 900 mg IV q8h + gentamicin loading dose IV or IM (2 mg/kg of body weight), followed by a maintenance dose (1.5 mg/kg) q8h. Daily dosing (3 to 5 mg/kg) can be substituted.
  - Preferred "oral" regimen includes the following:
    ○ Ceftriaxone 250 mg IM once + doxycycline, 100 mg PO BID for 14 days
    ○ With or without metronidazole, 500 mg PO BID for 14 days
- Disseminated infection in adults (1–3)[A]
  - Ceftriaxone 1 g IM or IV q24h until 24 to 48 hours after improvement begins, then switch to cefixime 400 mg PO BID to complete at least 1 week of antibiotic treatment. *Also treat for chlamydial infection.*
- Meningitis and endocarditis (1–3)[A]
  - Ceftriaxone 1 to 2 g IV q12h 10 to 14 days for meningitis; 4 weeks for endocarditis
- *Contraindications:* Doxycycline is *contraindicated in pregnancy and young children.*

Pediatric Considerations

- Children >45 kg same dosing as adults (1–3)[A]
- Children <45 kg: uncomplicated urethral, cervical, rectal or pharyngeal gonococcal infections (1–3)[A]
  - Ceftriaxone 125 mg IM in single dose
  - Disseminated infections: ceftriaxone 50 mg/kg IV or IM daily (max dose 1 g) in single dose; bacteremia: 7 days; meningitis: 10 to 14 days; endocarditis: 4 weeks
- Ophthalmic neonatorum prophylaxis: single application of erythromycin 0.5% ophthalmic ointment to each eye immediately after delivery (1–3)[A]
- Neonatal conjunctivitis: ceftriaxone 25 to 50 mg/kg IV or IM in a single dose (not to exceed 125 mg) (1–3)[A]
- *Conjunctival exudates should be cultured for definitive diagnosis (1–3)[A].*
- Scalp abscesses (from scalp electrodes) (1–3)[A]
  - Ceftriaxone 25 to 50 mg/kg/day IV or IM in a single daily dose for 7 days, with duration of 10 to 14 days if meningitis is documented.

- Asymptomatic infants born to mothers with untreated gonorrhea (1–3)[A]
  - Ceftriaxone 25 to 50 mg/kg IV or IM, not to exceed 125 mg in a single dose

Pregnancy Considerations

Pregnant women should be treated with cephalosporin or recommended alternative (1–4)[A].

- Azithromycin 2 g orally in single dose for women intolerant to cephalosporin
- Treat concurrently with azithromycin or amoxicillin for presumed *C. trachomatis* coinfection.
- Women with 1st-trimester gonococcal infection should be retested within 3 to 6 months.
- High-risk uninfected pregnant women should be retested during the 3rd trimester.

Second Line

- Due to antimicrobial resistance, combination therapy using two agents with different mechanisms of action improves treatment efficacy and decreases resistance to cephalosporins (1–3)[A].
  - Use of a second antimicrobial (azithromycin as a single 1-g oral dose or doxycycline 100 mg orally twice daily for 7 days) is recommended for use with ceftriaxone (1–3)[A].
  - Azithromycin as the second antimicrobial is preferred to doxycycline because of convenience and compliance of single-dose therapy as well as higher resistance with tetracyclines (1–3)[A].
- For additional treatment options, see CDC STD treatment guidelines: http://www.cdc.gov/std/tg2015/

INPATIENT CONSIDERATIONS

Admission Criteria/Initial Stabilization

- Hematogenously disseminated infection
- Pneumonia or eye infection in infants
- PID: if unable to take oral medications, significant tubo-ovarian abscess, or patient is pregnant

 ONGOING CARE

FOLLOW-UP RECOMMENDATIONS

Patient Monitoring

U.S. Preventive Services Task Force (USPSTF) (4)[A]

- Screen all sexually active women, including those who are pregnant if they are at increased risk of infection (*young or have other individual/population risk factor*): **Grade B recommendation**
- Insufficient evidence to recommend for or against screening men at increased risk of infection: **Grade I recommendation**
- No routine screening in men and women who are low risk for infection: **Grade D recommendation**
- Insufficient evidence to recommend for or against screening in pregnant women who are not at increased risk for infection: **Grade I recommendation**
- Prophylactic ocular topical medication for *all* newborns: **Grade A recommendation**
- Report cases of gonorrhea to public health authorities (3,4)[A]

PATIENT EDUCATION

- Counseling concerning risk reduction, condom use, future fertility, and full STI testing
- Encourage patient to notify partners (from past 60 days); consider EPT.

PROGNOSIS

Complete cure with return to normal function with adequate and timely treatment

COMPLICATIONS

- Infertility
- Urethral stricture
- Corneal scarring
- Destruction of joint articular surfaces
- Cardiac valvular damage

Pediatric Considerations

Vertical transmission to newborn infants is a significant risk among patients with gonococcal infection at the time of delivery (1,2)[A].

REFERENCES

1. Mayor MT, Roett MA, Uduhiri KA. Diagnosis and management of gonococcal infections. *Am Fam Physician.* 2012;86(10):931–938.
2. Centers for Disease Control and Prevention. 2010 sexually transmitted diseases treatment guidelines: gonococcal infections. http://www.cdc.gov/std/treatment/2010/gonococcal-infections.htm
3. Centers for Disease Control and Prevention. Update to CDC's sexually transmitted diseases treatment guidelines, 2010: oral cephalosporins no longer a recommended treatment for gonococcal infections. *MMWR Morb Mortal Wkly Rep.* 2012;61(31):590–594.
4. U.S. Preventive Services Task Force. Chlamydia and Gonorrhea: Screening, September 2014. http://www.uspreventiveservicestaskforce.org/Page/Document/UpdateSummaryFinal/chlamydia-and-gonorrhea-screening?ds=1&s=Gonorrhea

 SEE ALSO

Chlamydia Infection (Sexually Transmitted); HIV/AIDS; Pelvic Inflammatory Disease; Syphilis

CODES

ICD10

- A54.9 Gonococcal infection, unspecified
- A54.31 Gonococcal conjunctivitis
- A54.03 Gonococcal cervicitis, unspecified

CLINICAL PEARLS

- Due to frequent coinfection, treatment for uncomplicated gonorrhea should include two drugs, one of which is effective against chlamydia.
- Screen patients with gonorrhea for chlamydia, syphilis, HIV, and hepatitis.

G

GOUT

Ryan B. Feeney, PharmD • Michael C. Barros, PharmD, BCPS, BCACP • Paul N. Williams, MD, FACP

 BASICS

DESCRIPTION
- Gout is an inflammatory arthritis related to a hyperuricemia (serum uric acid [SUA] level >6.8 mg/dL) (1).
- Acute gouty arthritis can affect ≥1 joints; the first metatarsophalangeal joint is most commonly involved at presentation (podagra).
- Although hyperuricemia is necessary for the development of gout, it is not the only determining factor.
- Characterized by deposition of monosodium urate (MSU) crystals that accumulate in joints and soft tissues, resulting in acute and chronic arthritis, soft-tissue masses called tophi, urate nephropathy, and uric acid nephrolithiasis
- After an initial flare, a second flare occurs in ~60% of patients within 1 year and 78% within 2 years of the initial attack (2).
- Management involves treating acute attacks and preventing recurrent disease by long-term reduction of SUA levels through pharmacology and lifestyle adjustments

EPIDEMIOLOGY
Incidence
Annual incidence of gout (3):
- Uric acid 7 to 8.9 mg/dL is 0.5%.
- Uric acid >9 mg/dL is 4.5%.

Prevalence
- Increasing prevalence over the past decades (3)
- 2007 to 2008 prevalence of gout in the United States (3)
  - Men 5.8% (6.1 million)
  - Women 2.0% (2.2 million)
- 2008 prevalence of hyperuricemia in the United States (3)
  - Men 21.2% (SUA >7.0 mg/dL)
  - Women 21.6% (SUA >5.7 mg/dL)

ETIOLOGY AND PATHOPHYSIOLOGY
- Hyperuricemia results from urate overproduction, underexcretion, or often a combination of the two.
- Gout occurs when MSU, a product of purine metabolism, precipitates out of solution and accumulates in joints and soft tissues.
- Transient changes in urate solubility caused by local temperature decrease, trauma, or acidosis may lead to an acute gouty attack.
- Urate crystals that precipitate trigger an immune response.
- Left untreated, this crystal deposition leads to permanent joint damage and tophus formation.

Genetics
- Phosphoribosyl pyrophosphate (PRPP) deficiency and hypoxanthine-guanine-phosphoribosyltransferase (HGPRT) deficiency (Lesch-Nyhan syndrome) are inherited enzyme defects associated with overproduction of uric acid.
- Polymorphisms in the URAT1 and SLC 2A9 (GLUT9) renal transporters are hereditary enzyme defects resulting in primary underexcretion of uric acid.

RISK FACTORS
- Age >40 years
- Male gender
- Increased purine uptake (meats and seafood)
- Alcohol intake (especially beer)
- High fructose intake
- Obesity

- Hyperuricemia
- Congestive heart failure
- Coronary artery disease
- Dyslipidemia
- Renal disease
- Organ transplant
- Hypertension
- Hyperinsulinemia
- Metabolic syndrome
- Diabetes mellitus
- Urate-elevating medications:
  - Thiazide diuretics: ethambutol
  - Loop diuretics (less of a risk vs. thiazides)
  - Niacin
  - Calcineurin inhibitors (cyclosporine and tacrolimus)
  - Acetylsalicylic acid (*not* recommended in high doses)

GENERAL PREVENTION
- Maintain optimal weight.
- Regular exercise
- Diet modification (purine-rich foods)
- Reduce alcohol consumption (beer and liquor).
- Maintain fluid intake and avoid dehydration.

COMMONLY ASSOCIATED CONDITIONS
- Hypertension
- Dyslipidemia
- Nontraumatic joint disorders
- Heart disease
- Urinary tract disease
- Diabetes mellitus
- Metabolic syndrome
- Obesity
- Renal disease

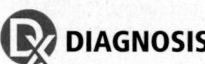 **DIAGNOSIS**

HISTORY
- Classic presentation of acute gouty arthritis:
  - Intense pain and tenderness in the first metatarsophalangeal joint (podagra)
  - Can occur in the midtarsal, ankle, or knee joints
  - Joint may be swollen, warm, and red
  - Often awakes patients from sleep due to an intolerance to contact with clothing or bed sheets
  - There is a rapid onset of intense pain, often beginning in the early morning and progressing rapidly over 12 to 24 hours.
  - In the absence of treatment, flares can last up to 10 days.
- Fever can be seen.
- SC or intraosseous nodules, referred to as tophi
- Pain with urination secondary to uric acid renal stones

PHYSICAL EXAM
- Examine suspected joint(s) for tenderness, swelling, and range of motion (ROM).
- Assess for presence of firm nodules known as tophi.
- In patients with chronic gout, tophi can frequently be found in the helix of the ear, over the olacrenon process, or on the Achilles tendon.
- Patients with untreated chronic gout can have evidence of joint inflammation and deformity.

DIFFERENTIAL DIAGNOSIS
Acute bursitis, tendonitis, septic arthritis, pseudogout (calcium pyrophosphate deposition disease), cellulitis, osteoarthritis

DIAGNOSTIC TESTS & INTERPRETATION
- SUA (may be normal during an acute flare)
- CBC (can see elevation of WBC during an acute gout flare)
- Synovial fluid analysis: urate crystals (negatively birefringent under polarizing microscopy), cell count (WBC usually 2,000 to 5,000 cells/mm³); culture to rule out infection. Some guidelines suggest that gout can be diagnosed clinically without synovial fluid analysis.
- Screen for uric acid overproduction—24-hour urinary uric acid in those patients with gout onset before the age of 25 years or had a history of urolithiasis (1)[C].
- Radiograph is normal early in disease but can reveal
  - Swelling in acute gout
  - Periarticular erosions with periosteum overgrowth in chronic gout
- Urate kidney stones are radiolucent and thus invisible on radiograph.

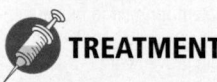 **TREATMENT**

GENERAL MEASURES
Topical ice as needed (4)[B]

MEDICATION
- Acute treatment
  - General principles:
    - Acute gouty arthritis attacks should be treated with pharmacologic therapy (4)[C].
    - Pharmacologic treatment should be initiated within 24 hours of acute gout attack onset (4)[C].
    - Ongoing pharmacologic urate-lowering therapy should not be interrupted during an acute gout attack (4)[C].
    - Choice of agent is based on severity of pain and the number of joints involved (4).
  - Mild/moderate gout severity (≤6 of 10 on visual analog pain scale, particularly for an attack involving only one or a few small joints or one to two large joints)
    - NSAIDs:
      - Naproxen (Naprosyn, Anaprox, Aleve): 750 mg followed by 250 mg q8h for 5 to 8 days (4)[A]
      - Indomethacin (Indocin): 50 to 150 mg/day for 2 to 7 days (4)[A]
      - Sulindac (Clinoril): 200 mg BID for 7 to 10 days (4)[A]
      - Celecoxib (Celebrex)
      - Not FDA approved but can be considered in selected patients with contraindications or intolerance to NSAIDs (4)[B].
        - Dose at 800 mg once followed by 400 mg on day 1, then 400 mg BID for 1 week (4)[B]
    - Corticosteroids
      - Those with an acute flare involving one to two large joints can consider intra-articular corticosteroids; can consider using PO corticosteroids in combination.
      - For other acute flares, use PO corticosteroids:
        - Prednisone (Sterapred): 0.5 mg/kg/day for 5 to 10 days followed by discontinuation (4)[A] or alternately 2 to 5 days at full dose followed by tapering for 7 to 10 days and then discontinuing (4)[C]
        - Methylprednisolone (Medrol) dose pack (4)[C]
        - Triamcinolone acetonide (Trivaris): 60 mg IM single dose followed by oral corticosteroids (4)[C]

- Colchicine (Colcrys)
  - Used for gout attacks where the onset was <36 hours prior to treatment initiation (4)[A]
  - Begin a loading dose of 1.2 mg followed by 0.6 mg 1 hour later, followed by 0.6 mg once or twice daily 12 hours later, until the gout attack resolves (4)[C].
  - Dose reduction recommended in moderate to severe kidney disease and in those on inhibitors of cytochrome P450 3A4 and P-glycoprotein (clarithromycin, erythromycin, cyclosporine, and disulfiram) (4).
- Severe gout (≥7 of 10 on visual analog pain scale, involving ≥4 joints with arthritis involving >1 region, or involving three separate large joints)
  - Initial combination therapy is an option and includes the use of full doses of the following (4)[C]:
    - Colchicine and NSAIDs
    - PO corticosteroids and colchicine
    - Intra-articular steroids with all other modalities
- For patients not responding to initial pharmacologic monotherapy, add a second agent (4)[C].
- Chronic treatment
  - Indications for pharmacologic urate-lowering therapy include any patient with
    - Tophus or tophi by clinical exam or imaging study (1)[A]
    - Frequent attacks of acute gouty arthritis (≥2 attacks/year) (1)[A]
    - Chronic kidney disease (CKD) stage 2 or worse (1)[C]
    - Past urolithiasis (1)[C]
  - Treat to the serum urate:
    - Minimum serum urate target is <6 mg/dL (1)[A].
    - Serum urate target may need to be <5 mg/dL to improve gout signs and symptoms (1)[B].
  - Urate-lowering agents can be prescribed during an acute attack provided that effective anti-inflammatory prophylaxis has been initiated prior to urate-lowering therapy (1)[C].
  - Anti-inflammatory prophylaxis required when initiating urate-lowering therapy include the following:
    - First line
      - Low-dose colchicine: 0.6 mg once or twice daily (4)[A]
      - Low-dose NSAIDs with proton pump inhibitor if indicated: naproxen 250 mg PO BID (4)[C]
    - Second line: Use of colchicine and NSAIDs both are not tolerated, contraindicated, or ineffective:
      - Low-dose prednisone or prednisolone at ≤10 mg/day (4)[C]
    - Treatment duration for the greater of
      - At least 6 months (4)[A] or
      - 3 months after achieving serum urate appropriate for the patient with no tophi on exam (4)[B], or for 6 months after achieving serum urate appropriate for the patient with ≥1 tophi on exam (4)[C]
  - Pharmacologic urate-lowering agents:
    - Allopurinol (Zyloprim): xanthine oxidase inhibitor (1)[A]
      - Starting dose should be no higher than 100 mg/day (1)[B]
      - Starting dose should be 50 mg/day in stage 4 CKD or worse
      - Gradually titrate the dose upward q2–5wk to appropriate maximum dose (1)[C]

- Dose can be >300 mg/day, even with renal impairment, as long as accompanied by patient education and monitoring of drug toxicity; maximum FDA-approved dosage is 800 mg/day (1)[B].
- Regularly monitor for allopurinol hypersensitivity syndrome (AHS), pruritus, rash, elevated hepatic transaminases, and eosinophilia.
- Screening for the HLA-B*5801 allele for AHS should be performed in those of Korean descent with stage 3 CKD or worse and Han Chinese or Thai descent irrespective of renal function (1)[A].
- Febuxostat (Uloric): selective xanthine oxidase inhibitor (1)[A]
  - No renal or hepatic adjustments needed for mild-to-moderate hepatic or renal impairment
  - Starting dose 40 mg/day; may be titrated to 80 mg/day
  - In select instances, may dose up to 120 mg/day (not FDA approved) (1)[A]
- Probenecid: uricosuric agent (1)[B]
  - Alternative first line urate-lowering therapy; use if at least one xanthine oxidase inhibitor is contraindicated or not tolerated (1)[B].
  - May be used in addition to allopurinol or febuxostat if serum urate target not achieved
  - Multiple drug interactions exist, as well as risk of urolithiasis with this agent.
  - Not recommended if creatinine clearance (CrCl) is <50 or with patient history of urolithiasis (1)[C].
  - Starting dose is 250 mg BID; gradually titrate to 2,000 mg/day
- Other treatment
  - Acute treatment: adrenocorticotropic hormone (ACTH): 25 to 40 IU SC (4)[A]; especially in those NPO
  - Pegloticase in select severe instances (1)

SURGERY/OTHER PROCEDURES
Large tophi that are infected or interfering with joint motion may need to be surgically removed.

 ## ONGOING CARE

FOLLOW-UP RECOMMENDATIONS
Patient Monitoring
- SUA q2–5wk while titrating urate-lowering treatment to goal (1)[C]
- Regularly monitor CBC, renal function, liver function test, and urinalysis.

DIET
- General lack of evidence regarding specific recommendations, although the American College of Rheumatology has outlined the following (1)[C]:
- General measures:
  - Weight loss for obese patients
  - Healthy overall diet
  - Exercise
  - Smoking cessation
  - Stay well hydrated
- Avoid
  - Organ meats high in purine content (sweetbreads, liver, kidney) (1)[A]
  - High-fructose corn syrup–sweetened sodas, other beverages, or foods
  - Alcohol overuse (>2 servings per day for men and >1 serving per day for women) (1)[A]
  - Any alcohol use in gout during periods of frequent gout attacks or advanced gout under poor control

- Limit
  - Serving sizes of beef, lamb, pork, and seafood with high purine content such as sardines and shellfish (1)[B]
  - Servings of naturally sweetened fruit juices
  - Table sugar and sweetened beverages and desserts
  - Table salt, including in sauces and gravies
  - Alcohol (particularly beer) in all gout patients (1)[B]
- Encourage
  - Low-fat or nonfat dairy products
  - Vegetables

PATIENT EDUCATION
- Dietary and lifestyle modifications (1)[B]
- Patient instructions on initiating treatment on signs and symptoms of an acute gout attack without the need to consult health care provider for each attack (1)[B]
- Discussion that gout is caused by excess uric acid and that effective urate-lowering therapy is essential treatment (1)[B]

PROGNOSIS
Gout can usually be successfully managed with proper treatment.

COMPLICATIONS
- AHS
- Increased susceptibility to infection
- Urate nephropathy
- Renal stones

REFERENCES
1. Khanna D, Fitzgerald JD, Khanna PP, et al. 2012 American College of Rheumatology guidelines for management of gout. Part 1: systematic nonpharmacologic and pharmacologic therapeutic approaches to hyperuricemia. *Arthritis Care Res*. 2012;64(10):1431–1446.
2. Doghramji PP. Managing your patient with gout: a review of treatment options. *Postgrad Med*. 2011;123(3):56–71.
3. Zhu Y, Pandya BJ, Choi HK. Prevalence of gout and hyperuricemia in the US general population: the National Health and Nutrition Examination Survey 2007–2008. *Arthritis Rheum*. 2011;63(10):3136–3141.
4. Khanna D, Khanna PP, Fitzgerald JD, et al. 2012 American College of Rheumatology guidelines for management of gout. Part 2: therapy and antiinflammatory prophylaxis of acute gouty arthritis. *Arthritis Care Res*. 2012;64(10):1447–1461.

 ## CODES

ICD10
- M10.9 Gout, unspecified
- M10.00 Idiopathic gout, unspecified site
- M10.30 Gout due to renal impairment, unspecified site

CLINICAL PEARLS
- MSU crystals found in synovial fluid aspirate are pathognomonic for gout.
- Acute gout and sepsis can coexist.
- Asymptomatic hyperuricemia does not require treatment.
- Losartan possesses uricosuric properties, therefore it may be an excellent agent if patient is hypertensive.

GRANULOMA ANNULARE

Mary Iaculli, DO • Joanne Wilkinson, MD, MSc

 BASICS

DESCRIPTION
A benign skin condition characterized by grouped, flesh-colored, or erythematous papules, which typically occur in an annular (ring-like) pattern. Five variants have been described; the most common of which is localized granuloma annulare (GA). The other types are generalized, patch type, subcutaneous (SC) (deep dermal), and perforating.

EPIDEMIOLOGY
Incidence
- GA is not common, although exact prevalence in the general population is unknown.
- Predominant sex: female > male (2.5:1)
- Most lesions resolve in 2 to 24 months but may last up to 5 to 10 years. 2/3 of patients are <30 years, and the age distribution varies by type, as follows:
  – Localized: children and adults <30 years
  – Generalized: bimodal: children <10 years and adults 30 to 60 years
  – Patch type: adults >30 years
  – SC: children 2 to 10 years
  – Perforating: typically children but also young adults

Prevalence
Among cases of GA, the approximate distribution is as follows:
- Localized: 75%
- Generalized: 10–15%
- Patch type: <5%
- Subcutaneous: <5%
- Perforating: <5% (perhaps higher in Hawaii)

ETIOLOGY AND PATHOPHYSIOLOGY
The cause of GA remains unknown, although it is hypothesized to be a delayed-type hypersensitivity to an unknown antigen. Lymphohistiocytic infiltrates, degeneration of collagen, and mucin deposition are characteristic histopathologic features of GA.

Genetics
There is some evidence for a possible hereditary component. Increased frequency of HLA-B35 in patients with generalized GA were reported in two studies (1,2).

RISK FACTORS
No definite risk factors have been identified. There is some evidence for possible associations with diabetes mellitus; TB; HIV, EBV, and other viral infections (including HSV); interferon-α therapy; trauma; insect bites; borreliosis; and malignancies (most commonly lymphoma).

GENERAL PREVENTION
There are no established strategies for preventing GA.

COMMONLY ASSOCIATED CONDITIONS
- Diabetes mellitus: There are conflicting reports about the association of GA with diabetes mellitus, and methodological design for these studies is weak. One retrospective study of 557 aged-matched patients found a higher incidence in localized GA with insulin-dependent diabetes mellitus (3). Another retrospective study reported higher incidence of diabetes mellitus in generalized GA versus localized GA (4). In contrast, two small studies, one is a case control and one is a prospective study, did not reveal an association between these disorders (5,6).
- Malignancy: There is a possible association with GA and malignancy; however, data is severely lacking. Cases linked with malignancy most commonly had an atypical presentation of GA with lymphoma (7).
- Dyslipidemia: Dyslipidemia may be associated with GA. A case-control study of 140 adults showed a statistically significant increase in elevated lipids in patients with GA, most commonly generalized GA (8).
- HIV: There are many case reports suggesting an association between GA and HIV. Generalized GA is most common pattern with HIV.
- For all associations, weak evidence exists through poorly designed, underpowered studies. More investigations are necessary.

 DIAGNOSIS

HISTORY
Cutaneous lesions of GA are generally asymptomatic. They may persist for months or years; longer duration is more often seen in the generalized subtype. They typically resolve spontaneously and may recur.

PHYSICAL EXAM
- Localized: asymptomatic, flesh-colored, or erythematous annular or arciform plaque with a moderately firm, rope-like border and central clearing, ranging from 5-mm to 5-cm in diameter. Small 1- to 2-mm papules may be noted in periphery, often not in continuous border. The most common locations are the dorsal aspects of the distal extremities. Involvement of palms is rare. 50% will have multiple lesions.
- Generalized: similar to localized but a higher number of lesions (>10), which are more diffuse distribution, often larger, and typically persist longer
- Patch type: erythematous macules and patches distributed symmetrically on the extremities and trunk. The typical annular configuration may or may not be present; often involves proximal extremities.
- SC: firm, nontender, SC nodule, which tends to grow rapidly; usually solitary but may occur in groups. Most common location is scalp or lower extremities, especially pretibial; other sites include upper extremities and buttocks.
- Perforating: Damaged collagen from dermis is extruded onto skin surface. Papules may be up to 4 mm and display yellowish umbilication, crusting, or scale. Lesions are often generalized and may occur anywhere. Lesions often heal with scar.

DIFFERENTIAL DIAGNOSIS
- Localized: tinea corporis, annular lichen planus, necrobiosis lipoidica, pityriasis rosea, erythema migrans of Lyme disease, leprosy
- Generalized: sarcoidosis, lichen planus, cutaneous metastases, mycosis fungoides
- Patch type: erythema migrans
- SC: rheumatoid nodule
- Perforating: molluscum contagiosum, sarcoidosis, insect bites

DIAGNOSTIC TESTS & INTERPRETATION
Initial Tests (lab, imaging)
- Diagnosis is typically established by history and physical, so lab investigations are rarely needed. Skin scraping/KOH test may be useful for excluding a fungal process.
- May consider work up for dyslipidemia, DM, HIV, and malignancy if clinically indicated

Diagnostic Procedures/Other
Skin punch biopsy is useful to confirm the diagnosis and designate subtype. Immunohistochemical streptavidin-biotin-horseradish peroxidase (HRP) analysis for CD68/KP-1, which is a marker for histiocytic differentiation, may aid in the diagnosis.

Test Interpretation
Dermal granulomatous infiltrate demonstrating foci of degenerative collagen associated with palisading around an anuclear dermis with mucin deposition. Histologic variants include interstitial (histiocytic infiltrate between collagen fibers), classic (palisading dermal granulomas), and epithelioid (tuberculoid and sarcoidal granulomas).

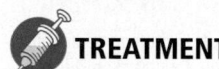 TREATMENT

GENERAL MEASURES
GA is a self-limited, asymptomatic condition that is likely to regress spontaneously. The clinician's primary role after diagnosis is to educate the patient regarding the anticipated natural history and to provide reassurance.

MEDICATION

- No strong evidence supports therapeutic intervention for GA. Reassurance with observation may be an adequate treatment for localized, asymptomatic disease.
- The trauma induced by biopsy alone can cause involution of the lesions through an unknown mechanism.
- The following therapies have been tried with variable success, and the possible benefit of treatment must be weighed against the significant toxicities of these treatments.

First Line
Corticosteroids (9)

- High-potency topical, with or without occlusion
- Intralesional triamcinolone: 2.5 to 5 mg/mL

Second Line
- Methotrexate: 15 mg IM weekly (10)
- Rifampin: 600 mg, ofloxacin 400 mg, with minocycline 100 mg once daily (11)
- Pimecrolimus 1% cream BID
- Isotretinoin: 0.5 to 0.75 mg/kg/day
- Dapsone: 100 mg/day
- Chloroquine: 3 mg/kg/day
- Hydroxychloroquine: 3 to 6 mg/kg/day
- Cyclosporine: 3 to 4 mg/kg/day
- Niacinamide: 500 mg TID
- TNF-α inhibitors, such as infliximab 5 mg/kg IV weeks 0, 2, and 6 and monthly thereafter for 10 months or adalimumab 80 mg SC × 1 for the 1st week then 40 SC × 1 for weeks 2 to 4

ADDITIONAL THERAPIES
- Fractional thermolysis (Er:YAG fractionated laser)
- Psoralen ultraviolet A (PUVA)
- Cryotherapy
- Surgical excision for SC GA

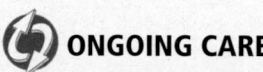

ONGOING CARE

FOLLOW-UP RECOMMENDATIONS
Routine follow-up is not required unless treatment is initiated. Then follow-up may be important to monitor for possible adverse effects associated with treatment. Referral to a dermatologist is prudent in cases of generalized GA and in those cases that persist despite conservative therapy.

PATIENT EDUCATION
The patient should be educated that GA is a benign, self-limited condition that may persist a long time, resolve, and/or recur.

PROGNOSIS
>50% of cases resolve spontaneously within 2 months to 2 years; although recurrence, typically at the original site, is common (>40%). Patients <39 years have been shown to have a shorter duration of illness.

COMPLICATIONS
Complications of treatment are much more likely than complications from GA.

REFERENCES

1. Friedman-Birnbaum R, Haim S, Gideone O, et al. Histocompatibility antigens in granuloma annulare. Comparative study of the generalized and localized types. *Br J Dermatol*. 1978;98(4):425–428.
2. Friedman-Birnbaum R, Gideoni O, Bergman R, et al. A study of HLA antigen associated in localized and generalized granuloma annulare. *Br J Dermatol*. 1986;115(3):329–333.
3. Muhlemann MF, Williams DR. Localized granuloma annulare is associated with insulin-dependent diabetes mellitus. *Br J Dermatol*. 1984;111(3):325–329.
4. Dabski K, Winkelmann RK. Generalized granuloma annulare: clinical and laboratory findings in 100 patients. *J Am Acad Dermatol*. 1989;20(1):39–47.
5. Nebesio CL, Lewis C, Chuang TY. Lack of an association between granuloma annulare and type 2 diabetes mellitus. *Br J Dermatol*. 2002;146(1):122–124.
6. Gannon TF, Lynch PJ. Absence of carbohydrate intolerance in granuloma annulare. *J Am Acad Dermatol*. 1994;30(4):662–663.
7. Li A, Hogan DJ, Sanusi ID, et al. Granuloma annulare and malignant neoplasms. *Am J Dermatopathol*. 2003;25(2):113–116.
8. Wu W, Robinson-Bostom L, Kokkotou E, et al. Dyslipidemia in granuloma annulare: a case-control study. *Arch Dermatol*. 2012;148(10):1131–1136.
9. Cyr PR. Diagnosis and management of granuloma annulare. *Am Fam Physician*. 2006;74(10):1729–1734.
10. Plotner AN, Mutasim DF. Successful treatment of disseminated granuloma annulare with methotrexate. *Br J Dermatol*. 2010;163(5):1123–1124.
11. Marcus DV, Mahmoud BH, Hamzavi IH. Granuloma annulare treated with rifampin, ofloxacin, and minocycline combination therapy. *Arch Dermatol*. 2009;145(7):787–789.

ADDITIONAL READING

- Browne F, Turner D, Goulden V. Psoralen and ultraviolet A in the treatment of granuloma annulare. *Photodermatol Photoimmunol Photomed*. 2011;27(2):81–84.
- Duarte AF, Mota A, Pereira MA, et al. Generalized granuloma annulare—response to doxycycline. *J Eur Acad Dermatol Venereol*. 2009;23(1):84–85.
- Liu A, Hexsel CL, Moy RL, et al. Granuloma annulare successfully treated using fractional photothermolysis with a 1,550-nm erbium-doped yttrium aluminum garnet fractionated laser. *Dermatol Surg*. 2011;37(5):712–715.
- Mazzatenta C, Ghilardi A, Grazzini M. Treatment of disseminated granuloma annulare with allopurinol: case report. *Dermatol Therapy*. 2010;(23 Suppl 1):S24–S27.
- Misago N, Narisawa Y. Subcutaneous granuloma annulare with overlying localized granuloma annulare. *J Dermatol*. 2010;37(8):755–757.
- Plotner AN, Mutasim DF. Successful treatment of disseminated granuloma annulare with methotrexate. *Br J Dermatol*. 2010;163(5):1123–1124.
- Shanmuga SC, Rai R, Laila A, et al. Generalized granuloma annulare with tuberculoid granulomas: a rare histopathologic variant. *Indian J Dermatol Venereol Leprol*. 2010;76(1):73–75.
- Werchau S, Enk A, Hartmann M. Generalized interstitial granuloma annulare—response to adalimumab. *Int J Dermatol*. 2010;49(4):457–460.
- Wu W, Robinson-Bostom L, Kokkotou E, et al. Dyslipidemia in granuloma annulare: a case-control study. *Arch Dermatol*. 2012;148(10):1131–1136.

 CODES

ICD10
L92.0 Granuloma annulare

CLINICAL PEARLS

- This condition is benign and often self resolves. Consider risk-benefit with patient when discussing treatment.
- In cases of suspected tinea that lack scaling, consider GA.
- Consider lipid testing, especially in those with generalized subtype.

G

GRANULOMA, PYOGENIC

Eddie Needham, MD, FAAFP

 BASICS

DESCRIPTION
- Pyogenic granulomas (PG) are benign, acquired, and solitary vascular proliferations that occur most often on the head and neck, the lips and oral cavity, the trunk, and the extremities (1).
- They are friable and tend to bleed easily due to the vascular nature of the lesion.
- Smooth, red to purple, sessile or pedunculated, grow rapidly over several weeks
- Synonym(s): Given that PG are neither pyogenic nor granulomatous, another term is lobular capillary hemangioma.

EPIDEMIOLOGY
The peak incidence of PG are the 2nd and 3rd decades of life (2).

Incidence
- In children, PG accounts for <1% of all skin lesions.
- 42% of all cases occur by age 5 years (2).
- 2% of pregnant women in the United States develop a PG by 5 months' pregnancy (3).

Prevalence
Relatively common condition

ETIOLOGY AND PATHOPHYSIOLOGY
- Thought to be an aberrant healing response to minor trauma in many cases
- May be related to hormonal changes in pregnancy
- Not caused by bacterial infection but associated with capillary proliferation
- Not considered as a hemangioma or neoplasm

- Associated with acute and chronic trauma, peripheral nerve injury, inflammatory systemic diseases, infection, drugs (systemic steroids, protease inhibitors, retinoids, epidermal growth factor receptor inhibitors)

RISK FACTORS
- Pregnancy
- Trauma
- Intraoral trauma or surgery
- Inflammatory systemic diseases

GENERAL PREVENTION
Good oral hygiene may be helpful.

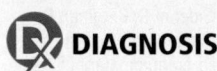 **DIAGNOSIS**

HISTORY
- Solitary lesion that develops rapidly from days to weeks after minor trauma
- Tends to bleed easily
- Grows early in pregnancy and partially regresses postpartum

PHYSICAL EXAM
- Most commonly located at the head, neck, and upper extremities, especially in children
- Among oral lesions, gingiva is the most common location.
- Usually a bright red, friable papule; can also be purple, yellow, or brown
- Moist and sometimes scaly-appearing surface
- Usually <1 cm but ranges from a few millimeters to 2 to 3 cm in diameter

- Giant lesions may occur on areas such as the foot (rare).
- Soft; pedunculated or sessile
- Solitary red papule, grows rapidly, forming a stalk, may bleed, and ulcerate.
- On diascopy, red structureless areas surrounded by a white collarette intersected by white lines
- Erythematous, soft compressible papule with serosanguineous crusting and sharp demarcation

DIFFERENTIAL DIAGNOSIS
- Benign lesions
  - Cherry/infantile hemangioma (4)
  - Fibrous papule (1,4)
  - Bacillary angiomatosis, from by *Bartonella* (1)
- Malignant lesions
  - Basal cell carcinoma (1)
  - Squamous cell carcinoma (1)
  - Amelanotic melanoma (1)
  - Kaposi sarcoma (1)
  - Cutaneous metastases (1)

DIAGNOSTIC TESTS & INTERPRETATION

Initial Tests (lab, imaging)
No labs are necessary for the diagnosis.

Diagnostic Procedures/Other
- Excisional/shave biopsy
- Send for pathology.

Test Interpretation
Microscopic examination reveals
- Small, endothelial-lined vascular spaces
- Loose/dense connective tissue stroma
- Acute and chronic inflammatory cells

- *No true granuloma formation*
- Abundant mitotic activity
- Resembles granulation tissue in an edematous matrix, showing immature capillaries with interspersed tissue

TREATMENT

When feasible, surgical excision is best to yield material for histopathologic analysis (1,5).

MEDICATION

- Cryotherapy with liquid nitrogen (recur 2%) (6)[B]
- Laser (recur 5%) (6)[B]
- Topical imiquimod (recur 0%) (6)[B]
- Silver nitrate (recur 15%) (6)[A]
- Topical 1.5% phenol solution may be used for periungual lesion (6)[B].
- Perform excision for bx if recurrent.

SURGERY/OTHER PROCEDURES

- Excisional biopsy should be tried in all situations, if possible, to ensure a proper diagnosis (i.e., not missing malignancies such as amelanotic melanoma or basal cell carcinoma) (recur 2–3%) (6)[B]. For smaller lesions in noncosmetically sensitive areas, surgical excision with simple closure gives the best result with least recurrence (6)[B].
- Liquid nitrogen may be nonsurgical option with the lowest recurrence rate (recur 2%) (6)[B].
- Shave excision with cautery may be optimal treatment for a lesion on fingertips (recur 7–9%) (6)[B].
- Electrosurgery: electrodesiccation and curettage (recur 7–9%) (6)[B]
- Excision must be adequate to avoid recurrence. Even a small fragment of tissue left behind may lead to recurrence.

ONGOING CARE

PATIENT EDUCATION
Patient should avoid trauma to area following excision.

PROGNOSIS
- Some lesions spontaneously resolve on their own (usually within 6 months).
- Complete resolution is expected with adequate excision.

COMPLICATIONS
Recurrence: After removal or destruction of solitary lesion, multiple satellite lesions can form around original treatment site.

REFERENCES

1. Lin RL, Janniger CK. Pyogenic granuloma. *Cutis.* 2004;74(4):229–233.
2. Harris MN, Desai R, Chuang TY, et al. Lobular capillary hemangiomas: an epidemiologic report, with emphasis on cutaneous lesions. *J Am Acad Dermatol.* 2000;42(6):1012–1016.
3. Kroumpouzos G, Cohen LM. Dermatoses of pregnancy. *J Am Acad Dermatol.* 2001;45(1):1–19.
4. Pagliai KA, Cohen BA. Pyogenic granuloma in children. *Pediatr Dermatol.* 2004;21(1):10–13.
5. Gilmore A, Kelsberg G, Safranek S. Clinical inquiries. What's the best treatment for pyogenic granuloma? *J Fam Pract.* 2010;59(1):40–42.
6. Lee J, Sinno H, Tahiri Y, et al. Treatment options for cutaneous pyogenic granulomas: a review. *J Plast Reconstr Aesthet Surg.* 2011;64(9):1216–1220.

ADDITIONAL READING

- Greene AK. Management of hemangiomas and other vascular tumors. *Clin Plast Surg.* 2011;38(1):45–63.
- Losa Iglesias ME, Becerro de Bengoa Vallejo R. Topical phenol as a conservative treatment for periungual pyogenic granuloma. *Dermatol Surg.* 2010;36(5):675–678.
- Piraccini BM, Bellavista S, Misciali C, et al. Periungual and subungual pyogenic granuloma. *Br J Dermatol.* 2010;163(5):941–953.
- Zalaudek I, Kreusch J, Giacomel J, et al. How to diagnose nonpigmented skin tumors: a review of vascular structures seen with dermoscopy: part II. Nonmelanocytic skin tumors. *J Am Acad Dermatol.* 2010;63(3):377–386.

CODES

ICD10
- L98.0 Pyogenic granuloma
- K06.8 Oth disrd of gingiva and edentulous alveolar ridge
- K13.4 Granuloma and granuloma-like lesions of oral mucosa

CLINICAL PEARLS

- Benign, acquired, usually rapidly growing, solitary vascular proliferation that involves exposed areas, such as distal extremities and face, as well as in the oral cavity
- Excision must be adequate to avoid recurrence.
- Excisional biopsy recommended to ensure proper diagnosis (and to not miss a malignant lesion)
- Excision with primary closure or excision with cautery should be the first choice for treatment in most lesions.

G

GRAVES DISEASE

Jasmine S. Beria, DO, MPH • Oksana Davydov, MD

BASICS

DESCRIPTION
Autoimmune disease in which thyroid-stimulating antibodies cause increased thyroid function; most common cause of hyperthyroidism. Classic findings are goiter, ophthalmopathy (orbitopathy), and occasionally dermopathy (pretibial or localized myxedema).

EPIDEMIOLOGY
Prevalence
- Overall prevalence of hyperthyroidism in United States: ~2% for women and 0.2% for men
- More common in white and Hispanic populations in comparison to the black population
- Graves disease accounts for 60–80% of all cases of hyperthyroidism.
- Hyperthyroidism occurs in 0.2% of pregnancies, of which 95% is due to Graves disease.
- Predominant age: 30 to 40 years
- Synonym(s): Basedow disease

ETIOLOGY AND PATHOPHYSIOLOGY
- Excessive production of thyroid-stimulating hormone (TSH) receptor antibodies from B cells primarily within the thyroid, likely due to genetic clonal lack of suppressor T cells
- Binding of these antibodies to TSH receptors in the thyroid activates the receptor, stimulating thyroid hormone synthesis and secretion as well as thyroid growth (leading to goiter).
- Binding to similar antigen in retro-orbital connective tissue causes ocular symptoms.

Genetics
Higher risk with personal or family history of any autoimmune disease, especially Hashimoto thyroiditis

RISK FACTORS
- Female gender
- Postpartum period
- Stressful life events
- Medications: iodine, amiodarone, lithium, highly active antiretroviral (HAART); rarely, immune-modulating medications (e.g., interferon therapy)
- Smoking (higher risk of developing ophthalmopathy)

GENERAL PREVENTION
Screening TSH in asymptomatic patients is not recommended. No data conclusively show that treatment of subclinical thyroid dysfunction improves quality of life or clinical outcome measures.

COMMONLY ASSOCIATED CONDITIONS
- Mitral valve prolapse
- Type 1 diabetes mellitus
- Addison disease, hypokalemic periodic paralysis
- Vitiligo, alopecia areata
- Other autoimmune disorders (myasthenia gravis, celiac disease)

DIAGNOSIS

Hyperthyroid patients appear hypermetabolic with increased adrenergic tone.

HISTORY
- Tachycardia, palpitations
- Tremor, restlessness
- Hyperactivity, anxiety, emotional lability, insomnia
- Sweating, heat intolerance
- Pruritus, skin changes
- Weight loss with increased appetite
- Fatigue, dyspnea (due to muscle weakness)
- Oligo-/amenorrhea (women), loss of libido, erectile dysfunction (men), gynecomastia
- Loose, frequent stools
- Blurred vision or diplopia, lacrimation, photophobia, gritty sensation in eyes (ocular dryness), retro-orbital discomfort, painful eye movement, loss of color vision or visual acuity
- Worsening of chronic medical conditions (anxiety, bipolar disorder, glucose intolerance, heart failure, or angina)

Geriatric Considerations
Elderly patients may not display classic symptoms; may present with atrial fibrillation, weight loss, or shortness of breath (1)[B].

PHYSICAL EXAM
- Ophthalmologic (present in 50% of cases): Grittiness/discomfort in the eyes, retrobulbar pressure/pain, lid lag/retraction, proptosis, ophthalmoplegia, papilledema, and loss of color vision may signify optic neuropathy.
- Thyroid: enlarged (goiter), nontender, and without nodules; possible bruit (increased blood flow)
- Integumentary: fine hair, warm skin, onycholysis, palmar erythema, possible pretibial myxedema (orange peel appearance), possible hyperpigmented plaques (dermopathy)
- Cardiac: resting tachycardia, hyperdynamic circulation, possible atrial fibrillation
- Extremities: fine tremor, hyperreflexia, proximal myopathy; rarely, soft tissue edema of extremities and clubbing of digits (acropachy)

DIFFERENTIAL DIAGNOSIS
- Toxic multinodular goiter (multiple hormone-producing nodules)
- Toxic adenoma (single hormone-producing nodule)
- Thyroiditis (hormone leakage)
  - Subacute, usually postviral (thyroid will be tender)
  - Lymphocytic, including postpartum
  - Hashimoto thyroiditis (antithyroperoxidase [TPO] antibodies may stimulate TSH receptors)
- Iatrogenic (treatment-induced)
  - Iodine-induced (dietary, radiographic contrast, or medications)
  - Amiodarone
  - Thyroid hormone overreplacement (accidental or intentional)
- Tumor
  - Pituitary adenoma producing TSH
  - Human chorionic gonadotropin (hCG)-producing tumors (stimulate TSH receptors)
  - Extraglandular thyroid hormone production (e.g., struma ovarii or metastatic thyroid cancer)

DIAGNOSTIC TESTS & INTERPRETATION
Initial Tests (lab, imaging)
- TSH is initial test: Suppressed (low or undetectable) TSH confirms hyperthyroidism.
- Free T_4 level will be high in Graves disease.
- After confirming suppressed TSH and high T_4, perform radioactive iodine uptake (RAIU) and scan. Patients with Graves disease will have diffuse, elevated RAIU (vs. localized/nodular elevated uptake in adenoma and multinodular goiter and decreased uptake in thyroiditis or exogenous thyroid hormone).

Pregnancy Considerations
Increase in serum T_4-binding globulin concentration and initial stimulation of TSH by hCG results in a total T_4 and T_3 rise during first half of pregnancy. The TSH level is decreased throughout pregnancy and should be compared to the trimester-specific ranges for pregnancy. Measurement of thyrotropin receptor antibody (TRAb) is positive in 95% of patients with Graves and should be used if diagnosis is unclear in pregnancy (2)[B].

TREATMENT

MEDICATION
Goal is to correct hypermetabolic state with the fewest side effects and lowest incidence of posttreatment hypothyroidism.

First Line
- β-Blockers provide prompt control of adrenergic symptoms; start while workup is in progress. Long-acting propranolol is used most commonly and titrated to symptom control (40 to 320 mg/day). Calcium channel blockers are an alternative in patients who cannot take β-blockers (3)[C].
- Radioactive iodine (RAI)
  - Concentrates in the thyroid gland and destroys thyroid tissue
  - Radioiodine plus prednisone therapy might have the least probability of leading to an exacerbation or new appearance of ophthalmopathy, and radioiodine therapy might have the least probability of causing a recurrence (4)[A].
  - Treatment of choice for definitive therapy of hyperthyroidism, in the absence of moderate or severe orbitopathy (4)[A]
  - High cure rate with single treatment, especially with high-dose regimen
  - Risks: side effects (neck soreness, flushing, decreased taste); worsening ophthalmopathy (15% incidence, higher in smokers); posttreatment hypothyroidism (80% incidence, not dosage-dependent); radiation thyroiditis (1% incidence); need to adhere to safety precautions until radiation is eliminated from the body
  - May worsen Graves orbitopathy (GO): Symptoms are usually mild and transient in those patients with no or mild ophthalmopathy; however, treatment for patients with moderate to severe GO is still guided by expert opinion pending further study (5)[C].
  - Pretreatment with antithyroid medication should be considered in patients with severe disease and the elderly, to reduce risk of posttreatment transient hyperthyroidism and posttreatment radiation thyroiditis as well as quicker return to normal thyroid function. Controversy remains regarding whether pretreatment results in treatment failure, and no definitive data support use (6)[C].
  - May be repeated in as soon as 3 months but usually after 6 months if not euthyroid

Pregnancy Considerations
RAI is contraindicated in pregnancy and during breastfeeding.

- Antithyroid drugs: methimazole (MMI) and propylthiouracil (PTU)
  - Compete with the thyroid for iodine, thereby decreasing the synthesis of thyroid hormone; PTU blocks peripheral conversion of T_4 to T_3.

- Treatment of choice for children and for adults who refuse RAI
- May use as pretreatment for older or cardiac patients before RAI or surgery
- MMI is now almost exclusively used because of its longer duration of action, allowing for once daily dosing, more rapid efficacy, and lower incidence of side effects (2)[A].
- No improvement in remission rates were noted with higher dose MMI; lowest effective dose should be used (7)[B].
- Minor side effects (<5% incidence): controlled by switching from one agent to another: rash, fever, arthralgias, GI side effects
- Major side effects necessitating change in treatment: polyarthritis (1–2%), agranulocytosis (<0.5%), and cholestasis/jaundice (rare)
- Discontinue treatment after 1 year if patient is euthyroid.
- 60% remission rate with 2 years of treatment (standard regimen); newer studies suggest no increased benefit to treatment beyond 18 months (8)[B].
- Relapse rates up to 50% in patients who respond initially; higher rates if smoker, large goiter, or positive thyroid-stimulating antibodies at end of treatment.

Pregnancy Considerations
PTU is preferred in 1st trimester of pregnancy due to teratogenic effects of MMI. Switch to MMI in 2nd and 3rd trimesters due to risk of PTU-induced hepatotoxicity (9)[A].

ISSUES FOR REFERRAL
- Endocrinologist for RAI therapy; if patient is pregnant or breastfeeding
- Graves ophthalmopathy
- Surgery if failed drug therapy or refusing RAI; obstruction or cosmesis

ADDITIONAL THERAPIES
- Symptom control may be achieved with iodides, which block conversion of T_4 to T_3 and inhibit TSH release. Use for pregnant patients who do not tolerate antithyroid medication or in conjunction with antithyroid medications; should not be used long term (may cause paradoxical increase in TSH release) or in combination with radioactive iodine.
- For corneal protection: tinted glasses when outdoors, artificial tears, patching/taping the lids at night
- For orbitopathy: Mild cases can be treated with lubricants, nocturnal ointments, botulinum toxin injection for upper lid retraction, and smoking cessation (10)[C]. Moderate to severe cases should be treated with pulse-dose IV glucocorticoid if no contraindications (11)[C]. Alternative is PO steroid (prednisone 60 to 80 mg/day for 2 to 4 weeks, then taper off).
- For dermopathy, medium- to high-potency topical corticosteroid

SURGERY/OTHER PROCEDURES
With regard to ophthalmopathy progression, postoperative bleeding, permanent hypoparathyroidism, temporary and permanent recurrent laryngeal nerve palsy—total thyroidectomy (TT) is consistent with subtotal thyroidectomy (ST) in patients with Graves disease. However, TT is associated with a reduced incidence of recurrent hyperthyroidism and results in an increase in temporary hypoparathyroidism (12)[A].

COMPLEMENTARY & ALTERNATIVE MEDICINE
Nutritional supplementation with L-carnitine may act as an antagonist of thyroid hormone and reduce hyperthyroid symptoms as well as decrease bone demineralization.

INPATIENT CONSIDERATIONS
Indications for hospital admission:
- Thyroid storm (rare but a life-threatening complication): Admit to ICU.
- Ophthalmopathy with visual impairment: severe cardiac symptoms (heart failure, rapid atrial fibrillation, angina)

 ONGOING CARE

FOLLOW-UP RECOMMENDATIONS
Patient Monitoring
- Monitoring is for the resolution of hyperthyroidism and for the development of hypothyroidism.
- Check TSH and T_4 levels every 1 to 2 months for the first 6 months after treatment, then every 3 months for a year, then every 6 to 12 months thereafter. For patients on treatment with PTU and MMI, check CBC yearly. Also, check anti-TSH receptor antibodies at 12 months of treatment to determine possibility of discontinuing medication.

Pregnancy Considerations
Postpartum exacerbation of hyperthyroidism is common for women not currently under treatment, so TSH and symptoms should be monitored.

PATIENT EDUCATION
Adherence to both follow-up surveillance and medication regimens is the most important way to achieve a good outcome and promote lifelong health.

PROGNOSIS
- Generally good with treatment
- May have irreversible ocular, cardiac, and psychiatric consequences
- Increased morbidity and mortality due to osteoporosis, atherosclerotic disease, insulin resistance and obesity, and endothelial cell dysfunction (thromboembolic risk)

COMPLICATIONS
Hypothyroidism is the most common consequence of treatment (25–80%, depending on treatment modality). Patients should be monitored annually, even if asymptomatic.

REFERENCES
1. Bartalena L. The dilemma of how to manage Graves' hyperthyroidism in patients with associated orbitopathy. *J Clin Endocrinol Metab*. 2011;96(3):592–599.
2. Bahn Chair RS, Burch HB, Cooper DS, et al. Hyperthyroidism and other causes of thyrotoxicosis: management guidelines of the American Thyroid Association and American Association of Clinical Endocrinologists. *Thyroid*. 2011;21(6):593–646.
3. Reid JR, Wheeler SF. Hyperthyroidism: diagnosis and treatment. *Am Fam Physician*. 2005;72(4):623–630.
4. Ren Z, Qin L, Wang JQ, et al. Comparative efficacy of four treatments in patients with Graves' disease: a network meta-analysis. *Exp Clin Endocrinol Diabetes*. 2015;123(5):317–322.
5. Boelaert K, Torlinska B, Holder RL, et al. Older subjects with hyperthyroidism present with a paucity of symptoms and signs: a large cross-sectional study. *J Clin Endocrinol Metab*. 2010;95(6):2715–2726.
6. Cooper DS, Rivkees SA. Putting propylthiouracil in perspective. *J Clin Endocrinol Metab*. 2009;94(6):1881–1882.
7. Helfand M. Screening for subclinical thyroid dysfunction in nonpregnant adults: a summary of the evidence for the U.S. Preventive Services Task Force. *Ann Intern Med*. 2004;140(2):128–141.
8. Maugendre D, Gatel A, Campion L, et al. Antithyroid drugs and Graves' disease—prospective randomized assessment of long-term treatment. *Clin Endocrinol*. 1999;50(1):127–132.
9. Stagnaro-Green A, Abalovich M, Alexander E, et al. Guidelines of the American Thyroid Association for the diagnosis and management of thyroid disease during pregnancy and postpartum. *Thyroid*. 2011;21(10):1081–1125.
10. Melcescu E, Horton WB, Kim D, et al. Graves orbitopathy: update on diagnosis and therapy. *South Med J*. 2014;107(1):34–43.
11. Zang S, Ponto KA, Kahaly GJ. Clinical review: intravenous glucocorticoids for Graves' orbitopathy: efficacy and morbidity. *J Clin Endocrinol Metab*. 2011;96(2):320–332.
12. Guo Z, Yu P, Liu Z, et al. Total thyroidectomy vs bilateral subtotal thyroidectomy in patients with Graves' diseases: a meta-analysis of randomized clinical trials. *Clin Endocrinol*. 2013;79(5):739–746.

 SEE ALSO

Algorithms: Anxiety; Cardiac Arrhythmias; Weight Loss, Unintentional

CODES

ICD10
- E05.00 Thyrotoxicosis w diffuse goiter w/o thyrotoxic crisis
- E05.01 Thyrotoxicosis w diffuse goiter w thyrotoxic crisis or storm
- E05.20 Thyrotxcosis w toxic multinod goiter w/o thyrotoxic crisis

CLINICAL PEARLS
Thyroid hormone controls metabolic rate and affects many organ systems. Hyperthyroid patients appear hypermetabolic, with symptoms and signs of increased adrenergic tone.

GUILLAIN-BARRÉ SYNDROME

Simon B. Griesbach, MD • Grant M. Reed, DO

 BASICS

DESCRIPTION
- A group of acquired autoimmune disorders causing acute peripheral neuropathy and ascending paralysis that progressively worsens for up to 4 weeks followed by a slow spontaneous recovery of function.
- Subtypes classified by pattern of neural injury:
  - *Acute inflammatory demyelinating polyradiculo-neuropathy (AIDP)*: progressive limb weakness with areflexia (~95% of GBS cases in Europe and North America)
  - Axonal subtypes:
    - *Acute motor axonal neuropathy (AMAN)*: Pure motor neuropathy strongly associated with *Campylobacter jejuni* and a higher rate of respiratory failure. (~5% of cases in Europe and North America but 30–47% of cases in China, Japan, and Central and South America.)
    - *Acute motor-sensory axonal neuropathy (AMSAN)*: combined motor–sensory neuropathy; poor prognosis with prolonged course
  - Regional subtypes:
    - *Miller Fisher syndrome (MFS)*: triad with opthalmoplegia, ataxia, and areflexia; antibodies to GQ1b present in 90% of patients with MFS.
    - *Bickerstaff encephalitis*: possible variant of MFS with encephalopathy, ophthalmoplegia, ataxia, and hyperreflexia
    - *Pharyngeal-cervical-brachial GBS*: Parasympathetic and cholinergic dysfunction leads to neck, arm, and oropharyngeal weakness along with upper extremity areflexia.
  - Sensory subtypes:
    - *Acute pandysautonomia*: orthostatic hypotension, gastroparesis, ileus, constipation/diarrhea, sudomotor/pupillary abnormalities, and neuropathic pain
    - *Acute sensory ataxic neuropathy (ASAN)*: controversial variant with sensory loss and ataxia
- *Polyneuritis cranialis*: Bilateral cranial nerve involvement and severe peripheral sensory loss associated with CMV infections.
- Synonym(s): GBS, acute inflammatory demyelinating polyneuropathy; Landry-Guillain-Barré-Strohl syndrome, acute inflammatory idiopathic polyneuritis; acute autoimmune neuropathy; Landry ascending paralysis

ALERT
Rapidly progressing paralysis and respiratory failure occurs in 25–30% of patients. Some require mechanical ventilation within 48 hours.

ALERT
Areflexia is a red flag for GBS in patients with rapidly progressive limb weakness.

ALERT
A history of weakness preceded by respiratory or GI infection suggests GBS.

EPIDEMIOLOGY
Incidence
- Most common acute paralytic disease in Western countries at 0.6 to 4.0/100,000 worldwide
- U.S. incidence: 1.6 to 1.8/100,000, with 4,954 new cases reported from 2000 to 2004.

- Increases with age: 0.8/100,000 in children <18 years of age; 3.2/100,000 in adults >60 years of age
- 1.8 times higher incidence in males compared to females.

ETIOLOGY AND PATHOPHYSIOLOGY
- Autoimmune targeting of Schwann cell surface membrane, myelin, and/or gangliosides causing destruction and demyelination of peripheral nerves.
- Pathogenesis thought to involve molecular mimicry (i.e., an immune response to antigenic targets that are coincidentally shared by infectious organisms and host peripheral nerve tissue).

Genetics
Host factors appear to play a role in GBS, but no clear genetic risk has been identified.

RISK FACTORS
- Influenza vaccinations
  - Inactivated seasonal flu vaccines associated with a small increase in GBS risk equivalent to 1 case/million vaccines above background incidence. This compares to 17 cases of GBS per million people infected with influenza virus.
  - Incidence of GBS associated with influenza vaccine has steadily decreased over time.
  - *Of historical note*: Increased incidence during 1976 U.S. National H1N1 Immunization Program had vaccine-attributable risk of 8.8 per million recipients compared to 1.6 per million recipients in the 2009 H1N1 vaccination campaign.

COMMONLY ASSOCIATED CONDITIONS
- Infection of the respiratory (22–53%) or GI tract (6–26%) in preceding 6 weeks
  - *C. jejuni*: most common precipitant of GBS, (21–32% of cases):
    - Associated with axonal degeneration, slower recovery, more severe residual disability
  - Cytomegalovirus (CMV): Primary CMV infection precedes 10–22% of cases.
  - Rarely associated with *Mycoplasma pneumoniae*, influenza infection, Epstein-Barr virus, varicella-zoster virus, and HIV infection

 DIAGNOSIS

HISTORY
- AIDP presents with onset of progressive limb weakness that reaches its worst within 4 weeks (73% reach a functional nadir in 1 week).
- Preceding respiratory or gastrointestinal infection
- Earliest symptoms include pain, numbness, paresthesias, or limb weakness. These typically affect distal extremities and spread proximally.
- Neuropathic pain, sometimes severe, occurs in 40–50%, commonly in the back and lower extremities.
- Purely sensory symptoms effectively excludes GBS.

PHYSICAL EXAM
Diagnostic criteria for typical GBS:
- Required for diagnosis:
  - Progressive weakness reaching nadir between 12 hours and 28 days
  - Affects >1 limb
  - Areflexia/hyporeflexia
- Strongly supportive:
  - Paresthesias with only mild changes in objective sensory function (e.g., pinprick, light touch)

- Relative symmetry
- Cranial nerve involvement, especially bilateral/symmetric weakness of facial muscles
- Recovery beginning within 4 weeks after progression ceases
- Autonomic dysfunction
- Absence of fever at onset

DIFFERENTIAL DIAGNOSIS
Differential diagnosis of acute flaccid paralysis:
- Brain: basilar artery stroke, brainstem encephalitis
- Spinal cord: transverse myelitis, cord compression
- Motor neuron: poliomyelitis
- Peripheral neuropathy other than GBS: vasculitis, critical illness polyneuropathy, infectious (e.g., diphtheria, Lyme disease), CIDP, acute intermittent porphyria
- Neuromuscular junction: myasthenia gravis, Eaton-Lambert, botulism, toxins (e.g., heavy metals, inhalant abuse, organophosphates)
- Muscle: electrolyte disturbance (hypokalemia, hypophosphatemia), inflammatory myopathy, critical illness myopathy, acute rhabdomyolysis, trichonosis, periodic paralysis
- Psychological causes of weakness

DIAGNOSTIC TESTS & INTERPRETATION
Initial Tests (lab, imaging)
- Studies to establish the diagnosis:
  - Lumbar puncture (LP): Increased CSF protein (>0.55 g/L) without pleocytosis is present in ~80% of cases (CSF protein is often normal within the first 48 hours of symptom onset).
  - Nerve conduction study (NCS): *Most useful confirmatory test*; conduction velocities abnormal in 85% of patients with demyelination, even early in the disease. If nondiagnostic, repeat after 1 to 2 weeks.
- Imaging generally not required. MRI demonstrates spinal nerve root and/or cauda equina enhancement.
- Studies to find underlying cause:
  - Stool culture and serology for *C. jejuni*
  - Acute and convalescent serology for CMV, EBV, HIV, and *M. pneumoniae*
  - Anti-GQ1b antibodies in MFS variant

Follow-Up Tests & Special Considerations
- Analyze CSF prior to treatment with intravenous immunoglobulin (IVIG), which can cause aseptic meningitis.
- A repeat NCS 3 to 8 weeks after onset can classify the subtype of GBS (1)[B].

Diagnostic Procedures/Other
Sural nerve biopsy not indicated except to rule out vasculitis or amyloidosis

 TREATMENT

GENERAL MEASURES
- Pain treatment: NSAIDs helpful but often insufficient. Gabapentin and carbamazepine decrease opiate requirements in patients with GBS. One is not superior to the other (2)[A].
- DVT prophylaxis recommended in nonambulatory patients (3)[C].
- Neostigmine or erythromycin may be effective for ileus, if present (3)[C].

MEDICATION

First Line
- IVIG 0.4 g/kg/day for 5 days
  - In severe disease, IVIG started within 2 weeks of onset hastens recovery as much as plasma exchange (PE) (4)[A].
  - In children, IVIG likely hastens recovery compared with supportive care alone (4)[A].
  - Treatment with IVIG after PE confers no clinically significant extra benefit (4)[A].
- Plasma exchange (PE):
  - Compared with supportive treatment alone, those treated with PE have a quicker to recover walking (NNT 7), less requirement and shorter duration for mechanical ventilation (NNT 8), recover full muscle strength more quickly (NNT 8), and have fewer severe sequelae at 1 year (NNT 17) (5)[A].
  - Higher risks of relapse found with PE versus supportive care with no difference in severe infection or mortality (5)[A].
  - In mild GBS, two sessions of PE are superior to none. In moderate GBS, four sessions are superior to two. In severe GBS, six sessions are not significantly better than four (5)[A].
  - PE is most beneficial if started within 7 days of disease onset. It is still helpful until up to 30 days (5)[A].
  - The value of PE in children <12 years old is unknown.

Second Line
- Corticosteroids: not beneficial as monotherapy; do not significantly hasten recovery or affect long-term outcome. Low-quality evidence suggests they delay recovery (6)[A].
- CSF filtration is no different than PE in one small RCT (7)[B].
- Interferon β and brain-derived neurotrophic factor no different than placebo (7)[B]

ADDITIONAL THERAPIES
- Physical and occupational therapy improve fatigue and functional abilities (3)[C].
- Speech and language therapy improve swallowing function, if affected (3)[C].

COMPLEMENTARY & ALTERNATIVE MEDICINE
Tripterygium polyglycoside hastened recovery significantly more than corticosteroids (NNT 4), in one small trial (7)[A].

INPATIENT CONSIDERATIONS

Admission Criteria/Initial Stabilization
- Admit all patients suspected of having GBS.
- Closely monitor respiratory status with serial measurement of vital capacity (VC) and static inspiratory/expiratory pressures (PI_{max} and PE_{max}).
- Predictors of respiratory failure:
  - Rapid progression: ≥3 days between onset of weakness and hospital admission
  - Facial and/or bulbar weakness
  - VC decrease >30%
  - Medical Research Council (MRC) sum score indicating muscle weakness: 0 to 5/5 muscle strength grading for bilateral upper arm abductors, elbow flexors, wrist extensors, hip flexors, knee extensors, and foot dorsal flexors totaling 60 points.

- Indications for intubation:
  - VC <20 mL/kg
  - PI_{max} <30 cm H_2O
  - PE_{max} <40 cm H_2O

Nursing
- Prevent complications of immobilization with DVT prophylaxis and frequent turning.
- Respiratory care, aspiration precautions, pulmonary toilet
- Monitor bowel and bladder function for ileus and urinary retention.

Discharge Criteria
Mildly affected patients who can walk unaided and are stable for >2 weeks are unlikely to experience disease progression and may be managed as outpatients. Monitor bowel and bladder function for ileus and urinary retention.

ONGOING CARE

FOLLOW-UP RECOMMENDATIONS

Patient Monitoring
- Patients require close monitoring of respiratory, cardiac, and hemodynamic function, typically in the ICU setting.
- Pulmonary function testing (VC, respiratory frequency) q2–6h in the progressive phase and q6–12h in the plateau phase
- Monitor bulbar weakness and ability to handle airway secretions.
- Telemetry in patients with severe disease

PATIENT EDUCATION
Emphasize expectation for significant recovery and explain phases of illness.

PROGNOSIS
- If untreated, three phases of illness:
  - Initial progressive phase up to 4 weeks with highest risk of death and complication
  - Variable plateau phase
  - Recovery phase (weeks to months): return of proximal then distal strength
- 80% recover within 6 to 12 months with maximum 18 months past onset
- 20% with residual disability after 1 year:
  - Bilateral footdrop, intrinsic hand muscle wasting, sensory ataxia, dysesthesia
  - Half with severe disability
- Factors associated with poor functional outcome:
  - Age >60 years, rapid progression, severe disease indicated by GBS disability score or MRC sum score, preceding diarrhea, positive *C. jejuni* or CMV serology, axonal degeneration, need for mechanical ventilation

COMPLICATIONS
- 3% mortality at 6 months and 4% at 1 year. Older patients, those with severe disease have highest risk.
- 25–30% require mechanical ventilation.
- 70% develop autonomic dysfunction with hemodynamic instability, urinary retention, ileus, and anhidrosis.
- 10% have relapse
- ~2% develop relapsing chronic inflammatory demyelinating polyradiculoneuropathy (CIDP).

REFERENCES
1. Shahrizaila N, Goh KJ, Abdullah S, et al. Two sets of nerve conduction studes may suffice in reaching a reliable electrodiagnosis in Guillain-Barré syndrome. *Clin Neurophysiol.* 2013;124(7):1456–1459.
2. Liu J, Wang LN, McNicol ED. Pharmacological treatment for pain in Guillain-Barré syndrome. *Cochrane Database Syst Rev.* 2015;(4):CD009950.
3. Hughes RA, Wijdicks EF, Benson E, et al. Supportive care for patients with Guillain-Barré syndrome. *Arch Neurol.* 2005;62(8):1194–1198.
4. Hughes RA, Swan AV, van Doorn PA. Intravenous immunoglobulin for Guillain-Barré syndrome. *Cochrane Database Syst Rev.* 2014;(9):CD002063.
5. Raphaël JC, Chevret S, Hughes RA, et al. Plasma exchange for Guillain-Barré syndrome. *Cochrane Database Syst Rev.* 2012;(7):CD001798.
6. Hughes RA, van Doorn PA. Corticosteroids for Guillain-Barré syndrome. *Cochrane Database Syst Rev.* 2012;(8):CD001446.
7. Hughes RA, Pritchard J, Hadden RD. Pharmacological treatment other than corticosteroids, intravenous immunoglobulin and plasma exchange for Guillain-Barré syndrome. *Cochrane Database Syst Rev.* 2013;(2):CD008630.

ADDITIONAL READING
- Rinaldi S. Update on Guillain-Barré syndrome. *J Peripher Nerv Syst.* 2013;18(2):99–112.
- Sejvar JJ, Baughman AL, Wise M, et al. Population incidence of Guillain-Barré syndrome: a systematic review and meta-analysis. *Neuroepidemiology.* 2011;36(2):123–133.
- van den Berg B, Bunschoten C, van Doorn PA, et al. Mortality in Guillain-Barré syndrome. *Neurology.* 2013;80(18):1650–1654.
- Vellozzi C, Iqbal S, Broder K. Guillain-Barré syndrome, influenza, and influenza vaccination: the epidemiologic evidence. *Clin Infect Dis.* 2014;58(8):1149–1155.
- Walgaard C, Lingsma HF, Ruts L, et al. Prediction of respiratory insufficiency in Guillain-Barré syndrome. *Ann Neurol.* 2010;67(6):781–787.

CODES

ICD10
G61.0 Guillain-Barré syndrome

CLINICAL PEARLS
- Suspect GBS in cases of ascending flaccid paralysis with areflexia and antecedent history of viral respiratory illness or gastroenteritis.
- When GBS is suspected, evaluate VC and inspiratory force for signs of respiratory compromise.
- Uncomplicated GBS has a slow spontaneous recovery. Treatment with IVIG or PE speeds rate of recovery and reduces disability.
- Most useful diagnostic tests are nerve conduction studies and LP.
- GBS risk following influenza infection is 40 to 70 times greater than after seasonal influenza vaccination.

G

GYNECOMASTIA

Christine C. Zacharia, MD • Geetha Gopalakrishnan, MD

 BASICS

DESCRIPTION
- Benign glandular proliferation of male breast tissue
- Increase in estrogens relative to androgens leads to the development of gynecomastia.
- Gynecomastia can be transient and represent the normal physiologic changes that occur in utero or in adolescence. However, gynecomastia presenting or persisting in adulthood is typically pathologic in nature.

EPIDEMIOLOGY
- 60–90% of infants have transient gynecomastia (1).
- 48–64% of pubertal males have mild transient gynecomastia (onset at 10 to 12 years of age and resolution by age 18 years in most individuals) (1).
- 24–65% of men between 50 and 80 years of age report gynecomastia (2).

ETIOLOGY AND PATHOPHYSIOLOGY
Increase in estrogen activity relative to androgen activity leads to the development of gynecomastia (3). Estrogen stimulates ductal cell hyperplasia, facilitates ductal branching and lengthening, increases vascularity, and results in the proliferation of periductal fibroblasts. These changes occur within 12 months and are followed by fibrosis in the later stages of gynecomastia. Multiple factors can alter the estrogen to androgen ratio and precipitate gynecomastia:
- Decrease in androgen production
- Increase in estrogen production
- Increase in peripheral conversion to estrogen
- Inhibition of the androgen receptor
- Increase in the level of sex hormone–binding globulin (SHBG) or the affinity of androgens to SHBG (decreases free or bioavailable testosterone)
- Displacement of estrogen relative to testosterone from SHBG due to medications

RISK FACTORS
Gynecomastia can be physiologic or pathologic in nature.
- Physiologic gynecomastia presents in infants and adolescent boys and resolves spontaneously.
  - Neonatal gynecomastia: The placenta converts dehydroepiandrosterone (DHEA) and dehydroepiandrosterone sulfate (DHEA-S) to estrone and estradiol resulting in transient gynecomastia.
  - Adolescent gynecomastia: Transient increases in estradiol levels at the onset of puberty leads to gynecomastia.
- Pathologic gynecomastia refers to persistent or adult-onset gynecomastia. Multiple medications and medical conditions can alter the estrogen to androgen ratio and precipitate gynecomastia. However, 25% of cases are idiopathic in nature.
  - Medications: spironolactone, calcium channel blockers, proton pump inhibitors, cimetidine, efavirenz, ketoconazole, phenytoin, cytotoxic drugs, antidepressants, antiandrogen, estrogen, gonadotropin-releasing hormone (GnRH) agonists, 5-alpha reductase inhibitors, growth hormone (4,5)

ALERT
Illicit drugs (most common cause): marijuana, heroin, methadone, alcohol, amphetamines, over the counter body building supplements

- Primary or secondary hypogonadism

- Testicular tumor: germ cell (secrete human chorionic gonadotropin or hCG), Leydig cell (secrete estrogen), Sertoli cell (excessive aromatization to estrogens)
- Adrenal tumors (secrete DHEA-S and estrogens)
- Ectopic hCG tumors (hepatoblastoma, gastric tumors, renal cell carcinomas)
- Prolactinemia: leads to secondary hypogonadism and gynecomastia. Prolactin can stimulate milk production in breast tissue.
- Hyperthyroidism
- Cirrhosis
- Renal disease or dialysis
- Malnutrition/starvation
- Androgen insensitivity syndromes (defect in the androgen receptor)
- True hermaphroditism (both testicular and ovarian tissue present)
- Aromatase excess syndrome (increased peripheral conversion of androgens to estrogen)
- Idiopathic: most likely secondary to age-associated decline in free testosterone and adipose tissue–mediated aromatase activity

Pediatric Considerations
Transient gynecomastia is seen in neonates or pubertal boys. Typically resolves within 6 to 24 months.

Geriatric Considerations
Age-associated decline in testosterone production and increase in SHBG production leads to low free testosterone levels in the elderly population. Furthermore, the increased ratio of fat mass to lean mass noted with aging leads to adipose tissue–mediated peripheral conversion of androgens to estrogen. Both factors contribute to the development of idiopathic gynecomastia in the elderly. Medications also play a significant role in the development of gynecomastia in this population.

COMMONLY ASSOCIATED CONDITIONS
- Peutz-Jeghers syndrome—autosomal dominant disorder associated with Sertoli cell tumors, benign hamartomatous polyps, and mucocutaneous hyperpigmentation
- Carney complex—autosomal dominant disorder associated with Sertoli cell tumors, myxoma, hyperpigmentation of the skin (lentiginosis), and endocrine disorders like Cushing syndrome
- Prostate carcinoma—treatment with estrogen and antiandrogen leads to gynecomastia in 50% of patients
- Klinefelter syndrome—congenital abnormality leads to primary hypogonadism and gynecomastia. These patients are at risk for breast cancer and need regular breast exams.

DIAGNOSIS

HISTORY
- Inquire about duration of breast growth, increase in breast tissue size, and associated breast pain and discharge.
- If suspicious of hypogonadism, ask about erectile dysfunction, muscle mass, and decreased shaving frequency and libido.
- Obtain a complete medical history including headache, loss of vision, loss of appetite, weight loss, malignancy, thyroid disorders, liver disease, renal disease, and genetic abnormalities.
- Obtain a family history including Carney complex and Peutz-Jeghers syndrome.
- Review medication list extensively and inquire about the use of illicit substances.

PHYSICAL EXAM
- Careful breast exam to evaluate characteristics:
  - Firm, concentric glandular tissue beneath the nipple and areola palpable by pinching the thumb and forefinger together from either side of the breast toward the nipple
  - May involve one or both breasts
  - Usually asymptomatic but may be painful or tender if it is of recent onset
  - Off center, hard, fixed mass is concerning for malignancy while palpation of subareolar fat is more consistent with pseudogynecomastia.
  - Breast discharge should raise concern for malignancy or prolactinemia. In the latter, the discharge is typically clear or milky.
- Thyroid exam (evaluate for diffuse enlargement and palpable nodules and check extremities for tremor and brisk reflexes)
- Abdominal exam (evaluate for masses and liver size)
- Genitourinary exam (evaluate for testicular size, hair pattern, and presence of ovary or uterus)
- Visual field exam (evaluate for peripheral field defect)

DIFFERENTIAL DIAGNOSIS
- Pseudogynecomastia—fat deposition without glandular proliferation often seen in obesity
- Breast cancer—on exam the lesion is typically unilateral, firm, eccentric to the nipple, and associated with skin dimpling, nipple retraction/discharge, and lymphadenopathy
- Lipomas
- Sebaceous cyst
- Dermoid cyst
- Mastitis
- Hematoma
- Hamartoma

DIAGNOSTIC TESTS & INTERPRETATION
- Laboratory and radiologic investigations should be tailored to fit history and physical exam findings.
- Idiopathic gynecomastia is a diagnosis of exclusion and therefore, laboratory tests to rule out medical conditions associated with gynecomastia is recommended.

Initial Tests (lab, imaging)
- Luteinizing hormone (LH)—elevated in primary hypogonadism and decreased in secondary hypogonadism (6)[C]
- Morning total and free testosterone—decreased testosterone level in hypogonadism (6)[C]
- Human chorionic gonadotropin (hCG)—elevated in germ cell tumors and ectopic hCG tumors (6)[C]
- Estradiol—elevated in Leydig cell tumors, Sertoli cell tumors, adrenal tumors, and with increased aromatase activity (6)[C]
- Urine for drugs of abuse (UDA)
- Other tests to consider include creatinine, liver function test, thyroid function tests, and prolactin.

Follow-Up Tests & Special Considerations
Consider imaging studies based on laboratory findings.
- Testicular ultrasound (testicular tumor)
- Chest x-ray (CXR) and abdominal CT/MRI (extragonadal germ cell tumor, ectopic hCG tumor, and adrenal tumor)
- MRI of pituitary (pituitary tumor)

Diagnostic Procedures/Other
Based on physical exam findings, consider biopsy of breast mass to rule out malignancy (i.e., off center, hard, fixed, discharge).

Test Interpretation
- **Elevated hCG:** Check testicular ultrasound. If positive for a mass, likely a testicular germ cell tumor. If the ultrasound is negative, consider extragonadal germ cell tumor or hCG-secreting neoplasm and order a CXR and CT abdomen (6)[C].
- **Elevated LH:** if in relation to low testosterone, likely primary hypogonadism. If elevated in relation to high testosterone, check thyroid-stimulating hormone (TSH) and free thyroxine (FT4). If FT4 elevated and TSH is suppressed, likely hyperthyroidism; if TSH and FT4 are normal, likely androgen resistance (6)[C].
- **Normal or decreased LH in relation to low testosterone:** Check prolactin level. If prolactin is elevated, likely due to a prolactin-secreting pituitary tumor; if normal, likely due to secondary hypogonadism (6)[C]
- **Normal or decreased LH in relation to increased estradiol:** Check testicular ultrasound. If positive for a mass, likely Leydig or Sertoli cell tumor. If negative for mass, check CT abdomen to evaluate the adrenals. If mass is present, possible adrenal neoplasm versus adenoma; if no mass is detected, then likely due to increased aromatase activity in extraglandular tissue (6)[C]
- **hCG, LH, testosterone, and estradiol are normal:** likely idiopathic or medication/drug-induced gynecomastia (6)[C]

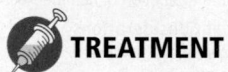
TREATMENT

GENERAL MEASURES
- Gynecomastia usually regresses spontaneously within 6 months of onset. This is true even for adult males. Therefore, patients can be monitored for the first 6 months and treatment considered if gynecomastia persists.
- The histologic changes early in the disease process can be reversed with medical therapy. However, with the development of fibrotic tissue, surgery is typically required. Typically, 1 to 2 years after the onset of gynecomastia, fibrotic changes can be seen and medical intervention is less effective (7)[C].
- Neonatal and pubertal gynecomastia spontaneously resolves within 6 to 24 months. Persistent pubertal gynecomastia (>24 months) occurs in 8% of pubertal boys. In adult males, 75% of gynecomastia is secondary to persistent pubertal gynecomastia, medications, and idiopathic conditions. Only 25% is related to an underlying medical condition.
- All illicit drug use and offending medications should be stopped if appropriate, and patients monitored for clinical improvement.
- Underlying medical conditions need to be treated (i.e., testosterone replacement for hypogonadal men, dopamine agonist for prolactinoma, appropriate treatment for thyrotoxicosis, and tumor resection).
- Medical and surgical therapy to reduce gynecomastia should be considered in patients with significant physical or psychological discomfort.

MEDICATION
- There are no FDA-approved medications for the treatment of gynecomastia but clinical trials involving selective estrogen receptor modulators and aromatase inhibitors demonstrate partial regression and symptom relief (i.e., breast tenderness).

  – Selective estrogen receptor modulators (SERMs): Clinical trials of both tamoxifen (10 to 20 mg/day) and raloxifene (60 mg/day) showed partial reduction in pubertal gynecomastia in 90% of study participants after 3 to 9 months but 40% of patients in both treatment groups were not

satisfied with the final results and underwent surgical removal (7)[B]. Tamoxifen has also been shown to reduce breast tenderness and prevent the development of gynecomastia in prostate cancer patients on androgen deprivation therapy. Therefore, SERMs (particularly tamoxifen) can be considered in men with 6 to 12 months of severe, painful gynecomastia symptoms.
  – Aromatase inhibitors block peripheral conversion of androgens to estrogens. In clinical trials, anastrozole (1 mg daily) has shown mixed results with one study reporting reduced breast volume in pubertal males and others not reporting a benefit. In prostate cancer patients, anastrozole prevented the development of gynecomastia in patients undergoing androgen deprivation therapy (8,9)[B].

ISSUES FOR REFERRAL
- Refer patients to an endocrinologist if abnormally elevated hormone levels are confirmed.
- If patients have refractory gynecomastia despite medical therapy and have prolonged gynecomastia characterized by the late fibrotic stage or symptoms concerning for breast cancer, referral to a surgeon would be appropriate.

ADDITIONAL THERAPIES
In clinical trials, prophylactic radiotherapy (10 to 15 Gy in one fraction over 3 days) prevented the development of gynecomastia in prostate cancer patients on androgen deprivation therapy. Higher doses (20 Gy in five fractions) improved pain symptoms in the same population. More studies are needed to evaluate the use of radiation therapy in other populations.

SURGERY/OTHER PROCEDURES
Surgery to remove breast tissue is recommended if:
- Gynecomastia does not regress within 12 months either spontaneously or after medical therapy
- Significant discomfort (i.e., pain, tenderness)
- Causes embarrassment or anxiety
- Biopsy suspicious for malignancy

FOLLOW-UP RECOMMENDATIONS
Patient Monitoring
- Every 3 to 6 months for 24 months; consider medical therapy (i.e., tamoxifen) if severe, painful symptoms persist after 6 to 12 months and surgery after 12 to 24 months. In individuals with asymptomatic or mild disease, routine yearly breast and physical exam is recommended.
- Patients with Klinefelter syndrome are at increased risk of breast cancer and should have routine breast exams done.

PATIENT EDUCATION
Patients should be encouraged to do periodic breast examination and to alert their clinical provider if a nodule is palpated in the breast or axilla, skin discoloration occurs, or nipple discharge develops.

PROGNOSIS
- Good in physiologic cases, as they often regress spontaneously within 3 to 6 months (6)
- Majority of patients experience regression once underlying disorder is treated or offending agents are eliminated (6).
- In patients who undergo surgery, majority are satisfied with the postop cosmetic appearance (10).

REFERENCES
1. Bembo SA, Carlson HE. Gynecomastia: its features, and when and how to treat it. *Cleve Clin J Med.* 2004;71(6):511–517.
2. Cuhaci N, Polat SB, Evranos B, et al. Gynecomastia: clinical evaluation and management. *Indian J Endocrinol Metab.* 2014;18(2):150–158.
3. Boccardo F, Rubagotti A, Battaglia M, et al. Evaluation of tamoxifen and anastrozole in the prevention of gynecomastia and breast pain induced by bicalutamide monotherapy of prostate cancer. *J Clin Oncol.* 2005;23(4):808–815.
4. Bowman JD, Kim H, Bustamante JJ. Drug-induced gynecomastia. *Pharmacotherapy.* 2012;32(12):1123–1140.
5. Jover F, Cuadrado JM, Roig P, et al. Efavirenz-associated gynecomastia: report of five cases and review of the literature. *Breast J.* 2004;10(3):244–246.
6. Braunstein GD. Clinical practice. Gynecomastia. *N Eng J Med.* 2007;357(12):1229–1237.
7. Lawrence SE, Faught KA, Vethamuthu J, et al. Beneficial effects of raloxifene and tamoxifen in the treatment of pubertal gynecomastia. *J Pediatr.* 2004;145(1):71–76.
8. Mauras N, Bishop K, Merinbaum D, et al. Pharmacokinetics and pharmacodynamics of anastrozole in pubertal boys with recent-onset gynecomastia. *J Clin Endocrinol Metab.* 2009;94(8):2975–2978.
9. Plourde PV, Reiter EO, Jou HC, et al. Safety and efficacy of anastrozole for the treatment of pubertal gynecomastia: a randomized, double-blind, placebo-controlled trial. *J Clin Endocrinol Metab.* 2004;89(9):4428–4433.
10. Gioffrè Florio MA, Alfio AR, Famà F, et al. Evaluation of complications and long-term results after surgery for gynaecomastia [in Italian]. *Chir Ital.* 2004;56(1):113–116.

ADDITIONAL READING
Eckman A, Dobs A. Drug-induced gynecomastia. *Expert Opin Drug Saf.* 2008;7(6):691–702.

 SEE ALSO

Algorithm: Gynecomastia

 CODES

ICD10
N62 Hypertrophy of breast

CLINICAL PEARLS
- Gynecomastia can be transient and represents the normal physiologic changes in neonates or adolescents. However, gynecomastia presenting or persisting in adulthood is typically pathologic in nature.
- Thorough history and physical exam should be performed on all patients and offending medications eliminated.
- Lab and radiologic studies should be conducted to rule out medical conditions associated with gynecomastia including thyrotoxicosis, prolactinemia, hypogonadism, testicular tumors, adrenal tumors, and ectopic hCG tumors. Treatment should be tailored to exam findings.
- ~25% of gynecomastia is idiopathic in nature and treatment should focus on symptom control.
- Clinical trials of SERMs, aromatase inhibitors, and radiation therapy seem promising. Surgery is the treatment of choice for refractory gynecomastia.

G

HAMMER TOES

Nicole Nelson, DO • David Bode, MD

 BASICS

Deformities of digits 2 to 5 ("lesser" digits) of the foot.

DESCRIPTION

- Plantar flexion deformity of the proximal inter-phalangeal (PIP) joint with varying degrees of hyperextension of the metatarsophalangeal (MTP) and distal interphalangeal (DIP) joint; primarily in sagittal plane (1)
- Can be flexible, semirigid, or fixed
  - Flexible: passively correctable to neutral position
  - Semirigid: partially correctable to neutral position
  - Fixed: not correctable to neutral position without intervention

EPIDEMIOLOGY

Most common deformity of lesser digits, typically affecting only one or two toes:

- Second toe is the most commonly involved.

Incidence

- Undefined
- Increases with age, duration of deformity (from flexible to rigid)

Prevalence

- Predominant sex: female > male (2)
  - Female predominance from 2.5:1 to 9:1, depending on age group
- Can range from 1% to 20% of population studied
- Blacks are more often affected than whites (2).

ETIOLOGY AND PATHOPHYSIOLOGY

- Can be congenital or acquired
- Biomechanical dysfunction results in loss of function of extensor digitorum longus (EDL) tendon at the PIP joint and the flexor digitorum longus (FDL) tendon at the MTP joint; the intrinsic muscles sublux dorsally as the MTP hyperextends. This results in plantar flexion of the PIP joint and hyperextension of the MTP joint (2).
- Specific pathomechanics vary by etiology:
  - Toe length discrepancy or narrow footwear toe box induces PIP joint flexion by forcing digit to accommodate shoe.
    - May also lead to MTP joint synovitis secondary to overuse, with elongation of plantar plate and MTP joint hyperextension
  - Rheumatoid arthritis (RA) causes MTP joint destruction and resultant subluxation.
  - Any condition that compromises intra-articular and periarticular tissues, such as second ray longer than first, inflammatory joint disease, neuromuscular conditions, improper-fitting shoes, and trauma (3)
  - Damage to joint capsule, collateral ligaments, or synovia leads to unstable PIP joint or MTP joint.

Genetics

- Significant heritability rates of 49–90% (4)
- Specific genetic markers are not identified.

RISK FACTORS

- Pes cavus, pes planus
- Hallux valgus
- Metatarsus adductus
- Ankle equinus
- Neuromuscular disease (rare)
- Trauma; improperly fitted shoes (narrow toe box) and/or tight hosiery
- Abnormal metatarsal and/or digit length
- Inflammatory joint disease (e.g., RA)
- Connective tissue disease
- Diabetes mellitus

GENERAL PREVENTION

- Proper fitting of shoes. Use of pressure-dispersive footwear helps reduce pain.
- Foot orthoses modulate biomechanical dysfunction and muscular imbalance, preventing progression (2).
- Control of predisposing factors (e.g., inflammatory joint disease) may also slow progression.

COMMONLY ASSOCIATED CONDITIONS

- Hallux valgus
- Cavus foot
- Metatarsus adductus
- Dorsal callus

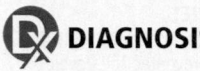 **DIAGNOSIS**

History and physical exam are typically sufficient for diagnosis of hammer toes. Additional tests are available to exclude other conditions.

HISTORY

- Location, duration, severity, and rate of progression of foot deformity
- Type, location, duration of pain
  - Patients often relate sensation of lump on plantar aspect of MTP joint.
- Degree of functional impairment
- Improving/exacerbating factors
- Type of footwear and hosiery worn
- Peripheral neurologic symptoms
- Any prior treatment rendered

PHYSICAL EXAM

- Note MTP joint hyperextension, PIP joint flexion, and DIP joint extension.
- Observe any adjacent toe deformities (e.g., hallux valgus, flexion contractures).
- Assess degree of flexibility and reducibility of deformity in both weight-bearing and non–weight-bearing positions (2)[C].
- Note any hyperkeratosis over the joint, ulcers, clavi (dorsal PIP joint, metatarsal head), adventitious bursa, erythema, or skin breakdown (2)[C].
- Palpate for pain over dorsal aspect of PIP joint or MTP joint.
- Drawer test of MTP joint
- Palpate web spaces to exclude interdigital neuroma.
- Neurovascular evaluation (e.g., pulses, sensation, muscle bulk)

DIFFERENTIAL DIAGNOSIS

- Hammer toe: hyperextension of the MTP and DIP joints and plantar flexion of the PIP joint
- Claw toe: dorsiflexion of MTP joint and plantar flexion of the DIP joint
- Mallet toe: fixed or flexible deformity of the DIP joint of the toe
- Overlapping fifth toe
- Interdigital neuroma
- Plantar plate rupture
- Nonspecific synovitis of MTP joint
- Fracture; exostosis
- Arthritis (e.g., rheumatoid, psoriatic)

DIAGNOSTIC TESTS & INTERPRETATION

Initial Tests (lab, imaging)

- Not required unless clinically indicated to rule out suspected metabolic or inflammatory arthropathies (2)[C]: rheumatoid factor, antinuclear antibodies (ANA), HLA-B27 serologies for inflammatory disease
- Weight-bearing x-rays of affected foot in antero-posterior (AP), lateral, and oblique views (2)[C]:
  - AP view superior for assessing MTP subluxation or dislocation
  - Lateral view is best for the evaluation of hammer toe.

Follow-Up Tests & Special Considerations

MRI or bone scan if osteomyelitis is suspected

Diagnostic Procedures/Other

- Nerve conduction studies or EMG if neurologic disorder is suspected
- Doppler or plethysmography if impaired circulation and surgery is considered
- Computerized weight-bearing pressure testing is indicated only in setting of neuromuscular deficiencies.

Test Interpretation

Histologic evaluation is not necessary before treatment.

 TREATMENT

- Goal of treatment is to relieve symptoms and help patients return to their normal activity level.
- Surgical and nonsurgical interventions are available.
- Mild cases may not require treatment.

GENERAL MEASURES

Nonsurgical (conservative) treatments include

- Shoe modifications (wider and/or deeper toe box) to accommodate the deformity and decrease the pressure over osseous prominences. Avoid high-heeled shoes (2)[C].
- Toe sleeve or orthodigital padding of the hammer toe prominence (5)[C]
- Hammer toe–straightening orthotics or taping to reduce flexible deformities

- Débridement of hyperkeratotic lesions can reduce symptoms. Topical keratolytics may be helpful (2)[C].
- Shoe orthotics mitigate abnormal biomechanics.
- Physical therapy for stretching and strengthening of the toes helps preserve flexibility.

MEDICATION
For pain relief

First Line
NSAIDs may be helpful in managing symptoms of pain as well as soft tissue and joint inflammation.

ISSUES FOR REFERRAL
If nonsurgical (conservative) treatment is unsuccessful and/or impractical or patient has combined deformity of MTP joint, PIP joint, and/or DIP joint, then patient may be referred to an orthopedic surgeon or surgical podiatrist.

SURGERY/OTHER PROCEDURES
- Surgical procedures for the correction of hammer toes depend on the degree and flexibility of the contracture(s) and related abnormalities.
- Surgical interventions for *flexible* hammer toes include (1,3,5,6)[C]
  - PIP joint arthroplasty (most common)
  - Flexor tendon lengthening/flexor tenotomy
  - Extensor tendon lengthening/tenotomy/MTP joint capsulotomy
  - Flexor to extensor tendon transfer
  - Exostosectomy
  - Implant arthroplasty
- Surgical interventions for semirigid/rigid hammer toes include (1,3,5)[C]
  - PIP joint resection arthroplasty or arthrodesis
  - Girdlestone-Taylor flexor-to-extensor transfer
  - Metatarsal shortening (Weil osteotomy)
  - Exostosectomy
  - Diaphysectomy of the proximal phalanx (less common)
  - Middle phalangectomy (less common)
  - Soft tissue releases/lengthening
- Procedures may be performed as isolated operations or in conjunction with other procedures.
- Contraindications for surgery: active infection, inadequate vascular supply, and desire for cosmesis alone

 ONGOING CARE

FOLLOW-UP RECOMMENDATIONS
- Obtain radiographs immediately following surgery or at the first postoperative visit; subsequent x-rays as needed.
- Full weight-bearing in a postoperative (surgical) shoe or other device based on the procedure(s) performed and the individual patient
- Elevate the foot to minimize swelling.
- Return to regular shoe wear after pain is controlled, swelling has subsided, and wounds have healed.
- Role and efficacy of postoperative physical therapy (3 times a week for 2 to 3 weeks) unclear

Patient Monitoring
In the absence of complications, the patient should be seen initially within the 1st week following the procedure(s). Frequency of subsequent visits is determined based on the procedure(s) performed and the postoperative course.

PATIENT EDUCATION
- Patients should be aware of mild to moderate swelling and plantar foot discomfort that may persist for many (1 to 6) months after surgery and may limit footwear options until resolved.
- MTP joint and PIP joint may remain stiff for extended periods of time.
- "Molding" of the operative toe (assuming the contours of adjacent toes) is common.
- Encourage patients to wear shoes of adequate size with "roomy" (rounded or squared) toe box.

PROGNOSIS
- Nonoperative (conservative) treatment usually alleviates pain; however, the deformity may progress.
- Surgical treatment of flexible hammer toe deformity reliably corrects the deformity and alleviates pain. Recurrence and progression are common, especially if the patient continues to wear ill-fitting shoes.
- Surgical treatment of fixed hammer toe deformity provides reliable deformity correction and pain relief. Recurrence is uncommon.

COMPLICATIONS
- Common complications specific to digital surgery include but are not limited to
  - Persistent edema
  - Recurrence of deformity
  - Residual pain
  - Excessive stiffness
  - Metatarsalgia
- Less common complications include
  - Numbness (e.g., digital nerve palsy)
  - Flail toe
  - Symptomatic osseous regrowth
  - Malposition of toe
  - Malunion/nonunion
  - Infection
  - Vascular impairment (e.g., toe ischemia, gangrene)

REFERENCES

1. Shirzad K, Kiesau CD, DeOrio JK, et al. Lesser toe deformities. *J Am Acad Orthop Surg.* 2011;19(8): 505–514.
2. Thomas JL, Blitch EL IV, Chaney DM, et al. Diagnosis and treatment of forefoot disorders. Section 1: digital deformities. *J Foot Ankle Surg.* 2009;48(3):418.e1–418.e9.
3. Zelen CM, Young NJ. Digital arthrodesis. *Clin Podiatr Med Surg.* 2013;30(3):271–282.
4. Hannan MT, Menz HB, Jordan JM, et al. High heritability of hallux valgus and lesser toe deformities in adult men and women. *Arthritis Care Res (Hoboken).* 2013;65(9):1515–1521.
5. Smith BW, Coughlin MJ. Disorders of the lesser toes. *Sports Med Arthrosc.* 2009;17(3):167–174.
6. Kwon JY, De Asla RJ. The use of flexor to extensor transfers for the correction of the flexible hammer toe deformity. *Foot Ankle Clin.* 2011;16(4): 573–582.

ADDITIONAL READING

- Marx RC, Mizel MS. What's new in foot and ankle surgery. *J Bone Joint Surg Am.* 2013;95(10): 951–957.
- Miller JM, Blacklidge DK, Ferdowsian V, et al. Chevron arthrodesis of the interphalangeal joint for hammertoe correction. *J Foot Ankle Surg.* 2010;49(2):194–196.

 SEE ALSO

Algorithm: Foot Pain

 CODES

ICD10
- M20.40 Other hammer toe(s) (acquired), unspecified foot
- M20.41 Other hammer toe(s) (acquired), right foot
- M20.42 Other hammer toe(s) (acquired), left foot

CLINICAL PEARLS
- Hammer toe is a plantar flexion deformity of the PIP joint.
- Initial management of hammer toe deformity is conservative. Consider surgery if pain persists or the deformity worsens.
- Properly fitting footwear helps minimize recurrence. Patients should be aware of mild to moderate swelling and plantar foot discomfort that may persist for months after surgery and may limit footwear options until resolved.

H

HAND-FOOT-AND-MOUTH DISEASE

Lee J. Herskowitz, DO, MBA

BASICS

DESCRIPTION
- Common acute viral illness affecting mostly children
- Characterized by vesicles on the buccal mucosa and tongue and peripherally distributed small, tender cutaneous lesions on the hands, feet, buttocks, and (less commonly) genitalia
- Group A coxsackieviruses are the most common causative agent (1).
- Synonym(s): herpangina (when affecting oral mucosa and posterior pharynx)

EPIDEMIOLOGY
- Self-limiting illness resolves in 7 to 10 days.
- Moderately contagious
- Infection is spread by direct contact with nasal discharge, saliva, blister fluid, or stool. .
- Infected individuals are most contagious during the 1st week of the illness. Some exposed individuals (especially adults) may be asymptomatic but still contagious.
- The viruses that cause hand-foot-and-mouth disease (HFM) can persist for weeks after symptoms have resolved, most commonly in stool, allowing transmission following resolution of symptoms.
- The incubation period is 3 to 7 days (1).

Incidence
- Children <5 years of age are most commonly affected, especially in day care facilities (1,2).
- Can occur as isolated cases, outbreaks, or epidemics
- Occurs worldwide
- Mother-to-fetus transmission is possible.
- Most large outbreaks occur in Southeast Asia.

ETIOLOGY AND PATHOPHYSIOLOGY
- HFMS is not the same as foot (hoof) and mouth found in cattle, and there is no cross species infectious concern (3).
- Transmission by the fecal–oral route or contact with skin lesions or oral secretions; caused by viruses that belong to the Enterovirus genus and replicated in the GI tract (3)
- Most commonly coxsackievirus A16
- Also coxsackieviruses A5, A7, A9, A10, B2, B5, and Enterovirus 71

GENERAL PREVENTION
- Hand washing, especially around food handling or diaper changes
- Exclusion of children from group settings during the first few days of the illness in the presence of open lesions in the mouth or on the skin may reduce the spread of infection.
- Hand hygiene measures are effective in reducing transmission.
- Pregnant woman should avoid contact with infected individuals.

DIAGNOSIS

HISTORY
- 1- to 2-day prodrome of fever, anorexia, malaise, abdominal pain, upper respiratory symptoms
- Fever may last 3 to 4 days
- Sore throat (follows fever)
- Painful mouth lesions (often preceding skin lesions)
- Rash on hands and feet
- Often history of sick contacts

PHYSICAL EXAM
- Tender vesicles or ulcers on buccal mucosa, sides of tongue, and palate
- Begin as small red papules and evolve into vesicles and then ulcerations
- May persist for up to 1 week
- Cutaneous vesicles 3 to 5 mm in diameter start as painful maculopapular eruptions, occur typically on dorsal aspect of fingers and toes.
- May also occur on the palms, soles, buttocks, and groin
- Adults are less likely to have cutaneous findings.

DIFFERENTIAL DIAGNOSIS
- Herpes simplex
- Herpes zoster
- Scarlet fever
- Roseola infantum
- Fifth disease
- Other enteroviral infections
- Kawasaki disease
- Viral pharyngitis
- Varicella
- Rickettsial infection (RFSF)

DIAGNOSTIC TESTS & INTERPRETATION
Typically clinically diagnosed

Initial Tests (lab, imaging)
Culture for responsible virus (virus isolation) can be obtained from oral lesions, cutaneous vesicles, nasopharyngeal swabs, stool, and CSF, although not typically performed. PCR of throat swabs and vesicle fluid is the most efficient test if enterovirus 71 is suspected (3).

TREATMENT

- Symptomatic
- Avoid spicy or acidic foods to limit oral pain.
- Numbing sprays or cautious use of viscous lidocaine can be used for oral pain, especially for pharyngitis (use oral topical analgesics)
- IV fluids may be required in more severe cases of dehydration.

MEDICATION

- Symptomatic care using ibuprofen or acetaminophen for pain from oral ulcers or fever
- Soothing mouthwashes ("MAGIC MOUTHWASH") can be compounded by the parents or pharmacy containing equal amounts of viscous lidocaine, diphenhydramine, and Maalox. Instruct to swish and spit (caution in young children due to risk of lidocaine toxicity).

Pediatric Considerations
Avoid aspirin use in treating febrile illness in children.

INPATIENT CONSIDERATIONS

- Patients with CNS manifestations or autonomic dysregulation should require hospitalization.
- Admit those with dehydration unable to maintain adequate oral hydration.

ONGOING CARE

DIET

- Encourage cold liquids (e.g., ice cream, popsicles) to prevent dehydration.
- Avoid acidic, salty, and spicy foods, as they will increase pain.

COMPLICATIONS

- Dehydration most common due to painful oral ulcerations
- Rarely, aseptic meningitis or other neurologic complications
- Fever >3 days and lethargy are associated with CSF pleocytosis.
- Concomitant CNS disease may occur when HFM syndrome is caused by Enterovirus 71. In Southeast Asia, this results in a mortality rate of 3 deaths per 10,000 cases.
- Cardiopulmonary complications include myocarditis, pneumonitis, and pulmonary edema.
- Temporary loss of fingernails or toenails may occur rarely.

REFERENCES

1. Centers for Disease Control and Prevention. Hand, Foot, and Mouth Disease (HFMD). http://www.cdc.gov/hand-foot-mouth/
2. Centers for Disease Control and Prevention. Notes from the field: severe hand, foot, and mouth disease associated with coxsackievirus A6—Alabama, Connecticut, California, and Nevada, November 2011-February 2012. *MMWR Morb Mortal Wkly Rep.* 2012;61(12):213–214.
3. A Guide to Clinical Management and Public Health Response for Hand, Foot and Mouth disease (HFMD) World Health Organization: Western Pacific Region. http://www.wpro.who.int/publications/docs/GuidancefortheclinicalmanagementofHFMD.pdf

CODES

ICD10

- B08.4 Enteroviral vesicular stomatitis with exanthem
- B34.1 Enterovirus infection, unspecified
- B08.5 Enteroviral vesicular pharyngitis

CLINICAL PEARLS

- Most common: May to October
- Children <5 years of age tend to have worse symptoms than older children.
- Hand-foot-and-mouth disease is the most common cause of mouth sores in pediatric patients.
- Usually self-limiting, resolving in 7 to 10 days
- Careful handwashing to limit dissemination.

H

HEADACHE, CLUSTER

Jeffrey Phillips, MD

BASICS

DESCRIPTION
- Primary headache disorder
- Multiple attacks of unilateral, excruciating, sharp, searing, or piercing pain. Typically localized in the periorbital area and temple accompanied by signs of ipsilateral autonomic features
- Autonomic symptoms: parasympathetic hyperactivity signs (ipsilateral lacrimation, eye redness, nasal congestion) and sympathetic hypoactivity (ipsilateral ptosis and miosis)
- Patients often pace, rubbing their heads to try to alleviate the pain.
- Symptoms usually remain on the same side during a single cluster attack.
- Individual attacks last 15 to 180 minutes if untreated and occur from once every other day to 8 times per day.
- Attacks usually occur in series (cluster periods) lasting for weeks or months separated by remission periods usually lasting months or years. However, about 10–15% of patients have chronic symptoms without remissions.

EPIDEMIOLOGY
Incidence
1-year incidence: 53/100,000

Prevalence
- Lifetime prevalence 124/100,000 (~0.1%)
- Predominant sex: male > female (4.3:1)
- Mean age of onset: between 29.6 and 35.7 years
- Episodic/chronic ratio 6:1

ETIOLOGY AND PATHOPHYSIOLOGY
- Complex and incompletely understood
- Proposed mechanisms include the following:
  - Activation of posterior hypothalamus may trigger an attack, causing activation of the trigeminal nerve, leading to intense pain symptoms.
  - Autonomic symptoms: activation of craniofacial parasympathetic nerve fibers secondary to pathologic activation of trigemino-autonomic brainstem reflex

Genetics
- Usually sporadic: autosomal dominant in 5% of cases; autosomal recessive or multifactorial in other families
- Evidence varies: first-degree relatives carry 5- to 8-fold; second degree, 1- to 3-fold increased relative risk of disease

RISK FACTORS
- Male gender
- Age (70% onset before age 30 years)
- Cigarette smoking
- Family history of cluster headache (CH)
- Head trauma
- Alcohol induces attacks during a cluster but not during remission.
- Small amounts of vasodilators (e.g., alcohol, nitroglycerin, sildenafil)
- Strong odors

COMMONLY ASSOCIATED CONDITIONS
- Depression (24%)
- Increased risk of suicide secondary to the extreme nature of the pain
- Medication-overuse headache

- Asthma (9%)
- History of migraine, frequently in female patients
- Sleep apnea (14%)
- Increased prevalence of cardiac right-to-left shunt and patent foramen ovale (relationship unclear)

DIAGNOSIS

- Diagnosis is clinical.
- *International Classification of Headache Disorders* (2nd edition) criteria: at least five attacks of severe or very severe unilateral orbital, supraorbital, or temporal pain lasting 15 to 180 minutes if untreated
- At least one of the following:
  - Ipsilateral
    - Conjunctival injection and/or lacrimation
    - Nasal congestion and/or rhinorrhea
    - Eyelid edema
    - Forehead and facial sweating
    - Miosis and/or ptosis
  - Sense of restlessness or agitation
- Attack frequency: one every other day to eight per day
- Episodic CH: at least two cluster periods lasting 7 days to 1 year, separated by a pain-free interval of >1 month (80–90% of cases)
- Chronic CH: cluster-free interval of <1 month in a ≥12-month period

HISTORY
- Episodic periods of headache described as excruciating, unilateral, sharp, searing, or piercing pain, typically localized in the periorbital area.
- Eye redness, tearing, nasal discharge, sweating
- Timing of headaches often circadian in nature

PHYSICAL EXAM
- Usually patients seen between attacks
- Acute distress, crying, screaming, restless, and/or agitated during attacks
- Ipsilateral lacrimation, injected conjunctivae, ptosis, and miosis
- Nasal stuffiness or rhinorrhea
- Bradycardia or tachycardia

DIFFERENTIAL DIAGNOSIS
- Paroxysmal hemicrania, short-lasting unilateral neuralgiform headache attacks with conjunctival injection and tearing (SUNCT)
- Hemicrania continua, hypnic headaches, trigeminal and other facial neuralgias, migraine, temporal arteritis, herpes zoster
- Secondary CH:
  - Vertebral or carotid artery dissection, brain arteriovenous malformations, intracranial artery aneurysms
  - Pituitary tumors
  - Nasopharyngeal carcinoma
  - Maxillary sinus with foreign body/sinusitis
  - Cavernous hemangioma
  - Meningiomas/carcinomas/metastases

DIAGNOSTIC TESTS & INTERPRETATION
- Diagnosis is primarily clinical.
- Diagnosis is often delayed (>40% report 5-year delay in diagnosis).
- Consider neuroimaging (MRI/CT head and vascular imaging of brain):
  - Abnormal neurologic exam
  - Suspect secondary CH

TREATMENT

Many of the medications discussed in the following section are used off-label in the treatment of CH.

GENERAL MEASURES
- Avoid major changes in sleep habits.
- Stop smoking.
- Avoid use of alcohol during cluster period.
- Avoid extreme changes in altitude due to changes in oxygen levels.
- Avoid exposure to chemical agents/solvents.

MEDICATION
- Avoid pain therapy, especially narcotic analgesics, for acute attacks.
- Goal is abortion of acute attack and prophylaxis for expected duration of the cluster.
- Assess cardiovascular risk before instituting a vasoactive drug, such as triptans or ergot derivatives.

First Line
For acute attacks:
- Oxygen
  - 100% at 6 to 12 L/min for 15 minutes via nonrebreathing mask provides relief within 15 minutes (1)[A].
  - Avoid in severe chronic obstructive pulmonary disease (COPD) as might affect hypoxic respiratory drive.
- Sumatriptan (Imitrex)
  - 6 mg SC, max 12 mg/24 hr with at least 1 hour between injections is most effective medication for acute attacks. NNT (needed to treat) 2.4 for headache relief in 15 minutes. Sumatriptan nasal spray: 20 mg. May repeat in 2 hours, max dose 40 mg/24 hr NNT 3.2 for headache relief at 30 minutes (2)[A].
- Zolmitriptan
  - Nasal spray: 5- and 10-mg dosage both effective. May repeat in 2 hours, max 10 mg/24 hr. NNT 12 and 4.9 for headache relief in 15 minutes for 5 and 10 mg, respectively. Zolmitriptan tablet: 5- and 10-mg dosage both effective. May repeat in 2 hours, max dose 10 mg/24 hr. NNT 6.7 and 4.5 for headache relief in 30 minutes for 5 and 10 mg, respectively (2)[A].

ALERT
Triptans are contraindicated in ischemic cardiac disease, stroke, uncontrolled hypertension, prinzmetal angina, basilar migraine, hemiplegic migraine, ischemic bowel disease, and peripheral vascular disease.

- Prophylaxis: used at start of cluster period to prevent and shorten further attacks. Start as soon as possible:
  - Verapamil
    - Can start at 240 mg/day and increase by 40 to 80 mg every 10 to 14 days. Short- or long-acting equivalent. Most patients respond to daily dose of 200 to 480 mg but up to 960 mg/day may be needed. NNT = 1.2 (3)[A]
    - ECG monitoring for doses/increments >480 mg/day required because of risk of bradycardia (q3mo used as a guideline)
    - Similar efficacy to lithium, but fewer adverse effects and faster onset make it the preferred choice.
    - Often used in conjunction with another agent

Second Line
- Acute attack
  - Lidocaine/**cocaine**: 10 mg (1 mL) of lidocaine or 40 to 50 mg of 10% cocaine intranasal. No well-controlled randomized controlled trials (RCTs) done. Most common side effects are nasal congestion, unpleasant taste (4)[B].
  - Octreotide: SC 100 μg. Can be considered in patients when triptans are contraindicated. Main side effect is GI upset (5)[A].
  - Ergotamine/dihydroergotamine (DHE): original treatments for CH. Now rarely used because of significant side effects. No controlled trials done. Still used for transitional prophylaxis (see below)
- Prophylaxis
  - Lithium: Start 300 mg BID, titrate to therapeutic range of 0.8 to 1.1 mEq/L. Most patients benefit from 600 to 1,200 mg/day. Widely used without formal evidence of efficacy. Retrospective case series show that lithium led to >50% reduction in attack frequency within 2 weeks in 77% of the patients with episodic CH. Must monitor levels of liver, renal, and thyroid function. Caution with nephrotoxic drugs, diuretics. Inferior to verapamil (6)[B]
  - Melatonin: 10 mg in the evening showed reduction in headache frequency versus placebo in small RCT. No side effects were reported.
  - Antiepileptics: topiramate, sodium valproate, gabapentin: Open studies showed reduction of cluster duration and frequency of headache, but RCT did not show superiority to placebo. Significant adverse effects
  - Civamide: 100 μL of 0.025% into each nostril daily. Only studied in episodic CH in one trial of 28 patients. Not available in the United States. Most common side effects were nasal burning, lacrimation, pharyngitis, and rhinorrhea.
  - Capsaicin: 0.025% ipsilateral nostril for 7 days, shows benefit in small RCT.
  - Methysergide: No studies available to confirm efficacy. Has serious adverse effects, including pulmonary and retroperitoneal fibrosis. Cannot be given with triptans and ergots
  - Pizotifen: Modest benefit limited by fatigue and weight gain

ADDITIONAL THERAPIES
Transitional preventive treatment are as follows:
- Used until longer-term preventive treatment becomes effective. Longer term maintenance agents are started concurrently:
  - Steroids: Several open studies suggested benefit, but no rigorous trials to prove efficacy. Studies support at least 40 mg/day (up to 80 mg/day) prednisone with a 10- to 30-day taper provides benefit to 60–90% patients. Adverse effects for short-term use: insomnia, psychosis, hyponatremia, edema, hyperglycemia, peptic ulcer

ALERT
Ergots are contraindicated in patients with cardiovascular disease and cannot be used with triptans.

Pregnancy Considerations
Collaboration between headache specialist, obstetrician, and pediatrician strongly encouraged. Patient should be informed of treatment benefits and risks as well as drug's potential teratogenic effect. For abortive treatment, oxygen is most appropriate first-line therapy. Nasal lidocaine (pregnancy Category B) can be used as second-line therapy. As preventive therapy, verapamil (pregnancy Category C) and steroids (pregnancy Category C) remain the preferred options. Use of SC or intranasal sumatriptan (pregnancy Category C) should be limited as much as possible. Avoid ergotamines (pregnancy Category X).

ISSUES FOR REFERRAL
Consider a neurology or headache center referral for refractory or complicated patients.

SURGERY/OTHER PROCEDURES
- Surgery may be considered only for patients who are refractory to, or have contraindications to, medical therapy.
- Various techniques focus on stimulation or ablation of segments of trigeminal nerve root and sphenopalatine ganglion. Other techniques are aimed at decreasing pain and inflammation surrounding the greater occipital nerve.
- Greater occipital nerve steroid injection: A retrospective analysis showed ~80% of patients with partial or complete response. Effect lasted 3.5 weeks; 21 mg of betamethasone and 2 mL of 2% lidocaine were used. One class I RCT showed benefit within 72 hours in 85% of lidocaine/betamethasone group compared with none in lidocaine/saline group. Cortivazol injection reduced severity and frequency of headache compared with placebo in an RCT (7)[A].
- No evidence for Botox or hyperbaric oxygen treatment
- Neurostimulation
  - Occipital nerve stimulation (ONS) was shown to reduce severity and attack frequency in chronic CH patients.
  - Deep brain stimulation (DBS) of the posterior inferior hypothalamus shows moderate therapeutic effect.
  - Currently investigating sphenopalatine ganglion stimulation

INPATIENT CONSIDERATIONS
Suicidal ideation, unwilling to contract for safety

ONGOING CARE

FOLLOW-UP RECOMMENDATIONS
Patient Monitoring
- Anticipate cluster bouts and initiate early prophylaxis.
- Monitor for depression.
- Watch for adverse medication response and side effects, such as unmasking of underlying cardiovascular disorder when using medications to treat CH.

PROGNOSIS
- Unpredictable course. With aging, attack frequency often decreases.
- Poor prognosis associated with older age of onset, male gender, disease duration of >20 years for episodic form
- Possibility of transformation of episodic cluster to chronic cluster and occasionally chronic cluster to episodic cluster

COMPLICATIONS
- Depression and suicide
- Side effects of medication, including unmasking of coronary artery disease
- Potential for drug abuse/misuse

REFERENCES
1. Cohen AS, Burns B, Goadsby PJ. High-flow oxygen for treatment of cluster headache: a randomized trial. *JAMA.* 2009;302(22):2451–2457.
2. Law S, Derry S, Moore RA. Triptans for acute cluster headache. *Cochrane Database Syst Rev.* 2010;(4):CD008042.
3. Leone M, D'Amico D, Frediani F, et al. Verapamil in the prophylaxis of episodic cluster headache: a double-blind study versus placebo. *Neurology.* 2000;54(6):1382–1385.
4. Costa A, Pucci E, Antonaci F, et al. The effect of intranasal cocaine and lidocaine on nitroglycerin-induced attacks in cluster headache. *Cephalalgia.* 2000;20(2):85–91.
5. Matharu MS, Levy MJ, Meeran K, et al. Subcutaneous octreotide in cluster headache: randomized placebo-controlled double-blind crossover study. *Ann Neurol.* 2004;56(4):488–494.
6. Stochino ME, Deidda A, Asuni C, et al. Evaluation of lithium response in episodic cluster headache: a retrospective case series. *Headache.* 2012;52(7):1171–1175.
7. Leroux E, Valade D, Taifas I, et al. Suboccipital steroid injections for transitional treatment of patients with more than two cluster headache attacks per day: a randomised, double-blind, placebo-controlled trial. *Lancet Neurol.* 2011;10(10):891–897.

ADDITIONAL READING
- Ashkenazi A, Schwedt T. Cluster headache—acute and prophylactic therapy. *Headache.* 2011;51(2):272–286.
- Beck E, Sieber WJ, Trejo R. Management of cluster headache. *Am Fam Physician.* 2005;71(4):717–724.
- Fontaine D, Lanteri-Minet M, Ouchchane L, et al. Anatomical location of effective deep brain stimulation electrodes in chronic cluster headache. *Brain.* 2010;133(Pt 4):1214–1223.
- Hainer BL, Matheson EM. Approach to acute headache in adults. *Am Fam Physician.* 2013;87(10):682–687.
- International Headache Society: http://www.ihs-headache.org

 SEE ALSO

Algorithm: Headache, Chronic

CODES

ICD10
- G44.009 Cluster headache syndrome, unspecified, not intractable
- G44.019 Episodic cluster headache, not intractable
- G44.029 Chronic cluster headache, not intractable

CLINICAL PEARLS
- CHs are rare but disabling. Patients are often agitated and restless during the attack.
- Oxygen and triptans, not narcotics, are first-line therapy for acute attacks.
- Abortive, transitional, and prophylaxic treatment must all be considered.

H

HEADACHE, MIGRAINE

Benjamin N. Schneider, MD

BASICS

DESCRIPTION
Recurrent headache disorder manifesting in attacks lasting 4 to 72 hours. Typical characteristics are unilateral location, pulsating quality, moderate or severe intensity, aggravation by physical activity, and association with nausea and/or photophobia and phonophobia (1).

- Most frequent subtypes of migraine (1):
  - Without aura (common migraine): defining >80% of attacks, often associated with nausea, vomiting, photophobia, and/or phonophobia
  - With aura (classic migraine): visual or other types of fully reversible neurologic phenomenon lasting 5 to 60 minutes
  - Chronic (transformed) migraine: chronic headache pattern evolving from episodic migraine. Migraine-like attacks are superimposed on a daily or near-daily headache pattern (e.g., tension headaches), >15 headache days/month for at least 3 months.
  - Menstrual-related (moliminal) migraine: associated with onset of menstrual period
- Rare but important subtypes (1):
  - Status migrainosus: debilitating migraine lasting >72 hours
  - With brainstem aura (basilar migraine): brainstem symptoms—dysarthria, vertigo, tinnitus, or ataxia, which are fully reversible and lasting 5 to 60 minutes.
  - Hemiplegic migraine: aura consisting of fully reversible hemiplegia and/or hemiparesis
  - Recurrent painful ophthalmoplegic neuropathy (ophthalmoplegic migraine): neuralgia accompanied by paresis of an ocular cranial nerve with ipsilateral headache
  - Retinal: repeated attacks of monocular visual disturbance, including scintillations, scotomata, or blindness, associated with migraine headache

EPIDEMIOLOGY
Female > male (3:1)

Prevalence
- Affects >28 million Americans
- Adults: women 18%; men 6%

ETIOLOGY AND PATHOPHYSIOLOGY
- No longer believed to be primarily vascular in etiology; rather, cortical spreading depolarization/depression
- Trigeminovascular hypothesis: hyperexcitable trigeminal sensory neurons in brainstem are stimulated and release neuropeptides, such as substance P and calcitonin gene–related peptide (CGRP), leading to vasodilation and neurogenic inflammation.

Genetics
- >80% of patients have a positive family history.
- Familial hemiplegic migraine has been shown to be linked to chromosomes 1, 2, and 19 (1).

RISK FACTORS
- Family history of migraine
- Female gender
- Stress
- Menstrual cycle, hormones
- Sleep pattern disruption
- Diet: skipped meals (40–56%), alcohol (29–35%), chocolate (19–22%), cheese (9–18%), caffeine overuse (14%), monosodium glutamate (MSG)

(12%), and artificial sweeteners (e.g., aspartame, sucralose)
- Medications: estrogens, vasodilators

GENERAL PREVENTION
- Avoid precipitants of attacks.
- Biofeedback, education, and psychological intervention
- Lifestyle modifications are the cornerstone of prevention: sleep hygiene, stress management, healthy diet, and regular exercise.
- Prophylactic medication if attacks are frequent, severely debilitating, or not controlled by acute interventions

COMMONLY ASSOCIATED CONDITIONS
- Depression, psychiatric disorders
- Sleep disturbance (e.g., sleep apnea)
- Cerebral vascular disease
- Peripheral vascular disease
- Seizure disorders
- Irritable bowel syndrome
- Obesity
- Patent foramen ovale (PFO)
- Medication overuse headache (MOH)

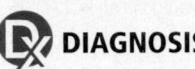

DIAGNOSIS

Migraine is a clinical diagnosis; thorough history and neuro examination are usually all that are necessary.

HISTORY
- Screening mnemonic "POUND": **P**ulsating, duration of 4 to 72 h**O**urs, **U**nilateral, **N**ausea, **D**isabling
  - + Likelihood ratio (LR) = 24 for migraine diagnosis if 4 of 5 criteria are present
  - + LR = 0.41 for migraine diagnosis if ≤2 criteria are present (2)
    - Headache usually begins with mild pain escalating into unilateral (30–40% bilateral) throbbing (40% nonthrobbing) pain lasting 4 to 72 hours.
    - Intensified by movement and associated with systemic manifestations: nausea (87%), vomiting (56%), diarrhea (16%), photophobia (82%), phonophobia (78%), muscle tenderness (65%), lightheadedness (72%), and vertigo (33%)
    - May be preceded by aura
  - Visual disruptions are most common—scotoma, hemianopsia, fortification spectra, geometric visual patterns, and occasionally hallucinations.
  - Somatosensory disruption in face or arms
  - Speech difficulties
    - Obtain headache profile: number of headaches per month; number of days per month headaches limit daily activities; and frequency and amount of all headache medications used.
    - Migraine disability assessment (MiDAS) is a useful tool to assess level of disability and correlates well with headache diaries.
    - Identify possible triggers (e.g., stress, sleep disturbance, food, caffeine, alcohol).

PHYSICAL EXAM
Neurologic exam should be performed including fundoscopy; abnormalities consistent with other causes to severe headaches MIGHT include the following:
- Gait abnormalities and other new cerebellar findings
- Loss of gross and/or fine motor function
- Altered mental status including possible hallucinations (visual, auditory, olfactory)
- Short-term memory loss

DIFFERENTIAL DIAGNOSIS
- Other primary headache syndromes
- If focal neurologic signs/symptoms are present, consider transient ischemic attack (TIA) or stroke.
- Secondary headaches: tumor, infection, vascular pathology, prescription or illicit drug use (MOH)
- Psychiatric disease
- Rarely, atypical forms of epilepsy

DIAGNOSTIC TESTS & INTERPRETATION
Neuroimaging is appropriate ONLY with suspicious symptomatology and/or an abnormality on physical examination (3). Other red flags include the following:
- New onset in patient >50 years of age
- Change in established headache pattern
- Atypical pattern or unremitting/progressive neurologic symptoms
- Prolonged or bizarre aura
- Type of imaging: Data are insufficient to make evidence-based recommendations regarding relative sensitivity of MRI compared with CT in the evaluation of migraine or other nonacute headache
- EEG is NOT indicated unless evaluating loss of consciousness or altered mental status.

Pregnancy Considerations
- Frequency may decrease in 2nd and 3rd trimesters.
- Nonpharmacologic methods are mainstay of treatment.
- No treatment drug has an FDA approval during pregnancy.
  - Acetaminophen (Category C) triptans, antiemetics, and short-acting opioids can be considered for acute headaches during pregnancy.
  - Ergotamines are contraindicated (Category X).
  - Avoid herbal remedies.
  - Sumatriptan, naratriptan and opiates are pregnancy Category C—risk cannot be rule out but early data suggest no increase in birth defects.
  - Sumatriptan by injection is ideal for breastfeeding women with disabling migraines.
  - Propranolol (Category C) is effective for prophylaxis during pregnancy and lactation.

TREATMENT

GENERAL MEASURES
- Most patients manage attacks with self-care.
- Cold compresses to area of pain
- Withdrawal from stressful surroundings
- Sleep is desirable.
- See also "General Prevention."

MEDICATION
- **First-line abortive treatments**
  - Mild to moderate attacks:
    - NSAIDs, such as ibuprofen, naproxen, and diclofenac are inexpensive and effective in up to 60% of cases.
    - Aspirin 500 mg–acetaminophen 500 mg–caffeine 130 mg (AAC) combination (e.g., Excedrin Migraine) is an inexpensive, nonprescription, and FDA-approved treatment.
  - Moderate to severe attacks:
    - Triptans are preferred when OTC agents fail for mild/moderate attacks OR as initial treatment for moderate to severe attacks:
    - All triptans have similar efficacy and tolerability, but some patients may respond better to one triptan over another.

○ Early intervention with triptans during the aura, prior to onset of pain, prevent headache 89% of the time.

– Common adverse drug reactions include chest pressure, flushing, weakness, dizziness, feeling of warmth, and paresthesia.
  ○ Suggested initial doses (refer to individual labeling for more detailed dosing instructions)
  ○ Sumatriptan 100 mg PO; 6 mg SQ; 20 mg intranasal
  ○ SQ route quickest onset but most side effects
  ○ Eletriptan 40 mg PO
  ○ Rizatriptan 10 mg PO
  ○ Zolmitriptan 2.5 mg PO; 5 mg intranasal
  ○ Naratriptan 2.5 mg PO
  ○ Frovatriptan 2.5 mg PO
    ■ 44–77% of patients taking triptans report complete pain relief within 2 hours.
    ■ Frovatriptan and naratriptan have slow onset but long half-lives.
– Combination triptan and NSAID: sumatriptan 85 mg/naproxen 500 mg PO at onset of HA show improved efficacy over either alone.
– Antiemetics: Consider antinausea medications that antagonize dopamine receptors:
  ○ Metoclopramide, prochlorperazine
  ○ Emergency therapy; 10 to 25 mg single dose (4)[A]

- **Contraindications to treatments**
  – Avoid 5-HT-1 agonists (triptans) and ergots in coronary artery disease, peripheral vascular disease, uncontrolled hypertension, and complicated migraine (e.g., brainstem or hemiplegic migraine).
  – Triptans should not be used with ergots, MAOI, or other triptans.
  – Avoid opioids or butalbital in patients with frequent migraines.
- **Precautions**
  – Frequent use of acute-treatment drugs may lead to increase in migraine patterns and medication overuse headache.
- **Second-line abortive treatment**
  – Acetaminophen 1,000 mg or aspirin 975 mg plus the addition of a dopamine antagonist (e.g., metoclopramide 10 mg) may be as effective as PO sumatriptan 100 mg for acute migraine.
  – Ergotamines (e.g., dihydroergotamine SC, Migranal intranasal): drug of choice in status migrainosus and nonpregnant patients but limited use due to side effects and replaced by triptans
  – Opiate use is controversial and can contribute to medication overuse or chronic daily headache with use as few as 8 days per month (5).
    ○ IV dexamethasone: Use as adjunctive
- **First-line preventative treatment**
  – Prevention should not be limited to pharmacologic agents. Trigger reduction, biofeedback, relaxation techniques, and cognitive behavioral therapy have evidence of efficacy.
  – Lifestyle modifications should be recommended for all migraine sufferers.
  – ~38% of migraineurs need preventative therapy, but only 3–13% use it (6). Trial and error is needed to determine optimal therapy.
- The American Migraine Prevalence and Prevention Study recommendations suggest prophylactic treatment when:
  – Quality of life is severely impaired.
  – ≥6 headache days/month of any severity, ≥4 headache days/month of moderate severity, or ≥2 headache days/month of severe impairment.

– Migraine unresponsive to abortive treatment.
– Frequent, very long, or uncomfortable auras occur.

- For prevention of *episodic migraine*, divalproex, valproate, topiramate, metoprolol, and timolol are effective for migraine prevention and should be offered to patients to reduce attack frequency and severity (6)[A].
  – NSAIDs are probably effective for migraine prevention, especially for people with predictable triggers (menses, etc.) but pose a risk for MOH.
- For treatment/prevention of *chronic migraine*, the FDA has approved botulinum toxin A (Botox), as it significantly reduced the frequency of headache days in chronic migraineurs.

ISSUES FOR REFERRAL
- Obscure diagnosis, concomitant medical conditions, significant psychopathology
- Unresponsive to usual treatment
- Analgesic-dependent headache patterns

COMPLEMENTARY & ALTERNATIVE MEDICINE
- Butterbur (*Petasites hybridus*; Petadolex): 50 to 75 mg BID
  – Use caution with CYP3A4 meds.
- Riboflavin (vitamin B_2): 400 mg/day
- Magnesium: 400 mg/day
- MIG-99 (feverfew): 6.25 mg TID
- Histamine SC: 1 to 10 ng twice weekly
- Acupuncture is at least as effective as, or possibly more effective than prophylactic drug treatment and has fewer adverse effects.

INPATIENT CONSIDERATIONS
Admission Criteria/Initial Stabilization
Consider if diagnosis not clear; status migrainosus; may need to exclude intracranial bleeds, TIA, stroke; monitor vital signs and patient comfort.

IV Fluids
Fluids are a necessary part of inpatient management.

Discharge Criteria
Judgment based on patient's overall clinical status and patient's ability to tolerate PO medications

 ONGOING CARE

FOLLOW-UP RECOMMENDATIONS
- Early intervention is key at the onset of an attack.
- Preventative treatment should aim to decrease frequency and severity of acute attacks, make acute treatments more efficacious, and minimize adverse drug reactions.

Patient Monitoring
- Monitor frequency of attacks, pain behaviors, and medication usage via headache diary.
- Encourage lifestyle modifications. Counsel patients and manage expectations.

PATIENT EDUCATION
Educate patients about migraine triggers.

PROGNOSIS
- With increasing age, there may be a reduction in severity, frequency, and disability of attacks.
- Most attacks subside within 72 hours.

COMPLICATIONS
- Status migrainosus (>72 hours)
- Cerebral ischemic events (rare)
- Medication overuse headache (MOH): Headache occurring 10 or more days/month for >3 months as a consequence of regular overuse of an acute or symptomatic headache medication. Likelihood with butalbital > opiates > triptans > NSAIDs.

REFERENCE
1. Headache Classification Committee of the International Headache Society. The International Classification of Headache Disorders, 3rd edition (beta version). *Cephalalgia*. 2013;33(9):629–808.
2. Detsky ME, McDonald DR, Baerlocher MO, et al. Does this patient with headache have a migraine or need neuroimaging? *JAMA*. 2006;296(10):1274–1283.
3. Loder E, Weizenbaum E, Frishberg B, et al. Choosing wisely in headache medicine: the American Headache Society's list of five things physicians and patients should question. *Headache*. 2013;53(10):1651–1659.
4. Gilmore B, Michael M. Treatment of acute migraine headache. *Am Fam Physician*. 2011;83(3):271–280.
5. Taylor FR, Kaniecki RG. Symptomatic treatment of migraine: when to use NSAIDs, triptans, or opiates. *Curr Treat Options Neurol*. 2011;13(1).15–27.
6. Silberstein SD, Holland S, Freitag F, et al. Evidence-based guideline update: pharmacologic treatment for episodic migraine prevention in adults: report of the Quality Standards Subcommittee of the American Academy of Neurology and the American Headache Society. *Neurology*. 2012;78(17):1337–1345.

 SEE ALSO

Algorithm: Headache, Chronic

CODES
ICD10
- G43.909 Migraine, unsp, not intractable, without status migrainosus
- G43.109 Migraine with aura, not intractable, w/o status migrainosus
- G43.409 Hemiplegic migraine, not intractable, w/o status migrainosus

CLINICAL PEARLS
- Migraine is a chronic headache disorder of unclear etiology often characterized by unilateral, throbbing headaches that may be associated with additional neurologic symptoms.
- Accurate diagnosis of migraine is crucial.
- Consider nonspecific analgesics for milder attacks; migraine-specific treatments (triptans) for more severe attacks.
- Avoid opiates and barbiturates as well as frequent (>8/month) use of triptans or NSAIDs to avoid creating an MOH.
- All patients should be counseled on lifestyle modifications and trigger identification.
- Those with frequent or highly debilitating migraines prophylactic treatment should be encouraged.

HEADACHE, TENSION

Kaelen C. Dunican, PharmD • Brandi Hoag, DO

 BASICS

DESCRIPTION

- Typically characterized by bilateral mild to moderate pain and pressure; may be associated with pericranial tenderness at the base of the occiput
- Two types
  - Episodic tension–type headache (ETTH) divided into
    - Infrequent: <1 day per month
    - Frequent: ≥1 but <15 days per month
  - Chronic tension–type headache (CTTH): ≥15 days per month for >3 months
- Synonym(s): muscle contraction headache; stress headache

EPIDEMIOLOGY
Most common type of primary headache

Prevalence
- Global prevalence in adults is 42% (1).
- Lifetime prevalence is 79%.
- More prevalent among women
- Prevalence of CTTH is 3%.
- Prevalence of ETTH decreases with age, whereas the prevalence of CTTH increases with age.

ETIOLOGY AND PATHOPHYSIOLOGY
- Debatable: peripheral and/or central mechanisms
- Activation of peripheral nociceptors leads to muscle tenderness in ETTH.
- Central sensitization is associated with CTTH:
  - Nitric oxide may play an important role in central sensitization.
  - Debatable: low-platelet serotonin
- Peripheral: may provoke the central mechanism leading from ETTH to CTTH
- Stress is the most frequently reported precipitating factor.

Genetics
An increased genetic risk has been suggested by studies, particularly for CTTH.

RISK FACTORS
Associated with triggers/precipitating factors
- Stress (mental or physical)
- Change in sleep regimen
- Skipping meals
- Certain foods (caffeine, alcohol, chocolate)
- Dehydration
- Physical exertion
- Environmental factors (sun glare, odors, smoke, noise, lighting)
- Poor or sustained posture
- Female hormonal changes
- Medications (e.g., nitrates, SSRIs, antihypertensives)
- Overuse of abortive headache medication

GENERAL PREVENTION
- Identify and avoid triggers/precipitating factors.
- Minimize emotional stress.
- Encourage relaxation techniques:
  - Biofeedback, relaxation therapy, and physical therapy
  - Consider counseling/psychotherapy.

COMMONLY ASSOCIATED CONDITIONS
- 83% of patients with migraine headaches also suffer from tension-type headaches.
- Debatable: increased prevalence of comorbid anxiety and depression

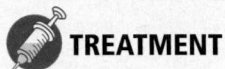 **DIAGNOSIS**

HISTORY
Obtain a thorough headache history to rule out other headache disorders, including severity, symptoms, onset, location, and radiation of pain; quality of pain; concurrent medical conditions and medications; and recent trauma or other procedures.

Diagnosis is based on clinical symptoms.

- Diagnostic criteria provided by the International Headache Society:
  - Headache lasting 30 minutes to 7 days
  - At least two of the following:
    - Bilateral location
    - Pressing/tightening (nonpulsating) quality
    - Mild or moderate intensity
    - Not aggravated by routine physical activity
  - Not associated with nausea or vomiting (chronic type may be associated with nausea)
  - No more than one of the following: photophobia or phonophobia
- Headache not due to another disorder
- Fronto-occipital or generalized pain (dull, pressing, or bandlike)
- Associated symptoms:
  - Fatigue
  - Irritability
  - Difficulty concentrating
  - Muscular tightness, tenderness, or stiffness in neck, occipital, and frontal regions

PHYSICAL EXAM
- General physical exam: vital signs, funduscopic and cardiovascular assessment, palpation of the head and neck
- Neurologic exam: mental status, pupillary responses, motor-strength testing, deep tendon reflexes, sensation, cerebellar function, gait testing, signs of meningeal irritation

DIFFERENTIAL DIAGNOSIS
- Migraine headache
- Cluster headache
- Head trauma
- Subarachnoid hemorrhage
- Subdural hematoma
- Unruptured vascular malformation
- Ischemic cerebrovascular disease
- Temporal arteritis
- Arterial hypertension (HTN)
- Cerebral venous thrombosis
- Benign intracranial HTN
- Intracranial neoplasm, infection, or meningitis
- Low CSF pressure
- Medication (nonprescription analgesic dependency, nitrates)
- Caffeine dependency
- Metabolic disorders (hypoxia, hypercapnia, hypoglycemia)

- Toxic effects from drugs or fumes
- Temporomandibular joint syndrome
- Eyes: glaucoma, refractive errors
- Sinusitis or middle ear infection
- Cervical spondylosis
- Severe anemia or polycythemia
- Uremia and hepatic disorders
- Paget disease of bone

DIAGNOSTIC TESTS & INTERPRETATION
Labs and neuroimaging (CT or MRI) are only necessary when a secondary cause is suspected:
- Atypical pattern of headache (does not fit specific category such as migraine, cluster, or tension)
- Rapid increase in frequency (2)[C]
- Focal neurologic findings
- New onset after age 40 years
- Sudden onset or worsening with exertion CT scan, with and without contrast, is as sensitive as MRI and is the test of choice.
- Use MRI when lesions of the posterior fossa or an aneurysm is suspected.

![syringe icon] **TREATMENT**

- NSAIDs, acetaminophen (APAP), and aspirin (ASA) are effective for short-term pain relief of ETTH (3,4)[B].
- Amitriptyline should be considered first line for prophylaxis of CTTH (3,4)[B].

GENERAL MEASURES
Relief measures: relaxation routines; rest in quiet, dark room; hot bath or shower; massage of back of neck and temples

MEDICATION
Choice of simple analgesic is based on patient-specific parameters:
- NSAIDs may be more effective than APAP for ETTH (3)[C]:
  - Ibuprofen and naproxen may be preferred due to better GI tolerability.
- APAP should be considered for patients taking warfarin, unable to tolerate NSAIDs, or allergic to ASA or NSAIDs.

First Line
- For acute attack (ETTH): NSAIDs, APAP, or ASA:
  - NSAIDs:
    - Ibuprofen (Motrin, Advil): 400 to 800 mg; may repeat q8h PRN (max 3.2 g/day)
    - Naproxen (Naprosyn): 375 to 500 mg or naproxen sodium (Aleve, Anaprox) 440 to 550 mg; may repeat q8–12h PRN (max 1,250 mg base/day)
    - Ketoprofen (Orudis): 12.5 to 50 mg; may repeat q6–8h PRN (max 300 mg/day)
    - Diclofenac (Voltaren, Cataflam): 50 to 100 mg; may repeat q8h PRN (max 150 mg/day)
    - Contraindications: ASA or NSAID allergy or bronchospasm, renal disease, bleeding disorders, increased risk of cardiovascular events (myocardial infarction [MI], stroke, new onset, or worsening of HTN)
    - Drug interactions: antihypertensives, anti-coagulants, antiplatelet drugs, ASA, lithium, methotrexate
    - Adverse effects: epigastric distress, peptic ulcer

- APAP (Tylenol): 1,000 mg; may repeat q6h PRN (max 4 g/day):
  - Adverse effects (rare): rash, pancytopenia, liver damage
  - Precaution: hepatic impairment, consumption of ≥3/day alcoholic beverages
- Aspirin: 500 to 1,000 mg; may repeat q6h PRN (max 4 g/day):
  - Contraindication: ASA or NSAID allergy or bronchospasm, bleeding disorders
  - Drug interactions: anticoagulants, antiplatelet drugs, ACE inhibitors, β-blockers, corticosteroids, NSAIDs, sulfonylureas
  - Adverse effects: GI irritation/bleeding, thrombocytopenia
- Prophylaxis for CTTH: tricyclic antidepressants (TCAs) (amitriptyline [Elavil]) 10 to 75 mg/day:
  - Not FDA approved for CTTH
  - Contraindications: acute recovery phase of MI, use of monamine oxidase inhibitors (MAOIs) within 14 days
  - Drug interactions: clonidine, MAOIs, quinolone antibiotics, SSRIs, sympathomimetics, azole antifungals, valproic acid
  - Adverse effects: drowsiness, dry mouth, tachycardia, heart block, blurred vision, urinary retention, seizure

Second Line
- For acute attack (ETTH):
  - Caffeine combinations: 130 mg caffeine with 500 mg APAP and/or 500 mg ASA q6h PRN (3)[C]
  - Narcotic analgesics (rarely indicated; consider secondary causes of headache or secondary gain such as drug-seeking behavior for personal use or diversion/sale)
  - Ketorolac: 60 mg IM, single dose
- For CTTH prophylaxis:
  - Mirtazapine: 15 to 30 mg/day (not FDA approved for CTTH) (3,4)[B]
  - Venlafaxine XR (Effexor XR): 37.5 to 300 mg/day (not FDA approved for CTTH) (3,4)[B]

ALERT
Use of abortive agents >2 days/week may lead to *medication-overuse headaches*; must withdraw acute treatment to diagnose.

Pediatric Considerations
ASA and antidepressants are contraindicated.

ADDITIONAL THERAPIES
- The combination of stress management therapy and a TCA (amitriptyline) may be most effective for CTTH.
- Maprotiline: 75 mg/day (not FDA approved for CTTH) (3)[C]
- Topiramate: 100 mg/day (limited clinical evidence for prevention of CTTH; not FDA approved for CTTH)
- Alternative TCAs (although limited evidence of benefit, all are widely used for prophylaxis) (5)[B]
  - Desipramine (Norpramin): 50 to 100 mg/day
  - Imipramine (Tofranil): 50 to 100 mg/day
  - Nortriptyline (Pamelor): 25 to 50 mg/day
  - Protriptyline (Vivactil): 25 mg/day

- Drugs with conflicting clinical evidence for CTTH (not FDA approved for CTTH):
  - Tizanidine: 2 to 6 mg TID
  - Memantine: 20 to 40 mg/day
- Botulinum toxin type A is not likely to be effective for ETTH or CTTH (6)[A].

COMPLEMENTARY & ALTERNATIVE MEDICINE
- Electromyographic (EMG) biofeedback may be effective and is enhanced when combined with relaxation therapy (3,7)[C].
- Cognitive-behavioral therapy may be helpful (3,7)[C].
- Physical therapy, including positioning, ergonomic instruction, massage, transcutaneous electrical nerve simulation, and application of heat/cold may help.
- Alternative agents (not FDA approved for TTH)
  - Tiger Balm or peppermint oil applied topically to the forehead may be effective for ETTH.
  - Limited evidence for use of acupuncture and physical therapy (7)[B]
- Chiropractic spinal manipulation cannot be recommended for the management of ETTH; recommendations cannot be made for CTTH (8)[B].

INPATIENT CONSIDERATIONS
Admission Criteria/Initial Stabilization
Outpatient treatment

 ## ONGOING CARE

FOLLOW-UP RECOMMENDATIONS
- Regulate sleep schedule.
- Regular exercise

DIET
- Identify and avoid dietary triggers.
- Regulate meal schedule.

PATIENT EDUCATION
For additional information, contact:
- National Headache Foundation: http://www.headaches.org
- American Council for Headache Education: http://www.achenet.org

PROGNOSIS
- Usually follows a chronic course when life stressors are not changed
- Most cases are intermittent.

COMPLICATIONS
- Lost days of work and productivity (more with CTTH)
- Cost to health system
- Dependence/addiction to narcotic analgesics
- GI bleeding from NSAID use

REFERENCES
1. Ferrante T, Manzoni GC, Russo M, et al. Prevalence of tension-type headache in adult general population: the PACE study and review of the literature. *Neurol Sci.* 2013;34(Suppl 1):S137–S138.
2. Freitag F. Managing and treating tension-type headache. *Med Clin North Am.* 2013;97(2):281–292.
3. Bendtsen L, Jensen R. Treating tension-type headache—an expert opinion. *Expert Opin Pharmacother.* 2011;12(7):1099–1109.
4. Bendtsen L, Evers S, Linde M, et al. EFNS guideline on the treatment of tension-type headache—report of an EFNS task force. *Eur J Neurol.* 2010;17(11):1318–1325.
5. Verhagen AP, Damen L, Berger MY, et al. Lack of benefit for prophylactic drugs of tension-type headache in adults: a systematic review. *Fam Pract.* 2010;27(2):151–165.
6. Jackson JL, Kuriyama A, Hayashino Y. Botulinum toxin A for prophylactic treatment of migraine and tension headaches in adults: a meta-analysis. *JAMA.* 2012;307(16):1736–1745.
7. Sun-Edelstein C, Mauskop A. Complementary and alternative approaches to the treatment of tension-type headache. *Curr Pain Headache Rep.* 2012;16(6):539–544.
8. Bryans R, Descarreaux M, Duranleau M, et al. Evidence-based guidelines for the chiropractic treatment of adults with headache. *J Manipulative Physiol Ther.* 2011;34(5):274–289.

 ## SEE ALSO

Algorithm: Headache, Chronic

 ## CODES

ICD10
- G44.209 Tension-type headache, unspecified, not intractable
- G44.219 Episodic tension-type headache, not intractable
- G44.229 Chronic tension-type headache, not intractable

CLINICAL PEARLS
- Tension-type headache may be difficult to distinguish from migraine without aura. A tension-type headache is typically described as bilateral, mild to moderate, and dull pain, whereas a migraine is typically pulsating, unilateral, and associated with nausea, vomiting, and photophobia or phonophobia.
- Evidence suggests that NSAIDs may be more effective than APAP for ETTH. Consider APAP for patients who cannot tolerate, or have a contraindication, to NSAIDs. Initial dose of APAP should be 1,000 mg (500 mg may not be as effective).
- CTTH is difficult to treat, and these patients are more likely to develop medication-overuse headache. Clinical evidence supports the use of amitriptyline + stress-management therapy for CTTH.
- Medication-overuse headaches must be avoided by limiting use of abortive agents to no more than 2 days/week.
- A headache diary may be useful to identify triggers, response to treatment, and medication-overuse headaches.

H

HEARING LOSS

Scott A. Wiltz, MD, MPH, FAAFP

 BASICS

DESCRIPTION
- Decrease in the ability to comprehend sound. It can be partial, complete, unilateral, or bilateral.
- Types of hearing loss include conductive hearing loss (CHL or air–bone gap), sensorineural hearing loss (SNHL), or mixed hearing loss.
- System(s) affected: auditory; external and middle ear (CHL) or inner ear (SNHL)

EPIDEMIOLOGY
- All ages affected; common in children (CHL) and elderly (SNHL)
- Usually more severe at an earlier age in men

Incidence
- 37% of people >60 years of age
- At least 1.4 million children (≤18 years of age)
- Sudden sensorineural hearing loss (SSHL) occurs in 5 to 20 per 100,000 persons.

Prevalence
Hearing loss has increased in individuals aged ≥3 years from 13.2 million in 1971 to 37.5 million in 2004.

Geriatric Considerations
- ~80% of people aged >85 years have hearing loss.
- Hearing aids are underused.
- Loss of communication is a source of emotional stress and a physical risk for the elderly.

Pediatric Considerations
- Congenital hearing loss
  - 1 to 6/1,000 infants have hearing loss.
  - Mandatory screening in >97% of newborns with otoacoustic emission (OAE) and auditory brainstem response (BR) testing
- Audiologic testing after major intracranial infection (meningitis)

Pregnancy Considerations
- Otosclerosis can worsen during pregnancy.
- Maternal infections cause permanent pediatric hearing loss.

ETIOLOGY AND PATHOPHYSIOLOGY
- CHL: Hearing loss can result from middle ear effusion, obstruction of canal (cerumen/foreign body, osteomas/exostoses, cholesteatoma, tumor), loss of continuity (ossicular discontinuity), stiffening of the components (myringosclerosis, tympanosclerosis, and otosclerosis), and loss of the pressure differential across the tympanic membrane (TM) (perforation).
- SNHL: damage along the pathway from oval window, cochlea, auditory nerve, and brainstem. Examples include vascular/metabolic insult, mass effect, infection and inflammation, and acoustic trauma.
  - Noise-induced hearing loss is caused by acoustic insult that affects outer hair cells in the organ of Corti, causing them to be less stiff. Over time, severe damage occurs with fusion and loss of stereocilia; eventually may progress to inner hair cells and auditory nerve as well.
- Large vestibular aqueduct or superior canal dehiscence: Third mobile window shunts acoustic energy away from cochlea.

Genetics
- Connexin 26 (13q11–13q12): most common cause of nonsyndromic genetic hearing loss
- Mitochondrial disorders (may predispose to aminoglycoside ototoxicity)
- Otosclerosis: familial
- Most common congenital syndromes
  - Hemifacial microsomia
  - Stickler syndrome
  - Congenital cytomegalovirus
  - Usher syndrome
  - Branchio-oto-renal syndrome
  - Pendred syndrome
  - CHARGE association
  - Neurofibromatosis type 2
  - Waardenburg syndrome

RISK FACTORS
- Conductive
  - Chronic sinusitis; allergy
  - Cigarette smoking
  - Sleep apnea with continuous positive airway pressure (CPAP) use
  - Adenoid hypertrophy; nasopharyngeal mass
  - Eustachian tube dysfunction
  - Neuromuscular disease
  - Family history/heredity
  - Prematurity and low birth weight
  - Craniofacial abnormalities (e.g., cleft palate, Down syndrome)
  - Third mobile window (superior canal dehiscence or large vestibular aqueduct)
- Sensorineural
  - Aging/older age
  - Loud noise/acoustic trauma
  - Dizziness/vertigo: especially Ménière disease or history of labyrinthitis
  - Medications (aminoglycosides, loop diuretics, quinine, aspirin, chemotherapeutic agents)
  - Bacterial meningitis
  - Head trauma
  - Atherosclerosis
  - Vestibular schwannoma/skull base neoplasm
  - Previous ear surgery
- Sensorineural, pediatric specific
  - Postnatal asphyxia
  - Mechanical ventilation lasting ≥5 days
  - In utero infections (toxoplasmosis, other agents, rubella, cytomegalovirus, herpes simplex [TORCH] syndrome)
  - Toxemia of pregnancy
  - Maternal diabetes
  - Rh incompatibility
  - Prematurity or birth weight <1,500 g
  - Hyperbilirubinemia; exchange transfusions
  - Anomalous temporal bone (Mondini or large vestibular aqueduct)
  - Infectious diseases: chickenpox, measles, encephalitis, influenza, mumps

GENERAL PREVENTION
- Limit noise exposure; use hearing protection.
- Avoid ear canal instrumentation (e.g., cotton swabs).
- Limit ototoxic medications.

DIAGNOSIS

HISTORY
- There is an indeterminate evidence per the U.S. Preventive Services Task Force for universal screening of hearing loss in adults.
- Social problems and comments from friends and family members are often the first presentation of presbycusis, as patients are often not aware of the degree of hearing loss they experience and how it affects their life. Onset is gradual.
- Difficulty hearing
  - Rapid versus gradual decline: Rapid loss (<3 days) is a medical emergency. Urgent ENT referral and steroid therapy is recommended.
  - Difficulty with discrimination of sounds, hearing in crowds, or turning up the volume of television sets
  - Frequently having to ask speakers to repeat
  - Friends/family complain of hearing loss
- Tinnitus, bilateral or unilateral
- Otalgia
- Otorrhea, clear or purulent
- Dizziness or vertigo
- Ear fullness
- Autophony (hearing own voice louder or echoing)
- Depression or anxiety
- History of ear infections or ear surgeries
- History of trauma or noise exposure
- Family history of hearing loss
- History of recent viral infection
- Nasal obstruction
- Frequent epistaxis

PHYSICAL EXAM
- A simple 512-Hz tuning fork test lateralizes to unaffected ear in sudden SNHL (emergency) and lateralizes to the affected ear in CHL (not an emergency).
- Whispering screen: A whisper heard from ~2 feet away is a good screen for intact hearing. Patients with SNHL have difficulty with this because their hearing loss is usually in the high frequency range.
- 512-Hz tuning fork tests:
  - Sensorineural loss
    ○ Placed on the forehead: lateralizes to nonaffected ear (Weber test)
    ○ Base of tuning fork placed on the mastoid and then fork end placed next to ear; heard louder next to ear (Rinne test)
  - Conductive loss
    ○ Placed on the forehead or teeth lateralizes to affected or symptomatic ear
    ○ Placed on the mastoid and then next to ear; heard louder behind the ear on the side of conductive deficit
- Otoscopy: Assess for deformity, canal patency, and otorrhea; TM integrity/retraction/mobility with insufflation, canal, or middle ear mass.
- Facial symmetry
- Cranial nerve exam
- Nasopharyngoscopy: adenoid hypertrophy or nasopharyngeal mass (mandatory in adult patient with new unilateral serous effusion)
- Pediatric: Survey for syndromic anomalies.

DIFFERENTIAL DIAGNOSIS
- Conductive
  - Cerumen impaction/foreign body
  - Perforation of TM
  - Middle ear fluid (serous otitis media)
  - Acute otitis media/adhesive otitis media
  - Ossicular erosion (infection, cholesteatoma)
  - Myringosclerosis/tympanosclerosis
  - Temporal bone fracture
  - Otosclerosis
  - Glomus tumor
- Sensorineural
  - Presbycusis (hearing loss related to aging)
  - Noise-induced (recreational, occupational)
  - Ménière disease
  - Ototoxicity (aspirin, aminoglycosides)
  - Viral labyrinthitis
  - Cerebellopontine angle tumor
  - Large vestibular aqueduct syndrome
  - Syndromic hearing loss
  - Congenital cochlear malformation
  - Syphilis
  - Cytomegalovirus; rubella
  - Temporal bone fracture
  - Metabolic (hyper-/hypothyroidism)
  - Paget disease
  - Perilymphatic (inner ear) fistula

DIAGNOSTIC TESTS & INTERPRETATION
Often, labs are not needed. If indicated
- MRI of the brain and brainstem with gadolinium to evaluate SNHL in congenital, early onset, and asymmetric hearing loss
- Fine-cut CT temporal bones without contrast may help in the evaluation of CHL.
- Any pediatric patient with SNHL: Consider genetic testing for connexin 26, mitochondrial studies.
- TORCH screening (congenital infection)
- Rapid plasma reagin (RPR) or Venereal Disease Research Laboratory (VDRL) confirmed by fluorescent treponemal antibody absorption (FTA-ABS)
- Lyme titer in endemic areas
- Antinuclear antibodies and sedimentation rate as a screen for autoimmune disease
- Pendred syndrome (goiter, mental retardation + SNHL): perchlorate test, thyroid function tests
- Alport syndrome (nephritis + SNHL): urinalysis, renal function tests
- Jervell and Lange-Nielsen syndrome (syncope, family history of sudden death + profound SNHL): ECG

Diagnostic Procedures/Other
- Audiometry: pure tone (air and bone), speech testing, and impedance (middle ear pressure) testing
- Tympanometry: Type B or C tympanograms indicate fluid or retraction, respectively. Negative middle ear peak pressures were seen even with normal (type A) tympanograms.
- Other tests
  - Auditory brainstem response
  - OAEs: "echo" of the cochlea
  - Behavioral (visual reinforcement) audiometry; used in children 6 months to 5 years old
- Myringotomy and tubes can be considered for persistent fluid with hearing loss.

Test Interpretation
Varies depending on etiology

TREATMENT
Hearing rehabilitation:
- Personal amplifiers, situation-specific amplification (e.g., amplified phone), or personal hearing aids can be considered for any individual who has significant communication difficulties due to hearing loss.
- Cochlear implants for patients with bilateral severe to profound hearing loss who no longer derive benefit from hearing aids

MEDICATION
- Depends on cause
- Any sudden SNHL (usually unilateral) is a medical emergency; obtain a hearing testing and start steroid therapy.
- Treatment should begin ASAP, ideally within 1 to 2 weeks of onset with high-dose oral steroids: 1 mg/kg or 60 to 100 mg/day prednisone or 12 to 16 mg/day dexamethasone for 7 to 14 days, followed by a taper: For patients who cannot tolerate systematic steroids, intratympanic steroids are equally effective (1)[A].
  - Clinical practical guidelines for sudden hearing loss include the following (2)[C]:
    - Distinguishing SNHL from CHL; testing for bilateral sudden hearing loss in patients with unilateral sudden hearing loss; obtaining an MRI, auditory brainstem response, or audiometric follow-up to evaluate for retrocochlear pathology; offer intratympanic steroid perfusion for refractory cases after initial management fails to treat idiopathic sudden SNHL (ISSNHL) and follow-up within 6 months of diagnosis.
    - May offer corticosteroids as initial therapy to patients with ISSNHL and hyperbaric oxygen within 3 months of ISSNHL diagnosis
    - Recommended against prescribing antivirals, thrombolytics, vasodilators, vasoactive substances, or antioxidants to patients with ISSNHL
    - Also recommended against routine laboratory tests in patients with ISSNHL

ISSUES FOR REFERRAL
- Audiology: If hearing loss is suspected, refer to audiology for formal evaluation. Audiologists also provide hearing aid options and maintenance.
- Genetics: if congenital syndrome or familial hearing loss is suspected
- Speech therapist: if speech delay or speech impediment is present
- Endocrinology: Pendred syndrome, other associated endocrine disorder (hypo-/hyperthyroidism)
- Cardiology: Jervell and Lange-Nielsen syndrome
- Ophthalmology: Usher syndrome
- Neurology and neurosurgery: cerebellopontine angle (CPA) lesion, intracranial complication of middle ear disease

SURGERY/OTHER PROCEDURES
- CHL often has surgical options for repair.
  - Tympanostomy and tube placement
  - Tympanoplasty
  - Mastoidectomy
  - Ossicular chain reconstruction
  - Stapedectomy/stapedotomy
  - Canaloplasty
- Those with profound bilateral SNHL may qualify for cochlear implantation.

ONGOING CARE

FOLLOW-UP RECOMMENDATIONS
Patient Monitoring
Audiogram and clinical exam are the primary means of monitoring patient. Patients with hearing assistive devices benefit from audiology involvement.

DIET
Salt restriction to 2 g/day is helpful for patients with Ménière disease.

PATIENT EDUCATION
National Institute on Deafness and Other Communication Disorders (NIDCD): http://www.nidcd.nih.gov/health/hearing/Pages/Default.aspx

PROGNOSIS
- SNHL is usually permanent and may be progressive. However, amplification devices (e.g., hearing aids) may help improve functionality.
- ISSNHL may recover spontaneously in 32–70% of cases, but urgent referral and treatment is recommended to maximize recovery. No factors have been proven to predict recovery (3).

COMPLICATIONS
Acute middle ear problems may become chronic (perforations, cholesteatoma).

REFERENCES
1. Spear SA, Schwartz SR. Intratympanic steroids for sudden sensorineural hearing loss: a systematic review. *Otolaryngol Head Neck Surg*. 2011;145(4):534–543.
2. Stachler RJ, Chandrasekhar SS, Archer SM, et al. Clinical practice guideline: sudden hearing loss. *Otolaryngol Head Neck Surg*. 2012;146(3 Suppl):S1–S35.
3. Walling AD, Dickson GM. Hearing loss in older adults. *Am Fam Physician*. 2012;85(12):1150–1156.

CODES

ICD10
- H91.90 Unspecified hearing loss, unspecified ear
- H90.2 Conductive hearing loss, unspecified
- H90.5 Unspecified sensorineural hearing loss

CLINICAL PEARLS
- In sudden hearing loss, if a 512-Hz tuning fork test (Weber test) lateralizes to the *unaffected ear*, suspect sensorineural causes (emergent evaluation needed), but if it lateralizes to the *affected* ear, the diagnosis is CHL (not an emergency).
- ~80% of people aged >85 years have hearing loss, encourage screening and treatment, especially in patients with early dementia.

H

HEART FAILURE, ACUTELY DECOMPENSATED

Bruce L. Lovins, MD • Jennifer M. Slowik, DO, MS • Christopher J. Snyder, MD

BASICS

DESCRIPTION
Acute decompensated heart failure (ADHF) is a heterogeneous syndrome of acute impairment in cardiac pump function resulting in inefficient perfusion to bodily tissues. This may be due to structural or functional cardiac disorders and may represent a new diagnosis or worsening of preexisting chronic HF.

EPIDEMIOLOGY

Incidence
- Medicare spends more to diagnose and treat HF than any other medical condition. In 2012, the total cost of HF approached $30.7 billion. In the United States, there are 870,000 new cases annually. HF is the primary cause of >55,000 deaths each year and a contributing factor in >280,000 deaths.
- 1 million hospital discharges/year and about half of people who have HF die within 5 years of diagnosis.

Prevalence
- ~5.7 million people over the age of 20 in the United States carry an HF diagnosis; prevalence is expected to increase 46% from 2012 to 2030 resulting in more than 8 million cases.
- Primarily a disease of the elderly; 75% of hospital admissions for HF are in persons >65 years of age.

ETIOLOGY AND PATHOPHYSIOLOGY
- Two physiologic components explain most of the clinical findings of ADHF.
  - Systolic dysfunction: an *inotropic* abnormality, often due to myocardial infarction (MI) or dilated or ischemic cardiomyopathy, resulting in diminished systolic emptying (ejection fraction <45%)
  - Diastolic dysfunction: a *compliance* abnormality, often due to hypertensive cardiomyopathy, in which the ventricular relaxation is impaired (ejection fraction >45%).
- Common causes of ADHF
  - Exacerbation of chronic HF caused by dietary or medication nonadherence, infection, or any of the following as cause of new HF or exacerbation
  - Coronary artery disease (CAD), MI (especially new-onset ADHF)
  - Arrhythmia: atrial fibrillation, tachyarrhythmias, high-grade heart block
  - Valvular and vascular abnormalities: aortic stenosis or regurgitation, rheumatic heart disease (mitral and aortic valvular disease)
  - Uncontrolled hypertension (HTN), pulmonary HTN
  - High-output states: hyperthyroidism, anemia
  - Medications: cardiac depressants (β-blocker overdose), chemotherapeutic agents
  - Others: infiltrative disease, Chagas disease, pericardial disease, postpartum cardiomyopathy, wet beriberi, sepsis, COPD, pulmonary embolism

Genetics
Familial cardiomyopathy predisposes to development of HF (rare).

RISK FACTORS
- History of chronic HF
- CAD and MI
- HTN, systemic or pulmonary
- Valvular heart disease
- Diabetes mellitus
- Cardiotoxic medications
- Chronic kidney disease and acute kidney injury (AKI)
- Arrhythmia
- Infection

GENERAL PREVENTION
Control BP and other risk factors. Thiazide diuretics and ACE inhibitors are superior to other agents in preventing development of HF. Treat cardiovascular disease.

COMMONLY ASSOCIATED CONDITIONS
- Dysrhythmia followed by pump failure is the leading cause of death in ADHF. Most patients have >5 comorbidities (especially CAD, chronic kidney disease, and diabetes) and take >5 medications.
- Cardiogenic shock
- Hyponatremia and altered mental status, especially in the elderly

DIAGNOSIS

Clinical diagnosis, no gold standard: ED diagnosis of ADHF is incorrect 10–20% of the time.

HISTORY
- History of HF, prior MI, uncontrolled HTN
- Dyspnea on exertion, deteriorating exercise capacity, fatigue, general weakness, chest pain/discomfort if acute coronary syndrome (ACS) is present.
- Paroxysmal nocturnal dyspnea, orthopnea, nocturnal nonproductive cough, sometimes frothy or pink sputum, wheezing (especially nocturnal) in absence of history of asthma or infection (cardiac asthma)
- Edema, abdominal bloating (ascites), anasarca, cyanosis, weight gain (>2 kg/week)

PHYSICAL EXAM
- S_3 and/or jugular venous distension most useful positive finding, although no vital sign/PE finding has sensitivity >70%
- Peripheral edema, cool extremities, cyanosis, hepatomegaly, hepatojugular reflux, cardiac murmur, hypotension, laterally displaced apical impulse
- Lung exam: rales (crackles) and sometimes wheezing, Cheyne-Stokes respirations

DIFFERENTIAL DIAGNOSIS
Pulmonary embolism, exertional asthma, acute MI, cardiac ischemia with angina, chronic obstructive pulmonary disease (COPD), pneumonia, constrictive pericarditis, tamponade, tension pneumothorax, high-output states (anemia, sepsis, hyperthyroidism, ARDS)

DIAGNOSTIC TESTS & INTERPRETATION
Laboratory data are adjunctive and indicative of complications.

Initial Tests (lab, imaging)
- Cardiac troponins, EKG to evaluate for ACS (1)[C]
- Echocardiogram: Determining ejection fraction (EF) is critical to proper diagnosis and management of heart failure, but may not be necessary in the acute setting if performed recently. Formal echocardiographic study is most useful single test to determine EF and valvular abnormalities; may be repeated if change suspected in underlying cardiac status. Echocardiogram: EF <45% is HF with reduced EF, EF >45% is HF with preserved EF, valvular abnormalities, tamponade (1)[C].
- B-type natriuretic peptide (BNP) and/or N-type pro-BNP (BT-BNP) may be helpful to differentiate the cause of dyspnea if diagnosis is not certain, but is not indicated in routine care of ADHF. Both tests have been shown to have similar specificities and sensitivities in identifying ADHF (2)[A].
- BNP <100 essentially rules out HF as a cause of dyspnea with negative predictive value of ~99%. Most dyspneic patients with ADHF have BNP >400.

- BNP values of 100 to 400 are more problematic, as they may indicate HF or may be due to conditions such as pulmonary embolism, AKI, ACS, atrial fibrillation, and pulmonary HTN.
- BNP may be higher in the elderly, lower in the obese
- NT-proBNP values >450 pg/mL for people below age 50, >900 pg/mL ages 50 to 75 years, and >1,800 pg/mL for people older than 75 years are highly suggestive of HF (sensitivity 90%, specificity of 84%) (3)[B].
- Chest x-ray (changes lag clinical symptoms by up to 6 hours): increased heart size (cardiothoracic ratio >50%), vascular redistribution (cephalization) with "butterfly" pattern of pulmonary edema, interstitial and alveolar edema, Kerley B lines, pleural effusions
- Other labs that may help identify the cause of the decompensation: TSH (hypothyroidism), CBC (anemia), serum creatinine (renal disease) (1)[C]
- Respiratory alkalosis and dilutional hyponatremia (poor prognosis) may also be present.

Follow-Up Tests & Special Considerations
Please see "Heart Failure, Chronic" topic.

Diagnostic Procedures/Other
Cardiac catheterization may be considered when CAD is suspected. Pulmonary artery catheterization may be performed to guide therapy in severe cases with cardiogenic shock.

Test Interpretation
Cardiac pathology depends on the etiology of HF. Please refer to "Heart Failure, Chronic" topic.

TREATMENT

Approach is to improve symptoms, hemodynamics, and renal function, to minimize myocardial damage and hospital length of stay, and to identify the etiology or precipitating factors. See "Heart Failure, Chronic" chapter as well.

MEDICATION

ALERT
Many medications have been shown to improve hemodynamics and symptoms in ADHF but do not decrease mortality. Diuretics are used initially in fluid overload ADHF, with nitrates added if needed. Nitrates have been used historically to treat ischemic ADHF, but there is no solid evidence-based for this practice, although evidence is sparse (4)[A]. Once ADHF is stabilized, an ACE inhibitor and β-blocker should be started in those with reduced systolic function (5)[A]. Avoid NSAIDs. Avoid use of diltiazem and verapamil in patients with systolic dysfunction.

First Line
- Loop diuretics initially for fluid-overloaded ADHF in hemodynamically stable patients (contraindicated if SBP <90 mm Hg, severe hyponatremia, acidosis) (6)[A]; be cautious of electrolyte abnormalities if kidney disease is present. Avoid if possible diagnosis of pneumonia. Continuous infusion is not better than bolus, and high dose is not significantly better than low dose (5)[B].
  - Furosemide (Lasix): 40 mg IV
  - If on Lasix chronically, initial IV dose should be equal or exceed chronic oral daily dose (max 180 mg). Monitor for appropriate urine output.
  - Metolazone (Zaroxolyn): 2.5 to 20 mg/day PO, more useful if reduced creatinine clearance
- Thiazides in combination with loop diuretics may be useful if resistant to diuresis (HCTZ 25 mg PO).

Thiazides and spironolactone or eplerenone (25 to 50 mg PO) may be used in combination with loop diuretics if excessive volume overload

- Vasodilators: no change in outcomes but may reduce dyspnea in patients with severe HTN, mitral regurgitation, or acute pulmonary edema; don't use if SBP <90 mm Hg, history of aortic stenosis, or phosphodiesterase inhibitor use (5)[A]
  - IV nitroglycerin may be of short-term benefit to decrease preload, afterload, and systemic resistance (IV 10 to 20 μg/min).
  - IV nitroprusside: Administer with caution, infusion rate 5 to 10 μg/min. Consider an arterial line.
- Morphine: IV boluses 2.5 to 5 mg IV helps with chest pain and restlessness. Monitor respirations.

Second Line
- Tolvaptan (an oral vasopressin antagonist), for treatment of cognitive symptoms of severe hypervolemic hyponatremia refractory to water restriction and maximum medical therapy (5)[B]

- Inotropes: consider adding if reduced systolic function and signs of hypoperfusion. Withdraw as soon as hemodynamic parameters improve, as these may increase short- and medium-term mortality.
  - Phosphodiesterase inhibitors (milrinone, enoximone) decrease pulmonary resistance; may be used for patients on β-blockers but may increase medium-term mortality in CAD patients
  - Dobutamine infusion requires close BP monitoring; avoid in cardiogenic shock or with tachyarrhythmias.
  - Low-dose dopamine infusion may be considered.
  - Levosimendan (calcium sensitizer) improves hemodynamic parameters but not survival compared to placebo while improving hemodynamic parameters and survival compared to dobutamine
- Nesiritide, a BNP analog, is not recommended for most hospitalized patients with ADHF; higher rates of hypotension, no benefit on death, or rehospitalization rates

ADDITIONAL THERAPIES
- Oxygen: begin treatment early; ideally, arterial oxygen saturation >92% (90% if COPD). For acute cardiogenic pulmonary edema, noninvasive positive pressure ventilation decreases early mortality compared to standard therapy (7)[A].
- No significant difference between continuous positive airway pressure (CPAP) and noninvasive positive pressure ventilation (NIPPV). If possible, avoid mechanical ventilation for patients with right HF (7)[A].
- Treat anemia with transfusion: conservative trigger Hgb <8; target Hgb 10.
- For patients with new-onset arrhythmias, consider pacing and/or antiarrhythmics.
- For patients with HF with preserved EF, achieve BP control; no mortality benefit demonstrated with any specific class of medications
- For severe cardiogenic shock, consider intra-aortic balloon pump or percutaneous or surgically implanted ventricular assist devices (VADs).
- Please refer to "Heart Failure, Chronic" for maintenance treatments.

SURGERY/OTHER PROCEDURES
- Heart valve surgery if defective heart valve is responsible
- PCI/CABG for patients with CAD/MI if applicable
- Cardiac transplantation considered in patients <55 years of age and without other disqualifying

medical problems who are developing chronic decompensated HF unresponsive to other therapeutic maneuvers and who are considered to have a life expectancy of >1 year.

INPATIENT CONSIDERATIONS
Postdischarge appointment, left ventricular EF assessment, and start on ACE inhibitor (or ARB) and β-blocker if left ventricular systolic dysfunction present

Admission Criteria/Initial Stabilization
See earlier discussion.

- Acute change in HF, with pulmonary edema accompanied by decreased oxygenation, change in mental status, AKI, or significant hyponatremia
- Consider observation unit stay for hemodynamically stable patients with preexisting HF and the following:
  - No acute interventions needed for comorbid condition
  - SBP >120 mm Hg, BUN <40, creatinine <3.0, absence of elevated troponins/ischemic EKG changes
  - Respiratory rate <32 breaths/min without needing noninvasive ventilation
  - No actively titrated vasoactive IV infusions
  - Partial improvement in vital signs and/or increased urine output with initial treatment
  - Clinical impression that patient could be discharged in the next 24 hours and rapid outpatient follow-up is available.

IV Fluids
1.5 to 2 L/day fluid restriction may be useful to reduce congestive symptoms, especially in the case of hyponatremia (5)[C].

Discharge Criteria
Subjective improvement, resting heart rate (HR) <100 bpm, systolic BP >80 mm Hg, HF outpatient education

 ONGOING CARE

FOLLOW-UP RECOMMENDATIONS
Patient education performed at all outpatient and inpatient visits. Please see "Heart Failure, Chronic" topic.

Patient Monitoring
Rapid office follow-up after hospitalization and home health monitoring by specially trained nurses have both been shown to decrease frequency of hospitalizations.

DIET
Reduce sodium (2 g); maintain cardiac or diabetic diet if these comorbidities are present.

PATIENT EDUCATION
- Definition and etiology: Understand the cause of HF and why symptoms occur.
- Prognosis: Understand important prognostic factors and make realistic decisions.
- Symptom monitoring and self-care: recognize signs/symptoms, record daily weight, know how and when to contact a health care provider; may increase diuretic dose with >1 kg in a day, >2 kg weight gain in 5 days or dyspnea/contact health care provider
- Pharmacologic treatment: Understand indications, dosing, effects, and side effects of drugs.
- Adherence: Understand the importance of maintaining the treatment plan.
- Alcohol, smoking, and drugs: Abstinence is recommended in patients with alcohol-induced cardiomyopathy. Otherwise, normal alcohol guidelines apply. Smoking and illicit drug cessation.
- Exercise: Understand the benefits of exercise.

PROGNOSIS
- The ADHERE risk tree stratifies ADHF patients for inpatient mortality using systolic blood pressure, BUN, and creatinine.
- S_3 on physical exam correlates with poor prognosis.
- After diagnosis, 1-year survival ~75%, 5-year survival <50%, 10-year survival <25%

COMPLICATIONS
Arrhythmia, pulmonary edema, hyponatremia, death

REFERENCES

1. McMurray JJ, Adamopoulos S, Anker SD, et al. ESC guidelines for the diagnosis and treatment of acute and chronic heart failure 2012: the Task Force for the Diagnosis and Treatment of Acute and Chronic Heart Failure 2012 of the European Society of Cardiology. Developed in collaboration with the Heart Failure Association (HFA) of the ESC. *Eur Heart J.* 2012;33(14):1787–1847.
2. Worster A, Balion CM, Hill SA, et al. Diagnostic accuracy of BNP and NT-proBNP in patients presenting to acute care settings with dyspnea: a systematic review. *Clin Biochem.* 2008;41(4–5):250–259.
3. Januzzi JL, van Kimmenade R, Lainchbury J, et al. NT-proBNP testing for diagnosis and short-term prognosis in acute destabilized heart failure: an international pooled analysis of 1256 patients: the International Collaborative of NT-proBNP Study. *Eur Heart J.* 2006;27(3):330–337.
4. Wakai A, McCabe A, Kidney R, et al. Nitrates for acute heart failure syndromes. *Cochrane Database Syst Rev.* 2013;(8): CD005151.
5. Yancy CW, Jessup M, Bozkurt B, et al. 2013 ACCF/AHA guideline for the management of heart failure: executive summary: a report of the American College of Cardiology Foundation/American Heart Association Task Force on practice guidelines. *Circulation.* 2013;128(16):1810–1852.
6. Felker GM, Lee KL, Bull DA, et al. Diuretic strategies in patients with acute decompensated heart failure. *N Engl J Med.* 2011;364(9):797–805.
7. Mariani J, Macchia A, Belziti C, et al. Noninvasive ventilation in acute cardiogenic pulmonary edema: a meta-analysis of randomized controlled trials. *J Card Fail.* 2011;17(10):850–859.

ADDITIONAL READING

Mozaffarian D, Benjamin EJ, Go AS, et al. Heart disease and stroke statistics—2015 update: a report from the American Heart Association. *Circulation.* 2015;131(4):e29-e322.

CODES

ICD10
- I50.9 Heart failure, unspecified
- I50.21 Acute systolic (congestive) heart failure
- I50.31 Acute diastolic (congestive) heart failure

CLINICAL PEARLS
- BNP is overused diagnostically and is best reserved for situations in which diagnosis of ADHF is unclear.
- Look for underlying cause of each episode of ADHF.
- IV diuretics are used initially in fluid-overload acute HF, with nitrates added if needed.
- Using early noninvasive ventilation for the treatment of pulmonary edema can bridge care while awaiting the effects of diuretics, and can decrease morbidity and mortality associated with intubation.

HEART FAILURE, CHRONIC

Jeffrey Shih, MD • David DeNofrio, MD

BASICS

DESCRIPTION
- Heart failure (HF) is the condition resulting from inability of the heart to fill and/or pump blood sufficiently to meet tissue metabolic needs. Alternatively, HF may occur when adequate cardiac output can be achieved only at the expense of elevated filling pressures. It is the principal complication of heart disease.
- HF is the preferred term over congestive heart failure because patients are not always congested (fluid overloaded).
- HF may involve the left heart, the right heart, or be biventricular. The New York Heart Association (NYHA) classification is a subjective grading scale used for classifying patients with HF: NYHA I: asymptomatic; NYHA II: symptomatic with moderate exertion; NYHA III: symptomatic with mild exertion and may limit activities of daily living; NYHA IV: symptomatic at rest. For acute HF, see "Heart Failure, Acutely Decompensated."

EPIDEMIOLOGY
The annual direct and indirect cost of HF in the United States is ~$34.4 billion.

Incidence
In the United States, 550,000 new cases diagnosed annually with >250,000 deaths per year.

Prevalence
- ~5.7 million people in the United States have HF; <1% in those age <50 years, increasing to 10% of those age >80 years
- Primarily a disease of the elderly; 75% of hospital admissions for HF are for persons >65 years of age.

ETIOLOGY AND PATHOPHYSIOLOGY
Two physiologic components explain most of the clinical findings of HF and result in classifications of patients in four general categories:
- HF with reduced ejection fraction (HFrEF) or systolic HF: an *inotropic* abnormality, often due to myocardial infarction (MI) or dilated cardiomyopathy, resulting in diminished systolic emptying (ejection fraction [EF] ≤40%)
- HF with preserved ejection fraction (HFpEF) or diastolic HF: a *compliance* abnormality, often due to hypertensive cardiomyopathy, in which the ventricular relaxation is impaired (EF ≥50%)
- Borderline HFpEF (EF 41–49%): mild systolic dysfunction but clinically behaves like HFpEF
- Improved HFpEF (EF >40%): previously HFrEF but with improvement in systolic function
- Patients with systolic dysfunction may also have diastolic dysfunction.
- Most common etiologies: coronary artery disease (CAD)/MI and hypertension (HTN)
- Myocarditis and cardiomyopathy (CM): alcoholic, viral, long-standing HTN, drugs (e.g., chemotherapeutic agents), muscular dystrophy, infiltrative (e.g., amyloidosis, sarcoidosis), postpartum state, infectious (e.g., Chagas disease, HIV), hypertrophic CM (HCM), inherited familial dilated CM, left ventricular noncompaction
- Valvular and vascular abnormalities: any valvular stenosis or regurgitation, rheumatic heart; renal artery stenosis, usually bilateral, may cause recurrent "flash" pulmonary edema, especially in setting of severe chronic HTN
- Chronic lung disease and pulmonary HTN (cor pulmonale)
- Iatrogenic volume overload (requires extreme overload in patients with normal hearts and kidneys)
- Arrhythmias (atrial fibrillation and other tachyarrhythmias, high-grade heart block)
- Miscellaneous: high-output states: hyperthyroidism, anemia; cardiac depressants (β-blocker overdose), stress-induced
- Idiopathic: 20–50% of idiopathic dilated cardiomyopathies are familial.
- HF is progressive—manifested by the remodeling (altered heart geometry) process.

Genetics
Multiple genetic abnormalities responsible for a variety of phenotypes have been identified (HCM, arrhythmogenic right ventricular [RV] dysplasia, left ventricular [LV] noncompaction, dilated CM). Consider genetic screening for first-degree relatives of HCM and arrhythmogenic RV dysplasia.

RISK FACTORS
For development of HF: CAD/MI, HTN (80% of cases of HF in the United States caused by either CAD or HTN), valvular heart disease, diabetes mellitus, cardiotoxic medications (e.g., anthracyclines, tyrosine-kinase inhibitors, TNF-α inhibitors), obesity, older age

GENERAL PREVENTION
Control HTN and other risk factors. Thiazide diuretics and angiotensin-converting enzyme inhibitors (ACE-I) are superior to other agents in preventing development of HF.

COMMONLY ASSOCIATED CONDITIONS
Sudden cardiac death and progressive pump failure are the leading causes of death. Most patients have >5 comorbid medical conditions and take >5 medications.

DIAGNOSIS

HISTORY
- Dyspnea on exertion: *cardinal sign of left-sided HF*. Deteriorating exercise capacity: easily fatigued, general weakness
- Nocturnal nonproductive cough, orthopnea, and paroxysmal nocturnal dyspnea; sometimes frothy or pink sputum. Wheezing, especially nocturnal, in absence of history of asthma or infection (cardiac asthma); Cheyne-Stokes respirations
- Anorexia and/or fullness or dull pain in right upper quadrant (hepatic congestion). Nausea and poor appetite may indicate advanced HF.

PHYSICAL EXAM
- Increased filling pressures: rales (crackles) and sometimes wheezing, peripheral edema, S_3 gallop, hepatomegaly, jugular venous distension, hepatojugular reflux, ascites
- Remodeling: enlarged or displaced point of maximal impulse
- Poor cardiac output: hypotension, pulsus alternans, tachycardia, narrow pulse pressure, cool extremities, cyanosis

DIFFERENTIAL DIAGNOSIS
Simple dependent edema, pulmonary embolism, exertional asthma, cardiac ischemia, asthma/COPD, constrictive pericarditis, nephrotic syndrome, cirrhosis, venous occlusive disease with subsequent peripheral edema, high-output states: anemia, sepsis, hyperthyroidism, lymphedema, tamponade

DIAGNOSTIC TESTS & INTERPRETATION
Diagnosis should be primarily clinical, with laboratory data as adjunctive and indicative of complications.

Initial Tests (lab, imaging)
- β-type natriuretic peptide (BNP) and N-type pro-BNP (NT-BNP) helpful in the acute setting to differentiate the cause of dyspnea (BNP <100 essentially rules out HF; most dyspneic patients with HF have a BNP >400) (1)[A]. Other, non-HF conditions, such as pulmonary embolism, renal failure, and acute coronary syndromes, may cause elevated BNP. Obesity may lower BNP levels. The use of BNP-guided therapy in chronic HF and acutely decompensated HF is not well-established.
- Lab findings include respiratory alkalosis, mild azotemia, decreased ESR, proteinuria (usually <1 g/day), elevated creatinine (cardiorenal syndrome), dilutional hyponatremia (poor prognosis), hyperuricemia, and hyperbilirubinemia.
- Chest x-ray (changes lag clinical symptoms by up to 6 hours): increased heart size, vascular redistribution (cephalization) with "butterfly" pattern of pulmonary edema, interstitial and alveolar edema, Kerley B lines, and pleural effusions. Findings of pulmonary edema may be absent in long-standing HF.

Diagnostic Procedures/Other
Determination of left ventricular ejection fraction (LVEF) is critical to proper diagnosis and management:
- Echocardiogram is the most useful test to determine LVEF, RV function, diastolic dysfunction, ventricular size, wall thickness, and valvular abnormalities. May be repeated if change suspected in underlying cardiac status
- Nuclear imaging to estimate ventricular sizes, assess for ischemia or infarction and systolic function
- Cardiac MRI can be considered in select circumstances: suspicion of cardiac sarcoidosis, arrhythmogenic RV CM, acute myocarditis, amyloidosis, and hemochromatosis. It is also useful for differentiating restrictive CM and constrictive pericarditis.
- Cardiac catheterization is important for excluding CAD as an etiology in the setting of risk factors.
- Endomyocardial biopsy should not be performed routinely, only in special circumstances (e.g., suspected giant cell myocarditis) that may change therapy (1)[C].

Test Interpretation
Cardiac pathology depends on underlying etiology.

TREATMENT

GENERAL MEASURES
Correct and treat risk factors for HF. The treatment of chronic HF is focused on improving hemodynamics, relieving symptoms, and blocking the neurohormonal response to hopefully improve survival.

MEDICATION
Diuretics are used initially in fluid overload acute HF. The addition of ACE-I and aldosterone antagonists can be added at any time. Once acute HF is stabilized, a β-blocker should be started. Avoid nonsteroidal anti-inflammatory drugs (NSAIDs), which markedly worsen HF. Avoid use of diltiazem and verapamil in patients with systolic dysfunction as they may increase mortality and have negative inotropic effects.

First Line
- ACE-I: used to decrease afterload. Shown to increase survival, improve symptoms and overall

exercise capacity in patients in all NYHA classifications; benefit greatest for patients with systolic dysfunction and post-MI. Number needed to treat (NNT) ~25 per year for mortality. All ACE-I considered equally effective. Initiate at low doses and titrate as tolerated to target doses.

- Angiotensin receptor blockers (ARBs) are indicated for those who are intolerant to ACE-I. They are probably slightly less effective than ACE-I. Avoid combination of ACE-I and ARB.

- β-Blockers: used in systolic or diastolic HF (Note: initiate in hemodynamically stable/compensated patients at low dose and titrate upward slowly); NNT = 25 for mortality. Mortality decreased in systolic HF. Evidence for titration to heart rate rather than specific dose (1)[A].

  – Carvedilol: 3.125 mg PO BID to a target of 25 mg PO BID; metoprolol succinate extended release: 12.5 mg/day PO to a target of 200 mg/day PO or bisoprolol 1.25 to 10 mg once daily (currently not FDA approved for the treatment of HF)

- Diuretics are helpful to manage volume overload/reduce preload.

  – Furosemide (Lasix): 20 to 320 mg/day IV/IM/PO divided dose; bumetanide (Bumex): 0.5 mg to 10 mg/day IV/PO divided dose; torsemide (Demadex): 10 to 200 mg/day PO divided dose (1)[C]
  – Metolazone (Zaroxolyn): 2.5 to 20 mg/day PO divided dose; hydrochlorothiazide: 12.5 to 100 mg/day PO divided dose; chlorothiazide (Diuril): 250 to 2,000 mg/day IV/PO divided dose
  – Spironolactone, eplerenone (improve mortality when added to standard therapy in NYHA class II–IV + EF <35%): spironolactone 12.5 to 25 mg/day PO; maximum 50 mg/day PO; eplerenone 25 to 50 mg/day. Caution regarding hyperkalemia and chronic kidney disease (CKD) (1)[A]

- Digoxin reduces symptoms but has not clearly shown any positive effect on mortality: In patients with preserved renal function (creatinine clearance >50 mL/min), the recommended dose is 0.125 mg/day. Levels lower than used for atrial fibrillation are effective and safer (1)[B].

- The combination of hydralazine (75 mg/day divided BID or TID) and isosorbide dinitrate (40 mg QID) is effective for African Americans (1)[A] or if unable to take ACE-I or an ARB (1)[B].

- Ivabradine (Corlanor) is FDA approved to reduce hospitalization from worsening HF based on the SHIFT trial (2). Ivabradine is contraindicated in ADHF, hypotension (<90/50 mm Hg), severe hepatic impairment, pacemaker-dependence, bradyarrhythmias, or strong CYP3A4 inhibitors. It should not be administered to patients that are currently in atrial fibrillation and should be discontinued if atrial fibrillation develops (2)[A].

- Sacubitril/valsartan (Entresto) was approved by the FDA in July of 2015. It is indicated to reduce the risk of CV death and HF hospitalizations in patients with NYHA class II–IV symptoms due to HFrEF based on the PARADIGM HF trial. This medication is used in place of an ACE inhibitor or ARB and in conjunction with other HF therapies (3)[A].

- Anticoagulation is not recommended in patients with HFrEF unless there are other indications such as atrial fibrillation, cardioembolism, or intracardiac thrombus (4)[A].

- In diastolic HF, no medical therapy has improved survival (1,5)[A]. ARBs and spironolactone can be used to potentially reduce hospitalizations (1)[A], (6)[B].

ADDITIONAL THERAPIES
Device therapy including implantable cardioverter defibrillators (ICD) and cardiac resynchronization therapy (CRT) shown to improve outcomes

- CRT is recommended for patients in sinus rhythm with a QRS width ≥150 ms due to left bundle branch block (LBBB) and LVEF ≤35% and persistent mild to moderate HF (NYHA II–III) despite optimal medical therapy. CRT may be considered for ambulatory NYHA class IV patients in sinus rhythm with a QRS width ≥150 ms, LBBB, and LVEF ≤35% (1)[A].
- CRT may be considered for patients with LVEF ≤35%, sinus rhythm, QRS width ≥150 ms, non-LBBB pattern, and NYHA III or ambulatory NYHA IV symptoms (1)[A].
- CRT may also be considered for patients with a QRS width between 120 and 150 ms, LBBB, LVEF ≤35%, and persistent mild to severe HF (NYHA II–IV) despite optimal medical therapy (1)[B].
- ICDs are recommended for primary prevention in patients with *nonischemic* CM and *ischemic* CM who are at least 40 days post-MI; LVEF ≤35%, NYHA class II or III HF (1)[A], or LVEF ≤30%, NYHA I HF (1)[B]; and on optimal medical therapy and >1 year estimated survival. Generally not indicated in American Heart Association (AHA) stage D (end-stage) HF
- CRT is recommended in patients with reduced LVEF and chronic RV pacing or with bradyarrhythmias and an anticipated need for a pacemaker (7)[A].

SURGERY/OTHER PROCEDURES
- Heart valve surgery if defective heart valve is responsible; mitral valve repair especially helpful if mitral regurgitation is the primary issue and not functional.
- Advanced therapies such as cardiac transplantation and LV assist device (LVAD) implantation can be considered in patients with HF refractory to conventional medical/device therapies without other disqualifying medical and psychosocial conditions. Cardiac transplantation is generally considered for patients ≤70 years old with a predicted 1-year survival worse than that afforded by transplantation. Indications for LVAD implantation are generally similar to cardiac transplantation but are evolving.

INPATIENT CONSIDERATIONS
Admission Criteria/Initial Stabilization
- See "Heart Failure, Acutely Decompensated."
- Admit patients with hemodynamic/respiratory compromise, hypoxia/hypoxemia, change in mental status, acute renal insufficiency, significant volume overload, and significant electrolyte abnormalities (e.g., hyponatremia).

Discharge Criteria
Subjective improvement, euvolemia on clinical assessment, resting heart rate (HR) <100 bpm, systolic BP >80 mm Hg, HF outpatient education performed

 ## ONGOING CARE

FOLLOW-UP RECOMMENDATIONS
- Critical patient education performed at all outpatient and inpatient physician visits
- Rapid office follow-up (1 to 2 weeks) after hospitalization.

Patient Monitoring
Home health monitoring by specially trained nurses have both been shown to decrease frequency of hospitalizations. Readmissions remain problematic.

DIET
Reduce sodium load (<1.5 to 2 g/day). Optimal level is unknown.

PATIENT EDUCATION
AHA: www.americanheart.org

PROGNOSIS
After diagnosis: 1-year survival ~75%, 5-year survival <50%, and 10-year survival <25%

COMPLICATIONS
Sudden death (arrhythmic), acute pulmonary edema, death, progressive pump failure

REFERENCES
1. Yancy CW, Jessup M, Bozkurt B, et al. 2013 ACCF/AHA guideline for the management of heart failure: a report of the American College of Cardiology Foundation/American Heart Association Task Force on Practice Guidelines. *J Am Coll Cardiol*. 2013;62(16):e147–e239.
2. Swedberg K, Komajda M, Böhm M, et al. Ivabradine and outcomes in chronic heart failure (SHIFT): a randomised placebo-controlled study. *Lancet*. 2010;376(9744):875–885.
3. McMurray JJ, Packer M, Desai AS, et al. Angiotensin-neprilysin inhibition versus enalapril in heart failure. *N Engl J Med*. 2014;371(11):993–1004.
4. Homma S, Thompson JL, Pullicino PM, et al. Warfarin and aspirin in patients with heart failure and sinus rhythm. *N Engl J Med*. 2012;366(20):1859–1869.
5. Massie BM, Carson PE, McMurray JJ, et al. Irbesartan in patients with heart failure and preserved ejection fraction. *N Engl J Med*. 2008;359(23):2456–2467.
6. Pitt B, Pfeffer MA, Assmann SF, et al. Spironolactone for heart failure with preserved ejection fraction. *N Engl J Med*. 2014;370(15):1383–1392.
7. Curtis AB, Worley SJ, Adamson PB, et al. Biventricular pacing for atrioventricular block and systolic dysfunction. *N Engl J Med*. 2013;368(17):1585–1593.

ADDITIONAL READING
Nohria A, Lewis E, Stevenson LW. Medical management of advanced heart failure. *JAMA*. 2002;287(5):628–640.

 ## SEE ALSO

Algorithms: Congestive Heart Failure: Differential Diagnosis

CODES

ICD10
- I50.9 Heart failure, unspecified
- I50.1 Left ventricular failure
- I50.22 Chronic systolic (congestive) heart failure

CLINICAL PEARLS
- Have patients weigh themselves daily and report weight gains of >2 lb in a day or 5 lb above dry weight.
- β-Blockers, ACE-I, and aldosterone antagonists are the core medications for management of chronic HF.
- Consider referral for biventricular pacing in patients with LBBB and ICD in those with low EF.
- Refer to an HF specialist if frequently hospitalized.

H

HEAT EXHAUSTION AND HEAT STROKE

Sean C. Robinson, MD • Brian Frank, MD

 BASICS

DESCRIPTION

- A continuum of increasingly severe heat illnesses caused by dehydration, electrolyte losses, and failure of the body's thermoregulatory mechanisms when exposed to elevated environmental temperatures.
  - Heat exhaustion is a mild to moderate form of heat illness displaying dehydration type symptoms with a normal to elevated temperature <104°F (1).
  - Heat stroke is characterized by an elevated core temperature >104°F with central nervous system abnormalities (1,2).
- System(s) affected: endocrine/metabolic, nervous, hepatic, hematologic
- Synonym(s): heat illness; heat injury; hyperthermia; heat collapse; heat prostration

Geriatric Considerations
Elderly persons are more susceptible.

Pediatric Considerations
Children are more susceptible.

Pregnancy Considerations
Pregnant women may be more susceptible to volume depletion with heat stress.

EPIDEMIOLOGY
- Predominant age: more likely in children or elderly
- Predominant sex: male = female

Incidence
- Depends on intensity of heat; estimate of 20/100,000 persons per season (3)
- Concern for increasing incidence of disease if ambient environmental temperatures continue to rise

Prevalence
- Depends on predisposing conditions in combination with environmental factors
- Roughly 600 deaths/year in the United States

ETIOLOGY AND PATHOPHYSIOLOGY
- Direct cellular toxicity of heat, imbalance between inflammatory and anti-inflammatory cytokines, and vascular endothelial damage causing end-organ dysfunction
- Interplay between failure of heat-dissipating mechanisms, an overwhelming heat stress, and an exaggerated acute-phase inflammatory response

RISK FACTORS
- Poor acclimatization to heat or poor physical conditioning
- Salt or water depletion
- Obesity
- Acute febrile or GI illnesses
- Chronic illnesses: uncontrolled diabetes mellitus or hypertension, cardiac disease
- Alcohol and other substance abuse
- High heat and humidity, poor air circulation in environment
- Heavy, restrictive clothing
- Nutritional supplementation that includes ephedra (2)
- Medications (α-adrenergics, anticholinergics, antihistamines, antipsychotics, benzodiazepines, β-blockers, calcium channel blockers, clopidogrel, diuretics, laxatives, neuroleptics, phenothiazines, thyroid agonists, tricyclic antidepressants) (1)

GENERAL PREVENTION
- The most important factor in preventing heat stress is adequate fluid replacement.
- Allow acclimatization to hot weather through proper conditioning and activity modification.
- Dress appropriately with loose-fitting, open-weaved, light-colored clothing.
- Avoid dehydration by consuming a proper amount of fluids during activity or exercise.
- Never leave children unattended in cars during hot weather.
- Try to gain access to air-conditioned environments during hot weather.

PROGNOSIS
- The prognosis is good when mental function is not altered and when serum enzymes are not elevated; recovery is within 24 to 48 hours in most cases.
- The mortality rate for heat stroke (10–80%) is directly related to the duration and intensity of hyperthermia, as well as to the speed and effectiveness of diagnosis and treatment (3).

COMPLICATIONS
- May involve failure of any major organ system
- Cardiac arrhythmias or infarction
- Pulmonary edema, acute respiratory distress syndrome
- Coma, seizures
- Acute renal failure
- Rhabdomyolysis
- Disseminated intravascular coagulopathy (DIC)
- Hepatocellular necrosis

 DIAGNOSIS

- Heat exhaustion: Symptoms are milder than in heat stroke, with no severe CNS derangements:
  - Fatigue and lethargy
  - Weakness
  - Dizziness
  - Nausea, vomiting
  - Myalgias
  - Headache
  - Profuse sweating
  - Tachycardia
  - Hypotension
  - Lack of coordination
  - Agitation
  - Intense thirst
  - Hyperventilation
  - Paresthesias
  - Core temperature usually elevated but can be normal, if elevated <104°F (40°C)
- Heat stroke: divided into two categories, classic and exertional:
  - Classic: caused by environmental exposure, primarily in elderly or chronically ill patients, and may develop gradually over days
    ○ Delirium
    ○ Confusion
    ○ Coma
    ○ Core temperature >104°F (>40°C)
    ○ Hot, flushed, dry skin
  - Exertional: typically younger, very active patients; rapid onset
    ○ Exhaustion
    ○ Confusion, disorientation
    ○ Delirium
    ○ Coma
    ○ Hot, flushed skin, typically with sweating
    ○ Core temperature >104°F (>40°C) (1,2)

DIFFERENTIAL DIAGNOSIS
- Other causes of elevated temperature, dehydration, or circulatory collapse
- Febrile illnesses, sepsis
- Drug-induced fluid loss
- Cardiac arrhythmia or infarction
- Acute cocaine intoxication
- Neuroleptic malignant syndrome
- Malignant hyperthermia (an autosomally inherited disorder of skeletal and cardiac muscle in which patients have abnormal muscle metabolism on exposure to halothane or skeletal muscle reactants)

DIAGNOSTIC TESTS & INTERPRETATION
Used primarily to detect end-organ damage

Initial Tests (lab, imaging)
- Electrolytes, urinalysis
- Creatinine, BUN
- Liver enzymes, muscle enzymes (creatine phosphokinase)
- CBC
- Increased urine-specific gravity
- Results of these studies may indicate hypernatremia, hyperchloremia, and hemoconcentration.
- Drugs that may alter lab results: diuretics

Diagnostic Procedures/Other
Rectal temperature monitoring (do not rely on oral temperature) (1,2)[A]

 TREATMENT

GENERAL MEASURES
- Fluid and electrolyte replacement with normal saline gradually; avoid hypotonic fluids (1,2)[C].
- Consider CVP monitoring.
- Body immersion in ice water, careful consideration of airway protection (1,3)[C]
- Evaporative cooling: spraying water over the patient and facilitating evaporation and convection with the use of fans (1,3)[C]
- Immersing the hands and forearms in cold water (3)[C]
- Use of ice or cold packs on the neck, groin, and axillae (1,2)[C]
- No clear superiority of any one method (1).

MEDICATION
First Line
No medications are required in the initial management. Use isotonic saline solution to rehydrate (1,3)[C].

Second Line
- Consider immunomodulators such as corticosteroids.
- Iced gastric, bladder, or peritoneal lavage (3)[C]
- In DIC, consider appropriate replacement therapy.

INPATIENT CONSIDERATIONS
Admission Criteria/Initial Stabilization
- Important to cool patient before transport if you suspect heat stroke
- Rapid cooling: Remove clothing, wet patient down, and apply ice packs.
- Emergency treatment; best in a hospital setting

 ONGOING CARE

FOLLOW-UP RECOMMENDATIONS
Rest with legs elevated (3)[C].

Patient Monitoring
- Rectal temperature monitoring: Cooling may be discontinued when the core temperature drops to 102°F (38.9°C) and stabilizes.
- Heat stroke patients may require airway management, hemodynamic monitoring, and careful fluid and electrolyte administration and monitoring.
- Consider CVP monitoring.

DIET
- Cool or cold clear liquids only (noncarbonated)
- Avoid caffeine.
- Unrestricted sodium

PATIENT EDUCATION
- The key to prevention is proper hydration.
- Stress the importance of proper conditioning and acclimatization.
- Instruct patients to recognize heat stress signs and symptoms.
- Maintain as much skin exposure as possible in hot, humid conditions while using proper sunblock protection.

REFERENCES
1. Lipman GS, Eifling KP, Ellis MA, et al. Wilderness Medical Society practice guidelines for the prevention and treatment of heat-related illness: 2014 update. *Wilderness Environ Med*. 2014;25(4 Suppl):S55–S65.
2. Becker JA, Stewart LK. Heat-related illness. *Am Fam Physician*. 2011;83(11):1325–1330.
3. Yeo TP. Heat stroke: a comprehensive review. *AACN Clin Issues*. 2004;15(2):280–293.

ADDITIONAL READING
- Armstrong LE, Casa DJ, Millard-Stafford M, et al. American College of Sports Medicine position stand. Exertional heat illness during training and competition. *Med Sci Sports Exerc*. 2007;39(3):556–572.
- Atha WF. Heat-related illness. *Emerg Med Clin North Am*. 2013;31(4):1097–1108.
- Bouchama A, Dehbi M, Chaves-Carballo E. Cooling and hemodynamic management in heatstroke: practical recommendations. *Crit Care*. 2007;11(3):R54
- Smith JE. Cooling methods used in the treatment of exertional heat illness. *Br J Sports Med*. 2005;39(8):503–507.

 CODES

ICD10
- T67.5XXA Heat exhaustion, unspecified, initial encounter
- T67.0XXA Heatstroke and sunstroke, initial encounter
- T67.3XXA Heat exhaustion, anhydrotic, initial encounter

CLINICAL PEARLS
- The diagnosis of heat stroke relies on both hyperthermia and CNS dysfunction (e.g., irritability, ataxia, confusion, seizures, or coma).
- Start the cooling process immediately when heat exhaustion or heat stroke is recognized, beginning with wetting the skin with a cool mist and giving oral rehydration solutions containing saline, if the patient is alert and oriented.
- If in the field (e.g., sporting events, wilderness), cooling should be priority prior to transport
- Do not rely on oral temperature.

H

HEMATURIA

Tracy O. Middleton, DO

 BASICS

DESCRIPTION

- Gross (visible) or microscopic (nonvisible) blood in the urine
- Symptomatic or asymptomatic

EPIDEMIOLOGY

Prevalence

- Microscopic hematuria in school-aged children: 0.4–4%
- Microscopic hematuria in asymptomatic adults varies from 0.19% to 31%, depending on population (1).

ETIOLOGY AND PATHOPHYSIOLOGY

- Trauma
  - Exercise-induced (resolves with rest)
  - Abdominal trauma or pelvic fracture with renal, bladder, or ureteral injury
  - Iatrogenic from abdominal or pelvic surgery; chronic indwelling catheters
  - Foreign body, physical/sexual abuse
- Neoplasms
  - Urologic malignancies
  - Benign tumors
  - Endometriosis of the urinary tract (suspect in females with cyclic hematuria)
- Inflammatory causes
  - UTI: most common cause of hematuria in adults
  - Renal diseases: radiation nephritis and cystitis, acute/chronic tubulointerstitial nephritis (due to drugs, infections, systemic disease)
  - Glomerular disease
    - ○ Goodpasture syndrome (antiglomerular basement membrane disease; autoimmune; associated pulmonary hemorrhage)
    - ○ IgA nephropathy
    - ○ Lupus nephritis
    - ○ Henoch-Schönlein purpura
    - ○ Membranoproliferative, poststreptococcal, or rapidly progressive glomerulonephritis (GN)
    - ○ Wegener granulomatosis
  - Endocarditis/visceral abscesses
  - Other infections: schistosomiasis, TB, syphilis
- Metabolic causes
  - Stones (85% have hematuria)
    - ○ Hypercalciuria: a common cause of both gross and microscopic hematuria in children
    - ○ Hyperuricosuria
- Congenital/familial causes
  - Cystic disease: polycystic, solitary renal cyst
  - Benign familial hematuria or thin basement membrane nephropathy (autosomal dominant)
  - Alport syndrome (X-linked in 85%; hematuria, proteinuria, hearing loss, corneal abnormalities)
  - Fabry disease (X-linked recessive inborn error of metabolism; vascular kidney disease)
  - Nail-patella syndrome (autosomal dominant; nail and patella hypoplasia; hematuria in 33%)
  - Renal tubular acidosis type 1 (autosomal dominant or autoimmune)
- Hematologic causes
  - Bleeding dyscrasias (e.g., hemophilia)
  - Sickle cell anemia/trait (renal papillary necrosis)
- Vascular causes
  - Hemangioma
  - Arteriovenous malformations (rare)
  - Nutcracker syndrome: compression of left renal vein and subsequent renal parenchymal congestion
  - Renal artery/vein thrombosis
  - Arterial emboli to kidney
- Chemical causes
  - Aminoglycosides, cyclosporine, analgesics, oral contraceptives, Chinese herbs
- Obstruction
  - Strictures or posterior urethral valves
  - Hydronephrosis from any cause
  - Benign prostatic hyperplasia: Rule out other causes of hematuria.
- Other causes: loin pain hematuria (most often in young women on oral contraceptives)

RISK FACTORS

- Smoking
- Occupational exposures (dyes, rubber, or tire manufacturing)
- Analgesic abuse (e.g., phenacetin)
- Medications (e.g., cyclophosphamide)
- Pelvic irradiation
- Chronic infection, especially with calculi
- Recent upper respiratory tract infection
- Positive family history of renal diseases (stones, GN)
- Underlying primary renal disorder
- Chronic indwelling foreign body

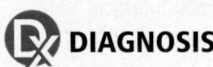 **DIAGNOSIS**

HISTORY

Considerations

- Burning, urgency, frequency: UTI
- Dark cola–colored urine: glomerular origin
- Clots: extraglomerular bleeding
- Arthritis/arthralgias/rash: lupus, vasculitis, Henoch-Schönlein purpura
- Flank pain: stones, infarction, pyelonephritis
- Recent upper respiratory infection (URI): poststreptococcal GN, membranoproliferative GN
- Concurrent URI: IgA nephropathy
- Excessive vitamin use: stones
- Marathon runner: traumatic, rhabdomyolysis
- Travel: schistosomiasis, TB
- Painless hematuria and/or weight loss: malignancy
- Family history: Alport disease (hereditary nephritis), sickle cell, polycystic, IgA nephropathy, thin basement membrane disease, von Willebrand

PHYSICAL EXAM

Considerations

- Elevated BP, edema, and weight gain: glomerular disease
- Fever: infection
- Palpable kidney: neoplasm, polycystic
- Genitalia: Look for meatal erosion, lesions

DIAGNOSTIC TESTS & INTERPRETATION

- A hematuria risk index may assist in stratifying patients at risk for urothelial malignancies who require more intensive testing. High-risk indicators are gross hematuria, age >50 years, male gender, and smoking (2)[B].
- Studies are ongoing using urinary biomarkers + clinical factors to predict the likelihood of bladder cancer (3)[B].

- American Urological Association (AUA) suggests upper urinary tract imaging in all adults with unexplained hematuria (4)[C].

Initial Tests (lab, imaging)

- Urine dipstick (sensitivity 91–100%; specificity 65–99%)
  - False negatives are rare but can be caused by high-dose vitamin C.
  - False positives: oxidizers (povidone, bacterial peroxidases, bleach), myoglobin, alkaline urine (>9), semen, food coloring, food (beets, blackberries) (1)
  - Phenazopyridine may discolor the dipstick, making interpretation difficult.
- Microscopic urinalysis should always be done to confirm dipstick findings and quantify RBCs.
  - AUA defines clinically significant microscopic hematuria as ≥3 RBCs/HPF on a properly collected urinary specimen when there is not an obvious benign cause (4)[C].
  - Positive dipstick but a negative microscopic exam should be followed by 3 repeat tests. If any 1 is positive, proceed with a workup (4)[C].
  - Exclude factitious or nonurinary causes, such as menstruation, mild trauma, exercise, poor collection technique, or chemical/drug causes, through cessation of activity/cause and a repeat urinalysis in 48 hours (1)[C].
  - RBC casts are pathognomonic for glomerular origin; dysmorphic cells are also suggestive.
- Voided urine cytology
  - No longer recommended by AUA for routine evaluation of hematuria (4)[C]
  - Some still consider cytology in those with risk factors for urinary malignancy (1)[C].
- Renal function tests (eGFR, BUN, creatinine) to differentiate intrinsic renal disease and to evaluate for risks for imaging contrast dye or certain medications
  - Indicators of renal disease are: significant (>500 mg/day) proteinuria, red cell casts, dysmorphic RBCs, increased creatinine, and albumin:creatinine ratio ≥30 mg/mmol (4)[C],(5)[A].
- Urine culture if suspected infection/pyuria (1)[C]
- PT/INR for patients on warfarin or suspected of abusing warfarin
- Multidetector CT urography (MDCTU); sensitivity 91–100%, specificity 94–97% (1)[C]
  - The initial imaging of choice in nonpregnant adults with unexplained hematuria (1,6)[C]
  - Highly specific and relatively sensitive for the diagnosis of upper urinary tract neoplasms, especially when >1 cm (6)[C]
  - Higher radiation dose; weigh risk of disease versus risk of radiation exposure.
  - Does not obviate the need for cystoscopy, particularly in high-risk patients (6)[C]
  - Presence of calculi on noncontrast does not exclude another diagnosis or need for contrast phase.
  - Visualization of ureters is discontinuous.
  - Less cost-efficient
- CT
  - Perform unenhanced helical CT for suspected stone disease in children if US is negative (7)[C].
  - Perform CT abdomen and pelvis with contrast in children with traumatic hematuria (7)[C].
- Renal ultrasound
  - Best for differentiating cystic from solid masses
  - Sensitive for hydronephrosis
  - No radiation or iodinated contrast exposure
  - Cost-efficient
  - Poor sensitivity for renal masses <3 cm

- Point of care US in the emergency room may help patients with suspected stones avoid CT (8)[B].
- US can be used first line in patients with contraindications to CTU or at low risk of malignancy (6)[C].
- Main disadvantage is inability to thoroughly evaluate the urothelium for transitional cell cancer.
- Magnetic resonance urography (MRU)
  - High sensitivity/specificity for renal parenchyma; less useful for collecting system or stones
  - Can be used in patients with contraindications to MDCTU (4,6)[C]
- IV urography (IVU)
  - Limited sensitivity for small renal masses and for differentiating cystic from solid masses
  - Addition of US or CT often necessary to evaluate renal parenchyma, so IVU is rarely used.
  - Potential reactions to IV iodine contrast media
- MRI
  - Similar to CT in sensitivity for renal masses
  - No radiation exposure
  - Least cost-efficient
  - Limited ability to reliably detect urinary tract calcifications (6)[C]
  - Can be combined with retrograde pyelogram (RPG) for patients who cannot tolerate MDCTU or MRU (4)[C]

Diagnostic Procedures/Other
- Flexible cystoscopy
  - Best for evaluation of bladder pathology, especially small urothelial lesions; negative predictive value for bladder tumors is 99% (1)[C].
  - AUA recommends all patients with hematuria who are ≥35 years of age and all patients with risk factors for bladder cancer regardless of age to receive cystoscopy in addition to imaging (4)[C].
- Renal biopsy
  - Not routine but may be necessary to diagnose GN or in the face of increasing renal insufficiency
- RPG
  - Reserved for patients in which findings on MDCTU are equivocal or in addition to US or noncontrast studies in patients who are contraindicated for contrast or MRI (4,6)[C]
  - Sensitive for small lesions of supravesicular collecting system
  - Requires cystoscopy
- Ureteroscopy/pyeloscopy
  - For visualization of suspected supravesical collecting system lesions
  - Biopsy, excision, fulguration, or extraction of lesions/stones possible
  - Requires anesthesia
  - Requires cystoscopy
  - Risk of injury to collecting system

Follow-Up Tests & Special Considerations
- Other tests depend on suspected etiology: STD testing, antineutrophil cytoplasmic antibody (ANCA), C3, C4, antistreptolysin O (ASO) titer, hemoglobin electrophoresis (9)[C].
- Consider genetic testing in patients suspected of having familial hematuria (10)[C].
- Insufficient evidence to recommend routine use of urinary tumor markers
- Malignancies are detected in up to 5% of patients with microscopic hematuria and up to 40% of patients with gross hematuria (1)[C].

Pregnancy Considerations
Renal US is initial imaging choice for pregnant patients (6)[C]. MRU or RPG combined with either MRI or US are alternatives (4)[C].

Pediatric Considerations
- Consider GN, Wilms tumor, child abuse, and hypercalciuria.
- Isolated asymptomatic microscopic hematuria may not need full workup; these patients rarely need cystoscopy; observe for development of hypertension, gross hematuria, or proteinuria (9)[C].
- Gross or symptomatic hematuria needs a full workup.
  - If eumorphic RBCs, consider US (rule out stones, congenital abnormalities) and urinary Ca:Cr ratio. Urine Ca:Cr ratio >0.2 is suggestive of hypercalciuria in children >6 years of age (9)[C].
- If dysmorphic RBCs, consider renal consult.
- Renal US identifies most congenital and malignant conditions; CT is reserved for cases of suspected trauma (with contrast) or stones (without contrast) (7,9)[C].

TREATMENT

MEDICATION
None indicated for undiagnosed hematuria

ISSUES FOR REFERRAL
Prompt nephrology referral for proteinuria, red cell casts, elevated serum creatinine, and albumin: creatinine ratio ≥30 mg/mmol (4,5)[A].

SURGERY/OTHER PROCEDURES
Gross hematuria: Clots may require continuous bladder irrigation with a large-bore Foley catheter (2- or 3-way catheter may be helpful) to prevent clot retention.

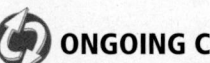

ONGOING CARE

FOLLOW-UP RECOMMENDATIONS
Patient Monitoring
Some experts still recommend periodic urinalysis; recent literature suggests that, after thorough initial negative investigations (imaging, cystoscopy), no follow-up is indicated for the asymptomatic patient with microscopic hematuria unless symptoms or frank hematuria develop. AUA recommends annual urinalyses in these patients, until two consecutive are negative and the consideration for a repeat workup at 3 to 5 years if hematuria is persistent (1,4)[C].

DIET
Increased fluids for stones or clots

PROGNOSIS
- Generally excellent for common causes of hematuria
- Poorer for malignant tumors and certain types of nephritis
- Persistent asymptomatic microscopic hematuria is associated with an increased risk of end-stage renal disease in patients aged 16 to 25 years.

REFERENCES

1. Sharp VJ, Barnes KT, Erickson BA. Assessment of asymptomatic microscopic hematuria in adults. *Am Fam Physician*. 2013;88(11):747–754.
2. Loo RK, Lieberman SF, Slezak JM, et al. Stratifying risk of urinary tract malignant tumors in patients with asymptomatic microscopic hematuria. *Mayo Clin Proc*. 2013;88(2):129–138.
3. Lotan Y, Svatek RS, Krabbe LM, et al. Prospective external validation of a bladder cancer detection model. *J Urol*. 2014;192(5):1343–1348.
4. Davis R, Jones JS, Barocas DA, et al. Diagnosis, evaluation and follow-up of asymptomatic microhematuria (AMH) in adults: AUA guideline. *J Urol*. 2012;188(6 Suppl):2473–2481.
5. Carville S, Wonderling D, Stevens P. Early identification and management of chronic kidney disease in adults: summary of updated NICE guidance. *BMJ*. 2014;349:g4507.
6. Shen L, Raman SS, Beland MD, et al. *Expert Panel on Urologic Imaging. ACR Appropriateness Criteria® Hematuria*. Reston, VA: American College of Radiology; 2014.
7. Dillman JR, Coley BD, Karmazyn B, et al. *Expert Panel on Pediatric Imaging. ACR Appropriateness Criteria® Hematuria—Child*. Reston, VA: American College of Radiology; 2012. http://www.guideline.gov/content.aspx?id=43874. Accessed 2015.
8. Smith-Bindman R, Aubin C, Bailitz J, et al. Ultrasonography versus computed tomography for suspected nephrolithiasis. *N Engl J Med* 2014;371(12):1100–1110.
9. Massengill SF. Hematuria. *Pediatr Rev*. 2008;29(10):342–348.
10. Taylor J, Flinter F. Familial haematuria: when to consider genetic testing. *Arch Dis Child*. 2014;99:857–861.

 SEE ALSO

Algorithm: Hematuria

 CODES

ICD10
- R31.9 Hematuria, unspecified
- R31.1 Benign essential microscopic hematuria
- R31.0 Gross hematuria

CLINICAL PEARLS

- Screening asymptomatic patients for microscopic hematuria is an "I" recommendation from the USPSTF (1)[B].
- Asymptomatic hematuria and hematuria persisting after treatment of UTIs must be evaluated.
- Patients with bladder cancer can have intermittent microscopic hematuria; a thorough evaluation in high-risk patients is needed after just one episode.
- Routine use of anticoagulants should not cause hematuria unless there is an underlying urologic abnormality (1)[C].
- Signs of underlying renal disease indicate the need for a nephrologic workup, but a urologic evaluation is still needed in the presence of persistent hematuria (4)[C].

H

HEMOCHROMATOSIS

Robert A. Marlow, MD, MA

 BASICS

DESCRIPTION

Hemochromatosis is a hereditary disorder in which the small intestine absorbs excessive iron (1,2).

- Early clinical features include arthralgia, fatigue, and decreased libido.
- Late effects include cirrhosis of the liver, diabetes, hypermelanotic pigmentation of the skin, and heart failure.
- Because there is no mechanism to excrete excess iron, the excess is stored in muscle and in organs, including the liver, pancreas, and heart, eventually resulting in severe damage to the affected organs.
- Liver damage ultimately may result in hepatocellular carcinoma.
- System(s) affected: endocrine/metabolic
- Synonym(s): bronze diabetes; Troisier-Hanot-Chauffard syndrome

EPIDEMIOLOGY

Incidence

- Predominant age: Metabolic abnormality is congenital, but symptoms usually present in the 5th and 6th decades.
- Predominant sex: gene frequency: male = female, although clinical signs are more frequent in men (3)

Prevalence

- 3/1,000 people (heterozygote frequency, 1/10) (4)
- The most common genetic abnormality in the United States

Pediatric Considerations

Rarely, iron overload may occur as early as 2 years of age. The disorder can be diagnosed before iron overload is clinically apparent.

ETIOLOGY AND PATHOPHYSIOLOGY

- Type 1 hemochromatosis is caused by mutations in the *HFE* gene, type 2 by mutations in either the *HFE2* gene or *HAMP* gene, type 3 by mutations in the *TFR2* gene, and type 4 by mutations in the *SLC40A1* gene. The cause of neonatal hemochromatosis is unknown.
- The mechanism for increased iron absorption in the face of excessive iron stores is not clear. Iron metabolism appears normal in this disease except for a higher level of circulating iron.
- Iron overload may be caused by thalassemia, sideroblastic anemia, liver disease, excess iron intake, or chronic transfusion.

Genetics

- Genetically heterogeneous disorder of iron overload; types 1, 2, and 3 are autosomal recessive; type 4 is autosomal dominant. Neonatal hemochromatosis is rare.
- Penetrance is incomplete; expressivity is variable.
- Factors contributing to variable expressivity include different mutations in the same gene, mitigating or exacerbating genes, and environmental factors.

RISK FACTORS

- The disease is a genetic disorder.
- Affected individuals should not ingest iron supplements, eat raw shellfish, or eat large quantities of iron-rich food, such as red meat.
- Alcohol increases the absorption of iron. (As many as 41% of patients with symptomatic disease are alcoholic.)
- Loss of blood, such as that which occurs during menstruation and pregnancy, delays the onset of symptoms.

GENERAL PREVENTION

- Family members of affected individuals should be screened.
- Pregnant women with the disorder should avoid iron supplements.

ALERT

Screening of population is *not* recommended because the vast majority of those with homozygous hemochromatosis will remain asymptomatic and have a normal life span (5,6)[A].

COMMONLY ASSOCIATED CONDITIONS

See "Complications."

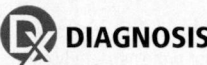 DIAGNOSIS

HISTORY

- Weakness (83%)
- Abdominal pain (58%)
- Arthralgia (43%)
- Loss of libido or potency (38%)
- Amenorrhea (22%)
- Dyspnea on exertion (15%)
- Neurologic symptoms (6%)
- Symptoms of diabetes

PHYSICAL EXAM

- Hepatomegaly (83%)
- Increased skin pigmentation (75%)
- Loss of body hair (20%)
- Splenomegaly (13%)
- Peripheral edema (12%)
- Jaundice (10%)
- Gynecomastia (8%)
- Ascites (6%)
- Testicular atrophy
- Hepatic tenderness

DIFFERENTIAL DIAGNOSIS

- Repeated transfusions
- Hereditary anemias with ineffective erythropoiesis
- Alcoholic cirrhosis
- Porphyria cutanea tarda
- Atransferrinemia
- Excessive ingestion of iron (rare)

DIAGNOSTIC TESTS & INTERPRETATION

- Transferrin saturation (serum iron concentration ÷ total iron-binding capacity × 100): >70% is virtually diagnostic of iron overload; ≥45% warrants further evaluation. Iron supplements and transfusions may elevate serum iron.
- Serum ferritin: >300 μg/L for men and postmenopausal women and 200 μg/L for premenopausal women (7); may be elevated by inflammatory reactions, other forms of liver disease, certain tumors (e.g., acute granulocytic leukemia), and rheumatoid arthritis
- After the diagnosis is established
  - Obtain an oral glucose tolerance test or hemoglobin A1C to rule out diabetes and an echocardiogram to rule out cardiomyopathy.
  - Consider abdominal US to assess for cirrhosis.
  - Decreased FSH
  - Decreased LH
  - Decreased testosterone
  - Increased serum glutamic-oxaloacetic transaminase
  - Hypoalbuminemia
- If the diagnosis is uncertain after laboratory testing, MRI may be helpful to assess hepatic iron (1).

Diagnostic Procedures/Other

- Liver biopsy for stainable iron is the standard for diagnosis. Presence or absence of cirrhosis also can be ascertained. However, with the availability of genetic testing, liver biopsy is not frequently necessary to confirm the diagnosis (7)[C].
- DNA PCR testing for *HFE* gene mutations C282Y and H63D: present in 85–90% of patients
- Homozygosity for the C282Y mutation or compound heterozygosity for C282Y and H63D with biochemical evidence for iron overload can confirm the diagnosis (8).

Test Interpretation

- Increased hepatic parenchymal iron stores
- Hepatic fibrosis and cirrhosis with hepatomegaly
- Pancreatic enlargement
- Excess hemosiderin in liver, pancreas, myocardium, thyroid, parathyroid, joints, skin
- Cardiomegaly
- Joint deposition of iron

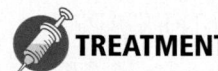 TREATMENT

MEDICATION

- None. Only when phlebotomy is not feasible or in the presence of severe heart disease should the iron-chelating agent deferoxamine (Desferal) be considered.
- Hepatitis A and hepatitis B immunizations should be done if there is no evidence of previous exposure (9).

GENERAL MEASURES

- Remove excess iron by repeated phlebotomy once or twice weekly to establish and maintain a mild anemia (hematocrit of 35–39%) (7)[C].
- When the patient finally becomes iron-deficient, a lifelong maintenance program of 2 to 6 phlebotomies a year to keep storage iron normal; maintain serum ferritin 50 to 100 μg/L.

INPATIENT CONSIDERATIONS

Admission Criteria/Initial Stabilization

Outpatient treatment

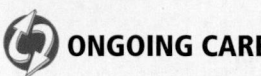 ONGOING CARE

FOLLOW-UP RECOMMENDATIONS

Full activity unless there is significant heart disease

Patient Monitoring

- Measure hematocrit before each phlebotomy; skip phlebotomy if hematocrit is <36%.
- Schedule an additional phlebotomy when hematocrit is >40%.
- When anemia becomes refractory, repeat transferrin saturation and serum ferritin to confirm depletion of iron stores.
- When iron stores are depleted, 2 to 6 phlebotomies a year should keep iron stores normal; maintain serum ferritin 50 to 100 μg/L.
- During maintenance therapy, measure transferrin saturation and serum ferritin yearly.

DIET

- An iron-poor diet is not of significant benefit.
- Avoid alcohol, iron-fortified foods, iron-containing supplements, and uncooked shellfish (increased susceptibility to *Vibrio* sp.).
- Restrict vitamin C to small doses between meals.
- Tea chelates iron and may be drank with meals.

PATIENT EDUCATION

- Iron Disorders Institute, PO Box 675, Taylors, SC 29687
- American Hemochromatosis Society, Inc., PO Box 950871, Lake Mary, FL 32795-0871

PROGNOSIS

- Patients diagnosed before cirrhosis develops and treated with phlebotomy have a normal life expectancy.
- Life expectancy is reduced in patients with cirrhosis and DM and in those who require >18 months of phlebotomy therapy to return iron stores to normal.
- Patients with ferritin levels <1,000 μg/L are unlikely to have cirrhosis (3,10).

COMPLICATIONS

- Cirrhosis
- Hepatoma (only in patients with cirrhosis)
- DM
- Cardiomyopathy
- Arthritis
- Hypogonadism

REFERENCES

1. van Bokhoven MA, van Deursen CT, Swinkels DW. Diagnosis and management of hereditary haemochromatosis. *BMJ*. 2011;342:c7251.
2. Sood R, Bakashi R, Hegade VS, et al. Diagnosis and management of hereditary haemochromatosis. *Br J Gen Pract*. 2013;63(611):331–332.
3. Allen KJ, Gurrin LC, Constantine CC, et al. Iron-overload-related disease in HFE hereditary hemochromatosis. *N Engl J Med*. 2008;358(3): 221–230.
4. Brandhagen DJ, Fairbanks VF, Baldus W. Recognition and management of hereditary hemochromatosis. *Am Fam Physician*. 2002;65(5): 853–860.
5. Bacon BR, Adams PC, Kowdley KV, et al. Diagnosis and management of hemochromatosis: 2011 practice guideline by the American Association for the Study of Liver Diseases. *Hepatology*. 2011;54(1):328–343.
6. Crownover BK, Covey CJ. Hereditary hemochromatosis. *Am Fam Physician*. 2013;87(3):183–190.
7. Qaseem A, Aronson M, Fitterman N, et al. Screening for hereditary hemochromatosis: a clinical practice guideline from the American College of Physicians. *Ann Intern Med*. 2005;143(7):517–521.
8. Cherfane CE, Hollenbeck RD, Go J, et al. Hereditary hemochromatosis: missed diagnosis or misdiagnosis? *Am J Med*. 2013;126(11):1010–1015.
9. Alexander J, Kowdley KV. Hereditary hemochromatosis: genetics, pathogenesis, and clinical management. *Ann Hepatol*. 2005;4(4):240–247.
10. Janssen MC, Swinkels DW. Hereditary haemochromatosis. *Best Pract Res Clin Gastroenterol*. 2009;23(2):171–183.

ADDITIONAL READING

- Bardou-Jacquet E, Brissot P. Diagnostic evaluation of hereditary hemochromatosis (HFE and non-HFE). *Hematol Oncol Clin North Am*. 2014;28(4):625–635.
- Ekanayake D, Roddick C, Powell LW. Recent advances in hemochromatosis: a 2015 update: a summary of proceedings of the 2014 conference held under the auspices of Hemochromatosis Australia. *Hepatol Int*. 2015;9(2):174–182.
- Salgia RJ, Brown K. Diagnosis and management of hereditary hemochromatosis. *Clin Liver Dis*. 2015;19(1):187–198.
- U.S. Preventive Services Task Force. Screening for hemochromatosis: recommendation statement. *Ann Intern Med*. 2006;145(3):204–208.

CODES

ICD10

- E83.110 Hereditary hemochromatosis
- E83.118 Other hemochromatosis
- E83.111 Hemochromatosis due to repeated red blood cell transfusions

CLINICAL PEARLS

- The best laboratory tests available to screen a patient initially for hemochromatosis are serum ferritin and transferrin saturation. An elevated transferrin saturation is the earliest abnormality in hemochromatosis. Ferritin is a sensitive measure of iron overload but can be elevated in a variety of infectious and inflammatory conditions without iron overload being present.
- Liver biopsy need not be done to confirm the diagnosis or to check for cirrhosis if the patient is homozygous for C282Y or is heterozygous for C282Y/H63D. If the patient's serum ferritin is <1,000 μg/L, LFTs are normal, and hepatomegaly is not present, cirrhosis is very unlikely, so liver biopsy is not needed.
- Initially, a patient with hemochromatosis should have a phlebotomy weekly until the serum ferritin is 50 to 100 μg/L, and the transferrin saturation falls to <30%. Then, lifelong maintenance therapy of 2 to 6 phlebotomies a year is mandatory to keep the ferritin 50 to 100 μg/L and the transferrin saturation <50%.
- Most patients with hemochromatosis go undiagnosed. Because treatment with phlebotomy will prevent all complications when begun early, physicians should consider the diagnosis of hemochromatosis much more frequently. However, the U.S. Preventive Services Task Force recommends against routine screening of asymptomatic average-risk populations.

H

HEMOPHILIA

Katie L. Westerfield, DO • Bryan Malave, MD

 BASICS

DESCRIPTION

- Deficiency of factor VIII (hemophilia A) or factor IX (hemophilia B) coagulation proteins leading to bleeding tendencies in affected individuals. The majority of cases are due to inherited genetic mutations in factor VIII or factor IX coagulation proteins. However, an estimated 30% of all hemophilia cases result from spontaneous mutations.
- Hemophilia A and B are clinically indistinguishable, but can be differentiated by assays that detect levels of factors VIII and IX, respectively.
- Disease severity correlates with the relative levels of coagulation factors present in serum analysis:
  - Severe: frequent spontaneous bleeding (factor activity <1%)
  - Moderate: bleeding with mild to moderate trauma (factor activity 1–5%)
  - Mild: bleeding with major trauma, tooth extraction, or surgery (factor activity 5–40%)
- Frequency of bleeding is similar when levels of severity are comparable in hemophilia A and B.
- Synonym(s): Christmas disease (hemophilia B)

EPIDEMIOLOGY

- Worldwide, an estimated 400,000 people are affected with hemophilia. Estimated frequency of 1 in 10,000 births (1).
- Hemophilia A represents 80–85% of the total hemophilia population; hemophilia B comprises the remaining 15–20%.

ETIOLOGY AND PATHOPHYSIOLOGY

- Damage to vascular endothelium leads to exposure of subendothelial tissue factors, which interact with platelets, plasma proteins, and coagulation factors to produce a localized platelet plug contributing to hemostasis. Complexes involving factors VIII and IX participate in the intrinsic coagulation pathway to activate factor X, FXa. Downstream interactions involving FXa culminate in the conversion of prothrombin to thrombin, mediating platelet activation and fibrin deposition necessary for stabilization of the platelet plug.
- Deficiencies of factor VIII or factor IX result in decreased production of FXa, leading to an unstable platelet plug and impaired hemostasis.

Genetics

- Exhibits an X-chromosome linked inheritance pattern. Males are almost exclusively affected; females are asymptomatic carriers, unless their factor activity is <40% of normal.
- Carriers with symptomatically low clotting factor levels are treated similarly to patients with the trait:
  - May bleed at the time of surgery
- Males within the same family share similar deficiencies and level of severity owing to the same genetic defect.

GENERAL PREVENTION

- Patients should carry medical ID tags listing their bleeding disorder or factor deficiency, inhibitor status, type of treatment products used, and initial treatment doses for mild, moderate, or severe bleeding.
- Immediate family members of affected patients should have factor VIII and IX levels checked prior to invasive procedures, childbirth, and if bleeding tendencies occur.
- Genetic testing should be offered to at-risk female family members to facilitate genetic counseling.

 DIAGNOSIS

- History and initial presentation
  - 2/3 of presenting hemophilic patients have a positive family history. All male infants born to known carriers should have factor level testing.
  - Prolonged bleeding with circumcision, dental work, surgery, or injury
  - Excessive or easy bruising in early childhood
  - Spontaneous bleeding, especially in joints, muscle, or soft tissue
  - Typical presentation times: mild (36 months), moderate (8 months), severe (1 month)
  - *Pregnancy Considerations*: Treat all males born to a carrier as if they have hemophilia. Test at birth. Avoid vacuum/forceps deliveries (2)[B].
  - Cord blood can be used for testing (3)[A].
- Life-threatening bleeds
  - Intracranial hemorrhage: generally resulting from trauma; incidence of 1:10; fatal in 30% of cases
  - Hematomas of bowel wall can cause obstruction or intussusception as well as pain mimicking appendicitis.
  - Neck or throat bleeds: can lead to airway obstruction
- Serious bleeds
  - Hemarthrosis, most commonly of ankles, elbows, and knees
    - Infants may present with irritability or decreased use of limb.
    - Adults may have prodromal stiffness, acute pain, and swelling of joint.
    - Arthropathy results from repeated bleeding into joints, damaging cartilage, and subchondral bone:
      - Can result in fixed joints, muscle wasting, and significantly impaired mobility
  - Muscular hematomas most commonly occur in quadriceps, iliopsoas, and forearm:
    - May result in compartment syndrome and ischemic nerve damage, such as femoral nerve neuropathy due to undetected retroperitoneal hemorrhage
  - Mucous membrane bleeding, such as in the genitourinary tract, leading to hematuria
  - Pseudotumor syndrome: untreated hemorrhage causing a hematoma, which calcifies (named because it can be mistaken for cancer)

DIFFERENTIAL DIAGNOSIS

- Von Willebrand disease
- Vitamin K deficiency, anticoagulant (warfarin, rivaroxaban, argatroban, heparin, enoxaparin) therapy (factor IX is vitamin K–dependent)
- Other factor deficiencies: afibrinogenemia, dysfibrinogenemia, fibrinolytic defects, platelet disorders
- Child abuse

DIAGNOSTIC TESTS & INTERPRETATION

Initial Tests (lab, imaging)

- CBC with platelet count, PT, aPTT, platelet function (preferred) or bleed time, vWF, factor VIII:C assay, factor IX assay. Prolonged aPTT: corrected when mixed with pooled normal plasma in absence of inhibitors
- PT, platelet count, and platelet function are normal.
- Diagnosis based on factor VIII:C or IX activity
  - Normal factor levels: 50 to 150 IU/dL
  - Mild: 5 to 40 IU/dL
  - Moderate: 1 to 5 IU/dL
  - Severe: <1 IU/Dl

Follow-Up Tests & Special Considerations

Inhibitors to factor VIII and IX (see "Complications"):

- Should be periodically measured using the Nijmegen or Bethesda assay, which quantifies the alloantibody titer
- Screen before invasive procedures and at regular intervals.

Diagnostic Procedures/Other

Prenatal diagnosis: genetic testing of a sample of chorionic villus or fluid obtained at amniocentesis. Not recommended (2)[B]

Test Interpretation

In affected joints: synovial hemosiderosis, articular cartilage degeneration, thickening of periarticular tissues, bony hypertrophy

TREATMENT

GENERAL MEASURES

- Avoid aspirin or other NSAIDs.
- Treat early; symptoms may occur before bleeding is clinically apparent. Acute bleeds should be treated as quickly as possible, preferable within 2 hours (1)[A].
- For surgical prophylaxis
  - If major surgery is undertaken, factor levels should be maintained at >50% for at least 2 to 3 weeks after the procedure:
    - Fibrin glue products may be beneficial for oozing.
  - Dental extractions: Antifibrinolytics (Amicar, tranexamic acid) may be used.
  - Minor procedures: may use desmopressin (DDAVP)
- Hepatitis A and B vaccinations are recommended.
- Encourage physical activity for normal neuromuscular development: Patients should avoid high-impact contact sports; restrict activities in proportion to degree of factor deficiency. Organized sports should be encouraged as opposed to unstructured activities (1)[B].

MEDICATION

First Line

- Principles of therapy

  - Primary prophylaxis: administration of specific factor replacement therapy in the absence of bleeding to maintain adequate baseline plasma levels sufficient for hemostasis in all categories of severity (1)[A]

    - Lower frequency of acute bleeds and episodes of life-threatening hemorrhage compared to on-demand therapy
    - Standard of care for children with severe hemophilia A to prevent joint bleeds and joint degeneration
    - Dosing, frequency, duration of therapeutic regimens tailored to individual patient needs in clinical practice
  - On-demand therapy: treatment administered in response to occurrence of bleeding
    - Amount and duration of factor replacement depends on location and severity of bleeding:
      - Mild bleeds correct to a factor level of >30% major hemorrhages and large muscle bleeds require correction to levels between 50% and 100%.
      - Life-threatening bleeds require levels between 80% and 100%, sustained with bolus dosing or continuous infusion.

- Specific agents:
  - Hemophilia A: Replacement with factor VIII concentrates is the treatment of choice:
    ○ Two sources for the factor available:
      ▪ Purified plasma-derived factor VIII: Donor pool is screened and the plasma-derived factor is treated to inactivate viruses (HIV, hepatitis B, and hepatitis C). Theoretical risks still exist.
      ▪ Recombinant factor VIII
        □ Dosing: 1 IU of factor VIII (the amount in 1 mL of plasma)/kg body weight administered will raise the plasma level of the recipient by 2%.
        □ Most FVIII products have short half-lives, requiring frequent injections novel recombinant factor VIII, rFVIIIFc, dosed prophylactically 1 to 2 times per week (4)[B].
  - Hemophilia B: Replacement with factor IX concentrates is the treatment of choice:
    ○ Plasma-derived factor IX and recombinant factor IX (preferred) are commercially available.
      ▪ Dosing: 1 IU/kg body weight administered will raise plasma factor IX levels 1%.
- Hemophilia patients with inhibitors (neutralizing alloantibodies to factors VIII or IX)
  - Inhibitor formation should be suspected when replacement with the deficient factor fails to correct coagulopathy.
  - Low-titer (<5 BU/mL) patients: Replace with high doses of the deficient factor to overcome the circulating inhibitor concentration.
  - High-titer patients: Treat using products that *bypass* the factor neutralized by the alloantibody, or emergently with high doses of the specific deficient factor:
    ○ Two bypassing agents are available; both are efficacious at providing 80% of bleeding episodes:
      ▪ Anti-inhibitor coagulation complex (AICC)
      ▪ Recombinant activated factor VII (rFVIIa)
- Immune tolerance induction (ITI): protocols to promote immune tolerance through repeated exposure to high-dose factor VIII therapy over 12 to 18 months, with or without immunosuppressive therapy (corticosteroids, cyclophosphamide, rituximab). Success rates are 60–80%.
  - Home therapy allows immediate access to clotting factor, resulting in decreased pain, dysfunction, and long term disability (2)[B].

Second Line
- Cryoprecipitate and fresh frozen plasma (FFP) can be used in instances where the specific factor concentrate is unavailable for *emergent hemostasis*.
  - FFP: contains all coagulation factors but generally difficult to attain high levels of factors VIII or IX
    ○ Starting dose: 15 to 20 mL/kg
  - Cryoprecipitate: derived from precipitates of cooled FFP; contains significant levels of factor VIII (up to 100 IU/bag) but *not* factor IX:
    ○ Dosing: 1 mL cryoprecipitate has ~3 to 5 IU factor VIII.
- Desmopressin (DDAVP): synthetic vasopressin; stimulates endogenous release of factor VIII (and *vWF*) from endothelial stores; used in mild to moderate hemophilia
  - IV or SC: 0.3 μg/kg infused 30 minutes prior to procedure; may repeat if needed

- Intranasal (150 μg/spray): adult dose, 1 spray to each nostril (300 μg total). Alternate dose if <50 kg: 150 μg once.
  - Adverse effect: hyponatremic seizures, especially in children; restrict fluids and watch sodium levels and urine output.
- Antifibrinolytic agents: inhibit plasminogen activation, thereby stabilizing the clot
  - Effective in controlling mucosal bleeding, such as bleeding in oral cavity, epistaxis, and menorrhagia; can also be used prophylactically (e.g., prior to tooth extractions)
    ○ Tranexamic acid (25 mg/kg PO q6–8h or 10 mg/kg IV q6–8h)
    ○ Aminocaproic acid (Amicar) is less frequently used.

ONGOING CARE

FOLLOW-UP RECOMMENDATIONS
Patient Monitoring
Regular evaluations every 6 to 12 months, including a musculoskeletal evaluation, an inhibitor screen, liver tests, and tests for antibodies to hepatitis viruses and HIV

PATIENT EDUCATION
- National Hemophilia Foundation: http://www.hemophilia.org/
- World Federation of Hemophilia: http://www.wfh.org/

PROGNOSIS
- Survival is normal for those with mild disease; mortality is increased 2- to 6-fold in those with moderate to severe disease.
- Intracranial hemorrhage is a leading cause of death in hemophilia.
- Hemophilic arthropathy is the main cause of morbidity in patients with severe hemophilia.

COMPLICATIONS
- Hemophilic arthropathy: Symptoms include pain, limitation of motion, and contractures.
- Theoretical transmission of bloodborne infections, such as hepatitis A, B, C, and D and HIV; this risk has been greatly reduced with current testing of blood products.
- Development of inhibitor autoantibodies
  - More common in hemophilia A (20–30% of patients compared to 5% in hemophilia B) and in patients with severe disease requiring multiple transfusions
  - Risk factors for inhibitor development:
    ○ Specific genetic defect (family history); null mutations have higher inhibitor incidence.
    ○ Very low or no circulating factor, therefore requiring multiple transfusions
    ○ Age of first exogenous factor exposure; previous studies report a higher incidence of developing antibodies in those exposed to exogenous factor at <6 months of age, but new studies show this may be due to severity of disease.
    ○ Concurrent inflammation/infection when administering factor (e.g., surgical prophylaxis)
    ○ Duration of factor exposure
  - No increased risk of bleeding, but when bleeding occurs, it is more difficult to achieve hemostasis due to decreased response to factor replacement.

REFERENCES
1. Srivastava A, Brewer AK, Mauser-Bunschoten EP, et al. Guidelines for the management of hemophilia. *Haemophilia*. 2013;19(1):e1–e47.
2. Tsui NB, Kadir RA, Chan KC, et al. Noninvasive prenatal diagnosis of hemophilia by microfluidics digital PCR analysis of maternal plasma DNA. *Blood*. 2011;117(13):3684–3691.
3. National Hemophilia Foundation. MASAC guidelines for perinatal management of women with bleeding disorders and carriers of hemophilia A nd B. https://www.hemophilia.org/Researchers-Healthcare-Providers/Medical-and-Scientific-Advisory-Council-MASAC/MASAC-Recommendations/MASAC-Guidelines-for-Perinatal-Management-of-Women-with-Bleeding-Disorders-and-Carriers-of-Hemophilia-A-and-B. Accessed June 4, 2015.
4. Mahlangu J, Powell JS, Ragni MV, et al. Phase 3 study of recombinant factor VIII Fc fusion protein in severe hemophilia A. *Blood*. 2014;123(3):317–325.

ADDITIONAL READING
- Benson G, Auerswald G, Elezović I, et al. Immune tolerance induction in patients with severe hemophilia with inhibitors: expert panel views and recommendations for clinical practice. *Eur J Haematol*. 2012;88(5):371–379.
- Berntorp E, Shapiro AD. Modern haemophilia care. *Lancet*. 2012;379(9824):1447–1456.
- Fischer K. Prophylaxis for adults with haemophilia: one size does not fit all. *Blood Transfus*. 2012;10(2):169–173.
- Franchini M, Mannucci PM. Past, present and future of hemophilia: a narrative review. *Orphanet J Rare Dis*. 2012;7:24.
- Gater A, Thomson TA, Strandberg-Larsen M. Haemophilia B: impact on patients and economic burden of disease. *Thromb Haemost*. 2011;106(3):398–404.
- Kulkarni R, Soucie JM, Lusher J, et al. Sites of initial bleeding episodes, mode of delivery and age of diagnosis in babies with haemophilia diagnosed before the age of 2 years: a report from the Centers for Disease Control and Prevention's (CDC) Universal Data Collection (UDC) project. *Haemophilia*. 2009;15(6):1281–1290.
- Leissinger C, Gringeri A, Antmen B, et al. Anti-inhibitor coagulant complex prophylaxis in hemophilia with inhibitors. *N Engl J Med*. 2011;365(18):1684–1692.
- Ragni MV, Fogarty PJ, Josephson NC, et al. Survey of current prophylaxis practices and bleeding characteristics of children with severe haemophilia A in US haemophilia treatment centres. *Haemophilia*. 2012;18(1):63–68.

 CODES

ICD10
- D66 Hereditary factor VIII deficiency
- D67 Hereditary factor IX deficiency
- Z14.01 Asymptomatic hemophilia A carrier

H

HEMORRHOIDS

Juan Qiu, MD, PhD

 BASICS

DESCRIPTION
- Varicosities of the hemorrhoidal venous plexus
- External hemorrhoids
  - Located below the dentate line (painful)
  - Covered by squamous epithelium
- Internal hemorrhoids
  - Located above the dentate line (painless)
- Both types of hemorrhoids often coexist.
- Classification of internal hemorrhoids (1–3)
  - 1st-degree: Hemorrhoids do not prolapse.
  - 2nd-degree: prolapse through the anus on straining but reduce spontaneously
  - 3rd-degree: protrude and require digital reduction
  - 4th-degree: cannot be reduced
- Hemorrhoids often progress from itching, bleeding stage to protrusion with easy reduction; then difficult reduction; and finally, rectal prolapse. Thrombosis may occur at any protrusion stage. External hemorrhoids cause pain; internal hemorrhoids generally do not (2,3).

Geriatric Considerations
Hemorrhoids are more common in elderly, as is rectal prolapse.

Pediatric Considerations
- Uncommon in infants and children; when discovered, look for underlying cause (e.g., vena caval or mesenteric obstruction, cirrhosis, portal hypertension [HTN]).
- Occasionally, as in adults, hemorrhoids may result from chronic constipation, fecal impaction, and straining at stool. Surgery is rarely required in children.

Pregnancy Considerations
- Common in pregnancy
- Usually resolves after pregnancy
- No treatment required, unless extremely painful.

EPIDEMIOLOGY
- Predominant age: adults; peak from 45 to 65 years
- Predominant sex: male = female

Incidence
Common

Prevalence
~4–5% in general population in the United States

ETIOLOGY AND PATHOPHYSIOLOGY
- There are three primary hemorrhoidal cushions typically located in left lateral, right anterior, and right posterior positions. Hemorrhoidal cushions augment anal closure pressure and protect the anal sphincter during stool passage. During Valsalva, intra-abdominal pressure increases raising pressure within the hemorrhoidal cushions helping to preserve anal closure. Mechanisms implicated in symptomatic hemorrhoidal disease include the following:
  - Dilated veins of hemorrhoidal plexus
  - Tight internal anal sphincter
  - Abnormal distention of the arteriovenous anastomosis
  - Prolapse of the cushions and the surrounding connective tissues

Genetics
No known genetic pattern

RISK FACTORS
- Pregnancy
- Pelvic space-occupying lesions
- Liver disease; portal HTN
- Constipation
- Occupations that require prolonged sitting
- Loss of perianal muscle tone due to old age, rectal surgery, birth trauma/episiotomy, anal intercourse
- Obesity
- Chronic diarrhea

GENERAL PREVENTION
- Avoid constipation by consuming high-fiber diet (>30 g/day) and ensuring proper hydration.
- Maintain appropriate weight.
- Avoid prolonged sitting or straining on the toilet.

COMMONLY ASSOCIATED CONDITIONS
- Liver disease; portal HTN
- Pregnancy
- Constipation

 DIAGNOSIS

Diagnosis is typically straightforward through history and inspection of the perineum, rectal exam, and anoscopy.

HISTORY
- Internal/external hemorrhoids
  - Classically, bright red blood per rectum
    - May range from scant blood on toilet paper to copious blood in the toilet bowl
  - Constipation or diarrhea
  - Straining with defecation
- Small or minimal external hemorrhoids
  - Episodic bleeding on stool or toilet paper, pruritus and pain
- More extensive internal hemorrhoids
  - Feeling of incomplete evacuation
  - Thrombosed hemorrhoids present as an acute painful mass (2,3).

PHYSICAL EXAM
- Anorectal exam including anoscopy (2,3)
- Inspection following straining at stool
- For protruding hemorrhoids: mass, more prominent bleeding. If not reducible, increased risk of strangulation and/or thrombosis with acute pain
- Abdominal exam to exclude mass
- Peripheral stigmata of cirrhosis and portal hypertension (caput, telangiectasias, palmar erythema)

DIFFERENTIAL DIAGNOSIS
- Rectal or anal neoplasia
- Condyloma
- Skin tag
- Inflammatory bowel disease
- Anal fistula, fissure, or abscess

DIAGNOSTIC TESTS & INTERPRETATION
Diagnostic Procedures/Other
Sigmoidoscopy or colonoscopy depending on risk factors for malignancy in patients with rectal bleeding (3)[A]

 TREATMENT

Prevention
- Fiber supplements
- Stool softeners

GENERAL MEASURES
- Hemorrhoids are a recurrent disease, even after surgical excision. Preventive measures should be continued indefinitely.
- For mild symptoms or prevention (3)[A]
  - Avoid prolonged sitting during bowel movements.
  - Avoid straining.
  - Avoid constipation by eating a high-fiber diet or by taking fiber supplements; if necessary, take regular stool softeners.
  - Regular exercise
- For pain, Sitz baths warm water or hypertonic Epsom salts (1 cup per 2 quarts of water)
- Pruritus or mild discomfort after stooling responds well to topical hydrocortisone ointment, anesthetic ointments or sprays, and warm Sitz baths.
- Constipation relief, anal hygiene, local ointments, and Sitz baths are effective through the stage of easy reduction (stage 2). More severe stages often require ligation or surgery (3)[A].

MEDICATION
First Line
- Dietary modification with adequate fluid (generally ≥2 L water/day) and fiber (≥30 g/day) is the primary first-line, nonoperative therapy for symptomatic hemorrhoids (3)[A].
- Pain
  - Hydrocortisone ointment (0.5–1%)
  - Analgesic sprays or ointments: benzocaine and dibucaine (Nupercainal). Use sprays with caution, as they may contain alcohol that can cause burning sensation when applied.
- Pruritus: hydrocortisone (Anusol-HC, Cortifoam) ointment
- Bleeding
  - Astringent suppositories (Preparation H)
  - Hydrocortisone (Anusol-HC, Cortifoam) ointment

Second Line
Treatment for special cases
- Thrombosed external hemorrhoids: common complication of hemorrhoidal disease. With conservative treatment, the thrombus will be absorbed over the course of weeks, and pain improves within 2 to 3 days (1–3)[A].
- With severe acute pain, prompt excision should be performed under local anesthetics and the wound left open without packing. Use Sitz baths, topical anesthetics, and mild pain relievers for the first 7 to 10 days after excision (1–3)[A].
- Strangulated hemorrhoid: from irreducible 3rd- or 4th-degree hemorrhoid. If untreated, it can progress to ulceration and thrombosis. Treatment requires urgent or emergent hemorrhoidectomy.
- Acute hemorrhoidal bleeding associated with portal HTN can be life-threatening. Treatment should be suture of the bleeding site with incorporation of the mucosa, submucosa, and internal sphincter. Coagulopathy should be corrected.

SURGERY/OTHER PROCEDURES

- Indications: failure of medical and nonoperative therapy, symptomatic stage 3 or stage 4 symptoms in presence of a concomitant anorectal condition requiring surgery, or patient preference (1–3)[A]
- Incision of thrombosed hemorrhoid: for severe pain
- Severe protruding hemorrhoids
  - Rubber band ligation (internal hemorrhoids only) (1–3)[A]
  - Sclerotherapy: for symptomatic prolapsed stage I or II hemorrhoids; care must be taken not to inject near periprostatic parasympathetic nerves. Not for advanced disease or if evidence of infection, inflammation, and ulceration is present
    - Cryotherapy is no longer recommended due to high rate of complications.
  - Prolapsed rectum
    - Requires surgical correction
  - Surgical resection
    - Gold standard: Conventional hemorrhoidectomy should be considered for grade III hemorrhoids not responding to banding, mixed internal and external, grade IV hemorrhoids, or when complicated by fissures, fistula, or extensive skin tags (1–3)[A].
- Newer techniques reduce surgical time, early postoperative pain, urinary retention, and time to return to normal activity.
  - Transanal hemorrhoidal dearterialization (THD): fewer complications and can be used in cases of recurrent diseases (2,3)[A],(4)[B]
  - Stapled hemorrhoidopexy: less painful than traditional surgery but higher incidence of skin tags and recurrent prolapse (2)[A],(4)[B]
  - LigaSure hemorrhoidectomy: reduces operating time, is superior in patient tolerance, and is equally effective as conventional hemorrhoidectomy in long-term symptom control (5,6)[B],(7,8)[A]

COMPLEMENTARY & ALTERNATIVE MEDICINE

Aloe vera cream on the surgical site after hemorrhoidectomy reduces postoperative pain and decreases healing time and analgesic requirements.

 ONGOING CARE

FOLLOW-UP RECOMMENDATIONS

- Encourage physical fitness, weight management, and dietary compliance.
- Avoid prolonged sitting and straining on the toilet.

Patient Monitoring

As needed, depending on treatment

DIET

High-fiber with a target of 30 g of insoluble fiber/day through sources such as wheat bran cereals, oatmeal, peanuts, artichokes, beans, corn, peas, spinach, potatoes, apples, apricots, blackberries, raspberries, prunes, pears, bananas; adequate fluids (6 to 8 glasses of water/day); avoid excessive caffeine.

PATIENT EDUCATION

High-fiber diet: Today's Dietitian Top Fiber-Rich Foods List. http://www.todaysdietitian.com/newarchives/063008p28.shtml

PROGNOSIS

- Spontaneous resolution
- Recurrence

COMPLICATIONS

- Thrombosis
- Ulceration
- Anemia (rare)
- Incontinence
- Pelvic sepsis following hemorrhoidectomy

REFERENCES

1. Klein JW. Common anal problems. *Med Clin North Am.* 2014;98(3):609–623.
2. Hall JF. Modern management of hemorrhoidal disease. *Gastroenterol Clin North Am.* 2013;42(4):759–772.
3. Ganz RA. The evaluation and treatment of hemorrhoids: a guide for the gastroenterologist. *Clin Gastroenterol Hepatol.* 2013;11(6):593–603.
4. Ratto C. THD Doppler procedure for hemorrhoids: the surgical technique. *Tech Coloproctol.* 2014;18(3):291–298.
5. Michalik M, Pawlak M, Bobowicz M, et al. Long-term outcomes of stapled hemorrhoidopexy. *Wideochir Inne Tech Maloinwazyjne.* 2014;9(1):18–23.
6. Chen CW, Lai CW, Chang YJ, et al. Results of 666 consecutive patients treated with LigaSure hemorrhoidectomy for symptomatic prolapsed hemorrhoids with a minimum follow-up of 2 years. *Surgery.* 2013;153(2):211–218.
7. Nienhuijs S, de Hingh I. Conventional versus LigaSure hemorrhoidectomy for patients with symptomatic hemorrhoids. *Cochrane Database Syst Rev.* 2009;(1):CD006761.
8. Xu L, Chen H, Lin G, et al. Ligasure versus Ferguson hemorrhoidectomy in the treatment of hemorrhoids: a meta-analysis of randomized control trials. *Surg Laparosc Endosc Percutan Tech.* 2015;25(2):106–110.

ADDITIONAL READING

- Reese GE, von Roon AC, Tekkis PP. Haemorrhoids. *BMJ Clin Evid.* 2009;2009:0415.
- Rivadeneira DE, Steele SR, Ternent C, et al. Practice parameters for the management of hemorrhoids (revised 2010). *Dis Colon Rectum.* 2011;54(9):1059–1064.

 SEE ALSO

Colorectal Cancer; Portal Hypertension

 CODES

ICD10

- K64.9 Unspecified hemorrhoids
- K64.0 First degree hemorrhoids
- K64.1 Second degree hemorrhoids

CLINICAL PEARLS

- Hemorrhoids are a very common clinical condition. Internal hemorrhoids are painless. External hemorrhoids are typically painful.
- Anal hygiene and symptomatic pain relief are the treatments of choice for stage 1 and 2 hemorrhoids. Sitz baths with warm water or hypertonic Epsom salts (1 cup per 2 quarts of water) are effective for pain relief.
- All patients should be encouraged to eat a high-fiber diet with 30 g of insoluble fiber per day.
- More advanced hemorrhoidal disease requires intervention with ligation or surgery.

H

HENOCH-SCHÖNLEIN PURPURA

Shani I. Muhammad, MD

 BASICS

DESCRIPTION
- Henoch-Schönlein purpura (HSP) is a nonthrombo-cytopenic, predominantly IgA-mediated, small vessel vasculitis that affects multiple organ systems and occurs in both children and adults.
- HSP is often self-limited, with the greatest morbidity and mortality attributable to long-term renal damage.
- Characterized by a tetrad of purpuric skin lesions, arthralgia, abdominal pain, and nephropathies

EPIDEMIOLOGY
Incidence
- Annual incidence: 135/1 million children and 3.4 to 14.3/1 million adults
- Mean age of patients affected is 6 years; 90% <10 years of age but has been reported in patients age 6 months to 75 years old
- Gender: Male-to-female ratio is 1.2:1.
- Race/ethnicity: most common in Caucasians and Asians, less common among African Americans

Prevalence
- Annual prevalence: 10 to 22/100,000 persons
- Year-round occurrence; more common in late fall to early spring

ETIOLOGY AND PATHOPHYSIOLOGY
- Autoimmune disorder in which IgA production is increased in response to trigger(s), IgA1 immune complexes then activate the complement pathway, leading to production of inflammatory cytokines and chemokines.
- Immune complex deposition results in small vessel inflammation; fibrosis; and necrosis within skin, intestinal mucosa, joints, and kidneys.
- No single etiologic agent has been identified.
- Known triggers include infection, drugs, vaccinations, and insect bites.
- Infectious antigens include (but are not limited to) group A *Streptococcus* (may be present in up to 30% of HSP-associated nephritis), parvovirus B19, *Bartonella henselae*, *Helicobacter pylori*, *Haemophilus parainfluenzae*, coxsackievirus, adenovirus, hepatitis A and B viruses, Mycoplasma, Epstein-Barr virus, varicella, *Campylobacter*, methicillin-resistant *Staphylococcus aureus*.
- Drugs: acetaminophen, quinolones, etanercept, codeine, clarithromycin
- Vaccinations: MMR (measles, mumps, rubella), pneumococcal, meningococcal, influenza, hepatitis B

Genetics
Associated with α_1-antitrypsin deficiency, familial Mediterranean fever, HLA-DRB1*01, HLA-B35

COMMONLY ASSOCIATED CONDITIONS
- Malignancy (rare): Greatest association is with solid tumors, including lymphoma, prostate cancer, and non–small cell lung cancer, but also associated with multiple myeloma.
- Studies suggest a possible relationship with *H. pylori* infection (1)[A].

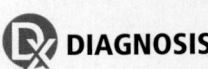 **DIAGNOSIS**

Palpable purpura and *at least one* of the following:
- Diffuse abdominal pain
- Biopsy with predominant IgA deposition

- Arthralgia or arthritis
- Renal involvement (hematuria or proteinuria)
- Direct immunofluorescence showing IgA deposition (2)[A]

HISTORY
- History of exposure to known trigger, including recent infection (particularly upper respiratory infection), vaccination, or offending drug
- Rash (most common presenting symptom): purpuric, palpable; distribution often symmetric on lower extremities and buttocks; may present on upper extremities, trunk, and face; typical duration 3 to 10 days; no definitive temporal association with other symptoms
- Fatigue
- Low-grade fever
- Nausea/vomiting
- Abdominal pain (diffuse, colicky, may be transient or constant)
- Hematochezia/melena
- Polyarthritis (often symmetric involvement of knees and ankles)
- Gross hematuria
- Rare symptoms: periorbital or scrotal swelling, headache, neuropathy, hemoptysis

PHYSICAL EXAM
- Rash (96% of cases, 74% primary presenting symptom):
  – May start as urticaria, develops into nonblanching purpura, with or without petechiae and ecchymoses, may also be bullous
  – Distribution usually symmetric, most commonly involving the lower extremities but may involve the face and trunk
- Abdominal tenderness (66% of cases, 12% primary presenting symptom):
  – Evidence of GI hemorrhage (28% of cases)
- Joint tenderness (64% of cases, 15% primary presenting symptom):
  – Mainly affects knees or ankles; may have associated warmth and limited range of motion, less commonly effusion; erythema is absent.
  – Mostly nonmigratory, transient, and nondeforming
- Orchitis (5%):
  – Presents as scrotal swelling and tenderness, may have associated torsion
- Renal disease (<1% primary presenting symptom):
  – Hypertension may be present.
- Rarely, patients present with CNS or pulmonary involvement, which may manifest as signs of cerebral hemorrhage or diffuse interstitial pneumonia, respectively.

DIFFERENTIAL DIAGNOSIS
- Infection:
  – Meningococcemia
  – Rocky Mountain spotted fever
  – Bacterial endocarditis
  – Rheumatic fever
- Immune-mediated:
  – Polyarteritis nodosa
  – Wegener granulomatosis
  – Systemic lupus erythematosus
  – Kawasaki disease
- Other:
  – Inflammatory bowel disease
  – Idiopathic thrombocytopenic purpura
  – Juvenile rheumatoid arthritis
  – Leukemia
  – Acute surgical abdomen
  – Child abuse

DIAGNOSTIC TESTS & INTERPRETATION
- No single lab test confirms the diagnosis of HSP.
- Labs directed toward excluding other illnesses and assessing degree of renal involvement

Initial Tests (lab, imaging)
The following are generally accepted as initial labs for HSP:
- CBC:
  – Leukocytosis and thrombocytosis may occur. Thrombocytopenia indicates an alternative cause of purpura.
  – Hemoglobin is variable, depending on whether GI hemorrhage occurs.
- Basic serum chemistry panel (electrolytes, BUN, creatinine:
  – Electrolyte imbalances or elevated creatinine indicate renal dysfunction.
- Urinalysis:
  – Gross or microscopic hematuria, proteinuria, and red cell casts indicate renal dysfunction.
- PT and PTT:
  – Normal in HSP
- Imaging is not part of the routine workup for HSP but may be performed to rule out alternative etiologies or for evaluation of suspected complications, particularly in cases of GI and renal involvement. Initial imaging modalities to consider include the following:
  – Abdominal radiographs, with or without barium enema: evaluate for free abdominal air suggestive of bowel perforation
  – Abdominal ultrasound: sensitive for the detection of intramural bleeding in HSP and may also show thickened bowel wall, reduced peristalsis, intussusception
- Renal ultrasound: evaluates for hydronephrosis in cases of renal failure

Follow-Up Tests & Special Considerations
The following labs are also useful in diagnosing HSP:
- Blood culture:
  – To rule out sepsis/bacteremia when diagnosis is unclear
- Acute phase reactants:
  – Expect mild elevation.
- IgA level:
  – Often elevated, although nonspecific, nonsensitive
- Visfatin levels (3)
- Degree of elevation correlates with disease severity and likelihood of renal involvement (3).
- Complement levels:
  – Normal; sometimes decreased
- Antinuclear antibody/antineutrophil cytoplasmic antibody:
  – Negative
- Antistreptolysin-O titer:
  – Evaluates for preceding streptococcal infection
- Stool guaiac if suspected GI hemorrhage
- CT arteriography may be necessary to identify the location of bleeding in patients with GI hemorrhage.

Diagnostic Procedures/Other
- Renal biopsy: Obtain if diagnosis is uncertain or if nephrotic range proteinuria shows mesangial IgA deposition, mesangial proliferation, or, in severe cases, crescentic glomerulonephritis.
- Skin biopsy of purpura: IgA deposition in the dermis on immunofluorescence (2)[A]

- Endoscopy may be considered in cases of GI hemorrhage given symptomatic overlap of HSP with inflammatory bowel disease.
- Barium enema may be therapeutic in some instances of intussusception, although surgical correction is commonly needed.

TREATMENT

GENERAL MEASURES
Rest and elevation of affected areas may limit purpura.

MEDICATION
- In the absence of renal dysfunction or complication, HSP is usually self-limited and best managed with supportive care.
- NSAIDs are effective for symptomatic treatment of joint pain. Caution is advised in cases of GI hemorrhage; avoid use in cases of renal involvement and consider acetaminophen as an alternative.
- Steroids given early in disease course using oral prednisone 1 to 2 mg/kg/day for 1 to 2 weeks decrease both duration of abdominal pain and severity of joint pain and may have benefit in preventing GI bleeding and causes of surgical abdomen, including intussusception.
- Steroids have benefit in treatment of severe and/or bullous purpura.
- Steroids given early in disease are effective for the acute treatment of crescentic nephritis and may prevent chronic renal disease in such patients.
- Early intervention with steroids has no effect on the prevention or development of renal involvement after 1 year.
- High-dose IV pulse steroids (500 mg to 1 g) may be considered in cases of mesenteric vasculitis and severe renal impairment. Evidence is very limited to support use of cyclophosphamide, plasmapheresis, and intravenous immunoglobulin (IVIG) for severe renal and GI involvement, as well as colchicine for severe skin lesions.
- Mycophenolate mofetil (MMF) could be valuable in the treatment of complicated HSP (3,4)[A].

ISSUES FOR REFERRAL
- Consider nephrology referral for renal biopsy if nephrotic range proteinuria at any time or proteinuria >100 mg/mmol for 3 months after diagnosis.
- Dermatology referral for skin biopsy

INPATIENT CONSIDERATIONS
Admission Criteria/Initial Stabilization
- Insufficient oral intake
- Renal insufficiency
- Severe abdominal pain
- Severe GI bleeding
- Altered mental status
- Mobility restriction due to arthritis
- HTN
- Nephrotic syndrome

IV Fluids
Hydration should be maintained.

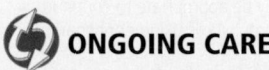

ONGOING CARE

FOLLOW-UP RECOMMENDATIONS
Patient Monitoring
- Patients should be seen weekly during the acute illness. Visits should include history and physical exam to include BP measurement and urinalysis.

- Because ~100% of patients who develop renal involvement will do so within 6 months of HSP diagnosis, all patients should be followed at least monthly with BP and urinalysis for a duration of no <6 months.
- Women with a history of HSP should be monitored for proteinuria and HTN during pregnancy.
- Consider workup for occult malignancy in patients with adult-onset HSP.

PATIENT EDUCATION
- American Family Physician handout on HSP available at: http://www.aafp.org/afp/1998/0801/p411.html
- National Kidney and Urologic Diseases Information Clearinghouse (NKUDIC): http://www.niddk.nih.gov/health-information/health-topics/kidney-disease/henoch-sch%C3%B6nlein-purpura-hsp/Pages/facts.aspx

PROGNOSIS
- Long-term prognosis heavily dependent on presence and severity of nephritis
- HSP is self-limited in 94% of children and 89% of adults.
- Most cases of HSP resolve within 4 weeks of diagnosis. Recurrence rate within 6 months of diagnosis is 33%.
- Factors associated with poorer prognosis include age >8 years, fever at presentation, purpura above the waist, elevated ESR or IgA concentration, and increasing severity of renal histology grade.
- Chronic renal disease occurs in up to 20% of children with nephritic and nephrotic syndrome compared with 50% of adults who had any renal involvement. Risk of long-term renal failure is ≤5%.
- Risk factors that may result in renal failure include old age, HTN, elevated serum creatinine, and nephrotic and mixed nephritic–nephrotic syndrome at the onset of disease (3)[A].

COMPLICATIONS
- Nephrotic/nephritic syndrome and renal failure
- HTN
- Hemorrhagic cystitis
- Ureteral obstruction
- Intestinal infarction, perforation, obstruction, stricture
- GI hemorrhage
- Intussusception
- Alveolar hemorrhage
- CNS complications, including cerebral hemorrhage and seizure
- Anterior uveitis
- Myocarditis
- Orchitis
- Testicular torsion

REFERENCES
1. Kutlubay Z, Zara T, Engin B, et al. *Helicobacter pylori* infection and skin disorders. *Hong Kong Med J*. 2014;20(4):317–324.
2. Mysorekar VV, Sumathy TK, Shyam Prasad AL. Role of direct immunofluorescence in dermatological disorders. *Indian Dermatol Online J*. 2015;6(3):172–180.
3. Nikibakhsh AA, Mahmoodzadeh H, Karamyyar M, et al. Treatment of severe henoch-schonlein purpura nephritis with mycophenolate mofetil. *Saudi J Kidney Dis Transpl*. 2014;25(4):858–863.
4. Antoon JW, Keane MW. Migratory polyarthritis in a child. *Clin Pediatr (Phila)*. 2012;51(4):401–403.

ADDITIONAL READING
- Batu ED, Ozen S. Pediatric vasculitis. *Curr Rheumatol Rep*. 2012;14(2):121–129.
- Boulis E, Majithia V, McMurray R. Adult-onset Henoch-Schonlein purpura with positive c-ANCA (anti-proteinase 3): case report and review of literature. *Rheumatol Int*. 2013;33(2):493–496.
- Cao N, Chen T, Guo ZP, et al. Elevated serum levels of visfatin in patients with henoch-schönlein purpura. *Ann Dermatol*. 2014;26(3):303–307.
- Dillon MJ, Ozen S. A new international classification of childhood vasculitis. *Pediatr Nephrol*. 2006;21(9):1219–1222.
- González LM, Janniger CK, Schwartz RA. Pediatric Henoch-Schönlein purpura. *Int J Dermatol*. 2009;48(11):1157–1165.
- Hoyer PF. Prevention of renal disease in Henoch-Schönlein purpura: clear evidence against steroids. *Arch Dis Child*. 2013;98(10):750–751.
- Jithpratuck W, Elshenawy Y, Saleh H, et al. The clinical implications of adult-onset Henoch-Schonelin purpura. *Clin Mol Allergy*. 2011;9(1):9.
- Kawasaki Y. The pathogenesis and treatment of pediatric Henoch-Schonlein purpura nephritis. *Clin Exp Nephrol*. 2011;15(5):648–657.
- McCarthy HJ, Tizard EJ. Clinical practice: diagnosis and management of Henoch-Schönlein purpura. *Eur J Pediatr*. 2010;169(6):643–650.
- Ozen S, Pistorio A, Iusan SM, et al. EULAR/PRINTO/PRES criteria for Henoch-Schönlein purpura, childhood polyarteritis nodosa, childhood Wegener granulomatosis and childhood Takayasu arteritis: Ankara 2008, part II: final classification criteria. *Ann Rheum Dis*. 2010;69(5):798–806.
- Reamy BV, Williams PM, Lindsay TJ. Henoch-Schönlein purpura. *Am Fam Physician*. 2009;80(7):697–704.
- Sohagia AB, Gunturu SG, Tong TR, et al. Henoch-Schonlein purpura—a case report and review of the literature. *Gastroenterol Res Pract*. 2010;2010:597648.
- Trnka P. Henoch-Schönlein purpura in children. *J Paediatr Child Health*. 2013;49(12):995–1003.
- Weiss PF, Klink AJ, Localio R, et al. Corticosteroids may improve clinical outcomes during hospitalization for Henoch-Schönlein purpura. *Pediatrics*. 2010;126:674–681.

 CODES

ICD10
D69.0 Allergic purpura

CLINICAL PEARLS
- HSP is a systemic small vessel vasculitis characterized by clinical tetrad of palpable purpura, abdominal pain, arthralgia, and renal dysfunction.
- The main form of treatment is supportive care, but oral corticosteroids are beneficial in certain circumstances.
- In all patients with HSP, regardless of renal involvement at presentation, it is reasonable to check BP and urinalysis at weekly to monthly intervals for no <6 months after diagnosis to monitor for developing renal dysfunction.

H

HEPARIN-INDUCED THROMBOCYTOPENIA

Tipsuda Junsanto-Bahri, MD • Maria A. Pino, PhD, MS, RpH

BASICS

DESCRIPTION
- Unexplained decrease in platelet count in a patient treated with heparin
  - Minimum platelet count falls between 30 and 50% from baseline.
- Antibody-mediated prothrombotic disorder initiated by heparin administration
- Unlike other thrombocytopenias, heparin-induced thrombocytopenia (HIT) is an idiosyncratic reaction that produces thrombosis rather than bleeding.
- Two types: nonimmune heparin-associated thrombocytopenia (previously called HIT type I) and HIT (immune induced; previously called HIT type II)
  - Nonimmune heparin-associated thrombocytopenia: more common, onset 1 to 4 days after starting heparin, mild thrombocytopenia (>100,000), few complications
  - HIT: less common, onset 5 to 14 days after primary exposure to heparin, thrombocytopenia often <100,000 but usually >20,000; high risk of thrombosis
    - Presentation of thrombocytopenia can be immediate with recent heparin exposure (within past 100 days).

EPIDEMIOLOGY
Incidence
- 10–15% of heparin-treated patients will experience decrease in platelet count.
- 0.3–3% will develop HIT.

ETIOLOGY AND PATHOPHYSIOLOGY
- Nonimmune heparin-associated thrombocytopenia: potentially a result of direct platelet membrane binding with heparin
- HIT: Heparin can cause an increase in the blood concentration of platelet factor 4 (PF4), a chemokine. PF4 will form a complex with heparin.
- Heparin/PF4 complex can, in turn, stimulate the production of specific antiheparin/PF4 complex antibodies. These antibodies cause platelet activation and a prothrombotic state. Ultimately, this hypercoagulable state leads to thromboembolic complications in many patients.

RISK FACTORS
- Postsurgical > medical > obstetric
  - Postcardiopulmonary bypass is the most significant risk factor.
- Bovine unfractionated heparin (UFH) > porcine UFH > low-molecular-weight heparin (LMWH)
- Female > male
- Heparin duration >4 days

GENERAL PREVENTION
- Inquire about recent heparin exposure and any history of HIT.
- Use of LMWH (vs. unfractionated), for a shorter duration, reduce the risk of developing HIT.
- Properly document past HIT reactions in patient's medical record. Develop a HIT recognition and treatment protocol (1)[A].
- No form of heparin should be administered once the diagnosis of HIT is confirmed.

COMMONLY ASSOCIATED CONDITIONS
- Venous thrombosis: deep venous thrombosis (DVT), pulmonary embolism (PE), adrenal vein thrombosis with hemorrhagic infarction
- Arterial thrombosis
- Skin lesions (skin necrosis at site of injection)
- Acute systemic reactions

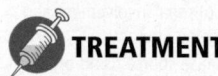

DIAGNOSIS

- Nonimmune heparin-associated thrombocytopenia: asymptomatic drop in platelet count
- HIT: thrombocytopenia or thrombosis with the presence of heparin-dependent antibodies
  - The foundation for diagnosis is based on both clinical and serologic findings.

HISTORY
- Duration of current heparin therapy
- Previous exposure to heparin, including heparin flushes and heparin-coated catheters
- In patients being treated with heparin for thrombosis, in which thrombosis recurs during therapy, consider HIT as a potential cause.
- Pretest probability for HIT can be calculated using the "4 Ts" methodology:
  - Thrombocytopenia of new onset
  - Timing of thrombocytopenia (5 to 10 days after exposure)
  - Thrombosis of new onset
  - Thrombocytopenia by other causes is ruled out.
- The HIT Expert Probability score is an effective pretest probability tool (2)[B].

PHYSICAL EXAM
- Signs of venous or arterial thrombosis
- Skin necrosis (begins with erythema, progresses to ecchymosis and necrosis)
- Ischemic changes (signs of limb, renal, splenic, mesenteric ischemia)
- Bleeding (less common)
- Acute systemic reactions after IV bolus of heparin (e.g., signs of anaphylaxis)

DIFFERENTIAL DIAGNOSIS
Other potential causes of thrombocytopenia include (list is not all-inclusive)
- Sepsis and other infections
- Drug reactions
- Autoimmune
- Transfusion reactions
- Physical destruction (e.g., during cardiopulmonary bypass)

DIAGNOSTIC TESTS & INTERPRETATION
- Serial platelet counts in patients receiving heparin who have a possible risk of HIT >1%: Check platelets at baseline and then every 2 to 3 days from days 4 to 14 of heparin therapy (3)[B]:
  - Withhold platelet monitoring for patients receiving heparin with risk of HIT <1%
- Confirmatory lab tests needed for a clinical diagnosis can be divided into two major categories:
  - Antigen assay to detect presence of HIT antibodies:
    - ELISA: up to 99% sensitive, poor specificity; thus, has an excellent negative predictive value for HIT

- Functional assay to detect evidence of platelet activation in the presence of heparin:
  - Serotonin release assay (SRA), gold standard for diagnosis: high specificity and high sensitivity
  - Heparin-induced platelet activation (HIPA): high specificity and low sensitivity
- Antigenic assay should be the initial test.
  - Either a functional assay or an antigenic assay alone may not be adequate for clinical diagnosis; their use in combination is usually recommended.
- The diagnostic interpretation of these laboratory tests must be made in the context of the clinical estimation of the pretest probability because HIT is a clinicopathologic syndrome. Patients may form heparin-dependent antibodies and still not develop HIT.

TREATMENT

Treatment is by prompt withdrawal of heparin and replacement with a suitable alternative anticoagulant.

GENERAL MEASURES
- Discontinue all heparin products, including flushes and heparin-coated catheters.
- All patients with a diagnosis of HIT should receive alternative anticoagulation as they are of high thrombotic risk.
- Nonimmune heparin-associated thrombocytopenia generally resolves when heparin is stopped:
  - Consider a nonheparin alternative such as fondaparinux if pharmacologic DVT prophylaxis is warranted (3)[C].
- Platelet transfusions can increase thrombosis. Give platelet transfusions only if bleeding or during an invasive procedure with a high risk of bleeding.
- Warfarin should not be administered until platelet recovery. If warfarin has been administered, vitamin K should be given (reference, Warkentin TE).
- Adverse reaction to heparin should be clearly documented in the medical record with instruction to avoid all heparin products.

- For patients with a documented history of HIT, under special circumstances only (such as the need for cardiopulmonary bypass), the use of heparin for a short duration may be acceptable if the absence of heparin/PF4 complex antibodies can be documented. Patients who develop antibodies to the heparin/PF4 complex have a significantly higher rate of postoperative thrombotic events than patients who lack these antibodies (4)[B].

MEDICATION
- Most patients require anticoagulation because of
  - Preexisting thrombosis *or*
  - Risk of thrombosis during 30 days after HIT diagnosis (consider anticoagulation for 30 days)
- Dosing of anticoagulant depends on indication (prophylaxis vs. treatment):
  - In cases with a clinically low suspicion/pretest probability of HIT and laboratory confirmation is pending, it may be appropriate to continue antithrombotic prophylaxis using nonheparin anticoagulants.
  - In cases with high suspicion/pretest probability of HIT and laboratory confirmation is pending, it is appropriate to begin anticoagulation treatment with a nonheparin product (5)[B].

- Direct thrombin inhibitors (DTIs) (argatroban and bivalirudin)
  - Reduce relative risk of thrombosis by 30% and are associated with a 5–10% risk of important bleeding.
  - Can produce misleading elevation in international normalized ratio (INR) (most likely an in vitro reaction)
    - Argatroban > bivalirudin (3)[B]
  - Argatroban
    - Initial dose, 2 μg/kg/min by continuous IV infusion; decrease dose with reduced hepatic function or with critical illness.
    - Dose adjustments based to achieve activated partial thromboplastin time (aPTT) 1.5 to 3 times the baseline.
  - Bivalirudin
    - Favorable pharmacologic profile; however, evidence for use is insufficient compared to argatroban (limited to case series).
    - Reduced risk of bleeding in patients undergoing percutaneous artery interventions (PCIs) and other cardiac procedures
    - Initial dose of 0.15 mg/kg/hr followed by adjustments to keep aPTT 1.5 to 2.5 times the baseline. Reduced dose with renal insufficiency (creatinine clearance [CrCl] <30 mL/min)
    - Dose adjustments based on aPTT
- Factor Xa inhibitor (fondaparinux)
  - Reports of its use are theorized to be useful; however, minimal data support its efficacy for HIT, and an ideal dose has yet to be determined.
  - Association with the development of HIT has been reported.
  - Optional agent for thromboembolic prophylaxis when practitioner wants to avoid heparin
  - Contraindicated in patients with renal dysfunction (CrCl <30 mL/min) (5)[C]
- Warfarin
  - Must anticoagulate with an immediate-acting agent before starting warfarin
  - Use of warfarin without other anticoagulants should be avoided because it can cause thrombosis.
  - Begin warfarin after platelet count is >150,000.
  - Discontinue other anticoagulant and continue only warfarin after INR is therapeutic (2 to 3) for at least 5 days. This management differs from the normal heparin-to-warfarin transition in other conditions requiring anticoagulation (5,6)[C].
- LMWH
  - Although LMWH has a lower risk of initiating a HIT reaction, it should *not* be used when antibodies are already present. These antibodies can cross-react with LMWH and induce thrombosis and thrombocytopenia.

INPATIENT CONSIDERATIONS
Nursing
- Avoid heparin flushes.
- Avoid platelet transfusion.
- Clearly document reaction in all medical records to control the future use of heparin.

ONGOING CARE

FOLLOW-UP RECOMMENDATIONS
- The transition period of anticoagulation with a DTI and warfarin in patients with HIT can be problematic.
- The INR while administering both a DTI and warfarin should be therapeutic (2 to 3) for at least 5 days before discontinuing the DTI.
- Warfarin therapy should not be commenced until the platelet count has stabilized within a normal range.
- Warfarin therapy should continue for a minimum of 3 months.
- DTIs can prolong INR; therefore, if INR is <4 while on both warfarin and a DTI, temporarily hold the DTI for 4 to 6 hours and recheck INR; this second INR will represent only the anticoagulant effect of warfarin.
- Monitor use of concurrent drugs with warfarin.

Patient Monitoring
- Serial platelet counts
- Monitor PTT or INR as determined by the anticoagulation agent.

PATIENT EDUCATION
- Patient should inform all health care providers of any previous adverse reaction to heparin.
- HIT information available at: http://medlibrary.org/medwiki/Heparin-induced_thrombocytopenia

PROGNOSIS
- Thrombosis in HIT has 20–30% mortality, with additional morbidity from stroke and limb ischemia.
- Platelet counts normalize within weeks after stopping heparin.
- Risk of delayed thrombosis, especially in the first 30 days

REFERENCES

1. Smythe MA, Mehta TP, Koerber JM, et al. Development and implementation of a comprehensive heparin-induced thrombocytopenia recognition and management protocol. *Am J Health Syst Pharm*. 2012;69(3):241–248.
2. Cuker A, Arepally G, Crowther MA, et al. The HIT Expert Probability (HEP) Score: a novel pre-test probability model for heparin-induced thrombocytopenia based on broad expert opinion. *J Thromb Haemost*. 2010;8(12):2642–2650.
3. Bakchoul T, Greinacher A. Recent advances in the diagnosis and treatment of heparin-induced thrombocytopenia. *Ther Adv Hematol*. 2012;3(4):237–251.
4. Zhang R, Huang Y, Zhang M, et al. Serum antibodies to the heparin/platelet factor 4 complex are an independent predictor of thrombotic complications following pediatric fontan surgery. *Clin Appl Thromb Hemost*. 2012;18(5):448–452.
5. Linkins LA, Dans AL, Moores LK, et al. Treatment and prevention of heparin-induced thrombocytopenia: Antithrombotic Therapy and Prevention of Thrombosis, 9th ed: American College of Chest Physicians Evidence-Based Clinical Practice Guidelines. *Chest*. 2012;141(2 Suppl):e495S–e530S.
6. Shantsila E, Lip GY, Chong BH. Heparin-induced thrombocytopenia: a contemporary clinical approach to diagnosis and management. *Chest*. 2009;135(6):1651–1664.

ADDITIONAL READING

- Dager WE, Dougherty JA, Nguyen PH, et al. Heparin-induced thrombocytopenia: treatment options and special considerations. *Pharmacotherapy*. 2007;27(4):564–587.
- Lo GK, Juhl D, Warkentin TE, et al. Evaluation of pretest clinical score (4 T's) for the diagnosis of heparin-induced thrombocytopenia in two clinical settings. *J Thromb Haemost*. 2006;4(4):759–765.
- Stone GW, Ware JH, Bertrand ME, et al. Antithrombotic strategies in patients with acute coronary syndromes undergoing early invasive management: one-year results from the ACUITY trial. *JAMA*. 2007;298(21):2497–2506.
- Warkentin TE. Heparin-induced thrombocytopenia: diagnosis and management. *Circulation*. 2004;110(18):e454–e458.
- Warkentin TE, Greinacher A, Craven S, et al. Differences in the clinically effective molar concentrations of four direct thrombin inhibitors explain their variable prothrombin time prolongation. *Thromb Haemost*. 2005;94(5):958–964.
- Warkentin TE, Maurer BT, Aster RH. Heparin-induced thrombocytopenia associated with fondaparinux. *N Engl J Med*. 2007;356(25):2653–2655.

 ## CODES

ICD10
D75.82 Heparin induced thrombocytopenia (HIT)

CLINICAL PEARLS

- Heparin exposure through virtually any preparation (including LMWH), any dose, or any route can cause HIT, a life-threatening condition which is associated with severe and extensive thromboembolism.
- LMWH is contraindicated in HIT; although LMWH is less likely to cause HIT. Once HIT is present, the antibodies will cross-react and continue to cause a HIT reaction.
- If a patient is suspected of HIT (with or without confirmatory testing), immediately discontinue all forms of heparin.
- Patients will require anticoagulation either because of preexisting thrombosis or the risk of thrombosis in first 30 days after HIT.
- A direct thrombin inhibitor (DTI) should be used until a patient's INR is therapeutic (2 to 3) on warfarin for at least 5 days.
- The key to avoiding sequelae from HIT is awareness, vigilance, and a high degree of suspicion.

H

HEPATIC ENCEPHALOPATHY

Walter M. Kim, MD, PhD • Jyoti Ramakrishna, MD

BASICS

DESCRIPTION

- Reversible altered mental and neuromotor functioning occurring in association with acute or chronic liver disease and/or portal systemic shunting
- The prominent features are confusion, impaired arousability, and a "flapping tremor" (asterixis).
- System(s) affected: gastrointestinal; nervous
- Synonym(s): portosystemic encephalopathy; hepatic coma; liver coma

EPIDEMIOLOGY

Predominant sex: male = female (reflecting underlying liver disease)

Prevalence

- Overt HE occurs in 30–45% of cirrhotic patients.
- Occurs in all cases of fulminant hepatic failure
- Present in nearly 1/2 of patients who require liver transplantation.
- Parallels the age predominance of fulminant liver disease: peaks in the 40s; cirrhosis peaks in the late 50s; may occur at any age

ETIOLOGY AND PATHOPHYSIOLOGY

- There is no defined pathophysiology for the development of HE. Three classifications have been proposed (1):
  - Type A: resulting from acute liver failure
  - Type B: resulting from portosystemic bypass or shunting
  - Type C: resulting from cirrhosis
- Several metabolic factors have been implicated in HE based on the failure of the liver to detoxify agents noxious to the CNS (e.g., ammonia, mercaptan, fatty acids).
- Increased aromatic and reduced branched chain amino acids in blood may act as false neurotransmitters, possibly interacting with the γ-aminobutyric acid (GABA) receptor and causing clinical symptoms.
- HE presents most commonly in long-standing cirrhosis with spontaneous shunting of intestinal blood through collateral vessels or surgically constructed portacaval shunts.
- Transjugular intrahepatic portosystemic shunt (TIPS), a widely used radiologically inserted shunt to lower portal pressure, is associated with HE in some cases.
- Asterixis is the inability to maintain a particular posture due to metabolic encephalopathy. Abnormal diencephalic function leads to the characteristic liver flap noted when the arms and wrists are held in extension. Asterixis is also present in patients with uremia, barbiturate toxicity, and some cases of pulmonary disease. As such, asterixis is not pathognomonic for HE.

Genetics

- Unknown
- Conditions such as cystic fibrosis, α-1-antitrypsin deficiency, and Wilson disease can contribute to HE.

RISK FACTORS

In patients with underlying liver disease, precipitating factors include the following:

- Infection (overt or occult, including spontaneous bacterial peritonitis)
- GI hemorrhage
- Use of sedative or opiate drugs.
- Fluid or electrolyte disturbance (Na^+, K^+, Mg^{2+}, or other electrolyte depletion)

- TIPS
- Constipation

GENERAL PREVENTION

- Recognize early signs and seek prompt treatment.
- Avoid nonessential medications, particularly opiates, benzodiazepines, and sedatives.

COMMONLY ASSOCIATED CONDITIONS

- May occur as a complication of acute fatty liver of pregnancy
- Occurs rarely in patients with a portacaval shunt but normal liver function

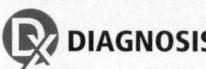

DIAGNOSIS

HISTORY

- Preexisting liver disease
- Confusion; altered mental status
- Impaired arousability

PHYSICAL EXAM

- Age 10 to 60 years
  - Prominent signs of underlying liver disease (50%); jaundice most common, ascites second most common
  - GI hemorrhage with hematemesis or melena (20%)
  - Systemic infection, urinary tract infection, or pulmonary infection (20%)
  - Five grades (West Haven classification) of confusion and degree of obtundation (1):
    - Minimal: psychometric or neuropsychological alterations without mental status changes
    - Grade I: lack of awareness, anxiety, shortened attention span, impairment of arithmetic, altered sleep rhythm
    - Grade II: asterixis, lethargy, disorientation to time, personality change, inappropriate behavior
    - Grade III: somnolence, confusion, gross disorientation, bizarre behavior
    - Grade IV: coma
- Age >60 years
  - Signs of underlying liver disease diminish (25%)
  - Confusion more prominent
  - Precipitating GI hemorrhage or infection is less often identified.
  - Progression is slower.
- Age <10 years
  - Signs of underlying liver disease prominent; usually fulminant hepatic failure or advanced cirrhosis
  - Progression is very rapid, often 6 to 12 hours.
  - Wilson disease can imitate HE.
- Vital signs:
  - Bradycardia
  - Increased blood pressure suggestive of increased intracranial pressure
- Jaundice, ascites, and other correlates of liver disease
- CNS exam pertaining to stage of HE: Assess short-term memory and presence of asterixis ("liver flap"—a flapping of the wrist when arms are held in extension with the wrist fully extended)

DIFFERENTIAL DIAGNOSIS

- Metabolic encephalopathy related to anoxia, hypoglycemia, hypokalemia, hypo- or hypercalcemia, or uremia
- Head trauma, concussion, subdural hematoma

- Transient ischemic attack (TIA), ischemic stroke
- Alcohol intoxication
- Alcohol withdrawal syndrome
- Confusion due to medications or illicit drugs
- Meningitis, encephalitis
- Wilson disease
- Reye syndrome

DIAGNOSTIC TESTS & INTERPRETATION

- Clinical findings yield diagnosis in 80% of cases.
- Response to treatment often confirms the diagnosis.
- EEG: symmetric slowing of basic (α) rhythm (common with other metabolic encephalopathies-limited utility) (2)
- Visual evoked potential: specific in grades II to IV
- Number connection test, line drawing test, clicker flicker frequency (CFF) test, continuous reaction time (CRT) test, inhibitory control test (ICT), and other psychometric tests may be used to assess for minimal HE.

Initial Tests (lab, imaging)

- Liver tests, including aspartate aminotransferase (AST), alanine aminotransferase (ALT), and serum albumin to evaluate severity of liver disease
- Prothrombin time (PT) and international normalized ratio (INR) are elevated in liver failure due to impaired hepatic synthesis of coagulation factors.
- Serum ammonia level is elevated in 90% of patients with HE; levels affected by infusion of amino acid solutions, opiate administration (constipation), uremia, tissue breakdown, burns, trauma, or infection
- CBC-anemia and leukocytosis
- Complete metabolic profile to identify hypokalemia, hyperbilirubinemia, altered calcium concentration, hypomagnesemia, and hypoglycemia
- BUN: Creatinine >20 suggests dehydration or GI bleeding.
- Blood, urine, and ascitic fluid cultures to identify infection, if clinically indicated
- Consider arterial blood gas measurement.
- Toxicology screen for illicit drugs.
- Head CT to identify frontal cortical atrophy and mild general edema.
- MRI may demonstrate increased T1 signal in globus pallidus.

Tests Interpretation

- Brain edema in 100% of fatal cases
- Glial hypertrophy in chronic encephalopathy

TREATMENT

GENERAL MEASURES

- Identify and treat precipitating causes: GI bleeding, infection, electrolyte imbalance. Eliminate offending medications.
- Grade I or higher: Ensure adequate fluid intake and at least 1,000 kcal (4.19 MJ) daily; avoid hypoglycemia.
- Administer initial enema to all patients who don't have diarrhea.
- If clumsiness and poor judgment are prominent, avoid falls and other accidents.
- Avoid sedatives, opiates, diphenoxylate, and atropine.

MEDICATION

First Line

- Lactulose syrup (nonabsorbable disaccharide whose laxative action decreases colonic transit time while bacterial digestion acidifies the colon, thereby promoting excretion of ammonia): 30 to 45 mL PO up to every hour for goal of 3 to 6 bowel movements per day. Diminish to 15 to 30 mL BID when ≥3 bowel movements occur daily (3)[A].

- Lactulose enema (for patients who cannot tolerate oral lactulose or have suspected ileus): 300 mL lactulose plus 700 mL tap water, retained for 1 hour

- If worsening occurs acutely or there is no improvement in 2 days, add antibiotics:

  - Rifaximin: 400 mg PO TID or 550 mg PO BID (nonabsorbable antibiotic); highly effective in reversing minimal HE and preventing HE recurrence (4)[B]

- Contraindications:
  - Total ileus
  - Hypersensitivity reaction
- Precautions:
  - Hypokalemia
  - Electrolyte imbalance
  - Renal failure

Second Line

- Neomycin: 1 to 2 g/day PO divided q6–8h, if renal function is within normal limits
- Polyethylene glycol has recently been studied for acute hepatic encephalopathy and appears to be effective.
- Metronidazole is an alternative antibiotic.
- Flumazenil may be of benefit in select patients.

ISSUES FOR REFERRAL

Refer early to a transplant center.

SURGERY/OTHER PROCEDURES

- Artificial liver perfusion devices are useful in fulminant hepatic failure as a bridge until a donor liver is available for transplantation.
- Consider liver transplant in grade II to IV patients.

COMPLEMENTARY & ALTERNATIVE MEDICINE

Probiotics and prebiotics have been associated with improvement of HE through modulation of gut flora (5)[C].

INPATIENT CONSIDERATIONS

Admission Criteria/Initial Stabilization

- Monitor clinical status closely in grades I and II when diagnosis is clear, and watch for progression.
- Evaluate patients with grade II to IV HE in fulminant hepatic failure for liver transplantation

ONGOING CARE

FOLLOW-UP RECOMMENDATIONS

Activity as tolerated once resolved

Patient Monitoring

- Trail-making test (a pencil/paper connect-the-dots according to numbers) can help monitor HE patients. Period evaluation helps determine how much maintenance treatment is needed and what diet is appropriate. The test should be run daily at first and then at each visit when changes in drugs and diet are made.

- Patients with changed findings on the trail-making test should be seen twice weekly.
- Stable patients should be seen monthly.
- Number connection test or line drawing test at each office visit also help with patient monitoring.
- In cirrhosis, evaluate for transplantation and periodically monitor Model for End-stage Liver Disease (MELD) score.

DIET

- Integrate with underlying disease.
- Regular protein diet (1.2 to 1.5 g/kg/day) (6)[C]; vegetable protein diets are better tolerated than animal protein diets in patients with advanced cirrhosis; special IV/enteral formulations with increased branched chain amino acids are available.
- Grades III to IV patients need parenteral nutrition or jejunal feeds.

PATIENT EDUCATION

American Association for the Study of Liver Diseases, 1729 King Street, Suite 200, Alexandria, VA 22314; 703-299-9766; www.aasld.org

PROGNOSIS

- With adequate aggressive treatment, HE resolves without residue or recurrence
- Chronic disease
  - Coma returns.
  - With each recurrence, HE is more difficult to treat—the degree of improvement with treatment is less and the mortality rate approaches 80%.

COMPLICATIONS

- Recurrence
- With many recurrences, permanent basal ganglion injury (non-Wilsonian hepatolenticular degeneration)
- Hepatorenal syndrome

REFERENCES

1. Vilstrup H, Amodio P, Bajaj J, et al. Hepatic encephalopathy in chronic liver disease: 2014 Practice Guideline by the American Association for the Study of Liver Diseases and the European Association for the Study of the Liver. *Hepatology.* 2014;60(2):715–735.
2. Saxena N, Bhatia M, Joshi YK, et al. Electrophysiological and neuropsychological tests for the diagnosis of subclinical hepatic encephalopathy and prediction of overt encephalopathy. *Liver.* 2002;22(3):190–197.
3. Als-Nielsen B, Gluud LL, Gluud C. Non-absorbable disaccharides for hepatic encephalopathy: systematic review of randomised trials. *BMJ.* 2004; 328(7447):1046.
4. Bass NM, Mullen KD, Sanyal A, et al. Rifaximin treatment in hepatic encephalopathy. *N Engl J Med.* 2010;362(12):1071–1081.
5. Liu Q, Duan ZP, Ha DK, et al. Synbiotic modulation of gut flora: effect on minimal hepatic encephalopathy in patients with cirrhosis. *Hepatology.* 2004; 39(5):1441–1449.
6. Córdoba J, López-Hellín J, Planas M, et al. Normal protein diet for episodic hepatic encephalopathy: results of a randomized study. *J Hepatol.* 2004; 41(1):38–43.

ADDITIONAL READING

- Agrawal A, Sharma BC, Sharma P, et al. Secondary prophylaxis of hepatic encephalopathy in cirrhosis: an open-label, randomized controlled trial of lactulose, probiotics, and no therapy. *Am J Gastroenterol.* 2012;107(7):1043–1050.
- Blei AT, Córdoba J; Practice Parameters Committee of the American College of Gastroenterology. Hepatic encephalopathy. *Am J Gastroenterol.* 2001;96(7):1968–1976.
- Ellul MA, Gholkar SA, Cross TJ. Hepatic encephalopathy due to liver cirrhosis. *BMJ.* 2015;351:h4187.
- McGee RG, Bakens A, Wiley K, et al. Probiotics for patients with hepatic encephalopathy. *Cochrane Database Syst Rev.* 2011;(11):CD008716.
- Ong JP, Aggarwal A, Krieger D, et al. Correlation between ammonia levels and the severity of hepatic encephalopathy. *Am J Med.* 2003;114(3):188–193.
- Quero Guillén JC, Herrerías Gutiérrez JM. Diagnostic methods in hepatic encephalopathy. *Clin Chim Acta.* 2006;365(1–2):1–8.
- Sidhu SS, Goyal O, Mishra BP, et al. Rifaximin improves psychometric performance and health-related quality of life in patients with minimal hepatic encephalopathy (the RIME Trial). *Am J Gastroenterol.* 2011;106(2):307–316.

 SEE ALSO

Algorithm: Delirium

 CODES

ICD10

- K72.90 Hepatic failure, unspecified without coma
- K72.91 Hepatic failure, unspecified with coma

CLINICAL PEARLS

- HE includes a spectrum of neuropsychiatric findings that occur in patients with significant alterations in hepatic function.
- Lactulose is a cornerstone of therapy for HE.
- Asterixis ("liver flap") is the classic physical finding associated with HE.

HEPATITIS A

Daniel J. Stein, MD, MPH • Stephen K. Lane, MD, FAAFP

BASICS

DESCRIPTION
One of the world's most common diseases, hepatitis A is an infection with the hepatitis A virus (HAV) primarily involving the liver (1).

EPIDEMIOLOGY
Pediatric Considerations
- Disease is often milder or asymptomatic in children; severity increases with age.
- Infections are asymptomatic in 70% of children age <6 years.
- In 2009, <50% of 13- to 17-year-olds in the United States had been vaccinated.

Pregnancy Considerations
- Pregnant women with HAV have increased risk of complications including preterm labor (2).
- Vertical transmission has been reported; fecal-oral transmission during birth is possible.
- Breastfeeding is not contraindicated.

Incidence
- HAV is cause of roughly 50% of reported cases of viral hepatitis in the United States (3).
- 1.4 million cases globally each year
- Since the hepatitis A vaccine has been in routine use (1995), the incidence of HAV has decreased by 95%.
- Approximately 3,000 HAV infections in 2009, lowest ever recorded in the United States (1)
- Incidence in the United States: 0.5/100,000 (1)
- No difference based on sex
- As many as 1/2 of current HAV infections in the United States are acquired from travel to endemic countries.

Prevalence
Serologic evidence of prior HAV infection: 1/3 of United States population. Anti-HAV prevalence related to age, ranging from 9% in children ages 6 to 11 years to 75% of those >70 years. Related inversely to income

ETIOLOGY AND PATHOPHYSIOLOGY
- HAV is a single-stranded linear RNA enterovirus of the *Picornaviridae* family.
- Infection is limited to liver hepatocytes and macrophages.
- HAV is excreted into the bile and then stool, providing major route of spread.
- Primary transmission is fecal-oral.
- Humans are the only natural host.
- Incubation is 2 to 6 weeks (mean 4 weeks).
- Greatest infectivity is during 2 weeks before and one week after the onset of clinical illness.
- Infection occurs primarily after consuming food or water contaminated with HAV, or via direct contact with HAV-infected person with poor hygiene.
- Outbreaks can occur related to a common food or water source with multiple individuals exposed
- Virus is stable in water and on surfaces, but is easily killed with high heat or cleaning agents.
- Shellfish (clams and oysters) may be contaminated if harvested from waters contaminated with HAV.
- Blood-borne transmission is rare.
- HAV is not a chronic disease, but can last for months.

Genetics
Autoimmune hepatitis is rarely associated with human leukocyte antigen class II; DR3 and DR4 after active infection with HAV.

RISK FACTORS
- Travel to developing countries accounts for >50% of cases in North America and Europe.
- Employment in health care
- Household exposure
- Intimate exposure, especially men who have sex with men
- Injection of illicit drugs
- Child care centers, schools
- Institutionalized individuals
- Clotting factor disorders, such as hemophilia
- Blood exposure/transfusion (rare)
- No identifiable risk factor in 50%

GENERAL PREVENTION
- Proper sanitation and personal hygiene (including hand washing), especially for food handlers, health care, and daycare workers
- Active immunization: HAV vaccines: Havrix and Vaqta; Twinrix-combination HAV and HBV
- Vaccine is recommended for (1)[C],(4)[A]:
  - All children aged 12 to 23 months, with catch-up administration until 18 years old
  - All travelers to countries with a high endemic rate of hepatitis A
  - Men who have sex with men
  - Illicit IV drug users
  - Anyone with chronic liver disease (including pre- and postliver transplant)
  - Individuals with a clotting factor disorder
  - Household members and close contacts of children adopted from countries with a high HAV prevalence (prior to arrival)
  - Anyone exposed during an outbreak
- Per the CDC, routine vaccination is no longer routinely recommended for food service, child care, or health care workers (1)[C].
- HIV-infected patients who are negative for HAV IgG should receive HAV vaccine series, preferably early in course of HIV infection
  - If CD4 count is <200 cells/mm³ or the patient has symptomatic HIV disease, defer vaccination until several months after initiation of antiretroviral (ARV) therapy to maximize the antibody response to the vaccine.
- HAV is *not* killed by freezing.
- HAV is killed by
  - Heating to 185°F for 60 seconds
  - Chlorine
  - Iodine

DIAGNOSIS

HISTORY
- Onset is often abrupt. Common symptoms include nausea, emesis and diarrhea, and headache
- Symptom severity increases with age
- Pediatric cases (under 6) frequently asymptomatic
- Other symptoms:
  - Fever, malaise, fatigue, myalgias, anorexia
  - Dark urine (bilirubinuria)
  - Right upper abdominal pain
  - Pruritus (can suggest cholestasis)

PHYSICAL EXAM
- Fever (variable)
- Jaundice and icterus present in >70% of adults and older children
- Hepatomegaly is also common; splenomegaly is less common.
- Right upper quadrant abdominal tenderness
- Rarely can have lymphadenopathy (cervical), arthritis, or rash
- Asterixis can indicate acute hepatic failure.

DIFFERENTIAL DIAGNOSIS
- Hepatitis B, C, D, E. Not clinically distinguishable from other forms of viral hepatitis; diagnosis may be suspected with typical symptoms during an outbreak.
- Drug-induced hepatitis; toxin-induced hepatitis
- Alcoholic hepatitis
- Hemochromatosis (adults) or Wilson disease
- Autoimmune hepatitis
- Malaria
- Infectious mononucleosis, cytomegalovirus (CMV)
- Primary or secondary hepatic malignancy
- Ischemic hepatitis or Budd-Chiari syndrome
- Nonhepatobiliary disease (elevated AST/ALT): celiac disease, congestive heart failure, thyroid disease
- Bacterial infections (Q fever, leptospirosis, syphilis, Rocky Mountain spotted fever)
- Parasites (liver flukes or toxocariasis)

DIAGNOSTIC TESTS & INTERPRETATION
Initial Tests (lab, imaging)
- Anti-HAV IgM: positive at time of onset of symptoms sensitivity and specificity >95%. Primary test used to diagnose acute infection.
- Anti-HAV IgG: appears soon after IgM and generally persists from years to lifetime
- AST and ALT elevated ~500 to 5,000: ALT usually > AST (3)
- Alkaline phosphatase: mildly elevated
- Bilirubin: conjugated and unconjugated fractions usually increased. Usually follows rises in ALT/AST, consistent with hepatocellular injury pattern
- Prothrombin time and partial thromboplastin time usually remain normal or near normal.
  - Significant rises should raise concern of possible acute hepatic failure or coexistent chronic liver disease
- CBC: mild leukocytosis; aplasia and pancytopenia are rare.
  - Thrombocytopenia may predict illness severity.
  - Autoimmune hemolytic anemia (rare)
- Albumin, electrolytes, and glucose to evaluate for hepatic and renal function (rare renal failure)
- Urinalysis (not clinically necessary): bilirubinuria
- Consider ultrasound (US) to rule out biliary obstruction only if lab pattern is cholestatic.

Follow-Up Tests & Special Considerations
Illness usually resolves within 4 weeks from onset of symptoms. Repeat labs are not generally indicated unless symptoms persist or new ones develop.

Diagnostic Procedures/Other
Liver biopsy is usually not necessary. US can evaluate other causes (e.g., thrombosis or concurrent cirrhosis)

Tests Interpretation
- Positive serum markers in hepatitis A
  - Acute disease: anti-HAV IgM only
  - Recent disease (last 6 months): anti-HAV IgM and IgG positive
  - Previous disease: anti-HAV IgM negative and IgG positive
- If liver biopsy obtained, shows portal inflammation; immunofluorescent stains for HAV antigen positive

 TREATMENT

GENERAL MEASURES
- Maintain appropriate nutrition/hydration.
- Avoid alcohol.
- Attend to personal hygiene to prevent spread.
- Monitor coagulation defects, fluid and electrolytes, acid–base imbalance, hypoglycemia, and impairment of renal function.
- Report to local public health department.
- Laboratory evaluation including coagulation factors is important to rule out fulminant hepatic failure.
- Referral to liver transplant center for fulminant failure (rare)

MEDICATION
- Preexposure vaccination should be given according to recommended guidelines.

- Give postexposure prophylaxis to persons within 2 weeks of exposure to HAV who have not previously received HAV vaccine (5)[A],(6)[C].
  - Administer hepatitis A vaccine to healthy persons between the ages of 1 and 40 years at age-appropriate dose (7)[A].
  - Administer immunoglobulin (0.02 mL/kg) to persons <1 or >40 years of age, or to patients with significant comorbidities (immunosuppression, liver disease) who are at risk for poor immune response (5)[A],(6)[C].
- Use immunoglobulin for passive preexposure prophylaxis in those not eligible for the vaccine (5)[A],(6)[C].

  - 0.02 mL/kg provides 1 to 2 months of coverage; 0.06 mL/kg provides 3 to 5 months of coverage
  - Long-term prophylaxis should be with 0.06 mL/kg every 5 months for sustained risk (e.g., travelers)
  - Use immunoglobulin with the vaccine in cases where travelers need immediate protection and are older than 40 years.
  - Use immunoglobulin alone in children under 1 year old and unvaccinated pregnant women who will be traveling.
  - Do not give immunoglobulin with the MMR or varicella vaccines.

First Line
- No antiviral medications indicated; spontaneous resolution occurs in almost all patients.
- Limit acetaminophen use to 2 g/day or less.
- Avoid hepatoxic agents.

Second Line
- Antiemetics (e.g., ondansetron)
- IV fluids
- Pruritus: diphenhydramine 50 mg PO IM q6h, consider cholestyramine 4 g BID if cholestasis

ISSUES FOR REFERRAL
- Dictated by severity of illness
- Hepatic failure, refer to a high-volume liver transplant program

SURGERY/OTHER PROCEDURES
Liver transplant in fulminant hepatic failure—rare

COMPLEMENTARY & ALTERNATIVE MEDICINE
Avoid botanicals with potential hepatotoxicity, including barberry, comfrey, golden ragwort, groundsel, huang qin, kava kava, pennyroyal, sassafras, senna, valerian, wall germander, and wood sage.

INPATIENT CONSIDERATIONS
Admission Criteria/Initial Stabilization
Treatment is usually outpatient unless signs of liver failure; dictated by severity of illness

IV Fluids
Treat dehydration and any noted electrolyte imbalances.

Nursing
Enteric isolation. Private rooms, gowns, and masks are not necessary. Frequent hand washing. Use gloves when handling material potentially contaminated with feces.

 ONGOING CARE

FOLLOW-UP RECOMMENDATIONS
Return to work/school 10 to 14 days after onset of symptoms with diligence to hygiene (patients remain infectious for up to 4 weeks from symptom onset).

Patient Monitoring
Monitor coagulation defects, fluid and electrolytes, acid–base imbalance, hypoglycemia, and renal function.

DIET
- Adequate balanced nutrition
- Avoid alcohol.

PATIENT EDUCATION
- Segregate food handlers with HAV.
- HAV immunity persists after infection
- CDC Hepatitis A FAQs Link: http://www.cdc.gov/hepatitis/hav/afaq.htm

PROGNOSIS
- Excellent; mortality is 0.3% (1)
- Risk increased with underlying chronic liver disease and in the elderly (1.8% mortality age >50) (1)

COMPLICATIONS
- Coagulopathy, encephalopathy, and renal failure
- Relapsing HAV: usually milder than the initial case
- Positive anti-HAV IgM. Total duration is usually <9 months.
- Prolonged cholestasis: characterized by protracted periods of jaundice and pruritus (>3 months), resolves without intervention (supportive care only)

- Autoimmune hepatitis: can be seen after HAV infection; good response to steroids
- Hepatic failure: rare (1–2%)
- Postviral encephalitis, Guillain-Barré syndrome, pancreatitis, aplastic or hemolytic anemia, agranulocytosis, thrombocytopenic purpura, pancytopenia, arthritis, vasculitis, and cryoglobulinemia (all rare)

REFERENCES
1. Centers for Disease Control and Prevention. Hepatitis A questions and answers for health professionals. http://www.cdc.gov/hepatitis/hav/havfaq.htm. Accessed August 18, 2015.
2. Almashhwari AA, Ahmed KT, Rahman RN, et al. Liver diseases in pregnancy: diseases not unique to pregnancy. *World J Gastroenterol*. 2013;19(43): 7630–7638.
3. Matheny SC, Kingery JE. Hepatitis A. *Am Fam Physician*. 2012;86(11):1027–1034.
4. Irving GJ, Holden J, Yang R, et al. Hepatitis A immunisation in persons not previously exposed to hepatitis A. *Cochrane Database Syst Rev*. 2012;(7):CD009051.
5. Liu JP, Nikolova D, Fei Y. Immunoglobulins for preventing hepatitis A. *Cochrane Database Syst Rev*. 2009;(2):CD004181.
6. Fiore AE, Wasley A, Bell BP. Prevention of hepatitis A through active or passive immunization: recommendations of the Advisory Committee on Immunization Practices (ACIP). *MMWR Recomm Rep*. 2006;55(RR-7):1–23.
7. Victor JC, Monto AS, Surdina TY, et al. Hepatitis A vaccine versus immune globulin for postexposure prophylaxis. *N Engl J Med*. 2007;357(17):1685–1694.

 SEE ALSO

- Hepatitis B; Hepatitis C
- Algorithm: Hyperbilirubinemia, Cirrhosis, and Jaundice

CODES

ICD10
B15.9 Hepatitis A without hepatic coma

CLINICAL PEARLS
- HAV disease severity directly correlates with age; children are often asymptomatic.
- HAV vaccine is indicated for all children, travelers, those at elevated risk of disease, and anyone with liver impairment.
- Check HAV IgG in all HIV-positive patients; provide HAV vaccine to those who are negative.
- Treatment of acute disease is supportive
- Give postexposure prophylaxis to eligible patients within 14 days of exposure

HEPATITIS B
Jason Chao, MD, MS

BASICS

DESCRIPTION
Systemic viral infection associated with acute and chronic liver disease and hepatocellular carcinoma (HCC)

EPIDEMIOLOGY
Incidence
- Predominant age: can infect patients of all ages
- Predominant sex: fulminant hepatitis B virus (HBV): male > female (2:1)
- In the United States, estimated 38,000 new infections in 2009, 70% due to IV drug use
- African Americans have the highest rate of acute HBV infection in the United States.
- Overall rate of new infections is down 82% since 1991 (due to national immunization strategy).
- U.S. vaccine coverage for the birth dose of HBV increased from 68.6% in 2011 to 71.6% in 2012.

Prevalence
- In the United States, 800,000 to 1.4 million people have chronic HBV.
- Asia and the Pacific Islands have the largest populations at risk for HBV.
- Chronic HBV worldwide: 350 to 400 million persons
  - 1 million deaths annually
    - Second most important carcinogen (behind tobacco)
    - Of chronic carriers with active disease, 25% die due to complications of cirrhosis or HCC.
    - Of chronic carriers, 75% are Asian.

ETIOLOGY AND PATHOPHYSIOLOGY
HBV is a DNA virus of the *Hepadnaviridae* family. Highly infectious via blood and secretions for at least a week outside the body.

Genetics
Family history of HBV and/or HCC

RISK FACTORS
- Screen the following high-risk groups for HBV with HBsAg/sAb. Vaccinate if seronegative (1)[A]:
  - Persons born in endemic areas (45% of world)
  - Hemodialysis patients
  - IV drug users (IVDUs), past or present
  - Men who have sex with men (MSM)
  - HIV- and HCV-positive patients
  - Household members of HBsAg carriers
  - Sexual contacts of HBsAg carriers
  - Inmates of correctional facilities
  - Patients with chronically elevated aspartate aminotransferase/alanine aminotransferase (AST/ALT)
- Additional risk factors:
  - Needle stick/occupational exposure
  - Recipients of blood/products; transplanted organ recipients
  - Intranasal drug users
  - Body piercing/tattoos
  - Survivors of sexual assault

Pediatric Considerations
- Shorter acute course; fewer complications
- 90% of vertical/perinatal infections become chronic.

Pregnancy Considerations
- Screen all prenatal patients for HBsAg (1)[A].
- Consider treating patients with high viral load at 28 weeks with oral nucleos(t)ide medicines beginning at 32 weeks to reduce perinatal transmission (2)[C].

Marker	Acute Infection	Chronic Infection	Inactive Carrier	Resolved Infection	Susceptible to Infection	Vaccinated
HBsAg	+	+	+	−	−	−
HBsAb	−	−	−	+	−	+
HBcAb	+IgM	−IgM; +total/IgG	+	+	−	−
HBeAg	+	±	−	−	−	−
HBeAb	−	±	+	±	−	−
HBV DNA	Present	Present	Low–negative	−	−	−
ALT	Marked elevation	Normal to mildly elevated	Normal	Normal	Normal	Normal

- Infants born to HBV-infected mothers require HB immune globulin (HBIg) (0.5 mL) and HBV vaccine within 12 hours of birth.
- Breastfeeding is safe if HBIg and HBV vaccine are administered and the areolar complex is without fissures or open sores. Oral nucleos(t)ide medications are not recommended during lactation.
- HIV coinfection significantly increases risk of vertical transmission.
- Continue medications if pregnancy occurs while on an oral antiviral therapy to prevent acute flare.

GENERAL PREVENTION
Most effective: HBV vaccination series (three doses)
- Vaccinate
  - All infants at birth and during well-child care visits
  - All at-risk patients (see "Risk Factors")
  - Health care and public safety workers
  - Sexual contacts of HBsAg carriers
  - Household contacts of HBsAg carriers
- Proper hygiene/sanitation by health care workers, IVDU, and tattoo/piercing artists
  - Barrier precautions, needle disposal, sterilize equipment, cover open cuts
- Do not share personal items exposed to blood (e.g., nail clipper, razor, toothbrush).
- Safe sexual practices (condoms)
- HBsAg carriers cannot donate blood or tissue.
- Postexposure (e.g., needle stick): HBIg 0.06 mL/kg in <24 hours in addition to vaccination

COMMONLY ASSOCIATED CONDITIONS
HIV coinfection, hepatitis C coinfection

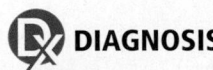

DIAGNOSIS

HISTORY
- Exposure: detailed family and social history
- Acute HBV
  - Fever, malaise, fatigue, arthralgias, myalgias
  - Anorexia, nausea, vomiting
  - Jaundice, scleral icterus
  - Dark urine, pale stools
  - Right upper quadrant (RUQ) abdominal pain
- Chronic HBV: typically asymptomatic

PHYSICAL EXAM
Acute: ill; jaundice/scleral icterus; RUQ tenderness; hepatomegaly

DIFFERENTIAL DIAGNOSIS
- Epstein-Barr virus (EBV); cytomegalovirus (CMV); hepatitis A, C, or E
- Drug-induced, alcoholic, or autoimmune hepatitis
- Wilson disease or rheumatologic/immunologic disorders

DIAGNOSTIC TESTS & INTERPRETATION
Initial Tests (lab, imaging)
- AST/ALT: markedly elevated in acute HBV (particularly ALT), with levels in the hundreds to several thousand IU/mL. Transaminases may be normal or mildly elevated in chronic HBV:
  - Transaminases elevate before bilirubin
- Bilirubin (conjugated/unconjugated): normal to markedly elevated in acute HBV
  - Last test to normalize as acute infection resolves
- Alkaline phosphatase: mild elevation
- HBcAb IgM may be the only early finding ("window period," before HBsAg turns positive)
- For acute hepatitis:
  - Monitor PT, albumin, electrolytes, glucose, and CBC.
  - If severe acute HBV, check for superinfection with hepatitis D (HDV Ag and HDV Ab)
  - Hepatitis B serologic markers
- Hepatitis B e-antigen (HBeAg+) indicates high replication/infectivity; confirmed with high HBV DNA (≥10^5 copies/mL); these patients benefit from medical therapy.
- HBV precore mutants have undetectable HBeAg despite active viral replication (confirm with HBV DNA level) as well as antibody to e-antigen (HBeAb+).
- Screen for HDV, HIV, HCV, and immunity to hepatitis A virus (HAV Ab total/IgG).
- Ultrasound to document ascites, organomegaly, signs of portal hypertension, hepatic or portal obstruction, and to screen for HCC
- Contrast CT or MRI if ultrasound is abnormal or if α-fetoprotein (AFP) is elevated.

Follow-Up Tests & Special Considerations
HBsAg+ persistence >6 months defines chronic HBV:
- Measure HBV DNA level and ALT every 3 to 6 months.
- If age >40 years and ALT borderline or mildly elevated, consider liver biopsy.
- Measure baseline AFP.
- Follow HBeAg for elimination (every 6 to 12 months)
- Lifetime monitoring for progression, need for treatment, and screening for HCC

Diagnostic Procedures/Other
- Liver biopsy
- Noninvasive tests (Hepascore, Fibrotest) or measure of elastography (Fibroscan) to assess for hepatic fibrosis.

Test Interpretation
Liver biopsy in chronic HBV may show interface hepatitis and inflammation, necrosis, cholestasis, fibrosis, cirrhosis, or chronic active hepatitis.

TREATMENT

GENERAL MEASURES
- Vaccinate for HAV if seronegative
- Monitor CBC, coagulation, electrolytes, glucose, renal function, and phosphate.
- Monitor ALT and HBV DNA; increased ALT and reduced DNA implies response to therapy.
- Screen for HCC if HBsAg+.

MEDICATION
First Line
- Acute HBV
  - Supportive care; spontaneously resolves in 95% of immunocompetent adults
  - Antiviral therapy not indicated except for fulminant liver failure or immunosuppressed.

Chronic Hepatitis B Therapy

HBeAg	HBV DNA viral load	ALT*	Recommend
(+)	≥20,000 IU/mL	Elevated	Treat with antiviral or interferon
(−)	≥2,000 IU/mL	Elevated	Consider biopsy or serum fibrosis marker and treatment.
(+)	≤20,000 IU/mL	Any	Monitor q6–12mo
(−)	≥2,000 IU/mL	Normal	Biopsy; treat if disease
(+)	≥20,000 IU/mL	Normal	Observe, consider treatment if ALT elevated. Biopsy if age >40 years or ALT is high normal to mild elevation.
(−)	≤2,000 IU/mL	Any	Monitor q6–12mo
Cirrhosis	Any	Any	Treat with mono or combination treatment.
Liver failure	Any	Any	Treat + refer for transplant

*ALT elevated if >2 × ULN; ULN for male = 30 IU/mL and for female = 19 IU/mL.

- Chronic HBV: Treatment is based on HBeAg status:
  - FDA-approved drugs: lamivudine 100 mg, adefovir 10 mg, entecavir 0.5 to 1 mg, telbivudine 600 mg, or tenofovir 300 mg, all given PO every day (dose based on renal function); pegylated interferon (peg-IFN) α2a, α2b SC weekly (3)[A]
- Entecavir, tenofovir, and peg-IFN are preferred first-line agents (3)[A].
- Extended oral agents regimens indicated (3)[A]:
  - If HBeAg+, treat 6 to 12 months post loss of HBeAg and gain of HBeAb, and monitor after cessation.
  - If HBeAg−, treat indefinitely or until HBsAg clearance and HBsAb development.
- Change/add drug based on resistance:
  - Confirm patient adherence with medications before assuming resistance.
  - Adherence to therapy lowers rate of resistance.
- Adjust dosing for renal function
- Peg-IFN preferred to standard interferon:
  - Weekly peg-IFN (Pegasys) injections for 48 weeks
  - Most efficacious for genotype A
  - Contraindicated if decompensated cirrhosis
- Goals of therapy: undetectable HBV DNA, normal ALT, loss of HBeAg, gain of HBeAb; loss of HBsAg and gain of HBsAb
- Precautions:
  - Oral drugs: renal insufficiency
  - Peg-IFN: coagulopathy, myelosuppression, depression/suicidal ideation

Second Line
Emtricitabine suppresses viral load; not FDA approved.

ISSUES FOR REFERRAL
- Refer all persistent HBsAg+ patients to have them evaluated for antiviral therapy.
- Refer immediately to liver transplant program if fulminant acute hepatitis, end-stage liver disease, or HCC

SURGERY/OTHER PROCEDURES
Liver transplantation, operative resection, radiofrequency ablation for HCC

INPATIENT CONSIDERATIONS
Admission Criteria/Initial Stabilization
- Worsening course (marked increase in bilirubin, transaminases, or symptoms)
- Hepatic failure (high PT, encephalopathy)

ONGOING CARE

FOLLOW-UP RECOMMENDATIONS
Patient Monitoring
- Monitor serial ALT and HBV DNA:
  - High ALT + low HBV DNA associated with favorable response to therapy
- Serologic markers: See table.
- CBC to monitor WBC and platelets for patients on interferon therapy
- Monitor HBV DNA q3–6mo during therapy:
  - Undetectable DNA at week 24 of oral drug therapy associated with low resistance at year 2
- Monitor for complications (ascites, encephalopathy, variceal bleed) in cirrhosis.
- Recommend vaccination for all household contacts and sexual partners.
- Ultrasound q6–12mo to screen for HCC starting at age 40 years in men and age 50 in women (3)[B].

DIET
Avoid alcohol.

PATIENT EDUCATION
- Acute HBV
  - Review transmission precautions.
- Chronic HBV
  - Alcohol and tobacco use accelerate progression
  - Strict medication compliance to prevent flare

- Patient education materials in English and others, including many Asian languages, available at http://www.cdc.gov/hepatitis/Resources/PatientEdMaterials.htm

PROGNOSIS
- Acute infection: 95% of adults recover
- Severity of encephalopathy predicts survival in fulminant hepatic failure
- Acute HBV: mortality 1%
- Acute HBV + HDV: mortality 2–20%
- Chronic HBV
  - Spontaneous resolution: 0.5% per year
  - Premature death from cirrhosis or HCC: 25%
  - Risk of HCC rises with rate of viral replication, even if no cirrhosis

COMPLICATIONS
- Acute or subacute hepatic necrosis; cirrhosis; hepatic failure
- HCC (all chronic HBV patients are at risk)
- Severe flare of chronic HBV with corticosteroids and other immunosuppressants: Avoid if possible.
- Reactivation of resolved infection if immunosuppressed (e.g., chemotherapy): premedicate prophylactically if HBsAg+ or if HBcAb+ and receiving systemic chemotherapy (1)[A]

REFERENCES
1. Weinbaum CM, Williams I, Mast EE, et al. Recommendations for identification and public health management of persons with chronic hepatitis B virus infection. *MMWR Recomm Rep.* 2008;57(RR-8):1–20.
2. Borgia G, Carleo MA, Gaeta GB, et al. Hepatitis B in pregnancy. *World J Gastroenterol.* 2012;18(34):4677–4683.
3. McMahon BJ. Chronic hepatitis B virus infection. *Med Clin North Am.* 2014;98(1):39–54.

ADDITIONAL READING
Centers for Disease Control and Prevention. Updated CDC recommendations for the management of hepatitis B virus–infected health-care providers and students. *MMWR Recomm Rep.* 2012;61(RR-3):1–12.

SEE ALSO
- Cirrhosis of the Liver; Hepatitis A; Hepatitis C
- Algorithm: Hyperbilirubinemia, Cirrhosis, and Jaundice

CODES

ICD10
- B19.10 Unspecified viral hepatitis B without hepatic coma
- B16.9 Acute hepatitis B w/o delta-agent and without hepatic coma
- B18.1 Chronic viral hepatitis B without delta-agent

CLINICAL PEARLS
- All patients born in endemic countries should be screened for HBV infection with HBsAg.
- Patients with chronic HBV need lifetime monitoring for disease progression and HCC.
- HBV is the second most common worldwide carcinogen (behind tobacco).

HEPATITIS C

Christopher Lin-Brande, MD • Amy M. Davis, MD • Krunal Patel, MD

BASICS

DESCRIPTION
Systemic viral infection (acute and chronic) primarily involving liver

EPIDEMIOLOGY
- Highest incidence ages 20 to 39; highest prevalence ages 40 to 59
- Males and non-Hispanic blacks more likely to be infected (1).

Geriatric Considerations
Age >60 years less likely to respond to therapy; treat earlier if able.

Pregnancy Considerations
- Routine HCV testing is not indicated.
- Vertical transmission occurs in 6 of every 100 births in HCV-positive mothers; risk increases 2 to 3 times if HIV coinfection.
- Breastfeeding is safe if no fissures.

Pediatric Considerations
- Prevalence: 0.3%
- Test children born to HCV-positive mothers with HCV Ab after 18 months or HCV RNA at 1 to 2 months for early diagnosis.
- Fewer symptoms; fewer abnormal liver tests; more likely to clear spontaneously; slower rate of progression

Incidence
In 2013, CDC estimated there were 29,718 total new cases of hepatitis C. 2,138 of these were new acute cases.

Prevalence
- ~3.6 million in the United States (1.3%) are HCV Ab-positive.
- Prevalence is highest in persons born between 1945 and 1965 (2.6%) (1).
- 2.7 million have chronic HCV (HCV RNA-positive).
- HCV-related deaths are more common than HIV-related deaths.
- Most common cause of chronic liver disease and transplantation in the United States
- Six genotypes (GT) were known. GT 1 is predominant form in the United States (75%). GT does not change during infection and predicts response to treatment.

ETIOLOGY AND PATHOPHYSIOLOGY
Single-stranded RNA virus of *Flaviviridae* family

RISK FACTORS
- Exposure risks
  - Chronic hemodialysis
  - Blood/blood product transfusion or organ transplantation before July 1992
  - Hemophilia treatment before 1987
  - Household or health care–related exposure to HCV-infected body fluids (1.8% risk)
  - Children born to HCV-positive mothers
  - Adults born between 1945 and 1965
- Risk behaviors and/or medical conditions
  - Prior history of injection drug use
  - Intranasal illicit drug use
  - History of incarceration
  - Tattooing in unregulated settings
  - Current sexual partners of HCV-positive persons
  - HIV and hepatitis B infection

GENERAL PREVENTION
- *Primary prevention*
  - Do not share razors/toothbrushes/nail clippers.
  - Use and dispose needles properly through harm-reduction programs.
  - Practice safer sex.
  - Cover cuts and sores.
- *Secondary prevention*
  - No vaccine or postexposure prophylaxis available
  - Substance abuse treatment
  - Reinforce use of barrier contraception for HIV-seropositive coinfected with HCV.
  - Assess for degree of liver fibrosis/cirrhosis.

COMMONLY ASSOCIATED CONDITIONS
Diabetes, metabolic syndrome, iron overload, depression, substance abuse/recovery, autoimmune and hematologic disease, HIV, and hepatitis B coinfection

DIAGNOSIS

HISTORY
- Determine exposure risk: *detailed* social history including alcohol and IV drug use, psychiatric and medical comorbidities, coinfections
- Chronic HCV: Most cases are mildly symptomatic (nonspecific fatigue) or asymptomatic elevated ALT/aspartate aminotransferase (AST).
- Acute HCV: *If* symptoms develop (rare)
  - Onset typically 4 to 12 weeks postexposure
  - Jaundice, dark urine, steatorrhea, nausea, abdominal pain (right upper quadrant), fatigue, low-grade fevers, myalgias, arthralgias
  - 15–40% resolve; rest progress to chronic hepatitis C

PHYSICAL EXAM
- Typically normal unless advanced fibrosis/cirrhosis
- May have right upper quadrant (RUQ) tenderness/hepatomegaly
- General signs of chronic liver disease: spider angioma, caput medusa, palmar erythema, jaundice, gynecomastia, Terry nails, ascites
- Extrahepatic manifestations: arthralgias/myalgias, neuropathy, glomerulonephritis, livedo reticularis, lichen planus, pruritus, sicca syndrome, cold agglutinin disease

DIFFERENTIAL DIAGNOSIS
Hepatitis A or B; Epstein-Barr virus (EBV), cytomegalovirus (CMV); alcoholic hepatitis; nonalcoholic steatohepatitis (NASH); hemochromatosis; Wilson disease, α1–antitrypsin deficiency; ischemic, drug-induced, or autoimmune hepatitis

DIAGNOSTIC TESTS & INTERPRETATION
Initial Tests (lab, imaging)
- Screening is recommended for adults born between 1945 and 1965, anyone with exposure risks, current and former IV drug users, HIV-positive individuals, especially men who have sex with men (MSM) and patients with persistently elevated ALT.
- CDC algorithm
  - HCV Ab
    - If nonreactive, no further action unless recent exposure is suspected (HCV RNA).
    - If reactive, test HCV RNA and genotype.
  - HCV RNA
    - If not detected, no current HCV infection. No further action in most cases but can repeat either test if recent exposure suspected
    - If detected, that there is current HCV infection, counsel and treat.
- HCV Ab can be detected 4 to 10 weeks after infection.
- HCV RNA can be detected 2 to 3 weeks after infection.
- RNA detectability precedes ALT elevation.

- AST/ALT: often normal but may be persistently elevated in chronic HCV; ALT usually is 1 to 2 times upper limit of normal; AST may be normal/elevated, but typically less so than ALT.
  - Acute hepatitis C can cause elevation of transaminases and bilirubin (direct and indirect).
- AST/ALT ratio ≥1 associated with cirrhosis
  - If AST/ALT ratio >2, rule out alcohol abuse.
- Persistent HCV RNA >6 months = chronic HCV

Follow-Up Tests & Special Considerations
- Platelets, creatinine, TSH, vitamin D (may predict treatment response)
- Liver function panel, coagulation factors
- HCV GT
- IL28B testing: C/C homozygote more likely to clear
- HBV (hepatitis panel) and HIV coinfection
- Vaccinate if seronegative for hepatitis A/B.
- Pneumococcal polysaccharide vaccine (PPSV23)

Diagnostic Procedures/Other
Evaluate for advanced hepatic fibrosis.
- Indirect markers: AST-to-platelet ratio index (APRI), FIB-4, FibroIndex, Forns index, HepaScore/FibroScore, FibroSure
  - Factors such as age, gender, AST, ALT, platelets, bilirubin, estimate fibrosis.
- Direct markers: FIBROSpect II
- Liver imaging: US, CT scan, MRI, transient ultrasound elastography, MR elastography
- Liver biopsy (gold standard)
  - Indications: discordant indirect marker results, concurrent non-HCV liver disease, elastography not available
  - Not necessary to diagnose hepatocellular carcinoma if diagnosis is clear based on imaging

Test Interpretation
- Biopsy measures grade (degree of inflammation) and stage (amount of existing fibrosis)
- Scoring systems: Batts and Ludwig, METAVIR, International Association for the Study of the Liver (IASL)

TREATMENT

GENERAL MEASURES
- Report acute cases of HCV to health department.
- Consider treating all patients with virologic evidence of HCV.
- Pretreatment counseling should include thorough behavioral health and substance abuse history.
- Optimize medical therapy for comorbid conditions prior to treatment.
- Discuss treatment plan and likelihood of success based on individual factors such as BMI, genotype, race, stage of fibrosis, and viral load.
- Treatment evolution of HCV (2)
  - Pegylated-interferon (PEG) plus ribavirin (RBV) regimens in the 1990s: ~50% cure (may still be used for directly-acting antiviral agent [DAA] nonresponders)
  - Combination PEG/RBV plus DAA in early 2000s: ~75% cure
  - All-oral DAAs in the last 4 years: >95% cure
- New therapies increasingly all-oral, including DAAs and host-targeting antiviral agents (HTAs)
- Goal is sustained virologic response (SVR): undetectable HCV RNA after 12 to 24 weeks of treatment.
- HCV cascade: Of those with chronic HCV, only 50% are diagnosed, 25% are HCV RNA confirmed, 15% are prescribed treatment, and 10% achieve SVR (3).

MEDICATION

First Line

Acute HCV: Treatment may be delayed 12 to 16 weeks after suspected inoculation to allow chance for spontaneous clearance. Regimen is same as for chronic HCV.

Genotype	Drug Regimen
1a[a]	Ledipasvir/sofosbuvir (Harvoni) for 12 weeks
	Ombitasvir/paritaprevir/ritonavir plus dasabuvir (Viekira Pak) and weight-based RBV (Rebetol) for 12 weeks (no cirrhosis) or 24 weeks (cirrhosis)
	Sofosbuvir (Sovaldi) plus simeprevir (Olysio) with or without weight-based RBV for 12 weeks (no cirrhosis) or 24 weeks (cirrhosis)
1b[a]	Ledipasvir/sofosbuvir for 12 weeks
	Ombitasvir/paritaprevir/ritonavir plus dasabuvir for 12 weeks (no cirrhosis) or with the addition of weight-based RBV for 24 weeks (cirrhosis)
	Sofosbuvir plus simeprevir for 12 weeks (no cirrhosis) or 24 weeks (cirrhosis)
2	Sofosbuvir plus weight-based RBV for 12 weeks (no cirrhosis) or for 16 weeks (cirrhosis)
3	Sofosbuvir plus weight-based RBV for 24 weeks
4[a]	Ledipasvir/sofosbuvir for 12 weeks
	Ombitasvir/paritaprevir/ritonavir plus dasabuvir and weight-based RBV for 12 weeks
	Sofosbuvir plus weight-based RBV for 24 weeks
5	Sofosbuvir plus pegylated interferon plus weight-based RBV for 12 weeks
6	Ledipasvir/sofosbuvir for 12 weeks

AASLD, American Association for the Study of Liver Diseases; RBV, ribavirin.

[a]Three options with similar effectiveness.

ISSUES FOR REFERRAL

- Involve a physician experienced with HCV therapy in all cases.
- Refer to liver transplant program if fulminant acute hepatitis, at first complication of end-stage disease, MELD score ≥12 or at diagnosis of HCC.

COMPLEMENTARY & ALTERNATIVE MEDICINE

No evidence for effective complementary therapy in HCV/cirrhosis/HCC. Milk thistle (silymarin) safe; may reduce ALT, does not eradicate virus or improve outcomes; avoid on IFN.

ONGOING CARE

FOLLOW-UP RECOMMENDATIONS

- Treat early to prevent fibrosis. If cirrhosis is already present, treatment may not prevent decompensation.
- If treatment is deferred, screen patients with annual LFTs, monitor for disease progression, and maintain sobriety (if alcohol dependence involved).
- Monitor serial viral load only if on antiviral therapy.
- Abdominal ultrasound every 6 to 12 months to monitor for hepatocellular carcinoma (expert opinion). AFP is no longer in AASLD guidelines.

Patient Monitoring

- Serial ALT/AST; fasting glucose and CBCs
- Follow electrolytes, thyroid-stimulating hormone (TSH), renal function, PT.
- For 12-week course, follow-up 4 weeks after starting therapy and 12 weeks after completing therapy
  - 4-week HCV RNA: If detectable, recheck at week 6. If RNA has increased >10 times, stop therapy.
  - SVR12: Undetectable HCV RNA 12 weeks after completing therapy generally translates to long-term cure (goal of therapy).
- SVR decreases risk of portal hypertension, hepatic decompensation, and hepatocellular carcinoma (HCC). Monitor for decompensation (low albumin, ascites, encephalopathy, GI bleed).

DIET

- Low-fat, high-fiber diet and exercise to treat obesity/fatty liver
- Extra protein and fluids while on IFN therapy

PATIENT EDUCATION

- Avoid alcohol, tobacco, and illicit drugs (including marijuana); refer to rehabilitation/12-step program and monitor for relapse as appropriate.
- Warn against claims of false cures.
- Caution with nutritional supplements and hepatotoxic medications (may contain hepatotoxins).
- http://www.cdc.gov/knowmorehepatitis/

PROGNOSIS

- For every 100 persons infected with HCV
  - 75 to 85 will develop chronic infection.
  - 60 to 70 will develop chronic liver disease.
  - 10 to 20 will develop cirrhosis over 20 to 30 years (more rapid if older age at infection, male gender, alcohol/substance abuse, HIV/HBV coinfection, or diabetes/insulin resistance).
    - 1–5% annual risk of HCC
    - 3–6% annual risk of hepatic decompensation
- Chronic HCV is curable in ~70% of cases; in non-cirrhotic genotype 2 or 3, cure rate is ~90%.

COMPLICATIONS

- Fibrosis and cirrhosis typically develop within the first 5 to 10 years of infection.
- Acute/subacute hepatic necrosis, liver failure, hepatocellular carcinoma, transplant and complications, death
- Risk factors for cirrhosis: age, white race, hypertension, alcohol use, anemia. Risk for decompensation: diabetes, hypertension, anemia

REFERENCES

1. Denniston MM, Jiles RB, Drobeniuc J, et al. Chronic hepatitis C virus infection in the United States, National Health and Nutrition Examination Survey 2003 to 2010. Ann Intern Med. 2014;160(5): 293–300.
2. Lange CM, Jacobson IM, Rice CM, et al. Emerging therapies for the treatment of hepatitis C. EMBO Mol Med. 2014;6(1):4–15.
3. Yehia BR, Schranz AJ, Umscheid CA, et al. The treatment cascade for chronic hepatitis C virus infection in the United States: a systematic review and meta-analysis. PLoS One. 2014;9(7):e101554.

ADDITIONAL READING

- American Association for the Study of Liver Diseases. HCV guidelines: recommendations for testing, managing, and treating hepatitis c. http://www.hcvguidelines.org/
- Centers for Disease Control and Prevention. Viral hepatitis—hepatitis c information. http://www.cdc.gov/hepatitis/hcv/

SEE ALSO

Hepatitis A; Hepatitis B; Cirrhosis of the Liver; HIV/AIDS

CODES

ICD10

- B19.20 Unspecified viral hepatitis C without hepatic coma
- B17.10 Acute hepatitis C without hepatic coma
- B18.2 Chronic viral hepatitis C

CLINICAL PEARLS

- 1 of every 10 patients with hepatitis C has no identifiable risk factors.
- 15–25% of HCV-infected persons spontaneously resolve infection without specific treatment.
- Look for coinfections (HBV/HIV) and comorbid substance abuse in patients infected with HCV.

H

HERNIA
Margaret Fairhurst, DO

 BASICS

DESCRIPTION
Hernias are areas of weakness or frank disruption of the fibromuscular tissues of the body wall through which intracavity structures pass.

- Types
  - Inguinal
    - Direct inguinal: acquired; herniation through defect in transversalis fascia of abdominal wall medial to inferior epigastric vessels; increased frequency with age as fascia weakens
    - Indirect inguinal: congenital; herniation lateral to the inferior epigastric vessels through internal inguinal ring into inguinal canal. A "complete hernia" is one that descends into the scrotum, whereas an "incomplete hernia" remains within the inguinal canal.
  - Pantaloon: combination of direct and indirect inguinal hernia with protrusion of abdominal wall on both sides of the epigastric vessels
  - Femoral: herniation that descends through the femoral canal deep to the inguinal ligament. Because of the narrow neck of a femoral hernia, this type of hernia is especially prone to incarceration and strangulation.
  - Incisional or ventral: herniation through a defect in the anterior abdominal wall at the site of a prior surgical incision
  - Congenital: herniation through fascial defect in abdominal wall, secondary to collagen deficiency disease
  - Umbilical: Defect occurs at umbilical ring tissue.
  - Epigastric: protrusion through the linea alba above the level of the umbilicus. These may develop at exit points of small paramidline nerves and vessels, or through an area of congenital weakness in the linea alba.
  - Interparietal (e.g., Spigelian hernia): Hernia sac insinuates itself between layers of the abdominal wall; strangulation common, often mistaken for tumor or abscess.
  - Other: obturator, sciatic, perineal
- Definitions
  - Reducible: Extruded sac and its contents can be returned to original intra-abdominal position, either spontaneously or with gentle manual manipulation.
  - Irreducible/incarcerated: Extruded sac and its contents cannot be returned to original intra-abdominal position.
  - Strangulated: Blood supply to hernia sac contents is compromised.
  - Richter: Partial circumference of the bowel is incarcerated or strangulated. Partial wall damage may occur, increasing potential for bowel rupture and peritonitis.
  - Sliding: wall of a viscus forms part of the wall of the inguinal hernia sac (i.e., R-cecum, L-sigmoid colon)

Geriatric Considerations
Abdominal wall hernias increase with advancing age, with significant increase in risk during surgical repair.

Pregnancy Considerations
- Increased intra-abdominal pressure and hormone imbalances with pregnancy may contribute to increased risk of abdominal wall hernias.
- Umbilical hernias are associated with multiple, prolonged deliveries.

EPIDEMIOLOGY
Incidence
- 75–80% groin hernias: inguinal and femoral
- 2–20% incisional/ventral, depending on whether a prior surgery was associated with infection or contamination
- 3–10% umbilical, considered congenital
- 1–3% other
- Groin
  - 6–27% lifetime risk in adult men
  - Two-peak theory: most inguinal hernias present before 1 year of age or after 55 years of age
  - ~50% of children <2 years of age will have a patent processus vaginalis, decreasing to 40% after age 2 years. Only between 25% and 50% will become clinically significant.
  - Inguinal hernia found in <5% of newborns but male-to-female ratio is 10:1.
  - Increased incidence in premature infants
  - Increased incidence in patients with abdominal aortic aneurysms
  - Femoral <10% of all groin hernias, 40% present as a surgical emergency
- Incisional/ventral: ~10–23% of abdominal surgeries complicated by an incisional hernia, most common in upper midline incisions.
- Incidence ratio: male = female
- Umbilical: 10–20% of newborns; most close by 5 years of age

Prevalence
- Groin and inguinal hernias are more prevalent in men.
- Femoral and umbilical hernias are more prevalent in women.
- Most inguinal hernias are indirect in both genders.
- Incisional/ventral hernias are more prevalent in obese persons, as well as in smokers. The opposite may be true for inguinal hernias.

ETIOLOGY AND PATHOPHYSIOLOGY
Loss of tissue strength and elasticity, especially with aging or congenital defect in abdominal fascia resulting in a defect in the fascia of the abdominal wall. Most pediatric hernias are congenital defects (e.g., patent processus vaginalis), whereas most adult hernias are a result of acquired weakness in the tissues of the anterior abdominal wall.

Genetics
No known genetic pattern

RISK FACTORS
- Increased abdominal pressure, coughing, heavy lifting, constipation, pregnancy, ascites, prostatism, obesity, advancing age (loss of tissue turgor), smoking, steroid use, low birth weight, prematurity
- Age: Femoral and scrotal hernias, along with recurrent groin hernias, are associated with increased risk for acute hernia surgery.

COMMONLY ASSOCIATED CONDITIONS
Obesity, chronic obstructive pulmonary disease, multiple abdominal surgeries, pregnancy, advanced age, Ehlers-Danlos syndrome, Marfan syndrome, polycystic kidney disease (PKD), osteogenesis imperfecta, Down syndrome, abdominal aortic aneurysm

 DIAGNOSIS

HISTORY
- Pain, nausea, vomiting, bloating; relieved with reclining; many are asymptomatic.
- May observe protrusion through abdominal wall during increased intra-abdominal pressure (Valsalva maneuver or cough)

PHYSICAL EXAM
- Exam should initially occur with patient standing. During palpation, the patient should be instructed to cough, strain, or perform Valsalva maneuver so the extent of intracavity content movement can be appreciated. Exam should also be performed with patient in supine position.
- Inguinal (superior to inguinal ligament)
  - Direct inguinal hernia: Finger in inguinal canal finds defect of the transversalis fascia as a deep (posterior to anterior) bulge palpated by pad of finger with increased intra-abdominal pressure.
  - Indirect inguinal hernia: Finger in inguinal canal finds a persistent process vaginalis as a bulge (lateral to medial) palpated by fingertip; it may extend down into scrotum.
- Femoral (inferior to inguinal ligament): bulge in upper middle thigh; neck of the sac will protrude lateral to and below a finger placed on the pubic tubercle.
- Umbilical: palpable protrusion at umbilicus
- Incisional/ventral: palpable protrusion at site of prior abdominal incision or midline superior to the umbilicus
- Epigastric: palpable protrusion that occurs off midline above umbilicus

DIFFERENTIAL DIAGNOSIS
Lymphadenopathy, hydrocele, lipoma, varices, cryptorchidism, abscess, tumor, sports hernia (athletic pubalgia), pelvic fractures, adductor tears, omphalomesenteric duct, urachal cyst

DIAGNOSTIC TESTS & INTERPRETATION
Hernia evaluation rarely requires imaging; reserve for suspected abdominal hernia or unclear diagnosis. Plain radiographs to rule out obstruction
- Ultrasound (US) can be used to assess inguinal hernias.
- CT or tangential radiography for incisional and abdominal wall hernias and postsurgical patients with complaints of abdominal pain
- Herniography is no longer recommended.

Pediatric Considerations
There is insufficient evidence for contralateral exploration in pediatric patients, except using US.

Follow-Up Tests & Special Considerations
For occult hernias not well appreciated on exam or with imaging, diagnostic laparoscopy may be beneficial.

 TREATMENT

- Elective setting
  - Elective surgical repair is associated with significantly lower morbidity and mortality.
- Acute setting
  - Pain management is recommended for symptomatic hernias.
  - Strangulated hernias should be surgically repaired as early as possible to prevent complications such as necrosis and viscus perforation.

– Manual reduction of incarcerated hernia improves outcomes by allowing for elective repair after reduction of acute swelling and inflammation.
– Complication rate is nearly 20 times greater in emergent repair of pediatric inguinal hernias than elective procedure.
– Acute hernia repair carries a higher morbidity and lower survival rate.
– Laparoscopic repair of incisional/ventral hernia (IVH) is safe, with fewer complications and shorter hospital stays and possibly a shorter surgical time. However, postoperative pain and recurrence rates are similar for both techniques.
– For patients undergoing repair, operative times are shorter for laparoscopic totally extraperitoneal repair then with open mesh repair and without any difference in complication rates (1)[B].

MEDICATION
- Antibiotics: Antibiotic prophylaxis did not reduce wound infections after groin hernia repairs.
- Pain: Local anesthetic during surgical repair results in significant reduction of postoperative pain. Tension-free procedures, such as Lichtenstein, may be performed under local anesthesia.

ADDITIONAL THERAPIES
Geriatric Considerations
Use of a truss (external supportive device) for direct inguinal hernias is common; no data exist regarding efficacy.

ISSUES FOR REFERRAL
Warn patients of symptoms or signs of incarceration or strangulation (acute abdominal pain, fever, bloody bowel movements), which mandate immediate self-referral to emergency room.

SURGERY/OTHER PROCEDURES
All inguinal hernias should be surgically repaired, but watchful waiting in the asymptomatic patient is a safe option if significant comorbidities may compromise emergent repair.

- Incarceration and strangulation are absolute indications for hernia repair.
- Contraindications: patients who are not surgical candidates based on cardiovascular risk factors
  – Elective repair should be avoided in pregnant patients or those with active infections.
- Special considerations
  – Umbilical hernias <0.5 cm usually obliterate and can be managed by observation.
  – Umbilical hernias in children age 2 to 4 years may be observed, as there is a high rate of spontaneous closure.
  – Operative times and complication rates are similar when comparing single-incision laparoscopic inguinal hernia repair versus traditional multiport laparoscopic repair (2)[B].
  – "Watchful waiting" is recommended in pregnancy. Elective postpartum hernia repair provided similar results to the nonpregnant population without increased risk of incarceration or strangulation before or during delivery.
  – Women had lower recurrence rates with laparoscopic methods than with Lichtenstein open method.
  – Ascites is not a strict contraindication for surgical repair. There is a greater risk of strangulation and complication without repair than the increased risks associated with repair in the presence of ascites.
  – The more emergent hernia operations can be performed using the same methods for nonacute situations. However, incarceration with strangulation may require laparotomy with partial bowel resection.

- Gold standard
  – Inguinal hernia
    ○ Open: Lichtenstein with mesh (37%) or mesh plug (34%): decreased recurrence rates
    ○ Laparoscopic (14%) with mesh: decreased hospital stay and postoperative pain
      ■ Requires general anesthesia
      ■ Transabdominal preperitoneal (TAPP) versus total extraperitoneal (TEP)
    ○ Pediatric: Laparoscopic percutaneous repair is an efficient, safe, and effective alternative to open repair. It is associated with reduced operative times without an increase in complication or recurrence rates (3)[B].
  – Incisional/ventral
    ○ Laparoscopic repair is effective for most patients with primary or recurrent ventral hernias; it is associated with a <10% recurrence rate.
  – Umbilical
    ○ Pediatric: open excision and closure with suture
    ○ Adult: Open repair with mesh or plug may reduce hernia recurrence.
- Newer techniques
  – Prolene hernia system
  – Biologic wound closure system: reduced recurrence in contaminated procedures
- Complications
  – Recurrence
  – Seromas
  – Postoperative pain, temporary or chronic: improved in laparoscopic approach versus open
  – Wound infection
  – Injury to cord structures in inguinal herniorrhaphy; with nerve injury, most symptoms will resolve.

 ONGOING CARE

PATIENT EDUCATION
- Cleveland Clinic: http://my.clevelandclinic.org/disorders/hernia/hic_hernia.aspx
- Umbilical hernias: Boston Children's Hospital: http://www.childrenshospital.org/az/Site1018/mainpageS1018P0.html

PROGNOSIS
- Groin (pediatric): low recurrence rates (<3%) with surgical treatment; may spontaneously resolve in infants
- Groin (adult): ≥1% per year risk of bowel strangulation without surgical treatment; 0–10% postoperative recurrence rates, depending on surgeon's experience level and method
- Incisional/ventral: 3–5% postoperative occurrence: 2–17% postrepair recurrence, increased to 20–46% in larger hernias
- Umbilical (pediatric)
  – High rate of spontaneous resolution
  – Hernia less likely to close further in older children and in children with larger defects
- Umbilical (adult): up to 11% postoperative recurrence rate
- Epigastric: most will ultimately become incarcerated and/or strangulated without surgical treatment. Recurrence is high due to frequency of missed defects during repair.

REFERENCES
1. Winslow ER, Quasebarth M, Brunt LM. Perioperative outcomes and complications of open vs laparoscopic extraperitoneal inguinal hernia repair in a mature surgical practice. *Surg Endosc.* 2004:18(2): 221–227.
2. Buckley FP III, Vassaur H, Monsivais S, et al. Comparison of outcomes for single-incision laparoscopic inguinal herniorrhaphy and traditional three-port laparoscopic herniorrhaphy at a single institution. *Surg Endosc.* 2014;28(1):30–35.
3. Timberlake MD, Herbst KW, Rasmussen S, et al. Laparoscopic percutaneous inguinal hernia repair in children: review of technique and comparison with open surgery [published online ahead of print May 13, 2015]. *J Pediatr Urol.* 2015;11(5): 262.e1–262.e6

ADDITIONAL READING
- Abi-Haidar Y, Sanchez V, Itani KM. Risk factors and outcomes of acute versus elective groin hernia surgery. *J Am Coll Surg.* 2011;213(3):363–369.
- Brandt ML. Pediatric hernias. *Surg Clin North Am.* 2008;88(1):27–43, vii–viii.
- Buch KE, Tabrizian P, Divino CM. Management of hernias in pregnancy. *J Am Coll Surg.* 2008;207(4): 539–542.
- Matthews RD, Neumayer L. Inguinal hernia in the 21st century: an evidence-based review. *Curr Probl Surg.* 2008;45(4):261–312.
- Ng TT, Hamlin JA, Kahn AM. Herniography: analysis of its role and limitations. *Hernia.* 2009;13(1):7–11.
- Rosemar A, Angerås U, Rosengren A. Body mass index and groin hernia: a 34-year follow-up study in Swedish men. *Ann Surg.* 2008;247(6):1064–1068.
- Sajid MS, Bokhari SA, Mallick AS, et al. Laparoscopic versus open repair of incisional/ventral hernia: a meta-analysis. *Am J Surg.* 2009;197(1):64–72.
- Snyder CL. Current management of umbilical abnormalities and related anomalies. *Semin Pediatr Surg.* 2007;16(1):41–49.

 SEE ALSO

Algorithms: Abdominal Pain, Lower; Intestinal Obstruction; Pelvic Pain

CODES
ICD10
- K46.9 Unspecified abdominal hernia without obstruction or gangrene
- K40.90 Unil inguinal hernia, w/o obst or gangr, not spcf as recur
- K41.90 Unil femoral hernia, w/o obst or gangrene, not spcf as recur

CLINICAL PEARLS
- Inguinal
  – Direct inguinal: acquired; herniation through defect in transversalis fascia of abdominal wall medial to inferior epigastric vessels
  – Indirect inguinal: congenital; herniation lateral to the inferior epigastric vessels; a "complete hernia" descends into the scrotum; an "incomplete hernia" remains within the inguinal canal.
- Pantaloon: combination of direct and indirect inguinal hernia
- Femoral: descends through the femoral canal deep to the inguinal ligament
- Incisional or ventral: iatrogenic; herniation through a defect at site of a prior surgical incision
- Umbilical: Defect occurs at umbilical ring tissue.

H

HERPES EYE INFECTIONS

Rachel Marinch Carpenter, MD • William Fosmire, MD

BASICS

DESCRIPTION

- Eye infection (blepharitis, conjunctivitis, keratitis, stromal keratitis, uveitis, retinitis, glaucoma, or optic neuritis) caused by herpes simplex virus (HSV) types 1 or 2 or varicella-zoster virus (VZV, also known as human herpes virus type 3 [HHV3])
- Categories
  – HSV: can affect many parts of the eye but most often affects the cornea (herpes keratoconjunctivitis); HSV1 > HSV2; can be further divided into primary and recurrent
  – VZV: when VZV is reactivated and affects the ophthalmic division of the 5th cranial nerve, this is known as herpes zoster ophthalmicus (HZO), a type of shingles
- System(s) affected: eye, skin, CNS (neonatal)

EPIDEMIOLOGY

- Predominant age: HSV-mean age of onset 37.4 years but can occur at any age, including primary infection in newborns; VZV usually advancing age (>50 years)
- Predominant sex: HSV—male = female; HZO—female > male

Incidence

- HSV keratitis: In the United States, approximated at 18.2 per 100,000 person-years. Incidence is 1.5 million per year worldwide (1).
- VZV: 1 million new cases of shingles per year in the United States; 25–40% develop ophthalmic complications. Temporary keratitis is most common.

Prevalence

- Ocular HSV prevalence estimated at 500,000 in the United States (1)
- VZV: Prevalence of herpes zoster infection is 20–30%. Ocular involvement in 50% if not treated with antivirals (2). Overall lifetime prevalence of HZO: 1%

ETIOLOGY AND PATHOPHYSIOLOGY

- HSV and VZV are *Herpesviridae* dsDNA viruses
- HSV: primary infection from direct contact with infected person via saliva, genital contact, or birth canal exposure (neonates)
  – Primary infection may lead to severe disease in neonates, including eye, skin, CNS, and disseminated disease.
  – Recurrent infection is more common overall cause of herpetic eye infections.
- VZV: Primary infection from direct contact with infected person may cause varicella ("chickenpox") and/or lead to a latent state within trigeminal ganglia.
  – Reactivation of the virus may affect any dermatome (resulting in herpes zoster or "shingles"), including the ophthalmic branch (HZO).

RISK FACTORS

- HSV: personal history of HSV or close contact with HSV-infected person
  – General risk factors for reactivation: stress, trauma, fever, UV light exposure, other viral infections
  – Risk factors for HSV keratitis: UV laser eye treatment, some topical ocular medications such as prostaglandin analogues and primary/secondary immunosuppression
- HZO
  – History of varicella infection, advancing age (>50 years), sex (female > male), acute/painful prodrome, trauma, stress, immunosuppression (1,3)

GENERAL PREVENTION

- Contact precautions with active lesions (HSV and VZV)
- VZV can be spread to those who have not had chickenpox and are not immunized.
- Varicella vaccination (Zostavax) (VZV only): single 0.65 mL SC dose; no booster. Recommended by the CDC for all persons age ≥60 years. Reduces incidence of herpes zoster by 51% and HZO for 49%; also significantly decreases rates of post-herpetic neuralgia (PHN) (4)
- Acyclovir can be used prophylactically to prevent recurrence of ocular HSV.
- HSV immunization currently being researched (1)

Pregnancy Considerations

- Pregnant women without history of chickenpox should avoid contact with persons with active zoster.
- Pregnancy increases risk of recurrence of HSV/VZV.
- Live vaccine (Zostavax) is contraindicated during pregnancy.

COMMONLY ASSOCIATED CONDITIONS

Primary and secondary immunocompromised states

DIAGNOSIS

HISTORY

- Varies according to the virus and the ocular structures involved
- History of varicella or herpes simplex infection
- Acute onset, eye pain, headache, photophobia, tearing, ocular redness, decreased or blurry vision (3)[A]
- May present with a prodromal period of fever, malaise, headache, and eye pain before skin eruptions and eye lesions (HZO) (3)[A]

PHYSICAL EXAM

- Varies according to the virus and ocular structures involved
  – HSV most commonly affects the corneal epithelium (1)[A].
  – VZV most commonly affects corneal stroma and uvea (3)[A].
- Typically unilateral in presentation
  – HZO presents as early as 1 to 2 days after unilateral vesicular eruption in a dermatomal pattern (3)[A].
- Decreased visual acuity
- Conjunctival injection near the limbus
- Decreased corneal sensation
- Slit-lamp exam
  – Fluorescein and rose bengal stain: Dendritic corneal lesions most often seen in HSV, followed by stromal keratitis, corneal edema, or infiltrate (2)[C].
  – Stromal keratitis often seen in HZO, although dendritic lesions may form (2)[A].

- Hutchinson sign: vesicular lesion on nose from VZV indicates an increased risk of HZO due to involvement of nasociliary branch of trigeminal nerve, which also innervates the eye (3)[A].

DIFFERENTIAL DIAGNOSIS

- Any other cause of red, painful eye
  – Bacterial, fungal, allergic, or other viral conjunctivitis
  – Acute angle-closure glaucoma
- Corneal abrasion, recurrent corneal erosion, toxic conjunctivitis
- Temporal arteritis
- Trigeminal neuralgia

DIAGNOSTIC TESTS & INTERPRETATION

Initial Tests (lab, imaging)

- Typically none needed, as diagnosis is primarily based on history and physical exam (3)[A]
- Other
  – Corneal swab for HSV DNA by polymerase chain reaction (PCR) (PPV = 96%)
  – If vesicle present, can perform a Tzanck smear for VZV or HSV (multinucleated giant cells)
  – Antibody titers to assess exposure only; DFA (direct fluorescent antibody); tissue culture

TREATMENT

GENERAL MEASURES

- Avoid contact with nonimmune people.
- No contact lenses should be worn during treatment period.
- Cool compresses
- Artificial tears
- Oral pain medications

MEDICATION

First Line

- HSV corneal epithelial disease
  – Trifluridine 1%: apply 1 drop q2h while awake to a max of 9 drops daily until reepithelialization occurs, then 1 drop q4h for another 7 days
  – Acyclovir: 400 mg PO 5 times per day for 10 days
  – Ganciclovir 0.15% gel: apply 1 drop in eye q3h while awake, ~5 times daily, until reepithelialization occurs, then 1 drop q8h for 7 days
  – Vidarabine 3% ointment (Vira-A): apply 0.5 inch into lower conjunctival sac 5 times daily q3h, until reepithelialization occurs.
  – Trifluridine and acyclovir cure about 90% of treated eyes within 2 weeks with no significant differences in effectiveness (5)[A].
  – Evidence conflicting as to whether ganciclovir is as good as or better than acyclovir (5)[A].
  – Epithelial débridement by an ophthalmologist: may accelerate healing in combination with treatment as above (5)[A]
  – Avoid topical steroids.

- Utility of PO antivirals unclear HSV stromal keratitis or uveitis (without epithelial disease): combination of antiviral and steroid treatment; requires ophthalmology evaluation
  - Prednisolone acetate: 1% drops QID with slow taper (6)[A]
  - Consider systemic steroids in severe uveitis (6)[A].
  - Trifluorothymidine: 1% drops QID for prophylaxis while on topical steroids
- HZO
  - Valacyclovir (Valtrex) 1 g PO TID for 7 to 10 days or famciclovir (Famvir) 500 mg PO TID for 7 to 10 days or acyclovir 800 mg PO 5 times a day for 7 to 10 days
  - Valacyclovir and famciclovir result in significant reduction in PHN compared to acyclovir (number needed to treat [NNT] = 3) with equivalent efficacy (7)[A]
  - Topical antibiotic ophthalmic ointment to protect ocular surfaces (e.g., Bacitracin, Polymyxin): 0.5-inch ribbon BID to TID for 7 to 10 days (8)[C]
  - If immunocompromised: acyclovir 10 to 15 mg/kg IV q8h for 10 days
  - Prednisolone acetate: 1% drops QID with slow taper with an ophthalmologist (8)[C]
- Cycloplegic agent if anterior uveitis present; intraocular pressure-lowering agent if necessary

Second Line
- HSV: acyclovir 2 g/day PO in divided doses over 10 days in patients intolerant of topical antivirals
- Topical idoxuridine, acyclovir, brivudine, although approved internationally, are not approved for use in the United States.
- Concomitant treatment with interferon may also improve outcomes but is not currently available.

ALERT
- HZO: Antiviral therapy is most effective within the first 72 hours of rash onset but should still be initiated >72 hours after onset because of the possible complications of HZO (2)[C].
- Topical antiviral agents
  - Toxic to corneal epithelium, especially after 10 to 14 days of continuous use
- Acyclovir: reduce dosage in renal insufficiency
- Topical steroids
  - Should only be prescribed by an ophthalmologist
  - Contraindicated with active corneal epithelial disease, which is best monitored with a slit lamp
  - Can increase intraocular pressure, cause corneal thinning, and, with long-term use, cause cataracts
- Prednisone: caution in immunocompromised patients

ISSUES FOR REFERRAL
Emergent or urgent ophthalmology referral, depending on severity of disease

ADDITIONAL THERAPIES
- Recurrent HSV requires suppressive therapy:
  - Acyclovir 400 mg PO every day or BID or valacyclovir 500 mg PO daily (9)[C]
- HZO leading to PHN is very common and can be treated with gabapentin or pregabalin, TCAs, opioids, and/or lidocaine gel.

SURGERY/OTHER PROCEDURES
Corneal transplantation for severe scarring or perforation

INPATIENT CONSIDERATIONS
Admission Criteria/Initial Stabilization
- Severe systemic VZV disease
- Systemic HSV in neonates —see "Herpes Simplex Virus, Pediatric"

Discharge Criteria
Resolution of systemic disease

 ## ONGOING CARE

FOLLOW-UP RECOMMENDATIONS
Patient Monitoring
- Monitor with slit-lamp exam q1–2d until improvement, then q3–4d until epithelial defect resolves.
- Weekly after epithelial disease resolves until off topical antivirals

PATIENT EDUCATION
Educate patients about the importance of early recognition of recurrent symptoms and need for prompt evaluation and treatment.

PROGNOSIS
- Many cases are self-limited but, depending on the ocular structure involved, can lead to permanent blindness, especially in the setting of recurrent disease.
- Ocular HSV is the number one cause of infectious blindness worldwide (1).
- Recurrent ocular HSV
  - HSV epithelial disease without treatment
  - Without sequelae, 40% resolve.
  - With treatment, 90–95% resolve without complication.

Pediatric Considerations
- Neonatal primary HSV often disseminated, with high mortality rate; 37% develop vision worse than 20/200
- Pediatric cases more likely to be bilateral (26%); recurrent (48% in 15 months); and may cause amblyopia

COMPLICATIONS
- Recurrence
- Corneal neovascularization and scarring resulting in poor vision
- Neurotrophic ulcer with perforation
- Secondary bacterial or fungal infection
- Secondary glaucoma in 10%
- Post-herpetic neuralgia in 20–40% with VZV, typically longer lasting in older patients
- Vision loss from optic neuritis or chorioretinitis

 ## REFERENCES
1. Faroog AV, Shukla D. Herpes simplex epithelial and stromal keratitis: an epidemiologic update. *Surv Opththalmol*. 2012;57(5):448–462.
2. Carter WP III, Germann CA, Baumann MR. Ophthalmic diagnoses in the ED: herpes zoster ophthalmicus. *Am J Emerg Med*. 2008;26(5):612–617.
3. Liesegang TJ. Herpes zoster ophthalmicus natural history, risk factors, clinical presentation, and morbidity. *Ophthalmology*. 2008;115(2 Suppl):S3–S12.
4. Gelb LD. Preventing herpes zoster through vaccination. *Ophthalmology*. 2008;115(2 Suppl):S35–S38.
5. Wilhelmus KR. Antiviral treatment and other therapeutic interventions for herpes simplex virus epithelial keratitis. *Cochrane Database Syst Rev*. 2015;(1):CD002898.
6. Knickelbein JE, Hendricks RL, Charukamnoetkanok P. Management of herpes simplex virus stromal keratitis: an evidence-based review. *Surv Ophthalmol*. 2009;54(2):226–234.
7. McDonald EM, de Kock J, Ram FS. Antivirals for management of herpes zoster including ophthalmicus: a systematic review of high-quality randomized controlled trials. *Antivir Ther*. 2012;17(2):255–264.
8. Dworkin RH, Johnson RW, Breuer J, et al. Recommendations for the management of herpes zoster. *Clin Infect Dis*. 2007;44(Suppl 1):S1–S26.
9. de Rojas Silva MV, Díez-Feijóo E, Javaloy J, et al. Prophylactic perioperative antiviral therapy for LASIK in patients with inactive herpetic keratitis. *J Refract Surg*. 2006;22(4):404–406.

ADDITIONAL READING
Rowe AM, St Leger AJ, Jeon S, et al. Herpes keratitis. *Prog Retin Eye Res*. 2013;32:88–101.

 ## SEE ALSO
- Algorithm: Eye Pain
- Topic: Herpes Simplex
- Topic: Herpes Simplex Virus, Pediatric
- Topic: Herpes Zoster

CODES
ICD10
- B00.50 Herpesviral ocular disease, unspecified
- B02.30 Zoster ocular disease, unspecified
- B00.52 Herpesviral keratitis

CLINICAL PEARLS
- HSV and VZV can lead to a wide array of ocular manifestations, ranging from self-limited disease to potentially vision-threatening disease and complications.
- A slit-lamp exam with fluorescein stain should be performed on all patients with possible HSV keratitis or HZO.
- Topical antiviral treatment is appropriate for HSV, but systemic PO antiviral treatment is necessary for HZO.
- An ophthalmologist should be consulted before prescribing topical steroids. All HZO patients should be referred to an ophthalmologist.
- Hutchinson sign (vesicular lesion on nose from VZV) is a strong indicator of HZO.
- Zostavax is effective at preventing zoster and HZO as well as decreasing the duration of PHN.

H

HERPES SIMPLEX

Sonia Rivera-Martinez, DO, FACOFP • Sharon L. Koehler, DO, FACS

 BASICS

DESCRIPTION
- Characteristic vesicular rash primarily located in oral and genital regions as the result of infection with
  - Herpes simplex virus (HSV)-1 is primarily associated with blisters on lips, in mouth, face, eyes.
  - HSV-2 is the primary source of genital herpes, although cross-reactivity is common (HSV-1 can cause genital sores through oral–genital contact).
- Associated with a wide range of sequelae. Complexity and variation of presentation depends on the age and immune status of host, whether the infection is primary or recurrent and the degree of dissemination.
- Viral shedding is typically greatest in the first (primary) infection and lessens with recurrences.
- Meningitis/encephalitis and pneumonia are serious systemic manifestations associated with HSV infection.

EPIDEMIOLOGY
- Predominant age: Affects all ages; however, most HSV-1 is acquired in childhood, and most HSV-2 is acquired in young–middle adulthood.
- Predominant sex: male = female

Incidence
- Over 1,000,000 new cases of HSV per year
- HSV can reactivate, causing recurrent disease.

Prevalence
- Widespread; 0.65–25% of adults may shed HSV-1 or HSV-2 at any given time. Many are unaware of their infection status.
- Prevalence of antibodies to HSV-1 is 90% by adulthood in the general population. 30% of adults have antibodies to HSV-2.

ETIOLOGY AND PATHOPHYSIOLOGY
HSV-1 and 2 are double-stranded DNA viruses from the family *Herpesviridae*. HSV-1 and 2 are transmitted by contact with infected skin during periods of viral shedding. Transmission also occurs vertically during childbirth. Most often, HSV-1 is associated with oral lesions and HSV-2 with genital lesions.

RISK FACTORS
- Immunocompromised state
  - Chemotherapy, malignancy/chronic disease states such as diabetes or AIDS, old age
- Atopic eczema, especially in children
- Prior HSV infection
- Sexual intercourse with infected person (condoms help minimize HSV transmission, but lesions outside condom-protected areas can spread virus)
- Occupational exposure
  - Dental professionals at higher risk for HSV-1 and resulting herpetic whitlow
- Neonatal herpes simplex: Primary infection is life-threatening and usually acquired by vaginal birth to an infected mother; fetal and neonatal risk are greatest in mothers with primary genital herpes infection; incubation is usually from 5 to 7 days (rarely 4 weeks); cutaneous, mucous membrane, or ocular signs seen in only 70%.

GENERAL PREVENTION
- If active lesions are present, avoid direct contact with immunocompromised people, elderly, and newborns.
- Hand hygiene
- Kissing, sharing beverages, and sharing utensils/toothbrushes can transmit HSV.
- Genital herpes: Avoid sexual contact if active lesions (herpes simplex is also transmitted when disease appears to be inactive), discuss condom benefits and limits, consider antiviral therapy to reduce viral shedding, encourage safe sex.
- Topical microbicides (not yet commercially available) may prevent transmission of HSV-2.

COMMONLY ASSOCIATED CONDITIONS
- Erythema multiforme: 50% of associated cases are caused by HSV-1 or -2.
- Screen all severe, unusual locations, or treatment-resistant HSV cases for HIV.

 DIAGNOSIS

HISTORY
- Many patients are unaware of a known exposure.
- Prodrome of fatigue, low-grade fever, itching, tingling, or hot skin for several days immediately prior to outbreak of characteristic vesicular rash
- Herpes labialis is precipitated by sunlight, fever, trauma, menses, and stress; prodrome of pain, burning, and itching commonly occur 6 to 48 hours before vesicles appear.

PHYSICAL EXAM
- Vesicles are often clustered and become painful ulcerated lesions, often with erythematous base.
- Primary genital herpes: See "Herpes, Genital."
- Primary herpetic gingivostomatitis and pharyngitis: usually in early childhood; incubation from 2 to 12 days, followed by fever, sore throat, pharyngeal edema, and erythema
  - Small vesicles develop on pharyngeal and oral mucosa, rapidly ulcerate, and increase in number to involve soft palate, buccal mucosa, tongue, floor of mouth, lips, and cheeks; tender, bleeding gums; cervical adenopathy; fever, general toxicity, poor oral intake, and excess salivation contribute to dehydration; autoinoculation of other sites may occur; resolves in 10 to 14 days
- Primary herpes keratoconjunctivitis: unilateral conjunctivitis with regional adenopathy, blepharitis with vesicles on lid marginal keratitis with dendritic lesions, or with punctate opacities; lasts 2 to 3 weeks; systemic involvement prolongs process
- Eczema herpeticum: diffuse pox-like eruption complicating atopic dermatitis; sudden appearance of lesions in typical atopic areas (upper trunk, neck, head); high fever, localized edema, adenopathy
- Herpetic whitlow: localized infection of affected finger with intense itching and pain, followed by vesicles that may coalesce with swelling and erythema. Mimics pyogenic paronychia; neuralgia and axillary adenopathy are possible; heals in 2 to 3 weeks

- Congenital infection through transplacental transfer may present with jaundice, hepatosplenomegaly, disseminated intravascular coagulation (DIC), encephalitis, seizures, temperature instability, chorioretinitis, and conjunctivitis with or without vesicles.
- Recurrent diseases from endogenous reactivation
  - Herpes labialis: recurrent lesions with HSV-1; usually <1 recurrence/6 months, but 5–25% may have >1 attack/month; vesicles often at vermilion border, then ulcerate and crust within 48 hours; heal within 8 to 10 days; may have local adenopathy
  - Ocular herpes: May recur as keratitis, blepharitis, or keratoconjunctivitis; dendritic ulcers, decreased corneal sensation, decreased visual acuity; uveitis may cause permanent visual loss.

DIFFERENTIAL DIAGNOSIS
- Impetigo: honey-crusted vesicles
- Aphthous stomatitis: grayish, shallow erosions with ring of hyperemia of anterior in mouth and lips
- Herpes zoster: unilateral dermatome distribution
- Syphilitic chancre: painless ulcer
- Folliculitis: may mimic "shave bumps" in genital area
- Herpangina: Vesicles predominate on anterior tonsillar pillars, soft palate, uvula, and oropharynx but not more anteriorly on lips/gums (usually caused by group A coxsackievirus).
- Stevens-Johnson syndrome

DIAGNOSTIC TESTS & INTERPRETATION
- Screen for other sexually transmitted infections (STIs) in patients with primary genital herpes.
- Viral: HIV, hepatitis B and C, and human papillomavirus (HPV) have crossover
- Bacterial: Screen for concurrent gonorrhea, chlamydia in new primary genital outbreaks.

Initial Tests (lab, imaging)
- Tzanck smear shows multinucleated giant cells often with eosinophilic intranuclear inclusions (scrape material from lesion to slide, fix with ethanol/methanol, stain with Giemsa or Wright stain); varicella (herpes zoster) has identical findings.
- HSV culture: Swab and plate on viral-specific media. Sample may need to be refrigerated; can take up to 6 days to be positive. Highly specific, hence, reliable if positive but has 20% false–negative rate.
- HSV type-specific antibody tests distinguish between HSV-1 and HSV-2.
  - Polymerase chain reaction (PCR), direct fluorescent antibody (DFA), ELISA, and Western blot
  - 3 weeks after infection, 50% of those infected test positive; 70%, 6 weeks after infection; by 16 weeks nearly all infected test positive

Diagnostic Procedures/Other
Biopsy is occasionally needed to confirm diagnosis.

Test Interpretation
- Intraepithelial edema (ballooning degeneration) and intracellular edema
- Brain biopsy (in encephalitis) shows hemorrhagic necrosis of gray and white matter with acute and chronic inflammation, thrombosis, and fibrinoid necrosis of parenchymal vessels; intranuclear inclusions in astrocytes, oligodendroglia, and neurons

TREATMENT

GENERAL MEASURES
- Cool dressings moistened with aluminum acetate solution
- Painful urination and inability to void due to painful genital lesions is helped by pouring a cup of warm water over genitals while urinating or by sitting in a warm bath while urinating (sitz baths).
- Children with gingivostomatitis who resist oral intake due to pain or extensive skin disease (eczema herpeticum) may require IV hydration.

MEDICATION
First Line
- Begin treatment promptly, preferably in prodromal phase.
- Acyclovir (generic)
  - Mucocutaneous (or genital) HSV
    - Primary/first infection: 400 mg TID or 200 mg 5 times per day for 7 to 10 days
    - If severe, start with IV q8h dosing for the first few days, then complete 10-day course PO route.
    - Recurrence: 400 mg PO TID for 5 days *or* 800 mg BID for 5 days *or* 800 mg TID for 2 days
    - Suppression: 400 mg BID daily (1)[B]
  - Keratitis HSV: 400 mg PO 5 times per day; however, topical treatment is preferred as first line.
  - Pediatric dosing: neonatal herpes simplex or encephalitis: 60 mg/kg/day IV divided q8h for 14 to 21 days (2)[B]
    - Older (>3 months of age) immunocompetent is weight-based dosing (40 to 80 mg/kg/day [max 1,000 mg/day] divided q8h for 5 to 7 days).
  - Safe in pregnancy and lactation—Category B
  - Recurrent herpes labialis: 800 to 1,600 mg/day for prevention (3–5)[B]
- Penciclovir (Denavir): 1% cream. Apply to oral lesions q2h during waking hours for 4 days (6)[B].
- Valacyclovir (Valtrex)
  - Primary genital herpes: 1 g PO BID for 7 to 10 days. Recurrent genital herpes: 500 mg PO BID for 3 days; suppression: 500 to 1,000 mg PO daily (depending on frequency of outbreaks); labialis HSV (cold sores/oral lesions): 2,000 mg PO q12h for 1 day (3–5)[B]
  - 500-mg daily dose if suppression is needed/desired
  - Recurrent herpes labialis: 500 mg/day for 4 months for prevention (3,4)[B]
- Famciclovir (Famvir)
  - Primary genital herpes: 250 mg PO TID for 7 to 10 days
  - Recurrence: 125 mg PO BID for 5 days or 1,000 mg PO BID for 1 day
  - Suppression: 250 mg PO BID
- Precautions
  - Renal dosing for all oral antivirals
  - Significant possible interactions: Probenecid with IV acyclovir and possibly probenecid with valacyclovir may reduce renal clearance and elevate antiviral drug levels.

Second Line
- Foscarnet
  - Drug of choice for acyclovir resistance in immunocompromised persons with systemic HSV
  - 40 mg/kg IV q8h (assume valacyclovir and famciclovir resistance also if acyclovir resistance occurs)

- Other topicals
  - Ophthalmic preparations for herpes keratoconjunctivitis; acyclovir, vidarabine (Vira-A), ganciclovir, trifluridine
  - Topical acyclovir and penciclovir improve recurrent herpes labialis healing times by ~10% (3)[B].
  - Topical analgesics: Lidocaine 2% or 5% helps reduce pain associated with vulvar and penile outbreaks.
- Over-the-counter topical antivirals: docosanol

ISSUES FOR REFERRAL
Refer recurrent cases of herpes keratoconjunctivitis to an ophthalmologist.

INPATIENT CONSIDERATIONS
Admission Criteria/Initial Stabilization
- Pregnancy considerations
  - Caesarean section and/or acyclovir are indicated if any active genital lesions (or prodrome) present at time of delivery; consider cesarean delivery if primary genital herpes is suspected within previous 4 weeks (6)[B].
  - Daily oral antivirals from 36 weeks onward in women with history of recurrent genital herpes to prevent outbreak near to/at time of delivery
  - Avoid fetal scalp electrodes, forceps, vacuum extractor, and artificial rupture of membranes if mother has history of genital HSV.
  - Risk of viral shedding at delivery from asymptomatic recurrent genital HSV is low (~1.6%).
- Pediatric considerations
  - Neonates with likely exposure (high index of suspicion) to HSV at birth or those who exhibit signs of HSV infection should have all body fluids cultured and immediately start treatment with IV acyclovir.

ONGOING CARE

FOLLOW-UP RECOMMENDATIONS
- For most cases, follow-up is not necessary. Lesions and symptoms resolve rapidly within 10 days. Extensive cases should be rechecked in 1 week; monitor for secondary bacterial infections.
- Consider long-term suppression.

DIET
If oral lesions are present, avoid salty, acidic, or sharp foods (e.g., snack chips, orange juice).

PATIENT EDUCATION
- Explain the natural history that timing of exposure is difficult to determine and that the virus will remain in the body indefinitely. Minimize psychological impact of the diagnosis to reduce stigma.
- Emphasize personal hygiene to avoid self-spreading to other body areas (autoinoculation) or exposing others. Frequent hand washing; avoid scratching; cover active, moist lesions.
- Reinforce safe sexual practices.

PROGNOSIS
- Usual duration of primary disease is 5 days to 2 weeks.
- Antiviral treatment shortens duration, reduces complications, and mitigates recurrences (if used for suppression).
- Viral shedding during recurrence is briefer than with primary disease; frequency of recurrence is variable and depends on individual host factors.

- Newborns/immunocompromised individuals are at highest risk for major morbidity/mortality.
- HSV is never eliminated from the body but stays dormant in dorsal root ganglia and can reactivate, causing recurrent symptoms and lesions.

COMPLICATIONS
- Herpes encephalitis: Brain biopsy may be needed for diagnosis.
- Herpes pneumonia

REFERENCES
1. Gupta R, Warren T, Wald A. Genital herpes. *Lancet.* 2007;370(9605):2127–2137.
2. Pinninti SG, Kimberlin DW. Neonatal herpes simplex virus infections. *Pediatr Clin North Am.* 2013;60(2): 351–365. doi:10.1016/j.pcl.2012.12.005.
3. Rahimi H, Mara T, Costella J, et al. Effectiveness of antiviral agents for the prevention of recurrent herpes labialis: a systematic review and meta-analysis. *Oral Surg Oral Med Oral Pathol Oral Radiol.* 2012;113(5):618–627.
4. Harmenberg J, Oberg B, Spruance S. Prevention of ulcerative lesions by episodic treatment of recurrent herpes labialis: a literature review. *Acta Derm Venereol.* 2010;90(2):122–130.
5. Cernik C, Gallina K, Brodell RT. The treatment of herpes simplex infections: an evidence-based review. *Arch Intern Med.* 2008;168(11):1137–1144.
6. Obiero J, Mwethera PG, Wiysonge CS. Topical microbicides for prevention of sexually transmitted infections. *Cochrane Database Syst Rev.* 2012;(6):CD007961.

ADDITIONAL READING
Wang X, Zhou F, Zhao J, et al. Elevated risk of opportunistic viral infection in patients with Crohn's disease during biological therapies: a meta analysis of randomized controlled trials. *Eur J Clin Pharmacol.* 2013;69(11):1891–1899.

SEE ALSO
- Herpes, Genital
- Algorithm: Genital Ulcers

CODES
ICD10
- B00.9 Herpesviral infection, unspecified
- A60.00 Herpesviral infection of urogenital system, unspecified
- B00.1 Herpesviral vesicular dermatitis

CLINICAL PEARLS
- 25–30% of the U.S. population has evidence of genital herpes (HSV-2), and >80% is seropositive for HSV-1.
- Most individuals are unaware they are infected. This allows for asymptomatic passage of the virus.
- Viral suppression therapy for patients with frequent recurrences reduces transmission and decreases outbreak frequency.

H

HERPES ZOSTER (SHINGLES)

Robert J. Hyde, MD, MA, NRP, FACEP

BASICS

DESCRIPTION
- Results from reactivation of latent varicella-zoster virus (human herpesvirus type 3) infection
- Postherpetic neuralgia (PHN) is defined as pain persisting at least 1 month after rash has healed. The term *zoster-associated pain* is more clinically useful.
- Usually presents as a painful unilateral vesicular eruption with a dermatomal distribution
- System(s) affected: nervous; integumentary; exocrine
- Synonym(s): shingles

EPIDEMIOLOGY
Predominant sex: male = female

Incidence
- Incidence increases with age. 2/3 of cases occur in adults age ≥50 years. Incidence is increasing overall as the U.S. population ages.
- Herpes zoster: 4/1,000 person-years (1)
- PHN: 18% in adult patients with herpes zoster; 33% in patients ≥79 years of age

Prevalence
Nearly 1 million new cases of herpes zoster annually

Pregnancy Considerations
May occur during pregnancy

Geriatric Considerations
- Increased incidence of zoster outbreaks
- Increased incidence of PHN

Pediatric Considerations
- Occurs less frequently in children
- Has been reported in newborns infected in utero

ETIOLOGY AND PATHOPHYSIOLOGY
Reactivation of varicella-zoster virus from dorsal root/cranial nerve ganglia. Upon reactivation, the virus replicates within neuronal cell bodies, and virions are carried along axons to dermatomal skin zones, causing local inflammation and vesicle formation.

RISK FACTORS
- Increasing age
- Immunosuppression (malignancy or chemotherapy)
- HIV infection
- Use of immunosuppressant drugs (e.g., following organ transplant surgery)
- Spinal surgery

GENERAL PREVENTION
- Herpes zoster vaccination (Zostavax) is recommended by Advisory Committee on Immunization Practices (ACIP) for patients ≥60 years (FDA-approved for patients >50 years) (2–4):
  - Vaccine reduces cases of zoster and the incidence of PHN (5,6).
- Patients with active zoster may transmit disease-causing varicella virus (chickenpox) to susceptible persons.

COMMONLY ASSOCIATED CONDITIONS
Immunocompromised individuals, HIV infection, posttransplantation, immunosuppressive drugs, and malignancy

DIAGNOSIS

HISTORY
- Prodromal phase (sensations over involved dermatome prior to rash)
  - Tingling, paresthesias
  - Itching
  - Boring "knifelike" pain
- Acute phase
  - Constitutional symptoms (e.g., fatigue, malaise, headache, low-grade fever) are variable.
  - Dermatomal rash

PHYSICAL EXAM
- Acute phase
  - Rash: initially erythematous and maculopapular; evolves rapidly to grouped vesicles
  - Vesicles become pustular and/or hemorrhagic in 3 to 4 days.
  - Weakness (1% have weakness in distribution of rash)
  - Resolution of rash, with crusts separating by 14 to 21 days
- Possible sine herpete (zoster without rash) and other chronic disorders associated with varicella-zoster virus without the typical rash
  - Herpes zoster ophthalmicus (HZO). Vesicles on tip of the nose (Hutchinson sign) indicate involvement of the external branch of cranial nerve V; associated with increased incidence of ocular zoster.
- Chronic phase
  - PHN (15% overall; increases with age)
  - A small percentage (1–5%) may affect the motor nerves, causing weakness (*zoster motorius*); facial nerve (e.g., Ramsay Hunt syndrome); spinal motor radiculopathies.

DIFFERENTIAL DIAGNOSIS
- Rash
  - Herpes simplex virus
  - Coxsackievirus
  - Contact dermatitis
  - Superficial pyoderma
- Pain
  - Cholecystitis
  - Appendicitis
  - Nephrolithiasis
  - Pleuritis
  - Myocardial infarction
  - Diabetic neuropathy

DIAGNOSTIC TESTS & INTERPRETATION
Initial Tests (lab, imaging)
Rarely necessary because clinical appearance is sufficiently distinctive

Follow-Up Tests & Special Considerations
- Viral culture
- Tzanck smear (does not distinguish from herpes simplex, and false-negative results occur)
- Polymerase chain reaction
- Immunofluorescent antigen staining
- Varicella-zoster–specific IgM

Test Interpretation
- Multinucleated giant cells with intralesional inclusion
- Lymphatic infiltration of sensory ganglia with focal hemorrhage and nerve cell destruction

TREATMENT

GENERAL MEASURES
- Treatment is directed to control symptoms and prevent complications.
- Antiviral therapy decreases viral replication, lessens inflammation and nerve damage, and reduces the severity and duration of long-term pain.
- Prompt analgesic control may shorten the duration of zoster-associated pain.
- Lotions, such as calamine and colloidal oatmeal, may help reduce itching and burning sensation.

MEDICATION
First Line
- Acute treatment
  - Antiviral agents initiated within 72 hours of skin lesions help relieve symptoms, speed resolution, and prevent or mitigate PHN (7)[A].
  - Valacyclovir: 1,000 mg PO TID for 7 days
  - Famciclovir: 500 mg PO TID for 7 days
  - Acyclovir: 800 mg q4h (5 doses daily) for 7 days
- Analgesics (acetaminophen, NSAIDs)
- Corticosteroids given acutely during zoster infection do not prevent PHN (8).
  - Tricyclic antidepressants (TCAs; amitriptyline 25 mg at bedtime and other low-dose TCAs) relieve pain acutely and may reduce pain duration; dose may be titrated up to 75 to 150 mg/day as tolerated.
  - Lidocaine patch 5% (Lidoderm) applied over painful areas (limit 3 patches simultaneously or trim a single patch) for up to 12 hours may be effective.
  - Gabapentin: 100 to 600 mg TID for pain and other quality-of-life indicators; limited by adverse effects

- Capsaicin cream and other analgesics may be useful adjuncts. Use opioids sparingly.
- Pregabalin: 50 to 100 mg TID reduces pain, but usefulness is limited by side effects.

• Prevention of PHN and zoster-associated pain: No treatment has been shown to prevent PHN completely, but treatment may shorten duration and/or reduce severity of symptoms (9)[A].

- Antiviral therapy with valacyclovir, famciclovir, or acyclovir given during acute skin eruption may decrease the duration of pain.
- Low-dose amitriptyline (25 mg at bedtime) started within 72 hours of rash onset and continued for 90 days may reduce PHN incidence/duration.
- Insufficient evidence to suggest that corticosteroids reduce incidence, severity, or duration of PHN (8)

• Precautions
- Assess renal function prior to using valacyclovir, famciclovir, or acyclovir.
- Valacyclovir, famciclovir, and acyclovir are pregnancy Category B.

Second Line
Numerous therapies have been advocated, but supporting evidence to routinely recommend is lacking.

COMPLEMENTARY & ALTERNATIVE MEDICINE
Studies on cupping therapy (traditional Chinese medicine) show potential benefit, but evidence is conflicting (10)[A].

INPATIENT CONSIDERATIONS
Admission Criteria/Initial Stabilization
Outpatient treatment, unless disseminated or occurring as complication of serious underlying disease requiring hospitalization

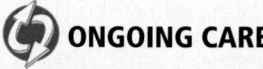

ONGOING CARE

FOLLOW-UP RECOMMENDATIONS
Referral to ophthalmology if concern for involvement of ophthalmic branch of the trigeminal nerve

Patient Monitoring
Follow duration of symptoms—particularly PHN. Consider hospitalization if symptoms are severe; patients are immunocompromised; >2 dermatomes are involved; serious bacterial superinfection, disseminated zoster, or meningoencephalitis develops.

DIET
No special diet

PATIENT EDUCATION
• The duration of rash is typically 2 to 3 weeks.
• Encourage good hygiene and proper skin care.
• Warn of potential for dissemination (dissemination must be suspected with constitutional illness signs and/or spreading rash).
• Warn of potential PHN.
• Warn of potential risk of transmitting illness (chickenpox) to susceptible persons.
• Seek medical attention if any eye involvement.

PROGNOSIS
• Immunocompetent individuals should experience spontaneous and complete recovery within a few weeks.
• Acute rash typically resolves within 14 to 21 days.
• PHN may occur in patients despite antiviral treatment.

COMPLICATIONS
• PHN
• Herpes zoster ophthalmicus: 10–20%
• Superinfection of skin lesions
• Meningoencephalitis
• Disseminated zoster
• Hepatitis; pneumonitis; myelitis
• Cranial and peripheral nerve palsies
• Acute retinal necrosis

REFERENCES

1. Yawn BP, Saddier P, Wollan PC, et al. A population-based study of the incidence and complication rates of herpes zoster before zoster vaccine introduction. *Mayo Clin Proc.* 2007;82(11):1341–1349.
2. Hales CM, Harpaz R, Ortega-Sanchez I, et al. Update on recommendations for use of herpes zoster vaccine. *MMWR Morb Mortal Wkly Rep.* 2014;63(33):729–731.
3. Schmader KE, Levin MJ, Gnann JW Jr, et al. Efficacy, safety, and tolerability of herpes zoster vaccine in persons aged 50-59 years. *Clin Infect Dis.* 2012;54(7):922–928.
4. Harpaz R, Ortega-Sanchez IR, Seward JF, et al. Prevention of herpes zoster: recommendations of the Advisory Committee on Immunization Practices (ACIP). *MMWR Recomm Rep.* 2008;57(RR-5):1–30.
5. Chen N, Li Q, Zhang Y, et al. Vaccination for preventing postherpetic neuralgia. *Cochrane Database Syst Rev.* 2011;(3):CD007795.
6. Langan SM, Smeeth L, Margolis DJ, et al. Herpes zoster vaccine effectiveness against incident herpes zoster and post-herpetic neuralgia in an older US population: a cohort study. *PLoS Med.* 2013;10(4):e1001420.
7. McDonald EM, de Kock J, Ram FS. Antivirals for management of herpes zoster including ophthalmicus: a systematic review of high-quality randomized controlled trials. *Antivir Ther.* 2012;17(2):255–264.
8. Chen N, Yang M, He L, et al. Corticosteroids for preventing postherpetic neuralgia. *Cochrane Database Syst Rev.* 2010;(12):CD005582.
9. Li Q, Chen N, Yang J, et al. Antiviral treatment for preventing postherpetic neuralgia. *Cochrane Database Syst Rev.* 2009;(2):CD006866.
10. Cao H, Li X, Liu J. An updated review of the efficacy of cupping therapy. *PLoS One.* 2012;7(2):e31793.

 SEE ALSO

• Bell Palsy; Chickenpox (Varicella Zoster); Herpes Eye Infections; Herpes Simplex
• Algorithm: Genital Ulcers

 CODES

ICD10
• B02.9 Zoster without complications
• B02.29 Other postherpetic nervous system involvement

CLINICAL PEARLS
• Zoster vaccine is recommended for patients ≥60 years of age and is approved for patients >50 years.
• Patients with herpes zoster should begin antiviral therapy within 72 hours of the onset of rash to be most effective.
• Patients with active herpes zoster can transmit clinically active disease (chickenpox) to susceptible individuals.

H

HERPES, GENITAL

Cecilia M. Kipnis, MD

 BASICS

DESCRIPTION
- Chronic, recurrent infection of any area innervated by the sacral ganglia
- Due to herpes simplex virus (HSV) type 1 or 2
- HSV-1 causes anogenital and orolabial lesions.
- HSV-2 causes anogenital lesions.
- Primary episode: occurs in the absence of pre-existing antibodies to HSV-1 or HSV-2 (may be asymptomatic)
- 1st episode nonprimary: initial genital eruption (likely due to HSV-2); preexisting antibodies to HSV-1 are present.
- Reactivation: recurrent episodes
- Synonym(s): herpes genitalis

EPIDEMIOLOGY
- Predominant age: 15 to 65 years; cases increase with age due to cumulative effect
- Predominant sex: female > male
- Predominant race: non-Hispanic blacks

Incidence
>700,000 new cases per year

Prevalence
- 50–70% in developed countries, approaches 100% in developing countries (1)
- Overall prevalence of HSV-2 is 10–40% in the general population and up to 60–95% in the HIV-positive population (1).
- Up to 90% of seropositive persons do not have formal diagnosis.
- >50 million are infected with HSV-2 in the United States.

ETIOLOGY AND PATHOPHYSIOLOGY
- HSV is a double-stranded DNA virus of the Herpetoviridae family (1).
- Spread via genital-to-genital contact, oral-to-genital contact, and via maternal–fetal transmission. Viral shedding continues in the absence of lesions (2).
- Incubation is 2 to 12 days after exposure.

RISK FACTORS
- Risk increases with age, number of lifetime partners, history of sexually transmitted infections (STIs), sexual encounters before the age of 17 years, and partner with HSV-1 or HSV-2.
- Infection with HSV-1 increases the risk of being infected with HSV-2 by 3-fold.
- Immunosuppression, fever, stress, and trauma increases risk of reactivation.

COMMONLY ASSOCIATED CONDITIONS
Syphilis, HIV, chlamydia, gonorrhea, and other STIs

 DIAGNOSIS

HISTORY
- Many patients are asymptomatic (74% of HSV-1 and 63% of HSV-2) or do not recognize clinical manifestations of disease (2).
- Symptoms often more severe, associated with constitutional symptoms and longer in duration with primary episode.
- Common presenting symptoms (primary episode): multiple genital ulcers, dysuria, pruritus, fever, tender inguinal lymphadenopathy, headache, malaise, myalgias, cervicitis/dyspareunia, urethritis (watery discharge)
- 1st episode, nonprimary: less severe symptoms than a primary episode due to preexisting antibodies to HSV-1 which have some activity against HSV-2
- Common presenting symptoms for recurrent episodes: prodrome of tingling, burning, or shooting pain (2 to 24 hours before lesion appears); single ulcer; dysuria; pruritus (last 4 to 6 days on average)
- Less common presentations: constipation (from anal involvement causing tenesmus), proctitis, stomatitis, pharyngitis, sacral paresthesias

PHYSICAL EXAM
- Impossible to differentiate primary, 1st episode nonprimary, recurrent disease, or type of virus (HSV-1 or HSV-2) based on symptoms or exam
- Lesions occur in "boxer short" distribution and within anus, vagina, and on cervix.
- Lesion may appear as papular, vesicular, pustular, ulcerated, or crusted; can be in various stages.
- Inguinal lymphadenopathy
- Extragenital manifestations include meningitis, recurrent meningitis (Mollaret syndrome), sacral radiculitis/paresthesias, encephalitis, transverse myelitis, and hepatitis

Pediatric Considerations
- Neonatal infection occurs in 20 to 50/100,000 live births; 80% of infections result from asymptomatic maternal viral shedding during an undiagnosed primary infection in the 3rd trimester.
- Transmission ranges from 30–50% if the primary episode is near time of delivery. High morbidity and mortality
- Suspect sexual abuse with genital lesions in children

DIFFERENTIAL DIAGNOSIS
- Primary syphilis
- Chancroid
- Herpes zoster
- Ulcerative balanitis
- Granuloma inguinale
- Lymphogranuloma venereum
- HIV
- Cytomegalovirus; Epstein-Barr virus
- Drug eruption
- Trauma
- Behçet syndrome
- Neoplasia

DIAGNOSTIC TESTS & INTERPRETATION
Initial Tests (lab, imaging)
- Viral isolation from lesion (swab or scraping)
  - Culture and PCR are preferred (3)[A].
  - Use Dacron or polyester-tipped swabs with plastic shafts (cotton tips/wood shafts inhibit viral growth and/or replication) (1).
  - Culture by unroofing vesicle to obtain fluid sample. Specificity >99%, sensitivity depends on sample: 52–93% for vesicle, 41–72% for ulcer, 19–30% for crusted lesion (1,3)
  - Culture requires timely transport of live virus to the laboratory in appropriate medium at 4°C.
  - PCR has the greatest sensitivity (98%) and specificity (>99%) but is also expensive and not readily available. It can increase detection rates by up to 70% (4). Used primarily for CSF (1)
- Type-specific serologic assays
  - Western blot (gold standard) and type-specific IgG antibody (glycoprotein G) enzyme-linked immunosorbent assay (ELISA) are used to discriminate between HSV-1 and HSV-2 (3)[B].
  - Western blot is >97–99% sensitive and specific but labor intensive and not readily available (1,3).
  - ELISA is 81–100% sensitive and 93–100% specific (1).
  - Seroconversion occurs 10 days to 4 months after infection (3). Antibody testing is not necessary if a positive culture or PCR has been obtained.
  - IgM antibody testing is not useful because HSV IgM is often present with recurrent disease and does not distinguish new from old infection.
  - Screening with type-specific antibody in the general population is not recommended (3) but may be considered in
    - Asymptomatic patients with HIV infection
    - Discordant couples (one partner with known HSV, the other without)

TREATMENT

GENERAL MEASURES
- Cool compresses with aluminum acetate (Domeboro)
- Ice packs to perineum, sitz baths, topical anesthetics
- Analgesics, NSAIDs

MEDICATION
Antiviral medications should be started within 72 hours of onset of symptoms (including prodrome). If presentation is >72 hours, antivirals may be helpful if new lesions continue to form or patient is experiencing significant pain.

First Line

- Acyclovir (4)[A]: the most studied antiviral in genital herpes. Decreases pain, duration of viral shedding, and time to full resolution
  - Primary episode
    - 400 mg PO TID for 7 to 10 days
    - 200 mg PO 5 times a day for 7 to 10 days
    - Longer if needed for incomplete healing
  - Episodic therapy
    - 200 mg 5 times per day for 5 days
    - 400 mg TID for 5 days
    - 800 mg BID for 5 days
    - 800 mg TID for 2 days
  - Daily suppression
    - 400 mg BID
  - Severe, complicated infections requiring IV therapy
    - 5 to 10 mg/kg/dose q8h until clinical improvement; switch to PO therapy to complete a 10-day course.
  - HIV infection: 400 mg PO 3 to 5 times per day until clinical resolution is attained
  - Precautions
    - Modify dose in renal insufficiency.
- Valacyclovir (Valtrex) (4)[A]: prodrug of acyclovir, improved bioavailability, less frequent dosing
  - Primary episode
    - 1 g PO BID for 7 to 10 days
  - Episodic therapy
    - 500 mg PO BID for 3 to 5 days
    - 1 g PO daily for 5 days
  - Daily suppression
    - 500 mg PO daily
    - 1 g PO daily
- Famciclovir (Famvir) (4)[A]
  - Primary episode
    - 250 mg PO TID for 7 to 10 days
  - Episodic therapy
    - 125 mg PO BID for 5 days
    - 1 g PO BID for 1 day
  - Daily suppression: 250 mg PO BID

Second Line

- Used for acyclovir-resistant HSV
- Foscarnet: 40 mg/kg/dose IV q8h in severe disease
  - Associated with significant toxicity
- Cidofovir topical: 0.1–0.3% gel for 5 days

Pregnancy Considerations

ACOG Clinical Management Guidelines (4)[A],(5)[C]:

- SCREENING: Pregnant women who test antibody negative for HSV-1 and HSV-2 should avoid sexual contact in the 3rd trimester if their partner is antibody positive.
- SUPPRESSIVE THERAPY: Pregnant women with a history of genital herpes should be offered suppression treatment starting at 36 gestational weeks until delivery to decrease reactivation rate. Goal is to reduce the risk of neonatal infection and C-section. Recommended regimens to continue until delivery:
  - Acyclovir 400 mg PO TID
  - Valacyclovir 500 mg PO BID
- Monitor for outbreaks during pregnancy and examine for any lesions at the onset of labor. C-section is recommended if prodromal symptoms or lesions are present at onset of labor to reduce neonatal transmission.

Pediatric Considerations

- High-risk infants include those with active symptoms or lesions, those delivered vaginally with maternal lesions present, and those born during a primary maternal episode. Monitor closely, obtain diagnostic laboratory specimens (HSV PCR and ocular, nasal, anal, and oral cultures), and treat with acyclovir 20 mg/kg IV q8h for 10 to 14 days (4)[A].
- Low-risk infants who are asymptomatic can be observed while obtaining serum HSV PCR and ocular, nasal, anal, and oral cultures.
- Infants with possible HSV infection should be isolated from other neonates; maternal separation is not necessary and breastfeeding is not contraindicated.

ONGOING CARE

GENERAL PREVENTION

- Use barrier contraception, daily suppressive antiviral therapy, and avoid sexual contact when symptoms are present to decrease transmission.
- Abstinence is the only means of complete protection.

FOLLOW-UP RECOMMENDATIONS

- Avoid sexual contact when symptoms or lesions are present.
- Alert partners of herpes status prior to sexual activity.
- Concordant couples (i.e., both partners with the same type of herpes [HSV-1 or HSV-2]) may have sex without worry of triggering outbreaks.

Patient Monitoring

Test for other STIs if initial HSV infection

PATIENT EDUCATION

- Herpes Resource Center: http://www.ashasexualhealth.org/stdsstis/herpes/
- Warren T. *The Good News About the Bad News: Herpes: Everything You Need to Know.* Oakland, CA: New Harbinger Publications; 2009.
- Centers for Disease Control and Prevention: http://www.cdc.gov/

PROGNOSIS

- Resolution of signs/symptoms: 3 to 21 days
- Average recurrence rate is one to four episodes per year (2).
- Antivirals do not eliminate virus from body but can reduce transmission, shedding, and outbreaks.

Pediatric Considerations

Neonatal infection survival rates: localized >95%, CNS 85%, systemic 30%

COMPLICATIONS

Behavioral issues include lowered self-esteem, guilt, anger, depression, fear of rejection, and fear of transmission to partner.

REFERENCES

1. LeGoff J, Péré H, Bélec L. Diagnosis of genital herpes simplex virus infection in the clinical laboratory. *Virol J.* 2014;11:83.
2. Hofstetter AM, Rosenthal SL, Stanberry LR. Current thinking on genital herpes. *Curr Opin Infect Dis.* 2014;27(1):75–83.
3. Geretti AM. Genital herpes. *Sex Transm Infect.* 2006;82(Suppl 4):iv31–iv34.
4. Centers for Disease Control and Prevention. 2010 sexually transmitted diseases treatment guidelines. http://www.cdc.gov/std/treatment/2010/. Accessed 2014.
5. ACOG Committee on Practice Bulletins. ACOG practice bulletin. Clinical management guidelines for obstetrician-gynecologists. No. 82 June 2007. Management of herpes in pregnancy. *Obstet Gynecol.* 2007;109(6):1489–1498.

ADDITIONAL READING

- Money D, Steben M. SOGC clinical practice guidelines: guidelines for the management of herpes simplex virus in pregnancy. Number 208, June 2008. *Int J Gynaecol Obstet.* 2009;104(2):167–171.
- Tavares F, Cheuvart B, Heineman T, et al. Meta-analysis of pregnancy outcomes in pooled randomized trials on a prophylactic adjuvanted glycoprotein D subunit herpes simplex virus vaccine. *Vaccine.* 2013;31(13):1759–1764.
- Tobian AA, Grabowski MK, Serwadda D, et al. Reactivation of herpes simplex virus type 2 after initiation of antiretroviral therapy. *J Infect Dis.* 2013;208(5):839–846.

SEE ALSO

Algorithm: Genital Ulcers

CODES

ICD10

- A60.00 Herpesviral infection of urogenital system, unspecified
- A60.04 Herpesviral vulvovaginitis
- A60.09 Herpesviral infection of other urogenital tract

CLINICAL PEARLS

- Genital herpes infections can be caused by HSV-1 and HSV-2.
- Many seropositive individuals are unaware that they are infected.
- Most primary episodes are asymptomatic.
- Viral shedding occurs in the absence of lesions.

H

HICCUPS

Vanessa W. McNair, MD, MPH • Jeannette M. McIntyre, MD • Steven B. Sapida, DO

BASICS

DESCRIPTION
- Hiccups are caused by a repetitive sudden involuntary contraction of the inspiratory muscles (predominantly the diaphragm) terminated by abrupt closure of the glottis, which stops the inflow of air and produces a characteristic sound.
- Hiccups are classified based on their duration: Acute hiccups last <48 hours; persistent hiccups last >48 hours but <1 month; intractable hiccups last for >1 month.
- System(s) affected: nervous, pulmonary
- Synonym(s): hiccoughs; singultus

Geriatric Considerations
Can be a serious problem, particularly among the elderly

Pregnancy Considerations
- Fetal hiccups are noted as rhythmic fetal movements (confirmed sonographically) that can be confused with contractions.
- Fetal hiccups are a sign of normal neurologic development (1).

EPIDEMIOLOGY
- Predominant age: all ages (including fetus)
- Predominant sex: male > female (4:1)

Prevalence
Self-limited hiccups are extremely common, as are intra- and postoperative hiccups.

ETIOLOGY AND PATHOPHYSIOLOGY
- Results from stimulation of ≥1 limbs of the hiccup reflux arc (vagus and phrenic nerves) with a "hiccup center" located in the upper spinal cord and brain (2)
- In men, >90% have an organic basis; whereas in women, a psychogenic cause is more common.
- Specific underlying causes include the following:
  - Alcohol abuse
  - CNS lesions (brain stem tumors, vascular lesions, Parkinson disease, multiple sclerosis, syringomyelia, hydrocephalus)
  - CNS infections (encephalitis, meningitis)
  - Seizure disorder
  - Diaphragmatic irritation (tumors, pericarditis, eventration, splenomegaly, hepatomegaly, peritonitis)
  - Irritation of the tympanic membrane
  - Pharyngitis, laryngitis
  - Mediastinal and other thoracic lesions (pneumonia, aortic aneurysm, tuberculosis [TB], myocardial infarction [MI], lung cancer, rib exostoses)
  - Esophageal lesions (reflux esophagitis, achalasia, Candida esophagitis, carcinoma, obstruction)
  - Gastric lesions (ulcer, distention, cancer)
  - Hepatic lesions (hepatitis, hepatoma)
  - Pancreatic lesions (pancreatitis, pseudocysts, cancer)
  - Inflammatory bowel disease
  - Cholelithiasis, cholecystitis
  - Prostatic disorders
  - Appendicitis
  - Postoperative, abdominal procedures
  - Toxic metabolic causes (uremia, hyponatremia, gout, diabetes)
  - Drug-induced (dexamethasone, methylprednisolone, anabolic steroids, benzodiazepines, α-methyldopa, propofol)
  - Psychogenic causes (hysterical neurosis, grief, malingering)
  - Idiopathic

RISK FACTORS
- General anesthesia; conscious sedation
- Postoperative state
- Genitourinary disorders
- Irritation of the vagus and phrenic nerve (or branches)
- Gastroesophageal reflux
- Structural, vascular, infectious, neoplastic, or traumatic CNS lesions

GENERAL PREVENTION
- Identify and correct the underlying cause if possible.
- Avoid gastric distention.
- Acupuncture shows promise in comparison to chronic drug therapy to control hiccups (3).

COMMONLY ASSOCIATED CONDITIONS
See "Etiology."

DIAGNOSIS

- Hiccup attacks usually occur at brief intervals and last only a few seconds or minutes. Persistent bouts lasting >48 hours often imply an underlying physical or metabolic disorder.
- Intractable hiccups may occur continuously for months or years (4).
- Hiccups usually occur with a frequency of 4 to 60 per minute (4).
- Persistent and intractable hiccups warrant further evaluation.

HISTORY
- Recent surgery (especially genitourinary)
- General anesthesia
- Behavioral health history
- Medications
- Alcohol use/illicit drug use
- GI, cardiac, neurologic, or pulmonary disorders (see "Etiology")

PHYSICAL EXAM
- Correlate exam with potential etiologies (e.g., rales with pneumonia; organomegaly with splenic or hepatic disease).
- Examine the ear canal for foreign bodies.
- Head and neck exam to look for neck masses and lymphadenopathy
- Complete neurologic exam

DIFFERENTIAL DIAGNOSIS
Hiccups may rarely be confused with burping (eructation).

DIAGNOSTIC TESTS & INTERPRETATION
- If history suggests an underlying etiology, consider condition-specific testing as appropriate (e.g., CBC, metabolic panel, chest x-ray).
- Fluoroscopy is useful to determine whether one hemidiaphragm is dominant.

Diagnostic Procedures/Other
- Upper endoscopy; colonoscopy; CT scan (or other imaging) of brain, thorax, abdomen, and pelvis looking for underlying causes
- The extent of the workup is often in proportion to the duration and severity of the hiccups (2,5).

TREATMENT

- Outpatient (usually)
- Inpatient (if elderly, debilitated, or intractable hiccups)
- Many hiccup treatments are purely anecdotal.

GENERAL MEASURES
- Seek medical attention for frequent bouts or persistent hiccups.
- Treat any specific underlying cause when identified (2,4,5)[C]
  - Dilate esophageal stricture or obstruction.
  - Treat ulcers or reflux disease.
  - Remove hair or foreign body from ear canal.
  - Angostura bitters for alcohol-induced hiccups
  - Catheter stimulation of pharynx for operative and postoperative hiccups
  - Antifungal treatment for Candida esophagitis
  - Correct electrolyte imbalance.
- Medical measures
  - Relief of gastric distention (gastric lavage, nasogastric aspiration, induced vomiting)
  - Counterirritation of the vagus nerve (supraorbital pressure, carotid sinus massage, digital rectal massage)—use with caution
  - Respiratory center stimulants (breathing 5% CO_2)
  - Behavioral health modification (hypnosis, meditation, paced respirations)
  - Phrenic nerve block or electrical stimulation (or pacing) of the dominant hemidiaphragm
  - Acupuncture
  - Miscellaneous (cardioversion)

MEDICATION

First Line

Possible drug remedies (5–7)[B]
- Baclofen, a GABA analog: 5 to 10 mg PO TID (2,4,5,8)[B]

- Chlorpromazine (FDA approved for hiccups): 25 to 50 mg PO/IV TID
- Haloperidol: 2 to 5 mg PO/IM followed by 1 to 2 mg PO TID
- Phenytoin: 200 to 300 mg PO HS

- Metoclopramide: 5 to 10 mg PO QID
- Nifedipine: 10 to 20 mg PO daily to TID
- Amitriptyline: 10 mg PO TID
- Viscous lidocaine 2%: 5 mL PO daily to TID
- Gabapentin (Neurontin): 300 mg PO HS; may increase up to 1,800 mg/day PO in divided doses (4)[B]; 1,200 mg/day PO for 3 days, then 400 mg/day PO for 3 days in patients undergoing stroke rehabilitation or in the palliative care setting where chlorpromazine adverse effects are undesirable (4)[B].
- Combination of lansoprazole 15 mg PO daily, clonazepam 0.5 mg PO BID, and dimenhydrinate 25 mg PO BID (6)[B].
- Contraindications: Refer to manufacturer's literature.
  – Baclofen is not recommended in patients with stroke or other cerebral lesions or in severe renal impairment.
- Precautions: Refer to manufacturer's literature.
  – Abrupt withdrawal of baclofen should be avoided.

Second Line
Possible drug therapies (2,6,8–10)[C]
- Amantadine, carbidopa-levodopa in Parkinson disease
- Steroid replacement in Addison disease
- Antifungal agent in *Candida* esophagitis
- Ondansetron in carcinomatosis with vomiting
- Nefopam (a nonopioid analgesic with antishivering properties related to antihistamines and antiparkinsonian drugs) is available outside the United States in both IV and oral formulations.
- Olanzapine 10 mg QHS
- Pregabalin 375 mg/day

ISSUES FOR REFERRAL
For acupuncture or phrenic nerve crush, block, or electrostimulation; cardioversion

SURGERY/OTHER PROCEDURES
- Phrenic nerve crush or transaction or electrostimulation of the dominant diaphragmatic leaflet
- Resection of rib exostoses

COMPLEMENTARY & ALTERNATIVE MEDICINE
- Acupuncture is increasingly used to manage persistent or intractable hiccups, especially in cancer patients (3,4)[A].
- Simple home remedies (2,7)[C]
  – Swallowing a spoonful of sugar
  – Sucking on hard candy or swallowing peanut butter
  – Holding breath and increasing pressure on diaphragm (Valsalva maneuver)
  – Tongue traction
  – Lifting the uvula with a cold spoon
  – Inducing fright
  – Smelling salts
  – Rebreathing into a paper (not plastic) bag
  – Sipping ice water
  – Rubbing a wet cotton-tipped applicator between hard and soft palate for 1 minute

INPATIENT CONSIDERATIONS
Admission Criteria/Initial Stabilization
Most patients can be managed as outpatients; those with severe intractable hiccups may require rehydration, pain control, IV medications, or surgery.

 ## ONGOING CARE

FOLLOW-UP RECOMMENDATIONS
Patient Monitoring
Until hiccups cease

DIET
Avoid gastric distension from overeating, carbonated beverages, and aerophagia.

PATIENT EDUCATION
See "General Measures."

PROGNOSIS
- Hiccups often cease during sleep.
- Most acute benign hiccups resolve spontaneously or with home remedies.
- Intractable hiccups may last for years or decades.
- Hiccups have persisted despite bilateral phrenic nerve transection.

COMPLICATIONS
- Inability to eat
- Weight loss
- Exhaustion, debility
- Insomnia
- Cardiac arrhythmias
- Wound dehiscence
- Death (rare)

REFERENCES
1. Witter F, Dipietro J, Costigan K, et al. The relationship between hiccups and heart rate in the fetus. *J Matern Fetal Neonatal Med.* 2007;20(4): 289–292.
2. Calsina-Berna A, García-Gómez G, González-Barboteo J, et al. Treatment of chronic hiccups in cancer patients: a systemic review. *J Palliat Med.* 2012;15(10):1142–1150.
3. Ge AX, Ryan ME, Giaccone G, et al. Acupuncture treatment for persistent hiccups in patients with cancer. *J Altern Complement Med.* 2010;16(7):811–816.
4. Thompson DF, Brooks KG. Gabapentin therapy of hiccups. *Ann Pharmacother.* 2013;47(6): 897–903.
5. Ramírez FC, Graham DY. Treatment of intractable hiccup with baclofen: results of a double-blind randomized, controlled, cross-over study. *Am J Gastroenterol.* 1992;87(12):1789–1791.
6. Maximov G, Kamnasaran D. The adjuvant use of lansoprazole, clonazepam and dimenhydrinate for treating intractable hiccups in a patient with gastritis and reflux esophagitis complicated with myocardial infarction: a case report. *BMC Res Notes.* 2013;6:327.
7. Lewis JH. Hiccups and their cures. *Clin Perspect Gastroenterol.* 2000;3(5):277–283.
8. Moretto EN, Wee B, Wiffen PJ, et al. Interventions for treating persistent and intractable hiccups in adults. *Cochrane Database Syst Rev.* 2013;(1):CD008768.
9. Marinella MA. Diagnosis and management of hiccups in the patient with advanced cancer. *J Support Oncol.* 2009;7(4):122–127, 130.
10. Matsuki Y, Mizogami M, Shigemi K. A case of intractable hiccups successfully treated with pregabalin. *Pain Physician.* 2014;17(2):E241–E242.

ADDITIONAL READING
- Berger TJ. A rash case of hiccups. *J Emerg Med.* 2013;44(1):e107–e108.
- Chang FY, Lu CL. Hiccup: mystery, nature and treatment. *J Neurogastroenterol Motil.* 2012;18(2): 123–130.
- Choi TY, Lee MS, Ernst E. Acupuncture for cancer patients suffering from hiccups: a systematic review and meta-analysis. *Complement Ther Med.* 2012;20(6):447–455.
- Hurst DF, Purdom CL, Hogan MJ. Use of paced respiration to alleviate intractable hiccups (Singultus): a case report. *Appl Psychophysiol Biofeedback.* 2013;38(2):157–160.
- Lewis JH. Hiccups: causes and cures. *J Clin Gastroenterol.* 1985;7(6):539–552.
- Rizzo C, Vitale C, Montagnini M. Management of intractable hiccups: an illustrative case and review. *Am J Hosp Palliat Care.* 2014;31(2):220–224.

 ## CODES

ICD10
- R06.6 Hiccough
- F45.8 Other somatoform disorders

CLINICAL PEARLS
- Most hiccups resolve spontaneously.
- An organic cause for persistent hiccups is more likely to be found in men and individuals with intractable hiccups.
- Rule out a foreign body in the ear canal as hiccup trigger.
- Baclofen and gabapentin are the only pharmacologic agents proven effective in a clinical trial.
- Acupuncture may be effective for persistent hiccups.

H

HIDRADENITIS SUPPURATIVA

Travis C. Geraci, MD • Siva Vithananthan, MD, FACS

BASICS

DESCRIPTION
- Chronic follicular occlusive disease manifested as recurrent inflammatory nodules, abscesses, sinus tracts, and complex scar formation
- Lesions are tender, malodorous, often with exudative drainage.
- Common in intertriginous skin regions: axillae, groin, perianal, perineal, inframammary skin
- System affected: skin
- Synonym(s): acne inversa; Verneuil disease; apocrinitis; hidradenitis axillaris

Geriatric Considerations
Rare after menopause

Pediatric Considerations
Rarely occurs before puberty; occurrence in children is associated with premature adrenarche.

Pregnancy Considerations
No Accutane (isotretinoin) or tetracycline treatment during pregnancy. Disease may ease during pregnancy and rebound after parturition.

EPIDEMIOLOGY
Predominant sex: female > male (3:1)

Incidence
Peak onset during 2nd and 3rd decades of life

Prevalence
0.3–4%

ETIOLOGY AND PATHOPHYSIOLOGY
- Not fully understood; previously considered a disorder of apocrine glands
- Inflammatory disorder of the hair follicle triggered by follicular plugging within apocrine gland–bearing skin.
- Hormonally induced ductal keratinocyte proliferation leads to a failure of follicular epithelial shedding, causing follicular occlusion.
- Mechanical stress on skin (intertriginous regions) precipitates follicular rupture and immune response.
- Bacterial involvement is a secondary event.
- Rupture and reepithelialization cause sinus tracts to form.
- Obesity and smoking are major risk factors in disease onset and severity.

Genetics
- Familiar occurrences suggest single gene transmission (autosomal dominant), but the condition may also be polygenic.
- Estimated 40% of patients have an affected family member.

RISK FACTORS
- Obesity
- Smoking
- Hyperandrogenism, oral contraceptive pills (OCPs)
- Lithium may trigger onset of or exacerbate this condition.

GENERAL PREVENTION
- Lose weight if overweight or obese.
- Smoking cessation
- Avoid constrictive clothing/synthetic fabrics, frictional trauma, heat exposure, excessive sweating, shaving, depilation, and deodorants.
- Use of antiseptic soaps.

COMMONLY ASSOCIATED CONDITIONS
- Acne vulgaris, acne conglobate
- Perifolliculitis capitis abscedens et suffodiens (dissecting cellulitis of scalp)
- Pilonidal disease
- Arthritis and spondyloarthritis (seronegative)
- Obesity (with diabetes, atopy, acanthosis)
- Irritable bowel disease (Crohn disease)
- Squamous cell carcinoma
- PAPASH syndrome (pyogenic arthritis, pyoderma gangrenosum, acne, suppurative hydradenitis)

DIAGNOSIS

HISTORY
- Diagnostic criteria adopted by the 2nd International Conference on Hidradenitis Suppurativa, 2009 (1)[C]
- All three criteria must be present for diagnosis:
  - Typical lesions: painful nodules, abscesses, draining sinus, bridged scars, and "tombstone" double-ended pseudocomedones in secondary lesions
  - Typical topography: axillae, groins, perineal and perianal region, buttocks, infra- and intermammary folds
  - Chronicity and recurrences, commonly refractory to initial treatments.

PHYSICAL EXAM
- Tender nodules (dome-shaped) 0.5 to 3 cm in size are present.
  - Location corresponds with the distribution of apocrine-related mammary tissue and terminal hair follicles dependent on low androgen concentrations.
  - Sites ordered by frequency of occurrence: axillary, inguinal, perianal and perineal, mammary and inframammary, buttock, pubic region, chest, scalp, retroauricular, eyelid
  - Large lesions are often fluctuant; comedones may be present.
  - Possible malodorous discharge
- Hurley clinical staging system
  - Stage I: abscess formation (singular or multiple) without sinus tracts or scarring
  - Stage II: widely separated, recurrent abscesses with tract formation and scarring
  - Stage III: diffuse, multiple interconnected tracts and abscesses
- Sartorius clinical staging system (points attributed)
  - Anatomic region
  - Quantity and quality of lesions
  - Distance between lesions
  - Presence or absence of normal skin between lesions

DIFFERENTIAL DIAGNOSIS
- Acne vulgaris, conglobate
- Furunculosis/carbuncles
- Infected Bartholin or sebaceous cysts
- Lymphadenopathy/lymphadenitis
- Cutaneous Langerhans cell histiocytosis
- Actinomycosis
- Granuloma inguinale
- Lymphogranuloma venereum
- Apocrine nevus
- Crohn disease with anogenital fistula(s) (may coexist with hidradenitis suppurativa)
- Cutaneous tuberculosis
- Fox-Fordyce disease

DIAGNOSTIC TESTS & INTERPRETATION

Initial Tests (lab, imaging)
- Cultures of skin or aspirates of boils are most commonly negative. When positive, cultures are often polymicrobial and commonly grow Staphylococcus aureus and Staphylococcus epidermidis.
- Lesion biopsy usually unnecessary. Useful to rule out other disorders such as squamous cell carcinoma.
- May note increased erythrocyte sedimentation rate (ESR), leukocytosis, decreased serum iron, normocytic anemia, or changes in serum electrophoresis pattern.

Follow-Up Tests & Special Considerations
- Consider biopsy of concerning lesions due to increased risk of squamous cell carcinoma.
- If the patient is female, overweight, and/or hirsute, consider evaluating the following:
  - Dehydroepiandrosterone sulfate
  - Testosterone: total and free
  - Sex hormone-binding globulin
  - Progesterone

Diagnostic Procedures/Other
- Incision and drainage, culture and biopsy
- Ultrasound may be useful in planning an excision to identify the full extent of sinus tracts.

Test Interpretation
- Dermis shows granulomatous inflammation and inflammatory cells, giant cells, sinus tracts, subcutaneous abscesses, and extensive fibrosis.
- Hair follicular dilatation and occlusion by keratinized stratified squamous epithelium

TREATMENT

Despite the prevalence of this condition, few large-scale randomized controlled trials have explored the safety and efficacy of treatment. Evidence is generally of poor quality (2)[A]. Treatment goals: Reduce extent of disease, prevent new lesions, remove chronic disease, and limit scar formation.

- Conservative treatment includes all items under general prevention, plus use of warm compresses, sitz baths, topical antiseptics for inflamed lesions, and nonopioid analgesics.
- Weight loss and smoking cessation result in marked improvement.
- For stage I–II, attempt medical treatment.
- Short medical trial may be appropriate in stage III prior to moving on to surgical therapies.
- No medications are curative; relapse is almost inevitable, but the disease may be controlled.

GENERAL MEASURES
- Education and psychosocial support
- Appropriate hygiene including avoidance of shearing stress to skin (light clothing), daily cleansing with antibacterial soap
- Diet: Avoid dairy and high glycemic loads.
- Symptomatic treatment for acute lesions
- Improve environmental factors that cause follicular blockage (see "General Prevention").
- Smoking cessation and weight loss

MEDICATION

First Line

• Stage I disease: Consider either systemic or topical antibiotics.

– Topical antibiotics (clindamycin has the most evidence) (3)[B]

  ○ Clindamycin 1% solution BID for 12 weeks with or without Benzoyl peroxide 5–10% solution
  ○ Chlorhexidine 4% solution
– Systemic antibiotics (initial 7- to 10-day course)
  ○ Tetracycline 500 mg BID
  ○ Doxycycline 100 mg q12h
  ○ Augmentin 875 mg q8–12h
  ○ Clindamycin 300 mg BID (4)[B]

• Stage II–III disease
– Address overlying bacterial infection with broad-spectrum coverage. Base antibiotic selection on disease location, characteristics; longer durations (3 to 6 months) may be required.
– Tetracycline 500 mg BID
– Minocycline 100 mg BID
– Doxycycline 100 mg BID
– Minor surgical procedures (punch débridement, local unroofing) to treat individual lesions or sinus tracts
• Other modalities (rarely used)

– Hormonal therapy: antiandrogenic therapy such as cyproterone acetate (may not be available in the United States), estrogen/norgestrel oral contraceptive, finasteride (5 mg daily) (5)[B]

• Intralesional corticosteroids: accelerates healing, although efficacy not formally evaluated (triamcinolone acetonide 5 to 10 mg/mL)

Second Line

• Combination of antibiotic regimens
– Clindamycin and rifampin
– Rifampin, moxifloxacin, and metronidazole
• Dapsone 50 to 150 mg daily (6)[C]

• Metformin: significant reduction in Sartorius score (7)[B]
• Oral retinoids (Isotretinoin): poor efficacy, limited therapeutic effect (8)[B]

• TNF-α inhibitors:

– Infliximab: a majority of patients in the treatment group had a 50% or greater decrease in disease (9)[B]
– Etanercept: no difference versus placebo (10)[A]

– Adalimumab: limited efficacy

ISSUES FOR REFERRAL

• Lack of response to treatment, stage II–III disease, or concern for malignancy (squamous cell carcinoma) is a reason to refer for surgical excision or radiation/laser treatment (stage II).
• If significant psychosocial stress exists secondary to disease, refer for stress management or psychiatric evaluation.
• Suspicion of hyperandrogenic states (e.g., polycystic ovary syndrome [PCOS]) should prompt investigation or referral.
• Severe perianal/perivulvar disease or otherwise very extensive disease may prompt referral to plastic surgeon or reconstructive urologist.

SURGERY/OTHER PROCEDURES

• Important mode of treatment
• Could be used in conjunction with antibiotics or if first-line therapy fails

• Various surgical approaches have been used for stage II–III disease (11,12)[B]:

– Incision and drainage: may be necessary to treat as a temporizing method for acute flare-ups

– Deroofing and marsupialization of the sinus tracts is often beneficial primarily for Hurley stage I–II disease, as healing time is reduced. Recurrences remain common but usually are smaller than original lesions (13)[B].

– Wide full-thickness excision with healing by granulation or flap placement is the most definitive treatment and rarely has local recurrence if all sinus tracts are excised. Rates of local recurrence (within 3 to 72 months): axillary (3%), perianal (0%), inguinoperineal (37%), submammary (50%)
• Laser therapy for Hurley stage I–II disease (rarely used)

– Consider monthly treatments with neodymium-doped yttrium aluminum garnet (Nd:YAG) laser for 3 to 4 months.
– CO_2 laser ablation with healing by secondary intention
• Cryotherapy and photodynamic therapy have shown variable results, they are not routinely recommended.

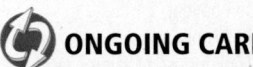 ONGOING CARE

FOLLOW-UP RECOMMENDATIONS

Follow up monthly or sooner to evaluate progress and to assist with symptom management.

DIET

• Avoid dairy, high glycemic loads.
• Healthy diet that promotes weight loss.
• May benefit from zinc supplementation

PATIENT EDUCATION

• Severity can range from only 2 to 3 papules per year to extensive draining sinus tracts.
• Medications are temporizing measures, rarely curative. Attempts at local surgical "cures" do not affect recurrence at other sites.
• Smoking cessation and weight loss can improve symptoms significantly. Hidradenitis Suppurativa Foundation: www.hs-foundation.org

PROGNOSIS

• Individual lesions heal slowly in 10 to 30 days.
• Recurrences may last for several years.
• Relentlessly progressive scarring and sinus tracts are likely with severe disease.
• Radical wide-area excision, with removal of all hair-bearing skin in the affected area, shows the greatest chance for cure.

COMPLICATIONS

• Contracture and stricturing of the skin after extensive abscess rupture, scarring, and healing; or at sites of surgical excisions
• Lymphatic obstruction, lymphedema
• Psychosocial: anxiety, malaise, depression, self-injury
• Anemia, amyloidosis, and hypoproteinemia (due to chronic suppuration)
• Lumbosacral epidural abscess, sacral bacterial osteomyelitis
• Squamous cell carcinoma may develop in indolent sinus tracts.
• Disseminated infection or septicemia (rare)
• Urethral, rectal, or bladder fistula (rare)

REFERENCES

1. Hidradenitis Suppurativa Foundation. http://www.hs-foundation.org.
2. Rambhatla PV, Lim HW, Hamzavi I. A systematic review of treatments for hidradenitis suppurativa. *Arch Dermatol.* 2012;148(4):439–446.
3. Jemec GB, Wendelboe P. Topical clindamycin versus systemic tetracycline in the treatment of hidradenitis suppurativa. *J Am Acad Dermatol.* 1998;39(6):971–974.
4. van der Zee HH, Boer J, Prens EP, et al. The effect of combined treatment with oral clindamycin and oral rifampicin in patients with hidradenitis suppurativa. *Dermatology.* 2009;219(2):143–147.
5. Searles GE. Daily oral finasteride 5 mg for hidradenitis suppurativa. Paper presented at: Annual Meeting of the Canadian Dermatology Association; July 3, 2009; Vancouver, British Columbia, Canada.
6. Kaur MR, Lewis HM. Hidradenitis suppurativa treated with dapsone: a case series of five patients. *J Dermatolog Treat.* 2006;17(4):211–213.
7. Verdolini R, Clayton N, Smith A, et al. Metformin for the treatment of hidradenitis suppurativa: a little help along the way. *J Eur Acad Dermatol Venereol.* 2013;27(9):1101–1108.
8. Soria A, Canoui-Poitrine F, Wolkenstein P, et al. Absence of efficacy of oral isotretinoin in hidradenitis suppurativa: a retrospective study based on patients' outcome assessment. *Dermatology.* 2009;218(2):134–135.
9. Grant A, Gonzalez T, Montgomery MO, et al. Infliximab therapy for patients with moderate to severe hidradenitis suppurativa: a randomized, double-blind, placebo-controlled crossover trial. *J Am Acad Dermatol.* 2010;62(2):205–217.
10. Adams DR, Yankura JA, Fogelberg AC, et al. Treatment of hidradenitis suppurativa with etanercept injection. *Arch Dermatol.* 2010;146(5):501–504.
11. Blok JL, van Hattem S, Jonkman MF, et al. Systemic therapy with immunosuppressive agents and retinoids in hidradenitis suppurativa: a systematic review. *Br J Dermatol.* 2013;168(2):243–252.
12. Kagan RJ, Yakuboff KP, Warner P, et al. Surgical treatment of hidradenitis suppurativa: a 10-year experience. *Surgery.* 2005;138(4):734–740; discussion 740–741.
13. van der Zee HH, Prens EP, Boer J. Deroofing: a tissue-saving surgical technique for the treatment of mild to moderate hidradenitis suppurativa lesions. *J Am Acad Dermatol.* 2010;63(3):475–480.

ADDITIONAL READING

• Alikhan A, Lynch PJ, Eisen DB. Hidradenitis suppurativa: a comprehensive review. *J Am Acad Dermatol.* 2009;60(4):539–561.
• Jemec GB. Clinical practice. Hidradenitis suppurativa. *N Engl J Med.* 2012;366(2):158–164.
• Mandal A, Watson J. Experience with different treatment modules in hidradenitis suppuritiva: a study of 106 cases. *Surgeon.* 2005;3(1):23–26.
• Slade DE, Powell BW, Mortimer PS. Hidradenitis suppurativa: pathogenesis and management. *Br J Plast Surg.* 2003;56(5):451–461.

 CODES

ICD10

L73.2 Hidradenitis suppurativa

CLINICAL PEARLS

• Chronic inflammatory disease of the skin, often difficult to control with behavior changes and medication alone
• First-line treatment for mild disease is topical and/or systemic antibiotics.
• For patients with refractory or severe disease, wide local excision provides the only chance at a cure. Success rates depend on the location and extent of excision.

H

HIRSUTISM

Laura Novak, MD • Imola K. Osapay, MD

 BASICS

DESCRIPTION
- Presence of excessive terminal (coarse, pigmented) hair of body and face, in a male pattern, in women of reproductive age
- May be present in normal adults as an ethnic characteristic or may develop as a result of androgen excess
- Often seen in polycystic ovarian syndrome (PCOS) which is characterized by hirsutism, acne, menstrual irregularities, and obesity
- System(s) affected: dermatologic, endocrine/metabolic, reproductive

Pregnancy Considerations
- May have related infertility. Offer intervention, if desired.
- As hormone balance improves, fertility may increase; provide contraception, as needed.
- Several medications used for treatment are contraindicated in pregnancy.

EPIDEMIOLOGY
Prevalence
5–10% of adult women

ETIOLOGY AND PATHOPHYSIOLOGY
- Hirsutism is due to increased androgenic (male) hormones, either from increased peripheral binding (idiopathic) or increased production from the ovaries, adrenals, or fat.
- Exogenous medications can also cause hirsutism.

Genetics
Multifactorial

RISK FACTORS
- Family history
- Ethnicity—increased in Ashkenazi Jews and Mediterranean backgrounds
- Anovulation

GENERAL PREVENTION
- Women with late-onset congenital adrenal hyperplasia (CAH) should be counseled that they may be carriers for the severe early-onset childhood disease.
- Avoid quackery.

COMMONLY ASSOCIATED CONDITIONS
- PCOS: most common cause of hirsutism. Variable presentation but commonly presents with a combination of excess androgen, abnormal menses, and insulin resistance. It is estimated that 75% of hirsute women have PCOS (1).
- Associated insulin resistance or PCOS can increase the risk of heart disease.
- Prolonged amenorrhea and anovulation:
  - Prolonged amenorrhea may, over time, put the patient at risk for endometrial hyperplasia or carcinoma.

- Hypothyroidism or hyperprolactinemia
- Late-onset CAH (21-hydroxylase deficiency): a genetic enzyme deficiency associated with more severe and earlier onset hirsutism; present in <2% of hirsute, amenorrheic patients
- Tumor: rare (<0.2%); ovarian or adrenal; especially if associated with virilization (rapid onset, clitoromegaly, balding, deepening voice) (2)
- Cushing syndrome: rare; characterized by central obesity, moon facies, striae, hypertension

 DIAGNOSIS

HISTORY
- Severity, duration, and age of onset of hirsutism
- Psychosocial impact on patient
- Menstrual and fertility history
- Medication history: Look for use of valproic acid, testosterone, danazol, glucocorticoids, and athletic performance drugs.
- The presence of galactorrhea

PHYSICAL EXAM
- Increased hair growth on face, chest, and groin
- Check skin for acne, striae, acanthosis nigricans (velvety black skin in the axilla or neck).
- Virilization: Deep voice, male pattern balding, and clitoromegaly indicate risk of tumor.
- The Ferriman-Gallwey scale (an instrument that rates hair growth in nine areas on a scale of 0 to 4, with >8 being positive) may be used for diagnosis but underrates patient's perception of hirsutism and altered by previous cosmetic treatment (1).

DIFFERENTIAL DIAGNOSIS
- Idiopathic hirsutism—hirsutism with normal androgen levels
- PCOS—irregular menses, elevated androgens, polycystic ovaries on US, infertility, insulin resistance
- Late-onset CAH presents in adolescence with severe hirsutism and irregular menses.
- Androgen-secreting tumor—rapid onset, virilization, resistance to treatment
- Thyroid dysfunction
- Hyperprolactinemia if accompanied by galactorrhea or amenorrhea
- Rare endocrine disorders—Cushing (central obesity, stria, and hypertension), acromegaly (enlarging extremities and facial deformity)

DIAGNOSTIC TESTS & INTERPRETATION
- Diagnosis is clinical. Empiric treatment without lab workup is an acceptable option in mild–moderate hirsutism (2)[C].
- PCOS is diagnosed by having two out of three signs: menstrual dysfunction, clinical or biochemical hyperandrogenemia, polycystic ovaries on US (2)[C].
- Lab testing is performed to rule out underlying tumor and pituitary diseases, which are rare.

Initial Tests (lab, imaging)
- Basic workup of mild–moderate hirsutism is a total testosterone level +/− a thyroid screen (1–3)[C]. Testosterone: random total testosterone level is usually sufficient. A morning free testosterone is slightly more sensitive, but the difference is not clinically relevant (1,4).
- If testosterone is >150 (some use 200) ng/dL, consider ovarian or adrenal tumor (2,3).
- Testosterone is made by both the ovaries and adrenals, so both areas should be imaged. US is best for the ovaries, and CT is best for the adrenals.
- If testosterone is not in the tumor range, treat clinicallyTSH-elevation indicates hypothyroidism.
- The workup of PCOS recommended by ACOG (the American Congress of Obstetricians and Gynecologists) includes the above plus:
  - Screening for metabolic syndrome with a fasting and 2-hour glucose after 75-g glucose load, lipid panel, waist circumference, and blood pressure (3)[C]
- Ovarian US
- If the patient is amenorrheic, check prolactin, FSH, LH, and a pregnancy test.

Follow-Up Tests & Special Considerations
- 17-hydroxyprogesterone (17-OHP)
  - Elevations of 17-OHP (>300) can indicate late-onset CAH; rare (<2%)
  - Consider in patients with onset in early adolescence or high-risk group (Ashkenazi Jews) (2)[C].
  - If elevated, do corticotropin stimulation test.
- If prolactin level is high, MRI the pituitary
- If PCOS is diagnosed, ACOG recommends screening for dyslipidemia and DM type 2 (3)[C].
- Dehydroepiandrosterone sulfate (DHEA-S) is no longer recommended routinely but should be checked in virilization (4)[C].
  - Levels >700 may indicate adrenal tumor.

TREATMENT

GENERAL MEASURES
- Treatment in mild hirsutism depends on patient preference and psychosocial effect.
- If patient desires pregnancy, induction of ovulation may be necessary.
- Provide contraception, as needed.
- Encourage patient to maintain ideal weight with lifestyle modification.
- Treat accompanying acne.

MEDICATION

First Line
- Treatment goal is to decrease new hair growth and improve metabolic disorders.
- Oral contraceptives are first line to manage menstrual abnormalities and hirsutism/acne (5)[B]; it will decrease androgens, improve metabolic syndrome, and slow but not reverse hair growth. It take 6 months to show effect and are continued for years; any preparation is effective; however, those containing the progestins, norgestimate, desogestrel, or drospirenone may have more androgen-blocking effects, but also are associated with more DVTs (3)[C].
- Progesterone (depot or intermittent oral) can be used if estrogens are contraindicated (3)[C].
- Eflornithine (Vaniqa) HCl cream: apply BID at least 8 hours apart; reduces facial hair in 40% of women (must be used indefinitely to prevent regrowth). Only FDA-approved hirsutism treatment.

Second Line
- Antiandrogenic drugs will further reduce hirsutism to 15–25%. Usually begun 6 months after first-line therapy if results are suboptimal. Must be used in combination with oral contraceptives to prevent menorrhagia and potential fetal toxicity. All should be avoided in pregnancy (2,4)[C].
  - Spironolactone, 50 to 200 mg/day: onset of action is slow; use with oral contraceptives to prevent menorrhagia. Watch for hyperkalemia, especially with drospirenone-containing OCP (Yasmin); avoid use in pregnancy.
  - Finasteride: 5 mg/day decreases androgen binding; not approved by FDA. Use with contraception (pregnancy Category X).
  - Cyproterone, not available in the United States: 12.5 to 100 mg/day for days 5 to 15 of cycle combined with ethinyl estradiol 20 to 50 μg days 5 to 25 of cycle
  - Flutamide is not recommended (2).
- Insulin sensitizers (metformin, thioglitazones): mildly effective but less so than oral contraceptives. May be used in diabetes or if oral contraceptives are contraindicated. Metformin is more effective than thioglitazones (2)[A].
- Steroids: used in late-onset CAH
  - Dexamethasone: 2 mg/day
- Cosmetic treatment: includes many methods of hair removal
  - Temporary: shaving, chemical depilation, plucking, waxing
  - Permanent: Laser epilation and photoepilation are preferred to electrolysis (3)[C].

COMPLEMENTARY & ALTERNATIVE MEDICINE
Several herbals including spearmint tea, saw palmetto, licorice, fennel, and soy have been shown in small (<50 people) and short (<12 weeks) studies to decrease hair size or lower androgen levels (5)[C].

 ONGOING CARE

FOLLOW-UP RECOMMENDATIONS
No special activity

Patient Monitoring
Monitor for known side effects of medications.

DIET
No special diet

PATIENT EDUCATION
- Hormonal treatment stops further hair growth and will improve but not reverse present hair.
  - Treatment takes 6 months to effect and may need to be lifelong.
- Cosmetic measures may be needed for the present hair (see above).

PROGNOSIS
- Good (with long-term therapy) for halting further hair growth
- Moderate to poor for reversing current hair growth

COMPLICATIONS
- If PCOS is present, dysfunctional uterine bleeding may lead to anemia.
- If PCOS is present, anovulation may increase uterine cancer risk.
- Androgenic excess may adversely affect lipid status, cardiac risk, and bone density.
- Poor self-image

REFERENCES

1. Azziz R, Carmina E, Dewailly D, et al. The androgen excess and PCOS society criteria for the polycystic ovary syndrome: the complete task force report. *Fertil Steril*. 2009;91(2):456–488.
2. Martin KA, Chang RJ, Ehrmann DA, et al. Evaluation and treatment of hirsutism in premenopausal women: an endocrine society clinical practice guideline. *J Clin Endocrinol Metab*. 2008;93(4):1105–1120.
3. ACOG Committee on Practice Bulletins—Gynecology. ACOG practice bulletin no. 108: polycystic ovary syndrome. *Obstet Gynecol*. 2009;114(4):936–949. Reaffirmed 2013.
4. Rosenfeld RL. Clinical practice. Hirsutism. *N Eng J Med*. 2005;353(24):2578–2588.
5. Anjum F, Mubeen U, Tabasum H, et al. Physiological perspectives of hirsutism in Unani medicine: An overview and update. *IJHM*. 2013;1(3):79–85.

ADDITIONAL READING

- Bode D, Seehusen DA, Baird D. Hirsutism in women. *Am Fam Physician*. 2012;85(4):373–380.
- Brown J, Farquhar C, Lee O, et al. Spironolactone versus placebo or in combination with steroids for hirsutism and/or acne. *Cochrane Database Syst Rev*. 2009;(2):CD000194.
- Harborne L, Fleming R, Lyall H, et al. Metformin or antiandrogen in the treatment of hirsutism in polycystic ovary syndrome. *J Clin Endocrinol Metab*. 2003;88(9):4116–4123.
- National Institute of Health. Evidence-based methodology workshop on PCOS. https://prevention.nih.gov/docs/programs/pcos/FinalReport.pdf.
- Somani N, Harrison S, Bergfeld WF. The clinical evaluation of hirsutism. *Dermatol Ther*. 2008;21(5):376–391.
- Swiglo BA, Cosma M, Flynn DN, et al. Clinical review: antiandrogens for the treatment of hirsutism: a systematic review and metaanalyses of randomized controlled trials. *J Clin Endocrinol Metab*. 2008;93(4):1153–1160.

 SEE ALSO

Acne Vulgaris; Infertility; Polycystic Ovarian Syndrome (PCOS)

CODES

ICD10
- L68.0 Hirsutism
- E28.2 Polycystic ovarian syndrome

CLINICAL PEARLS
- PCOS is the most common cause of hirsutism (two out of three: menstrual dysfunction, clinical or biochemical hyperandrogenemia, polycystic ovaries on US)
- Treatment is long term and often lifelong.
- Associated insulin resistance and DM is common and need to be treated.

H

HIV/AIDS

Meera Shah, MD, MS, AAHIVS

 BASICS

DESCRIPTION

HIV is a retrovirus (subgroup lentivirus) that integrates into CD4 T-lymphocytes, altering cell-mediated immunity and causing cell death, severe immunodeficiency, opportunistic infections, and malignancies if untreated.

- Because of treatment advances, HIV is now classified as a chronic disease.
- The natural history of untreated HIV infection includes viral transmission, acute retroviral syndrome, recovery and seroconversion, asymptomatic chronic HIV infection, and symptomatic HIV infection or AIDS.
- Without treatment, the average patient progresses to AIDS about 10 years after acquiring the virus.
- All HIV-infected persons with CD4 <200 cells/mm³ or with AIDS-defining illnesses are categorized as living with AIDS.

EPIDEMIOLOGY

Incidence

In the United States, HIV incidence has remained relatively stable at about 50,000 infections per year since the mid-1990s.

Prevalence

- Estimated 1.2 million persons in the United States are living with HIV/AIDS as of 2012; 12.8% are unaware of their status (1).
- HIV/AIDS cases are disproportionately high among racial/ethnic minority populations.
- Transmission of drug-resistant HIV is rising.

ETIOLOGY AND PATHOPHYSIOLOGY

- HIV primarily infects CD4+ cells. HIV is a single-stranded, positive-sense, enveloped RNA virus. After entering target cells, through the process of reverse transcription, viral RNA is transcribed to DNA and imported to the host cell nucleus and encoded into the cellular DNA. The virus can become latent or produce new viral RNA and proteins that are released to infect other CD4+ cells. Host CD8+ cells are activated to produce the seroconversion response.
- There are two types of HIV. HIV-1 is the virus that was first described and is more virulent. It causes the majority of HIV infections worldwide. HIV-2 is less infective and seen primarily in West Africa or countries with economic ties to West Africa.

Genetics

People who have a mutation in CCR5, a cell-surface chemokine coreceptor, are resistant to HIV infection.

RISK FACTORS

- Sexual activity (70% of transmission): Ulcerative urogenital lesions promote transmission (2).
- Male-to-male sexual contact accounts for most (63%) newly diagnosed HIV/AIDS cases (1).
- Injection drug abuse (IDA)
- Children of HIV-infected women
  - Maternal HIV-1 RNA level predicts transmission.
  - HIV testing and treatment in pregnancy: With ARV prophylaxis, scheduled C-section and avoiding breastfeeding, HIV transmission rates have declined to <2% in the US and Europe (3)[B].
  - HIV can also be transmitted in breastmilk. HIV+ women should not breastfeed their infants.

- Recipients of blood products prior to 1985
- Occupational exposure (health care workers)

GENERAL PREVENTION

- Avoid unprotected, high-risk sexual intercourse and intravenous drug use, particularly with shared needles.
- Preexposure prophylaxis (PrEP) is recommended for individuals at high risk for transmission (4)[A].

COMMONLY ASSOCIATED CONDITIONS

- Syphilis may be more aggressive in HIV-infected.
- Tuberculosis (TB) is coepidemic with HIV; test all persons with HIV for TB (and vice versa). Dually infected patients have 100 times greater risk of developing active TB.
- Patients coinfected with hepatitis C or hepatitis B have a more rapid progression to cirrhosis.

 DIAGNOSIS

- Acute retroviral syndrome: CD4 lymphocyte count declines with increase in viral load 1 to 4 weeks after transmission; confirmed by demonstrating a high-HIV RNA in the absence of HIV antibody
- Acute retroviral syndrome presents as a mononucleosis-like syndrome including:
  - Fever (97%)
  - Adenopathy
  - Pharyngitis (73%)
  - Rash (77%)
  - Myalgias/arthralgia (58%)
  - Less common symptoms include headache, diarrhea, nausea, vomiting, weight loss, thrush, and neurologic symptoms (12%).
  - Seroconversion: Positive HIV antibody test occurs 4 weeks to 6 months after exposure.
- Clinical latency (asymptomatic): variable duration (average is 8 to 10 years) accompanied by a gradual decline in CD4 cell counts and relatively stable HIV RNA levels (the viral "set point"). Patients often develop persistent generalized lymphadenopathy (>1 cm in ≥2 extrainguinal sites) and may develop fever, weight loss, myalgias, and gastrointestinal problems if the diagnosis is unrecognized.
- Symptomatic conditions:
  - Fever or diarrhea >1 month, bacillary angiomatosis, thrush, persistent candidal vulvovaginitis, cervical dysplasia or carcinoma in situ, oral hairy leukoplakia, herpes zoster, idiopathic thrombocytopenic purpura, pelvic inflammatory disease, peripheral neuropathy or myelopathy
- AIDS: defined by a CD4 cell count <200, a CD4 cell percentage of total lymphocytes <14%, or one of several AIDS-related opportunistic infections: *Pneumocystis jiroveci (carinii)* pneumonia, cryptococcal meningitis, recurrent bacterial pneumonia, candida esophagitis, CNS toxoplasmosis, TB and non-Hodgkin lymphoma (NHL), progressive multifocal encephalopathy, HIV nephropathy, Kaposi sarcoma, NHL, Hodgkin lymphoma, invasive cervical cancer
- Advanced HIV disease: CD4 cell count <50. Most AIDS-related deaths occur at this time. Common late opportunistic infections: cytomegalovirus (CMV) disease (retinitis, colitis) or disseminated *Mycobacterium avium* complex as well as HIV wasting syndrome (>10% weight loss) and HIV encephalopathy/dementia/cognitive–motor disorder.

HISTORY

- Complete medical history, including risk exposures and social/occupational history
- Review of systems: fever, chills, night sweats, diarrhea, weight loss, fatigue, adenopathy, oral sores, odynophagia (esophageal candidiasis), cough, shortness of breath and dyspnea on exertion (early *P. jiroveci* pneumonia), visual changes (CMV retinitis), skin rash, neurologic symptoms (CNS infection, malignancy, or dementia), sinusitis
- Review immunization record.

PHYSICAL EXAM

Focus on weight, skin, retinal exam, oropharynx, lymph nodes, liver, spleen, mental status, sensation, genital, and rectal examinations.

DIFFERENTIAL DIAGNOSIS

Burkitt lymphoma; candidiasis; coccidioidomycosis; cryptococcus; CMV; herpes simplex; lymphoma; toxoplasmosis, influenza

DIAGNOSTIC TESTS & INTERPRETATION

Initial Tests (lab, imaging)

- Screening: Rapid oral test available and FDA approved. Two FDA-approved home testing kits are also available.
- Obtain HIV RNA if acute HIV infection is suspected.
- 4th-generation HIV testing combines antibody/antigen immunoassay for HIV-1, HIV-2 (5)
  - Can be positive within 2 to 3 weeks of exposure
  - Is considered a confirmatory test
- CD4 cell count and percentage (5)[A]
- HIV RNA viral load (5)[A]
- CBC with differential
- Serum chemistry
- Serologies: hepatitis A, B, and C; syphilis
- Urine screen for STIs (*Neisseria gonorrhoeae, Chlamydia trachomatis*)
- Oral and anal screen for STIs (*N. gonorrhoeae, C. trachomatis*)
- Cervical cytology at diagnosis, after 6 months and then annually in women with a cervix
- Anal cytology in HIV-positive men who have sex with men and women with abnormal cervical cytology
- Purified protein derivative (PPD) or QuantiFERON-TB Gold to screen for latent TB infection, chest x-ray if pulmonary symptoms or positive PPD
- Glucose-6-phosphate levels
- HLAB*5701 testing if abacavir is considered for treatment.
- Lipids at baseline and during highly active antiretroviral therapy (HAART)
- Genotypic tests for resistance to antiretrovirals for patients with pretreatment HIV RNA >1,000 copies/mL. Transmitted resistance to at least one drug can be seen in 6–16% of individuals (5)[A].
- Tropism assay if considering CCR5 antagonist therapy

 TREATMENT

- Initiate antiretroviral therapy in all patients with HIV to reduce risk of disease progression (AI to BIII) and to prevent the risk of transmission (AI to AIII) (5).

- Several conditions increase the urgency for therapy including pregnancy (AI), AIDS-defining conditions (AI), acute opportunistic infections, CD4 <200 (AI), HIV-associated nephropathy (AII), acute/early infection (BII), HIV/HBV coinfection (AII), HIV/HCV coinfection (BII), rapidly declining CD4 counts (>100 cells/mm³ per year) (AIII), and high viral loads (>100,000 copies/mL) (BII) (5)
- Genotypic testing is recommended to guide therapy in patients who are naïve to antiretroviral therapy.
- Tenofovir/emtricitabine or Truvada (300 mg/200 mg PO daily) FDA-approved for PrEP in adults at high risk (4)

GENERAL MEASURES
- The main goal of HAART is to reduce viral load (ideally below limits of assay detection) and delay immune suppression. Viral load is the most important indicator of response to HAART.
- Check for transmitted drug resistance before starting HAART (5)[A].
- Prevent HIV-associated complications, short- and long-term adverse drug reactions, HIV transmission and drug resistance, and preservation of HIV treatment options.
- Assess substance abuse, economic factors (unstable housing, food insecurity), social support, mental illness, comorbidities, high-risk behaviors, and factors known to impair adherence and promote transmission.
- Prophylactic antimicrobial agents and vaccines:
  - *P. jiroveci prophylaxis*: trimethoprim/sulfamethoxazole (TMP-SMX) 1 DS (160 mg/800 mg) tab PO daily indicated if CD4 <200 cells/mm³, prior *P. jiroveci*, thrush, or unexplained fever for >2 weeks
  - *Mycobacterium tuberculosis*: Treat for latent TB if positive PPD or QuantiFERON-Gold without prior prophylaxis or treatment, with negative CXR, recent TB contact, or history of inadequately treated TB that healed.
  - *Toxoplasma gondii prophylaxis*: 33% per year risk of infection in untreated patients with CD4 <100 cells/mm³; prophylaxis: TMP-SMX 1 DS tab daily
  - *M. avium complex prophylaxis:* 20–40% risk with CD4 <50 and no HAART. Preferred prophylaxis is azithromycin 1,200 mg PO weekly.
  - *Streptococcus pneumoniae*: 50 to 100 times increased risk of invasive infection compared with general population; Prevnar and Pneumovax at least 8 weeks apart, every 5 years
  - Influenza vaccine annually
  - Hepatitis A and B vaccines
  - Tdap vaccination every 10 years. Substitute one-time dose of Tdap vaccine at time of next booster.

MEDICATION
- Recommended regimens for ARV-naïve (5):
  - Integrase strand transfer inhibitor-based regimens:
    ○ Dolutegravir/abacavir/lamivudine (50 mg/600 mg/300 mg PO daily)—only for patients who are HLA-B*5701 negative (AI)
    ○ Dolutegravir (50mg PO daily) plus tenofovir disoproxil fumarate/emtricitabine (300 mg/200 mg PO daily) (AI)
    ○ Elvitegravir/cobicistat/tenofovir/emtricitabine (150 mg/150 mg/300 mg/200 mg PO daily)—only for patients with preantiretroviral therapy CrCl >70 mL/min (AI)
    ○ Raltegravir (400 mg PO BID) plus tenofovir/emtricitabine (300 mg/200 mg PO daily) (AI)

  - Protease inhibitor-based regimen:
    ○ Darunavir and ritonavir (800 mg PO daily and 100 mg PO daily) plus tenofovir/emtricitabine (300 mg/200 mg PO daily) (AI)
- Alternative regimens
  - Based on a patient's individual needs and genotype, an alternative regimen may be chosen, which have been outlined in the DHHS guidelines.
- Drug failure: Before selecting regimen, review clinical symptoms, history of HAART, and adherence. Perform resistance testing.
- Protease inhibitors (PI) can cause metabolic syndrome.
- HAART, especially the protease inhibitors, have interactions with other medications, such as antacids, steroids, contraceptives

 ONGOING CARE

FOLLOW-UP RECOMMENDATIONS
Patient Monitoring
- If HIV RNA is detectable at 2 to 8 weeks, repeat every 4 to 8 weeks until suppressed to less than level of detection, then follow every 3 to 6 months (5).
- Monitor HIV RNA, CD4, CBC every 3 to 4 months (5). CD4 monitoring may be spaced out after long-term virologic control.
- Test fasting lipids and fasting glucose annually; basic chemistry, aspartate aminotransferase, alanine aminotransferase, T/D bilirubin every 6 to 12 months (5)
- HLA-B 5701 if considering abacavir (5)
- Pregnancy test women of childbearing age (5)
- Urinalysis every 6 to 12 months or as clinically indicated (5)
- Hepatitis C as clinically indicated (5)

DIET
- Encourage good nutrition.
- Discuss unknown and potentially harmful effects of supplement use including drug–drug interactions.
- Avoid raw eggs and unpasteurized milk. Severely immunocompromised patients should boil tap water to prevent *Cryptosporidium*.

PATIENT EDUCATION
- Provide nonjudgmental, sex-positive prevention counseling, reviewing high-risk behaviors and viral transmission.
- Emphasize importance of adherence to HAART to prevent resistance.
- National AIDS Hotline: 800-342-2437 [Spanish 800-342-7432]
- National Institute of Health AIDS Clinical Trials Group: 800-874-2572
- American Foundation for AIDS Research: 212-719-0033 (new treatments and research) www.aidsinfo.nih.gov

PROGNOSIS
- Untreated HIV infection leading to the diagnosis of AIDS has an associated life expectancy of about 3 years, and if the patient has an OI, the life expectancy is about 1 year.
- AIDS-defining opportunistic infections usually do not develop until CD4 <200.
- Adherence failure—not drug resistance—is the most common cause of treatment failure (1)[B].

COMPLICATIONS
- Immunodeficiency
- Opportunistic infections
- Malignancy, including cervical or anal cancer

REFERENCES
1. Centers for Disease Control and Prevention. HIV/AIDS Statistics Overview. http://www.cdc.gov/hiv/statistics/overview/index.html. Accessed 2015.
2. Quinn TC, Wawer MJ, Sewankambo N, et al. Viral load and heterosexual transmission of human immunodeficiency virus type 1. Rakai Project Study Group. *N Engl J Med*. 2000;342(13):921–929.
3. U.S. Department of Health and Human Services. Recommendations for the use of antiretroviral drugs in pregnant HIV-1-infected women for maternal health and interventions to reduce perinatal HIV transmission in the United States. https://aidsinfo.nih.gov/contentfiles/lvguidelines/perinatalgl.pdf. Accessed 2015.
4. Centers for Diease Control and Prevention. Preexposure prophylaxis for the prevention of HIV infection in the United States—2014. A clinical practice guideline. http://www.cdc.gov/hiv/guidelines/index.html. Accessed 2015.
5. U.S. Department of Health and Human Services. Guidelines for the use of antiretroviral agents in HIV-1 infected adults and adolescents. http://aidsinfo.nih.gov/contentfiles/lvguidelines/adultandadolescentgl.pdf. Accessed 2015.

ADDITIONAL READING
Aberg JA, Gallant JE, Ghanem KG, et al. Primary care guidelines for the management of persons infected with HIV: 2013 update by the HIV medicine association of the Infectious Diseases Society of America. *Clin Infect Dis*. 2014;58(1):e1–e34.

CODES

ICD10
- Z21 Asymptomatic human immunodeficiency virus infection status
- B20 Human immunodeficiency virus [HIV] disease
- R75 Inconclusive laboratory evidence of human immunodef virus

CLINICAL PEARLS
- Acute HIV seroconversion illness mimics mononucleosis and is characterized by fever, sore throat, adenopathy, myalgias, and rash.
- Transmitted drug resistance is increasing. Evaluate patients for resistance before initiating HAART.
- Appropriate vaccination and prophylactic antibiotics should be administered to HIV+ patients based on clinical history and CD4 count.
- Discuss prevention strategies, including PrEP, with individuals who are at high risk of HIV infection.

H

HODGKIN LYMPHOMA

Jennifer J. Gao, MD   Fred J. Schiffman, MD

 BASICS

DESCRIPTION
Historical background:

- Described in 1832 by Thomas Hodgkin in "On some morbid appearance of the absorbent glands and spleen"
- First neoplasm to be (i) defined by cytologic grounds based on presence of Reed-Sternberg (RS) cells, (ii) clinically staged neoplastic disease, and (iii) treated with chemotherapy and/or radiotherapy
- Neoplastic RS cells of monoclonal lymphoid B-cell origin within inflammatory background of lymphocytes (T-helper type 2 and regulatory T cells), eosinophils, histiocytes, and plasma cells (1,2)
- Two subtypes: classic Hodgkin lymphoma (CHL, 95% of cases) and nodular lymphocyte predominant Hodgkin lymphoma (NLPHL, 3–8% of cases) (1)
  - NLPHL: B cells, neoplastic luteinizing hormone (LH) cells with multilobulated nuclei, small nucleoli, and popcorn-like appearance
  - CHL histologic subdivisions: nodular sclerosing (60%), mixed cellularity (30%), lymphocyte depleted (<10%), lymphocyte rich (<10%)
  - Frequency of lymph node involvement: cervical > mediastinal > axillary > paraaortic

EPIDEMIOLOGY
- Incidence: 2.8/100,000/year
- Predominance: 8% of lymphoid malignancies (1)

Geriatric Considerations
Poorer prognosis if present at ≥60 years:
- Less likely to tolerate intensive chemotherapy
- Less likely to be included in clinical trial

Pediatric Considerations
Young females (<30 years of age) treated with thoracic radiation are at high risk for breast cancer, and early breast cancer screening is recommended.

Pregnancy Considerations
- Abdominal ultrasonography to detect subdiaphragmatic disease
- Treatment:
  - Delay until after delivery if asymptomatic and early-stage
  - ABVD safely used in 2nd and 3rd trimesters
  - Vinblastine monotherapy to control symptoms
  - 1st trimester: ABVD may or may not cause fetal malformations.

Incidence
- ~9,000 new cases in the United States annually
- Mean age at diagnosis: 38 years
- Hodgkin is most common in early adulthood (15 to 40) and then again after age 55 years.

Prevalence
~190,000 living with Hodgkin lymphoma in the United States in 2012

ETIOLOGY AND PATHOPHYSIOLOGY
- RS cells likely derived from germinal center B cells with mutations in immunoglobulin variable chain
- Seasonal features and higher frequencies with Epstein-Barr virus (EBV) suggest environmental factors.
- T-lymphocyte defects persist even after successful treatment.
- Human leukocyte antigen (HLA) is strongly associated with increased risk (2).

- EBV positivity associated with increased risk (2)
- Genome-wide association studies identified 19p13.3 at intron 2 of *TCF3*.

Genetics
- First-degree relative: 3 to 9 times risk
- Siblings of younger patients: 7 times risk
- Weak correlation between familial HL and HLA class I regions containing HLA A1, B5, B8, B18 alleles

RISK FACTORS
- Immunodeficiency (inherited or acquired)
- Autoimmune disorders
- EBV (2)
- Seasonal factors

COMMONLY ASSOCIATED CONDITIONS
In HIV:
- AIDS-defining illness
- Predominantly mixed-cellularity or lymphocyte-depleted histologic subtypes
- At diagnosis: widespread disease, extranodal involvement, systemic symptoms

 DIAGNOSIS

HISTORY
- Asymptomatic lymphadenopathy (cervical/supraclavicular)
- Pel-Ebstein fever
- Constitutional symptoms: night sweats, weight loss, fatigue, anorexia
- Alcohol-induced pain
- Pruritus

PHYSICAL EXAM
Focus on lymph nodes, spleen, and liver.

DIFFERENTIAL DIAGNOSIS
Non-Hodgkin lymphoma, infectious lymphadenopathy, solid tumor metastases, sarcoidosis, autoimmune disease, AIDS/HIV, drug reaction

DIAGNOSTIC TESTS & INTERPRETATION

Initial Tests (lab, imaging)
- CBC and electrolytes
- LFT, including hepatitis serologies
- HIV
- Pregnancy test
- Pulmonary function tests (diffusion capacity of the lung for carbon monoxide for ABVD or BEACOPP)
- Chest x-ray
- CT of chest, abdomen, and pelvis
- PET: for initial staging, midtreatment decision making, and end-of-treatment evaluation
- Bone scan, gallium scan, abdominal ultrasound
- EBV (2)

Follow-Up Tests & Special Considerations
- Fertility considerations:
  - Semen cryopreservation if chemotherapy or pelvic radiation therapy
  - In vitro fertilization or ovarian tissue/oocyte cryopreservation
- Radiation therapy (RT) considerations:
  - Splenic RT: pneumococcal, *Haemophilus influenzae*, meningococcal vaccine

Diagnostic Procedures/Other
- Excisional lymph node biopsy
- Immunohistochemistry
- Bone marrow biopsy
- Liver biopsy (in selected cases)

Test Interpretation
RS cell characteristics include the following:
- Diameter: 20 to 50 μm
- Abundant acidophilic cytoplasm
- Bi- or polylobulated nucleus
- Acidophilic nucleoli
- CD30+, CD15+, CD45−, CD3−, CD20+ in 40% of cases
- RS cells necessary but not sufficient for diagnosis (needs inflammatory background)

 TREATMENT

- Ann Arbor staging with Cotswold modification
  - Stage I: single lymph node or of a single extralymphatic organ or site
  - Stage II: ≥2 lymph node regions on the same side of diaphragm alone or with involvement of extralymphatic organ or tissue
  - Stage III: node groups on both sides of the diaphragm
  - Stage IV: dissemination involving extranodal organs (except the spleen, which is considered lymphoid tissue)
  - Subclasses: A = no systemic symptoms; B = systemic symptoms (fever, night sweats, weight loss >10% body weight); X = bulky disease (widened mediastinum, > intrathoracic diameter, or >10-cm nodal mass)
  - Pathologic stage at given site denoted by: M = bone marrow, H = liver, L = lung, O = bone, P = pleura, D = skin:
    ○ Splenectomy, liver biopsy, lymph node biopsy, bone marrow biopsy mandatory for pathologic staging
- Goal: Aim for cure.
- All subsequent treatment and follow-up care recommendations based on National Comprehensive Cancer Network (NCCN) consensus. Please refer to NCCN Practice Guidelines in Oncology for Hodgkin lymphoma.

MEDICATION

First Line
- ABVD: doxorubicin, bleomycin, vinblastine, dacarbazine:
  - Highly emetic, severe phlebitis
  - Monitor cardiac function on doxorubicin.
  - Dacarbazine cannot be omitted without loss of efficacy (3).
- BEACOPP: bleomycin, etoposide, doxorubicin, cyclophosphamide, vincristine, procarbazine, prednisone:
  - Bleomycin: risk of pulmonary toxicity, death; test dose may be administered prior to first cycle
- Stage I/II with no risk factors: two cycles ABVD followed by 20 Gy involved field radiotherapy (IFRT)
- Stage I/II with risk factors (large mediastinal mass, unfavorable histology, age, extranodal disease, erythrocyte sedimentation rate (ESR), B symptoms, number of nodal areas): four cycles chemotherapy (BEACOPP and/or ABVD) followed by 30 Gy IFRT
- Stage III/IV: four to six cycles chemotherapy (BEACOPP and/or ABVD) and consider autologous stem cell transplant (SCT) or radiotherapy

- Relapsed and refractory: high-dose conditioning therapy (HDCT) followed by autologous SCT:
  – Maintenance therapy: trials with brentuximab vedotin (anti-CD30) and lenalidomide under way
  – Brentuximab vedotin: anti-CD30, use in relapsed HL after two prior lines of treatment have been tried, side effects include peripheral neuropathy, nausea, fatigue, neutropenia, diarrhea (4)
  – Allogeneic SCT to be considered if failed autologous SCT (used in trials only)
  – Consolidation with brentuximab vedotin after autologous SCT improves progression free survival in those at risk for relapse or progression after transplantation (5).

Second Line
- Median survival <3 years if fail second-line therapy, including SCT
- SCT in progressive disease or relapse:
  – High-dose chemotherapy and autologous stem cell transplant (HDCT/autoSCT): improved event-free and progression-free survival compared with conventional chemotherapy but not overall survival; can achieve disease-free survival in 30–40% of patients after alloSCT (6,7)
  – Reduced intensity conditioning (RIC) with bis-chloroethylnitrosourea (BCNU), etoposide, cytarabine, melphalan (BEAM) followed by allogeneic transplant (alloSCT) to induce graft-versus-tumor (GVT) effect in patients who have relapsed after autoSCT, complete response seen in 81%, non-relapse mortality of 13% at 1 year, 1-year relapse rate of 36% (6,8)
- Rituximab: excellent activity against lymphocyte-predominant variant due to CD20+ lymphocytes
- Brentuximab vedotin: anti-CD30 chimeric antibody conjugated to synthetic antimicrotubule agent monomethyl auristatin E:
  – Approved by the U.S. Food and Drug Administration (FDA) in 2011 for patients who failed/not candidate for SCT or failure of two prior multiagent chemotherapy regimens
- Nivolumab: anti-PD1 therapy with response in 20 out of 23 patients (9)
- Novel agents undergoing studies: NF-κB inhibitors (bortezomib), mammalian target of rapamycin (mTOR) inhibitors (everolimus), immunomodulators (lenalidomide), cell signaling targets histone deacetylase (HDAC) inhibitors (vorinostat, panobinostat, mocetinostat)

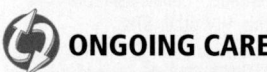 ONGOING CARE

FOLLOW-UP RECOMMENDATIONS
Patient Monitoring
- During therapy: CBC, nutrition, and hydration
- Restage with PET after two to four cycles of chemotherapy: sensitive prognostic indicator
- Posttreatment monitoring:
  – History and physical (H&P): q2–4mo for first 2 years, then q3–6mo for next 3 to 5 years
  – Laboratory studies
    ○ CBC, platelets, ESR, chemistry profile q2–4mo for 1 to 2 years, then q3–6mo for next 3 to 5 years
    ○ Thyroid-stimulating hormone (TSH) annually if radiation to neck
  – Imaging:
    ○ Chest: chest x-ray or CT q6–12mo during first 2 to 5 years

- ○ Abdominal/pelvic: CT q6–12mo during first 2 to 3 years
  ○ Annual breast mammogram or MRI beginning 8 to 10 years after therapy or at age 40 years if chest or axillary irradiation
  ○ Surveillance PET should not be done routinely due to risk of false-positive findings.
- Splenic irradiation or splenectomy as part of Hodgkin treatment increases risk of secondary cancers (leukemia, myelodysplastic syndrome, non-Hodgkin lymphoma, solid cancers) (10).

PATIENT EDUCATION
- Reproductive impact
- Risks of secondary malignancy
- Oral and dental care during therapy
- Leukemia & Lymphoma Society (http://www.lls.org/)

PROGNOSIS
- Cure rate for classic Hodgkin lymphoma: 80%
- Relapse or progression of disease rate: 5–20%
- Overall survival rates:
  – 1-year survival: 92%
  – 5-year survival: 85%
  – 10-year survival: 81%
- International prognostic score for advanced disease:
  – Age ≥45 years
  – Male gender
  – Albumin <4 g/dL
  – Hemoglobin <10.5 g/dL
  – Lymphocytopenia: <600 lymphocyte cells/dL or lymphocytes <8% of WBC
  – WBC ≥15,000 cells/dL
  – Stage IV disease
- Main cause of death
  – Initial 5 years: Hodgkin lymphoma
  – After 5 to 10 years: leukemia, myelodysplastic syndrome
  – After 20 years: second primary malignancy, cardiovascular disease

REFERENCES

1. Goel A, Fan W, Patel AA, et al. Nodular lymphocyte predominant Hodgkin lymphoma: biology, diagnosis and treatment. *Clin Lymphoma Myeloma Leuk*. 2014;14(4):261–270.
2. Cozen W, Timofeeva MN, Li D, et al. A meta-analysis of Hodgkin lymphoma reveals 19p13.3 TCF3 as a novel susceptibility locus. *Nat Commun*. 2014;5:3856.
3. Behringer K, Goergen H, Hitz F, et al. Omission of dacarbazine or bleomycin, or both, from the ABVD regimen in treatment of early-stage favourable Hodgkin's lymphoma (GHSG HD13): an open-label, randomised, non-inferiority trial. *Lancet*. 2015;385(9976):1418–1427.
4. Siddiqi T, Thomas SH, Chen R. Role of brentuximab vedotin in the treatment of relapsed or refractory Hodgkin lymphoma. *Pharmgenomics Pers Med*. 2014;7:79–85.
5. Moskowitz CH, Nademanee A, Masszi T, et al. Brentuximab vedotin as consolidation therapy after autologous stem-cell transplantation in patients with Hodgkin's lymphoma at risk of relapse or progression (AETHERA): a randomised, double-blind, placebo-controlled, phase 3 trial. *Lancet*. 2015;385(9980):1853–1862.
6. Lim AB, Ritchie DS. Hodgkin lymphoma, allogeneic transplant and the graft-versus-tumor effect: size does matter. *Leuk Lymphoma*. 2014;55(6):1223–1224.
7. Rancea M, von Tresckow B, Monsef I, et al. High-dose chemotherapy followed by autologous stem cell transplantation for patients with relapsed or refractory Hodgkin lymphoma: a systematic review with meta-analysis. *Crit Rev Oncol Hematol*. 2014;92(1):1–10.
8. Sobol U, Rodriguez T, Smith S, et al. Seven-year follow-up of allogeneic transplant using BCNU, etoposide, cytarabine and melphalan chemotherapy in patients with Hodgkin lymphoma after autograft failure: importance of minimal residual disease. *Leuk Lymphoma*. 2014;55(6):1281–1287.
9. Ansell SM, Lesokhin AM, Borrello I, et al. PD-1 blockade with nivolumab in relapsed or refractory Hodgkin's lymphoma. *N Engl J Med*. 2015;372(4):311–319.
10. Mosalpuria K, Loberiza F Jr. Splenectomy and second malignancies in patients with Hodgkin lymphoma: is there a causal relationship? *Leuk Lymphoma*. 2015;56(1):10–11.

ADDITIONAL READING
- Armitage JO. Early-stage Hodgkin's lymphoma. *N Engl J Med*. 2010;363(7):653–662.
- Borchmann P, Eichenauer DA, Engert A. State of the art in the treatment of Hodgkin lymphoma. *Nat Rev Clin Oncol*. 2012;9(8):450–459.
- Czuczman M, Straus D, Gribben J, et al. Management options, survivorship, and emerging treatment strategies for follicular and Hodgkin lymphomas. *Leuk Lymphoma*. 2010;51(Suppl 1):41–49.
- Dinner S, Advani R. Targeted therapy in relapsed classical Hodgkin lymphoma. *J Natl Compr Canc Netw*. 2013;11(8):968–976.
- National Cancer Institute. Surveillance, Epidemiology, and End Results Program. SEER stat fact sheet: Hodgkin lymphoma. http://seer.cancer.gov/statfacts/html/hodg.html.
- National Comprehensive Cancer Network. NCCN clinical practice guidelines in oncology. Hodgkin lymphoma. Version 2. 2013. http://www.nccn.org/.
- von Tresckow B, Engert A. Refractory Hodgkin lymphoma. *Curr Opin Oncol*. 2013;25(5):463–469.

 CODES

ICD10
- C81.90 Hodgkin lymphoma, unspecified, unspecified site
- C81.91 Hodgkin lymphoma, unsp, lymph nodes of head, face, and neck
- C81.92 Hodgkin lymphoma, unspecified, intrathoracic lymph nodes

CLINICAL PEARLS
- Neoplastic disease of lymphatics
- RS cells of monoclonal lymphoid B-cell origin within inflammatory background of lymphocytes
- Two subtypes: CHL, 95% of cases and NLPHL, 5% of cases
- Cure rate for CHL: 80%
- 5-year survival: ~86%
- Relapse or progression of disease rate: 5–20%
- Immunotherapy with PD1 blockade currently underway and promising

H

HOMELESSNESS

Dana Sprute, MD, MPH, FAAFP • Lauren Engelmann, MD

 BASICS

DESCRIPTION

"Homeless" or "homeless individual or homeless person" includes the following: (i) an individual who lacks a fixed, regular, and adequate nighttime residence; and (ii) an individual who has a primary nighttime residence that is (a) a supervised publicly or privately operated shelter designed to provide temporary living accommodations (including welfare hotels, congregate shelters, and transitional housing for the mentally ill); (b) an institution that provides a temporary residence for individuals intended to be institutionalized; and (c) a public or private place not designed for, or ordinarily used as, a regular sleeping accommodation for human beings.

EPIDEMIOLOGY

Prevalence

As of January 2014, on any given night there are 578,424 homeless individuals in the United States: 37% are homeless families; 15% are chronically homeless individuals; 48% are not chronically homeless individuals; and 33% are children (1)[A].

- From 2013 to 2014, overall homelessness decreased by 2.3%; targeted federal assistance has increased. Risk for becoming homeless remains high (1)[A].
- Although many homeless individuals reside in temporary housing or shelters, 42% live on the streets (1,2)[A].
- Homelessness continues to decrease due to increases in targeted federal funding for rapid rehousing/permanent housing; 2015 fiscal year $4.5 billion (highest in history to date) (2)[A].

RISK FACTORS

- Economic factors
  - Poverty
    - 2015 federal poverty definition: $24,250 annual income for 4-person household in the lower 48 states and District of Columbia, slightly higher in Alaska and Hawaii (3)[A].
    - In 2013, 15% of the U.S. population fell below federal poverty definition (4)[A].
  - Unemployment: U.S. rate 5.3% in July 2015 (U.S. Bureau of Labor Statistics, accessed August 4, 2015)
  - Lack of affordable health care: In 2015, 13.2% of people in United States are without health insurance (4)[A].
    - Young adults (ages 19 to 34 years) are disproportionately uninsured (27%) compared with the average for all ages (13%); the uninsured rate for ages 19 to 25 years decreased by 7.4% since between 2009 and 2013, following Affordable Care Act provision allowing individuals in this age group to stay on their parents' insurance plans (4)[A].
    - Access to insurance has markedly improved because of the introduction of the Affordable Care Act; the number of uninsured Americans has dropped 35% since October 2013 (4)[A].
  - Lack of affordable housing: housing is considered affordable if ≤30% of household income
    - Over 6.5 million households are defined by HUD as "severely housing cost burdened" (≥50% of income is spent on housing) (5)[A].

- At-risk populations: intimate partner violence, victims of violence; youth (particularly those aging out of foster care); veterans; rural; addiction; psychiatric illness; disabled due to chronic medical disease, psychiatric illness, or substance use disorder; reentry after incarceration/prison
  - Intimate partner violence (IPV): 63% of homeless women experience IPV; in many cases, IPV leads directly to homelessness (6)[A].
  - Youth: Each year, 550,000 unaccompanied youths (up to age 24 years) experience an episode of homelessness lasting longer than a week (6)[A].
  - Veterans: 11% of homeless adults; homelessness rate decreased between 2009 and 2014 (1) [A].
  - Addiction disorders: 46% of homeless individuals report alcohol and/or drug use as a major factor contributing to homelessness (6)[A].
  - Psychiatric illness: 45% of homeless report indicators of a mental health issue in the past year; 25% of homeless adults suffer from chronic mental illness (6)[A].
  - Reentry after incarceration: 30–50% of parolees are homeless at any given time (6)[A].
- Fundamental issues in homelessness and health care that require ongoing consideration (7)[C]:
  - Unstable housing, limited access to nutritious food and water, lack of transportation
  - Higher risk for abuse and violence
  - Physical/cognitive impairments, behavioral health problems
  - Developmental discrepancies for children: speech delay, chronic ear infection, insufficient opportunity to practice gross and fine motor skills
  - Higher risk for communicable disease
  - Lack of health insurance/resources, discontinuous/inaccessible health care, lack of a medical home, barriers to disability assistance
  - Cultural/linguistic barriers: racial and ethnic groups overrepresented in homeless population
  - Limited education/literacy
  - Lack of social supports: Alienation from family and friends precipitates homelessness.
  - Criminalization of homelessness: frequent arrests for loitering, sleeping in public places

GENERAL PREVENTION

- Policy and funding for community programs that provide emergency/rapid housing, housing stabilization, and case management services to address risk factors.
- Affordable Care Act (ACA): In 2010, increased Medicaid eligibility for homeless and expanded home- and community-based services and case management for the homeless population (8)[A].
- Department of Housing and Urban Development (HUD): increasing permanent supportive housing units, increasing services for veterans and those with disabilities (8)[A]
- Social Justice Policy Recommendations: permanent affordable housing, foreclosure and homelessness prevention, increased funds for HUD McKinney-Vento programs (emergency, transitional, and permanent housing), rural homeless assistance, universal health care, universal livable income, employment/workforce services, prevention of hate crimes against the homeless, decriminalization of homelessness

COMMONLY ASSOCIATED CONDITIONS

- Hunger
- Medical conditions
  - Worsening of chronic conditions: lack of healthy food, places to store medications, or medical equipment; inability to get restful sleep; decreased health literacy (7)[C]
  - Infectious diseases
    - Tuberculosis (TB), HIV/AIDS, STI (7)[C]
    - Skin/nail infections and infestation (lice and scabies)
    - Liver disease (e.g., hepatitis B or C, or alcohol-related)
- Cognitive impairment: traumatic brain injury (TBI), cerebrovascular accident (CVA), substance use
- Dental problems
- Exposure-related conditions (frostbite, heatstroke)
- Psychiatric illness (7)[C]
- Trauma: increased risk of assault, victims of hate crimes

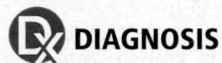 **DIAGNOSIS**

HISTORY

- Living conditions: location, access to food, restrooms, place to store medicines, safety
- Prior homelessness: what precipitated it, first time, chronic
- Individual/family history of reactive airway disease (RAD), chronic otitis media, anemia, diabetes, cardiovascular disease (CVD), TB, HIV/STIs, hospitalizations
- Family members, especially dependent children
- Medications: include OTC medication, dietary supplements, medication "borrowed" from others
- Prior providers: oral health, primary care, current medical home
- Mental health: stress, anxiety, appetite, sleep, concentration, mood, speech, memory, thought process and content, suicidal/homicidal ideation, insight, judgment, impulse control, social interactions; symptoms of brain injury (headaches, seizures, memory loss, lability, irritability, dizziness, insomnia, poor organizational/decision-making skills)
- Alcohol/nicotine/drug use: amount, frequency, duration
- Gender identity/orientation, behaviors, rape, pregnancies, hepatitis, HIV, other STIs
- History or current abuse: emotional, physical, sexual; patient safety
- Legal problems/violence: history of incarceration
- Regular/strenuous activities: routines (treatment feasibility); level of strenuous activity
- Work: previous types of jobs, length held, veteran status, occupational injuries/toxic exposures; vocational skills, interest
- Education: highest level; ever in special education; assess ability to read/language skills/English fluency.
- Nutrition/hydration: diet, food resources, preparation skills, liquid intake
- Cultural heritage/affiliations: family, friends, faith community, other sources of support
- Strengths: coping skills, resourcefulness, abilities, interests

PHYSICAL EXAM

- Comprehensive exam: height/weight, BMI, especially: liver, dermatologic, oral, feet, neurologic, mental status

- Focused exams: for patients uncomfortable with full-body, unclothed exam at first visit
- Dental assessment: age-appropriate teeth, obvious caries, dental/referred pain, diabetes, CVD

DIAGNOSTIC TESTS & INTERPRETATION
- Mental health: Patient Health Questionnaire (PHQ-9, PHQ-2), MHS-III, MDQ
- Cognitive assessment: Mini-Mental Status Exam (MMSE), Traumatic Brain Injury Questionnaire (TBIQ), Repeatable Battery for the Assessment of Neuropsychological Status (RBANS)
- Developmental assessment: Ages & Stages Questionnaires, Parents' Evaluation of Developmental Status (PEDS), Denver II, or other standard screening tool
- Interpersonal violence: IPV, sexual assault, TBI
- Forensic evaluation: if indicated by history
- Baseline labs: as needed to address suspected medical concerns
- TB screening: PPD
- STI screening: HIV, chlamydia, gonorrhea, syphilis, hepatitis B, hepatitis C, trichomonas, bacterial vaginosis, monilia
- Substance abuse: SSI-AOD (Simple Screening Instrument for Alcohol and Other Drugs), urine drug screen

Follow-Up Tests & Special Considerations
- **Reproductive health care and STIs:** Obtain detailed sexual history (sexual identity, orientation, behaviors/sexual practices, number of partners). Consider possible exploitation of patient, especially if mental illness/developmental disability suspected. Communicate willingness to initiate contraception first visit without exam. Genital exam recommended, but be sensitive to patient needs, if possible sexual abuse history. If pelvic exam is refused, consider empiric treatment for STI (and possibility of multiple orifice infection). Dispense medications on site; ask if partner needs treatment.
- **Pediatric care:** complete exam every visit, use each visit to identify/address problems and provide vaccinations as homeless families may not see a medical provider unless child is sick. Vision and hearing screening at every visit and refer for abnormalities.

TREATMENT
- Establish rapport: sensitivity to prior negative health care experiences
- Enlist resources: mental health and substance abuse programs, free clinics, case management
- Health care maintenance: vaccinations (hepatitis A and B, Pneumovax, TdaP, influenza) cancer and chronic disease screening for adults; Early Periodic Screening, Diagnosis, and Treatment Program (EPSDT) screening and vaccinations for children
- Care plan
  - Basic needs: Food, clothing and housing may be higher priorities than health care.
  - Patient goals and priorities: immediate/long-term health needs. Address patient wants first.
  - Action plan: simple language, portable pocket card
  - After hours: extended clinic hours
  - Safety plan: for violence and abuse suspected; mandatory reporting requirements
  - Emergency plan: location of nearest emergency department (ED), preparation for evacuation
  - Adherence plan: Use of interpreter; identification of potential barriers

MEDICATION
- Simple regimen: low pill count, once-daily dosing
- Dispensing: small amounts on-site to promote follow-up, decrease loss/theft/misuse risk. Determine resources for written prescriptions.
- Storage of medications: If no access to refrigeration, avoid medications requiring it.
- Patient assistance: free/low-cost drugs if readily available for continuous use; seek local options for assistance
- Aids to adherence: harm reduction, outreach/case management, directly observed therapy
- Side effects: primary reason for nonadherence (diarrhea, polyuria, nausea, disorientation)
- Analgesia/symptomatic treatment: Consider pain contract, single provider for pain medication refills.
- Dietary supplements: multivitamins with minerals, nutritional supplements
- Managed care: generics, if possible; assistance getting prescription filled
- Lab monitoring: Monitor patients on antipsychotic medications for metabolic disorders.

ADDITIONAL THERAPIES
- Associated problems/complications
  - Fragmented care: multiple providers. Use electronic medical record (EMR); list prescribed medication on wallet-sized card.
  - Masked symptoms/misdiagnosis: for example, weight loss, dementia, edema, lactic acidosis
  - Focus on immediate concerns, not possible future consequences
  - Integrated treatment for concurrent mental illness/substance use disorders
  - Support for parent of child abused by others and for abused parent
- Follow-up
  - Reliable phone/e-mail contact for patient/friend/family/case manager
  - Frequent follow-up, incentives, nonjudgmental care regardless of adherence
  - Anticipate/accommodate unscheduled clinic visits.
  - Provide car fare, tokens, and help with transportation services.
  - Monitor school attendance and address health/developmental problems with family/school.

INPATIENT CONSIDERATIONS
Admission Criteria/Initial Stabilization
Homeless likely to benefit from admission if living conditions are suboptimal to treat medical, psychiatric, and substance use disorders.

Discharge Criteria
- Bed rest, extended periods of elevation, rest, or icing are not feasible in most instances.
- Plans requiring multiple return visits likely to fail if no transportation.
- Admission to inpatient rehabilitation if appropriate and possible

ONGOING CARE

FOLLOW-UP RECOMMENDATIONS
- Patients with a history of nonadherence need additional support (e.g., case manager, outreach) to succeed in ongoing care after hospital discharge.
- Limited access to telephones to schedule appointments; may be unable to receive telephone messages with test results or rescheduled appointment times.

- Arrange appointments prior to discharge.
- Document the best way to contact the individual.
- Refer to health care agency designed to address needs of people who are homeless with integrated physical/mental health services and substance use treatment.

PROGNOSIS
Mortality rates for homeless adults are 3 to 4 times higher compared with general U.S. population (9)[C].

REFERENCES
1. U.S. Department of Housing and Urban Development, Office of Community Planning and Development. The 2014 point-in-time annual homeless assessment report to congress. https://www.hudexchange.info/resources/documents/2014-AHAR-Part1.pdf. Accessed August 22, 2015.
2. National Alliance to End Homelessness. The state of homelessness in America, 2015. http://www.endhomelessness.org/page/files/State_of_Homelessness_2015_FINAL_online.pdf. Accessed August 22, 2015.
3. U.S. Department of Health and Human Services. 2015 poverty guidelines. http://aspe.hhs.gov/2015-poverty-guidelines. Accessed August 22, 2015.
4. U.S. Department of Health and Human Services. Health Insurance Coverage and the Affordable Care Act. http://www.hhs.gov/healthcare. Accessed August 22, 2015.
5. U.S. Department of Housing and Urban Development. Affordable Housing. http://portal.hud.gov/hudportal/HUD?src=/program_offices/comm_planning/affordablehousing. Accessed August 22, 2015.
6. National Alliance to End Homelessness. www.endhomelessness.org. Accessed August 22, 2015.
7. Bonin E, Brehove T, Carlson T, et al. *Adapting Your Practice: General Recommendations for the Care of Homeless Patients*. Nashville, TN: Health Care for the Homeless Clinicians' Network, National Health Care for the Homeless Council, Inc.; 2010.
8. United States Interagency Council on Homelessness. Opening doors: federal strategic plan to prevent and end homelessness, update 2013. http://usich.gov/opening_doors/annual-update-2013. Accessed August 22, 2015.
9. Maness DL, Khan M. Care of the homeless: an overview. *Am Fam Physician*. 2014;89(8):634–640.

CODES

ICD10
- Z59.0 Homelessness
- Z59.1 Inadequate housing
- Z59.8 Other problems related to housing and economic circumstances

CLINICAL PEARLS
- Ending homelessness requires permanent housing, supportive services, and implementing policies to prevent chronic homelessness.
- Assistance in gaining access to benefits or meeting basic needs may decrease stress, improve therapeutic relationship, and allow individuals to direct attention to physical health.

HORDEOLUM (STYE)

Konstantinos E. Deligiannidis, MD, MPH, FAAFP

BASICS

DESCRIPTION
- An acute inflammation or infection of the eyelid margin involving the sebaceous gland of an eyelash (external hordeolum) or a meibomian gland (internal hordeolum)
- System(s) affected: skin/exocrine
- Synonym(s): internal hordeolum; external hordeolum; Zeisian stye; meibomian stye; stye

EPIDEMIOLOGY
- Predominant age: none
- Predominant sex: male = female

Incidence
Unknown: Although external hordeolum is common, internal hordeolum is rare.

ETIOLOGY AND PATHOPHYSIOLOGY
- Bacterial infection of sebaceous or meibomian glands, causing an acute inflammatory reaction
- In an internal hordeolum, the meibomian gland may become obstructed, leading to a pustule on the conjunctival surface as opposed to the margin of the eyelid.
- Most commonly caused by *Staphylococcus aureus* (~90–95% of all cases) or by *Staphylococcus epidermidis*
- Seborrhea can predispose to infections of the eyelid.

Genetics
No known genetic pattern

RISK FACTORS
- Poor eyelid hygiene
- Previous hordeolum
- Contact lens wearers
- Application of makeup
- Predisposing blepharitis (low-grade infections of the eyelid margin)
- Ocular rosacea

GENERAL PREVENTION
Eyelid hygiene

COMMONLY ASSOCIATED CONDITIONS
- Acne
- Seborrhea
- An association may exist between hordeolum during childhood and developing rosacea in adulthood.

DIAGNOSIS

HISTORY
- Localized inflammation (vs. involvement of the entire eyelid or surrounding skin)
- Foreign body sensation in the eye
- Prior episodes are common.

PHYSICAL EXAM
- Localized inflammation of the eyelashes or a small pustule at the margin of the eyelid
- Localized swelling and tenderness on the internal or external aspect of the eyelid with an opening to either side
- To determine if an internal hordeolum is obstructed, the eyelid should be gently everted to examine for a pustule on the tarsal conjunctiva.
- Itching or scaling of the eyelids; collection of discharge, redness, and irritation leading to localized tenderness and pain
- The size of the swelling usually correlates to the severity of the hordeolum.

DIFFERENTIAL DIAGNOSIS
- Chalazion
- Blepharitis
- Eyelid neoplasms
- Periorbital cellulitis
- Dacryocystitis

DIAGNOSTIC TESTS & INTERPRETATION
Culture of the eyelid margins usually is not necessary.

Diagnostic Procedures/Other
History and eye exam

Test Interpretation
Bacterial contamination and white cells in eyelid discharge

TREATMENT

GENERAL MEASURES
- The hordeolum should not be expressed.
- Warm compresses to the area of inflammation can help increase blood supply and encourage spontaneous drainage.
- Good personal hygiene with attention to cleansing the eyelids on a daily basis helps to prevent recurrent infections.

MEDICATION
First Line
- A Cochrane review found no evidence for or against nonsurgical treatment of internal hordeolum. External hordeola were not considered (1)[A].

- Usually, a hordeolum spontaneously drains, aided by warm compresses to the area.
- Also, lid scrubs, digital massage, and alternative medicine have been used to reduce healing time and relieving symptoms.
- Application of an antibiotic ointment (e.g., erythromycin) to the margin of the eyelid after proper cleansing (except in children age <12 years, in whom there is a risk of blurred vision and amblyopia) helps reduce bacterial proliferation. There is little evidence that any topical therapy is effective. Erythromycin ophthalmic ointment may be applied up to 6 times per day for 7 to 10 days or an antibiotic ointment containing bacitracin (2,3)[C].
- Treat underlying dry eye with artificial tears.

Second Line
- Occasionally, the use of an aminoglycoside ophthalmic ointment, such as gentamicin or tobramycin, may be necessary if condition is refractory to simpler treatment (case reports).
- Oral dicloxacillin or cephalexin for 2 weeks if refractory to topical antibiotics

ISSUES FOR REFERRAL
Consider referral if unresponsive to oral antibiotics.

SURGERY/OTHER PROCEDURES
- If the infection becomes localized to a single gland, incision, drainage, or curettage sometimes is necessary. This is an in-office procedure with a local anesthetic: Exercise caution because ocular perforation has been reported with the injection of an anesthetic to an infected lid.
- Use of combined antibiotic ointment (neomycin sulfate, polymyxin B sulfate, and gramicidin) after surgery was not shown to have any statistically significant benefit compared with artificial tears.

COMPLEMENTARY & ALTERNATIVE MEDICINE
Broncasma berna is a polyvalent antigen vaccine that may be useful in the treatment of recurrent hordeolum.

INPATIENT CONSIDERATIONS
Admission Criteria/Initial Stabilization
Outpatient

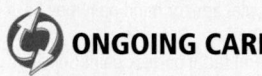 ONGOING CARE

FOLLOW-UP RECOMMENDATIONS
No restrictions

Patient Monitoring
The patient should be seen within several weeks to assess the effectiveness of therapy or should at least call the physician's office with a progress report.

DIET
No special diet

PATIENT EDUCATION
- The patient should be instructed in proper cleansing of the eyelids using a solution of tap water and baby shampoo or a commercially prepared hypoallergenic cleanser.
- The stye should not be squeezed or incised.

PROGNOSIS
- Usually responds well to good hygiene and warm compresses
- Inflammation usually improves within a week.
- Hordeolum tends to recur in some patients, usually due to incomplete elimination of bacteria.

COMPLICATIONS
An internal hordeolum, if untreated, may lead to chalazion, infections of adjacent glands, or generalized cellulitis of the lid.

REFERENCES

1. Lindsley K, Nichols JJ, Dickersin K. Interventions for acute internal hordeolum. *Cochrane Database Syst Rev*. 2013;(4):CD007742.
2. Wald ER. Periorbital and orbital infections. *Pediatr Rev*. 2004;25(9):312–320.
3. Mueller JB, McStay CM. Ocular infection and inflammation. *Emerg Med Clin North Am*. 2008;26(1):57–72.

ADDITIONAL READING

- Bamford JT, Gessert CE, Renier CM, et al. Childhood stye and adult rosacea. *J Am Acad Dermatol*. 2006;55(6):951–955.

- Hirunwiwatkul P, Wachirasereechai K. Effectiveness of combined antibiotic ophthalmic solution in the treatment of hordeolum after incision and curettage: a randomized, placebo-controlled trial: a pilot study. *J Med Assoc Thai*. 2005;88(5):647–650.
- Kim JH, Yang SM, Kim HM, et al. Inadvertent ocular perforation during lid anesthesia for hordeolum removal. *Korean J Ophthalmol*. 2006;20(3):199–200.
- Nakatani M. Treatment of recurrent hordeolum with Broncasma Berna. *Eye (Lond)*. 1999;13(Pt 5):692.
- Wald ER. Periorbital and orbital infections. *Infect Dis Clin North Am*. 2007;21(2):393–408, vi.

 CODES

ICD10
- H00.019 Hordeolum externum unspecified eye, unspecified eyelid
- H00.029 Hordeolum internum unspecified eye, unspecified eyelid
- H00.039 Abscess of eyelid unspecified eye, unspecified eyelid

CLINICAL PEARLS
- A hordeolum should not be expressed.
- Warm compresses to the area of inflammation can encourage spontaneous drainage.
- Application of an antibiotic ointment (e.g., erythromycin) to the margin of the eyelid after proper cleansing helps reduce bacterial proliferation but may have no effect on the healing of the stye.
- Good personal hygiene with attention to cleansing the eyelids on a daily basis can prevent recurrent infections.

H

HORNER SYNDROME

Deborah A. Lardner, DO, DTM&H • Michael Passafaro, DO, DTM&H, FACEP, FACOEP

 BASICS

DESCRIPTION

- Horner syndrome presents as a classic triad of ipsilateral miosis, eyelid ptosis, and/or anhidrosis of the face and neck (with iris heterochromia in children).
- It is caused by the interruption of sympathetic nerve supply to the head, neck, and eye.
  - Central or preganglionic lesion (complete syndrome): 1st- or 2nd-order neuron
  - Peripheral postganglionic lesion (incomplete syndrome, no anhidrosis): 3rd-order neuron
- System(s) affected: nervous, skin/exocrine
- Synonym(s): Bernard-Horner syndrome; Bernard syndrome; Horner's syndrome; cervical sympathetic syndrome; oculosympathetic syndrome; oculosympathetic paralysis; oculosympathetic deficiency; oculosympathetic paresis

EPIDEMIOLOGY

- Predominant age: none
- Predominant sex: male = female

Incidence
Unknown

Prevalence
Unknown

ETIOLOGY AND PATHOPHYSIOLOGY

- Constellation of signs produced when sympathetic innervation to the head, neck, and eye is interrupted somewhere along the three-neuron arc
  - Absence of innervation of iris dilator and Müller muscles leads to miosis and slight ptosis, respectively.
  - Sympathetic innervation also controls sweat glands; interruption causes anhidrosis.
- Oculosympathetic pathway
  - 1st-order neuron: Sympathetic nerve fibers originate in the hypothalamus, descend through the brainstem, and synapse at the ciliospinal center (of Budge) located at approximately the C8–T2 levels of the spinal cord.
  - 2nd-order neuron: exits the spinal column at the T1 level primarily, arches over the apex of the lung and under the subclavian artery, ascending to the superior cervical ganglion at the level of the carotid bifurcation and angle of the jaw
  - 3rd-order neuron: ascends along the adventitia of the internal carotid artery, through the cavernous sinus in proximity to cranial nerve [CN] VI, and joins CN VI to innervate the iris dilator muscle and Müller muscle in the eye
- Sympathetic fibers innervating sweat glands and vasodilatory muscles branch off before the cervical sympathetic ganglion traveling along the external carotid artery, so distal lesions will not result in anhidrosis.
- Lesions anywhere along this pathway will lead to ipsilateral Horner syndrome.
- Idiopathic (40%), congenital, or acquired
- Best classified by which order neuron is affected and by age (pediatric vs. adult)
- 1st-order neuron (13%)
  - Arnold-Chiari malformation
  - Basal meningitis (e.g., syphilis)
  - Basal skull tumors

- Cerebral vascular accident: lateral medullary (Wallenberg) syndrome
  - Cervical cord trauma
  - Demyelinating disease (multiple sclerosis)
  - Intrapontine hemorrhage
  - Neck trauma
  - Pituitary tumor
  - Syringomyelia
  - Unintended subdural placement of lumbar epidural catheter
- 2nd-order neuron (44%)
  - Aneurysm/dissection of aorta
  - Central venous catheterization
  - Chest tubes
  - First rib fracture
  - Lymphadenopathy (Hodgkin, leukemia, tuberculosis, mediastinal tumors, sarcoid)
  - Mandibular tooth abscess
  - Neurofibromatosis types I and II
  - Pancoast tumor or infection of lung apex
  - Proximal common carotid artery dissection
  - Trauma/surgical injury
- 3rd-order neuron lesions (43%)
  - Carotid cavernous fistula or other pathology
  - Carotid endarterectomy or carotid artery stenting
  - Cluster headaches
  - Internal carotid artery dissection
  - Herpes zoster
  - Lesions of the middle ear (acute otitis media)
  - Lyme disease
  - Nasopharyngeal cancer
  - Tonsillectomy
  - Raeder paratrigeminal syndrome
- Drugs: acetophenazine, alseroxylon, bupivacaine, butaperazine, carphenazine, chloroprocaine, deserpidine, diacetylmorphine, diethazine, ethopropazine, etidocaine, guanethidine, influenza virus vaccine, levodopa, lidocaine, mepivacaine, mesoridazine, methdilazine, methotrimeprazine, oral contraceptives, perazine, prilocaine, procaine, prochlorperazine, promazine, propoxycaine, reserpine, thioproperazine, thioridazine, trifluoperazine

Genetics
Rare autosomal dominant inheritance

RISK FACTORS

- Most common: apical bronchogenic carcinoma (Pancoast tumor) in smokers
- Aneurysm of the carotid or subclavian artery
- Injuries to the carotid artery high in the neck
- Dissection of the carotid arteries
- Carotid artery occlusion
  - 15% of patients with carotid artery occlusion develop ipsilateral Horner syndrome.
  - May occur without evidence of cerebral ischemia, neck injuries, or operative procedures
- Cluster headaches
  - 20% have an ipsilateral Horner syndrome.

Pediatric Considerations
2nd-order neuron lesion is the most common etiology: birth trauma to neck and shoulder, chest surgery, neuroblastoma (paraspinal), and vascular anomalies of the carotid arteries.

COMMONLY ASSOCIATED CONDITIONS
- Wallenberg syndrome
- Pancoast tumor
- C8 radiculopathy

 DIAGNOSIS

HISTORY

- Ptosis (typically mild; 1 to 2 mm)
- Miosis (with an associated dilation lag)
- Anhidrosis or hypohidrosis (often not appreciated by patients or clinicians):
  - Ipsilateral side of the body: central (1st-order neuron)
  - Ipsilateral face: preganglionic (2nd-order neuron)
  - Medial portion of forehead and side of nose: postganglionic (3rd-order neuron after vasomotor and sudomotor fiber have branched off)

Pediatric Considerations
In infants and children, loss of facial flushing is appreciated more than anhidrosis (harlequin sign).

ALERT
Horner syndrome in the presence of pain merits special consideration:

- Axial, shoulder, scapula, arm, or hand pain may be related to Pancoast tumor.
- Acute-onset, ipsilateral facial or neck pain: Consider carotid artery dissection until proven otherwise.
- Paratrigeminal syndromes:
  - Raeder paratrigeminal syndrome type I: orbital pain, miosis, ptosis, with associated ipsilateral lesions of CN III–VI; suspect middle cranial fossa mass lesion.
  - Raeder paratrigeminal syndrome type II: episodic retrobulbar or orbital pain, miosis, ptosis with no CN lesions; suspect migraine variant, syphilis, herpes zoster, hypertension.

PHYSICAL EXAM

- Measure pupillary diameter in dim and bright light and reactivity to light and accommodative response:
  - Anisocoria is greatest in dark, with affected pupil failing to dilate.
  - Redilation (after light is removed) may lag 15 to 20 seconds on the affected side.
- Examine the upper lids for ptosis (<2 mm).
- Examination of the lower lids for "upside-down ptosis": elevation of lower lid due to Müller muscle weakness
  - Illusion of enophthalmos secondary to narrowing of palpebral fissure
- Ipsilateral impaired flushing may be found.
- Loss of ciliospinal reflex. Pinching the skin on back of the neck normally produces ipsilateral pupil dilation (unreliable).
- Biomicroscopic exam of the papillary margin and iris structure and color
  - In congenital Horner syndrome, long-standing Horner syndrome, or Horner syndrome that occurs in children <2 years: Iris shows reduced pigmentation, blue-gray, and mottling of the affected eye (heterochromia iridis) because formation of iris pigment early in life is under sympathetic control.
- Observe for the presence of nystagmus, facial swelling, lymphadenopathy, or vesicular eruptions.
- Ophthalmoparesis, specifically CN VI palsy with Horner syndrome, is suggestive of cavernous sinus lesion.
- Neurologic and chest exams for associated physical findings

DIFFERENTIAL DIAGNOSIS
- Neurologic diseases
- 3rd nerve palsy
- Unilateral use of miotics
- Unilateral use of mydriatics
- Adie tonic pupil
- Iris sphincter muscle damage

DIAGNOSTIC TESTS & INTERPRETATION
Initial Tests (lab, imaging)
CBC, fluorescent treponemal antibody absorption test, venereal disease research laboratory, purified protein derivative; vanillylmandelic acid, homovanillic acid to rule out neuroblastoma in pediatric patients
- Chest x-ray if patient is a smoker (apical bronchogenic carcinoma)
- CT/MRI/MRA of the brain, chest, and spinal cord
  - If painful, order MRI/MRA to evaluate for carotid artery dissection emergently.
- Ultrasound may be considered for evaluation of internal carotid artery

Pediatric Considerations
In a child of any age without contributory history, MRI brain, neck, and chest to exclude a mass lesion (1)[B]

DIAGNOSTIC PROCEDURES/OTHER
- Confirmation of Horner syndrome
  - Topical 0.5% apraclonidine (2)[A],(3,4)[B]
  - 4–10% topical cocaine
    - Used to confirm diagnosis of Horner syndrome but will not identify location of lesion
    - If the diagnosis is clear clinically, this test is not required.
    - A normal pupil will dilate. The miotic pupil in Horner syndrome (regardless of location of lesion) will not dilate or will dilate poorly after 45 minutes because of the absence of norepinephrine at the nerve endings of the 3rd-order neuron (2)[A].
    - Positive test is anisocoria of ≥1 mm.
    - Cocaine blocks the reuptake of norepinephrine by the neuron.
- Distinguishing a 3rd-order neuron disorder from a 1st- or 2nd-order neuron disorder:
  - Topical 1% hydroxyamphetamine (2)[A]
    - If there is a 1st- or 2nd-order neuron lesion, dilation will take place.
    - Failure of the pupil to dilate, or poor dilation, indicates a 3rd-order neuron lesion (positive when anisocoria increases by ≥1 mm).
    - No pharmacologic test exists to differentiate between a 1st- and 2nd-order neuron lesion.
    - Hydroxyamphetamine causes release of endogenous norepinephrine stored in the postganglionic neuron.
    - Alternative test: 1% topical pholedrine
- Must wait >24 hours between the cocaine and hydroxyamphetamine tests.

Pediatric Considerations
Due to transsynaptic degeneration in children, the hydroxyamphetamine test is not reliable.

Test Interpretation
- Brainstem lesion
- Massive hemisphere lesion
- Cervical cord lesion
- Root lesion
- Sympathetic chain lesion

TREATMENT

GENERAL MEASURES
- Horner syndrome in itself does not produce any disability or necessarily require treatment.
- Treat the underlying etiology.
- Search for a tumor or other compressive lesion.

MEDICATION
Carotid artery dissection: Pharmacologic treatment options include thrombolysis, antithrombotic therapy with anticoagulation, or antiplatelet therapy. No randomized control trials have compared these treatment options (5)[C].

ISSUES FOR REFERRAL
- Neurologic, neuro-ophthalmic, oculoplastic
- Neurologic or vascular surgery: interventional in cases of suspected carotid artery dissection or aneurysm
- Neurosurgery, surgical oncology, oncology, or radiotherapy consultation depends on the particular etiology.

SURGERY/OTHER PROCEDURES
- Surgical care depends on etiology.
- Consider ptosis repair surgery (oculoplastics).

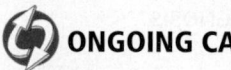

ONGOING CARE

PROGNOSIS
- Postganglionic: usually benign
- Central and preganglionic: poorer prognosis

COMPLICATIONS
- Chronic pupillary constriction
- Cosmesis

REFERENCES
1. Al-Moosa A, Eggenberger E. Neuroimaging yield in isolated Horner syndrome. *Curr Opin Ophthalmol*. 2011;22(6):468–471.
2. Antonio-Santos AA, Santo RN, Eggenberger ER. Pharmacological testing of anisocoria. *Expert Opin Pharmacother*. 2005;6(12):2007–2013.
3. Koc F, Kavuncu S, Kansu T, et al. The sensitivity and specificity of 0.5% apraclonidine in the diagnosis of oculosympathetic paresis. *Br J Ophthalmol*. 2005;89(11):1442–1444.
4. Chen PL, Chen JT, Lu DW, et al. Comparing efficacies of 0.5% apraclonidine with 4% cocaine in the diagnosis of Horner syndrome in pediatric patients. *J Ocul Pharmacol Ther*. 2006;22(3):182–187.
5. Patel RR, Adam R, Maldjian C, et al. Cervical carotid artery dissection: current review of diagnosis and treatment. *Cardiol Rev*. 2012;20(3):145–152.

ADDITIONAL READING
- Ahmadi O, Saxena P, Wilson BK, et al. First rib fracture and Horner's syndrome: a rare clinical entity. *Ann Thorac Surg*. 2013;95(1):355.
- Almog Y, Gepstein R, Kesler A. Diagnostic value of imaging in Horner syndrome in adults. *J Neuroophthalmol*. 2010;30(1):7–11.
- Bazari F, Hind M, Ong YE. Horner's syndrome—not to be sneezed at. *Lancet*. 2010;375(9716):776.
- Davagnanam I, Fraser CL, Miszkiel K, et al. Adult Horner's syndrome: a combined clinical, pharmacological, and imaging algorithm. *Eye (Lond)*. 2013;27(3):291–298.
- Kong YX, Wright G, Pesudovs K, et al. Horner syndrome. *Clin Exp Optom*. 2007;90(5):336–344.
- Lee JH, Lee HK, Lee DH, et al. Neuroimaging strategies for three types of Horner syndrome with emphasis on anatomic location. *AJR Am J Roentgenol*. 2007;188(1):W74–W81.
- Lyrer PA, Brandt T, Metso TM, et al. Clinical import of Horner syndrome in internal carotid and vertebral artery dissection. *Neurology*. 2014;82(18):1653–1659.
- Mahoney NR, Liu GT, Menacker SJ, et al. Pediatric Horner syndrome: etiologies and roles of imaging and urine studies to detect neuroblastoma and other responsible mass lesions. *Am J Ophthalmol*. 2006;142(4):651–659.
- Martin TJ. Horner's syndrome, pseudo-Horner's syndrome, and simple anisocoria. *Curr Neurol Neurosci Rep*. 2007;7(5):397–406.
- Reede DL, Garcon E, Smoker WR, et al. Horner's syndrome: clinical and radiographic evaluation. *Neuroimaging Clin N Am*. 2008;18(2):369–385.

CODES

ICD10
- G90.2 Horner's syndrome
- S14.5XXA Injury of cervical sympathetic nerves, initial encounter

CLINICAL PEARLS
- Horner syndrome triad: ipsilateral miosis, eyelid ptosis, and anhidrosis caused by a lesion of the oculosympathetic pathway
- Ptosis is mild, usually <2 mm.
- Red flags: If associated with pain, suspect central or preganglionic lesion.
- Confirm the diagnosis clinically with topical cocaine to the affected eye.
- Use hydroxyamphetamine to differentiate which order neuron is affected.
- Order imaging studies based on history and physical and hydroxyamphetamine testing.
- Horner syndrome in the presence of acute-onset, ipsilateral facial or neck pain: Consider carotid artery dissection until proven otherwise.

H

HYDROCELE

Jared M. Patton, MD, MS • John E. Laird, MD, FAAFP

BASICS

DESCRIPTION
A collection of fluid between the parietal and visceral layers of the tunical vaginalis within the scrotum
- Communicating hydrocele (patent processus vaginalis)
  - Direct communication with the peritoneal cavity
  - Contains peritoneal fluid
  - Almost always with associated indirect inguinal hernia
  - Decreases in size with recumbent position
- Noncommunicating hydrocele (the processus vaginalis is not patent)
  - No direct connection to the peritoneal cavity
  - Fluid contained is from the mesothelial lining.
  - Can be isolated to the cord with the distal and proximal portions of the processus vaginalis closed
- Acute hydrocele: fluid collection resulting from an acute process within the tunica vaginalis, typically involving only the scrotum
- System(s) affected: Urogenital

Pediatric Considerations
In a communicating hydrocele, consider contralateral inguinal exploration to rule out an occult indirect hernia.

EPIDEMIOLOGY
Predominant age: childhood (1)

Incidence
Estimated at 0.7–4.7% of male infants

Prevalence
- 1,000/100,000
- Estimated at 1% of adult men

ETIOLOGY AND PATHOPHYSIOLOGY
- Incomplete closure of the processus vaginalis trapping peritoneal fluid anywhere along the length of the tunica vaginalis
- Failure of closure of the processus vaginalis maintaining a communication to the peritoneal cavity
- Imbalance of the secretion and reabsorption of fluid from the lining of the tunica vaginalis
- Infection
- Tumors
- Trauma
- Ipsilateral renal transplantation

RISK FACTORS
- Ventriculoperitoneal shunt
- Exstrophy of the bladder
- Cloacal exstrophy
- Ehlers-Danlos syndrome
- Peritoneal dialysis

COMMONLY ASSOCIATED CONDITIONS
- Testicular tumors
- Scrotal trauma
- Ventriculoperitoneal shunt
- Nephrotic syndrome
- Renal failure with peritoneal dialysis

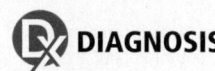
DIAGNOSIS

HISTORY
- Acute, subacute, or chronic swelling of the scrotum or inguinal canal
- Frequent changes in size of the hydrocele with position change or activity (indicative of communicating)
- Usually painless unless acute onset
- Sensation of heaviness or pressure in the scrotum
- Pain radiating to the flank/back

PHYSICAL EXAM
- Swelling in the scrotum or inguinal canal
- Scrotal mass, usually fluctuant
- Fluctuation in size with change of position (communicating hydrocele)
- Scrotal mass that transilluminates

DIFFERENTIAL DIAGNOSIS
- Indirect inguinal hernia
- Orchitis
- Epididymitis
- Varicocele
- Traumatic testicular injury
- Testicular torsion or torsion of appendix testes
- Testicular neoplasm

DIAGNOSTIC TESTS & INTERPRETATION
- Inguinoscrotal ultrasound (US): can demonstrate the presence of bowel (e.g., distinguish incarcerated hernia from a hydrocele of the cord) as well as the presence of testicular torsion
- Testicular MRI when US is unable to distinguish etiology
- Doppler US or testicular nuclear scan can distinguish testicular torsion.

Diagnostic Procedures/Other

ALERT
Aspiration of a hydrocele for diagnosis is not indicated and may lead to severe complications if herniated bowel is present.

Test Interpretation
Patent processus vaginalis on imaging in communicating hydroceles

TREATMENT

ISSUES FOR REFERRAL
- Urology referral for symptomatic adults or if underlying diagnosis is unclear
- Pediatric urology/surgery referral for children with symptomatic noncommunicating hydrocele
- Children with communicating hydroceles can be expectantly managed until at least 2 years of age to allow time for spontaneous resolution unless there is a concern for inguinal hernia (1)[C].

- New-onset hydrocele in late childhood and preadolescent patients typically resembles the adult type hydrocele pathology (2)[B].

SURGERY/OTHER PROCEDURES
- Children: Surgical treatment is generally deferred until 2 years of age as many hydroceles will spontaneously resolve. Some evidence shows that delaying longer than 2 years may be appropriate and decrease unnecessary surgery (1)[C].
  - When surgery is indicated, children with communicating hydroceles may undergo either open or laparoscopic approach.

    - Open inguinal approach involves ligation of the processus vaginalis and excision, distal splitting, or drainage of hydrocele sac (in a hydrocele of cord, the sac can be completely removed) (3)[B]
    - Open scrotal approach involves ligation and removal of the processus vaginalis. The benefit of this approach is improved cosmesis and decreased operative time (4)[B].
    - Laparoscopic repair offers the benefit of contralateral exploration and repair with low long-term recurrence rates and similar operative times as open procedures (5)[B].

- Adults: No therapy is needed unless the hydrocele causes discomfort or unless there is a significant underlying cause such as a tumor (6).
  - If resection is indicated, a scrotal approach with resection of hydrocele sac has the highest complication rate but lowest recurrence rate (7)[C].
  - Jaboulay-Winkelmann procedure (for a thick hydrocele sac): The hydrocele sac is wrapped posteriorly around cord structures (7)[C],(8)[A].
  - Lord procedure (for a thin hydrocele sac): Radial sutures are used to gather the hydrocele sac posterior to testis and epididymis (7)[C],(8)[A].
  - Aspiration of the hydrocele with instillation of a sclerosing agent has been successfully used in adults.
    - Aspiration with instillation of 1 to 4 mg of polidocanol has demonstrated a cure rate of 56% after the first treatment and 89% after the second treatment (9)[A].
    - The benefit of aspiration versus surgery is a decrease in cost and operative complications. (9)[A].
  - Hydrocelectomy may be performed endoscopically via a transscrotal approach; it involves cauterization of the entire parietal surface of the tunical vaginalis (10)[A].

INPATIENT CONSIDERATIONS
Admission Criteria/Initial Stabilization
- Open inguinal or scrotal approach is typically performed as an outpatient.
- Laparoscopic approach may require 24-hour admission for postoperative monitoring.
- Sclerotherapy is a same-day office procedure.

ONGOING CARE

FOLLOW-UP RECOMMENDATIONS
Patient Monitoring
- Depending on method of treatment, initial follow-up is generally in the first 4 to 6 weeks.
- With sclerotherapy follow-up for confirmation of resolution or to proceed with retreatment
- Postoperative follow-up at 2 to 4 weeks and subsequent 2- to 3-month intervals until resolution of any postoperative complications

COMPLICATIONS
- Complication rate for a scrotal approach may reach 30% (6)[C].
- Postoperative traumatic hydrocele is common and usually resolves spontaneously.
- Injury to vas deferens or spermatic vessels
- Suture granuloma
- Hematoma
- Wound infection
- Recurrence

REFERENCES
1. Hall NJ, Ron O, Eaton S, et al. Surgery for hydrocele in children—an avoidable excess? *J Pediatr Surg.* 2011;46(12):2401–2405.
2. Koutsoumis G, Patoulias I, Kaselas C. Primary new-onset hydroceles presenting in late childhood and pre-adolescent patients resemble the adult type hydrocele pathology. *J Pediatr Surg.* 2014;49(11):1656–1658.
3. Gahukamble DB, Khamage AS. Prospective randomized controlled study of excision versus distal splitting of hernial sac and processus vaginalis in the repair of inguinal hernias and communicating hydroceles. *J Pediatr Surg.* 1995;30(4):624–625.
4. Alp BF, Irkilata HC, Kibar Y, et al. Comparison of the inguinal and scrotal approaches for the treatment of communicating hydrocele in children. *Kaohsiung J Med Sci.* 2014;30(4):200–205.
5. Yang XD, Wu Y, Xiang B, et al. Ten year experience of laparoscopic repair of pediatric hydrocele and the long-term follow-up results [published online ahead of print July 14, 2015]. *J Pediatr Surg.*
6. Swartz MA, Morgan TM, Krieger JN. Complications of scrotal surgery for benign conditions. *Urology.* 2007;69(4):616–619.
7. Ku JH, Kim ME, Lee NK, et al. The excisional, plication and internal drainage techniques: a comparison of the results for idiopathic hydrocele. *BJU Int.* 2001;87(1):82–84.
8. Miroglu C, Tokuc R, Saporta L. Comparison of an extrusion procedure and eversion procedures in the treatment of hydrocele. *Int Urol Nephrol.* 1994;26(6):673–679.
9. Lund L, Kloster A, Cao T. The long-term efficacy of hydrocele treatment with aspiration and sclerotherapy with polidocanol compared to placebo: a prospective, double-blind, randomized study. *J Urol.* 2014;191(5):1347–1350.
10. Emir L, Sunay M, Dadali M, et al. Endoscopic versus open hydrocelectomy for the treatment of adult hydroceles: a randomized controlled clinical trial. *Int Urol Nephrol.* 2011;43(1):55–59.

 CODES

ICD10
- N43.3 Hydrocele, unspecified
- N43.2 Other hydrocele
- P83.5 Congenital hydrocele

CLINICAL PEARLS
- A hydrocele can usually be diagnosed by physical exam and transillumination. If there is any concern for other underlying process, a formal US is recommended.
- Aspirating a hydrocele is not indicated as the primary treatment due to high recurrence rate.
- Attempted aspiration of an unconfirmed hydrocele could lead to bowel injury in an undiagnosed inguinal hernia.
- Laparoscopic repair in children offers the benefit of contralateral exploration and repair.
- Expectant management of children with hydrocele until >2 years of age is acceptable to allow sufficient time for spontaneous resolution.

H

HYDROCEPHALUS, NORMAL PRESSURE

Dennis E. Hughes, DO, FACEP

 BASICS

DESCRIPTION
- Normal pressure hydrocephalus (NPH) is a clinical triad of gait instability, incontinence, and dementia (mnemonic: *wet, wobbly, wacky*). Originally described by Hakim in 1957, it occurs rarely but is potentially treatable.
- Two forms of the disorder: idiopathic and secondary (to trauma)
- Absence of papilledema on clinical exam and normal CSF pressures at lumbar puncture

ALERT
Idiopathic NPH primarily affects persons >60 years; extremely rare before 40 years

EPIDEMIOLOGY

Incidence
- No formal epidemiologic data exist regarding NPH because of the lack of consensus-derived diagnostic criteria. The natural history of untreated NPH has not been studied.
- Idiopathic (iNPH) form primarily affects elderly, at least >40 years of age.
- Secondary form can occur at any age.
- Male = female

Prevalence
- 3.3/100,000 age 50 to 59 years to 11.7/100,000 age 70 to 79 years for iNPH and increases to upwards of 5.9% in those ≥80 years
- Estimated to be a contributing factor in 6% of all cases of dementia

ETIOLOGY AND PATHOPHYSIOLOGY
- Idiopathic form is a communicating hydrocephalus, a disorder of decreased CSF absorption (not over-production). In iNPH, the leading theory suggests that poor venous compliance impairs the subarach-noid granulations' ability to maintain baseline removal of CSF. In secondary NPH, scarring is likely.
- The result is a pressure gradient between the subarachnoid space and ventricular system.
- CSF production decreases in the face of an in-creased pressure set-point (but still in excess of the amount of CSF absorbed).
- Elevated pressure distends ventricles and com-presses the brain parenchyma.

- As a result of compression, ischemic changes occur in the parenchymal vasculature with subsequent tissue damage and loss.
- Some believe that the idiopathic form is a result of persistently insufficient removal of CSF by immature subarachnoid granulations from childhood.
- Secondary NPH may result from the following:
  – Head trauma (most common)
  – Subarachnoid hemorrhage
  – Resolved acute meningitis
  – Chronic meningitis (tuberculosis, syphilis)
  – Paget disease of the skull

RISK FACTORS
- Idiopathic risk is unknown (case reports suggest a possible genetic link but unsubstantiated).
- Secondary form is due to head trauma, subarach-noid hemorrhage, meningitis, or encephalitis.

 DIAGNOSIS

Detailed history and careful examination is the key to early diagnosis.

HISTORY
- Insidious and usually progressive gait instability usually manifests initially, followed by changes in mentation, and eventually, urinary incontinence.
- Behavioral changes noted in many cases: Depres-sion, mania, and psychotic features in many cases precede the physical findings and respond poorly to usual treatment (1)[B].
- Difficulty with initiation of movement: Feet appear "glued to the floor." Gait is wide-based, shuffling, and turning appears "en bloc."
- Inattention, forgetfulness, and lack of spontaneity often are seen with the subcortical dementia of NPH.
- Urinary urgency initially, followed by lack of inhibi-tion and then frank incontinence.
- A minimum duration of at least 3 to 6 months of symptoms and progression over time
- A remote trauma or infection suggests secondary versus the idiopathic form.
- A lack of psychiatric, neurologic, or other medical conditions to explain the symptoms (including structural reasons for CSF flow restriction) (2)
- Because memory impairment may be present, it is important to include a knowledgeable informant who is familiar with the patient's premorbid state.
- Frontal lobe function is affected disproportionately to the memory impairment (objective testing may lead to an early diagnosis).

PHYSICAL EXAM
- Decreased step height and length
- Reduced speed of walking (cadence)
- Widened standing base
- Swaying of trunk during walking
- Decreased fine motor speed and accuracy
- Recall impaired for recent events
- Impaired ability to do multistep tasks or interpret abstractions

DIFFERENTIAL DIAGNOSIS
- Alzheimer disease (may be a comorbid condition in as many as 75%)
- Parkinson disease
- Chronic alcoholism
- Intracranial infection
- Multi-infarct dementia
- Subdural hematoma
- Carcinomatous meningitis
- Collagen vascular disorders
- Depression
- Syphilis
- B_{12} deficiency
- Urologic disorders
- Other hydrocephalus disorders

DIAGNOSTIC TESTS & INTERPRETATION

Initial Tests (lab, imaging)
- Thyroid-stimulating hormone (TSH)
- Syphilis serology
- CBC
- Serum B_{12}, folate
- Metabolic profile
- Blood alcohol, analysis for drugs of abuse
- Urinalysis
- CSF analysis, including an opening pressure <245 mm H_2O (a value greater than this rules out iNPH by definition)
- Imaging is essential.

  – Either CT or MRI shows the ventriculomegaly (particularly lateral and 3rd ventricles) with preservation of the cerebral parenchyma (as opposed to ventricular enlargement seen in other forms of dementia where brain atrophy is present). A narrow subarachnoid space ("tight convexity") was recently shown to correlate to probable or definite iNPH (3)[A].
  – MRI can allow detection of other features, such as signs of altered brain water content and callosal angles. However, these supportive findings are not independently diagnostic of NPH.

Diagnostic Procedures/Other

CSF removal aids in the definitive diagnosis as well as predicting response to surgical treatment.

- High-volume (30 to 70 mL) CSF removal via spinal tap on 3 successive days or continuous spinal drainage (150 to 200 mL/day) for 3 days
- Comparison of gait analysis before and after CSF removal (a ≥20% improvement indicates a positive test) especially when combined with coexisting executive function improvement (4)[B]

TREATMENT

MEDICATION

- No medication is significantly helpful.
- Use of carbonic anhydrase inhibitors (acetazolamide) with repeat lumbar punctures has provided mild and transient relief but is only supported by anecdotal evidence.
- Use of levodopa to rule out Parkinson disease may be helpful (NPH will display little, if any, significant improvement to dopamine agonist).

ISSUES FOR REFERRAL

- Neurology or neurosurgical consultation is helpful in suspected cases when other reversible medical conditions are ruled out.
- Recent cohort studies have demonstrated clinical improvement after surgical shunts. Perimeters of urinary continence, gait stability, and cognitive scores all improved at 1-year post shunt.

ADDITIONAL THERAPIES

Gait training and use of ambulation assist devices, as indicated, but limited efficacy

SURGERY/OTHER PROCEDURES

- Current therapy is limited to placement of ventriculoperitoneal or ventriculoatrial shunt from a lateral ventricle tunneled SC and drained into the peritoneal cavity (or right atrium). There is no compelling evidence (no randomized controlled trial [RCT]) that this therapy is effective.
- Patients whose symptoms have been present for a shorter period (<2 years) have a greater chance of improvement with shunting. Also, patients with a known cause of NPH tend to respond more favorably. However, improvement has been seen in patients with symptoms present for a long time (5)[B].

INPATIENT CONSIDERATIONS

Admission Criteria/Initial Stabilization

Usually only for planned surgical treatment

ONGOING CARE

FOLLOW-UP RECOMMENDATIONS

- Assessment and modification of environment for fall risks
- Evaluation for ability to operate a motor vehicle safely (if driving)

Patient Monitoring

- Repeat neuropsychological testing to evaluate the status of the dementia after treatment.
- Improvement in the incontinence and walking speed can also be objectively measured.

PATIENT EDUCATION

Information at: http://www.ninds.nih.gov/disorders/normal_pressure_hydrocephalus/normal_pressure_hydrocephalus.htm

PROGNOSIS

Natural history is progressive deterioration. Patient's axial skeletal stability worsens with inability to walk, stand, sit, or turn over in bed.

COMPLICATIONS

- In patients treated surgically, cerebral infarcts, hemorrhage, infection, and seizures (in addition to the usual surgical risks): all usual age-related illnesses (as NPH is a condition affecting those age >65 years)
- Shunt malfunction (especially when symptoms recur after successful shunt placement)
- Falls due to gait instability
- UTIs
- Skin breakdown, pressure ulcers, infections as movement dysfunction progresses

REFERENCES

1. Oliveira MF, Oliveira JR, Rotta JM, et al. Psychiatric symptoms are present in most of the patients with idiopathic normal pressure hydrocephalus. *Arq Neuropsiquiatr*. 2014;72(6):435–438.
2. Williams MA, Relkin NR. Diagnosis and management of idiopathic normal-pressure hydrocephalus. *Neuro Clin Pract*. 2013;3(5):375–385.
3. Hashimoto M, Ishikawa M, Mori E, et al. Diagnosis of idiopathic normal pressure hydrocephalus is supported by MRI-based scheme: a prospective cohort study. *Cerebrospinal Fluid Res*. 2010;7:18.
4. Allali G, Laidet M, Beauchet O, et al. Dual-task related gait changes after CSF tapping: a new way to identify idiopathic normal pressure hydrocephalus. *J Neuroeng Rehabil*. 2013;10:117.
5. Razay G, Vreugdenhil A, Liddell J. A prospective study of ventriculo-peritoneal shunting for idiopathic normal pressure hydrocephalus. *J Clin Neurosci*. 2009;16(9):1180–1183.

ADDITIONAL READING

- Andrén K, Wikkelsø C, Tisell M, et al. Natural course of idiopathic normal pressure hydrocephalus. *J Neurol Neurosurg Psychiatry*. 2014;85(7):806–810.
- Ghosh S, Lippa C. Diagnosis and prognosis in idiopathic normal pressure hydrocephalus. *Am J Alzheimers Dis Other Demen*. 2014;29(7):583–589.
- Jaraj D, Rabiei K, Marlow T, et al. Prevalence of idiopathic normal-pressure hydrocephalus. *Neurology*. 2014;82(16):1449–1454.

 SEE ALSO

Algorithm: Ataxia

 CODES

ICD10

- G91.2 (Idiopathic) normal pressure hydrocephalus
- G91.0 Communicating hydrocephalus
- G91.3 Post-traumatic hydrocephalus, unspecified

CLINICAL PEARLS

- Consider in unexplained dementia or behavioral change
- Poor prognosis without therapy

H

HYDRONEPHROSIS

Pang-Yen Fan, MD

 BASICS

DESCRIPTION

- Hydronephrosis refers to a structural finding—dilatation of the renal calyces and pelvis.
  - May occur with urinary tract infection (UTI), vesicoureteric reflux (VUR), high urine output, or physiologic changes in pregnancy
  - Sometimes accompanied with hydroureter
  - Presentation varies from incidental finding to discovery during workup for UTI or for flank or abdominal pain.
- Hydronephrosis should not be used interchangeably with obstructive uropathy, which refers to the damage to renal parenchyma resulting from urinary tract obstruction (UTO).

EPIDEMIOLOGY

- UTO is more common in men than women and in children than adults (congenital anomalies).
- Acute unilateral obstruction is more common than bilateral.

ETIOLOGY AND PATHOPHYSIOLOGY

- Hydronephrosis develops with increased pressure in the urinary collecting system.
- Increased pressure within the renal collecting system can cause calyceal fornix rupture and urinary extravasation.
- Over time, pressures return to normal, but kidney function declines from intense renal vasoconstriction.
- With concomitant urinary infection, bacteria can enter the renal vasculature, resulting in sepsis.
- UTO: may be acute/chronic, partial/complete, uni-/bilateral
  - Intraluminal obstruction: calculi, sloughed renal papillae, blood clot, fungal ball
  - Intrinsic abnormality of the urinary collecting system: transitional cell carcinomas, benign prostatic hypertrophy, prostate cancer, congenital ureteropelvic junction (UPJ) obstruction, uretero-cele, neurogenic bladder (functional obstruction), urethral stricture or tuberculosis (TB) (can cause ureteral narrowing)
  - Extrinsic compression of the urinary collecting system: extraurinary malignancy (lymphoma, colon, cervix), aortic/iliac aneurysm, retroperitoneal fibrosis, uterine prolapse (15% affected), endometriosis, ovarian vein syndrome, IgG4-related disease
  - Transplant hydronephrosis: Consider BK virus.
- UTO in transplanted kidneys is commonly due to ureteral strictures, lymphoceles (ureteral compression and bladder dysfunction).
- VUR resulting in varying degrees of hydroureteronephrosis
- Physiologic hydronephrosis of pregnancy
- Hydronephrosis due to high urine output (e.g., diabetes insipidus, psychogenic polydipsia)
- Hydronephrosis of infection: due to bacterial toxins inhibiting smooth muscle contraction of the renal pelvis and ureter

Pediatric Considerations
- Antenatal hydronephrosis is diagnosed in 1–5% of pregnancies, usually by US, as early as the 12th to 14th week of gestation.
- Children with antenatal hydronephrosis are at greater risk of postnatal pathology.
- Postnatal evaluation begins with US exam; further studies, such as voiding cystourethrogram (VCUG), based on the severity of postnatal hydronephrosis
- In neonates, it is the most common cause of abdominal mass.
- Common etiologies in children are VUR, congenital UPJ obstruction, neurogenic bladder, and posterior urethral valves.
- Pediatric diagnostic algorithm differs from adult due to different differential diagnosis necessitating age-appropriate testing.

Pregnancy Considerations
- Physiologic hydronephrosis in pregnancy is more prominent on the right than left and can be seen in up to 80% of pregnant women.
- Dilatation is caused by hormonal effects, external compression from expanding uterus, and intrinsic changes in the ureteral wall.
- Despite high incidence, most cases are asymptomatic.
- If symptomatic and refractory to medical management, ureteric calculus should be considered and urinary infection must be excluded.

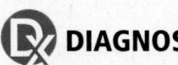 **DIAGNOSIS**

Symptoms vary according to cause, chronicity, location, and degree of obstruction.

HISTORY

- Although often asymptomatic, hydronephrosis can be associated with pain ranging from vague, intermittent discomfort to severe renal colic.
- Nausea and vomiting may be associated with severe pain or infection.
- Fever, chills with coexisting infection
- Polyuria may occur due to impaired urinary concentration in partial obstruction, postobstructive diuresis.
- Anuria, if complete bilateral obstruction or complete obstruction of a solitary kidney
- Symptoms of chronic kidney disease (CKD): anorexia, malaise, weight gain, edema, shortness of breath, mental state changes, tremors from long-standing bilateral obstruction
- Dietl crisis: sudden attack of flank pain due to distension of renal pelvis caused by rapid ingestion of large amount of liquid or kinking of a ureter, producing temporary occlusion of urine flow
- Symptoms of bladder outlet obstruction: weak urine stream, nocturia, straining to void, overflow incontinence, urgency, and frequency
- General medical and surgical history: malignancy (extrinsic compression), radiotherapy (ureteric stricture/fibrosis), surgery (iatrogenic obstruction), trauma (hematoma or fibrosis), gynecologic disease (endometriosis, ovarian masses, uterine prolapse), smoking (urothelial cancer), drugs (methysergide-induced retroperitoneal fibrosis)

PHYSICAL EXAM

- General signs
  - Volume overload (edema, rales, hypertension [HTN]) from renal failure
  - Diaphoresis, tachycardia, tachypnea with pain
  - High-grade fever, if infection
- Abdominal exam: CVA tenderness, palpable bladder, rarely palpable abdominal mass (may be visible, particularly in thin children)
- Pelvic exam: pelvic mass, uterine prolapse, palpable enlarged prostate (cancer or benign), urethral meatal stenosis, phimosis

DIAGNOSTIC TESTS & INTERPRETATION

- Urinalysis with microscopy: hematuria, proteinuria, crystalluria, pyuria
- Midstream urine culture and sensitivity: Exclude UTI.
- Basic metabolic panel: Elevated urea and creatinine may indicate obstructive uropathy. Hyperkalemic nonanion gap metabolic acidosis may indicate type 4 distal RTA due to obstruction.
- CBC: Anemia of CKD, leukocytosis; if infection, check platelet count prior to considering ureteral instrumentation.
- Prostate-specific antigen (PSA): adult males age >50 years or with abnormal digital rectal exam or bladder outlet obstruction signs or symptoms
- Urine cytology: for malignant cells in urothelial malignancies
- US and noncontrast CT scan are effective in diagnosing presence and cause of obstruction in most cases.
- US: screening test of choice for hydronephrosis
  - Sensitivity 90%, specificity 84.5% compared with IVU. Does not assess function and rarely detects cause and level of obstruction. Degree of hydronephrosis does not correlate with duration or severity of the obstruction.
  - Advantages: detects renal parenchymal disease (decreased renal size, increased cortical echogenicity, cortical thinning, cysts); no exposure to radiation or contrast; safe in pregnancy, contrast allergy, and renal dysfunction
  - False-positive findings 15.5% (for UTO): normal extrarenal pelvis, parapelvic cysts, VUR, excessive diuresis
  - False-negative findings 10%: dehydration, acute obstruction, calyceal dilatation misinterpreted as renal cortical cysts, and retroperitoneal fibrosis
- Noncontrast helical CT (NHCT): test of choice for suspected nephrolithiasis
  - Reported sensitivity 94–96%, specificity 94–100%. Stone is most commonly found at levels of ureteric luminal narrowing: UPJ, pelvic brim, and the vesicoureteric junction.
  - Typical findings in acute obstruction are hydronephrosis with hydroureter proximal to the level of obstruction, perinephric stranding, and renal swelling. If chronic, renal atrophy may be noted.
  - Advantages: no contrast exposure, time-saving, cost-effective, identifies extraurinary pathology
  - Disadvantages: does not assess function or degree of obstruction; higher radiation exposure, although low radiation dose protocols have shown comparable accuracy

- DTPA or MAG-3 radionuclide renal scan (diuretic renal scintigraphy)
  - Indicated only for evaluation of hydronephrosis without apparent obstruction
  - Determines presence of true obstruction as well as total and split (right vs. left) renal function
  - Furosemide is given 20 minutes after the tracer and the T1/2 for the tracer's washout is measured. T1/2; <10 minutes is unobstructed, >20 minutes is obstructed, and 10 to 20 minutes is equivocal; some experts consider <15 minutes normal.
  - Advantages: no contrast exposure, safe in contrast allergy and renal dysfunction
  - False-positive findings: delayed excretion due to renal failure, massive dilatation causing a water-reservoir effect of delayed excretion without obstruction
  - False-negative findings: dehydration or inadequate diuretic challenge
- Multiphase contrast-enhanced CT
  - Nonenhanced phase detects stones and swelling.
  - Parenchymal phase demonstrates decreased enhancement of renal parenchyma with acute obstruction; can identify extraurinary causes of obstruction and determine the relative glomerular filtration rate (GFR) of each kidney with accuracy equal to radionuclide renal scan
  - Delayed phase allows visualization of the collecting system and soft tissue filling defects (e.g., urothelial cancer).
- Magnetic resonance urography (MRU): indicated when US and NHCT are nondiagnostic
  - Provides anatomic, functional, and prognostic information. Sensitivity not superior to US or NHCT for nephrolithiasis (70%) but superior for soft tissue causes including strictures.
  - Advantages: no radiation exposure, safe in young children and pregnant women
  - Disadvantages: more expensive and time-consuming (35 vs. 5 minutes) and less available compared with CT. Gadolinium is contraindicated in renal failure due to risk of nephrogenic systemic fibrosis.

Diagnostic Procedures/Other

Cystoscopy, retrograde pyelogram ± ureteroscopy, and biopsy are occasionally used to determine the cause of obstruction (e.g., small urothelial cancer missed on imaging) or to confirm a normal distal ureter prior to pyeloplasty. In addition, such procedures are often needed to establish a definitive pathologic diagnosis for mass lesions.

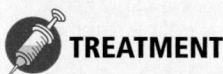

TREATMENT

GENERAL MEASURES

- Medical treatment: correction of fluid and electrolyte abnormalities, pain control, antibiotics as an adjunct to drainage if infection present
- Relief of obstruction: prompt drainage indicated in the presence of UTI, compromised renal function, or uncontrollable/persistent pain
  - Bladder outlet obstruction: urethral or suprapubic catheter
  - Ureteric obstruction: retrograde (cystoscopic) or antegrade (percutaneous) stenting

- VUR is often managed conservatively with antibiotics; surgical management required in severe cases in children or women of childbearing age
- Medical expulsive therapy (MET) with α-blockers or calcium channel blockers indicated for urethral stones <10 mm in patients with controlled pain, no signs of sepsis, with good renal function

SURGERY/OTHER PROCEDURES

- Hydronephrosis due to obstruction
  - Congenital UPJ obstruction: Pyeloplasty (open or laparoscopic) and minimally invasive stricture incision (endopyelotomy) are used with comparable results.
  - Nephrolithiasis: Extracorporeal shock wave lithotripsy (ESWL) is the initial treatment of choice for management of impacted upper urethral stones ≤2 cm. Ureteroscopy with or without intracorporeal lithotripsy has lower retreatment but higher complication rates and longer hospital stay. Ureteral stenting pre-ESWL or postureteroscopy associated with no additional benefit and more discomfort and morbidity (1)[A]
  - Transitional cell cancer: nephroureterectomy
  - Idiopathic retroperitoneal fibrosis: ureterolysis (frees ureters from inflammatory mass)
  - Prostate disorders: various treatment modalities, including transurethral resection of the prostate (TURP) and radical prostatectomy
- Nonobstructed hydronephrosis
  - VUR: ureteric reimplantation, endoscopic suburethral injection

INPATIENT CONSIDERATIONS

Admission Criteria/Initial Stabilization

Obstruction coexisting with infection (pyonephrosis) is a true urologic emergency requiring urgent drainage. Typically, this requires placement of percutaneous nephrostomy tube(s), as retrograde (cystoscopic) stenting is often difficult, but both are equally effective.

 ONGOING CARE

FOLLOW-UP RECOMMENDATIONS

- Serial monitoring of kidney function (electrolytes, BUN, and creatinine) and BP until renal function stabilizes. Frequency of monitoring depends on severity of renal dysfunction.
- Follow-up US after stabilization of renal function to assess for resolution of hydronephrosis. If hydronephrosis persists, consider diuretic radionuclide study to rule out persistent obstruction.

PROGNOSIS

- Recovery of renal function depends on etiology, presence or absence of UTI, and degree and duration of obstruction.
- Significant recovery can occur despite days of complete obstruction, although some irreversible injury may develop within 24 hours. Delays in therapy can lead to irreversible renal damage (2).
- Diagnostic testing is of poor predictive value. Course of incomplete obstruction is highly unpredictable.

COMPLICATIONS

- Urine stasis: increased risk of infection and stones formation
- Obstruction causes progressive atrophy of kidney with irreversible loss of function.
- Spontaneous rupture of a calyx may occur with urine extravasation in the perinephric space.
- Postobstructive diuresis: marked polyuria after relief of obstruction:
  - Caused mostly by fluid and solute overload but may be exacerbated by impaired renal tubular concentrating ability. Urine output may be >500 mL/hr.
  - Replace urine losses with hypotonic fluid (usually with 0.45% NaCl) and only enough to avoid volume depletion. Replacement of urine output with equal amounts of saline will perpetuate the diuresis.

REFERENCES

1. Aboumarzouk OM, Kata SG, Keeley FX, et al. Extracorporeal shock wave lithotripsy (ESWL) versus ureteroscopic management for ureteric calculi. *Cochrane Database Syst Rev.* 2011;(12):CD006029.
2. Cohen EP, Sobrero M, Roxe DM, et al. Reversibility of long-standing urinary tract obstruction requiring long-term dialysis. *Arch Intern Med.* 1992;152(1):177–179.

ADDITIONAL READING

- Ramsey S, Robertson A, Ablett MJ, et al. Evidence-based drainage of infected hydronephrosis secondary to ureteric calculi. *J Endourol.* 2010;24(2):185–189.
- Seitz C, Liatsikos E, Porpiglia F, et al. Medical therapy to facilitate the passage of stones: what is the evidence? *Eur Urol.* 2009;56(3):455–471.
- Shen P, Jiang M, Yang J, et al. Use of ureteral stent in extracorporeal shock wave lithotripsy for upper urinary calculi: a systematic review and meta-analysis. *J Urol.* 2011;186(4):1328–1335.
- Worster A, Preyra I, Weaver B, et al. The accuracy of noncontrast helical computed tomography versus intravenous pyelography in the diagnosis of suspected acute urolithiasis: a meta-analysis. *Ann Emerg Med.* 2002;40(3):280–286.

 CODES

ICD10

- N13.30 Unspecified hydronephrosis
- N13.39 Other hydronephrosis
- Q62.0 Congenital hydronephrosis

CLINICAL PEARLS

- US and noncontrast CT identify most causes of hydronephrosis.
- Relief of obstruction, when present, is the primary treatment.

HYPERCHOLESTEROLEMIA

Sebastian T. Tong, MD, MPH • Wendy Brooks Barr, MD, MPH, MSCE

BASICS

DESCRIPTION
- Serum total cholesterol >240 mg/dL
- Lipoprotein subtypes:
  - Low-density lipoproteins (LDL): primary target of therapy, atherogenic
  - High-density lipoproteins (HDL): atheroprotective
  - Triglycerides (TG)
- High cholesterol is a significant risk factor for atherosclerotic cardiovascular disease (ASCVD).
- System(s) affected: cardiovascular (CV)

EPIDEMIOLOGY
Age: increases with age

Prevalence
27.9% of men and 27.5% of women in the United States with total cholesterol >240 mg/dL

ETIOLOGY AND PATHOPHYSIOLOGY
- Pathophysiology
  - Deposition of cholesterol in vascular walls creating fatty streaks that become fibrous plaques
  - Inflammation causes plaque instability, leading to plaque rupture
- Etiology
  - Primary: diet, lack of physical activity, obesity
  - Secondary: excessive alcohol intake, hypothyroidism, diabetes, nephrotic syndrome, liver disease, chronic renal failure, medications (thiazide diuretics, carbamazepine, cyclosporine, progestins, anabolic steroids, corticosteroids, protease inhibitors)

Genetics
- Familial hypercholesterolemia (FH)
  - Elevated LDL levels from birth
  - Prevalence = 1/500 in the United States
  - Predisposed to atherosclerotic disease in early adulthood and high coronary heart disease (CHD) risk in 40s to 50s
  - Tendon xanthomas on Achilles and extensor tendons of hands are common.
  - Early lipid-lowering drug therapy is shown to reduce ASCVD risk.
- Early cholesterol testing of first-degree relatives is beneficial.

RISK FACTORS
Obesity (BMI >30 kg/m²), physical inactivity, heredity. Traditionally, diet rich in saturated fat and cholesterol is considered to be risk factors for hypercholesterolemia and vascular disease. This has become somewhat controversial, with emphasis now on trans-fats as more atherogenic. Relationship of diet to disease is very complex.

GENERAL PREVENTION
- Reduced intakes of saturated fat and cholesterol
- Regular physical activity
- Weight control (see "Ongoing Care")

COMMONLY ASSOCIATED CONDITIONS
Hypertension, diabetes mellitus (DM), obesity

DIAGNOSIS

Screening recommendations:
- U.S. Preventive Services Task Force (USPSTF): total cholesterol and HDL cholesterol (HDL-C) every 5 years
  - All men age ≥35 years
  - Women ≥45 years if at increased risk for ASCVD
  - Men aged 20 to 35 years and women aged 20 to 45 years if at increased risk for ASCVD (1)[A]
- American Diabetic Association: yearly dyslipidemia screening for diabetics

Pediatric Considerations
National Heart, Lung, and Blood Institute (NHLBI): recommended lipid screening on all children between 9 and 11 years. However, these recommendations are highly controversial and not supported by most other organizations (2)[C].

HISTORY
- Review possible secondary etiologies.
- Review medications that may change lipid levels.
- Assess other ASCVD risk factors.

PHYSICAL EXAM
Nonspecific findings

DIAGNOSTIC TESTS & INTERPRETATION
Initial Tests (lab, imaging)
- Fasting lipid panel: total cholesterol (TC), LDL, HDL, TG: LDL is usually a calculated value and is accurate if TG <350 mg/dL.
- If elevated LDL or other form of hyperlipidemia, clinical/laboratory assessment before initiating lipid-lowering therapy: ALT, diabetes screening
- Consider genetic etiology in very high LDL (>190 mg/dL).

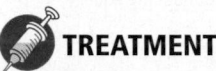

TREATMENT

ALERT
2013 American College of Cardiology/American Heart Association (ACC/AHA) cholesterol guidelines no longer recommend treatment to an LDL goal. Review of evidence suggests there was never a strong evidence to support specific LDL targets.

United States: ACC/AHA cholesterol guidelines (3)[C]
- Four groups benefit from statin therapy:
  - Clinical ASCVD
    - <75 years old: high-intensity statin
    - >75 years old or not candidate for high-intensity statin: moderate-intensity statin
  - Primary elevation of LDL-C >190 mg/dL: high-intensity statin
  - Diabetes (type 1 or 2) ages 40 to 75 years with LDL-C 70 to 189 mg/dL:
    - 10-year ASCVD risk <7.5%: moderate-intensity statin
    - 10-year ASCVD risk >7.5%: high-intensity statin
  - Without above but estimated 10-year ASCVD risk >7.5% based on Pooled Cohort Equations (http://my.americanheart.org/professional/StatementsGuidelines/PreventionGuidelines/Prevention-Guidelines_UCM_457698_SubHomePage.jsp): Consider moderate- to high-intensity statin.

- Definition of clinical ASCVD:
  - Acute coronary syndrome or history of MI
  - Stable or unstable angina
  - Coronary or other arterial revascularization
  - Stroke or TIA
  - Peripheral arterial disease
- Significant controversy over recommendation to treat patients with >7.5% 10-year ASCVD risk:
  - Concern that Pooled Cohort Equations significantly overestimate ASCVD risk.
  - Concern for significant overtreatment: one study showing 96% of men and 66% of women >55 years of age on statins based on recommendations
- Many more patients treated and medications used in the United States than elsewhere in the world without substantial evidence for improved outcomes

United Kingdom: National Institute for Health and Care Excellence (NICE) cholesterol guidelines (4)[C]
- No history of CV disease: if 10-year risk of CVD >10%, start atorvastatin 20 mg
- If eGFR <60 or type I diabetes, start atorvastatin 20 mg regardless of risk.
- History of CV disease: Start atorvastatin 80 mg.
- 10-year risk to be calculated using QRISK2: http://www.qrisk.org/
- Nonfasting lipid panel before treatment initiation and at 3 months of treatment: goal reduction of 40% in non-HDL cholesterol

European: European Society of Cardiology/European Atherosclerosis Society (ESC/EAS) cholesterol guidelines (5)[C]
- Risk stratification to low, moderate, high, and very high risk based on SCORE charts
- High- and very high-risk patients should be offered drug therapy.

ALERT
Elevated serum TG
- If >500, TG lowering becomes primary target until TG <500 to prevent acute pancreatitis.
  - Therapeutic life changes + statin + fibrate

MEDICATION
- Therapeutic lifestyle changes are cornerstone therapies to be attempted before drug therapy (diet and regular exercise; see "Ongoing Care").
- Check fasting lipoprotein profile 4 to 12 weeks after starting medication to evaluate response/compliance.
  - High-intensity statin: should lower LDL-C >50%
  - Moderate-intensity statin: should lower LDL-C 30–50%

First Line
HMG-CoA reductase inhibitors (statins)
- Categorized based on intensity
  - High intensity
    - Atorvastatin 40 to 80 mg/day
    - Rosuvastatin 20 to 40 mg/day
  - Moderate intensity
    - Atorvastatin 10 to 20 mg/day
    - Rosuvastatin 5 to 10 mg/day
    - Simvastatin 20 to 40 mg/day
    - Pravastatin 40 to 80 mg/day
    - Lovastatin 40 mg/day

○ Fluvastatin XL 80 mg/day
○ Fluvastatin 40 mg BID
○ Pitavastatin 2 to 4 mg/day
– Low intensity
○ Simvastatin 10 mg/day
○ Pravastatin 10 to 20 mg/day
○ Lovastatin 20 mg/day
○ Fluvastatin 20 to 40 mg/day
○ Pitavastatin 1 mg/day
• To be taken in the evening or at bedtime for best effect (exception: atorvastatin, rosuvastatin)
• Effect is greatest in lowering LDL-C; shown to decrease CHD incidence and all-cause mortality, although number needed to treat may be high in primary prevention.
• Contraindications: pregnancy, lactation, or active liver disease
• Drug interactions: cyclosporine, macrolide antibiotics, various antifungal agents, HIV protease inhibitors, fibrates/nicotinic acid (to be used with caution)
• Adverse reactions:
– Mild myalgia is common.
– Liver transaminase elevations: ALT before therapy to establish baseline; if ALT >3 times upper limit of normal, do not start statin; routine monitoring is not recommended; reasonable to measure hepatic function if symptoms suggesting hepatotoxicity occur.
– Association with increased cases of diabetes: 0.1 excess cases of diabetes per 100 persons on moderate-intensity statin and 0.3 excess cases per 100 persons on high-intensity statin
– Myopathies (considered rare but not well studied):
○ Creatine kinase (CK) baseline reasonable for those at increased risk for adverse muscle events; routine monitoring not needed unless muscle symptoms occur
○ Instruct patients to report immediately any muscle pain, muscle weakness, or brown urine.
○ If myopathy or rhabdomyolysis is suspected, discontinue statin use and draw serum CK, creatinine, urine analysis.
○ Can rechallenge statin at lower dose or different type after resolution of symptoms

ALERT
FDA alert: Simvastatin should no longer be prescribed at 80 mg/day doses due to increased risk of myopathy. Patients who have been at this drug dosage for >1 year can continue if no signs of myopathy. Dose restrictions to reduce myopathy risk include the following:

• Do not exceed simvastatin 10 mg/day with amiodarone, verapamil, and diltiazem.
• Do not exceed simvastatin 20 mg/day with amlodipine and ranolazine.

ALERT
Avoid grapefruit juice with statins.

Pregnancy Considerations
• Statins contraindicated during pregnancy: class X
• Lactation: possibly unsafe

Second Line
• Second-line drugs are no longer recommended in any guidelines.

• Ezetimibe
– Can be taken by itself or in combination with a statin: monotherapy (Zetia 10 mg/day) or ezetimibe/simvastatin (Vytorin 10/10, 10/20, 10/40)
– Effect: Lowers LDL-C; one recent RCT shows combination therapy with statin has small benefit in reducing CV events and CV-related mortality after acute coronary syndromes (6).
– Adverse reactions: generally well tolerated
• Fibrates
– Types: Gemfibrozil (Lopid) 600 mg BID, fenofibrate (Antara, Lofibra, Tricor, Triglide)
– Effect: most effective in lowering TG with moderate effect in lowering LDL and raising HDL. More recent studies fail to show benefit in most patients.
– Contraindications: severe hepatic or renal insufficiency
– Possible interactions: potentiates effects of warfarin and oral hypoglycemic agents
– Adverse reactions: GI complaints; increased likelihood of gallstones
• Nicotinic acid: raises HDL but no evidence for improved outcomes in recent trials and significant potential harms; should no longer be used in routine practice
• Bile acid sequestrant: causes significant GI side effects, no evidence for improved outcomes, rarely used
• Proprotein Convertase Subtilisin/Kexin Type 9 (PCSK9) inhibitors (7):
– Drug currently in approval process showing significant reduction in all-cause mortality, CV mortality and CV events
– Requires SC injections every 2 to 4 weeks to administer and will be very expensive

COMPLEMENTARY & ALTERNATIVE MEDICINE
• Omega-3 fatty acids and fish oil intake: Sources are fish oil (salmon), plant sources (flaxseed, canola oil, soybean oil, nuts); mainly lower TG level but has some benefit in lowering LDL and raising HDL although overall CV benefit and mortality reduction is uncertain. Supplements do not reduce overall or cardiovascular mortality. Patients should be advised to eat a variety of oily fish twice a week.
• β-Sitosterols and red yeast rice (contains natural lovastatin-analogue) can reduce total cholesterol and LDL.
• Garlic: appears to have some lipid-lowering effect, but more studies are needed; effective dose not established but generally 1 to 2 cloves of raw garlic/day, 300 mg dried garlic powder tablet BID or TID, or 7.2 g of aged garlic extract/day

 ## ONGOING CARE

FOLLOW-UP RECOMMENDATIONS
Exercise: sustained exercise for 30 minutes, 3 to 4 times per week: increases HDL, lowers total cholesterol, and helps control weight

Patient Monitoring
• Initially, lipid panel in 4 to 12 weeks after starting therapy, routine monitoring of LDL levels in patients on statin is not necessary.
• Routine monitoring of LFTs is no longer recommended if initial ALT is within normal range.

REFERENCES
1. U.S. Preventive Services Task Force. Lipid disorders in adults (cholesterol, dyslipidemia): screening. http://www.uspreventiveservicestaskforce.org/Page/Document/UpdateSummaryFinal/lipid-disorders-in-adults-cholesterol-dyslipidemia-screening. 2008.
2. National Heart, Lung, and Blood Institute. Integrated guidelines for cardiovascular health and risk reduction in children and adolescents. http://www.nhlbi.nih.gov/health-pro/guidelines/current/cardiovascular-health-pediatric-guidelines. 2011.
3. Stone NJ, Robinson JG, Lichtenstein AH, et al. 2013 ACC/AHA guideline on the treatment of blood cholesterol to reduce atherosclerotic cardiovascular risk in adults: a report of the American College of Cardiology\American Heart Association Task Force on Practice Guidelines. *Circulation*. 2014;129(25 Suppl 2):S1–S45.
4. National Institute for Health and Care Excellence. NICE Clinical Guideline (CG181): lipid modification: cardiovascular risk assessment and the modification of blood lipids for the primary and secondary prevention of cardiovascular disease. 2014. http://www.nice.org.uk/guidance/cg181
5. Reiner Z, Catapano AL, De Backer G, et al. ESC/EAS guidelines for the management of dyslipidaemias: the Task Force for the management of dyslipidaemias of the European Society of Cardiology (ESC) and the European Atherosclerosis Society (EAS). *Eur Heart J*. 2011;32(14):1769–1818.
6. Cannon CP, Blazing MA, Giugliano RP, et al. Ezetimibe added to statin therapy after acute coronary syndromes. *N Engl J Med*. 2015;372(25):2387–2397.
7. Navarese EP, Kolodziejczak M, Schulze V, et al. Effects of proprotein convertase subtilisin/kexin type 9 antibodies in adults with hypercholesterolemia: a systematic review and meta-analysis. *Ann Intern Med*. 2015;163(1):40–51.

ADDITIONAL READING
Taylor F, Huffman MD, Macedo AF, et al. Statins for the primary prevention of cardiovascular disease. *Cochrane Database Syst Rev*. 2013;(1):CD004816.

 ## SEE ALSO
• Hypothyroidism, Adult
• Algorithm: Hypercholesterolemia

CODES

ICD10
E78.0 Pure hypercholesterolemia

CLINICAL PEARLS
• Hypercholesterolemia is a significant risk factor for ASCVD, but ASCVD is a multifactorial disease with many different risk factors.
• Diet and exercise should be tried before pharmaceutical interventions.
• Statins are considered first-line medications for hypercholesterolemia. Other medications show little evidence of benefit.

H

HYPEREMESIS GRAVIDARUM

Emma Brooks, MD

BASICS

DESCRIPTION
- Hyperemesis gravidarum is persistent vomiting in a pregnant woman that interferes with fluid and electrolyte balance as well as nutrition:
  - Usually associated with the first 8 to 20 weeks of pregnancy
  - Believed to have biomedical and behavioral aspects
  - Associated with high estrogen and human chorionic gonadotropin (hCG) levels
  - Symptoms usually begin ∼2 weeks after first missed period.
- System(s) affected: endocrine/metabolic; gastrointestinal; reproductive
- Synonym(s): morning sickness

Pregnancy Considerations
Common condition during pregnancy, typically in the 1st and 2nd trimesters but may persist into the 3rd trimester.

EPIDEMIOLOGY
Incidence
Hyperemesis gravidarum occurs in 1–2% of pregnancies.

Prevalence
Hyperemesis gravidarum is the most common cause of hospitalization in the first half of pregnancy and the second most common cause of hospitalization of pregnant women.

ETIOLOGY AND PATHOPHYSIOLOGY
- Unknown
- Possible psychologic factors
- Hyperthyroidism
- Hyperparathyroidism
- Gestational hormones
- Liver dysfunction
- Autonomic nervous system dysfunction
- CNS neoplasm
- Addison disease

RISK FACTORS
- Obesity
- Nulliparity
- Multiple gestations
- Gestational trophoblastic disease
- Gonadotropin production stimulated
- Altered GI function
- Hyperthyroidism
- Hyperparathyroidism
- Liver dysfunction

- Female fetus
- *Helicobacter pylori* infection (1)

GENERAL PREVENTION
Anticipatory guidance in 1st and 2nd trimesters regarding dietary habits in hopes of avoiding dehydration and nutritional depletion.

Pregnancy Considerations
- 2% of pregnancies have electrolyte disturbances.
- 50% of pregnancies have at least some GI disturbance.

COMMONLY ASSOCIATED CONDITIONS
Hyperthyroidism

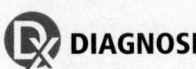
DIAGNOSIS

HISTORY
- Hypersensitivity to smell
- Alteration in taste
- Excessive salivation
- Poor appetite
- Nausea
- Vomiting with retching
- Decreased urine output
- Fatigue
- Dizziness with standing

DIAGNOSTIC TESTS & INTERPRETATION
Initial Tests (lab, imaging)
- Urinalysis: may see glucosuria, albuminuria, granular casts, and hematuria (rare); ketosis more common
- Thyroid-stimulating hormone (TSH), T4
- Electrolytes, BUN, creatinine:
  - Electrolyte abnormalities due to nausea and vomiting and subsequent dehydration
  - Acidosis
- Calcium
- Uric acid
- Hypoalbuminemia
- No imaging is indicated for the diagnosis of hyperemesis gravidarum unless there is concern for hydatidiform mole or multiple gestation, in which case ultrasound may be obtained.

Follow-Up Tests & Special Considerations
- If hypercalcemia, consider checking parathyroid hormone (PTH) for hyperparathyroidism.
- Drugs are unlikely to alter lab results.

Diagnostic Procedures/Other
Indicated only if it is necessary to rule out other diagnoses, as listed in the following section

DIFFERENTIAL DIAGNOSIS
Other common causes of vomiting must be considered:
- Gastroenteritis
- Gastritis
- Reflux esophagitis
- Peptic ulcer disease
- Cholelithiasis
- Cholecystitis
- Pyelonephritis
- Anxiety
- Hyperparathyroidism
- *H. pylori* infection

TREATMENT

Pyridoxine and doxylamine (pregnancy Category A) are first-line treatments for hyperemesis gravidarum (2)[C]. This is followed by metoclopramide or ondansetron (pregnancy Category B), then prochlorperazine (pregnancy Category C), methylprednisolone (pregnancy Category C), or promethazine (pregnancy Category C).

GENERAL MEASURES
- Patient reassurance
- Bed rest
- If dehydrated, IV fluids, either normal saline or 5% dextrose normal saline (with consideration for potential thiamine deficiency). Repeat if there is a recurrence of symptoms following initial improvement.
- For severe cases, consider PO thiamine 25 to 50 mg TID or IV 100 mg in 100 mL of normal saline over 30 minutes once weekly and potential parental nutrition if needed.
- Ondansetron carries an FDA warning regarding concerns for QT prolongation, but this is in the setting of high-dose IV administration and in patients with heart disease. It has unclear risk in the setting of pregnancy. The majority of the current studies appear to show no increased risk of fetal malformation with the use of ondansetron, but this is still an area of controversy (3)[C],(4)[B].

MEDICATION
- Pyridoxine (vitamin B$_6$) 25 mg PO or IV every 8 hours
- Antihistamines (e.g., diphenhydramine [25 to 50 mg q4–6h] or doxylamine [12.5 mg PO BID]) (5)[C]
- Combination product Diclegis (sustained-release pyridoxine 10 mg and doxylamine 10 mg) dosed (start 2 tabs PO q hs; if sx persist, increase to 1 tab in AM & 2 hs; if sx still persist, take 1 tab q AM, 1 mid day, and 2 hs; max 4 tablets/day)

- Phenothiazines (e.g., promethazine or prochlorperazine):
  – Precautions: Phenothiazines are associated with prolonged jaundice, extrapyramidal effects, and hyper- or hyporeflexia in newborns.
- Meclizine 25 mg PO q6h
- Metoclopramide 10 mg PO q6 to 8h
- Methylprednisolone 16 mg PO/IV q8h for 2 to 3 days, then taper over 2 weeks if initial 3-day treatment is effective.
- Ondansetron 4 to 8 mg PO q8h

Pregnancy Considerations
All medications taken during pregnancy should balance the risks and benefits both to the mother and the fetus.

COMPLEMENTARY & ALTERNATIVE MEDICINE
- Ginger 350 mg PO TID may help (6)[A].
- Motion sickness wristbands are another nonpharmacologic intervention that may improve symptoms. Evidence is mixed regarding the impact of acupressure and acupuncture in treating hyperemesis gravidarum (7)[C].
- Medical hypnosis may be a helpful adjunct to the typical medical treatment regimen, but further study is needed (8)[C].

INPATIENT CONSIDERATIONS
Admission Criteria/Initial Stabilization
- Typically outpatient therapy
- In some severe cases, parenteral therapy in the hospital or at home may be required.
- Enteral volume and nutrition repletion may be indicated.

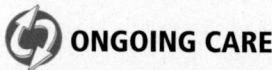 ONGOING CARE

FOLLOW-UP RECOMMENDATIONS
Activity as tolerated after improvement

Patient Monitoring
- In severe cases, follow-up on a daily basis for weight monitoring.
- Special attention should be given to monitor for ketosis, hypokalemia, or acid–base disturbances due to hyperemesis.

DIET
- NPO for first 24 hours if patient is ill enough to require hospitalization.
- For outpatient: a diet rich in carbohydrates and protein, such as fruit, cheese, cottage cheese, eggs, beef, poultry, vegetables, toast, crackers, rice. Limit intake of butter. Patients should avoid spicy meals and high-fat foods. Consider cold foods. Encourage small amounts at a time every 1 to 2 hours.

PATIENT EDUCATION
- Attention should be given to psychosocial issues, such as possible ambivalence about the pregnancy.
- Patients should be instructed to take small amounts of fluid frequently to avoid volume depletion.
- Avoid individual foods known to be irritating to the patient.
- Wet-to-dry nutrients (sherbet, broth, gelatin to dry crackers, toast)

PROGNOSIS
- Self-limited illness with good prognosis if patient's weight is maintained at >95% of prepregnancy weight.
- With complication of hemorrhagic retinitis, mortality rate of pregnant patient is 50%.

COMPLICATIONS
- Patients with >5% weight loss are associated with intrauterine growth retardation and fetal anomalies.
- Poor weight gain is associated with slightly increased risk for small gestational age infant <2,500 g and premature birth <37 weeks (9)[A].
- Hemorrhagic retinitis
- Liver damage
- CNS deterioration, Wernicke encephalopathy secondary to thiamine deficiency, coma

REFERENCES
1. Li L, Li L, Zhou X, et al. *Helicobacter pylori* infection is associated with an increased risk of hyperemesis gravidarum: a meta-analysis. *Gastroenterol Res Pract.* 2015;2015:278905.
2. Maltepe C, Koren G. The management of nausea and vomiting of pregnancy and hyperemesis gravidarum—a 2013 update. *J Popul Ther Clin Pharmacol.* 2013;20(2):e184–e192.
3. Doggrell SA, Hancox JC. Cardiac safety concerns for ondansetron, an antiemetic commonly used for nausea linked to cancer treatment and following anaesthesia. *Expert Opin Drug Saf.* 2013;12(3):421–431.
4. Pasternak B, Svanström H, Hviid A. Ondansetron in pregnancy and risk of adverse fetal outcomes. *N Engl J Med.* 2013;368(9):814–823.
5. Boelig RC, Berghella V, Kelly AJ, et al. Interventions for treating hyperemesis gravidarum. *Cochrane Database of Syst Rev.* 2013;(6):CD010607.
6. Viljoen E, Visser J, Koen N, et al. A systematic review and meta-analysis of the effect and safety of ginger in the treatment of pregnancy-associated nausea and vomiting. *Nutr J.* 2014;13:20.
7. Xu J, MacKenzie IZ. The current use of acupuncture during pregnancy and childbirth. *Curr Opin Obstet Gynecol.* 2012;24(2):65–71.
8. McCormack D. Hypnosis for hyperemesis gravidarum. *J Obstet Gynaecol.* 2010;30(7):647–653.
9. Veenendaal MV, van Abeelen AF, Painter RC, et al. Consequences of hyperemesis gravidarum for offspring: a systematic review and meta-analysis. *BJOG.* 2011;118(11):1302–1313.

ADDITIONAL READING
- Abas MN, Tan PC, Azmi N, et al. Ondansetron compared with metoclopramide for hyperemesis gravidarum: a randomized controlled trial. *Obstet Gynecol.* 2014;123(6):1272–1279.
- Anderka M, Mitchell AA, Louik C, et al. Medications used to treat nausea and vomiting of pregnancy and the risk of selected birth defects. *Birth Defects Res A Clin Mol Teratol.* 2012;94(1):22–30.
- Jarvis S, Nelson-Piercy C. Management of nausea and vomiting in pregnancy. *BMJ.* 2011;342:d3606.
- Matthews A, Haas DM, O'Mathúna DP, et al. Interventions for nausea and vomiting in early pregnancy. *Cochrane Database Syst Rev.* 2014;(3):CD007575.
- McCarthy FP, Lutomski JE, Greene RA. Hyperemesis gravidarum: current perspectives. *Int J Womens Health.* 2014;6:719–725.
- Tan PC, Omar SZ. Contemporary approaches to hyperemesis during pregnancy. *Curr Opin Obstet Gynecol.* 2011;23(2):87–93.

 ## CODES

ICD10
- O21.9 Vomiting of pregnancy, unspecified
- O21.0 Mild hyperemesis gravidarum
- O21.1 Hyperemesis gravidarum with metabolic disturbance

CLINICAL PEARLS
- Do not allow patients to become volume depleted. Once this occurs, it is more difficult to interrupt the process.
- Do not be hesitant to use medications to assist the patient, as this may help avoid volume depletion.
- Consider secondary causes of hyperemesis if it develops after 12 weeks of gestation.

H

HYPERKALEMIA

Merima Bucaj, DO • Roselyn Jan Wuthrich Clemente-Fuentes, MD

BASICS

DESCRIPTION
- Hyperkalemia is a common electrolyte disorder that may be defined as a plasma potassium (K) concentration >5.5 mEq/L (>5 mmol/L).
- Hyperkalemia depresses cardiac conduction and can lead to fatal arrhythmias.
- Normal K regulation
  - Ingested K enters portal circulation; pancreas releases insulin in response. Insulin facilitates K entry into cells.
  - K in renal circulation causes renin release from juxtaglomerular cells, leading to activation of angiotensin I, which is converted to angiotensin II in lungs. Angiotensin II acts in adrenal zona glomerulosa to stimulate aldosterone secretion. Aldosterone, at the renal collecting ducts, causes K to be excreted and sodium to be retained.
- Four major causes
  - Increased load: either endogenous from tissue release or exogenous from a high intake, usually in association with impaired excretion
  - Decreased excretion: due to decreased glomerular filtration rate
  - Cellular redistribution: shifts from intracellular space (majority of K is intracellular) to extracellular space
  - Pseudohyperkalemia: related to red cell lysis during collection or transport of blood sample, thrombocytosis, or leukocytosis

Geriatric Considerations
Increased risk for hyperkalemia because of decreases in renin and aldosterone as well as comorbid conditions

EPIDEMIOLOGY
Prevalence
- 1–10% of hospitalized patients
- 2–3% in general population but as high as 50% in patients with chronic kidney disease (1)
- Predominant sex: male = female
- No age-related predilection

ETIOLOGY AND PATHOPHYSIOLOGY
- Pseudohyperkalemia
  - Hemolysis of red cells in phlebotomy tube (spurious result is most common)
  - Thrombolysis
  - Leukocytosis
  - Thrombocytosis
  - Hereditary spherocytosis
  - Infectious mononucleosis
  - Traumatic venipuncture or fist clenching during phlebotomy (spurious result)
- Transcellular shift (redistribution)
  - Metabolic acidosis
  - Insulin deficiency
  - Hyperglycemia (diabetic ketoacidosis or hyperosmolar hyperglycemic state)

- Tissue damage (rhabdomyolysis, burns, trauma) (2)
- Tumor lysis syndrome (3)
- Cocaine abuse
- Exercise with heavy sweating
- Mannitol
- Impaired K excretion
  - Renal insufficiency/failure
  - Addison disease
  - Mineralocorticoid deficiency
  - Primary hyporeninemia, primary hypoaldosteronism
  - Type IV renal tubular acidosis (hyporeninemic hypoaldosteronism)
- Medication-induced
  - Excess K supplementation
  - Statins
  - ACE inhibitors
  - Angiotensin receptor blockers
  - β-Blockers
  - Cyclosporine
  - Digoxin toxicity
  - Ethinyl estradiol/drospirenone
  - Heparin
  - NSAIDs
  - Penicillin G potassium
  - Pentamidine
  - Spironolactone
  - Succinylcholine
  - Tacrolimus
  - Trimethoprim, particularly with other medications associated with hyperkalemia (4,5)

Genetics
Associated with some inherited diseases and conditions
- Familial hyperkalemic periodic paralysis
- Congenital adrenal hyperplasia

RISK FACTORS
- Impaired renal excretion of K
- Acidemia
- Massive cell breakdown (rhabdomyolysis, burns, trauma)
- Use of K-sparing diuretics.
- Excess K supplementation

GENERAL PREVENTION
Diet and oral supplement compliance in those at risk

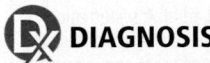

DIAGNOSIS

HISTORY
- Neuromuscular cramps
- Diarrhea
- Abdominal pain
- Myalgias
- Numbness
- Muscle weakness or paralysis

PHYSICAL EXAM
- Decreased deep tendon reflexes
- Flaccid paralysis of extremities

DIAGNOSTIC TESTS & INTERPRETATION
- Serum electrolytes
- Renal function: BUN, creatinine
- Urinalysis: K, creatinine, osmoles (to calculate fractional excretion of K and transtubular K gradient; both assess renal handling of K)
- Disorders that may alter lab results
  - Acidemia: K shifts from the intracellular to extracellular space
  - Insulin deficiency
  - Hemolysis of sample
- Cortisol and aldosterone levels to check for mineralocorticoid deficiency when other causes are ruled out

Diagnostic Procedures/Other
EKG abnormalities usually occur when K ≥7 mEq/L
- Peaked T wave with shortened QT interval in precordial leads (most common, usually earliest EKG change) (6)
- Lengthening of PR interval
- Loss of P wave
- Widened QRS
- Sine wave at very high K
- Can eventually lead to arrhythmias including ventricular fibrillation and asystole

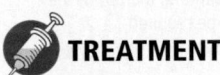

TREATMENT

MEDICATION
- Stabilize myocardial membranes. Initial treatment with calcium gluconate IV 1,000 mg (10 mL of 10% solution) over 2 to 3 minutes
  - With constant cardiac monitoring
  - Can repeat after 5 minutes if needed
  - Effect begins within minutes, but only lasts 30 to 60 minutes and should be used in conjunction with definitive therapies
  - Can also use calcium chloride (3 times as concentrated; however, it needs central or deep vein to avoid tissue necrosis)
- Drive extracellular potassium into cells
  - Nebulized albuterol (at 10 to 20 mg/4 mL saline over 10 minutes—4 to 8 times bronchodilation dose) and other β-agonists have an additive effect with insulin and glucose
  - Dextrose 50% 1 amp (if plasma glucose <250 mg/dL) and insulin 10 U IV may drive K intracellularly but does not decrease total body K and may result in hypoglycemia (close monitoring advised, especially 1 to 2 hours postinjection).
  - Sodium bicarbonate not routinely recommended but some possible benefits in severe metabolic acidosis (7)[C]

- Remove excess potassium from body.
  - Cation exchange resins definitive treatment but require several doses and best used with rapidly acting transient therapies above and when dialysis not readily available (8)[A]
  - Sodium polystyrene sulfonate (Kayexalate): 15 g PO or 30 g rectally
    - This requires 1 to 4 hours to lower K. This may be repeated q6h, if necessary.
    - Enema has faster effect than PO.
  - Hemodialysis is the definitive therapy when other measures are not effective. This may be required particularly when conditions such as digitalis toxicity, rhabdomyolysis, end-stage renal disease, severe chronic kidney disease, or acute kidney injury, are present. Should watch for postdialysis rebound
  - Little clinical evidence for the use of diuretics (loop and thiazides), however, can consider for control of chronic hyperkalemia (2)[B].
  - Zirconium cyclosilicate and patiromer calcium are promising therapies in development which bind potassium in intestinal tract (9)[C].

ALERT
- Sodium polystyrene sulfonate provides a sodium load that may exacerbate fluid overload in patients with cardiac or renal failure.
- Avoid sodium polystyrene sulfonate use in patients who are postoperative or with a bowel obstruction or ileus due to high risk of intestinal necrosis.
- Rapid administration of calcium in patients with suspected digitalis toxicity may result in a fatal dysrhythmia. Calcium should be administered slowly over 20 to 30 minutes in 5% dextrose with extreme caution.

INPATIENT CONSIDERATIONS
Admission Criteria/Initial Stabilization
- If hyperkalemia is severe, treat first, and then do diagnostic investigations.
- IV calcium to stabilize myocardium (caution in setting of digoxin toxicity, when calcium may worsen effects of toxicity)
- Insulin (usually 10 U IV, given with 50 mL of 50% glucose (if serum glucose <250 mg/dL) to avoid hypoglycemia; consider repeating if elevation persists.
- Inhaled β_2-agonist (nebulized albuterol)
- Discontinue any medications that may increase K (e.g., K-sparing diuretics, exogenous K).
- Admit for cardiac monitoring if EKG changes are present or if K is >6 mEq/L (6 mmol/L).

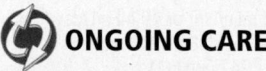 ## ONGOING CARE

FOLLOW-UP RECOMMENDATIONS
Patient Monitoring
- Reduction of plasma K should begin within the first hour of treatment initiation.

- Serum K levels should be rechecked every 2 to 4 hours until the patient has stabilized, and recurrent hyperkalemia is no longer a threat.
- Identification and elimination of possible causes and risk factors for hyperkalemia are essential.

DIET
≤80 mEq (≤80 mmol) of K/24 hours. Many foods contain K. Those that are particularly high in K (>6.4 mEq/serving) include bananas, orange juice, other citrus fruits and their juices, tomatoes, tomato juice, cantaloupe, honeydew melon, peaches, potatoes, and salt substitutes. Multiple herbal medications can also increase K levels, including alfalfa, dandelion, horsetail nettle, milkweed, hawthorn berries, toad skin, oleander, foxglove, and ginseng.

PATIENT EDUCATION
Consult with a dietitian about a low-K diet.

PROGNOSIS
- Associated with poor prognosis in patients with heart failure and chronic kidney disease
- Associated with poor prognosis in disaster medicine, with trauma, tissue necrosis, K^+ supplementation, metabolic acidosis, if calcium gluconate administered for treatment of hyperkalemia, if AKI, or if prolonged duration of hyperkalemia (2,7)

COMPLICATIONS
- Life-threatening cardiac arrhythmias
- Hypokalemia
- Potential complications of the use of ion-exchange resins for the treatment of hyperkalemia include volume overload and intestinal necrosis (8)[C].

REFERENCES

1. Palmer BF, Clegg DJ. Hyperkalemia. *JAMA*. 2015;314(22):2405–2406.
2. Zimmerman JL, Shen MC. Rhabdomyolysis. *Chest*. 2013;144(3):1058–1065.
3. Howard SC, Jones DP, Pui CH. The tumor lysis syndrome. *N Engl J Med*. 2011;364(19):1844–1854.
4. Antoniou T, Gomes T, Juurlink DN, et al. Trimethoprim-sulfamethoxazole–induced hyperkalemia in patients receiving inhibitors of the renin-angiotensin system: a population-based study. *Arch Intern Med*. 2010;170(12):1045–1049.
5. Weir MA, Juurlink DN, Gomes T, et al. Beta-blockers, trimethoprim-sulfamethoxazole, and the risk of hyperkalemia requiring hospitalization in the elderly: a nested case-control study. *Clin J Am Soc Nephrol*. 2010;5(9):1544–1551.
6. Wong R, Banker R, Aronowitz P. Electrocardiographic changes of severe hyperkalemia. *J Hosp Med*. 2011;6(4):240.
7. Khanagavi J, Gupta T, Aronow WS, et al. Hyperkalemia among hospitalized patients and association between duration of hyperkalemia and outcomes. *Arch Med Sci*. 2014;10(2):251–257.
8. Sterns RH, Rojas M, Bernstein P, et al. Ion-exchange resins for the treatment of hyperkalemia: are they safe and effective? *J Am Soc Nephrol*. 2010;21(5):733–735.
9. Ingelfinger JR. A new era for the treatment of hyperkalemia? *N Engl J Med*. 2015;372(3):275–277.

ADDITIONAL READING

- Bosch X, Poch E, Grau JM. Rhabdomyolysis and acute kidney injury. *N Engl J Med*. 2009;361(1):62–72.
- Hall AB, Salazar M, Larison DJ. The sequencing of medication administration in the management of hyperkalemia. *J Emerg Nurs*. 2009;35(4):339–342.
- Hollander-Rodriguez JC, Calvert JF Jr. Hyperkalemia. *Am Fam Physician*. 2006;73(2):283–290.
- Jain N, Kotla S, Little BB, et al. Predictors of hyperkalemia and death in patients with cardiac and renal disease. *Am J Cardiol*. 2012;109(10):1510–1513.
- Noori N, Kalantar-Zadeh K, Kovesdy CP, et al. Dietary potassium intake and mortality in long-term hemodialysis patients. *Am J Kidney Dis*. 2010;56(2):338–347.
- Pepin J, Shields C. Advances in diagnosis and management of hypokalemic and hyperkalemic emergencies. *Emerg Med Pract*. 2012;14(2):1–17.
- Riccardi A, Tasso F, Corti L, et al. The emergency physician and the prompt management of severe hyperkalemia. *Intern Emerg Med*. 2012;7(Suppl 2):S131–S133.

 ## SEE ALSO

- Addison Disease; Hypokalemia
- Algorithm: Hyperkalemia

 ## CODES

ICD10
E87.5 Hyperkalemia

CLINICAL PEARLS

- Emergency and urgent management of hyperkalemia takes precedent to a thorough diagnostic workup. Urgent treatment includes stabilization of the myocardium with calcium gluconate to protect against arrhythmias and pharmacologic strategies to move K from the extracellular (vascular) space into cells.
- Calcium and dextrose/insulin are only temporizing measures and do not actually lower total body K levels. Definitive treatment with either dialysis or cation exchange resin (sodium polystyrene sulfonate) necessary.
- To lower a patient's risk of developing hyperkalemia, have the patient follow a low-K diet, use selective β_1-blockers, such as metoprolol or atenolol, instead of nonselective β-blockers such as carvedilol. Avoid NSAIDs. Concomitant use of kaliuretic loop diuretics may be useful.

HYPERNATREMIA

Nilgun Ozturk, MD • Pang-Yen Fan, MD

 BASICS

DESCRIPTION
- Serum sodium (Na) concentration >145 mEq/L (1)
- Usually represents a state of hyperosmolality (1)
- Na concentration reflects balance between total body water (TBW) and total body Na. Hypernatremia occurs from deficit of water relative to Na.
- Hypernatremia results from net water loss or, more rarely, from primary Na gain (1).
- May exist with hypo-, hyper-, or euvolemia, although hypovolemia is by far most common type
  - Hypovolemic: occurs with a decrease in TBW and a proportionately smaller decrease in total body Na
  - Euvolemic: no change in TBW with a proportionate increase in total body Na
  - Hypervolemic: increase in TBW and a proportionately greater increase in total body Na
- It has been shown to be an indicator for higher mortality in critically ill patients and patients with chronic kidney disease (CKD) (2)[B].

EPIDEMIOLOGY
Incidence
- More common in elderly and young
- Occurs in 1% of hospitalized elderly patients (3)
- Seen in about 9% of ICU patients (3). Gastroenteritis with diarrhea is the most common cause of hypernatremia in infants.
- Women are at an increased risk due to decreased TBW, as compared with men.

ETIOLOGY AND PATHOPHYSIOLOGY
- Pure water loss (total body Na normal) resulting from the following:
  - Adipsia/hypodipsia (e.g., impaired thirst regulation, decreased access to water) (4)
  - Nephrogenic diabetes insipidus (DI) (congenital or due to renal dysfunction, hypercalcemia, hypokalemia, medication-related, particularly lithium)
  - Central DI (due to head trauma, stroke, meningitis) (3)
  - Increased insensible water loss (e.g., fever, hyperventilation, hypermetabolic state, heat exposure, newborns under radiant warmers)
- Hypotonic fluid loss (total body Na decreased) resulting from the following:
  - Loss of fluid containing relatively more water than Na (e.g., excessive sweating, severe burns)
  - Urinary loss
    - Osmotic diuresis: hyperglycemia, mannitol
    - Diuretics, especially loop diuretics
    - Diabetes mellitus, particularly new presentation/decompensated
    - Post acute tubular necrosis (ATN) or post obstructive diuresis
    - Intrinsic renal disease
  - Gastrointestinal loss
    - Diarrhea, especially in children
    - Vomiting, nasogastric (NG) lavage
    - Enterocutaneous fistula
- Excess Na (increase in total body Na) resulting from the following:
  - IV NaCl or $NaHCO_3$ during cardiopulmonary resuscitation, metabolic acidosis, or hyperkalemia (3)
  - Sea water ingestion
  - Excessive use of $NaHCO_3$ antacid.

- Incorrect infant formula preparation
- Intrauterine NaCl for abortion
- Excessive Na in dialysate solutions
- Disorders of the adrenal axis (Cushing syndrome, Conn syndrome, congenital adrenal hyperplasia)
- Tube feeding

With acute hypernatremia, the rapid decrease in brain volume can cause rupture of the cerebral veins, leading to focal intracerebral and subarachnoid hemorrhages and possibly irreversible neurologic damage (5).

Genetics
Some forms of DI may be hereditary.

RISK FACTORS
- Patients at increased risk include those with an impaired thirst mechanism or restricted access to water, as well as those with increased water loss
- Infants/children
- Elderly patients (may also have a diminished thirst response to osmotic stimulation via an unknown mechanism)
- Patients who are intubated/have altered mental status.
- Diabetes mellitus
- Prior brain injury
- Surgery
- Diuretic therapy, especially loop diuretics
- Lithium treatment

GENERAL PREVENTION
- Treatment/prevention of underlying cause
- Properly prepare infant formula and never add salt to any commercial infant formula.
- Keep patients well hydrated.

COMMONLY ASSOCIATED CONDITIONS
- Gastroenteritis
- Altered mental status
- Burns
- Hypermetabolic conditions
- Head injury
- Renal dysfunction

 DIAGNOSIS

HISTORY
- Excessive thirst, nausea, vomiting, diarrhea, oliguria, polyuria
- Fever, myalgia, muscle weakness
- Neurologic symptoms common: altered mental status, seizure (especially if rapid development of hypernatremia), twitching, lethargy, irritability, coma, anophthalmos
- Severe symptoms are likely to occur with acute increases in plasma Na levels or at concentrations >160 mEq/L.
- Obtain list of current and recent medications.
- Review recent illnesses and activities.

PHYSICAL EXAM
- Sinus tachycardia, hypotension, orthostatic hypotension, poor O_2 saturation
- Dry mucous membranes, cool/gray skin
- Neurologic abnormalities: lethargy, weakness, focal deficits (in cases of intracerebral bleeding/lesion), confusion, coma, seizures

DIFFERENTIAL DIAGNOSIS
- DI
- Hyperosmotic coma
- Salt ingestion
- Hypertonic dehydration
- Hypothyroidism
- Cushing syndrome

DIAGNOSTIC TESTS & INTERPRETATION
Initial Tests (lab, imaging)
- Serum Na, potassium, BUN, creatinine, calcium, and osmolality (serum lithium if appropriate)
- Urine Na and osmolality
  - DI: urine osmolality (usually <300 mosmol/kg) < serum osmolality, and urine Na usually low normal/slightly low (due to dilution) (4)
  - Osmotic diuresis: urine osmolality intermediate, urine Na low/low-normal, total daily osmole excretion high
  - Salt ingestion: increased urine osmolality (above 600 mosmol/kg) and high urine Na
  - Hypertonic dehydration: increased urine osmolality and decreased urine Na
- Serum glucose
- Special tests for DI
  - Water deprivation test: In DI, urine osmolality does not increase as it normally should when hypernatremic.
  - Antidiuretic hormone (ADH) stimulation: distinguishes central versus nephrogenic DI
    - Urine osmolality does not increase after ADH or desmopressin (DDAVP) in nephrogenic DI.
- Head CT/MRI in DI to rule out craniopharyngioma, other brain tumor or masses, or median cleft syndrome

Diagnostic Procedures/Other
History, physical, laboratory studies, family history for central DI

TREATMENT

GENERAL MEASURES
- The treatment of hypernatremia involves treating the underlying cause and correcting the water deficit.
- Goal for corrected Na is 145 mEq/L (1).
- Speed of correction depends on symptom severity/rate of development of hypernatremia. Avoid rapid correction to prevent development of cerebral edema if chronic hypernatremia (>24 hours):
  - Maximum of 0.5 mEq/L/hr or 10 mEq/L/day (6)[C]
  - May correct at up to 1 mEq/L/hr if acute hypernatremia (<24 hours) (1)
- Treat volume depletion first, then hypernatremia:
  - Restore intravascular volume with IV fluids to normalize serum Na levels.
- Replace water orally if patient is conscious.
- Important formulas in determining rate of fluid administration
  - TBW = coefficient × wt (kg), where coefficient = 0.6 for children, 0.5 for nonelderly women and elderly men, 0.45 for elderly women

- Calculated free water deficit (liters) = TBW × [1 − (Na_t/Na_m)], where Na_t = target Na+, and Na_m = measured Na+. Note: wt = weight in kilograms.
  - Change in serum Na per 1 L infusate = [(infusate Na + infusate K) − serum Na]/[TBW + 1]
- Account for ongoing fluid losses during calculation of rate of fluid administration.
- Dialysis can be considered if acute kidney injury is present concomitantly and if conventional treatment has failed (7)[B].

MEDICATION

First Line
- See "General Measures" for overall approach.
- Volume depletion: Use isotonic fluids initially if signs of hemodynamic compromise, then change to hypotonic fluids when stable:
  - Hypotonic fluids (0.45% NaCl or dextrose 5% in water)
    ○ Important not to decrease serum Na by >10 mEq/L/day to prevent cerebral edema (4)[C]
- Hypervolemia: Give furosemide along with hypotonic fluids. Dose varies depending on desired urine output. Loop diuretics with fluid restriction worsen hypernatremia (4)[C].
- Central DI
  - DDAVP acetate: Use parenteral form for acute symptomatic patients, and use intranasal or oral form for chronic therapy (4).
  - Free water replacement: may use 2.5% dextrose in water if giving large volumes of water in DI to avoid glycosuria
  - May consider sulfonylureas/thiazide diuretics for chronic, but not acute, treatment
- Nephrogenic DI
  - Treat with diuretics and NSAIDs.
  - Lithium-induced nephrogenic DI: hydrochlorothiazide 25 mg PO BID or indomethacin 50 mg PO TID, or amiloride hydrochloride 5 to 10 mg PO BID (8)
- Precautions
  - Rapid correction of hypernatremia can cause cerebral edema, central pontine myelinosis, seizures, or death (9).
  - Hypocalcemia and more rarely acidosis can occur during correction.
  - DI: High rates of dextrose 5% in water can cause hyperglycemia and glucose-induced diuresis.

Second Line
- Consider NSAIDs in nephrogenic DI.
- Modalities requiring further investigations
- Continuous renal replacement therapy (CRRT): Multiple case reports and case series have shown success and safety in using CRRT to treat hypernatremia in critically ill patients with CHF and severe burns (7,10).

ISSUES FOR REFERRAL
Underlying renal involvement associated with hypernatremia would benefit from a nephrology referral.

INPATIENT CONSIDERATIONS

Admission Criteria/Initial Stabilization
Symptomatic patient with serum Na >155 mEq/L requires IV fluid therapy.

IV Fluids
Refer to "Medication" section.

Nursing
Bed rest until stable or underlying condition resolved/controlled

Discharge Criteria
Stabilization of serum Na level and symptoms are minimal.

 ONGOING CARE

FOLLOW-UP RECOMMENDATIONS

Patient Monitoring
- Frequent reexams in an acute setting
- Frequent electrolytes and blood glucose: initially q4–6h
- Urine osmolality and urine output in DI
- Ensure adequate ingestion of calories because patients may ingest so much water that they feel full and do not eat.
- Measure ongoing losses of water and solute and replace as needed.
- Daily weights

DIET
- Ensure proper nutrition during acute phase.
- After resolution of acute phase, may want to consider Na-restricted diet for patient
- Low-salt, low-protein diet in nephrogenic DI

PATIENT EDUCATION
Patients with nephrogenic DI must avoid salt and drink large amounts of water.

PROGNOSIS
Most recover but neurologic impairment can occur.

COMPLICATIONS
- CNS thrombosis/hemorrhage
- Seizures
- Mental retardation
- Hyperactivity
- Chronic hypernatremia: >2 days duration has higher mortality
- Serum Na >180 mEq/L (>180 mmol/L): often results in residual CNS damage
- More common if rapid development of hypernatremia

REFERENCES

1. Adrogué HJ, Madias NE. Hypernatremia. *N Engl J Med*. 2000;342(20):1493–1499.
2. Kovesdy CP, Lott EH, Lu JL, et al. Hyponatremia, hypernatremia, and mortality in patients with chronic kidney disease with and without congestive heart failure. *Circulation*. 2012;125(5): 677–684.
3. Bagshaw SM, Townsend DR, McDermid RC. Disorders of sodium and water balance in hospitalized patients. *Can J Anaesth*. 2009;56(2): 151–167.
4. Hannon MJ, Finucane FM, Sherlock M, et al. Clinical review: disorders of water homeostasis in neurosurgical patients. *J Clin Endocrinol Metab*. 2012;97(5):1423–1433.
5. Sterns RH. Disorders of plasma sodium—causes, consequences, and correction. *N Engl J Med*. 2015;372(1):55–65.
6. Al-Absi A, Gosmanova EO, Wall BM. A clinical approach to the treatment of chronic hypernatremia. *Am J Kidney Dis*. 2012;60(6):1032–1038.
7. Huang C, Zhang P, Du R, et al. Treatment of acute hypernatremia in severely burned patients using continuous veno-venous hemofiltration with gradient sodium replacement fluid: a report of nine cases. *Intensive Care Med*. 2013;39(8):1495–1496.
8. Libber S, Harrison H, Spector D. Treatment of nephrogenic diabetes insipidus with prostaglandin synthesis inhibitors. *J Pediatr*. 1986;108(2):305–311.
9. Mastrangelo S, Arlotta A, Cefalo MG, et al. Central pontine and extrapontine myelinolysis in a pediatric patient following rapid correction of hypernatremia. *Neuropediatrics*. 2009;40(3): 144–147.
10. Park HS, Hong YA, Kim HG, et al. Usefulness of continuous renal replacement therapy for correcting hypernatremia in a patient with severe congestive heart failure. *Hemodial Int*. 2012;16(4):559–563.

ADDITIONAL READING
Waite MD, Fuhrman SA, Badawi O, et al. Intensive care unit–acquired hypernatremia is an independent predictor of increased mortality and length of stay. *J Crit Care*. 2013;28(4):405–412.

 SEE ALSO
- Diabetes Insipidus
- Algorithm: Hypernatremia

 CODES

ICD10
E87.0 Hyperosmolality and hypernatremia

CLINICAL PEARLS
- Occurs from water deficit in comparison to total body Na stores
- Common causes include dehydration, DI, impaired access to fluids
- Determine if the patient has hypervolemic, euvolemic, or hypovolemic hypernatremia in the differential diagnosis of etiology; most commonly hypovolemic; other entities rare
- Avoid rapid correction of hypernatremia to prevent development of cerebral edema when hypernatremia is chronic (goal rate is 10 meq/L in 24 hours).
- Use hypotonic fluids unless patient has hemodynamic compromise, which necessitates use of isotonic fluids.
- Use oral replacement in conscious patients if possible.
- Use the estimated water deficit, desired rate of correction, and estimation of ongoing free water losses to calculate a fluid repletion regimen.

H

HYPERPARATHYROIDISM

Aleta Paschal, MD   Cassandra White, MD

 BASICS

DESCRIPTION

A dysfunction of the body's normal regulatory feedback mechanisms resulting in excess production of parathyroid hormone (PTH)

- Primary hyperparathyroidism (HPT): intrinsic parathyroid gland dysfunction resulting in excessive secretions of PTH with a lack of response to feedback inhibition by elevated calcium
- Secondary HPT: excessive secretion of PTH in response to hypocalcemia, which can be caused by vitamin D deficiency or renal failure
- Tertiary HPT: autonomous hyperfunction of the parathyroid gland in the setting of long-standing secondary HPT

EPIDEMIOLOGY

Incidence
Predominant sex: female > male (2:1)

Prevalence
Primary HPT: 1/1,000 in the United States

ETIOLOGY AND PATHOPHYSIOLOGY

- PTH is synthesized by the four parathyroid glands, which are located behind the four poles of the thyroid gland (locations can vary).
- Ectopic (abnormal locations and most common is the thymus) or supernumerary glands (more than four glands) (1)
- Blood supply: inferior thyroid artery
- PTH releases calcium from bone by osteoclastic stimulation (bone resorption).
- PTH increases reabsorption of calcium in the distal tubules of the kidneys.
- PTH stimulates conversion of 25-hydroxycholecalciferol (25[OH]D) to 1,25-dihydroxycholecalciferol (1,25[OH]$_2$D or active vitamin D) in the kidneys.
  - 1,25(OH)$_2$D increases calcium absorption from the GI tract, increases calcium and phosphate reabsorption in the kidneys, and stimulates osteoclastic activity and bone resorption.
- Primary HPT: unregulated PTH production and release, causing increase in serum calcium
  - Solitary adenoma (89%)
  - Double adenomas (5%)
  - Diffuse hyperplasia (6%) caused by multiple adenomas, multiple endocrine neoplasia (MEN) types 1 and 2a, and familial hypocalciuric hypercalcemia
  - Parathyroid carcinoma (<2%)
- Secondary HPT: adaptive parathyroid gland hyperplasia and hyperfunction
  - Dietary: vitamin D or calcium deficiency
  - Chronic renal disease resulting in the following:
    ○ Renal parenchymal loss causing hyperphosphatemia
    ○ Impaired calcitriol production causing hypocalcemia
    ○ General skeletal and renal resistance to PTH
- Tertiary HPT: autonomous oversecretion of PTH following prolonged parathyroid stimulation

Genetics
- MEN types 1 and 2a: Patients with multiple gland hyperplasia in the absence of renal disease should be screened for MEN-1 gene mutation.

- Neonatal severe primary HPT
- HPT—jaw tumor syndrome
- Familial hypocalciuric hypercalcemia (FHH): autosomal dominant
- Familial isolated HPT

RISK FACTORS
Chronic kidney disease, increasing age, poor nutrition, radiation, and/or family history

GENERAL PREVENTION
Adequate intake of calcium and vitamin D may help prevent secondary HPT.

COMMONLY ASSOCIATED CONDITIONS
- MEN syndromes types 1 and 2a
- Chronic renal failure

℞ DIAGNOSIS

HISTORY
- History of present illness
  - 50% of patients are asymptomatic.
  - Bone, abdominal, and flank pain as well as psychosis, which are all classic complaints of hypercalcemia
- Past medical history
  - The following conditions may be associated with HPT:
    ○ MEN syndrome (MEN-associated conditions include pancreatic cancer, pituitary adenomas, medullary thyroid cancer, and pheochromocytoma), nephrolithiasis (in 20–30%), nephrocalcinosis, pancreatitis, gastroduodenal ulcer, hypertension, short QT interval, left ventricular hypertrophy, osteitis fibrosa cystica, cystic bone lesions, spontaneous fracture, vertebral collapse, osteoporosis, gout, pseudogout, anxiety, depression, psychosis, coma, conjunctivitis, band keratopathy, conjunctival calcium deposits, radiation to the neck
- Medications: thiazides or lithium
- Review of systems
  - Possible symptoms include polydipsia, polyuria, flank pain, abdominal pain, constipation, vomiting, anorexia, weight loss, muscle fatigue, pain, weakness, hypotonia, arthralgia, bone pain, fatigue, apathy, and somnolence.

PHYSICAL EXAM
Limited usefulness; 70–80% of patients have no obvious symptoms or signs of disease.
- Physical findings may found related to underlying cause of HPT.

DIFFERENTIAL DIAGNOSIS
- Increased PTH: ectopic PTH production
- Nonparathyroid causes
  - Malignancy: lung (squamous cell) carcinoma, breast carcinoma, multiple myeloma, lymphoma, leukemia, prostate cancer, Paget disease
  - Granulomatous disease: sarcoidosis, tuberculosis, berylliosis, histoplasmosis, coccidioidomycosis
  - Drugs: thiazide diuretics, vitamin D intoxication, vitamin A excess, lithium, milk-alkali syndrome, exogenous calcium intake

  - Endocrine: hyperthyroidism, acute adrenal insufficiency
  - Familial: hypocalciuric hypercalcemia

DIAGNOSTIC TESTS & INTERPRETATION

Initial Tests (lab, imaging)
- Disease is often detected by an incidental finding of hypercalcemia.
- Order serum calcium level and albumin
  - Calculate serum calcium on 2 occasions using: (0.8 × [Normal Albumin − Pt's Albumin]) + Serum Ca. If corrected calcium is above your lab's normal range (normally >2.65 mmol/L), consider this true hypercalcemia which is consistent with hyperparathyroidism.
- If hypercalcemia is confirmed, follow with intact PTH level (2)[B].
  - High PTH (>3.0 pmol/L) suggests primary HPT.
  - Low PTH (<3.0 pmol/L) suggests non–PTH-mediated hypercalcemia.
- If elevated calcium is inconsistent, elevated ionized serum calcium in the setting of high PTH confirms diagnosis. Other findings may include low serum phosphate, elevated serum chloride, decreased serum CO_2, and abnormal 24-hour urine calcium excretion.
- Normocalcemic primary HPT found in 2009; consistent with normal calcium, low bone mineral density, and elevated PTH(must r/o secondary HPT) (3)
- In secondary HPT, an elevated phosphorus suggests chronic renal failure; a low phosphorus suggests another cause, most commonly vitamin D deficiency.

Follow-Up Tests & Special Considerations
- A 24-hour urine calcium concentration to creatinine clearance ratio >0.02 suggests primary HPT; a ratio <0.01 may be normal or indicate FHH; important because FHH does not require surgery (2)[C]
- Routine measurement of 25(OH)D levels is recommended in all patients with primary HPT. In case of vitamin D deficiency (<20 ng/mL or <50 nmol/L), defer management decisions until levels are maintained >20 ng/mL (50 nmol/L) (4)[C].
- Intraoperative measurement of intact PTH and/or γ-probe localization of abnormal glands with technetium-99m sestamibi scan has aided focused resections for patients with single-gland etiology (5)[C].
- Screening for kidney stones is not recommended in patients without a history of nephrolithiasis (5)[B].

Diagnostic Procedures/Other
- Consider EKG to assess for short QT interval.
- Imaging is not required for diagnosis. It is required for surgical planning, especially for minimally invasive parathyroidectomy (MIP) (6)[C].
  - Imaging is also indicated to localize hyperplasia or an ectopic parathyroid gland in repeat surgery.
- Imaging options for presurgical localization
  - Technetium-99m sestamibi with single-photon emission computed tomography (SPECT)
    ○ Has had the greatest reported success in localizing single parathyroid adenomas (7)[B]
  - US
    ○ Painless, noninvasive, inexpensive, and does not expose the patient to radiation; however, its accuracy is very operator-dependent (8)[C].

- Positron emission tomography (PET) using C-methionine (MET-PET) is comparable to US and technetium-99m sestamibi with SPECT in terms of diagnostic use (6)[B].
- Four-dimensional CT (4D-CT) may be more effective for primary localization than both US and sestamibi-SPECT (9)[B].
- CT and MRI are mostly used to localize ectopic mediastinal glands.
- Comprehensive cervical US (CCU) used for further localization following a negative sestamibi scan often reveals a single adenoma (10)[C].
  - A negative sestamibi scan likely indicates parathyroid hyperplasia/multiglandular disease and thus requires open neck exploratory surgery.
  - CCU after negative sestamibi result allows more patients who were previously excluded to be candidates for MIP.

TREATMENT

MEDICATION
- Primary HPT: Operative management is curative. For those awaiting or unable to have surgery
  - Bisphosphonates (alendronate): reduces bone turnover and helps to maintain bone density; avoid in kidney disease.
  - Calcimimetics (cinacalcet): Further studies needed to establish long-term benefit in primary HPT.
  - Selective estrogen receptor modulator therapy (raloxifene)
  - Hormone replacement therapy with estrogens is not recommended as first-line treatment; must weigh benefit with risks of known systemic effects
    - Can be used in postmenopausal women who do not undergo or refuse surgery
- Secondary HPT
  - Calcium replacement
  - Vitamin D analogues (paricalcitol and calcitriol)
  - Phosphorus-binding agents (sevelamer)
  - Calcimimetic (cinacalcet) (2,11)[A]: activates calcium-sensing receptor in parathyroid gland thereby inhibiting PTH secretion
- Tertiary HPT
  - Medical treatment is not curative and generally not indicated.

SURGERY/OTHER PROCEDURES
- Operative management is curative for patients with primary HPT in 95–98% of patients.
- Indications for parathyroidectomy
  - Symptomatic primary HPT
    - Nephrolithiasis
    - Nephrocalcinosis
    - Osteitis fibrosa cystica
  - Asymptomatic primary HPT
    - Serum Ca^+ level >1 mg/dL above normal
    - Age <50 years
    - GFR <60 mL/min/1.73 m^2 or creatinine clearance reduced to <60 mL/min
    - Bone density loss with a T score ≤ -2.5 at the lumbar spine, femoral neck, total hip, or 33% radius
- Tertiary HPT
- Surgical removal of diseased gland or tissue is only proven curative therapy for HPT.

- Surgical options include the following:
  - Bilateral open neck exploratory surgery
  - MIP using preoperative sestamibi scan with SPECT/US and intraoperative PTH levels (high sensitivity 79–95% to predict location of single parathyroid adenoma) (11) which result in decreased pain, smaller incisions, improved cosmetic results, lower morbidity, and decreased length of hospital stay when compared with open neck exploratory surgery.
- Follow postoperative serum calcium level (hypocalcemia in "hungry bone" syndrome); patients also at risk for bleeding and airway compromise; keep injectable calcium and seizure medications at bedside.
- Monitor renal function closely.

INPATIENT CONSIDERATIONS
Admission Criteria/Initial Stabilization
Critical hypercalcemia requires IV fluid rehydration, IV bisphosphonate therapy, and SC calcitonin (4 U/kg q12h) for severe symptoms.

ONGOING CARE

FOLLOW-UP RECOMMENDATIONS
Asymptomatic patients with primary HPT require serial monitoring of calcium and PTH.

Patient Monitoring
In patients with primary HPT who are asymptomatic, measurements of serum calcium and creatinine annually and bone density scan every 1 to 2 years is sufficient.

DIET
- In the presence of hypercalciuria or elevated 1,25(OH)$_2$D levels, dietary calcium restriction is recommended. Otherwise, daily calcium intake should be maintained at up to 1,000 mg.
- Restrict dietary phosphate in secondary HPT.

PATIENT EDUCATION
- Importance of periodic lab testing
- Signs of severe hypercalcemia

PROGNOSIS
Prognosis after surgery is excellent in primary HPT, with resolution of many of the preoperative symptoms.

COMPLICATIONS
Related to high levels of PTH and/or elevated calcium

REFERENCES

1. Bliss RD, Gauger PG, Delbridge LW. Surgeon's approach to the thyroid gland: surgical anatomy and the importance of technique. *World J Surg.* 2000;24(8):891–897.
2. Fraser WD. Hyperparathyroidism. *Lancet.* 2009;374(9684):145–158.
3. Lowe H, McMahon DJ, Rubin MR, et al. Normocalcemic primary hyperparathyroidism: further characterization of a new clinical phenotype. *J Clin Endocrinol Metab.* 2007;92(8):3001–3005.
4. Eastell R, Arnold A, Brandi ML, et al. Diagnosis of asymptomatic primary hyperparathyroidism: proceedings of the third international workshop. *J Clin Endocrinol Metab.* 2009;94(2):340–350.
5. Bilezikian JP, Khan AA, Potts JT Jr, et al. Guidelines for the management of asymptomatic primary hyperparathyroidism: summary statement from the third international workshop. *J Clin Endocrinol Metab.* 2009;94(2):335–339.
6. Caldarella C, Treglia G, Isgrò MA, et al. Diagnostic performance of positron emission tomography using ^{11}C-methionine in patients with suspected parathyroid adenoma: a meta-analysis. *Endocrine.* 2013;43(1):78–83.
7. Caldarella C, Treglia G, Pontecorvi A, et al. Diagnostic performance of planar scintigraphy using ^{99}mTc-MIBI in patients with secondary hyperparathyroidism: a meta-analysis. *Ann Nucl Med.* 2012;26(10):794–803.
8. Udelsman R, Pasieka JL, Sturgeon C, et al. Surgery for asymptomatic primary hyperparathyroidism: proceedings of the third international workshop. *J Clin Endocrinol Metab.* 2009;94(2):366–372.
9. Cheung K, Wang TS, Farrokhyar F, et al. A meta-analysis of preoperative localization techniques for patients with primary hyperparathyroidism. *Ann Surg Oncol.* 2012;19(2):577–583.
10. Kandil E, Malazai AJ, Alrasheedi S, et al. Minimally invasive/focused parathyroidectomy in patients with negative sestamibi scan results. *Arch Otolaryngol Head Neck Surg.* 2012;138(3):223–225.
11. Kunstman JW, Kirsch JD, Mahajan A, et al. Clinical review: parathyroid localization and implications for clinical management. *J Clin Endocrinol Metab.* 2013;98(3):902–912.

CODES

ICD10
- E21.3 Hyperparathyroidism, unspecified
- E21.0 Primary hyperparathyroidism
- E21.1 Secondary hyperparathyroidism, not elsewhere classified

CLINICAL PEARLS

- 50% of patients with primary HPT are asymptomatic.
- HPT is often detected by an incidental finding of hypercalcemia on a routine serum chemistry analysis.
- Classic symptoms of hypercalcemia include painful bones, renal stones, abdominal pains, and behavioral changes ("stones, bones, moans, and groans").
- Repeat calcium (elevated), correct for serum albumin, and obtain intact PTH levels to make an initial diagnosis.
- The two most commonly used imaging modalities in HPT are technetium-99m sestamibi scan and US.
- Surgery is curative for most cases of primary HPT.

H

HYPERPROLACTINEMIA

D'Ann Somerall, DNP, FNP-BC • William E. Somerall, Jr., MD, MEd

BASICS

DESCRIPTION
Hyperprolactinemia is an abnormal elevation in the serum prolactin level with multiple possible etiologies.

EPIDEMIOLOGY
Prevalence
- Predominant age: reproductive age
- Predominant sex: female > male
- More readily detected in females because a slight elevation in prolactin causes changes in menstruation and galactorrhea

ETIOLOGY AND PATHOPHYSIOLOGY
- Prolactin, which is produced by lactotrophs in the anterior pituitary, is regulated by:
  - Inhibitory factors, primarily dopamine, produced in the hypothalamus and delivered via the hypothalamic-pituitary vessels in the pituitary stalk
  - Stimulatory factors, primarily thyrotropin-releasing hormone (TRH)
- Causes of hyperprolactinemia include the following:
  - Physiologic
    - Pregnancy due to increased estrogen
    - Breastfeeding
    - Nipple stimulation
    - Stress, including postoperative state
  - Medications
    - Dopamine (D_2) blockers: prochlorperazine, metoclopramide
    - Dopamine depleters: α-methyldopa, reserpine
    - Antidepressants: selective serotonin reuptake inhibitors (SSRIs), tricyclic antidepressants (SSRIs do not appear to cause clinically significant hyperprolactinemia)
    - Verapamil (but no other calcium channel blockers; thought to decrease hypothalamic synthesis of dopamine)
    - Antipsychotics: haloperidol, fluphenazine, risperidone
  - Hypothyroidism (due to elevated TRH)
  - Chest wall conditions:
    - Herpes zoster
    - After thoracotomy
    - Trauma
  - Prolactin-secreting adenoma (anterior pituitary), categorized:
    - Microadenoma: <1 cm
    - Macroadenoma: >1 cm
  - Pituitary stalk compression/disruption:
    - Craniopharyngioma
    - Rathke cleft cyst
    - Meningioma
    - Astrocytoma
    - Metastases
    - Head trauma
    - Infiltrative/inflammatory disorders
  - Diminished prolactin clearance:
    - Chronic renal failure
    - Cirrhosis
- Cocaine

DIAGNOSIS

HISTORY
- Galactorrhea
- Amenorrhea
- Oligomenorrhea
- Infertility
- Osteoporosis/osteopenia
- Decreased libido, impotence
- Weight gain
- Also may have signs and symptoms of pituitary enlargement:
  - Headache
  - Visual field impairment (bitemporal hemianopsia)
  - Hypopituitarism (secondary to tumor pressure on surrounding structures)
- Also may have signs and symptoms of associated conditions:
  - Hypothyroidism
  - Cushing disease
  - Acromegaly
  - Multiple endocrine neoplasia (MEN)-1 syndrome

PHYSICAL EXAM
- Visual field testing
- Cranial nerve exam

DIFFERENTIAL DIAGNOSIS
Macroprolactinemia: Macroprolactin, a polymer of several units of prolactin, is detected by immunologically based lab tests but is not biologically active. If patient is asymptomatic but found to have elevated prolactin (PRL), consider this diagnosis and notify the lab. No treatment is required.

DIAGNOSTIC TESTS & INTERPRETATION
- Serum prolactin (most accurate results if checked fasting, in morning) <25 μg/L normal; >25 μg/L abnormal; >250 μg/L often indicates a prolactinoma (1)[A]

- Pregnancy test
- Thyroid-stimulating hormone (TSH)
- Luteinizing hormone (LH)/follicle-stimulating hormone (FSH) if amenorrheic
- Chemistry, renal function
- LFTs

Initial Tests (lab, imaging)
A single measurement of serum prolactin; a level above the upper limit of normal confirms the diagnosis.
- Pituitary MRI: single best imaging
- CT scan if MRI is contraindicated
- Levels should be drawn prior to breast exam.

Follow-Up Tests & Special Considerations
Formal visual field testing if pituitary adenoma is suspected

TREATMENT

GENERAL MEASURES
- Discontinue offending medications, if any (1)[A].
- Treat underlying causes (1)[A].
- For asymptomatic patients with mild PRL elevations, observation alone may be considered (1,2)[A].
- Medications indicated for (1)[A]:

  - Symptoms of hypogonadism, such as decreased libido
  - Galactorrhea (if bothersome to patient)
  - Restoration of fertility
  - Pituitary adenoma
  - Prevention of osteoporosis

MEDICATION
Dopamine agonists: decrease serum prolactin concentrations and decrease the size of most lactotroph adenomas

- Cabergoline (Dostinex): This is now a first-line choice due to efficacy and favorable side effect profile (1,3)[A]: dosed twice weekly. Cabergoline was more effective than bromocriptine in reducing persistent hyperprolactinemia, galactorrhea, and amenorrhea/oligomenorrhea (2)[A]. Has recently been reported to be associated with significant improvements in the body mass index, total HDL and LDL cholesterol levels, and insulin sensitivity; decrease in proinflammatory markers; and carotid intima media thickness, indicated with bromocriptine failure or resistance; has been shown to reduce erectile dysfunction in hyperprolactinemic men (1)[A]

  - Adverse effects (better tolerated if start with low dose, slow titration, given at night with food):
    - Nausea/vomiting
    - Headache
    - Dizziness
    - Fatigue
    - Light-headedness

    - Postural hypotension (2)[A]
- Bromocriptine (Parlodel): This has the longest clinical history: dosed BID; preferred by some clinicians when infertility is an indication for treatment (2,4)[A].
- Both are effective for reducing tumor size and improving symptoms (2)[A].
- SE less with cabergoline than bromocriptine (2)[A]. Pergolide (Permax) is no longer used in the United States. If patient is still on med, do not withdraw abruptly.

ADDITIONAL THERAPIES

Patients with medically and surgically refractory prolactinomas; radiotherapy produced a reduction in prolactin levels in nearly all patients and normalization in over a quarter of patients with low complication rates (2)[A].

SURGERY/OTHER PROCEDURES

- For adenomas, medical treatment will be successful in 80–90% of patients. In some cases, surgery is indicated (1).
- Indications
  - Intolerance or resistance to medical treatment
  - Headache
  - Visual field loss
  - CSF leak due to tumor apoplexy or shrinkage
  - Cranial nerve deficit
- Risks
  - High recurrence rate (up to 40%)
  - CSF leakage
  - Meningitis
  - Transient diabetes insipidus (5)
- Pituitary insufficiency

ONGOING CARE

FOLLOW-UP RECOMMENDATIONS

Patient Monitoring

- Depends on etiology
- After at least 2 years of treatment, no tumor and prolactin levels normal may consider decreasing and stopping medication. Must be followed closely, as tumor may grow back (1).
- Consider:
  - Formal visual field testing yearly (4)[A]
  - Serial MRIs if clinically indicated (4)[A]

Pregnancy Considerations

- If pregnancy is desired in a woman with hyperprolactinemia, dopamine agonists are not approved during pregnancy and should be discontinued once pregnancy is confirmed, but their use is recommended if neurologic findings are present (1)[A].
- With microprolactinoma: Treat with bromocriptine if symptomatic; monthly pregnancy tests; discontinue bromocriptine when pregnancy is confirmed.

- With macroprolactinomas: a definitive, individualized plan is made. Options include discontinuation of bromocriptine at conception and careful monitoring of PRL levels and VS, with or without MRI scan evidence of tumor enlargement; prepregnancy transsphenoidal surgery with debulking of tumor; continuation of bromocriptine throughout gestation, with a risk to the fetus.
- Careful monitoring of visual fields in each trimester. No need to monitor prolactin levels, as they are normally high due to pregnancy (1)[A].

PATIENT EDUCATION

- Discuss risks of untreated hyperprolactinemia:
  - Headache
  - Visual field loss
  - Decreased bone density
  - Infertility
- Patient guide to hyperprolactinemia diagnosis and treatment

PROGNOSIS

- Tends to recur after discontinuation of medical therapy (1)
- Over 10 years, 7% chance of progression of prolactin-secreting microadenoma (4)

COMPLICATIONS

- Depends on underlying cause
- If pituitary adenoma, risk of permanent visual field loss

REFERENCES

1. Hoffman AR, Melmed S, Schlechte J. Patient guide to hyperprolactinemia diagnosis and treatment. *J Clin Endocrinol Metab.* 2011;96(2):35A–36A.
2. Wang AT, Mullan RJ, Lane MA, et al. Treatment of hyperprolactinemia: a systematic review and meta-analysis. *Syst Rev.* 2012;1:33.
3. Wong A, Eloy JA, Couldwell WT, et al. Update on prolactinomas. Part 2: treatment and management strategies. *J Clin Neurosci.* 2015;22(10): 1568–1574.
4. Casanueva FF, Molitch ME, Schlechte JA, et al. Guidelines of the Pituitary Society for the diagnosis and management of prolactinomas. *Clin Endocrinol (Oxf).* 2006;65(2):265–273.
5. Bloomgarden E, Molitch ME. Surgical treatment of prolactinomas: cons. *Endocrine.* 2014;47(3):730–733.
6. Sun GE, Pantalone KM, Gupta M, et al. Is chronic nipple piercing associated with hyperprolactinemia? *Pituitary.* 2013;16(3):351–353.

ADDITIONAL READING

- Inancli SS, Usluogullari A, Ustu Y, et al. Effect of cabergoline on insulin sensitivity, inflammation, and carotid intima media thickness in patients with prolactinoma. *Endocrine.* 2013;44(1):193–199.
- Inder WJ, Castle D. Antipsychotic-induced hyperprolactinaemia. *Aust N Z J Psychiatry.* 2011;45(10):830–837.
- Jackson J, Safranek S, Daugird A. Clinical inquiries. What is the recommended evaluation and treatment for elevated serum prolactin? *J Fam Pract.* 2006;54(10):897–899.
- Klibanski A. Clinical practice. Prolactinomas. *N Engl J Med.* 2010;362(13):1219–1226.
- Melmed S, Casanueva FF, Hoffman AR, et al. Diagnosis and treatment of hyperprolactinemia: an Endocrine Society clinical practice guideline. *J Clin Endocrinol Metab.* 2011;96(2):273–288.
- Molitch ME. Pituitary gland: can prolactinomas be cured medically? *Nat Rev Endocrinol.* 2010;6(4): 186–188.

 CODES

ICD10

E22.1 Hyperprolactinemia

CLINICAL PEARLS

- If a cause for hyperprolactinemia cannot be found by history, examination, and routine laboratory testing, an intracranial lesion might be the cause and brain MRI with specific pituitary cuts and intravenous contrast media should be performed.
- Treatment of hyperprolactinemia should be targeted at correcting the cause (hypothyroidism, discontinuation of offending medications, etc.).
- There is a difference among antipsychotics in influencing prolactin levels. In general, those with the highest potency D_2 antagonism are most likely to elevate prolactin levels. Among the newer atypical antipsychotics, risperidone has been identified as more likely to elevate prolactin.
- Chronic nipple piercing has not been shown to cause hyperprolactinemia (6).
- High prolactin levels decrease testosterone by inhibiting gonadotropin-releasing hormone (GnRH), LH, and FSH secretion and by decreasing central dopamine activity, both of which are important in mediating sexual arousal.

H

HYPERSENSITIVITY PNEUMONITIS
Han Q. Bui, MD, MPH

BASICS

- Hypersensitivity pneumonitis (HP) is also called extrinsic allergic alveolitis (EAA).
- HP is a diffuse inflammatory disease of the lung parenchyma caused by an immunologic reaction to aerosolized antigenic particles found in a variety of environments. Classification depends on time frame involved:
  - Acute: fever, chills, diaphoresis, myalgias, nausea; cough and dyspnea common but not necessarily present. Occurs 4 to 12 hours after heavy exposure to an inciting agent. Symptoms subside within 12 hours to several days after removal from exposure. Complete resolution occurs within weeks.
  - Subacute: mainly caused by continual low-level antigen exposure, could have a low-grade fever in first week; cough, dyspnea, fatigue, anorexia, weight loss—develops over days to weeks
  - Chronic: from recurrent exposure either acute or subacute cases, prolonged and progressive cough, dyspnea, fatigue, weight loss, could lead to fibrosis and respiratory failure
- Farmer's lung is an old term of this disease, a type of HP, particular to the farmer population; causative agent is a bacterium found in moldy hay or straw. Farmer's lung now has new and different etiologies due to modernization of farming practices (1,2).

EPIDEMIOLOGY
- Not well defined. Tends to occur in adults as a result of occupation-related exposure, but some home environmental exposures are also seen.
- HP is increasingly recognized as an important cause of fibrotic interstitial lung disease (3).

Incidence
0.9 per 100,000

Prevalence
- Farmers: 1–19% exposed farmers
- Bird fanciers: 6–20% exposed individuals
- Others: 1–8% exposed

ETIOLOGY AND PATHOPHYSIOLOGY
- Hypersensitivity reaction involving immune complexes: inhaled antigens bind to IgG, triggering complement cascade (types III and IV immunologic reactions) (4)
- Cellular-mediated reaction: T cell–mediated immune inflammatory response
- Farming, vegetable, or dairy cattle workers (1,2)
  - Moldy hay, grain, silage: thermophilic actinomycetes, such as *Faenia rectivirgula*
  - Mold on pressed sugar cane: *Thermoactinomyces sacchari*, *Thymus vulgaris*
  - Tobacco plants: *Aspergillus* sp., *Scopulariopsis brevicaulis*
  - Mushroom worker's lung: *Saccharopolyspora rectivirgula*, *T. vulgaris*, *Aspergillus* spp.
  - Potato riddler's lung: Thermophilic actinomycetes, *T. vulgaris*, *Faenia rectivirgula*, *Aspergillus* sp.
  - Wine maker's lung: *Mucor stolonifer*

- Cheese washer's lung: *Penicillium casei*, *Aspergillus clavatus*
- Coffee worker's lung: coffee bean dust
- Tea grower's lung: tea plants
- Ventilation and water-related contamination (1,2)
  - Contaminated humidifiers and air conditioners: amoebae, nematodes, yeasts, bacteria
  - Unventilated shower: *Epicoccum nigrum*
  - Hot-tub lung: *Cladosporium* sp., *Mycobacterium avium complex*
  - Sauna taker's lung: *Aureobasidium* sp.
  - Summer-type pneumonitis: *Trichosporon cutaneum*
  - Swimming pool lung (lifeguard) lung: aerosolized endotoxin and *M. avium complex*
  - Contaminated basement pneumonitis: *Cephalosporium* and *Penicillium* spp.
- Bird and poultry handling (1)
  - Bird fancier's lung: droppings, feathers, serum proteins
  - Poultry worker's lung: serum proteins
  - Turkey-handling disease: serum proteins
  - Canary fancier's lung: serum proteins
  - Duck fever: feathers, serum proteins
- Veterinary work and animal handling (1,2)
  - Laboratory worker's lung: urine, serum, pelts, proteins
  - Pituitary snuff taker's disease: dried, powdered neurohypophysis
  - Furrier's lung: animal pelts
  - Bat lung: bat serum protein
  - Fish meal worker's lung: fish meal
  - Coptic lung: cloth wrapping of mummies
  - Mollusc shell HP: sea-snail shell
  - Pearl oyster shell pneumonitis: oyster shells
- Grain and flour (1,2)
  - Grain measurer's lung: cereal grain, grain dust
  - Miller's lung: *Sitophilus granarius*
  - Malt worker's disease: *A. fumigatus*, *A. clavatus*
- Lumber milling, construction, wood stripping, paper, wallboard manufacture (1,2)
  - Wood dust pneumonitis: *Alternaria* sp., *Bacillus subtilis*
  - Sequoiosis: *Graphium*, *Pullularia*, *Trichoderma* sp., *Aureobasidium pullulans*
  - Maple bark disease: *Cryptostroma corticale*
  - Wood trimmer's disease: *Rhizopus* sp., *Mucor* sp.
  - Wood pulp worker's disease: *Penicillium* sp.
  - Suberosis: *T. viridis*, *P. glabrum*
- Plastic manufacturing, painting, electronics, chemicals (1)
  - Chemical HP: diphenyl diisocyanate, toluene diisocyanate
  - Detergent worker's lung: *B. subtilis* enzymes
  - Pauli reagent alveolitis: sodium diazobenzene sulfate
  - Vineyard sprayer's lung: copper sulfate
  - Pyrethrum: *Pyrethrum*
  - Epoxy resin lung: phthalic anhydride
  - Bible printer's lung: moldy typesetting water
  - Machine operator's lung: *Pseudomona fluorescens*, aerosolized metal working fluid

- Textile workers
  - Byssinosis: cotton mill dust
  - Velvet worker's lung: nylon, tannic acid, potato starch
  - Upholstery fabric: aflatoxin-producing fungus, *Fusarium* sp.
  - Lycoperdonosis: puffball spores

Genetics
No evidence of clear genetic susceptibility. Possible genetic predisposition involving tumor necrosis factor alpha (TNF-α) and major histocompatibility complex (MHC) class II genes (1,4)[B]

RISK FACTORS
- Contact with organic antigens increases the risk of developing HP. Viral infection at time of exposure could also increase risk (5).
- Nonsmokers have an increased incidence of HP compared with smokers (nicotine could have a protective effect) (5).
  - Smokers have a diminished antibody response to inhaled antigens.
  - However, smokers that develop disease tend to have the chronic form, and mortality is higher.

GENERAL PREVENTION
Avoidance of offending antigen and/or use of protective equipment

COMMONLY ASSOCIATED CONDITIONS
Constrictive bronchiolitis

DIAGNOSIS

- Diagnosis criteria most widely used but not validated: (i) history and physical and pulmonary function tests (PFTs) indicating restriction or diffusion disease, (ii) radiologic imaging consent with interstitial lung disease, (iii) exposure to a recognized cause, (iv) proof of sensitization in BAL fluids (serum precipitins and/or lymphocytosis) (2)
- Six significant predictors: exposure to a known antigen, positive precipitating antibodies, recurrent episodes of symptoms, inspiratory crackles, symptoms 4 to 8 hours after exposure, weight loss (6)
- Acute form: develops 4 to 12 hours following exposure. Cough, dyspnea without wheezing, fever, chills, diaphoresis, headache, nausea, malaise, chest tightness. Symptoms last hours to days.
- Sequela (prior subacute, chronic): gradual or progressive productive cough, dyspnea, fatigue, anorexia, weight loss can lead to respiratory failure; develops over days, weeks to months.
- Symptomatic improvement when away from work or home

PHYSICAL EXAM
- Acute: fever, tachypnea, diffuse fine rales
- Sequela or chronic: inspiratory crackles, progressive hypoxia, weight loss, diffuse rales, clubbing, rarely wheezing

DIAGNOSTIC TESTS & INTERPRETATION

- Testing for antibodies (Ab) is NOT diagnostic as up to 40% may have positive AB without disease. Antigens that cover most cases: pigeon and parakeet sera, dove feather, *Aspergillus sp.*, *Penicillium*, *S. rectivirgula*, and *T. viridans*.
- PFTs: Typical profile is a restrictive pattern with low diffusing capacity, could also have an obstructive pattern (6).
- Bronchoalveolar lavage (BAL) with serum precipitins and lymphocytosis: usually with low CD4-to-CD8 ratio. Findings not unique to HP (1,6)
- Positive antigen–specific inhalation challenge testing: reexposure to the environment, inhalation challenge to the suspected antigen in a hospital setting but it lacks standardization (7)
- Chest x-ray (CXR): used to rule out other diseases
  - Acute: ground-glass infiltrates, nodular or striated patchy opacities, interstitial pattern in a variety of distributions in lung field. Up to 20% could be normal.
  - Sequela/chronic: upper lobe fibrosis, nodular or ground-glass opacities, volume loss, emphysematous changes
- CT scan of chest. Patterns not specific to HP:
  - Acute: ground-glass opacities, poorly defined centrilobular nodules and ground-glass opacities and air trapping on expiratory images (7,8)
  - Chronic: fibrosis, ground-glass attenuation, irregular opacities, bronchiectasis, loss of lung volume, honeycombing, emphysematous changes (7,8)
- High-resolution CT (HRCT) mid-to-upper zone predominance of centrilobular ground glass or nodular opacities with signs of air trapping (7).
- Usually start with CXR; may progress to HRCT based on findings (1,7)

Diagnostic Procedures/Other

Lung biopsy:

- Transbronchial: reveals small, poorly formed noncaseating granulomas near respiratory or terminal bronchioles, large foam cells, peribronchial fibrosis
- Open lung biopsy: highest yield in advanced disease. Reveals varying patterns of organizing pneumonia, centrilobular and perilobular fibrosis, multinucleated giant cells with clefts

DIFFERENTIAL DIAGNOSIS

- Acute: acute infectious pneumonia: influenza (or other viral pneumonia), mycoplasma, *Pneumocystis jiroveci* pneumonia, asthma, aspiration (4)
- Chronic: sarcoidosis, chronic bronchitis, chronic obstructive pulmonary disease, tuberculosis, collagen vascular disease, idiopathic pulmonary fibrosis, lymphoma, fungal infections, *P. jiroveci* pneumonia (4)

ALERT

HP in farmers must be distinguished from febrile, toxic reactions to inhaled dusts (organic dust toxic syndrome [ODTS]). Nonimmunologic reactions occur 30–50% more commonly than HP in farmers. ODTS is associated with intense exposure occurring on a single day.

 TREATMENT

GENERAL MEASURES

Outpatient, except for acute pneumonitis cases and admission for workup (BAL, lung biopsy)

First Line

- Avoidance of offending antigen is primary therapy and results in disease regression (1,2).
- Corticosteroids: help control the symptoms of exacerbations but do not improve long-term outcomes
  - Prednisone: 20 to 50 mg daily (6)
  - For severe symptomatic patients, initial course of 1 to 2 weeks with taper (6)

Second Line

- Bronchodilators and inhaled corticosteroids may symptomatically improve patients with wheeze and chest tightness (5,6)[B].

- Oxygen may be needed in advanced cases.
- Lung transplantation may be the last resort in severe cases unresponsive to therapy.

ISSUES FOR REFERRAL

Referral to pulmonologist/immunologist

INPATIENT CONSIDERATIONS

Admission Criteria/Initial Stabilization

Supportive management, as needed, to maintain oxygenation and ventilation:

- Unstable ventilation, oxygen requirement, mental status changes
- Need for invasive evaluation (lung biopsy)

 ONGOING CARE

FOLLOW-UP RECOMMENDATIONS

Patient Monitoring

- Initial follow-up should be weekly to monthly, depending on severity and course
- Follow treatments with serial CXR, PFTs, and circulating antibody levels

DIET

No dietary restrictions

PATIENT EDUCATION

Note that chronic exposure may lead to a loss of acute symptoms with exposure (i.e., the patient may lose awareness of exposure–symptom relationship).

PROGNOSIS

- Presence of fibrosis is a poor prognosis factor (1,2).
- Acute: good prognosis with reversal of pathologic findings if elimination of offending antigen early in disease (2,5)
- Sequela/chronic: Corticosteroids have been found to improve lung function acutely but offer no significant difference in long-term outcome (5,6)[C].

COMPLICATIONS

- Progressive interstitial fibrosis with eventual respiratory failure
- Cor pulmonale and right-sided heart failure

REFERENCES

1. Girard M, Cormier Y. Hypersensitivity pneumonitis. *Curr Opin Allergy Clin Immunol*. 2010;10(2): 99–103.
2. Costabel U, Bonella F, Guzman J. Chronic hypersensitivity pneumonitis. *Clin Chest Med*. 2012;33(1):151–163.
3. Glazer CS. Chronic hypersensitivity pneumonitis: important considerations in the work-up of this fibrotic lung disease. *Curr Opin Pulm Med*. 2015;21(2):171–177.
4. Grunes D, Beasley MB. Hypersensitivity pneumonitis: a review and update of histologic findings. *J Clin Pathol*. 2013;66(10):888–895.
5. Selman M, Buendía-Roldán I. Immunopathology, diagnosis, and management of hypersensitivity pneumonitis. *Semin Respir Crit Care Med*. 2012;33(5):543–554.
6. Lacasse Y, Girard M, Cormier Y. Recent advances in hypersensitivity pneumonitis. *Chest*. 2012;142(1):208–217.
7. Ohshimo S, Bonella F, Guzman J, et al. Hypersensitivity pneumonitis. *Immunol Allergy Clin North Am*. 2012;32(4):537–556.
8. Hirschmann JV, Pipavath SN, Godwin JD. Hypersensitivity pneumonitis: a historical, clinical, and radiologic review. *Radiographics*. 2009;29(7):1921–1938.

ADDITIONAL READING

Girard M, Lacasse Y, Cormier Y. Hypersensitivity pneumonitis. *Allergy*. 2009;64(3):322–334.

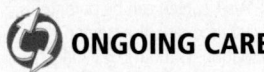 CODES

ICD10

- J67.9 Hypersensitivity pneumonitis due to unspecified organic dust
- J67.0 Farmer's lung
- J67.2 Bird fancier's lung

CLINICAL PEARLS

- Skin testing is not useful for the diagnosis of HP.
- Diagnosis should be suspected in every patient with unexplained cough and dyspnea on exertion, functional impairment (restriction or diffusion defect), and unclear fever, especially if exposure to potential antigens is known (workplace, domestic bird keeping, moldy walls in the home) (2).
- Once the disease is established, smoking does not appear to attenuate its severity, and it may predispose to more chronic and severe course.
- Use of protective gear on individual with high-risk exposure occupations can prevent HP.
- Chronic hypersensitivity pneumonitis is increasingly recognized as an important mimic of other fibrotic lung diseases (3).

H

HYPERSPLENISM

Shadi Hamdeh, MD • Adil Abdalla, MD

 BASICS

DESCRIPTION
- Hypersplenism is defined as overactivity of the spleen and presents as the following:
  - Splenomegaly (commonly but not always)
  - Cytopenias with respective bone marrow hyperplasia of precursors
  - Resolution of cytopenias with splenectomy
- Splenomegaly is not synonymous with hypersplenism. Overactivity of the spleen can occur without enlargement, as is seen in immune thrombocytopenic purpura (ITP) and autoimmune hemolytic anemia. Similarly, splenomegaly is not always associated with hypersplenism.

EPIDEMIOLOGY
May be as common as 30–70% in patients with cirrhosis and portal hypertension (HTN)

ETIOLOGY AND PATHOPHYSIOLOGY
Enlargement of the spleen results in sequestration of formed blood elements, leading to peripheral cytopenias and concomitant bone marrow precursor hyperplasia.

Many of the common etiologies are listed below. Almost any process involving the spleen or the hematologic system can result in hypersplenism:
- Infectious
  - Tuberculosis
  - Brucellosis
  - Malaria
  - Leishmaniasis
  - Ehrlichiosis
  - Schistosomiasis
  - Histoplasmosis
  - Candidiasis
  - Viral
  - Syphilis
  - Infective endocarditis
- Hematologic
  - Myeloproliferative disorders
  - Polycythemia vera
  - Primary hypersplenism
  - ITP
  - Hemolytic anemias
- Neoplastic
  - Hematologic malignancies
  - Melanoma
  - Various carcinomas
  - Metastatic cancers
- Storage diseases
  - Gaucher disease
  - Niemann-Pick disease
  - Amyloidosis
  - Glycogen storage disease
- Inflammatory
  - Sarcoidosis
  - Systemic lupus erythematosus
  - Felty syndrome

- Congestive
  - Cirrhosis
  - Heart failure
  - Portal or splenic vein thrombosis
  - Congenital malformations of the portal vein

 DIAGNOSIS

HISTORY
- Patients may complain of abdominal fullness or protrusion of the spleen through the abdominal wall; may complain of early satiety if the spleen is compressing stomach
- Patients may complain of tenderness in the left upper quadrant, especially with viral infections. In lymphoproliferative disorders, spleen may be enlarged but asymptomatic unless there is splenic infarction. Given location of the spleen next to the diaphragm, a sense of fullness may be referred through the phrenic nerve to the C3–C5 dermatomes in the left shoulder.
- Symptoms related to the underlying cause of hypersplenism may be present.

PHYSICAL EXAM
Splenomegaly
- The normal spleen is not palpable. A palpable spleen always indicates underlying abnormality such as splenomegaly and, in turn, hypersplenism in the appropriate clinical context or may indicate a wandering spleen. Also, spleen can be palpated in chronic obstructive pulmonary disease and acute asthma exacerbation, without coexisting splenomegaly.
- Begin by percussing Traube semilunar space, demarcated laterally by left anterior axillary line, inferiorly by the left costal margin, and superiorly by the left 6th rib. This space is usually hollow. Splenic enlargement may cause dullness to percussion in this area. Other processes that may cause dullness include pleural or pericardial effusions. Additionally, if the patient recently ate a large meal, this area may be dull to percussion.
- With patient supine, rest hand gently on the abdomen to prevent sudden tensing of the abdominal musculature, which may obscure palpation. Better abdominal relaxation can be obtained by flexing the knees toward the abdomen. As the spleen enlarges, it moves caudally and medially. Start by palpating in the right lower quadrant and moving toward the umbilicus, toward the left upper quadrant. If there is doubt about whether the spleen has moved beyond the costal margin, ask patient to take a large breath, which will push the diaphragm, and, in turn, the spleen toward the examiner's hands.
- Jaundice: if hemolytic anemia is present or in advanced cirrhosis
- Petechiae, purpura, or ecchymosis: if thrombocytopenia is present
- Lymphadenopathy: in hematologic or solid organ malignancies. It also can be seen in infectious etiologies.

DIAGNOSTIC TESTS & INTERPRETATION
On CBC, any and all cell lines may be decreased, resulting in the following:
- Anemia
- Leukopenia
- Thrombocytopenia

Initial Tests (lab, imaging)
- CBC
- Reticulocyte count if anemia
- If there is hemolysis, there should be an elevated reticulocyte count, elevated LDH, decreased haptoglobin, along with evidence of hyperbilirubinemia (unconjugated).
- US
- CT
- Tc-99m sulfur colloid scintigraphy
- PET
- MRI

Follow-Up Tests & Special Considerations
Based on other historical and exam findings, testing for specific infectious etiologies may be warranted:
- Blood parasite smear for malaria and other parasitic infections
- EBV serologies
- HIV ELISA with Western blot
- JAK2 mutation in polycythemia vera
- PPD for tuberculosis
- Hgb electrophoresis in hereditary hemoglobinopathies

Diagnostic Procedures/Other
- Bone marrow biopsy
- Liver biopsy for cirrhosis and storage diseases

Test Interpretation
Hyperplasia of bone marrow precursors, especially those correlating with the patient's individual cytopenias

 TREATMENT

MEDICATION
- No specific medication can be recommended for patients with hypersplenism. The most important intervention is to treat the underlying disorder.
- If ITP is the cause, the patient may benefit from the following:
  - Prednisone or methylprednisolone
  - IVIG
  - Rituximab
- If an infectious cause is discovered, treatment with appropriate antibiotic therapy may help to improve the cytopenias.

SURGERY/OTHER PROCEDURES
- Many patients with severe uncontrolled cytopenias undergo splenectomy.
- Laparoscopic splenectomy is preferred over open splenectomy (1)[A].

ALERT

- If this cannot be done (i.e., in cases of emergent splenectomy), wait at least 14 days postsplenectomy to immunize.
  – Pneumococcal vaccine
    ○ Pneumococcal polyvalent-23 vaccine (PPSV23) for use in adults and fully immunized children ≥2 years of age
    ○ Pneumococcal polyvalent-13 vaccine (PCV13) for infants and young children ≥2 months of age as part of routine immunization schedule (3)[A]
    ○ PCV13 for children >2 years of age, adolescents and adults in addition to PPSV23; refer to CDC for timing of administration
    ○ Current guidelines recommend single revaccination of PPSV23 5 years after the initial dose and again at age of ≥65 years, at least 5 years after the previous dose.
  – *H. influenzae* vaccine
    ○ All unvaccinated individuals ≥5 years of age should be given 1 dose of *H. influenzae* type B (Hib) conjugate vaccine.
    ○ Children <5 years old should also be vaccinated. Refer to CDC for timing.
    ○ Vaccinated individuals can also be given additional dose of vaccine (4)[A].
  – Meningococcal vaccine (5)[A]
    ○ Meningococcal conjugate vaccine (MCV4) for use in patients between 2 and 55 years
    ○ Meningococcal polysaccharide vaccine (MPSV4) for use in patients >55 years of age
    ○ Revaccination is recommended every 5 years.
  – Influenza vaccine should be administered yearly based on prevalent circulating strains. Although patients are not at higher risk from influenza itself, infection with influenza may place patients at higher risk for secondary bacterial infections.
- Radiofrequency ablation (RFA) is becoming more available and can be successful at preventing recurrence of hypersplenism. It is not currently known whether there are differences between RFA and splenectomy in terms of postprocedure infectious risks. Other alternatives to splenectomy include total and partial splenic embolization and shunting, although these techniques are evolving and additional studies are needed to evaluate efficacy and morbidity as compared to splenectomy.

INPATIENT CONSIDERATIONS

Admission Criteria/Initial Stabilization

- Hypersplenism alone generally does not warrant admission. However, all patients should be monitored closely for complications of the resulting cytopenias, including bleeding and infection, as well as complications of splenomegaly, including increased risk of splenic rupture. In some patients, the large spleen compresses the stomach and prevents adequate oral intake.

- Splenectomized patients are at increased risk of infection and postsplenectomy sepsis, especially with *Streptococcus pneumoniae*. Fevers, chills, or pain concerning for underlying infection warrant immediate attention as clinical decompensation can occur within hours. Empiric broad-spectrum antibiotics should not be delayed while evaluation is ongoing. Common empiric regimens include the following:
  – Ceftriaxone: 2g IV q24h and vancomycin 1 g IV q12h
  – Levofloxacin: 750 mg IV q24h and vancomycin 1 g IV q12h in β-lactam–allergic patients

 ## ONGOING CARE

- Adult patients who are splenectomized should be advised to monitor closely for fever or rigors at home, which may be an early sign of bacteremia. They should be instructed to begin antibiotics immediately prior to proceeding to a medical facility for evaluation. Early antibiotics have been shown to reduce the mortality from overwhelming postsplenectomy sepsis.
- Controlled trials have not been performed, but some regimens include the following:
  – Amoxicillin-clavulanate: 875 mg PO twice daily
  – Cefuroxime axetil: 500 mg PO twice daily
- Patients allergic to β-lactam antibiotics can be given an extended-spectrum fluoroquinolone such as levofloxacin 750 mg PO *or* moxifloxacin 400 mg PO daily.
- In children with splenectomy, daily antibiotic prophylaxis for overwhelming postsplenectomy sepsis with penicillin VK or amoxicillin is recommended until age 5 or at least 3 years after splenectomy:
  – Age 2 months to 5 years: 125 mg PO BID
  – >5 years old: 250 mg PO BID

PATIENT EDUCATION

Patients who are splenectomized should be counseled extensively about the risk of overwhelming postsplenectomy sepsis and the need to obtain prompt medical evaluation in the event of fevers, chills, or any other concerning symptoms.

REFERENCES

1. Bai YN, Jiang H, Prasoon P. A meta-analysis of perioperative outcomes of laparoscopic splenectomy for hematological disorders. *World J Surg.* 2012;36(10):2349–2358.
2. Advisory Committee on Immunization Practices. Recommended adult immunization schedule: United States, 2012. *Ann Intern Med.* 2012;156(3):211–217.
3. American Academy of Pediatrics. Children with asplenia or functional asplenia. In: Pickering LK, Baker CJ, Kimberlin DW, et al, eds. *Red Book: 2009 Report of the Committee on Infectious Diseases.* 28th ed. Elk Grove Village, IL: American Academy of Pediatrics; 2009:72.
4. American Academy of Pediatrics Committee on Infectious Diseases. *Haemophilus influenzae* type b conjugate vaccines: recommendations for immunization with recently and previously licensed vaccines. *Pediatrics.* 1993;92(3):480–488.
5. Centers for Disease Control and Prevention. Updated recommendations for use of meningococcal conjugate vaccines—Advisory Committee on Immunization Practices (ACIP), 2010. *MMWR Morb Mortal Wkly Rep.* 2011;60(3):72–76.

ADDITIONAL READING

- Abdella HM, Abd-El-Moez AT, Abu El-Maaty ME, et al. Role of partial splenic arterial embolization for hypersplenism in patients with liver cirrhosis and thrombocytopenia. *Indian J Gastroenterol.* 2010;29(2):59–61.
- Di Sabatino A, Carsetti R, Corazza GR. Post-splenectomy and hyposplenic states. *Lancet.* 2011;378(9785):86–97.
- Feng K, Ma K, Liu Q, et al. Randomized clinical trial of splenic radiofrequency ablation versus splenectomy for severe hypersplenism. *Br J Surg.* 2011;98(3):354–361.
- Iriyama N, Horikoshi A, Hatta Y, et al. Localized, splenic, diffuse large B-cell lymphoma presenting with hypersplenism: risk and benefit of splenectomy. *Intern Med.* 2010;49(11):1027–1030.
- Jandl JH, Aster RH, Forkner CE, et al. Splenic pooling and the pathophysiology of hypersplenism. *Trans Am Clin Climatol Assoc.* 1967;78:9–27.
- Kapoor P, Singh E, Radhakrishnan P, et al. Splenectomy in plasma cell dyscrasias: a review of the clinical practice. *Am J Hematol.* 2006;81(12):946–954.
- Mourtzoukou EG, Pappas G, Peppas G, et al. Vaccination of asplenic or hyposplenic adults. *Br J Surg.* 2008;95(3):273–280.
- Shatz DV, Schinsky MF, Pais LB, et al. Immune responses of splenectomized trauma patients to the 23-valent pneumococcal polysaccharide vaccine at 1 versus 7 versus 14 days after splenectomy. *J Trauma.* 1998;44(5):760–765.

 ## SEE ALSO

Anemia, Autoimmune Hemolytic; Malaria; Polycythemia Vera; Tuberculosis

 ## CODES

ICD10

D73.1 Hypersplenism

CLINICAL PEARLS

- Splenectomy is not necessary to make the diagnosis.
- Avoid splenectomy in patients unless absolutely necessary. Splenectomized patients are at lifelong risk for overwhelming postsplenectomy infection and sepsis.
- If splenectomy is to be performed, give immunization for pneumococcus, meningococcus, *Haemophilus*, and influenza at least 14 days prior to surgery. Otherwise, wait until the 14th postop day to immunize.

H

HYPERTENSION, ESSENTIAL

Lisa M. Schroeder, MD • Luma Dababneh, MD

 BASICS

DESCRIPTION
- Hypertension (HTN) is defined (JNC VIII) as ≥2 elevated BPs
  - Age 60 years or older: systolic BP (SBP) ≥150 mm Hg and/or diastolic BP (DBP) ≥90 mm Hg at ≥2 visits (1)
  - Age <60 years with chronic kidney disease (CKD) or diabetes: SBP ≥140 mm Hg and/or DBP ≥90 mm Hg at ≥2 visits (1)
- HTN is a strong risk factor for cardiovascular disease and strokes.
- Synonym(s): benign, chronic, idiopathic, familial, or genetic HTN; high BP

Geriatric Considerations
- Isolated systolic HTN is common.
- Therapy has been shown to be effective and beneficial at preventing stroke, although target SBP is higher than in younger patients (~150 mm Hg systolic), and adverse reactions to medications are more frequent. The benefit of therapy has been conclusively demonstrated in older patients for SBP ≥160 mm Hg.

Pediatric Considerations
- Measure BP during routine exams for >3 years of age.
- Defined as SBP or DBP ≥95th percentile on repeated measurements (2)
- Pre-HTN: SBP or DBP between 90th and 95th percentile (2)

Pregnancy Considerations
- Elevated BP during pregnancy may be either chronic HTN or pregnancy-induced preeclampsia. ACE inhibitors and angiotensin II receptor blockers (ARBs) are contraindicated.
- Maternal and fetal mortality benefit from treatment of severe HTN. Evidence is not clear for mild HTN (see topic "Preeclampsia").

EPIDEMIOLOGY
Incidence
- Lifetime risk for men and women aged 55 to 65 years by age 80 to 85 years is >90%.
- Predominant age: essential (primary, benign, idiopathic) onset usually in the 20s to 30s
- Predominant sex: male > female; males tend to run higher than females and have a significantly higher risk of cardiovascular disease at any given pressure.

Prevalence
In 2009 to 2010, prevalence in adults was 28.6% (2009–2010 National Health and Nutrition Examination Survey [NHANES])

ETIOLOGY AND PATHOPHYSIOLOGY
- >90% of HTN has no identified cause.
- Secondary causes of HTN (see "Hypertension, Secondary and Resistant"): renal parenchymal: glomerulonephritis, pyelonephritis, polycystic kidneys; endocrine: primary hyperaldosteronism, pheochromocytoma, hyperthyroidism, Cushing syndrome; vascular: coarctation of aorta, renal artery stenosis; chemical: commonly, oral contraceptives, NSAIDs, decongestants, corticosteroids; sleep apnea, black licorice, caffeine

Genetics
BP levels are strongly familial, but no clear genetic pattern exists. Familial risk for cardiovascular diseases should be considered.

RISK FACTORS
Family history, obesity, alcohol use, excess dietary sodium, stress, physical inactivity, tobacco abuse, insulin resistance

 DIAGNOSIS

HISTORY
- HTN is asymptomatic except in extreme cases or after related cardiovascular complications develop.
- Headache can be seen with higher BP, often present on awakening and occipital in nature.

PHYSICAL EXAM
- Retinopathy: narrowed arteries, arteriovenous (AV) nicking, copper or silver wiring of retinal arterioles
- Increased/louder S_2 (aortic component heart sound)
- Synchronous radial and femoral pulse can help to rule out coarctation of the aorta.

DIFFERENTIAL DIAGNOSIS
- Secondary HTN: Because of the low incidence of reversible secondary HTN, special tests should be considered only if the history, physical exam, or basic laboratory evaluation indicate the possibility. (See "Hypertension, Secondary and Resistant.")
- White coat hypertension: elevation of BP in office setting and normal BP outside office

DIAGNOSTIC TESTS & INTERPRETATION
MEASURING BP:
- Caffeine, exercise and smoking avoided >30 minutes before measurement.
- Patient seated quietly for 5 minutes with feet on floor.
- Patient's arm supported at heart level.
- Correct cuff size
- Average of two or more measurements

Initial Tests (lab, imaging)
- Hemoglobin and hematocrit or CBC
- Complete urinalysis (may reveal proteinuria)
- Potassium, calcium, creatinine, and uric acid
- Lipid panel (total, HDL, LDL, triglyceride [TG])
- Fasting blood glucose, hemoglobin A1c
- ECG to evaluate possible presence of left ventricular hypertrophy (LVH) or rhythm abnormalities affecting therapy

Follow-Up Tests & Special Considerations
- Special tests (only if history, physical, or labs indicates) (See "Hypertension, Secondary and Resistant.")
- Ambulatory (24-hour) BP monitoring if "white coat" HTN is suspected, episodic HTN or autonomic dysfunction
- Home BP monitoring is effective, especially if white coat HTN is a consideration; elevated home BPs correlate with adverse outcomes, possibly more so than office BPs, and normal readings are reassuring.

Diagnostic Procedures/Other
- Age 60 years or older: SBP (SBP) ≥150 mm Hg and/or DBP ≥90 mm Hg) at ≥2 visits
- Age <60 years with CKD or diabetes: SBP ≥140 mm Hg and/or DBP ≥90 mm Hg at ≥2 visits
- The Joint National Committee (JNC) 8 recommends emphasis on
  - Family or personal history of HTN; cardiovascular, cerebrovascular, renal disease, and diabetes
  - Previous elevated BPs
  - Previous treatment for HTN

- History of weight gain, exercise activities, sodium and fat intake, and alcohol use
- Symptoms suggesting secondary HTN
- Psychosocial and environmental factors affecting BP and risk for cardiovascular disease
- Other cardiovascular risk factors, such as obesity, smoking, hyperlipidemia, and diabetes, OSA
- Funduscopic exam for arteriolar narrowing, AV compression, hemorrhages, exudates, and papilledema
- Body mass index (BMI)
- Waist circumference
- BP in both arms
- Complete cardiac and peripheral pulse exam: Compare radial and femoral pulse for differences in volume and timing, auscultation for carotid and femoral bruits.
- Abdominal exam for masses and bruits: Listen high in the flanks over the kidneys.
- Neurologic assessment

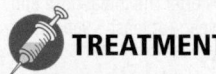 **TREATMENT**

GENERAL MEASURES
- Benefit of pharmacologic treatment of low-risk patients with Class I hypertension (SBP 140 to 150 mm Hg, DBP 90 to 99 mm Hg) remains uncertain (3)[A].
- Treating patients age <60 years or with CKD or diabetes to lower-than-standard BP targets, ≥140/90 mm Hg, does not further reduce mortality or morbidity. Individualize goal pressures based on risk factors.
- Target SBP at or just below 150 mm Hg in patients >60 years of age is acceptable in the general population (1).
- Although primary focus is SBP goal, treatment should accommodate patient preferences (1). Majority of treatment benefit is attained with initial 2 to 3 medications. Striving for small additional drops in BP to achieve a "target" is less clinically beneficial and more likely to cause side effects.
- Lower DBP targets were not associated with decreased morbidity/mortality (4).
- Aerobic exercise (30 minutes of aerobics 4 to 5 days per week), weight reduction for obese patients
- Smoking cessation
- Reduce salt intake <2.4 g/day.
- Risk stratification from JNC 7 no longer addressed in JNC 8 (1)
  - Age 60 years or older: SBP ≥150 mm Hg and/or DBP ≥90 mm Hg at ≥2 visits
  - Age <60 years with CKD or diabetes: SBP ≥140 mm Hg and/or DBP ≥90 mm Hg at ≥2 visits
  - Assess overall risk and individualize decision to treat.
- Choose from one of four classes of medications: (1)[A] ACE inhibitors, ARBs, calcium channel blockers (CCBs), or diuretics.

MEDICATION
- Multiple drugs at submaximal dose may achieve target BP with fewer side effects. In patients on >1 medication, divide between morning and nighttime for better 24-hour antihypertensive effect.
- Sequential monotherapy attempts might be tried with different classes because individual responses vary.
- Many patients will require multiple medications.

- First-line agents for uncomplicated essential HTN include thiazide diuretics, ACE inhibitors, ARBs, and long-acting CCBs (amlodipine, felodipine) (1,5)[A].
- If concomitant conditions, choose first-line agent based on comorbidity.
- Combination first-line agents: Benazepril combined with amlodipine may be superior to combination with HCTZ in high-risk patients. Some suggest that ACE/ARB + dihydropyridine CCB is the first choice after monotherapy.
- β-Blockers had been strongly recommended until recent meta-analyses. Atenolol may be particularly *ineffective* in reducing adverse outcomes of HTN (except in patients with left ventricle hypertrophy undergoing dialysis).
- β-Blockers might benefit patients with ischemic heart disease, CHF, or migraine post ST segment elevation myocardial infarction (STEMI). ACE inhibitors should be used in patients with diabetes, proteinuria, atrial fibrillation, or heart failure with reduced ejection fraction (HFrEF) but *not in pregnancy*.
- α-Adrenergic blockers are not the first choice for monotherapy but remain as second line after combination therapy of first-line agents; might benefit males with benign prostatic hypertrophy (BPH).
- CCB could be considered in patients with isolated systolic HTN, atherosclerosis, angina, migraine, or asthma; well-documented to reduce risk of stroke
- Thiazide diuretics or CCB preferred as first line in the general black population.

First Line
- Thiazide diuretics (4)[A]
  - Chlorthalidone: 12.5 to 25 mg/day (more potent than hydrochlorothiazide but causes more hyponatremia and hypokalemia)
  - Hydrochlorothiazide:12.5 to 50 mg/day
  - Indapamide: 1.25 to 2.5 mg/day
- ACE inhibitors
  - Lisinopril: 10 to 40 mg/day
  - Enalapril: 5 to 40 mg/day
  - Ramipril: 2.5 to 20 mg/day
  - Benazepril: 10 to 40 mg/day
- CCB
  - Diltiazem CD: 180 to 360 mg/day
  - Nifedipine (sustained release): 30 to 90 mg/day
  - Verapamil (sustained release): 120 to 480 mg/day
  - Amlodipine: 2.5 to 10 mg/day
- ARBs
  - Losartan: 25 to 100 mg in 1 or 2 doses; has unique but modest uricosuric effect
  - Valsartan: 80 to 320 mg daily
  - Irbesartan: 75 to 300 mg daily
  - Candesartan: 4 to 32 mg daily
  - Renin inhibitor: aliskiren 150 to 300 mg daily
- Contraindications
  - Diuretics may worsen gout.
  - β-Blockers (relative) in reactive airway disease, heart block, diabetes, and peripheral vascular disease; probably should be avoided in patients with metabolic syndrome or insulin-requiring diabetes
  - Diltiazem or verapamil: Do not use with systolic dysfunction or heart block.
  - ACE inhibitors can worsen bilateral renovascular disease and are pregnancy Category D.

Second Line
- Many may be combined. Choose additional medications with complementary effects (i.e., ACE inhibitors/ARBs with diuretic or a vasodilator with a diuretic or β-blocker).
- Medication-refractory HTN or suspected aldosteronism: spironolactone: 25 to 100 mg/day

- Centrally acting α-2 agonists: clonidine: 0.1 to 1.2 mg BID or weekly patch 0.1 to 0.3 mg/day; guanfacine: 1 to 3 mg daily; or methyldopa: 250 to 2,000 mg BID
- α-Adrenergic antagonists: prazosin: 1 to 10 mg BID; terazosin: 1 to 20 mg/day; or doxazosin: 1 to 16 mg/day
- Peripherally acting adrenergic inhibitors: rarely used: reserpine: 0.1 to 0.25 mg/day
- Vasodilators
  - Hydralazine: 10 to 25 mg QID; risk of tachycardia, so generally combined with β-blocker; also drug-induced systemic lupus erythematosus (SLE)
  - Minoxidil: rarely used due to adverse effects. May be more effective than other medications in renal failure and refractory HTN
- Loop diuretics (for volume overload): furosemide: 20 to 320 mg/day or bumetanide: 0.5 to 2 mg/day
- K⁺-sparing diuretics in patients with hypokalemia while taking thiazides: amiloride: 5 to 10 mg/day or triamterene: 50 to 150 mg/day

COMPLEMENTARY & ALTERNATIVE MEDICINE
Biofeedback and relaxation exercise

 ## ONGOING CARE

FOLLOW-UP RECOMMENDATIONS
Patient Monitoring
- Reevaluate patients q3–6mo until stable, then q6–12mo. Consider use of home self-BP monitoring; quality-of-life issues including sexual function should be considered.
- Poor medication adherence is a leading cause of apparent medication failure.
- Annual urinalysis, creatinine, and potassium

DIET
- ~20% of patients will respond to reduced-salt diet (<100 mmol/day; <6 g NaCl or <2.4 g Na).
- Consider Dietary Approaches to Stop Hypertension (DASH) diet: http://www.nhlbi.nih.gov/files/docs/public/heart/hhp_low.pdf
- Limit alcohol consumption to <1 oz/day.
- Dietary supplements such as garlic, cocoa, vitamin C, coenzyme Q10, omega 3, and magnesium have been suggested for lowering BP but evidence is lacking.

PATIENT EDUCATION
- Emphasize the asymptomatic nature of HTN and importance of lifetime treatment.
- Printed aids for high BP education available: http://www.nhlbi.nih.gov/health/resources/heart

COMPLICATIONS
Heart failure, renal failure, LVH, myocardial infarction, retinal hemorrhage, stroke, hypertensive heart disease, drug side effects

REFERENCES
1. James PA, Oparil S, Carter BL, et al. 2014 evidence-based guideline for the management of high blood pressure in adults: report from the panel members appointed to the Eighth Joint National Committee (JNC 8). *JAMA*. 2014;311(5):507–520.
2. Riley M, Bluhm B. High blood pressure in children and adolescents. *Am Fam Physician*. 2012;85(7):693–700.
3. Diao D, Wright JM, Cundiff DK, et al. Pharmacotherapy for mild hypertension. *Cochrane Database Syst Rev*. 2012;(8):CD006742.
4. Arguedas JA, Perez MI, Wright JM. Treatment blood pressure targets for hypertension. *Cochrane Database Syst Rev*. 2009;(3):CD004349.
5. Chobanian AV, Bakris GL, Black HR, et al. The seventh report of the Joint National Committee on prevention, detection, evaluation, and treatment of high blood pressure: the JNC 7 report. *JAMA*. 2003;289(19):2560–2572.

ADDITIONAL READING
- ALLHAT Officers and Coordinators for the ALLHAT Collaborative Research Group. Major outcomes in high-risk hypertensive patients randomized to angiotensin-converting enzyme inhibitor or calcium channel blocker vs diuretic: the Antihypertensive and Lipid-Lowering Treatment to Prevent Heart Attack Trial (ALLHAT). *JAMA*. 2002;288(23):2981–2997.
- Cushman WC, Evans GW, Byington RP, et al. Effects of intensive blood-pressure control in type 2 diabetes mellitus. *N Engl J Med*. 2010;362(17):1575–1585.
- Dorsch MP, Gillespie BW, Erickson SR, et al. Chlorthalidone reduces cardiovascular events compared with hydrochlorothiazide: a retrospective cohort analysis. *Hypertension*. 2011;57(4):689–694.
- Mancia G, Fagard R, Narkiewicz K, et al. 2013 ESH/ESC guidelines for the management of arterial hypertension: the Task Force for the Management of Arterial Hypertension of the European Society of Hypertension (ESH) and of the European Society of Cardiology (ESC). *Eur Heart J*. 2013;34(28):2159–2219.
- National Institute for Health and Care Excellence. NICE guidelines [CG127]. Hypertension in adults: diagnosis and management. https://www.nice.org.uk/guidance/cg127.

 ## SEE ALSO
Hypertension, Secondary and Resistant; Hypertensive Emergencies; Polycystic Kidney Disease

 ## CODES
ICD10
I10 Essential (primary) hypertension

CLINICAL PEARLS
- Treatment of HTN reduces risk of many serious medical conditions with numbers needed to treat to prevent one serious event (e.g., stroke or myocardial infarction) ranging from ~20 patients per year for severe HTN to more than several hundred per year for mild HTN.
- Multiple submaximal doses are likely to have fewer side effects and more effectiveness than fewer maximum-dosed drugs.
- In older patients, measure BP standing to avoid overtreatment and syncope.

H

HYPERTENSION, SECONDARY AND RESISTANT

George H. Maxted, MD

 BASICS

DESCRIPTION

Uncontrolled hypertension (HTN) comprises the following entities (see "Alert" below):

- Resistant HTN: defined as blood pressure that remains above goal in spite of the concurrent use of three antihypertensive agents of different classes. Ideally, one of the three agents should be a diuretic, and all agents should be prescribed at optimal dose amounts (1–3)[C].
- Secondary HTN: elevated BP that results from an identifiable underlying mechanism (1–3)
- Both the recent Eighth Joint National Committee (JNC 8) and AHA/ACC/CDC guidelines recommend a goal BP of <140/90 mm Hg, although JNC 8 allows for a goal of <150/90 mm Hg for patients older than age 60 years (4,5)[C].

Geriatric Considerations

- Onset of HTN in adults >60 years of age is a strong indicator of secondary HTN.
- In patients >80 years of age, consider a higher target systolic blood pressure (SBP) of ≥150 mm Hg. Be cautious to avoid excessive diastolic lowering.
- Elderly may be particularly responsive to diuretics and dihydropyridine calcium channel blockers.
- Systolic HTN is particularly problematic in the elderly.
- Secondary causes more common in the elderly include sleep apnea, renal disease, renal artery stenosis, and primary aldosteronism.

ALERT
Pseudoresistance

- Inaccurate measurement of BP
  – Cuff too small
  – Patient not at rest; sitting quietly for 5 minutes
- Poor adherence: In primary care settings, this has been estimated to occur in 40–60% of patients with HTN.
- White coat effect: prevalence 20–40%. Do not make clinical decisions about HTN based solely on measurement in the clinic setting. Home BP monitoring and/or ambulatory BP monitoring is more reliable.
- Inadequate treatment

EPIDEMIOLOGY

- Predominant age: In general, HTN has its onset between ages 30 and 50 years. Patients with resistant HTN are more likely to experience the combined outcomes of death, myocardial infarction, congestive heart failure (CHF), stroke, or chronic kidney disease.
- Depending on etiology, age of onset can vary. Age of onset <20 or >50 years increases likelihood of a secondary cause for HTN.
- The strongest predictors for resistant HTN are age (>75 years), presence of left ventricular hypertrophy (LVH), obesity (body mass index [BMI] >30), and high baseline systolic BP. Other predictors include chronic kidney disease, diabetes, living in the southeastern United States, African American race (especially women), and excessive salt intake.

Prevalence

- Prevalence of resistant HTN is unknown. NHANES analysis indicates only 53% of adults are controlled to a BP of <140/90 mm Hg.
- Secondary HTN occurs in about 5–10% of adults with chronic HTN.

ETIOLOGY AND PATHOPHYSIOLOGY

- Obstructive sleep apnea (OSA): one study diagnosed OSA in 83% of treatment-resistant hypertensives.
- Primary hyperaldosteronism (17–22% of resistant HTN cases)
- Chronic renal disease (2–5% of hypertensives)
- Renovascular disease (0.2–0.7%, up to 35% of elderly, 20% of patients undergoing cardiac catheterization)
- Cushing syndrome (0.1–0.6%)
- Pheochromocytoma (0.04–0.1% of hypertensives)
- Other rare causes: hyperthyroidism, hyperparathyroidism, aortic coarctation, intracranial tumor
- Drug-related causes
  – Medications, especially NSAIDs (may also blunt effectiveness of ACE inhibitors), decongestants, stimulants (e.g., amphetamines, attention deficient hyperactivity disorder [ADHD] medications), anorectic agents (e.g., modafinil, ephedra, guarana, ma huang, bitter orange), erythropoietin, natural licorice (in some chewing tobacco), yohimbine, glucocorticoids
  – Oral contraceptives: unclear association; mainly epidemiologic and with higher estrogen pills
  – Cocaine, amphetamines, other illicit drugs; drug and alcohol withdrawal syndromes
- Lifestyle factors: Obesity and dietary salt may negate the beneficial effect of diuretics. Excessive alcohol may cause or exacerbate HTN. Physical inactivity also contributes.

RISK FACTORS

A recent large cohort study revealed that those with resistant HTN (16.2%) were more likely to be male, Caucasian, older, and diabetic. They were also more likely to be taking β-blockers, calcium channel blockers, and α-adrenergic blockers compared with other drug classes. Factors predictive of resistant or secondary HTN: female sex, African American race, obesity, diabetes, worsening of control in previously stable hypertensive patient, onset in patients age <20 years or >50 years, lack of family history of HTN, significant target end-organ damage, stage 2 HTN (systolic BP >160 mm Hg or diastolic BP >100 mm Hg), renal disease, and alcohol or drug use (3)[A]

GENERAL PREVENTION

The prevention of resistant and secondary HTN is thought to be the same as for primary or essential HTN: Adopting a Dietary Approaches to Stop Hypertension (DASH) diet, a low-sodium diet, weight loss in obese patients, exercise, limitation of alcohol intake, and smoking cessation may all be of benefit. Relaxation techniques may be of help, but data are limited.

Dx DIAGNOSIS

HISTORY

- Ask or review at every visit: "The Big Four" SANS mnemonic: (i) Salt intake, (ii) Alcohol intake, (iii) NSAID use, (iv) Sleep (author's suggestion, based on reference listed).
- Review home BP readings; consider ambulatory BP monitoring.
- History will vary with etiology of HTN
  – Pheochromocytoma: episodes of headache, palpitations, sweating
  – Cushing syndrome: weight gain, fatigue, weakness, easy bruising, amenorrhea

  – OSA: loud snoring while asleep, daytime somnolence
  – Increased intravascular volume: swelling

PHYSICAL EXAM

- Ensure that the BP is measured correctly. The patient should be sitting quietly with back supported for 5 minutes before measurement. Proper cuff size: bladder encircling at least 80% of the arm. Support arm at heart level. Minimum of two readings at least 1 minute apart. Check BP in both arms. Also check standing BP for orthostasis.
- Attention to findings related to possible etiologies: renovascular HTN: systolic/diastolic abdominal bruit. Pheochromocytoma: diaphoresis, tachycardia. Cushing syndrome: hirsutism, moon facies, dorsal hump, purple striae, truncal obesity. Thyroid disease: enlarged thyroid, tremor, exophthalmos, tachycardia. Coarctation of the aorta: upper limb HTN with decreased or delayed femoral pulses
- Funduscopic exam

DIAGNOSTIC TESTS & INTERPRETATION

- ECG performed as part of the initial workup; LVH is an important marker of resistant HTN.
- Sleep study if history and physical indicate. The Epworth Sleepiness Scale is recommended.
- Home-based polysomnography has been shown to be accurate in screening for OSA. Overnight oximetry is not helpful.

Initial Tests (lab, imaging)

Initial limited diagnostic testing should include urinalysis, CBC, potassium, sodium, glucose, creatinine, lipids, thyroid-stimulating hormone (TSH), and calcium. 50% of patients with hyperaldosteronism may have normal potassium levels.

- Imaging tests listed are necessary only if history, physical, or lab data indicate.
- Abdominal US: if renal disease is suspected
- MR angiography (MRA) of renal vasculature: Preferred test for renovascular HTN. Sensitive but low specificity. Conventional angiography or CT angiography second line after MRA to look at distal renal artery. Renal arteriography remains the gold standard for renovascular disease.
- Adrenal "incidentaloma" frequently arises in this era of multiple CT studies. If present in the setting of resistant HTN, consider hyperaldosterone or hyperadrenalcorticoid states.

Follow-Up Tests & Special Considerations

Further testing for primary aldosteronism (PA) may be considered.

- Empiric treatment with an aldosterone inhibitor may be preferable and more clinically relevant: Spironolactone or eplerenone. Amiloride may be more effective in African Americans.
- Plasma aldosterone-to-renin ratio (ARR) is the preferred lab test, *but* the test is difficult to perform and interpret properly. Consult your reference lab and interpret results with caution.
  – Further testing for pheochromocytoma: plasma
  – Other tests to consider for resistant or secondary HTN: 24-hour urine for free cortisol, calcium, parathyroid hormone (PTH), overnight 1-mg dexamethasone suppression test, urine toxicology screen

Diagnostic Procedures/Other
Consider 24-hour ambulatory BP monitoring, especially if white coat effect is suspected. Home BP monitor results predict mortality, stroke, and other target organ damage better than office BP. Optimal protocol involves two paired measurements: morning and evening (four measurements) over 4 to 7 days.

- Oscillometric, electronic, upper arm, fully automatic device with memory; average multiple readings over several days
- See http://www.dableeducational.org/ for validated monitors.

TREATMENT

- Treatment modality depends on etiology of HTN. Please see each etiology listed for information on proper treatment.
- Emphasize Adherence to JNC 8 and/or AHA/ACC guidelines, with emphasis on lifestyle modification. (4,5)[C]
  - Obese patients, African Americans, and elderly may be particularly responsive to diuretics.
  - Tolerance to diuretics may occur: long-term adaptation to thiazides or the "braking effect." Consider increasing the dose of thiazide or adding an aldosterone inhibitor.
- Treatment specific to certain secondary etiologies
  - Primary aldosteronism: aldosterone receptor antagonist: spironolactone or eplerenone
  - Cushing syndrome: aldosterone receptor antagonist
  - OSA: continuous positive airway pressure (CPAP) ± oxygen, surgery, weight loss.
    - Mandibular advancement devices may be equally effective in some patients.
  - Nocturnal hypoxia: oxygen supplementation
- Earlier studies had suggested benefit from renal sympathetic denervation, but a recent sham study, SYMPLICITY HTN-3, was not supportive (6)[B].

MEDICATION
- Follow treatment guidelines and algorithms by JNC8 and AHA/ACC/CDC, understanding the differences between them (4,5)[C].
- Aldosterone antagonists may offer significant benefit (7,8)[B].
- Central-acting agents (e.g., clonidine) are effective at reducing BP, but outcome data are lacking.

ALERT
- Agents specific for treatment of HTN emergencies should be initiated under a situation in which immediate BP reduction will prevent or limit end-organ damage (see "Hypertensive Emergencies").
- Renovascular HTN: Angioplasty is the treatment of choice for fibromuscular dysplasia of a renal artery.
- The recent CORAL study concluded that in patients with atherosclerotic renovascular disease and HTN, renal artery stenting did not improve outcomes over medical therapy alone (9).
- Referral to an HTN specialist or clinic: Retrospective studies indicate improved control rates for patients with resistant HTN referred to special HTN clinics.

First Line
See "Hypertension."

INPATIENT CONSIDERATIONS
Admission Criteria/Initial Stabilization
Hospitalization may be necessary for hypertensive urgency or emergency general measures.

 ONGOING CARE

FOLLOW-UP RECOMMENDATIONS
Encourage aerobic activity of 30 min/day, depending on patient condition.

DIET
- Reduced salt may lower BP.
- Recommend the Mediterranean diet or DASH.

PATIENT EDUCATION
Home BP monitoring is recommended.

REFERENCES
1. Calhoun DA, Jones D, Textor S, et al. Resistant hypertension: diagnosis, evaluation, and treatment. A scientific statement from the American Heart Association Professional Education Committee of the Council for High Blood Pressure Research. *Hypertension.* 2008;51(6):1403–1419.
2. Sarafidis PA, Bakris GL. Resistant hypertension: an overview of evaluation and treatment. *J Am Coll Cardiol.* 2008;52(22):1749–1757.
3. Daugherty SL, Powers JD, Magid DJ, et al. Incidence and prognosis of resistant hypertension in hypertensive patients. *Circulation.* 2012;125(13):1635–1642.
4. James PA, Oparil S, Carter BL, et al. 2014 evidence-based guideline for the management of high blood pressure in adults: report from the panel members appointed to the Eighth Joint National Committee (JNC 8). *JAMA.* 2014;311(5):507–520.
5. Go AS, Bauman MA, Coleman King SM, et al. An effective approach to high blood pressure control: a science advisory from the American Heart Association, the American College of Cardiology, and the Centers for Disease Control and Prevention. *Hypertension.* 2014;63(4):878–885.
6. Bhatt DL, Kandzari DE, O'Neill WW, et al. A controlled trial of renal denervation for resistant hypertension. *N Engl J Med.* 2014;370(15):1393–1401.
7. Calhoun DA. Low-dose aldosterone blockade as a new treatment paradigm for controlling resistant hypertension. *J Clin Hypertens (Greenwich).* 2007;9(1 Suppl 1):19–24.
8. Gaddam KK, Nishizaka MK, Pratt-Ubunama MN, et al. Characterization of resistant hypertension: association between resistant hypertension, aldosterone, and persistent intravascular volume expansion. *Arch Intern Med.* 2008;168(11):1159–1164.
9. Cooper CJ, Murphy TP, Cutlip DE, et al. Stenting and medical therapy for atherosclerotic renal-artery stenosis. *N Engl J Med.* 2014;370(1):13–22.

ADDITIONAL READING
- Agarwal R, Bills JE, Hecht TJ, et al. Role of home blood pressure monitoring in overcoming therapeutic inertia and improving hypertension control: a systematic review and meta-analysis. *Hypertension.* 2011;57(1):29–38.
- Aronow WS, Fleg JL, Pepine CJ, et al. ACCF/AHA 2011 expert consensus document on hypertension in the elderly: a report of the American College of Cardiology Foundation Task Force on Clinical Expert Consensus documents developed in collaboration with the American Academy of Neurology, American Geriatrics Society, American Society for Preventive Cardiology, American Society of Hypertension, American Society of Nephrology, Association of Black Cardiologists, and European Society of Hypertension. *J Am Coll Cardiol.* 2011;57(20):2037–2114.
- Basner RC. Cardiovascular morbidity and obstructive sleep apnea. *N Engl J Med.* 2014;370(24):2339–2341.
- Ernst ME, Moser M. Use of diuretics in patients with hypertension. *N Engl J Med.* 2009;361(22):2153–2164.
- Johansson JK, Niiranen TJ, Puukka PJ, et al. Optimal schedule for home blood pressure monitoring based on a clinical approach. *J Hypertens.* 2010;28(2):259–264.
- Powers BJ, Olsen MK, Smith VA, et al. Measuring blood pressure for decision making and quality reporting: where and how many measures? *Ann Intern Med.* 2011;154(12):781–788.
- Rimoldi SF, Scherrer U, Messerli FH. Secondary arterial hypertension: when, who, and how to screen? *Eur Heart J.* 2014;35(19):1245–1254.

 SEE ALSO

Aldosteronism, Primary; Coarctation of the Aorta; Cushing Disease and Cushing Syndrome; Hyperparathyroidism; Hypertension, Essential; Hyperthyroidism; Pheochromocytoma

CODES

ICD10
- I15.9 Secondary hypertension, unspecified
- I15.8 Other secondary hypertension
- I15.0 Renovascular hypertension

CLINICAL PEARLS
- Onset of HTN in adults >60 years of age is a strong indicator of secondary HTN.
- Common causes of resistant HTN: obstructive sleep apnea, excessive salt intake, medication nonadherence
- Common secondary causes include sleep apnea, renal disease, renal artery stenosis, and primary aldosteronism.
- Home BP monitoring predicts outcomes better than office monitoring of BP.

H

HYPERTHYROIDISM

Anup K. Sabharwal, MD, MBA, FACE, CCD • Atil Y. Kargi, MD

BASICS

Hyperthyroidism or thyrotoxicosis is composed of a spectrum of clinical findings consistent with thyroid hormone excess. The former describes excess from the thyroid gland, whereas the latter can be produced from another source.

DESCRIPTION

- Graves disease (GD): the most common form; diffuse goiter and thyrotoxicosis are common characteristics. Infiltrative orbitopathy is seen in up to 50% of patients. Infiltrative dermopathy is rare. Autoantibodies are directed at the thyrotropin-stimulating hormone (TSH) receptors.
- Toxic multinodular goiter (TMNG): second most common; most common cause of hyperthyroidism in patients > age 65; patients >40 years, insidious onset, frequent in iodine-deficient areas
- Toxic adenoma (Plummer disease): younger patients, autonomously functioning nodules
- Iodine-induced hyperthyroidism
- Thyroiditis: transient autoimmune process:
  - Subacute thyroiditis/De Quervain: granulomatous giant cell thyroiditis, benign course; viral infections have been involved.
  - Postpartum thyroiditis
  - Drug-induced thyroiditis: amiodarone, interferon-α, interleukin-2, lithium
  - Miscellaneous: thyrotoxicosis factitia, TSH-secreting pituitary tumors, and functioning trophoblastic tumors (1)[B]
- Subclinical hyperthyroidism: suppressed TSH with normal thyroxine (T_4); may be associated with osteoporosis and atrial fibrillation
- Thyroid storm: rare hyperthyroidism; fever, tachycardia, gastrointestinal symtoms, CNS dysfunction (e.g., coma); up to 50% mortality

Geriatric Considerations
- Characteristic symptoms and signs may be absent.
- Atrial fibrillation is common when TSH <0.1 mIU/L (2)[A].

Pediatric Considerations
- Neonates and children are treated with antithyroids for 12 to 24 months.
- Radioactive iodine treatment is controversial in patients <15 to 18 years.

Pregnancy Considerations
Propylthiouracil (PTU) is currently the drug of choice during 1st trimester of pregnancy and methimazole (MMI) is preferred in the 2nd and 3rd trimester. Treat with lowest effective dose. Avoid treatment-induced hypothyroidism. Radioiodine therapy is contraindicated.

EPIDEMIOLOGY
- 1.3% of population
- Predominant sex: female > male (7 to 10:1)
- Predominant age: autoimmune thyroid disease (GD) in 2nd and 3rd decades. TMNG more common in patients >40 years.

Incidence
- Female: 1/1,000
- Male: 1/3,000

ETIOLOGY AND PATHOPHYSIOLOGY
- GD: autoimmune disease
- TMNG: 60% TSH receptor gene abnormality; 40% unknown

- Toxic adenoma: point mutation in TSH receptor gene with increased hormone production
- Thyroiditis:
  - Hashitoxicosis: autoimmune destruction of the thyroid; antimicrosomal antibodies present
  - Subacute/de Quervain thyroiditis: granulomatous reaction; genetic predisposition in specific human leukocyte antigens; viruses, such as coxsackievirus, adenovirus, echovirus, and influenza virus, have been implicated; self-limited course, 6 to 12 months
  - Suppurative: infectious
  - Drug-induced thyroiditis: Amiodarone produces an autoimmune reaction and a destructive process. Lithium, interferon-α, and interleukin-2 cause an autoimmune thyroiditis.
  - Postpartum thyroiditis: autoimmune thyroiditis that lasts up to 8 weeks and, in 60% of patients, hypothyroidism manifests in the future

Genetics
Concordance rate for GD among monozygotic twins is 35%.

RISK FACTORS
- Positive family history, especially in maternal relatives
- Female
- Other autoimmune disorders
- Iodide repletion after iodide deprivation, especially in TMNG

COMMONLY ASSOCIATED CONDITIONS
- Autoimmune diseases
- Down syndrome
- Iodine deficiency

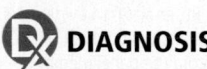

DIAGNOSIS

HISTORY
- Thyrotoxicosis is a hypermetabolic state in which energy production exceeds needs, causing increased heat production, diaphoresis, and even fever.
- Thyrotoxicosis affects several different systems:
  - Constitutional: fatigue, weakness, increased appetite, weight loss
  - Neuropsychiatric: agitation, anxiety, emotional lability, psychosis, coma and poor concentration and memory
  - GI: increased appetite, hyperdefecation
  - Gynecologic: oligomenorrhea, amenorrhea
  - Cardiovascular: tachycardia (most common) and chest discomfort that mimics angina

Geriatric Considerations
Apathetic hyperthyroidism in the elderly

PHYSICAL EXAM
- Adults:
  - Skin: warm, moist, pretibial myxedema (GD only)
  - Head, eye, ear, nose, throat (HEENT): exophthalmos, lid lag
  - Endocrine: hyperhidrosis, heat intolerance, goiter, gynecomastia, low libido, and spider angiomata (males)
  - Cardiovascular: tachycardia, atrial fibrillation, cardiomegaly
  - Musculoskeletal: skeletal demineralization, osteopenia, osteoporosis, fractures
  - Neurologic: tremor, proximal muscle weakness, anxiety and lability, brisk deep tendon reflexes
  - Rarely: thyroid acropathy (clubbing), localized dermopathy

- Children:
  - Linear growth acceleration
  - Ophthalmic abnormalities more common

DIFFERENTIAL DIAGNOSIS
- Anxiety
- Malignancy
- Diabetes mellitus
- Pregnancy
- Menopause
- Pheochromocytoma
- Depression
- Carcinoid syndrome

DIAGNOSTIC TESTS & INTERPRETATION
- 95% have suppressed TSH and elevated free T_4. Total T_4 and triiodothyronine (T_3) represent the bound hormone and can be affected by pregnancy and hepatitis (1)[A].

- T_3: elevated, especially in T_3 toxicosis or amiodarone-induced thyrotoxicosis: presence of TSH receptor antibody or thyroid-stimulating immunoglobulin is diagnostic of GD
- Free thyroxine index (FTI): calculated from T_4 and thyroid hormone–binding ratio; corrects for misleading results caused by pregnancy and estrogens
- Inappropriately normal or elevated TSH with high T_4 suspicious for pituitary tumor or thyroid hormone resistance
- Drugs may alter lab results: estrogens, heparin, iodine-containing compounds (including amiodarone and contrast agents), phenytoin, salicylates, steroids (e.g., androgens, corticosteroids)
- Drug precautions: Amiodarone and lithium may induce hyperthyroidism; MMI may cause warfarin resistance.
- Other findings that can occur: anemia, granulocytosis, lymphocytosis, hypercalcemia, transaminase, and alkaline phosphate elevations

Initial Tests (lab, imaging)
- TSH, free T_4, T_4, T_3, thyroid-stimulating immunoglobin (TSI)
- TSH receptor antibodies (TSH-R Abs): The routine assay is the TSH-binding inhibitor immunoglobulin assay (TBII). TSH-R Abs are useful in the prediction of postpartum Graves thyrotoxicosis and neonatal thyrotoxicosis.
- Thyroxine/triiodothyronine ratio: The T_4-to-T_3 ratio may be a useful tool when the iodine uptake testing is not available/contraindicated. ~2% of thyrotoxic patients have "T_3 toxicosis."
- Nuclear medicine uptake and scanning (^{123}I or ^{131}I): The reference-range values for 24-hour radioiodine uptake is between 5% and 25%.
- Increased thyroid iodine uptake is seen with TMNG, toxic solitary nodule, and GD.
- GD shows a diffuse uptake and can have a para-doxical finding of high uptake at 4 to 6 hours but normal uptake at 24 hours because of the rapid clearance.
- TMNG will show a heterogeneous uptake, whereas solitary toxic nodule will show a warm or "hot" nodule.
- In iodine-deficient areas, an increased uptake is associated with low urine iodine levels.

- Causes of thyrotoxicosis with low iodine uptake:
  - Acute thyroiditis, thyrotoxicosis factitia, and iodine intoxication with amiodarone or contrast material can cause low-uptake transient thyrotoxicosis. After thyroiditis resolves, the patient can become euthyroid or hypothyroid.
  - Iodine loading can cause iodine trapping and decreased iodine uptake (Wolff-Chaikoff effect).
  - Thyrotoxicosis factitia: Thyroglobulin levels are low in exogenous intake and high in endogenous production.
  - Other extrathyroidal causes include struma ovarii and metastatic thyroid carcinoma.
  - Technetium-99m scintigraphy: controversial because it has a 33% discordance rate with radioactive iodine scanning

Follow-Up Tests & Special Considerations
In severe cases, such as thyroid storm, hospitalize until stable, especially if >60 years of age, because of the risk of atrial fibrillation.

Diagnostic Procedures/Other
Neck US will show increased diffuse vascularity in GD.

Test Interpretation
- GD: hyperplasia
- Toxic nodule: nodule formation

TREATMENT

- Decision of which patients to treat and how to treat should be individualized.
- Observation may be appropriate for patients with mild hyperthyroidism (TSH >0.1 or with no symptoms) especially those who are young and with low risk of complications (Afib, osteoporosis).
- Antithyroid medication is contraindicated in patients with thyroiditis. Treatment for subacute thyroiditis is supportive with NSAIDs and β-blockers. Steroids can be used for 2 to 3 weeks (3). GD or TNMG can be managed by either antithyroid medication, RAIT, or thyroidectomy.
- Radioactive iodine therapy (RAIT): most common definitive treatment used in United States for GD and TMNG
- Pretreatment with antithyroid drugs is preferred to avoid worsening thyrotoxicosis after RAIT. MMI is preferred over PTU as pretreatment because of decreased relapse, but it is held 3 to 5 days before therapy (3)[A].
- Usually patients become hypothyroid 2 to 3 months after RAIT; therefore, antithyroid medications are continued after ablation.
- Glucocorticoids: reduce the conversion of active T_4 to the more active T_3. In Graves ophthalmopathy, the use of prednisone before and after RAIT prevents worsening ophthalmopathy (3)[B].
- Smoking in GD patients is a risk factor for ophthalmopathy, especially after RAIT.
- For GD, due to the chance of remission, 12- to 18-month trial of antithyroid medications may be considered prior to offering RAIT.
- For TMNG, the treatment of choice is RAIT. Medical therapy with antithyroid medications has shown a high recurrence rate. Surgery is considered only in special cases (3)[B].

- For amiodarone-induced thyrotoxicosis (AIT) type I, the treatment is antithyroid drugs and β-blockers. Thyroidectomy is the last option. AIT type II is self-limited but may use glucocorticoids.

MEDICATION
First Line
- Antithyroid drugs: MMI and PTU are thionamides that inhibit iodine oxidation, organification, and iodotyrosine coupling. PTU can block peripheral conversion of T_4 to active T_3. Both can be used as primary treatment for GD and prior to RAIT or surgery (1)[A].
- Duration of treatment: 12 to 18 months; 50–60% relapse after stopping; treatment beyond 18 months did not show any further benefit on remission rate. The most serious side effects are hepatitis (0.1–0.2%), vasculitis, and agranulocytosis; baseline CBC recommended:
  - MMI (preferred): adults: 10 to 15 mg q12–24h; children aged 6 to 10 years: 0.4 mg/kg/day PO once daily
  - PTU: adults (preferred in thyroid storm and 1st trimester of pregnancy): 100 to 150 mg PO q8h, not to exceed 200 mg/day during pregnancy
- β-Adrenergic blocker: Propranolol in high doses (>160 mg/day) inhibits T_3 activation by up to 30%. Atenolol, metoprolol, and nadolol can be used.
- Glucocorticoids: reduce the conversion of active T_4 to the more active T_3
- Cholestyramine: anion exchange resin that decreases thyroid hormone reabsorption in the enterohepatic circulation; dose: 4 g QID (1)[B]
- Other agents:
  - Lithium: inhibits thyroid hormone secretion and iodotyrosine coupling; use is limited by toxicity
  - Lugol solution or saturated solution of potassium iodide (SSKI); blocks release of hormone from the gland but should be administered at least 1 hour after thionamide was given; otherwise, acts as a substrate for hormone production (Jod-Basedow effect)
  - RAIT: See "Treatment" section.

ISSUES FOR REFERRAL
Patients with Graves ophthalmopathy should be referred to an experienced ophthalmologist.

SURGERY/OTHER PROCEDURES
Thyroidectomy for compressive symptoms, masses, and thyroid malignancy may be performed in the 2nd trimester of pregnancy only.

ONGOING CARE

FOLLOW-UP RECOMMENDATIONS
Patient Monitoring
- Repeat thyroid tests q3mo, CBC and LFTs on thionamide therapy; continue therapy with thionamides for 12 to 18 months.
- After RAIT, thyroid function tests at 6 weeks, 12 weeks, 6 months, and annually thereafter if euthyroid; TSH may remain undetectable for months even after patient is euthyroid; follow T_3 and T_4.

DIET
Sufficient calories to prevent weight loss

PROGNOSIS
Good (with early diagnosis and treatment)

COMPLICATIONS
- Surgery: hypoparathyroidism, recurrent laryngeal nerve damage, and hypothyroidism
- RAIT: postablation hypothyroidism
- GD: high relapse rate with antithyroid drug as primary therapy
- Graves ophthalmopathy, worsening heart failure if cardiac condition, atrial fibrillation, muscle wasting, proximal muscle weakness, increased risk of cerebrovascular accident (CVA) and cardiovascular mortality

REFERENCES
1. Bahn Chair RS, Burch HB, Cooper DS, et al. Hyperthyroidism and other causes of thyrotoxicosis: management guidelines of the American Thyroid Association and the American Association of Clinical Endocrinologists. *Thyroid*. 2011;21(6):593–646.
2. Cappola AR, Fried LP, Arnold AM, et al. Thyroid status, cardiovascular risk, and mortality in older adults. *JAMA*. 2006;295(9):1033–1041.
3. Abraham P, Avenell A, Park CM, et al. A systematic review of drug therapy for Graves' hyperthyroidism. *Eur J Endocrinol*. 2005;153(4):489–498.

CODES

ICD10
- E05.90 Thyrotoxicosis, unspecified without thyrotoxic crisis or storm
- E05.20 Thyrotxcosis w toxic multinod goiter w/o thyrotoxic crisis
- E06.1 Subacute thyroiditis

CLINICAL PEARLS
- Not all thyrotoxicoses are secondary to hyperthyroidism.
- GD presents with hyperthyroidism, ophthalmopathy, and goiter.
- Medical treatment for GD has a high relapse rate after stopping medications.
- Thyroid storm is a medical emergency that needs hospitalization and aggressive treatment.
- Serum TSH level may be misleading and remain low in the early period after initating treatment, even when T_4 and T_3 levels have decreased.

HYPERTRIGLYCERIDEMIA

S. Lindsey Clarke, MD, FAAFP

BASICS

DESCRIPTION
- Hypertriglyceridemia is a common form of dyslipidemia characterized by an excess fasting plasma concentration of triglycerides (TG).
  - TG are fatty molecules made of glycerols that are esterified by fatty acids at all three hydroxyl groups.
  - They occur naturally in vegetable oils and animal fats.
  - In humans, TG are major sources of dietary energy; they are packaged into chylomicrons and very-low-density lipoproteins.
  - Hypertriglyceridemia is independently associated with cardiovascular disease risk, but the degree to which excess TG cause atherosclerosis is uncertain and debatable.
- Hypertriglyceridemia is a biomarker of risk for premature coronary artery disease in both men and women at levels ≥200 mg/dL and for pancreatitis at levels ≥1,000 mg/dL.
- Classifications of TG levels in adults after a 12-hour fast:
  - Normal: <150 mg/dL (1.7 mmol/L)
  - Borderline to high: 150 to 199 mg/dL
  - High: 200 to 499 mg/dL
  - Very high: ≥500 mg/dL
  - Divide by 88.5 to convert to millimoles per liter.
- TGs are considered high in children when TG exceed the 95th percentiles for age and sex.
  - 143 mg/dL for adolescent boys, 126 mg/dL for adolescent girls
  - 111 mg/dL for preadolescent boys, 120 mg/dL for preadolescent girls

EPIDEMIOLOGY
- Predominant gender: male > female
- Predominant race: Hispanic, white > black

Prevalence
- 33% of U.S. population has TG levels ≥150 mg/dL.
- 1.7% has TG levels ≥500 mg/dL.
- Highest prevalence at age 50 to 70 years
- The most common genetic syndromes with hypertriglyceridemia are familial combined hyperlipidemia and familial hypertriglyceridemia (≤1% of general population each).

ETIOLOGY AND PATHOPHYSIOLOGY
- Primary
  - Familial
  - Acquired (sporadic)
- Secondary
  - Obesity and overweight
  - Physical inactivity
  - Cigarette smoking
  - Excess alcohol intake
  - Very high carbohydrate diets (>60% of total caloric intake)

- Certain medications
  - Interferon-α
  - Atypical antipsychotics
  - β-Blockers other than carvedilol
  - Bile acid sequestrants
  - Corticosteroids
  - Oral estrogens
  - Protease inhibitors
  - Raloxifene
  - Retinoic acid
  - Tamoxifen
  - Thiazides
- Medical conditions
  - Type 2 diabetes mellitus
  - Hypothyroidism
  - Chronic renal failure, nephrotic syndrome
  - Autoimmune disorders (e.g., systemic lupus erythematosus)
  - Paraproteinemias (e.g., macroglobulinemia, myeloma, lymphoma, lymphocytic leukemia)
  - Pregnancy (usually physiologic and transient)

Genetics
- Familial hypertriglyceridemia: autosomal dominant
- Familial dysbetalipoproteinemia: autosomal recessive
- Familial combined hyperlipidemia: unknown

RISK FACTORS
- Genetic susceptibility
- Obesity, overweight
- Lack of exercise
- Diabetes
- Alcoholism
- Certain medications (see "Etiology and Pathophysiology")
- Medical conditions (see "Etiology and Pathophysiology")

GENERAL PREVENTION
- Weight reduction
- Moderation of dietary fat and carbohydrates
- Regular aerobic exercise

COMMONLY ASSOCIATED CONDITIONS
- Coronary artery disease
- Diabetes mellitus type 2 and insulin resistance
- Dyslipidemias
  - Decreased high-density lipoprotein (HDL) cholesterol
  - Increased low-density lipoprotein (LDL), non-HDL, and total cholesterol
  - Small, dense LDL particles
- Metabolic syndrome (three of the following):
  - Abdominal obesity (waist circumference >40 inches in men, >35 inches in women)
  - TG ≥150 mg/dL
  - Low HDL cholesterol (<40 mg/dL in men, <50 mg/dL in women)
  - BP ≥130/85 mm Hg
  - Fasting glucose ≥100 mg/dL

- Nonalcoholic steatohepatitis (NASH)
- Pancreatitis
- Polycystic ovary syndrome

DIAGNOSIS

HISTORY
- Usually asymptomatic
- Patients with chylomicronemia syndrome can have memory loss, headache, vertigo, dyspnea, and paresthesias.
- Pancreatitis: epigastric pain, nausea, and vomiting
- Assess for other cardiac risk factors.
- Family history of coronary artery disease

PHYSICAL EXAM
- Obesity, overweight (body mass index ≥25 kg/m^2)
- Eruptive cutaneous, tuberous, and striate palmar xanthomas
- Lipemia retinalis
- Epigastric tenderness in pancreatitis
- Hepatomegaly in NASH and chylomicronemia

DIFFERENTIAL DIAGNOSIS
Primary and secondary hypertriglyceridemia

DIAGNOSTIC TESTS & INTERPRETATION
Initial Tests (lab, imaging)
- Serum: turbid with milky supernatant
- Fasting lipid profile (12-hour fast)
  - Routine screening every 5 years beginning at age 35 years for men and age 45 years for women
  - Begin screening earlier in those at higher risk for coronary heart disease.
  - For interpretation, see "Description."
- Secondary causes
  - Glycosylated hemoglobin, fasting or postprandial glucose for type 2 diabetes mellitus
  - Creatinine, urinary protein measurement for nephrotic syndrome, renal failure
  - Thyroid-stimulating hormone for hypothyroidism
  - Human chorionic gonadotropin for pregnancy
- Atherosclerosis: cardiac stress imaging, coronary angiography, CT arteriography
- Pancreatitis: CT scan, US of pancreas

Follow-Up Tests & Special Considerations
- Repeat lipid panel after 2 months of therapy.
- High levels of apolipoprotein (APO) B (≥90 mg/dL) are a strong predictor of coronary death in patients whose LDL cannot be calculated because of very high TGs. However, evidence for routine clinical use is lacking.

Test Interpretation
- Chylomicronemia syndrome: lipid-laden macrophage (foam cell) infiltration of visceral organs, bone marrow, and skin
- Atherosclerosis
- Pancreatitis

TREATMENT

GENERAL MEASURES
- Therapeutic lifestyle changes, first-line interventions for all patients, can reduce TG by as much as 50% (1)[C]:
  - Dietary modifications can reduce TG by 20–50% (see "Diet").
  - Moderate-intensity physical activity can reduce TG by 20–30%.
  - Weight loss of 5–10% can reduce TG by 20%.
  - Persons with very high TG should abstain from alcohol.
- Search for correctable secondary causes, treat underlying illness, or remove offending drug.
- Improve glycemic control if diabetic.
- Control other cardiac risk factors such as hypertension, diabetes mellitus, and smoking.
- Primary hypertriglyceridemia: Screen other family members.
- Cardiovascular risk reduction through LDL lowering should be prioritized over TG lowering unless patient is at risk for pancreatitis because of very high TG (≥500 mg/dL) (1)[C]. Usually outpatient; see "Admission Criteria/Initial Stabilization."

MEDICATION
First Line
- Statins: the most effective agents for reducing cardiovascular risk; primarily affect LDL but also have modest TG-lowering effect; dosing depends on intensity of statin desired based on 10-year cardiovascular risk; 2013 ACC/AHA guidelines recommend initiating therapy for 7.5% 10-year risk and other clinical factors (2)[C]:
  - Atorvastatin (Lipitor): 10 to 80 mg/day
  - Pravastatin (Pravachol): 10 to 80 mg/day
  - Rosuvastatin (Crestor): 5 to 40 mg/day
  - Simvastatin (Zocor): 5 to 40 mg nightly
  - Adverse reactions: myalgias, myopathy, rhabdomyolysis (especially if combined with fibrates); contraindicated in pregnancy and lactation
- Fibrates: the most effective agents for reducing TG; used primarily to reduce risk of pancreatitis when TGs very high (≥500 mg/dL); have been shown to decrease nonfatal myocardial infarction but not all-cause mortality (1)[C],(3)[A]:
  - Fenofibrate (Tricor, others): 35 to 200 mg daily
  - Gemfibrozil (Lopid): 600 mg BID
  - Adverse reactions: GI upset, hepatotoxicity, cholelithiasis, myalgias, rhabdomyolysis (when combined with a statin), gemfibrozil–warfarin interaction (enhanced anticoagulation)
  - Gemfibrozil should be avoided in combination with statins due to high risk of muscle injury. If combination therapy is needed, use fenofibrate.

Second Line
- Omega-3 fatty acids
  - Lovaza: 4 g daily or 2 g BID
  - Epanova: 2 to 4 g daily (4)[C]
  - Vascepa: 2 g BID with food (5)[C]
  - Safe, well-tolerated but limited outcomes data

- Niacin (6)[A]. Clinical use of niacin should be very limited, as it fails to show outcome benefit in statin users:
  - 1,000 to 3,000 mg IR daily divided BID–TID; 500 to 2,000 mg ER nightly
  - Adverse reactions: flushing, pruritus, peptic ulcer disease, hepatotoxicity, fulminant hepatic necrosis (with ER forms), hyperuricemia and gout, hyperglycemia, and toxic amblyopia
  - Pretreatment with aspirin reduces flushing.

ISSUES FOR REFERRAL
- Hypertriglyceridemia refractory to treatment
- Familial hypertriglyceridemia syndromes

INPATIENT CONSIDERATIONS
Admission Criteria/Initial Stabilization
- Acute pancreatitis
- Acute coronary syndrome
- In medical emergencies such as acute hypertriglyceridemic pancreatitis with TG levels >1,000 mg/dL, TG can be lowered rapidly and safely by apheresis or insulin infusion.

Discharge Criteria
Stabilization of acute complicating illness

 ONGOING CARE

FOLLOW-UP RECOMMENDATIONS
2 months after initiation or modification of therapy (repeat fasting lipid profile)

Patient Monitoring
- Fasting lipid profile q6–12mo
- Maintain TG <1,000 mg/dL to reduce risk of acute pancreatitis (possibly effective, unproven).
- Hepatic transaminases
- Creatine phosphokinase if patient has myalgias

DIET
- Restrict dietary fat to 30% of total caloric intake; restrict further to 15% of caloric intake if TG ≥1,000 mg/dL (1)[C].
- Limit carbohydrates (especially simple carbohydrates and sugars) to 60% of total caloric intake.
- Mediterranean-style diet reduces TG 10–15% more than a low-fat diet.
- Increase marine-derived omega-3 polyunsaturated fatty acids (4 g/day reduces TG by 25–30%, dose–response relationship).
- Eliminate trans fatty acids.
- Increase dietary fiber.
- Avoid concentrated sugars such as fructose.
- Moderate alcohol intake (<1 oz/day or complete abstinence if TGs are very high)

PATIENT EDUCATION
Smoking cessation

PROGNOSIS
- Good with correction of TG levels
- Patients with primary hypertriglyceridemia usually require lifelong treatment.

COMPLICATIONS
- Atherosclerosis
- Chylomicronemia syndrome
- Pancreatitis

REFERENCES

1. Miller M, Stone NJ, Ballantyne C, et al. Triglycerides and cardiovascular disease: a scientific statement from the American Heart Association. *Circulation.* 2011;123(20):2292–2333.
2. Stone NJ, Robinson JG, Lichtenstein AH, et al. 2013 ACC/AHA guideline on the treatment of blood cholesterol to reduce atherosclerotic cardiovascular risk in adults: a report of the American College of Cardiology/American Heart Association Task Force on Practice Guidelines. *Circulation.* 2014;129(25)(Suppl 2):S1–S45.
3. Wi J, Kim JY, Park S, et al. Optimal pharmacologic approach to patients with hypertriglyceridemia and low high-density lipoprotein-cholesterol: randomized comparison of fenofibrate 160 mg and niacin 1500 mg. *Atherosclerosis.* 2010;213(1):235–240.
4. Kastelein JJ, Maki KC, Susekov A, et al. Omega-3 free fatty acids for the treatment of severe hypertriglyceridemia: the EpanoVa fOr Lowering Very high triglyceridEs (EVOLVE) trial. *J Clin Lipidol.* 2014;8(1):94–106.
5. Maki KC, Orloff DG, Nicholls SJ, et al. A highly bioavailable omega-3 free fatty acid formulation improves the cardiovascular risk profile in high-risk, statin-treated patients with residual hypertriglyceridemia (the ESPRIT trial). *Clin Ther.* 2013;35(9):1400–1411.e1–e3.
6. Abourbih S, Filion KB, Joseph L, et al. Effect of fibrates on lipid profiles and cardiovascular outcomes: a systematic review. *Am I Med.* 2009;122(10):962.e1–962.e8.

ADDITIONAL READING
- Berglund L, Brunzell JD, Goldberg AC, et al. Evaluation and treatment of hypertriglyceridemia: an Endocrine Society clinical practice guideline. *J Clin Endocrinol Metab.* 2012;97(9):2969–2989.
- Pharmacist's Letter. PL Detail-Document. Strategies for lowering triglycerides. *Pharmacist's Letter/Prescriber's Letter.* June 2011.

 SEE ALSO

- Hypercholesterolemia; Pancreatitis, Acute
- Algorithm: Hypertriglyceridemia

 CODES

ICD10
E78.1 Pure hyperglyceridemia

CLINICAL PEARLS
- Hypertriglyceridemia is a risk factor for coronary artery disease at levels ≥200 mg/dL and for pancreatitis at levels ≥1,000 mg/dL.
- Diet and exercise are first-line interventions for all patients who have hypertriglyceridemia.
- In patients with TG levels <500 mg/dL, the primary treatment for cardiovascular risk management is statins.
- For patients with TG levels ≥500 mg/dL, the greatest amount of TG lowering is achieved with fibrates, although magnitude of clinical benefit is uncertain.

H

HYPOGLYCEMIA, DIABETIC

Joseph A. Florence, MD • Emily K. Flores, PharmD, BCPS

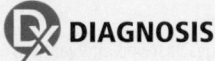

BASICS

DESCRIPTION
- Abnormally low concentration of glucose in circulating blood of a patient with diabetes mellitus (DM); often referred to as an *insulin reaction*
- Classification includes the following (1)[A]:
  - Severe hypoglycemia: an event requiring assistance of another person to actively administer treatment
  - Documented symptomatic hypoglycemia: an event during which typical symptoms are accompanied by a measured plasma glucose of <70 mg/dL (3.9 mmol/L)
  - Asymptomatic hypoglycemia: an event not accompanied by symptoms but a measured glucose of <70 mg/dL (3.9 mmol/L)
  - Probable symptomatic hypoglycemia: event with symptoms but glucose not tested
  - Pseudohypoglycemia: an event with typical symptoms but glucose ≥70 mg/dL (3.9 mmol/L)
- Hypoglycemia is the leading limiting factor in the glycemic management of type 1 diabetes mellitus (T1DM) and type 2 diabetes mellitus (T2DM). Severe or frequent hypoglycemia requires modification of treatment regimens, including higher treatment goals.

ALERT
Hypoglycemia unawareness

- Major risk factor for severe hypoglycemic reactions
- Most commonly found in patients with long-standing T1DM and children age <7 years

EPIDEMIOLOGY
Incidence
- From the Accord Study, the annual incidence of hypoglycemia was the following (2)[A]:
  - 3.14% in the intensive treatment group
  - 1.03% in the standard group
  - Increased risk among women, African Americans, those with less than high school education, aged participants, and those who used insulin at trial entry
- From the RECAP-DM study (3)[A]: Hypoglycemia was reported in 35.8% of patients with T2DM who added a sulfonylurea or thiazolidinedione to metformin therapy during the past year.

ETIOLOGY AND PATHOPHYSIOLOGY
- Loss of hormonal counterregulatory mechanism in glucose metabolism
- Diet: too little food (skipping or delaying meals), decreased carbohydrate (CHO) intake
- Medication: too much insulin or oral hypoglycemic agent (improper dose, timing, or erratic absorption)
- Exercise/physical activity: unplanned or excessive
- Alcohol consumption
- Vomiting or diarrhea

RISK FACTORS
- Nearly 3/4 of severe hypoglycemic episodes occur during sleep.
- Autonomic neuropathy
- Illness, stress, and unplanned life events
- Duration of DM >5 years, advanced age, renal/liver disease, congestive heart failure (CHF), hypothyroidism, hypoadrenalism, gastroenteritis, gastroparesis (unpredictable CHO delivery)

- Starvation or prolonged fasting
- Alcoholism: Alcohol consumption may increase risk of delayed hypoglycemia, especially if on insulin or insulin secretagogues. Evening consumption of alcohol is associated with an increased risk of nocturnal and fasting hypoglycemia, especially in patients with T1DM.
- Current smokers with T1DM
- Insulin secretagogues: Sulfonylureas (glyburide, glimepiride, glipizide, etc.) and glinide derivatives (repaglinide, nateglinide) stimulate insulin secretion.
- Hypoglycemia is rare in diabetics not treated with insulin or insulin secretagogues.
- Other antidiabetes medications such as glucagon-like peptide-1 (GLP-1) agonist and sodium-glucose contransporter-2 (SGLT-2) agents carry a lower but present risk of hypoglycemia.
- Severe hypoglycemia is associated with comorbid conditions in patients aged ≥65 years and in users of a long-acting sulfonylurea.
- Intensive insulin therapy (further lowering A1C from 7% to 6%) is associated with higher rate of hypoglycemia.

Geriatric Considerations
American Geriatric Society Beers criteria recommend avoiding glyburide and chlorpropamide due to their prolonged half-life in older adults and risk for prolonged hypoglycemic episodes. Medications should be dosed for age and renal function.

Pediatric Considerations
Children may not realize when they have hypoglycemia, needing increased supervision during times of higher activity. Children may have higher glycemic goals for this reason. Caregivers should be instructed in use of glucagon (1,4)[A].

Pregnancy Considerations
Hypoglycemia management and avoidance education should be reemphasized and blood glucose monitoring increased due to more stringent glycemic goals and increased risk in early pregnancy.

GENERAL PREVENTION
- Maintain routine schedule of diet (consistent CHO intake), medication, and exercise (4)[A].
- Regular self-monitoring of blood glucose (SMBG), if taking insulin or secretagogue
  - ≥3 times daily testing if multiple injections of insulin, insulin pump therapy, or pregnant diabetic; frequency and timing dictated by needs and treatment goals
  - Particularly helpful for asymptomatic hypoglycemia
- Diabetes treatment and teaching programs (DTTPs) especially for high-risk type 1 patients, which teach flexible insulin therapy to enable dietary freedom
- Hypoglycemia may be prevented with use of insulin analogs, continuous SC insulin infusion (CSII) pumps, and continuous glucose monitoring (CGM) systems.
- If preexercise glucose is <100 mg/dL and taking insulin or secretagogue, then CHO consumption or reduction in medication may prevent hypoglycemia.

COMMONLY ASSOCIATED CONDITIONS
- Autonomic dysfunction
- Neuropathies
- Cardiomyopathies
- Older type 2 diabetics with severe hypoglycemia have a higher risk of dementia.

DIAGNOSIS

HISTORY
- Discuss frequency and cause of hypoglycemia (4)[A].
- Symptoms vary considerably between individuals.
- Adrenergic symptoms
  - Hunger, trembling, pallor, sweating, shaking, pounding heart, anxiety
- Neurologic symptoms
  - Dizziness, poor concentration, drowsiness, weakness, confusion, lightheadedness, slurred speech, blurred vision, double vision, unsteadiness, poor coordination
  - Hypoglycemia causes a significant deterioration in reading span and subject-verb agreement, demonstrating that language processing is impaired during moderate hypoglycemia (5)[A].
- Behavioral symptoms
  - Tearfulness, confusion, fatigue, irritability, aggressiveness
- If altered cognition, consider hypoglycemia

PHYSICAL EXAM
- General: confusion, lethargy
- HEENT: diplopia
- Coronary: tachycardia
- Neurologic: tremulousness, weakness, paresthesias, stupor, seizure, or coma
- Mental status: irritability, inability to concentrate, or short-term memory loss
- Skin: pale, diaphoresis
- End-organ damage: microvascular, macrovascular, ophthalmologic, neurologic, renal

DIFFERENTIAL DIAGNOSIS
Hypoglycemia not associated with DM may be seen in:
- Chronic alcoholics and binge drinkers
- GI dysfunction causing postprandial hypoglycemia or alimentary reactive hypoglycemia
- Hormonal deficiency states (hormonal reactive hypoglycemia)
- Hypoglycemia of sepsis
- Islet cell tumors
- Factitious hypoglycemia from surreptitious injection of insulin

DIAGNOSTIC TESTS & INTERPRETATION
- Plasma, serum, or whole-blood glucose <70 mg/dL
- SMBG and CGM are especially useful for asymptomatic hypoglycemia (1)[A].
- A hypoglycemic reading from a CGM sensor should be verified by SMBG fingerstick glucose testing prior to treatment (4)[A].
- Suspect hypoglycemic unawareness in T1DM with low/normal HgbA1c (1)[A].
- Chronic hypoglycemia is indicated by low HgbA1c level.
- Disorders that may alter lab results
  - Conditions that affect erythrocyte turnover, such as hemolysis or blood loss, and hemoglobin variants may alter HbgA1c (4)[A].

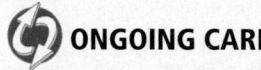 TREATMENT

GENERAL MEASURES

- Glucose: preferred; any form of CHO that contains glucose should be effective (see "Medication" section below) (4)[A].
- Glucagon should be prescribed to patients at significant risk of severe hypoglycemia. People in close contact with these individuals should be instructed in using an emergency glucagon kit (4)[A].

- Alpha-glucosidase inhibitors (acarbose, precise) prevent digestion of complex CHOs; therefore, hypoglycemia must be treated with monosaccharides, such as glucose tablets.

- Patients with severe hypoglycemia combined with hypoglycemic unawareness should have glycemic targets raised to avoid hypoglycemia (4)[A].
- Patients with T1DM should use insulin analogs to reduce hypoglycemia risk (4)[A].
- CGM augmented CSII with automated insulin suspension when blood glucose falls below a threshold value reduces the combined rate of severe and moderate hypoglycemia in T1DM and reduces nocturnal hypoglycemia without increasing A1c levels in patients >16 years old (4,6)[A].

MEDICATION

- Conscious patients (4)[A]:
  - Glucose (15 to 20 g) is preferred, although any form of CHO may be used.
    - Any sugar-containing food or beverage that can be rapidly absorbed: juice or nondiet soda (4 to 5 oz), candy (5 to 6 pieces of hard candy), or OTC glucose tablets (4 tablets = 16 g CHO)
    - Takes ~15 minutes for CHOs to be digested and enter bloodstream as glucose
    - Blood glucose value may correct prior to symptoms resolving.
    - "Rule of 15": 15 to 20 g CHO (~60 to 80 calories simple CHO) repeated q15min until blood sugar is ≥70 mg/dL
  - Once sugar has normalized, a meal or snack should be consumed to prevent recurrence of hypoglycemia.
- Loss of consciousness at home (6)[A]:
  - Administer glucagon
  - IM or SC in the deltoid or anterior thigh
    - Age <6 years and/or weight <20 to 25 kg: 0.50 mg
    - Age ≥6 years and/or weight >20 to 25 kg: 1 mg
    - May repeat dose in 15 minutes if needed
- In unconscious, with emergency medical personnel present or patient hospitalized (6)[A]:
  - Give 25 g IV 50% dextrose every 5 to 10 minutes until patient awakens.
  - Then, feed orally and/or administer 5% dextrose IV at level that will maintain blood glucose >100 mg/dL.
  - Patients with hypoglycemia secondary to oral hypoglycemics should be monitored for 24 to 48 hours because hypoglycemia may recur after apparent clinical recovery.
- Significant possible interactions:
  - Overtreatment may cause hyperglycemia.
  - Clearance of certain oral hypoglycemics may be prolonged in persons with renal or liver disease.

ISSUES FOR REFERRAL

- Frequent or recurring episodes that do not readily respond to treatment
- Consultant pharmacists in long-term care facilities

INPATIENT CONSIDERATIONS

Admission Criteria/Initial Stabilization

- Any doubt of cause
- Expectation of prolonged hypoglycemia (e.g., caused by sulfonylurea drug)
- Inability to drink
- Treatment has not resulted in prompt sensory recovery.
- Seizures, coma, or altered behavior (e.g., ataxia, disorientation, unstable motor coordination, dysphasia) secondary to documented or suspected hypoglycemia

Discharge Criteria

Normoglycemia and risk of severe hypoglycemia is negligible.

 ONGOING CARE

FOLLOW-UP RECOMMENDATIONS

Rest until glucose is normal.

Patient Monitoring

SMBG

DIET

- If alcohol consumed, combine with food to reduce risk of hypoglycemia.

- CHO sources high in protein should not be used to treat or prevent hypoglycemia (4)[A].
- Fats may slow absorption of CHOs and may retard and then prolong the acute glycemic response (6)[A].

PATIENT EDUCATION

- Always have access to quick-acting CHO.
- For planned exercise, consider a reduced insulin dose; additional CHOs are needed for unplanned exercise.
- Educate patients and their relatives, close friends, teachers, and supervisors to be aware of DM diagnosis and signs/symptoms of hypoglycemia and treatment.
- Teach SMBG and self-adjustment for insulin therapy, diet control, and exercise regimen.
- Wear medical alert identification bracelet or necklace.

PROGNOSIS

Full recovery usually depends on rapidity of diagnosis and treatment.

COMPLICATIONS

- Coma, seizure, myocardial infarction, stroke (especially in elderly)
- Prolonged or severe hypoglycemia may cause permanent neurologic damage and/or cognitive impairment.
- Children with T1DM have a greater vulnerability to neurologic manifestations of hypoglycemia.

ALERT

The ACCORD trial (adults with T2DM) demonstrated that intensively lowering blood glucose below current recommendations increased the risk of death versus standard treatment strategy (2)[A].

REFERENCES

1. Seaquist ER, Anderson J, Childs B, et al. Hypoglycemia and diabetes: a report of a workgroup of the American Diabetes Association and The Endocrine Society. *J Clin Endocrinol Metab*. 2013;98(5):1845–1859.
2. Gerstein HC, Miller ME, Byington RP, et al. Effects of intensive glucose lowering in type 2 diabetes. *N Engl J Med*. 2008;358(24):2545–2559.
3. Alvarez Guisasola F, Tofé Povedano S, Krishnarajah G, et al. Hypoglycaemic symptoms, treatment satisfaction, adherence and their associations with glycaemic goal in patients with type 2 diabetes mellitus: findings from the Real-Life Effectiveness and Care Patterns of Diabetes Management (RECAP-DM) Study. *Diabetes Obes Metab*. 2008;10(Suppl 1):25–32.
4. American Diabetes Association. Standards of medical care in diabetes–2015: summary of revisions. *Diabetes Care*. 2015;38(Suppl):S4.
5. Allen KV, Pickering MJ, Zammitt NN, et al. Effects of acute hypoglycemia on working memory and language processing in adults with and without type 1 diabetes. *Diabetes Care*. 2015;38(6):1108–1115.
6. Cryer PE, Axelrod L, Grossmann AB, et al. Evaluation and management of adult hypoglycemic disorders: an Endocrine Society Clinical Practice Guideline. *J Clin Endocrinol Metab*. 2009;94(3):709–728.

ADDITIONAL READING

Thompson AE. JAMA patient page. Hypoglycemia. *JAMA*. 2015;313(12):1284.

 SEE ALSO

- Diabetes Mellitus, Type 1
- Algorithm: Hypoglycemia

CODES

ICD10

- E11.649 Type 2 diabetes mellitus with hypoglycemia without coma
- E10.649 Type 1 diabetes mellitus with hypoglycemia without coma
- E13.649 Oth diabetes mellitus with hypoglycemia without coma

CLINICAL PEARLS

- Address hypoglycemia in every visit with patients at risk.
- Best treatment includes:
  - Patient education and empowerment
  - Frequent SMBG
  - Flexible insulin (or other drug) regimens
  - Regular professional guidance and support
  - Individualized glycemic goals based in part on the risk of hypoglycemia.
- Hypoglycemia unawareness should be recognized and addressed by less aggressive glycemic goals.
- Any form of CHO that contains glucose should be effective, such as sugar-containing food or beverage that can be rapidly absorbed:
  - Using the "rule of 15" is an easy way to teach patients to manage hypoglycemia at home. "Rule of 15": 15 to 20 g CHO (~60 to 80 calories simple CHO) repeated q15min until blood sugar is ≥70 mg/dL.

H

HYPOGLYCEMIA, NONDIABETIC

Matthew A. Silva, PharmD, RPh, BCPS • Pablo I. Hernandez Itriago, MD, MS, FAAFP

BASICS

DESCRIPTION
- Hypoglycemia defined by the Whipple triad
  - Low plasma glucose level (≤60 mg/dL) with hypoglycemic symptoms that are relieved when glucose is corrected.
  - Occurs commonly in patients with diabetes receiving sulfonylurea or insulins; less commonly in patients without diabetes
- Reactive hypoglycemia occurs in response to a meal, drugs, herbal substances, or nutrients and may occur 2 to 3 hours postprandially or later (1).
  - Symptoms are generally observed with serum glucose ≤60 mg/dL, lower in patients with hypoglycemic unawareness.
  - Also seen after GI surgery (in association with dumping syndrome in some patients)
- Spontaneous (fasting) hypoglycemia may be associated with primary conditions including hypopituitarism, Addison disease, myxedema, or disorders related to hepatic dysfunction or renal failure (1,2).
  - If hypoglycemia presents as a primary disorder, consider hyperinsulinism and extrapancreatic tumors.

EPIDEMIOLOGY
Incidence
- True incidence is unknown.
- 0.5–8.6% of hospitalized patients ≥65 years (3–5)
  - Asymptomatic in 25% of cases

Prevalence
True prevalence is unknown:
- Predominant age: older adult
- Predominant sex: female > male

ETIOLOGY AND PATHOPHYSIOLOGY
- Reactive, postprandial
  - Alimentary hyperinsulinism
  - Meals high in refined carbohydrate
  - Certain nutrients, including fructose, galactose, leucine
  - Glucose intolerance (prediabetes)
  - GI surgery
  - Idiopathic (unknown cause)
- Spontaneous
  - Fasting
  - Alcohol or prescription medication–associated (6) (insulin, sulfonylureas, thiazolidinediones, incretin mimetics, DPP-IV inhibitors, β-blockers, salicylates, quinine, hydroxychloroquine, fluoroquinones, doxycycline, sertraline, disopyramide, pentamidine)
  - Nonprescription over-the-counter (OTC) agents, including performance-enhancing agents. Adulterated versions of phosphodiesterase inhibitors and performance-enhancing agents are routinely imported and may contain sulfonylureas and other hypoglycemic agents.
  - Consider medication errors as a source of unexplained hypoglycemia even in patients without diabetes.
  - Surreptitious drug use (self-injection of insulin or ingestion of oral hypoglycemic medications in patients with diabetes)
  - Natural medicines or herbs (bitter melon, caffeine, cassia cinnamon, chromium, fenugreek, ginseng, guarana, mate, stevia, vanadium)

- Postsurgical (e.g., gastrectomy, Roux-en-Y) hypoglycemia/dumping syndrome
  - Islet cell hyperplasia or tumor (insulinoma)
  - Extrapancreatic insulin-secreting tumor
  - Hepatic disease
  - Glucagon deficiency
  - Adrenal insufficiency
  - Catecholamine deficiency
  - Hypopituitarism
  - Hypothyroidism
  - Eating disorders
  - Exercise
  - Fever
  - Pregnancy
  - Renal glycosuria
  - Large tumors
  - Ketotic hypoglycemia of childhood
  - Enzyme deficiencies or defects
  - Severe malnutrition
  - Sepsis
  - Total parenteral nutrition therapy
  - Hemodialysis

Genetics
Some aspects may involve genetics (e.g., hereditary fructose intolerance).

RISK FACTORS
Refer to "Etiology and Pathophysiology."

GENERAL PREVENTION
- Follow dietary and exercise guidelines.
- Patient recognition of early symptoms and knowledge of corrective action

Pediatric Considerations
- Usually divided into two syndromes:
  - Transient neonatal hypoglycemia
  - Hypoglycemia of infancy and childhood
- Screening infants for hypoglycemia is appropriate when pregnancy was complicated by maternal diabetes.
- Cases of hypoglycemia observed in children taking propranolol for infantile hemangioma
- Associated with indomethacin when treating patent ductus arteriosus

Geriatric Considerations
- More likely to have underlying disorders or be caused by medications
- Iatrogenic hypoglycemia is common in the hospitalized elderly with renal insufficiency.

COMMONLY ASSOCIATED CONDITIONS
- Severe liver disease; alcoholism
- Addison disease; adrenocortical insufficiency
- Myxedema
- Malnutrition (patients with renal failure)
- GI surgery
- Panhypopituitarism
- Insulinoma

DIAGNOSIS

HISTORY
- CNS (neuroglycopenic) symptoms predominate with gradual glucose reduction:
  - Headache
  - Confusion
  - Light-headedness

  - Fatigue and weakness
  - Visual disturbances
  - Changes in personality
- Adrenergic symptoms: more prominent in acute drop in glucose
  - Anxiety
  - Tremulousness
  - Dizziness
  - Diaphoresis
  - Warmth/flushing
  - Heart palpitations
- GI symptoms
  - Hunger
  - Nausea
  - Belching

PHYSICAL EXAM
- CNS (neuroglycopenic) symptoms predominate with gradual glucose reduction:
  - Convulsions
  - Coma
  - Hypotension
- Adrenergic symptoms: more prominent in acute drop in glucose
  - Tremulousness
  - Diaphoresis
  - Warmth/flushing
  - Heart palpitations

DIFFERENTIAL DIAGNOSIS
CNS disorders

- Psychogenic
- Pseudohypoglycemia: Symptoms of hypoglycemia or self-diagnosis in patients in whom low blood glucose may not be detectable and may be impossible to convince that they do not suffer from hypoglycemia after all tests are found to be normal.

DIAGNOSTIC TESTS & INTERPRETATION
Initial Tests (lab, imaging)
- Blood glucose ≤45 mg/dL (≤2.5 mmol/L) when symptomatic followed by symptom resolution with feeding (2)[C]
- Plasma glucose overnight fasting: ≤60 mg/dL (≤3.33 mmol/L); confirm on ≥2 occasions (2)[C].
- Plasma glucose 72-hour fasting: ≤45 mg/dL (≤2.5 mmol/L) for females; ≤55 mg/dL (≤3.05 mmol/L) for males; fasting may be ended when Whipple triad is achieved or hypoglycemia is demonstrated (2)[C].
- Abdominal CT to rule out abdominal tumor

Follow-Up Tests & Special Considerations
- Misinterpretation of glucose tolerance tests may lead to misdiagnosis of hypoglycemia; ≥1/3 of normal patients have hypoglycemia, with or without symptoms, during the 4-hour glucose tolerance test. These patients may be at future risk for type 2 diabetes.
- C-peptide measurement (2)[C]
- Check liver studies, serum insulin, adrenocorticotrophic hormone (ACTH), and cortisol. Serum insulin should be suppressed when glucose is <60 mg/dL.
- Serum β-hydroxybutyrate (2)[C]
- Insulin radioimmunoassay: Elevated insulin levels suggest islet cell hyperplasia or tumor.
- Drugs that may alter lab results: Many drugs can affect glucose levels; refer to drug or laboratory reference.

Diagnostic Procedures/Other
- For definitive diagnosis, patient should have
  - Documented low glucose levels
  - Symptoms when glucose levels are low
  - Evidence that symptoms are relieved specifically by ingestion of sugar or other food
  - Identification of the specific type of hypoglycemia
- Serum β-hydroxybutyrate <2.7 mg/dL in the presence of high serum insulin, C-peptide, and low serum glucose suggests excessive insulin production (2)[C].

 ## TREATMENT

GENERAL MEASURES
- Outpatient except for severe cases; may also be inpatient for testing
- Oral carbohydrate for alert patient without drug overdose (2 to 3 tbsp of sugar in glass of water or fruit juice, 1 to 2 cups of milk, piece of fruit, or several soda crackers)
- If unable to swallow: Use glucagon IM or SC.
- If caused by medication or nutrients: Avoid or control causative agents.
- If triggered by meals: Try high-protein diet with carbohydrate restriction.
- Nonhypoglycemic hypoglycemia or pseudohypoglycemia
  - Many patients (often women aged 20 to 45 years) present with diagnosis of reactive hypoglycemia (self-diagnosed or misinterpretation of tests).
  - Symptoms may pertain to chronic fatigue and somatic complaints (stress often plays a role in these symptoms).
  - Management difficult; listening is important. Try 120-g carbohydrate diet.
  - Counseling may be useful for stress and other problems.

MEDICATION
- Once diagnosis is established, begin therapy appropriate for underlying disorder.
- If unable to swallow: glucagon 1 mg (1 unit) IM or SC. If no response, give IV bolus of 25 to 50 g of 50% glucose solution followed by continuous infusion until patient able to take by mouth.
- Postsurgical gastrectomy patients unresponsive to dietary changes may benefit from propantheline, psyllium, fiber, or oat bran, which delays gastric emptying.
- Insulinoma

SURGERY/OTHER PROCEDURES
If islet cell tumor (insulinoma) or other insulin-secreting tumor, surgery is treatment of choice; if inoperable, diazoxide may relieve symptoms (1)[C].

INPATIENT CONSIDERATIONS
Admission Criteria/Initial Stabilization
Hypoglycemia unresponsive to oral intake

 ## ONGOING CARE

FOLLOW-UP RECOMMENDATIONS
- Exercise routine or daily activity may need to be reevaluated.
- Patients with recurrent hypoglycemia should have glucose source at hand for immediate ingestion during symptoms.

Patient Monitoring
- Depends on type and severity of symptoms and treatment of underlying cause
- Hypoglycemia from sulfonylureas can last for hours to days depending on half-life and renal function.

DIET
- High protein, high fiber, complex carbohydrates from multigrain, and whole foods in moderation
- Frequent small feedings (six daily)
- Avoid fasting.

PATIENT EDUCATION
- Dietary instruction
- Counseling for stress, if appropriate
- Recognition of early symptoms of hypoglycemia and how to take corrective action

PROGNOSIS
Favorable, with appropriate treatment

COMPLICATIONS
- Insulinoma: If tumor identified and removed, some surgical risk is involved.
- Organic brain syndrome: may occur with extensive, prolonged hypoglycaemia

REFERENCES
1. Guettier JM, Gorden P. Hypoglycemia. *Endocrinol Metab Clin North Am.* 2006;35(4):753–766.
2. Service FJ. Hypoglycemic disorders. *N Engl J Med.* 1995;332(17):1144–1152.
3. Kagansky N, Levy S, Rimon E, et al. Hypoglycemia as a predictor of mortality in hospitalized elderly patients. *Arch Intern Med.* 2003;163(15):1825–1829.
4. Mannucci E, Monami M, Mannucci M, et al. Incidence and prognostic significance of hypoglycemia in hospitalized non-diabetic elderly patients. *Aging Clin Exp Res.* 2006;18(5):446–451.
5. Nirantharakumar K, Marshall T, Hodson J, et al. Hypoglycemia in non-diabetic in-patients: clinical or criminal? *PLoS One.* 2012;7(7):e40384.
6. Ben Salem C, Fathallah N, Hmouda H, et al. Drug-induced hypoglycaemia: an update. *Drug Saf.* 2011;34(1):21–45.

ADDITIONAL READING
- Bharmal SV, Moyes V, Ahmed S, et al. Hypoglycaemia: possible mediation by chromium salt medication. *Hormones (Athens).* 2010;9(2):181–183.
- Cansu DU, Korkmaz C. Hypoglycaemia induced by hydroxychloroquine in a non-diabetic patient treated for RA. *Rheumatology (Oxford).* 2008;47(3):378–379.
- Chan TY. Outbreaks of severe hypoglycaemia due to illegal sexual enhancement products containing undeclared glibenclamide. *Pharmacoepidemiol Drug Saf.* 2009;18(12):1250–1251.
- Lawrence KR, Adra M, Keir C. Hypoglycemia-induced anoxic brain injury possibly associated with levofloxacin. *J Infect.* 2006;52(6):e177–e180.
- Pollak PT, Mukherjee SD, Fraser AD. Sertraline-induced hypoglycemia. *Ann Pharmacother.* 2001;35(11):1371–1374.
- Singh M, Jacob JJ, Kapoor R, et al. Fatal hypoglycemia with levofloxacin use in an elderly patient in the post-operative period. *Langenbecks Arch Surg.* 2008;393(2):235–238.
- Yamada C, Nagashima K, Takahashi A, et al. Gatifloxacin acutely stimulates insulin secretion and chronically suppresses insulin biosynthesis. *Eur J Pharmacol.* 2006;553(1–3):67–72.

 ## SEE ALSO
- Hypoglycemia, Diabetic; Insulinoma
- Algorithm: Hypoglycemia

 ## CODES

ICD10
- E16.2 Hypoglycemia, unspecified
- E16.1 Other hypoglycemia
- P70.4 Other neonatal hypoglycemia

CLINICAL PEARLS
- Symptoms coincide with low blood glucose levels and resolve with PO/IV glucose or glucagon.
- Avoid known agents/nutrients that trigger hypoglycemia.
- Treat underlying cause.

H

HYPOKALEMIA

Joanne Dannenhoffer, MD • Frank J. Domino, MD

 BASICS

DESCRIPTION

Hypokalemia is defined as a serum potassium concentration <3.5 mEq/L (normal range, 3.5 to 5.0 mEq/L).

- Mild hypokalemia (serum potassium 3.0 to 3.5 mEq/L)
- Moderate hypokalemia (serum potassium 2.5 to 3.0 mEq/L)
- Severe hypokalemia (serum potassium <2.5 mEq/L)

EPIDEMIOLOGY

Predominant sex: male = female

Incidence

- Electrolyte abnormality is commonly encountered in clinical practice and in the elderly (1).
- Found in >20% of hospitalized patients (when defined as potassium <3.6 mEq/L)
- Higher incidence (5–20%) in individuals with eating disorders
- >10% of inpatients with alcoholism
- Higher incidence in patients with AIDS
- Higher incidence in patients receiving diuretics
- Associated risk after bariatric surgery

ETIOLOGY AND PATHOPHYSIOLOGY

Most common causes:

- Decreased intake: deficient diet in alcoholics and elderly; anorexia nervosa
- GI loss: vomiting, diarrhea, nasogastric tubes, laxative abuse, fistulas, villous adenoma, ureterosigmoidostomy, malabsorption, chemotherapy, radiation enteropathy, bulimia
- Intracellular shift of potassium: metabolic alkalosis, insulin excess, β-adrenergic catecholamine excess (acute stress, β_2-agonists), hypokalemic periodic paralysis, intoxications (theophylline, caffeine, barium, toluene)
- Renal potassium loss
  – Drugs: diuretics (especially loop and thiazides), amphotericin B, aminoglycosides
  – Mineralocorticoid excess states: primary hyperaldosteronism; secondary hyperaldosteronism (congestive heart failure [CHF], cirrhosis, nephrotic syndrome, malignant hypertension, renin-producing tumors); renovascular hypertension; Bartter syndrome; Gitelman syndrome; congenital adrenogenital syndromes; exogenous mineralocorticoids (glycyrrhizic acid in licorice, carbenoxolone, steroids in nasal sprays); Liddle syndrome; vasculitis
  – Osmotic diuresis (e.g., poorly controlled diabetes)
  – Renal tubular acidosis (type I and II)
  – Magnesium depletion
- Glucocorticoid excess states: Cushing syndrome, exogenous steroids, ectopic adrenocorticotrophic hormone production, II-β-hydroxysteroid dehydrogenase deficiency, refeeding syndrome

Genetics

Some rare, familial disorders can cause hypokalemia.

- Familial hypokalemic periodic paralysis: hypokalemia after a high-carbohydrate or high-sodium meal or after exercise
- Congenital adrenogenital syndromes
- Liddle syndrome: increases K+ secretion
- Familial interstitial nephritis

GENERAL PREVENTION

When initiating a diuretic, especially loop and thiazide diuretics, advice patients to increase their dietary potassium intake (see "Diet").

COMMONLY ASSOCIATED CONDITIONS

- Acute GI illnesses with severe vomiting or diarrhea
- Increased risk of cardiac arrhythmias; atrial fibrillation (2,3)
- Hypokalemia is a predictor of development of severe alcohol withdrawal syndrome (SWAS) (4).

 DIAGNOSIS

- Patients with hypokalemia often have no symptoms, especially if the hypokalemia is mild (serum potassium 3.0 to 3.5 mEq/L).
- Neuromuscular (most prominent manifestations)
  – Skeletal muscle weakness (proximal > distal muscles, lower limbs > upper limbs) may range from mild weakness to total paralysis, including respiratory muscles; it may lead to rhabdomyolysis and/or respiratory arrest in severe cases.
  – Smooth muscle involvement may lead to GI hypomotility, producing ileus and constipation.
- Cardiovascular
  – Ventricular arrhythmias; higher risk if underlying CHF, left ventricular failure (LVF), cardiac ischemia
  – Increased risk of atrial fibrillation
  – Hypotension
  – Cardiac arrest
- Renal: polyuria, polydipsia, nocturia owing to impaired ability to concentrate, myoglobinuria
- Metabolic: hyperglycemia

HISTORY

Muscle weakness, hypotension, vomiting, diarrhea, polyuria, polydipsia

PHYSICAL EXAM

Decreased skin turgor in dehydration, hypotension, orthostasis, pulmonary congestion/rales, peripheral edema in heart failure

DIFFERENTIAL DIAGNOSIS

- Spurious hypokalemia occurs when blood with high WBC count (>100,000/mm^3) is allowed to stand at room temperature (WBCs extract potassium from plasma).
- Thyrotoxicosis

DIAGNOSTIC TESTS & INTERPRETATION

- Serum potassium <3.5 mEq/L (<3.5 mmol/L)
- Disorders that may alter lab results: leukemia and other conditions with high WBCs

Initial Tests (lab, imaging)

- EKG
- If source of potassium loss not likely to be medications or GI tract: serum electrolytes, urinary potassium
- Calculate plasma anion gap normal (anion gap = Na − [Cl + HCO$_3$]); normal values, 12 ± 4 mEq/L. Must correct calculated anion gap for hypoalbuminemia. Increase calculated anion gap by 2.5 mEq/L for each 1 g/dL decrease in albumin <4 g/dL.
- CT scan of adrenal glands if there is evidence of mineralocorticoid excess

Follow-Up Tests & Special Considerations

- If excessive renal potassium loss (>20 mEq/day) and hypertension, plasma renin and aldosterone levels should be determined to differentiate adrenal from nonadrenal causes of hyperaldosteronism. If hypertension is absent and the patient is acidotic, renal tubular acidosis should be considered.
- If hypertension is absent and serum pH is normal to alkalotic
  – High urine chloride (>10 mEq/day [>10 mmol/day])—diuretics or Bartter syndrome
  – Low urine chloride (<10 mEq/day [<10 mmol/day])—GI losses likely
- ECG
  – Hypokalemia increases the myocyte resting potential, which increases the refractory period; this can lead to arrhythmias.
  – Flattening or inversion of T waves
  – Increased prominence of U waves (small, positive deflection after T wave, best seen in V$_2$ and V$_3$)
  – Depression of ST segment
  – Ventricular ectopia

Test Interpretation

In severe hypokalemia, necrosis of cardiac and skeletal muscle

 TREATMENT

GENERAL MEASURES

- Underlying cause of hypokalemia should be identified.
- For asymptomatic patients treated with oral replacement, outpatient follow-up is sufficient.
- Patients with cardiac manifestations require IV replacement with cardiac monitoring in an intensive care setting.

MEDICATION

- Nonemergent conditions (serum potassium >2.5 mEq/L [>2.5 mmol/L], no cardiac manifestations)
  - Oral therapy preferred: 40 to 120 mEq/day (40 to 120 mmol/day) in divided doses usually is adequate.
  - IV potassium should be given only when oral administration is not feasible (e.g., vomiting, postoperative state). Rate should not exceed 10 mEq/hr, and concentration should not exceed 40 mEq/L. Up to 40 mEq in 100 mL over 1 hour can be given safely through a central venous line. The patient's cardiac rhythm should be closely monitored.
  - Potassium chloride is suitable for all forms of hypokalemia.
  - Other potassium salts may be indicated if a co-existing disorder is present: potassium bicarbonate or bicarbonate precursor (gluconate, acetate, or citrate) in metabolic acidosis or phosphate in phosphate deficiency
- Emergent situations (serum potassium <2.5 mEq/L [<2.5 mmol/L], arrhythmias), IV replacement: Rate of administration should not exceed 20 mEq/hr (20 mmol/hr); maximum recommended concentration, 60 mEq/L (60 mmol/L) of saline for peripheral administration. Administration through central venous lines preferred for rates above 20 mEq/hr.
- Check serum magnesium and replace, if needed; cannot adequately replace potassium in a setting of low magnesium.
- Precautions
  - Any form of potassium replacement carries the risk of hyperkalemia.
  - Serum potassium should be checked more frequently in groups at higher risk: the elderly, diabetic patients, and patients with renal insufficiency.
  - Patients receiving digitalis and patients with diabetic ketoacidosis in whom intracellular shift in potassium is expected after insulin therapy is initiated must have more aggressive replacement.
- Significant possible interactions: Concomitant administration of potassium-sparing diuretics (spironolactone, triamterene, amiloride, ACE inhibitors) magnifies risk of hyperkalemia.

Geriatric Considerations
May need to correct magnesium depletion

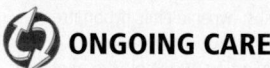 ONGOING CARE

FOLLOW-UP RECOMMENDATIONS
Patient Monitoring
- Patients receiving IV therapy should have cardiac monitoring and serum potassium level checked frequently (q4–6h).
- Patients requiring potassium supplements should have serum potassium studied at intervals and magnesium level dictated by clinical judgment and patient compliance (5)[C].

DIET
In patients with mild hypokalemia (potassium, 3.0 to 3.5 mEq/L [3.0 to 3.5 mmol/L]) not caused by GI losses, dietary supplementation may be sufficient; potassium-rich foods include oranges, bananas, cantaloupes, prunes, raisins, dried beans, dried apricots, and squash.

PATIENT EDUCATION
- Instructions for appropriate diet
- If potassium supplementation is necessary, stress the need for compliance.

PROGNOSIS
- Associated with higher morbidity and mortality because of cardiac arrhythmias
- Ease of correction of hypokalemia and need for prolonged treatment rest on the primary cause; if it can be eliminated (e.g., resolution of diarrhea, discontinuation of diuretics, removal of adrenal tumor), hypokalemia can be expected to resolve and no further treatment is indicated.

COMPLICATIONS
- Hyperkalemia can occur during the course of treatment.
- Increased risk of digoxin toxicity
- Increased risk of atrial fibrillation (2,3)[B]

REFERENCES

1. Hanlon JT, Semla TP, Schmader KE. Medication misadventures in older adults: literature from 2013. *J Am Geriatr Soc.* 2014;62(10):1950–1953.
2. Krijthe BP, Heeringa J, Kors JA, et al. Serum potassium levels and the risk of atrial fibrillation: the Rotterdam Study. *Int J Cardiol.* 2013;168(6): 5411–5415.
3. Tran CT, Bundgaard H, Ladefoged SD, et al. Potassium dynamics are attenuated in hyperkalemia and a determinant of QT adaptation in exercising hemodialysis patients. *J Appl Physiol (1985).* 2013; 115(4):498–504.
4. Goodson CM, Clark BJ, Douglas IS. Predictors of severe alcohol withdrawal syndrome: a systematic review and meta-analysis. *Alcohol Clin Exp Res.* 2014;38(10):2664–2677.
5. Unwin RJ, Luft FC, Shirley DG. Pathophysiology and management of hypokalemia: a clinical perspective. *Nat Rev Nephrol.* 2011;7(2):75–84.

ADDITIONAL READING

- Arsenault KA, Yusuf AM, Crystal E, et al. Interventions for preventing post-operative atrial fibrillation in patients undergoing heart surgery. *Cochrane Database Syst Rev.* 2013;(1):CD003611.
- Asmar A, Mohandas R, Wingo CS. A physiologic-based approach to the treatment of a patient with hypokalemia. *Am J Kidney Dis.* 2012;60(3):492–497.

- Ben Salem C, Hmouda H, Bouraoui K. Drug-induced hypokalaemia. *Curr Drug Saf.* 2009;4(1):55–61.
- Chan KE, Lazarus JM, Hakim RM. Digoxin associates with mortality in ESRD. *J Am Soc Nephrol.* 2010;21(9):1550–1559.
- Ernst ME, Moser M. Use of diuretics in patients with hypertension. *N Engl J Med.* 2009;361(22): 2153–2164.
- Facchini M, Sala L, Malfatto G, et al. Low-K+ dependent QT prolongation and risk for ventricular arrhythmia in anorexia nervosa. *Int J Cardiol.* 2006; 106(2):170–176.
- Jones E. Hypokalemia. *N Engl J Med.* 2004;350(11): 1156.
- Osadchii OE. Mechanisms of hypokalemia-induced ventricular arrhythmogenicity. *Fundam Clin Pharmacol.* 2010;24(5):547–559.
- Palmer BF. A physiologic-based approach to the evaluation of a patient with hypokalemia. *Am J Kidney Dis.* 2010;56(6):1184–1190.
- Zietse R, Zoutendijk R, Hoorn EJ. Fluid, electrolyte and acid-base disorders associated with antibiotic therapy. *Nat Rev Nephrol.* 2009;5(4):193–202.

SEE ALSO

- Hyperkalemia
- Algorithm: Hypokalemia

CODES

ICD10
E87.6 Hypokalemia

CLINICAL PEARLS

- In patients without heart disease, a low potassium level will rarely cause cardiac disturbances. In an otherwise healthy patient, gentle repletion using oral potassium or an increase in potassium-rich foods should be adequate.
- In patients with cardiac ischemia, heart failure, or left ventricular hypertrophy, even mild to moderate hypokalemia can cause arrhythmias. These patients should receive potassium repletion as well as cardiac monitoring.
- To safely prevent hypokalemia in diabetic and renal insufficiency patients, ensure adequate dietary potassium intake with foods rich in potassium, including spinach, tomatoes, broccoli, squash, potatoes, bananas, cantaloupe, and oranges. Avoid potassium-sparing diuretics, if possible.
- Uncorrected hypomagnesemia can hinder the correction of hypokalemia. Check magnesium levels and replete as necessary.

H

HYPONATREMIA
Ruben Peralta, MD, FACS

 BASICS

DESCRIPTION
- Hyponatremia is a plasma sodium (Na) concentration of <135 mEq/L. Hyponatremia itself does not provide information about the "total body water" state of the patient. Patients with hyponatremia may be fluid overloaded, hypovolemic, or euvolemic.
- System(s) affected: endocrine/metabolic

EPIDEMIOLOGY
Incidence
- Most common electrolyte disorder seen in the general hospital population
- Predominant age: all ages
- Predominant sex: male = female

Prevalence
2.5% of hospitalized patients

Geriatric Considerations
The elderly have lower total body water, a decreased thirst mechanism, and decreased urinary concentrating ability; their kidneys are less responsive to antidiuretic hormone (ADH), and they show decreased renal mass, renal blood flow, and glomerular filtration rate, making them at higher risk for hyponatremia.

ETIOLOGY AND PATHOPHYSIOLOGY
- Hypovolemic hyponatremia: Decrease in total body water and greater decrease in total body Na; decreased extracellular fluid volume; orthostatic hypotension and other changes consistent with hypovolemia are present.
- Euvolemic hyponatremia: Increase in total body water with normal total body Na; extracellular fluid volume is minimally to moderately increased but with no edema.
- Hypervolemic hyponatremia: Increase in total body Na and greater increase in total body water; extracellular fluid increased markedly; edema is present.
- Redistributive hyponatremia: shift of water from intracellular compartment to extracellular compartment with resulting dilution of Na; total body water and total body Na unchanged; occurs with hyperglycemia
- Pseudohyponatremia: dilution of aqueous phase by excessive proteins, glucose, or lipids; total body water and total body sodium unchanged; occurs in hypertriglyceridemia or multiple myeloma
- Low Na creates an osmotic gradient between plasma and cells and fluid shifts into cells, causing edema and increased intracranial pressure.
- Hypovolemic hyponatremia: extrarenal loss of sodium (Na <30 mmol/L in urine)
  - GI loss: vomiting, diarrhea
  - Third spacing: peritonitis, pancreatitis, burns, rhabdomyolysis
  - Skin loss: burns, sweating, cystic fibrosis
  - Heat-related illnesses

- Hypovolemic hyponatremia: renal loss of sodium (Na >30 mmol/L in urine)
  - Cerebral salt wasting syndrome
  - Adrenal pathology (e.g., Addison disease, hemorrhage, tuberculosis)
  - Diuretics
  - Osmotic diuresis
- Euvolemic hyponatremia (Na >30 mmol/L in urine)
  - Hypothyroidism
  - Hypopituitarism or other cause of glucocorticoid deficiency
  - Medications (e.g., carbamazepine, clofibrate, cyclosporine, levetiracetam, opiates, oxcarbazepine, phenothiazines, SSRIs, tricyclic antidepressants, vincristine) (1)
  - Primary polydipsia
  - Syndrome of inappropriate antidiuretic hormone secretion (SIADH)
  - Iatrogenic (e.g., excess hypotonic IV fluids)
- Hypervolemic hyponatremia (Na <30 mmol/L in urine, except chronic renal failure)
  - Nephrotic syndrome
  - Cirrhosis
  - Congestive heart failure (CHF)
  - Chronic renal failure
- Redistributive hyponatremia
  - Hyperglycemia
  - Mannitol infusion
  - Hypertriglyceridemia
- Multiple myeloma

Genetics
- Polymorphisms have been demonstrated.
- Mutations have been associated with nephrogenic syndrome of inappropriate antidiuresis (NSIAD; SIADH).

GENERAL PREVENTION
Depends on underlying condition

COMMONLY ASSOCIATED CONDITIONS
- Hypothyroidism
- Hypopituitarism
- Adrenocortical hormone deficiency
- HIV patients
- SIADH is associated with cancers, pneumonia, tuberculosis, encephalitis, meningitis, head trauma, cerebrovascular accident, HIV infection.
- Acute neurologic patients, brain injury
- Marathon runners in hot environments

 DIAGNOSIS

- Symptoms related to the rate of fall in serum Na and the degree of hyponatremia
- Mild (130 to 135 mEq/L): usually asymptomatic
- Moderate (120 to 130 mEq/L): nausea, vomiting, malaise
- Severe: (115 to 120 mEq/L): headache, lethargy, restlessness, disorientation

- Severe/rapid decreases can cause seizure, coma, and respiratory arrest and may be fatal.
- Other signs and symptoms: weakness, muscle cramps, anorexia, hiccups, depressed deep tendon reflexes, hypothermia, positive Babinski responses, cranial nerve palsies, orthostatic hypotension

PHYSICAL EXAM
- Volume status: skin turgor, jugular venous pressure, heart rate, orthostatic BP
- Exam for underlying illness: signs of CHF, cirrhosis, hypothyroidism

DIFFERENTIAL DIAGNOSIS
See "Etiology and Pathophysiology."

DIAGNOSTIC TESTS & INTERPRETATION
Initial Tests (lab, imaging)
- Comprehensive metabolic profile (BUN, creatinine, glucose, electrolytes, liver function studies, etc.)
- Thyroid-stimulating hormone (TSH)
- Lipid panel
- Serum osmolality
- Urine sodium and osmolality
- Chest x-ray to rule out pulmonary pathology if SIADH is diagnosed

Follow-Up Tests & Special Considerations
- CT scan of head if pituitary problem is suspected or if SIADH from CNS problem is suspected
- Interpretation of labs: Suspect hypovolemic hyponatremia.
  - Plasma osmolality is low.
  - BUN-to-Cr ratio > 20:1
  - If urine Na >20 mEq/L (>20 mmol/L): renal loss
  - If urine Na <10 mEq/L (<10 mmol/L): extrarenal loss
  - Serum potassium >5 mEq/L (>5 mmol/L): Consider mineralocorticoid deficiency.
- Interpretation of labs: Suspect euvolemic hyponatremia.
  - Plasma osmolality low
  - BUN-to-Cr ratio < 20:1
  - Urine Na >20 mEq/L (>20 mmol/L)
  - TSH to rule out hypothyroidism
  - Consider 1-hour cosyntropin-stimulation test to rule out adrenal insufficiency.
- Interpretation of labs: hypervolemic hyponatremia
  - Plasma osmolality is low.
  - Urine Na <10 mEq/L (<10 mmol/L) in nephrotic syndrome, CHF, cirrhosis
  - Urine Na >20 mEq/L (>20 mmol/L) in acute and chronic renal failure
- Redistributive hyponatremia
  - Plasma osmolality is normal or high.
  - Glucose or mannitol levels are elevated.
- Pseudohyponatremia
  - Plasma osmolality is normal.
  - Triglyceride, glucose, or protein levels are elevated.

TREATMENT

GENERAL MEASURES
- Assess all medications patient is taking.
- Institute seizure precautions.

MEDICATION

ALERT
Rapid correction of severe symptomatic hyponatremia has been associated with central pontine myelinolysis, a neurologic disorder in which loss of myelin and supportive structures in pons and occasionally in other areas of the brain occurs (2)[C]. This results in irreversible injury. Symptoms are apparent 2 to 6 days after injury and include seizure, coma, spastic paraparesis, dysarthria, and dysphagia.

- Treatment tailored to clinical situation: The degree of hyponatremia, how rapidly the hyponatremia developed, and whether the patient is symptomatic influence the urgency of correction. Some general principles apply
  - Expected change in serum Na with selected infusates: $\Delta Na = [(\text{infusate Na} + \text{infusate K} - \text{serum Na})/(TBW + 1)]$ where TBW = a coeff × weight (wt) as in the following text:

Table 1. Total Body Water

Children	0.6 × weight
Women	0.5 × weight
Men	0.6 × weight
Elderly women	0.45 × weight
Elderly men	0.5 × weight

- Formula to determine correction available at http://www.medcalc.com/sodium.html
- Asymptomatic, euvolemic patients can be treated with fluid restriction; the underlying cause also must be addressed.
- For severely hyponatremic/symptomatic patients, it is generally considered safe to increase the serum Na by 0.6 to 2 mEq/L/hr, not to exceed 8 mEq/24 hr.
- For mild to moderate hyponatremia, use isotonic saline solution (0.9%). For moderate to severe hyponatremia, consider specialist consultation for use of hypertonic saline (3%) via central line access at a rate of 1 to 2 mL/kg body weight/hr; increasing serum sodium levels by 0.5 mmol/L/hr and monitoring frequently the plasma sodium level (~q2h).
- In patients with severe hyponatremia (euvolemic and hypervolemic state) who do not respond to the above-mentioned approach, consider the use of vasopressin V2-receptor antagonists, such as tolvaptan or conivaptan (3)[A].
- Treat underlying condition: heart failure, cirrhosis, and so forth.
- Chronic hyponatremia resulting from SIADH: demeclocycline (inhibits ADH action at the collecting duct) if fluid restriction alone is not effective
  - Contraindication: can cause nephrotoxicity in patients with liver disease
  - In doses of 600 to 1,200 mg/day, the drug produces a nephrogenic diabetes insipidus.
  - Significant possible interactions: oral anticoagulants, oral contraceptives, penicillin

ALERT
Caution: If severe, consider hypertonic saline (3% Na chloride) with central line access, exercise extreme caution, and monitor serum Na as frequently as q1–2h.

INPATIENT CONSIDERATIONS
Admission Criteria/Initial Stabilization
- Admission is mandatory if the patient has acute hyponatremia or is symptomatic; acute hyponatremia (developing over <48 hours) carries the risk of cerebral edema.
- Admission is advised if patient is asymptomatic and has a serum Na <125 mEq/dL.

ONGOING CARE

DIET
- Euvolemic hyponatremia: Restrict water to 1 L/day.
- Hypervolemic hyponatremia: water and Na restriction

PROGNOSIS
- In hospitalized patients, hyponatremia is associated with an elevated risk of adverse clinical outcomes and higher mortality (4,5)[B].

- Recently, in community-dwelling, middle-aged, and elderly adults, mild hyponatremia has been shown to be an independent predictor of death.
- Associated with poor prognosis in patients with acute pulmonary embolism
- Associated with poor prognosis in patients with liver cirrhosis and those waiting for liver transplant; it is associated with significant postop risk and short-term graft loss.

COMPLICATIONS
- Occult tumor may present if SIADH is identified.
- Hypervolemia if saline is used
- Osmotic demyelination (central pontine and extrapontine irreversible myelinolysis) (2,6)[C]
- Hyponatremia is the cause in 30% new onset seizures in intensive care settings.
- Chronic hyponatremia is associated with increased odds of osteoporosis.

REFERENCES

1. Meulendijks D, Mannesse CK, Jansen PA, et al. Antipsychotic-induced hyponatraemia: a systematic review of the published evidence. *Drug Saf*. 2010;33(2):101–114.
2. Singh TD, Fugate JE, Rabinstein AA. Central pontine and extrapontine myelinolysis: a systematic review. *Eur J Neurol*. 2014;21(12):1443–1450.
3. Rozen-Zvi B, Yahav D, Gheorghiade M, et al. Vasopressin receptor antagonists for the treatment of hyponatremia: systematic review and meta-analysis. *Am J Kidney Dis*. 2010;56(2):325–337.
4. Bavishi C, Ather S, Bambhroliya A, et al. Prognostic significance of hyponatremia among ambulatory patients with heart failure and preserved and reduced ejection fractions. *Am J Cardiol*. 2014;113(11):1834–1838.
5. Basu A, Ryder RE. The syndrome of inappropriate antidiuresis is associated with excess long-term mortality: a retrospective cohort analyses. *J Clin Pathol*. 2014;67(9):802–806.
6. Esposito P, Piotti G, Bianzina S, et al. The syndrome of inappropriate antidiuresis: pathophysiology, clinical management and new therapeutic options. *Nephron Clin Pract*. 2011;119(1):c62–c73.

ADDITIONAL READING

- Abraham WT, Hensen J, Gross PA, et al. Lixivaptan safely and effectively corrects serum sodium concentrations in hospitalized patients with euvolemic hyponatremia. *Kidney Int*. 2012;82(11):1223–1230.
- Cowtan T. Thiazide diuretics. *N Engl J Med*. 2010; 362(7):659.
- De Picker L, Van Den Eede F, Dumont G, et al. Antidepressants and the risk of hyponatremia: a class-by-class review of literature. *Psychosomatics*. 2014 55(6):536–547.
- Ernst ME, Moser M. Use of diuretics in patients with hypertension. *N Engl J Med*. 2009;361(22): 2153–2164.
- Friedman B, Cirulli J. Hyponatremia in critical care patients: frequency, outcome, characteristics, and treatment with the vasopressin V2-receptor antagonist tolvaptan. *J Crit Care*. 2013;28(2):219. e1–219.e12.
- Lim YJ, Park EK, Koh HC, et al. Syndrome of inappropriate secretion of antidiuretic hormone as a leading cause of hyponatremia in children who underwent chemotherapy or stem cell transplantation. *Pediatr Blood Cancer*. 2010;54(5):734–737.
- Sood L, Sterns RH, Hix JK, et al. Hypertonic saline and desmopressin: a simple strategy for safe correction of severe hyponatremia. *Am J Kidney Dis*. 2013;61(4):571–578.
- Spasovski G, Vanholder R, Allolio B, et al. Clinical practice guideline on diagnosis and treatment of hyponatraemia. *Eur J Endocrinol*. 2014;170(3): G1–G47.
- Sterns RH, Hix JK, Silver SM. Management of hyponatremia in the ICU. *Chest*. 2013;144(2):672–679.

SEE ALSO

Algorithm: Hyponatremia

CODES

ICD10
E87.1 Hypo-osmolality and hyponatremia

CLINICAL PEARLS

- Alcohol-dependent individuals with vitamin deficiencies, elderly women taking thiazide diuretics, and people with hypokalemia or burns are at increased risk of central pontine myelinolysis. A longer duration of hyponatremia is also a risk factor.
- Bronchogenic carcinoma, pancreas, duodenal, prostate, thymoma, lymphoma, and mesothelioma are neoplastic diseases associated with SIADH.
- Formulas have been developed (Adrogue and Madias) for safe correction of hyponatremia and are available online (see http://www.medcalc.com/sodium.html).

H

HYPOPARATHYROIDISM

Christina Kelly, MD, FAAFP

 BASICS

DESCRIPTION
- Deficient secretion of parathyroid hormone (PTH)
- Usually asymptomatic
- Acute hypoparathyroidism: tetany that is mild (muscle cramps, peri-oral numbness, paresthesias of hands and feet) or severe (carpopedal spasm, laryngospasm, heart failure, seizures, stridor)
- Chronic: lethargy, anxiety/depression, urolithiasis and renal impairment, dementia, blurry vision from cataracts or keratoconjunctivitis, parkinsonism or other movement disorders, mental retardation, dental abnormalities, and dry, puffy, coarse skin
- System(s) affected: endocrine/metabolic, musculoskeletal, nervous, opthomalogic, renal

Pediatric Considerations
- May occur in premature infants
- Neonates born to hypercalcemic mothers may experience suppression of developing parathyroid glands.
- Congenital absence of parathyroids
- May appear later in childhood as autoimmune or APS-1

Geriatric Considerations
Hypocalcemia is fairly common in elderly; however, rarely secondary to hypoparathyroidism

Pregnancy Considerations
- Use of magnesium as a tocolytic may induce functional hypoparathyroidism.
- For women with hypoparathyroidism, calcitriol requirements decrease during lactation.

EPIDEMIOLOGY
More common in women; affects all ages

Incidence
Most common after surgical procedure of the anterior neck. Transient hyperparathyroidism is seen after 6.9–46% of thyroidectomies, whereas permanent hypoparathyroidism, 0.9–1.6% at experienced centers.

Prevalence
Wide variation. Autosomal dominant hypocalcemia with hypercalciuria (ADHH): 1/70,000 typically in infancy with hypocalcemic seizures

ETIOLOGY AND PATHOPHYSIOLOGY
- PTH is involved in the control of serum-ionized calcium levels:
  - Mobilizes calcium and phosphorus from bone stores
  - Stimulates formation of 1,25-dihydroxy-vitamin D
  - Stimulates reabsorption of calcium in the distal convoluted tubule and phosphate excretion in proximal tubule
- Loss of PTH action results in hypocalcemia, hyperphosphatemia, and hypercalciuria.
- Magnesium is crucial for PTH secretion and activation of the PTH receptor; hypo- or hypermagnesemia may result in functional hypoparathyroidism.
- Acquired hypoparathyroidism
  - Surgical: removal or damage to parathyroid glands or their blood supply; thyroid, parathyroid, or radical neck surgery for head and neck cancers (1)

- Autoimmune: isolated or combined with other endocrine deficiencies in polyglandular autoimmune (PGA) syndrome
- Deposition of heavy metals in gland: copper (Wilson disease) or iron (hemochromatosis, thalassemias), radiation-induced destruction, and metastatic infiltration
- Functional hypoparathyroidism: associated with hypomagnesemia; hypermagnesemia
- Congenital
  - Calcium-sensing receptor (CaSR) abnormalities: hypocalcemia with hypercalciuria
  - HDR or Barakat syndrome: deafness, renal dysplasia
  - Familial: mutations of the *TBCE* gene; abnormal PTH secretions
  - 22q11.2 deletion syndrome
- Autoimmune: genetic gain-of-function mutation in CaSR
- Infiltrative: metastatic carcinoma, hemochromatosis, Wilson disease, granulomas
- Hypo- (alcoholics) or hypermagnesemia: chronic iron overloads

Genetics
- Genetic defects may result in X-linked or in autosomal recessive hypoparathyroidism due to abnormal parathyroid gland development; associated with mutations in the transcription factor glial cell missing B (BCMB)
- Mutations in transcription factors or regulators of parathyroid gland development
  - Component of a larger genetic syndrome (APS-1 or DiGeorge syndrome) or in isolation (X-linked hypoparathyroidism) (2)
  - May be autosomal dominant (DiGeorge), autosomal recessive (APS-1), or X-linked recessive (X-linked hypoparathyroidism) (2)
  - Congenital syndromes
    - 22q11.2 deletion syndrome, familial hypomagnesemia, hypoparathyroidism with lymphedema (2)
    - Hypoparathyroidism with sensorineural deafness
    - ADHH: mutations gain-of-function of the *CaSR* gene suppressing the parathyroid gland, without elevation of PTH
  - PGA syndrome type I: mucocutaneous candidiasis, hypoparathyroidism, and Addison disease

RISK FACTORS
Neck surgery and neck trauma, neck malignancies, family history of hypocalcemia, PGA syndrome

GENERAL PREVENTION
Intraoperative identification and preservation of parathyroid tissue

COMMONLY ASSOCIATED CONDITIONS
- DiGeorge syndrome
- PGA syndrome type I
- Multiple endocrine deficiency autoimmune candidiasis (MEDAC) syndrome
- Juvenile familial endocrinopathy
- Addison disease
- Moniliasis (HAM) syndrome: a polyglandular deficiency syndrome, possibly genetic, characterized by hypoparathyroidism

 DIAGNOSIS

HISTORY
Often asymptomatic; ask about previous neck trauma or surgery, head or neck irradiation, family history of hypocalcemia, or presence of other autoimmune endocrinopathies.
- Fatigue, circumoral or distal extremity paresthesias
- Muscle cramps, seizures, neuropsychiatric symptoms

PHYSICAL EXAM
- Surgical scar on neck
- Chvostek sign: ipsilateral twitching of the upper lip on tapping the facial nerve on the cheek. 10% of normal people have positive Chvostek sign.
- Trousseau sign: painful carpal spasm after 3-minute occlusion of brachial artery with BP cuff. BP cuff inflated to > systolic BP for 3 minutes leads to carpal spasm (flexion of metacarpophalangeal [MCP] joints, extension of interphalangeal [IP] joints, adduction of fingers and thumb).
- Tetany, laryngo- or bronchospasm, cardiac arrhythmias, refractory heart failure, dyspnea, edema
- Dry, coarse, puffy hair; brittle nails
- Loss of deep tendon reflexes
- Dysrhythmias (secondary hypocalcemia)
- Cataracts
- Tooth enamel defects

DIFFERENTIAL DIAGNOSIS
- Vitamin D deficiency/resistance
- Pseudohypoparathyroidism, which presents in childhood, kidney and bone unresponsiveness to PTH; characterized by hypocalcemia, hyperphosphatemia, and, in contrast to hypoparathyroidism, elevated rather than reduced PTH concentrations
- Hypoalbuminemia, renal failure, malabsorption, familial hypocalcemia, hypomagnesemia

DIAGNOSTIC TESTS & INTERPRETATION
Initial Tests (lab, imaging)
- Calcium: ionized (low) and total (low) (correct serum calcium level for albumin)
  - Corrected serum calcium = total serum calcium + 0.8 (4 − serum albumin)
- Phosphorus (high)
- Intact or "whole" PTH (low or inappropriately normal)
- Magnesium (low may be cause of hypoparathyroidism; may also be normal)
- BUN, creatinine, 25-OH vitamin D level (especially in elderly)
- Urinary calcium (normal or high)
- Calcium should be monitored after thyroid or parathyroid surgery.
- Radiographs may show absent tooth roots, calcification of cerebellum, choroid plexus, or cerebral basal ganglia.

Follow-Up Tests & Special Considerations
- ECG: prolongation of ST and QTc intervals nonspecific repolarization changes, dysrhythmias

- Urine calcium: Creatinine ratio (normal 0.1 to 0.2) may be low before treatment but should be monitored to prevent stones due to hypercalciuria.
- Gene sequencing: Evaluation of other hormone levels may be required to diagnose APS-1.
- Hungry bone syndrome (transient hypoparathyroidism after parathyroid surgery)
  - Hypocalcemia due to hungry bone syndrome may persist despite recovery of PTH secretion from the remaining normal glands. Thus, serum PTH concentrations may be low, normal, or even elevated.
- Infiltrative: osteoblastic metastasis of prostate, breast, or lung cancer
- Metabolic/nutritional: renal failure, neonatal hypocalcemia, hypoalbuminemia, malabsorption, calcium (Ca^{++}) chelators, hypomagnesemia
- Familial hypocalcemia, acute hyperphosphatemia (rare), vitamin D deficiency
- Autoantibodies against NACHT leucine-rich-repeat protein 5 (NALPS) found in 49% of 73 patients with APS-1 and hypoparathyroidisms

Test Interpretation
Parathyroid gland parenchymal tissue completely or almost completely replaced by fat

 TREATMENT

GENERAL MEASURES
- Monitor ECG during calcium repletion.
- Maintenance therapy: may require lifelong treatment with calcium and calcitriol
  - Maintain serum calcium in low normal range: 8 to 8.5 mg/dL (2 to 2.12 mmol/L).
- If hypercalcemia occurs, hold therapy until calcium returns to normal. Treat magnesium deficiency if present.
- Phosphate binders are required if high calcium-phosphate product.
- Thiazide diuretics combined with a low-salt diet may be used to prevent hypercalciuria, nephrocalcinosis, and nephrolithiasis.
- Oral calcium administration and vitamin D supplementation after thyroidectomy may reduce the risk for symptomatic hypocalcemia after surgery.

MEDICATION
Acute Hypoparathyroidism
- Hypoparathyroid with severe symptoms (tetany, seizures, cardiac failure, laryngospasm, bronchospasm)
  - IV calcium gluconate: 1 or 2 g, each infused over a period of 10 minutes. Central venous catheter is preferred because calcium-containing solutions can irritate surrounding tissues. Follow with infusion of 10 g calcium gluconate in 1 L 5% dextrose water at a rate of 1 to 3 mg calcium gluconate/kg body weight/hr (1)[B].
- Hypomagnesemia: acutely: 1 to 2 g IV q6h. Long-term magnesium oxide tablets (600 mg) once or twice per day
- Maintenance: See "First Line" treatment for chronic hypoparathyroidism.

Chronic Hypoparathyroidism
First Line
- Adults
  - Oral calcium: calcium salts: 1 to 3 g/day PO. For geriatric patients, consider using calcium citrate instead of calcium carbonate.
  - Calcitriol: (vitamin D 1, 25-dihydroxycholecalciferol): 0.25 µg/day. Doses 0.5 to 2.0 µg/day are usually required (2)[A].
- Children
  - Oral elemental calcium: 25 to 50 mg/kg daily
  - Calcitriol: 0.25 µg daily for age >1 year

Second Line
Cholecalciferol 10,000 to 50,000 U duration of action 4 to 8 weeks

ISSUES FOR REFERRAL
Endocrinologist, nephrologist, ophthalmologist

ADDITIONAL THERAPIES
Parathyroid hormone 1 to 34 and 1 to 84 SC
- Improved well-being and increased bone mineral density have been shown with PTH therapy, but other long-term benefits have not (3).

SURGERY/OTHER PROCEDURES
Autotransplantation of cryopreserved parathyroid tissue: restores normocalcemia in 23% of cases

INPATIENT CONSIDERATIONS
Admission Criteria/Initial Stabilization
Laryngospasm, seizures, tetany, QT prolongation

Discharge Criteria
Resolution of hypocalcemic symptoms, patient educated on hypoparathyroidism and treatment

 ONGOING CARE

FOLLOW-UP RECOMMENDATIONS
Patient Monitoring
- Goal is a total corrected serum calcium level in low normal range (8 to 8.5 mg/dL or 2 to 2.12 mmol/L), 24-hour urine calcium <300 mg, and calcium-phosphate product <55.
- Outpatient measurement of serum calcium, phosphate, magnesium, and creatinine weekly to monthly during initial management; for changes in medication, check weekly or every other week; when stable, measure every 3 to 6 months (3)[A].
- Measure 24-hour urinary calcium secretion yearly.
- If symptoms of renal stone disease or increasing Cr, get renal imaging (3)[A].
- Annual slit-lamp and ophthalmologic evaluations are recommended.
- DEXA scan (2)[A]

DIET
Low-phosphate diet in patients with hyperphosphatemia

PATIENT EDUCATION
https://www.hypopara.org/

PROGNOSIS
Hypoparathyroidism following neck surgery is often transient. Length of required treatment may vary depending on origin.

COMPLICATIONS
- Reversible: due to low calcium levels, most likely to improve with adequate treatment
  - Neuromuscular symptoms: Paresthesias (circumoral, fingers, toes), tetany, seizures, parkinsonian symptoms; pseudotumor cerebri has been described.
  - Renal: hypercalciuria, nephrocalcinosis, nephrolithiasis
  - Cardiovascular: heart failure, arrhythmias
- Irreversible: when condition starts early in childhood and will not improve with calcium and vitamin D treatment
  - Stunting of growth
  - Enamel defects and hypoplasia of teeth
  - Atrophy, brittleness, and ridging of nails
  - Cataracts and basal ganglia calcifications

REFERENCES
1. Al-Azem, Khan A. Hypoparathyroidism. *Best Pract Res Clin Endocrinol Metab.* 2012;26(4):517–522.
2. Bilezikian JP, Khan A, Potts JT Jr, et al. Hypoparathyroidism in the adult: epidemiology, diagnosis, pathophysiology, target-organ involvement, treatment, and challenges for future research. *J Bone Miner Res.* 2011;26(10):2317–2337.
3. Bollerslev J, Rejnmark L, Marcocci C, et al. European Society of Endocrinology Clinical Guideline: treatment of chronic hypoparathyroidism in adults. *Eur J Endocrinol.* 2015;173(2):G1–G20.

ADDITIONAL READING
- Michels TC, Kelly KM. Parathyroid disorders. *Am Fam Physician.* 2013;88(4):249–257.
- National Institute of Child Health and Human Development. Hypoparathyroidism: For researchers and health care practitioners. https://www.nichd.nih.gov/health/topics/hypopara/resources/pages/providers.aspx

 CODES

ICD10
- E20.9 Hypoparathyroidism, unspecified
- P71.4 Transitory neonatal hypoparathyroidism
- E89.2 Postprocedural hypoparathyroidism

CLINICAL PEARLS
Often asymptomatic; consider if hypocalcemic with fatigue and circumoral or distal extremity paresthesias.
- Correct the serum calcium level for albumin level.
- Monitor calcium after thyroid or parathyroid surgery.
- Serum levels of magnesium and 25-OH should be measured to rule out deficiency that could contribute to reduced serum calcium levels.

H

HYPOTHERMIA

Scott T. Henderson, MD

 BASICS

DESCRIPTION
- A core temperature of <35°C (95°F)
- May take several hours to days to develop
- Patients with cold-water immersion can appear to be dead but can still be resuscitated.
- System(s) affected: all body systems
- Synonym(s): accidental hypothermia

EPIDEMIOLOGY
- Predominant age: very young and the elderly
- Predominant sex: male > female

Geriatric Considerations
More common due to lower metabolic rate, impaired ability to maintain normal body temperature, and impaired ability to detect temperature changes

Prevalence
Estimates vary widely due to lack of pathologic evidence, and it is typically a secondary cause when diagnosing disorders.

ETIOLOGY AND PATHOPHYSIOLOGY
- Overwhelming environmental cold stress
- Decreased heat production
- Increased heat loss
- Impaired thermoregulation

RISK FACTORS
- Alcohol consumption
- Bronchopneumonia
- Cardiovascular disease
- Cold-water immersion
- Dermal dysfunction (burns, erythrodermas)
- Drug intoxication
- Endocrinopathies (myxedema, severe hypoglycemia)
- Excessive fluid loss
- Hepatic failure
- Hypothalamic and central nervous system (CNS) dysfunction
- Malnutrition
- Mental illness; Alzheimer disease
- Prolonged cardiac arrest
- Prolonged environmental exposure
- Renal failure
- Sepsis
- Trauma (especially head)
- Uremia

GENERAL PREVENTION
- Appropriate clothing, with particular attention to head, feet, and hands
- For outdoor activities, carry survival bags with rescue foil blanket for use if stranded or injured.
- Avoid alcohol.
- Alertness to early symptoms and initiating preventive steps (e.g., drinking warm fluids)
- Identify medications that may predispose to hypothermia (e.g., neuroleptics, sedatives, hypnotics, tranquilizers).

COMMONLY ASSOCIATED CONDITIONS
- Addison disease
- CNS dysfunction
- Congestive heart failure
- Diabetes
- Hypopituitarism
- Hypothyroidism
- Ketoacidosis
- Pulmonary infection
- Sepsis
- Uremia

 DIAGNOSIS

HISTORY
Presentation varies with the temperature of the patient at the time of presentation.

ALERT
History of prolonged exposure to cold may make the diagnosis obvious, but hypothermia may be overlooked in other situations, especially in comatose patients.

PHYSICAL EXAM
Esophageal temperature is most accurate, minimally invasive method of assessing core temperature (1)[C].
- Must have secure airway
- Probe inserted into lower third of esophagus
Exam findings vary with the temperature of the patient at the time of presentation.
- Mild (32–35°C)
  - Lethargy and mild confusion
  - Shivering
  - Tachypnea
  - Tachycardia
  - Loss of fine motor coordination
  - Increased BP
  - Peripheral vasoconstriction
- Moderate (28–32°C)
  - Delirium
  - Bradycardia
  - Hypotension
  - Hypoventilation
  - Cyanosis
  - Arrhythmias (prolonged PR interval, AV junctional rhythm, accelerated idioventricular rhythm, prolonged QT interval, altered T waves)
  - Semicoma and coma
  - Muscular rigidity
  - Generalized edema
  - Slowed reflexes
- Severe (<28°C)
  - Very cold skin
  - Rigidity
  - Apnea
  - Bradycardia
  - No pulse: ventricular fibrillation or asystole
  - Areflexia
  - Unresponsive
  - Fixed pupils

ALERT
Use specially designed thermometers that can record low temperatures and measure core temperatures.

Pediatric Considerations
- Infants may present with bright red, cold skin and very low energy.
- A child's body temperature drops faster than an adult does when immersed in cold water.

DIFFERENTIAL DIAGNOSIS
- Cerebrovascular accidents
- Intoxication
- Drug overdose
- Complications of diabetes, hypothyroidism, hypopituitarism

DIAGNOSTIC TESTS & INTERPRETATION
Initial Tests (lab, imaging)
- Arterial blood gases (corrected for temperature)
- CBC and platelet counts
- Serum electrolytes
- Urinalysis
- Coagulation studies
- Fibrinogen levels
- Blood culture
- BUN/creatinine
- Glucose
- Amylase
- Liver function studies
- Cardiac enzymes
- Calcium
- Magnesium
- Alcohol level
- Drug screen
- Cervical spine, chest, and abdomen x-rays, if appropriate

Follow-Up Tests & Special Considerations
Serum cortisol and TSH if underlying endocrine dysfunction (hypothalamus stimulates release of hormones in response to hypothermia)

Diagnostic Procedures/Other
EKG

Test Interpretation
Serum potassium >12 mmol/L associated with nonsurvival

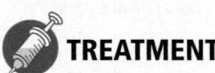 **TREATMENT**

GENERAL MEASURES
- Prehospital (1)[C]
  - Factors to guide treatment
    - Level of consciousness
    - Shivering intensity
    - Cardiovascular stability based on blood pressure and cardiac rhythm.
    - ABCs of basic life support
    - Remove wet garments.
      - Dry patient.
    - Protect against heat loss and wind chill.
    - If far from definitive care, begin active rewarming but do not delay transport.
      - Mild hypothermic patients with shivering ability will have improved comfort and might have a reduced cold-stress response with active rewarming (2)[B].
    - Give warm humidified oxygen if available.
- See "Admission Criteria/Initial Stabilization."

MEDICATION
- For sepsis or bacterial infections: Antibiotics based on site and etiology.
- For hypoglycemia: D50W at a dose of 1 mg/kg
- Thiamine: 100 mg, if alcoholic or cachectic
- Naloxone: 2 mg
- Levothyroxine: 150 to 500 μg for myxedema
- For severe acidosis: sodium bicarbonate

- Precautions
  - Medications including epinephrine, lidocaine, and procainamide can accumulate to toxic levels if used repeatedly. Should be avoided until core temperature is >30°C:
    - When temperature reaches >30°C, IV medications are indicated but at longer than the standard intervals.
  - It may be reasonable to consider vasopressors during cardiac arrest according to standard ACLS algorithm with concurrent rewarming.
- Significant possible interactions:
  - Use all drugs cautiously due to impaired metabolism and renal elimination.
- Once rewarming has occurred, there is mobilization of depot stores.
- Routine use of steroids or antibiotics does not increase survival or decrease postresuscitative damage.

INPATIENT CONSIDERATIONS
Admission Criteria/Initial Stabilization
- Rewarming depends on severity of hypothermia and presence of cardiac arrest.
- If no cardiac arrest, consider active external rewarming (3)[B].
- If cardiac arrest is present, consider active internal rewarming (3)[B].
- Warm center of body first (4)[C].
- The rate of rewarming is determined by whether a perfusing cardiac output is present.
  - If a perfusing cardiac output is present, 1–2°C/hr is appropriate.
  - If not, then a faster rate of >2°C/hr should be used.
- Monitor core temperature; use a consistent method.
- Monitor BP and cardiac rhythm.
- Correct metabolic acidosis.
- Evaluate for frostbite and other trauma.
- Mild hypothermia
  - Passive rewarming
  - Administration of heated IV solutions
  - Provide warm fluids by mouth if fully alert.
- Moderate hypothermia
  - Active external rewarming with forced warm air systems
- Severe hypothermia (active internal [core] rewarming)
  - Minimally invasive
  - Heated IV fluids
  - Heated humidified oxygen
  - Body cavity lavage
    - Thoracic cavity lavage (40–45°C)
    - Peritoneal lavage (40–45°C)
  - Extracorporeal blood rewarming
    - Cardiopulmonary bypass
    - Extracorporeal membrane oxygenation
    - Continuous arteriovenous rewarming
    - Hemodialysis and hemofiltration
- Cardiac arrhythmias
  - Atrial fibrillation and sinus bradycardia are common, but patients usually convert to normal sinus rhythm with rewarming.
  - If ventricular fibrillation is present, it should be treated with one shock. If patient does not respond, consider deferring further attempts until rewarm has occurred.
  - Do not treat transient ventricular arrhythmias.
  - If cardiac pacing required, preferable to use external noninvasive pacemaker.
- Admit patients, preferably to the ICU, with underlying disease, physiologic abnormalities, or core temperature <32°C.

IV Fluids
- Normal saline is preferred (1)[C].
- Heat IVs from 40°C to 45°C when possible, but should be no colder than the patient's core temperature.

ALERT
- Avoid fluid overload.
- Avoid overheating dextrose solutions; dextrose caramelizes at 60°C.
- Avoid lactated Ringer solution because of decreased lactate metabolism.

Nursing
Because of the cold, heart is irritable and susceptible to arrhythmias; take special care in moving and transporting.

Discharge Criteria
Discharge from emergency department once normothermic, if mild hypothermia and no predisposing conditions or complications, and has suitable place to go.

 ONGOING CARE

FOLLOW-UP RECOMMENDATIONS
Patient Monitoring
- During acute episode
  - Monitor cardiac rhythm.
  - Monitor electrolytes and glucose frequently.
  - Monitor urinary output.
  - Follow blood gases.
- Following acute episode
  - Continued therapy for any underlying disorder

DIET
Warm fluids only if alert and able to swallow
- Alcohol intake increases risk of becoming hypothermic in cold conditions.
- Encourage persons with cardiovascular disease to avoid outdoor exercise in cold weather.
- Refer to social service agency for help with adequate housing, heat, and/or clothing, if appropriate.

PROGNOSIS
- Mortality rates are decreasing due to increased recognition and advanced therapy.
- Mortality usually depends on the severity of underlying cause and comorbidities.
- In previously healthy individuals, recovery is usually complete.
  - Mortality rate in healthy patients is <5%.
- Mortality rate in patients with coexisting illness is >50%.

Geriatric Considerations
Mortality rates increase with increasing age.

COMPLICATIONS
- Core temperature after drop
- Cardiac arrhythmias
- Hypotension
- Hyperkalemia
- Hypoglycemia
- Rhabdomyolysis
- Sepsis
- Pneumonia (aspiration and broncho)
- Pulmonary edema
- Acute respiratory distress syndrome
- Pancreatitis
- Peritonitis
- GI bleeding

- Ileus
- Acute tubular necrosis
- Bladder atony
- Intravascular thromboses/disseminated intravascular coagulation
- Metabolic acidosis
- Gangrene of extremities
- Compartment syndromes
- Seizures
- Cerebral ischemia
- Delirium

REFERENCES
1. Zafren K, Giesbrecht GG, Danzl DF, et al. Wilderness Medical Society practice guidelines for the out-of-hospital evaluation and treatment of accidental hypothermia: 2014 update. *Wilderness Environ Med.* 2014;25(4)(Suppl):S66–S85.
2. Lundgren P, Henriksson O, Naredi P, et al. The effect of active warming in prehospital trauma care during road and air ambulance transportation—a clinical randomized trial. *Scand J Trauma Resusc Emerg Med.* 2011;19:59.
3. Kempainen RR, Brunette DD. The evaluation and management of accidental hypothermia. *Respir Care.* 2004;49(2):192–205.
4. van der Ploeg GJ, Goslings JC, Walpoth BH, et al. Accidental hypothermia: rewarming treatments, complications and outcomes from one university medical centre. *Resuscitation.* 2010;81(11):1550–1555.

ADDITIONAL READING
- Brown DJ, Brugger H, Boyd J, et al. Accidental hypothermia. *N Engl J Med.* 2012;367(20):1930–1938.
- Petrone P, Asensio JA, Marini CP. Management of accidental hypothermia and cold injury. *Curr Probl Surg.* 2014;51(10):417–431.

 SEE ALSO

- Frostbite; Near Drowning
- Algorithm: Hypothermia

 CODES

ICD10
- T68.XXXA Hypothermia, initial encounter
- T68.XXXD Hypothermia, subsequent encounter
- T68.XXXS Hypothermia, sequela

CLINICAL PEARLS
- Most common cause of hypothermia in the United States is cold exposure due to alcohol intoxication.
- With a severely decreased core temperature, one should assume resuscitation, if possible, unless there are obvious lethal injuries. Continue resuscitation and rewarm to 33–35°C ("not dead until warm and dead").
- ECG changes are associated with hypothermia: slowing of sinus rate with T-wave inversion; QT, QRS, and PR interval prolongation; atrial and ventricular arrhythmias; hypothermic J waves (Osborn waves) characterized by a notching of the QRS complex and ST segment

H

HYPOTHYROIDISM, ADULT

Adithi Naidu, MD • Faraz Ahmad, MD • Jason Chao, MD, MS

 BASICS

DESCRIPTION

- Clinical and metabolic state resulting from decreased levels of free thyroid hormone or from resistance to hormone action
- Primary (intrinsic thyroid disease) >95% of cases or central (secondary or tertiary resulting from hypothalamic-pituitary disease)
- Subclinical or overt
- Subclinical: serum TSH above the upper reference limit with a normal free T_4 and normal hypothalamic-pituitary-thyroid axis (1)[A]
- Overt: elevated TSH, usually >10 mIU/L with a subnormal free T_4

EPIDEMIOLOGY

Incidence

- Women: 3.5 per 1,000 persons per year
- Men: 0.6 per 1,000 persons per year
- Risk of developing hypothyroidism in women with positive antibodies and elevated TSH was 4% per year and 2–3% per year in those with either alone (1)[A].

Prevalence

- The National Health and Nutrition Examination Survey III (NHANES III), SHypo (Subclinical hypothyroidism) 9.3%, overt 0.3% in an unselected U.S. population over age 12 years, between 1988 and 1994 with upper limit TSH 4.5
- Framingham study, 5.9% of women and 2.3% of men over age 60 years had a serum TSH >10 mIU/L.
- British Whickham survey, 9.3% of women and 1.2% of men had a serum TSH >10 (1)[A].

ETIOLOGY AND PATHOPHYSIOLOGY

- Primary: abnormality at the thyroid gland (>95% of cases)
- Most common cause worldwide: environmental iodine deficiency (1) [A]
- Most common cause in the United States: Hashimoto thyroiditis (autoimmune thyroid disease [AITD])
  - AITD is characterized pathologically by infiltration of the thyroid with sensitized T lymphocytes and serologically by circulating thyroid antibodies.
  - Autoimmunity to the thyroid gland is an inherited defect in immune surveillance, leading to abnormal regulation of immune responsiveness or alteration of presenting antigen in the thyroid (1)[A].
- Postablative/posttherapeutic: follows radioactive iodine therapy or thyroid surgery for hyperthyroidism, thyroid cancer, benign nodular thyroid disease or neck malignancies
- Transient hypothyroidism during the course of subacute or painless thyroiditis (silent thyroiditis, most common during postpartum period) and subacute granulomatous thyroiditis
- Drug use: propylthiouracil, methimazole, lithium, amiodarone, and newer chemotherapeutic agents such as tyrosine kinase inhibitors (sunitinib), interleukin-2, or interferon-α
- Central: Hypothyroidism due to insufficient stimulation by TSH of an otherwise normal thyroid gland.
- Can be secondary (level of the pituitary) or tertiary (level of the hypothalamus)
- Etiology involves genetic defects, tumors, vascular, empty sella syndrome, inflammatory, infiltrative, iatrogenic, posttrauma, or drug related.

RISK FACTORS

- Women >60 years of age
- Personal or family history of autoimmune diseases, including type 1 diabetes mellitus, Addison disease, Hashimoto thyroiditis, vitiligo, pernicious anemia
- Pregnant women or those with previous postpartum thyroiditis
- Previous head or neck irradiation
- Past history of thyroid dysfunction or thyroid surgery
- Abnormal thyroid examination, presence of goiter and/or TPOAb positivity
- Treatment with amiodarone, lithium, interferon-α, sunitinib, or sorafenib
- Those with Down syndrome or Turner syndrome

COMMONLY ASSOCIATED CONDITIONS

- Type 1 diabetes
- Pernicious anemia
- Primary adrenal failure (Addison disease)
- Myasthenia gravis
- Celiac disease
- Rheumatoid arthritis
- Systemic lupus erythematosis
- Vitiligo
- Depression
- Genetic syndromes that have multiple autoimmune endocrinopathies (MAE) such as type 1 MAE and type 2 MAE.

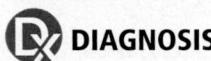 **DIAGNOSIS**

HISTORY

- Weakness/fatigue
- Cold intolerance
- Slowed thinking
- Hearing impairment
- Constipation
- Muscle cramps, arthralgias, paresthesias
- Modest weight gain (10 lb [4.5 kg])
- Menstrual disturbances
- Depression
- Change in voice (hoarseness)
- Carpal tunnel syndrome

PHYSICAL EXAM

- Dry, coarse, thickened skin
- Hair loss/brittle hair
- Coarsening of voice
- Periorbital puffiness
- Swelling of hands and feet (nonpitting)
- Bradycardia
- Reduced systolic BP; increased diastolic BP
- Delayed relaxation of deep tendon reflexes
- Macroglossia
- Goiter (particularly in patient with Hashimoto thyroiditis)

Geriatric Considerations

- Characteristic signs and symptoms frequently nonspecific, changed, or absent
- Normal serum thyrotropin ranges are higher (in those over 65 years of age)

DIFFERENTIAL DIAGNOSIS

- Chronic fatigue syndrome
- Depression
- Euthyroid sick syndrome
- Congestive heart failure
- Primary amyloidosis
- Dementia from other causes
- Primary adrenal insufficiency
- Thyrotropin-secreting pituitary adenoma

DIAGNOSTIC TESTS & INTERPRETATION

- Primary hypothyroidism
  - Elevated TSH (>4.5 mIU/L)
  - Decreased serum free T_4
  - Normal TRH stimulation test
- Central (secondary or tertiary) hypothyroidism
  - Assess only free T_4 or free T_4 index, not TSH (1)[A].
  - Decreased serum free T_4
  - Abnormal TRH stimulation test
  - Antithyroid antibodies absent
  - Imaging of the hypothalamus and pituitary gland
- Subclinical hypothyroidism
  - Elevated serum TSH (>4.5 mIU/L)
  - Normal serum free T_4 (2)[A]
  - Note: Serum free triiodothyronine (T_3) or total T_3 should not be done to diagnose hypothyroidism (1)[A].

Follow-Up Tests & Special Considerations

- Antithyroid antibodies may define the cause of primary hypothyroidism but are not necessary in all settings.
- Drugs that may alter lab results:
  - Drugs that decrease TSH:
    ○ Thyroid supplement, cortisone, dopamine, octreotide
  - Drugs that increase TSH:
    ○ Phenytoin, amiodarone, dopamine antagonist (metoclopramide/domperidone, salicylates, oral colecystographic dyes [sodium ipodate]), or estrogen or androgen in excess
- Disorders that may alter lab results
  - Any severe illness, pregnancy, chronic protein malnutrition, hepatic failure, or nephrotic syndrome

Test Interpretation

SCREENING

- Patient with risks factors as described above
- Patient with laboratory or imaging abnormalities
  - Substantial hyperlipidemia or change in lipid pattern
  - Hyponatremia, often resulting from inappropriate production of antidiuretic hormone
  - High serum muscle enzyme concentrations
  - Macrocytic anemia
  - Pericardial or pleural effusion
  - Pituitary or hypothalamic disorder
- Pregnant women
  - Personal or family history of thyroid disease
  - DM type 1
  - H/o recurrent miscarriage, morbid obesity, or infertility; thyroid peroxidase antibody (TPOAb) should be considered (1)[A].
  - Universal screening not recommended for patients pregnant or planning pregnancy
- U.S. Preventive Services Task Force does not recommend routine screening for children or adults (1)[A].

- Recommendations by expert groups:
  - ATA recommend screening in all adults at age 35 years and every 5 years thereafter.
  - AACE recommend screening older patients, especially women.
  - AAFP recommend screening patients 60 years and older.
  - ACOG recommends women with h/o autoimmune disease or strong family h/o thyroid disease should be screened at age 19 years.

TREATMENT

MEDICATION
First Line
- Levothyroxine (Synthroid, Levothroid)
  - 1.6 μg/kg/day; increase by 12.5 to 25 μg/day every 4 to 8 weeks until TSH in normal range
  - Dosage requirements may vary with age, gender, residual secretory capacity of thyroid gland, other drugs being taken by patient, and intestinal function (1)[A].
  - Elderly patients may require 2/3 of dose used in young adults because clearance is decreased.
  - Levothyroxine should be taken on an empty stomach, ideally an hour before breakfast. Administering at bedtime may result in higher levels than administering in the morning (3)[A]
  - Medications that interfere with its absorption should be taken 4 hours after the T_4 dose: ferrous sulfate, proton pump inhibitors, calcium carbonate, bile acid resins.
- Contraindications
  - Thyrotoxic heart disease
  - Uncorrected adrenocorticoid insufficiency
  - MI, acute
  - TSH suppression, preexisting
- Precautions
  - Start with lower doses, such as 12.5 to 25 μg, in elderly and in patients with heart disease.
  - Diabetic patients may need readjustment of hypoglycemic agents with institution of thyroxine (T_4).
  - Dosage of oral anticoagulants may need adjustment; monitor prothrombin time while initiating treatment.
  - Elderly patients more susceptible to AFib and osteoporotic fracture with thyroid hormone excess
  - Patients requiring doses that are higher than expected should be evaluated for GI disorders (*H. pylori*, celiac disease).
- Significant possible interactions
  - Oral anticoagulants, insulin, oral hypoglycemic, estrogen, OCP, PPI, cholestyramine
  - Ferrous sulfate, calcium carbonate, antacids, laxatives, colestipol, sucralfate, ciprofloxacin, and cholestyramine may decrease absorption.
- Controversy exists whether subclinical hypothyroidism should be treated. Cochrane Review found no improvement in survival, cardiovascular morbidity, or health-related quality of life. Some evidence indicates improvement in lipid profiles and left ventricular function. Subclinical hypothyroidism should be treated in patients with iron deficiency anemia and in patients with TSH >10 (2,4,5)[B].
- If surgery is elective, render patient euthyroid prior to procedure.
- If surgery is urgent, proceed with individualized replacement therapy preoperatively and postoperatively.

Pregnancy Considerations
- Replacement therapy may need adjustment; average dose increase from 25–50% (6)[A].
- TSH levels should be monitored monthly during 1st trimester; goal TSH of 2 to 2.5 mIU/L for 1st trimester, <3.0 mIU/L for 2nd trimester, and <3.5 mIU/L for 3rd trimester (6)[A].
- Postpartum: Check TSH levels at 6 weeks (6)[A].
- Painless subacute thyroiditis may occur in postpartum period, leading to transient hypothyroidism lasting 3 months. Treatment with replacement therapy may be warranted. Up to 30% of these individuals develop permanent hypothyroidism.

Second Line
- No benefit to adding triiodothyronine (T_3) to T_4 (6)[A]
- Desiccated thyroid hormone is not recommended for the treatment of hypothyroidism (1).

ISSUES FOR REFERRAL
- Children and infants
- Pregnancy or women planning conception
- Patient in whom it is difficult to maintain a euthyroid state
- Cardiac disease
- Presence of goiter, nodule, or other structural changes in the thyroid gland
- Presence of adrenal or pituitary disorders (1)[C]

INPATIENT CONSIDERATIONS
Admission Criteria/Initial Stabilization
- Myxedema coma (decompensated severe untreated hypothyroidism)
- True clinical emergency (requires ICU care)
- Profound hypothermia and unconsciousness
- Increased risk of shock and potentially fatal arrhythmias

ONGOING CARE

FOLLOW-UP RECOMMENDATIONS
Patient Monitoring
- Monitor TSH and free T_4 every 4 to 8 weeks after initiating treatment or after change in dose. Once stabilized, periodic TSH level should be done after 6 months and then at 12-month intervals or more frequently if the clinical situation dictates otherwise (1)[B].
- Follow cardiac status closely in older patients.
- Check TSH more frequently in pregnancy, initiation of estrogen supplementation, or after large changes in body weight.
- In central hypothyroidism, TSH unreliable; must monitor free T_4 and T_3
- Thyroid hormones should not be used to treat obesity in euthyroid patients (1)[A].

PATIENT EDUCATION
- Stress importance of compliance with thyroid replacement therapy.
- Explain need for lifelong treatment.
- Further education required for patients taking multiple medications that may interact
- Instruct to report to physician any signs of infection or heart problems.
- Describe signs of thyrotoxicity.
- High-bulk diet may help avoid constipation.

PROGNOSIS
- Return to normal state is the rule.
- Relapses will occur if treatment is interrupted.
- If untreated, may progress to myxedema coma

COMPLICATIONS
- Hypothyroid patients (mild to moderate) tolerate surgery, with mortality and complications similar to euthyroid patients.
- Myxedema coma: mortality 30–60%
- Increased susceptibility to infection
- Megacolon
- Sexual dysfunction
- Organic psychosis with paranoia
- Infertility
- Hypersensitivity to opiates
- Treatment over long periods can lead to bone demineralization.
- Iatrogenic thyrotoxicosis can lead to AFib and osteoporosis.
- Can lead to adrenal crisis with vigorous treatment, especially in patients with undiagnosed polyendocrine syndromes
- Treatment-induced congestive heart failure in people with coronary artery disease
- Subclinical hypothyroidism is associated with increased ischemic heart disease and increased all-cause mortality in men but not in women.

REFERENCES
1. Garber JR, Cobin RH, Gharib H, et al. Clinical practice guidelines for hypothyroidism in adults: cosponsored by the American Association of Clinical Endocrinologist and the American Thyroid Association. *Thyroid.* 2012;22(12):1200–1235.
2. Cooper DS, Biondi B. Subclinical thyroid disease. *Lancet.* 2012;379(9821):1142–1154.
3. Khandelwal D, Tandon N. Overt and subclinical hypothyroidism: who to treat and how. *Drugs.* 2012;72(1):17–33.
4. Jonklaas J, Bianco AC, Bauer AJ, et al. Guidelines for the treatment of hypothyroidism: prepared by the American Thyroid Association Task Force on thyroid hormone replacement. *Thyroid.* 2014;24(12):1670–1751.
5. Villar HC, Saconato H, Valente O, et al. Thyroid hormone replacement for subclinical hypothyroidism. *Cochrane Database Syst Rev.* 2007;(3):CD003419.
6. Alexander EK, Marqusee E, Lawrence J, et al. Timing and magnitude of increases in levothyroxine requirements during pregnancy in women with hypothyroidism. *N Engl J Med.* 2004;351(3):241–249.

CODES

ICD10
- E03.9 Hypothyroidism, unspecified
- E06.3 Autoimmune thyroiditis
- E89.0 Postprocedural hypothyroidism

CLINICAL PEARLS

- Monitor TSH and free T_4 every 4 to 8 weeks after initiating treatment or after change in dose. Once stabilized, periodic TSH level should be done after 6 months and then at 12-month intervals, or more frequently if the clinical situation dictates otherwise (1)[B].
- Screening test: TSH levels (1)[A]
- Serum free T_3 or total T_3 should not be done to diagnose hypothyroidism (1)[A].
- Dosage requirements may vary with age, gender, residual secretory capacity of thyroid gland, other drugs being taken by patient, and intestinal function (1)[A].

H

Sahil Mullick, MD • Naureen Bashir Rafiq, MBBS, MD

BASICS

DESCRIPTION

A generalized skin reaction associated with various infectious (fungal, bacterial, viral, or parasitic) or inflammatory cutaneous conditions distant from the primary disease site (1)

- "Id" is often combined with a root to reflect the causative factor (i.e., bacterid, syphilid, and tuberculid). Dermatophytid is the most frequently referenced id reaction. A dermatophytid is an autosensitization reaction in which a secondary cutaneous reaction occurs at a site distant to a primary fungal infection. The eruption typically begins within 1 to 2 weeks of the onset of the main lesion or following exacerbation of the main lesion.
- Most commonly localized vesicular lesions, erythema nodosum, and erythema multiforme
- System(s) affected: skin/exocrine
- Synonym(s): dermatophytid, trichophytid, autoeczematization

EPIDEMIOLOGY

- Predominant age: all ages
- Predominant sex: male = female
- Predominant race: all races

Incidence
Unknown

Prevalence
Common

ETIOLOGY AND PATHOPHYSIOLOGY

Precise pathophysiology is uncertain. Circulating antigens may react with antibodies at sensitized areas of the skin. An abnormal immune recognition of autologous skin antigens may also occur. Inflammation may lower the irritation threshold of the skin, and hematogenous spread of cytokines from the primary site of inflammation may also play a role (1).

- Etiology
  - Infectious
    ○ Fungal infections: *Trichophyton mentagrophytes*, *Trichophyton rubrum*, *Epidermophyton floccosum*, and *Candida* spp.
    ○ Bacterial infections: *Streptococcus pyogenes*, *Staphylococcus aureus*, and *Mycobacterium tuberculosis*
    ○ Viral infections: HSV, *Molluscum contagiosum*, orf, and milker's nodules
    ○ Parasitic infections: *Sarcoptes scabiei* and *Leishmania* spp.
  - Allergic
    ○ Id reactions occur in patients with nickel and aluminum allergy.
  - Miscellaneous
    ○ Id reaction rarely develop due to retained postoperative sutures, ionizing radiation, and blunt trauma.
    ○ Rarely, id reaction has been documented in patients receiving intravesical BCG live therapy for transitional cell carcinoma.

RISK FACTORS

- Fungal infection of the skin, especially tinea pedis
- Stasis dermatitis

GENERAL PREVENTION

- Good skin hygiene (particularly in intertriginous areas) to minimize risk of developing fungal infections
- Promptly treat any developing fungal infection.

COMMONLY ASSOCIATED CONDITIONS

- Primary fungal infection
- Stasis dermatitis

DIAGNOSIS

HISTORY

Itchy rash: Inquire about presence of lesions (typically fungal or bacterial) that could have incited the id reaction in the preceding days to weeks.

PHYSICAL EXAM

- Common
  - Symmetric, pruritic vesicles on the palms and, most commonly, on lateral aspects of fingers
  - Tinea infection on the feet; contact or other eczematous dermatosis; bacterial, fungal, or viral infection of the skin
- Less common
  - Papules
  - Lichenoid eruption
- Eczematoid eruption

DIFFERENTIAL DIAGNOSIS

- Pompholyx (dyshidrotic eczema)
- Contact dermatitis
- Drug eruptions
- Pustular psoriasis
- Folliculitis
- Scabies

DIAGNOSTIC TESTS & INTERPRETATION

- Potassium hydroxide (KOH) or fungal culture of primary lesion
- No fungal elements are present at the site of the id reaction.
- Special tests: Skin shows a positive trichophyton reaction. A wheal >10 mm at 20 minutes and induration >5 mm at 72 hours is a positive response.

Follow-Up Tests & Special Considerations

- The id reaction resolves with successful eradication of the primary skin condition.
- It is important to distinguish dermatophytids from drug-induced allergic reactions, as continued treatment is essential to clear the underlying infection.

Test Interpretation
Histology

- Vesicles in the upper dermis
- Superficial perivascular lymphohistiocytic infiltrate with small numbers of eosinophils and increased granular cell layer
- No infectious agents present in biopsy specimen

TREATMENT

GENERAL MEASURES

- Outpatient treatment of the underlying infection or eczematous dermatitis
- Symptomatic treatment of pruritus with antihistamines and/or topical steroids if needed (may require class 1 or 2 steroid)
- Treatment for secondary bacterial infection

MEDICATION

First Line
- PO antihistamines for pruritus (2)
  - Chlorpheniramine: 4 mg PO q4–6h PRN; max 24 mg/24 hr; (pediatric: 6 to 11 years 2 mg PO q4–6h PRN; max 12 mg/24 hr; ≥12 years, refer to adult dosing)
  - Diphenhydramine: 25 to 50 mg PO q4–6h PRN; max 400 mg/24 hr; (pediatric: 5 mg/kg/24 hr divided q6h PRN; 2 to 5 years max 37.5 mg/24 hr; 6 to 11 years max 150 mg/24 hr; ≥12 years, refer to adult dosing)
  - Hydroxyzine: 25 to 100 mg PO q6–8h PRN; max 600 mg/24 hr; (pediatric: 2 mg/kg/24 hr divided q6h PRN)
- Topical treatments for pruritus
  - Triamcinolone 0.1% ointment TID
  - Hydrocortisone 0.5%, 1%, 2.5%: up to QID
  - Capsaicin 0.025%, 0.075% cream: Apply TID–QID; EMLA (2.5% lidocaine + 2.5% prilocaine) applied 30 to 60 minutes prior to capsaicin may minimize burning.
  - Doxepin 5% cream: Apply QID for up to 8 days (to max of 10% of the body).
  - Permethrin 5% cream (for scabies)
    ◦ Apply from neck down after bath.
    ◦ Wash off thoroughly with water in 8 to 12 hours.
    ◦ May repeat in 7 days
  - Permethrin 1% cream rinse (for lice)
    ◦ Shampoo, rinse, towel dry, saturate hair and scalp (or other affected area), leave on 10 minutes, then rinse.
    ◦ May repeat in 7 days
  - White petroleum emollients: Apply after short bath/shower in warm (not hot) water.
- Systemic steroids only if reaction is severe or generalized (e.g., prednisone 20 mg)

Second Line
- Topical and/or systemic antifungals for identified associated fungal infection (common)
  - Tinea cruris/corporis
    ◦ Topical azole antifungal compounds econazole (Spectazole) and ketoconazole (Nizoral): usually applied BID for 2 to 4 weeks
    ◦ Terbinafine (Lamisil): over-the-counter (OTC) compound; can be applied daily or BID for 1 to 2 weeks
    ◦ Butenafine (Mentax): applied once daily for 2 weeks; also very effective
  - Tinea capitis
    ◦ PO griseofulvin for *Trichophyton* and *Microsporum* sp.; microsized preparation available; dosage 20 to 25 mg/kg/day divided BID or as a single dose daily for 6 to 12 weeks
    ◦ PO terbinafine can be used for *Trichophyton* sp. at 62.5 mg/day in patients weighing 10 to 20 kg, 125 mg/day if weight 20 to 40 kg, 250 mg/day if weight >40 kg, and use for 4 to 6 weeks.
- Topical or systemic antibiotics for any secondary bacterial infection
- Treatment with antiviral agents for erythema multiforme associated with HSV is required.

 ONGOING CARE

PATIENT EDUCATION
Avoid hot, humid conditions that promote fungal growth. Aerate susceptible body areas (e.g., wear sandals or open footwear). If possible, wear loose-fitting clothing and undergarments, dry wet skin after bathing, and use powders and antiperspirants to discourage fungal growth. Treat primary dermatitis promptly.

PROGNOSIS
After appropriate treatment, complete resolution in days to weeks

COMPLICATIONS
- Secondary bacterial infection (cellulitis)
- After resolution of dermatophytid, postinflammatory hyperpigmentation is common and disappears without treatment in 1 month.

REFERENCES
1. Ilkit M, Durdu M, Karakaş M. Cutaneous id reactions: a comprehensive review of clinical manifestations, epidemiology, etiology, and management. *Crit Rev Microbiol*. 2012;38(3):191–202.
2. Cotes ME, Swerlick RA. Practical guidelines for the use of steroid-sparing agents in the treatment of chronic pruritus. *Dermatol Ther*. 2013;26(2): 120–134.

ADDITIONAL READING
- Elmariah SB, Lerner EA. Topical therapies for pruritus. *Semin Cutan Med Surg*. 2011;30(2):118–126.
- Paulsen LL, Geller DD, Guggenbiller M. Symmetrical vesicular eruption on the palms. *Am Fam Physician*. 2012;85(8):811–812.
- Stachler RJ, Al-khudari S. Differential diagnosis in allergy. *Otolaryngol Clin North Am*. 2011;44(3): 561–590, vii–viii.
- Veien NK. Acute and recurrent vesicular hand dermatitis. *Dermatol Clin*. 2009;27(3):337–353, vii.
- Yosipovitch G, Bernhard JD. Clinical practice. Chronic pruritus. *N Engl J Med*. 2013;368(17):1625–1634.

 CODES

ICD10
- L30.2 Cutaneous autosensitization
- B35.9 Dermatophytosis, unspecified

CLINICAL PEARLS
- When one skin eruption follows another closely in time, consider an id reaction.
- When assessing an itchy rash, inquire about potential fungal or bacterial lesions in the preceding days to weeks as a potential prelude to the id reaction.

IMMUNE THROMBOCYTOPENIA (ITP)

William A. Stevens, MD • Khalid A. Jaboori, MD, MPH

 BASICS

DESCRIPTION
- Immune thrombocytopenia (ITP) is a condition characterized by the immunologic destruction of platelets and/or impaired thrombopoiesis in response to an unknown stimulus.
- ITP is classified by the following:
  - Age: adult or pediatric
  - Phases: newly diagnosed (<3 months), persistent, and chronic (>12 months)
  - Etiology: primary (idiopathic) or secondary when occurring in association with another disorder
- ITP is a relatively common disease of childhood that typically follows a viral infection. Onset is within 1 week, and spontaneous resolution occurs within 2 months in 83% of patients.
- In adults, ITP is usually a chronic disease and spontaneous remission is rare.
- System(s) affected: heme, lymphatic, immunologic
- Synonym(s): idiopathic thrombocytopenic purpura; immune thrombocytopenic purpura; and Werlhof disease

EPIDEMIOLOGY
- Peak age
  - Pediatric ITP: 2 to 4 years
  - Chronic ITP: >50 years with incidence two times higher in persons 60 years than those <60 years of age
- Predominant gender
  - Pediatric ITP: male = female
  - Chronic ITP: female > male (1.2 to 1.7:1)

Incidence
- Pediatric acute ITP: 1.9 to 6.4/100,000 children/year (1)
- Adult ITP: 3.3/100,000 per year

Prevalence
Limited data. In one population (in Oklahoma) (2):
- Overall prevalence of 11.2/100,000 persons
- In children (<16 years): 8.1/100,000 with average age of 6 years
- In adults (>16 years): 12.1/100,000 persons with average age of 55 years

ETIOLOGY AND PATHOPHYSIOLOGY
- Accelerated platelet uptake and destruction by reticuloendothelial phagocytes results from action of IgG autoantibodies against platelet membrane glycoproteins IIb/IIIa. There is also cell-mediated platelet destruction by CD8+ T cells.
- Autoantibodies interfere with megakaryocyte maturation, resulting in decreased production.

RISK FACTORS
- Autoimmune thrombocytopenia (e.g., Evan syndrome)
- Common variable immune deficiency
- Drug side effect (e.g., quinidine, gold, penicillin, procainamide, methyldopa, sulfamethoxazole)
- Infections: *Helicobacter pylori*, hepatitis C, HIV, CMV, and varicella zoster
- Vaccination side effect
- Bone marrow transplantation side effect
- Connective tissue disease, such as systemic lupus erythematosus, antiphospholipid antibody syndrome
- Lymphoproliferative disorders

COMMONLY ASSOCIATED CONDITIONS
- Viral infections, such as measles, rubella, varicella, influenza, and EBV
- Live virus vaccinations carry a lower risk than natural viral infection: 2.6/100,000 cases MMR vaccine doses versus 6 to 1,200/100,000 cases of natural rubella or measles infections

 DIAGNOSIS

A careful history, physical exam, and review of CBC and peripheral blood smear remain the key components of the diagnosis of ITP.

HISTORY
- Often asymptomatic; found incidentally on routine CBC
- Posttraumatic bleeding occurs at counts of 40 to 60×10^9/L.
- With counts <30×10^9/L, bruising tendency, epistaxis, menorrhagia, and gingival bleeding are common.
- GI bleeding, hematuria, and hemoptysis are less common.
- Spontaneous bleeding may occur with platelet count <20×10^9/L.
- Intracerebral bleeding is rare and may occur with counts <20×10^9/L and associated trauma or vascular lesions, resulting in neurologic symptoms.
- Constitutional symptoms are absent. Symptoms are varied and most are asymptomatic at time of diagnosis.

PHYSICAL EXAM
- Ecchymoses, petechiae, epistaxis, and bleeding from the gums are common.
- Abnormal uterine bleeding may be present.
- Hemorrhagic bullae on buccal mucosa reflect acute, severe thrombocytopenia.
- Absence of splenomegaly, hepatomegaly, lymphadenopathy, stigmata of congenital disease

DIFFERENTIAL DIAGNOSIS
- Acute leukemia
- Thrombotic thrombocytopenic purpura
- Hemolytic uremic syndrome
- Factitious: platelet clumping on peripheral smear
- Thrombocytopenia secondary to sepsis
- Myelodysplastic syndrome, particularly in older patients
- Decreased marrow production: malignancy, drugs, viruses, megaloblastic anemia
- Posttransfusion
- Gestational thrombocytopenia
- Isoimmune neonatal purpura
- Congenital thrombocytopenias
- Disseminated intravascular coagulation
- Alcohol-induced thrombocytopenic purpura

DIAGNOSTIC TESTS & INTERPRETATION
Initial Tests (lab, imaging)
- CBC with differential and peripheral smear:
  - Isolated decreased platelet count <100×10^9/L
  - Giant platelets are usually present.
  - Normal red and white blood cell morphology
- For patients with history, exam, CBC, and peripheral smear typical of ITP, consider the following:
  - PT/PTT is normal.

- In adults, serologies for hepatitis B, hepatitis C, and HIV infections are recommended (3)[B].
- In pediatric ITP, immunoglobulin levels to exclude common variable immunodeficiency are commonly obtained (3)[B].
- Other tests are not necessary for patients with typical ITP presentation: antiplatelet, antinuclear, antiphospholipid antibodies; *H. pylori* testing; thrombopoietin; platelet parameters; direct antiglobulin test; reticulocyte count; urinalysis; and thyroid function tests (3)[C]

Diagnostic Procedures/Other
- Imaging is not necessary.
- Bone marrow aspiration/biopsy
  - Not necessary for diagnosis (pediatric (3)[B]; adult (3)[C])
  - Can be considered for a patient with atypical symptoms, such as fever and weight loss and multiple abnormalities in blood count

Test Interpretation
- Peripheral smear: normal red and white cells with large or giant platelets but diminished in number
- Marrow reveals abundant megakaryocytes with normal erythroid and myeloid precursors.

 TREATMENT

GENERAL MEASURES
- Management with observation alone in children with no or mild bruising or petechiae regardless of platelet count (3)
- Outpatient management unless patient has platelet count <20×10^9/L and is at risk for bleeding (3).
- Admit patients with active bleeding.

MEDICATION
First Line
- Pediatric
  - First-line treatment:
    - For children with no or mild bleeding (bruising and petechiae only with no mucosal bleeding), observation alone regardless of platelet count (3)[B]
    - For children with significant bleeding
      - Single-dose intravenous immunoglobulin (IVIG) 0.8 to 1 g/kg, especially when a more rapid increase in platelet count is desired (3)[B]. Do not administer in patients with IgA deficiencies because of anaphylaxis risk.
      - A short course of corticosteroids (e.g., PO prednisone 2 mg/kg/day for 2 weeks with 3 weeks taper) (3)[B]
      - For nonsplenectomized children who are Rh-positive, single dose of anti-Rho(D) immunoglobulin (anti-D), 50 to 75 g/kg. Do not use in children with low hemoglobin or evidence of hemolysis (3)[B].
  - Second and other treatments for pediatric and adolescent persons with ITP (3)
    - Splenectomy for chronic or persistent ITP (3)[B]
    - Rituximab (Rituxan) 375 mg/m² weekly for 4 weeks (3)[C]
    - High-dose dexamethasone 0.6 mg/kg/day for 4 days every 4 weeks (3)[C]
    - Others without adequate data: azathioprine, cyclosporin A, danazol, mycophenolate mofetil, anti-CD52 monoclonal antibody, and interferon

- Adult
  - First line, adult ITP
    - Treatment is recommended for newly diagnosed patients with platelet count $<30 \times 10^9$/L (3)[C].
    - PO prednisone 1 to 2 mg/kg/day for 21 days then tapered (3)[B]
    - PO dexamethasone 40 mg daily for 4 days given every 2 to 4 weeks until platelets above 50×10^9/L (3)[B]
    - If corticosteroids are contraindicated:
      - IVIG: 1 to 2 g/kg once, repeating as necessary (3)[C]
      - OR anti-D: 50 to 75 μg/kg once, repeating as necessary for Rh$^+$, nonsplenectomized patients. Do not use anti-D in patients with low hemoglobin or evidence of hemolysis (3)[C].
  - Second line, adult ITP
    - Splenectomy for patients who failed corticosteroid therapy (3)[B]
    - For patients whom splenectomy is contraindicated, thrombopoietin receptor agonists (3)[B]: eltrombopag (Promacta), 50 mg/day PO OR romiplostim (Nplate), 1 μg/kg SC weekly; may be used for patients at high risk of bleeding.
    - Rituximab: 375 mg/m^2 IV weekly for 4 weeks, for patients at high risk of bleeding who have failed one line of therapy or post splenectomy (3)[C]
    - Consider combination therapy with dexamethasone and rituximab (4)[C].
    - Thrombopoietin receptor agonists can be considered for patients at risk of bleeding who failed first line of therapy (3)[C].
    - Others to consider: azathioprine, cyclosporine A, cyclophosphamide, danazol, dapsone, mycophenolate mofetil, and vincristine
- ITP in pregnancy
  - Preeclampsia or gestational thrombocytopenia may cause thrombocytopenia unrelated to ITP.
  - Corticosteroids or IVIG are considered safe and are considered first line (4)[C].
  - DO NOT USE danazol or cyclophosphamide
  - ITP management at time of delivery is based on maternal bleeding risks, and mode of delivery should be based on obstetric indications (4)[C]. Platelet autoantibodies can cross the placenta and cause neonatal thrombocytopenia.
  - Caesarean section can be considered if platelet count $>50 \times 10^9$/L.
  - Prednisone and/or IVIG may be considered 2 to 3 weeks prior to delivery.
- ITP secondary to HIV
  - Antivirals should be considered before other treatment (3)[C].
  - If treatment is required, corticosteroids, IVIG, or anti-D are first-line options; and splenectomy is a second-line option (3)[C].
- ITP secondary to HCV
  - Antivirals should be considered before other treatment (3)[C].
  - If treatment required, IVIG is initial treatment (3)[C].
- EMERGENCY TREATMENT
  - Patients with intracranial or GI bleeding, massive hematuria, internal hematoma, or who need emergent surgery.
  - IV corticosteroids (e.g., IV methylprednisolone, 1 g/day for 3 doses (3)[B] with caution in patients with GI bleeding and/or IVIG 1 g/kg, repeat following day for count $<50 \times 10^9$/L (3)[B].
  - Platelet transfusions with IVIG may also be considered for significant bleeding (3)[C].

- Other agents that may be considered: Recombinant factor VIIa (3)[C] not only promotes hemostasis but also increases risk of thrombosis. Efficacy of antifibrinolytic agents, aminocaproic acids, and tranexamic acid, is unproved; they may be used as adjunctive treatments only. Emergent splenectomy has been reported.

ISSUES FOR REFERRAL
Hematology consultation is recommended for acute bleeding or for those who fail to respond to first-line therapies.

ADDITIONAL THERAPIES
Proprietary traditional Chinese medicines: Dihuang Zhixue (blend of Rehmannia root and others herbs) showed benefit for childhood refractory ITP in a single, small, randomized controlled trial (5); limited evidence for Kami-kihi-to, minor decoction of *Bupleurum*, replenishing qi and tonifying kidney, roasted licorice decoction, Sairei-to, Shengxueling, and Zhinu-I and Zhinu-II (6). Unclear evidence for active hexose correlated compound, berberine, dong quai, ginseng, licorice, melatonin, and periwinkle (7).

SURGERY/OTHER PROCEDURES
Splenectomy

- Mortality rate is very low ($<1\%$) even in patients with severe thrombocytopenia.
- Necessary vaccinations prior to splenectomy: polyvalent pneumococcal vaccine and quadrivalent meningococcal vaccine every 3 to 5 years and one-time *Haemophilus influenzae B* (Hib).
- Consider lifelong prophylactic antibiotics with penicillin or erythromycin.
- Should raise the platelet count to at least 20×10^9/L prior to surgery
- Reported 5- to 10-year efficacy is ~65% for all patients.
- Laparoscopic splenectomy has similar long-term outcomes compared to open splenectomy and has better short-term outcomes (8)[C].

 ONGOING CARE

FOLLOW-UP RECOMMENDATIONS
Patient Monitoring
Platelet counts weekly for patients on prednisone and monthly for stable patients are reasonable.

DIET
- Evidence demonstrating benefit of an anti-inflammatory diet in ITP is lacking.
- The following foods and supplements can cause significant bleeding: garlic, ginger, *Ginkgo biloba*, and saw palmetto
- Some foods and supplements that may inhibit platelets: evening primrose oil, fish oil, feverfew, ginseng, licorice, soy, vitamin C, vitamin E, and wintergreen
- Partial list of foods and supplements with coumarin or salicylate components: alfalfa, angelica, anise, asafetida, aspen bark, birch, black cohosh, celery, chamomile, cinnamon, dandelion, fenugreek, heartsease, horse chestnut, meadowsweet, poplar, prickly ash, *Quassia*, sarsaparilla, sweet birch, sweet clover, and willow bark.

PATIENT EDUCATION
- Modified activity to prevent injury or bruising; avoid contact sports.
- Avoid anticoagulants, aspirin and other platelet-inhibiting drugs, and NSAIDs.

PROGNOSIS
- Acute ITP
  - ~80–85% of patients completely recover within 2 months.
  - 15% proceed to chronic ITP.
- Chronic ITP
  - ~10–20% of the patients recover spontaneously.
  - Remainder with diminished platelets for months to years
  - May see spontaneous remissions (5%) and relapses
- ~10% are refractory (fail medical therapy and splenectomy).

COMPLICATIONS
- Related to thrombocytopenia: 1% mortality due to intracranial hemorrhage and severe blood loss
- Related to treatment: for example, corticosteroid adverse effects, anaphylaxis and renal failure with IVIG, hepatotoxicity with eltrombopag, reports of progressive multifocal leukoencephalopathy with rituximab, hemolysis with anti-D, and septicemia for splenectomized patients

REFERENCES
1. Terrell DR, Beebe LA, Vesely SK, et al. The incidence of immune thrombocytopenic purpura in children and adults: a critical review of published reports. *Am J Hematol*. 2010;85(3):174–180.
2. Terrell DR, Beebe LA, Neas BR, et al. Prevalence of primary immune thrombocytopenia in Oklahoma. *Am J Hematol*. 2012;87(9):848–852.
3. Neunert C, Lim W, Crowther M, et al. The American Society of Hematology 2011 evidence-based practice guideline for immune thrombocytopenia. *Blood*. 2011;117(16):4190–4207.
4. Gudbrandsdottir S, Birgens HS, Frederiksen H, et al. Rituximab and dexamethasone vs dexamethasone monotherapy in newly diagnosed patients with primary immune thrombocytopenia. *Blood*. 2013;121(11):1976–1981.
5. Liu QC, Wu WH, Wu DY, et al. Clinical observation on the treatment of childhood refractory idiopathic thrombocytopenic purpura with Dihuang Zhixue Capsule. *Chin J Integr Med*. 2008;14(2):132–136.
6. Platelet Disorder Support Association. http://www.pdsa.org/. Accessed August 10, 2014.
7. Natural Standard. https://naturalmedicines.therapeuticresearch.com/databases.aspx. Accessed August 10, 2014.
8. Qu Y, Xu J, Jiao C, et al. Long-term outcomes of laparoscopic splenectomy versus open splenectomy for idiopathic thrombocytopenic purpura. *Int Surg*. 2014;99(3):286–290.

CODES

ICD10
D69.3 Immune thrombocytopenic purpura

CLINICAL PEARLS
- ITP: platelet counts of $<100 \times 10^9$/L caused by accelerated destruction and/or impaired thrombopoiesis by antiplatelet antibodies
- Pediatric ITP: relatively common, with spontaneous remission in 2 months
- Adult ITP: usually persistent; requires treatment, with rare spontaneous remission

IMPETIGO
Elisabeth L. Backer, MD

 BASICS

DESCRIPTION

- A contagious, superficial, intraepidermal infection occurring prominently on exposed areas of the face and extremities, most often seen in children
- Infected patients usually have multiple lesions.
- Cultures are positive in >80% cases for *Staphylococcus aureus* either alone or combined with group A β-hemolytic streptococci; *S. aureus* is the more common pathogen since the 1990s.
- Nonbullous impetigo: most common form of impetigo. Formation of vesiculopustules that rupture, leading to crusting with a characteristic golden appearance; local lymphadenopathy may occur.
- Bullous impetigo: staphylococcal impetigo that progresses rapidly from small to large flaccid bullae (newborns/young children) caused by epidermolytic toxin release; less lymphadenopathy; trunk more often affected; <30% of patients
- Folliculitis: considered by some to be *S. aureus* impetigo of hair follicles
- Ecthyma: a deeper, ulcerated impetigo infection often with lymphadenitis
- System(s) affected: skin/exocrine
- Synonym(s): pyoderma; impetigo contagiosa; impetigo vulgaris; fox impetigo

EPIDEMIOLOGY

Incidence
- Predominant sex: male = female
- Predominant age: children ages 2 to 5 years

Prevalence
In the United States: not reported but common

Pediatric Considerations
- Poststreptococcal glomerulonephritis may follow impetigo (in young children).
- Impetigo neonatorum may occur due to nursery contamination.

ETIOLOGY AND PATHOPHYSIOLOGY
- Coagulase-positive staphylococci: pure culture ~50–90%; more contagious via contact
- β-Hemolytic streptococci: pure culture only ~10% of the time (primarily group A)

- Mixed infections of streptococci and staphylococci are common; data suggest increasing importance of staphylococci over the past 20 years.
- Direct contact or insect vector
- Can result from contamination at trauma site
- Regional lymphadenopathy

RISK FACTORS
- Warm, humid environment
- Tropical or subtropical climate
- Summer or fall season
- Minor trauma, insect bites, breaches in skin
- Poor hygiene, poverty, crowding, epidemics, wartime
- Familial spread
- Poor health with anemia and malnutrition
- Complication of pediculosis, scabies, chickenpox, eczema/atopic dermatitis
- Contact dermatitis (*Rhus* spp.)
- Burns
- Contact sports
- Children in daycare
- Possibly tobacco exposure
- Carriage of group A *Streptococcus* and *Staphylococcus aureus*

GENERAL PREVENTION
- Close attention to family hygiene, particularly hand washing among children
- Covering of wounds
- Avoidance of crowding and sharing of personal items
- Treatment of atopic dermatitis

COMMONLY ASSOCIATED CONDITIONS
- Malnutrition and anemia
- Crowded living conditions
- Poor hygiene
- Neglected minor trauma
- Any chronic/underlying dermatitis

 DIAGNOSIS

HISTORY
- Lesions are often described as painful.
- May be slow and indolent or rapidly spreading
- Most frequent on face around mouth and nose or at site of trauma

PHYSICAL EXAM
- Tender red macules or papules as early lesions (contact dermatitis presents with pruritic lesions)
- Thin-roofed vesicles to bullae: usually nontender
- Pustules
- Weeping, shallow, red ulcers
- Honey-colored crusts
- Satellite lesions
- Often multiple sites
- Bullae on buttocks, trunk, face

DIFFERENTIAL DIAGNOSIS
- Nonbullous
  - Contact dermatitis
  - Chickenpox
  - Herpes
  - Folliculitis
  - Erysipelas
  - Insect bites
  - Severe eczematous dermatitis
  - Scabies
  - Tinea corporis
- Bullous
  - Burns
  - Pemphigus vulgaris
  - Bullous pemphigoid
- Stevens-Johnson syndrome

DIAGNOSTIC TESTS & INTERPRETATION

Initial Tests (lab, imaging)
- None usually done; cultures of pus/bullae fluid may be helpful if no response to empiric therapy.
  - Culture: taken from the base of lesion after removal of crust will grow both staphylococci and group A streptococci
  - Antistreptolysin-O (ASO) titer: can be weak positive for streptococci but overall not useful
  - Antideoxyribonuclease B (anti-DNase B) and antihyaluronidase (AHT) response more reliable than ASO response
  - Streptozyme: positive for streptococci
- Disorders that may alter lab results: Streptococcal pharyngitis will alter streptococcal enzyme tests.

Follow-Up Tests & Special Considerations
- Monitor for spread of disease and systemic manifestations.
- Serologic testing is helpful in context of impetigo with subsequent poststreptococcal glomerulonephritis.

TREATMENT

GENERAL MEASURES
- Treatment speeds healing and avoids spread of disease.
- Prevent with mupirocin or triple antibiotic ointment TID to sites of minor skin trauma.
- Remove crusts; clean with gentle washing 2 to 3 times daily; and clean with antibacterial soap, chlorhexidine, or Betadine.
- Washing of entire body may prevent recurrence at distant sites.

MEDICATION
- In 2005, the Infectious Diseases Society of America (IDSA) recommended topical treatment for limited lesions and oral medication when the disease is more severe/extensive (1)[A].
- Optimal treatment is unclear due to limited quality of evidence. Treatment reduces spread of infection and enhances resolution (2)[C].
- Penicillin and macrolide therapy is no longer recommended. Fluoroquinolones are not indicated due to resistance patterns.
- Consult the local hospital or health department for microbial resistance information.
- Nonbullous (minor spread, treat 7 days; widespread, treat 10 days); bullous (treat 10 days)
  - Retapamulin 1% ointment to be applied BID for 5 days
  - Mupirocin (Bactroban) 2% topical ointment applied TID for 5 to 7 days (nonbullous only); not as effective on scalp as around mouth
  - Dicloxacillin: adult 250 mg PO QID; pediatric <40 kg: 12 to 25 mg/kg/day divided q6h; >40 kg: 125 to 250 q6h
- Dicloxacillin, cephalexin, topical mupirocin, and fusidic acid are effective unless local staphylococcal strains are resistant. (For methicillin-resistant *S. aureus* [MRSA] infections, treatment options include clindamycin, tetracyclines, or trimethoprim-sulfamethoxazole.) Oral doses given for 7 days are usually sufficient (3)[C].
- 1st-generation cephalosporins
  - Children
    - Cephalexin 25 to 50 mg/kg/day divided, q6–12h
    - Cefaclor 20 to 40 mg/kg/day divided q8h
    - Cephradine 25 to 50 mg/kg/day divided q6–12h
    - Cefadroxil 30 mg/kg/day divided BID
  - Adults
    - Cephalexin 250 mg up to QID
    - Cefaclor 250 mg TID
    - Cephradine 500 mg BID
    - Cefadroxil 1 g/day in divided doses
- Clindamycin 300 mg q6–8h
- Severe bullous disease may require IV therapy such as nafcillin or cefazolin.

ISSUES FOR REFERRAL
If resistant or extensive infections occur, especially in immunocompromised patients

ADDITIONAL THERAPIES
Monitor for microbial resistance patterns.

ONGOING CARE

FOLLOW-UP RECOMMENDATIONS
- Athletes are restricted from contact sports.
- School and daycare contagious restrictions
- Children can return to school 24 hours after initiation of antimicrobial treatment.

Patient Monitoring
If not clear within 7 to 10 days, culture the lesions.

PATIENT EDUCATION
Avoidance of infection spread is the key; hand washing is vital, especially for reducing spread in children.

PROGNOSIS
- Complete resolution in 7 to 10 days with treatment
- Antibiotic treatment will not prevent or halt glomerulonephritis, as it will rheumatic fever.
- If not clear within 7 to 10 days, culture is necessary to find resistant organism.
- Recurrent impetigo: Evaluate for carriage of *S. aureus* in nares (also perineum, axillae, toe web). Apply mupirocin ointment to nares BID for 5 days for clearance/decolonization.

COMPLICATIONS
- Ecthyma
- Erysipelas
- Poststreptococcal acute glomerulonephritis
- Cellulitis
- Bacteremia
- Osteomyelitis
- Septic arthritis
- Pneumonia
- Lymphadenitis

REFERENCES
1. Koning S, van der Sande R, Verhagen AP, et al. Interventions for impetigo. *Cochrane Database Syst Rev*. 2012;(1):CD003261.
2. Stevens DL, Bisno AL, Chambers HF, et al. Practice guidelines for the diagnosis and management of skin and soft-tissue infections: 2014 update by the Infectious Diseases Society of America. *Clin Infect Dis*. 2014;59(2):147–159.
3. Del Giudice P, Hubiche P. Community-associated methicillin-resistant *Staphylococcus aureus* and impetigo. *Br J Dermatol*. 2010;162(4):905.

ADDITIONAL READING
- George A, Rubin G. A systematic review and meta-analysis of treatments for impetigo. *Br J Gen Pract*. 2003;53(491):480–487.
- Parish LC, Jorizzo JL, Breton JJ, et al. Topical retapamulin ointment (1%, wt/wt) twice daily for 5 days versus oral cephalexin twice daily for 10 days in the treatment of secondarily infected dermatitis: results of a randomized controlled trial. *J Am Acad Dermatol*. 2006;55(6):1003–1013.
- Stanley JR, Amagai M. Pemphigus, bullous impetigo, and the staphylococcal scalded-skin syndrome. *N Engl J Med*. 2006;355(17):1800–1810.

SEE ALSO

Algorithm: Rash, Focal

CODES

ICD10
- L01.00 Impetigo, unspecified
- L01.01 Non-bullous impetigo
- L01.03 Bullous impetigo

CLINICAL PEARLS
- Superficial, intraepidermal infection
- Predominantly staphylococcal in origin
- Microbial resistance patterns need to be monitored.
- Topical treatment is recommended for limited lesions and oral medication only when the disease is more severe/extensive.

INCONTINENCE, FECAL

Kalyanakrishnan Ramakrishnan, MD

BASICS

Continuous or recurrent involuntary passage of fecal material for >1 month in individual at least 4 years of age

- Involves recurrent, involuntary loss of solid/liquid stool
- Requires careful rectal exam to assess rectal tone, voluntary squeeze, and rule out overflow incontinence from fecal impaction
- Endorectal ultrasound (EUS) is the simplest, most reliable and least invasive method to detect anatomic anal sphincter defects.
- The goal of treatment is to restore continence and/or improve quality of life.

DESCRIPTION
Major incontinence is the involuntary evacuation of feces. Minor incontinence (fecal soilage) includes incontinence to flatus and occasional seepage of liquid stool.

Geriatric Considerations
- The prevalence of fecal incontinence increases with age. It is an important cause of nursing home placement among the elderly.
- Idiopathic fecal incontinence is more common in older women.

EPIDEMIOLOGY
Incidence
Patients will not report fecal incontinence unless specifically queried ("silent affliction"). The number of patients affected is likely significantly underestimated.

Prevalence
- In younger persons: women > men
- 8% of adults
- 15% of adults age >70 years
- 56–66% of hospitalized older patients and >50% of nursing home residents
- 50–70% of patients who have urinary incontinence also suffer from fecal incontinence.

Pregnancy Considerations
Obstetric injury to the pelvic floor may result in either temporary incontinence or persistent incontinence.

Geriatric Considerations
- Fecal impaction and overflow diarrhea leading to fecal incontinence is common in older patients.
- Surgical history—particularly anal surgery, including hemorrhoidectomy, anal fissure repair (sphincterotomy), anal dilatation, or prior pelvic floor surgeries

ETIOLOGY AND PATHOPHYSIOLOGY
- Continence requires complex orchestration of pelvic musculature, nerves, and reflex arcs.
- Stool volume and consistency, colonic transit time, anorectal sensation, rectal compliance, anorectal reflexes, external and internal sphincter muscle tone, puborectalis muscle function, and mental capacity each play a role in maintaining fecal continence.
- Disease processes or structural defects impacting any of these factors may contribute to fecal incontinence.
- Diabetes is the most common metabolic disorder leading to fecal incontinence through pudendal nerve neuropathy.
- Congenital: spina bifida and myelomeningocele with spinal cord damage
- Trauma: anal sphincter damage from vaginal delivery or surgical procedures

- Medical: diabetes, stroke, spinal cord trauma, degenerative disorders of the nervous system, inflammatory conditions, rectal neoplasia

RISK FACTORS
- Functional status—older age, female sex, obesity, limited physical activity contribute to poor functional status
- Neuropsychiatric conditions (dementia, depression)
- Multiple sclerosis, spinal cord injury, stroke, diabetic neuropathy
- Prostatectomy, radiation
- Trauma: Risk factors for perineal trauma at the time of vaginal delivery include occipitoposterior presentation, prolonged second stage of labor, assisted vaginal delivery (forceps or vacuum-assist), and episiotomy.
- Diarrhea, inflammatory bowel disease (IBD), irritable bowel syndrome (IBS), menopause, smoking, constipation
- Potential association with child abuse and sexual abuse
- Congenital abnormalities, such as imperforate anus/rectal prolapse
- Fecal impaction

GENERAL PREVENTION
- Behavioral and lifestyle changes: Obesity, limited physical activity/exercise, poor diet, and smoking are modifiable risk factors.
- Postmeal bowel regimen—defecate regularly after meals to maximize effect of gastrocolic reflex.
- Pelvic floor muscle training during and after pregnancy and pelvic surgery
- Increase fiber intake (>30 g/day)

COMMONLY ASSOCIATED CONDITIONS
- Age >70 years
- Urinary incontinence/pelvic organ prolapse
- Chronic medical conditions—diabetes mellitus, dementia, stroke, spinal cord compression, depression, immobility, chronic obstructive pulmonary disease, IBS, and IBD
- Perineal trauma (obstetric)
- Anorectal surgery
- History of pelvic/rectal irradiation

DIAGNOSIS

Diagnosis is based on history and physical findings.

HISTORY
- Patients seldom volunteer information about fecal incontinence. Direct questioning is important.
- Problem-specific history includes (1)[C]:
  - Severity of soiling by liquid stool or gross incontinence of solid stool
  - Onset and duration (recent onset vs. chronic)
  - Frequency, presence of constipation/diarrhea
- Medication review
- Review diet, medical and obstetric history, lifestyle, and mobility.
- Evaluate for social withdrawal and depression.

PHYSICAL EXAM
- Inspect the perineum for chemical dermatitis, hemorrhoids, fistula, surgical scars, skin tags, rectal prolapse, soiling, and ballooning of the perineum (sarcopenia of pelvic musculature).
- A patulous anal orifice may indicate myopathy or a neurologic disorder.

- Evaluate the external sphincter response to perineal skin stimulation (anal wink). Absence suggests neuropathy.
- Ask the patient to bear down, preferably in standing position, to assess for rectal prolapse.
- Digital rectal exam to assess anal canal pressure sphincter tone, rectal bleeding, hemorrhoids, neoplasm, fecal consistency, and diarrhea/distal fecal impaction.
- General neurologic examination, including perianal sensation (1)[C]
- Evaluate mental status.

DIFFERENTIAL DIAGNOSIS
- Anorectal disorders
  - Inflammatory/infectious disorders
  - Neoplasms, radiation proctitis, ischemic colitis, fistulas
  - Prolapsed internal hemorrhoids; rectal prolapse
  - Trauma: obstetric, surgical, radiation, accidental, sexual
- Neurologic disorders
  - Stroke, dementia, neoplasms, spinal cord injury, and/or diseases causing altered level of consciousness
  - Pudendal neuropathy, neurosyphilis, multiple sclerosis, diabetes mellitus
- Miscellaneous causes
  - Infectious diarrhea, fecal impaction and overflow, IBS, laxative abuse, IBD, short bowel syndrome, myopathies, senescence and frailty, collagen vascular disease, psychological and behavioral problems

DIAGNOSTIC TESTS & INTERPRETATION
The approach to fecal incontinence in older patients should be individualized, minimally invasive, and practically feasible. History and physical exam are generally sufficient for diagnosis. If uncertainty remains, consider the following:

- EUS is the most reliable and least invasive test for defining anatomic defects in the external and internal anal sphincters, rectal wall, and the puborectalis muscle (1)[B]. EUS can predict therapeutic response to sphincteroplasty.

- Plain abdominal x-ray (impaction, constipation)
- Sigmoidoscopy/anoscopy/colonoscopy (colitis, neoplasm)

Initial Tests (lab, imaging)
- If history of travel, antibiotics, tube feedings, or signs and symptoms of sepsis, consider stool studies:
  - Culture
  - Ova and parasites
  - *Clostridium difficile* toxin assay
- Thyroid-stimulating hormone (TSH), electrolytes, and BUN in elderly patients
- EUS may demonstrate structural abnormalities of the anal sphincters, rectal wall, or puborectalis muscle.
- EUS may detect a sphincter injury in over 1/3 of primiparous vaginal deliveries and nearly half of multiparous vaginal deliveries.

Follow-Up Tests & Special Considerations
- Defecography can measure the anorectal angle, evaluate pelvic descent, and detect occult/overt rectal prolapse (2)[C].
- MRI defecography (dynamic MRI) can further define pelvic floor anatomy.

- Anorectal manometry: Measures parameters such as maximal resting anal pressure, amplitude and duration of squeeze pressure, the rectoanal inhibitory reflex, threshold of conscious rectal sensation, rectal compliance, and anorectal pressures during straining.
- Pudendal nerve terminal motor latency (PNTML): This technique is operator-dependent and has poor correlation with clinical and histologic findings.
- Electromyography: can assess neurogenic/myopathic damage

 TREATMENT

GENERAL MEASURES

- In ambulatory patients, scheduled (or prompted) defecation is effective, particularly in patients with overflow incontinence.
- Kegel exercises to strengthen pelvic floor
- If bed-bound, scheduled osmotic or stimulant laxatives for constipation
- Enemas, laxatives, and suppositories may help promote more complete bowel emptying in impacted patients while minimizing postdefecation leakage.
- Scheduled toileting and use of stool deodorants (Periwash, Derifil, Devrom).

MEDICATION

Limited evidence that antidiarrheals (loperamide, codeine) and drugs enhancing sphincter tone (phenylephrine gel, sodium valproate) are of benefit (3)[B]. Cholestyramine, colestipol useful in diarrhea following malabsorption or cholecystectomy; alosetron in diarrhea due to IBS, amitriptyline in idiopathic fecal incontinence

First Line
Specific treatment of underlying disorder (e.g., infectious diarrhea/IBD) may improve fecal continence.

Second Line
- Increasing dietary fiber in milder forms of fecal incontinence reduces symptoms (1)[B]. Stool-bulking agents include high-fiber diet, psyllium products, or methylcellulose.
- Antidiarrheal agents, such as adsorbents or opium derivatives, may reduce fecal incontinence (1)[C].
- Disimpact patients with fecal impaction and overflow incontinence and treat with a bowel regimen to prevent recurrence.

ADDITIONAL THERAPIES
- Biofeedback: initial treatment modality in motivated patients with some voluntary sphincter control (1)[C]; teaches patients to recognize rectal distension and contract the external anal sphincter while keeping intra-abdominal pressure low
- Biofeedback plus electrical stimulation is more effective than either alone.
- Patients with systemic neurologic disorders, anal deformities, or frequent episodes of incontinence respond poorly.

SURGERY/OTHER PROCEDURES
- Surgery should be considered only when nonsurgical approaches have failed.
- Sphincter repair should be offered for highly symptomatic patients with well-defined defect of external anal sphincter (1)[A].
- Injectable therapy (tissue-bulking agent injected into the anorectal submucosa or the intersphincteric space) appears safe and effective for patients with internal anal sphincter dysfunction (4)[B].

- Artificial anal sphincter implantation/dynamic graciloplasty (where gracilis muscle transposed into anus as modified sphincter) may be considered in patients with severe fecal incontinence and irreparable sphincter damage (5)[B].
- Stoma (colostomy/ileostomy) creation may be appropriate in patients with disabling fecal incontinence when other available therapeutic options have failed or if preferred by patient (1)[B].
- Anal plugs are available to minimize fecal leakage in patients who do not benefit from other treatment modalities, especially immobilized, institutionalized, or neurologically disabled patients; often poorly tolerated (6)[C].
- Sacral nerve stimulation (neuromodulation) via implantation of SC electrodes delivering low-amplitude electrical stimulation to sphincter muscles improves overall rectal tone, especially in patients with a coexistent sphincter defect (7)[B].
- SECCA PROCEDURE (radiofrequency anal sphincter remodeling)—temperature-controlled radiofrequency energy delivered to the anorectal junction distal to the dentate line causing tissue damage, scarring, and anal canal narrowing. Minimally invasive, ambulatory procedure useful in mild-to-moderate fecal incontinence (8)[C].
- Magnetic anal sphincter (MAS) devices—series of interlinked titanium beads (14 to 20) with internal magnetic cores placed to form a flexible ring that encircles the external anal sphincter 3 to 5 cm from the anal verge. During expulsion of feces, the beads separate allowing evacuation. After evacuation, the beads approximate and close the canal (9)[B]. Useful in moderate and severe incontinence

INPATIENT CONSIDERATIONS

Admission Criteria/Initial Stabilization
If secondary to fecal impaction, manual evacuation of fecal mass (after lubrication with lidocaine jelly)

Nursing
- Avoid catharsis.
- No hot water, soap, or hydrogen peroxide enemas.

Discharge Criteria
Outpatient care

 ONGOING CARE

FOLLOW-UP RECOMMENDATIONS
Periodic rectal exam

Patient Monitoring
Consider impaction if there is <1 bowel movement every other day with fecal incontinence.

DIET
- High fiber (20 to 30 g/day) and at least 1.5 L fluid daily
- Avoid precipitants (caffeine).

PATIENT EDUCATION
Kegel/sphincter training exercises are necessary but not sufficient for treating fecal incontinence.

PROGNOSIS
- Reimpaction likely if bowel regimen discontinued
- 50% failure rate over 5 years following overlapping sphincteroplasty

COMPLICATIONS
- Depression and social isolation
- Skin ulcerations
- Artificial bowel sphincter: infection, erosion, mechanical failure

REFERENCES

1. Tjandra JJ, Dykes SL, Kumar RR, et al. Practice parameters for the treatment of fecal incontinence. *Dis Colon Rectum*. 2007;50(10):1497–1507.
2. Vitton V, Vignally P, Barthet M, et al. Dynamic anal endosonography and MRI defecography in diagnosis of pelvic floor disorders: comparison with conventional defecography. *Dis Colon Rectum*. 2011;54(11):1398–1404.
3. Omar MI, Alexander CE. Drug treatment for faecal incontinence in adults. *Cochrane Database Syst Rev*. 2013;(6):CD002116.
4. Maeda Y, Laurberg S, Norton C. Perianal injectable bulking agents as treatment for faecal incontinence in adults. *Cochrane Database Syst Rev*. 2013;(2):CD007959.
5. Chapman AE, Geerdes B, Hewett P, et al. Systematic review of dynamic graciloplasty in the treatment of faecal incontinence. *Br J Surg*. 2002;89(2):138–153.
6. Deutekom M, Dobben AC. Plugs for containing faecal incontinence. *Cochrane Database Syst Rev*. 2012;(4):CD005086.
7. Ratto C, Litta F, Parello A, et al. Sacral nerve stimulation in faecal incontinence associated with an anal sphincter lesion: a systematic review. *Colorectal Dis*. 2012;14(6):e297–e304.
8. Frascio M, Mandolfino F, Imperatore M, et al. The SECCA procedure for faecal incontinence: a review. *Colorectal Dis*. 2014;16(3):167–172.
9. Lehur PA, McNevin S, Buntzen S, et al. Magnetic anal sphincter augmentation for the treatment of fecal incontinence: a preliminary report from a feasibility study. *Dis Colon Rectum*. 2010; 53(12):1604–1610.

ADDITIONAL READING

- Rao SSC. Current and emerging treatment options for fecal incontinence. *J Clin Gastroenterol*. 2014;48(9):752–764.
- Rao SSC. Fecal incontinence. In: Feldman M, Friedman LS, Brandt LJ, eds. *Sleisenger and Fordtran's Gastrointestinal and Liver Disease*. 9th ed. Philadelphia, PA: Saunders/Elsevier; 2010:247–258.

 CODES

ICD10
- R15.9 Full incontinence of feces
- R15.2 Fecal urgency
- R15.0 Incomplete defecation

CLINICAL PEARLS
- New onset fecal incontinence may indicate spinal cord compression if accompanied by other neurologic signs or symptoms.
- Differentiate true incontinence from pseudoincontinence (overflow or functional incontinence).
- Scheduled defecation after meals, bulking agents, and scheduled enemas minimize impaction and are helpful in mild/moderate fecal incontinence.

INCONTINENCE, URINARY ADULT FEMALE

Cara Marshall, MD

 BASICS

DESCRIPTION
- Urinary incontinence: involuntary loss of urine that is objectively demonstrable and is of medical, financial, social, or hygienic concern
- Stress incontinence: associated with increased intra-abdominal pressure such as coughing, laughing, sneezing, or exertion
- Urge incontinence: sudden uncontrollable loss of urine (also known as overactive bladder or detrusor overactivity)
- Mixed incontinence: loss of urine from a combination of stress and urge incontinence
- Overflow incontinence: high residual or chronic urinary retention leading to urinary spillage from an overdistended bladder
- Functional incontinence: loss of urine due to deficits of cognition and/or mobility
- Total incontinence: continuous leakage of urine; leakage without awareness

EPIDEMIOLOGY
- Affects 25% of young women and up to 57% of women aged 40 to 60 years. Women 19 to 64 years of age have predominantly stress incontinence (12–28%), followed by mixed (7–12%), and urge (5–10%) incontinence.
- Prevalence in women >75 years is 75%, and 6% of nursing home admissions are directly attributable to incontinence (1).
- Severe or large-volume incontinence is primarily mixed (37%), followed by urge (27%) and stress (15%) (2).

ETIOLOGY AND PATHOPHYSIOLOGY
- Stress incontinence: occurs with increased intra-abdominal pressure. Two types:
  - Anatomic: due to urethral hypermobility from lack of pelvic support
  - Intrinsic sphincter deficiency (ISD): impaired closure of urethra. Urethral mucosal seal and inherent closure from collagen, fibroelastic tissue, smooth and striated muscles, and so forth, may be lost secondary to surgical scarring, radiation, or hormonal and senile changes.
- Urge incontinence: may be due to detrusor overactivity or may be idiopathic
- Overflow incontinence: urinary retention (usually from neurogenic bladder)
- Total incontinence: constant loss of urine. Ectopic ureters in females usually open in the urethra distal to the sphincter or in the vagina, causing continuous leakage. May also occur with fistulous connections between bladder, ureters, or urethra, and vagina or uterus.

RISK FACTORS
Advanced age, impaired functional status, obesity (BMI >30), history of gestational diabetes, pregnancy, vaginal childbirth, pelvic surgery or radiation, urethral diverticula, genital prolapse, smoking, chronic obstructive pulmonary disease (COPD), cognitive impairment, constipation, caffeine, and pelvic floor dysfunction

GENERAL PREVENTION
Obesity avoidance, smoking cessation, high-fiber diet to reduce constipation

COMMONLY ASSOCIATED CONDITIONS
Pelvic organ prolapse, UTI, COPD, diabetes mellitus, neurologic disease, obesity, chronic constipation, depression, low libido, dyspareunia, and any disease that results in chronic cough

 DIAGNOSIS

HISTORY
- Age: Stress incontinence is more common in women aged 19 to 64 years, whereas mixed incontinence is more common in women >65 years. Onset from childhood indicates congenital causes (e.g., ectopic ureter).
- Amount and frequency of leakage
- Stress incontinence: Occurs in small spurts; patients typically remain dry at night in bed.
- Urge incontinence: sudden urge followed by leakage of large amounts, usually associated with frequency and nocturia. Sensory stimuli may trigger (e.g., cold).
- Continuous slow leakage in between regular voiding indicates ectopic ureter, urinary fistula, and so forth.
- Pain: Suprapubic pain with dysuria implies urinary infection, dyspareunia, interstitial cystitis, and so forth.
- Medical history
  - Neurologic conditions or suggestive symptomatology: cerebrovascular accident, parkinsonism, multiple sclerosis, myelodysplasia, diabetes, spinal cord injury
  - Radiation to pelvic and vaginal areas: causes ISD, overactive bladder, fibrotic changes of pelvic floor musculature, and low bladder compliance
  - Obstetric history: Weakness of the pelvic floor is more likely in multiparous women.
  - History of smoking and COPD with a chronic cough can aggravate incontinence.
  - Constipation can aggravate incontinence.
- Medications
  - Sympatholytic α-blockers (terazosin, prazosin, doxazosin, tamsulosin, alfuzosin, silodosin) can cause or worsen incontinence.
  - Sympathomimetic agents, tricyclic antidepressants, anticholinergics, and opioids can cause retention with overflow incontinence.
- Surgical history: Pelvic surgery, including gynecologic and bowel surgery, can injure the pelvic floor musculature and affect neurologic function.

PHYSICAL EXAM
- General status
  - Obesity (BMI)
- General neurologic examination
  - Mental status, speech, intellectual performance
  - Motor status: gait, generalized or focal weakness, rigidity, tremor
  - Sensory status: impairment of perineal–sacral area sensation
- Urologic examination
  - Abdomen: masses, incisional scars of previous surgeries
  - Suprapubic tenderness: may indicate cystitis
  - Palpable, distended bladder: chronic urinary retention

- Pelvic examination
  - Examination of the perineum and external genitalia, including tissue quality and sensation
  - Vaginal (half-speculum) examination for prolapse
  - Bimanual pelvic and anorectal examination for pelvic masses, fecal impaction, pelvic floor function, and so forth
    - Urethral hypermobility: gauged by palpation of the descent of the proximal urethra on straining
    - Assessment of pelvic floor resting tone and function (ability to isolate and contract pelvic floor musculature) (3)[C]
  - Stress test for urinary incontinence: Patient is asked to cough or strain to reproduce stress incontinence.
  - Cystocele: if evident, stage (grade 0 to 4)
  - Rectocele: if evident, stage (stage 0 to IV)

DIFFERENTIAL DIAGNOSIS
- Nocturnal enuresis: idiopathic, detrusor overactivity, neurogenic, cardiogenic, or sleep apnea
- Continuous leakage: ectopic ureter, urinary fistulas
- Postvoid dribbling: urethral diverticulum, idiopathic, iatrogenic, surgical
- Pelvic pain/dyspareunia: interstitial cystitis
- Pelvic organ prolapse
- Hematuria/recurrent UTI/pelvic mass: malignancy (4)

DIAGNOSTIC TESTS & INTERPRETATION
- Urinalysis and urine culture
- Renal function assessment: recommended if renal impairment is suspected

Initial Tests (lab, imaging)
- Unnecessary in uncomplicated patients
- Bladder scan to evaluate postvoid residual if overflow is suspected (<50 to 100 mL expected) (4)
- Upper tract imaging if upper tract involvement is suspected: scan or renal ultrasound (US)
- International Consultation of Incontinence Modulator Questionnaire (ICIQ) is highly recommended for assessment of patient's perspective of symptoms of incontinence and his or her impact on quality of life.
- 3IQ questionnaire helps differentiate between stress and urge incontinence (http://www.overactivebladder.com/sites/g/files/g10016541/f/201502/3IQ_updated.pdf) (2).
- 3-day voiding diary to evaluate fluid intake, caffeine intake, timing of leakage, and patient habits

Follow-Up Tests & Special Considerations
Asymptomatic bacteriuria is common. With a positive urine culture, initial treatment is indicated; however, if this is ineffective, repeat treatment is not indicated (3).

Diagnostic Procedures/Other
Urodynamic studies (not indicated in initial workup):
- Cystometric study of detrusor function
- Results on urodynamic testing are not predictive of treatment or surgery success (5)[A].

 TREATMENT

GENERAL MEASURES
- Treat correctable causes (e.g., UTI).
- Encourage weight loss in obese patients.
- Aggressively correct constipation.
- Treat mixed for primary symptom type (4)[C].

MEDICATION

First Line
- Stress incontinence
  - Lifestyle changes
    - Reduce BMI to <25 (5)[A].
    - Reduce caffeine to <1 cup coffee/day (5)[B].
    - Aggressive treatment of constipation: Limit medications that may induce constipation, polyethylene glycol 3350 (PEG 3350), increased fluid intake, and so forth.
  - Kegel exercises
    - Pelvic floor muscle training, at least eight contractions TID (3)[A].
    - Proper technique should be confirmed on exam; training by physical therapists.
    - Maintain treatment for at least 3 months (2).
    - 5 times as effective as placebo (1)[A]
- Urge incontinence
  - Supervised bladder training/scheduled voiding (1)[C]

Second Line
- Stress incontinence
  - Surgical management for stress incontinence:
    - Midurethral sling (preferred surgical intervention) (4)[A]
      - Women with moderate to severe stress incontinence have better outcomes at 1 year with midurethral slings than pelvic floor muscle training (6)[A].
      - Retropubic (more perioperative complications)
      - Transobturator (more pain/dyspareunia)
      - Single incision sling (MiniArc, SOLYX)
    - Abdominal approaches: Marshall-Marchetti-Krantz cystourethropexy, Burch colposuspension, laparoscopic colposuspension (4)[A]
    - Periurethral injection of bulking agents (may provide symptom relief but not permanent cure): silicone particles, carbon beads, calcium hydroxylapatite (5)[B]
- Urge incontinence: anticholinergic agents (1)[A]

  - Tolterodine (Detrol LA): 2 to 4 mg/day PO
  - Oxybutynin (Ditropan XL): 5 to 30 mg/day PO
  - Solifenacin (VESIcare): 5 to 10 mg/day PO
  - Darifenacin (Enablex): 7.5 to 15 mg/day PO
  - Trospium chloride (Sanctura XR): 60 mg/day PO
  - Transdermal oxybutynin gel (Gelnique): 10% applied daily
  - Transdermal oxybutynin patch (Oxytrol): twice weekly—available over the counter (OTC)
  - Fesoterodine (Toviaz): 4 to 8 mg/day PO
  - Dry mouth, dry eyes, constipation, impaired cognitive function, and other anticholinergic side effects can limit use.

  - Avoid with narrow-angle glaucoma, urinary retention (postvoid residual [PVR] >250 mL), impaired gastric emptying, and frail elders (3)[A]. No single agent has been shown to be overall superior (1)[A].
  - Fesoterodine achieves incontinence > tolterodine, at the expense of greater adverse effects (1)[B].
  - Extended-release and transdermal medications cause fewer side effects (5)[B].
  - β-3 agonist: mirabegron (Myrbetriq ER): 25 to 50 mg/day PO (1)[B]; onset of action delayed ~8 weeks; increases BP (avoid use in those with uncontrolled HTN)

Third Line
- Stress incontinence
- Duloxetine (Cymbalta) may have some limited efficacy (1)[C].

- Estrogen may be beneficial in topical form, but transdermal estrogen may worsen symptoms (1)[B].

  - Biofeedback and electrostimulation of pelvic floor muscles
  - Occlusive and supportive devices (e.g., cones, pessaries, and super tampons)
  - Acupuncture (in selected cases)
- Urge incontinence

  - Intradetrusor onabotulinumtoxinA **100 to 200 U** (urinary retention common, temporary self-catheterization may be needed) (4)[A]
  - Sacral nerve stimulation: 50% reduction in episodes in 2/3 of patients who have failed other treatments. Invasive with frequent complications (4)[B]

  - Percutaneous tibial nerve stimulation: office-based therapy, requires frequent visits (3)
  - Bladder augmentation (4)[C]

 ONGOING CARE

FOLLOW-UP RECOMMENDATIONS
Patient Monitoring
- Postoperative assessment: Rule out UTI, check postvoid residual, check suture lines.
- Periodic long-term follow-up with outcome-based questionnaire surveys

PATIENT EDUCATION
Instructions on self-care and warning signs are available at PubMed Health: Urinary Incontinence: https://www.nlm.nih.gov/medlineplus/urinaryincontinence.html

PROGNOSIS
Significant improvements are usually obtained with most patients.

COMPLICATIONS
- Prolonged exposure to urine causes skin breakdown and dermatitis, which may lead to ulceration and secondary infection.
- Inability for self-care is the precipitating factor for many nursing home admissions.
- Social isolation/depression
- Weight gain (due to self-limiting exercise from fear of leakage)
- Impaired sexual function
- Impaired quality of life

REFERENCES

1. Qaseem A, Dallas P, Forciea MA, et al. Nonsurgical management of urinary incontinence in women: a clinical practice guideline from the American College of Physicians. *Ann Intern Med*. 2014;161(6):429–440.
2. Myers DL. Female mixed urinary incontinence: a clinical review. *JAMA*. 2014;311(19):2007–2014.
3. Smith A, Bevan D, Douglas HR, et al. Management of urinary incontinence in women: summary of updated NICE guidance. *BMJ*. 2013;347:f5170.
4. Lucas M, Bedretdinova D, Bosch J, et al. Guidelines on urinary incontinence. European Association of Urology; 2014. http://uroweb.org/guideline/urinary-incontinence/?type=summary-of-changes
5. Wood LN, Anger JT. Urinary incontinence in women. *BMJ*. 2014;349:g4531.
6. Labrie J, Berghmans BL, Fischer K, et al. Surgery versus physiotherapy for stress urinary incontinence. *N Engl J Med*. 2013;369(12):1124–1133.

ADDITIONAL READING

- Abrams P, Andersson KE, Birder L, et al. Fourth International Consultation on Incontinence Recommendations of the International Scientific Committee: evaluation and treatment of urinary incontinence, pelvic organ prolapse, and fecal incontinence. *Neurourol Urodyn*. 2010;29(1):213–240.
- Gormley EA, Lightner DJ, Burgio KL, et al. Diagnosis and treatment of overactive bladder (non-neurogenic) in adults: AUA/SUFU guideline. *J Urol*. 2012;188(6 Suppl):2455–2563.
- Nygaard I. Clinical practice. Idiopathic urgency urinary incontinence. *N Engl J Med*. 2010;363(12):1156–1162.
- Visco AG, Brubaker L, Richter HE, et al. Anticholinergic therapy vs. onabotulinumtoxina for urgency urinary incontinence. *N Engl J Med*. 2012;367(19):1803–1813.

CODES

ICD10
- R32 Unspecified urinary incontinence
- N39.3 Stress incontinence (female) (male)
- N39.41 Urge incontinence

CLINICAL PEARLS

- Urinary incontinence is the involuntary loss of urine that is objectively demonstrable; markedly detrimental to quality of life; and is of medical, financial, social, or hygienic concern.
- Stress incontinence: associated with increased intra-abdominal pressure such as coughing, laughing, sneezing, or exertion
- Urge incontinence: sudden uncontrollable urgency, leading to leakage of urine (also known as overactive bladder or detrusor overactivity)
- Rule out UTI or STI by culture.
- Aggressively treat constipation.
- Assume that the majority of women can be significantly helped by treatment.
- For stress incontinence, physical therapy/pelvic floor rehabilitation and midurethral sling surgeries are most commonly used.
- For urge incontinence, if anticholinergic agents fail, intradetrusor onabotulinumtoxinA is often beneficial.

INCONTINENCE, URINARY ADULT MALE

Amar Talati, DO • David O. Parrish, MS, MD, FAAFP

BASICS

DESCRIPTION
- Urinary incontinence (UI) refers to the involuntary loss of urine that presents a medical, financial, social, or hygienic problem; the five main types of incontinence include stress, urge, mixed, overflow (urinary retention), and functional UI (1).
- Stress incontinence: involuntary urine leaks secondary to increased intra-abdominal pressure being greater than the sphincter can control; may be precipitated by sneezing, laughing, coughing, exertion
- Urge incontinence: Involuntary leakage of urine associated with urgency is believed to be secondary to uncontrolled contraction of the urinary bladder. It is also called detrusor overactivity.
- Mixed incontinence: involuntary leakage of urine with urgency and with stress, such as sneezing, laughing, coughing, exertion
- Overflow incontinence: Also known as urinary retention; this occurs with bladder overdistention due to impaired detrusor contraction or bladder outlet obstruction (due to benign prostatic hyperplasia [BPH], bladder stones, bladder tumors, pelvic tumors, urethral strictures or spasms).
- Functional UI: urine leakage variable, often due to environmental or physical barriers to toileting (i.e., reduced mobility).
- Other causes transient UI often due to infection, medication side effects, or psychological disorder, in addition to postmicturition dribbling associated with BPH
- Polyuria is defined by excessive amounts of urine ($\geq$2.5 to 3 L) over 24 hours
- Nocturnal polyuria is where >33% of total daily urine output occurs during sleeping hours.

EPIDEMIOLOGY
- Stress incontinence in men is rare, unless it is attributable to prostate surgery, neurologic disease, or trauma.
- Detrusor overactivity may be spontaneous or provoked, but involuntary, and may be neurogenic in cause or idiopathic.
- Reported rates of incontinence range from 1% after transurethral resection to 2–66% after radical prostatectomy, and 1–15% following transvesical prostatectomy, although rates decline with time (1).

Prevalence
- 12.4% prevalence of UI in community dwelling adult men in the United States as based on the National Health and Nutrition Examination Survey (NHANES) as of 2008.
- 4.5% reported moderate to severe UI, of which 48.6% experienced urge, 23.5% experienced other UI, 15.4% experienced mixed, and 12.5% experienced stress incontinence as per the NHANES report in 2010.
- UI is common in nursing home patients, with a prevalence of about 70% in the Southeastern United States from 1999 to 2002.
- Major depression, hypertension, and benign prostatic hypertrophy associated with UI.
- Incontinence in men of all ages is approximately half as prevalent as it is in women; however, after 80 years of age, both sexes are affected equally (1).

ETIOLOGY AND PATHOPHYSIOLOGY
- Incontinence secondary to bladder abnormalities
  - Detrusor overactivity results in urge incontinence.
  - Detrusor overactivity commonly is associated with bladder outlet obstruction from benign prostatic hyperplasia (BPH).
- Incontinence secondary to outlet abnormalities
  - Sphincteric damage secondary to pelvic surgery or radiation
  - Sphincteric dysfunction secondary to neurologic disease
  - Commonly associated with BPH due to compression of the urethra, affecting urinary flow
- Mixed incontinence is caused by abnormalities of both the bladder and the outlet overflow or by enlarged prostate/bladder neck contracture from prostate surgery.
- Stress incontinence is caused by weakened urethral sphincter and/or pelvic floor weakness.

RISK FACTORS
- Age
- Hypertension
- Neurologic disease
- Prostate surgery
- Pelvic trauma
- History of urinary tract infections
- Major depression
- Diabetes

GENERAL PREVENTION
Proper management of conditions, such as symptomatic bladder outlet obstruction caused by BPH early in the course may prevent continence problems later in life; no evidence for screening in men unless patient is experiencing symptoms using The 3 Incontinence Questions tool to evaluate the type of UI (2)[C].

COMMONLY ASSOCIATED CONDITIONS
- Neurologic disease (cerebrovascular accident, parkinsonism, multiple sclerosis, myelodysplasia, spinal cord injury)
- Pelvic radiation
- Pelvic trauma
- BPH
- Prostate surgery

DIAGNOSIS

HISTORY
- Voiding symptoms
  - Duration and characteristics of incontinence
  - Stress, urge, mixed, overflow, functional, transient
  - Precipitants, severity, timing, and associated symptoms
  - Use of pads, briefs, diapers
  - Fluid intake
  - Alteration in bowel habits
  - Previous treatments and effect on incontinence
  - BPH symptoms
- Diabetes mellitus
- Associated conditions, such as neurologic disease, cardiopulmonary disorders, renal disorders, sleep disturbance, mental health or cognitive impairment, erectile dysfunction
- Elderly patients: Assess cognitive levels (dementia/delirium), psychological disorders, mobility problems—69% did not seek help for UI due to perception of normal part of aging or that it was not a major issue.

- Medication use: diuretics, drugs for BPH
- Alcohol and drug use, including caffeine
- Radical pelvic surgery/radiation
  - Abdominoperineal resection
  - Prostatectomy: radical for cancer, open/transurethral for benign disease
- **Red flag symptoms** requiring rapid referral to specialist management
  - Pain, hematuria, recurrent urinary tract infection, history of prostate irradiation, history of radical pelvic surgery (i.e., prostate surgery), constant leakage suggesting fistula, voiding difficulty, suspected neurologic disease

PHYSICAL EXAM
- Abdominal examination
  - Suprapubic mass suggests retention.
  - Suprapubic tenderness suggests UTI.
  - Surgical scars suggesting pelvic surgery.
  - Skin lesions associated with neurologic disease (e.g., neurofibromatosis and café au lait spots)
- External genitalia
- Prostate
- Spine/back
- Skeletal deformities
- Scars from previous spinal surgery
- Sacral abnormalities may be associated with neurogenic bladder dysfunction
  - Cutaneous signs of spinal dysraphism
    - SC lipoma
    - Vascular malformation, tuft of hair, or skin dimple on lower back
  - Cutaneous signs of sacral agenesis
    - Low, short gluteal cleft
    - Flattened buttocks
    - Coccyx is not palpable.
- Focal neurologic exam
  - Motor function
    - Inspect muscle bulk for atrophy.
    - Tibialis anterior (L4–S1): dorsiflexion of foot
    - Gastrocnemius (L5–S2): plantarflexion of foot
    - Toe extensors (L5–S2): toe extension
- Sensory function
- Reflexes
  - Anal reflex (S2–S5)
    - Gently stroke mucocutaneous junction of circumanal skin.
    - Absent visible contraction (wink) suggests peripheral nerve/sacral (conus medullaris) abnormality.
  - Bulbocavernosus reflex (BCR) (S2–S4)
    - Elicited by squeezing glans to cause reflex contraction of anal sphincter
    - Absence of BCR suggests sacral nerve damage.

DIFFERENTIAL DIAGNOSIS
- Urge incontinence
- Stress incontinence
- Mixed incontinence
- Overflow incontinence
- Functional UI
- Transient UI

DIAGNOSTIC TESTS & INTERPRETATION
- Urinalysis and urine culture to check for glucosuria, pyuria, proteinuria, and/or blood
- Voiding diary, The 3 Incontinence Questions
- Pad test if quantity of leakage or objective outcome measure is desired.
- Do not routinely perform urodynamics before conservative treatment for UI (EAU Grade B).

- Postvoid residual (PVR) volume if difficulty voiding or other lower urinary tract symptoms using ultrasound (US) to measure postvoid residual: PVR persistently ≥100 mL indicates voiding dysfunction.
- Uroflowmetry
- PSA only if diagnosis of prostate cancer will influence treatment or if levels can help decision-making for patients at risk for BPH.
- Renal function if renal impairment or hydronephrosis is suspected, or if considering surgical treatment for lower urinary tract symptoms
- Voiding cystogram in select cases

Diagnostic Procedures/Other
- Urodynamics is useful for confirming bladder outlet obstruction as a possible cause of detrusor overactivity and may reduce surgical treatment of symptoms and persistence of objective obstruction following surgery compared to immediate transurethral resection of prostate in men with voiding dysfunction (level 2 [mid-level] evidence)
- Prostate US and biopsy if indicated by physical exam or PSA
- Urethrocystoscopy to exclude suspected bladder or urethral pathology or before invasive therapies if findings might influence treatment
- Imaging of upper and lower urinary tract is not routinely indicated as part of UI assessment.
- Consider US (preferred) or MRI of lower urinary tract if indicated.
  - US is rarely required to diagnose or rule out BPH in patients with UI as digital rectal exam can diagnose and guide treatment in most patients. Consider US of prostate if it assists with choice of drug therapy for lower urinary tract symptoms.
  - Consider US of prostate to assess for intravesical prostatic protrusion (IPP) if considering surgical treatment.
  - Consider US of upper urinary tract in patients with large postvoid residual, hematuria, or history of urolithiasis.

TREATMENT

- Best managed by combining lifestyle modification and medication; rule out transient causes of UI.
- Lifestyle changes: Manage diabetes, weight loss (especially if overweight), limit fluids (especially at night), toilet on a scheduled basis, eliminate certain foods that may make symptoms worse (e.g., caffeine, acidic foods, alcohol), reduce use of medications that may cause UI or nocturnal diuresis.
- Treat reversible causes if symptomatic (i.e., UTI), if not symptomatic in elderly, do not treat.
- Before and after radical prostatectomy, it is best to offer pelvic floor muscle training to improve recovery and reduce long-term UI (level 2 evidence).

GENERAL MEASURES
- Bladder diaries are invaluable in helping patients understand patterns of incontinence.
- Time voiding to avoid significant bladder distention.
- Techniques of relaxed voiding and double voiding
- Urethral milking to prevent postmicturition dribble
- Distraction and behavioral techniques to take mind off the bladder and toilet
- Treat for constipation if applicable.

MEDICATION
First Line
- Urge incontinence: Antimuscarinic agents are first line, caution in those with bladder outlet obstruction

and PVR >250 to 300 mL. In men with urgency associated with BPH, consider α-blockers (i.e., tamsulosin, alfuzosin, silodosin) as monotherapy or in combination with antimuscarinic for residual overactive bladder (3).
- Review efficacy and side effects <30 days after treatment.
  - Oxybutynin (Ditropan XL) 5 to 15 mg PO every day
  - Tolterodine (Detrol LA) 2 to 4 mg PO every day
  - Darifenacin (Enablex) 7.5 to 15 mg PO every day
  - Solifenacin (VESIcare) 5 to 10 mg PO every day
  - Trospium chloride (Sanctura XR) 60 mg PO every day
  - Transdermal oxybutynin (Gelnique) 10% apply daily (EAU Grade B)—no dry mouth
  - Fesoterodine (Toviaz) 4 to 8 mg PO every day
- Stress incontinence
  - No generally accepted drug therapy
  - Mixed stress and urge incontinence, ER formulations are preferred due to reduced side effects.

Second Line
- Urge incontinence
- Tricyclic antidepressants
  - Imipramine 10 to 25 mg PO BID/TID
- Desmopressin (DDAVP) for occasional short-term relief of UI
  - 25 to 50 μg PO or intranasal at bedtime
- Intradetrusor botulinum toxin injections 100 U intravesical injections (not FDA-approved)
- Mirabegron (Myrbetriq) new β3 agonist (FDA-approved) 25 to 50 mg PO daily. *Caution*: HTN
- Duloxetine for temporary improvements of incontinence with dose titration (mixed stress/urge)

Geriatric Considerations
- Anticholinergics and tricyclics may result in significant cognitive impairment in elderly patients.
- DDAVP should be avoided in patients with known/potential cardiac disease.

ADDITIONAL THERAPIES
- Pelvic floor rehabilitation (Kegel exercises) may significantly reduce both stress and urge incontinence in male patients and should be considered a part of initial management for stress UI.
- Timed voiding is a useful therapy for patients with urge incontinence.
- Overflow incontinence is usually caused by poor bladder contractility with urinary retention.
  - Indwelling catheter
  - Intermittent catheterization
  - Evaluate for outlet obstruction.

SURGERY/OTHER PROCEDURES
- Urge incontinence
  - Sacral nerve stimulation with behavioral therapy
  - Augmentation cystoplasty and urinary diversion
  - Botulinum toxin injection via cystoscopy
- Stress incontinence (4)[B]
  - Urethral bulking agents: modest success rates with low cure rates
  - Male sling procedures: promising short-term and intermediate results but no long-term studies
  - Artificial urinary sphincter implant has excellent long-term continence rates and is considered gold standard (5).

COMPLEMENTARY & ALTERNATIVE MEDICINE
- Acupuncture in selected cases
- Physical therapy in selected cases

ONGOING CARE

FOLLOW-UP RECOMMENDATIONS
Patient Monitoring
Must monitor residual volume after voiding in patients taking anticholinergic medications; monitor side effects.

PROGNOSIS
Continence can be improved in almost all patients.

COMPLICATIONS
- Dermatitis
- Candidiasis
- Skin breakdown
- Social isolation
- Avoidance of sex
- Weight gain

REFERENCES

1. Khandelwal C, Kistler C. Diagnosis of urinary incontinence. *Am Fam Physician*. 2013;87(8):543–550.
2. Gravas S, Bachmann A, Descazeaud A, et al. *EAU guidelines on the management of non-neurogenic male lower urinary tract symptoms (LUTS), including benign prostatic obstruction (BPO)*. Arnhem: The Netherlands; European Association of Urology; 2014.
3. Gormley EA, Lightner DJ, Burgio KL, et al. Diagnosis and treatment of overactive bladder (non-neurogenic) in adults: AUA/SUFU guideline. *J Urol*. 2012;188(6 Suppl):2455–2463.
4. Lucas MG, Bedretdinova D, Bosch JL, et al. *EAU Guidelines on urinary incontinence*. Arnhem: The Netherlands; European Association of Urology; 2014.
5. Herschorn S, Bruschini H, Comiter C, et al. Surgical treatment of stress incontinence in men. *Neurourol Urodyn*. 2010;29(1):179–190.

ADDITIONAL READING

- Bauer RM, Bastian PJ, Gozzi C, et al. Postprostatectomy incontinence: all about diagnosis and management. *Eur Urol*. 2009;55(2):322–333.
- Markland AD, Goode PS, Redden DT, et al. Prevalence of urinary incontinence in men: results from the national health and nutrition examination survey. *J Urol*. 2010;184(3):1022–1027.

CODES

ICD10
- R32 Unspecified urinary incontinence
- N39.3 Stress incontinence (female) (male)
- N39.41 Urge incontinence

CLINICAL PEARLS

- Think "outside" the lower urinary tract: Comorbid medical illness and impairments are independently associated with UI; treat contributing comorbidities and rule out secondary causes.
- Always check PVR to rule out overflow incontinence.
- Have patient complete the International Prostate Symptom Score and do uroflow, PSA if indicated.
- Urodynamics if conservative management fails
- Pelvic floor rehabilitation handouts may have a significant effect for male patients than physical therapy-mediated pelvic floor rehabilitation.

INFECTIOUS MONONUCLEOSIS, EPSTEIN-BARR VIRUS INFECTIONS

Dennis E. Hughes, DO, FACEP

 BASICS

DESCRIPTION

- Epstein-Barr virus (EBV) is a member of the herpes virus family.
  - Two subtypes: ST1 predominates in Western Hemisphere, Southeast Asia; ST1 and ST2 equally prevalent in Africa
- Primary infection typically occurs in childhood; responsible for infectious mononucleosis (most common disease association) and numerous cancers.
- WHO classified EBV as "tumor virus" in 1997 due to association with cancer induction (1).

EPIDEMIOLOGY

Incidence
Worldwide, infects >90% of people (antibody-positive)

Prevalence
Primary EBV infection

- Military, college students, and others living in cloistered and crowded populations have the highest infection rate.
- Predominant age of primary infection is 10 to 19 years.
  - Primary clinical manifestation is infectious mononucleosis (IM).
  - Early childhood infections are usually asymptomatic.
- By ~20 years of age, 60–90% of persons have a persistent (lifelong) anti-EBV antibody.
- Seroconversion occurs later in childhood in developed countries; there is suggestion of race/ethnicity disparity in the United States with higher seroprevalence in non-Hispanic black, Asian, and Hispanic populations (2).

ETIOLOGY AND PATHOPHYSIOLOGY

- After inoculation, the virus replicates in the nasopharyngeal epithelium with resulting cell lysis, virion spread and viremia. The reticuloendothelial system is affected, resulting in a host response and the appearance of atypical lymphocytes in the peripheral blood.
- A polyclonal B-cell proliferative response follows. Relatively few circulating lymphocytes are infected by EBV (<0.1% of circulating mononuclear cells in the acute illness).
- A persistent (asymptomatic) state ensues with the EBV genome sequestered.
- A subsequent coinfection increases risk of developing an EBV-associated condition (e.g., malignancy).
- Either by B-cell stimulation or diminished EBV-specific immune modulation, the previously latent EBV-infected B cells replicate, allowing clinical manifestation of the EBV genome. The proteins produced may either modify host response to or contribute directly to the subsequent malignancy (3,4).
- Immunosuppression (organ transplant/acquired immune deficiency) can result in transformation and lymphoproliferative disorders.

RISK FACTORS

- Age
- Sociohygienic level
- Geographic location
- Close, intimate contact
- Immunosuppression

GENERAL PREVENTION

- Avoid close physical contact with persons known to be currently symptomatic with EBV/IM
- Hand washing and personal hygiene
- General precautions with potential blood exposure (EBV can be transmitted via blood contamination, and marrow/organ transplant)
- EBV vaccines are currently undergoing study.

COMMONLY ASSOCIATED CONDITIONS

- Infectious mononucleosis: Symptomatic primary EBV infection common in otherwise healthy older children, adolescents, and young adults.
  - Clinical features vary in severity and duration: In children age <10 years, generally mild; in adolescents and adults, symptoms can be more severe and protracted.
  - Incubation period is 30 to 50 days.
- X-linked lymphoproliferative syndrome (XLP-rare inherited extreme vulnerability to EBV infection)
- Lymphoproliferative syndromes due to EBV infections in transplant recipients
- Lymphomas (B-cell lymphoblastic, T-cell)
- Lymphocytic interstitial pneumonitis
- Hairy leukoplakia of the tongue, leiomyosarcoma, and CNS lymphomas in patients with AIDS
- Burkitt lymphoma (most common childhood tumor in Africa and Papua New Guinea where malaria is also endemic and may be a cofactor)
- Nasopharyngeal carcinoma (particularly in Southeast China)
- Parotid carcinoma
- Hodgkin lymphoma (most common EBV-associated malignancy in United States, European Union)
- Postulated to be associated with multiple sclerosis (2 to 3 times incidence in EBV-positive individuals)
- Chronic active Epstein-Barr Virus (CAEBV) due to loss of host control of viral replication

![Dx] DIAGNOSIS

HISTORY

- May begin abruptly or insidiously
- Syndrome of fatigue, malaise, and odynophagia
- In adults, fever to 103°F (39.4°C) with gradual fall over a variable period of 7 to 10 days; in severe cases, temperature elevations of 104–105°F (40.0–40.6°C) may persist for 2 weeks.
- Children typically with low-grade fever or completely afebrile
- Chest pain (myocarditis and pericarditis)

PHYSICAL EXAM

- Fever, lymphadenopathy, pharyngitis in >50%, with palatal petechiae and hepatosplenomegaly in ~10%
- Tender lymphadenopathy (cervical nodes are most commonly enlarged)
- Splenomegaly in 50%
- Diffuse hyperemia and hyperplasia of oropharyngeal lymphoid tissue
- Gelatinous, grayish-white exudative tonsillitis persists for 7 to 10 days in 50%.
- Petechiae develop at border of hard and soft palates in 60%.
- Axillary, epitrochlear, popliteal, inguinal, mediastinal, and mesenteric lymphadenopathy (95% of patients)
- Lymph node enlargement subsides over days/weeks
- Skin manifestations in 3–16%
  - Erythematous macular/maculopapular rash
  - Petechial and purpuric exanthems have been reported.
  - Rash location: trunk and upper arms; occasionally, the face and forearms are involved.

DIFFERENTIAL DIAGNOSIS

- Streptococcal pharyngitis and tonsillitis
- Diphtheria
- Blood dyscrasias
- Rubella, measles
- Viral hepatitis
- Cytomegalovirus, toxoplasmosis

DIAGNOSTIC TESTS & INTERPRETATION

Initial Tests (lab, imaging)

- CBC with differential
- Lymphocytes and atypical lymphocytes
  - Increased numbers of lymphocytes (especially atypical lymphocytes; may be up to 70% of leukocytes) in peripheral blood
  - In 1st week after onset, WBC count is normal/moderately decreased.
    - By the 2nd week, lymphocytosis develops with >10% atypical lymphocytes.
  - During early illness, atypical lymphocytes are B cells transformed by the EBV; later, atypical cells are primarily T cells.
- Antibodies
  - Heterophile antibodies in 80–90% of adults
  - Heterophile antibody is an IgM response, which appears during the 1st and 2nd week of illness and disappears in 4 to 6 weeks.
  - In general, agglutinin titer is higher in infectious mononucleosis than in other disorders; an unabsorbed heterophile titer >1:128 and ≥1:40 after absorption is significant.
- Specific antibodies to EBV-associated antigens
  - Viral capsid-specific IgM and IgG are present early
  - Viral capsid-IgM disappears after several weeks, viral capsid-IgG persists for life.
- Liver tests: hypertransaminasemia, hyperbilirubinemia are common; jaundice is rare.

- Atypical lymphocytes are not specific for EBV infections and may be present in other clinical conditions, including rubella, infectious hepatitis, allergic rhinitis, asthma, and primary atypical pneumonia.
- Abdominal ultrasound to monitor for splenic enlargement is not routinely indicated. Consider ultrasound for those wishing to return to strenuous activity/contact sports at day 21 of illness to ensure resolution of splenomegaly.

Follow-Up Tests & Special Considerations
- Abnormal hepatic enzymes persist in 80% of patients for several weeks; hepatomegaly in 15–20%
- In transplant recipients, quantitative polymerase chain reaction (PCR) used to monitor EBV loads

Diagnostic Procedures/Other
Chest x-ray
- Hilar adenopathy may be observed in infectious mononucleosis with extensive lymphoid hyperplasia.

Test Interpretation
- Mononuclear infiltrations involve lymph nodes, tonsils, spleen, lungs, liver, heart, kidneys, adrenal glands, skin, and CNS.
- Bone marrow hyperplasia with small granulomas formation may be present; these findings are nonspecific and have no prognostic significance.

TREATMENT

GENERAL MEASURES
- Treatment is mostly supportive.
- NSAIDs or acetaminophen
- During acute stage, limit activity for 4 weeks to reduce potential complications (e.g., splenic rupture).
- Transplant recipients who develop EBV infection may require reduction in immunosuppression as well as administration of monoclonal anti-CD20 (rituximab).

MEDICATION
- In primary infections:

  – Antimicrobial agents (usually penicillin) only if throat culture is positive for group A β-hemolytic streptococci. Previously, ampicillin rash in presumed group B *Streptococcus* (GBS) was thought to be highly suggestive of infectious mononucleosis. Incidence of rash much lower than historically thought (4)[B].

  – Warm saline gargles for oropharyngeal pain
  – Corticosteroids
    ○ May provide some symptomatic relief but no improvement in resolution of illness
    ○ Consider in severe pharyngotonsillitis with oropharyngeal edema and airway encroachment. Dexamethasone 0.3 mg/kg/day for 1 to 3 days.
    ○ Consider steroids for patients with marked toxicity or major complications (e.g., hemolytic anemia, thrombocytopenic purpura, neurologic sequelae, myocarditis, pericarditis) (5)[B].

- Antiviral medications (acyclovir) have been evaluated in small randomized controlled trials (RCTs) and found to shorten recovery time and improve subjective symptoms in acute EBV infection. They are not routinely used.

ISSUES FOR REFERRAL
Most cases can be managed as an outpatient without the need for specialty referral. Consider referral for complications such as oropharyngeal edema with airway compromise needing intubation or ventilator support.

SURGERY/OTHER PROCEDURES
- With profound thrombocytopenia, refractory to corticosteroid therapy, splenectomy may be necessary.
- Only current effective treatment for XLP is hematopoietic stem cell transplantation.
- Inability to tolerate oral intake (solid or liquid)
- Immunosuppression
- Splenic rupture

ONGOING CARE

FOLLOW-UP RECOMMENDATIONS

ALERT
Splenic rupture may be fatal if not recognized. Occurrence is estimated at 0.1%.

Patient Monitoring
- Avoid contact sports, heavy lifting, and excess exertion until spleen and liver have returned to normal size (ultrasound can verify in athletic populations).
- Eliminate alcohol and exposure to other hepatotoxic drugs or herbal supplements until LFTs normalize.
- Closely monitor patients during the first 2 to 3 weeks after the onset of symptoms since complication rates are highest during this period.
- Alert patients that symptoms (malaise, fatigue, intermittent sore throat, lymphadenopathy) may persist for months.

DIET
No restrictions. Hydration during acute phase is important.

PROGNOSIS
- Most recover in ~4 weeks.
- Fatigue may persist for months.

COMPLICATIONS
- Neurologic (rare)
  – Aseptic meningitis, meningoencephalitis
  – Bell palsy; Guillain-Barré syndrome
  – Transverse myelitis
  – Cerebellar ataxia
  – Acute psychosis
- Hematologic (rare)
  – Thrombocytopenia, slight to moderate, early in illness
  – Hemolytic anemia with marked neutropenia during early weeks
  – Aplastic anemia
  – Agammaglobulinemia
- Pneumonitis
- Splenic rupture
  – Rare, but most often occurs in the first 21 days of illness

REFERENCES
1. Grywalska E, Rolinski J. Epstein-Barr virus-associated lymphomas. *Semin Oncol.* 2015; 42(2):291–303.
2. Dowd JB, Palermo T, Brite J, et al. Seroprevalence of Epstein-Barr virus infections in U.S. children ages 6–19, 2003–2010. *PLoS One.* 2013;8(5): e64921.
3. Thorley-Lawson DA, Hawkins JB, Tracy SI, et al. The pathogenesis of Epstein-Barr virus persistent infection. *Curr Opin Virol.* 2013;3(3):227–232.
4. Chovel-Sella A, Ben Tov A, Lahav E, et al. Incidence of rash after amoxicillin treatment in children with infectious mononucleosis. *Pediatrics.* 2013;131(5):e1424–e1427.
5. Odumade OA, Hogquist KA, Balfour HH Jr. Progress and problems in understanding and managing primary Epstein-Barr virus infections. *Clin Microbiol Rev.* 2011;24(1):193–209.

ADDITIONAL READING
- Almohmeed YH, Avenell A, Aucott L, et al. Systematic review and meta-analysis of the sero-epidemiological association between Epstein Barr virus and multiple sclerosis. *PLoS One.* 2013;8(4):e61110.
- Klein G, Klein E, Kashuba E. Interaction of Epstein-Barr virus (EBV) with human B-lymphocytes. *Biochem Biophys Res Commun.* 2010;396(1):67–73.

 CODES

ICD10
- B27.00 Gammaherpesviral mononucleosis without complication
- B27.09 Gammaherpesviral mononucleosis with other complications
- B27.01 Gammaherpesviral mononucleosis with polyneuropathy

CLINICAL PEARLS
- In cases of acute symptomatic infectious mononucleosis, 98% present with fever, sore throat, cervical node enlargement, and tonsillar hypertrophy.
- False-negative monospot (heterophile antibody) common in the first 10 to 14 days of illness. 90% will have heterophile antibodies by week 3 of illness.
- Lymphocytosis (not monocytosis) is common in infectious mononucleosis.

INFERTILITY

Sharon L. Koehler, DO, FACS • Sonia Rivera-Martinez, DO, FACOFP

BASICS

DESCRIPTION
Definition: failure of a couple to conceive after ≥12 months of regular unprotected intercourse or after ≥6 months if the woman is ≥35 years. Primary: Couple has never been pregnant. Secondary: Couple has been pregnant. Fecundability: the probability of achieving pregnancy in one menstrual cycle.

EPIDEMIOLOGY

Incidence
Incidence is the probability of achieving a pregnancy within 1 year. ~85% of couples will conceive within 12 months of unprotected intercourse.

Prevalence
- In the United States, 5–15% of women currently trying to conceive are infertile.
- ~11.5% of married couples between ages 15 and 34 years and 42% between ages 35 and 44 years meet the criteria for being infertile.
- May increase as more women delay childbearing; 20% of women in the United States have their first child >35 years.

ETIOLOGY AND PATHOPHYSIOLOGY
- Most cases multifactorial: Approximately 50% of cases due to female factors (of which 20% are due to ovulatory dysfunction and 30% due to tubal and pelvic pathology), 30% due to male factors and 20% are of unknown etiology.
- Acquired: Most common cause of infertility in the United States is pelvic inflammatory disease (PID) secondary to chlamydia, endometriosis, polycystic ovary syndrome (PCOS), premature ovarian failure, and increased maternal age.
- Diminished ovarian reserve (DOR): low fertility due to low quantity or functional quality of oocytes.
- Congenital: anatomic and genetic abnormalities.

Genetics
- Higher incidence of genetic abnormalities among infertile population, including Klinefelter syndrome (47XXY), Turner syndrome (45X or mosaic), and fragile X syndrome.
- Y chromosomal microdeletions are associated with isolated defects of spermatogenesis → found in 16% of men with azoo-/severe oligospermia.
- Cystic fibrosis transmembrane conductance regulator (CFTR) gene mutation causing congenital bilateral absence of vas deferens (CBAVD).

RISK FACTORS
- Female
- Gynecologic history: irregular/abnormal menses, sexually transmitted infections (STIs), dysmenorrhea, fibroids, prior pregnancy
- Medical history: endocrinopathy, autoimmune disease, undiagnosed celiac disease (1), collagen vascular diseases (2), thrombophilia, obesity, and cancer
- Surgical history: appendicitis, pelvic surgery, intrauterine surgery, tubal ligation.
- Social history: smoking, alcohol/substance abuse, eating disorders, exercise, advanced maternal age
- Male
- Medical history: STI, prostatitis, medication use (i.e., β-blockers, calcium channel blocker, antiulcer medication), endocrinopathy, cancer
- Surgical history: orchiopexy, hernia repair, vasectomy with/without reversal

- Social: smoking, alcohol/substance abuse, anabolic steroids, environmental exposures, occupations leading to increased scrotal temperature

GENERAL PREVENTION
Normal diet and exercise, avoid smoking and other substance abuse, prevention of STIs

COMMONLY ASSOCIATED CONDITIONS
- Sexual behavior increasing risk for STIs
- Pelvic pathology: endometriosis, ovarian cysts, endometrial polyps, and uterine fibroids
- Endocrine dysfunction (thyroid, glucose metabolism, menstrual cycle abnormalities, prolactin)
- Anovulation is commonly associated with hyperandrogenism and PCOS.

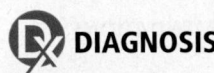

DIAGNOSIS

HISTORY
- Complete reproductive history:
  - Age at menarche, regularity of menstrual cycle, physical development, previous methods of contraception, history of abnormal Pap smears and treatment
  - History of abortion, D&Cs, bilateral tubal ligation, vasectomy, or other pelvic/abdominal surgery
- Frequency of intercourse and sexual dysfunction
- Abdominal pain or other abdominal symptoms
- STI
- History of endocrine abnormalities
- History of malignancy or chronic illness
- Family history: close relatives with congenital abnormalities or mental retardation; infertility or early menopause in close relatives of female partner
- Medications: drug abuse, allergies, occupation, and exposure to environmental hazards

PHYSICAL EXAM
- BMI and distribution of body fat
- Female
  - Pubertal development with Tanner staging
  - Signs of PCOS: androgen excess, obesity, signs of insulin resistance
  - Breast exam: galactorrhea
  - Vaginal exam: describe rugation, discharge, anatomic variation
  - Uterine size/shape, mobility, tenderness
  - Adnexal tenderness infection or mass
- Male
  - Abnormalities of the penis or urethral meatus
  - Testes: volume, symmetry, masses (varicocele, hydrocele), presence/absence of vas deferens

DIAGNOSTIC TESTS & INTERPRETATION

Initial Tests (lab, imaging)
Evaluation is directed by history:
- Assessment of ovulation
  - Irregular or infrequent menses, not accompanied by consistent premenstrual or moliminal characteristics, which are inconsistent in flow and duration, are indicative of ovulatory dysfunction.
  - Luteal-phase progesterone ≥3 ng/mL confirms ovulation has recently occurred but does not indicate when it occurred.
  - Luteinizing hormone (LH) testing kit: identifies mid-cycle LH surge, which occurs approximately 14 to 26 hours prior to ovulation. Greatest fertility on day of LH surge until 2 days after. Predicts time of ovulation in advance so couples can time intercourse.

  - Basal body temperature (BBT): ~1 degree increase in BBT taken upon wakening indicates ovulation has occurred: Greatest fertility spans 7 days PRIOR to rise in BBT. Not preferred
- Assessment of ovarian reserve
  - Follicle-stimulating hormone (FSH)/estradiol (E₂): FSH and E₂ levels on cycle days (CD) 2 to 5 are used to predict response to ovulation induction and pregnancy. High FSH levels >10 mIU/mL and high estradiol (>80 pg/mL) indicate a low chance of pregnancy with in vitro fertilization (IVF).
  - Anti-müllerian hormone (AMH) and antral follicle counts (AFCs): The number of antral follicles measured by transvaginal ultrasound (US) at any one time in the ovary is termed the "antral follicle count." AMH is secreted by the granulosa cells of the antral follicles and decreases as a woman approaches menopause. AMH <0.7 μ/dL and total AFC <10 between both ovaries during the follicular phase indicate DOR.
  - Clomiphene challenge test: Measure FSH on CD 3, administer 100 mg clomiphene CDs 5 to 9, recheck FSH on CD 10. FSH ≥10 mIU/mL on CDs 3 or 10 indicates DOR; may increase the sensitivity of the standard day 3 FSH test
- Semen analysis
  - Warranted in all infertile couples. Semen analysis alone is not used to predict male fertility potential: normal results in 6–27% of infertile males, abnormal results in fertile males
  - Semen collection: collected after 2 to 5 days of abstinence. Repeat test 2 to 3 times due to inherent variability within the same individual.
  - Parameters for male subfertility: sperm concentration <13.5 mill/mL, sperm motility <32%, sperm morphology <9% normal
- Additional labs
  - Prolactin, thyroid-stimulating hormone, 17-hydroxyprogesterone, androgen levels
  - HIV, HSV 1 and 2, chlamydia gonorrhea antibody, RPR, hepatitis B and C, CMV
  - Genetic testing based on family history
- Transvaginal US for anatomic abnormality
- Hysterosalpingogram (HSG) to evaluate patency of tubes and contour of the cavity; may be both diagnostic and therapeutic.
- Sonohysterography (SHG) may provide a more detailed evaluation of the uterine cavity, if indicated.

Follow-Up Tests & Special Considerations
- Abnormal lab values warrant reevaluation/referral.
- Abnormal imaging may require surgical evaluation.

Diagnostic Procedures/Other
- Hysteroscopy: gold standard, used to directly visualize the endometrial cavity; may be indicated to evaluate filling defects on HSG or SHG
- Laparoscopy: used to directly visualize the peritoneal cavity and may be indicated to evaluate abnormal findings on HSG. It is the only way to definitively diagnose endometriosis.

TREATMENT

GENERAL MEASURES
- Be aware of insurance coverage for each patient. Be mindful of the couple's emotional state: depression, anger, anxiety, and marital discord are common. Many patients benefit from counseling and support measures.

- All female fertility patients should be taking folate supplementation.
- New evidence is suggesting beneficial effects of antioxidants in decreasing time to pregnancy. Additionally, dietary carotenoids in males may improve sperm quality (3,4).
- IVF is the most effective infertility treatment available:
  - Eggs are removed from the female and fertilized outside the body. The embryo is monitored for 3 to 5 days and then implanted into the uterus on day 3 or day 5.
  - Anatomic causes should be referred immediately for IVF, although surgical consult may be required.
  - Fewer complications have been reported for individuals undergoing IVF for anatomic causes rather than ovulatory dysfunction (low APGAR scores, DM) (5)[A].
  - Donor eggs may be obtained.
- Male factor
  - Consider lifestyle changes.
  - Intrauterine insemination (IUI): Sperms are placed via a catheter directly in the uterus. IUI effectively increases the sperm count.
  - Intracytoplasmic sperm injection (ICSI) is performed in conjunction with IVF for males with severe abnormalities (i.e., <5 million sperm) or those who have failed to conceive with IUI. A single sperm is injected directly into the cytoplasm of the egg. Fertilization occurs ~70% of the time.
  - Donor sperm may be obtained.

MEDICATION
First Line
- Treatment of infertility depends on the etiology.
- Anovulation: must determine if HYPOgonadotrophic or NORMOgonadotrophic.
  - Hypogonadotrophic patients: Standard treatment to induce ovulation consists of daily injections of both FSH and LH, which need to be carefully monitored to avoid overstimulation, resulting in ovarian hyperstimulation syndrome (OHSS).
  - Normogonadotrophic patients: most commonly due to PCOS. Ovulation induction with clomiphene citrate (Clomid). Regimen: 50 mg/day for 5 days beginning typically on CD 5 after spontaneous or progestin-induced withdrawal bleed. If no ovulation, increase dose to 100 mg/day in subsequent cycles; maximum, 150 mg/day. Some will increase dose with ovulation but no pregnancy. Most effective with ~10% body weight loss if obese.
- Unexplained infertility: IVF most effective; IUI, clomiphene, or LH/FSH yield minor improvements; better outcomes in combination
- Coital or cervical problems: IUI
- Endometriosis: either IVF or surgery; medical therapy does not increase pregnancy rates.

Second Line
- If clomiphene fails to induce ovulation:
  - Aromatase inhibitors (i.e., letrozole) may produce a better response.
  - Metformin beneficial in anovulatory women with PCOS; initiate with 500 mg daily and increase to ~1,500 mg/day; monitor renal function. Metformin may take up to 3 months to be effective. Consider also oral contraceptive pills (OCPs) for ≥2 cycles, and then retry the clomiphene immediately after stopping the OCPs.

- Generally in subspecialty care: Gonadotropin therapies (injectable FSH or FSH + LH) are effective, but riskier, treatments for infertility. They are effective for hypothalamic dysfunction for which clomiphene generally is not.

ISSUES FOR REFERRAL
Reproductive endocrinology and/or urology: Specialized lab prep is needed for IUI. FSH + LH therapies and IVF warrant referral in most cases.

ADDITIONAL THERAPIES
Consider using surrogate pregnancy if couple is amenable and female cannot conceive.

SURGERY/OTHER PROCEDURES
Reproductive surgery may be necessary in those with anatomic causes of infertility. Polypectomy could be beneficial for large polyps obstructing the lumen of the uterus. Myomectomy may increase pregnancy success rates for intramural fibroids that obstruct or distort the uterine cavity. Salpingectomy is recommended and increases fertility in those with hydrosalpinx.

COMPLEMENTARY & ALTERNATIVE MEDICINE
Acupuncture may increase live birth rates with IVF.

INPATIENT CONSIDERATIONS
Admission Criteria/Initial Stabilization
Rarely needed; however, may be needed occasionally for problems in early pregnancy and OHSS

 ONGOING CARE

FOLLOW-UP RECOMMENDATIONS
Patients should be referred to a specialist and consider more aggressive options if not successful after 3 to 6 cycles of oral ovulation induction.

Patient Monitoring
Cycle monitoring may decrease risks. US can show the number of developing follicles per cycle, which may help to predict OHSS and risk of multiple gestations.

DIET
A diet with sufficient calories to maintain a BMI permissive for ovulation. If obese, weight loss is recommended.

PATIENT EDUCATION
- Knowledge of women of reproductive age is lacking regarding the adverse effects of STI, irregular menses, and obesity on reproduction. Infertility treatment should focus on patient education (6)[A].
- American Society for Reproductive Medicine (http://www.asrm.org)
- Resolve: Patient advocacy group (http://www.resolve.org)

PROGNOSIS
Excellent; most couples will achieve a pregnancy. Without therapy, ~50% of couples not yet pregnant will conceive during the second and third years of trying.

COMPLICATIONS
Anxiety (stress levels are high during treatment), multiple pregnancy (rates increase with all medical ovulation induction therapies), OHSS (very rare with oral medications but more common with FSH treatments). Couples with infertility may have a slightly increased risk of congenital abnormalities in offspring.

REFERENCES
1. Tersigni C, Castellani R, de Waure C, et al. Celiac disease and reproductive disorders: meta-analysis of epidemiologic associations and potential pathogenic mechanisms. *Hum Reprod Update*. 2014;20(4):582–593.
2. Hurst BS, Lange SS, Kullstam SM, et al. Obstetric and gynecologic challenges in women with Ehlers-Danlos syndrome. *Obstet Gynecol*. 2014;123(3):506–513.
3. Ruder EH, Hartman TJ, Reindollar RH, et al. Female dietary antioxidant intake and time to pregnancy among couples treated for unexplained infertility. *Fertil Steril*. 2014;101(3):759–766.
4. Zareba P, Colaci DS, Afeiche M, et al. Semen quality in relation to antioxidant intake in a healthy male population. *Fertil Steril*. 2013;100(6):1572–1579.
5. Grigorescu V, Zhang Y, Kissin DM, et al. Maternal characteristics and pregnancy outcomes after assisted reproductive technology by infertility diagnosis: ovulatory dysfunction versus tubal obstruction. *Fertil Steril*. 2014;101(4):1019–1025.
6. Lundsberg LS, Pal L, Gariepy AM, et al. Knowledge, attitudes, and practices regarding conception and fertility: a population-based survey among reproductive-age United States women. *Fertil Steril*. 2014;101(3):767–774.

ADDITIONAL READING
- Fritz MA. The modern infertility evaluation. *Clin Obstet Gynecol*. 2012;55(3):692–705.
- Pavone ME, Hirshfeld-Cytron JE, Kazer RR. The progressive simplification of the infertility evaluation. *Obstet Gynecol Surv*. 2011;66(1):31–41.
- Practice Committee of American Society for Reproductive Medicine. Diagnostic evaluation of the infertile female: a committee opinion. *Fertil Steril*. 2012;98(2):302–307.
- Practice Committee of American Society for Reproductive Medicine. Diagnostic evaluation of the infertile male: a committee opinion. *Fertil Steril*. 2012;98(2):294–301.

 SEE ALSO
- Endometriosis; Amenorrhea; Infertility; Metabolic Syndrome; Polycystic Ovarian Syndrome (PCOS)
- Algorithm: Infertility

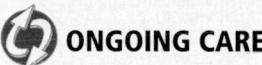 **CODES**

ICD10
- N97.9 Female infertility, unspecified
- N46.9 Male infertility, unspecified
- N97.1 Female infertility of tubal origin

CLINICAL PEARLS
- Women <35 years of age should be evaluated for infertility after failing to conceive after 1 year of unprotected intercourse; those ≥35 years should receive evaluation after 6 months, and those ≥40 years should receive assistance immediately.
- Medical therapy for endometriosis does not increase pregnancy rates, but surgical treatment does.

INFLUENZA

Katherine M. Tromp, PharmD • Hershey S. Bell, MD, MS, FAAFP

BASICS

DESCRIPTION
- Acute, typically self-limited, febrile infection caused by orthomyxovirus influenza types A and B
- Marked by inflammation of nasal mucosa, pharynx, conjunctiva, and respiratory tract
- Outbreaks have varying degrees of severity and generally peak in winter.
- Influenza virus can undergo antigenic shift (abrupt change) leading to strains of virus to which little immunologic resistance exists in a population, potentially resulting in pandemic outbreak. Minor seasonal variations are called *antigenic drift*.
- System(s) affected: typical cases: head/eyes/ears/nose/throat; pulmonary; complicated cases: cardiac and CNS involvement
- Synonym(s): flu; grippe; acute catarrhal fever

EPIDEMIOLOGY
- Predominant age: children (3 months to 16 years) and young adults
  - Morbidity: seasonal morbidity and rates of hospitalization highest in very young (preschool), elderly (>75 years of age), and individuals with comorbid illness (lung disease, malignancy)
- Predominant sex: male = female

Incidence
- Seasonal influenza in preuniversal vaccination: 95 million cases per year, typically fall/winter
- Attack rates in healthy children: 10–40% each year, prior to routine influenza vaccination

ETIOLOGY AND PATHOPHYSIOLOGY
Orthomyxovirus (influenza types A [majority] and B). Influenza A virus subtypes HxNx based on hemagglutinin and neuraminidase.
- Incubation is 1 to 4 days; infected persons are most contagious during peak symptoms.
- Spread by aerosolized droplets or contact with respiratory secretions
- Hemagglutinin binds to columnar respiratory epithelium where replication occurs, and neuraminidase protein facilitates spread along respiratory epithelium.

RISK FACTORS
- For contracting disease
  - Crowded environments such as nursing homes, barracks, schools, and correctional facilities
- For complications
  - Neonates, infants, elderly
  - Pregnancy, especially in 3rd trimester
  - Chronic pulmonary diseases
  - Cardiovascular diseases, including valvular problems and congestive heart failure (CHF)
  - Metabolic disease, morbid obesity
  - Hemoglobinopathies
  - Malignancy; immunosuppression
  - Neuromuscular diseases that limit respiratory function and ability to handle secretions
  - Patients <19 years of age who are on long-term aspirin therapy.

GENERAL PREVENTION
- Vaccination: All persons >6 months should be vaccinated annually, with very few exceptions as follows:
  - Inactivated influenza vaccine (IIV) is available with either 3 (IIV3) or 4 (IIV4) strains of influenza. IIV also is available as high-dose, intradermal, cell

culture-based (ccIIV3), and recombinant hemagglutinin influenza vaccine (RIV3).
  - Live attenuated influenza vaccine (LAIV) is an intranasal quadrivalent vaccine.
- IIV recommended annually for the following:
  - All persons aged ≥6 months
  - Vaccine should be administered annually as soon as the vaccine is available.
  - Protection occurs 1 to 2 weeks after immunization.
  - Typically mild side effects include low-grade fever and local reaction at vaccination site.
  - Inactivated IM dose: ≥3 years of age: 0.5 mL; children 6 to 35 months of age: 0.25 mL
  - Intradermal formulation for 18- to 64-year-olds uses a short 30-gauge needle in a single-use prefilled syringe with 0.1 mL vaccine; somewhat higher local reactions when given intradermal
  - Single dose every year except for children <9 years of age, who should receive 2 doses (4 weeks apart) the first year they receive influenza vaccine.
  - Vaccine contraindication: Severe allergy such as anaphylaxis to eggs or other IIV components; hives from eggs are not considered a contraindication to IIV due to very low ovalbumin dose in current IIV and good safety information; observe egg-allergic patients for 30 minutes after vaccination; no skin testing with influenza vaccine is needed in egg-allergic patients. Egg allergy is a contraindication to LAIV. RIV is safe in patients with an egg allergy.
  - Precaution: Guillain-Barré syndrome within 6 weeks after a previous dose of influenza vaccine
- LAIV recommended annually for the following:
  - Healthy persons 2 to 49 years old
  - Vaccine contraindications: anaphylaxis to eggs or other vaccine components, immunocompromising conditions, pregnancy, high-risk conditions including asthma or other chronic cardiopulmonary conditions, history of Guillain-Barré syndrome, chronic aspirin therapy in children
  - Single dose every year except for children <9 years of age, who should receive 2 doses (4 weeks apart) the first year they receive influenza vaccine
- IIV-HD: high-dose trivalent IIV
  - Contains 4 times the antigen concentration of IIV
  - Licensed for persons ≥65 years of age
  - Results in higher antibody levels but somewhat higher rates of local reactions
  - Advisory Committee on Immunization Practices does not express a preference for or against IIV-HD.
- Antiviral prophylaxis depends on current resistance patterns each year; see http://www.cdc.gov/flu/ for the current patterns or check with local health department.
  - In high-risk groups that have not been vaccinated or need additional control measures during epidemics. *Not* a substitute for vaccination unless vaccine is contraindicated (1)[A].
  - During influenza season, for those with contraindications to vaccine who have been exposed to the virus (1)[A]
  - For staff and residents in nursing home outbreaks
  - For immune-deficient persons who are expected not to respond to vaccination after exposure to the virus

Pediatric Considerations
- Vaccinate children 6 to 23 months old with IIV
- Either IIV or LAIV in healthy children 2 to 18 years of age
- For prophylaxis, oseltamivir dosage varies by weight and is recommended by the CDC for prophylaxis for children ≥3 months; zanamivir is approved for prophylaxis for children ≥5 years of age at a dosage of 2 inhalations per day. For prophylaxis, the dosage of amantadine and of rimantadine is 5 mg/kg/day up to 150 mg in 2 divided doses. Currently, amantadine and rimantadine are not recommended due to resistance.

Pregnancy Considerations
- The CDC recommends vaccinating all women who will be pregnant during influenza season.
- If unvaccinated at the time of flu season, pregnant women should receive IIV.
- Oseltamivir, zanamivir, peramivir, rimantadine, and amantadine are pregnancy Category C.

COMMONLY ASSOCIATED CONDITIONS
Bacterial pneumonia

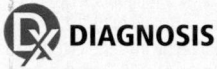

DIAGNOSIS

Rule out influenza by the ABSENCE of the following:
- Systemic symptoms
- Cough
- Not being able to cope with daily activities
- Being confined to bed

HISTORY
Sudden onset of the following:
- Fever (37.7–40.0°C), especially if combined with presenting within 3 days of illness onset
- Anorexia
- Chills, sweats, malaise, myalgia, arthralgia
- Headache
- Sore throat/pharyngitis
- Nonproductive cough
- Rhinorrhea, nasal congestion

PHYSICAL EXAM
- Physical exam is not specific for influenza.
- Physical examination should exclude complications such as otitis media, pneumonia, sinusitis, and tracheobronchitis.

DIFFERENTIAL DIAGNOSIS
- Respiratory viral infections including respiratory syncytial virus, parainfluenza, adenovirus, enterovirus ("influenza-like illness")
- Infectious mononucleosis
- Coxsackievirus infections
- Viral or streptococcal tonsillitis
- Atypical mycoplasmal pneumonia
- *Chlamydia pneumoniae*
- Q fever
- Less likely possibilities include severe acute respiratory syndrome, primary HIV infection, acute myeloid leukemia, tuberculosis, anthrax, and malaria

DIAGNOSTIC TESTS & INTERPRETATION

Initial Tests (lab, imaging)

- During influenza season, base diagnosis solely on clinical findings. If additional testing is needed
  - Reverse transcription polymerase reaction (RT-PCR) from nasopharyngeal swab or aspirate is the gold standard for diagnostic confirmation.
  - CBC: typically shows normal WBC count or mild leukopenia. Leukocytosis may indicate bacterial complications.
  - Direct fluorescent antibody or indirect fluorescent antibody staining for influenza antigen; results available in hours (dependent on lab expertise)
  - Commercial rapid enzyme-linked immunosorbent assay antigen tests are available. Some rapid tests diagnose influenza A, whereas others diagnose A and B. Sensitivity and specificity vary by manufacturer, strain of influenza, and age of patient. False negatives are fairly common particularly during periods of peak influenza activity in the population being tested.
  - Viral isolation not particularly useful except in periods of low influenza activity when making the correct diagnosis is critical.
- Imaging
  - Chest x-ray if pneumonia is suspected

 TREATMENT

- Symptomatic treatment is typically all that is required (saline nasal spray, analgesic gargle, antipyretics, analgesics).
- Cool-mist or ultrasonic humidifier to increase moisture of inspired air
- Droplet precautions: See http://www.cdc.gov/HAI/settings/outpatient/basic-infection-control-prevention-plan-2011/transmission-based-precautions.html#c
- 5 days is the average period of viral shedding in immunocompetent hosts.
- Hospitalized patients may require oxygen or ventilatory support.
- Tobacco cessation

MEDICATION

- Antiviral treatment depends on current resistance patterns each year; check http://www.cdc.gov/flu/ or local health department for current patterns. Antivirals are most effective if administered within first 48 hours in those with laboratory-confirmed (or highly suspected based on clinical findings) influenza illness.
- Antivirals within 48 hours of symptom onset are recommended if at risk of complications (i.e., diabetes, CHD, COPD, asthma, etc.) (1)[A].
- Antivirals are recommended if hospitalized (2)[A].
- Antivirals include amantadine, rimantadine, oseltamivir, zanamivir, and peramivir.
- Antivirals may be considered for persons not at increased risk of complications from influenza whose onset of symptoms is within the past 48 hours and who wish to shorten the duration of illness and further reduce their relatively low risk of complications (1)[A].
- Symptomatic treatment is preferred for those patients *without risk factors* and *without* signs of lower respiratory tract infection 2.

- Effect is 24-hour reduction of symptoms and a reduction in complication rates.
  - Zanamivir dose: 2 inhalations BID for 5 days (age ≥7 years)
  - Rimantadine dose: 100 mg BID for ages 13 to 64 years; 100 mg/day for >65 years of age
  - Amantadine dose: 100 mg BID for ages 13 to 64 years; 100 mg/day for >65 years of age
  - Oseltamivir dose: 75 mg PO BID for 5 days (age ≤13 years)
  - If severe renal impairment, 75 mg/day PO
  - Oseltamivir for children ≥1 year of age
    - <15 kg, 30 mg BID
    - >15 to 23 kg, 45 mg BID
    - >23 to 40 kg, 60 mg BID
    - >40 kg, 75 mg BID
  - Oseltamivir for children <1 year of age: 3 mg/kg/dose BID
- Peramivir dose: 600 mg IV infusion over 15 to 30 minutes for adults ≥18 years of age
- Antipyretics
  - Acetaminophen: in children
- Precautions
  - Zanamivir may cause bronchospasm if the patient has COPD or asthma; the patient should have a bronchodilator available.
  - Amantadine has anticholinergic properties and should be used with caution in those with psychiatric, addiction, or neurologic disorders, as it may increase risk for suicide attempts or increase neurologic symptoms.
  - Rimantadine may increase the risk of seizures in those with an underlying seizure disorder.
  - Oseltamivir may cause nausea and vomiting; may be less severe if taken with food.
  - Peramivir may cause serious skin reactions.
- *Amantadine and rimantadine are currently not recommended due to resistance.*
- Decrease dose of certain antivirals if creatinine clearance <30 mL/min.
- Ibuprofen or other NSAIDs for symptomatic relief
- Aspirin: should not be used in children <16 years due to risk of Reye syndrome
- Outpatient treatment is sufficient except for cases with severe complications or in high-risk groups.

 ONGOING CARE

FOLLOW-UP RECOMMENDATIONS

- Mild cases: Usually, no follow-up is required.
- Moderate or severe cases: Follow up until symptoms and any secondary sequelae resolve.

DIET

Increase fluid intake

PATIENT EDUCATION

CDC: http://www.cdc.gov/flu/

PROGNOSIS

Good

COMPLICATIONS

- Otitis media
- Acute sinusitis
- Croup
- Bronchitis
- Pneumonia (primary viral or secondary bacterial)
- Apnea in neonates
- Reye syndrome

- Rhabdomyolysis/myositis
- Postinfluenza asthenia
- COPD or CHF exacerbation
- Encephalopathy, death

Geriatric Considerations

Complications are more likely in elderly who are also more likely to require hospitalization.

REFERENCES

1. Centers for Disease Control and Prevention. Influenza antiviral medications: summary for clinicians. http://www.cdc.gov/flu/professionals/antivirals/summary-clinicians.htm.
2. Harper SA, Bradley JS, Englund JA, et al. Seasonal influenza in adults and children—diagnosis, treatment, chemoprophylaxis, and institutional outbreak management: clinical practice guidelines of the Infectious Diseases Society of America. *Clin Infect Dis*. 2009;48(8):1003–1032.

ADDITIONAL READING

- Centers for Disease Control and Prevention. Influenza. Available at http://www.cdc.gov/flu/index.htm.
- Ebell MH, White LL, Casault T. A systematic review of the history and physical examination to diagnose influenza. *J Am Board Fam Pract*. 2004;17(1):1–5.
- Grayson ML, Melvani S, Druce J, et al. Efficacy of soap and water and alcohol-based hand-rub preparations against live H1N1 influenza virus on the hands of human volunteers. *Clin Infect Dis*. 2009;48(3):285–291.
- Lalezari J, Campion K, Keene O, et al. Zanamivir for the treatment of influenza A and B infection in high-risk patients: a pooled analysis of randomized controlled trials. *Arch Intern Med*. 2001;161(2):212–217.
- Osterholm MT, Kelley NS, Sommer A, et al. Efficacy and effectiveness of influenza vaccines: a systematic review and meta-analysis. *Lancet Infect Dis*. 2012;12(1):36–44.

CODES

- J11.1 Influenza due to unidentified influenza virus with other respiratory manifestations
- J10.1 Flu due to oth ident influenza virus w oth resp manifest
- J11.00 Flu due to unidentified flu virus w unsp type of pneumonia

CLINICAL PEARLS

- Influenza is an acute, (typically) self-limited, febrile infection caused by influenza virus types A and B.
- With rare exceptions, all persons >6 months should be vaccinated against influenza on an annual basis.
- Complications from influenza are most common in the very young, very old, and those with preexisting comorbidities.
- Hand hygiene either with soap and water (slightly superior) or with alcohol-based hand rubs and covering coughs are simple ways to reduce the spread of influenza.

INGROWN TOENAIL

Andrew Richardson, MD • Rae Adams, MD

BASICS

DESCRIPTION
- In an ingrown toenail, the distal margin of the nail plate grows into the lateral nail fold, causing irritation, inflammation, and sometimes bacterial or fungal infection:
  - Stage 1 (inflammation): erythema, edema, tenderness to palpation of lateral nail fold
  - Stage 2 (abscess): increased pain, erythema, and edema as well as drainage (purulent or serous)
  - Stage 3 (granulation): chronic inflammation leads to further erythema, edema, and pain, often with granulation tissue growing over the nail plate and significant nail fold hypertrophy
- Can be recurrent
- Synonym(s): onychocryptosis, unguis incarnatus

EPIDEMIOLOGY
- Great toenail is most often affected.
- Lateral edge of nail is more commonly affected than the medial edge.
- Most common in males aged 16 to 25 years
- More common in elderly females than in elderly males
- More common in those with lower incomes

Prevalence
- 24.5/1,000 overall
- 50/1,000 ≥65 years

ETIOLOGY AND PATHOPHYSIOLOGY
- Nail plate penetrates the nail fold causing a foreign body reaction (inflammation).
- Bacteria or fungi may enter through the opening in the nail fold, causing infection and abscess formation.
- The inflamed and infected area leads to granulation tissue and hypertrophy of the nail fold.

RISK FACTORS
- Genetic factors
  - Increased nail fold width
  - Decreased nail thickness
  - Medial rotation of the toe
- Many others proposed; none proven, including the following:
  - Distorted, thickened nail (onychogryphosis)
  - Fungal infection (onychomycosis)
  - Hyperhidrosis
  - Improper trimming of the lateral nail plate
  - Poorly fitting shoes
  - Trauma to nail or nail fold
  - Conditions that predispose to pedal edema (i.e., thyroid dysfunction, diabetes, obesity, heart failure, renal disease)

GENERAL PREVENTION
- Properly fitting shoes
- Proper nail trimming (see "Patient Education")

DIAGNOSIS

HISTORY
- Pain
- Redness
- Swelling
- Drainage

PHYSICAL EXAM
- Nail fold tenderness
- Erythema
- Edema
- Drainage (serous or purulent)
- Granulation tissue
- Lateral nail fold hypertrophy

DIFFERENTIAL DIAGNOSIS
- Cellulitis
- Felon (pulp abscess on plantar aspect of toe)
- Onychogryphosis (gross thickening and hardening of the nail)
- Onycholysis (separation of nail from nail bed)
- Onychomycosis (fungal infection of the nail)
- Osteomyelitis
- Paronychia
- Subungual exostosis (osteochondroma beneath the nail)

DIAGNOSTIC TESTS & INTERPRETATION
Initial Tests (lab, imaging)
None needed unless patient appears septic. Then consider CBC and blood cultures.
- Consider MRI, x-ray, or bone scan if osteomyelitis is suspected.
- Consider x-ray if subungual exostosis is suspected.

TREATMENT

- Surgical interventions are more effective than nonsurgical interventions in preventing recurrence (1,2)[A].
- The use of phenol for nail bed ablation is probably more effective than nail avulsion alone in preventing recurrence (1,2)[A].
- Nail avulsion techniques (described in the following section) are more effective than nail fold debulking techniques (not described in this topic) (2)[A].
- Nonsurgical interventions, such as a flexible gutter splint, are another option for treatment of stage 2 or 3 ingrown nails (3,4)[B].

GENERAL MEASURES
For stage 1:
- Warm, soapy water soaks for 10 to 20 minutes twice daily until symptoms resolve (5)
- Proper nail trimming
- Properly fitted shoes

MEDICATION
- Neither oral nor topical antibiotics are useful as an adjunct to surgical treatment.
- NSAIDs are usually adequate for analgesia.

ADDITIONAL THERAPIES
- For stage 1 ingrown nails, several treatments are available:
  - Cotton wool
    - Bluntly insert a wisp of cotton under the ingrown portion of the nail using a small curette or nail elevator.
    - Instruct the patient to reinsert new cotton if the other comes out until the nail grows beyond the nail fold.
    - Consider adding silver nitrate cautery to the nail fold, which the patient then repeats at home.
  - Dental floss
    - Bluntly insert some dental floss to lift the nail away from the lateral nail fold.
    - Instruct the patient to replace the floss as necessary if it comes out or gets dirty.
    - Keep floss in place until the nail grows beyond the nail fold.
  - Taping
    - Apply surgical tape to both sides of toe.
    - Use another piece of tape from one side to the other to pull the lateral nail fold away from the nail plate.
    - Instruct the patient to keep taping until the nail grows beyond the fold.
  - Cryotherapy of the lateral nail fold
- For stage 2 ingrown nails, consider attempting conservative treatment, as above, especially cotton wool, or cryotherapy.

SURGERY/OTHER PROCEDURES
- For stage 2 ingrown nails where conservative treatment has failed, stage 3 ingrown nails, or recurrent ingrown nails, consider either
  - Partial avulsion of the nail with phenol nail matrix ablation
    - Achieve local anesthesia as described in the following text.
    - May consider placing a tourniquet around the base of the toe to assist with hemostasis (caution in patients with diabetes or peripheral vascular disease)
    - Elevate the ingrown part of the nail from the nail bed with a periosteal (Freer) elevator or hemostat.

○ Incise the nail longitudinally with scissors or a nail splitter a few millimeters from the ingrown border, starting at the distal edge and proceeding to the matrix.

○ Grasp the avulsed fragment with a hemostat and pull this portion gently out with a hemostat, utilizing longitudinal traction, as well as rotation if needing.

○ Remove the tourniquet once hemostasis is attained.

○ Dip a urethral swab in 80–88% phenol solution.

○ Apply the phenol for 1 minute to the nail matrix under the proximal nail fold. Use multiple swabs if necessary.

○ Wash the area with isopropyl (rubbing) alcohol to neutralize phenol.

– Flexible gutter splint

○ Cut a 1- to 2-cm long piece of sterilized plastic tube, such as IV tubing, 2 to 3 mm in diameter (alternatively, you may use a cap from a 29-gauge needle).

○ Make a slit in the tubing lengthwise and cut the end off at an angle.

○ Apply local anesthesia (see below).

○ Release the ingrown edge of the nail from the nail fold with a hemostat.

○ Slide the tube, angled end first, along the ingrown edge of the nail.

○ Consider fixing the tube in place with self-curing formable acrylic resin (used for dentures and sculptured nails), tape, or a single suture through the nail plate.

○ Leave the tube in place until nail has grown beyond the nail fold.

• Other options for nail matrix ablation include the following:

– Sodium hydroxide (NaOH)

– Cryotherapy

– Electrocautery with a special flattened tip coated with Teflon on one side to protect the proximal nail fold

– Radiofrequency ablation

– Carbon dioxide laser

– Curettage

– Surgical excision

• Local anesthesia can be achieved with either

– Distal wing block: Infuse 1% lidocaine without epinephrine near the junction of the proximal and lateral nail folds. Continue infusing until the nail folds and the tip of the digit under the distal nail are white from the pressure of the anesthetic.

– Digital ring block: Infuse 1% lidocaine without epinephrine on the medial and lateral surfaces of the involved digit to anesthetize the plantar and dorsal digital nerves. Lidocaine with epinephrine may be used in selected patients (no peripheral vascular disease, diabetes, cardiac problems, or any evidence of digital infection, gangrene, or bone fracture) (6).

 ONGOING CARE

FOLLOW-UP RECOMMENDATIONS

• Dress with antibiotic ointment or sterile petroleum jelly; cover with sterile gauze and tube gauze.

• Postop instructions should include the following:

– Rest and elevate the foot for 12 to 24 hours.

– Take NSAIDs for discomfort.

– Change dressing and wash with soap and water at least daily for 1 to 2 weeks following procedure.

– Expect a sterile exudate for 2 to 6 weeks.

– Avulsed nails may take 6 to 12 months to grow completely out (if no matrix ablation).

– Call for increasing pain, redness, or swelling.

– Average time to return to normal activities is 2 weeks.

• Patients treated conservatively should be followed up in the office every 7 to 10 days until marked improvement is noted.

PATIENT EDUCATION

• Trim nails straight across perpendicular to long axis of the nail (do not round corners) and not too short.

• Wear properly fitting, comfortable shoes.

COMPLICATIONS

• Cellulitis after surgical procedure (uncommon)

• Damage to fascia or periosteum from overly aggressive matrix ablation

• Damage to nail bed

• Distal toe ischemia due to prolonged use of a tourniquet during surgery (rare)

• Nail plate deformity (due to nail matrix damage)

• Osteomyelitis (rare)

• Permanent narrowing of nail (if partial matrix ablation is performed)

• Persistent postoperative wound drainage

• Recurrence (40–80% with avulsion alone, 0.6–14% with matrix ablation, 6–13% with gutter splint)

REFERENCES

1. Eekhof JA, Van Wijk B, Knuistingh Neven A, et al. Interventions for ingrowing toenails. *Cochrane Database Syst Rev*. 2012;(4):CD001541.

2. Park DH, Singh D. The management of ingrowing toenails. *BMJ*. 2012;344:e2089.

3. Arai H, Arai T, Nakajima H, et al. Formable acrylic treatment for ingrowing nail with gutter splint and sculptured nail. *Int J Dermatol*. 2004;43(10): 759–765.

4. Nazari S. A simple and practical method in treatment of ingrown nails: splinting by flexible tube. *J Eur Acad Dermatol Venereol*. 2006;20(10): 1302–1306.

5. Heidelbaugh J, Lee H. Management of the ingrown toenail. *Am Fam Physician*. 2009;79(4):303–308.

6. Altinyazar HC, Demirel CB, Koca R, et al. Digital block with and without epinephrine during chemical matricectomy with phenol. *Dermatol Surg*. 2010;36(10):1568–1571.

ADDITIONAL READING

• Bos AM, van Tilburg MW, van Sorge AA, et al. Randomized clinical trial of surgical technique and local antibiotics for ingrowing toenail. *Br J Surg*. 2007;94(3):292–296.

• Chapeskie H. Ingrown toenail or overgrown toe skin?: alternative treatment for onychocryptosis. *Can Fam Physician*. 2008;54(11):1561–1562.

• Reyzelman AM, Trombello KA, Vayser DJ, et al. Are antibiotics necessary in the treatment of locally infected ingrown toenails? *Arch Fam Med*. 2000;9(9):930–932.

• Richert B. Basic nail surgery. *Dermatol Clin*. 2006;24(3):313–322.

• Woo SH, Kim IH. Surgical pearl: nail edge separation with dental floss for ingrown toenails. *J Am Acad Dermatol*. 2004;50(6):939–940.

 SEE ALSO

For a video of this Nail Avulsion and Matrixectomy procedure, go to http://5minuteconsult.com /procedure/1508006.

 CODES

ICD10
L60.0 Ingrowing nail

CLINICAL PEARLS

• The best treatment for a stage 1 ingrown toenail is to insert a wisp of cotton or dental floss between the nail plate and lateral nail fold.

• The best treatment for a stage 3 ingrown toenail is partial nail avulsion with phenol matrix ablation.

• Patients can prevent ingrown toenails by trimming nails properly and wearing properly fitting shoes.

• Oral and topical antibiotics are not useful in the treatment of ingrown nails in conjunction with surgical treatment.

INJURY AND VIOLENCE

Jonathan R. Ballard, MD, MPH, MPhil

BASICS

DESCRIPTION
- Injury, intentional or not, is considered predictable and preventable (1).
- Unintentional injuries are no longer considered "accidents" given that injuries are preventable (1).
- Unintentional injury is the fifth leading cause of death and intentional self-harm is the 10th leading cause of death in 2010 in the United States (2).
- Injury is the leading cause of death of people aged 1 to 44 years and a leading cause of disability for people of all ages, regardless of sex, race/ethnicity, or socioeconomic status (1).
- Violence-related deaths account for 54,103 deaths in the United States in 2009 (3) with 61% suicide, 25% homicide, and 14% deaths of undetermined intent (4).

EPIDEMIOLOGY
Incidence

Leading Cause of Death by Age Group, United States, 2011 (5)

Age	Most Common	Number of Deaths
<1	Congenital anomalies	5,013
1–44	**Unintentional injury**	46,050
45–64	Malignant neoplasm	161,469
65+	Heart disease	475,097

- Children mostly die of unintentional injuries: (in order) motor vehicle accidents (MVAs), fire/burn, drowning, and suffocation (6)
- MVAs are the most common type of unintentional injury in adolescents, followed by firearm-associated injuries (7).
- Suicide is the second leading cause of death for adolescents and young adults age 15 to 34 years (5).
- Poisoning is particularly deadly for young adults ages 15 to 59 years for whom it is the leading cause of unintentional home injury deaths (6).
- Unintentional death by firearm is fourth common cause of death in children ages 5 to 14 years, third common cause for adolescents and adults ages 15 to 29 years (6).
- Homicide is the third leading cause of death in 2011 for persons between ages 1 to 4 and 15 to 34 in the United States (5).
- *Watch for homicide as cause of unexplained death in young children.*

ETIOLOGY AND PATHOPHYSIOLOGY
Multifactorial

RISK FACTORS
- MVAs:
  - MVAs account for 35,303 deaths in 2010 in the United States, with an age-adjusted rate of 11 deaths per 100,000 persons (3).
  - More than 2.3 million adult drivers and passengers were treated in emergency departments from MVAs in 2009 (8).
  - Young adults (18 to 24 years old) have the highest crash-related injury rates of all adults (8).

- Motorcyclists are found to be 37 times more likely to die in a motor vehicle crash than passenger car occupants and 9 times more likely to be injured (9).
  - Risk factors for involvement in an MVA include high speed, teenage drivers, alcohol consumption, distracted driving including hand-held mobile phones and inadequate visibility (10).
  - Risk of death by an MVA increases with male driver, inexperience, nighttime driving, speeding, tailgating, driving with other teenagers, cell phones, unrestrained occupants, use of older cars, nonuse of crash helmets, alcohol, and drug use. In elderly—poor vision, medical conditions, and comorbidities increases risk of death by an MVA (8,10).
- Pedestrians:
  - 4,280 pedestrians were killed by motor vehicles in 2010 and about 70,000 were injured in 2010 (8).
  - Pedestrians are 1.5 more times likely than passenger vehicle occupants to be killed in a car crash on each trip (8).
- Bicycles:
  - Risk of death increased from crash with motor vehicle if speed >30 km/hr (~18 mph) and cyclist impact with front of vehicle (10).
  - Risk factors for cyclist injury include alcohol consumption, shared use motorways, poor visibility, lack of understanding of road safety, and design/type of impacting vehicle (10).
- Suffocation: increased risk for children <1 year, unsafe sleeping environments (11)
- Drowning: increased risk for African American children, unattended children in bathtubs, access to swimming pools, and recreational water activities (11)
- Homicide:
  - Third leading cause of death for children 1 to 4 years and adolescents and young adults ages 15 to 34 years (5).
  - Lack of access to social capital, community organization, and economic resources; familial instability; community and family violence; access to firearms (4)
  - Homicide and suicide: access to firearms, mental health, alcohol and drug use, exposure to suicidal behavior, history of aggressive behavior, cognitive deficits, poor supervision, exposure to violence, parental drug and alcohol use, poor peer-to-peer interaction, academic failure, poverty, lower socioeconomic class (4)
- Adolescent violence:
  - 33% of students are involved in fights annually; 13% of students participated in ≥1 fights at school in the last year (11).
  - 17% of students have carried a weapon in the last 30 days; 6.1% of students have carried a weapon to school; 9% of students have been injured by a weapon at school (11).
- Injury (sports-related):
  - High school athletes are at increased risk (12).
  - High school students sustained 1.2 million injuries during the 2008 to 2009 school year (12).
- Bullying:
  - Prevalence is 30% for children either bullying and/or being bullied in 6th to 10th graders (13)
  - Bullying associated with low self-esteem, social isolation, and depression (13)
  - 1:9 middle school students report being cyberbullied (via the Internet or cell phones); ~50% of victims don't know perpetrator's identity (13).

- Interpersonal violence (IPV):
  - 40–70% of female homicides killed by boyfriends or husbands (14)
  - Nearly 31% of women and 26% of men report having some form of IPV in their lifetime (14).
  - Dating violence: Prevalence has been reported to range from 9% to 46% (14).
  - Female, young (33% of rapes occur prior to 12 years of age; 50% by 18 years), history of IPV or sexual assault or child abuse, drugs, marital difficulties, unemployment, depression, minority status, income or educational disparity, poverty, weak legal sanctions (14)
- Falls: poor vision, psychotropic medications and diuretics, arthritis, impaired mobility, inappropriate footwear and walking aids, cognitive impairment, gait imbalance, environmental risk factors (9)
- Poisonings:
  - Poisonings are the second leading cause of unintentional home injury deaths for ages 15 to 59 years (6).
  - Prescription drug overdose is a leading cause of accidental death in adults (6).
  - A significant increase in opioid-associated deaths has occurred from 2000 to 2008 (6).
  - Combined use of other sedating drugs (6)
  - Watch for opioid-induced poisonings in unexplained altered mental status.

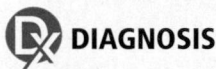

DIAGNOSIS

HISTORY
- Mechanism, timing, and location of injury:
  - Blunt versus penetrating; intentional versus unintentional; others injured versus isolated injury; circumstances (weather, substance use, restrained vs. unrestrained)
  - Does history correlate with level of injury (i.e., level of suspicion for abuse [elderly, child, or partner])?
  - Is further evaluation required (blood and/or urine testing, response to opioid receptor antagonists, imaging)?
- IPV: neurologic deficits, seizures, chronic pain, GI, STI, pregnancy, psychiatric presentations

  - In January 2013, USPSTF recommends that clinicians screen women of childbearing age for intimate partner violence, such as domestic violence, and provide or refer women who screen positive to intervention services (15)[B].

TREATMENT

- Prevention: The primary focus for reducing injury and violence is specific individually tailored preventive measures based on risk factors and population-level prevention (1). Prevention efforts have been framed as "the 5 E's": enhanced education, engineering strategies, economic incentives, and enforcement/enactment of laws (1,9)[C].
- Prevention by level of intervention: primary (i.e., prevent crash), secondary (i.e., prevent injury upon crash), and tertiary (i.e., prevent poor outcomes upon injury) (1,9)[C]
- Acute setting: Follow Basic Life Support (BLS), Advanced Trauma Life Support (ATLS), Advanced Cardiovascular Life Support (ACLS) and Pediatric Advanced Life Support (PALS) guidelines (1,16)[A].

- Motor vehicle injuries:

  - Infants, toddlers, and children: age-appropriate child safety seats and passenger restraints with distribution programs, education programs for parents and caregivers, safety seat checkpoints, harsh penalties for drivers transporting children under the influence of drugs and/or alcohol, legislation regarding restraint of motor vehicle occupants (9)[A]
  - Adolescents and adults: graduated driver licensing programs, blood alcohol concentration laws, minimum drinking age laws, sobriety checkpoints, programs for alcohol servers, zero alcohol tolerance laws for young drivers, school-based education programs on drinking and driving. Emergency medical services (EMS) response times, engineering cars for rapid extraction, organized trauma systems; collapsible automobile steering columns have been shown to decrease injury mortality and morbidity (9)[B].
  - Older adults: alternative transportation programs, screening for high-risk drivers, gradual curtailment of driving privileges, more frequent license renewal process (9)[B]
  - Bicycle helmets can reduce risk of head injury by 63–88%. Canadian helmet legislation decreased mortality by 52% (9)[B].
  - Pedestrian injury: pedestrian safety education, reflective clothing, use of crosswalks, limit mobile phone use while crossing roads (9)[B]. Street lighting for pedestrians (9)[A]. Fluorescent clothing for pedestrians and cyclists (9)[A]
  - Cyclists injury: flashing lights and reflectors at night (9)[B]. Helmet use (9)[A]. Cyclists separation to motor vehicles (9)[B]

- Falls:

  - Home safety assessments, installation of handrails and grab bars, removal of tripping hazards, nonslip mats, exercise programs such as Tai Chi to improve strength and balance, night lights, cataract surgery, gradual withdrawal of psychotropic medication (9)[B]
  - In May 2012, USPSTF recommended exercise or physical therapy and vitamin D supplementation to prevent falls in community-dwelling adults aged 65 years or older who are at increased risk for falls (15)[B].
  - The USPSTF does not recommend automatically performing an in-depth multifactorial risk assessment in conjunction with comprehensive management of identified risks to prevent falls in community-dwelling adults aged 65 years or older because the likelihood of benefit is small (15)[C].

- Drowning:

  - Improved supervision of young children, especially for those with epilepsy. Swimming lessons in those >4 years old, trained lifeguard supervision, fencing, locked gates and pool alarms, no use of alcohol in recreation aquatic activities, personal floatation devices, and boating safety awareness; parental and caregiver certification in CPR (9)[B]

- Violence (homicide, suicide, assaults):
  - Primary prevention: Most effective strategies focus on younger age groups to change individual attitudes and risk-taking behaviors (9)[C].

  - Secondary prevention: Detect and identify violence in early stages (9)[B]. The USPSTF recommends that clinicians screen women of childbearing age for intimate partner violence, such as domestic violence, and provide or refer women who screen positive to intervention services (15)[B].
  - Tertiary prevention: IPV reduced by alcoholism treatment for partner, intense advocacy interventions of >12 hours (9)[A]

  - Suicide: access to mental health services, improved family and community support, development of healthy coping and problem-solving skills

  - USPSTF recommends screening adults for depression when depression care supports are in place to assure accurate diagnosis, effective treatment, and follow-up (15)[B].
  - Dating violence: self-reported dating violence reduced by school and community-based programs for prevention of dating violence (9)[A]

- Sports-related injuries:

  - Proper equipment. Helmets can prevent bicyclist head injuries and mortality (9)[A].
  - Plan of action for dealing with concussion and head injury in young athletes, with guidelines regarding if or when it is safe to return to play (17)[B].

- Poisonings:

  - Follow acute care guidelines. Contact Poison Control Center hotline immediately after discovered ingestion of toxin for recommendations (18)[A].

ONGOING CARE

COMPLICATIONS
Social burden of injury: loss of productivity, emotional loss, nonmedical expenditures, reduced quality of life, litigation, rehabilitation, mental health costs, altered family and peer relationships, chronic pain, substance use and abuse, changes in lifestyle (1,9)

REFERENCES

1. Sleet DA, Dahlberg LL, Basavaraju SV, et al. Injury prevention, violence prevention, and trauma care: building the scientific base. *MMWR Surveill Summ*. 2011;60(Suppl 4):78–85.
2. Murphy SL, Xu J, Kochanek KD. Deaths: final data for 2010. *Natl Vital Stat Rep*. 2013;61(4):1–117.
3. Centers for Disease Control and Prevention. National Center for Injury Prevention and Control. Web-based Injury Statistics Query and Reporting System (WISQARS). http://www.cdc.gov/injury/wisqars.
4. Centers for Disease Control and Prevention. Division of Violence Prevention Annual Report 2011. http://www.cdc.gov/violenceprevention/pdf/dvp_annualreport_2011.pdf.
5. Centers for Disease Control and Prevention, National Center for Injury Prevention and Control. Leading Causes of Death 2011. http://www.cdc.gov/injury/wisqars/pdf/leading_causes_of_death_by_age_group_2011-a.pdf.
6. Mack KA, Rudd RA, Mickalide AD, et al. Fatal unintentional injuries in the home in the U.S., 2000–2008. *Am J Prev Med*. 2013;44(3):239–246.
7. Centers for Disease Control and Prevention. National Suicide Statistics at a Glance. www.cdc.gov/ViolencePrevention/suicide/statistics/index.html.
8. Centers for Disease Control and Prevention. Injury Prevention and Control: Motor Vehicle Safety. http://www.cdc.gov/Motorvehiclesafety.
9. Curry P, Ramaiah R, Vavilala MS. Current trends and update on injury prevention. *Int J Crit Illn Inj Sci*. 2011;1(1):57–65.
10. World Health Organization. *World Report on Road Traffic Injury and Prevention*. Geneva, Switzerland: World Health Organization; 2004. http://whqlibdoc.who.int/publications/2004/9241562609.pdf?ua=1.
11. Committee on Injury, Violence, and Poison Prevention. Policy statement—role of the pediatrician in youth violence prevention. *Pediatrics*. 2009;124(1):393–402.
12. Centers for Disease Control and Prevention, National Center for Injury Prevention and Control. *National Action Plan for Child Injury Prevention*. Atlanta, GA: CDC, NICP; 2012. www.cdc.gov/safechild/pdf/National_Action_Plan_for_Child_Injury_Prevention.pdf
13. Donnerstein E. Internet bullying. *Pediatr Clin North Am*. 2012;59(3):623–633.
14. Moyer VA. Screening for intimate partner violence and abuse of elderly and vulnerable adults: U.S. Preventive Services Task Force recommendation statement. *Ann Intern Med*. 2013;158(6):478–486.
15. U.S. Preventive Services Task Force. Recommendations. www.uspreventiveservicestaskforce.org/Page/Name/recommendations.
16. Field JM, Hazinski MF, Sayre MR, et al. Part 1: executive summary: 2010 American Heart Association guidelines for cardiopulmonary resuscitation and emergency cardiovascular care. *Circulation*. 2010;122(18)(Suppl 3):S640–S656.
17. Armstrong C. Evaluation and management of concussion in athletes: recommendations from the AAN. *Am Fam Physician*. 2014;89(7):585–587.
18. Mowry JB, Spyker DA, Cantilena LR Jr, et al. 2012 annual report of the American Association of Poison Control Centers' National Poison Data System (NPDS). *Clin Toxicol*. 2013;51(10):949–1229.

CODES

ICD10
- T14.90 Injury, unspecified
- T14.8 Other injury of unspecified body region
- R29.6 Repeated falls

CLINICAL PEARLS

- Injury and violence are predictable and preventable.
- Unintentional injury is the fifth leading cause of death.
- Injury is the primary source of lost years of productive life for individuals younger than age 44 years.
- MVAs cause most deaths in children and adolescents.
- Children die of unintentional injuries (in order): MVA, drowning, fire/burn, and suffocation
- Nearly 31% of women and 26% of men report having some form of IPV in their lifetime.

INSOMNIA

Susanne Wild, MD

BASICS

DESCRIPTION
- Difficulty initiating or maintaining sleep or non-restorative sleep despite adequate opportunity and circumstances for sleep
- Causes at least one of the following forms of daytime impairment related to nighttime sleep difficulty:
  – Fatigue or malaise
  – Attention, concentration, or memory impairment
  – Social or vocational dysfunction or poor school performance
  – Mood disturbance or irritability
  – Daytime sleepiness
  – Motivation, energy, or initiative reduction
  – Proneness for errors or accidents at work or while driving
  – Tension, headaches, or GI symptoms in response to sleep loss
  – Concerns or worries about sleep

EPIDEMIOLOGY
- Predominant age: increases with age
- Predominant sex: female > male (5:1)

Prevalence
- Insomnia (transient and chronic): 5–35% of the population; 10–15% associated with daytime impairment
- Chronic insomnia: 10% middle-aged adults; 1/3 of people >65 years

ETIOLOGY AND PATHOPHYSIOLOGY
- Transient/intermittent (<30 days)
  – Stress/excitement/bereavement
  – Shift work
  – Medical illness
  – High altitude
- Chronic (>30 days)
  – Medical: gastroesophageal reflux disease, sleep apnea, chronic pain, congestive heart failure, Alzheimer disease, Parkinson disease, chronic fatigue syndrome, irritable bowel syndrome
  – Psychiatric: mood, anxiety, psychotic disorders
  – Primary sleep disorder: idiopathic, psychophysiologic (heightened arousal and learned sleep-preventing associations), paradoxical (sleep state misperception)
  – Circadian rhythm disorder: irregular pattern, jet lag, delayed/advanced sleep phase, shift work
  – Environmental: light (liquid crystal display [LCD] clocks), noise (snoring, household, traffic), movements (partner/young children/pets)
  – Behavioral: poor sleep hygiene, adjustment sleep disorder
  – Substance induced
  – Medications: antihypertensives, antidepressants, corticosteroids, levodopa-carbidopa, phenytoin, quinidine, theophylline, thyroid hormones

Pregnancy Considerations
Transient insomnia occurs secondary to change of sleep position, nocturia, gastritis, back pain, anxiety.

RISK FACTORS
- Age
- Female gender
- Medical comorbidities
- Unemployment
- Psychiatric illness
- Impaired social relationships
- Lower socioeconomic status
- Shift work
- Separation from spouse or partner
- Drug and substance abuse

GENERAL PREVENTION
- Practice consistent sleep hygiene:
  – Fixed wake-up times and bedtimes regardless of amount of sleep obtained (weekdays and weekends)
  – Go to bed only when sleepy.
  – Avoid naps.
  – Sleep in a cool, dark, quiet environment.
  – No activities or stimuli in bedroom associated with anything but sleep or sex.
  – 30-minute wind-down time before sleep
  – If unable to sleep within 20 minutes, move to another environment and engage in quiet activity until sleepy.
- Limit caffeine intake to mornings.
- No alcohol after 4 PM.
- Fixed eating times
- Avoid medications that interfere with sleep.
- Regular moderate exercise

COMMONLY ASSOCIATED CONDITIONS
- Psychiatric disorders
- Painful musculoskeletal conditions
- Obstructive sleep apnea
- Restless leg syndrome
- Drug or alcohol addiction/dependence

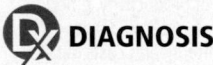

DIAGNOSIS

HISTORY
- Daytime sleepiness and napping
- Unintended sleep episodes (driving, working)
- Insomnia history
  – Duration, time of problem
  – Sleep latency, difficulty in maintaining sleep (repeated awakening), early morning awakening, nonrestorative sleep, or patterns (weekday vs. weekend, with or without bed partner, home vs. away)
- Sleep hygiene
  – Bedtime/wakening time
  – Physical environment of sleep area: LED clocks, TV, room lighting, ambient noise
  – Activity: nighttime eating, exercise, sexual activity
  – Intake: caffeine, alcohol, herbal supplements, diet pills, illicit drugs, prescriptions, over-the-counter (OTC) sleep aids
- Symptoms or history of depression, anxiety, obsessive-compulsive disorder, or other major psychological symptomatology
- Symptoms of restless leg syndrome and periodic limb movement disorder
- Symptoms of heightened arousal
- Snoring and other symptoms of sleep apnea
- Symptoms or history of drug or alcohol abuse
- Current medication use
- Chronic medical conditions
- Acute change or stressors such as travel or shift work
- Sleep diary: sleep log for 7 consecutive days

DIFFERENTIAL DIAGNOSIS
- Sleep-disordered breathing such as obstructive sleep apnea
- CNS hypersomnias (e.g., narcolepsy)
- Circadian rhythm sleep disturbances
- Sleep-related movement disorders (e.g., restless leg syndrome)
- Substance abuse
- Insomnia due to medical or neurologic disorder
- Mood and anxiety disorders such as depression or anxiety

DIAGNOSTIC TESTS & INTERPRETATION
- Diagnostic testing usually not required; consider polysomnography if sleep apnea or periodic limb movement disorder is suspected (1)[C].
- Primary insomnia
  – Symptoms for at least 1 month: difficulty in initiating/maintaining sleep or nonrestorative sleep
  – Impairment in social, occupational, or other important areas of functioning
  – Does not occur exclusively during narcolepsy, breathing-related sleep disorder, circadian rhythm sleep disorder, or parasomnia
  – Does not occur exclusively during major depressive disorder, generalized anxiety disorder, delirium
  – Is not secondary to physiologic effects of substance or general medical condition
  – Sleep disturbance (or resultant daytime fatigue) causes clinically significant distress.
- Secondary insomnia
  – Due to substance abuse, medication induced (diuretics, stimulants, etc.), primary depressive disorder, generalized anxiety disorder or phobias, acute situational stress, posttraumatic stress disorder, pain

Initial Tests (lab, imaging)
Testing to consider based on history and physical exam:
- Thyroid-stimulating hormone
- Urine toxicology

Diagnostic Procedures/Other
Polysomnography or multiple sleep latency test not routinely indicated but may be considered if
- Initial diagnosis is uncertain.
- Treatment interventions have proven unsuccessful.

TREATMENT

- Transient insomnia
  – May use medications for short-term use only; benzodiazepines favored
  – Self-medicating with alcohol can increase awakenings and sleep-stage changes.
- Chronic insomnia
  – Treatment of underlying condition (major depressive disorder, generalized anxiety disorder, medications, pain, substance abuse)
  – Advise good sleep hygiene.
  – Cognitive-behavioral therapy is the first-line treatment for chronic insomnia, especially in >60 years population, especially when sedatives are not advantageous (2)[A].
  – Behavioral therapy is an effective treatment for insomnia and a potentially more effective long-term treatment than pharmacotherapy (3)[B].
  – Ramelteon is the only agent without abuse potential (4)[B].

MEDICATION

- Reserved for transient insomnia such as with jet lag, stress reactions, transient medical condition
- Nonbenzodiazepine hypnotics
  – Act on benzodiazepine receptor so have abuse potential
    ○ Zaleplon (Sonata) 5 to 20 mg; half-life 1 hour
    ○ Zolpidem (Ambien) 5 to 10 mg (males); 5 mg (females); half-life 2.5 to 3 hours
    ○ Zolpidem (Ambien CR) 6.25 to 12.5 mg (males); 6.25 mg (females); half-life 2.5 to 3 hours
    ○ Eszopiclone (Lunesta) 1 to 3 mg; half-life 6 hours
- Benzodiazepine hypnotics
  – Short acting
    ○ Triazolam (Halcion) 0.25 mg; half-life 1.5 to 5.5 hours
  – Intermediate acting
    ○ Temazepam (Restoril) 7.5 to 30 mg; half-life 8.8 hours long-acting:
      ▪ Lorazepam (Ativan) 1 to 4 mg; half-life 14 hours
      ▪ Diazepam (Valium) 5 to 10 mg; half-life 30 to 60 hours
      ▪ Estazolam (Prosom) 1 to 2 mg; half-life 10 to 24 hours
- Contraindications/precautions:
  – Not indicated for long-term treatment due to risks of tolerance, dependency, daytime attention and concentration compromise, incoordination, rebound insomnia
  – Long-acting benzodiazepines associated with higher incidence of daytime sedation and motor impairment
  – Avoid in elderly, pregnant, breastfeeding, substance abusers, and patients with suicidal or parasuicidal behaviors.
  – Avoid in patients with untreated obstructive apnea and chronic pulmonary disease.
  – No good evidence for benzodiazepines for patients undergoing palliative care (5)[A]
  – Nonbenzodiazepine receptor agonists may occasionally induce parasomnias (sleepwalking, sleep eating, sleep driving).
- Melatonin receptor agonist
  – Ramelteon 8 mg; half-life 1 to 2.6 hours
    ○ Effective to reduce sleep time onset for short- and long-term use in adults, without abuse potential; no comparative studies with older agents have been completed. Onset of effect may take up to 3 weeks (4)[B].
- Serotonergic antidepressants
  – Trazodone 25 to 200 mg; half-life 3 to 9 hours
  – Doxepin 10 to 50 mg; half-life 15 hours
    ○ New formulation of medication is available at dosage 3 to 6 mg QHS.
  – Amitriptyline 25 to 50 mg; half-life 10 to 26 hours
  – Mirtazapine 7.5 to 15 mg; half-life 20 to 40 hours
- Sedating antihistamines are not recommended and should be used conservatively for insomnia due to insufficient evidence of efficacy and significant concerns about risks of these medications.

Geriatric Considerations

Caution (risk of falls and confusion) when prescribing benzodiazepines or other sedative hypnotics; if absolutely necessary, use short-acting nonbenzodiazepine agonists at half the dosage or melatonin agonists for short-term treatment.

ADDITIONAL THERAPIES

Associated with hypertension, congestive heart failure, anxiety and depression, and obesity; management of these chronic conditions will help with incidence and symptoms of insomnia.

COMPLEMENTARY & ALTERNATIVE MEDICINE

- Melatonin: decreases sleep latency when taken 30 to 120 minutes prior to bedtime, but there is no good evidence for efficacy in insomnia, and long-term effects are unknown (6)[B]
- Valerian: Inconsistent evidence supporting efficacy and its slow onset of action (2 to 3 weeks) makes it unsuitable for the acute treatment of insomnia.
- Acupuncture: insufficient evidence on effect of needle acupuncture and its variants (7)
- Antihistamines: insufficient evidence; should not be recommended for use
- Cognitive-behavioral therapy (including relaxation therapy): effective and considered more useful than medications; recommended initial treatment for patients with chronic insomnia
- Mindfulness awareness practices: improved sleep quality and sleep-related daytime impairment for older adults per small randomized trial (8)

 ## ONGOING CARE

FOLLOW-UP RECOMMENDATIONS
- Daily exercise improves quality of sleep and may be more effective than medication.
- Avoid exercise within 4 hours of bedtime.

Patient Monitoring
- Reassess need for medications periodically; avoid standing prescriptions.
- Caution patients that nonbenzodiazepine agonists (zolpidem, zaleplon, eszopiclone), as well as benzo-diazepines, can be habit forming.
- Studies suggest an association between receiving a hypnotic prescription and a >3-fold increase in hazards of death, even when prescribed <18 pills per year (9)[B].

DIET
- Avoid caffeine or reserve for morning only.
- Avoid heavy late-night snacks (light snack at bedtime may help).
- Avoid alcohol within 6 hours of bedtime.

PROGNOSIS
- Situational insomnia should resolve with time.
- Treatment of underlying etiology and consistent sleep hygiene are the mainstays of treatment.

COMPLICATIONS
- Transient insomnia can become chronic.
- Daytime sleepiness, cognitive dysfunction
- Pulmonary hypertension if chronic sleep apnea left untreated
- Sleep apnea may lead to hypertension, stroke, or cardiac ischemia.

REFERENCES

1. Kushida CA, Littner MR, Morgenthaler T, et al. Practice parameters for the indications for polysomnography and related procedures: an update for 2005. *Sleep.* 2005;28(4):499–521.
2. Montgomery P, Dennis J. Cognitive behavioural interventions for sleep problems in adults aged 60+. *Cochrane Database Syst Rev.* 2003;(1): CD003161.
3. Ebben MR, Spielman AJ. Non-pharmacological treatments for insomnia. *J Behav Med.* 2009;32(3): 244–254.
4. Reynoldson JN, Elliott E Sr, Nelson LA. Ramelteon: a novel approach in the treatment of insomnia. *Ann Pharmacother.* 2008;42(9):1262–1271.
5. Hirst A, Sloan R. Benzodiazepines and related drugs for insomnia in palliative care. *Cochrane Database Syst Rev.* 2002;(4):CD003346.
6. Verster GC. Melatonin and its agonists, circadian rhythms, and psychiatry. *Afr J Psychiatry (Johannesbg).* 2009;12(1):42–46.
7. Cheuk DK, Yeung WF, Chung KF, et al. Acupuncture for insomnia. *Cochrane Database Syst Rev.* 2012;(9): CD005472.
8. Black DS, O'Reilly GA, Olmstead R, et al. Mindful-ness meditation and improvement in sleep quality and daytime impairment among older adults with sleep disturbances: a randomized clinical trial. *JAMA Intern Med.* 2015;175(4):494–501.
9. Kripke DF, Langer RD, Kline LE. Hypnotics' association with mortality or cancer: a matched cohort study. *BMJ Open.* 2012;2(1):e000850.

ADDITIONAL READING

Glass J, Lanctôt KL, Herrmann N, et al. Sedative hypnotics in older people with insomnia: meta-analysis of risks and benefits. *BMJ.* 2005;331 (7526):1169.

 ## SEE ALSO

- Anxiety; Depression; Fibromyalgia; Sleep Apnea, Obstructive
- Algorithms: Anxiety; Insomnia, Chronic; Restless Legs Syndrome (RLS)

 ## CODES

ICD10
- G47.00 Insomnia, unspecified
- F51.02 Adjustment insomnia
- F51.01 Primary insomnia

CLINICAL PEARLS

- Treatment of underlying etiology of the insomnia and consistent sleep hygiene are key.
- Most medications are indicated for short-term use only.
- Sedative hypnotics are not recommended in the elderly because risks may outweigh benefits.
- Patients with chronic insomnia benefit from cognitive-behavioral therapy.

INTELLECTUAL DISABILITY (INTELLECTUAL DEVELOPMENTAL DISORDER)

Jennifer L. Ayres, PhD

BASICS

- Intellectual disability (ID) is a global deficit in cognitive functioning evidenced by a significant difference between one's mental and chronologic ages (also known as *intelligence quotient* [IQ]) and significantly impaired adaptive functioning (1).
- Although these cognitive issues typically have a pervasive impact, patients with ID will display highly variable levels of functioning and subsequent service needs.
- Patients must be evaluated individually. Treatment plans must be tailored to specific needs.
- The term *mental retardation* was deleted from the *DSM-5* and replaced with "intellectual disability" or "intellectual developmental disorder." The rationale was that the term mental retardation is considered pejorative and culturally insensitive.

DESCRIPTION
- ID is defined as an IQ ≤70 + 5 and a significant impairment in intellectual functioning, including verbal and nonverbal reasoning, planning, academic learning, problem solving, and experiential learning. The intellectual functioning is confirmed by both IQ testing and clinical assessment (1).
- A diagnosis of ID also requires deficits in adaptive functioning, such as communication, socialization, and independent living (1).
- By definition, ID is a neurodevelopmental disorder that is typically present from birth or determined during early childhood (1).
- Currently, ID is subgrouped according to the patient's level of adaptive functioning and level of support needed. Severity levels: *mild* (typical development in some domains, mild impairment in others), *moderate* (skills are markedly behind same-age peers), *severe* (skills are quite limited, compared to peers), profound (very limited awareness of concepts, language, dependent on others for all aspects of adaptive functioning) (1).
- The three most common causes of ID are Down syndrome, fragile X syndrome, and fetal alcohol syndrome (FAS).
- If the ID reflects a loss of previously acquired intellectual skills, comorbid diagnoses of ID and neurocognitive disorder may be appropriate.

ALERT
For some causes of ID, prenatal testing is available.

EPIDEMIOLOGY
Incidence
- 1 of 6 children (2)
- Predominant sex: male > female: 1.6:1 for mild ID, 1.2:1 for severe ID (1)

Prevalence
In the United States, 1% of the general population. The prevalence for severe ID is 6/1,000 (1).

ETIOLOGY AND PATHOPHYSIOLOGY
- Causes:
  - Maternal substance abuse (e.g., alcohol); FAS is a leading environmental cause of ID.
  - Maternal infections: TORCH viruses (toxoplasma, other infections, rubella, cytomegalovirus, and herpes simplex)
  - Down syndrome

- Sex chromosome abnormalities: fragile X, Turner syndrome, Klinefelter syndrome
- Autosomal dominant conditions: neurocutaneous syndromes (e.g., neurofibromatosis, tuberous sclerosis)
- Autosomal recessive conditions:
  - Amino acid metabolism (e.g., phenylketonuria, maple syrup urine disease)
  - Carbohydrate metabolism (e.g., galactosemia, fructosuria)
  - Lipid metabolism
  - Tay-Sachs disease
  - Gaucher disease
  - Niemann-Pick disease (e.g., mucopolysaccharidosis)
  - Purine metabolism (e.g., Lesch-Nyhan disease)
  - Other (e.g., Wilson disease)
- Maternal use of prescription medications (e.g., Accutane, dilantin)
- Perinatal factors:
  - Prematurity
  - Birth injuries
  - Perinatal anoxia
- Postnatal factors:
  - Childhood diseases (e.g., meningitis, encephalitis, hypothyroidism, seizure disorders)
  - Trauma (e.g., accidents, physical abuse, hypoxia)
  - Severe deprivation
  - Poisoning (e.g., lead, carbon monoxide, household products)

Genetics
A number of genetic and epigenetic causes are known, and more are under investigation (3).

RISK FACTORS
- Maternal substance abuse during pregnancy
- Maternal infection during pregnancy
- For some causes, family history

GENERAL PREVENTION
- Public health efforts to reduce alcohol and drug use by pregnant women
- Prenatal folic acid supplementation

COMMONLY ASSOCIATED CONDITIONS
- Seizures
- Mood disorders
- Behavioral disorders
- Constipation

DIAGNOSIS

A diagnosis of ID should be made only through a psychodiagnostic assessment conducted by a mental health provider who is trained and licensed to conduct formal psychological testing.

HISTORY
- Children with profound/severe ID are typically diagnosed at birth or during the newborn period and may have dysmorphic features.
- Children with ID are often identified because they fail to meet motor/language milestones.

PHYSICAL EXAM
Careful examination by a physician trained in the assessment of morphologic features suggestive of a specific etiology for ID (e.g., microcephaly) (4)

DIFFERENTIAL DIAGNOSIS
- Brain tumors
- Auditory, visual, and/or speech/language impairment
- Autism spectrum disorder (language and social skills are more affected than other cognitive abilities); however, 75% of individuals with an autistic disorder may meet criteria for a comorbid diagnosis of ID.
- Expressive/receptive language disorders
- Cerebral palsy
- Emotional/behavioral disturbance
- Learning disorders (reading, math, written expression)
- Auditory/sensory processing difficulties
- Lack of environmental opportunities for appropriate development

DIAGNOSTIC TESTS & INTERPRETATION
- Visual and hearing tests to rule out these etiologies as a cause of impairment and provide an assessment of visual and auditory functioning, which are often impaired in children and adults with ID.
- Formal testing of intellectual and adaptive functioning:
  - A child's communication skills must be considered in test selection. For example, a patient with auditory processing issues/limited expressive/receptive language skills may need to be assessed using a nonverbal IQ test, such as the Leiter-R, Test of Nonverbal Intelligence, or other nonverbal measures.
  - Commonly used intelligence tests (e.g., Bayley Scales of Infant Development, Stanford-Binet Intelligence Scale, Wechsler Intelligence Scales) are determined by age/developmental level of the child.
  - Common tests of adaptive functioning include the Vineland Adaptive Behavior Scales, 2nd ed., and Adaptive Behavior Assessment System, 2nd ed. These tests assess areas of functioning such as age-appropriate communication, social skills, activities of daily living, and motor skills.
- Metabolic screening is not routine unless history and physical suggest or no newborn screening done (5).

Initial Tests (lab, imaging)
- Lead (5)[B]
- Thyroid-stimulating hormone if systemic features present/no newborn screening (5)[B]
- Routine cytogenetic testing (karyotype) (5)[B]:
  - Fragile X screening (FMR1 gene), particularly with a family history of ID
  - Rett syndrome (MECP2 gene) in women with unexplained moderate to severe ID (5)
- Molecular screening, such as array comparative genomic hybridization, is used increasingly and may yield a diagnosis in 10% of undiagnosed cases (4)[B].
- Neuroimaging (MRI more sensitive than CT) is routinely recommended. The presence of physical findings (microcephaly, focal motor deficit) will increase the yield of a specific diagnosis (5)[B].
- MRI may show mild cerebral abnormalities but is unlikely to establish etiology of ID (4).

Follow-Up Tests & Special Considerations
- Electroencephalogram is not routine unless epilepsy or a specific epileptiform syndrome is present (5)[C].
- Assessment of quality of life provides salient information about a patient's general sense of well-being and life satisfaction; however, quality of life may be difficult to assess when significant behavioral issues confound an individual's self-report and socialization.

TREATMENT

- Early intervention services tailored to the individual's specific needs
- Caregiver support, including:
  - Training caregiver(s) to address behavioral issues, discipline, and support socialization development
  - Encouraging caregivers to create a structured home environment that is based on the child's developmental level and specific needs rather than age-appropriate expectations.
  - Providing caregiver(s) with an opportunity to address their reactions to the diagnosis and their child's special needs
  - Informing caregivers about advocacy groups and available community, state, and national resources (6–8)
  - Encouraging caregiver(s) to seek social support to increase overall sense of well-being
  - Encouraging caregivers to seek respite care as needed to ensure that they have an opportunity to engage in health self-care.
- Individualized education plans and, depending on the level of impairment, social skills and behavioral plans/training
- Refer to job training programs and independent living opportunities, if appropriate.
- Notice all changes in behavior, which may be indicative of pain/illness, particularly in individuals with limited communication skills.
- Assess for abuse and neglect.

MEDICATION

Medication may be appropriate for comorbid conditions (e.g., anxiety, ADHD, depression).

ONGOING CARE

The physician should match his or her communication of exam procedures, test results, and treatment recommendations to the patient's level of cognitive functioning and receptive language skills.

- Most patients with ID will fall within the mild range and are fully capable of understanding information if it is provided at the appropriate level.
- Provide oral and written explanations directly to the patient instead of solely to his or her caregivers. The dignity of the patient must be respected at all times. This includes providing honest information, responding to patient's questions with respect, and not infantilizing the patient due to his or her ID.

FOLLOW-UP RECOMMENDATIONS

- Many adults and children with ID exhibit poor physical fitness. Preliminary studies suggest structured exercise programs are effective to engage this population in healthy activities (9)[A].
- Linkage to community-based resources for job training, independent living, caregiver support, school-based services

Patient Monitoring

- Primary care with attention to associated medical conditions
- Vision testing at least once before age 40 years (age 30 years in Down syndrome) and every 2 years thereafter (10)[B]

- Hearing evaluations every 5 years after age 45 years (every 3 years throughout life in Down syndrome) (10)[B]
- Screen for sexual activity and offer contraception and testing for STIs (10)[B].
- Abuse and neglect of people with ID are common. Screen at least annually and if behavior change is noted. Report abuse/neglect to appropriate protective agencies (10)[B].
- Dysphagia and aspiration are common; consider speech pathology evaluation and swallowing study (11)[B].
- Monitor for and treat constipation (11)[B].
- Osteoporosis: common; low threshold to order imaging studies after traumatic injury (11)[B]

DIET

No restrictions, except in cases of metabolic and storage disorders (e.g., phenylketonuria)

PATIENT EDUCATION

- The Arc of the United States (The Arc): www.thearc.org
- American Association of Intellectual and Developmental Disabilities: www.aaidd.org
- Family support groups (Parent to Parent, local Down Syndrome, or Autism Association)
- Special Olympics: www.specialolympics.org

PROGNOSIS

Although ID is a lifelong diagnosis, individuals with ID are capable of living a fulfilling, purposeful life that includes having a career, living independently, marrying/participating in a committed relationship, and becoming a parent. Also, the level of severity and support needed may vary over the course of the individual's life.

COMPLICATIONS

- Constipation is a commonly overlooked problem and can lead to significant morbidity.
- Polypharmacy, often associated with psychotropic medication use to control behaviors, should be addressed to minimize adverse side effects.

REFERENCES

1. American Psychiatric Association. *Diagnostic and Statistical Manual of Mental Disorders*. 5th ed. Arlington, VA: American Psychiatric Association; 2013.
2. Centers for Disease Control and Prevention. Developmental disabilities. http://www.cdc.gov/ncbddd/developmentaldisabilities/index.html. Accessed 2014.
3. Grant ME. The epigenetic origins of mental retardation. *Clin Genet*. 2008;73(6):528–530.
4. van Karnebeek CD, Jansweijer MC, Leenders AG, et al. Diagnostic investigations in individuals with mental retardation: a systematic literature review of their usefulness. *Eur J Hum Genet*. 2005;13(1):6–25.
5. Shevell M, Ashwal S, Donley D, et al. Practice parameter: evaluation of the child with global developmental delay: report of the Quality Standards Subcommittee of the American Academy of Neurology and the Practice Committee of the Child Neurology Society. *Neurology*. 2003;60(3):367–380.

---

6. Shogren KA, Bradley VJ, Gomez SC, et al. Public policy and the enhancement of desired outcomes for persons with intellectual disability. *Intellect Dev Disabil*. 2009;47(4):307–319.
7. Rizzolo MC, Hemp R, Braddock D, et al. Family support services for persons with intellectual and developmental disabilities: recent national trends. *Intellect Dev Disabil*. 2009;47(2):152–155.
8. Samuel PS, Hobden KL, LeRoy BW, et al. Analysing family service needs of typically underserved families in the USA. *J Intellect Disabil Res*. 2012;56(1):111–128.
9. Heller T, Hsieh K, Rimmer JH. Attitudinal and psychosocial outcomes of a fitness and health education program on adults with down syndrome. *Am J Ment Retard*. 2004;109(2):175–185.
10. Sullivan WF, Heng J, Cameron D, et al. Consensus guidelines for primary health care of adults with developmental disabilities. *Can Fam Physician*. 2006;52(11):1410–1418.
11. Prater CD, Zylstra RG. Medical care of adults with mental retardation. *Am Fam Physician*. 2006;73(12):2175–2183.

CODES

ICD10

- F79 Unspecified intellectual disabilities
- F70 Mild intellectual disabilities
- F71 Moderate intellectual disabilities

CLINICAL PEARLS

- The term mental retardation may be interpreted as culturally insensitive and disrespectful to patients and their caregivers. ID or intellectual developmental disorder is the correct diagnosis.
- Overall functioning with ID is highly variable and influenced by multiple factors, including appropriateness of school placement/special education services, exposure to early intervention, behavioral therapy, parent training, self-esteem, and social skills.
- Previous stereotypes of people with ID (e.g., always happy, poor prognosis, unable to function independently) have been refuted. People with ID are showing a level of functioning variability that parallels what is found in the non-ID population.
- Be aware of the unique parenting needs that caregivers may face. Link families to community and national resources that can provide practical and emotional support when appropriate.
- Because children with developmental disabilities are at higher risk of being abused than their peers without developmental disabilities, discuss with caregivers how to educate children about safety precautions in a developmentally appropriate manner.

I

INTERSTITIAL CYSTITIS

Rebecca R. Yeager, MD • Montiel T. Rosenthal, MD

BASICS

DESCRIPTION
- A condition of pain or discomfort in the bladder associated with a need to urinate frequently and urgently
- A disease of unknown cause, probably representing a final common pathway from several etiologies
- Likely, pathogenesis is disruption of urothelium, impaired lower urinary tract defenses and loss of bladder muscular wall elasticity. The symptoms in many patients are insidious, and the disease progresses for years before diagnosis is established.
- Newer research implicates urine and serum inflammatory proteins antiproliferative factor, epidermal growth factor, heparin-binding epidermal growth factor, glycosaminoglycans, and bladder nitric oxide as contributing factors.
- Mild: normal bladder capacity under anesthesia; ulceration, cracking, or glomerulation of mucosa (or not) with bladder distention under anesthesia; no incontinence symptoms wax and wane and may not progress. Interstitial cystitis is a bladder sensory problem.
- Severe: progressive bladder fibrosis; small true bladder capacity under anesthesia; poor bladder wall compliance. In 5–10% of cases, Hunner ulcers present at cystoscopy; may have overflow incontinence and/or chronic bacteriuria unresponsive to antibiotics.
- System(s) affected: renal/urologic
- Synonym(s): urgency frequency syndrome; IC/bladder pain syndrome (BPS)

Pregnancy Considerations
Unpredictable symptom improvement or exacerbation during pregnancy; no known fetal effects from interstitial cystitis; usual problems of unknown effect on fetus with medications taken during pregnancy

EPIDEMIOLOGY
- Occurs predominantly among whites
- Predominant sex: female > male (10:1)
- Patients <30 years have predominant symptoms: dysuria, frequency, urinary urgency, pain in external genitals, and dyspareunia; and those >60 years more commonly have nocturia, urinary incontinence, or Hunner ulcer disease.
- Predominant age
  - Mild: 20 to 40 years
  - Severe: 20 to 70 years
- Pediatric considerations
  - <10 years old and again at 13 to 17 years
  - Daytime enuresis, dysuria without infection

Prevalence
In the United States:
- Up to 1 million affected, but many cases likely are unreported
- 0.052% but may be higher up to 10%

ETIOLOGY AND PATHOPHYSIOLOGY
- Unknown but is not primarily psychosomatic
- Possible causes
  - Subclinical urinary infection
  - Damage to glycosaminoglycan mucus layer increasing bladder wall permeability to irritants such as urea
  - Autoimmune
  - Mast cell histamine release
- Neurologic upregulation/stimulation

RISK FACTORS
Unknown

COMMONLY ASSOCIATED CONDITIONS
- Fibromyalgia
- Allergies
- Chronic fatigue syndrome
- Depression
- Vulvodynia
- Sexual dysfunction
- Sleep disturbance
- Migraines
- Syncope
- Dyspepsia
- Chronic prostatitis
- Chronic pelvic pain
- Irritable bowel syndrome
- Anal/rectal disease

DIAGNOSIS

- Frequent, urgent, relentless urination day and night; >8 voids in 24 hours
- Pain with full bladder that resolves with bladder emptying (except if bacteriuria is present)
- Urge urinary incontinence if bladder capacity is small
- Sleep disturbance
- Dyspareunia, especially with full bladder
- Secondary symptoms from chronic pain and sleeplessness, especially depression

HISTORY
- Pelvic Pain and Urgency/Frequency Patient Symptom Scale: self-reporting questionnaire for screening potential interstitial cystitis patients (1)[B] (http://wgcaobgyn.com/files/urgency_frequency_pt_symptom_scale.pdf)
- Frequent UTIs, vaginitis, or symptoms during the week before menses
- O'Leary/Sant Voiding and Pain Indices (http://www.ichelp.org/wp-content/uploads/2015/06/OLeary_Sant.pdf)

PHYSICAL EXAM
- Perineal/prostatic pain in men
- Anterior vaginal wall pain in women

DIFFERENTIAL DIAGNOSIS
- Uninhibited bladder (urgency, frequency, urge incontinence, less pain, symptoms usually decrease when asleep)

- Urinary infection: cystitis, prostatitis
- Bladder neoplasm
- Bladder stone
- Neurologic bladder disease
- Nonurinary pelvic disease (STIs, endometriosis, pelvic relaxation)

DIAGNOSTIC TESTS & INTERPRETATION

Initial Tests (lab, imaging)
- Urinalysis: normal except with chronic bacteriuria (rare)
- Urine culture from catheterized specimen: normal except with chronic bacteriuria (rare) or partial antibiotic treatment
- Urine cytology
  - Normal: reserve for men >40 years old and women with hematuria

Diagnostic Procedures/Other
- Cystoscopy (especially in men >40 years old or women with hematuria)
  - Bladder wall visualization
  - Hydraulic distention: no improved diagnostic certainty over history and physical alone
- No role for urodynamic testing
- Intravesical lidocaine can help to pinpoint the bladder as the source of pain in patients with pelvic pain; this can be both diagnostic and therapeutic.
- Potassium sensitivity test
  - Insert catheter, empty bladder, instill 40 mL H_2O over 2 to 3 minutes, rank urgency on scale of 0 to 5 in intensity, rank pain on scale of 0 to 5 in intensity, drain bladder, instill 40 mL potassium chloride (KCl) 0.4 mol/L solution:
    - If immediate pain, flush bladder with 60 mL H_2O and treat with bladder instillations.
    - If no immediate pain, wait for 5 minutes and rate the urgency and pain.
  - If urgency or pain >2, treat as above.
- Pain or urgency >2 is considered a positive test and strongly correlates with interstitial cystitis if no radiation cystitis or acute bacterial cystitis is present.

Test Interpretation
- Nonspecific chronic inflammation on bladder biopsies
- Urine cytology negative for dysplasia and neoplasia
- Possible mast cell proliferation in mucosa

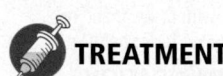

TREATMENT

GENERAL MEASURES
- Appropriate health care: outpatient
- Self-care (eliminate foods and liquids that exacerbate symptoms on individual basis, fluid management) (2)[C]
- Biofeedback bladder retraining (2)[C]

MEDICATION
- Randomized controlled trials of most medications for interstitial cystitis demonstrate limited benefit over placebo; there are no clear predictors of what will benefit an individual. Prepare the patient that treatment may involve trial and error.

- Behavioral therapy combined with oral agents found improved outcomes compared to medications alone.
- Intravesical injections of botulinum toxin are not effective in the treatment of ulcer-type interstitial cystitis.

First Line
- Note: AUA consensus states medicines should be considered second-line therapy after patient education, stress reduction, behavior modification, and self-care (2)[C].
- Pentosan polysulfate (Elmiron) 100 mg TID on empty stomach; may take several months (3 to 6) to become effective; rated as modestly beneficial in systematic drug review (only FDA-approved treatment for interstitial cystitis) (3)[C]
- Amitriptyline: Most effective at higher doses (≥50 mg/day); however, initiate with lower doses to minimize side effects (4)[B].
- Hydroxyzine 25 to 50 mg HS
- Sildenafil 25 mg/day (5)[B]
- Cimetidine 400 mg BID (2)[C]
- Triple-drug therapy: 6 months of pentosan, hydroxyzine, doxepin
- Antibacterials for bacteriuria
- Oxybutynin, hyoscyamine, tolterodine, and other anticholinergic medications decrease frequency.
- Prednisone (only for ulcerative lesions)
- Montelukast has shown some benefit.
- NSAIDs for pain and any inflammatory component
- Bladder instillations
  - Lidocaine, sodium bicarbonate, and heparin or pentosan polysulfate sodium
  - Dimethyl sulfoxide (DMSO) every 1 to 2 weeks for 3 to 6 weeks, then PRN
  - Heparin sometimes added to DMSO
  - Intravesical liposomes
  - Other agents: steroids, silver nitrate, oxychlorosene (Clorpactin)
- Contraindication
  - No anticholinergics for patients with close-angle glaucoma
- Significant possible interaction
  - Refer to manufacturer's profile of each drug.

Second Line
- Phenazopyridine, a local bladder mucosal anesthetic, usually is not very effective.
- Intravesicular injection of botulinum type A for nonulcer interstitial cystitis
- Cyclosporin A (2)[C]

ISSUES FOR REFERRAL
- Need for clarity with respect to diagnosis
- Surgical intervention

ADDITIONAL THERAPIES
Myofascial physical therapy (targeted pelvic, hip girdle, abdominal trigger point massage) (6)[B]

SURGERY/OTHER PROCEDURES
- Hydraulic distention of bladder under anesthesia: symptomatic but transient relief
- Cauterization of bladder ulcer

- Augmentation cystoplasty to increase bladder capacity and decrease pressure with or without partial cystectomy. Expected results in severe cases: much improved, 75%; with residual discomfort, 20%; unchanged, 5%
- Urinary diversion with total cystectomy only if disease is completely refractory to medical therapy
- Sacral neuromodulation

COMPLEMENTARY & ALTERNATIVE MEDICINE
Guided imagery

 ONGOING CARE

FOLLOW-UP RECOMMENDATIONS
Patient Monitoring
Not specifically needed unless symptoms are unresponsive to treatment

DIET
- Variable effects from person to person
- Common irritants include caffeine, chocolate, citrus, tomatoes, carbonated beverages, potassium-rich foods, spicy foods, acidic foods, and alcohol.

PATIENT EDUCATION
Interstitial Cystitis Association, 110 Washington St. Suite 340, Rockville, MD 20850; 1-800-HELPICA: http://www.ichelp.org/

PROGNOSIS
- Mild: exacerbations and remissions of symptoms; may not be progressive; does not predispose to other diseases
- Severe: progressive problems that usually require surgery to control symptoms

COMPLICATIONS
Severe, with long-term, continuous high bladder pressure could be associated with renal damage.

REFERENCES

1. Parsons CL, Dell J, Stanford EJ, et al. Increased prevalence of interstitial cystitis: previously unrecognized urologic and gynecological cases identified using a new symptom questionnaire and intravesical potassium sensitivity. *Urology*. 2002;60(4):573–578.
2. Hanno PM, Erickson D, Moldwin R, et al. Diagnosis and treatment of interstitial cystitis/bladder pain syndrome: AUA guideline amendment. *J Urol*. 2015;193(5):1545–1553.
3. Dancel R, Mounsey A, Handler L. Medications for treatment of interstitial cystitis. *Am Fam Physician*. 2015;91(2):116–118.
4. Foster HE Jr, Hanno PM, Nickel JC, et al. Effect of amitriptyline on symptoms in treatment naïve patients with interstitial cystitis/painful bladder syndrome. *J Urol*. 2010;183(5):1853–1858.
5. Chen H, Wang F, Chen W, et al. Efficacy of daily low-dose sildenafil for treating interstitial cystitis: results of a randomized, double-blind, placebo-controlled trial—treatment of interstitial cystitis/painful bladder syndrome with low-dose sildenafil. *Urology*. 2014;84(1):51–56.
6. FitzGerald MP, Payne CK, Lukacz ES, et al. Randomized multicenter clinical trial of myofascial physical therapy in women with interstitial cystitis/painful bladder syndrome and pelvic floor tenderness. *J Urol*. 2012;187(6):2113–2118.

ADDITIONAL READING
Rais-Bahrami S, Friedlander JI, Herati AS, et al. Symptom profile variability of interstitial cystitis/painful bladder syndrome by age. *BJU Int*. 2012;109(9):1356–1359.

 SEE ALSO

- Urinary Tract Infection (UTI) in Females
- Algorithm: Pelvic Girdle Pain (Pregnancy or Postpartum Pelvic Pain)

CODES

ICD10
- N30.10 Interstitial cystitis (chronic) without hematuria
- N30.11 Interstitial cystitis (chronic) with hematuria

CLINICAL PEARLS
- The potassium sensitivity test has been the most useful in confirming an initial diagnosis of interstitial cystitis.
- Potassium sensitivity test
  - Insert catheter, empty bladder, instill 40 mL H_2O over 2 to 3 minutes; rank urgency on scale of 0 to 5 in intensity; rank pain on scale of 0 to 5 in intensity; drain bladder; and instill 40 mL KCl 0.4 mol/L solution.
- Submucosal petechial hemorrhages and/or ulceration at the time of bladder distention and cystoscopy further support the diagnosis.
- At present, there is no definitive treatment for interstitial cystitis.
- Most patients with severe disease receive multiple treatment approaches. Regular multidisciplinary follow-up, pharmacologic therapy, avoidance of symptom triggers, and psychological and supportive therapy are all important because this disease tends to wax and wane. Monitor patients for comorbid depression.
- Empowering patients to manage their symptoms, communicate regularly with their physicians, and learn as much as they can about this disease which may help them to optimize their outcome.

I

INTERSTITIAL NEPHRITIS

Roger P. Holland, MD, PhD

 BASICS

DESCRIPTION
- Acute and chronic tubulointerstitial diseases result from the interplay of renal cells and inflammatory cells and their products. Lethal or sublethal injury to renal cells leads to expression of new local antigens, inflammatory cell infiltration, and activation of pro-inflammatory and chemoattractant cytokines. These cytokines are produced by macrophages and lymphocytes and also by the renal cells (i.e., proximal tubule, vascular endothelial cells, interstitial cells, fibroblasts). The outcome can be acute interstitial nephritis (AIN) or chronic interstitial nephritis (CIN).
- AIN presents as acute kidney injury (AKI) after the use of offending drugs or agents (OFA) and is associated with typical findings of proteinuria, hematuria, and white cell casts. Less frequently, AIN is secondary to infection or systemic diseases (e.g., sarcoidosis, mixed connective tissue disease [MCTD], SLE, Sjögren syndrome).
- System(s) affected: renal/urologic, endocrine/metabolic, immunologic
- Synonym(s): acute interstitial allergic nephritis

EPIDEMIOLOGY
Pediatric Considerations
- Children with history of lead poisoning are more likely to develop CIN as young adults.
- Tubulointerstitial nephritis with uveitis (TINU) presents in adolescent females.

Incidence
- AIN and CIN accounts for 10–15% of kidney disease.
- Peak incidence in women 60 to 70 years of age

Geriatric Considerations
The elderly (≥65 years) have more severe disease and increased risk of permanent damage due to their increased use of OFA, specifically more drug-induced AIN (87% vs. 64%), proton pump inhibitor–induced AIN (18% vs. 6%) but less AIN due to autoimmune or systemic causes (7% vs. 27%) than younger adults (1)[B].

ETIOLOGY AND PATHOPHYSIOLOGY
- AIN
  - Delayed drug hypersensitivity reactions
  - Causes AKI
  - Renal dysfunction generally is usually partially or completely reversible, possibly reflecting the regenerative capacity of tubules with a preserved basement membrane.
  - Hypersensitivity to drugs (75%): not dose dependent. The three top drug causes were omeprazole (12%), amoxicillin (8%), and ciprofloxacin (8%) in a recent case series (2)[C].
    - Antibiotics (e.g., penicillins, cephalosporins, sulfonamides, tetracycline, vancomycin, fluoroquinolones, macrolides, TB meds)
    - Proton pump inhibitors
    - Antivirals (Indinavir)
    - NSAIDs (all, including Cox-2 inhibitors)
    - Diuretics (thiazide, loop, and triamterene)
    - Miscellaneous (allopurinol, H_2 blockers, diphenylhydantoin, and 5-aminosalicates such as Azulfidine and mesalamine)
  - Infections: *Legionella, Leptospira,* streptococci, CMV, *Mycobacterium tuberculosis* (5–10%)
  - Autoimmune disorders (e.g., SLE, Sjögren syndrome, sarcoidosis, Wegener granulomatosis, cryoglobulinemia) (10–15%)
  - Toxins (e.g., snake bite venom)

- CIN
  - Follows long-term exposure to OFA (e.g., heavy metals, especially lead)
  - Often found on routine labs or evaluation for hypertension (HTN)
  - Characterized by interstitial scarring, fibrosis, and tubular atrophy, resulting in progressive chronic kidney disease (CKD)

GENERAL PREVENTION
- Early recognition and prompt discontinuation of OFA
- Avoid further nephrotoxic substances.

COMMONLY ASSOCIATED CONDITIONS
CIN
- Chronic pyelonephritis
- Abuse of analgesics
- Lithium use
- Gout and gout therapy
- Immune disorders
- Malignancy (lymphoma, multiple myeloma)
- Amyloidosis
- Exposure to heavy metals (e.g., lead, cadmium)
- Renal papillary necrosis

 DIAGNOSIS

- AIN: suspected in a patient who presents with non-specific signs and symptoms of AKI (e.g., malaise, fever, nausea, vomiting) with an elevated serum creatinine and an abnormal urinalysis
  - AKI
    - Elevated creatinine, BUN, and electrolyte abnormalities (e.g., hyperkalemia, low serum bicarbonate)
    - Decreased urine output (oliguria in 51%)
    - Signs of fluid overload or depletion
  - Signs of systemic allergy (e.g., fever [27%], maculopapular rash [15%], peripheral eosinophilia [23%], arthralgias [45%], but less commonly found when NSAIDs are the OFA)
  - White cells, red cells, and white cell casts
- CIN
  - HTN
  - Decreased urine output or polyuria
  - Inability to concentrate urine
  - Polydipsia
  - Metabolic acidosis
  - Anemia
  - Fanconi syndrome

HISTORY
- Medications: Onset of AIN following drug exposure ranges from 3 to 5 days (as occurs with a second exposure to an OFA) to as long as several weeks to many months (the latter with NSAIDs, especially) (2)[B].
- Infections: may have symptoms related to an associated infection or systemic condition
- TINU patients present with interstitial nephritis and uveitis and occasionally systemic findings.
- Exposure to heavy metals
- Post organ transplant

PHYSICAL EXAM
- Increased BP
- Fluid retention/extremity swelling/weight gain
- Rash accompanying renal findings in acute AIN
- Lung crackles if fluid is overloaded
- Pericardial rub if uremic pericarditis

DIFFERENTIAL DIAGNOSIS
- AKI secondary to other causes:
  - Prerenal (e.g., hypovolemia, shock, sepsis, renal artery emboli)
  - Intrarenal (e.g., acute tubular necrosis, hypertensive nephropathy, DM nephropathy)
  - Postrenal (e.g., obstructive uropathy)
  - Some OFA that cause AIN can produce other forms of AKI as well:
    - NSAIDs can exacerbate prerenal disease.
    - Aminoglycosides can cause acute tubular necrosis.
- CKD secondary to long-standing HTN, diabetes, and chronic pyelonephritis

DIAGNOSTIC TESTS & INTERPRETATION
- Chemistry
  - Elevated plasma creatinine: seen in all patients, with 40% requiring dialysis
  - Hyperkalemia and acidosis
- CBC
  - Eosinophilia (80%): NSAID-induced AIN is only associated with eosinophilia in ~15% of cases.
  - Anemia
- Urinalysis with urine electrolytes
  - Hematuria (95%)
  - Mild and variable proteinuria: usually <1 g/24 hr, except in AIN-associated with NSAIDs where it is significantly higher (3)[B]
  - Urine sediment: white cells, red cells, white cell casts. Red blood cell casts are rare.
  - Eosinophiluria but has no clinical utility specific for AIN (4)[C]
  - Fractional excretion of sodium (FENa >1%) indicative of tubular damage
  - Normal urinalysis does not rule out AIN.
- CXR to evaluate for pulmonary tuberculosis, sarcoidosis, and other infections
- Serologic testing for immunologic disease (e.g., sarcoidosis, Sjögren syndrome, Wegener granulomatosis, Behçet syndrome) or infectious causes (e.g., histoplasmosis, coccidiomycosis, toxoplasmosis, EBV)
  - Serum levels of angiotensin-converting enzyme and serum Ca^{++} for sarcoidosis
  - Antinuclear antibody (ANA) and dsDNA to exclude SLE
  - Urinary antigen to exclude *Legionella* infection
  - Anti-Ro/SSA, anti-La/SSB antibodies, CRP, and rheumatoid factor to exclude Sjögren syndrome
- Liver function tests: elevated serum transaminase levels in patients with associated drug-induced liver injury
- Renal US may demonstrate kidneys that are normal to enlarged in size with increased cortical echogenicity, but no US findings will reliably confirm or exclude AIN versus other causes of AKI.
- IV pyelography (IVP) and CT scans with contrast are relatively contraindicated because of the associated nephrotoxicity and limited diagnostic yield.

Follow-Up Tests & Special Considerations
Patients who do not recover renal function and those with CIN should receive long-term follow-up care to protect kidneys from further potentially nephrotoxic therapies.

Diagnostic Procedures/Other
- Renal biopsy is the definitive method of establishing the diagnosis of AIN. Ideally, it should be performed to:
  - Patients treated with an OFA known to cause AIN but have normal urinalysis

– Patients who are being considered for steroid therapy
– Patients who are not on glucocorticosteroid therapy initially and do not have spontaneous recovery following cessation of the OFA
– Patients with advanced renal failure of recent onset (<3 months)
– Patients with any features (e.g., high-grade proteinuria) that makes the diagnosis of AIN uncertain
• Contraindications: Renal biopsy is contraindicated in bleeding diathesis, solitary kidney, end-stage renal disease (ESRD) with small kidneys, uncontrolled HTN and sepsis, or renal parenchymal infection.

Test Interpretation
• Acute
– Marked interstitial infiltrate consisting of T lymphocytes and monocytes. Eosinophils, plasma cells, and neutrophils also may be found.
– In general, the urinary findings will distinguish AIN from other causes (e.g., acute tubular necrosis, glomerulonephritis).
• Chronic: CIN is characterized by tubular atrophy, fibrosis, and cellular infiltration with mononuclear cells.

TREATMENT

For AIN, data on corticosteroids' efficacy have been limited (5)[B].

GENERAL MEASURES
• Discontinue offending agent. If topical NSAIDs are in use, discontinue these as well.
• Reduce exposure to other nephrotoxic agents (e.g., furosemide, aminoglycosides).
• Supportive measures:
– Maintain adequate hydration.
– Symptomatic relief for fever, rash, and so forth
– Control of BP and anemia
– Correct acidosis and electrolyte imbalances.
– Possible short-term dialysis until recovery of renal function (5)[B]

MEDICATION
• Mainstay of treatment is supportive therapy.
• If patient is taking multiple offending agents, a reasonable clinical approach should include substitution of the suspected drug with another medication.
• If AKI persists after removing the offending agent, attempt medication therapy.

First Line
• Optimal therapy of AIN is unknown because there are no randomized controlled trials (RCTs) or large observational studies.
• Immunosuppressive therapy is employed if no subsequent improvement within 3 to 7 days after discontinuation of OFA.
• A renal biopsy is preferred to confirm AIN and to exclude other possible diseases or CIN, where immunosuppressive Rx is not indicated.
• Prednisone 1 mg/kg/day PO or equivalent IV dose to a max of 40 to 60 mg/day for 1 to 2 weeks, beginning a gradual taper after serum creatinine has returned to near baseline for a duration of 2 to 3 months, followed by a gradual taper over 3 to 4 weeks (6)[B]. Complete recover is noted in 49% and partial in 39% (1)[C].
– Steroids started within 7 days of withdrawal of offending agent are more likely to recover function than those who started later (odds ratio [OR] 6.6).

Second Line
• There is a limited experience with treating AIN in patients who are steroid-dependent (i.e., relapse during prednisone taper), steroid-resistant (as with NSAID-induced disease), or cannot tolerate steroids.
• Mycophenolate mofetil may be considered in these patients who have biopsy-proven AIN (7)[C]. Rx may need to be continued for 1 to 3 years.
• Lead toxicity: Chelation may improve function.
– Succimer 10 mg/kg (max 500 mg) PO q8h for 5 days, then q12h for 14 days, or
– EDTA 2 g IV/IM; if IM, use with 2% lidocaine.
• SLE nephritis: steroids + cyclophosphamide or azathioprine
• Urate nephropathy: urate-lowering agents
– Allopurinol starting at 100 mg/day, increasing to 300 mg/day to achieve serum urate level <6 mg/dL
– Dose may need to be adjusted down depending on the level of renal impairment.
– Allopurinol itself can be a cause of AIN.
– Discontinue thiazide.
• Lithium-induced nephritis: Use amiloride as adjunct.
• Indinavir-induced nephritis: Use probenecid as adjunct.

ISSUES FOR REFERRAL
Most patients presenting with AKI, proteinuria, and acid–base and/or electrolyte disorders require consultation with a nephrologist.

INPATIENT CONSIDERATIONS
Patients with AKI and/or with serious electrolyte or acid–base disorders may require inpatient care until stabilization or resolution.

Admission Criteria/Initial Stabilization
• Persistent oliguria or anuria
• Severe acidosis and/or electrolyte abnormalities
• ECG changes

Discharge Criteria
• Stable vitals; correction of all electrolyte imbalances, including magnesium; and resolution of acute ECG changes
• Normal urine production

ONGOING CARE

FOLLOW-UP RECOMMENDATIONS
Patient Monitoring
If patients must remain on nephrotoxic agents, measure renal function, electrolytes, and phosphorus frequently.

DIET
• Low potassium (<2 g/day)
• Low sodium
• Low protein

PATIENT EDUCATION
Printed materials for patients are available at the National Kidney Disease Education Program (NKDEP), (866) 4-KIDNEY, http://www.niddk.nih.gov/health-information/health-communication-programs/nkdep/Pages/default.aspx.

PROGNOSIS
• If the associated AIN is detected early (within 1 week of the rise in serum creatinine) and the offending agent is discontinued promptly, the long-term outcome is favorable for a return to baseline or near baseline serum creatinine levels, except in the instance of NSAID-induced AIN.
• Renal biopsy reveals extent of damage.

• AIN
– Recovery within weeks to months (8)[C]
– Acute dialysis is needed for 1/3 of patients before resolution.
– Rarely progresses to ESRD
• CIN: can progress to ESRD
– Renal disease may remit in 1 year if untreated.
– TINU has relapsing course, requiring systemic corticosteroids.
• Untreated severe AKI has 45–70% mortality.

COMPLICATIONS
• Chronic tubulointerstitial disease may progress to ESRD, requiring dialysis or transplantation.
• Analgesics increase the risk of transitional cell cancers of the uroepithelium.

REFERENCES

1. Muriithi AK, Leung N, Valeri AM, et al. Clinical characteristics, causes and outcomes of acute interstitial nephritis in the elderly. *Kidney Int.* 2015;87(2):458–464.
2. Muriithi AK, Leung N, Valeri AM, et al. Biopsy-proven acute interstitial nephritis, 1993–2011: a case series. *Am J Kidney Dis.* 2014;64(4):558–566.
3. Clive DM, Stoff JS. Renal syndromes associated with nonsteroidal antiinflammatory drugs. *N Engl J Med.* 1984;310(9):563–572.
4. Muriithi AK, Nasr SH, Leung N. Utility of urine eosinophils in the diagnosis of acute interstitial nephritis. *Clin J Am Soc Nephrol.* 2013;8(11):1857–1862.
5. Koselj M, Kveder R, Bren AF, et al. Acute renal failure in patients with drug-induced acute interstitial nephritis. *Ren Fail.* 1993;15(1):69–72.
6. Clarkson MR, Giblin L, O'Connell FP, et al. Acute interstitial nephritis: clinical features and response to corticosteroid therapy. *Nephrol Dial Transplant.* 2004;19(11):2778–2783.
7. Preddie DC, Markowitz GS, Radhakrishnan J, et al. Mycophenolate mofetil for the treatment of interstitial nephritis. *Clin I Am Soc Nephrol.* 2006;1(4):718–722.
8. Rossert J. Drug-induced acute interstitial nephritis. *Kidney Int.* 2001;60(2):804–817.

ADDITIONAL READING
• Braden GL, O'Shea MH, Mulhern JG. Tubulointerstitial diseases. *Am J Kidney Dis.* 2005;46(3):560–572.
• Fouque D, Laville M. Low protein diets for chronic kidney disease in non diabetic adults. *Cochrane Database Syst Rev.* 2009;(3):CD001892.

CODES

ICD10
• N12 Tubulo-interstitial nephritis, not spcf as acute or chronic
• N10 Acute tubulo-interstitial nephritis
• N11.9 Chronic tubulo-interstitial nephritis, unspecified

CLINICAL PEARLS
• First step in treatment is to remove OFA.
• Most common OFA in elderly is PPIs and antibiotics.
• A renal biopsy is preferred to confirm AIN.
• Immunosuppressive therapy is employed if no subsequent improvement within 3 to 7 days after discontinuation of OFA.

IRRITABLE BOWEL SYNDROME

Mark B. Stephens, MD, MS, FAAFP, CAPT, MC, USN

 BASICS

DESCRIPTION
- A functional gastrointestinal disorder characterized by
  - Chronic abdominal pain associated with
    - Alteration in bowel habits
    - Absence of organic pathology
- May be characterized as diarrhea-predominant or constipation-predominant or may alternate between the two
- Synonym(s): spastic colon; irritable colon

EPIDEMIOLOGY
Irritable bowel syndrome (IBS) accounts for up to 50% of visits to gastroenterologists:
- Second only to upper respiratory infection as cause of lost workdays

Prevalence
Pooled estimate of 11% IBS prevalence internationally; ranges from South Asia (7%) to South America (21%) (1)
- Predominant age: 20 to 39 years
- If age >50 years, consider other diagnoses.
- Predominant sex: in the United States, female > male (2:1)
- More common in low socioeconomic communities

ETIOLOGY AND PATHOPHYSIOLOGY
- The etiology is unknown, associated with intestinal motility abnormalities and enhanced sensitivity to visceral stimuli.
- The trigger may be luminal or environmental.
- Evidence for the role of small intestine bacterial overgrowth (SIBO) in IBS and association with antibiotic therapy is conflicting; older age and female gender are predictors of SIBO in IBS patients.

Genetics
Unknown, but more common in families of IBS patients

RISK FACTORS
- Other family members with similar GI disorder
- History of childhood sexual abuse
- Sexual/domestic abuse (primarily in women)
- Depression
- Gastrointestinal infection

Pregnancy Considerations
No risk to mother or fetus

GENERAL PREVENTION
See "Diet."

COMMONLY ASSOCIATED CONDITIONS
- Chronic migraine
- Urinary frequency and urgency
- Fibromyalgia
- Chronic fatigue syndrome
- Sleep disorders
- Dyspareunia
- Depression
- Posttraumatic stress disorder

 DIAGNOSIS

HISTORY
- Rome III criteria: recurrent pain or discomfort in the abdomen at least 3 days per month over the past 3 months associated with at least two other criteria:
  - Symptoms improve with defecation.
  - Onset is associated with a change in stool frequency.
  - Onset is associated with a change in the form or appearance of the stool.
- Symptoms can also include:
  - Mucus in stools
  - Constipation, bloating, diarrhea, abdominal distension
  - Upper abdominal discomfort after eating
  - Straining for normal consistency stools
  - Urgency of defecation
  - Feelings of incomplete evacuation
  - Abnormal stool form
  - Nausea, vomiting (rarely)
- May have history of abuse or depression
- Patient may note worsening of symptoms with stress or around menses.
- IBS is unlikely in patients with a history of:
  - Weight loss
  - Bleeding
  - Nocturnal diarrhea
  - Fever
  - Anemia

PHYSICAL EXAM
- Generally normal
- Perform to exclude other causes.
- Vital signs typically are normal.
- Generally, there is an absence of jaundice and organomegaly but may have tenderness to palpation.

DIFFERENTIAL DIAGNOSIS
- Inflammatory bowel disease
- Lactose intolerance; fructose malabsorption
- Infections (*Giardia lamblia*, *Entamoeba histolytica*, *Salmonella*, *Campylobacter*, *Yersinia*, *Clostridium difficile*)
- Celiac sprue
- Microscopic colitis
- Laxative abuse
- Magnesium-containing antacids
- Hypo-/hyperthyroidism
- Pancreatic insufficiency
- Depression
- Small bowel bacterial overgrowth
- Somatization
- Villous adenoma
- Endocrine tumors
- Diabetes mellitus
- Radiation damage to colon or small bowel

DIAGNOSTIC TESTS & INTERPRETATION
- With a typical history and no danger signs (anemia or weight loss), obtain baseline labs to rule out other causes and begin treatment.
- In patients who do not respond to treatment, further evaluation with imaging and/or endoscopy is warranted to exclude organic pathology.

Initial Tests (lab, imaging)
Rule out pathology specific to the patient's symptoms:
- Diarrhea-predominant: ESR, CBC, tissue transglutaminase, thyroid-stimulating hormone (TSH), and stool for ova and parasites (2)
- Constipation-predominant: CBC, TSH, electrolytes, calcium (2)
- Abdominal pain: LFTs and amylase
- Abdominal CT scan or abdominal ultrasound to evaluate pain is generally normal.
- Consider small bowel series or video capsule endoscopy to rule out Crohn disease (will be normal).
- Sitz Marker study may be used to evaluate colonic transit in patients with constipation.

Follow-Up Tests & Special Considerations
Consider lactulose breath test to assess for small bowel bacterial overgrowth associated with IBS (2)[C].

Diagnostic Procedures/Other
Sigmoidoscopy/colonoscopy may be used to rule out inflammatory bowel disease or microscopic colitis.

ALERT
Screen all persons >50 for colorectal cancer.

Test Interpretation
None

TREATMENT

- Goals: Relieve symptoms and improve quality of life (3).
  - Determine if diarrhea predominant, constipation predominant, or mixed type
- Lifestyle modification
  - Exercise 3 to 5 times per week decreases severity (3).
  - Food diary to determine triggers (3)
- Medications
  - Fiber supplementation (psyllium) increases stool bulk; does not typically relieve abdominal pain; may be used for all types (3,4)[B]
- Medications that improve abdominal pain, global symptoms, and symptom severity in all types:
  - Antispasmodics such as hyoscyamine 0.125 to 0.25 mg PO/SL q4h PRN and dicyclomine 20 to 40 mg PO BID can be used for all types but have adverse effects such as dry mouth, dizziness, and blurred vision (3).
  - Probiotics such as *Lactobacillus*, *Bifidobacterium*, and *Streptococcus* (5)[C]
  - Serotonin antagonists 5-HT3 and 5-4T agonists (alosetron, cilansetron) have been shown to improve IBS symptoms (versus placebo) (6).

- Diarrhea predominant
  - Antidiarrheal such as loperamide 4 to 8 mg/day orally divided into once a day to 3 times a day as needed to decrease stool frequency and increase stool consistency; does not help with abdominal pain; may also use diphenoxylate/atropine (3)
  - Antibiotics such as 2-week course of rifaximin improve bloating, pain, and stool consistency (7).
  - Alosetron (Lotronex 0.5 mg orally twice a day), used for women with severe symptoms but associated with ischemic colitis, constipation, and death in a small number of patients (8)
- Constipation-predominant
  - Laxatives such as polyethylene glycol (MiraLAX) may improve stool frequency but not pain.
  - Antibiotics such as neomycin and selective chloride channel activators such as lubiprostone (Amitiza) 8 mg twice a day can improve global symptoms and severity (3,9)[B].
  - Linaclotide (guanylate cyclase-C agonist) has been shown to improve bowel function and reduces abdominal pain and overall severity in adults only (10).
- Mixed
  - Use medications above based on symptoms (3).
- Treat underlying behavioral issues:
  - Use of SSRIs such as Prozac, sertraline, Paxil, and tricyclic antidepressants such as imipramine can improve abdominal pain and symptom score (4).
  - Tricyclic antidepressants can help control IBS symptoms in moderate to severe cases (11)[B].
  - Behavioral therapy helps reduce symptoms (7).

ISSUES FOR REFERRAL
- Behavioral health referral may help with management of affective or personality disorders.
- Gastroenterology referral for difficult to control cases

ADDITIONAL TREATMENT
Probiotics use may result in reducing IBS symptoms and decreasing pain and flatulence. There is no difference among *Lactobacillus, Streptococcus, Bifidobacterium*, and combinations of probiotics.

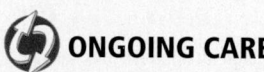

ONGOING CARE

FOLLOW-UP RECOMMENDATIONS
Patient Monitoring
The IBS Severity Score is a validated measure to assess the severity of IBS symptoms and can help monitor response to treatment.

IBS Severity Score:
- How severe has your abdominal pain been over the last 10 days?
- On how many of the last 10 days did you get pain?

- How severe has your abdominal distension (bloating, swollen, or tight) been over the last 10 days?
- How satisfied have you been with your bowel habit (frequency, ease, etc.) over the last 10 days?
- How much has your IBS been affecting/interfering with your life in general over the last 10 days?

DIET
Low FODMAPs diet: This diet contains fermentable oligosaccharides, disaccharides, monosaccharides, and polyols that are carbohydrates (sugars) found in foods. FODMAPs are osmotic, so they may not be digested or absorbed well and could be fermented upon by bacteria in the intestinal tract when *eaten in excess*.

A low FODMAP diet may help reduce symptoms, which will limit foods high in fructose, lactose, fructans, galactans, and polyols.

- Increase fiber slowly to avoid excess intestinal gas production.
- During initial evaluation, may wish to try 2 weeks of lactose-free diet to rule out lactose intolerance.
- Avoid large meals, fatty foods, and caffeine, which can exacerbate symptoms.
- A gluten-free diet resolves symptoms for some patients (especially diarrhea predominant IBS) despite negative testing for celiac disease.

PATIENT EDUCATION
IBS is not a psychiatric illness.

PROGNOSIS
- IBS is a functional disorder that reduces quality of life. Many patients have behavioral health issues. IBS does not increase mortality (1).
- Expect recurrences, especially when under stress.
- Evidence suggests that "symptom shifting" occurs in some patients, whereby resolution of functional bowel symptoms is followed by the development of functional symptoms in another system (1).

REFERENCES
1. Canavan C, West J, Card T. The epidemiology of irritable bowel syndrome. *Clin Epidemiol.* 2014;6:71–80.
2. Reddymasu SC, Sostarich S, McCallum RW. Small intestinal bacterial overgrowth in irritable bowel syndrome: are there any predictors? *BMC Gastroenterol.* 2010;10:23.
3. Wilkins T, Pepitone C, Alex B, et al. Diagnosis and management of IBS in adults. *Am Fam Physician.* 2012;86(5):419–426.
4. Ruepert L, Quartero AO, de Wit NJ, et al. Bulking agents, antispasmodics and antidepressants for the treatment of irritable bowel syndrome. *Cochrane Database Syst Rev.* 2011;(8):CD003460.
5. Ciorba MA. A gastroenterologist's guide to probiotics. *Clin Gastroenterol Hepatol.* 2012;10(9):960–968.
6. Ford AC, Brandt LJ, Young C, et al. Efficacy of 5-HT3 antagonists and 5-HT4 agonists in irritable bowel syndrome: systematic review and meta-analysis. *Am J Gastroenterol.* 2009;104(7):1831–1843.
7. Schey R, Rao SS. The role of rifaximin therapy in patients with irritable bowel syndrome without constipation. *Expert Rev Gastroenterol Hepatol.* 2011;5(4):461–464.
8. Rahimi R, Nikfar S, Abdollahi M. Efficacy and tolerability of alosetron for the treatment of irritable bowel syndrome in women and men: a meta-analysis of eight randomized, placebo-controlled, 12-week trials. *Clin Ther.* 2008;30(5):884–901.
9. Drossman DA, Chey WD, Johanson JF, et al. Clinical trial: lubiprostone in patients with constipation-associated irritable bowel syndrome—results of two randomized, placebo-controlled studies. *Aliment Pharmacol Ther.* 2009;29(3):329–341.
10. Videlock EJ, Cheng V, Cremonini F. Effects of linaclotide in patients with irritable bowel syndrome with constipation or chronic constipation: a meta-analysis. *Clin Gastroenterol Hepatol.* 2013;11(9):1084.e3–1092.e3.
11. Rahimi R, Nikfar S, Rezaie A, et al. Efficacy of tricyclic antidepressants in irritable bowel syndrome: a meta-analysis. *World J Gastroenterol.* 2009;15(13):1548–1553.

 SEE ALSO

Algorithm: Diarrhea, Chronic

 CODES

ICD10
- K58.9 Irritable bowel syndrome without diarrhea
- K58.0 Irritable bowel syndrome with diarrhea

CLINICAL PEARLS
- Use Rome III criteria for diagnosis.
- Goals of treatment are to relieve symptoms and improve quality of life.
- If patient does not respond to initial treatment, consider further evaluation to exclude organic pathology.

KAWASAKI SYNDROME

Alicia D. Evans, MD • Scott P. Grogan, DO, MBA, FAAFP

 BASICS

DESCRIPTION

- Kawasaki syndrome (KS) is a self-limited acute, febrile, systemic vasculitis of small- and medium-sized arteries that predominantly affects patients age 6 months to 5 years and is the most prominent cause of acquired coronary artery disease in pediatric populations.
  - Vasculitis of coronary arteries resulting in aneurysms/ectasia, further leading to myocardial infarction (MI)/ischemia or sudden death
- System(s) affected: cardiovascular, gastrointestinal, hematologic/lymphatic/immunologic, musculoskeletal, nervous, pulmonary, renal/urologic, skin/exocrine
- Synonym(s): mucocutaneous lymph node syndrome (MCLS), infantile polyarteritis, Kawasaki disease

ALERT
KS should be considered in any child with extended high fever unresponsive to antibiotics or antipyretics, rash, and nonexudative conjunctivitis.

EPIDEMIOLOGY
Incidence
- Worldwide: affects all races but most prevalent in Asia; Japan annual incidence rate 216/100,000 in children <5 years of age
- In the United States, the annual incidence in children <5 years is 19/100,000. In comparison to Caucasians, African Americans have a 1.5 times risk, and Asian Americans have a 2.5 times increased risk. Highest state incidence is in Hawaii.
- Leading cause of acquired heart disease in children in developed countries
  - Predominant age: 1 to 5 years
  - 85% of cases are children <5 years of age and 50% <2 years of age.
  - Male-to-female ratio = 1.5:1

Prevalence
- Highest to lowest prevalence: Asians > African Americans > Hispanics > Caucasians
- Seasonal variation: increased in winter and early spring in temperate places, summer in Asia, and outbreaks at 2- to 3-year intervals

ETIOLOGY AND PATHOPHYSIOLOGY
- Acute KS causes inflammation in the smooth muscle layer of medium extraparenchymal arteries, especially the coronary arteries.
- Inflammatory cells in the media secrete cytokines (TNF-α), interleukins, and matrix metalloproteases that cause fragmentation of the internal elastic lamina.
- A prominence of IgA plasma cells and IgA deposits are characteristic features and may be found in the lungs.
- As the process resolves, active inflammatory cells are replaced by fibroblasts and monocytes; tissue repair/remodeling may cause vascular fibrosis and stenosis.
- Unknown; believed to be an exaggerated immune response to infectious agent due to the acute, self-limited nature; community-wide outbreaks; age distribution; seasonality; and laboratory features indicating respiratory route of entry

Genetics
- Siblings of patients in Japan have a 10- to 30-fold increased risk, and >50% develop KS within 10 days of first case. Increased occurrence of KS in children whose parents also had illness in childhood.

- Populations at higher risk and family link suggest a genetic predisposition.

GENERAL PREVENTION
No preventive measures available

 DIAGNOSIS

≥5 days of fever and ≥4 of the following 5 principal clinical features; or <4 features and presence of coronary artery disease on 2D echocardiography:
- Bilateral conjunctival injection with limbic sparing
- Erythematous mouth and pharynx, tongue, and lips
- A polymorphous, generalized, erythematous rash
- Changes in the skin of the peripheral extremities
- Cervical lymphadenopathy

Pediatric Considerations
- Prolonged fever without rash and treated with antibiotics may cause clinicians to believe that later rash development is due to a drug reaction.
- Can be diagnosed on day 4 of illness if ≥4 principal features are present
- Incomplete KS
  - ≥5 days of fever, 2 to 3 principal clinical features, labs indicating systemic inflammation, and exclusion of other diseases
  - Incomplete cases that exhibit <4 clinical criteria often occur in infants ≤6 months of age or older children/adolescents. The frequency of coronary artery aneurysms (CAAs) is often higher in patients with missed diagnosis/delayed treatment. Therefore, in infants with prolonged fever and few or no clinical features, consider echocardiography and inflammatory labs.

HISTORY
- Fever is the first sign during the acute phase.
- Symptoms may not occur all at once, but usually occur in close proximity.

PHYSICAL EXAM
- High-spiking and remittent fever for ≥5 days
  - Fever is high (102–105°F [39.4–40.5°C]) and unresponsive to antibiotics.
  - May be prolonged up to 3 to 4 weeks
  - Extreme irritability is a very common feature.
- Bilateral, painless, nonpurulent, conjunctival injection without corneal ulceration or edema. Limbic sparing is usually seen.
- Changes in lips and oral cavity
  - Redness and swelling of lips in the acute stage; cracking, fissuring, bleeding in subacute phase
  - Strawberry/erythematous tongue
- Extensive erythematous polymorphous rash: within 5 days of fever
  - Morbilliform is most common. May be maculopapular, scarlatiniform; can resemble erythema multiforme, erythroderma, urticarial exanthem; rarely micropustular
  - Perineal desquamation, especially in skin folds
- Extremity changes
  - Reddened palms and soles on days 3 to 5
  - Edema of hands and feet on days 4 to 7; painful induration
  - Desquamation of fingers and toes that begins in periungual area at 2 to 3 weeks
- Acute, unilateral cervical lymphadenopathy (least common symptom)
  - ≥1 lymph nodes >1.5 cm, firm, nonfluctuant, and usually with no to slight tenderness

- Cardiac exam: tachycardia, gallop rhythms, hyperdynamic precordium, innocent flow murmurs, depressed contractility
- Other organ system involvement
  - Cardiovascular: myocarditis; pericarditis (often subclinical), CAAs, and other medium-sized arterial aneurysms
  - Gastrointestinal: anorexia, abdominal pain, vomiting/diarrhea, acute gallbladder hydrops, hepatic enlargement, jaundice
  - Renal: proteinuria, sterile pyuria
  - Joints: polyarthritis of small joints in acute phase; weight-bearing joints affected after 10th day from onset of fever
  - Neurologic: irritability, aseptic meningitis, peripheral neuropathy (unilateral facial palsy), transient high-frequency hearing loss

DIFFERENTIAL DIAGNOSIS
- Bacterial: staphylococcal scalded-skin syndrome, toxic shock syndrome, scarlet fever, bacterial cervical lymphadenitis, *Mycoplasma* infection, leptospirosis, Lyme disease, Rocky Mountain spotted fever
- Viral: measles, adenovirus, Epstein-Barr virus
- Toxoplasmosis
- Reiter syndrome
- Hypersensitivity drug reactions (erythema multiforme minor, Stevens-Johnson syndrome)
- Juvenile rheumatoid arthritis
- Acrodynia (mercury poisoning)

DIAGNOSTIC TESTS & INTERPRETATION
- Initial workup: CBC with differential, urinalysis (UA)/culture, blood culture; lumbar puncture if signs of meningitis or if <90 days old
  - Leukocytosis (12,000 to 40,000 cells/mm^3) with immature and mature granulocytes
  - Anemia: normochromic, normocytic
  - Thrombocytosis (500,000 to >1,000,000/mm^3) in second and third week. Thrombocytopenia during acute phase is associated with CAA and MI.
- Elevated C-reactive protein (CRP) (>35 mg/L in 80% cases), erythrocyte sedimentation rate (ESR) (>60 mm/hr in 60% cases), and α_1-antitrypsin

ALERT
ESR can be artificially high after intravenous immunoglobulin (IVIG) therapy.

- Hyponatremia
- Moderately elevated AST, ALT, GGT, and bilirubin
- Decreased albumin and protein
- CSF pleocytosis may be seen (lymphocytic with normal protein and glucose).
- *N*-terminal brain natriuretic peptide might be elevated in acute phase.
- Sterile pyuria but not seen in suprapubic collection
- Nasal swab to rule out adenovirus

Initial Tests (lab, imaging)
- If KS is suspected, obtain ECG and echocardiogram.
  - ECG may show arrhythmias, prolonged PR interval, and ST/T wave changes.
  - Echocardiography has a high sensitivity and specificity for detection of abnormalities of proximal left main coronary artery, and right coronary artery may show perivascular brightening, ectasia, decreased left ventricular contractility, pericardial effusion, or aneurysms.
  - Cardiac stress test if CAA seen on echocardiogram
- Baseline chest x-ray (CXR): may show pleural effusion, atelectasis, and congestive heart failure (CHF)

- Hydrops of the gallbladder may be associated with abdominal pain or may be asymptomatic.

Diagnostic Procedures/Other
- No laboratory study is diagnostic; diagnosis rests on constellation of clinical features and exclusion of other illnesses.
- Magnetic resonance coronary angiography is non-invasive modality to visualize coronary arteries for stenosis, thrombi, and intimal thickening (1).
- Patients with complex coronary artery lesions may benefit from coronary angiography after the acute inflammatory process has resolved; generally recommended in 6 to 12 months

 TREATMENT

GENERAL MEASURES
Use antibiotics until bacterial etiologies are excluded (e.g., sepsis or meningitis).

MEDICATION
- Optimal therapy is IVIG 2 g/kg IV over 10 to 12 hours with high-dose aspirin preferably within 7 to 10 days of fever, followed by low-dose aspirin until follow-up echocardiograms indicate a lack of coronary abnormalities.
  - IVIG lowers the risk of CAA and may shorten fever duration.
  - The extreme irritability often resolves very quickly after IVIG is given.
- Retreatment with IVIG if clinical response is incomplete or fever persists/returns >36 hours after start of IVIG treatment.
  - ≥10% of patients do not respond to initial IVIG treatment. 2/3 of nonresponders respond to the second dose of IVIG.
  - Nonresponders tend to have ↑ bands, ↓ albumin, and an abnormal echo.
- Aspirin, 80 to 100 mg/kg/day in 4 doses beginning with IVIG administration. Switch to low-dose aspirin (3 to 5 mg/kg/day) when afebrile for 48 to 72 hours, or continue until day 14 of illness. Maintain low dose for 6 to 8 weeks until follow-up echocardiogram is normal and CRP and/or ESR are normal. Continue salicylate regimen in children with coronary abnormalities long term or until documented regression of aneurysm (2)[C].
- Aspirin does not appear to reduce CAA (3)[B].
- Contraindications
  - IVIG: documented hypersensitivity, IgA deficiency, anti-IgE/IgG antibodies, severe thrombocytopenia, coagulation disorders
  - Aspirin: vitamin K deficiency, bleeding disorders, liver damage, documented hypersensitivity, hypoprothrombinemia
- Precautions
  - No statistically significant difference is noted between different preparations of IVIG.
  - High-dose aspirin therapy can result in tinnitus, decrease of renal function, and increased transaminases.
  - Do not use ibuprofen in children with CAAs who are taking aspirin for antiplatelet effects.
  - Significant possible interactions: Aspirin therapy has been associated with Reye syndrome in children who develop viral infections, especially influenza B and varicella. Yearly influenza vaccination thus is recommended for children requiring long-term treatment with aspirin. Delay any live vaccines for 11 months after IVIG treatment.

Second Line
- Corticosteroids should be used only if ≥2 IVIG treatments have failed. The addition of corticosteroids to IVIG and aspirin during initial treatment might improve CAA outcomes but lacks consistent evidence (4)[C].
- In patients refractory to IVIG and steroids, consider infliximab or cyclosporine (5)[B].
- Plasma exchange may decrease likelihood of CAA in IVIG nonresponders (6)[B].

ISSUES FOR REFERRAL
Pediatric cardiologist if abnormalities on echo or if extensive stenosis

ADDITIONAL THERAPIES
- Treatment and prevention of thrombosis are crucial.
- Antiplatelet agents (clopidogrel, dipyridamole), heparin, low-molecular-weight heparin, or warfarin are sometimes added to the low-dose aspirin regimen, depending on severity of coronary involvement.

SURGERY/OTHER PROCEDURES
- Rarely needed; coronary artery bypass grafting for severe obstruction/recurrent MI. Younger patients have a higher mortality rate.
- Coronary revascularization via percutaneous coronary intervention for patients with evidence of ischemia on stress testing

INPATIENT CONSIDERATIONS
IV Fluids
Normal saline (NS) for rehydration and 1/2 NS for maintenance

Discharge Criteria
Discharge if afebrile after IVIG treatment for 24 hours.

 ONGOING CARE

FOLLOW-UP RECOMMENDATIONS
With aneurysms, contact and high-risk sports should be avoided.

Patient Monitoring
- Repeat ECG and echocardiogram at 6 to 8 weeks. If abnormal, repeat at 6 to 12 months.
- Patients with complex coronary artery lesions may benefit from coronary angiography at 6 to 12 months.

PROGNOSIS
- Usually self-limited
- Moderate-sized aneurysms usually regress in 1 to 2 years, resolving in 50–66% of cases.
- Recurrence (3% in Japan, <1% in the United States)
- Sudden death in early adulthood (rare)

COMPLICATIONS
- 15–25% of untreated patients develop CAAs in convalescent phase.
- 2–7% of treated patients develop aneurysms. 1% develop giant aneurysms.
- Risk factors for aneurysm
  - Male, <1 year of age, ↑ ESR >4 weeks, fever >2 weeks, fever >48 hours after IVIG treatment
- Mortality of 0.08–0.17% is due to cardiac disease.

REFERENCES
1. JCS Joint Working Group. Guidelines for diagnosis and management of cardiovascular sequelae in Kawasaki disease (JCS 2008)—digest version. Circ J. 2010;74(9):1989–2020.
2. Baumer JH, Love SJ, Gupta A, et al. Salicylate for the treatment of Kawasaki disease in children. Cochrane Database Syst Rev. 2006;(4):CD004175.
3. Lee G, Lee SE, Hong YM, et al. Is high-dose aspirin necessary in the acute phase of Kawasaki disease? Korean Circ J. 2013;43(3):182–186.
4. Chen S, Dong Y, Yin Y, et al. Intravenous immunoglobulin plus corticosteroid to prevent coronary artery abnormalities in Kawasaki disease: a meta-analysis. Heart. 2013;99(2):76–82.
5. Patel RM, Shulman ST. Kawasaki disease: a comprehensive review of treatment options. J Clin Pharm Ther. 2015;40(6):620–625.
6. Hokosaki T, Mori M, Nishizawa T, et al. Long-term efficacy of plasma exchange treatment for refractory Kawasaki disease. Pediatr Int. 2012;54(1):99–103.

ADDITIONAL READING
- Huang SK, Lin MT, Chen HC, et al. Epidemiology of Kawasaki disease: prevalence from national database and future trends projection by system dynamics modeling. J Pediatr. 2013;163(1):126.e1–131.e1.
- Kobayashi T, Saji T, Otani T, et al. Efficacy of immunoglobulin plus prednisolone for prevention of coronary artery abnormalities in severe Kawasaki disease (RAISE study): a randomised, open-label, blinded-endpoints trial. Lancet. 2012;379(9826):1613–1620.
- Newburger JW, Takahashi M, Gerber MA, et al. Diagnosis, treatment, and long-term management of Kawasaki disease: a statement for health professionals from the Committee on Rheumatic Fever, Endocarditis and Kawasaki Disease, Council on Cardiovascular Disease in the Young, American Heart Association. Circulation. 2004;110(17):2747–2771.
- Oates-Whitehead RM, Baumer JH, Haines L, et al. Intravenous immunoglobulin for the treatment of Kawasaki disease in children. Cochrane Database Syst Rev. 2003;(4):CD004000.
- Rowley AH, Shulman ST. Pathogenesis and management of Kawasaki disease. Expert Rev Anti Infect Ther. 2010;8(2):197–203.
- Takahashi K, Oharaseki T, Yokouchi Y. Update on etio and immunopathogenesis of Kawasaki disease. Curr Opin Rheumatol. 2014;26(1):31–36.
- Uehara R, Belay ED. Epidemiology of Kawasaki disease in Asia, Europe, and the United States. J Epidemiol. 2012;22(2):79–85.

CODES

ICD10
M30.3 Mucocutaneous lymph node syndrome [Kawasaki]

CLINICAL PEARLS
- The diagnosis of KS rests on a constellation of clinical features.
- Once KS is suspected, all patients need an inpatient cardiac evaluation, including ECG and echocardiogram.
- Expert recommendations for optimal therapy is IVIG 2 g/kg IV over 10 hours, with high-dose aspirin 80 to 100 mg/kg/day in 4 doses.

K

KERATOACANTHOMA

Carl Bryce, MD, Capt, USAF • Matthew J. Snyder, DO

 BASICS

DESCRIPTION
- Rapidly proliferating, solitary, dome-shaped, erythematous or flesh-colored papule or nodule with a central keratinous plug, typically reaching 1 to 2 cm in diameter
- Highly debated as to whether keratoacanthoma (KA) is a benign or malignant variant of squamous cell carcinoma (SCC). Majority are benign and resolve spontaneously, but lesions do have the potential for invasion and metastasis; therefore require treatment.
- Three clinical stages of KAs (1):
  - Proliferative: rapid growth of the lesion over weeks to several months
  - Maturation/stabilization: Lesion stabilizes and growth subsides.
  - Involution: spontaneous resolution of the lesion, leaving a hypopigmented, depressed scar; most but not all lesions will enter this stage.
- System(s) affected: integumentary

EPIDEMIOLOGY
- Greatest incidence over the age of 50 years but may occur at any age
- Presentation increased during summer and early fall seasons
- Most frequently on sun-exposed, hair-bearing skin but may occur anywhere
- Predominant sex: male > female (2:1)
- Most commonly in fair-skinned individuals; highest rates in Fitzpatrick I–III
- 104 cases per 100,000 individuals

ETIOLOGY AND PATHOPHYSIOLOGY
- Derived from an abnormality causing hyperkeratosis within the follicular infundibulum
- Squamous epithelial cells proliferate to extend upward around the keratin plug and proceed downward into the dermis; followed by invasion of elastic and collagen fibers
- Cellular mechanism responsible for the hyperkeratosis is currently unknown; role of human papillomavirus has been discussed but has no established causality (2).
- Regression may be due to immune cytotoxicity or terminal differentiation of keratinocytes.
- Multiple etiologies have been suggested:
  - UV radiation
  - May be provoked by surgery, cryotherapy, chemical peels or laser therapy
  - Viral infections: human papillomavirus (HPV) or Merkel cell polyomavirus
  - Genetic predisposition: Muir-Torre syndrome, xeroderma pigmentosum, Ferguson-Smith syndrome
  - Immunosuppression
  - Chemical carcinogen exposure

Genetics
- Mutation of *p53* or H-*ras*
- Ferguson-Smith (AD)
- Witten-Zak (AD)
- Muir-Torre (AD)
- Xeroderma pigmentosum (AR)
- Gzybowski (sporadic)
- Incontinentia pigmenti (XLD)

RISK FACTORS
- UV exposure/damage: outdoor and/or indoor tanning
- Fitzpatrick skin type I–III
- Trauma (typically appears within 1 month of injury): laser resurfacing, surgery, cryotherapy, tattoos
- Chemical carcinogens: tar, pitch, and smoking
- Immunocompromised state
- Discoid lupus erythematosus

GENERAL PREVENTION
Sun protection

COMMONLY ASSOCIATED CONDITIONS
- Frequently, the patient has concurrent sun-damaged skin: solar elastosis, solar lentigines, actinic keratosis, nonmelanoma skin cancers (basal cell carcinoma, SCC)
- In Muir-Torre syndrome, KAs are found with coexisting sebaceous neoplasms and malignancy of the GI and GU tracts.

DIAGNOSIS

HISTORY
- Lesion begins as a small, solitary, pink macule that undergoes a rapid growth phase; classically reaching a diameter of 1 to 2 cm; size may vary.
- Once the proliferative stage has subsided, lesion size remains stable.
- May decrease in size, indicating regression
- Asymptomatic, occasionally tender
- If multiple lesions present, important to elicit a family history and recent therapies or treatments.
- If sebaceous neoplasms present, must review history for signs/symptoms of GI or GU malignancies

PHYSICAL EXAM
- Firm, solitary, erythematous or flesh-colored, dome-shaped papule or nodule with a central keratin plug, giving a crateriform appearance
- Surrounding skin and borders of lesion may show telangiectasia, atrophy, or dyspigmentation.
- Solitary; although multiple lesions can occur.
- Most commonly seen on sun-exposed areas: face, neck, scalp, dorsum of upper extremities, and posterior legs
- May also be seen on areas without sun exposure: buttocks, anus, subungual, mucosal surfaces

- Subungual KAs are very painful and seen on the first 3 digits of the hands.
- Examine for regional lymphadenopathy due to chance of lesion invasion and metastasis.

- Dermoscopy (3)[B]
  - Central keratin
  - White circles, blood spots
  - Cannot reliably distinguish between AK and SCC

DIFFERENTIAL DIAGNOSIS
- SCC
- Nodular or ulcerative basal cell carcinoma
- Cutaneous horn
- Hypertrophic actinic keratosis
- Amelanotic melanoma
- Merkel cell carcinoma
- Metastasis to the skin
- Molluscum contagiosum
- Prurigo nodularis
- Verruca vulgaris
- Verrucous carcinoma
- Sebaceous adenoma
- Hypertrophic lichen planus
- Hypertrophic lupus erythematosus
- Deep fungal infection
- Atypical mycobacterial infection
- Nodular Kaposi sarcoma

DIAGNOSTIC TESTS & INTERPRETATION
- Excisional biopsy including the center of the lesion as well as the margin is the best diagnostic test (2)[C].
- A shave biopsy may be insufficiently deep to distinguish KA from an SCC.
- If unable to perform an excisional biopsy, a deep shave (saucerization) of the entire lesion, extending into the subcutaneous fat, can be done.
- Punch biopsies should be avoided because they give an insufficient amount of tissue to represent the entire lesion.

Initial Tests (lab, imaging)
- Subungual KA: radiograph of the digit to monitor for osteolysis (cup-shaped radiolucent defect)
- Aggressive tumors may need CT with contrast for evaluation of lymph nodes and MRI if there is concern of perineural invasion.
- Most lesions do not need any form of imaging.

Test Interpretation
- Pathology of biopsy: a well-demarcated central core of keratin surrounded by well-differentiated, mildly pleomorphic, atypical squamous epithelial cells with a characteristic glassy eosinophilic cytoplasm
- May see elastic and collagen fibers invading into the squamous epithelium

- Histologic differentiation of a KA from an SCC may be difficult and unreliable, although immunochemical staining for cellular protein Ki-67 may help do this (4).
- KAs have a greater tendency than SCC to display fibrosis and intraepidermal abscesses of neutrophils and eosinophils.
- Regressing KA shows flattening and fibrosis at base of lesion.

TREATMENT

- Treatment of choice is an excisional procedure plus electrodessication and curettage; however, there are many treatment options available (2)[C].
- Aggressive tumors (>2 cm) or lesions in cosmetically sensitive areas (face, digits, genitalia) that require tissue sparing, consider Mohs micrographic surgery
  – Mohs is the treatment of choice in cases with perineural or perivascular invasion.
- Small lesions (<2 cm) of the extremities may undergo electrodessication and curettage.
- Immunocompromised patients should receive immediate surgical treatment.

MEDICATION

- Nonsurgical management is a viable and relatively cost-effective option in these select cases not amenable to surgery due to lesion number, size, or location; also for patients with multiple comorbidities who are unwilling or unable to withstand surgery
- Evidence for the following treatments based on case reports and retrospective reviews:

  – Intralesional methotrexate 12.5 to 25 mg in 0.5 mL normal saline every 2 to 3 weeks for one to four treatment sessions (5)[B]

    o Monitor for pancytopenia with complete blood count (5)[C].

  – 5% Imiquimod cream 3 times per week for 11 to 13 weeks (5)[B]
  – Topical 5% 5-fluorouracil cream daily, 61–92% cure rate (5)[B]
  – Intralesional 5-fluorouracil of 50 mg/mL on a weekly basis for three to eight treatment sessions—98% cure rate (5)[B]
  – Intralesional IFN a-2a or a-2b (83%, 100% cure rate, respectively) (5)[B]
  – Intralesional bleomycin—100% cure rate (5)[B]

  – Isotretinoin oral 0.5 to 1 mg/kg/day

ISSUES FOR REFERRAL

Dermatology referral if lesions are >2 cm, numerous, mucosal, or subungual

ADDITIONAL THERAPIES

- Photodynamic therapy with methyl aminolevulinic acid and red light, successful case reports (6)[B] but also reported aggravation following treatment

- Cryotherapy
- Argon or YAG lasers

- Radiotherapy, primary or adjuvant: KAs may regress with low doses of radiation but may require doses up to 25 to 50 Gy in low-dose (5 to 10 Gy) fractions for possible SCC (7)[B].
- Erlotinib (EGFR inhibitor) 150 mg daily for 21 days, single case report (8)[B]

SURGERY/OTHER PROCEDURES

Excisional and office-based procedures as discussed above.

ONGOING CARE

FOLLOW-UP RECOMMENDATIONS

After the surgical site has healed or lesion has resolved, patient should be seen every 6 months due to increased risk of developing new lesions or skin cancers, annually at minimum (3)[C].

Patient Monitoring

- Skin self-exams should be routinely performed with detailed instructions (see "Additional Reading").
- If multiple KAs are present in patient or family members, evaluate for Muir-Torre syndrome and obtain a colonoscopy beginning at age 25 years, as well as testing for genitourinary cancer (3)[C].

PATIENT EDUCATION

- Sun protection measures: sun block with SPF >30, wide-brimmed hats, long sleeves, dark clothing, avoiding indoor tanning
- Arc welding may produce harmful UV radiation and skin should not be exposed.
- Tar, pitch, and smoking should be avoided.

PROGNOSIS

- Atrophic scarring and hypopigmentation can occur with self-resolution but may be significantly reduced by intervention.
- 52 of 445 cases (12%) spontaneously regressed without treatment and none of these recurred (2).
- 393 (88%) regressed following medical or excisional treatment (2).
- 445 cases reported with no metastases or deaths attributable to the KA (2).
- 4–8% recurrence
- Mucosal and subungual lesions do not regress, must undergo treatment

REFERENCES

1. Zalaudek I, Bonifazi E, Ferrara G, et al. Keratoacanthomas and spitz tumors: are they both "self-limiting" variants of malignant cutaneous neoplasms? *Dermatology*. 2009;219(1):3–6.
2. Savage JA, Maize JC Sr. Keratoacanthoma clinical behavior: a systematic review. *Am J Dermatopathol*. 2014;36(5):422–429.
3. Rosendahl C, Cameron A, Argenziano G, et al. Dermoscopy of squamous cell carcinoma and keratoacanthoma. *Arch Dermatol*. 2012;148(12):1386–1392.
4. Scola N, Segert HM, Stücker M, et al. Ki-67 may be useful in differentiating between keratoacanthoma and cutaneous squamous cell carcinoma. *Clin Exp Dermatol*. 2014;39(2):216–238.
5. Chitwood KL, Etzkorn J, Cohen G. Topical and intralesional treatment of nonmelanoma skin cancer: efficacy and cost comparisons. *Dermatol Surg*. 2013;39(9):1306–1316.
6. Jeon HC, Choi M, Paik SH, et al. Treatment of keratoacanthoma with 5% imiquimod cream and review of the previous report. *Ann Dermatol*. 2011;23(3):357–361.
7. Bruscino N, Corradini D, Campolmi P, et al. Superficial radiotherapy for multiple keratoacanthomas. *Dermatol Ther*. 2014;27(3):163–167.
8. Reid DC, Guitart J, Agulnik M, et al. Treatment of multiple keratoacanthomas with erlotinib. *Int J Clin Oncol*. 2010;15(4):413–415.

ADDITIONAL READING

- The American Academy of Dermatology: https://www.aad.org/spot-skin-cancer/learn-about-skin-cancer/types-of-skin-cancer
- The Skin Cancer Foundation: http://www.skincancer.org/

SEE ALSO

Squamous Cell Carcinoma, Cutaneous

CODES

ICD10

- D23.9 Other benign neoplasm of skin, unspecified
- D48.5 Neoplasm of uncertain behavior of skin
- L85.8 Other specified epidermal thickening

CLINICAL PEARLS

- Suspect KA with a solitary, dome-shaped, erythematous or flesh-colored papule or nodule with a central keratinous plug.
- If KA is in the differential diagnosis, elicit time frame of onset during patient encounter; rapid onset supports diagnosis.
- Due to the broad differential diagnosis of a suspected KA and unreliable clinical differentiation between these, strongly consider surgical excision as first-line diagnostic test and therapy.
- Medical and radiation therapies are reasonable and effective options available for patients who are not surgical candidates or for lesions that are not amenable for surgery.

K

KERATOSIS, ACTINIC

Zoltan Trizna, MD, PhD

BASICS

DESCRIPTION
- Common, usually multiple, premalignant lesions of sun-exposed areas of the skin. Many resolve spontaneously, and a small proportion progress to squamous cell carcinoma
- Common consequence of excessive cumulative ultraviolet (UV) light exposure
- Synonym(s): solar keratosis

Geriatric Considerations
Frequent problem

Pediatric Considerations
Rare (if child, look for freckling and other stigmata of xeroderma pigmentosum)

EPIDEMIOLOGY
Incidence
- Rates vary with age group and exposure to sun.
- Predominant age: ≥40 years; progressively increases with age
- Predominant sex: male > female
- Common in those with blonde and red hair; rare in darker skin types

Prevalence
- Age-adjusted prevalence rate for actinic keratoses (AKs) in U.S. Caucasians is 6.5%.
- For 65- to 74-year-old males with high sun exposure: ~55%; low sun exposure, ~18%

ETIOLOGY AND PATHOPHYSIOLOGY
- The epidermal lesions are characterized by atypical keratinocytes at the basal layer with occasional extension upward. Mitoses are present. The histopathologic features resemble those of squamous cell carcinoma (SCC) in situ or SCC, and the distinction depends on the extent of epidermal involvement.
- Cumulative UV exposure

Genetics
The p53 chromosomal mutation has been shown consistently in both AKs and SCCs. Many new genes have been shown recently to have similar expression profiles in AKs and SCCs.

RISK FACTORS
- Exposure to UV light (especially long-term and/or repeated exposure due to outdoor occupation or recreational activities, indoor or outdoor tanning)

- Skin type: burns easily, does not tan
- Immunosuppression, especially organ transplantation

GENERAL PREVENTION
Sun avoidance and protective techniques are helpful.

COMMONLY ASSOCIATED CONDITIONS
- SCC
- Other features of chronic solar damage: lentigines, elastosis, and telangiectasias

DIAGNOSIS

HISTORY
- The lesions are frequently asymptomatic; symptoms may include pruritus, burning, and mild hyperesthesia.
- Lesions may enlarge, thicken, or become more scaly. They also may regress or remain unchanged.
- Most lesions occur on the sun-exposed areas (head and neck, hands, forearms).

PHYSICAL EXAM
- Usually small (<1 cm), often multiple red, pink, or brown macules, papules, or plaques that are rough to palpation
- Yellow or brown adherent scale is often present on top of the lesion.
- Several clinical variants exist.
  - Atrophic: dry, scaly macules with indistinct borders and an erythematous base
  - Hypertrophic: Overlying hyperkeratosis (in an extreme form, cutaneous horn) may be impossible to differentiate from SCC clinically.
  - Pigmented: smooth tan/brown plaque, spreading centrifugally
  - Bowenoid: red scaly plaques with distinct borders
  - Actinic cheilitis: inflammatory lesion involving usually the lower lip

DIFFERENTIAL DIAGNOSIS
- SCC (hypertrophic type)
- Keratoacanthoma
- Bowen disease
- Basal cell carcinoma
- Verruca vulgaris
- Less likely: verrucous nevi, warty dyskeratoma, lichenoid keratoses, seborrheic keratoses, porokeratoses, seborrheic dermatitis or psoriasis (near hairline), lentigo maligna, solar lentigo, discoid lupus erythematosus

DIAGNOSTIC TESTS & INTERPRETATION
Diagnostic Procedures/Other
- The diagnosis is usually made clinically, except where there is a suspicion of carcinoma.
- Skin biopsy is especially recommended if large, ulcerated, indurated, or bleeding; or if the lesions are nonresponsive to treatment.

Test Interpretation
- Dysplastic keratinocytes in lower levels of epidermis with a dermal lymphocytic infiltrate
- Neoplastic cells, mostly found in the lower epidermal layers, are cytologically identical to those of SCCs.
- If neoplastic cells extend throughout entire epidermis or into the dermis, the lesions will qualify as an SCC in situ or invasive SCC, respectively.
- Malignant cells are sparse except of the bowenoid variety.
- Hypertrophic, atrophic, bowenoid, acantholytic, and pigmented varieties show the corresponding epidermal findings.

TREATMENT

First-line treatment is cryotherapy (technically, this is considered surgery, especially by insurance companies) (1,2)[A]. Medical therapy is usually reserved for extensive AKs ("field therapy").

GENERAL MEASURES
- Sun-protective techniques
- Sunscreens and physical sun protection recommended.

MEDICATION
First Line
- Topical treatments target both visible and subclinical lesions.
- With the exception of generic 5-fluorouracil, medication cost is high ($600 to $1,200 per course).
- Topical fluorouracil (Efudex, Carac, Fluoroplex cream, Fluoroplex solution)
  - Every day—BID for 3 to 6 weeks, depending on the brand, concentration, and formulation
  - Can be very irritating
  - May be most effective of the topical treatments (3)[A] listed in this section.

- Topical imiquimod (Aldara) 5% cream
  - Apply 2 days per week at HS for up to 16 weeks to an area not larger than the forehead or one cheek.
  - Can be irritating
- Topical imiquimod (Zyclara) 3.75% cream
  - Apply once a day for 2 weeks, followed by no treatment for the next 2 weeks; then apply once a day for another 2 weeks.
  - Can be irritating
- Topical ingenol mebutate (Picato) 0.015% and 0.05% gel
  - Apply to the face and scalp once a day for 3 consecutive days.
  - Apply to the trunk and extremities once a day for 2 consecutive days.
    - It should only be used on one contiguous skin area of not more than 25 cm^2.
    - Cases of severe allergic reactions (including anaphylaxis) and herpes zoster reactivation unrelated to application errors have been reported.
- Diclofenac (Solaraze) 3% gel
  - Apply BID for 60 to 90 days.

Second Line
- Topical tretinoin (Retin-A) or tazarotene (Tazorac): may be used to enhance the efficacy of topical fluorouracil
- Systemic retinoids: used infrequently

ADDITIONAL THERAPIES
Close monitoring with no treatment is an appropriate option for mild lesions.

SURGERY/OTHER PROCEDURES
- Cryosurgery ("freezing," liquid nitrogen)
  - Most common method for treating AK
  - Cure rate: 75–98.8%
  - May leave scars
  - May be superior to photodynamic therapy for thicker lesions
- Photodynamic therapy with a photosensitizer (e.g., aminolevulinic acid) and "blue light"
  - May clear >90% of AKs
  - Less scarring than cryotherapy
  - May be superior to cryotherapy, especially in the case of more extensive skin involvement

- Curettage and electrocautery (electrodesiccation and curettage [ED&C]; "scraping and burning")
- Medium-depth peels, especially for the treatment of extensive areas
- CO_2 laser therapy
- Dermabrasion
- Surgical excision (excisional biopsy)

 ONGOING CARE

FOLLOW-UP RECOMMENDATIONS
Patient Monitoring
Depends on associated malignancy and frequency with which new AKs appear

PATIENT EDUCATION
- Teach sun-protective techniques.
  - Limit outdoor activities between 10 AM and 4 PM.
  - Wear protective clothing and wide-brimmed hat.
  - Proper use (including reapplication) of sunscreens with SPF >30, preferably a preparation with broad-spectrum (UV-A and UV-B) protection
- Teach self-examination of skin (melanoma, squamous cell, basal cell).
- Patient education materials
  - http://dermnetnz.org/lesions/solar-keratoses.html
  - www.skincarephysicians.com/actinickeratosesnet/index.html
  - www.skincancer.org/Actinic-Keratosis-and-Other-Precancers.htm

PROGNOSIS
Very good. A significant proportion of the lesions may resolve spontaneously (4), with regression rates of 20–30% per lesion per year.

COMPLICATIONS
- AKs are premalignant lesions that may progress to SCCs. The rate of malignant transformation is unclear; the reported percentages vary (4) but range from 0.1% to a few percent per year per lesion.
- Patients with AKs are at increased risk for other cutaneous malignancies.
- Approximately 60% of SCCs arise from an AK precursor.

REFERENCES
1. Helfand M, Gorman AK, Mahon S, et al. *Actinic Keratoses*. Rockville, MD: Agency for Healthcare Research and Quality; 2001.
2. de Berker D, McGregor JM, Hughes BR. Guidelines for the management of actinic keratoses. *Br J Dermatol*. 2007;156(2):222–230.
3. Gupta AK, Paquet M. Network meta-analysis of the outcome "participant complete clearance" in nonimmunosuppressed participants of eight interventions for actinic keratosis: a follow-up on a Cochrane review. *Br J Dermatol*. 2013;169(2):250–259.
4. Criscione VD, Weinstock MA, Naylor MF, et al. Actinic keratoses: natural history and risk of malignant transformation in the Veterans Affairs Topical Tretinoin Chemoprevention Trial. *Cancer*. 2009;115(11):2523–2530.

ADDITIONAL READING
- Kanellou P, Zaravinos A, Zioga M, et al. Genomic instability, mutations and expression analysis of the tumour suppressor genes p14(ARF), p15(INK4b), p16(INK4a) and p53 in actinic keratosis. *Cancer Lett*. 2008;264(1):145–161.
- Rossi R, Mori M, Lotti T. Actinic keratosis. *Int J Dermatol*. 2007;46(9):895–904.

 CODES

ICD10
L57.0 Actinic keratosis

CLINICAL PEARLS
- AKs are premalignant lesions.
- Often more easily felt than seen
- Therapy-resistant lesions should be biopsied, especially on the face.

KERATOSIS, SEBORRHEIC
Jelaun Newsome, DO

 ## BASICS

DESCRIPTION
- One of the most common benign tumors of the epidermis
- Formed from keratinocytes
- Frequently appears in multiples on the head, neck, and trunk of older individuals but may occur on any hair-bearing area of the body. Lesions spare the palms and soles.
- Typically are light brown to black, sharply demarcated, round, or elongated lesions with a velvety, verrucous-like, "stuck-on" appearance; lesions may also appear waxy yellow or pink.
- Clinical variants include the following:
  - Common seborrheic keratosis
  - Dermatosis papulosa nigra
  - Stucco keratosis
  - Flat seborrheic keratosis
  - Pedunculated seborrheic keratosis
- System(s) affected: integumentary
- Synonym(s): verruca seborrhoica; seborrheic wart; senile wart; basal cell papilloma; verruca senilis; basal cell acanthoma; benign acanthokeratoma

EPIDEMIOLOGY
Incidence
- Predominant age
  - Usually appear after the 3rd decade
  - Most commonly seen during middle and older age
  - Can occasionally arise as early as adolescence
- Predominant sex: male = female
- Most common among Caucasians, except for the dermatosis papulosa nigra variant, which usually presents in darker skinned individuals

Prevalence
- 69–100% in patients >50 years of age
- The prevalence rate increases with advancing age.

ETIOLOGY AND PATHOPHYSIOLOGY
- Seborrheic keratoses are monoclonal tumors.
- Etiology still is largely unclear.
- Ultraviolet (UV) light and genetics are thought to be involved.
- The role of human papillomavirus is uncertain.

Genetics
An autosomal dominant inheritance pattern is suggested.

RISK FACTORS
- Advanced age
- Exposure to UV light and genetic predisposition are possible factors (1).

GENERAL PREVENTION
Sun protection methods may help prevent seborrheic keratoses from developing.

COMMONLY ASSOCIATED CONDITIONS
- Sign of Leser-Trélat: A paraneoplastic syndrome characterized by a sudden eruption of multiple seborrheic keratoses in association with an internal malignancy, most commonly stomach or colon adenocarcinoma. Usually represents a poor prognosis. The validity of this syndrome as a marker for internal malignancy is controversial (2)[B].
- Documentation of other cutaneous lesions, such as basal cell carcinoma, malignant melanoma, Bowen disease, or squamous cell carcinoma, growing adjacent to or within a seborrheic keratosis, has been reported. The exact relationship between lesions is unclear.

DIAGNOSIS

HISTORY
- Usually asymptomatic
- Trauma or irritation of the lesion may result in pruritus, erythema, bleeding, pain, and/or crusting.

PHYSICAL EXAM
- Typically begin as oval- or round-shaped, flat, dull, sharply demarcated patches
- As they mature, may develop into thicker, elevated, uneven, verrucous-like papules, plaques, or peduncles with a waxy or velvety surface, and appear "stuck on" to the skin (3)
- Commonly appear on sun-exposed areas of the body, predominately the head, neck, or trunk but may appear on any hair-bearing skin
- Vary in color from black, brown, tan, gray to white, or skin-colored, and range in size, from 1 mm to 4 cm
- Usually occur as multiples, with patients having >100 is not uncommon.
- May grow along folds on truncal skin, forming a "Christmas tree" pattern
- If irritated, may be bleeding, inflamed, painful, pruritic, or crusted
- Common clinical variants include the following (4):
  - Common seborrheic keratoses: on hair-bearing skin, usually on the face, neck, and trunk; verrucous-like, waxy, or velvety lesions that appear "stuck on" to the skin
  - Dermatosis papulosa nigra: Small black papules that usually appear on the face, neck, chest, and upper back; most common in darker skinned individuals, more common in females; most have a positive family history.
  - Stucco keratoses: small gray-white, rough, verrucous papules; usually occur in large numbers on the lower extremities or forearms; more common in men
  - Flat seborrheic keratoses: oval-shaped, brown patches or macules on face, chest, and upper extremities; increases with age
  - Pedunculated seborrheic keratoses: Hyperpigmented peduncles appear on areas of friction (neck, axilla).

DIFFERENTIAL DIAGNOSIS
Consider the following diagnoses if the seborrheic keratosis is:
- Pigmented
  - Malignant melanoma
  - Melanocytic nevus
  - Angiokeratoma
  - Pigmented basal cell carcinoma
- Lightly pigmented
  - Basal cell carcinoma
  - Bowen disease
  - Condyloma acuminatum
  - Fibroma
  - Verruca vulgaris
  - Eccrine poroma
  - Invasive squamous cell carcinoma
  - Acrochordon
  - Acrokeratosis verruciformis of Hopf
  - Follicular infundibulum tumor
- Flat
  - Solar lentigo
  - Verrucae planae juveniles
- Hyperkeratotic
  - Actinic keratosis

DIAGNOSTIC TESTS & INTERPRETATION
Initial Tests (lab, imaging)
Not needed unless internal malignancy is suspected

Diagnostic Procedures/Other
- The diagnosis can usually be made based on clinical appearance.
- Dermoscopy
  - Can aid in diagnosis
  - Common findings are comedo-like openings, fissures, ridges, sharply demarcated borders, milia-like cysts, pseudofollicular openings, hairpin vessels, and horn pseudocysts (5,6).
- Biopsy and histologic exam should be performed if the seborrheic keratosis
  - Is atypical
  - Has inflammation
  - Recently changed in appearance
  - Diagnosis remains unclear.

Test Interpretation
- Histologic findings include the following:
  - Acanthosis and papillomatosis due to basaloid cell proliferation
  - "Squamous eddies" or squamous epithelial cell clusters
  - Hyperpigmentation
  - Hyperkeratosis
  - Horn cysts
  - Pseudocysts
- Several histologic variants exist.

TREATMENT
- Treatment is not usually necessary due to the benign nature of the lesions.
- Removal of seborrheic keratoses may be indicated if
  - Symptomatic
  - Aesthetically displeasing or undesirable (common)
  - There is a question of malignancy.

MEDICATION
Current topical treatments of seborrheic keratoses are less effective than a surgical approach.

ISSUES FOR REFERRAL
- New seborrheic keratoses appear abruptly.
- A seborrheic keratosis becomes inflamed or changes in appearance.

SURGERY/OTHER PROCEDURES
- A surgical approach to treatment is preferred.
- Choice depends on physician preference and availability of the treatment.
- The following procedures are used:
  - Cryotherapy (liquid nitrogen)
    - Spray flat lesions for 5 to 10 seconds; may require more time or additional treatments if the seborrheic keratosis is thicker
    - Possible complications include scarring, hypopigmentation, recurrence.
  - Curettage
  - Electrodessication
  - Shave excision
  - Excisional biopsy
  - Chemical peel
- Use of following laser treatments have been reported:
  - Ablative CO_2
  - Ablative erbium-YAG
  - Argon
  - 492 nm
  - 510 nm
  - Alexandrite lasers
- No statistically significant differences were found in patient's ratings of cosmetic appearance between cryotherapy and curettage. The majority of patients preferred cryotherapy over curettage due to decreased postoperative wound care, despite the increased discomfort experienced and increased frequency of seborrheic keratosis remaining after cryotherapy when compared to curettage (7)[B].

ONGOING CARE

FOLLOW-UP RECOMMENDATIONS
Patient Monitoring
After initial diagnosis, follow-up is not usually required unless
- Inflammation or irritation develops.
- There is a change in appearance.
- New seborrheic keratoses suddenly appear.

PATIENT EDUCATION
- Sun-protective methods may help reduce seborrheic keratosis development.
- Patient education materials
  - http://www.aad.org/dermatology-a-to-z/diseases-and-treatments/q–t/seborrheic-keratoses
  - www.cdc.gov/cancer/skin/basic_info/prevention.htm

PROGNOSIS
- Seborrheic keratoses generally do not become malignant.
- Sign of Leser-Trélat usually represents a poor prognosis.

COMPLICATIONS
- Irritation and inflammation due to mechanical irritation (i.e., from clothing, jewelry)
- Possible complications of surgical treatment include hypopigmentation, hyperpigmentation, scarring, incomplete removal, and recurrence.
- Misdiagnosis (rare)

REFERENCES
1. Saeed AK, Salmo N. Epidermal growth factor receptor expression in mice skin upon ultraviolet B exposure — seborrheic keratosis as a coincidental and unique finding. Adv Biomed Res. 2012;1:59.
2. Ponti G, Luppi G, Losi L, et al. Leser-Trélat syndrome in patients affected by six multiple metachronous primitive cancers. J Hematol Oncol. 2010;3:2.
3. Luba MC, Bangs SA, Mohler AM, et al. Common benign skin tumors. Am Fam Physician. 2003;67(4):729–738.
4. Noiles K, Vender R. Are all seborrheic keratoses benign? Review of the typical lesion and its variants. J Cutan Med Surg. 2008;12(5):203–210.
5. Marghoob AA, Usatine RP, Jaimes N. Dermoscopy for the family physician. Am Fam Physician. 2013;88(7):441–450.
6. Takenouchi T. Key points in dermoscopic diagnosis of basal cell carcinoma and seborrheic keratosis in Japanese. J Dermatol. 2011;38(1):59–65.
7. Wood LD, Stucki JK, Hollenbeak CS, et al. Effectiveness of cryosurgery vs curettage in the treatment of seborrheic keratoses. JAMA Dermatol. 2013;149(1):108–109.

ADDITIONAL READING
- Culbertson GR. 532-nm diode laser treatment of seborrheic keratoses with color enhancement. Dermatol Surg. 2008;34(4):525–528.
- Draelos ZD, Rizer RL, Trookman NS. A comparison of postprocedural wound care treatments: do antibiotic-based ointments improve outcomes? J Am Acad Dermatol. 2011;64(Suppl 3):S23–S29.
- Garcia MS, Azari R, Eisen DB. Treatment of dermatosis papulosa nigra in 10 patients: a comparison trial of electrodesiccation, pulsed dye laser, and curettage. Dermatol Surg. 2010;36(12):1968–1972.
- Georgieva IA, Mauerer A, Groesser L, et al. Low incidence of oncogenic EGFR, HRAS, and KRAS mutations in seborrheic keratosis. Am J Dermatopathol. 2014;36(8):635–642.
- Hafner C, Vogt T. Seborrheic keratosis. J Dtsch Dermatol Ges. 2008;6(8):664–677.
- Herron MD, Bowen AR, Krueger GG. Seborrheic keratoses: a study comparing the standard cryosurgery with topical calcipotriene, topical tazarotene, and topical imiquimod. Int J Dermatol. 2004;43(4):300–302.
- Krupashankar DS. Standard guidelines of care: CO2 laser for removal of benign skin lesions and resurfacing. Indian J Dermatol Venereol Leprol. 2008;74(Suppl):S61–S67.
- Rajesh G, Thappa DM, Jaisankar TJ, et al. Spectrum of seborrheic keratoses in South Indians: a clinical and dermoscopic study. Indian J Dermatol Venereol Leprol. 2011;77(4):483–488.
- Taylor SC, Averyhart AN, Heath CR. Postprocedural wound-healing efficacy following removal of dermatosis papulosa nigra lesions in an African American population: a comparison of a skin protectant ointment and a topical antibiotic. J Am Acad Dermatol. 2011;64(3 Suppl):S30–S35.

CODES
ICD10
- L82.1 Other seborrheic keratosis
- L82.0 Inflamed seborrheic keratosis

CLINICAL PEARLS
- Seborrheic keratoses are one of the most common benign tumors of the epidermis.
- Prevalence increases with age.
- Underlying internal malignancy should be considered if large numbers of seborrheic keratoses appear suddenly.

K

KNEE PAIN

Jeff Wang, MD, MPH • J. Herbert Stevenson, MD

BASICS

DESCRIPTION
Knee pain is a common outpatient complaint with a broad differential diagnosis.
- Knee pain may be acute, chronic, or an acute exacerbation of a chronic condition.
- Trauma, overuse, and degenerative change are frequent causes.
- A detailed history, including patient age, pain onset and location, mechanism of injury, and associated symptoms can help narrow the differential diagnosis.
- A thorough and focused examination of the knee (as well as the back, hips, and ankles) helps to establish the correct diagnosis and appropriate treatment.

EPIDEMIOLOGY
Incidence
- Knee pain accounts for 1.9 million primary care visits annually.
- The incidence of knee osteoarthritis is 240 cases/100,000 person/year.

Prevalence
- The knee is a common site of lower extremity injury.
  - Patellar tendonopathy and patellofemoral syndrome are the most common causes of knee pain in runners (1).
- Osteoarthritis (OA) is one of the leading causes of disability in the United States.

ETIOLOGY AND PATHOPHYSIOLOGY
- Trauma (ligament or meniscal injury, fracture, dislocation)
- Overuse (tendinopathy, patellofemoral syndrome, bursitis, apophysitis)
- Age-related (arthritis, degenerative conditions, apophysis [young])
- Rheumatologic (rheumatoid arthritis [RA], gout, pseudogout)
- Infectious (bacterial, postviral, Lyme disease)
- Referred pain (hip, back)
- Vascular: popliteal artery aneurysm, deep vein thrombosis
- Others: tumor, cyst, plica

RISK FACTORS
- Obesity
- Malalignment
- Poor flexibility, muscle imbalance, or weakness
- Rapid increases in training frequency and intensity
- Improper footwear, training surfaces, technique
- Activities that involve cutting, jumping, pivoting, deceleration, kneeling
- Previous injuries

GENERAL PREVENTION
- Maintain normal body mass index.
- Use appropriate exercise training principles; avoid overtraining.
- Correct postural strength and flexibility imbalances.
- Proper activity-specific techniques and equipment

COMMONLY ASSOCIATED CONDITIONS
- Fracture, contusion
- Effusion, hemarthrosis
- Patellar dislocation/subluxation
- Meniscal or ligamentous injury
- Tendinopathy, bursitis
- Osteochondral injury
- OA, septic arthritis
- Muscle strain

DIAGNOSIS

HISTORY
- Pain:
  - Diffuse pain: OA, patellofemoral pain syndrome (chondromalacia)
  - Pain ascending/descending stairs: meniscal injury, patellofemoral pain syndrome
  - Pain with prolonged sitting, standing from sitting: patellofemoral pain syndrome
  - Mechanical symptoms (locking): meniscal injury
- Mechanism of injury:
  - Hyperextension, deceleration, cutting: anterior cruciate ligament (ACL) injury
  - Hyperflexion, fall on flexed knee, "dashboard injury": posterior cruciate ligament (PCL) injury
  - Lateral force (valgus load): medial collateral injury
  - Twisting on planted foot: meniscal injury
- Effusion:
  - Rapid onset (2 hours): ACL tear, patellar subluxation, tibial plateau fracture. Hemarthrosis is common.
  - Slower onset (24 to 36 hours), smaller: meniscal injury, ligament sprain
  - Swelling behind the knee: popliteal cyst. Prepatellar: bursitis

PHYSICAL EXAM
- Observe gait (antalgia), patellar tracking.
- Inspect for malalignment, atrophy, swelling, ecchymosis, or erythema.
- Palpate for effusion, warmth, and tenderness.
- Evaluate active and passive range of motion (ROM) and flexibility of quadriceps and hamstrings.
- Evaluate strength and muscle tone.
- Note joint instability, locking, and catching.
- Evaluate hip ROM, strength, and stability.
- Special tests:
  - Patellar apprehension test: patellar instability. Patellar grind test: patellofemoral pain or OA (1)
  - Lachman test (more sensitive and specific), pivot shift, anterior drawer: ACL integrity
  - Posterior drawer, posterior sag sign: PCL integrity
  - Valgus/varus stress test: medial/lateral collateral ligament (MCL/LCL) integrity
  - McMurray test, Apley grind, Thessaly test: meniscal injury
  - Ober test: Iliotibial band (ITB) tightness
  - Dial test: positive with posterolateral corner laxity
  - Patellar tilt test and squatting may help suggest patellofemoral pain syndrome, but there is not yet one definitive test.
  - Patella facet tenderness suggests OA or patellofemoral pain syndrome (1)[A].

DIFFERENTIAL DIAGNOSIS
- Acute onset: fracture, contusion, cruciate or collateral ligament tear, meniscal tear, patellar dislocation/subluxation. If systemic symptoms: septic arthritis, gout, pseudogout, Lyme disease, and osteomyelitis
- Insidious onset: patellofemoral pain syndrome/chondromalacia, ITB syndrome, OA, RA, bursitis, tumor, tendinopathy, loose body, bipartite patella, degenerative meniscal tear
- Anterior pain: patellofemoral pain syndrome, patellar injury, patellar tendinopathy, pre- or suprapatellar bursitis, tibial apophysitis, fat pad impingement, quadriceps tendinopathy, OA (1)
- Posterior pain: PCL injury, posterior horn meniscal injury, popliteal cyst or aneurysm, hamstring or gastrocnemius injury, deep venous thrombosis (DVT)
- Medial pain: MCL injury, medial meniscal injury, pes anserine bursitis, medial plica syndrome, OA
- Lateral pain: LCL injury, lateral meniscal injury, ITB syndrome, OA

DIAGNOSTIC TESTS & INTERPRETATION
Initial Tests (lab, imaging)
- Suspected septic joint, gout, pseudogout:
  - Arthrocentesis with cell count, Gram stain, culture, protein/glucose, synovial fluid analysis
- Suspected RA:
  - CBC, erythrocyte sedimentation rate (ESR), rheumatoid factor
- Consider Lyme titer.
- Radiographs to rule out fracture in patients with acute knee trauma (Ottawa rules):
  - Age >55 years *or*
  - Tenderness at the patella or fibular head *or*
  - Inability to bear weight 4 steps *or*
  - Inability to flex knee to 90 degrees
- Radiographs help diagnose OA, osteochondral lesions, patellofemoral pain syndrome:
  - Weightbearing, upright anteroposterior, lateral, merchant/sunrise, notch/tunnel views

Follow-Up Tests & Special Considerations
- MRI is a "gold standard" for soft tissue imaging.
- Ultrasound may help diagnose tendonopathy (2)[B].
- CT can further elucidate fracture.

Diagnostic Procedures/Other
Arthroscopy may be beneficial in the diagnosis of certain conditions, including meniscus and ligament injuries.

Geriatric Considerations
OA, degenerative meniscal tears, and gout are more common in middle-aged and elderly populations.

Pediatric Considerations
- 3 million pediatric sports injuries occur annually.
- Look for physeal/apophyseal and joint surface injuries in skeletally immature:
  - Acute: patellar subluxation, avulsion fractures, ACL tear
  - Overuse: patellofemoral pain syndrome, apophysitis, osteochondritis dissecans, patellar tendonitis, stress fracture
  - Others: neoplasm, juvenile RA, infection, referred pain from slipped capital femoral epiphysis

TREATMENT

GENERAL MEASURES
Acute injury: PRICEMM therapy (**p**rotection, **r**elative rest, **i**ce, **c**ompression, **e**levation, **m**edications, **m**odalities)

MEDICATION

First Line
- Oral medications:
  - Acetaminophen: up to 3 g/day. Safe and effective in OA
  - Nonsteroidal anti-inflammatory drugs (NSAIDs):
    - Ibuprofen: 200 to 800 mg TID
    - Naproxen: 250 to 500 mg BID:
      - Useful for acute sprains, strains
      - Useful for short-term pain reduction in OA. Long-term use is not recommended due to side effects.
      - Not recommended for fracture, stress fracture, chronic muscle injury; may be associated with delayed healing; low dose and brief course only if necessary
  - Tramadol/opioids: not recommended as first-line treatment; can be used with acute injuries
  - Celecoxib: 200 mg QID may be effective in OA with less GI side effects than NSAIDs (3)[A].
- Topical medications:
  - Topical NSAIDs may provide pain relief in OA and are more tolerable than oral medications.
  - Topical capsaicin may be an adjuvant for pain management in OA.
- Injections:
  - Intra-articular corticosteroid injection may provide short-term benefit in knee OA (2)[A].
  - Viscosupplementation may reduce pain and improve function in patients with OA (2)[A], particularly those wishing to delay joint replacement.

ISSUES FOR REFERRAL
- Acute trauma, young athletic patient
- Joint instability
- Lack of improvement with conservative measures
- Salter-Harris physeal fractures (pediatrics)

ADDITIONAL THERAPIES
- Physical therapy is recommended as initial treatment for patellofemoral pain (4) and tendonopathies (2)[A].
- Muscle strengthening improves outcome in OA.
- Foot orthoses, taping, acupuncture
- May need bracing for stability (4)
- Plate-rich plasma injection in early OA (5)[B]
- Botulinum toxin A for patellofemoral pain syndrome (6)[B]

SURGERY/OTHER PROCEDURES
- Surgery may be indicated for certain injuries (e.g., ACL tear in competitive athletes).
- Chronic conditions refractory to conservative therapy may require surgical intervention.

COMPLEMENTARY & ALTERNATIVE MEDICINE
May reduce pain and improve function in early OA:
- Glucosamine sulfate (500 mg TID) (7)
- Chondroitin (400 mg TID) (7)
- S-adenosylmethionine (SAMe), ginger extract, methylsulfonylmethane: less reliable improvement with inconsistent supporting evidence (8)
- Acupuncture

 ONGOING CARE

FOLLOW-UP RECOMMENDATIONS
- Activity modification in overuse conditions
- Rehabilitative exercise in OA:
  - Low-impact exercise: walking, swimming, cycling
  - Strength, ROM, and proprioception training

Patient Monitoring
- Rehabilitation after initial treatment of acute injury.
- In chronic and overuse conditions, assess functional status, rehabilitation adherence, and pain control at follow-up visit.

DIET
Weight reduction for overweight patient with OA

PATIENT EDUCATION
- Review activity modifications.
- Encourage active role in the rehabilitation process.
- Review medication risks and benefits.

PROGNOSIS
Varies with diagnosis, injury severity, chronicity of condition, patient motivation to participate in rehabilitation, and whether surgery is required

COMPLICATIONS
- Disability
- Arthritis
- Chronic joint instability
- Deconditioning

REFERENCES
1. Hong E, Kraft MC. Evaluating anterior knee pain. *Med Clin North Am.* 2014;98(4):697–717.
2. Ayhan E, Kesmezacar H, Akgun I. Intraarticular injections (corticosteroid, hyaluronic acid, platelet rich plasma) for the knee osteoarthritis. *World J Orthop.* 2014;5(3):351–361.
3. Bijlsma JW, Berenbaum F, Lafeber FP. Osteoarthritis: an update with relevance for clinical practice. *Lancet.* 2011;377(9783):2115–2126.
4. Bolgla LA, Boling MC. An update for the conservative management of patellofemoral pain syndrome: a systematic review of the literature from 2000 to 2010. *Int J Sports Phys Ther.* 2011;6(2):112–125.
5. Campbell KA, Saltzman BM, Mascarenhas R, et al. Does intra-articular platelet-rich plasma injection provide clinically superior outcomes compared with other therapies in the treatment of knee osteoarthritis? A systematic review of overlapping meta-analyses. *Arthroscopy.* 2015;31(11):2213–2221.
6. Chen JT, Tang AC, Lin SC, et al. Anterior knee pain caused by patellofemoral pain syndrome can be relieved by Botulinum toxin type A injection. *Clin Neurol Neurosurg.* 2015;129(Suppl 1):S27–S29.
7. Henrotin Y, Marty M, Mobasheri A. What is the current status of chondroitin sulfate and glucosamine for the treatment of knee osteoarthritis? *Maturitas.* 2014;78(3)184–187.
8. Debbi EM, Agar G, Fichman G, et al. Efficacy of methylsulfonylmethane supplementation on osteoarthritis of the knee: a randomized controlled study. *BMC Complement Altern Med.* 2011;11:50.

ADDITIONAL READING
- Collins NJ, Bisset LM, Crossley KM, et al. Efficacy of nonsurgical interventions for anterior knee pain: systematic review and meta-analysis of randomized trials. *Sports Med.* 2012;42(1):31–49.
- Derry S, Moore RA, Rabbie R. Topical NSAIDs for chronic musculoskeletal pain in adults. *Cochrane Database Syst Rev.* 2012;(9):CD007400.
- Lopes AD, Hespanhol Júnior LC, Yeung SS, et al. What are the main running-related musculoskeletal injuries? A systematic review. *Sports Med.* 2012;42(10):891–905.
- Nunes GS, Stapait EL, Kirsten MH, et al. Clinical test for diagnosis of patellofemoral pain syndrome: systematic review with meta-analysis. *Phys Ther Sport.* 2013;14(1):54–59.
- Ziltener JL, Leal S, Fournier PE. Non-steroidal anti-inflammatory drugs for athletes: an update. *Ann Phys Rehabil Med.* 2010;53(4):278–282.

 SEE ALSO

Algorithms: Knee Pain; Popliteal Mass

 CODES

ICD10
- M25.569 Pain in unspecified knee
- M17.9 Osteoarthritis of knee, unspecified
- M76.50 Patellar tendinitis, unspecified knee

CLINICAL PEARLS
- Consider ligamentous injury, meniscal tear, and fracture for patients presenting with acute knee pain.
- Consider OA, patellofemoral pain, syndrome, tendinopathy, bursitis, and stress fracture in patients presenting with more chronic symptoms.
- Consider physeal, apophyseal, or articular cartilage injury in young patients presenting with knee pain.
- The presence of an effusion in a patient <30 years of age indicates a significant injury.
- Referred pain from the hip (slipped capital femoral epiphysis, Legg-Calvé-Perthes disease) can present as knee pain.

K

LABYRINTHITIS

Mary S. Lindholm, MD

 BASICS

DESCRIPTION
- The sudden and persistent onset of vertigo, often accompanied by hearing loss, caused by acute inflammation or infection of the labyrinth
- Labyrinthitis is a clinical diagnosis in absence of neurologic deficits.
- Typically presents with false sense of motion or room-spinning vertigo lasting for hours or days and often sudden unilateral hearing loss
- Often associated with vestibular hypofunction of the involved ear. Peripheral vertigo improves over time with central compensation.
- System(s) affected: nervous, special sensory (auditory and vestibular)
- Synonym(s): acute peripheral vestibulopathy; vestibular neuronitis (vertigo/dizziness only); vestibular neuritis (vertigo/dizziness only)

ALERT
- "Vertigo" and "dizziness" are commonly used terms. Clarify symptoms by giving options of alternative descriptions such as light-headedness, disequilibrium, room-spinning vertigo, or imbalance.
- Hearing loss and duration of symptoms can help narrow the differential diagnosis in patients with vertigo.
- Benign paroxysmal positional vertigo (BPPV) is the most common cause of vertigo. Unlike labyrinthitis, BPPV is episodic, with severe symptoms lasting <1 minute. BPPV is diagnosed using the Dix-Hallpike maneuver. Unlike labyrinthitis, it is not associated with hearing loss.
- Ménière disease presents with the classic triad of episodic vertigo, tinnitus, and sensorineural hearing loss that is often fluctuant (1)[C].

Geriatric Considerations
- Elderly are less likely to compensate fully and may report symptoms of disequilibrium lasting weeks to months after resolution of the acute vertigo.
- Avoid excessive use of scopolamine, meclizine, and other vestibular suppressants following the initial event, as this will delay central compensation.
- Benzodiazepines are preferred vestibular suppressant treatment but do increase the risk of falls in older persons.

Pediatric Consideration
Less common in children, incidence of vestibular vertigo in 10-year-olds estimated to be 5.7% (2)[C]

EPIDEMIOLOGY
- 10% of all patients seen for dizziness
- Most common in 30 to 50 years of age (3)
- Predominant sex: female = male

Incidence
- Viral labyrinthitis is the most common etiology.
- Suppurative or serous labyrinthitis secondary to otitis media is increasingly rare.

Prevalence
In the United States, 2nd most common cause of dizziness due to persistent peripheral vestibular hypofunction (9%); benign positional vertigo (40%) is most common. More than 1/3 of adults see a health care provider for vertigo in their lifetimes (4).

ETIOLOGY AND PATHOPHYSIOLOGY
- Acute inflammation or damage to the inner ear, involving both branches of the vestibulocochlear nerve
- Viruses pass via hematogenous spread into the labyrinth or directly from the middle ear to labyrinth via the round/oval window.
- Bacterial toxins and host inflammatory mediators from a middle ear infection may reach the inner ear.
- Ischemia: ischemic or thromboembolic events involving the labyrinthine artery can cause symptoms that mimic acute labyrinthitis. Often presents with associated neurologic symptoms
- Autoimmune: Local or systemic inflammatory processes may affect the inner ear via autoantibodies vasculitis of the labyrinthine artery.
  - Wegener granulomatosis, Cogan syndrome, systemic lupus erythematous, polyarteritis nodosa, Behçet disease
- Infections
  - Common viral: cytomegalovirus, mumps, varicella zoster, rubeola, influenza, parainfluenza, herpes simplex, adenovirus, coxsackievirus, respiratory syncytial virus, HIV
  - Common bacterial: *Streptococcus pneumoniae*, *Haemophilus influenzae*, *Moraxella catarrhalis*, *Neisseria meningitidis*, *Streptococcus* spp., *Staphylococcus* spp., *Borrelia burgdorferi*
  - Treponemal: *Treponema pallidum*
- Ototoxic drugs (e.g., aspirin, aminoglycosides, loop diuretics, cisplatin)

Genetics
No known genetic link

RISK FACTORS
- Viral upper respiratory infection
- Otitis media
- Vestibulotoxic/ototoxic medications
- Head trauma
- History of allergies
- Meningitis
- Cerebrovascular disease
- Other risk factors include autoimmune disease, herpes zoster infection, excessive alcohol consumption, and smoking.

GENERAL PREVENTION
- Scheduled immunizations (to prevent common viral pathogens)
- Prevent maternal transmission of pathogens, including syphilis and HIV.

COMMONLY ASSOCIATED CONDITIONS
- Viral upper respiratory infection
- Allergies
- Otitis media
- Cholesteatoma
- Head injury

DIAGNOSIS

HISTORY
- Vertigo *AND* (often) hearing loss in one ear
- Vertigo is acute in onset and lasts days to weeks.
- Nausea and vomiting are common.

- Fullness of affected ear
- Tinnitus of affected ear (roaring, ringing)
- Upper respiratory tract infection symptoms
- Otorrhea or otalgia (not common with viral causes)
- Severe headache, fever, and nuchal rigidity in the setting of meningitis
- Recurrent symptoms should raise suspicion for autoimmune causes.
- Profound imbalance or associated focal neurologic signs are not typical and should prompt imaging.

PHYSICAL EXAM
- Nystagmus
  - Fast-beating nystagmus toward affected ear (acutely)
  - Fast-beating nystagmus away from affected ear (chronically)
- Symptoms abate in supine position and with eyes closed or with visual fixation.
- Otologic exam may be unremarkable in the setting of viral labyrinthitis.
- Serous/purulent effusion may be present in the middle ear.
- Retraction of the tympanic membrane and keratinaceous debris may be present with cholesteatoma.

DIFFERENTIAL DIAGNOSIS
- Vestibular neuritis/neuronitis (vertigo without hearing loss)
- BPPV: episodic, vertigo lasting seconds/minutes, worse when lying down or looking up
- Ménière disease: episodic vertigo lasting minutes to hours, associated with the triad of episodic vertigo, tinnitus, and hearing loss
- Vestibular migraine
- Autoimmune inner ear disease
- Postconcussive syndrome
- Acute otitis media
- Ototoxicity
- Cardiovascular accident (CVA)/brainstem infarct
- Cerebellopontine-angle tumors (e.g., vestibular schwannoma)
- Less common etiologies: parainfectious encephalomyelitis or cranial polyneuritis, Ramsay Hunt syndrome, HIV infection, syphilis, temporal lobe epilepsy, perilymphatic fistula, superior canal dehiscence, idiopathic sudden single-sided deafness, multiple sclerosis, vasculitis (cerebral or systemic)

DIAGNOSTIC TESTS & INTERPRETATION
- Routine lab studies are not helpful in making the diagnosis unless an autoimmune cause is highly suspected.
- Consider culture of otorrhea or middle ear fluid to direct antibiotic choice.
- Consider lumbar puncture only if meningitis is suspected.
- Consider screening for syphilis or HIV when clinically indicated by risk factors or clinical history.
- Imaging is not required for the diagnosis of acute labyrinthitis.
- If associated neurologic symptoms or sensorineural hearing loss are present, an MRI and MR angiography of brain and brainstem are recommended.
- Vertigo usually spontaneously resolves, and there is a low risk of developing Ménière disease or migraines.

Follow-Up Tests & Special Considerations
Labyrinthitis ossificans is fibrosis of the internal auditory canal following bacterial meningitis and is thought to occur due to a suppurative labyrinthitis. This can occur rapidly, especially after *S. pneumoniae* meningitis.

Diagnostic Procedures/Other
- Audiogram should be obtained.
- Vestibular tests are not typically indicated in the acute setting. If vertigo and dizziness persist after expected resolution of symptoms, electronystagmography should be used.

Test Interpretation
- Audiogram may show varying degrees of both hearing loss and discrimination.
- Caloric testing may show relative weakness of the horizontal semicircular canal of the affected side. Sensitivity and specificity of this test are variable within literature.

TREATMENT

- Symptom management and reassurance
- Vestibular rehabilitation is the mainstay of treatment and has been shown to be safe and effective management for unilateral peripheral vestibular dysfunction (5)[A].
- Patients should begin exercises as soon as the acute phase resolves and movement is tolerable, generally within 2 to 3 days of onset.
- Vestibular suppressants as needed (see "Medication") for severe acute attacks of vertigo only. Patients should be advised *NOT* to use these medications as scheduled medications or for prophylaxis without symptoms.
- Sudden single-sided hearing loss (onset within 2 weeks) should be managed with high-dose oral steroids as soon as possible.
- Auricular acupuncture and Ginkgo biloba may be emerging adjunctive therapies to reduce vertiginous symptoms, although research is limited (6)[B],(7)[C].
- For suppurative labyrinthitis, appropriate antibiotics to eradicate infection

GENERAL MEASURES
Vestibular exercises for prolonged symptoms and unilateral vestibular loss have been shown to alleviate postural control.

MEDICATION
Use of the following drugs should be on a PRN basis. Benzodiazepines can also assist with the anxiety associated with vertigo. No patient should take vestibular suppressants as a chronic medication, as they can block central compensation.
- Vestibular suppressants
  - Lorazepam (Ativan): 0.5 to 2 mg sublingual (SL)/PO BID PRN or diazepam (Valium) 2 to 5 mg QID PO PRN
  - Meclizine (Antivert, Bonine, Zentrip [dissolvable]) 12.5 to 25 mg PO BID–TID PRN
  - Dimenhydrinate (Dramamine) 25 to 50 mg PO q4–6h PRN

- Antiemetics
  - Ondansetron (Zofran) 4 to 8 mg PO TID PRN or granisetron (Kytril) 1 mg PO TID PRN
  - Meclizine (Antivert, Bonine) 12.5 to 25 mg PO q4h PRN
  - Promethazine (Phenergan) 12.5 to 25 mg PO/PR QID PRN or prochlorperazine (Compazine) 25 mg PR BID PRN
  - Metoclopramide (Reglan) 10 mg PO TID PRN
- Antivirals
  - Acyclovir 800 mg PO 5 times per day for 7 days can be used in cases associated with herpes.
- Steroids
  - Adults: methylprednisolone initially 100 mg PO daily, then tapered to 10 mg PO daily over 3 weeks
  - Pediatrics: prednisone 1 mg/kg PO daily 3 times per week, then taper over 3 weeks
  - Given early in the setting of bacterial meningitis, may decrease the otologic sequelae, specifically labyrinthitis ossificans
  - Used in treatment of labyrinthitis for associated sudden sensorineural hearing loss

Pregnancy Considerations
Dimenhydrinate, diphenhydramine, ondansetron, granisetron, and metoclopramide are pregnancy Category B.

First Line
- Benzodiazepines, which are better vestibular suppressants, are preferred over antihistamine/anticholinergics such as meclizine. Sublingual benzodiazepines are very effective for vertigo and should be considered first-line therapy.
- Urgent steroid treatment in acute setting

ISSUES FOR REFERRAL
- Consider neuro-otology referral for other peripheral causes of vertigo or unremitting vertigo.
- Consider neurology referral for suspected central causes of vertigo or dizziness.
- Consider otolaryngology referral for progressive bilateral hearing loss and vertigo after preliminary laboratory workup excluding rheumatologic causes.

INPATIENT CONSIDERATIONS
Admission Criteria/Initial Stabilization
- Patients with systemic infection, young age, or intractable vertigo with nausea and vomiting may need to be hospitalized for intravenous fluids and medications.
- Usually outpatient management

ONGOING CARE

FOLLOW-UP RECOMMENDATIONS
Patient Monitoring
Follow hearing loss weekly with audiograms until hearing stabilizes. Acute vertiginous symptoms may last up to 6 weeks. Residual symptoms have been documented to last months or year (8)[C].

DIET
Avoid alcohol, as this may exacerbate symptoms.

PATIENT EDUCATION
Lie still with eyes closed in a darkened room during acute attacks. Otherwise, encourage activity as tolerated. Minimize rapid head movement until symptoms resolve.

PROGNOSIS
Prognosis depends on cause of labyrinthitis.

COMPLICATIONS
Permanent hearing loss, more common with bacterial causes, and chronic impairment of balance

REFERENCES
1. Post RE, Dickerson LM . Dizziness: a diagnostic approach. *Am Fam Physician.* 2010;82(4):361–368.
2. Jahn K, Langhagen T, Schroeder AS, et al. Vertigo and dizziness in childhood—update on diagnosis and treatment. *Neuropediatrics.* 2011;42(4):129–134.
3. Neuhauser HK, Lempert T . Vertigo: epidemiologic aspects. *Semin Neurol.* 2009;29(5):473–481.
4. Wipperman J . Dizziness and vertigo. *Prim Care.* 2014;41(1):115–131.
5. Hillier SL, McDonnell M . Vestibular rehabilitation for unilateral peripheral vestibular dysfunction. *Cochrane Database Syst Rev.* 2011;(2):CD005397.
6. Sokolova L, Hoerr R, Mischenko T. Treatment of vertigo: a randomized, double blind trial comparing efficacy and safety of Ginkgo biloba extract EGb 761 and betahistine. *Int J Otolaryngol.* 2014;2014:682439.
7. Romoli M, Allais G, Airola G, et al. Ear acupuncture and fMRI: a pilot study for assessing the specificity of auricular points. *Neurol Sci.* 2014;35(Suppl 1):189–193.
8. Lee HK, Ahn SK, Jeon SY, et al. Clinical characteristics and natural course of recurrent vestibulopathy: a long-term follow-up study. *Laryngoscope.* 2012;122(4):883–886.

 SEE ALSO

Ménière Disease; Postconcussive Syndrome; (Mild Traumatic Brain Injury) Tinnitus

 CODES

ICD10
- H83.09 Labyrinthitis, unspecified ear
- H83.01 Labyrinthitis, right ear
- H83.02 Labyrinthitis, left ear

CLINICAL PEARLS
- Ask patients to describe symptoms in their own words, alternative symptoms include light-headedness, vertigo, disequilibrium, or imbalance.
- Benzodiazepines are better vestibular suppressant and are preferred over antihistamine/anticholinergics such as meclizine.
- Episodic vertigo tends to be caused by BPPV or Ménière disease, whereas persistent vertigo is more consistent with labyrinthitis.

L

LACRIMAL DISORDERS (DRY EYE SYNDROME)

Kinder K. Fayssoux, MD • Mark Minot, MD

 BASICS

DESCRIPTION

- Diseases and abnormalities of tear production and maintenance of tear film
- The most common lacrimal disorder is dry eye syndrome, which is often referred to as dysfunctional tear syndrome.
- Lacrimal duct disorders usually result in overflow tearing.
- System(s) affected: skin/exocrine

EPIDEMIOLOGY

Prevalence

Very common throughout the United States; more often seen in arid climates:

- Predominant gender: female > male
- Predominant age: Dry eye symptoms increase with age and are most often seen in the elderly.

ETIOLOGY AND PATHOPHYSIOLOGY

- Tear film is composed of three layers:
  - Mucin layer: allows spread of aqueous tears
  - Thick aqueous layer: produced by lacrimal gland
  - Lipid layer: controls tear evaporation
- Results from poor tear production, rapid tear evaporation, and/or an abnormal concentration of mucin or lipid in tear film
- Most common cause of dry eye symptoms is aqueous tear deficiency.
- Decreased androgens are thought to contribute to a decrease in tear production.

RISK FACTORS

- Exposure to dry environments (e.g., high altitudes)
- Contact lens wear
- Female gender
- Computer use
- Hormonal diseases
- History of collagen vascular disease such as rheumatoid arthritis, Sjögren syndrome, thyroid disease, rosacea, Bell palsy, eyelid abnormalities
- Medications, including oral contraceptives, diuretics, β-blockers, anticholinergics, antihistamines, and antidepressants
- Smoking
- Vitamin A deficiency
- Eye surgery: blepharoplasty, cataract, laser vision correction
- Artificial tears (with preservatives)

GENERAL PREVENTION

- Prevent exposure to eye irritants from pollution, cigarette smoke, and sun exposure.
- Ensure adequate vitamin A intake through diet or as a supplement.
- Patients with prior laser vision correction should wait at least 6 months before undergoing blepharoplasty because of the effects on corneal sensation, tear production, and tear film alteration (1)[C].
- Increasing awareness of this condition among people residing in dry environments
- Decrease or stop contact lens wear.

COMMONLY ASSOCIATED CONDITIONS

- Sjögren syndrome
- Rheumatoid arthritis
- Thyroid disease
- Rosacea
- Pregnancy
- Menopause
- Malnutrition

 DIAGNOSIS

HISTORY

- Dry sensation in eyes
- Foreign body sensation
- Blurry vision
- Itching
- Ocular pain
- Photophobia
- Burning
- Occasional tearing due to excessive reflex tearing
  - Patient's symptoms usually worsen in dry, smoky environments, while reading, driving, or using a computer for extended periods.

Pediatric Considerations

Lacrimal duct obstruction should be suspected in an infant presenting with excessive tearing (epiphora).

PHYSICAL EXAM

- Slit-lamp exam reveals decreased tear film and may reveal punctate epithelial defects on cornea.
- Schirmer test can be used to assess tear production.
- Ocular staining may reveal epithelial defects.

DIFFERENTIAL DIAGNOSIS

- Ocular: allergy, conjunctivitis, contact lens complication, exposure keratopathy
- Other: ocular rosacea, thyroid ophthalmopathy, ocular manifestation of HIV, Bell palsy, vitamin A deficiency

DIAGNOSTIC TESTS & INTERPRETATION

Initial Tests (lab, imaging)

Tear production can be measured using a Schirmer filter strip after instillation of topical anesthetic. Wetting of <10 mm of the slip after 5 minutes is indicative of insufficient tear production.

Diagnostic Procedures/Other

- Staining of the ocular surface with fluorescein will show areas of abnormal uptake and patches of drying. It allows the tear break-up time (TBUT) to be calculated. A TBUT of <10 seconds is abnormal.
- Rose bengal will be taken up by dead or dying epithelial cells, and it may be a more sensitive test.

Test Interpretation

In Sjögren syndrome, infiltration of the lacrimal gland with inflammatory cells may be evident.

 TREATMENT

GENERAL MEASURES

- Those with systemic illnesses predisposed to dry eye should be informed and instructed in the appropriate use of artificial tear supplements. Some artificial tear supplements with preservatives may exacerbate the condition.
- Symptoms of dry eye may decrease with an increase in home humidification and hydration.

MEDICATION

First Line

- Preservative-free artificial tears: 1 drop in each eye several times a day to prevent discomfort (2)[A],(3)[C].
- Ophthalmic lubricating ointment may be used in each eye at bedtime (4)[B].

Second Line

- Dry eye has been identified as having an inflammatory component that responds in refractory cases to topical immunosuppressives such as cyclosporine 0.05% (Restasis), 1 drop to each eye BID (5–7)[A].
- Emerging therapies include topical androgens, secretagogues (e.g., oral pilocarpine), cytokine-blocking agents, and a P2Y2 receptor agonist (diquafosol).

ISSUES FOR REFERRAL
Rheumatology referral if systemic collagen vascular disease is suspected

ADDITIONAL THERAPIES
Lid massage and warm compresses several times a day

Pediatric Considerations
For most babies born with nasolacrimal duct obstructions, the obstructions will clear spontaneously during the 1st year of life. On occasion, surgical probing is necessary.

SURGERY/OTHER PROCEDURES
Punctal occlusion, with either punctal plugs or laser, is used in moderate to severe dry eye if medical therapy fails.

COMPLEMENTARY & ALTERNATIVE MEDICINE
- Fatty acid (omega-3), linoleic acid, and γ-linoleic acid supplements (8)[B]
- Acupuncture has been studied with inconclusive results (9)[A].

 ONGOING CARE

FOLLOW-UP RECOMMENDATIONS
Patient Monitoring
- Monitor early to assess efficacy of treatment.
- The viscosity of artificial tears and frequency of use can be increased for symptom relief.

DIET
- Diet rich in omega-3 fatty acids and/or linoleic acids may benefit some patients.
- Adequate vitamin A intake

PATIENT EDUCATION
All individuals with systemic illnesses predisposed to dry eye, postmenopausal women, residing in arid climates, or those >60 years of age should be instructed in the use of artificial tear supplements to combat dry eye symptoms.

PROGNOSIS
- Lacrimal disorders can be adequately managed with artificial tear supplements.
- Blocked tear ducts can be managed with probing and punctal dilation and/or dacryocystorhinostomy procedures in more severe cases.

COMPLICATIONS
Severe dry eye may lead to the following:
- Corneal breakdown
- Secondary invasion by bacteria
- Eye infections

REFERENCES
1. Lee WB, McCord CD Jr, Somia N, et al. Optimizing blepharoplasty outcomes in patients with previous laser vision correction. *Plast Reconstr Surg.* 2008;122(2):587–594.
2. Ousler GW, Michaelson C, Christensen MT. An evaluation of tear film breakup time extension and ocular protection index scores among three marketed lubricant eye drops. *Cornea.* 2007;26(8):949–952.
3. Karadayi K, Ciftci F, Akin T, et al. Increase in central corneal thickness in dry and normal eyes with application of artificial tears: a new diagnostic and follow-up criterion for dry eye. *Ophthalmic Physiol Opt.* 2005;25(6):485–491.
4. Tauber J. Efficacy, tolerability and comfort of a 0.3% hypromellose gel ophthalmic lubricant in the treatment of patients with moderate to severe dry eye syndrome. *Curr Med Res Opin.* 2007;23(11):2629–2636.
5. Hardten DR, Brown MJ, Pham-Vang S. Evaluation of an isotonic tear in combination with topical cyclosporine for the treatment of ocular surface disease. *Curr Med Res Opin.* 2007;23(9):2083–2091.
6. Roberts CW, Carniglia PE, Brazzo BG. Comparison of topical cyclosporine, punctal occlusion, and a combination for the treatment of dry eye. *Cornea.* 2007;26(7):805–809.
7. Sall K, Stevenson OD, Mundorf TK, et al. Two multicenter, randomized studies of the efficacy and safety of cyclosporine ophthalmic emulsion in moderate to severe dry eye disease. CsA Phase 3 Study Group. *Ophthalmology.* 2000;107(4):631–639.
8. Barabino S, Rolando M, Camicione P, et al. Systemic linoleic and gamma-linoleic acid therapy in dry eye syndrome with an inflammatory component. *Cornea.* 2003;22(2):97–101.
9. Lee MS, Shin BC, Choi TY, et al. Acupuncture for treating dry eye: a systematic review. *Acta Ophthalmol.* 2011;89(2):101–106.

ADDITIONAL READING
- Dogru M, Nakamura M, Shimazakie J, et al. Changing the trends in the treatment of dry-eye disease. *Expert Opin Investig Drugs.* 2013;22(12):1581–1601.
- Galor A, Feuer W, Lee DJ, et al. Prevalence and risk factors of dry eye syndrome in a United States veterans affairs population. *Am J Ophthalmol.* 2011;152(3):377.e2–384.e2.
- Gilbard J. The diagnosis and management of dry eyes. *Otolaryngol Clin North Am.* 2005;38(5):871–885.
- Tong L, Petznick A, Lee S, et al. Choice of artificial tear formulation for patients with dry eye; where do we start? *Cornea.* 2012;31(Suppl 1):S32–S36.

 SEE ALSO

Sjögren Syndrome

 CODES

ICD10
- H04.129 Dry eye syndrome of unspecified lacrimal gland
- H04.9 Disorder of lacrimal system, unspecified
- H04.122 Dry eye syndrome of left lacrimal gland

CLINICAL PEARLS
- Dry eye syndrome is common in the United States, affecting postmenopausal women more than any other population.
- Symptoms are usually adequately managed with preservative-free artificial tears and humidified environments.
- Dry eye symptoms that are refractory to medical treatment and/or punctal plugs should raise suspicion of an underlying systemic condition, and a rheumatology consult should be considered.

L

LACTOSE INTOLERANCE

Nihal K. Patel, MD

 BASICS

DESCRIPTION
- Inability to digest lactose into constituent components (glucose and galactose) due to low levels of lactase in the brush border of the small intestinal mucosa, causing bloating, borborygmi (audible stomach "rumblings"), abdominal pain, and diarrhea
  - Congenital lactose intolerance: very rare
  - Primary lactose intolerance: common in adults who develop low lactase levels after childhood
  - Secondary lactose intolerance: inability to digest lactose caused by any condition injuring the intestinal mucosa (e.g., infectious enteritis, celiac disease, eosinophilic gastroenteritis, or inflammatory bowel disease) or a reduction of available mucosal surface (e.g., resection)
- Lactase activity peaks at birth then decreases after the first few months of life, declining continuously during lifetime. 75% of adults' worldwide exhibit decline in lactase activity. *However, only 50% of lactase activity is needed to digest lactose without causing symptoms of lactose intolerance.*
- Lactose malabsorption also results from reduction of lactase activity. It is asymptomatic, and is as common in healthy patients as in those with functional bowel disorders.
- System(s) affected: endocrine/metabolic, gastrointestinal

Pediatric Considerations
- Primary lactose intolerance usually begins in late childhood.
- No consensus exists on whether young children (<5 years of age) should avoid lactose following diarrheal illness.
- Lactose-free formulas are available.
- Exclude milk protein allergy.

EPIDEMIOLOGY
Incidence
- ≥50% of infants with acute or chronic diarrheal disease have lactose intolerance. Particularly common with rotavirus infection.
- Lactose intolerance is common with giardiasis, ascariasis, irritable bowel syndrome (IBS), tropical and nontropical sprue, and the AIDS malabsorptive syndrome.

Prevalence
- In South America, Africa, and Asia, rates of lactose intolerance are >50%.
- In the United States, the prevalence is 15% among whites, 53% among Hispanic Americans, and 80% among African Americans.
- In Europe, lactose intolerance varies from 15% in Scandinavian countries to 70% in Italy.
- Predominant age:
  - Primary: teenage and adult
  - Secondary: depends on underlying condition
- Predominant sex: male = female

ETIOLOGY AND PATHOPHYSIOLOGY
- Primary lactose intolerance: Normal decline in the lactase activity in the intestinal mucosa is genetically controlled and permanent after weaning from breastmilk.
- Secondary lactose intolerance: associated with gastroenteritis in children and with nontropical and tropical sprue, regional enteritis, abetalipoproteinemia, cystic fibrosis, inflammatory bowel disease, celiac disease, and immunoglobulin deficiencies in both adults and children

Genetics
- In Caucasians, lactase deficiency has been associated with a single nucleotide polymorphism (SNP) consisting of a nucleotide switch of T for C 13.910. bp on chromosome 2. This results in variants of CC-13910 (lactase nonpersistence) *OR* CT-13910/TT-13910 (lactase persistence) (1).
- SNP (C/T-13910) is associated with lactase persistence in northern Europeans.
- Other SNPs (G/C-14010, T/G-13915, and C/G-13907) have been linked to lactase persistence in Africans.

RISK FACTORS
- Adult-onset lactase deficiency has wide geographic variation.
- Age:
  - Signs and symptoms usually do not become apparent until after age 6 to 7 years.
  - Symptoms may not be apparent until adulthood, depending on dietary lactose intake and rate of decline of intestinal lactase activity.
  - Lactase activity correlates with age, regardless of symptoms.

GENERAL PREVENTION
Lactose avoidance relieves symptoms. Patients can learn what level of lactose is tolerable in their diet.

COMMONLY ASSOCIATED CONDITIONS
- Tropical or nontropical sprue
- Giardiasis
- Inflammatory bowel disease
- Immunoglobulin deficiencies
- Celiac disease
- Cystic fibrosis

Dx DIAGNOSIS

- Lactose intolerance is defined by a positive lactose hydrogen breath test result plus accompanying clinical symptoms.
- Lactose intolerance can mimic symptoms of functional gastrointestinal disorders. Lactose intolerance can also be a coexisting condition.

HISTORY
- Assess patient's daily lactose consumption. A single dose of lactose (12 g, equivalent to 1 cup of milk) consumed alone produces no or minor symptoms in persons with lactose intolerance or maldigestion.

- Lactose doses of 15 to 18 g are well tolerated with other nutrients. Doses >18 g cause progressively more symptoms, and quantities >50 g elicit symptoms in most individuals.
- Symptoms may arise 30 minutes to 2 hours after consumption of lactose-containing products.
- Symptoms include bloating, cramping, abdominal discomfort, vomiting diarrhea or loose stools, and flatulence.
- Symptoms tend to appear 30 minutes to 2 hours after eating.
- Abdominal pain may be crampy in nature and often is localized to the periumbilical area or lower quadrant.
- Stools usually are bulky, frothy, and watery
- Only 1/3 to 1/5 of individuals with lactose malabsorption develop symptoms.

PHYSICAL EXAM
Borborygmi may be audible on physical examination and to the patient. The exam is otherwise typically nonspecific.

DIFFERENTIAL DIAGNOSIS
- Sucrase deficiency
- Cow's milk protein allergy
- IBS
- Bacterial overgrowth
- Celiac disease
- Inflammatory bowel disease

DIAGNOSTIC TESTS & INTERPRETATION
Initial Tests (lab, imaging)

- The lactose breath hydrogen test (LBT) is the best diagnostic test for lactose intolerance. It is noninvasive, easy to perform, and cost effective. It is limited by suboptimal sensitivity (2)[B]. Intestinal bacteria digest carbohydrates and produce hydrogen and methane that are measurable in expired air:

  - Oral lactose is administered in the fasting state, (2 g/kg; max dose 25 g). Breath hydrogen is sampled at baseline and at 30-minute intervals for 3 hours. The postlactose and baseline values are compared. A breath hydrogen value of 10 ppm is normal. Values between 10 and 20 ppm may be indeterminate unless accompanied by symptoms; values >20 ppm are considered diagnostic of lactose malabsorption.
- The biochemical assay of lactase activity on duodenal sampling is as sensitive as LBT in detecting lactase deficiency. It is more accurate than LBT in predicting the clinical response to a lactose-free diet. Cost and invasiveness limit clinical utility
- For patients with symptoms of lactose intolerance who are undergoing endoscopy for other reasons, a biochemical assay on duodenal biopsies can rule out lactose malabsorption
- A positive LBT confirms lactose malabsorption but does not define the etiology.

Diagnostic Procedures/Other

Lactose absorption test is an alternative to LBT in adults (more invasive and equivalent in sensitivity and specificity to breath test). Following oral administration of a 50-g test dose in adults (2 g/kg in children), blood glucose levels are monitored at 0, 60, and 120 minutes. An increase in blood glucose of <20 mg/dL (1.1 mmol/L) with the concurrent development of symptoms is diagnostic. False-negative results may occur in patients with diabetes or bacterial overgrowth.

Test Interpretation

Lactase deficiency in intestinal mucosa may be patchy or focal.

 TREATMENT

There is insufficient evidence on treatments (including probiotics, colonic adaptation, and other supplements) to recommend any as definitive first-line.

- Treatment of lactose malabsorption in the absence of a correctable underlying disease includes four general principles (3)[B].
  - Patients should avoid milk and dairy products in order to improve symptoms.
  - Up to 12 to 15 g of lactose can be tolerated in patients with lactose intolerance without significant symptoms (1 cup of milk).
  - Lactose should be gradually reintroduced along with other nutrients until the patient's threshold for symptoms is reached. Spreading lactose servings throughout the day instead of a single dose has been shown to improve tolerance.
  - If symptoms persist, patients can substitute fermented and matured milk products for lactose.
- Certain strains, concentrations, and preparations of probiotics may alleviate symptoms.
- Incrementally increasing doses of lactose to induce colonic adaptation have met with limited success.
- To date, insufficient scientific evidence exists to strongly recommend lactose-reduced or hydrolyzed milk, lactase supplements taken with milk, probiotics, or colonic adaptation to treat lactose intolerance. Use of these supplements should be considered on a case-by-case fashion.
- Maintain calcium and vitamin D intake.

MEDICATION

First Line

Lactase (Lactaid, Lactrase):

- Commercially available "lactase" preparations are bacterial or yeast β-galactosidases.
- Take 1 to 2 capsules or tablets prior to ingesting milk products.
- Vary in effectiveness at preventing symptoms
- Can add tablets or contents of capsules to milk (1 to 2 caps/tabs per quart of milk) before drinking; also available in milk in some areas
- Not effective for all people with lactose intolerance
- High-quality, large, randomized controlled trials showing efficacy and safety are lacking.

COMPLEMENTARY & ALTERNATIVE MEDICINE

Certain probiotic formulations taken with meals may alleviate some symptoms of lactose intolerance (4)[B].

 ONGOING CARE

DIET

- Reduce or restrict dietary lactose to control symptoms. This is patient-specific and done as "trial-and-error."
- Yogurt and fermented products such as hard cheese are often better tolerated than milk.
- Supplement calcium (e.g., calcium carbonate)
- Prehydrolyzed milk (Lactaid) is available.

PATIENT EDUCATION

- Patients must learn to read labels on commercial products because milk sugar is used in many products and may cause symptoms.
- Lactose-intolerant patients may tolerate whole milk or chocolate milk better than skim milk due to slower rate of gastric emptying.
- Lactose consumed with other food products is better tolerated than when consumed with milk alone.
- Primary lactase deficiency is permanent; secondary lactose intolerance usually is temporary, although it may persist for months after the inciting event.
- 20% of prescription drugs and 6% of over-the-counter (OTC) medicines use lactose as a base.
- Most patients can tolerate 12 to 15 g of lactose, despite lactose intolerance or malabsorption.

PROGNOSIS

- Normal life expectancy
- Symptoms can be controlled through diet alone if lactase tablets are ineffective.

COMPLICATIONS

Calcium deficiency: Avoidance of milk and other dairy products can lead to reduced calcium intake, which may increase the risk for osteoporosis and fracture.

REFERENCES

1. Mattar R, de Campos Mazo DF, Carrilho FJ. Lactose intolerance: diagnosis, genetic, and clinical factors. *Clin Exp Gastroenterol*. 2012;5:113–121.
2. Law D, Conklin J, Pimentel M. Lactose intolerance and the role of the lactose breath test. *Am J Gastroenterol*. 2010;105(8):1726–1728.
3. Shaukat A, Levitt MD, Taylor BC, et al. Systematic review: effective management strategies for lactose intolerance. *Ann Intern Med*. 2010;152(12):797–803.
4. Levri KM, Ketvertis K, Deramo M, et al. Do probiotics reduce adult lactose intolerance? A systematic review. *J Fam Pract*. 2005;54(7):613–620.

ADDITIONAL READING

- Almeida CC, Lorena SL, Pavan CR, et al. Beneficial effects of long-term consumption of a probiotic combination of Lactobacillus casei Shirota and Bifidobacterium breve Yakult may persist after suspension of therapy in lactose-intolerant patients. *Nutr Clin Pract*. 2012;27(2):247–251.
- Boettcher E, Crowe SE. Dietary proteins and functional gastrointestinal disorders. *Am J Gastroenterol*. 2013;108(5):728–736.
- Fernández-Bañares F. Reliability of symptom analysis during carbohydrate hydrogen-breath tests. *Curr Opin Clin Nutr Metab Care*. 2012;15(5):494–498.
- Furnari M, Bonfanti D, Parodi A, et al. A comparison between lactose breath test and quick test on duodenal biopsies for diagnosing lactase deficiency in patients with self-reported lactose intolerance. *J Clin Gastroenterol*. 2013;47(2):148–152.
- Tan-Dy CR, Ohlsson A. Lactase treated feeds to promote growth and feeding tolerance in preterm infants. *Cochrane Database Syst Rev*. 2013;(3):CD004591.

 CODES

ICD10

- E73.9 Lactose intolerance, unspecified
- E73.8 Other lactose intolerance
- E73.1 Secondary lactase deficiency

CLINICAL PEARLS

- The diagnosis of lactose intolerance is based on clinical history and typically confirmed by hydrogen breath testing.
- Most lactose intolerant patients can tolerate 12 to 15 g of lactose per day.
- Lactose-intolerant patients may tolerate yogurt and fermented products better than milk and cheese.
- A food diary helps identify problematic foods.
- Patients should read ingredient labels to look for milk, lactose, whey, and curd.
- Lactose-intolerant patients may tolerate whole milk or chocolate milk better than skim milk due to a slower rate of gastric emptying.
- Many patients with lactose intolerance unnecessarily avoid all dairy products, causing inadequate intake of calcium and vitamin D, which may predispose them to osteoporosis.

L

LARYNGITIS

Hugh Silk, MD, MPH, FAAFP • Sheila O. Stille, DMD • Anne M. Barnard, MD

BASICS

DESCRIPTION
- Laryngitis is the inflammation, erythema, and edema of the mucosa of the larynx and/or vocal cords characterized by hoarseness, loss of voice, throat pain, coughing, and often a negative impact on a person's quality of life and daily activities
- There is a range of severity, but most cases are acute and are associated with viral upper respiratory infection, irritation, or acute vocal strain.
- System(s) affected: pulmonary; ears, eyes, nose, throat (ENT)
- Synonym(s): acute laryngitis; chronic laryngitis; croup or laryngotracheitis (in children)

EPIDEMIOLOGY
- Predominant age: affects all ages
- Children more susceptible than adults due to increased risk of symptomatic inflammation from smaller airways
- Predominant sex: male = female

Incidence
Common

Prevalence
Common

ETIOLOGY AND PATHOPHYSIOLOGY
- Misuse or abuse of voice
- Infectious
  - Viral: influenza A, B; parainfluenza; adenovirus; coronavirus; rhinovirus; human papillomavirus; cytomegalovirus; varicella-zoster virus; herpes simplex virus; respiratory syncytial virus; coxsackievirus
  - Fungal: uncommon, but thought to be underdiagnosed, potentially accounting for up to 10% of presentations in both immunocompromised and immunocompetent patients; risk factors include recent antibiotic or inhaled corticosteroid use (1): histoplasmosis, blastomycosis, *Coccidioides*, *Cryptococcus*, and *Candida*
  - Bacterial: (uncommon): β-hemolytic streptococcus, *Streptococcus pneumoniae*, *Haemophilus influenzae*, tuberculosis (TB), leprosy, *Moraxella catarrhalis*, *Mycoplasma pneumoniae*, *Chlamydophila pneumoniae*
  - Secondary syphilis if left untreated
  - Leprosy (in 30–55% of those with leprosy, larynx is affected; tropical and warm countries)
- Irritants
  - Inhalation of irritating substances (e.g., air pollution, cigarette smoke)
  - Aspiration of caustic chemicals
  - Gastroesophageal reflux disease (GERD)/laryngopharyngeal reflux disease (LPRD)
  - Excessively dry environment
  - Allergy exposures (including pollens)
- Anatomic
  - Aging changes: muscle atrophy, loss of moisture in larynx, and bowing of vocal cords
  - Vocal cord nodules/polyps ("singer's nodes")
  - Local cancer

- Iatrogenic: inhaled steroids such as those used to treat asthma; surgical injury; endotracheal intubation injury
- Idiopathic
- Neuromuscular disorder (e.g., myasthenia gravis); stroke
- Rheumatoid arthritis
- Trauma (e.g., blunt or penetrating trauma to neck)

RISK FACTORS
- Acute:
  - Upper respiratory tract infection
  - Voice overuse—excess talking, singing, or shouting
  - Pneumonia
  - Influenza
  - Lack of immunization for pertussis or diphtheria
  - Immunocompromised
  - Recent endotracheal intubation or local surgery
- Chronic:
  - Allergies
  - Chronic rhinitis/sinusitis
  - Voice abuse
  - GERD/LPRD (rare) (2,3)[A]
  - Smoking: primary or secondhand
  - Excessive alcohol use
  - Stroke
  - Constant exposure to dust or other irritants such as chemicals at workplace; environmental pollution
  - Medications: inhaled steroids, anticholinergics, antihistamines, anabolic steroids (4)[B]

Geriatric Considerations
May be more ill, slower to heal

Pediatric Considerations
- Common in this age group
- Consider congenital/anatomic causes.

GENERAL PREVENTION
- Avoid overuse of voice (voice training is helpful for vocal musicians/public speakers).
- Influenza virus vaccine is suggested for high-risk individuals.
- Quit smoking, and avoid secondhand smoke.
- Limit or avoid alcohol/caffeine/acidic foods.
- Control GERD/LPRD.
- Maintain proper hydration status.
- Avoid allergens.
- Wear mask around chemical/environmental irritants.
- Good hand washing (infection prevention)

COMMONLY ASSOCIATED CONDITIONS
- Viral pharyngitis
- Diphtheria (rare): Membrane can descend into the larynx.
- Pertussis: larynx involved as part of the respiratory system
- Bronchitis
- Pneumonitis
- Croup, epiglottitis, in children

Dx DIAGNOSIS

HISTORY
- Hoarseness, throat tickling, dry cough, and rawness
- Dysphonia (abnormal-sounding voice)
- Constant urge to clear the throat
- Possible fever
- Malaise
- Dysphagia/odynophagia
- Regional cervical lymphadenopathy
- Stridor or possible airway obstruction in children (5)[C]
- Cough may be worse at night in children.
- Hemoptysis
- Laryngospasm or sense of choking
- Allergic rhinitis/rhinorrhea/postnasal drip (PND)
- Occupation or other reasons for voice overuse
- Smoking history
- Blunt or penetrating trauma to neck
- GERD/LPRD

PHYSICAL EXAM
- Head and neck exam, including airway patency, cervical nodes; cranial nerve exam
- Visualization of the larynx: preferably with a flexible or rigid endoscope, or with an indirect mirror examination as a screening technique to dictate further appropriate testing (6)
- Note quality of voice (i.e., hoarse, breathy, wet, "hot potato like," asthenic [weak], strained).

DIFFERENTIAL DIAGNOSIS
- Diphtheria
- Vocal nodules or polyps
- Laryngeal malignancy
- Thyroid malignancy
- Upper airway malignancy
- Epiglottitis
- Pertussis
- Laryngeal nerve trauma/injury
- Foreign body (in children)
- Autoimmune (rheumatoid arthritis) (7)

DIAGNOSTIC TESTS & INTERPRETATION
- Rarely needed
- WBCs elevated in bacterial laryngitis
- Viral culture (seldom necessary)

Follow-Up Tests & Special Considerations
- Barium swallow, only if needed for differential diagnosis
- CT scan if foreign body suspected

Diagnostic Procedures/Other
- Fiber-optic or indirect laryngoscopy: looking for red, inflamed, and occasionally hemorrhagic vocal cords; rounded edges and exudate (Reinke edema)
- Consider otolaryngologic evaluation and biopsy: laryngitis lasting >2 weeks in adults with history of smoking or alcohol abuse to rule out malignancy

- pH probe (24-hour): no difference in incidence of pharyngeal reflux as measured by pH probe between patients with chronic reflux laryngitis and healthy adults (8)[C]
- Strobovideo laryngoscopy for diagnosis of subtle lesions (e.g., vocal cord nodules or polyps)

 TREATMENT

- Limited but good evidence that treatment beyond supportive care is ineffective.
- Antibiotics appear to have no benefit, as etiologies are predominantly viral (9)[A].
- Corticosteroids in severe cases of laryngitis to reduce inflammation such as croup
- May need voice training, if voice overuse
- Nebulized epinephrine reduces croup symptoms 30 minutes posttreatment; evidence does not favor racemic epinephrine or L-epinephrine, or IPPB over simple nebulization. Racemic epinephrine reduces croup symptoms at 30 minutes, but effect lasts only 2 hours (10)[A].

GENERAL MEASURES
- Acute:
  - Usually a self-limited illness lasting <3 weeks and not severe
  - Antibiotics of no value (9)[A]
  - Avoid excessive voice use, including whispering.
  - Steam inhalations or cool-mist humidifier
  - Increase fluid intake, especially in cases associated with excessive dryness.
  - Avoid smoking (or secondhand exposure).
  - Warm saltwater gargles
- Chronic:
  - Symptomatic treatment as above
  - Voice therapy (for patients with intermittent dysphagia and vocal abuse)
  - Smoking cessation
  - Reduction or cessation of alcohol intake
  - Occupational change or modification, if exposure-driven
  - Allergen avoidance
  - Consider discontinuing offending medication.
- Reflux laryngitis: Elevate head of bed, diet changes, other antireflux lifestyle change management; proton pump inhibitors

MEDICATION
Usually none

First Line
- Analgesics
- Antipyretics (rare)
- Cough suppressants
- Throat lozenges
- Plenty of fluids

Second Line
- Inhaled corticosteroids (consider only if allergy induced)
- Oral corticosteroids: only if urgent need in adults (presenter, singer, actor)
- Oral corticosteroids: Evidence of benefit has been studied with single-dose dexamethasone in children ages 6 months to 5 years for moderate-severity croup; reduces symptoms within 6 hours, reduces hospitalizations, hospital length of stay, and revisits to office (11)[A].
- Standard of care is to prescribe proton pump inhibitors for chronic laryngitis if GERD or LPRD is suspected; however, evidence suggests only a modest benefit, if any (12,13)[C].
- Treat nonviral infectious underlying causes.
- Candidal laryngitis:
  - Mild cases: oral antifungal (fluconazole)
  - Amphotericin B or echinocandin can be given in life-threatening cases.

ISSUES FOR REFERRAL
- Immediate emergency ENT referral for patients with stridor or respiratory distress
- ENT referral for persistent symptoms (>2 to 3 weeks) or concern for foreign body
- Consider otolaryngologic evaluation and biopsy for laryngitis lasting >2 weeks in adults, especially in those with history of smoking or alcohol abuse to rule out malignancy.
- Consider GI consult to rule out GERD/LPRD.

SURGERY/OTHER PROCEDURES
- Vocal cord biopsy of hyperplastic mucosa and areas of leukoplakia if cancer or TB is suspected
- Removal of nodules or polyps if voice therapy fails

COMPLEMENTARY & ALTERNATIVE MEDICINE
The following, although not well studied, have been recommended by some experts:

- Barberry, black currant, echinacea, eucalyptus, German chamomile, goldenrod, goldenseal, warmed lemon and honey, licorice, marshmallow, peppermint, saw palmetto, slippery elm, vitamin C, zinc

 ONGOING CARE

PATIENT EDUCATION
- Educate on the importance of voice rest, including whispering.
- Provide assistance with smoking cessation.
- Help the patient with modification of other predisposing habits or occupational hazards.

PROGNOSIS
Complete clearing of the inflammation without sequelae

COMPLICATIONS
Chronic hoarseness

REFERENCES

1. Merati AL. Acute and chronic laryngitis. In: Flint PW, Haughey BH, Lund VL, et al, eds. *Cummings otolaryngology head and neck surgery*. 5th ed. Philadelphia, PA: Mosby Elsevier, 2010.
2. Hawkshaw MJ, Pebdani P, Sataloff RT. Reflux laryngitis: an update, 2009–2012. *J Voice*. 2013;27(4):486–494.
3. Hom C, Vaezi MF. Extraesophageal manifestations of gastroesophageal reflux disease. *Gastroenterol Clin North Am*. 2013;42(1):71–91.
4. Ray S, Masood A, Pickles J, et al. Severe laryngitis following chronic anabolic steroid abuse. *J Laryngol Otol*. 2008;122(3):230–232.
5. Gallivan GJ, Gallivan KH, Gallivan HK. Inhaled corticosteroids: hazardous effects on voice—an update. *J Voice*. 2007;21(1):101–111.
6. Tulunay OE. Laryngitis—diagnosis and management. *Otolaryngol Clin North Am*. 2008;41(2):437–451.
7. Hamdan AL, Sarieddine D. Laryngeal manifestations of rheumatoid arthritis. *Autoimmune Dis*. 2013;2013:103081.
8. Johnson DA. Medical therapy of reflux laryngitis. *J Clin Gastroenterol*. 2008;42(5):589–593.
9. Reveiz L, Cardona AF. Antibiotics for acute laryngitis in adults. *Cochrane Database Syst Rev*. 2015;(5):CD004783.
10. Bjornson C, Russell KF, Vandermeer B, et al. Nebulized epinephrine for croup in children. *Cochrane Database Syst Rev*. 2013;(10):CD006619.
11. Russell KF, Liang Y, O'Gorman K, et al. Glucocorticoids for croup. *Cochrane Database Syst Rev*. 2011;(1):CD001955.
12. Wood JM, Athanasiadis T, Allen J. Laryngitis. *BMJ*. 2014;349:g5827.
13. Kim JH, Sung IK, Hong SN, et al. Is the proton pump inhibitor test helpful in patients with laryngeal symptoms? *Dig Dis Sci*. 2013;58(6):1663–1667.

 CODES

ICD10
- J04.0 Acute laryngitis
- J37.0 Chronic laryngitis
- J04.2 Acute laryngotracheitis

CLINICAL PEARLS
- Laryngitis is usually self-limited and needs only comfort care. Standard treatment is voice rest.
- Refer to ENT for direct visualization of vocal cords for prolonged laryngitis.
- Corticosteroids have some benefits for children with moderately severe croup.
- Voice training useful for chronic

L

LAXATIVE ABUSE

Matthew E. Bryant, MD

 BASICS

DESCRIPTION
- A chronic watery diarrhea caused by intentional or unintentional misuse of laxatives due to self-medication or provider error
- System(s) affected: gastrointestinal, nervous, psychiatric, skin, and renal
- Synonym(s): factitious diarrhea; cathartic colon; as part of Münchausen syndrome (self or by proxy)—most dramatic form

EPIDEMIOLOGY
- Predominant age: 18 to 40 years associated with bulimia or anorexia nervosa
- Common in the elderly as a result of treatment for constipation, either by health care professional or self-directed (*unintentional*)
- Associated with athletes in sports with weight limits (wrestling)
- Predominant sex (*intentional abuse*): female (90%) > male
- More common in upper socioeconomic classes

Prevalence
Laxative abuse in different groups
- 0.7–5.5% in the general population
- As many as 15% undergoing evaluation for chronic diarrhea
- Unexplained chronic diarrhea after routine investigations: 4–7%
- Up to 70% of patients with binging/purging anorexia and bulimia nervosa abuse laxatives but rarely as the sole method of purging.
- Chronic use of constipating medications (opioids)

Pediatric Considerations
Children may be given excess laxatives by caregivers (Münchausen syndrome by proxy).

Geriatric Considerations
Elderly in nursing homes are at increased risk for laxative overuse (usually inadvert).

ETIOLOGY AND PATHOPHYSIOLOGY
- Four types of chronic diarrhea: secretory, osmotic, inflammatory, and fatty. Rule out other causes, laxative abuse is a diagnosis of exclusion (1).
- Chronic ingestion of any laxative agent
  - Stimulant (most common, rapid onset of action)
    - Diphenylmethane (Bisacodyl)
    - Anthraquinones (Senna, Cascara, Castor oil)
  - Saline and osmotic products (sodium phosphate, magnesium sulfate/citrate and hydroxide, lactulose, polyethylene glycol)
  - Bulking agents (psyllium)
  - Surfactants (docusate)
- Psychologic factors
  - Bulimia or anorexia nervosa (associated with behavioral pathology)
  - Secondary gain (attention-seeking): disability claims or need for concern, caring from others
  - Inappropriate perceptions of "normal" bowel habits

RISK FACTORS
In patients with eating disorders
- Longer duration of illness
- Comorbid psychiatric diagnoses (e.g., major depression, obsessive-compulsive disorder, posttraumatic stress disorder, anxiety, borderline personality disorder)
- Early age of eating disorder symptoms

GENERAL PREVENTION
- Educate patients about proper nutrition, normal bowel function, potential adverse effects of excessive laxative use, and medications (e.g., magnesium-containing antacids) that can cause diarrhea.
- Ask patients specifically about laxative use; inadvertent overuse is common.

COMMONLY ASSOCIATED CONDITIONS
- Anorexia nervosa, bulimia nervosa
- Use of constipating medications (opioids, iron supplements).
- Any chronic disorder associated with constipation
- Depression and anxiety
- Borderline personality
- Self-injurious behaviors/suicidal ideation
- Impulsive behavior
- Münchausen syndrome/Münchausen syndrome by proxy (children) may have associated factitious symptoms involving diverse organ systems.
- Fictitious disorders
- Patient is dependent on a caregiver.

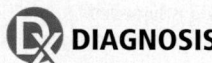 **DIAGNOSIS**

HISTORY
- Suspect in patients with undiagnosed, refractory chronic diarrhea.
- Assess over-the-counter medication use, and take thorough dietary history (2).
- Signs and symptoms: increasing frequency of bowel movements; large volume, watery diarrhea; nocturnal bowel movements (typically absent in osmotic diarrhea or in irritable bowel syndrome) (2,3).
- Additional symptoms: abdominal pain, rectal pain, nausea, vomiting, weight loss, malaise, muscle weakness, or chronic constipation
- Assess "doctor shopping" and potential factitious symptoms.

PHYSICAL EXAM
- No specific findings but may include cachexia, evidence of dehydration, abdominal pain or distension, and edema; fever may be due to self-infected wounds or thermometer manipulation (2).
- Bulimics or anorexics who purge may have Russell sign (excoriation of fingers from repeated self-induced retching) (4); clubbing, cyclic edema, skin pigmentation changes, parotid hypertrophy
- Rarely, severe cases may be associated with renal failure, cardiac arrhythmias, skeletal muscle paralysis, anemia from blood-letting or self-induced skin wounds.

DIFFERENTIAL DIAGNOSIS
Any etiology of chronic diarrhea, especially in high-risk groups

DIAGNOSTIC TESTS & INTERPRETATION
If patient has not had an initial workup for chronic diarrhea, rule out infectious, inflammatory, and malignant causes based on patient demographics and risk factors.

Initial Tests (lab, imaging)
- Serum electrolytes hypokalemia, hypernatremia, hyperphosphatemia
  - Acute diarrhea: metabolic acidosis (hypovolemia)
  - Chronic diarrhea: metabolic alkalosis secondary to hypokalemia-induced inhibition of chloride uptake with inhibited bicarbonate secretion
- CBC, stool cultures, *Clostridium difficile* polymerase chain reaction (PCR) to rule out infectious cause if history is suspicious (fecal leukocytes, ova and parasites (O&P)—check for giardia, isospora, and cryptosporidia specifically) (2,3).
- Colonoscopy, small-bowel endoscopy, or imaging studies are not usually necessary but help to evaluate other causes of chronic diarrhea (2).
- *Melanosis coli* on sigmoidoscopy or colonoscopy indicate overuse of anthracene laxatives.

Follow-Up Tests & Special Considerations
The following algorithm can be used to confirm diagnosis and determine what laxative is being used (1,5)[B].

- Collect 24-hour stool: If stool is solid, workup is over.
- Obtain stool osmolality, stool electrolytes, and calculate osmolal gap $[-290 -2 (Na^+ + K^+)]$, Na^+ and K^+ are stool concentrations.
  - If osmolality >400 mOsm/kg, rule out urine contamination of stool. Measure urea and creatinine of sample.
  - If osmolality <250 to 400 mOsm/kg, rule out water added to stool (colon cannot dilute stool to osmolality of plasma).
  - If osmolality = 250 to 400 mOsm/kg, measure osmolal gap.
    - Gap >50: unmeasured solute; check fecal fat and stool magnesium levels.
    - Gap <50: Rule out use of secretory laxative; urinalysis and stool analysis for laxative titers. Do not obtain serum laxative titers, as they peak 1 to 2 hours after ingestion. Urine titers can be 10 times as high as plasma titers.
- Confirm diagnosis with multiple stool analyses before addressing patient with concern for intentional abuse.

 TREATMENT

GENERAL MEASURES
- Behavioral support is essential in intentional use.
- Wean patient off laxatives and supplements; substitute high-fiber diet and bulk preparations or short-term saline enemas
- Treat secondary constipation (3)[C].
- Treat metabolic abnormalities.

MEDICATION

Replace needed fluid, vitamins, electrolytes, and minerals.

First Line

- Patient education on normal bowel habits
- Nonstimulant laxatives (if needed) to treat constipation (3)[C]
  - Polyethylene glycol (3)[C]
  - Lactulose (3)[C]
  - High-fiber diet
- Precautions: Patients may be manipulative to deny problem; may hide laxatives in hospital rooms.
- Significant possible interactions
  - Increased rate of intestinal motility may affect rate of absorption of medications (e.g., antibiotics, hormones).
  - Docusate sodium may potentiate hepatotoxicity of other drugs.
  - Consider loperamide to improve anal tone and promote rectal inhibitory reflex (6)[C].

ISSUES FOR REFERRAL

In cases of Münchausen syndrome by proxy, legal proceedings must be considered, because most victims are children. Behavioral health support for patients with significant psychological comorbidities

SURGERY/OTHER PROCEDURES

Avoid exploratory surgery and repetitive evaluations or invasive procedures.

INPATIENT CONSIDERATIONS

Admission Criteria/Initial Stabilization

- Persistent diarrhea with hemodynamic instability
- Electrolyte/metabolic complications, including lactic acidosis
- Cardiac arrhythmias

IV Fluids

Resuscitate based on clinical presentation. If patient is hemodynamically stable and without significant abnormalities in serum sodium, give normal saline boluses or oral replacement to correct metabolic alkalosis (chronic) or acidosis (acute) as needed. If patient is hemodynamically unstable, treat volume status as in hypovolemic shock, while monitoring serum electrolytes closely (especially sodium, potassium, and bicarbonate (6,7)[C].

Nursing

If stable, patient does not need continuous telemetry. Depending on psychiatric history, patient may need one-on-one or line-of-sight observation. Special care must be taken to ensure adequate nutrition and control access to laxatives. If surreptitious laxative ingestion is suspected, do not perform unauthorized room searches due to legal constraints.

Discharge Criteria

- Psychological evaluation, support, and follow-up
- Diet and bowel programs
- Resolution of electrolyte abnormalities/dehydration

ONGOING CARE

FOLLOW-UP RECOMMENDATIONS

Patient Monitoring

- Ongoing behavioral counseling
- Careful medical support; frequent visits as needed
- Assess serum electrolytes.

DIET

Ensure good nutritional habits.

- Increase fiber intake.
- Avoid constipating substances.
- Adequate calories, especially with bulimia

PROGNOSIS

- Natural history is unclear and varied depending on underlying cause.
- Prognosis is related to underlying behavioral disorders in intentional abuse or underlying organic disease (if present).
- Prognosis is poor with anorexia nervosa; very poor in Münchausen syndrome.
- Cathartic colon is commonly refractory to treatment (7)[C].

COMPLICATIONS

- Risk of multiple tests, procedures, and surgeries (intentional use)
- Malnutrition
- Electrolyte imbalances (hypokalemia, hypermagnesemia, phosphate nephropathy) (3)
- Renal failure
- Cardiac arrhythmias/sudden death (3)
- Renal calculi
- Cathartic colon with constipation as a consequence of prolonged irritant laxative use (7)
- Fecal impaction in elderly
- Recurrences are common for factitious abuse, even after confrontation.
- Rebound edema (7)

REFERENCES

1. Thomas PD, Forbes A, Green J, et al. Guidelines for the investigation of chronic diarrhoea, 2nd edition. *Gut*. 2003;52(Suppl 5):v1–v15.
2. Schiller LR. Definitions, pathophysiology, and evaluation of chronic diarrhoea. *Best Pract Res Clin Gastroenterol*. 2012;26(5):551–562.
3. Roerig JL, Steffen KJ, Mitchell JE, et al. Laxative abuse: epidemiology, diagnosis and management. *Drugs*. 2010;70(12):1487–1503.
4. Sim LA, McAlpine DE, Grothe KB, et al. Identification and treatment of eating disorders in the primary care setting. *Mayo Clin Proc*. 2010;85(8):746–751.
5. Fine KD, Santa Ana CA, Fordtran JS. Diagnosis of magnesium-induced diarrhea. *N Engl J Med*. 1991;324(15):1012–1017.
6. Kent AJ, Banks MR. Pharmacologic management of diarrhea. *Gastroenterol Clin North Am*. 2010;39(3):495–507.
7. Neims DM, McNeill J, Giles TR, et al. Incidence of laxative abuse in community and bulimic populations: a descriptive review. *Int J Eat Disord*. 1995;17(3):211–228.

ADDITIONAL READING

- Abraham BP, Sellin JH. Drug-induced, factitious, and idiopathic diarrhea. *Best Pract Res Clin Gastroenterol*. 2012;26(5):633–648.
- Bytzer P, Stokholm M, Andersen I, et al. Prevalence of surreptitious laxative abuse in patients with diarrhoea of uncertain origin: a cost benefit analysis of a screening procedure. *Gut*. 1989;30(10):1379–1384.
- Shelton JH, Santa Ana CA, Thompson DR, et al. Factitious diarrhea induced by stimulant laxatives: accuracy of diagnosis by a clinical reference laboratory using thin layer chromatography. *Clin Chem*. 2007;53(1):85–90.
- Sweetser S. Evaluating the patient with diarrhea: a case-based approach. *Mayo Clin Proc*. 2012;87(6):596–602.
- Tozzi F, Thornton LM, Mitchell J, et al. Features associated with laxative abuse in individuals with eating disorders. *Psychosom Med*. 2006;68(3):470–477.

SEE ALSO

Algorithm: Diarrhea, Chronic

CODES

ICD10

F55.2 Abuse of laxatives

CLINICAL PEARLS

- Laxative abuse may be intentional or unintentional.
- When associated with eating disorders, laxative abuse is associated with more severe disease.
- Consider laxative abuse in patients with watery diarrhea, especially if unexplained or refractory.
- As many as 15% of patients referred to tertiary care centers for unexplained chronic diarrhea abuse laxatives.
- Presentation is diverse and nonspecific including weight loss, weakness, and hypotension.
- Patients often won't acknowledge diarrhea if laxative abuse is intentional.

L

LEAD POISONING

Jason Chao, MD, MS

 BASICS

DESCRIPTION
- Consequence of a high body burden of lead (Pb), an element with no known physiologic value
- Synonym(s): lead poisoning, inorganic

EPIDEMIOLOGY
- Predominant age: 1 to 5 years, adult workers
- Predominant sex: male > female (1:1 in childhood)

Prevalence
- 2007 to 2010: Centers for Disease Control and Prevention (CDC) estimated that 2.6% of U.S. children aged 1 to 5 years had blood Pb levels >5 μg/dL, but levels are variable among communities and populations.
- Sporadic cases in adults

ETIOLOGY AND PATHOPHYSIOLOGY
- Inhalation of Pb dust or fumes, or ingestion of Pb
- Pb replaces calcium in bones. Pb interferes with heme synthesis, causes interstitial nephritis, and interferes with neurotransmitters, especially glutamine; high levels affect blood–brain barrier and lead to encephalopathy, seizures, and coma.
- Early life Pb exposure causes methylation changes leading to epigenetic alterations that may lead to brain dysfunction.

RISK FACTORS
- Children with pica or with iron-deficiency anemia
- Residence in or frequent visitor to deteriorating pre-1960 housing with lead-painted surfaces or recent renovation
- Soil/dust exposure near older homes, Pb industries, or urban roads
- Sibling or playmate with current or past Pb poisoning
- Dust from clothing of Pb worker or hobbyist
- Pb dissolved in water from Pb or Pb-soldered plumbing
- Pb-glazed ceramics especially with acidic food or drink
- Recent refugee
- Folk remedies and cosmetics
  - Mexico: Azarcon, Greta
  - Dominican Republic: Litargirio, a topical agent
  - Asia and Middle East: Chuifong tokuwan, pay-loo-ah, ghasard, bali goli, kandu, ayurvedic herbal medicine from South Asia, kohl (alkohl, ceruse), surma, saoott, cebagin
- Hobbies: glazed pottery making, target shooting, Pb soldering, preparing Pb shot or fishing sinkers, stained-glass making, car or boat repair, home remodeling
- Occupational exposure: plumbers, pipe fitters, Pb miners, auto repairers, glass manufacturers, shipbuilders, printer operators, plastic manufacturers, Pb smelters and refiners, steel welders or cutters, construction workers, rubber product manufacturers, battery manufacturers, bridge reconstruction workers
- Dietary: zinc or calcium deficiency
- Imported toys with Pb

Pediatric Considerations
- Children are at increased risk because of incomplete development of the blood–brain barrier at <3 years of age, allowing more Pb into the CNS; ingested Pb has 40% bioavailability in children compared with 10% in adults.
- Common childhood behaviors such as frequent hand-to-mouth activity and pica (repeated ingestion of nonfood products), greatly increase the risk of ingesting Pb.

GENERAL PREVENTION
- Family should receive counseling on potential sources of Pb and methods to decrease Pb exposure. Children at high risk should receive blood Pb screening (1)[C].
- Warn parents about the dangers posed by unsafe renovation methods.
- Wet mopping and dusting with a high-phosphate solution (e.g., powdered automatic dishwasher detergent with 1/4 cup/gallon of water) will help to control Pb-bearing dust. But high-phosphate detergent is no longer available in some states.
- Pregnant women with community-specific or any individual risk factor for Pb poisoning should be screened for Pb toxicity (2)[C].

COMMONLY ASSOCIATED CONDITIONS
Iron-deficiency anemia

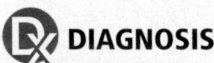 **DIAGNOSIS**

HISTORY
- Often asymptomatic
- Mild-to-moderate toxicity
  - May cause myalgia or paresthesia, fatigue, irritability, lethargy
  - Abdominal discomfort, arthralgia, difficulty concentrating, headache, tremor, vomiting, weight loss, muscular exhaustibility
- Severe toxicity three major clinical syndromes:
  - Alimentary type: anorexia, metallic taste, constipation, severe abdominal cramps due to intestinal spasm and sometimes associated with abdominal wall rigidity
  - Neuromuscular type (characteristic of adult plumbism): peripheral neuritis, usually painless and limited to extensor muscles
  - Cerebral type or Pb encephalopathy (more common in children): seizure, coma, and long-term sequelae, including neurologic defects, delayed mental development, and chronic hyperactivity
- Chronic exposure may cause renal failure.

PHYSICAL EXAM
Often normal, but abdominal tenderness may be severe. Neurologic exam may reveal neuropathy or encephalopathy.

DIFFERENTIAL DIAGNOSIS
- Alimentary type may be confused with acute abdomen.
- Neuromuscular type may be confused with other polyneuropathies.
- Cerebral type may be confused with ADD, mental retardation, autism, dementia, and other causes of seizures.

- Elevated erythrocyte protoporphyrin may be caused by iron-deficiency anemia or, less commonly, hemolytic anemia.
- Erythropoietic protoporphyria produces a very high erythrocyte protoporphyrin level.

DIAGNOSTIC TESTS & INTERPRETATION
- Blood Pb >5 μg/dL (0.24 μmol/L) collected with Pb-free container
- Use a laboratory that can achieve routine performance within 2 μg/dL.
- In 2012, CDC recommended using a reference value as the basis for management, currently >5 μg/dL
- Screening capillary Pb levels >5 μg/dL (0.24 μmol/L) should be confirmed with a venous sample.
- Hemoglobin and hematocrit slightly low; eosinophilia or basophilic stippling on peripheral smear may be seen but is not diagnostic of Pb toxicity.
- Renal function is decreased in late stages.
- Abdominal radiograph for Pb particles in gut if recent ingestion is suspected.
- Radiograph of long bones may show lines of increased density in the metaphyseal plate resulting from growth arrest but does not usually alter management and is not routinely recommended.
- X-ray fluorescence for the total body burden of Pb is experimental.

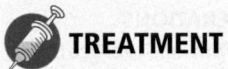 **TREATMENT**

Blood level (μg/dL)	Time to confirmation testing
≥ref value–9	1–3 months
10–44	1 week–1 month
45–59	48 hours
60–69	24 hours
≥70	Urgently as emergency test

ALERT
- For any blood Pb levels persistently >15 μg/dL, contact local public health department for home inspection.
- If Pb level is between 5 and 45 μg/dL, the higher the Pb level, the more urgent the need for confirmation testing.
- For all elevated levels: Educate family on sources of Pb (3)[C].
- Pb level > ref level to <45: Complete history and physical exam, follow-up Pb monitoring; complete inspection of home or workplace to determine source of Pb and Pb-hazard reduction; neurodevelopmental monitoring: iron status, Hgb, or Hct (4)[C].
- Pb level 45 to 69: Actions for lower level plus free erythrocyte protoporphyrin, oral chelation therapy, or hospitalization if Pb-safe environment cannot be ensured (4)[C].
- Pb >70: Hospitalize for chelation therapy (5)[C]

MEDICATION
- Consider oral chelation for asymptomatic and Pb >45 and <70; chelation (preferably parenteral) for Pb >70 or symptomatic Pb <70 (5)[C].
- Do not begin chelation until Pb particles present in gut are cleared (5)[C].

First Line

- Oral chelation: Succimer (Chemet), dimercaptosuccinic acid (DMSA) 10 mg/kg q8h for 5 days; then 10 mg/kg q12h for 2 weeks. This may be repeated after 2 weeks off if Pb levels are not stabilized at <15 μg/dL (<0.72 μmol/L) (5)[C].
- Parenteral chelation (begin after establishment of adequate urine output):
  - Dimercaprol (British anti-Lewisite [BAL]) 75 mg/m² given deep IM; then BAL 450 mg/m²/day divided q4h for 5 days plus Ca edetate calcium disodium (EDTA) 1,500 mg/m²/day continuous IV infusion for 5 days. If rebound Pb level ≥45 μg/dL (≥2.17 μmol/L), chelation may be repeated after 2-day interval if symptomatic or after 5-day interval if asymptomatic.
  - Ca EDTA 1,000 mg/m²/day for 5 days; may be repeated after 5 to 7 days
- Diazepam for initial control of seizures; further control maintained with paraldehyde
- Contraindications: BAL should not be given to patients allergic to peanuts (the drug solution contains peanut oil).
- Precautions
  - Succimer: GI upset, rash, nasal congestion, muscle pains, elevated liver function tests
  - Ca EDTA: renal failure, increased excretion of zinc, copper, and iron
  - BAL: nausea, vomiting, fever, headache, transient hypertension, hepatocellular damage
- Significant possible interactions
  - Vitamins should not be given concurrently with oral chelation.
  - BAL may precipitate hemolytic crisis in a patient with glucose-6-phosphate dehydrogenase deficiency.

Second Line

Oral chelation with penicillamine (D-penicillamine, Depen, Cuprimine) (5)[C]

- Penicillin-allergic patient should not receive penicillamine (cross-sensitivity is common).
- 10 to 15 mg/kg/day given BID mixed in apple juice/sauce on empty stomach (*not* approved by the FDA)
- Penicillamine may cause GI upset, renal failure, granulocytopenia, liver dysfunction, iron deficiency, and drug-induced lupus-like syndrome.

ISSUES FOR REFERRAL

Consider consultation if parenteral chelation is required.

ADDITIONAL THERAPIES

Remove patient from potential source of Pb or Pb level >45 until complete home inspection is performed.

INPATIENT CONSIDERATIONS

Admission Criteria/Initial Stabilization

- Blood Pb level >70 μg/dL
- If symptomatic, blood Pb level >35 μg/dL
- Outpatient care unless parenteral chelation is required or immediate removal from contaminated environment.

Discharge Criteria

- If Pb source is in the home, the patient must reside elsewhere until the abatement process is completed.
- Avoid visit to any site of potential contamination.

 ONGOING CARE

FOLLOW-UP RECOMMENDATIONS

Patient Monitoring

- After chelation, check for rebound Pb level in 7 to 10 days. Follow with regular monitoring, initially biweekly or monthly.
- Correct iron deficiency or any other nutritional deficiencies present.
- Once Pb <35 μg/dL, repeat testing every 1 to 3 months until level <25 μg/dL is achieved. Then monitor every 3 to 6 months until level <10 μg/dL. Once <9 μg/dL, test every 6 to 9 months (4)[C].

DIET

- If symptomatic, avoid excessive fluids.
- Avoid pica.
- Adequate calcium, iron, zinc, and vitamin C to reduce absorption and retention of Pb (6)[B]

PATIENT EDUCATION

- Needleman HL, Landrigan PJ. *Raising Children Toxic Free: How to Keep Your Child Safe From Lead, Asbestos, Pesticides, and Other Environmental Hazards.* New York, NY: Farrar, Straus and Giroux; 1995.
- National Lead Information Center, 422 South Clinton Avenue, Rochester, NY 14620; 800-424-5323; www.epa.gov/lead/
- National Safety Council, 1121 Spring Lake Drive, Itasca, IL 60143-3201; 800-621-7615; http://www.nsc.org/learn/safety-knowledge/Pages/Lead-Poisoning-Prevention.aspx

PROGNOSIS

- Symptomatic Pb poisoning without encephalopathy generally improves with chelation, but subtle CNS toxicity may be long lasting or permanent.
- If encephalopathy occurs, permanent sequelae (e.g., mental retardation, seizure disorder, blindness, and hemiparesis) occurs in 25–50%.

COMPLICATIONS

- CNS toxicity may be long lasting or permanent.
- Long-term Pb exposure may cause chronic renal failure (Fanconi-like syndrome), gout, or Pb line (blue–black) on gingival tissue.
- Pb exposure in pregnancy is associated with reduced birth weight and premature birth.
- Pb is an animal teratogen.

REFERENCES

1. Wengrovitz AM, Brown MJ. Recommendations for blood lead screening of Medicaid-eligible children aged 1–5 years: an updated approach to targeting a group at high risk. *MMWR Recomm Rep.* 2009; 58(RR-9):1–11.
2. Centers for Disease Control and Prevention. *Guidelines for the Identification and Management of Lead Exposure in Pregnant and Lactating Women.* Atlanta, GA: Centers for Disease Control and Prevention; 2010.
3. Binns HJ, Campbell C, Brown MJ, et al. Interpreting and managing blood lead levels of less than 10 microg/dL in children and reducing childhood exposure to lead: recommendations of the Centers for Disease Control and Prevention Advisory Committee on Childhood Lead Poisoning Prevention. *Pediatrics.* 2007;120(5):e1285–e1298.
4. Centers for Disease Control and Prevention. *Low Level Lead Exposure Harms Children: A Renewed Call for Primary Prevention.* Atlanta, GA: Centers for Disease Control and Prevention; 2012.
5. American Academy of Pediatrics Committee on Drugs. Treatment guidelines for lead exposure in children. *Pediatrics.* 1995;96(1, Pt 1):155–160.
6. Woolf AD, Goldman R, Bellinger DC. Update on the clinical management of childhood lead poisoning. *Pediatr Clin North Am.* 2007;54(2):271–294, viii.

ADDITIONAL READING

- American Academy of Pediatrics Committee on Environmental Health. Lead exposure in children: prevention, detection, and management. *Pediatrics.* 2005;116(4):1036–1046.
- Chandramouli K, Steer CD, Ellis M, et al. Effects of early childhood lead exposure on academic performance and behaviour of school age children. *Arch Dis Child.* 2009;94(11):844–848.
- Senut MC, Cingolani P, Sen A, et al. Epigenetics of early-life lead exposure and effects on brain development. *Epigenomics.* 2012;4(6): 665–674.

 SEE ALSO

Anemia, Iron Deficiency

 CODES

ICD10

- T56.0X4A Toxic effect of lead and its compounds, undetermined, init
- T56.0X1A Toxic effect of lead and its compounds, accidental, init

CLINICAL PEARLS

- The following children should have Pb screening:
  - 6 to 11 months of age with ≥1 risk factors:
    - Live in or visit a house built before 1960 with peeling paint or recent renovation
    - Sibling/playmate with elevated Pb
    - Live with adult with job or hobby involving Pb
    - Live near industry likely to release Pb
  - Children living in high-risk communities (>12% elevated Pb) should be tested yearly from ages 1 to 5.
  - Newly arrived refugees
  - Children in low-risk areas should be screened by a questionnaire containing the above risk factors.
- There is no clear safe Pb level. Many experts consider Pb levels >4 μg/dL as elevated.
- There are no studies that show benefit of chelation for asymptomatic children with Pb <45. Removal of sources of Pb is paramount.

L

LEGIONNAIRES' DISEASE

Sean R. Wise, MD • Alex P. Houser, DO

 BASICS

DESCRIPTION
- *Legionnaires' disease* was named for an epidemic of lower respiratory tract disease at an American Legion convention in Philadelphia in 1976. The causative bacterium was previously unrecognized. It was isolated, identified, and named *Legionella pneumophila*. The organism primarily causes pneumonia and flulike illness. *Legionella* preferentially colonizes man-made water systems (e.g., hotels, hospitals, air conditioning cooling towers).
  - Among the three most common clinical pneumonias
  - Most common atypical pneumonia
- System(s) affected: gastrointestinal, pulmonary
- Synonym(s): Legionella pneumonia; legionellosis

EPIDEMIOLOGY
- Predominant age: 15 months to 84 years; 74–91% of patients are >50 years old
- Predominant gender: male > female

Incidence
- Reported cases in the United States from 2000 to 2009 increased from 3.9 to 11.5 cases per million.
- Outbreaks occur most often at the end of the summer and early fall.
- Represents 2–9% of all cases of pneumonia in the United States.

ETIOLOGY AND PATHOPHYSIOLOGY
- *L. pneumophila* is a weak gram-negative aerobic saprophytic freshwater bacterium. It is widely distributed in soil and water. Bipolar flagella provide motility; grows optimally at 40–45°C
- Exists as an intracellular protozoan parasite, colonizing surfaces and growing in biofilms, which persist in nematodes.
- Serogroups 1 to 6 account for clinical disease.
- Serogroup 1 represents 70–92% of all clinical cases of *Legionella* in the United States.
- In the lung, *Legionella* infects alveolar macrophages.
- The organism is transmitted by aspiration, direct transmission (e.g., contaminated respiratory equipment), and (most importantly) by airborne dissemination and aerosolization of contaminated water sources (e.g., contaminated shower water—felt responsible for the inaugural Philadelphia outbreak).
- Recently, community outbreaks have been associated with whirlpools, spas, fountains, and also aboard cruise ships.

RISK FACTORS
- Impaired cellular immunity (*Legionella* are intracellular pathogens)
- Male gender
- Smoking
- Alcohol abuse
- Immunosuppression/HIV
- Chronic cardiopulmonary disease
- Advanced age
- Transplant recipients
- Diabetes mellitus
- Use of antimicrobials within the past 3 months.

GENERAL PREVENTION
- *Not transmitted person to person* (respiratory isolation is unnecessary.)

- Superheat and flush water systems: Heat water to 70°C, and flush outlets with hot water for 30 minutes (1)[C].
- Ultraviolet light or copper–silver ionization are bactericidal.
- Monochloramine disinfection of municipal water supplies decreases risk for *Legionella* infection.
- No person-to-person transmission has been previously documented.

COMMONLY ASSOCIATED CONDITIONS
Pontiac fever: self-limited flulike illness without pneumonia caused by *Legionella* species

 DIAGNOSIS

- Illness ranges from asymptomatic seroconversion and mild febrile illness to severe pneumonia.
- Wound infections with *Legionella* have also been reported.
- Incubation period is 2 to 14 days.

HISTORY
- Signs and symptoms (with associated percentage):
  - Dry cough: 92%, (may occassionally become productive)
  - Fever/chills: 90%
  - Dyspnea: 62%
  - Pleuritic chest pain: 35%
  - Headache: 48%
  - Myalgia/arthralgia: 40%
  - Watery diarrhea: 50%
  - Nausea and vomiting: 49%
  - Neuropsychiatric symptoms such as encephalopathy, confusion, disorientation, obtundation, depression, hallucinations, insomnia, seizure: 53%
- History of immunosuppression increases risk.

PHYSICAL EXAM
- Fever
- Relative bradycardia (key sign)
  - Defined as a temperature ≥102°F with an inappropriately low pulse pressure <100 beats/minute (normal compensatory reaction to fever is tachycardia >110 beats/minute)
- Rales and signs of consolidation (egophony; tactile fremitus)

DIFFERENTIAL DIAGNOSIS
- Other bacterial pneumonias, especially atypical pneumonias: *Mycoplasma pneumoniae*, Q fever (*Coxiella burnetii*), *Chlamydophila pneumoniae*, *Chlamydophila psittaci*, *Francisella tularensis*
- Viral pneumonias, such as adenovirus, influenza (human, avian, swine), cytomegalovirus (CMV)

DIAGNOSTIC TESTS & INTERPRETATION
Initial Tests (lab, imaging)
- Diagnosis:
  - Gold standard is sputum culture for *Legionella*. Alert lab about diagnostic possibility (sample needs buffered charcoal yeast extract agar). Variable sensitivity (10–80%) and time consuming (up to 7 days for results). Hampered by lack of sputum production in >50% of patients.

- Urinary antigen test (UAT) detects serogroup 1 (which causes most human disease). UATs are highly specific (95–100%) but variably sensitive. *Legionella* antigenuria can be detected 1 to 2 days after onset of disease and persists for up to 10 months. Limited by only detecting serogroup 1 (may miss 40% of cases) (2)[C].
  - Indications for UAT: severe pneumonia, ICU admission, failure of outpatient antibiotic treatment, current alcohol abuse, recent travel (within past 2 weeks), pleural effusion
- Combination of respiratory cultures and urine *Legionella* antigen is optimal for diagnosis (3)[C].
- Monoclonal direct fluorescence assay (DFA) on respiratory secretions is diagnostic:
  - Sensitivity 25–75%
  - Limited by lengthy (4 to 6 weeks) seroconversion
- Silver/Gimenez stains used for lung specimens.
- Disorders that may alter lab results: Direct immunofluorescence can cross-react with *Pseudomonas* and *Bacteroides* sp., *Escherichia coli*, and *Haemophilus* sp.
- Other lab abnormalities (seen less commonly with other forms of pneumonia):
  - Hyponatremia
  - Hypophosphatemia (transient)
  - Lymphopenia
  - Mildly elevated serum transaminases
  - Elevated LDH
  - Elevated creatinine kinase
  - Microscopic hematuria
  - Highly elevated C-reactive protein (CRP) (>30)
  - Highly elevated ferritin (≥2 times normal)
- Chest radiograph
  - Not specific for *Legionella*
  - Commonly shows unilateral lower lobe patchy alveolar infiltrate with consolidation
  - Cavitation and abscess formation is more common in immunocompromised patients.
  - Pleural effusion occurs in up to 50%.
  - May take 1 to 4 months for radiographic findings to resolve. Progression of infiltrate on x-ray can be seen despite antibiotic therapy.

Diagnostic Procedures/Other
Transtracheal aspiration/bronchoscopy occasionally necessary for sputum/lung samples

Test Interpretation
- Multifocal pneumonia with alveolitis and bronchiolitis, and fibrinous pleuritis; may have serous or serosanguineous pleural effusion
- Abscess formation occurs in up to 20% of patients.
- Progression of infiltrates on x-ray (despite appropriate therapy) suggests Legionnaires' disease. Radiographic improvement may not correlate with clinical findings (longer lag times).

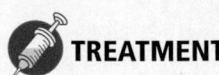 TREATMENT

GENERAL MEASURES
- Severity of illness and available support dictate the appropriate site for care.
- Supportive care:
  - Oxygenation, hydration, and electrolyte balance with antibiotic therapy

- Extrapulmonary complications and higher mortality in patients with AIDS.
- In severe pneumonia, guidelines recommend obtaining a UAT and starting empiric antibiotics to include coverage for *Legionella* (4)[C].

MEDICATION

First Line

- Antibiotics that achieve high intracellular concentrations (e.g., macrolides, tetracyclines, fluoroquinolones) are most effective; first-line treatment is levofloxacin; however, no prospective randomized controlled trials have compared fluoroquinolones to macrolides for the treatment of *Legionella*. Levofloxacin was associated with more rapid defervescence, fewer complications, decreased hospital stay by 3 days, and decreased mortality (4% vs. 10.9%) compared with macrolide antibiotics (4)[A].

- Start antibiotics parenterally if sufficiently ill due to the GI symptoms associated with *Legionella*:
  - Levofloxacin is the preferred agent:
    ○ Levofloxacin 750 mg/day IV (switch to PO when patient is afebrile/tolerating PO) for 5 days or 500 mg/day for 10 to 14 days
  - Azithromycin may also be used first line. It requires a shorter duration of treatment than levofloxacin due to a longer half-life:
    ○ Azithromycin 500 mg/day IV (switch to PO when afebrile/tolerating PO) for 7 to 10 days
- Contraindications: hypersensitivity reactions
- Precautions: liver disease
- Significant possible interactions:
  - Can increase theophylline, carbamazepine, and digoxin levels; can increase activity of oral anticoagulants
  - May decrease the effectiveness of digoxin, quinidine, oral contraceptives, and hypoglycemic agents
- Longer courses of treatment (up to 21 days) may be needed in immunocompromised patients.

Second Line

- Doxycycline 100 mg IV/PO q12h for total 14 days; for severe infections, initial dose is 200 mg IV/PO q12h.
- Doxycycline cannot be used in pregnant patients and is not approved for children <8 years of age.

INPATIENT CONSIDERATIONS

Admission Criteria/Initial Stabilization

- Inability to tolerate oral antibiotics
- Hypoxemia
- Criteria for direct admission to the ICU:
  - Any of the major criteria for severe CAP:
    ○ Septic shock requiring vasopressor support
    ○ Acute respiratory failure requiring intubation and/or mechanical ventilation
  - Three or more of the minor criteria for severe CAP:
    ○ RR ≥30 breaths/min; PaO₂:FiO₂ ratio ≤250; multilobular infiltrates; confusion/disorientation; uremia (BUN ≥20 mg/dL); leukopenia (WBC <4,000 cells/mm³); thrombocytopenia (PLT <100,000 cells/mm³); hypothermia (temperature <36°C); hypotension requiring aggressive fluid resuscitation

Discharge Criteria

- Afebrile
- Able to tolerate oral antibiotics
- Normal oxygen saturation

 ONGOING CARE

FOLLOW-UP RECOMMENDATIONS

Patient Monitoring

- Monitor respiratory status, hydration, and electrolyte status closely.
- Chest radiography does not help with monitoring clinical response.

PATIENT EDUCATION

- Disease prevention: Eliminate pathogens from water supplies, low-emission cleaning procedures of cooling towers with control measurements of water and air samples.
- *Legionella* is not spread person-to-person.

PROGNOSIS

- Improved prognosis when appropriate antibiotics are started early in the disease course.
- Recovery is variable:
  - Patients may clinically worsen despite appropriate treatment early in the course of therapy (first 1 to 2 days).
  - Improvement with defervescence in 3 to 5 days and complete recovery in 6 to 10 days is typical. Some may have a more protracted course.
- Mortality in nosocomial infections ranges between 15 and 34%.

COMPLICATIONS

- Dehydration
- Hyponatremia
- Respiratory insufficiency requiring ventilator support
- Bacteremia/abscess formation in immunocompromised patients
- Extrapulmonary diseases:
  - Encephalitis
  - Cellulitis
  - Sinusitis
  - Pancreatitis
  - Pyelonephritis
  - Endocarditis (most common extrapulmonary site)
  - Pericarditis
  - Perirectal abscess
- Renal failure
- Disseminated intravascular coagulation
- Multiple organ dysfunction syndrome (MODS)
- Coma
- Death occurs in 8–12% of treated immunocompetent patients and in up to 80% of untreated immunocompromised patients.

REFERENCES

1. Walser SM, Gerstner DG, Brenner B, et al. Assessing the environmental health relevance of cooling towers—a systematic review of legionellosis outbreaks. *Int J Hyg Environ Health.* 2014;217(2–3):145–154.
2. Bartlett JG. Diagnostic tests for agents of community-acquired pneumonia. *Clin Infect Dis.* 2011;52(Suppl 4):S296–S304.
3. Tronel H, Hartemann P. Overview of diagnostic and detection methods for legionellosis and *Legionella* spp. *Lett Appl Microbiol.* 2009;48(6):653–656.
4. Burdet C, Lepeule R, Duval X, et al. Quinolones versus macrolides in the treatment of legionellosis: a systematic review and meta-analysis. *J Antimicrob Chemother.* 2014;69(9):2354–2360.

ADDITIONAL READING

- Cunha BA, Klein NC, Strollo S, et al. Legionnaires' disease mimicking swine influenza (H1N1) pneumonia during the "herald wave" of the pandemic. *Heart Lung.* 2010;39(3):242–248.
- Mandell LA, Wunderink RG, Anzueto A, et al. Infectious Diseases Society of America/American Thoracic Society consensus guidelines on the management of community-acquired pneumonia in adults. *Clin Infect Dis.* 2007;44(Suppl 2):S27–S72.
- Mercante JW, Winchell JM. Current and emerging *Legionella* diagnostics for laboratory and outbreak investigations. *Clin Microbiol Rev.* 2015;28(1): 95–133.
- Phin N, Parry-Ford F, Harrison T, et al. Epidemiology and clinical management of Legionnaires' disease. *Lancet Infect Dis.* 2014;14(10):1011–1021.
- Shimada T, Noguchi Y, Jackson JL, et al. Systemic review and metaanalysis: urinary antigen tests for legionellosis. *Chest.* 2009;136(6):1576–1585.

 SEE ALSO

Pneumonia, Bacterial

CODES

ICD10

- A48.1 Legionnaires' disease
- A48.2 Nonpneumonic Legionnaires' disease [Pontiac fever]

CLINICAL PEARLS

- Consider Legionnaires' disease in patients with pneumonia, extrapulmonary findings (atypical CAP) and relative bradycardia, and any three of the following: relative lymphopenia, mildly elevated serum transaminases (aspartate aminotransferase/alanine aminotransferase), highly increased ferritin levels, or hypophosphatemia.
- Consider Legionnaires' disease in cases of nosocomial pneumonia.
- *Legionella* is an intracellular organism that must be grown on buffered charcoal yeast extract agar.
- Because an increase in *Legionella* antibody titers cannot be detected >3 to 4 weeks, serology is not useful in early stages of the disease.
- Respiratory specimen cultures combined with urine *Legionella* antigen testing is the preferred strategy for definitive diagnosis.

L

LEUKEMIA, ACUTE LYMPHOBLASTIC IN ADULTS (ALL)

Richard A. Larson, MD

BASICS

DESCRIPTION
- ALL in adults is a malignant proliferation and accumulation of immature lymphocytes.
- ALL is the most common malignancy in children (see "Acute Lymphoblastic Leukemia, Pediatric")
- System(s) affected: hemic/lymphatic/immunologic
- Synonym(s): acute lymphocytic leukemia

Pregnancy Considerations
Many chemotherapy drugs are teratogenic.

EPIDEMIOLOGY
- Predominant age in adults: Median age, 35 to 40 years; incidence increases with age.
- Predominant sex: male > female (slightly)

Incidence
In the United States: 3,000 adult cases per year

ETIOLOGY AND PATHOPHYSIOLOGY
- Unknown
- Epstein-Barr virus is implicated in Burkitt leukemia/lymphoma.

Genetics
- Increased incidence in children with Down syndrome or in rare familial diseases such as ataxia-telangiectasia, Bloom syndrome, Fanconi anemia, Klinefelter syndrome, and neurofibromatosis (1)
- With P53 mutation in Li-Fraumeni syndrome
- Can rarely occur in adult identical twins

RISK FACTORS
- Age >60 years
- Incidence seems to increase after exposure to chemical agents such as benzene or to radiation, but acute myeloid leukemia (AML) is more common.
- May follow aplastic anemia

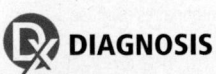

DIAGNOSIS

HISTORY
- Anemia: fatigue, shortness of breath, light-headedness, angina, headache
- Thrombocytopenia: easy bruising
- Neutropenia: fever, infection
- Lymphocytosis: bone pain
- CNS: confusion

PHYSICAL EXAM
- Thrombocytopenia: petechiae, ecchymoses, epistaxis, retinal hemorrhages
- Anemia: pallor
- Neutropenia: fever, infection
- Lymphocytosis: lymphadenopathy, splenomegaly; less often, hepatomegaly
- CNS: cranial nerve palsies, confusion

DIFFERENTIAL DIAGNOSIS
- Malignant disorders: other leukemias, especially AML; chronic myeloid leukemia in lymphoid blast phase; prolymphocytic leukemia; malignant lymphomas; multiple myeloma; bone marrow metastases from solid tumors (breast, prostate, lung, renal); myelodysplastic syndromes
- Nonmalignant disorders: aplastic anemia, myelofibrosis, autoimmune diseases (Felty syndrome, lupus), infectious mononucleosis, pertussis, autoimmune thrombocytopenic purpura, leukemoid reaction to infection

DIAGNOSTIC TESTS & INTERPRETATION
Initial Tests (lab, imaging)
CBC with differential, liver function tests, uric acid, anemia: normochromic, normocytic
- Thrombocytopenia
- Peripheral blood lymphoblasts (B-cells or T-cells)
- Elevated lactate dehydrogenase
- Elevated uric acid

Follow-Up Tests & Special Considerations
Special tests
- Immunophenotyping of marrow/blood lymphoblasts: B lineage (CD19, CD20, CD22, CD24); T lineage (CD2, cCD3, CD5, CD7); common ALL antigen (CD10); human leukocyte antigen (HLA)-DR; terminal deoxynucleotidyl transferase (TdT); aberrant myeloid antigens (CD13, CD33); stem cell antigen (CD34)
- Cytochemical stains: Myeloperoxidase, negative; Sudan black B, usually negative; TdT, positive; periodic acid–Schiff ± is variable, depending on subtype.
- Cytogenetics: Specific recurring chromosomal abnormalities have independent diagnostic and prognostic significance (hyperdiploidy >50 chromosomes or t[14q11q13] are favorable; the Philadelphia chromosome, t[9;22], t[4;11], −7 and +8 are unfavorable). A translocation t(8;14) or t(2;8) or t(8;22) identifies Burkitt-type mature B-cell leukemia that requires specific therapy.
- Reverse transcription polymerase chain reaction for rapid diagnosis of BCR/ABL+ ALL
- Genomic analysis by next-generation sequencing: detection of mutations associated with Ph-like ALL
- HLA typing of patient and siblings for hematopoietic cell transplantation
- Chest CT scan and/or chest radiograph to evaluate for mediastinal mass or hilar adenopathy and for pulmonary infiltrates suggestive of infection
- US exam to assess splenomegaly or renal enlargement suggestive of leukemic infiltration

Diagnostic Procedures/Other
- Bone marrow examination with aspiration, biopsy, immunophenotyping, cytochemistry, cytogenetics, and molecular diagnostics
- Lymph node biopsy is rarely necessary but can be diagnostic.
- Lumbar puncture is typically done both for diagnosis of CNS involvement and for intrathecal chemotherapy. It should be done at diagnosis and immediately if neurologic symptoms or signs are present. Repeat lumbar puncture after bone marrow remission is achieved to evaluate occult CNS involvement and continue prophylactic CNS treatment.

Test Interpretation
Diffuse replacement of marrow and lymph node architecture by sheets of malignant lymphoblasts

TREATMENT

GENERAL MEASURES
- Appropriate health care
  - Inpatient care during remission induction chemotherapy
  - Postremission therapy is usually outpatient.
- Protective isolation from infection
- Adequate calcium and vitamin D supplementation may reduce bone injury from corticosteroids and avascular necrosis of large joints.

MEDICATION
First Line
Optimal therapy is not yet known (2)[B]. ALL should be treated at a comprehensive oncology center. All treatment regimens are still investigational but clearly effective for some fraction of patients. Younger adults (<40 years old) benefit from pediatric-inspired regimens (3,4)[B]. The modified Cancer and leukemia Group B protocol 9111 is an example of therapy for older adults (5)[B]:

- Remission induction
  - Cyclophosphamide: 1,200 mg/m^2 IV on day 1 (800 mg/m^2 if ≥60 years old)
  - Daunorubicin: 45 mg/m^2 IV on days 1, 2, and 3 (30 mg/m^2 if ≥60 years old)
  - Vincristine: 2 mg IV on days 1, 8, 15, and 22
  - Pegylated asparaginase 2,000 U/m^2 (max 3,750 U) given on day 5. 1,000 U/m2 may be better tolerated.
  - Dexamethasone 10 mg/m^2 on days 1 to 7 and 15 to 21
  - Filgrastim, G-CSF: 5 μg/kg/day SC starting on day 4 has been shown to shorten the duration of neutropenia and improve the complete remission rate, especially in older patients.
  - Imatinib mesylate: 600 to 800 mg/day (or dasatinib 70 mg BID) are effective alone and in combination with chemotherapy for Philadelphia chromosome-positive ALL (6)[B].
- Consolidation (repeat twice in 8 weeks)
  - Cyclophosphamide: 1,000 mg/m^2 IV day 1
  - Intrathecal (IT) methotrexate: 15 mg with hydrocortisone 50 mg on day 1
  - Mercaptopurine (6-mercaptopurine): 60 mg/m^2/day on days 1 to 14
  - Cytarabine: 75 mg/m^2/day SC on days 1 to 4 and 8 to 11
  - Vincristine: 2 mg IV on days 15 and 22
  - Pegylated asparaginase 2,000 U/m^2 (maximum 3,750 U) on day 15
- CNS prophylaxis and interim maintenance: 24 Gy cranial irradiation
  - IT-methotrexate: 15 mg with hydrocortisone 50 mg on days 1, 8, 15, 22, and 29
  - Mercaptopurine: 60 mg/m^2/day on days 1 to 70, taken in the evening
  - Oral methotrexate: 20 mg/m^2 on days 36, 43, 50, 57, and 64
- Late intensification
  - Doxorubicin: 30 mg/m^2 IV on days 1, 8, and 15
  - Vincristine: 2 mg IV on days 1, 8, and 15
  - Dexamethasone: 10 mg/m^2 on days 1 to 14
  - Cyclophosphamide: 1,000 mg/m^2 IV on day 29
  - Thioguanine (6-thioguanine): 60 mg/m^2 on days 29 to 42
  - Cytarabine: 75 mg/m^2 SC on days 29 to 32 and 36 to 39
- Prolonged maintenance
  - Vincristine: 2 mg/m^2 IV for 16 months
  - Prednisone: 60 mg/m^2 for 5 days with the vincristine or dexamethasone 10 mg/m^2 on days 1 to 5
  - Mercaptopurine: 60 mg/m^2/day for 16 months, taken in the evening
  - Oral methotrexate: 20 mg/m^2/week for 16 months
  - Special: Philadelphia chromosome–positive ALL (6,7)[B]
    - Imatinib mesylate (400 to 800 mg/day) is effective alone and in combination with chemotherapy.

○ Dasatinib (70 mg BID) is effective in combination with dexamethasone or with chemotherapy (7)[B].

– Contraindications: Doses and schedule may need to be altered for older patients and for concurrent infection and organ toxicity (8)[C].

– Precautions

○ Tumor lysis syndrome (elevated uric acid, potassium, and phosphate with decreased calcium, leading to renal failure, disseminated intravascular coagulation, and cardiac arrhythmias) may be prevented by administering allopurinol 300 mg/day. Begin 2 days before chemotherapy begins. Reduce doses if used with mercaptopurine or azathioprine. Give increased fluids; IV urate oxidase (rasburicase) can be used to treat hyperuricemia rapidly.

○ Oral sulfamethoxazole-trimethoprim or aerosolized pentamidine is given for *Pneumocystis jiroveci* prophylaxis.

○ Profound immunosuppression: Take appropriate precautions when patient is neutropenic.

○ High-dose cyclophosphamide causes severe nausea and vomiting. Use appropriate antiemetic regimen to prevent.

○ Neurotoxicity, ileus with vincristine

○ Asparaginase may cause severe allergic reactions as well as impaired pancreatic and liver function. Monitor serum glucose concentrations frequently and carefully. Pancreatitis or thrombosis may occur. Peg-asparaginase is preferred now and can be used IV, SC, or IM in place of native *Escherichia coli* asparaginase.

○ Avascular (osteo) necrosis (AVN) of bone may occur in adolescents and young adults after alkylating agents and corticosteroids.

○ Rituximab (anti-CD20 monoclonal antibody) appears to improve the outcome of patients with ALL if CD20 is expressed on >20% of their blast cells.

○ Also note: Burkitt leukemia/lymphoma (mature B-cell ALL-L3)

■ The outcome is clearly better if high-dose methotrexate and alkylating agents are used as part of initial therapy.

■ Only 18 weeks of treatment are required.

■ Rituximab (anti-CD20 monoclonal antibody) improves the outcome of patients with Burkitt leukemia when added to chemotherapy (9)[B].

Second Line

• Clofarabine has been approved for relapsed childhood ALL. Nelarabine has been approved as a single agent for relapsed T-cell ALL. Pegylated asparaginase (IV or IM) is now used in place of *E. coli*–derived L-asparaginase. Liposomal vincristine has been approved for single-agent use for the treatment of relapsed ALL in adults.

• Immunoconjugates such as inotuzumab ozogamicin are under investigation.

• The bifunctional antiCD19/antiCD3 antibody blinatumomab is approved for relapsed/refractory ALL (10)[B].

• Allogeneic hematopoietic stem cell transplantation is recommended for any patient with relapsed ALL or during first remission if high-risk genetic features are present (11)[B],(12)[A].

ISSUES FOR REFERRAL

ALERT

ALL can become a fatal disorder quickly. As soon as the diagnosis is suspected, patients should be referred immediately to an appropriate oncology center.

SURGERY/OTHER PROCEDURES

Surgical placement of a percutaneous, silastic, double-lumen central venous catheter or a percutaneous intravenous central catheter (PICC)

COMPLEMENTARY & ALTERNATIVE MEDICINE

Unproven; may result in adverse drug interactions with chemotherapy

 ONGOING CARE

FOLLOW-UP RECOMMENDATIONS

Ambulatory as tolerated

Patient Monitoring

• Daily during induction chemotherapy for metabolic and infectious complications

• Weekly during remission consolidation chemotherapy

• Monthly during maintenance therapy

• Every 3 months thereafter

DIET

• Nutritional support; if needed IV hyperalimentation

• Avoid alcohol.

• Calcium and vitamin D

PATIENT EDUCATION

• Risks of infection, transfusion, chemotherapy

• Stop smoking.

PROGNOSIS

• ~80–95% of adults <60 years will achieve a complete remission, and 35–60% will remain free of disease at 5 years.

• Older patients (>60 years) do less well, but 80% may achieve a complete remission.

• Patients with unfavorable cytogenetic subtypes (especially t[9;22] and t[4;11]) should undergo allogeneic stem cell transplantation in first remission if an HLA-identical donor is available. Autologous stem cell transplantation should be considered for Ph+ ALL patients who become reverse transcriptase polymerase chain reaction negative for BCR/ABL and lack an allogeneic donor.

COMPLICATIONS

• Infections (*Pneumocystis carinii* pneumonia, bacterial pneumonia or sepsis, fungal pneumonia)

• Bleeding

• Coagulopathy (deep vein thrombosis) from asparaginase therapy

• Need for transfusions

• Sterility from treatment

• Arachnoiditis and CNS effects from intrathecal chemotherapy, high-dose methotrexate and irradiation

• Pancreatitis and liver dysfunction from chemotherapy

• Osteonecrosis of joints (avascular necrosis) related to corticosteroids

• Relapse of ALL in marrow or extramedullary sites (CNS, testis)

REFERENCES

1. Mullighan CG. The molecular genetic makeup of acute lymphoblastic leukemia. *Hematology Am Soc Hematol Educ Program*. 2012;2012:389–396.

2. Bassan R, Hoelzer D. Modern therapy of acute lymphoblastic leukemia. *J Clin Oncol*. 2011;29(5): 532–543.

3. Stock W, La M, Sanford B, et al. What determines the outcomes for adolescents and young adults with acute lymphoblastic leukemia treated on cooperative group protocols? A comparison of Children's Cancer Group and Cancer and Leukemia Group B studies. *Blood*. 2008;112(5):1646–1654.

4. Curran E, Stock W. How I treat acute lymphoblastic leukemia in older adolescents and young adults. *Blood*. 2015;125(24):3702–3710.

5. Larson RA, Dodge RK, Linker CA, et al. A randomized controlled trial of filgrastim during remission induction and consolidation chemotherapy for adults with acute lymphoblastic leukemia: CALGB study 9111. *Blood*. 1998;92(5):1556–1564.

6. Chalandon Y, Thomas X, Hayette S, et al. Randomized study of reduced-intensity chemotherapy combined with imatinib in adults with Ph-positive acute lymphoblastic leukemia. *Blood*. 2015;125(24):3711–3719.

7. Foà R, Vitale A, Vignetti M, et al. Dasatinib as first-line treatment for adult patients with Philadelphia chromosome-positive acute lymphoblastic leukemia. *Blood*. 2011;118(25): 6521–6528.

8. Gökbuget N. How I treat older patients with ALL. *Blood*. 2013;122(8):1366–1375.

9. Rizzieri DA, Johnson JL, Byrd JC, et al. Improved efficacy using rituximab and brief duration, high intensity chemotherapy with filgrastim support for Burkitt or aggressive lymphomas: cancer and Leukemia Group B study 10 002. *Br J Haematol*. 2014;165(1):102–111.

10. Topp MS, Gökbuget N, Stein AS, et al. Safety and activity of blinatumomab for adult patients with relapsed or refractory B-precursor acute lymphoblastic leukaemia: a multicentre, single-arm, phase 2 study. *Lancet Oncol*. 2015;16(1):57–66.

11. Mattison RJ, Larson RA. Role of allogeneic hematopoietic cell transplantation in adults with acute lymphoblastic leukemia. *Curr Opin Oncol*. 2009;21(6):601–608.

12. Oliansky DM, Larson RA, Weisdorf D, et al. The role of cytotoxic therapy with hematopoietic stem cell transplantation in the treatment of adult acute lymphoblastic leukemia: update of the 2006 evidence-based review. *Biol Blood Marrow Transplant*. 2012;18(1):16–17.

 CODES

ICD10

• C91.00 Acute lymphoblastic leukemia not having achieved remission

• C91.01 Acute lymphoblastic leukemia, in remission

• C91.02 Acute lymphoblastic leukemia, in relapse

CLINICAL PEARLS

ALL can become fatal quickly; as soon as diagnosis is suspected, refer the patient to an oncology center. Optimal therapy is not yet known. ALL should be treated at a comprehensive oncology center. All treatment regimens are still investigational but clearly are effective for a large fraction of patients.

L

LEUKEMIA, ACUTE MYELOID

Jan Cerny, MD, PhD

BASICS

DESCRIPTION
- Acute myeloid leukemia (AML) is characterized by proliferation and accumulation of abnormal immature myeloid progenitors (blasts) with reduced capacity to differentiate into more mature cellular elements. This leads to bone marrow failure and results in a variety of systemic symptoms.
- Previously, the French–American–British (FAB) classification system divided AML based on the cell morphology with the addition of cytogenetics (subtypes M0–M7).
- The World Health Organization (WHO) classification attempts to provide more meaningful prognostic information.
  - AML with characteristic genetic abnormalities: translocation t(8;21), t(15;17), and inversion in chromosome 16 inv(16)
  - AML with multilineage dysplasia: presence of a prior myelodysplastic syndrome (MDS) or myeloproliferative neoplasm (MPN) that transformed into AML
  - AML and MDS, therapy related
  - AML not otherwise categorized
  - Acute leukemias of ambiguous lineage (*biphenotypic acute leukemia*)

EPIDEMIOLOGY
- ~13,500 cases diagnosed in 2007; second most common type of leukemia in adults
- Predominant sex: male ≥ female

Incidence
The incidence of AML increases with age, and median age is >70 years.

ETIOLOGY AND PATHOPHYSIOLOGY
Precise causes unknown, but some risk factors have been identified (see "Risk Factors").

Genetics
- Unknown; some are familial.
- Cytogenetics and genetics play an important role in diagnosis and prognosis of AML and have implications for therapy.
- Three risk groups
  - Good risk: inv(16), t(8;21), t(15;17)
  - Standard risk: normal karyotype
  - Poor risk: monosomy 5 and 7 (typically secondary AML), deletion 5q, abnormalities of 11q23 or complex karyotype
- *FLT3* gene mutations, especially internal transmembrane duplications (FLT3-ITD), have been associated with poor survival in AML. These and growing list of (onco)gene (e.g., *NPM1*, *DNMT3A*, and *P53*) mutations have been studied to further risk-stratify patients (1,2)[A].

RISK FACTORS
- Genetic predisposition (e.g., Down syndrome); other familial disorders are Bloom syndrome (~25% develop AML), Fanconi anemia (52%), neurofibromatosis, Li-Fraumeni syndrome, Wiskott-Aldrich syndrome, Kostmann syndrome, and Diamond-Blackfan anemia

- Radiation exposure
- Immunodeficiency states
- Chemical and drug exposure (nitrogen mustard and alkylating agents; benzene)
- MDS
- Cigarette smoking

GENERAL PREVENTION
None currently identified, but treatment of high-risk MDS with demethylating agents (Vidaza, 5-azacitidine) has been shown to prolong time to transformation from MDS into AML (3)[A].

COMMONLY ASSOCIATED CONDITIONS
The following are oncologic emergencies:
- Disseminated intravascular coagulopathy (DIC) especially in acute promyelocytic leukemia (APL) but may be seen in any AML
- Leukostasis (high blast number and increased adhesive ability of blasts)
- Tumor lysis syndrome (TLS): spontaneous or in response to chemotherapy

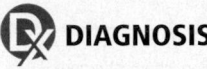

DIAGNOSIS

HISTORY
Fatigue (anemia or tumor burden); bleeding (low platelets or DIC); difficulty clearing infections (neutropenia or immune dysregulation)

PHYSICAL EXAM
- Mostly nonspecific and related to marrow or tissue infiltration
  - Fever
  - Bleeding
  - Pallor
  - Splenomegaly
  - Hepatosplenomegaly
  - Lymphadenopathy (usually reactive)
- If CNS is involved, symptoms of increased intracranial pressure can be present.
- Occasionally, patients will present with prominent extramedullary sites of leukemia (e.g., skin infiltration or ultimately as a myeloid sarcoma).

DIFFERENTIAL DIAGNOSIS
- Virus-induced cytopenia, lymphadenopathy, and organomegaly
- Immune cytopenias (including systemic lupus erythematosus [SLE])
- Drug-induced cytopenias
- Other marrow failure and infiltrative diseases (e.g., aplastic anemia, paroxysmal nocturnal hemoglobinuria, MDSs, Gaucher disease)

DIAGNOSTIC TESTS & INTERPRETATION
- CBC shows subnormal RBCs, neutrophils, and platelets.
- Bone marrow for histology, flow cytometry, and cytogenetics to establish diagnosis and prognosis
- ESR
- Lactate dehydrogenase (LDH) and uric acid can be elevated (e.g., TLS).
- Coagulation profile can be normal or prolonged (e.g., DIC).

- Drugs that may alter lab results: chemotherapy agents, corticosteroids
- Other special tests: Spinal tap may reveal fluid with leukemic cells.
- Ultrasonography or CT scan of the abdomen may discover organomegaly.

Diagnostic Procedures/Other
Bone-marrow studies are usually necessary to make the diagnosis.
- Aspirates: for cell morphology, cytochemistries, immunophenotyping (can confirm differentiation stage of AML); cytogenetics: chromosomal aberration (prognostic value; see "Genetics")
- Biopsies provide valuable information for cellularity, architecture, and so forth.

Test Interpretation
- Marrow is usually hypercellular and the normal architecture effaced; leukemic blast count is 20% or more.
- Liver and spleen may be infiltrated with leukemic cells.

TREATMENT

- Chemotherapy is the backbone of AML therapy; it consists of induction and consolidation phase ± maintenance (APL).
- Bone marrow transplantation (BMT) for high-risk AML
- Only modest improvements have been made in AML induction chemotherapy. Supportive care has improved significantly.

GENERAL MEASURES
- Ongoing assessment of bone marrow, liver, heart, and kidney functions during therapy
- Close monitoring of coagulation parameters (risk for DIC)
- Supportive therapy with
  - Good hydration
  - Transfusions of packed RBCs and platelets based on patient's needs (threshold as for platelets as low as 5,000); use leuko-reduced, irradiated blood products, as all patients can be considered for BMT.
  - Avoid antiplatelet agents (e.g., aspirin products).
  - Follow febrile neutropenic guidelines in neutropenic patient who becomes febrile (even low-grade fever).

Geriatric Considerations
- Older patients (>60 to 65 years of age) remain a therapeutic challenge. These patients are offered so-called reduced-intensity or nonmyeloablative BMT.
- Adding growth factors (granulocyte-colony stimulating factor [G-CSF]) may reduce toxicity in older patients (but is not broadly accepted).
- Hypomethylating agent, such as 5-azacitidine, significantly prolongs survival in older adults with low marrow blast count (<30%).

Pediatric Considerations
Tolerate intense treatments better

Pregnancy Considerations
Chemotherapy is a viable option in the 2nd and 3rd trimesters.

MEDICATION
First Line
- APL (APL, AML with t[15;17])
  - All-trans retinoic acid (ATRA) and arsenic trioxide both promote maturation to granulocytes.
  - Idarubicin is often added to induction therapy.
- Treatment of AML in younger adults: AML (other than APL)
  - Induction (daunorubicin or idarubicin [anthracycline and cytarabine]): The generally accepted combination is 3 + 7 (anthracycline is given for 3 days and cytarabine for 7 days) or more intensive regimens with high dose of cytarabine (HiDAC) or high dose of anthracycline.
- Remission is typically consolidated in younger patients by the following:
  - In good-risk AML, 3 to 4 cycles of HiDAC and BMT is reserved for time of recurrence.
  - In poor-risk patients, 1 to 2 cycles of HiDAC (until donor is identified) are followed by allogeneic BMT.
  - Intermediate-risk AML should be treated based on individual patient's features, donor availability, and access to clinical trials. A meta-analysis showed that even intermediate-risk patients benefit from allogeneic BMT (4)[A].
- Treatment of AML in older adults (>65 years of age) remains a challenge. These patients have poor performance status, more likely secondary AML, higher incidence of unfavorable cytogenetics, comorbidities, shorter remissions, and shorter overall survival.
  - Intensive chemotherapy may be feasible for patients with good performance status; alternative regimens with mitoxantrone, fludarabine, and clofarabine. New drugs (hypomethylating agents as above, FLT3 inhibitors, monoclonal antibodies, etc.) are being studied in clinical trials (5)[A].
- Contraindications: comorbidities; therapy has to be individualized.
- Precautions
  - If organ failure, some drugs may be avoided or dose reduced (e.g., no anthracyclines in patients with preexisting cardiac problems).
  - Patients will be immunosuppressed during treatment. Avoid live vaccines. Administer varicella-zoster or measles immunoglobulin as soon as exposure of patient occurs.
- Significant possible interactions: Allopurinol accentuates the toxicity of 6-mercaptopurine.

Second Line
Healthy, younger patients usually are offered reinduction chemotherapy and allogeneic BMT.

ISSUES FOR REFERRAL
- AML should be managed by specialized team led by a hematologist/oncologist.
- Refer patient to a transplant center early because a search for a donor may be necessary.

SURGERY/OTHER PROCEDURES
- BMT: Decision between myeloablative and nonmyeloablative approach should be based on patient's performance status, comorbidities, and AML risk factors.
  - Allogeneic BMT is acceptable in first remission in intermediate- or high-risk AML or in second remission in all other AML patients. Matched related donor used to be preferred over matched unrelated donor (lower risk of graft-versus-host disease); recent data suggest equal outcomes, as allogeneic transplant regimens and posttransplant care have improved significantly.
- Haploidentical transplants and cord blood may be used as alternative sources of hematopoietic stem cells for adults.
- Autologous BMT may be acceptable in specific situations (e.g., no donor is available).

INPATIENT CONSIDERATIONS
Admission Criteria/Initial Stabilization
Induction treatment for AML requires inpatient care, usually on a specialized ward. Episodes of febrile neutropenia typically require admission and IV antibiotics.

IV Fluids
Appropriate hydration to prevent TLS

Nursing
IV may lead to chemical burns in the event of extravasation.

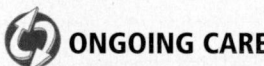 ONGOING CARE

FOLLOW-UP RECOMMENDATIONS
Ambulatory, as tolerated; no intense or contact sports; no aspirin due to risk of bleeding.

Patient Monitoring
- Repeat bone marrow studies to document remission and also if a relapse is suspected.
- Follow CBC with differential, coagulation studies, uric acid level, and other chemistries related to TLS (creatinine, potassium, phosphate, calcium); monitor urinary function at least daily during induction phase and less frequently later.
- Physical evaluation, including weight and BP, should be done frequently during treatment.

DIET
Ensure adequately balanced calorie/vitamin intake. Total parenteral nutrition (TPN) in case of severe mucositis

PATIENT EDUCATION
- Leukemia Society of America, 600 Third Avenue, New York, NY 10016, 212-573-8484
- National Cancer Institute, Bethesda, MD, has pamphlets and telephone education.
- Baker LS. *You and Leukemia: A Day At a Time.* Philadelphia, PA: Saunders; 1978.

PROGNOSIS
AML remission rate is 60–80%, with only 20–40% long-term survival. The wide variable prognosis is due to prognostic group (age, cytogenetics, and genetics).

COMPLICATIONS
- Acute side effects of chemotherapy, including febrile neutropenia
- TLS
- DIC
- Late-onset cardiomyopathy in patients treated with anthracyclines
- Chronic side effects of chemotherapy (secondary malignancies)
- Graft-versus-host disease in patients who have received allogeneic BMT

REFERENCES
1. Döhner H, Estey EH, Amadori S, et al. Diagnosis and management of acute myeloid leukemia in adults: recommendations from an international expert panel, on behalf of the European LeukemiaNet. *Blood.* 2010;115(3):453–474.
2. Patel JP, Gönen M, Figueroa ME, et al. Prognostic relevance of integrated genetic profiling in acute myeloid leukemia. *N Engl J Med.* 2012;366(12):1079–1089.
3. Fenaux P, Mufti GJ, Hellstrom-Lindberg E, et al. Efficacy of azacitidine compared with that of conventional care regimens in the treatment of higher-risk myelodysplastic syndromes: a randomised, open-label, phase III study. *Lancet Oncol.* 2009;10(3):223–232.
4. Koreth J, Schlenk R, Kopecky KJ, et al. Allogeneic stem cell transplantation for acute myeloid leukemia in first complete remission: systematic review and meta-analysis of prospective clinical trials. *JAMA.* 2009;301(22):2349–2361.
5. Fenaux P, Mufti GJ, Hellström-Lindberg E, et al. Azacitidine prolongs overall survival compared with conventional care regimens in elderly patients with low bone marrow blast count acute myeloid leukemia. *J Clin Oncol.* 2010;28(4):562–569.

ADDITIONAL READING
O'Donnell MR, Appelbaum FR, Coutre SE, et al. Acute myeloid leukemia. *J Natl Compr Canc Netw.* 2008;6(10):962–993.

 SEE ALSO

Disseminated Intravascular Coagulation; Leukemia, Acute Lymphoblastic in Adults (ALL); Leukemia, Chronic Myelogenous; Myelodysplastic Syndromes; Myeloproliferative Neoplasms

 CODES

ICD10
- C92.00 Acute myeloblastic leukemia, not having achieved remission
- C92.01 Acute myeloblastic leukemia, in remission
- C92.02 Acute myeloblastic leukemia, in relapse

CLINICAL PEARLS
- Prognosis of leukemia depends on the cytogenetic and molecular profile of the disease.
- Allogeneic transplant remains the only therapy with curative potential for patients with intermediate- and high-risk AML.

L

LEUKEMIA, CHRONIC LYMPHOCYTIC

Jan Cerny, MD, PhD

BASICS

DESCRIPTION
- Chronic lymphocytic leukemia (CLL) is a monoclonal disorder characterized by a progressive accumulation of mature but functionally incompetent lymphocytes.
- CLL should be distinguished from prolymphocytic leukemia (PLL); based on percentage of prolymphocytes, the disease may be regarded as CLL (<10% prolymphocytes), PLL (>55% prolymphocytes), or CLL/PLL (>10% and <55% prolymphocytes).
- Small lymphocytic lymphoma is a lymphoma variant of CLL.
- System(s) affected: hematologic, lymphatic, immunologic

EPIDEMIOLOGY
Incidence
- With 15,000 to 17,000 new cases reported every year, CLL *represents the most common form of leukemia in adults in the United States.*
- In 2013, an estimated 4,580 adults in United States will die from CLL, which makes it the second leading cause of death among adults with leukemia in United States after acute myeloid leukemia (1)[A].
- Predominant age: CLL primarily affects elderly individuals, median age of diagnosis being 70 years. The incidence continues to rise in those age >55 years.
- Predominant sex: male > female (1.7:1)
- The incidence is higher among whites than among African Americans.

ETIOLOGY AND PATHOPHYSIOLOGY
- The cell of origin in CLL is a clonal B cell arrested in the B-cell differentiation pathway, intermediate between pre–B cells and mature B cells. In the peripheral blood, these cells resemble mature lymphocytes and typically show B-cell surface antigens: CD19, CD20, CD21, and CD23. In addition, they express CD5 (usually found on T cells).
- The BCL-2 protooncogene is overexpressed in B-CLL. BCL-2 is a known suppressor of apoptosis (programmed cell death), resulting in extremely long life of the affected lymphocytes.
  - Unknown, but genetic mutations leading to disrupted function and prolonged survival of affected lymphocytes are suspected.

Genetics
CLL is an acquired disorder, and reports of truly familial cases are exceedingly rare. CLL has been shown, however, to occur at higher frequency among first-degree relatives of patients with the disease, and several somatic gene mutations have been identified at significantly higher rates among CLL patients.

RISK FACTORS
- As in the case of most malignancies, the exact cause of CLL is uncertain.
- Possible chronic immune stimulation is suspected but is still being elucidated.
- Monoclonal B-cell lymphocytosis: 1% risk progression to CLL

GENERAL PREVENTION
Unknown

COMMONLY ASSOCIATED CONDITIONS
- Immune system dysregulation is common.
- Autoimmune hemolytic anemia (AIHA) may accompany CLL.
- Immune thrombocytopenic purpura (ITP) may accompany CLL.
- Pure red cell aplasia (PRCA) may accompany CLL.

DIAGNOSIS

HISTORY
- Insidious onset; it is not unusual for CLL to be discovered incidentally. Up to 40% of patients are asymptomatic at the time of diagnosis.
- Others may have the following:
  - Repetitive infections (e.g., not only pneumonia but also mucocutaneous herpetic infections)
  - Enlarged lymph nodes
  - Early satiety and/or abdominal discomfort related to an enlarged spleen
  - Mucocutaneous bleeding and/or petechiae due to thrombocytopenia
  - Fatigue-related and/or other symptoms of anemia
  - Fevers, night sweats, >10% weight loss (B symptoms)

PHYSICAL EXAM
- Localized or generalized lymphadenopathy
- Splenomegaly (30–40%)
- Hepatomegaly (20%)
- Mucocutaneous bleeding (thrombocytopenia)
- Skin petechiae (thrombocytopenia)
- Pallor

DIFFERENTIAL DIAGNOSIS
- Infectious causes are the following:
  - Bacterial (tuberculosis)
  - Viral (mononucleosis)
- Malignant causes are the following:
  - Leukemic phase of non-Hodgkin lymphomas
  - Hairy cell leukemia
  - Waldenstrom macroglobulinemia
  - Large granular lymphocytic leukemia

DIAGNOSTIC TESTS & INTERPRETATION
Initial Tests (lab, imaging)
- CBC with differential shows B cell absolute lymphocytosis with >5,000 B lymphocytes/μL. The blood smear also shows ruptured lymphocytes ("smudge" cells) and morphologically mature-appearing small lymphocytes.
- Exam of the blood smear is important in diagnosis of CLL.
- Diagnosis can be confirmed by immunophenotyping: CLL cells are positive for CD19, CD20, and CD24 as well as CD5. They have low levels of surface membrane immunoglobulin (Ig) M or IgD. The monoclonality is proven by the presence of a single immunoglobulin light chain (κ or λ). FMC7 is absent.

- CBC shows anemia and/or thrombocytopenia.
- Plasma β_2-microglobulin may be elevated.
- Serum protein electrophoresis (some patients may have monoclonal gammopathy)
- Lactate dehydrogenase (LDH) may be elevated (due to disease activity or to AIHA).
- Hypogammaglobulinemia
- In cases associated with AIHA, labs consistent with hemolysis may be present (elevated LDH, total bilirubin; reticulocyte count does not have to be elevated due to bone marrow infiltration).
- Liver/spleen ultrasound may demonstrate organomegaly and may also detect enlarged abdominal lymph nodes.
- CT scan of chest/abdomen/pelvis typically is not necessary for staging. However, it may help to identify compression of organs or internal structures from enlarged lymph nodes.
- Positron emission tomography (PET) scan might be helpful to guide biopsy if Richter transformation is suspected (see below).

Follow-Up Tests & Special Considerations
Frequency and type of follow-up depend on severity of symptoms as well as risk factors (see "Prognosis").

Diagnostic Procedures/Other
- Although bone marrow biopsy has its prognostic value (diffuse infiltration is a risk factor), it is not done routinely.
- Consider a lymph node biopsy if lymph node(s) begins to enlarge rapidly in a patient with known CLL to assess the possibility of transformation to a high-grade lymphoma (Richter syndrome), especially when accompanied by fever, weight loss, and pain.

Test Interpretation
- A bone marrow aspirate usually shows >30% lymphocytes.
- Cytogenetic (fluorescence in situ hybridization) may show chromosomal changes, which are prognostic (i.e., del[13q], del[11q], del[17p], trisomy 12, and del[6q]).
- *SF3B1* mutation is associated with rapid disease progression and shorter survival in CLL (2)[A].

TREATMENT

GENERAL MEASURES
Patients with frequent infections associated with hypogammaglobulinemia are likely to benefit from monthly infusions of intravenous immunoglobulin (IVIG).

MEDICATION
First Line
- Most patients are asymptomatic and do not need active treatment unless they have generalized (so-called B) symptoms, progressive marrow failure, AIHA or thrombocytopenia, progressive splenomegaly, massive lymphadenopathy, or progressive lymphocytosis (increase >50% in 2 months or a doubling time of <6 months).

- Low-risk disease, Rai stage 0, and Binet stage A require only periodic follow-up.
- Intermediate-risk group, Rai stages I and II, and Binet stage B could be observed until evidence of disease progression or development of symptoms.
- Treatment should be initiated in high-risk patients, Rai stage III and IV, and Binet stage C.
- Early treatment in low-risk group is not recommended.
- Three main groups of drugs used are alkylating agents (chlorambucil and, recently, bendamustine), purine analogues (fludarabine and pentostatin), and monoclonal antibodies (rituximab and alemtuzumab).
- Single-agent (fludarabine, bendamustine, or chlorambucil) or combination regimens commonly used
- Fludarabine-based regimens are FC (in combination with cyclophosphamide), FR (fludarabine + rituximab), and FCR (fludarabine + cyclophosphamide + rituximab).
- FCR is the widely used regimen of choice if patient can tolerate it.
- Steroids (prednisone) are useful in patients with autoimmune manifestations of CLL (e.g., AIHA, ITP).

Second Line
- Combinations of chemotherapeutic agents that patient did not fail yet. Occasionally, some patients can be retreated with a drug used previously.
- Ibrutinib, is a Bruton tyrosine kinase (BTK) inhibitor from a novel class of agents, which has a high level of activity in CLL (3)[A].
- Newer agents, like ofatumumab (novel anti-CD20), lenalidomide, and others, have shown promising activity.
- Alemtuzumab (anti-CD52) has shown activity in relapsed and refractory disease.
- Consider splenectomy (surgery/radiation) if massive splenomegaly causes significant anemia and thrombocytopenia.
- Allogenic and autologous stem cell transplant can be considered in high-risk and younger patients (limited data available).

ISSUES FOR REFERRAL
- Surgical consultation for splenectomy in selected patients
- Bone marrow transplant in young patients with refractory disease (however, still considered experimental therapy)
  - Allogeneic hematopoietic stem cell transplant (HSCT) with nonmyeloablative conditioning offers lower treatment-related mortality and may be appropriate for certain patients.

ADDITIONAL THERAPIES
Patients requiring therapy who are high-risk for tumor lysis syndrome should be given allopurinol to prevent uric acid nephropathy.

SURGERY/OTHER PROCEDURES
- Splenectomy in selected patients with splenomegaly and refractory cytopenia
- Radiation (if compression symptoms from bulky lymphadenopathy)

INPATIENT CONSIDERATIONS
Admission Criteria/Initial Stabilization
No specific criteria but due to complications of disease (e.g., AIHA) or of therapy (e.g., febrile neutropenia) or significant tumor lysis syndrome after initiation of chemotherapy

 ONGOING CARE

FOLLOW-UP RECOMMENDATIONS
Patient Monitoring
Patients with low-risk CLL and/or patients in remission
- CBC with differential (lymphocytosis) every 3 to 6 months, LDH, β_2-microglobulin, IgG level
- Physical exam (lymphadenopathy, splenomegaly)

DIET
- Ensure adequately balanced calorie/vitamin intake.
- Follow weight.

PATIENT EDUCATION
Leukemia and Lymphoma Society has educational pamphlets: http://www.webmd.com/cancer/tc/leukemia-topic-overview.

PROGNOSIS
There are two staging systems used: the Rai in the United States and the Binet in Europe. Neither is completely satisfactory.
- Rai staging system
  - Stage 0: lymphocytosis only; median survival of 120 months
  - Stage I: lymphocytosis and adenopathy; median survival of 95 months
  - Stage II: lymphocytosis and splenomegaly and/or hepatomegaly; median survival of 72 months
  - Stage III: lymphocytosis and anemia (hemoglobin <10 g/dL); median survival of 30 months
  - Stage IV: lymphocytosis and thrombocytopenia (platelets <100 × 10^9/L); median survival of 30 months
- Binet staging system
  - Stage A: hemoglobin ≥10 g/dL, platelets 100 × 10^9, and <3 lymph node areas involved (Rai stages 0, I, and II); survival >120 months
  - Stage B: Hemoglobin and platelet levels as in stage A and 3 or more lymph node areas involved (Rai stages I and II); survival is 61 months.
  - Stage C: Hemoglobin <100 g/L, platelets <100 × 10^9, or both (Rai stages III and IV); survival is 32 months.
- Adverse risk factors
  - Advanced Rai or Binet stage
  - Peripheral lymphocyte doubling time <12 months
  - Diffuse marrow infiltration
  - Increased number of prolymphocytes or cleaved cells
  - Poor response to chemotherapy
  - High β_2-microglobulin and thymidine kinase levels and low micro RNAs (miRNAs)
  - Abnormal karyotyping: deletion 17p (del[17p] *P53* mutation or deletion) and del(11q)
  - New IgVH unmutated status (expression of ZAP-70 >20% or CD38 >30% evaluated by immunophenotyping are surrogate markers)
  - NOTCH1 mutation (also associated with unmutated IgVH)

COMPLICATIONS
- Acute or long-term effects of chemotherapy
- Richter syndrome (above)
- AIHA (in some cases may be related to the use of fludarabine)
- Slightly increased risk of solid tumors (especially Kaposi sarcoma, malignant melanoma, laryngeal cancers, lung cancers)
- Infection (especially gram negative and encapsulated organisms)
- Membranoproliferative glomerulonephritis (MPGN) or other glomerular pathology

REFERENCES
1. Siegel R, Naishadham D, Jemal A. Cancer statistics, 2013. *CA Cancer J Clin*. 2013;63(1):11–30.
2. Wan Y, Wu CJ. *SF3B1* mutations in chronic lymphocytic leukemia. *Blood*. 2013;121(23):4627–4634.
3. Advani RH, Buggy JJ, Sharman JP, et al. Bruton tyrosine kinase ibrutinib (PCI-32765) has significant activity in patients with relapsed/refractory B-cell malignancies. *J Clin Oncol*. 2013;31(1):88–94.

ADDITIONAL READING
- Chiorazzi N, Rai KR, Ferrarini M. Chronic lymphocytic leukemia. *N Engl J Med*. 2005;352(8):804–815.
- National Comprehensive Cancer Network guidelines: http://www.nccn.org/
- Shanafelt TD, Kay NE. Comprehensive management of the CLL patient: a holistic approach. *Hematology Am Soc Hematol Educ Program*. 2007:324–331.

 CODES

ICD10
- C91.10 Chronic lymphocytic leuk of B-cell type not achieve remis
- C91.11 Chronic lymphocytic leukemia of B-cell type in remission
- C91.12 Chronic lymphocytic leukemia of B-cell type in relapse

CLINICAL PEARLS
- CLL represents the most common form of leukemia in adults in the United States.
- Predominant age: CLL primarily affects elderly individuals, median age of diagnosis being 70 years. The incidence continues to rise in those age >55 years.
- Clinical monitoring of asymptomatic and low-risk patients is a reasonable approach ("watch and wait").
- High-risk patients, bulky disease, or patients who fail fludarabine- and rituximab-based therapies have typically poor prognosis and may require intensive therapies, including allogeneic transplantation.
- Median survival is 3 to 10 years, depending on stage.

L

LEUKEMIA, CHRONIC MYELOGENOUS

Jan Cerny, MD, PhD

BASICS

DESCRIPTION
- Chronic myelogenous leukemia (CML) is a myeloproliferative neoplasm characterized by clonal proliferation of myeloid precursors in the bone marrow with continuing differentiation into mature granulocytes.
- Hallmark of CML is Philadelphia chromosome (translocation t[9;22]).
- Natural history of the disease evolves in three clinical phases: a chronic phase, an accelerated phase, and blast phase or crisis (transformation to acute leukemia).

EPIDEMIOLOGY
Incidence
- Per year, 1.6 cases/100,000 persons
- Predominant age: 50 to 60 years
- Predominant sex: male > female (1.3:1)

Prevalence
Accounts for 15–20% of adult leukemias

ETIOLOGY AND PATHOPHYSIOLOGY
Philadelphia chromosome is a balanced translocation between *BCR* (on chromosome 22) and *ABL* (on chromosome 9) genes t(9;22)(q34;q11). This fusion gene, *BCR-ABL*, codes for an abnormal constitutively active tyrosine kinase that affects numerous signal transduction pathways, resulting in uncontrolled cell proliferation and reduced apoptosis.

Genetics
Acquired genomic changes

RISK FACTORS
Ionizing radiation exposure (uncommon)

GENERAL PREVENTION
None currently identified

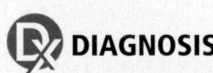
DIAGNOSIS

85–90% of patients present in the chronic phase, and the disease can be found accidentally during routine screening.

HISTORY
- Chronic phase: fatigue, weight loss, night sweats, abdominal fullness owing to enlarged spleen, early satiety, dyspnea, bleeding. Rare: Bruising, left upper quadrant abdominal pain, sternal pain (owing to expanding bone marrow), and gouty arthritis; up to 30% of patients are asymptomatic.
- Accelerated phase: Progressive splenomegaly and left upper quadrant abdominal pain occasionally referred to the left shoulder (owing to splenic infarction or rupture), progressive weight loss and sweats, unexplained fever or bone pain, chloromas (extramedullary tumors).
- Blast phase: bleeding, bruising, infections, prominent constitutional symptoms

PHYSICAL EXAM
- Splenomegaly (50–90%), hepatomegaly (up to 50%)
- Less common: splenic friction rub, lymphadenopathy

DIFFERENTIAL DIAGNOSIS
- Chronic myelomonocytic leukemia, chronic neutrophilic leukemia, chronic eosinophilic leukemia, juvenile myelomonocytic leukemia, infectious mononucleosis, leukemoid reaction, polycythemia vera, and treatment with granulocyte-stimulating factors
- Acute myelogenous leukemia resembles blast crisis with myeloid blasts, and acute lymphoblastic leukemia resembles blast crisis with lymphoid blasts.
- Atypical CML is a chronic myeloproliferative disorder with a clinical hematologic picture similar to CML, but it lacks Philadelphia chromosome and *BCR-ABL* rearrangement.

DIAGNOSTIC TESTS & INTERPRETATION
- CBC
  - Hematocrit: may be normal, slightly increased, or decreased
  - WBC count: markedly increased (50,000 to 100,000/μL), with granulocytes in all stages of development, including occasional blasts <10% in chronic phase, basophilia, eosinophilia
  - Platelets: normal, elevated (34%), or occasionally low
  - In accelerated phase: anemia, 10–19% blood or marrow blasts, basophils plus eosinophils >20%, thrombocytopenia
  - Blast phase: blood or marrow blasts >20%
- Genetics
  - Demonstration of the Philadelphia chromosome, t(9;22), by cytogenetic techniques, fluorescence in situ hybridization (FISH), or reverse transcription-polymerase chain reaction (RT-PCR)
  - Additional cytogenetic abnormalities occur in the accelerated and blast phases (monosomy 7, t[3;21], trisomies 8 and 19, Philadelphia chromosome duplication, abnormalities of chromosome 17 such as monosomy, trisomy, and isochromosome mutations). These may contribute to resistance to tyrosine kinase inhibitors (TKIs; e.g., imatinib). Further molecular testing (mutations within *BCR-ABL*) is suggested in case of loss of response to therapy.
- Others:
  - Low or absent leukocyte alkaline phosphatase in neutrophils
  - High lactate dehydrogenase (LDH)
  - Elevated uric acid

Initial Tests (lab, imaging)
- CBC, LDH, uric acid, bone marrow biopsy and aspiration, cytogenetics on bone marrow, and FISH for *BCR-ABL*, RT-PCR, LFTs
- Abdominal ultrasound or CT scan shows splenomegaly; not mandatory.

Follow-Up Tests & Special Considerations
- Mutation analysis of tyrosine kinase domain of *ABL* kinase, as they may cause resistance to therapy with TKIs
- HLA-A*02 positive is associated with CML, and a protective effect is seen with the HLA-B*35 allele (pooled odds ratio 0.64, 95% confidence interval 0.48 to 0.86).

Diagnostic Procedures/Other
Bone marrow aspiration and biopsy

Test Interpretation
Myeloid hyperplasia with elevated myeloid: erythroid ratio, normal maturation, marrow basophilia, and increased reticulin fibrosis

TREATMENT

MEDICATION
- TKIs (e.g., imatinib) provide durable, long-term control of disease.
- The response to TKIs is assessed at specific time points from the beginning of treatment and is categorized as follows:
  - Complete hematologic response (CHR): normalization of peripheral counts, no disease symptoms, no immature cells
  - Minor/partial/complete cytogenetic response (CCR): 1–34%, 35–90%, no Philadelphia-positive metaphases
  - Major molecular response (MMR): decreased level of *BCR-ABL* transcript by PCR 3-log
  - Complete molecular response (CMR): *BCR-ABL* transcript is undetectable by PCR.

First Line
- Imatinib mesylate (Gleevec), an oral TKI, 400 mg/day
- Side effects: thrombocytopenia, anemia, elevated liver enzymes, edema, GI disturbances, rash
- International Randomized Study of Interferon versus STI571 (IRIS) established imatinib as first-line therapy (1)[A].
- Imatinib dose can be increased to 600 and 800 mg/day if only suboptimal response is achieved with standard dose.
- 2nd-generation TKIs have shown higher efficacy and fewer side effects and are approved for first-line therapy of chronic phase CML: nilotinib (Tasigna) and dasatinib (Sprycel) (2,3)[A].

Second Line
- Dasatinib, 2nd-generation TKI; active against most of *BRC-ABL* mutants; not active in *T315I* mutation
  - 100 mg/day in patients resistant or intolerant to imatinib and 70 mg BID for patients in accelerated or blastic phase
  - Side effects: pleural effusions, cytopenias
- Nilotinib, also 2nd-generation TKI; highly selective and more potent *BCR-ABL* TKI; active against most *BRC-ABL* mutants; not active in *T315I* mutation
  - 400 mg PO BID in patients resistant or intolerant to imatinib in chronic or accelerated phase
  - Side effects: cytopenias, QTc prolongation, pancreatitis
- Bosutinib and omacetaxine are now approved for patient who failed or did not tolerate two TKIs previously. Ponatinib has now more restricted approval, but together with omacetaxine, they are the only effective agents in patients with *T315I* mutation. Agents targeting leukemic stem cells are being developed for clinical use.

ISSUES FOR REFERRAL
All patients with CML should be referred to a hematologist. Patients with inadequate response to TKIs or with *T315I* mutation should consult with a bone marrow transplant physician.

SURGERY/OTHER PROCEDURES
Allogenic bone marrow transplant (BMT)

- It is the only known cure; however, 71% of patients who achieve CCR with imatinib maintain that response for 7 years, and no patient progressed on the trial between years 5 and 6 of treatment.
- Most effective in patients <50 years of age who are in the chronic phase
- Initial mortality is higher (related to the use of myeloablative regimens) than medical management but provided higher rates of survival in pre-TKI era.
- Significant improvement in transplant techniques leading to better outcomes, such as alternative sources of stem cells; nonmyeloablative regimens have shown improvements in transplant-related mortality.
- Transplant option should be thoroughly discussed with young patients in chronic phase and considered an alternative to TKIs especially if the patient does not tolerate TKIs or disease is not responding.
- Can be considered in patients who fail to achieve CHR by 3 months, have no cytogenetic response or cytogenetic relapse, or have *T315I* mutation

INPATIENT CONSIDERATIONS
Admission Criteria/Initial Stabilization
Acute abdominal symptoms (infarcted or ruptured spleen); tumor lysis syndrome owing to initial therapy; complications of BMT

- Hydroxyurea might be given, with the goal of reduction of the WBC count, but it has minimal impact on patient response to TKIs.
- Induction chemotherapy (for acute leukemia) in setting of blastic phase
- Allopurinol to prevent tumor lysis syndrome in patients with very high counts; however, probably not necessary when TKIs are used

Discharge Criteria
Abatement of acute symptoms

 ONGOING CARE

FOLLOW-UP RECOMMENDATIONS
- Frequency depends on stage at presentation and response to first-line therapy
- Although splenomegaly persists, avoid contact sports or trauma to abdomen.

Patient Monitoring
- CBC with differential: weekly until blood counts stable, then every 2 to 4 weeks during CHR; once in CCR and stable, patient can be followed less frequently (3-month intervals)
- Bone marrow cytogenetics (evaluation for clonal evolution) every 6 months while in CHR, every 12 to 18 months while in complete cytogenic response, MMR, CMR
- Quantitative RT-PCR every 3 months (peripheral blood)
- ECGs (concern for QT prolongation), LFTs while on TKIs. Nilotinib, bosutinib, and ponatinib can cause pancreatitis.

PROGNOSIS
- With treatment and good response, the survival is similar to the normal population.
- Without treatment: CML invariably will progress to accelerated phase within 2 to 5 years and blast phase within several months of the accelerated phase.
- Poor prognosis: patients presenting in accelerated or blastic phase or presenting with very large spleen size, platelets >700,000/μL, and patients resistant to TKIs (*T315I* mutation)

COMPLICATIONS
- Splenic infarct or rupture
- Progression to accelerated or blastic phase
- Thrombotic events owing to elevated platelets
- Bleeding owing to low or dysfunctional platelets
- Sequelae of anemia

REFERENCES
1. O'Brien SG, Guilhot F, Goldman JM, et al. International randomized study of interferon versus STI571 (IRIS) 7-year follow-up: sustained survival, low rate of transformation and increased rate of major molecular response (MMR) in patients (pts) with newly diagnosed chronic myeloid leukemia in chronic phase (CML-CP) treated with imatinib (IM). *ASH Ann Meeting Abstracts.* 2008;112:186.
2. Saglio G, Kim DW, Issaragrisil S, et al. Nilotinib versus imatinib for newly diagnosed chronic myeloid leukemia. *N Engl J Med.* 2010;362(24):2251–2259.
3. Kantarjian H, Shah NP, Hochhaus A, et al. Dasatinib versus imatinib in newly diagnosed chronic-phase chronic myeloid leukemia. *N Engl J Med.* 2010;362(24):2260–2270.

ADDITIONAL READING
- Kantarjian HM, Baccarani M, Jabbour E, et al. Second-generation tyrosine kinase inhibitors: the future of frontline CML therapy. *Clin Cancer Res.* 2011;17(7):1674–1683.
- Kantarjian H, Pasquini R, Hamerschlak N, et al. Dasatinib or high-dose imatinib for chronic-phase chronic myeloid leukemia after failure of first-line imatinib: a randomized phase 2 trial. *Blood.* 2007;109(12):5143–5150.
- Naugler C, Liwski R. Human leukocyte antigen class I alleles and the risk of chronic myelogenous leukemia: a meta-analysis. *Leuk Lymphoma.* 2010;51(7):1288–1292.

 CODES

ICD10
- C92.10 Chronic myeloid leukemia, BCR/ABL-positive, not having achieved remission
- C92.11 Chronic myeloid leukemia, BCR/ABL-positive, in remission
- C92.12 Chronic myeloid leukemia, BCR/ABL-positive, in relapse

CLINICAL PEARLS
- CML belongs to the myeloproliferative disorders group
- The gold standard for diagnosis of CML is detection of the Philadelphia chromosome or its products, *BCR-ABL* mRNA, and fusion protein.
- TKIs provide durable, long term control of the disease and have dramatically altered treatment.
- Atypical CML is a form of clinically typical CML but without the presence of the typical *BCR-ABL* translocation.
- Blast crisis is a form of acute leukemia that is a possible complication of CML.

LEUKOPLAKIA, ORAL

Christine K. Jacobs, MD, FAAFP

BASICS

DESCRIPTION
- Oral leukoplakia is defined by the World Health Organization as white plaques of questionable risk having excluded (other) known diseases or disorders that carry no increased risk for cancer (1)[C].
- System(s) affected: gastrointestinal

EPIDEMIOLOGY
- Develops in middle age, increases with age
- Most common in India, where more people smoke and chew tobacco and areca nuts

Prevalence
- 1–3% of the adult population is affected.
- Usual age of onset is over 40 years old with peak in the 60s.
- Males twice as often as females

Geriatric Considerations
Malignant transformation to carcinoma is more common in older patients.

ETIOLOGY AND PATHOPHYSIOLOGY
Hyperkeratosis or dyskeratosis of the oral squamous epithelium
- Tobacco use in any form
- Alcohol consumption/alcoholism
- Oral infections
- Candida albicans infection may induce dysplasia and increase malignant transformation (2)[B].
- Human papillomavirus, types 11 and 15
- Sunlight
- Vitamin deficiency
- Syphilis
- Dental restorations/prosthetic appliances
- Estrogen therapy
- Chronic trauma or irritation
- Epstein-Barr virus (oral hairy leukoplakia)
- Areca nut/betel (Asian populations)
- Mouthwash preparations and toothpaste containing the herbal root extract sanguinaria

Genetics
- Dyskeratosis congenital and epidermolysis bullosa increase the likelihood of oral malignancy (1)[B].
- P53 overexpression correlates with leukoplakia and particularly squamous cell carcinoma (3)[B].

RISK FACTORS
- 70–90% of oral leukoplakia is related to tobacco, particularly smokeless tobacco or areca/betel nut use.
- Alcohol increases risk 1.5-fold
- Repeated or chronic mechanical trauma from dental appliances or cheek biting

- Chemical irritation to oral regions
- Diabetes
- Age
- Socioeconomic status
- Risk factors for malignant transformation of leukoplakia
  - Female
  - Long duration of leukoplakia
  - Nonsmoker (idiopathic leukoplakia)
  - Located on tongue or floor of mouth
  - Size >200 mm²
  - Nonhomogenous type
  - Presence of epithelial dysplasia

GENERAL PREVENTION
- Avoid tobacco of any kind, alcohol, habitual cheek biting, tongue chewing.
- Use well-fitting dental prosthesis.
- Regular dental check-ups to avoid bad restorations
- Diet rich in fresh fruits and vegetables may help to prevent cancer.
- HPV vaccination may be preventive.

COMMONLY ASSOCIATED CONDITIONS
- HIV infection is closely associated with hairy leukoplakia.
- Erythroplakia in association with leukoplakia, "speckled leukoplakia," or erythroleukoplakia is a marker for underlying dysplasia.

DIAGNOSIS

Leukoplakia is an asymptomatic white patch on the oral mucosa.

HISTORY
- Usually asymptomatic
- History of tobacco or alcohol use or oral exposure to irritants

PHYSICAL EXAM
- Location
  - 50% on tongue, mandibular alveolar ridge, and buccal mucosa
  - Also seen on maxillary alveolar ridge, palate, and lower lip
  - Infrequently seen on floor of the mouth and retromolar areas
  - Floor of mouth, ventrolateral tongue, and soft palate complex are more likely to have dysplastic lesions.
- Appearance
  - Varies from homogeneous, nonpalpable, faintly translucent white areas to thick, fissured, papillomatous, indurated plaques
  - May feel rough or leathery
  - Lesions can become exophytic or verruciform.
  - Color may be white, gray, yellowish white, or brownish gray.
  - Cannot be wiped or scraped off

- World Health Organization classification (1)
  - Homogeneous refers to color
    - Flat, corrugated, wrinkled, or pumice
  - Nonhomogeneous refers to color and texture (more likely to be dysplastic or malignant).
    - Erythroleukoplakia (mixture of red and white)
    - Exophytic: papillary or verrucous texture

DIFFERENTIAL DIAGNOSIS
- White oral lesions that can be wiped away: acute pseudomembranous candidiasis
- White oral lesions that cannot be rubbed off (1)
  - Morsicatio buccarum (habitual cheek-biting), generally benign (4)[C]
  - Chemical injury
  - Acute pseudomembranous candidiasis
  - Traumatic or frictional keratosis (e.g., linea alba)
  - Leukoedema (benign milky opaque lesions that disappear with stretching)
  - Aspirin burn (from holding aspirin in cheek)
  - Lichen planus (bilateral fairly symmetric lesions, reticular pattern of slightly raised gray-white lines)
  - Lichenoid reaction
  - Verrucous carcinoma
  - Discoid lupus erythematosus
  - Skin graft (known history)
  - Squamous cell carcinoma
  - Oral hairy leukoplakia, commonly on the lateral border of the tongue with a bilateral distribution (in HIV patients with Epstein-Barr virus infection)
  - Smoker's palate (leukokeratosis nicotina palati)
  - White sponge nevus (congenital benign spongy lesions)
  - Syphilitic oral lesion
  - Dyskeratosis congenita (a rare inherited multisystem disorder)

DIAGNOSTIC TESTS & INTERPRETATION
Biopsy to rule out carcinoma if lesion is persistent, changing, or unexplained

Initial Tests (lab, imaging)
- Laboratory tests generally are not indicated
  - Consider saliva culture if C. albicans infection is suspected.
- No imaging is indicated.

Follow-Up Tests & Special Considerations
- Biopsy is necessary to rule out carcinoma if lesion is persistent, changing, or unexplained (1).
- Consider CBC, rapid plasma reagin (RPR).

Diagnostic Procedures/Other
- Oral cytology is superior to conventional oral examination (5)[A].
- Computer-assisted cytology or liquid-based cytology is not superior to oral cytology (5)[A].

- Noninvasive brush biopsy and analysis of cells with DNA–image cytometry constitute a sensitive and specific screening method.
- Patients with dysplastic or malignant cells on brush biopsy should undergo more formal excisional biopsy (1).
- Excisional biopsy is definitive procedure.

Test Interpretation
- Biopsy specimens range from hyperkeratosis to invasive carcinoma.
- At initial biopsy, 6% are invasive carcinoma.
- 0.13–6% subsequently undergo malignant transformation
- Location is important: 60% on floor of mouth or lateral border of tongue are cancerous; buccal mucosal lesions are generally not malignant but require biopsy if not resolving.

TREATMENT
- All oral leukoplakias should be treated.
- Treatment may include the following:
  - For 2 to 3 circumscribed lesions, surgical excision
  - For multiple or large lesions where surgery would cause unacceptable deformity, consider cryosurgery or laser surgery (6)[C].
  - Removal of predisposing habits (alcohol and tobacco)
- Complete excision is standard treatment for dysplasia or malignancy.
- After treatment, up to 30% of leukoplakia recurs, and some leukoplakia still transforms to squamous cell carcinoma (6)[B].
- Oral hairy leukoplakia may be treated with podophyllin with acyclovir cream (7)[A].

GENERAL MEASURES
- Eliminate habitual lip biting.
- Correct ill-fitting dental appliances, bad restorations, or sharp teeth.
- Stop smoking and using alcohol.
- Some small lesions may respond to cryosurgery.
- β-carotene, lycopene, retinoids, and cyclooxygenase 2 (COX-2) inhibitors may cause partial regression.
- For hairy tongue: tongue brushing

MEDICATION
Carotenoids, vitamins A, C, and K, bleomycin, and photodynamic therapy ineffective to prevent malignant transformation and recurrence (8)[A]

ISSUES FOR REFERRAL
Consider otolaryngologist or oral surgery referral for extensive disease

SURGERY/OTHER PROCEDURES
- Scalpel excision, laser ablation, electrocautery, or cryoablation
- Cryotherapy slightly less effective than photodynamic therapy response (73% vs. 90%) and recurrence (27% vs. 24%) (9)[A]
- CO_2 laser had 20% recurrence and 10% malignant transformation within 5 years (10)[B].

INPATIENT CONSIDERATIONS
Admission Criteria/Initial Stabilization
- Eliminate etiologic factors.
- Reevaluate in 7 to 14 days.
- Biopsy if lesion is persistent.

ONGOING CARE

FOLLOW-UP RECOMMENDATIONS
Patient Monitoring
- Regular, close follow-up, even after successful treatment
- Biopsy as needed

DIET
Regular

PATIENT EDUCATION
- If biopsy is negative, stress importance of periodic and careful follow-up.
- Initiate a dental referral to eliminate dental factors.
- Stress importance of stopping tobacco and alcohol use.
- Encourage participation in smoking cessation program.

PROGNOSIS
- Most leukoplakia is benign.
- Leukoplakia may regress, remain stable, or progress.
- 0.13–6% of initially benign lesions subsequently develop into cancer.
- More likely to be cancerous if on floor of mouth or lateral border of tongue

COMPLICATIONS
- New lesions may develop after treatment.
- Risk of malignant transformation to squamous cell carcinoma is approximately 5–17% (11)[B].
- Larger lesions and nonhomogeneous leukoplakia are associated with higher rates of malignant transformation.

REFERENCES

1. Warnakulasuriya S, Johnson NW, van der Waal I. Nomenclature and classification of potentially malignant disorders of the oral mucosa. *J Oral Pathol Med*. 2007;36(10):575–580.
2. Cao J, Liu HW, Jin JQ. The effect of oral candida to development of oral leukoplakia into cancer [In Chinese]. *Zhonghua Yu Fang Yi Xue Za Zhi*. 2007;41(Suppl):90–93.
3. Duarte EC, Ribeiro DC, Gomez MV, et al. Genetic polymorphisms of carcinogen metabolizing enzymes are associated with oral leukoplakia development and p53 overexpression. *Anticancer Res*. 2008;28(2A):1101–1106.
4. Cam K, Santoro A, Lee JB. Oral frictional hyperkeratosis (morsicatio buccarum): an entity to be considered in the differential diagnosis of white oral mucosal lesions. *Skinmed*. 2012;10(2):114–115.
5. Fuller C, Camilon R, Nguyen S, et al. Adjunctive diagnostic techniques for oral lesions of unknown malignant potential: systematic review with meta-analysis. *Head Neck*. 2015;37(5):755–762. doi:10.1002/hed.23667.
6. Feller L, Lemmer J. Oral leukoplakia as it relates to HPV infection: a review. *Int J Dent*. 2012;2012:540561.
7. Moura MD, Haddad JP, Senna MI, et al. A new topical treatment protocol for oral hairy leukoplakia. *Oral Surg Oral Med Oral Pathol Oral Radiol Endod*. 2010;110(5):611–617.
8. Ribeiro AS, Salles PR, da Silva TA, et al. A review of the nonsurgical treatment of oral leukoplakia. *Int J Dent*. 2010;2010:186018.
9. Kawczyk-Krupka A, Waśkowska J, Raczkowska-Siostrzonek A, et al. Comparison of cryotherapy and photodynamic therapy in treatment of oral leukoplakia. *Photodiagnosis Photodyn Ther*. 2012;9(2):148–155.
10. Jerjes W, Upile T, Hamdoon Z, et al. CO2 laser of oral dysplasia: clinicopathological features of recurrence and malignant transformation. *Lasers Med Sci*. 2012;27(1):169–179.
11. Rhodus NL, Kerr AR, Patel K. Oral cancer: leukoplakia, premalignancy, and squamous cell carcinoma. *Dent Clin North Am*. 2014;58(2):315–340.

ADDITIONAL READING

- Nair DR, Pruthy R, Pawar U, et al. Oral cancer: premalignant conditions and screening—an update. *J Cancer Res Ther*. 2012;8(Suppl 1):S57–S66.
- Reamy BV, Derby R, Bunt CW. Common tongue conditions in primary care. *Am Fam Physician*. 2010;81(5):627–634.
- Warnakulasuriya S, Dietrich T, Bornstein MM, et al. Oral health risks of tobacco use and effects of cessation. *Int Dent J*. 2010;60(1):7–30.
- Yardimci G, Kutlubay Z, Engin B, et al. Precancerous lesions of oral mucosa. *World J Clin Cases*. 2014;2(12):866–872.

SEE ALSO

Infectious Mononucleosis, Epstein-Barr Virus Infections; HIV/AIDS

CODES

ICD10
- K13.21 Leukoplakia of oral mucosa, including tongue
- K13.3 Hairy leukoplakia

CLINICAL PEARLS
- Excisional biopsy is indicated for any undiagnosed leukoplakia.
- After treatment, up to 30% of leukoplakia recurs, and some leukoplakia still transforms to squamous cell carcinoma; thus, long-term surveillance is essential.
- To lessen risk of malignant transformation, encourage tobacco and alcohol cessation and consider *C. albicans* eradication.

L

LICHEN PLANUS

Mercedes E. Gonzalez, MD, FAAD • Herbert P. Goodheart, MD

 BASICS

Lichen planus (LP) is an idiopathic eruption with characteristic shiny, flat-topped (Latin: *planus,* "flat") purple (violaceous) papules and plaques on the skin, often accompanied by characteristic mucous membrane lesions. Itching may be severe.

DESCRIPTION

- Classic (typical) LP is a relatively uncommon inflammatory disorder of the skin and mucous membranes; hair and nails may also be affected.
  - Skin lesions are small, flat, angular, red-to-violaceous, shiny, pruritic papules and/or plaques with overlying fine, white lines (called Wickham striae), or gray-white puncta; most commonly seen on the flexor surfaces of the upper extremities, extensor surfaces of the lower extremities, the genitalia, and on the mucous membranes
  - On the oral mucosa, lesions typically appear as raised white lines in a lacelike pattern seen most often on the buccal mucosa.
  - Onset is abrupt or gradual. Course is unpredictable; may resolve spontaneously, recur intermittently, or persist for many years
- Drug-induced LP
  - Clinical and histopathologic findings may mimic those of classic LP. Lesions usually lack Wickham striae (see in the following text) and oral involvement is rare.
  - There is generally a latent period of months from drug introduction until lesions appear.
  - Lesions resolve when the inciting agent is discontinued, often after a prolonged period.
- LP variants
  - Follicular: also called lichen planopilaris; typically seen on the scalp, can lead to scarring alopecia
  - Annular: Papules spread centrifugally as central area resolves; occur on glans penis, axillae, and oral mucosa
  - Linear: may be an isolated finding
  - Hypertrophic: itchy, hyperkeratotic, thick plaques on dorsal legs and feet
  - Atrophic: rare, most often the result of resolved lesions
  - Bullous LP: Intense inflammation in the dermis leads to blistering of epidermis.
  - LP pemphigoides: a combination of LP and bullous pemphigoid (IgG autoantibodies to collagen 17)
  - Nail LP: affects the nail matrix, lateral thinning, longitudinal ridging, and fissuring
- System(s) affected: skin/exocrine
- Synonym(s): lichenoid eruptions

EPIDEMIOLOGY

- Predominant age: 30 to 60 years old; rare in children and the geriatric population
- Predominant sex: female > male

Prevalence

In the United States, 450/100,000

ETIOLOGY AND PATHOPHYSIOLOGY

LP is considered to be a T-cell–mediated autoimmune response to self-antigens on damaged keratinocytes.

RISK FACTORS

Exposure to certain drugs or chemicals

- Thiazides, furosemide, β-blockers, sulfonylureas, antimalarials, penicillamine, gold salts, and angiotensin-converting enzyme inhibitors
- Rarely: photo-developing chemicals, dental materials, tattoo pigments

COMMONLY ASSOCIATED CONDITIONS

- An association has been noted between LP and hepatitis C virus infection, particularly in certain geographic regions (Asia, South America, the Middle East, Europe) (1). Hepatitis should be considered in patients with widespread presentations of LP and those with primarily oral disease.
- In addition, chronic active hepatitis, lichen nitidus, and primary biliary cirrhosis have been noted to coexist with LP.
- Association with dyslipidemia has been reported (2)[B].
- LP has also been reported in association with other diseases of altered immunity, more often than would be expected by chance.
  - Bullous pemphigoid
  - Alopecia areata
  - Myasthenia gravis
  - Vitiligo
  - Ulcerative colitis
  - Graft-versus-host reaction
  - Lupus erythematosus (lupus erythematosus–LP overlap syndrome)
  - Morphea and lichen sclerosis et atrophicus

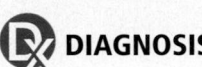 **DIAGNOSIS**

LP is most commonly diagnosed by its appearance despite its range of clinical presentations. A skin biopsy should be performed if the diagnosis is in doubt.

HISTORY

A minority of patients have a family history of LP. Affected families have an increased frequency of human leukocyte antigen B7 (HLA-B7). A thorough drug history should be performed.

PHYSICAL EXAM

- Skin (often severe pruritus)
  - Papules: 1 to 10 mm, shiny, flat-topped (planar) lesions that occur in crops; lesions may have a fine scale.
  - Evidence of scratching (i.e., crusts and excoriations) is usually absent.
  - Color: violaceous, with white lacelike pattern (Wickham striae) on surface of papules. Wickham striae are best seen after topical application of mineral oil and, if present, are virtually pathognomonic for LP.
  - Shape: polygonal or oval. Annular lesions may appear on trunk and mucous membranes. Various shapes and sizes may be noted (polymorphic).
  - Arrangement: may be grouped, linear, or scattered individual lesions
  - Koebner phenomenon (isomorphic response): New lesions may be noted at sites of minor injuries, such as scratches or burns.

- Distribution: ventral surface of wrists and forearms, dorsa hands, glans penis, dorsa feet, groin, sacrum, shins, and scalp. Hypertrophic (verrucous) lesions may occur on lower legs and may be generalized.
- Postinflammatory hyperpigmentation: Lesions typically heal, leaving darkly pigmented macules in their wake.
- Mucous membranes (40–60% of patients with skin lesions; 20% have mucous membrane lesions without skin involvement)
  - Most commonly asymptomatic, nonerosive, milky-white lines with an elegant, lacy, netlike streaked pattern
  - Usually seen on buccal mucosa but may appear on tongue, gingiva, palate, or lips
  - Less commonly, LP may be erosive; rarely bullous
  - Painful, especially if ulcers present
  - Lesions may develop into squamous cell carcinoma (1–3%).
  - Glans penis, labia minora, vaginal vault, and perianal areas may be involved.
- Hair/scalp
  - LP of the hair follicle (lichen planopilaris) presents with keratotic plugs at the follicle orifice with a violaceous rim; may result in atrophy and permanent destruction of hair follicles (scarring alopecia)
- Nails (10%)
  - Involvement of nail matrix may cause proximal-to-distal linear grooves and partial or complete destruction of nail bed with pterygium formation.

DIFFERENTIAL DIAGNOSIS

- Skin
  - Lichen simplex chronicus
  - Eczematous dermatitis
  - Psoriasis
  - Discoid lupus erythematosus
  - Other lichenoid eruptions (those that resemble LP)
  - Pityriasis rosea
  - Lichen nitidus
- Oral mucous membranes
  - Leukoplakia
  - Oral hairy leukoplakia
  - Candidiasis
  - Squamous cell carcinoma (particularly in ulcerative lesions)
  - Aphthous ulcers
  - Herpetic stomatitis
  - Secondary syphilis
- Genital mucous membranes
  - Psoriasis (penis and labia)
  - Nonspecific balanitis, Zoon balanitis
  - Fixed drug eruption (penis)
  - Candidiasis (penis and labia)
  - Pemphigus vulgaris, bullous pemphigoid, and Behçet disease (all rare)
- Hair and scalp
  - Scarring alopecia (central centrifugal cicatricial alopecia)

DIAGNOSTIC TESTS & INTERPRETATION

If suggested by history

- Serology for hepatitis
- Liver function tests

Diagnostic Procedures/Other
- Skin biopsy
- Direct immunofluorescence helps to distinguish LP from discoid lupus erythematosus.

Test Interpretation
- Dense, bandlike (lichenoid) lymphocytic infiltrate of the upper dermis
- Vacuolar degeneration of the basal layer
- Hyperkeratosis and irregular acanthosis, increased granular layer
- Basement membrane thinning with "saw-toothing"
- Degenerative keratinocytes, known as colloid or Civatte bodies, are found in the lower epidermis.
- Melanin pigment in macrophages

 TREATMENT

Although LP can resolve spontaneously, treatment is usually requested by patients who may be severely symptomatic or troubled by its cosmetic appearance.

GENERAL MEASURES
- Goal is to relieve itching and resolve lesions.
- Asymptomatic oral lesions require no treatment.

MEDICATION
First Line
- Skin
- Superpotent topical steroids (e.g., 0.05% clobetasol propionate) twice daily.
  - Potent topical steroids such as triamcinolone acetonide 0.1% or fluocinonide 0.05% under occlusion
  - Intralesional corticosteroids (e.g., triamcinolone [Kenalog] 5 to 10 mg/mL) for recalcitrant and hypertrophic lesions
  - Antihistamines (e.g., hydroxyzine, 25 mg PO q6h) have limited benefit for itching but may be helpful for sedation at bedtime.
  - "Soak and smear" technique: can lead to a rapid improvement of symptoms in even 1 to 2 days and may obviate the need for systemic steroids. Soaking allows water to hydrate the stratum corneum and allows the anti-inflammatory steroid in the ointment to penetrate more deeply into the skin. Smearing of the ointment traps the water in the skin because water cannot move out through greasy materials.
    - Soaking is done in a bathtub using lukewarm plain water for 20 minutes, then, without drying the skin, the affected area is immediately smeared with a thin film of the steroid ointment containing clobetasol or another superpotent topical steroid.
    - Soak and smear may be done for 4 to 5 days or longer, if necessary. The treatments are best done at night because the greasy ointment applied to the skin gets on pajamas (instead of on daytime clothes) and the ointment is on the skin during sleep. A topical steroid cream is applied thereafter during the daytime hours, if necessary.
- Mucous membranes
  - For oral, erosive, painful LP, a Cochrane review found at best weak evidence for the effectiveness of any intervention (3)[A].
    - Topical corticosteroids (0.1% triamcinolone [Kenalog] in Orabase) or 0.05% clobetasol propionate ointment BID
    - Intralesional corticosteroids

  - Topical 0.1% tacrolimus (Protopic ointment) BID or 1% pimecrolimus (Elidel) cream BID. A Cochrane review found no evidence that calcineurin inhibitors are better than placebo (4)[A].
  - Topical retinoids (e.g., 0.05% tretinoin [retinoic acid] in Orabase)

Pediatric Considerations
Children may absorb a proportionally larger amount of topical steroid because of larger skin surface-to-weight ratio.

Second Line
Skin and mucous membranes
- Intralesional corticosteroids
- Topical 0.1% tacrolimus (Protopic ointment) BID or topical 1% pimecrolimus (Elidel) cream BID
- Oral prednisone: used only for a short course (e.g., 30 to 60 mg/day for 2 to 4 weeks) or IM triamcinolone (Kenalog) 40 to 80 mg every 6 to 8 weeks
  - Precautions with systemic steroids
    - Systemic absorption of steroids may result in hypothalamic-pituitary-adrenal axis suppression, Cushing syndrome, hyperglycemia, or glucosuria.
    - Increased risk with high-potency topical steroids (i.e., use over large surface area, prolonged use, occlusive dressings)
    - In pregnancy: usually safe, but benefits must outweigh the risks
- Oral retinoids: Isotretinoin in doses of 10 mg PO daily for 2 months, acitretin 30 mg, or alitretinoin 30 mg PO daily have resulted in improvement in some refractory cases. Observe carefully for resultant dyslipidemia.
- Oral metronidazole 500 mg BID for 20 to 60 days can be given as a safer alternative to systemic corticosteroids.
- Cyclosporine may be used in severe cases, but cost and potential toxicity limit its use; topical use for severe oral involvement refractory to other treatments
- Thalidomide
- Psoralen ultraviolet-A (PUVA), broad- or narrow-band ultraviolet B (UVB) (5)[A]
- Griseofulvin (5)[A]
- Azathioprine
- Mycophenolate mofetil
- Metronidazole

ALERT
Avoid oral and topical retinoids during pregnancy.

INPATIENT CONSIDERATIONS
Admission Criteria/Initial Stabilization
Outpatient care

 ONGOING CARE

FOLLOW-UP RECOMMENDATIONS
Patient Monitoring
Serial oral examinations for erosive/ulcerative lesions

PATIENT EDUCATION
- Oral, erosive, or ulcerative LP: annual follow-up to screen for malignancy (6)[A]
- Avoid spicy foods, cigarettes, and excessive alcohol.
- Avoid dry crispy foods such as corn chips, pretzels, and toast.

PROGNOSIS
- Spontaneous resolution in weeks is possible, but disease may persist for years, especially oral lesions and hypertrophic lesions on the shins.
- There is a tendency toward relapse.
- Recurrence in 12–20%, especially in those with generalized involvement

COMPLICATIONS
- Alopecia
- Nail destruction
- Squamous cell carcinoma of the mouth or genitals

REFERENCES
1. Shengyuan L, Songpo Y, Wen W, et al. Hepatitis C virus and lichen planus: a reciprocal association determined by a meta-analysis. *Arch Dermatol*. 2009;145(9):1040–1047.
2. Arias-Santiago S, Buendía-Eisman A, Aneiros-Fernández J, et al. Cardiovascular risk factors in patients with lichen planus. *Am J Med*. 2011;124(6):543–548.
3. Cheng S, Kirtschig G, Cooper S, et al. Interventions for erosive lichen planus affecting mucosal sites. *Cochrane Database Syst Rev*. 2012;(2):CD008092.
4. Thongprasom K, Carrozzo M, Furness S, et al. Interventions for treating oral lichen planus. *Cochrane Database Syst Rev*. 2011;(7):CD001168.
5. Atzmony L, Reiter O, Hodak E, et al. Treatments for cutaneous lichen planus: a systematic review and meta-analysis. *Am J Clin Dermatol*. 2016;17(1):11–22.
6. Fitzpatrick SG, Hirsch SA, Gordon SC. The malignant transformation of oral lichen planus and oral lichenoid lesions: a systematic review. *J Am Dent Assoc*. 2014;145(1):45–56.

ADDITIONAL READING
- Fazel N. Cutaneous lichen planus: a systematic review of treatments. *J Dermatolog Treat*. 2015;26(3):280–283.
- Kolios AG, Marques Maggio E, Gubler C, et al. Oral, esophageal and cutaneous lichen ruber planus controlled with alitretinoin: case report and review of the literature. *Dermatology*. 2013;226(4):302–310.

CODES

ICD10
- L43.9 Lichen planus, unspecified
- L43.0 Hypertrophic lichen planus
- L43.1 Bullous lichen planus

CLINICAL PEARLS
- Remember the 7 P's of LP: **p**urple, **p**lanar, **p**olygonal, **p**olymorphic, **p**ruritic (not always), **p**apules that heal with **p**ostinflammatory hyperpigmentation.
- Serial oral or genital exams are indicated for erosive/ulcerative LP lesions to monitor for the development of squamous cell carcinoma.
- An association has been noted between LP and hepatitis C virus infection, chronic active hepatitis, and primary biliary cirrhosis.
- The "soak and smear" technique can lead to a rapid improvement of symptoms in 1 to 2 days and may obviate the need for systemic steroids.

L

LICHEN SIMPLEX CHRONICUS

Geoffrey Strider Farnsworth, MD

 BASICS

DESCRIPTION
- Lichen simplex chronicus (LSC) is a chronic dermatitis resulting from chronic, repeated rubbing or scratching of the skin. Skin becomes thickened with accentuated lines ("lichenification").
- System(s) affected: skin
- Synonym(s): LSC; lichen simplex; localized neurodermatitis; neurodermatitis circumscripta

EPIDEMIOLOGY

Geriatric Considerations
Most common in middle aged and elderly

Pediatric Considerations
Rare in preadolescents

Incidence
- Common
- Peak incidence 35 to 50 years
- Predominant sex: females > males (2:1)

Prevalence
Common

ETIOLOGY AND PATHOPHYSIOLOGY
- Itch–scratch cycle leads to a chronic dermatosis. Repeated scratching or rubbing causes inflammation and pruritus, which leads to continued scratching.
- Primary LSC: Scratching secondary to nonorganic pruritus, habit or a conditioned response to stress/anxiety
- Common triggers are excess dryness of skin, heat, sweat, and psychological stress.
- Secondary LSC: begins as a pruritic skin disease that evolves into neurodermatitis, which persists after resolution of the primary condition. Precursor dermatoses include atopic dermatitis, contact dermatitis, lichen planus, stasis dermatitis, psoriasis, tinea, and insect bites.
- There is a possible relation between disease development and underlying neuropathy, particularly radiculopathy or nerve root compression.
- Pruritus-specific C neurons are temperature sensitive, which may explain itching that occurs in warm environments.

RISK FACTORS
- Anxiety disorders
- Dry skin
- Insect bites
- Pruritic dermatosis

GENERAL PREVENTION
Avoid common triggers such as psychological distress, environmental factors such as heat and excessive dryness, skin irritation, and the development of pruritic dermatoses.

COMMONLY ASSOCIATED CONDITIONS
- Prurigo nodularis is a nodular variety of the same disease process.
- Atopic dermatitis
- Anxiety, depression, and obsessive-compulsive disorders

 DIAGNOSIS

HISTORY
- Gradual onset
- Begins as a localized area of pruritus
- Most patients acknowledge that they respond with vigorous rubbing, itching, or scratching, which brings temporary satisfaction.
- Pruritus is typically paroxysmal, worse at night, and may lead to scratching during sleep.
- Can be asymptomatic with patient scratching at night while asleep

PHYSICAL EXAM
- Well-circumscribed lichenified plaques with varying amounts of overlying excoriation or scaling
- Lichenification: accentuation of normal skin lines
- Hyperpigmentation or hypopigmentation can be seen.
- Scarring is uncommon with typical LSC; can be seen following ulcer formation or secondary infection.
- Most commonly involves easily accessible areas
  - Lateral portions of lower legs/ankles
  - Nape of neck (lichen simplex nuchae)
  - Vulva/scrotum/anus
  - Extensor surfaces of forearms
  - Palmar wrist
  - Scalp

DIFFERENTIAL DIAGNOSIS
- Lichen sclerosis
- Psoriasis
- Atopic dermatitis
- Contact, irritant, or stasis dermatitis
- Extramammary Paget disease
- Lichen planus
- Mycosis fungoides
- Lichen amyloidosis
- Tinea
- Nummular eczema

DIAGNOSTIC TESTS & INTERPRETATION

Initial Tests (lab, imaging)
- No specific diagnostic test
- Microscopy (i.e., KOH prep) and culture preparation may be helpful in identifying possible bacterial or fungal infection.

Diagnostic Procedures/Other
- Skin biopsy if diagnosis is in question.
- Patch testing may be used to rule out a contact dermatitis.

Test Interpretation
- Hyperkeratosis
- Acanthosis
- Lengthening of rete ridges
- Hyperplasia of all components of epidermis
- Mild to moderate lymphohistiocytic inflammatory infiltrate with prominent lichenification

 TREATMENT

GENERAL MEASURES
- Patient education is critical.
- Low likelihood of resolution if patient unable to avoid scratching.
- Treatment aimed at reducing inflammation and pruritus.

MEDICATION

First Line
- Reducing inflammation
  - Topical steroids are first-line agents (1,2)[C].
  - High-potency steroids alone, such as 0.05% betamethasone dipropionate cream or 0.05% clobetasol propionate cream, can be used initially but should be avoided on the face, anogenital region, or intertriginous areas. They should be used on small areas only, for no longer than 2 weeks except under the close supervision of a physician.
  - Switch to intermediate- or low-potency steroids as response allows.
  - An intermediate-potency steroid, such as 0.1% triamcinolone cream, may be used for initial, brief treatment of the face and intertriginous areas, and for maintenance treatment of other areas.
  - A low-potency steroid, such as 1% hydrocortisone cream, should be used for maintenance treatment of the face and intertriginous areas.
  - Steroid tape, flurandrenolide, has optimized penetration and provides a barrier to continued scratching. Change tape once daily.
  - Intralesional steroids, such as triamcinolone acetate, are also safe and effective for severe cases.
- Preventing scratching
  - Topical antipruritic agents
  - 1st-generation oral antihistamines such as diphenhydramine and hydroxyzine for antipruritic and sedative effects
  - Sedating tricyclics, such as doxepin and amitriptyline, for nighttime itching
  - Itching may occur at night while the patient is asleep; occlusive dressings may be helpful in these cases.

ALERT
High-dose and prolonged treatment with topical steroids can cause dermal/epidermal atrophy as well as pigmentary changes and should not be used on the face, intertriginous areas, or anogenital region. Duration of treatment on other parts of the body should not exceed 3 weeks without close physician supervision.

Second Line
All recommendations
- Topical aspirin has been shown to be helpful in treating neurodermatitis (3)[C].
- Topical 5% doxepin cream has significant antipruritic activity (3)[C].
- Topical capsaicin cream can be helpful for treatment of early disease manifestations (3)[C].

- 0.1% tacrolimus applied twice daily over 6 weeks for as an effective alternative treatment (4)[C]
- Gabapentin was found to decrease symptoms in patients who are nonresponsive to steroids.
- Topical lidocaine can be effective in decreasing neuropathic pruritus (3)[C].
- Intradermal botulinum toxin injections has been reported to improve symptoms in patients with recalcitrant pruritus.
- Transcutaneous electrical nerve stimulation may relieve pruritus in patients for whom topical steroids were not effective (5)[C].
- A case report showed NB-UVB as a possible off-label treatment of refractory LSC (6)[C].
- SSRIs may be effective in controlling compulsive scratching secondary to psychiatric diagnosis.

ISSUES FOR REFERRAL
- No response to treatment
- Presence of signs and symptoms suggestive of a systemic cause of pruritus
- Consultation with a psychiatrist for patients with severe stress, anxiety, or compulsive scratching
- Consultation with an allergist for patients with multisystem atopic symptoms

ADDITIONAL THERAPIES
- Cooling of the skin with ice or cold compresses
- Soaks and lubricants to improve barrier layer function
- Occlusion of lesion with bandages or Unna boots.
- Nail trimming
- Silk underwear to decrease friction in genital LSC.

COMPLEMENTARY & ALTERNATIVE MEDICINE
- Acupuncture has been shown as an effective treatment for pruritus (7)[C].
- Cognitive-behavioral therapy may improve awareness and help to identify coping strategies.
- Hypnosis may be beneficial in decreasing pruritus and preventing scratching.
- Homeopathic remedies (i.e., thuja and graphite) have been used.

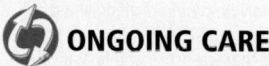 ONGOING CARE

FOLLOW-UP RECOMMENDATIONS
Patient Monitoring
Patients should be followed for response to therapy, complications from therapy (especially topical steroids), and secondary infections.

DIET
Regular balanced diet

PATIENT EDUCATION
- Patients should understand the cause of this disease and the critical role they play in its resolution:
  – Emphasize that scratching and rubbing must stop for lesions to heal. Medications ineffective if scratching continues
- Stress reduction techniques can be useful for patients for whom stress plays a role.
- Avoid exposure to known triggers.

PROGNOSIS
- Often chronic and recurrent
- Good prognosis if the itch–scratch cycle can be broken
- After healing, the skin should return to normal appearance but may also retain accentuated skin markings or post inflammatory pigmentary changes that may be slow to resolve.

COMPLICATIONS
- Secondary infection
- Scarring is rare without ulceration or secondary infection.
- Complications related to therapy, as mentioned in medication precautions
- Squamous cell carcinoma within affected regions is rare.

REFERENCES
1. Lynch PJ. Lichen simplex chronicus (atopic/neurodermatitis) of the anogenital region. *Dermatol Ther*. 2004;17(1):8–19.
2. Datz B, Yawalkar S. A double-blind, multicenter trial of 0.05% halobetasol propionate ointment and 0.05% clobetasol 17-propionate ointment in the treatment of patients with chronic, localized atopic dermatitis or lichen simplex chronicus. *J Am Acad Dermatol*. 1991;25(6 Pt 2):1157–1160.
3. Patel T, Yosipovitch G. Therapy of pruritus. *Expert Opin Pharmacother*. 2010;11(10):1673–1682.
4. Tan ES, Tan AS, Tey HL. Effective treatment of scrotal lichen simplex chronicus with 0.1% tacrolimus ointment: an observational study. *J Eur Acad Dermatol Venereol*. 2015;29(7):1448–1449.
5. Mohammad Ali BM, Hegab DS, El Saadany HM. Use of transcutaneous electrical nerve stimulation for chronic pruritus. *Dermatol Ther*. 2015;28(4):210–215.
6. Virgili A, Minghetti S, Borghi A, et al. Phototherapy for vulvar lichen simplex chronicus: an 'off-label use' of a comb light device. *Photodermatol Photoimmunol Photomed*. 2014;30(6):332–334.
7. Ma C, Sivamani RK. Acupuncture as a treatment modality in dermatology: a systematic review. *J Altern Complement Med*. 2015;21(9):520–529.

ADDITIONAL READING
- Aschoff R, Wozel G. Topical tacrolimus for the treatment of lichen simplex chronicus. *J Dermatolog Treat*. 2007;18(2):115–117.
- Engin B, Tufekci O, Yazici A, et al. The effect of transcutaneous electrical nerve stimulation in the treatment of lichen simplex: a prospective study. *Clin Exp Dermatol*. 2009;34(3):324–328.
- Gencoglan G, Inanir I, Gunduz K. Therapeutic hotline: treatment of prurigo nodularis and lichen simplex chronicus with gabapentin. *Dermatol Ther*. 2010;23(2):194–198.
- Goldstein AT, Parneix-Spake A, McCormick CL, et al. Pimecrolimus cream 1% for treatment of vulvar lichen simplex chronicus: an open-label, preliminary trial. *Gynecol Obstet Invest*. 2007;64(4):180–186.

- Heckmann M, Heyer G, Brunner B, et al. Botulinum toxin type A injection in the treatment of lichen simplex: an open pilot study. *J Am Acad Dermatol*. 2002;46(4):617–619.
- Hercogová J. Topical anti-itch therapy. *Dermatol Ther*. 2005;18(4):341–343.
- Kirtak N, Inaloz HS, Akçali C, et al. Association of serotonin transporter gene-linked polymorphic region and variable number of tandem repeat polymorphism of the serotonin transporter gene in lichen simplex chronicus patients with psychiatric status. *Int J Dermatol*. 2008;47(10):1069–1072.
- Konuk N, Koca R, Atik L, et al. Psychopathology, depression and dissociative experiences in patients with lichen simplex chronicus. *Gen Hosp Psychiatry*. 2007;29(3):232–235.
- Lotti T, Buggiani G, Prignano F. Prurigo nodularis and lichen simplex chronicus. *Dermatol Ther*. 2008;21(1):42–46.
- Shenefelt PD. Biofeedback, cognitive-behavioral methods, and hypnosis in dermatology: is it all in your mind? *Dermatol Ther*. 2003;16(2):114–122.
- Solak O, Kulac M, Yaman M, et al. Lichen simplex chronicus as a symptom of neuropathy. *Clin Exp Dermatol*. 2009;34(4):476–480.
- Wu M, Wang Y, Bu W, et al. Squamous cell carcinoma arising in lichen simplex chronicus. *Eur J Dermatol*. 2010;20(6):858–859.
- Yosipovitch G, Sugeng MW, Chan YH, et al. The effect of topically applied aspirin on localized circumscribed neurodermatitis. *J Am Acad Dermatol*. 2001;45(6):910–913.
- Yüksek J, Sezer E, Aksu M, et al. Transcutaneous electrical nerve stimulation for reduction of pruritus in macular amyloidosis and lichen simplex. *J Dermatol*. 2011;38(6):546–552.

 CODES

ICD10
L28.0 Lichen simplex chronicus

CLINICAL PEARLS
- LSC is a chronic inflammatory condition that results from repeated scratching and rubbing.
- Primary LSC originates de novo, whereas secondary LSC occurs in the setting of a preexisting pruritic dermatologic condition.
- LSC is a clinical diagnosis based on history and skin examination with biopsy only indicated in difficult or unclear cases.
- Stopping the itch–scratch cycle through patient education, skin lubrication, and topical medications is key.
- Treatment aimed at decreasing both inflammation and pruritus utilizing topical steroids and antipruritics.

L

LIPOMA
Bradley M. Turner, MD, MPH, MHA

BASICS

DESCRIPTION
- Lipomas are the most common soft tissue tumor (benign or malignant).
- One of several distinct benign lipomatous tumors. In its most conventional (simple) form, lipomas are composed of mature adipose tissue, typically enveloped by a well-defined thin fibrous capsule.
- Not distinguishable histologically from normal adipose tissue
- Several nonconventional forms of lipomas (less commonly encountered) have been described, which may present in multiple locations, contain varying amounts of both adipose and nonadipose tissue, and/or have more atypical cytologic features.
- These nonconventional variants include chondroid lipoma, myolipoma, lipoblastoma, angiolipoma, spindle cell lipoma/pleomorphic lipoma, intramuscular/intermuscular lipoma, lipoma of tendon sheath and joint, lipoma arborescens, lipomatosis of nerve, diffuse lipomatosis, multiple symmetric lipomatosis, adiposis dolorosa, and hibernoma.
- Typically slow growing, superficial (subcutaneous), and asymptomatic; less commonly presents as a painful (angiolipoma) or deep-seated lesion
- May present as an infiltrative lesion (cellular angiolipoma, diffuse lipomatosis, multiple symmetric lipomatosis (Madelung disease), and adiposis dolorosa (Dercum disease)
- Often found in the upper trunk, especially the shoulders, back, neck, and head; but can be found anywhere in the body
- Lipomas have been reported in anatomic locations as varied as cardiac, intrathoracic, endobronchial, retroperitoneal, breast, calf, thigh, scapular, intraosseous, fingers, palmar, toe, epidural, spinal, intra-articular (knee), parapharyngeal, nasopharyngeal, adrenal, inguinal, bladder, scrotal, ovarian, intracranial, intraneural, and GI tract (most often in the ileum).
- Lipomas can cause respiratory distress due to bronchial obstruction of major airways, GI obstruction or bleeding, neuropathic symptoms from compression in locations such as the forearm or ankle, or cord compression if in dural/medullary components of the spinal cord.
- Must be differentiated from other tumors, particularly liposarcomas, as treatment protocols differ.

EPIDEMIOLOGY
- Lipomas can occur at any age but most commonly occur in middle-aged adults, typically in the 40- to 60-year-old age group.
- Hibernomas typically present in the 3rd decade.
- Conventional lipomas and most variants are rare in children; however, lipoblastoma and diffuse lipomatosis typically present in children <3 years of age.
- No clear gender predilection in conventional lipomas and most variants.
- Females reportedly more commonly diagnosed with chondroid lipoma, myolipoma, and adiposis dolorosa.
- Males reportedly more commonly diagnosed with spindle cell/pleomorphic lipoma, intramuscular/intermuscular lipoma, lipoblastoma, and multiple symmetric lipomatosis.
- Approximately 5% of patients have multiple lipomas.

Incidence
Has been reported as 2.1 per 1,000 individuals per year; however, incidence is difficult to accurately estimate.

Prevalence
Has been reported as present in ~1% the population; however, as with incidence, prevalence is difficult to accurately estimate and is most likely underestimated.

ETIOLOGY AND PATHOPHYSIOLOGY
- The etiology and pathogenesis of lipomas is unclear.
- A pathogenetic link between soft tissue trauma and the formation of lipomas has been suggested.
- Two potential explanations to correlate soft tissue trauma and adipose tissue tumor growth have been proposed:
  - Formation of so-called posttraumatic pseudolipomas by prolapsing adipose tissue through fascia resulting from direct impact
  - Lipoma formation as a result of preadipocyte differentiation and proliferation mediated by cytokine release following soft tissue trauma and hematoma formation

Genetics
- Approximately 2/3 of lipomas demonstrate chromosomal aberrations.
- The most common chromosomal aberrations are rearrangements of the chromatin remodeling gene *HMGA2* on chromosome 12q15 (67%).
- Less common chromosomal aberrations include anomalies of the 13q12–22 region (15%) and rearrangements of the 6p21 region (5%).
- Frequent association of chromosomal aberrations in the long arm of chromosomes 13 and 16 with spindle cell/pleomorphic lipomas
- Consistent chromosomal aberrations identified in the long arm of chromosome 11 with hibernomas
- Various case reports of other chromosomal aberrations exist.

RISK FACTORS
- Because the pathogenesis of lipomas is unclear, risk factors are difficult to qualify.
- Possible risk factors include obesity, alcohol abuse, liver disease, glucose intolerance, and soft tissue trauma (see "Etiology and Pathophysiology").

COMMONLY ASSOCIATED CONDITIONS
May appear as part of a hereditary syndrome: Dercum disease, Madelung syndrome (also known as Launois-Bensaude syndrome), Gardner syndrome, Cowden syndrome, and Bannayan-Riley-Ruvalcaba syndrome (children)

DIAGNOSIS

HISTORY
- Useful questions on history are duration, associated symptoms, tenderness, recurrence, progression, similar lesions, and weight loss.
- Lipomas are generally slow growing—if the presenting lesion is fast growing, suspect another diagnosis.

PHYSICAL EXAM
- Lipomas are usually soft, homogenous, oval, and nontender, with a rubbery or doughy consistency; if hard, suspect another diagnosis.
- The overlying skin is typically mobile and normal in appearance; if erythematous, suspect another diagnosis such as infection.

- Lipomas are commonly ≤5 cm in diameter. If larger, this raises suspicion for liposarcoma (1), although lipomas can be >10 cm (2,3).

DIFFERENTIAL DIAGNOSIS
- Differential diagnosis includes a variety of benign and malignant tumors (1,4).
- The most common considerations include epidermal inclusion cyst, trichilemmal cysts, hematoma, vasculitis, panniculitis, rheumatic nodules, abscess/infection, and malignant disease.
- Trichilemmal cysts can often be differentiated from lipomas by their characteristic central punctum and surrounding induration.
- An abscess typically has pain, along with overlying induration and erythema.
- Diagnosis may be more challenging with other lesions, particularly deeper-seated lesions.
- Imaging, core needle biopsy, or excision can be useful in further clarifying the diagnosis (1–4).

DIAGNOSTIC TESTS & INTERPRETATION
Patients presenting with smaller (≤5 cm) subcutaneous lesions that are clinically considered lipomas typically will not receive preoperative imaging. Larger lesions with irregular shape and/or suggestion of myofascial involvement should receive preoperative imaging (1)[A].

Initial Tests (lab, imaging)
- Because of differences in treatment, prognosis, and long-term follow-up, it is important to preoperatively distinguish lipomas from liposarcomas and other malignant lesions (2–6). If there is doubt regarding nature of the lipoma, further testing is indicated.
- US, MRI, or CT can be used in the suspected diagnosis of lipoma (1,2).
- US may be limited with larger lesions or lesions which have atypical patterns (2).
- MRI is the most sensitive imaging modality for lipomatous masses, has a high negative predictive value (1)[A], and can be useful when US is equivocal (2)[A].
- MRI can be extremely helpful in distinguishing a lipoma from a liposarcoma (1,2)[B], although lipoma variants may show characteristics of a liposarcoma due to the presence of decreased adipose tissue, nonadipose tissue, and/or irregular margins.
- MRI findings suggestive of liposarcoma include nonadipose areas, a partially ill-defined margin, neurovascular involvement, enhancing thick/nodular septum, a bright signal intensity on T1-weighted images that are not completely suppressed on T1 fat suppression images, and a high T2 signal within the lesion (1–3).

Diagnostic Procedures/Other
- If diagnosis is in doubt, an open surgical incisional biopsy has traditionally been considered the "gold standard" to obtain a histologic diagnosis (4).
- A core-needle biopsy has been proposed as a preferred biopsy method that can provide accurate diagnosis and assessment of malignant potential if examined by an experienced pathologist (4)[C].
- Fine needle aspiration cytology is not considered appropriate for the initial diagnostic evaluation of mesenchymal tumors (4).

Test Interpretation

- Pathologic interpretation is still generally considered as the "gold standard" of diagnosis (1,4).
- Lipomas are typically composed of benign adipose tissue, with inconspicuous nuclei, and varying amounts of connective tissue.
- Lipomas are typically surrounded by a fibrous, well-defined thin capsule that is separate from the surrounding tissue; however, this may not be present on the microscopic tissue due to sampling bias.
- Atypical features such as prominent or atypical nuclei, inflammation, fibrosis, and necrosis may be present and may be mistaken for atypical features seen in atypical lipomatous tumor/well-differentiated liposarcoma (ALT/WDL) (5).
- Pathologists may overcall a diagnosis of ALT/WDL in lipomas with atypical features (1,5,6).
- Complementary molecular testing may augment histologic diagnosis in challenging cases, as *MDM2* gene amplification is not present in benign lipomas but has been reported to be a highly sensitive marker in ALT/WDL (3,5,6)[B].

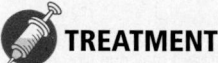

TREATMENT

- If diagnostically certain that the lesion is a benign lipoma, observation is a consideration.
- Treatment of lipoma typically consists of surgical excision; however, advances in medical treatment can shrink lipomas (1)[A].
- Treatments like steroid injection or liposuction can be cosmetically useful in superficial lesions, particularly in locations where scars should be avoided (1)[A], although liposuction has not always been associated with the best aesthetic outcomes (1)[C].
- A successful trial of lipomas treated with subcutaneous deoxycholate injections has been reported, suggesting that low-concentration deoxycholate may be a relatively safe and effective treatment for small collections of adipose tissue (1)[C].
- Indications for removal of a suspected lipoma include diagnostic uncertainty, cosmetic concerns, nerve impingement, pain, increase in size, irregular characteristics, size >5 cm, samples of a core needle biopsy consistent with atypical features, or features consistent with a sarcoma (1)[A].

SURGERY/OTHER PROCEDURES

- Surgical removal techniques include enucleation/excisional biopsy and open incisional biopsy (1,4).
- In uncomplicated cases, the excision can be performed in the office or in the minor procedure room under local anesthetic.
- Plan the incision to follow skin lines, if possible, to minimize scarring. Use a surgical marker to draw out the palpable margins of the lipoma and the planned incision. The incision should be ~50–75% of the length of the lipoma along Langer lines (defined as parallel skin creases correlating with the direction of least elasticity) (1)[C].
- After anesthetizing the skin with a local anesthetic, a linear incision is carried out down to the level of the capsule using a number 11 or 15 blade.
- Blunt dissection (curved hemostat) and sharp dissection (iris scissor) are used to separate the fibrous capsule from the surrounding soft tissue. Care must be taken not to invade the capsule to maintain proper aesthetics (1).

- As the lobule is lifted, the dissection is continued to free up the entire tumor.
- Apply pressure to the outside of the lipoma to express it through the skin opening. In many cases, the lipoma will simply pop out. If not, more dissection may be needed, or the incision may need to be lengthened.
- After the lipoma is out, pressure with gauze is usually all that is needed to obtain good hemostasis. If bleeding persists, use electrocoagulation before closing the incision (1).
- If necessary, dead space may be closed with deep absorbable sutures. The skin may be closed with nonabsorbable simple interrupted sutures or skin adhesive.
- A minimal scar technique to facilitate removal from a small incision using segmental dissection of the lipoma has been described (1)[B].
- It is advisable to send all biopsied tissue to pathology (1)[C].

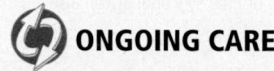 ONGOING CARE

FOLLOW-UP RECOMMENDATIONS
Usual surgical follow-up is needed to monitor for any complications.

PATIENT EDUCATION
Handout: "What are lipomas?" *Am Fam Physician*. 2002;65(5):905. Available at: http://www.aafp.org/afp/20020301/905ph.html

PROGNOSIS
Most lipomas grow very slowly, are asymptomatic, and remain stable. Recurrence after excision is rare (1–2%), unless the excision was incomplete.

COMPLICATIONS
- Hematoma and seroma formation are the most common complications.
- Infection is rare but possible.
- The risk of recurrence is greatest with intramuscular lipomas and lipomas with infiltrating tendencies (cellular angiolipoma, diffuse lipomatosis, multiple symmetric lipomatosis, and adiposis dolorosa).
- Occasionally, a bilobar lipoma may be missed, resulting in "recurrence."

REFERENCES

1. Pandya KA, Radke F. Benign skin lesions: lipomas, epidermal inclusion cysts, muscle and nerve biopsies. *Surg Clin North Am*. 2009;89(3):677–687.
2. Strauss DC, Qureshi YA, Hayes AJ, et al. The role of core needle biopsy in the diagnosis of suspected soft tissue tumours. *J Surg Oncol*. 2010;102(5):523–529.
3. Jaovisidha S, Suvikapakornkul Y, Woratanarat P, et al. MR imaging of fat-containing tumours: the distinction between lipoma and liposarcoma. *Singapore Med J*. 2010;51(5):418–423.
4. Brisson M, Kashima T, Delaney D, et al. MRI characteristics of lipoma and atypical lipomatous tumor/well-differentiated liposarcoma: retrospective comparison with histology and MDM2 gene amplification. *Skeletal Radiol*. 2013;42(5):635–647.
5. Zhang H, Erickson-Johnson M, Wang X, et al. Molecular testing for lipomatous tumors: critical analysis and test recommendations based on the analysis of 405 extremity-based tumors. *Am J Surg Pathol*. 2010;34(9):1304–1311.
6. Weaver J, Downs-Kelly E, Goldblum JR, et al. Fluorescence in situ hybridization for MDM2 gene amplification as a diagnostic tool in lipomatous neoplasms. *Mod Pathol*. 2008;21(8):943–949.

ADDITIONAL READING

- Aust MC, Spies M, Kall S, et al. Posttraumatic lipoma: fact or fiction? *Skinmed*. 2007;6(6):266–270.
- Bancroft LW, Kransdorf MJ, Peterson JJ, et al. Benign fatty tumors: classification, clinical course, imaging appearance, and treatment. *Skeletal Radiol*. 2006;35(10):719–733.
- Gaskin CM, Helms CA. Lipomas, lipoma variants, and well-differentiated liposarcomas (atypical lipomas): results of MRI evaluations of 126 consecutive fatty masses. *AJR Am J Roentgenol*. 2004;182(3):733–739.
- Liang CW, Mariño-Enríquez A, Johannessen C, et al. Translocation (Y;12) in lipoma. *Cancer Genetics*. 2011;204(1):53–56.
- Macchia G, Nord KH, D'Alessandro G, et al. Rearrangements of chromosome bands 15q12-q21 are secondary to HMGA2 deregulation in conventional lipoma. *Oncol Rep*. 2014;31(2):807–811.
- Rotunda AM, Ablon G, Kolodney MS. Lipomas treated with subcutaneous deoxycholate injections. *J Am Acad Dermatol*. 2005;53(6):973–978.
- Salam GA. Lipoma excision. *Am Fam Physician*. 2002;65(5):901–904.

 CODES

ICD10
- D17.9 Benign lipomatous neoplasm, unspecified
- D17.79 Benign lipomatous neoplasm of other sites
- D17.1 Benign lipomatous neoplasm of skin, subcu of trunk

CLINICAL PEARLS

- Lipomas are slow growing, often asymptomatic, and typically diagnosed without imaging or biopsy.
- Asymptomatic subcutaneous lipomas can be followed clinically unless there is diagnostic uncertainty, they are causing cosmetic or pain problems, are large (>5 cm) or growing rapidly, or causing compression of vital organs/nerves.
- Most symptomatic lipomas are removed surgically. With the appropriate indications, nonsurgical options are available.
- In uncomplicated cases, excision can be performed in the office setting and do not require preoperative testing.
- Consider referral to a subspecialist if a lipoma is in a delicate anatomic location or if there is a concern that the lesion might be malignant.

L

LONG QT INTERVAL
Carl Bryce, MD, Capt, USAF • Matthew J. Snyder, DO

 BASICS

DESCRIPTION
- QT interval: electrocardiogram (ECG) measurement that measures the duration of repolarization of myocardial cells. Measured from the onset of the QRS complex to the end of the T wave
- Corrected QT interval (QTc): QT interval corrected for heart rate (interval shortens with increased rate). See formulas.
- Prolonged QTc is generally defined as >470 ms for adult males and >480 ms for adult females (1):
  - 440 to 460 ms considered borderline in men
  - 440 to 470 ms considered borderline in women
  - 440 to 460 ms considered borderline in children aged 1 to 15 years old (2)
- Most cases of prolonged QT are acquired, but genetic mutations can also cause hereditary long QT syndromes (LQTS).
- Prolonged QTc from any cause can precipitate polymorphic ventricular tachycardia (VT) called torsade de pointes (TdP), leading to dizziness, syncope, and sudden cardiac death from ventricular fibrillation (VF).

EPIDEMIOLOGY
Incidence
Incidence of medication-induced QTc prolongation and TdP varies with medication and a host of other factors. Exact incidences are difficult to estimate but may be 1:2,000 to 1:2,500. (1).

Prevalence
- Hereditary LQTS is estimated to occur in 1/2,500 to 1/7,000 births.
- Five thousand people across the United States may die yearly due to LQTS-related cardiac arrhythmia (2).

ETIOLOGY AND PATHOPHYSIOLOGY
- Acquired
  - Electrolyte abnormalities such as hypokalemia, hypomagnesemia
  - Hypothyroidism
  - Underlying heart disease
  - Medications (3)[A]
    - Antiarrhythmic medications (quinidine, procainamide, dofetilide, sotalol, disopyramide, and amiodarone)
    - Antipsychotic medications, especially if given IV (haloperidol*, chlorpromazine*, thioridazine*, pimozide*)
    - Many antidepressants (SSRIs, SNRIs, trazodone, TCAs)
    - Antibiotics/antivirals/antifungals (clarithromycin*, erythromycin* which are also CYP3A4 inhibitors)
    - Antiemetics (metoclopramide, ondansetron, promethazine)
    - Opioids (methadone*, buprenorphine)
    - Antihistamines (cetirizine, hydroxyzine, diphenhydramine)
    - Decongestants (pseudoephedrine, phenylephrine)
    - Stimulants (albuterol, phentermine)
    - Misc: chloroquine*, pentamidine*
    - *Denote "high-risk" medication for TdP.
- Congenital
  - Defective membrane proteins that work as channels for sodium and potassium in myocytes

- Pathophysiology
  - Depolarization of the myocardium results from the rapid influx of sodium through sodium channels and causes myocyte contraction, with resulting cardiac muscle contraction and systole (seen on ECG as the QRS complex).
  - During repolarization, there is an efflux of potassium from the cell through both rapid (I_{Kr}) and slow (I_{Ks}) potassium channels. The T wave on an ECG represents myocyte repolarization.
  - Drug-induced QT prolongation due to blockade of I_{Kr} leading to delayed repolarization (2).
  - Medications, medical conditions, electrolyte disturbances, and genetic mutations that affect functioning of these membrane channels can cause delayed repolarization.
  - Delayed repolarization can lead to a propensity for reentry and initiate TdP.
  - TdP type rhythm may be self-limited but symptomatic (syncope or near syncope). It can also degrade into VF.

Genetics
- 12 different genes have been linked to LQTS (3).
- Incomplete penetrance makes both diagnosis and management of asymptomatic disease challenging.
- LQTS 1 (42–54%) is the most common. Mutation causes a defect in the I_{Ks} transport protein. Arrhythmias can be triggered by tachycardia due to exercise (swimming seems to be especially problematic) and other high catecholamine states.
- LQTS 2 (35–45%) is a defect in the I_{Kr} transport protein that is sensitive to catecholamine surges. Sudden loud noises or emotional arousal can provoke arrhythmias.
- LQTS 3 (8%) is a defect in the sodium channel that allows an excess of sodium into the cell, increasing repolarization time. Arrhythmias tend to manifest more during rest or sleep.
- Jervell and Lange-Nielsen syndrome: Autosomal recessive form of LQTS that features homozygous mutations affect the I_{Ks} channel and presents with severe form of LQTS 1. Features also include deafness.
- Romano-Ward syndrome: autosomal dominant form of LQTS with variable penetrance. Hearing is normal.

RISK FACTORS
For the feared complication, TdP, risk factors include the following (3):
- Female (~2 times increased risk)
- QTc >500 ms (2 to 3 times increased risk)
- QTc >60 ms over previous baseline
- History of syncope or presyncope
- History of TdP
- Bradycardia
- Liver or kidney disease (by increasing blood levels of QT prolonging medications)
- Medications that cause QTc prolongation
  - High doses
  - Fast infusions
  - Combination of medications
- Electrolyte abnormalities
  - Hypokalemia
  - Hypomagnesemia
  - Hypocalcemia
- For hereditary LQTS
  - Catecholamine surges from exercise (especially swimming), emotional stress, loud noises

GENERAL PREVENTION
- Avoid (or use with caution) causative medications, including combinations with potentially additive effects. Replete electrolytes (goal Mg >2, K 4.5 to 5.0) (4)[C]
- Treat underlying medical disease (hypothyroidism, cardiac disease).
- Avoid strenuous sports in LQTS.
- Avoid sudden loud noises in LQTS (alarm clocks, doorbells, telephones).
- 36th Bethesda Conference recommends restriction of athletes from participation to class 1A activities (e.g., bowling, golf, riflery) although evidence regarding safe participation is emerging (1)[C].

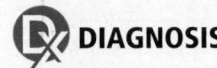 **DIAGNOSIS**

HISTORY
- Evaluate for syncope, near syncope, and associated precipitating events (such as emotional triggers, swimming, diving).
- Evaluate for history of seizures in patient or in family (tonic–clonic movement may due to cerebral hypoperfusion during episodes of ventricular arrhythmia or due to seizure-like activity during a syncopal episode.).
- Detailed medication history
- Evaluate for family history of sudden death and syncope.
- Congenital deafness

PHYSICAL EXAM
- Usually normal physical exam
- If underlying cardiac disease present, may have findings specific to cardiac condition
- Evaluate for signs of hypothyroidism.
- Congenital deafness may be present in some forms of LQTS.

DIAGNOSTIC TESTS & INTERPRETATION
Initial Tests (lab, imaging)
- ECG
- Metabolic panel
- Calcium level
- Magnesium level
- TSH

Follow-Up Tests & Special Considerations
- Echocardiogram to evaluate for cardiomyopathy
- Outpatient cardiac rhythm monitoring
- Consider provocative testing (epinephrine infusion, exercise stress testing) to evaluate for QTc interval changes and/or to evaluate for coronary artery disease (2)[C].
  - Genetic testing for LQTS mutations

Test Interpretation
- QTc calculation using ECG is best done by measuring the QT interval in lead II and measuring the RR interval immediately preceding this QT interval. The Bazett formula is commonly used, although it overcorrects for tachycardia and undercorrects for bradycardia (2).
- Bazett formula: $QTc = QT/\sqrt{(RR)}$ (all measurements in seconds, and RR obtained by direct measurement or 60/heart rate)
- Fridericia formula is similar to Bazett but uses a cube root instead of a square root of the RR interval. $QTc = QT/(RR)^{1/3}$

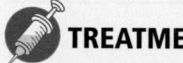 **TREATMENT**

GENERAL MEASURES
- VT, TdP, and VF should be treated emergently as per ACLS guidelines.
- Cardiac pacing may be needed emergently for drug-induced TdP to prevent bradycardia.
- Withdraw offending agents, correct electrolytes (2)[C].

MEDICATION
First Line
- For Tdp: magnesium sulfate 2 g infused over 2 to 15 minutes, followed by continuous infusion of 2 to 4 mg/min if needed. Monitor for magnesium toxicity in those with renal insufficiency (2)[C].
- For hereditary LQTS, to prevent life-threatening arrhythmias: Propranolol or nadolol are generally regarded as the best β-blockers for management of LQTS, though rigorous studies are lacking (4)[B].
- β-Blockers are effective in decreasing but not eliminating the risk of fatal arrhythmias.
- For high-risk patients or those who remain symptomatic on a β-blocker, implantable cardiac defibrillators (ICDs) with or without pacemaker is an important consideration (2)[B].

Second Line
- Atenolol or metoprolol may be used, although switching from other β-blockers may precipitate lethal or near-lethal events (4)[B].

ISSUES FOR REFERRAL
- Refer to cardiologist for establishing diagnosis, especially for hereditary LQTS.
- Symptomatic prolonged QT

SURGERY/OTHER PROCEDURES
- ICD for those with a history of major cardiac events
- Left cervical-thoracic sympathetic denervation was used for symptomatic LQTS prior to the advent of β-blockers. It is still an option for those patients with LQTS who are refractory to β-blocker therapy (3)[B].

INPATIENT CONSIDERATIONS
Admission Criteria/Initial Stabilization
- Patients with TdP, VT, and VF should be promptly treated as per ACLS guidelines. Correct electrolytes on an emergent basis. Evaluate for acquired QT prolongation. If no cause is found, consider hereditary LQTS.
- Patients with prolonged QTc and syncope/near syncope should be monitored on telemetry during evaluation.
- Monitor ECG if initiating medications or combining medications that may prolong QT, suggest at baseline, within 30 days, and then annually (3)[C].
- Monitor electrolytes and urgently treat hypomagnesemia and hypokalemia in those with significantly prolonged QT, and discontinue or change offending medications (5)[C].

Nursing
- Avoid sudden loud noises or emotional stress for those who have LQTS.
- Review adherence to β-blocker therapy.
- Notify others if telemetry monitoring reveals prolonged QT interval in hospitalized patients—they are at risk for poor outcomes (6).

 ONGOING CARE

FOLLOW-UP RECOMMENDATIONS
On routine visits, ask about syncope, presyncope, and palpitations in those who have QTc prolongation.
- Patient monitoring: Consider ECG and/or outpatient cardiac rhythm monitoring with any medication additions or dosage changes that may cause further prolongation of the QTc.
- For those who may have symptomatic QTc prolongation of any cause, prompt evaluation is warranted.
- Check labs for electrolyte imbalances, correct as needed.

PATIENT EDUCATION
- Educate patients with QTc prolongation about medications side effects and possibility of medication interactions.
- Patients with congenital forms of LQTS should be aware of, and avoid situations that may trigger torsade (depending on their specific gene mutation)
- Large emotional and psychological impact of diagnosis. Additional reading by Fortescue shares personal impact of LQTS.
- Information and support from groups listed (see "Additional Reading") may be helpful.

PROGNOSIS
Untreated, quite poor. Perhaps 20% of untreated patients presenting with syncope die within 1 year, 50% within 10 years (3).

REFERENCES
1. Abrams DJ, Macrae CA. Long QT syndrome. *Circulation*. 2014;129(14):1524–1529.
2. Kallergis EM, Goudis CA, Simantirakis EN, et al. Mechanisms, risk factors, and management of acquired long QT syndrome: a comprehensive review. *ScientificWorldJournal*. 2012;2012:212178.
3. Clarke CJ, McDaniel GM. The risk of long QT syndrome in the pediatric population. *Curr Opin Pediatr*. 2009;21(5):573–578.
4. Wilde AA, Ackerman MJ. Beta-blockers in the treatment of congenital long QT syndrome: is one beta-blocker superior to another? *J Am Coll Cardiol*. 2014;64(13):1359–1361.
5. QT prolongation, torsades de pointes, and medication safety. *Pharmacist's Letter/Prescriber's Letter*. 2010;26(4):260421.
6. Laksman Z, Momciu B, Seong YW, et al. A detailed description and assessment of outcomes of patients with hospital recorded QTc prolongation. *Am J Cardiol*. 2015;115(7):907–911.

ADDITIONAL READING
- Chockalingam P, Crotti L, Girardengo G, et al. Not all beta-blockers are equal in the management of long QT syndrome types 1 and 2: higher recurrence of events under metoprolol. *J Am Coll Cardiol*. 2012;60(20):2092–2099.
- Fortescue EB. A piece of my mind. Keeping the pace. *JAMA*. 2014;311(23):2383–2384.
- Levine E, Rosero SZ, Budzikowski AS, et al. Congenital long QT syndrome: considerations for primary care physicians. *Cleve Clin J Med*. 2008;75(8):591–600.
- Morita H, Wu J, Zipes DP. The QT syndromes: long and short. *Lancet*. 2008;372(9640):750–763.
- van Noord C, Eijgelsheim M, Stricker BH. Drug- and non-drug-associated QT interval prolongation. *Br J Clin Pharmacol*. 2010;70(1):16–23.
- Webster G, Berul CI. Congenital long-QT syndromes: a clinical and genetic update from infancy through adulthood. *Trends Cardiovasc Med*. 2008;18(6):216–224.
- Yap YG, Camm AJ. Drug induced QT prolongation and torsades de pointes. *Heart*. 2003;89(11):1363–1372.
- http://www.crediblemeds.org (Medication lists and additional resources related to long QT and torsade de pointes)
- Cardiac Arrhythmias Research and Education Foundation (http://www.longqt.org)
- Sudden Arrhythmia Death Syndromes Foundation (http://www.sads.org)

 SEE ALSO

Algorithms: Cardiac Arrhythmias; Arrhythmias, Torsade de Pointes Ventricular Tachycardia

 CODES

ICD10
I45.81 Long QT syndrome

CLINICAL PEARLS
- Evaluate for acquired causes before making a diagnosis of hereditary LQTS.
- For accurate diagnosis, calculate QTc manually.
- The ideal management of TdP is prevention; avoid multiple "stacking" risk factors and seek alternates to high-risk medications, correct electrolytes, and monitor treatment with serial ECGs if no alternatives exist.
- Magnesium sulfate is the treatment of choice during ACLS for TdP.
- β-Blockers are initial treatment of choice for hereditary LQTS.

LUNG, PRIMARY MALIGNANCIES
Maryann R. Cooper, PharmD, BCOP • Gerald Gehr, MD

BASICS

DESCRIPTION
- Lung cancers (primary) are the leading cause of cancer-related death in the United States (estimated 159,260 deaths in 2015, 27% of all cancer-related deaths).
- Divided into two broad categories
  - Non–small cell lung cancer (NSCLC) (>85% of all lung cancers)
    - Adenocarcinoma (~40% of NSCLC): Most common type in the United States, most common type in nonsmokers, metastasizes earlier than squamous cell, poor prognosis; bronchoalveolar, a subtype of adenocarcinoma has better prognosis.
    - Squamous cell carcinoma (<25% of NSCLC): dose-related effect with smoking; slower growing than adenocarcinoma
    - Large cell (~10% of NSCLC): prognosis similar to adenocarcinoma
  - Small cell lung cancer (SCLC) (16% of all lung cancers): centrally located, early metastases, aggressive
- Other: mesothelioma, carcinoid tumor, and sarcoma
- Staging
  - NSCLC: staged from 0 to IV based on: primary tumor (T), lymph node status (N), and presence of metastasis (M)
  - SCLC: staged based on disease location: limited to ipsilateral hemithorax (stages I–IIIB); extensive if metastatic beyond hemithorax (stages IIIB and IV)
- Tumor locations: upper: 60%; lower: 30%; middle: 5%; overlapping and main stem: 5%
- May spread by local extension to involve chest wall, diaphragm, pulmonary vessels, vena cava, phrenic nerve, esophagus, or pericardium
- Most commonly metastasize to lymph nodes (pulmonary, mediastinal), then liver, adrenal, bone (osteolytic), kidney, brain

EPIDEMIOLOGY
Incidence
- Estimated 224,210 new cases in the United States in 2015
- Predominant age: >40 years; peak at 70 years
- Predominant sex: male > female

Prevalence
- Most common cancer worldwide
- Lifetime probability: men: 1 in 13; women: 1 in 16

ETIOLOGY AND PATHOPHYSIOLOGY
Multifactorial; see "Risk Factors."

Genetics
NSCLC
- Oncogenes: Ras family (H-ras, K-ras, N-ras)
- Tumor suppressor genes: retinoblastoma, *p53*

RISK FACTORS
- Smoking (relative risk [RR] 10 to 30)
- Secondhand smoke exposure
- Radon
- Environmental and occupational exposures
  - Asbestos exposure (synergistic increase in risk for smokers)
  - Air pollution
  - Ionizing radiation
  - Mutagenic gases (halogen ethers, mustard gas, aromatic hydrocarbons)
  - Metals (inorganic arsenic, chromium, nickel)

- Lung scarring from tuberculosis
- Radiation therapy to the breast or chest

GENERAL PREVENTION
- Smoking cessation and prevention programs
- Screening recommended by USPSTF but remains controversial; the risks of screening (e.g., radiation, biopsy) may offset the benefit (1)[A].
- Annual screening with low-dose computed tomography in adults ages 55 to 80 years who have a 30 pack-year smoking history and currently smoke or have quit within the past 15 years
- Screening should be discontinued once a person has not smoked for 15 years or develops a health problem that substantially limits life expectancy or the ability or willingness to have curative lung surgery.
- Prevention via aggressive smoking cessation counseling and therapy; a 20–30% risk reduction occurs within 5 years of cessation.
- Avoid supplemental β-carotene and vitamin E in smokers.
- Avoid hormone replacement therapy in postmenopausal smokers or former smokers (increased risk of death from NSCLC).

COMMONLY ASSOCIATED CONDITIONS
- Paraneoplastic syndromes: hypertrophic pulmonary osteoarthropathy, Lambert-Eaton syndrome, Cushing syndrome, hypercalcemia from ectopic parathyroid-releasing hormone, syndrome of inappropriate antidiuretic hormone (SIADH)
- Hypercoagulable state
- Pancoast syndrome
- Superior vena cava syndrome
- Pleural effusion
- Chronic obstructive pulmonary disease (COPD), other sequelae of cigarette smoking

DIAGNOSIS

HISTORY
- May be asymptomatic for most of course
- Pulmonary
  - Cough (new or change in chronic cough)
  - Wheezing and stridor
  - Dyspnea
  - Hemoptysis
  - Pneumonitis (fever and productive cough)
- Constitutional
  - Malaise
  - Bone pain (metastatic disease)
  - Fatigue
  - Weight loss, anorexia
  - Fever
  - Anemia
  - Clubbing of digits
- Other presentations:
  - Chest pain (dull, pleuritic)
  - Shoulder/arm pain (Pancoast tumors)
  - Dysphagia
  - Plethora (redness of face or neck)
  - Hoarseness (involvement of recurrent laryngeal nerve)
  - Horner syndrome
  - Neurologic abnormalities (e.g., headaches, syncope, weakness, cognitive impairment)
  - Pericardial tamponade (pericardial invasion)

PHYSICAL EXAM
- General: pain, performance status, weight loss
- Head, eye, ear, nose, throat (HEENT): Horner syndrome, dysphonia, stridor, scleral icterus
- Neck: supraclavicular/cervical lymph nodes, mass
- Lungs: effusion, wheezing, airway obstruction, pleural effusion
- Abdomen/groin: hepatomegaly or lymphadenopathy
- Extremities: signs of hypertrophic pulmonary osteoarthropathy, deep venous thrombosis (DVT)
- Neurologic: Rule out cognitive and focal motor defects.

DIFFERENTIAL DIAGNOSIS
- COPD (may coexist)
- Granulomatous (tuberculosis, sarcoidosis)
- Cardiomyopathy
- Congestive heart failure (CHF)

DIAGNOSTIC TESTS & INTERPRETATION
Initial Tests (lab, imaging)
- CBC
- BUN, serum creatinine
- Liver function tests (LFTs), lactate dehydrogenase (LDH)
- Electrolytes
  - Hypercalcemia (Paraneoplastic syndrome)
  - Hyponatremia (SIADH)
- Sputum cytology
- Chest x-ray (CXR) (compare with old films)
  - Nodule or mass, especially if calcified
  - Persistent infiltrate
  - Atelectasis
  - Mediastinal widening
  - Hilar enlargement
  - Pleural effusion
- CT scan of chest (with IV contrast material)
  - Nodule or mass (central or peripheral)
  - Lymphadenopathy
- Evaluation for metastatic disease
  - Brain MRI: Lesions may be necrotic, bleeding.
  - CT abdomen: hepatic, adrenal, renal masses
- Positron emission tomography (PET) scan: to evaluate metastasis
- Bone scan: advanced disease or bone pain

Follow-Up Tests & Special Considerations
CBC, BUN, serum creatinine, LFTs prior to each cycle of chemotherapy

Diagnostic Procedures/Other
- Biopsy with pathology review
- In patients with advanced NSCLC, determination of epidermal growth factor receptor (EGFR)-activating mutations, *KRAS/NRAS* mutations, and *ALK* gene rearrangements in patients with nonsquamous or mixed squamous histology
- Pulmonary function tests
- Enlarged mediastinal lymph nodes necessitate staging by mediastinoscopy, video-assisted thoracoscopy, or fine needle aspiration.
- Transbronchial biopsy (Wang needle)
- Bronchoscopy for surgical planning
- Bone marrow aspirate (small cell)
- Cervical mediastinoscopy (the upper, middle peritracheal, and subcarinal lymph nodes)
- Anterior mediastinotomy (the posterior mediastinum and peritracheal, subazygous, hilar, and aortopulmonary window nodal regions)
- Video-assisted thoracoscopy (associated pleural disease and suspected mediastinal nodal spread)

Test Interpretation

Pathologic changes from smoking are progressive: basal cell proliferation, development of atypical nuclei, stratification, metaplasia of squamous cells, carcinoma in situ, and then invasive disease.

 TREATMENT

GENERAL MEASURES

- NSCLC
  - Stage I, stage II, and selected stage III tumors are surgically resectable. Neoadjuvant or adjuvant therapy is recommended for many patients with high risk IB, II, and III NSCLC. Patients with resectable disease who are not surgical candidates may receive curative radiation therapy.
  - Patients with unresectable or N2, N3 disease are treated with concurrent chemoradiation. Selected patients with T3 or N2 disease can be treated effectively with surgical resection and either pre- or postoperative chemotherapy or chemoradiation therapy.
  - Patients with distant metastases (M1) can be treated with radiation therapy or chemotherapy for palliation or best supportive care alone.
- SCLC
  - Limited stage: concurrent chemoradiation
  - Extensive stage: combination chemotherapy
  - Consider prophylactic cranial irradiation (PCI) in patients achieving a complete or partial response (2)[A].
- Quality-of-life assessments: Karnofsky performance scale (KPS), Eastern Cooperative Oncology Group (ECOG)
- Discussions with patient and family about end-of-life care

MEDICATION

- Chemotherapy is the mainstay of treatment.
- Adjuvant chemotherapy following surgery improves survival in patients with fully resected stage II–III NSCLC.
- Palliative measures: analgesics
- Dyspnea: oxygen, morphine

First Line

- NSCLC
  - Stages II–III: neoadjuvant or adjuvant chemotherapy (3,4)[A]
    - Cisplatin-based doublets (combination with paclitaxel, etoposide, vinorelbine, docetaxel, gemcitabine)
    - Carboplatin alternative for patients unlikely to tolerate cisplatin
    - Cisplatin plus pemetrexed (nonsquamous cell)
  - Unresectable stage IIA, IIIB
    - Concurrent chemoradiation
      - Cisplatin plus etoposide, vinblastine, or pemetrexed (nonsquamous cell) plus concurrent radiation
      - Carboplatin plus pemetrexed (nonsquamous cell) plus concurrent radiation
- Stage IV
  - No chemotherapy regimen can be recommended for routine use.
  - Cisplatin or carboplatin-based doublets (5)[A]
  - +/− bevacizumab (nonsquamous cell)
  - Erlotinib or afatinib for patients with EGFR mutations
  - Crizotinib for patients with EML4-ALK translocations
    - Ceritinib for patients that fail or are intolerant to crizotinib

- Maintenance therapy after 4 to 6 cycles in patients achieving a response or stable disease
  - Continuation of bevacizumab, pemetrexed (nonsquamous cell), gemcitabine, erlotinib, or crizotinib or switch to pemetrexed (nonsquamous cell), erlotinib (EGFR mutations), docetaxel or observation
- SCLC
  - Cisplatin or carboplatin plus etoposide

Second Line

- NSCLC
  - Cisplatin-based doublets +/− bevacizumab (nonsquamous cell) if not previously used
  - Docetaxel, pemetrexed (nonsquamous cell), erlotinib, gemcitabine, ramucirumab plus docetaxel, or nivolimab (squamous cell)
- SCLC
  - Topotecan or CAV (cyclophosphamide, doxorubicin, vincristine), gemcitabine, docetaxel, paclitaxel

ADDITIONAL THERAPIES

- Smoking cessation counseling
- Consider IV bisphosphonates or denosumab in patients with bone metastases to reduce skeletal-related events.

SURGERY/OTHER PROCEDURES

- Resection for NSCLC, for stages I, II, and IIIa, if medically fit to undergo surgery
- Resection of isolated, distant metastases has been achieved and may improve survival.
- Resection involves lobectomy in 71%, wedge in 16%, and complete pneumonectomy in 18%.
- Resection should be accompanied by lymph node dissection for pathologic staging.

 ONGOING CARE

FOLLOW-UP RECOMMENDATIONS

Patient Monitoring

- Depends on clinical history; in general, postoperative visits every 3 to 6 months in the year after surgery with physical exam and CXR
- Follow-up CT scans, as indicated

PATIENT EDUCATION

- http://www.cancer.gov/about-cancer
- http://smokefree.gov/

PROGNOSIS

- For combined, all types and stages, 5-year survival rate is 16% (NSCLC: 17%; SCLC 6%).
- NSCLC
  - Localized disease (stages I and II): 49%
  - Regional disease: 16%
  - Distant metastatic disease: 2%
- SCLC
  - Without treatment: median survival from diagnosis of only 2 to 4 months
  - Limited-stage disease: median survival of 16 to 24 months; 5-year survival rate: 14%
  - Extensive-stage disease: median survival of 6 to 12 months; long-term disease-free survival is rare.

COMPLICATIONS

- Development of metastatic disease, especially to brain, bones, adrenals, and liver
- Local recurrence of disease
- Postoperative complications
- Side effects of chemotherapy or radiation

REFERENCES

1. Aberle DR, Adams AM, Berg CD, et al. Reduced lung-cancer mortality with low-dose computed tomographic screening. N Engl J Med. 2011;365(5):395–409.
2. Slotman B, Faivre-Finn C, Kramer G, et al. Prophylactic cranial irradiation in extensive small-cell lung cancer. N Engl J Med. 2007;357(7): 664–672.
3. Pignon JP, Tribodet H, Scagliotti GV, et al. Lung adjuvant cisplatin evaluation: a pooled analysis by the LACE Collaborative Group. J Clin Oncol. 2008;26(21):3552–3559.
4. Gilligan D, Nicolson M, Smith I, et al. Preoperative chemotherapy in patients with resectable non-small cell lung cancer: results of the MRC LU22/NVALT 2/EORTC 08012 multicentre randomised trial and update of systematic review. Lancet. 2007;369(9577):1929–1937.
5. Delbaldo C, Michiels S, Rolland E, et al. Second or third additional chemotherapy drug for non-small cell lung cancer in patients with advanced disease. Cochrane Database Syst Rev. 2007;(4):CD004569.

ADDITIONAL READING

- Collins LG, Haines C, Perkel R, et al. Lung cancer: diagnosis and management. Am Fam Physician. 2007;75(1):56–63.
- Detterbeck FC, Lewis SZ, Diekemper R, et al. Executive summary: diagnosis and management of lung cancer, 3rd ed: American College of Chest Physicians evidence-based clinical practice guidelines. Chest. 2013;143(Suppl 5):7S–37S.
- National Cancer Institute. General information about non-small cell lung cancer (NSCLC). http://www.cancer.gov/types/lung/hp/non-small-cell-lung-treatment-pdq#section/_4
- National Cancer Institute. Small cell lung cancer treatment—for health professional (PDQ). http://www.cancer.gov/types/lung/hp/small-cell-lung-treatment-pdq#section/_1CODES

CODES

ICD10

- C34.90 Malignant neoplasm of unsp part of unsp bronchus or lung
- C34.10 Malignant neoplasm of upper lobe, unsp bronchus or lung
- C34.30 Malignant neoplasm of lower lobe, unsp bronchus or lung

CLINICAL PEARLS

- Prognosis and treatment of lung cancer differs greatly between small cell- and non–small cell histologies.
- Adjuvant cisplatin-based chemotherapy improves survival in patients with completely resected stage II–III NSCLC.
- Chemotherapy, with or without radiation, can be offered to patients with advanced NSCLC or SCLC.
- There is little role for surgery in the treatment of SCLC.

L

LUPUS ERYTHEMATOSUS, SYSTEMIC (SLE)

Katherine M. Tromp, PharmD • Hershey S. Bell, MD, MS, FAAFP

 BASICS

DESCRIPTION
- Systemic lupus erythematosus (SLE) is a multisystem autoimmune inflammatory disease characterized by a chronic relapsing/remitting course; can be mild to severe and may be life-threatening (CNS and renal forms)
- System(s) affected: mucocutaneous; musculoskeletal; renal; nervous; pulmonary; cardiac; hematologic; vascular; gastrointestinal (GI)
- Synonym(s): SLE; lupus

ALERT
Women with SLE have a 7- to 50-fold increased risk of coronary artery disease and may present with atypical/nonspecific symptoms.

EPIDEMIOLOGY
Predominant age: 15 to 45 years

Incidence
- Per year, 1.6 to 7.6/100,000 and increasing due to better diagnosis
- Most common: African American women (8.1 to 11.4/100,000/year)
- Least common: Caucasian men (0.3 to 0.9/100,000/year)

Prevalence
Occurs in 30 to 50/100,000 and increasing due to increased survival

ETIOLOGY AND PATHOPHYSIOLOGY
- Skin: photosensitivity; scaly erythematous, plaques with follicular plugging, dermal atrophy, and scarring; nonscarring erythematous psoriasiform/annular rash; alopecia; mucosal ulcers
- Musculoskeletal: nonerosive arthritis; ligament and tendon laxity, ulnar deviation, and swan neck deformities; avascular necrosis
- Renal: glomerulonephritis
- Pulmonary: pleuritis, pleural effusion, alveolar hemorrhage, pneumonitis, interstitial fibrosis, pulmonary hypertension, pulmonary embolism (PE)
- Cardiac: nonbacterial verrucous endocarditis, pericarditis, myocarditis, atherosclerosis
- CNS: thrombosis of small intracranial vessels ± perivascular inflammation resulting in micro- or macroinfarcts ± hemorrhage
- Peripheral nervous system: mononeuritis multiplex, peripheral neuropathy
- GI: pancreatitis, peritonitis, colitis
- Hematologic: hemolytic anemia, thrombocytopenia, leukopenia, lymphopenia
- Vascular: vasculitis, thromboembolism
- Most cases are idiopathic with possible environmental factors.
- Drug-induced lupus: hydralazine, D penicillamine, quinidine, procainamide, minocycline, isoniazid, etc

Genetics
- Identical twins: 24–58% concordance
- Fraternal twins and siblings: 2–5% concordance
- 8-fold risk if first-degree relative with SLE
- Major histocompatability complex associations: HLA-DR2, HLA-DR3
- Deficiency of early complement components, especially C1q, C1r/s, C2, and C4

- Immunoglobulin receptor polymorphisms: *FC-γR2A, FC-γR3A,* and others
- Polymorphism in genes associated with regulation of programmed cell death, protein tyrosine kinases, and interferon production

RISK FACTORS
- Race: African Americans, Hispanics, Asians, and Native Americans
- Predominant sex: females > males (8:1)
- Environmental: UV light, infectious agents, stress, diet, drugs, hormones, vitamin D deficiency, and tobacco

COMMONLY ASSOCIATED CONDITIONS
- Overlap syndromes: rheumatoid arthritis (RA), Sjögren syndrome, scleroderma
- Antiphospholipid syndrome; coronary artery disease; nephritis; depression

 DIAGNOSIS

Consider SLE in multisystem disease including fever, fatigue, and signs of inflammation.

HISTORY
- Fever, fatigue, malaise, weight loss, headache
- Rash (butterfly/*hyperpigmented ears* or *scalp*), photosensitivity, alopecia
- Oral/nasal ulcers (usually painless)
- Arthritis, arthralgia, myalgia, weakness
- Pleuritic chest pain, cough, dyspnea, hemoptysis
- Early stroke (age <50 years), seizure, psychosis, cognitive deficits
- Proteinuria, cellular casts
- Hemolytic anemia, leukopenia, lymphopenia, thrombocytopenia
- Abdominal pain, anorexia, nausea, vomiting
- Raynaud phenomenon

PHYSICAL EXAM
- Vital signs: fever, hypertension
- Malar, discoid, psoriasiform, or annular rash, alopecia
- Oral/nasal ulcers (*often minimally symptomatic*)
- Lymphadenopathy, splenomegaly
- Acrocyanosis
- Inflammatory arthritis, tenosynovitis
- Pleural/pericardial rub, heart murmur
- Bibasilar rales
- Cranial/peripheral neuropathies

DIFFERENTIAL DIAGNOSIS
Undifferentiated connective tissue disease, Sjögren syndrome, fibromyalgia, RA, vasculitis, idiopathic thrombocytopenia purpura, antiphospholipid antibody syndrome, drug-induced lupus

DIAGNOSTIC TESTS & INTERPRETATION

Initial Tests (lab, imaging)
- Antinuclear antibody (ANA)
  - High sensitivity (98%), low specificity
  - False-positive rate of 5–30%: elderly, autoimmune thyroid/liver disease, chronic infection, etc
  - Low titers <1:160 of limited clinical use
- Anti–double-stranded DNA (dsDNA) and anti-Smith antibodies: high specificity for SLE; predictor of nephritis and hemolytic anemia
  - Correlates with disease activity
- RNA protein antibodies (anti-RNP, anti-Ro, anti-La): less specific for SLE

- False-positive Venereal Disease Research Laboratory (VDRL) test: high sensitivity, low specificity. Surrogate marker of cardiolipin antibody presence
- Low serum complement levels: C3, C4
- Erythrocyte sediment rate (ESR): nonspecific, often high in active disease
- CBC: hemolytic anemia, thrombocytopenia, leukopenia, or lymphopenia
- Serum creatinine: elevated in lupus nephritis
- Urinalysis (UA): proteinuria, hematuria, cellular cast
- Phospholipid antibodies: cardiolipin immunoglobulin (Ig) G/IgM, lupus anticoagulant, β_2-glycoprotein IgG/IgM
- Anti-P (ribosomal autoantibodies) is associated with SLE arthritis and disease activity.
- Initial imaging is dependent on presenting symptoms.
- Radiograph of involved joints
- Chest x-ray: infiltrates, pleural effusion, low lung volumes
- Chest CT scan, ventilation-perfusion (V-Q) scan, duplex ultrasound for PE or deep vein thrombosis
- Head CT scan: ischemia, infarct, hemorrhage
- Brain MRI: focal areas of increased signal intensity
- Echocardiogram: pericardial effusion, valvular vegetations, pulmonary hypertension
- Contrast angiography for medium-size artery vasculitis: mesenteric/limb ischemia, CNS symptom

Follow-Up Tests & Special Considerations
- Hemolytic anemia: elevated reticulocyte count and indirect bilirubin, low haptoglobin, positive direct Coombs test
- Confirm positive phospholipid antibodies results in 12 weeks.
- If phospholipid antibodies are initially negative, but symptoms arise, repeat, as they may become positive over time.
- 24-hour urine collection/spot protein/creatinine to quantify proteinuria
- Histone antibodies present in >95% of drug-induced lupus (vs. 80% of idiopathic SLE)
- Fasting lipid panel and glucose
- Follow vitamin D[25(O)H] levels and replenish PRN.

Diagnostic Procedures/Other
- Renal biopsy to diagnose lupus nephritis (if UA abnormal)
- Skin biopsy with immunofluorescence on involved and uninvolved non–sun-exposed skin (*lupus band test*) may help differentiate SLE rash from others.
- Lumbar puncture in patients with fever and CNS/meningeal symptoms
- EEG for seizures/global CNS dysfunction
- Neuropsychiatric testing for cognitive impairment
- EMG/nerve conduction study (NCS) for peripheral neuropathy and myositis
- Nerve and/or muscle biopsy
- ECG, cardiac enzymes, stress tests
- American College of Rheumatology classification (not diagnostic) criteria: any 4 of the 11 listed (95% specificity and 85% sensitivity):
  - Malar (butterfly) rash
  - Discoid rash
  - Photosensitivity: by patient history/physician observation
  - Oral/nasopharyngeal ulcers
  - Nonerosive arthritis: involving ≥2 peripheral joints
  - Pleuritis *OR* pericarditis
  - Renal disorder: proteinuria (>0.5 g/day or >3+)

OR cellular casts (red cell, hemoglobin, granular, tubular, or mixed)
- Neurologic disorder: psychosis/seizures
- Hematologic disorder: hemolytic anemia, leukopenia (<4,000/mm^3 on ≥2 tests), lymphopenia (<1,500/mm^3 on ≥2 tests), thrombocytopenia (<100,000/mm^3)
- Immunologic disorder: anti-DNA, anti-Sm, anticardiolipin IgG/IgM, lupus anticoagulant, or false–positive VDRL findings
- Positive ANA in absence of drugs known to cause positive ANA

Test Interpretation
- Skin: vascular/perivascular inflammation, immune-complex deposition at dermal–epidermal junction, mucinosis, basal layer vacuolar changes
  - Similar findings seen in other connective tissue disorders such as dermatomyositis
- Renal: mesangial hypercellularity/matrix expansion, subendothelial/subepithelial immune deposits, glomerular sclerosis, fibrous crescents
  - Vary depending on degree of involvement
- Vascular: immune-complex deposition in vessel walls with fibrinoid necrosis and perivascular mononuclear cell infiltrates, intraluminal fibrin thrombi

TREATMENT

GENERAL MEASURES
- Education, counseling, and support
- Influenza/pneumococcal vaccines are safe; avoid live vaccines in immunocompromised patients.
- Low-estrogen oral contraceptives safe in mild SLE

MEDICATION
First Line
- *Antimalarial agents and NSAIDs are first-line therapy for patients with mild SLE* (1)[A].
  - Hydroxychloroquine for constitutional and musculoskeletal symptoms, rash, mild serositis; may reduce flares and increase long-term survival (2,3)[A]. NSAIDs for musculoskeletal manifestations, mild serositis, headache, and fever (2)[C]
- Systemic glucocorticoids (prednisone or equivalent)
  - Low dose (<0.5 mg/kg) for minor disease activity not responsive to NSAIDs or when NSAIDs are contraindicated (2)[A]
  - High-dose (1 to 2 mg/kg/day) (2)[A] or IV pulse methylprednisolone for organ-threatening disease, particularly CNS and renal; often combined with immunosuppressive agent (2)[A]
- Topical glucocorticosteroids for skin manifestations

Second Line
- Belimumab as adjunct for preventing flares in patients with active lupus despite first-line therapy (4)[A]
  - 10 mg/kg IV every 2 weeks × 3 doses, then monthly
- Methotrexate (2)[A], azathioprine (2)[B], mycophenolate mofetil (2)[C], or leflunomide as steroid-sparing agent for persistent active disease or to maintain remission
  - Requires laboratory monitoring for toxicity
- Treatments under investigation: rituximab, epratuzumab, abatacept, interferon-α inhibitors
- Immunosuppressive agents for severe disease
  - Cyclophosphamide (2)[A]: adequate hydration to reduce risk of hemorrhagic cystitis
  - Mycophenolate mofetil (2)[A]: more efficacious for lupus nephritis (1)[A]

SURGERY/OTHER PROCEDURES
Renal transplant for end-stage renal disease

COMPLEMENTARY & ALTERNATIVE MEDICINE
Biofeedback, visual imagery, cognitive therapy

INPATIENT CONSIDERATIONS
Admission Criteria/Initial Stabilization
- Difficult to differentiate SLE flare from infection; may need to treat both pending full evaluation
- IV pulse Solu-Medrol 1 g/day for 3 to 5 days for life- or organ-threatening disease (2)[A]

ONGOING CARE

FOLLOW-UP RECOMMENDATIONS
Patient Monitoring
- Clinical evaluation for signs and symptoms
  - Weekly to monthly for active disease
  - Every 3 to 6 months for mild/inactive disease
- Measures of disease activity and damage: Systemic Lupus Erythematosus Disease Activity Index, British Isles Lupus Assessment Group Index, European Consensus Lupus Activity Measure
- Laboratory studies
  - CBC with differential
  - Serum creatinine, UA
  - Vitamin D
  - Declining C3/C4 and rising DS-DNA and ESR may correlate with disease activity.
- Monitor for adverse effects of treatment
  - NSAIDs: GI bleeding and/or ulceration
  - Glucocorticoids: glucose, lipids, bone density
  - Hydroxychloroquine: ophthalmologic exam every 6 to 12 months
  - Methotrexate: CBC, creatinine, albumin, aspartate aminotransferase (AST), alanine aminotransferase (ALT) every 2 months
  - Azathioprine and mycophenolate mofetil: CBC every 1 to 3 months
  - Cyclophosphamide
    - CBC, creatinine, UA every 2 weeks, and liver function tests monthly during treatment
    - UA every 6 to 12 months for life

DIET
- No special diet unless for complications such as renal failure, diabetes, hyperlipidemia (2)[C]
- Adequate calcium/vitamin D intake in patients on corticosteroids (2)[A]
- Low glycemic index or calorie-restricted diet in patients on corticosteroids

PATIENT EDUCATION
- Avoid UV light exposure: sunscreens (SPF ≥30), protective clothing (2)[B]
- Weight control, smoking cessation, exercise (2)[C]
- Stress avoidance/management

PROGNOSIS
- Permanent treatment-free remission is uncommon.
- 5-year survival after diagnosis is 95%.
- Poor prognostic factor: major organ involvement
- Drug-induced lupus resolves within weeks to months after discontinuation of the offending drug.

COMPLICATIONS
Infections, neoplasms, cardiac disease, nephritis, neuropsychiatric lupus; depression

Pregnancy Considerations
- Exacerbations during pregnancy are less common when in remission for 6 months prior to conception.
- Fetal loss is increased, especially in those with active lupus/antiphospholipid antibodies.
- A 2% risk of congenital heart block if anti-SS-A (Ro) or anti-SS-B (La) antibodies are present.
- See "Antiphospholipid Antibody Syndrome" for recommendations regarding use of aspirin and heparin to prevent pregnancy complications.

REFERENCES
1. Yildirim-Toruner C, Diamond B. Current and novel therapeutics in the treatment of systemic lupus erythematosus. *J Allergy Clin Immunol*. 2011;127(2):303–312.
2. Bertsias G, Ioannidis JP, Boletis J, et al. EULAR recommendations for the management of systemic lupus erythematosus. Report of a task force of the EULAR Standing Committee for International Clinical Studies Including Therapeutics. *Ann Rheum Dis*. 2008;67(2):195–205.
3. Ruiz-Irastorza G, Ramos-Casals M, Brito-Zeron P, et al. Clinical efficacy and side effects of antimalarials in systemic lupus erythematosus: a systematic review. *Ann Rheum Dis*. 2010;69(1):20–28.
4. Navarra SV, Guzmán RM, Gallacher AE, et al. Efficacy and safety of belimumab in patients with active systemic lupus erythematosus: a randomised, placebo-controlled, phase 3 trial. *Lancet*. 2011;377(9767):721–731.

ADDITIONAL READING
Lisnevskaia L, Murphy G, Isenberg D. Systemic lupus erythematosus. *Lancet*. 2014;384(9957):1878–1888.

SEE ALSO
Antiphospholipid Antibody Syndrome

CODES

ICD10
- M32.9 Systemic lupus erythematosus, unspecified
- M32.10 Systemic lupus erythematosus, organ or system involv unsp
- M32.14 Glomerular disease in systemic lupus erythematosus

CLINICAL PEARLS
- *Aggressiveness of therapy should reflect intensity of disease.*
- Most important diagnostic test is the UA: if abnormal, order kidney biopsy; *serum and urine lab values often do not reveal extent of kidney disease.*
- Atherosclerotic and atheroembolic complications are the major cause of death; address modifiable cardiovascular risk factors.

LUPUS NEPHRITIS

Neena R. Gupta, MD

BASICS

DESCRIPTION
- The renal manifestation of systemic lupus erythematosus (SLE)
- American College of Rheumatology (ACR) criteria: persistent proteinuria >500 mg/day or ≥3 on dipstick and/or presence of cellular casts. Alternatively, spot urine protein-to-creatinine ratio >0.5 and "active urinary sediment" (>5 RBC/hpf, >5 WBC/hpf in absence of infection, or cellular casts—RBC or WBC casts) (1)
- Clinical manifestations are primarily due to immune complex–mediated glomerular disease. Tubulointerstitial and vascular involvement often seen. Diagnosed based on clinical findings, urine abnormalities, autoantibodies, and renal biopsy.
- Treatment and prognosis depend on International Society of Nephrology/Renal Pathology Society (ISN/RPS) histologic class—risk of end-stage renal disease (ESRD) highest in class IV.
- Delay in diagnosis/treatment increases risk of ESRD.

EPIDEMIOLOGY
- Peak incidence of SLE is 15 to 45 years of age.
- Predominant sex: female > male (10:1)
- Once SLE develops, lupus nephritis (LN) affects both genders equally; it is more severe in children and men and less severe in older adults.

Incidence
- SLE: 1.4 to 21.9/100,000 (2)
- Up to 60% of SLE patients develop LN over time, and 25–50% of SLE patients have nephritis as the initial presentation.

Pediatric Considerations
LN is more common and more severe in children: 60–80% have LN at or soon after SLE onset.

Prevalence
SLE: 7.4 to 159.4/100,000 (2)

ETIOLOGY AND PATHOPHYSIOLOGY
- Immune complex–mediated inflammation injures glomeruli, tubules, interstitium, and vasculature.
- Glomeruli: varying degrees of mesangial proliferation, crescent formation (see "Test Interpretation"), and fibrinoid necrosis causing reduced glomerular filtration rate (GFR)
- Persistence of inflammation (chronicity) leads to sclerosis and glomerular loss.
- Tubulointerstitial injury (edema, inflammatory cell infiltrate acutely; tubular atrophy in chronic phase) with or without tubular basement membrane immune complex deposition leads to reduced renal function.
- Vascular lesions: immune complex deposition and noninflammatory necrosis in arterioles
- SLE is a multifactorial disease, with a multigenic inheritance; exact etiology remains unclear.
- Defective T-cell autoregulation and polyclonal B-cell hyperactivity contribute to dysregulated apoptosis. Impaired clearance of apoptotic cells inhibits self-tolerance to nuclear antigen
- Anti-DNA, anti-C1q, anti-α-actin, and other nuclear component autoantibodies develop.
- Deposition of circulating immune complexes or autoantibodies attaching to local nuclear antigens leads to complement activation, inflammation, and tissue injury.
- Interaction of genetic, hormonal, and environmental factors leads to great variability in LN severity.

Genetics
Multigenic inheritance; clustering in families, ~25% concordance in identical twins

RISK FACTORS
Younger age, African American or Hispanic race, more ACR criteria for SLE, longer disease duration, hypertension, lower socioeconomic status, family history of SLE, anti-dsDNA antibodies

COMMONLY ASSOCIATED CONDITIONS
Skin, hematologic, cerebral, pulmonary, GI, and cardiopulmonary systems are often involved in SLE.

DIAGNOSIS

HISTORY
Assess for risk factors and other signs/symptoms of SLE: rash, photosensitivity, arthritis, neurologic complaints, fever, weight loss, alopecia.

PHYSICAL EXAM
- Hypertension, fever
- Pleural/pericardial rub
- Skin rash
- Edema
- Arthritis

DIFFERENTIAL DIAGNOSIS
- Primary glomerular disease
- Secondary renal involvement in other systemic disorders such as antineutrophil cytoplasmic autoantibody (ANCA) associated vasculitis, Henoch-Schönlein purpura (HSP), antiglomerular basement membrane disease, and viral infections
- Mixed connective tissue disorder may have glomerulonephritis indistinguishable from LN.

DIAGNOSTIC TESTS & INTERPRETATION
- Renal biopsy is the gold standard for diagnosing and classifying LN.
- Combine clinical data with serologic and renal biopsy patterns to differentiate LN from other processes.
- Active urine sediment suggests nephritis.
- Autoantibodies, low C3, C4, and CH50 complement levels support LN diagnosis.

Initial Tests (lab, imaging)
- Urinalysis may show hematuria, proteinuria, and active urine sediment (3)[C].
- Serum electrolytes, BUN, creatinine, albumin, routine serologic markers of SLE such as antinuclear antibody (ANA), anti-dsDNA, anti-Ro, anti-La, anti-RNP, anti-Sm, antiphospholipid antibody, C3, C4, CH50, CBC with differential, and C-reactive protein (CRP) (3)[C]
- CBC may show anemia, thrombocytopenia, and leukopenia.
- Renal ultrasound (3)[C]

Follow-Up Tests & Special Considerations
- Monitor disease activity q3mo (3)[C]: urinalysis for hematuria and proteinuria; blood for C3, C4, anti-dsDNA, serum albumin, and creatinine.
- Patients with estimated glomerular filtration rate (eGFR) of <60 mL should be managed according to the National Kidney Foundation guidelines for chronic kidney disease. http://www.kdigo.org/clinical_practice_guidelines/pdf/CKD/KDIGO_2012_CKD_GL.pdf

Pregnancy Considerations
- Pregnancy leads to worsening of renal function in LN. Risk factors include renal impairment at baseline, active disease, hypertension, and proteinuria.
- Risk factors for fetal loss include elevated serum creatinine, heavy proteinuria, hypertension, and anticardiolipin antibodies.

Test Interpretation
- Adequate renal biopsy (at least 10 glomeruli for light microscopy or total 20 to 25 glomeruli) is essential. Light, immunofluorescence, and electron microscopy are needed for accurate classification.
- On immunofluorescence microscopy: Immune complex deposits consisting of IGG, IGA, IGM, C1q, and C3 ("full house") are highly suggestive of LN.
- Revised ISN/RPS histologic classification guides therapeutic decisions. http://jasn.asnjournals.org/content/15/2/241.full.pdf
- LN is classified as purely mesangial (classes I and II), focal proliferative: <50% glomeruli (class III), diffuse proliferative: ≥50% (class IV), membranous (class V), and advanced sclerosis (class VI). Subdivisions for activity (A) and chronicity (C) in class III/IV and for segmental (S) or global (G) glomerular involvement in class IV (Class III A, C, A/C and class IV S[A], G[A], S[A/C], S[C], G[C]).
- LN may change to another class over time or with therapy.
- Focal and diffuse proliferative LN (classes III and IV) are common and most likely to progress to ESRD.

TREATMENT

GENERAL MEASURES
- Monitor bone density; optimize vitamin D and calcium intake in patients on glucocorticoid therapy.
- Low-salt diet for hypertension and edema. For eGFR <60 mL: Follow National Kidney Foundation guidelines for chronic kidney disease.
- Avoid sun or ultraviolet light exposure.

MEDICATION
Note: Other than methylprednisolone and prednisone, no other medications listed below are FDA approved for lupus nephritis.

First Line
- **Class I + II LN:** No specific therapy is needed, as long-term renal prognosis is good. Renin-angiotensin system blockade (ACE inhibitors or angiotensin receptor blockers) to manage BP and proteinuria. There are many drugs in this class (e.g., lisinopril 5 to 40 mg/day PO, losartan 25 to 100 mg/day PO).
- **Proliferative LN (Class III, IV, V + III/IV):** Induce remission by steroids + IV cyclophosphamide or mycophenolate mofetil (MMF) and maintenance of remission by low-dose steroids and azathioprine (AZA) or MMF (1).
- Principles of treatment:
  - Avoid delay in treatment.
  - Inducing remission quickly (3 to 6 months)
  - Maintaining response and avoiding iatrogenic morbidity (5 to 10 years)

- **INDUCTION**: steroids + immunosuppressive agent (for mild class III, high-dose steroids may be sufficient):
  - Glucocorticoids: methylprednisolone pulse 0.5 to 1 g/day for 3 days followed by oral prednisone 0.5 to 1 mg/kg/day PO (max 60 mg/day, taper after 4 to 8 weeks) (4,5)[A] AND
  - Cyclophosphamide (CYC): IV CYC (high dose = 0.5 to 1 g/m^2 monthly for 6 doses—NIH regimen; low dose = 0.5 g q2wk for 6 doses—Euro-Lupus regimen) OR
  - Mycophenolate mofetil (MMF): 1 to 3 g/day PO divided BID (target 3 g/day as tolerated) for 6 months. MMF is as effective as CYC in achieving remission with fewer side effects (6)[A].
- **MAINTENANCE:**
  - Glucocorticoids: oral prednisone tapered to low doses (generally <10 mg/day by 6 months) AND
  - MMF 1 to 2 g/day divided BID PO OR AZA (azathioprine): 1 to 2.5 mg/kg/day PO (4,5)[A]
  - In the ALMS (Aspreva Lupus Management Study) MMF shown to be superior than AZA for maintenance therapy in a varied population (7)[A].
  - In the MAINTAIN nephritis trial, MMF shown to be equal to AZA for maintenance therapy in mostly Caucasian population (8)[A].
  - Cyclophosphamide IV quarterly for 1 to 2 year after renal remission; not used now due to availability of less toxic regimen
- **Class V LN**: good prognosis in general, treatment not standardized
  - For subnephrotic patients, no specific treatment except renin-angiotensin system blockade.
    Options for nephrotic patients include steroids with either calcineurin inhibitors, IV CYC, AZA, or MMF (5)[B].
  - Class V LN with presence of class III or class IV biopsy findings needs aggressive combination regimen as for class III/IV.

Second Line
Other treatments in selected patients: rituximab, plasma exchange, IVIG, calcineurin inhibitors. Belimumab was approved by FDA in 2011, but trials excluded patients with severe active LN (9)[C].

ISSUES FOR REFERRAL
Nephrology consults for initial management and relapses

ADDITIONAL THERAPIES
- KDIGO 2012 guidelines for LN state that all patients with LN of any class be treated with hydroxychloroquine (maximum daily dose of 6 to 6.5 mg/kg ideal body weight), unless they have a specific contraindication to this drug.
- BP control; treat dyslipidemia and other modifiable cardiovascular risk factors.
- Anticoagulation for symptomatic antiphospholipid antibody syndrome

SURGERY/OTHER PROCEDURES
- Renal transplant for ESRD when indicated
- Patient and graft survival rates are similar to non-SLE patients (2)[C].
- Risk of recurrent LN in renal transplant recipients ranges between 0% and 30%; graft loss due to recurrence is rare.

INPATIENT CONSIDERATIONS
Admission Criteria/Initial Stabilization
- Uncontrolled hypertension, acute kidney injury
- Severe extrarenal manifestation
- Control hypertension and proteinuria, if present.
- Labs to help confirm SLE/LN, renal ultrasound
- Nephrology for manage input and renal biopsy

IV Fluids
Patients who have nephrotic syndrome or acute kidney injury should be fluid restricted.

Discharge Criteria
Once the patient is stabilized and renal biopsy is performed, manage safely as an outpatient.

 ONGOING CARE

FOLLOW-UP RECOMMENDATIONS
Patient Monitoring
- Monitor urine protein-to-creatinine ratio, urine microscopy, serum albumin and creatinine, antibody titers (especially anti-dsDNA), C3, C4, BP at least every 3 months for first 2 to 3 years (3)[C].
- Once stable on maintenance therapy with no active disease, follow-up every 6 to 12 months (3)[C].
- Cyclophosphamide: CBC, ensure adequate hydration
- MMF: CBC, LFT, SrCr
- Azathioprine: CBC

DIET
Low-salt diet. For eGFR <60 mL: Follow National Kidney Foundation guidelines for chronic kidney disease.

PATIENT EDUCATION
Medication adherence and self-monitoring for relapse

PROGNOSIS
- 10-year survival of 88% and 94% in SLE patients with and without renal involvement (1)
- Relapse rate is ~35%. 10–20% of patients progress to ESRD within 10 years (10).
- 5-year renal survival of class IV LN <30% before 1970 has improved to >80% in last 2 decades (2).
- Early and complete remission with treatment is the best prognostic factor. Predictors of remission include low baseline proteinuria, normal creatinine, Caucasian race, and treatment initiation within 3 months of clinical diagnosis.
- Indicators of poor prognosis: diffuse proliferative LN (especially crescentic), higher activity/chronicity index, African American race, lower socioeconomic status, poor response to treatment, high creatinine at baseline, uncontrolled hypertension, and relapse

COMPLICATIONS
- Risks from immunosuppression: infections, malignancy
- Treatment side effects: Cyclophosphamide causes primary amenorrhea.
- MMF may cause GI upset and nausea and is a teratogen (azathioprine recommended for women who desire pregnancy).
- Risk of vascular thromboses (hypercoagulable state from antiphospholipid antibodies)
- About 10–20% of patients develop ESRD from progressive disease refractory to treatment requiring dialysis/kidney transplantation.

REFERENCES
1. Hahn BH, McMahon MA, Wilkinson A, et al. American College of Rheumatology guidelines for screening, treatment, and management of lupus nephritis. *Arthritis Care Res (Hoboken)*. 2012;64(6): 797–808.
2. Ortega LM, Schultz DR, Lenz O, et al. Review: lupus nephritis: pathologic features, epidemiology and a guide to therapeutic decisions. *Lupus*. 2010;19(5):557–574.
3. Mosca M, Tani C, Aringer M, et al. European League Against Rheumatism recommendations for monitoring patients with systemic lupus erythematosus in clinical practice and in observational studies. *Ann Rheum Dis*. 2010;69(7):1269–1274.
4. Ponticelli C, Glassock RJ, Moroni G. Induction and maintenance therapy in proliferative lupus nephritis. *J Nephrol*. 2010;23(1):9–16.
5. Bomback AS, Appel GB. Updates on the treatment of lupus nephritis. *J Am Soc Nephrol*. 2010;21(12): 2028–2035.
6. Henderson LK, Masson PM, Craig JC, et al. Induction and maintenance treatment of proliferative lupus nephritis: a meta-analysis of randomized controlled trials. *Am J Kidney Dis*. 2013;61(1):74–87.
7. Dooley MA, Jayne D, Ginzler EM, et al. Mycophenolate versus azathioprine as maintenance therapy for lupus nephritis. *N Engl J Med*. 2011;365(20): 1886–1895.
8. Morris HK, Canetta PA, Appel GB. Impact of ALMS and MAINTAIN trials on the management of lupus nephritis. *Nephrol Dial Transplant*. 2013;28(6): 1371–1376.
9. Lo MS, Tsokos GC. Treatment of systemic lupus erythematosus: new advances in targeted therapy. *Ann N Y Acad Sci*. 2012;1247:138–152.

ADDITIONAL READING
- Kidney Disease: Improving Global Outcomes (KDIGO) Glomerulonephritis Work Group. KDIGO clinical practice guideline for glomerulonephritis. *Kidney Inter*. 2012;2(Suppl):139–274.
- Ward MM. Recent clinical trials in lupus nephritis. *Rheum Dis Clin North Am*. 2014;40(3):519–535.
- Weening JJ, D'Agati VD, Schwartz MM, et al. The classification of glomerulonephritis in systemic lupus erythematosus revisited. *J Am Soc Nephrol*. 2004; 15(2):241–250.

 CODES

ICD10
M32.14 Glomerular disease in systemic lupus erythematosus

CLINICAL PEARLS
- Early diagnosis, correct classification (requires renal biopsy), and rapid treatment improve renal survival in patients with LN.
- Treat proliferative/progressive LN with a short induction course followed by maintenance therapy using glucocorticoids and immunosuppressants.
- Survival rates for patients with LN have improved dramatically over the past several decades.

L

LYME DISEASE

Felix B. Chang, MD, DABMA, FAAMA

BASICS

DESCRIPTION

- A multisystem infection caused by *Borrelia* spirochetes, transmitted primarily by ixodid ticks
  - *Ixodes scapularis* (deer ticks) in the New England and Great Lakes areas
  - *Ixodes pacificus* in the West (blacklegged ticks and Western blacklegged ticks)
  - *Ixodes ricinus* in Europe
  - *Ixodes persuladas* in Asia and Russia
- Early localized Lyme disease includes a characteristic expanding skin rash (erythema migrans [EM]) (70%) and constitutional flulike symptoms.
- Disseminated Lyme disease presents with involvement of ≥1 organ systems. Neurologic, cardiac, and pauciarticular arthritis are the most common.
- Post-Lyme disease syndrome includes arthritis (50%) and chronic neurologic syndromes.
- System(s) affected: hemic/lymphatic/immunologic; musculoskeletal; skin/exocrine; cardiac; neurologic
- Synonym(s): Lyme arthritis; Lyme borreliosis

EPIDEMIOLOGY

Incidence

- 96% of U.S. cases in 2011 were reported from 13 states: New England, New York, New Jersey, Delaware, Pennsylvania, Maryland, Minnesota, and Wisconsin (1).
- In states where Lyme disease is endemic, the incidence is 0.5 per 1,000 but can be substantially higher in local areas.
- Cases have been reported from all 50 states.
- From 2003 to 2012, a total of 279,509 cases of Lyme disease were reported in the United States.
- Currently the seventh most common reportable disease in the United States

Prevalence

- The most reported vector-borne illness in the United States
- Predominant age: most common in children ages 5 to 14 years and in adults aged 55 to 70 years of age
- Predominant sex: male > female in the United States

ETIOLOGY AND PATHOPHYSIOLOGY

- Infection with spirochete *Borrelia burgdorferi* in the United States, or *Borrelia afzelii* or *Borrelia garinii* in Europe, transmitted by the bite of ixodid ticks (2)[A]
- Approximately 90% of cases are transmitted during the nymph stage of the tick life cycle.
- If a tick is infected, the chance of transmission increases with time attached: 12% at 48 hours, 79% at 72 hours, and 94% at 96 hours of attachment.
- Primary animal reservoir is the white-footed mouse.
- Spirochetes multiply and spread within dermis. Host response results in characteristic (EM) rash. Hematogenous dissemination results in disease within CNS, cardiovascular, or other organ systems.
- Star ticks (*Amblyomma americanum*), the American dog tick (*Dermacentor variabilis*), the Rocky Mountain wood tick (*Dermacentor andersoni*), and the brown dog tick (*Rhipicephalus sanguineus*) are not known to transmit Lyme disease.

Genetics

Human leukocyte antigen: Patients with haplotype DR4 or DR2 may be more susceptible to prolonged arthritis.

RISK FACTORS

- Exposure in tick-infested area, particularly from April to November
- Those who reside or are employed in endemic areas where ixodid ticks are found are at increased risk.
- Ixodid ticks are commonly found on deer. Hunters may be at an increased risk.

GENERAL PREVENTION

- "Tick checks": Examine skin after outdoor activities.
- Remove ticks within 36 hours to limit transmission.
- Wear clothing covering the ankles in endemic areas.
- Use insect repellents containing DEET.
- Apply permethrin to clothes, shoes, and tents.
- Antibiotic prophylaxis is recommended for the prevention of Lyme disease in endemic areas following an *Ixodes* tick bite.
- Prophylactic treatment with 1 dose of 200 mg of doxycycline within 72 hours of a tick bite in highly endemic areas is 87% effective. Contraindicated in pregnancy and in children; no prophylactic agent is approved for these groups (2)[A].

COMMONLY ASSOCIATED CONDITIONS

- Coinfection with babesiosis has been reported. Suggested by high fever
- Southern tick–associated rash illness may be mistaken for Lyme disease. It is seen in the Southeastern and South Central United States and is associated with the bite of the lone star tick, *A. americanum.*

DIAGNOSIS

HISTORY

- History of a tick bite followed by EM and/or illness (3).
- Early Lyme disease: incubation period 3 to 30 days
  - Some patients may be asymptomatic (4).
  - Fever; headache; myalgias; arthralgias
- Disseminated Lyme disease
  - Carditis (pleuritic chest pain; palpitations)
  - Facial palsies or other cranial neuropathies
  - Joint pain (polyarthritis/algias; late disease: monoarthritis-like knee)
  - Iritis, conjunctivitis
  - Migratory musculoskeletal pain
- Late untreated Lyme disease
  - Recurrent synovitis
  - Recurrent tendonitis and bursitis
  - Encephalopathic symptoms
    - Headaches
    - *Cognitive slowing*
    - Confusion
    - Profound fatigue

- Symptoms mimicking other CNS diseases
  - Multiple sclerosis–like symptoms
  - Stroke-like symptoms
  - Transverse myelitis
- Peripheral neuropathic symptoms; motor, sensory, or autonomic neuropathies
- Meningitis

PHYSICAL EXAM

- Early Lyme disease
  - EM (4)[A]
- Disseminated Lyme disease
  - Multiple EM
  - Facial palsies or other cranial neuropathies
  - Heart block—irregular pulse
  - Pericarditis—friction rub
  - Arthritis
  - Other focal neurologic findings

DIFFERENTIAL DIAGNOSIS

- Other rickettsial disease (Rocky Mountain spotted fever [RMSF])
- Juvenile rheumatoid arthritis; systemic lupus erythematosus (SLE); rheumatoid arthritis (RA)
- Viral syndromes
- Contact dermatitis; cellulitis; granuloma annulare (mimic EM)
- Syphilis
- AV block

DIAGNOSTIC TESTS & INTERPRETATION

Initial Tests (lab, imaging)

- Testing and treatment not indicated if tick attached for <48 hours (3)
- Diagnosis is based mainly on clinical findings in endemic areas (4).
- Serology: enzyme-linked immunosorbent assay (ELISA) for immunoglobulin (Ig) M and IgG *B. burgdorferi* antibodies, followed by a Western blot test if positive or equivocal, or an indirect immunofluorescence assay
- Culture of CSF for *B. burgdorferi*
- Plasma polymerase chain reaction (PCR) testing is of little value (only exception is synovial fluid analysis).
- No imaging routinely indicated.

Follow-Up Tests & Special Considerations

Disorders that may alter lab results: False-positive response has been seen with RMSF, syphilis, SLE, and RA.

- Arthritis: Serology + PCR of synovial fluid is both sensitive and specific.
- Neuroborreliosis: serology + CSF pleocytosis (PCR of CSF has a very low sensitivity)
- Late-stage disease with negative serology may be seen in patients who received early antibiotic treatment.
- After an infection, antibodies may persist for months to years. *Serologic tests do not distinguish active from past infection.*
- Antibodies are not protective.

Diagnostic Procedures/Other
Lumbar puncture when neurologic findings are present, with ELISA of CSF for *B. burgdorferi* antibodies. Xenodiagnosis in humans (5)

Test Interpretation
Culture of *B. burgdorferi* from blood or skin biopsy has a very low yield.

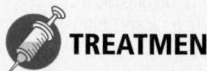
TREATMENT

GENERAL MEASURES
Early and disseminated Lyme disease can usually be treated as an outpatient except when complicated by carditis or meningitis (requires parenteral antibiotics).

MEDICATION
First Line
- EM

  – Doxycycline (Vibramycin) 100 mg PO BID for 10 to 21 days (do not use in children <8 years old or in pregnant women) (2,6)[A]; *or*

  – Amoxicillin 500 mg PO TID for 14 to 21 days (pediatric dose 50 mg/kg/day); *or*

  – Cefuroxime axetil 500 mg PO BID for 14 to 21 days
    ○ Doxycycline has the advantage of covering other tick-borne infections such as ehrlichiosis, anaplasmosis, and RMSF.
    ○ Alternative: azithromycin 500 mg QD for 7 to 10 days or clarithromycin 500 mg BID for 14 to 21 days

- Neurologic disease

  – Normal CSF, treat for 14 to 21 days (2)[A].

  – Doxycycline 100 mg PO BID or amoxicillin 500 mg PO TID

  – Abnormal CSF, treat for 4 weeks: ceftriaxone 2 g QD IV, cefotaxime 2 g q8h, *or* penicillin G 5 mIU q6h

  – Cardiac disease
    ○ Mild (first-degree AV block, PR <300 ms): doxycycline 100 mg PO BID or amoxicillin 500 mg PO TID for 14 to 21days
    ○ More serious: ceftriaxone 2 g QD IV for 30 days

- Arthritis without neurologic disease (2)[A]

  – Oral treatment for 28 days with doxycycline 100 mg BID or amoxicillin 500 mg TID

  – If oral treatment fails, repeat oral regimen for 28 days or begin IV treatment with ceftriaxone 2 g QD for 2 to 4 weeks.

- Contraindications
  – Allergy to specific medication
  – Doxycycline is contraindicated in children and in women who are pregnant or breastfeeding.

- Precautions
  – In ~15% of patients treated with IV therapy, a Jarisch-Herxheimer–type reaction develops within 24 hours of initiation of therapy.

- Significant possible interactions
  – Oral anticoagulants may require dose adjustments.
  – Oral contraceptives may be less effective.

Pediatric Considerations
- Amoxicillin is the drug of choice in children.
- Tetracyclines are contraindicated.

Pregnancy Considerations
- Because *B. burgdorferi* can cross the placenta, pregnant patients with active disease should be treated with parenteral antibiotics.
- Doxycycline should not be used in pregnancy.

Second Line
- Azithromycin, 500 mg PO daily for 7 days, can be used for those allergic to β-lactams and unable to take tetracyclines but is less effective (2).
- There is no evidence for meaningful clinical benefit from prolonged treatment or retreatment of patients with persistent unexplained symptoms despite previous antibiotic treatment of Lyme disease.

INPATIENT CONSIDERATIONS
Admission Criteria/Initial Stabilization
- Admission is recommended for patients with Lyme carditis and symptoms of chest pain, syncope, or dyspnea, and for those with second- or third-degree heart block or first-degree heart block of ≥300 ms.
- Admission is also recommended for patients with symptoms of meningitis.

ONGOING CARE

FOLLOW-UP RECOMMENDATIONS
Patient Monitoring
Based on the severity of symptoms, patients with Lyme carditis, neurologic syndromes, or arthritis may require prolonged follow-up.

DIET
No restrictions

PATIENT EDUCATION
- In endemic areas, patients should be advised to protect themselves against tick exposure.
- https://www.rheumatology.org/Practice/Clinical/Patients/Diseases_And_Conditions/Lyme_Disease/
- Prevention
  – Use repellents that contains 20–30% DEET (N,N-diethyl-meta-toluamide) on exposed skin and clothing for protection that last up to several hours.
  – Use 0.5% permethrin on clothing.
  – Bathe or shower as soon as possible after coming indoors (preferably within 2 hours) and perform tick check after outdoor activities.

PROGNOSIS
- Early treatment with antibiotics can shorten the duration of symptoms and prevent later disease.
- Response of late-stage disease to treatment is variable. Symptoms may take weeks to resolve after beginning treatment.

COMPLICATIONS
- Recurrent synovitis, tendonitis, bursitis (7)[A]
- Chronic neurologic symptoms
- Peripheral neuropathies
- Posttreatment Lyme disease syndrome: 10–20% lingering symptoms of fatigue, pain, or joint and muscle aches. Can last for 6 months (8)[A]

REFERENCES
1. Centers for Disease Control and Prevention. Statistics on Lyme disease. http://www.cdc.gov/lyme/stats/index.html. Accessed 2015.
2. Wright WF, Riedel DJ, Talwani R, et al. Diagnosis and management of Lyme disease. *Am Fam Physician*. 2012;85(11):1086–1093.
3. Duncan CJ, Carle G, Seaton RA. Tick bite and early Lyme borreliosis. *BMJ*. 2012;334:e3124.
4. Marques A, Telford SR III, Turk SP, et al. Xenodiagnosis to detect *Borrelia burgdorferi* infection: a first-in-human study. *Clin Infect Dis*. 2014;58(7):937–945. doi:10.1093/cid/cit939.
5. Klempner MS, Baker PJ, Shapiro ED, et al. Treatment trials for post-Lyme disease symptoms revisited. *Am J Med*. 2013;126(8):665–669.
6. Nadelman RB, Hanincová K, Mukherjee P, et al. Differentiation of reinfection from relapse in recurrent Lyme disease. *N Engl J Med*. 2012;367(20):1883–1890.
7. Marques A. Chronic Lyme disease: a review. *Infect Dis Clin North Am*. 2008;22(2):341–360.
8. Wormser GP, Dattwyler RJ, Shapiro ED, et al. The clinical assessment, treatment, and prevention of Lyme disease, human granulocytic anaplasmosis, and babesiosis: clinical practice guidelines by the Infectious Diseases Society of America. *Clin Infect Dis*. 2006;43(9):1089–1134.

ADDITIONAL READING
Tickborne Diseases of the United States. A Reference Manual for Health Care Providers. Third edition, 2015. www.cdc.gov/lyme/resources/tickbornediseases.pdf

CODES
ICD10
- A69.20 Lyme disease, unspecified
- A69.23 Arthritis due to Lyme disease
- A69.21 Meningitis due to Lyme disease

CLINICAL PEARLS
- The presence of EM following a tick bite in an endemic area is an indication for empiric treatment for Lyme disease.
- Repeat episodes of EM in appropriately treated patients are due to reinfection and not relapse.
- Lyme disease during pregnancy may lead to infection of the placenta and possible stillbirth. Amoxicillin is the preferred treatment during pregnancy.
- Ticks must be attached for at least 24 hours or more to transmit Lyme disease.
- There is no evidence that Lyme disease can be transmitted by breastfeeding or close personal contact.
- Vaccines for Lyme disease is no longer available.

LYMPHANGITIS

Amar Kapur, DO, CPT, MC, USA

 BASICS

DESCRIPTION

Acute or chronic inflammation of lymphatic channels due to a skin breach or local trauma. Presents as red, tender streaks along lymphatic channels and extending to regional lymph nodes

- May result from compromised lymphatic drainage due to surgical procedures
- May be infectious or noninfectious

ETIOLOGY AND PATHOPHYSIOLOGY

- Acute infection
  - Usually caused by group A β-hemolytic *Streptococcus*
  - Less commonly caused by:
    ○ *Staphylococcus aureus*
    ○ *Pasteurella multocida*
    ○ *Erysipelothrix*
    ○ *Spirillum minus* (rat bite disease)
    ○ *Pseudomonas*
    ○ Other *Streptococcus* sp.
    ○ Immunocompromised patients can be infected with gram-negative rods, gram-negative bacilli, or fungi.
    ○ In fresh water exposures, *Aeromonas hydrophila*
- Nodular lymphangitis
  - Also known as sporotrichoid lymphangitis
  - Presents as painful or painless nodular subcutaneous swellings along lymphatic vessels
  - Lesions may ulcerate with accompanying regional lymphadenopathy.
  - Typical of infections from the following: *Sporothrix schenckii*, *Nocardia brasiliensis*, *Mycobacterium marinum*, leishmaniasis, tularemia, and systemic mycoses
  - Pathology may show granulomas.
- Noninfectious granulomatous lymphangitis
  - Rare-acquired lymphedema of the genitalia in children
  - May be due to atypical Crohn disease or sarcoidosis (1)[C]
- Filarial lymphangitis
  - Mosquito bites transmit parasites causing inflammation and dilatation in the lymphatic vessels; can predispose to secondary bacterial infection
  - Usually caused by nematodes *Wuchereria bancrofti*. Other causes are *Brugia malayi* and *Brugia timori*.
- Lymphangitis due to surgery
  - May occur after surgical procedures and lymph node dissection
- Cutaneous lymphangitis carcinomatosa is rare. Represents ~5% of all skin metastases; caused by occlusion of lymphatic channels of dermis by neoplastic cells (2)
- Sclerosing lymphangitis of the penis
  - Swelling around coronal sulcus of penis usually resulting from vigorous sexual activity or masturbation

RISK FACTORS

- Impaired lymphatic drainage due to surgery, nodal dissection, or irradiation
- Diabetes mellitus
- Chronic steroid use
- Peripheral venous catheter
- Varicella infection
- Immunocompromising condition
- Human, animal, or insect bites
- Fungal, bacterial, or mycobacterial skin infections
- Any trauma to the skin
- IV drug abuse
- Residence in endemic areas of filariasis

GENERAL PREVENTION

- Reduce chronic lymphedema with compression devices or by treating underlying process
- Insect repellant
- Proper wound and skin care

COMMONLY ASSOCIATED CONDITIONS

- Lymphedema
- Prior lymph node dissection
- Tinea pedis (athlete's foot)
- Sporotrichosis
- Cellulitis, erysipelas
- Filarial infection (*W. bancrofti*)

 DIAGNOSIS

HISTORY

- History of trauma to skin, cut, abrasion, or fungal infection
- Systemic symptoms:
  - Malaise
  - Fever and chills
  - Loss of appetite
  - Headache
  - Muscle aches
- Travel to a tropical region or region with known filariasis

PHYSICAL EXAM

Local signs:

- Erythematous, macular linear streaks from site of infection toward the regional lymph nodes
- Tenderness and warmth over affected skin or lymph nodes
- May have blistering of affected skin
- Fluctuance, swelling, or purulent drainage
- Nodular lymphangitis can present with subcutaneous swellings along the lymphatic channels.
- Sporotrichosis may present with papulonodular lesions that may ulcerate.
- Sites may be nonpainful.

DIFFERENTIAL DIAGNOSIS

- Superficial thrombophlebitis
  - Thrombus or infection within the thrombosis (septic thrombophlebitis)
- Contact dermatitis
- Allergic reaction: less likely to be allergic if >24 hours after exposure (e.g., insect bite)
- Lymphangitis carcinomatosa
- Malignancy-related inflammation

DIAGNOSTIC TESTS & INTERPRETATION

- CBC may show leukocytosis; blood smear may show filarial infection.
- Blood or wound cultures
- Biopsy cultures
- FNAC for filariasis of testiculoscrotal swelling but not for other superficial locations (3)

Initial Tests (lab, imaging)

Plain radiology unnecessary; may consider lymphangiography for lymphedema (4)[C]

Diagnostic Procedures/Other

- Swab, aspirate, and/or biopsy primary site, purulent discharge, nodule or distal ulcer for culture, acid fast staining, histology, and microscopy
- Blood cultures if systemically ill
- Serology (e.g., *Francisella tularensis*, histoplasma)
- Blood film/smear (e.g., filaria)
- Lymphangiography to determine lymphedema or lymphatic obstruction

TREATMENT

GENERAL MEASURES

- Hot, moist compresses to affected area
- If lymphedema is involved, compression garments and weight loss may help.
- Abstinence from sexual activity (for sclerosing lymphangitis)

MEDICATION

- Treat common organisms empirically. Use culture and susceptibility to guide subsequent antibiotic treatment (5)[B].

- If mild disease, use outpatient oral antibiotics.
- If no improvement after 48 hours of oral antibiotics, reassess and consider IV antibiotics and/or hospitalization.
- If systemic involvement, start IV antibiotics.
- If necrotizing fasciitis due to group A β-hemolytic *Streptococcus* is suspected, treat aggressively with antibiotics and surgical intervention.

First Line

- Antibiotics for group A streptococcal infection
  - Amoxicillin (if patient known to have only group A *Streptococcus*)
    ○ Dosing
      ■ Adults
        □ Mild to moderate: 500 mg PO q12h
        □ Severe: 875 mg PO q12h or 500 mg PO q8h

- Children <3 months: 30 mg/kg/day PO divided q12h
- Children ≥3 months, ≤40 kg
  - Mild to moderate: 25 mg/kg/day PO divided q12h or 20 mg/kg/day divided q8h
  - Severe: 45 mg/kg/day PO divided q12h or 40 mg/kg/day divided q8h
- Children ≥40 kg same as adult dosing
  - Common adverse effects
    - Diarrhea
  - Serious adverse effects
    - Anaphylaxis, Stevens-Johnson syndrome (SJS), toxic epidermal necrolysis (TEN)
  - Drug interactions
    - Methotrexate, venlafaxine, warfarin, hormonal contraceptives
  - Contraindications
    - Hypersensitivity to penicillin
- Ampicillin/sulbactam
  - Dosing
    - Adults and children ≥40 kg: 1.5 to 3 g (ampicillin + sulbactam component) IV/IM q6h
    - Children <40 kg: 200 mg/kg/day IV infusion, in divided doses q6h; maximum 8 g ampicillin per day
  - Common adverse effects
    - Diarrhea, injection site reactions
  - Serious adverse effects
    - *Clostridium difficile* diarrhea, pseudomembranous enterocolitis
  - Drug interactions
    - Hormonal contraceptives
  - Contraindications
    - Hypersensitivity reactions
- Ceftriaxone
  - Dosing
    - Adults: 1 to 2 g IV/IM q24h
    - Children: 50 to 75 mg/kg/day IV/IM once daily or in divided doses q12h; maximum 2 g/day
  - Common adverse effects
    - Injection site reactions, diarrhea
  - Serious adverse effects: same as amoxicillin or ampicillin
  - Drug interactions
    - Do not administer calcium-containing solutions in the same IV line.
  - Contraindications
    - Hypersensitivity to cephalosporins
    - Concurrent calcium-containing IV fluids
    - Increased risk of kernicterus, salt precipitation in lungs and kidneys in neonates <28 days (use cefotaxime instead)
- Cephalexin
  - Dosing
    - Adults: 500 mg PO q12h
    - Children: 25 to 50 mg/kg/day divided q12h
  - Common adverse effects
    - Diarrhea
  - Serious adverse effects
    - SJS, TEN, interstitial nephritis, renal failure, pseudomembranous enterocolitis, anaphylaxis
  - Contraindications
    - Hypersensitivity to cephalosporins

- Azithromycin (if penicillin or cephalosporin allergy)
  - Dosing
    - Adults: 500 mg PO on day 1 followed by 250 mg/day PO on days 2 to 5
    - Children ≥2 years: 12 mg/kg/day PO (maximum dose: 500 mg/day) once daily for 5 days (FDA off-label use for skin infections in children)
  - Common adverse effects
    - Abdominal pain, nausea, vomiting, diarrhea, headache
  - Serious adverse effects
    - Prolonged QT interval, torsades de pointes, liver failure, Lambert-Eaton syndrome, myasthenia gravis, corneal erosion, anaphylaxis
  - Drug interactions
    - Nelfinavir, warfarin, other medications with potential to prolong QT interval
  - Contraindications
    - Hepatic dysfunction or cholestatic jaundice with prior treatment
    - Hypersensitivity to macrolide (azithromycin, erythromycin, clarithromycin)
- Diethylcarbamazine, ivermectin, albendazole, and doxycycline are used to treat filarial infection.
- Acetaminophen or ibuprofen (NSAIDs) for pain and fever

SURGERY/OTHER PROCEDURES

- Incision and drainage of abscess if present
- Necrotizing fasciitis needs surgical evaluation and likely débridement
- Nodular lymphangitis may benefit from I&D
- With severe lymphedema, consider surgical drainage

INPATIENT CONSIDERATIONS

Admission Criteria/Initial Stabilization

- Admit for signs of serious illness: fluids if in hypotensive shock.
- Fever, chills, systemic toxicity
- IV antibiotics
- ICU or surgery as indicated

Discharge Criteria

Patient can be discharged on oral antibiotics after systemic symptoms resolve. Home IV antibiotics are an option depending on clinical setting.

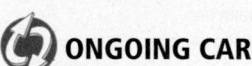 ONGOING CARE

FOLLOW-UP RECOMMENDATIONS

- Elevate affected area.
- 48-hour follow-up to ensure improvement
- Recurrent lymphangitis should prompt workup to ascertain underlying cause (other infectious organism, anatomic abnormality, etc.).

Patient Monitoring

Close follow-up to ensure decreasing inflammation

PATIENT EDUCATION

Instruct patients on proper wound and skin care.

PROGNOSIS

- Good prognosis for uncomplicated cases
- Antimicrobial therapy is effective in 90% of patients.
- Untreated, can spread rapidly, especially group A *Streptococcus*

COMPLICATIONS

Sepsis, cellulitis, necrotizing fasciitis, myositis

REFERENCES

1. Taylor MJ, Hoerauf A, Bockarie M. Lymphatic filariasis and onchocerciasis. *Lancet*. 2010;376(9747):1175–1185.
2. Prat L, Chouaid C, Kettaneh A, et al. Cutaneous lymphangitis carcinomatosa in a patient with lung adenocarcinoma: case report and literature review. *Lung Cancer*. 2013;79(1):91–93.
3. Khare P, Kala P, Jha A, et al. Incidental diagnosis of filariasis in superficial location by FNAC: a retrospective study of 10 years. *J Clin Diagn Res*. 2014;8(12):FC05–FC08.
4. Falagas ME, Bliziotis IA, Kapaskelis AM. Red streaks on the leg. Lymphangitis. *Am Fam Physician*. 2006;73(6):1061–1062.
5. Badger C, Seers K, Preston N, et al. Antibiotics/anti-inflammatories for reducing acute inflammatory episodes in lymphoedema of the limbs. *Cochrane Database Syst Rev*. 2004;(2):CD003143.

ADDITIONAL READING

- Babu AK, Krishnan P, Andezuth DD. Sclerosing lymphangitis of penis—literature review and report of 2 cases. *Dermatol Online J*. 2014;20(7):9.
- Edlich RF, Winters KL, Britt LD, et al. Bacterial diseases of the skin. *J Long Term Eff Med Implants*. 2005;15(5):499–510.
- Raja A, Seshadri RA, Sundersingh S. Lymphangitis carcinomatosa: report of a case and review of literature. *Indian J Surg Oncol*. 2010;1(3):274–276.
- Schubach A, Barros MB, Wanke B. Epidemic sporotrichosis. *Curr Opin Infect Dis*. 2008;21(2):129–133.

 CODES

ICD10

- I89.1 Lymphangitis
- L03.91 Acute lymphangitis, unspecified
- N48.29 Other inflammatory disorders of penis

CLINICAL PEARLS

- Lymphangitis classically presents with erythematous linear streaks of the skin from the inciting site (e.g., bite, cut, abrasion) to regional lymph nodes.
- Patients with prior surgical lymph node dissection are predisposed to lymphangitis.
- Patients with severe systemic symptoms should be admitted and treated with IV antibiotics.
- Parasitic or fungal infections can cause acute or chronic lymphangitis.
- Treatment of underlying skin infection (such as tinea pedis) may prevent recurrence.

LYMPHEDEMA

Jon S. Parham, DO, MPH

 BASICS

DESCRIPTION
- Accumulation of lymphatic fluid in the interstitial tissue causing swelling
- Lymphedema can develop when lymphatic vessels are missing or impaired (primary) or when lymph vessels are damaged or lymph nodes are removed (secondary).
- Most common in the lower limb (80%) but also can occur in the arms, face, trunk, and external genitalia

EPIDEMIOLOGY
Incidence
- Predominant sex: female > male
- Predominant age: any age
- 13% of patients with breast cancer treated with surgery; 42% of those treated with surgery and radiation therapy; 25% after GYN cancer surgery
- Milroy disease presents at birth; estimated to be between 1/6,000 and 1/300 live births
- Meige disease develops during puberty.

Prevalence
- 120 million people worldwide are affected with lymphatic filariasis in 73 countries but no primary infections in United States.
- 10 million people are affected by nonfilarial secondary lymphedema in the United States.

ETIOLOGY AND PATHOPHYSIOLOGY
Secondary lymphedema:
- Postoperative: gradual failure of distal lymphatics, which have to "pump" lymph at a greater pressure through damaged proximal ducts
- Risk is higher with postoperative radiation because radiation reduces regrowth of ducts due to fibrous scarring.
- Trauma; recurrent infection; malignancy, including metastatic disease, and marked obesity
- Developing countries: Most common cause is filariasis (*Wucheria bancrofti*).

Genetics
- Milroy disease: autosomal dominant; diagnosed either at birth or the 1st year of life
- Lymphedema praecox has onset between the ages of 1 and 35 years.
- Lymphedema tarda occurs in those >35 years of age.

RISK FACTORS
- Filariasis: most common cause worldwide
- Mastectomy
- Prior trauma, infection of affected limb
- History of prior surgical (particularly if lymph nodes were removed) or radiation therapy for malignancy (radiation can damage lymph nodes and cause skin dermatitis)
- Long history of venous insufficiency
- Obesity, DVT

GENERAL PREVENTION
Healthy body weight maintenance; treatment of congestive heart failure (CHF) and venous insufficiency

COMMONLY ASSOCIATED CONDITIONS
Venous disease

 DIAGNOSIS

HISTORY
Recent surgery: Vein stripping can significantly exacerbate mild lymphedema (1)[B]:
- First symptom: painless swelling
- Feeling of heaviness in the limb, especially at the end of the day and in hot weather

PHYSICAL EXAM
- Initial: pitting edema, can spread proximally
- Later: nonpitting; after first year, does not spread proximally/distally but spreads radially
- Hyperkeratosis (thicker skin)
- Papillomatosis (rough skin)
- Increase in skin turgor
- Positive Stemmer sign (inability to pinch the skin of the dorsum of the second toe between the thumb and forefinger): must exclude heart failure

DIFFERENTIAL DIAGNOSIS
- CHF, renal failure, lipidemia
- Hypoalbuminemia, protein-losing nephropathy
- DVT, chronic venous disease
- Postoperative complications following ipsilateral surgery
- Cellulitis, Baker cyst, idiopathic edema

DIAGNOSTIC TESTS & INTERPRETATION
- Lack of response to elevation or diuretic therapy may indicate a lymphatic insufficiency (2)[B].
- Diuretics increase excretion of salt and water, thereby decreasing plasma volume, venous capillary pressure, and filtration. Diuretics improve filtration edema but do not improve lymph drainage over the long term.
- Some relevant protein biomarkers for lymphedema have been identified and show promise for early- and latent-stage diagnosis (3)[B].

Initial Tests (lab, imaging)
- Comprehensive chemistry panel: evaluates for hepatic or renal impairment
- Urinalysis: protein-losing nephropathy
- Ultrasound: evaluates for acute/chronic DVT; gives information about soft tissue changes but does not tell about truncal anatomy of the lymphatics (1)[B]
- Duplex ultrasound: Lymphedema causes gradual impedance of venous return that aggravates the edema; 82% of patients with unexplained limb edema were diagnosed using a combination of duplex ultrasound and lymphoscintigram (4)[A].

Follow-Up Tests & Special Considerations
- Lymphangiogram: direct cannulation of lymphatics through the skin; risk for infection, local inflammation; not used commonly (4)[C]
- Fluorescence microlymphography may be highly sensitive (91.4%) and specific (85.7%), atraumatic and is without radiation in diagnosis of leg lymphedema (5)[B]

- Lymphoscintigram: radiolabeled protein technetium-99m–labeled colloid
  - Measures lymphatic function, lymph movement, lymph drainage, and response to treatment
  - Sensitivity, 73–97%; specificity, 100%
  - Best to use 1 hour and delayed images together (4)[A]
- Indocyanine green lymphography: reported
  - Superior to lymphoscintigraphy in early diagnosis of arm (6)[B]
  - Accurately screens post surgically for subclinical lymphedema (7)[B]
- CT scan: calf skin thickening, thickening of the SC compartment, increased fat density, thickened perimuscular aponeurosis; typical honeycomb appearance (4)[B]
- MRI: circumferential edema, increased volume of SC tissue, honeycomb pattern above the fascia between the muscle and subcutis; cannot differentiate primary from secondary lymphedema (4)[B]

TREATMENT

GENERAL MEASURES
- Seek optimal weight, early treatment of cellulitis, avoid trauma to affected area (direct injury, venipunctures, inept nail care, extreme heat/cold).
- Achieve mechanical reduction and maintenance of limb size: compression garments via professionals.
- Elevate affected limb/area, but avoid stasis.
- Avoid BP cuffs in affected limbs.
- Prevent skin infection with daily cleansing, inspection, and skin care (with emollients).
- Treatment of varicose veins may benefit some.

MEDICATION
- Diuretics of limited benefit and may lead to volume depletion
- Benzopyrenes (flavonoids and coumarin) (not available for prescription use in the United States)
  - Micronized purified flavonoid fraction (Daflon 500 mg) is effective in decreasing venous stasis and idiopathic cyclic edema, chronic venous insufficiency, and postmastectomy lymphedema. It also reduces capillary permeability and the inflammatory component (8)[C].
- Coumarin reduces edema fluid by increasing the number of macrophages and enhancing proteolysis, resulting in the removal of protein, increasing softness in the limbs, and decreasing elevated skin temperature with subsequent symptom improvement and decreased secondary infection. Some reports of hepatotoxicity (8)[C].

ISSUES FOR REFERRAL
- Refer to physical therapist with lymphedema training for manual decongestive therapy.
  - In patients with recurrent or metastatic disease, discuss with oncologist prior to initiation of complete decongestive therapy in order not to promote the spread of cancer.
- Provide education for patient/family for self-administration of therapy in future.
- Education for family about bandaging
- Fitting for compression garments

ADDITIONAL THERAPIES

- Exercise: Lymph flow occurs as a result of inspiratory reduction in the intrathoracic pressure associated with inspiration. Best results are achieved with combination of flexibility, strength, and aerobic training (4)[B]. Compression with custom-made elastic stocking (minimum pressure is 40 mm Hg).

  – Protection against external incidental trauma
  – Decreases the intrinsic trauma on the skin due to chronically increased interstitial pressures, which cause stretch of the skin and SC tissues
  – No data on preference of custom-made versus prefabricated

  – Replace every 3 to 6 months or when starting to lose elasticity (1)[B].
- Multilayer bandaging: inner layer of tubular stockinette followed by foam and padding to protect the joint flexures and to even out the contours of the limb so that pressure is distributed evenly; outer layer of at least two short-stretch extensible bandages; more effective than hosiery alone (1)[B]
- Pneumatic pumps: development of high pressure up to 150 mm Hg; can reduce limb girth by 37–68.6%; wear a compression stocking when not using pump; high risk of genital edema; no metastasis in limb due to risk of spread (1)[B]

- Thai "Schnogh", a novel, intense tourniquet technique, has initially shown at least 50% limb volume reduction (9)[C]

SURGERY/OTHER PROCEDURES

- Bypass procedures: creation of lymphatic–venous anastomosis or lymph node transplantation (most effective) via microsurgery showed a reduction in use of conservative compression therapy (10)[B]: reserved for refractory cases only. In a pilot study, low-level laser therapy was shown not to be inferior to manual lymphatic drainage or the combination of the two in arm volume reduction in breast cancer–related lymphedema and required ≤1/2 the treatment time (11)[C].
- Thoracic sympathetic ganglion block for breast cancer–related lymphedema, a new treatment showed better life quality and arm size reduction >50% (11)[B]

- Debulking procedures (Charles procedure): radical excision of SC tissue with primary or staged skin grafting (8)[C]
  – Men had less improvement than women.
  – Main risk is infection and necrosis of the skin graft.
  – Liposuction is cosmetically preferred to debulking.

COMPLEMENTARY & ALTERNATIVE MEDICINE

Heat therapy: Hot water immersion, microwave, and electromagnetic irradiation may be helpful (1)[C].

INPATIENT CONSIDERATIONS
Admission Criteria/Initial Stabilization
Systemic signs of infection
- May admit to specialized rehabilitation unit for combination treatment in patients with heart failure or severe pulmonary disease
- IV antibiotics for infection

Nursing
- Leg elevation
- Encourage patient mobilization/exercise.
- Patient education for bandaging/wound care

Discharge Criteria
- Resolution of signs/symptoms of infection (e.g., elevated WBC count, fever, abnormal vital signs)
- Clinical improvement in wound appearance

 ## ONGOING CARE

FOLLOW-UP RECOMMENDATIONS
Lymphedema will return in several days if patient stops wearing compression garments during the day and bandaging at night.

Patient Monitoring
- Daily visit to therapist for acute treatment
- Monthly visits for maintenance care

DIET
Low sodium; weight loss–oriented if needed

PATIENT EDUCATION
- Use compression garments, especially when exercising.
- Avoid affected limb(s) being dependant for long period of time: Patient should perform daily skin examination.
- http://www.nlm.nih.gov/medlineplus/lymphedema.html

PROGNOSIS
No cure, but treatment can produce good results with daily care

COMPLICATIONS
- Infection (local vs. systemic): common
- Risk of wound formation (venous wounds/abrasions) that are difficult to heal: common
- Lymphangiosarcoma: Found in lymphedematous arms of patients following radical mastectomy; also in patients with Milroy disease. Treatment is radiotherapy with surgery, reserved for patients with discrete nonmetastatic disease.

REFERENCES

1. Warren AG, Brorson H, Borud LJ, et al. Lymphedema: a comprehensive review. *Ann Plast Surg*. 2007;59(4):464–472.
2. Mortimer PS. Implications of the lymphatic system in CVI-associated edema. *Angiology*. 2000;51(1):3–7.
3. Lin S, Kim J, Lee MJ, et al. Prospective transcriptomic pathway analysis of human lymphatic vascular insufficiency: identification and validation of a circulating biomarker panel. *PLoS One*. 2012;7(12):e52021.
4. Brennan MJ, Miller LT. Overview of treatment options and review of the current role and use of compression garments, intermittent pumps, and exercise in the management of lymphedema. *Cancer*. 1998;83(12 Suppl):2821–2827.
5. Keo HH, Husmann M, Groechenig E, et al. Diagnostic accuracy of fluorescence microlymphography for detecting limb lymphedema. *Eur J Vasc Endovasc Surg*. 2015;49(4):474–479.
6. Mihara M, Hara H, Araki J, et al. Indocyanine green (ICG) lymphography is superior to lymphoscintigraphy for diagnostic imaging of early lymphedema of the upper limbs. *PloS One*. 2012;7(6):e38182.
7. Akita S, Mitsukawa N, Rikihisa N, et al. Early diagnosis and risk factors for lymphedema following lymph node dissection for gynecologic cancer. *Plast Reconstr Surg*. 2013;131(2):283–290.
8. Tiwari A, Cheng KS, Button M, et al. Differential diagnosis, investigation, and current treatment of lower limb lymphedema. *Arch Surg*. 2003;138(2):152–161.
9. Chanwimalueang N, Ekataksin W, Piyaman P, et al. Twisting Tourniquet(©) Technique: introducing Schnogh, a novel device and its effectiveness in treating primary and secondary lymphedema of extremities. *Cancer Med*. 2015;4(10):1514–1524.
10. Basta MN, Gao LL, Wu LC. Operative treatment of peripheral lymphedema: a systematic meta-analysis of the efficacy and safety of lymphovenous microsurgery and tissue transplantation. *Plast Reconstr Surg*. 2014;133(4):905–913.
11. Ridner SH, Poage-Hooper E, Kanar C, et al. A pilot randomized trial evaluating low-level laser therapy as an alternative treatment to manual lymphatic drainage for breast cancer-related lymphedema. *Oncol Nurs Forum*. 2013;40(4):383–393.

 ## CODES

ICD10
- I89.0 Lymphedema, not elsewhere classified
- Q82.0 Hereditary lymphedema
- I97.89 Oth postproc comp and disorders of the circ sys, NEC

CLINICAL PEARLS
- Use short-stretch bandages for wrapping (not ACE wraps).
- Avoid heat/whirlpool: typically worsens condition.
- Much higher risk for cutaneous-sourced infections than patients with only venous insufficiency
- Lymphoscintigram is a standard diagnostic, but consider Indocyanine green lymphography or fluorescence microlymphography.

MACULAR DEGENERATION, AGE-RELATED

Richard W. Allinson, MD

 BASICS

DESCRIPTION
- Age-related macular degeneration (ARMD) results in pigmentary changes in the macula or typical drusen associated with visual loss to the 20/30 level or worse, not caused by cataract or other eye disease, in individuals >50 years of age, although some definitions exclude age or visual acuity criteria.
- Leading cause of irreversible, severe visual loss in persons age >65 years
- Stages
  - Atrophic/nonexudative
  - Neovascular/exudative
- System(s) affected: nervous
- Synonym(s): senile macular degeneration; subretinal neovascularization

EPIDEMIOLOGY
- Neovascular/exudative form is rare in blacks and more common in whites.
- Predominant sex: female

Incidence
- In the Framingham Eye Study (FES), drusen were noted in 25% of all participants who were ≥52 years of age. ARMD-associated visual loss was noted in 5.7%.
- Atrophic/nonexudative stage accounts for 20% of cases of severe visual loss
- Neovascular/exudative stage accounts for 80% of cases of severe visual loss

Prevalence
Per FES study:
- People 65 to 74 years old: 11%
- People ≥75 years old: 27.9%

ETIOLOGY AND PATHOPHYSIOLOGY
- Breaks in the Bruch membrane allow choroidal neovascular membranes (CNVMs) to invade the retinal pigment epithelium (RPE) and grow into the subretinal space.
- Atrophic/nonexudative: drusen and/or pigmentary changes in the macula
- Neovascular/exudative: growth of blood vessels underneath the retina
- Visible light can result in the formation and accumulation of metabolic by-products in the RPE, a pigment layer underneath the retina that normally helps remove metabolic by-products from the retina. Excess accumulation of these metabolic by-products interferes with the normal metabolic activity of the RPE and can lead to the formation of drusen.
- Neovascular stage generally arises from the atrophic stage.
- Most do not progress beyond the atrophic/non-exudative stage; however, those who do are at a greater risk of severe visual loss.

Genetics
- Genetic susceptibility may be a factor in ARMD: ~25% genetically determined.
- Complement factor H is an important susceptibility gene for ARMD.
- Although the development of ARMD may be predicted by specific alleles, the clinical response to antivascular endothelial growth factor is not (1)[A].

RISK FACTORS
- Obesity
- Ethnicity: non-Hispanic whites
- Cigarette smoking
- *Chlamydia pneumoniae* infection
- Family history
- Excess sunlight exposure
- Blue or light iris color
- Hyperopia
- History of cardiovascular disease
- Short stature
- Aspirin use
- Female sex

GENERAL PREVENTION
- Ultraviolet (UV) protection for eyes
- Routine ophthalmologic visits
  - Every 2 to 4 years for patients age 40 to 64 years
  - Every 1 to 2 years after age 65 years
- Patients who take statins, which modify lipid profiles, may have a reduced risk.

COMMONLY ASSOCIATED CONDITIONS
- Presumed ocular histoplasmosis syndrome
- Exudative retinal detachment
- Vitreous hemorrhage
- Other causes of CNVMs

 DIAGNOSIS

HISTORY
- Patients frequently notice distortion of central vision.
- Patients may notice straight lines appear crooked (e.g., telephone poles).

PHYSICAL EXAM
- Atrophic/nonexudative stage retinal exam
  - Drusen (small yellowish white lesions)
    - Subtypes: hard drusen and soft drusen
  - Atrophy of the RPE
- Neovascular/exudative stage retinal exam
  - Blood vessels growing underneath the retina from the choroid are called *CNVMs* or *subretinal neovascularization* (SRN). The choroid is the vascular layer underneath the RPE.
  - Subretinal fluid or hemorrhage
  - Exudates
  - On Amsler grid testing, the horizontal or vertical lines may become broken, distorted, or missing.
- Disciform scar: an advanced stage resulting in a fibrovascular scar

DIFFERENTIAL DIAGNOSIS
- Idiopathic SRN
- Presumed ocular histoplasmosis syndrome
- Diabetic retinopathy
- Hypertensive retinopathy

DIAGNOSTIC TESTS & INTERPRETATION
Diagnostic Procedures/Other
- Amsler grid testing
- Fluorescein angiography
  - Detection of CNVMs
  - Differentiate between atrophic and neovascular ARMD.
- Indocyanine green video angiography: may identify occult or hidden CNVMs
- Optical coherence tomography (OCT) may be useful in identifying CNVMs, subretinal fluid, and retinal thickening.
  - Fluorescein angiography is better than time-domain OCT in detecting new-onset CNVMs

Test Interpretation
Drusen: deposits of hyaline material between the RPE and Bruch membrane (the limiting membrane between the RPE and the choroid)

 TREATMENT

MEDICATION
First Line
- Ranibizumab (Lucentis)
  - Antibody fragment that inhibits all active forms of vascular endothelial growth factor (VEGF)
  - Approved for neovascular (wet) ARMD
  - Injected intravitreally, at a dose of 0.5 mg, every 4 weeks
  - 1 year after treatment, up to 40% of patients treated with ranibizumab gained at least three lines of vision and ~95% maintained vision.
  - Ranibizumab is superior to verteporfin in the treatment of predominately classic CNVMs.
  - The PrONTO study demonstrated OCT-guided, variable-dosing regimen with ranibizumab resulted in similar results to the MARINA and ANCHOR studies with monthly injections.
  - When comparing ranibizumab and bevacizumab in a multicenter study, both treatments were effective in stabilizing visual loss, and no difference was found in the visual outcome between the two treatment groups. A slightly higher rate of serious systemic adverse events was noted in the bevacizumab group (2)[A].
    - In this study treatment as needed resulted in less gain in visual acuity, whether instituted at enrollment or after 1 year of monthly treatment.
  - Eyes with ≥50% of the lesion composed of blood had a similar visual prognosis compared to other treated eyes in the Comparison of Age-related Macular Degeneration Treatmenst Trials (CATT). Neovascular ARMD lesions composed of >50% blood can be managed similarly to those with less or no blood (3)[A].
  - The treat and extend regimen (TER) is commonly used to decrease the treatment burden. Once no signs of CNVM activity are detected, patient follow-ups and treatments are then extended by intervals of 2 weeks as long as no signs of CNVM activity are present, up to a maximum interval of 12 weeks. If examination shows any sign of recurrence, the interval is shortened by 2 weeks at a time, until the disease is considered to be inactive. Interval extension is then restarted, with the maximum final interval being 2 weeks less than the period when the previous recurrence was observed.
  - Ranibizumab and bevacizumab had equivalent effects on visual acuity at 1 year using the TER. The visual acuity results at 1 year were comparable to those of other clinical trials with monthly treatment (4)[A]
- VEGF Trap-Eye/aflibercept (Eylea)
  - A decoy VEGF receptor that inhibits all isoforms of VEGF-A and placental growth factor (PlGF), the members of the VEGF family in mammals primarily involved in ocular neovascularization
  - Approved for neovascular (wet) ARMD
  - Injected intravitreally, at a dose of 2 mg, every 4 weeks for 12 weeks then every 8 weeks

– Dosed as needed after the 12-week fixed dosing schedule resulted in a 5.3-letter gain in best corrected visual acuity at 52 weeks (5)[B].
– Routine use of prophylactic antibiotics after intravitreal injections may be unnecessary (6)[B].

– Maybe beneficial in patients who are not responding to ranibizumab or bevacizumab (7)[C]

Second Line
• Bevacizumab (Avastin) is a full-length antibody to VEGF, administered intravitreally at a dose of 1.25 mg; it is being evaluated in the treatment of neovascular ARMD. Widely used off-label because of its lower cost.
• Agents that block platelet-derived growth factor (PDGF) are being investigated.

GENERAL MEASURES
Low-vision aids may be helpful.

SURGERY/OTHER PROCEDURES
• Laser treatment for CNVMs located ≥200 microns from the center of the macula has been evaluated in the Macular Photocoagulation Study (MPS).
– Anti-VEGF treatment is first-line therapy for subfoveal CNVM's.
• Vitrectomy has been used to remove CNVMs, but this is generally not recommended.
• CNVMs can bleed spontaneously, leaving blood underneath the retina. Vitrectomy to remove subretinal blood may be of benefit and should be performed within 7 days of the bleed. Tissue plasminogen activator (tPA) instilled in the eye, may help remove a subretinal hemorrhage. In some cases, intravitreal gas with or without tPA may displace submacular blood:
– Intravitreal anti-VEGF monotherapy may be helpful in the treatment of neovascular ARMD associated with a submacular hemorrhage (8)[C].
• Photodynamic therapy (PDT) with verteporfin reduces vision loss in patients with >50% "classic" subfoveal CNVMs. Verteporfin is administered IV, and a diode laser at 689 nm is applied to the CNVM.
– Patients should be informed of a <4% risk of acute, severe vision loss after PDT.
– Ranibizumab has greater clinical efficacy than PDT.
– Combination treatment with intravitreal ranibizumab and PDT appears to offer similar gain in visual acuity when compared with ranibizumab monotherapy (9)[B].
– Combination treatment with ranibizumab and PDT may reduce the number of ranibizumab retreatments.
• Stereotactic radiotherapy is being investigated in the treatment of neovascular ARMD.
• Laser photocoagulation to treat drusen is not recommended.

COMPLEMENTARY & ALTERNATIVE MEDICINE
Free radical formation in the retina, induced by visible light, may play a role in cellular damage that results in atrophic/nonexudative macular degeneration. The Age-Related Eye Disease Study (AREDS) found that a high-dose regimen of antioxidant vitamins and mineral supplements reduced progression of ARMD in some cases.
• Recommended daily doses: vitamin C 500 mg, vitamin E 400 IU, β-carotene 15 mg, zinc oxide 80 mg, and cupric oxide 2 mg
• Exercise caution with β-carotene use in smokers due to potential link to lung cancer.

• The Age-Related Eye Disease Study 2 (AREDS2) found the addition of lutein with zeaxanthin alone or in combination with omega-3 fatty acids had no overall effect in further reducing the risk of progression to advanced ARMD (10)[A].

 ONGOING CARE

FOLLOW-UP RECOMMENDATIONS
Patient Monitoring
• Amsler grid can aid in discovering visual disturbances.
• Patients with soft drusen or pigmentary changes in the macula are at an increased risk of visual loss. They should monitor their vision, such as by daily Amsler grid testing, and subjective measures of visual acuity, such as reading ability. If no new symptoms, follow-up examination in 6 to 12 months

DIET
• Eating dark green, leafy vegetables (spinach/collard greens), which are rich in carotenoids, may decrease the risk of developing the neovascular/exudative stage.
• Fish consumption with omega-3 fatty acid intake reduces the risk of ARMD.
• A Western type diet characterized by higher intake of red meat, processed meat, high-fat dairy products, French fries, refined grains, and eggs increases the risk of ARMD as compared to an Oriental type diet characterized by higher intake of vegetables, legumes, fruit, whole grains, tomatoes, and seafood which decreases the risk of ARMD (11)[A].

PATIENT EDUCATION
Instruct visually impaired patients to check with the local low-vision center for aids.

PROGNOSIS
• Patients with bilateral soft drusen and pigmentary changes in the macula, but no evidence of exudation, have an increased likelihood of developing CNVMs and subsequent visual loss.
• Patients with bilateral drusen carry a cumulative risk of 14.7% over 5 years of suffering significant visual loss in one eye from the neovascular stage of ARMD.
• Patients with neovascular stage in one eye and drusen in the opposite eye are at an annual risk of 5–14% of developing the neovascular stage in the opposite eye with drusen.
• High incidence of recurrence after thermal laser treatment for CNVMs

COMPLICATIONS
• Blindness
• The intraocular pressure should be monitored in eyes receiving intravitreal anti-VEGF injections.

REFERENCES
1. Hagstrom SA, Ying GS, Pauer GJ, et al. Pharmacogenetics for genes associated with age-related macular degeneration in the Comparison of AMD Treatment Trials (CATT). *Ophthalmology*. 2013;120(3):593–599.
2. Martin DF, Maguire MG, Fine SL, et al. Ranibizumab and bevacizumab for treatment of neovascular age-related macular degeneration: two-year results. *Ophthalmology*. 2012;119(7):1388–1398.
3. Altaweel MM, Daniel E, Martin DF, et al. Outcomes of eyes with lesions composed of >50% blood in the Comparison of Age-related Macular Degeneration Treatments Trials (CATT). *Ophthalmology*. 2015;122(2):391.e5–398.e5.
4. Berg K, Pedersen TR, Sandvik L, et al. Comparison of ranibizumab and bevacizumab for neovascular age-related macular degeneration according to LUCAS treat-and-extend protocol. *Ophthalmology*. 2015;122(1):146–152.
5. Heier JS, Boyer D, Nguyen QD, et al. The 1-year results of CLEAR-IT 2, a phase 2 study of vascular endothelial growth factor trap-eye dosed as-needed after 12-week fixed dosing. *Ophthalmology*. 2011;118(6):1098–1106.
6. Yin VT, Weisbrod DJ, Eng KT, et al. Antibiotic resistance of ocular surface flora with repeated use of a topical antibiotic after intravitreal injection. *JAMA Ophthalmol*. 2013;131(4):456–461.
7. Chang AA, Li H, Broadhead GK, et al. Intravitreal aflibercept for treatment-resistant neovascular age-related macular degeneration. *Ophthalmology*. 2014;121(1):188–192.
8. Shienbaum G, Garcia Filho CA, Flynn HW Jr, et al. Management of submacular hemorrhage secondary to neovascular age-related macular degeneration with anti-vascular endothelial growth factor monotherapy. *Am J Ophthalmol*. 2013;155(6):1009–1013.
9. Larsen M, Schmidt-Erfurth U, Lanzetta P, et al. Verteporfin plus ranibizumab for choroidal neovascularization in age-related macular degeneration: twelve-month MONT BLANC study results. *Ophthalmology*. 2012;119(5):992–1000.
10. Age-Related Eye Disease Study 2 Research Group. Lutein + zeaxanthin and omega-3 fatty acids for age-related macular degeneration: the Age-Related Eye Disease Study 2 (AREDS2) randomized clinical trial. *JAMA*. 2013;309(19): 2005–2015.
11. Chiu CJ, Chang ML, Zhang FF, et al. The relationship of major American dietary patterns to age-related macular degeneration. *Am J Ophthalmol*. 2014;158(1):118.e1–127.e1.

CODES
ICD10
• H35.30 Unspecified macular degeneration
• H35.32 Exudative age-related macular degeneration
• H35.31 Nonexudative age-related macular degeneration

CLINICAL PEARLS
• Patients frequently notice distortion of central vision.
• Patients may notice straight lines appear crooked (e.g., telephone poles).
• Hyperopia is a risk factor for ARMD.
• The AREDS study found that a high-dose regimen of antioxidant vitamins and mineral supplements reduces progression of ARMD in some cases.
• Tobacco cessation should be strongly encouraged.

M

MALARIA
Paul M. Arguin, MD

 BASICS

DESCRIPTION
- Acute or chronic infection transmitted to humans by *Anopheles* spp. mosquitoes
- Most morbidity and mortality is caused by *Plasmodium falciparum*. An estimated 198 million cases occur annually, including 584,000 deaths, most of which occur in children <5 years of age in sub-Saharan Africa (1).
- Nonimmune individuals are most susceptible to rapid progression to severe disease.
- System(s) affected: cardiovascular, hematologic, renal, respiratory, cerebral, lymphatic, immunologic

EPIDEMIOLOGY
- Cases imported to the United States: 58% *P. falciparum*; 17% *Plasmodium vivax*; 3% *Plasmodium malariae*; 3% *Plasmodium ovale*; 1% mixed; 17% unknown
- Occurs worldwide in tropical latitudes: *P. falciparum, P. malariae, P. vivax,* and *P. ovale. P. knowlesi* in parts of Southeast Asia.

Incidence
- Most U.S. cases (>99%) are imported.
- ~1,500 cases and 5 deaths per year in the United States (2)

Prevalence
- Predominant age: all ages
- Predominant sex: male = female

ETIOLOGY AND PATHOPHYSIOLOGY
- Malarial parasites digest red blood cell (RBC) proteins and alter the RBC membrane, thereby causing hemolysis, increased splenic clearance, and anemia.
- RBC lysis stimulates release of cytokines and tumor necrosis factor-α (TNF-α) causing fever and systemic symptoms.
- *P. falciparum* alters RBC viscosity, causing obstruction and end-organ ischemia.

Genetics
Unknown genetic predilection but inherited conditions may affect disease severity and susceptibility (glucose-6-phosphate dehydrogenase deficiency, sickle cell disease or trait, and hereditary elliptocytosis)

RISK FACTORS
- Travel/migration from endemic areas (primarily sub-Saharan Africa)
- Rarely, blood transfusion, mother-to-fetus transmission, and local autochthonous transmission

GENERAL PREVENTION
- Mosquito avoidance measures: Use of insect repellent, wear clothing that covers exposed skin, use mosquito nets treated with permethrin, and avoid outdoor activity from dusk to dawn.
- *Malarial chemoprophylaxis when in endemic area*
  – Mefloquine: begin at least 2 weeks before arrival and continue for 4 weeks after leaving area. Adults, 250 mg (1 tablet) weekly; children ≤9 kg, 5 mg/kg; children >9 to 19 kg, 1/4 tablet weekly; children >19 to 30 kg, 1/2 tablet weekly; children >30 to 45 kg, 3/4 tablet weekly; children >45 kg as adult
    ○ Caution: mefloquine-resistant areas
  – Atovaquone/proguanil: begin 1 to 2 days before arrival and continue for 1 week after leaving area.

Adults, 1 adult tablet daily; children 5 to 8 kg, 1/2 pediatric tablet daily; children 9 to 10 kg, 3/4 pediatric tablet daily; children 11 to 20 kg, 1 pediatric tablet daily; children 21 to 30 kg, 2 pediatric tablets daily; children 31 to 40 kg, 3 pediatric tablets daily; children >40 kg, 1 adult tablet daily
  – Doxycycline: begin 1 to 2 days before arrival and continue for 4 weeks after leaving area. Adults, 100 mg daily; children, 2 mg/kg up to 100 mg daily (not for children <8 years old)
  – Chloroquine: begin 1 to 2 weeks before arrival and continue for 4 weeks after leaving area. Adults, 500 mg (300-mg base) weekly; children, 8.3 mg/kg (5-mg base/kg) weekly up to 300 mg
    ○ Caution: chloroquine-resistant areas
  – Primaquine: begin 1 to 2 days before arrival and continue for 1 week after leaving area; adults, 30 mg/day; children, 0.5 mg/kg/day up to adult dose
    ○ For use only in areas predominantly endemic for *P. vivax*
    ○ Caution: Glucose-6-phosphate dehydrogenase deficiency must be excluded prior to first use.

COMMONLY ASSOCIATED CONDITIONS
Bacterial coinfections sometimes occur.

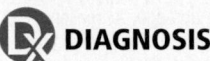 **DIAGNOSIS**

HISTORY
- Initial symptoms of malaria are nonspecific. Suspect malaria in ill patients returning from endemic area presenting with
  – Fever, malaise, myalgias, chills, headache, nausea, splenomegaly (with chronic infection), hypotension, anemia (with chronic or severe disease), thrombocytopenia, jaundice, vomiting, and/or diarrhea (resembling gastroenteritis)
- *P. falciparum*
  – Incubation usually 12 to 14 days, symptoms within 1 month of infection in most individuals (partially immune individuals such as immigrants may become ill up to 1 year after last exposure)
  – Severe disease and complications: vascular collapse, CNS impairment, renal failure, and acute respiratory distress syndrome
- *P. vivax* and *P. ovale*
  – Incubation period 12 to 18 days for primary infection and up to 12 months (and longer) for relapses; generally presents with fevers
  – Dormant parasites may remain in liver and reactivate years after initial infection.
  – Can be severe
- *P. malariae*
  – Incubation period ~35 days
  – May become chronic; untreated can persist asymptomatically in human host for years
- *P. knowlesi*
  – Incubation period ~12 days
  – Possibly severe

PHYSICAL EXAM
- Often not specific
- General: elevated temperature, fatigue, tachycardia, tachypnea, jaundice
- Neurologic: mental status and motor–sensory exam (cerebral malaria)

- Cardiopulmonary exam: hemodynamic stability and signs of vascular leak (effusion)
- Skin exam: pallor, rash
- Abdominal exam: organomegaly

DIFFERENTIAL DIAGNOSIS
- Infections (disseminated or localized): abscess, viral, gastroenteritis, typhoid/paratyphoid, other bacteremias, rickettsial disease, mycobacteria
- Collagen vascular disease (systemic lupus erythematosus [SLE], vasculitides)
- Neoplasms (lymphoma, leukemia, other blood dyscrasias, other tropical causes of splenomegaly)
- Severe malaria infection may mimic hepatitis, pneumonia, stroke, or sepsis.

DIAGNOSTIC TESTS & INTERPRETATION
- Malarial smear thick and thin preparations (3)[A]
  – Microscopy to evaluate for presence of parasite forms, determine species, and quantify the percentage of RBCs that are infected. Relatively easy to perform with proper training.
  – Test should be performed on site, immediately, with results quickly available.
    ○ Rapid antigen capture enzyme: can detect the presence of malaria parasites within minutes. Cannot determine species or quantify parasitemia. Positive and negative results must always be confirmed by microscopy.
    ○ Other tests: species-specific PCR; species confirmation by PCR is encouraged.
- General laboratory findings (nonspecific)
  – In uncomplicated infection
    ○ Elevated liver function tests and lactate dehydrogenase
    ○ Thrombocytopenia, anemia, and leukopenia
- Note: a low to low-normal platelet count or a slightly high bilirubin should alert the clinician to the diagnosis after exposure in an endemic setting.
- Note: Antimalarial prophylaxis may reduce parasitemia.

Initial Tests (lab, imaging)
- CBC with differential and platelets
- Basic chemistry panel including bilirubin
- Malaria thick and thin blood films (if negative, repeat q12–24h for at least three sets)
- Imaging necessary only for respiratory disease (chest x-ray) or cerebral malaria (CT scan prior to lumbar puncture)

Follow-Up Tests & Special Considerations
- Nonimmune individuals with suspected or confirmed *P. falciparum* should be hospitalized.
- Clinical specimens from suspected or confirmed malaria cases in the United States can be submitted to the Centers for Disease Control and Prevention (CDC) for diagnostic confirmation, speciation, and drug resistance surveillance free of charge.

Test Interpretation
Interpretation of microscopy. Blood is obtained from the patient and spread on a microscope slide as a thick/thin prep and stained with Giemsa (most commonly). The slide is viewed under 100X oil immersion to examine for ring, gametocyte, trophozoite, and schizont forms. The thick film is better for detecting parasites. The thin film is used to determine species and calculating the percentage of RBCs infected. Both should always be performed.

TREATMENT

MEDICATION

First Line

- For uncomplicated chloroquine-resistant *P. falciparum* (most *P. falciparum*), chloroquine-resistant *P. vivax*, or when species is unknown, the following regimens are recommended (4)[A]:

  - Atovaquone-proguanil (Malarone): adult tablet: 250 mg atovaquone and 100 mg proguanil. Pediatric tablet: 62.5 mg atovaquone and 25 mg proguanil. Adults: 4 adult tablets once per day for 3 days. Children 5 to 8 kg: 2 pediatric tablets once per day for 3 days; children 9 to 10 kg: 3 pediatric tablets once per day for 3 days; children 11 to 20 kg: 1 adult tablet once per day for 3 days; children 21 to 30 kg: 2 adult tablets once per day for 3 days; children 31 to 40 kg: 3 adult tablets once per day for 3 days; children >40 kg: 4 adult tablets once per day for 3 days
  - Artemether-lumefantrine (Coartem): tablet contains 20 mg artemether and 120 mg lumefantrine. Persons 5 to <15 kg: 1 tablet BID for 3 days; persons 15 to <25 kg: 2 tablets BID for 3 days; persons 25 to <35 kg: 3 tablets BID for 3 days; persons ≥35 kg: 4 tablets BID for 3 days
  - Quinine sulfate plus doxycycline or clindamycin: adults: quinine sulfate 650 mg (salt) TID for 3 days (should be extended to 7 days for infections acquired in Southeast Asia). Doxycycline 100 mg BID for 7 days. Clindamycin 20 mg (base)/kg/day divided TID for 7 days. Children: quinine sulfate 10 mg (salt)/kg TID for 3 days (should be extended to 7 days for infections acquires in Southeast Asia) plus clindamycin dosed as above.
  - Mefloquine: adults: 750 mg followed by 500 mg 8 hours later. Children: 15 mg/kg followed by 10 mg/kg 8 hours later (maximum total dose: 1,250 mg)
- PO therapy for *P. ovale*, *P. malariae*, chloroquine-sensitive *P. falciparum* (rare), and chloroquine-sensitive *P. vivax* (New Guinea has highest rates of chloroquine-resistant *P. vivax*); in addition to the treatment regimens listed above, other options are as follows:
  - Chloroquine: adults: 1 g (600-mg base) followed by 500 mg (300-mg base) at 6, 24, and 48 hours after first dose. Children: 16.6 mg/kg (10-mg base/kg) on day 1 (max 1,000 mg [600-mg base]), then 8.3 mg/kg (5-mg base) at 6, 24, and 48 hours after first dose
  - Primaquine (should be added to the acute treatment regimen for cure of dormant forms of *P. vivax* and *P. ovale*): adults: 30-mg base (52.6 mg) daily for 2 weeks. Children: 0.6-mg base/kg/day for 2 weeks
- Therapy for severe malaria
  - Clinical features defining severe malaria:
    - Impaired level of consciousness (LOC)
    - Respiratory distress, jaundice
    - Repeated convulsions, shock
    - Renal failure
  - Laboratory features:
    - Parasitemia >5%
    - Hypoglycemia
    - Acidosis (usually lactic acidosis)
- Parenteral therapy
  - Quinidine gluconate 10 mg/kg in normal saline over 1 to 2 hours followed by 0.02 mg/kg/min continuous infusion
  - Intensive care monitoring is necessary, especially when initiating quinidine therapy.

- In severe malaria, contact the CDC for assistance; CDC Malaria Branch: 770-488-7100; http://www.cdc.gov/Malaria/
- In 2007, the CDC made artesunate available in the United States for severe malaria in special circumstances under an investigational protocol. Contact the CDC for assistance.

ISSUES FOR REFERRAL

Infectious disease or tropical medicine consultation advised. Malaria is a reportable disease (http://www.cdc.gov/malaria/features/new_report_form.html).

ADDITIONAL THERAPIES

None

Pediatric Considerations

- Children are particularly susceptible to severe disease.
- All children, even infants, should receive chemoprophylaxis if traveling to an endemic area.
- Malaria commonly resembles acute gastroenteritis in children.
- Children with severe disease are particularly prone to hypoglycemia. Use IV fluids with glucose for maintenance and monitor blood glucose frequently.

Pregnancy Considerations

- Chloroquine is safe in the doses recommended for prevention and treatment of malaria; FDA pregnancy Category C.
- Mefloquine is safe in the doses recommended for prevention and treatment of malaria; FDA pregnancy Category B.
- Atovaquone-proguanil (Malarone) has not been studied in pregnant women; it has not been shown to cause birth defects or other problems in animal studies; FDA pregnancy Category C.
- No primaquine (FDA class undetermined) or tetracyclines (FDA pregnancy Category D) in pregnancy
- Quinine/Quinidine (FDA pregnancy Category C, respectively) should be used during pregnancy because benefit outweighs risk.

COMPLEMENTARY & ALTERNATIVE MEDICINE

None. Deaths have resulted from using unapproved alternatives to recommended medications.

SURGERY/OTHER PROCEDURES

Rarely, splenectomy must be performed in patients with splenic rupture.

INPATIENT CONSIDERATIONS

Admission Criteria/Initial Stabilization

- Inpatient care for all cases of *P. falciparum* malaria. Hospitalize patients with signs of severe illness, regardless of species; outpatient care for others.
- Nonimmune patients with *P. falciparum* may progress from mild symptoms to death within 12 hours.
- All patients treated on outpatient basis should have follow-up within 24 hours.

IV Fluids

Maintenance IV fluids with glucose because of risk of hypoglycemia are recommended if unable to tolerate fluids by mouth. Excess fluids may result in iatrogenically induced pulmonary edema.

Nursing

Observe for fluid excess, renal insufficiency (urine output), and hypoglycemia

Discharge Criteria

Clinical improvement and ability to tolerate oral medications and fluids, with documented decreasing parasitemia levels

 ONGOING CARE

PATIENT EDUCATION

- Malarial chemoprophylaxis prior to travel
- Travel information may be obtained at the CDC travel Web site: http://www.cdc.gov/travel
- http://www.cdc.gov/malaria/new_info/2014/malaria_ebola.htm

PROGNOSIS

Malaria infection (particularly *P. falciparum*) can carry a high mortality if untreated. If diagnosed early and treated appropriately, the prognosis is excellent.

COMPLICATIONS

- If not treated early: cerebral malaria, acute renal failure, acute gastroenteritis, respiratory distress syndrome, and massive hemolysis
- Other complications: seizures, anuria, delirium, coma, dysentery, algid malaria, blackwater fever, hyperpyrexia
- *P. malariae*: Nephrotic syndrome may develop in patients with chronic infection.

REFERENCES

1. World Health Organization. *World Malaria Report 2014*. Geneva, Switzerland: WHO Press; 2014.
2. Cullen KA, Arguin PM. Malaria surveillance—United States, 2012. *MMWR Surveill Summ*. 2014;63(12):1–22.
3. Centers for Disease Control and Prevention. Guidance for malaria diagnosis in patients suspected of ebola infection in the United States. http://www.cdc.gov/malaria/new_info/2014/malaria_ebola.htm. Updated January 15, 2015.
4. Griffith KS, Lewis LS, Mali S, et al. Treatment of malaria in the United States: a systematic review. *JAMA*. 2007;297(20):2264–2277.

ADDITIONAL READING

- Centers for Disease Control and Prevention. Guidelines for treatment of malaria in the United States. http://www.cdc.gov/malaria/resources/pdf/treatmenttable.pdf. Updated July 1, 2013.
- Steinhardt LC, Magill AJ, Arguin PM. Review: malaria chemoprophylaxis for travelers to Latin America. *Am J Trop Med Hyg*. 2011;85(6):1015–1024.

CODES

ICD10

- B54 Unspecified malaria
- B50.9 Plasmodium falciparum malaria, unspecified
- B51.9 Plasmodium vivax malaria without complication

CLINICAL PEARLS

- Consider malaria in travelers returning from endemic areas who present with fever or nonspecific flulike illness.
- Early identification and aggressive treatment, particularly of nonimmune persons with suspected or confirmed *P. falciparum* malaria, is important.
- Patients who develop clinical malaria despite chemoprophylaxis should be treated with medication that is different from their chemoprophylaxis drug.
- *P. falciparum* malaria can be rapidly fatal and should be cared for in the inpatient setting.

M

MARFAN SYNDROME

Rayna Goldstein, MD • Michele Roberts, MD, PhD

BASICS

DESCRIPTION

- Marfan syndrome (MFS) is an inherited disorder of connective tissue.
- Because many features of MFS appear in the general population, specific diagnostic criteria (Ghent nosology) were established and revised, recognizing a constellation of features with major and minor criteria for establishing the diagnosis (1,2).
- System(s) affected: musculoskeletal, cardiovascular, ocular, pulmonary, skin/integument, connective tissue (dura)

Pediatric Considerations
Careful monitoring, as described. Early surgical intervention may reduce the degree of scoliosis.

Pregnancy Considerations
- Manage pregnancy in MFS as high risk, with a cardiologist; prepregnancy evaluation: screening transthoracic echocardiogram for aortic root dilation
- Consider β-blockers in all pregnancies to minimize risk of aortic dilation throughout the pregnancy.
- 1% complication rate if aortic root diameter <40 mm; 10% if >40 mm. Consider elective surgery before pregnancy if >47 mm.
- Avoid spinal anesthesia due to risk of dural ectasia.

EPIDEMIOLOGY
- Congenital; although clinical manifestations may be apparent in infancy, affected individuals may not present until adolescence or young adulthood.
- No gender, ethnic, or racial predilection; with advanced paternal age, a slightly increased risk of de novo mutation resulting in MFS in offspring

Prevalence
1/5,000 to 1/10,000

ETIOLOGY AND PATHOPHYSIOLOGY
Genetic abnormality; mutations of the *FBN1* (fibrillin) gene. Fibrillin is an extracellular matrix protein widely distributed in elastic and nonelastic connective tissue.

Genetics
- Mutations of the fibrillin-1 (*FBN1*) gene on chromosome 15q21.1 OMIM 154700.
- MFS is an autosomal dominant condition with complete penetrance and variable expressivity. Apparent nonpenetrance may be due to lack of recognition of MFS in a mildly affected individual.
- Each child of an affected parent has a 50% chance of inheriting MFS and may be more or less severely affected. 25% of cases result from de novo mutation.

GENERAL PREVENTION
Prenatal diagnosis is possible in families with a known mutation.

COMMONLY ASSOCIATED CONDITIONS
- High prevalence of obstructive sleep apnea in MFS; may be a risk factor for aortic root dilatation
- Increased prevalence of migraine in MFS

DIAGNOSIS

- In the revised Ghent nosology:
  - Cardiovascular manifestations (aortic root aneurysm/dissection) and ectopia lentis have more weight.
  - Molecular genetic testing for *FBN1* plays a more prominent diagnostic role but is not required.

- Less specific manifestations were removed or made less influential, thus avoiding obligate thresholds that were not evidence based. Careful follow-up diminishes risk of missed diagnosis.
- New criteria explicitly allow for alternative diagnoses, when additional features warrant: Shprintzen-Goldberg syndrome (SGS), Loeys-Dietz syndrome (LDS), or vascular-type Ehlers-Danlos syndrome (vEDS).
- *Z*-score calculator for aortic root enlargement: http://www.marfan.org/
- In the absence of a family history of MFS:
  - Aortic root dilatation or dissection ($Z \geq 2$) (Ao) *and* ectopia lentis (EL): unequivocal diagnosis of MFS, irrespective of systemic features, except when they are diagnostic of SGS, LDS, or vEDS.
  - Ao *and* a bona fide *FBN1* mutation: diagnostic of MFS, even in the absence of EL
  - Where Ao is present but EL is absent and the *FBN1* status is negative (or unknown), diagnosis of MFS requires systemic findings score of ≥7 points using new scoring system (see below) and exclusion of SGS, LDS, and vEDS.
  - With EL but without Ao, *FBN1* mutation previously associated with Ao is required for diagnosis of MFS.
- Systemic features, scoring system (see "Physical Exam"):
  - Wrist *and* thumb sign +3 (thumb protrudes from clenched fist); wrist *or* thumb sign +1 (encircles wrist with little finger and thumb of opposite hand)
  - Pectus carinatum deformity +2; pectus excavatum or chest asymmetry +1
  - Hindfoot deformity +2; pes planus +1
  - Pneumothorax +2
  - Dural ectasia +2
  - Protrusio acetabuli +2 by x-ray, CT, or MRI
  - Reduced upper-to-lower segment ratio (US/LS) *and* increased arm/height *and* no severe scoliosis +1
  - Scoliosis or thoracolumbar kyphosis +1
  - Reduced elbow extension +1
  - Facial features (3/5) +1
  - Skin striae +1
  - Myopia >3 diopters +1
  - Mitral valve prolapse (all types) +1
- Maximum: 20 points; score ≥7 indicates systemic involvement.
- Positive family history requires a family member independently diagnosed using above criteria.
- With a positive family history, MFS can be diagnosed with ectopia lentis, *or* systemic score ≥7, *or* aortic root dilatation with $Z \geq 2$ in persons >20 years old, *or* $Z \geq 3$ in persons <20 years old.
- In persons <20 years old who have negative family history and suggestive findings but who do not meet Ghent criteria, "nonspecific connective tissue disorder" is diagnosed; close follow-up is recommended.
- In the presence of a relevant *FBN1* mutation, "potential MFS" is diagnosed and close follow-up is recommended.
- In adults who have suggestive findings but who do not meet Ghent criteria, consider alternative diagnoses: ectopia lentis syndrome, mitral valve prolapse syndrome, MASS (**M**itral valve prolapse, **A**ortic dilation, **S**kin, and **S**keletal) phenotype.

PHYSICAL EXAM
- Facial features: dolichocephaly (head length longer than expected compared with width), enophthalmos, down-slanting palpebral fissures, malar hypoplasia, micrognathia

- High-arched, narrow palate
- Thumb sign: distal phalanx of thumb protrudes from clenched fist; wrist sign: thumb and 5th digit overlap when circling wrist.
- Pectus carinatum deformity: pectus excavatum or chest asymmetry beyond normal variation
- Hindfoot valgus with forefoot abduction and lowering of the midfoot; distinguish from pes planus
- Height may be normal or may be ≥3.3 *SD* >mean.
- Reduced upper segment-to-lower segment (US/LS) ratio: 0.93 in unaffected individuals versus ≤0.85 in affected white adults, ≤0.78 in affected black adults. US is measured from the top of the head to the top of the midpubic bone; LS from the top of the pubic bone to the sole of the foot. In children, abnormal US/LS: US/LS <1, age 0 to 5 years; US/LS <0.95, 6 to 7 years; US/LS <0.9, 8 to 9 years; <0.85, age ≥10 years.
- Increased arm span to height ratio >1.05
- Scoliosis or thoracolumbar kyphosis is diagnosed if, on bending forward, there is a vertical difference ≥1.5 cm between the ribs of the left and right hemithorax.
- Reduced elbow extension if angle between upper and lower arm measures ≤170 degrees on full extension
- Skin: Striae atrophicae are significant if not associated with significant weight changes (or pregnancy) and if located on midback, lumbar region, upper arm, axilla, or thigh.
- Because of lack of specificity, joint hypermobility, high-arched palate, and recurrent or incisional herniae were removed from diagnostic criteria (1).

DIFFERENTIAL DIAGNOSIS
Clinical manifestations overlapping with MFS in cardiovascular, ocular, and skeletal systems:

- Ectopia lentis syndrome: no aortic root dilatation
- Mitral valve prolapse syndrome: MVP; limited systemic features may include pectus excavatum, scoliosis, mild arachnodactyly; aortic enlargement and ectopia lentis preclude this diagnosis.
- MASS phenotype: mitral valve prolapse; myopia; borderline, nonprogressive aortic enlargement ($Z < 2$); and nonspecific skeletal and skin involvement. Aortic involvement in MASS usually nonprogressive; some risk for more severe vascular involvement.
- Shprintzen-Goldberg, Loeys-Dietz, Ehlers-Danlos, Stickler syndromes; congenital contractural arachnodactyly; Weill-Marchesani syndrome, multiple endocrine neoplasia type 2B, fragile X
- Homocystinuria: Marfanoid habitus, thrombosis, mental retardation; urine amino acid analysis is diagnostic; lens dislocates downward.
- Familial thoracic aortic aneurysm
- Aortopathy NGS panel likely to play a more prominent role, especially as VUS are classified (3)

DIAGNOSTIC TESTS & INTERPRETATION
- Sequencing of *FBN1* is the preferred method for molecular diagnosis. Mutations can be found in 95% of patients meeting diagnostic criteria for MFS.
- Specific criteria have been established (1) for *FBN1* mutations causative of MFS. *FBN1* mutation is a valuable marker for risk or aortic dissection (4).
- Echocardiography: Measure aortic root at the level of sinuses of Valsalva; check for mitral valve prolapse. The Marfan Foundation has nomograms to calculate aortic root Z-score in children (http://www.marfan.org/).

- In patients whose physical exam is suggestive of MFS, measure urinary homocystine to rule out homocystinuria, an inborn error of metabolism.
- Anteroposterior (AP) radiograph: protrusio acetabuli
- Scoliosis: Cobb angle ≥20 degrees on radiographs; imaging for MFS diagnosis or as per clinical exam
- Hindfoot valgus with forefoot abduction and lowering of the midfoot: anterior and posterior views
- MRI or CT to evaluate for dural ectasia and if symptomatic, symptoms highly variable, nonspecific, and include lower back pain

Diagnostic Procedures/Other
- Ectopia lentis is diagnosed on slit-lamp examination after maximal dilatation of the pupil (60%); lens dislocation is most often upward and temporal.
- Myopia: Common in the general population; myopia >3 diopters contributes to MFS systemic score.
- Elongated globe, keratoconus, increased risk of vitreous or retinal detachment, glaucoma, and early cataract formation

Test Interpretation
- Cystic medial necrosis of the aorta: descriptive, not pathognomonic
- Myxomatous degeneration of cardiac valves

 TREATMENT

MEDICATION
- Prevention of aortic complications: β-adrenergic blockers. Dosage adjusted to target heart rate (resting rate 60 bpm, increase to ≤110 bpm after moderate exertion or <100 bpm after submaximal exercise) (1)[C]
- If β-blockers are contraindicated: Calcium channel blockers, ACE inhibitors, and ARBs may retard aortic dilation in children and adolescents (5)[B].
- Consider antibiotic prophylaxis for dental procedures in presence of mitral or aortic regurgitation (http://www.marfan.org/resource/fact-sheet/endocarditis-prophylaxis-people-marfan-syndrome#.VhMqKvlViko).
- Recent studies support losartan plus β-blockers to prevent progressive aortic root dilatation (6)[B].

ISSUES FOR REFERRAL
Genetics, cardiology, orthopedics, ophthalmology

SURGERY/OTHER PROCEDURES
- When cardiac symptoms develop or aortic root diameter is ≥5 cm, consider surgical intervention (7). Many MFS patients will ultimately require reconstructive cardiovascular surgery:
  - Dissection of ascending aorta (type A) is a surgical emergency. Consider prophylactic surgery when diameter of sinus of Valsalva approaches 5 cm, rate of change approaches 1 cm/year, and with progressive aortic regurgitation (3); other risk factors: family history, other cardiac pathology, pregnancy.
  - Dissection of descending thoracic aorta (type B): Surgical indications include intractable pain, limb or organ ischemia, and aortic diameter >5.5 cm (or rapidly increasing) (1).
- Mitral valve repair: for severe mitral valve regurgitation or progressive LV dilatation or dysfunction, or in patients undergoing valve-sparing root replacement (1)
- Lens subluxation: Incidence of glaucoma is high, so surgery is performed only if the condition cannot be treated with corrective lenses; surgical removal of lens for opacity, impending complete luxation, lens-induced glaucoma or uveitis, or anisometropia or refractive error not amenable to optical correction (1)

- Severe pectus excavatum may interfere with pulmonary or cardiac function and require surgery.
- Scoliosis: bracing for curves 20 to 40 degrees until growth is complete or surgery if >40 degrees
- Surgery for only most severe cases of dural ectasia
- Hip replacement in middle age or later if protrusio acetabuli has led to severe arthritic change

 ONGOING CARE

FOLLOW-UP RECOMMENDATIONS
- Avoid sports that can increase aortic root enlargement or pneumothorax; in general, avoid contact sports, Valsalva, breathing against resistance, and exhaustion (8)[C].
- Exercise restrictions: Follow recommendation from the National Marfan Foundation (http://www.marfan.org/) and guidelines from the American Heart Association/American College of Cardiology Task Forces.

Patient Monitoring
Exams at least twice/year while patient is growing, with attention to the cardiovascular system and to scoliosis.
- Cognitive ability is usually normal, but visual and medical difficulties may interfere with learning (8)[C].
- Cardiac
  - Aortic root dilatation in MFS is usually progressive, warrants vigilance even when not seen on initial examination; age <20 years, yearly echocardiogram; adults with repeatedly normal aortic root measurements, echo every 2 to 3 years (1)[C].
  - Yearly echocardiograms (initially), more frequent if aortic diameter is increasing rapidly (≥5 cm/year) or is approaching surgical threshold (≥4.5 cm in adults)
  - Regular imaging after surgical repair of aorta
- Musculoskeletal
  - Excessive linear growth of long bones, extremities disproportionately long, paucity of muscle mass, peak growth velocity 2 years early. Growth curves for MFS are available (8)[C].
  - Clinical evaluation for scoliosis earlier than in general population; plain radiographs of spine during growth years
  - Evaluate for scoliosis, joint laxity, and pectus deformity every visit to age 1 year, annually age 1 to 5 years, semiannually age 6 to 18 years, and yearly thereafter.
  - Bone age in preadolescence: Consider hormonal therapy if with large discrepancy (8)[C].
  - Scoliosis or pectus deformity may progress more rapidly than in those without MFS.
  - Excellent prognosis for scoliosis curves <30 degrees; bracing may be effective for curves <35 degrees; rapid progression likely if curve >50 degrees (8)[C]
- Annual ophthalmologic evaluation: ectopia lentis, myopia, cataract, glaucoma, and retinal detachment; myopia is very common in MFS with early onset, rapid progression, and high degree of severity; early monitoring, aggressive refraction to prevent amblyopia (1)[C]
- Respiratory: pulmonary function tests (PFTs) for pulmonary complaints; obstructive sleep apnea
- Review diagnosis, examine family members, offer support group information at diagnosis and PRN.
- Provide genetic counseling at diagnosis, discuss pregnancy risks in adolescence, discuss activity restrictions starting age 6 years, transition planning in early adolescence. Review symptoms of potential catastrophic events: aortic dissection, vision changes, and pneumothorax starting age 6 years.

PATIENT EDUCATION
- National Marfan Foundation, http://www.marfan.org/
- NLM Genetics Home Reference: Marfan syndrome http://ghr.nlm.nih.gov/condition/marfan-syndrome

PROGNOSIS
Life-threatening complications involve cardiovascular dysfunctions. In 1972, lifespan was 32 years. Currently, lifespan is nearly normal.

COMPLICATIONS
Bacterial endocarditis, aortic dissection, aortic or mitral valve insufficiency, dilated cardiomyopathy, retinal detachment, glaucoma, pneumothorax

REFERENCES
1. Loeys BL, Dietz HC, Braverman AC, et al. The revised Ghent nosology for the Marfan syndrome. J Med Genet. 2010;47(7):476–485.
2. Faivre L, Collod-Beroud G, Callewaert B, et al. Pathogenic FBN1 mutations in 146 adults not meeting clinical diagnostic criteria for Marfan syndrome: further delineation of type 1 fibrillinopathies and focus on patients with an isolated major criterion. Am J Med Genet A. 2009;149A(5):854–860.
3. Wooderchak-Donahue W, VanSant-Webb C, Tvrdik T, et al. Clinical utility of a next generation sequencing panel assay for Marfan and Marfan-like syndromes featuring aortopathy. Am J Med Genet A. 2015;167A(8):1747–1757.
4. Faivre L, Collod-Beroud G, Child A, et al. Contribution of molecular analyses in diagnosing Marfan syndrome and type I fibrillinopathies: an international study of 1009 probands. J Med Genet. 2008;45(6):384–390.
5. Williams A, Davies S, Stuart AG, et al. Medical treatment of Marfan syndrome: a time for change. Heart. 2008;94(4):414–421.
6. Groenink M, den Hartog AW, Franken R, et al. Losartan reduces aortic dilatation rate in adults with Marfan syndrome: a randomized controlled trial. Eur Heart J. 2013;34(45):3491–3500.
7. Benedetto U, Melina G, Takkenberg JJ, et al. Surgical management of aortic root disease in Marfan syndrome: a systematic review and meta-analysis. Heart. 2011;97(12):955–958.
8. Tinkle BT, Saal HM. Health supervision for children with Marfan syndrome. Pediatrics. 2013;132(4):e1059–e1072.

 CODES

ICD10
- Q87.40 Marfan's syndrome, unspecified
- Q87.43 Marfan's syndrome with skeletal manifestation
- Q87.418 Marfan's syndrome with other cardiovascular manifestations

CLINICAL PEARLS
- Because many features of MFS appear in the general population, diagnostic criteria have been established. Molecular diagnostic testing for FBN1 mutations will play an increasing role.
- Screen very tall athletes for aortic root dilatation.
- Early diagnosis of homocystinuria is important because clinical complications can be minimized with appropriate diet and medication.
- Ectopia lentis and aortic root dilatation are best discrimination features, but height ≥3.3 SD above the mean is a simple discriminant in primary care.

M

MARIJUANA (CANNABIS) USE DISORDER

Kara C. Farley, MD • Dustin K. Smith, DO

BASICS

DESCRIPTION

Marijuana or cannabis use disorder is classified in *DSM-5* in different categories (mild, moderate, or severe) depending on how many symptoms are present. Mild: 2 to 3; Moderate: 4 to 5; Severe: 6+ (1). The definition is used leading to clinically significant impairment or distress, manifested by two or more of the following symptoms within a 12-month period:

- Taken in larger amounts and over a longer period of time than intended
- Persistent desire or unsuccessful efforts to cut down or control amount used
- A great deal of time spent in activities is necessary to obtain, use, or recover.
- Presence of craving for the substance
- Recurrent use resulting in failure to fulfill major role obligations at work, school, or home
- Continued use despite having persistent or recurrent social or interpersonal problems due to cannabis use
- Important social, occupational, or recreational activities are given up or reduced.
- Recurrent use in physically hazardous situations
- Use is continued despite knowledge of having a persistent physical or psychological problem caused or exacerbated by cannabis.
- Tolerance, defined by using increased amounts of cannabis to achieve the desired effect or intoxication or diminished effect with continued use of the same amount of cannabis
- Withdrawal

EPIDEMIOLOGY

- The United States is ranked first among 17 European and North American countries by the World Health Organization for prevalence of marijuana use.
- Cannabis is the most widely used illicit psychoactive substance in the United States (2).
- ~42% of teens will have tried marijuana by the time they graduate from high school.
- Approximately 30% of students report having used marijuana at college entry (3).
- In the United States, 10% of those who ever used marijuana become daily users, and 20–30% became weekly users.
- In the United States, some states have approved medical marijuana use, and two states (Washington and Colorado) have approved recreational use of marijuana.
- Other states in the United States are currently trying to pass legislation to legalize the use of recreational marijuana.

ETIOLOGY AND PATHOPHYSIOLOGY

- Main active ingredient in marijuana: delta-9-tetrahydrocannabinol (THC)
- When marijuana is smoked, THC rapidly passes from the lungs into the blood and to the brain, where it binds to cannabinoid receptors (CBRs).
- CBRs are responsible for memory, thinking, concentration, sensory and time perception, pleasure, movement, and coordination.
- THC artificially stimulates the CBRs, disrupting the function of endogenous cannabinoids. A marijuana "high" results from overstimulation of these receptors.
- Over time, overstimulation alters the function of CBRs, which can lead to addiction and to withdrawal symptoms when drug use stops.
- Effects of smoked marijuana occur within minutes and can last 1 to 3 hours.
- Effects from marijuana consumed in foods or beverages appear later, usually in 30 minutes to 1 hour but can last up to 4 hours.
- Smoking marijuana delivers significantly more THC into the bloodstream than eating or drinking the drug.

RISK FACTORS

- Age (highest use among those 18 to 25 years)
- Male sex
- Comorbid psychiatric disorders (i.e., bipolar disorder, posttraumatic stress disorder [PTSD])
- Other substance use (i.e., alcohol, cocaine)
- Lower educational achievement (rates of dependence is lowest among college graduates)

DIAGNOSIS

- Screen for marijuana use along with other lifestyle questions such as tobacco and alcohol use.
- Ask for frequency and amount used (e.g., "How long does a nickel bag last you?").
- Unexplained deterioration in school or work performance may be a red flag for abuse.
- Problems with, or changes in, social relationships (e.g., spending more time alone or with persons suspected of using drugs) and recreational activities (e.g., giving up activities that were once pleasurable) may indicate abuse.
- If available, information from concerned parents or spouses should be obtained.

HISTORY

- Clinical presentation of acute intoxication:
  - Euphoria, elation, laughter, heightened sensory perception, altered perception of time, increased appetite
  - Poor short-term memory, concentration
  - Fatigue, depression
  - Occasionally, distrust, fear, anxiety, panic
  - With large doses, acute psychosis: delusions, hallucinations, loss of sense of personal identity (4)
- Withdrawal symptoms include the following:
  - Nausea
  - Weight loss
  - Decreased appetite
  - Insomnia
  - Depressed mood

PHYSICAL EXAM

- Evaluate for:
  - Conjunctival injection
  - Xerostomia
  - Nystagmus
  - Increased heart rate
  - Altered pulmonary status
  - Altered body temperature
  - Reduced muscle strength
  - Decreased coordination
- Withdrawal findings include the following:
  - Restlessness/agitation
  - Irritability
  - Tremor
  - Diaphoresis
  - Increased body temperature

DIAGNOSTIC TESTS & INTERPRETATION

Positive urine drug screen; cannabinoids can be detected in urine weeks to months after marijuana use.

TREATMENT

- Several methods of behavioral-based interventions:
  - Cognitive-behavioral therapy
  - Motivational interviewing
  - Counseling
  - Contingency management
  - Social network behavior therapy
  - Twelve-step approach
  - Family-oriented therapy
  - Brief intervention
  - Relapse prevention
  - Community reinforcement approach
- No intervention to date has proved consistently effective for marijuana abuse.
- Despite this, trials on cognitive-behavioral therapy and contingency management have shown better outcomes in reducing marijuana use and maintaining abstinence (5).
- Trials also show that addition of a comprehensive parenting training curriculum did not further enhance efficacy (5).
- With marijuana abuse, most prevalent among patients suffering from other psychiatric disorders, studies indicate that treating the mental health disorder may help reduce marijuana use, particularly among heavy users and those with more chronic mental disorders.
- Advice to give to patients for management of withdrawal:
  - Gradually reduce amount of marijuana used before cessation.
  - Delay first use of marijuana until later in the day.
  - Consider use of nicotine replacement therapy if planning to stop, separate tobacco use at the same time.
  - Relaxation, distraction
  - Avoid cues and triggers associated with cannabis use.

- Prescribe short-term analgesia and sedation for withdrawal symptoms, if required.
- If irritability and restlessness are marked, consider prescribing very-low-dose diazepam for 3 to 4 days.
- Provide user and family members with information regarding marijuana abuse and withdrawal to increase understanding of the abuse and reduce likelihood of relapse.
- Withdrawal symptoms peak on day 2 or 3, and most are over by day 7. Sleep and vivid dreams can continue for 2 to 3 weeks.

MEDICATION

- No effective medication for the treatment of marijuana abuse
- One study suggested oral THC could be used to abate marijuana withdrawal in individuals who are trying to quit.
- Another study concluded medications used to treat other drug use disorders, such as buspirone, lithium, and fluoxetine, may have therapeutic benefit.

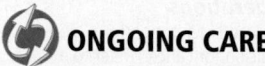 ONGOING CARE

FOLLOW-UP RECOMMENDATIONS

- Monitor cessation of marijuana use with urine tests over several weeks for the inactive metabolite of cannabis (carboxy-THC).
- Heavy smokers may continue to be positive for marijuana for up to 6 weeks.

PATIENT EDUCATION

To learn more about marijuana abuse, visit the National Institute on Drug Abuse (NIDA) Web site at www.drugabuse.gov. Other NIDA Web sites include the following:

- https://drugpubs.drugabuse.gov/promotions/back-to-school
- http://www.drugabuse.gov/drugs-abuse/marijuana
- https://teens.drugabuse.gov/

COMPLICATIONS

- Acute adverse effects
  - Anxiety and panic, especially in naïve users, depression
  - Psychotic symptoms at high doses
  - Motor vehicle accidents if a person drives while intoxicated
  - Chronic adverse effects: abnormal brain development; diminished lifetime achievement
  - Chronic bronchitis and impaired respiratory function in regular smokers
  - Psychotic symptoms and disorders in heavy users, especially those with a history of psychotic symptoms or a family history of these disorders (schizophrenia)
  - Addiction to marijuana and other substances

REFERENCES

1. American Psychiatric Association. Substance-related and addictive disorders. *Diagnostic and Statistical Manual of Mental Disorders*. 5th ed. Arlington, VA: American Psychiatric Association; 2013. http://dx.doi.org/10.1176/appi.books.9780890425596.dsm16. Accessed December 2015.
2. Suerken CK, Reboussin BA, Sutfin EL, et al. Prevalence of marijuana use at college entry and risk factors for initiation during freshman year. *Addict Behav*. 2014;39(1):302–307.
3. Hall W, Degenhardt L. Adverse health effects of non-medical cannabis use. *Lancet*. 2009;374(9698):1383–1391.
4. Abayomi O, Adelufosi AO. Psychosocial interventions for cannabis abuse and/or dependence among persons with co-occurring cannabis use and psychotic disorders. *Cochrane Database Syst Rev*. 2015;(1):CD011488.
5. Stanger C, Ryan SR, Scherer EA, et al. Clinic- and home-based contingency management plus parent training for adolescent cannabis use disorders. *J Am Acad Child Adolesc Psychiatry*. 2015;54(6):445–453.e2.

ADDITIONAL READING

- Budney AJ, Vandrey RG, Hughes JR, et al. Oral delta-9-tetrahydrocannabinol suppresses cannabis withdrawal symptoms. *Drug Alcohol Depend*. 2007;86(1):22–29.
- Denis C, Lavie E, Fatséas M, et al. Psychotherapeutic interventions for cannabis abuse and/or dependence in outpatient settings. *Cochrane Database Syst Rev*. 2006;(3):CD005336.
- Fergusson DM, Boden JM. Cannabis use and later life outcomes. *Addiction*. 2008;103(6):969–976.
- Freeman MJ, Rose DZ, Myers MA, et al. Ischemic stroke after use of the synthetic marijuana "spice." *Neurology*. 2013;81(24):2090–2093.
- Hooper SR, Woolley D, De Bellis MD. Intellectual, neurocognitive, and academic achievement in abstinent adolescents with cannabis use disorder. *Psychopharmacology (Berl)*. 2014;231(8):1467–1477.
- Hubbard JR, Franco SE, Onaivi ES. Marijuana: medical implications. *Am Fam Physician*. 1999;60(9):2583–2593.
- National Institute on Drug Abuse. *Research Report Series: Marijuana Abuse*. Bethesda, MD: U.S. Department of Health and Human Services and National Institute of Health; 2010.
- Vandrey R, Haney M. Pharmacotherapy for cannabis dependence: how close are we? *CNS Drugs*. 2009;23(7):543–553.

- Winstock AR, Ford C, Witton J. Assessment and management of cannabis use disorders in primary care. *BMJ*. 2010;340:c1571.

 CODES

ICD10

- F12.10 Cannabis abuse, uncomplicated
- F12.20 Cannabis dependence, uncomplicated
- F12.288 Cannabis dependence with other cannabis-induced disorder

CLINICAL PEARLS

- Marijuana abuse may result in poor performance in school or work, legal problems, and arguments with family.
- Patients with schizophrenia are frequently found to be using marijuana and their use hindering the treatment for schizophrenia. Management of these dual diagnoses is important for the successful treatment of schizophrenia.
- Patients should be screened for marijuana use and asked about frequency and amount used.
- Effects of smoked marijuana can last 1 to 3 hours. Effects from foods or beverages containing marijuana appear later, usually in 30 minutes to 1 hour but can last up to 4 hours.
- Smoking marijuana delivers significantly more THC into the bloodstream than eating or drinking the drug.
- Acute marijuana intoxication is manifested by conjunctival injection, increased heart rate, euphoria, heightened sensory perception, altered perception of time, increased appetite, poor short-term memory and concentration, and fatigue. Large doses may result in acute psychosis, delusions, or hallucinations.
- Inquire all patients about their use of marijuana. Changes in values and attitudes have made marijuana use more mainstream, and patients do not consider marijuana a substance of abuse.
- Withdrawal symptoms include nausea, weight loss, decreased appetite, insomnia, and depressed mood. Peaks on day 2 or 3 and most are over by day 7.
- Cognitive-behavioral therapy, motivational interviewing, motivational enhancement therapy, and contingency management are four methods of behavioral-based interventions used in the treatment of marijuana abuse.
- Some recent research finds that adolescents with cannabis use disorder may not be susceptible to THC neuropsychological deficits once they achieve remission from all drugs for at least 30 days.

M

MASTALGIA

Eduardo Lara-Torre, MD • Amanda B. Murchison, MD • Patrice M. Weiss, MD, FACOG

BASICS

DESCRIPTION
- Painful breast tissue, often bilateral, which can be cyclic or noncyclic
  - 2/3 of breast pain is cyclic and usually associated with hormonal changes related to menses, external hormones, pregnancy, or menopause.
  - 1/3 is noncyclic and often is related to a breast or chest wall lesion.
- Synonym(s): mastodynia; breast pain

EPIDEMIOLOGY
Incidence
- Predominant sex: most common in women but occurs occasionally in men
- Predominant age: generally seen from adolescence to menopause
- Frequency of breast cancer with those reporting breast pain ranges from 1.2% to 6.7%.
- Up to 70% of women report some degree of breast pain at some point in their lives.
- Most describe mild pain, but 11% describe pain as moderate to severe.
- Higher incidence in the older population, larger breasted individuals, and those who are less fit and active (1)[B].

ETIOLOGY AND PATHOPHYSIOLOGY
- Causative pathophysiology remains unclear but is thought to be related to hormonal or nutritional factors.
- When fibrocystic disease is the source, growth and distension of the cyst with hormonal fluctuation can cause pain.
- Hormonal factors (e.g., hormone-replacement therapy, oral contraceptives, pregnancy, menses, puberty, and menopause) may influence the diverse conditions that cause mastalgia or may themselves cause breast tenderness and pain.
- Benign breast disorders (e.g., fibrocystic changes)
- Trauma (including sexual abuse/assault)
- Diet and lifestyle (e.g., poor-fitting exercise breast support)
- Lactation problems (e.g., engorgement, mastitis, breast abscess)
- Breast masses, including breast cancer
- Hidradenitis suppurativa
- Costochondritis (Tietze syndrome)
- Postthoracotomy syndrome
- Spinal and paraspinal disorders
- Potential side effects of medications
- Postradiation effects
- Referred pain (e.g., pulmonary, cardiac, or gallbladder disease)
- Ductal ectasia

Genetics
Familial tendency

RISK FACTORS
- Diet high in saturated fats
- Cigarette smoking
- Recent weight gain
- Pregnancy
- Large, pendulous breasts (caused by stretching of Cooper ligaments)
- Exogenous hormones
- Caffeine has been shown not to be a risk factor (2)[A].

GENERAL PREVENTION
- Avoid exposure to risk factors.
- Properly fitted bra support

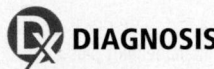

DIAGNOSIS

HISTORY
- Location, duration, frequency, severity, associated symptoms, related activities (e.g., trauma), and aggravating and ameliorating factors
- Complete medical history with focus on gynecologic/obstetric history
- Complete systematic review of systems
- Diet/smoking history
- Detailed family history for risk assessment for breast cancer
- There may be an association with other pain syndromes such as fibromyalgia (3)[B].

PHYSICAL EXAM
- Examine breasts systematically in both standing and sitting positions.
- Assess for skin changes, breast symmetry and contour, dimpling, localized tenderness, bruising, masses, nipple discharge, and lymphadenopathy. Look for signs that are suggestive of breast malignancy.

DIFFERENTIAL DIAGNOSIS
- The most important disease to rule out is breast cancer (although uncommon), particularly if pain is localized.
- Manipulation or trauma also can worsen symptoms.
- Chest wall pain or referred pain resulting from splenomegaly also must be differentiated from mastalgia.
- Sometimes, cyclic pain is concurrent with premenstrual syndrome.
- Ductal ectasia of the breast

DIAGNOSTIC TESTS & INTERPRETATION
Initial Tests (lab, imaging)
- If galactorrhea is found, check a fasting prolactin level.
- Consider thyroid-stimulating hormone (TSH).
- Consider an ultrasound in women with focal, persistent breast pain.
- Mammogram ± ultrasound in women aged ≥30 to 35 years

Pediatric Considerations
Ultrasound is the imaging test of choice for children and adolescents. A mammogram is not useful.

Diagnostic Procedures/Other
- Cysts may need to be aspirated to relieve symptoms or verify diagnosis.
- Biopsies may be indicated based on the results of examination, ultrasound, or mammography.

Pediatric Considerations
In children and adolescents, do not perform biopsies unless there is a suspicion for cancer. Refer to a specialist in pediatric breast disease.

Test Interpretation
- Normal breast tissue
- Benign: fibrocystic changes, duct ectasia, solitary papillomas, simple fibroadenomas
- Small increased risk of breast cancer: ductal hyperplasia without atypia, sclerosing adenosis, diffuse papillomatosis, complex fibroadenomas
- Moderate increased risk: atypical ductal hyperplasia, atypical lobular hyperplasia
- Breast cancer

TREATMENT

GENERAL MEASURES
- Stop or modify the current hormonal therapy.
- A repeat examination may help to establish any cyclic nodularity pattern.
- Wear a properly fitted support bra (may be fitted by a professional).
- Reassurance (sufficient for most patients)
- Weight loss for obese patients
- Smoking cessation
- Relaxation training

MEDICATION
First Line
Acetaminophen or NSAIDs, either oral or topical (e.g., diclofenac sodium or piroxicam) (4)[B]

Second Line

- Oral contraceptives may help some patients prevent fibrocystic disease but may worsen pain in some sensitive patients.
- If the patient is on an oral contraceptive, switch to the one that has a lower estrogen component.
- In some patients with mastalgia only during their menses, menstrual suppression with continuous oral contraceptives may be of benefit.
- Oral progesterone: 10 mg PO daily
- Other possibilities for patients with refractory symptoms, used infrequently because of potential side effects, include the following:
  - Danazol: 100 mg BID (possibly lower doses) may be the most effective; major adverse effects include menstrual irregularities, weight gain, acne, hirsutism, and voice change; *may be used during luteal phase only*; approved by the FDA for this indication
  - Toremifene: 30 mg PO daily (5)[B]
  - Bromocriptine: 5 mg PO daily and cabergoline 0.5 mg PO weekly, both during the 2nd half of the menstrual cycle are equally effective, but cabergoline has fewer side effects (6)[B].
  - Tamoxifen or Centchroman: Selective estrogen receptor modulators (SERM) may be used with a dose of 10 mg or 30 mg daily respectively (7)[A].

ADDITIONAL THERAPIES

If the patient is breastfeeding, correct any breastfeeding difficulties; treat underlying mastitis or breast abscess.

Pediatric Considerations

Children and adolescents may require referrals to a specialist.

SURGERY/OTHER PROCEDURES

Some patients may need surgical breast reduction.

COMPLEMENTARY & ALTERNATIVE MEDICINE

- Vitamin E and evening primrose oil have not been found to be of benefit for chronic mastalgia (2)[A].
- Flaxseed oil is not effective for the treatment of mastalgia (2)[C].

 ONGOING CARE

FOLLOW-UP RECOMMENDATIONS

As needed

Patient Monitoring

- As needed for patients not receiving pharmacotherapy
- Time of follow-up will vary by type of pharmacotherapy and patient's particular problems.

DIET

- Decrease fat intake to 20% of total calories.
- No evidence suggests that reduction in caffeine intake may help to decrease the severity or incidence of the disease (3)[A].

PATIENT EDUCATION

Avoid or adjust risk factors.

PROGNOSIS

- Premenstrual mastalgia increases with age and then generally stops at menopause unless the patient is receiving hormone therapy (HT).
- Most patients can control symptoms without receiving HT.
- Several months of HT may provide several more months of relief, but mastalgia may recur.
- Cyclic mastalgia responds better than noncyclic mastalgia to treatment.
- Effects of long-term HT are unknown.

REFERENCES

1. Scurr J, Hedger W, Morris P, et al. The prevalence, severity, and impact of breast pain in the general population. *Breast J*. 2014;20(5):508–513.
2. Chase C, Wells J, Eley S. Caffeine and breast pain: revisiting the connection. *Nurs Womens Health*. 2011;15(4):286–294.
3. Genc V, Genc A, Ustuner E, et al. Is there an association between mastalgia and fibromyalgia? Comparing prevalence and symptom severity. *Breast*. 2011;20(4):314–318.
4. Ahmadinejad M, Delfan B, Haghdani S, et al. Comparing the effect of diclofenac gel and piroxicam gel on mastalgia. *Breast J*. 2010;16(2):213–214.
5. Gong C, Song E, Jia W, et al. A double-blind randomized controlled trial of toremifen therapy for mastalgia. *Arch Surg*. 2006;141(1):43–47.
6. Aydin Y, Atis A, Kaleli S, et al. Cabergoline versus bromocriptine for symptomatic treatment of premenstrual mastalgia: a randomised, open-label study. *Eur J Obstet Gynecol Reprod Biol*. 2010;150(2):203–206.
7. Jain BK, Bansal A, Choudhary D, et al. Centchroman vs tamoxifen for regression of mastalgia: a randomized controlled trial. *Int J Surg*. 2015;15:11–16.

ADDITIONAL READING

- Ader DN, Shriver CD. Cyclical mastalgia: prevalence and impact in an outpatient breast clinic sample. *J Am Coll Surg*. 1997;185(5):466–470.
- Blommers J, de Lange-De Klerk ES, Kuik DJ, et al. Evening primrose oil and fish oil for severe chronic mastalgia: a randomized, double-blind, controlled trial. *Am J Obstet Gynecol*. 2002;187(5):1389–1394.
- Brennan M, Houssami N, French J. Management of benign breast conditions. Part 1—painful breasts. *Aust Fam Physician*. 2005;34(3):143–144.
- Colak T, Ipek T, Kanik A, et al. Efficacy of topical nonsteroidal antiinflammatory drugs in mastalgia treatment. *J Am Coll Surg*. 2003;196(4):525–530.
- Miltenburg DM, Speights VO Jr. Benign breast disease. *Obstet Gynecol Clin North Am*. 2008;35(2):285–300.
- Olawaiye A, Withiam-Leitch M, Danakas G, et al. Mastalgia: a review of management. *J Reprod Med*. 2005;50(12):933–939.
- Rosolowich V, Saettler E, Szuck B. *SOGC Clinical Practice Guideline: Mastalgia*. Ottawa, Canada: Society of Obstetricians and Gynaecologists of Canada; 2006. http://sogc.org/guidelines/mastalgia/
- Smith RL, Pruthi S, Fitzpatrick LA. Evaluation and management of breast pain. *Mayo Clinic Proc*. 2004;79(3):353–372.

 SEE ALSO

- Premenstrual Syndrome (PMS) and Premenstrual Dysphoric Disorder (PMDD)
- Algorithms: Breast Discharge; Breast Pain

 CODES

ICD10

N64.4 Mastodynia

CLINICAL PEARLS

- When evaluating a patient with breast pain, always rule out cancer first.
- In the adolescent population, do not biopsy; instead, refer to a pediatric specialist.
- Premenstrual mastalgia increases with age and then generally stops at menopause unless the patient is receiving HT.

M

MASTITIS

Anne Claire Adams, MD • Montiel T. Rosenthal, MD

 BASICS

DESCRIPTION
- Mastitis is an inflammation of the breast parenchyma and possibly associated tissues (areola, nipple, subcutaneous [SC] fat).
- Usually associated with bacterial infection (and milk stasis in the postpartum mother)
- Usually an acute condition but can become chronic cystic mastitis

EPIDEMIOLOGY
- Predominantly affects females
- Mostly in the puerperium; epidemic form rare in the age of reduced hospital stays for mothers and newborns
- Neonatal form
- Posttraumatic: ornamental nipple piercing increases risk of transmission of bacteria to deeper breast structures: *Staphylococcus aureus* is the predominant organism.

Incidence
- 3–20% of breastfeeding mothers develop nonepidemic mastitis.
- Greatest incidence among breastfeeding mothers 2 to 6 weeks postpartum
- Neonatal form occurs at 1 to 5 weeks of age, with equal gender risk and unilateral presentation.
- Pediatric form
- Around or after puberty
- 82% of cases in girls

ETIOLOGY AND PATHOPHYSIOLOGY
- Microabscesses along milk ducts and surrounding tissues
- Inflammatory cell infiltration of breast parenchyma and surrounding tissues
- Nonpuerperal (infectious)
  - *S. aureus, Bacteroides* sp., *Peptostreptococcus, Staphylococcus* (coagulase neg.), *Enterococcus faecalis*
  - *Histoplasma capsulatum*
  - *Salmonella enterica*
  - Rare case of *Actinomyces europaeus*
- Puerperal (infectious)
  - *Staphylococcus aureus, Streptococcus pyogenes* (group A or B), *Corynebacterium* sp., *Bacteroides* sp., *Staphylococcus* (coagulase neg.), *Escherichia coli, Salmonella* sp.
  - Methicillin-resistant *S. aureus* (MRSA)
- Rare secondary site for tuberculosis in endemic areas (1% of mastitis cases in these areas): single breast nodule with mastalgia
- *Corynebacterium* sp. associated with greater risk for development of chronic cystic mastitis
- Granulomatous mastitis
  - Idiopathic
    - Predilection for Asian and Hispanic women
    - Association with α-1-antitrypsin deficiency, hyperprolactinemia with galactorrhea, oral contraceptive use, *Corynebacterium* sp. infection, and breast trauma
    - Most women have a history of lactation in previous 5 years.
  - Lupus; autoimmune

- Puerperal
  - Retrograde migration of surface bacteria up milk ducts
  - Bacterial migration from nipple fissures to breast lymphatics
  - Secondary monilial infection in the face of recurrent mastitis or diabetes
  - Seeding from mother to neonate in cyclical fashion
- Nonpuerperal
  - Ductal ectasia
  - Breast carcinoma
  - Inflammatory cysts
  - Chronic recurring SC or subareolar infections
  - Parasitic infections: *Echinococcus*; filariasis; Guinea worm in endemic areas
  - Herpes simplex
  - Cat-scratch disease
- Lupus

RISK FACTORS
- Breastfeeding
- Milk stasis
  - Inadequate emptying of breast
    - Scarring of breast due to prior mastitis
    - Scarring due to previous breast surgery (breast reduction, biopsy, or partial mastectomy)
  - Breast engorgement: interruption of breastfeeding
- Nipple trauma increases risk of transmission of bacteria to deeper breast structures: *S. aureus* predominant organism
- Neonatal colonization with epidemic *Staphylococcus*
- Neonatal
  - Bottle-fed babies
  - Manual expression of "witch's milk"
  - Can predispose to lethal necrotizing fasciitis
- Maternal diabetes
- Maternal HIV
- Maternal vitamin A deficiency (in animal models)

GENERAL PREVENTION
Regular emptying of both breasts and nipple care to prevent fissures when breastfeeding. Also good hygiene including hand washing and washing breast pumps after each use (1)[A].

COMMONLY ASSOCIATED CONDITIONS
Breast abscess

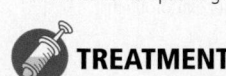 **DIAGNOSIS**

- Fever >38.5°C and malaise
- Nausea ± vomiting
- Localized breast tenderness, heat, swelling, and redness
- Possible breast mass

HISTORY
- Breast pain
- "Hot cords burning in chest wall"
- Consider yeast infection if nipple pain and burning and/or infant with thrush

PHYSICAL EXAM
- Breast tenderness
- Localized breast induration, redness, and warmth
- Peau d'orange appearance to overlying skin

DIFFERENTIAL DIAGNOSIS
- Abscess (bacterial, idiopathic granulomatous mastitis, fungal, tuberculosis)
- Tumor
  - Idiopathic granulomatous mastitis
  - Inflammatory breast cancer
  - Wegener granulomatosis
  - Sarcoidosis
  - Foreign body granuloma
  - Vasospasm (may be presentation for Reynaud) (2)[B]
- Ductal cyst (ductal ectasia)
- Consider monilial infection in lactating mother, especially if mastitis is recurrent.

DIAGNOSTIC TESTS & INTERPRETATION
Initial Tests (lab, imaging)
Mastitis is typically a clinical diagnosis. Labs rarely needed. In those ill enough to need hospitalization, consider the following:
- CBC
- Blood culture
- In epidemic puerperal mastitis
  - Milk leukocyte count
  - Milk culture
  - Neonatal nasal culture
- No imaging required for postpartum mastitis in a breastfeeding mother that responds to antibiotic therapy.
- Mammography for women with nonpuerperal mastitis
- Breast ultrasound to rule out abscess formation in women
  - Special consideration for this in women with breast implants who have mastitis

Follow-Up Tests & Special Considerations
Lactating mothers produce salty milk from affected side (higher Na and Cl concentrations) as compared with unaffected side. Consider breast milk culture if suspect MRSA. Also consider testing for tuberculosis as may be initial presentation.

Diagnostic Procedures/Other
Options if further progression to abscess formation
- Needle aspiration
- Incision and drainage
- Excisional biopsy
- US-guided core needle biopsy is diagnostic method of choice for idiopathic granulomatous mastitis

TREATMENT

A recent Cochrane review found that insufficient evidence exists to confirm or refute the effectiveness of antibiotic therapy for the treatment of lactational mastitis (3)[A]. If present <24 hours and symptoms are mild, conservative management with milk removal and supportive measures is recommended.

MEDICATION
- Prioritized on the basis of likelihood of MRSA as etiologic factor and clinical severity of condition.
- Treat for 10 to 14 days.
- For idiopathic granulomatous mastitis and localized infection, usually resolves with antibiotics and drainage

First Line
- Outpatient
  - Effective milk removal is the most important management step (4)[A].
  - Dicloxacillin 500 mg QID
  - Cephalexin 500 mg QID
  - Trimethoprim/sulfamethoxazole (TMP/SMX); DS BID (if mastitis not improving within 48 hours after starting first-line treatment consider MRSA)
  - *Lactobacillus fermentum* or *Lactobacillus salivarius* 9 log 10 CFU/day
- Inpatient
  - Nafcillin 2 g q4h
  - Oxacillin 2 g q4h
  - Vancomycin 1 g q12h (MRSA possible)
- Breastfeeding beyond 1 month
  - Penicillin, ampicillin, or erythromycin

If idiopathic granulomatous mastitis, consider corticosteroids ± methotrexate (5)[B]

Pediatric Considerations
TMP/SMX given to breastfeeding mothers with mastitis can potentiate jaundice for neonates.

Second Line
- If mastitis is odoriferous and localized under areola, add metronidazole 500 mg TID IV or PO.
- If yeast is suspected in recurrent mastitis, add topical and oral nystatin.

ISSUES FOR REFERRAL
- Abscess formation
- Need for breast biopsy

ADDITIONAL THERAPIES
- Warm packs to improve blood flow and milk let down and/or ice packs to reduce inflammation to affected breast for comfort
- The use of a breast pump may aid in breast emptying, especially if the infant is unable to assist in doing this.
- Wear supporting bra that is not too tight.

SURGERY/OTHER PROCEDURES
In cases of biopsy-proven idiopathic granulomatous mastitis, surgical removal can result in a 5–50% chance of recurrence, fistula formation, and poor wound healing.

INPATIENT CONSIDERATIONS
If a new mother is admitted to the hospital for treatment of her mastitis, rooming-in of the infant with the mother is mandatory so that breastfeeding can continue (4)[C]. In some hospitals, rooming-in may require hospital admission of the infant.

Admission Criteria/Initial Stabilization
- Failure of outpatient/oral therapy
  - Patient unable to tolerate oral therapy
  - Patient noncompliant with oral therapy
  - Severe illness without adequate supportive care at home
- Neonatal mastitis
- Antibiotics
- Frequent emptying of breasts, if breastfeeding
- Analgesics for pain
  - Ibuprofen
  - Acetaminophen

Nursing
- Breastfeeding/pumping of breasts encouraged
- Start infant with feedings on affected side.
- Abscess drainage is not a contraindication for breastfeeding.
- Massage in direction from blocked area toward nipple.
- Positioning infant at breast with chin or nose pointing to blockage will help drain affected area.

Discharge Criteria
- Afebrile
- Tolerating oral antibiotics well

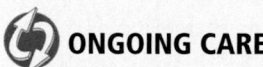 ONGOING CARE

FOLLOW-UP RECOMMENDATIONS
Rest for lactating mothers, up to bathroom

DIET
- Encourage oral fluids.
- Multivitamin, including vitamin A

PATIENT EDUCATION
- Encourage oral fluids.
- Rest is essential
- Regular emptying of both breasts with breastfeeding
- Nipple care to prevent fissures

PROGNOSIS
- Puerperal
  - Good with prompt (within 24 hours of symptom onset) antibiotic treatment and breast emptying; 96% success rate
  - 11% risk of abscess if left untreated with antibiotics
  - Antibodies develop in breast glands within first few days of infection, which may provide protection against infection or reinfection.
- Rare risk of abscess formation beyond 6 weeks postpartum if no recurrent mastitis

COMPLICATIONS
- Breast abscess 3% of women with puerperal mastitis
- Recurrent mastitis with resumption of breastfeeding or with breastfeeding after next pregnancy
- Bacteremia
- Sepsis

REFERENCES
1. Crepinsek MA, Crowe L, Michener K, et al. Interventions for preventing mastitis after childbirth. *Cochrane Database Syst Rev.* 2012;(10):CD007239.
2. Buck ML, Amir LH, Cullinane M, et al. Nipple pain, damage, and vasospasm in the first 8 weeks postpartum. *Breastfeed Med.* 2014;9(2):56–62.
3. Jahanfar S, Ng CJ, Teng CL. Antibiotics for mastitis in breastfeeding women. *Cochrane Database Syst Rev.* 2013;(2):CD005458.
4. Amir LH. ABM clinical protocol #4: mastitis, revised March 2014. *Breastfeed Med.* 2014;9(5):239–243.
5. Sheybani F, Sarvghad MR, Naderi HR, et al. Treatment for and clinical characteristics of granulomatous mastitis. *Obstet Gynecol.* 2015;125(4):801–807.

ADDITIONAL READING
Spencer JP. Management of mastitis in breastfeeding women. *Am Fam Physician.* 2008;78(6):727–731.

 SEE ALSO

Algorithms: Breast Discharge; Breast Pain

 CODES

ICD10
- N61 Inflammatory disorders of breast
- O91.22 Nonpurulent mastitis associated with the puerperium
- O91.23 Nonpurulent mastitis associated with lactation

CLINICAL PEARLS
- Complete emptying of the breasts on a regular schedule, avoiding constrictive clothing or bras that might obstruct breast ducts, meticulous attention to nipple care, "adequate rest," and a liberal intake of oral fluids for the mother can all reduce the risk of a breastfeeding mother's developing mastitis.
- First-line treatment for puerperal mastitis is dicloxacillin 500 mg PO QID for 10 to 14 days. Most mastitis can be treated with oral therapy.
- Among breastfeeding mothers, if the symptoms of mastitis fail to resolve within several days of appropriate management, including antibiotics, further investigations may be required to confirm resistant bacteria, abscess formation, an underlying mass, or inflammatory or ductal carcinoma.
- More than two recurrences of mastitis in the same location or with associated axillary lymphadenopathy warrant evaluation with ultrasound or mammography to rule out an underlying mass.

M

MASTOIDITIS

Adam Anglyn, DO • Robert M. Hasty, DO, FACOI, FACP

 BASICS

An inflammatory process of the mastoid air cells or posterior process of the temporal bone, most commonly a suppurative complication of acute otitis media (AOM)

DESCRIPTION
- Acute mastoiditis typically presents following AOM or may be the first sign of AOM. Symptoms are present for <1 month.
- Subdivided into two stages
  - Acute mastoiditis with periostitis: involves the mastoid periosteum with purulence in the mastoid air cells
  - Acute mastoid osteitis (coalescent mastoiditis): destruction of bony septae separating air cells; leading to empyema and more serious head/neck complications
- Subacute mastoiditis (masked mastoiditis): indolent process, may occur with insufficiently treated AOM
- Chronic mastoiditis: due to failed treatment of chronic otitis media. Usually associated with cholesteatoma; symptoms last months to years.

EPIDEMIOLOGY
- Children > adults
- Most common in children <2 years of age
- In children: males > females
  - Incidence is reduced after introduction of antibiotics but may again be increasing with rise of antibiotic-resistant *Streptococcus pneumoniae*. Introduction of PVC 13 vaccine may mitigate this rise (1)[C].

Incidence
1 to 4 cases/100,000 persons/year (2)

ETIOLOGY AND PATHOPHYSIOLOGY
- Subclinical stage begins with AOM causing inflammation of mastoid air cells (likely present in all cases of AOM)
- Obstruction of the aditus ad antrum (connecting the tympanic cavity and mastoid)
  - Blocks outflow tract of mastoid air cells
  - Edema and accumulation of purulent material with penetration of periosteum (acute mastoiditis with periostitis)
- Increased pressure from fluid within the air cells leads to destruction of bony septae (acute mastoid osteitis/acute coalescent mastoiditis).
- Acute mastoid osteitis can spread to adjacent areas in head and neck with abscess formation:
  - Subperiosteal abscess (most common complication), Bezold abscess, suppurative labyrinthitis, suppurative CNS complications
- AOM: *Haemophilus influenzae, S. pneumoniae*
- Acute mastoiditis: *Streptococcus pneumoniae* (most common), *Streptococcus pyogenes, H. influenzae, Staphylococcus aureus* (including methicillin-resistant *Staphylococcus aureus* [MRSA])
- Chronic mastoiditis: *Pseudomonas aeruginosa, S. aureus,* Enterobacteriaceae, anaerobic bacteria, polymicrobials (3)

Genetics
No known genetic pattern

RISK FACTORS
- Cholesteatoma
- Recurrent AOM or chronic suppurative otitis media
- Immunocompromised state

GENERAL PREVENTION
- Pneumococcal conjugate vaccine
- Early referral to ENT for chronic otitis media
- Appropriate diagnosis and treatment of AOM
- Prevention of recurrent AOM
- Treat chronic eustachian tube dysfunction (pressure equalization tubes).
- Identify cholesteatoma early.

 DIAGNOSIS

HISTORY
- Most common symptoms in infancy (2)[A]

  - Lethargy/malaise/irritability
  - Fever
  - Poor feeding/decreased appetite
- Otalgia/possible otorrhea
- Hearing loss
- Headache
- Pain/redness/swelling noted over mastoid.
- At the time of admission (2)[A]

  - 42% of children have history of otologic disease.
  - 54% on antibiotic therapy
  - Average duration of symptoms: 10 days
- Suspicion for mastoiditis increases when symptoms of AOM persist >2 weeks.

PHYSICAL EXAM
- Postauricular changes: erythema, tenderness, edema, and/or fluctuance (81–85%) (2)[A]
- Bulging, erythematous, or dull tympanic membrane (60–71%)
- Protrusion of auricle (79%)
- Fever (76%)
- Otorrhea if tympanic membrane is perforated
- Edema of external auditory canal
- Tympanic membrane (TM) can be normal in 10% of patients.

DIFFERENTIAL DIAGNOSIS
- Postauricular cellulitis or inflammatory adenopathy
- Severe otitis externa
- Benign neoplasm: aneurysmal bone cyst, fibrous dysplasia
- Malignant neoplasm: rhabdomyosarcoma, neuroblastoma
- Deep neck space infections
- Parotitis

DIAGNOSTIC TESTS & INTERPRETATION
Initial Tests (lab, imaging)
- CBC with differential: increased WBC count (4)[C]
- Elevated erythrocyte sedimentation rate (ESR) and C-reactive protein (CRP) (3,4)
- Blood cultures
- Myringotomy/tympanocentesis: Send for cultures, Gram stain, acid-fast stain (2)[B].
- Mastoiditis is often a clinical diagnosis. CT confirms diagnosis and identifies regional complications.
- If obvious physical exam and/or historical findings are absent, temporal bone imaging is recommended for patients with cervical or postauricular findings (5).
- Plain radiographs of mastoid have low diagnostic yield but may show distortion of mastoid outline or clouding of mastoid air cells. These changes are not diagnostic and can also be seen in AOM.
- CT findings (97% sensitivity; 94% positive predictive value) (6)
  - Clouding/opacification of air cells (also in AOM)
  - Mastoid air cell coalescence
  - Cortical bone erosion
  - Rim-enhancing fluid collections
- CT of temporal bone with contrast helps identify suppurative extension (5)[C].
- Technetium-99m bone scan is more sensitive to osteolytic changes than CT.
- Indications for CT scan in children (6)[C]
  - Neurologic signs
  - Vomiting/lethargy
  - Suspected cholesteatoma
  - Fever after 48 to 72 hours of therapy
  - Concern for local disease progression
- MRI use increasing; may see increased fluid signal of mastoid air cells on T2-weighted MRI—an incidental finding in the absence of clinical signs

Follow-Up Tests & Special Considerations
Interpret normal WBC with caution in symptomatic immunocompromised patients.

Diagnostic Procedures/Other
- Tympanocentesis to obtain middle ear fluid for culture and sensitivity (2)[B]
- Myringotomy with culture (also therapeutic)
- Audiography if suspected hearing loss
- Obtain CSF if intracranial extension suspected.
- Biopsy tissue protruding through TM or tympanostomy tube

 TREATMENT

- IV antibiotics and myringotomy (± tympanostomy tubes) is the preferred treatment for uncomplicated acute mastoiditis (reflecting a shift away from more invasive surgical treatment).
- Simple mastoidectomy is recommended for patients not responding to treatment after 3 to 5 days to avoid intracranial complications (7)[C].

GENERAL MEASURES
- Inpatient care during acute phase for IV antibiotics
- Keep the affected ear dry.

MEDICATION
First Line
- Empiric antibiotics against most common organisms: *Streptococcus pneumoniae* (including multiple resistant strains), *Streptococcus pyogenes*, *Staphylococcus aureus* (including MRSA), *P. aeruginosa*
- Use combination therapy with 3rd generation cephalosporin (ceftriaxone or cefotaxime) plus clindamycin with additional coverage for resistant strains (5,7)[C].
- Ceftriaxone 1 to 2 g IV q24h
  - Pediatric dosing: 50 to 75 mg/kg/day IV divided q12–24h
  - Precaution: Adjust dose with renal impairment.
- Clindamycin for coverage of ceftriaxone-resistant *S. pneumoniae* in pediatric patients (5)[C]:
  - Clindamycin pediatric dosing: 20 to 40 mg/kg/day IV divided q6–8h
- Cefotaxime 1 to 2 g IV q4–8h, depending on severity
  - Pediatric dosing: 100 to 200 mg/kg/day divided q6–8h
- Add vancomycin 30 to 60 mg/kg/day divided q8–12h if concerned for MRSA:
  - Pediatric dosing: 15 mg/kg/dose q6–8h
  - Precaution: Adjust dose with renal impairment.
- For patients with a history of recurrent AOM or recent antibiotic administration, treat with piperacillin–tazobactam 3.375 g IV q6h:
  - Pediatric dosing: 300 mg/kg/day based on piperacillin component divided q6–8h
- For other significant contraindications, precautions, or interactions, please refer to the manufacturer's literature.

Second Line
- Oral antibiotics are given after 7 to 10 days of IV antibiotics and once myringotomy/blood cultures identify pathogen and sensitivities. Common oral antibiotics include:
  - Amoxicillin–clavulanate (Augmentin) or clindamycin + 3rd-generation cephalosporin for 3 weeks or total treatment duration of 4 weeks
- For chronic mastoiditis: Use topical drops, ofloxacin otic solution (0.3%) or neomycin, polymyxin B, hydrocortisone three drops, 3 to 4 times per day.

ISSUES FOR REFERRAL
Consult ENT for mastoiditis in adults and children.

SURGERY/OTHER PROCEDURES
- Perform tympanocentesis to obtain cultures and guide antibiotic choice (2)[B].
- Myringotomy and tympanostomy tubes allow drainage of middle ear (7)[C].
- Mastoidectomy is a definitive treatment for patients who fail to improve within 24 to 48 hours despite IV antibiotics and myringotomy and for those with meningeal or intracranial complications (6,7)[C].
- Simple mastoidectomy is most effective for management of subperiosteal abscesses, if a trial of conservative therapy with drainage, myringotomy, and IV antibiotics fails (8)[C].

- Clean ear canal under microscope to ensure pressure-equalization tube patency and adequate drainage of middle ear.
- Topical antibiotic drops usually used after insertion of pressure-equalization tubes.

INPATIENT CONSIDERATIONS
Admission Criteria/Initial Stabilization
- Clinical or imaging evidence of acute mastoiditis
- Hospitalize patients with acute mastoiditis and start IV antibiotics immediately.

Nursing
Avoid getting affected ear wet.

Discharge Criteria
- Afebrile for 48 hours before IV antibiotics are discontinued
- Clinical improvement
- Able to take oral antibiotics

 ONGOING CARE

FOLLOW-UP RECOMMENDATIONS
- Oral antibiotics for 3 weeks following course of IV antibiotics (total duration of antibiotics is 4 weeks)
- For chronic mastoiditis, consider several months of antimicrobial prophylaxis with amoxicillin.

Patient Monitoring
- Assess for hearing loss postoperatively (audiogram) after acute condition has subsided.
- Follow-up with ENT, particularly patients with intracranial complications or hearing loss

PATIENT EDUCATION
Avoid getting the affected ear wet.

PROGNOSIS
- Depends on severity and stage of disease
- Conductive hearing loss may require reconstructive surgery.
- Most cases of mastoiditis recover fully if the diagnosis is made early and treated appropriately.

COMPLICATIONS
Total estimated complication rate is 18% (3).
- Extracranial
  - Subperiosteal abscess (most common)
  - Bezold abscess (abscess of sternocleidomastoid muscle, insidious, risk of mediastinitis)
  - Citelli abscess (osteomyelitis of the calvaria)
  - Osteomyelitis of the temporal bone
  - Suppurative labyrinthitis (resulting in deafness)
  - Facial nerve paralysis
- Intracranial
  - Intracranial abscess: epidural/subdural/cerebral
  - Meningitis/cerebritis/periostitis
  - Gradenigo syndrome (palsy of the 6th cranial nerve, draining ear, and retro-orbital pain)
  - Sigmoid sinus thrombophlebitis
  - Central venous sinus thrombosis

REFERENCES
1. Tamir SO, Roth Y, Dalal I, et al. Acute mastoiditis in the pneumococcal conjugate vaccine era. *Clin Vaccine Immunol.* 2014;21(8):1189–1191.
2. van den Aardweg MT, Rovers MM, de Ru JA, et al. A systematic review of diagnostic criteria for acute mastoiditis in children. *Otol Neurotol.* 2008;29(6):751–757.
3. Chien JH, Chen YS, Hung IF, et al. Mastoiditis diagnosed by clinical symptoms and imaging studies in children: disease spectrum and evolving diagnostic challenges. *J Microbiol Immunol Infect.* 2012;45(5):377–381.
4. Bilavsky E, Yarden-Bilavsky H, Samra Z, et al. Clinical, laboratory, and microbiological differences between children with simple or complicated mastoiditis. *Int J Pediatr Otorhinolaryngol.* 2009;73(9):1270–1273.
5. Lin HW, Shargorodsky J, Gopen Q. Clinical strategies for the management of acute mastoiditis in the pediatric population. *Clin Pediatr (Phila).* 2010;49(2):110–115.
6. Bakhos D, Trijolet JP, Morinière S, et al. Conservative management of acute mastoiditis in children. *Arch Otolaryngol Head Neck Surg.* 2011;137(4):346–350.
7. Psarommatis IM, Voudouris C, Douros K, et al. Algorithmic management of pediatric acute mastoiditis. *Int J Pediatr Otorhinolaryngol.* 2012;76(6):791–796.
8. Psarommatis I, Giannakopoulos P, Theodorou E, et al. Mastoid subperlosteal abscess in children: drainage or mastoidectomy? *J Laryngol Otol.* 2012;126(12):1204–1208.

ADDITIONAL READING
- Minks DP, Porte M, Jenkins N. Acute mastoiditis—the role of radiology. *Clin Radiol.* 2013;68(4):397–405.
- Pritchett CV, Thorne MC. Incidence of pediatric acute mastoiditis: 1997–2006. *Arch Otolaryngol Head Neck Surg.* 2012;138(5):451–455.

CODES

ICD10
- H70.90 Unspecified mastoiditis, unspecified ear
- H70.009 Acute mastoiditis without complications, unspecified ear
- H70.099 Acute mastoiditis with other complications, unspecified ear

CLINICAL PEARLS
- Suspect mastoiditis when symptoms of AOM persist >2 weeks despite a normal-appearing TM.
- Hospitalize all patients with acute mastoiditis for IV antibiotics. Consult ENT for drainage procedure.
- Treat with broad-spectrum IV antibiotics; collect middle ear fluid cultures to guide-specific therapy.
- If conservative treatment fails after 3 to 5 days, perform mastoidectomy to avoid intracranial complications.

M

MEASLES (RUBEOLA)

Herbert L. Muncie, Jr., MD

 BASICS

DESCRIPTION
- A highly communicable, acute viral illness characterized by an exanthematous maculopapular rash that begins at the head and spreads inferiorly to the trunk and extremities
- Rash is preceded by fever and the classic triad of cough, coryza, and conjunctivitis (3 Cs). Koplik spots are pathognomonic lesions of the oral mucosa.
- Public health problem in the developing world, with significant morbidity and mortality
- System(s) affected: hematologic; lymphatic; immunologic; pulmonary; skin
- Synonym(s): rubeola

EPIDEMIOLOGY
- Transmission: direct contact with infectious droplets; highly contagious; 90% of nonimmune close contacts likely to become infected on exposure.
  - Droplets can remain in the air for hours.
- Infectivity is greatest during the prodromal phase.
  - Patients are considered contagious from 4 days before symptoms until 4 days after rash appears.
  - Immunocompromised patients are considered contagious for the entire duration of disease.
- Incubation period: averages 12.5 days from exposure to onset of prodromal symptoms (1)[B]
- Predominant age: varies based on local vaccine practices and disease incidence. In developing countries, most cases occur in children <2 years.

Incidence
- United States: no longer considered an endemic disease by the CDC; isolated outbreaks still occur.
- In the first half of 2015, the CDC reported 159 confirmed cases of measles. Of these cases, 111 (70%) were associated with an outbreak that originated in Disney theme parks in Orange County, California.
  - Many cases were in vaccine-eligible patients who declined due to philosophic or religious beliefs.
  - Children aged 6 to 23 months traveling abroad are at increased risk if unvaccinated.
- Worldwide: An estimated 20 million measles cases occur each year, with 122,000 measles deaths in 2012. Over 95% of measles deaths occur in poor countries with limited health infrastructure (2).

ETIOLOGY AND PATHOPHYSIOLOGY
Measles virus enters through the respiratory mucosa and replicates locally. It spreads to regional lymphatic tissues and other reticuloendothelial sites via the bloodstream.
- Measles virus is a spherical, enveloped, nonsegmented, single-stranded, negative-sense RNA virus of genus *Morbillivirus*, family *Paramyxoviridae*.
- Humans are the only natural host.

RISK FACTORS
- For developing measles:
  - Lack of adequate vaccination (two doses)
  - Travel to countries where measles is endemic
  - Contact with exposed individuals, travelers, or immigrants
- For severe measles or measles complications:
  - Immunodeficiency
  - Malnutrition
  - Pregnancy
  - Vitamin A deficiency
  - Age <5 years or >20 years

GENERAL PREVENTION
- 100% preventable with proper vaccination (3)[A]
- Measles vaccine (active immunization)
  - Vaccine is usually given in combination with mumps and rubella (MMR) or with added varicella (MMR-V; ProQuad)
  - Primary vaccination requires two doses
    ○ First dose given at 12 to 15 months of age; 95% develop immunity.
    ○ Second dose given at time of school entry (4 to 6 years of age) or any time >4 weeks after first measles vaccine; the 5% of initial nonresponders almost always develop immunity after the second dose.
    ○ Health care workers should have immunity verified and if not immune, should receive the vaccine if not contraindicated.
  - Common adverse reactions to vaccine
    ○ Fever
    ○ Febrile seizures are rare (<5%) and occur 6 to 12 days after vaccination. Risk of febrile seizures increases if initial immunization is delayed past age 15 months (4)[B].
    ○ Transient, mild, measles-like rash 7 to 10 days after vaccination (2%, with decreasing incidence during second vaccination)
    ○ If hypersensitivity reaction occurs, test for immunity; if immune, second dose is not needed.
    ○ There is no substantiated link between MMR vaccine and autism (5)[A].
  - Contraindications
    ○ Live viral vaccines are contraindicated in immunosuppressed patients. For MMR, however, asymptomatic HIV-infected children with adequate CD4 count should be vaccinated.
    ○ Pregnancy: Live vaccine is contraindicated (theoretical risk of fetal infection).
    ○ Anaphylactic reaction to gelatin or neomycin; consult allergist before vaccination.
    ○ Egg anaphylaxis is not considered a contraindication.

COMMONLY ASSOCIATED CONDITIONS
- Immunosuppression
- Malnutrition

DIAGNOSIS

HISTORY
- Prodromal period: usually 2 to 3 days before rash (may be up to 8 days)
  - Fever
    ○ May begin 8 to 12 days after exposure; can persist until 2 to 3 days after rash onset
    ○ Temperature often >102°F (39–40.5°C); can precipitate febrile seizures
    ○ Fever onset >3 days after rash suggests complicated course
  - "3 Cs" triad: cough, coryza, and conjunctivitis
  - Cough may persist for 2 weeks.
  - Prodromal symptoms typically intensify over 2 to 4 days, peaking on first day of rash before subsiding.
- Other symptoms include loose stools, malaise, irritability, photophobia (from iridocyclitis), sore throat, headache, and abdominal pain.

PHYSICAL EXAM
- Koplik spots
  - Pathognomonic of prodromal measles
  - 2- to 3-mm, gray–white, raised lesions on erythematous base on buccal mucosa
  - Occur ~48 hours before measles exanthem
- Exanthematous rash (characteristic but not pathognomonic)
  - Maculopapular blanching rash
  - Begins at ears and hairline and spreads head to toe, reaching hips by day 2
  - Discrete erythematous patches become confluent over time, particularly on the upper body.
  - Clinical improvement usually occurs within 48 hours after rash appears.
  - Rash fades in 3 to 4 days changing to a brownish color, followed by fine desquamation.
- Lymphadenopathy and pharyngitis may be seen during exanthematous period.

DIFFERENTIAL DIAGNOSIS
- Drug eruptions
- Rubella
- *Mycoplasma pneumoniae* infection
- Infectious mononucleosis
- Parvovirus B19 infection, roseola
- Enteroviruses
- Rocky Mountain spotted fever, dengue
- Toxic shock syndrome
- Meningococcemia
- Kawasaki disease

DIAGNOSTIC TESTS & INTERPRETATION
Initial Tests (lab, imaging)
- Obtain serum sample and throat (or nasopharyngeal) swab. Molecular testing of serum and respiratory specimens is the most accurate method to confirm measles infection. IgM assay and measles RNA by real-time polymerase chain reaction (RT-PCR)
- Measles virus–specific IgM assay from serum and saliva. Antibodies may be undetectable on first day of exanthema but are usually detectable by day 3.
  - Sensitivity: 77% within 72 hours of rash onset; 100% within 4 to 11 days after rash onset. If negative but rash lasts >72 hours, repeat.
  - IgM falls to undetectable levels 4 to 8 weeks after rash onset.
- Measles virus–specific IgG may be undetectable up to 7 days after exanthem; levels peak 14 days after exanthem.
  - A 4-fold increase in IgG titers 14 days after an initial titer that was measured at least 7 days after rash onset is confirmatory.
- Viral cultures for measles are not usually performed.
- Mild neutropenia is common.
- Liver transaminases and pancreatic amylase may be elevated, particularly in adults.
- Chest x-ray if concern for secondary pneumonia

ALERT
Report suspected measles cases to public health authorities.

TREATMENT

GENERAL MEASURES

- Place all patients with measles in respiratory isolation until 4 days after onset of rash; immunocompromised patients should be isolated for duration of illness.
- Supportive therapy (i.e., antipyretics, antitussives, humidification, increased oral fluid consumption)

MEDICATION

- No approved antiviral therapy is available. Immuno-suppressed children with severe measles have been treated with IV or aerosolized **ribavirin**. No controlled trial data exist, and this use is not FDA approved.
- Vitamin A: WHO recommends daily dosages for two consecutive days:
  – Children <6 months of age 50,000 IU
  – Children 6 to 12 months of age 100,000 IU
  – Children >12 months of age 200,000 IU
- Antibiotics

  – Reserved for patients with clinical signs of bacterial superinfection (pneumonia, purulent otitis, pharyngitis/tonsillitis) (6)[B]
  – A small randomized, double-blinded trial resulted in an 80% (number needed to treat [NNT] = 7) decrease in measles-associated pneumonia with prophylactic antibiotics; consider antibiotic use prophylactically in patients with a high risk of complications (7)[B].

- Outbreak control
  – *A single case of measles constitutes an outbreak.*
  – Immunize contacts (individuals exposed or at risk of having been exposed) within 72 hours.
    o Monovalent vaccine may be given to infants 6 months to 1 year of age, but two further doses of vaccine after 12 months must be given for adequate immunization.
    o Monovalent or combination vaccine may be given to all measles-exposed susceptible individuals age >1 year if not contraindicated.
    o Individuals not immunized within 72 hours of exposure should be excluded from school, child care, and health care settings (social quarantine) until 2 weeks after onset of rash in last case of measles.
  – Immunoglobulin therapy (passive immunity) may be necessary for the following high-risk individuals exposed to measles for whom vaccine is inappropriate:
    o Children age <1 year (infants 6 to 12 months of age may receive MMR vaccine in place of IG if given within 72 hours of exposure)
    o Pregnant women
    o Individuals with severe immunosuppression
    o IM immunoglobulin should be given within 6 days of measles exposure; CDC recommends 0.25 mL/kg to maximum of 15 mL for infants and pregnant women; immunocompromised individuals receive 0.5 mL/kg to a maximum of 15 mL.

INPATIENT CONSIDERATIONS

Outpatient care is appropriate, except where complications develop (e.g., encephalitis, pneumonia).

 ONGOING CARE

FOLLOW-UP RECOMMENDATIONS

Signs of complications needing close follow-up include:

- Difficulty breathing or noisy breathing
- Changes in vision
- Changes in behavior, confusion
- Chest or abdominal pain

PATIENT EDUCATION

- Adhere to recommended immunization schedules.
- Avoid exposure, particularly to unimmunized children and adults, pregnant women, and immunocompromised persons, until 4 days after rash onset.
- Avoid contact with potential sources of secondary bacterial pathogens until respiratory symptoms resolve.
- Centers for Disease Control and Prevention. Measles. www.cdc.gov/measles/about/index.html

PROGNOSIS

- Typically self-limited; prognosis good
- High fatality rates may be seen among malnourished or immunocompromised children, particularly in developing countries.

COMPLICATIONS

- Otitis media (5–15%)
- The immune response to measles infection para-doxically depresses response to non–measles-virus antigens, which renders individuals more susceptible to pneumonia and diarrhea.
- Respiratory complications:
  – Bronchopneumonia (5–10%)
    o Accounts for most measles-related deaths
    o May be viral or bacterial
  – Interstitial pneumonitis (immunocompromised patients)
  – Laryngotracheobronchitis ("measles croup"): occurs in younger age group (<2 years)
- GI complications: diarrhea (may lead to dehydration)
- Neurologic complications
  – Febrile seizures
  – Acute disseminated encephalomyelitis with seizures and neurologic abnormalities (occurs in 1/1,000 cases): presents within 2 weeks of rash, probably an autoimmune response
  – Inclusion body encephalitis is rare but fatal in those with defective cellular immunity.
  – Subacute sclerosing panencephalitis
    o Rare degenerative CNS disease resulting from persistent measles infection following natural disease; usually fatal
    o Presents 5 to 15 years after infection
    o Most often in persons infected before age 2 years
- Ocular complications
  – Keratitis
    o Can lead to permanent scarring, blindness
    o Vitamin A deficiency predisposes to more severe keratitis and its complications.
- Other secondary bacterial infections
- Death: results from complications, mainly pneumonia, rather than the virus itself. CDC statistics show that for every 1,000 children who get measles, 1 or 2 will die.

REFERENCES

1. Lessler J, Reich NG, Brookmeyer R, et al. Incubation periods of acute respiratory viral infections: a systematic review. *Lancet Infect Dis*. 2009;9(5):291–300.
2. Orenstein W, Seib K. Mounting a good offense against measles. *N Engl J Med*. 2014;371(18): 1661–1663.
3. Althouse BM, Bergstrom TC, Bergstrom CT. Evolution in health and medicine Sackler colloquium: a public choice framework for controlling transmissible and evolving diseases. *Proc Natl Acad Sci U S A*. 2010;107(Suppl 1):1696–1701.
4. Rowhani-Rahbar A, Fireman B, Lewis E, et al. Effect of age on the risk of fever and seizures following immunization with measles-containing vaccines in children. *JAMA Pediatr*. 2013;167(12):1111–1117.
5. Demicheli V, Jefferson T, Rivetti A, et al. Vaccines for measles, mumps and rubella in children. *Cochrane Database Syst Rev*. 2005;(4):CD004407.
6. Kabra SK, Lodha R. Antibiotics for preventing complications in children with measles. *Cochrane Database Syst Rev*. 2013;(8):CD001477.
7. Garly ML, Balé C, Martins CL, et al. Prophylactic antibiotics to prevent pneumonia and other complications after measles: community based randomised double blind placebo controlled trial in Guinea-Bissau. *BMJ*. 2006;333(7581):1245.

ADDITIONAL READING

- Mulholland EK, Griffiths UK, Biellik R. Measles in the 21st century. *N Engl J Med*. 2012;366(19): 1755–1757.
- Papania MJ, Wallace GS, Rota PA, et al. Elimination of endemic measles, rubella, and congenital rubella syndrome from the western hemisphere: the US experience. *JAMA Pediatr*. 2014;168(2):148–155.

 CODES

ICD10

- B05.9 Measles without complication
- B05.2 Measles complicated by pneumonia
- B05.89 Other measles complications

CLINICAL PEARLS

- **There is no substantiated link between MMR vaccine and autism.**
- Measles is a highly communicable viral disease whose natural transmission has been halted in the United States by mass immunization.
- A single case of measles constitutes an outbreak.
- Suspected measles cases must be reported to state or local health departments to contain outbreak.
- Immunization requires two doses: one at 12 to 15 months of age and one at school age (4 to 6 years of age).
- Presentation includes a prodrome of fever, cough, coryza, and conjunctivitis, followed by a descending maculopapular rash beginning on the face and progressing to the chest and lower body (centrifugal).
- Consider measles in the differential diagnosis of a febrile rash illness (especially in unvaccinated individuals with recent international travel).
- Measles-associated pneumonia is the most common cause of mortality.

M

MEASLES, GERMAN (RUBELLA)
Mark B. Stephens, MD, MS, FAAFP, CAPT, MC, USN

 BASICS

DESCRIPTION
- A mild, generally self-limited exanthematous viral infection of children and adults, with rare complications. Nonimmune women who become infected with rubella while pregnant may have devastating fetal effects. Up to 50% of rubella infections may be asymptomatic (1,2)[A].
- System(s) affected: hematologic; nervous; pulmonary; exocrine; ophthalmologic; skeletal
- Synonym(s): German measles; 3-day measles

Pregnancy Considerations
- Pregnancy-associated rubella infection may lead to congenital rubella syndrome (CRS) with potentially devastating fetal outcomes.
- CRS is present in up to 90% of fetuses exposed during the 1st trimester (2)[A].
- Screening pregnant women for rubella immunity and vaccinating nonimmune women is the most effective means to prevent CRS (2)[A].
- Although no case of vaccine-associated CRS has been reported, women should not become pregnant for at least 28 days after vaccination because the vaccine-type virus can cross the placenta (2)[A].
- Polymerase chain reaction (PCR) detection of viral RNA in amniotic fluid and fetal blood sampling allow for rapid diagnosis of fetal infection after 15 weeks' gestation (3)[B].

EPIDEMIOLOGY
- 50- to 70-nm RNA togavirus of genus *Rubivirus* (1)[A]
- 13 genotypes have been identified (4)[A].
- Live attenuated vaccine available in United States. since 1969—primarily to prevent CRS
- Since 2004, all cases of rubella in United States have been imported, typically in travelers with inadequate immunity (1)[A].
- Average incubation: 14 days; range 12 to 23 days
- Infectious period between 7 days before and 5 to 7 days after rash onset
- Transmitted by respiratory droplets
- Most common in late winter and early spring
- Humans are only natural hosts (1)[A].

Incidence
- U.S. incidence: <10/100,000 since 2001
- From 2004 to 2012, six cases of CRS reported in United States (5).
- Still occurs worldwide in developing countries: 100,000 cases of CRS annually worldwide

ETIOLOGY AND PATHOPHYSIOLOGY
- Virus invades the respiratory epithelium, replicates in nasopharynx and regional lymph nodes, and spreads hematogenously. Infected patients shed virus from the nasopharynx 3 to 8 days after inoculation. Shedding lasts 7 or more days after onset of rash.
- Disease progresses from a prodromal stage (1 to 5 days) to lymphadenopathy (5 to 10 days) and finally to an exanthematous, pruritic, and maculopapular rash. Rash starts on the face and spreads to the trunk and extremities, sparing the palms and soles (14 to 17 days after onset of initial symptoms).

- Rubella first described by German scientists in the early 1800's as a variant of measles or scarlet fever
- 1962 to 1965: global pandemic resulting in an estimated 12.5 million cases in the United States, with 2,000 cases of encephalitis; 11,250 cases of therapeutic or spontaneous abortions; 2,100 neonatal deaths; and 20,000 infants born with CRS (1)[A]

Genetics
Children with CRS and children with type 1 diabetes share a high frequency of HLA-DR3 histocompatibility Ag and a high prevalence of islet cell Ab.

RISK FACTORS
Inadequate immunization, inadequate immunity after prior vaccination, immunodeficiency states, immunosuppressive therapy, crowded living/working conditions, international travel (1)[A]

GENERAL PREVENTION
- Vaccination is the most effective preventive strategy.
- Available combined with measles and mumps (MMR) or with varicella (MMR-V). Single rubella vaccine is not available in the United States.
  - A 2-dose schedule combined MMR vaccine recommended for those born after 1957. The 1st dose recommended at ages 12 to 15 months; 2nd dose recommended either at 4 to 6 years or at 11 to 12 years of age. Children with HIV should receive MMR vaccine at 12 months of age if no contraindications exist. In the event of an outbreak, immediate vaccination for infants 6 to 11 months old is recommended (2)[A].
  - Vaccine is recommended for nonimmune people in the following groups: prepubertal boys and girls, all women of reproductive age, college students, daycare personnel, health care workers, and military personnel.
- Contraindicated: pregnancy, immunodeficiency (except HIV infection), within 3 months of IVIG or blood administration, severe febrile illness, or hypersensitivity to vaccine components. Patients who receive rubella vaccine do not transmit rubella to others, although the virus can be isolated from the pharynx. Breastfeeding is not a contraindication to vaccination (1)[A].
- During outbreaks, serologic screening before vaccination is *NOT* recommended because rapid mass vaccination is necessary to stop disease spread (2)[A].
- The MMR vaccine *is not associated with autism* (6)[A],(7)[B].
- Children who receive the MMR-V vaccine have a 2-fold increase in risk of febrile seizures compared with those who receive MMR and varicella vaccines separately (7)[B].
- Routine rubella antibody screening is recommended during pregnancy by the CDC and ACOG (6)[A].

 DIAGNOSIS

Council of State and Territorial Epidemiologists (CSTE) Case Definition Classifications of Rubella (1)[A]

- Clinical case definition
  - Acute onset of pink, coalescent macules on the face spreading to the trunk and extremities, becoming discrete macules then fading in previously affected areas

---

- Temperature >99°F (37.2°C; if measured)
- Arthralgia or arthritis, lymphadenopathy, or conjunctivitis
- Laboratory criteria for diagnosis
  - Isolation of virus from throat or nasopharynx, serum, CSF, urine, or cataracts (postmortem)
  - 4-fold rise in acute- and convalescent-phase titers of serum IgG Ab
  - Positive serologic test for IgM Ab
  - PCR positive for virus

HISTORY
- Most cases of postnatal rubella are due to inadequately immunized travelers returning from endemic areas.
- Rubella can spread quickly among persons residing in close quarters.
- Postnatal rubella: low-grade fever, sore throat, nausea, anorexia, arthritis, arthralgia, malaise. 50% may be asymptomatic.
- CRS: parental concerns about hearing or vision impairment, jaundice, or developmental delay
- Deafness could be the only manifestation and not be noticed until 2nd year of life (2)[A].

PHYSICAL EXAM
- Postnatal rubella: low-grade fever, lymphadenopathy (posterior auricular, occipital, posterior cervical), exanthem (mild, pink, discrete 1- to 4-mm maculopapular rash), soft palate petechiae (Forchheimer sign) (20%) (1)[A]
- CRS: microcephaly, large anterior fontanelle, sensorineural hearing loss (58%), cataracts, glaucoma, microphthalmia, pigmentary retinopathy, purpuric ("blueberry muffin") skin lesions, murmur (50%) consistent with patent ductus arteriosus (PDA), hepatosplenomegaly, jaundice, cryptorchidism, inguinal hernia, radiolucent bone disease (2)[A]

DIFFERENTIAL DIAGNOSIS
- Postnatal rubella
  - Measles virus (rubeola)
  - Scarlet fever (strep A)
  - Infectious mononucleosis
  - Erythema infectiosum (parvovirus B19)
  - Roseola infantum (i.e., exanthem subitum)
  - Toxoplasmosis
  - Drug eruptions
  - Other exanthematous enteroviral infections
- Congenital rubella
  - Measles
  - Parvovirus B19
  - Human herpesvirus 6
  - Other exanthematous entero- or arboviruses

DIAGNOSTIC TESTS & INTERPRETATION
- Because 50% of cases are subclinical, laboratory testing is best to confirm the diagnosis (1,2)[A].
- Detection of wild-type virus is gold standard (1)[A].
- Enzyme immunoassay (EIA): preferred testing for IgM antibodies, which may not be detectable before 5 days after the onset of rash (1)[A]
- Hemagglutination inhibition (HAI) test: A 4-fold increase of IgG Ab levels from acute to convalescent phase is diagnostic for recent infection (1)[A].
- Latex agglutination (LA) test: sensitive and specific but dependent on experience of lab personnel (1)[A]

- Immunofluorescent antibody (IFA) assay: used for detection of viral IgG and IgM Ab (1)[A]
- Avidity test: not routinely used. Should only be performed in reference labs. Used to distinguish between recent and past infections (1)[A]
- Serum collection should be performed within 7 to 10 days after illness onset. When testing for IgM, repeat collection may be necessary if the sample was taken before day 5. When testing for seroconversion, a 2nd IgG sample should be collected 2 to 3 weeks after the first (acute to convalescent phase). In most cases, IgG is detectable 8 days after rash onset (1)[A].
- Virus may be isolated from 1 week prior to 2 weeks after the onset of rash. Maximal viral shedding occurs up to day 4 after rash onset. Best results are from throat swabs (1)[A].
- Epidemiologically, viral genotyping by reverse transcription (RT)-PCR helps determine the country of origin. Throat swabs should be collected 4 days after the rash onset and sent to the CDC (1)[A].
- Viral cultures of CSF are reserved for suspected cases of CRS or rubella encephalitis (1)[A].
- If a pregnant female is exposed, amniotic fluid PCR or fetal blood sampling may be done at 15 weeks' gestation for viral detection. Placental biopsy (less common) may be done at 12 weeks' gestation. If positive, offer genetic counseling (1)[A].
- As the incidence of rubella decreases, the positive predictive value (PPV) of IgM results decreases. False-positive findings occur in patients with parvovirus B19, mononucleosis, and positive rheumatoid factor (1)[A].
- After reexposure, a person with a low level of Ab from past infection or prior vaccination may experience an acute, small rise in Ab levels. This is not associated with a high incidence of contagious to others or of fetal risk (1)[A].

Follow-Up Tests & Special Considerations
- Reporting: state-dependent. Samples should be sent to the CDC for genotyping. Cases of CRS are reported to the National Congenital Rubella Syndrome Registry (1,2)[A].
- Infants with CRS may shed virus up to 1 year. Observe contact isolation during all hospitalizations until child turns 1 year old (unless child has two negative throat cultures and urine specimens a month apart after 3 months of age) (2)[A].

 TREATMENT

- Supportive for mild cases
- Isolate patients for 5 to 7 days after rash onset.

- Postnatal rubella: mild and self-limited; treat symptomatically. Hospitalize for complications: idiopathic thrombocytopenic purpura (ITP) or encephalitis (1)[A].
- CRS: supportive care unless neurologic or hemorrhagic complications develop; phototherapy may be indicated for jaundice; multidisciplinary management of long-term complications (2)[A]

MEDICATION
No specific therapy available for mild cases.

First Line
- Age- and dose-appropriate antipyretics
- NSAIDs can be used for arthritis and arthralgias in adults and infants age >6 months.
- IVIG can be given for severe thrombocytopenia—most cases, however, are self-limited.

 ONGOING CARE

FOLLOW-UP RECOMMENDATIONS
Patient Monitoring
- Individuals immune to rubella through natural infection or vaccine may be reinfected when reexposed; such infection is usually asymptomatic and detectable only by serology. Those who have received the vaccine have lower measurable IgG levels than those who had the natural disease.

- In CRS, it is important to detect auditory and visual impairment early (2)[A].
- 2/3 of internationally adopted children have no written record of immunizations (4)[A].

PATIENT EDUCATION
http://www.cdc.gov/rubella/

PROGNOSIS
- Postnatal rubella: Complete recovery is typical.
- CRS

  – Varied and unpredictable spectrum, ranging from stillbirth to normal infancy/childhood (1,2)[A]
  – Detectable levels of IgG persist for years and then may decline (does not drop at the expected 2-fold dilution/month). By age 5 years, 20% have no detectable antibody (2)[A].
  – IgM may not be detectable until 1 month after birth and may persist for 6 to 12 months (2)[A].
  – Overall mortality (up to 10%) is greatest during first 6 months.
  – 70% of encephalitis cases develop residual neurologic defects, including autistic syndrome.
  – Prognosis is excellent if only minor congenital defects are present.

COMPLICATIONS
- Postinfectious encephalitis (1/5,000 cases)
- Thrombocytopenic purpura (1/3,000 cases)
- CRS: incidence dependent on trimester exposed
- Rubella vaccine may rarely cause encephalitis or ITP.
  – ITP is self-limited and is not a contraindication to vaccination.

REFERENCES

1. Centers for Disease Control and Prevention. Chapter 14—rubella. In: McLean H, Redd S, Abernathy E, et al, eds. *Manual for the Surveillance of Vaccine-Preventable Diseases*. 5th ed. Atlanta, GA: Centers for Disease Control and Prevention; 2014. http://www.cdc.gov/vaccines/pubs/surv-manual/chpt14-rubella.html. Accessed January 21, 2016.
2. Centers for Disease Control and Prevention. Chapter 15—congenital rubella syndrome. In: McLean H, Redd S, Abernathy E, et al, eds. *Manual for Surveillance of Vaccine-Preventable Diseases*. 5th ed. Atlanta, GA: Centers for Disease Control and Prevention; 2014. http://www.cdc.gov/vaccines/pubs/surv-manual/chpt15-crs.html. Accessed January 21, 2016.
3. Tang JW, Aarons E, Hesketh LM, et al. Prenatal diagnosis of congenital rubella infection in the second trimester of pregnancy. *Prenat Diagn*. 2003;23(6):509–512.
4. Abernathy ES, Hubschen JM, Muller CP, et al. Status of global virologic surveillance for rubella viruses. *J Infect Dis*. 2011;204(Suppl 1):S524–S532.
5. Centers for Disease Control and Prevention. Three cases of congenital rubella syndrome in the postelimination era—Maryland, Alabama, and Illinois, 2012. *MMWR Morb Mortal Wkly Rep*. 2013;62(12):226–229.
6. McLean HQ, Fiebelkorn AP, Temte JL, et al. Prevention of measles, rubella, congenital rubella syndrome, and mumps, 2013: summary recommendations of the Advisory Committee on Immunization Practices (ACIP). *MMWR Recomm Rep*. 2013;62(RR-04):1–34.
7. Lai J, Fay KE, Bocchini JA. Update on childhood and adolescent immunizations: selected review of US recommendations and literature: part 2. *Curr Opin Pediatr*. 2011;23(4):470–481.

ADDITIONAL READING

- Centers for Disease Control and Prevention. Rubella. In: Atkinson W, Wolfe C, Hamborsky J, eds. *Epidemiology and Prevention of Vaccine-Preventable Diseases*. 13th ed. Atlanta, GA: Centers for Disease Control and Prevention; 2012. www.cdc.gov/vaccines/pubs/pinkbook/rubella.html. Accessed January 21, 2016.
- Mongua-Rodriguez N, Díaz-Ortega JL, García-García L, et al. A systematic review of rubella vaccination strategies implemented in the Americas: impact on the incidence and seroprevalence rates of rubella and congenital rubella syndrome. *Vaccine*. 2013;31(17):2145–2151.
- Walling A. Measles, mumps, and rubella in pregnant women. *Am Fam Physician*. 2006;73(5):907–908.

 CODES

ICD10
- B06.9 Rubella without complication
- B06.00 Rubella with neurological complication, unspecified
- P35.0 Congenital rubella syndrome

CLINICAL PEARLS
- Rubella is typically a self-limited viral exanthematous infection of children and adults.
- Nonimmune women who are infected with rubella while pregnant may have devastating fetal effects (CRS).

M

MEDIAL TIBIAL STRESS SYNDROME (MTSS)/SHIN SPLINTS

Michael Y. Yang, MD • Marc W. McKenna, MD

 BASICS

DESCRIPTION

- Medial tibial stress syndrome (MTSS) is preferred nosologically to "shin splints." Aching pain along the inner edge of the tibial shaft develops when the musculature and/or periosteum in the (lower) leg become irritated by repetitive activity. The condition is part of a continuum of stress-related injuries to the lower leg. MTSS does not encompass pain from ischemia (compartment syndrome) or stress fractures.
- Tendonitis/periostitis of the medial soleus muscles, anterior tibialis, and posterior tibialis muscles
- Synonyms: tibial stress reaction; anterior muscle syndrome; periostitis; perimyositis; shin splints

EPIDEMIOLOGY

Incidence
Common, can account for between 5% and 35% of novice-running injuries. Frequently occurs bilaterally (1).

Pediatric Considerations
MTSS may account for up to 31% of all overuse injuries in high school athletes (2).

ETIOLOGY AND PATHOPHYSIOLOGY

- Multifactorial anatomic and biomechanical factors
  - Overuse injuries causing or limited by
    - Microtrauma from repetitive motion leading to periosteal inflammation
    - Overpronation of the subtalar joint and tight gastrocnemius/soleus complex with increased eccentric loading of musculature inserting along the medial shin
    - Interosseous membrane pain
    - Periostitis
    - Tears of collagen fibers
    - Enthesopathy
  - Anatomic structures affected include the following:
    - Flexor hallucis longus
    - Tibialis anterior
    - Tibialis posterior
    - Soleus
    - Crural fascia
- Pathogenesis: theorized to be due to persistent repetitive loading, which leads to inadequate bone remodeling and possible microfissures causing pain without evidence of fracture or ischemia

RISK FACTORS

- Intrinsic or personal risk factors:
  - Greater internal and external ranges (>65 degrees) of hip motion
  - Significant overpronation at the ankle
  - Imbalance of inverters and everter musculature of the ankle and foot

- Female gender
- Leaner calf girth
- Femoral neck anteversion
- Navicular drop
- Genu varum
- External or environmental factors
  - Lack of physical fitness
  - Inexperienced runners—particularly those with rapid increases in mileage and inadequate prior conditioning
  - Excessive overuse or distance running, particularly on hard or inclined (crowned) surfaces
  - Prior injury
  - Equipment (shoe) failure
- Other risk factors
  - Elevated BMI
  - Lower bone mineral density
  - Tobacco use
- Those typically affected include the following:
  - Runners
  - Military personnel—common in recruit/boot camp
  - Gymnasts, soccer, and basketball players
  - Ballet dancers

GENERAL PREVENTION

- Proper technique for guided calf stretching and lower extremity strength training
- Rehabilitation for prior injuries
- Other suggested recommendations
  - Gait analysis and retraining, particularly for overpronation
  - Orthotic footwear inserts

COMMONLY ASSOCIATED CONDITIONS

- Rule out stress fracture and compartment syndrome.
- Pes planus (flat feet)

 DIAGNOSIS

HISTORY

- Patients typically describe dull, sharp, or deep pain along the lower leg that is resolved with rest.
- Patients are often able to run through the pain in early stages.
- Pain is commonly associated with exercise (also true with compartment syndrome), but in severe cases, pain may persist with rest.

PHYSICAL EXAM

- Tenderness to palpation is typically elicited along the posteromedial border of the middle-to-distal third of the tibia.
- Pain with plantar flexion
- Ensure neurovascular integrity of the lower extremity, examining distal pulses, sensation, reflexes, and muscular strength.

DIFFERENTIAL DIAGNOSIS

- Bone
  - Tibial stress fractures
    - Typically, pain persists at rest or with weight-bearing activities.
    - Focal tenderness over the anterior tibia
- Muscle/soft tissue injury
  - Strain, tear, tendinopathy
  - Muscle hernia
- Fascial
  - Chronic exertional compartment syndrome (3)[C]
    - Pain without direct tenderness on exam
    - Pain increases with exertion and resolves at rest.
    - Pain is described as cramping or squeezing.
    - Pain with possible weakness or paresthesias on exam
  - Interosseous membrane tear
- Nerve
  - Spinal stenosis
  - Lumbar radiculopathy
  - Common peroneal nerve entrapment
- Vascular
  - DVT
  - Popliteal arterial entrapment (4)[B]
    - Rare but limb-threatening disease
    - History of intermittent unilateral claudication
    - MRI reveals compression of the artery by the medial head of the gastrocnemius muscle.
- Infection
  - Osteomyelitis
- Malignancy
  - Bone tumors

DIAGNOSTIC TESTS & INTERPRETATION

- Plain radiographs help rule out stress fractures if >2 weeks of symptoms (5).
- Bone scintigraphy
  - Diffuse linear vertical uptake in the posterior tibial cortex on the lateral view.
  - Stress fractures demonstrate a focal ovoid uptake.
- High-resolution MRI reveals abnormal periosteal and bone marrow signals, which are useful for early discrimination of tibial stress fractures.
- Increased pain and localized tenderness warrants further imaging with MRI due to concern for tibial stress fracture.
- Exclude compartment syndrome using intracompartmental pressure testing.

TREATMENT

GENERAL MEASURES

- Activity modification with a gradual return to training based on improvement of symptoms
- Patients should maintain fitness with low-impact activities such as swimming and cycling.
- Continue activity modification until patients are pain-free on ambulation.
- Good supportive footwear is recommended.

MEDICATION

- Analgesia with acetaminophen or other oral nonsteroidal anti-inflammatory agent
- Cryotherapy (ice massage) is also advised to relieve acute-phase symptoms (6)[C].

ADDITIONAL THERAPIES

- Stretching of the gastrocnemius, soleus, and peroneal muscles are treatment mainstays (6)[C].
- Calf stretch, peroneal stretch, TheraBand exercises, and eccentric calf raises may improve endurance and strength.
- Compression stockings have been used to treat MTSS with mixed results.
- Structured running programs with warm up exercises have not been demonstrated to reduce pain in young athletes (7)[B].

SURGERY/OTHER PROCEDURES

- Surgical intervention includes a posterior medial fascial release in individuals with both
  - Severe limitation of physical activity and
  - Failure of 6 months of conservative treatment
    - Patient should be counseled that complete return of activity to sport may not be always achieved postoperatively. Surgical risks include infection and hematoma formation.
- Extracorporeal shock wave therapy (ESWT) may decrease recovery time when added to a running program (8)[B].

COMPLEMENTARY & ALTERNATIVE MEDICINE

- Individualized polyurethane orthoses may help chronic running injuries (9)[A].
- Special insoles, shock-absorbing running shoes, and knee braces have not been shown to decrease the incidence of MTSS (6)[C].
- Ultrasound, acupuncture, aquatic therapy, electrical stimulation, whirlpool baths, cast immobilization, taping, and steroid injection may help improve pain.
- Physical therapy approaches including Kinesio tape and fascial distortion massage may yield quicker return to activity (10)[B].

 ONGOING CARE

FOLLOW-UP RECOMMENDATIONS
Patient Monitoring
- Patients should avoid prematurely resuming preinjury running pace.
- Stretching and strengthening exercises should be added.
- Preinjury training errors should be identified and corrected with a gradual return to activity dictated by symptoms (pain).

PROGNOSIS
The condition is usually self-limiting, and most patients respond well with rest and nonsurgical intervention.

COMPLICATIONS
- Stress fractures and compartment syndrome
- Undiagnosed MTSS or chronic exertional compartment syndrome can lead to a complete fracture or tissue necrosis, respectively.

REFERENCES

1. Fullem BW. Overuse lower extremity injuries in sports. *Clin Podiatr Med Surg.* 2014;32(2): 239–251.
2. Cuff S, Loud K, O'Riordan MA. Overuse injuries in high school athletes. *Clin Pediatr (Phila).* 2010;49(8):731–736.
3. Hutchinson M. Chronic exertional compartment syndrome. *Br J Sports Med.* 2011;45(12): 952–953.
4. Politano AD, Bhamidipati CM, Tracci MC, et al. Anatomic popliteal entrapment syndrome is often a difficult diagnosis. *Vasc Endovascular Surg.* 2012;46(7):542–545.
5. Chang GH, Paz DA, Dwek JR, et al. Lower extremity overuse injuries in pediatric athletes: clinical presentation, imaging findings, and treatment. *Clin Imaging.* 2013;37(5):836–846.
6. Fields KB, Sykes JC, Walker KM, et al. Prevention of running injuries. *Curr Sports Med Rep.* 2010; 9(3):176–182.
7. Moen MH, Holtslag L, Bakker E, et al. The treatment of medial tibial stress syndrome in athletes; a randomized clinical trial. *Sports Med Arthrosc Rehabil Ther Technol.* 2012;4:12.
8. Moen MH, Rayer S, Schipper M, et al. Shockwave treatment for medial tibial stress syndrome in athletes; a prospective controlled study. *Br J Sports Med.* 2012;46(4):253–257.
9. Hirschmüller A, Baur H, Müller S, et al. Clinical effectiveness of customised sport shoe orthoses for overuse injuries in runners: a randomised controlled study. *Br J Sports Med.* 2011;45(12): 959–965.
10. Schulze C, Finze S, Bader R, et al. Treatment of medial tibial stress syndrome according to the fascial distortion model: a prospective case control study. *ScientificWorldJournal.* 2014;2014:790626.

ADDITIONAL READING

- Abelson B. The Tibialis Anterior Stretch–Kinetic Health. https://www.youtube.com/watch?v= 6Z6XM63x2TM. June 19, 2014.
- Cosca DD, Navazio F. Common problems in endurance athletes. *Am Fam Physician.* 2007;76(2):237–244.
- Hamstra-Wright KL, Bliven KC, Bay C. Risk factors for medial tibial stress syndrome in physically active individuals such as runners and military personnel: a systematic review and meta-analysis. *Br J Sports Med.* 2015;49(6):362–369.

CODES

ICD10
- S86.899A Other injury of other muscle(s) and tendon(s) at lower leg level, unspecified leg, initial encounter
- S86.891A Other injury of other muscle(s) and tendon(s) at lower leg level, right leg, initial encounter
- S86.892A Other injury of other muscle(s) and tendon(s) at lower leg level, left leg, initial encounter

CLINICAL PEARLS

- MTSS is the preferred term for "shin splints."
- Diagnosis is based on the history of repetitive overuse accompanied by characteristic shin pain.
- Pain that is worsened with activity and relieved with rest is commonly described along the middle and distal third of the posteromedial tibial surface.
- Treatment includes ice, activity modification, analgesics, eccentric stretching, gait retraining, and a gradual return to activity.

M

MELANOMA

Carl Bryce, MD, Capt, USAF • Matthew J. Snyder, DO

 BASICS

DESCRIPTION
- Melanoma is a tumor arising from malignant transformation of cells from the melanocytic system.
  - Most arise in the skin but may also present as a primary lesion in any tissue: ocular, GI, GU, lymph node, and leptomeninges.
  - Metastatic spread to any site in the body
- Main types of cutaneous melanoma include the following (1):
  - Superficial-spreading melanoma: 50–80% cases; occurs in sun-exposed areas (trunk, back, and extremities); most ~6 mm diameter at diagnosis; when seen in younger patients, presents as a flat, slow growing, irregularly bordered lesion
  - Nodular: 20–30%, present in older patients, often ulcerate and hemorrhage, most commonly thick and pigmented
  - Lentigo maligna (subtype of melanoma in situ): slowest growing; older population; occurs in sun-exposed areas (head, neck, forearms). Lentigo maligna melanoma (LMM) is its invasive counterpart.
  - Amelanotic melanoma (<5%): can be missed and diagnosed at a later stage, as it can mimic benign skin conditions
  - Acral-lentiginous: 2–8% of all melanomas; however, most common melanoma in black or Asian patients, found in palmar, plantar, and subungual areas.
  - Subungual melanoma (0.7–3.5%): dark longitudinal band in nail bed; Hutchinson sign when proximal nail fold involved
  - Desmoplastic melanoma (~1%): sarcoma-like tendencies with increased hematogenous spread
- System(s) affected: skin/exocrine

Geriatric Considerations
Lentigo maligna, slowly enlarging pigmented lesion, is most common in elderly patients. This type is usually found on face, beginning as a circumscribed macular patch of mottled pigmentation showing shades of dark brown, tan, or black.

Pediatric Considerations
Large congenital nevi (>5 cm) are risk factors and have a >2% lifetime risk of malignant conversion. Blistering sunburns in childhood significantly increase risk.

Pregnancy Considerations
No increased risk of melanoma in pregnancy. However, it is suggested waiting 1 to 2 years if further pregnancy is desired in case of recent melanoma. Melanoma can spread to the placenta.

EPIDEMIOLOGY
Incidence
- In 2015, an estimated 73,870 Americans were diagnosed with melanoma, with 9,940 expected deaths (2).
- Predominant age: median age: 62 and 54 years for men and women respectively, >50% of all individuals with melanoma are between 20 and 40 years of age.
- Predominant sex: male > female (1.5 times)
- Incidence among whites greater than that among minority groups; ~20 times higher than blacks (1)
- Minority groups demonstrate increased rates of metastasis, advanced stages at diagnosis, thicker initial lesions, earlier age at diagnosis, and overall poorer outcomes.
- Low socioeconomic status associated with higher incidence of melanoma

Prevalence
- Lifetime risk: men: 1/37; female: 1/56
- 2% of all cancer deaths
- The most common cancer affecting women age 25 to 29 years of age and second only to breast cancer in women 30 to 34 years of age (1).

ETIOLOGY AND PATHOPHYSIOLOGY
- DNA damage by UV-A/UV-B exposure
- Tumor progression: initially may be confined to epidermis with lateral growth, may then grow into dermis with vertical growth

Genetics
- Dysplastic nevus syndrome is a risk factor for development of melanoma. Close surveillance is warranted.
- 8–12% of patients with melanoma have a family history of disease.
- Mutation in CDKN2A (p16) is found in 1/3 of patients with family incidence of melanoma.
- Mutations in BRAF (V600E) implicated in 50–60% of cutaneous melanomas
- Familial Atypical Mole Malignant Melanoma (FAMMM) syndrome characterized by >50 atypical moles, +FH of melanoma, clinical diagnosis (3)

RISK FACTORS
- Genetic predisposition
- UV-A and UV-B exposure
- History of >5 sunburns during lifetime
- History of intense intermittent sun exposure
- Previous pigmented lesions (especially dysplastic melanocytic nevi)
- Fair complexion, freckling, blue eyes, and blond/red hair
- Highest predictor of risk is increased number of nevi (>100).
- Family/personal history of melanoma
- Tanning bed use: 75% increased risk if 1st exposure before age 35 years
- Changing nevus
- Large (>5 cm) congenital nevi
- Other skin cancers
- Chronic immunosuppression (chronic lymphocytic leukemia, non-Hodgkin lymphoma, AIDS, or posttransplant)
- Blistering sunburns in childhood
- Living at high altitude (>700 meters or 2,300 feet above sea level)
- Occupational exposure to ionizing radiation

GENERAL PREVENTION
- Avoidance of sunburns, especially in childhood
- Use of sunscreen with at least SPF 30 to all skin exposed to sunlight, reapplying regularly and after toweling or swimming
- Avoid tanning beds; class 1 carcinogen by World Health Organization (WHO).
- Screening of high-risk individuals, especially males >50 years
- Education for proper diagnosis plays a large factor in prevention.
- Any suspicious lesions should be biopsied with a narrow excision encompassing the entire breadth plus sufficient depth of the lesion. Options include elliptical excisions, punch, or shave biopsies.

COMMONLY ASSOCIATED CONDITIONS
- Dysplastic nevus syndrome
- >50 nevi. These individuals have higher lifetime risk of melanoma than the general population, as 50% of all melanoma arise in preexisting nevi.
- Giant congenital nevus: 6% lifetime incidence of melanoma
- Xeroderma pigmentosum is a rare condition associated with an extremely high risk of skin cancers, including melanoma.
- Psoriasis after psoralen-UV-A (PUVA) therapy

 DIAGNOSIS

HISTORY
- Change in a pigmented lesion: either hypo- or hyperpigmentation, bleeding, scaling, ulceration, or changes in size or texture
- Obtain family and personal history of melanoma or nonmelanoma skin cancer.
- Obtain social history on sunbathing, tanning, and other sun exposure.

PHYSICAL EXAM
- ABCDE: Asymmetry, Border irregularity, Color variegation (especially red, white, black, blue), Diameter >6 mm, Evolution over time
- Any new and/or changing nevus, bleeding/ulcerated
- Location on Caucasians is primarily back and lower leg, on African Americans is the hands, feet, and nails.
- May include mucosal surfaces (nasopharynx, conjunctiva)
- Individuals at high risk for melanoma should have careful ocular exam to assess for presence of melanoma in the iris and retina.

DIFFERENTIAL DIAGNOSIS
- Dysplastic and blue nevi
- Vascular skin tumor
- Pigmented actinic keratosis
- Traumatic hematoma
- Pigmented squamous cell and basal cell carcinomas, seborrheic keratoses, other changing nevi

DIAGNOSTIC TESTS & INTERPRETATION
- Lactate dehydrogenase (LDH), chest/abdomen/pelvic CT, MRI, and/or PET CT at baseline and in monitoring progression in metastatic disease (stage IV) (5)
- Imaging studies only helpful in detecting and evaluating for progression of metastatic disease

Diagnostic Procedures/Other
- Dermoscopy allows for magnification of lesions, allowing for a decreased number of biopsies of benign skin lesions in addition to providing increased sensitivity in detecting melanoma and basal cell carcinoma (4)[B].
- Surgical biopsy remains the standard of care. Any suspicious nevus should be excised, either by elliptical excision; a scoop shave (saucerization) technique may be appropriate, as long as a full-thickness can be achieved (1)[C].
- Sentinel lymph node biopsy, a staging procedure, remains an important factor for prognosis (5)[A].

Test Interpretation
- Nodular melanoma is primarily vertical growth, whereas the other three types are horizontal.
- Estimated that 1/10,000 dysplastic nevi become melanoma annually.
- Immunohistochemical testing increases sensitivity of lymph node biopsies.
- Staging is based on the tumor-node-metastasis (TNM) criteria by 2010 American Joint Committee on Cancer (AJCC) criteria (5).

TREATMENT

GENERAL MEASURES
Full surgical excision of melanoma is the standard of care. See below for recommended surgical margins.

MEDICATION
- For stages I to III, surgical excision is curative in most cases; in patients with stage IV disease, systemic treatment with chemotherapy is recommended.
- Preferred regimens (5)[A] include the following:
  - Ipilimumab (monoclonal antibody against CTLA-4) in combination with Nivolumab (anti-PD-1 monoclonal antibody) demonstrated 61% response versus ipilimumab alone (6)[A].
  - Vemurafenib (Zelboraf) or Dabrafenib are BRAF inhibitors approved for metastatic, unresectable melanoma expressing BRAF V600E or V600K mutations.
  - High-dose interleukin-2 controversial (significant toxicity, 1–2% mortality related to treatment)
  - Referral for enrollment in clinical trials
- Additional active regimens (e.g., dacarbazine [DTIC], temozolomide, paclitaxel, carmustine [BCNU], cisplatin, carboplatin, vinblastine); often limited to those who are not candidates to preferred regimens.
- Imatinib (Gleevec) in tumors with C-KIT mutation
- Interferon-α as adjuvant therapy received FDA approval in 1995 (high dose) and 2011 (pegylated) to treat stage IIB to III melanoma; shown to improve 4-year relapse rate but no overall effect on survival; 1/3 of patients will discontinue due to toxicity (granulocytopenia, hepatotoxicity). Biochemotherapy is advocated by some (i.e., chemo + immunotherapy combination), although optimal regimen remains uncertain given disease heterogeneity (5)[B].

ISSUES FOR REFERRAL
- Consultation with oncologist for consideration of chemotherapeutic options
- Plastic surgery sometimes needed after final excision

ADDITIONAL THERAPIES
Immunotherapy using various vaccine preparations has produced mixed results and remains an area for further research (7)[B].

SURGERY/OTHER PROCEDURES
- Standard of care for melanoma includes early surgical excision with the following recommended margins (5)[A]:
  - In situ tumors: 0.5 cm margin has been the standard of care but may be insufficient in lentigo maligna (8)[B].
  - Thickness of 1.01 to 2.00 mm: 1 to 2 cm margins
  - Thickness of >2.00 mm: 2 cm margins
- Sentinel lymph node biopsy is indicated in patients with T2-, T3-, and T4-staged melanomas.
  - Selected patients with stage T1b melanoma should also be considered for sentinel lymph node biopsy.
  - Not recommended in melanoma in situ or T1a
- Mohs surgery is often used for lesions with ill-defined borders or lesions of head and neck.
- Radiotherapy can be used to treat lentigo maligna in addition to certain head and neck lesions.
- Palliative radiation therapy can be used with metastatic melanoma.

COMPLEMENTARY & ALTERNATIVE MEDICINE
Molecular and mouse tumor model studies support role of topical silymarin (milk thistle derivative) in decreasing UV radiation–induced inflammation, oxidative stress, and carcinogenesis (8)[B].

INPATIENT CONSIDERATIONS
Admission Criteria/Initial Stabilization
Most treatments are done as outpatients with no stabilization needed.

 ONGOING CARE

FOLLOW-UP RECOMMENDATIONS
After diagnosis and treatment, close follow-up and skin protection (i.e., sunblock, UV protective clothing) are highly advised.

Patient Monitoring
- Routine screening clinical skin examination annually for all persons >40 years is controversial and without proven benefit.
- Total body photography and dermoscopy should be used for surveillance of skin lesions, most commonly used for patients with >5 atypical nevi.
- For patients with a history of cutaneous melanoma, specialty guidelines suggest every 3 to 12 months depending on recurrence risk (5)[C], general agreement to plan annual examinations after 5 years stable (9)[A].
- Lab and imaging tests after diagnosis and treatment of stage I to II melanoma are low yield, have high false-positive rates, and are not recommended (5)[B].

DIET
No data to support specific dietary manipulations; general recommendations from American Cancer Society for cancer prevention

PATIENT EDUCATION
- Teach patients who are at risk, or have had melanoma, the principles of ABCDE examinations.
- High-risk patients should perform monthly skin self-examinations and be taught to examine inaccessible areas.
- Patients with a history of melanoma or dysplastic nevus syndrome should have regular total body examinations.

PROGNOSIS
- Breslow depth (thickness) in millimeters remains among strongest predictors of prognosis.
- Median age at death 68 years
- Highest survival seen in women <45 years of age at diagnosis
- Metastatic melanoma has an average survival of 6 to 9 months; 15–20% 5-year survival with current treatment.
- Stages I and II, appropriately treated, have 20-year survival rates of 90% and 80%, respectively.

COMPLICATIONS
- Metastatic spread
- Unsatisfactory cosmetic results following the primary surgery

REFERENCES
1. Shenenberger D. Cutaneous malignant melanoma: a primary care perspective. *Am Fam Physician*. 2012;85(2):161–168.
2. American Cancer Society. What are the key cancer statistics about melanoma skin cancer? http://www.cancer.org/cancer/skincancer-melanoma/detailedguide/melanoma-skin-cancer-key-statistics. Accessed June 2015.
3. Bichakjian CK, Halpern AC, Johnson TM, et al. Guidelines of care for the management of primary cutaneous melanoma. *J Am Acad Dermatol*. 2011;65(5):1032–1047.
4. Marghoob AA, Usatine RP, Jaimes N. Dermoscopy for the family physician. *Am Fam Physician*. 2013;88(7):441–450.
5. Coit DG, Andtbacka R, Anker CJ, et al. Melanoma, version 2.2013: featured updates to the NCCN guidelines. *J Natl Compr Canc Netw*. 2013;11(4):395–407.
6. Postow MA, Chesney J, Pavlick AC, et al. Nivolumab and ipilimumab versus ipilimumab in untreated melanoma. *New Engl J Med*. 2015;372(21):2006–2017.
7. Ozao-Choy J, Lee DJ, Faries MB. Melanoma vaccines: mixed past, promising future. *Surg Clin North Am*. 2014;94(5):1017–1030.
8. Erickson C, Miller SJ. Treatment options in melanoma in situ: topical and radiation therapy, excision and Mohs surgery. *Int J Dermatol*. 2010;49(5):482–491.
9. Cromwell K, Ross MI, Xing Y, et al. Variability in melanoma post-treatment surveillance practices by country and physician specialty: a systematic review. *Melanoma Res*. 2012;22(5):376–385.

ADDITIONAL READING
- American Joint Committee on Cancer offers an online calculator to predict survival outcome from initial diagnosis. http://melanomaprognosis.org
- Perkins A, Duffy RL. Atypical moles: diagnosis and management. *Am Fam Physician*. 2015;(91):762–767.
- Tuong W, Cheng LS, Armstrong AW. Melanoma: epidemiology, diagnosis, treatment, and outcomes. *Dermatol Clin*. 2012;30(1):113–124.

 SEE ALSO

Dysplastic Nevus Syndrome

 CODES

ICD10
- C43.9 Malignant melanoma of skin, unspecified
- C43.30 Malignant melanoma of unspecified part of face
- C43.4 Malignant melanoma of scalp and neck

CLINICAL PEARLS
- Remember that amelanotic melanomas exist; pigmentation is not required.
- 80% of cutaneous melanomas arise in existing nevi. Any changing nevi should be considered for full-thickness biopsy.
- Excellent prognosis in early detection and treatment, as well as being a common cancer affecting young adult women, require a high clinical suspicion and low threshold for thorough evaluation.

M

MÉNIÈRE DISEASE

Jason E. Cohn, DO, MS • Nadir Ahmad, MD, FACS • Thomas C. Spalla, MD

BASICS

DESCRIPTION

- An inner ear (labyrinthine) disorder characterized by recurrent attacks of hearing loss, tinnitus, vertigo, and sensations of aural fullness due to an increase in the volume and pressure of the inner ear endo-lymph fluid (endolymphatic hydrops)
- Often unilateral initially, nearly half become bilateral over time.
- Severity and frequency of vertigo may diminish with time, but hearing loss is often progressive and/or fluctuating.
- Usually idiopathic (Ménière disease) but may be secondary to another condition causing endolymphatic hydrops (Ménière syndrome)
- System(s) affected: nervous
- Synonym(s): Ménière syndrome; endolymphatic hydrops

EPIDEMIOLOGY

- Predominant age of onset: 40 to 60 years
- Predominant gender: female > male (1.3:1)
- Race/ethnicity: white, Northern European > blacks

Incidence

Estimates 1 to 150/100,000 per year

Prevalence

Varies from 7.5 to >200/100,000

ETIOLOGY AND PATHOPHYSIOLOGY

- Not fully understood; theories include increased pressure of the endolymph fluid due to increased fluid production or decreased resorption. This may be caused by endolymphatic sac pathology, abnormal development of the vestibular aqueduct, or inflammation caused by circulating immune complexes. Increased endolymph pressure may cause rupture of membranes and changes in endolymphatic ionic gradient.
- Ménière *syndrome* may be secondary to injury or other disorders (e.g., reduced middle ear pressure, allergy, endocrine disease, lipid disorders, vascular, viral, syphilis, autoimmune). Any disorder that could cause endolymph hydrops could be implicated in Ménière *syndrome*.

Genetics

Some families show increased incidence, but genetic and environmental influences are incompletely understood.

RISK FACTORS

May include

- Stress
- Allergy
- Increased salt intake
- Caffeine, alcohol, or nicotine
- Chronic exposure to loud noise
- Family history of Ménière
- Certain vascular abnormalities (including migraines)
- Certain viral exposures (especially herpes simplex virus [HSV])

GENERAL PREVENTION

Reduce known risk factors: stress; salt, alcohol, and caffeine intake; smoking; noise exposure; ototoxic drugs (e.g., aspirin, quinine, aminoglycosides).

COMMONLY ASSOCIATED CONDITIONS

- Anxiety (secondary to the disabling symptoms)
- Migraines
- Hyperprolactinemia

DIAGNOSIS

Diagnosis is clinical.

HISTORY

Symptomatic episodes are typically spontaneous but may be preceded by an aura of increasing fullness in the ear and tinnitus. These may occur in clusters, with long periods of symptom-free remissions.

- Formal criteria for diagnosis from American Academy of Otolaryngology–Head and Neck Surgery:
  - At least two episodes of rotational-horizontal vertigo >20 minutes in duration
  - Tinnitus or aural fullness
  - Hearing loss: Low frequency (sensorineural) is confirmed by audiometric testing.
  - Other causes (e.g., acoustic neuroma) excluded.
  - During severe attacks: pallor, sweating, nausea, vomiting, falling, prostration
  - Symptoms are exacerbated by motion.

PHYSICAL EXAM

- Physical exam rules out other conditions; no finding is unique to Ménière disease.
- Horizontal nystagmus may be seen during attacks.
- Otoscopy is typically normal.
- Triggering of attacks in the office with Dix-Hallpike maneuver suggests diagnosis of benign paroxysmal positional vertigo, not Ménière disease.

DIFFERENTIAL DIAGNOSIS

- Acoustic neuroma or other CNS tumor
- Syphilis
- Third window syndromes
- Endolymphatic sac tumor
- Viral labyrinthitis
- Transient ischemic attack (TIA), migraine
- Vertebrobasilar disease
- Other labyrinthine disorders (e.g., Cogan syndrome, benign positional vertigo, temporal bone trauma)
- Diabetes or thyroid dysfunction
- Vestibular neuronitis
- Medication side effects
- Otitis media
- Autoimmune inner ear disease
- Autosomal dominant sensorineural hearing loss

DIAGNOSTIC TESTS & INTERPRETATION

Testing is done to rule out other conditions but does not necessarily confirm or exclude Ménière disease.

Initial Tests (lab, imaging)

- Consider serologic tests specific for *Treponema pallidum* in at-risk populations.
- Thyroid, fasting blood sugar, and lipid studies
- Consider MRI to rule out acoustic neuroma or other CNS pathology, including tumor, aneurysm, and multiple sclerosis (MS).
- MRI can help diagnosis Ménière disease by identifying endolymphatic hydrops (1,2)[B].

Diagnostic Procedures/Other

- Auditory
  - Audiometry using pure tone and speech to show low-frequency sensorineural (nerve) loss and impaired speech discrimination. Usually shows low-frequency sensorineural hearing loss
  - Tuning fork tests (i.e., Weber and Rinne) ABR or MRI to rule out acoustic neuroma
  - Electrocochleography may be useful to confirm etiology.
- Vestibular
  - Caloric testing: Electronystagmography may show reduced caloric response. Can obtain reasonably comparable information with use of 0.8 mL of ice water caloric testing. Reduced activity on either side is consistent with Ménière diagnosis but is not itself diagnostic.

Test Interpretation

- Histologic temporal bone analysis (at autopsy). Dilation of inner ear fluid system, neuroepithelial damage with hair cell loss, basement membrane thickening, and perivascular microvascular damage
- Cytochemical analysis can reveal altered AQP4 and AQP6 expression in the supporting cell, altered cochlin, and mitochondrial protein expression (3)[B].

TREATMENT

- Usually managed in outpatient setting
- A paucity of evidence-based guidelines exist; therefore, there is no gold standard treatment.
- Medications are primarily for symptomatic relief of vertigo and nausea.
- During attacks, bed rest with eyes closed prevents falls. Attacks rarely last >4 hours.

MEDICATION

First Line

- Acute attack: Initial goal is stabilization and symptom relief. For severe episodes
  - Benzodiazepines (such as diazepam): decrease vertigo and anxiety
  - Antihistamines (meclizine/dimenhydrinate): decrease vertigo and nausea
  - Anticholinergics (transdermal scopolamine): reduces nausea and emesis associated with motion sickness
  - Antidopaminergic agents (metoclopramide, (promethazine): decrease nausea, anxiety
  - Rehydration therapy and electrolyte replacement
  - Steroid taper for acute hearing loss
- Maintenance (goal is to prevent/reduce attacks)
  - Lifestyle changes (e.g., low-salt diet) are needed.
  - Diuretics may help reduce attacks by decreasing endolymphatic pressure and volume; there is insufficient evidence to recommend routine use:
    - ○ Hydrochlorothiazide; hydrochlorothiazide/triamterene (Dyazide, Maxzide)
    - ○ Acetazolamide (Diamox)
- Contraindications/warnings:
  - Atropine: cardiac disease, especially supraventricular tachycardia and other arrhythmias, prostatic enlargement
  - Scopolamine: children and elderly, prostatic enlargement
  - Diuretics: electrolyte abnormalities, renal disease

- Precautions:
  - Sedating drugs should be used with caution, particularly in the elderly. Patients are cautioned not to operate motor vehicles or machinery. Atropine and scopolamine should be used with particular caution.
  - Diuretics: Monitor electrolytes.
- Significant possible interactions: transdermal scopolamine: anticholinergics, antihistamines, tricyclic antidepressants, other

Second Line
- Steroids, both intratympanic and systemic (PO or IV) have been used for longer treatment of hearing loss:
  - Intratympanic administration results in higher steroid levels in the inner ear and may be more effective and safer than systemic (2)[C].
  - Addition of prednisone 30 mg/day to diuretic treatment reduced severity and frequency of tinnitus and vertigo in one pilot study.
- In Europe, betahistine, a histamine agonist is routinely used (unavailable in the United States). Other vasodilators, such as isosorbide dinitrate, niacin, and histamine, have also been used; evidence of their effectiveness is incomplete.
- Evidence is lacking for routine use of Famvir, may improve hearing more than balance.
- Intratympanic gentamicin has shown to improve vertigo (4–6)[B].

ISSUES FOR REFERRAL
- Consider ear, nose, throat/neurology referral.
- Patients should have formal audiometry to confirm hearing loss.

ADDITIONAL THERAPIES
- Application of intermittent pressures via a myringotomy using a Meniett device has been shown to relieve vertigo (7)[B]:
  - Safe; requires a long-term tympanostomy tube
- Vestibular rehabilitation may be beneficial for patients with persistent vestibular symptoms:
  - Safe and effective for unilateral vestibular dysfunction

SURGERY/OTHER PROCEDURES
- Interventions that preserve hearing:
  - Endolymphatic sac surgery, either decompression or drainage of endolymph into mastoid or subarachnoid space
    - Less invasive; may decrease vertigo; may influence hearing/tinnitus
  - Endolymphatic sac surgery is effective in controlling vertigo in short- and long-term follow-up in at least 75% of patients with Ménière disease who failed medical therapy (8)[A].
  - Vestibular nerve section (intracranial procedure)
    - More invasive
    - Decreases vertigo and preserves hearing
  - Tympanostomy tube: may decrease symptoms by decreasing the middle ear pressure
- Interventions for patients with no serviceable hearing:
  - Labyrinthectomy: very effective at controlling vertigo but causes deafness
  - Vestibular neurectomy

- Cochlear implantation has shown to improve tinnitus and quality of life (9)[B].
- There are new surgeries on the rise, for example, endolymphatic duct blockage, which in one study proved to be superior to endolymphatic sac decompression (10)[B].

COMPLEMENTARY & ALTERNATIVE MEDICINE
Insufficient evidence to support effectiveness, but many integrative techniques have been tried, including the following:
- Acupuncture, acupressure, tai chi
- Niacin, bioflavonoids, Lipoflavonoids, ginger, ginkgo biloba, and other herbal supplements

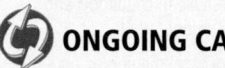 ONGOING CARE

FOLLOW-UP RECOMMENDATIONS
Patient Monitoring
Due to the possibility of progressive hearing loss despite decrease in vertiginous attacks, it is important to monitor changes in hearing and to monitor for more serious underlying causes (e.g., acoustic neuroma).

DIET
- Diet is usually not a factor, unless attacks are brought on by certain foods.
- A low salt is often recommended but not proven effective in randomized controlled trials.

PROGNOSIS
- Alert patients about the nature of alternating attacks and remission.
- Between attacks, patient may be fully active but is often limited due to fear or lingering symptoms. This can be severely disabling.
- 50% resolve spontaneously within 2 to 3 years.
- Some cases last >20 years.
- Severity and frequency of attacks diminish, but hearing loss is often progressive.
- 90% can be treated successfully with medication; 5–10% of patients require surgery for incapacitating vertigo.
- There is a mental illness burden associated with Ménière disease (11)[B].

COMPLICATIONS
Loss of hearing; injury during attack; inability to work

REFERENCES
1. Wu Q, Dai C, Zhao M, et al. The correlation between symptoms of definite Ménière disease and endolymphatic hydrops visualized by magnetic resonance imaging [published ahead of print August 29, 2015]. *Laryngoscope*.
2. Gu X, Fang ZM, Liu Y, et al. Diagnostic advantages of intratympanically gadolinium contrast-enhanced magnetic resonance imaging in patients with bilateral Ménière's disease. *Am J Otolaryngol*. 2015;36(1):67–73.
3. Ishiyama G, Lopez IA, Sepahdari AR, et al. Meniere's disease: histopathology, cytochemistry, and imaging. *Ann N Y Acad Sci*. 2015;1343:49–57.
4. Marques P, Manrique-Huarte R, Perez-Fernandez N. Single intratympanic gentamicin injection in Ménière's disease: VOR change and prognostic usefulness. *Laryngoscope*. 2015;125(8):1915–1920.
5. Rah YC, Han JJ, Park J, et al. Management of intractable Ménière's disease after intratympanic injection of gentamicin. *Laryngoscope*. 2015;125(4):972–978.
6. Casani AP, Cerchiai N, Navari E, et al. Intratympanic gentamicin for Meniere's disease: short- and long-acting follow-up of two regimens of treatment. *Otolaryngol Head Neck Surg*. 2014;150(5):847–852.
7. Ahsan SF, Standring R, Wang Y. Systematic review and meta-analysis of Meniett therapy for Ménière's disease. *Laryngoscope*. 2015;125(1):203–208.
8. Sood AJ, Lambert PR, Nguyen SA, et al. Endolymphatic sac surgery for Ménière's disease: a systematic review and meta-analysis. *Otol Neurotol*. 2014;35(6):1033–1045.
9. Mick P, Amoodi H, Arnoldner C, et al. Cochlear implantation in patients with advanced Ménière's disease. *Otol Neurotol*. 2014;35(7):1172–1178.
10. Saliba I, Gabra N, Alzahrani M, et al. Endolymphatic duct blockage: a randomized controlled trial of a novel surgical technique for Ménière's disease treatment. *Otolaryngol Head Neck Surg*. 2015;152(1):122–129.
11. Furukawa M, Kitahara T, Horii A, et al. Psychological condition in patients with intractable Ménière's disease. *Acta Otolaryngol*. 2013;133(6):584–589.

ADDITIONAL READING
- Long AF, Xing M, Morgan K. Exploring the evidence base for acupuncture in the treatment of Ménière's syndrome—a systematic review. *Evid Based Complement Alternat Med*. 2011;2011:429102.
- Lopez-Escamez JA, Carey J, Chung WH, et al. Diagnostic criteria for Ménière's disease. *J Vestib Res*. 2015;25(1):1–7.

 SEE ALSO

Hearing Loss; Labyrinthitis; Tinnitus

 CODES

ICD10
- H81.09 Meniere's disease, unspecified ear
- H81.01 Meniere's disease, right ear
- H81.02 Meniere's disease, left ear

CLINICAL PEARLS
- Ménière disease is characterized by vertigo, hearing loss, and tinnitus +/− aural fullness.
- There is a wide differential diagnosis for Ménière disease; therefore, one must fully investigate symptoms.
- Multiple medical, surgical, and rehabilitative treatments are available to decrease the severity and frequency of attacks.

M

MENINGITIS, BACTERIAL

Felix B. Chang, MD, DABMA, FAAMA

BASICS

DESCRIPTION
- A potentially life-threatening bacterial infection of the meninges
- System affected: nervous

EPIDEMIOLOGY
- Predominant age: neonates, infants, and elderly
- Predominant sex: male = female

Incidence
Varies with age (1)[C]
- <2 months: 80/100,000
- 2 to 23 months: 7/100,000
- 2 to 10 years: 0.5/100,000
- 11 to 17 years: 0.4/100,000
- 18 to 34 years: 0.66/100,000
- 35 to 49 years: 0.95/100,000
- ≥65 years: 1.92/100,000

Varies with pathogen
- *Streptococcus pneumoniae*: 0.81/100,000
- Group B *Streptococcus*: 0.25/100,000
- *Neisseria meningitidis*: 0.19/100,000
- *Haemophilus influenzae*: 0.08/100,000
- *Listeria monocytogenes*: 0.05/100,000

ETIOLOGY AND PATHOPHYSIOLOGY
Bacterial infection causes inflammation of the pia mater, arachnoid, and the fluid of the ventricles. Age groups with likely pathogens guide empiric choice of antibiotics. Guide therapy by culture whenever possible (1):
- Newborns (<2 months)
  - Group B *Streptococcus*
  - *Escherichia coli*
  - *L. monocytogenes*
- Infants and children
  - *S. pneumoniae*
  - *N. meningitidis*
  - *H. influenzae*
- Adolescents and young adults
  - *N. meningitidis*
  - *S. pneumoniae*
- Immunocompromised adults
  - *S. pneumoniae, L. monocytogenes*, gram-negative bacilli such as *Pseudomonas aeruginosa*
- Older adults
  - *S. pneumoniae* 50%
  - *N. meningitidis* 30%
  - *L. monocytogenes* 5%
  - 10% gram-negatives bacilli: *E. coli, Klebsiella, Enterobacter, P. aeruginosa*

Genetics
Navajo Indians and American Eskimos appear to have genetic or acquired susceptibility to invasive disease.

RISK FACTORS
- Immune compromise
- Alcoholism, diabetes, chronic disease
- Neurosurgical procedure/head injury
- Abdominal surgery
- Neonates: prematurity, low birth weight, premature rupture of membranes, maternal peripartum infection, and urinary tract abnormalities
- Abnormal communication between nasopharynx and subarachnoid space (congenital, trauma)
- Parameningeal source of infection: otitis, sinusitis, mastoiditis
- Trauma: skull fracture

GENERAL PREVENTION
- Treat infections appropriately.
- Strict aseptic techniques for patients with head wounds or skull fractures
- Consider CSF fistula in patients with recurrent meningitis.
- Meningitis caused by *H. influenzae* type B has decreased 55% with routine vaccination.
- Conjugate vaccines against *S. pneumoniae* may reduce the burden of disease in childhood and produce herd immunity among adults.
- Close contacts meningococcal meningitis patients should receive chemoprophylaxis (2)[A].

COMMONLY ASSOCIATED CONDITIONS
Conditions associated with a worse prognosis:
- Alcoholism, old age, infancy
- Diabetes mellitus, multiple myeloma
- Head trauma, seizures
- Coma, bacteremia, sepsis
- Bacteremia, sepsis, sinusitis

DIAGNOSIS

HISTORY
- Antecedent upper respiratory infection
- Fever, headache, vomiting, photophobia
- Seizures, confusion, nausea, rigors
- Profuse sweats, weakness
- Elderly: subtle findings including confusion
- Infants: irritability, lethargy, poor feeding
- Altered mental status

PHYSICAL EXAM
The triad of fever, neck stiffness, and altered mental status has low sensitivity (44%) (3)[C]. 95% of patients present with at least two of the following four symptoms: headache, fever, neck stiffness, and altered mental status.
- Meningismus
- Focal neurologic deficits
- Meningococcal rash: macular and erythematous at first, then petechial or purpuric
- Papilledema
- Brudzinski sign: Passive flexion of neck elicits involuntary flexing of knees in supine patients.
- Kernig sign: resistance or pain to knee extension following 90-degree hip flexion by clinician in supine patients

DIFFERENTIAL DIAGNOSIS
- Bacteremia, sepsis, brain abscess
- Seizures, other nonbacterial meningitides
- Aseptic meningitis
- Drug-induced: NSAIDs, cotrimoxazole, amoxicillin, cephalosporin, isoniazid
- Inflammatory noninfectious: Behçet disease, systemic lupus erythematosus (SLE), sarcoidosis
- Stroke

DIAGNOSTIC TESTS & INTERPRETATION
Initial Tests (lab, imaging)
- Prompt lumbar puncture (1)[A]
  - Head CT first if focal neuro findings, papilledema, or altered mentation
- Typical CSF analysis: turbid
  - Adults
    - >500 cells/mL WBCs
    - Glucose <40 mg/dL
    - <2/3 blood-to-glucose ratio
    - CSF protein >200 mg/dL
    - CSF opening pressure >30 cm
    - Suspect ruptured brain abscess when WBC count is unusually high (>100,000).
- CSF Gram stain and cultures
- Polymerase chain reaction (PCR) of CSF (particularly in suspected viral meningitis)
- Bacterial antigen tests should be reserved for cases in which the initial CSF Gram stain is negative and CSF culture is negative at 48 hours of incubation.
- Serum blood cultures, serum electrolytes
- Evaluate clotting function if petechiae or purpura are present.
- Chest radiograph may reveal pneumonitis or abscess.
- Later in course: head CT if hydrocephalus, brain abscess, subdural effusions, and subdural empyema are suspected or if no clinical response after 48 hours of appropriate antibiotics
- C-reactive protein (CRP): Normal CRP has high negative, predictive value for bacterial meningitis (3)[B].

Diagnostic Procedures/Other
Lumbar puncture
- Head CT first if concern for increased intracranial pressure or warning signs of space-occupying lesion (new-onset seizure, papilledema, or brain herniation) or focal neurologic deficit
- IDSA CT recommendations: immunocompromised, history of central nervous system disease (stroke, mass lesion, focal infection), papilledema, focal neurologic defect including fixed dilated pupil, gaze palsy, weakness of extremity, visual field cut, new-onset seizure <12 week prior to presentation, abnormal level of consciousness (3)[C]
- Contraindications to LP: signs of increased intracranial pressure (decerebrate posturing, papilledema), skin infection at site of lumbar puncture, CT or MRI evidence of obstructive hydrocephalus, cerebral edema, herniation

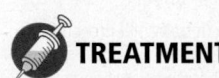

TREATMENT

GENERAL MEASURES
- Initiate empiric antibiotic therapy immediately after lumbar puncture (LP > Abx), or if head CT scan is needed, then immediately after blood cultures (Abx > CT > LP).
- Vigorous supportive care to ensure prompt recognition of seizures and prevention of aspiration

MEDICATION
Empiric IV therapy (with dexamethasone when indicated) until culture results are available
- Consider local patterns of bacterial sensitivity.

First Line
- Neonates
- Ampicillin: 150 mg/kg/day divided q8h *AND*
- Cefotaxime 150 mg/kg/day divided q8h
- Infants >4 weeks of age (3,4)[A]
  - Ceftriaxone: 100 mg/kg/day divided q12–24h or cefotaxime 225 to 300 mg/kg/day divided q6–8h *AND*
  - Vancomycin: 60 mg/kg/day divided q6h
- Adults (3,4)[A]
  - Vancomycin: loading dose 25 to 30 mg/kg IV then 15 to 20 mg/kg q8–12h with goal trough of 15 to 20 *AND*
  - Ceftriaxone: 2 g IV q12h *OR*
  - Cefotaxime: 2 g IV q4–6h
  - >50 years, add ampicillin: 2 g IV q4h for *Listeria*
  - Immunocompromised use vancomycin, ampicillin, ceftazidime, and acyclovir.
- Precaution: aminoglycoside ototoxicity
- Penicillin-allergic patients (3,4)[A]
  - Chloramphenicol: 1 g IV q6h *AND*
  - Vancomycin: loading dose 25 to 30 mg/kg IV then 15 to 20 mg/kg q8–12h (goal trough of 15 to 20)
- Treatment duration
  - *S. pneumoniae*: 10 to 14 days
  - *N. meningitidis*, *H. influenzae*: 7 to 10 days
  - Group B *Streptococcus* organisms, *E. coli*, *L. monocytogenes*: 14 to 21 days
  - Neonates: 12 to 21 days or at least 14 days after a repeated culture is sterile
- Corticosteroids (5)[A]
  - Pediatrics
    - Early treatment with dexamethasone (0.15 mg/kg IV q6h for 2 to 4 days) decreases mortality and morbidity for patients >1 month of age with acute bacterial meningitis with no increased risk of GI bleeding.
    - Corticosteroids are associated with lower rates of severe hearing loss, any hearing loss, and neurologic sequelae.
  - Adults
    - Initiate in adults, then only continue if CSF Gram stain is gram-positive diplococcus or if blood or CSF positive for *S. pneumoniae*.
    - Dexamethasone: 10 mg IV q6h started 15 to 20 minutes before or with antibiotic for 4 days

Second Line
Antipseudomonal penicillins
- Aztreonam
- Quinolones (e.g., ciprofloxacin)
- Meropenem

ISSUES FOR REFERRAL
Consultation from infectious disease and/or critical care specialist

INPATIENT CONSIDERATIONS
Admission Criteria/Initial Stabilization
Bacterial meningitis requires hospitalization.
- Nursing
- ICU monitoring may be needed.
- Patients with suspected meningococcal infection require respiratory isolation for 24 hours.

Discharge Criteria
Consider home therapy to complete IV antibiotics once clinically stable and culture/sensitivity results are known.

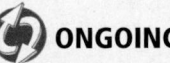 ONGOING CARE

FOLLOW-UP RECOMMENDATIONS
Patient Monitoring
- Brainstem auditory—evoked response hearing test for infants before hospital discharge
- Vaccinations
  - *Hib* conjugate vaccine is recommended during infancy for 4 doses.
  - Meningococcal conjugate vaccine quadrivalent (MCV4) is given to children aged 11 to 12 years with a booster at 16 years.
  - Immunizing infants <3 months old with MCV4 does not reduce morbidity or mortality, and vaccinating pregnant women does not reduce infant infections.
  - Administer 2 doses MCV4 at least 2 months apart to adults with the following:
    - HIV, functional asplenia
    - Persistent complement deficiencies
  - Administer 1 dose of meningococcal vaccine to:
    - Military recruits
    - Microbiologists routinely exposed to isolates of *N. meningitidis*
    - Those who travel to or live in countries where meningitis is hyperendemic or epidemic.
    - 1st year college students up through age 21 years who live in residence halls if they have not received a dose on or after their 16th birthday
  - MCV4 is preferred for adults with any of the preceding indications who are ≤55 years of age; meningococcal polysaccharide vaccine (MPSV4) is preferred for adults aged ≥56 years.
  - Revaccination with MCV4 every 5 years is recommended for adults previously vaccinated with MCV4 or MPSV4 who are at increased risk.
- Prophylaxis (2)[A]
  - Only for close contacts of patients
  - Rifampin is effective in eradicating *N. meningitidis* up to 4 weeks after treatment but may lead to resistance.
  - Rifampin: 600 mg PO BID for 2 days
    - Ciprofloxacin and ceftriaxone are effective up to 2 weeks after treatment without leading to resistance.
    - Ciprofloxacin: 500 mg PO for 1 dose
    - Ceftriaxone: 250 mg IM for 1 dose

DIET
Regular, as tolerated, except with syndrome of inappropriate secretion of antidiuretic hormone.

PROGNOSIS
Overall case fatality: 21%
- Fatality rate increases linearly with age.

COMPLICATIONS
- Seizures: 20–30%; focal neurologic deficit
- Cranial nerve palsies (III, VI, VII, VIII)
  - Comprises 10–20% of the cases
  - Usually disappear within a few weeks
- Sensorineural hearing loss: 10% in children
- Neurodevelopmental sequelae: 30% subtle learning deficits

- Obstructive hydrocephalus, subdural effusion
- Syndrome of inappropriate secretion of antidiuretic hormone
- Elevated intracranial pressure: herniation, brain swelling

REFERENCES
1. Centers for Disease Control and Prevention. Meningitis. www.cdc.gov/meningitis/bacterial.html. Accessed September 9 2015.
2. Zalmanovici Trestioreanu A, Fraser A, Gafter-Gvili A, et al. Antibiotics for preventing meningococcal infections. *Cochrane Database Syst Rev*. 2013;(10): CD004785.
3. Smith L. Management of bacterial meningitis: new guidelines from the IDSA. *Am Fam Physician*. 2005;71(10):2003–2008.
4. Liu C, Bayer A, Cosgrove SE, et al. Clinical practice guidelines by the Infectious Diseases Society of America for the treatment of methicillin-resistant *Staphylococcus aureus* infections in adults and children. *Clin Infect Dis*. 2011;53(3):319.
5. Brouwer MC, McIntyre P, Prasad K, et al. Corticosteroids for acute bacterial meningitis. *Cochrane Database Syst Rev*. 2013;(6):CD004405.

ADDITIONAL READING
- Kulik DM, Uleryk EM, Maguire JL. Does this child have bacterial meningitis? A systematic review of clinical prediction rules for children with suspected bacterial meningitis. *J Emerg Med*. 2013;45(4):508–519.
- van de Beek D, Brouwer MC, Thwaites GE, et al. Advances in treatment of bacterial meningitis. *Lancet*. 2012;380(9854):1693–1702.
- Wall EC, Ajdukiewicz KM, Heyderman RS, et al. Osmotic therapies added to antibiotics for acute bacterial meningitis. *Cochrane Database Syst Rev*. 2013;(3):CD008806.

CODES

ICD10
- G00.9 Bacterial meningitis, unspecified
- G00.2 Streptococcal meningitis
- G00.8 Other bacterial meningitis

CLINICAL PEARLS
- Initiate antibiotic therapy immediately (following diagnostic lumbar puncture) if meningitis is suspected.
- Corticosteroids reduce hearing loss and neurologic sequelae but not overall mortality.
- Repeat lumbar puncture if patients don't respond to antimicrobial therapy after 48 hours.
- Classic triad of fever, neck stiffness, and altered mental status has low sensitivity for bacterial meningitis. Meningeal signs are unreliable for diagnosis or ruling out meningitis.
- Rapidly evolving petechial rash (purpura fulminans) is more common in meningococcal meningitis.
- 50–90% of patients with bacterial meningitis have positive blood cultures. Mixed bacterial infections are rare.

M

MENINGITIS, VIRAL
Christine M. Broszko, MD • James E. Hougas, III, MD, Maj, USAF, MC

 BASICS

DESCRIPTION
- A clinical syndrome characterized by signs/symptoms of acute meningeal inflammation
- Viral meningitis (VM) is the most common cause of aseptic meningitis.
- Aseptic meningitis has no identifiable bacterial pathogen in CSF.
- System(s) affected: nervous

EPIDEMIOLOGY
Incidence
- Estimated 30,000 to 75,000 VM cases annually in United States
- Estimated 26,000 to 42,000 VM hospitalizations annually in United States
- Most common form of infectious meningitis
  - Annual incidence of VM is higher than all other causes of meningitis combined.
- Peaks June 1 to October 31
  - Non-polio enteroviruses and arthropod-borne viruses predominate in warm months (70% of cases July to October).
  - Mumps usually occurs in the winter and spring, often in epidemics.
- Occurs in both outbreak and sporadic forms

ETIOLOGY AND PATHOPHYSIOLOGY
- First described by Wallgren in 1925
- In immunocompetent hosts, VM is generally caused by a systemic viral infection with neurotropic predilection.
- Less commonly, direct neural transmission occurs from an acute flare of a chronic viral illness (such as HSV) already present in an immunocompetent host.
- 85–95% of cases are caused by enterovirus family; (often transmitted by the fecal–oral route) including coxsackievirus A and B, echovirus, and non-polio E variants: E9 and E30. Most recently, outbreak of E68 in 2014
- Less common: HSV-1, HSV-2, varicella-zoster virus (VZV), adenovirus, lymphocytic choriomeningitis virus (LCMV), cytomegalovirus (CMV), Epstein-Barr virus (EBV), HIV, parvovirus B19, and mumps virus
- Parechovirus 3 is the most common cause of viral meningitis in infants <90 days old.
- Arthropod-borne viruses: West Nile virus, St. Louis encephalitis virus, California encephalitis virus
- Recurrent benign lymphocytic (Mollaret) meningitis-80% associated with HSV-2.

Genetics
None identified

RISK FACTORS
- Close contact with known cases of VM
- Age (common in children <5 years)
- Immunocompromised hosts may be more susceptible to CMV, HSV, and adenovirus in particular.
- LCMV is transmitted via exposure to rodent feces, bite, bodily fluids, or nesting materials.

Geriatric Considerations
Cases of VM in the elderly are rare; consider alternative diagnoses (e.g., carcinomatous meningitis, NSAID- or medication-induced meningitis).

GENERAL PREVENTION
Limit exposure to known hosts. Observe hand washing and general hygiene procedures.

COMMONLY ASSOCIATED CONDITIONS
Encephalitis; neurologic deficits; myopericarditis; neonatal enteroviral sepsis

---

DIAGNOSIS

HISTORY
Predominant symptoms include acute onset (hours to days) of:
- Fever (in 76–100% of patients)
- Headache (prominent early symptom)
- Photophobia
- Myalgias
- Nausea, vomiting
- Malaise
- Nuchal rigidity (>50%)
- Mental status changes
  - Encephalitis is associated with other neurologic dysfunction, such as behavioral change, focal neurologic deficits, seizure. There is a continuum between meningitis and encephalitis that can be labeled as one or the other according to predominant symptom type, or jointly labeled "meningoencephalitis."

Also document the following:
- Travel and exposure history
- Sexual activity (e.g., HSV, HIV)
- Outdoor activities (Lyme disease)
- Exposure to rodent feces and/or urine (LCMV)
- Solid-organ transplant (LCMV, CMV)
- Immunocompromised host (CMV, HSV, adenovirus)
- History of varicella-zoster infection (VZV)
- Immunization status (mumps virus)

PHYSICAL EXAM
- Altered mental status (AMS)
  - AMS is more common in encephalitis than meningitis.
- Fever (>100.4°F/38°C)
- Meningeal signs (should not be used exclusively to diagnose or rule out meningitis):
  - Nuchal rigidity
  - Brudzinski sign: Neck flexion elicits involuntary hip and knee flexion in supine patient.
  - Kernig sign: resistance to knee extension following flexion of hips to 90 degrees by physician
  - Jolt accentuation test: Rapid horizontal rotation of the head accentuates the headache.
- Genital lesions (HSV2: can precede meningeal symptoms by up to a week)
- Parotitis (mumps)
- Asymmetric flaccid paralysis (West Nile virus)
- Mucocutaneous findings
  - Vesicular rash in hand, foot, and mouth disease (coxsackie)
  - Herpangina (coxsackie A)
  - Herpes zoster rash (VZV)
  - Erythema chronicum migrans or cranial neuropathy (Lyme disease [*Borrelia burgdorferi*])
  - Generalized maculopapular rash (Echovirus 9)
  - Oropharyngeal thrush (HIV)
  - Petechial rash (*Neisseria meningitidis*)

DIFFERENTIAL DIAGNOSIS
- Bacterial meningitis (BM)
- Encephalitis
- Other infectious agents:
  - Tuberculosis; syphilis; leptospirosis; Lyme disease; Rocky Mountain spotted fever; ehrlichiosis; *Coccidioides*; *Cryptococcus neoformans*; amebiasis; Rickettsial infection
- Parameningeal infections (e.g., subdural empyema)
- Postinfectious encephalomyelitis
- Viral syndrome (e.g., influenza)
- Leukemia or carcinomatous meningitis

- Migraine/tension headache
- Acute metabolic encephalopathy
- Chemical meningitis
- Drug-induced meningitis (NSAIDs, IVIG, Bactrim)
- Brain/epidural abscess

DIAGNOSTIC TESTS & INTERPRETATION
Initial Tests (lab, imaging)
- Rule out BM:
  - There is debate over whether patients with low suspicion of BM need a lumbar puncture (LP). Some authors contend that if meningeal symptoms have been present >48 hours with a normal neurologic exam in an immunocompetent patient with confirmed normal level of alertness, BM is extremely unlikely and LP is not warranted. Others contend that BM cannot be excluded clinically and to exercise caution discharging meningitic patients without LP.
  - Bacterial Meningitis Score (BMS): The BMS is a validated clinical decision rule to identify at very low risk of BM. Low-risk features include negative CSF Gram stain, CSF absolute neutrophil count (ANC) <1,000 cells/μL, CSF protein <80 mg/dL, peripheral blood ANC <10,000 cells/μL, and no seizure around the time of initial presentation.
  - CSF bacterial culture is positive in 80–90% of BM patients who haven't received antibiotics for 2 to 4 hours prior to LP.
- LP is the standard of care for suspected BM:
  - If BM is suspected, start antibiotics immediately.
  - Contraindications for LP: signs of increased intracranial pressure (e.g., focal neurologic findings, papilledema, altered mental status, vomiting), known ventricular obstruction, new onset seizure, immunocompromised state, local infection over potential LP site or suspected epidural abscess, use of anticoagulation or coagulopathy, and possibility of cardiorespiratory compromise due to patient positioning during procedure
  - Post-LP headache: occurs in 37% of patients within 48 hours
  - CSF analysis: glucose, protein, WBC count with differential, RBC count, Gram stain, culture; consider CSF lactate:
    - ○ CSF lactate elevation can differentiate BM from VM (decreased sensitivity if pretreated with antibiotics) (1,2)[A].
- Typical CSF findings in VM
  - Elevated WBC count: 10 to 1,000/mm³, classically lymphocyte predominance (less consistent in younger patients); may show neutrophil predominance in first 48 hours
  - Decreased or normal glucose (relative to concurrent serum glucose)
  - Protein normal to slightly elevated (<150 mg/dL)
  - Negative Gram stain and bacterial culture
  - Elevated opening pressure
  - RBCs in CSF (Consider HSV meningitis/encephalitis.)
  - Pathogen identification
    - ○ Gold standard: CSF viral culture for enteroviruses, HSV, and mumps has low sensitivity (<6%); viral culture may yield no additional information over nucleic acid amplification alone.
    - ○ Polymerase chain reaction (PCR): has a sensitivity of 95–100% for HSV-1 and -2, EBV, and enterovirus
    - ○ RT PCR test is approved by the FDA for enteroviral meningitis. Results in 2 to 3 hours
    - ○ Serology can be performed for many arthropod-borne viruses.

- Other labs: CBC, blood culture, blood glucose; consider serum CRP and procalcitonin (PCT).
  – CBC: normal or mildly elevated WBCs
  – Multiple studies show PCT correlation with BM. PCT levels of >0.25 to 2.13 are 90% sensitive and 98% specific for BM. Elevated serum CRP was 82% sensitive and 81% specific (1,3)[B].
- Consider EEG if concern for encephalitis.
- Indication for imaging depends on clinical scenario. Perform CT prior to LP if papilledema, spinal cord trauma, altered mental status, or focal neurologic findings. CT scan not typically clinically necessary in the absence of risk factors.

Follow-Up Tests & Special Considerations
Disorders that may alter lab results:

- Diabetes: Consider current blood sugar level to correlate with CSF glucose level.
- Preexisting neurologic diseases (e.g., intracranial neoplasm, demyelinating disease)

 TREATMENT

GENERAL MEASURES
Management is largely supportive care (e.g., pain control, IV fluids).

MEDICATION

First Line

- Analgesics (adult doses; titrate doses to pain relief)
  – Morphine 2.5 to 5 mg IV
  – Hydromorphone (Dilaudid) 1 to 2 mg IV
  – Hydrocodone (Norco) 5/325 mg 1 to 2 tablets PO q6h OR oxycodone (Percocet) 5/325 mg 1 to 2 tablets PO q4–6h
- Antiemetics
  – Ondansetron (Zofran) 4 to 8 mg IV q8h
  – Metoclopramide (Reglan) 10 to 20 mg IV/IM q4–6h
- Antipyretics: acetaminophen (Tylenol) 650 mg PO or rectal suppository q4h
- Antiviral agents: Initiate empiric acyclovir at 10 mg/kg IV q8h for patients with CSF pleocytosis, negative Gram stain, and suspicion for HSV while awaiting results of definitive (e.g., HSV PCR) testing.
- Antibiotics
  – Not indicated for treatment of VM
  – If unclear etiology, treat symptomatically and follow the patient closely in the hospital setting while awaiting laboratory results.
  – If in doubt, initiate an IV broad-spectrum antibiotic with good CSF penetration. Consider especially in elderly, <3 month old, or immunocompromised patient. Empiric treatment for BM in otherwise healthy patient
    ○ If <1 month, consider ampicillin PLUS gentamicin OR cefotaxime. All dosing dependent on age and size.
    ○ If 1 month to 17 years old, consider vancomycin PLUS ceftriaxone OR cefotaxime. Dosing dependent on age and size.
    ○ If 18 years to 49 years old, consider vancomycin (15 to 20 mg/kg/dose q8–12h; also consider loading dose of 25 to 30 mg/kg) PLUS ceftriaxone (2g q12h) OR cefotaxime (2g q4–6h).
    ○ In >50 years old, consider vancomycin (15 to 20 mg/kg/dose q8–12h; also consider loading dose of 25 to 30 mg/kg) PLUS ampicillin (150 to 250 mg/kg/day divided q3–4h) PLUS ceftriaxone (2g q12h) OR cefotaxime (2g q4–6h).
- If concern for BM, consider corticosteroids along with antibiotic therapy.

INPATIENT CONSIDERATIONS

Admission Criteria/Initial Stabilization
Generally, VM is treated as outpatient. Patients with VM and complications (encephalitis) may be hospitalized. Hospitalize for empiric antibiotic therapy, pain/fluid control, immunocompromised patient, or <1 year old.

- Study of ED visits found that most children diagnosed with VM were hospitalized (91%).

IV Fluids
Crystalloid bolus or continuous infusion, based on hydration status and clinical presentation

Nursing

- Neurologic monitoring for changes in mental status, fever, and other clinical indicators to assess disease progression
- Contact precautions until BM is ruled out
- Private room indicated with sterile precautions
- Encourage hand washing.

Discharge Criteria
Discharge depends on likelihood of BM, CSF, WBC count, and clinical parameters such as dehydration, functional level, social circumstances, and ability to follow up.

 ONGOING CARE

FOLLOW-UP RECOMMENDATIONS
Primary care follow up to ensure resolution.

Patient Monitoring

- Monitor for relapse or exacerbation of symptoms.
- Monitor for neurologic/neuroendocrine complications:
  – Seizures, cerebral edema, syndrome of inappropriate antidiuretic hormone (SIADH)
  – Assess ability to have companion monitor change in mental/neurologic status if patient discharged.

DIET
Consider NPO if nausea or vomiting. Advance to clear fluids/regular diet as tolerated.

PATIENT EDUCATION

- Discuss low probability of transmission to contacts.
- Expected duration of illness is 5 to 10 days.
- Recurrence of headache, myalgia, weakness is possible over 2 to 3 weeks

PROGNOSIS

- Complete recovery generally within 7 to 10 days
- Headaches and other neurologic symptoms may persist intermittently for weeks to months.
- Only 0.6% of hospitalizations for VM result in death.
- European studies suggest potential residual post-meningeal cognitive impairment.

COMPLICATIONS
Fatigue, irritability, muscle weakness, seizures/abscess/mastoiditis (rare)

REFERENCES

1. Viallon A, Desseigne N, Marjollet O, et al. Meningitis in adult patients with a negative direct cerebrospinal fluid examination: value of cytochemical markers for differential diagnosis. *Crit Care.* 2011;15(3):R136.
2. Sakushima K, Hayashino Y, Kawaguchi T, et al. Diagnostic accuracy of cerebrospinal fluid lactate for differentiating bacterial meningitis from aseptic meningitis: a meta-analysis. *J Infect.* 2011;62(4):255–262.
3. Vikse J, Henry BM, Roy J, et al. The role of serum procalcitonin in the diagnosis of bacterial meningitis in adults: a systematic review and meta-analysis. *Int J Infect Dis.* 2015;38:68–76.

ADDITIONAL READING

- Ciovacco WA, Baraff LJ. Lumbar puncture is not needed for all patients suspected to have viral meningitis. *Ann Emerg Med.* 2012;59(3):228–229.
- Mohseni MM, Wilde JA. Viral meningitis: which patients can be discharged from the emergency department? *J Emerg Med.* 2012;43(6):1181–1187.
- Nigrovic LE, Fine AM, Monuteaux MC, et al. Trends in the viral management of viral meningitis at United States children's hospitals. *Pediatrics.* 2013;131(4):670–676.
- Polage CR, Petti CA. Assessment of the utility of viral culture of cerebrospinal fluid. *Clin Infect Dis.* 2006;43(12):1578–1579.
- Studahl M, Lindquist L, Eriksson BM, et al. Acute viral infections of the central nervous system in immunocompetent adults: diagnosis and management. *Drugs.* 2013;73(2):131–158.
- Swadron SP. Pitfalls in the management of headache in the emergency department. *Emerg Med Clin North Am.* 2010;28(1):127–147.
- Talan DA. Bacterial cause of suspected meningitis cannot be safely excluded without cerebrospinal fluid analysis. *Ann Emerg Med.* 2012;59(3):227–228.
- Thomas KE, Hasbun R, Jekel J, et al. The diagnostic accuracy of Kernig's sign, Brudzinski's sign, and nuchal rigidity in adults with suspected meningitis. *Clin Infect Dis.* 2002;35(1):46–52.

 SEE ALSO

Algorithm: Delirium

 CODES

ICD10

- A87.9 Viral meningitis, unspecified
- A87.1 Adenoviral meningitis
- A87.0 Enteroviral meningitis

CLINICAL PEARLS

- Viral meningitis cannot always be reliably distinguished from BM based on clinical findings. Potential cases of BM should be hospitalized for evaluation and treatment pending laboratory results.
- VM is more common than BM in children.
- Antibiotic administration >2 to 4 hours prior to CSF analysis may result in "partially treated" BM that mimics VM.
- IV acyclovir should be administered if there is high clinical suspicion for HSV.
- If BM is suspected, broad-spectrum antibiotics should be administered until BM has been ruled out.
- Morbidity with VM is low but increases if there is associated encephalitis.

M

MENINGOCOCCAL DISEASE

Han Q. Bui, MD, MPH

 BASICS

DESCRIPTION
- Meningococcemia is a blood-borne infection caused by *Neisseria meningitidis*.
- Bacteremia without meningitis: Patient is acutely ill and may have skin manifestations (rashes, petechiae, and ecchymosis) and hypotension.
- Bacteremia with meningitis: sudden onset of fever, nausea, vomiting, headache, decreased ability to concentrate, and myalgias
- Disease progresses rapidly within a matter of hours.
- Meningococcal bacteremia rarely occurs without frank sepsis.
- Skin findings and hypotension may be present.
  - A petechial rash appears as discrete lesions 1 to 2 mm in diameter; most frequently on the trunk and lower portions of the body and will be seen in >50% of patients on presentation.
  - Purpura fulminans is a severe complication of meningococcal disease and occurs in up to 25% of cases. It is characterized by acute onset of cutaneous hemorrhage and necrosis due to vascular thrombosis and disseminated intravascular coagulopathy.

EPIDEMIOLOGY
Incidence
- The mortality rate is ~13%.
  - 11–19% of survivors suffer serious sequelae, including deafness, neurologic deficit, or limb loss due to peripheral ischemia.
- Disease is seasonal, peaking in December/January.
- Annually, ~1,000 cases of invasive meningococcal disease occur in the United States (1).
  - Most common in adolescents and young adults, followed by infants <1 year

ETIOLOGY AND PATHOPHYSIOLOGY
- *N. meningitidis* is a gram-negative diplococcus with at least 13 serotypes.
- *N. meningitidis* has an outer coat that produces disease—causing endotoxin.
- Major serogroups in the United States are B, C, Y, and W-135
  - Serogroup B is the predominant cause of meningococcemia in children <1 year.
  - Serogroup C is the most common cause of meningococcal disease in the United States.
  - Serogroup Y is the predominant cause of meningococcemia in the elderly (2).
- Major serogroups worldwide are A, B, C, Y, and W-135
  - W-135 is the major cause of disease in the "meningitis belt" of sub-Saharan Africa.

Genetics
Late complement component deficiency has an autosomal recessive inheritance.

RISK FACTORS
- Age: 3 months to 1 year
- Late complement component deficiency (C5, C6, C7, C8, or C9)
- Asplenia (1)
- Living in close quarters (e.g., household contacts, nursery/daycare centers, dormitories, military barracks)
- Exposure to active and passive tobacco smoke (1)

GENERAL PREVENTION
- Two vaccines are currently licensed for use in the United States. Each contains antigens to serogroups A, C, Y, and W-135. Neither provides immunity against serotype B, which is responsible for 1/3 of U.S. cases (3)
  - Meningococcal polysaccharide vaccine (MPSV4): recommended for patients ≥55 years who are at elevated risk (1)
    ○ Duration of protection is short: 1 to 3 years for patients <5 years; 3 to 5 years for adolescents and adults (3)
    ○ Often used for patients requiring short duration of protection—traveling to endemic areas, college freshmen, community outbreaks (3)
  - Meningococcal conjugate vaccine (MCV4): recommended for patients 2 to 55 years (1)
- In October 2014, the Food and Drug Administration (FDA) licensed the first serogroup B meningococcal (MenB) vaccine (MenB-FHbp) as a 3-dose series. In January 2015, FDA licensed a second MenB vaccine (MenB-4C) as a 2-dose series. Both vaccines were approved for use in persons aged 10 to 25 years. Individuals aged ≥10 years who are at increased risk for meningococcal disease due to persistent complement component deficiencies, anatomic or functional asplenia should receive MenB vaccine (3).
- Protective levels of antibody are achieved ~7 to 10 days after primary immunization (2).
- Vaccine is recommended for all persons 11 to 18 years and persons 19 to 55 years at increased risk for the disease.
  - Guillain-Barré syndrome has been associated with the MCV4 vaccine, so a personal history of Guillain-Barré is a relative contraindication for receiving this vaccine.
- CDC International Travel Advisory
  - Vaccine is required by the government of Saudi Arabia for Hajj pilgrims >2 years of age.
  - The vaccine should be given to travelers to sub-Saharan Africa ("meningitis belt").

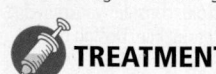 **DIAGNOSIS**

HISTORY
- Symptoms
  - Sudden onset of fever, nausea, vomiting, headache, myalgias, chills, rigor, and/or sore throat (nonsuppurative)
    ○ Pharyngitis may be mistaken for streptococcal pharyngitis.
    ○ Myalgia may be mistaken for severe "flu," with a peak incidence coinciding in winter months.
  - Changes in mental status, decreased ability to concentrate, stiff neck, convulsions
  - Atypical presentations include acute arthritis or neuritis (4).
- Assess possible exposures.

PHYSICAL EXAM
- Fever, hypotension, tachycardia
- Neurologic: nuchal rigidity, focal neurologic findings, coma, seizure
  - Focal neurologic findings and seizures are more commonly seen with *Haemophilus influenzae* or *Streptococcus pneumoniae*.
- Cardiopulmonary: signs of heart failure with pulmonary edema—gallop, rales
- Dermatologic: maculopapular rash, petechiae, ecchymosis, purpura

- Median time of onset of specific meningitis symptoms (e.g., neck stiffness, photophobia, bulging fontanelle) is as fast as 12 to 15 hours after onset of illness (4).
- Late signs of meningitis (e.g., unconsciousness, delirium, or seizures) occur ~15 hours in infants <1 year and ~24 hours in older children (5).

DIFFERENTIAL DIAGNOSIS
- Sepsis; bacterial meningitis (other organisms)
- Gonococcemia
- Acute bacterial endocarditis
- Rocky mountain spotted fever
- Hemolytic uremic syndrome
- Gonococcal arthritis dermatitis syndrome
- Influenza

DIAGNOSTIC TESTS & INTERPRETATION
ALERT
- Isolation of *N. meningitidis* from a sterile site (blood or CSF) is the gold standard for diagnosing systemic meningococcal infection.
- Antibiotic administration may render blood and/or CSF culture negative within 2 hours. Treat, then test.

Initial Tests (lab, imaging)
- CBC with differential
  - Leukocytosis (left shift; toxic granulation) or leukopenia, thrombocytopenia
- Lactic acidosis
- Coagulation studies
  - Prolonged prothrombin time/partial thromboplastin time
  - Low fibrinogen
  - Elevated fibrin degradation products
- Blood culture
  - Blood culture positive for *N. meningitidis*
  - Cultures positive in 50–60% of cases
- CSF
  - Grossly cloudy
  - Increased WBCs with polymorphonuclear predominance
  - Gram stain showing gram-negative diplococci
  - Glucose-to-blood glucose ratio <0.4
  - Protein >45 mg/dL
  - Positive for *N. meningitidis* antigen (MAT or PCR)
  - CSF culture for *N. meningitidis*: positive in 80–90% of cases
- CT scan of head if concern for space-occupying lesions

Test Interpretation
- Disseminated intravascular coagulation (DIC)
- Exudates on meninges
- Polymorphonuclear infiltration of meninges
- Hemorrhage of adrenal glands

TREATMENT

MEDICATION
First Line
- Antibiotics
  - Begin treatment as soon as meningococcal meningitis is suspected.

- Age influences empiric treatment based on common etiologic organisms.
  - Preterm to <1 month: ampicillin plus cefotaxime or ampicillin plus gentamicin
    - Cefotaxime
      - 0 to7 days: 50 mg/kg q12h
      - 8 to 28 days: 50 mg/kg q8h
    - Ampicillin
      - >2,000 g
        - 0 to 7 days: 50 mg/kg q8h
        - 8 to 28 days: 50 mg/kg q6h
      - <2,000 g
        - 0 to 7 days: 50 mg/kg q12h
        - 8 to 28 days: 50 mg/kg q8h
  - 1 month to 50 years: cefotaxime or ceftriaxone plus vancomycin
    - If severe penicillin allergy: chloramphenicol plus trimethoprim-sulfamethoxazole (TMP-SMX) plus vancomycin
  - >50 years of age or patients with alcoholism, debilitating disease, or impaired immunity: ampicillin plus ceftriaxone plus vancomycin
    - Ampicillin: 2 g IV q4h
    - Ceftriaxone: 2 g IV q12h
    - Vancomycin: 30 to 45 mg/kg/day IV divided q6h
    - If severe penicillin allergy: TMP-SMX plus vancomycin
- Penicillin G
  - Effective if the isolate is penicillin sensitive
  - Penicillin can be used if the isolate has a penicillin minimum inhibitory concentration (MIC) of <0.1 μg/mL.
  - For isolates with a penicillin MIC of 0.1 to 1 μg/mL, treatment with high-dose penicillin is effective, but a 3rd-generation cephalosporin is preferred (5).
  - Penicillin G: 4 million units IV q4h (pediatric dose: 0.25 mU/kg/day IV divided q4–6h) OR ampicillin: 2 g IV q4h (pediatric dose: 200 to 300 mg/kg/day IV divided q6h)
- Duration of treatment: 7 days (6)
- Dexamethasone
  - Indications
    - Known or suspected pneumococcal meningitis in selected adults
    - Children with H. influenzae type B meningitis
- Dexamethasone is often given initially in adults and children with suspected bacterial meningitis while awaiting microbiologic data.
- Dexamethasone has not been shown to be of benefit in meningococcal meningitis and should be discontinued once this diagnosis is established.
- Dosage
  - Infants and children >6 weeks: IV 0.15 mg/kg/dose q6h for the first 2 to 4 days of antibiotic treatment
  - Start 10 to 20 minutes before or with the first dose of antibiotic.
- Chemoprophylaxis
  - Indications
    - Close contacts: Those who have had prolonged (>8 hours) contact while in close proximity (<3 feet) to the patient or who have been directly exposed to the patient's oral secretions between 1 week before the onset of the patient's symptoms and until 24 hours after initiation of appropriate antibiotic therapy (2).
      - Examples: household members and personnel in nurseries, daycare centers, nursing homes, dormitories, military barracks, correctional facilities, and other closed institutional settings

- No chemoprophylaxis is indicated for casual contacts, including most health care workers, unless there is exposure to respiratory secretion.
  - Timing
    - Ideally <24 hours after case identification
    - Chemoprophylaxis should not be administered if identified >14 days after exposure.
  - Prophylactic regimens
    - Rifampin, ciprofloxacin, and ceftriaxone
      - Ceftriaxone
        - Recommended for pregnant women
        - Adults: 250 mg IM as a single dose
      - Rifampin (meningococcal meningitis prophylaxis)
        - Adult: 600 mg IV or PO q12h for 2 days
        - Pediatric
          - <1 month: 10 mg/kg/day in divided doses q12h for 2 days
          - Infants and children: 20 mg/kg/day in divided doses q12h for 2 days (max 600 mg/dose)
      - Ciprofloxacin
        - Adults: 500 mg PO as a single dose (7)[B]
- Vaccination
  - For household contacts (if the case is from a vaccine-preventable serogroup)
- Precautions
  - Adjust the dosage of medications in patients with severe renal dysfunction.

Second Line
- For meningitis
  - Chloramphenicol: 1 g IV q6h (pediatric dose: 75 to 100 mg/kg/day divided q6h) or ceftriaxone 2 g IV q12h (pediatric dose: 80 to 100 mg/kg/day divided q12–24h)
  - In large outbreaks, a single dose of long-acting chloramphenicol has been used. Single-dose ceftriaxone shows equal efficacy in one randomized controlled trial.
- Precautions
  - Ceftriaxone should not be used in patients with a history of anaphylactic reactions to penicillin (e.g., hypotension, laryngeal edema, wheezing, hives).
  - Chloramphenicol may cause aplastic anemia.

ISSUES FOR REFERRAL
Potential complications
- Seizure activity
- DIC
- Acute respiratory distress syndrome
- Renal failure
- Adrenal failure
- Multisystem organ failure

INPATIENT CONSIDERATIONS
Admission Criteria/Initial Stabilization
- If meningitis is suspected, initiate antibiotics (± corticosteroids), and proceed immediately to lumbar puncture.
- Droplet isolation for 24 hours from the beginning of antibiotic therapy

IV Fluids
Replace volume as needed; with septic shock, large volumes of crystalloid may be required.

 ONGOING CARE

PATIENT EDUCATION
Educate family and close contacts regarding the risk of contracting meningococcal infections.

PROGNOSIS
Overall mortality is 13%.

COMPLICATIONS
- DIC
- Acute tubular necrosis
- Neurologic: sensorineural hearing loss, cranial nerve palsy, seizures
- Obstructive hydrocephalus
- Subdural effusions
- Acute adrenal hemorrhage
- Waterhouse-Friderichsen syndrome

REFERENCES
1. Centers for Disease Control and Prevention. Factsheet: meningococcal disease and meningococcal vaccine. http://www.cdc.gov/meningococcal/clinical-info.html. Accessed 2014.
2. Gardner P. Clinical practice. Prevention of meningococcal disease. N Engl J Med. 2006;355(14):1466–1473.
3. Folaranmi T, Rubin L, Martin SW, et al. Use of serogroup B meningococcal vaccines in persons aged ≥10 years at increased risk for serogroup B meningococcal disease: recommendations of the Advisory Committee on Immunization Practices, 2015. MMWR Morb Mortal Wkly Rep. 2015;64(22):608–612.
4. Rodríguez CL, Octavio JG, Isea C, et al. Acute polyarthritis as sole manifestation of meningococcal disease. J Clin Rheumatol. 2012;18(1):42–43.
5. Thompson MJ, Ninis N, Perera R, et al. Clinical recognition of meningococcal disease in children and adolescents. Lancet. 2006;367(9508):397–403.
6. Tunkel AR, Hartman BJ, Kaplan SL, et al. Practice guidelines for the management of bacterial meningitis. Clin Infect Dis. 2004;39(9):1267–1284.
7. Fraser A, Gafter-Gvili A, Paul M, et al. Antibiotics for preventing meningococcal infections. Cochrane Database Syst Rev. 2005;(1):CD004785.

ADDITIONAL READING
- Visintin C, Mugglestone MA, Fields EJ, et al. Management of bacterial meningitis and meningococcal septicaemia in children and young people: summary of NICE guidance. BMJ. 2010;340:c3209.
- Wright C, Wordsworth R, Glennie L. Counting the cost of meningococcal disease: scenarios of severe meningitis and septicemia. Paediatr Drugs. 2013;15(1):49–58.

 CODES

ICD10
- A39.4 Meningococcemia, unspecified
- A39.0 Meningococcal meningitis
- A39.2 Acute meningococcemia

CLINICAL PEARLS
- Invasive meningococcal disease can be rapidly fatal. Therefore, rapid identification of cases with early treatment is essential for good clinical outcomes. Treat then test in suspected cases
- Provide chemoprophylaxis to close contacts.
- Vaccinate at-risk populations as a preventive measure.

M

MENISCAL INJURY

Jennifer B. Schwartz, MD

BASICS

DESCRIPTION
- The menisci are fibrocartilaginous intra-articular structures located between the medial and lateral femoral condyles and tibial plateau.
- Each meniscus has a body, anterior horn, and posterior horn
- The menisci help stabilize the knee, distribute forces across the joint, and aid joint lubrication.
- After age 10 years, the menisci begin to devascularize
  - In adults, the outer 1/3 remains vascularized.
  - The inner 2/3 is avascular and heals poorly.

Geriatric Considerations
Meniscal tears in older patients are typically due to chronic degeneration.

Pediatric Considerations
- Meniscal injuries are rare in children <10 years old (prior to physial fusion).
- Meniscal tears in young children are often due to a *discoid meniscus* (anatomic variant with thicker and wider meniscus—usually the lateral meniscus).
- MRI is less sensitive and specific for diagnosing meniscal tears in children <12 years of age.

EPIDEMIOLOGY
- More common in the 3rd to 5th decades of life
- More common in males

Incidence
- Medial meniscus more commonly injured
- Injuries can be *acute* or *degenerative*.
  - Acute tears more likely <40 years old and due to trauma
  - Degenerative tears more likely >40 years old

Prevalence
One of the most common musculoskeletal injuries

ETIOLOGY AND PATHOPHYSIOLOGY
- Acute tears typically occur due to a twisting motion of the knee with foot planted.
- Degenerative tears occur with minimal trauma.

Genetics
A congenital abnormality leading to discoid meniscus increases the risk of meniscal tear among children. No specific gene locus has been identified.

RISK FACTORS
- Increased age (>60 years), male
- Obesity
- High degree of physical activity (especially cutting sports like soccer, football, basketball, and rugby)
- Anterior cruciate ligament (ACL), posterior cruciate ligament (PCL) insufficiency:
  - Waiting >12 months between ACL injury and surgery increases risk of medial meniscal tear (1)[C].

GENERAL PREVENTION
- Treatment and rehabilitation of previous knee injuries, particularly ACL injuries
- Strengthening and increased flexibility of quadriceps and hamstring muscles

COMMONLY ASSOCIATED CONDITIONS
- ACL is concomitantly torn in 1/3 of cases.
- Medial and lateral collateral ligament tears
- Tibial plateau or femoral shaft fractures
- Baker cyst—strong association with medial meniscal tears (2)[C]

DIAGNOSIS

HISTORY
- Noncontact twisting or hyperflexion mechanism
- Delayed swelling, typically >24 hours postinjury
- Knee pain (on affected side):
  - Increased with knee flexion (i.e., stairs, squatting)
  - Increased with weight bearing
- Locking, catching, popping
- Sensation of buckling or giving out

PHYSICAL EXAM
- Pertinent findings on physical exam are the following:
  - Effusion (mild–moderate)
  - Joint line tenderness
  - Decreased range of motion, locking
  - Pain with full flexion (posterior horn tear) or extension (anterior horn tear)
- Accuracy of special tests varies (3)[C]
  - Positive McMurray test: pain, clicking of meniscus being stressed
  - Positive Apley grind test is neither sensitive nor specific.
  - Positive Thessaly test: Patient rotates knee and body three times with knee flexed 20 degrees; has pain along joint line.

DIFFERENTIAL DIAGNOSIS
- ACL or collateral ligament tear
- Pathologic plica
- Osteochondritis dissecans
- Loose body or fracture
- Osteoarthritis (OA)—symptoms of OA may be caused by meniscal tears (4)[C]
- Patellofemoral syndrome
- Gout, pseudogout, rheumatoid arthritis

DIAGNOSTIC TESTS & INTERPRETATION
- Laboratory evaluation not indicated unless signs of septic arthritis.
- Plain radiographs can detect fractures, loose bodies, or arthritic changes.
- Ultrasound may help screen for meniscal tears. Less helpful for lateral tears (5)[C]

Follow-Up Tests & Special Considerations
- MRI is the primary study to diagnose meniscal tears.
  - Increased signal within a meniscus corresponds to degenerative changes; signal contacting the articular surface indicates an acute tear.
- Meniscal tears are often found incidentally on MRI and may not be the cause of patient's symptoms.
  - 36–76% of meniscal tears found on MRI were asymptomatic. Asymptomatic tears increase with age and in the setting of OA.
  - Patients with synovitis and displacement of meniscus on MRI may benefit from intervention (6)[C].

Diagnostic Procedures/Other
Arthroscopy may be needed if the MRI is indeterminate.

TREATMENT

GENERAL MEASURES
- Treatment depends on the type/location/extent of the tear, as well as age and activity level of the patient
- Conservative treatment (RICE [rest, ice, compression, elevation], activity modification, physical therapy, intra-articular corticosteroid injections) are effective first-line options for many patients, especially those with degenerative tears.
  - No increased benefit from surgery versus physical therapy for symptomatic meniscal tears in patients with mild to moderate OA (7)[C].
  - Small, partial thickness, or peripheral tears may heal on their own or remain asymptomatic.
- Consider surgical intervention if:
  - Mechanical symptoms, locking
  - Concurrent injuries (i.e., ACL tear)
  - Persistent symptoms following 3 to 6 months of conservative treatment
  - Young patients (<30 years) or very active patients with an acute tear

MEDICATION
First Line
NSAIDs, opioid analgesics if severe pain

ISSUES FOR REFERRAL
Surgical consult for patients meeting operative criteria or wishing surgical repair

ADDITIONAL THERAPIES
- Rehabilitation is required for both surgical and nonsurgical patients.
- Electrical stimulation may help improve recovery when coupled with physical therapy.
- Weight control: Weight gain is associated with increased cartilage loss and pain in adults with medial meniscal tears.
- Platelet-rich plasma (PRP) may or may not improve symptoms of meniscal tears (8)[C].

SURGERY/OTHER PROCEDURES

- Most surgeries can be performed arthroscopically.
- Meniscectomy (partial or total) removes the injured portion of the meniscus.
  - Can lead to articular cartilage degeneration and OA. Higher risk if 40 years of age, high BMI, valgus malalignment (9)[C]
- Meniscal repairs decrease future OA and often have better outcomes than meniscectomy (10)[C].

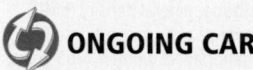 ONGOING CARE

FOLLOW-UP RECOMMENDATIONS

- Return to play requires that the patient be pain-free, have full range of motion, and full strength.
- Following meniscal repair, patients can generally return to all activities in 3 to 6 months.
- Combined ACL and meniscal repair requires 6 months of postoperative rehabilitation before the patient can return to sports.

PATIENT EDUCATION

Patients should be aware of the risks and benefits of surgery compared with conservative treatment.

PROGNOSIS

Prognosis better if surgery is done within 8 weeks, patient is <30 years of age, or tear is peripheral/lateral <2.5 cm.

COMPLICATIONS

- Meniscectomies may eventually lead to OA. Consequently, meniscal repair is preferred to meniscectomy whenever possible.
- Risk of developing OA increases 6-fold 20 years after a meniscectomy.

REFERENCES

1. Snoeker BA, Bakker EW, Kegel CA, et al. Risk factors for meniscal tears: a systematic review including meta-analysis. *J Orthop Sports Phys Ther*. 2013;43(6):352–367.
2. Artul S, Jabaly-Habib A, Artoul F, et al. The association between Baker's cyst and medial meniscal tear in patients with symptomatic knee using ultrasonography. *Clin Imaging*. 2015;39(4):659–661.
3. Smith BE, Thacker D, Crewesmith A, et al. Special tests for assessing meniscal tears within the knee: a systematic review and meta-analysis. *Evid Based Med*. 2015;20(3):88–97.
4. Kamimura M, Umehara J, Takahashi A, et al. Medial meniscus tear morphology and related clinical symptoms in patients with medical knee osteoarthritis. *Knee Surg Sports Traumatol Arthrosc*. 2015;23(1):158–163.
5. Akatsu Y, Yamaguchi S, Mukoyama S, et al. Accuracy of high-resolution ultrasound in the detection of meniscal tears and determination of the visible area of menisci. *J Bone Joint Surg Am*. 2015;97(10):799–806.
6. Troupis JM, Batt MJ, Pasricha SS, et al. Magnetic resonance imaging in knee synovitis: clinical utility in differentiating asymptomatic and symptomatic meniscal tears. *J Med Imaging Radiat Oncol*. 2015;59(1):1–6.
7. Katz JN, Brophy RH, Chaisson CE, et al. Surgery versus physical therapy for a meniscal tear and osteoarthritis. *N Engl J Med*. 2013;368(18):1675–1684.
8. Pujol N, Salle De Chou E, Boisrenoult P, et al. Platelet-rich plasma for open meniscal repair in young patients: any benefit? *Knee Surg Sports Traumatol Arthrosc*. 2015;23(1):51–58.
9. Hulet C, Menetrey J, Beaufils P, et al. Clinical and radiographic results of arthroscopic partial lateral meniscectomies in stable knees with a minimum follow up of 20 years. *Knee Surg Sports Traumatol Arthrosc*. 2015;23(1):225–231.
10. Xu C, Zhao J. A meta-analysis comparing meniscal repair with meniscectomy in the treatment of meniscal tears: the more meniscus, the better outcome? *Knee Surg Sports Traumatol Arthrosc*. 2015;23(1):164–170.

ADDITIONAL READING

- El Ghazaly SA, Rahman AA, Yusry AH, et al. Arthroscopic partial meniscectomy is superior to physical rehabilitation in the management of symptomatic unstable meniscal tears. *Int orthop*. 2015;39(4):769–775.
- Goossens P, Keijsers E, van Geenen RJ, et al. Validity of the Thessaly test in evaluating meniscal tears compared with arthroscopy: a diagnostic accuracy study. *J Orthop Sports Phys Ther*. 2015;45(1):18–24.
- Griffin JW, Hadeed MM, Werner BC, et al. Platelet-rich plasma in meniscal repair: does augmentation improve surgical outcomes? *Clin Orthop Relat Res*. 2015;473(5):1665–1672.
- Guenther ZD, Swami V, Dhillon SS, et al. Meniscal injury after adolescent anterior cruciate ligament injury: how long are patients at risk? *Clin Orthop Relat Res*. 2014;472(3):990–997.
- Hall M, Juhl CB, Lund H, et al. Knee extensor muscle strength in middle-aged and older individuals undergoing arthroscopic partial meniscectomy: a systematic review and meta-analysis [published online ahead of print March 16, 2015]. *Arthritis Care Res (Hoboken)*.
- Katz JN, Brophy RH, Chaisson CE, et al. Surgery versus physical therapy for a meniscal tear and osteoarthritis. *N Engl J Med*. 2013;368(18):1675–1684.
- Vermesan D, Prejbeanu R, Laitin S, et al. Arthroscopic debridement compared to intra-articular steroids in treating degenerative medial meniscal tears. *Eur Rev Med Pharmacol Sci*. 2013;17(23):3192–3196.

 SEE ALSO

Algorithm: Knee Pain

 CODES

ICD10

- S83.209A Unsp tear of unsp meniscus, current injury, unsp knee, init
- S83.249A Oth tear of medial meniscus, current injury, unsp knee, init
- S83.289A Oth tear of lat mensc, current injury, unsp knee, init

CLINICAL PEARLS

- Degenerative meniscal tears are common in patients >40 years of age and generally do not require surgical repair.
- MRI is imaging modality of choice to identify meniscal tears.
- Functional outcomes following meniscal injury are improved with a comprehensive plan of rehabilitation involving strengthening and stretching of knee musculature.
- In patients opting for surgery, meniscal preservation should be the goal. Meniscal repairs have a better functional outcome and decreased risk of OA compared with meniscectomy.
- Improving core strength, proprioception, and quadricep/hamstring flexibility may prevent knee injuries, especially in female athletes.

M

MENOPAUSE

Anjie Li, MD • Julia V. Johnson, MD

BASICS

DESCRIPTION
- Natural menopause: defined retrospectively after 12 consecutive months of amenorrhea in a non-pregnant woman ≥40 years of age:
  - Results from loss of ovarian activity
  - Not associated with a pathologic etiology
- Perimenopause/menopausal transition (MT): defined as the period from the onset of irregular menses to the final menstrual cycle. Begins on average 4 years before menopause. Starts at mean age of 47 years.
- Postmenopause: usually >1/3 of a woman's life
- Primary ovarian insufficiency: irregular or cessation of menses before age 40

EPIDEMIOLOGY
- The median age of menopause is 51 years.
- 5% of women undergo menopause after age 55 years; another 5% between ages 40 and 45 years (1)[B].
- Occurs earlier in Hispanic women and later in Japanese-American women as compared with Caucasians (2)[B]

Incidence
In the United States, 1.3 million women reach menopause annually.

ETIOLOGY AND PATHOPHYSIOLOGY
Normal physiologic process:
- As women age, the number of ovarian follicles decreases: Ovarian production of estrogen varies and then decreases. Follicle-stimulating hormone (FSH) production varies and then increases.
- Inadequate estradiol production leads to absence of the luteinizing hormone (LH) surge and failure to ovulate. These cycles result in anovulation and lack of progesterone production.
- Eventual failure to produce estradiol leads to thinning of endometrial lining and eventual menses cessation.
- Surgical menopause: Removal of functioning ovaries leads to immediate menopause.

RISK FACTORS
- Aging
- Oophorectomy
- Hysterectomy
- Sex chromosome abnormalities (e.g., Turner syndrome and fragile X syndrome)
- Family history of early menopause
- Smoking (earlier age of onset by 2 years)
- Chemotherapy and/or pelvic radiation (permanent or reversible)

GENERAL PREVENTION
Menopause is physiologic event. Increased risk of long term medical issues include cardiovascular disease (CVD) and osteoporotic fractures:
- Decrease risk of CVD by:
  - Increased exercise
  - Avoid smoking.
  - Maintain healthy diet and lose weight.
  - Treat hyperlipidemia, diabetes, and hypertension.
  - Take daily low-dose aspirin.
- Decrease risk of osteoporotic fractures by:
  - Weight-bearing exercise
  - Avoid smoking.
  - Avoid excessive alcohol intake.
  - Dietary calcium of 1,200 mg/day
  - Adequate vitamin D (800 to 1,200 IU daily)
  - Fall prevention

DIAGNOSIS

HISTORY
- Cessation of menses:
  - Generally preceded by a period of irregular cycles with heavy vaginal bleeding followed by diminished vaginal bleeding
- Vasomotor symptoms: sudden feeling of warmth, most commonly over face, neck, and chest, with average duration of ~3 minutes, intervals unpredictable

  - Most commonly reported symptom; reported by over 80% of women (3)[B].
  - Frequency and duration varies. 87% of women who report flushes experience them daily, ~33% have >10 per day. Mean duration of symptoms lasts 4 to 10.2 years and may begin during MT and extend well past menopause (4)[A].

  - Varies with ethnicity; greatest in African and Hispanic women and least in Asian women
  - More common in obese women
- Urogenital atrophy in up to 50% (5)[B]:

  - Vaginal/vulvar dryness discharge, itch, dyspareunia, and possible sexual dysfunction
  - Alkaline vaginal pH and atrophy increases risk of vaginal infections and UTIs
  - Persists or worsens with aging
  - Urologic symptoms (urgency, frequency, dysuria, incontinence) not clearly correlated with MT
- Anxiety, depression: Some studies show a new diagnosis of depression is 2.5 times more likely to occur during the MT as compared to premenopause.
- Sleep disturbance: Arousal from sleep and chronic insomnia may be linked with vasomotor symptoms.
- Joint pain with unclear link to loss of estrogen
- Change in intensity and severity of migraines
- Skin thinning, mild hirsutism, brittle nails

Geriatric Considerations
Vaginal bleeding in postmenopausal women is abnormal; endometrial cancer/endometrioid adenocarcinoma (EAC) must be ruled out.

PHYSICAL EXAM
- Decrease in breast size and change in breast texture
- External, speculum, and bimanual pelvic exams: atrophic vulva and vaginal mucosa; increased risk for uterine prolapse

DIFFERENTIAL DIAGNOSIS
Pregnancy, hyperthyroidism and other thyroid disease, pituitary adenoma, Sheehan syndrome, hypothalamic dysfunction, anorexia nervosa, Asherman syndrome, obstruction of uterine outflow tract

DIAGNOSTIC TESTS & INTERPRETATION
Initial Tests (lab, imaging)
- U.S. Preventive Service Task Force (USPSTF) recommends mammogram every 2 years from ages 50 to 74.
- Lab testing for menopause is not required; the patient's age and symptoms establish the diagnosis.
- If laboratory confirmation is desired:
  - Elevated serum FSH level >30 mIU/mL indicates ovarian failure.
  - Symptoms may precede lab changes.
  - Infertility evaluation: may use elevated day 3 FSH, decreased anti-müllerian hormone levels, and decreased antral follicle count to predict decreased ovarian reserve
- Estrogens, androgens, and oral contraceptive pills (OCPs) may alter lab results.

Follow-Up Tests & Special Considerations
- Pregnancy test
- TSH and prolactin level if pituitary disease is suspected
- Vaginal bleeding in a postmenopausal patient should be evaluated by transvaginal ultrasound (TVUS) and/or endometrial biopsy (EMB). If endometrial stripe is <5 mm on TVUS, EAC is unlikely.
- USPSTF recommends bone mineral density (BMD) screening with dual energy x-ray absorptiometry (DEXA) scan in postmenopausal women >65 years, or <65 years if the risk for fracture is equivalent to that of a 65-year-old woman (using the FRAX tool to assess, http://www.shef.ac.uk/FRAX/). Risk factors include a previous history of fractures, low body weight, cigarette smoking, and family history of osteoporotic fracture.

Test Interpretation
- Abnormal BMD and DEXA scan results:
  - T-score on DEXA of −1 to −2.5 = osteopenia
  - T-score < −2.5 = osteoporosis
  - Defer to femoral neck T-score over spine T-score
- Z-score measures age-matched mean bone density (not clinically useful).

TREATMENT

MEDICATION
First Line
Hormone therapy (HT): developing an individual risk–benefit profile is essential. Treatment goal is to minimize menopausal symptoms to improve quality of life.
- The primary indication for HT is the treatment of moderate to severe vasomotor symptoms.

  - Oral estrogen or estrogen-progestin mix can reduce weekly hot flush frequency ~75% (4)[A].
- HT also helpful with sleep disorders, urogenital atrophy, and lowers risk of osteoporotic fractures and colorectal cancer. May help with mood symptoms
- In women with an intact uterus, give estrogen with progestin as unopposed estrogen carries an increased risk of EAC.
- Treatment regimens include, but are not limited to:
  - Standard dose: conjugated equine estrogen (CEE) 0.625 mg/day OR micronized estradiol 17β 1.0 mg/day OR transdermal estradiol 17β 0.0375 to 0.05 mg/day
  - Low dose: CEE 0.3 to 0.45 mg/day OR micronized estradiol 17β 0.5 mg/day OR transdermal estradiol 17β 0.025 mg/day
  - Ultra-low dose: micronized estradiol 17β 0.025 mg/day OR transdermal estradiol 17β 0.014 mg/day
  - Micronized progesterone 100 mg/day can be used as progestin. Alternative: medroxyprogesterone acetate (MPA) 2.5 mg/day. Combination estradiol/progestin transdermal treatments have either levonorgestrel or norethindrone as progestin source. Although NOT approved for postmenopausal women, the levonorgestrel intrauterine system (IUS) has been used.
  - Bazedoxifene + conjugated estrogens for relief of vasomotor symptoms and bone loss prevention
- American Congress of Obstetricians and Gynecologists (ACOG) recommends HT should be individualized with lowest effect dose given for the shortest duration of time needed to relieve vasomotor symptoms. Lower doses have similar symptom reduction profiles for many patients (6)[A]. Results of ultra-low dose regimens are mixed (7)[A].

- Although generally well tolerated, side effects of HT include breast tenderness, vaginal bleeding, bloating, and headaches.
- Precautions:
  - Women's Health Initiative (WHI) study demonstrate of every 10,000 women who take CEE with MPA, each year, there were 7 more CHD events, 8 more strokes, 8 more PEs, and 8 more invasive breast cancers independent of mammography screening frequency. Absolute risk reductions revealed 6 fewer colorectal cancers and 5 fewer hip fractures (8)[A].
  - Breast cancer risk not seen until 5 years of use
  - Cardiovascular risks not seen until after age 60 or 10 years from menopause.
  - Women on estrogen alone had no increased risk of breast cancer in the 8 years of the study and showed later cardiovascular risk compared to estrogen + progestin.
  - HT should NOT be used for cardioprotective benefit as risk outweighs benefit (9)[A].
  - Higher doses of estrogen can cause hypercoagulability, breast tenderness, gallbladder disease, and hypertension (HTN).
  - Contraindications to HT:
    - Estrogen-dependent malignancies
    - Unexplained uterine bleeding
    - History of thromboembolism or stroke
    - CAD
    - Active liver disease
- For osteoporosis: women with a history of hip or vertebral fracture, or personal history of osteoporosis should be treated with one of the following:
  - Bisphosphonates to inhibit osteoclast action and resorption of bone:
    - Alendronate: 70 mg/week or 10 mg/day
    - Risedronate: 35 mg once a week or 5 mg/day
    - Zoledronic acid: 5 mg IV annually
    - Ibandronate:150 mg/month PO or 3 mg IV q3mo
  - Selective estrogen receptor modulators (SERMs) selectively inhibit or stimulate estrogen-like action with stimulation of osteoblasts:
    - Raloxifene: 60 mg/day
      - Decreases the risk of vertebral fracture, but failed to demonstrate a decrease in the risk of extravertebral fractures
    - Bazedoxifene + conjugated estrogens (0.45 mg/20 mg)
      - FDA approved for moderate to severe vasomotor symptoms and osteoporosis.
  - Denosumab (60 mg SC every 6 months) is a monoclonal antibody prevents RANKL (receptor activator of nuclear factor kappa-B ligand) from accelerating osteoclast generation. Reduces incidence of vertebral and hip fractures in postmenopausal women.
  - Parathyroid hormone—rarely used due to the adverse effect on bone, but shown to reduce fracture risk in menopausal women with osteoporosis.
- For vulvar/vaginal atrophy:
  - Topical estrogen therapy (ET) reverses vaginal atrophy, enhances blood flow, and reduces UTI. Continue for as long as distressing symptoms remain. Initiate treatment daily for 1 to 2 weeks, then decreased to 2 times weekly. Comes as estradiol cream, tablet, or ring. Apply vaginally:
    - Estradiol cream 0.01% (1 g), conjugated estrogen 0.625 mg/g (0.5 g), vaginal tablet (10 μg) used twice weekly, or vaginal ring (7.5 μg daily lasting for 3 months)
    - Ospemifene: 60 mg PO daily. SERM for moderate to severe dyspareunia associated with vaginal atrophy.

- Although there is no increased risk of endometrial hyperplasia or EAC, women with bleeding on these treatments should be evaluated with TVUS or EMB. Patients with h/o hormone-dependent cancer should meet with a gynecologist before using medication.

Second Line
Nonhormonal treatments may be helpful to treat vasomotor symptoms in women who wish to or need to avoid HT (e.g., breast cancer):
- Paroxetine (7.5 mg/day) is approved for treatment of vasomotor symptoms. This SSRI demonstrated modest decrease in hot flushes.
- Other SSRI/SSNIs: venlafaxine (37.5 to 75 mg/day), or fluoxetine (20 mg/day), and citalopram (20 mg/day) shown to reduce hot flushes as compared to placebo
- Gabapentin (300 to 900 mg/day) shown to have an effect on lowering hot flushes compared to placebo.
- Clonidine (.05 mg BID) may be used to treat mild hot flashes, less effective than SSRI/SRNIs.
- Note that most trials of second-line therapies have been brief (i.e., a few months).

COMPLEMENTARY & ALTERNATIVE MEDICINE
Trials of nonprescribed therapies are difficult to interpret due to variability of components and doses:
- Soy isoflavone in placebo-controlled trials showed a mixed effect in reducing hot flashes.
- Red clover, black cohosh, reflexology, aerobics, and magnet therapy showed no impact on hot flashes when compared with placebo.
- Small clinical trials of evening primrose, dong quai, ginseng, and wild yam do not support use for relief of hot flashes.

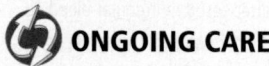 ONGOING CARE

FOLLOW-UP RECOMMENDATIONS
Patient Monitoring
A DEXA scan is indicated at age 65 for all women, and for younger women with risk equivalent to age 65.

DIET
Calcium-rich diet and vitamin D supplementation (800–1,200 IU/day). Calcium supplements may have adverse effects including increased risk of kidney stone and increased risk of cardiac events.

PATIENT EDUCATION
Encourage lifestyle modifications:
- Smoking cessation
- Weight-bearing exercise >30 minutes, 3 times weekly
- Healthy diet to maintain appropriate weight
- Avoid excess alcohol.
- Address cardiovascular risk factor modification.

PROGNOSIS
If untreated:
- Ultimate disappearance of vasomotor symptoms
- Worsening of vaginal/vulvar atrophy
- Osteoporosis: possible fractures of the hip, vertebrae, and wrists

COMPLICATIONS
- Osteoporosis: At menopause, women have accelerated bone loss up to 3–5% per year for 5 to 7 years.
- Increased risk of CVD following menopause

REFERENCES

1. McKinlay SM, Brambilla DJ, Posner JG. The normal menopause transition. *Maturitas*. 1992;14(2): 103–115.
2. Henderson KD, Bernstein L, Henderson B, et al. Predictors of the timing of natural menopause in the Multiethnic Cohort Study. *Am J Epidemiol*. 2008;167(11):1287–1294.
3. Feldman BM, Voda A, Gronseth E. The prevalence of hot flash and associated variables among perimenopausal women. *Res Nurs Health*. 1985;8(3):261–268.
4. MacLennan AH, Broadbent JL, Lester S, et al. Oral oestrogen and combined oestrogen/progestogen therapy versus placebo for hot flushes. *Cochrane Database Syst Rev*. 2004;(4):CD002978.
5. Dennerstein L, Dudley EC, Hopper JL, et al. A prospective population-based study of menopausal symptoms. *Obstet Gynecol*. 2000;96(3):351–358.
6. Notelovitz M, Lenihan JP, McDermott M, et al. Initial 17beta-estradiol dose for treating vasomotor symptoms. *Obstet Gynecol*. 2000;95(5):726–731.
7. Diem S, Grady D, Quan J, et al. Effects of ultralow-dose transdermal estradiol on postmenopausal symptoms in women aged 60 to 80 years. *Menopause*. 2006;13(1):130–138.
8. Rossouw JE, Anderson GL, Prentice RL, et al. Risks and benefits of estrogen plus progestin in healthy postmenopausal women: principal results from the Women's Health Initiative randomized controlled trial. *JAMA*. 2002;288(3):321–333.
9. Marjoribanks J, Farquhar C, Roberts H, et al. Long term hormone therapy for perimenopausal and postmenopausal women. *Cochrane Database Syst Rev*. 2012;(7):CD004143.

ADDITIONAL READING

- ACOG Practice Bulletin No. 141: management of menopausal symptoms. *Obstet Gynecol*. 2014;123(1):202–216.
- Grady D. Clinical practice. Management of menopausal symptoms. *N Engl J Med*. 2006;355(22):2338–2347.
- Mørch LS, Løkkegaard E, Andreasen AH, et al. Hormone therapy and ovarian cancer. *JAMA*. 2009;302(3):298–305.
- National Guideline Clearinghouse. Menopause. www.guideline.gov
- Nelson HD. Commonly used types of postmenopausal estrogen for treatment of hot flashes: scientific review. *JAMA*. 2004;291(13):1610–1620.
- North American Menopause Society. The 2012 hormone therapy position statement of: the North American Menopause Society. *Menopause*. 2012;19(3):257–271.
- Screening for Breast Cancer, Topic Page. July 2010. U.S. Preventive Services Task Force. http://www.uspreventiveservicestaskforce.org/uspstf/uspsbrca.htm

 CODES

ICD10
- N95.1 Menopausal and female climacteric states
- Z78.0 Asymptomatic menopausal state
- E28.310 Symptomatic premature menopause

CLINICAL PEARLS
- Menopause is usually diagnosed by history alone.
- HT can be used short term for relief of moderate to severe vasomotor symptoms, but should not be used for long-term prevention of cardiovascular disease.

M

MENORRHAGIA (HEAVY MENSTRUAL BLEEDING)

Brian D. Bates, MD • Joanne Wilkinson, MD, MSc

 BASICS

DESCRIPTION

- The current preferred terminology for menorrhagia is "heavy menstrual bleeding" (HMB), a subcategory of "abnormal uterine bleeding" (AUB) (1).
- HMB is an excessive amount (≥80 mL/cycle, compared with normal average of 30 to 60 mL/cycle) or duration of menstrual flow at predictable intervals.
- HMB applies only to ovulatory menses.
- Other patterns of AUB which may overlap with HMB include:
  - Intermenstrual bleeding: bleeding between regular menses
  - Irregular bleeding: typically due to ovulatory dysfunction (encompassing the previously used terms metrorrhagia and oligomenorrhea)
  - Polymenorrhea: menstrual cycle length <21 days
- System affected: reproductive

EPIDEMIOLOGY

Prevalence
- AUB, including HMB, is thought to affect between 9% and 14% of women between menarche and menopause (2).
- AUB is more common close to menarche and menopause.

Pediatric Considerations
- Genital bleeding before puberty is not menstrual bleeding by definition and requires further evaluation.
- HMB presenting in adolescence is more likely related to a bleeding disorder, and patients should be evaluated for a bleeding disorder (3).
- Postmenarchal patients may have heavy and irregular menstrual bleeding related to an immature hypothalamic-pituitary axis.

Pregnancy Considerations
Bleeding in pregnancy is not menstrual bleeding by definition and requires further evaluation. Pregnancy test should be obtained as part of the evaluation of abnormal uterine bleeding.

Geriatric Considerations
Menopause is diagnosed after 12 months of amenorrhea in the absence of other causes and is typically preceded by irregular bleeding. All postmenopausal bleeding requires additional workup for malignancy.

ETIOLOGY AND PATHOPHYSIOLOGY
- No cause is identified in about 1/2 of patients.
- Bleeding disorders
  - Von Willebrand disease (present in about 13% of patients) (2)
  - ITP and other platelet disorders
  - Factor deficiencies

- Medication side effect most commonly related to anticoagulants including warfarin
  - Renal failure leading to uremic platelet dysfunction
  - Cirrhosis leading to coagulopathy
- Uterine fibroids, typically submucosal
- Endometrial polyps
- Hypothyroidism
- Iatrogenic causes including copper IUD
- Endometriosis
- Adenomyosis
- Pelvic inflammatory disease
- Some causes more typically presenting as irregular menstrual bleeding include:
  - Polycystic ovarian syndrome (PCOS)
  - Hypothalamic-pituitary dysfunction, often postmenarchal or during menopausal transition
  - Endometrial or ovarian neoplasia
  - Some forms of hormonal birth control
  - Hyperthyroidism
  - Hyperprolactinemia
- HMB has been associated with increased production and sensitivity to prostaglandins.

GENERAL PREVENTION
- Combined oral contraceptives may prevent HMB, particularly when progesterone is dominant. Lower estrogen doses result in less menstrual bleeding
- NSAIDs including ibuprofen inhibit prostaglandin production and result in decreased blood loss and pain during menses.
- Progesterone-only contraceptives may reduce overall blood loss but often result in irregular bleeding.

COMMONLY ASSOCIATED CONDITIONS
Iron deficiency anemia

DIAGNOSIS

HISTORY
- Although HMB is defined as menstrual bleeding >80 mL/cycle, patient assessment of menstrual volume is highly inaccurate and the diagnosis is often based on a patient's subjective concerns (4).
- Suggestive historical features for HMB:
  - Bleeding substantially heavier than patient's usual flow
  - Changing pads or tampons every 1 to 2 hours as quantified by patient
  - Menses lasting >7 days
  - Significant clots
- Symptoms that suggest bleeding is ovulatory:
  - Regular menstrual interval
  - Midcycle pain (mittelschmerz)
  - Premenstrual symptoms: breast soreness, mood changes

- Abdominal pain or cramps at other times of the cycle may be associated with structural causes:
  - Polyps
  - Adenomyosis
  - Leiomyoma
  - Ovarian tumors
- Symptoms that suggest an underlying bleeding disorder include:
  - Epistaxis
  - Mucosal bleeding (e.g., gums)
  - Easy bruising
  - Family history of bleeding disorder
- Review of medications, with particular attention to contraceptive and anticoagulant medication
- Other medical conditions that may relate to HMB:
  - Renal or hepatic disease
  - Thyroid disease
- Evaluate for symptoms of anemia including fatigue and dyspnea

PHYSICAL EXAM
- Prompt assessment for signs of hemodynamic instability (5)
- Thyroid nodule or goiter suggests thyroid disease.
- Signs of a bleeding disorder include petechiae and ecchymoses.
- Pelvic examination, including speculum and bimanual examination, may reveal the following:
  - Cervical or vaginal source of bleeding
  - Pelvic or adnexal mass
  - Evidence of reproductive tract infection such as cervical motion tenderness
  - Uterine enlargement
- Hirsutism, acne, and obesity are suggestive of PCOS.

DIFFERENTIAL DIAGNOSIS
- Normal menses
- Anovulatory bleeding
- Intermenstrual bleeding
- Complications of pregnancy
  - Spontaneous abortion
- Other sources of bleeding:
  - Cervical
  - Vaginal
  - Gastrointestinal

DIAGNOSTIC TESTS & INTERPRETATION
Initial Tests (lab, imaging)
- Pregnancy test
- CBC to assess for:
  - Anemia
  - Thrombocytopenia
  - Leukocytosis may suggest infection
- Thyroid-stimulating hormone (TSH) test

- Labs to consider in select cases:
  - Coagulation panel for evaluation for bleeding disorder in adolescent or adult with history suggestive of bleeding disorder
  - Workup of anovulatory bleeding may also include prolactin, androgens, FSH, LH, and estrogen.
  - Appropriate cervical cancer screening
  - Evaluation for infection including gonorrhea and chlamydia
- Imaging should be obtained based on clinician judgment and should begin with transvaginal ultrasonography.
- Transabdominal ultrasonography should be performed if transvaginal approach does not provide full assessment of anatomy.

Follow-Up Tests & Special Considerations
- Saline infusion sonohysterography recommended if ultrasound suggests intracavitary pathology and is more sensitive and specific than transvaginal ultrasound (2)[C]
- Hysteroscopy can be performed if direct visualization is desired.

Diagnostic Procedures/Other
Endometrial biopsy to assess for malignancy and hyperplasia is recommended in some situations including (5):
- Any AUB, including HMB, after age 45 years in an ovulatory (premenopausal) woman
- Woman <45 years with persistent or refractory AUB, risk factors such as unopposed estrogen exposure, or concerning endometrial imaging

TREATMENT

GENERAL MEASURES
Treat underlying conditions (e.g., hypothyroidism) when possible.

MEDICATION
First Line
- For acute control of severe bleeding (6):
  - Obtain IV access and consider blood transfusion or clotting factor administration.
  - Estrogen, conjugated equine: 25 mg IV every 4 to 6 hours for 24 hours
  - Monophasic combined oral contraceptive that contains 35 μg ethinyl estradiol: 3 times per day for 7 days
  - Medroxyprogesterone acetate: 20 mg orally 3 times per day for 7 days
  - Tranexamic acid: 1.3 g orally or 10 mg/kg IV 3 times per day for 5 days, antifibrinolytic agent
- For less severe bleeding (typical case) or after control of acute bleeding has been achieved (2):
  - Levonorgestrel intrauterine device (Mirena IUD): typically results in light bleeding or amenorrhea with patient satisfaction similar to hysterectomy and endometrial ablation (7)[A]

- Combination estrogen-progestin oral contraceptive: may be prescribed in cyclic, extended, or continuous dosing and typically results in regular, lighter, and less painful menses
- Depot medroxyprogesterone acetate: 150 mg/1mL IM every 3 months, typically results in amenorrhea or light irregular bleeding
- Tranexamic acid: 1.3 g orally for 5 days during menses; antifibrinolytic agent that is an option for women who desire nonhormonal treatment NSAIDs (e.g., naproxen, mefenamic acid, ibuprofen) can reduce blood loss and dysmenorrheal (2)[B].

Second Line
- Noncontraception estrogen-progestin oral contraceptives (ultra-low-dose estrogen): may be considered when a relative contraindication to estrogen is present
- Oral progestins: multiple formulations and dosing, typically used in women who have contraindications to estrogen or are trying to conceive

SURGERY/OTHER PROCEDURES
- Dilation and curettage can be considered in the setting of acute severe bleeding.
- For women who desire fertility, myomectomy may be considered for treatment of uterine leiomyomas (fibroids).
- For women who do not desire fertility, consider endometrial ablation, uterine artery embolization, or hysterectomy.
  - Endometrial ablation shows similar outcomes to levonorgestrel IUD, patients still require contraception.
  - Uterine artery embolization is used to treat uterine leiomyomas.
  - Hysterectomy is curative but with significant complications and long recovery, typically reserved for failure of medical management or presence of another indication such as malignancy.

ONGOING CARE

DIET
Iron supplementation may help correct for increased blood loss.

PATIENT EDUCATION
Patient and provider should engage in informed decision making with understanding of treatment risks and benefits.

PROGNOSIS
Most patients respond well to medical management, and hysterectomy is a curative option in appropriate cases.

COMPLICATIONS
- Iron deficiency anemia
- Acute severe blood loss

REFERENCES

1. Munro MG, Critchley HO, Broder MS, et al. FIGO classification system (PALM-COEIN) for causes of abnormal uterine bleeding in nongravid women of reproductive age. *Int J Gynaecol Obstet*. 2011; 113(1):3–13.
2. Sweet MG, Schmidt-Dalton TA, Weiss PM, et al. Evaluation and management of abnormal uterine bleeding in premenopausal women. *Am Fam Physician*. 2012;85(1):35–43.
3. Diaz A, Laufer MR, Breech LL. Menstruation in girls and adolescents: using the menstrual cycle as a vital sign. *Pediatrics*. 2006;118(5):2245–2250.
4. Matteson KA, Munro MG, Fraser IS. The structured menstrual history: developing a tool to facilitate diagnosis and aid in symptom management. *Semin Reprod Med*. 2011;29(5):423–435.
5. Matthews ML. Abnormal uterine bleeding in reproductive-aged women. *Obstet Gynecol Clin North Am*. 2015;42(1):103–115.
6. American College of Obstetricians and Gynecologists. ACOG Committee Opinion No. 557: management of acute abnormal uterine bleeding in nonpregnant reproductive-aged women. *Obstet Gynecol*. 2013; 121(4):891–896.
7. Lethaby A, Hussain M, Rishworth JR, et al. Progesterone or progestogen-releasing intrauterine systems for heavy menstrual bleeding. *Cochrane Database Syst Rev*. 2015;(4):CD002126.

CODES

ICD10
- N92.0 Excessive and frequent menstruation with regular cycle
- N92.3 Ovulation bleeding
- N92.2 Excessive menstruation at puberty

CLINICAL PEARLS
- Women with heavy menstrual bleeding are at high risk for iron deficiency anemia.
- A thorough menstrual history is critical to differentiate heavy menstrual bleeding from similar conditions including anovulatory bleeding.
- Teenagers presenting with heavy menstrual bleeding should be evaluated for an underlying bleeding disorder.
- All postmenopausal bleeding and bleeding during pregnancy requires additional workup.
- The Levonorgestrel (Mirena) intrauterine device may be used for heavy menstrual bleeding and is associated with high patient satisfaction rates.

M

MESENTERIC ADENITIS

Anne Walsh, MMSc, PA-C, DFAAPA • Kashyap Trivedi, MD

BASICS

Inflammation of the mesenteric lymph nodes. A common cause of self-limited RLQ abdominal pain.

DESCRIPTION
- Characterized by benign inflammation of the mesenteric lymph nodes; can be acute or chronic
- May clinically mimic acute appendicitis

EPIDEMIOLOGY
- Commonly misdiagnosed, making definitive incidence unknown
- Most common cause of appendicitis-like pain in children (1)
  - 20% in patients presenting for appendectomy (2)
- More common in children <15 years old than in adults
  - Primary adenitis is more common in children.
  - Secondary adenitis is more common in adults.
    - Rule out diverticulitis, appendicitis, Crohn disease, or systemic infectious/inflammatory disease (e.g., HIV, SLE).

Prevalence
Affects males and females equally.
- Adenitis secondary to *Yersinia* infection is more prevalent in boys than girls.
  - *Yersinia enterocolitica* is most common in North America, Eastern Europe, and Australia.

ETIOLOGY AND PATHOPHYSIOLOGY
- Primary: underlying inflammatory process not present; presumed due to acute infectious gastroenteritis (specifically, terminal ileitis)
- Secondary: underlying inflammatory process present (see "Commonly Associated Conditions")
- In infectious etiologies, pathogens are ingested, translocate through the intestinal epithelium via Peyer patches, and gain access to mesenteric lymph nodes. An inflammatory reaction within mesenteric lymph nodes causes symptoms and clinical disease. Infectious agents include:
  - *Y. enterocolitica*
  - *Campylobacter jejuni*
  - *Salmonella typhi*
  - β-Hemolytic *Streptococcus* spp.
  - *Staphylococcus* spp.
  - *Streptococcus viridans*
  - *Escherichia coli*
  - *Mycobacterium tuberculosis*
  - *Giardia lamblia*
  - Epstein-Barr virus (EBV)
  - Acute HIV infection
  - Rubeola virus
  - Cat-scratch disease
  - Adenovirus species

Genetics
No known genetic susceptibility

RISK FACTORS
- Typically preceded by URI or pharyngitis
- History of ingesting undercooked pork particularly in areas where *Yersinia* is endemic (parts of Europe).

GENERAL PREVENTION
Minimize risk by fully cooking foods, especially meat.

COMMONLY ASSOCIATED CONDITIONS
- Appendicitis
- Diverticulitis
- Crohn disease
- Celiac disease
- Other systemic inflammatory/autoimmune disease

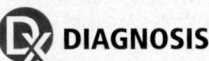

DIAGNOSIS

HISTORY
The onset of symptoms is variable; nausea or abdominal pain is usually the initial presenting symptom. Symptoms are often nonspecific.
- Nausea and vomiting (may precede abdominal pain)
- Abdominal pain: periumbilical, RLQ
- Diarrhea
- Fever, malaise, fatigue, anorexia
- Recent history of upper respiratory tract infection

PHYSICAL EXAM
- Fever; can have toxic appearance
- Abdominal tenderness; (with or without rebound and often in the RLQ)
- Peripheral/generalized lymphadenopathy
- Rectal tenderness
- Rhinorrhea
- Pharyngeal hyperemia

DIFFERENTIAL DIAGNOSIS
- Appendicitis, intussusception, intestinal duplication, regional enteritis (Crohn disease), Meckel diverticulitis, ulcerative colitis
- Epiploic appendagitis, mesenteric ischemia
- UTI, pyelonephritis
- Salpingitis, PID, ectopic pregnancy
- Neoplasm (e.g., lymphoma)

DIAGNOSTIC TESTS & INTERPRETATION
Initial Tests (lab, imaging)
- CBC: leukocytosis with left shift
- Basic metabolic panel may show electrolyte disturbances and azotemia if dehydrated and/or alkalotic from recalcitrant vomiting.
- β-HCG in women of childbearing potential
- Stool cultures if diarrhea
- Serologies if specific infectious agent suspected
- Blood cultures if septic
- CT scan: enlarged mesenteric lymph nodes (larger in size, number, and distribution than appendicitis)
  - Specific CT appearance includes ≥3 clustered lymph nodes measuring at least 5 mm in the short axis, most commonly to the right of the psoas muscle (3)[B].
  - May or may not have evidence of ileal or ileocecal wall thickening
  - Appendix appears normal.
- Ultrasound: less sensitive; used for exclusion of other potential diagnoses
  - Preferred in children and women (1)[C]
  - Used to evaluate for signs of appendicitis (96% positive predictive value in children) (2)[B]

Diagnostic Procedures/Other
Lymph node biopsy: only for those undergoing laparotomy can isolate the causative organism

Test Interpretation
- Lymph nodes are enlarged and soft.
- Adjoining mesentery may be edematous.
- Microscopically, lymph nodes display nonspecific hyperplasia. If a suppurative infection is present, lymph nodes may contain necrotic material with pus formation.
  - Lymphatic sinuses may be enlarged.
  - If *Y. enterocolitica* infection, lymph node capsule may be thickened, with surrounding edema; lymph node hyperplasia, with plasma cell infiltration also occur.

TREATMENT

MEDICATION
First Line
- Supportive and symptomatic treatment for uncomplicated cases
- IV fluid resuscitation if hypovolemic
- Correct underlying electrolyte aberrations.
- Pain control

Second Line
- Broad-spectrum antibiotic therapy for moderately to severely ill patients if diagnosis is unclear pending workup and/or surgical evaluation
- Treatment duration varies based on cause and severity of illness. For uncomplicated cases, antibiotic treatment is not necessary.

SURGERY/OTHER PROCEDURES
Surgery is usually indicated in cases of suppuration and/or abscess formation, with signs of peritonitis, or if acute appendicitis cannot be excluded with certainty.

INPATIENT CONSIDERATIONS
Admission Criteria/Initial Stabilization
- Admit patients with complications and/or hemodynamic instability.

- Volume resuscitation and correction of underlying electrolyte abnormalities

IV Fluids
- IV fluids may be indicated for patients who cannot tolerate PO intake due to nausea or vomiting.
- Aggressive fluid hydration is indicated if there is any evidence of sepsis.

Discharge Criteria
Hemodynamic stability, able to tolerate PO diet, able to follow up in the outpatient setting

 ONGOING CARE

FOLLOW-UP RECOMMENDATIONS
Patient Monitoring
Close outpatient monitoring is needed to ensure total resolution of symptoms.

DIET
There are no specific dietary recommendations. Hold oral intake as necessary until nausea and vomiting resolve. Advance diet slowly as tolerated.

PATIENT EDUCATION
In cases of *Yersinia* infection, patients should avoid unpasteurized milk, raw pork, and contaminated water.

PROGNOSIS
- Generally self-limiting and benign condition
- Increased morbidity/mortality for patients presenting with sepsis

COMPLICATIONS
- Increased GI losses leading to hypovolemia and electrolyte imbalance
- Abscess formation, peritonitis, sepsis
- Latent extraintestinal manifestations, including arthralgias, truncal and extremity rashes, and erythema nodosum with *Y. enterocolitica* infection

- Postinfectious chronic complications of *Yersinia* infection including reactive arthritis, conjunctivitis, urethritis; postinfectious irritable bowel syndrome

REFERENCES
1. Millet I, Alili C, Pages E, et al. Infection of the right iliac fossa. *Diagn Interv Imaging*. 2012;93(6): 441–452.
2. Toorenvliet B, Vellekoop A, Bakker R, et al. Clinical differentiation between acute appendicitis and acute mesenteric lymphadenitis in children. *Eur J Pediatr Surg*. 2011;21(2):120–123.
3. Purysko AS, Remer EM, Filho HM, et al. Beyond appendicitis: common and uncommon gastrointestinal causes of right lower quadrant abdominal pain at multidetector CT. *Radiographics*. 2011;31(4): 927–947.

ADDITIONAL READING
Patlas MN, Alabousi A, Scaglione M, et al. Cross-sectional imaging of nontraumatic peritoneal and mesenteric emergencies. *Can Assoc Radiol J*. 2013;64(2):148–153.

 CODES

ICD10
I88.0 Nonspecific mesenteric lymphadenitis

CLINICAL PEARLS
- Mesenteric adenitis is an inflammatory process that mimics appendicitis. Diagnosis requires imaging to distinguish from acute appendicitis.
- The condition is more common in children, often following a URI.
- The treatment is generally supportive care.

MESOTHELIOMA

Holli K. Neiman-Hart, MD, FAAFP

 BASICS

DESCRIPTION

- Mesothelioma is a rare, aggressive malignancy of the mesothelial or serous tissues primarily found in the pleura (65–70%) or peritoneum (20–33%), tunica vaginalis (1–2%) or pericardium (1–2%) (1).
- Inhalation of asbestos is the predominant cause of mesothelioma, most often from occupational exposure.

EPIDEMIOLOGY

Incidence

- The incidence in the United States is decreasing, but it is increasing in other countries, particularly Great Britain and Australia.
- It is expected that rates of mesothelioma will start to drop after 2015 to 2025 related to reduced exposure and better understanding of the process of development of mesothelioma after exposure to asbestos (2).
- The incidence increases with age, peaking in the 6th decade, with 70% of pleural disease occurring in males. Peritoneal involvement is slightly higher in women.
- Main risk factor is asbestos exposure, but tumors have arisen after prior radiation or exposure to talc, erionite or mica, or in patients with familial Mediterranean fever and diffuse lymphocytic leukemia.

Prevalence

There are 3,300 cases of mesothelioma diagnosed in the United States annually (3).

ETIOLOGY AND PATHOPHYSIOLOGY

- The predominant cause of mesothelioma is exposure to asbestos (hydrated magnesium silicate fibrous minerals).
- There is a long latent period of up to 44 years between exposure and development of mesothelioma (2).
- Inhaled or ingested asbestos fibers become trapped in pleural or peritoneal membranes causing changes of irritation and inflammation.

Genetics

Loss of nuclear deubiquitinase BAP1 is associated with incidence of mesothelioma in some families as well as with other cancers such as melanoma.

RISK FACTORS

- The predominant risk factor is exposure to asbestos.
- Occupational exposures involve mining or milling of fibers, work with textiles, cement, friction materials, insulation, or shipbuilding.
- Nonoccupational exposures include renovation or destruction of asbestos-containing buildings, exposure to industrial sources in the community or natural geologic sources, or exposure to soiled clothing of asbestos workers (1,3,4).
- Radiation exposure, smoking, proximity to naturally occurring asbestos deposits, or inhalation of other fibrous silicates can contribute to malignant mesothelioma.

GENERAL PREVENTION

- Avoidance of asbestos exposure
- Strict adherence to protective protocols for workers in buildings where asbestos is found.
- Continued aggressive remediation of asbestos-affected buildings and homes

DIAGNOSIS

HISTORY

- Symptoms are usually nonspecific and occur when disease is advanced. General fatigue, night sweats, and weight loss may be present.
- Pleural mesothelioma presents with gradual onset of pulmonary symptoms, chest pain, dyspnea, and cough.
- Peritoneal disease presents with vague abdominal pain, increased abdominal girth, nausea, anorexia, and weight loss

PHYSICAL EXAM

- Pulmonary findings of decreased breath sounds, dullness to percussion, asymmetric chest wall expansion
- Abdominal findings include distension, fluid wave with ascites, and tenderness.

DIFFERENTIAL DIAGNOSIS

- Pleural mesothelioma differential diagnosis includes inflammatory reactions (empyema, pleural effusion), metastatic tumor from other sites, fibrosarcoma, malignant fibrous histiocytoma, sarcomatoid carcinoma, or synovial sarcoma.
- Peritoneal mesothelioma differential diagnosis includes peritoneal carcinomatosis, serous peritoneal carcinoma, ovarian carcinoma in women, lymphomatosis, tuberculous peritonitis

DIAGNOSTIC TESTS & INTERPRETATION

Initial Tests (lab, imaging)

- At present, there is no tumor marker or serum chemistry that is of value in establishing the diagnosis of mesothelioma.
- Biomarkers that may be elevated in mesothelioma include fibulin-3, mesothelin, and osteopontin. However, they do not have an established role in diagnosis or monitoring response to therapy (2)[A].
- Pleural mesothelioma diagnosis requires tissue. Thoracentesis for cytology and closed pleural biopsy may be adequate, but often, more invasive procedures such as video-assisted thoracoscopic surgery (VATS) is needed to obtain an adequate specimen (1,2)[A].

Follow-Up Tests & Special Considerations

Seeding of biopsy sites and tracks may occur in mesothelioma, which can be prevented with prophylactic radiation therapy to the scar or biopsy site (5)[A].

Diagnostic Procedures/Other

- CT, MRI, PET, or integrated PET-CT helps with clinical staging in pleural and peritoneal disease (1–4),(5)[A].
- Mediastinoscopy, bronchoscopy, and laparoscopy can assist in full surgical staging of pleural disease (2)[A].
- Endobronchial ultrasound for staging is under investigation for pleural disease.

Test Interpretation

- The tumor, node, metastasis (TNM) staging system is most commonly used although some centers use other staging systems.
- Butchart staging system is the oldest and still used in some parts of the world.
- Brigham staging system attempts to define resectability and lymph node involvement.

TREATMENT

GENERAL MEASURES

- A multidisciplinary team is important in management and should include thoracic surgery, oncology, pathology, pulmonary, and radiology for patient specific planning of management.
- Pain assessment and control should follow principles of cancer pain management (5).

MEDICATION

First Line

- In pleural disease, combined therapy with cisplatin + gemcitabine or cisplatin + pemetrexed are associated with longer median survival than cisplatin alone (2),(4)[A].
- Vinflunine is showing some potential for first-line treatment in pleural disease (2)[A].
- Hyperthermic intraoperative or early postoperative intraperitoneal chemotherapy can decrease increase drug concentration to the peritoneum and decrease systemic side effects. Use cisplatin, mitomycin C, fluorouracil, doxorubicin, and/or paclitaxel (1,2),(3)[A].

Second Line

- Palliative benefit in pleural disease with mitomycin C, vinblastine, cisplatin, and pemetrexed alone or in combination with carboplatin (2,3),(4)[A]
- Systemic therapy for peritoneal disease may include pemetrexed + cisplatin; vinorelbine or gemcitabine alone or in combination (1),(5)[A].

ISSUES FOR REFERRAL

- Pulmonary, oncology, and surgical follow-up after discharge as indicated
- Anger and depression may require psychological or psychiatric services (5).

ADDITIONAL THERAPIES

- Immunotherapy in pleural disease uses humanized anti-CB3 AB (OKT3), cytotoxic T lymph (CTL), interferon α-2a, and autovaccine in advanced disease (1–5).
  - Gene therapy
  - Photodynamic therapy
  - Radiotherapy in some cases of pleural disease
  - Vascular endothelial growth factor (anti-VEGF-2) in combination with chemotherapy (2)
    - Vaccines are under study (5).

SURGERY/OTHER PROCEDURES

- For pleural mesothelioma, the role of surgery is not as clear cut. Pleurectomy with tumor decortication and extrapleural pneumonectomy reduce the tumor load, but there remains no clear effect on mortality (2,4,5).
- Radical resection of the peritoneum and cytoreductive surgery is associated with a better prognosis (1).

INPATIENT CONSIDERATIONS

Admission Criteria/Initial Stabilization

Based on overall condition

IV Fluids

As indicated by general condition

Nursing

As indicated by condition

Discharge Criteria

As indicated by general condition

ONGOING CARE

FOLLOW-UP RECOMMENDATIONS

- Smoking cessation
- Immunization for pneumococcal pneumonia and influenza

Patient Monitoring

Monitor for paraneoplastic phenomenon including fever, thrombocytosis, malignancy-related thrombosis, hypoglycemia, and rare Coombs-positive hemolytic anemia.

DIET

No specific restrictions

PROGNOSIS

- Prognosis is based on gender, stage, and level of completeness of cytoreduction.
- Poorly differentiated tumor grade, failure to undertake surgical resection, advanced age, and male gender are all independent predictors of poorer prognosis (2,3).
- Average survival is 17 to 92 months, with 5-year survival rate at 63%.

COMPLICATIONS

Relapses and progression, infection, dysphagia

Geriatric Considerations

Age >65 years is associated with significantly increased morbidity and mortality.

Pediatric Considerations

Rarely a pediatric issue, as most disease occurs after the 5th decade of life.

Pregnancy Considerations

Rarely an issue with pregnancy, as most disease occurs after the 5th decade of life.

REFERENCES

1. Bridda A, Padoan I, Mencarelli R, et al. Peritoneal mesothelioma: a review. *MedGenMed*. 2007; 9(2):32.
2. Weder W. Mesothelioma. *Ann Oncol*. 2010; 21(Suppl 7):vii326–vii333.
3. Mott FE. Mesothelioma: a review. *Ochsner J*. 2012; 12(1):70–79.
4. Fuhrer G, Lazarus AA. Mesothelioma. *Dis Mon*. 2011;57(1):40–54.
5. van Meerbeck JP, Scherpereel A, Surmont VF, et al. Malignant pleural mesothelioma: the standard of care and challenges for future management. *Crit Rev Oncol Hematol*. 2011;78(2):92–111.

CODES

ICD10

- C45.9 Mesothelioma, unspecified
- C45.0 Mesothelioma of pleura
- C45.1 Mesothelioma of peritoneum

CLINICAL PEARLS

- Mesothelioma remains a rare but universally fatal disease in part due to long latency.
- Multimodal treatment has decreased recurrence rates and has extended survival time.

M

METABOLIC SYNDROME

Naomi Parrella, MD

BASICS

DESCRIPTION

- A constellation of metabolic abnormalities that confer increased risk for type 2 diabetes mellitus (T2DM), cardiovascular disease, stroke, fatty liver, and certain cancers and includes metabolic derangement manifesting with at least three of the following:
  1. Increased abdominal circumference
  2. Elevated BP
  3. Elevated triglycerides
  4. Decreased High denstiy lipoprotein (HDL)
  5. Elevated fasting glucose
- Also involves the following metabolic abnormalities:
  - Insulin resistance with or without impaired glucose tolerance
  - Proinflammatory state
  - Prothrombotic state

EPIDEMIOLOGY

- Predominant age: >60 years old (~50% of cases)
- Predominant sex: male = female
- Ethnicity: Mexican Americans (highest risk)

Prevalence

- Affects 34% of U.S. adults aged >20 years; increasing with the aging population and the prevalence of obesity (1)
- Data vary among race and ethnicity with different trends for women and men. The available literature suggests that metabolic syndrome is a rapidly growing epidemic worldwide.

Pediatric Considerations

- Obese children and adolescents are at high risk of metabolic syndrome (prevalence of 6.4% in the United States). Risk factors in children and adolescents include heredity, low birth weight, childhood weight gain and obesity, endocrine abnormalities, hostility, maternal gestational diabetes, and poor health habits.
- International Diabetes Federation consensus report defined criteria in three age groups (6 to ≤10 years; 10 to ≤16 years; 16+ years, adult criteria applicable) (2)[C]. Obesity defined by waist circumference ≥90th percentile; rest of the diagnostic criteria (triglycerides [TGs], high-density lipoprotein cholesterol [HDL-C], hypertension [HTN], and fasting blood sugar/T2DM) are largely the same as in adults for children ≥10 years, with some exceptions, and warrant treatment. Clinical significance of metabolic syndrome in pediatric population is not well established using these criteria (2). BMI used alone is as accurate as using IDF criteria to predict adult MetSyn, subclinical atherosclerosis and diabetes mellitus type 2 (3)[C]. Focus on promoting healthy lifestyle habits and weight management rather than diagnosis.

ETIOLOGY AND PATHOPHYSIOLOGY

- Increase in intra-abdominal and visceral adipose tissue
- Adipose tissue dysfunction and insulin resistance
- Decreased levels of adiponectin, an adipocytokine, known to protect against T2DM, HTN, atherosclerosis, and inflammation
- Abnormal fatty acid metabolism, endothelial dysfunction, systemic inflammation, oxidative stress, elevated renin-angiotensin system activation, and a prothrombotic state (increased tissue plasminogen activator inhibitor-1) are also associated.

- The main etiologic factors are the following:
  - Obesity (particularly abdominal)/excess visceral adipose tissue
  - Insulin resistance
  - Other contributing factors:
    - Advancing age
    - Proinflammatory state
    - Genetics
- Endocrine (e.g., postmenopausal state)

Genetics

Genetic factors contribute significantly to causation. Most identified genes are transcription factors or regulators of transcription and translation. It is a multifactorial disease with evidence of complex interactions between genetics and environment.

RISK FACTORS

- Obesity/intra-abdominal obesity
- Childhood obesity
- Insulin resistance
- Older age
- Ethnicity
- Family history
- Physical inactivity
- High-carbohydrate diet
- Sugar-sweetened beverages daily
- Smoking
- Postmenopausal status
- Low socioeconomic status
- Alteration of gut flora

GENERAL PREVENTION

- Effective weight loss and maintenance of normal body weight long term
- Regular and sustained physical activity
- Diet low in saturated fats and simple sugars

COMMONLY ASSOCIATED CONDITIONS

- Polycystic ovary syndrome
- Nonalcoholic fatty liver disease (NAFLD)
- Acanthosis nigricans
- Chronic renal disease
- Depression
- Cognitive impairment
- Obstructive sleep apnea
- Gallstones (cholesterol)
- Erectile dysfunction (in men)
- Hyperuricemia and gout

DIAGNOSIS

HISTORY

- Not necessary for diagnosis of metabolic syndrome
- Family history of metabolic syndrome, T2DM, and cardiovascular disease
- Symptoms indicating cardiovascular disease or diabetes
- Comprehensive lifestyle history:
  - Diet, including intake of carbohydrates and fats
  - Weight history, including onset of obesity and previous weight loss attempts
  - Exercise regimen
  - Alcohol intake
- Cigarette smoking
- Assess cardiovascular risk with Framingham risk assessment tool.

PHYSICAL EXAM

Various criteria-based definitions have been proposed and in 2009, harmonized (4). A diagnosis of metabolic syndrome can be made when ≥3 of the following 5 characteristics are present:

- Abdominal obesity: men >102 cm, women >88 cm (ATP III recommends lowering threshold in population susceptible to insulin resistance, especially Asian Americans)
- BP ≥130/85 mm Hg or treatment
- TGs ≥150 mg/dL or treatment
- HDL: men >40 mg/dL, women <50 mg/dL or treatment
- Fasting glucose ≥100 mg/dL or treatment

DIFFERENTIAL DIAGNOSIS

Individual components of the syndrome may be present without fulfilling all the diagnostic criteria. Obstructive sleep apnea, thyroid abnormalities, Cushing syndrome, medication effect (especially psychotropic, chronic steroids, β-blockers and thiazide diuretic [5] medications) may also be considered in the differential.

DIAGNOSTIC TESTS & INTERPRETATION

Initial Tests (lab, imaging)

- Fasting lipids (particularly TGs and HDL)
- Fasting glucose

Follow-Up Tests & Special Considerations

- Formal 75-mg oral glucose tolerance test or Hemoglobin A1C for diagnosis of impaired glucose tolerance (IGT)
- Liver function tests
- Measurement of fasting insulin levels is controversial.
- None necessary to diagnose metabolic syndrome

Diagnostic Procedures/Other

- Home BP monitoring or 24-hour BP monitoring may be used to rule out white coat hypertension.
- ECG, stress test, and coronary angiography may be used for diagnosis of cardiovascular disease arising as a complication of the syndrome.

Test Interpretation

- Microalbuminuria
- Increased WBC count
- Increased C-reactive protein
- Increased fibrinogen
- Increased proinflammatory cytokines (e.g., tumor necrosis factor-α)
- Increased uric acid
- Increased homocysteine
- T2DM
- Fatty liver (complicated by end-stage liver disease and hepatocellular carcinoma)
- Hypertensive and/or diabetic eye disease
- Renal impairment/failure
- Peripheral vascular disease
- Coronary artery disease
- Cerebrovascular disease

TREATMENT

Primary therapeutic goal is to prevent or reduce obesity and risk factors. Aggressive lifestyle modification (diet and exercise) is considered first-line therapy and most clinically effective (6)[C].

GENERAL MEASURES
- Aggressive treatment of individual risk factors
- Increase daily physical activity.
- Avoid or stop smoking.
- Avoid excess alcohol intake.
- Avoid sugar sweetened beverages.
- Increase leafy green vegetables.

MEDICATION
- Daily treatment with aspirin is recommended for patients with cardiovascular disease or those at high risk.
- Consult clinical guidelines for treatment of dyslipidemia, hypertension, IGT, and diabetes.
- Multiple medications usually are required to achieve adequate BP control.
- Diagnosis and treatment of insulin resistance is controversial.

First Line
Lifestyle modification alone as initial strategy is applicable to individuals with low 10-year risk for coronary artery disease (CAD). In individuals with higher 10-year risk, more aggressive risk factor–based approach is recommended in addition to lifestyle modifications:

- Obesity: Lifestyle changes are the cornerstone of treatment. Aim for a ~5–10% weight reduction. Any amount of weight loss is associated with significant benefits.
  - Phentermine–topiramate (delayed release) (Qsymia) (7)[A] and lorcaserin (Belviq) (8)[A] have been approved by the FDA for nonpregnant, nonlactating adults for management of obesity with promising outcomes on weight, BP, dyslipidemia, and other metabolic/glycemic parameters.
- Physical activity: Endurance exercise may reverse metabolic syndrome (9)[A]. 30 to 60 minutes of moderate-intensity aerobic activities such as brisk walking 5 to 7 days/week; increase in daily lifestyle activities and resistance training 1 to 2 days/week (10)[A]. In patients with established CAD, assess detailed history of physical activity and exercise tolerance to guide activity prescription. Advise medically supervised programs for high-risk population (recent acute coronary syndrome [ACS], congestive heart failure, recent revascularization). Cumulative exercise time over the day contributes to health benefit.
- Dyslipidemia: Drug therapy can be commenced after 6 weeks of lifestyle modification. See section on "Dyslipidemia."
- HTN: Aim for similar targets to patients with diabetes (<140/80 mm Hg based on ADA guidelines). See section on "Hypertension."
  - ACE inhibitor or angiotensin receptor blocker (e.g., losartan 50 mg/day if ACE inhibitor intolerance) is usually prescribed for patients with diabetes.
- Impaired glucose tolerance
  - Current guidelines emphasize that treatment should be with diet and exercise. The role of oral hypoglycemic agents to prevent diabetes in patients with the metabolic syndrome is unclear. Metformin, 500 mg to 1 g, 1 to 2 times daily, may be considered.
- If CAD or T2DM is already evident, treat as per guidelines. Use ASA 81 mg for primary prevention as indicated per USPSTF if benefits outweigh bleeding risk.

ISSUES FOR REFERRAL
- Obesity management
- Nutrition
- Exercise program
- Smoking cessation

SURGERY/OTHER PROCEDURES
- Bariatric surgery to treat obesity in severely obese patients who have failed trials of lifestyle modification and pharmacotherapy; surgery is recommended in appropriate individual if body mass index (BMI) >40 or BMI >35 with obesity-related comorbidities.
- Liposuction of abdominal adipose tissue does not reduce insulin resistance or cardiovascular risk factors.

COMPLEMENTARY & ALTERNATIVE MEDICINE
Fish oils and plant sterol esters for cardioprotective effects

INPATIENT CONSIDERATIONS
Management usually does not require admission.

Admission Criteria/Initial Stabilization
Serious complications (e.g., ACS, hypertensive crisis, diabetic coma)

ONGOING CARE

FOLLOW-UP RECOMMENDATIONS
- Regular 30-minute exercise will improve all components of the metabolic syndrome. Cumulative small periods of exercise over the day provide significant health benefits.
- Encourage changing sedentary activity choices (e.g., driving car, taking elevator, and the like) to more active ones (e.g., walking, cycling).
- Regular monitoring of weight, abdominal circumference measurements, BP, fasting lipids, and sugar levels

Patient Monitoring
- Regular monitoring of weight, abdominal circumference measurements, BP, fasting lipids, and sugar levels
- Fasting lipids, fasting sugar, and/or oral glucose tolerance test should be checked annually.

DIET
- Weight reduction to correct abdominal obesity is a primary goal achieved by dietary modification and increased physical activity.
- Dietary recommendations may include limiting simple carbohydrates in diet, eating a Mediterranean or DASH (Dietary Approaches to Stop Hypertension) diet.
- Increased consumption of leafy green vegetables may decrease risk of developing T2DM (11)[A]. Encourage increasing intake of vegetables and fiber, and keep fruit and alcohol in moderation.
- Avoid sugar-sweetened beverages.

PROGNOSIS
Increased risk of T2DM (~5-fold), CAD (~1.5 to 3-fold), acute myocardial infarction (~2.5-fold), and all-cause mortality (~1.5-fold)

COMPLICATIONS
Long-term complications are primarily CAD and T2DM. Recent evidence demonstrates an increased risk of NAFLD, stroke, and an increased risk of developing certain cancers, especially breast cancer in postmenopausal women.

REFERENCES
1. Ford ES, Li C, Zhao G. Prevalence and correlates of metabolic syndrome based on a harmonious definition among adults in the US. *J Diabetes.* 2010;2(3):180–193.
2. Zimmet P, Alberti KG, Kaufman F, et al. The metabolic syndrome in children and adolescents—an IDF consensus report. *Pediatr Diabetes.* 2007;8(5):299–306.
3. Magnussen CG, Koskinen J, Chen W, et al. Pediatric metabolic syndrome predicts adulthood metabolic syndrome, subclinical atherosclerosis, type 2 diabetes mellitus but is no better than body mass index alone: the Bogalusa Heart Study and the Cardiovascular Risk in Young Finns Study. *Circulation.* 2010;122(16):1604–1611.
4. Alberti KG, Eckel RH, Grudy SM, et al. Harmonizing the metabolic syndrome: a joint interim statement of the International Diabetes Federation Task Force on Epidemiology and Prevention; National Heart, Lung, and Blood Institute; American Heart Association; World Heart Federation; International Association for the Study of Obesity. *Circulation.* 2009;120(16):1640–1645.
5. Wofford MR, King DS, Harrell TK. Drug-induced metabolic syndrome. *J Clin Hypertens (Greenwich).* 2006;8(2):114–119.
6. Dunkley AJ, Charles K, Gray LJ, et al. Effectiveness of interventions for reducing diabetes and cardiovascular disease risk in people with metabolic syndrome: systematic review and mixed treatment comparison meta-analysis. *Diabetes Obes Metab.* 2012;14(7):616–625.
7. Shin JH, Gadde KM. Clinical utility of phentermine/topiramate (Qsymia™) combination for the treatment of obesity. *Diabetes Metab Syndr Obes.* 2013;6:131–139.
8. Chan EW, He Y, Chui CS, et al. Efficacy and safety of lorcaserin in obese adults: a meta-analysis of 1-year randomized controlled trials (RCTs) and narrative review of short-term RCTs. *Obes Rev.* 2013;14(5):383–392.
9. Pattyn N, Cornelissen VA, Eshghi SR, et al. The effect of exercise on the cardiovascular risk factors constituting the metabolic syndrome: a meta-analysis of controlled trials. *Sports Med.* 2013;43(2):121–133.
10. Lakka TA, Laaksonen DE. Physical activity in prevention and treatment of the metabolic syndrome. *Appl Physiol Nutr Metab.* 2007;32(1):76–88.
11. Carter P, Gray LJ, Troughton J, et al. Fruit and vegetable intake and incidence of type 2 diabetes mellitus: systematic review and meta-analysis. *BMJ.* 2010;341:c4229.

ADDITIONAL READING
Samson SL, Garber AJ. Metabolic syndrome. *Endocrinol Metab Clin North Am.* 2014;43(1):1–23.

CODES

ICD10
E88.81 Metabolic syndrome

CLINICAL PEARLS
- Abdominal circumference should be measured as part of a cardiovascular risk assessment.
- Recognizing metabolic syndrome in the clinic can help prioritize treatment goals and guidance to work to reduce associated risk factors.
- Prevention or reduction of obesity is the cornerstone of management of metabolic syndrome.
- Increasing cumulative physical activity over the day significantly adds to the benefit of regular 30 to 60-minute exercise regimen.
- Aggressive lifestyle modification is the first-line lifelong treatment for all patients.

M

METATARSALGIA

Michael Y. Yang, MD • Marc W. McKenna, MD

BASICS

DESCRIPTION
- Metatarsalgia is a generic term referring to pain in the forefoot in the region of the metatarsal heads.
- System affected: musculoskeletal

EPIDEMIOLOGY

Incidence
Especially common in athletes engaging in high-impact sports (running, jumping, dancing), in rock climbers (12.5%), and in older active adults.

Prevalence
Common

ETIOLOGY AND PATHOPHYSIOLOGY
- The 1st metatarsal head bears significant weight when walking or running. A normal metatarsal arch ensures this balance. The 1st metatarsal head normally has adequate padding to accommodate increased forces.
- Reactive tissue can build a callus around the metatarsal head, compounding the pain.
  - Excessive or repetitive stress. Forces are transmitted to the forefoot during several stages (midstance and push-off) of walking and running. These forces are translated across the metatarsal heads at nearly three times the body weight (1)[C].
  - A pronated splayfoot disturbs this balance, causing equal weight bearing on all metatarsal heads.
  - Any foot deformity changes distribution of weight, impacting areas of the foot that do not have sufficient padding.
  - Soft tissue dysfunction: intrinsic muscle weakness, laxity in the Lisfranc ligament
  - Abnormal foot posture: forefoot varus or valgus, cavus or equinus deformities, loss of the metatarsal arch, splayfoot, pronated foot, inappropriate footwear
  - Dermatologic: warts, calluses (2)[C]
- Great toe
  - Hallux valgus (bunion), either varus or rigidus
- Lesser metatarsals
  - Freiberg infraction (i.e., aseptic necrosis of the metatarsal head usually due to trauma in adolescents who jump or sprint)
  - Hammer toe or claw toe
  - Morton syndrome (i.e., long 2nd metatarsal)

RISK FACTORS
- Obesity
- High heels, narrow shoes, or overly tight-fitting shoes (rock climbers typically wear small shoes)
- Competitive athletes in weight-bearing sports (e.g., ballet, basketball, running, soccer, baseball, football)
- Foot deformities or changes in ROM (e.g., pes planus, pes cavus, tight Achilles tendon, tarsal tunnel syndrome, hallux valgus, prominent metatarsal heads, excessive pronation, hammer toe deformity, tight toe extensors) (2)[C]

Geriatric Considerations
- Concomitant arthritis
- Metatarsalgia is common in older athletes.
- Age-related atrophy of the metatarsal fat pad may increase the risk for metatarsalgia.

Pediatric Considerations
- Muscle imbalance disorders (e.g., Duchenne muscular dystrophy) cause foot deformities in children.
- In adolescent girls, consider Freiberg infraction.
- Salter I injuries may affect subsequent growth and healing of the epiphysis.

Pregnancy Considerations
- Forefoot pain during pregnancy usually results from change in gait, center of mass, and joint laxity.
- Wear properly fitted, low-heeled shoes.

GENERAL PREVENTION
- Wear properly fitted shoes with good padding.
- Start weight-bearing exercise programs gradually.

COMMONLY ASSOCIATED CONDITIONS
- Arthritis
- Morton neuroma
- Sesamoiditis
- Plantar keratosis–callous formation

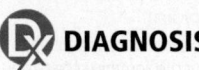

DIAGNOSIS

HISTORY
- Pain gradually develops and persists over the heads of one or more metatarsals. Pain is usually on the plantar surface and worse during midstance gait phase.
- Pain is often chronic.
- Predisposition with pes cavus and hyperpronation
- Pain often described as walking with a pebble in the shoe; aggravated during midstance or propulsion phases of walking or running.

PHYSICAL EXAM
- Point tenderness over plantar metatarsal heads
- Pain in the interdigital space or a positive metatarsal squeeze test suggests Morton neuroma.
- Plantar keratosis
- Tenderness of the metatarsal head(s) with pressure applied by the examiner's finger and thumb
- Erythema and swelling (occasionally)

DIFFERENTIAL DIAGNOSIS
- Stress fracture (most commonly 2nd metatarsal)
- Morton neuroma (i.e., interdigital neuroma)
- Tarsal tunnel syndrome
- Sesamoiditis or sesamoid fracture
- Salter I fracture in children
- Arthritis (e.g., gouty, rheumatoid, inflammatory, osteoarthritis, septic, calcium pyrophosphate dihydrate crystal deposit disease [CPPD])

- Lisfranc injury
- Avascular necrosis of the metatarsal head
- Ganglion cyst
- Foreign body
- Vasculitis (diabetes)
- Bony tumors

DIAGNOSTIC TESTS & INTERPRETATION

Initial Tests (lab, imaging)
- Weight-bearing radiographs: anteroposterior, lateral, and oblique views:
  - Occasionally, metatarsal or sesamoid axial films (to rule out sesamoid fracture) or skyline view of the metatarsal heads to assess the plantar declination of the metatarsal heads: obtained with the metatarsophalangeal joints in dorsiflexion (to evaluate alignment)
- Ultrasound and MRI in recalcitrant cases especially if concern for stress fracture (3)[C]
- MR arthrography of the metatarsophalangeal (MTP) joint can delineate capsular tears, typically of the distal lateral border of the plantar plate (an often underrecognized cause of metatarsalgia.
- Only if diagnosis is in question
  - Erythrocyte sedimentation rate or C-reactive protein
  - Rheumatoid factor
  - Uric acid
  - Glucose
  - CBC with differential

Diagnostic Procedures/Other
Plantar pressure distribution analysis may help distinguish pressure distribution patterns due to malalignment.

TREATMENT

Treatment for metatarsalgia is typically conservative.
- Relieve pain
- Ice initially
- Rest: temporary alteration of weight-bearing activity; use of cane or crutch. For more physically active patients, suggest an alternative exercise or cross-training:
  - Moist heat later
  - Taping or gel cast
  - Stiff-soled shoes will act as a splint.
- Relieve the pressure beneath the area of maximal pain by redistributing the pressure load of the foot, which can be achieved by weight loss.

MEDICATION
Nonsteroidal anti-inflammatory medications for 7 to 14 days if no contraindications toward use

ISSUES FOR REFERRAL
High-level athletes may benefit from early podiatric or orthopedic evaluation.

ADDITIONAL THERAPIES
- Physical therapy to restore normal foot biomechanics
- Low-heeled (<2 cm height) wide-toe-box shoes
- Metatarsal bars, pads, and arch supports. Metatarsal bars are often more effective than pads.
- Orthotics/rocker bar (prescriptive orthotics have been shown to be effective treatment)
- Thick-soled shoes
- Shaving the callus may provide temporary relief. Callus excision is not recommended.
- Corticosteroid injection may benefit interdigital neuritis but should be used with caution as it may cause MTP instability and fat pad atrophy.
- Improve flexibility and strength of the intrinsic muscles of the foot with:
  - Exercises (e.g., towel grasps, pencil curls)
  - Physical therapy to maintain range of motion and restore normal biomechanics

SURGERY/OTHER PROCEDURES
- If no improvement with conservative therapy for 3 months, refer to foot/ankle orthopedic surgeon or podiatrist.
- Surgery may help correct anatomic abnormality: bunionectomy, partial osteotomy, or surgical fusion. Success rates vary depending on procedure.
- Direct plantar plate repair (grade II tear) combined with Weil osteotomy can restore normal alignment of the MTP joint, leading to diminished pain with improved functional scores.
- The Weil osteotomy (distal metatarsal oblique osteotomy) is safe and effective for metatarsalgia.
- Callus removal is generally not recommended (callus is a response to pressure change—not the cause).
- Morton neurectomy or ultrasound-guided alcohol ablation of Morton neuroma are options (4)[C].
- Surgery only as a last resort if no anatomic abnormality is present.

COMPLEMENTARY & ALTERNATIVE MEDICINE
Magnetic insoles are not effective for chronic non-specific foot pain.

INPATIENT CONSIDERATIONS
Admission Criteria/Initial Stabilization
Patients generally admitted only for surgery

 ## ONGOING CARE

FOLLOW-UP RECOMMENDATIONS
Patient Monitoring
If stress fracture has been ruled out and patient's condition has not improved >3 months of conservative treatment, consider surgical evaluation.

PATIENT EDUCATION
- Instruct about wearing proper shoes and gradual return to activity.
- Cross-training until symptoms subside. Goal is to restore normal foot biomechanics, relieve abnormal pressure on the plantar metatarsal heads, and relieve pain (5)[C].

PROGNOSIS
Outcome depends on the severity of the problem and whether surgery is required to correct it.

COMPLICATIONS
- Back, knee, and hip pain due to change in gait
- Transfer metatarsalgia following surgical intervention, which subsequently transfers stress to other areas.

REFERENCES

1. Hockenbury RT. Forefoot problems in athletes. *Med Sci Sports Exerc*. 1999;31(7 Suppl):S448–S458.
2. DiPreta JA. Metatarsalgia, lesser toe deformities, and associated disorders of the forefoot. *Med Clin North Am*. 2014;98(2):233–251.
3. Iagnocco A, Coari G, Palombi G, et al. Sonography in the study of metatarsalgia. *J Rheumatol*. 2001;28(6):1338–1340.
4. Musson RE, Sawhney JS, Lamb L, et al. Ultrasound guided alcohol ablation of Morton's neuroma. *Foot Ankle Int*. 2012;33(3):196–201.
5. Espinosa N, Brodsky JW, Maceira E. Metatarsalgia. *J Am Acad Orthop Surg*. 2010;18(8):474–485.

ADDITIONAL READING

- Birbilis T, Theodoropoulou E, Koulalis D. Forefoot complaints—the Morton's metatarsalgia. The role of MR imaging. *Acta Medica (Hradec Kralove)*. 2007;50(3):221–222.
- Buda R, Di Caprio F, Bedetti L, et al. Foot overuse diseases in rock climbing: an epidemiologic study. *J Am Podiatr Med Assoc*. 2013;103(2):113–120.
- Burns J, Landorf KB, Ryan MM, et al. Interventions for the prevention and treatment of pes cavus. *Cochrane Database Syst Rev*. 2007;(4):CD006154.

- Deshaies A, Roy P, Symeonidis PD, et al. Metatarsal bars more effective than metatarsal pads in reducing impulse on the second metatarsal head. *Foot (Edinb)*. 2011;21(4):172–175.
- Janisse DJ, Janisse E. Shoe modification and the use of orthoses in the treatment of foot and ankle pathology. *J Am Acad Orthop Surg*. 2008;16(3):152–158.
- Ko PH, Hsiao TY, Kang JH, et al. Relationship between plantar pressure and soft tissue strain under metatarsal heads with different heel heights. *Foot Ankle Int*. 2009;30(11):1111–1116.
- Pace A, Scammell B, Dhar S. The outcome of Morton's neurectomy in the treatment of metatarsalgia. *Int Orthop*. 2010;34(4):511–515.
- Thomas JL, Blitch EL IV, Chaney DM, et al. Diagnosis and treatment of forefoot disorders. Section 2. Central metatarsalgia. *J Foot Ankle Surg*. 2009;48(2):239–250.

 ## SEE ALSO

Morton Neuroma (Interdigital Neuroma)

CODES

ICD10
- M77.40 Metatarsalgia, unspecified foot
- G57.60 Lesion of plantar nerve, unspecified lower limb
- M77.42 Metatarsalgia, left foot

CLINICAL PEARLS
- Metatarsalgia refers to pain of the plantar surface of the forefoot in the region of the metatarsal heads.
- Metatarsalgia is common in athletes who participate in high-impact sports involving the lower extremities.
- Patients describe as "walking with a pebble in the shoe." Pain is worse during midstance or propulsion phases of walking or running.
- The most common physical finding is point tenderness over plantar metatarsal heads.
- Pregnant patients should wear properly fitted, low-heeled shoes to reduce incidence of metatarsalgia.

METHICILLIN-RESISTANT *STAPHYLOCOCCUS AUREUS* (MRSA) SKIN INFECTIONS

Stephen A. Martin, MD, EdM • Paul P. Belliveau, PharmD, RPh

 BASICS

DESCRIPTION
- Community-acquired methicillin-resistant *Staphylococcus aureus* (CA-MRSA) has unique properties allowing the organism to cause skin and soft tissue infections (SSTIs) in healthy hosts:
  - CA-MRSA has a different virulence and disease pattern than hospital-acquired MRSA (HA-MRSA).
- CA-MRSA infections impact patients who have not been recently (<1 year) hospitalized or had a medical procedure (e.g., dialysis, surgery, catheters).
- *The prevalence of CA-MRSA is rapidly increasing in the United States.*
- CA-MRSA typically causes mild to moderate SSTIs, particularly abscesses, furuncles, and carbuncles:
  - Severe or invasive disease from CA-MRSA is less frequent but can include the following:
    - Necrotizing pneumonia with abscesses
    - Necrotizing fasciitis
    - Septic thrombophlebitis
    - Sepsis
    - Osteomyelitis
- Although less frequent, HA-MRSA can still cause SSTIs in the community. One study showed no significant difference in hospitalization rates among CA-MRSA, HA-MRSA, and methicillin-sensitive *S. aureus* (MSSA) infections.
- System(s) affected: skin, soft tissue

EPIDEMIOLOGY
- Predominant age: all ages, generally younger
- Predominant sex: female > male

Incidence
- 316/100,000/year (2004 to 2005)
- 46/100,000/year pediatric MRSA SSTI hospitalizations (2009)

Prevalence
- Significantly affected by local epidemiology
- 25–30% of U.S. population are colonized with *S. aureus*; up to 7% are colonized with MRSA.
- CA-MRSA isolated in ~60% of SSTIs presenting to emergency departments (range 15–74%). In 1993, 1.5 million SSTIs were seen in U.S. emergency rooms. In 2005, this had increased to 3.4 million. Hospital admissions for SSTIs increased 29% between 2000 and 2004.
- CA-MRSA accounts for up to 75% of all community staphylococcal infections in children.

ETIOLOGY AND PATHOPHYSIOLOGY
- First noted in 1980. Current U.S. CA-MRSA epidemic began in 1999. The United States 300 clone is predominant.
- CA-MRSA is distinguished from HA-MRSA by
  - Lack of a multidrug-resistant phenotype
  - Presence of exotoxin virulence factors
  - Type IV *Staphylococcus* cassette cartridge (contains the methicillin-resistance gene *mecA*)

RISK FACTORS
- ~50% of patients with CA-MRSA do not have an obvious risk factor
- Use of any antibiotic in the past month.
- Presence of an abscess

- Reported "spider bite"
- History of MRSA infection
- Close contact with a similar infection
- Children, particularly in daycare centers
- Competitive athletes
- Incarceration
- Hospitalization in the past 12 months (although *S. aureus* can colonize for years)

GENERAL PREVENTION
- Colonization (particularly of the anterior nares) is a risk factor for subsequent *S. aureus* infection. It is not clear whether this is the case for CA-MRSA. Oropharyngeal and inguinal colonization are equally prevalent.
- CA-MRSA may be transmitted more easily through environmental and household contact (1)[B].
- Health care workers are a primary MRSA vector for hospitalized patients, reinforcing the need for meticulous cleaning of hands and equipment.
- Research for a vaccine is underway.
- CDC guidance for prevention of MRSA in athletes: http://www.cdc.gov/mrsa/community/team-hc-providers/advice-for-athletes.html

COMMONLY ASSOCIATED CONDITIONS
Many patients are otherwise healthy.

 DIAGNOSIS

HISTORY
- Review potential risk factors.
- "Spider bite" is commonly confused with MRSA—patients may report an unclear history of spider bite.
- Prior MRSA skin infection
- Risk factors alone cannot rule in or rule out a CA-MRSA infection.

PHYSICAL EXAM
- Furuncles and/or carbuncles, sometimes with surrounding cellulitis. A nonsuppurative cellulitis is also possible, although it is a less common presentation of CA-MRSA.
- Erythema, warmth, tenderness, swelling
- Fluctuance
- Folliculitis, pustular lesions
- Appearance like an insect or spider bite
- Tissue necrosis

DIFFERENTIAL DIAGNOSIS
SSTIs due to another cause

DIAGNOSTIC TESTS & INTERPRETATION
Initial Tests (lab, imaging)
- Wound cultures establish definitive diagnosis. Recent guidelines recommend cultures only when a purulent lesion is accompanied by systemic signs of illness or immunocompromise (2)[B].
- Susceptibility testing; many labs use oxacillin instead of methicillin.
- A "D-zone disk-diffusion test" evaluates for inducible clindamycin resistance in CA-MRSA resistant to erythromycin.

- In unclear cases, ultrasound may help identify abscesses (3,4)[A].
- Although CT or MRI may show fascial plane edema in necrotizing fasciitis, do not delay surgical intervention waiting for imaging, particularly in ill patients.

Diagnostic Procedures/Other
Purulent lesions should be incised and drained (I&D); needle aspiration is not recommended (2).

TREATMENT
- Recent guidelines recommends treating with antibiotics active against MRSA for patients with carbuncles or abscesses who failed initial antibiotic treatment, have markedly impaired host defenses, or present with systemic inflammatory response (SIRS) and hypotension (2).
- Routine use of agents to eliminate MRSA colonization for patients with active infection or their close contacts is not currently recommended.
- Most CA-MRSA infections are localized SSTIs and not requiring hospitalization or vancomycin.
- Initial empirical antibiotic coverage should be based on local CA-MRSA prevalence and individual patient risk factors.
- http://www.cdc.gov/mrsa/pdf/Flowchart_pstr.pdf

GENERAL MEASURES
- Modify therapy based on culture and susceptibility.
- Determine if household or other close contacts have SSTI or other infections and evaluate accordingly.
- Treat underlying condition (e.g., tinea pedis).
- Restrict contact if wound cannot be covered.
- Elevate affected area.

MEDICATION
ALERT
For purulent infections, consider surgical drainage and debulking, wound culture, and narrow-spectrum antimicrobials:

- Successful I&D may have more impact than antibiotics in mild cases for both adults and children.
- Moist heat may work for small furuncles.
- Patients with an abscess are frequently cured by incision and drainage alone.

- Packing does not appear to improve outcomes (3)[A].

First Line
CA-MRSA SSTIs: 7- to 14-day course (depends on severity and clinical response):
- Trimethoprim/sulfamethoxazole (TMP-SMX): DS (160 mg TMP and 800 mg of SMX) 1 to 2 tablet(s) PO BID daily (8 to 12 mg/kg/day of trimethoprim component in 2 divided doses for children)
- Doxycycline or minocycline: 100 mg PO BID (children >8 years and <45 kg; 2 to 5 mg/kg/day PO in 1 to 2 divided doses, not to exceed 200 mg/day; children >8 years and >45 kg, use adult dosing), taken with a full glass of water

- Clindamycin: 300 to 450 mg PO QID (30 to 40 mg/kg/day PO in 3 divided doses for children), taken with full glass of water. Check D-zone test in erythromycin-resistant, clindamycin-susceptible *S. aureus* isolates (a positive test indicates induced resistance—choose a differnt antibiotic).
- CA-MRSA is resistant to β-lactams (including oral cephalosporins and antistaphylococcal penicillins) and often macrolides, azalides, and quinolones.
- Although most CA-MRSA isolates are susceptible to rifampin, this drug should *never* be used as a single agent because of concerns regarding resistance. The role of combination therapy with rifampin in CA-MRSA SSTIs is not clearly defined.
- There has been increasing resistance to clindamycin, both initial (~33%) and induced.
- Although CA-MRSA isolates are susceptible to vancomycin, oral vancomycin cannot be used for CA-MRSA SSTIs due to limited absorption.

Second Line
Treat severe CA-MRSA SSTIs requiring hospitalization and HA-MRSA SSTIs using:

- Vancomycin: Generally, 1 g IV q12h (30 mg/kg/day IV in 2 divided doses; in children: 40 mg/kg/day IV in 4 divided doses) vancomycin-like antibiotics that require only 1 or 2 doses may soon be more broadly available (5)[A].
- Linezolid: 600 mg IV/PO BID uncomplicated: children <5 years of age, 30 mg/kg/day in 3 divided doses; 20 mg/kg/day IV/PO in 2 divided doses for children 5 to 11 years of age; children >11 years, use adult dosing. Complicated: birth to 11 years, 30 mg/kg/day IV/PO in 3 divided doses; older, use adult dosing)
  - Linezolid seems to be more effective than vancomycin for treating people with SSTIs, but current studies have high risk of bias.
- Clindamycin: 600 mg IV TID; in children, 10 to 13 mg/kg/dose q6–8h up to 40 mg/kg/day
- Daptomycin: 4 mg/kg/day IV (safety/efficacy not established in patients <18 years of age) if no pulmonary involvement
- Ceftaroline 600 mg BID IV (for adults)

Pediatric Considerations
- Tetracyclines not recommended <8 years of age
- TMP-SMX not recommended <2 months

Pregnancy Considerations
- Tetracyclines are contraindicated.
- TMP-SMX not recommended in 1st or 3rd trimester

Geriatric Considerations
A recent review notes no prospective trials in this age group and recommends use of general adult guidelines.

ISSUES FOR REFERRAL
Consider consultation with infectious disease in cases of
- Refractory CA-MRSA infection
- Plan to attempt decolonization

SURGERY/OTHER PROCEDURES
Progression to serious SSTIs, including necrotizing fasciitis, is possible and mandates prompt surgical evaluation.

INPATIENT CONSIDERATIONS
Admission Criteria/Initial Stabilization
Consider admission if:
- Systemically ill (e.g., febrile) with stable comorbidities
- Systemically well with comorbidities that may delay or complicate resolution of SSTI
- Presence of SSTI complications (sepsis, necrotizing fasciitis) and comorbidities
- If indicated, alternatives to inpatient admission include observation units and outpatient parenteral antimicrobial therapy (OPAT) programs

Nursing
Contact precautions

Discharge Criteria
If admitted for IV therapy, assess the following before discharge:
- Afebrile for 24 hours
- Clinically improved
- Able to take oral medication
- Has adequate social support and is available for outpatient follow-up

 ONGOING CARE

FOLLOW-UP RECOMMENDATIONS
Patient Monitoring
For outpatients:
- Return promptly with systemic symptoms, worsening local symptoms, or failure to improve within 48 hours. Consider a follow-up within 48 hours of initial visit to assess response and review culture.

PATIENT EDUCATION
- Keep wounds that are draining covered with clean, dry bandages.
- Clean hands regularly with soap and water or alcohol-based gel. Hot soapy shower daily.
- Do not share items that may be contaminated (including razors or towels).
- Clean clothes, towels, and bed linens
- National MRSA Education Initiative: www.cdc.gov/mrsa/
- A mixture of 1/4-cup household bleach diluted in 1 gallon of water can be used to clean surfaces.

PROGNOSIS
In outpatients, improvement should occur within 48 hours.

COMPLICATIONS
- Necrotizing pneumonia or empyema (after an influenza-like illness)
- Necrotizing fasciitis
- Sepsis syndrome
- Pyomyositis and osteomyelitis
- Purpura fulminans
- Disseminated septic emboli
- Endocarditis

REFERENCES

1. Uhlemann AC, Dordel J, Knox JR, et al. Molecular tracing of the emergence, diversification, and transmission of *S. aureus* sequence type 8 in a New York community. *Proc Natl Acad Sci U S A*. 2014;111(18):6738–6743.
2. Stevens DL, Bisno AL, Chambers HF, et al. Practice guidelines for the diagnosis and management of skin and soft tissue infections: 2014 update by the Infectious Diseases Society of America. *Clin Infect Dis*. 2014;59(2):e10–e52.
3. Mistry RD. Skin and soft tissue infections. *Pediatr Clin North Am*. 2013;60(5):1063–1082.
4. Singer AJ, Talan DA. Management of skin abscesses in the era of methicillin-resistant *Staphylococcus aureus*. *N Engl J Med*. 2014;370(11):1039–1047.
5. Chambers HF. Pharmacology and the treatment of complicated skin and skin-structure infections. *N Engl J Med*. 2014;370(23):2238–2239.

ADDITIONAL READING
- Amin AN, Cerceo EA, Deitelzweig SB, et al. Hospitalist perspective on the treatment of skin and soft tissue infections. *Mayo Clin Proc*. 2014;89(10):1436–1451.
- Chen LF, Chastain C, Anderson DJ. Community-acquired methicillin-resistant *Staphylococcus aureus* skin and soft tissue infections: management and prevention. *Curr Infect Dis Rep*. 2011;13(5): 442–450.
- Fenster DB, Renny MH, Ng C, et al. Scratching the surface: a review of skin and soft tissue infections in children. *Curr Opin Pediatr*. 2015;27(3):303–307.
- Fitch MT, Manthey DE, McGinnis HD, et al. Videos in clinical medicine. Abscess incision and drainage. *N Engl J Med*. 2007;357(19):e20.
- Gurusamy KS, Koti R, Toon CD, et al. Antibiotic therapy for the treatment of methicillin-resistant *Staphylococcus aureus* (MRSA) infections in surgical wounds. *Cochrane Database Syst Rev*. 2013;(8):CD009726.
- Holmes NE, Howden BP. What's new in the treatment of serious MRSA infection? *Curr Opin Infect Dis*. 2014;27(6):471–478.
- Ramakrishnan K, Salinas RC, Agudelo Higuita NI. Skin and soft tissue infections. *Am Fam Physician*. 2015;92(6):474–483.

 CODES

ICD10
- A49.02 Methicillin resis staph infection, unsp site
- A41.02 Sepsis due to Methicillin resistant Staphylococcus aureus
- J15.212 Pneumonia due to Methicillin resistant Staphylococcus aureus

CLINICAL PEARLS
- Incise and drain purulent lesions and send for wound culture if abscess is present.
- Local susceptibility patterns of CA-MRSA dictate antibiotic treatment. The CDC has a helpful algorithm for outpatient treatment of CA-MRSA: http://www.cdc.gov/mrsa/pdf/Flowchart_pstr.pdf
- CA-MRSA skin lesions are commonly misidentified as "spider bites".

M

MILD COGNITIVE IMPAIRMENT

Birju B. Patel, MD, FACP, AGSF • N. Wilson Holland, MD, FACP, AGSF

 BASICS

DESCRIPTION

- Mild cognitive impairment (MCI) is defined as significant cognitive impairment in the absence of dementia, as measured by standard memory tests:
  - Concern regarding change in cognition
  - Preservation of independence in functional activities (ADLs)
  - Impairment in ≥1 cognitive domains (attention, executive dysfunction, memory, visuospatial, language) (1)
  - Other terms used in the literature relating to MCI: isolated memory impairment; cognitive impairment not dementia (CIND); predementia; mild cognitive disorder; age-associated memory impairment; age-related cognitive decline; benign senescent forgetfulness. Some of these conditions do not progress to dementia (i.e., benign senescent forgetfulness, age-associated memory impairment, age-related cognitive decline). *DSM-5* mentions "mild neurocognitive disorder" (NCD) which may be a precursor to Alzheimer disease and has many of the same features as MCI (2).
- Annual rates of conversion of MCI to dementia are 2–15% in the elderly.

EPIDEMIOLOGY

Incidence

- Predominant sex: male > female (3)
- Predominant age:
  - Higher in older persons and in those with less education
  - 12 to 15/1,000 person-years in those age ≥65 years
  - 54/1,000 person-years in those age ≥75 years

Prevalence

- MCI is more prevalent than dementia in the United States.
- 3–5% for those age ≥60 years
- 15% for those age ≥75 years

ETIOLOGY AND PATHOPHYSIOLOGY

- Subtypes of MCI:
  - Single-domain amnestic
  - Multiple-domain amnestic
  - Nonamnestic single-domain
  - Nonamnestic multiple-domain
- The amnestic subtype is higher risk for progression to Alzheimer disease (4).
- Vascular, degenerative, traumatic, metabolic, psychiatric, or a combination

Genetics

Apolipoprotein (APO) E4 genotype: Various pathways exist leading to amyloid accumulation and deposition thought to be associated with dementia.

RISK FACTORS

- Age
- Diabetes
- Hypertension
- Hyperlipidemia
- Cerebrovascular disease
- Smoking
- Sleep apnea
- APO E4 genotype

COMMONLY ASSOCIATED CONDITIONS

See "Risk Factors" (5).

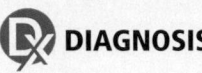 DIAGNOSIS

HISTORY

- Focus on cognitive deficits and impairment.
- Review all medications that may affect cognition; give particular emphasis to anticholinergic medications (patients on these may mistakenly be classified as having MCI).
- Rule out depression.
- Assess function (ADLs, instrumental ADLs) and subtle changes in daily function (e.g., in the workplace).
- Impact on interpersonal relationships and caregiver stress
- Assess vascular risk factors (hypertension, diabetes, hyperlipidemia, and cerebrovascular disease).
- Assess behavioral changes.

PHYSICAL EXAM

- A general exam focusing on clinical clues to identifying vascular disease (e.g., bruits, abnormal BP)
- Neurologic exam to rule out reversible CNS causes cognitive impairment or other causes of cognitive impairment (e.g., Parkinson disease).
- Office measures of cognitive function, depression, and functional status

DIFFERENTIAL DIAGNOSIS

- Delirium
- Dementia
- Depression
- "Reversible" cognitive impairment
  - Medications (anticholinergics and medications with anticholinergic properties)
  - Hypothyroidism
  - Vitamin B$_{12}$ deficiency
- Reversible CNS conditions
- Give consideration to sleep conditions, especially sleep apnea, that can contribute to cognitive deficits.

DIAGNOSTIC TESTS & INTERPRETATION

Initial Tests (lab, imaging)

- CBC
- Comprehensive metabolic profile
- Thyroid-stimulating hormone
- Vitamin B$_{12}$
- Lipids
- Consider HIV testing in the appropriate risk setting.
- Imaging tests are helpful when there are focal neurologic deficits or rapid or atypical presentations:
  - CT scan can detect structural CNS conditions leading to cognitive impairment:
    - Subdural hematoma
    - Normal pressure hydrocephalus
    - Metastatic disease
  - MRI further evaluates vascular, infectious, neoplastic, and inflammatory conditions.
- Cognitive testing is important (e.g., Montreal Cognitive Assessment [MOCA] and Saint Louis University Mental Status [SLUMS]); MOCA may be more sensitive for detecting and following MCI.
- Neuropsychological testing for complex and atypical presentations
- Vascular risk factor reduction and treatment

Follow-Up Tests & Special Considerations

- Document progression of functional impairment, cognitive decline, concurrent depression, and comorbid conditions.
- Advanced planning while patient is competent.
- Early education of caregivers on safety, maintaining structure, managing stress, and future planning

Test Interpretation

- Little is known about MCI pathology due to a lack of longitudinal studies.
- Alzheimer dementia pathophysiology:
  - Neurofibrillary tangles in hippocampus
  - Senile plaques (amyloid deposition)
  - Neuronal degeneration
- Those with MCI have intermediate amounts of pathologic findings of Alzheimer disease with amyloid deposition and neurofibrillary tangles in the mesial temporal lobes compared with those with dementia.
- Amnestic MCI is associated with white matter hyperintensity volume on MRI, whereas nonamnestic MCI is associated with infarcts.

TREATMENT

GENERAL MEASURES
Atherosclerotic risk factors should be treated aggressively.

MEDICATION
The use of cholinesterase inhibitors (ChEIs) in MCI is not associated with any delay in the onset of Alzheimer disease or dementia. Moreover, the safety profile showed that the risks associated with ChEIs are significant. Therefore, ChEIs are not routinely recommended (6)[A],(7)[C].

ISSUES FOR REFERRAL
Consider referral to a memory specialist (i.e., geriatrician, neurologist, geropsychiatrist, neuropsychologist) to evaluate and differentiate subtypes of MCI and specific cognitive deficits.

ADDITIONAL THERAPIES
There may be benefit in terms of improvement in performance on tests for global cognitive functioning with cognitive training and physical exercise (2)[C]

COMPLEMENTARY & ALTERNATIVE MEDICINE
• No evidence suggests the efficacy of vitamin E in the prevention or treatment of people with MCI. More research is needed to identify the role of vitamin E, if any, in the management of cognitive impairment.

• Long-term use of ginkgo biloba extract has shown to have no benefit in the treatment of MCI and in terms of progression to dementia. In addition, ginkgo biloba can be associated with increase in bleeding risk including CNS bleeds (8)[B].

INPATIENT CONSIDERATIONS
• Delirium is more common in patients hospitalized with all forms of cognitive impairment.
• Avoid medications that may worsen or precipitate cognitive decline (e.g., anticholinergics, antihistamines).
• Patients may be extremely sensitive to the hospital environment:
  – Moderate level of stimulation is best.
  – Avoid sensory deprivation. Make sure that patients have access to hearing aids and eyeglasses.
  – Use frequent cueing and have caregivers or family in the room whenever possible with patient.
  – Frequently orient patients to date and time.

ONGOING CARE

FOLLOW-UP RECOMMENDATIONS
Patients should be reevaluated every 6 to 12 months to determine if symptoms are progressing.

Patient Monitoring
Appropriate cognitive and functional testing should be used to evaluate progression, along with clinical history and exam. If a medication is started, patients need to be followed more frequently to evaluate for efficacy, side effects, dose titration, and so forth. Declining executive function may be an early marker to progression of MCI to dementia, and clinicians should monitor and advise patients and families proactively to look for this. Impairments in ADL function is a good clue to progression to dementia from MCI.

DIET
Diets that are promoted by the American Heart Association to minimize atherosclerotic risk factors should be emphasized.

PATIENT EDUCATION
• Encourage lifestyle changes:
  – Physical activity, such as walking 30 minutes daily on most days of the week
  – Mental activity that stimulates language skills and psychomotor coordination should be encouraged. Computer activities, reading books, crafts, crossword puzzles, and games may be linked to decreased risk of development of MCI (9)[C],(10)[B].
• Cognitive rehabilitation strategies may be beneficial in helping with daily activities relating to memory tasks in MCI.
• Participation in exercise programs modestly improved some measures of cognition in some studies.
• Treatment of vascular risk factors (hypertension, diabetes, cerebrovascular disease, and hyperlipidemia) is important in lowering risk of progression to dementia.

PROGNOSIS
• Conversion rates from MCI to dementia range from 5% to 15% annually.
• Amnestic subtypes of MCI are most likely to progress to dementia.
• MCI has prognostic value in that once it is diagnosed, there is a higher risk of progression to dementia (11)[B].

REFERENCES

1. Petersen RC. Clinical practice. Mild cognitive impairment. *N Engl J Med.* 2011;364(23):2227–2234.
2. Petersen RC, Caracciolo B, Brayne C, et al. Mild cognitive impairment: a concept in evolution. *J Intern Med.* 2014;275(3):214–228.
3. Petersen RC, Roberts RO, Knopman DS, et al. Prevalence of mild cognitive impairment is higher in men. The Mayo Clinic Study of Aging. *Neurology.* 2010;75(10):889–897.
4. Albert MS, DeKosky ST, Dickson D, et al. The diagnosis of mild cognitive impairment due to Alzheimer's disease: recommendations from the National Institute on Aging-Alzheimer's Association workgroups on diagnostic guidelines for Alzheimer's disease. *Alzheimers Dement.* 2011;7(3):270–279.
5. Li J, Wang YJ, Zhang M, et al. Vascular risk factors promote conversion from mild cognitive impairment to Alzheimer disease. *Neurology.* 2011;76(17):1485–1491.
6. Russ TC, Morling JR. Cholinesterase inhibitors for mild cognitive impairment. *Cochrane Database Syst Rev.* 2012;(9):CD009132.
7. Patel BP, Holland NW. Adverse effects of acetylcholinesterase inhibitors clinical geriatrics. *Clin Geriatr.* 2011;19:27–30.
8. Vellas B, Coley N, Ousset PJ, et al. Long-term use of standardised ginkgo biloba extract for the prevention of Alzheimer's disease (GuidAge): a randomised placebo-controlled trial. *Lancet Neurol.* 2012;11(10):851–859.
9. Marshall GA, Rentz DM, Frey MT, et al. Executive function and instrumental activities of daily living in mild cognitive impairment and Alzheimer's disease. *Alzheimers Dement.* 2011;7(3):300–308.
10. Nagamatsu LS, Handy TC, Hsu CL, et al. Resistance training promotes cognitive and functional brain plasticity in seniors with probable mild cognitive impairment. *Arch Intern Med.* 2012;172(8):666–668.
11. Roberts RO, Knopman DS, Mielke MM, et al. Higher risk of progression to dementia in mild cognitive impairment cases who revert to normal. *Neurology.* 2014;82(4):317–325.

CODES

ICD10
G31.84 Mild cognitive impairment, so stated

CLINICAL PEARLS
• Amnestic MCI affects primarily memory and is more likely to progress to Alzheimer dementia.
• Screen for reversible factors, particularly anticholinergic medications, depression, and sleep disorders.
• Look closely at vascular risk factors and modify them as best as possible.
• ChEIs should not be used routinely unless memory complaints are affecting quality of life in patients. Potential side effects of these medications should be thoroughly discussed with patients and their families. A baseline EKG should be done prior to initiation of ChEIs due to risk of bradycardia and syncope.
• Encourage both physical and mental exercises.

M

MITRAL REGURGITATION

Yongkasem Vorasettakarnkij, MD, MSc

BASICS

DESCRIPTION
- Disorder of mitral valve (MV) closure, either primary or secondary (functional), resulting in a backflow of the left ventricular (LV) stroke volume into the left atrium (LA); uncompensated, this leads to LV and LA enlargement, elevated pulmonary pressures, atrial fibrillation, heart failure, and sudden cardiac death
- Types of mitral regurgitation (MR):
  - Acute versus chronic
  - Primary versus secondary (functional)
    - Primary: MV structures include not only the mitral annulus, MV leaflets, chordae tendineae, and papillary muscles but also posterior LA wall and LV wall.
    - Secondary: No valvular abnormalities are found. The abnormal and dilated LV causes papillary muscle displacement, resulting in leaflet tethering with annular dilatation that prevents coaptation.
- System(s) affected: cardiac; pulmonary

EPIDEMIOLOGY
Moderate to severe MR affects 2.5 million people in the United States (2000 data). It is the most common valvular disease, and its prevalence is expected to double by 2030 (1).

Prevalence
- By severity on echocardiography:
  - Mild MR: 19% (up to 40% if trivial jets included)
  - Moderate MR: 1.9%
  - Severe MR: 0.2%
- By category (1)
  - Degenerative (myxomatous disease, annular calcification): 60–70%
  - Ischemic: 20%
  - Endocarditis: 2–5%
  - Rheumatic: 2–5%

ETIOLOGY AND PATHOPHYSIOLOGY
- Acute MR: acute damage to MV leads to sudden LA and LV volume overload. Sudden rise in LV volume load without compensatory LV remodeling results in impaired forward cardiac output and possible cardiogenic shock.
- Chronic MR: LV eccentric hypertrophy compensates for increased regurgitant volume to maintain forward cardiac output and alleviate pulmonary congestion. However, ongoing LV remodeling can result in LV dysfunction. Simultaneously, LA compensatory dilatation for the larger regurgitant volume predisposes patients to develop atrial fibrillation (AF).
- Ischemic MR: papillary muscle rupture, ischemia during acute myocardial infarction (MI), and incomplete coaptation of valve leaflets or restricted valve movement resulting from ischemia
- Acute MR
  - Flail leaflet: myxomatous disease, infective endocarditis, or trauma
  - Ruptured chordae tendineae: trauma, spontaneous rupture, infective endocarditis, or rheumatic fever
  - Ruptured or displaced papillary muscle: acute MI, severe myocardial ischemia, or trauma
- Chronic MR
  - Primary
    - Degenerative: mitral annular calcification, mitral valve prolapse (MVP)
    - Infective endocarditis
    - Rheumatic heart disease (RHD)
    - Inflammatory diseases: lupus, eosinophilic endocardial disease

- Anorectic drugs
- Congenital (cleft leaflet)
- Secondary (functional)
  - Ischemic: coronary artery disease (CAD)/MI
  - Nonischemic: cardiomyopathy, LV dysfunction from any cause, hypertrophic cardiomyopathy

RISK FACTORS
Age, hypertension, RHD, endocarditis, anorectic drugs

GENERAL PREVENTION
- Risk factor modification for CAD
- Antibiotic prophylaxis for poststreptococcal RHD
- Endocarditis prophylaxis for MR is no longer recommended.

COMMONLY ASSOCIATED CONDITIONS
MVP with MR common in Marfan syndrome

DIAGNOSIS

HISTORY
- Associated conditions: RHD, prior MI, connective tissue disorder
- Acute MR
  - Sudden onset of dyspnea
  - Orthopnea, paroxysmal nocturnal dyspnea
  - Chronic MR
    - Exertional dyspnea
    - Fatigue
    - Palpitation: paroxysmal/persistent AF

PHYSICAL EXAM
- Acute MR
  - Rapid and thready pulses
  - Sign of poor tissue perfusion with peripheral vasoconstriction
  - Hyperdynamic precordium without apical displacement
  - S_3 and S_4 (if in sinus rhythm)
  - Systolic murmur at left sternal border and base
    - Early, middle, or holosystolic murmur
    - Often soft, low-pitched decrescendo murmur
  - Rales
- Chronic MR
  - Brisk upstroke of arterial pulse
  - Leftward displaced LV apical impulse
  - Systolic thrill at the apex (suggests severe MR)
  - Soft S_1 and widely split S_2, S_3 gallop
  - Loud P_2 (if pulmonary hypertension)
  - Holosystolic murmur at apex that radiates to axilla
  - Ankle edema, jugular venous distension, and ascites, if development of right-sided heart failure

DIFFERENTIAL DIAGNOSIS
- Aortic stenosis (AS): usually midsystolic but can be long; difficult to distinguish from holosystolic, at apical area, and radiating to the carotid arteries (unlike MR)
- Tricuspid regurgitation: holosystolic but at left lower sternal border; does not radiate to axilla or increase in intensity with inspiration (unlike MR)
- Ventricular septal defect (VSD): harsh holosystolic murmur at lower left sternal border but radiates to right sternal border (not axilla)

DIAGNOSTIC TESTS & INTERPRETATION
- Chest x-ray (CXR)
  - Acute MR: pulmonary edema, normal heart size
  - Chronic MR: LA and LV enlargement
- ECG
  - Acute MR
    - Varies depending on etiologies (e.g., acute MI)

- Chronic MR
  - P mitrale from LA enlargement, AF
  - LV hypertrophy
  - Q waves from prior MI

Initial Tests (lab, imaging)
- Cardiac enzymes and brain natriuretic peptide (BNP), if appropriate
- Transthoracic echocardiogram (TTE)
  - Indications for TTE (2)
    - Baseline evaluation of LV size and function, right ventricular function and LA size, pulmonary artery pressure, and severity of MR
    - Delineation of mechanism of MR
    - Surveillance of asymptomatic moderate to severe LV dysfunction (ejection fraction [EF] and end-systolic dimension [ESD])
    - Evaluate MV apparatus and LV size and function after a change in signs/symptoms in a patient with MR.
    - Evaluate after MV repair or replacement.
  - Findings in acute MR
    - Evidence of etiology: flail leaflet or infective vegetations
    - Normal LA and LV size
  - Findings in chronic MR
    - Evidence of degenerative, rheumatic, ischemic, congenital, and other causes
    - Enlarged LA and LV

Follow-Up Tests & Special Considerations
- Intervals for follow up TTE: See "Follow-Up Recommendations."
- Cardiovascular magnetic resonance (CMR):
  - TTE results are not satisfactory to assess LV and RV volumes, function, or MR severity (2)[C].
- Transesophageal echocardiogram (TEE)
  - Intraoperatively to define the anatomic basis of MR and to guide repair (2)[C]
  - Nondiagnostic information about severity, mechanism of MR, and/or status of LV function from noninvasive imaging (2)[C]
- Exercise hemodynamics with either doppler echo or cardiac catheterization (2)[C]
  - Discrepancy between symptoms and the severity of MR from resting TTE in symptomatic patients with chronic primary MR
- Exercise treadmill testing (2)[C]
  - To establish symptom status and exercise tolerance in asymptomatic patients with chronic primary MR.
- Noninvasive imaging (stress nuclear/position emission tomography, CMR, stress echocardiography), cardiac CT angiography, or cardiac catheterization, including coronary angiography
  - To establish etiology of chronic secondary MR and/or to assess myocardial viability (2)[C]

Diagnostic Procedures/Other
Cardiac catheterization (2)
- Left ventriculography and hemodynamic measurement
  - Noninvasive tests are inconclusive regarding severity of MR, LV function, or the need for surgery.
- Coronary angiography: prior to MV surgery in patients at risk for CAD

Test Interpretation
Quantification of severe MR requires integration of the following:
- Structural parameters
  - LA size: dilated, unless acute
  - LV size: dilated, unless acute

– Leaflets: abnormal
– Doppler parameters
– Quantitative parameter

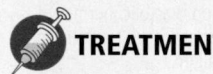 **TREATMENT**

MEDICATION

• Acute, severe MR
  – Medical therapy has a limited role and is aimed primarily to stabilize hemodynamics preoperatively.
  – Vasodilators (nitroprusside, nicardipine): to improve hemodynamic compensation but is often limited by systemic hypotension (2)
• Chronic MR
  – Primary
    ○ Asymptomatic: no proven long-term medical therapy
    ○ Symptomatic: diuretics, β-blockers (carvedilol, metoprolol), angiotensin-converting enzyme inhibitors (ACEIs) or angiotensin receptor blockers (ARBs), and possibly aldosterone antagonists as indicated in standard therapy for heart failure (2)[C]
  – Secondary: LV dysfunction or symptomatic (stages B–D)
    ○ ACEIs or ARBs, β-blockers, and/or aldosterone antagonists as indicated in standard therapy for heart failure (2)[C]

SURGERY/OTHER PROCEDURES

• Isolated MV surgery is not indicated for patients with mild to moderate MR.
• Acute, severe MR secondary to acute MI
  – Acute rupture of papillary muscle: emergency MV repair/replacement
  – Papillary muscle displacement
    ○ Aggressive medical stabilization and intra-aortic balloon pump
    ○ Valve surgery usually required in addition to revascularization.
• Chronic severe MR
  – MV repair in an experienced center is recommended over MV replacement in most circumstances (3):
    ○ Survival rate: early and overall mortality were lower after MV repair than after MV replacement
    ○ 10-year rate of stroke: 10% (repair) versus 12% (bioprosthetic valve replacement) versus 23% (mechanical valve replacement)
    ○ Risk of endocarditis: 1.5% at 15 years versus 0.3–1.2% per year
    ○ Overall rates of reoperation are similar.
  – Severe primary MR (2)
    ○ MV surgery
      ▪ Symptomatic patients (stage D)
        □ Absence of severe LV dysfunction (EF ≥30%) (2)[B]
        □ Severe LV dysfunction (EF <30%) (2)[C]
      ▪ Asymptomatic patients
        □ Mild to moderate LV dysfunction (EF 30–60% and/or ESD ≥40 mm, stage C2) (2)[B]
        □ MV repair is reasonable for asymptomatic patients (stage C1) with preserved LV function (EF >60% and ESD <40 mm):
          • The likelihood of successful repair without residual MR is >95% and expected mortality <1% when performed at a heart valve center of excellence (2)[C].

• Nonrheumatic MR with new onset AF or resting pulmonary hypertension (pulmonary artery systolic pressure [PASP] >50 mm Hg) and the likelihood of a successful and durable repair is high (2)[C].
  ○ Transcatheter MV repair:
    ▪ May be considered for severely symptomatic patients (NYHA class III/IV) despite optimal GDMT for HF, who have a reasonable life expectancy but a prohibitive surgical risk because of severe comorbidities (2)[C]
  – Severe secondary MR (2)
    ○ MV surgery
      ▪ Undergoing coronary artery bypass graft (CABG) or aortic valve replacement (AVR) (2)[C]
      ▪ Persistent symptom (NYHA class III-IV) despite optimal GDMT for HF (2)[C]
    ○ Cardiac resynchronization therapy with biventricular pacing is recommended for symptomatic patients (stage B–D) who meet the indications for device therapy (2)[C].

Geriatric Considerations
• Medical therapy alone for patients >75 years of age with MR is preferred, owing to increased operative mortality and decreased survival (compared with those with AS), especially with preexisting CAD or need for MV replacement.
• MV repair is preferable than MV replacement.

INPATIENT CONSIDERATIONS

Admission Criteria/Initial Stabilization
Acute MR: Stabilize ABCs (airway, breathing, circulation). Initiate IV, O₂, and monitoring. Nitroprusside (+dobutamine and/or aortic balloon counterpulsation if hypotensive). Treat underlying causes (e.g., MI). Treat acute pulmonary edema with furosemide and morphine. Obtain urgent surgical consultation.

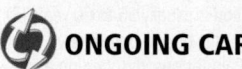 **ONGOING CARE**

FOLLOW-UP RECOMMENDATIONS
Chronic MR: asymptomatic

• Mild MR with normal LV size and function and no pulmonary hypertension: Annual clinical evaluation to assess symptom progression and TTE every 3 to 5 years to assess MR severity, LV size and function.
• Moderate MR: annual clinical evaluation and TTE every 1 to 2 years
• Severe MR: clinical evaluation and TTE every 6 to 12 months
• Consider serial CXRs and ECGs, and consider stress test if exercise capacity is doubtful.

PATIENT EDUCATION
• Exercise after MV repair: Avoid sports with risk for bodily contact or trauma. Low-intensity competitive sports are allowed.
• Competitive athletes with MR
  – Asymptomatic with normal LV size and function, normal pulmonary artery pressures, and sinus rhythm: no restrictions
  – Mildly symptomatic and those with LV dilatation: Activities with low to moderate dynamic and static cardiac demand allowed
• AF and anticoagulation: no contact sports

PROGNOSIS
• Acute, severe MR: Mortality risk with surgery is 50%; mortality risk with medical therapy alone is 75% in first 24 hours and 95% at 2 weeks.
• Chronic MR: asymptomatic severe MR with normal LVEF: 10% yearly rate of progression to symptoms and subnormal resting LVEF. Symptomatic severe MR: 8-year survival rate, 33% without surgery; mortality rate, 5% yearly

Pregnancy Considerations
MR with NYHA functional class III–IV at high risk for maternal and/or fetal risk

COMPLICATIONS
Acute pulmonary edema, CHF, AF, bleeding risk with anticoagulation, endocarditis, sudden cardiac death

REFERENCES
1. Enriquez-Sarano M, Akins CW, Vahanian A. Mitral regurgitation. *Lancet*. 2009;373(9672):1382–1394.
2. Nishimura RA, Otto CM, Bonow RO, et al. 2014 AHA/ACC guideline for the management of patients with valvular heart disease: a report of the American College of Cardiology/American Heart Association Task Force on practice guidelines. *Circulation*. 2014;129(23):e521–e643.
3. Foster E. Clinical practice. Mitral regurgitation due to degenerative mitral-valve disease. *N Engl J Med*. 2010;363(2):156–165.

ADDITIONAL READING
• Acker MA, Parides MK, Perrault LP, et al. Mitral-valve repair versus replacement for severe ischemic mitral regurgitation. *N Engl J Med*. 2014;370(1):23–32.
• Feldman T, Young A. Percutaneous approaches to valve repair for mitral regurgitation. *J Am Coll Cardiol*. 2014;63(20):2057–2068.
• Vahanian A, Alfieri O, Andreotti F, et al. Guidelines on the management of valvular heart disease (version 2012). *Eur Heart J*. 2012;33(19):2451–2496.
• Yancy CW, Jessup M, Bozkurt B, et al. 2013 ACCF/AHA guideline for the management of heart failure: a report of the American College of Cardiology Foundation/American Heart Association Task Force on practice guidelines. *Circulation*. 2013;128(16):e240–e327.

 CODES

ICD10
• I34.0 Nonrheumatic mitral (valve) insufficiency
• I05.1 Rheumatic mitral insufficiency
• Q23.3 Congenital mitral insufficiency

CLINICAL PEARLS
• Follow-up for mild to moderate MR: serial exam and/or echo unless LV structural changes
• Severe MR is usually managed with MV repair.
• Endocarditis prophylaxis is not recommended.

M

MITRAL STENOSIS

Zeeshan Hussain, MD • Nirmanmoh Bhatia, MD • Marcus F. Stoddard, MD

BASICS

DESCRIPTION
- Mitral stenosis (MS) presents as resistance to diastolic filling of the left ventricle (LV) due to narrowing of mitral valve (MV) orifice.
- Normal valve orifice 4 to 6 cm^2; symptoms typically seen when orifice is <2.5 cm^2.
- Hemodynamic consequences are due to passive transmission of left atrial (LA) pressure to the pulmonary circulation; may coexist with mitral regurgitation and aortic valvulopathies
- Stages vary from A (with risk factors), B (hemodynamically obstruction), C (severe but no symptoms), to D (symptomatic) (1)

EPIDEMIOLOGY
- Most common acquired valvular disease secondary to rheumatic heart disease (60% of cases)
- Predominant age: Symptoms primarily occur in 4th to 7th decades.
- Predominant sex: female > male (2:1)

Incidence
Decreased incidence of MS is seen in the United States because of decreased incidence of rheumatic fever (primarily shift in prevalence away from rheumatogenic strains of group A streptococci [GAS] and also treatment of GAS infection). However, global burden remains significant (2).

ETIOLOGY AND PATHOPHYSIOLOGY
- Obstruction between LA and LV impairs LV filling during diastole and leads to increased LA pressure.
- Increased LA pressure is transmitted passively ("back pressure") to the pulmonary circulation; over time, pulmonary hypertension (HTN) results.
- Over time, LA pressure overload can dilate the chamber and interrupt the cardiac conduction system, resulting in atrial fibrillation.
- Pulmonary HTN can also cause increased collateralization between pulmonary and bronchial circulation, resulting in intraparenchymal hemorrhage with hemoptysis.
- Rheumatic fever: most common (see "Risk Factors")
- Aging (extension of mitral annular calcification)
- Rare causes
  - Congenital (associated with mucopolysaccharidoses)
  - Autoimmune: systemic lupus erythematosus (SLE), rheumatoid arthritis
  - Malignant carcinoid
  - Other acquired: LA myxoma, LA thrombus, endomyocardial fibrosis

RISK FACTORS
- Rheumatic fever is the greatest risk factor.
  - 30–40% of rheumatic fever patients eventually develop MS, presenting an average of 20 years after diagnosis of rheumatic fever.
  - Acute rheumatic fever occurs 2 to 3 weeks after episode of untreated GAS pharyngitis caused by rheumatogenic organism in a genetically susceptible host.
  - Low socioeconomic status (i.e., crowded conditions) favors the spread of streptococcal infection.
- Aging (increasing valvular calcification)
- Chest irradiation (increasing tissue fibrosis)

GENERAL PREVENTION
- Prompt recognition and treatment of GAS infection; recognition of cardinal signs and symptoms of acute rheumatic fever via Jones criteria

- Modified Jones criteria for acute rheumatic fever: Diagnosis requires evidence of streptococcal infection plus two major criteria or one major plus two minor criteria.

Evidence of streptococcal infection	Antistreptolysin O titer or positive throat culture
Major criteria	Carditis, polyarthritis, Sydenham chorea, erythema marginatum, subcutaneous nodules
Minor criteria	Migratory arthralgias, fever, acute phase reactants (elevated erythrocyte sedimentation rate [ESR], leukocytosis), prolonged PR interval on ECG

COMMONLY ASSOCIATED CONDITIONS
- Atrial fibrillation (30–40% of symptomatic patients)
- Associated valve lesions due to chronic inflammation (aortic stenosis, aortic insufficiency)
- Pulmonary congestion and pulmonary HTN
- Right heart failure
- Systemic embolism, pulmonary embolism (10%)
- Infection, including infectious endocarditis (1–5%)

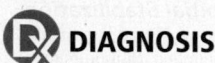
DIAGNOSIS

HISTORY
- History of rheumatic fever
- Severity of presentation depends on valve area; most early cases will be asymptomatic.
- Mean age of presentation is usually 50 to 60 years (3).
- Presenting features usually due to pulmonary vascular congestion: Palpitations, dyspnea on exertion, fatigue, pulmonary edema, and paroxysmal nocturnal dyspnea may cause chest pain.
- Atrial fibrillation, embolic event
- In advanced disease, symptoms of HTN and right heart failure predominate: jugular venous distention, hepatomegaly, ascites, and peripheral edema
- Other presentations: hemoptysis, hoarseness (compression of recurrent laryngeal nerve by enlarged pulmonary artery or LA), dysphagia (compression), rarely as infective endocarditis
- Infection, atrial fibrillation with rapid rate, exercise, or pregnancy may exacerbate symptoms.

PHYSICAL EXAM
- Reduced peripheral pulses
- Auscultation
  - Classic murmur: accentuated S$_1$, opening snap, apical early decrescendo diastolic rumble with presystolic accentuation
  - Murmur variability seen in severe stenosis
    - With mobile, noncalcified valve, murmur persists throughout diastole and S$_1$, and the opening snap remains loud.
    - With a heavily calcified valve, murmur often is difficult to hear. S$_1$ and the opening snap may be soft to absent.
    - In contrast to tricuspid stenosis, the intensity of the murmur from MS increases with inspiration and a prominent *a* wave in jugular venous pulse.

- If HTN is present: Right ventricle (RV) lift, increased P$_2$, high-pitched decrescendo diastolic murmur of pulmonic insufficiency (Graham Steell murmur) may have signs of right heart failure.
- May also find associated aortic or, less commonly, tricuspid murmurs due to aortic or tricuspid valve involvement from rheumatic heart disease

DIAGNOSTIC TESTS & INTERPRETATION
Initial Tests (lab, imaging)
- ECG (4,5)[C]
  - LA enlargement (manifested by broad, notched P waves in lead II [P mitrale] with a negative terminal deflection of the P wave in lead V$_1$)
  - Atrial fibrillation is common.
  - Right ventricular hypertrophy (RVH), right axis deviation, and a large R wave in V$_1$ are possible.
- Chest radiograph (4,5)[C]
  - LA enlargement, straightening of the left heart border, a "double density," and elevation of the left main stem bronchus
  - Prominent pulmonary arteries at the hilum with rapid tapering, RVH
  - Pulmonary edema pattern with Kerley B lines (late presentation)

- ECG indications (1)[B],(5)[C]
  - Class I
    - Diagnosis of MS
    - Assess severity.
    - Reassess after change in symptoms.
    - Exercise Doppler for discrepancies between symptoms and echo findings.
    - During evaluation for commissurotomy
    - TEE when transthoracic echo nondiagnostic, to exclude thrombus in left atrium or to evaluate severity of MR (1)[B]
  - Class II
    - Reassess asymptomatic patients.
    - Very severe (<1.0 cm^2) MS: yearly
    - Severe (≤1.5 cm^2) MS: every 1 to 2 years
    - Mild or moderate MS: every 3 to 5 years
  - Class III
    - Satisfactory result of transthoracic echo
- ECG findings
  - MV anterior leaflet doming, immobility of the posterior leaflet
  - Echo can demonstrate alternative causes of MS if not rheumatic.
  - MV area defined (1)
    - Normal: 4 to 6 cm^2
    - Progressive MS: >1.5 cm^2
    - Severe MS: <1.5 cm^2
    - Very severe: <1.0 cm^2
- Cardiac catheterization indications (1,5)[C]
  - Class I recommendations
    - When echo is inconclusive
    - Discrepancy between echo and symptoms
    - Discrepancy between echo and valve area
  - Class II recommendations
    - To assess response of LA and pulmonary artery pressures to exercise when symptoms and echo findings do not match
    - Assess cause of severe HTN out of proportion to echo results.
  - Class III recommendations: satisfactory result of echo

Follow-Up Tests & Special Considerations
- If valve area >1.5 cm^2 and mean pressure gradient <5 mm Hg, then no further initial workup is needed.
- If valve area is <1.5 cm^2, then do further workup prior to surgical correction.

Diagnostic Procedures/Other

Exercise or dobutamine stress test (1,5)[C].

- When symptoms are severe but echo findings are mild
- To determine if surgery is needed

Test Interpretation

Rheumatic fever–induced pathologic changes: leaflet thickening, leaflet calcification, commissural fusion, chordal shortening

 TREATMENT

GENERAL MEASURES

- Exercise
  - Patients with mild MS are usually asymptomatic even with strenuous exercise.
  - Usually recommend low-level aerobic exercise, limited by symptoms of dyspnea (5)[C]
- Counsel patients that MS usually is slowly progressive but can have sudden onset of atrial fibrillation, which could become rapidly fatal. Call 911 for marked worsening of symptoms.
- Atrial fibrillation accompanying MS impairs LV filling, especially with a rapid ventricular response.
  - Rate control with β-blockers or calcium channel blockers (1)[C]
  - Cardioversion for medical failure or if patient is unstable (6)[B]
  - If the atrial fibrillation has been present for >24 to 48 hours, then anticoagulate for 3 weeks then cardiovert, or alternatively, heparinize, perform TEE, and if no atrial thrombus, then cardiovert (6)[B].
  - After cardioversion, patient needs long-term anticoagulation.
  - These patients can critically decompensate due to loss of atrial contractility, causing an inability to fill the LV.

MEDICATION

First Line

- Because MS is a mechanical anomaly, medical management is always considered adjunctive to interventional management when the latter is indicated.
- Antibiotic prophylaxis against rheumatic fever and/or carditis is recommended for patients with history of rheumatic fever (1)[C].
  - Penicillin V PO or penicillin G IM: IM is more effective than PO (7)[A].
  - Sulfadiazine
  - Macrolides: Take antibiotic continuously to prevent recurrence of rheumatic fever or carditis.
  - Duration of rheumatic fever prophylaxis
    - Rheumatic fever without carditis: Take for 5 years or until age 21 years, whichever is longer.
    - Rheumatic fever with carditis but no residual heart disease: Take for 10 years or well into adulthood, whichever is longer.
    - Rheumatic fever with carditis plus residual heart disease: Take for 10 years or until 40 years old, whichever is longer.
- Antibiotic prophylaxis against infective endocarditis is not routinely recommended (1)[B].
- β-Blockers or calcium channel blockers for tachycardia or exertional symptoms (1)[B]
- Diuretics for congestive symptoms (5)[C]
- Digitalis for atrial fibrillation if LV or RV dysfunction (5)[C]
- Anticoagulation (1)[B]
  - Class I recommendations
    - MS and atrial fibrillation or history of atrial fibrillation

    - MS and prior embolic event
    - MS and LA thrombus
  - Class IIB recommendations
    - Asymptomatic MS but with severe MS and LA dimension >54 mm by echo
    - Severe MS, enlarged LA and spontaneous contrast on echo
- Warfarin (international normalized ratio) range 2 to 3
- Heparin in the acute atrial fibrillation setting
- The new oral anticoagulants (factor Xa inhibitor and direct thrombin inhibitor) are not approved for use in atrial fibrillation that is secondary to MS.

Second Line

Amiodarone for rate control if β-blockers or calcium channel blockers cannot be used (5)[C]

SURGERY/OTHER PROCEDURES

- Balloon valvotomy: symptomatic patients with NYHA class II, III, or IV symptoms with valves that look favorable and with favorable comorbidities (1)[A]
- MV surgery: when MS is severe and balloon valvotomy is contraindicated due to unfavorable anatomy (1)[B],(8)[C]

Pregnancy Considerations

Volume expansion during pregnancy can exacerbate heart failure symptoms. Hence, MS often presents during the intrapartum period. For patients with known severe MS, intervention should be pursued before pregnancy. Such patients have a high rate of both maternal and fetal complications, including death. Percutaneous balloon valvotomy can be performed in symptomatic pregnant patients.

 ONGOING CARE

FOLLOW-UP RECOMMENDATIONS

- Ascertain the valve gradient and pulmonary arterial pressure with ECG.
- Follow-up will depend on the severity of the MS and the patient's symptoms.
  - Asymptomatic patients: annual history and examination; follow-up serial echocardiography based on the severity of MS
  - Symptomatic patients are reviewed according to individual therapy, symptoms, and signs; ECG to evaluate for changes (1)[C]

DIET

Salt restriction for pulmonary congestion

PROGNOSIS

Natural history

- Asymptomatic latent period after rheumatic fever for 10 to 30 years. 10-Year survival for asymptomatic or minimally symptomatic patients is 80%. 10-Year survival after onset of symptoms is 50–60%.
- Symptoms typically become debilitating 10 years after onset.
- 10-Year survival after onset of debilitating symptoms is only 0–15%.
- Mean survival with significant HTN is <3 years.
- The severity of MS progresses over time in almost all patients. There are no known definitive medical therapies, apart from prevention of recurrent rheumatic fever, that alter its natural history. When symptoms develop, balloon valvotomy, open mitral commissurotomy, or closed mitral commissurotomy provides effective means of reducing stenosis but is not curative. Restenosis sometimes occurs and can be early (<5 years) or late (>20 years).

- Appropriate medical treatment can delay necessity for surgery, and surgical treatment substantially prolongs survival in patients with severe MS.

COMPLICATIONS

Left and right heart failure, atrial fibrillation and systemic embolization, pulmonary HTN, bacterial endocarditis

REFERENCES

1. Nishimura RA, Otto CM, Bonow RO, et al. 2014 AHA/ACC guideline for the management of patients with valvular heart disease: a report of the American College of Cardiology/American Heart Association Task Force on Practice Guidelines. *J Thorac Cardiovasc Surg*. 2014;148(1):e1–e132.
2. Ray S. Changing epidemiology and natural history of valvular heart disease. *Clin Med (Lond)*. 2010;10(2):168–171.
3. Ramakrishna CD, Khadar SA, George R, et al. The age-specific clinical and anatomical profile of mitral stenosis. *Singapore Med J*. 2009;50(7):680–685.
4. Maganti K, Rigolin VH, Sarano ME, et al. Valvular heart disease: diagnosis and management. *Mayo Clin Proc*. 2010;85(5):483–500.
5. Bruce CJ, Nishimura RA. Newer advances in the diagnosis and treatment of mitral stenosis. *Curr Probl Cardiol*. 1998;23(3):125–192.
6. Anderson JL, Halperin JL, Albert NM, et al. Management of patients with atrial fibrillation (compilation of 2006 ACCF/AHA/ESC and 2011 ACCF/AHA/HRS recommendations): a report of the American College of Cardiology/American Heart Association Task Force on Practice Guidelines. *J Am Coll Cardiol*. 2013;61(18):1935–1944.
7. Manyemba J, Mayosi BM. Penicillin for secondary prevention of rheumatic fever. *Cochrane Database Syst Rev*. 2002;(3):CD002227.
8. Zakkar M, Amirak E, Chan KM, et al. Rheumatic mitral valve disease: current surgical status. *Prog Cardiovasc Dis*. 2009;51(6):478–481.

ADDITIONAL READING

- Chandrashekhar Y, Westaby S, Narula J. Mitral stenosis. *Lancet*. 2009;374(9697):1271–1283.
- Guérios EE, Bueno R, Nercolini D, et al. Mitral stenosis and percutaneous mitral valvuloplasty (part 1). *J Invasive Cardiol*. 2005;17(7):382–386.

 CODES

ICD10

- I05.0 Rheumatic mitral stenosis
- I05.8 Other rheumatic mitral valve diseases
- I34.2 Nonrheumatic mitral (valve) stenosis

CLINICAL PEARLS

- Asymptomatic patients may be followed clinically with yearly exams for development of symptoms with periodic echo to evaluate valve area.
- Once symptoms of MS develop, initiate appropriate medical therapy but advise patient that, for most, surgical therapy will be needed to prolong survival. Almost all cases of MV stenosis progress in severity over time.
- MS often presents during the intrapartum period. For patients with known severe MS, intervention should be pursued prior to pregnancy. Pregnancy in a patient with severe MS has a high rate of both maternal and fetal complications, including death.

M

MITRAL VALVE PROLAPSE

Zeeshan Hussain, MD • Wasiq Faraz Rawasia, MD • Marcus F. Stoddard, MD

BASICS

DESCRIPTION
- Mitral valve prolapse (MVP) is a systolic billowing of one or both mitral leaflets into the left atrium (LA) during systole ± mitral regurgitation (MR).
- More specifically, MVP is a single or bileaflet prolapse of at least 2 mm superior displacement into the LA during systole on the parasternal long-axis annular plane of the valve on echocardiogram ± leaflet thickening.
  – Classic: prolapse with >5 mm of leaflet thickening
  – Nonclassic: prolapse with <5 mm of leaflet thickening (1)
- Synonym(s): systolic click-murmur syndrome; billowing mitral cusp syndrome; myxomatous mitral valve; floppy valve syndrome; redundant cusp syndrome; Barlow syndrome

EPIDEMIOLOGY
Incidence
- Predominant age: MVP has been described in all age groups.
- Initial descriptions based on clinical examinations suggested a 2:1 female predominance. Using modern echocardiogram criteria, men and women are affected equally (2).
- The most serious consequences of hemodynamically significant MR occur in men age >50 years.

Prevalence
MVP is the most common valvular abnormality, affecting 1.0–2.5% of the general population, depending on the precise definition (2,3).

ETIOLOGY AND PATHOPHYSIOLOGY
- The pathology causing MVP is multifactorial and includes the following:
  – Abnormal valve tissue
    ○ Myxomatous degeneration: redundant layers of leaflet "hooding" the cords, chordal elongation, and annular dilatation
    ○ Myxoid leaflets are more elastic and less stiff than normal valves.
    ○ Chordal rupture is more common.
  – Disparity in size between the mitral valve and the left ventricle (LV)
  – Connective tissue disorders (1)
- MVP is often associated with variable degrees of MR.
- Frequently, there is enlargement of the LA and LV.
- Mitral annulus is often dilated.
- Involvement of other valves may occur (tricuspid valve prolapse 40%, pulmonic prolapse and aortic prolapse 2–10%).
- Possible increased vagal tone
- Possible increased urine epinephrine and norepinephrine
- MVP patients often have orthostatic hypotension and tachycardia.
- Genetics causes proliferation of the spongiosa layer of the leaflets (3).
- Fibrosis on surface of leaflets (3)
- Thinning and elongation of chordae tendineae
- The mitral valve differentiates during days 35 to 42 of fetal development, the same time as differentiation of the vertebrae and ribs.

Genetics
- Familial MVP is inherited as an autosomal dominant trait but with variable expressivity and incomplete penetrance.
- Two genetic loci identified
  – MMVP1 on chromosome 16p11.2–p12.1
  – MMVP2 on chromosome 11p15.4

RISK FACTORS
- MVP is a primary cardiovascular disorder.
- MVP is more likely to occur in patients with connective tissue disorders (see "Commonly Associated Conditions").
- Physical characteristics associated with MVP
  – Straight thoracic spine
  – Pectus excavatum
  – Asthenic body habitus
  – Low body mass index (BMI)
  – Scoliosis or kyphosis
  – Hypermobility of the joints
  – Arm span > height
  – Narrow anteroposterior (AP) diameter of the chest

COMMONLY ASSOCIATED CONDITIONS
- Marfan syndrome (91% of Marfan syndrome patients have MVP, although large majority of MVP patients do not meet criteria for Marfans.) (1)
- Ehlers-Danlos syndrome
- Hypertrophic cardiomyopathy
- Pseudoxanthoma elasticum
- Osteogenesis imperfecta
- von Willebrand disease
- Primary hypomastia

DIAGNOSIS

Physical exam and echocardiography

HISTORY
- Most patients are asymptomatic.
- The most frequent symptom is palpitations.
- Symptoms related to autonomic dysfunction
  – Anxiety and panic attacks
  – Arrhythmias
  – Exercise intolerance
  – Palpitations and chest pains that are atypical for coronary artery disease (CAD)
  – Fatigue
  – Orthostasis, syncope, or presyncope
  – Neuropsychiatric symptoms
- Symptoms related to progression of MR
  – Fatigue
  – Dyspnea
  – Exercise intolerance
  – Orthopnea
  – Paroxysmal nocturnal dyspnea
  – Congestive heart failure (CHF)
- Symptoms occur as a result of an associated complication (stroke, arrhythmia).

PHYSICAL EXAM
- Auscultatory examination
  – Mid to late systolic click
    ○ May vary in timing and intensity based on ventricular beat-to-beat volume variations
    ○ At low ventricular volumes, the valve may prolapse earlier during systole and further into the LA than during volume overload.
    ○ It may or may not be followed by a high-pitched, mid to late systolic murmur at the cardiac apex.

  – Murmur: a mid to late crescendo systolic murmur best heard at apex, middle- to high-pitched, occasionally musical or honking in quality
  – Occasionally, only the ejection click is present.
  – The duration of the murmur corresponds with the severity of MR.
- Dynamic auscultation
  – Maneuvers that move the click and murmur toward S_1
    ○ Arterial vasodilation
    ○ Amyl nitrite
    ○ Valsalva
    ○ Augmented contractility
    ○ Decreased venous return (which can be induced by standing up)
  – Maneuvers that move the click and murmur toward S_2
    ○ Squatting
    ○ Leg raise
    ○ Isometric exercise
  – Valsalva maneuver may help differentiate hypertrophic obstructive cardiomyopathy (HOCM) from MVP because it increases the intensity of the murmur in HOCM whereas it makes it longer but not louder in MVP.

DIFFERENTIAL DIAGNOSIS
- MR
- Tricuspid regurgitation
- Tricuspid valve prolapse
- Papillary muscle dysfunction
- Hypertrophic cardiomyopathy
- Ejection clicks (do not change timing with systole)

DIAGNOSTIC TESTS & INTERPRETATION
Initial Tests (lab, imaging)
- Echocardiogram (test of choice) (4)[B],(5)[C]
  – In asymptomatic individuals with physical signs of MVP, an echocardiogram is indicated for diagnosis (4)[B].
  – Follow-up echocardiograms are not indicated for asymptomatic patients who have MVP with no changes clinically, even if they had mild MR (4,5)[C].
  – Parasternal long-axis view is most specific for diagnosis (4).
  – Findings that may be seen with MVP
    ○ Anterior leaflet billowing
    ○ Leaflet thickening of ≥5 mm
    ○ Leaflet redundancy
    ○ MR
    ○ Posterior leaflet displacement
  – Nondiagnostic transthoracic echocardiogram: ≤10%
  – Transesophageal echocardiography particularly with 3D imaging may be considered to further visualize the anatomy if an intervention is being planned (6)[B].
  – Stress echocardiograms may reveal exercise-induced MR or latent LV dysfunction (1,5)[C].
- Angiography
  – Rarely used for diagnostic purposes
  – MVP may be incidentally seen on a catheterization.
- ECG is usually normal.
  – May be nonspecific ST-T wave changes
  – T-wave inversions, prominent Q waves, or prolonged QT may also occur.

- A chest x-ray (CXR) is not necessary for diagnosis.
  - Typically, the CXR is normal.
  - Other findings
    - Possible pulmonary edema: Pulmonary edema may be asymmetric with acute chordal rupture and flail leaflet.
    - Possible calcification of the mitral annulus
- Holter monitoring is optional if patient has palpitations. Order Holter monitoring as usual for syncope or dizziness
- Tilt table testing may be of value in patients with MVP who presents with syncope of unknown etiology.

Follow-Up Tests & Special Considerations
Patients with a family history of MVP should be screened with echocardiography (4)[B].

Test Interpretation
- Myxomatous proliferation of the middle layer (spongiosa) of the valve, resulting in increased mucopolysaccharide deposition and myxomatous degeneration
- By electron microscopy, the collagen fibers in the valve leaflets are disorganized and fragmented.
- With increased stroma deposition, the valve leaflets enlarge and become redundant.
- The endothelium is usually noncontiguous and a frequent site for thrombus or infective vegetation.

 TREATMENT

GENERAL MEASURES
Treat MVP with orthostatic symptoms by liberalizing fluid and salt intake. If severe, mineralocorticoids may rarely be used. Support stockings may also be beneficial.

MEDICATION
- Asymptomatic MVP is treated with reassurance; normal lifestyle and regular exercise is encouraged.
- MVP and transient ischemic attacks are treated with aspirin 75 to 325 mg daily (Class I recommendation) (4)[C].
- MVP with history of cryptogenic stroke, or atrial fibrillation with CHADS$_2$ (acronym for **C**ongestive heart failure, **H**ypertension, **A**ge >75 years, **D**iabetes mellitus, and prior **S**troke or transient ischemic attack) score <2, is generally treated with aspirin 75 to 325 mg daily (4)[C].
- MVP with atrial fibrillation with CHADS$_2$ score ≥2 is treated with warfarin (4)[C].
- MVP with high-risk echocardiographic features (thickening >5 mm or valve redundancy) and a history of stroke, warfarin therapy may be considered (4)[C].
- MVP with palpitations is treated with β-blockers and/or recommendation to discontinue alcohol, cigarettes, and caffeine (5)[C].

ADDITIONAL THERAPIES
- Endocarditis prophylaxis is no longer recommended for MVP.
- Patients with prior endocarditis undergoing dental, respiratory tract, infected skin, or musculoskeletal procedures should receive prophylaxis for endocarditis with amoxicillin 30 to 60 minutes prior to procedure. Ampicillin, cefazolin, or ceftriaxone IM or IV may be used if unable to tolerate oral medications (4)[B].

SURGERY/OTHER PROCEDURES
- Referral for surgery is recommended for patients with severe MR with impaired LV systolic function or flail leaflet owing to ruptured chordae tendineae (4)[C].
- Minimally invasive mitral valve repair patients have shorter postoperative hospital stay compared with conventional median sternotomy open repair for patients with bileaflet prolapse and severe MR (7)[B].
- Surgical repair of MR due to isolated posterior leaflet prolapse is associated with a low reoperation rate (8)[A].
- Asymptomatic patients with atrial fibrillation or pulmonary hypertension should be considered for intervention as well (3)[C].

 ONGOING CARE

FOLLOW-UP RECOMMENDATIONS
- Asymptomatic MVP patients with no significant MR can be followed clinically every 3 to 5 years (4)[C].
- Patients who are symptomatic or have high-risk features on initial echocardiogram, including moderate to severe MR, may need serial echocardiograms and should be followed clinically once per year (4)[C].
- Patients with MVP and severe MR may require coronary angiography and transesophageal echocardiography if cardiac surgical referral is planned (4)[C].

PATIENT EDUCATION
- No contraindication to pregnancy
- Restriction from competitive sports if patient has MVP with one of the following features (9):
  - A history of syncope associated with document arrhythmia
  - A family history of MVP-related sudden cardiac death
  - Sustained or repetitive and nonsustained supraventricular tachycardia or frequent and/or complex ventricular tachyarrhythmias on ambulatory Holter monitoring
  - Severe MR
  - A prior embolic event
  - LV systolic dysfunction
- Explain the hereditary nature of familial MVP.

PROGNOSIS
- Excellent prognosis for asymptomatic patients
- For patients with severe MR or reduced ejection fraction, the prognosis is similar to that for nonischemic MR.

COMPLICATIONS
- Sudden cardiac death: not clearly established. May be secondary to ventricular arrhythmias especially if significant MR is present (1,5).
- Chordae rupture with acute mitral insufficiency (higher risk of cardiac death; up to 2% per year)
- Infectious endocarditis (risk increased if murmur present) (5)
- Cerebrovascular ischemic event (1)
- Fibrin emboli
- Heart failure with progressive MR
- Arrhythmias such as atrial and ventricular premature beats, paroxysmal supraventricular tachycardias may all be seen. Risk increases with coexistent MR (5).
- Pulmonary hypertension

REFERENCES
1. Hayek E, Gring CN, Griffin BP. Mitral valve prolapse. *Lancet*. 2005;365(9458):507–518.
2. Freed LA, Levy D, Levine RA, et al. Prevalence and clinical outcome of mitral-valve prolapse. *N Engl J Med*. 1999;341(1):1–7.
3. Verma S, Mesana TG. Mitral-valve repair for mitral-valve prolapse. *N Engl J Med*. 2009;361(23): 2261–2269.
4. Bonow RO, Carabello BA, Chatterjee K, et al. 2008 focused update incorporated into the ACC/AHA 2006 guidelines for the management of patients with valvular heart disease: a report of the American College of Cardiology/American Heart Association Task Force on Practice Guidelines (Writing Committee to revise the 1998 guidelines for the management of patients with valvular heart disease). Endorsed by the Society of Cardiovascular Anesthesiologists, Society for Cardiovascular Angiography and Interventions, and Society of Thoracic Surgeons. *J Am Coll Cardiol*. 2008;52(13):e1–e142.
5. Sims JM, Miracle VA. An overview of mitral valve prolapse. *Dimens Crit Care Nurs*. 2007;26(4): 145–149.
6. Shah PM. Current concepts in mitral valve prolapse—diagnosis and management. *J Cardiol*. 2010;56(2):125–133.
7. Speziale G, Nasso G, Esposito G, et al. Results of mitral valve repair for Barlow disease (bileaflet prolapse) via right minithoracotomy versus conventional median sternotomy: a randomized trial. *J Thorac Cardiovasc Surg*. 2011;142(1):77–83.
8. Johnston DR, Gillinov AM, Blackstone EH, et al. Surgical repair of posterior mitral valve prolapse: implications for guidelines and percutaneous repair. *Ann Thorac Surg*. 2010;89(5):1385–1394.
9. Maron BJ, Ackerman MJ, Nishimura RA, et al. Task Force 4: HCM and other cardiomyopathies, mitral valve prolapse, myocarditis, and Marfan syndrome. *J Am Coll Cardiol*. 2005;45(8):1340–1345.

ADDITIONAL READING
Zuppiroli A, Mori F, Favilli S, et al. Arrhythmias in mitral valve prolapse: relation to anterior mitral leaflet thickening, clinical variables, and color Doppler echocardiographic parameters. *Am Heart J*. 1994;128(5):919–927.

 CODES

ICD10
I34.1 Nonrheumatic mitral (valve) prolapse

CLINICAL PEARLS
- MVP patients may have orthostatic hypotension and tachycardia.
- Asymptomatic MVP patients with no significant MR can be followed clinically every 3 to 5 years. Patients who are symptomatic or have high-risk features on initial echocardiogram, including moderate to severe MR, may need serial echocardiograms and should be followed clinically once per year.
- Endocarditis prophylaxis is no longer recommended for MVP.

M

MOLLUSCUM CONTAGIOSUM

Erica F. Crannage, PharmD, BCPS, BCACP • Rupal Trivedi, MD

 BASICS

DESCRIPTION
Molluscum contagiosum is a common, benign, viral (poxvirus) skin infection, characterized by small (2 to 5 mm), waxy white or flesh-colored, dome-shaped papules with central umbilication. When lesions are opened, a creamy, white-gray material can be expressed. Molluscum contagiosum is highly contagious and spreads by autoinoculation, skin-to-skin contact, sexual contact, and shared clothing/towels. Molluscum contagiosum is a self-limited infection in immunocompetent patients but can be difficult to treat and disfiguring in immunocompromised patients.

EPIDEMIOLOGY
Prevalence
- 1% in the United States, occurring mainly in children 2 to 15 years and sexually active young adults
- 5–18% HIV population

ETIOLOGY AND PATHOPHYSIOLOGY
- DNA virus; Poxviridae family
- Four genetic virus types, clinically indistinguishable
- Virions invade and replicate in cytoplasm of epithelial cells causing abnormal cell proliferation
- Genome encodes proteins to evade host immune system.
- Incubation period: 2 to 6 weeks
- Time to resolution: 6 to 24 months
- Not associated with malignancy
- No cross-hybridization or reactivation by other poxviruses

RISK FACTORS
- Skin-to-skin contact with infected person
- Contact sports
- Swimming
- Eczema, atopic dermatitis
- Sexual activity with infected partner
- Immunocompromised: HIV, chemotherapy, corticosteroid therapy, transplant patients

GENERAL PREVENTION
- Avoid skin-to-skin contact with host (e.g., contact sports, sexual activity).
- Avoid sharing clothing and towels.

COMMONLY ASSOCIATED CONDITIONS
- Atopic dermatitis
- Immunosuppression medications: corticosteroids, chemotherapy
- HIV/AIDS

 DIAGNOSIS

HISTORY
- Contact with known infected person
- Participation in contact sports
- Sexual activity

PHYSICAL EXAM
- Perform thorough skin exam including conjunctiva and anogenital area
- Discrete, firm papules with a central umbilication
- Umbilication is not obvious in small children.
- White curdlike core under umbilicated center
- Lesions are flesh, pearl, or red in color.
- May have surrounding erythema or dermatitis
- Immunocompetent hosts: average of 11 to 20 lesions, 2 to 5 mm diameter (range: 1 to 10 mm)
- Hosts with HIV/AIDS: hundreds of widespread lesions
- Children: trunk, extremities, face, anogenital region
- Sexually active: inner thighs, anogenital area

Pediatric Considerations
- Infants <3 months, consider vertical transmission
- Children: fever, >50 lesions, limited response to therapy, consider immunodeficiency
- Children: anogenital lesions, consider autoinoculation/possible sexual abuse

DIFFERENTIAL DIAGNOSIS
- AIDS patients: cryptococcus, penicilliosis, histoplasmosis, coccidioidomycosis
- Basal cell carcinoma
- Benign appendageal tumors: syringomas, hydrocystomas, ectopic sebaceous glands
- Condyloma acuminatum
- Dermatofibroma
- Eyelid: abscess, chalazion, foreign-body granuloma
- Folliculitis/furunculosis
- Keratoacanthoma
- Oral squamous cell carcinoma
- Trichoepithelioma
- Verruca vulgaris
- Warty dyskeratoma

DIAGNOSTIC TESTS & INTERPRETATION
Initial Tests (lab, imaging)
- Virus cannot be cultured.
- Culture lesion if concern is secondary infection
- Sexual transmission: Test for other sexually transmitted infections, including HIV.

- Microscopy: scrape lesion
  - Core material has characteristic Henderson-Paterson intracytoplasmic viral inclusion bodies.
  - Crush prep with 10% potassium hydroxide will show characteristic inclusion bodies as well.
  - Alternatively, hematoxylin-eosin-stained formalin-fixed tissue shows same confirmatory features.

Diagnostic Procedures/Other
Clinical; using magnifying lens

Tests Interpretation
Molluscum cytoplasmic inclusion bodies within keratinocytes

TREATMENT

GENERAL MEASURES
- In healthy patients, molluscum contagiosum is generally self-limited and heals spontaneously.
- No single intervention is shown to be convincingly more effective than any other in treating molluscum contagiosum (1)[B].
- No treatment is FDA-approved for treatment of molluscum contagiosum.
- Three categories of treatment: destructive, immune-enhancing, and antiviral

MEDICATION
First Line
- Cantharidin 0.7–0.9% solution: In office application to lesions, cover with dressing; wash off in 2 to 6 hours or sooner if blistering. Repeat treatment every 2 to 4 weeks until lesions resolve (1)[B],(2,3)[C].
  - Not commercially available in the United States but may be obtained from Canada
  - Adverse effects: blistering, erythema, pain, pruritus
  - Precautions: Do not use on face or on genital mucosa.

Second Line
- Benzoyl peroxide 10% cream: Apply to each lesion twice daily for 4 weeks (1)[B].
  - Inexpensive
  - Adverse effects: mild dermatitis
- For immunocompromised patients with refractory lesions, consider
  - Starting or maximizing HAART therapy in patients with HIV/AIDS (4)[C]

- Cidofovir
  - 3% cream applied to lesions once daily, 5 days/week for 8 weeks (4)[C]
  - 1% cream applied to lesions once daily, 5 days/week for 2 weeks, repeat in 1 month, if necessary (4)[C]
  - Adverse effects with topical use: erythema, pain, pruritus, erosions
  - 3 to 5 mg/kg IV weekly for 1 to 2 weeks, followed by IV infusions every other week, until clinical clearance or up to 9 infusions (5)[C]
  - Adverse effects with IV use: nephrotoxicity, neutropenia
  - Monitoring with IV use: renal function and complete blood counts prior to and 24 to 48 hours after infusions
  - Precaution: Must coadminister oral probenecid and provide IV hydration with each IV infusion; refer to cidofovir manufacturer's recommendations on dosing.
- Ingenol mebutate 0.015% gel applied to lesions once daily for 3 days; may repeat once if needed (6)[C] very expensive
  - Adverse effects: erythema, irritation

SURGERY/OTHER PROCEDURES
Considered first line

- Cryotherapy: 5 to 10 seconds with 1- to 2-mm margins; repeat every 3 to 4 weeks as needed until lesions disappear (7)[B].
  - Adverse effects: erythema, edema, pain, blistering
  - Contraindications: cryoglobulinemia, Raynaud disease
- Curettage under local or topical anesthesia (1)[A],(8)[B]
  - Adverse effects: pain, scarring

COMPLEMENTARY & ALTERNATIVE MEDICINE

- Australian lemon myrtle oil: Apply 10% solution once daily for 21 days (9)[B].
- Potassium hydroxide 5–10% solution: Apply 1 to 2 times a day until the lesions disappeared completely (10)[B].

Pediatric Considerations
- Surgical interventions: Second line in small children due to associated pain
- Pain control: Pretreat with topical lidocaine or EMLA before surgical treatment.
- Note: Adverse effect:
  - Lidocaine or EMLA over large body surface area: Methemoglobinemia and CNS toxicity. Refer to manufacturer's recommendations on dosing and use in children.

Pregnancy Considerations
Safe in pregnancy: curettage, cryotherapy, incision, and expression

 ONGOING CARE

FOLLOW-UP RECOMMENDATIONS
Patient Monitoring
Depends on type of treatment

PATIENT EDUCATION
- Cover lesions to prevent spread.
- Avoid scratching.
- Avoid contact sports.
- Avoid sharing towels and clothing.
- Avoid sexual activity when lesions present.

PROGNOSIS
- Immunocompetent: self-limited, resolves in 3 to 12 months (range: 2 months to 4 years)
- Immunocompromised: lesions difficult to treat; may persist for years

COMPLICATIONS
- Secondary infection
- Scarring, hyper-/hypopigmentation

REFERENCES

1. van der Wouden JC, Menke J, Gajadin S, et al. Interventions for cutaneous molluscum contagiosum. *Cochrane Database Syst Rev.* 2006;(2):CD004767.
2. Moye V, Cathcart S, Burkhart CN, et al. Beetle juice: a guide for the use of cantharidin in the treatment of molluscum contagiosum. *Dermatol Ther.* 2013;26(6):445–451.
3. Silverberg NB, Sidbury R, Mancini AJ. Childhood molluscum contagiosum: experience with cantharidin therapy in 300 patients. *J Am Acad Dermatol.* 2000;43(3):503–507.
4. Chen X, Anstey AV, Bugert JJ. Molluscum contagiosum virus infection. *Lancet Infect Dis.* 2013;13(10):877–888.
5. Erikson C, Driscoll M, Gaspari A. Efficacy of intravenous cidofovir in the treatment of giant molluscum contagiosum in a patient with human immunodeficiency virus. *Arch Dermatol.* 2011;147(6):652–654.
6. Javed S, Tyring SK. Treatment of molluscum contagiosum with ingenol mebutate. *J Am Acad Dermatol.* 2014;70(5):e105.
7. Al-Mutairi N, Al-Doukhi A, Al-Farag S, et al. Comparative study on the efficacy, safety, and acceptability of imiquimod 5% cream versus cryotherapy for molluscum contagiosum in children. *Pediatr Dermatol.* 2010;27(4):388–394.
8. Hanna D, Hatami A, Powell J, et al. A prospective randomized trial comparing the efficacy and adverse effects of four recognized treatments of molluscum contagiosum in children. *Pediatr Dermatol.* 2006;23(6):574–579.
9. Burke BE, Baillie JE, Olson RD. Essential oil of Australian lemon myrtle (*Backhousia citriodora*) in the treatment of molluscum contagiosum in children. *Biomed Pharmacother.* 2004;58(4):245–247.
10. Can B, Topaloglu F, Kavlale M, et al. Treatment of pediatric molluscum contagiosum with 10% potassium hydroxide solution. *J Dermatolog Treat.* 2014;25(3):246–248.

ADDITIONAL READING

- Brown J, Janniger CK, Schwartz RA, et al. Childhood molluscum contagiosum. *Int J Dermatol.* 2006;45(2):93–99.
- Dohil MA, Lin P, Lee J, et al. The epidemiology of molluscum contagiosum in children. *J Am Acad Dermatol.* 2006;54(1):47–54.
- Olsen JR, Gallacher J, Piguet V, et al. Epidemiology of molluscum contagiosum in children: a systematic review. *Fam Pract.* 2014;31(2):130–136.
- Ting PT, Dytoc MT. Therapy of external anogenital warts and molluscum contagiosum: a literature review. *Dermatol Ther.* 2004;17(1):68–101.

 CODES

ICD10
B08.1 Molluscum contagiosum

CLINICAL PEARLS

- Natural resolution is preferred treatment in healthy patients.
- Reassure parents that lesions will heal naturally and generally resolve without scarring.
- No specific treatment has been identified as superior to any other.
- Consider topical corticosteroids for pruritus or associated dermatitis.

M

MORTON NEUROMA (INTERDIGITAL NEUROMA)
Catherine Mygatt, MD • J. Herbert Stevenson, MD

 BASICS

DESCRIPTION
- Perineural fibrosis of the common digital nerve as it passes between metatarsals
  - The interspace between the 3rd and 4th metatarsals is most commonly affected.
  - Between the 2nd and 3rd metatarsals is the next most common site.
- System(s) affected: musculoskeletal, nervous
- Synonym(s): plantar digital neuritis; Morton metatarsalgia; intermetatarsal neuroma

EPIDEMIOLOGY
Prevalence
- Unknown
- Mean age: 45 to 50 years
- Predominant sex: female > male (8:1)

ETIOLOGY AND PATHOPHYSIOLOGY
- Lateral plantar nerve joins a portion of medial plantar nerve, creating a nerve with a larger diameter than those going to other digits.
- Nerve lies in SC tissue, deep to the fat pad of foot, just superficial to the digital artery and vein.
- Overlying, the nerve is the strong, deep transverse metatarsal ligament that holds the metatarsal bones together.
- With each step the patient takes, the inflamed nerve becomes compressed between the ground and the deep transverse metatarsal ligament. This can generate perineural fibrotic reaction with subsequent neuroma formation.

RISK FACTORS
- High-heeled shoes
  - Transfer more weight to the forefoot.
- Shoes with tight toe boxes
  - Cause lateral compression
- Pes planus (flat feet)
  - Pulls nerve medially, increasing irritation
- Obesity
- Female gender
- Ballet dancing, basketball, aerobics, tennis, running, and similar activities

GENERAL PREVENTION
- Wear properly fitting shoes.
- Avoid high heels and shoes with narrow toe boxes.

 DIAGNOSIS

HISTORY
- Most common complaint is pain localized to interspace between 3rd and 4th toes.
- Pain is less severe when not bearing weight.
- Pain, cramping, or numbness of the forefoot during weight bearing or immediately after strenuous foot exertion
- Radiation of pain to the toes
- Pain is relieved by removing shoes and massaging the foot.
- Patients often complain of "walking on a marble."
- Burning pain in the ball of the foot radiating to the toes
- Tingling or numbness in the toes
- Aggravated by wearing tight or narrow shoes

PHYSICAL EXAM
- Intense pain when pressure applied between metatarsal heads, sometimes with a palpable nodule
- Assess midfoot motion and digital motion to determine if arthritis or synovitis.
- Palpate along metatarsal shafts to assess for metatarsalgia or stress fractures.

DIFFERENTIAL DIAGNOSIS
- Stress fracture
- Hammer toe
- Metatarsophalangeal synovitis
- Metatarsalgia
- Arthritis
- Bursitis
- Foreign body

DIAGNOSTIC TESTS & INTERPRETATION
Initial Tests (lab, imaging)
- Predominantly a clinical diagnosis; imaging should be reserved for when the diagnosis is unclear or more than one web space is involved (1)[A],(2)[B].
- Radiographs may help to rule out osseous pathology if diagnosis is in question, but films usually are normal in patients with a Morton neuroma (1)[A].
- US has 79% specificity and 99% sensitivity for Morton neuromas but is poor at assessing the size of the lesion. Specificity declines to 50% for lesions <6 mm (1)[A].
- MRI can rule out an osseous tumor and help determine how much of the nerve to resect surgically; it has a sensitivity of 83% and a specificity of 99% (1)[A].

Diagnostic Procedures/Other
- Five special tests have been described: thumb index finger squeeze test, Mulder sign, foot squeeze test, plantar percussion test, and toe tip sensation deficit.

  - Thumb index finger squeeze test is the most sensitive and specific (96% and 96%, respectively). Positive when pain elicited by squeezing the symptomatic intermetatarsal space between the index finger and thumb (3)[B].
  - Mulder sign is a painful "click" produced by squeezing the metatarsal heads together while compressing the neuroma between the thumb and index finger of the other hand; sensitivity 40–84% (1)[A].
  - Foot squeeze test is positive when pain is induced in the symptomatic web space when the metatarsal heads are compressed by grasping the foot; sensitivity 40% (3)[B].

  - Plantar and dorsal percussion tests are positive when percussion of the affected webspace is painful.
  - Toe tip sensation deficit exists when the sensation of the toe distal to the affected web space is decreased relative to the other toes.

- More than one of the above tests being positive increases the diagnostic accuracy (4)[B].

Test Interpretation
Chronic fibrosis and thickening of the digital nerve

TREATMENT

GENERAL MEASURES
- Wear flat shoes with a roomy toe box.
- Plantar pads may help with alignment of metatarsal heads and provide relief.
- NSAIDs for temporary symptom relief

MEDICATION
First Line
Injectable steroids (e.g., betamethasone phosphate/ acetate or methylprednisolone): use if general measures fail; number needed to treat (NNT) for significant benefit over conservative measures = 2.3 (5,6)[A].

Second Line

- US-guided alcohol ablation therapy to sclerose the nerve is safe, reduces pain, and may offer an alternative to surgery (7,8)[B].
- A pilot study has demonstrated that injection with onabotulinumtoxina is of possible usefulness to relieve the pain and improve function in Morton neuroma (9)[B].
- There is no evidence for the use of supinatory insoles (10)[A].

ISSUES FOR REFERRAL

Continued pain despite conservative treatments and injections.

SURGERY/OTHER PROCEDURES

Surgical removal of the neuroma or shortening of the metatarsals, with or without release of the transverse metatarsal ligament, have a 61–100% success rate defined by satisfaction scores (11)[A].

 ONGOING CARE

FOLLOW-UP RECOMMENDATIONS

At diagnosis, or if no improvement after 3 months of conservative treatment, consider corticosteroid injection.

- May repeat injection if no improvement after 2 to 4 weeks, or consider referring for surgical management.
- 21–51% of patients receiving a single corticosteroid injection require surgical intervention within 2 to 4 years (12)[B].
- Size >5 mm and younger patients are more likely to undergo invasive treatment (12)[B].

PATIENT EDUCATION

Wear properly fitting comfortable shoes.

PROGNOSIS

- 40–50% improve with 3 months of conservative treatment.
- 45–60% improve with steroid injection (6)[A].
- 96% improve with surgery.

COMPLICATIONS

Hip and knee pain related to gait changes

REFERENCES

1. Sharp RJ, Wade CM, Hennessy MS, et al. The role of MRI and ultrasound imaging in Morton's neuroma and the effect of size of lesion on symptoms. *J Bone Joint Surg Br.* 2003;85(7):999–1005.
2. Pastides P, El-Sallakh S, Charalambides C. Morton's neuroma: a clinical versus radiological diagnosis. *Foot Ankle Surg.* 2012;18(1):22–24.
3. Mahadevan D, Venkatesan M, Bhatt R, et al. Diagnostic accuracy of clinical tests for Morton's neuroma compared with ultrasonography. *J Foot Ankle Surg.* 2015;54(4):549–553.
4. Owens R, Gougoulias N, Guthrie H, et al. Morton's neuroma: clinical testing and imaging in 76 feet, compared to a control group. *Foot Ankle Surg.* 2011;17(3):197–200.
5. Saygi B, Yildirim Y, Saygi EK, et al. Morton's neuroma: comparative results of two conservative methods. *Foot Ankle Int.* 2005;26(7):556–559.
6. Thomson CE, Beggs I, Martin DJ, et al. Methyl-prednisolone injections for the treatment of Morton neuroma: a patient-blinded randomized trial. *J Bone Joint Surg Am.* 2013;95(9):790–798.
7. Musson RE, Sawhney JS, Lamb L, et al. Ultrasound guided alcohol ablation of Morton's neuroma. *Foot Ankle Int.* 2012;33(3):196–201.
8. Hughes RJ, Ali K, Jones H, et al. Treatment of Morton's neuroma with alcohol injection under sonographic guidance: follow-up of 101 cases. *AJR Am J Roentgenol.* 2007;188(6):1535–1539.
9. Climent JM, Mondéjar-Gómez F, Rodríguez-Ruiz C, et al. Treatment of Morton neuroma with botulinum toxin A: a pilot study. *Clin Drug Investig.* 2013;33(7):497–503.
10. Thomson CE, Gibson JN, Martin D. Interventions for the treatment of Morton's neuroma. *Cochrane Database Syst Rev.* 2004;(3):CD003118.
11. Akermark C, Crone H, Skoog A, et al. A prospective randomized controlled trial of plantar versus dorsal incisions for operative treatment of primary Morton's neuroma. *Foot Ankle Int.* 2013;34(9):1198–1204.
12. Mahadevan D, Salmasi M, Whybra N, et al. What factors predict the need for further intervention following corticosteroid injection of Morton's neuroma? *Foot Ankle Surg.* In press.

ADDITIONAL READING

- Jain S, Mannan K. The diagnosis and management of Morton's neuroma: a literature review. *Foot Ankle Spec.* 2013;6(4):307–317.
- Schreiber K, Khodaee M, Poddar S, et al. Clinical inquiry. What is the best way to treat Morton's neuroma? *J Fam Pract.* 2011;60(3):157–158, 168.

 CODES

ICD10

- G57.60 Lesion of plantar nerve, unspecified lower limb
- G57.61 Lesion of plantar nerve, right lower limb
- G57.62 Lesion of plantar nerve, left lower limb

CLINICAL PEARLS

- Morton neuroma is usually a clinical diagnosis.
- Footwear modification is the mainstay of treatment.
- Corticosteroid injection into, or US-guided alcohol ablation of the neuroma may be helpful.
- Neurectomy is the definitive treatment. Patients should be aware of the likelihood of postoperative dysesthesias.

M

MOTION SICKNESS

Courtney I. Jarvis, PharmD • Allison Hargreaves, MD

 BASICS

DESCRIPTION

- Motions sickness is not a true sickness but a normal response to a situation in which sensory conflict about body motion exists among visual receptors, vestibular receptors, and body proprioceptors.
- Also can be induced when patterns of motion differ from those previously experienced
- System affected: nervous
- Synonym(s): car sickness; sea sickness; air sickness; space sickness; physiologic vertigo

EPIDEMIOLOGY

Incidence
Predominant sex: female > male

Prevalence
Estimation is complex; syndrome occurs in ~25% due to travel by air, ~29% by sea, and ~41% by road. Estimates for vomiting are 0.5% by air, 7% by sea, and 2% by road.

ETIOLOGY AND PATHOPHYSIOLOGY

- Precise etiology unknown; thought to be due to a mismatch of vestibular and visual sensations
- Rotary, vertical, and low frequency motions produce more symptoms than linear, horizontal, and high-frequency motions.
- Nausea and vomiting occur as a result of increased levels of dopamine and acetylcholine, which stimulate chemoreceptor trigger zone and vomiting center in CNS.

Genetics
Heritability estimates range from 55% to 75%.

RISK FACTORS

- Motion (auto, plane, boat, amusement rides)
- Travel
- Visual stimuli (e.g., moving horizon)
- Poor ventilation (fumes, smoke, carbon monoxide)
- Emotions (fear, anxiety)
- Zero gravity
- Pregnancy, menstruation, oral contraceptive use
- History of migraine headaches, especially vestibular migraine
- Other illness or poor health

GENERAL PREVENTION
See "General Measures."

Pediatric Considerations
- Rare in children <2 years of age
- Incidence peaks between 3 and 12 years of age.
- Antihistamines may cause excitation in children.

Geriatric Considerations
- Age confers some resistance to motion sickness.
- Elderly are at increased risk of anticholinergic side effects from treatment.

Pregnancy Considerations
- Pregnant patients are more likely to experience motion sickness.
- Treat with medications is thought to be safe during morning sickness (e.g., meclizine, dimenhydrinate).

COMMONLY ASSOCIATED CONDITIONS
- Migraine headache
- Vestibular syndromes

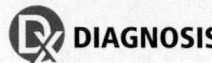 DIAGNOSIS

HISTORY
Presence of the following signs and symptoms in the context of a typical stimulus (1)[C]:

- Nausea
- Vomiting
- Stomach awareness (feeling of fullness in epigastrium)
- Diaphoresis
- Facial and perioral pallor
- Hypersalivation
- Yawning
- Hyperventilation
- Anxiety
- Panic
- Malaise
- Fatigue
- Weakness
- Confusion
- Dizziness

PHYSICAL EXAM
No specific findings

DIFFERENTIAL DIAGNOSIS
- Mountain sickness
- Vestibular disease, central and peripheral
- Gastroenteritis
- Metabolic disorders
- Toxin exposure

DIAGNOSTIC TESTS & INTERPRETATION
None indicated

 TREATMENT

- Follow guidelines under "General Measures" section to prevent motion sickness (1)[C].
- Premedicate before travel with antidopaminergic, anticholinergic, or antihistamine agents (1)[A]:
  - For extended travel, consider treatment with scopolamine transdermal patch (2)[A].
  - 2nd-generation (nonsedating) antihistamines are not effective at preventing motion sickness (3)[B].
  - Serotonin (5-HT3) antagonists (e.g., ondansetron) are not effective in preventing motion sickness (4)[B].
- Conflicting data exist on the efficacy of acupressure for nausea and vomiting associated with motion sickness (5)[B].
- Benzodiazepines suppress vestibular nuclei but would not be considered first line due to sedation and addiction potential (6)[C].
- Serotonin receptor agonist (rizatriptan) may be effective for migraineurs with motion sickness (7)[C].

GENERAL MEASURES
- Avoid noxious types of motions.
- Choose locations within vehicle that minimizes motion (airplanes: over the wing; automobiles: driver's or front passenger seat, facing forward; boat: facing towards the waves, away from rocking bow, near surface of the water; buses: near the front, at lowest level, facing forward; trains: at lowest level, facing forward).
- Improve ventilation; avoid noxious stimuli.
- Use semirecumbent seating or lay supine.
- Fix vision on horizon; avoid fixation on moving objects; keep eyes fixed on still, distant objects.
- Avoid reading while actively traveling.
- Frequent and graded exposure to stimulus that triggers nausea (habituation).
- Eat before travel, avoid empty stomach; eat light, soft, bland, low-fat, and low-acid foods; avoid alcohol.
- Increase airflow around face.
- Acupressure on point PC6 has been shown to reduce feelings of nausea but not the incidence of vomiting during pregnancy, after surgery, and in cancer chemotherapy. However, conflicting evidence of efficacy has been found for motion sickness. Point PC6 (*Neiguan* on pericardium meridian): 2 cm proximal of transverse crease of palmar side of wrist between tendons of the palmaris longus and the flexor carpi radialis (5)[B]

MEDICATION

First Line

- Scopolamine transdermal patch (Transderm Scop): Apply 2.5-cm^2 (4 mg) patch behind ear at least 4 hours (preferably 6 to 12 hours) before travel, and replace every 3 days (2)[A].

- Dimenhydrinate (Dramamine): take 30 to 60 minutes before travel
  - Adults and adolescents: 50 to 100 mg q4–6h, maximum 400 mg/day
  - Children 6 to 12 years of age: 25 to 50 mg q6–8h, maximum 150 mg/day
  - Children 2 to 5 years of age: 12.5 to 25 mg q6–8h, maximum 75 mg/day
- Meclizine (Antivert): take 60 minutes before travel
  - Adults and adolescents >12 years of age: 25 to 50 mg q24h
  - Children <12 years of age: not recommended
- Diphenhydramine (Benadryl): take 30 to 60 minutes before travel
  - Adults and adolescents: 25 to 50 mg q6–8h, maximum 300 mg/day
  - Children 6 to 12 years of age: 5 mg/kg or 12.5 to 25 mg q6–8h, maximum 300 mg/day
- Promethazine (Phenergan): take 30 to 60 minutes before travel
  - Adults and adolescents: 25 mg q12h; 25 to 50 mg IM if already developed severe motion sickness
  - Children 2 to 12 years of age: 0.5 mg/kg q12h, maximum 25 mg BID. *Caution*: increased risk of dystonic reaction in this age group
- Contraindications: patients at risk for acute angle-closure glaucoma
- Precautions:
  - Young children
  - Elderly
  - Pregnancy
  - Urinary obstruction
  - Pyloric-duodenal obstruction
- Adverse reactions:
  - Drowsiness
  - Dry mouth
  - Blurred vision
  - Confusion
  - Headache
  - Urinary retention
- Significant possible interactions:
  - Sedatives (antihistamines, alcohol, antidepressants)
  - Anticholinergics (belladonna alkaloids)

Second Line

- Benzodiazepines: take 1 to 2 hours before travel
  - Diazepam 2 to 10 mg PO q6–12h
  - Lorazepam 1 to 2 mg PO q8h
- Contraindications:
  - Severe respiratory dysfunction
  - Severe liver dysfunction
- Precautions:
  - Alcohol/drug abuse
  - Elderly
  - Sedation
  - Addiction is possible.

COMPLEMENTARY & ALTERNATIVE MEDICINE

Ginger: 940 mg or 1 g; take 4 hours before travel (evidence controversial) (8)[B]

 ## ONGOING CARE

DIET

- Eat before travel, avoid empty stomach; eat light, soft, bland, low-fat, and low-acid foods.
- Avoid alcohol.

PROGNOSIS

- Symptoms should resolve when motion exposure ends.
- Resistance to motion sickness seems to increase with age.

COMPLICATIONS

- Hypotension
- Dehydration
- Depression
- Panic
- Syncope

REFERENCES

1. Brainard A, Gresham C. Prevention and treatment of motion sickness. *Am Fam Physician*. 2014;90(1):41–46.
2. Spinks AB, Wasiak J, Villanueva EV, et al. Scopolamine (hyoscine) for preventing and treating motion sickness. *Cochrane Database Syst Rev*. 2007;(3):CD002851.
3. Cheung BS, Heskin R, Hofer KD. Failure of cetirizine and fexofenadine to prevent motion sickness. *Ann Pharmacother*. 2003;37(2):173–177.
4. Hershkovitz D, Asna N, Shupak A, et al. Ondansetron for the prevention of seasickness in susceptible sailors: an evaluation at sea. *Aviat Space Environ Med*. 2009;80(7):643–646.
5. Streitberger K, Ezzo J, Schneider A. Acupuncture for nausea and vomiting: an update of clinical and experimental studies. *Auton Neurosci*. 2006;129 (1–2):107–117.
6. Zajonc TP, Roland PS. Vertigo and motion sickness. Part II: pharmacologic treatment. *Ear Nose Throat J*. 2006;85(1):25–35.
7. Furman JM, Marcus DA, Balaban CD. Rizatriptan reduces vestibular-induced motion sickness in migraineurs. *J Headache Pain*. 2011;12(12):81–88.
8. White B. Ginger: an overview. *Am Fam Physician*. 2007;75(11):1689–1691.

ADDITIONAL READING

Murdin L, Golding J, Bronstein A. Managing motion sickness. *BMJ*. 2011;343:d7430.

 ## SEE ALSO

Algorithm: Dizziness

 ## CODES

ICD10

T75.3XXA Motion sickness, initial encounter

CLINICAL PEARLS

- The scopolamine patch should be applied at least 4 hours before travel, although it may be more effective if placed 6 to 12 hours before departure.
- Oral medications should be administered 30 to 60 minutes before departure.
- Although acupressure wristbands have been found to be effective by systematic reviews in postoperative and chemotherapy-induced nausea and vomiting, conflicting data exist for motion sickness.

M

MULTIPLE MYELOMA

Jasmine S. Beria, DO, MPH • Maria M. Plummer, MD

 BASICS

DESCRIPTION
- Multiple myeloma (MM) is a clonal proliferation of malignant plasma cells.
- This clonal proliferation in the bone marrow can cause extensive skeletal destruction with osteolytic lesions and pathologic fractures.
- The malignant plasma cells produce monoclonal protein in the blood and urine.
- MM is also characterized by hypercalcemia, increased susceptibility to infections, renal impairment, and end-organ damage.
- Monoclonal gammopathy of undetermined significance (MGUS) is a common disorder with limited monoclonal plasma cell proliferation that progresses to MM at rate of ~1% per year.
- MGUS progresses to smouldering or asymptomatic MM and eventually to symptomatic MM.
- Synonym(s): plasma cell myeloma; plasma cell leukemia

EPIDEMIOLOGY
- Accounts for ~1% of all cancers and slightly >10% of hematologic malignancies in the United States
- Median age of diagnosis is 69 years.
- Slight male predominance. Blacks about 2 to 3 times more commonly affected than whites; less common in Asians.

Incidence
4 to 5 new cases/100,000 annually

Prevalence
In 2012, there were 89, 658 cases in the United States (1).

ETIOLOGY AND PATHOPHYSIOLOGY
- Clonal proliferation of plasma cells derived from postgerminal center B cells (2)
- Plasma cells undergo multiple chromosomal mutations to progress to MM.
- Genetic damage in developing B lymphocytes at time of isotype switching, transforming normal plasma cells into malignant cells, arising from single clone
- Earliest chromosomal translocations involve immunoglobulin heavy chains on chromosome 14q32, with the translocation at t(4;14), t(14;16), t(14;20), and deletion, del(17p) having a poorer prognosis.
- Malignant cells multiply in bone marrow, suppressing normal bone marrow cells and producing large quantities of monoclonal immunoglobulin (M) protein.
- Malignant cells stimulate osteoclasts that cause bone resorption and inhibit osteoblasts that form new bone, causing lytic bone lesions.

Genetics
Rare family clusters; the hyperphosphorylated form of Paratarg-7, a protein of unknown significance, is inherited as an autosomal dominant trait in familial cases of MM and MGUS, suggesting a potential pathogenic role.

RISK FACTORS
- Most cases have no known risks associated.
- Older age; immunosuppression; and chemicals like dioxin, herbicides, insecticides, petroleum, heavy metals, plastics, and ionizing radiation increase the risk of MM.
- MGUS stage consistently precedes MM.

COMMONLY ASSOCIATED CONDITIONS
Secondary amyloidosis commonly due to MM

 DIAGNOSIS

HISTORY
- 34% of patients are asymptomatic at the time of presentation.
- Hypercalcemia (28%): anorexia, nausea, somnolence, and polydipsia
- Renal failure (20–50%)
- Anemia (73%)
- Bony lesions (80%): lytic lesions causing bone pain (58%) (3), osteoporosis or pathologic fracture (26–34%)
- Other symptoms: fatigue (32%), peripheral neuropathy, weight loss (24%), recurrent infections, hyperviscosity syndrome, and cord compression

PHYSICAL EXAM
- Dehydration
- Skin findings of amyloidosis: waxy papules, nodules, or plaques that may be evident in the eyelids, retroauricular region, neck, or inguinal and anogenital regions; petechiae and ecchymosis; "pinch purpura"
- Extramedullary plasmacytomas can present as large, purplish, subcutaneous masses.
- Hyperviscosity syndrome in 7%: retinal hemorrhages, prolonged bleeding, neurologic changes
- Tender bones and masses

DIFFERENTIAL DIAGNOSIS
- MGUS
- Smoldering MM
- Metastatic carcinoma (kidney, breast, non–small cell lung cancer)
- Waldenström macroglobulinemia
- AL amyloidosis
- Solitary plasmacytoma
- Polyneuropathy, organomegaly, endocrinopathy, M protein, skin changes (POEMS) syndrome

DIAGNOSTIC TESTS & INTERPRETATION
Criteria for diagnosis: The diagnosis of MM requires the following (2)[A]:

- Bone marrow (BM) involvement with ≥10% of plasma cells (PC) or the presence of a plasmacytoma
- Monoclonal protein (M-spike) in the blood and/or urine
- Presence of one or more of the following: calcium elevation (>11 g/dL), renal insufficiency (creatinine >2 mg/dL), anemia (hemoglobin <10 g/dL or >2 g/dL below normal), bone disease

Initial Tests (lab, imaging)
- CBC with differential to evaluate anemia and other cytopenias with evaluation of peripheral blood smear
- BUN, creatinine (elevated creatinine due to myeloma cast nephropathy)
- Serum electrolytes, serum albumin, serum calcium
- Serum lactate dehydrogenase (LDH), β_2-microglobulin
- Serum protein electrophoresis (SPEP), serum immunofixation electrophoresis (SIFE): M protein level elevated
- Quantitative serum immunoglobulin levels: immunoglobulin (Ig) G, IgA, and IgM

- Quantitative serum free light chain (FLC) levels: κ and λ chains
- Elevated ESR, C-reactive protein
- Urine analysis: 24-hour urine for protein, urine protein electrophoresis (UPEP), urine immunofixation electrophoresis (UIFE); 20% positive urine protein (2)[A]:
  – Urinalysis dip is often negative for protein, as this test identifies albumin, and the protein in MM is Bence-Jones (BJ) monoclonal protein.
- Bone marrow aspirate and biopsy for histology, immunohistochemistry, flow cytometry, cytogenetics, and fluorescence in situ hybridization (FISH)
- Skeletal survey: for lytic bone lesions, osteopenia, osteoporosis, or compression fractures
- MRI for any back pain or earliest signs/symptoms of spinal cord compression

Follow-Up Tests & Special Considerations
- CT scan: if high suspicion for bone lesions despite normal skeletal survey; can differentiate malignant from benign vertebral compression fractures in patients who are not MRI candidates
- PET scans: used if bone involvement is suspected despite a normal skeletal survey, MRI, and CT
- Baseline bone densitometry may be indicated (2)[A].
- Bone marrow aspiration and biopsy to monitor response to treatment
- SPEP with SIFE: M protein helps to track progression of myeloma and response to treatment.
- Serum immunoglobulins and free light chains can be used to monitor response or relapse.
- Plasma cell labeling index may be helpful to identify the fraction of the myeloma cell population that is proliferating (2)[A].

Diagnostic Procedures/Other
Staging:
- Durie Salmon stage
  – Stage I: low cell mass: $<0.6 \times 10^{12}$ cells/m^2 plus all of the following: hemoglobin >10 g/dL, M protein <5 g/dL if IgG or <3 g/dL if IgA, normal serum calcium, urine BJ protein <4 g/24 hr, no generalized lytic bone lesions
  – Stage II: neither stage I nor stage III
  – Stage III: high cell mass: $>1.2 \times 10^{12}$ cells/m^2 plus one or more of the following: hemoglobin <8.5 g/L, serum calcium >12 mg/dL, bone lesions, M protein > 7g/dL if IgG and >5 g/dL if IgA, urine BJ protein >12 g/24 hr, advanced lytic bone lesions
- International staging system (ISS)
  – Stage I: albumin ≥3.5 g/dL and β_2-microglobulin <3.5 μg/mL
  – Stage II: neither stage I nor stage III
  – Stage III: β_2-microglobulin ≥5.5 μg/Ml
- Mayo Clinic risk stratification (mSMART)
  – Standard risk: t(11:14), t(6:14), and hyperdiploidy
  – Intermediate risk: t(4:14), del(13q) by cytogenetics, hypodiploidy
  – High risk: t(14:16), t(14:20), del(17 p), and plasma cell labeling index >3%

Test Interpretation
Bone marrow involvement with plasma cells ≥10%; Russell bodies

TREATMENT

- Treatment varies depending on level of disease activity and stage of MM.
- Treatment for smoldering MM is close monitoring at 3-month intervals. Early treatment with lenalidomide and dexamethasone delays progression and increases overall survival (3)[B].
- Key determinant factor in choosing chemotherapy regimen is to establish if the patient is an autologous stem cell transplant (ASCT) candidate or not.
- Treatment protocols vary by institution and patient.
- ASCT following induction chemotherapy is standard of care for patients with symptomatic disease.

GENERAL MEASURES

Maintain adequate hydration to prevent renal insufficiency. All patients receiving primary melanoma therapy should be given bisphosphonates initially (2)[A].

MEDICATION

- Induction chemotherapy for ASCT-eligible patients (4)[C]:
  - Standard risk: (lenalidomide/low-dose dexamethasone)
  - Intermediate risk: (bortezomib/cyclophosphamide/dexamethasone)
  - High risk: (bortezomib/lenalidomide/dexamethasone)
  - After ASCT, maintenance can include a bortezomib compound for the high- or intermediate-risk group; lenalidomide can be considered for the standard group. Maintenance lenalidomide after ASCT has shown to improve progression-free survival (PFS) of 41 versus 23 months with placebo and has shown to be an effective treatment for MM (5,6)[A].
- Induction chemotherapy for ASCT-ineligible patients:
  - Same regimens as ASCT-eligible patients, however, the number of treatment cycles are increased (4)[C].

First Line

- Bortezomib
  - A proteasome inhibitor; it blocks the ubiquitin-proteasome catalytic pathway in cells by binding to the 20S proteasome complex.
  - Toxicity: peripheral neuropathy, cytopenia, nausea
  - Consider herpes simplex virus (HSV) prophylaxis.
- Cyclophosphamide
  - Nitrogen mustard–derivative alkylating agent
  - Often used in combination with prednisone or thalidomide in cases of relapsed disease
  - Toxicity: cytopenia, anaphylaxis, interstitial pulmonary fibrosis, secondary malignancy, impaired fertility
- Immunomodulators
  - Thalidomide and lenalidomide
    - Works by antiangiogenesis inhibition, immunomodulation, and inhibition of tumor necrosis factor
    - Toxicity: birth defects, deep vein thrombosis (DVT), neuropathy, rash, nausea, bradycardia
    - DVT prophylaxis, usually with aspirin
- Dexamethasone
  - Low doses (40 mg/week) superior to higher doses
  - Increases risk of DVT
- Bisphosphonates (7)[A]
  - No effect on mortality but decrease pain, pathologic vertebral fractures, and fractures of other bones
  - IV pamidronate or zoledronic acid can be used; evidence that zoledronic acid may be superior in preventing skeletal-related events.
  - Dose-adjust/monitor renal function.
  - Monitor for osteonecrosis of jaw.

- Alternative options:
  - As first-line treatment for transplant-ineligible patients with newly diagnosed MM, bortezomib/melphalan/prednisone was associated with significantly increased PFS compared with melphalan/prednisone (8)[A].

Second Line

- May be treated with any of the agents not already used
- The following agents can be used as salvage therapy to treat relapsed or refractory MM:
  - Bortezomib/lenalidomide
  - Liposomal doxorubicin
  - Carfilzomib: 2nd-generation selective proteasome inhibitor
- Emerging options: pomalidomide, thalidomide analog
- Bortezomib is a highly effective option in previously treated/relapse patients and is well-tolerated (9)[A].
- Interferon-α may be appropriate in selected patients, but because of its toxicity and availability of better alternatives, it has a limited role in treating MM.

ISSUES FOR REFERRAL

For spinal or other bone pathology, refer to orthopedics for support.

ADDITIONAL THERAPIES

- Local radiation therapy for bone pain
- Effective pain management: Avoid NSAIDs due to nephrotoxicity.
- Kyphoplasty/vertebroplasty: consider for symptomatic vertebral compressions
- Plasmapheresis: for hyperviscosity syndrome (a rare complication)
- Erythropoietin: for selected patients with anemia
- Patients should receive vaccines for pneumococcus and influenza.
- Do not administer zoster vaccine and other live-virus vaccines.

INPATIENT CONSIDERATIONS

Admission Criteria/Initial Stabilization

Indications: pain, infections, cytopenia, renal failure, bone complications, spinal cord compression

- Avoid IV radiographic contrast materials due to risk for contrast-induced nephropathy.
- Adequate hydration
- Manage hypercalcemia and control hyperuricemia.

 ONGOING CARE

PATIENT EDUCATION

- http://myeloma.org/Main.action
- http://www.nccn.org/patients/guidelines/myeloma/index.html

PROGNOSIS

- Median survival overall is 3 years. The 5-year survival rate is around 35%.
- Median survival by ISS stage:
  - Stage I: 62 months
  - Stage II: 44 months
  - Stage III: 29 months
- Median survival in patients with high-risk multiple myeloma (see staging for definition) is <2 to 3 years, even after ASCT; standard risk have median overall survival of 6 to 7 years.

COMPLICATIONS

Many; including infection, pain, lytic bone lesions, hypercalcemia, hyperuricemia, spinal cord compression, anemia, hyperviscosity syndrome, amyloidosis, renal insufficiency

REFERENCES

1. Howlader N, Noone AM, Krapcho M, et al. *SEER Cancer Statistics Review, 1975–2012*. Bethesda, MD: National Cancer Institute. http://seer.cancer.gov/csr/1975_2012/. Accessed 2015.
2. Mhaskar R, Redzepovic J, Wheatley K, et al. Bisphosphonates in multiple myeloma: a network meta-analysis. *Cochrane Database Syst Rev*. 2012;(5):CD003188.
3. Mateos MV, Hernández MT, Giraldo P, et al. Lenalidomide plus dexamethasone for high-risk smoldering multiple myeloma. *N Engl J Med*. 2013;369(5):438–447.
4. Palumbo A, Anderson K. Multiple myeloma. *N Engl J Med*. 2011;364(11):1046–1060.
5. Palumbo A, Hajek R, Delforge M, et al. Continuous lenalidomide treatment for newly diagnosed multiple myeloma. *N Engl J Med*. 2012;366(19):1759–1769.
6. Yang B, Yu RL, Chi XH, et al. Lenalidomide treatment for multiple myeloma: systematic review and meta-analysis of randomized controlled trials. *PLoS One*. 2013;8(5):e64354.
7. Rajkumar SV. Multiple myeloma: 2013 update on diagnosis, risk-stratification, and management. *Am J Hematol*. 2013;88(3):226–235.
8. San Miguel JF, Schlag R, Khuageva NK, et al. Persistent overall survival benefit and no increased risk of second malignancies with bortezomib-melphalan-prednisone versus melphalan-prednisone in patients with previously untreated multiple myeloma. *J Clin Oncol*. 2013;31(4):448–455.
9. Knopf KB, Duh MS, Lafeuille MH, et al. Meta-analysis of the efficacy and safety of bortezomib re-treatment in patients with multiple myeloma. *Clin Lymphoma Myeloma Leuk*. 2014;14(5):380–388.

ADDITIONAL READING

- Grass S, Preuss KD, Thome S, et al. Paraproteins of familial MGUS/multiple myeloma target family-typical antigens: hyperphosphorylation of autoantigens is a consistent finding in familial and sporadic MGUS/MM. *Blood*. 2011;118(3):635–637.
- National Comprehensive Cancer Network. NCCN multiple myeloma clinical practice guidelines in oncology (Version 2.2014). National Comprehensive Cancer Network Web site. Published 2014. http://www.nccn.org/. Accessed 2014.

CODES

ICD10

- C90.00 Multiple myeloma not having achieved remission
- C90.01 Multiple myeloma in remission
- C90.02 Multiple myeloma in relapse

CLINICAL PEARLS

- MM is a plasma cell malignancy that causes end-organ damage.
- Look for presence of "CRAB" (hypercalcemia, renal insufficiency, anemia, and bone lesions).
- Suspect MM if high total protein-to-albumin ratio is present.
- Maintain high index of suspicion for spinal cord compression.
- Avoid nephrotoxins (radiographic contrast material, NSAIDs, dehydration).
- Patients with MM are immunocompromised.

M

MULTIPLE SCLEROSIS

Adam W. Kowalski, MD • Vernon Wheeler, MD, FAAFP

 BASICS

DESCRIPTION
- An autoinflammatory disease causing demyelin-ation, neuronal loss, and scarring within the white matter of the brain and spinal cord.
- Four recognized forms of multiple sclerosis (MS) (1):
  - Relapsing-remitting multiple sclerosis (RRMS): episodic flare-ups occurring over days to weeks between periods of neurologic stability. During attacks, new symptoms may present, whereas previous symptoms may worsen. Complete recovery or residual deficits may ensue following each bout.
  - Secondary progressive multiple sclerosis (SPMS): beginning as RRMS, progressive deterioration of neurologic function ensues; not associated with attacks, (progression may continue or halt). ~2% risk per year of RRMS becoming SPMS
  - Primary progressive multiple sclerosis (PPMS): steady decline of neurologic function from onset of disease without episodic flares
  - Progressive relapsing multiple sclerosis (PRMS): steady decline of neurologic function from onset of disease with episodic flare-ups

Pregnancy Considerations
- Most patients experience lower exacerbation rates during pregnancy. Following delivery, the immune system reverts and MS flares become more likely.
- Breastfeeding does not affect the risk of MS relapse.
- Relapse during postpartum can be safely treated by IVIG and corticosteroids (2)[C].

EPIDEMIOLOGY
- Age: Peak incidence ages 15 to 45 years, mean age 28 to 31 (slightly earlier in women than men)
- Gender: Studies suggest F:M between 1.4:1 and 3:1
- Latitude: Prevalence tends to rise with increasing distance from the equator, although newer data reveals this latitude gradient may be declining (3,4).

Incidence
- Women (worldwide): 3.6 cases/100,000 person-years
- Men (worldwide): 2.0 cases/100,000 person-years

Prevalence
- United States: ~350,000 MS patients
- Worldwide: ~2,500,000 MS patients

ETIOLOGY AND PATHOPHYSIOLOGY
- MS lesions: Inflammatory cells, mainly T lymphocytes and macrophages, surround vasculature within the CNS, creating sites of inflammation. These cells then disrupt the blood–brain barrier and infiltrate the surrounding white matter, meanwhile preserving the vessel wall. B lymphocytes, as well as myelin-specific autoantibodies also infiltrate the CNS and cause degeneration of the myelin sheaths.
- Following demyelination, faster salutatory nerve conduction velocities (impulses jumping between nodes of Ranvier) are replaced with considerably slower continuous nerve velocities.
- Astrocytes begin to proliferate and cause gliosis.
- Oligodendrocytes, which have survived, or are some formed from precursor cells, are able to partially re-myelinate stripped axons, producing irreversible scars.
- In each MS lesion, axonal damage may occur, but it is the cumulative axonal loss over time that is responsible for the progressive and irreversible neurologic disability seen in MS patients.
- Most axons are typically lost from the lateral corti-cospinal (motor) tracts of the spinal cord.

Genetics
- Strong predisposition: HLA DRB1 (5)
- Proposed predisposition: IL2RA and IL7RA
- Race: Caucasian > Africans or Asians

RISK FACTORS
- Genetic: DRB1 locus on chromosome 6 has strongest MS risk association; DRB1*15 and *16 produce major histocompatibility complexes (MHC) with high binding affinity to myelin basic proteins (MBPs) (3,5).
- Geographic: Previously distance from equator showed association with increased risk, though now declining. However, sun exposure (ultraviolet B (UVB) radiation necessary for endogenous vitamin D production) appears to have inverse relation to MS incidence (3).
- Infectious: viral infections (especially EBV, HHV) (3,5)
- Race: Caucasian > African, Asian, Native American, although this is decreasing (5)
- Others: tobacco smoking (6)

GENERAL PREVENTION
Further research is required to determine prevention from environmental risk factors. A goal of therapy is to prevent new attacks and disability.

COMMONLY ASSOCIATED CONDITIONS
- Internuclear ophthalmoplegia (INO): Injury to the medial longitudinal fasciculus (MLF) causes impaired adduction to the affected eye.
- Optic neuritis: inflammation of optic nerve resulting in loss of vision
- Uhthoff phenomenon: Symptoms worsen with exposure to higher than usual temperature.
- Lhermitte sign: electric-like shocks extending down the spine caused by neck movement, especially flexion

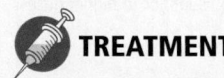 DIAGNOSIS

- A person with MS can present with a number of neurologic signs and symptoms depending on the locations of the lesions within the CNS (5)[C].
- Clinical diagnosis: ≥2 attacks; objective clinical evidence of ≥2 lesions or objective clinical evidence of 1 lesion with history of a previous episode. Flare-up duration must be at least >24 hours. Relapses must be separated by ≥1 month. ≥1 out of 2 neurologic signs must be present. The second clinical sign may be obtained through an abnormal paraclinical exam such as MRI or evoked potentials or may be supported by an abnormal paraclinical exam (5,7)[C].
- For patients with steady decline of neurologic function for ≥6 months without flares, intrathecal IgG may be used to support the diagnosis (5)[C].

HISTORY
Symptoms may include fatigue, depression, emotional instability, epilepsy, memory loss, diplopia, sudden vision loss, facial palsy, dysarthria, dysphagia, muscle weakness or spasms, ataxia, vertigo, falls, hyperesthesia or paresthesia, pain, bowel or bladder incontinence, urinary frequency or retention or impotence (5)[C].

PHYSICAL EXAM
- Optic disc swelling or pallor
- INO
- Nystagmus in abducting eye
- Ataxia
- Intention tremor
- Hypesthesia or paresthesia
- Cerebellar dysarthria (scanning speech)
- Spasticity (especially in lower extremities)

DIFFERENTIAL DIAGNOSIS
- Lyme disease
- Systemic lupus erythematosus (SLE)
- Antiphospholipid antibody syndrome
- Epilepsy
- Progressive multifocal leukoencephalopathy (PML)
- CNS neoplasms
- Guillain-Barré syndrome
- Metachromatic leukodystrophy
- Sarcoidosis
- Stroke
- Vascular malformation
- HIV, neurosyphilis
- Cobalamin (vitamin B_{12}) deficiency
- Acute disseminated encephalomyelitis (ADEM)
- Behçet disease
- Normal pressure hydrocephalus

DIAGNOSTIC TESTS & INTERPRETATION
- CSF: Increased monocyte cell count and intrathecally formed IgG levels. Total protein within CSF may be normal or increased. The presence of oligoclonal bands (OCB) is used to determine amount of IgG in-trathecally synthesized. ≥2 OCBs is diagnostic (5)[B]
- Tests used for exclusion of alternative diagnoses: antinuclear antibodies (ANAs), serum cobalamin level, erythrocyte sedimentation rate (ESR), and testing for syphilis
- MRI of head/spine (more sensitive than CT):
  - T_2 (spin-echo) image: hyperintense lesions
  - T_2 image: hypointense lesions
  - Gadolinium (Gd): Given IV, leakage of Gd into the parenchyma represents an increase in BBB perme-ability due to vascular breakdown.
- McDonald criteria (5):
  - Dissemination in space: ≥1 T_2 lesion on MRI in at least 2 out of 4 CNS regions typically affected by MS: periventricular, juxtacortical, infratentorial, or spinal cord or by waiting for another clinical attack implying a different CNS location
  - Dissemination in time: simultaneous presentation of asymptomatic Gd-enhanced and nonenhanc-ing lesions at any moment or a new T_2 and/or Gd-enhanced lesion on an MRI when compared baseline scans.

Diagnostic Procedures/Other
Evoked potentials (EPs): Assess function in visual, auditory, and somatosensory or motor CNS pathways by measuring CNS electric potentials evoked by stimu-lation of either the brain or selected peripheral nerves; a marked delay in a provoked CNS EP, without a clinical manifestation, is suggestive of a demyelinating disorder (5).

TREATMENT

GENERAL MEASURES
- Three main categories currently exist for MS treatment: treatment for acute relapses, treatment for reducing MS-related activity using disease-modifying agents, and symptomatic therapy (2,5)[B]
- For apparent acute relapse, rule out infectious etiology prior to treatment.

MEDICATION

- Acute relapses (2)[B]

  – Methylprednisolone 1 g/day IV for 3 to 5 days; without subsequent oral tapering; a second course may be given.
    - ○ Adverse effects: fluid retention, potassium loss, weight gain, GI disturbances, acne, and emotional lability
- Reduction of MS biologic activity, interferon-β (IFN-β) (1,5,8)
  – Avonex (IFN-β_{1a}) 30 μg IM weekly
  – Rebif (IFN-β_{1a}) 22 or 44 μg SC 3 times per week
  – Betaseron (IFN-β_{1b}) 0.25 mg SC every other day
  – Extavia (IFN-β_{1b}) 0.25 mg SC every other day
    - ○ CBC w/ diff., Plt, LFTs at 1, 3, and 6 months after starting Tx
    - ○ TFTs every 6 months if Hx of thyroid dysfunction Reduction of MS biologic activity, non-IFN-β (1,5,8)
    - ○ Glatiramer acetate (Copaxone) 20 mg SC daily or 40 mg 3 times per week
      - ■ Common adverse reactions: injection site reaction, nausea, chest pain, hypertonia, diaphoresis
      - ■ No recommended routine tests
  – Natalizumab (Tysabri): 300 mg IV every 4 weeks
    - ○ Restricted distribution in the United States; call 1-800-456-2255 for more info.
    - ○ MRI at baseline
  – Alemtuzumab (Lemtrada) 12 mg IV daily for 5 days, then 12 months later 12 mg IV for 3 days
    - ○ Premedicate with corticosteroids (methyl-prednisolone 1,000 mg) first 3 days of each treatment. Also consider antihistamines, antipyretics; antiviral prophylaxis (for herpetic viral infections) beginning on the first day of treatment and continue at least 2 months and until CD4+ lymphocyte count is ≥200/mm^3
  – Fingolimod (Gilenya): 0.5 mg PO daily
    - ○ EKG at baseline
    - ○ Serious adverse reactions: QT prolongation, AV block; 6-hour observation following first dose
  – Teriflunomide (Aubagio): 7 to 14 mg PO daily
    - ○ Avoid pregnancy, teratogenic; pregnancy test at baseline
    - ○ Use reliable contraception during Tx.
- Symptomatic therapies (5)[B]:

  – Ataxia: clonazepam, propranolol, ondansetron
  – Spasticity: baclofen, diazepam, tizanidine, dantrolene, cyclobenzaprine hydrochloride
  – Pain: NSAIDs, carbamazepine, gabapentin, phenytoin, amitriptyline, mexiletine
  – Bladder dysfunction: (urgency) propantheline bromide, oxybutynin, tolterodine tartrate; (retention) phenoxybenzamine, terazosin hydrochloride, bethanechol
  – Constipation: high-fiber diets, fluids, natural or other laxatives, stool softeners, bulk-producing agents, suppositories
  – Sexual dysfunction: tadalafil, sildenafil, vardenafil
  – Weakness/fatigue: dalfampridine, amantadine, methylphenidate
  – Tremors: clonazepam, β-blockers, primidone
  – Depression: fluoxetine, other SSRIs, tricyclic antidepressants, nontricyclic antidepressants

ADDITIONAL THERAPIES

- Cognitive behavioral therapy
- Physical and occupational therapy
- Water therapy: Swimming, in cool water, is typically well-tolerated.
- Strenuous physical activity appears to confer protective benefit and slow the disease progression in pediatric patients.

COMPLEMENTARY & ALTERNATIVE MEDICINE

- Omega-3: immunomodulary properties
- Vitamin D supplementation, sunlight exposure

 ONGOING CARE

FOLLOW-UP RECOMMENDATIONS

Treat relapses with corticosteroids to minimize disease progression and duration of relapse. Maintain regular activity, but avoid overwork and fatigue. Rest during periods of acute relapse (2)[B].

Patient Monitoring

Assessing the severity of neurologic impairment from MS can be done using the Kurtzke Expanded Disability Status Score (EDSS): 0 indicates a normal neurologic exam and 10 indicates death due to MS. The EDDS uses a functional status (FS) score, covering the following: pyramidal symptoms, cerebellar, brainstem, sensory, bowel and bladder, visual/optic, and cerebral/mental functions. EDDS scoring system (9)[C]:

- 1.0 – No disability, minimal signs in 1 FS
- 2.0 – Minimal disability in 1 FS
- 3.0 – Moderate disability in 1 FS or mild disability in 3 to 4 FS, but fully ambulatory
- 4.0 – Ambulatory without aid or rest for ∼500 m
- 5.0 – Ambulatory without aid or rest for ∼200 m
- 6.0 – Intermittent/constant unilateral assistance (cane, crutch, or brace) must be able to walk 100 m
- 7.0 – Unable to walk beyond 5 m even with aid; essentially restricted to wheelchair, wheels self and transfers alone; active in wheelchair for ∼12 hrs/day
- 8.0 – Essentially restricted to bed, chair, or wheelchair; may be out of bed most of the day; retains self-care functions, generally effective use of arms
- 9.0 – Helpless, bed-bound; but patient can communicate, eat
- 10.0 – Death due to MS

DIET

High fiber, bulk laxatives, fluids to prevent constipation

PATIENT EDUCATION

National Multiple Sclerosis Society: 1-800-344-4867 or www.nationalmssociety.org/

PROGNOSIS

- Differs in each individual; depends on the form of MS, the individual's sex and age, the initial presentation of the disease, and the amount of disability
- Average life expectancy is 5 to 10 years less than unaffected people.
- Specific clinical features suggesting more favorable course: early onset, RRMS form, female sex, <2 relapses within first year of diagnosis, and minimal functional decline after 5 years (5).
- Mortality secondary to MS relapse is unusual; death more commonly associated with a complication of MS such as infection in a person with more disability.

COMPLICATIONS

Depression or emotional instability, paraplegia, chronic pain, sexual dysfunction, delirium, impaired vision (9)

REFERENCES

1. Compston A, Coles A. Multiple sclerosis. *Lancet.* 2008;372(9648):1502–1517.
2. Thrower BW. Relapse management in multiple sclerosis. *Neurologist.* 2009;15(1):1–5.
3. Ascherio A, Munger KL. Environmental risk factors for multiple sclerosis. Part I: the role of infection. *Ann Neurol.* 2007;61(4):288–299.
4. Alonso A, Hernán MA. Temporal trends in the incidence of multiple sclerosis: a systematic review. *Neurology.* 2008;71(2):129–135.
5. Rejdak K, Jackson S, Giovannoni G. Multiple sclerosis: a practical overview for clinicians. *Br Med Bull.* 2010;95:79–104.
6. Ascherio A, Munger KL. Environmental risk factors for multiple sclerosis. Part II: noninfectious factors. *Ann Neurol.* 2007;61(6):504–513.
7. Polman CH, Reingold SC, Banwell B, et al. Diagnostic criteria for multiple sclerosis: 2010 revisions to the McDonald criteria. *Ann Neurol.* 2011;69(2):292–302.
8. Zintzaras E, Doxani C, Mprotsis T, et al. Network analysis of randomized controlled trials in multiple sclerosis. *Clin Ther.* 2012;34(4):857–869.e9.
9. Kurtzke JF. Rating neurologic impairment in multiple sclerosis: an expanded disability status scale (EDSS). *Neurology.* 1983;33(11):1444–1452.
10. Grover SA, Aubert-Broche B, Fetco D, et al. Lower physical activity is associated with higher disease burden in pediatric multiple sclerosis [published online ahead of print August 12, 2015]. *Neurology.* 2015;85(19):1663–1669.
11. Fazekas F, Lublin FD, Li D, et al. Intravenous immunoglobulin in relapsing-remitting multiple sclerosis: a dose-finding trial. *Neurology.* 2008; 71(4):265–271.
12. Reston JT, Uhl S, Treadwell JR, et al. Autologous hematopoietic cell transplantation for multiple sclerosis: a systematic review. *Mult Scler.* 2011; 17(2):204–213.

ADDITIONAL READING

Hauser SL. Hematopoietic stem cell transplantation for MS: extraordinary evidence still needed. *JAMA.* 2015;313(3):251–252.

 CODES

ICD10

G35 Multiple sclerosis

CLINICAL PEARLS

- Immune-mediated inflammatory disease causing demyelination, neuronal loss, and scarring within the white matter of the CNS
- Charcot classical MS triad: nystagmus, intention tremor, and dysarthria
- Acute relapses are treated with steroids; disease-modifying medications are used for chronic treatment; currently, there is no treatment for promoting remyelination or neuronal repair.
- Based on limited clinical data, IVIG is not thought to be effective therapy for relapsing remitting MS (10).
- Autologous stem cell transplantation for MS shows promise, but more rigorous research is needed (11,12).

M

MUMPS

Frances Yung-tao Wu, MD

BASICS

An acute, generalized paramyxovirus infection typically presenting with unilateral or bilateral parotitis

DESCRIPTION
- Up to 1/3 of individuals with mumps are asymptomatic.
- Painful parotitis occurs in 95% of symptomatic mumps cases. Epidemics in late winter and spring. Transmission by respiratory secretions.
- Incubation period is 14 to 24 days.
- System(s) affected: hematologic/lymphatic/immunologic, reproductive, skin, exocrine
- Synonym(s): epidemic parotitis; infectious parotitis

EPIDEMIOLOGY
- Predominant age: 85% of mumps case occur before age 15 years:
  - Adult cases are typically more severe.
- Predominant sex: male = female
- Geriatric population: Most adults are immune.
- Acute epidemic mumps
  - Most cases occur in unvaccinated children between ages 5 and 15 years.
  - Recent (2006) U.S. epidemic in vaccinated college students aged 18 to 24 years: 5,700 U.S. cases:
    - Another U.S. epidemic in 2009 to 2010 in New York/New Jersey: >1,500 cases
- Mumps is unusual in children <2 years of age and most infants <1 year are immune.
  - Period of maximal communicability is 24 hours before to 72 hours after onset of parotitis

Incidence
- 1,151 cases in the United States in 2014 (1)
- Occasional epidemic outbreaks in a given region

Prevalence
- 0.0064/100,000 persons
- 90% of adults are seropositive even without history.

ETIOLOGY AND PATHOPHYSIOLOGY
Mumps virus replicates in glandular epithelium of parotids, pancreas, and testes, leading to interstitial edema and inflammation.
- Interstitial glandular hemorrhage may occur.
- Pressure caused by edema of the testes against the tunica albuginea can lead to necrosis and loss of function.

RISK FACTORS
- Foreign travel: Many other nations do *not* vaccinate for mumps, including most of Africa and South Asia.
- Crowded environments such as dormitories, barracks, or detention facilities increase risk of transmission.

- Immunity wanes after single-dose vaccination:
  - When receiving two doses, immunity drops from 95% to 86% after 9 years.
  - Genotypic variation from original vaccine strain may have a role in decreased vaccine efficacy (2).

GENERAL PREVENTION
- Vaccination
  - Two doses of live mumps vaccine or measles-mumps-rubella (MMR) vaccine are recommended, first at 12 to 15 months and second at 4 to 6 years of age.
  - 95% effective in clinical studies, but field trials show 68–95% efficacy, which may be below level for herd immunity to prevent spread.
  - Scandinavian data suggest prevention may require 95% first dose and >80% second dose adherence.
  - Adverse effects: most common proven effect is idiopathic thrombocytopenic purpura (ITP), with incidence of 3.3/100,000 doses
  - *No relationship between MMR vaccine and autism*
- Immunoglobulin (Ig) is not effective in preventing mumps.
- Postexposure vaccination does not protect from recent exposure (3)[B]
- Isolate hospitalized patients for 5 days after onset.
- Isolate nonimmune individuals for 26 days after last case onset (social quarantine).

Pregnancy Considerations
- Live viral vaccines are typically contraindicated in pregnancy; however, vaccination of children should not be delayed due to a pregnant family member.
- Immunization of contacts protects against future (but not current) exposures.

DIAGNOSIS

HISTORY
- Parotid swelling peaks in 1 to 3 days and lasts 3 to 7 days.
- Clinical diagnosis (swelling of one or both parotid glands):
  - Lasting ≥2 days
  - No other apparent cause
  - Rare presentation of meningitis without parotitis (1–10%)
- Up to 1/3 of individuals with mumps are asymptomatic.
- Rare prodrome of fever, neck muscle ache, and malaise
- Sour foods cause pain in parotid gland region.
- Moderate fever, usually not >104°F (40°C):
  - High fever frequently is associated with complications.

PHYSICAL EXAM
- Painful parotid swelling (unilateral or bilateral) obscures angle of mandible and elevates earlobe
- Meningeal signs in 15%, encephalitis in 0.5%
- Rarely arthritis, orchitis, thyroiditis, mastitis, pancreatitis, oophoritis, myocarditis
- Rare maculopapular, erythematous rash
- Up to 50% of cases may be very mild.
- Redness at opening of Stensen duct but no pus
- Swelling in sternal area; rare, but pathognomonic of mumps

DIFFERENTIAL DIAGNOSIS
- If not epidemic, other viruses are more common: parainfluenza parotitis, Epstein-Barr virus, coxsackievirus, adenovirus, parvovirus B19
- Suppurative parotitis: often associated with *Staphylococcus aureus* (presence of Wharton duct pus on massaging parotid gland essentialy excludes diagnosis of mumps)
- Recurrent allergic parotitis
- Salivary calculus with intermittent swelling
- Lymphadenitis from any cause, including HIV infection
- Cytomegalovirus parotitis in immunocompromised patients
- Mikulicz syndrome: chronic, painless parotid and lacrimal gland swelling of unknown cause that occurs in tuberculosis, sarcoidosis, lupus, leukemia, lymphosarcoma, and salivary gland tumors
- Sjögren syndrome, diabetes mellitus, uremia, malnutrition
- Drug-related parotid enlargement (iodides, guanethidine, phenothiazine)
- Other causes of the complications of mumps (meningoencephalitis, orchitis, oophoritis, pancreatitis, polyarthritis, nephritis, myocarditis, prostatitis)
- Mumps orchitis must be differentiated from testicular torsion and from chlamydial or bacterial orchitis. (Testicular sonogram can be useful.)

DIAGNOSTIC TESTS & INTERPRETATION
- Three special tests used to confirm an outbreak—if positive, report to health department (1)[A]

  - IgM titer (positive by day 5 in 100% of non-immunized patients)
  - Swab of parotid duct or other affected salivary ducts for viral culture
  - Rise in IgG titer samples; test should be ordered if patient previously immunized: 1st sample within 5 days of onset, and 2nd, 2 weeks later.
- Other potential findings: elevated serum amylase; CSF leukocytosis, or leukopenia.
- Testicular ultrasound may help differentiate mumps orchitis from testicular torsion.

Diagnostic Procedures/Other
If meningitis is present, lumbar puncture to exclude bacterial process. CSF pleocytosis, usually lymphocytes, is found in 65% of patients with parotitis.

Test Interpretation
Periductal edema and lymphocytic infiltration in affected glands on biopsy

 TREATMENT

- No specific antiviral therapy, only supportive care (1)[A],(4)[C]

- Analgesics to relieve pain
- Avoid corticosteroids for mumps orchitis because they can reduce testosterone concentrations and increase testicular atrophy.
- IVIG only successful for certain autoimmune-based sequelae:
  – Postinfectious encephalitis
  – Guillain-Barré syndrome
  – ITP
- Interferon-α2b improved severe bilateral orchitis but did not decrease testicular atrophy in small studies (5)[B].

GENERAL MEASURES
- Rarely need to hospitalize patients with high fever, pancreatitis, or CNS symptoms for supportive care, steroids, or interferon using appropriate isolation precautions
- Orchitis
  – Ice packs to scrotum can help to relieve pain.
  – Scrotal support with adhesive bridge while recumbent and/or athletic supporter while ambulatory

MEDICATION
First Line
- Analgesics and anti-inflammatory medications (acetaminophen, nonsteroidal anti-inflammatory drugs [NSAIDs]) may diminish pain and swelling in acute orchitis and arthritis mumps.
- May use acetaminophen for fever and/or pain
- Precautions: Avoid aspirin for pain in children as previously associated with Reye syndrome.

Second Line
- Interferon-α2b
- Chinese medicinal herbs and acupuncture have not shown benefit in randomized controlled trials (6,7).

INPATIENT CONSIDERATIONS
Admission Criteria/Initial Stabilization
- Hospitalize only if CNS symptoms occur.
- Outpatient supportive care if no complications

IV Fluids
If severe nausea or vomiting accompanies pancreatitis

 ONGOING CARE

FOLLOW-UP RECOMMENDATIONS
Mumps orchitis:

- Bed rest and local supportive clothing (e.g., two pairs of briefs) or adhesive-tape bridge
- Withhold from school until no longer contagious (9 days after onset of pain)

Patient Monitoring
Most cases will be mild. Monitor hydration status.

DIET
Liquid diet if unable to chew

PATIENT EDUCATION
Orchitis is common in older children but rarely results in sterility, even if bilateral.

PROGNOSIS
- Complete recovery is typical; immunity is lifelong.
- Transient sensorineural hearing loss in 4% of adults
- Recurrence after 2 weeks may be nonepidemic parotitis.

COMPLICATIONS
- May precede, accompany, or follow salivary gland involvement and may occur (rarely) without primary involvement of the parotid gland
- Orchitis is common (30%) in postpubertal boys:
  – It starts within 8 days after parotitis.
  – Impaired fertility in 13%; absolute sterility is rare.
- Meningitis (1–10%) or encephalitis (0.1%) may present 5 to 10 days after first symptoms of illness. Aseptic meningitis is typically mild, but meningoencephalitis may lead to seizures, paralysis, hydrocephalus, or (in 2% of cases), death.
- Acute cerebellar ataxia has been reported after mumps infections; self-resolving in 2 to 3 weeks.
- Oophoritis in 7% of postpubertal females; no decreased fertility
- Pancreatitis, usually mild
- Nephritis, thyroiditis, and arthralgias are rare.
- Myocarditis: usually mild, but may depress ST segment; may be linked to endocardial fibroelastosis
- Deafness: 1/15,000 unilateral nerve deafness; may not be permanent
- Inflammation about the eye (keratouveitis) is rare.
- Dacryoadenitis, optic neuritis

Pediatric Considerations
- Orchitis is more common in adolescents.
- Young children are less likely to develop complications.
- Most complications occur in postpubertal group.
- Avoid aspirin use in children with viral symptoms.

Pregnancy Considerations
Disease may increase the rate of spontaneous pregnancy loss in 1st trimester. Perinatal mumps often has a benign course.

REFERENCES
1. Centers for Disease Control and Prevention. Overview of mumps. http://www.cdc.gov/mumps/about/index.html
2. Gouma S, Sane J, Gijselaar D, et al. Two major mumps genotype G variants dominated recent mumps outbreaks in the Netherlands (2009–2012). *J Gen Virol*. 2014;95(Pt 5):1074–1082.
3. Fiebelkorn AP, Lawler J, Curns AT, et al. Mumps postexposure prophylaxis with a third dose of measles-mumps-rubella vaccine, Orange County, New York, USA. *Emerg Infect Dis*. 2013;19(9):1411–1417.
4. Davis NF, McGuire BB, Mahon JA, et al. The increasing incidence of mumps orchitis: a comprehensive review. *BJU Int*. 2010;105(8):1060–1065.
5. Yapanoglu T, Kocaturk H, Aksoy Y, et al. Long-term efficacy and safety of interferon-alpha-2B in patients with mumps orchitis. *Int Urol Nephrol*. 2010;42(4):867–871.
6. Shu M, Zhang YQ, Li Z, et al. Chinese medicinal herbs for mumps. *Cochrane Database Syst Rev*. 2012;(9):CD008578.
7. He J, Zheng M, Zhang M, et al. Acupuncture for mumps in children. *Cochrane Database Syst Rev*. 2012;(9):CD008400.

ADDITIONAL READING
- Flaherty DK. The vaccine-autism connection: a public health crisis caused by unethical medical practices and fraudulent science. *Ann Pharmacother*. 2011;45(10):1302–1304.
- MacDonald N, Hatchette T, Elkout L, et al. Mumps is back: why is mumps eradication not working? *Adv Exp Med Biol*. 2011;697:197–220.
- Shirts BH, Welch RJ, Couturier MR. Seropositivity rates for measles, mumps, and rubella IgG and costs associated with testing and revaccination. *Clin Vaccine Immunol*. 2013;20(3):443–445.
- Zamir CS, Schroeder H, Shoob H, et al. Characteristics of a large mumps outbreak: clinical severity, complications and association with vaccination status of mumps outbreak cases. *Hum Vaccin Immunother*. 2015;11(6):1413–1417.

 CODES

ICD10
- B26.9 Mumps without complication
- B26.1 Mumps meningitis
- B26.2 Mumps encephalitis

CLINICAL PEARLS
- Mumps is a clinical diagnosis based on swelling of ≥1 parotid glands for ≥2 days without other obvious cause. Confirmatory testing must be done in epidemic settings.
- Ultrasound is useful to distinguish testicular torsion from testicular pain related to mumps orchitis.
- A history of vaccination with MMR does not exclude mumps. The MMR vaccine is 68–95% effective after a series of two immunizations. Immunity commonly wanes over time.

M

MUSCULAR DYSTROPHY
Nimmy Thakolkaran, MD • George G.A. Pujalte, MD, FACSM

BASICS

- Primary inherited myopathies caused by dysfunctional proteins of muscle fibers and extracellular matrix
- Distribution of weakness, other associated symptoms, and disease prognosis depend on the specific gene affected and severity of the mutation.

DESCRIPTION
- Duchenne muscular dystrophy (DMD)
  - Highest incidence muscular dystrophy, X-linked inheritance, early onset, progressive
  - Patients are wheelchair-dependent prior to age 13 years.
- Becker muscular dystrophy (BMD)
  - Less severe phenotype than Duchenne, also caused by mutation in *DMD* gene; later onset and milder clinical course
  - Distinction from DMD is clinical: Patients are usually wheelchair-dependent after age 16 years.
  - Collectively referred to as dystrophinopathies
- Myotonic muscular dystrophy (MMD)
  - Myotonia (slow relaxation after muscle contraction), distal and facial weakness
  - Second most common inherited muscle disease.
- Facioscapulohumeral muscular dystrophy (FSHMD)
  - Facial and shoulder muscles most affected
  - Third most common inherited muscle disease.
- Limb-girdle muscular dystrophy (LGMD)
  - Proximal weakness and atrophy, variable prognosis with many different identified mutations
- Oculopharyngeal muscular dystrophy (OPMD)
  - Usually adult-onset, affects extraocular and pharyngeal muscles. Presents with ptosis and dysphagia
- Emery-Dreifuss muscular dystrophy (EDMD)
  - Triad of early development of joint contractures, slowly progressive muscle wasting, and cardiomyopathy. Can present as sudden death in apparently healthy young adults
- Congenital muscular dystrophies (CMD)
  - Heterogeneous group of autosomal recessive myopathic diseases presenting in infancy with generally poor prognosis
  - Includes Fukuyama CMD, Ullrich CMD, Walker-Warburg syndrome, muscle-eye-brain disease

EPIDEMIOLOGY
Incidence
- Duchenne: 1/3,600 male births (1)
- Myotonic dystrophy: 1/10,000 births
- Other muscular dystrophies vary widely by population but are generally rare.

ETIOLOGY AND PATHOPHYSIOLOGY
Mutations affect proteins connecting cytoskeleton to cell membrane and extracellular matrix, causing muscle fibers to become fragile and easily damaged; muscle weakness and atrophy result.
- DMD/BMD
  - Defective protein is dystrophin, product of the largest human gene, *DMD*; Duchenne phenotype results from mutations that cause profound loss of dystrophin, the protein involved in calcium transport in muscle cells and stabilizing fibers during contraction.
  - Becker phenotype results from less severe mutations in *DMD* gene; patients have low but detectable levels of functional dystrophin.
- MMD: Trinucleotide repeat expansion in the untranslated region of the gene *DMPK* on chromosome 19; encodes myotonin–protein kinase

- LGMD: mutations in genes encoding proteins associated with dystrophin: calpain-, dysferlin-, and fukutin-related proteins are affected most commonly.
- EDMD: Dysfunctional proteins are associated with the nuclear membrane in muscle fibers; emerin in X-linked form, lamin A/C in autosomal forms
- OPMD: Trinucleotide repeat expansion in *PABPN1* results in nuclear inclusions in muscle cells by hampering normal transport of mRNA from the nucleus.
- FSHMD: Deletion in untranslated region of chromosome 4; function of deleted genes is unclear, although the most accepted concept is that they likely affect the expression of multiple genes by epigenetic effects.

Genetics
- X-linked
  - Duchenne and Becker muscular dystrophies
  - Gene located at Xp21
    - 30% of affected males have a de novo mutation (mother is not a carrier).
    - 20% of female carriers have some manifestation of the mutation (usually mild muscle weakness or cardiomyopathy).
- Autosomal dominant
  - Generally later onset and less severe than diseases with recessive or X-linked inheritance
  - FSHMD, OPMD, some forms of LGMD and EDMD
  - Myotonic dystrophy
    - Trinucleotide repeat expansion with more severe phenotype in subsequent generations due to accumulation of repeats
- Autosomal recessive
  - Most types of CMD

GENERAL PREVENTION
Genetic counseling for carriers and prenatal diagnosis

COMMONLY ASSOCIATED CONDITIONS
- Decreased IQ: on average, 1 *SD* below the mean in DMD; speech and language delay
- Dilated cardiomyopathy and conduction abnormalities
  - Can be severe in EDMD
  - Can affect otherwise asymptomatic female carriers of DMD
  - Progressive scoliosis

DIAGNOSIS

HISTORY
- DMD: normal attainment of early motor milestones with subsequent abnormal gait and slowing gross motor development: clumsiness, waddling gait, frequent falls, difficulty running or climbing stairs
- BMD: progressive difficulty with ambulation and frequent falls in later childhood
- MMD: slurred speech, muscle wasting, difficulty with ambulation; often with family history
- LGMD: back pain, lordosis/inability to rise from a chair, climb stairs, and use arms overhead
- FSHMD: facial weakness, inability to close eyes completely
- EDMD: contractures of elbows and ankles, difficulty with ambulation in teenage years
- OPMD: ptosis and dysphagia; often with family history

PHYSICAL EXAM
- DMD/BMD
  - Proximal muscle weakness; Gower sign: use of arms to push upper body into standing posture from lying prone
  - Trendelenburg gait (hip waddling)

  - Hyporeflexia/areflexia
  - Winged scapulae and lordosis
  - Pseudohypertrophy of the calf (caused by replacement of muscle with fibroadipose tissue)
  - Contractures of lower extremity joints and elbows
- MMD
  - Characteristic facial appearance: narrow face, open triangular mouth, high-arched palate, concave temples, drooping eyelids, frontal balding in males
  - Myotonia: inability to relax muscles after contraction
  - Distal muscle weakness and wasting
- CMD
  - Arthrogryposis (multiple joint contractures); diffuse hypotonia and muscle wasting in an infant

DIFFERENTIAL DIAGNOSIS
- Glycogen storage diseases and other metabolic myopathies
- Mitochondrial myopathies: MELAS (**M**itochondrial **E**ncephalopathy, **L**actic **A**cidosis, and **S**troke-like episodes), MERRF (**M**yoclonus with **E**pilepsy and **R**agged-**R**ed Fibers)
- Inflammatory myopathies: polymyositis, dermatomyositis, inclusion-body myositis
- Neuromuscular junction diseases: myasthenia gravis, Lambert-Eaton syndrome
- Motor neuron diseases: amyotrophic lateral sclerosis, spinal muscular atrophy
- Charcot-Marie-Tooth disease
- Friedreich ataxia

DIAGNOSTIC TESTS & INTERPRETATION
Initial Tests (lab, imaging)
- Creatine kinase (CK): initial screening test if MD is suspected (2)[A]
- Elevated in DMD (10 to 100 times); elevated at birth, peaks at time of presentation, and falls during illness
- Initial detected lab abnormality may be elevated aspartate transaminase/alanine transaminase (AST/ALT) originating from muscle.
- Genetic testing/molecular diagnosis
  - For definitive diagnosis in patient with characteristic presentation and elevated CK
  - Deletion and duplication analysis (MLPA or CGH) will identify most patients; followed by genomic sequencing of *DMD* gene for point mutations (3)[A].
  - Genetic testing is available clinically for most other muscular dystrophies.

Diagnostic Procedures/Other
- Muscle biopsy: rarely performed in DMD (dystrophin protein absent); may be helpful in other cases (4)[A]
- Electromyography and nerve conduction studies are not necessary unless considering alternative diagnoses.
- ECG: abnormalities found in >90% of males and up to 10% of female carriers of DMD; Q waves in anterolateral leads, tall R waves in V1, shortened PR interval, arrhythmias, resting sinus tachycardia

Test Interpretation
- Heterogenic muscle fibers: atrophy and hypertrophy of fibers with proliferation of connective tissue in muscle
- Immunohistochemical staining for dystrophin protein
  - DMD: no detectable dystrophin in most fibers; occasional revertant fibers with normal dystrophin
  - BMD: highly variable staining for dystrophin throughout muscle

TREATMENT

Trials of agents that affect gene expression, such as antisense oligonucleotides, and small molecules that cause skipping of premature stop codons (ataluren) are ongoing; however, steroid treatment is the only clinically available therapy that affects disease progression.

GENERAL MEASURES
- Ambulation prolonged by knee-ankle-foot orthoses
- Serial casting to treat contractures
- Diagnose sleep apnea with polysomnography; treat with noninvasive ventilation.
- Adaptive devices to improve function
- Avoid overexertion and strenuous exercise.

MEDICATION
- Prednisone 0.75 mg/kg/day (4)[A]

  - Slows the decline in muscle function, progression to scoliosis, and degradation of pulmonary function; prolongs functional ambulation; prolongs lifespan; improved cardiac outcomes
  - Therapy should be initiated when there is no longer progress in motor skills, but prior to decline (2).
  - Monitor adverse effects.
    ○ Bisphosphonates should be considered for preventing loss of bone density; annual exam for cataracts; hypertension should be monitored; no NSAIDs due to risk of peptic ulcer disease (PUD); stress-dose steroids during surgeries and illnesses due to adrenal suppression.
    ○ Patients should be aware of immune suppression and notify emergency providers.
- Deflazacort (0.9 mg/kg) is an alternative oral steroid that is also considered first-line therapy in DMD; it acts on muscle regeneration and differentiation; not available in the United States (3)
- ACE inhibitors
  - Treatment of cardiomyopathy; may be used in conjunction with β-blockers

ISSUES FOR REFERRAL
- Refer to neuromuscular diseases center for definitive diagnosis and coordinated multidisciplinary care (4).
- Cardiology for management of cardiomyopathy
- Pulmonology for monitoring of pulmonary function and clearance regimen
- Physical medicine and rehabilitation for management of adaptive devices
- Nutrition/swallowing: for normal weight gain, attention for dysphagia
- Psychosocial: learning/behavior and coping assessment, social development (2)

ADDITIONAL THERAPIES
Novel medication: Ataluren interferes with premature stop codons, allowing expression of dystrophin protein. In DMD patients with nonsense mutation; FDA approved orphan drug designation (3)

SURGERY/OTHER PROCEDURES
- Spinal surgery for scoliosis—diminishes rate of deformity progression (5),(6)[A].
- Scapular fixation for scapular winging may be beneficial; also lacking clinical trials
- Consider surgical treatment of ankle/knee contractures.
- Surgical procedures should be performed at a center experienced in DMD; total IV anesthesia should be used.

ONGOING CARE

- Individualized education plan and developmental evaluation for school accommodations
- Maintenance of current influenza and pneumococcal vaccination status

FOLLOW-UP RECOMMENDATIONS
Patient Monitoring
- Electrocardiogram (ECG), echocardiogram, and consultation with a cardiologist at diagnosis and annually after age 10 years
  - Female carriers of DMD mutation should be monitored every 5 years.
- Annual spinal radiography for scoliosis
- Dual-energy x-ray absorptiometry (DEXA) scanning and serum marker testing for osteoporosis
- Pulmonary function testing twice yearly if no longer ambulatory
- Psychosocial: coping, emotional adjustment, depression

DIET
- Obesity is common due to steroid treatment and wheelchair confinement: Weight control can improve quality of life.
- Diet may be limited by dysphagia; swallow evaluation can determine appropriate foods; may require gastrostomy
- Calcium and vitamin D supplementation for patients on steroids; monitor vitamin D levels.

PATIENT EDUCATION
- Muscular Dystrophy Association: http://www.mda.org
- Parent Project Muscular Dystrophy: http://www.endduchenne.org

PROGNOSIS
- DMD/BMD
  - Progressive weakness, contractures, inability to walk
  - Kyphoscoliosis and progressive decline in respiratory vital capacity with recurrent pulmonary infections.
  - Significantly shortened lifespan (DMD: 16 ± 4 years; BMD: 42 ± 16 years). Respiratory failure cause of death in 90%; remaining due to myocardial disease (heart failure and dysrhythmia) (5)
- Other types: slow progression and near-normal lifespan with functional limitations

COMPLICATIONS
- Cardiac arrhythmia, cardiomyopathy
- Dysphagia, gastroesophageal reflux disease (GERD), constipation
- Scoliosis, joint contractures
- Obstructive sleep apnea
- Malignant hyperthermia–like reaction to anesthesia
- Respiratory failure and early death

REFERENCES

1. Chung J, Smith AL, Hughes SC, et al. Twenty-year follow-up of newborn screening for patients with muscular dystrophy [published online ahead of print August 11, 2015]. *Muscle Nerve*. doi:10.1002/mus.24880.
2. Bushby K, Finkel R, Birnkrant DJ, et al. Diagnosis and management of Duchenne muscular dystrophy, part 1: diagnosis, and pharmacological and psychosocial management. *Lancet Neurol*. 2010;9(1):77–93.
3. Falzarano MS, Scotton C, Passarelli C, et al. Duchenne muscular dystrophy: from diagnosis to therapy. *Molecules*. 2015;20(10):18168–18184.
4. Bushby K, Finkel R, Birnkrant DJ, et al. Diagnosis and management of Duchenne muscular dystrophy, part 2: implementation of multidisciplinary care. *Lancet Neurol*. 2010;9(2):177–189.
5. Roberto R, Fritz A, Hagar Y, et al. The natural history of cardiac and pulmonary function decline in patients with Duchenne muscular dystrophy. *Spine (Phila Pa 1976)*. 2011;36(15):E1009–E1017.
6. van Ruiten HJ, Straub V, Bushby K, et al. Improving recognition of Duchenne muscular dystrophy: a retrospective case note review. *Arch Dis Child*. 2014;99(12):1074–1077.

ADDITIONAL READING

- American Academy of Pediatrics Section on Cardiology and Cardiac Surgery. Cardiovascular health supervision for individuals affected by Duchenne or Becker muscular dystrophy. *Pediatrics*. 2005;116(6):1569–1573.
- Cheuk DKL, Wong V, Wraige E, et al. Surgery for scoliosis in Duchenne muscular dystrophy. *Cochrane Database Syst Rev*. 2013;(2):CD005375.
- Cossu G, Sampaolesi M. New therapies for Duchenne muscular dystrophy: challenges, prospects and clinical trials. *Trends Mol Med*. 2007;13(12):520–526.
- Emery AE. The muscular dystrophies. *Lancet*. 2002;359(9307):687–695.
- Fairclough RJ, Bareja A, Davies KE. Progress in therapy for Duchenne muscular dystrophy. *Exp Physiol*. 2011;96(11):1101–1113.
- Manzur AY, Kuntzer T, Pike M, et al. Glucocorticoid corticosteroids for Duchenne muscular dystrophy. *Cochrane Database Syst Rev*. 2008;(1):CD003725.
- Orrell RW, Copeland S, Rose MR. Scapular fixation in muscular dystrophy. *Cochrane Database Syst Rev*. 2010;(1):CD003278.
- Schram G, Fournier A, Leduc H, et al. All-cause mortality and cardiovascular outcomes with prophylactic steroid therapy in Duchenne muscular dystrophy. *J Am Coll Cardiol*. 2013;61(9):948–954.
- Takami Y, Takeshima Y, Awano H, et al. High incidence of electrocardiogram abnormalities in young patients with Duchenne muscular dystrophy. *Pediatr Neurol*. 2008;39(6):399–403.
- van der Kooi EL, Lindeman E, Riphagen I. Strength training and aerobic exercise training for muscle disease. *Cochrane Database Syst Rev*. 2005;(1):CD003907.

CODES

ICD10
- G71.0 Muscular dystrophy
- G71.11 Myotonic muscular dystrophy
- G71.2 Congenital myopathies

CLINICAL PEARLS

- Primary care providers should have a low threshold to obtain serum CK as a screening test in the face of gross motor delay/muscular weakness, especially in boys.
- Steroids should be initiated in patients with DMD when gross motor function ceases to progress.
- High-quality care of patients requires a medical home; a multidisciplinary team of physicians, therapists, and other providers; and extensive patient and family support.

M

MYASTHENIA GRAVIS

Melody A. Jordahl-Iafrato, MD

BASICS

DESCRIPTION
Primary disorder of neuromuscular transmission characterized by fluctuating muscle weakness:

- Ocular myasthenia gravis (MG) (15%): weakness limited to eyelids and extraocular muscles
- Generalized MG (85%): commonly affects ocular as well as a variable combination of bulbar, proximal limb, and respiratory muscles
- 50% of patients who present with ocular symptoms develop generalized MG within 2 years.
- Onset may be sudden and severe, but it is typically mild and intermittent over many years, maximum severity reached within 3 years for 85%.
- System(s) affected: neurologic; hematologic; lymphatic; immunologic; musculoskeletal

EPIDEMIOLOGY
Occurs at any age but a bimodal distribution to the age of onset:
- Female predominance: 20 to 40 years
- Male predominance: 60 to 80 years

Incidence
Estimated annual incidence 2 to 21/1 million

Prevalence
In the United States, 200/1 million; increasing over the past 5 decades

Pediatric Considerations
A transient form of neonatal MG seen in 10–20% of infants born to mothers with MG. It occurs as a result of the transplacental passage of maternal antibodies that interfere with function of the neuromuscular junction; resolves in weeks to months.

ETIOLOGY AND PATHOPHYSIOLOGY
- Reduction in the function of acetylcholine receptors (AChR) at muscle endplates, resulting in insufficient neuromuscular transmission
- Antibody-mediated autoimmune disorder
- Antibodies are present in most cases of MG.
  - Seropositive/antiacetylcholine receptor (anti-AChR): a humoral, antibody-mediated, T-cell–dependent attack of the AChRs or receptor-associated proteins at the postsynaptic membrane of the neuromuscular junction. Found in 85% of generalized MG and 50% of ocular MG. Thymic abnormalities common (1)
  - Muscle-specific kinase (MuSK). 5% of generalized MG patients. Typically females. Is a severe form, respiratory and bulbar muscles involved. Thymic abnormalities are rare (1).
  - In remainder of seronegative, 12–50% with anti-LRP4, a molecule that forms a complex with MuSK, clinical phenotype not well defined (1)
  - Seronegative MG (SNMG): 5%; may have anti-AChR detectable by cell-based assay. Clinically similar to anti-AChR, thymic hyperplasia may be present (1).
- Also documented immediately after viral infections (measles, Epstein-Barr virus [EBV], HIV, and human T-lymphotropic virus [HTLV])

Genetics
- Congenital MG syndrome describes a collection of rare hereditary disorders. This condition is not immune-mediated but instead, results from the mutation of a component of the neuromuscular junction (autosomal recessive).
- Familial predisposition is seen in 5% of cases.

RISK FACTORS
- Familial MG
- D-penicillamine (drug-induced MG)
- Other autoimmune diseases

COMMONLY ASSOCIATED CONDITIONS
- Thymic hyperplasia (60–70%)
- Thymoma (10–15%)
- Autoimmune thyroid disease (3–8%)

DIAGNOSIS

Myasthenia Gravis Foundation of America Clinical Classification (2)[C]:

- Class I: any eye muscle weakness, possible ptosis, no other evidence of muscle weakness elsewhere
- Class II: eye muscle weakness of any severity; mild weakness of other muscles:
  - Class IIa: predominantly limb or axial muscles
  - Class IIb: predominantly bulbar and/or respiratory muscles
- Class III: eye muscle weakness of any severity; moderate weakness of other muscles:
  - Class IIIa: predominantly limb or axial muscles
  - Class IIIb: predominantly bulbar and/or respiratory muscles
- Class IV: eye muscle weakness of any severity; severe weakness of other muscles:
  - Class IVa: predominantly limb/axial muscles
  - Class IVb: predominantly bulbar and/or respiratory muscles (can also include feeding tube without intubation)
- Class V: intubation needed to maintain airway

HISTORY
The hallmark of MG is fatigability.

- Fluctuating weakness, often subtle, that worsens during the day and after prolonged use of affected muscles, may improve with rest
- Early symptoms are transient with asymptomatic periods lasting days or weeks.
- With progression, asymptomatic periods shorten, and symptoms fluctuate from mild to severe.
- >50% of patients present with ocular symptoms (ptosis and/or diplopia). Eventually, 90% of patients with MG develop ocular symptoms.
- Ptosis might be unilateral, bilateral, or shifting from eye to eye.
- 15% present with bulbar symptoms.
- <5% present with proximal limb weakness alone.

ALERT
Myasthenic crisis: respiratory muscle weakness producing respiratory insufficiency and pending respiratory failure

PHYSICAL EXAM
- Ptosis may worsen with propping of opposite eyelid (curtain sign) or sustained upward gaze.
- "Myasthenic sneer," in which the midlip rises but corners of mouth do not move.
- Muscle weakness is usually proximal and symmetric.
- Test for muscle fatigability by repetitive or prolonged use of individual muscles.
- Important to test and monitor respiratory function.

DIFFERENTIAL DIAGNOSIS
- Thyroid ophthalmopathy
- Oculopharyngeal muscular dystrophy
- Myotonic dystrophy
- Kearns-Sayre syndrome
- Chronic progressive external ophthalmoplegia
- Brainstem and motor cranial nerve lesions
- Botulism
- Motor neuron disease (e.g., amyotrophic lateral sclerosis [ALS])
- Lambert-Eaton myasthenic syndrome
- Drug-induced myasthenia
- Congenital myasthenic syndrome
- Dermatomyositis/polymyositis
- Neurosarcoidosis
- Tolosa-Hunt syndrome

DIAGNOSTIC TESTS & INTERPRETATION
Initial Tests (lab, imaging)
- Anti-AChR antibody (74–85% are seropositive):
  - Generalized myasthenia: 75–85%
  - Ocular myasthenia: 50%
  - MG and thymoma: 98–100%
  - Poor correlation between antibody titer and disease severity (1)[C]
  - False-positive results in thymoma without MG, Lambert-Eaton myasthenic syndrome, small cell lung cancer, and rheumatoid arthritis treated with penicillamine
- Anti-MuSK antibody:
  - Used if MG is suspected, patient seronegative
  - Strong correlation between titer and disease severity (1)[C]
- LRP4 and clustered anti-AChR:
  - Used if MG suspected, patient seronegative
- Thyroid and other autoimmune testing antistriated muscle (anti-SM) antibody:
  - Present in 84% of patients with thymoma who are <40 years of age
  - Can be present without thymoma in patients >40 years of age
- Chest radiographs or CT scans may identify a thymoma.
- MRI of brain and orbits to rule out other causes of cranial nerve deficit

Diagnostic Procedures/Other
- Tensilon (Edrophonium) test:
  - Initial 2-mg IV dose, followed by another 2 mg every 60 seconds up to a maximum dose of 10 mg
  - A positive test shows improvement of strength within 30 seconds of administration.
  - Sensitivity 80–90% (3)[C]

– Cardiac disease and bronchial asthma are relative contraindications, especially in elderly.
– Atropine: 0.4 to 0.6 mg IV may rarely be required as antidote; must be available.
– Can also do trial of other cholinesterase inhibitors (neostigmine or oral) and monitor response
• Ice pack test:
– Ice pack applied to closed eyelid for 60 seconds, then removed; extent of ptosis immediately assessed.
– Ice will decrease the ptosis induced by MG.
– Sensitivity 80% in patients with prominent ptosis
• Electrophysiology testing:
– Repetitive nerve stimulation (RNS):
  ○ Widely available, most frequently used
  ○ Moderately sensitive for both generalized MG (75%) and ocular MG (50%) (3)[C]
– Single-fiber electromyogram (SFEMG):
  ○ Assesses temporal variability between two muscle fibers within same motor unit (jitter)
  ○ Sensitive (90–95%) but less specific
  ○ Technically difficult to perform; limited availability, use if suspected and negative RNS (3)[C]

Test Interpretation
• Lymphofollicular hyperplasia of thymic medulla occurs in 65% of patients with MG, thymoma in 15%.
• Immunofluorescence: IgG antibodies and complement on receptor membranes in seropositive patients

TREATMENT

GENERAL MEASURES
• Treatment based on age, gender, and disease severity and progression
• Three basic approaches: symptomatic, immunosuppressive, and supportive. Few should receive a single therapeutic modality.

MEDICATION
First Line
Symptomatic treatments (anticholinesterase agents)
• Pyridostigmine bromide (Mestinon):
  – *Most commonly prescribed because available in oral tablet*
  – Starting dose of 30 mg PO TID with food
  – Maximum dose: 120 mg q3–4h
  – Long-acting available, but effect not consistent
• Neostigmine methylsulfate (Prostigmin):
  – Starting dose of 0.5 mg SC or IM q3h
  – Titrate dosage to clinical need.
• Patients with anti-MuSK may not respond well to these meds.

Second Line
• Immunosuppressants: Oral corticosteroids are the first choice of drugs when immunosuppression is necessary.
– Prednisone: Start as inpatient with a 60 mg/day PO; taper the dosage every 3 days; switch to alternate-day regimen within 2 weeks. Taper very slowly to establish the minimum dosage necessary to maintain remission (4)[B].
– Cyclophosphamide: adults: 1 to 5 mg/kg/day PO; children: 2 to 8 mg/kg/day PO (5)[B]
– Cyclosporine: adults: 5 mg/kg/day PO (nephrotoxicity and drug interactions) (5)[B]

– Mycophenolate: 1 g PO or IV BID
– Azathioprine: 100 to 200 mg/day PO (5)[B]
  ○ *Most frequently used for long-term immunomodulation*, similar efficacy to steroids and IVIG
  ○ Benefit may not be apparent for up to 18 months after initiation of therapy.
  ○ Prednisolone + azathioprine may be effective when used as a corticosteroid-sparing agent.
• Acute immunomodulating treatments:
– Plasmapheresis: bulk removal of 2 to 3 L of plasma 3 times per week, repeated until rate of improvement plateaus (6)[B]
  ○ Improves weakness in nearly all and can last up to 3 months
– Immunoglobulin: 2 g/kg IV over 2 to 5 days (5)[B]
– *Plasmapheresis and immunoglobulin have comparable efficacy in treating moderate to severe MG (6)[C].*
– Rapid onset of effect but short duration of action
– Used for acute worsening of MG to improve strength prior to surgery, prevent acute exacerbations induced by corticosteroids, and as a chronic intermittent treatment to provide relief in refractory MG.
• Other immunosuppressant therapies:
– Tacrolimus
– Rituximab:
  ○ Seronegative MuSK-antibody positive MG patients may have better response to rituximab than conventional therapies.

ALERT
Use caution with drugs that can precipitate weakness: aminoglycosides, fluoroquinolones, β-blockers, calcium channel blockers, neuromuscular blockers, statins, diuretics, oral contraceptives, gabapentin, phenytoin, lithium, among others.

SURGERY/OTHER PROCEDURES
• Thymectomy recommended for patients with thymic abnormalities
• May be beneficial for patients without thymic abnormalities in those <60 years of age

Pediatric Considerations
• Infants with severe weakness from transient neonatal myasthenia may be treated with oral pyridostigmine; general support is necessary until the condition clears.
• Corticosteroids limited only to severe disease

INPATIENT CONSIDERATIONS
Admission Criteria/Initial Stabilization
• Management of pulmonary infections
• Myasthenic/cholinergic crises
• Plasmapheresis
• IV γ-globulin

ONGOING CARE

PATIENT EDUCATION
MG Foundation of America (MGFA): http://www.myasthenia.org/

PROGNOSIS
• Overall good but highly variable
• Myasthenic crisis associated with substantial morbidity and 4% mortality
• Seronegative patients are more likely to have purely ocular disease, and those with generalized SNMG have a better outcome after treatment.

COMPLICATIONS
Acute respiratory arrest; chronic respiratory insufficiency

REFERENCES
1. Berrih-Aknin S, Frenkian-Cuvelier M, Eymard B. Diagnostic and clinical classification of autoimmune myasthenia gravis. *J Autoimmun.* 2014;48–49:143–148.
2. Jaretzki A III, Barohn RJ, Ernstoff RM, et al. Myasthenia gravis: recommendations for clinical research standards. Task Force of the Medical Scientific Advisory Board of the Myasthenia Gravis Foundation of America. *Neurology.* 2000;55(1):16–23.
3. Meriggioli MN, Sanders DB. Myasthenia gravis: diagnosis. *Semin Neurol.* 2004;24(1):31–39.
4. Schneider-Gold C, Gajdos P, Toyka KV, et al. Corticosteroids for myasthenia gravis. *Cochrane Database Syst Rev.* 2005;(2):CD002828.
5. Hart IK, Sathasivam S, Sharshar T. Immunosuppressive agents for myasthenia gravis. *Cochrane Database Syst Rev.* 2007;(4):CD005224.
6. Barth D, Nabavi Nouri M, Ng E, et al. Comparison of IVIg and PLEX in patients with myasthenia gravis. *Neurology.* 2011;76(23):2017–2023.

ADDITIONAL READING
• Angelini C. Diagnosis and management of autoimmune myasthenia gravis. *Clin Drug Investig.* 2011;31(1):1–14.
• Meriggioli MN. Myasthenia gravis: immunopathogenesis, diagnosis, and management. *Continuum Lifelong Learn Neurol.* 2009;15(1):35–62.

 CODES

ICD10
• G70.00 Myasthenia gravis without (acute) exacerbation
• G70.01 Myasthenia gravis with (acute) exacerbation
• P94.0 Transient neonatal myasthenia gravis

CLINICAL PEARLS
• An autoimmune disease, marked by abnormal fatigability and weakness of selected muscles, which is relieved by rest
• Anticholinesterase medication and a thymectomy lessen symptom severity.
• Steroid therapy, plasma exchange, or immunoglobulin can be used in severely affected patients.

M

MYELODYSPLASTIC SYNDROMES

Richard A. Larson, MD

 BASICS

DESCRIPTION

Myelodysplastic syndromes (MDSs) constitute a heterogeneous group of acquired hematopoietic stem cell disorders characterized by cytologic dysplasia in the bone marrow and blood and by various combinations of anemia, neutropenia, and thrombocytopenia.

- The natural progression of disease evolves as cellular maturation becomes more arrested and blast cells accumulate. There is an overlap between arbitrary diagnostic subgroups (1)[C],(2)[A],(3)[C].

- World Health Organization (WHO) classification
  - Refractory cytopenia with unilineage dysplasia
    - Refractory anemia (RA); refractory neutropenia; refractory thrombocytopenia
    - <5% blasts and <15% ring sideroblasts in marrow; <1% blasts in blood
  - Refractory anemia with ring sideroblasts (RARS)
    - <5% blasts in marrow; ≥15% of erythroid precursors are ring sideroblasts; no blasts in blood
    - Also known as acquired idiopathic sideroblastic anemia
  - RARS and marked thrombocytosis
  - Refractory cytopenia with multilineage dysplasia:
    - Marked trilineage dysplasia but without excess blasts in marrow; no Auer rods; <1% blasts in blood
  - Refractory cytopenia with multilineage dysplasia and ring sideroblasts
  - RA with excess blasts-1 (RAEB-1):
    - 5–9% blasts in marrow; no Auer rods; <5% blasts in blood; <1,000 monocytes/mm³
  - RAEB-2
    - 10–19% blasts in marrow; 5–19% blasts in blood; ±Auer rods; <1,000 monocytes/mm³
  - MDS associated with isolated del(5q)
    - RA with erythroid hyperplasia, increased megakaryocytes with hypolobated nuclei, and normal or increased platelets; <5% blasts in marrow; <1% blasts in blood
  - Acute MDS with sclerosis:
    - RAEB with marked myelosclerosis
  - Chronic myelomonocytic leukemia (CMMoL) is now grouped with myelodysplastic/myeloproliferative disorders:
    - <20% blasts and promonocytes in marrow and blood with >1,000 monocytes/mm³
  - RAEB in transformation is now considered acute myeloid leukemia (AML):
    - 20–30% blasts in marrow; >20% blasts in blood
    - Incidence: 2:1 (female > male)
  - Therapy-related MDS (t-MDS):
    - Seen 3 to 7 years after treatment with alkylating agents and/or radiotherapy
    - Evolves to AML over ~6 months
    - Classified by the WHO as therapy-related myeloid neoplasm
- System(s) affected: hematologic, lymphatic, immunologic
- Synonym(s): dysmyelopoietic syndrome; hemopoietic dysplasia; preleukemia; smoldering or subacute myeloid leukemia

Pediatric Considerations
Pediatric presentations of MDS
- Monosomy 7 syndrome
- Juvenile chronic myelogenous leukemia

EPIDEMIOLOGY
- Predominant age: median age, >65 years; uncommon in children and young adults
- Predominant sex: male = female

Incidence
Apparent increased incidence (1 to 2/100,000 per year) in recent years may be due to improved diagnosis; incidence increases markedly with older age.

Genetics
- Most are clonal neoplasms by cytogenetics, G6PD isoenzyme analysis, or restriction fragment length polymorphism analysis.
- Mutations in *RAS* oncogene
- Mutations in *RPS14* gene on chromosome 5q
- Mutations in *TET2, SF3B1, SRSF2, U2AF1, DNMT3A, ASXL1*

RISK FACTORS
- Primary MDS is associated with older age, occupational exposure to petroleum solvents (benzene, gasoline), and smoking.
- Secondary (therapy-related) MDS is associated with prior treatment with alkylating agents or radiotherapy.

COMMONLY ASSOCIATED CONDITIONS
- Anemia
- Neutropenia
- Thrombocytopenia
- Pancytopenia
- Opportunistic infections
- Bleeding, bruising
- Sweet syndrome (neutrophilic dermatosis)

 DIAGNOSIS

HISTORY
- Fatigue
- Fever
- Easy bruising

PHYSICAL EXAM
- Anemia
  - Fatigue
  - Shortness of breath
  - Light-headedness
  - Angina
- Leukopenia
  - Fever
  - Infection
- Thrombocytopenia
  - Ecchymoses
  - Petechiae
  - Epistaxis
  - Purpura
- Splenomegaly (uncommon)
  - Mild to moderate enlargement may be encountered, particularly in CMMoL.
- Skin infiltrates
  - Sweet syndrome

DIFFERENTIAL DIAGNOSIS
- Other malignant disorders
  - Evolving AML or erythroleukemia
  - Chronic myeloproliferative disorders
  - Polycythemia vera
  - Myeloid metaplasia with myelofibrosis
  - Malignant lymphoma
  - Metastatic carcinoma
- Nonmalignant disorders
  - Aplastic anemia
  - Autoimmune disorders (Felty syndrome, lupus, hemolytic anemia)
  - Nutritional deficiencies (vitamin B₁₂, pyridoxine, copper, protein malnutrition)
  - Heavy metal intoxication
  - Alcoholism
  - Chronic liver disease
  - Hypersplenism
  - Chronic inflammation
  - Recent cytotoxic therapy or irradiation
  - HIV infection
  - Paroxysmal nocturnal hemoglobinuria

DIAGNOSTIC TESTS & INTERPRETATION
Initial Tests (lab, imaging)
- CBC with differential and peripheral smear
- Reticulocyte count and serum erythropoietin level if anemia were present
- Review of the peripheral blood smear for the presence of dysplasia
- Liver/spleen scan or CT, although rarely necessary, may disclose occult splenomegaly or lymphadenopathy.
- Cytogenetics
  - At least 50% of patients with primary MDS and nearly all with t-MDS have clonal chromosomal abnormalities: +8, −7, del(5q), del(7q), del(20q), iso(17p), various others, and complex karyotypes.
  - Detection of clonal abnormality establishes a diagnosis of neoplasm and rules out a nutritional, toxic, or autoimmune disorder.
  - Cytogenetic analysis of metaphase cells from a bone marrow aspiration provides more information than fluorescence in situ hybridization analysis on blood cells.
- Granulocyte function tests: abnormal in 50% (decreased myeloperoxidase activity, phagocytosis, chemotaxis, and adhesion)
- Platelet function tests: impaired aggregation
- Marrow colony assays in vitro
  - Results are variable and correlate poorly with clinical course.
  - Poor clonal growth may suggest more rapid evolution to AML.
- Immunophenotyping
  - Nonspecific myeloid markers are present.
  - Occasionally, evidence can be found for concomitant lymphoproliferative disorder.
  - Loss of CD59 expression suggests paroxysmal nocturnal hemoglobinuria (PNH).

Follow-Up Tests & Special Considerations
- Anemia: often macrocytic; occasional poikilocytosis, anisocytosis; variable reticulocytosis
- Granulocytopenia: hypogranular or agranular neutrophils with poorly condensed chromatin; Pelger-Huet anomaly with hyposegmented nuclei
- Thrombocytopenia: occasionally giant platelets or hypogranular platelets
- Fetal hemoglobin may be elevated.
- Flow cytometry to detect loss of CD59 on RBCs, CD16 on granulocytes, and CD14 on monocytes; typical of PNH
- Direct antiglobulin (Coombs) test
- Paraprotein: present in some
- Erythropoietin: usually normally elevated given the degree of anemia unless renal failure is present
- Increased serum and tissue iron (ferritin), especially if anemia has been long-standing
- Serum copper level

Diagnostic Procedures/Other
- Review peripheral blood smear.
- Bone marrow aspiration, biopsy, and cytogenetics
- Myeloid gene mutation array

Test Interpretation
- Ineffective hematopoiesis with dysplasia in one or more cell lineages dominates the bone marrow picture in MDS.
- Marrow cellularity usually is normal or increased for the patient's age but may be hypoplastic in ~10%.
- Reticulin fibrosis usually is minimal except in t-MDS and acute MDS with sclerosis.
- Myeloblasts may be clustered in the intertrabecular spaces with abnormal localization of immature precursors.

 TREATMENT

GENERAL MEASURES
- Immunize for pneumococcal pneumonia, pertussis, influenza, and hepatitis B (4)[C].
- RBC transfusions to alleviate symptoms
- Platelet transfusions only for bleeding or before surgery to avoid alloimmunization
- Early use of antibiotics for fever, even while culture results are pending, due to quantitative and qualitative granulocyte disorder
- Iron chelation therapy to avoid iron overload from chronic transfusions

MEDICATION
First Line
- Epoetin alfa or darbepoetin can increase hemoglobin levels in MDS patients who have low serum erythropoietin levels at baseline (5)[C].
- Only azacitidine, decitabine, and lenalidomide have been approved by the FDA for MDS.
- Azacitidine and decitabine have been proven in randomized controlled trials to be more effective for these heterogeneous disorders than only supportive care, with antibiotics, and transfusions.
- Vitamins, iron, corticosteroids, androgens, or thyroid hormone are rarely helpful, unless evidence of a specific deficiency exists.
- Clinical trials show azacitidine, 75 mg/m²/day SC for 7 days and repeated every 28 days, decreases RBC transfusion requirements, yields longer times to AML or death, and improves quality of life.
- Decitabine was approved with a continuous IV schedule that usually requires hospitalization. More commonly, it is given at 20 mg/m² IV over 1 hour daily for 5 days as an outpatient, repeated every 4 weeks.
- Lenalidomide, 10 mg PO daily for 21 days every 4 weeks has yielded complete remission in patients with MDS and del(5q). It is less effective in patients with MDS without del(5q) (6)[B].
- Intensive chemotherapy
  - Younger patients with MDS may benefit from AML chemotherapy, especially if Auer rods are present, but toxicity may be severe for older patients.
  - Remission durations are variable (median, ~1 year).
- Allogeneic hematopoietic stem cell transplantation:
  - Recommended for younger patients with HLA antigen–matched donors to eradicate the malignant clone and resupply normal hematopoietic stem cells (7)[A].

- Aminocaproic acid (epsilon-aminocaproic acid) or tranexamic acid may benefit patients with chronic, severe thrombocytopenia and bleeding.
- Contraindications: Cytotoxicity of chemotherapy may increase the risk of bleeding and infection and the need for transfusion support.
- Precautions: Aspirin, salicylates, and NSAIDs should be avoided.

Second Line
- Danazol or prednisone may be of benefit for concomitant autoimmune thrombocytopenia.
- Investigational agents
  - Low doses of cytarabine, tretinoin (all-trans retinoic acid), 13-cis retinoic acid, arsenic trioxide, histone/protein deacetylase inhibitors, interferon, cyclosporine, antithymocyte globulin, filgrastim, and interleukin-3
  - Agents, such as thalidomide, that inhibit the production of tumor necrosis factor in the marrow.
- Amifostine may stimulate the proliferation of normal hematopoiesis.

ISSUES FOR REFERRAL
- Refer younger adults for allogeneic hematopoietic cell transplantation.
- Refer patients with symptoms or transfusion requirements for clinical trials.

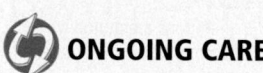 ONGOING CARE

FOLLOW-UP RECOMMENDATIONS
Usually outpatient, except when necessary to hospitalize for the treatment of infection, blood transfusions, or intensive chemotherapy

Patient Monitoring
- At least monthly during supportive care
- More frequently if receiving treatment

DIET
Reduce alcohol use and iron intake (unless patient is iron-deficient).

PATIENT EDUCATION
- Stop smoking.
- Seek early medical attention for fever, bleeding, or symptoms of anemia.
- Advise about the risks of chronic transfusion therapy.

PROGNOSIS
- Median survival for RA and RARS is 5 years, but it may extend much longer (8)[B].
- RA with del(5q) syndrome is favorable.
- Median survival for RAEB, RCMD, and CMMoL is ~1 year; 50% of patients evolve to AML and the other 50% die of infection or bleeding.

COMPLICATIONS
- Infection
- Bleeding
- Complications of anemia and transfusions

REFERENCES
1. Malcovati L, Hellström-Lindberg E, Bowen D, et al. Diagnosis and treatment of primary myelodysplastic syndromes in adults: recommendations from the European LeukemiaNet. *Blood*. 2013;122(17): 2943–2964.
2. Swerdlow SH, Campo E, Harris NL, et al., eds. *WHO Classification of Tumours of Haematopoietic and Lymphoid Tissues*. 4th ed. Lyon, France: IARC Press; 2008.
3. Greenberg PL. The multifaceted nature of myelodysplastic syndromes: clinical, molecular, and biological prognostic features. *J Natl Compr Canc Netw*. 2013;11(7):877–884.
4. Larson RA. Myelodysplasia: when to treat and how. *Best Pract Res Clin Haematol*. 2006;19(2):293–300.
5. Fenaux P, Adès L. How we treat lower-risk myelodysplastic syndromes. *Blood*. 2013;121(21): 4280–4286.
6. List A, Dewald G, Bennett J, et al. Lenalidomide in the myelodysplastic syndrome with chromosome 5q deletion. *N Engl J Med*. 2006;355(14): 1456–1465.
7. Koreth J, Pidala J, Perez WS, et al. Role of reduced-intensity conditioning allogeneic hematopoietic stem-cell transplantation in older patients with de novo myelodysplastic syndromes: an international collaborative decision analysis. *J Clin Oncol*. 2013;31(21):2662–2670.
8. Voso MT, Fenu S, Latagliata R, et al. Revised International Prognostic Scoring System (IPSS) predicts survival and leukemic evolution of myelodysplastic syndromes significantly better than IPSS and WHO Prognostic Scoring System: validation by the Gruppo Romano Mielodisplasie Italian Regional Database. *J Clin Oncol*. 2013;31(21):2671–2677.

ADDITIONAL READING
- Cheson BD, Greenberg PL, Bennett JM, et al. Clinical application and proposal for modification of the International Working Group (IWG) response criteria in myelodysplasia. *Blood*. 2006;108(2):419–425.
- Larson RA, Le Beau MM. Therapy-related myeloid leukaemia: a model for leukemogenesis in humans. *Chem Biol Interact*. 2005;153–154:187–195.
- Nybakken GE, Bagg A. The genetic basis and expanding role of molecular analysis in the diagnosis, prognosis, and therapeutic design for myelodysplastic syndromes. *J Mol Diagn*. 2014;16(2):145–158.
- Singh ZN, Huo D, Anastasi J, et al. Therapy-related myelodysplastic syndrome: morphologic subclassification may not be clinically relevant. *Am J Clin Pathol*. 2007;127(2):197–205.

 CODES

ICD10
- D46.9 Myelodysplastic syndrome, unspecified
- D46.4 Refractory anemia, unspecified
- D46.B Refract cytopenia w multilin dysplasia and ring sideroblasts

CLINICAL PEARLS
- MDS constitutes a heterogeneous group of acquired, hematopoietic stem cell disorders characterized by cytologic dysplasia in the bone marrow and blood and by various combinations of anemia, neutropenia, and thrombocytopenia.
- The natural progression of this malignant disease evolves as cellular maturation becomes more arrested and blast cells accumulate.

M

699

MYELOPROLIFERATIVE NEOPLASMS

Tarsheen K. Sethi, MBBS • Sanjay Mohan, MD, MSCI

BASICS

DESCRIPTION
- Myeloproliferative neoplasms (MPNs) are a group of diseases that share a common cell of origin in the pluripotent hematopoietic stem cell.
- MPNs are characterized by proliferation of a specific stem cell lineage such as myeloid, erythroid, or megakaryocytic; resulting in granulocytosis, erythrocytosis, or thrombocytosis, respectively.
- The "classic" MPNs include chronic myelogenous leukemia (CML), polycythemia vera (PV), essential thrombocythemia (ET), and primary myelofibrosis (PMF). The World Health Organization (WHO) classification also includes chronic neutrophilic leukemia, chronic eosinophilic leukemia not otherwise specified (CEL-NOS), systemic mastocytosis, and myeloproliferative neoplasm unclassifiable. This topic focuses on the classic MPNs.
- CML is characterized by the presence of Philadelphia-chromosome (reciprocal translocation between chromosomes 9 and 22 resulting in a BCR-ABL fusion gene). This results in an uninhibited proliferation of myeloid precursor stem cells resulting in granulocytosis and elevation of various granulocyte precursors.
- The following three MPNs are characterized by varying degree of presence of JAK 2 mutation.
  - PMF: MPN characterized by marrow fibrosis, extramedullary hematopoiesis, and splenomegaly
  - ET: MPN characterized by a clonal proliferation of megakaryocytes, leading to thrombocytosis
  - PV: MPN characterized by trilineage growth of hematopoietic stem cells with erythroid precursors predominating, leading to erythrocytosis

EPIDEMIOLOGY
Incidence
- CML: 0.6 to 2.0/100,000/year; median age at diagnosis 66 years; male > female (1.6:1)
- PMF: 0.5 to 1.5/100,000/year; median age at diagnosis 65 years; male = female
- ET: 0.6 to 2.5/100,000/year; median age at diagnosis 60 years, second peak in younger patients at ~30 years; female > male (2:1)
- PV: 1 to 2/100,000/year; male > female (1.3:1)

ETIOLOGY AND PATHOPHYSIOLOGY
- CML: BCR-ABL1 gene leads to increased and unrestrained activity of the ABL tyrosine kinase resulting in an unchecked activation of downstream signaling pathways which have an antiapoptotic effect on the hematopoietic cells.
- PMF: Progenitor hematopoietic stem cells undergo a clonal proliferation independent of growth factors likely due to activation of downstream intracellular pathways. The fibroblasts are nonclonal, and the increased fibrosis is likely driven by growth factors released by hematopoietic cells especially megakaryocytes.
- ET: Thrombopoietin-induced megakaryocyte proliferation is uncontrolled due to a combination of increased sensitivity to thrombopoietin and decreased feedback regulation of the thrombopoietin levels which is usually inversely proportional to the platelet mass.
- PV: Gain-of-function mutation (JAK2) leads to increased erythrocyte production due to a downstream activation of proteins involved in cell proliferation and resistance to apoptosis. The JAK2 tyrosine kinase is downstream of the erythropoietin receptor and thus its constitutive activation makes the hematopoietic progenitor cell independent of erythropoietin.

Genetics
- Philadelphia chromosome (BCR-ABL1 gene): translocation and fusion of the BCR gene on chromosome 22 and the ABL gene on chromosome 9; seen in all patients with CML
- JAK2 mutations: point mutations in the tyrosine kinase domain of JAK2, causing a substitution of phenylalanine for valine at position 617 (JAK2V617F); leading to unrestrained JAK2 activation with a deactivation of typical feedback mechanism
- Seen in >95% of PV cases; 50% of ET and PMF cases
- CALR mutation: Calreticulin (CALR) is an endoplasmic reticulum chaperone protein directing proper folding of proteins. This mutation may be seen in up to a third of patients of ET and PMF. These patients are seen to have a higher platelet count but lower risk of thrombosis.
- Myeloproliferative leukemia virus (MPL) gene: Mutations found in 5–10% of patients with PMF and in 3–5% of those with ET. This encodes the thrombopoietin receptor MPL.
- JAK2, CALR, and MPL mutations are mutually exclusive and together account for 85% of cases of ET and PMF.

RISK FACTORS
- Rare familial cases have been reported.
- CML: exposure to ionizing radiation

COMMONLY ASSOCIATED CONDITIONS
- Progression to acute myeloid leukemia; most common with CML
- Thrombosis/hemorrhage

DIAGNOSIS

HISTORY
- Many MPN cases are found incidentally on routine blood work.
- CML: Most patients are asymptomatic at time of diagnosis.
  - Fatigue, malaise, weight loss, excessive perspiration, abdominal fullness, early satiety, bleeding episodes
- PMF: Symptoms depend on the degree of anemia and splenomegaly.
  - Fatigue, shortness of breath, early satiety, constitutional symptoms, cachexia, Budd-Chiari syndrome, splenic infarcts, osteosclerosis resulting in bone pains.
- ET: characterized by thrombotic and hemorrhagic events
  - Thrombotic events (deep vein thrombosis, pulmonary embolism, Budd-Chiari syndrome), microvascular occlusive events (digital ischemia, erythromelalgia), major/minor hemorrhagic events; headaches, dizziness, syncope, tingling, visual changes, transient ischemic attacks
- PV: Symptoms are due to level of erythrocytosis and the resultant increased blood viscosity.
  - Erythromelalgia, pruritus after hot baths, headaches, tinnitus, paresthesias, gout attacks

PHYSICAL EXAM
- CML: splenomegaly, hepatomegaly
- PMF: splenomegaly seen in nearly all patients; hepatomegaly, pallor
- ET: possible petechiae, purpura, ecchymosis; splenomegaly
- PV: cyanotic blush (lips, nose, ears, distal extremities), increased blood pressure, splenomegaly, epistaxis, ecchymosis

DIFFERENTIAL DIAGNOSIS
- CML: leukemoid reaction (elevated LAP), juvenile myelomonocytic leukemia, chronic myelomonocytic leukemia (CMML), chronic eosinophilic leukemia, chronic neutrophilic leukemia
- PMF: other MPNs, lymphoma, hairy cell leukemia; secondary myelofibrosis (malignant or nonmalignant)
- ET: reactive thrombocytosis, CML, PV, PMF, and myelodysplastic syndromes
- PV: hypoxic states (e.g., chronic obstructive pulmonary disease [COPD], anemia), renal cell carcinoma, Wilms tumor, hepatoma, polycystic kidney disease, exogenous androgens

DIAGNOSTIC TESTS & INTERPRETATION
- CML: White blood cell count >10,000 × 10^9/L with differential showing increased mature and immature neutrophils and an increased percentage of myelocytes, metamyelocytes, and band forms; neutrophils have decreased leukocyte alkaline phosphatase; platelet count >600,000 × 10^9/L and a normochromic, normocytic anemia. Basophilia is common.
- PMF (1)[A] (WHO criteria): Diagnosis requires meeting all three major criteria and two or more minor criteria:
  - Major criteria: (i) megakaryocyte proliferation and atypia accompanied by either reticulin or collagen fibrosis; (ii) not meeting WHO criteria for CML, PV, MDS, or other myeloid neoplasm; (iii) demonstration of JAK2V617F or other clonal marker or absence of marker with no evidence of secondary marrow fibrosis
  - Minor criteria: (i) leukoerythroblastosis, (ii) increased serum lactate dehydrogenase level, (iii) anemia, and (iv) palpable splenomegaly
- ET (1)[A] (WHO criteria): Diagnosis requires meeting all four major criteria:
  - Major criteria: (i) thrombocytosis with persistent platelet level ≥450 × 10^9/L; (ii) megakaryocyte proliferation with large and mature morphology; (iii) not meeting the WHO criteria for CML, PV, PMF, MDS, or other myeloid neoplasm; and (iv) demonstration of JAK2V617F or other clonal marker or absence of clonal marker with no evidence of reactive thrombocytosis
- PV (1)[A] (WHO criteria): Diagnosis requires either both major criteria and one minor criterion or the first major criterion and two of the minor criteria:
  - Major criteria: (i) hemoglobin >18.5 g/dL in men, >16.5 g/dL in women or other evidence of increased red cell volume and (ii) presence of JAK2V617F or other functionally similar mutation (e.g., JAK2 exon 12 mutation) (1)[B]
  - Minor criteria: (i) bone marrow biopsy showing hypercellularity for age with trilineage myeloproliferation, (ii) low serum erythropoietin level, (iii) endogenous erythroid colony formation in vitro

Initial Tests (lab, imaging)
If clinical suspicion of MPN, obtain a CBC and peripheral blood smear; if suggestive, obtain bone marrow biopsy.

- PMF: radiographic osteosclerosis in 25–66%

Diagnostic Procedures/Other

- CML: diagnosis with identification of Philadelphia chromosome: Fluorescence in situ hybridization is more sensitive than karyotyping and is routinely used. Polymerase chain reaction (P210) is done at baseline to help monitor response to tyrosine kinase inhibitors.
  - Bone marrow biopsy: increased cellularity and increased myeloid to erythroid ratio
- PMF, ET, and PV: genotypic analysis and bone marrow biopsy as described in earlier WHO criteria; "dry tap" is common in PMF.
- Risk stratification
  - CML: three phases of CML
    - (i) Chronic phase (85% patients at diagnosis; <5% blast counts); (ii) accelerated phase (poorly controlled splenomegaly regardless of treatment, 10–19% blast counts, worsening anemia, basophil ≥20%); and (iii) blast crisis (resembles acute myeloid leukemia or lymphoid leukemia, >20% blast counts)
  - PMF: International Prognostic Scoring System (IPSS) at diagnosis and Dynamic IPSS (DIPSS-plus) throughout disease
    - IPSS: age >65 years, constitutional symptoms, hemoglobin <10 g/dL, leukocyte count >25 × 10^9, circulating blasts >1%
      - Low risk = 0 of above; intermediate-1 risk = 1 of above; intermediate-2 risk = 2 of above; high risk = ≥3 of above
    - DIPSS-plus: same 5 risk factors in the IPSS + the need for red cell transfusion, platelets <100 × 10^9/L and unfavorable karyotype
      - Low risk = 0 of above; intermediate-1 risk = 1 of above; intermediate-2 risk = 2–3 of above; high risk = ≥4 of above
  - ET: low risk = age <40 years, no prior thromboembolic events, no cardiovascular risk factors, platelet count <1,500 × 10^9/L; intermediate risk = age 40 to 59 years, presence of cardiovascular risk factors, platelet count <1,500 × 10^9/L; high risk = age ≥60 years and/or prior thromboembolic or hemorrhagic episode and/or platelet count >1,500 × 10^9/L
  - PV: low risk = age <60 years, no history of thrombosis/cardiovascular risk factors; intermediate risk = platelets >1,000 × 10^9/L and cardiovascular risk factors; high risk = age >60 years or a history of thrombosis

TREATMENT

GENERAL MEASURES
Low-dose aspirin for ET and PV

MEDICATION

First Line
- CML
  - Chronic phase: Imatinib mesylate (Gleevec): 400 mg/day, a tyrosine kinase inhibitor (TKI). Dasatinib and nilotinib are also approved for use in the first line (1).
  - Accelerated or blast phase: Increase imatinib to 800 mg/day or switch to 2nd- of 3rd-generation TKIs like nilotinib and dasatinib.
  - While awaiting confirmation of diagnosis, hydroxyurea can be used to lower the WBC count.
- PMF: Main goal is symptomatic relief:
  - Low and intermediate-1 risk: no drug therapy indicated, symptom-directed therapy
  - Intermediate-2 and high risk: hydroxyurea or consider allogeneic SCT

- JAK2 inhibitor ruxolitinib is approved for intermediate or high-risk myelofibrosis. It is also approved for post-PV and post-ET myelofibrosis (2).
  - Supportive treatment
    - Anemia: transfusions, erythropoiesis-stimulating agents, androgens, danazol, thalidomide, or lenalidomide
    - Splenomegaly: hydroxyurea, splenectomy, or IV cladribine for refractory cases
    - Thrombosis: hydroxyurea and low-dose aspirin
- ET low and intermediate risk: "Watch and wait" + low-dose aspirin if microvascular disturbances are present and no contraindications; high risk: hydroxyurea 15 mg/kg/day in divided doses to reduce platelet count to <450 × 10^9/L (2).
- PV
  - Low and intermediate risk: phlebotomy and low-dose aspirin
  - High risk (or those who do not tolerate phlebotomy): hydroxyurea 500 to 1,000 mg/day (2).

Second Line
- CML: Only curable treatment is aSCT; reserved for accelerated/blast phase due to high rates of morbidity and mortality with aSCT
  - 2nd-generation TKIs: dasatinib, nilotinib, and bosutinib; increasing evidence for improved, deeper responses with these medication resulting in use of 2nd-generation TKIs for first-line therapy. Ponatinib is a 3rd-generation TKI that has activity in cases of TKI resistance due to a T315I mutation for which all the other available TKIs are ineffective.
- PMF: Only curable treatment is allogeneic SCT; reserved for intermediate-2 or high-risk patients
  - If unresponsive to hydroxyurea, use pegylated interferon-α; tolerance may be an issue.
- ET: If resistant/intolerant to hydroxyurea, use anagrelide.
  - If resistant/intolerant to hydroxyurea or anagrelide, pregnant or age <40 years: Use interferon-α.
- PV: if resistant or intolerant to hydroxyurea, can use ruxolitinib

ISSUES FOR REFERRAL
Patients with MPNs are usually referred to hematology/oncology.

SURGERY/OTHER PROCEDURES
May require splenectomy/palliative radiation for foci of extramedullary hematopoiesis

INPATIENT CONSIDERATIONS

Admission Criteria/Initial Stabilization
Severe cachexia; renal failure and hepatomegaly secondary to extramedullary hematopoiesis; massive splenomegaly requiring treatment; severe thrombotic/hemorrhagic episodes; anemia; tumor lysis syndrome

IV Fluids
Optimal hydration to prevent tumor lysis syndrome

ONGOING CARE

PROGNOSIS
- CML: 10-year survival rate ~80% from time of diagnosis; 85% will die in blast crisis; 12- to 18-month median survival for accelerated phase; 3- to 6-month median survival for blast phase
- PMF: worst prognosis of the MPNs; drug therapy does not modify disease course but treats the symptoms; median survival for IPSS

low risk = 135 months, intermediate-1 risk = 95 months; intermediate-2 risk = 48 months; high risk = 27 months
- PV: median survival often >10 years
- ET: near-normal life expectancy

COMPLICATIONS
- CML: blast crisis, transformation to acute leukemia, gout, or nephropathy due to hyperuricemia
- PMF: 10% develop acute myeloid leukemia; anemia, massive hepatosplenomegaly, thrombohemorrhagic events, osteosclerosis, secondary gout, splenic infarcts, paraspinal/epidural extramedullary hematopoiesis
- ET: <10% develop post-ET myelofibrosis, 2% develop acute myeloid leukemia; thrombohemorrhagic events
- PV: 15–20% develop post-PV myelofibrosis, 5% develop leukemia; erythromelalgia, pruritus, secondary gout, headaches, vascular occlusive events

REFERENCES
1. Fava C, Rege-Cambrin G, Saglio G. The choice of first-line chronic myelogenous leukemia treatment. *Ann Hematol.* 2015;94(Suppl 2):S123–S131.
2. Geyer HL, Mesa RA. Therapy for myeloproliferative neoplasms: when, which agent, and how? *Blood.* 2014;124(24):3529–3537.

ADDITIONAL READING
- Cervantes F, Dupriez B, Pereira A, et al. New prognostic scoring system for primary myelofibrosis based on a study of the International Working Group for Myelofibrosis Research and Treatment. *Blood.* 2009;113(13):2895–2901.
- Druker BJ, Guilhot F, O'Brien SG, et al. Five-year follow-up of patients receiving imatinib for chronic myeloid leukemia. *N Engl J Med.* 2006;355(23):2408–2417.
- Vannucchi AM, Kiladjian JJ, Griesshammer M, et al. Ruxolitinib versus standard therapy for the treatment of polycythemia vera. *N Engl J Med.* 2015;372(5):426–435.
- Verstovsek S, Mesa RA, Gotlib J, et al. A double-blind, placebo-controlled trial of ruxolitinib for myelofibrosis. *N Engl J Med.* 2012;366(9):799–807.

 SEE ALSO

Leukemia, Chronic Myelogenous; Polycythemia Vera

 CODES

ICD10
- D47.1 Chronic myeloproliferative disease
- C92.10 Chronic myeloid leukemia, BCR/ABL-positive, not having achieved remission
- D45 Polycythemia vera

CLINICAL PEARLS

Ruxolitinib has a role in amelioration of constitutional and splenomegaly-related symptoms in myelofibrosis.

M

NARCOLEPSY

Jennifer M. Slowik, DO, MS • Kevin A. Carter, DO, FAASM

 BASICS

DESCRIPTION

- Disorder characterized by excessive daytime sleepiness often associated with cataplexy (sudden bilateral weakness of skeletal muscles) and other rapid eye movement (REM) sleep phenomena, such as sleep paralysis and hypnagogic hallucinations (e.g., vivid auditory or visual perceptions without an external stimulus that occur as one is falling asleep).
- Frequently overlooked disorder, with an average of 15 years of symptoms prior to diagnosis
- System affected: nervous

EPIDEMIOLOGY

Incidence

- Onset usually in teenage years
- Bimodal distribution peak at 15 and 35 years of age
- Predominant sex: male > female (1.6:1)
- Incidence: 0.74/100,000 persons/year

Prevalence

- Narcolepsy type 1 (with cataplexy): 25 to 50/100,000 people
- Narcolepsy type 2 (without cataplexy): 20 to 34/100,000 people

ETIOLOGY AND PATHOPHYSIOLOGY

- Narcolepsy type 1 is a neurodegenerative disorder resulting from selective loss of neurons containing hypocretin (orexin) in the hypothalamus; may be autoimmune (associated with influenza A, H1N1 vaccine, and *Streptococcus pyogenes*).
- Orexin neurons also regulate metabolism, feeding, reward and autonomic tone; weight gain especially in children from reduction of metabolism
- 90–95% of patients with narcolepsy type 1 have low hypocretin in CSF
- The cause of narcolepsy type 2 is not well established.
- Possible involvement of immune system and environmental influences

Genetics

- Increased incidence in families with positive history: 1–2% in first-degree relative of index case (10 to 40 times the general population)
- Twin concordance is 25–31% (suggests environmental contribution).
- Most are sporadic
- 85–95% of patients with narcolepsy and cataplexy have human leukocyte antigen (HLA) DQB1*0602; 45% of patients with narcolepsy without cataplexy express this antigen. HLA DQB1*0602 is present in 24% of the general population.
- Autosomal-recessive inheritance pattern
- 12% of Asians, 25% of Whites, and 38% of African Americans are gene carriers.

RISK FACTORS

- Obesity
- Head trauma
- CNS infectious disease
- Anesthesia
- Psychological stress
- Family history
- Recent influenza A, streptococcal infection, or H1N1 vaccine

COMMONLY ASSOCIATED CONDITIONS

Obstructive sleep apnea (up to 25%), obesity, anxiety

 DIAGNOSIS

HISTORY

- Classic tetrad of excessive daytime sleepiness, cataplexy, sleep paralysis, and hypnagogic hallucinations (four most common symptoms): Only 10–20% of patients have all four symptoms
- 3 general forms
  - Narcolepsy type 1: 40%
  - Narcolepsy type 2: 60%
  - Secondary narcolepsy due to a medical condition (e.g., Parkinson disease with sleep disturbance, myotonic dystrophy, CNS tumors, Prader-Willi syndrome, Niemann-Pick disease type C)
- Excessive daytime sleepiness and sleep attacks (cardinal symptom)
  - Primary symptom and required for diagnosis
  - Instantaneous, irresistible REM sleep
  - First and most disabling symptom
  - Tendency to take naps lasting 5 to 10 minutes
  - Episodes last minutes and rarely more than an hour
  - 1 to 8 naps/day but normal 24-hour sleep duration
  - Associated with dreaming
  - Nap restores wakefulness for several hours
  - More likely in a monotonous, warm environment, after a large meal, or with strong emotions
- Cataplexy: auxiliary symptom (60%; cardinal symptom)
  - Pathognomonic if present
  - Sudden bilateral weakness of skeletal muscles
  - Provocation by sudden strong emotions
  - Consciousness and memory are not impaired.
  - Short duration (seconds to minutes)
  - Can be limited to a particular muscle group (e.g., jaw droop with inability to speak; arm, neck, or leg weakness; respiratory and eye muscles not affected)
  - Status cataplecticus is a rare, prolonged episode of cataplexy (lasting hours) that is more likely in children or on withdrawal of drugs.
- Sleep paralysis: auxiliary symptom (25–50%)
  - When falling asleep or on awakening, the patient wants to but cannot move; this can end abruptly when the patient is touched or spoken to.
  - Brain wakes from sleep while body remains paralyzed in REM sleep
  - Lasts seconds to minutes
  - Patients are aware of events around them but cannot open eyes or move.
  - Can be preceded by hallucinatory phenomena
  - 50% of the normal population have had at least one of these episodes (thus, this symptom is nonspecific)
- Hypnagogic hallucinations: auxiliary symptom (30–60%)
  - Vivid, frightening visual, auditory or tactile illusions or hallucinations at onset of sleep
  - Dreamlike experiences that occur during wakefulness or suddenly at sleep onset
  - Characteristic hallucinations include seeing human or animal faces or feeling that someone else is in the room.
- Disturbed nocturnal sleep (66%)
  - Normal total sleep with decreased sleep efficiency
  - More frequent transitions from wakefulness to sleep
  - Retrograde amnesic and automatic behavior lasting minutes to hours

  - Increased periodic leg movements (50%)
  - Depression (18–37%)
  - Automatic behavior: activity without memory of the event
  - Panic attacks and social phobias (20%)

PHYSICAL EXAM

- A complete exam is useful to rule out other causes of hypersomnia.
- If cataplexy is witnessed, examiner will be unable to elicit deep tendon reflexes.

DIFFERENTIAL DIAGNOSIS

Excessive daytime sleepiness is present in 4% of the general population, although most individuals are not narcoleptic. Possible etiologies include the following:

- Sleep apnea syndromes (40–50% of those with excessive somnolence); increased incidence in narcolepsy, up to 26% prevalence
- Epileptic seizures and syncope
- Idiopathic hypersomnia (5–10% of those with excessive somnolence)
- Psychiatric (depression, substance abuse/withdrawal)
- Sleep related movement disorders (restless leg syndrome, periodic limb movements of sleep)
- Iatrogenic secondary to medication (benzodiazepines, opioids, antihistamines, β-blockers, and some antipsychotics, antidepressants, and anticonvulsants)
- Poor sleep hygiene and habits leading to sleep deficit
- Circadian rhythm disorders (jet lag, shift work, delayed or advanced sleep phase disorders)
- Seizures
- Niemann-Pick type C
- Hypersomnia related to a medical condition, such as Parkinson disease
- Kleine-Levin syndrome (recurrent hypersomnia that lasts days to weeks and recurs months later)
- Menstrual-associated hypersomnia

Pediatric Considerations

Narcolepsy is rare before the age of 5 years. Excessive daytime sleepiness is more often attributable to obstructive sleep apnea (OSA), poor sleep hygiene, and the increased sleep requirements early in life. Recommended amount of sleep decreases with age: newborns 16 to 18 hr/day; preschool-aged children 11 to 12 hr/day; school aged children and teens 10 hr/day; adults 7 to 8 hr/day.

DIAGNOSTIC TESTS & INTERPRETATION

Initial Tests (lab, imaging)

- Epworth Sleepiness Scale: score ranges from 0 to 24 and >10 is suggestive of a sleep disorder rather than generalized fatigue (1)[A].
- Stanford Sleepiness Scale: patients select one of seven statements that best describe energy level, concentration, and sleepiness. Statements 4 to 7 may indicate excessive sleepiness.
- Nighttime polysomnography (PSG): Monitoring of patients in a sleep laboratory will usually document fragmented sleep with a normal amount of REM sleep but rapid onset REM (within 15 minutes of sleep onset) and decreased sleep efficiency (2)[A]. The PSG is useful to rule out other causes of excessive daytime sleepiness, including sleep apnea syndromes and nocturnal myoclonus.

- Multiple sleep latency test (MSLT): begins ≥90 minutes after nighttime test (2)[A]
  - The patient is monitored during 4 to 5, 20 minute naps taken at 2-hour intervals; rapidity of sleep onset and type of sleep pattern are documented. The supportive test includes mean sleep latency (time to fall asleep) of ≤8 minutes and ≥2 sleep-onset REM periods.
  - Sensitivity 77%; specificity 97%; positive predictive value 73%
- Maintenance of Wakefulness Test (MWT): used to assess ability to remain awake to determine restrictions (e.g., driving), assess treatment response. Not usually performed during the initial evaluation.

Follow-Up Tests & Special Considerations
- HLA typing for DQB1 in ambiguous cases
- Low CSF hypocretin-1 level: 99% specificity, 87% sensitivity in patients with cataplexy; useful in children when unable to do an MSLT

Diagnostic Procedure/Other
- Narcolepsy type 1 (2)[C]
  - Excessive daytime sleepiness daily for ≥3 months
  - One of the following:
    - Cataplexy with sleep latency ≤8 minutes with ≥2 sleep-onset REM periods within 15 minutes of the onset of sleep (SOREMP)
    - Low CSF hypocretin-1 level <110 pg/mL or <1/3 of mean values in normal subjects
- Narcolepsy type 2 (2)[C]
  - All above without the cataplexy and low hypocretin-1
- Diagnosis of exclusion

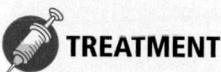

TREATMENT

GENERAL MEASURES
- None of the currently available medications enables people with narcolepsy to consistently maintain a fully normal state of alertness.
- Drug therapy should be supplemented by various behavioral strategies: Avoid shift work, heavy meals, and caffeine later in the day.
- Well-timed 20-minute naps may be helpful.
- Avoid sedating drugs and alcohol.
- Use safety precautions, particularly when driving. People with untreated narcoleptic symptoms are involved in automobile accidents roughly 10 times more frequently than the general population. However, accident rates are at normal levels among patients who have received appropriate medication therapy.

MEDICATION
First Line
- Excessive daytime sleepiness (EDS)
  - Modafinil (Provigil) (3)[A]:
    - Structurally distinct from amphetamines
    - 200 to 400 mg/day divided BID; start with 100 mg/day and increase over 3 to 4 days; maximum of 300 mg/dose, 400 mg/day 3.
    - First-line treatment: 60% effective and 20% partially effective
    - Half-life of 14 hours, can dose daily
    - Fewest adverse effects (headache, GI upset, increased metabolism of oral contraceptives) with less rebound hypersomnia and does not affect BP; tolerance limited
    - No decrease in cataplexy

  - Armodafinil (Nuvigil):
    - Enantiomeric form of modafinil with slightly longer half-life of 15 hours
    - 150 to 250 mg every morning
- Cataplexy:
  - Sodium oxybate (Xyrem):
    - 2.5 to 9 g; may take 3 months for full response
    - Preferred treatment for narcolepsy with cataplexy and disturbed nocturnal sleep
    - Give 1/2 dose once in bed and 1/2 dose 2 to 4 hours later.
    - Date rape drug; abuse potential (3)[A]
    - Can use with modafinil in severe cases
    - May worsen sleep-disordered breathing in patients with OSA
    - Expensive with short half-life
  - Tricyclic antidepressants
    - Protriptyline: 5 to 60 mg/day
    - Clomipramine: 10 to 150 mg/day
    - High side-effect profile: dry mouth, sedation, urinary retention, impotence
  - Serotonin-norepinephrine reuptake inhibitors
    - Venlafaxine: 37.5 to 75 mg BID
    - Fluoxetine: 20 to 80 mg/day
    - Work by suppressing REM sleep
  - The patient may develop a tolerance to the anti-cataplectic drugs and can have rebound cataplexy when a drug is withdrawn.
  - Although often used, quality evidence is lacking to demonstrate improvement in cataplexy symptoms from antidepressants (4)[A].
- Auxiliary symptoms (e.g., hypnagogic hallucination, sleep paralysis) require treatment less often than EDS and cataplexy but anticataplectics are useful when symptoms are problematic (4)[C].

Second Line
- EDS
  - Amphetamines
    - Methylphenidate (Ritalin): initial dose 10 to 60 mg/day divided BID or TID; maximum dose 60 mg/day (3)[B], short-acting, most potent amphetamine available. Can be used in combination with modafinil and armodafinil.
    - Dextroamphetamine: initial dose 10 mg/day; can increase by 10 mg weekly to a maximum dose 60 mg/day divided BID or TID (3)[B]
    - Contraindicated in patients with HTN
    - Adverse reactions: headaches, irritability, hypertension (HTN), psychosis, anorexia, habituation, rebound hypersomnia
    - If the patient develops a tolerance to stimulants, switch drugs rather than increase dose; there is little cross-tolerance
- Cataplexy
  - Selegiline: selective MAO-B inhibitor
    - Anticataplectic effective for excessive daytime sleepiness; 20 to 40 mg/day divided morning and noon (3)[B]
    - Doses >20 mg require a low-tyramine diet because the drug begins to lose selectivity.

ISSUES FOR REFERRAL
- Unresponsive to primary medications
- Patient support groups can be very beneficial.

ONGOING CARE

FOLLOW-UP RECOMMENDATIONS
Patient Monitoring
Frequent BP checks and regular follow-ups (approximately every 6 months) are recommended.

DIET
Selegiline: Doses >20 mg require a low-tyramine diet because the drug begins to lose selectivity.

PATIENT EDUCATION
- Narcolepsy information from the National Institute of Neurological Disorders and Stroke at www.ninds.nih.gov/disorders/narcolepsy/narcolepsy.htm
- Narcolepsy Network, Inc., North Kingstown, RI 02852; www.narcolepsynetwork.org

PROGNOSIS
Narcolepsy is a lifelong disease. Symptoms can worsen with aging. In women, symptoms can improve after menopause.

REFERENCES
1. Johns MW. A new method for measuring daytime sleepiness: the Epworth sleepiness scale. *Sleep* 1991;14(6):540–545.
2. American Academy of Sleep Medicine. *International Classification of Sleep Disorders: Diagnostic and Coding Manual*. 3rd ed. Darien, IL: American Academy of Sleep Medicine; 2014.
3. Mohsenin V. Narcolepsy—master of disguise: evidence-based recommendations for management. *Postgrad Med*. 2009;121(3):99–104.
4. Vignatelli L, D'Alessandro R, Candelise L. Antidepressant drugs for narcolepsy. *Cochrane Database Syst Rev*. 2008;(1):CD003724.

ADDITIONAL READING
- Leschziner G. Narcolepsy: a clinical review. *Pract Neurol*. 2014;14(5):323–331.
- Zaharna M, Dimitriu A, Guilleminault C. Expert opinion on pharmacotherapy of narcolepsy. *Expert Opin Pharmacother*. 2010;11(10):1633–1645.

CODES

ICD10
- G47.419 Narcolepsy without cataplexy
- G47.411 Narcolepsy with cataplexy
- G47.429 Narcolepsy in conditions classified elsewhere w/o cataplexy

CLINICAL PEARLS
- Narcolepsy is a frequently missed disorder, with an average of 15 years of symptoms before a definitive diagnosis is made.
- The classic tetrad of symptoms includes excessive daytime sleepiness, cataplexy, sleep paralysis, and hypnagogic hallucinations but only cataplexy is pathognomonic for the disorder.
- The International Classification of Sleep Disorders has specific diagnostic criteria for narcolepsy.
- Medications are helpful but not curative.

N

NASAL POLYPS

Katherine Holmes, MD • Daniel Young, MD

BASICS

- Chronic inflammatory lesion of nasal mucosa
- Appearance of edematous pedunculated mass in the nasal cavity or within the paranasal sinus
- Often causes symptoms of blockage, discharge, or loss of smell
- Most commonly bilateral; suspect tumor, such as inverted papilloma, if unilateral
- Estimated to be ~1–4% in adults
- Much rarer in children: ~0.1%
- Increases with age
- Predominant sex: female > male (2:1)
- Asthma is present in 65% of patients, 25% of patients have undiagnosed asthma.

- No clearly delineated pathway; research has demonstrated separate TH1- and TH2-driven pathways (1,2)[B].
- Development of condition remains unclear; multiple inflammatory and infectious pathways resulting from chronic rhinosinusitis is most common (1,3)[B].

- Chronic sinusitis
- Allergic fungal sinusitis
- Aspirin sensitivity
- Primary ciliary dyskinesia (Kartagener syndrome)

- Laryngopharyngeal reflux (4)[B]

GENERAL PREVENTION
Use of intranasal corticosteroids after polyp removal surgery has shown effectiveness against recurrence.

COMMONLY ASSOCIATED CONDITIONS
- Bronchial asthma
- Aspirin hypersensitivity

- Allergic rhinitis (4)[B]

- Cigarette smoking promotes eosinophilic inflammation.

DIAGNOSIS

- Two or more symptoms, one of which is either nasal blockage/obstruction/congestion OR nasal discharge (5)[A].
- Nasal obstruction/restricted nasal airflow: persistent mouth breathing (5)[A]

- Nasal discharge:
  - Anterior discharge—rhinorrhea
  - Postnasal drip
- Reduction/loss of smell
- Dull headaches
- Facial pain/pressure

- Symptoms of acute, recurrent, or chronic rhinosinusitis (5)[A]

- Anterior rhinoscopy looking for a pale translucent mass of tissue
  - Most commonly from lateral wall of middle meatus

  - Otoscope with nasal speculum or even otologic speculum is typically used (5)[A].
- Flexible/rigid endoscopy is required to assess the nasal cavity fully (5)[A].

  - Endoscopy is the gold standard for diagnosis.
  - Topical anesthesia nasal spray should be used prior to the endoscopy if patient is awake.

- Tympanic membrane examination for eustachian tube dysfunction secondary to large posterior nasal polyps (5)[A]
- Examine the posterior pharynx via oral cavity for large posterior polyps (5)[A].

- Antrochoanal polyp
- Benign or malignant tumor:
  - Papilloma
  - Intranasal glioma
  - Encephalocele
  - Rhabdomyosarcoma
  - Mycetoma

- Allergy testing (3)[B]:

  - Skin prick test
  - Immunocap testing
  - Radioallergosorbent test (RAST)

- Testing for cystic fibrosis in children with multiple benign polyps: sweat test: often requires repeat tests (3)[B]
- CT scanning (3)[B]:

  - May be helpful to corroborate history and endoscopic findings
  - Unable to differentiate polyp from other soft tissue masses

- MRI (3)[B]:

  - May aid in unilateral polyposis if concern for neoplasia, mycetoma, or encephalocele
Histologic exam to exclude malignancy if unilateral polyp

- Diagnosis is made by the combination of rhinoscopy, endoscopy, and CT scanning.

- CT reveals extent of disease and is necessary to formulate a plan for surgical intervention (3)[B].

- Ciliated pseudostratified columnar epithelium: with areas of transitional or squamous epithelium
- Chronic infiltration of inflammatory cells

- Eosinophils are the predominant cells in most patients (4)[B].

TREATMENT

- Intranasal corticosteroid use has been demonstrated to reduce polyp size and recurrence, as well as improvement in nasal congestion based on controlled studies (2,5)[A],(6)[B].
- Treat for a minimum of 12 weeks; minimal systemic absorption, side effects rare—minor nose bleeding is most common (2,5)[A].

  - Budesonide 256 μg/day
  - Beclomethasone dipropionate 320 μg/day
  - Fluticasone propionate 400 μg/day
  - Mometasone furoate 200 μg BID
  - For children mometasone furoate is preferred:
    - 100 μg BID ages 6 to 12

    - 200 μg BID for ages 12 to 17 (7)[A]
- Oral systemic corticosteroids: less definitive benefit; more systemic adverse effects; use with caution in patients with diabetes mellitus, hypertension, or peptic ulcer disease (2,5)[A]

- Prednisolone
  - Weight-based dosing burst with taper
- Perioperative use oral prednisone 30 mg daily 5 to 7 days prior to surgery (2)[A]
  - Decrease nasal mucosa inflammation
  - Improves surgical field
  - Shorter surgical time
  - Improves postop results
  - Weight-based dosing burst with taper

ISSUES FOR REFERRAL

Patients with severe obstruction symptoms should be referred for surgery (5)[A].

ADDITIONAL THERAPIES

Antileukotrienes: clinical improvement without aspirin hypersensitivity (2,5)[A],(3)[B]:

- Aspirin desensitization may have a role in reducing recurrence of nasal polyposis.
- Anti-interleukin-5 immunomodulators: may benefit those with T_H2 eosinophilic disease process
- Oral antibiotics: doxycycline for 3 to 4 weeks or oral macrolide for 12 weeks is an option for disease unresponsive to steroids alone with mixed results of therapy (8)[C]
- Indicated for patients with four or more episodes in 1 year of acute rhinosinusitis refractory to medical therapy (5)[A]
  - Disease must be documented endoscopically or on CT during symptomatic period prior to surgical intervention.
- Most surgeries are approached endonasally.
  - Endoscopic sinus surgery has become the mainstay of treatment.
  - The external (Caldwell-Luc) approach is used for more difficult cases but carries higher risk of complications.
- Functional endonasal sinus surgery has slightly lower revision rate than intranasal polypectomy. Both modalities provide effective symptom relief.
- Postoperative use of nasal corticosteroids delay the recurrence of nasal polyps and hence the timing of revision surgery (2)[A],(6)[B].
- Postoperative use of steroid releasing stents to prevent polyp recurrence by decreasing mucosal inflammation (2)[A],(6)[B].
- Intrapolyp steroid injection may be considered in cases refractory to other interventions but has risk of visual loss.

 ONGOING CARE

- Acute/chronic sinus infection
- Heterotropic bone formation within the sinus cavity
- Recurrence:
  - Of patients, 5–10% with severe disease
  - Twice as likely in those with asthma (4)[B]

REFERENCES

1. Tomassen P, Van Zele T, Zhang N, et al. Pathophysiology of chronic rhinosinusitis. *Proc Am Thorac Soc.* 2011;8(1):115–120.
2. Poetker DM, Jakubowski LA, Lal D, et al. Oral corticosteroids in the management of adult chronic rhinosinusitis with and without nasal polyps: an evidence-based review with recommendations. *Int Forum Allergy Rhinol.* 2013;3(2):104–120.
3. DeMarcantonio MA, Han JK. Nasal polyps: pathogenesis and treatment implications. *Otolaryngol Clin North Am.* 2011;44(3):685–695, ix.
4. Kariyawasam H, Rotiroti G. Allergic rhinitis, chronic rhinosinusitis and asthma: unravelling a complex relationship. *Curr Opin Otolaryngol Head Neck Surg.* 2013;21(1):79–86.
5. Fokkens WJ, Lund VJ, Mullol J, et al. EPOS 2012: European position paper on rhinosinusitis and nasal polyps 2012. A summary for otorhinolaryngologists. *Rhinology.* 2012;50(1):1–12.
6. Rudmik L, Schlosser RJ, Smith TL, et al. Impact of topical nasal steroid therapy on symptoms of nasal polyposis: a meta-analysis. *Laryngoscope.* 2012;122(7):1431–1437.
7. Chur V, Small CB, Stryszak P, et al. Safety of mometasone furoate nasal spray in the treatment of nasal polyps in children. *Pediatr Allergy Immunol.* 2013;24(1):33–38.
8. Schlosser RJ, Soler ZM. Evidence-based treatment of chronic rhinosinusitis with nasal polyps. *Am J Rhinol Allergy.* 2013;27(6):461–466.

ADDITIONAL READING

- Aouad RK, Chiu AG. State of the art treatment of nasal polyposis. *Am J Rhinol Allergy.* 2011;25(5):291–298.
- Bachert C. Evidence-based management of nasal polyposis by intranasal corticosteroids: from the cause to the clinic. *Int Arch Allergy Immunol.* 2011;155(4):309–321.

- Håkansson K, Thomsen SF, Konge L, et al. A comparative and descriptive study of asthma in chronic rhinosinusitis with nasal polyps. *Am J Rhinol Allergy.* 2014;28(5):383–387.
- Hopkins C, Slack R, Lund V, et al. Long-term outcomes from the English national comparative audit of surgery for nasal polyposis and chronic rhinosinusitis. *Laryngoscope.* 2009;119(12):2459–2465.
- Lee KI, Kim DW, Kim EH, et al. Cigarette smoke promotes eosinophilic inflammation, airway remodeling, and nasal polyps in a murine polyp model. *Am J Rhinol Allergy.* 2014;28(3):208–214.
- Rimmer J, Fokkens W, Chong LY, et al. Surgical versus medical interventions for chronic rhinosinusitis with nasal polyps. *Cochrane Database Syst Rev.* 2014;(12):CD006991.
- Sharma R, Lakhani R, Rimmer J, et al. Surgical interventions for chronic rhinosinusitis with nasal polyps. *Cochrane Database Syst Rev.* 2014;(11):CD006990.

 CODES

ICD10

- J33.9 Nasal polyp, unspecified
- J33.0 Polyp of nasal cavity
- J33.8 Other polyp of sinus

CLINICAL PEARLS

- Intranasal corticosteroid use has been demonstrated to reduce polyp size and recurrence, as well as improvement in nasal congestion.
- Asthma is a common concominant diagnosis and is often previously undiagnosed.
- Aggressive medical and surgical treatment improves asthma outcomes.
- Treat for a minimum of 12 weeks
- Allergy testing can be helpful.
- Nasal polyposis associated with asthma and aspirin hypersensitivity known as Samter triad or aspirin exacerbated respiratory disease (AERD) (1,3)[B]
- Patients with severe obstruction should be referred for surgery.
- Unilateral nasal polyp needs malignancy workup (MRI).

N

NEAR DROWNING/NONFATAL DROWNING

Stephen L. Cook, MD • Matthew Kendall Hawks, MD

 BASICS

DESCRIPTION
- Survival for at least 24 hours following respiratory impairment due to submersion in liquid
- System(s) affected: cardiovascular, nervous, pulmonary, renal
- Synonym(s): submersion injury; drowning with or without morbidity

EPIDEMIOLOGY
Incidence
- From 2009 to 2013, an average of 4,268 deaths/year occurred from drowning in the United States (1).
- Three age-related peaks: toddlers and young children (1 to 5 years), adolescents and young adults (15 to 25 years), and the elderly
- 80% of people who die from drowning are male (2).
- Greater incidence in minorities; African Americans age 5 to 14 years old are affected at 3 times the Caucasian rate (2).

Prevalence
- From 2009 to 2013, drowning was the second most common cause of death among children age 1 to 4 years old and was the fifth most common cause of accidental death among all ages overall (1).
- For every child age <15 years who dies from drowning, five more children are seen in the emergency room for nonfatal submersion injuries.

ALERT
Proper water safety techniques are critical in avoiding morbidity and mortality from drowning.

ETIOLOGY AND PATHOPHYSIOLOGY
Hypoxemia via aspiration and/or reflex laryngospasm causing cerebral hypoxia and multisystem organ involvement
- 10–20% of victims drown without aspiration; likely due to prolonged laryngospasm, previously termed "dry lungs."
- Bathtub and bucket drowning in children <1 year of age
- Swimming pool drowning in children and young adults
- Motor vehicle accidents (e.g., automobile submerged in water)
- Head trauma while swimming or diving
- Suicide
- Pulmonary: morbidity primarily as a result of hypoxia. Aspiration also causes dilution of surfactant with decreased gas transfer across alveoli, atelectasis, development of intrapulmonary right-to-left shunting; acute respiratory distress syndrome (ARDS); obstruction due to laryngospasm and bronchospasm
- Cardiac: hypoxic-ischemic injury and arrhythmia (primary or secondary)
- Renal: acute tubular necrosis from hypoxemia, shock, hemoglobinuria, myoglobinuria
- Neurologic: hypoxic-ischemic brain injury with damage especially to the hippocampus, insular cortex, and basal ganglia; cerebral edema
- Coagulation: hemolysis and coagulopathy

RISK FACTORS
- Alcohol ingestion
- Use of illicit drugs
- Seizure disorder
- Inability to swim

- Hyperventilation prior to underwater swimming
- Risk-taking behavior
- Inadequate physical barriers surrounding pools
- Boating mishaps and trauma during water sports, particularly when not wearing a life jacket
- Scuba diving
- Inadequate adult supervision of children
- Concomitant stroke or myocardial infarction (MI)
- Hypothermia
- Cardiac arrhythmias: familial long QT and polymorphic ventricular tachycardia (VT)
- Residence within sunbelt states
- African Americans
- Low socioeconomic status
- Lack of instruction regarding swimming and supervision

GENERAL PREVENTION
- Periodic education/reinforcement of supervision with an emphasis on drowning prevention for caretakers of young children
- Consistent practice of proper adult supervision of children
- Knowledge of water safety guidelines
- Mandatory physical barriers surrounding pools
- Pool alarms
- Fences higher than 54 inches (137 cm) for home pools
- Avoidance of alcohol or recreational drugs around water
- Swimming instruction at an early age
- Cardiopulmonary resuscitation (CPR) instruction for pool owners and parents
- Boating safety knowledge
- Personal flotation device (e.g., preserver, if necessary)

Pediatric Considerations
Children should never be left alone near water. Young children can drown in very small amounts of water, such as in bathtubs, buckets, and toilets.

COMMONLY ASSOCIATED CONDITIONS
- Trauma
- Seizure disorder
- Alcohol or illicit drug use
- Hypothermia
- Concomitant stroke or MI
- Cardiac arrhythmias: familial long QT and familial polymorphic VT
- Hyperventilation

 DIAGNOSIS

HISTORY
- Victim found in or near water
- Duration of submersion
- Loss of consciousness
- Period of apnea
- Artificial ventilation/CPR performed
- History of associated trauma
- Approximate water temperature
- Recent use of alcohol or drugs
- Known seizure disorder
- Known cardiac disease, including arrhythmia or prolonged QT
- Preceding syncope or history of medical condition predisposing to syncope

PHYSICAL EXAM
- Airway status and degree of respiratory effort and/or distress
- Pulse: absent, weak, or normal
- Vital signs, including pulse oximetry
- Glasgow Coma Scale (GCS)
- Wheezing
- Evidence of trauma

DIFFERENTIAL DIAGNOSIS
Syncopal event, head trauma, arrhythmia, seizure, MI, stroke, alcohol or other substance overdose, nonaccidental trauma

DIAGNOSTIC TESTS & INTERPRETATION
Initial Tests (lab, imaging)
May be unnecessary if initial GCS and pulse oximetry are normal and remain that way for 6 to 8 hours.
- CBC with differential
- Arterial blood gases (ABGs): hypoxia, hypercarbia, acidosis
- Electrolytes: hypokalemia, hyponatremia, hypernatremia
- Blood glucose: May be low if the cause of near drowning; increased levels may impair neurologic recovery after ischemic brain injury.
- BUN, creatinine: acute tubular necrosis
- EKG, cardiac monitoring, and serial troponin: MI
- Creatine kinase (CK) and urine myoglobin: rhabdomyolysis
- Coagulation studies: coagulopathy
- Urinalysis/urine drug screen
- Blood alcohol level
- A chest x-ray (CXR) may be unnecessary for patients with all of the following:
  – Normal initial GCS and pulse oximetry
  – No evidence of respiratory distress
  – No change after 6 to 8 hours of observation
- For others, a CXR may show evidence of aspiration, atelectasis, pneumothorax, or ARDS.
- Head CT and/or C-spine imaging as needed for associated trauma.

Follow-Up Tests & Special Considerations
- Patients with an initial GCS of 15 and pulse oximetry >95% should be observed for 6 to 8 hours in the emergency department (ED).
- CXR findings may be minimal or absent on early imaging.

Diagnostic Procedures/Other
- Continuous cardiac monitoring
- Continuous pulse oximetry
- Continuous core temperature monitoring if hypothermic
- ECG
- Central venous pressure (CVP) monitoring for critically ill patients with hypotension refractory to IV fluids
- Electroencephalogram (EEG) if suspect seizure as cause

TREATMENT

Early resuscitation and reversal of hypoxemia optimizes outcome.

GENERAL MEASURES
- Prehospital
  – Never approach a struggling victim alone.

- Initially evaluate as per Basic Life Support (BLS) and Advanced Cardiovascular Life Support (ACLS) (3).
- Rescue breathing may be helpful while the victim is in the water and not able to be immediately removed from the water, but chest compressions in the water may not be effective and may even harm the rescuer and the victim (3)[C].
- Remove the victim from the water and begin effective resuscitation as quickly as possible (4).
- Early CPR that emphasizes effective chest compressions and rapid defibrillation as indicated.
- Start CPR if pulse is not definitely felt within 10 seconds, even in the hypothermic victim whose heart rate may be severely bradycardic (3)[C].
- Routine cervical collar use and spinal precautions are not needed unless a high suspicion for trauma exists (5)[C].
- Supplemental oxygen and early intubation, as needed (5)[A].
- If patient is breathing on his or her own and does not need spinal precautions, consider placing in the right lateral decubitus position to prevent aspiration of vomit or gastric contents (4).
- ED
- Oxygen, as needed, to maintain saturation >94%.
- Continuous positive airway pressure (PAP), BiPAP, or intubation if supplemental O_2 alone is unsuccessful
- If intubation is indicated, employ lung-protective vent settings (lower end-inspiratory airway pressures, lower tidal volumes of 6 mL/kg, higher positive end-expiratory pressures of 6 to 12 cm H_2O) to avoid lung barotrauma (6)[A].
- Indications for intubation
  ○ Neurologic deterioration
  ○ Inability to protect the airway
  ○ Inability to maintain oxygen saturation >90% or PaO_2 >60 mm Hg on high-flow supplemental oxygen
  ○ $PaCO_2$ >50 mm Hg
- Remove wet clothing and initiate rewarming.
- Core temperature reading for possible hypothermia
- Rewarming with minimally invasive core rewarming such as warm IV fluids, warm/humidified oxygen, and external rewarming
- Active core rewarming reserved for refractory cases and only when extracorporeal blood warming is unavailable, depending on physician comfort level, due to major complications that can develop including core temperature after drop, rewarming acidosis, and rewarming shock.

MEDICATION

First Line

- High-flow oxygen, as needed (4)[A]
- For bronchospasm: aerosolized bronchodilator (4)[C]: albuterol (Proventil, Ventolin), 3 mL of 0.083% solution or 0.5 mL of 0.5% solution diluted in 3 mL of saline
- Pressors, as needed, for hypotension refractory to IV fluid resuscitation
- Prophylactic antibiotics and steroids are not helpful (5)[B].

Second Line

For pneumonia: antibiotics based on sputum or endotracheal lavage culture (5)[A]

INPATIENT CONSIDERATIONS

Admission Criteria/Initial Stabilization

- All symptomatic patients
- Patients with abnormalities in vital signs, mental status, oxygenation, CXR, or laboratory analysis

IV Fluids

To maintain adequate intravascular volume (4)[C]

Nursing

- Continuous cardiac monitoring
- Continuous pulse oximetry monitoring
- Frequent monitoring of vital signs and clinical reassessment
- Careful monitoring of neurologic status

Discharge Criteria

Patients can be discharged from the ED after 6 to 8 hours of observation if the following criteria are met:

- GCS = 15
- Normal CXR, if indicated
- Lack of clinical evidence of respiratory difficulty
- Normal lung exam
- Normal vital signs
- Oxygen saturation ≥95% on room air (5)

 ## ONGOING CARE

FOLLOW-UP RECOMMENDATIONS

Appropriate follow up with primary care provider, orthopedic, neurologic, cardiac, pulmonary, and additional specialists as indicated

Patient Monitoring

- Continuous cardiac monitoring
- Continuous pulse oximetry monitoring
- Frequent monitoring of vital signs and clinical reassessment
- Careful monitoring of neurologic status
- ABG monitoring, as indicated (5)
- A pulmonary artery catheter may be needed for hemodynamic monitoring in unstable patients (4)[C].
- Intracranial pressure monitoring in selected patients (4)[C]
- Serum electrolyte determinations (5)

DIET

NPO until mental status normalizes

PATIENT EDUCATION

Re-emphasize preventive measures on discharge from hospital. Educate parents regarding supervision and preventive practices.

PROGNOSIS

- 75% of drowning victims survive; 6% of these with residual neurologic deficits
- Patients with an initial GCS ≥13 and an oxygen saturation ≥95% have a low risk of complications and an excellent chance for a full recovery.
- Patients who are comatose or receiving CPR at the time of presentation, as well as those who have dilated and fixed pupils and no spontaneous respiratory activity have a more guarded and often poor prognosis, often secondary to neurologic sequelae.
- Neurogenic pulmonary edema may occur within 48 hours of initial presentation.

COMPLICATIONS

- Early
  - Bronchospasm
  - Vomiting/aspiration
  - Hypoglycemia
  - Hypothermia
  - Seizure

- Hypovolemia
- Electrolyte abnormalities
- Arrhythmia from hypoxia or hypothermia (rarely from electrolyte imbalance)
- Hypotension
- Late
- ARDS
- Anoxic encephalopathy
- Pneumonia
- Lung abscess/empyema
- Renal failure
- Coagulopathy
- Sepsis
- Barotrauma
- Seizure

REFERENCES

1. Centers for Disease Control and Prevention. Fatal injury reports. http://www.cdc.gov/injury/wisqars/fatal_injury_reports.html
2. Centers for Disease Control and Prevention. Unintentional drowning: get the facts. www.cdc.gov/HomeandRecreationalSafety/Water-Safety/waterinjuries-factsheet.html/
3. Berg R, Hemphill R, Abella BS, et al. Part 5: adult basic life support: 2010 American Heart Association guidelines for cardiopulmonary resuscitation and emergency cardiovascular care. *Circulation*. 2010;122(18)(Suppl 3):S685–S705.
4. Orlowski JP, Szpilman D. Drowning. Rescue, resuscitation, and reanimation. *Pediatr Clin North Am*. 2001;48(3):627–646.
5. Salomez F, Vincent JL. Drowning: a review of epidemiology, pathophysiology, treatment and prevention. *Resuscitation*. 2004;63(3):261–268.
6. Sutherasan Y, Vargas M, Pelosi P. Protective mechanical ventilation in the non-injured lung: review and meta-analysis. *Crit Care*. 2014;18(2):211.

 ## CODES

ICD10

- T75.1XXA Unsp effects of drowning and nonfatal submersion, init
- T75.1XXD Unsp effects of drowning and nonfatal submersion, subs
- T75.1XXS Unsp effects of drowning and nonfatal submersion, sequela

CLINICAL PEARLS

- The single most important treatment for near-drowning victims is prompt reversal of the hypoxic state. This should form the cornerstone for all other treatment modalities. Without oxygenation, other treatment is futile.
- Family physicians and pediatricians should review water safety tips and guidelines with parents and children at yearly visits. Encourage pool owners and parents with young children to become CPR-certified. Prevention of drowning can save many lives each year.
- Despite successful resuscitation, patients are at risk for ARDS due to delayed pulmonary edema that may start hours after their submersion incident. For this reason, careful monitoring of every resuscitated patient is essential.
- Patients requiring intubation should be treated with lung-protective vent settings to prevent barotrauma.
- Patients with an initial GCS ≥13 and an oxygen saturation ≥95% have a low risk of complications and an excellent chance for a full recovery.

N

NEPHROTIC SYNDROME

Jeremy D. DeFoe, DO • Karen S. Phelps, MD

BASICS

DESCRIPTION
- A clinical syndrome of heavy proteinuria (>3.5 g/1.73 m^2/24 hr), hypoalbuminemia, hyperlipidemia, and edema
- Includes both primary and secondary forms
- Associated with many types of kidney disease

EPIDEMIOLOGY
Based on definitive diagnosis
- Diabetic nephropathy: most common cause of secondary nephrotic syndrome (1)
- Minimal change disease (MCD)
  - Most common nephrotic syndrome in children, peaks at 2 to 8 years
  - Associated with drugs or lymphoma in adults
- Amyloidosis: rare
- Lupus nephropathy (LN): Adult women are affected about 10 times more often than men.
- Focal segmental glomerulosclerosis (FSGS)
  - 25% of nephrotic syndrome in adults
  - Most common primary nephrotic syndrome in African Americans
  - Has both primary and secondary forms
- Membranous nephropathy
  - Most common primary nephrotic syndrome in Caucasians
  - Associated with malignancy and infection
- Membranoproliferative glomerulonephritis (MGN)
  - May be primary or secondary
  - May present in the setting of a systemic viral or rheumatic illness

ETIOLOGY AND PATHOPHYSIOLOGY
- Increased glomerular permeability to protein molecules, especially albumin
- Edema results primarily from renal salt retention, with arterial underfilling from decreased plasma oncotic pressure playing an additional role.
- Hyperlipidemia is thought to be a consequence of increased hepatic synthesis resulting from low oncotic pressure and urinary loss of regulatory proteins.
- The hypercoagulable state that can occur in some nephrotic states is likely due to loss of antithrombin III in urine.
- Primary renal disease:
  - MCD
  - FSGS
  - MGN
  - IgA nephropathy
- Secondary renal disease (associated primary renal disease are shown in parentheses):
  - Diabetic nephropathy
  - Amyloidosis
  - LN
  - FSGS
  - Infections (MGN)
  - Cancer (MCD or MGN)
  - Drugs (MCD or MGN)

Genetics
Genetic factors are likely to play a role in susceptibility to the various nephrotic syndromes, although these have not been sufficiently defined to be useful clinically.

RISK FACTORS
- Drug addiction (e.g., heroin [FSGS])
- Hepatitis B and C, HIV, other infections
- Immunosuppression
- Nephrotoxic drugs
- Vesicoureteral reflux (FSGS)
- Cancer (usually MGN, may be MCD)
- Chronic analgesic use/abuse
- Preeclampsia
- Diabetes mellitus

GENERAL PREVENTION
In general, there are few preventive measures, except avoidance of known causative medications.

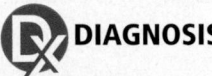

DIAGNOSIS

HISTORY
- Inquire about signs or symptoms of systemic disease: joint complaint, rash, edema, infectious complaint, fevers, anorexia, oliguria, foamy urine, acute flank pain, hematuria.
- Obtain a recent drug history for medications that may be causative, especially NSAIDs.
- Assess for risk factors.

PHYSICAL EXAM
A complete physical exam may discover clues to systemic disease as a potential cause and/or may suggest the severity of disease.
- Fluid retention: abdominal distention, abdominal fluid shift, extremity edema, puffy eyelids, scrotal swelling, weight gain, shortness of breath. Pericardial rub and decreased breath sounds with pleural effusions may develop.
- Hypertension
- Orthostatic hypotension

ALERT
The potential for thromboembolic disease leading to pulmonary embolism is one of the most life-threatening aspects of a patient who is actively nephrotic.

DIFFERENTIAL DIAGNOSIS
- Edema and proteinuria: see "Etiology and Pathophysiology."
- Edema alone: Other diseases to rule out in patients who have edema without proteinuria include congestive heart failure, cirrhosis, hypothyroidism, nutritional hypoalbuminemia, protein-losing enteropathy.

DIAGNOSTIC TESTS & INTERPRETATION
Initial Tests (lab, imaging)
- Confirm proteinuria if present: by urine dipstick initially, and then quantitate by 24-hour urine or spot urine protein-to-creatinine ratio.
- Rule out urine infection with urine culture.
- Full blood count and coagulation screen
- Renal function tests: BUN, creatinine with estimated glomerular filtration rate (GFR)
- Glucose to rule out overt diabetes
- Consider blood cultures to rule out a postinfectious process.
- Lipid panel
- Liver function tests to exclude liver disease or infection

- Look for autoimmune disease.
  - Antinuclear antibody and/or antidouble-stranded DNA positivity suggest lupus.
  - Complement levels: A low C3 may suggest a postinfectious or membranoproliferative process, whereas both low C3 and C4 point to lupus.
- Serum protein electrophoresis/urine immune electrophoresis to rule in a paraproteinemia
- Hepatitis B and C screen
- HIV and syphilis testing
- Urinalysis to evaluate for the presence of cellular casts
- Renal US to verify the presence of 2 kidneys of normal shape and size
- Chest x-ray to detect presence of pleural effusion or infection
- If thrombosis is suspected:
  - Doppler US of the legs
  - MRI or venography for renal vein thrombosis
  - Ventilation/perfusion nuclear medicine lung scan and/or CT may be required to rule out pulmonary embolism.

Diagnostic Procedures/Other
Renal biopsy
- Rarely done in children with first episode of nephrotic syndrome, as MCD is common and empiric steroid therapy is the standard of care.
- Required to confirm the clinical diagnosis in adults and assist with making a treatment plan (1)

Test Interpretation
- Light microscopy
  - May see nothing (e.g., MCD)
  - Sclerosis (e.g., FSGS or diabetic nodules in diabetes)
  - Diffuse hypercellularity suggests a proliferative disease such as IgA nephropathy, LN, or postinfectious glomerulonephritis (GN).
- Immunofluorescence: Mesangial IgA suggests IgA nephropathy, Henoch-Schönlein; other staining patterns are specific for other disease processes.
- Electron microscopy: The location of immunoglobulin deposits is useful in pointing to a particular diagnosis.

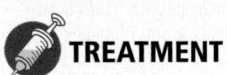

TREATMENT

MEDICATION
First Line
- Edema: salt restriction and salt-wasting diuretics (loop and thiazide diuretics):
  - Salt restriction to <2 g sodium per day
  - Restrict fluid intake to <1.5 L/day if hyponatremic.
  - Target weight loss of 0.5 to 1 kg/day (1 to 2 lb/day)
- Statins have been shown to improve endothelial function (2)[A] and may decrease proteinuria (3)[A], but effect on GFR and preservation of renal function is small. The major role for statin use is in cardiovascular risk reduction.
- ACE inhibitors or angiotensin II receptor blockers are thought to reduce proteinuria, hyperlipidemia, thrombotic tendencies, progression of renal failure, and to control hypertension, if present (2,4)[A].
- For steroid-responsive disease (MCD and FSGS), steroids dosed in consultation with nephrologist

Second Line

- Many of the nephrotic diseases will require escalation in therapy above steroids. These include rapidly relapsing forms, as well as MGN, LN, and IgA nephropathy. Bolus steroids and other immunosuppressives are required in this circumstance (cyclophosphamide, mycophenolate mofetil, chlorambucil, cyclosporine) (5)[A].
- Rituximab, combined with steroids or other immunosuppressive agents, has demonstrated early promise in the treatment of refractory nephrotic syndrome (6)[B].
- Randomized controlled data have been insufficient to determine which patients require prophylactic anticoagulation (7)[A]. Common practice is to anticoagulate with heparin and then warfarin in patients who have persistent nephrotic-range proteinuria. This decision is made based on the patient's history of edema, hypoalbuminemia, thromboembolism, or immobility.
- Hypocalcemia from vitamin D loss should be treated with oral vitamin D.

ISSUES FOR REFERRAL

Consultation with a nephrologist is often required to assist with renal biopsy to confirm diagnosis and to assist with management of edema. Cytotoxic medications may be called for, depending on the disease process, and this may best be handled by a nephrologist.

ADDITIONAL THERAPIES

Ambulation or range-of-motion exercises to lower risk of deep vein thrombosis (DVT)

INPATIENT CONSIDERATIONS

Admission Criteria/Initial Stabilization

Respiratory distress, sepsis/severe infection, thromboses, renal failure, hypertension, or other complications

Discharge Criteria

Hemodynamically, stable patients without complications may be managed as outpatients.

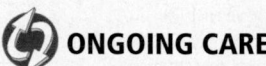 **ONGOING CARE**

FOLLOW-UP RECOMMENDATIONS

Patient Monitoring

- Frequent monitoring is required for relapse, disease progression, and for detecting signs of toxicity of medical management.
- Reevaluate for azotemia, urine protein, hypertension, edema, loss of renal function, cholesterol, and weight.

DIET

- Normal protein (1 g/kg/day)
- Low fat (cholesterol)
- Reduced sodium
- Supplemental multivitamins and minerals, especially vitamin D and iron
- Fluid restriction if hyponatremic

PATIENT EDUCATION

- Printed material for patients: National Kidney Foundation, 30 E. 33rd Street, Suite 1100, New York, NY 10016; 800-622-9010
  - Childhood nephrotic syndrome
  - Diabetes and kidney disease
  - Focal glomerulosclerosis
- Web site: National Institutes of Health: nephrotic syndrome

PROGNOSIS

Nephrotic syndrome in children (MCD) is typically self-limited and carries a good prognosis. In the adult, the prognosis is variable. Complete remission is expected if the basic disease is treatable (infection, malignancy, drug-induced); otherwise, a relapsing and remitting course is possible, with progression to dialysis seen in more aggressive forms (diabetic glomerulosclerosis).

COMPLICATIONS

- Thromboembolism:
  - Deep vein, renal vein, or central venous thrombosis may occur.
  - The risk appears to be greater the lower the serum albumin.
  - Pulmonary embolism is a known complication.
- Pleural effusion
- Ascites
- Hyperlipidemia, cardiovascular disease
- Acute renal failure, progressive renal failure
- Protein malnutrition/muscle wasting
- Infection secondary to low serum IgG concentrations, reduced complement activity, and depressed T-cell function: peritonitis, pneumonia, or cellulitis
- Loss of vitamin D (vitamin D–binding protein loss in urine) leading to bone disease

REFERENCES

1. Kodner C. Nephrotic syndrome in adults: diagnosis and management. *Am Fam Physician*. 2009;80(10): 1129–1134.
2. Gruppo Italíano dí Studí Epidemíologící ín Nefrología. Randomised placebo-controlled trial of effect of ramipril on decline in glomerular filtration rate and risk of terminal renal failure in proteinuric, non-diabetic nephropathy. *Lancet*. 1997;349(9069):1857–1863.
3. Fried LF, Orchard TJ, Kasiske BL. Effect of lipid reduction on the progression of renal disease: a meta-analysis. *Kidney Int*. 2001;59(1):260–269.
4. Kunz R, Friedrich C, Wolbers M, et al. Meta-analysis: effect of monotherapy and combination therapy with inhibitors of the renin angiotensin system on proteinuria in renal disease. *Ann Intern Med*. 2008;148(1):30–48.
5. Hodson EM, Willis NS, Craig JC. Interventions for idiopathic steroid-resistant nephrotic syndrome in children. *Cochrane Database Syst Rev*. 2010;(11): CD003594.
6. Kamei K, Okada M, Sato M, et al. Rituximab treatment combined with methylprednisolone pulse therapy and immunosuppressants for childhood steroid-resistant nephrotic syndrome. *Pediatr Nephrol*. 2014;29(7):1181–1187.
7. Kulshrestha S, Grieff M, Navaneethan SD. Interventions for preventing thrombosis in adults and children with nephrotic syndrome (protocol). *Cochrane Database Syst Rev*. 2006;(2):CD006024.

ADDITIONAL READING

- Cadnapaphornchai MA, Tkachenko O, Shchekochikhin D, et al. The nephrotic syndrome: pathogenesis and treatment of edema formation and secondary complications. *Pediatr Nephrol*. 2014;29(7):1159–1167.
- Madaio MP, Harrington JT. The diagnosis of glomerular diseases: acute glomerulonephritis and the nephrotic syndrome. *Arch Intern Med*. 2001;161(1): 25–34.
- Meyrier A. An update on the treatment options for focal segmental glomerulosclerosis. *Expert Opin Pharmacother*. 2009;10(4):615–628.

 SEE ALSO

Amyloidosis; Diabetes Mellitus, Type 1; Diabetes Mellitus, Type 2; Glomerulonephritis, Acute; HIV/AIDS; Lupus Erythematosus, Discoid; Multiple Myeloma; Acute Kidney Injury (Acute Renal Failure)

 CODES

ICD10

- N04.9 Nephrotic syndrome with unspecified morphologic changes
- N04.1 Nephrotic syndrome w focal and segmental glomerular lesions
- N04.2 Nephrotic syndrome w diffuse membranous glomerulonephritis

CLINICAL PEARLS

- Nephrotic syndrome is a clinical syndrome of >3.5 g/day proteinuria, hypoalbuminemia, hyperlipidemia, and edema often associated with diabetes and NSAIDs use.
- Pediatric nephrotic syndrome typically carries a good prognosis and is more easily treated with steroids, although recurrences are common.
- Nondiabetic adults with nephrotic syndrome will require a renal biopsy to determine cause.
- Have a high index of suspicion for symptoms that may represent an embolic event in patients with nephrotic syndrome.

NEUROFIBROMATOSIS TYPE 1

Rayna Goldstein, MD • Michele Roberts, MD, PhD

BASICS

DESCRIPTION

- Neurofibromatosis types 1 (NF1) and 2 (NF2) are neurocutaneous syndromes (phakomatoses). Although they share a name, they are distinct and unrelated conditions with genes on different chromosomes.
  - NF2 is a rare condition that causes bilateral vestibular schwannomas.
  - NF1 is a multisystem disorder that may affect any organ. It is the most common of the phakomatoses.
- System(s) affected: musculoskeletal, nervous, skin/exocrine, cardiovascular, neuroophthalmologic
- Synonym(s): von Recklinghausen disease, formerly peripheral NF

EPIDEMIOLOGY

Incidence
- Predominant sex for NF1: male = female
- Birth incidence NF1: 1:2,500 to 3,000

Prevalence
1:3,000 to 1:4,000

ETIOLOGY AND PATHOPHYSIOLOGY

- Neurofibromin is a guanosine triphosphatase–activating protein that acts as a tumor suppressor by downregulating a cellular protooncogene, *p21-ras*, which enhances cell growth and proliferation.
- Neurofibromata are benign tumors composed of Schwann cells, fibroblasts, mast cells, and vascular components that develop along nerves.
- The two-hit hypothesis has been invoked to explain malignant transformation in *NF1*.

Genetics
- Online Mendelian Inheritance in Man 162200
- Caused by a mutation in the *NF1* gene on chromosome 17q11.2; autosomal dominant inheritance; protein product is called *neurofibromin*.
- 50% of cases are due to de novo mutations, mostly paternal; likelihood increases with paternal age
- Prenatal diagnosis is possible if mutation is known.
- Penetrance is nearly 100%; expressivity is highly variable, even within a family.
- Gene is large, with a variety of mutations causing NF1. Molecular technology can detect 95% of clinically important *NF1* mutations, but clinical diagnosis frequently can be made in childhood.
- ~5% of individuals with NF1 have a large deletion of the entire *NF1* gene (or nearly so); they usually have a more severe phenotype.
- *Segmental NF* is limited to a single body region and is caused by mosaicism for the *NF1* mutation.

RISK FACTORS
- Having an affected first-degree relative is a diagnostic criterion for NF1, although relatives may be unaware of their condition.
- Affected individuals with a positive family history, as well as those with a new mutation, have a 50% risk of transmitting NF1 to each of their offspring; 1 in 12 will be severely affected.
- Individuals with segmental NF1 may have gonadal mosaicism and may be at risk for transmission of the mutated gene.

COMMONLY ASSOCIATED CONDITIONS
Congenital heart disease, pulmonary stenosis, hypertension, renal artery stenosis

DIAGNOSIS

- NF1 can be diagnosed by routine exam by age 4 years, with attention to skin stigmata; diagnostic criteria include ≥2 of the following (1):
  - ≥6 café au lait (light brown) macules, ≥5 mm in prepubertal individuals or ≥15 mm in adults
  - ≥2 neurofibromata of any type or 1 plexiform (noncircumscribed) neurofibroma
  - Axillary or inguinal freckling
  - ≥2 Lisch nodules (benign iris hamartomas, asymptomatic)
  - Optic glioma by MRI
  - Characteristic osseous lesions: sphenoid dysplasia, long-bone cortical thinning, ribbon ribs, angular scoliosis
  - First-degree relative with NF1 by above criteria
- Prenatal diagnosis is possible with known mutation or by linkage testing (with positive family history), although not predictive of clinical course.

HISTORY
- Family history of a first-degree relative with NF1
- Manifestations generally are not visible at birth, although plexiform neurofibromata usually are congenital and tibial bowing is congenital.
- In addition to cutaneous lesions, NF1 may present with painful neurofibromata, pathologic fractures, or headaches secondary to hypertension caused by pheochromocytomas.
- Optic gliomata may present as involuntary eye movement, squinting, loss of vision, or as diencephalic syndrome.

PHYSICAL EXAM
- Skin
  - Café au lait macules develop during the first 3 years of childhood and are usually the presenting feature of NF1. Evenly pigmented, irregularly shaped (coast-of-California), light brown macules present in 97% of patients with NF1; many unaffected individuals have one to three such macules.
  - Neurofibromata can be cutaneous, subcutaneous, or plexiform and may be soft or firm; buttonhole invagination is pathognomonic. Cutaneous neurofibromata usually begin to appear during late childhood or adolescence.
  - Plexiform neurofibromata are present in up to 50% of individuals with NF1
    - Usually congenital; may be subtle in infancy
    - Freckling or hypertrichosis may be present over plexiform neurofibromata; may affect underlying structures or cause focal hyperplasia
    - Many are internal, not obvious on exam.
    - Most grow slowly over many years but can have rapid growth, especially in early childhood.
  - Evaluate for new lesions and progression of pre-existing ones. Rapidly growing cutaneous lesions should be evaluated thoroughly.
  - Axillary freckling (Crowe sign) or inguinal freckling (91%)
- Ophthalmologic
  - Lisch nodules (benign iris hamartomas) in 30%: well-defined, dome-shaped, gelatinous hamartomatous lesions projecting from the iris, varying from clear yellow to brown
  - Essentially unique to NF, Lisch nodules are asymptomatic; significant only for diagnosis.
  - Pallor or atrophy of optic disc, bulging of orbit, loss of vision may be signs of optic glioma.

- Skeletal
  - Scoliosis and vertebral angulation
  - Localized bone hypertrophy, especially of the face
  - Limb abnormalities:
    - Pseudoarthrosis of the tibia
    - Tibial dysplasia (anterolateral bowing of the tibia) is congenital, if present.
    - Nonossifying fibromas of the long bones in adolescents and adults are uncommon but can increase risk of fracture.
- Pay particular attention to neurologic examination or new focal pain.
- Measure BP yearly. Hypertension is more common in patients with NF1 and could be secondary to renal artery stenosis, aortic stenosis, and pheochromocytoma.
- Evaluate neurodevelopmental progress in children. Learning disabilities occur in 50–75%.

DIFFERENTIAL DIAGNOSIS
Familial café au lait spots (autosomal dominant, no other NF1 features), Legius syndrome, constitutional mismatch repair deficiency syndrome (CMMRD), NF2, Watson syndrome, LEOPARD syndrome, McCune-Albright syndrome, neurocutaneous melanosis, proteus syndrome, lipomatosis, Jaffe–Campanacci syndrome

Geriatric Considerations
In NF1, cutaneous lesions and tumors increase in size and number with age.

Pediatric Considerations
- Children who have inherited the *NF1* gene of an affected parent usually are identified by age 1 year, but external stigmata may be subtle. If there are no stigmata by age 2 years, NF is unlikely, but the child should be reexamined within the next few years. Definite diagnosis can be made by age 4 years using National Institute of Health (NIH) criteria (1).
- Young children with multiple café au lait spots, but no other stigmata after careful physical and ophthalmologic evaluation, should be followed clinically as if they have NF1 (2).
- Molecular confirmation may be appropriate, especially with atypical presentation (3).

DIAGNOSTIC TESTS & INTERPRETATION
- DNA sequence and deletion/duplication analysis of the *NF1* gene can identify mutations in ~96% of those with a clinical diagnosis.
- Molecular genetic testing is available, although often not necessary for diagnosis. Diagnostic laboratory information: https://www.genetests.org/
- Confirmatory genetic testing is appropriate in those who are suspected of having NF1 but do not fulfill diagnostic criteria or for prenatal diagnosis or preimplantation genetic diagnosis (PGD) (4).

Initial Tests (lab, imaging)
- Characteristic radiographic findings: sphenoid dysplasia, long bone cortical thinning, ribbon ribs, and angular scoliosis. Screening radiographs of the knees in adolescents is controversial. CT can demonstrate bony changes.
- MRI findings of the orbits, brain, or spine (86%). Routine head MRI scanning in asymptomatic individuals with NF1 is controversial. Optic gliomata (seen on MRI, 11–15%) may lead to blindness. Although areas of increased T_2 signal intensity (unidentified bright objects) are common on brain MRI, they are not diagnostic of NF1 and likely are of no clinical significance.

- The NIH Consensus Development Conference does not recommend routine neuroimaging as a means of establishing a diagnosis, although modification of diagnostic criteria is discussed (1)[C].

Diagnostic Procedures/Other
- Ophthalmologic evaluation, including slit-lamp exam of the irides; visual field testing to evaluate optic gliomata
- Neuropsychological testing: Intelligence usually normal but may have significant deficits in language, visuospatial skills, and neuromotor skills.

TREATMENT

MEDICATION

First Line
There are no specific therapeutic agents approved; individual aspects are treated as they arise (e.g., anticonvulsants for seizures, medications for ADHD, management of blood pressure).

Second Line
- In case studies, Sirolimus, a mammalian target of rapamycin [mTOR] inhibitor, did not shrink nonprogressive plexiform neurofibromas, but did relieve pain and retard progression of inoperable plexiform neurofibromas (5)[C].
- Multiple clinical trials for NF1 are recruiting patients (see https://www.clinicaltrials.gov/).

ISSUES FOR REFERRAL
- Patients with more than minimal manifestations of NF1: Refer to a multidisciplinary NF clinic.
- Referral for psychosocial issues of family and affected individuals
- Educational intervention for children with learning disabilities or ADHD (40%)
- Early referral to orthopedics for congenital tibial bowing

ADDITIONAL THERAPIES
- Occupational therapy for children with NF1 who present with fine motor difficulties
- There is no evidence supporting laser therapy for café au lait spots.
- The Children's Tumor Foundation (CTF) has established the NF Clinical Trials Consortium and the CTF NF Clinic Network to facilitate future clinical trials and help identify best practices (6).

SURGERY/OTHER PROCEDURES
Surgical treatment for severe scoliosis, plexiform neurofibromata, or malignancy

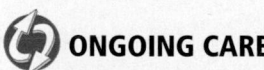

ONGOING CARE

FOLLOW-UP RECOMMENDATIONS
NF1 health supervision 2008 guidelines:
- Infancy to 1 year (7)[C]
  - Growth and development: mild short stature, macrocephaly (increased brain volume); aqueductal stenosis/obstructive hydrocephalus, hydrocephalus
  - Check for focal neurologic signs or asymmetric neurologic exam.
  - Skeletal abnormalities, especially spine and legs
  - Neurodevelopmental progress
- 1 to 5 years (7)[C]
  - Café au lait spots and axillary freckling have no clinical significance.
  - Annual ophthalmologic exam
  - Brain MRI for visual changes, persistent headaches, seizures, marked increase in head size, plexiform neurofibroma of the head

- Assess speech and language: hypernasal speech due to velopharyngeal insufficiency and delayed expressive language development.
- Developmental evaluation of learning and motor abilities; may benefit from speech/language and/or motor therapy, and special education
- Monitor BP annually.
- 5 to 13 years (7)[C]
  - Evaluate for skin tumors causing disfigurement and obtain consultation if surgery is desired to improve appearance or function.
  - Evaluate for premature or delayed puberty. If sexual precocity is noted, evaluate for an optic glioma or hypothalamic lesion. Review the effects of puberty on NF.
  - Evaluate for learning disabilities and ADHD.
  - Evaluate social adjustment, development, and school placement.
  - Monitor ophthalmologic status yearly until age 8 years; complete eye exam every 2 years.
  - Monitor BP annually.
  - Refer patient to a clinical psychologist or child psychiatrist for problems with self-esteem.
  - Discuss growth of neurofibromata during adolescence and pregnancy.
  - Counsel parents about discussing diagnosis with child.
- 13 to 21 years (7)[C]
  - Examine the adolescent for abnormal pubertal development.
  - Thorough skin examination for plexiform neurofibromata and a complete neurologic exam for findings suggestive of deep plexiform neurofibromata; seek surgical consultation for signs of pressure on deep structures.
  - Continue to monitor BP yearly.
  - Continue ophthalmologic examination every 2 years until age 18 years.
  - Discuss genetics of NF1 or refer for genetic counseling.
  - Discuss sexuality, contraception, and reproductive options.
  - Discuss effects of pregnancy on NF1, if appropriate. Neurofibromata may enlarge and new tumors may develop during pregnancy.
  - Review prenatal diagnosis or refer the patient to a geneticist.

PATIENT EDUCATION
- Genetic counseling and patient education regarding future complications about family planning
- Support groups are important: http://www.ctf.org/.

PROGNOSIS
Variable; most patients have a mild expression of NF1 and lead normal lives.

COMPLICATIONS
- Disfigurement: Skin neurofibromata develop primarily on exposed areas. The number tends to increase with puberty or pregnancy.
- Scoliosis: 10–30% (most cases mild); bowing of long bones, 2%; osteopenia and osteoporosis
- A large head is common but rarely associated with hydrocephalus.
- Increased risk of malignancy: malignant peripheral nerve sheath tumor (MPNST) (5–10%) usually in adults (1), especially within the field of previous radiotherapy for plexiform neurofibroma
- CNS tumors (5–15%), especially optic pathway glioma (most common CNS tumor), most often asymptomatic, but if symptomatic, usually presents before age 6 years. Symptomatic lesions are usually stable or only slowly progressive.

- High relative risk (RR) for some uncommon malignancies
- Increased risk for pheochromocytoma, rhabdomyosarcoma, leukemia, Wilms tumor
- Relative risk for cancer of the esophagus (3.3), stomach (2.8), colon (2.0), liver (3.8), lung (3.0), bone (19.6), thyroid (4.9), malignant melanoma (3.6), non-Hodgkin lymphoma (3.3), chronic myeloid leukemia (6.7), female breast (2.3), and ovary (3.7)
- Learning disability: ~50%; may be associated with ADHD; mental retardation in 4–8%
- GI neurofibromata may cause GI disturbances.
- Seizures: 6–7%
- Hypertension is a frequent finding in adults and may occur during childhood.
- Disorders of puberty

Pregnancy Considerations
Increased risk of perinatal complications, stillbirth, intrauterine growth constriction; risk of cord compression, and outlet obstruction by pelvic neurofibromata

REFERENCES

1. DeBella K, Szudek J, Friedman JM. Use of the National Institutes of Health Criteria for diagnosis of neurofibromatosis 1 in children. *Pediatrics*. 2000;105(3 Pt 1):608–614.
2. Nunley KS, Gao F, Albers AC, et al. Predictive value of café au lait macules at initial consultation in the diagnosis of neurofibromatosis type 1. *Arch Dermatol*. 2009;145(8):883–887.
3. Burkitt Wright EM, Sach E, Sharif S, et al. Can the diagnosis of NF1 be excluded clinically? A lack of pigmentary findings in families with spinal neurofibromatosis demonstrates a limitation of clinical diagnosis. *J Med Genet*. 2013;50(9):606–613.
4. National Institutes of Health Consensus Development Conference statement: neurofibromatosis. Bethesda, Md., USA, July 13–15, 1987. *Neurofibromatosis*. 1988;1(3):172–178.
5. Hua C, Zehou O, Decassou S, et al. Sirolimus improves pain in NF1 patients with severe plexiform neurofibromas. *Pediatrics*. 2014:133(6): e1792–e1797.
6. Williams VC, Lucas J, Babcock MA, et al. Neurofibromatosis type 1 revisited. *Pediatrics*. 2009;123(1):124–133.
7. Hersh JH. Health supervision for children with neurofibromatosis. *Pediatrics*. 2008;121(3):633–642.

 SEE ALSO

Tuberous Sclerosis Complex; Von Hippel-Lindau Syndrome

 CODES

ICD10
Q85.01 Neurofibromatosis, type 1

CLINICAL PEARLS
- Marked clinical variability. External stigmata may be subtle or absent in young children. Minimally affected children may become severely affected adults.
- A single café au lait spot is of no concern in a child, but having ≥6 is a diagnostic criterion for NF1.

N

NEUROPATHIC PAIN

Janet Grotticelli, DO, MBA, CHSE

 BASICS

DESCRIPTION

- Defined as pain caused by a lesion or disease that leads to an abnormal and dysfunctional somatosensory system (1)
- A complex state that arises from abnormal neural activity secondary to disease, injury, or dysfunction of the peripheral or central nervous system
- Can exist without ongoing disease
- Can arise from damage to the nerve pathways at any point from the terminals of the peripheral nociceptors to the cortical neurons in the brain
- May be triggered by direct nerve injury, infection, metabolic dysfunction, autoimmune disease, neoplasm, drugs, radiation, and neurovascular disorders
- May reflect abnormal central nervous system activity rather than a manifestation of any underlying pathology itself (i.e., phantom limb pain, complex regional pain syndrome [CRPS])

EPIDEMIOLOGY

Incidence
Data is challenging due to the diversity of related clinical entities.
- Includes various chronic conditions that together, affect up to 8% of the population (2)

Prevalence
- Approximately 20% of people with cancer have cancer-related neuropathic pain as a result of either the disease or its treatment (3).
- The lifetime incidence of herpes zoster (shingles) is ~25%. Studies in the United States and Netherlands found 2.6% and 10%, respectively, will develop chronic postherpetic neuralgia (3).
- 33 million people infected with HIV across the world; ~35% have neuropathic pain (3)
- Up to 50% of people with diabetes have some form of neuropathy.

ETIOLOGY AND PATHOPHYSIOLOGY
- Positive symptoms due to changes in peripheral nerves, loss of inhibitory mechanisms in CNS, and central sensitization
- Negative symptoms (sensory deficits) reflecting neural damage
- Associated with a predisposing factor
- Risk factors:
  - Demyelinating disorders (multiple sclerosis, Guillain-Barré)
  - Neoplasm (primary/metastatic)
  - Neurovascular (central poststroke syndrome, diabetes, trigeminal neuralgia)
  - Autoimmune disease (Sjögren syndrome, polyarteritis nodosa)
  - Structural disease (herniated disc disease) (4)

RISK FACTORS
- General risk factors include older age, female gender, physical inactivity, manual occupation
- There is growing evidence of genetic factors
- Includes factors that increase the risk of underlying conditions, as well as those that increase the risk of pain when these conditions are present:
  - Diabetes
  - Herpes zoster
  - Trigeminal neuralgia
  - HIV
  - Lyme disease
  - Cancer and chemotherapy
  - Stroke
  - Multiple sclerosis
  - Trauma
  - Surgery
  - Limb amputation
  - Nutritional deficiencies
  - Medications

COMMONLY ASSOCIATED CONDITIONS
- Depression/anxiety
- Insomnia
- Drug dependence

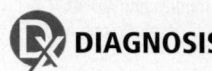 **DIAGNOSIS**

The diagnosis is based primarily on history (e.g., underlying disorder and distinct pain qualities) and the findings on physical examination (e.g., pattern of sensory disturbance); however, several tests may sometimes be helpful (2,5)[A].

HISTORY
- Careful history that includes:
  - Onset and duration of symptoms: this is a chronic condition, location, intensity, character, temporal profile, and possible exacerbating factors. Concomitant symptoms should also be questioned. Past medical and surgical history, psychosocial history, and functional history (i.e., the impact of symptoms on level of mobility, activities of daily living, relation with others, sleep, and mood) are also important.
  - Sensory descriptors: numbness, weakness, reduced sensation to touch, pinprick, temperature, or vibration; decreased proprioception
- Pain is often described as burning, shock-like, tingling (2,4)[A].
- No single feature is diagnostic (1).

PHYSICAL EXAM
- Positive signs/symptoms (2,6)[A]
  - Hypoesthesia (abnormally reduced sensation of a tactile stimulus) to touch or cold
  - Hypoalgesia (abnormally reduced pain sensation to a noxious stimulus)
  - Hyperalgesia: (abnormally increased pain sensation to a noxious stimulus) to pinprick, blunt pressure, heat, or cold
  - Allodynia: (pain sensation to a nonnoxious stimulus) for example, pain evoked by light touch, clothing, bed sheets
- Motor signs and symptoms: may include hypotonia, tremor, dystonia, ataxia, hypo-/hyperreflexia, or motor neglect. Motor symptoms include weakness, fatigability, decreased range of motion, joint stiffness, and spontaneous muscle spasm (4)[A].
- Sensory examination
  - Light touch, pinprick, vibration sense, and proprioception may be diminished or absent in the involved nerve territory.
  - Sensory disturbance may aberrantly extend beyond a discrete nerve territory.
- Skin examination
  - Alterations in temperature, color, sweating, and hair growth suggestive of CRPS
  - Residual dermatomal scars consistent with previous herpes zoster (shingles) infection
  - Characteristic skin changes consistent with diabetes mellitus

DIFFERENTIAL DIAGNOSIS
- Nociceptive pain: induced by transmission impulses along peripheral nociceptors usually due to tissue damage
- Differentiate by clinical signs and symptoms, mechanisms and therapeutic management

DIAGNOSTIC TESTS & INTERPRETATION
For definite diagnosis, the abnormal sensory findings are confirmed to the innervation territory of the lesioned nervous system structure AND diagnostic test(s) confirming a nervous system lesion or disease that could explain neuropathic pain (1)[A].

Initial Tests (lab, imaging)
None specifically for neuropathic pain but can rule in or out a cause of symptoms
- Neuroimaging based on affected area
- Blood and cerebrospinal fluid samples
  - Structural tests:
    - Skin biopsy analyses
    - Sural nerve biopsy
    - Structural imaging tests
- Serum B_{12}
- 25-hydroxyvitamin D
- Thyroid-stimulating hormone (TSH)
- Rapid plasma reagin (RPR) or Venereal Disease Research Laboratory (VDRL) test
- Fasting glucose, creatinine Lyme serology

Follow-Up Tests & Special Considerations
- Nerve conduction study (NCS): The standard electrodiagnostic tool for assessing peripheral nerve fiber function (2)[A].
- Electromyography (2)[A]
- Evoked potentials (2)[A]
- Quantitative Sensory Testing (2)[A]
- Thermography (2)[A]
- CSF samples (2)[A]

 TREATMENT

GENERAL MEASURES
- Generally resistant to acetaminophen or NSAIDs
- Learn ways to relax body and mind

MEDICATION
- The efficacy of systemic drug treatments is generally not dependent on the etiology of the underlying disorder (2,7).
- Combined therapy (polypharmacy) may be more effective.
- Treatment needs to be individualized

First Line
- Calcium channel alpha-2-delta ligands
  - Gabapentin (2,8)[A]
    - Dosing: 1,200 to 3,600 mg in three divided doses
    - Precautions: reduce dosages in renal insufficiency
    - Common side effects: sedation, dizziness, peripheral edema, weight gain
  - Pregabalin (2,8)[A]
    - Used for the treatment of PDN, spinal cord injury, PHN, fibromyalgia (3)[A]
    - Dosing: 300 to 600 mg in two doses
    - Precautions: reduce dosages in renal insufficiency
    - Common side effects: sedation, dizziness, peripheral edema, weight gain

- Tricyclic antidepressants (2,8)[A]
  - Nortriptyline, desipramine, amitriptyline, clomipramine, imipramine
    - Dosing: start at 10 to 25 mg at bedtime, then increase by 10 to 25 mg every 4 to 7 days up to 150 mg/day to efficacy and side effects
    - Precautions: cardiac disease, glaucoma, prostatic adenoma, seizure, tramadol use
    - Geriatric considerations: patients (dose ≤75 mg daily)
    - Common side effects: somnolence, anticholinergic effects, weight gain
- Serotonin-norepinephrine reuptake inhibitors (SNRIs) (2,8)[A]
  - Duloxetine
    - Dosing: 30 mg once daily/60 mg twice daily. Effective doses 60 to 120 mg daily
    - Precautions: hepatic disorder, tramadol use, hypertension
    - Common side effects: nausea
  - Venlafaxine
    - Dosage: 37.5 mg once or twice daily/225 mg daily. Effective doses 150 to 225 mg daily
    - Precautions: cardiac disease, hypertension; tramadol use
    - Common side effects: nausea, hypertension at high dosages
- Topical lidocaine (first line for elderly, frail patients only)
  - Lidocaine, 5% plasters (2,8)[A]
    - Dosage: 1 to 3 patches/3 patches for 12 hours to cover the painful area
    - Precautions: none
    - Common side effects: local erythema, itch, rash
  - Carbamazepine (9)[A]

Second Line

- Topical treatments (2)[A]
  - Lidocaine patches
    - (See "Topical Lidocaine")
  - Capsaicin high-concentration patches (8%)
    - Dosage: 1 to 4 patches to cover the painful area, repeat every 3 months; 30 minutes application to feet, 60 minutes application to remainder of body; avoid use on face
    - Precautions: caution in progressive neuropathy
    - Common side effects: pain, erythema, itching, rare hypertension (initial increase in pain)
- Tramadol (2)[A]
  - Dosage: 50 mg once or twice daily/400 mg daily as long-acting drug. Increase by 50 to 100 mg every 3 to 7 days
  - Precautions: history of substance abuse, suicide risk
  - Geriatric considerations: use of antidepressant in elderly patients.
  - Common side effects: nausea, vomiting, constipation, dizziness, somnolence

Third Line

- Opioids (2)[A]
  - Morphine, oxycodone
    - Dosage: 10 to 15 mg morphine every 4 hours or as needed (equianalgesic doses for other opioids)/up to 300 mg morphine has been used
    - Precautions: history of substance abuse, suicide risk, risk of misuse on long-term use
  - Botulinum toxin type A
    - Dosage: 50 to 300 units subcutaneously to the painful area; repeat every 3 months
    - Precautions: infection of area
    - Common side effects: pain at injection site

ISSUES FOR REFERRAL

Referral to pain clinic if refractory to initial treatment or additional therapies below are warranted.

ADDITIONAL THERAPIES

- Cannabinoids (dronabinol and nabilone): The appropriateness of medical marijuana for a patient should be comprehensive assessments that revolve around risk-benefit discussion (8,10).
- Neural stimulation (11)
- Spinal cord stimulation (SCS): Pain that is continuous and unchanging responds best. The most common indication is failed back surgery syndrome with leg pain. Less common indications are peripheral nerve injury, CRPS, and painful peripheral neuropathy (11).
- Dorsal root ganglion stimulation to treat challenging pain syndromes that do not respond to conventional SCS (11).
- Peripheral nerve stimulation (PNS): indications include pain in the distribution of an accessible peripheral nerve. The most common nerves treated are the supraorbital, infraorbital, greater occipital, ulnar, median, suprascapular, intercostal, ilioinguinal, iliohypogastric, genitofemoral, lateral femoral cutaneous, saphenous, sciatic, posterior tibial, superficial peroneal, and sural nerves (11).
- Intrathecal drug delivery considered invasive and labor intensive, may be used when other conservative therapies fail (11).
- Transcutaneous electrical nerve stimulation is widely used, evidence is poor in supporting the efficacy (11).
- Osteopathic manipulative treatment should be offered to all patients. Myofascial trigger point release can be an effective primary technique. Indirect or passive myofascial techniques may be used to address all regions of tissue texture change (12).
- Hypnosis can reduce pain and anxiety related to the pain.
- Acupuncture

SURGERY/OTHER PROCEDURES

Nerve destructive procedures haven't shown effectiveness and may cause additional insult/injury (an exception is treatment of terminal cancer) (11).

- Sympathectomy dorsal root entry zone lesion (dorsal rhizotomy)
- Lateral cordotomy
- Trigeminal nerve ganglion ablation (13)[A]

 ONGOING CARE

FOLLOW-UP RECOMMENDATIONS

- Multidisciplinary team
- Periodic evaluation to rule out other treatable conditions (2)

Patient Monitoring

- Pain management requires ongoing evaluation, patient education, and reassurance
- Patient compliance and adequacy of analgesic drug titrations should be continually evaluated and documented.

PROGNOSIS

Chronic course of pain symptoms often requires management with numerous medications and adjunctive therapies.

COMPLICATIONS

Long-term disability and drug addiction are possible.

REFERENCES

1. Haanpää M. Clinical Examination of a Patient with Possible Neuropathic Pain. International Association for the Study of Pain, 2014 Refresher Courses: 15th World Congress on Pain.
2. Gilron I, Baron R, Jensen T. Neuropathic pain: principles of diagnosis and treatment. Mayo Clin Proc. 2015;90(4):532–545.
3. van Hecke O, Austin SK, Khan RA, et al. Neuropathic pain in the general population: a systematic review of epidemiological studies. Pain. 2014;155(4):654–662.
4. Finnerup NB, Sindrup SH, Jensen TS. The evidence for pharmacological treatment of neuropathic pain. Pain. 2010;150(3):573–581.
5. Gilron I, Watson CP, Cahill CM, et al. Neuropathic pain: a practical guide for the clinician. CMAJ. 2006;175(3):265–275.
6. Kerstman E, Ahn S, Battu S, et al. Neuropathic pain. Handb Clin Neurol. 2013;110:175–187.
7. Finnerup NB, Attal N, Haroutounian S, et al. Pharmacotherapy for neuropathic pain in adults: a systematic review and meta-analysis. Lancet Neurol. 2015;14(2):162–173.
8. Attal N, Bouhassira D. Pharmacotherapy of neuropathic pain: which drugs, which treatment algorithms? Pain. 2015;156(Suppl 1):S104–S114.
9. Zhou M, Chen N, He L, et al. Oxcarbazepine for neuropathic pain. Cochrane Database Syst Rev. 2013;(3):CD007963.
10. Hill KP. Medical marijuana for treatment of chronic pain and other medical and psychiatric problems: a clinical review. JAMA 2015;313(24):2474–2483.
11. Wallace M. Interventional and Nonpharmacological Therapies for Neuropathic Pain. International Association for the Study of Pain, 2014 Refresher Courses: 15th World Congress on Pain.
12. Galluzzi KE. Managing neuropathic pain. J Am Osteopath Assoc. 2007;107(10)(Suppl 6): ES39–ES48.
13. Straube S, Derry S, Moore RA, et al. Cervico-thoracic or lumbar sympathectomy for neuropathic pain and complex regional pain syndrome. Cochrane Database Syst Rev. 2013;(9):CD002918.

CODES

ICD10

- M79.2 Neuralgia and neuritis, unspecified
- E10.40 Type 1 diabetes mellitus with diabetic neuropathy, unsp
- E11.40 Type 2 diabetes mellitus with diabetic neuropathy, unsp

CLINICAL PEARLS

- Neuropathic pain is a chronic pain syndrome, affecting between 2% and 8% of people with a major impact on quality of life.
- The ongoing challenge for clinicians (and patients) is being able to determine which treatment is most likely to work for any one individual.
- The first line of treatment is pharmacologic and may be more beneficial with additional therapies.
- Generally resistant to acetaminophen or NSAIDs

N

NEUROPATHY, PERIPHERAL

Amy Chen, MD, PhD • David N. Herrmann, MBBCh

 BASICS

DESCRIPTION

- Peripheral neuropathy (PN) is a functional or structural disorder of the peripheral nervous system (PNS).
- PN affects any combination of motor, sensory, or autonomic nerves.
- The motor PNS comprises spinal cord motor neurons, their nerve roots that combine to form plexus, and branches that form individual nerves innervating skeletal muscles. Peripheral motor involvement causes muscle atrophy, weakness, cramps, and fasciculations.
- The sensory PNS consists of sensory organs, which transmit touch, vibration, and position sensation in large-diameter myelinated fibers; pain and temperature in small-diameter, lightly myelinated and unmyelinated C fibers to the dorsal root ganglia. Sensory signals are relayed to the central nervous system (CNS) for integration. Disorders of sensory nerves produce negative phenomena (loss of sensibility, lack of balance) or heightened phenomena (tingling or pain). Large sensory fiber dysfunction impairs touch and vibration sensation, whereas small fiber sensory neuropathy (SFN) affects pin and thermal sensation and causes neuropathic pain.
- The autonomic nervous system (ANS) includes the sympathetic and parasympathetic systems. ANS dysfunction causes cardiovascular, gastrointestinal, and sudomotor symptoms.
- The PNS can be affected from the cell body (sensory ganglionopathy or motor neuronopathy), root (radiculopathy), or plexus (plexopathy) to the nerve (demyelinating or axonal neuropathy).

EPIDEMIOLOGY

Prevalence

Approximately 2.4% of general population or 8% of people >55 years old, are affected by distal symmetric PN, the most common form of PN.

ETIOLOGY AND PATHOPHYSIOLOGY

- PN can be acquired or hereditary.
- The most common cause of acquired PN is diabetes.
- Other categories of acquired PN with illustrative examples are the following:
  - Vascular: ischemia, vasculitis
  - Infectious: HIV, hepatitis C, cryoglobulinemia, Lyme disease
  - Traumatic: compression, crush, or transection
  - Autoimmune: rheumatoid arthritis, Sjögren, postinfectious Guillain-Barré syndrome (GBS), chronic inflammatory demyelinating polyneuropathy (CIDP)
  - Metabolic: diabetes, renal failure, hypothyroidism, vitamin B_{12} deficiency, celiac disease
  - Iatrogenic/toxic: chemotherapy, platinum, taxanes, metronidazole, colchicine, infliximab, alcoholism
  - Idiopathic: 30% of PN
  - Neoplastic/paraneoplastic: paraproteinemia, Waldenstrom macroglobulinemia, multiple myeloma, amyloidosis, neurofibromatosis
- PN occurs due to demyelination or axonal degeneration.
- Demyelination results from Schwann cell dysfunction, mutations in myelin protein genes, or direct damage to myelin sheaths.
- Axonal degeneration occurs when injury/dysfunction occurs at the cell body or axon.

Genetics

- Approximately 50% of undiagnosed PN is hereditary.
- Currently, there are over 70 known genetic causes of hereditary PN.
- Charcot-Marie-Tooth (CMT) neuropathies: the most common hereditary PN
  - CMT1A (duplication of the *PMP22* gene) is the most common CMT.
  - A *PMP22* deletion causes hereditary neuropathy with liability to pressure palsy (HNPP)

RISK FACTORS

Systemic disorders predispose to PN.

GENERAL PREVENTION

- Healthy nutrition and avoidance of alcoholism and of pressure at nerve entrapment sites
- Surveillance for glucose dysmetabolism and tight glycemic control may prevent diabetic PN.

DIAGNOSIS

HISTORY

- A detailed inquiry for symptoms of sensory, motor, or autonomic dysfunction:
  - Numbness, tingling, prickling, burning pain, a "tightly wrapped" sensation, and an "unsteady gait"
  - Distal weakness manifests as foot drop (tripping, foot slapping) or difficulty with grip; proximal weakness (e.g., difficulty arising from a chair) is less common.
  - Orthostatic dizziness, abnormal sweating, constipation, or voiding difficulties
- Symptom onset:
  - Acute: Consider infection (e.g., Lyme disease), postinfectious dysimmune process (e.g., GBS), ischemia (e.g., vasculitis), toxin, or trauma.
  - Subacute: Consider metabolic, neoplastic, paraneoplastic, or dysimmune processes.
  - Chronic: Consider dysimmune process (CIDP), idiopathic, or hereditary.
- Progression: stable or indolent; slowly or rapidly progressive; monophasic or relapsing or remitting
- Anatomic pattern: focal, multifocal, diffuse

PHYSICAL EXAM

- Based on exam, a functional (*sensory*: small-fiber vs. large-fiber vs. mixed, *sensorimotor*, *motor*, *autonomic*) and anatomic pattern of PN (*distal symmetric*, *multifocal*, or *focal*) should be established.
- Cognition preserved in isolated PN.
- Cranial nerves may be involved with focal or multifocal PN (e.g., bifacial weakness may occur with GBS, Lyme disease, sarcoidosis, among other causes).
- Stocking/glove sensory loss is typical of distal symmetric sensory PN (e.g., diabetes).
- Isolated reduced pin or thermal sensation or allodynia suggests a pure SFN.
- Reduced vibration and joint position sense suggests large-fiber sensory neuropathy; when severe, a Romberg sign is present, and gait is wide-based or ataxic.
- Distal muscle atrophy and weaknesses of toe extension and finger abduction are often present with distal symmetric axonal PN.
- In acquired demyelinating PN (e.g., GBS or CIDP), weakness is commonly both proximal and distal.

- Deep tendon reflexes may be reduced or absent, distally at the ankles in large-fiber axonal PN, or diffusely in demyelinating PN.
- High arched or flat feet or hammer toes suggest hereditary PN.

ALERT
Hemibody deficits or sensory loss below a spinal cord level suggest a CNS process.

ALERT
Hyperreflexia and spasticity are upper motor neuron signs not seen with isolated PN.

DIFFERENTIAL DIAGNOSIS

The following categories of PN can be identified (differential diagnosis [DDx] listed when applicable):

- Pure sensory neuropathy
  - DDx: SFN, sensory ganglionopathy, polyradiculopathy
- Distal symmetric sensorimotor axonal PN
  - Most common type of PN
  - DDx: distal acquired demyelinating symmetric PN (DADS)
- Motor predominant PN
  - DDx: motor neuron disease, polyradiculopathy, immune-mediated multifocal motor neuropathy (MMN)
- Mononeuropathy
  - Most likely due to compression, entrapment, or trauma
  - DDx: monoradiculopathy
- Mononeuropathy multiplex
  - DDx: plexopathy, polyradiculopathy

DIAGNOSTIC TESTS & INTERPRETATION

Initial Tests (lab, imaging)

- Nerve conduction studies and electromyography (NCS/EMG)
  - Best performed by physicians with specialty training in electrodiagnostic medicine
  - Delineate axonal versus demyelinating, anatomic pattern, chronicity, and severity of PN.
- Blood tests
  - CBC, BUN, creatinine, fasting glucose, HgA1C, vitamin B_{12}, serum protein electrophoresis, and immunofixation
- Specialized skin biopsy
  - In clinically suspected SFN if NCS/EMG is normal
  - Analysis of lower limb epidermal nerve fiber density (ENFD) (1)[A]
- Autonomic tests
  - Not routinely done but useful to characterize autonomic PN
- Neuroimaging
  - Generally not indicated in evaluation of PN but useful in evaluation of brachial plexopathies, radiculopathies, or where findings are attributable to the CNS

Follow-Up Tests & Special Considerations

- Additional blood tests are done based on the medical history, the PN type, and NCS/EMG findings.
- Genetic testing for diagnosis of hereditary PN should be ordered by neurologists with expertise in PN.
- Screen patients with distal symmetric PN for unhealthy alcohol use with CAGE-AID or AUDIT-C.

Diagnostic Procedures/Other
- Nerve biopsy (sural or superficial peroneal nerve): useful if vasculitis, amyloidosis, granulomatous disorders, or neoplastic infiltration is suspected; rarely helpful in late-onset chronic, slowly progressive distal symmetric PN
- Lumbar puncture
  - Cytoalbuminologic dissociation in GBS or CIDP
  - Infection, inflammation, or neoplasia in polyradiculopathies

Test Interpretation
- Demyelinating PN: disproportionate slowing of conduction velocities or prolonged distal latencies on NCS
- Axonal PN: reduced amplitude in sensory or motor responses, with relatively preserved conduction velocities on NCS
- Reduced ENFD on distal leg skin biopsies is supportive of SFN.

TREATMENT

GENERAL MEASURES
Manage associated medical conditions; disease-modifying therapy for specific forms of PN (e.g., CIDP); symptomatic relief of pain and dysautonomia; rehabilitation to optimize function.

MEDICATION
First Line
- Treatment of neuropathic pain: evidence of efficacy derived from clinical trials in diabetic painful neuropathy (DPN) and postherpetic neuralgia (PHN):
- Pregabalin: for DPN and PHN
- Duloxetine: for DPN
- Lidocaine patch: for PHN
- Gabapentin: (off-label) for DPN
- Tricyclic antidepressants: (off-label) for DPN
- Venlafaxine: (off-label) for DPN
- Tramadol: (off-label) for DPN
- Targeted treatment for underlying systemic conditions:
  - Glycemic control, thyroid hormone supplementation, vitamin supplementation, antimicrobial therapy (e.g., Lyme disease, HIV), glucocorticoids for sarcoidosis, and cytotoxic therapy for vasculitis
- Immunotherapy for dysimmune PN

- Intravenous immunoglobulin (IVIG): within the first 2 weeks of GBS to hasten recovery (2)[A]; as a first-line alternative to corticosteroids for treatment of CIDP (3)[A]; and for prevention of secondary axonal loss in MMN (4)[A]
  - Loading dose 2 g/kg body weight divided into 2 to 5 days; maintenance regimen variable for CIDP and MMN
  - Adverse effects (AE): headache, fever, hypertension, and rarely, pulmonary embolism

- Plasma exchange: first agent shown to improve functional outcome for patients with GBS (5)[A]; short-term benefit in CIDP (6)[A]
  - AE: catheter complication, hypotension, and others

- Corticosteroids: a first-line option in treatment of CIDP (7)[C]; oral or pulsed IV regimen can induce remission
- Treatment of autonomic symptoms
  - Compression stockings, hydration, midodrine, and fludrocortisone for orthostatic hypotension
  - Pyridostigmine for immune-mediated dysautonomia (off-label)

ISSUES FOR REFERRAL
- Rapidly progressive symptoms, suspected demyelinating PN, or hereditary PN should be referred to a neurologist with expertise in neuromuscular disorders.
- Patients with vasculitic PN should be referred to rheumatology.
- Patients with paraproteinemia should have a skeletal bone survey and be referred to hematology.
- Patients with imbalance, ataxia, or falls should be referred to physical therapy for gait and balance training.

ADDITIONAL THERAPIES
- Combination therapy (e.g., gabapentin with TCA or venlafaxine or tramadol) can be more effective than monotherapy for neuropathic pain.
- Long-acting opiates can be considered for refractory neuropathic pain.
- Additional immunosuppressant agents (e.g., cyclophosphamide) may be used in refractory chronic dysimmune PN.

SURGERY/OTHER PROCEDURES
- Decompressive surgery for entrapment neuropathy (e.g., carpal tunnel syndrome)
- Foot and ankle surgery to improve symptoms or function in hereditary PN
- Radiation, surgery, or bone marrow transplantation for plasmacytoma or osteosclerotic myeloma or POEMS syndrome
- Liver transplantation for amyloidotic PN

COMPLEMENTARY & ALTERNATIVE MEDICINE
Low-intensity transcutaneous electrical nerve stimulation (TENS), acupuncture, mediation

INPATIENT CONSIDERATIONS
Admission Criteria/Initial Stabilization
- Patients with suspected GBS should be admitted for diagnosis, monitoring (30–60% may develop cardiovascular or respiratory failure), and for acute treatment.
- Elective intubation may be required in GBS when forced vital capacity is <15 mL/kg body weight.
- Other rapidly progressive undiagnosed PNs that impair independent ambulation may require admission.

ONGOING CARE

FOLLOW-UP RECOMMENDATIONS
- Physical therapy and gait assistive devices as needed
- Flu vaccination should be avoided in the first year following GBS.

PROGNOSIS
- Late-onset idiopathic distal symmetric axonal PN are indolent
- 80% of GBS have a near complete or good recovery. 80% of CIDP have moderate or good response with treatment but can be relapsing.

REFERENCES
1. Lauria G, Hsieh ST, Johansson O, et al. European Federation of Neurological Societies/Peripheral Nerve Society Guideline on the use of skin biopsy in the diagnosis of small fiber neuropathy. Report of a joint task force of the European Federation of Neurological Societies and the Peripheral Nerve Society. *Eur J Neurol.* 2010;17(7):903–912, e44–e49.
2. Hughes RA, Swan AV, van Doorn PA. Intravenous immunoglobulin for Guillain-Barré syndrome. *Cochrane Database Syst Rev.* 2014;(9):CD002063.
3. Nobile-Orazio E, Cocito D, Jann S, et al. Intravenous immunoglobulin versus intravenous methylprednisolone for chronic inflammatory demyelinating polyradiculoneuropathy: a randomised controlled trial. *Lancet Neurol.* 2012;11(6):493–502.
4. Cats EA, van der Pol WL, Piepers S, et al. Correlates of outcome and response to IVIg in 88 patients with multifocal motor neuropathy. *Neurology.* 2010;75(9):818–825.
5. Plasmapheresis and acute Guillain-Barré syndrome. The Guillain-Barré syndrome Study Group. *Neurology.* 1985;35(8):1096–1104.
6. Dyck PJ, Daube J, O'Brien P, et al. Plasma exchange in chronic inflammatory demyelinating polyradiculoneuropathy. *N Engl J Med.* 1986;314(8):461–465.
7. Dyck PJ, O'Brien PC, Oviatt KF, et al. Prednisone improves chronic inflammatory demyelinating polyradiculoneuropathy more than no treatment. *Ann Neurol.* 1982;11(2):136–141.

CODES

ICD10
- G62.9 Polyneuropathy, unspecified
- G60.9 Hereditary and idiopathic neuropathy, unspecified
- G60.8 Other hereditary and idiopathic neuropathies

CLINICAL PEARLS
- There are many causes of PN. Diagnosis is made by history and physical exam, targeted laboratory testing, NCS/EMG, skin biopsy, or ANS testing.
- Consider hereditary neuropathy if patient has an early age of PN symptom onset, family history of PN, or foot deformity.
- GBS is monophasic and progresses for up to 4 weeks; CIDP progresses beyond 8 weeks, and if untreated, usually has a progressive course.

N

NICOTINE ADDICTION

Benjamin N. Schneider, MD • Kamala Nyamathi, MD

 BASICS

DESCRIPTION
Nicotine addiction is the constellation of signs of dependence and compulsive use despite knowledge of its adverse effects.

EPIDEMIOLOGY
Incidence
20–25% of the U.S. population use nicotine.

Prevalence
70 million people in the United States ≥12 years of age reported current use of tobacco (58.7 million smoked cigarettes, 13.3 million cigars, 2.1 million pipes, and 8.6 million used smokeless tobacco) (1).

Pediatric Considerations
Nicotine use is common and underrecognized in this population. Use of cigarettes; smokeless tobacco; and now, e-cigarettes in the past month: 8th graders: 4%, 3%, and 8.7%; 10th graders: 7.2%, 5.3%, and 16.2%; 12th graders: 13.6%, 8.4%, and 17% (2).

ETIOLOGY AND PATHOPHYSIOLOGY
- Similar to other addictive drugs, nicotine affects neural pathways that control reward and pleasure.
- Nicotinic acetylcholine receptors (nAChRs) are thought to play a major role in nicotine's effect on brain chemistry via their influence of glutamate, GABA, dopamine, serotonin, acetylcholine, and norepinephrine.
- Through these neurotransmitters, nicotine induces euphoria, assists in information processing, and reduces anxiety and fatigue.
- Polymorphisms in neuronal nAChR genes are associated with increased susceptibility to dependence.
- Specific genes associated with nicotine dependence have been linked with decreased activity of CYP2B86 (an enzyme that breaks down brain nicotine) and are thought to cause increased cravings. These patients are 1.5 times more likely to fail treatment.

RISK FACTORS
- Mental illness (depression, posttraumatic stress disorder, bipolar disorder, and schizophrenia)
- Low socioeconomic status
- Low educational status
- Early first-hand nicotine experience
- Concurrent substance abuse
- Home and peer influence

GENERAL PREVENTION
- The U.S. Preventive Services Task Force (USPSTF) strongly recommends clinicians screen all:
  - Adults for tobacco use and provide cessation interventions for those who screened positive (Grade A).
  - Pregnant women for tobacco use and provide pregnancy-tailored counseling to those who screened positive (Grade A).
- The USPSTF recommends that clinicians provide interventions, including education or brief counseling to prevent initiation of tobacco use among school-aged children and adolescents (Grade B).

Pregnancy Considerations
- Carbon monoxide and nicotine interfere with fetal oxygen supply, resulting in decreased birth weights and possible intrauterine growth restriction
- Maternal smoking adversely affects fetal lung development, with lifelong decreases in pulmonary function and increased asthma risk.
- Smoking is associated with increased risk of spontaneous abortion, sudden infant death syndrome, learning and behavioral problems, and increased risk of childhood obesity.

COMMONLY ASSOCIATED CONDITIONS
- Chronic obstructive pulmonary disease (COPD) (emphysema and chronic bronchitis)
- Cancers (lung, oral/pharyngeal, kidney, bladder, cervical, anal)
- Atherosclerotic disease
- Periodontal disease

 DIAGNOSIS

HISTORY
- Identify types of nicotine products used.
- Amount and duration of nicotine use
- Previous attempts to quit (methods and efficacy)

PHYSICAL EXAM
- Cardiovascular exam
- Pulmonary exam

DIFFERENTIAL DIAGNOSIS
Not applicable

DIAGNOSTIC TESTS & INTERPRETATION
- Low-dose CT scan: recommended by The American College of Chest Physicians for individuals age 55 to 75 years old with a history of 30+ pack years who are currently smoking or have quit within the past 15 years (unless they have comorbidities that are anticipated to limit life expectancy)
- Spirometry: not recommended for routine screening, only if COPD is suspected

TREATMENT

COUNSELING (3)[A]
- Advice from providers improves quit rate number needed to treat [NNT] 75.
- Providing brief, simple advice about cessation increases the likelihood of sustained cessation at 12 months.
- More intensive advice (i.e., motivational interviewing) may result in higher rates of quitting.
- Providing follow-up support may increase quit rates slightly.
- Brief strategies to help the patient willing to quit tobacco use—the "5 As" (4)[A]
  - Ask patient if he or she uses nicotine.
  - Advise him or her to quit.
  - Assess willingness to make a quit attempt.
  - Assist those willing to make a quit attempt.
  - Arrange for follow-up contact to prevent relapse.
- Enhancing motivation to quit—the "5 Rs" (4)[A]
  - Relevance: Encourage patient to indicate why quitting is personally relevant.
  - Risks: Ask patient to identify potential negative consequences of use.
  - Rewards: Ask patient to identify potential benefits of cessation.
  - Roadblocks: Ask patient to identify barriers or impediments to quitting and provide treatment (e.g., problem-solving counseling or medication) that could address barriers.
  - Repetition: This motivational intervention should be repeated each visit.
- Users should be given a choice of quitting methods.
- Quit rates are equivalent for tapering nicotine use versus abrupt cessation. Patient preference should be part of the plan.

MEDICATION
- Seven FDA-approved medications exist: nicotine replacement therapy (NRT), both long acting (i.e., patch) and short acting (i.e., gum, inhaler, lozenge, nasal spray), and non-NRT meds like bupropion SR and varenicline.
- With few exceptions, the choice of a first-line medication depends on patient preference.
- Combination NRT: All forms of NRT increase quit rate (5)[A] 50–70%. Combining long-acting and short-acting NRTs is more effective than using any single method alone. Heavier users may need higher doses. Starting NRT before planned quit date may increase the chances of success.
- Nicotine replacement (Gum: pregnancy Category C all other formulations are pregnancy Category D).
  - Nicotine transdermal (NicoDerm CQ): For >10 cigarettes/day, start with 21 mg patch/day for 6 weeks, then 14 mg patch/day for 2 weeks, then 7 mg patch/day for 2 weeks; for use of <10 cigarettes/day, start with 14 mg patch/day for 6 weeks, then 7 mg patch/day for 2 weeks. Extending use of the patch beyond 8 to 10 weeks may improve abstinence rates.

ALERT
May cause insomnia or vivid dreams when left on overnight. Patients may remove the patch overnight to curb these symptoms (rates of smoking cessation don't differ between continuous use vs. overnight removal).

  - Nicotine gum (Nicorette): For >25 cigarettes/day habit, use 4 mg gum q1–2h for 6 weeks; for <25 cigarettes/day habit, use 2 mg gum q1–2h for 6 weeks; decrease dosing by q1–2h for 3 weeks; chew then tuck between cheek and gingiva once nicotine flavor is released, repeat up to 30 minutes then discard.
  - Nicotine lozenge (Commit): for patients who smoke their first cigarette within 30 minutes of waking, 4 mg lozenge PO q1–2h for 6 weeks; first cigarette >30 minutes after waking, 2 mg lozenge PO q1–2h for 6 weeks; decrease dosing by q1–2h for 3 weeks
  - Nicotine nasal (Nicotrol NS): 1 to 2 sprays (0.5 mg/spray) each nostril q1h for 8 weeks, then taper; max 10 sprays/hr and 80 sprays/day
  - Nicotine inhaler (Nicotrol inhaler): 6 to 16 cartridges inhaled (4 mg/cartridge) per day for 6 to 12 weeks, then taper; incorporates the behavioral and sensory aspects of smoking
- Varenicline is a nicotinic acetylcholine partial agonist. Trials have suggested this agent may be more efficacious than bupropion (6)[A]. Longer term therapy (up to 24 weeks) may delay or prevent relapse:
  - Starter pack: 0.5 mg/day for 3 days, 0.5 mg BID for 4 days, 1 mg/day starting on day 7
    ○ Maintenance pack 1 mg BID continue for 12 weeks total; if successful in quitting, may continue for another 12 weeks.

ALERT
Varenicline carries a black box warning for risks of serious neuropsychiatric events. Use only with extreme caution in patients with serious psychiatric disorders, as use may exacerbate these conditions. Varenicline may also increase the risk of cardiovascular events in patients with known CVD, although data is limited and of unclear significance.

- Varenicline + bupropion has not been shown to be more effective than either agent alone but with increased side effects.
- Varenicline + nicotine replacement has been shown to be more effective at 6 months than varenicline alone (NNT 6 [B]).
- Bupropion SR is an atypical antidepressant and norepinephrine-dopamine reuptake inhibitor.
  – Start 1 week before a target quit date due to time needed to reach steady state.
  – Use 150 mg/day for 3 days, then 150 mg twice a day for 7 to 12 weeks.

ALERT
1:1,000 risk of seizure, its use is contraindicated in patients with a history of epilepsy.

- Nortriptyline is a tricyclic antidepressant.
  – Start 25 mg/day, gradually increase to target dose of 75 to 100 mg/day and continue for 12 weeks.
  – Stop smoking 2 to 4 weeks after starting treatment.

ALERT
Contraindicated in narrow-angle glaucoma or heart disease (acute myocardial infarction, atrioventricular or bundle-branch block, long QT)

ADDITIONAL THERAPIES
- Users who get support from partners and others are more likely to quit.
- Group programs double cessation rates compared to self-help materials. It is unclear whether groups are better than individual counseling or other advice, but they are more effective than no treatment. Not all users making a quit attempt want to attend meetings, but for those who do, they are likely to be helpful.
- E-cigarettes improve abstinence at 1 month versus placebo, but this effect is lost at 3- and 6-month follow up. Adverse effects include dry cough (26–32%), throat irritation (7–32%), and shortness of breath (2–20%) (7).
- New data suggest that certain e-cigarette flavorings may alter lung functioning on a cellular level (8).

Pregnancy Considerations
- Smoking is associated with decreased intrauterine growth restriction, placenta previa, abruptio placentae, decreased maternal thyroid function, preterm premature rupture of membranes, low birth weight, perinatal mortality, and ectopic pregnancy.
- Quitting smoking before 15 weeks' gestation provides the greatest benefit for both the woman and fetus, but quitting any time is beneficial.
- There is still insufficient data regarding the safety and efficacy of NRT in pregnancy (gum is considered as Category C, while remaining NRTs are Category D).
- Similarly, little is known about the effects of varenicline and bupropion on fetal development (Category C).
- It is recommended that pregnant women be offered behavioral therapy and education with NRT and medications reserved for patients in need of additional assistance (9).
- NRT is metabolized faster in pregnant women, so higher doses may be required.

COMPLEMENTARY & ALTERNATIVE MEDICINE
- Acupuncture: no consistent evidence of efficacy
- Hypnotherapy: no consistent evidence of efficacy

INPATIENT CONSIDERATIONS
- Programs to stop use that begin during hospitalization and include follow-up support after discharge are effective.
- Programs are effective for all hospitalized users, regardless of admitting diagnosis (10)[A].
- Consider NRT for all inpatients who use nicotine to decrease withdrawal symptoms (10)[A].

 ONGOING CARE

FOLLOW-UP RECOMMENDATIONS
- Patients motivated to quit smoking and who have initiated therapy should follow up 1 to 2 weeks after initiation of therapy to monitor response and observe for any medication side effects.
- Encourage routine exercise as a component of smoking-cessation treatment.

DIET
Weight gain (4 to 5 kg over 10 years) possible after smoking cessation

PATIENT EDUCATION
- http://smokefree.gov/
- http://women.smokefree.gov/
- http://teen.smokefree.gov
- http://www.nicotine-anonymous.org
- https://quitnet.meyouhealth.com/#/
- 1-877-44U-QUIT (1-877-448-7848)

PROGNOSIS
- >85% of those who try to quit on their own relapse, most within a week.
- Approximately 50–60% of women who quit smoking in pregnancy return to smoking within 1-year postpartum.
- Cessation medications and techniques listed above significantly improve cessation.

REFERENCES

1. National Institute on Drug Abuse. *Tobacco Addiction*. NIH Publication Number 09-4342. Bethesda, MD: National Institute of Health; 2009.
2. Johnston LD, O'Malley PM, Bachman JG, et al. *Monitoring the Future, National Results on Adolescent Drug Use: Overview of Key Findings, 2011*. Ann Arbor, MI: Institute for Social Research, University of Michigan; 2012.
3. Stead LF, Bergson G, Lancaster T. Physician advice for smoking cessation. *Cochrane Database Syst Rev*. 2008;(2):CD000165.
4. National Guideline Clearinghouse (NGC). Guideline synthesis: Tobacco use cessation. In: *National Guideline Clearinghouse (NGC)*. Rockville, MD: Agency for Healthcare Research and Quality (AHRQ); 2001. http://www.guideline.gov.
5. Stead LF, Perera R, Bullen C, et al. Nicotine replacement therapy for smoking cessation. *Cochrane Database Syst Rev*. 2011;(11):CD000146.
6. Cahill K, Stead LF, Lancaster T. Nicotine receptor partial agonists for smoking cessation. *Cochrane Database Syst Rev*. 2012;(4):CD006103.
7. Allehebi RO, Khan MH, Stanbrook MB. Efficacy and safety of electronic cigarettes for smoking cessation: a systematic review. *Am J Respir Crit Care Med*. 191;2015:A3715.
8. Rowell TR, Lee s, Tarran R. Select e-cigarette flavors alter calcium signaling, cell viability and proliferation in lung epithelia. *Am J Respir Crit Care Med*. 191;2015:A2896.
9. American College of Obstetricians and Gynecologists. Committee Opinion No. 471: smoking cessation during pregnancy. 2010;116(5):1241–1244.
10. Rigotti NA, Clair C, Munafò MR, et al. Interventions for smoking cessation in hospitalised patients. *Cochrane Database Syst Rev*. 2012;(5):CD001837.

ADDITIONAL READING

- Benowitz NL. Nicotine addiction. *N Engl J Med*. 2010;362(24):2295–2303.
- Centers for Disease Control and Prevention. Smoking and tobacco use: http://www.cdc.gov/tobacco/index.htm.
- Clinical Practice Guideline Treating Tobacco Use and Dependence 2008 Update Panel, Liaisons, and Staff. A clinical practice guideline for treating tobacco use and dependence: 2008 update. A U.S. Public Health Service Report. *Am J Prev Med*. 2008;35(2):158–176.
- Civljak M, Stead LF, Hartmann-Boyce J, et al. Internet-based interventions for smoking cessation. *Cochrane Database Syst Rev*. 2013;(7):CD007078.
- The Health Consequences of Smoking- 50 years of Progress: A Report of the Surgeon General, 2014 http://www.surgeongeneral.gov/library/reports/50-years-of-progress/. Especially Appendix 14.4, *Treatment for Tobacco Use and Dependence*.
- Wilson JF. In the clinic. Smoking cessation. *Ann Intern Med*. 2007;146(3):ITC2-1–ICT2-16.

CODES

ICD10
- F17.200 Nicotine dependence, unspecified, uncomplicated
- F17.201 Nicotine dependence, unspecified, in remission
- F17.203 Nicotine dependence unspecified, with withdrawal

CLINICAL PEARLS
- Nicotine and particularly smoking cessation should be encouraged for all patients who use.
- Consider NRT for all hospitalized patients who smoke to decrease withdrawal symptoms.
- Treatments, including but not limited to medications significantly increase the rate of long-term abstinence.
- No single type of NRT/medication is best; thus, the choice should be based on patient preference and risk factors for side effects.
- Nicotine dependence is a chronic disease and will often require repeated interventions and multiple cessation attempts.

N

NONALCOHOLIC FATTY LIVER DISEASE (NAFLD)

Jill T. Wei, MD • Daniel T. Lee, MD, MA

 BASICS

- A spectrum of fatty liver diseases not due to excess alcohol consumption ranging from nonalcoholic fatty liver (NAFL) to steatohepatitis and cirrhosis with hepatocyte injury with/without fibrosis.
- Leading cause of chronic liver disease; implicated in up to 90% of patients with asymptomatic, mild aminotransferase elevation not caused by alcohol, viral hepatitis, or medications

DESCRIPTION
- NAFL (1)
  – Reversible condition in which large vacuoles of triglyceride fat accumulate in hepatocytes
  – Liver biopsy: fatty deposits in >30% of cells, no hepatocyte ballooning, no necrosis, no fibrosis
  – Alanine aminotransferase/aspartate aminotransferase (ALT/AST) enzymes usually normal but may be elevated, rarely >3 to 4 times ULN
  – Minimal risk of progression to cirrhosis and liver failure
  – Synonym: steatosis
- Nonalcoholic steatohepatitis (NASH): progressive form of NAFL (1)
  – Liver biopsy: fatty deposits in >50% of cells with ballooning, acute/chronic inflammation, ± fibrosis
  – ALT and AST elevated, generally <3 to 4 times ULN
  – May progress to cirrhosis, liver failure, and rarely hepatocellular cancer; 30% with NASH may progress to fibrosis over 5 years.
- NASH cirrhosis (1)
  – Presence of cirrhosis with current or previous histologic evidence of steatosis or steatohepatitis

EPIDEMIOLOGY
- NAFLD: most common chronic liver disease globally; usually benign, asymptomatic
- Predicted to become the most frequent indication for liver transplantation by 2030 (2)
- NASH may be symptomatic with progressive inflammation and fibrosis.
  – Predominant age: 40s to 50s; can occur in children
  – Predominant sex: male > female (slight)

Incidence
Estimates vary widely from 31 to 86 cases of NAFLD per 10,000 person-years to 29/100,000 person-years (1)

Prevalence
- United States estimate: 30–40% (3)
- Worldwide: 6–33%, median 20% (1)
- Present in 58–74% of obese persons (BMI >30) and 90% of morbidly obese persons (BMI >39) (1)
- Among individuals with T2DM, rate of 69–87%; in patients with dyslipidemia, rate of 50% (1)

ETIOLOGY AND PATHOPHYSIOLOGY
Primary mechanism is *insulin resistance*, which leads to increased lipolysis, triglyceride synthesis, and increased hepatic uptake of fatty acids.
- NAFLD: excessive triglyceride accumulation in the liver and an impaired ability to remove fatty acids
- NASH: "2-hit" hypothesis: (i) macrovesicular steatosis due to increased hepatic lipid synthesis, reduced transfer of lipids, and increased insulin resistance with hepatic oxidative stress and (ii) mitochondrial damage leading to impaired restoration of ADT stores, lipid peroxidation, and resultant inflammatory injury (1)

- Other possible mechanism is lipotoxicity. Free fatty acid metabolites cause endoplasmic reticular stress, hepatocyte apoptosis, necrosis, and inflammation. Hepatocellular injury triggers fibrogenesis and inflammation, hastening disease progression (3).

Genetics
Largely unknown: Some familial clustering and increased heritability. NAFL: more first-degree relatives with cirrhosis than matched controls; NASH: 18% with affected first-degree relative. Carriers of hemochromatosis gene are more likely to be affected. Patatin-like phospholipase domain-containing 3 (PNPLA3) I148M polymorphism may play a role in NAFLD, hypertriglyceridemia, and insulin resistance (1,2).

RISK FACTORS
- Obesity (BMI >30), visceral obesity (waist circumference >102 cm for men or >88 cm for women), hypertension, dyslipidemia, high serum triglycerides and low serum high-density lipoprotein (HDL) levels, metabolic syndrome
- Type 2 diabetes, cardiovascular disease, and chronic kidney disease (2)
- Possible associations with hypothyroidism, hypopituitarism, hypogonadism, obstructive sleep apnea, pancreatoduodenal resection, osteoporosis, psoriasis, and polycystic ovary syndrome (2)
- Increasing age associated with increased prevalence, severity, advanced fibrosis, and mortality
- High fructose intake linked to intestinal dysbiosis and metabolic stress (4)
- Protein–calorie malnutrition; total parenteral nutrition (TPN) >6 weeks
- Severe weight loss (starvation, bariatric surgery)
- Organic solvent exposure (e.g., chlorinated hydrocarbons, toluene); vinyl chloride; hypoglycin A
- Gene for hemochromatosis/other conditions with increased iron stores
- Smoking (5)
- Drugs: tetracycline, glucocorticoids, tamoxifen, methotrexate, valproic acid, fialuridine, many chemotherapy regimens, and nucleoside analogues

Pregnancy Considerations
Acute fatty liver of pregnancy: Rare but serious complication in 3rd trimester. 50% of cases are associated with preeclampsia (6).
- Symptoms: nausea, vomiting, headache, fatigue, right upper quadrant or epigastric gain, jaundice
- Elevated ALT and AST >300 IU/L but usually <1,000 IU/L; elevated bilirubin
- Liver biopsy confirms diagnosis but should not delay treatment.
- Early recognition and prompt delivery is key
- Recurrence is rare (6)

Pediatric Considerations
- Increasing prevalence of NAFLD among children parallels rise in pediatric obesity.
- Reports of NAFLD as early as age 2 years and NASH-related cirrhosis as early as age 8 years
- Treat with intensive lifestyle modification. Vitamin E may be of possible benefit.
- Reye syndrome: fatty liver syndrome with encephalopathy usually following viral illness
  – Vomiting with dehydration
  – Confusion, progressive CNS damage
  – Hepatomegaly with extensive fatty vacuolization
  – Hypoglycemia (7)
- Etiology unknown; viral URIs and drugs (especially salicylates) have been implicated.

- Mortality rate: 50%
- Treat with mannitol, IV glucose, and FFP.

GENERAL PREVENTION
- Avoid excess alcohol: ≤3 standard drinks/day (men); ≤2 standard drinks/day (women)
- Maintain appropriate BMI.
- Prevention and optimal management of diabetes
- Avoid hepatotoxic medications.
- HAV and HBV vaccination if not immune
- Pneumococcal and annual influenza vaccinations

COMMONLY ASSOCIATED CONDITIONS
Central obesity; HTN; type 2 diabetes; insulin resistance; hyerlipidemia; preeclampsia in pregnancy; CVD; hypothyroidism; hypogonadism; OSA (2)

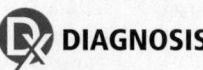 DIAGNOSIS

- Routine screening not recommended
- Consider NAFLD in patients with asymptomatic aminotransferase elevations (1)[A].
- Can occur with normal AST/ALT levels (1)[A]
- NAFLD has no distinguishing historical/lab features to distinguish from other chronic liver disorders.
- Index of suspicion is higher with risk factors such as metabolic syndrome, insulin resistance, or obesity.
- May present as cryptogenic cirrhosis
- Noninvasive biomarkers of steatosis/fibrosis are not sufficiently reliable. Liver biopsy is the definitive diagnostic test but should only be considered when results are likely to change management.

HISTORY
- Typically asymptomatic
- Possible fatigue and/or abdominal fullness
- Vague right upper quadrant pain
- History of medications, alcohol use, family history

PHYSICAL EXAM
Most common signs (all are infrequent)
- Liver tenderness
- Mild to marked hepatomegaly
- Splenomegaly
- In advanced cases: cutaneous stigmata of chronic liver disease or portal hypertension, for example, palmar erythema, spider angiomata, ascites

DIFFERENTIAL DIAGNOSIS
- Viral hepatitis
- Alcoholic fatty liver
- Drug- or toxin-induced hepatitis
- Metabolic liver disease
- Autoimmune hepatitis
- Celiac disease
- Muscle disease, if nonhepatic cause of elevated enzymes are possible

DIAGNOSTIC TESTS & INTERPRETATION
- Both ALT and AST may be elevated.
  – Nonalcoholic, usually ALT:AST >1
  – If alcohol-induced, usually AST:ALT ≥2
  – Nonspecific enzyme abnormalities may exist or may be normal with advanced cirrhosis (1).
- Level of enzyme elevation does NOT correlate with degree of fibrosis (1).
- Serum ferritin (1.5 times normal), alkaline phosphatase (2 to 3 times normal), and total and direct bilirubin may be elevated (1).

- Severity and chronicity are characterized by defects in ability to produce plasma proteins (serum albumin, PT) and thrombocytopenia (1).
- Lipids abnormalities are common and include elevated cholesterol, low-density lipoprotein (LDL), and triglyceride and decreased HDL (1).
- Biomarkers of inflammation, increased oxidative stress, or hepatocyte apoptosis such as leptin, adiponectin, CRP, serum caspase, and cytokeratin 18 may help differentiate NASH from NAFLD (1)[B].
- Serologic studies to exclude other etiologies of liver disease, for example, celiac, α-1-antitrypsin, iron, copper, HepA IgG, HepB SAg, HepC SAb, anti-smooth muscle antibody, ANA, serum gammaglobulin (1)[B]
- Ultrasound (US) is first-line imaging modality for assessing liver chemistry abnormalities: fatty liver is hyperechoic on US. MRI/CT may also be used (1)[B].

Follow-Up Tests & Special Considerations

- Imaging modalities such as FibroScan (which detects tissue elasticity in cases of suspected hepatic fibrosis) and MR spectroscopy (to assess changes in hepatic fat) are currently being evaluated to better characterize NAFLD (8)[B].
- No imaging modality can distinguish simple steatosis from steatohepatitis.

Diagnostic Procedures/Other

- Liver biopsy is the gold standard for diagnosis. To perform procedure, biopsy must have likelihood of changing management (1)[B].
- NAFLD fibrosis score age (>50 years), BMI (>30), platelet count, albumin, and AST/ALT ratio identifies patients at risk of developing fibrosis/cirrhosis (9)[B].

Test Interpretation

- Liver biopsy is the gold standard for prognosis (1).
- In NASH, steatosis, ballooning, and lobular inflammation are minimal criteria for diagnosis. Other common findings include mild to moderate portal inflammation, acidophil bodies, perisinusoidal zone 3 fibrosis, megamitochondria, and Mallory-Denk bodies (hyaline) in hepatocytes (1).
- Staging is based largely on the extent of fibrosis (1).

TREATMENT

- Sustained weight loss through lifestyle modification of at least 3–5% of body weight is most successful treatment (1,9)[A].
- Foregut bariatric surgery not yet proven to specifically treat NASH (1)[B]
- Aerobic exercise 3 to 5 times weekly for 20 to 45 minutes with reduced calorie intake/diet modifications (1)[B]
- Tight control of diabetes (1,9)[B]
- Treatment of metabolic syndrome—hypertension, dyslipidemia, and obesity (1,9)[B]
- Limit alcohol consumption (<21 drinks/week for men and <14 drinks/week for women) (9)[A].
- Avoid hepatotoxic medications (1)[B].

MEDICATION

Currently no effective medication treatment (1,9)[A]

Several promising agents include the following:

- Thiazolidinediones (pioglitazone) (1)[B]
- Vitamin E (1)[B]

- Other drugs studied in small studies (1,9,10)[B,C]
  - Statins, but study excluded cases with AST and AST >1.5 times normal limit
  - Gemfibrozil; omega-3 fatty acids
  - Angiotensin receptor blockers; probiotics
  - Obeticholic acid (bile acid derivative)
  - Ursodeoxycholic acid

ISSUES FOR REFERRAL

Persistent AST/ALT elevations 2 to 3 times above upper limit of normal without diagnosis or those with fibrosis on biopsy benefit from hepatology evaluation (1)[A].

SURGERY/OTHER PROCEDURES

Bariatric procedures: NAFLD is not a contraindication in otherwise eligible obese patients. There is a lack of data to definitively assess benefits and harms of surgery in treating patients with NASH (1)[B].

ONGOING CARE

FOLLOW-UP RECOMMENDATIONS

- Annual monitoring of LFTs (1,9)[B]
- Consider surveillance monitoring with US or CT scan to evaluate disease progression/improvement (9)[B]. Improvements can provide motivation for ongoing lifestyle changes.
- Routine liver biopsy is not recommended but may be repeated 5 years after baseline biopsy if progression of fibrosis is suspected (1,9)[B].
- Hepatic fibrosis staging is the strongest predictor for all-cause and disease-specific mortality in patients with histologically confirmed NAFLD (2)[B].

DIET

Low in saturated and trans fat; low in simple carbohydrates; avoid excessive alcohol (protective or worsening effect of light/moderate consumption inconclusive).

PATIENT EDUCATION

Extensive counseling on sustained lifestyle changes in nutrition, exercise, and alcohol use.

PROGNOSIS

Within the spectrum of NALFD, only NASH has been shown to be progressive, potentially leading to cirrhosis, hepatocellular carcinoma, cholangiocarcinoma, and/or liver failure (11):

- Cirrhosis develops in up to 15–20% of patients. Approximately 2–3% of patients with cirrhosis will develop HCC each year (3).
- Transplantation is effective, but NASH may recur after transplantation due to ongoing risk factors.

COMPLICATIONS

Progressive disease may lead to decompensated cirrhosis and portal hypertension with complications such as ascites, encephalopathy, bleeding varices, and hepatorenal or hepatopulmonary syndromes.

REFERENCES

1. Chalasani N, Younossi Z, Lavine JE, et al. The diagnosis and management of non-alcoholic fatty liver disease: practice guideline by the American Gastroenterological Association, American Association for the Study of Liver Diseases, and American College of Gastroenterology. *Gastroenterology.* 2012;142(7):1592–1609.
2. Byrne CD, Targher G. NAFLD: a multisystem disease. *J Hepatol.* 2015;62(1)(Suppl):S47–S64.
3. Spengler EK, Loomba R. Recommendations for diagnosis, referral for liver biopsy, and treatment of nonalcoholic fatty liver disease and nonalcoholic steatohepatitis. *Mayo Clin Proc.* 2015;90(9):1233–1246.
4. Sharma M, Mitnala S, Vishnubhotla RK, et al. The riddle of nonalcoholic fatty liver disease: progression from nonalcoholic fatty liver to nonalcoholic steatohepatitis. *J Clin Exp Hepatol.* 2015;5(2):147–158.
5. Than NN, Newsome PN. A concise review of non-alcoholic fatty liver disease. *Atherosclerosis.* 2015;239(1):192–202.
6. Ahmed KT, Almashhrawi AA, Rahman RN, et al. Liver diseases in pregnancy: diseases unique to pregnancy. *World J Gastroenterol.* 2013;19(43):7638–7646.
7. Hurwitz ES, Nelson DB, Davis C, et al. National surveillance for Reye syndrome: a five-year review. *Pediatrics.* 1982;70(6):895–900.
8. Browning JD. New imaging techniques for non-alcoholic steatohepatitis. *Clin Liver Dis.* 2009;13(4):607–619.
9. Nascimbeni F, Pais R, Bellentani S, et al. From NAFLD in clinical practice to answers from guidelines. *J Hepatol.* 2013;59(4):859–871.
10. Ratziu V, Goodman Z, Sanyal A. Current efforts and trends in the treatment of NASH. *J Hepatol.* 2015;62(1)(Suppl):S65–S75.
11. White DL, Kanwal F, El-Serag HB. Association between nonalcoholic fatty liver disease and risk for hepatocellular cancer, based on systematic review. *Clin Gastroenterol Hepatol.* 2012;10(12):1342–1359.e2.

ADDITIONAL READING

- Rinella ME. Nonalcoholic fatty liver disease: a systematic review. *JAMA.* 2015;313(22):2263–2273.
- Schwimmer JB, Pardee PE, Lavine JE, et al. Cardiovascular risk factors and the metabolic syndrome in pediatric nonalcoholic fatty liver disease. *Circulation.* 2008;118(3):277–283.
- Thoma C, Day CP, Trenell MI. Lifestyle interventions for the treatment of non-alcoholic fatty liver disease in adults: a systematic review. *J Hepatol.* 2012;56(1):255–266.

SEE ALSO

Alcohol Abuse and Dependence; Cirrhosis of the Liver; Diabetes Mellitus, Type 2; Metabolic Syndrome

CODES

ICD10
K76.0 Fatty (change of) liver, not elsewhere classified

CLINICAL PEARLS

- NAFLD: major cause of liver disease. Spectrum ranges from NAFL to NASH, advanced fibrosis, and cirrhosis.
- NAFLD: most common chronic liver disease in children; parallel rise in childhood obesity and NAFLD
- Lifestyle changes with targeted weight loss are the cornerstones of therapy for NAFLD.
- NAFLD is a common cause of asymptomatic mild serum aminotransferase elevation.

N

NOSOCOMIAL INFECTIONS

Cheryl Durand, PharmD • Edward L. Yourtee, MD, FACP

 BASICS

DESCRIPTION

- Health care–associated infections (HAIs)
- Infection must not have been present or incubating on admission to a health care facility.
- CDC categories:
  – Catheter-associated urinary tract infection (CAUTI)
  – Surgical site infection (SSI)
  – Ventilator-associated pneumonia (VAP)
  – Central line–associated bloodstream infection (CLABSI)
  – *Clostridium difficile* infection (C. diff, *C. difficile*, CDAD, CDI)
- The National Healthcare Safety Network (NHSN) at www.cdc.gov/nhsn monitors emerging HAI pathogens and their mechanisms of resistance to promote current prevention strategies.
- *Medicare and Medicaid will not pay for the treatment of certain HAI including CAUTIs, CLABSIs, and SSIs.*

EPIDEMIOLOGY

- General
  – 13/1,000 patient-days in the ICU (1)
  – 7/1,000 patient-days in high-risk nurseries
  – 2.6/1,000 patient-days in nurseries (1)
  – Estimated cost of HAIs is $20 billion per year (2).
- Infection specific
  – CAUTI
    ○ Hospital stay increased by 1 to 3 days.
    ○ Cost up to $600/infection
  – VAP
    ○ Hospital stay increased by 6 days.
    ○ Cost up to $5,000/infection
  – CLABSI
    ○ Hospital stay increased by 7 to 20 days.
    ○ Cost up to $56,000/infection
  – SSI
    ○ Hospital stay increased by 7.3 days.
    ○ Cost >$3,000/infection
    ○ May not be apparent until 1 month after surgery
  – *C. difficile* infection (see topic "*Clostridium difficile* Infection")

Incidence

- 1 out of 25 inpatients in the United States has at least one HAI (3).
  – 722,000 HAIs in U.S. acute care hospitals in 2011 (3)
  – UTI: 13% of HAIs (3)
  – Pneumonia: 22% of HAIs (3)
  – Bloodstream infection: 10% of HAIs (3)
  – SSI: 22% of HAIs (3)
  – 107,000 *C. difficile* cases in 2011(4)[A]
- Infections caused by gram-negative rods resistant to almost all antibiotics are increasing. Up to 70% of nosocomial infections are resistant to at least one previously active antimicrobial.

ETIOLOGY AND PATHOPHYSIOLOGY

- Endogenous spread: Patient host flora causes invasive disease (most common).
- Exogenous spread: Flora acquired from within health care facility.
- Causative organisms
  – UTI: *Escherichia coli*, *Klebsiella* spp., *Serratia* spp., *Enterobacter*, *Pseudomonas aeruginosa*, *Enterococcus* spp., *Candida albicans* (3)
  – Pneumonia: aerobic gram-negative bacilli, *Staphylococcus aureus*, *P. aeruginosa*, *Streptococcus* spp. (3)
  – Bloodstream infection: *Staphylococcus* spp., *Candida* spp., *Enterococcus* spp., gram-negative bacilli (3)

– SSI: *S. aureus*, gram-negative bacilli, *Enterococcus* spp., *Streptococcus* spp., *Enterobacter* spp., *Bacteroides* spp. (3)

RISK FACTORS

- Extremes of age
- Invasive surgical procedures (abdominal surgeries, orthopedic surgeries, urogynecologic surgeries, neurosurgery)
- Use of indwelling medical devices.
- Chronic disease (including diabetes, renal failure, and malignancy)
- Immunodeficiency
- Malnutrition
- Medications (recent antibiotics, proton pump inhibitors, and sedatives)
- Colonization with pathogenic strains of flora
- Breakdown of mucosal/cutaneous barriers, including trauma and battle wounds
- Anesthesia
- Lack of attention to detail with universal precautions

GENERAL PREVENTION

- Prevention should target both patient-specific and facility-related risk factors.
- Hand hygiene—thoroughly wash hands (5)[C]
  – On entering and leaving any patient room (5)
  – After contact with blood, excretions, body fluids, wound dressings, nonintact skin, mucous membranes (5)
  – Before using and after removing gloves (gloves are permeable to bacteria)
  – When moving hands from contaminated to clean body site (5)
  – Alcohol-based products are satisfactory when hands are not visibly soiled (5).
  – Soap and water should be used when surfaces are visibly soiled or when contact with spores is anticipated.
- Antibiotic stewardship—appropriate selection of antimicrobial therapy includes the following:
  – Judicious use of antibiotics to reduce the emergence of multidrug-resistant organisms and the occurrence of *C. difficile* infection (2).
  – Use of narrow-spectrum early-generation antibiotics when possible.
  – Taking an antibiotic "time out" at 72 hours to review the patient's clinical status and culture results, and eliminate ("streamline") any redundant or unnecessary antibiotics
  – Use shorter courses of antibiotics when appropriate.
- Hospital-based surveillance programs and antibiograms
- Infection control programs with specially trained employees (5)[C]
- Employee education on HAIs (5)[C]
- Disinfection of hospital rooms with hydrogen peroxide vapor or UV irradiation in addition to standard cleaning reduces environmental contamination and the risk of infection with multidrug-resistant organisms.
- Minimize invasive procedures.
- Caregiver stethoscope cleaning
  – Stethoscope bacterial contamination is common. Regular cleaning with alcohol-based preparations reduces bacterial load. Evidence is lacking to confirm whether stethoscope contamination causes nosocomial infections.
- Isolation of known pathogen carriers (5)[A]
  – Contact precautions
    ○ Institute for known pathogens spread by direct contact including methicillin-resistant *S. aureus*

(MRSA), vancomycin-resistant *Enterococcus* (VRE), *C. difficile*, extended-spectrum β-lactamase–producing gram-negative rods, and carbapenemase-producing gram-negative rods.
    ○ Glove when entering room (5)[B]
    ○ Gown if clothing will touch patient or environment (5)[B]
  – Droplet precautions
    ○ Infectious particles measure >5 μm.
    ○ Institute for pathogens shed via talking, coughing, sneezing, mucosal shedding, airway suctioning, and bronchoscopy. These include *Neisseria meningitidis*, influenza, *Haemophilus influenzae*, *Corynebacterium diphtheriae*, and *Bordetella pertussis*.
    ○ Mask when entering room (5)[B]
  – Airborne precautions
    ○ Infectious particles measure <5 μm.
    ○ Institute for pathogens shed via coughing including tuberculosis, varicella-zoster virus, and measles.
    ○ Fit-tested National Institute of Occupational Safety and Health (NIOSH)–approved ≥ N-95 respirator on entering room (5)[B]
- Infection-specific measures
  – CAUTI
    ○ Employee education on urinary catheters (indications, placement, maintenance)
    ○ Sterile catheter placement technique (6)[C]
    ○ Closed urine collection system (6)[C]
    ○ Use catheter only for necessary duration and remove as early as possible (6)[B].
    ○ Use of nurse-driven protocols for guideline-driven catheter removal.
    ○ Do not confuse catheter-associated asymptomatic bacteriuria with CAUTI.
    ○ Do not screen for bacteriuria by routinely performing a urine culture when the catheter is withdrawn.
  – VAP
    ○ Intubate only when clinically necessary (7)[C]
    ○ Perform oral decontamination with oral chlorhexidine (8)[A].
    ○ Avoid nasotracheal intubation (7)[B].
    ○ Inline suctioning (7)[C]
    ○ Elevate head to 30 to 45 degrees (7)[C].
  – CLABSI
    ○ Educate staff about appropriate use of IV catheters (indications, placement, maintenance) (9)[A].
    ○ Place catheters using sterile technique (including chlorhexidine prep and maximal barrier precautions) (9)[A].
    ○ Use order "bundles" to improve adherence to catheter insertion guidelines.
    ○ Remove catheter promptly when no longer clinically indicated (9)[A].
    ○ Hand hygiene in addition to glove use (9)[A]
    ○ Regularly monitor catheter site (9)[A].
    ○ With introduction of these measures, CLASBI rates fell 46% between 2008 and 2011 (10)[A].
  – SSI
    ○ Proper surgical hand hygiene (2)[B]
    ○ Prophylactic antibiotic therapy when indicated (2)[A]; eliminate underlying infections before surgery if possible (2)[A].

○ Remove hair with electric clippers/depilatory agent prior to incision (2)[B].

○ Poor postoperative blood sugar control increases risk of infection.

– C. difficile infection

○ Gloves combined with hand hygiene with soap and water (spores are resistant to alcohol-based products) (2)

○ Restrict use of fluoroquinolones, cephalosporins, and clindamycin when possible (2).

○ C. difficile is associated with the use of proton pump inhibitors: H₂ blockers is preferred for acid suppression (11)[A].

○ Probiotics may reduce nonspecific antibiotic-associated diarrhea; the effectiveness of probiotics for prevention of C. difficile is unclear (11).

– Bloodstream infections

○ Use of chlorhexidine-impregnated washcloths to bathe ICU patients reduces bloodstream infections by 28% (12)[B].

○ Routine surveillance for systemic inflammatory response syndrome (SIRS) using established criteria

DIAGNOSIS

Consistent with nature of infection

HISTORY
- Exposure to health care facility
- Recent surgery/open wounds
- History of invasive procedure
  - Urinary catheter placement
  - Indwelling vascular catheter
- Recent intubation/mechanical ventilation
- History of past infections (MRSA, VRE, etc.)

PHYSICAL EXAM
Consistent with nature of infection; site-specific exam for infections of skin, catheter sites, wounds, signs of sepsis, or pneumonia

DIFFERENTIAL DIAGNOSIS
- Community-acquired infection
- Sepsis/SIRS
- Other causes of infectious diarrhea

DIAGNOSTIC TESTS & INTERPRETATION
Specific to condition
- CBC, blood culture
- Wound culture
- Urine culture
- Chest x-ray
- Stool culture

Test Interpretation
Consistent with underlying infection

TREATMENT

GENERAL MEASURES
- Treat with appropriate antibiotics.
- Order bundles improve adherence to sepsis guidelines and improves survival.
- UTI: Remove urinary catheters.
- CLABSI: Remove IV catheter.
- C. difficile: Stop all antibiotics not being used to treat C. difficile infection.

MEDICATION
First Line
- Targeted antimicrobial therapy
- Several agents have been recently approved for the treatment of antibiotic-resistant infections and should be considered for second-line therapy.
  – Daptomycin, telavancin, dalbavancin, ceftaroline, oritavancin, tedizolid, ceftolozane-tazobactam, and ceftazidime-avibactam

ISSUES FOR REFERRAL
- Failure to respond to initial therapy
- Some emerging resistant gram-negative infections are resistant to nearly all antibiotics and require expert consultation for management.

SURGERY/OTHER PROCEDURES
- Screening for nasal carriage and isolation reduce the nosocomial spread of MRSA.
- Treating proven nasal carriers of Staphylococcus or MRSA with mupirocin prevents S. aureus nosocomial infections after surgery, as long as the prevalence of mupirocin resistance is low (13)[B].

INPATIENT CONSIDERATIONS
IV Fluids
As needed for hemodynamic support

Nursing
- Hand washing should be performed on entering and exiting the patient room even when there is no direct contact with the patient.
- Isolation precautions as indicated

Discharge Criteria
When infection has resolved or patient is stable and not an infectious risk

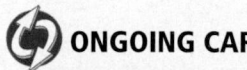

ONGOING CARE

FOLLOW-UP RECOMMENDATIONS
Patient Monitoring
Risk for recurrence is generally low in immunocompetent patients. Manage underlying comorbidities (risk factors).

PROGNOSIS
- 99,000 deaths in 2002 in the United States (1)
- Bloodstream infection mortality: 27%
- Pneumonia mortality: 33–50%
- SSI mortality: 11%

COMPLICATIONS
Related to specific nature of infection

REFERENCES

1. Klevens RM, Edwards JR, Richards CL Jr, et al. Estimating health care-associated infections and deaths in U.S. hospitals, 2002. Public Health Rep. 2007;122(2):160–166.
2. Yokoe DS, Mermel LA, Anderson DJ, et al. A compendium of strategies to prevent healthcare-associated infections in acute care hospitals. Infect Control Hosp Epidemiol. 2008;29(Suppl 1):S12–S21.
3. Magill SS, Edwards JR, Bamberg W, et al. Multistate point-prevalence survey of health care-associated infections. N Engl J Med. 2014;370(13): 1198–1208.
4. Lessa FC, Mu Y, Bamberg WM, et al. Burden of Clostridium difficile infection in the United States. N Engl J Med. 2015;372(9):825–834.
5. Siegel JD, Rhinehart E, Jackson M, et al. 2007 guideline for isolation precautions: preventing transmission of infectious agents in health care settings. Am J Infect Control. 2007;35(10)(Suppl 2): S65–S164.
6. Hooton TM, Bradley SF, Cardenas DD, et al. Diagnosis, prevention, and treatment of catheter-associated urinary tract infection in adults: 2009 international clinical practice guidelines from the Infectious Diseases Society of America. Clin Infect Dis. 2010;50(5):625–663.
7. Tablan OC, Anderson LJ, Besser R, et al. Guidelines for preventing health-care associated pneumonia, 2003: recommendations of CDC and the Healthcare Infection Control Practices Advisory Committee. MMWR Recomm Rep. 2004;53(RR-3):1–36.
8. Chan EY, Ruest A, Meade MO, et al. Oral decontamination for prevention of pneumonia in mechanically ventilated adults: systematic review and meta-analysis. BMJ. 2007;334(7599):889.
9. O' Grady NP, Alexander M, Burns LA, et al. 2011 Guidelines for the Prevention of Intravascular Catheter-Related Infections. www.cdc.gov/hicpac /BSI/01-BSI-guidelines-2011.html. Accessed 2011.
10. Centers for Disease Control and Prevention. 2013 National and State Healthcare-Associated Infections Progress Report. www.cdc.gov/hai /progress-report/index.html.
11. Surawicz CM, Brandt LJ, Binion DG, et al. Guidelines for diagnosis, treatment, and prevention of Clostridium difficile infections. Am J Gastroenterol. 2013;108(4).478–498.
12. Climo MW, Yokoe DS, Warren DK, et al. Effect of daily chlorhexidine bathing on hospital-acquired infection. N Engl J Med. 2013;368(6):533–542.
13. van Rijen M, Bonten M, Wenzel R, et al. Mupirocin ointment for preventing Staphylococcus aureus infections in nasal carriers. Cochrane Database Syst Rev. 2008;(4):CD006216.

CODES

ICD10
- T83.51XA Infect/inflm reaction due to indwell urinary catheter, init
- T81.4XXA Infection following a procedure, initial encounter
- J95.851 Ventilator associated pneumonia

CLINICAL PEARLS

- Nosocomial infections increase mortality, length of hospital stay, and cost of hospitalization.
- Preventive efforts should address patient-specific and facility-related risk factors.
- Proper hand hygiene, using an alcohol-based hand product or soap and water should be carried out before and after each patient encounter, even when gloves are used. Alcohol-based hand rubs are not effective for killing spores formed by C. difficile. Hand washing with soap and water is preferred in this situation.
- Adherence to contact, droplet, or airborne precautions reduces the spread of infection.
- The risk of developing a resistant nosocomial infection can be reduced by antibiotic streamlining, use of narrow-spectrum antibiotics, and frequent patient reevaluation to ensure the necessity of continuing antibiotics.

N

OBESITY

Maya Leventer-Roberts, MD, MPH

 BASICS

DESCRIPTION
- Obesity is the state of excess adipose tissue, frequently characterized in adults by body mass index (BMI), body weight (kg)/(body height [m^2]), of $\geq$30 kg/m^2.
- Obesity is associated with negative health outcomes (1), and the concurrent presence of abdominal obesity increases the risk of morbidity and mortality.
- System(s) affected: endocrine/metabolic, cardiac, respiratory, gastrointestinal, musculoskeletal, dermatologic, mental health
- Synonym(s): overweight; adiposity

Geriatric Considerations
Note: Underweight BMI ($\leq$18) is associated with an increased risk of mortality. The most likely explanation is that this is a secondary effect; severe chronic conditions can cause anorexia and weight loss.

EPIDEMIOLOGY
- Predominant age: Incidence rises in the early 20s.
- Predominant sex: female > male

Prevalence
- Mean prevalence of obesity among adults is 35% in the United States (2,3).
- Overweight: 40% of men and 25% of women
- Obese: 20% of men and 25% of women

Pediatric Considerations
- Pediatric obesity is defined as have a BMI at $\geq$95th percentile, as by age and sex specific WHO or CDC growth curves.
- Obesity during adolescence and young adulthood is strongly associated with obesity in adulthood.

ETIOLOGY AND PATHOPHYSIOLOGY
- Obesity is caused by an imbalance among food intake, absorption, and energy expenditure.
- Underlying organic causes include psychiatric disturbances, hypothyroidism, hypothalamic disorders, insulinoma, and Cushing syndrome.
- Medications can contribute to obesity, including corticosteroids, neuroleptics (particularly atypical antipsychotics), and antidepressants.

Genetics
- Genetic syndromes such as Prader-Willi and Bardet-Biedl are found in a minority of people with obesity.
- Studies are insufficiently powered to isolate specific genes as independent predictors of obesity.

RISK FACTORS
- Parental obesity
- Sedentary lifestyle
- Consumption of calorie-dense food
- Low socioeconomic status
- >2 hours per day of television viewing

GENERAL PREVENTION
- Encourage at least 1 hour of daily exercise, limited television viewing, and moderation in portion size.
- Avoid calorie-dense and nutrient-poor foods such as sweetened beverages and processed foods.

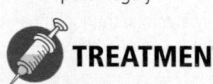 **DIAGNOSIS**

HISTORY
- Diet and exercise habits
- Prior attempts at weight loss
- Reported readiness to change lifestyle
- Social support and resources
- Comorbidities: diabetes mellitus type 2, hypertension, hyperlipidemia, sleep apnea
- Psychiatric history
- Symptoms suggesting hypothyroidism, Cushing syndrome, and genetic syndromes

PHYSICAL EXAM
- Elevated BMI:
  - Overweight: BMI = 25 to 29.9 kg/m^2
  - Obese: BMI 30 to 39.9 kg/m^2
  - Morbid obesity: BMI $\geq$40 kg/m^2
- Abdominal circumference:
  - Measuring around the abdomen at the level of the umbilicus.
    - Elevated:
      - Male: >40 inches (102 cm)
      - Female: >35 inches (88 cm)

DIAGNOSTIC TESTS & INTERPRETATION
- Yearly screening and laboratory assessment (4)[C]
- Screen for underlying physiologic causes as well as associated comorbid conditions.
- Labs should be done while fasting (nonfasting labs within normal limits are considered adequate).
- Preserved glucose, total insulin, hemoglobin A1C
- Serum lipid panel
- Thyroid function tests
- LFTs
- Imaging interpretation
  - Hypertrophy and/or hyperplasia of adipocytes
  - Cardiomegaly
  - Hepatomegaly

TREATMENT

GENERAL MEASURES
- Begin with the following assessment:
  - Motivation to lose weight (5)[A]
  - Patient-specific goals of therapy
  - Referral for intensive counseling for diet, exercise, and behavior modification
  - Long-term follow-up plan
- Goal for therapy is to achieve and sustain long-term weight loss up of at least 10% of body weight.
- Tracking of caloric intake and exercise
- Use of commercial weight loss programs (e.g., Weight Watchers) can be more effective than "standard of care" counseling (6)[B].
- Behavior therapy and cognitive-behavioral methods can result in modest weight loss but are most effective when combined with dietary and exercise treatments.

MEDICATION
- National Institute of Health guidelines suggest nonpharmacologic treatment for at least 6 months (5)[C].
- Medication treatment may be initiated for unsatisfactory weight loss in those with:
  - BMI $\geq$30
  - BMI $\geq$27 combined with associated risk factors (e.g., coronary artery disease, diabetes, sleep apnea, hypertension, hyperlipidemia)
- Diet, exercise, and behavior therapy *must* be included with pharmacologic treatment for those without comorbid conditions.
- Relapse may occur after discontinuation of medication.
- Treatment for comorbidities (such as diabetes and hyperlipidemia) should be considered.

First Line
- Medications may produce modest weight loss (7)[B].
- The lipase inhibitor orlistat (Xenical) decreases the absorption of dietary fat. Dose: 120 mg PO TID with meals containing fat; omit dose if meal is skipped or does not contain fat. Patients must avoid taking fat-soluble vitamin supplements within 2 hours of taking orlistat. The FDA has approved orlistat (Alli) 60 mg PO TID to be sold over the counter as a weight loss aid (8)[B]; adverse effects mainly GI (cramps, flatus, fecal incontinence)

- Contraindications
  - Orlistat: chronic malabsorption syndromes, cholestasis, pregnancy

Second Line
- Appetite suppressants recommended for short-term treatment ($\leq$6 months) (9)[A]

- Only beneficial in patients who exercise and eat reduced calorie diet
  - Naltrexone/bupropion (Contrave): 8 mg naltrexone/90 mg bupropion per tablet; slow titration up to 2 tablets PO BID by week 4; contraindicated if uncontrolled HTN, seizure disorder, chronic opioid use, pregnancy
  - Liraglutide (Saxenda): 1.203 mg SC once daily; GLP-1 agonist recently approved for obesity; discontinue if weight loss is <4% after 16 weeks.
  - Topiramate: Initiate with 25 mg BID and increase by 50 mg/week up to 100 mg PO BID; not FDA-approved for the treatment of obesity; tolerance is a concern (paresthesias, somnolence, difficulty concentrating).
- Schedule IV drugs
  - Lorcaserin (Belviq) 10 mg PO BID (D/C if weight loss is <5% after 12 weeks); works as serotonin agonist; avoid in those with CrCl <30 mL/min; contraindicated in pregnancy; avoid use with other serotonergic drugs.
  - Phentermine: 15, 30, 37.5 mg PO every morning; discontinue if tolerance or no response after 4 weeks; contraindicated if history of CV disease, hyperthyroidism, history of substance abuse, pregnancy

- Phentermine/topiramate (3.75 to 23 mg, 7.5 to 46 mg, 11.25 to 69 mg, 15 to 92 mg); initiate 3.75 to 23 mg PO once daily; requires enrollment into Risk Evaluation and Mitigation Strategy (REMS); women of childbearing age require negative pregnancy test prior to initiation and monthly thereafter
- Diethylpropion: 25 mg PO before meals TID; discontinue if no response after 4 weeks. Contraindicated if severe HTN, hyperthyroidism, history of substance abuse

Pregnancy Considerations
During pregnancy, obese women should gain fewer pounds than recommended for nonobese women.

SURGERY/OTHER PROCEDURES
Patients meeting criteria should be evaluated for gastric bypass or lap band procedures (10)[C].

- Requires complex presurgical evaluation, surgery, and follow-up in a skilled treatment center.

- Surgical treatment is the most effective long-term weight-loss treatment available for morbidly obese patients, but there is insufficient evidence on long-term outcomes (11)[A].

 ONGOING CARE

FOLLOW-UP RECOMMENDATIONS
- Exercise is an integral part of any weight loss program, yet exercise alone rarely results in significant weight loss.
- Combination of weight training and aerobic activity is preferred over aerobic activity alone.

Patient Monitoring
Long-term routine follow-up may prevent relapse after weight loss or further weight gain.

DIET
- Long-term studies suggest net calorie reduction of 500 to 1,000 kcal/day and ease of use are more important than the diet composition for long-term results (12)[A]:
  - A reduction of 500 kcal/day intake can result in ~1 lb (0.45 kg) weight loss per week.
  - Portion-controlled servings are recommended.
- Very low-calorie diet (400 to 800 kcal/day consumption)
  - Can result in more rapid weight loss than higher calorie diets but are less effective in the long term
  - Complications can include dehydration, orthostatic hypotension, fatigue, muscle cramps, constipation, headache, cold intolerance, and relapse after discontinuation
  - Contraindications: recent myocardial infarction or cerebrovascular accident, renal disease, cancer, pregnancy, insulin-dependent diabetes mellitus, and some psychiatric disturbances

PATIENT EDUCATION
- Emphasize the value of a healthy BMI.
- Recommended Web site:
  - www.nal.usda.gov/fnic/foodcomp/search for the FDA nutritional content in common foods

PROGNOSIS
- Lowest mortality associated with a BMI of 22
- Long-term maintenance of weight loss is difficult to achieve.
- A motivated patient is most likely to achieve successful weight loss (13).

COMPLICATIONS
- Cardiovascular disease
- Stroke (in men)
- Thromboembolism
- Heart failure
- Hypertension
- Hypoventilation and sleep apnea syndromes
- Higher death rates from cancer: colon, breast, prostate, endometrial, gallbladder, liver, kidney
- Diabetes mellitus
- Skin changes
- Hyperlipidemia
- Gallbladder disease
- Osteoarthritis
- Gout
- Poor self-esteem
- Discrimination
- Increased sick leave

REFERENCES
1. Flegal K, Graubard B, Williamson D, et al. Excess deaths associated with underweight, overweight, and obesity. *JAMA.* 2005;293(15):1861–1867.
2. Ogden CL, Carroll MD, Flegal KM. Prevalence of obesity in the United States. *JAMA.* 2014;312(2):189–190.
3. Ogden CL, Carroll MD, Fryar CD, et al. Prevalence of obesity among adults and youth: United States, 2011-2014. *NCHS Data Brief.* 2015;(219):1–8.
4. National Heart, Lung and Blood Institute, National Institutes of Health, U.S. Department of Health and Human Services. *Clinical guidelines on the identification, evaluation, and treatment of overweight and obesity in adults: the evidence report.* Bethesda, MD: National Institutes of Health; 1998. NIH Publication 98-4083.
5. Shaw K, O'Rourke P, Del Mar C, et al. Psychological interventions for overweight or obesity. *Cochrane Database Syst Rev.* 2005;(2):CD003818.
6. Jebb SA, Ahern AL, Olson AD, et al. Primary care referral to a commercial provider for weight loss treatment versus standard care: a randomised controlled trial. *Lancet.* 2011;378(9801):1485–1492.
7. Padwal R, Li SK, Lau DC. Long-term pharmacotherapy for obesity and overweight. *Cochrane Database Syst Rev.* 2004;(3):CD004094.
8. Kramer CK, Leitão CB, Pinto LC, et al. Efficacy and safety of topiramate on weight loss: a meta-analysis of randomized controlled trials. *Obes Rev.* 2011;12(5):e338–e347.
9. Dombrowski SU, Knittle K, Avenell A, et al. Long term maintenance of weight loss with non-surgical interventions in obese adults: systematic review and meta-analyses of randomised controlled trials. *BMJ.* 2014;348:g2646. doi:10.1136/bmj.g2646.
10. Colquitt J, Clegg A, Loveman E, et al. Surgery for morbid obesity. *Cochrane Database Syst Rev.* 2005;(4):CD003641.
11. Puzziferri N, Roshek TB III, Mayo HG, et al. Long-term follow-up after bariatric surgery: a systematic review. *JAMA.* 2014;312(9):934–942.
12. Thomas DE, Elliott EJ, Baur L. Low glycaemic index or low glycaemic load diets for overweight and obesity. *Cochrane Database Syst Rev.* 2007;(3):CD005105.
13. Ogden LG, Stroebele N, Wyatt HR, et al. Cluster analysis of the national weight control registry to identify distinct subgroups maintaining successful weight loss. *Obesity (Silver Spring).* 2012;20(10):2039–2047.

 CODES

ICD10
- E66.9 Obesity, unspecified
- E66.3 Overweight
- R63.5 Abnormal weight gain

CLINICAL PEARLS
- Drug treatment with a first-line medication may be indicated when nonpharmacologic treatment for 6 months has been ineffective and the patient has a BMI >30 or a BMI >27 with associated risk factors. Medications may achieve a modest long-term weight loss.
- Surgical treatment may be indicated in patients with a BMI >40 who have failed more conservative treatment, particularly when there are associated risk factors, such as diabetes mellitus.
- No convincing evidence supports a specific diet method.

OBSESSIVE-COMPULSIVE DISORDER (OCD)

Amar Kapur, DO, CPT, MC, USA

 BASICS

DESCRIPTION
- A psychiatric condition classified as an anxiety disorder characterized by pathologic obsessions (recurrent intrusive thoughts, ideas, or images) and compulsions (repetitive, ritualistic behaviors or mental acts) causing significant patient distress
- Not to be confused with obsessive-compulsive personality disorder

EPIDEMIOLOGY
Incidence
- Predominant age: mean age of onset 22 to 36 years
  - Male = female (males present at younger age)
  - Child/adolescent onset in 33% of cases
  - 1/3 of cases present by age 15 years
  - 85% of cases present at <35 years of age
  - Diagnosis rarely made at >50 years of age
- Predominant gender: female > males but males more commonly affected in childhood

Pediatric Considerations
Insidious onset; consider brain insult in acute presentation of childhood obsessive-compulsive disorder (OCD).

Geriatric Considerations
Consider neurologic disorders in new-onset OCD in the elderly.

Prevalence
- 2.3% lifetime in adults
- 1–2.3% prevalence in children/adolescents

ETIOLOGY AND PATHOPHYSIOLOGY
- Exact pathophysiology is unknown.
- Dysregulation of serotonergic pathways
- Dysregulation of corticostriatal-thalamic-cortico (CSTC) pathway
- Exact etiology unknown
- Genetic and environmental factors
- Pediatric autoimmune disorder associated with streptococcal infections

Genetics
- Greater concordance in monozygotic twins
- Positive family history: prevalence rates of 7–15% in first-degree relatives of children/adolescents with OCD

RISK FACTORS
- Exact cause of OCD is not fully elucidated.
- Combination of biologic and environmental factors likely involved the following:
  - Link between low serotonin levels and development of OCD
  - Link between brain insult and development of OCD (i.e., encephalitis, pediatric streptococcal infection, or head injury)

GENERAL PREVENTION
- OCD cannot be prevented.
- Early diagnosis and treatment can decrease patient's distress and impairment.

COMMONLY ASSOCIATED CONDITIONS
- Major depressive disorder
- Panic disorder
- Phobia/social phobia
- Tourette syndrome/tic syndromes and other movement disorders
- Substance abuse
- Eating disorder/body dysmorphic disorder

 DIAGNOSIS

HISTORY
- Patient presents with either obsessions or compulsions, which cause marked distress, are time-consuming (>1 hr/day) and cause significant occupational/social impairment.
- Four criteria support diagnosis of obsessions:
  - Patients are aware that they are thinking the obsessive thoughts; thoughts are not imposed from outside (as in thought insertion).
  - Thoughts are not just excessive worrying about real-life problems.
  - Recurrent thoughts are persistent, intrusive, and inappropriate, causing significant anxiety and distress.
  - Attempts to suppress intrusive thoughts are made with some other thought/activity.
- Two criteria support a diagnosis of compulsions:
  - The response to an obsession is to perform repetitive behaviors (e.g., hand washing) or mental acts (e.g., counting silently) rigidly.
  - Although done to reduce stress, the responses are either not realistically connected with the obsession or they are excessive.
  - In children, check for precedent streptococcal infection.

PHYSICAL EXAM
- Dermatologic problems caused by excessive hand washing may be observed.
- Hair loss caused by compulsive pulling/twisting of the hair (trichotillomania) may be observed.

DIFFERENTIAL DIAGNOSIS
- Obsessive-compulsive personality disorder
  - In personality disorder, traits are ego-syntonic and include perfectionism and preoccupation with detail, trivia, or procedure and regulation. Patients tend to be rigid, moralistic, and stingy. These traits are often rewarded in the patient's job as desirable.
- Impulse-control disorders: compulsive gambling, sex, or substance abuse: The compulsive behavior is not in response to obsessive thoughts, and the patient derives pleasure from the activity.
- Major depressive disorder
- Eating disorder
- Tics (in tic disorder) and stereotyped movements
- Schizophrenia: Patient perceives thought to be true and coming from an external source.
- Generalized anxiety disorder, phobic disorders, separation anxiety: similar response on heightened anxiety, but presence of obsessions and rituals signifies OCD diagnosis
- Anxiety disorder due to a general medical condition: Obsessions/compulsions are assessed to be a direct physiologic consequence of a general medical condition.

DIAGNOSTIC TESTS & INTERPRETATION
According to *DSM-5*, diagnostic criteria for OCD are (1)[C]:
- Presence of obsessions, compulsions, or both
- Obsessions are defined by:
  - Recurrent or persistent thoughts, urges, or images that are experienced at some time during the disturbance, as intrusive and unwanted, and that in most individuals cause marked anxiety or distress
  - The individual attempts to ignore or suppress such thoughts, urges, or images or to neutralize them with some other thought or actions (i.e., by performing compulsion).

- Compulsions are defined by the following:
  - Repetitive behavior (e.g., hand washing, ordering, checking) or mental acts (e.g., praying, counting, repeating words silently) that the individual feels driven to perform in response to an obsession or according to rules that must be applied rigidly.
  - The behavior or mental acts are aimed at preventing or reducing anxiety or distress or preventing some dreaded event or situation. However, these behavior or mental acts are not connected in a realistic way with what they are designed to neutralize or prevent or are clearly excessive.
- The obsessions or compulsions are time-consuming (e.g., take >1 hr/day) or cause clinically significant distress or impairment in social, occupational, or other important areas of functioning.
- The obsessive-compulsive symptoms are not attributable to the physiologic effects of a substance (e.g., a drug of abuse, a medication, or other medical condition).
- The disturbance is not better explained by the symptoms of another mental disorder (e.g., excessive worries, as in generalized anxiety disorder, preoccupation with appearance, as in body dysmorphic disorder or skin picking etc.).
- Specify if:
  - With good or fair insight: The individual recognizes the OCD beliefs are definitely or probably not true or that they may or may not be true.
  - With poor insight: The individual thinks that OCD beliefs are probably true.
  - With absent insight/delusional beliefs: The individual is completely convinced that OCD beliefs are true.
- Specify if:
  - Tic related: The individual has a current or past history of tic disorder.

Diagnostic Procedures/Other
- Yale-Brown Obsessive-Compulsive Scale (Y-BOCS) or CY-BOCS for children (2)[C]
- Maudsley Obsessive-Compulsive Inventory (MOCI) (3)[C]

Test Interpretation
- Compulsions are designed to relieve the anxiety of obsessions; they are not inherently enjoyable (ego-dynastic) and do not result in completion of a task.
- Common obsessive themes
  - Harm (i.e., being responsible for an accident)
  - Doubt (i.e., whether doors/windows are locked or the iron is turned off)
  - Blasphemous thoughts (i.e., in a devoutly religious person)
  - Contamination, dirt, or disease
  - Symmetry/orderliness
- Common rituals or compulsions
  - Hand washing, cleaning
  - Checking
  - Counting
  - Hoarding
  - Ordering, arranging
  - Repeating
- Neither obsessions nor compulsions are related to another mental disorder (i.e., thoughts of food and presence of eating disorder).
- 80–90% of patients with OCD have obsessions and compulsions.
- 10–19% of patients with OCD are pure obsessional.

TREATMENT

GENERAL MEASURES

- Combined medications and cognitive-behavioral therapy (CBT) is most effective (1,2)[A].
- Family psychoeducation
- Parent behavior management training if patient is a child/adolescent
- Brain modulation available for severe OCD includes electroconvulsive therapy and transcranial magnetic stimulation in small groups of patients.

MEDICATION

First Line

- Adequate trial at least 10 to 12 weeks
- Doses may exceed typical doses for depression.
- Optimal duration for pediatrics unknown but recommended minimum of maintenance treatment: 6 months

- SSRIs recommended first-line agents (4,5)[A]

  - Fluoxetine (Prozac)
    - Adults: 20 mg/day; increase by 10 to 20 mg every 4 to 6 weeks until response; range: 20 to 80 mg/day
    - Children (7 to 17 years of age): 10 mg/day; increase 4 to 6 weeks until response; range: 20 to 60 mg/day
  - Sertraline (Zoloft)
    - Adults: 50 mg/day; increase by 50 mg every 4 to 7 days until response; range: 50 to 200 mg/day; may divide if above 100 mg/day
    - Children (6 to 17 years of age): 25 mg/day; increase by 25 mg every 7 days until response; range: 50 to 200 mg/day
  - Paroxetine (Paxil)
    - Adults: 20 mg/day; increase by 10 mg every 4 to 7 days until response; range: 40 to 60 mg/day
    - Children: Safety and effectiveness in patients <18 years have not been established.
  - Fluvoxamine (Luvox)
    - Adult: 100 mg/day; increase by 50 mg every 4 to 7 days until response; range: 200 to 300 mg/day
    - Children (8 to 17 years of age): 25 mg/day; increase by 25 mg every 4 to 7 days until response; range: 50 to 200 mg/day
- Absolute SSRI contraindications
  - Hypersensitivity to SSRIs
  - Concomitant use within 14 days of monoamine oxidase inhibitor (MAOI)
- Relative SSRI contraindications
  - Severe liver impairment
  - Seizure disorders (lower seizure threshold)
- Precautions
  - Watch for suicidal behavior/worsening depression during first few months of therapy/after dosage changes with antidepressants, particularly in children, adolescents, and young adults.
  - Long half-life of fluoxetine (>7 days) may be troublesome if patient has an adverse reaction.
  - May cause drowsiness and dizziness when therapy was initiated; warn patients about driving and heavy equipment hazards.

Pregnancy Considerations

All SSRIs are pregnancy Category C, except paroxetine, which is Category D.

Second Line

- Try switching to another SSRI.
- 40–60% of patients will remain refractory to SSRI

- Tricyclic acid (TCA), clomipramine (Anafranil)
  - Adults: 25 mg/day; increase gradually over 2 weeks to 100 mg/day, then to 250 mg/day (max dose) over next several weeks, as tolerated.
  - Children (10 to 17 years of age): 25 mg/day; titrate as needed and tolerated up to 3 mg/kg/day or 200 mg/day (whichever is less).
  - Absolute clomipramine contraindications
    - Within 6 months of a myocardial infarction (MI)
    - Hypersensitivity to clomipramine or other TCA
    - Concomitant use within 14 days of an MAOI
    - 3rd-degree atrioventricular (AV) block
  - Relative clomipramine contraindications
    - Narrow-angle glaucoma (increased intraocular pressure)
    - Prostatic hypertrophy (urinary retention)
    - 1st- or 2nd-degree AV block, bundle-branch block, and congestive heart failure (proarrhythmic effect)
    - Pregnancy Category C
  - Precautions
    - Dangerous in overdose
    - Pretreatment ECG for patients >40 years of age
    - Watch for suicidal behavior/worsening depression during first few months of therapy or after dosage changes with antidepressants, particularly in children, adolescents, and young adults.
    - May cause drowsiness and dizziness when therapy is initiated; warn patients about driving and heavy equipment hazards.

ISSUES FOR REFERRAL

- Psychiatric referral for CBT (in vivo exposure and prevention of compulsions)
- Psychiatric evaluation if obsessions and compulsions significantly interfere with patient's functioning in social, occupational, or educational situations

ADDITIONAL THERAPIES

Dopamine receptor antagonists (antipsychotic agents) alone are not effective in treatment of OCD. They can be used as augmentation to SSRI therapy for treatment-resistant OCD; they also can worsen OCD symptoms (4)[C]. Some evidence show that addition of quetiapine or risperidone to antidepressants will increase efficacy; data with olanzapine are too limited to draw conclusions (4)[A].

- Risperidone (Risperdal): initial dose: 0.5 mg/day; target dose: 0.5 to 2 mg/day
- Quetiapine (Seroquel): initial dose: 25 mg/day; target dose: 600 mg/day

 ## ONGOING CARE

FOLLOW-UP RECOMMENDATIONS

Y-BCOS or MOCI surveys to track progress

Patient Monitoring

Monitor for decrease in obsessions and time spent performing compulsions.

DIET

No dietary modifications/restrictions recommended

PATIENT EDUCATION

- Importance of medication adherence
- Importance of psychotherapy (CBT)
- International OCD Foundation, Boston, MA 617-973-5801: https://iocdf.org/
- Obsessive Compulsive Anonymous, New Hyde Park, NY: http://obsessivecompulsiveanonymous.org

PROGNOSIS

- Chronic waxing and waning course in most patients:
  - 24–33% fluctuating course
  - 11–14% phasic periods of remission
  - 54–61% chronic progressive course
- Early onset a poor predictor

COMPLICATIONS

- Depression in 1/3 patients with OCD
- Avoidant behavior (phobic avoidance)
  - Children may drop out of education.
  - Adults may become homebound.
- Anxiety and panic-like episodes associated with obsessions

REFERENCES

1. American Psychiatric Association. *Diagnostic and Statistical Manual of Mental Disorders.* 5th ed. Washington, DC: American Psychiatric Association.
2. Sánchez-Meca J, Lopez-Pina JA, Lopez-Lopez JA, et al. The Maudsley Obsessive-Compulsive Inventory. *Int J Clin Health Psychol.* 2011;11(3):473–493.
3. Gava I, Barbui C, Aguglia E, et al. Psychological treatments versus treatment as usual for obsessive compulsive disorder (OCD). *Cochrane Database Sys Rev.* 2007;(2):CD005333.
4. Stein DJ, Denys D, Gloster AT, et al. Obsessive-compulsive disorder: diagnostic and treatment issues. *Psychiatr Clin North Am.* 2009;32(3):665–685.
5. Kakhi S, Soomro GM. Obsessive compulsive disorder in children and adolescents: duration of maintenance drug treatment [published ahead of print June 3, 2015]. *BMJ Clin Evid.*
6. Komossa K, Depping AM, Meyer M, et al. Second-generation antipsychotics for obsessive compulsive disorder. *Cochrane Database Sys Rev.* 2010;(12):CD008141.

ADDITIONAL READING

Ruscio AM, Stein DJ, Chiu WT, et al. The epidemiology of obsessive-compulsive disorder in the National Comorbidity Survey Replication. *Mol Psychiatry.* 2010;15(1):53–63.

CODES

ICD10

- F42 Obsessive-compulsive disorder
- F63.9 Impulse disorder, unspecified
- F63.3 Trichotillomania

CLINICAL PEARLS

- CBT is the initial treatment of choice for mild OCD.
- CBT plus an SSRI or an SSRI alone is the treatment choice for more severe OCD.
- The majority of patients with OCD respond to first SSRI treatment.
- Improvement in symptoms however, is often incomplete, ranging from 25% to 60%.

OCULAR CHEMICAL BURNS

Robert J. Hyde, MD, MA, NRP, FACEP • Patricia Ruth Atchinson, DO

 ## BASICS

DESCRIPTION
- Chemical exposure to the eye can result in rapid, devastating, and permanent damage and is one of the true emergencies in ophthalmology.
- Separate alkaline from acid chemical exposure
  - Alkali burns: more severe. Alkaline compounds are lipophilic, penetrating rapidly into eye tissue; saponification of cells leads to necrosis and may produce injury to lids, conjunctiva, cornea, sclera, iris, and lens (cataracts).
  - Acid burns: Acid usually does not damage internal structures because its associated anion causes protein denaturation, creating a barrier to further acid penetration. (Hydrofluoric acid is an exception to this rule; see below.) Injury is often limited to lids, conjunctiva, and cornea.
- System(s) affected: nervous, skin/exocrine
- Synonym(s): chemical ocular injuries

EPIDEMIOLOGY
- Predominant age: can occur at any age, peak from 20 to 40 years of age
- Predominant sex: male > female

Incidence
- Estimated 300/100,000 per year
- Alkali burns twice as common as acid burns

ETIOLOGY AND PATHOPHYSIOLOGY
- Acidic compounds
  - Anion leads to protein denaturing and protective barrier formation by coagulation necrosis forming an eschar. This more superficial mechanism of injury tends to have prominent scarring that may lead to vision loss:
    - Hydrofluoric acid is an exception. In its nonionized form, it behaves like an alkaline substance, capable of penetrating the corneal stroma and leading to extensive anterior segment lesions. When ionized, it may combine with intracellular calcium and magnesium to form insoluble complexes, leading to potassium ion movements and cell death. Once systemically absorbed, severe hypocalcemia can occur.
- Alkaline compounds
  - Lipophilic compounds that penetrate into deep structures on disassociation into cations and hydroxide
  - Hydroxide causes saponification of fatty acids in cell membranes, leading to cell death.
  - Cation causes hydration of glycosaminoglycans, leading to corneal opacification and hydration of collagen, resulting in rapid shortening and thickening of collagen fibrils that leads to an acute elevation in intraocular pressure secondary to shrinking and contraction of the cornea and sclera.
  - Long-term elevation in intraocular pressure may occur from accumulation of inflammatory debris within the trabecular meshwork.
  - Penetration into deep structures may also affect perfusing vessels, leading to ischemia of affected area.

Sources of Alkaline and Acidic Compounds

Alkaline Compounds	Typical Sources
Calcium hydroxide (lime)	Cement, whitewash
Sodium hydroxide (lye)	Drain cleaner, airbags
Potassium hydroxide (lye)	Drain cleaner
Ammonia	Cleaning agents
Ammonium hydroxide	Fertilizers
Acidic Compounds	**Typical Sources**
Sulfuric acid	Car batteries
Sulfurous acid	Bleach
Hydrochloric acid	Chem labs, swimming pools
Acetic acid	Vinegar
Hydrofluoric acid	Glass polish

RISK FACTORS
- Construction work (plaster, cement, whitewash)
- Use of cleaning agents (drain cleaners, ammonia)
- Automobile battery explosions (sulfuric acid)
- Industrial work, including work in industrial chemical laboratories
- Alcoholism
- Any risk factor for assault (~10% of injuries due to deliberate assault)

GENERAL PREVENTION
Safety glasses to safeguard eyes

COMMONLY ASSOCIATED CONDITIONS
Facial (including eyelids) cutaneous chemical or thermal burns

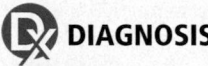 ## DIAGNOSIS

HISTORY
- Most often complaints of pain, photophobia, blurred vision, and a foreign body sensation
- In alkali burns, can have initial pain that later diminishes
- Mild burns: pain and blurred vision
- Moderate to severe burns: severe pain and markedly reduced vision

PHYSICAL EXAM
- Acidic compound may present with a ground-glass appearance secondary to superficial scar formation.
- Alkaline compounds may present with corneal opacification secondary to glycosaminoglycan hydration; however, severe acid burns may also present with this finding.
- Mild burns
  - Blurry vision
  - Eyelid skin erythema and edema
  - Corneal epithelial defects or superficial punctate keratitis
  - Conjunctival chemosis, hyperemia, and hemorrhages without perilimbal ischemia
  - Mild anterior chamber reaction
- Moderate to severe burns
  - Reduced vision
  - 2nd- and 3rd-degree burns of eyelid skin
  - Corneal edema and opacification
  - Corneal epithelial defects
  - Marked conjunctival chemosis and perilimbal blanching
  - Moderate anterior chamber reaction
  - Increased intraocular pressure
  - Local necrotic retinopathy

DIFFERENTIAL DIAGNOSIS
- Thermal burns
- Ocular cicatricial pemphigoid
- Other causes of corneal opacification
- Ultraviolet radiation keratitis

DIAGNOSTIC TESTS & INTERPRETATION
Not necessary unless suspicion of intraocular or orbital foreign body is present. In this case, CT should be used and MRI is contraindicated.

Diagnostic Procedures/Other
- Measure pH of tear film with litmus paper or electronic probe:
  - Irrigating fluid with nonneutral pH (e.g., normal saline has pH of 4.5) may alter results.
- Careful slit-lamp exam, fundus ophthalmoscopy, tonometry, and measurement of visual acuity
- Full extent of damage from alkali burns may not be apparent until 48 to 72 hours after exposure.

Test Interpretation
- Corneal epithelial defects or superficial punctate keratitis, edema, opacification
- Conjunctival chemosis, hyperemia, and hemorrhages
- Perilimbal ischemia
- Anterior chamber reaction
- Increased intraocular pressure

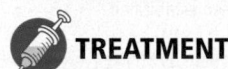 ## TREATMENT

Copious irrigation and removal of corneal or conjunctival foreign bodies are always the initial treatment (1–3)[A]:

- Passively open patient's eyelid and have patient look in all directions while irrigating.
- Be sure to remove all reservoirs of chemical from the eyes.
- Continue irrigation until the tear film and superior/inferior cul-de-sac is of neutral pH (7 ± 0.1) and pH is stable (2)[C]:
  - Severe burns should be irrigated for at least 15 minutes to as much as 2 to 4 hours; this irrigation should not be interrupted during transportation to hospital (2)[C].
  - Irrigation via Morgan lens (polymethylmethacrylate scleral lens) is a good way to achieve continuous irrigation over a prolonged period of time.
  - It is impossible to overirrigate.
- Initial pH testing should be done on both eyes even if the patient claims to only have unilateral ocular pain/irritation so that a contralateral injury is not neglected.

- Use whatever nontoxic fluid is available for irrigation on scene. In hospital, sterile water, normal saline, normal saline with bicarbonate, balanced salt solution (BSS), or lactated Ringer solution may be used:
  - No therapeutic difference in effectiveness has been noted between types of solutions (1)[C].
- A topical anesthetic can be used to provide patient comfort (e.g., proparacaine, tetracaine).
- Sweep the conjunctival fornices every 12 to 24 hours to prevent adhesions (2)[C].
- Eye patching may relieve pain but has not been shown to improve outcomes (4)[C].

MEDICATION
First Line
- Further treatment (depending on severity and associated conditions)
  - Topical prophylactic antibiotics: any broad-spectrum agent (e.g., bacitracin–polymyxin B [Polysporin] ointment q2–4h, ciprofloxacin [Ciloxan] drops q2–4h, chloramphenicol [Chloroptic] ointment q2–4h) (1)[C]:
    ○ Some experts suggest that systemic tetracycline 250 mg PO q6h and especially derivatives such as doxycycline 100 mg PO BID may be beneficial to encourage healing of persistent corneal epithelial defects by inhibiting metalloproteinases (5)[C].
  - Tear substitutes: hydroxypropyl methylcellulose (HypoTears PF, Refresh Plus) drops q4h, carboxymethylcellulose (Refresh PM) ointment at bedtime (1)[C]:
    ○ Most beneficial in those with impaired tear production (elderly patients)
  - Cycloplegics for photophobia and/or uveitis: cyclopentolate 1% TID or scopolamine 1/4% BID (1)[C]
  - Antiglaucoma for elevated intraocular pressure: latanoprost (Xalatan) 0.005% q24h, timolol (Timoptic) 0.5% BID, or levobunolol (Betagan) 0.5% BID, and/or acetazolamide (Diamox) 125 to 250 mg PO q6h, or methazolamide (Neptazane) 25 to 50 mg PO BID, and/or IV mannitol 20% 1 to 2 g/kg as needed (1)[C]
  - Corticosteroids for intraocular inflammation: prednisolone (Pred-Forte) 1% or equivalent q1–4h for 7 to 10 days; if severe, prednisone 20 to 60 mg PO daily for 5 to 7 days. Taper rapidly if epithelium is intact by this time (1)[C]:
    ○ Use of corticosteroids >10 days may do harm by inhibiting repair and cause corneoscleral melt (1,6)[C].
  - Vitamin C (ascorbic acid) 500 mg PO QID and topical 10% ascorbate solution in artificial tears reduces the incidence of corneal thinning and ulceration (2)[C].
  - Acetylcysteine (Mucomyst) 10–20% topically q4h to promote wound healing (2)[C]
- Precautions
  - Timolol and levobunolol: history of heart failure (HF) or chronic obstructive pulmonary disease (COPD)
  - Acetazolamide and methazolamide: history of nephrolithiasis or metabolic acidosis
  - Mannitol: history of HF or renal failure
  - Scopolamine: history of urinary retention
  - Topical corticosteroids must be used with caution in the presence of damaged corneal epithelium because iatrogenic infection can occur. Daily follow-up or consultation with an ophthalmologist is recommended.

SURGERY/OTHER PROCEDURES
- Goal of subacute treatment is restoration of the normal ocular surface anatomy, control of glaucoma, and restoration of corneal clarity.
- Surgical options include the following:
  - Débridement of necrotic tissue (1)[C]
  - Conjunctival/tenon advancement (tenoplasty) to restore vascularity in severe burns (1)[C]
  - Tissue adhesive (e.g., isobutyl cyanoacrylate) for impending or actual corneal perforation of
    ○ Tectonic keratoplasty for acute perforation >1 mm (1)[C]
  - Limbal autograft transplantation for epithelial stem cell restoration (1)[C]
  - Amniotic membrane transplantation (6)[C] or umbilical cord serum drops (*)[B] to promote epithelial regeneration (6)[C]
  - Conjunctival or mucosal membrane transplant to restore ocular surface in severe injury (1)[C]
  - Lamellar or penetrating keratoplasty for tectonic stabilization or visual rehabilitation (1)[C]

INPATIENT CONSIDERATIONS
Admission Criteria/Initial Stabilization
Based on ophthalmologic consultation and concomitant burn injuries

 ONGOING CARE

FOLLOW-UP RECOMMENDATIONS
Patient Monitoring
- Depending on severity of ocular injury
  - From daily to weekly visits initially
- May be inpatient
- If on mannitol or prednisone, consider frequent serum electrolytes.

PATIENT EDUCATION
- Safety glasses
- Need for immediate ocular irrigation with any available water following chemical exposure to the eyes

PROGNOSIS
- Depends on severity of initial injury: Increased limbal involvement in clock hours and greater percentage of conjunctival involvement correlate with poorer prognosis (Dua classification system).
- For mildly injured eyes, complete recovery is the norm.
- For severely injured eyes, permanent loss of vision is not uncommon.

COMPLICATIONS
- Orbital compartment syndrome
- Persistent epitheliopathy
- Fibrovascular pannus
- Corneal ulcer/perforation
- Corneal scarring
- Progressive symblepharon
- Neurotrophic keratitis
- Lid malposition secondary to cicatricial ectropion and entropion
- Glaucoma
- Cataract
- Hypotony
- Phthisis bulbi
- Blindness

REFERENCES
1. Wagoner MD. Chemical injuries of the eye: current concepts in pathophysiology and therapy. *Surv Ophthalmol.* 1997;41(4):275–313.
2. Singh P, Tyagi M, Kumar Y, et al. Ocular chemical injuries and their management. *Oman J Ophthalmol.* 2013;6(2):83–86.
3. Eslani M, Baradaran-Rafii A, Movahedan A, et al. The ocular surface chemical burns. *J Ophthalmol.* 2014;2014:196827.
4. Chau JP, Lee DT, Lo SH. A systematic review of methods of eye irrigation for adults and children with ocular chemical burns. *Worldviews Evid Based Nurs.* 2012;9(3):129–138.
5. Spector J, Fernandez WG. Chemical, thermal, and biological ocular exposures. *Emerg Med Clin North Am.* 2008;26(1):125–136.
6. Ralph RA. Tetracyclines and the treatment of corneal stromal ulceration: a review. *Cornea.* 2000;19(3):274–277.

ADDITIONAL READING
- Fish R, Davidson RS. Management of ocular thermal and chemical injuries, including amniotic membrane therapy. *Curr Opin Ophthalmol.* 2010;21(4):317–321.
- Gicquel JJ. Management of ocular surface chemical burns. *Br J Ophthalmol.* 2011;95(2):159–161.
- Lin A, Patel N, Yoo D, et al. Management of ocular conditions in the burn unit: thermal and chemical burns and Stevens-Johnson syndrome/toxic epidermal necrolysis. *J Burn Care Res.* 2011;32(5):547–560.
- Roblin I, Urban M, Flicoteau D, et al. Topical treatment of experimental hydrofluoric acid skin burns by 2.5% calcium gluconate. *J Burn Care Res.* 2006;27(6):889–894.
- Sharma N, Lathi SS, Sehra SV, et al. Comparison of umbilical cord serum and amniotic membrane transplantation in acute ocular chemical burns. *Br J Ophthalmol.* 2015;99(5):669–673.

 SEE ALSO

Burns

 CODES

ICD10
- T26.50XA Corrosion of unsp eyelid and periocular area, init encntr
- T26.60XA Corrosion of cornea and conjunctival sac, unsp eye, init
- S05.00XA Inj conjunctiva and corneal abrasion w/o fb, unsp eye, init

CLINICAL PEARLS
- Prompt irrigation of all chemical burns, even prior to arrival to the emergency department, is essential to ensure best outcomes. It is impossible to overirrigate.
- All patients with chemical injuries to their eyes should have urgent ophthalmology consultation and/or referral.

ONYCHOMYCOSIS

Lauren M. Simon, MD, MPH, FAAFP, FACSM

 BASICS

DESCRIPTION
- Fungal infection of fingernails/toenails
- Caused mostly by dermatophytes but also yeasts and nondermatophyte molds
- Toenails are more commonly affected than fingernails.
- System(s) affected: skin, exocrine
- Synonym(s): tinea unguium; ringworm of the nail

EPIDEMIOLOGY
Prevalence
- Occurs in 2–10% of general population
- Predominant age: 20% in adults >60 years of age
- Rare before puberty
- Prevalence 15–40% in persons with human immunodeficiency infection (1)

ETIOLOGY AND PATHOPHYSIOLOGY
- Dermatophytes: *Trichophyton* (*Trichophyton rubrum* most common), *Epidermophyton*, *Microsporum*
- Yeasts: *Candida albicans* (most common), *Candida parapsilosis*, *Candida tropicalis*, *Candida krusei*
- Molds: *Scopulariopsis brevicaulis*, *Hendersonula toruloidea*, *Aspergillus* sp., *Alternaria tenuis*, *Cephalosporium*, *Scytalidium hyalinum*
- Dermatophytes cause 90% of toenail and most of fingernail onychomycoses.
- Fingernail onychomycosis is more often caused by yeasts, especially *Candida*.
- Dermatophytes can invade normal keratin, whereas nondermatophyte molds invade altered keratin (dystrophic/injured nails).

RISK FACTORS
- Older age
- Tinea pedis
- Occlusive footwear
- Cancer/diabetes/psoriasis
- Peripheral vascular disease
- Cohabitation with others with onychomycosis
- Immunodeficiency
- Communal swimming pools
- Smoking
- Peripheral vascular disease
- History of nail trauma
- Autosomal dominant genetic predisposition

COMMONLY ASSOCIATED CONDITIONS
- Immunodeficiency/chronic metabolic disease (e.g., diabetes)
- Tinea pedis/manuum

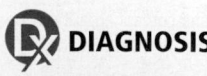 DIAGNOSIS

PHYSICAL EXAM
- Dermatophytes: commonly preceded by dermatophyte infection at another site; 80% involve toenails, especially hallux; simultaneous infection of fingernails and toenails is rare. Five clinical forms occur.
  - Distal/lateral subungual onychomycosis (most common): mainly due to *T. rubrum*. Spreads from distal/lateral margins to nail bed to nail plate; subungual hyperkeratosis; onycholysis; nail dystrophy; discoloration—yellow-white or brown-black, yellow streaking laterally; can progress proximally, *bois vermoulu* ("worm-eaten wood"); onychomadesis

- Proximal subungual onychomycosis (rare <1% of cases): hands/feet; leukonychia—begins at proximal part of nail plate, appearing to occur from the proximal underside of the nail (or direct invasion of the nail plate from above); spreads to nail plate and lunula; seen with immunosuppressive conditions
  - Superficial (formerly known as superficial white onychomycosis) about 10% of cases: hallux is preferentially affected; infection of outer surface of nail plate; opaque white spots on nail plate eventually merge to involve entire surface of the nail. Most commonly due to *Trichophyton mentagrophytes*
  - Endonyx onychomycosis involves interior of nail plate, sparing nail bed. Nail develops milky white appearance with indentations. Subungual hyperkeratosis is absent.
  - Totally dystrophic onychomycosis causes complete destruction of nail plate by fungus, resulting in thickened and ridged nail bed covered with keratotic debris.
- Candidal
  - Hands, 70%, especially for the dominant hand
  - Middle finger is most common.
  - Pain is mild, unless secondarily infected.
  - Increases on prolonged contact with water
  - Primarily affects tissue surrounding nail
  - Begins with cuticle detachment
  - White or white-yellow nail discoloration
  - Secondary ungual changes: convex, irregular, striated nail plate with dull, rough surface
  - Onycholysis, especially on hands
  - Distal subungual onychomycosis may occur.
  - Primary involvement of the nail plate is uncommon (thin, crumbly, opaque, brownish nail plate deformed by transverse grooves).
  - Periungual edema/erythema may occur (club-shaped, bulbous fingertips).
- Molds (nondermatophyte)
  - More common in those >60 years of age
  - More common in nails of hallux
  - Resembles distal and lateral onychomycosis

Pediatric Considerations
- Candidal infection presents more commonly as superficial onychomycosis.
- The U.S. Food and Drug Administration (FDA) has not approved any systemic antifungal agents for treatment of onychomycosis in children. Efficacy and safety profiles in children for some systemic antifungals are similar to those previously reported in adults (2).

DIFFERENTIAL DIAGNOSIS
- Psoriasis (most common alternate diagnosis)
- Traumatic dystrophy
- Lichen planus
- Onychogryphosis ("ram's horn nails")
- Eczematous conditions
- Hypothyroidism
- Drugs and chemicals
- Yellow nail syndrome
- Neoplasms (0.7–3.5%) of all melanoma cases are subungual. In a brownish yellow nail, if dark pigment extends into periungual skin fold, consider subungual melanoma.

DIAGNOSTIC TESTS & INTERPRETATION
- Accurate diagnosis requires both laboratory and clinical evidence.
- About 50% of nail dystrophy seen on visual inspection is not fungal in origin, so laboratory assessment improves diagnostic accuracy.

- If onychomycosis is suspected clinically and initial diagnostic laboratory tests are negative, the tests should be repeated.
- A nail plate biopsy or partial/full removal of nail with culture is needed to diagnose proximal subungual onychomycosis.

Initial Tests (lab, imaging)
- Direct microscopy with potassium hydroxide (KOH) preparation (1)[C]
  - Clean nail with 70% isopropyl alcohol.
  - Using sterile clippers, remove diseased, discolored nail plate.
  - Collect debris from stratum corneum of most proximal area (beneath nail or crumbling nail itself) with 1-mm curette/scalpel.
  - Place sample on microscope slide with drop of 5–10% KOH. View after 5 minutes.
  - Gentle heat applied to slide can enhance keratin breakdown.
  - High sensitivity if >2 preparations were examined
  - Look for hyphae, pseudohyphae, or spores.
- Cultures: False-negative finding in 30% (secondary to loss of dermatophyte viability; improved by immediate culture on Sabouraud cell culture medium); results may take 3 to 6 weeks.
- In office dermatophyte test, medium culture indicates dermatophyte growth with yellow-to-red color change of the medium; results in 3 to 7 days; limited studies.
- Histologic examination of nail clippings/nail plate punch biopsy: proximal lesions; stain both with periodic acid–Schiff (PAS) stain (1)[C].
- KOH-treated nail clipping stained with PAS: significantly higher rates of detection of onychomycosis as compared with standard methods of KOH preparation and fungal culture (3)[C]
- Polymerase chain reaction (PCR) increases sensitivity of detection of dermatophytes in nail specimen, results available within 3 days can be used as complementary to direct microscope exam and fungal culture; not widely available.
- Fluorescence microscopy can be used as a rapid screening tool for identification of fungi in nail specimens.
- Commercial laboratories may use KOH with calcofluor white stain to improve view of fungal elements in fluorescent microscopy.
- Discontinue all topical medication for at least 1 week before obtaining a sample.

Test Interpretation
Pathogens within the nail keratin

 TREATMENT

GENERAL MEASURES
- Avoid factors that promote fungal growth (i.e., heat, moisture, occlusion, tight-fitting shoes).
- Treat underlying disease risk factors.
- Treat secondary infections.

MEDICATION
Pregnancy Considerations
Oral antifungals and ciclopirox are pregnancy Category B (terbinafine, ciclopirox) or C (itraconazole, fluconazole, and griseofulvin). Griseofulvin is not advised in pregnancy due to risks of teratogenicity and conjoined twins. Ideally postpone treatment of onychomycosis until after pregnancy.

First Line

- Oral antifungals are preferred due to higher rates of cure but have systemic adverse effects and many drug–drug interactions.

- Terbinafine: 250 mg/day PO for 6 weeks for fingernails and 12 weeks for toenails; most effective in cure and prevention of relapse compared with other antifungals and with itraconazole pulse in meta-analysis for toenail onychomycosis I (4)[A]

- Itraconazole pulse: 200 mg PO BID for 1 week, then 3 weeks off, repeat for two cycles for fingernails and three to four cycles for toenails; does not need to monitor liver function tests (LFTs) with pulse dosing

- Itraconazole continuous: 200 mg/day PO for 6 weeks for fingernails and 12 weeks for toenails (less effective than itraconazole pulse for dermatophytes, more effective than terbinafine for *Candida* and molds)

Second Line

- Fluconazole pulse: 150 to 300 mg PO weekly for 6 months (lower cure rate); not FDA-approved for onychomycosis

- Griseofulvin: 500 to 1,000 mg/day PO for up to 18 months (lower cure rate, continue until the diseased nail is replaced)

- Posaconazole: 100, 200, or 400 mg once daily for 24 weeks; 400 mg once daily for 12 weeks; higher cost

- Topical agents: Use limited to disease not involving the lunula (proximal nail plate). Topical therapy does not cause systemic toxicity but is less effective than oral therapy. Head-to-head comparison of efficacy of available agents is generally not available.

- Ciclopirox: 8% nail lacquer (available generically): Apply once daily to affected nails (if without lunula involvement) for up to 48 weeks; remove lacquer with alcohol every 7 days, then file away loose nail material and trim nails (low-cure rate, avoids systemic adverse effects, less cost-effective). Application after PO treatment may reduce recurrences. Systematic review >60% failure rate after 48 weeks of use (5)[A],(6)

- Tavaborole 5% solution, a topical oxaborole antifungal is indicated for onychomycosis of the toenails due to *Trichophyton rubrum* or *Trichophyton mentagrophytes*. Complete or almost-complete cure 15–18% after 48 weeks (NNT compared to vehicle approx 7)

- Efinaconazole solution 10% (7). Complete or almost-complete cure after 48 weeks in range of 15–18% (NNT compared to vehicle 7 to 10)

- Contraindications for oral antifungals
  - Hepatic disease
  - Pregnancy (see "Pregnancy Considerations")
  - Current/history of congestive heart failure (CHF) (itraconazole)
  - Ventricular dysfunction (itraconazole)
  - Porphyria (griseofulvin)

- Precautions/adverse effects
  - Oral antifungals
    - Hepatotoxicity/neutropenia
    - Hypersensitivity
    - Photosensitivity, lupus-like symptoms, proteinuria (griseofulvin)
    - Chronic kidney disease (avoid terbinafine for patients with creatine clearance [CrCl] <50 mL/min, decrease fluconazole dose)
    - CHF, peripheral edema, pulmonary edema (itraconazole)
    - Rhinitis (itraconazole)

- Ciclopirox: rash, nail disorders; avoid contact with skin except along nail edge; caution with broken skin or vascular compromise

- Oral agents: numerous significant drug–drug interactions. Need to check each medication:
  - Terbinafine (inhibits cytochrome P450 2D6 isozyme [CYP2D6]): for example, β-blockers, monoamine oxidase inhibitors (MAOIs), SSRIs, tricyclic antidepressants (TCAs), warfarin, oxycodone
  - Itraconazole, fluconazole (inhibit CYP3A4): for example, antiarrhythmics, benzodiazepines, ergot alkaloids, 3-hydroxy-3-methylglutaryl coenzyme A (HMG-CoA) reductase inhibitors, calcium channel blockers, corticosteroids, hydrochlorothiazide, hypoglycemics, oral contraceptives (OCPs), warfarin, zolpidem
  - Griseofulvin: for example, OCPs, salicylates, warfarin

SURGERY/OTHER PROCEDURES

- Nail débridement to remove infected keratin (efficacy not well studied): Use for few nails involved or if not, for candidate of systemic therapy.
  - Mechanical: Soften with occlusive dressing with 40% urea gel; detach from nail bed with tweezers, file with abrasive stone or curette.
  - Chemical: Protect peripheral tissue with adhesive strips; apply ointment of 30% salicylic acid, 40% urea, or 50% potassium iodide under occlusive dressing.
  - Débridement may be combined with topical antifungal therapy.
  - Surgical avulsion if few nails are involved; for pain control.

- Laser treatment has shown some positive results but limited efficacy data (7).

- Photodynamic therapy using topical photosensitizing agents and irradiation with appropriate light source some success for treatment of superficial nail infections; limited data.

COMPLEMENTARY & ALTERNATIVE MEDICINE

- *Melaleuca alternifolia* (tea tree oil) Cochrane review found no evidence of benefit (5).

- Vicks VapoRub application to nails daily for 48 weeks has been found safe, but efficacy is uncertain.

 ONGOING CARE

FOLLOW-UP RECOMMENDATIONS

- Formation of a new fingernail takes 4 to 6 months, and a new toenail takes 12 to 18 months.
- Cure defined as:
  - Clinical cure, 100% absence of clinical signs, and/or
  - Mycotic cure, negative mycology with ≥1 of the following clinical signs:
    - Distal subungual hyperkeratosis/onycholysis leaving <10% of the nail plate affected
    - Nail plate thickening that does not improve with treatment because of comorbid condition

Patient Monitoring

- Topical agents: Slow response is expected; visits every 6 to 12 weeks.
- Terbinafine, griseofulvin: baseline, and as needed, LFTs and CBC
- Itraconazole continuous: baseline, and as needed, LFTs

PATIENT EDUCATION

- Advise patient to:
  - Keep affected area clean and dry.
  - Avoid rubber/other occlusive, tight-fitting footwear.
  - Wear absorbent cotton socks.
  - Launder clothing and towels frequently in hot water.
  - Avoid sharing nail implements or use on both normal and abnormal nails.
- Cure of all toenails may not be attainable.
- Nails may not appear normal after cure.

PROGNOSIS

- Complete clinical cure in 25–50% (higher mycologic cure rates) with oral therapy
- Recurrence is 10–50% (relapse/reinfection).
- Poor prognostic factors
  - Areas of nail involvement >50%
  - Significant proximal/lateral disease
  - Subungual hyperkeratosis >2 mm
  - White/yellow or orange/brown streaks in the nail (includes dermatophytoma)
  - Total dystrophic onychomycosis (with matrix involvement)
  - Nonresponsive organisms (e.g., *Scytalidium* mold)
  - Patients with immunosuppression
  - Diminished peripheral circulation

COMPLICATIONS

- Secondary infections with progression to soft tissue infection/osteomyelitis
- Toenail discomfort/pain that can limit physical mobility or activity
- Anxiety, negative self-image

REFERENCES

1. Westerberg DP, Voyack MJ. Onychomycosis: current trends in diagnosis and treatment. *Am Fam Physician.* 2013;88(11):762–770.
2. Gupta AK, Paquet M. Systemic antifungals to treat onychomycosis in children: a systematic review. *Pediatr Dermatol.* 2013;30(3):294–302.
3. Eisman S, Sinclair R. Fungal nail infection: diagnosis and management. *BMJ.* 2014;348:g1800.
4. Gupta AK, Ryder JE, Johnson AM. Cumulative meta-analysis of systemic antifungal agents for the treatment of onychomycosis. *Br J Dermatol.* 2004;150(3):537–544.
5. Crawford F, Hollis S. Topical treatments for fungal infections of the skin and nails of the foot. *Cochrane Database Syst Rev.* 2007;(3):CD001434.
6. Gupta AK, Paquet M, Simpson FC. Therapies for the treatment of onychomycosis. *Clin Dermatol.* 2013;31(5):544–554.
7. Ameen M, Lear J, Madan V, et al. British Association of Dermatologists' guidelines for the management of onychomycosis 2014. *Br J Dermatol.* 2014; 171(5):937–958.

CODES

ICD10
- B35.1 Tinea unguium
- B37.2 Candidiasis of skin and nail

CLINICAL PEARLS

- Psoriasis and chronic nail trauma are commonly mistaken for fungal infection.
- Diagnosis should be based on both clinical and mycologic laboratory evidence.

OPTIC NEURITIS

Olga M. Cerón, MD • Pablo I. Hernandez Itriago, MD, MS, FAAFP

 BASICS

DESCRIPTION

- Inflammation of the optic nerve (cranial nerve II)
- Most common form is acute demyelinating optic neuritis (ON), but other causes include infectious disease and systemic autoimmune disorders.
- Optic disc may be normal in appearance at onset (retrobulbar ON, 67%) or swollen (papillitis, 33%).
- Key features:
  – Abrupt visual loss (typically monocular)
  – Periorbital pain with eye movement (90%)
  – Pain in the distribution of the first division of the trigeminal nerve
  – Dyschromatopsia: color vision deficits
  – Relative afferent pupillary defect (RAPD)
- Usually unilateral in adults; bilateral disease is more common in children.
- Presenting complaint in 25% of patients with multiple sclerosis (MS)
- In children, headaches are common.
- System(s) affected: nervous
- Synonym(s): papillitis; demyelinating optic neuropathy; retrobulbar ON

EPIDEMIOLOGY

Incidence

- 1 to 5/100,000 cases per year
- More common in northern latitudes
- More common in whites than in other races
- Predominant age: 18 to 45 years; mean age 30 years
- Predominant sex: female > male (3:1)

ETIOLOGY AND PATHOPHYSIOLOGY

- In both MS-associated and isolated monosymptomatic ON, the cause is presumed to be a demyelinating autoimmune reaction.
- Possible mechanisms of inflammation in immune-mediated ON are the cross-reaction of viral epitopes and host epitopes and the persistence of a virus in CNS glial cells.
- Neuromyelitis optica (NMO) IgG autoantibody, which targets the water channel aquaporin-4
- Primarily idiopathic
- MS
- Viral infections: measles, mumps, varicella-zoster, coxsackievirus, adenovirus, hepatitis A and B, HIV, herpes simplex virus, cytomegalovirus
- Nonviral infections: syphilis, tuberculosis, meningococcus, cryptococcosis, cysticercosis, bacterial sinusitis, streptococcus B, *Bartonella*, typhoid fever, Lyme disease, fungus
- Systemic inflammatory disease: sarcoidosis, systemic lupus erythematosus, vasculitis
- Local inflammatory disease: intraocular or contiguous with the orbit, sinus, or meninges
- Toxic: lead, methanol, arsenic, radiation
- Vascular lesions affecting the optic nerve
- Posterior uveitis (i.e., birdshot retinochoroidopathy, toxoplasmosis, toxocariasis)
- Tumors

- Medications: ethambutol, chloroquine, isoniazid, chronic high-dose chloramphenicol, tumor necrosis factor α-antagonist, infliximab (Remicade), adalimumab (Humira), etanercept (Enbrel)

COMMONLY ASSOCIATED CONDITIONS

- MS (common): ON is associated with an increased risk of MS.
- Other demyelinating diseases: Guillain-Barré syndrome, Devic NMO, multifocal demyelinating neuropathy, acute disseminated encephalomyelitis

 DIAGNOSIS

HISTORY

- Decreased visual acuity, deteriorating in hours to days, usually reaching lowest level after 1 week
- Usually unilateral but can also be bilateral
- Brow ache, globe tenderness, deep orbital pain exacerbated by eye movement (92%)
- Retro-orbital pain may precede visual loss.
- Desaturation of color vision (dull or faded colors), especially red tones
- Apparent dimness of light intensities
- Impairment of depth perception (80%); worse with moving objects (Pulfrich phenomenon)
- Transient increase in visual symptoms with increased body temperature and exercise (Uhthoff phenomenon)
- May present with a recent flulike viral syndrome
- Detailed history and review of systems, looking for a history of demyelinating, infectious, or systemic inflammatory disease

PHYSICAL EXAM

Complete general exam, full neurologic exam, and ophthalmologic exam looking for the following:

- Decreased visual acuity and color perception
- Central, cecocentral, arcuate, or altitudinal visual field deficits
- Papillitis: swollen disc ± peripapillary flame-shape hemorrhage or often normal disc exam
- Temporal disc pallor seen later at 4 to 6 weeks (1)[A]
- RAPD (Marcus-Gunn pupil): The pupil of the affected eye dilates with a swinging light test unless disease is bilateral.

DIFFERENTIAL DIAGNOSIS

- Demyelinating disease, especially MS
- Infectious/systemic inflammatory disease
- Neuroretinitis: virus, toxoplasmosis, *Bartonella*
- Toxic or nutritional optic neuropathy
- Acute papilledema (bilateral disc edema)
- Compression:
  – Orbital tumor/abscess compressing the optic nerve
  – Intracranial tumor/abscess compressing the afferent visual pathway
  – Orbital pseudotumor
  – Carotid–ophthalmic artery aneurysm

- Temporal arteritis or other vasculitides
- Trauma or radiation
- NMO (Devic disease)
- Anterior ischemic optic neuropathy
- Leber hereditary optic neuropathy
- Kjer-type autosomal dominant optic atrophy
- Severe systemic hypertension
- Diabetic papillopathy

DIAGNOSTIC TESTS & INTERPRETATION

Initial Tests (lab, imaging)

- In typical presentations, ESR is standard, but other labs are unnecessary. Antinuclear antibodies (ANAs), angiotensin-converting enzyme level, fluorescent treponemal antibody absorption (FTA-ABS), and chest radiograph have been shown to have no value in typical cases (1)[A].

- In atypical presentations, including absence of pain, a very swollen optic nerve, >30 days without recovery or retinal exudates, labs may be indicated to rule out underlying disorders:
  – CBC
  – ANA test
  – Rapid plasma reagin test
  – FTA-ABS test
- MRI of brain and orbits: thin cuts (2 to 3 mm) gadolinium-enhanced and fat-suppression images to look for Dawson fingers of MS (periventricular white matter lesions oriented perpendicular to the ventricles) and also to look for enhancement of the optic nerve
- CT scan of chest to rule out sarcoidosis if clinical suspicion is high.
- Ocular coherence tomography (OCT) of the retinal nerve fiber layer (RNFL); a noninvasive imaging technique of the optic nerve. May serve as a diagnostic tool to quantify thickness of the nerve fiber layer objectively and, thus, monitor structural change (axonal loss) of the optic nerve in the course of the disease.

Follow-Up Tests & Special Considerations

- Visual field test (Humphrey 30–2) to evaluate for visual field loss: diffuse and central visual loss more predominant in the affected eye at baseline (2)[A]

- Low-contrast visual acuity (as a measure of disease progression)
- A novel blood test called *NMO-IgG* checks for antibodies for NMO.

Diagnostic Procedures/Other

- In atypical cases, including bilateral deficits, young age, or suspicion of infectious etiology, lumbar puncture (LP) with neurology consultation is indicated.

- LP for suspected MS is a physician-dependent decision. Some studies indicate that it may not add value to MRI for MS detection (1)[A] but no consensus on the subject exists.

TREATMENT

Most persons with ON recover spontaneously.

MEDICATION
First Line
- IV methylprednisolone has been shown to speed up the rate of visual recovery but without significant long-term benefit; consider for patients who require fast recovery (i.e., monocular patients or those whose occupation requires high-level visual acuity). For significant vision loss, parenteral corticosteroids may be considered on an individualized basis: Optic Neuritis Treatment Trial (ONTT):
  - Observation and corticosteroid treatment are both acceptable courses of action.
  - High-dose IV methylprednisolone (250 mg q6h for 3 days) followed by oral corticosteroids (1 mg/kg/day PO for 11 days, taper over 1 to 2 weeks) (3)[A]
- Others use IV Solu-Medrol infusion (1 g in 250 mL D_5 1/2 normal saline infused over 1 hour daily for 3 to 5 days):
  - No evidence of long-term benefit (1)[A],(4)[B]
  - May decrease recovery time (3)[A],(4)[B]
  - May decrease risk of MS at 2 years but not 5 years (3)[A]
- Give antiulcer medications with steroids.

Second Line
- Disease-modifying agents, such as interferon-β1a (IFN-β1a; Avonex, Rebif) and IFN-β1b (Betaseron), are used to prevent or delay the development of MS in people with ON who have ≥2 brain lesions evident on MRI.
  - These medications have been proposed for use in patients with one episode of ON (clinically isolated syndrome) at high risk of developing MS (1+ lesion on brain MRI).
- The Controlled High Risk Avonex Multiple Sclerosis (CHAMPS) trial study has shown that IFN-β1a reduces the conversion to clinically definite MS in high-risk patients by ~50% (5)[A].
- Decisions should be made individually with neurology consultation.

ALERT
Never use oral prednisone alone as the primary treatment because this may increase the risk for recurrent ON (3)[A].

Pediatric Considerations
- No systematic study defining high-dose corticosteroids in children with ON have been conducted.
  - Consensus recommends: 3 to 5 days of IV methylprednisolone (4 to 30 mg/kg per day), followed by a 2 to 4 week taper of oral steroids (6)[C]
- Optic disc swelling and bilateral disease are more common in children as is severe loss of visual acuity (20/200 or worse).
- Consider infectious and postinfectious causes of optic nerve impairment.

ISSUES FOR REFERRAL
Referral to a neurologist and/or ophthalmologist

 ONGOING CARE

FOLLOW-UP RECOMMENDATIONS
Patient Monitoring
Monthly follow-up to monitor visual changes and steroid side effects

PATIENT EDUCATION
- Provide reassurance about recovery of vision.
- If the disease is believed to be secondary to demyelinating disease, patient should be informed of the risk of developing MS.
- For patient education materials favorably reviewed on this topic, contact:
  - National Eye Institute, Information Officer, Department of Health and Human Services, 9000 Rockville Pike, Bethesda, MD 20892, 301-496-5248
  - North American Neuro-Ophthalmology Society (NANOS), 5841 Cedar Lake Road, Suite 204, Minneapolis, MN 55416, 952-646-2037, fax: 952-545-6073, http://www.nanosweb.org/i4a/pages/index.cfm?pageid=3280

PROGNOSIS
- Orbital pain usually resolves within 1 week.
- Visual acuity
  - Rapid spontaneous improvement at 2 to 3 weeks and continues for several months (may be faster with IV corticosteroids)
  - Often returns to normal or near-normal levels (20/40 or better) within 1 year (90–95%), even after near blindness
- Other visual disturbances (e.g., contrast sensitivity, stereopsis) often persist after acuity returns to normal.
- Recurrence risk of 35% within 10 years: 14% affected eye, 12% contralateral, 9% bilateral; recurrence is higher in MS patients (48%).
- ON is associated with an increased risk of developing MS; 35% risk at 7 years, 58% at 15 years (7)[A]:
  - Brain MRI helps to predict risk:
    - 0 lesions: 16%
    - 1 to 2 lesions: 37%
    - 3+ lesions: 51%
- Poor prognostic factors:
  - Absence of pain
  - Low initial visual acuity
  - Involvement of intracanalicular optic nerve
- Children with bilateral visual loss have a better prognosis than adults.

COMPLICATIONS
Permanent loss of vision

REFERENCES

1. Vedula SS, Brodney-Folse S, Gal RL, et al. Corticosteroids for treating optic neuritis. *Cochrane Database Syst Rev.* 2007;(1):CD001430.
2. Keltner JL, Johnson CA, Cello KE, et al. Visual field profile of optic neuritis: a final follow-up report from the optic neuritis treatment trial from baseline through 15 years. *Arch Ophthalmol.* 2010;128(3):330–337.
3. Simsek I, Erdem H, Pay S, et al. Optic neuritis occurring with anti-tumour necrosis factor alpha therapy. *Ann Rheum Dis.* 2007;66(9):1255–1258.
4. Gleicher NB, ed. *Principles and Practice of Medical Therapy in Pregnancy.* 3rd ed. Norwalk, CT: Appleton & Lange; 1998:1396–1399.
5. Galetta SL. The controlled high risk Avonex multiple sclerosis trial (CHAMPS Study). *J Neuroophthalmol.* 2001;21(4):292–295.
6. Bonhomme GR, Mitchell EB. Treatment of pediatric optic neuritis. *Curr Treat Options Neurol.* 2012;14(1):93–102.
7. Optic Neuritis Study Group. Visual function 15 years after optic neuritis: a final follow-up report from the Optic Neuritis Treatment Trial. *Ophthalmology.* 2008;115(6):1079.e5–1082.e5.
8. Kaufman DI, Trobe JD, Eggenberger ER, et al. Practice parameter: the role of corticosteroids in the management of acute monosymptomatic optic neuritis. Report of the Quality Standards Subcommittee of the American Academy of Neurology. *Neurology.* 2000;54(11):2039–2044.
9. Arnold AC. Evolving management of optic neuritis and multiple sclerosis. *Am J Ophthalmol.* 2005;139(6):1101–1108.
10. Balcer LJ. Clinical practice. Optic neuritis. *N Engl J Med.* 2006;354(12):1273–1280.

 SEE ALSO

Multiple Sclerosis

 CODES

ICD10
- H46.9 Unspecified optic neuritis
- H46.00 Optic papillitis, unspecified eye
- H46.10 Retrobulbar neuritis, unspecified eye

CLINICAL PEARLS
- MRI is the procedure of choice for determining relative risk and possible therapy for MS prevention.
- The ONTT showed that high-dose IV methylprednisolone followed by oral prednisone accelerated visual recovery but did not improve the 6-month or 1-year visual outcome compared with placebo, whereas treatment with oral prednisone alone did not improve the outcome and was associated with an increased rate of recurrence of ON (1,2,8)[A], (9)[B],(10)[C].

OSGOOD-SCHLATTER DISEASE (TIBIAL APOPHYSITIS)

David P. Sealy, MD • Robert J. Tiller, MD, FAAFP

 BASICS

DESCRIPTION
- Osgood-Schlatter Disease (OSD) is a syndrome associated with traction apophysitis and patellar tendinosis that is most common in adolescent boys and girls.
  - Patients present with pain and swelling of the anterior tibial tubercle
- System(s) affected: musculoskeletal
- Synonym: Tibial tubercle apophysitis

EPIDEMIOLOGY
Incidence
Incidence in girls increasing with increased participation in organized youth sports; still more common in boys

Prevalence
- A common apophysitis in childhood and adolescence affecting athletes (21%) and nonathletes (4.5%) (1)[B]
- Approximately 10% remain symptomatic as adults (2)[C].
- 10% of all adolescent knee pain is due to OSD.

ETIOLOGY AND PATHOPHYSIOLOGY
Traction apophysitis of the tibial tubercle due to repetitive strain on the secondary ossification center of the tibial tuberosity, concurrent patellar tendinosis, and disruption of the proximal tibial apophysis
- Basic etiology unknown, exacerbated by exercise
  - Jumping and pivoting sports place highest strain on the tibial tubercle. Repetitive trauma is the most likely inciting factor.
- Possible association with tight hip flexors and tight quadriceps; increased quadriceps strength in adolescence relative to hamstring strength
- Early sports specialization increases the risk for OSD 4-fold (3)[B].

RISK FACTORS
- Affects children and adolescents most commonly from the ages of 8 to 18 years
  - Girls 8 to 14 years
  - Boys 10 to 18 years
- OSD is slightly more common in boys.
- Rapid skeletal growth
- Participation in repetitive-jumping sports and sports with heavy quadriceps activity (football, volleyball, basketball, hockey, soccer, skating, gymnastics)
- Ballet (2-fold risk compared with nonathletes)
- Potential increased risk of OSD in adolescents with ADD/ADHD (4)[C]

GENERAL PREVENTION
- Avoid sports with heavy quadriceps loading (especially deceleration activities—eccentric loading).
- Patients may compete if pain is minimal.
- Increase hamstring and quadriceps flexibility.

COMMONLY ASSOCIATED CONDITIONS
- Shortened (tight) rectus femoris found in 75% with OSD
- Possible association with ADD/ADHD; adolescents with ADD/ADHD are at risk for other musculoskeletal injuries.
- Sinding-Larsen-Johansson apophysitis

 DIAGNOSIS

HISTORY
- Unilateral or bilateral (30%) pain of the tibial tuberosity
- Pain exacerbated by exercise, especially jumping and landing after jumping
- Pain upon kneeling on the affected side(s)
- Antalgic or straight-legged gait

PHYSICAL EXAM
- Knee pain with squatting or crouching
- Absence of effusion or condyle tenderness
- Tibial tuberosity swelling and tenderness
- Pain increased with resisted knee extension or kneeling
- Erythema over tibial tuberosity
- Functional testing: Single-leg squat (SLS) and standing broad jump reproduce pain (3)[C].

DIFFERENTIAL DIAGNOSIS
- Stress fracture of the proximal tibia
- Pes anserinus bursitis
- Quadriceps tendon avulsion
- Patellofemoral stress syndrome
- Chondromalacia patellae (retropatellar pain)
- Proximal tibial neoplasm
- Osteomyelitis of the proximal tibia
- Tibial plateau fracture
- Sinding-Larsen-Johansson syndrome (patellar apophysitis)—pain over inferior patellar tendon
- Patellar fracture
- Infrapatellar bursitis
- Patellar tendinitis—pain over inferior patellar tendon and inferior pole of patella

DIAGNOSTIC TESTS & INTERPRETATION
Initial Tests (lab, imaging)
- Generally a clinical diagnosis. No tests are indicated unless other diagnoses are under consideration.
- Radiographic imaging of the proximal tibia and knee may show heterotopic calcification in the patellar tendon:
  - X-rays are rarely diagnostic, but appearance of a separate fragment at the tibial tuberosity identifies candidates for potential surgical intervention.
  - Calcified thickening of the tibial tuberosity with irregular ossification at tendon insertion on the tibial tubercle (5)[B]

Diagnostic Procedures/Other
- Bone scan may show increased uptake in the area of the tibial tuberosity:
  - Increased uptake in apophysis is normal in children, but with OSD, there *may be more uptake on the opposite side*.
- Ultrasound is an excellent alternative, showing thickening of the distal patellar tendon and infrapatellar bursa effusion.
- MRI shows fragmentation of the tibial tubercle and bone edema.

Test Interpretation
Biopsy is not necessary but would show osteolysis and fragmentation of the tibial tubercle.

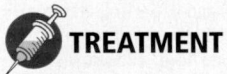 **TREATMENT**

GENERAL MEASURES
- Frequent ice applications 2 to 3 times per day for 15 to 20 minutes
- Rest and activity modification—avoid activities that increase pain and/or swelling.
- Physical therapy helps with hamstring and quadriceps strengthening and stretching.
- Open- and closed-chain eccentric quadriceps strengthening
- Avoid aggressive stretching if pain is significant to avoid risk of tibial tubercle avulsion (1)[B].
- Consult orthopedic surgery for tibial tuberosity fracture or complete avulsion.
- Electrical stimulation and iontophoresis may be beneficial (1)[B].
- Patients with marked pronation may benefit from orthotics.
- A single study showed benefit from an infrapatellar strap and many experts recommend the use of a knee brace with an H- or U-shaped buttress (1)[C].

MEDICATION

First Line
- Any analgesic may be considered.
- NSAIDs may help control pain.
- Opioids are not recommended as first line.

Second Line
- More potent analgesics, such as opioids, may be considered for short-term use in extreme situations.
- Corticosteroid injections are not recommended.
- Hypertonic glucose and/or Xylocaine injections have shown recent benefit (6)[C].

ISSUES FOR REFERRAL
When conservative therapy is unsuccessful, consider surgical referral.

SURGERY/OTHER PROCEDURES
- Débridement of a thickened, cosmetically unsatisfactory tibial tubercle (rare) or removal of mobile heterotopic bone
- Surgical excision of a painful tibial tubercle is rarely needed (<5%) and may be successfully done with bursoscopy instead of an open procedure (5)[C].
- Recent report of successful pain elimination in OSD with percutaneous screw fixation of the tibial tuberosity (2)[C]
- 75% return to normal sport activity and 89% are not restricted from competition due to recurrent pain.

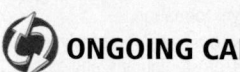 ONGOING CARE

FOLLOW-UP RECOMMENDATIONS
- Athletes may return to play if pain is controlled.
- Presence of pain does not preclude competition.

Patient Monitoring
With worsening of symptoms only

PATIENT EDUCATION
- Avoid jumping sports or reduce activities that increase pain and swelling.
- Assure family that symptoms and findings will diminish with time and rest.
- Patients can safely play sports with mild pain.
- Quadriceps stretching and strengthening are important.

PROGNOSIS
- Except in rare cases, this is a self-limiting illness that resolves within 2 years of full skeletal maturation.
- 10% of patients with OSD as adolescents will have symptoms in adulthood. Up to 60% of adults with prior OSD report occasional symptoms and pain with kneeling.
- Most patients with OSD have residual "knots" of tibial tubercles that never completely resolve.

COMPLICATIONS
- Rarely, a heavily fragmented and inflamed tibial ossicle will avulse and require surgery.
- Rare complications in adulthood include pseudoarthrosis of the tibial tubercle, genu recurvatum, patella alta, and ossicle fragmentation possibly leading to osteoarthritis of the knee.

REFERENCES
1. Kabiri L, Tapley H, Tapley S. Evaluation and conservative treatment for Osgood-Schlatter disease: a critical review of the literature. *Intl J Ther Rehab*. 2014;21(2):91–96.
2. Narayan N, Mitchell PD, Latimer MD. Complete resolution of the symptoms of refractory Osgood-Schlatter disease following percutaneous fixation of the tibial tuberosity [published online ahead of print February 12, 2015]. *BMJ Case Rep*.
3. Hall R, Barber Foss K, Hewett TE, et al. Sports specialization's association with an increased risk of developing anterior knee pain in adolescent female athletes. *J Sport Rehabil*. 2015;24(1):31–35.
4. Guler F, Kose O, Koparan C, et al. Is there a relationship between attention deficit/hyperactivity disorder and Osgood-Schlatter disease? *Arch Orthop Trauma Surg*. 2013;133(9):1303–1307.
5. Eun SS, Lee SA, Kumar R, et al. Direct bursoscopic ossicle resection in young and active patients with unresolved Osgood-Schlatter disease. *Arthroscopy*. 2015;31(3):416–421.
6. Topol GA, Podesta LA, Reeves KD, et al. Hyperosmolar dextrose injection for recalcitrant Osgood-Schlatter disease. *Pediatrics*. 2011;128(5):e1121–e1128.

ADDITIONAL READING
- Kaya DO, Toprak U, Baltaci G, et al. Long-term functional and sonographic outcomes in Osgood-Schlatter disease. *Knee Surg Sports Traumatol Arthrosc*. 2013;21(5):1131–1139.
- Nierenberg G, Falah M, Keren Y, et al. Surgical treatment of residual Osgood-Schlatter disease in young adults: role of the mobile osseous fragment. *Orthopedics*. 2011;34(3):176.
- Pihlajamäki HK, Visuri TI. Long-term outcome after surgical treatment of unresolved Osgood-Schlatter disease in young men: surgical technique. *J Bone Joint Surg Am*. 2010;92(Suppl 1, Pt 2):258–264.
- Sailly M, Whiteley R, Johnson A. Doppler ultrasound and tibial tuberosity maturation status predicts pain in adolescent male athletes with Osgood-Schlatter's disease: a case series with comparison group and clinical interpretation. *Br J Sports Med*. 2013;47(2):93–97.

 CODES

ICD10
- M92.50 Juvenile osteochondrosis of tibia and fibula, unsp leg
- M92.51 Juvenile osteochondrosis of tibia and fibula, right leg
- M92.52 Juvenile osteochondrosis of tibia and fibula, left leg

CLINICAL PEARLS
- Infrapatellar pain in an adolescent athlete undergoing a rapid growth spurt is OSD, patellar tendinosis, or Sinding-Larsen-Johansson syndrome.
- Always consider lumbar disc disease, osteogenic sarcoma, or hip pathology in the differential diagnosis of OSD.
- OSD is generally self-limited. Athletes should modify activity based on pain. Mild pain is not a contraindication to athletic participation.
- Treatment focuses on strengthening and stretching of the hamstrings and quadriceps.
- 10% of adolescents with OSD will be symptomatic as adults.

OSTEOARTHRITIS

Patrick Wakefield Joyner, MD, MS, LCDR

 BASICS

DESCRIPTION

- Progressive loss of articular cartilage with reactive changes at joint margins and in subchondral bone
- Primary
  - Idiopathic: categorized by clinical features (localized, generalized, erosive)
- Secondary
  - Posttraumatic
  - Childhood anatomic abnormalities (e.g., congenital hip dysplasia, slipped capital femoral epiphysis [SCFE], Legg-Calvé-Perthes disease)
  - Inheritable metabolic disorders (e.g., Wilson disease, alkaptonuria, hemochromatosis)
  - Neuropathic arthropathy (Charcot joints)
  - Hemophilic arthropathy
  - Endocrinopathies: acromegalic arthropathy, hyperparathyroidism, hypothyroidism
  - Paget disease
  - Noninfectious inflammatory arthritis (e.g., rheumatoid arthritis [RA], spondyloarthropathies)
  - Gout, calcium pyrophosphate deposition disease (pseudogout)
  - Septic or tuberculous arthritis
- System(s) affected: musculoskeletal
- Synonym(s): osteoarthrosis; degenerative joint disease (DJD)

EPIDEMIOLOGY

- Symptomatic osteoarthritis (OA) is most common in patients >40 years of age.
- Leading cause of disability in patients >65 years old
- Radiographic evidence of OA: 33–90% in those >65 years old
- Predominant sex: male = female
- 90% of hip OA is primary. Hip OA is more common in whites.

Prevalence

- ~60 million patients
- Increases with age; radiographic evidence of OA is nearly universally present in patients >65 years old.
- Moderate to severe hip OA in 3–6% of whites; <1% in East Indians, blacks, Chinese, and Native Americans

ETIOLOGY AND PATHOPHYSIOLOGY

- Failure of chondrocytes to maintain the balance between degradation and synthesis of extracellular collagen matrix. Collagen loss results in alteration of proteoglycan matrix and increased susceptibility to degenerative change.
- Biomechanical, biochemical, inflammatory, and immunologic factors contribute to cartilage loss. Attempts at repair most commonly manifest as osteophyte formation.

Genetics

- Up to 65% of OA may have a genetic link.
- The heritability of end-stage hip OA has been estimated to be as high as 27%.
- Twin studies in women show 50% (hip; knee) to 65% (hip) heritability rates of OA.

RISK FACTORS

- Increasing age: >50 years
- The effect of age as a risk factor is greatest for hip and knee OA, especially after 70 years of age.
- Hand OA is most common in postmenopausal women.
- Obesity (weight-bearing joints)
- Prolonged occupational or sports stress
- Injury to a joint from trauma, infection, or preexisting inflammatory arthritis
- Female gender (knee and hand)

 DIAGNOSIS

HISTORY

- Distinguish OA from other types of arthritis by:
  - Absence of systemic findings
  - Minimal articular inflammation
  - Distribution of involved joints (e.g., distal and proximal interphalangeal joints)
- OA characterized by slowly developing joint pain. Pain often described as aching or burning in nature. Anecdotally, many patients describe pain changes with alterations in weather conditions.
- Transient stiffness (especially after awakening in morning and after sitting) that tends to lessen 10 to 15 minutes after joint movement.
- OA is more commonly affects hands, spine, and large weight-bearing joints (hip, knee).

PHYSICAL EXAM

- Joint bony enlargement (Heberden nodes of distal interphalangeal joints; Bouchard nodes of proximal interphalangeal joints)
- Decreased range of motion of affected joints
- Tenderness usually absent; may occur along joint margin if synovitis is persistent
- Crepitation is a late sign.
- Weakness and wasting of muscles around the joint
- Local pain and stiffness with OA of spine. Radicular pain (if compression of nerve roots)
- Changes in joint alignment (genu varum [bow-legs] and genu valgum [knock-knees])

DIFFERENTIAL DIAGNOSIS

- Crystalline arthropathies (gout; pseudogout): inflammatory arthritides (RA); spondyloarthropathies (reactive arthritis; psoriatic arthritis); septic arthritis
- Fibromyalgia; avascular necrosis; Lyme disease

DIAGNOSTIC TESTS & INTERPRETATION

Initial Tests (lab, imaging)

- Routine chemistries are not helpful in diagnosis.
- X-rays are usually normal early in disease process.
- As OA progresses, plain films show:
  - Narrowed, asymmetric joint space
  - Osteophyte formation
  - Subchondral bony sclerosis
  - Subchondral cyst formation
- Erosions may occur on surface of distal and proximal interphalangeal joints (erosive OA).

Follow-Up Tests & Special Considerations

- May be useful in monitoring treatment with NSAIDs (renal insufficiency and GI bleeding)
- In secondary OA, underlying disorder may have abnormal lab results (e.g., hemochromatosis [abnormal iron studies]).

Diagnostic Procedures/Other

Joint aspiration

- May help to distinguish OA from chronic inflammatory arthritis
- OA: cell count usually <500 cells/mm^3, predominantly mononuclear
- Inflammatory: cell count usually >2,000 cells/mm^3, predominantly neutrophils
- Birefringent crystals in gout (−) and pseudogout (+)

Test Interpretation

- Macroscopic patchy cartilage damage and bony hypertrophy
- Histologic phases:
  - Extracellular matrix edema and cartilage microfissures
  - Subchondral fissuring and pitting
  - Erosion and formation of osteocartilaginous loose bodies
- Subchondral bone trabecular microfractures and sclerosis with osteophyte formation
- Degradation secondary to release of proteolytic and collagenolytic enzymes, prostaglandins, and associated immune response.

 TREATMENT

GENERAL MEASURES

- Weight management
- Heat or cold applications for symptomatic relief
- Physical therapy to maintain or regain joint motion and muscle strength
  - Quadriceps-strengthening exercises relieve knee pain and disability.
- Muscle strengthening improves pain in general.
- Aerobic exercise improves long-term functional outcomes.
- Exercise must be maintained; benefits are lost 6 months after exercise cessation.
- Protect joints from overuse; ambulatory aides are beneficial (e.g., cane, crutches, walker) as is proper fitting footwear.
- Assess for bracing, joint supports, or insoles in patients with biomechanical joint pain or instability:
  - Bracing is more beneficial in patients with unicompartmental disease of the knee.
- For knee OA in particular, **nonpharmacologic modalities are strongly recommended**: aerobic, aquatic, and/or resistance exercise and weight loss.
- Nonpharmacologic modalities that are conditionally recommended for knee OA include medial wedge insoles for valgus knee OA, subtalar strapped lateral insoles for varus knee OA, medially directed patellar taping, manual therapy, walking aids, thermal agents, tai chi, self-management programs, and psychosocial intervention.

MEDICATION

First Line

- Manage pain and inflammation:
  - Acetaminophen up to 1,000 mg TID–QID: effective for pain relief in OA of knee and hip
  - Topical NSAID gels, creams have short-term (<4 weeks) benefits. Topical NSAIDs should be a core treatment for knee and hand OA.
  - If acetaminophen or topical NSAIDs are insufficient, consider an oral NSAID/COX-2 inhibitor. Use the lowest effective dose for the shortest time possible. Use is associated with renal insufficiency, hypertension, edema, and GI bleeding.
  - May use nonacetylated salicylates (e.g., salsalate, choline-magnesium salicylate) or low-dose ibuprofen ≤1,600 mg/day
  - Topical NSAIDs and capsaicin is effective as adjuncts and alternatives to PO analgesic/anti-inflammatory agents in knee OA.
- NSAID contraindications:
  - All PO NSAIDs/COX-2 inhibitors have analgesic effects of a similar magnitude but vary in their potential GI and cardiorenal toxicity.
  - NSAIDs should be avoided in patients with renal disease, CHF, HTN, active peptic ulcer disease, and previous hypersensitivity to an NSAID or aspirin (asthma, nasal polyps, hypotension, urticaria/angioedema).
  - Combination of NSAIDs and full strength aspirin (325 mg) is contraindicated due to risk of adverse reactions.
  - In patients at high cardiovascular risk: Combination of a nonselective NSAID and low-dose aspirin (81 mg) is recommended.
  - Oral or parenteral corticosteroids are contraindicated.
- Precautions:
  - If PO NSAID/COX-2 inhibitor use is necessary for a patient aged >65 years or a patient <65 years with increased GI-bleeding risk factors, proton-pump inhibitors are recommended.
  - Significant possible interactions:
    - NSAIDs reduce effectiveness of ACE inhibitors and diuretics.
    - Aspirin and NSAIDs (except COX-2 inhibitors) may increase effects of anticoagulants.
    - Salicylates reduce effectiveness of spironolactone (Aldactone) and uricosurics.
    - Corticosteroids and some antacids increase salicylate excretion, whereas ascorbic acid and ammonium chloride reduce salicylate excretion and may cause toxicity.

Pregnancy Considerations

- ASA and NSAIDs have reported fetal risk during 1st and 3rd trimesters of pregnancy.
- Compatible with breastfeeding

Second Line

- Topical capsaicin is an adjunct therapy for knee and hand OA; may cause local burning
- Topical NSAIDs (e.g., diclofenac gel) can lower gastric and renal risks associated with oral NSAIDs.
- Rubefacients (e.g., oil of wintergreen) are not recommended.
- Physical therapy: Core strengthening for hip OA and knee muscle strengthening for knee OA decrease joint reactive forces on the affected joint and can relieve pain.
- Bracing; Medial and lateral unloader braces are effective; long leg alignment x-rays can help determine the appropriate brace (1).

Third Line

- Intra-articular corticosteroid injections can be used for acute flares and for patients failing first- and second-line treatments. Minimize injections (<2/joint/year).
- Current recommendations do not support the use of viscosupplementation injections for OA.
- Platelet-rich plasma (PRP) is more effective than HA injections for early stage knee OA (2).
- PRP injections appear to be more effective for early OA when done in a series of three (3).
- Glenohumeral joint OA managed with HA injections and corticosteroid injection have similar outcomes (4).
- TENS is effective for pain relief in large joint OA.
- Ultrasound improves injection accuracy.

ADDITIONAL THERAPIES

Address psychosocial factors (i.e., self-efficacy, coping skills). Screen for and appropriately treat anxiety and depression. Improve social support.

SURGERY/OTHER PROCEDURES

Surgery (e.g., osteotomy, débridement, removal of loose bodies, joint replacement, fusion) may be indicated in advanced disease.

COMPLEMENTARY & ALTERNATIVE MEDICINE

- Nutritional supplements (glucosamine and chondroitin sulfate) may benefit some patients and have low toxicity. There is lack of standardized outcome assessments. Trial results using glucosamine and chondroitin have been mixed. If no response is apparent within 6 months, treatment should be discontinued.
- TENS units and acupuncture have shown benefit.

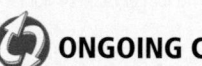 ## ONGOING CARE

FOLLOW-UP RECOMMENDATIONS

Patient Monitoring

- Regularly assess joint range of motion and functional status.
- Monitor for GI blood loss, cardiac, renal, and mental status in older patients on NSAIDs or aspirin.
- Periodic CBC, renal function tests, stool for occult blood in patients on chronic NSAID therapy

PATIENT EDUCATION

- American College of Rheumatology: http://www.rheumatology.org/public/factsheets/index.asp?aud=pat
- Arthritis Foundation: http://www.arthritis.org

PROGNOSIS

- Progressive disease: early in course, pain relieved by rest; later, pain may persist at rest and at night.
- Joint effusions and enlargement may occur (especially in knees), as disease progresses.
- Osteophyte (spur) formation, especially at joint margins
- Advanced stage with full-thickness loss of cartilage at which point joint replacement is a consideration

COMPLICATIONS

- Leading cause of musculoskeletal pain and disability
- Decompensated CHF, GI bleeding, decreased renal function on chronic NSAID or aspirin therapy

REFERENCES

1. Dessery Y, Belzile EL, Turmel S, et al. Comparison of three knee braces in the treatment of medial knee osteoarthritis. *Knee.* 2014;21(6):1107–1114.
2. Guler O, Mutlu S, Isyar M, et al. Comparison of short-term results of intraarticular platelet-rich plasma (PRP) and hyaluronic acid treatments in early-stage gonarthosis patients. *Eur J Orthop Surg Traumatol.* 2015;25(3):509–513.
3. Görmeli G, Görmeli CA, Ataoglu B, et al. Multiple PRP injections are more effective than single injections and hyaluronic acid in knees with early osteoarthritis: a randomized, double-blind, placebo-controlled trial [published online ahead of print August 2, 2015]. *Knee Surg Sports Traumatol Arthrosc.*
4. Colen S, Geervliet P, Haverkamp D, et al. Intra-articular infiltration therapy for patients with glenohumeral osteoarthritis: a systematic review of the literature. *Int J Shoulder Surg.* 2014;8(4):114–121.

ADDITIONAL READING

- Chen WL, Hsu WC, Lin YJ, et al. Comparison of intra-articular hyaluronic acid injections with transcutaneous electric nerve stimulation for the management of knee osteoarthritis: a randomized controlled trial. *Arch Phys Med Rehabil.* 2013;94(8):1482–1489.
- Jiang L, Tian W, Wang Y, et al. Body mass index and susceptibility to knee osteoarthritis: a systematic review and meta-analysis. *Joint Bone Spine.* 2012;79(3):291–297.
- Shimizu M, Higuchi H, Takagishi K, et al. Clinical and biochemical characteristics after intra-articular injection for the treatment of osteoarthritis of the knee: prospective randomized study of sodium hyaluronate and corticosteroid. *J Orthop Sci.* 2010;15(1):51–56.

 ## CODES

ICD10

- M19.90 Unspecified osteoarthritis, unspecified site
- M19.91 Primary osteoarthritis, unspecified site
- M19.93 Secondary osteoarthritis, unspecified site

CLINICAL PEARLS

- Patients with OA typically have morning stiffness lasting for <15 minutes.
- OA most commonly affects the hips, knees, and hands (PIP and DIP joints).
- Intra-articular steroid injections should be limited to no more than 2 per joint per year (if used at all).
- Consider PRP for early stage knee OA.
- American Academy of Orthopaedic Surgeons (AAOS) recommends against the use of HA injections for OA.
- Long-term therapy should be based on individual patient goals and expectations, particularly regarding pain management and activity level.

OSTEOMYELITIS
Tricia Elaine VanWagner, MD

 BASICS

DESCRIPTION
- An acute or chronic infection and inflammation of the bone; can occur as a result of hematogenous seeding, contiguous spread of infection, or direct inoculation into intact bone (trauma or surgery)
- Two major classification systems:
  - Lew and Waldvogel classification
    - Classified according to duration (acute or chronic) and the mechanism of infection (hematogenous, contiguous)
  - Cierny-Mader classification
    - Based on the portion of bone affected, the physiologic status of the host, and other risk factors
    - Stage 1: medullary bone (typically monomicrobial)
    - Stage 2: bony surface (deep soft tissue infection or ulcer)
    - Stage 3: advance local infection (polymicrobial); often associated with open fracture or infected orthopedic hardware
    - Stage 4: Extensive disease (multiple tissue layers) requires combination medical and surgical therapy.
    - Class A host: otherwise normal
    - Class B host: immunocompromised
    - Class C host: Treatment risk outweighs benefit.
- Special situations
  - Vertebral osteomyelitis
    - Acute, subacute, or chronic
    - May result from hematogenous seeding, direct inoculation, or contiguous spread
    - Back pain is most common initial symptom.
    - Lumbar spine is most commonly involved, followed by thoracic spine.
  - Infections of prosthetic joints
    - Obtaining specific diagnosis and targeted therapy quicker (easy access)
    - X-ray, then 3-phase bone scan, as MRI/CT is limited use in this circumstance
    - Treat with combination of antibiotics, including rifampin.
  - Posttraumatic infections
    - Depends on type of fracture, level of contamination, and severity of tissue injury
    - Tibia is the most commonly involved.
- System(s) affected: musculoskeletal

EPIDEMIOLOGY
- Predominant age: more common in older adults
- Predominant sex: male > female
- Hematogenous osteomyelitis
  - Adults (most >50 years of age): vertebral
  - Children: long bones
- Contiguous osteomyelitis: related to trauma and surgery in younger adults and decubitus ulcers and infected total joint arthroplasties in older adults

Incidence
Generally low; normal bone is resistant to infection.

Prevalence
Up to 66% of diabetics with foot ulcers

ETIOLOGY AND PATHOPHYSIOLOGY
- Infection is caused by biofilm bacteria (protects bacteria from antimicrobial agents and host immune responses).
- Acute: suppurative infection of bone with edema and vascular compromise leading to sequestra

---

- Chronic: presence of necrotic bone or sequestra or recurrence of previous infection
- Hematogenous osteomyelitis (typically monomicrobial)
  - *Staphylococcus aureus* (most common)
  - Coagulase-negative staphylococci and aerobic gram-negative bacteria
  - *Salmonella* sp. (sickle cell disease)
  - *Mycobacterium tuberculosis* and fungi (rare) in endemic areas or in immunocompromised hosts
- Contiguous focus osteomyelitis (commonly polymicrobial)
  - Diabetes or vascular insufficiency
    - Coagulase-positive and coagulase-negative staphylococci
    - Streptococci, gram-negative bacilli, anaerobes (*Peptostreptococcus* sp.)
  - Prosthetic device
    - Coagulase-negative staphylococci and *S. aureus*

RISK FACTORS
- Diabetes mellitus
- Recent trauma/surgery
- Foreign body (e.g., prosthetic implant)
- Neuropathy and vascular insufficiency
- Immunosuppression
- Sickle cell disease
- Injection drug use
- Previous osteomyelitis

GENERAL PREVENTION
- Antibiotic prophylaxis
  - Clean bone surgery
    - Administer IV antibiotics within an hour of skin incision and continue no longer than 24 hours after the procedure.
  - Closed fractures
    - Cefazolin, cefuroxime, clindamycin (β-lactam allergy), or vancomycin (β-lactam allergy or MRSA infection)
  - Open fractures
    - In patients who can receive antibiotics within 3 hours of injury with prompt operative treatment, 1st-generation cephalosporins are preferred (clindamycin or vancomycin if allergy exists). Add aminoglycoside if type III fracture and penicillin for anaerobic coverage if farm injury or possible bowel contamination.
- All diabetic patients should have an annual foot examination.

COMMONLY ASSOCIATED CONDITIONS
See "Risk Factors."

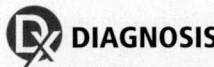 **DIAGNOSIS**

HISTORY
- Fever, chills, lethargy (particularly in children)
- Pain, swelling, erythema in affected area
- Hematogenous osteomyelitis
  - Elicit a history of conditions predisposing to bacteremia (diabetes, renal insufficiency, invasive procedures, IV drug use)
- Contiguous osteomyelitis and vascular insufficiency
  - Recent trauma/surgery within 1 to 2 months
  - Presence of prosthetic device
  - History of diabetes
- Chronic osteomyelitis
  - History of acute osteomyelitis

PHYSICAL EXAM
- Fever
- Restriction of movement of the involved extremity or refusal to bear weight
- Pain or tenderness in the infected area
- Signs of localized inflammation
- Motor and sensory deficits (vertebral infection)
- Visible defect: probe to bone
- Ulcer >2-cm wide and >2-cm deep increases likelihood in diabetic foot ulcers.
- In patients with diabetes, classic signs and symptoms of infection may be masked due to vascular disease and neuropathy.

DIFFERENTIAL DIAGNOSIS
- Systemic infection from other source
- Aseptic bone infarction
- Localized inflammation or infection of overlying skin and soft tissues (e.g., gout)
- Brodie abscess (subacute osteomyelitis)
- Neuropathic joint disease (Charcot foot)
- Fractures/trauma
- Tumor

DIAGNOSTIC TESTS & INTERPRETATION
Initial Tests (lab, imaging)
Labs
- WBC is not reliable (can be normal with infection).
- CRP is usually elevated but nonspecific.
- ESR is high in most cases:
  - ESR >70 mm/hr increases likelihood.
- Antimicrobial agents given prior to culture may alter culture results.
- Disorders that may alter lab results: immunosuppression (including diabetes), chronic inflammatory disease, other/adjacent sites of infection (1)[C]
- Routine radiography is first-line imaging: Classic triad for osteomyelitis is demineralization, periosteal reaction, and bone destruction:
  - Bone destruction is not apparent on plain films until after 10 to 21 days of infection.
  - Bone must undergo 30–50% destruction before damage is evident on films.
  - Bone scan is typically first test after plain x-ray in setting of joint prosthesis.
- Radionuclide scanning (e.g., technetium, indium, or gallium) is useful when diagnosis is ambiguous or extent of disease is in question but is limited by low sensitivity and specificity.
- MRI
  - Best for visualization of septic arthritis, spinal infection, and diabetic foot infections (1)[C]
  - T1-weighted image: low signal intensity
  - T2-weighted image: high signal intensity
  - MRI with gadolinium: sensitivity and specificity range from 60–100% to 50–90%, respectively
  - MRI is not helpful in assessing the response to therapy due to persistence of bony edema.
- CT
  - Better than standard radiography in fragments and sequestration, but inferior to MRI in soft tissue and bone marrow assessment
  - Helps define soft tissues and identify sequestra

Follow-Up Tests & Special Considerations
- A persistently elevated CRP (4 to 6 weeks) can be associated with persistent osteomyelitis.
- Patients receiving prolonged antimicrobial therapy should be monitored with:
  - Weekly CBC
  - Liver and kidney function tests

Diagnostic Procedures/Other
- Cultures
  - Definitive diagnosis is made by blood culture (hematogenous) or by needle aspiration/bone biopsy, with identification of the microorganism by culture and sensitivity or histology.
  - Patients with positive blood cultures and with radiographic evidence of osteomyelitis may not need bone culture.
  - Wound swabs and sinus tract cultures correlate well with the presence of *S. aureus* in deep cultures.
- Image-guided bone biopsy for vertebral osteomyelitis (unless positive blood culture and positive radiographic evidence)

Test Interpretation
Inflammatory process of bone with pyogenic bacteria, necrosis

TREATMENT

GENERAL MEASURES
- Adequate nutrition
- Smoking cessation
- Control diabetes

MEDICATION
- Direct empiric therapy toward probable organism and tailor once culture results are available.
- Optimal antimicrobial concentration at infection site is essential (consider vascular perfusion to site).
- Antibiotic dosing altered for renal function
- Duration of therapy 4 to 6 weeks for acute osteomyelitis and generally >8 weeks for chronic osteomyelitis or MRSA infection
- In children, early transition from IV to oral therapy, (after 3 to 4 days if responding well) followed by oral therapy for 3 weeks may be as effective as longer courses for uncomplicated acute osteomyelitis (2)[B].

First Line
- *S. aureus* or coagulase-negative staphylococci
  - MSSA: β-lactam at high dose (nafcillin or oxacillin 2 g IV q4h) *or* cefazolin 2 g IV q8h
  - MRSA: vancomycin 15 mg/kg IV q8–12h (use q8h interval if CrCl >70 mL/min) with target trough of 15 to 20 μg/mL
- *Streptococcus* sp.
  - Ceftriaxone 2 g IV q24h or cefazolin 2 g IV q8h
- *Enterobacter* sp.
  - Fluoroquinolone (levofloxacin 750 mg IV/PO q24h) *or* ceftriaxone 2 g IV q24h
- *Pseudomonas aeruginosa*
  - Ciprofloxacin 750 mg PO BID or levofloxacin 750 mg PO q24h

- Anaerobes
  - Clindamycin 600 mg IV q8h (300 to 450 mg PO q6–8h)

Second Line
- *S. aureus*
  - MSSA: fluoroquinolone plus rifampin (levofloxacin 750 mg IV/PO q24h plus rifampin 300 mg PO q12h *or* 600 mg PO q24h)
  - MRSA: linezolid 600 mg PO/IV q12h *or* daptomycin 6 mg/kg IV q24h
- *Streptococcus* sp.
  - Penicillin G 4 million U q4–6h
- *Enterobacter* sp. (quinolone-resistant, including extended-spectrum β-lactamase–producing *Escherichia coli*)
  - Carbapenem (imipenem/cilastatin) 500 mg IV q6h
- *P. aeruginosa*
  - Cefepime or ceftazidime 2 g IV q8h (consider adding aminoglycoside)
- Anaerobes
  - Metronidazole 500 mg IV/PO q6–8h

ADDITIONAL THERAPIES
- Hyperbaric oxygen therapy may be a useful adjunct.
- Negative pressure wound therapy is a possible adjunctive treatment.

SURGERY/OTHER PROCEDURES
Surgical drainage, dead space management, adequate soft tissue coverage, restoration of blood supply, and removal of necrotic tissues improve cure rates.

Pediatric Considerations
Medullary osteomyelitis (stage 1) in children may be treated without surgical intervention (2)[B].

INPATIENT CONSIDERATIONS

Admission Criteria/Initial Stabilization
Correct electrolyte imbalances, hyperglycemia, azotemia, and acidosis; control pain.

Nursing
Bed rest and immobilization of the involved bone and/or joint

Discharge Criteria
Clinical and laboratory evidence of resolving infection and appropriate outpatient therapy

ONGOING CARE

FOLLOW-UP RECOMMENDATIONS
Patient Monitoring
Blood levels of antimicrobial agents, ESR, CRP, and repeat plain radiography as clinical course dictates

PATIENT EDUCATION
Diabetic glycemic control and foot care

PROGNOSIS
- Superficial and medullary osteomyelitis treated with antimicrobial and surgical therapy have a response rate of 90–100%.
- Up to 36% recurrence rate in diabetics
- Increased mortality after amputation

COMPLICATIONS
- Abscess formation
- Bacteremia
- Fracture/nonunion
- Loosening of prosthetic implant
- Postoperative infection
- Sinus tract formation can be associated with neoplasms, especially in presence of long-standing infection.

REFERENCES
1. Malhotra R, Chan CS, Nather A. Osteomyelitis in the diabetic foot. *Diabet Foot Ankle*. 2014;5. doi:10.3402/dfa.v5.24445.
2. Howard-Jones AR, Isaacs D. Systematic review of duration and choice of systemic antibiotic therapy for acute haematogenous bacterial osteomyelitis in children. *J Paediatr Child Health*. 2013;49(9):760–768.

ADDITIONAL READING
- Bhavan KP, Marschall J, Olsen MA, et al. The epidemiology of hematogenous vertebral osteomyelitis: a cohort study in a tertiary care hospital. *BMC Infect Dis*. 2010;10:158.
- Dinh MT, Abad CL, Safdar N. Diagnostic accuracy of the physical examination and imaging tests for osteomyelitis underlying diabetic foot ulcers: meta-analysis. *Clin Infect Dis*. 2008;47(4):519–527.
- Fraimow IIS. Systemic antimicrobial therapy in osteomyelitis. *Semin Plast Surg*. 2009;23(2):90–99.
- Stumpe KD, Strobel K. Osteomyelitis and arthritis. *Semin Nucl Med*. 2009;39(1):27–35.
- Vardakas KZ, Kontopidis I, Gkegkes ID, et al. Incidence, characteristics, and outcomes of patients with bone and joint infections due to community-associated methicillin-resistant *Staphylococcus aureus*: a systematic review. *Eur J Clin Microbiol Infect Dis*. 2013;32(6):711–721.
- Zimmerli W. Clinical practice. Vertebral osteomyelitis. *N Engl J Med*. 2010;362(11):1022–1029.

 CODES

ICD10
- M86.9 Osteomyelitis, unspecified
- M86.00 Acute hematogenous osteomyelitis, unspecified site
- M86.10 Other acute osteomyelitis, unspecified site

CLINICAL PEARLS
- Hematogenous osteomyelitis is usually monomicrobial, whereas osteomyelitis due to contiguous spread or direct inoculation is usually polymicrobial.
- Acute osteomyelitis typically presents with gradual onset of pain.
- Treatment of osteomyelitis often requires both surgical débridement and at least 6 weeks of antimicrobial therapy.

OSTEOPOROSIS

David A. Ross, MD • Rahul Kapur, MD, CAQSM

BASICS

DESCRIPTION
A skeletal disease characterized by low bone mass, deterioration of bone tissue, and disruption of bone architecture that leads to compromised bone strength and an increased risk of fracture.

EPIDEMIOLOGY
- Most common bone disease in humans
- Predominant age: elderly >60 years of age
- Predominant sex: female > male (80%/20%)

Incidence
Of persons age >50 years, 9% had osteoporosis at either the femoral neck or lumbar spine.

Prevalence
- >9.9 million Americans have osteoporosis.
- Women >50 years of age: 24%
- Men >50 years of age: 7.5%
- 50% of postmenopausal women will have an osteoporotic fracture during their lifetime and 15% will experience a hip fracture.
- Two million fractures are attributed to osteoporosis on an annual basis in the United States.

ETIOLOGY AND PATHOPHYSIOLOGY
- Imbalance between bone resorption and bone formation
- Aging
- Hypoestrogenemia

Genetics
- Familial predisposition
- More common in Caucasians and Asians than in African Americans and Hispanics

RISK FACTORS
- Nonmodifiable
  - Advanced age (>65 years)
  - Female gender and menopause
  - Caucasian or Asian
  - Family history of osteoporosis
  - History of atraumatic fracture
- Modifiable
  - Low body weight (58 kg or body mass index [BMI] <21)
  - Calcium/vitamin D deficiency
  - Inadequate physical activity
  - Cigarette smoking
  - Excessive alcohol intake (>3 drinks/day)
  - Medications: see "Commonly Associated Conditions"

GENERAL PREVENTION
The aim in the prevention and treatment of osteoporosis is to prevent fracture:

- Regularly perform weight-bearing exercise.
- Consume a diet that includes adequate calcium (1,000 mg/day for men aged 50 to 70; 1,200 mg/day for women aged 51+ years and men 70+ years) and vitamin D (800 to 1,000 IU/day).
- The USPSTF has concluded that vitamin D supplementation is effective in preventing falls in community-dwelling adults aged ≥65 years who are at increased risk for falls (1)[B].
- Evidence is insufficient to assess the balance of the benefits and harms of daily supplementation with >400 IU of vitamin D_3 and >1,000 mg of calcium for the primary prevention of fractures in noninstitutionalized postmenopausal women (1)[B].
- USPSTF recommends against daily supplementation with <400 IU of vitamin D_3 and <1,000 of calcium for the primary prevention of fractures in noninstitutionalized postmenopausal women (1)[B].
- Avoid smoking.
- Limit alcohol consumption (<3 drinks/day).
- Fall prevention (vitamin D supplementation, home safety assessment, correction of visual impairment)
- Screen (USPSTF recommendations):
  - All women ≥65 years of age (1)[B]
  - Women >50 years of age with ≥10-year fracture risk (using the WHO's Fracture Risk Assessment [FRAX] Tool) >9.3%
  - The current evidence is insufficient to assess the balance of benefits and harms of screening for osteoporosis in men; however, The National Osteoporosis Foundation recommends screening men age >70 years, especially if at increased risk.

COMMONLY ASSOCIATED CONDITIONS
- Malabsorption syndromes: gastrectomy, inflammatory bowel disease, celiac disease
- Hypoestrogenism: menopause, hypogonadism, eating disorders, female athlete triad
- Endocrinopathies: hyperparathyroidism, hyperthyroidism, hypercortisolism, diabetes mellitus
- Hematologic disorders: hemophilia, sickle cell disease, multiple myeloma, thalassemia, hemochromatosis
- Other disorders: multiple sclerosis, end stage renal disease, rheumatoid arthritis, lupus, chronic obstructive pulmonary disease (COPD), HIV/AIDS
- Medications: antiepileptics, aromatase inhibitors (raloxifene), chronic corticosteroids (>5 mg prednisone or equivalent for >3 months), medroxyprogesterone acetate, heparin, SSRI, thyroid hormone (in supraphysiologic doses), proton pump inhibitors

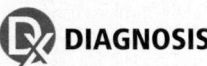

DIAGNOSIS

HISTORY
- Review modifiable and nonmodifiable risk factors
- Online risk factor assessment tools are available:
  - FRAX http://www.shef.ac.uk/FRAX/
- Assess for any commonly associated conditions.

PHYSICAL EXAM
- Thoracic kyphosis, poor balance, deconditioning
- Historical height loss >1.5 cm (difference between current height and peak height at age 20)
- Prospective height loss >2 cm (difference between current height and previously documented height)

DIFFERENTIAL DIAGNOSIS
- Multiple myeloma/other neoplasms
- Osteomalacia
- Type I collagen mutations
- Osteogenesis imperfecta

DIAGNOSTIC TESTS & INTERPRETATION
Dual-energy x-ray absorptiometry (DEXA) of the lumbar spine/hip is considered the gold standard for the diagnosis of osteoporosis.

Initial Tests (lab, imaging)
Consider in screening for secondary osteoporosis:
- Serum 25-hydroxyvitamin D and parathyroid hormone
- CBC

- Serum chemistry, including calcium, phosphorus, magnesium, total protein, albumin, liver enzymes, creatinine, alkaline phosphatase, and thyroid stimulating hormone
- Urinalysis (24-hour collection) for calcium, sodium, and creatinine (to identify calcium malabsorption of hypercalciuria)
- DEXA of the lumbar spine/hip is the gold standard for measuring bone mineral density (BMD).
- A BMD at the hip or lumbar spine that is ≤2.5 standard deviations (SDs) below the mean BMD of a young-adult reference population is diagnostic of osteoporosis.
- A minimum of 2 years may be needed to reliably measure a change in BMD.
- BMD is expressed in terms of T-scores and Z-scores:
  - T-score is the number of *SDs* a patient's BMD deviates from the mean for young, normal (age 25 to 40 years) control individuals of the same sex.
  - WHO defines normal BMD as a T-score ≥−1, osteopenia as a T-score between −1 and −2.5, and osteoporosis as a T-score ≤−2.5.
  - WHO thresholds can be used for postmenopausal women and men >50 years of age.
  - The *Z*-score is a comparison of the patient's BMD with an age-matched population.
  - A *Z*-score <−2 should prompt evaluation for causes of secondary osteoporosis.
- Quantitative ultrasound densitometry does not measure BMD directly but may be used clinically in predicting fractures in postmenopausal women and in men >65 (2).
- Plain radiographs lack sensitivity to diagnose osteoporosis, but an abnormality (e.g., widened intervertebral spaces, rib fractures, vertebral compression fractures) should prompt evaluation.

Follow-Up Tests & Special Considerations
Further labs depending on initial evaluation, Z-score −2.5 or lower or young age
- Iron and ferritin (hemochromatosis)
- Testosterone levels (hypogonadism in men)
- Serum protein electrophoresis and free κ and λ light chains (multiple myeloma)
- Urinary-free cortisol (Cushing disease)
- Tissue transglutaminase antibodies (celiac disease)
- Markers of bone resorption (urine *N*-telopeptides of type 1 collagen, serum C-telopeptides of type 1 collagen, serum *N*-terminal propeptide of type 1 procollagen): no prospective studies supporting use in osteoporosis diagnosis and management; potential role for identifying patients at high risk for fracture and monitoring response to therapy

Diagnostic Procedures/Other
Bone biopsy may be recommended for patients with bone disease and renal failure to establish the correct diagnosis as it can assess the degree of mineralization and microarchitecture and specific bone loss mechanisms.

Test Interpretation
- In osteoporosis can see reduced skeletal mass; trabecular bone thinned or lost more than cortical bone
- Can assess osteoclast and osteoblast relative activity
- Can rule out other metabolic bone diseases
- Can assess if bone marrow is normal or atrophic

TREATMENT

- All patients with a T-score ≤ −2.5 with no risk factors
- All postmenopausal women who have had an osteoporotic vertebral/hip fracture
- All postmenopausal women who have BMD values consistent with osteoporosis (T-score ≤2.5) at the lumbar spine, femoral neck, or total hip region
- Postmenopausal women with T-scores from −1.0 to −2.5 and a 10-year risk, based on FRAX calculator, of an osteoporotic fracture (spine, hip, shoulder, and wrist) of at least 20% or hip of at least 3%
- Treat men >50 years of age who present with a hip or vertebral fracture or a T-score < −2.5 after appropriate evaluation; however, evidence for the effectiveness of treatment of osteoporosis in men is limited.

MEDICATION
Calcium 1,200 mg/day and vitamin D 800 IU/day

First Line
- Bisphosphonates
  - Alendronate 10 mg PO daily or 70 mg PO weekly
  - Risedronate 5 mg PO daily, 35 mg PO weekly, 75 mg PO twice monthly, or 150 mg PO monthly
  - Ibandronate 150 mg PO once monthly or 3 mg IV every 3 months
  - Zoledronic acid 5 mg IV yearly
- These drugs become incorporated into skeletal tissue, where they inhibit the resorption of bone by osteoclasts (3,4).
- Alendronate, risedronate, and zoledronic acid reduce the incidence of vertebral and nonvertebral fractures while Ibandronate reduces vertebral fracture only.
- The side effects are similar for all bisphosphonates and include gastrointestinal problems such as difficulty swallowing and inflammation of the esophagus and stomach.
- Osteonecrosis of the jaw has been associated with bisphosphonates, particularly in patients with cancer who receive high doses (5).
- There is a possible risk of midfemur fractures in patients receiving bisphosphonates for >5 years (6).
- Avoid oral bisphosphonates in patients with
  - Delayed esophageal emptying
  - Inability to stand/sit upright for at least 30 to 60 minutes after taking the bisphosphonates
  - Hypocalcemia (correct prior to initiating therapy)
  - Severe renal impairment (creatine clearance [CrCl] ≤30 to 35 mL/min for alendronate, risedronate, and ibandronate and ≤35 mL/min for zoledronic acid)

Second Line
- Raloxifene 60 mg PO daily
  - Selective estrogen receptor modulator with positive effects on BMD and vertebral fracture risk but no stimulatory action on breasts/uterus
  - Nonvertebral or hip fracture efficacy has not been demonstrated; increases risk of thromboembolism.
  - Additional side effects include menopausal symptoms (hot flashes and night sweats).
- Teriparatide 20 mg SC daily
  - Recombinant formulation of PTH
  - Works anabolically to stimulate the growth of bone through osteoblastic activation
  - Studies have shown a reduction in the incidence of vertebral fractures by 65% and nonvertebral fractures by 53%.
  - No data exist on its safety and efficacy after >2 years of use (7).
- Denosumab: 60 mg SQ every 6 months
  - Human monoclonal antibody receptor activator of nuclear factor kappa-B ligand (RANKL) receptor
  - Inhibits osteoclast formation

- Estrogen 0.625 mg PO daily (with progesterone if patient has a uterus): effective in prevention and treatment of osteoporosis (34% reduction in hip and vertebral fractures after 5 years of use), but the risks (e.g., increased rates of myocardial infarction, stroke, breast cancer, pulmonary embolus, and deep vein thrombosis) must be weighed against the benefits
- Strontium 2 g PO daily
  - Appears to inhibit bone resorption and increase bone formation
  - Available for use in Europe
- Calcitonin
  - PTH antagonist that reduces osteoclastic activity, therefore decreasing bone turnover
  - FDA approved for treatment of osteoporosis in women who are at least 5 years postmenopausal when alternative treatments are not suitable.
  - Calcitonin reduces vertebral fracture occurence in those with prior vertebral.
  - Has been associated with an increased risk for malignancy

ISSUES FOR REFERRAL
Endocrinology for recurrent bone loss/fracture

ADDITIONAL THERAPIES
- Weight-bearing exercise 30 minutes 3 times per week
- Smoking cessation
- Physical therapy to help with muscle strengthening

SURGERY/OTHER PROCEDURES
Options for patients with painful vertebral compression fractures failing medical treatment:
- Vertebroplasty: Orthopedic cement is injected into the compressed vertebral body.
- Kyphoplasty: A balloon is expanded within the compressed vertebral body to reconstruct volume of vertebrae. Cement is injected into the space.

COMPLEMENTARY & ALTERNATIVE MEDICINE
- Isoflavones not better than placebo for fracture risk
- Beneficial effect of Chinese herbal medicines in improving BMD is still uncertain.

INPATIENT CONSIDERATIONS
Admission Criteria/Initial Stabilization
Inpatient care for pain control of acute back pain secondary to new vertebral fractures and for acute treatment of femoral and pelvic fractures

Discharge Criteria
Rehabilitation, nursing home, or home care may be needed following hospitalization for fractures.

ONGOING CARE

FOLLOW-UP RECOMMENDATIONS
Patient Monitoring
- Weight-bearing exercises, such as walking, jogging, stair climbing, and tai chi, have been shown to decrease falls and fracture risk.
- Yearly height measurement is essential to determination of osteoporosis treatment efficacy. Patients who lose >2 cm in height should have repeat vertebral imaging to determine if any new vertebral fractures have occurred (2).
- While there is no consensus, most recommendations suggest BMD testing by DEXA scanning retesting 2 years after starting bisphosphonate therapy.
- For many women, 3 to 5 years of treatment with a bisphosphonate is as good as 10 years of treatment.
- A comprehensive risk assessment should be performed after 3 to 5 years of treatment. Those at

high risk for vertebral fracture or with very low BMD may benefit by continuing treatment beyond 5 years.
- Physicians prescribing bisphosphonates should advise patients of the small risk of osteonecrosis and encourage dental examinations (2).

DIET
- Diet to maintain normal body weight
- Calcium and vitamin D (see "General Prevention")

PATIENT EDUCATION
National Osteoporosis Foundation: http://nof.org/

PROGNOSIS
- With treatment, 80% of patients stabilize skeletal manifestations, increase bone mass and mobility, and have reduced pain.
- 15% of vertebral and 20–40% of hip fractures may lead to chronic care and/or premature death.

COMPLICATIONS
Severe, disabling pain and recurrent fractures

REFERENCES

1. Christenson ES, Jiang X, Kagan R, et al. Osteoporosis management in post-menopausal women. *Minerva Ginecol.* 2012;64(3):181–194.
2. Cosman, F, de Beur SJ, LeBoff MS, et al. Clinician's guide to prevention and treatment of osteoporosis. *Osteoporos Int.* 2014;25(10):2359–2381.
3. Poole KE, Compston JE. Bisphosphonates in the treatment of osteoporosis. *BMJ.* 2012;344:e3211.
4. Heng C, Badner VM, Vakkas TG, et al. Bisphosphonate-related osteonecrosis of the jaw in patients with osteoporosis. *Am Fam Physician.* 2012;85(12):1134–1141.
5. McClung M, Harris ST, Miller PD, et al. Bisphosphonate therapy for osteoporosis: benefits, risk, and drug holiday. *Am J Med.* 2013;126(1):13–20.
6. Rao SS, Budhwar N, Ashfaque A. Osteoporosis in men. *Am Fam Physician.* 2010;82(5):503–508.
7. Gómez-de Diego R, Mang-de la Rosa M, Romero-Pérez MJ, et al. Indications and contraindications of dental implants in medically compromised patients: update. *Med Oral Patol Oral Cir Bucal.* 2014;19(5):e483–e489.

CODES

ICD10
- M81.0 Age-related osteoporosis w/o current pathological fracture
- M80.00XA Age-rel osteopor w current path fracture, unsp site, init
- M80.08XA Age-rel osteopor w current path fracture, vertebra(e), init

CLINICAL PEARLS

- Screen all women ≥65 years of age with DEXA scans.
- Premenopausal women with osteoporosis should be screened for secondary causes, such as malabsorption syndromes, hyperparathyroidism, hyperthyroidism, and medication sensitivity.
- Evaluate and treat all patients presenting with fractures from minimal trauma.
- Bisphosphonates are first line for treatment of osteoporosis in most patients.
- If the patient is not responding to treatment, consider screening for a secondary, treatable cause of osteoporosis.

OTITIS EXTERNA

Douglas S. Parks, MD

 BASICS

DESCRIPTION

Inflammation of the external auditory canal:

- Acute diffuse otitis externa: the most common form; an infectious process, usually bacterial, occasionally fungal (10%)
- Acute circumscribed otitis externa: synonymous with furuncle; associated with infection of the hair follicle, a superficial cellulitic form of otitis externa
- Chronic otitis externa: same as acute diffuse but of longer duration (>6 weeks)
- Eczematous otitis externa: may accompany typical atopic eczema or other primary skin conditions
- Necrotizing malignant otitis externa: an infection that extends into the deeper tissues adjacent to the canal; may include osteomyelitis and cellulitis; rare in children
- System(s) affected: skin/exocrine
- Synonym(s): swimmer's ear

EPIDEMIOLOGY

Incidence
- Unknown; higher in the summer months and in warm, wet climates
- Predominant age: all ages
- Predominant sex: male = female

Prevalence
- Acute, chronic, and eczematous: common
- Necrotizing: uncommon

ETIOLOGY AND PATHOPHYSIOLOGY
- Acute diffuse otitis externa
  - Traumatized external canal (e.g., from use of cotton swab)
  - Bacterial infection (90%): *Pseudomonas* (67%), *Staphylococcus*, *Streptococcus*, gram-negative rods
  - Fungal infection (10%): *Aspergillus* (90%), *Candida*, *Phycomycetes*, *Rhizopus*, *Actinomyces*, *Penicillium*
- Chronic otitis externa: bacterial infection: *Pseudomonas*
- Eczematous otitis externa (associated with primary skin disorder)
  - Eczema
  - Seborrhea
  - Psoriasis
  - Neurodermatitis
  - Contact dermatitis
  - Purulent otitis media
  - Sensitivity to topical medications
- Necrotizing otitis externa
  - Invasive bacterial infection: *Pseudomonas*, increasing incidence of methicillin-resistant *Staphylococcus aureus* (MRSA)
  - Associated with immunosuppression

RISK FACTORS
- Acute and chronic otitis externa
  - Traumatization of external canal
  - Swimming
  - Hot, humid weather
  - Hearing aid use
- Eczematous: primary skin disorder
- Necrotizing otitis externa in adults
  - Advanced age
  - Diabetes mellitus (DM)
  - Debilitating disease
  - AIDS
  - Immunosuppression
- Necrotizing otitis externa in children (rare)
  - Leukopenia
  - Malnutrition
  - DM
  - Diabetes insipidus

GENERAL PREVENTION
- Avoid prolonged exposure to moisture.
- Use preventive antiseptics (acidifying solutions with 2% acetic acid [white vinegar] diluted 50/50 with water or isopropyl alcohol, or 2% acetic acid with aluminum acetate [less irritating]) after swimming and bathing.
- Treat predisposing skin conditions.
- Eliminate self-inflicted trauma to canal with cotton swabs and other foreign objects.
- Diagnose and treat underlying systemic conditions.
- Use ear plugs when swimming.

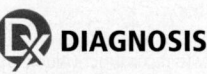 **DIAGNOSIS**

HISTORY
Variable-length history of itching, plugging of ear, ear pain, and discharge from ear

PHYSICAL EXAM
- Ear canal: red, containing purulent discharge and debris
- Pain on manipulation of the pinnae
- Possible periauricular adenitis
- Possible eczema of pinna
- Cranial nerve (VII, IX to XII) involvement (extremely rare)

DIFFERENTIAL DIAGNOSIS
- Idiopathic ear pain
- Otitis media with perforation
- Hearing loss
- Cranial nerve (VII, IX to XII) palsy with necrotizing otitis externa
- Wisdom tooth eruption
- Basal cell or squamous cell carcinoma

DIAGNOSTIC TESTS & INTERPRETATION
- Gram stain and culture of canal discharge (occasionally helpful)
- Antibiotic pretreatment may affect results.
- Radiologic evaluation of deep tissues in necrotizing otitis externa with high-resolution CT scan, MRI, gallium scan, and bone scan

Test Interpretation
- Acute and chronic otitis externa: desquamation of superficial epithelium of external canal with infection
- Eczematous otitis externa: pathologic findings consistent with primary skin disorder; secondary infection on occasion
- Necrotizing otitis externa: vasculitis, thrombosis, and necrosis of involved tissues; osteomyelitis

 TREATMENT

Outpatient treatment, except for resistant cases and necrotizing otitis externa

GENERAL MEASURES
- Cleaning the external canal may facilitate recovery.
- Analgesics as appropriate for pain
- Antipruritic and antihistamines (eczematous form)
- Ear wick (Pope) for nearly occluded ear canal

MEDICATION
- Resistance is an increasing problem. *Pseudomonas* is the most common bacteria, and it is more susceptible to fluoroquinolones such as ciprofloxacin or ofloxacin, whereas *Staphylococcus* is equally susceptible to both fluoroquinolones and polymyxin B combinations (1)[B]. If a patient has recurring episodes or is not improved in 2 weeks, change the class of antibacterial and consider cultures and sensitivities.
- There is evidence that using a topical antibiotic with a corticosteroid shortens time to symptom resolution, although there is no evidence that it increases overall cure rate. There is not enough evidence to demonstrate that any antibiotic regimen is clearly superior to any other (2)[B].
- Oral antibiotics are indicated only if there is associated otitis media. Oral antibiotics alone are not effective and markedly increase the risk of progressing to chronic otitis externa.
- Analgesics as needed; narcotics may be necessary. Recurrent otitis externa may be prevented by applying equal parts white vinegar and isopropyl alcohol (over-the-counter [OTC] rubbing alcohol) to external auditory canals after bathing and swimming.

First Line
- Acute bacterial and chronic otitis externa

  – Ciprofloxacin 0.3% and dexamethasone 0.1% suspension: 4 drops BID for 7 days or ofloxacin: 0.3% solution 10 drops once a day for 7 days (3)[A]. Less ototoxicity and reported antibiotic resistance (4)[A], but branded drugs are far more expensive.
  – Neomycin/polymyxin B/hydrocortisone (Cortisporin): 5 drops QID. If the tympanic membrane is ruptured, use the suspension; otherwise, the solution may be used; may be ototoxic and resistance-developing in *Staphylococcus* and *Streptococcus* sp. (5)[B]; least expensive.
  – Acetic acid 2% with hydrocortisone 1%: 3 to 5 drops q4–6h for 7 days; may cause minor local stinging. This is as effective as neomycin–polymyxin B (6)[B] but is expensive. It may take up to 2 days longer to achieve resolution of symptoms (2)[A]. A wick may be helpful in severe cases by keeping the canal open and keeping antibiotic solution in contact with infected skin (7)[C].

- Fungal otitis externa
  – Topical therapy, antiyeast for *Candida* or yeast: 2% acetic acid 3 to 4 drops QID; clotrimazole 1% solution; itraconazole oral
  – Parenteral antifungal therapy: amphotericin B
  – Patients with Ramsay-Hunt syndrome: acyclovir IV
- Eczematous otitis externa: topical therapy
  – Acetic acid 2% in aluminum acetate
  – Aluminum acetate (5%; Burow solution)
  – Steroid cream, lotion, ointment (e.g., triamcinolone 0.1% solution)
  – Antibacterial, if superinfected
- Necrotizing otitis externa
  – Parenteral antibiotics: antistaphylococcal and antipseudomonal
  – 4 to 6 weeks of therapy
  – Fluoroquinolones PO for 2 to 4 weeks

Second Line
- Acute bacterial and chronic otitis externa

  – Betamethasone 0.05% solution may be as effective as a polymyxin B combination without the risk of ototoxicity or antibiotic resistance. However, the data are not very robust, and more study is needed (2)[A].

- Azole antifungals for fungal otitis externa

ISSUES FOR REFERRAL
Resistant cases or those requiring surgical intervention

SURGERY/OTHER PROCEDURES
For necrotizing otitis externa or furuncle

COMPLEMENTARY & ALTERNATIVE MEDICINE
- OTC white vinegar; 3 drops in affected ear for minor case
- Tea tree oil in various concentrations has been used as an antiseptic (8)[B]. Ototoxicity has been reported in animal studies at very high doses.
- Grapefruit seed extract in various concentrations has been described as useful in the lay literature.

INPATIENT CONSIDERATIONS
Admission Criteria/Initial Stabilization
Necrotizing otitis media requiring parenteral antipseudomonal antibiotics

Discharge Criteria
Resolution of infection

 ONGOING CARE

FOLLOW-UP RECOMMENDATIONS
No restrictions

Patient Monitoring
- Acute otitis externa
  – 48 hours after therapy instituted to assess improvement
  – At the end of treatment
- Chronic otitis externa
  – Every 2 to 3 weeks for repeated cleansing of canal
  – May require alterations in topical medication, including antibiotics and steroids
- Necrotizing otitis externa
  – Daily monitoring in hospital for extension of infection
  – Baseline auditory and vestibular testing at beginning and end of therapy

DIET
No restrictions

PROGNOSIS
- Acute otitis externa: rapid response to therapy with total resolution
- Chronic otitis externa: With repeated cleansing and antibiotic therapy, most cases will resolve. Occasionally, surgical intervention is required for resistant cases.
- Eczematous otitis externa: Resolution will occur with control of the primary skin condition.
- Necrotizing otitis externa: usually can be managed with débridement and antipseudomonal antibiotics; recurrence rate is 100% when treatment is inadequate. Surgical intervention may be necessary in resistant cases or if there is cranial nerve involvement. Mortality rate is significant, probably secondary to the underlying disease.

COMPLICATIONS
- Mainly a problem with necrotizing otitis externa; may spread to infect contiguous bone and CNS structures
- Acute otitis externa may spread to pinna, causing chondritis.

REFERENCES

1. Dohar JE, Roland P, Wall GM, et al. Differences in bacteriologic treatment failures in acute otitis externa between ciprofloxacin/dexamethasone and neomycin/polymyxin B/hydrocortisone: results of a combined analysis. *Curr Med Res Opin.* 2009;25(2):287–291.
2. Rosenfeld RM, Schwartz SP, Cannon CR, et al. Clinical practice guideline: acute otitis externa. *Otolaryngol Head Neck Surg.* 2014;150(1 Suppl);S1–S24.
3. Kaushik V, Malik T, Saeed SR. Interventions for acute otitis externa. *Cochrane Database Syst Rev.* 2010;(1):CD004740.
4. Mösges R, Nematian-Samani M, Hellmich M, et al. A meta-analysis of the efficacy of quinolone containing otics in comparison to antibiotic-steroid combination drugs in the local treatment of otitis externa. *Curr Med Res Opin.* 2011;27(10):2053–2060.
5. Cantrell HF, Lombardy EE, Duncanson FP, et al. Declining susceptibility to neomycin and polymyxin B of pathogens recovered in otitis externa clinical trials. *South Med J.* 2004;97(5):465–471.
6. van Balen FA, Smit WM, Zuithoff NP, et al. Clinical efficacy of three common treatments in acute otitis externa in primary care: randomised controlled trial. *BMJ.* 2003;327(7425):1201–1205.
7. Block SL. Otitis externa: providing relief while avoiding complications. *J Fam Pract.* 2005;54(8):669–676.
8. Farnan TB, McCallum J, Awa A, et al. Tea tree oil: in vitro efficacy in otitis externa. *J Laryngol Otol.* 2005;119(3):198–201.

 SEE ALSO

Algorithm: Ear Pain

CODES

ICD10
- H60.90 Unspecified otitis externa, unspecified ear
- H60.339 Swimmer's ear, unspecified ear
- H60.509 Unsp acute noninfective otitis externa, unspecified ear

CLINICAL PEARLS
- Acute diffuse otitis externa is the most common form: bacterial (90%), occasionally fungal (10%).
- Acute circumscribed otitis externa is associated with infection of a hair follicle.
- Chronic otitis externa is the same as acute diffuse but of longer duration (>6 weeks).
- Eczematous otitis externa may accompany typical atopic eczema or other primary skin conditions.
- Necrotizing malignant otitis externa is an infection that extends into the deeper tissues adjacent to the canal. It may include osteomyelitis and cellulitis; it is rare in children.

OTITIS MEDIA
Paul George, MD, MHPE

 BASICS

DESCRIPTION
- Inflammation of the middle ear; usually accompanied by fluid collection
- Acute otitis media (AOM): inflammation of the middle ear. Rapid onset; cause may be infectious, either viral (AOM-v) or bacterial (AOM-b), but there is also a sterile etiology (AOM-s).
- Recurrent AOM: ≥3 episodes in 6 months or ≥4 episodes in 1 year with ≥ 1 in the past 6 months
- Otitis media with effusion (OME): fluid in the middle ear without signs or symptoms of infection
- Chronic otitis media with or without cholesteatoma
- System(s) affected: nervous, ENT
- Synonym(s): secretory or serous otitis media

EPIDEMIOLOGY
Incidence
- AOM
  - Predominant age: 6 to 24 months; declines >7 years; rare in adults
  - Predominant gender: male > female
  - By age 7 years, 93% of children have had ≥1 episodes of AOM; 39% have had ≥6.
  - Placement of tympanostomy tubes is second only to circumcision as the most frequent surgical procedure in infants.
  - Increased incidence in the fall and winter
- OME
  - By age 4 years, 90% of children have had at least one episode.

Prevalence
- Most common infection for which antibacterial agents are prescribed in the United States
- Diagnosed 5 million times per year in the United States

ETIOLOGY AND PATHOPHYSIOLOGY
- AOM-b (bacterial): usually, a preceding viral upper respiratory infection (URI) produces eustachian tube dysfunction
  - *Streptococcus pneumoniae*: 20–35%, *Haemophilus influenzae*: 20–30%, *Moraxella (B.) catarrhalis*: 15%, group A streptococci: 3%, *Staphylococcus aureus*: 12% produce β-lactamases that hydrolyze amoxicillin and some cephalosporins.
- AOM-v (viral): 15–44% of AOM infections are caused primarily by viruses (e.g., respiratory syncytial virus, parainfluenza, influenza, enteroviruses, adenovirus, human metapneumovirus, and parechovirus).
- AOM-s (sterile/nonpathogens): 25–30%
- OME: Eustachian tube dysfunction; allergic causes are rarely substantiated.

Genetics
- Strong genetic component in twin studies for recurrent and prolonged AOM
- May be influenced by skull configuration or immunologic defects

RISK FACTORS
- Age
- Bottlefeeding while supine
- Routine daycare attendance
- Frequent pacifier use after 6 months of age
- Environmental smoke exposure
- Male gender
- Absence of breastfeeding
- Low socioeconomic status
- Family history of recurrent otitis
- AOM before age 1 year is a risk for recurrent AOM
- Presence of siblings in the household
- Underlying ENT disease (e.g., cleft palate, Down syndrome, allergic rhinitis)

GENERAL PREVENTION
- Pneumococcal vaccine (PCV)-7 immunization reduces the number of cases of AOM by about 6–28% (however, evidence shows that this is offset by an increase in AOM caused by other bacteria). The effect of the introduction of the PCV-13 vaccine on the incidence of AOM has yet to be studied (1,2)[B].
- Influenza vaccine reduces AOM.
- Breastfeeding for ≥6 months is protective.
- Avoiding supine bottlefeeding, passive smoke, and pacifiers >6 months may be helpful.
- Secondary prevention: Adenoidectomy and adenotonsillectomy for recurrent AOM has limited short-term efficacy and is associated with its own adverse risks.
- Vitamin D supplementation (1,000 U/day to maintain vitamin D levels >30) may be helpful in reducing recurrent AOM (3)[B].

COMMONLY ASSOCIATED CONDITIONS
URI

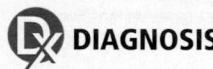 **DIAGNOSIS**

HISTORY
- AOM: acute history, signs, and symptoms of middle ear inflammation and effusion
  - Earache
  - Preceding or accompanying URI symptoms
  - Decreased hearing
- In adults, earache without fever or hearing loss may be the only presenting feature.

ALERT
- AOM in infants and toddlers:
  - May cause few symptoms in the first few months of life
  - Irritability may be the only symptom.
- OME: usually asymptomatic
  - Decreased hearing

PHYSICAL EXAM
- Infectious AOM:
  - Fever (not required for diagnosis)
  - Decreased eardrum mobility (with pneumatic otoscopy)
  - Moderate to severe bulging of tympanic membrane
  - Otorrhea
  - Redness alone is not a reliable sign.
- OME:
  - Eardrum often dull but not bulging
  - Decreased eardrum mobility (pneumatic otoscopy)
  - Presence of air-fluid level
  - Weber test is positive to affected ear for an ear with effusion.

DIFFERENTIAL DIAGNOSIS
- Tympanosclerosis
- Trauma
- Referred pain from the jaw, teeth, or throat
- TMJ in adults
- Otitis externa
- Otitis-conjunctivitis syndrome
- Temporal arteritis in adults

DIAGNOSTIC TESTS & INTERPRETATION
Initial Tests (lab, imaging)
WBC count may be higher in bacterial AOM than in sterile AOM, but this is almost never useful.

Diagnostic Procedures/Other
- To document the presence of middle ear fluid, pneumatic otoscopy can be supplemented with tympanometry and acoustic reflex measurement.
- Hearing testing is recommended when hearing loss persists for ≥3 months or at any time suspecting language delay, significant hearing loss, or learning problems.
- Language testing should be performed for children with hearing loss.
- Tympanocentesis for microbiologic diagnosis is recommended for treatment failures; may be followed by myringotomy.

 TREATMENT

- Significant disagreement exists about the usefulness of antibiotic treatment for this often self-resolving condition. Studies suggest that ~15 children need to be treated with antibiotics to prevent one case of persisting AOM pain at 1 to 2 weeks; the number needed to treat to cause harm (primarily diarrhea) is 8 to 10 (2)[B].
- If antibiotics are not used, 81% of patients >2 years of age are better in 1 week versus 94% if antibiotics are used.
- Delay of antibiotics found a modest increase in mastoiditis from 2/100,000 to 4/100,000.
- American Academy of Pediatrics/American Academy of Family Physicians (AAP/AAFP) guidelines recommend the following for observation versus antibacterial therapy, although these guidelines are not rigorously evidence-based (2)[B]:
  - <6 months of age: No recommendation (2004 guidelines suggest treatment with antibiotic therapy to any child diagnosed with otitis media < 6 months of age)
  - >6 months: Antibacterial therapy is recommended when the diagnosis with severe otitis media (i.e., moderate to severe otalgia or fever ≥39°C in the previous 24 hours) or otorrhea or bilateral otitis media between 6 months and 2 years of age
  - Observation is an option with nonsevere otitis media.
- OME: Watchful waiting for 3 months per AAP/AFPP guidelines for those not at risk (see "Complications"). Of these cases, 25–90% will recover spontaneously over this period. No benefit of antihistamines, decongestants, or antibiotics or systemic steroids (4)[A].

GENERAL MEASURES
- Assess pain.
- Although unusual in adults, the treatment is the same.
- Acetaminophen, ibuprofen, benzocaine drops (additional but brief benefit over acetaminophen)

MEDICATION

First Line
- AOM: AAP/AAFP consensus guideline recommends amoxicillin, 80 to 90 mg/kg/day in 2 divided doses; (5)[A] OR
- Amoxicillin-clavulanate 90 mg/kg/day of amoxicillin, with 6.4 mg/kg/day of clavulanate in 2 divided doses; recommended in children who have taken amoxicillin in the previous 30 days and those with concurrent conjunctivitis or history of AOM unresponsive to amoxicillin
- Treatment duration: 10-day course for children <2 years; 7-day course for children 2 to 5 years; 5- to 7-day course for children 6 years and older
- If penicillin allergic:
  – Non–type 1 hypersensitivity reaction: cefdinir, 14 mg/kg/day in 1 to 2 doses; cefpodoxime, 10 mg/kg/day BID; or cefuroxime 30 mg/kg/day BID
  – Type 1 hypersensitivity to penicillin: azithromycin (10 mg/kg/day [max dose 500 mg/day] as a single dose on day 1 and 5 mg/kg/day [max dose 250 mg/day] for days 2 to 5)
- A single dose of parenteral ceftriaxone (50 mg/kg) is as effective as a full course of antibiotics in uncomplicated AOM.
- A single dose of azithromycin has been approved by the FDA, but studies did not include otitis-prone children or have criteria for AOM diagnosis.
- Consider treatment of children between ages 6 months and 2 years with antibiotics to reduce duration of symptoms (6)[A].
- OME: See "General Measures"; no benefit to treatment. Medications promote transitory resolution in 10–15%, but the effect is short-lived.

Second Line
- Alternative antibiotics are indicated for the following AOM patients:
  – Persistent symptoms after 48 to 72 hours of amoxicillin
  – AOM within 1 month of amoxicillin therapy
  – Severe earache
  – Age <6 months with high fever
  – Immunocompromised
    ○ Amoxicillin-clavulanate, 90 mg/kg to 6.4 mg/kg/day, divided BID
    ○ Ceftriaxone, 50 mg/kg IM or IV q24h for 3 consecutive days can be reserved for those who are too sick to take oral medications or who unsuccessfully took amoxicillin-clavulanate. Neither erythromycin-sulfisoxazole nor trimethoprim-sulfamethoxazole should be used as a 2nd-line agent in treatment failures.
- Recurrent AOM: Antibiotic prophylaxis for recurrent AOM (>3 distinct, well-documented episodes in 6 months) is not recommended.

SURGERY/OTHER PROCEDURES
- Recurrent AOM: Consider referral for surgery if ≥3 episodes of well-documented AOM within 6 months, ≥4 episodes within 12 months with ≥1 episode in previous 6 months, or AOM episodes occur while on chemoprophylaxis.
- Tympanostomy tubes may be effective in selective patients, particularly children age <2 years with recurrent AOM (7)[A].

- Adenoidectomy has limited or no effect.
- Adenotonsillectomy reduced the rate of AOM by 0.7 episode per child only in the 1st year after surgery and had a 15% complications rate.
- OME: Referral for surgery for tympanostomy should be individualized. It can be considered if >4 to 6 months of bilateral OME and/or >6 months of unilateral OME and/or hearing loss >25 dB or for high-risk individuals at any time.
- Tympanostomy tubes may reduce recurrence of AOM minimally, but it does not lower the risk of hearing loss (8)[A].
- Adenoidectomy is indicated in specific cases; tonsillectomy or myringotomy is never indicated.

COMPLEMENTARY & ALTERNATIVE MEDICINE
- It is unclear whether alternative and homeopathic therapies are effective for AOM, including mixed evidence about the effectiveness of zinc supplementation of reducing AOM.
- Xylitol, probiotics, herbal ear drops, and homeopathic interventions may be beneficial in reducing pain duration, antibiotic use, and bacterial resistance.

INPATIENT CONSIDERATIONS

Admission Criteria/Initial Stabilization
Outpatient, except if surgery is indicated, or for AOM in febrile infants age <2 months or children requiring ceftriaxone who also require monitoring for 24 hours

 ONGOING CARE

FOLLOW-UP RECOMMENDATIONS
Patients with otitis media who do not respond within 48 to 72 hours should be reevaluated:
- If therapy was delayed and diagnosis is confirmed, start therapy with high-dose amoxicillin.
- If therapy was initiated, consider changing the antibiotic; options are limited because macrolides have limited benefit against *Haemophilus influenzae* over amoxicillin, and most oral cephalosporins have no improved outcomes.

Patient Monitoring
- AOM: Up to 40% may have persistent middle ear effusion at 1 month, with 10–25% at 3 months.
- OME: Repeat otoscopic or tympanometric exams at 3 months, as indicated, as long as OME persists or sooner if there are red flags (see earlier discussion).

PROGNOSIS
- See "General Measures."
- Recurrent AOM and OME: Usually subsides in school-aged children; few have complications.

COMPLICATIONS
- AOM: Serious complications are rare: tympanic membrane perforation/otorrhea, acute mastoiditis, facial nerve paralysis, otitic hydrocephalus, meningitis, hearing impairment.
- OME: Speech and language disabilities may occur. Hearing loss is not caused by OME, but in children who are at risk for speech, language, or learning problems (e.g., autism spectrum, syndromes, craniofacial disorders, developmental delay, and children already with speech/language delay), it could lead to further problems because they are less tolerant of a hearing impairment.
- Recurrent AOM and OME: atrophy and scarring of eardrum, chronic perforation and otorrhea, cholesteatoma, permanent hearing loss, chronic mastoiditis, other intracranial suppurative complications

REFERENCES
1. Rettig E, Tunkel DE. Contemporary concepts in the management of acute otitis media in children. *Otolaryngol Clin North Am.* 2014;47(5):651–672.
2. Harmes KN, Blackwood RA, Burrows HL, et al. Otitis media: diagnosis and treatment. *Am Fam Physician.* 2013;88 (7):435–440.
3. Marchioso P, Consonni D, Baggi E, et al. Vitamin D supplementation reduces the risk of acute otitis media in otitis-prone children. *Pediatr Infect Dis J.* 2013;32(10):1055–1060.
4. Coleman C, Moore M. Decongestants and antihistamines for acute otitis media in children. *Cochrane Database Syst Rev.* 2008;(3):CD001727.
5. Thanaviratananich S, Laopaiboon M, Vatanasapt P. Once or twice daily versus three times daily amoxicillin with or without clavulanate for the treatment of acute otitis media. *Cochrane Database Syst Rev.* 2008;(4):CD004975.
6. Hoberman A, Paradise JL, Rockette HE, et al. Treatment of acute otitis media in children under 2 years of age. *N Engl J Med.* 2011;364(2):105–115.
7. Kujala T, Alho OP, Luotonen J, et al. Tympanostomy with and without adenoidectomy for the prevention of recurrences of acute otitis media: a randomized controlled trial. *Pediatr Infect Dis J.* 2012;31(6):565–569.
8. Lous J, Burton MJ, Felding JU, et al. Grommets (ventilation tubes) for hearing loss associated with otitis media with effusion in children. *Cochrane Database Syst Rev.* 2005;(1):CD001801.

ADDITIONAL READING
Lieberthal AS, Carroll AE, Chonmaitree T, et al. The diagnosis and management of acute otitis media. *Pediatrics.* 2013;131(3):e964–e999.

 SEE ALSO

Algorithm: Ear Pain

 CODES

ICD10
- H66.90 Otitis media, unspecified, unspecified ear
- H66.40 Suppurative otitis media, unspecified, unspecified ear
- H65.199 Other acute nonsuppurative otitis media, unspecified ear

CLINICAL PEARLS
- Pneumatic otoscopy is the single most specific and clinically useful test for diagnosis.
- Consider a delay of antibiotics for 24 to 48 hours in uncomplicated presentations (>2 years of age) who do not have severe illness or otorrhea.
- First-line treatment is amoxicillin, 80 to 90 mg/kg/day for 10 days for children age <2 years; consider a 5- to 7-day course in >2 years of age.
- Erythema and effusion can persist for weeks.
- Antibiotics, antihistamines, and steroids are not indicated for OME.
- OME rarely develops in adults. Persistent unilateral effusion should be investigated to rule out neoplasm, particularly if there is a cranial nerve palsy.

OTITIS MEDIA WITH EFFUSION

Hobart Lee, MD, FAAFP

 BASICS

DESCRIPTION

- Also called serous otitis media, mucoid otitis media, or "glue ear"
- Otitis media with effusion (OME) is defined as the presence of fluid in the middle ear in the absence of acute signs or symptoms of infection.
- More commonly, a pediatric disease
- May occur spontaneously from poor eustachian tube function or as an inflammatory response after acute otitis media

EPIDEMIOLOGY

Incidence
Approximately 90% of children have OME before school age, mostly between the ages of 6 months and 4 years.

Prevalence
- Approximately 2.2 million new cases annually in the United States
- Less prevalent in adults and is usually associated with an underlying disorder

ETIOLOGY AND PATHOPHYSIOLOGY

- Chronic inflammatory condition where an underlying stimulus causes an inflammatory reaction with increased mucin production creating a functional blockage of the eustachian tube and thick accumulation of mucin-rich middle ear effusion
- Young children are more prone to OME due to shorter and more horizontal eustachian tubes, which become more vertical around 7 years of age.
- Biofilms, anatomic variations, and acute otitis media (AOM) caused by viruses or bacteria have been implicated as stimuli causing OME. The common pathogens causing AOM include nontypeable *Haemophilus influenzae*, *Streptococcus pneumoniae*, and *Moraxella catarrhalis*.
- In adults, OME is often associated with paranasal sinus disease (66%), smoking-induced nasopharyngeal lymphoid hyperplasia and adult onset adenoidal hypertrophy (19%), or head and neck tumors (4.8%).

RISK FACTORS

- Risk factors include a family history of OME, early daycare, exposure to cigarette smoke, bottlefeeding, and low socioeconomic status (1).
- Eustachian tube dysfunction may be a predisposing factor, although the evidence is unclear (2).
- Gastroesophageal reflux is associated with OME (2).

GENERAL PREVENTION
OME is generally not preventable, although lowering smoke exposure, breastfeeding, and avoiding daycare centers at an early age may decrease the risk (3).

 DIAGNOSIS

HISTORY

- OME is transient and asymptomatic in many pediatric patients.
- Most common reported symptom is hearing loss (2). There may be mild discomfort present in the ear, fullness, or "popping" (1).
- Infants may have ear rubbing, excessive irritability, sleep problems, or failure to respond appropriately to voices or sounds (1).
- Clinical features may include "a history of hearing difficulties, poor attention, behavioral problems, delayed speech and language development, clumsiness, and poor balance" (2).
- There may be a history of recent or recurrent episodes of acute otitis media or a recent upper respiratory tract infection (2).

PHYSICAL EXAM

- Cloudy tympanic membrane (TM) with distinctly impaired mobility. Air-fluid level or bubble may be visible in the middle ear (1,2).
- Color may be abnormal (yellow, amber, or blue), and the TM may be retracted or concave (2).
- Distinct redness of the tympanic membrane may be present in approximately 5% of OME cases (1).
- Clinical signs and symptoms of acute illness should be absent in patients with OME (1).

DIFFERENTIAL DIAGNOSIS

- Acute otitis media
- Bullous myringitis
- Tympanosclerosis (may cause decreased/absent motion of the TM)
- Sensorineural hearing loss

DIAGNOSTIC TESTS & INTERPRETATION

Diagnostic Procedures/Other
- The primary standard to make the diagnosis is pneumatic otoscopy, which demonstrates reduced/absent mobility of the TM secondary to fluid in the middle ear. Pneumatic otoscopy has 94% sensitivity and 80% specificity for diagnosing OME. Accuracy of diagnosis with an experienced examiner is between 70% and 79% (1)[C].

- Myringotomy is the gold standard but is not practical for clinical use (2)[C].
- Tympanometry may also be used to support or exclude the diagnosis in infants >4 months old, especially when the presence of middle ear effusion is difficult to determine (1)[C].
- Acoustic reflectometry (64% specificity and 80% sensitivity) may be considered instead of tympanometry (4)[B].
- Audiogram may show mild conductive hearing loss (2)[C].
- Hearing tests are recommended for OME lasting >3 months (1)[C].
- Language testing is recommended for children with abnormal hearing tests (1)[C].

 TREATMENT

- OME improves or resolves without medical intervention in most patients within 3 months, especially if secondary to AOM (1)[C].
- Current guidelines support a 3-month period of observation with optional serial exams, tympanometry, and language assessment during that wait time (1,2)[C].
- Adults found to have OME should be screened for an underlying disorder and treated accordingly (2)[C].

MEDICATION

- The 2004 AAFP/AAOHNS/AAP guideline and a 2012 Cochrane review recommend against routine use of antibiotics in treatment of OME. No long-term benefits of antibiotics have been proven, and often prescribed antibiotics have adverse side effects such as diarrhea, vomiting, rashes, and allergic reactions (1)[C],(5)[A].
- The 2004 AAFP/AAOHNS/AAP and a 2006 Cochrane review found that antihistamines and decongestants have no benefit over placebo in the treatment of OME with possible adverse side effects such as insomnia, hyperactivity, and drowsiness (1)[C],(5)[A].
- The 2004 AAFP/AAOHNS/AAP guideline recommends against administering oral or intranasal corticosteroids. No long-term benefit was shown and adverse side effects such as weight gain and behavioral changes are possible (1)[C].

- In adults, eustachian tube dysfunction secondary to allergic rhinitis or recent upper respiratory infection can be the cause of OME. It is unknown whether decongestants, antihistamines, or nasal steroids improve outcomes in adults.

ISSUES FOR REFERRAL

The following are indications for referral to a surgeon for evaluation of tympanostomy tube placement (6)[C]:

- Chronic bilateral OME (≥3 months) with hearing difficulty
- Chronic OME with symptoms (e.g., vestibular problems, poor school performance, behavioral issues, ear discomfort, or reduced quality of life)
- At-risk children (speech, language, or learning problems due to baseline sensory, physical, cognitive, or behavioral factors) with chronic OME or type B (flat) tympanogram

ADDITIONAL THERAPIES

- Hearing aids may be an acceptable alternative to surgery (2)[C].
- Autoinflation, which refers to the process of opening the eustachian tube by raising intranasal pressure (e.g., by forced exhalation with closed mouth and nose) may be beneficial in improving patients' tympanogram or audiometry results beyond 1 month (6)[A].

SURGERY/OTHER PROCEDURES

- Tympanostomy tubes are recommended as initial surgery. Risks include purulent otorrhea, myringosclerosis, retraction pockets, and persistent tympanic membrane perforations (1,2)[C].
- Adenoidectomy with myringotomy has similar efficacy to tympanostomy tubes in children >4 years of age but with added surgical and anesthetic risks (1)[C].
- Adenoidectomy should not be performed in children with persistent OME alone unless there is a distinct indication for the procedure for another problem (e.g., adenoiditis/chronic sinusitis/nasal obstruction) (1)[C].
- Adenoidectomy (and concurrent tube placement) may be considered when repeat surgery for OME is necessary (e.g., when effusion recurs after tubes have fallen out or are removed). In these cases, adenoidectomy has been shown to decrease the need for future procedures for OME (1,2)[C].
- Tonsillectomy or myringotomy alone is not recommended for treatment (1)[C].

 ONGOING CARE

FOLLOW-UP RECOMMENDATIONS

Patient Monitoring

- Children who are at risk for speech, language, or learning problems and whose OME persists for ≥3 months should undergo hearing evaluation (1)[C].
- Reevaluation and repeat hearing tests should be performed every 3 to 6 months until the effusion has resolved or until the child develops an indication for surgical referral (1)[C].

PROGNOSIS

Approximately 50% of children >3 years of age have OME resolution within 3 months.

COMPLICATIONS

- The most significant complication of OME is permanent hearing loss, leading to possible language, speech, and developmental delays.
- Underventilation of the middle ear can cause a cholesteatoma (1)[C].

REFERENCES

1. American Academy of Family Physicians, American Academy of Otolaryngology-Head and Neck Surgery, American Academy of Pediatrics Subcommittee on Otitis Media With Effusion. Otitis media with effusion. *Pediatrics.* 2004;113(5):1412–1429.
2. Qureishi A, Lee Y, Belfield K, et al. Update on otitis media—prevention and treatment. *Infect Drug Resist.* 2014;10:15–24.
3. Owen MJ, Baldwin CD, Swank PR, et al. Relation of infant feeding practices, cigarette smoke exposure, and group child care to the onset and duration of otitis media with effusion in the first two years of life. *J Pediatr.* 1993;123(5):702–711.
4. Shekelle P, Takata G, Chan LS, et al. Diagnosis, natural history, and late effects of otitis media with effusion. *Evid Rep Technol Assess (Summ).* 2002; (55):1–5.
5. Griffin G, Flynn CA. Antihistamines and/or decongestants for otitis media with effusion (OME) in children. *Cochrane Database Syst Rev.* 2011;(9): CD003423.
6. Perera R, Haynes J, Glasziou P, et al. Autoinflation for hearing loss associated with otitis media with effusion. *Cochrane Database Syst Rev.* 2006;(4): CD006285.

ADDITIONAL READING

- Browning GG, Rovers MM, Williamson I, et al. Grommets (ventilation tubes) for hearing loss associated with otitis media with effusion in children. *Cochrane Database Syst Rev.* 2010;(10):CD001801.
- Casselbrant ML, Mandel EM, Rockette HE, et al. Adenoidectomy for otitis media with effusion in 2-3-year-old children. *Int J Pediatr Otorhinolaryngol.* 2009;73(12):1718–1724.
- Rosenfeld RM, Schwartz SR, Pynnonen MA, et al. Clinical practice guideline: tympanostomy tubes in children. *Otolaryngol Head Neck Surg.* 2013;149 (1 Suppl):S1–S35.
- Simpson SA, Lewis R, van der Voort J, et al. Oral or topical nasal steroids for hearing loss associated with otitis media with effusion in children. *Cochrane Database Syst Rev.* 2011;(5):CD001935.
- van Zon A, van der Heijden GJ, van Dongen TM, et al. Antibiotics for otitis media with effusion in children. *Cochrane Database Syst Rev.* 2012;(9): CD009163.

 CODES

ICD10

- H65.90 Unspecified nonsuppurative otitis media, unspecified ear
- H65.00 Acute serous otitis media, unspecified ear
- H65.20 Chronic serous otitis media, unspecified ear

CLINICAL PEARLS

- Otitis media with effusion (OME) is defined as the presence of a middle ear effusion in the absence of acute signs of infection.
- In children, OME most often arises following an acute otitis media. In adults, it often occurs in association with eustachian tube dysfunction.
- The primary standard for diagnosis is pneumatic otoscopy.
- There is no benefit to the routine use of antibiotics, antihistamines, decongestants, or corticosteroids for the treatment of OME in children.
- Management includes watchful waiting and surgery (when indicated); which strategy is chosen depends on many factors, including the risk/presence of any associated speech, language, or learning delays and on the severity of any associated hearing loss.

OVARIAN CANCER

Celeste Straight, MD • Susan Zweizig, MD

BASICS

There are >22,000 new cases of ovarian cancer annually, and >15,000 women will die of their disease, making this the most lethal of gynecologic cancers.

DESCRIPTION
Malignancy that arises from the epithelium (90%), stroma, or germ cells of the ovary; also, tumors metastatic to the ovary; histologic types include the following:

- Epithelial
  - Serous (tubal epithelium)
  - Mucinous (cervical and GI mucinous epithelium)
  - Endometrioid (endometrial epithelium)
  - Clear cell (mesonephroid)
  - Brenner (transitional cell epithelium)
  - Carcinosarcoma
- Stromal
  - Granulosa cell tumor
  - Theca cell tumor
  - Sertoli–Leydig cell tumors
  - Gynandroblastoma
  - Lipid cell tumor
- Germ cell
  - Teratoma (immature)
  - Dysgerminoma
  - Embryonal carcinoma
  - Gonadoblastoma
  - Endodermal sinus tumor
  - Embryonal carcinoma
  - Choriocarcinoma
- Metastatic disease from the following:
  - Breast
  - Endometrium
  - Lymphoma
  - GI tract (Krukenberg tumor)
  - Primary peritoneal
- System(s) affected: GI, reproductive, endocrine, metabolic

EPIDEMIOLOGY
Incidence
- 21,990 new cases/year in the United States; 15,460 deaths/year
- Leading cause of gynecologic cancer death in women; mortality from ovarian cancer has decreased only slightly during the past 4 decades (1)[A].
- 75% diagnosed at advanced stage
- Predominant age
  - Epithelial: mid-50s
  - Germ cell malignancies: usually observed in patients <20 years of age

Prevalence
Lifetime risk for general population: 1 in 70 women develop ovarian cancer.

ETIOLOGY AND PATHOPHYSIOLOGY
- Malignant transformation of the ovarian epithelium from repeated trauma during ovulation may lead to this change. Many of these cancers originate in the distal fallopian tube.
- Most ovarian cancer (75%) presents as advanced disease. Metastatic disease may develop at the same time as the primary tumor (1).

Genetics
- Hereditary breast/ovarian cancer syndrome: early-onset breast or ovarian cancer, autosomal dominant transmission, usually associated with *BRCA-1* or *BRCA-2* mutation
- Lynch II syndrome: autosomal dominant inheritance; increased risk for colorectal, endometrial, stomach, small bowel, breast, pancreas, and ovarian cancers; defect in mismatch repair genes

RISK FACTORS
- 90% of ovarian cancer is sporadic and not inherited, but family history is the most significant risk factor. Multiple relatives with breast or ovarian cancer increases risk: Refer these patients for genetic counseling. Individuals in families with familial cancer syndromes have 20–60% risk of developing ovarian cancer.
- Nulligravidity (or infertility), early menarche, late menopause, endometriosis
- Environmental (talc, smoking, obesity)

GENERAL PREVENTION
For epithelial cancer, frequency of ovulation appears to be important. The following factors are protective (1)[A]:

- Use of oral contraceptives: 5 years of use decreases risk by 20%; 15 years by 50%.
  - The progestin component of oral contraceptive preparations (OCPs) may protect against ovarian cancer by regulating apoptosis of the ovarian epithelium (2)[A].
- Multiparity
- Breastfeeding
- Tubal ligation or hysterectomy
- Recent studies have shown no clear association exists between ovarian cancer and use of ovulation-induction agents such as clomiphene, but more long-term studies are necessary.
- NSAIDs and acetaminophen use have been shown to reduce risk of ovarian cancer.
- Recommendations for high-risk (family history of a hereditary ovarian cancer syndrome) population
  - Women should undergo pelvic examinations, CA-125 level measurement, and transvaginal US every 6 to 12 months beginning at age 25 to 35 years.
  - Women with family histories of ovarian cancer or premenopausal breast cancer should be referred for genetic counseling.
  - Prophylactic oophorectomy is advised for mutation carriers after childbearing is completed or by age 35 years.
    - Risk of primary peritoneal carcinoma is 1% after prophylactic oophorectomy.
- Screening: No effective screening exists for ovarian cancer (1)[A].
  - Routine use of CA-125 and transvaginal US for screening in women of average risk is discouraged. Annual pelvic examinations are recommended, particularly in postmenopausal women. An adnexal mass in a premenarchal female or a palpable adnexa in a postmenopausal female warrants further evaluation.

COMMONLY ASSOCIATED CONDITIONS
- Ascites
- Pleural effusion
- Decrease of serum albumin
- Breast carcinoma
- Bowel obstruction
- Carcinomatosis

DIAGNOSIS

HISTORY
- Bloating
- Early satiety, anorexia, dyspepsia
- Sense of abdominal fullness, increased abdominal size
- Abdominopelvic pain or cramping
- Urinary frequency or urgency in absence of infection
- Fatigue
- Dyspareunia
- Weight loss
- Severe pain secondary to ovarian rupture or torsion; most frequent in germ cell tumors
- Precocious puberty (choriocarcinoma, embryonal carcinoma) (3)[B]

PHYSICAL EXAM
- Ascites
- Cul-de-sac and/or pelvic nodularity
- Pelvic mass
- Pleural effusion
- Omental mass
- Cachexia
- Adenopathy
- Hirsutism in androgen-secreting germ cell tumors

DIFFERENTIAL DIAGNOSIS
- GI, fallopian, or endometrial malignances
- Irritable bowel syndrome
- Colitis
- Hepatic failure with ascites
- Diverticulitis
- Pelvic kidney
- Tubo-ovarian abscess or hydrosalpinx
- Uterine fibroids
- Endometriomas
- Physiologic cysts
- Benign or borderline neoplasms

DIAGNOSTIC TESTS & INTERPRETATION
Initial Tests (lab, imaging)
- Obtain only with confirmed or suspected disease.
- CA-125 (not specific for ovarian cancer, not to be used for screening)
- Liver function tests (LFTs) to rule out hepatic disease
- CBC
- Urinalysis
- Serum albumin
- Carcinoembryonic antigen (CEA) if GI primary suspected
- If nonepithelial tumor suspected: chorionic gonadotropin (β-hCG [dysgerminoma, choriocarcinoma, embryonal carcinoma]), α-fetoprotein (endodermal sinus tumor, embryonal carcinoma), lactate dehydrogenase (LDH [dysgerminoma]), or inhibin (granulosa cell tumor)
- Pelvic US
- CXR
- Abdominopelvic CT scan with contrast material

Follow-Up Tests & Special Considerations

Disorders that may alter lab results: CA-125 may be elevated from gynecologic causes (e.g., menses, pregnancy, endometriosis, peritonitis, myomas, pelvic inflammatory disease) and with ascites, pleural effusion, congestive heart failure (CHF), pancreatitis, systemic lupus erythematosus (SLE), or liver disease.

- Patients with ovarian cancer need current mammography.
- Barium enema or colonoscopy if a colon primary is suspected

Diagnostic Procedures/Other

- Endometrial biopsy if abnormal bleeding present
- Surgery is necessary for definitive diagnosis.
- Paracentesis if patient with symptomatic ascites and not an operative candidate

Test Interpretation

Epithelial ovarian cancer commonly involves the peritoneal surfaces of the abdomen and pelvis, especially the cul-de-sac, paracolic gutters, and diaphragmatic surfaces.

 TREATMENT

MEDICATION

First Line

- After surgery, most patients will require chemotherapy or adjuvant therapy. Stage 1a, grade 1 and most stage 1b, grade 1 tumors do not require adjuvant therapy. Patients with clear cell carcinomas, grade 3 tumors, or tumors staged 1c or worse do require adjuvant therapy. Patients should be encouraged to participate in clinical trials whenever possible.
- Paclitaxel (Taxol) or docetaxel are recommended in combination with platinum-based therapy (carboplatin or cisplatin) as the first-line treatment of epithelial ovarian cancer.
- Intraperitoneal (IP) chemotherapy in combination with IV chemotherapy improves survival in advanced ovarian cancer. IP chemotherapy is associated with more toxicity (4)[A].
- Germ cell cancers: bleomycin, etoposide, platinum agent
- Contraindications: poor functional status, excessive toxicity, hypersensitivity
- Precautions: All regimens cause bone marrow suppression. Cisplatin is associated with ototoxicity, renal toxicity, and peripheral neuropathy. Taxol can cause neutropenia and neuropathy.
- Antiemetic: ondansetron (Zofran), dronabinol (Marinol), metoclopramide (Reglan), prochlorperazine (Compazine), promethazine (Phenergan)

Second Line

- Liposomal doxorubicin
- Carboplatin/gemcitabine
- Topotecan
- Etoposide
- Bevacizumab
- Cyclophosphamide
- Tamoxifen may be used in recurrent disease when chemotherapy is not appropriate (5)[A].

ADDITIONAL THERAPIES

Some patients with advanced disease and poor functional status and/or extreme tumor burden are managed with preoperative chemotherapy (neoadjuvant treatment) followed by interval cytoreductive surgery. These patients receive more chemotherapy after tumor debulking.

SURGERY/OTHER PROCEDURES

- Surgical exploration with staging and debulking is critical. Maximal cytoreduction of tumor burden enhances effectiveness of adjuvant therapy and is associated with longer survival.
- For epithelial malignancies, careful staging, tumor excision/debulking includes the following:
  - Cytologic evaluation of peritoneal fluid (or washings from peritoneal lavage)
  - Bilateral salpingo-oophorectomy with hysterectomy and tumor reductive surgery
  - Excision of omentum
  - Inspection and palpation of peritoneal surfaces
  - Cytologic smear of right hemidiaphragmatic surface
  - Biopsy of adhesions or any suspicious areas
  - Biopsy of paracolic recesses, pelvic sidewalls, posterior cul-de-sac, and bladder peritoneum
  - Pelvic and para-aortic lymph node biopsies
- Germ cell cancers (less likely to be bilateral): salpingo-oophorectomy (unilateral if only one ovary involved) in young patient

 ONGOING CARE

FOLLOW-UP RECOMMENDATIONS

Patient Monitoring

- Physical exam every 3 months for the first 2 years after diagnosis; every 6 months until 5 years and then annually thereafter
- If CA-125 elevated at diagnosis, follow levels after treatment to detect recurrence (is often elevated 2 to 5 months before clinical detection of relapse).
- Germ cell/sex-cord stromal cancer: physical exam and tumor markers every 3 months for the first 2 years after diagnosis
  - Tumor markers for sex-cord stromal cancers should be checked every 6 months for 10 years, as recurrences can occur remote from initial diagnosis.
- CT scan of chest, abdomen, and pelvis and/or PET scan when recurrence suspected
- Screening with CXR, MRI, CT, or PET not recommended; insufficient data to support (6)[B]

PROGNOSIS

- Recurrence rates
  - Early-stage disease: 25%
  - Advanced disease: >80%
- 5-year survival rates for ovarian cancer based on International Federation of Gynecology and Obstetrics (FIGO) data
- For most recent FIGO staging criteria, see "References" (7)[A].

Stage I	a 90%	b 86%	c 83%
Stage II	a 71%	b 66%	c 71%
Stage III	a 47%	b 42%	c 33%
Stage IV	19%	—	—

COMPLICATIONS

- Pleural effusion
- Pseudomyxoma peritonei
- Ascites
- Toxicity of chemotherapy
- Bowel obstruction
- Malnutrition
- Electrolyte disturbances
- Fistula formation

REFERENCES

1. Schorge JO, Modesitt SC, Coleman RL, et al. SGO white paper on ovarian cancer: etiology, screening and surveillance. *Gynecol Oncol*. 2010;119(1):7–17.
2. Beral V, Doll R, Hermon C, et al. Ovarian cancer and oral contraceptives: collaborative reanalysis of data from 45 epidemiological studies including 23,257 women with ovarian cancer and 87,303 controls. *Lancet*. 2008;371(9609):303–314.
3. Goff BA, Mandel LS, Drescher CW, et al. Development of an ovarian cancer symptom index: possibilities for earlier detection. *Cancer*. 2007;109(2):221–227.
4. Armstrong DK, Bundy B, Wenzel L, et al. Intraperitoneal cisplatin and paclitaxel in ovarian cancer. *N Engl J Med*. 2006;354(1):34–43.
5. Orlando M, Costanzo MV, Chacon RD, et al. Randomized trial of combination chemotherapy (combo) versus monotherapy (mono) in relapsed ovarian carcinoma (ROC): a meta-analysis of published data. *J Clin Oncol*. 2007;25:5524.
6. Gadducci A, Cosio S, Zola P, et al. Surveillance procedures for patients treated for epithelial ovarian cancer: a review of the literature. *Int J Gynecol Cancer*. 2007;17(1):21–31.
7. Prat J. Staging classification for cancer of the ovary, fallopian tube, and peritoneum. *Int J Gynaecol Obstet*. 2014;124(1):1–5.

ADDITIONAL READING

- Salani R, Backes FJ, Fung MF, et al. Posttreatment surveillance and diagnosis of recurrence in women with gynecologic malignancies: Society of Gynecologic Oncologists recommendations. *Am J Obstet Gynecol*. 2011;204(6):466–478.
- Schumer ST, Cannistra SA. Granulosa cell tumor of the ovary. *J Clin Oncol*. 2003;21(6):1180–1189.

 CODES

ICD10

- C56.9 Malignant neoplasm of unspecified ovary
- C56.1 Malignant neoplasm of right ovary
- C56.2 Malignant neoplasm of left ovary

CLINICAL PEARLS

- Family history of ovarian cancer or early-onset breast cancer is the most significant risk factor for the development of ovarian cancer; yet, the vast majority of cases remain sporadic.
- The diagnosis of ovarian cancer should be suspected in women with persistent bloating, upper abdominal discomfort, or GI symptoms of unknown etiology.
- Surgery is the mainstay of diagnosis and treatment for ovarian cancer. Many patients benefit from adjuvant chemotherapy.
- The prognosis of advanced ovarian cancer is poor and requires close follow-up by physical exam, tumor markers, and imaging when indicated.

OVARIAN CYST, RUPTURED

Heather O'Connor Greer, MD • Patricia Beauzile, MD

BASICS

- Ovarian cysts are frequent in reproductive-aged women.
- Most ovarian cysts are benign physiologic follicles created by the ovary at the time of ovulation.
- Ovarian cysts can cause symptoms when they become enlarged and exert a mass effect on surrounding structures, or when they rupture and the cyst contents cause irritation of the peritoneum or nearby pelvic organs.
- Patients with a symptomatic ruptured cyst will usually complain of acute onset unilateral lower abdominal pain.
- Evaluation of the patient should include exclusion of ectopic pregnancy, ovarian torsion, and nongynecologic sources of acute unilateral lower abdominal pain.
- Once the diagnosis of a ruptured cyst is confirmed, most patients can be managed conservatively as outpatients with adequate pain control. Surgical intervention is rarely indicated.

DESCRIPTION
A suspected ruptured ovarian cyst should be treated as an unknown adnexal mass (mass of the ovary, fallopian tube, and surrounding tissue) until proven otherwise.

EPIDEMIOLOGY
- The actual incidence of ovarian cysts is difficult to calculate as many ruptured cysts are asymptomatic or found incidentally.
- Ovarian cysts can be seen on transvaginal ultrasounds in nearly all premenopausal women and in up to 18% of postmenopausal women. The vast majority of these cysts are benign or functional.
- Most ruptured ovarian cysts are self-limiting, and expectant management with pain control is usually sufficient.
- About 13% of ovarian masses in reproductive-aged women are malignant, as opposed to 45% in postmenopausal women.

RISK FACTORS
As benign physiologic cysts are a result of ovulation; medications or conditions associated with increased ovulation increase risk of cyst rupture. Examples include:
- Ovulation induction agents (i.e., Clomid, aromatase inhibitors, GnRH agonists)
- Tamoxifen increases the risk of ovarian cysts in reproductive-aged women.
- Rare risk factors for increased ovarian cyst formation include fibrous dysplasia/McCune-Albright syndrome.

GENERAL PREVENTION
Ovulation suppression with combined oral contraceptives is the mainstay therapy for prevention of recurrent ovarian cysts.

DIAGNOSIS

- When a ruptured ovarian cyst is suspected, a pregnancy test should be performed to rule out an ectopic pregnancy.
- Ultrasound imaging is standard for determining whether or not a patient with a ruptured cyst can be managed conservatively, or immediate intervention is indicated. Hemoperitoneum or hemodynamic instability is an indication for emergent intervention (1)[B].
- Sonographic imaging can also determine the characteristics of the cysts and can aid in separating malignant versus benign etiologies.
- Additionally, ultrasound is useful in confirming normal Doppler flow to affected ovary.

HISTORY
- A general past medical and surgical history should be reviewed.
- Specific questions that should be addressed if you suspect a ruptured cyst include:
  - Onset and characteristics of pain
  - Pain associated with sexual intercourse or strenuous activity
  - Date of last menstrual period
  - Vaginal bleeding
  - Nausea or vomiting
  - Shoulder pain
- Symptoms of circulatory collapse, including palpitation, shortness of breath, sensation of being hot or clammy, dizziness
- Additional information that will guide diagnosis should include patient age, symptom onset, particularly in relation to menstrual cycle, anatomic location, and imaging studies.

ALERT
Patients with bleeding diathesis or undergoing anticoagulation therapy may experience significant bleeding from hemorrhagic cysts.

PHYSICAL EXAM
- Vital signs are usually normal unless significant blood loss has occurred.
- Rupture characterized by significant blood loss may be present in the form of pallor, pale mucosal membranes, and tachycardia.
- Patient will have significant tenderness to palpation or an acute abdomen if the peritoneum is irritated or inflamed.

- On some occasions, a palpable adnexal mass can be felt on bimanual exam. Care should be taken not to cause further injury with a forceful exam.

DIFFERENTIAL DIAGNOSIS
Should include all causes of acute abdominal pain, both gynecologic and nongynecologic

ALERT
- Ectopic pregnancy should always be excluded with a negative pregnancy test.
- Benign nongynecologic causes of acute lower abdominal pain include:
  - Appendicitis
  - Diverticulitis
  - Infections of the urinary tract
  - Renal colic
- Malignant nongynecologic causes of acute lower abdominal pain can be attributed to neoplastic processes of the lower GI tract.
- Benign gynecologic etiologies include:
  - Functional ovarian cysts
  - Ovarian torsion
  - Ectopic pregnancy
  - Tubo-ovarian abscess
  - Teratomas
  - Fibroids
  - Endometrioma
  - Cystadenoma (mucinous or serous)
  - Hydrosalpinx
- Malignant gynecologic etiologies can usually be attributed to the various gynecologic cancers of the reproductive tract.

DIAGNOSTIC TESTS & INTERPRETATION
- Urinalysis, STD testing, and a complete blood count should be obtained to evaluate for infectious causes, PID, or symptomatic renal stones. There are no laboratory tests that can definitively diagnose ovarian cyst rupture (2)[C].
- A type and screen is indicated if surgical intervention is planned or blood products are being considered.
- Transvaginal ultrasound is helpful in determining the presence of an ovarian mass, its characteristics, and the presence of intraperitoneal fluid (1)[A].
- CT, MRI, or PET imaging are not indicated for initial evaluation; however, these modalities are useful if malignancy is suspected (1)[A].

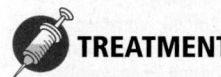

TREATMENT

GENERAL MEASURES
- Cyst rupture in a stable healthy patient can be managed conservatively with analgesia, bleeding and symptoms precautions, and outpatient follow-up (1)[A].

- For many patients, pain associated with a ruptured cyst will be transient and self-limiting.
- Scheduled NSAIDs or oral narcotics can be prescribed depending on pain severity.
- Unstable patients with hemodynamic compromise or patients with significant intraperitoneal fluid should be resuscitated, and laparoscopy or a laparotomy should be considered. Surgical exploration should also be considered if there is a concern for malignancy.

ISSUES FOR REFERRAL
- OB-GYN
  - Consider referral to an obstetrician if an adnexal mass is diagnosed during pregnancy. Such masses have a low risk of malignancy or acute complication for the pregnancy.
- GYNECOLOGIC ONCOLOGY
  - Referral to a gynecologic oncologist should be considered for complex adnexal masses with an elevated CA125 and associated symptoms concerning for malignancy such as ascites, early satiety, pleural effusion, enlarging abdominal mass, or bowel obstruction.
- GENERAL SURGERY
  - Acute lower abdominal pain that is nongynecologic and suspicious for bowel involvement should be referred to general surgery or a gastroenterologist.

SURGERY/OTHER PROCEDURES
- Although the need for surgical intervention is rare, it is usually of an emergent nature.
- In most cases, laparoscopy will be sufficient to evaluate intra-abdominal bleeding. The decision to proceed with cystectomy or oophorectomy should be made intraoperatively after a thorough evaluation of the intra-abdominal environment has been completed.
- The advantages of a laparoscopic approach include a shorter length of stay, and most patients can be discharged home the same day. Postoperative recovery time as well as patient satisfaction is significantly improved with a minimally invasive approach.
- Laparotomy should be performed in cases of critical hemodynamic instability or lack of laparoscopically trained surgeons. If there is concern for malignancy or metastases, laparotomy may be the preferred method of surgery.

INPATIENT CONSIDERATIONS
Patients who require inpatient management should be managed with serial abdominal exams, analgesia, and intravenous resuscitation as indicated by their initial presentation.

 ONGOING CARE

FOLLOW-UP RECOMMENDATIONS
- Follow up for patients managed conservatively should be scheduled 1 to 2 weeks from the initial onset of symptoms. Patients should present sooner for new or worsening symptoms.
- Patients with complete resolution of symptoms within a few days can follow-up as needed. However, these patients should be counseled on ovarian cysts and options for prevention.
- Patient in whom surgical intervention was indicated, postop follow-up should be scheduled 2 weeks from the date of surgery.
- Patients in whom an ovarian cyst was diagnosed incidentally should follow-up based on the size of their cyst.
- Simple cysts up to 10 cm in diameter on ultrasound findings are almost always benign and may safely be followed without intervention in pre- and postmenopausal patients. These patients should also be referred to a gynecologist (3)[B].

Pregnancy Considerations
Adnexal masses in pregnancy have a low risk of malignancy or acute complications to the pregnancy, so in most cases, they can be managed expectantly (1)[C].

PATIENT EDUCATION
Reassurance of the benign nature of most ovarian cysts is an important cornerstone of patient education.

REFERENCES
1. Prakash A, Li T, Ledger WL. The management of ovarian cysts in premenopausal women. *The Obstetrician and Gynecologist*. 2004;6:12–15.
2. McDonald JM, Modesitt SC. The incidental postmenopausal adnexal mass. *Clin Obstet Gynecol*. 2006;49(3):506–516.
3. Pavlik EJ, Ueland FR, Miller RW, et al. Frequency and disposition of ovarian abnormalities followed with serial transvaginal ultrasonography. *Obstet Gynecol*. 2013;122(2 Pt 1):210–217.

ADDITIONAL READING
- American College of Obstetricians and Gynecologists. ACOG practice bulletin. Management of adnexal masses. *Obstet Gynecol*. 2007;110(1): 201–214.
- Bottomley C, Bourne T. Diagnosis and management of ovarian cyst accidents. *Best Pract Res Clin Obstet Gynaecol*. 2009;23(5):711–724.

- Collins MT, Singer FR, Eugster E. McCune-Albright syndrome and the extraskeletal manifestations of fibrous dysplasia. *Orphanet J Rare Dis*. 2012;7 (Suppl 1):S4.
- Hoo WL, Yazbek J, Holland T, et al. Expectant management of ultrasonically diagnosed ovarian dermoid cysts: is it possible to predict outcome? *Ultrasound Obstet Gynecol*. 2010;36(2):235–240.
- Kaunitz AM. Oral contraceptive health benefits: perception versus reality. *Contraception*. 1999;59 (1 Suppl):29S–33S.
- Mimoun C, Fritel X, Fauconnier A, et al. Epidemiology of presumed benign ovarian tumors. *J Gynecol Obstet Biol Reprod (Paris)*. 2013;42(8):722–729.
- Møller LM. Complications of gynaecological operations. A one-year analysis of a hospital database. *Ugeskr Laeger*. 2005;167(49):4654–4659.
- Raziel A, Ron-El R, Pansky M, et al. Current management of ruptured corpus luteum. *Eur J Obstet Gynecol Reprod Biol*. 1993;50(1):77–81.
- Roch O, Chavan N, Aquilina J, et al. Radiological appearances of gynaecologic emergencies. *Insights Imaging*. 2012;3(3):265–275.
- Saunders BA, Podzielinski I, Ware RA, et al. Risk of malignancy in sonographically confirmed septated cystic ovarian tumors. *Gynecol Oncol*. 2010;118(3):278–282.
- Stany MP, Hamilton CA. Benign disorders of the ovary. *Obstet Gynecol Clin North Am*. 2008;35(2): 271–284.
- Suzuki S, Yasumoto M, Matsumoto R, et al. MR findings of ruptured endometrial cyst: comparison with tubo-ovarian abscess. *Eur J Radiol*. 2012;81(11):3631–3637.

 CODES

ICD10
- N83.20 Unspecified ovarian cysts
- N83.0 Follicular cyst of ovary
- N83.1 Corpus luteum cyst

CLINICAL PEARLS
- Functional ovarian cysts are very common in reproductive-age women and are usually self-limiting.
- Always exclude ectopic pregnancy.
- Management of symptomatic ruptured cysts is usually accomplished with outpatient pain control with follow-up.
- In cases where the patient with a ruptured cyst is unstable or presents with signs of an acute abdomen, surgical intervention is indicated.

OVARIAN TUMOR (BENIGN)

Kristin D'Orsi, DO • Mark J. Manning, DO, MsMEL

 BASICS

DESCRIPTION

- The ovaries are a source of many tumor types (benign, malignant, low malignant potential) because of the histologic variety of their constituent cells.
- Benign ovarian tumors create difficulties in differential diagnosis because of the need to identify malignancy and discriminate tumor from cysts, infectious lesions, ectopic pregnancy, and endometriomas.
- Tumors are often clinically silent until well developed; may be solid, cystic, or mixed; and they may be functional (producing sex steroids as with arrhenoblastomas and gynandroblastomas) or nonfunctional.
- System(s) affected: endocrine/metabolic, reproductive

Geriatric Considerations
Because incidence of malignancy increases with age, postmenopausal patients warrant comprehensive evaluation and follow-up.

Pediatric Considerations
Malignancy must be ruled out in premenarchal patients. Early neonatal cysts are rare.

EPIDEMIOLOGY

Incidence
- 30% of regularly cycling females
- 50% of women without regular cycles
- Predominant age: Premenarchal girls have a 6–11% risk of cancer in an ovarian tumor, and postmenopausal women have a 29–35% risk. A high percentage of ovarian tumors are malignant in girls <15 years of age.

ETIOLOGY AND PATHOPHYSIOLOGY
- Endometriosis with localized, repeated ovarian hemorrhage
- Physiologic cysts
- Tumorigenesis, with genetics as yet poorly defined

RISK FACTORS
- Cigarette smoking doubles the relative risk for developing functional ovarian cysts.
- Possible contributory factors are early menarche, obesity, infertility, and hypothyroidism.
- Tamoxifen increases risk of ovarian cyst formation (15–30%) (1).
- Risks for ovarian cancer include age >60 years; early menarche; late menopause; nulligravidity infertility; endometriosis; polycystic ovarian syndrome; family history of ovarian, breast, or colon cancer; a personal history of breast/colon cancer; or *BRCA* mutation.
- Risk for ovarian cancer is decreased in women who have used oral contraceptive pills (OCPs), are multiparous, have a history of a tubal ligation, or who have breastfed.

GENERAL PREVENTION
- OCPs do not appear to increase rates of cyst resolution, they do decrease the risk for forming new ovarian cysts (1).
- Resection of benign cysts has no impact on future risk for ovarian cancer.
- A case-control study of 299 women found no evidence that ovulation-induction treatment predisposes women to the development of borderline ovarian growths (2).

 DIAGNOSIS

- A careful history is important.
- Usually asymptomatic
- Pain is related to torsion, endometriosis, or rupture.

HISTORY
- Early satiety
- Dyspepsia/bloating
- Increased abdominal girth
- Bowel pressure or bladder pressure sensations
- Menstrual irregularities
- Dyspareunia
- Hormonal status (OCPs, hormone replacement therapy [HRT] or fertility drugs)

PHYSICAL EXAM
- Severe acne
- Examine lymph nodes for enlargement.
- Chest auscultation can reveal a pleural effusion.
- Abdominal exam may identify ascites, masses, or increased abdominal girth.
- Hirsutism/sexual precocity
- Pelvic exam
- Rectovaginal exam
- Virilization

DIFFERENTIAL DIAGNOSIS
- Ovarian malignancies
- Ovarian tumor of low malignant potential (Borderline tumor)
- Endometrioma
- Serous cystadenoma
- Mucinous cystadenoma
- Teratoma
- Hemorrhagic cyst
- Granulosa cell tumor
- Theca Lutein cyst
- Diverticulitis/bowel abscess
- Pelvic inflammatory disease (PID) with tubo-ovarian abscess
- Ectopic pregnancy
- Hydrosalpinx
- Paraovarian cyst
- Peritoneal inclusion cysts
- Functional cysts (follicular and corpus luteum cysts)
- Polycystic ovaries
- Ovarian fibroma
- Neoplasm metastatic to ovary

DIAGNOSTIC TESTS & INTERPRETATION
Initial Tests (lab, imaging)
- Serum β-human chorionic gonadotropin (β-hCG)
- CBC for WBCs is helpful if PID or ovarian torsion is suspected.
- Urinalysis
- Serum estrogens and androgens if signs of androgen excess (although only as part of polycystic ovarian [PCO] workup)
- Serum tumor markers may be considered but often confuse rather than help to resolve diagnosis; choose carefully (3)[B].
  - CA-125 should not be ordered in a premenopausal patient for screening purposes. If an ovarian tumor in a premenopausal patient is highly suspicious for cancer by ultrasound, a CA-125 level >200 U is concerning. In a postmenopausal patient, cancer must be ruled out and a CA-125 >35 U is concerning (value is lab dependent) (4)[B].
  - α-Fetoprotein and hCG can be ordered for suspected germ cell tumor.
  - Inhibin A and Inhibin B for suspected granulosa cell tumor
  - Lactate dehydrogenase (LDH) and α-fetoprotein (AFP) for suspected germ cell tumors
- Human epididymis protein 4 (HE4) may offer superior specificity compared to CA-125 for the differentiation of benign and malignant adnexal masses in premenopausal women (2)[B].
- Disorders that may alter lab results are the following:
  - CA-125: endometriosis, peritonitis, PID, Meigs syndrome, uterine fibroids, hepatitis, pancreatitis, systemic lupus erythematosus (SLE), diverticulitis
  - β-hCG: pregnancy, hydatidiform mole
  - α-Fetoprotein: hepatocellular carcinoma, hepatic cirrhosis, acute/chronic hepatitis
- Transvaginal ultrasound is the best means to determine the architecture of an ovarian cyst or mass (5)[B].
- Transvaginal ultrasonography may differentiate tumors from other pelvic lesions and identify features that place the patient at greater risk for malignancy (e.g., solid component; palpillations; multiple septations; ascites, bilaterality, fixed and irregular, rapidly enlarging, accompanied by cul-de-sac nodules).
- Transabdominal ultrasonography can help identify ascites.
- MRI can be helpful in better defining masses in women with low risk of ovarian cancer but who have an "indeterminant" mass on ultrasound. Usually not necessary, as decision for surgery can proceed without MRI if indicated; can add greatly to cost of care.
- Abdominopelvic CT scan with contrast material, if MRI is unavailable, although ultrasound still far superior (6)
- Mathematical models and calculators have been created to evaluate the risk of malignancy of ovarian tumors (7)[A].

Diagnostic Procedures/Other
- Exploratory laparoscopy or laparotomy
- Aspiration of cyst fluid (contraindicated in postmenopausal women)

Test Interpretation
- Ultrasound findings should include size and consistency of the mass such as cystic, solid, or mixed and if unilateral or bilateral.
- Thin-walled sonolucent, unilocular cysts with regular borders are most likely benign.
- Septations, mural nodules, papillary excrescences, or ascites are concerning for malignant etiology.
- Endometriomas (extrauterine endometrial tissue) are often homogeneous appearing cysts with low-level echoes.
- Cystic teratomas (dermoid cysts) are often hypoechoic with multiple small homogenous interfaces.
- Follicular cysts are the most common ovarian cysts in the premenopausal nonpregnant female.

Pregnancy Considerations
- Most cysts discovered during pregnancy are corpus luteum/follicular cysts.
- The two most commonly encountered tumors during pregnancy are cystadenomas (serous/mucinous) and dermoid cysts.

 TREATMENT

GENERAL MEASURES
- In premenopausal patients cystic lesions <10 cm in diameter, simple observation for 4 to 6 weeks is acceptable.
- Premenopausal women should have a repeat ultrasound ideally during their follicular phase (day 3 to 10 of cycle) (8)[C].
- In premenopausal patients, simple and hemorrhagic cysts <3 cm are not suspicious and do not likely need follow-up (8)[C].
- If a large cyst remains unchanged after 4 to 6 weeks of observation, then surgical exploration is indicated.
- In postmenopausal patients cysts <1 cm are likely benign (8)[C].

MEDICATION
First Line
- NSAIDs or opioids may be helpful for discomfort.

- Oral contraceptives do not hasten the resolution of functional ovarian cysts. Most cysts resolve without treatment within a few cycles (9)[B].

SURGERY/OTHER PROCEDURES
- Cystectomy/wedge resection for cyst with benign features
- Surgical removal of tumor to establish diagnosis when:
  - Premenopausal cysts >5 cm that persist >12 weeks
  - Mass is solid.
  - Mass is >10 cm.
  - Mass in a premenarchal/postmenopausal female
  - Suspicion of torsion/rupture
  - Postmenopausal cysts

- Cysts with worrisome features on ultrasound (e.g., papillations, septations)
- For masses that are worrisome for cancer, consider referral to a gynecologist/oncologist for initial surgery.
- Bilateral salpingo-oophorectomy may be appropriate in postmenopausal patients to reduce the risk of future pelvic surgery.

 ONGOING CARE

FOLLOW-UP RECOMMENDATIONS
Patient Monitoring
- Most require only yearly exams.
- Varies by diagnosis

PATIENT EDUCATION
A variety of excellent patient education materials (e.g., "Ovarian Cyst") can be downloaded from the American Association of Family Physicians and American College of Obstetricians and Gynecologists Internet sites: http://www.aafp.org/journals/afp.html?cmpid=_van_188 and http://www.acog.org/.

PROGNOSIS
Complete cure

COMPLICATIONS
Complications of untreated dermoid and mucinous cysts may include rupture, torsion, and pseudomyxoma peritonei.

REFERENCES
1. Cusidó M, Fábregas R, Pere BS, et al. Ovulation induction treatment and risk of borderline ovarian tumors. *Gynecol Endocrinol.* 2007;23(7):373–376.
2. Holcomb K, Vucetic Z, Miller MC, et al. Human epididymis protein 4 offers superior specificity in the differentiation of benign and malignant adnexal masses in premenopausal women. *Am J Obstet Gynecol.* 2011;205(4):358.e1–358.e6.
3. Maggino T, Gadducci A, D'Addario V, et al. Prospective multicenter study on CA 125 in postmenopausal pelvic masses. *Gynecol Oncol.* 1994;54(2):117–123.
4. National Institutes of Health Consensus Development Conference Statement. Ovarian cancer: screening, treatment, and follow-up. *Gynecol Oncol.* 1994;55(3 Pt 2):S4–S14.
5. Myers ER, Bastian LA, Havrilesky LJ, et al. Management of Adnexal Mass. Evidence Report/Technology Assessment No.130. Rockville, MD: Agency for Healthcare Research and Quality; 2006.
6. Iyer VR, Lee SI. MRI, CT, and PET/CT for ovarian cancer detection and adnexal lesion characterization. *AJR Am J Roentgenol.* 2010;194(2):311–321.
7. Van Calster B, Van Hoorde K, Valentin L, et al. Evaluating the risk of ovarian cancer before surgery using the ADNEX model to differentiate between benign, borderline, early and advanced stage invasive and secondary metastatic tumours: Prospective multicentre diagnostic study. *BMJ.* 2014;349:g5920.
8. Levine D, Brown DL, Andreotti RF, et al. Management of asymptomatic ovarian and other adnexal cysts imaged at US: Society of Radiologists in Ultrasound Consensus Conference Statement. *Radiology.* 2010;256(3):943–954.
9. Grimes DA, Jones LB, Lopez LM, et al. Oral contraceptives for functional ovarian cysts. *Cochrane Database Syst Rev.* 2014;(4):CD006134.

ADDITIONAL READING
- American College of Obstetricians and Gynecologists. ACOG Practice Bulletin. Management of adnexal masses. *Obstet Gynecol.* 2007;110(1):201–214.
- Crayford TJ, Campbell S, Bourne TH, et al. Benign ovarian cysts and ovarian cancer: a cohort study with implications for screening. *Lancet.* 2000;355(9209):1060–1063.
- Givens V, Mitchell GE, Harraway-Smith C, et al. Diagnosis and management of adnexal masses. *Am Fam Physician.* 2009;80(8):815–820.
- Kirilovas D, Schedvins K, Naessén T, et al. Conversion of circulating estrone sulfate to 17beta-estradiol by ovarian tumor tissue: a possible mechanism behind elevated circulating concentrations of 17beta-estradiol in postmenopausal women with ovarian tumors. *Gynecol Endocrinol.* 2007;23(1):25–28.
- Laberge PY, Levesque S. Short-term morbidity and long-term recurrence rate of ovarian dermoid cysts treated by laparoscopy versus laparotomy. *J Obstet Gynecol Can.* 2006;28(9):789–793.
- Marchesini AC, Magrio FA, Berezowski AT, et al. A critical analysis of Doppler velocimetry in the differential diagnosis of malignant and benign ovarian masses. *J Womens Health (Larchmt).* 2008;17(1):97–102.

 CODES

ICD10
- D27.9 Benign neoplasm of unspecified ovary
- D27.0 Benign neoplasm of right ovary
- D27.1 Benign neoplasm of left ovary

CLINICAL PEARLS
- In perimenopausal patients, follicles and simple cysts <3 cm are normal physiologic findings.
- Transvaginal pelvic ultrasound is the imaging test of choice to initially determine the architecture of an ovarian cyst or mass.
- Malignancy must be ruled out in both premenarchal and postmenopausal patients.
- Do not order CA-125 on premenopausal patients with an ovarian mass unless it is highly suspicious for cancer.

PALLIATIVE CARE

Erika Oleson, DO, MS

 BASICS

Palliative care is a specialty that focuses on preventing and alleviating suffering of patients (and their families) living with life-limiting illness at any stage of that illness.

DESCRIPTION
- Palliative care's principal aim is to prevent and alleviate suffering—whether physical (pain, breathlessness, nausea, etc.), emotional, social, or spiritual regardless of underlying diagnosis.
- The goal of palliative care is to improve or maintain quality of life of both patient and family despite serious illness.
- Palliative care is available for patients with serious, life-limiting illness, at any stage of their disease, with or without concurrent curative care.
- Location of care: Patients and their families may access palliative care services in hospital, rehabilitative or skilled nursing facility, and ambulatory setting.
- Hospice: In the United States, hospice is available for patients whose average life expectancy is 6 months or less and whose principal goal is to stay home (including long-term care or assisted living facility), avoid hospitalizations, and disease-directed care with a curative intent. Unlike regular nursing services in the home, hospice does not require a patient to be homebound and offers backup support for patients 24 hours a day and 7 days per week.

COMMONLY ASSOCIATED CONDITIONS
Symptoms/syndromes commonly treated in palliative care:
- Pain
  - Chronic pain
  - Headache
  - Neuropathic pain
  - Pain from bone metastases
  - Pruritus
- GI symptoms (~60% incidence)
  - Ascites
  - Anorexia/cachexia
  - Nausea (and vomiting)
    - Think of the underlying etiology and treat accordingly.
      - GI causes: constipation, bowel (full or partial) obstruction, ileus, heart burn, reflux, inflammation
      - Intrathoracic causes: cardiac, effusions (cardiac, pulmonary), mediastinal causes, esophageal
      - Autonomic dysfunction
      - Centrally mediated: intracranial pressure change, inflammation, cerebellar, vestibular, medication or metabolic cause stimulating vomiting center and/or chemoreceptor trigger zone
  - Bowel obstruction
  - Constipation and impaction of stool
  - Diarrhea
  - Dysphagia
  - Mucositis/stomatitis
  - Sialorrhea
- General medical
  - Delirium (40–85%)
- Pulmonary symptoms
  - Cough, chronic
  - Breathlessness or dyspnea (60%): often due to heart failure, COPD, lung cancer, and so forth
- Psychological symptoms
  - Anxiety
  - Depression
  - Insomnia
- Skin
  - Decubitus ulcer
  - Pruritus
  - Complex wounds (fungating tumors, etc.)

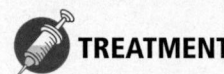 **DIAGNOSIS**

The PEACE tool evaluates the following (1):
- Physical symptoms
- Emotive and cognitive symptoms
- Autonomy and related issues
- Communication: contribution to others and closure of life affairs–related issues
- Economic burden and other practical issues, also transcendent and existential issues

HISTORY
A comprehensive palliative care assessment includes addressing the following:
- Underlying medical conditions and their associated physical symptoms
- Comprehensive pain and symptom assessment and review of systems (consider use of Edmonton Symptom Assessment Tool)
- Psychological symptom assessment
- Cultural, social, and practical concerns
- Spiritual and existential issues
  - FICA assessment (**F**aith, **I**mportance and influence, **C**ommunity, **A**ddress—how does the patient wish to be addressed?) (2)
  - HOPE (sources of **H**ope/strength/comfort, **O**rganized religion's role, **P**ersonal spirituality and practices, **E**ffects on medical care and end-of-life care) (3)
- Patient's identified presence and sources of suffering: personhood concerns
- Goals of care: including posthospital care, practical needs, hopes, and fears
- Prognosis: including functional status and patient's interest in knowing prognosis

PHYSICAL EXAM
Comprehensive physician examination is warranted, especially as directed by underlying diagnosis, symptoms, and functional decline.

DIAGNOSTIC TESTS & INTERPRETATION
Initial Tests (lab, imaging)
Per diagnosis and symptoms

TREATMENT

GENERAL MEASURES
- Targeted interventions to maximize quality of life and minimize symptom burden while taking into consideration the patient's values, goals, fears, and social setting.
- Treatment should involve an interdisciplinary team—addressing potential and realized suffering, whether physical, emotional, social, or spiritual.

MEDICATION
- Attempt to minimize polypharmacy
- Consider trimming medications that offer little improvement in the quality of life.
- Medication should focus on symptom management.
- Continue to use appropriate disease-modifying medications especially if they lessen symptom burden and enhance immediate quality of life.
- Improve compliance by addressing patient/caregiver understanding.

- *Pain* (4)[A]
  - Use immediate-release opioids PO/IV/SC and titrate to control.
  - Once pain is controlled, convert to long-acting **opioids** with short-acting agents made available as tolerance develops and/or patient develops breakthrough pain.
- Bone pain: NSAIDs added to narcotics are more effective than narcotics alone.

ALERT
Avoid morphine in patients with renal failure, can induce delirium, hyperalgesia, agitation, and seizures.

- *Vomiting* associated with a particular opioid may be relieved by substitution with an equianalgesic dose of another opioid or a sustained-release formulation (5).
  - Dopamine receptor antagonists (metoclopramide, prochlorperazine, promethazine) are commonly used. Haloperidol may help with nausea.
  - Droperidol: insufficient evidence to advise on the use for the management of nausea and vomiting
- *Constipation*: Consider prophylactic stool softeners (docusate) and stimulants (bisacodyl or senna) or osmotic laxatives (6)[A].

ALERT
Laxatives should be started when opioid treatment has begun to avoid constipation.

- SC methylnaltrexone is effective in inducing bowel movements without inducing withdrawal with opioid-induced constipation (7)[A].
- Dyspnea: Consider oxygen, if congestive heart failure (CHF); diuretics and/or long-acting nitrates, **benzodiazepines**
  - In addition to treating the underlying cause of breathlessness, as the disease advances, low-dose opioids may be beneficial to patients (4,8)[C]. Immediate-release **opioids** PO/IV treat dyspnea effectively and typically at doses lower than necessary for the relief of moderate pain.
- *Delirium*: lowest doses necessary of **benzodiazepines** or **antipsychotics** (haloperidol, etc.)
  - Monitor patient safety and use nonpharmacologic strategies to assist orientation (clocks, calendars, environment, and redirection).
  - Droperidol: When cause of delirium cannot be identified/corrected rapidly, consider neuroleptics (haloperidol or risperidone).

- Pruritus: no optimal therapy (9)[A]
- Anxiety: insufficient data for recommendations of specific medication, but anxiolytics and/or other agents may be tried (10)[A].
- Megestrol acetate improves appetite and slight weight gain in patients with anorexia-cachexia syndrome (11)[A].

ISSUES FOR REFERRAL
- Referral to palliative care
  - Any patient with a serious, life-limiting illness who could benefit from help with burdensome symptoms or suffering and/or complex goals of care discussion (12)[A].
  - Early referral to palliative care may improve quality of life and longevity for patients with advanced cancer (13)[A].
- Referral to hospice care
  - Any patient with an average life expectancy of 6 months or less. Consider the question, "Would you be surprised if the patient died within the next 6 months?" If the answer is no, they likely meet prognostic criteria for hospice.
    - Consider patients who have multiple hospitalizations and/or emergency department visits in the prior 6 months.
    - Refer to local hospice guidelines for additional disease-specific criteria.

REFERENCES

1. Okon TR, Evans JM, Gomez CF, et al. Palliative educational outcome with implementation of PEACE tool integrated clinical pathway. *J Palliat Med*. 2004;7(2):279–295.
2. Puchalski C, Romer AL. Taking a spiritual history allows clinicians to understand patients more fully. *J Palliat Med*. 2000;3(1):129–137.
3. Anandarajah G, Hight E. Spirituality and medical practice: using the HOPE questions as a practical tool for spiritual assessment. *Am Fam Physician*. 2001;63(1):81–89.
4. Lorenz KA, Lynn J, Dy SM, et al. Evidence for improving palliative care at the end of life: a systematic review. *Ann Intern Med*. 2008;148(2):147–159.
5. Smith HS, Smith JM, Smith AR. An overview of nausea/vomiting in palliative medicine. *Ann Palliat Med*. 2012;1(2):103–114.
6. Candy B, Jones L, Larkin PJ, et al. Laxative for the management of constipation in people receiving palliative care. *Cochrane Database Syst Rev*. 2015;(5):CD003448.
7. Candy B, Jones L, Goodman ML, et al. Laxatives or methylnaltrexone for the management of constipation in palliative care patients. *Cochrane Database Syst Rev*. 2011;(1):CD003448.
8. Ben-Aharon I, Gafter-Gvili A, Paul M, et al. Interventions for alleviating cancer-related dyspnea: a systematic review. *J Clin Oncol*. 2008;26(14):2396–2404.
9. Xander C, Meerpohl JJ, Galandi D, et al. Pharmacological intervention for pruritus in adult palliative care patients. *Cochrane Database Syst Rev*. 2013;(6):CD008320.
10. Candy B, Jackson KC, Jones L, et al. Drug therapy for symptoms associated with anxiety in adult palliative care patients. *Cochrane Database Syst Rev*. 2012;(10):CD004596.
11. Ruiz Garcia V, López-Briz E, Carbonell Sanchis R, et al. Megestrol acetate for treatment of anorexia-cachexia syndrome. *Cochrane Database Syst Rev*. 2013;(3):CD004310.
12. Weissman DE, Meier DE. Identifying patients in need of a palliative care assessment in the hospital setting: a consensus report from the Center to Advance Palliative Care. *J Palliat Med*. 2011;14(1):17–23.
13. Temel JS, Greer JA, Muzikansky A, et al. Early palliative care for patients with metastatic non-small-cell lung cancer. *N Engl J Med*. 2010;363(8):733–742.

 CODES

ICD10
Z51.5 Encounter for palliative care

CLINICAL PEARLS
- Early referral to palliative care may help enhance the quality of life and potential longevity of patients living with serious illness.
- Bone pain: NSAIDs added to narcotics are more effective than narcotics alone.
- Laxatives should be started when opioid treatment has begun to avoid constipation.

PANCREATIC CANCER

Alma M. Guerrero, MD • Edward Feller, MD, FACP, FACG

BASICS

DESCRIPTION
- Adenocarcinoma of the exocrine pancreas (85% of pancreatic cancers) is the fourth most common cause of cancer death in the United States (1).
- Rarely curable: overall 5-year relative survival rate of 6.7%
- 60–70% occurs in the head, 20% in the body and tail, 20% diffusely involve the gland.
- As few as 10% are localized at diagnosis. For localized, small cancers (<2 cm) with no lymph node metastases and no extension beyond the capsule, surgical resection has 5-year survival of about 25%.
- Majority of tumors have metastasized at diagnosis and are thus, largely incurable and have a 5-year survival rate of 2–3%.
- In apparently resectable disease, 20–40% have unresectable lesions at surgery.
- Ampullary, duodenal, or distal bile duct tumors may mimic pancreatic carcinoma and are more likely to be resectable and curable.
- For advanced or unresectable cancers, survival is <1% at 5 years; most patients die within 1 year.

EPIDEMIOLOGY
During 2003 to 2007, median age at diagnosis = 72 years; rare <45 years; after 45 years of age, occurrence rises (2).

Incidence
- An estimated 46,000 people diagnosed in 2014; 40,000 deaths (3)[A].
- More common in black and white races, 16.7 and 10.3 in 100,000 men and 14.4 and 10.3 in 100,000 women, respectively. Among Hispanic and Asian/Pacific Islanders, there is an incidence of 10.9 and 8.3 in 100,000 men and 10.1 and 8.3 in 100,000 women, respectively.

Prevalence
In 2008, in the United States, ~34,600 men and women (16,811 men and 17,846 women) were alive who had a history of pancreatic cancer.

RISK FACTORS
- Smoking: relative risk (RR) = 2 to 3; correlates with amount smoked
- Diabetes: RR = 2.1 (95% CI [1.6, 2.8]); 1 in 6 become diabetic within 6 months before diagnosis
- Prior partial gastrectomy or cholecystectomy: 2- to 5-fold increased risk 15 to 20 years after gastrectomy
- Familial aggregation/genetic factors: 5–10% of patients have a first-degree relative with the disease, which confers a 9-fold increase in risk versus the general population; subgroup may carry germline mutations of DNA repair genes (BRCA2).
- Hereditary chronic pancreatitis (autosomal dominant, highly penetrant): cumulative risk by ages 50 and 75 years is 10% and 54%, respectively.
- Peutz-Jeghers syndrome: RR 30 to 40
- Sporadic chronic pancreatitis

- Non-O blood type: RR 1 to 2
- High intake of dietary fat and obesity
- Alcohol: Recent data indicate a modest increase in risk confined to heavy alcohol consumers.
- Coffee intake and NSAID use NOT regarded as risk factors.

GENERAL PREVENTION
No effective screening modality exists to detect early cancer. Even with a strong family history or predisposition syndromes, use and cost-effectiveness of screening are unclear.

COMMONLY ASSOCIATED CONDITIONS
- Chronic pancreatitis, diabetes mellitus, cystic fibrosis (4)
- Subsets of familial pancreatic cancer involve germline cationic trypsinogen or PRSS1 mutations (hereditary pancreatitis), BRCA2 mutations (usually with hereditary breast–ovarian cancer syndrome), CDKN2 mutations (familial atypical mole, multiple melanoma), or DNA repair gene mutations (e.g., ATM and PALB2, apart from BRCA2).
- Majority of familial pancreatic cancers have no genetic underpinnings.
- Precursor lesions are potentially curable—pancreatic intraepithelial neoplasia, intraductal papillary mucinous neoplasia, and mucinous cystic neoplasms.

DIAGNOSIS

HISTORY
- Depends on tumor location; majority become symptomatic late in disease. Most pancreatic cancers develop in the pancreatic head and block the periampullary bile duct, causing obstructive jaundice.
- Weight loss 90%; pain 75% (progressive midepigastric dull ache that often radiates to the back); malnutrition 75%; jaundice 70%; anorexia 60%; pruritus 40%; diabetes mellitus 15%; weakness, fatigue, malaise 30–40%; alcoholic stools, dark urine, steatorrhea; depression is common.
- Pancreatic cancer is a consideration in acute pancreatitis in the elderly and with new-onset diabetes, but most new-onset diabetes is not associated with cancer; thus, evaluation for cancer is warranted only in selected cases.
- Uncommon: unexplained thrombophlebitis; acute pancreatitis from tumor obstruction of pancreatic duct; duodenal obstruction or GI bleeding

PHYSICAL EXAM
- Muscle wasting and malnutrition are common; skin lesions are indicative of pruritus. Exam can be normal.
- Palpable abdominal mass or ascites in 20%
- Jaundice: 70% if tumor obstructs bile duct; 10% with body or tail carcinoma
- Courvoisier sign (painless jaundice with a palpable gallbladder): uncommon; usually associated with pancreatic head tumors, periampullary or primary bile duct tumors; hepatomegaly in advanced disease

- Virchow node (left supraclavicular) and Sister Mary Joseph node (umbilical) in metastatic disease; palpable rectal shelf (nonspecific sign of carcinomatosis)
- Migratory thrombophlebitis (Trousseau sign) (uncommon) due to hypercoagulability in mucin-producing pancreatic cancer
- GI bleeding from tumor erosion into adjacent viscera (colon); portal hypertension-related bleeding (uncommon)
- Pancreatic panniculitis: subcutaneous areas of nodular fat necrosis

DIFFERENTIAL DIAGNOSIS
- Chronic pancreatitis, duodenal cancer, cholangiocarcinoma, lymphoma, islet cell tumor, sarcoma, cystic neoplasms, tumor metastatic to pancreas (rare)
- Nonmalignant conditions: choledocholithiasis, acute or chronic pancreatitis, biliary tract stricture, adenoma; chronic mesenteric ischemia
- Tuberculosis or fungal abscess in AIDS
- Patients may present with back pain mimicking musculoskeletal disease.

DIAGNOSTIC TESTS & INTERPRETATION
- Cross-sectional imaging (usually CT scan as first-line choice) to evaluate symptoms or abnormal lab results
- Endoscopic ultrasound-guided biopsy: best modality for tissue diagnosis; sensitivity 75–90%; specificity ~100% for diagnosis of a mass
- Routine laboratory tests may reveal elevated serum bilirubin and alkaline phosphatase (cholestasis), anemia, or decreased serum albumin (malnutrition).

Initial Tests (lab, imaging)
- Most patients do not require measurement of serum tumor markers (CA19-9) for diagnosis or management. Some evidence suggests use in predicting outcome and response to adjuvant chemotherapy.
- CEA and CA19-9 are not recommended as screening tests; useful in following patients with known disease (3)[A]
- Elevated CA19-9 antigen: 80% sensitivity; 90% specificity; individuals with Lewis-negative blood group antigen phenotype (5–10%) are unable to synthesize CA19-9; elevations can occur in benign pancreatic or biliary diseases and in nonpancreatic malignancy.

Follow-Up Tests & Special Considerations
- During therapy, increase in CA19-9 may identify progressive tumor growth. Normal CA19-9 does not exclude recurrence.
- CT scan (pancreatic protocol) using thin section, multiphase multidetector helical CT with a pancreatic protocol is the choice for diagnosis and staging: 85–90% sensitivity; 90–95% specificity; useful for evaluation of distant metastasis and prediction of resectability.
- Abdominal ultrasound: common initial test to assess jaundice and duct dilatation; less sensitive than CT for pancreatic masses

- Endoscopic ultrasound (EUS) is accurate for tissue biopsy, local tumor and node staging, predicting vascular invasion (90% specificity; 73% sensitivity), and when no mass is identified on CT.
- Endoscopic retrograde cholangiopancreatography (ERCP): 90% sensitivity; 95% specificity for ductal cancer; useful if endoscopic stent is indicated for biliary obstruction; generally confined to high probability for therapeutic intervention on biliary or pancreatic ductal systems
- MRI: no advantage over contrast-enhanced CT
- MR cholangiopancreatography: 90% sensitivity; 95% specificity. Preferred in specific settings: gastric outlet or duodenal stenosis or after surgical rearrangement (Billroth II) or ductal disruption; to detect bile duct obstruction, after attempted ERCP is unsuccessful or provides incomplete information
- Cystic pancreatic lesions may be benign or malignant; must be differentiated from pancreatic pseudocysts. Cystadenocarcinomas have better prognoses than typical pancreatic cancers.

Diagnostic Procedures/Other
- Percutaneous fine-needle biopsy with US or CT guidance: 80–90% sensitivity; 98–100% specificity
- EUS-guided biopsy: 85–90% sensitivity; virtually 100% specificity for pancreatic mass
- Staging laparoscopy and US: 92% sensitivity; 88% specificity; 89% accuracy
- Positive peritoneal cytology has a positive predictive value of 94%; specificity of 98%; sensitivity of 25% for determining unresectability.
- PET scan: 90% sensitivity but 70% specificity; limited anatomic information
- Tumor staging
  - Stage I: tumors limited to the pancreas
  - Stage II: regionally invasive; may involve lymph nodes but without celiac or mesenteric artery involvement
  - Stage III: direct involvement of celiac or superior mesenteric artery involvement
  - Stage IV: distant metastases

Test Interpretation
- Duct cell carcinoma: 90%
- Other less common tumors: acinar, papillary mucinous, signet ring, adenosquamous, mucinous, giant or small cell, cystadenocarcinoma, undifferentiated, unclassified carcinoma

ALERT
Chronic pancreatitis can present with similar pain, weight loss, jaundice, and an inflammatory mass on imaging.

TREATMENT

- Surgical resection: only chance of cure; no role for pancreatic resection in metastatic disease. As few as 15–20% are candidates for resection.
- Criteria for unresectability: extrapancreatic spread, encasement or occlusion of major vessels, distant metastases
- New combination chemotherapy regimens may offer advantages over gemcitabine. Standard therapies remain unsatisfactory; thus, patients should be considered for clinical trials (3).

MEDICATION
- Analgesics
- Stages I and II
  - Radical pancreatic resection plus chemotherapy
  - ESPAC-3 trial after resection: compared with 5-fluorouracil (5-FU) and folinic acid, gemcitabine did not improve overall survival.
  - Currently, postoperative gemcitabine alone or in combination with 5-FU–based chemoradiation is the current standard of care; preoperative neoadjuvant treatment trials are in progress.
- Stage III
  - Standard: Chemotherapy with gemcitabine-based regimens; added chemoradiation is controversial.
  - FLOFIRINOX and gemcitabine—nab-paclitaxel were recently shown to have a benefit in patients with metastatic disease; may be tried in patients with locally advanced disease
  - Palliation of biliary obstruction by endoscopic, surgical, or radiologic methods
  - Intraoperative radiation therapy and/or implantation of radioactive substances
- Stage IV
  - Chemotherapy: Gemcitabine with erlotinib, or paclitaxel, or a fluoropyrimidine may modestly prolong survival compared with gemcitabine alone.
  - Pain-relieving procedures (celiac or intrapleural block); supportive care; palliative decompression

ADDITIONAL THERAPIES
- For resected tumors: postoperative radiation therapy with other chemotherapeutic agents
- Intraoperative radiation therapy and/or implantation of radioactive substances (ongoing trials)
- Biliary decompression with endoprosthesis or transhepatic drainage for bile duct obstruction
- Celiac axis and intrapleural nerve blocks can provide effective pain relief for some patients.
- Opiates may be needed for pain control.

SURGERY/OTHER PROCEDURES
- Standard treatment options
  - Pancreaticoduodenectomy, Whipple procedure, en bloc resection of the head of the pancreas, distal common bile duct, duodenum, jejunum, and gastric antrum
  - Total pancreatectomy
  - Distal pancreatectomy for body and tail tumors
- Nonstandard surgeries
  - Pylorus-preserving pancreaticoduodenectomy, regional pancreatectomy
  - Palliative bypass
    - Biliary decompression; gastrojejunostomy for gastric outlet obstruction; duodenal endoprosthesis for obstruction

ONGOING CARE

DIET
- Anorexia, asthenia, pain, and depression may contribute to cachexia.
- Fat malabsorption due to exocrine pancreatic insufficiency may contribute to malnutrition; pancreatic enzyme replacement may help to alleviate symptoms.
- Fat-soluble vitamin deficiency may require replacement therapy.

PROGNOSIS
- 90% diagnosed with pancreatic cancer die from the disease, predominantly from metastatic disease (3).
- 5-year survival: ~30% if node-negative; 10% if node-positive. Median survival: 10 to 20 months
- Metastatic cancer: 1–2% 5-year survival
- For localized disease and small cancers (<2 cm) with no lymph node involvement and no extension beyond the capsule, complete surgical resection can yield a 5-year survival of 18–24%.
- Detection of curable precursor lesions is a focus of current efforts to improve diagnosis and prognosis.

COMPLICATIONS
- Diabetes mellitus, malabsorption, thrombophlebitis
- Duodenal or distal bile duct obstruction
- Surgical complications: intra-abdominal abscess, postgastrectomy syndromes, pancreaticojejunostomy, gastric and biliary anastomotic leaks; operative mortality varies.

REFERENCES
1. Chari ST, Kelly K, Hollingsworth MA, et al. Early detection of sporadic pancreatic cancer: summative review. Pancreas. 2015;44(5):693–712.
2. Yadav D, Lowenfels AB. The epidemiology of pancreatitis and pancreatic cancer. Gastroenterology. 2013;144(6):1252–1261.
3. Ryan DR, Hong TS, Bardeesy N. Pancreatic adenocarcinoma. N Engl J Med. 2014;371(11):1039–1049.
4. De La Cruz MS, Young AP, Ruffin MT. Diagnosis and management of pancreatic cancer. Am Fam Physician. 2014;89(8):626–632.

CODES

ICD10
- C25.9 Malignant neoplasm of pancreas, unspecified
- C25.0 Malignant neoplasm of head of pancreas
- C25.1 Malignant neoplasm of body of pancreas

CLINICAL PEARLS
- Sudden onset of diabetes mellitus in nonobese adults aged >40 years may warrant consideration of pancreatic cancer in selected cases.
- Cancer of the exocrine pancreas is rarely curable; overall 5-year survival rate of <4%. Fewer than 20% of cases are localized at diagnosis.
- Be wary of chronic pancreatitis, which can present with similar pain pattern, weight loss, jaundice, and an inflammatory mass on imaging.
- Because of the dismal prognosis on standard therapy, all patients with pancreatic cancer should be considered for appropriate clinical trials

PANCREATITIS, ACUTE
Robert L. Frachtman, MD, FACG • Marni Martinez, APRN

BASICS

DESCRIPTION
Acute inflammatory process of the pancreas with variable involvement of regional tissue or remote organ systems
- Inflammatory episode with symptoms related to intrapancreatic activation of enzymes with pain, nausea and vomiting, and associated intestinal ileus
- Varies widely in severity, complications, and prognosis, accounting for 280,000 hospital admissions per year in the United States
- Complete structural and functional recovery if there is no necrosis or pancreatic ductal disruption.

EPIDEMIOLOGY
Incidence
- 1 to 5/10,000
- Predominant age: none
- Predominant sex: male = female

Prevalence
Acute: 19/10,000

ETIOLOGY AND PATHOPHYSIOLOGY
- Alcohol
- Gallstones (including microlithiasis)
- Trauma/surgery
- Acute discontinuation of medications for diabetes or hyperlipidemia
- Following endoscopic retrograde cholangiopancreatography (ERCP)
- Medications (most common, not an exhaustive list)
  - ACE inhibitors
  - Angiotensin receptor blockers (ARBs)
  - Thiazide diuretics and furosemide
  - Antimetabolites (mercaptopurine and azathioprine) (1)
  - Corticosteroids
  - Glyburide
  - Exenatide (Byetta) (2)
  - Mesalamine
  - Pentamidine
  - Sulfamethoxazole/trimethoprim
  - Valproic acid
  - HMG-CoA reductase inhibitors, especially simvastatin (1)
  - Review all medications and continue only if the benefit outweighs risk, if medication is causally implicated.
- Metabolic causes
  - Hypertriglyceridemia (>1,000 mg/dL)
  - Hypercalcemia
  - Acute renal failure
  - Diet with high glycemic load (3)[B]
  - Systemic lupus erythematosus/polyarteritis
  - Autoimmune pancreatitis, associated with elevated IgG4
  - Infections (list not exhaustive)
    ○ Mumps, coxsackie, cryptosporidiosis
- Penetrating peptic ulcer (rare)
- Cystic fibrosis and *CFTR* gene mutations
- Tumors (e.g., pancreatic, ampullary) (4)
- Pancreas divisum
- Sphincter of Oddi dysfunction
- Scorpion venom
- Vascular disease
- Acute fatty liver of pregnancy

- Idiopathic/autoimmune
- Pathophysiology—enzymatic "autodigestion" of the pancreas, interstitial edema with severe interstitial acute fluid accumulation ("3rd spacing"), hemorrhage, necrosis, release of vasoactive peptides (within 6 weeks), pseudocyst or acute necrotic collection (>6 weeks), pancreatic ductal disruption, injury to surrounding vascular structures like splenic vein (thrombosis) and splenic artery (pseudoaneurysm)

Genetics
Hereditary pancreatitis is rare. Autosomal dominant

GENERAL PREVENTION
- Avoid excess alcohol consumption.
- Tobacco cessation
- Correct underlying metabolic processes (hypertriglyceridemia or hypercalcemia).
- Discontinue offending medications.
- Cholecystectomy (symptomatic cholelithiasis)
- Diet with low glycemic load (3)[B]

COMMONLY ASSOCIATED CONDITIONS
- Alcohol withdrawal, alcoholic hepatitis, diabetic ketoacidosis, and ascending cholangitis
- Obesity increases severity, local complications, and mortality (5).

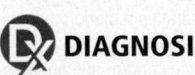

DIAGNOSIS

Symptoms do not always correlate directly with objective findings (imaging, amylase/lipase).

HISTORY
- Acute onset of "boring" epigastric pain, which may radiate posteriorly toward the back
- Nausea/vomiting
- Alcohol use
- Personal or family history of gallstones
- Medication use
- Abdominal trauma
- Recent significant rapid weight loss

PHYSICAL EXAM
- Vital signs—assess hemodynamic stability; fever
- Abdominal findings: epigastric tenderness, loss of bowel sounds
- Other findings: jaundice, rales/percussive dullness
- Rare (with hemorrhagic pancreatitis)
  - Flank discoloration (Grey-Turner sign) or umbilical discoloration (Cullen sign)

DIAGNOSTIC TESTS & INTERPRETATION
- Interpret laboratory and radiographic findings in the context of the clinical history, as false-positive and false-negative findings are common.
- American College of Gastroenterology require at least 2 of the 3 following elements to make a diagnosis of acute pancreatitis: characteristic abdominal pain, specific radiographic findings, and lipase level 3 times the ULN.
- Elevated serum amylase >3 times upper limit of normal (ULN) (severity is not related to degree of elevation)
- Elevated serum lipase >3 times ULN (may stay elevated longer than amylase in mild cases)
- Elevated total bilirubin. If >3 mg/dL, consider common bile duct obstruction.

- Transaminases rise quickly with acute bile duct obstruction. They also fall rapidly as alkaline phosphatase rises; a 3-fold elevation in the alanine aminotransferase (ALT) in the setting of acute pancreatitis has a 95% positive predictive value for gallstone pancreatitis. Triglyceride levels >1,000 mg/dL suggest hypertriglyceridemia as the cause.
- Glucose is increased in severe disease.
- Calcium is decreased in severe disease.
- WBC elevation to 10,000 to 25,000/μL possible and not indicative of active infection
- Rising hemoglobin is a poor prognostic sign (severe 3rd spacing-hemoconcentration). Rising blood urea nitrogen (BUN) and creatinine imply volume depletion or acute renal failure.

DIFFERENTIAL DIAGNOSIS
- Penetrating peptic ulcer
- Acute cholecystitis or cholangitis
- Macroamylasemia, macrolipasemia
- Mesenteric vascular occlusion and/or infarction
- Perforation of a viscus
- Intestinal obstruction
- Aortic aneurysm (dissecting or rupturing)
- Inferior wall myocardial infarction
- Lymphoma

Initial Tests (lab, imaging)
- Use follow-up labs to assess renal function, hydration, sepsis, biliary obstruction, and tissue oxygenation status.
- Plain film of abdomen helps rule out mechanical small bowel obstruction. Ileus is common.
- Chest x-ray (CXR) to evaluate for early acute respiratory distress syndrome (ARDS) and pleural effusion; can also rule out free subdiaphragmatic air.
- Ultrasound to rule out cholelithiasis; choledocholithiasis can occasionally be seen.
- CT scan
  - Confirms the diagnosis, assesses severity, establishes a baseline, and rules out other possibilities. CT does not rule out noncalcified cholelithiasis.
  - IV contrast is not essential on the initial CT scan and should be avoided in volume-depleted patients.
  - If not contraindicated, a CT scan with IV contrast at day 3 can assess the degree of necrosis when necrotizing pancreatitis is suspected because of O_2 saturation <90%, systolic BP <90 mm Hg, and so forth.
- MRCP helps assess for choledocholithiasis, pancreas divisum, a dilated pancreatic duct, and chronic ductal changes.
- Esophagogastroduodenoscopy (EGD) may be necessary to rule out a penetrating duodenal ulcer or an obstructing ampullary neoplasm if suggested by laboratory or imaging studies.
- ERCP may be necessary to decompress common bile duct due to an impacted stone.
- Endoscopic ultrasonography (EUS) is useful when a patient presents with "idiopathic pancreatitis" (4)[B].
- FNA may be added to EUS if autoimmune pancreatitis is suspected (6)[C].

Follow-Up Tests & Special Considerations
If renal function is stable, a contrast-enhanced CT scan at day 3 to assess for necrosis. Later in the course, if there is a spike in the temperature, CT-guided aspiration can help assess secondary infection.

TREATMENT

MEDICATION

First Line
- Analgesia: no consensus; guidelines vary widely on types and dosing for analgesia (7).
  - Hydromorphone (Dilaudid) 0.5 to 1 mg IV q1–2h PRN
  - AVOID Demerol due to the potential of accumulation of a toxic metabolite.
- Antibiotics
  - The use of prophylactic antibiotics is no longer recommended, even with necrotizing pancreatitis, in the absence of infection.
  - In patients with ascending cholangitis or necrotizing pancreatitis, β-lactam/β-lactamase inhibitor (e.g., piperacillin/tazobactam 4.5 g IV q8h) can be considered for initial treatment, before cultures (especially of aspirated collections) return, if there is a strong suspicion of active infection.
  - Levofloxacin 500 mg QD IV if cholangitis and there is an allergy to penicillin
  - Be vigilant for monilial superinfections when giving prophylactic antibiotics.

GENERAL MEASURES
Most cases of acute pancreatitis require hospitalization; ICU if multiorgan dysfunction or hypotension/respiratory failure. 15–20% of cases of acute pancreatitis progress from mild to severe (including persistent organ failure).
- Fluid resuscitation
  - Significant volume deficit due to 3rd spacing
  - Infuse bolus of 1,000 to 2,000 mL (lactated Ringers may be better than normal saline, unless hypercalcemic) (8)[C], followed by 250 to 300 mL/hr, adjusted on the basis of age, weight, hemodynamic response, and comorbid conditions.
  - Target urine output should be 0.5 to 1 mL/kg/hr. Lower infusion rate when this goal is achieved or once BUN decreases; 4 L should be the maximum fluid on day 1.
- Eliminate unnecessary medications, especially those potentially causing pancreatitis.
- Nasogastric (NG) tube for intractable emesis
- Follow renal function, volume status, calcium, and oxygenation. Organ failure is more important prognostic indicator than pancreatic necrosis.
- Intermittent pneumatic compression device
- Begin oral alimentation after pain, tenderness, and ileus have resolved; small amounts of high-carbohydrate, low-fat, and low-protein foods; advance as tolerated; NPO or NG tube if vomiting persists.
- Enteral nutrition at level of ligament of Treitz if oral feeding not possible within 5 to 7 days (preferable to total parenteral nutrition [TPN] due to decreased infection rate and decreased mortality). Discontinue with increases in pain, amylase/lipase levels, or fluid retention.
- TPN (without lipids if triglycerides are elevated) if oral or nasoenteric feedings are not tolerated (9).

ISSUES FOR REFERRAL
Refer to a tertiary center if pancreatitis is severe or actively evolving and when advanced imaging or endoscopic therapy is being considered.

SURGERY/OTHER PROCEDURES
- Consider cholecystectomy before discharge in patients with cholelithiasis and nonnecrotizing pancreatitis to reduce risk of recurrent acute gallstone pancreatitis.

- Necrosectomy should be performed nonsurgically for either infected or noninfected necrosis. Walled off necrosis should be observed for 4 weeks (treated with antibiotics if infected), followed by percutaneous or dual-modality drainage if available (10,11)[B].
- ERCP early if evidence of acute cholangitis or at 72 hours if evidence of ongoing biliary obstruction. ERCP with pancreatic ductal stent placement, if ductal disruption persists longer than 1 to 2 weeks.
- Resection or embolization for bleeding pseudoaneurysms
- Plasma exchange with insulin if necrotizing pancreatitis secondary to hypertriglyceridemia

INPATIENT CONSIDERATIONS

Discharge Criteria
- Pain controlled
- Tolerating oral diet
- Alcohol rehabilitation and tobacco cessation
- Low-grade fever and mild leukocytosis do not necessarily indicate infection and may take weeks to resolve. Infections may occur even after 10 days (33% of patients with necrotizing pancreatitis) due to secondary infection of necrotic material, requiring surgical débridement.

ONGOING CARE

FOLLOW-UP RECOMMENDATIONS
- Follow-up imaging studies in several weeks, if the original CT scan showed a fluid collection or necrosis or if the amylase/lipase continues to be elevated. Follow-up findings may include:
  - Pseudocyst (occurs in 10%) or abscess (sudden onset of fever): Conservative management is an option for asymptomatic pseudocysts up to 6 cm in diameter.
  - Splenic vein thrombosis (gastric variceal hemorrhage rarely occurs)
  - Pseudoaneurysm (splenic, gastroduodenal, intrapancreatic) hemorrhage can be life-threatening.
- Mild exocrine and endocrine dysfunction is usually subclinical. Patients with necrotizing pancreatitis, steatorrhea, or ductal obstruction should receive enzyme supplementation.

DIET
Continue to advance diet as tolerated. Dietary modification to reduce dietary fats, alcohol, and added sugars.

PROGNOSIS
85–90% of cases of acute pancreatitis resolve spontaneously; 3–5% mortality (17% in necrotizing pancreatitis)

REFERENCES
1. Nitsche CJ, Jamieson N, Lerch MM, et al. Drug induced pancreatitis. *Best Pract Res Clin Gastroenterol.* 2010;24(2):143–155.
2. Wang SQ, Li SJ, Feng QX, et al. Overweight is an additional prognostic factor in acute pancreatitis: a meta-analysis. *Pancreatology.* 2011;11(2):92–98.
3. Oskarsson V, Sadr-Azodi O, Orsini N, et al. High dietary glycemic load increases the risk of non-gallstone-related acute pancreatitis: a prospective cohort study. *Clin Gastroenterol Hepatol.* 2014;12(4):676–682.
4. Munigala S, Kanwal F, Xian H, et al. Increased risk of pancreatic adenocarcinoma after acute pancreatitis. *Clin Gastroenterol Hepatol.* 2014;12(7):1143–1150.e1.
5. Wu BU, Conwell DL. Acute pancreatitis part I: approach to early management. *Clin Gastroenterol Hepatol.* 2010;8(5):410–416.
6. Iwashita T, Yasuda I, Doi S, et al. Use of samples from endoscopic ultrasound-guided 19-gauge fine-needle aspiration in diagnosis of autoimmune pancreatitis. *Clin Gastroenterol Hepatol.* 2012;10(3):316–322.
7. Oláh A, Romics L Jr. Evidence-based use of enteral nutrition in acute pancreatitis. *Langenbecks Arch Surg.* 2010;395(4):309–316.
8. Hoque R, Farooq A, Ghani A, et al. Lactate reduces liver and pancreatic injury in toll-like receptor- and inflammasome-mediated inflammation via GPR81-mediated suppression of innate immunity. *Gastroenterology.* 2014;146(7):1763–1774.
9. Gravante G, Garcea G, Ong SL, et al. Prediction of mortality in acute pancreatitis: a systematic review of the published evidence. *Pancreatology.* 2009;9(5):601–614.
10. Trikudanathan G, Attam R, Arain MA, et al. Endoscopic interventions for necrotizing pancreatitis. *Am J Gastroenterol.* 2014;109(7):969–981.
11. Ross AS, Irani S, Gan SI, et al. Dual-modality drainage of infected and symptomatic walled-off pancreatic necrosis: long-term clinical outcomes. *Gastrointest Endosc.* 2014;79(6):929–935.

ADDITIONAL READING
- Fisher JM, Gardner TB. The "golden hours" of management in acute pancreatitis. *Am J Gastroenterol.* 2012;107(8):1146–1150.
- Lu X, Aoun E. Complications of acute pancreatitis. *Pract Gastroenterol.* 2012;36:11–22.
- Wu BU, Banks PA. Clinical management of patients with acute pancreatitis. *Gastroenterology.* 2013;144(6):1272–1281.

CODES

ICD10
- K85.9 Acute pancreatitis, unspecified
- K85.8 Other acute pancreatitis
- K85.2 Alcohol induced acute pancreatitis

CLINICAL PEARLS
- BISAP score is easier to apply than Ranson criteria and just as accurate in predicting mortality in acute pancreatitis.
- Review all medications upon admission and discontinue any that are implicated as causing pancreatitis.
- Patients with mild pancreatitis can progress to severe pancreatitis over the initial 48 hours, often due to inadequate fluid replacement.
- Referral to tertiary center is needed if acute pancreatitis is severe or evolving/worsening.

PANCREATITIS, CHRONIC

Robert L. Frachtman, MD, FACG • Marni Martinez, APRN

 BASICS

DESCRIPTION
- Long-standing and progressive destruction of the pancreas due to persistent inflammation
- Results in exocrine and/or endocrine insufficiency
- Major features
  - Pain
  - Malabsorption
  - Diabetes mellitus (type 3)
  - Increased risk of pancreatic cancer

EPIDEMIOLOGY
Incidence
Predominant age
- 35 to 45 years (usually related to alcohol)
- Predominant sex: male > female
- Hospitalization more common for blacks than whites

Prevalence
8/10,000

Genetics
Hereditary pancreatitis is a rare condition with an autosomal dominant inheritance pattern. Mutations in *PRSSI* gene and *SPINKI* gene

GENERAL PREVENTION
- Avoid tobacco.
- Avoid excess alcohol.

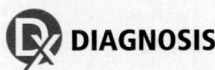 **DIAGNOSIS**

As with acute pancreatitis, symptoms and objective findings (imaging, amylase/lipase) do not always directly correlate.

HISTORY
- Epigastric pain, often radiating to the back
- Flare-ups may mimic acute pancreatitis.
- Persistent nausea and vomiting
- Chronic vague abdominal pain; may worsen postprandially or with alcohol consumption
- Alcohol use
- Cigarette smoking
- Steatorrhea and/or diarrhea
- Weight loss
- Children
  - Recurrent postprandial epigastric pain
  - Family history of chronic pancreatitis
  - Growth failure
  - Diabetes

PHYSICAL EXAM
- Acute superimposed on chronic pancreatitis
  - See "Pancreatitis, Acute"
  - Epigastric tenderness
  - Loss of bowel sounds
  - Fever
  - Tachycardia
  - Hypotension/shock
  - Jaundice
  - Rales/percussive dullness
- Chronic pancreatitis
  - Mild, diffuse tenderness
  - Ascites

DIAGNOSTIC TESTS & INTERPRETATION
Interpret laboratory and radiographic findings in chronic pancreatitis within the context of each patient presentation due to common false-positive and false-negative findings.

Initial Tests (lab, imaging)
Features and considerations
- Amylase and lipase usually normal or near normal
- Hyperglycemia
- Steatorrhea (fecal fat >7 g/day on 100 g of fat per day diet), with other malabsorptive consequences such as low B_{12} level
- Elevated alkaline phosphatase and bilirubin imply obstruction of the intrapancreatic common bile duct.
- Autoimmune pancreatitis: elevated serum IgG4 (type I, not type II), autoantibodies to lactoferrin and carbonic anhydrase (1)
- Pancreatic insufficiency: fecal elastase-1 <200 μg/g in moderate to severe pancreatic insufficiency
- Plain film of abdomen: pancreatic calcification if severe
- Ultrasound (US): helps assess common bile duct diameter, less useful for visualizing pancreas
- CT scan of abdomen: pseudocysts, pancreatic duct dilation, and calcifications, which are most commonly associated with alcohol, cigarette smoking, and hereditary pancreatitis and may take 5 to 10 years to develop (1)
- Magnetic resonance cholangiopancreatography (MRCP): pancreatic ductal deformities/strictures (with or without pancreatic ductal stones), retained common bile duct stones
- Endoscopic US (EUS): might help identify pancreatic cancer. Fine needle aspiration may be added if autoimmune pancreatitis is suspected (2)[B].

Follow-Up Tests & Special Considerations
Disorders that alter results for amylase or lipase
- Biliary tract disease
- Penetrating peptic ulcer
- Intestinal obstruction, ischemia, or infarction
- Ruptured ectopic pregnancy
- Renal insufficiency
- Burns
- Macroamylasemia; macrolipasemia

DIFFERENTIAL DIAGNOSIS
- Pancreatic cancer
- Lymphoma
- Other malabsorptive processes, such as bacterial overgrowth or celiac disease

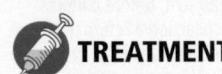 **TREATMENT**

MEDICATION
First Line
- Analgesics (no consensus on specific medications or doses)
  - Tramadol 50 mg q6h PO is commonly used as a first-line.
  - Chronic opioid (morphine, fentanyl) therapy may be required in some patients.
  - Gabapentin, pregabalin, SNRIs, or TCAs may be used as adjunctive therapy.
  - Traditional pancreatic enzyme supplements are microencapsulated and do not require acid inhibition for protection. Dosage is 25,000 to 40,000 IU at the beginning of the meal.
  - Uncoated enzymes (Viokase) may be more efficacious for pain control (when given with proton pump inhibitors [PPIs] to protect their integrity) compared with coated enzymes (3,4). There is a theoretical benefit to using PPIs, even with coated enzymes, in patients with vitamin deficiency to allow faster release of enzymes into the proximal duodenum where fat soluble vitamin absorption occurs (1).
  - Octreotide 25 to 50 μg/hr IV infusion can be supplemental therapy for pancreatic ductal fistulae, which can later be changed to long-acting SC administration.
  - Individualized doses of corticosteroids for autoimmune pancreatitis

GENERAL MEASURES
- Discontinue tobacco use, which can exacerbate chronic pancreatitis (5).
- Analgesia: Consider pain management consultation for chronic opioid management.

- Exocrine and endocrine replacement therapy (enzymes and insulin)
- Consider more advanced therapy for pain: celiac ganglion block via EUS and endoscopic or surgical decompression of partially obstructed pancreatic duct.

SURGERY/OTHER PROCEDURES

- Pseudocyst drainage
  - Conservative approach if asymptomatic
  - Endoscopic (via EUS) or surgical approach if mature wall
  - Percutaneous approach if rapidly enlarging or if thin wall
  - Endoscopic drainage and percutaneous drainage have similar clinical success rates, but percutaneous drainage requires more reintervention and longer hospital stay (6)[C].
- Pancreatic ascites with disruption of the main pancreatic duct
  - Endoscopic placement of pancreatic ductal stent is preferred, if possible.
  - Lateral pancreaticojejunostomy if endoscopic therapy is not possible
- Biliary obstruction (secondary to chronic pancreatitis, not choledocholithiasis)
  - Placement of retrievable metal stent or multiple plastic stents, if possible
  - Choledochojejunostomy if endoscopic therapy is not possible
- Pancreatic ductal obstruction by stone
  - Endoscopic pancreatic sphincterotomy with stone extraction
- Total pancreatectomy and islet autotransplantation
  - Favorable outcomes with pain reduction
  - Indication for timing of procedure uncertain
- Lithotripsy for chronic calcific pancreatitis may improve pain and decrease dependence on narcotic analgesics (7)[B].

INPATIENT CONSIDERATIONS
Discharge Criteria
- Pain control
- Resolution of problems secondary to ductal disruption, if present
- Alcohol rehab and smoking cessation, if needed

 ONGOING CARE

FOLLOW-UP RECOMMENDATIONS
Depends on the source of the pain and whether a ductal disruption exists

DIET
- Small meals high in protein, ~20 g/day of fat; adjust if diabetes is present. Patients with decreased endocrine function from chronic pancreatitis can be prone to hyper- or hypoglycemia (8)[C].
- Pancreatic enzyme replacement therapy (coated/microencapsulated for pancreatic insufficiency but noncoated with PPI for pancreatic pain)
- Vitamin A and vitamin E deficiency are not very common—levels should be checked and supplements provided only if deficiencies are noted (8)[C].

PROGNOSIS
- Patients with recurrent episodes of acute pancreatitis are more likely to develop chronic pancreatitis.
- May "burn out" with resolution of symptoms
- Narcotic addiction occurs frequently.
- Pancreatic exocrine and/or endocrine insufficiency may occur years later.
- Patients with chronic pancreatitis have an increased mortality, particularly from pancreatic cancer (9).
- 25% of patients with chronic pancreatitis have osteoporosis. Perform routine bone health assessment (10)[A].

REFERENCES

1. Forsmark CE. Management of chronic pancreatitis. *Gastroenterology*. 2013;144(6):1282.e3–1291.e3.
2. Iwashita T, Yasude I, Doi S, et al. Use of samples from endoscopic ultrasound-guided 19-gauge fine-needle aspiration in diagnosis of autoimmune pancreatitis. *Clin Gastroenterol Hepatol*. 2012;10(3):316–322.
3. Slaff J, Jacobson D, Tillman CR, et al. Protease-specific suppression of pancreatic exocrine secretion. *Gastroenterology*. 1984;87(1):44–52.
4. Puylaert M, Kapural L, Van Zundert J, et al. 26. Pain in chronic pancreatitis. *Pain Pract*. 2011;11(5):492–505.
5. Yadav D, Hawes RH, Brand RE, et al. Alcohol consumption, cigarette smoking, and the risk of recurrent acute and chronic pancreatitis. *Arch Intern Med*. 2009;169(11):1035–1045.
6. Akshintala VS, Saxena P, Zaheer A, et al. A comparative evaluation of outcomes of endoscopic versus percutaneous drainage for symptomatic pancreatic pseudocysts. *Gastrointest Endosc*. 2014;79(6):921–928.
7. Seven G, Schreiner MA, Ross AS, et al. Long-term outcomes associated with pancreatic extracorporeal shock wave lithotripsy for chronic calcific pancreatitis. *Gastrointest Endosc*. 2012;75(5):997.e1–1004.e1.
8. Duggan S, Conlon K. A practical guide to the nutritional management of chronic pancreatitis. *Pract Gastroenterol*. 2013;37:24–32.
9. Bang UC, Benfield T, Hyldstrup L, et al. Mortality, cancer, and comorbidities associated with chronic pancreatitis: a Danish nationwide matched-cohort study. *Gastroenterology*. 2014;146(4):989–994.
10. Duggan SN, Smyth ND, Murphy A, et al. High prevalence of osteoporosis in patients with chronic pancreatitis: a systematic review and meta-analysis. *Clin Gastroenterol Hepatol*. 2014;12(2):219–228.

ADDITIONAL READING

- Bornman PC, Botha JF, Ramos JM, et al. Guideline for the diagnosis and treatment of chronic pancreatitis. *S Afr Med J*. 2010;100(12 Pt 2):845–860.
- Bramis K, Gordon-Weeks AN, Friend PJ, et al. Systematic review of total pancreatectomy and islet autotransplantation for chronic pancreatitis. *Br J Surg*. 2012;99(6):761–766.
- Feurer M, Adler D. Evaluation and management of pancreatic pseudocysts. *Pract Gastroenterol*. 2014;38:12–25.
- Giuliano CA, Dehoorne-Smith ML, Kale-Pradhan PB. Pancreatic enzyme products: digesting the changes. *Ann Pharmacother*. 2011;45(5):658–666.
- Niemann T, Madsen LG, Larsen S, et al. Opioid treatment of painful chronic pancreatitis. *Int J Pancreatol*. 2000;27(3):235–240.
- Yadav D, O'Connell M, Papachristou GI. Natural history following the first attack of acute pancreatitis. *Am J Gastroenterol*. 2012;107(7):1096–1103.

 SEE ALSO

Choledocholithiasis; Peptic Ulcer Disease; Substance Use Disorders; Lupus Erythematosus, Systemic (SLE)

 CODES

ICD10
- K86.1 Other chronic pancreatitis
- K86.0 Alcohol-induced chronic pancreatitis

CLINICAL PEARLS
- EUS can help differentiate chronic pancreatitis from pancreatic cancer.
- Chronic pain management is an essential element of managing chronic pancreatitis.
- Pancreatic enzyme replacement therapy and the avoidance of tobacco and alcohol are cornerstone therapies for chronic pancreatitis.

PANIC DISORDER

Anub G. John, MD • Yash Kothari, MD • Hugh R. Peterson, MD, FACP

 BASICS

DESCRIPTION
- A classic panic attack that is characterized by rapid onset of a brief period of sympathetic nervous system hyperarousal accompanied by intense fear.
- In panic disorder, multiple panic attacks occur (including at least one without a recognizable trigger). Worried anticipation of additional attacks, which can be disabling, is present for at least 1 month, and often, maladaptive (e.g., avoidance) behaviors develop.

EPIDEMIOLOGY
Incidence
- Predominant age: All ages; in school-aged children, panic disorder can be confused with conduct disorder and school avoidance.
- Peak age of onset is early to mid-20s.
- Predominant sex: female > male (2:1)

Prevalence
- Lifetime prevalence: 4.7% (1)
- 4–8% of patients in a primary care practice population have panic disorder.
- Of patients presenting with chest pain in the emergency room, 25% have panic disorder.
- Chest pain is more likely due to panic if atypical, younger age, female, and known problems with anxiety.

ETIOLOGY AND PATHOPHYSIOLOGY
Unknown
- Biologic theories focus on limbic system malfunction in dealing with anxiety-evoking stimuli.
- Psychological theories posit deficits in managing strong emotions such as fear and anger.
- Noradrenergic neurotransmission from the locus coeruleus causes increased sympathetic stimulation throughout the body.
- Current neurobiologic research focuses on abnormal responses to anxiety-producing stimuli in the hippocampus, amygdala, and prefrontal cortex; for example, there appears to be limbic kindling in which an original frightening experience dominates future responses even when subsequent exposures are not objectively threatening.
- Brain pH disturbances (e.g., excess lactic acid) from normal mentation in genetically vulnerable patients may activate the amygdala and generate unexpected fear responses.

Genetics
Twin and family studies support a genetic predisposition.

RISK FACTORS
- Life stressors of any kind can precipitate attacks.
- History of sexual abuse and physical abuse, anxious and overprotective parents
- Substance abuse, bipolar disorder, major depression, obsessive-compulsive disorder (OCD), and simple phobia

COMMONLY ASSOCIATED CONDITIONS
- Of patients with panic disorder, >70% also have ≥1 other psychiatric diagnoses: PTSD (recalled trauma precedes panic attack), social phobia (fear of scrutiny precedes panic attack), simple phobia (fear of something specific precedes panic), major depression, bipolar disorder, substance abuse, OCD, separation anxiety disorder.
- Panic disorder is more common in patients with asthma, migraine headaches, hypertension, mitral valve prolapse, reflux esophagitis, interstitial cystitis, irritable bowel syndrome, fibromyalgia, nicotine dependence, and suicidality.

DIAGNOSIS

- Panic attack: an abrupt surge of intense fear, reaching a peak within minutes in which ≥4 of the following symptoms develop abruptly: (i) palpitations, pounding heart, or accelerated heart rate; (ii) sweating; (iii) trembling or shaking; (iv) sensations of shortness of breath or feeling smothered; (v) a choking sensation; (vi) chest pain or discomfort; (vii) nausea or abdominal distress; (viii) feeling dizzy, unsteady, lightheaded, or faint; (ix) derealization (feelings of unreality) or depersonalization (feeling detached from oneself); (x) fear of losing control or going crazy; (xi) fear of dying; (xii) paresthesias; (xiii) chills or hot flushes (2)[C]
- Panic disorder: recurrent unexpected panic attacks not better accounted for by another psychiatric condition (e.g., PTSD, OCD, separation anxiety disorder, social anxiety disorder, or specific phobia) and not induced by drugs of abuse, medical conditions, or prescribed drugs and with >1 month of at least one of the following: (i) worry about additional attacks; (ii) worry about the implications of the attack (e.g., losing control, having a heart attack, "going crazy"); and/or (iii) a significant maladaptive change in behavior related to the attacks (2)[C]
- Unlike *DSM-IV*, *DSM-5* defines agoraphobia as separate from panic disorder (2)[C].

HISTORY
- The best way to get a good history is through tactful, nonjudgmental questioning after the worst of the attack is over. Use open-ended questions and be unhurried. Interviewing family members may also be helpful.
- A thorough medication and substance abuse history is important.
- Patients must have a month of fear of out-of-the-blue panic attacks to diagnose panic disorder.

PHYSICAL EXAM
- During an attack, there will be tachycardia, hyperventilation, and sweating.
- Check the thyroid for fullness or nodules.
- Cardiac exam to check for a murmur or arrhythmias
- Lung exam to rule out asthma (limited airflow, wheezing)

DIFFERENTIAL DIAGNOSIS
- Medication use may mimic panic disorder and create anxiety: Antidepressants to treat panic may paradoxically initially cause panic; antidepressants in bipolar patients can cause anxiety/mania/panic; short-acting benzodiazepines (alprazolam), β-blockers (propranolol), and short-acting opioids can cause interdose rebound anxiety; benzodiazepine treatment causes panic when patients take too much and run out of these medicines early; bupropion, levodopa, amphetamines, steroids, albuterol, sympathomimetics, fluoroquinolones, and interferon can cause panic.
- Substances of abuse: alcohol withdrawal, benzodiazepine withdrawal, opioid withdrawal, caffeine, marijuana (panic with paranoia), amphetamine abuse, MDMA, hallucinogens (PCP, LSD), dextromethorphan abuse, synthetic cathinones (bath salts) abuse.
- Medical conditions: hypo-/hyperthyroidism, asthma/chronic obstructive pulmonary disease (COPD), reflux esophagitis with hyperventilation, tachyarrhythmias, premenstrual dysphoric disorder, menopause, pregnancy, hypoglycemia (in diabetes), hypoxia, inner ear disturbances (labyrinthitis), myocardial infarction, pulmonary embolus, transient ischemic attacks (TIAs), carcinoid syndrome, pre- and postictal states (e.g., in TLE), autoimmune disease, pheochromocytoma, Cushing syndrome, hyperaldosteronism, Wilson disease
- Psychiatric conditions that have overlapping symptomatology include mood, anxiety, and personality disorders such as major depression, bipolar disorder, PTSD, borderline personality disorder, social phobia, OCD, and generalized anxiety disorder. In PTSD, there is always a recollection or visual image that precedes the panic attack. In social phobia, fear of scrutiny precedes the panic attack. In bipolar disorder, major depression, borderline personality disorder, and particularly substance abuse, the patient often complains first of panic symptoms and anxiety and minimizes other potentially relevant symptoms and behaviors.
- Somatic symptom disorder is also an illness of multiple unexplained medical symptoms, but the presenting picture is usually one of chronic symptoms rather than the acute, dramatic onset of a panic attack. Somatic symptom disorder and panic disorder can be (and often are) diagnosed together.

DIAGNOSTIC TESTS & INTERPRETATION
Consider ECG and pulse oximetry to rule out certain serious causes of panic; consider Holter monitoring. No specific lab tests are indicated except to rule out conditions in the differential diagnosis.
- Finger-stick blood sugar in acute setting in a diabetic patient
- Thyroid-stimulating hormone (TSH), electrolytes, CBC
- Consider ordering echocardiogram if you suspect mitral valve prolapse.

Diagnostic Procedures/Other
If a medical cause of anxiety is strongly suspected, do the workup appropriate for that condition.

TREATMENT

Combined antidepressant therapy and psychotherapy is superior to either alone during initial treatment for panic disorder (3)[A]. Cognitive-behavioral therapy (CBT) provides long-lasting treatment, often without subsequent need for medications.

GENERAL MEASURES
CBT, tailored for panic disorder, consists of several steps: education, changing cognitions about the attack and the illness, relaxation and controlled breathing techniques, and, if appropriate, exposure to anxiety-provoking conditions coupled with in vivo relaxation exercises.

MEDICATION
- Medication management is indicated if psychotherapy is not successful (or not available) and may be combined with psychotherapy.
- Patient preference plays a big part in this decision.
- Because patients typically are anxious about their treatment, the therapeutic alliance is critical for the chronic care of this disorder.
- If medications are started, they should be maintained for at least 6 months after symptom control.

First Line
- FDA-approved choices for the treatment of panic disorder include sertraline, paroxetine, fluoxetine, alprazolam, and clonazepam, but avoid giving benzodiazepines to those with a history of substance abuse or who are currently abusing alcohol or benzodiazepines, unless following a detoxification protocol.
- Most antidepressants except bupropion may treat panic disorder, but fluoxetine and selegiline patch can cause more initial nervousness than other antidepressants.
- In nonbipolar patients, start a low-dose SSRI (e.g., 5 mg [escitalopram, 25 mg sertraline, 10 mg paroxetine) and consider doubling the dose after 2 or 3 weeks; while waiting for the antidepressant to work, schedule frequent visits, give the patient reassurance, teach a relaxation technique, encourage the patient to do vigorous aerobic exercise as soon as a panic attack begins (if medically appropriate and in an appropriate situation); refer the patient to a competent therapist for CBT (4)[A].
- In bipolar patients, panic symptoms often resolve when treated with a mood stabilizer rather than an antidepressant (which may cause mania).

Second Line
- Among serotonin–norepinephrine reuptake inhibitors, Venlafaxine extended release (ER) is effective. Start at 37.5 mg/day and titrate up to 75 mg/day after 7 days (maximum dose of 225 mg/day). Taper slowly over weeks to discontinue. Risk of hypertension at higher doses (5)[A].
- Tricyclic antidepressants, particularly imipramine (start 25 mg/day in the evening and increase up to 25 mg every 3 days to a maximum of 200 mg/day); slower titration and lower doses are often as effective. Imipramine is as efficacious as SSRIs in the treatment of panic disorder. Tricyclic antidepressants are considered second line because of difficulty in dosing, more side effects, and greater risk associated with overdose compared with SSRIs (6)[A].
- Benzodiazepines like alprazolam (start 0.5 mg TID and up to 5 mg/day) and (clonazepam (0.25 mg BID to target 1 mg/day) are FDA approved for panic disorder. Clonazepam has a longer half life, less interdose anxiety and lower abuse potential than alprazolam.

ISSUES FOR REFERRAL
Consider referral to a psychiatrist for panic disorder that is comorbid with bipolar disorder, borderline personality disorder, schizophrenia, suicidality, alcohol, or substance abuse.

ADDITIONAL THERAPIES
Aerobic exercise reduces symptoms better than placebo (7)[B].

INPATIENT CONSIDERATIONS
Admission Criteria/Initial Stabilization
- If certain life-threatening mimics of panic disorder have not been ruled out, such as a myocardial infarction (MI) or pulmonary embolus (PE), hospitalize patient to complete the evaluation.
- If a panic disorder patient has concrete suicidal ideation, a psychiatric admission is indicated.

ONGOING CARE

PATIENT EDUCATION
- www.nlm.nih.gov/medlineplus/panicdisorder.html
- Patient information handouts in *American Family Physician*. 2005;71:740 and 2006;74:1393.
- http://www.nimh.nih.gov/health/publications/panic-disorder-when-fear-overwhelms/index.shtml

PROGNOSIS
- Most patients recover with treatment.
- It can recur, but treatment of recurrence is usually successful.

COMPLICATIONS
- Iatrogenic benzodiazepine dependence
- Iatrogenic mania in bipolar patients treated for panic with unopposed antidepressants
- Misdiagnosis of more difficult-to-treat psychiatric conditions as panic and vice versa

REFERENCES

1. Kessler RC, Chiu WT, Demler O, et al. Prevalence, severity, and comorbidity of 12-month *DSM-IV* disorders in the National Comorbidity Survey Replication. *Arch Gen Psychiatry*. 2005;62(6):617–627.
2. American Psychiatric Association. *Diagnostic and Statistical Manual of Mental Disorders*. 5th ed. Arlington, VA: American Psychiatric Association; 2013.
3. Furukawa TA, Watanabe N, Churchill R. Combined psychotherapy plus antidepressants for panic disorder with or without agoraphobia. *Cochrane Database Syst Rev*. 2007;(1);CD004364.
4. Otto MW, Tuby KS, Gould RA, et al. An effect-size analysis of the relative efficacy and tolerability of serotonin selective reuptake inhibitors for panic disorder. *Am J Psychiatry*. 2001;158(12):1989–1992.
5. Pollack MH, Lepola U, Koponen H, et al. A double-blind study of the efficacy of venlafaxine extended-release, paroxetine, and placebo in the treatment of panic disorder. *Depress Anxiety*. 2007;24(1):1–14.
6. Bakker A, van Balkom AJ, Spinhoven P. SSRIs vs. TCAs in the treatment of panic disorder: a meta-analysis. *Acta Psychiatr Scand*. 2002;106(3):163–167.
7. Broocks A, Bandelow B, Pekrun G, et al. Comparison of aerobic exercise, clomipramine, and placebo in the treatment of panic disorder. *Am J Psychiatry*. 1998;155(5):603–609.

 SEE ALSO

Algorithm: Anxiety

CODES

ICD10
- F41.0 Panic disorder without agoraphobia
- F40.01 Agoraphobia with panic disorder
- F43.0 Acute stress reaction

CLINICAL PEARLS

Encouraging patients (who are medically able) to do 10 minutes of vigorous aerobic exercise the moment a panic attack seems to be starting is often a very effective way to help patients feel safe during panic attacks. Always evaluate a patient with panic for suicidality. Patients with panic disorder are at increased risk for suicide, particularly if depressed.

PARKINSON DISEASE

Theresa T. Vo, MD • C. Jack Fraim, MD

BASICS

DESCRIPTION
- Parkinson disease (PD) is a progressive neurodegenerative disorder caused by degeneration of dopaminergic neurons in the substantia nigra pars compacta.
- Cardinal symptoms include resting tremor, rigidity, bradykinesia, and postural instability.
- Diagnosis is based primarily on history and examination.

EPIDEMIOLOGY
Incidence
- Average age of onset: ~60 years
- Slightly more common in men than women

Prevalence
- Second most common neurodegenerative disease after Alzheimer disease
- 0.3% of general population and 1–2% of those ≥60 years of age and up to 4% of those ≥80 years of age
- Affects approximately 1 million people in the United States and 5 million worldwide

ETIOLOGY AND PATHOPHYSIOLOGY
Dopamine depletion in the substantia nigra and the nigrostriatal pathways results in the major motor complications of PD.
- Pathologic hallmark: selective loss of dopamine-containing neurons in the pars compacta of the substantia nigra
- Loss of neurons accompanied by presence of Lewy bodies, pale bodies (predecessor of the Lewy body), and Lewy neuritis

Genetics
Mutations in multiple autosomal dominant and autosomal recessive genes have been linked to PD/parkinsonian syndrome particularly when the age at symptom onset is <50 years. Genes investigated in PD include *SNCA*, Parkin, Pink-1, DJ-1and *LRRK2*.

RISK FACTORS
- Age and family history of PD or tremor are the greatest risk factors.
- History of smoking as well as coffee and caffeine intake may reduce risk.
- Weak association with exposure to toxins (herbicides and insecticides); however, relationship is not clear.

COMMONLY ASSOCIATED CONDITIONS
Non–motor-associated symptoms include cognitive abnormalities, autonomic dysfunction (e.g., constipation, urinary urgency), sleep disturbances, mental status changes (depression, psychosis, hallucinations, dementia), orthostatic hypotension, and pain.

DIAGNOSIS

- Diagnosis is based on clinical impression.
- Gold standard for diagnosis is neuropathologic exam.
- Generally, bradykinesia plus either tremor or rigidity must be present in order to make the diagnosis of idiopathic PD.

- Clinical features supportive of the diagnosis include unilateral onset, resting tremor, persistent asymmetry with the side of onset most affected, and significant response to dopaminergic therapy.

HISTORY
Symptoms often subtle or attributed to aging:
- Decreased emotion displayed in facial features
- General motor slowing and stiffness (one or both arms do not swing with walk)
- Resting tremor (often initially one hand)
- Speech soft/mumbling
- Falls/difficulty with balance (tends to occur with disease progression)

PHYSICAL EXAM
- Tremor
  - Resting tremor (4 to 6 Hz) that is often asymmetric.
  - Disappears with voluntary movement
  - Frequently emerges in a hand while walking and may present as pill rolling
  - May also present in jaw, chin, lips, tongue
- Bradykinesia
- Rigidity: cogwheel (catching and releasing) or lead pipe (continuously rigid)
- Postural instability

DIFFERENTIAL DIAGNOSIS
- Essential tremor: Bradykinesia is not present; often symmetric and occurs mostly during action or when holding hands outstretched
- SWEDD: scans without evidence of dopaminergic deficit; isolated upper extremity resting and postural tremor resembling PD but failing to progress to generalized PD; no akinesia
- Dementia with Lewy bodies: characterized clinically by visual hallucinations, fluctuating cognition, and parkinsonism, dementia occurs concomitantly with or before the development of parkinsonism
- Corticobasal degeneration: asymmetric parkinsonism, absence of tremor, no response to levodopa
- Multiple system atrophy: presets with parkinsonism but with varying degrees of dysautonomia, cerebellar involvement, and pyramidal signs
- Progressive supranuclear palsy: impairment in vertical eye movements (particularly down gaze), hyperextension of neck, and early falling; pseudobulbar palsy
- Idiopathic basal ganglia calcification
- Associated neurodegenerative disorders: late stages of Alzheimer disease, Huntington disease, frontotemporal dementia, spinocerebellar ataxias
- Secondary parkinsonism
  - Drug-induced: reversible; may take weeks/months after offending medication is stopped
    - Neuroleptics (most common cause)
    - Antiemetics (e.g., prochlorperazine and promethazine), metoclopramide
    - SSRIs
    - Calcium channel blockers (e.g., flunarizine and cinnarizine) metoclopramide
    - Amiodarone
    - Lithium
    - Cholinergics
    - Chemotherapeutics
    - Amphotericin B
    - Estrogens
    - Valproic acid

DIAGNOSTIC TESTS & INTERPRETATION
Initial Tests (lab, imaging)
- Diagnosis is mainly clinical and there are no physiologic or blood tests to confirm the diagnosis.
- Excellent response to an acute dopaminergic challenge test supports the diagnosis
- MRI of brain is nondiagnostic but can be used to rule out structural abnormalities.
- DaTscan: Striatal dopamine transporter imaging can distinguish PD and other parkinsonian syndromes but cannot differentiate between them.
- PET and single-photon emission CT may be helpful with diagnosis but are not required.

TREATMENT

GENERAL MEASURES
- Multidisciplinary rehabilitation with standard physical and occupational therapy components to improve functional outcomes.
- Physiotherapy to help with gait reeducation, enhancement of aerobic capacity, improvement in movement initiation, improvement in functional independence, and help with home safety

MEDICATION
- PD goal: Improve motor and nonmotor deficits.
- Agents are chosen based on patient age and symptoms present.
- No treatment shown to slow progression

First Line
- First-line agents in early PD: levodopa, dopamine agonists, monoamine oxidase B (MAO-B) inhibitors (1)[A]
  - Levodopa combined with carbidopa is still the most effective treatment for symptoms of PD, particularly bradykinesia.
  - Levodopa versus dopamine agonist is controversial (2)[B]:
    - Most patients eventually will develop motor fluctuations with levodopa. Younger patients are more likely to develop motor fluctuations. Some recommend delaying initiation of levodopa to decrease drug-induced motor fluctuations early in the disease.
    - Older patients often are less able to tolerate the adverse events of dopamine agonists.
    - All patients eventually will require levodopa.
  - MAO-B inhibitors (rasagiline) should be considered as initial monotherapy; investigated for potential neuroprotective effects (2)[B]
- Carbidopa + levodopa (carbidopa inhibits peripheral conversion of levodopa)
  - Immediate release (Sinemet)
    - Tablets (mg): 10/100, 25/100, 25/250
    - Usual initial maintenance dose: 25/100 mg PO TID. Most patients require 25 mg of carbidopa to inhibit peripheral conversion of levodopa.
    - Watch for nausea/vomiting, orthostatic hypotension, sedation, and vivid dreams.
  - Orally disintegrating (Parcopa)
    - Tablets (mg): 10/100, 25/100, 25/25
  - Sustained release (Sinemet CR):
    - Tablets (mg): 25/100, 50/200
    - Dose agents initially BID

- Carbidopa + levodopa + entacapone (Stalevo)
  - Tablets (mg): 12.5/50/200, 18.75/75/200, 25/100/200, 31.25/125/200, 37.5/150/200, 50/200/200
  - Addition of entacapone as a single agent should be initiated prior to use of this combination:
    o Once-daily dose of carbidopa/levodopa has been identified; may convert to Stalevo
    o Dose of levodopa may need to be decreased with the addition of entacapone.
  - Side effects are the same, plus diarrhea and brownish orange urine.
- Dopamine agonists (nonergot): side effects: nausea, vomiting, hypotension, sedation, edema, vivid dreaming, compulsive behavior, confusion, light-headedness, and hallucinations:
  - Pramipexole (Mirapex): tablets (mg): 0.125, 0.25, 0.5, 1, 1.5
    o Start with 0.125 mg TID, gradually increase every 5 to 7 days; usual maintenance of 0.5 to 1.5 mg TID
    o CrCl 30 to 59 mL/min 0.125 mg PO BID
    o CrCl 15 to 29 mL/min 0.125 mg PO daily
  - Pramipexole ER (Mirapex ER): tablets (mg): 0.375, 0.75, 1.5, 3, 4.5; start with 0.375 PO daily
  - Ropinirole (Requip): tablets (mg): 0.25, 0.5, 1, 2, 3, 4, 5; start with 0.25 mg TID, increase gradually to 3 to 8 mg TID
  - Requip XL: tablets (mg): 2, 4, 6, 8, 12; start at a 2-mg dose once daily, increase in 1 to 2 weeks
- Selective MAO-B inhibitors: side effects: insomnia, jitteriness, hallucinations; mostly found with selegiline; rasagiline similar adverse events as placebo in clinical trials. Rasagiline is metabolized via *CYP1A2*; caution with other medications using this enzyme system (e.g., ciprofloxacin):
  - Both agents contraindicated with meperidine and numerous other agents metabolized via *CYP1A2*
  - At therapeutic doses, unlikely to induce a "cheese reaction" (tyramine storm)
- Selegiline (Eldepryl)
  - Tablets: 5 mg; initiate 5 mg PO BID
  - Orally disintegrating tablet (Zelapar): 1.25 mg; 1.25 mg PO daily for 6 weeks; increase as needed to max of 2.5 mg daily
- Rasagiline (Azilect): tablets: 0.5 mg, 1.0 mg; initiate 0.5 to 1 mg daily

Second Line

- Second-line agents in early PD: β-adrenergic antagonists (postural tremor), amantadine, anticholinergics (young patients with tremor); there is lack of good evidence for symptom control (1)[A].
- Dopamine agonists (ergot): increased adverse event profile makes these agents nonpreferred to nonergot dopamine agonists; bromocriptine (Parlodel)
- Treatment of levodopa-induced motor complications
  - End of dose wearing off
    o Entacapone (with each levodopa dose) or rasagiline preferred (3)[B]
    o May also consider dopamine agonist, apomorphine, selegiline (4)[B]
  - Dyskinesias
    o Typically occur at peak dopamine level
    o Amantadine may be considered; however, its efficacy is questionable (1)[B].

- Anticholinergic agents: usually avoided due to lack of efficacy (only useful for tremor) and increased adverse event profile, including blurred vision, confusion, constipation, dry mouth, memory difficulty, sedation, and urinary retention
  - Trihexyphenidyl
    o Tablets: 2 mg, 5 mg
    o Start with 1 to 2 mg daily, increase by 2 mg every 3 to 5 days until usual dose is 6 to 10 mg in 3 to 4 divided doses
  - Benztropine (Cogentin)
    o Tablets: 0.5 mg, 1 mg, 2 mg
    o Start with 0.5 to 1 mg in 1 to 2 divided doses; increase by 0.5 mg every 5 to 6 days; usual dose is 1 to 2 mg/day in divided doses.
- *N*-methyl-D-aspartic acid antagonist: Exact mechanism is unknown and efficacy is questionable; however, it may be useful for dyskinesias. Side effects include confusion, dizziness, dry mouth, livedo reticularis, and hallucinations:
  - Amantadine (Symmetrel)
    o Tablets: 100 mg
    o Start with 100 mg BID; may increase to 300 mg daily in divided doses; renally adjusted
- Catechol-O-methyl transferase (COMT) inhibitors: entacapone preferred due to hepatotoxicity associated with tolcapone. Adverse events include nausea and orthostatic hypotension:
  - Entacapone (Comtan)
    o Tablets: 200 mg
    o 200 mg with each dose of carbidopa/levodopa; max dose, 1,600 mg/day
  - Tolcapone (Tasmar)
    o Tablets: 100 mg, 200 mg
    o Start 100 mg TID; max dose 600 mg/day; must be taken with carbidopa/levodopa
    o Requires LFT monitoring
- Apomorphine (Apokyn): nonergot-derived dopamine agonist given SC for off episodes in advanced disease; adverse events: nausea, vomiting, dizziness, hallucinations, orthostatic hypotension, somnolence
  - Only for "off" episodes with levodopa therapy
  - Requires initial "test" dose (2 mg); monitor for orthostatic hypotension after initial dose; this is a potent emetic, so initiate an antiemetic (e.g., trimethobenzamide) 3 days prior to start and continue for 2 months. Avoid ondansetron (combination contraindicated due to profound hypotension) and dopamine antagonists, such as prochlorperazine and metoclopramide.
  - Effective dose ranges from 2 to 6 mg/injection.

ISSUES FOR REFERRAL
Early specialty referral for patients with suspected PD for an accurate diagnosis and management

ADDITIONAL THERAPIES
- Emotional and psychological support of patient family
- Physical therapy and manual medicine has been shown to improve balance, muscle strength, and walking speed.
- Speech therapy: may be helpful in improving speech volume and maintaining voice quality

SURGERY/OTHER PROCEDURES
Deep brain stimulation (bilateral subthalamic nucleus/globus pallidus interna) is an effective therapeutic option for patients with motor complications refractory to best medical treatment who are healthy, have no significant comorbidities, are responsive to levodopa, and do not have depression or dementia.

 ## ONGOING CARE

DIET
- Increase dietary fluids and fiber and increase activity for constipation.
- For dysphagia, consider soft food, swallowing evaluation, and increased time for meals.
- Avoid large, high-fat meals that slow digestion and interfere with medication absorption.

PATIENT EDUCATION
- www.apdaparkinson.org
- www.parkinson.org
- www.michaeljfox.org

PROGNOSIS
- PD is a chronic progressive disease; prognosis varies based on patient-specific symptoms.
- Increased mortality in PD; on average, PD survival reduced by 5% every year of follow-up (4).

COMPLICATIONS
Most commonly the result of adverse effects of medications used to treat

REFERENCES
1. Gazewood JD, Richards DR, Clebak K. Parkinson disease: an update. *Am Fam Physician*. 2013; 87(4):267–273.
2. Nalls MA, Plagnol V, Hernandez DG, et al. Imputation of sequence variants for identification of genetic risks for Parkinson's disease: a meta-analysis of genome-wide association studies. *Lancet*. 2011;377(9766):641–649.
3. Pahwa R, Factor SA, Lyons KE, et al. Practice parameter: treatment of Parkinson disease with motor fluctuations and dyskinesia (an evidence-based review): report of the Quality Standards Subcommittee of the American Academy of Neurology. *Neurology*. 2006;66(7):983–995.
4. Diaz NL, Waters CH. Current strategies in the treatment of Parkinson's disease and a personalized approach to management. *Expert Rev Neurother*. 2009;9(12):1781–1789.

ADDITIONAL READING
Macleod AD, Taylor KS, Counsell CE. Mortality in Parkinson's disease: a systematic review and meta-analysis. *Mov Disord*. 2014;29(13):1615–1622.

 ## CODES

ICD10
- G20 Parkinson's disease
- G21.9 Secondary parkinsonism, unspecified
- G31.83 Dementia with Lewy bodies

CLINICAL PEARLS
- Emphasize the importance of exercise and movement to help preserve function.
- Pharmacotherapeutic regimens need to be individualized based on patient-specific symptoms and age.

PARONYCHIA

Nancy V. Nguyen, DO

 BASICS

DESCRIPTION

- Superficial inflammation of the lateral and posterior folds of skin surrounding the fingernail or toenail
  - Acute: characterized by pain, erythema, and swelling; usually a bacterial infection, appears after trauma. It can progress to abscess formation.
  - Chronic: characterized by swelling, tenderness, cuticle elevation, and nail dystrophy and separation lasting at least 6 weeks, or recurrent episodes of acute eponychial inflammation and drainage.
  - May be considered work-related among bartenders, waitresses, nurses, and others who often wash their hands
- System(s) affected: skin and nail bed
- Synonym(s): eponychia; perionychia

Pediatric Considerations
Less common in pediatric age groups. Thumb/finger-sucking is a risk factor (anaerobes and *Escherichia coli* may be present).

EPIDEMIOLOGY

Incidence
- Common in the United States
- Predominant age: all ages
- Predominant sex: female > male

ETIOLOGY AND PATHOPHYSIOLOGY
- Acute: *Staphylococcus aureus* (1) most common and *Streptococcus pyogenes* (1); less frequently, *Pseudomonas pyocyanea* and *Proteus vulgaris*. In digits exposed to oral flora especially in pediatric age group, consider *Eikenella corrodens*, *Fusobacterium*, and *Peptostreptococcus*.
- Chronic: eczematous reaction with secondary *Candida albicans* (~95%) (2)
- A paronychial infection commonly starts in the lateral nail fold.
- Recurrent inflammation, persistent edema, and fibrosis of nail folds cause nail folds to round up and retract, exposing nail grooves to irritants, allergens, and pathogens.
- Inflammation compromises ability of proximal nail fold to regenerate cuticle leading to decreased vascular supply. This can cause decrease efficacy of topical medications.
- Early in the course, cellulitis alone may be present. An abscess can form if the infection does not resolve quickly.

RISK FACTORS
- Acute: direct or indirect trauma to cuticle or nail fold, manicure/sculptured nails, nail biting, and thumb sucking and predisposing conditions such as diabetes mellitus (DM)

- Chronic: frequent immersion of hands in water with excoriation of the lateral nail fold (e.g., chefs, bartenders, housekeepers, swimmers, dishwashers, nurses), DM, immunosuppression (reported association with antiretroviral therapy for HIV and with use of epidermal growth factor inhibitors) (3)

GENERAL PREVENTION
- Acute: Avoid trauma such as nail biting; prevent thumb sucking.
- Chronic: Avoid allergens; keep fingers/hands dry; wear rubber gloves with a cotton liner. Prevent excoriation of the skin.
- Keep nails short. Avoid manicures. Apply moisturizer after washing hands.
- Good glycemic control in diabetic patients

COMMONLY ASSOCIATED CONDITIONS
- DM
- Eczema or atopic dermatitis
- Certain medications: antiretroviral therapy (3) (especially protease inhibitors, indinavir, and lamivudine, in which toes more commonly involved) (3)
- Immunosuppression (4)

 DIAGNOSIS

HISTORY
- Localized pain or tenderness, swelling, and erythema of posterior or lateral nail folds
  - Acute: fairly rapid onset
  - Chronic: 4 to 6 weeks' duration
- Previous trauma (bitten nails, ingrown nails, manicured nails)
- Contact with herpes infections
- Contact with allergens or irritants (frequent water immersion, latex) (4)

PHYSICAL EXAM
- Acute: red, warm, tender, tense posterior or lateral nail fold ± abscess
- Chronic: swollen, tender, boggy nail fold ± abscess
- Occasional elevation of nail bed
- Separation of nail fold from nail plate
- Red, painful swelling of skin around nail plate
- Fluctuance, purulence at the nail margin, or purulent drainage
- Secondary changes of nail platelike discoloration
- Suspect *Pseudomonas* if with green changes in nail (chloronychia) (5).
- Positive fluctuation when mild pressure over the area causes blanching and demarcation of the abscess

- Chronic: retraction of nail fold and absence of adjacent healthy cuticle, thickening of nail plate with prominent transverse ridges known as Beau lines and discoloration

DIFFERENTIAL DIAGNOSIS
- Felon (abscess of fingertip pulp; urgent diagnosis required)
- Contact dermatitis
- Herpetic whitlow (similar in appearance, very painful, often associated with vesicles)
- Acute osteomyelitis of the distal phalanx
- Psoriasis especially acute flare
- Allergic contact dermatitis (latex, acrylic)
- Reiter disease
- Pustular psoriasis
- Proximal/lateral onychomycosis (nail folds not predominantly involved)
- Malignancy: squamous cell carcinoma of the nail, malignant melanoma, metastatic disease

DIAGNOSTIC TESTS & INTERPRETATION
None required unless condition is severe; resistant to treatment or if recurrence or methicillin-resistant *S. aureus* (MRSA) is suspected, then
- Gram stain
- Culture and sensitivity
- Potassium hydroxide wet mount plus fungal culture especially in chronic
- Drugs that may alter lab results: Use of over-the-counter antimicrobials or antifungals.

Diagnostic Procedures/Other
- Incision and drainage recommended for suppurative cases or cases not responding to conservative management or empiric antibiotics
- Tzanck testing or viral culture in suspected viral cases
- Biopsy in cases not responding to conservative management or when malignancy suspected

 TREATMENT

GENERAL MEASURES
- Acute: warm compresses, elevation, splint protection if pain severe
- Chronic: Keep fingers dry; apply moisturizing lotion after hand washing; avoid exposure to irritants; improved diabetic control

MEDICATION

First Line
- Tetanus booster when indicated
- Acute (mild cases, no abscess formation)

  - Topical antibiotic cream alone or in combination with a topical steroid (6)[B]

- Antibiotic cream applied TID–QID after warm| soak (e.g., mupirocin or gentamicin/neomycin/ polymyxin B) for 5 to 10 days
- If eczematous: low-potent topical steroid applied BID (e.g., betamethasone 0.05% cream) for 7 to 14 days (7)[B]

- Acute (no exposure to oral flora)
  - Dicloxacillin 250 mg TID for 7 days
  - Cephalexin 500 mg TID–QID for 7 days
- Acute (suspected MRSA)
  - Trimethoprim/sulfamethoxazole 160 mg/800 mg BID for 7 days
  - Doxycycline 100 mg BID for 7 days
- Acute (exposure to oral flora)
  - Amoxicillin clavulanate: 875 mg/125 mg BID or 500 mg/125 mg TID for 7 days; pediatric, 45 mg/ kg q12h (for <40 kg)
  - Clindamycin 300 to 450 mg TID–QID for 7 days; pediatric, 10 mg/kg q8h; *plus* either doxycycline or trimethoprim/sulfamethoxazole
- Chronic
  - Topical steroids: betamethasone 0.05%; applied BID for 7 to 14 days (8)[B]
  - Topical antifungal: clotrimazole or nystatin; applied topically TID for up to 30 days
  - Other topical: Tacrolimus 0.1% ointment BID for up to 21 days has been shown to be effective but is more expensive.

Second Line
- Systemic antifungals (rarely needed, use if topical fails)
  - Itraconazole 200 mg for 90 days (may have longer action because it is incorporated into nail plate); pulse therapy may be useful (i.e., 200 mg BID for 7 days, repeated monthly for 2 months) (1)[C],(8)
  - Terbinafine 250 mg/day for 6 weeks (fingernails) or 12 weeks (toenails)
  - Fluconazole 100 mg daily for 7 to 14 days
  - Ciclopirox 0.77% topical suspension BID for 2 to 4 weeks along with strict irritant avoidance (7)[B]
- Antipseudomonal drugs (e.g., ceftazidime, aminoglycosides) when pseudomonas is suspected

ISSUES FOR REFERRAL
Chronic; in treatment failure, consider biopsy and/or, in cases of chronic paronychia, referral for possible partial excision of the nail fold or eponychial marsupialization with or without complete nail removal.

SURGERY/OTHER PROCEDURES
- Incision and drainage of abscess, if present
- A subungual abscess or ingrown nail requires partial or complete removal of nail with phenolization of germinal matrix.
- Recalcitrant cases may also need nail removal.

 ONGOING CARE

FOLLOW-UP RECOMMENDATIONS
Chronic: Avoid frequent immersion, triggers, allergens, or nail biting and finger sucking.

DIET
If patient is diabetic, consider appropriate dietary and medication changes for better control.

PATIENT EDUCATION
- Avoid trimming cuticles; avoid nail trauma; and stress importance of good diabetic control and diabetic education.
- Avoid contact irritants; use rubber gloves with cotton liners to avoid exposure to excess moisture.
- Use moisturizing lotion after washing hands; do not bite nails/suck on fingers.

PROGNOSIS
- With adequate treatment and prevention, healing can be expected in 1 to 2 weeks.
- Chronic paronychia may respond slowly to treatment, taking weeks to months.
- If no response in chronic lesions, rarely benign or malignant neoplasm may be present and referral should be considered.

COMPLICATIONS
- Acute: subungual abscess
- Chronic: nail thickening, discoloration of nail, and nail loss

REFERENCES

1. Rigopoulos D, Larios G, Gregoriou S, et al. Acute and chronic paronychia. *Am Fam Physician*. 2008;77(3):339–346.
2. Barlow AJ, Chattaway FW, Holgate MC, et al. Chronic paronychia. *Br J Dermatol*. 1970;82(5): 448–453.
3. Wollina U. Acute paronychia: comparative treatment with topical antibiotic alone or in combination with corticosteroid. *J Eur Acad Dermatol Venereol*. 2001;15(1):82–84.
4. Tosti A, Piraccini BM, D'Antuono A, et al. Paronychia associated with antiretroviral therapy. *Br J Dermatol*. 1999;140(6):1165–1168.
5. Rigopoulos D, Gregoriou S, Belyayeva E, et al. Efficacy and safety of tacrolimus ointment 0.1% vs. betamethasone 17-valerate 0.1% in the treatment of chronic paronychia: an unblinded randomized study. *Br J Dermatol*. 2009;160(4):858–860.
6. Tosti A, Piraccini BM, Ghetti E, et al. Topical steroids versus systemic antifungals in the treatment of chronic paronychia: an open, randomized double-blind and double dummy study. *J Am Acad Dermatol*. 2002;47(1):73–76.
7. Daniel CR III, Daniel MP, Daniel J, et al. Managing simple chronic paronychia and onycholysis with ciclopirox 0.77% and an irritant-avoidance regimen. *Cutis*. 2004;73(1):81–85.
8. Relhan V, Goel K, Bansal S, et al. Management of chronic paronychia. *Indian J Dermatol*. 2014;59(1): 15–20.

ADDITIONAL READING

- Chiriac A, Brzezinski P, Foia L, et al. Chloronychia: green nail syndrome caused by *Pseudomonas aeruginosa* in elderly persons. *Clin Interv Aging*. 2015;10:265–267.
- Hengge UR, Bardeli V. Images in clinical medicine. Green nails. *N Engl J Med*. 2009;360(11):1125.
- Iorizzo M. Tips to treat the 5 most common nail disorders: brittle nails, onycholysis, paronychia, psoriasis, onychomycosis. *Dermatol Clin*. 2015; 33(2):175–183.
- Rockwell PG. Acute and chronic paronychia. *Am Fam Physician*. 2001;63(6):1113–1116.
- Shroff PS, Parikh DA, Fernandez RJ, et al. Clinical and mycological spectrum of cutaneous candidiasis in Bombay. *J Postgrad Med*. 1990;36(2):83–86.

 SEE ALSO

Onychomycosis

 CODES

ICD10
- L03.019 Cellulitis of unspecified finger
- L03.039 Cellulitis of unspecified toe

CLINICAL PEARLS
- Consider tetanus booster when indicated.
- Consider incision and drainage when appropriate. Send culture.
- For chronic paronychia, topical steroid is first-line treatment. Consider other differentials in nonresponders (e.g., rare causes: Raynaud, metastatic cancer, psoriasis, drug toxicity)
- For chronic nonhealing lesion, consider dermatology referral.
- Consider possibility of cancer if chronic inflammatory process is unresponsive to treatment.
- Consider presence of more than one nail disease at the same time (e.g., paronychia and onychomycosis).

PAROTITIS, ACUTE AND CHRONIC
Colleen W. Meehan, MD, MPH • Kathleen Ferrer, MD, AAHIVS

BASICS

DESCRIPTION
- Parotitis is inflammation of the parotid gland caused by infection (viral or bacterial), noninfectious systemic illnesses, mechanical obstruction, or medications.
- Parotitis can be unilateral or bilateral, acute or chronic. Unilateral parotitis is usually associated with duct obstruction, whereas bilateral parotitis more commonly indicates a systemic cause.
- The parotid gland is the largest of the salivary glands, located lateral to the masseter muscle anteriorly and extending posteriorly over the sternocleidomastoid muscle behind the angle of the mandible. It produces exclusively serous secretions, which lack the bacteriostatic properties of mucinous secretions, making the parotid gland more susceptible to infection than other salivary glands.
- The parotid duct, also called Stensen duct, pierces the buccinator muscle to enter the buccal mucosa just opposite the second maxillary molar.
- The branches of the 7th cranial nerve or "facial nerve" divide the gland into lobes.
- The parotid gland contains lymph nodes.

EPIDEMIOLOGY
- Viral parotitis is the most common cause of parotitis in children, though the exact incidence is unknown and has decreased since the advent of the mumps vaccine.
- Acute bacterial parotitis occurs more frequently in elderly patients, neonates (especially preterm infants), and postoperative patients.
- Neonatal parotitis and juvenile recurrent parotitis are more common in males than females.
- Juvenile recurrent parotitis is the second most common inflammatory cause of parotitis in children in the United States; first episode usually occurs between the ages of 3 and 6 years.
- Chronic parotitis mainly affects adults, more often females. The average age of presentation is between 40 and 60 years.
- Chronic bilateral parotid enlargement is a common manifestation of HIV infection; for perinatally HIV-infected children, the average age of onset for parotid enlargement is 5 years.

RISK FACTORS
- Acute viral parotitis: lack of mumps, measles, rubella (MMR) vaccination
- Acute bacterial parotitis
  - Conditions that predispose to salivary stasis such as dehydration, debilitation, poor oral hygiene, Sjögren syndrome, cystic fibrosis, bulimia/anorexia, sialolithiasis (stones), ductal stenosis, trauma
  - Immunosuppression, HIV, chemotherapy, radiation, malnutrition, alcoholism
- Neonatal parotitis: prematurity, low birth weight, ductal obstruction, oral trauma, structural abnormalities, immunosuppression
- Juvenile recurrent parotitis: dental malocclusion, congenital duct malformation, genetic factors, immunologic anomalies
- Drug-induced parotitis: medications such as anticholinergics, antihistamines, diuretics, tricyclic antidepressants, antipsychotics, antineoplastic agents, and iodine
- Chronic parotitis: ductal stenosis, HIV, tuberculosis, Sjögren syndrome, and sarcoidosis

GENERAL PREVENTION
- MMR vaccination with the first dose between 12 and 15 months and second dose between 4 and 6 years of age; of note, mumps vaccination does not guarantee prevention, possibly due to waning immunity in adolescence
- Maintain adequate hydration and good dental hygiene.
- Suck on hard or sour candy and use hot compresses with parotid massages to stimulate salivary flow and prevent salivary stasis.
- Smoking cessation, abstinence from alcohol, and avoidance of chronic purging

ETIOLOGY AND PATHOPHYSIOLOGY
- Acute viral parotitis begins as a systemic infection that localizes to the parotid gland, resulting in inflammation and swelling of the gland.
  - Mumps, or paramyxovirus, has a predilection for the parotid gland and classically has been linked to parotitis.
- Acute bacterial parotitis results from stasis of salivary flow that allows retrograde introduction of bacterial pathogens into the parotid gland, resulting in localized infection.
- Acute parotitis pathogens
  - Viral
    - Paramyxovirus (mumps), parainfluenza virus types 1 and 3, influenza A, coxsackie viruses, Epstein-Barr virus (EBV)
    - Cytomegalovirus (CMV) and adenovirus have been seen in patients with HIV.
  - Bacterial
    - *Staphylococcus aureus* and anaerobes (oral flora) are most commonly seen.
    - *Streptococcus pneumoniae*, viridans streptococci, *Escherichia coli*, and *Haemophilus influenza* (less common)
    - Gram-negative rods such as *E. coli*, *Klebsiella*, *Enterobacter*, and *Pseudomonas* can be seen in chronically ill or hospitalized patients.
  - Fungal
    - *Candida* has been isolated in chronically ill or hospitalized patients.
    - *Actinomyces* can be found in patients with a history of trauma or dental caries.
- Acute, recurrent parotitis
  - Juvenile recurrent parotitis may be secondary to chronic inflammation; etiology is unknown, but a genetic predisposition may exist.
  - Mechanical: sialolithiasis, ductal stenosis; repeated sialolith formation can lead to ductal wall damage, fibrosis, and stricture formation, which further decreases salivary flow and perpetuates obstruction
  - Pneumoparotitis may occur when air is trapped in the ducts of the parotid gland; may be seen in wind instrument players, glass blowers, scuba divers, and with dental cleaning.
  - Medications: anticholinergics, antihistamines, tricyclic antidepressants, antipsychotics (especially phenylbutazone, thioridazine, clozapine), iodine (especially contrast media), and L-asparaginase (1)[C]
  - Other: diabetes, alcoholism, bulimia, "anesthesia mumps" (possible mechanisms include transient mechanical compression of Stensen duct by airway devices, loss of muscle tone around the Stensen orifice after neuromuscular relaxants, increased salivary secretion, and increased flexion or rotation of the head during general anesthesia)

- Chronic parotitis may occur due to chronic ductal stenosis but is often due to a chronic infectious or inflammatory condition
  - HIV
  - Tuberculosis, syphilis (rare)
  - Autoimmune: Sjögren syndrome (parotid enlargement, xerostomia, and keratoconjunctivitis)
  - Inflammatory: sarcoidosis
    - Heerfordt syndrome (parotid enlargement, facial palsy, and uveitis) is a rare manifestation of sarcoidosis.
- Chronic parotitis in HIV-infected patients can be due to the presence of benign lymphoepithelial cysts, follicular hyperplasia of parotid lymph nodes, or diffuse infiltrative lymphocytosis syndrome (DILS), causing infiltration of the parotid gland by CD8 cells.
  - Parotitis may also be secondary to immune reconstitution after initiation of combination antiretroviral therapy in HIV-infected patients.

COMMONLY ASSOCIATED CONDITIONS
HIV, Sjögren syndrome, sarcoidosis, sialolithiasis

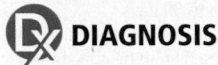

DIAGNOSIS

HISTORY
- Acute parotitis presents with sudden-onset pain and swelling of the cheek usually extending to and obscuring the angle of the mandible.
  - Viral parotitis is usually bilateral and accompanied by a prodrome of malaise, anorexia, headaches, myalgias, arthralgias, and fever; typically, overlying skin is not warm or erythematous, and no pus is reported at the opening of Stensen duct.
  - Bacterial parotitis is typically unilateral with induration, warmth, and erythema over the affected cheek; fever is often present.
  - Juvenile recurrent parotitis is usually unilateral; pain and swelling usually resolve within 2 weeks, and exacerbations occur until puberty; purulent exudate is not typical, but superinfection may occur.
  - Sialolithiasis is characterized by recurrent acute swelling and pain, exacerbated by eating; sialolithiasis affects the submandibular gland more frequently.
  - Other frequently reported symptoms include trismus (inability to open mouth), pain exacerbated by chewing or worsened by foods that stimulate production of saliva (i.e., sour candies), dry mouth with abnormal taste, difficulty with drinking/eating, anorexia, or dehydration.
- Chronic parotitis presents with recurrent or chronic nontender swelling of one or both parotid glands; can have periods of remission lasting weeks to years.
  - Sjögren syndrome, sarcoidosis, HIV, tuberculosis
  - Chronic parotitis may predispose to superinfection, which would present similarly to an acute parotitis.

PHYSICAL EXAM
- Parotitis is characterized by swelling or enlargement of the parotid gland(s) overlying the masseter muscle; it may obscure the angle of the mandible or cause the ear to protrude upward and outward.
- Palpation of the parotid gland is best done by using one hand to start at the attachment of the earlobe

and palpating anteriorly and inferiorly along the mandibular ramus while the other hand simultaneously palpates the Stensen duct orifice.
- Tender and bilateral suggests viral etiology, whereas tender, erythematous, warm, and unilateral suggests bacterial etiology.
- Nontender in HIV, tuberculosis, Sjögren sydrome, sarcoidosis
- Trismus may be noted.
- Pus from Stensen duct is suggestive of bacterial parotitis or superinfection; opening of duct may appear edematous and erythematous in both bacterial and viral parotitis.
- In juvenile recurrent parotitis, Stensen duct is often enlarged, dilated, erythematous, and swollen.
- Halitosis and dental decay are often associated with acute exacerbations.
- Facial nerve palsy can be seen in severe cases.

DIFFERENTIAL DIAGNOSIS
- Lymphoma, neoplasm, lymphangitis, cervical adenitis, otitis externa, dental abscess, odontogenic infections, Ludwig angina, and cellulitis should be considered in the differential.
- Parotid swelling or enlargement typically obscures the angle of the mandible (unlike cervical adenitis).
- Involvement of Stensen duct is unique to parotitis.

DIAGNOSTIC TESTS & INTERPRETATION
- History and physical exam are usually sufficient for diagnosis of parotitis.
- Performing aerobic culture and Gram stain of purulent drainage from Stensen duct or aerobic and anaerobic culture from needle aspiration of gland or abscess can be helpful to identify causative organism.
  - Anaerobic culture from Stensen duct will likely contain oropharyngeal contamination; hence, it is recommended to perform anaerobic cultures only from needle aspirate fluid.
- Acute bacterial parotitis often demonstrates an elevated white blood cell count and amylase.
- For suspected mumps, obtain mumps IgM antibody or mumps reverse transcription-polymerase chain reaction (RT-PCR). A 4-fold increase of mumps IgG antibody indicates infection.
- Consider sending EBV titers and respiratory virus PCR panel if viral parotitis suspected; CMV titers should be sent in immunocompromised patients.
- For chronic, recurrent, or nontender parotitis, obtain HIV test, PPD, SS-A SS-B antibodies, rheumatoid factor, and antinuclear antibodies to evaluate for underlying etiology.
- Consider obtaining ultrasound or CT scan of parotid area to assess for abscess, cystic masses, parotid tumors, ductal stenosis, or sialolithiasis if no response to initial treatment.
- Consider sialography with chronic parotitis to assess the anatomy and functional integrity of the gland; can be diagnostic and therapeutic.

Diagnostic Procedures/Other
Consider performing a biopsy or fine-needle aspiration of gland if there is suspicion for tuberculosis, Sjögren syndrome, or sarcoidosis.

Test Interpretation
- Findings characteristic of HIV are described in the "Etiology and Pathophysiology" section.
- Noncaseating granulomas may be seen in sarcoidosis, and caseating granulomas may be found in tuberculosis.

 TREATMENT

GENERAL MEASURES
- Usually a self-limiting course that requires primarily supportive treatment with rest, adequate hydration, analgesia, and antipyretics
  - Can stimulate glands to produce saliva by sucking on hard candies or glycerin swabs
  - Local heat and gentle massage of gland can provide symptomatic relief.
  - For chronic presentations, encourage good dental hygiene and treat underlying etiology of parotitis (HIV, Sjögren syndrome, etc.).
- Patients diagnosed with mumps should be isolated with standard and droplet precautions for 5 days after onset of parotid swelling.

MEDICATION
- Viral parotitis: with an uncertain diagnosis or toxic presentation, can empirically initiate antibiotics to cover *Staphylococcus aureus*, anaerobes (oral flora), and *Streptococcus pneumoniae*
- Acute bacterial parotitis
  - Outpatient management: amoxicillin/clavulanate, first-generation cephalosporin, clindamycin
  - Chronically ill or hospitalized: ampicillin/sulbactam or clindamycin and nafcillin; if methicillin resistance is probable, consider vancomycin or linezolid
- Pilocarpine and cevimeline can stimulate saliva production and inhibit ascending infection as well as provide symptomatic relief for patients with underlying Sjögren syndrome.

SURGERY/OTHER PROCEDURES
- Consider needle aspiration for bacterial parotitis with abscess formation or clinical deterioration with increasing pain, erythema, and swelling not responding to medication.
- May perform serial drainage for symptomatic cysts
- Consider superficial parotidectomy for severe recurrent parotid infections in patients with underlying predisposing etiology (such as Sjögren syndrome).
- Sialendoscopy with cortisone irrigation is effective and safe for the treatment of juvenile recurrent parotitis; cortisone irrigation alone may be just as effective (2)[A],(3)[C].
- For sialolithiasis, ductal stenosis, or for patients with >1 recurrence per year, consult otolaryngologist for possible duct ligation, ductoplasty, or parotidectomy.
- Sclerotherapy with methyl violet or tetracycline has been shown to be effective in the treatment of cysts in HIV parotitis and is also considered definitive treatment for chronic parotitis (4)[C].

INPATIENT CONSIDERATIONS
Admission is recommended for patients with comorbidities, systemic involvement, and inability to tolerate PO, as well as neonates and patients for whom close outpatient follow-up is not feasible.

 ONGOING CARE

FOLLOW-UP RECOMMENDATIONS
Antibiotic therapy initiated at diagnosis combined with adequate hydration should result in improvement within 48 hours. If not, patient should be reevaluated.

DIET
- Ensure adequate fluid intake.
- Hard or sour candies to promote salivary flow

PROGNOSIS
- Viral infection in immunocompetent individuals often resolves with excellent prognosis.
- Parotid cysts found in HIV-infected patients are usually benign lymphoepithelial lesions with infrequent malignant transformation.
- Increased incidence of malignant lymphoma or lymphoepithelial carcinoma may be seen in patients with Sjögren syndrome.

COMPLICATIONS
- For mumps, potential complications include orchitis, oophoritis, mastitis, meningitis, pancreatitis, sensorineural hearing loss, and nephritis.
- Untreated bacterial parotitis can lead to local extension, abscess formation, and facial paralysis.

REFERENCES
1. Brooks KG, Thompson DF. A review and assessment of drug-induced parotitis. *Ann Pharmacother*. 2012;46(12):1688–1699.
2. Ramakrishna J, Strychowsky J, Gupta M, et al. Sialendoscopy for the management of juvenile recurrent parotitis: a systematic review and meta-analysis. *Laryngoscope*. 2015;125(6):1472–1479.
3. Roby BB, Mattingly J, Jensen EL, et al. Treatment of juvenile recurrent parotitis of childhood: an analysis of effectiveness. *JAMA Otolaryngol Head Neck Surg*. 2015;141(2):126–129.
4. Berg EE, Moore CE. Office-based sclerotherapy for benign parotid lymphoepithelial cysts in the HIV-positive patient. *Laryngoscope*. 2009;119(5):868–870.

ADDITIONAL READING
- Armstrong MA, Turturro MA. Salivary gland emergencies. *Emerg Med Clin North Am*. 2013;31(2):481–499.
- Brook I. The bacteriology of salivary gland infections. *Oral Maxillofac Surg Clin North Am*. 2009;21(3):269–274.
- Capaccio P, Sigismund PE, Luca N, et al. Modern management of juvenile recurrent parotitis. *J Laryngol Otol*. 2012;126(12):1254–1260.

CODES

ICD10
- K11.20 Sialoadenitis, unspecified
- K11.21 Acute sialoadenitis
- K11.23 Chronic sialoadenitis

CLINICAL PEARLS
- History and physical exam are usually sufficient for diagnosis (parotid swelling and tenderness with or without purulent drainage from Stensen duct).
- In recurrent or chronic cases, consider other underlying etiologies such as HIV.
- *S. aureus* and anaerobes (oral flora) are the most common organisms isolated in acute bacterial parotitis.
- Encouraging good oral hygiene and adequate hydration in chronically ill, debilitated, and hospitalized patients can reduce parotitis occurrence.

PARVOVIRUS B19 INFECTION

David L. Anderson, MD • Thomas P. Garigan, MD, MA

 BASICS

DESCRIPTION
- Human parvovirus B19 is the primary cause of acute erythema infectiosum (EI, or fifth disease).
- Complications in susceptible individuals with increased RBC turnover (e.g., sickle cell anemia [SS]) include transient aplastic crisis (TAC). In immunocompromised individuals, pure red cell aplasia (PRCA) and chronic anemia are significant complications. In normal hosts, arthritis and arthralgias are common.
- System(s) affected: hematologic/lymphatic/ immunologic, musculoskeletal, skin/exocrine, possibly central nervous system, cardiac, renal

Pregnancy Considerations
A documented acute infection during pregnancy should prompt referral to a maternal–fetal medicine specialist. Maternal parvovirus B19 infection between 9 and 20 weeks' gestation may carry a significant fetal risk.

EPIDEMIOLOGY
- Infection is common in childhood.
- EI has an extremely low mortality rate.
- Peak age for EI is 4 to 12 years.
- Males and females are equally affected.
- Adult females are more likely to develop postinfectious arthritis.
- No known racial predilection
- In temperate climates, infections often occur from late winter to early summer.
- Local outbreaks may occur every 2 to 4 years.

Prevalence
Extremely common in the United States. Based on IgG serology:
- 1 to 5 years of age: 2–15% seropositive
- 6 to 15 years of age: 20–40% seropositive
- 16 to 40 years of age: 50–60% seropositive
- >40 years of age: 70–85% seropositive

ETIOLOGY AND PATHOPHYSIOLOGY
- Small (20 to 25 mm), nonenveloped, single-stranded DNA virus in *Parvoviridae* family
  - Only known parvovirus to infect humans; does not cross-infect dogs or cats
- Natural host of B19 is human erythroid progenitor.
- Respiratory, hematogenous, and vertical transmission are sources of human spread.
- 4- to 14-day incubation. Rash and joint symptoms occur 2 to 3 weeks after initial infection.
- Most contagious 5 to 10 days after exposure
- EI rash thought to be autoimmune due to IgM complexes concurrent with viral clearance.
- Cytotoxic infection of proerythroblasts reduces RBC production.

Genetics
Erythrocyte P antigen–negative individuals are resistant to infection.

RISK FACTORS
- School-related epidemic and nonimmune household contacts have a secondary attack rate of 20–50%.

- Highest secondary attack rates are for daycare providers and school personnel in contact with affected children.
- Those with increased cell turnover (e.g., hemoglobinopathy, SS, thalassemia) are at risk for TAC.
- Immunodeficiency (e.g., HIV, congenital) increases risk of PRAC and chronic anemia.
- As many as 40% of pregnant women are not immune. 1.5% seroconversion rate per year

GENERAL PREVENTION
- Respiratory spread. Standard measures include hand washing and barrier protection.
- Droplet precautions are recommended around patients with TAC, chronic infection, or anemia.
- Difficult to eliminate exposure because the period of maximal contagion occurs prior to the onset of clinical symptoms (rash).
- Pregnant health care workers should avoid caring for patients with TAC.
- No significant risk of infection based on occupational exposure. Exclusion from the workplace is neither necessary nor recommended.
- No preventive vaccine is available.

COMMONLY ASSOCIATED CONDITIONS
- Nondegenerative arthritis
  - In adults, 80% of patients may manifest polyarthritis and/or arthralgia (female > male).
  - In children, joint symptoms are less common.
  - Knees, hands, wrists, and ankles (frequently symmetric) are most commonly involved.
  - Joint symptoms usually subside within 3 weeks but may persist for months. Routine radiography is not necessary.
- TAC
  - Involves patients with increased RBC turnover (SS, spherocytosis, thalassemia) or decreased RBC production (iron deficiency anemia).
  - Patients present with fatigue, weakness, lethargy, and pallor (anemia).
  - Aplastic event may be life-threatening but is typically self-limited. Reticulocytes typically reappear in 7 to 10 days and full recovery in 2 to 3 weeks.
  - In children with sickle cell hemoglobinopathies and heredity spherocytosis, fever is the most common symptom (73%). Rash is uncommon in these patients.
- Chronic anemia
  - Seen in immunocompromised individuals (HIV, cancer, transplant) with poor IgM response
  - Usually no clinical manifestations (fever, rash, or joint symptoms)
- Fetal/neonatal infection (1)
  - Risk of transplacental spread of virus is ~33% in infected mothers.
  - Test pregnant women with a rash or arthralgias consistent with parvovirus B19.
  - Clinical manifestations vary. Many patients are seroconvert without symptoms and have a normal pregnancy. Other patients develop variable degrees of fetal hydrops. 2nd- and 3rd-trimester pregnancy loss can occur without hydrops.

- Suspect B19 infection in cases of nonimmune fetal hydrops.
  - Fetal bone marrow is primarily impacted. RBC survival is shortened, resulting in anemia and (potentially) high-output cardiac failure.
  - >95% of fetal complications (fetal hydrops and death) occur within 12 weeks of acute maternal parvovirus B19 infection.
  - Risk of fetal loss is highest (2–5%) in the 1st trimester.
  - Infants requiring intrauterine transfusions due to parvovirus B19 infection are at risk for long-term neurodevelopmental impairment.
- Papular purpuric gloves and socks syndrome (PPGSS) is an uncommon dermatosis associated with parvovirus B19 infection. It results in a petechial and ecchymotic rash of the hands and feet associated with febrile tonsillopharyngitis and oral ulcerations (2).

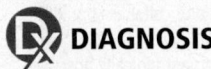 **DIAGNOSIS**

HISTORY
- Rash
- Headache
- Pharyngitis
- Coryza and rhinorrhea
- Arthralgias and arthritis
- Nausea and GI disturbances are more frequent and severe in adults (nonspecific flulike illness).
- Pruritus (especially soles of feet)
- Fever, myalgia, and malaise

PHYSICAL EXAM
- "Slapped cheek" appearance is a well-known facial rash that spares the nasolabial folds.
- A lacy, reticular rash on the trunk, buttocks, and limbs often follows 1 to 4 days later lasting 1 to 6 weeks.
- The rash may be pruritic and recurrent, exacerbated by bathing, exercise, sun exposure, heat, or emotional stress.
- B19 may manifest as painful pruritic papules and purpura on the hands and feet.

DIFFERENTIAL DIAGNOSIS
- Rubella
- Enteroviral disease
- Systemic lupus erythematosus
- Drug reaction
- Lyme disease
- Rheumatoid arthritis

DIAGNOSTIC TESTS & INTERPRETATION
Initial Tests (lab, imaging)
- No need for routine lab studies in typical cases. Diagnosis is clinical; illness is mild and self-limiting.
- IgG and IgM serology in immunocompetent patients
- B19-specific DNA polymerase chain reaction (PCR) testing for fetal infection (via cord blood or amniotic fluid) as well as for patients with chronic infection or those who are immunocompromised

- PCR increases diagnostic sensitivity and specificity to confirm infections in IgM-negative patients.
- For patients with TAC, CBC with reticulocyte count shows anemia and reticulocytopenia. IgM antibodies are present by day 3, and IgG antibodies are detectable at time of clinical recovery. PCR shows high levels of viremia.
- Pregnant women exposed to B19 require serial IgG and IgM serology to assess fetal risk.

Follow-Up Tests & Special Considerations
Fetal/neonatal infection (3)[C]

- To exclude congenital B19 in infants with negative B19 IgM, follow IgG serology over the 1st year of life.
- Maternal serum α-fetoprotein may be increased with hydrops fetalis.
- Documented acute maternal infection in the 1st trimester warrants serial fetal ultrasound to assess for hydrops: ascites, pericardial effusion, oligohydramnios, cardiomegaly, and placental thickening.
- Weekly peak systolic velocity measurements of the middle cerebral artery by Doppler US is recommended to evaluate for heart failure fetal anemia and the potential need for intrauterine transfusion (>1.5 MoM).
- Cerebral MRI to explore CNS damage in infected neonates with prolonged hydrops fetalis or hematocrit <15%.

Diagnostic Procedures/Other
- Skin biopsy is usually normal but may show mild inflammation consisting of perivascular infiltrations of mononuclear cells.
- In stillbirths related to maternal B19 infection, virus can be detected in all tissues.
- In hydrops fetalis, nucleated RBCs may have intranuclear inclusion bodies.

 TREATMENT

GENERAL MEASURES
- No therapy is usually needed (4)[C].
- Cessation of immunosuppressive therapy allows some patients to clear chronic infections.
- B19-associated anemia in HIV-positive patients may resolve with highly active antiretroviral therapy.

MEDICATION
First Line
- Anti-inflammatory agents for arthritic symptoms
- Antipyretics for fever. Avoid aspirin in children.

Second Line
- RBC transfusions for aplastic crisis
- Intravenous immunoglobulin (IVIG) for B19-related refractory anemia or PRAC, especially in immunodeficient states (5)[C]
- Intrauterine RBC transfusions reduce mortality in cases of fetal hydrops.

ISSUES FOR REFERRAL
- Acute infection during pregnancy should prompt referral to a maternal–fetal medicine specialist.
- TAC patients require treatment by a hematologist.
- Patients with chronic or abnormal B19 infections may benefit from consultation with immunology or infectious disease specialists.

INPATIENT CONSIDERATIONS
Admission Criteria/Initial Stabilization
- Outpatient management is typical for EI.
- Inpatient management for aplastic crisis, which may require RBC transfusions

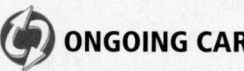 **ONGOING CARE**

FOLLOW-UP RECOMMENDATIONS
Patient Monitoring
Periodic blood counts for anemic patients

PATIENT EDUCATION
- Parvovirus B19 (fifth disease): http://www.cdc.gov/parvovirusB19/fifth-disease.html
- Parvovirus B19: What You Should Know: http://www.aafp.org/afp/2007/0201/p377.html
- Parvovirus B19 infection and pregnancy: http://www.cdc.gov/parvovirusB19/pregnancy.html
- March of Dimes Fifth Disease and Pregnancy: http://www.marchofdimes.org/complications/fifth-disease-and-pregnancy.aspx
- Counsel pregnant women regarding prevention of maternal B19 infection.
- Pregnant women should avoid exposure to patients with active/chronic infections. Exclusion of pregnant women from the workplace where EI is occurring is not recommended because they have likely been exposed.
- Children with typical rash are no longer infectious and may attend childcare or school.

PROGNOSIS
- Usually self-limited
- Joint symptoms subside in weeks (often by 2 weeks but may last months).
- ~20% of infections result in delayed virus elimination and viremia persisting for several months to years.
- Full recovery from aplastic crisis in 2 to 3 weeks

COMPLICATIONS
Conditions associated with B19 but where causality is unconfirmed.
- Chronic fatigue syndrome
- Glomerulonephritis, nephrotic syndrome, and other renal diseases
- Hepatitis
- Neurologic manifestations/stroke/meningoencephalitis
- Henoch-Schönlein purpura, idiopathic thrombocytopenic purpura, and vasculitis
- Myocarditis and pericarditis
- Hemophagocytic syndrome

REFERENCES
1. de Jong EP, de Haan TR, Kroes AC, et al. Parvovirus B19 infection in pregnancy. *J Clin Virol.* 2006;36(1):1–7.
2. Santonja C, Nieto-González G, Santos-Briz Á, et al. Immunohistochemical detection of parvovirus B19 in "gloves and socks" papular purpuric syndrome: direct evidence for viral endothelial involvement. Report of three cases and review of literature. *Am J Dermatopathol.* 2011;33(8):790–795.
3. de Jong EP, Walther FJ, Kroes AC, et al. Parvovirus B19 infection in pregnancy: new insights and management. *Prenat Diagn.* 2011;31(5):419–425.
4. Servey JT, Reamy BV, Hodge J. Clinical presentations of parvovirus B19 infection. *Am Fam Physician.* 2007;75(3):373–376.
5. Orange JS, Hossny EM, Weiler CR, et al. Use of intravenous immunoglobulin in human disease: a review of evidence by members of the Primary Immunodeficiency Committee of the American Academy of Allergy, Asthma and Immunology. *J Allergy Clin Immunol.* 2006;117(4 Suppl):S525–S553.

ADDITIONAL READING
- Azevedo KM, Setúbal S, Camacho LA, et al. Parvovirus B19 seroconversion in a cohort of human immunodeficiency virus-infected patients. *Mem Inst Oswaldo Cruz.* 2012;107(3):356–361.
- Beigi RH, Wiesenfeld HC, Landers DV, et al. High rate of severe fetal outcomes associated with maternal parvovirus B19 infection in pregnancy. *Infect Dis Obstet Gynecol.* 2008;2008:524601.
- Centers for Disease Control and Prevention. Risk associated with human parvovirus B19 infection. *MMWR Morb Mortal Wkly Rep.* 1989;38(6):81–88, 93–97.
- De Jong EP, Lindenburg IT, van Klink JM, et al. Intrauterine transfusion for parvovirus B19 infection: long-term neurodevelopmental outcome. *Am J Obstet Gynecol.* 2012;206(3):204.e1–204.e5.
- Heegaard ED, Brown KE. Human parvovirus B19. *Clin Microbiol Rev.* 2002;15(3):485–505.
- Lamont RF, Sobel JD, Vaisbuch E, et al. Parvovirus B19 infection in human pregnancy. *BJOG.* 2011;118(2):175–186.
- Snyder M, Wallace R. Clinical inquiry: what should you tell pregnant women about exposure to parvovirus? *J Fam Pract.* 2011;60(12):765–766.
- Young NS, Brown KE. Parvovirus B19. *N Engl J Med.* 2004;350(6):586–597.

 CODES

ICD10
- B34.3 Parvovirus infection, unspecified
- B08.3 Erythema infectiosum [fifth disease]

CLINICAL PEARLS
- Parvovirus B19 infection is usually a benign, self-limited illness with no long-term effects.
- The rash of EI, a "slapped cheek" appearance, signifies that the patient is no longer infectious.
- Patients with increased RBC turnover (SS, thalassemia) are at risk for TAC.
- Immunocompromised patients may be at risk for chronic anemia.
- Documentation of acute infection in pregnant women under 20 weeks' gestation merits maternal–fetal consultation.

PATELLOFEMORAL PAIN SYNDROME

Rathna Nuti, MD • Robert J. Dimeff, MD

BASICS

DESCRIPTION
- Pain in or around the patella that increases after prolonged sitting, squatting, kneeling, and stair climbing (1)
- System(s) affected: musculoskeletal

EPIDEMIOLOGY
Prevalence
- Most frequently diagnosed condition in patients <50 years old with knee complaints (1)
- Women have higher incidence than men (1,2).
- More predominant in female adolescents and physically active young adults (3)
- High incidence in physically active populations (3)
- Incidence of 15–25% in the general population (3)
- Accounts for 25% of all knee injuries (4)

ETIOLOGY AND PATHOPHYSIOLOGY
- Multifactorial etiology (1)
- Direct relationship with hip weakness and poor functional control of the femur during weight-bearing tasks (5)
- Structural anomalies and lower extremity malalignment also contribute (1).
- Shortened quadriceps results in increased contact time and force between the retropatellar cartilage and the trochlear groove (4).

Genetics
Unknown

RISK FACTORS
- Weak quadriceps (1)
- Female gender;
- Q angle >20 degrees (1)
- Limited quadriceps and gastrocnemius flexibility (6)
- Excessive knee valgus during landing (6)
- Subtalar hyperpronation (6)
- Tight iliotibial band and/or lateral retinaculum (6)
- Decreased strength (or timing) of (between) the medial quadriceps and the gluteus medius (6)
- Decreased hamstring flexibility (5)
- Decreased explosive strength (5)
- Improper training equipment (5)
- Decreased trochlear groove depth (5)
- Increased medial patellar mobility (5)
- Patella alta (5)
- Increased medial tibial intercondylar distance (5)

GENERAL PREVENTION
- Mitigate risk factors (1)
- Strengthening exercises (1)
- Reduce training volume (7)

COMMONLY ASSOCIATED CONDITIONS
- Overuse
- Knee ligament injury/surgery
- Patellar tendinopathy
- Prolonged synovitis
- Iliotibial band friction syndrome

DIAGNOSIS

HISTORY
- An accurate history should differentiate retropatellar pain from knee instability (e.g., pain quality, swelling, giving way, mechanical symptoms, and grinding, inciting events, overuse, and history of trauma)
- Most common symptom: anteromedial knee pain exacerbated by physical activity
- Pain often exacerbated when squatting (3)[A].
- Anterior knee pain when descending/ascending stairs, ambulating over uneven surfaces, or running
- Pain after activity as well as during activity

PHYSICAL EXAM
- Patellar tilt test: With patient supine, grasp patella between thumb and forefinger and try to lift up the outside edge of the patella using the thumb (3)[A].
- Squatting (3)[A]
- Vastus medialis coordination test: While patient is laying down supine, place fist under patient's knee and ask the patient to extend the knee slowly without pressing down or lifting away from you (3)[A].
- Apprehension sign: Compress the patella against the femur and ask the patient to contract quadriceps muscles; pain upon contraction is consistent with patellofemoral pain syndrome, although pain may be present in normal individuals as well (3)[A].
- Compression test: reproduction of pain with compression of patella against the trochlea (3)[A]

DIFFERENTIAL DIAGNOSIS
- Prepatellar bursitis; patellar and quadriceps tendinitis/tendinopathy
- Patellofemoral arthrosis; patellar subluxation and dislocation
- ACL, PCL, and meniscal pathology
- Soft tissue and bony tumors
- Iliotibial band syndrome
- Plica syndrome
- Patellar fat pad inflammation; patellofemoral osteoarthritis
- Chondromalacia patella/osteochondral defect
- Sinding-Larsen-Johansson syndrome
- Osgood-Schlatter disease
- Referred pain from hip or spine
- Traction apophysitis

DIAGNOSTIC TESTS & INTERPRETATION
- None indicated. *In general, imaging is unnecessary and not helpful in diagnosing patellofemoral pain syndrome.* If imaging is indicated because of severity, atypical symptoms, or persistence of symptoms despite treatment, four views (plain films) of the knee are recommended to view patellar tilt:
  - Lateral
  - Merchant (also called sunrise)
  - Standing anteroposterior
  - Posteroanterior tunnel views:
- Radiographic findings may not correlate with symptoms.

Follow-Up Tests & Special Considerations
Radiographic images may be normal until late stages, when the posterior patellar surface becomes irregular and cartilage erosion becomes radiographically detectable.

Test Interpretation
Generally a clinical diagnosis. Tests not necessary.

TREATMENT

Conservative therapy is the gold standard (5)[A].

GENERAL MEASURES

- Stretching and strengthening exercises, especially hip strengthening (5)[A]
- Taping and bracing (5)[A]
- Activity modification (5)[A]
- Cast immobilization (5)[A]
- NSAIDs for pain management (5)[A]
- Neuromuscular retraining interventions (especially with physical therapy) (5)[A]
- Supervised exercise therapy program including quadriceps training (1)[A]
- Foot orthoses (8)[A]
- Electrotherapy and biofeedback (8)[A]

MEDICATION

- NSAIDs for pain management (5)[A]

- The evidence for beneficial effects of glucosamine and chondroitin supplementation is conflicting and merits further investigation. They may have anti-inflammatory effects and function as articular cartilage and synovial fluid precursors.
- Nandrolone may be effective, but it is too controversial to recommend for treatment.

ISSUES FOR REFERRAL

Referral for surgery is a last resort after all conservative measures fail. Surgery is rarely needed.

ADDITIONAL THERAPIES

Ice packs after activity improve clinical symptoms.

SURGERY/OTHER PROCEDURES

- No additional benefits of surgery compared to conservative treatment (8)[A].
- Attempts to correct maltracking of the patellofemoral joint with a lateral retinacular release or tibial tubercle transposition have shown variable results (5)[A].

- Rarely indicated

 ONGOING CARE

PATIENT EDUCATION

Patient education and exercises: http://familydoctor .org/online/famdocen/home/healthy/physical/injuries/ 479.html

PROGNOSIS

- Patellofemoral pain syndrome often improves spontaneously with relative rest and physical therapy.
- Conversely, established chondromalacia patella, which involves actual injury to the patellofemoral joint cartilage has a poorer prognosis.

REFERENCES

1. Lankhorst NE, Bierma-Zeinstra SM, van Middelkoop M. Risk factors for patellofemoral pain syndrome: a systematic review. *J Orthop Sports Phys Ther*. 2012;42(2):81–94.
2. Lankhorst NE, Bierma-Zeinstra SM, van Middelkoop M. Factors associated with patellofemoral pain syndrome: a systematic review. *Br J Sports Med*. 2013;47(4):193–206.
3. Nunes GS, Stapait EL, Kirsten MH, et al. Clinical test for diagnosis of patellofemoral pain syndrome: systematic review with meta-analysis. *Phys Ther Sport*. 2013;14(1):54–59.
4. Barton CJ, Lack S, Malliaras P, et al. Gluteal muscle activity and patellofemoral pain syndrome: a systematic review. *Br J Sports Med*. 2013;47(4): 207–214.
5. Carry PM, Kanai S, Miller NH, et al. Adolescent patellofemoral pain: a review of evidence for the role of lower extremity biomechanics and core instability. *Orthopedics*. 2010;33(7):498–507.
6. Pappas E, Wong-Tom WM. Prospective predictors of patellofemoral pain syndrome: a systemic review with meta-analysis. *Sports Health*. 2012;4(2): 115–120.
7. Tenforde AS, Sayres LC, McCurdy ML, et al. Overuse injuries in high school runners: lifetime prevalence and prevention strategies. *PM R*. 2011;3(2): 125–131.
8. Peters JS, Tyson NL. Proximal exercises are effective in treating patellofemoral pain syndrome: a systematic review. *Int J Sports Phys Ther*. 2013;8(5): 689–700.

ADDITIONAL READING

- Callaghan MJ, Selfe J. Patellar taping for patellofemoral pain syndrome in adults. *Cochrane Database Syst Rev*. 2012;(4):CD006717.
- Collado H, Fredericson M. Patellofemoral pain syndrome. *Clin Sports Med*. 2010;29(3):379–398.
- Dixit S, DiFiori JP, Burton M, et al. Management of patellofemoral pain syndrome. *Am Fam Physician*. 2007;75(2):194–202.
- Fredericson M, Yoon K. Physical examination and patellofemoral pain syndrome. *Am J Phys Med Rehabil*. 2006;85(3):234–243.
- Frye JL, Ramey LN, Hart JM. The effects of exercise on decreasing pain and increasing function in patients with patellofemoral pain syndrome: a systematic review. *Sports Health*. 2012;4(3):205–210.
- Heintjes E, Berger MY, Bierma-Zeinstra SM, et al. Pharmacotherapy for patellofemoral pain syndrome. *Cochrane Database Syst Rev*. 2004;(3):CD003470.
- Waryasz GR, McDermott AY. Patellofemoral pain syndrome (PFPS): a systematic review of anatomy and potential risk factors. *Dyn Med*. 2008;7:9.

 SEE ALSO

Algorithm: Knee Pain

 CODES

ICD10

- M25.569 Pain in unspecified knee
- M25.561 Pain in right knee
- M25.562 Pain in left knee

CLINICAL PEARLS

- Patellofemoral pain syndrome is the most common cause of anterior knee pain in active adults. Women are more commonly affected.
- The diagnosis is made through an accurate history and physical exam. The apprehension sign is the most sensitive finding on physical exam.
- Well-designed exercises targeting quadriceps strengthening, hamstring, and IT band flexibility and hip stabilizer stretching/strengthening are the most effective evidence-based treatment.

PEDICULOSIS (LICE)

Kaelen C. Dunican, PharmD • Cynthia Jeremiah, MD

 BASICS

DESCRIPTION
- A contagious parasitic infection caused by ectoparasitic blood-feeding insects (lice)
- Two species of lice infest humans:
  - *Pediculus humanus* has two subspecies: the head louse (var. *capitis*) and the body louse (var. *corporis*). Both species are 1- to 3-mm long, flat, and wingless and have three pairs of legs that attach closely behind the head.
  - *Phthirus pubis* (pubic or crab louse): resembles a sea crab and has widespread claws on the second and third legs
- System(s) affected: skin/exocrine
- Synonym(s): lice; crabs

EPIDEMIOLOGY
Incidence
- In the United States: 6 to 12 million new cases per year
- Predominant age
  - Head lice: most common in children 3 to 12 years of age; more common in girls than boys
  - Pubic lice: most common in adults

Prevalence
Head lice: 1–3% in industrialized countries

ETIOLOGY AND PATHOPHYSIOLOGY
- Infestation by lice: *P. humanus* (var. *capitis*), *P. humanus* (var. *corporis*), or *P. pubis*
- Characteristics of lice:
  - Adult louse is dark grayish and moves quickly but does not jump or fly.
  - Eggs (nits) camouflage with the individuals' hair color and are cemented to the base of the hair shaft (within 4 mm of the scalp).
  - Nits (empty egg casings) appear white (opalescent) and remain cemented to the hair shaft.
  - Lice feed solely on human blood by piercing the skin, injecting saliva (anticoagulant properties to allow for blood meal), and then sucking blood.
  - Itching is a hypersensitivity reaction to the saliva of the feeding louse.
- Transmission: direct human-to-human contact
  - Head lice: direct head-to-head contact or contact with infested fomite (less likely)
  - Body lice: contact with contaminated clothing or bedding
  - Pubic lice: typically transmitted sexually (fomite transmission much less likely)

RISK FACTORS
- General: overcrowding and close personal contact
- Head lice
  - School-aged children, gender (girls; longer hair)
  - Sharing combs, hats (including helmets), clothing, and bed linens
  - African Americans rarely have head lice; theories include twisted hair shaft and increased use of pomades
- Body lice: poor hygiene, homelessness
- Pubic lice: promiscuity (very high transmission rate)

GENERAL PREVENTION
- Environmental measures: Wash, dry-clean, or vacuum all items that may have come in contact with infected individuals.
- Screen and treat affected household contacts.
- Head lice: Follow-up by school nurses may help to prevent recurrence and spread.
- Pubic lice: Limit the number of sexual partners (condoms do not prevent transmission nor does shaving pubic hair).
- Body lice: proper hygiene

COMMONLY ASSOCIATED CONDITIONS
Up to 1/3 of patients with pubic lice have at least one concomitant STI.

 DIAGNOSIS

HISTORY
- Pruritus is common, mostly at night.
- Often associated with "outbreak" in school settings
- Investigate contacts of infected individuals.

PHYSICAL EXAM
- Diagnosis is confirmed by visualization of live lice.
- *P. capitis* (head lice)
  - Found most often on the back of the head and neck and behind the ears (warmer areas)
  - Eyelashes may be involved.
  - Eggs, found cemented on the base of a hair shaft, are difficult to remove.
  - Pruritus may be accompanied by local erythema and small papules.
  - May see excoriations around hairline
  - Scratching can cause inflammation and secondary bacterial infection.
  - Pyoderma and lymphadenopathy may occur in severe infestation.
- *P. corporis* (body lice)
  - Poor general hygiene
  - Adult lice and nits in the seams of clothing
  - Intense pruritus involving area covered by clothing (trunk, axillae, and groin)
  - Uninfected bites present as erythematous macules, papules, and wheals.
  - Pyoderma and excoriation may be seen.
- *P. pubis* (pubic lice)
  - Pubic hair is the most common site, but lice may spread to hair around anus, abdomen, axillae, chest, beard, eyebrows, and eyelashes.
  - Eggs are present at the base of hair shafts.
  - Anogenital pruritus
  - Blue macules may be seen in surrounding skin.
  - Delay in treatment may lead to development of groin infection and regional adenopathy.

DIFFERENTIAL DIAGNOSIS
- Scabies and other mite species that can cause cutaneous reactions in humans
- Dandruff and other hair debris sometimes look like head lice eggs and nits but is less adherent.

DIAGNOSTIC TESTS & INTERPRETATION
- Diagnosis is based on visualization of live louse.
- Head lice: Comb hair thoroughly with a fine-toothed louse comb (0.2 to 0.3 mm between teeth) to identify live lice (1)[C]. Wet hair may limits static electricity. Simple visual inspection has same sensitivity as wet combing but is only ~25% as effective as dry combing with a metal comb (2).
- Body lice: Examine the seams of clothing to locate lice and eggs (3).
- Lice and eggs are more easily visualized under a microscope.
- In contrast to dandruff, eggs and nits cannot be removed easily from a hair shaft.

Follow-Up Tests & Special Considerations
- Empty nits remain on hair shafts for months after eradication of the live infestation. On Wood lamp exam, live nits fluoresce white and empty nits fluoresce gray.
- Pubic lice: Evaluate for concurrent STIs.

 TREATMENT

MEDICATION
Permethrin (over the counter [OTC]), synergized pyrethrin (OTC), spinosad (Rx), benzyl alcohol (Rx), malathion (Rx), and topical ivermectin (Rx) are all effective for head lice (1)[A],(2)[C]. Permethrin, synergized pyrethrin, and malathion are effective for pubic lice (2)[C]:

- Permethrin generally preferred because it has residual activity for up to 3 weeks. However, newer shampoos and conditioners may reduce the residual effect (1)[C].
- Malathion and spinosad are considered second line for head lice but may not require a second application due to ovicidal activity (1)[B],(2)[C].
- Ivermectin 0.5% lotion is also effective for head lice (2)[C].

First Line
- Head and pubic lice
- Pyrethrum insecticides: permethrin 1% cream rinse (Nix) or pyrethrins 0.33% with piperonyl butoxide 4% (synergized pyrethrin, Rid, Pronto): are first line unless there is proven resistance in the community.
  - Apply for 10 minutes, then wash.
  - Reapply synergized pyrethrin in 7 to 10 days (day 9 is optimal). Also be necessary with permethrin, if live lice are observed.
  - Side effects: application-site erythema, ocular erythema, and application-site irritation
- Body lice: best treated with synergized pyrethrin lotion applied once and left on for several hours
- Eyelash infestation: Apply petroleum jelly BID for 10 days.
- Precautions
  - Pyrethrin: Avoid in patients with ragweed allergy (may cause respiratory symptoms).
  - Pediculicides should never be used to treat eyelash infections.

Second Line
Head lice and pubic lice
- Malathion 0.5% lotion (Ovide)
  - Apply for 8 to 12 hours, then wash off
  - Excipients isopropyl alcohol (78%) and terpineol (12%) may contribute to its efficacy:
    ○ Flammable and has a bad odor
    ○ Despite ovicidal activity, a second application may be necessary after 7 to 10 days (day 9 is optimal) if live lice are observed.
  - Lindane 1% shampoo, no longer recommended by the American Academy of Pediatrics
    ○ Apply for 4 minutes, then wash (should *not* be repeated).
    ○ Side effects: neurotoxicity (seizures, muscle spasms), aplastic anemia
    ○ Contraindications: uncontrolled seizure disorder, premature infants

772

○ Precautions: Do not use on excoriated skin, in immunocompromised patients, conditions that increase seizure risk, or with medications that decrease seizure threshold.
○ Possible interactions: concomitant use with medications that lower the seizure threshold
- Head lice
  - Spinosad 0.9% lotion (Natroba)
    ○ Apply to dry hair and scalp for 10 minutes, then rinse with warm water. Repeat in 7 days if live lice are observed.
    ○ Side effects: application-site erythema, ocular erythema, and application-site irritation
  - Benzyl alcohol 5% lotion (Ulesfia)
    ○ Apply to dry hair using enough to saturate scalp and hair (amount depends on hair length), rinse after 10 minutes, and repeat in 7 days.
    ○ Side effects: pruritus, erythema, pyoderma, ocular irritation, application-site irritation
  - Ivermectin 0.5% lotion (Sklice)
    ○ Apply to dry hair by using enough to saturate the scalp and hair (max. 4 oz) then rinse after 10 minutes.
    ○ Side effects: burning sensation at application site, dandruff, dry skin, eye irritation
  - Mechanical removal of lice and nits by wetting hair and then systematically combing with a fine-toothed comb every 3 to 4 days for 2 weeks to remove all lice as they hatch

ALERT

Lindane: FDA black box warning of severe neurologic toxicity (use only when first-line agents have failed). The National Pediculosis Association strongly advises against using lindane at all.

GENERAL MEASURES

- Head lice: Clean items that have been in contact with the head of the infected individual within 48 hours.
- Wash all bedding, towels, clothes, headgear, combs, brushes, and hair accessories in hot water (60°C).
- Vacuum furniture and carpets
- Seal any personal articles that cannot be washed in hot water, dry cleaned, or vacuumed in a plastic bag and store for at least 2 weeks.
- Examine and treat household members and close contacts concurrently.
- Insecticide sprays are not necessary.
- Pubic lice: Avoid sexual activity until both partners are successfully treated.
- Nit and egg removal
  - Remove eggs that are within 1 cm of the scalp to prevent reinfestation.
  - After treatment with shampoo or lotion, eggs and nits remain in the scalp or pubic hair until mechanically removed. Hair conditioner facilitates nit removal.
  - Eggs and nits are best removed with a very fine nit comb.

Pediatric Considerations

- Avoid synergized pyrethrin and permethrin in infants <2 months of age. Avoid benzyl alcohol, topical ivermectin, and spinosad in children <6 months of age; and avoid malathion in children <2 years of age.
- Lindane: not recommended in patients <50 kg

Pregnancy Considerations

Permethrin, synergized pyrethrin, malathion, spinosad, and benzyl alcohol are pregnancy Category B. Lindane and topical ivermectin are Category C.

ADDITIONAL THERAPIES

- For "difficult to treat" cases of head lice, oral ivermectin 400 μg/kg (not approved by the FDA for lice), given twice at a 7-day interval, is superior to topical 0.5% malathion lotion (4,5)[B].

- Ivermectin: 200 μg/kg PO repeated in 10 days or 300 μg/kg PO repeated in 7 days
  - Should not be used in children <15 kg; pregnancy Category C
  - Not approved by the FDA for lice
- Dual therapy with 1% permethrin and oral trimethoprim/sulfamethoxazole (TMP/SMX) only for cases of multiple treatment failures or suspected cases of lice-related resistance to therapy (TMP/SMX is not approved by the FDA for lice).

- Permethrin 5% cream (Rx) is not FDA approved for lice and is unlikely to be effective for lice that are resistant to 1% cream rinse (1)[B].

COMPLEMENTARY & ALTERNATIVE MEDICINE

Head lice

- Dry-on, suffocation-based pediculicide: Cetaphil lotion
  - Apply thoroughly to hair, comb, dry with hair dryer, shampoo after 8 hours.
  - Repeat once a week until cured, up to a maximum of three applications.
  - Not approved by the FDA for lice
- Dimethicone 4% lotion: Apply to hair for 8 hours; repeat in 1 week (not approved by the FDA for lice).
- No home remedies (e.g., vinegar, isopropyl alcohol, olive oil, ylang ylang oil, mayonnaise, melted butter, and petroleum jelly) have been proven effective to treat head lice infestations.
- Herbal shampoos and pomades have not been evaluated in clinical trials and are not approved by the FDA for lice.
- Lavender oil and tea tree oil have been implicated in triggering prepubertal gynecomastia in boys and should not be used to treat lice.
- Electronic louse combs have not proven effective and are not approved by the FDA.

ONGOING CARE

FOLLOW-UP RECOMMENDATIONS

Children may return to school after completing topical treatment, even if nits remain in place. No-nit policies are not necessary.

Patient Monitoring

Drug resistance should be suspected if no dead lice are observed in 8 to 12 hours after treatment.

PATIENT EDUCATION

- National Pediculosis Association: http://www.headlice.org/
- CDC: http://www.cdc.gov/parasites/lice/
- http://www.guideline.gov/content.aspx?id=46429&search=lice

PROGNOSIS

- With appropriate treatment, >90% cure rate
- Recurrence is common, mainly from reinfection or treatment nonadherence. Resistance to synthetic pyrethroids is increasing.

COMPLICATIONS

- Poor sleep due to pruritus
- Persistent itching may be caused by too frequent use of the pediculicide.

- Missed school; social stigma
- Secondary bacterial infections
- Body lice can transmit typhus and trench fever.

REFERENCES

1. Devore CD, Schutze GE. Head lice. *Pediatrics*. 2015;135(5): e1355–e1365.
2. Burgess IF. Current treatments for pediculosis capitis. *Curr Opin Infect Dis*. 2009;22(2):131–136.
3. Gunning K, Pippitt K, Kiraly B, et al. Pediculosis and scabies: treatment update. *Am Fam Physician*. 2012;86(6):535–541.
4. Chosidow O, Giraudeau B, Cottrell J, et al. Oral ivermectin versus malathion lotion for difficult-to-treat head lice. *N Engl J Med*. 2010;362(10):896–905.
5. Feldmeier H. Treatment of pediculosis capitis: a critical appraisal of the current literature. *Am J Clin Dermatol*. 2014;15(5):401–412.

ADDITIONAL READING

- Cole SW, Lundquist LM. Spinosad for treatment of head lice infestation. *Ann Pharmacother*. 2011;45(7–8):954–959.
- Durand R, Bouvresse S, Berdjane Z, et al. Insecticide resistance in head lice: clinical, parasitological and genetic aspects. *Clin Microbiol Infect*. 2012;18(4): 338–344.
- Pariser DM, Meinking TL, Bell M, et al. Topical 0.5% ivermectin lotion for treatment of head lice. *N Engl J Med*. 2012;367(18):1687–1693.

 SEE ALSO

Arthropod Bites and Stings; Scabies

CODES

ICD10

- B85.0 Pediculosis due to Pediculus humanus capitis
- B85.1 Pediculosis due to Pediculus humanus corporis
- B85.3 Phthiriasis

CLINICAL PEARLS

- School-based no-nit policies are not necessary because empty nits may remain on hair shafts for months after successful eradication.
- Proper product application is essential; consider improper product application when assessing treatment failure.
- Prevalence of resistant infestations is increasing, so if no dead lice are observed in 8 to 12 hours after treatment, suspect resistance and use an alternative agent.
- Routine retreatment on day 9 is recommended for nonovicidal products (permethrin and synergized pyrethrin).
- With all treatment options, reinspect hair after 7 to 9 days and, if live lice are detected, repeat treatment on day 9.

PELVIC INFLAMMATORY DISEASE

Fozia Akhtar Ali, MD • Paula A. Shelton, MD

 BASICS

DESCRIPTION
- Pelvic inflammatory disease (PID) is an infectious and inflammatory disorder of the upper female genital tract, including the uterus, fallopian tubes, ovaries, and adjacent pelvic structures. It is community acquired from sexually transmitted organisms (1).
- Salpingitis is the most important component due to its impact on future fertility.
- Diagnosis may be challenging and incorrect in up to 1/3 of cases. No set of criteria is both sensitive and specific for the disease.
- System(s) affected: reproductive

EPIDEMIOLOGY
- Predominant age: 15 to 25 years; this number has remained constant since early 1900s.
- Predominant sex: female only (1)

Incidence
Over 770,000 cases of acute PID are diagnosed annually in the United States. Incidence decreased from 1885 to 2001. The CDC has estimated that more than 1 million women experience an episode of PID every year. The disease leads to approximately 2.5 million office visits, 200,000 hospitalizations, and 100,000 surgical procedures yearly. The cost of PID is approximately $2 billion annually; however, costs have decreased over the past decade (2).

ETIOLOGY AND PATHOPHYSIOLOGY
Multiple organisms may be etiologic agents in PID. Most cases are polymicrobial.
- *Chlamydia trachomatis*, *Neisseria gonorrhoeae*, genital tract mycoplasmas (particularly *Mycoplasma genitalium*), aerobic and anaerobic (*Bacteroides fragilis*), and vaginal flora (e.g., *Prevotella*, *Peptostreptococci*, *Gardnerella vaginalis*, *Escherichia coli*, *Haemophilus influenzae*) are recognized as etiologic agents (1,3,4).
- Many nongonococcal, nonchlamydial microorganisms recovered from upper genital tract in acute PID are associated with bacterial vaginosis (especially *Prevotella bivius*, *Prevotella disiens*, and *Prevotella capillosus*) (2).
- The precise mechanism by which microorganisms ascend from the lower genital tract is unclear. Possible mechanisms include the following: (i) travel from cervix to endometrium to salpinx to peritoneal cavity; (ii) lymphatic spread via infection of the parametrium (from an IUD); and (iii) hematogenous route, although this is rare.
- Of cases, 75% occur within 7 days of menses, when cervical mucus favors ascent of organisms.

RISK FACTORS
- Sexually active and age <25 years (5)
- First sexual activity at young age (<15 years)
- New/multiple sexual partners
- Nonbarrier contraceptive methods (i.e., oral contraceptive pills)
- Previous history of PID; 20–25% will have a recurrence.
- Cervical ectopy
- History of *C. trachomatis*; 10–40% will develop PID.
- History of gonococcal cervicitis; 10–20% will develop PID.

- Gynecologic procedures such as endometrial biopsy, curettage, and hysteroscopy break the cervical barrier, predisposing women to ascending infections.

GENERAL PREVENTION
- Educational programs about safer sex practices such as barrier contraceptives, especially condoms and spermicidal creams or sponges, provide some protection (5).
- The U.S. Preventive Services Task Force recommends screening for chlamydia in all sexually active women <25 years and in those 25 years and older at increased risk (new sex partner/multiple sex partners).
- Routine STI screening in pregnancy
- Early medical care with occurrence of genital lesions or abnormal discharge

COMMONLY ASSOCIATED CONDITIONS
- If PID is suspected in a patient with an IUD and a pelvic abscess is present; an *Actinomyces* infection requiring penicillin treatment may be present.
- Rupture of an adnexal abscess is rare but life-threatening. Early surgical exploration is mandatory (3).
- Chlamydial or gonococcal perihepatitis may occur with PID. This combination is called Fitz-Hugh-Curtis (FHC) syndrome and is characterized by severe pleuritic right upper quadrant pain. FHC syndrome complicates 10% of PID cases.
- Plasma cell endometritis has also been seen in the majority of females with PID; the density of plasma cell infiltration has been related to severity of symptoms (3).

 DIAGNOSIS

- The diagnosis of PID is based primarily on clinical evaluation. Clinical diagnosis alone is 87% sensitive and 50% specific.
- Physicians must consider PID in the differential diagnosis in women 15 to 44 years of age who present with lower abdominal or pelvic pain and cervical motion or pelvic tenderness, even if these symptoms are mild.
- The CDC recommends empiric treatment for PID if ≥1 of the following minimum criteria are present on pelvic exam in an at-risk patient: cervical motion tenderness, uterine tenderness, and adnexal tenderness in the presence of lower abdominal or pelvic pain.
- Additional criteria used to enhance specificity: fever >101°F, new/abnormal vaginal discharge, presence of abundant numbers of WBCs on wet prep, elevated ESR, and laboratory documentation of cervical infection with *N. gonorrhoeae* or *C. trachomatis* (1,6).
- Most specific criteria for diagnosing PID: Endometrial biopsy reveals endometritis/plasma cells; transvaginal ultrasound showing thickened, fluid-filled salpinges; and laparoscopic abnormalities consistent with PID (1).

HISTORY
- Lower abdominal or pelvic pain: typically described as dull, aching or crampy, bilateral, and constant; accentuated by motion, exercise, or coitus
- New/abnormal vaginal discharge (~75% of cases)

- Fever, chills, cramping, dyspareunia
- Low back pain
- Urinary discomfort
- Unanticipated vaginal bleeding, often postcoital, is reported in about 40% of cases.
- Recent hysterosalpingogram (HSG)
- IUD insertion within the past 21 days (1,3)

PHYSICAL EXAM
- Fever
- Lower abdominal pain and particularly cervical motion tenderness
- Findings of cervicitis with/without vaginal discharge (1)

DIFFERENTIAL DIAGNOSIS
- Appendicitis
- Constipation
- Gastroenteritis
- Ectopic pregnancy
- Ovarian tumor/torsion
- Hemorrhagic/ruptured ovarian cyst
- Endometriosis/dysmenorrhea
- Functional pelvic pain
- Inflammatory bowel disease
- Diverticulitis
- UTI/pyelonephritis
- Nephrolithiasis (1)

DIAGNOSTIC TESTS & INTERPRETATION
Initial Tests (lab, imaging)
- Pregnancy test must be performed to rule out ectopic pregnancy and complications of an intrauterine pregnancy.
- Specific testing for chlamydia and gonorrhea (usually nucleic acid amplification test [NAAT] and/or ligase chain reaction)
- Urinalysis (3,4)
- Saline microscopy of vaginal fluid (for WBC)
- Consider CBC: WBC count ≥10,500/mm³, although ≤50% of PID cases present with leukocytosis
- CRP (optional)
- Consider transvaginal ultrasound: not necessary for diagnosis; may show thickened, fluid-filled tubes (hydrosalpinges) ± free fluid, or tubo-ovarian abscess (TOA)

Follow-Up Tests & Special Considerations
- ESR >15 mm/hr or elevated C-reactive protein used in some diagnostic criteria
- Consider HIV testing in patients with PID.
- Follow-up ultrasound as outpatient for resolution of adnexal abscess.

Diagnostic Procedures/Other
- Culdocentesis with culture is rarely necessary.
- Laparoscopy is best used for confirming, as opposed to making, the diagnosis of PID and should be reserved for the following situations:
  - Ill patient with competing diagnosis (e.g., appendicitis)
  - Ill patient who has failed outpatient treatment.
  - Any patient not improving after 72 hours of inpatient treatment
- Endometrial biopsy (rarely indicated): reveals endometritis/plasma cells (3)

TREATMENT

- Outpatient treatment, if appropriate
- Criteria for hospitalization and parenteral treatment are described below.

GENERAL MEASURES
Avoid intercourse until treatment is completed (7)[C]. IUD removal is NOT required for mild PID.

MEDICATION
First Line
- Several antibiotic regimens are highly effective, with no single regimen of choice (3)[A].
- Outpatient treatment regimen
  – Ceftriaxone 250 mg IM single dose *plus*
  – Doxycycline 100 mg PO BID for 14 days ±
  – Metronidazole 500 mg PO BID for 14 days
- On the basis of the recent emergence of fluoroquinolone-resistant gonococci, the CDC no longer recommends the use of fluoroquinolones for the treatment of gonococcal infections and associated conditions such as PID.
- Metronidazole should be considered in cases where risk of infection with anaerobic organisms is considered high.

Second Line
- Because of emerging resistance in gonococcus, resistance testing and confirmation of treatment success is advisable (3).
- Outpatient treatment regimen
  – Cefoxitin 2 g IM single dose and probenecid 1 g PO administered concurrently in single dose *plus*
  – Doxycycline 100 mg PO BID for 14 days +/−
  – Metronidazole 500 mg PO BID for 14 days
- In persons with documented severe allergic reactions to penicillin or cephalosporins, azithromycin or spectinomycin might be an option for therapy of uncomplicated gonococcal infections.
- Special consideration
  – Refer sex partners for appropriate evaluation and treatment if they had sexual contact with patient during preceding 60 days or most recent sexual contact. Partners should be treated, irrespective of evaluation, with regimens effective against chlamydia and gonorrhea (3).

SURGERY/OTHER PROCEDURES
Reserved for failures of medical treatment and for suspected ruptured adnexal abscess with resulting acute surgical abdomen

INPATIENT CONSIDERATIONS
Admission Criteria/Initial Stabilization
- Hospitalization recommended in the following (3)[C]:
  – Surgical emergencies (e.g., appendicitis)
  – Suspected pelvic abscess
  – Pregnancy
  – Severe illness, nausea, vomiting, or high fever
  – Intolerance/inability to adhere to outpatient regimen
  – Failure to respond to outpatient therapy

- For inpatient treatment of PID, the CDC also lists two currently accepted treatment regimens (6):
  – Parenteral regimen A
    ○ Cefotetan 2 g IV q12h or cefoxitin 2 g IV q6h + doxycycline 100 mg PO or IV q12h (6)[A]
    ○ Parenteral therapy for 24 hours after clinical improvement (6)[C]. Continue doxycycline for a total of 14 days.
  – Parenteral regimen B
    ○ Clindamycin 900 mg IV q8h + gentamicin loading dose IV or IM (2 mg/kg of body weight) followed by a maintenance dose (1.5 mg/kg) q8h (6)[A]
    ○ Parenteral therapy for 24 hours after clinical improvement; continue doxycycline as aforementioned or clindamycin 450 mg PO QID for a total of 14 days.
- During pregnancy: PID is rare in pregnant patients; however, may appear prior to 12 weeks' gestation before mucous plug appears. Change doxycycline to azithromycin + second-generation cephalosporin (6).

ONGOING CARE

FOLLOW-UP RECOMMENDATIONS
Patient Monitoring
- Review at 72 hours is recommended particularly for patients with moderate or severe clinical presentation (8)[C].
- Close observation of clinical status, particularly for fever, symptoms, degree of peritonitis, serum WBC
- Retest for gonorrhea and chlamydia in 3 to 6 months. The likelihood of reinfection is high.
- Follow adnexal abscess size and position with serial ultrasound (6).

PATIENT EDUCATION
- Abstinence from any type of sexual contact until treatment of patient/partner (if necessary) is complete.
- Consistent and correct condom use should be enforced.
- Hepatitis B and human papilloma virus (HPV) vaccines should be given to patients who meet criteria.
- Advise comprehensive STI screening (6).

PROGNOSIS
- Wide variation with good prognosis if early effective therapy is instituted and further infection is avoided.
- Poor prognosis related to late therapy and continued high-risk sexual behavior
- Nongonococcal, nonchlamydial PID is more often associated with severe PID and with worse prognosis for future fertility (2).

COMPLICATIONS
- TOA will develop in ~7–16% of patients with PID.
- Recurrent infection occurs in 20–25% of patients.
- Risk of ectopic pregnancy is increased 7- to 10-fold among women with a history of PID.
- Tubal infertility occurs in 8%, 19.5%, and 40% of women after 1, 2, and 3 episodes of PID, respectively.
- Chronic pelvic pain occurs in 20% of cases and is related to adhesion formation, chronic salpingitis, or recurrent infection (1,2).

- Hydrosalpinx: After PID resolves, fallopian tube may fill with sterile fluid and become blocked; it may be associated with pain and infertility related to negative outcomes with IVF (9).

REFERENCES

1. Gradison M. Pelvic inflammatory disease. *Am Fam Physician*. 2012;85(8):791–796.
2. Lareau SM, Beigi RH. Pelvic inflammatory disease and tubo-ovarian abscess. *Infect Dis Clin North Am*. 2008;22(4):693–708, vii.
3. Judlin P. Current concepts in managing pelvic inflammatory disease. *Curr Opin Infect Dis*. 2010;23(1):83–87.
4. Weinstein SA, Stiles BG. A review of the epidemiology, diagnosis and evidence-based management of *Mycoplasma genitalium*. *Sex Health*. 2011;8(2):143–158.
5. Sweet RL. Treatment of acute pelvic inflammatory disease. *Infect Dis Obstet Gynecol*. 2011;2011:561909.
6. Workowski KA, Berman S; Centers for Disease Control and Prevention. Sexually transmitted diseases treatment guidelines, 2010. *MMWR Recomm Rep*. 2010;59(RR-12):1–110.
7. Brookoff D. Compliance with doxycycline therapy for outpatient treatment of pelvic inflammatory disease. *South Med J*. 1994;87(11):1088–1091.
8. Thompson SE, Brooks C, Eschenbach DA, et al. High failure rates in outpatient treatment of salpingitis with either tetracycline alone or penicillin/ampicillin combination. *Am J Obstet Gynecol*. 1985;152(6, Pt 1):635–641.
9. Camus E, Poncelet C, Goffinet F, et al. Pregnancy rates after in-vitro fertilization in cases of tubal infertility with and without hydrosalpinx: a meta-analysis of published comparative studies. *Hum Reprod*. 1999;14(5):1243–1249.

CODES

ICD10
- N73.9 Female pelvic inflammatory disease, unspecified
- N73.0 Acute parametritis and pelvic cellulitis
- N70.93 Salpingitis and oophoritis, unspecified

CLINICAL PEARLS

- Most often, PID starts with gonorrhea or chlamydia infection, but it can be polymicrobial.
- Physicians should treat on the basis of clinical judgment without waiting for confirmation from laboratory or imaging tests. PID is a common cause of infertility.
- Complications include hydrosalpinx, adhesions, pelvic pain, and 10-fold increased risk of ectopic pregnancy.
- Three major predictors of preserved post-PID fertility: (i) short duration of symptoms (<72 hours) prior to initiation of treatment, (ii) first episode of PID, and (iii) nongonococcal PID.

PEMPHIGOID, BULLOUS

John P. Fardal, DO • Lisa Clemons, MD

BASICS

DESCRIPTION

- Bullous pemphigoid (BP) is a chronic, acquired autoimmune subepidermal blistering skin disorder caused by linear deposition of autoantibodies against the epithelial basal membrane zone.
- Pruritic, tense, symmetric, localized, widespread bullae, or urticarial plaques
- Flexural surface (80%), axillary, inguinal folds, and abdomen (20%)
- Oral lesions develop in 10–20% of cases, rarely affecting mucosae of eyes, nose, pharynx, and anogenital zones.

EPIDEMIOLOGY

- Most common autoimmune blistering disease
- Typical between 60 and 80 years old, but juvenile bullous pemphigoid can occur
- Affects both females and males, possibly with higher incidence in females
- No association with race or geographic location

Incidence

- BP incidence increases with age (1).
- 6 to 13 new cases/million per year

ETIOLOGY AND PATHOPHYSIOLOGY

- Autoantibodies react against hemidesmosomal proteins: the 230-kDa BP antigen (BPAg1) within basal keratinocytes and 180-kDa (BPAg2 or type XVII collagen) in the basement membrane zone (BMZ).
- IgG is usually the predominant autoantibody leading to C3 complement activation, recruitment of inflammatory cells, and liberation of proteolytic enzymes that break down the dermoepidermal junction.
- The noncollagenous 16A domain (NC16A) located at the membrane proximal region of BP180 is considered the major target epitope and is recognized in 80–90% of BP patients.
- It has recently been shown that IgE antibodies correlate with a severe form of BP, and those who test positive for IgE anti-BP180 antibodies required longer duration for remission and therapy.

Genetics

- Certain class II antigens of the major histocompatibility complex (MHC) alleles DQB1*0301 predominate in the United States.
- Expression of this allele on antigen-presenting cells is thought to be involved in the presentation to autoreactive T cells in patients with BP.
- Molecular mimicry has been proposed as a mechanism by which exogenous agents may trigger the immune response.

RISK FACTORS

- Advanced age
- No clear precipitating factors but can be related to infections such as hepatitis B, hepatitis C, *Helicobacter pylori*, *Toxoplasma gondii*, cytomegalovirus (CMV)
- Associated with autoimmune disorders and inflammatory dermatoses like lichen planus, psoriasis, and other forms of bullous disease
- Increased risk in patients with neurologic disorders such as multiple sclerosis, dementia, stroke, Parkinson disease, and psychiatric disorders

- Although drug-induced BP is rare, chronic intake of neuroleptics, aldosterone antagonists, furosemide, dopaminergic drugs, opioids, salicylates, NSAIDs, and phenacetin have been associated.
- Less frequent: trauma, burns, surgical scars, UV radiation, and x-ray therapy

COMMONLY ASSOCIATED CONDITIONS

- Underlying malignancy can be found in patients with BP, but it may be age related, and the correlation is marginal.
- Several autoimmune disorders such as rheumatoid arthritis, Hashimoto thyroiditis, dermatomyositis, lupus erythematosus, inflammatory dermatoses–like psoriasis, and lichen planus have been reported but are rare.

DIAGNOSIS

HISTORY

- BP occurs sporadically without any obvious trigger factor.
- Prodromal nonbullous phase: mild to severe pruritus, associated with excoriated, eczematous, and often urticarial plaques
- Mucosal lesions can be mild, transient, and are often seen with extensive cutaneous disease.
- Bullous stage: single or numerous tense bullae on erythematous, noninflammatory, urticarial skin
- Unusual clinical presentations
  - Localized form: 30% of cases (e.g., disease limited to lower leg, anogenital region, site of trauma)
  - Vegetative form: uncommon, vegetating plaques in intertriginous areas
  - Lichen planus pemphigoides: rare variant, bullae on site of previously normal skin or mucosa, after the onset of lichen planus

PHYSICAL EXAM

- Lesions usually are 1 to 3 cm round or oval, tense blisters localized on either normal or inflamed skin.
- 80–90% appear in the lower trunk, axilla, and groin, and 10–20% in oral and intertriginous spaces.
- Blister rupture leads to painful erosions that may become crusted and occasionally invaded by organisms.
- Fluid is clear but sometimes presents with hemorrhagic exudates.
- Negative active acantholysis (Nikolsky sign) and no extension of bullae into the surrounding, unblistered skin when vertical pressure is applied to the top of the bulla (Asboe-Hansen sign) support the diagnosis.

DIFFERENTIAL DIAGNOSIS

- Blistering diseases with antibodies: pemphigus, cicatricial pemphigoid, pemphigoid gestationis, epidermolysis bullosa acquisita, linear IgA dermatosis, dermatitis herpetiformis, bullous erythema multiforme
- Blistering diseases without antibodies: erythema multiforme, toxic epidermal necrolysis, porphyria, epidermolysis bullosa, allergic contact dermatitis, bullous impetigo, staphylococcal scaled-skin syndrome, friction blisters

DIAGNOSTIC TESTS & INTERPRETATION

Initial Tests (lab, imaging)

- Diagnosis of BP is based on a combination of clinical features, and the key is immunopathologic findings on skin biopsy.
- Half of patients will have elevated total serum IgE.
- ~50% of patients have peripheral blood eosinophilia that does not correlate with serum IgE levels.
- Diagnosis of atypical and nonbullous variants relies on findings of direct and indirect immunofluorescence from specific circulating antibodies.
- Considerations
  - BP has a waxing and waning course with spontaneous remission in the absence of treatment.
  - ELISA for the NC16A domain of BP180 is available at some centers, reported sensitivity 82–94%; specificity 93–99.9%
  - Old age and poor general health along with presence of anti-BP180 have been related with poor prognosis.

Diagnostic Procedures/Other

- Diagnosis is made by skin biopsy with direct immunofluorescence exam.
- Histopathology: 4-mm punch biopsy from the edge of an intact bulla (perilesional skin). Staining shows subepidermal blister and multiple eosinophils.
- Immunohistochemistry: Studies have suggested that the detection of C3d deposits at the dermoepidermal junction in formalin-fixed tissue is helpful for the diagnosis and is the most consistent finding.
- Direct immunofluorescence (DIF): Second 4-mm perilesional punch biopsy will show linear deposition of IgG and/or C3 along BMZ.
- Serologic studies: Indirect immunofluorescence (IIF) and ELISA are done when DIF is negative, there is a strong suspicion of BP, and when the skin biopsy cannot be performed. Both detect circulating IgG antibodies against 230BP (specificity 96%) and 180BP (specificity 90%).

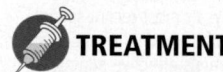

TREATMENT

GENERAL MEASURES

- Discontinue trigger factors.
- In oral lesions: Avoid hard consistency, spicy, and hot food. Soft and liquid meals should be given instead.
- Strict control of wounds to avoid complications.

MEDICATION

First Line

- Primary objectives are to control the skin eruption and minimize serious side effects of treatments, particularly in the elderly (2)[C].
- Potent topical corticosteroids are considered first line.
  - Topical clobetasol propionate 0.05% cream: 40 g/day used twice daily, noted to be as effective as 0.5 mg/kg prednisone (3)[B].
  - Side effects: skin atrophy, striae, hypertrichosis, acne, and ecchymosis

- Systemic therapy—has more side effects than topical
  - Oral prednisolone: 0.5 mg/kg/day for disease control. Goal is to achieve the lowest maintenance dosage that will prevent new lesion formation and reduce adverse reactions.
  - Clinical response is usually obtained within 1 to 2 weeks and is indicated by healing of existing lesions and cessation of new blister formation.
  - Evidence shows that higher doses >0.75 mg/kg/day do not improve healing rate but do increase mortality.
  - Taper the dose gradually within 1 to 2 years to avoid relapse; consider transition to steroid-sparing agent.
  - Side effects: cutaneous atrophy, osteoporosis, GI ulcers, Cushing syndrome, diabetes mellitus, hypertension
  - Tetracycline and nicotinamide may be beneficial in disease control and longer remission period (4)[C].

Second Line
- Although evidence is limited, immunosuppressive agents like azathioprine, mycophenolate mofetil, and methotrexate may be used in severe cases; especially in conjunction with systemic corticosteroids.
  - Addition of azathioprine to prednisone regimen reduces the total maintenance dose of prednisone by 45% without increasing serious side effects or mortality.
  - Azathioprine: 0.5 to 2.5 mg/kg/day, most common side effect: myelosuppression; caution for lethal hypersensitivity syndrome
  - Mycophenolate mofetil: 1.5 to 2 g/day, most common side effect: GI disturbance
- Methotrexate: 5 to 20 mg/week, low dose usually initiated (5 mg/week) plus folic acid replacement. Adverse effects: myelosuppression, hepatotoxicity. Higher rate of remission with the use of prednisone
- Dapsone: 25 to 50 mg daily, most common side effect: hemolytic anemia; watch for agranulocytosis.

Third Line
- Cyclosporine: caution with renal disease
- Plasmapheresis: Reduce the amount of prednisolone required to achieve disease control.
- Omalizumab: used in patients who have high levels of IgE antibodies
- IVIG: for patients who did not respond to first-line therapy or at risk of potentially fatal side effects from conventional therapy. The recommended dose is 1 to 2 g/kg divided over a 3- or 5-day cycle every 3 to 4 weeks.
- Rituximab has limited data (5)[C].

ISSUES FOR REFERRAL
- Dermatology for systemic management and/or scarring, which may suggest mucous membrane pemphigoid
- Gastroenterology, otorhinolaryngology referral in patients who have esophageal, pharyngeal, laryngeal involvement
- Ophthalmologic consult when patient complains of burning sensation, itching, visual changes, and in those patients who require high doses of steroids

INPATIENT CONSIDERATIONS
Admission Criteria/Initial Stabilization
Extensive denuding of skin, dehydration, and electrolyte imbalance requiring IV fluid reposition

 ONGOING CARE

FOLLOW-UP RECOMMENDATIONS
Patient Monitoring
- Taper medication when disease is stable and control side effects.
- Perform periodic skin examination for new lesions.
- Frequent bacterial cultures of cutaneous erosions are essential to identify early infections.

DIET
- Liquid or soft diet with active oral lesions
- After lesions are resolved, advance diet. Avoid hard or crunchy foods, as they may cause flare ups.
- Supplement with calcium and vitamin D for patients on systemic corticosteroids

PATIENT EDUCATION
- Symptoms of infection, worsening lesions
- Education in good skin hygiene and wound care
- Wash clothing and linens if they come in contact with oozing, crusting, or infected skin.
- Protect from sun exposure and physical trauma to the skin.

PROGNOSIS
- Disease length can persist from weeks to years even under treatment.
- Around 47% of patients experience relapse within 1 year of therapy, and ~50% of patients can achieve remission within 2.5 to 6 years.
- Yearly mortality varies from 6% to 40%.
- Poor prognosis and high mortality: old age, poor general condition, and the presence of antibodies in serum
- Other factors that may be included are age >80 years, prednisolone dose >37 mg/day after hospitalization, serum albumin levels of <3.6 g/dL, ESR >100 mm/hr.

COMPLICATIONS
- Most often secondary to medication: osteoporosis, cataracts, adrenal insufficiency, bone marrow suppression
- Skin infections
- Dehydration and electrolytes imbalance

REFERENCES
1. Marazza G, Pham HC, Schärer L, et al. Incidence of bullous pemphigoid and pemphigus in Switzerland: a 2-year prospective study. *Br J Dermatol*. 2009; 161(4):861–868.
2. Feliciani C, Joly P, Jonkman MF, et al. Management of bullous pemphigoid: the European Dermatology Forum consensus in collaboration with the European Academy of Dermatology and Venereology. *Br J Dermatol*. 2015;172(4) 867–877.
3. Joly P, Roujeau JC, Benichou J, et al. A comparison of oral and topical corticosteroids in patients with bullous pemphigoid. *N Engl J Med*. 2002;346(5):321–327.
4. Fivenson DP, Breneman DL, Rosen GB, et al. Nicotinamide and tetracycline therapy of bullous pemphigoid. *Arch Dermatol*. 1994;130(6):753–758.
5. Saouli Z, Papadopoulos A, Kaiafa G, et al. A new approach on bullous pemphigoid therapy. *Ann Oncol*. 2008;19(4):825–826.

ADDITIONAL READING
- García-Romero MT, Werth VP. Randomized controlled trials needed for bullous pemphigoid interventions. *Arch Dermatol*. 2012;148(2):243–246.
- Gürcan HM, Ahmed AR. Analysis of current data on the use of methotrexate in the treatment of pemphigus and pemphigoid. *Br J Dermatol*. 2009;161(4):723–731.
- Kirtschig G, Middleton P, Bennett C, et al. Interventions for bullous pemphigoid. *Cochrane Database Syst Rev*. 2010;(10):CD002292.
- Marzano AV, Tedeschi A, Berti E, et al. Activation of coagulation in bullous pemphigoid and other eosinophil-related inflammatory skin diseases. *Clin Exp Immunol*. 2011;165(1):44–50.
- Mutasim DF. Autoimmune bullous dermatoses in the elderly: an update on pathophysiology, diagnosis and management. *Drugs Aging*. 2010;27(1):1–19.
- Schmidt E, della Torre R, Borradori L. Clinical features and practical diagnosis of bullous pemphigoid. *Dermatol Clin*. 2011;29(3):427–438.
- Ujiie H, Nishie W, Shimizu H. Pathogenesis of bullous pemphigoid. *Dermatol Clin*. 2011;29(3):439–446.
- Venning VA, Taghipour K, Mohd Mustapa MF, et al. British Association of Dermatologists' guidelines for the management of bullous pemphigoid 2012. *Br J Dermatol*. 2012;167(6):1200–1214.

 CODES

ICD10
L12.0 Bullous pemphigoid

CLINICAL PEARLS
- Tense bullae differentiates the lesions of bullous pemphigoid from the flaccid bullae of pemphigus vulgaris.
- Low doses of potent topical steroid have been shown to be just as effective as larger amounts in the initial therapy of BP.

PEMPHIGUS VULGARIS

Byron M. Ingram, DO • Robert M. Hasty, DO, FACOI, FACP

BASICS

Pemphigus is derived from the Greek word *pemphix* meaning "bubble" or "blister." Pemphigus vulgaris is the most common form of pemphigus.

DESCRIPTION
- Rare, potentially fatal autoimmune mucocutaneous blistering disease due to loss of keratinocyte to keratinocyte adhesion that involves the skin and the mucous membranes
- Flaccid, painful, nonhealing bullae, pustules, or ulcerations that appear spontaneously on the skin and mucosal surfaces, typically begin in the oropharynx, and then may spread to the skin, having a predilection for the scalp, face, chest, axillae, groin, and pressure points.
- Patient often presents with erosions and no intact bullae.
- System(s) affected: skin, GI, genitourinary

EPIDEMIOLOGY
Incidence
- Disease of the middle-aged population, typically occurring after the age of 50 years, although some cases have been reported in younger adults and children
- Affects both sexes equally
- 0.1 to 3.2 cases per 100,000 individuals annually worldwide

Prevalence
- Uncommon, affects <200,000 people in the United States
- Seen more frequently in people of Mediterranean decent and Ashkenazi Jew

ETIOLOGY AND PATHOPHYSIOLOGY
- Autoantibodies (IgG) are directed against desmoglein (Dsg) 1 and 3 adhesion molecules. Dsgs interact with desmosomes, which hold epidermal cells together. The antibodies against Dsg molecules cause intraepidermal blister formation and acantholysis.
- Dsg 3 is predominantly expressed in oral epithelium, whereas both Dsg 1 and Dsg 3 are expressed in the skin.
- Dsg 1 is expressed more intensely in the superficial layer, whereas Dsg 3 is found more abundantly in basal and suprabasal layers.
- Additionally, autoantibodies against Dsg 4, the acetylcholine receptor, and pemphaxin have been identified in patients with pemphigus vulgaris (PV). The exact pathogenesis of pemphigus has yet to be fully explained and is likely a "multiple hit" process. Autoimmune; stimulus is unknown.
- Inducing factors include physical trauma, such as thermal burns, UV light, and ionizing radiation; neoplasm, emotional stress, drugs, and infections. Most patients lack a recognized inducing factor.

Genetics
Strong association with certain human leukocyte antigens (HLA), especially HLA DR4, DR14, DRB1, DQB1, DQ1, and DQ3, although the susceptibility gene differs depending on ethnic origin.

COMMONLY ASSOCIATED CONDITIONS
- Thymoma
- Myasthenia gravis
- Paraneoplastic pemphigus is a type of pemphigus defined by the fact that the patient has a malignancy at the time the pemphigus is diagnosed.
- Gastric adenocarcinoma

DIAGNOSIS

HISTORY
- Multiple, painful, nonhealing ulcers in the mouth—commonly the buccal and labial mucosa, palate, and tongue (1)[C]
- Progression (weeks to months) to small, clear fluid–filled blisters on the skin—commonly the scalp, face, and upper torso. Blisters rupture easily, forming ulcerations (1)[C].
- Consider laryngeal and nasal involvement in patients with hoarseness, odynophagia, or nasal congestion (1)[C].
- Drug-induced: penicillamine, ACE inhibitors, thiol-containing compounds, rifampin

PHYSICAL EXAM
- Mucosal lesions: Intact bullae are rare; commonly are ill-defined, irregularly shaped gingival, buccal, or palatine erosions that are painful and slow-healing; most often affected area is the oral cavity; may involve conjunctiva, oropharynx esophagus, labia, vagina, cervix, penis, urethra, and anus (1)[C].
- Cutaneous lesions: painful, flaccid blisters with clear fluid found on normal skin or on erythematous base; fragile bullae rupture easily, forming painful, superficial, coin-sized, sharply demarcated erosions (1)[C]. Pruritus is usually absent. Palms and soles are usually spared (2)[C]. Nails: Acute or chronic paronychia, onychomadesis, subungual hematomas, and nail dystrophies may be present.
- Nikolsky sign: involves application of pressure to skin causing intraepidermal cleavage that allows the superficial skin to slip free from the deeper layers, producing an erosion; can be elicited on normal skin or at the margin of a blister (1)[C]
- Asboe-Hansen sign: Lateral pressure on the edge of a blister may spread the blister into clinically unaffected skin.

DIFFERENTIAL DIAGNOSIS
- Predominance of oral mucous lesions: herpes simplex virus (HSV), aphthous ulcers, lichen planus, erythema multiforme
- Predominance of widespread cutaneous lesions: bullous pemphigoid, cicatricial pemphigoid, bullous drug eruptions, pemphigus erythematosus, pemphigus foliaceus, paraneoplastic pemphigus, impetigo, contact dermatitis, dermatitis herpetiformis, erythema multiforme, Stevens-Johnson syndrome, toxic epidermal necrolysis, pemphigoid gestationis, and linear IgA dermatosis

DIAGNOSTIC TESTS & INTERPRETATION
Diagnosis is achieved via different parameters: perilesional tissue biopsy, clinical, histologic, and immunologic examinations along with serologic findings. The clinical assessment should include a review of the patient's medications since clinical and laboratory studies cannot reliably distinguish between idiopathic pemphigus and drug-induced pemphigus.

Initial Tests (lab, imaging)
- Shave or 4-mm punch biopsy of edge of fresh bullous lesion
- A second 4-mm punch biopsy of the perilesional skin is sent for direct immunofluorescence (DIF).
- Serum for indirect immunofluorescence (IDIF) is positive for circulating autoantibodies against Dsgs in 80–90% if DIF is positive.

- ELISA testing can be used to distinguish pemphigus from the other blistering disorders. The sensitivity of ELISA exceeds 90% (3)[C]. In order to distinguish PV from BP, immunoblot assay is needed. These tests are not widely available so may not be accessible by all institutions.

Follow-Up Tests & Special Considerations
IDIF corresponds loosely to disease activity and may be useful to gauge disease activity.

Test Interpretation
- Light microscopy: intradermal blister; loss of cohesion between epidermal cells (acantholysis) with an intact basement membrane; "row of tombstones appearance"
- DIF looking for deposits of IgG between epidermal cells
- In women with cervical involvement, the histologic findings of pemphigus vulgaris may be mistaken for cervical dysplasia in Papanicolaou smears.

TREATMENT

Reduce inflammatory response and autoantibody production by suppression of the immune system to decrease blister formation and promote healing of blisters and erosions.

GENERAL MEASURES
- Minimize activities that may cause trauma to skin and precipitate blisters.
- Avoid use of dental plates, dental bridges, dental floss or contact lenses that may precipitate or exacerbate mucosal disease.
- Wound care: Daily gentle cleaning, topical agents to promote wound healing, and use of nonadhesive dressings. Clobetasol propionate 0.05% ointment 2 times daily in conjunction with systemic steroids for hard-to-treat lesions
- Oral analgesics: Use before eating for painful oral lesions (viscous lidocaine, Benadryl).

MEDICATION
First Line
- High-dose systemic glucocorticoids (e.g., prednisone 1 to 2 mg/kg/day) are the mainstay of treatment (4)[B],(5)[C],(6)[A].
- Glucocorticoids can be used alone; however, combination with other steroid-sparing immunosuppressive drugs is most effective (azathioprine—most commonly used [starting at 1 mg/kg/day and increasing by 0.5 mg/kg/day every 2 to 3 weeks to reach a maintenance dose of 2.5 mg/kg/day]; other nonsteroidal adjunctive therapies include dapsone [50 to 200 mg/day] or mycophenolate mofetil [MMF] [2 to 3 g/day]) (6)[A].
- Rituximab is becoming a first-line treatment and may be a safer alternative to steroids. Dosing: 4 weekly infusions 375 mg/m² or 1,000 mg ×2 separated by 2 weeks (5)[C]
- For mild to moderate disease: Combination therapy of nonsteroidal adjunctive treatment and prednisone is an effective treatment regimen to achieve rapid and complete control of PV. For those patients who fail treatment, rituximab is an efficacious alternative therapy (7)[C].

- Rapidly progressive lesions necessitate high prednisone dose (1.5 to 2.5 mg/kg/day) for early and adequate control of the disease. Patients with impaired physical status, especially those with relatively stable lesions at baseline, might safely and effectively be treated with low-dose oral prednisone on alternate days plus azathioprine every day (Lever's minitreatment [LMT]) for oral pemphigus (4)[B].

- For oropharyngeal disease: Perilesional/intralesional triamcinolone acetonide injections combined with conventional immunosuppressive therapy shortened the time of complete clinical remission and reduced the total amount of corticosteroids used.

Second Line
For refractory disease

- Rituximab alone or in combination with intravenous immunoglobulin (IVIG) is an effective therapy for patients with refractory PV (8)[A].
- Other options: methotrexate (10 to 20 mg/week), hydroxychloroquine, gold, plasmapheresis (5)[C]
- Cyclosporine (2.5 to 5 mg/kg/day) may be ineffective as a steroid-sparing agent (6)[A].
- Tumor necrosis factor (TNF)-α antagonist, etanercept, may be an effective therapeutic agent and may reduce healing time of skin lesions in PV and for patients presenting with recalcitrant disease (6)[A].
- IVIG is a recommended and effective treatment for patients who are not able to tolerate the standard treatment (9)[A].
- For persistent lesions: intralesional triamcinolone acetonide (20 mg/mL)

ISSUES FOR REFERRAL
- Ophthalmologist referral in suspected ocular involvement and prolonged use of high-dose steroids
- Referral to a dentist and/or otolaryngologist for patients with extensive oral disease

INPATIENT CONSIDERATIONS
Admission Criteria/Initial Stabilization
- Secondary infections requiring IV antibiotics
- Severe oral lesions leading to dehydration requiring fluid resuscitation

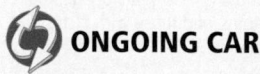 ONGOING CARE

A minority of (10%) achieve complete remission after initial treatment and do not need continued drug therapy; most require maintenance therapy to stay in remission.

FOLLOW-UP RECOMMENDATIONS
- Patients taking steroids long-term should be screened for osteopenia/osteoporosis, avascular necrosis, HPA-axis suppression, cataract, cushingoid features, hyperlipoproteinemia, myopathy, mood changes, and immunosuppression. Patients on systemic steroids should maintain adequate vitamin D and calcium intake through diet and supplements.
- Patients taking azathioprine should have CBC, Cr, and LFT checked at baseline and every 2 weeks, the first 3 months, then every 3 months after.
- PV can be exacerbated by sun exposure, dental work, trauma, stress, and radiographs. Patients undergoing dental work should be treated prophylactically with 20 mg of prednisone per day for 5 to 7 days in addition to their regular treatment regimen.
- Minimizing sun exposure, use of broad-spectrum sunscreen, and wearing protective clothing is recommended.

Patient Monitoring
Seek medical care for any unexplained blisters and if treated for PV and develop any of the following symptoms:
- Fever, chills
- General ill feeling
- Myalgias, joint pain
- New blisters or ulcers

DIET
- Patients with active oral lesions may benefit from liquid or soft diet and then advance as tolerated.
- Avoid spicy and acidic food when oral ulcers are present.
- Hard food that may cause mechanical trauma to epithelium, such as nuts, chips, and hard vegetables and fruits, may be best avoided in cases of active oral disease.

PATIENT EDUCATION
- Minimize activities that may cause trauma to skin and precipitate blisters, such as contact sports. Nontraumatic exercises, such as swimming, may be helpful.
- Explain wound care of erosions: daily gentle cleaning, covering open areas with clean petrolatum and nonadhesive dressings, as it will take longer for you to recover from infections if you are taking corticosteroids or immunosuppressants.
- Educate patients about the chronicity of the disease and the need for long-term follow up:
  – For oral pemphigus:
    ○ Soft diets and soft toothbrushes help to minimize local trauma.
    ○ Explain the need for meticulous oral hygiene to prevent dental decay. Encourage gentle tooth brushing, dental flossing, and visits to the dentist/dental hygienist at least every 6 months.
    ○ Discuss how dental plates, dental bridges, or contact lenses may precipitate or exacerbate mucosal disease.
    ○ Topical analgesics or anesthetics (e.g., benzydamine hydrochloride 0.15% or viscous lidocaine) may be useful in alleviating oral pain, particularly prior to eating or tooth brushing.
    ○ Patients may also contact the International Pemphigus & Pemphigoid Foundation (IPPF) for support groups.

PROGNOSIS
- Mortality rate with combination therapy is ~5%, with most deaths due to drug-induced complications, including sepsis.
- 10% of patients achieve complete remission after initial treatment; most require maintenance therapy to stay in remission.
- Morbidity and mortality are related to the extent of disease, the maximum dose of oral steroids required to induce remission, and the presence of other diseases. Prognosis is worse in older persons and patients with extensive disease.
- Most deaths occur during the first few years of the disease; if a patient survives 5 years, prognosis is good.

COMPLICATIONS
- Secondary infection, localized to skin or systemic, may occur because of impaired immune response due to use of immunosuppressive drugs. Most frequent cause of death is *Staphylococcus aureus* septicemia.
- Within the 1st year, patients are at the highest risk for the development of secondary infections. Older patients and potentially diabetic patients carry an increased risk.

- Consider secondary infections to include bacterial, fungal, and viral; particularly herpes simplex in nonhealing ulcers when the patient is receiving adequate treatment.
- Osteoporosis in patients requiring long-term systemic steroids
- Adrenal insufficiency has been reported following prolonged use of glucocorticoids.
- Bone marrow suppression and malignancies have been reported in patients receiving immunosuppressants, with an increased incidence of leukemia and lymphoma.
- Growth retardation has been reported in children taking systemic corticosteroids and immunosuppressants.

REFERENCES
1. Bystryn JC, Rudolph JL. Pemphigus. *Lancet*. 2005;366(9479):61–73.
2. Kavala M, Altintaş S, Kocatürk E, et al. Ear, nose and throat involvement in patients with pemphigus vulgaris: correlation with severity, phenotype and disease activity. *J Eur Acad Dermatol Venereol*. 2011;25(11):1324–1327.
3. Joly P, Litrowski N. Pemphigus group (vulgaris, vegetans, foliaceus, herpetiformis, brasiliensis). *Clin Dermatol*. 2011;29(4):432–436.
4. Chaidemenos G, Apalla Z, Koussidou T, et al. High dose oral prednisone vs. prednisone plus azathioprine for the treatment of oral pemphigus: a retrospective, bi-centre, comparative study. *J Eur Acad Dermatol Venereol*. 2011;25(2):206–210.
5. Santoro FA, Stoopler ET, Werth VP. Pemphigus. *Dent Clin North Am*. 2013;57(4):597–610.
6. Singh S. Evidence-based treatments for pemphigus vulgaris, pemphigus foliaceus, and bullous pemphigoid: a systematic review. *Indian J Dermatol Venereol Leprol*. 2011;77(4):456–469.
7. Strowd LC, Taylor SL, Jorizzo JL, et al. Therapeutic ladder for pemphigus vulgaris: emphasis on achieving complete remission. *J Am Acad Dermatol*. 2011;64(3):490–494.
8. Zakka LR, Shetty SS, Ahmed AR. Rituximab in the treatment of pemphigus vulgaris. *Dermatol Ther (Heidelb)*. 2012;2(1):17.
9. Ishii N, Hashimoto T, Zillikens D, et al. High-dose intravenous immunoglobulin (IVIG) therapy in autoimmune skin blistering diseases. *Clin Rev Allergy Immunol*. 2010;38(2–3):186–195.

ADDITIONAL READING

Leshem YA, Gdalevich M, Ziv M, et al. Opportunistic infections in patients with pemphigus. *J Am Acad Dermatol*. 2014;71(2):284–292.

 CODES

ICD10
L10.0 Pemphigus vulgaris

CLINICAL PEARLS

Pemphigus vulgaris is a rare, chronic, potentially fatal autoimmune vesiculobullous disease of the mucous membranes and skin. Biopsy immediately with rush processing. When clinical suspicion is high, initiate therapy without delay using systemic corticosteroids. Minimize activities that may cause trauma to skin and precipitate blisters, such as contact sports.

PEPTIC ULCER DISEASE

Fozia Akhtar Ali, MD • Paula A. Shelton, MD

BASICS

DESCRIPTION
- Duodenal ulcer
  - Most common form of peptic ulcer
  - Usually located in the proximal duodenum
  - Multiple ulcers or ulcers distal to the second portion of duodenum raise possibility of gastrinoma (Zollinger-Ellison syndrome).
- Gastric ulcer
  - Less common than duodenal ulcer in absence of NSAID use
  - Commonly located along lesser curvature of the antrum
- Esophageal ulcers
  - Located in the distal esophagus; usually secondary to gastroesophageal reflux disease (GERD); also seen with gastrinoma
- Ectopic gastric mucosal ulceration
  - May develop in those with Meckel diverticulum (1)

GENERAL PREVENTION
- NSAID ulcers: Avoid salicylates and NSAIDs (1).
  - Alternatives include acetaminophen and tramadol. COX-2 inhibitor use is controversial due to potential cardiac risks.
  - If NSAIDs are needed, adjust to decrease risk of ulcerogenesis, and add a proton pump inhibitor (PPI) or misoprostol.
  - To reduce ulcer risk, consider testing for and eradicating *Helicobacter pylori* before starting therapy with NSAIDs.
- Maintenance therapy with PPIs or H_2 blockers is indicated for patients with a history of ulcer complications, recurrences, refractory ulcers, or persistent *H. pylori* infection.
- Consider maintenance PPI treatment in patients with *H. pylori*–negative, non–NSAID-induced ulcer.
- Imbalance between aggressive factors (e.g., gastric acid, pepsin, bile salts, pancreatic enzymes) and defensive factors maintaining mucosal integrity (e.g., mucus, bicarbonate, blood flow, prostaglandins, growth factors, cell turnover)
- May be multifactorial
- *H. pylori* infection: 90% of duodenal ulcers and 70–90% of gastric ulcers
  - Lifetime risk for peptic ulcer disease (PUD) in *H. pylori*–infected people: 10–20%
  - Annual risk of developing duodenal ulcer in *H. pylori*–infected people: ≤1%
- Ulcerogenic drugs (e.g., NSAIDs)
- Hypersecretory syndromes (e.g., gastrinoma)
- Retained gastric antrum
- Less common: Crohn disease, vascular insufficiency, radiation therapy, cancer chemotherapy, smoking

EPIDEMIOLOGY

Incidence
- Predominant sex: male = female
- Predominant age
  - 70% of ulcers occur between ages 25 to 64 years.
  - Ulcer incidence increases with age.
- Peptic ulcer: 500,000 new cases/year
- Recurrence: 4 million/year
- Global incidence rate: 0.1–0.19%

Prevalence
- Peptic ulcer: 2% in the United States
- Lifetime prevalence is 5–10% for patients not infected with *H. pylori*; 10–20% if infected

Genetics
Increased incidence of PUD in families is likely due to familial clustering of *H. pylori* infection and inherited genetic factors reflecting response to the organism (1).

RISK FACTORS
- *H. pylori* infection (1)
- NSAID use (5–20%)
- Tobacco use
- Family history of ulcers
- Stress (after acute illness, ventilator support, extensive burns, head injury)
- Gastrinoma
- Alcohol use
- Medications: corticosteroids (high-dose and/or prolonged therapy), bisphosphonates, potassium chloride, chemotherapeutic agents (e.g., IV fluorouracil)

COMMONLY ASSOCIATED CONDITIONS
- Gastrinoma (Zollinger-Ellison syndrome)
- Multiple endocrine neoplasia type 1
- Carcinoid syndrome
- Chronic illness: Crohn disease, chronic obstructive pulmonary disease (COPD), chronic renal failure, hepatic cirrhosis, cystic fibrosis
- Hematopoietic disorders (rare): systemic mastocytosis, myeloproliferative disease, hyperparathyroidism, polycythemia rubra vera

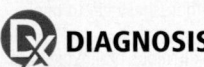

DIAGNOSIS

HISTORY
- Signs and symptoms:
  - Episodic gnawing or burning epigastric pain
  - Pain occurring after meals or on empty stomach
  - Nocturnal pain
  - Pain relieved by food intake (duodenal), antacids, or antisecretory agents
  - Nonspecific dyspeptic complaints: indigestion, nausea, vomiting, loss of appetite, and heartburn, epigastric fullness
- Alarm symptoms:
  - Anemia, hematemesis, melena, or heme-positive stool suggest bleeding
  - Vomiting and early satiety suggest obstruction.
  - Anorexia/weight loss
  - Persisting upper abdominal pain radiating to the back suggests penetration.
  - Severe, spreading upper abdominal pain suggests perforation.
  - Jaundice, dysphagia
  - Previous gastric surgery
- NSAID-induced ulcers are often silent; perforation or bleeding may be the initial presentation (1).

PHYSICAL EXAM
Physical exam for uncomplicated peptic ulcer may be unreliable and nonspecific: vital signs for hemodynamic stability, conjunctival pallor (anemia); epigastric tenderness (absent in at least 30% of older patients); guaiac-positive stool from occult blood loss (1)

DIFFERENTIAL DIAGNOSIS
Functional dyspepsia, gastritis, GERD, biliary colic, pancreatitis, cholecystitis, Crohn disease, intestinal ischemia, cardiac ischemia, GI malignancy

DIAGNOSTIC TESTS & INTERPRETATION

Initial Tests (lab, imaging)
- Lab tests to consider when evaluating PUD:
  - CBC: Rule out anemia.
  - Fecal occult blood test
  - If multiple/refractory ulcers: Consider fasting serum gastrin to rule out gastrinoma (1).
- Indications for *H. pylori* testing: new-onset PUD, prior history of PUD, persistent symptoms after empiric antisecretory therapy, gastric mucosa–associated lymphoid tissue (MALT) lymphoma, noninvestigated dyspepsia in patients <50 years of age without alarm symptoms (2)
- *H. pylori* diagnostic tests: False-negative results may occur if patient was recently treated with antibiotics, bismuth, or PPIs; or in patients with active bleeding. Diagnostic yield improved by checking 2 different tests:

  - Noninvasive tests (2)[A]:
    - Serology antibody: commonly used in primary care, slow to normalize after treatment, cannot be used to document successful eradication (sensitivity, 85%; specificity, 79%)
    - Urea breath test: identifies active *H. pylori* infection; also used for posttreatment testing (sensitivity, >95%; specificity, >90%)
    - Stool antigen: can be used for screening and posttreatment testing (sensitivity, 91%; specificity, 94%)
  - Invasive tests:
    - Upper endoscopy with gastric biopsy; Steiner stain for direct visualization of organism (sensitivity, >95%; specificity, >95%)
    - Rapid urease test: conducted on gastric biopsies (sensitivity, 93–97%; specificity, 95%)
- Barium or Gastrografin contrast radiography (double-contrast hypotonic duodenography): indicated when endoscopy is unsuitable or not feasible

Diagnostic Procedures/Other
Indications for upper endoscopy: patients with suspected peptic ulcers who are >55 years of age, those who have alarm symptoms, and those with ulcers that do not respond to treatment (3)[B]

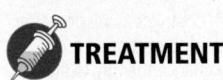

TREATMENT

MEDICATION

First Line
- Acid suppression: PPIs
  - Omeprazole 20 mg/day PO; lansoprazole 30 mg/day PO; rabeprazole 20 mg/day PO; esomeprazole 40 mg/day PO; pantoprazole 40 mg/day PO; dexlansoprazole 30 mg/day PO
  - Administer PPIs before breakfast.
- H_2 blockers: ranitidine or nizatidine 150 mg PO BID or 300 mg PO at bedtime; cimetidine 400 mg PO BID or 800 mg PO at bedtime; famotidine 20 mg PO BID or 40 mg PO at bedtime (4)
- Treat ulcers for 8 to 12 weeks or until healing is confirmed in patients with complicated ulcers (4).
- PPIs heal peptic ulcers more rapidly (4).
- Precautions:
  - Renal insufficiency: Decrease H_2 blocker dosage by 50% if CrCl <50 mL/min (2).
  - Cimetidine: Use caution with theophylline, warfarin, phenytoin, and lidocaine.
  - PPIs may decrease bone density. Obtain interval bone densitometry with long-term PPI use (5).

– PPIs may cause hypomagnesemia. Consider baseline and interval levels in patients, especially for long-term use and in patients taking diuretics.
– PPIs may be associated with increased risk of *Clostridium difficile* infection (5). Short-term use associated with development of community-acquired pneumonia; long-term use does not appear to have an increased risk.
– Despite earlier concerns, PPIs do not appear to decrease the efficacy of clopidogrel (5).
• NSAID-induced ulcers
– Discontinue NSAID use.
– Treat acutely with PPIs for 8 to 12 weeks; may use longer as maintenance for patients with recurrent, complicated, or idiopathic ulcers; or in patients who require long-term aspirin or NSAID use.
• *H. pylori*–induced ulcers
– *H. pylori* eradication regimens: Preferred duration of therapy is 14 days.
– Triple therapy: standard dose PPI given BID plus clarithromycin 500 mg PO BID plus amoxicillin 1 g PO BID or metronidazole 500 mg PO BID in patients with allergy to amoxicillin (2)
• Bacterial resistance: clarithromycin 10%; amoxicillin 1.4%; metronidazole 37%: Culture-guided choice of triple therapy is preferred (6).

Second Line
• For *H. pylori* eradication: Use second-line therapy if first-line fails (6):
– Bismuth quadruple therapy for 14 days
  ○ Bismuth subsalicylate 525 mg PO QID plus
  ○ Metronidazole 250 mg PO QID plus
  ○ Tetracycline 500 mg PO QID plus
  ○ Standard dose PPI PO twice daily
• Sequential therapy
– Standard-dose PPI PO twice daily plus amoxicillin 1,000 mg PO QID for 5 days followed by
– Standard-dose PPI PO twice daily plus clarithromycin 500 mg PO BID plus tinidazole (or metronidazole) 500 mg PO BID for 5 days
  ○ Levofloxacin 250 mg PO BID may be substituted in those with PCN allergy or in areas of high clarithromycin resistance rates.
– Another alternative salvage therapy:
  ○ Rifabutin 300 mg PO daily plus
  ○ Amoxicillin 1,000 mg PO BID plus
  ○ PPI orally BID
– Alternative ulcer-healing drugs:
  ○ Sucralfate and antacids are additional options; however, antisecretory options are preferred.
• Significant possible interactions:
– Cimetidine inhibits cytochrome P450 isozymes (avoid with theophylline, warfarin, phenytoin, and lidocaine).
– Omeprazole may prolong elimination of diazepam, warfarin, and phenytoin.
– Sucralfate reduces absorption of tetracycline, norfloxacin, ciprofloxacin, and theophylline; it leads to subtherapeutic levels.

Pregnancy Considerations
PPIs are *not* associated with an increased risk for major congenital birth defects, spontaneous abortions, or preterm delivery.

Breastfeeding
Both ranitidine and esomeprazole are secreted in breastmilk; however, at considerably lower doses than those used for treatment in infants with reflux disease. Use in breastfeeding women is generally safe (7).

SURGERY/OTHER PROCEDURES
• Endoscopy is indicated for patients age >50 years with new onset of dyspeptic symptoms, those who do not respond to treatment, and those of any age with alarm symptoms, such as bleeding and weight loss (8)[B].
• At endoscopy:
– Biopsy stomach for *H. pylori* testing (CLO test).
– Biopsy margin of gastric ulcer to exclude malignancy.
– Interventions to stop active bleeding or prevent rebleeding in those with certain stigmata include injection with epinephrine, heater probe treatment, or placement of endoscopic clips (3).
• Indications for surgery: Ulcers that are refractory to treatment and patients at high risk for complications (e.g., transplant recipients, patients dependent on steroids/NSAIDs); surgery also may be needed acutely to treat perforation and bleeding refractory to endoscopic therapy (8).
• Surgical options:
– Duodenal ulcers: truncal vagotomy and drainage (pyloroplasty/gastrojejunostomy), selective vagotomy (preserving the hepatic and/or celiac branches of the vagus) and drainage, or highly selective vagotomy (3)
– Gastric ulcers: partial gastrectomy, Billroth I or II
– Perforated ulcers: laparoscopy/open patching (3)

INPATIENT CONSIDERATIONS
Admission Criteria/Initial Stabilization
• Discontinue ulcerogenic agents (e.g., NSAIDs) (1).
• Bleeding peptic ulcers
– Stable: Give PPI to reduce transfusion requirements, need for surgery, and duration of hospitalization (9).
– Unstable: Fluid/packed RBC resuscitation followed by emergent esophagogastroduodenoscopy (EGD); use IV PPI.
– Insufficient evidence for concluding superiority, inferiority, or equivalence of high-dose PPI treatment over lower doses in peptic ulcer bleeding (5)[A]
• Oral PPIs are as effective as IV after endoscopic treatment (9).
• Perforated peptic ulcers: Free peritoneal perforation with bacterial peritonitis is a surgical emergency (3).

 ONGOING CARE

FOLLOW-UP RECOMMENDATIONS
Patient Monitoring
• *H. pylori* eradication: expected in >90% (with double antibiotic regimen): Confirm eradication by urea breath test.
• Acute duodenal ulcer: Monitor clinically.
• Acute gastric ulcer: Confirm healing via endoscopy after 12 weeks (if biopsy not done initially) to confirm that the lesion is benign.
• Tobacco cessation

PROGNOSIS
After *H. pylori* eradication (10):
• Low ulcer relapse rate; if relapse, consider surreptitious use of NSAIDs.
• Reinfection rates <1% per year
• Low risk of rebleeding
• Decreased NSAID ulcer recurrence (10)

COMPLICATIONS
• Hemorrhage: up to 25% of patients (initial presentation in 10%)
• Perforation: <5% of patients

• Gastric outlet obstruction: up to 5% of duodenal or pyloric channel ulcers; male predilection found
• Risk of gastric adenocarcinoma is increased in *H. pylori*–infected patients (2).
• Refractory peptic ulcer disease (5–10% after eradication of *H. pylori*, or completion of 12 weeks of PPI) (11)

REFERENCES

1. Ramakrishnan K, Salinas RC. Peptic ulcer disease. *Am Fam Physician*. 2007;76(7):1005–1012.
2. Saad R, Chey WD. A clinician's guide to managing *Helicobacter pylori* infection. *Cleve Clin J Med*. 2005;72(2):109–110,112–113,117–118.
3. Bertleff MJ, Lange JF. Perforated peptic ulcer disease: a review of history and treatment. *Dig Surg*. 2010;27(3):161–169.
4. Gill SK, O'Brien L, Einarson TR, et al. The safety of proton pump inhibitors (PPIs) in pregnancy: a meta-analysis. *Am J Gastroenterol*. 2009;104(6):1541–1545.
5. Neumann I, Letelier LM, Rada G, et al. Comparison of different regimens of proton pump inhibitors for acute peptic ulcer bleeding. *Cochrane Database Syst Rev*. 2013;(6):CD007999.
6. Luther J, Higgins PD, Schoenfeld PS, et al. Empiric quadruple vs. triple therapy for primary treatment of *Helicobacter pylori* infection: systematic review and meta-analysis of efficacy and tolerability. *Am J Gastroenterol*. 2010;105(1):65–73.
7. Marshall JK, Thompson AB, Armstrong D. Omeprazole for refractory gastroesophageal reflux disease during pregnancy and lactation. *Can J Gastroenterol*. 1998;12(3):225–227.
8. Laine L, Jensen DM. Management of patients with ulcer bleeding. *Am J Gastroenterol*. 2012;107(3):345–360.
9. Yen HH, Yang CW, Su WW, et al. Oral versus intravenous proton pump inhibitors in preventing re-bleeding for patients with peptic ulcer bleeding after successful endoscopic therapy. *BMC Gastroenterol*. 2012;12:66.
10. Gisbert JP, Calvet X, Cosme A, et al. Long-term follow-up of 1,000 patients cured of *Helicobacter pylori* infection following an episode of peptic ulcer bleeding. *Am J Gastroenterol*. 2012;107(8):1197–1204.
11. Yuan Y, Padol IT, Hunt RH. Peptic ulcer disease today. *Nat Clin Pract Gastroenterol Hepatol*. 2006;3(2):80–89.

CODES

ICD10
• K27.9 Peptic ulc, site unsp, unsp as ac or chr, w/o hemor or perf
• K26.9 Duodenal ulcer, unspecified as acute or chronic, without hemorrhage or perforation
• K25.9 Gastric ulcer, unspecified as acute or chronic, without hemorrhage or perforation

CLINICAL PEARLS
• In patients with PUD, *H. pylori* should be eradicated to assist in healing and to reduce the risk of gastric and duodenal ulcer recurrence.
• Upper endoscopy is indicated in patients with suspected peptic ulcers who are >55 years of age, those who have alarm symptoms, and those who do not respond to treatment.

PERFORATED TYMPANIC MEMBRANE

Timothy R. Takagi, MD

BASICS

DESCRIPTION
- The tympanic membrane (TM), or "ear drum" is a thin, trilaminar barrier that separates the external auditory canal (EAC) from the middle ear. Along with the ossicles of the middle ear, it transmits and amplifies sound vibrations to the cochlea.
- The TM consists of an outer squamous layer, contiguous with the EAC skin, the middle fibrous layer of both peripheral annular fibers and central radial fibers that provide support, and the inner mucosal layer, contiguous with the middle ear lining.
- Rupture of the TM can disrupt hearing and can allow pathogens access to the middle ear space from the EAC.
- Perforations may be classified by location:
  - *Central*: doesn't involve the annulus and is more likely to heal, spontaneously
  - *Marginal*: lies in the periphery, involves the annulus; may be associated with cholesteatoma; is less likely to heal and harder to repair
  - Involvement of the malleus decreases chance of healing.
  - Perforations of the posterior superior quadrant overly the ossicles and the cochlea and are associated with more extensive damage.
  - When a TM perforation heals, the mucosal and squamous layers reepithelialize, but the fibrous layer won't, resulting in a thinner membrane (paradoxically termed "monomeric")
- Classification of perforations by etiology:
  - Infectious: acute/chronic suppurative otitis media
  - Traumatic: barotrauma, (e.g., diving), acoustic trauma, (e.g., explosion), self-inflicted/penetrating (cotton tips)
  - Middle ear mass: cholesteatoma or neoplasm
  - Iatrogenic: persistent perforation after myringotomy tube placement or secondary acquired cholesteatoma
- The TM possesses the ability for spontaneous closure resulting in formation of a dimeric membrane (outer squamous and inner mucosal). However, if this does not occur, a persistent perforation will result.

EPIDEMIOLOGY
Incidence in the general population is unknown because many perforations heal spontaneously.

Genetics
Genetic susceptibility has been reported for recurrent acute otitis media (AOM) and chronic otitis media with effusion (COME), two of the etiologies of perforations (1).

GENERAL PREVENTION
Preservation of eustachian tube function, avoiding insertion of foreign bodies and objects into the EAC, and prompt treatment of significant infection and inflammation of the ear, reduces the chances of perforation.

RISK FACTORS
- Eustachian tube dysfunction and inability to equalize middle ear pressures
- Rapid changes in ambient pressures (air flight or diving)
- Insertion of objects into ears
- Head trauma, exposure to explosions

ETIOLOGY AND PATHOPHYSIOLOGY
- Barotrauma: Sudden of large changes in the pressure differential across the TM (such as in air flight or diving underwater)
- Direct penetration of the TM by a foreign object (e.g., cotton swab)
- Otitis media: Purulent, inflammatory process leads to ischemia and necrosis of the TM
- Inflammation and erosion results from neoplasm, cholesteatoma, and localized infection (e.g., otomycosis).

COMMONLY ASSOCIATED CONDITIONS
- Chronic eustachian tube (craniofacial abnormalities, such as cleft may predispose)
- OME
- Recurrent AOM
- Cholesteatoma
- Tympanosclerosis
- Ossicular chain damage (if traumatic perforation)

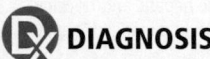
DIAGNOSIS

HISTORY
- Otorrhea/ear drainage (pus, blood, or clear fluid)
- Otalgia or earache consistent with AOM (perhaps associated with sudden relief)
- Tinnitus or buzzing
- Self-audible whistling from the ear with Valsalva maneuver or nose blowing
- Hearing loss or change
- Difficulty equalizing pressures, especially with altitude change or diving underwater
- Ear surgery (e.g., prior placement of PE tubes)
- Recurrent ear infections

PHYSICAL EXAM
- Otoscopic exam: Pay attention to location and size of any TM defect, as well as involvement of the annulus or the malleus. Also, inspect ear canal to look for evidence of otomycosis.
- Pneumatic otoscopy will reveal no motion because air passes freely into the middle ear space, and may induce vertigo (positive "fistula" sign).
- Fogging of the otoscope, in what otherwise appears to be a dry ear, may reveal occult perforation (2)[C].
- Note foreign bodies (cotton swabs, PE tubes). Batteries are a particular concern, due to the risk of acid leakage.
- Retraction pocket (chronic eustachian tube dysfunction and possible resulting cholesteatoma) typically in the posterosuperior quadrant
- Thinned TM segment indicates past, healed perforation.
- Keratin debris consistent with cholesteatoma (pearly white +/− chronic drainage)
- Mass in the middle ear space behind the TM (cholesteatoma, paragangliomas, CN VII schwannomas, etc.)
- An ulceration of the EAC, contiguous with the TM annulus, should lead to suspicion of squamous cell carcinoma.

- If history of hearing loss on that side: Weber (512-kHz tuning fork to center of forehead; if conductive hearing loss, sound should lateralize to the perforated side) and Rinne tests (place tuning fork to mastoid; when vibration no longer heard, transfer tuning fork next to outside ear canal; air conduction should be greater than bone conduction)
- Facial nerve palsy is uncommon to have with an isolated TM perforation. This is likely due to more occult pathology.
- Inspection of oropharynx for tonsillar asymmetry or neoplasm, that can cause eustachian tube obstruction.
- Hemotympanum

DIAGNOSTIC TESTS & INTERPRETATION
- Audiogram can reveal normal hearing or a mild conductive hearing loss:
  - A simple perforation will typically result in a low-frequency conductive hearing loss.
  - An audiogram that demonstrates a worse-than-expected conductive hearing loss or sensorineural hearing loss is more suspicious for ossicular chain damage or middle ear pathology.
- Tympanometry demonstrates an increased volume in the ear and decreased pressure (can demonstrate perforation even if not present on otoscopic exam); acoustic immittance demonstrates a volume >2 mL.
- MRI and CT imaging are not indicated for routine TM perforations.
- If there is suspicion for cholesteatoma or CN VII palsy, then obtain noncontrast CT of the temporal bone as initial imaging study.

DIFFERENTIAL DIAGNOSIS
- Tympanosclerosis may be confused with early cholesteatoma.
- Prior perforation (thin, healed membrane may be hard to discern)
- Cholesteatoma without perforation may still demonstrate chronic drainage.

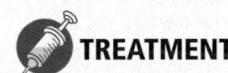
TREATMENT

GENERAL MEASURES
- Most TM perforations are nonurgent and do not require immediate evaluation by an otolaryngologist. Often, these can be managed with drops and pain control to decrease inflammation; ENT follow-up in few days to a week
- A significant portion of TM perforations heal spontaneously without additional intervention due to the TM's regenerative capacity.
- Observation of >3 months is a feasible option in select patients with uncomplicated, small perforations.
- Debate exists over dry ear precautions. But conservatively, patients should avoid getting water into the EAC and into middle ear space. Typical showering is less of an issue, but swimming in rivers/swimming pools should be avoided until the perforation has healed.

- Treatment of purulence with topical antibiotic drops will reduce otorrhea.
- If significant bleeding, topical Afrin can also be instilled in the ear canal.
- Most perforations are associated with minimal hearing loss (<40 dB) and lack vestibular complaints.
- Perforations with hearing loss >40 dB, any degree of ipsilateral facial weakness, those associated with vestibular symptoms, or those associated with cholesteatoma require referral to ENT; for traumatic perforation, obtain evaluation within 48 hours.
- For some patients with chronic eustachian tube dysfunction, having a perforated TM is a favorable situation because it allows for the equalization of pressure in the middle ear that would otherwise be more difficult because of the decreased eustachian tube function, thus obviating the need for tympanostomy tube placement later. For these patients, dry ear precautions are recommended.

MEDICATION
- Topical antibiotic and combined antibiotic/anti-inflammatory drops are the mainstay of treatment for AOM with perforation. These can be used for 5 to 7 days. Topical antibiotic drops should be continued if persistent otorrhea; may need evaluation by an otolaryngologist if drainage does not resolve with ototopical medication.
- Some topical antibiotics (gentamicin, neomycin sulfate, or tobramycin) may rarely cause ototoxicity with TM perforations because they absorb through the round window into the inner ear.
- While nonototoxic drops are preferred, cost and availability may be relevant considerations given the rarity of oto- and vestibulotoxicity (3)[C].
- Oral antibiotics are not recommended for AOM with perforations because antibiotic drops are more effective. Oral antibiotics should be used in AOM prior to perforation.
- Oral antibiotics are not indicated for the isolated TM perforation.

First Line
- Ciprofloxacin ear drops ± dexamethasone
- Ofloxacin ear drops

ADDITIONAL THERAPIES
- Dry ear precautions (cotton ball with petroleum jelly while showering and use of hairdryer to dry out ear if water enters the EAC)
- Dry ear precautions should be used if patients will be swimming in lakes/rivers, to minimize the introduction of pathogens into the EAC/middle ear cavity.
- Prevent infection primarily with eardrops or oral antibiotics as a secondary measure.

SURGERY/OTHER PROCEDURES
- For patients who participate in water sports as a part of daily life, such as swimmers and divers, repair is recommended to provide the patient a "safe ear."
- A case-by-case risk–benefit analysis must be performed in cases of conductive hearing loss because surgery entails the risk of hearing loss.

- Myringoplasty can be performed if the perforation is small and appears to be favorable. This is often performed with gel, paper patch, or other material (silk), which provides a scaffold across which the TM can heal.
- Tympanoplasty is performed for larger perforations, persistent perforations, or anteriorly based perforations. Perichondrium, fat, cartilage, pericranium, and temporalis fascia are often used in reconstructing the TM.
- A combined tympanoplasty/mastoidectomy surgery might be required for large perforations, chronic draining ears, presence of cholesteatoma, damage to the ossicular chain, or with evidence of mastoid disease.
- Surgery is often an outpatient procedure and may be done under sedation and local anesthesia. General anesthesia can also be used.
- Patients can receive mastoid compressive dressings and instructions for postoperative antibiotics.
- Potential major complications of surgery include worsening of hearing, facial nerve damage, CSF leak, bleeding, and repair failure.
- Ossiculoplasty might also be performed if pathology involves the ossicular chain; full repair of the ossicular chain can be performed as a primary procedure or as a second look.
  - If ossicular chain discontinuity is repaired, patients will require postoperative audiogram to evaluate airbone gap.

INPATIENT CONSIDERATIONS
The presence of comorbid disease like mastoiditis or meningitis would require inpatient stabilization with IV antibiotics/imaging and appropriate care for those disorders.

 ONGOING CARE

FOLLOW-UP RECOMMENDATIONS
Patient Monitoring
- Follow-up should be done to confirm TM healing and to obtain an audiogram.
- It is vital to reexamine the ear, especially after an episode of infection associated with a perforation, to rule out underlying cholesteatoma or chronic eustachian tube dysfunction, which may be contributing to the perforation.

DIET
No dietary restrictions

PATIENT EDUCATION
- Dry ear precautions
- Avoid cotton swabs in the ear.
- Call physician for worsening hearing loss, vertigo, **facial nerve palsy**, fever, or persistent drainage.

PROGNOSIS
- Most perforations will heal spontaneously; however, large perforations and those associated with a chronic draining ear often require surgery.
- Mortality associated with this condition is low, but there is a potential for infection to spread to the mastoid, leading to meningitis, if proper aural care is not maintained.

COMPLICATIONS
- Nonhealing perforation
- Infection (chronic suppurative otitis media, mastoiditis, meningitis)
- Conductive hearing loss
- Facial paralysis (rare and likely due to additional pathology)
- Ossicular chain disruption (traumatic induced)

REFERENCES
1. Rye MS, Blackwell JM, Jamieson SE. Genetic susceptibility to otitis media in childhood. *Laryngoscope*. 2012;122(3):665–675.
2. Naylor JF. Otoscope fogging: examination finding for perforated tympanic membrane. *BMJ Case Rep*. 2014;2014. doi: 10.1136/bcr-2013-200707.
3. Haynes DS, Rutka J, Hawke M, et al. Ototoxicity of ototopical drops—an update. *Otolaryngol Clin North Am*. 2007;40(3):669–683, xi.

ADDITIONAL READING
- Jensen RG, Koch A, Homøe P. Long-term tympanic membrane pathology dynamics and spontaneous healing in chronic suppurative otitis media. *Pediatr Infect Dis J*. 2012;31(2):139–144.
- Lou ZC, Lou ZH, Zhang QP. Traumatic tympanic membrane perforations: a study of etiology and factors affecting outcome. *Am J Otolaryngol*. 2012;33(5):549–555.
- Morris PS, Leach AJ. Acute and chronic otitis media. *Pediatr Clin North Am*. 2009;56(6):1383–1399.

 CODES

ICD10
- H72.90 Unsp perforation of tympanic membrane, unspecified ear
- H72.00 Central perforation of tympanic membrane, unspecified ear
- H72.2X9 Other marginal perforations of tympanic membrane, unsp ear

CLINICAL PEARLS
- To evaluate a patient with a suspected TM perforation, history and physical exam will usually suffice and does not require imaging.
- Nonhealing perforations associated with malodorous or recurrent infections are often associated with cholesteatoma and an otolaryngology consultation is recommended.
- Retraction pockets and history of AOM are suspicious for chronic eustachian tube dysfunction.
- Tympanoplasty surgery might be required for a perforation that does not spontaneously heal.
- Sudden sensorineural hearing loss warrants urgent referral and initiation of steroid therapy the same day.
- Sudden facial paralysis warrants urgent referral and initiation of steroid therapy ± antiviral treatment.

PERICARDITIS
Veronica J. Ruston, DO, Capt, USAF, MC • Angela M. Riegel, DO

 BASICS

DESCRIPTION
Inflammation of the pericardium, with or without associated pericardial effusion. Myopericarditis or perimyocarditis refers to cases that have myocardial involvement in addition to the pericardial sac.

EPIDEMIOLOGY
Incidence
Epidemiologic studies are lacking. Exact incidence is unknown but occurs in up to 5% of patients evaluated in the ER for chest pain without myocardial infarction (MI); appears to be a slightly increased prevalence in men.

ETIOLOGY AND PATHOPHYSIOLOGY
- Inflammation of the pericardial sac can be *acute* or *chronic* (recurrent). Chronic/recurrent inflammation may result in constrictive pericarditis.
- Can produce serous/purulent fluid/dense fibrinous material (depending on etiology), which may or may not lead to hemodynamic compromise

Genetics
No known genetic factors:
- Idiopathic: 85–90% of cases; likely related to viral infection, which may trigger immune-related process
- Infectious
  - Viral: coxsackievirus, echovirus, adenovirus, Epstein-Barr virus, cytomegalovirus, hepatitis viruses, influenza virus, HIV, measles, mumps, varicella
  - Bacterial: gram-positive and gram-negative organisms
  - Fungal (more common in immunocompromised populations): *Blastomyces dermatitidis*, *Candida* sp., *Histoplasma capsulatum*
  - Mycobacterial: *Mycobacterium tuberculosis*
  - Parasites: *Echinococcus*
- Noninfectious causes
  - Acute MI (2 to 4 days after MI), Dressler syndrome (weeks to months after MI)
  - Aortic dissection
  - Renal failure, uremia, dialysis-associated
  - Malignancy (e.g., breast cancer, lung cancer, Hodgkin disease, leukemia, lymphoma)
  - Radiation therapy
  - Trauma
  - Postpericardiotomy
  - After cardiac procedures (e.g., catheterization, pacemaker placement, ablation)
  - Autoimmune disorders: connective tissue disorders, systemic lupus erythematosus (SLE), rheumatoid arthritis, scleroderma, hypothyroidism, inflammatory bowel disease, spondyloarthropathies, Wegener granulomatosis
  - Sarcoidosis
- Medication induced: dantrolene, doxorubicin, hydralazine, isoniazid, mesalamine, methysergide, penicillin, phenytoin, procainamide, rifampin

COMMONLY ASSOCIATED CONDITIONS
Depends on etiology

 DIAGNOSIS

HISTORY
- Prodrome of fever, malaise, myalgias
- Acute, sharp, stabbing chest pain
- Duration typically hours to days

- Pleuritic pain
- Pain reduced by leaning forward, worsened by lying supine
- Shortness of breath

PHYSICAL EXAM
- Heart rate is usually rapid and regular.
- Pericardial friction rub: coarse, high-pitched sound best heard during end expiration at left lower sternal border with patient leaning forward. Highly specific for diagnosis (but not sensitive); may be transient and mono-, bi-, or triphasic
- New S_3 may suggest myopericarditis.
- Cardiac tamponade
- Diagnostic clinical criteria
  - Acute pericarditis (at least two of four criteria)
    ○ Typical (pleuritic) chest pain
    ○ Pericardial friction rub
    ○ ECG changes with widespread ST elevation
    ○ New/increasing pericardial effusion
  - Myopericarditis
    ○ Definite pericarditis *plus*
    ○ Symptoms (dyspnea, chest pain, or palpitations) *and* ECG changes not previously documented (ST/T wave abnormalities, supraventricular/ventricular tachycardia) *or* focal/diffuse depressed left ventricular (LV) function documented on imaging study
    ○ Absence of evidence of other cause
    ○ One of the following: elevated cardiac enzymes (creatine kinase [CK]-MB, troponin I or T) *or* new focal/diffuse depressed LV function *or* abnormal imaging consistent with myocarditis (MRI with gadolinium, gallium-67 scanning, antimyosin antibody scanning)
  - Case definitions
    ○ *Suspected myopericarditis*: criteria 1, 2, and 3
    ○ *Probable myopericarditis*: criteria 1, 2, 3, and 4
    ○ *Confirmed myopericarditis*: histopathologic evidence of myocarditis by endomyocardial biopsy (EMB) or autopsy (Note: In the clinical setting, for self-limited cases with predominantly pericarditis, EMB is rarely indicated.)

DIAGNOSTIC TESTS & INTERPRETATION
Initial Tests (lab, imaging)
- It is not necessary to order tests for uncomplicated cases or when the diagnosis is clear. Following labs may be helpful (1)[C]:
  - CBC: typically shows leukocytosis
  - Inflammatory markers: elevated erythrocyte sedimentation rate (ESR), C-reactive protein (CRP), and lactodehydrogenase (LDH)
  - Cardiac.biomarkers: typically elevated creatine kinase, troponins
    ○ Elevated troponins associated with younger age, male sex, pericardial effusion at presentation, and ST segment elevation on ECG
    ○ Adverse outcomes are not predicted by elevated troponin.
- ECG: Findings include widespread upward concave ST segment elevation and PR segment depression that may evolve through four stages. ECG may be normal/show nonspecific abnormalities:
  - Stage 1: diffuse ST segment elevation and PR segment depression
  - Stage 2: Normalization of the ST and PR segments and T waves begin to flatten and invert.
  - Stage 3: widespread T wave inversions
  - Stage 4: normalization of T waves; may have persistent inversions if chronic pericarditis

- ECG may demonstrate low voltage and electrical alternans with tamponade.
- Transthoracic echocardiogram is recommended to evaluate for the presence of pericardial effusion, tamponade, or myocardial disease (presence of effusion helps to confirm diagnosis of pericarditis) (1)[C].
- Chest x-ray (CXR) is performed to rule out pulmonary/mediastinal pathology. Enlarged cardiac silhouette suggests large pericardial effusion (at least 200 mL).
- CT and MRI allow visualization of pericardium to assess for complications or if initial workup is inconclusive (1)[C].
- Additional testing (if clinically appropriate based on history or atypical presentation or course) may include tuberculin skin test, sputum cultures, rheumatoid factor, antinuclear antibody, and HIV serology (1)[C].
- Viral cultures and antibody titers rarely clinically useful (1)[C]

Diagnostic Procedures/Other
- Pericardiocentesis indicated for cardiac tamponade; for suspected purulent, tuberculous, or neoplastic pericarditis; and for effusions >20 mm on echocardiography (2)[C]
- Surgical drainage with pericardial biopsy recommended if recurrent tamponade, ineffective pericardiocentesis, or hemodynamic instability (2)[C]

Test Interpretation
- Microscopic examination may reveal hyperemia, leukocyte accumulation, or fibrin deposition.
- Purulent fluid with neutrophilic predominance if bacterial etiology
- Lymphocytic predominance in viral, tuberculous, and neoplastic pericarditis

 TREATMENT

- Goal of treatment is to relieve pain and reduce complications (e.g., recurrence, tamponade, chronic restrictive pericarditis).
- Outpatient therapy is reported to be successful in 85% patients with low-risk features.

GENERAL MEASURES
Specific therapy directed toward underlying disorder for patients with identified cause other than viral/idiopathic disease.

MEDICATION
First Line
- NSAIDs are considered the mainstay of therapy for acute pericarditis:
  - Ibuprofen 400 to 800 mg TID for 1 to 2 weeks (2 to 4 weeks for recurrence) then taper (3)[C]
  - Aspirin 650 to 975 mg TID to QID for 1 to 2 weeks (2 to 4 weeks for recurrence) then taper; preferable for patients with recent MI because other NSAIDs impair scar formation in animal studies (4)[C]
  - Indomethacin 50 mg TID for 1 to 2 weeks (2 to 4 weeks for recurrence) then taper; should avoid in elderly due to flow restrictions to coronaries (3)[C]
  - Ketorolac 15 to 30 mg IV/IM q6h while inpatient; maximum duration of 5 days (3)[C]
  - GI protection should be provided (3)[C].

- Tapering should be done only if the patient is asymptomatic and CRP/ESR are normal and are done every 1 to 2 weeks (3)[C].
- Treatment duration using NSAIDs for initial attacks is 1 to 2 weeks, but for recurrences, consider 2 to 4 weeks of therapy (3)[C].
- Monitoring: NSAIDs: CBC and CRP at baseline and weekly until CRP normalizes
- Contraindications: hypersensitivity to aspirin or NSAIDs, active peptic ulcer/GI bleeding
- Precautions: Use with caution in patients with asthma, 3rd-trimester pregnancy, coagulopathy, and renal/hepatic dysfunction.

- Colchicine: common practice to use in combination with NSAIDs; 0.6 mg BID for up to 3 months (up to 6 months for recurrence); taper is not required. Efficacious as therapy for initial occurrence and if multiple recurrences. This is the only agent proven to prevent recurrences in RCTs. Adjunctive therapy can reduce rate of recurrence by 50% (2)[A]. Monitoring: Consider CBC, CRP, transaminases, creatine kinase, and creatinine at baseline and at least after 1 month.

- Pregnant: <20 weeks' gestation: Aspirin is first choice, but NSAIDs and prednisone are also allowed; >20 weeks' gestation: Prednisone is allowed with avoidance of NSAIDs, aspirin, and colchicine (1)[C].

Second Line
- Corticosteroid treatment is indicated in connective tissue disease, tuberculous pericarditis, or severe recurrent symptoms unresponsive to NSAIDs or colchicine; should be avoided in uncomplicated acute pericarditis. *Corticosteroid use alone has been found to be an independent risk factor for recurrence* (4)[C].
- If steroids are used, consider low dose (0.25 to 0.5 mg/kg/day for 2 weeks for first attack; 0.25 to 0.5 mg/kg/day for 2 to 4 weeks for recurrence); then slow taper (if >50 mg: 10 mg/day every 1 to 2 weeks; if 25 to 50 mg: 5 to 10 mg/day every 1 to 2 weeks; if 15 to 25 mg: 2.5 mg/day every 2 to 4 weeks; if <15 mg: 1 to 2.5 mg/day every 2 to 6 weeks) following remission. Remember adequate prophylaxis treatment for osteoporosis prevention (4)[C].
- If unable to taper from steroids, resume lowest steroid dose and begin slow taper of 1 to 2 mg every 2 to 4 weeks (3)[C].
- Intrapericardial administration of steroids may be effective and limits systemic side effects.

ISSUES FOR REFERRAL
- Refractory cases include those on unacceptably high long-term steroid doses (>25 mg/day).
- Consider trial of aspirin and/or NSAIDs plus steroid and colchicine.
- Uremic or dialysis-related cases require more frequent or urgent dialysis without significant benefit from pharmacologics (1)[C].

SURGERY/OTHER PROCEDURES
- Pericardiocentesis is indicated in cases of cardiac tamponade, high likelihood of tuberculous/purulent/neoplastic pericarditis, and large symptomatic effusions refractory to medical therapy.
- Pericardial biopsy may be considered for diagnosis in those with persistent worsening pericarditis without a definite diagnosis.
- Pericardioscopy for targeted diagnostic imaging may be performed at experienced tertiary referral centers in refractory and difficult cases.

- Pericardial window may be performed in cases of recurrent cardiac tamponade with large pericardial effusion despite medical therapy and severe symptoms.
- Pericardiectomy can be considered. The 2004 European Society of Cardiology guidelines recommend pericardiectomy (Class IIa) for frequent and highly symptomatic recurrences of pericarditis refractory to medical therapy. However, this is rarely performed in the United States and has high morbidity and mortality (1)[C].

INPATIENT CONSIDERATIONS
Admission Criteria/Initial Stabilization
Inpatient therapy recommended for pericarditis associated with clinical predictors of poor prognosis:
- Major predictors: fever >38°C, subacute onset, large pericardial effusion, cardiac tamponade, lack of response to NSAID/aspirin therapy after at least 1 week (5)[C]
- Minor predictors: immunosuppressed state, trauma, oral anticoagulation therapy, myopericarditis (5)[C]

IV Fluids
IV fluids considered for hypotension or in the setting of pericardial tamponade

Discharge Criteria
- Response to therapy with symptom improvement
- Hemodynamic stability

 ## ONGOING CARE

FOLLOW-UP RECOMMENDATIONS
- 7 to 10 days to assess response to treatment
- 1 month to check CBC and CRP and thereafter if symptoms continue to be present
- Those with clinical predictors of poor prognosis may require closer follow-up based on lab data and echocardiographic findings.

Patient Monitoring
Myopericarditis
- Use lower doses of anti-inflammatory drugs to control symptoms for 1 to 2 weeks while minimizing deleterious effects on myocarditic process.
- Exercise restrictions for 4 to 6 weeks or until symptoms resolved and biomarkers normalized (2)[C].
- Echocardiographic monitoring at 1, 6, and 12 months (especially in those with left ventricular dysfunction)

DIET
No restrictions

PROGNOSIS
Overall good prognosis; disease usually benign and self-limiting; purulent and tuberculosis pericarditis with high mortality

COMPLICATIONS
- Recurrent pericarditis: occurs in ~30% of patients, with most instances resulting from idiopathic, viral, or autoimmune pericarditis; inadequate treatment of the initial attack; and, less commonly, neoplastic etiologies. Recurrence usually within 1st weeks following initial episode but may occur months to years later; rarely associated with tamponade/constriction
- Cardiac tamponade: rare complication with increased incidence in neoplastic, purulent, and tuberculous pericarditis

- Effusive-constrictive pericarditis: Reported in 24% of patients undergoing surgery for constrictive pericarditis and in 8% of patients undergoing pericardiocentesis and cardiac catheterization for cardiac tamponade. Failure of right atrial pressure to fall by 50% or to a level below 10 mm Hg after pericardiocentesis is diagnostic.
- Constrictive pericarditis: rare complication in which rigid pericardium produces abnormal diastolic filling with elevated filling pressures. Pericardiectomy remains definitive therapy.

REFERENCES
1. Maisch B, Seferović PM, Ristić AD, et al. Guidelines on the diagnosis and management of pericardial diseases executive summary: the task force on the diagnosis and management of pericardial diseases of the European Society of Cardiology. *Eur Heart J.* 2004;25(7):587–610.
2. Imazio M, Brucato A, Belli R, et al. Colchicine for the prevention of pericarditis: what we know and what we do not know in 2014—systematic review and meta-analysis. *J Cardiovasc Med (Hagerstown).* 2014:15(12):840–846.
3. Lilly LS. Treatment of acute and recurrent pericarditis. *Circulation.* 2013;127(16):1723–1726.
4. Imazio M, Brucato A, Trinchero R, et al. Diagnosis and management of pericardial diseases. *Nat Rev Cardiol.* 2009;6(12):743–751.
5. Snyder MJ, Bepko J, White M. Acute pericarditis: diagnosis and management. *Am Fam Physician.* 2014;89(7):553–560.

ADDITIONAL READING
- Imazio M, Brucato A, Cemin R, et al. A randomized trial of colchicine for acute pericarditis. *N Engl J Med.* 2013;369(16):1522–1528.
- Imazio M, Spodick DH, Brucato A, et al. Controversial issues in the management of pericardial diseases. *Circulation.* 2010;121(7):916–928.
- Khandaker MH, Espinosa RF, Nishimura RA, et al. Pericardial disease: diagnosis and management. *Mayo Clin Proc.* 2010;85(6):572–593.

 ## CODES

ICD10
- I31.9 Disease of pericardium, unspecified
- I30.9 Acute pericarditis, unspecified
- I30.1 Infective pericarditis

CLINICAL PEARLS
- Consider *major* and *minor* predictors in deciding which patients should be admitted.
- Therapy aimed at symptomatic relief and NSAIDs are first-line treatment. Colchicine is recommended as an adjunct to NSAIDs.
- Pericardiocentesis is recommended in the setting of cardiac tamponade or possible purulent pericarditis.

PERIODIC LIMB MOVEMENT DISORDER

Donald E. Watenpaugh, PhD • John R. Burk, MD

 BASICS

DESCRIPTION
- Sleep-related movement disorder with these features:
  - Episodes of periodic limb movements (PLMs) during sleep
  - Movements consist of bilateral ankle dorsiflexion, sometimes with knee and hip flexion.
  - Arm or more generalized movements occur less commonly.
  - Movements may cause brief microarousals from sleep unbeknownst to the patient.
  - Complaints include insomnia, unrestorative sleep, daytime fatigue, and/or somnolence.
  - Bed partner may complain of movements.
  - Another sleep disorder (e.g., obstructive sleep apnea) does not cause the PLMs.
- System(s) affected: musculoskeletal, nervous
- Synonym(s): nocturnal myoclonus; sleep myoclonus; periodic leg movements of sleep

EPIDEMIOLOGY
Incidence
- Increases with age: 1/3 of patients >60 years exhibit PLMs but not necessarily periodic limb movement disorder (PLMD).
- Predominant sex: male = female
- PLMs in 15% of insomnia patients

Prevalence
- PLMs in sleep: common and often of no clinical consequence
- PLMs constituting PLMD (causing sleep complaints and/or daytime consequences) much less common: <5% of adults (but underdiagnosed)

ETIOLOGY AND PATHOPHYSIOLOGY
- Unstudied
- Primary: probable CNS dopaminergic impairment
- Secondary:
  - Iron deficiency
  - Peripheral neuropathy
  - Arthritis
  - Renal failure
  - Synucleinopathies (multiple-system atrophy)
  - Spinal cord injury
  - Pregnancy
  - Medications:
    - Most antidepressants (not bupropion or desipramine)
    - Some antipsychotic and antidementia medications
    - Antiemetics (metoclopramide)
    - Antihistamines

Genetics
Unstudied, but see "Restless Legs Syndrome" (RLS)

RISK FACTORS
- Family history of RLS
- Iron deficiency and associated conditions (e.g., pregnancy, gastric surgery, renal disease)
- Attention deficit hyperactivity disorder (ADHD)
- Aging
- Peripheral neuropathy
- Arthritis, orthopedic problems
- Chronic limb pain or discomfort

GENERAL PREVENTION
- Regular physical activity
- Adequate nightly sleep
- Avoid causes of secondary PLMD.
- Avoid causes of RLS.

COMMONLY ASSOCIATED CONDITIONS
- RLS
- Rapid eye movement (REM) sleep behavior disorder
- Narcolepsy
- Iron deficiency
- Renal failure
- Cardiovascular disease; stroke
- Gastric surgery
- Pregnancy
- Arthritis
- Synucleinopathies (multiple-system atrophy)
- Lumbar spine disease; spinal cord injury
- Peripheral neuropathy
- Insomnia, insufficient sleep
- ADHD
- Depression

Pediatric Considerations
- PLMD may precede overt RLS by years.
- Association with RLS is more common than in adults.
- Symptoms may be more consequential than in adults.
- Associated with ADHD

Pregnancy Considerations
- May be secondary to iron or folate deficiency
- Most severe in 3rd trimester
- Usually subsides after delivery

Geriatric Considerations
- May become a significant source of sleep disturbance
- May cause or exacerbate circadian disruption and "sundowning"
- Many medications given to the elderly cause or exacerbate PLMs, which can lead to PLMD or RLS.

 DIAGNOSIS

HISTORY
- Episodes of PLMs during sleep (often reported by bed partner) (1)[A]
- Insomnia: difficulty maintaining sleep
- Unrestorative sleep
- Daytime fatigue, tiredness, and/or somnolence
- Oppositional behaviors
- Memory impairment
- Depression
- ADHD, particularly in children

PHYSICAL EXAM
No specific findings

DIFFERENTIAL DIAGNOSIS
- When PLMs occur along with RLS, REM sleep behavior disorder, or narcolepsy, those disorders are diagnosed as "with PLMs," and PLMD is not diagnosed separately.
- Obstructive sleep apnea: Limb movements (LMs) occur during microarousals from apneas; treatment of sleep apnea eliminates these LMs.
- Sleep starts: nonperiodic, generalized, occur only at wake–sleep transition, <0.2 seconds duration
- Sleep-related leg cramps: isolated and painful
- Fragmentary myoclonus: 75 to 150 ms of EMG activity, minimal movement, no periodicity
- Nocturnal seizures: epileptiform EEG, motor pattern incongruent with PLMs
- Fasciculations, tremor: no sleep association
- Sleep-related rhythmic movement disorder: voluntary movement during wake–sleep transition; higher frequency than PLMs

DIAGNOSTIC TESTS & INTERPRETATION
- Polysomnography with finding of repetitive, stereotyped LMs (1)[A]:
  - Tibialis anterior electromyographic (EMG) activity lasting 0.5 to 10 seconds
  - EMG amplitude increases >8 μV from baseline.
  - Movements occur in a sequence of ≥4 at intervals of 5 to 90 seconds.
  - Children: ≥5 movements per hour; adults, 15
  - Movement may also involve arms.
  - Associated with heart rate variability from autonomic-level arousals
  - Most PLM episodes occur in the first hours of non-REM sleep.
  - Significant night-to-night PLM variability
- Serum ferritin to assess for iron deficiency

Diagnostic Procedures/Other
- Ankle actigraphy for in-home use
- EMG or nerve conduction studies for peripheral neuropathy/radiculopathy

Test Interpretation
Serum ferritin should be >75 ng/mL.

TREATMENT

Treatment paradigm similar to that for RLS, except that all medications are off-label for PLMD

GENERAL MEASURES
- Daily exercise
- Adequate nightly sleep
- Warm the legs (long socks, leg warmers, electric blanket, etc.).
- Hot bath before bedtime
- Avoid nicotine and evening caffeine and alcohol.

MEDICATION
- Use minimum effective dose.
- Consider risks, side effects, and interactions individually (e.g., benzodiazepines in elderly).
- Daytime sleepiness is unusual with the doses and timing employed for PLMD.

First Line
- Dopamine agonists: Take 1 hour before bed; titrate weekly to optimal dose (1,2)[B]:
  - Pramipexole (Mirapex): 0.125 to 0.5 mg; titrate by 0.125 mg
  - Ropinirole (Requip): 0.25 to 4 mg; titrate by 0.25 mg
  - Transdermal rotigotine (Neupro): 1 to 3 mg/24 hr patch; initiate with 1 mg/24 hr; titrate by 1 mg weekly to effectiveness.
- Avoid dopamine agonists in psychotic patients, especially if taking dopamine antagonists.

Second Line
- Anticonvulsants: useful for associated neuropathy (1,2)[B]:
  - Gabapentin enacarbil (Horizant): 600 mg/day
  - Pregabalin (Lyrica): 50 to 300 mg/day
- Opioids: low risk for tolerance with bedtime dose
  - Hydrocodone: 5 to 20 mg/day
  - Oxycodone: 2.5 to 20 mg/day
- Benzodiazepines and agonists (1,2)[B]:
  - Clonazepam (Klonopin): 0.5 to 3 mg/day
  - Zaleplon, zolpidem, temazepam, triazolam, alprazolam, diazepam

Pediatric Considerations
- First-line treatment is nonpharmacologic.
- Assess/correct iron deficiency.
- Consider low-dose clonidine or clonazepam.

Pregnancy Considerations
- Initial approach: iron supplementation, nonpharmacologic therapies
- Avoid medications class C or D.
- In 3rd trimester, low-dose clonazepam or opioids may be considered.

Geriatric Considerations
In weak or frail patients, avoid medications that may cause dizziness or unsteadiness.

ADDITIONAL THERAPIES
- If iron-deficient, iron supplementation:
  - 325 mg ferrous sulfate with 200 mg vitamin C between meals TID
  - Repletion may require months.
  - Symptoms continue without other treatment.
- Vitamin/mineral supplements, including calcium, magnesium, B_{12}, folate
- Clonidine: 0.05 to 0.1 mg/day
- Relaxis leg vibration device

SURGERY/OTHER PROCEDURES
Correction of orthopedic, neuropathic, or peripheral vascular problems

INPATIENT CONSIDERATIONS
- Control during recovery from orthopedic procedures
- Addition or withdrawal of medications that affect PLMD
- Changes in medical status may require medication changes (e.g., Mirapex contraindicated in renal failure and Requip contraindicated in liver disease).

IV Fluids
- Consider iron infusion when oral supplementation is ineffective, not tolerated, or contraindicated.
- When NPO, consider IV opiates.

Nursing
- Evening walks, hot baths, leg warming
- Sleep interruption risks prolonged wakefulness.

ONGOING CARE

FOLLOW-UP RECOMMENDATIONS
Patient Monitoring
- At monthly intervals until stable
- Annual and PRN follow-up thereafter
- If iron-deficient, remeasure ferritin to assess repletion.

DIET
Avoid caffeine and alcohol late in the day.

PATIENT EDUCATION
- National Sleep Foundation: http://sleepfoundation.org/
- American Academy of Sleep Medicine: http://www.sleepeducation.org/

PROGNOSIS
- Primary PLMD: lifelong condition with no current cure
- Secondary PLMD: may subside with resolution of cause(s)
- Current therapies usually control symptoms.
- PLMD often precedes emergence of RLS.

COMPLICATIONS
- Tolerance to medications requiring increased dose or alternatives
- Augmentation (increased PLMs and sleep disturbance, emergence of RLS) from prolonged use of dopamine agonists:
  - Higher doses increase risk.
  - Iron deficiency increases risk.
  - Add alternative medication, then detitrate dopaminergic agent.
- Iatrogenic PLMD (from antidepressants, etc.)

REFERENCES

1. Garcia-Borreguero D, Stillman P, Benes H, et al. Algorithms for the diagnosis and treatment of restless legs syndrome in primary care. *BMC Neurol*. 2011;11:28.
2. Aurora RN, Kristo DA, Bista SR, et al. The treatment of restless legs syndrome and periodic limb movement disorder in adults—an update for 2012: practice parameters with an evidence-based systematic review and meta-analyses: an American Academy of Sleep Medicine Clinical Practice Guideline. *Sleep*. 2012;35(8):1039–1062.

ADDITIONAL READING

Picchietti DL, Rajendran RR, Wilson MP, et al. Pediatric restless legs syndrome and periodic limb movement disorder: parent-child pairs. *Sleep Med*. 2009;10(8):925–931.

SEE ALSO

Restless Legs Syndrome

CODES

ICD10
G47.61 Periodic limb movement disorder

CLINICAL PEARLS

- Many patients with PLMs may not require treatment; however, when sleep disturbance from PLMs causes insomnia and/or daytime consequences, PLMD exists and should be treated.
- Many antidepressants and some antihistamines cause or exacerbate PLMs.
- Sleep disturbance, including that from PLMs, may cause or exacerbate ADHD.

PERIORAL DERMATITIS

Heather Summe, MD, MS • Nikki A. Levin, MD, PhD

 BASICS

DESCRIPTION
- A common facial eruption of women and children
- Presents as tiny, flesh-colored, or erythematous monomorphic papules or pustules around the mouth with characteristic sparing of the area immediately adjacent to the vermilion border
- May also involve the periocular, perinasal, and glabellar regions of the face
- Etiology is unknown, but a relation to topical steroid use has been suggested.
- Without treatment, the course is usually fluctuating and chronic.
- Variants in children include granulomatous periorificial dermatitis (GPD) and facial Afro-Caribbean childhood eruption.
- Synonym(s): periorificial dermatitis (POD); chronic papulopustular facial dermatitis; granulomatous perioral dermatitis; light-sensitive seborrhea; lupus-like perioral dermatitis; papulopustular facial dermatitis; rosacea-like dermatitis; stewardess disease

EPIDEMIOLOGY
- Occurs worldwide, especially in fair-skinned populations
- Predominantly affects children between 6 months and 16 years and women aged 17 to 45 years
- ~90% of adult cases are in women (1).
- 55% of childhood cases occur in females (2).
- All races are affected, but the granulomatous form is more common in African American and dark-skinned children.
- Some believe the number of cases peaked in the 1960s to 1970s and decreased in the 1980s to 1990s when the side effects of topical steroids were recognized. Others believe that cases are still increasing.

Incidence
- Peak incidence is in the 2nd and 3rd decades of life.
- In children, peak incidence is in the prepubertal period.

Prevalence
- Represents ~2% of patients presenting to dermatology clinics (3)
- ~3% of children using inhalational steroids develop some form of POD (4).

ETIOLOGY AND PATHOPHYSIOLOGY
- Exposure to an irritant results in breakdown of the epidermal barrier and subsequent water loss and sensation of dryness; this encourages use of facial products and corticosteroids, which may worsen the condition.
- This inflammatory cycle eventually leads to clinical features of the disease.
- The exact cause is unknown, and there may be more than one contributing factor.
- The most widely cited factor implicated in POD is use of potent topical corticosteroids on the face.
- Inhaled corticosteroids, especially when used with a spacer and nebulizer or mask, have also been reported to cause POD.
- Intranasal steroids have been associated with POD beginning in the nasolabial folds.
- Two cases associated with systemic steroid use have been reported in children (5).

- Use of foundation, moisturizer, and night cream was associated with a 13-fold increased risk of POD in one study (6).
- Other factors are implicated but not proven:
  - Drugs: oral contraceptives
  - Toothpastes: fluoridated, tartar control, whitening
  - Physical factors: UV light, heat, wind, salivary leakage
  - Infectious factors: fusiform bacteria, *Candida* species, *Demodex folliculorum*
  - Miscellaneous factors: atopy, GI disturbances, stress, contact allergy, lip-licking, immunosuppression, bubble gum, formaldehyde, varicella vaccination

Genetics
55% of pediatric patients with POD have a family history of atopy (6).

RISK FACTORS
See "Etiology and Pathophysiology."

GENERAL PREVENTION
- Avoid using potent topical corticosteroids on the face.
- Avoid using excessive foundation, moisturizer, and night cream.
- Avoidance of tartar-control and whitening toothpastes may also be helpful.

COMMONLY ASSOCIATED CONDITIONS
Atopic dermatitis

 DIAGNOSIS

HISTORY
- Patient reports a history of facial rash, which may improve with use of topical corticosteroids and flare with discontinuation.
- Affected skin may be pruritic or have a burning sensation.
- Course may be chronic and fluctuating.
- Recent topical, inhaled, or systemic steroid use in 72% of patients (7)
- May worsen with sun exposure

PHYSICAL EXAM
- Monomorphic, minute, flesh-colored to erythematous papules or pustules, sometimes surmounted with scale, in a perioral distribution, often asymmetrical, with sparing of the vermilion border 3 to 5 mm around the lips
- Granulomatous form can usually be distinguished clinically by the absence of pustules and the presence of yellow-brown papules.
- Common locations are alar creases, nasolabial folds, chin, periocular skin, eyelids, and glabella.
- Diameter of lesions is usually 1 to 2 mm.
- Distribution (3)
  - Perioral area (39%)
  - Perinasal (13%)
  - Periocular (1%)
  - Perioral and perinasal (14%)
  - Perioral and periocular (6%)
  - Perinasal and periocular (6%)
  - Perioral, perinasal, and periocular (10%)
- Lupus-like variant diagnosed by yellowish discoloration of lesions on diascopy

DIFFERENTIAL DIAGNOSIS
- Acne vulgaris
- Contact dermatitis
- Rosacea
- Seborrheic dermatitis
- Lip-licker's dermatitis
- Papular sarcoidosis
- *Demodex* infestation
- Acrodermatitis enteropathica
- Biotin deficiency
- Glucagonoma syndrome
- Xanthomas
- Eruptive syringomas
- Polymorphous light eruption
- Acne agminata
- Lupus miliaris disseminatus faciei
- Haber syndrome (familial rosacea-like dermatosis)

DIAGNOSTIC TESTS & INTERPRETATION
Diagnosis is usually clinical.
- No laboratory abnormalities are expected.
- Prick tests and IgE testing may show evidence of atopy but are not routinely done.
- Patch testing may be used to rule out contact dermatitis.
- Scrapings for *Demodex* mites

Diagnostic Procedures/Other
Skin biopsy is not routinely performed but can be helpful in atypical cases.

Test Interpretation
Histopathology of skin biopsy
- Mild, nonspecific inflammation with variable perifollicular or perivascular lymphohistiocytic infiltrate
- Eczematous changes, acanthosis, parakeratosis, and spongiosis
- Occasionally, follicular abscesses are seen.
- Older lesions may contain diffuse hypertrophy of connective tissue and hyperplasia of sebaceous follicles with occasional noncaseating granulomas in the dermis (1).
- Caseating granulomas are seen with granulomatous variant.

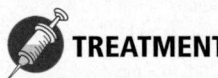 TREATMENT

GENERAL MEASURES
"Zero therapy" can be an effective treatment in adherent patients (3)[B]:

- Reduce use of facial soaps, makeup, and moisturizers, and wash with only water.
- Discontinue use of potent topical corticosteroids on the face.
  - This may result in a flare.
  - Flares may be decreased with use of less-potent topical steroids, calcineurin inhibitors, or IM steroid injection.
- Discontinue use of fluoridated, whitening, and tartar-control toothpaste.

MEDICATION

Based on disease severity and patient's tolerance for adverse effects

First Line

- Severe disease
  - Oral antibiotics
    - Tetracycline has been proven as an effective treatment (3)[A].
    - 250 to 500 mg BID for 8 to 10 weeks
    - Dose may be halved after 3 to 4 weeks if improvement is noted.
    - Contraindicated in children <8 years of age and pregnant women.
    - Common side effects: photosensitivity, GI upset, rash, candidiasis, headache, dizziness, and tinnitus
  - Doxycycline or minocycline (6)[C]
    - 50 to 100 mg BID for 6 to 8 weeks
    - Dose may be halved after 3 to 4 weeks if improvement is noted.
    - Contraindicated in children <8 years of age and pregnant women.
    - Common side effects of doxycycline: GI upset, esophagitis, joint pain, upper respiratory infection (URI) symptoms, rash, dysmenorrhea, candidiasis, headache, dizziness, photosensitivity, and elevated BUN
    - Common side effects of minocycline: GI upset, lightheadedness, vertigo, ataxia, headache, fatigue, tinnitus, rash, urticaria, candidiasis, and hyperpigmentation
  - Alternatively, doxycycline 40 mg/day modified-release capsule may achieve the anti-inflammatory effect without the microbial activity that promotes emergence of resistant bacterial strains (8)[C].
  - Erythromycin (6)[C] may be used when tetracycline are contraindicated or not tolerated.
    - 250 mg BID–TID for 6 to 8 weeks
    - Dose may be halved after 3 to 4 weeks if improvement noted.
    - May be used in children or pregnant women.
    - Common side effects: GI upset, diarrhea, rash, and urticaria
    - Rarer serious side effects: erythema multiforme, pancreatitis, convulsions, QT prolongation, and ventricular arrhythmias
- Moderate disease
  - Topical antibiotics
    - May be slower than systemic antibiotics in clearing lesions
    - Metronidazole cream 0.75% BID (3)[B]
    - Erythromycin 2% gel, solution, or ointment BID (3)[B]
    - Clindamycin 1% gel, lotion, or cream BID
- Mild disease
  - Zero therapy (see "General Measures") (3)[B]

Second Line

- Severe disease
  - Azithromycin (2) or clarithromycin (250 mg/day) may be used when tetracycline and erythromycin (3)[C] are contraindicated or not tolerated.
    - Common side effects: GI upset, headache, rash, abnormal taste sensation, and urticaria
  - Oral isotretinoin may be useful in granulomatous cases that are not responsive to a full dose of tetracycline (1)[C].
    - 0.2 mg/kg initially, followed by 0.1 mg/kg after notable improvement

  - Isotretinoin is a pregnancy Category X drug and may cause severe birth defects. Use with caution in women of reproductive age. Physician and patient must register with iPLEDGE program.
    - Common side effects: dry skin, cheilitis, arthralgias/myalgias, hypertriglyceridemia, elevated liver function tests (LFTs), hair loss, visual disturbances, depression, and tinnitus
  - Pimecrolimus 1% cream may accelerate healing (3)[A], and tacrolimus 0.1% ointment use has been reported with success (3).
    - Rare cases of lymphoma and skin malignancies have been reported. Avoid long-term use
- Moderate disease
  - Topical therapies
    - Other antiacne drugs, such as sodium sulfacetamide (2), azelaic acid, and adapalene (3), may be helpful.
    - Ichthyol (ammonium bituminosulfonate) (3)

ADDITIONAL THERAPIES

A number of other therapies have been reported in the literature, including photodynamic therapy with 5-aminolevulinic acid (3), radiotherapy, and liquid nitrogen. There has also been a case reported of oral metronidazole (250 mg BID) resulting in complete clearance of GPD without scarring after 1 month of use (9). Most recently, a randomized controlled trial showed significant improvement after 4 weeks of treatment with praziquantel 3% ointment BID (10).

COMPLEMENTARY & ALTERNATIVE MEDICINE

Compress with chamomile tea or physiologic solution may be used if the patient struggles with zero therapy (1).

ONGOING CARE

DIET

No restrictions

PATIENT EDUCATION

- Lesions may take many weeks to resolve.
- Symptoms may temporarily worsen, especially with discontinuance of steroids.
- Recurrence is rare.
- Topical corticosteroid use on the face should be avoided in the future.

PROGNOSIS

- Most cases resolve without recurrence.
- Oral or topical antibiotics usually lead to remission within 6 to 10 weeks.
- Untreated disease may persist for months to years and be characterized by unpredictable flares.
- Disease is not associated with significant morbidity.

COMPLICATIONS

- Most cases resolve without complications.
- Emotional stress can result from bothersome appearance of lesions and chronic course of disease.
- Scarring may be problematic with lupus-like variant.

REFERENCES

1. Lipozencic J, Ljubojevic S. Perioral dermatitis. *Clin Dermatol*. 2011;29(2):157–161.
2. Goel NS, Burkhart CN, Morrell DS. Pediatric periorificial dermatitis: clinical course and treatment outcomes in 222 patients. *Pediatr Dermatol*. 2015;32(3):333–336.
3. Wollenberg A, Bieber T, Dirschka T, et al. Perioral dermatitis [in English, German]. *J Dtsch Dermatol Ges*. 2011;9(5):422–427.
4. Henningsen E, Bygum A. Budesonide-induced periorificial dermatitis presenting as chalazion and blepharitis. *Pediatr Dermatol*. 2011;28(5):596–597.
5. Clementson B, Smidt AC. Periorificial dermatitis due to systemic corticosteroids in children: report of two cases. *Pediatr Dermatol*. 2012;29(3):331–332.
6. Vanderweil SG, Levin NA. Perioral dermatitis: it's not every rash that occurs around the mouth. *Dermatol Nurs*. 2009;21(6):317–320, 353.
7. Nguyen V, Eichenfield LF. Periorificial dermatitis in children and adolescents. *J Am Acad Dermatol*. 2006;55(5):781–785.
8. Rosso JQ. Management of papulopustular rosacea and perioral dermatitis with emphasis on iatrogenic causation or exacerbation of inflammatory facial dermatoses: use of doxycycline-modified release 40mg capsule once daily in combination with properly selected skin care as an effective therapeutic approach. *J Clin Aesthet Dermatol*. 2011;4(8):20–30.
9. Rodriguez-Caruncho C, Bielsa I, Fernandez-Figueras MT, et al. Childhood granulomatous periorificial dermatitis with a good response to oral metronidazole. *Pediatr Dermatol*. 2013;30(5):e98–e99.
10. Bribeche MR, Fedotov VP, Jillella A, et al. Topical praziquantel as a new treatment for perioral dermatitis: results of a randomized vehicle-controlled pilot study. *Clin Exp Dermatol*. 2014;39(4):448–453.

ADDITIONAL READING

- Hafeez ZH. Perioral dermatitis: an update. *Int J Dermatol*. 2003;42(7):514–517.
- Kim YJ, Shin JW, Lee JS, et al. Childhood granulomatous periorificial dermatitis. *Ann Dermatol*. 2011;23(3):386–388.
- Peralta L, Morais P. Perioral dermatitis—the role of nasal steroids. *Cutan Ocul Toxicol*. 2012;31(2):160–163.
- Weber K, Thurmayr R. Critical appraisal of reports on the treatment of perioral dermatitis. *Dermatology*. 2005;210(4):300–307.

CODES

ICD10

L71.0 Perioral dermatitis

CLINICAL PEARLS

- Suspect POD when an acneiform eruption involves the perioral, perinasal, or periocular areas with characteristic sparing of the skin immediately adjacent to the vermilion border.
- Ask patients about a history of recent corticosteroid use, facial product use, and use of fluoridated, whitening, or tartar-control toothpastes.
- Substitution of low-potency steroids may allow patients to discontinue higher potency steroids while avoiding a rebound flare.

PERIPHERAL ARTERIAL DISEASE

Zhen Lu, MD

 BASICS

DESCRIPTION
Peripheral arterial disease (PAD) is a manifestation of systemic atherosclerosis in which there is partial or total blockage in the arteries, exclusive of the coronary and cerebral vessels. Objectively, PAD is defined as a resting ankle-brachial index (ABI) of <0.90.

EPIDEMIOLOGY
- Predominant age: >40 years
- Predominant sex: male > female (2:1), based on the Framingham study
- Patients with symptomatic PAD have a 5-year mortality rate of 30%.
- Highly prevalent syndrome that affects 8 to 12 million individuals in the United States

Incidence
Incidence overall: 1 to 3/1,000/year

Prevalence
- U.S. prevalence: 2.7 to 4.1%
- Age-adjusted prevalence of PAD is close to 12%.
- Up to 29% among patients in primary care practices

ETIOLOGY AND PATHOPHYSIOLOGY
- In patients with PAD, arterial stenoses cause inadequate blood flow in distal limbs, which fails to meet the metabolic demand during exertion:
  - The degree of ischemia is proportional to the size and proximity of the occlusion to the end organ.
  - Acidic products of anaerobic metabolism build up within the muscle and result in claudication clinically.
  - Arterial occlusion also causes significantly diminished distal pressure in patients with PAD due to atherosclerotic lesions.
- Most common cause of arterial stenoses is atherosclerosis.

Genetics
Current NIH-funded research focuses on single-nucleotide polymorphisms in candidate genes that are regulated in the vasculature in an attempt to explore genetic factors responsible for PAD.

RISK FACTORS
- Age >40 years
- Cigarette smoking
- Diabetes mellitus
- Obesity
- Hypertension
- Hyperlipidemia
- Hyperhomocysteinemia

GENERAL PREVENTION
Control risk factors.

COMMONLY ASSOCIATED CONDITIONS
- See "Risk Factors."
- Associated with other common complications of atherosclerosis, including myocardial infarction (MI), transient ischemic attack (TIA), stroke, and limb amputation
- Occurs in ~40% of patients with cardiovascular disease

 DIAGNOSIS

HISTORY
- Intermittent claudication, with symptoms typically resolving within 2 to 5 minutes of rest (although it is regarded as the classic symptom for PAD, intermittent claudication is present in only 10% of patients with PAD)
- Rest leg pain (especially in a supine position)
- Skin ulceration (in advanced PAD)
- Gangrene (in advanced PAD)
- Impotence

PHYSICAL EXAM
- Skin pallor when leg is elevated above the level of the heart (in mild PAD)
- Dependent rubor
- Dry and scaly skin
- Poor nail growth
- Hair loss
- Reduced/absent extremity pulses (in advanced PAD)

DIFFERENTIAL DIAGNOSIS
- Arterial embolism
- Deep venous thrombosis
- Thromboangiitis obliterans (Buerger disease)
- Osteoarthritis
- Restless legs syndrome
- Peripheral neuropathy
- Spinal stenoses (pseudoclaudication)
- Intervertebral disc prolapse

DIAGNOSTIC TESTS & INTERPRETATION
Serum glucose is recommended screening for diabetes mellitus in suspected or confirmed PAD.

Initial Tests (lab, imaging)
- Fasting lipid profile is indicated for risk assessment of hyperlipidemia.
- Duplex ultrasonography and Doppler color-flow imaging, which are useful in detecting stenosed segments and assessing lesion severity, are initial imaging tests of choice.
- Magnetic resonance angiography, coupled with 3D reconstruction, is highly sensitive and specific for the localization of occluded lesions.
- CT scanning has a limited role in the evaluation of PAD.
- Angiography remains the gold standard in the diagnosis of PAD.

Diagnostic Procedures/Other
- Doppler ABI measures the ratio of the higher systolic BPs between the dorsalis pedis and the posterior tibial artery versus the higher of the systolic BPs in the two brachial arteries: Values for the ABI should be reported as "incompressible" if >1.40, "normal" if 1.00 to 1.40, "borderline" if 0.91 to 0.99, and "abnormal" if ≤0.90. ABI <0.4: severe ischemia
- Segmental limb pressures: usually obtained if abnormal ABI measurement is identified; a ≤20-mm Hg reduction in pressure is considered significant for PAD.

- Treadmill exercise test assesses the severity of claudication and the response to treatment.
- Segmental volume plethysmography: often used in conjunction with segmental limb pressures to measure the volume changes in an organ or limb; the study is indicated for calcified vessel when the ABI cannot be applied diagnostically.

TREATMENT

GENERAL MEASURES
- Claudication exercise rehabilitation program: patient to walk until symptoms develop, then rest and start again, for a total of 30 minutes initially; walking then is increased by 5 minutes until 50 minutes of intermittent walking is achieved.
- Modification of risk factors, including smoking cessation, diabetes mellitus, hypertension, and hyperlipidemia:
  - Weight loss is associated with a decrease in the risk of cardiovascular disease but has not been shown to improve PAD.
  - Antiplatelet therapy (aspirin) is recommended for patients with PAD when there is no other contraindication; however, neither the addition of an anticoagulant nor anticoagulant therapy alone has demonstrated superior outcome in PAD patients.
  - Lipid-lowering therapy with moderate-intensity statin; simvastatin (20 to 40 mg/day) has been shown to reduce the incidence of new intermittent claudication from 3.6% to 2.3% in patients with coronary artery disease (CAD).
  - No statistical significance for overall improvement of exercise performance or reduction in claudication symptoms for patients on niacin extended-release/lovastatin-combined therapy.
  - β-Adrenergic antagonists should be used with caution in individuals with severe PAD.
  - Smoking cessation is likely to reduce the severity of claudication.

MEDICATION
First Line
Antiplatelet therapy has been the mainstay treatment to prevent ischemic events in patients with PAD. However:

- The effect of aspirin on the risk reduction of overall ischemic events is inconclusive. Some suggest that aspirin delays disease progression and reduces the need for surgical intervention. AHA/ACCF guidelines (1)[A] note that the use of antiplatelet therapy to reduce cardiovascular risks in asymptomatic patients with borderline ABIs is characterized as "not well-established." Aspirin is recommended to reduce the risk of MI, stroke, and vascular death in symptomatic patients with PAD.

- Low-dose aspirin (75 to 150 mg/day) is as effective as higher doses of aspirin.

Second Line

- Clopidogrel (75 mg/day) is approved by the FDA for the secondary prevention of thrombotic events in patients with symptomatic lower extremity PAD and is recommended as an alternative to aspirin.
- Vorapaxar (Zontivity) 2.08 mg PO daily is a platelet aggregation inhibitor different in mechanism from existing antiplatelet drugs (TRAP inhibitor). It is contraindicated if history of CVA, TIA, or intracranial hemorrhage; concern for bleeding risk; and is expensive
- Other medications that may improve symptoms of claudication include pentoxifylline (1.2 g/day), cilostazol (100 mg BID), and naftidrofuryl (600 mg/day).
- Neither vasodilators nor anticoagulant therapy (e.g., heparin, low-molecular-weight heparin, or oral anticoagulant) has shown any clinically proven efficacy for the treatment of claudication and may be harmful.
- Cilostazol (100 mg BID) improves walking distance in people with intermittent claudication secondary to PAD. There is currently insufficient data on whether taking cilostazol results in a reduction of all-cause mortality and cardiovascular events or an improvement in quality of life (2)[A].
- Other medications that may reduce claudication include pentoxifylline (1.2 g/day), naftidrofuryl (600 mg/day), and prostaglandins (120 μg/day). Ticlopidine (250 mg BID) reduces the risk of MI, stroke, and death in patients with PAD, but it has a complication of thrombocytopenia in 2–3% of patients.

ADDITIONAL THERAPIES

- Weight reduction, smoking cessation, and BP control are essential in treating claudication.
- Exercise programs are of significant benefit compared with placebo or usual care in improving walking time and distance in people with leg pain from intermittent claudication who were considered to be fit for exercise intervention (3)[A]. A walking program should include walking at least 3 times per week for 30 to 60 minutes each time and has been shown to improve quality of life as much as or more so than medication.
- A healthy diet high in complex carbohydrates (e.g., whole grains and pastas), fruits and vegetables, and low in salt and animal fats

SURGERY/OTHER PROCEDURES

Surgical interventions, such as revascularization, are warranted for individuals who have debilitating intermittent claudication, ischemic rest pain, or tissue loss:

- Transluminal balloon angioplasty is a percutaneous method of dilating arterial stenoses or recanalizing occluded vessels with or without stents (reserved for short, isolated, and hemodynamically significant lesions of the iliac or proximal superficial femoral artery).
- Bypass surgery is the standard operative treatment for lower extremity peripheral occlusive disease.

COMPLEMENTARY & ALTERNATIVE MEDICINE

- Acupuncture, biofeedback, chelation therapy, and supplements such as *Ginkgo biloba*, omega-3 fatty acids, and vitamin E have been studied.
- *Ginkgo biloba* modestly reduces the symptoms of intermittent claudication (120 mg/day for up to 6 months) and can be considered as an adjunct to exercise therapy. Inconclusive evidence exists for the use of vitamin E.

 ONGOING CARE

FOLLOW-UP RECOMMENDATIONS

- An exercise training program composed of walking/ bicycle riding improves maximal treadmill walking distance and, therefore, enhances functional capacity.
- However, little added benefit exists from *Ginkgo biloba* treatment when added to supervised exercise training in patients with PAD as compared with patients in exercise training program alone.

DIET

A low-fat cardiac diet is recommended.

PROGNOSIS

- Among patients with intermittent claudication, 15–20% will experience worsening claudication; 5–10% will undergo lower extremity bypass surgery; and 2–5% will need primary amputation (rates for smokers and diabetics are much higher).
- 30,000 to 50,000 people in the United States undergo amputations annually because of PAD.

REFERENCES

1. Rooke TW, Hirsch AT, Misra S, et al. 2011 ACCF/AHA focused update of the guideline for the management of patients with peripheral artery disease (updating the 2005 guideline): a report of the American College of Cardiology Foundation/American Heart Association Task Force on Practical Guidelines. *J Am Coll Cardiol*. 2011;58(19):2020–2045.
2. Bedenis R, Stewart M, Cleanthis M, et al. Cilostazol for intermittent claudication. *Cochrane Database Syst Rev*. 2014;(10):CD003748.
3. Lane R, Ellis B, Watson L, et al. Exercise for intermittent claudication. *Cochrane Database Syst Rev*. 2014;(7):CD000990.

ADDITIONAL READING

- Duprez DA. Pharmacological interventions for peripheral artery disease. *Expert Opin Pharmacother*. 2007;8(10):1465–1477.
- Gey DC, Lesho EP, Manngold J. Management of peripheral arterial disease. *Am Fam Physician*. 2004; 69(3):525–532.
- Hankey GJ, Norman PE, Eikelboom JW. Medical treatment of peripheral arterial disease. *JAMA*. 2006;295(5):547–553.
- Hiatt WR, Hirsch AT, Creager MA, et al. Effect of niacin ER/lovastatin on claudication symptoms in patients with peripheral artery disease. *Vasc Med*. 2010;15(3):171–179.
- Wang J, Zhou S, Bronks R, et al. Supervised exercise training combined with ginkgo biloba treatment for patients with peripheral arterial disease. *Clin Rehabil*. 2007;21(7):579–586.

CODES

ICD10

- I73.9 Peripheral vascular disease, unspecified
- I70.209 Unsp athscl native arteries of extremities, unsp extremity
- I70.219 Athscl native arteries of extrm w intrmt claud, unsp extrm

CLINICAL PEARLS

- Screening of a general medical population for PAD is not recommended. Studies have indicated that screening for PAD among asymptomatic adults in the general population could lead to false-positive results and unnecessary workups. The prevalence among the general public who are asymptomatic is low.
- A patient already receiving medical treatment should be referred for further surgical evaluation for any of the following scenarios:
  - Unsatisfactory results despite medical therapy.
  - No definitive diagnosis can be made.
  - Critical limb ischemia is present, such as rest pain, gangrene, or ulceration.
- The clopidogrel (75 mg/day) versus aspirin (325 mg/ day) study in the patients at risk of ischemic events (CAPRIE) trial found a 23.8% relative risk ratio for MI, stroke, or cardiovascular death in PAD patients treated with clopidogrel compared with aspirin but no statistically significant difference in overall mortality reduction. Clopidogrel is much more expensive than aspirin.

PERITONITIS, ACUTE
Justin Thomas Ertle, BS, MD • Marie L. Borum, MD, EdD, MPH

 BASICS

DESCRIPTION
- Definition: inflammation of the peritoneum
- Classification:
  - Aseptic: due to chemical irritation or systemic inflammation of peritoneum
  - Bacterial: due to infection of peritoneal fluid
- Bacterial peritonitis types:
  - Primary/spontaneous bacterial peritonitis (SBP): infection of ascitic fluid without known source; typically monomicrobial
  - Secondary bacterial peritonitis: infection of peritoneal fluid from a detectable intra-abdominal source (i.e., perforation); typically polymicrobial
  - Tertiary bacterial peritonitis: persistent infection despite adequate therapy

EPIDEMIOLOGY
Incidence
- In patients with ascites, the incidence of SBP in a 1-year period is 10–25% (1).
- Secondary bacterial peritonitis correlates with incidence of the underlying pathology (e.g. colitis, appendicitis, diverticulitis, PUD).
- 57% of patients with secondary bacterial peritonitis progressed to tertiary peritonitis (2).
Prevalence
- SBP: In asymptomatic patients with cirrhosis and ascites, the prevalence is <3.5% in outpatients and 8–36% in the nosocomial setting (3).
- In patients with cirrhosis and ascites, 5% of peritonitis is secondary rather than SBP (4).

ETIOLOGY AND PATHOPHYSIOLOGY
- Mechanism
  - SBP:
    ○ Primary mechanism is bacterial translocation via lymphatic spread through mesenteric lymph nodes into ascitic fluid.
    ○ Cirrhotic patients have multiple secondary mechanisms:
      ■ Small intestinal bacterial overgrowth (SIBO) and increased intestinal mucosal permeability to bacteria both increase bacterial translocation.
      ■ Decreased cellular and humoral immunity increases susceptibility to bacterial translocation
  - Secondary bacterial peritonitis
    ○ Spillage/translocation of bacteria from inflamed or perforated intraperitoneal organs or introduction of bacterial through instrumentation—for example, peritoneal dialysis, intraperitoneal chemotherapy
  - Tertiary bacterial peritonitis
    ○ Occurs in secondary peritonitis with inadequacy of source control or altered host immunity
- Microbiology
  - SBP
    ○ *Escherichia coli* (46%), *Streptococcus* spp. (30%), *Klebsiella* (9%), and *Staphylococcus* (6%). Increasing rate of gram-positive and resistant organisms (e.g., extended-spectrum β-lactamase-producing [ESBL] *E. coli*, MRSA, enterococcus) in the nosocomial setting
  - Secondary bacterial peritonitis:
    ○ *E. coli, Klebsiella, Proteus, Streptococcus, Enterococcus, Bacteroides, Clostridium*

RISK FACTORS
- SBP: advanced cirrhosis with ascites, bacterascites, malnutrition, upper GI bleed, PPI usage, prior SBP
  - Acid suppression with PPIs been shown to promote SIBO increasing SBP, and hospitalized cirrhotics receiving PPIs are at increased risk of developing SBP (3).
  - 70% of cases of SBP are seen in patients with Child-Pugh class C cirrhosis (1).
- Secondary bacterial peritonitis: Factors associated with perforation or fluid translocation, for example, peritoneal dialysis, *H. pylori* and NSAIDs causing ulcers, vascular disease causing bowel ischemia, ETOH abuse causing pancreatitis

GENERAL PREVENTION
- SBP prophylaxis is beneficial when risk factors are present, including ascitic fluid protein concentration <1.0 g/dL, esophageal varices, or history of previous SBP
  - Prior SBP: prophylactic norfloxacin or TMP/SMX PO daily (5)[A].
  - Cirrhosis and GI bleed: 7-day course of ceftriaxone 2 g IV daily or norfloxacin BID, IV while bleeding, PO as tolerated (5)[A]
  - Cirrhotic ascites with low ascitic fluid protein (<1.5 g/dL) and either renal impairment (creatinine ≥1.2, BUN ≥25, or serum Na ≤130) or liver failure (Child score ≥9, bilirubin ≥3): prophylactic norfloxacin PO daily (3,5)[A]
- Limit use of PPIs to only proven indications, as PPIs increase incidence of SIBO (5)[B].

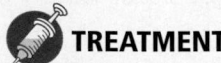 DIAGNOSIS

HISTORY
- SBP: history of cirrhosis or ascites, fever, mental status changes, abdominal pain, chills, nausea/vomiting, GI bleed
- Secondary bacterial peritonitis: history of perforation, abscess or peritoneal dialysis, acute abdominal pain, nausea, vomiting, anorexia, fever, mental status changes
- Tertiary: persistent signs and symptoms despite initial treatment, or history of recurrent peritonitis

ALERT
30% of patients are asymptomatic (1)[C].

Geriatric Considerations
Signs and symptoms are frequently absent, particularly in pediatric and elderly patients (1)[B].

PHYSICAL EXAM
- Tachycardia, fever, tachypnea, altered mental status
- Abdominal distention, ascites, abdominal wall guarding and rigidity, rebound tenderness, hypoactive/absent bowel sounds

DIFFERENTIAL DIAGNOSIS
- Liver disease: acute hepatitis, decompensated cirrhosis
- Luminal disease: abscess formation, ileus, volvulus, intussusception, mesenteric adenitis, pancreatitis, cholecystitis, malignancy, peritoneal carcinomatosis
- Extraluminal disease: ruptured ectopic pregnancy, tubo-ovarian abscess, PID, severe UTI, and/or pyelonephritis
- Systemic disease: tuberculosis, pneumonia, MI, porphyria, SLE

DIAGNOSTIC TESTS & INTERPRETATION
Initial Tests (lab, imaging)

ALERT
Early diagnosis is essential to reduce mortality. Paracentesis should be performed in any patient with new ascites, including suspected SBP (5)[B].

- Immediate evaluation
  - Perform paracentesis, blood, and urine cultures before administration of antibiotics (1,5)[B].
  - Ascitic fluid studies should minimally include culture (use aerobic and anaerobic blood culture bottles), Gram stain, cell count with differential, and albumin (1)[B]; if assessing for secondary peritonitis also include LDH, total protein and glucose.

ALERT
Lab interpretation: Ascitic fluid culture is negative in up to 50% of patients with SBP (1)[A].

- SBP: bacterascites and ascitic fluid PMN >250 cells/mm^3
- Culture-negative neutrocytic ascites: negative ascites culture, ascitic fluid PMN >250 cells/mm^3
- Nonneutrocytic bacterascites: positive ascites culture, ascitic fluid PMN <250 cells/mm^3
- Secondary peritonitis: PMN >250 cells/mm^3 on ascitic fluid analysis, with any of the following criteria:
  - Polymicrobial culture or two of the following: ascitic fluid total protein >1 g/dL, glucose <50 mg/dL, or LDH >225 mU/mL. Sensitivity for perforation 96%, sensitivity for nonperforation secondary peritonitis 50% (5)[B]
  - Secondary peritonitis with perforation is likely with alkaline phosphatase >240 U/l or CEA >5 ng/mL, sensitivity 92% (5)[B].

ALERT
Imaging: Criteria or clinical suspicion for secondary peritonitis necessitates emergent CT scan. CT diagnostic for secondary peritonitis in 85% (5)[B].

- Ultrasound or CT scan with enteral and IV contrast shows intra-abdominal mass, ascites, abscess, or extravasation of contrast in secondary peritonitis
- Abdominal or chest x-ray may show free air in peritoneal cavity, large/small bowel dilatation, intestinal wall edema in secondary peritonitis.

Follow-Up Tests & Special Considerations
- If asymptomatic bacterascites, recent antibiotic exposure, nosocomial atypical organism, or no clinical improvement, repeat paracentesis in 48 hours to resolution, defined as decrease in PMNs of 25% or negative cultures (1)[C].
- In hemorrhagic ascites, PMN count can be corrected by subtracting 1 PMN per 250 RBCs (3)[A].

TREATMENT

GENERAL MEASURES
- For SBP, control the effects of cirrhosis/ascites with salt restriction, spironolactone +/− furosemide, albumin infusion after large volume paracentesis, and/or lactulose for encephalopathy (5)[A].
- Avoid nephrotoxic medications (e.g., NSAIDs) or other renal insults (5)[C].

MEDICATION

- SBP empiric first-line treatment

  - Community-acquired SBP w/o recent β-lactam antibiotic use: 3rd-generation cephalosporins, preferably cefotaxime, 2 g IV q8h for 5 days (5)[A]
  - SBP in absence of previous quinolone use/prophylaxis, vomiting, shock, hepatic encephalopathy, or serum creatinine >3 mg/dL: Ofloxacin 400 mg PO can be substituted for cefotaxime (5)[B].
  - Nosocomial SBP or recent β-lactam antibiotic: Empiric therapy based on local susceptibility of patients with cirrhosis for resistant bacteria (e.g., ESBL Enterobacteriaceae, MRSA) (6)[B]
  - Symptomatic bacterascites with PMN count <250 cells/mm³: cefotaxime 2 g IV q8h while awaiting sensitivities (5)[B]

  - Second-line antibiotic regimens include fluoroquinolones (levofloxacin), piperacillin/tazobactam, or vancomycin (5)[C].

  - SBP with renal or hepatic impairment (serum creatinine >1 mg/dL, BUN >30 mg/dL, or total bilirubin >4 mg/dL): Add albumin 1.5 g/kg within 6 hours and 1 g/kg on day 3 (1)[A],(5)[B].

- Secondary bacterial peritonitis
  - Empiric broad spectrum antibiotic coverage for polymicrobial infection; IV cefotaxime or other 3rd- to 4th-generation cephalosporin plus metronidazole is one option for an initial regimen.

  - In peritoneal dialysis associated infection, intraperitoneal route superior to IV (6)[A]

- Tertiary bacterial peritonitis

  - If no unrepaired perforations or leaks, conservative medical management. This includes antibiotics (guided by prior susceptibilities if available) and early enteral nutrition to prevent atrophy and maintain immunocompetence (2)[B].
  - In recurrent or persistent peritoneal dialysis associated infection, removal of the PD catheter is warranted (6)[A].

SURGERY/OTHER PROCEDURES

- SBP
  - Medical management
- Secondary bacterial peritonitis

  - Emergent surgical management, including source control with open laparotomy to repair any perforated viscus and eradicate infected material, is the first-line treatment (2)[A],(5)[B].

- Tertiary bacterial peritonitis
  - If no unrepaired perforations or leaks, additional surgery for severe abdominal infection is correlated with deterioration and significant mortality (2).

ALERT

Mortality of SBP approaches 80% if the patient receives unnecessary exploratory laparotomy; conversely, mortality of secondary bacterial peritonitis approaches 100% if not treated surgically (1,3).

INPATIENT CONSIDERATIONS

Admission Criteria/Initial Stabilization

- Acute peritonitis typically warrants inpatient admission.
- In patients with cardiogenic or septic shock, invasive monitoring with early goal-directed fluid therapy
- Patients who present with peritonitis can be severely hypovolemic. In these cases, volume resuscitation is critical. In patients with significant renal or hepatic dysfunction, albumin decreases mortality (1)[A],(5)[B].

- Cirrhotic patients often take β-blockers as part of their outpatient regimen, but during an episode of SBP, β-blockers increase mortality, hepatorenal syndrome, and hospital stay in SBP patients (5)[B].
- Nasogastric tube placement can prevent aspiration in patients with vomiting or GI bleeding.

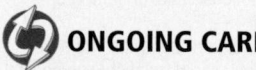 ONGOING CARE

FOLLOW-UP RECOMMENDATIONS

Patient Monitoring

Normalization of vital signs with resolution of leukocytosis indicates improvement.

- SBP: If follow-up paracentesis is performed after 48 hours to evaluate resolution, PMN decrease >25% is expected.
- Development of leukopenia indicates immune exhaustion and poor prognosis.

DIET

- NPO, total parental nutrition as necessary
- Resume enteral feeding after return of bowel function
- Sodium restriction can reduce future ascites (3)[A].

PROGNOSIS

- SBP
  - For inpatients with first episode of SBP, mortality ranges from 10% to 50% (3).
  - Prognosis is improved if antibiotics are started early, prior to onset of shock or renal failure.
  - Strongest negative prognostic indicator is renal insufficiency.
  - Other poor prognostic factors include nosocomial acquisition, old age, high Child-Pugh-Turcotte or MELD score, malnutrition, malignancy, peripheral leukopenia, and antibiotic resistance (3).
  - Patients with prior SBP have 1-year recurrence rate of 40–70% and 1-year mortality of 31–93% (1,3).
- Secondary bacterial peritonitis:
  - In-hospital mortality of treated patients is 67% (4).
  - Mortality approaches 100% if not treated surgically, especially if secondary to perforation (2,4).
  - Prognosis is worse in perforated etiologies.

COMPLICATIONS

- Renal failure, liver failure, encephalopathy, coagulopathy
- Secondary infection, iatrogenic infection, abscess, fistula formation, abdominal compartment syndrome
- Sepsis/septic shock, cardiovascular collapse, adrenal insufficiency, respiratory failure, ARDS

REFERENCES

1. Alaniz C, Regal RE. Spontaneous bacterial peritonitis: a review of treatment options. P T. 2009;34(4):204–210.
2. Panhofer P, Izay B, Riedl M, et al. Age, microbiology and prognostic scores help to differentiate between secondary and tertiary peritonitis. Langenbecks Arch Surg. 2009;394(2):265–271.
3. Wiest R, Krag A, Gerbes A. Spontaneous bacterial peritonitis: recent guidelines and beyond. Gut. 2012;61(2):297–310.
4. Soriano G, Castellote J, Alvarez C, et al. Secondary bacterial peritonitis in cirrhosis: a retrospective study of clinical and analytical characteristics, diagnosis and management. J Hepatol. 2010;52(1):39–44.
5. Runyon, B. Introduction to the revised American Association for the Study of Liver Diseases practice guideline management of adult patients with ascites due to cirrhosis 2012. Hepatology. 2013;57(4):1651–1653.
6. Ballinger A, Palmer SC, Wiggins KJ, et al. Treatment for peritoneal dialysis-associated peritonitis. Cochrane Database Syst Rev. 2014;(4):CD005284.

ADDITIONAL READING

- Bajaj JS, O'Leary JG, Wong F, et al. Bacterial infections in end-stage liver disease: current challenges and future directions. Gut. 2012;61(8):1219–1225.
- Cheong HS, Kang CI, Lee JA, et al. Clinical significance and outcome of nosocomial acquisition of spontaneous bacterial peritonitis in patients with liver cirrhosis. Clin Infect Dis. 2009;48(9):1230–1236.
- Deshpande A, Pasupuleti V, Thota P, et al. Acid-suppressive therapy is associated with spontaneous bacterial peritonitis in cirrhotic patients: a meta-analysis. J Gastroenterol Hepatol. 2013;28(2):235–242.
- Ghassemi S, Garcia-Tsao G. Prevention and treatment of infections in patients with cirrhosis. Best Pract Res Clin Gastroenterol. 2007;21(1):77–93.
- Jain P. Spontaneous bacterial peritonitis: few additional points. World J Gastroenterol. 2009;15(45):5754–5755.
- Koulaouzidis A, Bhat S, Karagiannidis A, et al. Spontaneous bacterial peritonitis. Postgrad Med J. 2007;83(980):379–383.
- Koulaouzidis A, Bhat S, Saeed AA. Spontaneous bacterial peritonitis. World J Gastroenterol. 2009;15(9):1042–1049.
- Mandorfer M, Bota S, Schwabl P, et al. Nonselective β blockers increase risk for hepatorenal syndrome and death in patients with cirrhosis and spontaneous bacterial peritonitis. Gastroenterology. 2014;146(7):1680.e1–1690.e1.

 SEE ALSO

Appendicitis, Acute; Cirrhosis of the Liver; Diverticular Disease; Peptic Ulcer Disease

 CODES

ICD10

- K65.0 Generalized (acute) peritonitis
- K65.2 Spontaneous bacterial peritonitis
- K65.8 Other peritonitis

CLINICAL PEARLS

- Maintain a high index of suspicion for SBP in cirrhotic patients with ascites. SBP occurs in preexisting ascites and carries a high mortality, especially if presenting with GI bleed.
- Early diagnosis and treatment reduces mortality.
- Paracentesis is necessary to diagnose SBP.
- Emergent CT scan should be performed if there is suspicion of secondary bacterial peritonitis.
- Distinguishing SBP from secondary bacterial peritonitis is essential, as SBP treatment consists of antibiotic therapy whereas secondary bacterial peritonitis necessitates emergent surgical intervention.
- Renal function is an important prognostic indicator for SBP. Albumin administration decreases the incidence of renal failure and mortality in patients with renal or hepatic impairment or large-volume paracentesis.

PERSONALITY DISORDERS

Moshe S. Torem, MD, DLFAPA

BASICS

DESCRIPTION

- Personality disorders (PDs) are a group of conditions, with onset at or before adolescence, characterized by enduring patterns of maladaptive and dysfunctional behavior that deviates markedly from one's culture and social environment, leading to functional impairment and distress to the individual, coworkers, and family.
  - These behaviors are perceived by patients to be "normal" and "right," and they have little insight as to their ownership, responsibility, and abnormal nature of these behaviors.
  - These conditions are classified based on the predominant symptoms and their severity.
- System(s) affected: nervous/psychiatric
- Synonym(s): character disorder; character pathology

Geriatric Considerations
Coping with the stresses of aging is challenging.

Pediatric Considerations
A history of childhood neglect, abuse, and trauma is not uncommon.

Pregnancy Considerations
Pregnancy adds pressures in coping with the activities of daily living (ADLs).

EPIDEMIOLOGY
Prevalence
- General population: 15% (1)
- Cluster A: 5.7%
- Cluster B: 6.0%
- Cluster C: 9.1%
- Outpatient psychiatric clinic: 3–30% (2)
- In male prisoners, the prevalence of antisocial personality disorder is ~60%.
- Predominant age: starts in adolescence and early 20s and persists throughout patient's life
- Predominant sex: male = female; some PDs are more common in females, and others are more common in males.

ETIOLOGY AND PATHOPHYSIOLOGY
- Environmental and genetic factors (3)
- Criteria for a PD includes an enduring pattern of the following:
  - Inner experience and behavior that deviates markedly from the expectations of one's culture in ≥2 of the following areas: cognition, affectivity, interpersonal functioning, or impulse control.
  - Inflexibility and pervasiveness across a broad range of personal and social situations
  - Significant distress or impairment in social or occupational functioning
  - The pattern is stable and of long duration.
  - The enduring pattern is not better explained as a manifestation of another psychiatric disorder.
  - The enduring pattern is not attributable to the effects of a drug or a medical condition.

- PDs are classified into three major clusters:
  - Cluster A: eccentricism and oddness
    - *Paranoid PD*: unwarranted suspiciousness and distrust of others
    - *Schizoid PD*: emotional, cold, or detached; socially isolated
    - *Schizotypal PD*: eccentric behavior, odd belief system/perceptions, social isolation, and general suspiciousness
  - Cluster B: dramatic, emotional, or erratic behavioral patterns
    - *Antisocial PD*: aggressive, impulsive, irritable, irresponsible, dishonest, deceitful
    - *Borderline PD:* unstable interpersonal relationships, high impulsivity from early adulthood, intense fear of abandonment, mood swings, poor self-esteem, chronic boredom, and feelings of inner emptiness
    - *Histrionic PD:* needs to be the center of attention, with self-dramatizing behaviors and attention seeking in a variety of contexts
    - *Narcissistic PD*: grandiose sense of self-importance and preoccupation with fantasies of success, power, brilliance, beauty, or ideal love; lack of empathy for other people's pain or discomfort, demanding to get their way
  - Cluster C: anxiety, excessive worry, fear, and unhealthy patterns of coping with emotions
    - *Avoidant PD*: social inhibition, feelings of inadequacy, hypersensitivity to negative evaluation, avoidance of occupational and interpersonal activities that involve the risk of criticism by others, views self as socially inept and personally unappealing or inferior to others
    - *Dependent PD*: excessive need to be taken care of, leading to submissive and clinging behavior with fears of separation, avoids expressing disagreements with others due to fear of losing support and approval, usually seeks out strong and confident people as friends or spouses and feels more secure in such relationships
    - *Obsessive-compulsive PD*: preoccupation with cleanliness, orderliness, perfectionism; preoccupation with excessive details, rules, lists, order, organization, and schedules to the extent that the major point of the activity is lost.
  - Personality change due to another medical condition. It is a persistent personality disturbance that is caused by the physiologic effects of a medical condition such as frontal lobe lesion, epilepsy, MS, Parkinson disease, lupus, head trauma, post encephalitis or meningitis, and so forth.
  - Other specified *PD and unspecified PD*: A category provided for two situations: (i) the individual's personality pattern meets the general criteria for PD and traits of several PDs are present, but the criteria for any specific PD are not met; (ii) the individual's personality pattern meets the general criteria for PD, but the individual is considered to have a PD that is not included in *DSM-5* classification such as passive-aggressive PD, depressive PD, masochistic PD, and dangerous and severe PD.

Genetics
Major character traits are inherited; others result from a combination of genetics and environment.

RISK FACTORS
- Positive family history
- Pregnancy risk factors
  - Nutritional deprivation
  - Use of alcohol or drugs.
  - Viral and bacterial infections
- Dysfunctional family with child abuse/neglect

COMMONLY ASSOCIATED CONDITIONS
Depression; other psychiatric disorders in patient and family members

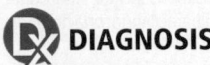

DIAGNOSIS

HISTORY
- Comprehensive interview and mental status examination
- Screen to rule out alcohol and drug abuse.
- Interview of relatives and friends is helpful in establishing an enduring pattern of behavior.

DIAGNOSTIC TESTS & INTERPRETATION
Psychological testing (e.g., MMPI-II)

Initial Tests (lab, imaging)
- CBC
- Comprehensive metabolic panel
- Thyroid-stimulating hormone
- HIV
- Toxicology screen for substance abuse

Follow-Up Tests & Special Considerations
- EEG to rule out a chronic seizure disorder
- CT and MRI of the brain may be necessary in newly developed symptoms to rule out organic brain disease (e.g., frontal lobe tumor).

DIAGNOSTIC TESTS & INTERPRETATION
- Medical disorders with behavioral changes
- Other psychiatric disorders with similar symptoms
  - In obsessive-compulsive disorder (OCD), symptoms are ego-dystonic (i.e., perceived as foreign and unwanted). In addition, OCD has a pattern of relapse and partial remission.
  - In obsessive-compulsive personality disorder (OCPD), symptoms are perceived as desirable behaviors (ego-syntonic) that the patient feels proud of and wants others to emulate. In addition, OCPD has a lifelong pattern (i.e., without significant relapse or remission).

TREATMENT

Psychotherapy with family involvement is the foundation of treatment. No specific drugs are indicated to treat PDs; some medications can reduce the intensity, frequency, and dysfunctional nature of certain behaviors (4)[B].

GENERAL MEASURES

- Long-term psychotherapy and cognitive-behavioral therapy (5)[B]
- Group therapy is helpful in the use of therapeutic confrontation and increasing one's awareness of and insight regarding the damaging effects of dysfunctional behavior patterns (6)[B].

MEDICATION

Medications are effective in the treatment of comorbid conditions such as anxiety and depression.

First Line

- Symptom management (7)[B]

  - Mini psychosis (associated with paranoid, schizoid, borderline, and schizotypal PDs): atypical antipsychotics: risperidone (Risperdal), quetiapine (Seroquel), olanzapine (Zyprexa), ziprasidone (Geodon), aripiprazole (Abilify), asenapine (Saphris), lurasidone (Latuda); start with a low dose, gradually adjusting to the patient's needs.
  - Anxiety: anxiolytics (benzodiazepines, buspirone [Buspar], and serotonin reuptake inhibitors)
  - Depressed mood: antidepressants
  - Many patients with borderline PD respond well to small doses of atypical neuroleptics and mood stabilizers (8)[B].

- Precautions: Some atypical neuroleptic drugs may be associated with hyperglycemia and insulin-resistant metabolic syndrome.

Second Line

Mood stabilizers: lithium carbonate, lamotrigine (Lamictal), carbamazepine (Tegretol, Equetro), and valproate (Depacon, Depakene, Depakote) (9)[B]

ISSUES FOR REFERRAL

- When psychiatric comorbidity of Axis I disorders is present (e.g., mood disorders, anxiety disorders, substance abuse, etc.)
- Suicidal ideation or attempts

ADDITIONAL THERAPIES

- Dialectical behavior therapy
- Psychoanalytic therapy
- Interactive psychotherapy
- Group therapy

INPATIENT CONSIDERATIONS

Admission Criteria/Initial Stabilization

Disorders with complications of suicide attempts

 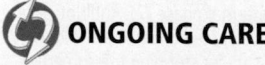

ONGOING CARE

FOLLOW-UP RECOMMENDATIONS

Continue outpatient treatment, potentially long term

Patient Monitoring

- Regular physical exercise (e.g., 30 to 45 min/day, helps with stress and improving the ADLs)
- If substance abuse is suspected, check drug screens.
- Infrequent sessions with relatives or friends are helpful in monitoring behavioral progress.

DIET

Emphasize variety of healthy foods; avoid obesity.

PATIENT EDUCATION

- Bibliotherapy and writing therapy, specific assignments, and watching certain movies to better understand the nature and origin of one's specific condition are helpful.
  - Kreger R. *The Essential Family Guide to Borderline Personality Disorder*. Center City, MN: Hazelden; 2008.
  - Mason PT, Kreger R. *Stop Walking on Eggshells*. Oakland, CA: New Harbinger Publishers; 2010.
- The movie *As Good as It Gets* illustrates someone with obsessive-compulsive behaviors and their impact on ADLs and relationships with family and friends.
- The movie series *The Godfather* includes several characters with antisocial PD and shows how this affects their interpersonal relationships and their own physical and mental health.
- The movie *What About Bob?* illustrates the challenges involved in treating certain patients with a borderline PD, especially in the management of boundaries in the doctor–patient relationship.
- The movie *A Streetcar Named Desire* illustrates an example of a woman with a histrionic PD.
- The movie *Wall Street* illustrates an example of a person with a narcissistic PD.
- The movie *The Caine Mutiny* illustrates an example of a person with a paranoid PD.
- The movie *Four Weddings and a Funeral* illustrates an example of a person with an avoidant PD.

PROGNOSIS

PDs are enduring patterns of behavior throughout one's lifetime and are not readily responsive to treatment.

COMPLICATIONS

- Disruptive family life with frequent divorces and separations, alcoholism, substance abuse, and drug addiction
- Disruptive behaviors in the workplace may cause absenteeism and loss of productivity.
- Violation of the law and disregard for the concerns and rights of others

REFERENCES

1. American Psychiatric Association. *Diagnostic and Statistical Manual of Mental Disorders*. 5th ed. Arlington, VA: American Psychiatric Association; 2013:645–684.
2. Angstman KB, Rasmussen NH. Personality disorders: review and clinical application in daily practice. *Am Fam Physician*. 2011;84(11):1253–1260.
3. Reichborn-Kjennerud T. Genetics of personality disorders. *Clin Lab Med*. 2010;30(4):893–910.
4. Hadjipavlou G, Ogrodniczuk JS. Promising psychotherapies for personality disorders. *Can J Psychiatry*. 2010;55(4):202–210.
5. Clarkin JF. An integrated approach to psychotherapy techniques for patients with personality disorder. *J Pers Disord*. 2012;26(1):43–62.
6. Livesley WJ. Integrated treatment: a conceptual framework for an evidence-based approach to the treatment of personality disorder. *J Pers Disord*. 2012;26(1):17–42.
7. Ripoll LH, Triebwasser J, Siever LJ. Evidence-based pharmacotherapy for personality disorders. *Int J Neuropsychopharmacol*. 2011;14(9):1257–1288.
8. Ripoll LH. Clinical psychopharmacology of borderline personality disorder: an update on the available evidence in light of the Diagnostic and Statistical Manual of Mental Disorders-5. *Curr Opin Psychiatry*. 2012;25(1):52–58.
9. Lieb K, Völlm B, Rücker G, et al. Pharmacotherapy for borderline personality disorder: cochrane systematic review of randomised trials. *Br J Psychiatry*. 2010;196(1):4–12.

ADDITIONAL READING

- Paris J. Modernity and narcissistic personality disorder. *Personal Disord*. 2014;5(2):220–226.
- Ronningstam E. Narcissistic personality disorder: a current review. *Curr Psychiatry Rep*. 2010;12(1):68–75.
- Stoffers J, Völlm BA, Rücker G, et al. Pharmacological interventions for borderline personality disorder. *Cochrane Database Syst Rev*. 2010;(6):CD005653.

 SEE ALSO

Obsessive-Compulsive Disorder (OCD)

 CODES

ICD10

- F60.9 Personality disorder, unspecified
- F60.0 Paranoid personality disorder
- F60.1 Schizoid personality disorder

CLINICAL PEARLS

- PDs are enduring patterns of behavior throughout one's lifetime and are not readily responsive to treatment.
- No specific drugs are effective to treat PDs; however, specific medications can reduce the intensity, frequency, and dysfunctional nature of certain behaviors, thoughts, and feelings.
- Most patients with a PD require a well-trained and experienced mental health professional.
- A stable, trustful alliance with the patient is the foundation for any therapeutic progress.
- Showing genuine interest in the patient as a whole person including the patient's life history and current life circumstances may be helpful in establishing a therapeutic and working alliance that are necessary for continuing treatment of PD patients.

PERTUSSIS

Mary Cataletto, MD, FAAP, FCCP • Margaret J. McCormick, MS, RN

BASICS

Highly contagious disease; aka whooping cough

DESCRIPTION
- Human host: adults most common reservoir
- Can affect all ages
- Worldwide distribution
- May be endemic or epidemic with outbreaks every 3 to 5 years
- Seasonality: can occur year-round; peaks late summer–autumn
- Transmission: person to person via aerosolized respiratory droplets
- Effective vaccine available but neither vaccine nor infection confer lifelong or 100% immunity.
- System(s) affected: respiratory
- Synonym(s): whooping cough

EPIDEMIOLOGY
Incidence
2012 was the most recent peak year with 48,277 reported cases in the United States (1)

ETIOLOGY AND PATHOPHYSIOLOGY
- Toxin mediated
- Infectious process with predilection for ciliated respiratory epithelium
- *Bordetella pertussis* (responsible for ~95% of cases)
- *Bordetella parapertussis*

RISK FACTORS
- Exposure to a confirmed case
- Non- or underimmunized infants and children
- Pregnancy
- Premature birth
- Chronic lung disease
- Immunodeficiency (e.g., AIDS)
- Infants <6 months of age account for ~90% pediatric pertussis hospitalizations (2).

GENERAL PREVENTION
- Public health measures
  - Surveillance activities
  - Prevention programs
  - Outbreak management
- Care of exposed persons
  - Household and close contacts
  - Child care workers
  - Health care workers
- Immunization
  - Vaccine products
  - Boosters
  - CDC and the Advisory Committee on Immunization Practices recommends one Tdap (tetanus toxoid, reduced diphtheria toxoid, and acellular pertussis) vaccination to all adolescents 11 to 12 years of age and one dose of Tdap for all adults age 18 years and older to provide increased herd immunity.

Pediatric Considerations
- Primary immunization series against pertussis followed by boosters
- Maternal immunization and cocooning are important strategies to help reduce neonatal pertussis (3).

ALERT
Tdap vaccine recommended with each pregnancy, preferably after 20 weeks' gestation regardless of Tdap/Td history (4)

Geriatric Considerations
The incidence of pertussis in individuals age 50 years and older has increased between 2006 and 2010 (5).

COMMONLY ASSOCIATED CONDITIONS
- Apnea
- Secondary bacterial pneumonia
- Sinusitis
- Seizures
- Encephalopathy
- Urinary incontinence

DIAGNOSIS

HISTORY
- Exposure to pertussis
- Incubation period 7 to 10 days (range 5 to 21 days)
- Classic symptoms are more common in adults and adolescents and include paroxysmal cough, posttussive whoop, and/or vomiting.
- Infants with pertussis may present with apnea or sudden death.

PHYSICAL EXAM
- Classic pertussis has three phases, which occur over 6 to 10 weeks:
  - Catarrhal phase: rhinorrhea, mild cough, low-grade fever
  - Paroxysmal phase: Cough occurs in bursts, with increased intensity and frequency, often followed by an inspiratory whoop and/or posttussive vomiting.
  - Convalescent phase: Coughing paroxysms decrease in frequency and intensity.
- In the absence of paroxysms or complications, the physical exam may be normal.

ALERT
Infants <6 months of age may have atypical presentations.

DIFFERENTIAL DIAGNOSIS
- *B. parapertussis*
- *Mycoplasma pneumoniae*
- *Chlamydia trachomatis*
- *Chlamydophila pneumoniae*
- *Bordetella bronchiseptica*
- Respiratory syncytial virus
- Adenovirus

DIAGNOSTIC TESTS & INTERPRETATION
Initial Tests (lab, imaging)
- Nasopharyngeal culture (gold standard): 100% specific and permits strain identification and antimicrobial resistance testing. Collect secretions from the back of the throat through the nose, using a Dacron or calcium alginate swab or syringe filled with saline. For best results, collect specimen during the first 2 weeks of cough—sensitivity decreases after 2 weeks (6)[C].
- Polymerase chain reaction (PCR) assays: Most commonly used because of improved sensitivity and turnaround time (6)[C].
- Specificity may vary between assays and must be interpreted within clinical context and local pertussis epidemiology. CDC "Best Practice" guidelines exist for PCR assays, although they have not yet received FDA approval. Six accurate results can be obtained during the first 3 weeks from onset of cough. Dacron swabs should be used as calcium alginate swabs are inhibitory to PCR (2,3).
- Serology: available commercially; however, there is no FDA-approved test or standardization
  - The CDC uses single point serology obtained between 2 and 8 weeks following cough onset when titers are expected to be at their peak (3).

Follow-Up Tests & Special Considerations
- Evaluation and follow-up for associated conditions and complications
- Chest radiograph (2 views) to evaluate for the presence of pneumonia
- EEG/neuroimaging may be considered in infant with seizures or acute life-threatening events (ALTEs).
- Infants <1 month of age who are treated with macrolides should be monitored for the possible development of hypertrophic pyloric stenosis.

TREATMENT

GENERAL MEASURES
Waiting rooms, during transport and procedures: Patients with suspected pertussis should wear masks.

MEDICATION
Pertussis illness may be less severe only if antibiotics are started early, that is, before the onset of paroxysms or during the catarrhal phase (2). Antibiotics can also help to prevent the spread of pertussis to close contacts and is necessary for stopping the spread of pertussis.

First Line
- Empiric antibiotic therapy should be initiated at the time diagnostic testing is performed if sufficient clinical suspicion for pertussis is present.

- Azithromycin is the first line of treatment for treatment and for postexposure prophylaxis (5-day course) (6)[C].
- If administered during catarrhal stage, these antibiotics may ameliorate disease.
- If administered after cough is established, antibiotics will have no individual benefit but may help to limit spread (6)[C].

ALERT
Risk of infantile hypertrophic pyloric stenosis has been associated with the use of macrolides in infants <1 month of age, but are still the drugs of choice. Consultation and monitoring are recommended.

ALERT
Due to reports of *fatal cardiac dysrhythmias* with azithromycin, consider alternate drugs in the elderly and in those with cardiovascular disease (7)[C].

Second Line
Trimethoprim-Sulfamethoxazole (TMP-SMX) (for persons >2 months of age) if:
- They cannot tolerate macrolides.
- They are infected with a macrolide-resistant strain.

ALERT
- TMP-SMX is *contraindicated* in infants <2 months of age (6)[C].
- Clarithromycin is not recommended in infants <1 month of age (6)[C].

ISSUES FOR REFERRAL
Evaluation and treatment of infants <6 months of age, especially those born prematurely, who are unimmunized and those who require hospitalization.

ADDITIONAL THERAPIES
Symptomatic treatment of the cough in pertussis (e.g., corticosteroids, β_2-adrenergic agonists, pertussis-specific immunoglobulin, antihistamine, and leukotriene receptor antagonist) have not shown consistent benefit (4)[B].

INPATIENT CONSIDERATIONS
Admission Criteria/Initial Stabilization
- Small, frequent meals may be necessary to ensure adequate nutrition.
- Correct fluid and electrolyte abnormalities.
- Infants may require IV fluids.

IV Fluids
Indicated for dehydration and when oral fluids are either contraindicated or poorly tolerated.

Nursing
- In addition to standard precautions, hospitalized patients should be isolated with respiratory precautions for 5 days after the initiation of effective antibiotic treatment and for 3 weeks after onset of paroxysms in older patients if antibiotics are not used.

- Gentle suctioning of nasal secretions
- Avoid stimuli that trigger paroxysms.
- Respiratory monitoring including pulse oximetry
- Educate each family about the importance of immunizations.
- Discuss chemoprophylaxis with each family.

Discharge Criteria
- Clinically stable
- Able to tolerate oral feedings

 ## ONGOING CARE

Supportive

FOLLOW-UP RECOMMENDATIONS
- Monitor infants who received EES or azithromycin for pyloric stenosis.
- Neurologic and/or pulmonary follow-up as necessary

Patient Monitoring
ICU care may be necessary for severely ill or compromised patients.

DIET
IV fluids/nutrition may be required to treat dehydration or supplement poor oral intake.

PATIENT EDUCATION
- American Academy of Pediatrics: http://www.aap.org
- Centers for Disease Control and Prevention: http://www.cdc.gov

PROGNOSIS
- Complete recovery in most cases
- Most severe morbidity and highest mortality in infants <6 months of age

COMPLICATIONS
- Highest and most severe in infants; may include apnea, cyanosis, and sudden death
- In children: may include conjunctival hemorrhage, inguinal hernia, pneumonia, and seizures
- More frequent in adults than adolescents: may include sinusitis, otitis media, pneumonia, weight loss, fainting, rib fracture, urinary incontinence, seizures, encephalopathy, and death

REFERENCES

1. Centers for Disease Control. 2013 Final pertussis surveillance report. Final 2013 reports of notifiable diseases. Updated August 15, 2014. http://www.cdc.gov/mmwr/preview/mmwrhtml/mm6332a6.htm. Accessed November 14, 2015.
2. Lopez MA, Cruz AT, Kowalkowski MA, et al. Trends in hospitalizations and resource utilization for pediatric pertussis. *Hosp Pediatr.* 2014;4(5):269–275.
3. Swamy GK, Wheeler SM. Neonatal pertussis, cocooning and maternal immunization. *Expert Rev Vaccines.* 2014;13(9):1107–1114.
4. Committee on Obstetric Practice. ACOG committee opinion no. 521: update on immunization and pregnancy: tetanus, diphtheria, and pertussis vaccination. *Obstet Gynecol.* 2012;119(3):690–691.
5. McGuiness CB, Hill J, Fonseca E, et al. The disease burden of pertussis in adults 50 years old and older in the United States: a retrospective study. *BMC Infect Dis.* 2013;13:32.
6. American Academy of Pediatrics. Pertussis (whooping cough). In: Kimberlin DW, Brady MT, Jackson MA, et al, eds. *Red Book: 2015 Report of the Committee on Infectious Diseases.* 30th ed. Elk Grove Village, Il: American Academy of Pediatrics; 2015:608–621
7. US Food and Drug Administration. Azithromycin: drug safety communication—risk of potentially fatal heart rhythms. http://www.fda.gov/Safety/Medwatch/SafetyInformation/SafetyAlertsforHumanMedicalProducts/ucm343350.htm. Accessed November 14, 2015.

ADDITIONAL READING

- Centers for Disease Control and Prevention. *Best Practices for Healthcare Professionals on the use of Polymerase Chain Reaction (PCR) for Diagnosing Pertussis.* Atlanta, GA: Centers for Disease Control and Prevention; 2011.
- Wang K, Bettiol S, Thompson MJ, et al. Symptomatic treatment of the cough in whooping cough. *Cochrane Database Syst Rev.* 2014;(9):CD003257.

CODES

ICD10
- A37.90 Whooping cough, unspecified species without pneumonia
- A37.80 Whooping cough due to other Bordetella species w/o pneumonia
- A37.10 Whooping cough due to Bordetella parapertussis w/o pneumonia

CLINICAL PEARLS

- Pertussis is a highly contagious infection.
- A high index of suspicion is needed. During the primary or catarrhal phase, the presentation may be nonspecific.
- Immunization (primary series and boosters), isolation, and early treatment of affected cases as well as chemoprophylaxis are key components to controlling the spread of pertussis.

PHARYNGITIS

Bryce L. Coombs, DO • David A. Moss, MD

 BASICS

DESCRIPTION
- Acute or chronic inflammation of the pharynx
- Most commonly caused by acute viral infection
- Group A *Streptococcus* (GAS) pharyngitis is a common clinical focus due to its potential for preventable suppurative (e.g., retropharyngeal or peritonsillar abscess) and nonsuppurative (e.g., rheumatic sequelae) complications.
- Synonym(s): sore throat; tonsillitis; "strep throat"
- Generally infection mediated but can be due to caustic injury, allergies, gastroesophageal reflux disease (GERD), smoking, endotracheal intubation, or trauma-related

EPIDEMIOLOGY
- Estimated 15 million cases diagnosed yearly
- Accounts for 1–2% of all outpatient visits and 6% of all pediatric visits to primary care physicians.
- Most commonly viral (40–60%)
- GAS is the most common bacterial cause of acute pharyngitis, accounting for 15–30% of pediatric and 5–15% of adult cases.
- Rheumatic fever is rare in the United States (incidence <1 per 100,000). Early antibiotic intervention has significantly diminished disease rates.
- All age groups, but some etiologies may predilect specific age groups
- No gender predilection

Pediatric Considerations
Rheumatic fever has its greatest incidence in children aged 5 to 18 years, but is currently a rare sequela of streptococcal pharyngitis in modern medicine.

ETIOLOGY AND PATHOPHYSIOLOGY
- Acute, viral (lower grade fever)
  - Rhinovirus
  - Adenovirus (associated with conjunctivitis)
  - Parainfluenza virus
  - Coxsackievirus (hand-foot-mouth disease)
  - Coronavirus
  - Echovirus
  - Herpes simplex virus (vesicular lesions)
  - Epstein-Barr virus (EBV/mononucleosis)
  - Cytomegalovirus
  - HIV
- Acute, bacterial (higher fevers)
  - Group A β-hemolytic streptococci
  - *Neisseria gonorrhoeae*
  - *Corynebacterium diphtheriae* (diphtheria)
  - *Haemophilus influenzae*
  - *Moraxella catarrhalis*
  - *Chlamydia pneumonia*
  - *Fusobacterium necrophorum* (20% young adult cases)
  - Group C or G *streptococcus*
  - *Arcanobacterium haemolyticum*
  - *Francisella tularensis* (tularemia)
- Acute, noninfectious
  - Various caustic, mechanical, or trauma-related (incl. endotracheal intubation)
- Chronic
  - More likely noninfectious
  - Chemical irritation (GERD)
  - Smoking
  - Neoplasms
  - Vasculitis
  - Radiation changes

Genetics
Patients with a positive family history of rheumatic fever have a higher risk of rheumatic sequelae following an untreated group A β-hemolytic streptococcal infection.

RISK FACTORS
- Epidemics of group A β-hemolytic streptococcal disease occurrence
- Cold and flu seasons
- Age (especially children/adolescents)
- Family history of rheumatic fever
- Close contact with infectious individuals (home, daycare, military barracks)
- Immunosuppression
- Fatigue
- Smoking/second-hand smoke exposure
- Acid reflux
- Oral sex
- Diabetes mellitus
- Recent illness (secondary postviral bacterial infection)
- Chronic colonization of bacteria in tonsils/adenoids

GENERAL PREVENTION
- Avoid close contact with infectious patients.
- Wash hands frequently.
- Avoid first- or second-hand smoke.
- Home humidifier at home
- Manage preventable causes (e.g., GERD).

 DIAGNOSIS

HISTORY
- Sore throat
- Difficulty swallowing (odynophagia)
- Cough (though rarely associated with GAS pharyngitis)
- Hoarseness
- Fever
- Anorexia
- Chills
- Malaise
- Contacts with similar symptoms or diagnosed infection

PHYSICAL EXAM
- Enlarged tonsils (tonsillar exudate or possible peritonsillar abscess/deep neck space infection)
- Pharyngeal erythema
- Cervical adenopathy
- Fever (higher in bacterial infections)
- Pharyngeal ulcers (CMV, HIV, Crohn, other autoimmune vasculitides)
- Scarlet fever rash: punctate erythematous macules with reddened flexor creases and circumoral pallor suggests streptococcal pharyngitis
- Tonsillar/soft palate petechiae suggests infectious mononucleosis (EBV/CMV).
- Gray oral pseudomembrane suggests diphtheria and occasionally infectious mononucleosis (EBV/CMV).
- Characteristic erythematous-based clear vesicles suggests HSV.
- Conjunctivitis suggests adenovirus.

DIFFERENTIAL DIAGNOSIS
- Viral syndrome
- Streptococcal infection
- Allergic rhinitis/postnasal drip
- GERD

- Malignancy (lymphoma or squamous cell carcinoma)
- Irritants/chemicals (detergent/caustic ingestion)
- Atypical bacterial (e.g., gonococcal, chlamydial, syphilis, pertussis, diphtheria)
- Oral candidiasis (patients typically complain mostly of dysphagia)

DIAGNOSTIC TESTS & INTERPRETATION
- Acute pharyngitis evaluation includes Prediction Rule Use to determine further testing (see below)
- Additional testing generally not needed if viral-like clinical features (e.g., cough, rhinorrhea, hoarseness, oral ulcers, diarrhea, conjunctivitis, rash) (1)[A].
- Avoid testing for GAS pharyngitis in children <3 years old as acute rheumatic flare is rare, unless there is a close sick contact who is GAS-positive (1)[B].
- Modified Centor clinical prediction rule for group A streptococcal infection (2)[A]:
  - +1 point: tonsillar exudates
  - +1 point: tender anterior chain cervical adenopathy
  - +1 point: absence of cough
  - +1 point: fever by history
  - +1 point: age <15 years
  - 0 point: age 15 to 45 years
  - −1 point: age >45 years
- Scoring:
  - If 4 points, positive predictive value of ~80%; treat empirically.
  - If 2 to 3 points, positive predictive value of ~50%, rapid strep antigen; treat if GAS-positive.
  - If 0 or 1 point, positive predictive value <20%; do not test; treat empirically with follow-up as needed.

Initial Tests (lab, imaging)
- Testing, if performed, is usually for the presence of group A β-hemolytic streptococci. Options include the following:
  - Rapid strep antigen test from throat swab with agglutination or molecular kits; provides quicker, more practical alternative to throat culture with 96% specificity and 86% sensitivity (though sensitivity varies by modality kit) (3)[A].
  - Blood agar throat culture from swab. Gold standard of diagnosis (3)[A]
  - Antistreptolysin-O (carrier state suspected if positive culture, and unchanged ASO titers)
- Special tests usually done only if history is suggestive of a different diagnosis.
  - Warm Thayer-Martin plate or antigen testing for *Neisseria gonorrhoeae*
  - Viral cultures for HSV and so forth, though expensive and often not indicated.
  - Monospot for EBV

Test Interpretation
Bacitracin disk sensitivity of hemolytic colonies suggests group A β-hemolytic streptococcus.

 TREATMENT

GENERAL MEASURES
Conservative therapy recommended for most cases, (unless bacterial etiology suspected):
- Salt water gargles
- Viscous lidocaine (2%) 5 to 10 mL PO q4h swish/spit
- Acetaminophen 10 to 15 mg/kg/dose q4h PRN pain or fever (pediatric). In adults, do not exceed >3 g per day.

- NSAIDs for pain or fever
- Anesthetic lozenges
- Cool-mist humidifier
- Hydration (PO or IV)

Pediatric Considerations
Opioids not recommended due to black box warnings.

MEDICATION
- Antibiotics (particularly penicillin) are chosen primarily to prevent rheumatic fever and peritonsillar abscess (quinsy) in streptococcal infections, though supportive data lacking.
  - 60–70% primary care visits by children with pharyngitis result in antibiotic prescriptions (4). Empiric therapy results in overuse of antibiotic.
  - Treatment duration generally 10 days (1)[A]
  - Antibiotics do not reduce risk of poststreptococcal glomerulonephritis.
  - Antibiotics shorten duration of symptoms by approximately 16 hours (5)
  - Antibiotics may prevent pharyngitis/fever by day 3 (NNT 4 if GAS-positive, 6.5 if GAS-negative, 14.4 if untested) (5)[A].
- Ulcers related to autoimmune diseases usually require systemic or intralesional injectable steroids.
- HIV-related ulcers are due to decreasing counts of CD4 and respond when patients' CD4 titers increase.

First Line
The following first-line therapies are recommended by 2012 IDSA guidelines (1)[A]:

- Penicillin V: children (<27 kg): 250 mg PO TID (BID dosing sufficient if good compliance); adolescents and adults (>27 kg): 250 mg PO QID or 500 mg PO BID
- Amoxicillin: 50 mg/kg PO once daily (max 1,000 mg/dose or 25 mg/kg PO BID (max = 500 mg/dose).

ALERT
Use with caution if diagnosis is unclear because using amoxicillin with EBV infection may induce rash.

- Penicillin G: children (<27 kg): 600,000 units IM injection times one dose; adolescents/adults (≥27 kg): 1.2 million units IM injection times one dose.

Second Line
- If no history of anaphylactic penicillin allergy:
  - Cephalexin 20 mg/kg PO BID or (children) 25 to 50 mg/kg/day divided BID or (adults) 1000 mg PO QID (max = 4 g/day)
  - Cefadroxil 30 mg/kg PO once daily (max = 1 g/day)
- If history of anaphylactic penicillin allergy:
  - Azithromycin 12 mg/kg PO once daily for 5 days (max = 500 mg/dose)
  - Clarithromycin 7.5 mg/kg PO BID (max = 250 mg/dose) or (adults) 250 to 500 mg PO BID
  - Clindamycin 7 mg/kg PO TID (max = 300 mg/dose) or (children) 10 to 30 mg/kg/day PO divided TID–QID or (adults) 150 to 450 mg PO TID–QID
- Penicillin is the most documented treatment to prevent rheumatic sequelae, but cephalosporins have a lower rate of antimicrobial failure against streptococcal pharyngitis.

- Newer macrolides, though effective against streptococcal pharyngitis, are more expensive and unproven at preventing rheumatic complications.
- Macrolide-resistant strains of GAS are currently <10% in the United States but more prevalent worldwide.

- IDSA recommends against adjunctive corticosteroid therapy (1)[B].

ISSUES FOR REFERRAL
Each GAS-confirmed episode should be documented to support the need for future tonsillectomy and adenoidectomy.

 ONGOING CARE

FOLLOW-UP RECOMMENDATIONS
- Patient should complete a full course of antibiotic therapy, regardless of symptom response.
- Patients are generally noninfectious after 24 hours of antibiotics.

- Follow-up culture for group A strep is not recommended (1)[A].

DIET
As tolerated. Encourage the consumption of fluids.

PROGNOSIS
- Streptococcal pharyngitis runs a 5- to 7-day course with peak fever at 2 to 3 days.
- Symptoms will resolve spontaneously without treatment, but rheumatic complications are still possible.

COMPLICATIONS
- Rheumatic fever (e.g., carditis, valve disease, arthritis)
- Poststreptococcal glomerulonephritis
- Peritonsillar abscess (a.k.a. quinsy tonsillitis): considered a clinical diagnosis and does not warrant ultrasound/computed tomography. Will generally require percutaneous/transoral drainage. Surgery may also involve a quinsy tonsillectomy, which is merely a tonsillectomy in the setting of acute infection. This is generally not advocated unless for special circumstances, as most otolaryngologists recommend infectious resolution before surgery.
- Acute airway compromise (rare) can typically be bypassed with nasal trumpets. Consult anesthesiologist/otolaryngologist.

- Repeated episodes of GAS pharyngitis may represent recurrent viral infections in a chronic pharyngeal GAS carrier (1)[B]. IDSA recommends against repeated diagnostic efforts/antibiotic therapy in a known chronic pharyngeal GAS carrier, as they are seldom contagious or at risk for serious complications.
- Evidence remains controversial for tonsillectomy as a treatment for chronic/recurrent throat infections. IDSA recommends against it (1)[A] while the American Academy of Otolaryngology proposes tonsillectomy only if there is also one of the following: fever, cervical adenopathy, tonsillar exudate, or confirmed GAS (6)[C]

REFERENCES

1. Shulman ST, Bisno AL, Clegg HW, et al. Clinical practice guideline for the diagnosis and management of group A streptococcal pharyngitis: 2012 update by the Infectious Diseases Society of America. *Clin Infect Dis.* 2012;55(10):1279–1282.
2. Fine AM, Nizet V, Mandl KD. Large-scale validation of the Centor and McIsaac scores to predict group A streptococcal pharyngitis. *Arch Intern Med.* 2012;172(11):847–852.
3. Lean WL, Arnup S, Danchin M, et al. Rapid diagnostic tests for group A streptococcal pharyngitis: a meta-analysis. *Pediatrics.* 2014;134(4):771–881.
4. Cohen CF, Cohen R, Levy C, et al. Selective testing strategies for diagnosing group A streptococcal infection in children with pharyngitis: a systematic review and prospective multicentre external validation study. *CMAJ.* 2015;187(1):23–32.
5. Spinks A, Glasziou PP, Del Mar CB. Antibiotics for sore throat. *Cochrane Database Syst Rev.* 2013;(11):CD000023.
6. Baugh RF, Archer SM, Mitchell RB, et al. Clinical practice guideline: tonsillectomy in children. *Otolaryngol Head Neck Surg.* 2011;144(1)(Suppl):S1–S30.

ADDITIONAL READING

- Kocher JJ, Selby TD. Antibiotics for sore throat. *Am Fam Physician.* 2014;90(1):23–24.
- Weber R. Pharyngitis. *Prim Care.* 2014;41(1):91–98.
- Zoorob R, Sidani MA, Fremont RD, et al. Antibiotic use in acute upper respiratory tract infections. *Am Fam Physician.* 2012;86(9):817–822.

 SEE ALSO

- Herpes Simplex; Infectious Mononucleosis, Epstein-Barr Virus Infections; Rheumatic Fever
- Algorithm: Pharyngitis

 CODES

ICD10
- J02.9 Acute pharyngitis, unspecified
- J02.0 Streptococcal pharyngitis
- J31.2 Chronic pharyngitis

CLINICAL PEARLS

- Most cases of pharyngitis are viral and do not require antibiotics.
- Risk of undiagnosed group A streptococcal infection is rheumatic sequelae—a rare complication.
- Use Modified Centor Score to guide testing and treatment.
- Penicillin is still first-line therapy for group A streptococcal infection.

PILONIDAL DISEASE

Tam Nguyen, MD, FAAFP

 BASICS

DESCRIPTION
- Pilonidal disease results from an abscess, or sinus tract, in the upper part of the natal (gluteal) cleft.
- Synonym(s): jeep disease

EPIDEMIOLOGY
Incidence
- 16 to 26/100,000 per year
- Predominant sex: male > female (3 to 4:1)
- Predominant age: 2nd to 3rd decades, rare >45 years
- Ethnic consideration: whites > blacks > Asians

Prevalence
Surgical procedures show male:female ratio of 4:1, yet incidence data are 10:1.

ETIOLOGY AND PATHOPHYSIOLOGY
Pilonidal means "nest of hair"; hair in the natal cleft allows hair to be drawn into the deeper tissues via negative pressure caused by movement of the buttocks (50%); follicular occlusion from stretching, and blocking of pores with debris (50%).
- Inflammation of SC gluteal tissues with secondary infection and sinus tract formation
- Polymicrobial, likely from enteric pathogens given proximity to anorectal contamination

Genetics
- Congenital dimple in the natal cleft/spina bifida occulta
- Follicular-occluding tetrad: acne conglobata, dissecting cellulitis, hidradenitis suppurativa, pilonidal

RISK FACTORS
- Sedentary/prolonged sitting
- Excessive body hair
- Obesity/increased sacrococcygeal fold thickness
- Congenital natal dimple
- Trauma to coccyx

GENERAL PREVENTION
- Weight loss
- Trim hair in/around gluteal cleft weekly
- Hygiene
- Ingrown hair prevention/follicle unblocking

 DIAGNOSIS

HISTORY
Three distinct clinical presentations
- Asymptomatic: painless cyst or sinus at the top of the gluteal cleft
- Acute abscess: severe pain, swelling, discharge from the top of the gluteal cleft that may or may not have drained spontaneously
- Chronic abscess: persistent drainage from a sinus tract at the top of the gluteal cleft

PHYSICAL EXAM
- Common: inflamed cystic mass at the top of the gluteal cleft with limited surrounding erythema ± drainage or a sinus tract
- Less common: significant cellulitis of the surrounding tissues near the gluteal cleft

DIFFERENTIAL DIAGNOSIS
- Furunculosis
- Hidradenitis suppurativa
- Anal fistula
- Perirectal abscess
- Crohn disease

DIAGNOSTIC TESTS & INTERPRETATION
Initial Tests (lab, imaging)
- Consider CBC and wound culture but generally not necessary for less-severe infections.
- MRI might be considered to differentiate between perirectal abscess and pilonidal disease.

 TREATMENT

GENERAL MEASURES
Shave area; remove hair from crypts weekly.

MEDICATION
- Antibiotics not indicated unless there is significant cellulitis (1).
- If antibiotics are needed, a culture to direct therapy might be useful.
- Cefazolin plus metronidazole or amoxicillin-clavulanate are often used empirically if cellulitis is suspected.

ISSUES FOR REFERRAL
- Patients who cannot comply with frequent dressing changes required after incision and drainage (I&D)
- Patients who have recurrence after I&D
- Patients who have complex disease with multiple sinus tracts

ADDITIONAL THERAPIES
- I&D with only enough packing to allow the cyst to drain; overpacking not indicated
- Antibiotics only if significant cellulitis; temporizing, not curative
- Negative pressure wound therapy (2)[A]
- Laser epilation of hair in the gluteal fold (3,4)[B]

SURGERY/OTHER PROCEDURES

Six levels of care based on severity or recurrence of disease; recent innovations in technique are aimed at expediting healing and minimizing recurrence

- I&D, remove hair, curette granulation tissue (5,6)[A].
- Excision of midline "pits" allows drainage of lateral sinus tracts (pit picking) (7,8)[A].
- Pilonidal cystotomy: Insert probe into sinus tract, excise overlying skin, and close wound (7,9)[B].
- Marsupialization: Excise overlying skin and roof of cyst, and suture skin edges to cyst floor (5,10)[B].
- Excision: use of flap closure. No clear benefit for open healing over surgical closure (11)[B]
- Off-midline surgical excision (cleft lift or modified Karydakis procedure): A systematic review showed a clear benefit in favor of off-midline rather than midline wound closure. When closure of pilonidal sinuses is the desired surgical option, off-midline closure should be the standard management (5,7,12)[A].

INPATIENT CONSIDERATIONS

Admission Criteria/Initial Stabilization
- Severe cellulitis
- Large area excision

 ## ONGOING CARE

FOLLOW-UP RECOMMENDATIONS
- Frequent dressing changes required after I&D
- Follow-up wound checks to assess for recurrence.

Patient Monitoring
Monitor for fever, more extensive cellulitis.

PATIENT EDUCATION
- Wash area briskly with washcloth daily.
- Shave the area weekly.
- Remove any embedded hair from the crypt.
- Avoid prolonged sitting.

PROGNOSIS
- Simple I&D has a 55% failure rate; median time to healing is 5 weeks.
- More extensive surgical excisions involve hospital stays and longer time to heal.

COMPLICATIONS
Malignant degeneration is a rare complication of untreated chronic pilonidal disease.

REFERENCES

1. Mavros MN, Mitsikostas PK, Alexiou VG, et al. Antimicrobials as an adjunct to pilonidal disease surgery: a systematic review of the literature. *Eur J Clin Microbiol Infect Dis*. 2013;32(7):851–858.
2. Farrell D, Murphy S. Negative pressure wound therapy for recurrent pilonidal disease: a review of the literature. *J Wound Ostomy Continence Nurs*. 2011;38(4):373–378.
3. Loganathan A, Arsalani Zadeh R, Hartley J. Pilonidal disease: time to reevaluate a common pain in the rear! *Dis Colon Rectum*. 2012;55(4):491–493.
4. Oram Y, Kahraman F, Karincaoğlu Y, et al. Evaluation of 60 patients with pilonidal sinus treated with laser epilation after surgery. *Dermatol Surg*. 2010;36(1):88–91.
5. Humphries AE, Duncan JE. Evaluation and management of pilonidal disease. *Surg Clin North Am*. 2010;90(1):113–124, Table of Contents.
6. Kement M, Oncel M, Kurt N, et al. Sinus excision for the treatment of limited chronic pilonidal disease: results after a medium-term follow-up. *Dis Colon Rectum*. 2006;49(11):1758–1762.
7. Al-Khamis A, McCallum I, King PM, et al. Healing by primary versus secondary intention after surgical treatment for pilonidal sinus. *Cochrane Database Syst Rev*. 2010;(1):CD006213.
8. Iesalnieks I, Deimel S, Kienle K, et al. Pit-picking surgery for pilonidal disease [in German]. *Chirurg*. 2011;82(10):927–931.
9. da Silva JH. Pilonidal cyst: cause and treatment. *Dis Colon Rectum*. 2000;43(8):1146–1156.
10. Aydede H, Erhan Y, Sakarya A, et al. Comparison of three methods in surgical treatment of pilonidal disease. *ANZ J Surg*. 2001;71(6):362–364.
11. Washer JD, Smith DE, Carman ME, et al. Gluteal fascial advancement: an innovative, effective method for treating pilonidal disease. *Am Surg*. 2010;76(2):154–156.
12. Ates M, Dirican A, Sarac M, et al. Short and long-term results of the Karydakis flap versus the Limberg flap for treating pilonidal sinus disease: a prospective randomized study. *Am J Surg*. 2011;202(5):568–573.

ADDITIONAL READING

- Aygen E, Arslan K, Dogru O, et al. Crystallized phenol in nonoperative treatment of previously operated, recurrent pilonidal disease. *Dis Colon Rectum*. 2010;53(6):932–935.
- Bradley L. Pilonidal sinus disease: a review. Part one. *J Wound Care*. 2010;19(11):504–508.
- Harlak A, Mentes O, Kilic S, et al. Sacrococcygeal pilonidal disease: analysis of previously proposed risk factors. *Clinics (Sao Paulo)*. 2010;65(2):125–131.
- Rao MM, Zawislak W, Kennedy R, et al. A prospective randomised study comparing two treatment modalities for chronic pilonidal sinus with a 5-year follow-up. *Int J Colorectal Dis*. 2010;25(3):395–400.
- Theodoropoulos GE, Vlahos K, Lazaris AC, et al. Modified Bascom's asymmetric midgluteal cleft closure technique for recurrent pilonidal disease: early experience in a military hospital. *Dis Colon Rectum*. 2003;46(9):1286–1291.

 ## CODES

ICD10
- L05.91 Pilonidal cyst without abscess
- L05.92 Pilonidal sinus without abscess
- L05.01 Pilonidal cyst with abscess

CLINICAL PEARLS

- Avoid prolonged sitting.
- Lose weight.
- Trim hair in gluteal cleft weekly.
- Refer recurring infections for more definitive surgical management.

PINWORMS

Jonathan MacClements, MD, FAAFP

BASICS

DESCRIPTION
- Intestinal infection with *Enterobius vermicularis*
  - Characterized by perineal and perianal itching
  - Usually worse at night
- System(s) affected: gastrointestinal; skin/exocrine
- Synonym(s): enterobiasis

EPIDEMIOLOGY
Predominant age: 5 to 14 years

Prevalence
- Most common helminthic infection in the United States
  - 20 to 42 million people harbor the parasite
- ~30% of children are infected worldwide.

Pediatric Considerations
More common in children, who are more likely to become reinfected.

ETIOLOGY AND PATHOPHYSIOLOGY
- Small white worms (2 to 13 mm) inhabit the cecum, appendix, and adjacent portions of the ascending colon following ingestion.
- Female worms migrate to the perineal areas at night to deposit eggs; this causes local irritation and itching.
- Scratching leads to autoingestion of the eggs and continuation of pinworm's life cycle within the host. Eggs incubate 1 to 2 months in the host small intestine. When mature, female pinworms migrate to the colon where they lay eggs around the anus at night and the lifecycle continues.
- Infestation by the intestinal nematode *E. vermicularis*

RISK FACTORS
- Institutionalization
- Crowded living conditions
- Poor hygiene
- Warm climate
- Handling of infected children's clothing or bedding

GENERAL PREVENTION
- Hand hygiene, especially after bowel movements
- Clip and maintain short fingernails.
- Wash anus and genitals at least once a day, preferably during shower.
- Avoid scratching anus and putting fingers near nose (pinworm eggs can also be inhaled) or mouth.

COMMONLY ASSOCIATED CONDITIONS
Pruritus ani

DIAGNOSIS

HISTORY
Many patients are asymptomatic. Common symptoms include the following:
- Perianal or perineal itching
- Vulvovaginitis
- Dysuria
- Abdominal pain (rare)
- Insomnia (typically due to pruritus)

PHYSICAL EXAM
Perineal and perianal exam. Particularly in early morning to look for evidence of migrating worms.

DIFFERENTIAL DIAGNOSIS
- Idiopathic pruritus ani (1)[A]
- Atopic dermatitis, contact dermatitis
- Psoriasis; lichen planus
- Human papillomavirus (HPV)
- Herpes simplex virus (HSV)
- Fungal infections; erythrasma
- Scabies
- Vaginitis; hemorrhoids

DIAGNOSTIC TESTS & INTERPRETATION
- Adhesive tape test (2)[A]
  - Place cellophane tape on the perianal skin in the early morning before bathing and affixed to a microscope slide to look for pinworm eggs.
  - If performed on three consecutive mornings, this test has 90% sensitivity
  - Alternatively, anal swabs or a pinworm paddle coated with adhesive material can be useful.
  - Scrapings from under fingernails of affected individuals can reveal pinworm eggs.
- Digital rectal exam with saline slide preparation of stool on gloved finger
- Stool samples are not helpful.
- *Routine stool examination for ova and parasites is positive in only 10–15% of infected patients.*

Test Interpretation
Identification of ova on low-power microscopy or direct visualization of the female worm (10-mm long); ova are asymmetric, flat on one side, and measure $56 \times 27 \ \mu m$.

TREATMENT

MEDICATION
First Line
- Treatment options include:
  - Mebendazole (Vermox): chewable 100-mg tablet as a single dose in adults and children >2 years of age; may repeat in 2 to 3 weeks; use with caution in children <2 years of age (3,4)[A].
  - Albendazole (Albenza): 400 mg PO as a single dose in adults and children >2 years of age; may repeat in 2 to 3 weeks; 200 mg PO as a single dose repeated in 7 days in children ≤2 years of age (3,4)[A].

– Pyrantel pamoate (Pin-X, Reese's Pinworm Medicine): oral liquid or tablet 11 mg/kg as a single dose in adults and children >2 years of age; maximum dose 1 g. Use with caution in children <2 years of age (3,4)[A].

- Repeat treatment after 2 weeks is often recommended due to the high frequency of reinfection. Refractory cases may (rarely) require retreatment every 2 weeks for 4 to 6 cycles.
- All symptomatic family members should be treated.

Pregnancy Considerations

Avoid drug therapy in pregnancy. Treat after delivery. Breastfeeding is OK during mebendazole therapy (3,4)[A].

 ## ONGOING CARE

FOLLOW-UP RECOMMENDATIONS

Unnecessary unless symptoms recur after initial therapy

PATIENT EDUCATION

- Take medicine with food.
- Practice good hygiene: hand washing and perianal hygiene; particularly after bowel movements
- Encourage frequent and careful hand washing.
- Clip fingernails.
- Wash clothing and bedding after diagnosis to prevent reinfection. Do not shake linen and clothing before laundering because this may spread the eggs.
- Do not share washcloths.
- Do not allow children to cobathe during treatment and for 2 weeks after; showering is preferred.

PROGNOSIS

- Asymptomatic carriers are common.
- Drug therapy is 90% curative.
- Reinfection is common, especially among children.

COMPLICATIONS

- Perianal scratching may lead to bacterial superinfection.
- Females: vulvovaginitis, urethritis, endometritis, and salpingitis (4,5)[A]
- UTIs
- Rarely, ectopic disease with granulomas of the pelvis, genitourinary tract, and appendix

REFERENCES

1. Stermer E, Sukhotnic I, Shaoul R. Pruritus ani: an approach to an itching condition. *J Pediatr Gastroenterol Nutr*. 2009;48(5):513–516.
2. Kucik CJ, Martin GL, Sortor BV. Common intestinal parasites. *Am Fam Physician*. 2004;69(5):1161–1168.
3. Enterobius vermicularis. In: *Drugs for Parasitic Infections. Treatment guidelines from The Medical Letter*. New Rochelle, NY: The Medical Letter, Inc.; 2010;8(Suppl). www.cdc.gov/parasites/pinworm/health_professionals/index.html
4. Dennie J, Grover SR. Distressing perineal and vaginal pain in prepubescent girls: an aetiology. *J Paediatr Child Health*. 2013;49(2):138–140.
5. Kashyap B, Samantray JC, Kumar S, et al. Recurrent paediatric pinworm infection of the vagina as a potential reservoir for *Enterobius vermicularis*. *J Helminthol*. 2014;88(3):381–383.

ADDITIONAL READING

Hamblin J, Connor PD. Pinworms in pregnancy. *J Am Board Fam Pract*. 1995;8(4):321–324.

 ## SEE ALSO

Pruritus Ani

 ## CODES

ICD10

B80 Enterobiasis

CLINICAL PEARLS

- Nocturnal or early morning perianal itch with restless sleep or insomnia (particularly in children), is hallmark of symptomatic pinworm infection.
- Treatment includes of mebendazole, albendazole, or pyrantel pamoate.
- Treat close contacts.
- Retreatment after 2 weeks is typically recommended.

PITUITARY ADENOMA

Anup K. Sabharwal, MD, MBA, FACE, CCD • Lewis S. Blevins, Jr., MD

BASICS

DESCRIPTION
Typically benign, slow-growing tumors that arise from cells in the pituitary gland
- Pituitary adenomas have been identified as the third most frequent intracranial tumor; accounts for 10–25%.
- Subtypes (hormonal): prolactinoma (PRL) 50%, non-functioning pituitary adenomas 30%, somatotroph adenoma (growth hormone [GH]) 15–20%, corticotroph adenoma (adrenocorticotrophic hormone [ACTH]) 5–10%, thyrotroph adenoma (thyroid-stimulating hormone [TSH]) <1%, gonadotropinoma (luteinizing hormone/follicle-stimulating hormone [LH/FSH]), mixed
- Defined as microadenoma <10 mm and macroadenoma ≥10 mm
- May secrete hormones and/or cause mass effects

EPIDEMIOLOGY
- Predominant age: Age increases incidence.
- Predominant sex: female > male (3:2) for microadenomas (often delayed diagnosis in men)

Incidence
- Autopsy studies have found microadenomas in 3–27% and macroadenomas in <0.5% of people without any pituitary disorders.
- MRI scans illustrate abnormalities consistent with pituitary adenoma in 1/10 persons.
- Clinically apparent pituitary tumors are seen in 18/100,000 persons.

ETIOLOGY AND PATHOPHYSIOLOGY
- Monoclonal adenohypophysial cell growth
- Hormonal effects of functional microadenomas often prompt diagnosis before mass effect.
- Prolactin increased by functional prolactinomas or inhibited dopaminergic suppression by stalk effect

Genetics
- Carney complex
- Familial isolated pituitary adenomas: ~15% have mutations in the aryl hydrocarbon receptor–interacting protein gene (AIP); present at a younger age and are larger in size (1)
- McCune-Albright syndrome
- Multiple endocrine neoplasia type 1 (MEN1)–like phenotype (MEN4): germline mutation in the cyclin-dependent kinase inhibitor 1B (CDKN1B) (1)

RISK FACTORS
Multiple endocrine neoplasias

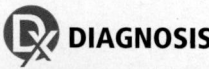
DIAGNOSIS

HISTORY
- Common
  - Hyperprolactinemia: infertility, amenorrhea, galactorrhea, gynecomastia, impotence
  - Headache (sellar expansion)
  - Visual disturbances: bitemporal hemianopsia
- Less common
  - Hypersomatotropinemia: acromegaly (coarse facial features, hand/foot swelling, carpal tunnel syndrome, hyperhidrosis, left ventricular hypertrophy)
  - Hyposomatotropinemia: failure to thrive (FTT) (children), asymptomatic (adults)
  - Intracranial pressure (ICP) elevation: headache, nausea, seizures

- Hypercorticotropinemia: Cushing disease (supraclavicular/dorsocervical fat pad thickening, moon face, hirsutism, acne, plethora, abdominal striae, centripetal obesity with thin limbs, easy bruising and bleeding, hyperglycemia)
- Rare
  - Apoplexy: headache, sudden collapse
  - Secondary hyperthyroidism: palpitations, diaphoresis, heat intolerance, diarrhea
  - Secondary adrenal insufficiency: weakness, irritability, anorexia, nausea/vomiting
- Hypothalamic compression: temperature, thirst/appetite disorders

PHYSICAL EXAM
- Common
  - Visual disturbances: bitemporal hemianopsia
  - Hyperprolactinemia: hypogonadism, galactorrhea, gynecomastia
  - Hypersomatotropinemia: acromegaly (coarse features, hand/foot swelling, diaphoresis)
  - Hyposomatotropinemia: FTT (children)
- Less common
  - ICP elevation: papilledema, dementia
  - Cushing disease: centripetal obesity, supraclavicular fat pad thickening, moon face, hirsutism, acne
- Rare
  - Apoplexy: hypotension, hypoglycemia, tachycardia, oliguria
  - Secondary hyperthyroidism: tachycardia, tachypnea, diaphoresis, warm/moist skin, tremor
  - Adrenal crisis: orthostatic hypotension
- Hypothalamic compression: temperature dysregulation, obesity, increased urination

DIFFERENTIAL DIAGNOSIS
Pituitary hyperplasia (e.g., pregnancy, primary hypothyroidism, menopause), Rathke cleft cyst, granulomatous disease (e.g., tuberculosis), lymphocytic hypophysitis, metastatic tumor, germinoma, craniopharyngioma

DIAGNOSTIC TESTS & INTERPRETATION
Select based on dysfunction(s) suspected
- Somatotrophic (GH secreting: 40 to 130/million)
  - Acromegaly/hypersomatotropinemia: serum IGF-1 elevated; oral glucose tolerance test with GH given at 0, 30, and 60 minutes (normally suppresses GH to <1 g/L)
  - Hyposomatotropinemia: low growth hormone–releasing hormone response
- Corticotropic
  - Cushing disease/hypercorticotropinemia
  - 24-hour urinary-free cortisol >50 μg
  - Overnight low-dose dexamethasone suppression test (DMST): normal free plasma cortisol (FPC) >1.8 μg/dL at 8 AM (after 1 mg given at 11 PM on night prior)
  - ACTH level assay (if DMST results abnormal): <20 pg/mL = adrenal tumor; ≥20 pg/mL = ectopic/pituitary source
  - Hypocorticotropinemia/secondary glucocorticoid deficiency: high-dose corticotropin stimulation test: FPC <10 g/dL at baseline, with an increase of <25% 1 hour after 250 μg; metyrapone test: 11-deoxycortisol <150 ng/L after 2 g given (prepare to give steroids because test may worsen insufficiency)
- Gonadotrophic/hypogonadotropinism: gonadotropin-releasing hormone stimulation of LH/FSH blunted in pituitary hypergonadism but increased in primary hypogonadism

- Lactotrophic (prolactin secreting): hyperprolactinemia: serum PRL >20 ng/mL
- Thyrotrophic (TSH secreting): hyper-/hypothyroidism: TSH and free T4 both increased for pituitary hyperthyroidism and both decreased for pituitary hypothyroidism

Initial Tests (lab, imaging)
- A typical panel for asymptomatic tumors: prolactin, GH, IGF-1, ACTH, 24-hour urinary-free cortisol or overnight DMST, β-HCG, FSH, LH, TSH, free T4
- Maintain the same GH and IGF-1 through patient management (2)[C].
- Screening for AIP mutations may be offered to families of patients with pituitary adenoma, where available.
- MRI preferred (>90% sensitivity and specificity) after biochemically confirmed
- Octreotide scintigraphy is useful in identifying tumors with somatostatin receptors (2)[B].

Diagnostic Procedures/Other
Inferior petrosal sinus sampling: ACTH sampled from inferior petrosal sinuses to distinguish Cushing disease (pituitary source) from ectopic ACTH

Test Interpretation
- Cell types identified by immunohistochemistry
- Light microscope: eosinophilic (GH, PRL), basophilic (FSH/LH, TSH, ACTH), chromophobic

TREATMENT

Medical therapy is primary therapy for prolactinomas and adjunct for other tumors.

MEDICATION
First Line
- Hyperprolactinemia: Dopamine agonists increase dopaminergic suppression of PRL.
  - Cabergoline (Dostinex): D2 receptor–specific
    - Initial dose: 0.25 mg PO once or twice weekly
    - Maintenance dose: Increase q4wk by 0.25 mg 2 times/week per PRL (max 2 mg/week).
    - Contraindications: hypersensitivity (ergots), uncontrolled hypertension (HTN), pregnancy
    - Precautions: caution with liver impairment
    - Interactions: may be inhibited by tricyclic antidepressants, phenothiazines, opiates
    - Adverse reactions: orthostatic hypotension, vertigo, dyspepsia, hot flashes
  - Bromocriptine (Parlodel): D2 receptor–specific
    - Initial dose: 1.25 to 2.5 mg PO daily (give with food)
    - Maintenance dose: increase by 2.5 mg/day q2–7d (max 15 mg/day)
    - Contraindications: hypersensitivity (ergots), uncontrolled HTN, pregnancy; preferred over cabergoline if required
    - Precautions: caution with liver impairment
    - Interactions: may be inhibited by tricyclic antidepressants, phenothiazines, opiates
    - Adverse reactions: orthostatic hypotension, seizures, hallucinations, stroke, myocardial infarction
- Somatotropinoma
  - Long-acting analogues of somatostatin (Sandostatin LAR and lanreotide Autogel)
    - Sandostatin LAR: 20 mg q28d (2)[A]; lanreotide Autogel 90 mg q28d; titrate per package insert.
    - Contraindication: hypersensitivity

○ Precautions: caution with biliary, thyroid, cardiac, liver, or kidney disease
○ Interactions: pimozide increases risk of QT prolongation; variable effects with β-blockers, diuretics, oral glycemic agents
○ Adverse reactions: ascending cholangitis, arrhythmias, congestive heart failure, glycemic instability
○ More effective as adjuvant than as primary treatment for somatotropinomas
○ Consider use of somatostatin analogue or pegvisomant in patients with severe residual disease (2)[A].
○ Consider use of cabergoline in patients with mild residual disease (3)[B].

– Pegvisomant (Somavert): GH receptor antagonist
  ○ Initial dose: 40 mg SC × 1, then 10 mg daily and titrate by 5 mg every 4 to 6 weeks based on IGF-1 levels (max 30 mg/day maintenance dose)
  ○ Contraindication: hypersensitivity
  ○ Precautions: caution if GH-secreting tumors, diabetes mellitus, impaired liver function
  ○ Interactions: NSAIDs, opiates, insulins, oral glycemic agents
  ○ Adverse reactions: hepatitis, tumor growth, GH secretion

• Corticotropinemia: peripheral inhibitors
  – Mitotane (Lysodren)
    ○ Initial dose: 2 to 6 g/day divided PO TID (max 19 g/day)
    ○ Maintenance dose: 2 to 16 g TID
    ○ Contraindication: hypersensitivity
    ○ Precautions: caution with liver dysfunction and brain damage
    ○ Interactions: contraindicated with rotavirus vaccine; caution with other vaccines
    ○ Adverse reactions: HTN, orthostatic hypotension, hemorrhagic cystitis, rash
  – Ketoconazole
    ○ Dosing: 200 mg PO TID (max 1,200 mg/day)
    ○ Contraindications: hypersensitivity, achlorhydria, fungal meningitis, impaired liver function
    ○ Precautions: caution with liver dysfunction
    ○ Interactions: contraindicated with dronedarone, methadone, statins, pimozide, sirolimus; caution with other antifungals
    ○ Adverse reactions: adrenal insufficiency, thrombocytopenia, hepatic failure, hepatotoxicity, anaphylaxis, leukopenia, hemolytic anemia
  – Signifor (pasireotide)
    ○ Dosing: initially, 0.6 to 0.9 mg twice daily, then 0.3 to 0.9 mg twice daily
    ○ Contraindication: none
    ○ Precautions: hypocortisolism, hyperglycemia, bradycardia or QT prolongation, liver test elevations, cholelithiasis, and other pituitary hormone deficiencies
  – Korlym (mifepristone):
    ○ Dosing: Administer PO once daily with a meal. The recommended starting dose is 300 mg once daily. Not to exceed 600 mg daily in renal impairment
  – Contraindication: pregnancy, use of simvastatin or lovastatin and CYP3A substrates with narrow therapeutic range, concurrent long-term corticosteroid use, women with history of unexplained vaginal bleeding, women with endometrial hyperplasia with atypia or endometrial carcinoma
  – Precautions: adrenal insufficiency, hypokalemia, vaginal bleeding and endometrial changes, QT interval prolongation, use of strong CYP3A inhibitors

– Interactions: potential interactions with drugs metabolized by CYP3A, CYP2C8/9, CYP2B6, and hormonal contraceptives. Nursing mothers should discontinue drug or discontinue nursing.
– Adverse reactions: most common adverse reactions in Cushing syndrome (≥20%): nausea, fatigue, headache, decreased blood potassium, arthralgia, vomiting, peripheral edema, HTN, dizziness, decreased appetite, endometrial hypertrophy
• Gonadotropinemia
  – Bromocriptine: See earlier discussion.
• Thyrotropinemia
  – Somatostatin analogues: See earlier discussion.

Second Line
• Corticotropinemia: peripheral inhibitors
  – Metyrapone
    ○ Dose: 250 mg PO QID
    ○ Contraindication: porphyria
    ○ Precautions: caution in liver/thyroid disease
    ○ Interactions: Dilantin increases metabolism.
    ○ Adverse reactions: nausea, hypotension
• Gonadotropinemia
  – Octreotide: See earlier discussion.

ISSUES FOR REFERRAL
• Neurosurgery consultation for symptomatic tumors (except for prolactinoma)
• Ophthalmologist evaluation prior to surgery

ADDITIONAL THERAPIES
• Fractionated radiotherapy: often effective as adjunctive when surgery is inadequate (3)[B]
• Stereotactic radiosurgery: alternative to surgery in high-risk patients or as adjunct (3)[B]

SURGERY/OTHER PROCEDURES
• Most are now done endoscopically via translabial/transsphenoidal approach (4)[A].

• Indications: symptoms or treatment-resistant
• Follow-up: serial neurologic/hormonal evaluations to evaluate complications (e.g., diabetes insipidus, CNS damage) and need for more treatment
• Remission rates: 72–87% for microadenoma but only 50–56% for macroadenomas

INPATIENT CONSIDERATIONS
Admission Criteria/Initial Stabilization
Outpatient management unless apoplexy or adrenal crisis

• Treat pituitary apoplexy immediately to prevent death (see "Complications") (4)[A].

• Consider stress-dose steroids in frail or hemodynamically unstable patients.
• Maintain BP with fluids and/or pressor agents.
• Check serum sodium, serum osmolality, and urine specific gravity if polyuric or electrolytes are imbalanced.
• Contact neurosurgery.

IV Fluids
• Diabetes insipidus: hyposmolar IV fluids
• Adrenal crisis: normal saline

Nursing
• Pituitary apoplexy: Monitor inputs/outputs (I/Os), central venous pressure and ICP, and do frequent neurologic checks.
• Adrenal crisis: Monitor BP and I/Os.

Discharge Criteria
Keep as inpatient postoperatively until diabetes insipidus and/or adrenal insufficiency is managed.

 ONGOING CARE

FOLLOW-UP RECOMMENDATIONS
Patient Monitoring
• Follow-up MRIs at 6 and 12 months after discharge
• Involved hormone(s) are followed postoperatively, especially after radiation because hypopituitarism may develop 10 to 15 years after treatment.

PROGNOSIS
Depends on type, size, symptoms, therapy

COMPLICATIONS
• Postoperative diabetes insipidus and/or hypogonadism (usually transient/common)
• Pituitary apoplexy (acute/uncommon): acute hemorrhagic pituitary infarction; adrenal crisis with severe headache; surgical decompression required to prevent shock, coma, and death
• Nelson syndrome (subacute/uncommon): rapid adenoma growth postadrenalectomy
• Pituitary hormone insufficiency (chronic/uncommon): often years after treatment
• Optic nerve neuropathy and brain necrosis after >60 Gy radiotherapy (chronic/rare)

REFERENCES
1. Georgitsi M, Raitila A, Karhu A , et al. Molecular diagnosis of pituitary adenoma predisposition caused by aryl hydrocarbon receptor-interacting protein gene mutations. *Proc Natl Acad Sci U S A.* 2007;104(10):4101–4105.
2. Tichomirowa MA, Daly AF, Beckers A. Treatment of pituitary tumors: somatostatin. *Endocrine.* 2005;28(1):93–100.
3. Mondok A, Szeifert GT, Mayer A, et al. Treatment of pituitary tumors: radiation. *Endocrine.* 2005;28(1): 77–85.
4. Buchfelder M. Treatment of pituitary tumors: surgery. *Endocrine.* 2005;28(1):67–75.

 SEE ALSO

Cushing Disease and Cushing Syndrome; Galactorrhea

 CODES

ICD10
D35.2 Benign neoplasm of pituitary gland

CLINICAL PEARLS
• An incidentaloma is an asymptomatic microadenoma found on imaging. General labs include PRL, GH, IGF-1, ACTH, 24-hour urinary-free cortisol/overnight DMST, β-subunit FSH, LH, TSH, and free T₄. Obtain follow-up MRIs at 6 and 12 months if normal, but consult endocrinology if not.
• Initial treatment selected for symptomatic pituitary adenoma includes a dopamine agonist for prolactinomas and surgical resection for all others.
• Pituitary apoplexy is a rapid hemorrhagic pituitary infarction due to compression of the blood supply. It is fatal within hours unless surgically decompressed.

PLANTAR FASCIITIS

Alan J. Williamson, MD, Lr Col, USAF, MC • Amber C. Taylor, MD

BASICS

DESCRIPTION
- Degenerative change of plantar fascia at origin on medial tuberosity of calcaneus
- Pain on plantar surface, usually at calcaneal insertion of plantar fascia upon weight bearing, especially in morning or on initiation of walking after prolonged rest

EPIDEMIOLOGY
Prevalence
- Lifetime: 10–15% of population
- Data suggest persistence with BMI >30.
- Condition is typically self-limiting, resolving within 10 months.

ETIOLOGY AND PATHOPHYSIOLOGY
- Repetitive microtrauma and collagen degeneration of plantar fascia
- Chronic degenerative change (-osis/-opathy rather than -itis) of plantar fascia generally at insertion on medial tuberosity of calcaneus

RISK FACTORS
- Dancers, runners, court sport athletes
- Obesity (BMI >30)
- Pes planus (flat feet), pes cavus (high arch), overpronation, leg length discrepancy
- Occupations with prolonged standing, especially on hard surfaces (nurses, letter carriers, warehouse/factory workers)
- Female, pregnancy
- Age (>40 to 60 years)
- Hamstring, calf tightness
- Decreased ankle range of motion in dorsiflexion (tight heel cord; <15 degrees of dorsiflexion)
- Systemic connective tissue disorders

GENERAL PREVENTION
- Maintain normal body weight.
- Avoid prolonged standing on bare feet, sandals, or slippers.
- Avoid training errors (increasing intensity, distance, duration, and frequency of high-impact activities too rapidly).
- Proper footwear (appropriate cushioning and arch support)
- Runners should replace footwear after every 250 to 500 miles.
- Avoid overtraining.

COMMONLY ASSOCIATED CONDITIONS
- Usually isolated
- Heel spurs common but not a marker of severity
- Posterior tibial neuropathy

DIAGNOSIS

HISTORY
- Pain on plantar surface of foot, usually at fascial insertion at calcaneus (medial calcaneal tubercle), but can have pain anywhere along length of plantar fascia
- Pain is typically worse with first few steps in the morning or after prolonged rest (poststatic dyskinesia).
- Pain typically improves after first few steps only to recur toward the end of the day.
- Pain can be dull and constant in chronic plantar fasciitis.
- Pain with prolonged ambulation or standing
- Limp with excessive toe walking
- Numbness and burning of medial hindfoot when associated with posterior tibial nerve compression

PHYSICAL EXAM
- Point tenderness on medial tuberosity of calcaneus at insertion of plantar fascia
- Pain along plantar fascia with dorsiflexion of foot
- Windlass test: pain with passive dorsiflexion of the toes; high specificity, low sensitivity; sensitivity improves (13.5→31.8%) if performed while standing.
- Decreased passive range of motion with dorsiflexion
- Evaluate for pes planus, pes cavus, and overpronation.
- Loss of heel fat pad suggests heel fat pad syndrome.
- Point tenderness on posterosuperior aspect of heel suggests Achilles tendinopathy.

DIFFERENTIAL DIAGNOSIS
- Calcaneal stress fracture
- Heel fat pad syndrome (painful or atrophic heel pad)
- Longitudinal arch strain
- Nerve entrapment (posterior tibial nerve—tarsal tunnel syndrome, medial calcaneal branch of posterior tibial nerve, abductor digiti quinti)
- Achilles tendinopathy
- Calcaneal contusion
- Plantar calcaneal bursitis
- Tendonitis of posterior tibialis
- Plantar fascia tear
- Calcaneal apophysitis (Sever disease)—adolescents

DIAGNOSTIC TESTS & INTERPRETATION
- None necessary; typically a clinical diagnosis
- Consider further imaging only if diagnosis is in question.
- Two radiographic views of foot can rule out fracture, tumor, cyst, periostitis, bony erosions; weight-bearing films preferred
- Ultrasound: hypoechoic at insertion, thickened plantar fascia (≥4 mm)
- MRI can evaluate for other soft tissue etiologies.
- CT or technetium-99 bone scan can rule out calcaneal stress fracture and evaluate for infection.
- Nerve conduction studies can rule out nerve entrapment.

TREATMENT

Nonoperative management is mainstay of treatment.

GENERAL MEASURES
- Supportive footwear with stable midfoot; avoid sandals or walking barefoot.
- Relative rest/activity modification
- Stretching: plantar fascial stretches more effective than Achilles tendon/gastrocnemius-soleus stretches
- Weight reduction if BMI >25
- Orthotics
  - Custom orthotics show no benefit over prefabricated orthotics and are more costly.
  - Improved effectiveness of night splints when used in association with orthotics.
- Strengthen calf and interosseous muscles, using the towel drag/pick-up exercise
- Night splints: can be uncomfortable for the first few nights but generally become less bothersome with time; especially effective with calf and Achilles tightness
- Ice (frozen water bottle roll)
- Massage (golf or tennis ball roll)

MEDICATION
First Line
Adjunct to control pain
- NSAIDs: naproxen 500 mg PO BID *or* ibuprofen 600 to 800 mg PO TID PRN for pain
- Acetaminophen 1,000 mg PO TID PRN for pain

Second Line
None

ISSUES FOR REFERRAL
- Podiatry, surgery: Consider referral if conservative measures fail after 3 to 6 months.
- Consider physical therapy for patient instruction on proper stretching and strengthening techniques.

ADDITIONAL THERAPIES
- Corticosteroid injections (1)[A]

  - Short-term pain relief for up to one month, benefit fades with time
  - Recommend ultrasound guidance when possible.
  - Risk for plantar fascial rupture and calcaneal fat pad atrophy with resultant permanent heel pain
  - Can cause injection and postinjection pain for up to 5 to 7 days

- Extracorporeal shock wave therapy (ESWT) (2,3)[B]

  - Growing body of evidence showing benefit
  - Multiple meta-analyses and systematic reviews show level I evidence of benefit; mixed recommendations on low- versus high-intensity ESWT.
  - Uncomfortable to patients but less risk than injection or surgery
  - Consider prior to surgery and (possibly) prior to steroid injection.
  - Delivery not yet standardized

- Low-dye and calcaneal taping
  - Limited, short-term evidence
  - Less effective in severe cases
- Promising therapies with inconsistent supporting evidence

  - Platelet-rich plasma injections (4)[B]: A systematic review demonstrated PRP improved baseline symptoms and was comparable to prolotherapy and better than corticosteroid injections in the short and long term (up to 12 months).
  - Prolotherapy (4)[B]: Comparable in efficacy to PRP for treatment of baseline symptoms, better than corticosteroid injections.

  - Low-level laser therapy
  - Botulinum toxin (BT) A injection (5)[B]

    ○ RCT comparing steroid injection to BT injection showed similar results in pain reduction and other measures of foot function at 1 month; improvements in these areas persisted at 6 months more so with BT than with steroid injection.
    ○ Randomized, multicenter, double-blind, placebo-controlled study comparing BT injection to placebo showed no statistical difference in pain and global assessment.

  - Radiofrequency nerve ablation (6)[B]: Prospective, RCT with sham treatment and crossover demonstrated efficacy; also, retrospective case series demonstrated benefit at 1 and 2 years after treatment.
  - Myofascial trigger point manual therapy
  - Intralesional autologous blood injection
  - Plantar iontophoresis

SURGERY/OTHER PROCEDURES
- Necessary in <10% of patients
- Recommended if conservative treatment fails after 6 to 12 months and pain is unrelenting.
- Open/endoscopic plantar fasciotomy (less risk and complications with endoscopic technique but requires specialized equipment and skills; is not widely used)
- Calcaneal spur resection
- More likely beneficial in severely obese
- No RCTs support surgery

COMPLEMENTARY & ALTERNATIVE MEDICINE
- Heel cup with magnet has proven ineffective.
- Acupuncture shows limited benefit in a few studies.

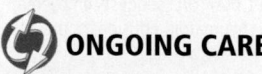 ONGOING CARE

FOLLOW-UP RECOMMENDATIONS
- Ensure patient adherence to proper stretching technique.
- Following 3 to 6 months of unsuccessful conservative treatment, consider additional therapies or referrals.

PATIENT EDUCATION
- Weight reduction if BMI >25
- Proper footwear (adequate cushion and arch support)

- Stretch plantar fascia: Pull toes into dorsiflexion prior to walking after prolonged sitting or sleep
- Ice the foot using a frozen water bottle: Roll foot over bottle for 10 minutes in the morning and after work.
- Massage plantar fascia: Roll foot over a golf ball.
- Strengthen foot muscles: Grab cloth or carpet by plantar flexing the toes.
- Decrease repetitive stress.

PROGNOSIS
- Generally good
- Self-limited (resolves within 2 years) in up to 85–90% of patients

COMPLICATIONS
- Rupture of plantar fascia (more common with repeated corticosteroid injections)
- Chronic pain
- Gait abnormality

REFERENCES

1. Li Z, Yu A, Qi B, et al. Corticosteroid versus placebo injection for plantar fasciitis: a meta-analysis of randomized controlled trials. *Exp Ther Med.* 2015;9(6):2263–2268.
2. Yin MC, Ye J, Yao M, et al. Is extracorporeal shock wave therapy clinical efficacy for relief of chronic, recalcitrant plantar fasciitis? A systematic review and meta-analysis of randomized placebo or active-treatment controlled trials. *Arch Phys Med Rehabil.* 2014;95(8):1585–1593.
3. Speed C. A systematic review of shockwave therapies in soft tissue conditions: focusing on the evidence. *Br J Sports Med.* 2014;48(21):1538–1542. doi:10.1136/bjsports-2012-091961.
4. Franceschi F, Papalia R, Franceschetti E, et al. Platelet-rich plasma injections for chronic plantar fasciopathy: a systematic review. *Br Med Bull.* 2014;112(1):83–95.
5. Jabbari B, Machado D. Treatment of refractory pain with botulinum toxins—an evidence-based review. *Pain Med.* 2011;12(11):1594–1606.
6. Landsman AS, Catanese DI, Wiener SN, et al. A prospective, randomized, double-blinded study with crossover to determine the efficacy of radiofrequency nerve ablation for the treatment of heel pain. *J Am Podiatr Med Assoc.* 2013;103(1):8–15.

ADDITIONAL READING

- Akşahin E, Doğruyol D, Yüksel HY, et al. The comparison of the effect of corticosteroids and platelet-rich plasma (PRP) for the treatment of plantar fasciitis. *Arch Orthop Trauma Surg.* 2012;132(6):781–785.
- Aqil A, Siddiqui MR, Solan M, et al. Extracorporeal shock wave therapy is effective in treating chronic plantar fasciitis: a meta-analysis of RCTs. *Clin Orthop Relat Res.* 2013;471(11):3645–3652.
- Chang KV, Chen SY, Chen WS, et al. Comparative effectiveness of focused shock wave therapy of different intensity levels and radial shock wave therapy for treating plantar fasciitis: a systematic review and network meta-analysis. *Arch Phys Med Rehabil.* 2012;93(7):1259–1268.

- Crawford F, Thomson CE. WITHDRAWN. Interventions for treating plantar heel pain. *Cochrane Database Syst Rev.* 2010;(1):CD000416.
- Erken HY, Ayanoglu S, Akmaz I, et al. Prospective study of percutaneous radiofrequency nerve ablation for chronic plantar fasciitis. *Foot Ankle Int.* 2014;35(2):95–103.
- Goff JD, Crawford R. Diagnosis and treatment of plantar fasciitis. *Am Fam Physician.* 2011;84(6):676–682.
- Hawke F, Burns J, Radford JA, et al. Custom-made foot orthoses for the treatment of foot pain. *Cochrane Database Syst Rev.* 2008;(3):CD006801.
- Healey K, Chen K. Plantar fasciitis: current diagnostic modalities and treatments. *Clin Podiatr Med Surg.* 2010;27(3):369–380.
- Huang YC, Wei SH, Wang HK, et al. Ultrasonographic guided botulinum toxin type A treatment for plantar fasciitis: an outcome-based investigation for treating pain and gait changes. *J Rehabil Med.* 2010;42(2):136–140.
- Jastifer JR, Catena F, Doty JF, et al. Low-level laser therapy for the treatment of chronic plantar fasciitis: a prospective study. *Foot Ankle Int.* 2014;35(6):566–571.
- Monto RR. Platelet-rich plasma efficacy versus corticosteroid injection treatment for chronic severe plantar fasciitis. *Foot Ankle Int.* 2014;35(4):313–318.
- Peterlein CD, Funk JF, Hölscher A, et al. Is botulinum toxin A effective for the treatment of plantar fasciitis? *Clin J Pain.* 2012;28(6):527–533.
- Ragab EM, Othman AM. Platelets rich plasma for treatment of chronic plantar fasciitis. *Arch Orthop Trauma Surg.* 2012;132(8):1065–1070.
- Uden H, Boesch E, Kumar S. Plantar fasciitis—to jab or to support? A systematic review of the current best evidence. *J Multidiscip Healthc.* 2011;4:155–164.

 SEE ALSO

Algorithm: Heel Pain

 CODES

ICD10
M72.2 Plantar fascial fibromatosis

CLINICAL PEARLS

- Plantar fasciitis is due to degeneration of plantar fascia at origin (medial calcaneal tuberosity) with characteristic pattern of pain.
- Pain with weight bearing (especially first few steps in the morning or after prolonged rest) is hallmark presentation.
- Conservative treatment is preferred. Wear supportive footwear to avoid excess pronation and provide adequate cushion. Modify activity, stretch plantar fascia, ice (water bottle roll), massage (golf ball roll), and provide arch support.

PLEURAL EFFUSION

Felix B. Chang, MD, DABMA, FAAMA

 BASICS

Abnormal accumulation of fluid in the pleural space

DESCRIPTION

Types: transudate, exudate

- Congestive heart failure 40%: transudate
- Pneumonia 25%, malignancy 15%, and pulmonary embolism (PE) 10% account for exudative effusions
- Malignant: lung cancer and metastases of breast, ovary, and lymphoma

EPIDEMIOLOGY

Incidence

Estimated 1.5 million cases/year in the United States; CHF: 500,000; pneumonia: 300,000; malignancy: 150,000; PE: 150,000; cirrhosis: 150,000; TB: 2,500; pancreatitis: 20,000; collagen vascular disease: 6,000

Prevalence

- Estimated 320 cases/100,000 people in industrialized countries; in hospitalized patients with AIDS, prevalence is 7–27%.
- No gender predilection: ~2/3 of malignant pleural effusions occurs in women.

ETIOLOGY AND PATHOPHYSIOLOGY

- Pleural fluid formation exceeds pleural fluid absorption.
- Transudates result from imbalances in hydrostatic and oncotic forces.
  - Increase in hydrostatic and/or low oncotic pressures; increase in pleural capillary permeability; lymphatic obstruction or impaired drainage; movement of fluid from the peritoneal or retroperitoneal space
- Transudates
  - CHF: 40% of transudative effusions; 80% bilateral. Constrictive pericarditis, atelectasis; superior vena cava syndrome
  - Cirrhosis (hepatic hydrothorax); nephrotic syndrome, hypoalbuminemia; myxedema
  - Urinothorax, central line misplacement; peritoneal dialysis
- Exudates
  - Lung parenchyma infection, bacterial (parapneumonic, tuberculous pleuritis), fungal, viral, parasitic (amebiasis, *Echinococcus*)
  - Cancer: lung cancer, metastases (breast, lymphoma, ovaries), mesothelioma
  - PE: 25% of PEs are transudate.
  - Collagen vascular disease: rheumatoid arthritis, systemic lupus erythematosus, Wegener granulomatosis, sarcoidosis, Churg-Strauss
  - GI: pancreatitis, esophageal rupture, abdominal abscess, after liver transplant. Chylothorax: thoracic duct tear, malignancy
  - Hemothorax: trauma, PE, malignancy, coagulopathy, aortic aneurysm
  - Others: after coronary artery bypass graft; Dressler syndrome; uremia, asbestos exposure, radiation; drug-induced: nitrofurantoin, bromocriptine, amiodarone, procarbazine, hydralazine, procainamide, quinidine, methotrexate, and methysergide

  - Meigs syndrome; yellow nail syndrome; ovarian stimulation syndrome; lymphangiomatosis; acute respiratory distress syndrome (ARDS)
  - Chylothorax: thoracic duct tear, malignancy, associated with lymphoma

RISK FACTORS

- Occupational exposures/drugs
- PE, TB, bacterial pneumonias
- Opportunistic infections (in HIV patients when CD4 count is <150 cells/μL)

COMMONLY ASSOCIATED CONDITIONS

Hypoproteinemia, heart failure, cirrhosis

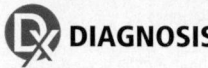 **DIAGNOSIS**

Presumptive diagnosis in 50% of cases. Small pleural effusions, radiographic area <2 intercostal spaces (<300 mL) are asymptomatic.

HISTORY

Dyspnea, fever, malaise, and weight loss; chest pain, cough, hemoptysis, and dull pain

PHYSICAL EXAM

- Pleural effusion >300 mL: tachypnea, asymmetric expansion of the thoracic cage; decrease/absent tactile fremitus; dullness to percussion; decreased/inaudible breath sounds, egophony, pleural friction rub
- Ascites suggest the following: hepatic hydrothorax, ovarian cancer, and Meigs syndrome.
- If associated with unilateral swelling in lower extremity, consider DVT with PE.

DIFFERENTIAL DIAGNOSIS

Empyema, malignancy, inflammatory, fungal, tuberculosis

DIAGNOSTIC TESTS & INTERPRETATION

Initial Tests (lab, imaging)

- Pleural fluid: appearance, pH, WBC differential, total protein, lactate dehydrogenase (LDH), glucose, Gram stain and culture, and acid-fast bacilli staining. Consider polymerase chain reaction (PCR) for *Mycobacterium tuberculosis* and *Streptococcus pneumoniae* (1,2)[A].
- If comorbidities implying risk, consider amylase, triglycerides, cholesterol, lupus erythematosus (LE) cells, cytology, antinuclear antibodies (ANAs), adenosine deaminase, tumor markers, rheumatoid factor, cytology, creatinine (2)[A]
- Light criteria, transudate versus exudate (98% sensitivity; 80% specificity); fluid is considered an exudate if any of the following (2)[A]:
  - Ratio of pleural fluid-to-serum protein levels >0.5; ratio of pleural fluid-to-serum LDH levels >0.6; pleural fluid LDH level >2/3 the upper limit for serum LDH level (1,3)[A]
- Other exudate criteria (4)[A]:

  - Serum-effusion albumin gradient ≤1.2 (sensitivity 87%; specificity 92%); cholesterol effusion >45 mg/dL and LDH effusion >200 mg/dL (sensitivity 90%; specificity 98%)

- Empyema: pus, putrid odor; culture. A putrid odor suggests an anaerobic empyema: LDH levels >1,000 IU/L (normal serum = 200 IU/L); glucose, <60 mg/dL; low pH
- Malignancy: cytology, red, bloody; glucose, normal to low, depending on the tumor burden; RBCs, >100,000/mm^3
- Lupus pleuritis: LE cells present; pleural fluid-to-serum ANAs ratio >1; glucose <60 mg/dL; pleural fluid-to-serum glucose ratio <0.5
- Fungal: positive KOH, culture; peritoneal dialysis: protein, <1 g/dL; glucose, 300 to 400 mg/dL
- Urinothorax: creatinine: pleural/blood >0.5; high LDH pleural fluid, with low protein levels
- Hemothorax: hematocrit: pleural/blood >0.5; benign asbestos effusion: unilateral, exudative; have elevated eosinophil count
- TB pleuritis: lymphocytes >80% predominance effusion; elevated levels of adenosine deaminase >50 U/L and interferon-γ >140 pg/mL; positive acid-fast bacillus (AFB) stain, culture; total protein >4 g/dL
- Chylothorax: milky; triglycerides >110 mg/dL; lipoprotein electrophoresis (chylomicrons)
- Amebic liver abscess: anchovy paste effusion; Waldenström macroglobulinemia and multiple myeloma: protein >7 g/dL
- Esophageal rupture: high salivary amylase; pleural fluid acidosis, pH <6; amylase-rich: acute pancreatitis, chronic pancreatic pleural effusion, malignancy, esophageal rupture; rheumatoid pleurisy: glucose <60 mg/dL; pleural fluid/serum glucose <0.5
- Lymphocytosis: tuberculous pleurisy, lymphoma, sarcoidosis, chronic rheumatoid pleurisy, yellow nail syndrome, or chylothorax (80–95% of the nucleated cells). Carcinomatosis in half of cases (50–70% are lymphocytes)
- Pleural fluid eosinophilia (>10% of total nucleated cells): pneumothorax, hemothorax, malignancy, drugs, pulmonary infarction, fungal (coccidiomycosis, cryptococcosis, histoplasmosis), benign asbestos pleural effusion
- Low glucose (<60 mg/dL): TB, malignancy, rheumatoid pleurisy, parapneumonic, empyema, hemothorax, paragonimiasis, Churg-Strauss syndrome
- RBC count >100,000/mm^3: trauma, malignancy, PE, injury after cardiac surgery, asbestos pleurisy, pancreatitis, TB
- Pleural fluid LDH >1,000 IU/L: suggests empyema, malignant effusion, rheumatoid effusion, or pleural paragonimiasis
- pH >7.3: rheumatoid pleurisy, empyema, malignant effusion, TB, esophageal rupture, or lupus nephritis
- Mesothelial cells in exudates: TB is unlikely if there are >5% of mesothelial cells.
- *Streptococcus pneumoniae* accounts for 50% of cases of parapneumonic effusions in AIDS patients, followed by *Staphylococcus aureus*, *Haemophilus influenzae*, *Mycoplasma pneumoniae*, *Legionella*, *Nocardia*, and *Bordetella bronchiseptica*. Exudate with low count of nucleated cells
- *Pneumocystis jirovecii* is an uncommon cause in HIV. Usually it is a small effusion, unilateral or bilateral, and serous to bloody in appearance. Demonstration of the trophozoite or cyst is mandatory.

- Cancer-related HIV pleural effusion: Kaposi sarcoma, Castleman disease, and primary effusion lymphoma. Kaposi sarcoma: mononuclear predominance, exudate, pH >7.4; LDH, 111 to 330 IU/L; glucose >60 mg/dL.
- Chest x-ray (CXR): posteroanterior–anteroposterior views
  - Upright x-rays show a concave meniscus in the costophrenic angle that suggests >250 mL of pleural fluid; homogeneous opacity, with visibility of pulmonary vessels through diffuse haziness and absence of air bronchogram; 75 mL of fluid will obliterate the posterior costophrenic sulcus.
  - Lateral x-rays show blunting of the posterior costophrenic angle and the posterior gutter; decubitus x-rays to exclude a loculated effusion and underlying pulmonary lesion or pulmonary thickening
  - Supine x-rays show costophrenic blunting, haziness, obliteration of the diaphragmatic silhouette, decreased visibility of the lower lobe vasculature, and widened minor fissure.
- Ultrasonography (US): detects as 5 to 50 mL of pleural fluid; identifies loculated effusions; site for thoracocentesis, pleural biopsy, or pleural drainage
- Chest CT scan with contrast for patients with undiagnosed pleural effusion. CT pulmonary angiography if PE is suspected.

Follow-Up Tests & Special Considerations
- 75% of patients with exudative effusions have a non-CHF cause.
  - NT-ProBNP: biomarker of CHF-associated effusion; >1,500 pg/mL; sensitivity and specificity 94% (2)[A]
  - Observation in uncomplicated asymptomatic patients (i.e., CHF, cirrhosis), viral pleurisy, thoracic or abdominal surgery

Diagnostic Procedures/Other
Diagnostic thoracentesis indicated for the following:
- Clinically significant pleural effusion (>10 mm thick on US or lateral decubitus x-ray with no known cause)
- CHF: asymmetric effusion, fever, chest pain, or failure to resolve after diuretics
- Parapneumonic effusions

 TREATMENT

Oxygen support

GENERAL MEASURES
- Therapeutic thoracentesis, if symptomatic

- Chest tube thoracostomy drainage: >1/2 hemithorax; complicated parapneumonic effusion (positive Gram stain or culture, pH <7.2, or glucose <60 mg/dL); empyema; hemothorax. Recommended limit is 1,000 to 1,500 mL in a single thoracentesis procedure (5)[B].

MEDICATION
First Line
CHF: diuretics (75% clearing in 48 hours); parapneumonic effusion: antibiotics; rheumatologic conditions/inflammation: steroids and NSAIDs

Second Line
Symptomatic nonmalignant effusions that are refractory to treatment may be managed with repeated therapeutic thoracentesis or pleurodesis.

ISSUES FOR REFERRAL
- Uncertain etiology; malignant effusion; high-risk diagnostic thoracentesis; decortication
- Video-assisted thoracoscopy for sclerosis; peritoneal shunts for symptomatic recurrence

ADDITIONAL THERAPIES
- Pleurodesis for symptomatic patients whose pleural effusion reaccumulates too quickly for repeat therapeutic thoracentesis
- Tunneled pleural catheter is the preferred treatment for patients with malignant pleural effusion and limited survival.
- Sclerosing agents for malignant effusions: doxycycline, bleomycin, talc, and minocycline; talc is more efficacious. The relative risk of nonrecurrent effusion was 1.34 (95% CI 1.16–1.55) in favor of talc compared with bleomycin, tetracycline, or mustine.

SURGERY/OTHER PROCEDURES
- Percutaneous pleural biopsy if a cause is not clear after thoracentesis
  - Close pleural biopsy: Pleura is diffusely involved (TB pleuritis, noncaseating granuloma in rheumatoid pleuritis).
  - CT-guided needle biopsy: pleural mass; video-assisted thoracoscopic pleural biopsy: negative percutaneous biopsy, patchy disease, or CT scan does not show obvious mass.
- Parapneumonic effusion should be sampled if free-flowing, but layer is >10 mm on a lateral decubitus film. Loculated, thickened pleura on a contrast-enhanced CT scan, clearly delineated by US open pleural biopsy by thoracotomy
- Contraindications for thoracocentesis: anticoagulation, bleeding diathesis, thrombocytopenia <20,000/mm³, mechanical ventilation
- Bronchoscopy: when malignancy is suspected (pulmonary infiltrate or mass on CXR or CT scan, hemoptysis, massive pleural effusion, or shift of the mediastinum toward the side of effusion)
- Thoracoscopy

INPATIENT CONSIDERATIONS
Admission Criteria/Initial Stabilization
Treat any underlying medical disorder.

 ONGOING CARE

FOLLOW-UP RECOMMENDATIONS
Patient Monitoring
- Check for the amount and quality of fluid drained, air leak (bubbling), and oscillation.
- Repeat a CXR when drainage decreases to <100 mL/day to evaluate complete clearing.
- For a large effusion, reevaluate catheter position; if positioned appropriately, consider fibrinolytics.

DIET
Cardiac diet in patients with heart failure; correct hypoproteinemia.

PROGNOSIS
- Malignant effusion: poor
- Low-pH malignant effusions have shorter survival and poorer response to chemical pleurodesis than those with pH >7.3.
- Low pleural fluid pH (≤7.15): high likelihood of pleural space drainage

COMPLICATIONS
- Pleural effusion: constrictive fibrosis, pleurocutaneous fistula
- Thoracentesis: pneumothorax (5–10%); hemothorax (~1%); empyema; spleen/liver laceration; reexpansion pulmonary edema (if >1.5 L is removed)

REFERENCES

1. Sahn SA, Huggins JT, San Jose E, et al. The art of pleural fluid analysis. *Clin Pulm Med*. 2013;20(2): 77–96.
2. Saguil A, Wyrick K, Hallgren J. Diagnostic approach to pleural effusion. *Am Fam Physician*. 2014;90(2): 99–104.
3. Light RW. Pleural effusions. *Med Clin North Am*. 2011;95(6):1055–1070.
4. Wilcox ME, Chong CA, Stanbrook MB, et al. Does this patient have an exudative pleural effusion? The rational clinical examination systematic review. *JAMA*. 2014;311(23):2422–2431.
5. Mahmood K, Wahidi MM. Straightening out chest tubes: what size, what type, and when. *Clin Chest Med*. 2013;34(1):63–71.

ADDITIONAL READING

Bielsa S, Porcel JM, Castellote J, et al. Solving the Light's criteria misclassification rate of cardiac and hepatic transudates. *Respirology*. 2012;17(4): 721–726.

CODES

ICD10
- J90 Pleural effusion, not elsewhere classified
- J91.0 Malignant pleural effusion
- J94.0 Chylous effusion

CLINICAL PEARLS

- Clinical presentation and pleural fluid analysis allow to diagnose the cause of effusion in 75% of patients at first evaluation.
- Bilateral pleural effusion suggest heart failure, malignancy in absence of cardiomegaly, and tuberculosis or parasitic infection in children.
- Loculation suggest pleural inflammation and may occur with the following: empyema, hemothorax, and TB.
- Parapneumonic effusion should be tapped ASAP.
- Ascites and pleural effusion suggest hepatic hydrothorax, ovarian cancer, or Meig syndrome
- Consider diagnostic thoracocentesis in patient with heart failure: fever, pleuritic chest pain, unilateral effusion or effusion of markedly disparate size, effusion not associated with cardiomegaly, effusion fails to respond to management of heart failure
- Most common cause of exudative effusion are pneumonia, neoplasms, and thromboembolism.

PNEUMONIA, BACTERIAL
Rahele Lameh, MD

 BASICS

Bacterial pneumonia is an infection of the pulmonary parenchyma by a bacterial organism.

DESCRIPTION
Bacterial pneumonia can be classified as the following:
- Community-acquired pneumonia (CAP): lower respiratory tract infection not acquired in a hospital, long-term care facility, or during other recent contact with the health care system
- Medical care–associated pneumonia
  - Hospital-acquired pneumonia (HAP): pneumonia within ≥48 hours after admission and did not appear to be incubating at time of admission
  - Ventilator-associated pneumonia (VAP): Pneumonia that develops >48 to 72 hours after endotracheal intubation.
  - Health care–associated pneumonia (HCAP): Pneumonia that occurs in a nonhospitalized patient with extensive health care contact, such as the following:
    ○ IV therapy/wound care within past 30 days
    ○ Residing in a nursing home/long-term care
    ○ Hospitalization in an acute care hospital for ≥2 days within the past 90 days
    ○ Visited a hospital/hemodialysis clinic within the past 30 days (1,2)

EPIDEMIOLOGY
- Influenza and pneumonia are the 8th leading cause of death in the United States, with about 53,692 deaths in 2010.
- In 2006, 55,477 people died of pneumonia (3).
- HAP is the leading cause of death among hospital-acquired infections and is the primary cause of death in the ICU.
- Rates of infection are three times higher in African Americans than in whites and are 5 to 10 times higher in Native American adults and 10 times higher in Native American children (2).
- Mortality rate in children is approximately 1.6 million a year (4). Hospitalization rate for children with CAP is still highest among the very young ages (<18 months). Respiratory viruses are the most commonly detected causes of pneumonia (5).

Incidence
- CAP: 5 to 11 cases/1,000 persons with increased incidence occurring in the winter months.
- HAP: 5 to 10 cases/1,000 admissions; incidence increase 6- to 20-fold in ventilated patients (6)[A].

ETIOLOGY AND PATHOPHYSIOLOGY
- Adults, CAP
  - Typical (85%): *Streptococcus pneumoniae, Haemophilus influenzae, Staphylococcus aureus,* group A *Streptococcus, Moraxella catarrhalis*
  - Atypical (15%): *Legionella* sp., *Mycoplasma pneumoniae, Chlamydophila pneumoniae*
- Adults, HCAP/HAP/VAP
  - Aerobic gram-negative bacilli: *Pseudomonas aeruginosa, Escherichia coli, Klebsiella pneumoniae,* and *Acinetobacter* sp.
  - Gram-positive cocci: *Streptococcus* sp. and *S. aureus* (including MRSA)
- Children
  - Birth to 20 days: *E. coli,* group B *Streptococci, Listeria monocytogenes*
  - 3 weeks to 3 months: *Chlamydia trachomatis, S. pneumoniae*

- 4 months to 18 years
  ○ Typical: *S. pneumoniae*
  ○ Atypical: *C. pneumoniae, M. pneumoniae*

RISK FACTORS
CAP
- Age >65 years
- HIV/immunocompromised
- Recent antibiotic therapy/resistance to antibiotics
- Asthma, CAD, COPD, chronic renal failure, CHF, diabetes, liver disease, VAP, HAP, HCAP
- Hospitalization for ≥2 days during past 90 days
- Severe illness
- Antibiotic therapy in the past 6 months
- Poor functional status as defined by activities of daily living score
- Immunosuppression (including steroid users)

GENERAL PREVENTION
- All children 2 to 59 months of age should be routinely vaccinated with pneumococcal conjugate (PCV13); given at 2, 4, and 6 months of age; a fourth dose at 12 to 15 months of age. PCV13 is also FDA approved for those >50 years of age.
- For adults aged 65 years or older who have not received any pneumonia vaccination, ACIP currently recommends PCV13 followed by pneumococcal polysaccharide (PPSV23) with 6 to 12 months interval. If they received PPSV23 vaccine before age 65 years, they should receive another dose of the vaccine at age 65 years or later if at least 5 years have passed since their previous dose.
- PPSV23 is also indicated at age 19 to 64 years who are immunocompromised, including asthma and cigarette smokers. A second dose of PPSV23 is recommended 5 years after the first dose for persons aged 19 to 64 years with functional or anatomic asplenia and for persons with immunocompromising conditions. ACIP does not recommend multiple revaccinations due to uncertainty about safety and benefit of revaccination.
- Annual influenza vaccine is recommended according to current guidelines.

 DIAGNOSIS

History
- Fever, chills, rigors, malaise, fatigue
- Dyspnea
- Cough, with/without sputum
- Pleuritic chest pain
- Myalgias
- GI symptoms

ALERT
High fever (>104°F [40°C]), male sex, multilobar involvement, and GI and neurologic abnormalities have been associated with CAP caused by *Legionella* infection.

Geriatric Considerations
Older adults with pneumonia often present with weakness, mental status change, or history of falls.

PHYSICAL EXAM
- Fever >100.4°F (38°C), tachypnea, tachycardia
- Rales, rhonchi, egophony, increased fremitus, bronchial breath sounds, dullness to percussion, asymmetric breath sounds, abdominal tenderness

DIFFERENTIAL DIAGNOSIS
Bronchitis, asthma exacerbation, pulmonary edema, lung cancer, pulmonary tuberculosis, pneumonitis

DIAGNOSTIC TESTS & INTERPRETATION
Initial Tests (lab, imaging)
- Routine laboratory testing to establish an etiology in outpatients with CAP is usually unnecessary.
- For hospitalized patients with CAP, a CBC, sputum Gram stain, and two sets of blood cultures
- More extensive diagnostic testing in patients with CAP is recommended if:
  - Blood cultures: ICU admission, cavitary infiltrates, leukopenia, alcohol abuse, severe liver disease, asplenia, positive pneumococcal urine antigen test (UAT), pleural effusion
  - Sputum Gram stain and cultures: ICU admission, failure of outpatient treatment, cavitary infiltrates, alcohol abuse, severe COPD/structural lung disease, positive *Legionella* UAT, positive pneumococcal UAT, pleural effusion
  - *Legionella* UAT: ICU admission, failure of outpatient treatment, alcohol abuse, travel in past 2 weeks, pleural effusion
  - Pneumococcal UAT: ICU admission, failure of outpatient treatment, leukopenia, alcohol abuse, severe liver disease, asplenia, pleural effusion
- A chest x-ray (CXR) is indicated when pneumonia is suspected or with an acute respiratory infection and
  - Vital signs: temperature >100°F (37.8°C); heart rate (HR) >100 beats/min; respiratory rate (RR) >20 breaths/min
  - At least two of the following clinical findings: decreased breath sounds, rales, no asthma
- Early in disease course, CXR may be negative.
- Evidence of necrotizing/cavitary pneumonia should raise suspicion for MRSA pneumonia, especially with history of prior MRSA skin lesions.

Diagnostic Procedures/Other
- For VAP/HAP: By bronchoscopic or nonbronchoscopic means, obtain a lower respiratory tract sample for culture prior to initiation/change of therapy. Serial evaluations may be needed (6)[A].
- Safe cessation of antibiotics can be done from a good quality negative sputum culture.

TREATMENT

MEDICATION
First Line
- Adults
  - CAP, outpatient
    ○ No significant differences in efficacy between antibiotic option in adults (7)[A]
    ○ Previously healthy, no antibiotics in past 3 months
      ■ Azithromycin 500 mg PO 1 time, then 250 mg PO daily for 4 days; clarithromycin 500 mg PO BID for 10 days; erythromycin 500 mg PO BID for 10 days, or
      ■ Doxycycline 100 mg PO BID for 10 days
    ○ Comorbid conditions, immunosuppressed, antibiotic use in past 3 months
      ■ Levofloxacin 750 mg PO daily for 5 days; moxifloxacin 400 mg PO daily for 10 days; or
      ■ Amoxicillin 1 g PO TID; amoxicillin-clavulanate 2 g PO BID + macrolide
      ■ Treatment may be stopped if
        □ Afebrile for >48 hours
        □ Supplemental oxygen no longer needed

□ No more than one of the following:
  • A. HR >100 beats/min
  • B. RR >24 breaths/min
  • C. Systolic BP ≤90 mm Hg
- CAP, inpatient (non-ICU)
  ○ IV antibiotics initially, then switch to oral after clinical improvement
  ○ Cefotaxime; ceftriaxone; ampicillin-sulbactam + macrolide (clarithromycin; erythromycin) for 14 days or
  ○ Moxifloxacin; levofloxacin for 14 days
  ○ If *Pseudomonas* is a consideration.
    ■ Piperacillin-tazobactam; cefepime; imipenem; meropenem + levofloxacin or
    ■ Piperacillin-tazobactam; cefepime; imipenem; meropenem + aminoglycoside and azithromycin or
    ■ Piperacillin-tazobactam; cefepime; imipenem; meropenem + aminoglycoside + levofloxacin
  ○ If MRSA is a consideration.
    ■ Add vancomycin or linezolid.
- HCAP/HAP/VAP
  ○ Use IV antibiotics.
  ○ Early onset (<5 days) and no risk factors for multidrug-resistant pathogens
    ■ Ceftriaxone; ampicillin-sulbactam; ertapenem or
    ■ Levofloxacin; moxifloxacin
  ○ Late onset (≥5 days) or risk factors for multidrug-resistant pathogens (antibiotic therapy in preceding 90 days; high frequency of antibiotic resistance in community/hospital; immunosuppressive disease/therapy; risk factors for HCAP)
    ■ MRSA coverage: linezolid or vancomycin + β-lactam cefepime; ceftazidime; imipenem; meropenem; piperacillin-tazobactam + either fluoroquinolone (levofloxacin) or aminoglycoside (amikacin; gentamicin; tobramycin) (level II)
    ■ Short-course versus prolonged-course antibiotic therapy for HAP in critically ill adults is only as effective and reduced recurrence of VAP-associated multidrug resistance (8).
    ■ Drug-resistant *S. pneumoniae* should be treated with high-dose amoxicillin, amoxicillin/clavulanate, cefpodoxime with a macrolide, or a respiratory fluoroquinolone.
- Adult IV antibiotic doses
  ○ β-Lactams (ampicillin-sulbactam 3 g q6h; aztreonam 2 g q6h; cefepime 1 to 2 g q8–12h; cefotaxime 1 g q6–8h; ceftazidime 2 g q8h; ceftriaxone 1 g daily; imipenem 500 mg q6h; meropenem 1 g IV q8h)
  ○ Aminoglycosides (amikacin 20 mg/kg daily; gentamicin 7 mg/kg daily; tobramycin 7 mg/kg daily)
  ○ Fluoroquinolones (levofloxacin 750 mg daily; moxifloxacin 400 mg daily)
  ○ Macrolides (azithromycin 500 mg daily; clarithromycin 500 mg daily; erythromycin 500 to 1,000 mg q6h)
  ○ Vancomycin 15 mg/kg q12h
  ○ Linezolid 600 mg q12h
  ○ Telavancin is an antibiotic which covers MRSA infection, and it was approved by FDA in 2013. Telavancin is approved for the treatment of HAP and VAP caused by *S. aureus*. This medication is indicated only when alternative agents cannot be used (3).
• Pediatric, outpatient (≥3 months)
  - Antibiotic treatment in preschool-aged children is not routinely required because viral pathogens are more common (9)[A].

- Oral antibiotics are as efficacious as IV in CAP (length of stay and oxygen requirement were reduced in those given oral antibiotics).
- Typical bacterial pneumonia
  ○ Amoxicillin 90 mg/kg/day PO BID (max 4 g/day) (9)[A]
  ○ Amoxicillin-clavulanate 90 mg/kg/day PO BID (max 4 g/day) (9)[A]
  ○ Alternative: levofloxacin 16 to 20 mg/kg/day PO BID for children 6 months to 5 years, 10 mg/kg/day daily for children ≥5 years (max 750 mg/day) (9)[C]
- Atypical bacterial pneumonia
  ○ Azithromycin 10 mg/kg PO on day 1 (max 500 mg), then 5 mg/kg/day (max 250 mg) on days 2 to 5 (8)[C]
  ○ Clarithromycin 15 mg/kg/day PO BID (max 1 g/day) (8)[C]
  ○ Erythromycin 40 mg/kg/day PO daily (8)[C]

INPATIENT CONSIDERATIONS
Admission Criteria/Initial Stabilization
• Clinical judgment and use of a validated severity of illness score are recommended to determine if inpatient management is indicated.
• The Pneumonia Severity Index (PSI) is a clinical prediction rule used to calculate the probability of morbidity and mortality among patients with CAP. PSI is risk stratified from I to V. PSI risk class from I to III can be treated as outpatients and IV to V should be hospitalized. PSI can be calculated at http://pda.ahrq.gov/clinic/psi/psicalc.asp
• The CURB-65 or CRB 65 (confusion, urea nitrogen-respiratory rate, blood pressure, age >65 years) (http://www.mdcalc.com/curb-65-severity-score-community-acquired-pneumonia/) is a severity of illness score for stratifying adults with CAP into different management groups (7).
• The SMART-COP (systolic BP, multilobar chest radiography, albumin, respiratory rate, tachycardia, confusion, oxygen level, and arterial pH) is a new method to predict which patients will require intensive respiratory/vasopressor support. A score of ≥3 has sensitivity of 92% to identify those patients who will receive intensive treatment (7).
• Patients with COPD or CHF are more likely to require ICU admission when suffering from CAP.
• Clinical prediction tools do not replace a physician's clinical judgment.

Pediatric Considerations
Inpatient treatment of children is recommended in the following settings: infants ≤3 to 6 months; presence of respiratory distress (tachypnea, dyspnea, retractions, grunting, nasal flaring, apnea, altered mental status, O_2 sat <90%); or if known to have CAP as result of a virulent pathogen such as community-associated MRSA should be hospitalized (10).

Discharge Criteria
Clinical stability: temperature ≤100°F (37.8°C); HR ≤100 beats/min; RR ≤24 beats/min; systolic BP ≤90 mm Hg; O_2 sat ≥90% or PaO_2 ≥60 mm Hg on room air; ability to maintain oral intake; normal mental status

ONGOING CARE

FOLLOW-UP RECOMMENDATIONS
Patient Monitoring
Consider chest CT if patient is failing to improve on current management.

PATIENT EDUCATION
Smoking cessation, vaccinations

COMPLICATIONS
Necrotizing pneumonia, respiratory failure, empyema, abscesses, cavitation, bronchopleural fistula, sepsis

REFERENCES
1. Marrie TJ, Huang JQ. Epidemiology of community-acquired pneumonia in Edmonton, Alberta: an emergency department-based study. *Can Respir J.* 2005;12(3):139–142.
2. Davidson M, Parkinson AJ, Bulkow LR, et al. The epidemiology of invasive pneumococcal disease in Alaska, 1986–1990—ethnic differences and opportunities for prevention. *J Infect Dis.* 1994;170(2):368–376.
3. FDA news release. FDA approves Vibativ for hospitalized patients with bacterial pneumonia. http://www.fda.gov/newsevents/newsroom/pressannouncements/ucm358209.htm. Accessed 2013.
4. Black RE, Cousens S, Johnson HL, et al. Global, regional, and national causes of child mortality in 2008: a systematic analysis. *Lancet.* 2010;375(9730):1969–1987.
5. Jain S, Williams DJ, Arnold SR, et al. Community-acquired pneumonia requiring hospitalization among U.S. children. *N Engl J Med.* 2015;372(9):835–845.
6. File TM Jr. Recommendations for treatment of hospital-acquired and ventilator-associated pneumonia: review of recent international guidelines. *Clin Infect Dis.* 2010;51(Suppl 1):S42–S47.
7. Watkins RR, Lemonovich TL. Diagnosis and management of community-acquired pneumonia in adults. *Am Fam Physician.* 2011;83(11):1299–1306.
8. Pugh R, Grant C, Cooke RP, et al. Short-course versus prolonged-course antibiotic therapy for hospital-acquired pneumonia in critically ill adults. *Cochrane Database Syst Rev.* 2011;(10):CD007577.
9. Bradley JS, Byington CL, Shah SS, et al. The management of community-acquired pneumonia in infants and children older than 3 months of age: clinical practice guidelines by the Pediatric Infectious Diseases Society and the Infectious Diseases Society of America. *Clin Infect Dis.* 2011;53(7):e25–e76.
10. Devitt M. PIDS and IDSA issue management guidelines for community-acquired pneumonia in infants and young children. *Am Fam Physician.* 2012;86(2):196–202.

CODES
ICD10
• J15.9 Unspecified bacterial pneumonia
• J15.4 Pneumonia due to other streptococci
• J14 Pneumonia due to Hemophilus influenzae

CLINICAL PEARLS
• Bacterial pneumonia can usually be treated empirically based on its classification as CAP or HCAP/HAP/VAP.
• A severity of illness score is helpful in determining the need for hospitalization of adult patients but does not replace a physician's clinical judgment.

PNEUMONIA, MYCOPLASMA

Jonathan D. Reves, DO • Robert M. Hasty, DO, FACOI, FACP

 BASICS

DESCRIPTION
- Bronchopulmonary infection caused by the *Mycoplasma* species, *Mycoplasma pneumoniae*
- Smallest free-living organism; fastidious and slow-growing; first isolated in cattle in 1898
- Most frequently affects children/young adults but can also occur in the elderly; often causes epidemics in close communities
- Infection may be asymptomatic, most often confined to the upper respiratory tract; however, may progress to pneumonia (5–10%).
- Course is usually acute with an incubation period of 2 to 3 weeks.
- Synonym(s): primary atypical pneumonia (PAP); Eaton agent pneumonia; cold agglutinin–positive pneumonia; walking pneumonia

Geriatric Considerations
Uncommonly isolated as a single agent in elderly patients

Pediatric Considerations
- Unusual in infants and children <5 years; (pneumonia <5 years is more commonly viral)
- Increased incidence of asthma exacerbation in older children
- All infants 3 to 6 months with suspected bacterial pneumonia should be hospitalized.

EPIDEMIOLOGY
Incidence
- Estimated 1 million cases per year in the United States
- Responsible for 20% of community-acquired pneumonia (CAP) requiring hospitalizations annually
- Infection occurs most frequently in fall/winter seasons but may develop year round.

Prevalence
- Predominant sex: male = female
- Predominant age group affected: 5 to 20 years
  - May occur at any age
  - Rare in children <5 years of age
- Responsible for 15–20% of all cases of CAP yearly
  - Most common cause of pneumonia in school children and young adults who do not have a chronic underlying condition

ETIOLOGY AND PATHOPHYSIOLOGY
- *M. pneumoniae* is a short-rod mucosal pathogen, which lacks a cell wall and thus not visible on Gram stain.
- Can grow under both aerobic and anaerobic conditions
- Highly contagious, *M. pneumoniae* is transmitted by contact and aerosols.
- Pathogenicity linked to its filamentous tips, which adhere selectively to respiratory epithelial cell membrane proteins with production of H_2O_2 and superoxide radicals, damaging cilia
- Many pathogenic features of infection are believed to be immune-mediated, not directly induced.
- Decreased ciliary movement produces prolonged paroxysmal, hacking cough.

ALERT
- Macrolide-resistant *M. pneumoniae* has emerged in cases of adult CAP and pediatric pneumonias in Asia, France, Italy, Israel, and the United States.
- Infection by *M. pneumoniae* has come to be recognized as a worldwide cause of CAP.
- *M. pneumonia* infection may worsen asthma symptoms as well as cause wheezing in children without asthma.

RISK FACTORS
- Immunocompromised state (e.g., HIV, transplant recipients, chemotherapy)
- Smoking
- Close community living (e.g., military bases, prisons, hospitals, fraternity houses, schools, household contacts)

GENERAL PREVENTION
Consider droplet isolation of active cases.

COMMONLY ASSOCIATED CONDITIONS
- Asthma exacerbations as a result of proinflammatory cytokine release
- Chronic obstructive pulmonary disease

 DIAGNOSIS

HISTORY
- Infection may be asymptomatic.
- Gradual onset of headache, malaise, low-grade fevers, chills
- Symptoms of upper respiratory infection then occur, including incessant, nonproductive, worsening cough (which may become mildly productive late in the disease); rhinorrhea; pharyngitis; and sinusitis (1)[A]
- Pneumonia may occur with associated pleural effusion; however, dyspnea is rare.
- The presence of pleuritic chest pain warrants a higher suspicion of *M. pneumoniae* (1)[A].
- Extrapulmonary findings may develop in 5–10% of patients, including arthralgias, skin rashes, cervical adenopathy, hemolysis, congestive heart failure (CHF), and cardiac conduction abnormalities.
- Neurologic symptoms develop more commonly in children and may include encephalitis, aseptic meningitis, cranial nerve palsies, cerebellar ataxia, ascending paralysis, and coma (2)[C].
- Persistent cough is common during convalescence; other sequelae are rare.

PHYSICAL EXAM
- Patients generally appear nontoxic.
- Hacking/pertussis-like cough may be present along with fever and lassitude.
- Normal lung findings with early infection, but rhonchi, rales, and/or wheezes may develop several days later (1)[A].
- Mild pharyngeal injection without exudates
- Minimal/no cervical adenopathy
- Erythematous tympanic membranes or bullous myringitis in patients >2 years of age is an uncommon but unique sign.
- Some patients may develop a pleural friction rub.
- Various exanthems, including erythema multiforme and Stevens-Johnson syndrome

DIFFERENTIAL DIAGNOSIS
- Viral/bacterial/fungal pneumonia
- Tuberculosis
- Other atypical pneumonias, including *Chlamydia pneumoniae*, *Chlamydophila psittaci*, *Coxiella burnetii* (Q fever), *Francisella tularensis* (tularemia), *Pneumocystis jiroveci*, *Legionella pneumophila*

DIAGNOSTIC TESTS & INTERPRETATION
- Microbial diagnosis is uncommon in outpatients as empiric treatment usually successful.

- PCR is the diagnostic test of choice, when available.
- No clinical or radiographical findings can differentiate between *M. pneumoniae* and other atypical pneumonia pathogens (*Chlamydia/Legionella*).

Initial Tests (lab, imaging)
- WBC count may be normal or elevated.
- Hemolytic anemia has been described but is rare.
- Elevated erythrocyte sedimentation rate (ESR) may be present but is nonspecific.
- When available, polymerase chain reaction (PCR) for *M. pneumoniae* DNA in respiratory secretions, CSF, and tissue samples may be the most sensitive and specific
- CXR shows reticulonodular pattern with patchy areas of lower lobe consolidation, although this is not specific. Small pleural effusion may be present in 10–15% cases.

Follow-Up Tests & Special Considerations
- Sputum Gram stains are not helpful because *M. pneumoniae* lacks a cell wall and cannot be stained.
- *M. pneumoniae* is difficult to culture and requires 7 to 21 days to grow; culturing is successful in 40–90% of cases but does not provide information to guide treatment, thus infrequently performed.
- Complement fixation serologic assay shows 4-fold rise in IgM antibody titer at 2 to 4 weeks after symptom onset; this is an older technique.
- Positive cold agglutinins (titer of ≥1:128 or rising 4-fold) in 50% of infections but can take 1 to 2 weeks to develop; not sensitive/specific; not routinely recommended
- CT of chest may show a combination of patchy tree-in-bud opacities with segmental ground glass opacities.

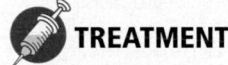 **TREATMENT**

GENERAL MEASURES
- Avoid sick contacts.
- Treatment is usually empiric and must be comprehensive to cover all likely pathogens in the context of the clinical setting.
- Calculation of pneumonia severity score (CAP score: www.mdcalc.com/psi-port-score-pneumonia-severity-index-adult-cap) may be helpful in determining inpatient versus outpatient treatment.

ALERT
There is insufficient evidence regarding the efficacy of antibiotics in pediatric patients infected with *M. pneumoniae*. However, some studies show benefit to treating with a macrolide and amoxicillin to cover *M. pneumoniae* in addition to other likely agents causing CAP (3,4)[A].

Pregnancy Considerations
- Azithromycin: pregnancy Category B (preferred treatment)
- Clarithromycin, levofloxacin, and moxifloxacin: pregnancy Category C
- Doxycycline: pregnancy Category D

MEDICATION
First Line
- Azithromycin
  - <3 months of age: not established
  - >3 months of age: day 1, 10 mg/kg PO × 1 (not to exceed 500 mg); days 2 to 5: 5 mg/kg PO daily (not to exceed 250 mg/day)

– Adults: 500 mg PO × 1 followed by 250 mg PO daily for 4 days (5)[A]

- Clarithromycin
  - Children <6 months of age: not established
  - Patients >6 months of age: 15 mg/kg/day PO divided q12h for 10 to 14 days
  - Adults: 250 to 500 mg PO BID for 10 to 14 days
- Erythromycin
  - Children: 20 to 50 mg/kg/day (base) PO divided q6–8h for 10 to 14 days
  - Adults: 500 mg (base) PO q6h for 10 to 14 days (5)[A],(6)[B]
- Doxycycline
  - Children <8 years of age: not recommended
  - Children >8 years of age (≤45 kg): 2 to 4 mg/kg/day up to 200 mg/day PO divided BID for 10 to 14 days
  - Children >8 years of age (≥45 kg): Refer to adult dosing.
  - Adults: 100 mg PO BID for 7 to 14 days (5)[A],(6)[B]
  - Useful in macrolide-resistant strains of *M. pneumoniae*.

Second Line
- Levofloxacin
  - Children <18 years of age: not recommended
  - Adults: 500 mg PO daily for 7 to 10 days (5)[A]
- Moxifloxacin
  - Children <18 years of age: not recommended
  - Adults: 400 mg/day PO for 7 to 10 days
- Levofloxacin and moxifloxacin show good activity against *M. pneumoniae*. Consider use with comorbid conditions and other pneumonia pathogens; also useful if macrolide resistance is suspected.

ADDITIONAL THERAPIES
- Albuterol inhaler: 2 puffs q4–6h as needed for wheezing
- Dexamethasone may downregulate cytokine release (7)[B].
- Acetaminophen/ibuprofen as needed for fever
- Up to 10.9% of hospitalized patients may require mechanical ventilation.
- Plasmapheresis in cases of severe hemolytic anemia.

INPATIENT CONSIDERATIONS
Admission Criteria/Initial Stabilization
- CAP score risk class IV/V
- Advanced age with comorbidities
- Complicating neoplastic disease
- Significant cerebrovascular, cardiac, renal, liver, or GI symptoms
- Altered mental status
- Inability to maintain oxygen saturation
- Tachycardia/tachypnea
- Hypotension
- Neurologic symptoms
- Signs of Stevens-Johnson syndrome
- Significant hemolysis (autoimmune hemolytic anemia, cold agglutinin disease)

Discharge Criteria
- Change from IV to PO antibiotic may be made when:
  - Respiratory distress and hypoxia have resolved.
  - Patients are tolerating oral hydration.
  - No significant complications are present.
- Generally, no need for 24-hour observation on PO antibiotics prior to discharge.

ONGOING CARE

FOLLOW-UP RECOMMENDATIONS
- Clearing of condition on CXR should be documented in patients >50 years of age (4)[A].
- In smokers, document a clear CXR in 6 to 8 weeks.
- Worsening symptoms/development of rash or meningeal/neurologic signs should prompt immediate presentation to medical attention.
- Antibiotic prophylaxis for exposed contacts is not routinely recommended.
- For household contacts who may be predisposed to severe mycoplasmal infection, macrolide or doxycycline prophylaxis should be used.

DIET
- No special diet considerations
- Ensure adequate hydration.

PATIENT EDUCATION
- Smoking cessation
- Contact and droplet precautions
- Adequate handwashing techniques

PROGNOSIS
- Symptoms usually resolve in 2 weeks.
- Some constitutional symptoms may persist for several weeks.
- With correct therapy, even most severe cases can expect complete recovery.

COMPLICATIONS
- All complications are rare, except reactive airway disease, hemolytic anemia, and erythema multiforme.
- Reactive airway disease may persist indefinitely and can cause acute chest syndrome in patients with sickle cell anemia.
- Meningoencephalitis
- Aseptic meningitis
- Peripheral neuropathy
- Transverse myelitis/acute transverse myelitis
- Cerebellar ataxia
- Acute disseminated encephalomyelitis
- Guillain-Barré syndrome
- Encephalitis (especially in children)
- Polyneuritis/polyarthritis
- Stevens-Johnson syndrome
- Pericarditis/myocarditis
- Respiratory distress syndrome
- Cerebral ataxia
- Thromboembolic phenomena
- Pleural effusion
- Nephritis
- Occasional deaths occur primarily among the elderly and persons with sickle cell disease.

REFERENCES

1. Wang K, Gill P, Perera R, et al. Clinical symptoms and signs for the diagnosis of *Mycoplasma pneumoniae* in children and adolescents with community-acquired pneumonia. *Cochrane Database Syst Rev.* 2012;(10):CD009175.
2. Meyer Sauteur PM, Jacobs BC, Spuesens EB, et al. Antibody responses to *Mycoplasma pneumoniae*: role in pathogenesis and diagnosis of encephalitis. *PLoS Pathog.* 2014;10(6):e1003983.
3. Mulholland S, Gavranich JB, Gillies MB, et al. Antibiotics for community-acquired lower respiratory tract infections secondary to *Mycoplasma pneumoniae* in children. *Cochrane Database Syst Rev.* 2012;(9):CD004875.
4. Bradley JS, Byington CL, Shah SS, et al. The management of community-acquired pneumonia in infants and children older than 3 months of age: clinical practice guidelines by the Pediatric Infectious Diseases Society and the Infectious Diseases Society of America. *Clin Infect Dis.* 2011;53(7):e25–e76.
5. Mandell LA, Wunderink RG, Anzueto A, et al. Infectious Diseases Society of America/American Thoracic Society consensus guidelines on the management of community-acquired pneumonia in adults. *Clin Infect Dis.* 2007; (44 Suppl 2):S27–S72.
6. Spindler C, Strålin K, Eriksson L, et al. Swedish guidelines on the management of community-acquired pneumonia in immunocompetent adults—Swedish Society of Infectious Diseases 2012. *Scand J Infect Dis.* 2012;44(12):885–902.
7. Remmelts HHE, Meijvis SCA, Biesma DH, et al. Dexamethasone downregulates the systemic cytokine response in patients with community-acquired pneumonia. *Clin Vaccine Immunol.* 2012;19(9):1532–1538.

ADDITIONAL READING

- Atkinson TP, Balish MF, Waites KB. Epidemiology, clinical manifestations, pathogenesis and laboratory detection of *Mycoplasma pneumoniae* infections. *FEMS Microbiol Rev.* 2008;32(6):956–973.
- Carbonara S, Monno L, Longo B, et al. Community-acquired pneumonia. *Curr Opin Pulm Med.* 2009;15(3):261–273.
- Chien S, Wells TG, Blumer JL, et al. Levofloxacin pharmacokinetics in children. *J Clin Pharmacol.* 2005;45(2):153–160.
- Eliakim-Raz N, Robenshtok E, Shefet D, et al. Empiric antibiotic coverage of atypical pathogens for community-acquired pneumonia in hospitalized adults. *Cochrane Database Syst Rev.* 2012;(9): CD004418.
- Kashyap S, Sarkar M. *Mycoplasma pneumonia*: clinical features and management. *Lung India.* 2010;27(2):75–85.
- Torres A, Blasi F, Peetermans WE, et al. The aetiology and antibiotic management of community-acquired pneumonia in adults in Europe: a literature review. *Eur J Clin Microbiol Infect Dis.* 2014;33(7):1065–1079.

CODES

ICD10
J15.7 Pneumonia due to Mycoplasma pneumoniae

CLINICAL PEARLS
- Most common atypical respiratory pathogens include *M. pneumoniae*, *C. pneumoniae*, and *L. pneumophila*.
- Atypical pneumonia is typically a clinical diagnosis; if labs are indicated, PCR is the mainstay of diagnosis with serology if PCR is not available.
- Watch closely for complicating symptoms that could indicate worsening disease.
- Atypical pneumonia with *M. pneumoniae* is typically self-limiting, difficult to identify, and usually responds to empiric treatment.
- Outbreaks of *M. pneumoniae* can be seen in close communities of young people.
- Onset of infection is typically have a gradual onset of symptoms, normal WBC, and less respiratory distress.

PNEUMONIA, PNEUMOCYSTIS JIROVECI
Cameron M. Shawver, DO • Marvin H. Sineath, Jr., MD, CAQSM

 BASICS

DESCRIPTION
- *Pneumocystis jiroveci* causes pneumonia primarily in immunocompromised patients.
- The fungus that causes this pneumonia in humans was previously called *Pneumocystis carinii*.
- The name was formally changed to *Pneumocystis jiroveci* in 2001, following the discovery that the fungus that infects humans is unique and distinctive from the fungus that infects animals (1).
- *P. jiroveci* is extremely resistant to traditional antifungal agents, including both amphotericin and azole agents (2).
- To prevent confusion, the term PCP, which used to represent *P. carinii* pneumonia, now represents *Pneumocystis* pneumonia (3).

ALERT
No combination of symptoms, signs, blood chemistries, or radiographic findings is diagnostic of *P. jiroveci* pneumonia (4).

EPIDEMIOLOGY
- *P. jiroveci* has a worldwide distribution, and most children have been exposed to the fungus by 2 to 4 years (5).
- The reservoir and mode of transmission for *P. jiroveci* is still unclear.
  - Human studies favor an airborne transmission model, with person-to-person spread being the most likely mode of infection acquisition (4).

Incidence
- Infants with HIV infection have a peak incidence of PCP between 2 and 6 months (5).
- HIV-infected infants have a high mortality rate, with a median survival of only 1 month.

Prevalence
- The prevalence of *P. jiroveci* colonization among healthy adults is 0–20% (2).
- Recent studies have demonstrated the transient nature of *P. jiroveci* colonization in asymptomatic, immunocompetent patients (4).
- 50% of patients with PCP are coinfected with ≥2 strains of *P. jiroveci* (5).
- There is evidence that distinct strains are responsible for each episode in patients who develop multiple episodes of PCP (5).

ETIOLOGY AND PATHOPHYSIOLOGY
Mode of transmission is unknown; likely respiratory from infected host

RISK FACTORS
Individuals at risk (4)
- Patients with HIV/AIDS infection, especially if not receiving prophylactic treatment for PCP
- Patients who are receiving high doses of glucocorticoids
- Patients who have an altered immune system not due to HIV
- Patients who are receiving chronic immunosuppressive medications
- Patients who have hematologic or solid malignancies resulting in malignancy-related immune depression

GENERAL PREVENTION
- Indications for prophylaxis
  - HIV-infected adults (5)
    - Should start when CD4 count is <200 cells/μL or if the patient develops oropharyngeal candidiasis
  - HIV-infected children (5)
    - Prophylaxis should be provided for children ≥6 years based on adult guidelines.
    - For children aged 1 to 5 years, start when CD4 count is <500 cells/μL.
    - For infants <12 months, start when the CD4 percentage is <15%.
  - Non–HIV-infected adults receiving immunosuppressive medications or with underlying immune system deficits should receive PCP prophylaxis, but currently there are no specific guidelines on when to start this.
- Medication
  - Trimethoprim-sulfamethoxazole (TMP-SMX)
    - Adults: 1 double-strength tablet daily or 1 double-strength tablet 3 times per week
    - Children >2 months: 150 mg TMP/m^2/day in divided doses q12h for 3 days per week
  - Atovaquone suspension
    - Adults: 1,500 mg PO once daily with food
    - Children: not to exceed 1,500 mg/day
      - 1 to 3 months: 30 mg/kg/day PO once daily
      - 4 to 24 months: 45 mg/kg/day PO once daily
      - >24 months: 30 mg/kg/day PO once daily
      - Adolescents ≥13 years: Refer to adult dosing.
  - Dapsone
    - Adults only: 50 mg BID or 100 mg once daily
  - Pentamidine
    - Adults only: 300 mg aerosolized every 4 weeks
- Discontinuation of prophylaxis
  - When CD4+ cell counts are >200 cells/μL for a period of 3 months in the adult population (2)[C]
  - There are no clear guidelines for discontinuation of prophylaxis in children.

COMMONLY ASSOCIATED CONDITIONS
- HIV/AIDS
- Chronic obstructive pulmonary disease (COPD)
- Interstitial lung disease
- Connective tissue diseases treated with corticosteroids
- Cancer and organ transplant patients on immunosuppressive medication

 DIAGNOSIS

HISTORY
- HIV-infected patients
  - Subacute onset over several weeks
    - Progressively worsening dyspnea
    - Tachypnea
    - Cough: nonproductive or productive of clear sputum
    - Low-grade fever, chills
    - Weakness, fatigue, malaise

- Non–HIV-infected immunocompromised patients
  - More acute onset with fulminant respiratory failure
    - Abrupt tachypnea, dyspnea
    - Fever
    - Dry cough

PHYSICAL EXAM
- Fever
- Tachypnea
- Tachycardia
- Lung exam is normal or near normal.

DIFFERENTIAL DIAGNOSIS
- Tuberculosis
- Bacterial pneumonia
- Fungal pneumonia
- Viral pneumonia

DIAGNOSTIC TESTS & INTERPRETATION
P. jiroveci cannot be cultured. Therefore, a diagnosis relies on detection of the organism by colorimetric or immunofluorescent stains or by polymerase chain reaction (PCR) (5)[C].
- ABG: reveals hypoxemia and increased alveolar–arterial gradient that varies with severity of disease
- LDH: Serum lactate dehydrogenase is frequently increased (nonspecific; likely due to underlying lung inflammation and injury).
- CD4 cell count is generally <200 cells/μL in HIV-infected patients with PCP.
- S-adenosylmethionine levels are significantly lower in a patient with PCP. The levels increase with successful treatment (6)[B].
- Comprehensive metabolic profile
- Chest x-ray (CXR) (4)[C]
  - Bilateral, symmetric, fine, reticular interstitial infiltrates involving perihilar areas; becomes more homogeneous and diffuse as severity of infection progresses
  - Less common patterns include upper lobe involvement in patients receiving aerosolized pentamidine, solitary or multiple nodular opacities, lobar infiltrates, pneumatoceles, and pneumothoraces.
  - May be normal in up to 30% of patients with PCP (3)[C]
- High-resolution CT is more sensitive than CXR.

Diagnostic Procedures/Other
- Fiber-optic bronchoscopy with bronchoalveolar lavage (BAL) is the preferred diagnostic procedure to obtain samples for direct fluorescent antibody staining.
  - Sensitivities range from 89% to >98%.
- *Pneumocystis* trophic forms or cysts obtained from induced sputum, BAL fluid, or lung tissue, which can be visualized using conventional stains
- PCR can detect *Pneumocystis* from respiratory sources, but the potential remains for false positives (4)[C].

TREATMENT

The recommended duration of therapy differs in patients who are with/without AIDS:

- In patients with PCP who do not have AIDS, the typical duration of therapy is 14 days.
- Treatment of PCP in patients who have AIDS was increased to 21 days due to the risk for relapse after only 14 days of treatment (4)[C].

MEDICATION
- TMP-SMX (2,4)[C]
- Adult dosing
  - TMP: 15 to 20 mg/kg/day, PO or IV, divided into 4 doses
- Pediatric dosing (>2 months) (4)[C]
  - TMP: 15 to 20 mg/kg/day in divided doses q6–8h
- Reduce doses of TMP-SMX in patients with renal failure.
- Treatment response to *Pneumocystis* therapy often requires at least 7 to 10 days before clinical improvement is documented (2)[C].
- Pregnancy risk factor: Category C (4)[C]
- Precautions
  - History of sulfa allergy
  - There is an emergence of drug-resistant PCP, especially against TMP-SMX.

Second Line
- Pentamidine (for moderate to severe cases)
  - Adults and children: 4 mg/kg IV or IM once daily
- Dapsone + trimethoprim (adults only)
  - Dapsone 100 mg PO once daily, *plus*
  - Trimethoprim 5 mg/kg PO TID
    - Check the glucose-6-phosphate dehydrogenase level before beginning dapsone, as hemolysis may result.
- Clindamycin + primaquine (adults only)
  - Clindamycin 600 to 900 mg IV q8h or 300 to 450 mg PO QID, *plus*
  - Primaquine 30 mg PO once daily
- Atovaquone
  - Adults: 750 mg PO BID (>13 years of age)
  - Children: 40 mg/kg/day PO divided BID (max 1,500 mg)
- Note: Pentamidine has greater toxicity than TMP-SMX: hypotension, hypoglycemia, pancreatitis (4)[C].

ADDITIONAL THERAPIES
Adjunctive corticosteroid (prednisone or methylprednisolone) (4)[C],(7)[A]

- Adjunctive corticosteroids are shown to provide benefits in patients who have AIDS and symptoms of moderate to severe PCP.
- Corticosteroids provide the greatest benefit to HIV patients who have hypoxemia manifested as a partial pressure of arterial oxygen <70 mm Hg or an alveolar–arterial gradient >35 mm Hg on room air.
- Adults and children >13 years of age: prednisone, 40 mg PO BID on days 1 to 5; 40 mg daily on days 6 to 11; 20 mg daily on days 12 to 21

INPATIENT CONSIDERATIONS
- No set criteria for hospital admission
- Five predictors of mortality in HIV-associated *Pneumocystis* pneumonia (8)
  - Increased age of the patient
  - Recent IV drug use
  - Total bilirubin >0.6 mg/dL
  - Serum albumin <3 g/dL
  - Alveolar–arterial oxygen gradient ≥50 mm Hg (8)[C]

ONGOING CARE

FOLLOW-UP RECOMMENDATIONS
In patients with HIV/AIDS: Patients with previous episodes of PCP should receive lifelong secondary prophylaxis unless they respond well to highly active antiretroviral therapy (HAART) and have a CD4 count >200 cells/μL for at least 3 months.

Patient Monitoring
Serum lactate dehydrogenase levels, pulmonary function test results, and ABG measurements generally normalize with treatment.

DIET
No special diet needed

PATIENT EDUCATION
- Centers for Disease Control and Prevention: www.cdc.gov/ncidod/dpd/parasites/pneumocystis/default.htm
- FamilyDoctor.org: http://familydoctor.org/familydoctor/en/diseases-conditions/hiv-and-aids/complications/pneumocystis-pneumonia-pcp-and-hiv.html

REFERENCES

1. Catherinot E, Lanternier F, Bougnoux ME, et al. *Pneumocystis jiroveci* pneumonia. *Infect Dis Clin North Am.* 2010;24(1):107–138.
2. Limper AH, Knox KS, Sarosi GA, et al. An official American Thoracic Society statement: treatment of fungal infections in adult pulmonary and critical care patients. *Am J Respir Crit Care Med.* 2011;183(1):96–128.
3. D'Avignon LC, Schofield CM, Hospenthal DR. *Pneumocystis* pneumonia. *Semin Respir Crit Care Med.* 2008;29(2):132–140.
4. Krajicek BJ, Thomas CF Jr, Limper AH. *Pneumocystis* pneumonia: current concepts in pathogenesis, diagnosis, and treatment. *Clin Chest Med.* 2009;30(2):265–278, vi.
5. Kovacs JA, Masur H. Evolving health effects of *Pneumocystis*: one hundred years of progress in diagnosis and treatment. *JAMA.* 2009;301(24):2578–2585.
6. Skelly MJ, Holzman RS, Merali S. S-adenosylmethionine levels in the diagnosis of *Pneumocystis carinii* pneumonia in patients with HIV infection. *Clin Infect Dis.* 2008;46(3):467–471.
7. Briel M, Bucher HC, Boscacci R, et al. Adjunctive corticosteroids for *Pneumocystis jiroveci* pneumonia in patients with HIV-infection. *Cochrane Database Syst Rev.* 2006;(3):CD006150.
8. Fei WM, Kim EJ, Sant CA, et al. Predicting mortality from HIV-associated *Pneumocystis* pneumonia at illness presentation: an observational cohort study. *Thorax.* 2009;64(12):1070–1076.

ADDITIONAL READING

- Benson CA, Kaplan JE, Masur H, et al. Treating opportunistic infections among HIV-infected adults and adolescents: recommendations from CDC, the National Institutes of Health, and the HIV Medicine Association/Infectious Disease Society of America. *MMWR Recomm Rep.* 2004;53(RR-15):1–112.
- Green H, Paul M, Vidal L, et al. Prophylaxis for *Pneumocystis* pneumonia (PCP) in non-HIV immunocompromised patients. *Cochrane Database Syst Rev.* 2007;(3):CD005590.
- Kaplan JE, Masur H, Holmes KK. Guidelines for preventing opportunistic infections among HIV-infected persons—2002. Recommendations of the U.S. Public Health Service and the Infectious Disease Society of America. http://www.cdc.gov/mmwr/preview/mmwrhtml/rr5108a1.htm.
- Shankar SM, Nania JJ. Management of *Pneumocystis jiroveci* pneumonia in children receiving chemotherapy. *Paediatr Drugs.* 2007;9(5):301–309.
- Stringer JR, Beard CB, Miller RF, et al. A new name (*Pneumocystis jiroveci*) for *Pneumocystis* from humans. *Emerg Infect Dis.* 2002;8(9):891–896.

SEE ALSO

HIV/AIDS

CODES

ICD10
B59 Pneumocystosis

CLINICAL PEARLS

- Colonization with *P. jiroveci* is common in the pediatric population.
- PCP only occurs in immunocompromised patients.
- Patients with HIV are at risk once their CD4 count is <200 cells/μL. At that time, TMP-SMX should be initiated as prophylaxis. Prophylaxis may end after HAART has been initiated and the CD4 count is >200 cells/μL for 3 months.
- Patients who are immunocompromised are also at risk. Currently, no clear clinical guidelines are available as to when to initiate or end prophylaxis.
- The first-line treatment is TMP-SMX. The typical duration of therapy is 14 days in non–AIDS-infected patients and 21 days in AIDS-infected patients.

PNEUMONIA, VIRAL

R. Aaron Lambert, MD

 BASICS

DESCRIPTION
- Inflammatory disease of the lungs due to a viral infection
- Most viral pneumonia results from exposure infection in the form of aerosolized secretions.
- Hematogenous and direct spread are also possible.

Geriatric Considerations
High rates of morbidity and mortality in the elderly

Pediatric Considerations
- Adenoviral infections in children are serious.
- More serious respiratory viral infections are almost always seen in infants and in immunocompromised patients.

Pregnancy Considerations
- Pregnant patients should avoid contact with anyone who has a viral infection.
- Influenza vaccination is recommended for all pregnant women during the influenza season.

EPIDEMIOLOGY
Incidence
- Predominant age: children <5 years
- Predominant sex: male = female

Prevalence
- Prevalence is variable with seasonal outbreaks, but the disease is more common during winter months.
- ~90% of all cases of childhood pneumonias have a viral cause.
- Between 4% and 39% of pneumonia diagnosed in adults has been attributed to viral causes.

ETIOLOGY AND PATHOPHYSIOLOGY
Overall: Influenza A and respiratory syncytial virus (RSV) are the leading causes followed by adenovirus and the parainfluenza viruses:
- Adults
  - Influenza A, B, and C
  - Influenza H1N1
  - Adenovirus
  - Parainfluenza
  - Coronavirus/SARS
- Children
  - Influenza A, B, and C
  - Influenza H1N1
  - Rhinovirus
  - Adenovirus
  - Parainfluenza
  - Rubeola (measles)
  - RSV (particularly for those born prematurely)
- Miscellaneous
  - Cytomegalovirus (CMV) (particularly in immuno-compromised patients)
  - Varicella
  - Herpes simplex virus (HSV)
  - Enterovirus
  - Rubeola
  - Epstein-Barr virus
  - Hantavirus
  - Human metapneumovirus

Genetics
No known genetic pattern has been recognized.

RISK FACTORS
- Seasonal: epidemic upper respiratory illness
- Living in close quarters
- Recent upper respiratory infection
- Travel to endemic area
- Nonvaccinated person
- Age >65 years or <5 years
- Altered mental status (due to dysphagia)
- Cardiac disease
- Chronic pulmonary disease (e.g., COPD, emphysema)
- Immunocompromised (HIV, transplant recipient, medication-induced)
- Cystic fibrosis
- Kartagener syndrome

GENERAL PREVENTION
- General hand-hygiene techniques are the first-line prevention in transmission of infectious particles.
- Influenza vaccination: Routine vaccination is now recommended for ALL persons aged ≥6 months.
  - Children who are 6 months to 8 years of age and receiving seasonal vaccination for the *first* time should receive two doses 4 weeks apart.
  - Children who are 6 months to 8 years of age who received two doses of the influenza vaccine should receive one dose of the seasonal influenza vaccine the following year.
  - See the CDC guidelines (1)[A] regarding the use of live attenuated vaccine versus inactivated vaccine.
- For those patients who are unable to receive influenza vaccine (e.g., with an egg allergy or other) and are at very high risk because of age, comorbid illness, or another risk factor, oseltamivir or zanamivir may be used for the duration of the season, with special recognition for potential viral resistance.
- For those who did not receive the vaccine and have been exposed to influenza, use of oseltamivir or zanamivir is recommended for up to 10 days following exposure.

COMMONLY ASSOCIATED CONDITIONS
- Rate of mixed viral–bacterial coinfection is ~20% and can lead to more severe illness or hospitalization.
- Fungal infection and *Pneumocystis jiroveci* pneumonia in immunocompromised patients

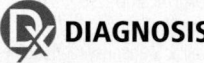 **DIAGNOSIS**

HISTORY
- Gradual onset
- Fever/chills
- Headache
- Myalgias
- Malaise
- Anorexia/decreased feeding in adults/infants

- Cough (with or without purulent sputum production)
- Dyspnea
- Rhinorrhea is predictive (OR 3.52) (2)[B].
- Pharyngitis
- Pleurisy
- Upper abdominal pain in children

PHYSICAL EXAM
- Fever
- Tachypnea
- Tachycardia
- Hypoxemia with severe disease
- Altered breath sounds (bronchophony, tactile fremitus, whispered pectoriloquy)
- Pulmonary rales and rhonchi
- Friction rub
- Possible associated rash (i.e., measles, HSV)

DIFFERENTIAL DIAGNOSIS
- Bacterial pneumonia (especially atypical etiologies: *Chlamydophila pneumoniae* and *C. psittaci*, *Mycoplasma pneumoniae*, *Legionella pneumophila*)
- Pulmonary edema
- *Pneumocystis pneumonia*/*P. jiroveci* pneumonia
- Aspiration pneumonia
- Hypersensitivity pneumonitis
- Bronchiolitis obliterans, with organizing pneumonia
- Pulmonary embolus/infarction
- Cystic fibrosis (in infants)
- Severe acute respiratory syndrome or severe acute respiratory syndrome–associated coronavirus

DIAGNOSTIC TESTS & INTERPRETATION
- No standard labs to diagnose viral pneumonia
- Specific lab investigations should be based on the clinical scenario.

Initial Tests (lab, imaging)
- CBC
  - Normal or near-normal granulocyte count, occasionally leukopenic with increased lymphocyte percentage
  - Hemoconcentration (hantavirus)
- Chest x-ray (CXR)
  - interstitial or alveolar infiltrates
  - peribronchial thickening
- Ground-glass opacities (GGO) are predictive (OR 4.68) (2)[B].
- ESR/CRP may be helpful in children.

Follow-Up Tests & Special Considerations
Clinicians can also consider additional testing, as clinically indicated:
- Appropriate direct fluorescent antibody or enzyme immunoassay from throat nasopharyngeal washings (children) or swab (adults), tracheal aspirate, or bronchoalveolar lavage specimens (HSV, varicella-zoster virus, influenza viruses A and B, RSV, adenovirus)

- Viral culture
  - Limitations: Results take 3 to 14 days. False-negative results occur with lower viral titers.
  - Rapid antigen detection: nasopharyngeal swab for rapid influenza testing
  - Cytopathology (cytoplasmic inclusion bodies [CMV], HSV, measles virus)
  - Serology (4-fold rise in acute compared with convalescent titers): Confirm diagnosis retrospectively but not clinically useful.
  - Serologic testing for hantavirus: enzyme immunoassay if available from health departments
  - Polymerase chain reaction (PCR) detection if modality is available:
    - Highly sensitive and specific, but a positive result does not imply causality.
- Sputum Gram stain and culture to identify bacterial copathogens, if present
- Chest CT may show consolidations surrounded by GGOs.

Diagnostic Procedures/Other
Bronchoscopy with bronchoalveolar lavage

TREATMENT

- Outpatient treatment for most patients
- Inpatient treatment for infants <4 months of age, elderly or for any patient with diffuse, severe infection (e.g., hypoxemia, hypercarbia, hypotension or shock, acute respiratory distress syndrome [ARDS]) or significant comorbidity (e.g., congestive heart failure [CHF], coronary artery disease, COPD)
- The Pneumonia Severity Index Calculator (3)[A] (http://www.mdcalc.com/psi-port-score-pneumonia-severity-index-adult-cap/) may be used to assess the need for hospitalization as well as mortality risk.
- Consider concomitant treatment for bacterial coinfection if severely ill or not responding to treatment.

MEDICATION
First Line
- Influenza viruses A and B
  - Oseltamivir (Tamiflu): adults and children >40 kg, 75 mg PO q12h for 5 days; dosage is adjusted to 75 mg PO q24h in cases where creatinine clearance rate is <30 mL/min. Children <40 kg, weight-based effectiveness is maximal when started within 48 hours of symptom onset.
  - Zanamivir (Relenza): patients >7 years of age, 2 inhalations (10 mg) q12h for 5 days
    - Shown to shorten symptoms by ~12 hours but not risk of complications (4)[B]
- Varicella-zoster virus
  - Acyclovir
    - Adults: for immunocompetent patients, 800 mg PO 5 times per day for 5 to 7 days
    - Children >2 years: for immunocompetent patients, 80 mg/kg/day PO divided q6h for 5 days. Start within 24 hours of symptom onset; immunocompromised patients 30 mg/kg/day PO divided q6h for 5 days. Start within 24 hours of symptom onset; immunocompromised patients 30 mg/kg/day IV divided q8h for 7 to 10 days.

- CMV or HSV
  - Acyclovir
    - Immunocompromised adults: 5 mg/kg IV q8h for 7 days
    - Children: Contact an infectious disease specialist or an experienced pharmacist regarding dosing.
  - Ganciclovir: Use should be in conjunction with infectious disease consultation.
- RSV
  - Ribavirin: Indicated in few, select cases (20 mg/mL via continuous aerosol administration for 12 to 18 hr/day for 3 to 7 days). Ribavirin is teratogenic and should not be administered by pregnant health care personnel: Its cost is high and benefits are marginal.

Second Line
- Influenza: Amantadine and rimantadine are no longer recommended due to high levels of resistance among circulating influenza A viruses (5)[B].
- Influenza: Peramivir 600 mg for 1 dose is an IV formulation available for acute illness in hospitalized patients (1).
- CMV, HSV, varicella virus infections
  - Foscarnet (Foscavir): 60 mg/kg/dose IV q8h in conjunction with infectious disease consultation

GENERAL MEASURES
- Most healthy individuals will only require symptomatic treatment.
- Encourage coughing and deep breathing exercises to clear secretions.
- Careful disposal of secretions/universal precautions.
- Hydration
- Respiratory isolation with negative pressure room for varicella virus, which is highly contagious

ONGOING CARE

FOLLOW-UP RECOMMENDATIONS
Patient Monitoring
- Physical exams
- Repeat a CXR only if warranted by clinical presentation. A CXR may take weeks to resolve after clinical illness has resolved.
- Oxygenation if illness severe enough for hospitalization

PATIENT EDUCATION
- For patient education materials on this topic, contact American Lung Association, 1301 Pennsylvania Avenue, NW, Suite 800, Washington, DC 20004; 800-LUNG-USA
- Centers for Disease Control and Prevention. Seasonal influenza (flu). http://www.cdc.gov/flu/

PROGNOSIS
- Usually favorable prognosis, with illness lasting several days to a week
- Postviral fatigue is common.
- Death can occur, especially in pediatric or bone marrow transplant recipients with adenovirus infections or in older people with influenza.
- The 2009 H1N1 influenza pandemic resulted in higher-than-usual mortality rates among the pediatric, young adult, and pregnant populations.

COMPLICATIONS
- Superimposed bacterial infections, such as *Streptococcus pneumoniae*, *Staphylococcus aureus*, *Haemophilus influenzae*, and others
- Respiratory failure requiring mechanical ventilation
- ARDS
- Reye syndrome after influenza in children (avoid aspirin)

REFERENCES

1. Centers for Disease Control and Prevention. Seasonal influenza (flu). http://www.cdc.gov/flu/.
2. Kim JE, Kim UJ, Kim HK, et al. Predictors of viral pneumonia in patients with community-acquired pneumonia. *PLoS One*. 2014;9(12):e114710.
3. MDCalc. PSI/PORT Score: Pneumonia Severity Index for CAP. http://www.mdcalc.com/psi-port-score-pneumonia-severity-index-adult-cap/. Accessed 2015.
4. Heneghan CJ, Onakpoya I, Thompson M, et al. Zanamivir for influenza in adults and children: systematic review of clinical study reports and summary of regulatory comments. *BMJ*. 2014;348:g2547.
5. Grohskoph LA, Sokolow LZ, Olsen SJ, et al. Prevention and control of influenza with vaccines: recommendations of the Advisory Committee on Immunization Practices, United States, 2015-16 influenza season. *MMWR Morb Mortal Wkly Rep*. 2015;64(30):818–825.

ADDITIONAL READING

- Marcos MA, Esperatti M, Torres A. Viral pneumonia. *Curr Opin Infect Dis*. 2009;22(2):143–147.
- Ruuskanen O, Lahti E, Jennings LC, et al. Viral pneumonia. *Lancet*. 2011;377(9773):1264–1275.

SEE ALSO

Bronchiolitis Obliterans and Organizing Pneumonia; Respiratory Distress Syndrome, Acute (ARDS)

CODES

ICD10
- J12.9 Viral pneumonia, unspecified
- J12.0 Adenoviral pneumonia
- J12.1 Respiratory syncytial virus pneumonia

CLINICAL PEARLS

- Laboratory testing may confirm the diagnosis of viral pneumonia, but this may not change therapy and must not replace clinical judgment.
- Influenza vaccination is recommended for all persons age ≥6 months.
- Most patients recover with conservative therapy.
- Monitor for concomitant bacterial infections.
- Amantadine and rimantadine are no longer recommended for use against influenza.

POLYARTERITIS NODOSA

Katherine S. Upchurch, MD • Rajandeep S. Paik, MD

BASICS

DESCRIPTION
- Polyarteritis nodosa (PAN) is an antineutrophil cytoplasmic antibody (ANCA)-negative necrotizing arteritis of medium or small arteries without glomerulonephritis or vasculitis of arterioles, capillaries, or venules (1).
- Involved systems include GI tract, peripheral nervous system (sensory and motor), central nervous system (CNS), renal (without glomerulonephritis), skin, testes/epididymis, heart (1–3).
- Features depend on location of vasculitis: mesenteric ischemia–related symptoms, new onset or worsening hypertension, mononeuritis multiplex, purpuric or nodular skin lesions, or livedo reticularis (3).
- Renal disease in PAN usually manifests as hypertension (HTN) and mild proteinuria with/without azotemia. Renal infarction may occur (3).
- PAN formerly encompassed several distinct entities (classic PAN, microscopic PAN, cutaneous PAN). With the advent of ANCA testing, microscopic PAN appears unrelated to the other two, pathophysiologically.
  - Patients with classic PAN are *typically ANCA-negative* (1,4).
  - Patients with microscopic PAN have ANCAs directed against myeloperoxidase (MPO) and (generally) involvement of small arterioles (microscopic polyangiitis [MPA]). This is now classified as ANCA-associated vasculitis (1).
  - Cutaneous (or limited) PAN is a chronic disease with cutaneous lesions with characteristic histopathologic features of PAN. There are few systemic manifestations, although myalgias and peripheral motor neuropathy (mononeuritis multiplex) or sensory neuropathy may be present. ANCA positivity is variable (5).
- Synonym(s): periarteritis; panarteritis; necrotizing arteritis

EPIDEMIOLOGY
Incidence
- Predominant age: Peak onset is in the 5th to 6th decade; incidence rises with age.
- 1.5:1 male predominance (6)

Prevalence
Rare: 2 to 33 cases/1 million adults (6)

ETIOLOGY AND PATHOPHYSIOLOGY
- Segmental, transmural, necrotizing inflammation of medium and small muscular arteries, with intimal proliferation, thrombosis, and ischemia of the organ/tissue supplied by the affected arteries. Aneurysm formation at vessel bifurcations (3)
- Hepatitis B–related PAN results in direct injury to the vessel due to viral replication or deposition of immune complexes, with complement activation and subsequent inflammatory response (3).
- Most cases are idiopathic; 20% are related to hepatitis B or C infection (7).
- In patients with PAN and hepatitis B, HBsAg has been recovered from involved vessel walls (7).

Genetics
Mutations of adenosine deaminase 2 (ADA 2) have been identified in families with PAN (8).

RISK FACTORS
Hepatitis B infection >> hepatitis C infection (cutaneous PAN) (7)

COMMONLY ASSOCIATED CONDITIONS
- Hepatitis B (strong association with classic PAN) (7)
- Hepatitis C (less strongly linked to cutaneous PAN)
- Hairy cell leukemia
- 27 existing case reports of systemic PAN following hepatitis B vaccination (9)
- Minocycline (symptoms resolve on stopping drug, reoccur if rechallenged) (10)
- Case reports also associating PAN with CMV infection, amphetamines, and interferon (11)

DIAGNOSIS

There are no formal diagnostic criteria for PAN (1,3). Suspect PAN in patients with the following:
- Acute, sometimes fulminant multisystem disease with a relatively short prodrome (i.e., weeks to months)
- Vasculitic skin rash with sensorimotor symptoms/findings
- Recent-onset HTN with systemic symptoms
- Unexplained sensory and/or motor neuropathy with systemic symptoms
- Hepatitis B infection with multisystem disease

HISTORY
General: systemic symptoms with multiorgan involvement (3)
- Constitutional symptoms (fever, weight loss, malaise)
- Organ-specific symptoms
  - Focal muscular weakness/extremity numbness
  - Myalgia and arthralgia
  - Rash
  - Recurrent postprandial pain, intestinal angina, nausea, vomiting, and bleeding
  - Altered mental status, headaches, mononeuritis multiplex
  - Testicular/epididymal pain, neurogenic bladder (rare)

PHYSICAL EXAM
Related to involved organ system (may dominate clinical picture and course) (2,3)
- Peripheral nervous system: peripheral neuropathy
- Renal: HTN
- Skin: purpura, urticaria, polymorphic rashes, subcutaneous nodules (uncommon, but characteristic), livedo reticularis; deep skin ulcers, especially in lower extremities; Raynaud phenomenon (rare); single digit gangrene (rare)
- GI: acute abdomen; rebound, guarding, tenderness
- CNS: seizures, altered mental status, papillitis
- Lung: signs of pleural effusion—dullness to percussion; decreased breath sounds
- Cardiac: signs of congestive heart failure and/or myocardial infarction—S3 gallop; pericarditis (friction rub is rare)
- Genitourinary: testicular/epididymal tenderness (can mimic testicular torsion)
- Musculoskeletal: arthritis (usually large joint in lower extremities)

DIFFERENTIAL DIAGNOSIS
- Other forms of vasculitis (ANCA-associated, such as GPA, Churg-Strauss syndrome, and MPA; Henoch-Schönlein purpura, drug-induced vasculitis, cryoglobulinemia, Goodpasture syndrome)
- Buerger disease
- Systemic lupus erythematosus (SLE)
- Embolic disease (atrial myxoma, cholesterol emboli)
- Thrombotic disease (antiphospholipid antibody syndrome)

- Dissecting aneurysm
- Ehlers-Danlos syndrome
- Multiple sclerosis, systemic amyloidosis
- Infection (subacute endocarditis, HIV infection, trichinosis, rickettsial diseases)

DIAGNOSTIC TESTS & INTERPRETATION
- No specific laboratory abnormalities. Confirm diagnosis with biopsy if possible (4)[C].
- Angiography (conventional, CT angiography, or MR angiography) may reveal microaneurysms and/or beading of bifurcating blood vessels.
- Avoid contrast in renal disease.
- Nonspecific laboratory abnormalities:
  - Elevated ESR and CRP
  - Mild proteinuria, elevated creatinine
  - Hepatitis B surface antigen positive in 10–50%
  - Hepatitis C antibody/hepatitis C virus RNA
  - ANCA, antiproteinase 3 (PR3), and anti-MPO are negative. Positive ANCA argues against PAN.
  - Rheumatoid factor may be positive.
  - Anemia of chronic disease (3,4)

Initial Tests (lab, imaging)
Lab tests performed to look for evidence of systemic disease and rule out other causes (3,4):
- CBC, ESR, CRP (elevated) (4)[C]
- Chemistries: elevated creatinine/BUN (4)[C]
- Hepatitis B serology: often positive; hepatitis C less commonly positive
- LFTs: abnormal if involving the liver/biliary tract
- Urinalysis: proteinuria/hematuria, generally no cellular casts or active urinary sediment (4)[C]
- ANA, cryoglobulins (4)[C]
- ANCA, anti-MPO, and anti-PR3 (4)[A]
- Complement levels (C3, C4)
- Angiographic demonstration of aneurysmal changes/beading of small and medium-sized arteries

Diagnostic Procedures/Other
- Electromyography and nerve conduction studies in patients with suspected mononeuritis multiplex. If abnormal, consider sural nerve biopsy.
- Arterial/tissue biopsy
- Skin biopsy from edges of ulcers; include deep dermis and subcutaneous (SC) fat to assess small muscular artery involvement (excisional *not* punch biopsy) (3,4)

Test Interpretation
- Necrotizing inflammation with fibrinoid necrosis of small and medium-sized muscular arteries; segmental, often at bifurcations and branchings. Venules not involved in classic PAN.
- Capillaritis/other lung parenchymal involvement by vasculitis *strongly suggests* another process (microscopic PAN, granulomatosis with polyangiitis [GPA; formerly known as Wegener granulomatosis], Churg-Strauss syndrome, or antiglomerular basement membrane disease).
- Acute lesions with infiltration of polymorphonuclear cells through vessel walls into perivascular area; necrosis, thrombosis, infarction of involved tissue
- Aneurysmal dilatations, including aortic dissection
- Peripheral nerves: 50–70% (vasa nervorum with necrotizing vasculitis)
- GI vessels: 50% (at autopsy) with bowel necrosis; gallbladder and appendix vasculature: 10%
- Muscle vessels: 50%

- Testicular vessels involved in symptomatic males
- *The key differences from other necrotizing vasculitides are lack of granuloma formation and sparing of veins and pulmonary arteries (2,3).*

TREATMENT

GENERAL MEASURES
Aggressively treat HTN to prevent associated complications (stroke, myocardial infarction, heart failure)

MEDICATION
First Line
- Severe (life-threatening) disease: corticosteroids (CS) (high-dose prednisone, methylprednisolone, or parenteral Solu-Medrol) (4,10)[A]
  - Only 50% of patients achieve and maintain remission with CS. Other patients require additional immunosuppressive therapy.
  - Cyclophosphamide (CTX) in combination with CS: Improves survival and spares use of chronic steroids in moderate/severe PAN (4,10)[A].
    - CTX has risk of infertility and malignancy.
  - Plasma exchange for refractory and renal disease (4,7)[A]
  - Rituximab use for refractory disease suggested by its efficacy in ANCA + vasculitis (4,12,13)[C].
- Less severe disease: CS alone ± other immunosuppressive agents (azathioprine, (4)[A] methotrexate, mycophenolate mofetil (4,10,14)[B])
- HBV-associated PAN: antiviral agents, short-term CS, plasma exchange (7,10)[C]

Second Line
- Tumor necrosis factor inhibitors anecdotally reported to be of use in PAN (15)
- PAN disease activity correlates with serum IL-6 levels; tocilizumab, an inhibitor of IL-6 approved for use in rheumatoid arthritis; no evidence-based data for PAN (16).

ADDITIONAL THERAPIES
- For patients receiving IV CTX, concurrent administration of mercaptoethane sulfonate reduces bladder exposure to carcinogenic metabolites (4)[C].
- Prophylactically treat patients on CTX for *Pneumocystis jiroveci (carinii)* pneumonia with trimethoprim sulfamethoxazole (use dapsone or atovaquone in intolerant/allergic patients) (4).

INPATIENT CONSIDERATIONS
Admission Criteria/Initial Stabilization
Depends on extent and involvement of specific organs

ONGOING CARE

FOLLOW-UP RECOMMENDATIONS
Patient Monitoring
- CBC, urinalysis, renal and hepatic function tests
- Acute-phase reactants (e.g., ESR, CRP) may help monitor disease activity
- Be alert for the following:
  - Treatment specific side effects of CS and immunosuppressant medications
  - Delayed appearance of neoplasms after treatment, especially bladder malignancy in patients treated with CTX. (Check annual U/A, urinary cytology with urologic evaluation if microscopic hematuria.) (4)[C]
  - Steroid-induced osteoporosis

DIET
Low salt (HTN)

PATIENT EDUCATION
- Patient education materials are available from the Arthritis Foundation, 1314 Spring St, NW, Atlanta, GA 30309; 800-283-7800
- ACR website: www.rheumatology.org

PROGNOSIS
- Expected course of untreated PAN is poor, with an estimated 5-year survival of 13% (17).
- Steroid and cytotoxic treatment increase 5-year survival rate to 75–80% (3,17).
- Survival is greater for hepatitis B–related PAN as a result of the introduction of antiviral treatments (7).
- Patients presenting with proteinuria, renal insufficiency, GI tract involvement, cardiomyopathy, or CNS involvement have a worse prognosis.

COMPLICATIONS
- End-organ damage from ischemia
- Complications from immunosuppressive agents

REFERENCES

1. Jennette JC, Falk RJ, Bacon PA, et al. 2012 revised International Chapel Hill Consensus Conference Nomenclature of Vasculitides. *Arthritis Rheum.* 2013;65(1):1–11.
2. Ebert EC, Hagspiel KD, Nagar M, et al. Gastrointestinal involvement in polyarteritis nodosa. *Clin Gastroenterol Hepatol.* 2008;6(9):960–966.
3. Pagnoux C, Seror R, Henegar C, et al. Clinical features and outcomes in 348 patients with polyarteritis nodosa: a systematic retrospective study of patients diagnosed between 1963 and 2005 and entered into the French Vasculitis Study Group Database. *Arthritis Rheum.* 2010;62(2):616–626.
4. Mukhtyar C, Guillevin L, Cid MC, et al. EULAR recommendations for the management of primary small and medium vessel vasculitis. *Ann Rheum Dis.* 2009;68(3):310–317.
5. Nakamura T, Kanazawa N, Ikeda T, et al. Cutaneous polyarteritis nodosa: revisiting its definition and diagnostic criteria. *Arch Dermatol Res.* 2009;301(1):117–121.
6. Phillip R, Luqmani R. Mortality in systemic vasculitis: a systematic review. *Clin Exp Rheumatol.* 2008;26(5)(Suppl 51):S94–S104.
7. Guillevin L, Mahr A, Callard P, et al. Hepatitis B virus-associated polyarteritis nodosa: clinical characteristics, outcome, and impact of treatment in 115 patients. *Medicine (Baltimore).* 2005;84(5):313–322.
8. Navon Elkan P, Pierce SB, Segel R, et al. Mutant adenosine deaminase 2 in a polyarteritis nodosa vasculopathy. *N Engl J Med.* 2014;370(10):921–931.
9. de Carvalho JF, Pereira RM, Shoenfeld Y. Systemic polyarteritis nodosa following hepatitis B vaccination. *Eur J Intern Med.* 2008;19(8):575–578.
10. Culver B, Itkin A, Pischel K. Case report and review of minocycline-induced cutaneous polyarteritis nodosa. *Arthritis Rheum.* 2005;53(3):468–470.
11. Bourgarit A, Le Toumelin P, Pagnoux C, et al. Deaths occurring during the first year after treatment onset for polyarteritis nodosa, microscopic polyangiitis, and Churg-Strauss syndrome: a retrospective analysis of causes and factors predictive of mortality based on 595 patients. *Medicine (Baltimore).* 2005;84(5):323–330.
12. de Menthon M, Mahr A. Treating polyarteritis nodosa: current state of the art. *Clin Exp Rheumatol.* 2011;29(1)(Suppl 4):S110–S116.
13. Stone JH, Merkel PA, Spiera R, et al. Rituximab versus cyclophosphamide for ANCA-associated vasculitis. *N Engl J Med.* 2010;363(3):221–232.
14. Specks U, Merkel PA, Seo P, et al. Efficacy of remission-induction regimens for ANCA-associated vasculitis. *N Engl J Med.* 2013;369(5):417–427.
15. Ribi C, Cohen P, Pagnoux C, et al. Treatment of polyarteritis nodosa and microscopic polyangiitis without poor-prognosis factors: a prospective randomized study of one hundred twenty-four patients. *Arthritis Rheum.* 2010;62(4):1186–1197.
16. Chan M, Lugmani R. Pharmacotherapy of vasculitis. *Expert Opin Pharmacother.* 2009;10(8):1273–1289.
17. Murakami M, Nishimoto N. The value of blocking IL-6 outside of rheumatoid arthritis: current perspective. *Curr Opin Rheumatol.* 2011;23(3):273–277.

ADDITIONAL READING

Kouchi M, Sato S, Kamono M, et al. A case of polyarteritis nodosa associated with cytomegalovirus infection. *Case Rep Rheumatol.* 2014;2014:604874.

 SEE ALSO

Hepatitis B; Hepatitis C

 CODES

ICD10
- M30.0 Polyarteritis nodosa
- M30.1 Polyarteritis with lung involvement [Churg-Strauss]
- M30.8 Other conditions related to polyarteritis nodosa

CLINICAL PEARLS

- PAN is a necrotizing vasculitis of small- to medium-sized muscular arteries with lack of granuloma formation that spares veins and pulmonary arteries.
- Clinical features of PAN depend on target organ involvement.
- Skin biopsies at ulcer edges (include deep dermis and SC fat) improve diagnostic yield.
- Check hepatitis B and C serologies.
- ANCA is negative in classic PAN.
- Treatment involves immunosuppression; choice of agent depends on extent and severity of disease.

POLYCYSTIC KIDNEY DISEASE

Maricarmen Malagon-Rogers, MD

 BASICS

DESCRIPTION

- A group of monogenic disorders that results in renal cyst development
- The most frequent are two genetically distinct conditions: autosomal dominant polycystic kidney disease (ADPKD) and autosomal recessive polycystic kidney disease (ARPKD).
- ADPKD is one of the most common human genetic disorders.

EPIDEMIOLOGY

- ADPKD is generally late onset.
  - Mean age of end-stage kidney disease (ESKD) 57 to 69 years
  - More progressive disease in men than in women
  - Up to 90% of adults have cysts in the liver.
- ARPKD usually present in infants.
  - A minority in older children and young adults may manifest as liver disease.
  - Nonobstructive intrahepatic bile dilatation is sometimes seen.
  - Found on all continents and in all races

Incidence

- Mean age of ESKD: *PKD1 mutation*, 54.3 years versus *PKD2 mutation*, 74 years
- ARPKD affects 1/20,000 live births; carrier level is 1/70.
- ADPKD affects 1/400 to 1,000 live births.

Prevalence

As ESKD, ADPKD: 8.7/1 million in the United States; 7/1 million in Europe

ETIOLOGY AND PATHOPHYSIOLOGY

- ADPKD
  - *PKD1* and *PKD2* mutations disrupt the function of polycystins on the primary cilium, forming fluid-filled cysts that progressively increase in size, leading to gross enlargement of the kidney, and distortion of the renal architecture.
  - Glomerular hyperfiltration compensates for the progressive loss of healthy glomeruli, and therefore, by the time GFR decline becomes detectable, as much as ½ of the original functional glomeruli are irreversibly lost.
  - The majority of patients with ADPKD ultimately progress to ESKD (1).
- ARPKD
  - *PKHD1* product fibrocystin is also located in cilia.
- ADPKD: Cysts arise from only 5% of nephrons:
  - Autosomal dominant pattern of inheritance but a molecularly recessive disease with the 2-hit hypothesis
  - Requires genetic and environmental factors
- ARPKD: Mutations are scattered throughout the gene with genotype–phenotype correlation.

Genetics

- ADPKD
  - Autosomal dominant inheritance
  - 50% of children of an affected adult are affected.
  - 100% penetrance; genetic imprinting and genetic anticipation are seen as well.
  - Two genes isolated
    - *PKD1* on chromosome 16p13.3 (85% of patients) encodes polycystin 1
    - *PKD2* on chromosome 4q21 (15% of patients) encodes polycystin 2

- ARPKD
  - Autosomal recessive inheritance
  - Siblings have a 1:4 chance of being affected; gene *PKHD1* on chromosome 6p21.1–p12 encodes fibrocystin.

RISK FACTORS

- Large inter- and intrafamilial variability
- A more rapidly progressive clinical course is predicted by onset of ESKD at <55 years, development of stage 3 CKD at <40 years old, onset of HTN at <18 years, total kidney volume greater than the expected for a given age, or presence of multiple complications (gross hematuria, microalbuminuria) (1).

GENERAL PREVENTION

Genetic counseling

COMMONLY ASSOCIATED CONDITIONS

- ADPKD
  - Cysts in other organs
    - Polycystic liver disease in 58% of young age group to 94% of 45-year-olds
    - Pancreatic cysts: 5%
    - Seminal cysts: 40%
    - Arachnoid cysts: 8%
  - Vascular manifestations
    - Intracerebral aneurysms in 6% of patients without family history and in 16% with family history
    - Aortic dissections
  - Cardiac manifestations: mitral valve prolapse: 25%
  - Diverticular disease
- ARPKD: liver involvement: affected in inverse proportion to renal disease; congenital hepatic fibrosis with portal HTN

 DIAGNOSIS

HISTORY

- ADPKD
  - Positive family history (15% are de novo mutations)
  - Flank pain: 60%
  - Hematuria
  - UTI
  - HTN: 50% aged 20 to 34 years; 100% with ESKD
  - Renal failure
  - Presymptomatic screening of ADPKD is not currently recommended for at-risk children (2).
    - Blood pressure should be routinely measured in these patients.
- ARPKD
  - 30% of affected neonates die:
    - Enlarged echogenic kidneys and oligohydramnios are diagnosed in utero.
    - Later in childhood: HTN
  - Adolescents and adults present with complications of portal HTN: esophageal varices
  - Hypersplenism

PHYSICAL EXAM

- HTN
- Flank masses

DIFFERENTIAL DIAGNOSIS

- ADPKD and ARPKD
- Tuberous sclerosis: prevalence 1/6,000
- Von Hippel-Lindau syndrome: prevalence 1/36,000
- Nephronophthisis: accounts for 10–20% of cases of renal failure in children; medullary cystic kidney disease
- Renal cystic dysplasias: multicystic dysplastic kidneys; grossly deformed kidneys; most common type of bilateral cystic diseases in newborns (prevalence: 1/4,000)
- Simple cysts: most common cystic abnormality
  - Localized or unilateral renal cystic disease
  - Medullary sponge kidney
  - Acquired renal cystic disease
- Renal cystic neoplasms: benign multilocular cyst (cystic nephroma)

DIAGNOSTIC TESTS & INTERPRETATION

Electrolytes, BUN/creatinine, urine analysis plus urinary citrate

Initial Tests (lab, imaging)

- ADPKD
  - Renal dysfunction
    - Impaired renal concentration (3), hypocitraturia aciduria
    - Hyperfiltration
    - Elevated creatinine
  - Urinalysis: hematuria and mild proteinuria
- ARPKD
  - Electrolyte abnormalities and renal insufficiency
  - Anemia, thrombocytopenia, leukopenia
- ADPKD
  - US: It is the easiest diagnostic method. However, it is suboptimal for disease exclusion at age <40 years (2)
    - Renal enlargement is universal.
    - In at-risk patients: By age 30 years, two renal cysts (bilateral or unilateral) are 100% diagnostic. In children, it sometimes appears similar to ARPKD; may be diagnosed in utero.
    - Presence of hepatic cysts in young adults is pathognomonic for ADPKD.
    - In the absence of family history, bilateral renal enlargement and cysts make the diagnosis.
  - CT scan/MRI ideally should be part of the initial evaluation (2).
    - Kidney volume assessed by CT or MRI is a main predictor of progression.
    - Helpful in identifying cysts in other organs
    - In subjects <40 years, fewer than five cysts by MRI excludes the diagnosis (2).
- ARPKD
  - US: Kidneys are enlarged, homogeneously hyperechogenic (cortex and medulla).
  - CT scan is more sensitive if diagnosis is in doubt.
  - Presence of hepatic fibrosis helps the diagnosis.

Follow-Up Tests & Special Considerations

- Diagnosis and prevention of secondary problems because of renal and liver abnormalities
- Follow-up of combined renal volume to assess disease severity
- Beyond age 2 years, renal size decreases in ARPKD but continues to grow in ADPKD at an average rate of 5.27% per year. Total kidney volume identifies patients with progressive disease (2).

Diagnostic Procedures/Other

- Genetic testing is available for *PKD1* and *PKD2* in ADPKD when imaging results are equivocal and for potential living related donors (4).
- For *PKHD1* in ARPKD, a prenatal diagnosis is feasible in about 72% of patients.

Test Interpretation

- ADPKD
  - Kidneys are diffusely cystic and, although enlarged, retain their general shape.
  - Cysts range from a few millimeters to several centimeters and are distributed evenly throughout the cortex and medulla.
  - They arise in all segments of the nephron, although they arise initially from the collecting ducts.
  - One kidney may be larger than the other.
- ARPKD
  - Disease is a spectrum, ranging from severe renal disease with mild liver damage to mild renal disease with severe liver damage.
  - Renal enlargement is due to fusiform dilatation of the collecting ducts in the cortex and medulla in the newborn period.
  - Liver lesion is diffuse but limited to fibrotic portal areas.

 TREATMENT

GENERAL MEASURES

- HTN: moderate sodium restriction, weight control, and regular exercise
- Medications: ACE inhibitors; angiotensin receptor blockers (ARBs)
- Pain: narcotics and other analgesics; bed rest; limit NSAIDs (they worsen renal function)
- Urolithiasis: treated with alkalinization of urine and hydration therapy; surgery as needed
- UTIs/Infections of cysts: lipid-soluble antibiotics more effective (e.g., trimethoprim-sulfamethoxazole and chloramphenicol); fluoroquinolones also useful
- Dialysis for ESKD patients
- Hematuria: Reduce physical activity.

MEDICATION

- No specific drug therapy is yet available for PKD, although several studies are being conducted for specific treatments (2,5).
- HTN: should be very well controlled to prevent complications. ACE inhibitors are preferred if no contraindications are present.
- The use of antihypertensive medications has been found to decrease mortality (6).
- Hyperlipidemia: statins preferred

ISSUES FOR REFERRAL

- Nephrologist primary management
- Urologic consultation for management of symptomatic/infected cysts
- Genetic counseling is critical.

SURGERY/OTHER PROCEDURES

- Indications for surgical intervention
  - Uncontrollable HTN
  - Severe back and loin pain, abdominal fullness
  - Renal deterioration due to enlarging cysts
  - Hematuria/hemorrhage or recurrent UTI

- Open and laparoscopic cyst unroofing: may decrease pain and narcotics requirements; has not been proven to prevent renal failure or to prolong current renal function
- Percutaneous cyst aspiration ± injection of sclerosing agent; not usually performed secondary to recurrent fluid accumulation
- Renal transplant for ESKD

INPATIENT CONSIDERATIONS

Admission Criteria/Initial Stabilization

Severe pain, gross hematuria with clots

 ONGOING CARE

FOLLOW-UP RECOMMENDATIONS

None in early stages of the disease; avoid vigorous activity if disease advances. Recurrent gross hematuria is secondary to trauma, associated with faster decline of renal function.

Patient Monitoring

- Monitor BP and renal function. Encourage hydration. Treat UTI and stone disease aggressively.
- Avoid nephrotoxic drugs.
- Creatinine and BP monitoring at least twice a year; more often as needed
- Screening for intracranial aneurysms (7)

DIET

- Low-protein diet may retard renal insufficiency.
- Limit caffeine because this might increase cyst growth.
- High water intake to decrease ADH >3 liters a day (5)

PROGNOSIS

- Renal failure in 2% by age 40 years; 23% by age 50 years; 48% by age 73 years
- ADPKD accounts for 10–15% of dialysis patients.
- No increased incidence of renal cell cancer

COMPLICATIONS

- Cyst rupture, infection, or hemorrhage
- Progression to renal failure
- Renal calculi

REFERENCES

1. Schrier RW, Brosnahan G, Cadnapaphornchai MA, et al. Predictors of autosomal dominant polycystic disease progression. *J Am Soc Nephrol*. 2014;25(11):2399–2418.
2. Chapman AB, Devuyst O, Eckardt KU, et al. Autosomal-dominant polycystic kidney disease (ADPKD): executive summary from a Kidney Disease: Improving Global Outcomes (KDIGO) Controversies Conference. *Kidney Int*. 2015;88(1):17–27. doi:10.1038/ki.2015.59.
3. Zittema D, Boertien WE, van Beek AP, et al. Vasopressin, copeptin, and renal concentrating capacity in patients with autosomal dominant polycystic kidney disease without renal impairment. *Clin J Am Soc Nephrol*. 2012;7(6):906–913.
4. Harris PC, Rossetti S. Molecular diagnostics for autosomal dominant polycystic kidney disease. *Nat Rev Nephrol*. 2010;6(4):197–206.
5. Mahnensmith RL. Novel treatments of autosomal dominant polycystic kidney disease. *Clin J Am Soc Nephrol*. 2014;9(5):831–836.
6. Patch C, Charlton J, Roderick PJ, et al. Use of antihypertensive medications and mortality of patients with autosomal dominant polycystic kidney disease: a population-based study. *Am J Kidney Dis*. 2011;57(6):856–862.
7. Rozenfeld MN, Ansari SA, Shaibani A, et al. Should patients with autosomal dominant polycystic kidney disease be screened for cerebral aneurysms? *AJNR Am J Neuroradiol*. 2014;35(1):3–9.

ADDITIONAL READING

- Chapman AB, Bost JE, Torres VE, et al. Kidney volume and functional outcomes in autosomal dominant polycystic kidney disease. *Clin J Am Soc Nephrol*. 2012;7(3):479–486.
- Harris PC, Torres VE. Polycystic kidney disease. *Annu Rev Med*. 2009;60:321–337.
- Torres VE, Chapman AB, Devuyst O, et al. Tolvaptan in patients with autosomal dominant polycystic kidney disease. *N Engl J Med*. 2012;367(25):2407–2418.
- Torres VE, Harris PC. Polycystic kidney disease in 2011: connecting the dots toward a polycystic kidney disease therapy. *Nat Rev Nephrol*. 2011;8(2):66–68.
- Torres VE, Harris PC, Pirson Y. Autosomal dominant polycystic kidney disease. *Lancet*. 2007;369(9569):1287–1301.
- Wilson PD. Polycystic kidney disease. *N Engl J Med*. 2004;350(2):151–164.

 SEE ALSO

Chronic Kidney Disease

 CODES

ICD10

- Q61.3 Polycystic kidney, unspecified
- Q61.19 Other polycystic kidney, infantile type
- Q61.2 Polycystic kidney, adult type

CLINICAL PEARLS

- Most PKD patients eventually develop ESKD. No specific treatment has been proven to prevent EKRD, but hydration and control of BP are reasonable goals and should be started soon.
- Patients may benefit from a nephrology consultation after the initial diagnosis to counsel regarding disease progression prevention. Then, they can be followed by primary care if the disease was an incidental finding or no significant kidney dysfunction is present.

POLYCYSTIC OVARIAN SYNDROME (PCOS)

Maria De La Luz Nieto, MD

 BASICS

DESCRIPTION

- Polycystic ovarian syndrome (PCOS) is a common endocrine disorder with heterogeneous manifestations that affects up to 7% of the U.S. population.
- Hyperandrogenism leading to anovulation, typically presenting as amenorrhea or oligomenorrhea
- Diagnosis is based on clinical assessment and ultrasound findings.
- Diagnostic clinical characteristics include menstrual dysfunction, infertility, hirsutism, acne, obesity, and metabolic syndrome. The ovaries are often polycystic on imaging.
- The etiology of PCOS is unknown but can be modified by lifestyle factors.
- System(s) affected: reproductive, endocrine/metabolic, skin/exocrine
- Synonym(s): Stein-Leventhal syndrome; polycystic ovary disease

ALERT
- Condition may begin at puberty.
- Pregnancy does not resolve the syndrome.
- Predisposes to and is associated with obesity, hypertension, diabetes, metabolic syndrome, hyperlipidemia, infertility, insulin-resistance syndrome

EPIDEMIOLOGY

Prevalence
- Incidence and prevalence are still highly debated due to a wide spectrum of diagnostic features: The National Institutes of Health (NIH) criteria require chronic anovulation in addition to clinical or biochemical signs of hyperandrogenism. The prevalence based on NIH criteria is 6.5–8%.
- Predominant age: reproductive age
- Predominant sex: females only

ETIOLOGY AND PATHOPHYSIOLOGY
- PCOS is a multifactorial functional disorder of unclear etiology.
- Recent evidence points to a primary role for insulin resistance with hyperinsulinemia.
- Androgenism: Ovaries are the main source of excess androgens. Polycystic ovaries have thickened thecal layers, which secrete excess androgens in response to luteinizing hormone (LH). LH receptors are overexpressed in thecal and granulosa cells of polycystic ovaries.
- Ovarian follicles: Abnormal androgen signaling may account for abnormal folliculogenesis causing polycystic ovaries. The mechanism that determines abnormal number of follicles is unknown but may be due to abnormal androgen signaling on the ovarian stroma.
- Insulin resistance: Women with PCOS have insulin resistance similar to that in type 2 diabetes. Elevated levels of insulin decrease sex hormone–binding protein (SHBG), increasing bioavailability of testosterone. Insulin may also act directly on adrenal, ovary, and hypothalamus to regulate androgen and gonadotropin release. Insulin resistance causes elevated insulin levels.
- Insulin resistance may cause the frequently associated metabolic syndrome and frank diabetes mellitus.

Genetics
Ultimate expression is likely a combination of polygenic and environmental factors.

RISK FACTORS
See "Commonly Associated Conditions"; cause and effect are difficult to extricate in this disorder.

GENERAL PREVENTION
None known; focus on early diagnosis and treatment to prevent long-term complications.

COMMONLY ASSOCIATED CONDITIONS
- Infertility
- Obesity
- Obstructive sleep apnea
- Hypertension
- Diabetes mellitus
- Endometrial hyperplasia/carcinoma
- Fatty liver disease
- Mood disturbances and depression

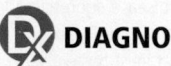 **DIAGNOSIS**

HISTORY
- A comprehensive history, including a family history of diabetes and premature onset of cardiovascular disease, is important in the differential diagnosis.
- Focus on the onset and duration of the various signs of androgen excess, menstrual history, and concomitant medications, including the use of exogenous androgens (1).

PHYSICAL EXAM
- Vital signs: body mass index (BMI), high BP
- General appearance: central obesity, deepened voice, hirsutism, acne
- Skin: hair pattern and growth, acne, seborrhea, acanthosis nigricans
- Genitalia: clitoromegaly and ovarian enlargement

ALERT
Look specifically for signs of virilization, such as hair pattern, deepened voice, and clitoromegaly.

DIFFERENTIAL DIAGNOSIS
- Cushing syndrome
- HAIR-AN syndrome
- Testosterone-producing ovarian or adrenal tumor
- Prolactin-producing pituitary adenoma
- Hyperthecosis
- Adult-onset adrenal hyperplasia
- Partial congenital adrenal hyperplasia (21-hydroxylase deficiency)
- 11β-hydroxylase deficiency
- 17β-hydroxysteroid dehydrogenase deficiency
- Acromegaly
- Drug-induced hirsutism, oligo-ovulation (e.g., danazol, steroids, valproic acid)
- Thyroid disease

DIAGNOSTIC TESTS & INTERPRETATION
- The value of measurement of circulating androgens to document PCOS is uncertain but should include measuring free testosterone concentration directly by equilibrium dialysis.

- Most common diagnostic criteria used is Rotterdam criteria (need 2 of 3):
  - Oligo- or anovulation
  - Clinical and/or biochemical signs of hyperandrogenism
  - Transvaginal ultrasonographic polycystic ovaries and exclusion of other etiologies; therefore, consider exclusion of Cushing disease, congenital adrenal hyperplasia, and androgen-secreting tumors.
- More recent criteria also focus on similar criteria while acknowledging that there may be forms of PCOS without overt evidence of hyperandrogenism (2,3)[C].

Initial Tests (lab, imaging)
- Screening workup should include human chorionic gonadotropin (hCG), TSH, prolactin, FSH (exclude premature ovarian failure), DHEAS, 17-OH progesterone, and testosterone level.
- LH determination may be ordered but is not usually necessary:
  - Hirsute women should have a testosterone or free testosterone determination and a DHEAS determination.
  - Consider 17-OH progesterone if congenital adrenal hyperplasia is a possibility.
- LH/FSH level ≥2.5 to 3/L in ~50% of women with PCOS, but LH testing is not generally necessary.
- Testosterone increased but <200 ng/dL (6.94 nmol/L).
- Typical findings in PCOS include mild elevation in DHEAS but <800 μg/dL (20.8 μmol/L), mild increase in 17-OH progesterone level, increased estrogen level, and decreased SHBG.
- Drugs that may alter lab results:
  - Oral contraceptives (OCs)
  - Steroids
  - Antidepressants
- Transvaginal ultrasound findings: one or both ovaries with ≥12 follicles measuring 2 to 9 mm or increased ovarian volume to 10 cm^3

Follow-Up Tests & Special Considerations
- Consider fasting serum glucose, insulin level, and plasminogen activator inhibitor-1 determinations to establish presence of insulin resistance and glucose intolerance, especially if diagnosis is in doubt.
- Overnight dexamethasone suppression test (Decadron 1 mg PO at 11:00 PM and fasting serum cortisol at 8:00 AM the next morning) to rule out Cushing syndrome in the appropriate setting
- Endometrial biopsy to rule out hyperplasia and/or carcinoma, if indicated
- If the syndrome is diagnosed, determination of fasting glucose and fasting lipid levels should be performed and formal glucose tolerance test is considered.

Test Interpretation
- Ovary usually enlarged with a smooth white glistening capsule
- Ovarian cortex lined with follicles in all stages of development, but most atretic
- Thecal cell proliferation with an increase in the stromal compartment

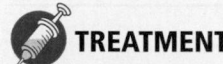 **TREATMENT**

GENERAL MEASURES
- No ideal treatment exists.
- Therapy must be individualized according to the needs and desires of each patient.

MEDICATION
Drug costs related to this condition are high.

First Line
- The goal of treatment in PCOS depends on symptoms and patient's goals for fertility.
- Treatment can be divided into five main categories: Lifestyle changes including appropriate nutrition and exercise to decrease body weight can restore ovulation and increase insulin sensitivity (4)[A],(5)[C].
- Menstrual irregularity when pregnancy not desired:
  – Low-dose OCs (30 to 35 μg); newer formulations containing progestins with lower androgenicity (e.g., norethindrone, desogestrel, norgestimate, drospirenone) may be particularly beneficial, but all OCs increase SHBG and decrease excess androgen and estrogen. If unable to tolerate OCs, then intermittent medroxyprogesterone (Provera) 10 mg PO for 10 days given every 1 to 2 months.
  – Metformin may help to correct metabolic abnormalities in women who are shown to be insulin resistant. Initial dose is 500 mg daily for 1 week, increasing by 500 mg/week to a total of 1,500 to 2,000 mg/day divided BID; take with food.
    ○ Overall, data support the usefulness of metformin on both cardiometabolic risk and reproduction assistance in PCOS women.
    ○ Thiazolidinediones may increase likelihood of ovulation and treat insulin resistance.
- If pregnancy is desired (6)[B]:
  – Ovulation induction with clomiphene (Clomid, Serophene) and/or exogenous gonadotropins. Birth rate with Clomid is 22.5%, 7.2% with metformin, and 26.8% in women who use both medications.
  – Metformin: 500 to 2,000 mg PO divided BID has been shown to improve hyperandrogenism and restore ovulation. Many times the drug is continued throughout the 1st trimester or the entire pregnancy if there is a history of spontaneous abortion or glucose intolerance. It does improve clinical pregnancy rates but does not improve live birth rates alone or in combination with clomiphene when used for ovulation induction.
  – Has been demonstrated that metformin reduces the incidence of gestational diabetes

Second Line
- Spironolactone for androgen excess hirsutism not addressed by OC therapy
- Cosmetic issues due to hyperandrogenism: Acne may respond best with OCs with low doses of cyproterone or drospirenone.
- Eflornithine hydrochloride 13.9% cream to inhibit hair growth

ADDITIONAL THERAPIES
Weight loss in overweight women results in biochemical and symptomatic improvement in most.

ISSUES FOR REFERRAL
- To reproductive endocrinologist for all women who cannot achieve pregnancy with Clomid
- High-risk pregnancies
- To endocrinologist if Cushing syndrome, congenital adrenal hyperplasia, or adrenal or ovarian tumors are found during the workup

SURGERY/OTHER PROCEDURES
- Ovarian wedge resection and laparoscopic laser drilling are controversial and rarely used today.
- Mechanical means of hair removal, including electrolysis, waxing, and depilatory, may improve cosmesis.

COMPLEMENTARY & ALTERNATIVE MEDICINE
Acupuncture assists with cycle normalization and weight loss.

 ONGOING CARE

FOLLOW-UP RECOMMENDATIONS
Follow-up at 6-month intervals to evaluate response to therapy and to monitor weight as well as medication side effects.

Patient Monitoring
- Counsel patient about the risk of endometrial and breast carcinoma, insulin resistance, and diabetes, as well as obesity and its role in infertility.
- See patient frequently throughout the menstrual cycle, depending on which drug combination is used to induce ovulation.

DIET
In overweight patients, weight loss is the most successful therapy because it improves cardiovascular risk, insulin sensitivity, and menstrual patterns: Counsel on lifestyle dietary changes; consider referral to nutritionist and weight center.

PATIENT EDUCATION
- Provide patient with information about PCOS, such as from http://www.acog.org/.
- Discuss the chronic nature of this condition and the risks and benefits and side effects of potential treatments.
- Review the importance of weight loss, if applicable. Modest weight loss of 5–10% of initial body weight has been demonstrated to improve many of the features of PCOS.

PROGNOSIS
- Fertility prognosis is good but may need assisted reproductive technologies.
- Proper follow-up and screening can prevent endometrial carcinoma.
- Early detection of diabetes may decrease morbidity and mortality associated with cardiovascular risk factor.

COMPLICATIONS
- Reproductive: infertility
- Metabolic: insulin resistance, diabetes mellitus, cardiovascular disease
- Psychosocial: increased anxiety, mood disorder, eating disorder, depression

REFERENCES
1. Azziz R, Carmina E, Dewailly D, et al. The Androgen Excess and PCOS Society criteria for the polycystic ovary syndrome: the complete task force report. *Fertil Steril*. 2009;91(2):456–488.
2. Carmina E, Oberfield SE, Lobo RA, et al. The diagnosis of polycystic ovary syndrome in adolescents. *Am J Obstet Gynecol*. 2010;203(3):201.e1–201.e5.
3. Chang RJ. A practical approach to the diagnosis of polycystic ovary syndrome. *Am J Obstet Gynecol*. 2004;191(3):713–717.
4. Tang T, Lord JM, Norman RJ, et al. Insulin-sensitising drugs (metformin, rosiglitazone, pioglitazone, D-chiro-inositol) for women with polycystic ovary syndrome, oligo amenorrhoea and subfertility. *Cochrane Database Syst Rev*. 2010;(1):CD003053.
5. Spritzer PM, Motta AB. Adolescence and polycystic ovary syndrome: current concepts on diagnosis and treatment. *Int J Clin Pract*. 2015;69(11):1236–1246.
6. Legro RS, Barnhart HX, Schlaff WD, et al. Clomiphene, metformin, or both for infertility in the polycystic ovary syndrome. *N Engl J Med*. 2007;356(6):551–566.

ADDITIONAL READING
- Diamanti-Kandarakis E, Economou F, Palimeri S, et al. Metformin in polycystic ovary syndrome. *Ann N Y Acad Sci*. 2010;1205:192–198.
- Lim CE, Wong WS. Current evidence of acupuncture on polycystic ovarian syndrome. *Gynecol Endocrinol*. 2010;26(6):473–478.
- Moran LJ, Misso ML, Wild RA, et al. Impaired glucose tolerance, type 2 diabetes and metabolic syndrome in polycystic ovary syndrome: a systematic review and meta-analysis. *Hum Reprod Update*. 2010;16(4):347–363.

 SEE ALSO

Algorithm: Amenorrhea, Secondary

 CODES

ICD10
- E28.2 Polycystic ovarian syndrome
- L68.0 Hirsutism

CLINICAL PEARLS
- In the United States, 40% of women with PCOS are not obese.
- Chronic anovulation should be treated because chronic estrogen stimulation in absence of progesterone may lead to endometrial hyperplasia.
- Specific therapies must be individualized according to the needs and desires of each patient.

POLYCYTHEMIA VERA

Richard D. Detheridge, MD • Roger P. Holland, MD, PhD

BASICS

DESCRIPTION
- Polycythemia vera (PV) is a chronic myeloproliferative clonal stem cell disorder marked by increased production of red blood cells (erythrocytosis) with excessive erythroid, myeloid, and megakaryocytic elements in the bone marrow.
- Morbidity and mortality are primarily related to complications from blood hyperviscosity or thrombosis development as well as malignant transformation.
- Myelofibrosis can develop in the bone marrow, leading to progressive hepatosplenomegaly.
- Synonym(s): primary polycythemia; Vaquez disease; Waldenstrom disease; primary PV; PV rubra; polycythemia, splenomegalic; Vaquez-Osler disease

EPIDEMIOLOGY
Incidence
- Predominant age: 50 to 75 years, 5% are <40 years
- Predominant sex: male > female (slightly)
- Incidence in the United States in 2012: 2.8/100,000 population of men and 1.3/100,000 population of women

Prevalence
In the United States in 2010, estimates ranged from 45 to 57 cases per 100,000 patients.

ETIOLOGY AND PATHOPHYSIOLOGY
JAK2 V617F mutation associated with clonal proliferative disorder

Genetics
JAK2 V617F (tyrosine kinase) mutation: >97% of patients with PV have an activating mutation; this is helpful in differentiating from secondary erythrocytosis. Homozygote carriers will have higher incidence of symptoms such as pruritus but will not have higher incidence of disease than heterozygotes.

RISK FACTORS
- PV is more prevalent among Jews of Eastern European descent than other Europeans or Asians.
- Familial history is rare.

COMMONLY ASSOCIATED CONDITIONS
- Budd-Chiari syndrome
- Mesenteric artery thrombosis
- Myocardial infarction
- Cerebrovascular accident or transient ischemic attack
- Venous thromboembolism and pulmonary embolism

DIAGNOSIS

HISTORY
- Patients may be asymptomatic or present with nonspecific complaints, including fatigue, malaise, and/or subjective weakness.
- Erythromelalgia (burning pain of feet/hands, occasionally with erythema, pallor, cyanosis, or paresthesias)
- Arterial and venous occlusive events
- Headaches
- Blurred vision or blind spots
- Pruritus, especially after the shower
- Spontaneous bruising/bleeding
- Peptic ulcer disease (due to alterations in gastric mucosal blood flow)
- Bone pain (ribs and sternum)
- Tinnitus

PHYSICAL EXAM
- Hypertension
- Facial plethora
- Splenomegaly
- Hepatomegaly
- Bone tenderness (especially ribs and sternum)
- Skin excoriations from significant pruritus
- Gouty tophi or arthritis

DIFFERENTIAL DIAGNOSIS
- Secondary polycythemias
- Hemoglobinopathy
- Ectopic erythropoietin production
- Spurious polycythemia

DIAGNOSTIC TESTS & INTERPRETATION
CBC; if suspicion is high, then obtain erythropoietin level and gene testing for *JAK2 V617F*.

Initial Tests (lab, imaging)
- 2008 World Health Organization diagnostic criteria requires two major criteria and one minor or the first major criterion with two minor criteria (1).
  - Major criteria:
    ○ Hemoglobin (Hgb) >18.5 g/dL (men); Hgb >16.5 g/dL (women); or Hgb >17 g/dL (men) or Hgb >15 g/dL (women) if associated with a sustained increase of ≥2 g/dL from baseline that cannot be attributed to correction of iron deficiency.
    ○ Presence of *JAK2 V617F* or similar mutation
  - Minor criteria:
    ○ Bone marrow trilineage myeloproliferation
    ○ Subnormal serum erythropoietin level
    ○ Endogenous erythroid colony (EEC) growth
- Diagnosis can be made reliably based on clinical symptoms, presence of *JAK2 V617* mutation, and low EPO (2).

- Other lab findings that are common but not specific
  - Hyperuricemia
  - Hypercholesterolemia
  - Elevated serum vitamin B_{12} levels
- CT or US to assess for splenomegaly, although not necessary for diagnosis
- Causes of secondary erythrocytosis:
  - Sleep apnea
  - Emphysema
  - Cigarette smoking
  - Renal artery stenosis
  - Carbon monoxide poisoning

Diagnostic Procedures/Other
- Bone marrow aspiration shows increased cellularity.
- Cytogenetic testing (*JAK2 V617F*)

Test Interpretation
- If *JAK2 V617F* mutation testing is negative and the erythropoietin level is normal or high, then PV is excluded; investigate causes of secondary erythrocytosis.
- Other causes of erythrocytosis such as ectopic erythropoietin production from a renal tumor, hypoxia from chronic lung, or cyanotic heart disease can be excluded with low or undetectable serum erythropoietin level and normal oxygen saturation.

TREATMENT

GENERAL MEASURES
- Risk factors: age, disease duration, disease phenotype, complications, disease activity
- Phlebotomy and low-dose aspirin is first-line therapy for low-risk patients.
- Phlebotomy reduces the blood hyperviscosity, improve platelet functions, restore systemic pressures, and decrease risk of thrombosis.
- Phlebotomy:
  - Reduce hematocrit to <45%; will significantly lower the rate of cardiovascular death and major thrombosis (3)[A].
  - Performed as often as every 2 to 3 days until normal hematocrit reached; phlebotomies of 250 to 500 mL. Reduce to 250 to 350 mL in elderly patients or patients with cerebrovascular disease.
  - May require concurrent myelosuppressive agent if at high risk for thrombosis
- Complications of phlebotomy: chronic iron deficiency (symptomatology: pica, angular stomatitis, and glossitis), possible muscle weakness, and dysphagia
- Other therapies:
  - Maintain hydration.
  - Pruritus therapy: H_1 and H_2 blockers, ataractics
  - Uric acid reduction therapy

MEDICATION

First Line

• Primary therapies:

- Low-dose aspirin 81 mg PO has been associated with a statistically nonsignificant reduction in the risk of fatal thrombotic events without increasing bleeding complications when used in conjunction with phlebotomy (4)[A].
- Hydroxyurea is recommended for patients at high risk for thrombosis (age >60 years or history of thrombotic event) and with splenomegaly and hepatomegaly. Common starting dose 500 to 1,500 mg PO daily, titrating to control hematocrit and platelet count. Be aware that hydroxyurea can lead to higher risk of leukemic transformation (5)[A].
- Radioactive phosphorous (^{32}P) may control Hgb level and platelet count by destroying overactive marrow cells. May take up to 3 months before affecting cells. Consider for patients intolerant or nonadherent to hydroxyurea or short expected survival due to mutagenic potential.
- Tyrosine kinase inhibitor imatinib 400 to 800 mg daily was shown to have moderate cytoreductive effects in PV (6)[B].
- Pegylated interferon-α-2a is effective in controlling erythrocytosis, although dosing is generally limited secondary to intolerable side effects (7)[B].
- Refer to hematologist/oncologist for further dosing and instructions.

• Symptomatic/adjunctive:

- Allopurinol 300 mg/day PO for uric acid reduction
- Cyproheptadine 4 to 16 mg PO daily as needed for pruritus
- H$_2$-receptor blockers or antacids for GI hyperacidity; cimetidine is also used for pruritus.
- SSRIs (paroxetine or fluoxetine) have shown some efficacy in controlling pruritus.
- Ultraviolet light may help with pruritus.

Second Line

Myelosuppression: chlorambucil or busulfan; busulfan at 2 to 4 mg daily may be effective option for elderly patients with advanced PV refractory or intolerant to hydroxyurea, but significant rate of transformation was observed.

ISSUES FOR REFERRAL

Referral to a hematologist to assist in diagnosis and management

ONGOING CARE

FOLLOW-UP RECOMMENDATIONS

Patient Monitoring

Monitor hematocrit often and phlebotomize as needed to maintain target goal.

DIET

• Avoid high-sodium diet, can cause fluid retention.
• Avoid iron supplement, a permissive chronic state of iron deficiency can help decrease blood production.

PATIENT EDUCATION

• Perform leg and ankle exercises to prevent clots.
• Continuous education regarding possible complications and seeking treatment early for any change or increase in symptoms

PROGNOSIS

• PV cannot be cured but can be controlled with treatment.
• Survival is >15 years with treatment.
• Patients are at risk for developing postpolycythemic myelofibrosis (PPMF) and an increased risk of malignant transformation.

COMPLICATIONS

• Splenomegaly or hepatomegaly
• Budd-Chiari syndrome
• Vascular thrombosis (major cause of death)
• Transformation to acute leukemia
• Transformation to myelofibrosis
• Hemorrhage
• Peptic ulcer
• Uric acid stones
• Secondary gout
• Increased risk for complications and mortality from surgical procedures. Assess risk/benefits and ensure optimal control of disorder before any elective surgery.

REFERENCES

1. Tefferi A, Thiele J, Vardiman JW. The 2008 World Health Organization classification system for myeloproliferative neoplasms: order out of chaos. *Cancer*. 2009;115(17):3842–3847.
2. Tefferi A. Polycythemia vera and essential thrombocythemia: 2013 update on diagnosis, risk-stratification, and management. *Am J Hematol*. 2013;88(6):507–516.
3. Marchioli R, Finazzi G, Specchia G, et al. Cardiovascular events and intensity of treatment in polycythemia vera. *N Engl J Med*. 2013;368(1):22–33.
4. Squizzato A, Romualdi E, Passamonti F, et al. Antiplatelet drugs for polycythaemia vera and essential thrombocythaemia. *Cochrane Database Syst Rev*. 2013;(4):CD006503.
5. Mascarenhas J, Mughal TI, Verstovsek S. Biology and clinical management of myeloproliferative neoplasms and development of the JAK inhibitor ruxolitinib. *Curr Med Chem*. 2012;19(26):4399–4413.
6. Merx K, Fabarius A, Erben P, et al. Effects of imatinib mesylate in patients with polycythemia vera: results of a phase II study. *Ann Hematol*. 2013;92(7):907–915.
7. Quintás-Cardama A, Kantarjian H, Manshouri T, et al. Pegylated interferon alfa-2a yields high rates of hematologic and molecular response in patients with advanced essential thrombocythemia and polycythemia vera. *J Clin Oncol*. 2009;27(32):5418–5424.

ADDITIONAL READING

• Passamonti F. How I treat polycythemia vera. *Blood*. 2012;120(2):275–284.
• Tefferi A, Fonseca R. Selective serotonin reuptake inhibitors are effective in the treatment of polycythemia vera-associated pruritus. *Blood*. 2002; 99(7):2627.

SEE ALSO

Myeloproliferative Neoplasms

CODES

ICD10

• D45 Polycythemia vera
• D75.1 Secondary polycythemia

CLINICAL PEARLS

• *JAK2* mutations are an important component of myeloproliferative disorders.
• Common complications include thrombosis, malignant transformation, and myelofibrosis.
• Phlebotomy is first-line treatment, and consultation with an experienced hematologist is recommended.

POLYMYALGIA RHEUMATICA

Ronald G. Chambers Jr., MD, FAAFP • Megan Babb, DO

BASICS

DESCRIPTION
- A clinical syndrome characterized by pain and stiffness (a term often used interchangeably by patients) of the shoulder, hip girdles, and neck (1).
- Primarily impacts the elderly, associated with morning stiffness and elevated markers of inflammation
- System(s) affected: musculoskeletal, hematologic/lymphatic/immunologic
- Synonym(s): senile rheumatic disease; polymyalgia rheumatica syndrome; pseudo-polyarthrite rhizomélique

Geriatric Considerations
- Incidence increases with age
- Average age of onset ~70 years

Pediatric Considerations
Rare in patients <50 years of age; peak incidence between 70 and 80 years of age (2)

EPIDEMIOLOGY
Incidence
- Incidence increases after 50. Incidence of PMR is 50/100,000 and incidence of giant cell arteritis (GCA) is 18/100,000 people in the United States.
- Predominant sex: female > male (2 to 3:1) (3)
- Most common in Caucasians, especially those of northern European ancestry

Prevalence
Prevalence in population >50 years old: 700/100,000

ETIOLOGY AND PATHOPHYSIOLOGY
- Unknown. Symptoms appear to be related to enhanced immune system activity and periarticular inflammatory activity.
- Pathogenesis
  - Polygenic; multiple environmental and genetic factors contribute
  - Histologic evidence of GCA and parvovirus B19 DNA in temporal artery specimen

Genetics
Associated with human leukocyte antigen determinants (HLA-DRB1*04 and DRB1*01 alleles) (4)

RISK FACTORS
- Age >50 years
- Presence of GCA

COMMONLY ASSOCIATED CONDITIONS
GCA (temporal arteritis) may occur in 15–30% of patients; more common in females than males with PMR.

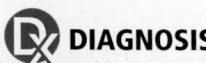

DIAGNOSIS

HISTORY
- Suspect PMR in elderly patients with new onset of proximal limb pain and stiffness (neck, shoulder, hip).
- Difficulty rising from chair or combing hair are signs of proximal muscle involvement.
- Nighttime pain
- Difficulty arising from a chair or raising the arms
- Systemic symptoms in ~25% (fatigue, weight loss, low-grade fever)

PHYSICAL EXAM
- Decreased range of motion (ROM) of shoulders, neck, and hips
- Muscle strength is usually normal, although it may be limited by pain and/or stiffness.
- Muscle tenderness
- Disuse atrophy
- Synovitis of the small joints and tenosynovitis
- Coexisting carpal tunnel syndrome

DIFFERENTIAL DIAGNOSIS
- Rheumatoid arthritis
- Palindromic rheumatism
- Late-onset seronegative spondyloarthropathies (e.g., psoriatic arthritis, ankylosing spondylitis)
- Systemic lupus erythematosus; Sjögren syndrome; fibromyalgia
- Polymyositis/dermatomyositis (check creatine phosphokinase, aldolase)
- Thyroid disease
- Hyperparathyroidism, hypoparathyroidism
- Hypovitaminosis D
- Viral myalgia
- Osteoarthritis
- Rotator cuff syndrome; adhesive capsulitis
- Remitting seronegative symmetrical synovitis with pitting edema (RS3PE) syndrome
- Occult infection or malignancy (e.g., lymphoma, leukemia, myeloma, solid tumor)
- Myopathy (e.g., steroid, alcohol, electrolyte depletion)
- Depression

DIAGNOSTIC TESTS & INTERPRETATION
Consider PMR in patients >50 years of age with proximal muscle pain and stiffness.
- Temporal artery biopsy if symptoms of GCA are present
- ESR (Westergren) elevation >40 mm/hr
  - ESR is typically elevated, sometimes >100 mm/hr
  - ESR normal (<40 mm/hr) in 7–22% of patients
- Elevated C-reactive protein
- Normochromic/normocytic anemia
- Anticyclic citrullinated peptide (anti-CCP) antibodies usually negative (in contrast to elderly-onset rheumatoid arthritis [RA])
- Rheumatoid factor: usually negative (5–10% of patients >60 years of age will have positive rheumatoid factor without RA)
- Mild elevations in liver function tests, especially alkaline phosphatase
- Antibodies to ferritin peptide
- Drugs that may alter lab results: prednisone
- Disorders that may alter lab results: other disorders causing elevation of the sedimentation rate (e.g., infection, neoplasm, renal failure)
- Normal EMG
- Normal muscle histology

Initial Tests (lab, imaging)
- ESR (usually >40 mm/hr); C-reactive protein; CBC
- MRI is not necessary for diagnosis but may show periarticular inflammation, tenosynovitis, and bursitis.
- US may show bursitis, tendinitis, and synovitis.
- MRI, PET, and temporal artery US may all play a role in diagnosis of PMR.

Diagnostic Procedures/Other
A temporal artery biopsy is indicated in patients with symptoms suggestive of GCA. Treat empirically pending biopsy results.

Test Interpretation
Scoring algorithm: morning stiffness >45 minutes (2 points), hip pain/limited ROM (1 point), absence of rheumatoid factor and anti-citrullinated protein antibody (ACPA) (2 points), and absence of peripheral joint pain (1 point). A score of >4 has 68% sensitivity and 78% specificity which increase with a positive temporal artery US.

TREATMENT

GENERAL MEASURES
- Address risk of steroid-induced osteoporosis.
  - Obtain dual energy x-ray absorptiometry and check 25-OH vitamin D levels if necessary.
  - Consider antiresorptive therapies (bisphosphonates) based on recommendations for treatment of corticosteroid-induced osteoporosis.
- Encourage adequate calcium (1,500 mg/day) and vitamin D (800 to 1,000 U/day) supplementation.
- Physical therapy for ROM exercises, if needed

MEDICATION
First Line
- Prednisone: 10 to 20 mg/day PO initially; expect a dramatic (diagnostic) response within days. 15 mg/day is an effective dose in most patients.
  - Increase to 20 mg/day if no immediate response.
  - If no response to 10 to 20 mg/day within a week, reconsider diagnosis.
- Divided-dose steroids (BID or TID) may be helpful (especially if symptoms recur in the afternoon).
- Consider using delayed-release prednisone at bedtime (may be more efficient in treating morning stiffness)
- Begin slow taper by 2.5 mg decrements every 2 to 4 weeks to a dose of 7.5 to 10 mg/day. Below this dose, taper by 1 mg/month to prevent relapse.
- Increase prednisone for recurrence of symptoms (relapse common).
- Corticosteroid treatment often lasts at least 1 to 2 years.
- May stop steroids at 6 to 12 months if patient is symptom-free and there is a normal ESR
- Contraindications
  - Use steroids with caution in patients with chronic heart failure, diabetes mellitus, immunocompromised conditions, and with systemic fungal or bacterial infection.
  - Treat infections concurrently.
- Precautions
  - Long-term steroid use (>2 years) is associated with sodium and water retention, exacerbation of chronic heart failure, hypokalemia, increased susceptibility to infection, osteoporosis, fractures, hypertension, cataracts, glaucoma, avascular necrosis, depression, and weight gain
  - Patients may develop temporal arteritis while on low-dose corticosteroid treatment for PMR. This requires an increase in dose to 40 to 60 mg.
  - Alternate-day steroids are not effective.

Second Line
- NSAIDs usually are not adequate for pain relief.
- Methotrexate has a modest effect in reducing relapse rate and lowering the cumulative dose of steroid therapy.
- There is conflicting evidence for antitumor necrosis factor agents (anti-TNF) (infliximab, etanercept) regarding steroid-sparing effects.
- Anti-interleukin (anti-IL) 6 therapy is under investigation for future use (5).
- Corticosteroid injections may reduce pain and stiffness and allow for increased levels of activity.

 ONGOING CARE

FOLLOW-UP RECOMMENDATIONS
Patient Monitoring
- Evaluate patients monthly initially and during medication taper; every 3 months otherwise.
- Follow ESR as steroids are tapered; both ESR and CRP should decline as symptoms improve.
- Follow-up for symptoms of GCA (e.g., headache, visual loss, and diplopia) and report immediately.
- Monitor side effects of corticosteroid therapy such as osteoporosis, hypertension, and hyperglycemia.
- Do not treat elevated ESR (do not increase the steroid dose to normalize the ESR If patient is asymptomatic).

DIET
- Regular diet
- Aim for adequate calcium and vitamin D.

PATIENT EDUCATION
- Review adverse effects of corticosteroids.
- Discuss the symptoms of GCA and instruct the patient to report them immediately should any occur.
- Contact physician if symptoms recur during steroid taper.
- Instruct patients to not discontinue steroids abruptly.
- Counsel patients on calcium and vitamin D requirements.
- Resources for patients
  - Arthritis Foundation: http://www.arthritis.org/
  - American College of Rheumatology: http://www.rheumatology.org/I-Am-A/Patient-Caregiver/Diseases-Conditions/Polymyalgia-Rheumatica

PROGNOSIS
- Most patients require at least 2 years of corticosteroid treatment.
- Prognosis is very good with proper treatment.
- Relapse is common (in 25–50% of patients), particularly if steroids are tapered too quickly.
- Higher age at diagnosis, female sex, high baseline ESR, increased plasma viscosity, increased levels of soluble IL-6 receptor, or high initial steroid dose have been associated with a prolonged disease course and greater number of disease flares.

COMPLICATIONS
- Complications related to chronic steroid use
- Exacerbation of disease with taper of steroids; development of GCA (may occur when PMR is being treated adequately)

REFERENCES

1. Mackie SL, Hughes R, Walsh M, et al. "An impediment to living life": why and how should we measure stiffness in polymyalgia rheumatica? *PLoS One*. 2015;10(5):e0126758.
2. Salvarani C, Gabriel SE, O'Fallon WM, et al. Epidemiology of polymyalgia rheumatica in Olmsted County, Minnesota, 1970-1991. *Arthritis Rheum*. 1995;38(3):369–373.
3. Liozon E, Ouattara B, Rhaiem K, et al. Familial aggregation in giant cell arteritis and polymyalgia rheumatica: a comprehensive literature review including 4 new families. *Clin Exp Rheumatol*. 2009;27(1 Suppl 52):S89–S94.
4. Weyand CM, Hunder NN, Hicok KC, et al. HLA-DRB1 alleles in polymyalgia rheumatica, giant cell arteritis, and rheumatoid arthritis. *Arthritis Rheum*. 1994;37(4):514–520.
5. Seitz M. Polymyalgia rheumatica: what is the current status? *Z Rheumatol*. 2015;74(6):507–510.

ADDITIONAL READING

- Aikawa NE, Pereira RM, Lage L, et al. Anti-TNF therapy for polymyalgia rheumatica: report of 99 cases and review of the literature. *Clin Rheumatol*. 2012;31(3):575–579.
- Buttgereit F, Gibofsky A. Delayed-release prednisone—a new approach to an old therapy. *Expert Opin Pharmacother*. 2013;14(8):1097–1106.
- Camellino D, Cimmino MA. Imaging of polymyalgia rheumatica: indications on its pathogenesis, diagnosis and prognosis. *Rheumatology (Oxford)*. 2012;51(1):77–86.

- Dasgupta B, Borg FA, Hassan N, et al. BSR and BHPR guidelines for the management of polymyalgia rheumatica. *Rheumatology (Oxford)*. 2010;49(1):186–190.
- Dasgupta B, Cimmino MA, Maradit-Kremers H, et al. 2012 provisional classification criteria for polymyalgia rheumatica: a European League Against Rheumatism/American College of Rheumatology collaborative initiative. *Ann Rheum Dis*. 2012;71(4):484–492.
- Hernández-Rodríguez J, Cid MC, López-Soto A, et al. Treatment of polymyalgia rheumatica: a systematic review. *Arch Intern Med*. 2009;169(20):1839–1850.
- Kreiner F, Galbo H. Effect of etanercept in polymyalgia rheumatica: a randomized controlled trial. *Arthritis Res Ther*. 2010;12(5):R176.
- Michet CJ, Matteson EL. Polymyalgia rheumatica. *BMJ*. 2008;336(7647):765–769.
- Régent A, Ly KH, Blet A, et al. Contribution of anti-ferritin antibodies to diagnosis of giant cell arteritis. *Ann Rheum Dis*. 2013;72(7):1269–1270.
- Spies CM, Burmester GR, Buttgereit F. Methotrexate treatment in large vessel vasculitis and polymyalgia rheumatica. *Clin Exp Rheumatol*. 2010;28 (5 Suppl 61):S172–S177.

 SEE ALSO

Arteritis, Temporal; Osteoarthritis; Arthritis, Rheumatoid (RA); Depression; Fibromyalgia; Polymyositis/Dermatomyositis

 CODES

ICD10
- M35.3 Polymyalgia rheumatica
- M31.5 Giant cell arteritis with polymyalgia rheumatica

CLINICAL PEARLS
- Consider PMR in patients >50 years of age presenting with proximal limb (hip, neck, shoulder) pain and stiffness.
- A normal ESR does not exclude PMR.
- If there is not a dramatic and rapid response to steroids, reconsider the diagnosis.
- Adjust steroid dosing according to patient symptoms, not the ESR.

POLYMYOSITIS/DERMATOMYOSITIS

Christopher M. Wise, MD

 BASICS

DESCRIPTION
- Systemic connective tissue disease characterized by inflammatory and degenerative changes in proximal muscles, sometimes accompanied by characteristic skin rash
  - If skin manifestations (Gottron sign [symmetric, scaly, violaceous, erythematous eruption over the extensor surfaces of the metacarpophalangeal and interphalangeal joints of the fingers]; heliotrope [reddish violaceous eruption on the upper eyelids]) are present, it is designated as dermatomyositis.
  - Different types of myositis include the following (1):
    - Idiopathic polymyositis
    - Idiopathic dermatomyositis
    - Polymyositis/dermatomyositis as an overlap (usually with lupus or systemic sclerosis or as part of mixed connective-tissue disease)
    - Myositis associated with malignancy
    - Necrotizing autoimmune myositis (often statin-associated) (2)
    - HIV-associated myopathy
- Inclusion-body myositis (IBM), a variant with atypical patterns of weakness and biopsy findings
- System(s) affected: cardiovascular, musculoskeletal, pulmonary, skin/exocrine
- Synonym(s): myositis; inflammatory myopathy; antisynthetase syndrome (subset with certain antibodies)

EPIDEMIOLOGY
Incidence
- Estimated at 1.2 to 19/million population/year (3)
- Predominant age: 5 to 15 years, 40 to 60 years, peak incidence in mid-40s
- Predominant sex: female > male (2:1)

Prevalence
2.4 to 33.8 patients/100,000 population (3)

Geriatric Considerations
Elderly patients with myositis or dermatomyositis are at increased risk of neoplasm.

Pediatric Considerations
Childhood dermatomyositis is likely a separate entity associated with cutaneous vasculitis and muscle calcifications.

ETIOLOGY AND PATHOPHYSIOLOGY
- Inflammatory process, mediated by T cells and cytokine release, leading to damage to muscle cells (predominantly skeletal muscles)
- In patients with IBM, degenerative mechanisms may be important.
- Unknown; potential viral, genetic factors

Genetics
Mild association with human leukocyte antigen (HLA)–DR3, HLA-DRw52

RISK FACTORS
Family history of autoimmune disease (e.g., systemic lupus, myositis) or vasculitis

COMMONLY ASSOCIATED CONDITIONS
- Malignancy (in 15–25%)
- Progressive systemic sclerosis
- Vasculitis
- Systemic lupus erythematosus (SLE)
- Mixed connective tissue disease

 DIAGNOSIS

HISTORY
- Symmetric proximal muscle weakness (1) causing difficulty when
  - Arising from sitting or lying positions
  - Climbing stairs
  - Raising arms
- Joint pain/swelling
- Dysphagia
- Dyspnea
- Rash on face, eyelids, hands, arms

PHYSICAL EXAM
Proximal muscle weakness
- Shoulder muscles
- Hip girdle muscles (trouble standing from seated or squatting position, weak hip flexors in supine position)
- Muscle swelling, stiffness, induration
- Distal muscle weakness is seen only in patients with IBM.
- Rash over face (eyelids, nasolabial folds), upper chest, dorsal hands (especially knuckle pads), fingers ("mechanic's hands")
- Periorbital edema
- Calcinosis cutis (childhood cases)
- Mesenteric arterial insufficiency/infarction (childhood cases)
- Cardiac impairment; arrhythmia, failure

DIFFERENTIAL DIAGNOSIS
- Vasculitis
- Progressive systemic sclerosis
- SLE
- Rheumatoid arthritis
- Muscular dystrophy
- Eaton-Lambert syndrome
- Sarcoidosis
- Amyotrophic lateral sclerosis
- Endocrine disorders
  - Thyroid disease
  - Cushing syndrome
- Infectious myositis (viral, bacterial, parasitic)
- Drug-induced myopathies:
  - Cholesterol-lowering agents (statins)
  - Colchicine
  - Corticosteroids
  - Ethanol
  - Chloroquine
  - Zidovudine
- Electrolyte disorders (magnesium, calcium, potassium)
- Heritable metabolic myopathies
- Sleep-apnea syndrome

DIAGNOSTIC TESTS & INTERPRETATION
- Diagnosis of muscle component (myositis) usually relies on four findings:
  - Weakness
  - Creatine kinase (CK) and/or aldolase elevation
  - Abnormal electromyogram (EMG)
  - Findings on muscle biopsy
- Presence of compatible skin rash of dermatomyositis

Initial Tests (lab, imaging)
- Increased CK, aldolase
- Increased serum AST (aspartate aminotransferase)

- Increased LDH (lactate dehydrogenase)
- Myoglobinuria
- Increased ESR
- Positive rheumatoid factor (<50% of patients)
- Positive antinuclear antibody (ANA) (>50% of patients)
- Leukocytosis (<50% of patients)
- Anemia (<50% of patients)
- Hyperglobulinemia (<50% of patients)
- Anti-HMGCR (3-hydroxy-3-methylglutaryl-coenzyme A reductase) seen in patient with statin-associated necrotizing autoimmune myositis
- Myositis-specific antibodies (antisynthetase antibodies) described in a minority of patients:
  - Anti-Jo-1 is the most common but has been found in <20% of patients.
  - Associated with an increased incidence of interstitial lung disease
- Chest radiograph as part of initial evaluation to assess for associated pulmonary involvement or malignancy

Follow-Up Tests & Special Considerations
- Changes in muscle enzymes (CK or aldolase) correlate with improvement and worsening.
- MRI to assess muscle edema and inflammation may be used in some patients to determine best biopsy site or response to therapy.

Diagnostic Procedures/Other
- EMG: muscle irritability, low-amplitude potentials, polyphasic action potentials, fibrillations
- Muscle biopsy (deltoid or quadriceps femoris)

Test Interpretation
- Microscopic findings:
  - Muscle fiber degeneration
  - Phagocytosis of muscle debris
  - Perifascicular muscle fiber atrophy
  - Inflammatory cell infiltrates in adult form
  - Via electron microscopy: inclusion bodies (IBM only)
  - Sarcoplasmic basophilia
- Muscle fiber increased in size
- Vasculopathy (childhood polymyositis/dermatomyositis)

TREATMENT

GENERAL MEASURES
General evaluation for malignancy in all adults, particularly with dermatomyositis, at initial evaluation and during follow up

MEDICATION
First Line
- Prednisone
  - 40 to 80 mg/day PO in divided doses (4)[B]
  - Consolidate doses and reduce prednisone slowly when enzyme levels are normal.
  - Probably need to continue 5 to 10 mg/day for maintenance in most patients.
- For steroid-refractory or steroid-dependent patients: azathioprine 1 mg/kg PO (arthritis dose) once daily or BID
  - Methotrexate 10 to 25 mg PO weekly, useful in most steroid-resistant patients

- Rash of dermatomyositis may require topical steroids or oral. hydroxychloroquine.
- Patients with IBM have very poor response to steroids and other first- and second-line drugs in general.

Second Line
- Other immunosuppressant drugs (e.g., cyclophosphamide, chlorambucil, cyclosporine, mycophenolate, tacrolimus) can be added to steroids.
- Combination methotrexate and azathioprine also may be useful in refractory cases.
- IVIG (5)[B] and rituximab (6)[B] have been reported to be helpful in a small series of patients with refractory disease.
- Contraindications: Methotrexate is contraindicated with previous liver disease, alcohol use, pregnancy, and underlying renal disease (use with extreme caution in patients with serum creatinine >1.5 mg/dL in general).
- Precautions
  - Prednisone: Adverse effects associated with long-term steroid use include adrenal suppression, sodium and water retention, hypokalemia, osteoporosis, cataracts, and increased susceptibility to infection.
  - Azathioprine: Adverse effects include bone marrow suppression, increased liver function tests, and increased risk of infection.
  - Methotrexate: Adverse effects include stomatitis, bone marrow suppression, pneumonitis, and risk of liver fibrosis and cirrhosis with prolonged use.

ISSUES FOR REFERRAL
- Diagnostic uncertainty, usually related to elevated muscle enzymes without typical symptoms of findings of muscle weakness
- Poor response to initial steroid therapy
- Excessive steroid requirement (unable to taper prednisone to <20 mg/day after 4 to 6 months)

SURGERY/OTHER PROCEDURES
None indicated, other than initial biopsy

INPATIENT CONSIDERATIONS
Admission Criteria/Initial Stabilization
- Inability to stand, ambulate
- Respiratory difficulty
- Fever or other signs of infection
- Inpatient evaluation seldom needed

 ONGOING CARE

FOLLOW-UP RECOMMENDATIONS
Patient Monitoring
- Follow muscle enzymes along with muscle strength and functional capacity.
- Monitor for steroid-induced complications (e.g., hypokalemia, hypertension, and hyperglycemia).
- Bone densitometry and consideration of calcium, vitamin D, and bisphosphonate therapy
- If azathioprine, methotrexate, or other immunosuppressant is used, appropriate laboratory monitoring should be done periodically (e.g., hematology, liver enzymes, and creatinine).
- Attempt to decrease and/or discontinue steroid dose as patient responds to therapy.

- Maintain immunosuppression until patient's muscle strength stabilizes for prolonged period depending on individual patient parameters, risks of medication, risk of relapse; time period undefined (months, years).

DIET
Moderation of caloric and sodium intake to avoid weight gain from corticosteroid therapy.

PATIENT EDUCATION
- Curtail excess physical activity in early phases when muscles enzymes are markedly elevated.
- Emphasize range-of-motion exercises.
- Gradually introduce muscle strengthening when muscle enzymes are normal or improved and stable (7)[B].

PROGNOSIS
- Residual weakness: 30%
- Persistent active disease: 20%
- 5-year survival 65–75%, but mortality is 3-fold higher than general population (8,9).
- Survival is worse for women and African Americans and those with dermatomyositis, IBM, or cancer.
- Most patients improve with therapy.
- Patients with IBM respond poorly to most therapies (10).
- 20–50% have full recovery.

COMPLICATIONS
- Pneumonia
- Infection
- Myocardial infarction
- Carcinoma (especially breast, lung)
- Severe dysphagia
- Respiratory impairment due to muscle weakness, interstitial lung disease
- Aspiration pneumonitis
- Steroid myopathy
- Steroid-induced diabetes, hypertension, hypokalemia, osteoporosis

REFERENCES

1. Dalakas MC. Inflammatory muscle diseases. *N Engl J Med*. 2015;372(18):1734–1747.
2. Mohassel P, Mammen AL. The spectrum of statin myopathy. *Curr Opin Rheumatol*. 2013;25(6):747–752.
3. Meyer A, Meyer N, Schaeffer M, et al. Incidence and prevalence of inflammatory myopathies: a systematic review. *Rheumatology (Oxford)*. 2015;54(1):50–63.
4. Aggarwal R, Oddis CV. Therapeutic approaches in myositis. *Curr Rheumatol Rep*. 2011;13(3):182–191.
5. Wang DX, Shu XM, Tian XL, et al. Intravenous immunoglobulin therapy in adult patients with polymyositis/dermatomyositis: a systematic literature review. *Clin Rheumatol*. 2012;31(5):801–806.
6. Oddis CV, Reed AM, Aggarwal R, et al. Rituximab in the treatment of refractory adult and juvenile dermatomyositis and adult polymyositis: a randomized, placebo-phase trial. *Arthritis Rheum*. 2013;65(2):314–324.
7. Alemo Munters L, Dastmalchi M, Andgren V, et al. Improvement in health and possible reduction in disease activity using endurance exercise in patients with established polymyositis and dermatomyositis: a multicenter randomized controlled trial with a 1-year open extension followup. *Arthritis Care Res*. 2013;65(12):1959–1968.
8. Marie I. Morbidity and mortality in adult polymyositis and dermatomyositis. *Curr Rheumatol Rep*. 2012;14(3):275–285.
9. Schiopu E, Phillips K, MacDonald PM, et al. Predictors of survival in a cohort of patients with polymyositis and dermatomyositis: effect of corticosteroids, methotrexate and azathioprine. *Arthritis Res Ther*. 2012;14(1):R22.
10. Machado P, Brady S, Hanna MG. Update in inclusion body myositis. *Curr Opin Rheumatol*. 2013;25(6):763–771.

 CODES

ICD10
- M33.20 Polymyositis, organ involvement unspecified
- M33.90 Dermatopolymyositis, unspecified, organ involvement unspecified
- M33.92 Dermatopolymyositis, unspecified with myopathy

CLINICAL PEARLS
- Corticosteroids alone may be sufficient in patients who have rapid improvement in weakness and muscle enzymes. However, most patients require azathioprine, methotrexate, or other immunosuppressive medications.
- The risk of associated malignancy is higher in patients >50 years and in those with cutaneous manifestations.
- Elevated muscle enzymes (e.g., CK and aldolase) are seen frequently as transient phenomena in patients with febrile illness and injuries; may return to normal on repeat.
- In patients with persistently elevated muscle enzymes and symptoms and findings of muscle weakness, EMG followed by muscle biopsy should be the initial studies considered.
- Suspect IBM in older patients with very slow onset and progression of symptoms, poor response to steroids and immunosuppressive therapy, and atypical patterns (asymmetric, sometimes distal) of muscle weakness.
- Suspect autoimmune necrotizing myositis in patients who develop myopathy while taking lipid-lowering drugs (statins) but fail to improve or worsen after withdrawal of statin therapy.

POPLITEAL (BAKER) CYST

Shane L. Larson, MD

 BASICS

DESCRIPTION

- A fluid-filled synovial sac arising in the popliteal fossa as a distention of (typically) the gastrocnemial-semimembranous bursa. Not a true cyst
- Can be unilateral or bilateral
- Most frequent cystic mass around the knee (1)
- Primary cysts are a distention of the bursa (arise independently without an intra-articular disorder).
- Secondary cysts occur if there is a communication between the bursa and knee joint, allowing articular fluid to fill the cyst.
- Associated with synovial inflammation

EPIDEMIOLOGY

Incidence
- Bimodal distribution
  - Children ages 4 to 7 years
  - Adults increasing with age
- Primary cysts usually seen in children <15 years
- Secondary cysts seen in adults

Prevalence
- Variable adult prevalence of 19–47% in symptomatic knees and 2–5% in asymptomatic knees.
- In children: 6.3% in symptomatic knees; 2.4% in asymptomatic knees

ETIOLOGY AND PATHOPHYSIOLOGY

Associated intra-articular pathology includes
- Meniscal tears, mostly of the posterior horn
- Anterior cruciate ligament (ACL) insufficiency
- Degenerative articular cartilage lesions
- Rheumatoid arthritis (20%)
- Osteoarthritis (50%)
- Osteochondritis
- Gout (14%)
- Other potential factors
  - Infectious arthritis
  - Polyarthritis
  - Villonodular synovitis
  - Lymphoma
  - Sarcoidosis
  - Connective tissue diseases (2)

- Extension or herniation of synovial membrane of the knee joint capsule or connection of normal bursa with the joint capsule
- May result from increased intra-articular pressure
- Commonly seen with knee effusions
- Direct trauma to the bursa is likely the primary cause in children because of no communication between the bursa and the joint.
- A valve-like mechanism allowing one-way passage of fluid from the joint to the bursal connection has been described.

RISK FACTORS

- Osteoarthritis of knee (most common) (3)[B]

- Rheumatoid arthritis
- Meniscal degeneration or tear
- Advancing age
- Ligamentous insufficiency

COMMONLY ASSOCIATED CONDITIONS

Any condition causing knee joint effusion

 DIAGNOSIS

HISTORY

- Painless mass arising in the popliteal fossa
- Most cysts are asymptomatic.
- Dull ache if cyst is large enough to impede joint motion—typically a restriction of flexion
- Painful if cyst ruptures
- Large cysts may cause entrapment neuropathy of the tibial nerve.
- Vascular compression, most commonly of the popliteal vein, may produce claudication or thrombophlebitis.
- Activity alters the cyst size.

PHYSICAL EXAM

- Examine in full extension and 90 degrees of flexion.
- Foucher sign: Mass increases with extension and disappears with flexion.
- Most commonly found in medial aspect of popliteal fossa lateral to the head of the gastrocnemius and medial to the neurovascular bundle

- Cyst is easiest to palpate when knee is slightly flexed and may occasionally be fluctuant or tender.
- Transillumination helps distinguish cyst from solid mass.
- Ruptured cysts are typically painful with associated swelling and bruising over the ipsilateral calf and ankle at the medial malleolus (Crescent sign).
- Ruptured cysts also are associated with pseudothrombophlebitis, and rarely, compartment syndrome (5).

DIFFERENTIAL DIAGNOSIS

- Infection/abscess
- Lipoma, liposarcoma
- Fibroma, fibrosarcoma
- Hematoma
- Deep venous thrombosis
- Vascular tumor
- Popliteal vein varices
- Xanthoma
- Aneurysm (rare)
- Ganglion cyst
- Thrombophlebitis
- Muscular herniation (rare, related to trauma)

DIAGNOSTIC TESTS & INTERPRETATION

Initial Tests (lab, imaging)
- CBC, ESR (if septic arthritis suspected)
- Ensure not a popliteal aneurysm prior to aspiration. Send aspirate for cell count and culture to determine if fluid is infectious, inflammatory, or mechanical.
- Ultrasound confirms presence and size; Doppler, can differentiate Baker cysts from popliteal vessel aneurysms, DVT, or soft tissue tumors (4).
- MRI helps assess derangements of internal joint structures and to identify cyst leakage.

Follow-Up Tests & Special Considerations
- Consider observation over invasive testing in children.
- Radiographs may show soft tissue density posteriorly.

- Arthrography may demonstrate communication with joint capsule or rupture.
- CT arthrography is superior for visualizing cystic details and can help distinguish lipomas, aneurysms, and malignancies from cysts.

 TREATMENT

GENERAL MEASURES
- No treatment if asymptomatic
- Treat any associated underlying conditions.
- Compressive wrap or sleeve for comfort.

MEDICATION
If etiology is identified from cellular fluid examination, treat the underlying condition.

First Line
Analgesics and NSAIDs for symptomatic relief

ADDITIONAL THERAPIES
- Physical therapy improves knee ROM and strength, particularly with coexisting pathology.
- Temporary relief with needle aspiration; recurrence common

- Improvement in joint ROM, knee pain, swelling, accompanied reduction in bursa size after aspiration, and intra-articular/intracystic corticosteroid injection (6)[B]
- A combination of physical therapy and corticosteroid injection leads to best improvements in pain, function, and reduction in cyst size (7)[A].
- Sclerotherapy injections of ethanol or dextrose/sodium morrhuate shown to have good results in small studies (8)[B].

SURGERY/OTHER PROCEDURES
- Consider excision when symptoms persist despite treatment or no etiology is found.
- Surgery usually not required in children
- Recurrence after standard surgery is common and is highest if chondral lesions are present.

- Arthroscopic surgery is highly successful if a valvular mechanism is identified and intra-articular pathology is treated (9,10)[B].
- A modified surgical technique in children has proved effective without recurrence (11)[B].
- Excision via arthroscopy or open procedure often requires concomitant treatment of underlying pathology (12)[B].

 ONGOING CARE

PROGNOSIS
- Variable; many cysts remain asymptomatic.
- Some cysts resolve with treatment of underlying etiology (e.g., gout, rheumatoid arthritis).
- In children, most cysts resolve without treatment.

COMPLICATIONS
- Compartment syndrome in ruptured cyst
- Thrombophlebitis from compression of the popliteal vein
- Infection of popliteal cyst
- Hemorrhage into cyst if on anticoagulants

REFERENCES

1. Marra MD, Crema MD, Chung M, et al. MRI features of cystic lesions around the knee. *Knee.* 2008;15(6):423–438.
2. Liao ST, Chiou CS, Chang CC. Pathology associated to the Baker's cysts: a musculoskeletal ultrasound study. *Clin Rheumatol.* 2010;29(9):1043–1047.
3. Chatzopoulos D, Moralidis E, Markou P, et al. Baker's cysts in knees with chronic osteoarthritic pain: a clinical, ultrasonographic, radiographic and scintigraphic evaluation. *Rheumatol Int.* 2008;29(2):141–146.
4. Roberts JR. Distinguishing Baker's cyst from DVT. *Emer Med News.* 2003;25(11):14–16.
5. Sanchez JE, Conkling N, Labropoulos N. Compression syndromes of the popliteal neurovascular bundle due to Baker cyst. *J Vasc Surg.* 2011;54(6):1821–1829.
6. Acebes JC, Sánchez-Pernaute O, Díaz-Oca A, et al. Ultrasonographic assessment of Baker's cysts after intra-articular corticosteroid injection in knee osteoarthritis. *J Clin Ultrasound.* 2006;34(3):113–117.
7. Di Sante L, Paoloni M, Dimaggio M, et al. Ultrasound-guided aspiration and corticosteroid injection compared to horizontal therapy for treatment of knee osteoarthritis complicated with Baker's cyst: a randomized, controlled trial. *Eur J Phys Rehabil Med.* 2012;48(4):561–567.
8. Centeno CJ, Schultz J, Freeman M. Sclerotherapy of Baker's cyst with imaging confirmation of resolution. *Pain Physician.* 2008;11(2):257–261.
9. Rupp S, Seil R, Jochum P, et al. Popliteal cysts in adults. Prevalence, associated intraarticular lesions, and results after arthroscopic treatment. *Am J Sports Med.* 2002;30(1):112–115.
10. Lie CW, Ng TP. Arthroscopic treatment of popliteal cyst. *Hong Kong Med J.* 2011;17(3):180–183.
11. Chen JC, Lu CC, Lu YM, et al. A modified surgical method for treating Baker's cyst in children. *Knee.* 2008;15(1):9–14.
12. Handy JR. Popliteal cysts in adults: a review. *Semin Arthritis Rheum.* 2001;31(2):108–118.

ADDITIONAL READING

- Akagi R, Saisu T, Segawa Y, et al. Natural history of popliteal cysts in the pediatric population. *J Pediatr Orthop.* 2013;33(3):262–268.
- Akgul O, Guldeste Z, Ozgocmen S. The reliability of the clinical examination for detecting Baker's cyst in asymptomatic fossa. *Int J Rheum Dis.* 2014;17(2):204–209.

 SEE ALSO

Algorithm: Knee Pain

 CODES

ICD10
- M71.20 Synovial cyst of popliteal space [Baker], unspecified knee
- M71.21 Synovial cyst of popliteal space [Baker], right knee
- M71.22 Synovial cyst of popliteal space [Baker], left knee

CLINICAL PEARLS
- Conservative treatment of Baker cysts is preferred in children, as most will spontaneously resolve.
- In adults, treatment of underlying cause may resolve Baker cysts.
- Pain, bruising, and swelling over the medial malleolus (crescent sign) suggests cyst rupture.

PORTAL HYPERTENSION
Walter M. Kim, MD, PhD • Jyoti Ramakrishna, MD

BASICS

DESCRIPTION
- Increased portal venous pressure >5 mm Hg that occurs in association with splanchnic vasodilatation, portosystemic collateral formation, and hyperdynamic circulation
- Most commonly secondary to elevated hepatic venous pressure gradient (HVPG; the gradient between portal and central venous pressures)
- Course is generally progressive, with risk of complications including acute variceal bleeding, ascites, encephalopathy, and hepatorenal syndrome.

EPIDEMIOLOGY
Incidence
- Prevalence: <200,000 persons in the United States
- Predominant age: adult
- Predominant sex: male > female

ETIOLOGY AND PATHOPHYSIOLOGY
- Causes generally classified as follows:
  - Prehepatic (portal vein thrombosis or obstruction)
  - Intrahepatic (most commonly cirrhosis)
  - Posthepatic (hepatic vein thrombosis, Budd-Chiari syndrome, right-sided heart failure)
- Cirrhosis accounts for 90% of intrahepatic cases; may be due to the following:
  - Virus (hepatitis B, hepatitis C, hepatitis D)
  - Alcoholism
  - Schistosomiasis
  - Wilson disease
  - Hemochromatosis
  - Primary biliary cirrhosis (PBC)
  - Sarcoidosis
- Increased HVPG results in venous collateral formation in the distal esophagus, proximal stomach, rectum, and umbilicus.
- Gastroesophageal variceal formation is found in 40% of patients with portal hypertension.
- Progression of portal hypertension results in splanchnic vasodilation and angiogenesis.

Genetics
No known genetic patterns except those associated with specific hepatic diseases that cause portal hypertension

RISK FACTORS
See "Etiology."

Pediatric Considerations
In children, portal vein thrombosis is the most common extrahepatic cause; intrahepatic causes are more likely to be biliary atresia, viral hepatitis, and metabolic liver disease.

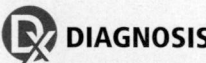

DIAGNOSIS

HISTORY
- Weakness/fatigue
- Jaundice
- Symptoms of heart failure including chest pain, shortness of breath, and/or edema
- Hematemesis
- Melena
- Oliguria
- History of chronic liver disease
- Alcoholic hepatitis
- Alcohol abuse

PHYSICAL EXAM
- Exam findings may be general or related to specific complications.
- General
  - Pallor
  - Icterus
  - Digital clubbing
  - Palmar erythema
  - Splenomegaly
  - Caput medusa
  - Spider angiomata
  - Umbilical bruit
  - Hemorrhoids
  - Gynecomastia
  - Testicular atrophy
- Gastroesophageal varices
  - Hypotension
  - Tachycardia
- Ascites
  - Distended abdomen
  - Fluid wave
  - Shifting dullness with percussion
- Hepatic encephalopathy
  - Confusion/coma
  - Asterixis
  - Hyperreflexia

DIFFERENTIAL DIAGNOSIS
Usually related to specific presentations
- Gastroesophageal varices with hemorrhage
  - Portal hypertensive gastropathy
  - Hemorrhagic gastritis
  - Peptic ulcer disease
  - Mallory-Weiss tear
- Ascites
  - Spontaneous bacterial peritonitis (SBP)
  - Pancreatic ascites
  - Peritoneal carcinomatosis
  - Tuberculous peritonitis
  - Nephrotic syndrome
  - Fluid overload from heart failure
  - Hepatic malignancy
- Hepatic encephalopathy
  - Delirium tremens
  - Intracranial hemorrhage
  - Sedative abuse
  - Uremia
- Hepatorenal syndrome
  - Drug nephrotoxicity
  - Renal tubular necrosis

DIAGNOSTIC TESTS & INTERPRETATION
Initial Tests (lab, imaging)
Direct calculation of HVPG (approximation of the gradient in pressure between portal vein and IVC):
- HVPG = wedged hepatic venous pressure (WHVP) − free hepatic venous pressure (FHVP)
- HVPG >10, esophageal varices generally develop.
- WHVP is estimated by occlusion of the hepatic vein by a balloon catheter and measurement of the proximal static column of blood.
- FHVP is estimated by direct measurement of the patent hepatic vein, intra-abdominal inferior vena cava, or right atrium.
- Nonspecific changes associated with underlying disease:
  - Hypersplenism: anemia (also may be due to malnutrition or bleeding), leukopenia, thrombocytopenia
  - Hepatic dysfunction
    - Hypoalbuminemia
    - Hyperbilirubinemia
    - Elevated alkaline phosphatase
    - Elevated liver enzymes (AST, ALT)
    - Abnormal clotting (prothrombin time, international normalized ratio, partial thromboplastin time)
  - GI bleeding
    - Iron deficiency anemia
    - Elevated serum ammonia
    - Fecal occult blood
    - Thrombocytopenia
  - Hepatorenal syndrome
    - Elevated serum creatinine (Cr), blood urea nitrogen (BUN)
    - Urine Na <5 mEq/L (<20 mmol/L)
  - US and CT scan/MRI may detect cirrhosis, splenomegaly, ascites, and varices.
  - US/duplex Doppler
    - Can determine presence and direction of flow in portal and hepatic veins
    - Useful in diagnosing portal vein thrombosis, shunt thrombosis, or the presence of ascites
  - CT scan/MRI: angiographic measurement of hepatic venous wedge pressure via jugular or femoral vein
    - Correlates with portal pressure
    - Risk of variceal bleeding is increased if hepatic venous pressure gradient >12 mm Hg.
  - Upper GI series may outline varices in esophagus and stomach.
  - Transient elastography is an emerging method to determine hepatic fibrosis and to predict portal hypertension (1).

Diagnostic Procedures/Other
Endoscopy can diagnose esophageal and gastric varices and portal hypertensive gastropathy.

Test Interpretation
Specific for underlying disease

TREATMENT

GENERAL MEASURES
- Avoid sedatives that may precipitate encephalopathy.
- Limit sodium intake because cirrhotic patients avidly retain sodium.

MEDICATION
Therapy for encephalopathy: See "Hepatic Encephalopathy."

First Line
- Prophylaxis against variceal bleeding (2,3)[A]:
  - Nonselective β-blockade
    - Propranolol: start with 10 to 20 mg/day PO BID to TID
    - Nadolol: 40 to 80 mg/day PO once-daily dosing
  - Doses may be titrated up as tolerated to maximum recommended doses; goal resting HR of 55 to 60 bpm

- Therapy for acute variceal hemorrhage:
  – Vasopressin: start with 0.2 to 0.4 U/min IV; increase to maximum dose 1 U/min as needed; pediatric dose: 0.002 to 0.005 U/kg/min; do not exceed 0.01 U/kg/min. After bleeding stops, continue at same dose for 12 hours and then taper off over 24 to 48 hours.
  – Octreotide: 50 μg IV bolus, followed by 25 to 50 μg/hr continuous infusion; pediatric dose: 1 μg/kg bolus followed by 1 μg/kg/hr is used traditionally; treat for up to 5 days.
- For prevention of recurrence and for overall reduction in mortality:
  – Propranolol: 10 to 60 mg/day PO BID to QID; pediatric dose: 0.5 to 1 mg/kg/day PO divided q6–8h
  – Nadolol: 40 to 80 mg/day PO reduces portal venous blood inflow by blocking the adrenergic dilatation of the mesenteric arterioles.
  – Tetrandrine, a calcium channel blocker, also has been found to reduce the rate of rebleeding with fewer side effects.
- Initial treatment for ascites (along with salt and fluid restriction):
  – Furosemide: 20 to 40 mg/day PO; pediatric dose: 1 to 2 mg/kg/dose PO ± IV albumin infusion
  – Spironolactone: 50 to 100 mg/day PO; pediatric dose: 1 to 3 mg/kg/day PO

Second Line
- Terlipressin (2 mg IV q4h; titrate down to 1 mg IV q4h once hemorrhage is controlled; may be used for up to 48 hours) is a more selective splanchnic vasoconstrictor and may be associated with fewer complications. It is currently used when standard therapy with somatostatin or octreotide fails.
- Addition of nitrates, such as nitroglycerin or isosorbide mononitrate, reduces portal pressures and bleeding rates and has been shown to reduce mortality. Because the risk–benefit ratio is not clear, nitrates are not considered first-line treatment.
- Studies are ongoing for possible benefits of other agents including simvastatin, clonidine, verapamil, and losartan.

ISSUES FOR REFERRAL
Patients with portal hypertension should be managed longitudinally by both a primary care physician and a gastroenterologist.

SURGERY/OTHER PROCEDURES
- Treatments available for specific complications of portal hypertension (in addition to or if refractory to medications):
  – Gastroesophageal varices with hemorrhage
    ○ Endoscopic variceal banding or sclerosis (the first-line treatment in many cases for acute hemorrhage) within 12 hours of presentation (4)[A]
    ○ Balloon tamponade (not used commonly when endoscopic treatment is available)
    ○ Transjugular intrahepatic portosystemic shunt (TIPS)
    ○ Portocaval shunting
  – Ascites refractory to medical management
    ○ Large-volume paracentesis
    ○ Peritoneovenous shunt
    ○ TIPS
- Liver transplantation should be considered for patients with advanced disease.

INPATIENT CONSIDERATIONS
- Acute GI bleeding should be managed in the inpatient setting, either on the regular medical floor if the patient is hemodynamically stable or occasionally in the ICU if the patient is unstable.
- Patients with mental status changes from encephalopathy need to be evaluated in the inpatient setting.

Admission Criteria/Initial Stabilization
- Acute bleeding from the intestinal tract, either vomiting or per rectum
- Acute confusional state/mental status changes
- If acute variceal bleeding:
  – Type and cross patient's blood.
  – Initial resuscitation with isotonic fluid until packed RBCs are available
  – Correct coagulopathy with vitamin K and fresh frozen plasma (FFP).
  – Endoscopy as soon as the patient is stabilized (for diagnosis and treatment)
- Avoid sedatives that may precipitate encephalopathy.
- Limit sodium administration because cirrhotic patients avidly retain sodium.
- Restrict protein only if encephalopathic.

ALERT
If the patient is an active alcohol drinker, watch for signs and symptoms of withdrawal. Follow inpatient protocols for alcohol withdrawal management.

IV Fluids
Use isotonic fluid for hydration.

Discharge Criteria
- For GI bleeding:
  – No active bleeding in 24 hours
  – Stable hemoglobin and hematocrit
  – Hemodynamically stable (especially heart rate)
- For encephalopathy: improvement in or resolution of mental status changes to baseline

ONGOING CARE

DIET
In patients with cirrhosis, sodium restriction is important because cirrhotic patients avidly retain sodium.

PATIENT EDUCATION
Refrain from drinking alcohol. Resources for patients who have difficulty with not drinking alcohol can be obtained from Alcoholics Anonymous at http://www.aa.org/.

PROGNOSIS
- Hepatic reserve defined by Child-Pugh classification: rating based on encephalopathy, ascites, bilirubin, albumin, prothrombin
- Variceal bleeding
  – 1/3 of patients with known varices will bleed eventually.
  – 50% rebleed, usually within 2 years, unless portal pressure is reduced by surgical or TIPS procedure.
  – 15–20% mortality rate
- Ascites and encephalopathy often recur.
- Prognosis of patients with ascites is poor: 50% 1-year survival without liver transplant (compared with 90% for patients with cirrhosis and no ascites)

REFERENCES
1. Llop E, Berzigotti A, Reig M, et al. Assessment of portal hypertension by transient elastography in patients with compensated cirrhosis and potentially resectable liver tumors. *J Hepatol.* 2012;56(1):103–108.
2. Hayes PC, Davis JM, Lewis JA, et al. Meta-analysis of value of propranolol in prevention of variceal haemorrhage. *Lancet.* 1990;336(8708):153–156.
3. Garcia-Tsao G, Sanyal AJ, Grace ND, et al. Prevention and management of gastroesophageal varices and variceal hemorrhage in cirrhosis. *Hepatology.* 2007;46(3):922–938.
4. De Franchis R, Baveno VI Faculty. Expanding consensus in portal hypertension: report of the Baveno VI Consensus Workshop: stratifying risk and individualizing care for portal hypertension. *J Hepatol.* 2015;63(3):743–752.

ADDITIONAL READING
- Abraldes JG, Angermayr B, Bosch J. The management of portal hypertension. *Clin Liver Dis.* 2005;9(4):685–713.
- Bloom S, Kemp W, Lubel J. Portal hypertension: pathophysiology, diagnosis and management. *Intern Med J.* 2015;45(1):16–26. doi:10.1111/imj.12590.
- Bosch J, Berzigotti A, Garcia-Pagan JC, et al. The management of portal hypertension: rational basis, available treatments and future options. *J Hepatol.* 2008;48(Suppl 1):S68–S92.
- Sanyal AJ, Bosch J, Blei A, et al. Portal hypertension and its complications. *Gastroenterology.* 2008;134(6):1715–1728.

CODES

ICD10
K76.6 Portal hypertension

CLINICAL PEARLS
- Portal hypertension can be diagnosed based on physical examination in the setting of known risk factors, specifically cirrhosis.
- Endoscopic treatment is successful for acute variceal hemorrhage 85% of the time.
- Prognosis of patients with ascites is poor: 50% 1-year survival without liver transplant (compared with 90% for patients with cirrhosis and no ascites).
- Advantages and disadvantages of balloon tamponade for acute variceal bleed:
  – Advantages include rapid and often effective control of bleeding (30–90%) and common availability of device.
  – Disadvantages include recurrence of bleeding when balloon is deflated, patient discomfort, and risk of esophageal perforation.

POSTCONCUSSION SYNDROME (MILD TRAUMATIC BRAIN INJURY)

Vicki R. Nelson, MD, PhD • Christopher L. Tangen, DO

 BASICS

DESCRIPTION
- Postconcussion syndrome (PCS) is a constellation of symptoms involving physical, cognitive, and/or behavioral symptoms that persist after a concussion (mild traumatic brain injury [MTBI]) and may continue for weeks to years (1)[C].
- It is unclear at what point postconcussive symptoms become postconcussive syndrome.
- Symptoms of PCS can include any symptom of concussion (1,2)[C]
  - Cognitive
    - Poor focus
    - Poor organization
    - Diminished academic/intellectual performance
    - Slowed response time
  - Physical
    - Headache
    - Nausea
    - Visual changes
    - Light and noise sensitivity
    - Tinnitus
    - Dizziness and balance problems
    - Fatigue and sleep disturbance
  - Behavioral
    - Depression
    - Irritability/emotional lability
    - Apathy
    - Increased sensitivity to alcohol
- Diagnosis is based on history and clinical symptoms.

EPIDEMIOLOGY
Incidence
The reported range of MTBI patients who develop PCS varies widely between 5% and 80%.
- The variation is due to difficulty in differentiating post-concussion *symptoms* from postconcussion *syndrome*.
- Consensus is that 80–90% of concussion victims recover from postconcussion *symptoms* within 7 to 10 days, slightly longer in children/adolescents (3)[C].

Prevalence
Predominant sex: Female > male, although female gender is not universally considered a risk factor.

ETIOLOGY AND PATHOPHYSIOLOGY
- Controversial; exact mechanism(s) unknown
- It is postulated that microscopic axonal injury from shearing forces leads to inflammation that causes secondary brain injury.
- There is conflicting data on structural brain damage and the correlation of imaging findings with physical symptoms (1,2,4–6)
- Because the pathophysiology of PCS is not well understood and because of symptom overlap with other psychiatric conditions, PCS remains a difficult condition to diagnose and to manage.
  - Only some people with MTBI develop PCS; it is unclear what causes PCS symptoms to occur and to persist (5,6).

– Psychiatric factors are commonly associated with, and may play a role in, the development of PCS. It can be a challenge to differentiate pure psychiatric dysfunction from true PCS (1,5,6)[C],(7)[B].

– Neuropsychiatry evaluation may be helpful to differentiate PCS from psychiatric disorders.

– Patient reported high symptom burden following MTBI is associated with increased risk of PCS (8)[B].

RISK FACTORS
- Amnesia, migraine, self-reported cognitive decline, noise and light sensitivity developing or worsening in the first day to weeks after MTBI (1)[C],(4)[B]
- Preexisting psychiatric disease including depression, anxiety, personality disorder, and posttraumatic stress disorder (PTSD)
- Preexisting expectation of poor outcomes in patients following concussion/MTBI (1)[C],(4)[B]
- Nonsport concussion
- Unclear if previous history of concussion(s) is a risk factor for PCS (2)[C].
- Low socioeconomic status

GENERAL PREVENTION
- Education of players, coaches, parents, and athletic trainers about concussion, PCS, and following game safety rules designed to protect players.
- Head injury precautions with activities are advised, but no good evidence that these decrease incidence of MTBI or PCS.
- Early screening and intervention(s) for anxiety and depression

COMMONLY ASSOCIATED CONDITIONS
- PTSD
- Anxiety/depression
- Fibromyalgia
- Personality disorders (namely, compulsive, histrionic, and narcissistic)
- *ADHD*

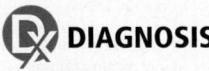 **DIAGNOSIS**

HISTORY
- Detailed history of recent impact/closed head injury, including the following:
  - Mechanism
  - Timing of injury related to symptoms
  - Previous head injuries, including concussion, and timing of those injuries
  - Previous medical, psychiatric, or social history
- Report of neurologic, cognitive, or behavioral symptoms by patient/family

PHYSICAL EXAM
Complete neurologic exam, including the following:
- Glasgow Coma Scale (GCS)
- Anxiety/depression screening
  - Patient Health Questionnaire-9 (PHQ-9)
  - GAD-7
- Sport Concussion Assessment Tool, NFL Sideline Concussion Assessment Tool, or computerized neuropsychological (CNP) testing both pre- and post-MTBI is common practice, although data are limited on validity (3)[C]. More info regarding CNP below

DIFFERENTIAL DIAGNOSIS
- Postconcussive symptoms
- PTSD
- Anxiety/depression
- Personality disorders
- Migraine headaches
- Chronic fatigue syndrome, fibromyalgia
- Evolving intracranial hemorrhage
- Exposure to toxins, including prescription and recreational drugs
- Endocrine/metabolic abnormality

DIAGNOSTIC TESTS & INTERPRETATION
Initial Tests (lab, imaging)
- If clinically warranted, consider evaluation for infection, intoxication, and endocrine/metabolic abnormality.
- Brain imaging both on initial evaluation of MTBI and PCS is generally neither fruitful nor indicated.
- Imaging to evaluate for bleeding may be helpful in patients with comorbid conditions or who are taking anticoagulation therapy.
- Recommend cervical imaging when concomitant cervical spine injury is suspected.

Follow-Up Tests & Special Considerations
- Several CNP testing programs can be used to guide decisions regarding return to play. If baseline testing is available, scores can be used as controls against scores achieved after MTBI.
- Formal neuropsychiatric evaluations are likely superior to CNP testing when available. None of these tests should be used alone in decision making, especially if a patient is still having symptoms despite improving or "baseline" scores (1,3)[C].
- Common neuropsychological testing programs for PCS
  - Immediate Post-Concussion Assessment and Cognitive Testing (ImPACT)
  - Axon Sports Computerized Cognitive Assessment Tool (CCAT)
  - Post Concussion Symptom Scale (PCSS)
  - Balance Error Scoring System (BESS)
  - Automated Neuropsychological Assessment Metrics (ANAM)

TREATMENT

GENERAL MEASURES
- Subthreshold exercise has been shown to help resolution and can start after 21 days (7)[B].
- Consider physical therapy for coexistent cervical or vestibular injury.
- Return to play
  - Persons with concussion or PCS should be restricted from sport activity until they are off all medications that may mask PCS symptoms and clinical symptoms have resolved (1,3)[C].
  - Return to full activity should progress according to step-wise concussion recommendations (1,3)[C].

MEDICATION
First Line
Headache/neck pain
- Nonopioid pain control (e.g., NSAIDs)
  - Sedation may obscure cognitive evaluation.
  - Possible association with use of opiates and increased risk of anxiety/depression in PCS patients (5)[B].
  - Consider occipital nerve block.

ALERT
Avoid opiates and benzodiazepines (5)[B].

- Depression/sleep disorders
  - Anxiety/depression screening starting in the first week post MTBI
    - Melatonin for sleep
    - Tricyclic antidepressants, or trazodone if there is concomitant sleep disturbance, may be beneficial.
    - SSRIs
  - Consider referral to mental health specialist(s).
- Cognitive disorders (6)
  - Evaluation by neuropsychiatrist
  - Methylphenidate may be considered (9)[A].
  - SSRIs may be considered, especially if concomitant anxiety/depression (9)[A].

ISSUES FOR REFERRAL
- Neuropsychiatric therapy including comprehensive cognitive evaluation for potential TBI rehabilitation
- Cognitive behavioral therapy for anxiety and depression symptoms
- Occupational therapy for vocational rehabilitation, if needed
- Physical therapy for vestibular rehabilitation
- Neurology referral if primary care interventions for seizures, headache, vertigo, or cognition are unsuccessful.
- Substance abuse counseling, if needed

COMPLEMENTARY & ALTERNATIVE MEDICINE
Massage therapy/osteopathic manipulative treatment for headache and neck pain

 ONGOING CARE

FOLLOW-UP RECOMMENDATIONS
Schedule regular follow-up to evaluate for persistent symptoms, efficacy of/need for neuropsychiatric evaluation, and the efficacy of/need for pharmacologic therapy.

Patient Monitoring
- Consider serial neuropsychological testing.
- Follow return to play guidelines (3)[C].

PATIENT EDUCATION
- Centers for Disease Control and Prevention: http://www.cdc.gov/headsup/
- Mayo Clinic Health Information: http://www.mayoclinic.com/health/post-concussion-syndrome/DS01020/
- Brain Injury Association of America: http://www.biausa.org/; (800) 444-6443

PROGNOSIS
- Prognosis generally is good.
- Adolescents may recover more slowly than adults.

COMPLICATIONS
- Repeat head injury or return to play before resolution of PCS can worsen/prolong symptoms.
- Case studies of second-impact syndrome, a rare but potentially fatal condition owing to a second head injury soon after the first, have been reported.

REFERENCES
1. Harmon KG, Drezner JA, Gammons M, et al. American Medical Society for Sports Medicine position statement: concussion in sport. *Br J Sports Med*. 2013;47(1):15–26.
2. Jotwani V, Harmon KG. Postconcussion syndrome in athletes. *Curr Sports Med Rep*. 2010;9(1):21–26.
3. McCrory P, Meeuwisse WH, Aubry M, et al. Consensus statement on concussion in sport: 4th International Conference on Concussion in Sport, Zurich, November 2012. *J Athl Train*. 2013;48(4):554–575.
4. Hou R, Moss-Morris R, Peveler R, et al. When a minor head injury results in enduring symptoms: a prospective investigation of risk factors for postconcussional syndrome after mild traumatic brain injury. *J Neurol Neurosurg Psychiatry*. 2012;83(2):217–223.
5. Silverberg ND, Iverson GL. Etiology of the post-concussion syndrome: physiogenesis and psychogenesis revisited. *NeuroRehabilitation*. 2011;29(4):317–329.
6. Meares S, Shores EA, Batchelor J, et al. The relationship of psychological and cognitive factors and opioids in the development of the postconcussion syndrome in general trauma patients with mild traumatic brain injury. *J Int Neuropsychol Soc*. 2006;12(6):792–801.
7. Leddy JJ, Willer B. Use of graded exercise testing in concussion and return-to-activity management. *Curr Sports Med Rep*. 2013;12(6):370–376.
8. Meehan WP III, Mannix R, Monuteaux MC, et al. Early symptom burden predicts recovery after sport-related concussion. *Neurology*. 2014;83(24):2204–2210.
9. Lee H, Kim SW, Kim JM, et al. Comparing effects of methylphenidate, sertraline and placebo on neuropsychiatric sequelae in patients with traumatic brain injury. *Hum Psychopharmacol*. 2005;20(2):97–104.

ADDITIONAL READING
- Barlow M, Schlabach D, Peiffer J, et al. Differences in change scores and the predictive validity of three commonly used measures following concussion in the middle school and high school aged population. *Int J Sports Phys Ther*. 2011;6(3):150–157.
- Leddy JJ, Kozlowski K, Donnelly JP, et al. A preliminary study of subsymptom threshold exercise training for refractory post-concussion syndrome. *Clin J Sport Med*. 2010;20(1):21–27.
- Leddy JJ, Sandhu H, Sodhi V, et al. Rehabilitation of concussion and post-concussion syndrome. *Sports Health*. 2012;4(2):147–154.
- Morgan CD, Zuckerman SL, Lee YM, et al. Predictors of postconcussion syndrome after sports-related concussion in young athletes: a matched case-control study. *J Neurosurg Pediatr*. 2015;15(6):589–598.

 SEE ALSO

Concussion (Mild Traumatic Brain Injury)

 CODES

ICD10
- F07.81 Postconcussional syndrome
- S06.9X0A Unsp intracranial injury w/o loss of consciousness, init
- S06.9X9A Unsp intracranial injury w LOC of unsp duration, init

CLINICAL PEARLS
- Imaging rarely useful for PCS; head CT scan is the test of choice for acute injury to exclude intracranial bleeding.
- Coordinate multidisciplinary treatment plans for patients with persistent symptoms.
- Return to play/activity should not occur until symptoms return to baseline and any pre-PCS medications are optimized by the prescribing clinician.

POSTTRAUMATIC STRESS DISORDER (PTSD)

Rachel Bramson, MD • Michael L. Brown, MD • Suzanne Shurtz, MLIS, AHIP

BASICS

DESCRIPTION
- Posttraumatic stress disorder (PTSD) is an anxiety disorder defined as a reaction that can occur after exposure to an extreme traumatic event involving death, threat of death, serious physical injury, or a threat to physical integrity.
- This reaction has three cardinal characteristics:
  - Reexperiencing the trauma
  - Avoidance of anything related to the traumatic event and/or numbing of general responsiveness
  - Increased arousal
- Traumatic events that may trigger PTSD include natural/human disasters, serious accidents, war, sexual abuse, rape, torture, terrorism, hostage-taking, or being diagnosed with life-threatening disease.
- PTSD can be:
  - Acute: symptoms lasting <3 months
  - Chronic: symptoms lasting ≥3 months
  - Delayed onset: 6 months (from event to symptom onset) in 25% of diagnosed cases

EPIDEMIOLOGY
- ~30% of men and women who have spent time in a war zone experience PTSD.
- Current estimates of PTSD in military personnel who served in Iraq range from 12–20%.
- 16% children and adolescents exposed to trauma develop PTSD (high in girls with interpersonal trauma 33%; low in boys with noninterpersonal trauma 8%) (1).

Incidence
~7.7 million American adults aged ≥18 years (3.5% of this age group) are diagnosed with PTSD each year.

Prevalence
Lifetime prevalence for PTSD is 8–9%.

ETIOLOGY AND PATHOPHYSIOLOGY
- During trauma, the locus coeruleus mediates sympathetic outflows to the amygdala (rapid effect) and adrenal medulla (sustained effect). The adrenal medulla then releases catecholamines, which stimulate peripheral afferent vagal β-receptors. Vagal afferents innervate the nucleus tractus solitarius (NTS) in the brainstem medulla. NTS fibers innervate the amygdala with norepinephrine (NE).
- With an increase in NE, the amygdala mediates coupling of emotional valence to declarative memories via long-term potentiation, forming deeply engraved trauma memories and leading to intrusive memories and emotions, potentially leading to PTSD.
- The orbitoprefrontal cortex (which usually exerts an inhibiting effect on this activation) appears less capable of inhibiting this activation due to stress-induced atrophy of specific nuclei in this region.

Genetics
- Monozygotic twins exposed to combat in Vietnam were at increased risk of the cotwin having PTSD compared with twins who were dizygotic.
- Some data suggest an association between dopamine transporter gene (DAT) *SLC6A3 3'* (VNTR) polymorphism, and PTSD.

RISK FACTORS
- Pretrauma environment:
  - Female sex
  - Younger age
  - Psychiatric history
  - Sexual abuse

- Peritrauma environment:
  - Severity of the trauma
  - Peritrauma emotionality
  - Perception of threat to life
  - Perpetration of the trauma
- Posttrauma environment:
  - Perceived injury severity
  - Medical complications
  - Perceived social support
  - Persistent dissociation from traumatic event
- Subsequent exposure to trauma-related stimuli

GENERAL PREVENTION
- There is moderate evidence for hydrocortisone (2) and some evidence for propranolol (3) reducing development of full posttraumatic syndrome.
- Compulsory psychological debriefing immediately after a trauma (critical incident stress management) does not prevent PTSD and may be harmful (4).

COMMONLY ASSOCIATED CONDITIONS
- Major depressive disorder
- Alcohol/substance abuse
- Panic disorder
- Obsessive-compulsive disorder
- Agoraphobia and/or social phobia
- Traumatic brain injury
- Smoking (especially with assaultive trauma)
- Major neurocognitive disorders, dementia, or amnesia

Pediatric Considerations
Oppositional defiant disorder and separation anxiety are common comorbid conditions.

DIAGNOSIS

HISTORY
Diagnosis is based on *DSM-V* criteria:
- Criterion A: exposure to trauma (≥1 of the following):
  - Direct experience of a traumatic event
  - In-person witnessing of a traumatic event
  - Learning of a traumatic event involving a close friend or family member
  - Repeated exposure to details of a traumatic event
- Criterion B: intrusive symptoms associated with the traumatic event (≥1 of the following):
  - Recurrent, involuntary, and intrusive distressing memories of the event
  - Recurrent distressing dreams related to the event
  - Dissociative reactions that simulate a recurrence of the event
  - Intense or prolonged distress to stimuli that resemble an aspect of the event
- Criterion C: avoidance of stimuli associated with the trauma (≥1 of the following):
  - Avoidance of memories, thoughts, or feelings about the event
  - Avoidance of external reminders that trigger memories, thoughts, or feelings about the event
- Criterion D: negative cognitive and mood changes associated with the trauma (≥2 of the following):
  - Inability to remember aspects of event
  - Persistent and exaggerated negative opinion of self, others, or the world
  - Distorted beliefs about the cause or consequences of the event
  - Negative emotional state
  - Diminished interest in significant activities
  - Feeling detached from others
  - Inability to experience positive emotions

- Criterion E: hyperarousal (≥2 of the following):
  - Difficulty sleeping/falling asleep
  - Decreased concentration
  - Hypervigilance
  - Outbursts of anger/irritable mood
  - Exaggerated startle response
  - Self-destructive behavior
- Criterion F: duration of the relevant criteria symptoms should be >1 month
- Criterion G: clinically significant distress/impairment in functioning
- Criterion H: relevant criteria not attributed to substance effects or other medical conditions

Pediatric Considerations
- Memories of the traumatic event may not appear distressing and may be seen as play reenactment.
- Frightening dreams of children may not have content attributable to the traumatic event.
- Reactions can include a fear of being separated from a parent, crying, whimpering, screaming, immobility and/or aimless motion, trembling, frightened facial expressions, excessive clinging, and regressive behavior.
- Older children may show extreme withdrawal, disruptive behavior, and/or an inability to pay attention. Regressive behaviors, nightmares, sleep problems, irrational fears, irritability, refusal to attend school, outbursts of anger, fighting, somatic complaints with no medical basis, and decline in schoolwork performance are often seen. Furthermore, depression, anxiety, feelings of guilt, and emotional numbing are often present.
- Parental posttraumatic stress has been shown to be a robust predictor of pediatric PTSD (5)[A].

PHYSICAL EXAM
- Patients may present with physical injuries from the traumatic event.
- Mental status examination:
  - Thoughts and perceptions (e.g., hallucinations, delusions, suicidal ideation, phobias)
  - General appearance: disheveled, poor hygiene
  - Behavior: agitation; startle reaction extreme
  - Psychological numbness
  - Orientation may be affected.
  - Memory: forgetfulness, especially concerning the details of the traumatic event
  - Poor concentration
  - Poor impulse control
  - Altered speech rate and flow
  - Mood and affect may be changed: depression, anxiety, guilt, and/or fear

Pediatric Considerations
Elevated heart rate immediately following trauma is associated with development of PTSD (5)[A].

DIFFERENTIAL DIAGNOSIS
- Acute stress disorder (symptoms <4 weeks)
- Generalized anxiety disorder
- Adjustment disorder
- Obsessive-compulsive disorder
- Schizophrenia
- Major depressive disorder
- Mood disorder with psychotic features
- Substance abuse
- Personality disorders
- Dissociative disorders
- Conversion disorder

TREATMENT

Better prognosis if treated with a combination of psychotherapy and pharmacotherapy, initiated soon after the trauma.

MEDICATION

First Line

- SSRIs: depression, panic attacks, startle response, sleep disruption (6)[A]. All commonly used SSRIs have been shown to be effective in the treatment of PTSD and are the first-line treatment:
  – Sertraline: 50 to 200 mg every day (FDA approved)
  – Paroxetine: starting dose: 10 mg every day; may be increased in 10 mg increments at intervals ≥1 week (FDA approved)
  – Fluoxetine: 20 mg every day/BID not to exceed 80 mg/day (demonstrates some efficacy for all three symptom clusters)
- Sleep disruption: Sleep disruption due to hyperarousal is ubiquitous in PTSD. Standard sedatives, such as trazodone 50 to 300 mg at bedtime, mirtazapine 7.5 to 30 mg qhs, or amitriptyline 25 to 100 mg qhs
- Nightmares/nighttime hyperarousal: prazosin 2 to 15 mg qhs (7)[A], clonidine 0.1 to 0.2 mg qhs, amitriptyline 25 to 100 mg qhs

Second Line

Refractory/residual symptoms: Consider augmentation with:

- Depression: mirtazapine 15 to 45 mg/day; consider switch to a serotonin-norepinephrine reuptake inhibitor (SNRI), such as venlafaxine XR 37.5 to 300 mg/day, duloxetine 60 to 120 mg/day, or desvenlafaxine 50 to 100 mg/day. Nefazodone 300 to 600 mg/day in divided doses can be very effective, but requires quarterly LFTs.
- Reexperiencing/intrusive thoughts: first-/second-generation antipsychotic medications: aripiprazole 5 to 15 mg/day, risperidone 0.5 to 2 mg/day, olanzapine 2.5 to 10 mg/day, quetiapine 50 to 400 mg/day (8)[A]. Second-generation Rx less prone to extrapyramidal symptoms (EPS): cognitive dulling
- Hyperarousal: clonidine, start 0.05 mg BID/TID; slowly titrate to as much as 0.45 mg/day divided doses; guanfacine 1 to 3 mg/day in divided doses (long-acting forms of both clonidine and guanfacine now available). Also consider second-generation antipsychotics quetiapine, risperidone, and olanzapine as above. Divided doses often more helpful.
- Impulsivity/explosiveness: anticonvulsants: valproic acid 500 to 2,000 mg/day, carbamazepine 200 to 600 mg/day, topiramate 50 to 200 mg/day
- Anxiety: benzodiazepines (see "ALERT"), including clonazepam, 1 to 4 mg/day in divided doses for a limited duration. Consider also hydroxyzine 25 to 50 mg TID/QID PRN or risperidone 0.25 to 0.5 mg TID PRN

ALERT

Given risk of substance abuse and questionable benefit in PTSD, recommended benzodiazepines be avoided (9)[A]. Short-acting benzodiazepines presents the greatest risk.

ADDITIONAL THERAPIES

- Psychotherapeutic interventions:
  – Exposure therapies have shown the highest effectiveness for treatment of PTSD (10)[A]:
    ◦ Behavioral and cognitive-behavioral therapy (CBT): Early CBT has been shown to speed recovery. CBT is currently considered the standard of care for PTSD by the U.S. Department of Defense.

◦ 1-week intensive CBT was as effective as 3-month weekly CBT in one study (11)[A].
◦ Internet-based CBT has shown benefit in reduction of PTSD symptoms.
◦ Prolonged exposure therapy: Reexperience distressing trauma-related memories and reminders to facilitate habituation and successful emotional processing of memory.
◦ EMDR (eye movement desensitization and reprocessing) has been shown to benefit patients with PTSD (12)[A].

– Stress-reduction techniques:
  ◦ Immediate symptom reduction (e.g., rebreathing in a bag for hyperventilation)
  ◦ Early recognition and removal from a stress
  ◦ Relaxation, meditation, and exercise techniques are also helpful in reducing the reaction to stressful events.

– Telemedicine-based collaborative care (with nurse case manager, pharmacy, psychology, and psychiatry) is more effective than usual care (13)[A].

- Interpersonal psychotherapy:
  – Supportive psychotherapy with an emphasis on the here and now
- Social:
  – Establish the social framework of the problem. Clarifying this allows the patient to begin viewing it within the proper context (e.g., change of job/relocation of adult-dependent offspring)

INPATIENT CONSIDERATIONS

Inpatient care is necessary only if the patient becomes suicidal/homicidal or for treatment of comorbid conditions (e.g., depression, substance abuse).

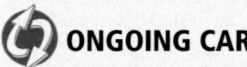 **ONGOING CARE**

PATIENT EDUCATION

National Center for PTSD: www.ptsd.va.gov

PROGNOSIS

- Varies significantly from patient to patient
- In 50% of cases, the symptoms spontaneously remit after 3 months; however, in other cases, symptoms may persist, often for many years, and cause long-term impairment in life functioning.
- Factors associated with a good prognosis include:
  – Rapid engagement of treatment
  – Early and ongoing social support
  – Avoidance of retraumatization
  – Positive premorbid function
  – Absence of other psychiatric disorders/substance abuse

COMPLICATIONS

- Increased risk for panic disorder, agoraphobia, obsessive-compulsive disorder, social phobia, specific phobia, major depressive disorder, somatization disorder; impulsive behavior, suicide, and homicide. Victims of sexual assault are at especially high risk for developing mental health problems and committing suicide.
- Benzodiazepines lead to abuse and dependence.
- Avoidance of stimuli associated with the trauma can generalize to wide-ranging avoidance. This leads to a far greater negative impact on the patient's life.

REFERENCES

1. Alisic E, Zalta AK, van Wesel F, et al. Rates of post-traumatic stress disorder in trauma-exposed children and adolescents: meta-analysis. *Br J Psychiatry*. 2014;204:335–340.

2. Amos T, Stein DJ, Ipser JC. Pharmacological interventions for preventing post-traumatic stress disorder (PTSD). *Cochrane Database Syst Rev*. 2014;(7):CD006239.
3. Searcy CP, Bobadilla L, Gordon WA, et al. Pharmacological prevention of combat-related PTSD: a literature review. *Mil Med*. 2012;177(6):649–654.
4. Rose S, Bisson J, Churchill R, et al. Psychological debriefing for preventing post traumatic stress disorder (PTSD). *Cochrane Database Syst Rev*. 2002;(2):CD000560.
5. Brosbe MS, Hoefling K, Faust J. Predicting posttraumatic stress following pediatric injury: a systematic review. *J Pediatr Psychol*. 2011;36(6):718–729.
6. Stein DJ, Ipser JC, Seedat S. Pharmacotherapy for post traumatic stress disorder (PTSD). *Cochrane Database Syst Rev*. 2006;(1):CD002795.
7. Writer BW, Meyer EG, Schillerstrom JE. Prazosin for military combat-related PTSD nightmares: a critical review. *J Neuropsychiatry Clin Neurosci*. 2014;26(1):24–33.
8. Han C, Pae CU, Wang SM, et al. The potential role of atypical antipsychotics for the treatment of posttraumatic stress disorder. *J Psychiatr Res*. 2014;56:72–81.
9. Jeffreys M, Capehart B, Friedman MJ. Pharmacotherapy for posttraumatic stress disorder: review with clinical applications. *J Rehabil Res Dev*. 2012;49(5):703–715.
10. Kornør H, Winje D, Ekeberg Ø, et al. Early trauma-focused cognitive-behavioural therapy to prevent chronic post-traumatic stress disorder and related symptoms: a systematic review and meta-analysis. *BMC Psychiatry*. 2008;8:81.
11. Ehlers A, Hackmann A, Grey N, et al. A randomized controlled trial of 7-day intensive and standard weekly cognitive therapy for PTSD and emotion-focused supportive therapy. *Am J Psychiatry*. 2014;171(3):294–304.
12. Goodson J, Helstrom A, Halpern JM, et al. Treatment of posttraumatic stress disorder in U.S. combat veterans: a meta-analytic review. *Psychol Rep*. 2011;109(2):573–599.
13. Fortney JC, Pyne JM, Kimbrell TA, et al. Telemedicine-based collaborative care for post-traumatic stress disorder: a randomized clinical trial. *JAMA Psychiatry*. 2015;72(1):58–67.

ADDITIONAL READING

American Psychiatric Association. *Diagnostic and Statistical Manual of Mental Disorders (DSM-V)*. 5th ed. Washington, DC: American Psychiatric Publishing; 2013.

 CODES

ICD10

- F43.10 Post-traumatic stress disorder, unspecified
- F43.11 Post-traumatic stress disorder, acute
- F43.12 Post-traumatic stress disorder, chronic

CLINICAL PEARLS

- Treatment is often best accomplished with a combination of psychotherapy and pharmacotherapy.
- The sooner therapy is initiated after the trauma, the better the prognosis.

PREECLAMPSIA AND ECLAMPSIA (TOXEMIA OF PREGNANCY)
Konstantinos E. Deligiannidis, MD, MPH, FAAFP

 BASICS

DESCRIPTION
- Preeclampsia is a disorder of pregnancy developing at the 20th week (or beyond), with new-onset hypertension (HTN) and new-onset proteinuria and/ or impaired organ function:
  - May progress from mild to life-threatening in hours to days
  - The disorder is reversible by delivery if at term or, if maternal/fetal health are in danger, by preterm delivery.
  - Eclampsia is defined as new-onset grand mal seizure activity in a patient with preeclampsia without underlying neurologic disease.
  - Most postpartum cases occur within 48 hours of delivery but can occur up to 4 weeks postpartum.
- System(s) affected: cardiovascular, renal, reproductive, fetoplacental, CNS, hepatic
- Synonym(s): toxemia of pregnancy

EPIDEMIOLOGY
Incidence
- Predominant age
  - Most cases occur in younger women because of the higher incidence of preeclampsia in younger (primiparous) women.
  - However, older (>40 years) patients with preeclampsia have 4 times the incidence of seizures compared with patients in their 20s.
- Preeclampsia: 5–8%
- Eclampsia develops in 1.6 to 10/10,000 deliveries in developed countries. In developing countries, estimates range from 6 to 157/10,000.
- 40% of eclamptic seizures occur before delivery; 16% occur >48 hours after delivery.

ETIOLOGY AND PATHOPHYSIOLOGY
Systemic derangements in eclampsia include the following:
- Cardiovascular: generalized vasospasm
- Hematologic: decreased plasma volume, increased blood viscosity, hemoconcentration, coagulopathy
- Renal: decreased glomerular filtration rate
- Hepatic: periportal necrosis, hepatocellular damage, subcapsular hematoma
- CNS: cerebral vasospasm and ischemia, cerebral edema, cerebral hemorrhage

Genetics
2 to 4 times increased risk in pregnant women with family history of preeclampsia

RISK FACTORS
Nulliparity; age >40 years; family history of preeclampsia; high body mass index; diabetes; chronic HTN, chronic renal disease, or both; multifetal pregnancy; previous preeclampsia; systemic lupus erythematosus; in vitro fertilization (1)

GENERAL PREVENTION
- Adequate prenatal care: Women who do not receive prenatal care are seven times more likely to die from complications.
- Good control of preexisting HTN
- Recent systematic reviews, meta-analyses, and task force recommendations show that low-dose aspirin (60 to 80 mg) started early in pregnancy may lower the risk of developing preeclampsia and the rate of preterm delivery and neonatal death in moderate- to high-risk patients and has no significant effect on the rate of placental abruption/neonatal bleeding complications. The number needed to treat (NNT) to prevent one case of preeclampsia ranges from 18 to 118 depending on risk population, but more info is required to see which women would benefit and when to start therapy (1)[C],(2–4)[A]. It may be recommended in those with preeclampsia in >1 prior pregnancy or with a history of preeclampsia and preterm delivery (1)[C].
- Low-dose calcium supplementation has been shown to reduce the risk and severity of preeclampsia (relative risk [RR] = 0.38) in calcium-deficient populations (1)[C],(5)[A].
- Although some evidence suggests vitamin C (1,000 mg/day) and vitamin E (400 U/day) may reduce the risk for preeclampsia, recent guidelines recommend against their use (1)[C],(6).

COMMONLY ASSOCIATED CONDITIONS
Abruptio placentae, placental insufficiency, fetal growth restriction, preterm delivery, fetal demise, maternal seizures (eclampsia), maternal pulmonary edema, maternal liver/kidney failure, maternal death

 DIAGNOSIS

Diagnosis depends on new-onset elevated BP (SBP ≥140 mm Hg or DBP ≥90 mm Hg on two occasions at least 4 hours apart, or ≥160/110 mm Hg) after 20 weeks of gestation AND EITHER proteinuria (>300 mg/24 hr or spot protein:creatinine ≥0.3), OR new-onset thrombocytopenia, renal insufficiency, impaired liver function, pulmonary edema, or cerebral/ visual symptoms (1)[C]. This 2013 ACOG guideline suggests defining preeclampsia as either without or with severe features. Older guidelines use the term "mild" and "severe." The term "mild" is discouraged because preeclampsia is an evolving process that must be frequently evaluated for severity (1)[C].

HISTORY
May be asymptomatic. In some cases, rapid excessive weight gain (>5 lb/week; >2.3 kg/week); more severe cases are associated with epigastric pain, headache, altered mental status, and visual disturbance.

PHYSICAL EXAM
- BP criteria:
  - Preeclampsia without severe features: Elevated BP ≥140/90 mm Hg on two occasions at least 4 hours apart, or more rapid diagnosis may be made with BP ≥160/110 mm Hg.
  - Preeclampsia with severe features: Elevated BP ≥160 systolic mm Hg or 110 mm Hg diastolic on two BP readings 4 hours apart while the patient is on bedrest, AND new onset of one or more of below:
    - Platelets <100,000/μL
    - >2 times normal liver transaminase levels, severe persistent right upper quadrant (RUQ)/ epigastric pain, or both
    - Creatinine >1.1 mg/dL, or doubling of serum creatinine levels
    - Pulmonary edema
    - Cerebral or visual symptoms
- Eclampsia: tonic-clonic seizure activity (focal/ generalized)
  - Note: headache, visual disturbance, and epigastric or RUQ pain often precede seizure
  - Seizures may occur once/repeatedly.
  - Postictal coma, cyanosis (variable)
  - Temperatures >39°C may be consistent with CNS hemorrhage.
  - Normal BP, even in response to treatment; does not rule out potential for seizures

DIFFERENTIAL DIAGNOSIS
- Chronic HTN: HTN before pregnancy; high BP before the 20th week
- Chronic HTN with superimposed preeclampsia
- Gestational HTN: Increased BP first discovered after 20 weeks, often close to term, with no proteinuria and without evidence of organ dysfunction. BP becomes normal by 12 weeks postpartum, or it is reclassified as chronic hypertension.
- Seizures in pregnancy: epilepsy, cerebral tumors, meningitis/encephalitis, ruptured cerebral aneurysm. Until other causes are proven, however, all pregnant women with convulsions should be considered to have eclampsia.

DIAGNOSTIC TESTS & INTERPRETATION
Initial Tests (lab, imaging)
- Routine spot urine testing for protein should be done at each prenatal visit in all hypertensive patients
- CBC, including platelets, creatinine, serum transaminase levels, and uric acid as baseline in hypertensive patients and if preeclampsia suspected or possible
- Coagulation profiles: abnormalities suggest severe disease.
- 24-hour urine or protein/creatinine ratio if urine protein dips 1+ on more than one occasion, or if preeclampsia is being considered
- Daily fetal movement monitoring by mother ("kick counts")
- US imaging is used to monitor growth and cord blood flow; perform, as indicated, based on clinical stability and laboratory findings.
- Nonstress test (NST) at diagnosis and then twice-weekly until delivery
- Biophysical profile if NST is nonreactive (1)[C]
- US imaging for growth progress every 3 weeks, and amniotic fluid volume at least once weekly (1)[C]
- With seizures, CT scan and MRI should be considered if focal findings persist or uncharacteristic signs/symptoms are present.

Follow-Up Tests & Special Considerations
Disseminated intravascular coagulation, thrombocytopenia, liver dysfunction, and renal failure can complicate preeclampsia associated with HELLP syndrome.

Test Interpretation
CNS: cerebral edema, hyperemia, focal anemia, thrombosis, and hemorrhage. Cerebral lesions account for 40% of eclamptic deaths.

 TREATMENT

- Preeclampsia without severe features:
  - Outpatient care
  - Maternal: daily home BP monitoring; daily weights; weekly labs (complete blood count [CBC], creatinine, liver function test [LFT])
  - Fetal:
    - Patient-measured: daily "kick counts"
    - Medical provider–measured: (see imaging section above)
    - Delivery at 37 weeks

- Preeclampsia with severe features:
  - Inpatient care if patient condition deteriorates (BP ≥160/110 mm Hg; severe headache; visual changes [scotoma or "flashing lights"]; impaired mentation; pulmonary edema; epigastric/RUQ pain; increasing LFTs; oliguria; thrombocytopenia) or if fetal status is deemed "nonreassuring"
  - Maternal: daily labs, adding coagulation tests; IV magnesium sulfate as seizure prophylaxis; IV labetalol **or** hydralazine and oral sustained-release nifedipine antihypertensive therapy titrated to keep systolic BP <160 mm Hg and diastolic BP <110 mm Hg (some recommend <150/100 mm Hg postpartum). Keep diastolic BP >90 mm Hg to avoid hypoperfusing the uterus.
  - Fetal: continuous heart monitoring; daily US with BP, amniotic fluid levels, fetal growth assessment as deemed necessary

GENERAL MEASURES
Management by gestational age of *severe* preeclampsia:

- <23 weeks: Offer to terminate pregnancy.
- At 23 to 34 weeks: Antihypertensives; evaluate maternal–fetal condition; steroids to enhance fetal lung maturity; plan delivery at 34 weeks with magnesium sulfate prophylaxis.
- If severe HTN, eclampsia, DIC, pulmonary edema, abnormal fetal test results/evaluation, or abruption placentae, then plan delivery once maternal condition is stable.
- If HELLP syndrome (full or partial), severe oligohydramnios, significant renal dysfunction, persistent symptoms, fetal growth restriction, ≥33 5/7 weeks' gestation, labor, or PROM, then steroids and then delivery after 48 hours.
- If the above do not apply, then expectant management until 34 weeks.
- At ≥34 weeks: magnesium sulfate and delivery (1)[C]

ALERT
- Regardless of gestational age, emergent delivery is recommended if there are signs of maternal hypertensive crisis, abruptio placentae, uterine rupture, or fetal distress.
- Seizures: control of convulsions, correction of hypoxia and acidosis, lowering of BP, steps to effect delivery as soon as convulsions are controlled
- Administer betamethasone 12 mg IM daily × 2 doses or dexamethasone 6 mg every 12 hours × 4 doses if delivery <34 weeks possible.

MEDICATION
First Line
- For seizure prophylaxis for women with severe preeclampsia: magnesium sulfate (MgSO$_4$): loading dose 4 g IV in 200 mL normal saline over 20 to 30 minutes; maintenance dose 1 to 2 g/hr IV continuous infusion (although recent guidelines suggest it not be universally administered for seizure prophylaxis to prevent eclampsia, the quality of the evidence is low, and the strength of the recommendation is qualified) (1)[C]
- For BP control
  - Antihypertensives are inadvisable for mildly elevated BP (without severe features).
  - Labetalol (IV): 20 mg over 2 minutes followed at 20 to 30 minutes intervals with doses of 20 to 80 mg titrated to keep BP <160/110 mm Hg; max of 300 mg/24 hr. (Contraindicated in asthma, heart disease, congestive heart failure.)
  - Hydralazine (IV): 5 to 10 mg over 2 minutes, followed at 20 minutes intervals with 5 to 10 mg

IV boluses; titrated to keep BP<160/110 mm Hg; max of 25 mg/24 hr.
  - Nifedipine sustained-release (PO) (used in the postpartum): 30 to 120 mg/day (caution with combination of nifedipine and magnesium sulfate resulting in hypotension and neuromuscular blockade)
- For eclampsia/seizures
  - In recent randomized trials, magnesium sulfate was found to be superior to phenytoin in the treatment and prevention of eclampsia and probably more effective and safer than diazepam.
  - Magnesium sulfate for seizures
    - 4 to 6 g IV over 15 to 20 minutes followed by 1 to 2 g/hr infusion
    - Further boluses of magnesium may be given for recurrent convulsions with the amount given based on the neurologic examination and patellar reflexes.
    - Contraindications: myasthenia gravis, renal failure, pulmonary edema
  - Levels of 6 to 8 mEq/mL are considered therapeutic, but clinical status is most important and must ensure that
    - Patellar reflexes are present.
    - Respirations are not depressed.
    - Urine output is ≥25 mL/hr.
  - May be given safely, even in the presence of renal insufficiency
- Fluid therapy
  - Ringer lactated solution with 5% dextrose at 60 to 120 mL/hr, with careful attention to fluid–volume status
- Precautions: Do not use diuretics. Carefully monitor neurologic status, urine output, respirations, and fetal status.
- Calcium carbonate (1 g, administered slowly IV) may reverse magnesium-induced respiratory depression.

Second Line
- Diazepam 2 mg/min until resolution or 20 mg given or
- Lorazepam 1 to 2 mg/min up to total of 10 mg or
- Phenytoin 15 to 20 mg/kg at a maximum rate of 50 mg/min or
- Levetiracetam 500 mg IV or oral, may be repeated in 12 hours (dose needs to be adjusted in renal impairment) or
- Phenobarbital 20 mg/kg infused at 50 mg/min; may repeat with additional 5 to 10 mg/kg after 15 minutes

ONGOING CARE

FOLLOW-UP RECOMMENDATIONS
- Without severe features: restricted activity; with severe features: restricted activity, in hospital
- Women with a history of preeclampsia should report this to physicians caring for them in later life. It is a potent cardiovascular disease risk factor.

DIET
- Salt restriction is inadvisable because the patient often is experiencing intravascular hypovolemia (1)[C].
- Calcium supplementation may be recommended for women who have low calcium intake (<600 mg/day) (1,6)[A].

PATIENT EDUCATION
American College of Obstetricians and Gynecologists, 409 12th St. SW, Washington, DC 20024-2188; (800) 762-ACOG; http://www.acog.org/

PROGNOSIS
- For nulliparous women with preeclampsia before 30 weeks of gestation, the recurrence rate for the disorder may be as high as 40% in future pregnancies.
- 25% of eclamptic women will have HTN during subsequent pregnancies, but only 5% of these will be severe and only 2% will be eclamptic again.
- Preeclamptic, multiparous women may be at higher risk for subsequent essential HTN; they also have higher mortality during subsequent pregnancies than do primiparous women.

COMPLICATIONS
- Most women do not have long-term sequelae from eclampsia, although many may have transient neurologic deficits.
- A history of preeclampsia is equivalent to traditional risk factors for cardiovascular disease. Women with a history of preeclampsia should be strongly advised to avoid obesity and smoking. Other signs of metabolic syndrome should be closely monitored as well.
- Maternal and/or fetal death

REFERENCES

1. American College of Obstetricians and Gynecologists, Task Force on Hypertension in Pregnancy. Hypertension in pregnancy. Report of the American College of Obstetricians and Gynecologists' Task Force on Hypertension in Pregnancy. *Obstet Gynecol.* 2013;122(5):1122–1131.
2. Gauer R, Atlas M, Hill J. Clinical inquiries. Does low-dose aspirin reduce preeclampsia and other maternal-fetal complications? *J Fam Pract.* 2008;57(1):54–56.
3. Villa PM, Kajantie E, Räikkönen K, et al. Aspirin in the prevention of pre-eclampsia in high-risk women: a randomised placebo-controlled PREDO Trial and a meta-analysis of randomised trials. *BJOG.* 2013;120(1):64–74.
4. Duley L, Henderson-Smart DJ, Meher S, et al. Antiplatelet agents for preventing pre-eclampsia and its complications. *Cochrane Database of Syst Rev.* 2007;(2):CD004659. doi:10.1002/14651858 .CD004659.pub2.
5. Hofmeyr GJ, Belizán JM, von Dadelszen P. Low-dose calcium supplementation for preventing pre-eclampsia: a systematic review and commentary. *BJOG.* 2014;121(8):951–957.
6. Magee LA, Helewa M, Moutquin JM, et al. Diagnosis, evaluation, and management of the hypertensive disorders of pregnancy. *J Obstet Gynaecol Can.* 2008;30(3 Suppl):S1–S48.

 ## CODES

ICD10
- O14.90 Unspecified pre-eclampsia, unspecified trimester
- O15.00 Eclampsia in pregnancy, unspecified trimester
- O14.00 Mild to moderate pre-eclampsia, unspecified trimester

CLINICAL PEARLS
- Management of preeclampsia depends on both the severity of the condition and the gestational age of the fetus.
- Diagnosis no longer requires presence of proteinuria.

PREMENSTRUAL SYNDROME (PMS) AND PREMENSTRUAL DYSPHORIC DISORDER (PMDD)

Courtney I. Jarvis, PharmD • Allison Hargreaves, MD

 BASICS

DESCRIPTION
- Premenstrual syndrome (PMS), a complex of physical and emotional symptoms sufficiently severe to interfere with everyday life, occurs cyclically during the luteal phase of menses.
- Premenstrual dysphoric disorder (PMDD) is a severe form of PMS characterized by severe recurrent depressive and anxiety symptoms, with premenstrual (luteal phase) onset, that remits a few days after the start of menses.
- PMDD is now included as a full diagnostic category in the 5th edition of the *Diagnostic and Statistical Manual of Mental Disorders (DSM-5)*.
- System(s) affected: endocrine/metabolic, nervous, reproductive

EPIDEMIOLOGY
Prevalence
- Many women have some physical and psychological symptoms before menses (this is not PMS).
- 30% of menstruating women suffer from PMS; 3–8% of menstruating women have PMDD.

ETIOLOGY AND PATHOPHYSIOLOGY
Not well understood. Leading theories postulate metabolites of progesterone interact with central neurotransmitter receptors (serotonin and γ-aminobutyric acid [GABA]), provoking downstream effects of decreased GABA-mediated inhibition and decreased serotonin levels. Women with PMS/PMDD have similar levels of progesterone but seem to have an increased sensitivity to its metabolites, compared with women without PMS/PMDD.

Genetics
- Role of genetic predisposition is controversial; however, twin studies do suggest a genetic component.
- Involvement of gene coding for the serotonergic *5HT1A* receptor and allelic variants of the estrogen receptor-α gene (*ESR1*) is suggested.

RISK FACTORS
- Age: usually present in late 20s to mid-30s
- History of mood disorder (major depression, bipolar disorder), anxiety disorder, personality disorder, or substance abuse
- Family history
- Low parity
- Tobacco use
- Psychosocial stressors/history of trauma
- High BMI

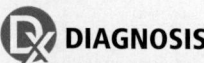 **DIAGNOSIS**

HISTORY
- *DSM-5* criteria (1)[A]
- Symptoms occur 1 week before menses, improve in the first few days after menses begin, and are minimal/absent in the week following menses (over most menstrual cycles during the past year).
- ≥5 of the following (1 must be among the first 4):
  - Marked depressed mood, feelings of hopelessness, or self-deprecating thoughts
  - Marked anxiety, tension, and/or feelings of being keyed up or on edge

- Marked affective lability (mood swings)
- Marked irritability or anger or increased interpersonal conflicts
- Decreased interest in usual activities and social withdrawal
- Lethargy, easy fatigability, or lack of energy
- Appetite change, overeating, food cravings
- Hypersomnia or insomnia
- Feeling out of control or overwhelmed
- Subjective difficulty concentrating
- Physical symptoms, such as abdominal bloating, breast tenderness, headaches, weight gain, and joint/muscle pain
- For PMDD, emotional symptoms must be sufficiently severe to interfere with work, school, usual social activities, or relationships with others.
- Symptoms may be superimposed on an underlying psychiatric disorder but may not be an exacerbation of another condition, such as panic disorder/major depression.
- Criteria should be confirmed by prospective patient record of symptoms for a minimum of two consecutive menstrual cycles (without confirmation, "provisional" should be noted with diagnosis).
- Use the Daily Record of Severity of Problems (available online at http://www.aafp.org/afp/2011/1015/p918-fig1.pdf) or similar inventory (2)[A].
- Symptoms should not be attributable to drug abuse, medications, or other medical conditions.

PHYSICAL EXAM
No specific physical exam required; may consider thyroid and pelvic exams if indicated by additional patient symptoms.

DIFFERENTIAL DIAGNOSIS
- Premenstrual exacerbation of underlying psychiatric disorder
- Psychiatric disorders (especially bipolar disorder, major depression, anxiety)
- Thyroid disorders
- Perimenopause
- Premenstrual migraine
- Chronic fatigue syndrome
- Irritable bowel syndrome (painful symptoms)
- Seizures
- Anemia
- Endometriosis (painful symptoms)
- Drug/alcohol abuse

DIAGNOSTIC TESTS & INTERPRETATION
- The repetitive nature of symptoms precludes need for labs if a classic history is present.
- Consider
  - Hemoglobin to rule out anemia
  - 25-OH vitamin D level to exclude deficiency, although precise relationship of deficiency with the disorder is unclear
  - Serum thyroid-stimulating hormone (TSH) to rule out hypothyroidism
- Imaging with pelvic ultrasound to diagnose causes of pelvic pain and dysmenorrhea may be needed.

 TREATMENT

GENERAL MEASURES
Although evidence is lacking for aerobic exercise in treating PMS/PMDD, it is often recommended as part of an integrated care plan.

MEDICATION
First Line
- SSRIs show a small to moderate effect in the treatment of physical, functional, and behavioral symptoms of PMS and PMDD compared to placebo (3)[A]:
  - Both intermittent luteal phase dosing and continuous full-cycle dosing are effective with no clear evidence of difference between modes of administration (3)[A].
  - All SSRIs tested appeared effective (3)[A].
  - SSRIs are effective at low doses. Higher doses have increased effect but are accompanied by increased side effects (3)[A].
- Fluoxetine (Prozac, Sarafem) 20 mg/day every day or 20 mg/day only during luteal phase, or 90 mg once a week for 2 weeks in luteal phase
- Sertraline (Zoloft) 50 to 150 mg/day every day or 50 to 150 mg/day only during luteal phase
- Citalopram (Celexa) 10 to 30 mg/day every day or 10 to 30 mg/day only during luteal phase
- Adverse effects (number needed to harm [NNH] with moderate-dose SSRI): nausea (NNH = 7), asthenia (NNH = 9), somnolence (NNH = 13), fatigue (NNH = 14), decreased libido (NNH = 14), and sweating (NNH = 14) (3)[A].
- Contraindications: patients taking monoamine oxidase inhibitors (MAOIs)
- Precautions
  - Increased risk of suicidal thinking and behavior in children and adolescents with depressive disorders; uncertain if this risk applies to those taking SSRIs for PMDD
  - Bipolar disorder
  - Seizure disorder
  - QTc prolongation (with citalopram)
  - Hepatic dysfunction
  - Renal dysfunction
- Possible interactions
  - MAOIs
  - Selegiline
  - Pimozide
  - Thioridazine
  - Cimetidine, omeprazole, and QTc prolonging agents (with citalopram)

Second Line
Alternative therapies should be considered if no response to SSRIs:
- Spironolactone (Aldactone) 50 to 100 mg/day for 7 to 10 days during luteal phase; helpful for fluid retention. Adverse reactions: lethargy, headache, irregular menses, hyperkalemia

- Oral contraceptive pills (OCPs)
  - OCPs can cause adverse effects similar to PMDD symptoms (4)[B].
  - Extended-cycle use of OCPs (e.g., 12 weeks on and 1 week off) or a shorter placebo interval (e.g., 24 active pills with 4 placebo days [24/4] compared with 21/7 preparations) may be beneficial (4)[B].
  - OCPs containing the progestin drospirenone (structurally similar to spironolactone) may improve physical symptoms and mood changes associated with PMDD (5)[A]. Caution: Risk of venous thromboembolism may be modestly higher than with other OCPs (4)[B].
  - Continuous administration of levonorgestrel/ethinyl estradiol may improve patient symptoms in PMDD (4)[B].
    - Suggested OCP formulations:
      - Ethinyl estradiol 0.02 to 0.03 mg/drospirenone 3 mg (Gianvi/Loryna/Nikki/Ocella/Syeda/Vestura/Yasmin/Yaz Zarah): 1 tablet/day
      - Ethinyl estradiol 0.02 to 0.03 mg/drospirenone 3 mg/levomefolate 0.451 mg (Beyaz/Safyral): 1 tablet/day
      - Levonorgestrel 90 μg/ethinyl estradiol 20 μg (Amethyst/Lybrel): 1 tablet/day
- Anxiolytics
  - Alprazolam (Xanax) 0.25 mg TID–QID only during luteal phase; taper at onset of menses (other benzodiazepines not studied for PMDD). Caution: addictive potential
  - Buspirone (BuSpar) 10 to 30 mg/day divided BID–TID in the luteal phase
- Ovulation inhibitors
  - Gonadotropin-releasing hormone (GnRH) agonists: leuprolide (Lupron) depot 3.75 mg/month IM
    - Precautions: Menopause-like side effects (e.g., osteoporosis, hot flashes, headaches, muscle aches, vaginal dryness, irritability) limit treatment to 6 months; may be first step if considering bilateral oophorectomy for severe, refractory PMDD
  - Danazol (Danocrine) 300 to 400 mg BID; adverse reactions: androgenic and antiestrogenic effects (e.g., amenorrhea, weight gain, acne, fluid retention, hirsutism, hot flashes, vaginal dryness, emotional lability)
  - Estrogen, transdermal preferred, 100 to 200 μg:
    - Precautions: increased risk of blood clot, stroke, heart attack, and breast cancer
    - Requires concomitant progesterone add-back therapy to protect against uterine hyperplasia and endometrial cancer
- Progesterone: insufficient evidence to support use (6)[A]

ISSUES FOR REFERRAL
Referral to psychiatrist may be indicated for mood/anxiety disorders if patient has no symptom-free period.

ADDITIONAL THERAPIES
Cognitive-behavioral therapy (CBT) is theoretically helpful for PMS/PMDD given its application for symptom reduction in other mood disorders, but direct evidence is lacking.

SURGERY/OTHER PROCEDURES
Bilateral oophorectomy, usually with concomitant hysterectomy, is an option for rare, refractory cases with severe, disabling symptoms.

COMPLEMENTARY & ALTERNATIVE MEDICINE
- Acupuncture demonstrated superiority to progestins, anxiolytics, and sham acupuncture with no evidence of harm (7)[A].
- Some data support the use of the following (8)[A]:
  - Calcium: 600 mg BID
  - Vitamin B$_6$: 50 to 100 mg/day
  - Chasteberry (Vitex agnus-castus): 4 mg/day of extract containing 6% of agnuside (or 20 to 40 mg/day of fruit extract)
  - Omega-3 fatty acids 2 g/day
- Data insufficient regarding the following (8)[A]:
  - Magnesium: 200 to 400 mg/day
  - Vitamin D: 2,000 IU/day
  - Vitamin E: 400 IU/day
  - Manganese: 1.8 mg/day
  - St. John's wort: 900 mg/day
  - Soy: 68 mg/day isoflavones
  - Ginkgo: 160 to 320 mg/day
  - Saffron: 30 mg/day
- Evidence supporting efficacy and/or safety of herbal products is lacking; the following products/interventions have *not* been found useful for PMS/PMDD, although not all studies are of high quality and able to eliminate possibility of benefit completely (8)[A]:
  - Evening primrose oil
  - Black currant oil
  - Black cohosh
  - Wild yam root
  - Dong quai
  - Kava kava
  - Light-based therapy

 ## ONGOING CARE

FOLLOW-UP RECOMMENDATIONS
Patient Monitoring
Increased risk of suicidal thinking and behavior in children and adolescents with depressive disorders on initiation of SSRIs; uncertain if this risk applies to those taking SSRIs for PMDD

DIET
- Reduce consumption of salt, sugar, caffeine, dairy products, and alcohol (anecdotal reports).
- Eat small, frequent portions of food high in complex carbohydrates (limited data).

PATIENT EDUCATION
- Counsel patients to eat a balanced diet rich in calcium, vitamin D, and omega-3 fatty acids and low in saturated fat and caffeine.
- Counsel women that they are not "crazy." PMDD is a real disorder with a physiologic basis.
- Although incompletely understood, successful treatment is often possible.

PROGNOSIS
- Many patients can have their symptoms adequately controlled. PMS disappears at menopause.
- PMS can continue after hysterectomy, if ovaries are left in place.

REFERENCES
1. American Psychiatric Association. *Diagnostic and Statistical Manual of Mental Disorders.* 5th ed. Washington, DC: American Psychiatric Association; 2013.
2. Borenstein JE, Dean BB, Yonkers KA, et al. Using the daily record of severity of problems as a screening instrument for premenstrual syndrome. *Obstet Gynecol.* 2007;109(5):1068–1075.
3. Marjoribanks J, Brown J, O'Brien PM, et al. Selective serotonin reuptake inhibitors for premenstrual syndrome. *Cochrane Database Syst Rev.* 2013;(6):CD001396.
4. Freeman EW, Halbreich U, Grubb GS, et al. An overview of four studies of a continuous oral contraceptive (levonorgestrel 90 mcg/ethinyl estradiol 20 mcg) on premenstrual dysphoric disorder and premenstrual syndrome. *Contraception.* 2012; 85(5):437–445.
5. Lopez LM, Kaptein AA, Helmerhorst FM. Oral contraceptives containing drospirenone for premenstrual syndrome. *Cochrane Database Syst Rev.* 2012;(2):CD006586.
6. Ford O, Lethaby A, Roberts H, et al. Progesterone for premenstrual syndrome. *Cochrane Database Syst Rev.* 2012;(3):CD003415.
7. Kim SY, Park HJ, Lee H, et al. Acupuncture for premenstrual syndrome: a systematic review and meta-analysis of randomised controlled trials. *BJOG.* 2011;118(8):899–915.
8. Whelan AM, Jurgens TM, Naylor H. Herbs, vitamins and minerals in the treatment of premenstrual syndrome: a systematic review. *Can J Clin Pharmacol.* 2009;16(3):e407–e429.

ADDITIONAL READING
- Biggs WS, Demuth RH. Premenstrual syndrome and premenstrual dysphoric disorder. *Am Fam Physician.* 2011;84(8):918–924.
- Nevatte T, O'Brien PM, Bäckström T, et al. ISPMD consensus on the management of premenstrual disorders. *Arch Womens Ment Health.* 2013;16(4): 279–291.
- Rapkin AJ, Akopians AL. Pathophysiology of premenstrual syndrome and premenstrual dysphoric disorder. *Menopause Int.* 2012;18(2):52–59.

 ## CODES

ICD10
N94.3 Premenstrual tension syndrome

CLINICAL PEARLS
- Have the patient keep a daily log of her symptoms and menses. Symptoms beginning in the week before menses and abating before the end of menses, occurring over at least 2 months, and sufficiently severe to interfere with daily functioning are diagnostic of PMS.
- The difference between PMS and PMDD is that PMDD is a severe form of PMS characterized by recurrent depressive and anxiety symptoms with luteal phase onset, sufficiently severe to disrupt social and occupational functioning. These symptoms remit a few days after the onset of menses.
- PMDD is not the same as more generalized depressive/anxiety disorders. PMDD-associated symptoms of depression and anxiety begin to resolve within the first few days of menses.
- Treatment only during the luteal phase is likely as effective as continuous-cycle treatment with SSRIs but has fewer adverse effects.

PRENATAL CARE AND TESTING
Fozia Akhtar Ali, MD • Teny Anna Philip, MD

BASICS

- The goal of prenatal care is to ensure the birth of a healthy baby with minimal risk for the mother by the following:
  - Identifying the patient who is at risk for complications
  - Estimating the gestational age (GA) as accurately as possible
  - Evaluating the health status of mother and fetus
  - Encouraging and empowering the patient to do her part to care for herself and her baby-to-be
  - Intervening when fetal abnormalities are present to prevent morbidity

GENERAL PREVENTION
- A recommended prenatal care schedule consists of the following:
  - Monthly visits to a health care professional for weeks 4 to 28 of pregnancy
  - Visits twice monthly from 28 to 36 weeks
  - Weekly after week 36 (delivery at week 38 to 40)
- Recommendations for use of dietary supplements in pregnancy
  - Folic acid supplementation (0.4 to 0.8 mg) prior to conception; 4 mg for secondary prevention
  - Calcium: 1,000 to 1,300 mg/day; supplement may be beneficial for women with high risk for gestational hypertension or communities with low dietary calcium intake.
  - Iron: Screen for anemia (Hgb/Hct) and treat if necessary. Recommend 30 mg/day of iron in pregnant women.
  - Vitamin A: Pregnant women in industrialized countries should limit to <5,000 IU/day.
  - Vitamin D: Consider supplementation in women with limited exposure to sunlight.
- Routine thyroid screening and vitamin D deficiency during pregnancy is not recommended.

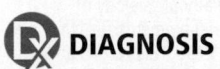

DIAGNOSIS

HISTORY
At the initial visit, a complete medical, obstetrical, family, and psychosocial history should be obtained and updated throughout the pregnancy.

- Assess and counsel as appropriate regarding the following:
  - Lifestyle, nutrition, safety of medications (teratogenicity, category); tobacco, alcohol, and drug use; toxins; relationship issues/domestic violence; stressors/supports; work environment; risk factors
- Domestic violence
  - ACOG guidelines recommend that physicians screen *all* pregnant patients for intimate partner domestic violence.
    - At the first prenatal visit
    - At least once per trimester
    - At the postpartum checkup

PHYSICAL EXAM
- A full physical exam should be performed at the first prenatal appointment.
- At each subsequent prenatal visit, the following should be recorded:
  - Weight: Total weight gain range (lb) should be 25 to 35 lb, except in obese women, for whom weight gain should be <15 lb.

- BP
  - ACOG defines hypertension as BP >140 mm Hg systolic or >90 mm Hg diastolic (1,2).
  - Monitor BP especially closely in patients with chronic hypertension (predating pregnancy), pre-eclampsia/eclampsia, or gestational hypertension.
- UA for glucose and protein; 24-hour protein excretion is the gold standard but not practical.
- Fundal height
- Fetal heart rate: usually audible by 12 weeks' GA with a Doppler instrument
- Routine fetal movement counts *not* recommended
- Fetal position by abdominal palpation at 36 weeks
- Pelvic/cervical exam if indicated

DIAGNOSTIC TESTS & INTERPRETATION
Cervical cancer screening

- A Pap smear should be obtained when indicated by standard Pap screening guidelines, regardless of gestation (ACOG, USPSTF, ASCCP, ACS, and ASCP guidelines state that women <21 years should not be screened regardless of age of sexual initiation or other risk factors).
- Squamous intraepithelial lesions can progress during pregnancy but often regress postpartum.
- LSIL in pregnancy: colposcopy preferred, but it is acceptable to defer colposcopy to postpartum (3).
- Colposcopy only to exclude the presence of invasive cancer in high-risk women
- Cervical biopsy should be avoided unless a malignancy is suspected. Endocervical sampling is contraindicated.
- First prenatal visit
  - Lab tests
    - Hematocrit or hemoglobin
    - Blood type: A, B, AB, or O
    - Rhesus type and antibody screen: Rh(+) or Rh(−)
    - Hemoglobin electrophoresis for patients at risk for sickle cell disease or thalassemia
    - Urine testing for glucose and protein
    - Urine culture
    - Rubella titer
    - Syphilis test
    - Gonorrhea/chlamydia screening
    - Hepatitis B surface antigen
    - HIV testing (patient may "opt out" if chooses to decline)
    - Routine screening for bacterial vaginosis, toxoplasmosis, CMV, and parvovirus not recommended
    - Cystic fibrosis screening (information should be made available to all couples)
      - Cystic fibrosis carrier screening should be offered before conception or early in pregnancy when one partner is of Caucasian, European, or Ashkenazi Jewish descent (4).
      - It is reasonable to offer cystic fibrosis carrier screening to all couples regardless of race or ethnicity as an alternative to selective testing.
- Screening tests (for birth defects), noninvasive
  - US nuchal translucency (NT): measures thickness at the back of the neck of the fetus
  - Blood screens: human chorionic gonadotropin (hCG), pregnancy-associated plasma protein A (PAPP-A), quad screen: α-fetoprotein (AFP), unconjugated estriol (UE3), hCG, inhibin-A (INH-A)
  - Cell-free DNA testing should be offered as an alternative noninvasive method of screening for fetal aneuploidies to high-risk pregnant women between 10 and 22 weeks' gestation. Women

---

who elect cell-free DNA testing will also need an AFP test for neural tube defects. The assay also allows screening for aneuploidy, rhesus typing in Rh(D) -negative women, and single-gene disorders (limited to detection of paternally inherited mutation). Because of a small but real risk for false-positive results, most experts advise using these assays as screening tests and confirming positive result with invasive prenatal diagnostics.
  - 1st-trimester screening between 11 and 14 weeks' GA using both NT and hCG/PAPP-A blood testing is an effective protocol in the general population and is more effective than NT alone, with an 83% detection rate for Down syndrome, with false-positive rate of 5%. Detects trisomy 21 (Down syndrome) and trisomy 18 (Edward syndrome). May be performed either as a single combined stand-alone test (US NT 1 blood [HCG and PAPP-A]) or as part of a sequential "step-by-step" 1st- and 2nd-trimester screening process (see the following discussion)
  - 2nd-trimester screening protocols
    - Obtain "multiple marker"/quad screen between 15 and 21 weeks' GA, optimally between 16 and 18 weeks; ~84% detection rate for trisomy 21, trisomy 18, and neural tube defects (NTDs), with false-positive rate of 5%, *or*
    - 2-step integrated screening protocol: combines information collected during the 1st and 2nd trimesters of the pregnancy to determine the risk of Down syndrome, trisomy 18, or open NTD:
      - Two options: stepwise sequential integrated screen (~91% detection rate with false-positive rate 3.3%):
        - 1st trimester: NT measurement, plus blood (hCG, PAPP-A):
          - If calculated risk for Down syndrome is ≥1:30, then additional steps are recommended (genetic counseling, US, and chorionic villi sampling [CVS]).
          - If calculated risk for Down syndrome is <1:30 *then*
        - 2nd-trimester quad screen (AFP, UE3, hCG, INH-A) is required, *or*
      - Serum integrated screen: 88% detection rate with false-positive rate of 4.5%; requires a 1st-trimester PAPP-A blood test without NT measurement, and a 2nd-trimester (16- to 18-week quad screen)
- Diagnostic tests (for birth defects), invasive
  - ACOG guidelines: All pregnant women, not just women ≥35 years, should be offered invasive prenatal diagnostic testing, such as CVS and amniocentesis to detect possible genetic abnormalities in their fetuses (5)[C].
  - Women found to be at increased risk of having a baby with Down syndrome with 1st-trimester screening should be offered genetic counseling and the option of CVS or midtrimester amniocentesis. If screening tests show increased risk of birth defect, there are two possible diagnostic tests:
    - CVS: 1st trimester: usually done after 10 weeks (10 to 12 weeks). Small sample of the placenta; chorionic tissue sample obtained either transcervical (TC) or transabdominal (TA). Complication: pregnancy loss rate of 1.0–1.5%
    - Amniocentesis
      - 1st trimester: usually at 11 to 13 weeks but higher rate of pregnancy loss and complication than either CVS or early 2nd-trimester procedures; therefore, not recommended

- 2nd trimester: usually done after 15 weeks (15 to 18 weeks). The prenatal diagnostic technique associated with the lowest risk of pregnancy loss. Small sample of amniotic fluid from the amniotic sac surrounding the developing fetus is obtained by an US-guided TA approach. Complication: pregnancy loss rate of ≤0.5%
- 24 to 28 weeks
  - Obtain diabetes screen (see the following discussion), repeat hematocrit or hemoglobin, and repeat antibody screen in Rh-negative mother prior to receiving prophylactic Rh immunoglobulin.
    - Gestational diabetes mellitus (GDM) screening: universal recommendation for ideal approach for screening and diagnosis of GDM remains elusive. In 2010, the International Association of Diabetes and Pregnancy Study Group proposed a new system in which diabetes in pregnancy is classified as overt versus gestational diabetes. The American Diabetes Association reaffirmed this in 2010 and 2013. Presently, this system is not endorsed by ACOG because there is no evidence that one-step screening using this criteria leads to clinically significant improvements in maternal and fetal outcomes but would lead to significant increase in health care costs.
    - Overt diabetes (test when women first present for prenatal care): fasting blood sugar ≥126 mg/dL or HbA1c ≥6.5%, or random ≥200 mg/dL that is confirmed with subsequent fasting blood sugar or HbA1c. (These thresholds were chosen due to correlation with adverse vascular events, e.g., retinopathy and CAD.)
    - Gestational diabetes: fasting plasma glucose >92 mg/dL but is <126 mg/dL at any GA. At 24 to 28 weeks of gestation, a 75 g 2-hour oral glucose tolerance test with at least 1 abnormal result: FBG ≥92 mg/dL, but <126 mg/dL or 1-hour >180 mg/dL, or 2-hour >153 mg/dL
    - The prevalence of gestational diabetes in the United States can be 2–25%, greater in African Americans, Hispanics, Native Americans, and Asians than in Caucasians. Using the IADPSG criteria for overt versus gestational diabetes, ~18% of women would be diagnosed with diabetes during pregnancy.
    - The following guidelines for GDM are established by ACOG:
      - Specified cutoffs define GDM
        - A value of >130 mg/dL will identify 90% of women with GDM, but 20–25% of all women screened will need to continue to the 3-hour oral glucose tolerance test (OGTT) (1,2).
        - Raising the value to >140 mg/dL will identify only 80% of women with GDM but decrease to 14–18% the number of women who will need to continue to the 3-hour OGTT (6).
      - Screening test: 1-hour OGTT (nonfasting)
        - 50 g PO glucose load with blood glucose testing 1 hour later
        - Carpenter and Coustan positive screen: >130 mg/dL
        - National Diabetes Data Group (NDDG) positive screen: >140 mg/dL

- Diagnostic test: 3-hour OGTT (fasting)
  - If abnormal 1-hour OGTT screening test, may be followed by a 3-hour OGTT
  - 100 g PO glucose load with blood drawn: fasting, 1, 2, and 3 hours after ingestion of glucose
  - Either the plasma or serum glucose level designated by Carpenter and Coustan or by the NDDG are appropriate to use:
    - *A positive diagnosis of GDM requires that ≥2 thresholds be exceeded.
      - Carpenter and Coustan standard
        - *>95 (fasting), >180 (1-hour), >155 (2-hour), >140 (3-hour)
      - National Diabetes Data Group standard:
        - *105 (fasting), >190 (1-hour), >165 (2-hour), >145 (3-hour)
- 35 to 37 weeks
  - Group B Streptococcus (GBS) culture: Universal screening for GBS colonization at 35 to 37 weeks of gestation remains the sole strategy for intrapartum antibiotic prophylaxis.
  - High-risk patients: High-risk patients should be screened again for gonorrhea, chlamydia, HIV, and syphilis.
- Postterm pregnancy
  - Rate of stillbirth increases with GA by 1/3,000 per week at 37 weeks; 3/3,000 per week at 42 weeks; and 6/3,000 at 43 weeks. In one meta-analysis, routine induction of labor at 41 weeks' gestation reduced rates of perinatal death without increased rates of cesarean delivery.
  - For gestational periods beyond 42 weeks, fetal well-being should be assessed with nonstress testing and US assessment of amniotic fluid volume.

 TREATMENT

ISSUES FOR REFERRAL
Abnormal screening labs or imaging may prompt referral to maternal–fetal medicine specialist or other medical specialist, as indicated.

 ONGOING CARE

PATIENT EDUCATION
- Immunizations during pregnancy. The following vaccines are considered safe per CDC (7):
  - Women should get (Tdap) during each pregnancy. Ideally, the vaccine should be given between 27 and 36 weeks of pregnancy—Hep B, and influenza; possibly include meningococcal, rabies. Contraindicated during pregnancy or safety not established:live vaccines including BCG, MMR, and varicella.
  - Patients should be made aware of the tests that are performed routinely, as well as other tests that might be elected (e.g., CVS or amniocentesis), as well as the choices that would be available if testing were abnormal (pregnancy termination, preparation for the birth of an infant with congenital anomalies, further testing).
- Prevention
  - Preconception counseling offers the opportunity to discuss individualized risks.

- To decrease the risks of NTDs, preconception folate supplementation is indicated.
- Recommendations
  - Airline travel: generally safe until up to 4 weeks from EDD. Lengthy trips associated with increased risk of thrombosis
  - Caffeine: Limit to <200 mg/day. Correlation between IUGR and miscarriage with caffeine is undetermined at this time.
  - Exercise: Healthy women with uncomplicated pregnancies should continue to exercise.
  - Seat belts/air bags: ACOG recommends that pregnant women wear lap and shoulder seatbelts and should not turn off air bags.
  - Sexual activity: Intercourse is not associated with adverse outcomes.
- Alcohol, cigarettes, and illicit drugs are injurious to fetal and maternal health.
  - Pregnancy-safe medications (teratogenicity)

REFERENCES

1. American College of Obstetricians and Gynecologists. Screening tools—domestic violence. http://www.acog.org/ACOG_Departments/Violence_Against_Women/Screening_Tools-Domestic-Violence. Accessed August 7, 2012.
2. Committee on Obstetric Practice. Committee Opinion no. 514: emergent therapy for acute-onset, severe hypertension with preeclampsia or eclampsia. *Obstet Gynecol.* 2011;118(6):1465–1468.
3. Massad LS, Einstein MH, Huh WK, et al. 2012 updated consensus guidelines for the management of abnormal cervical cancer screening tests and cancer precursors. *J Low Genit Tract Dis.* 2013;17(5)(Suppl 1):S1–S27.
4. American College of Obstetricians and Gynecologists Committee on Genetics. ACOG Committee Opinion no. 486: update on carrier screening for cystic fibrosis. *Obstet Gynecol.* 2011;117(4):1028–1031.
5. American College of Obstetricians and Gynecologists. ACOG Practice Bulletin no. 88, December 2007. Invasive prenatal testing for aneuploidy. *Obstet Gynecol.* 2007;110(6):1459–1467.
6. Berger H, Crane J, Farine D, et al. Screening for gestational diabetes mellitus [in English, French]. *J Obstet Gynaecol Can.* 2002;24(11):894–912.
7. Centers for Disease Control and Prevention. GBS prevention guidelines. http://www.cdc.gov/groupbstrep/guidelines/newdifferences.html.2010guidelines

 CODES

ICD10
- Z34.90 Encntr for suprvsn of normal pregnancy, unsp, unsp trimester
- Z36 Encounter for antenatal screening of mother
- Z34.00 Encntr for suprvsn of normal first pregnancy, unsp trimester

CLINICAL PEARLS

Prenatal care and screening are best accomplished using standardized flow sheets and checklists to ensure that the complex sequence of evaluations and education is performed consistently and properly.

PREOPERATIVE EVALUATION OF THE NONCARDIAC SURGICAL PATIENT

Andrew Grimes, MD • Stacy Jones, MD

 BASICS

DESCRIPTION
- Preoperative medical evaluation should determine the presence of established or unrecognized disease or other factors that may increase the risk of perioperative morbidity and mortality in patients undergoing surgery.
- Specific assessment goals include the following:
  - Conducting a thorough medical history and physical exam to assess the need for further testing and/or consultation
  - Recommending strategies to reduce risk and optimize patient condition prior to surgery
  - Encouraging patients to optimize their health for possible improvement of both perioperative and long-term outcomes
- Synonym(s): preoperative diagnostic workup; preoperative preparation; preoperative general health assessment

EPIDEMIOLOGY
Overall patient morbidity and mortality related to surgery is low. One large study of inpatients looking at 30-day mortality in the United States showed a rate of 1.32%. This rate varies by type of procedure and varies by country. Preoperative patient evaluation and subsequent optimization of perioperative care can reduce both postoperative morbidity and mortality.

RISK FACTORS
- Functional capacity (1): Exercise tolerance is one of the most important determinants of cardiac risk:
  - Self-reported exercise tolerance may be an extremely useful predictive tool when assessing risk. Patients unable to meet a 4 metabolic equivalent (MET) demand (defined in the "Diagnosis" section) during daily activities have increased perioperative cardiac and long-term risks.
  - Patients who report good exercise tolerance require minimal, if any, additional testing.
- Levels of surgical risk
  - An increased risk for major adverse cardiac events (MACE) is associated with procedures that are intrathoracic, intra-abdominal, or vascular procedures that are suprainguinal in nature (1).
- Clinical risk factors (1): history of ischemic heart disease, the presence of compensated heart failure or a history of prior congestive heart failure (CHF), cerebrovascular disease, diabetes mellitus (DM), and renal insufficiency; these risk factors plus surgical risk can dictate the need for further cardiac testing.
- Age: Patients >70 years of age are at higher risk for perioperative complications and mortality and have a longer length of stay in the hospital postoperatively. (likely attributed to increasing medical comorbidities with increasing age) Age alone should not be a deciding factor in the decision to proceed or not proceed with surgery.

 DIAGNOSIS

HISTORY
- Evaluate pertinent medical records and interview the patient. Many institutions provide standard patient questionnaires that screen for preoperative risk factors:
  - History of present illness and treatments
  - Past medical and surgical history
  - Patient and family anesthetic history and associated complications

- Current medications (including over-the-counter [OTC] medications, vitamins, supplements, and herbals) as well as reasons for use
- Allergies (including specific reactions)
- Social history: tobacco, alcohol, drug use, and cessation
- Family history: prior illnesses and surgeries
- Systems (both history and current status)
  - Cardiovascular: Inquire about exercise capacity.
    - 1 MET: can take care of self, eat, dress, and use toilet; walk around house indoors; walk a block or 2 on level ground at 2 to 3 mph
    - 4 METs: can climb flight of stairs or walk uphill, walk on level ground at 4 mph, run a short distance, do heavy work around house, participate in moderate recreational activities
    - 10 METs: can participate in strenuous sports such as swimming, singles tennis, football, basketball, or skiing
  - Note presence of CHF, cardiomyopathy, ischemic heart disease (stable vs. unstable), valvular disease, hypertension (HTN), arrhythmias, murmurs, pericarditis, history of pacemaker or implantable cardioverter defibrillator (ICD):
    - Rhythm management devices (pacemakers and automatic ICDs [AICD]) affect the perioperative course. Most importantly, the following information need to be available for proper management: name of cardiologist who manages the device, type of device, manufacturer, last interrogation, and any problems that have occurred recently. Based on this information and the location and type of surgery, a perioperative plan of management will be made (2).
    - Stents: Patients with coronary stents are maintained on antiplatelet therapy with a thienopyridine, such as clopidogrel, frequently in combination with aspirin. Premature discontinuation of antiplatelet therapy markedly increases the risk of acute stent thrombosis, the results of which can be catastrophic. Elective surgery should be delayed and antiplatelet therapy continued for 4 to 6 weeks after bare-metal stent placement and for at least 12 months after placement of drug-eluting stents. Even after this time period, any perioperative disruption in the patient's antiplatelet regimen should be discussed with the patient's cardiologist and surgeon. The risk of perioperative bleeding must be weighed against the risks associated with discontinuation of antiplatelet drugs prior to surgery.
  - Pulmonary: Chronic and active disease processes should be addressed: chronic infections, bronchitis, emphysema, asthma, wheezing, shortness of breath, cough (productive or otherwise):
    - Sleep apnea: Patients with obstructive sleep apnea (OSA) are at increased risk for perioperative adverse events. Because of the high incidence of undiagnosed sleep apnea in perioperative patients, many authors are recommending screening questionnaires such as the Berlin or STOP-BANG (3,4). The American Society of Anesthesiologists (ASA) has practice guidelines based on expert review that take into account the severity of sleep apnea, the invasiveness of surgery, and the projected need for postoperative opioids (5).
    - Patients with OSA frequently are at increased risk for obesity, coronary disease, HTN, atrial fibrillation, CHF, and pulmonary HTN.

Optimizing the management of these comorbidities may be the first important step in the preoperative management of patients with OSA. Often, patients with an existing diagnosis of OSA who use continuous positive airway pressure (CPAP) at night are asked to bring their CPAP machine to the hospital or surgery center when they are admitted for surgery.
- Some studies suggest that even short periods (3 weeks) of treatment with CPAP can improve some indices of ventilation and therefore may reduce postoperative morbidity.
- GI: hepatic disease, gastric ulcer, inflammatory bowel disease, hernias (especially hiatal), significant weight loss, nausea, vomiting, history of postoperative nausea and vomiting: Any symptoms consistent with gastroesophageal reflux disease (GERD) should be optimally treated.
- Hematologic: anemia, serious bleeding, clotting problems, blood transfusions, hereditary disorders
- Renal: kidney failure, dialysis, infections, stones, changes in bladder function
- Endocrine: nocturia, parathyroid, pituitary, adrenal disease, thyroid disease
  - Diabetes: Evidence that hyperglycemia in the perioperative period is associated with increased perioperative complications. Although recommendations vary, most experts recommend keeping perioperative blood glucose levels <180.
- Neurologic/psychiatric: seizures, stroke, paralysis, tremor, migraine headaches, nerve injury, multiple sclerosis, extremity numbness, psychiatric disorders (e.g., anxiety, depression)
- Musculoskeletal: arthritis, lower back pain
- Reproductive: possibility of pregnancy in women of childbearing potential
- Mouth/upper airway: dentures, crowns, partials, bridges, teeth (loose, chipped, cracked, capped)

PHYSICAL EXAM
- Assess vital signs, including arterial BP bilaterally.
- Check carotid pulses; auscultate for bruits.
- Examine lungs by auscultating all lung fields and listening for rales, rhonchi, wheezes, or other sounds indicating disease.
- Examine cardiovascular system by auscultating heart and noting any irregular rhythms or murmurs; precordial palpation.
- Palpate abdomen.
- Examine airway and mouth for ease of intubation, neck mobility, and size of tongue; note any lesions or dental deformities.
- If a regional anesthesia technique is being contemplated, perform a relevant, focused neurologic exam.

DIAGNOSTIC TESTS & INTERPRETATION
Initial Tests (lab, imaging)
- Laboratory testing should not be obtained routinely prior to surgery unless indicated (6)[C]. Specific tests should be requested if the evaluator suspects findings from the clinical evaluation that may influence perioperative patient management.
- Labs performed within the past 4 months prior to evaluation are reliable unless the patient has had an interim change in clinical presentation or is taking medications that require monitoring of plasma level or effect.

- CBC (6)[C]
  - Hemoglobin: if a patient has symptoms of anemia or is undergoing a procedure with major blood loss; extremes of age; liver or kidney disease
  - WBC count: if symptoms suggest infection or myeloproliferative disorder or the patient is at risk for chemotherapy-induced leukopenia
  - Platelet count: if history of bleeding, myelo-proliferative disorder, liver or renal disease, or the patient is at risk for chemotherapy-induced thrombocytopenia
- Serum chemistries (electrolytes, glucose, renal and liver function tests): should be obtained for extremes of age; in known renal insufficiency, CHF, liver dysfunction, or endocrine abnormalities; or the patient is on medications that alter electrolyte levels, such as diuretics
- PT/PTT: if history of a bleeding disorder, chronic liver disease, or malnutrition, or those with recent or chronic antibiotic or anticoagulant use
- Urinalysis: Routine urinalysis is not recommended preoperatively.
- Pregnancy test: controversial; should be *considered* for all female patients of childbearing age
- CXR is not generally indicated. It can be considered in patients with recent upper respiratory tract infection and in those with suspected cardiac or pulmonary disease (because there is a likelihood for unanticipated findings), but these indications are not considered unequivocal.

Diagnostic Procedures/Other

- ECG (1)[C]
  - Preoperative resting 12 lead ECG is reasonable for patients with known coronary disease, known peripheral vascular disease, significant arrhythmia, or known significant structural heart disease.
  - ECGs are not indicated for asymptomatic patients undergoing low-risk procedures.
- The AHA guidelines recommend using the Revised Cardiac Risk Index or the ACS NSQUIP online risk calculator to make an estimate of risk of MACE in the perioperative period. If the risk of MACE is low (<1%), then proceed with surgery. If the risk is >1%, the functional capacity needs to be considered. For patients with a functional capacity of >4 METS, then proceed with surgery. If the functional capacity is <4 METs or unknown, consider pharmacologic stress testing if it will change management (1).
- PFTs: Definitive data regarding the efficacy of preoperative testing are lacking. The most important factor is preoperative optimization of patients with chronic obstructive pulmonary disease (COPD) or reactive airways disease with indicated use of antibiotics, bronchodilators, and inhaled corticosteroids. Spirometry can help guide therapy. Upper abdominal and thoracic surgery have a higher risk of postoperative pulmonary complications.

TREATMENT

MEDICATION

- Reducing cardiac risk
  - Elective surgery should be delayed or canceled if the patient has any of the following: unstable coronary syndromes (unstable or severe angina), recent myocardial infarction (MI) (<30 days), decompensated heart failure, significant arrhythmias, or severe valvular disease.
  - Active HF should be treated with diuretics, afterload reduction, and β-adrenergic blockers.

- Perioperative β-blockade has been shown to reduce mortality and the incidence of perioperative MIs in high-risk patients. Studies conflict, however, in which patients need to be treated, the dosage and timing of treatment, and for what surgeries. *Patients chronically on β-blockers should have the medication continued in the perioperative period.* When β-blockers are discontinued in the perioperative period, 30-day mortality increases. β-Blockers are reasonable for vascular surgery patients with at least one clinical risk factor. It is not recommended to start β-blockers on the day of surgery in β-blocker naïve patients (1).
  - Perioperative statin use may have a protective effect on reducing cardiac complications. Currently, the American Heart Association (AHA) has a class I indication for perioperative statin therapy for patients already on statins prior to their surgery. There is also evidence that vascular surgery patients benefit from perioperative statins.
  - A recent review looked at prophylactic use of aspirin in the perioperative period and did not find a significant effect on perioperative mortality or risk for MI in patients undergoing noncardiac surgery and may be associated with an increased risk of perioperative bleeding. There were important exclusion criteria including patients with recent stent placement (7).
- Reducing pulmonary risk
  - Recommend cigarette cessation for at least 8 weeks prior to elective surgery.
  - Patients with asthma should not be wheezing and should have a peak flow of at least 80% of their predicted or personal-best value.
  - Treatment of COPD and asthma should focus on maximally reducing airflow obstruction and is identical to treatment of nonsurgical patients.
  - Lower respiratory tract infections (bacterial) should be treated with appropriate antibiotic therapy.

REFERENCES

1. Fleisher LA, Fleischmann KE, Auerbach AD, et al. 2014 ACC/AHA guideline on perioperative cardiovascular evaluation and management of patients undergoing non cardiac surgery: a report of the American College of Cardiology/American Heart Association Task Force on Practice Guidelines. Developed in collaboration with the American College of Surgeons, American Society of Anesthesiologists, American Society of Echocardiography, American Society of Nuclear Cardiology, Heart Rhythm Society, Society for Cardiovascular Angiography and Interventions, Society of Cardiovascular Anesthesiologists, and Society of Vascular Medicine Endorsed by the Society of Hospital Medicine. *J Nucl Cardiol.* 2015;22(1):162–215.
2. Crossley GH, Poole JE, Rozner MA, et al. The Heart Rhythm Society (HRS)/American Society of Anesthesiologists (ASA) Expert Consensus Statement on the perioperative management of patients with implantable defibrillators, pacemakers and arrhythmia monitors: facilities and patient management this document was developed as a joint project with the American Society of Anesthesiologists (ASA), and in collaboration with the American Heart Association (AHA), and the Society of Thoracic Surgeons (STS). *Heart Rhythm.* 2011;8(7):1114–1154.
3. Adesanya AO, Lee W, Greilich NB, et al. Perioperative management of obstructive sleep apnea. *Chest.* 2010;138(6):1489–1498.
4. Chung SA, Yuan H, Chung F. A systematic review of obstructive sleep apnea and its implications for anesthesiologists. *Anesth Analg.* 2008;107(5):1543–1563.
5. American Society of Anesthesiologists Task Force on Perioperative Management of Patients with Obstructive Sleep Apnea. Practice guidelines for the perioperative management of patients with obstructive sleep apnea: an updated report by the American Society of Anesthesiologists Task Force on Perioperative Management of patients with obstructive sleep apnea. *Anesthesiology.* 2014;120(2):268–286.
6. Apfelbaum JL, Connis RT, Nickinovich DG, et al. Practice advisory for preanesthesia evaluation: an updated report by the American Society of Anesthesiologists Task Force on Preanesthesia Evaluation. *Anesthesiology.* 2012;116(3):522–538.
7. Devereaux PJ, Mrkobrada M, Sessler DI, et al. Aspirin in patients undergoing noncardiac surgery. *N Engl J Med.* 2014;370(16):1494–1503.

ADDITIONAL READING

- Akhtar S, Barash PG, Inzucchi SE Scientific principles and clinical implications of perioperative glucose regulation and control. *Anesth Analg.* 2010;110(2):478–497.
- Chung F, Subramanyam R, Liao P, et al. High STOP-Bang score indicates a high probability of obstructive sleep apnoea. *Br J Anaesth.* 2012;108(5):768–775.
- Lander JS, Coplan NL. Statin therapy in the perioperative period. *Rev Cardiovasc Med.* 2011;12(1):30–37.
- Pearse RM, Moreno RP, Bauer P, et al. Mortality after surgery in Europe: a 7 day cohort study. *Lancet.* 2012;380 (9847):1059–1065.
- Semel ME, Lipsitz SR, Funk LM, et al. Rates and patterns of death after surgery in the United States, 1996 and 2006. *Surgery.* 2012;151(2):171–182.

 SEE ALSO

Algorithm: Preoperative Evaluation of the Noncardiac Surgical Patient

 CODES

ICD10

- Z01.818 Encounter for other preprocedural examination
- Z01.811 Encounter for preprocedural respiratory examination
- Z01.812 Encounter for preprocedural laboratory examination

CLINICAL PEARLS

- The preoperative evaluation should include medical record evaluation, patient interview, and physical exam.
- The minimum for the physical exam includes airway, pulmonary, and cardiovascular exams.
- Functional capacity, the level of surgical risk, and clinical risk factors determine if further cardiac testing is needed.
- No preoperative tests are routine.
- Active cardiac conditions should lead to delay or cancellation of nonemergent surgery.

PRESBYCUSIS

Matthew J. Richter, DO • John T. Ewing, DO

 BASICS

DESCRIPTION

- Age-related, bilateral sensorineural hearing loss (SNHL) typically symmetric
- Represents a lifetime of insults to the auditory system from toxic noise exposure and natural decline
- Initially presents as high-frequency SNHL with tinnitus (ringing)
- Impacts the "clarity" of sounds (i.e., ability to detect, identify, and localize sounds)
- Due to mild and progressive nature, presbycusis is often treated with amplification alone.
- Can lead to adverse effects on physical, cognitive, emotional, behavioral, and social function in the elderly (e.g., depression, social isolation)

EPIDEMIOLOGY

Incidence

According to an ongoing community-based epidemiologic study, the 10-year cumulative incidence rates of hearing loss (HL) are as follows (1):

- Age 48 to 59 years: M (31.7%), F (15.6%); all (21.8%)
- Age 60 to 69 years: M (56.8%), F (40.7%); all (45.5%)
- Age 70 to 79 years: M (87.1%), F (70.6%); all (73.7%)
- Age 80 to 92 years: M (100%), F (100%); all (100%)

Prevalence

- 10% of the population develops SNHL severe enough to impair communication.
- Increases to 40% in the population >65 years of age
- 80% of HL cases occur in elderly patients.
- Only 10–20% of older adults with HL have ever used hearing aids.
- Predominant sex: male > female
- Hearing levels are poorer in industrialized societies than in isolated or agrarian societies.

ETIOLOGY AND PATHOPHYSIOLOGY

- The external ear transmits sound energy to the tympanic membrane. The middle ear ossicles amplify and conduct the sound waves into the inner ear (cochlea) via the oval window. The organ of Corti, located in the cochlea, contains hair cells that detect these vibrations and depolarize, producing electrical signals that travel through the auditory nerve to the brain. Toxic noise exposure traumatizes the hair cells and leads to cell death and hearing loss. New research also suggests that overexcitation of the neurosynapses causes increased glutamate, which is also neurotoxic (2).
  - Sensory presbycusis: primary loss of the hair cells in the basal end of the cochlea (high frequency HL)
  - Neural presbycusis: loss of spiral ganglion cells (nerve cells induced by hair cells to produce action potentials to travel to the brainstem)
  - Strial (metabolic) presbycusis: atrophy of the stria vascularis (the cochlear tissue that generates the endocochlear electrical potential)
  - Cochlear conductive (mechanical) presbycusis: no morphologic findings (presumed stiffening of the basilar membrane)
  - Mixed presbycusis: combinations of hair cell, ganglion cell, and stria vascularis loss
  - Indeterminate presbycusis: no morphologic findings (presumed impaired cellular function)
- Presbycusis is caused by the accumulated effects of noise exposure, systemic disease, oxidative damage, ototoxic drugs, and genetic susceptibility.

Genetics

Presbycusis has a clear familial aggregation (3)[B]:

- Heritability estimates show 35–55% of the variance of sensory presbycusis is from genetic factors; even greater percentage in strial presbycusis
- Heritability is stronger among women than men.

RISK FACTORS

- Noise exposure (military, industrial, etc.)
- Ototoxic substances
  - Organic solvents
  - Heavy metals
  - Carbon monoxide
- Drugs
  - Aminoglycosides
  - Cisplatin
  - Salicylates
  - Diuretics
- Tobacco smoking
- Alcohol
- Lower socioeconomic status
- Family history of presbycusis
- Head trauma (temporal bone fractures)
- Cardiovascular disease (hypertension, atherosclerosis, hyperlipidemia); labyrinthine artery is terminal artery to the cochlea.
- Diabetes mellitus
- Autoimmune disease (autocochleitis/labyrinthitis)
- Metabolic bone disease
- Endocrine medical conditions: levels of aldosterone
- Alzheimer disease
- Otologic conditions (e.g., Ménière disease or otosclerosis)

GENERAL PREVENTION

- Avoid hazardous noise exposure.
- Use hearing protection.
- Maintain healthy diet and exercise.
- Screening

  - In the only published RCT on screening for HL, hearing aid use was significantly higher in three screened groups (4.1% in those using a questionnaire, 6.3% using handheld audiometry, and 7.4% using both modalities) versus unscreened control participants (3.3%) at 1-year follow-up (4)[B].
  - Based on a 2011 review, according to the USPSTF, there is insufficient evidence to assess the relative benefits and harms of HL screening in adults ≥50 years (5)[A].

 DIAGNOSIS

HISTORY

- Reduced hearing sensitivity and speech understanding in noisy/public environments
- Impaired localization of sound sources
- Increased difficulty understanding conversations, especially with women, due to higher frequency of spoken voice
- Presents bilaterally and symmetrically
- If unilateral hearing loss, alternative diagnosis should be pursued.
- Additional history if HL is suspected or detected (6)[B]
  - Time course of HL
  - Symptoms of tinnitus, otalgia, otorrhea, or vertigo
  - History of noise exposure, ear trauma, or head trauma
  - Presence of any neurologic deficit
- Reports from patient/family/caregiver (6)[B]
  - Confusion in social situations
  - Excessive volume of television/radio/computer
  - Social withdrawal
  - Anxiety in group settings

PHYSICAL EXAM

- Rinne and Weber tests are helpful for determining conductive versus sensorineural hearing loss but not recommended for general screening (7)[B].
- Pneumatic otoscopy to evaluate for simple middle ear effusion as cause of conductive hearing loss

DIFFERENTIAL DIAGNOSIS

- Acute noise-induced traumatic loss (explosion)
- Autoimmune HL
- Perilymph fistula (trauma/iatrogenic)
- Ménière disease
- Acoustic neuroma
- Complete canal occlusion (cerumen)
- Otitis externa
- Chronic otitis media or effusion
- Otosclerosis/osteogenesis imperfecta
- Large middle ear tumors (e.g., facial nerve schwannomas, paragangliomas)
- Vascular anomaly
- Cholesteatoma

DIAGNOSTIC TESTS & INTERPRETATION

- Handheld audiometry; insert probe in ear (sealing canal) and have patient indicate if tones can be heard.
  - Positive likelihood ratio (LR) range, 3.1 to 5.8; negative LR range, 0.03 to 0.40 (7)[B]
- Screening audiometry
  - Symmetric high-frequency hearing loss in descending slope pattern
  - SNHL frequencies >2 KHz initially
  - Essential to determine global clinical hearing status and if etiology is conductive hearing loss versus SNHL or pseudohypacusis (conversion)

TREATMENT

- Hearing aids (HAs)
  - Types
    - Analog HA: picks up sound waves through a microphone; converts them into electrical signals; amplifies and sends them through the ear canal to the tympanic membrane
    - Digital HA: programmable; may reduce acoustic feedback, reduce background noise, detect and automatically accommodate different listening environments, control multiple microphones
  - HAs have an average decibel gain of 16.3 dB
  - Associated with hypersensitivity to loud sounds ("loudness recruitment")
- Hearing-assistive technologies (HATs) (8)[A]
  - Can be used alone or in combination with HAs (for difficult listening conditions)
  - Addresses face-to-face communication, broadcast or other electronic media (radio, TV), telephone conversation, sensitivity to alerting signals and environment stimuli (doorbell, baby's cry, alarm clock, etc.)
  - Includes personal FM systems, infrared systems, induction loop systems, hardwired systems, telephone amplifier, telecoil, TDD (telecommunication device for the deaf), situation-specific devices (e.g., television), alerting devices
- Aural rehabilitation (also known as audiologic orientation or auditory training) (6)[A]
  - Adjunct to HA or HATs
  - Involves education regarding proper use of amplification devices, coaching on how to manage the auditory environment, training in speech perception and communication, and counseling for coping strategies to deal with the difficulties of HAs or HATs

ISSUES FOR REFERRAL

Refer to audiologist for formal evaluation and optimal fitting of HAs and/or HATs.

- Individuals receiving postfitting orientation/education have significantly fewer HA returns.
- Individuals receiving >2 hours of education and counseling report higher levels of satisfaction.

SURGERY/OTHER PROCEDURES

- Cochlear implants (CIs) (9,10)[B]
  - Indications include hearing no better than identifying ≤50% of key words in test sentences in the best aided condition in the worst ear and 60% in the better ear.
  - Works by bypassing the ear canal, middle ear, and hair cells in the cochlea to provide electric stimulation directly to the auditory nerve
  - Incoming sounds are received through the microphone in the audio processor component (resembles a small HA), which converts them into electrical impulses and sends them to the magnetic coil (located on the skin). The impulses transmit these across intact skin via radio waves to the implanted component (directly subjacent to the coil). The pulses travel to the electrodes in the cochlea and stimulate the cochlea at high rates.

  - Receiving a unilateral CI is most common; some may receive bilateral CIs (either sequentially or in the same surgery). Others may wear a CI in 1 ear and an HA in the contralateral ear (bimodal fit).
  - Younger age at CI placement derives greatest benefit (10)[A].
- Active middle ear implants (AMEIs) (9)[B]
  - Suitable for elderly adults who cannot wear conventional HAs for medical or personal (cosmetic) reasons and whose HL is not severe enough for a CI
  - Comes in different models and may include components that are implantable under the skin
- Electric acoustic stimulation: use of CI and HA together in one ear
  - Addresses the specific needs of patients presenting with good low-frequency hearing (a mild to moderate sensorineural HL in frequencies up to 1,000 Hz but poorer hearing in the high frequencies (sloping to 60 dB or worse HL above 1,000 Hz) (9)[B]
    - Contraindications: progressive HL, autoimmune disease; HL related to meningitis, otosclerosis, or ossification; malformation of the cochlea; a gap in air conduction and bone conduction thresholds of >15 dB; external ear contraindications, active infection, or unwillingness to use amplification devices (9)[B]

ONGOING CARE

FOLLOW-UP RECOMMENDATIONS
Patient Monitoring
- During follow-up visits, check for compliance of HA use.
  - 25–40% of adults will either stop wearing them or use them only occasionally.
- Assess perceived benefit of HA and, if ineffective, for indications for possible surgical treatments.
- Annual audiograms
- Can follow up with audiologists for HA fittings if HA becomes uncomfortable
- Asymmetric hearing loss should have evaluation via MRI for acoustic neuroma.
- Sudden SNHL is atypical and warrants urgent otolaryngologic evaluation/audiometry. The most recent recommendations by the American Academy of Otolaryngology recommend steroids empirically.

PATIENT EDUCATION
- Should be face-to-face; spoken clearly and unhurriedly, without competing background noise (e.g., radio, TV); and include a confirmation that the message is received.
- Formal speech reading classes may be beneficial; however, availability may be limited.

REFERENCES

1. Cruickshanks KJ, Nondahl DM, Tweed TS, et al. Education, occupation, noise exposure history and the 10-yr cumulative incidence of hearing impairment in older adults. *Hear Res.* 2010;264(1–2):3–9.
2. Yamasoba T, Lin FR, Someya S, et al. Current concepts in age-related hearing loss: epidemiology and mechanistic pathways. *Hear Res.* 2013;303:30–38.
3. Huang Q, Tang J. Age-related hearing loss or presbycusis. *Eur Arch Otorhinolaryngol.* 2010;267(8):1179–1191.
4. Yueh B, Collins MP, Souza PE, et al. Long-term effectiveness of screening for hearing loss: the screening for auditory impairment—which hearing assessment test (SAI-WHAT) randomized trial. *J Am Geriatr Soc.* 2010;58(3):427–434.
5. Chou R, Dana T, Bougatsos C, et al. Screening adults aged 50 years or older for hearing loss: a review of the evidence for the U.S. Preventive Services Task Force. *Ann Intern Med.* 2011;154(5):347–355.
6. Pacala JT, Yueh B. Hearing deficits in the older patient: "I didn't notice anything." *JAMA.* 2012;307(11):1185–1194.
7. Bagai A, Thavendiranathan P, Detsky AS. Does this patient have hearing impairment? *JAMA.* 2006;295(4):416–428.
8. Valente M. Summary guidelines: audiological management of adult hearing impairment. *Audio Today.* 2006;18:32–37.
9. Sprinzl GM, Riechelmann H. Current trends in treating hearing loss in elderly people: a review of the technology and treatment options—a mini-review. *Gerontology.* 2010;56(3):351–358.
10. Lin FR, Chien WW, Li L, et al. Cochlear implantation in older adults. *Medicine (Baltimore).* 2012;91(5):229–241.

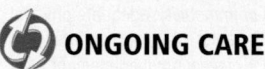 CODES

ICD10
- H91.10 Presbycusis, unspecified ear
- H91.13 Presbycusis, bilateral
- H91.11 Presbycusis, right ear

CLINICAL PEARLS

- Presbycusis is an age-related hearing loss (HL), showing increased incidence with age. It is often bilateral and initially begins as high-frequency HL. It presents as difficulty communicating in noisy conditions.
- There are more affected males than females.
- Compliance is only from 25–40% for those who own hearing aids (HA). A referral to an audiologist is key for optimal evaluation, fitting for HAs, and other assistive technologies or surgical treatment.
- Indication for CIs include hearing no better than identifying ≤50% key words in test sentences in the best aided condition in the worst ear and 60% in the better ear.
- Early audiology referral for individuals with suspected HL may improve treatment efficacy.

PRESSURE ULCER

Amy M. Zack, MD, FAAFP

 BASICS

DESCRIPTION

- A localized area of soft tissue injury resulting from pressure between an external surface and a bony prominence that causes local tissue breakdown classified in stages according to the National Pressure Ulcer Advisory Panel (NPUAP) classification.
  - Stage I: erythema of localized area, usually nonblanching over bony surface; may be painful, have consistency or temperature difference from surrounding tissue
  - Stage II: partial loss of dermal layer, resulting in pink ulceration; may be fluid-filled blister, or shiny, dry ulcer
  - Stage III: Full dermal loss often exposing subcutaneous tissue and fat.
  - Stage IV: Full-thickness ulceration exposing bone, tendon, or muscle. Osteomyelitis may be present.
- Synonym(s): decubitus ulcer; bed sores

EPIDEMIOLOGY

Incidence
2.5 million pressure ulcers treated yearly in United States in acute care facilities (1)

Prevalence
- Acute care 0.4–38%; long-term care 2.2–23.9%; home care 0–17%
- Majority occur in patients >65 years: 36% with hip fracture, 50% in ICU care (2)

ETIOLOGY AND PATHOPHYSIOLOGY

- Pathophysiology of pressure ulcers is changing, differs depending on stage of ulceration.
- Stages I to II result largely from prolonged moisture and friction and may not even be related to pressure and hypoxia, as previously believed (3).
- Stages III to IV likely begin with compressive forces, causing muscle damage and tissue hypoxia and leading to reperfusion injury of the deep tissue. The skin ulcer forms after significant deep tissue damage is already under way (3).
- Shearing and friction forces are also components of some ulcer formation, resulting in localized skin damage and early-stage ulcers (3).

RISK FACTORS

- Immobility: greatest risk factor regardless of patient, temporary or permanent immobility (4)
- Urinary and fecal incontinence present in >80% of immobile patients with pressure ulcers
- Poor nutritional status: Hypoalbuminemia and low BMI are markers for poor ulcer outcome (4).
- Poor skin perfusion, including vascular disease, diabetes, anemia, and tobacco use, increases risk.
- Extended stay in hospital/nursing home, inadequate staffing (5)
- Other risks include history of previous ulcer, age-related skin changes, immunocompromise, impaired skin sensation, and impaired awareness.

- Assessment scales commonly used for risk evaluation include Braden and Norton scales. The use of these does not decrease incidence, but they are more accurate than clinical judgment alone (6)[A].

GENERAL PREVENTION

- *Up to 95% are preventable*; identification of at-risk patients within 8 hours of admission, with early multidisciplinary care
- *Skin assessment*: policy in all health care settings (5)[B]
  - Increase frequency of assessments with decline in clinical condition (5)[C].
  - Include erythema, edema, skin temperature, and consistency in all evaluation (5)[B].
  - Assess around medical devices twice daily (5)[C].
- *Pressure relief*
  - Establish pressure relief schedule.
  - Proper patient positioning and the use of mattresses, cushions, heel protectors, and other devices to minimize pressure and friction
  - Regular turning of patients, including the use of angles and rotation of extremities, helps to minimize pressure.
- *Avoid positioning on area of erythema* (5)[C].
- *Minimize duration of immobility*: adequate physical and occupational therapies when appropriate
- *Aggressive moisture prevention*: management plan for incontinence (5)[C]
- *Nutrition*
  - Complete assessment of nutritional status and form plan, particularly protein intake and albumin levels.
  - Reassess with all changes in condition.
  - Develop individualized nutritional care plan for protein, calories, vitamins, and hydration (5)[C].
- *Manage skin health*: clean and dry with mild cleansers, skin protection where appropriate. Avoid massage or rubbing skin prone to ulcers (5)[C].
- *Microclimate control*: emerging therapy, control moisture, and temperature when selecting support structure. Avoid use of heating devices (5)[C].
- *Prophylactic dressings*: emerging therapy, apply foam dressing to bony prominences to avoid friction and shear (5)[B].
- *Textiles and fabrics*: Sheets and clothing should be silk-like rather than cotton or other abrasives.

COMMONLY ASSOCIATED CONDITIONS
See "Risk Factors."

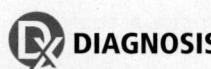 **DIAGNOSIS**

HISTORY
- Risk factors
- Date of ulcer diagnosis
- Treatment course

PHYSICAL EXAM

- Do full skin examination on admission to hospital or extended-care facility and repeatedly throughout admission, best with bathing/bed changes.
- 83% of hospitalized patients with decubitus ulcers develop them in first 5 days of hospitalization.
- Classify ulcer based on NPUAP stages (see "Description").
  - Focus on skin color, consistency, and temperature changes when classifying ulcer.
  - Assess and document location, category, size, tissue, color, edges, sinus tracts, exudate, odor.
  - Assess pain (5)[B].

DIFFERENTIAL DIAGNOSIS

- Venous stasis ulcers
- Arterial ulcers resulting from poor vascular supply
- Diabetic ulcers
- Pyoderma gangrenosum, cancers, vasculitides, and other dermatologic conditions

DIAGNOSTIC TESTS & INTERPRETATION

Initial Tests (lab, imaging)
- Wound culture: Do not culture surface drainage. If culture necessary, do deep tissue culture/bone biopsy.
- If systemic infection or that of bone, muscle is suspected, add infectious workup, including inflammatory markers, CBC, blood cultures, x-ray. MRI may be necessary to confirm osteomyelitis.
- Nutritional assessment: BMI, protein and calorie intake, albumin, prealbumin, CBC for anemia. No clear evidence in support of specific nutritional supplements including zinc and vitamin C (7)[A],(8)[B].

Follow-Up Tests & Special Considerations
Additional tests may be indicated when additional medical illness complicates assessment. This may include testing for diabetes, vascular disease, and other dermatologic diagnoses.

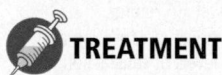 **TREATMENT**

GENERAL MEASURES

- Pressure reduction, minimize immobility, manage incontinence, and improve nutritional status and skin health (as described in "Prevention")
- Wound management by stage of ulcer
  - Stage I: aggressive preventive measures, thin film dressings for protection
  - Stage II: occlusive dressing to maintain healing, transparent films, hydrocolloids
  - Stages III to IV: débridement of necrotic tissue. Exudative ulcers will benefit from absorptive dressings such as calcium alginates, foams, hydrofibers. Dry ulcers require occlusive dressing to maintain moisture, including hydrocolloids, and hydrogels.

- Débridement: type depends on extent of necrosis or eschar, or presence of biofilm; incisional with scalpel when extensive dry. Mechanical with wet-dry dressings; enzymatic débridement is also frequently used. Débride only when there is adequate perfusion to wound.
- Surgical closure may be necessary in advanced wounds.
- Vacuum-assisted closure
  - Negative pressure reduces wound edema and improves local tissue perfusion.
  - Removes necrotic debris and reduces bacterial load
  - Literature review demonstrates the efficacy of negative-pressure wound therapy (9)[A].
- Dressings: mixed evidence for improvement (10)[B]
  - Select based on wound, exudate, ulcer stage.
  - Gauze: Avoid use, if no other options, wet-to-dry only.
  - Hydrocolloid: clean, shallow Stage II, not infected
  - Transparent: autolytic débridement, not for use on heavy exudate or over enzymatic debriding agents
  - Hydrogel: Stage II, shallow, minimal exudate, not infected
  - Alginate: Stage II to III, shallow with heavy exudate, infected, long duration dressing
  - Foam: Stage II to III, shallow with heavy exudate
  - Collagen-matrix: nonhealing Stage III to IV
  - Silver impregnated: infected or heavily colonized, high risk infection, short duration only
  - Honey impregnated: Stage II/III
  - Cadexomer iodine: Stage II/III with heavy exudate

MEDICATION

First Line
- See "General Measures" for first-line treatment.
- Pain control
- Aggressive management of contributing medical conditions
- Infection: If suspected, treat appropriately for cellulitis or osteomyelitis.
  - High index of suspicion for infection: poor healing, odor, pain, warmth, drainage, necrosis, diabetes, malnutrition, poor perfusion, immunosuppression, culture with $>10^5$ cfu/g or GBS presence
- Topical therapy
  - Débride as indicated
  - Nontoxic topical anesthetics including iodine, silver sulfadiazine, chlorhexidine (avoid hydrogen peroxide, Dakin solution) (5)[C]

Second Line
Nutritional interventions as determined by nutritional assessment. Weak evidence to support protein supplementation to reduce wound size (10)[C]

ISSUES FOR REFERRAL
- Vascular surgery is a consideration for improvement of blood flow to wound via vascular bypass.
- Plastic surgery is a consideration for skin graft/flap.

ADDITIONAL THERAPIES
- Alternative therapies
  - Light, laser, acoustic have little shown benefit.
  - Whirlpool contraindicated (5)[B]
  - Electrical stimulation shows some benefit (10)[B].

COMPLEMENTARY & ALTERNATIVE MEDICINE
- Nutritional support as needed
- Ultrasound and electrical stimulation create new vasculature in affected region (9)[C].

INPATIENT CONSIDERATIONS

Admission Criteria/Initial Stabilization
Refractory cellulitis, osteomyelitis, systemic infection, advanced nutritional decline, suspected patient mistreatment, inability to care for self

Nursing
- Dressing changes 1 to 3 times daily based on wound assessment and plan of care
- Assess risk factors according to scales.
- Assess for new or changing wounds.

Discharge Criteria
Clinical improvement in wound and systemic illness; when applicable, safe, and appropriate location for discharge

ONGOING CARE

FOLLOW-UP RECOMMENDATIONS
Weekly assessment by nurse with wound experience; biweekly assessment by physician

Patient Monitoring
- Home health nursing
- Change in plan of care if no improvement in 2 to 3 weeks

DIET
- 1 to 1.5 kg/day of protein
- Good glycemic control
- Include supply of micronutrients in diet or as supplements.

PATIENT EDUCATION
- Check skin regularly.
- Signs and symptoms of infection
- Report new or increased pain.
- Prevention of new wound where old wound healed
- Skin care, moisture prevention

PROGNOSIS
Variable, depending on the following:
- Removal of pressure
- Nutrition
- Wound care

COMPLICATIONS
- Infection
- Amputation

REFERENCES

1. Reddy M, Gill S, Rochon P. Preventing pressure ulcers: a systematic review. *JAMA*. 2006;296(8):974–984.
2. Baumgarten M, Margolis DJ, Orwig DL, et al. Pressure ulcers in elderly patients with hip fracture across the continuum of care. *J Am Geriatr Soc*. 2009;57(5):863–870.
3. Sibbald RG, Krasner DL, Woo KY. Pressure ulcer staging revisited: superficial changes & Deep Pressure Ulcer Framework. *Adv Skin Wound Care*. 2011;24(12):571–580.
4. Cakmak S, Gül U, Ozer S, et al. Risk factors for pressure ulcers. *Adv Skin Wound Care*. 2009:22(9):412–415.
5. European Pressure Ulcer Advisory Panel and National Pressure Ulcer Advisory Panel. *Prevention and Treatment of Pressure Ulcers: Quick Reference Guide*. Washington, DC: National Pressure Ulcer Advisory Panel, European Pressure Ulcer Advisory Panel, Pan Pacific Pressure Injury Alliance; 2014.
6. Pancorbo-Hidalgo PL, Garcia-Fernandez FP, Lopez-Medina IM, et al. Risk assessment scales for pressure ulcer prevention: a systematic review. *J Adv Nurs*. 2006;54(1):94–110.
7. Langer G, Schloemer G, Knerr A, et al. Nutritional interventions for preventing and treating pressure ulcers. *Cochrane Database Syst Rev*. 2003;(4):CD003216.
8. Jamshed N, Schneider E. Is the use of supplemental vitamin C and zinc for the prevention and treatment of pressure ulcers evidence based? *Ann Long-Term Care Med*. 2010;18(3):28–32.
9. Gregor S, Maegele M, Sauerland S, et al. Negative pressure wound therapy: a vacuum of evidence? *Arch Surg*. 2008;143(2):189–196.
10. Qaseem A, Humphrey LL, Forciea MA, et al. Treatment of pressure ulcers: a clinical practice guideline from the American College of Physicians. *Ann Intern Med*. 2015;162(5): 370–379.

ADDITIONAL READING

Stansby G, Avital L, Jones K, et al. Prevention and management of pressure ulcers in primary and secondary care: summary of NICE guidance. *BMJ*. 2014;348:g2592.

CODES

ICD10
- L89.95 Pressure ulcer of unspecified site, unstageable
- L89.91 Pressure ulcer of unspecified site, stage 1
- L89.92 Pressure ulcer of unspecified site, stage 2

CLINICAL PEARLS
- Create assessment and prevention protocols for all patients.
- Identify risk, reduce pressure, maximize nutrition, regular skin checks, and assess and treat wound appropriately.
- All care needs to be done in time-sensitive, patient-centered fashion.

PRETERM LABOR

Kara M. Coassolo, MD • John C. Smulian, MD, MPH

 BASICS

DESCRIPTION
Contractions occurring between 20 and 36 weeks' gestation at a rate of 4 in 20 minutes or 8 in 1 hour with at least one of the following: cervical change over time or dilation ≥2 cm

EPIDEMIOLOGY
Preterm birth is the leading cause of perinatal morbidity and mortality in the United States.

Incidence
10–15% of pregnancies experienced at least one episode of preterm labor.

Prevalence
~12% of all births in the United States are preterm (9% spontaneous preterm births and 3% indicated preterm births).

ETIOLOGY AND PATHOPHYSIOLOGY
- Premature formation and activation of myometrial gap junctions
- Inflammatory mediator–stimulated contractions
- Weakened cervix (structural defect or extracellular matrix defect)
- Abnormal placental implantation
- Systemic inflammation/infections (e.g., UTI, pyelonephritis, pneumonia, sepsis)
- Local inflammation/infections (intra-amniotic infections from aerobes, anaerobes, *Mycoplasma*, *Ureaplasma*)
- Uterine abnormalities (e.g., cervical insufficiency, leiomyomata, müllerian anomalies, diethylstilbestrol exposure)
- Overdistension (by multiple gestation or polyhydramnios)
- Preterm premature rupture of membranes
- Trauma
- Placental abruption
- Immunopathology (e.g., antiphospholipid antibodies)
- Placental ischemic disease (preeclampsia and fetal growth restriction)

Genetics
Familial predisposition

RISK FACTORS
- Demographic factors, including single parent, poverty, and black race
- Short interpregnancy interval
- No prenatal care
- Prepregnancy weight <45 kg (100 lb), body mass index <20
- Substance abuse (e.g., cocaine, tobacco)
- Prior preterm delivery (common)
- Previous 2nd-trimester dilation and evacuation (D&E)
- Cervical insufficiency or prior cervical surgery (cone biopsy or loop electrosurgical excision procedure [LEEP])
- Abdominal surgery/trauma during pregnancy
- Uterine structural abnormalities such as large fibroids or müllerian abnormalities
- Serious maternal infections/diseases

- Bacterial vaginosis
- Bacteriuria
- Vaginal bleeding during pregnancy
- Multiple gestation
- Select fetal abnormalities
- Intrauterine growth restriction
- Placenta previa
- Premature placental separation (abruption)
- Polyhydramnios
- Ehlers-Danlos syndrome

GENERAL PREVENTION
- Patient education at each visit in 2nd and 3rd trimesters for those at risk and periodically in the last two trimesters for the general population
- If previous preterm birth, evaluate if etiology is likely to recur and target intervention to specific condition.
  – Weekly injections of 17α-hydroxyprogesterone (250 mg IM every week) from 16 to 36 weeks if previous spontaneous preterm birth
  – Consider cerclage placement before 24 weeks' gestation for those at high risk because of cervical insufficiency or significant or progressive cervical shortening (1)[A],(2)[C].
  – For women with a short cervix in the 2nd trimester (<20 mm on transvaginal US), progesterone 200 mg/day per vagina for 24 to 34 weeks may decrease the risk of preterm delivery (3)[A].

 DIAGNOSIS

Diagnosis is generally based on a combination of significant cervical changes (such as dilation, effacement) with regular contractions. However, there is no single test that will reliably diagnose or predict true preterm labor. The diagnosis is based on a combination of physical findings and diagnostic tests that are interpreted in the context of the degree of risk to the patient.

HISTORY
- Address risk factors, especially etiologies of previous preterm birth.
- Regular uterine contractions or cramping
- Dull, low backache or pain
- Intermittent lower abdominal pain
- Increased low pelvic pressure
- Change in vaginal discharge
- Vaginal bleeding
- Fluid leakage

PHYSICAL EXAM
- Sterile speculum exam for membrane rupture evaluation, cultures, and cervical inspection
- Bimanual cervical exam if intact membranes: dilation of the cervix >1 cm and/or effacement of the cervix >50%

ALERT
Avoid bimanual examination when possible if rupture of the membranes is suspected.

DIFFERENTIAL DIAGNOSIS
- Braxton-Hicks contractions/false labor
- Round ligament pain
- Lumbosacral muscular back pain
- Urinary tract or vaginal infections
- Adnexal torsion
- Degenerating fibroid
- Appendicitis
- Dehydration
- Viral gastroenteritis
- Nephrolithiasis

DIAGNOSTIC TESTS & INTERPRETATION
Initial Tests (lab, imaging)
- In symptomatic women from 22 to 34 weeks' gestation with intact membranes and no intercourse or bleeding in past 24 hours, obtain a fetal fibronectin (FFN) swab from the posterior vaginal fornix (4)[C]. FFN must be obtained prior to digital cervical exam.
  – If results are positive (≥50 ng/mL), patient is at a modest increased risk of preterm birth (positive predictive value [PPV] 13–30% for delivery within 2 weeks).
  – If results are negative, >97% of patients will not deliver in 14 days, so can consider avoiding complicated or high-risk interventions.
- Urinalysis and urine culture
- Cultures for gonorrhea and chlamydia
- Wet prep for bacterial vaginosis evaluation (although evidence for improved outcomes with treatment is weak)
- Vaginal introitus and rectal culture for group B *Streptococcus*
- pH and ferning test of vaginal fluid to evaluate for rupture of membranes
- CBC with differential
- Drug screen when appropriate
- US to identify number of fetuses and fetal position, confirm gestational age, estimate fetal weight, quantify amniotic fluid, and look for conditions making tocolysis contraindicated.
- Transvaginal US to evaluate cervical length, funneling, and dynamic changes after obtaining FFN (if clinical assessment of the cervix is uncertain or if the cervix is closed on digital exam)

Follow-Up Tests & Special Considerations
- Repeat FFN as indicated by symptoms.
- After successful treatment, progressive changes of the cervix on repeat examination or US (in 1 to 2 weeks) may indicate need for hospitalization.

Diagnostic Procedures/Other
- Monitor contractions with external tocodynamometer.
- Consider amniocentesis at any preterm gestational age to evaluate for intra-amniotic infection (cell count with differential, glucose, Gram stain, aerobic, anaerobic, *Mycoplasma*, *Ureaplasma* cultures).

Test Interpretation
- Placental inflammation
  – Acute inflammation usually caused by infection
  – Chronic inflammation caused by immunopathology
- Abruption

TREATMENT

GENERAL MEASURES
- Treat underlying risk factors (e.g., antibiotics for infections, hydration for dehydration).
- Liquids only or NPO if delivery is imminent
- Hospitalization is necessary if the patient is on IV tocolysis.

MEDICATION

Tocolysis may allow time for interventions such as transfer to tertiary care facility and administration of corticosteroids but may not prolong pregnancy significantly (5)[A].

First Line
- Tocolysis
  - Nifedipine: 30 mg PO loading dose; then 10 to 20 mg q6h for 24 hours; then 10 to 20 mg PO q8h (do not use sublingual route); check BP often and avoid hypotension. Concurrent use with magnesium sulfate should be avoided to avoid theoretic risk of neuromuscular blockade.
  - Indomethacin: 50 to 100 mg PO initial dose; then 25 to 50 mg q6–8h for 24 hours (or, if available, 100-mg suppository per rectum q12h for 2 doses); then 25 mg q6–8h; use for no longer than 72 hours due to risk of premature closure of ductus arteriosus, oligohydramnios, and possibly neonatal necrotizing enterocolitis. Use with caution in patients with platelet dysfunction, liver dysfunction, or allergy to aspirin.
  - Contraindications to tocolysis: severe preeclampsia, hemorrhage, chorioamnionitis, advanced labor, intrauterine growth retardation, fetal distress, or lethal fetal abnormalities
- Antibiotics: antibiotics for group B *Streptococcus* prophylaxis if culture is positive or unknown
- Steroids: If mother is at 23 to 34 weeks' gestation with no evidence of systemic infection, give glucocorticoids to decrease neonatal respiratory distress, intraventricular hemorrhage, necrotizing enterocolitis, and overall perinatal mortality. Betamethasone 12 mg IM for 2 doses 24 hours apart (preferred choice) *or* dexamethasone 6 mg IM q12h for 4 doses (6)[A]

Second Line
- Magnesium sulfate by IV infusion has not been shown to be superior to placebo in prolonging pregnancy beyond 48 hours. The side effects are generally greater compared with calcium channel blockers or NSAIDs. Therefore, this agent should be used cautiously if at all (standard dosages for tocolysis start with a 4- to 6-g IV bolus over 20 minutes followed by 2 to 3 g/hr infusion until contractions stop) (7)[C].
  - Magnesium may decrease the risk of cerebral palsy when 12-hour course is given prior to an anticipated preterm birth.
  - Relative contraindications to magnesium sulfate include myasthenia gravis, hypocalcemia, renal failure, or concurrent use of calcium channel blockers.
- Terbutaline 0.25 mg SC q30min for up to 3 doses until contractions stop, then 0.25 mg SC q6h for 4 doses (optional); if contractions persist or pulse >120 bpm, change to another tocolytic agent (may be poorly tolerated by mothers).

- Terbutaline PO or by infusion pump has been used in the past for treatment or prevention of preterm labor. Due to reports of serious cardiovascular events and maternal deaths, PO or long-term SC administration of terbutaline should not be given.
- Significant possible interactions include pulmonary edema from crystalloid fluids and tocolytic agents, especially magnesium sulfate.
- PO maintenance therapy with any agent is ineffective and is not recommended.

ISSUES FOR REFERRAL
- If delivery is inevitable but not immediate, consider transport to a tertiary care center or hospital equipped with a neonatal ICU.
- Consider consultation with maternal–fetal medicine specialist.

ADDITIONAL THERAPIES
- Pelvic rest (e.g., no douching or intercourse) and activity restriction are often recommended; however, data to prove the efficacy are lacking. Some reduction in physical activity may be reasonable; this should be individualized.
- Strict bed rest has not been demonstrated to be effective in most situations.

SURGERY/OTHER PROCEDURES
- For malpresentation or fetal compromise, consider cesarean delivery if labor is progressing.
- Cerclage for cervical insufficiency (until 24 weeks' gestation)

INPATIENT CONSIDERATIONS
Admission Criteria/Initial Stabilization
Suspected/threatened preterm labor
- IV access
- Continuous fetal and contraction monitoring
- Assess cervix for dilatation and effacement.

IV Fluids
Hydrate with 500 mL 5% dextrose normal saline solution or 5% dextrose lactated Ringer solution for first half hour; then at 125 mL/hr.

Nursing
Monitor for fluid overload (input/output monitoring, symptoms, lung auscultation, pulse oximetry), especially with tocolysis and multiple gestations.

Discharge Criteria
- Regular contractions and cervical change resolve
- If cervix is dilated ≥3 cm or FFN is positive, individualize decision to discharge by gestational age and patient circumstances.

ONGOING CARE

FOLLOW-UP RECOMMENDATIONS
Patient Monitoring
- Weekly office visits with contraction monitoring, cervical checks, or cervical US if at high risk for recurrence
- Routine use of maintenance tocolysis is ineffective in preventing preterm birth.

DIET
Regular

PATIENT EDUCATION
Call physician or proceed to hospital whenever regular contractions last >1 hour, bleeding, increased vaginal discharge or fluid, decreased fetal movement.

PROGNOSIS
- If membranes are ruptured and no infection is confirmed, delivery often occurs within 3 to 7 days.
- If membranes are intact, 20–50% deliver preterm.

COMPLICATIONS
Labor resistant to tocolysis, pulmonary edema, infection with preterm rupture of membranes

REFERENCES
1. Tita AT, Rouse DJ. Progesterone for preterm birth prevention: an evolving intervention. *Am J Obstet Gynecol.* 2009;200(3):219–224.
2. Simhan HN, Caritis SN. Prevention of preterm delivery. *N Engl J Med.* 2007;357(5):477–487.
3. Berghella V, Rafael TJ, Szychowski JM, et al. Cerclage for short cervix on ultrasonography in women with singleton gestations and previous preterm birth: a meta-analysis. *Obstet Gynecol.* 2011;117(3):663–671.
4. Goldenberg RL, Goepfert AR, Ramsey PS. Biochemical markers for the prediction of preterm birth. *Am J Obstet Gynecol.* 2005;192(5)(Suppl):S36–S46.
5. Haas DM, Caldwell DM, Kirkpatrick P, et al. Tocolytic therapy for preterm delivery: systematic review and network meta-analysis. *BMJ.* 2012;345:e6226.
6. Roberts D, Dalziel S. Antenatal corticosteroids for accelerating fetal lung maturation for women at risk of preterm birth. *Cochrane Database Syst Rev.* 2006;(3):CD004454.
7. American College of Obstetricians and Gynecologists Committee on Obstetric Practice; Society for Maternal-Fetal Medicine. Committee Opinion No. 455: magnesium sulfate before anticipated preterm birth for neuroprotection. *Obstet Gynecol.* 2010;115(3):669–671.

CODES

ICD10
- O60.00 Preterm labor without delivery, unspecified trimester
- O60.02 Preterm labor without delivery, second trimester
- O60.03 Preterm labor without delivery, third trimester

CLINICAL PEARLS
- Treatment of preterm labor may delay delivery to facilitate short-term interventions.
- Steroids improve neonatal outcomes.
- Progesterone therapy can prevent recurrence of preterm birth in next pregnancy.

PRIAPISM

Shenelle Wilson, MD • Kelvin A. Moses, MD, PhD

BASICS

DESCRIPTION
- Penile erection that lasts for >4 hours and is unrelated to sexual stimulation or excitement.
- Classified into ischemic and nonischemic types
- Ischemic (low-flow) priapism is painful and requires urgent clinical intervention.
- Stuttering priapism is recurrent episodes of short-lived, self-limiting ischemic priapism over an extended period.
- Nonischemic (high-flow) priapism is painless, could be related to prior trauma, and does not require urgent treatment.
- Malignant priapism is a rare condition resulting most commonly from penile metastases from primary bladder, prostatic, rectosigmoid, and renal tumors.
- System(s) affected: reproductive

Pediatric Considerations
In children, nearly all priapism is caused either by sickle cell anemia or trauma (1).

EPIDEMIOLOGY
Incidence
In the United States, one study estimates 1,868 to 2,960 cases of priapism each year. They also noted an increasing incidence from 1998 to 2006, specifically in those from nonhematologic causes (2):
- Mean age: 33.7 years. There has been an age shift in recent years toward men in their 40s.
- Other studies have found the incidence of priapism to double in men aged >40 years (2.9 vs. 1.5/100,000 person-years) (3).
- Race: 61.1% black, 30% white, 6.3% Hispanic
- Associations: sickle cell anemia (41.9%), drug abuse (7.9%), sickle cell trait (2.5%)
- Anatomy and physiology
  - The penis consists of three longitudinally oriented corpora: two dorsolaterally paired corpora cavernosa that are responsible for penile erection and a single ventral corpus spongiosum that surrounds the glans penis and extends distally to form the glans penis
  - In general, the penile artery (which is a branch of the internal pudendal artery that, in turn, is a branch from the internal iliac artery) supplies the penis. It divides into three branches: dorsal artery, bulbar artery (supplies the corpus spongiosum), and cavernosal artery (the main blood supply to the erectile tissue).
  - During an erection, smooth muscle relaxation of the cavernosal arterioles results in high-volume inflow to the sinusoids, resulting in compression of the exiting venules. This leads to significant volume expansion of the corpora cavernosa.
  - During the flaccid resting state, the sympathetic nervous system is predominantly in control. Penile tumescence and erection are driven by the parasympathetic nervous system through the generation of nitric oxide (NO).
  - Smooth muscle relaxation occurs via usage of the phosphodiesterase type 5 (PDE-5A) pathway, which generates cyclic guanosine monophosphate (cGMP).

ETIOLOGY AND PATHOPHYSIOLOGY
- In ischemic priapism, decreased venous outflow results in increased intracavernosal pressure. This leads to erection, decreased arterial inflow, blood stasis, local hypoxia, and acidosis (a compartment syndrome). Eventually, penile tissue necrosis and fibrosis may occur. The exact mechanism is unknown and may involve trapping of erythrocytes in the veins, draining the erectile bodies.
- In nonischemic priapism, there is increased arterial flow without decreased venous outflow. There is increased inflow and outflow, which results in a sustained, nonpainful, partially rigid erection.
- Aberrations in the PDE-5A pathway have been proven in mice to be one mechanism of priapism (4).
- Ischemic priapism
  - Idiopathic, estimated to about 50% (1)
  - Intracavernosal injections of vasoactive drugs for erectile dysfunction
  - Oral agents for erectile dysfunction
  - Pelvic vascular thrombosis
  - Prolonged sexual activity
  - Sickle cell disease and trait
  - Leukemia from infiltration of the corpora
  - Other blood dyscrasias (G6PD deficiency, thrombophilia)
  - Pelvic hematoma or neoplasia (penis, urethra, bladder, prostate, kidney, rectal)
  - Cerebrospinal tumors
  - Asplenism
  - Fabry disease
  - Tertiary syphilis
  - Total parenteral nutrition, especially 20% lipid infusion (results in hyperviscosity)
  - Bladder calculus
  - Trauma to penis
  - UTIs, especially prostatitis, urethritis, cystitis
  - Several drugs suspected as causing priapism (e.g., chlorpromazine, prazosin, cocaine, trazodone, and some corticosteroids); anticoagulants (heparin and warfarin); phosphodiesterase inhibitors (sildenafil, others); immunosuppressants (tacrolimus); and antihypertensives (hydralazine, propranolol, guanethidine)
  - Intracavernous fat emulsion
  - Hyperosmolar IV contrast
  - Spinal cord injury
  - General or spinal anesthesia
  - Heavy alcohol intake or cocaine use
- Nonischemic priapism
  - The most common cause is penile or perineal trauma resulting in a fistula between the cavernous artery and the corpora.
  - Acute spinal cord injury
  - Rarely, iatrogenic causes for the management of ischemic priapism can result in nonischemic priapism.
  - Certain urologic surgeries have also resulted in nonischemic priapism.

RISK FACTORS
- Sickle cell anemia, lifetime risk of ischemic priapism 29–42% (1)
- Dehydration

GENERAL PREVENTION
- Avoid dehydration.
- Avoid excessive sexual stimulation.
- Avoid causative drugs (see "Etiology and Pathophysiology") when possible.
- Avoid genital and pelvic trauma.

COMMONLY ASSOCIATED CONDITIONS
- Sickle cell anemia or sickle cell trait
- Drug abuse
- G6PD deficiency
- Leukemia
- Neoplasm

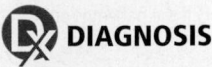

DIAGNOSIS

HISTORY
- Penile erection that is persistent, prolonged, painful, and tender (ischemic).
- Duration of erection, degree of pain
- Perineal or penile trauma
- Prior episodes of priapism
- Urination difficult during erection
- History of any hematologic abnormalities
- Cardiovascular disease
- Medications
- Recreational drugs
- Loss of erectile function if treatment is not prompt and effective.

PHYSICAL EXAM
- Ischemic priapism
  - Penis is fully erect, corpora cavernosa are rigid and tender, and corpora spongiosum and glans are flaccid. Usually associated with tenderness and pain
- Nonischemic priapism
  - Penis is partially erect and the corpora cavernosa are semirigid and nontender, with the glans and corpora spongiosum flaccid. Usually not tender or painful
- Perineum, abdomen, and lymph node exam also valuable to rule out underlying condition.
- A complete penile and scrotal exam is necessary. Determine if a penile prosthesis is present.

DIAGNOSTIC TESTS & INTERPRETATION
- CBC with reticulocyte count to detect leukemia or platelet abnormalities
- Sickling hemoglobin (Hgb) solubility test and Hgb electrophoresis
- Coagulation profile
- Platelet count
- Urinalysis
- Urine toxicology if illicit drugs suspected
- Corporal blood gas (CBG) should be used to distinguish ischemic from nonischemic priapism.
- A color duplex ultrasound of the penis and perineum may be necessary to differentiate ischemic from nonischemic priapism. In ischemic priapism, there is no blood flow in the cavernosal arteries, whereas in nonischemic patients, there is high blood flow (1); may also see fistulas or pseudoaneurysms suggestive of nonischemic priapism.
- Penile arteriography can be used to identify the presence and site of fistulas in patients with nonischemic priapism.

Diagnostic Procedures/Other
A physical exam is usually able to distinguish ischemic from nonischemic priapism; however, CBG is the most definitive method.

Test Interpretation
- Pelvic vascular thrombosis
- Partial thrombosis of corpora cavernosa of the penis
- Corpus spongiosum, glans penis: no involvement
- Arterial priapism will show arteriocavernous fistula.

TREATMENT

- Ischemic priapism requires immediate treatment to preserve future erectile function (a longer delay in treatment means a higher chance of future impotence).
  - Cavernosal aspiration with a large bore needle with irrigation (success rate ~30%) (1,5)
  - Cavernosal injection of phenylephrine (α-adrenergic sympathomimetic) with monitoring of patient's BP and pulse (success rate ~65%) (5). Inject q5–10min until detumescence.
  - Continue aspiration, irrigation, and phenylephrine for several hours. If this fails, shunt procedures are considered (first a distal shunt).
- Nonischemic priapism
  - Initial observation
  - If this fails, arteriography and embolization with absorbable materials (5% rate of impotence vs. 39% with permanent materials) or surgical ligation as a last resort (5)
- Treat the underlying condition (i.e., sickle cell disease). Do not delay intracavernous treatment.

GENERAL MEASURES

- Reassure the patient about the outcome, if warranted.
- Provide continuous caudal or spinal anesthesia if the etiology is neurogenic.
- Treat any underlying cause.
- In sickle cell anemia: IV hydration; supplemental oxygen; partial exchange or repeated transfusions to reduce percentage of sickle cells to <50%
- Relieve the patient's pain.
- Initiating proper management depends on whether the priapism is ischemic or nonischemic.

MEDICATION

- Opioids for pain, if needed
- Intracavernous injection of phenylephrine is recommended by the American Urological Association for ischemic priapism (5).
- Phenylephrine minimizes risk of cardiovascular side effects that are more common with other sympathomimetics; terbutaline has been studied and may be effective (uncontrolled trials showed a 65% resolution rate) for priapism caused by self-injection of agents to treat erectile dysfunction (5).
- Ketoconazole 200 mg TID and prednisone 5 mg daily for 2 weeks; then tapering to ketoconazole 200 mg nightly for 6 months has been shown to prevent recurrent ischemic priapism (6).
- For stuttering priapism, a trial of gonadotropin-releasing hormone (GnRH) agonists or antiandrogens is effective; self-injection of phenylephrine is also effective.
- PDE-5 inhibitors also have a role in the prevention of priapism in patients suffering from stuttering priapism (7).

ISSUES FOR REFERRAL

A urologist should be consulted in all cases of suspected priapism to ensure the highest likelihood of preserved erectile function.

SURGERY/OTHER PROCEDURES

- For ischemic priapism, introduction of 18- or 19-gauge needle into corpora cavernosa (best done by urologist if available) at 9 o'clock and 3 o'clock positions with aspiration of 20 to 30 mL of blood from corpus cavernosum. May follow with intracavernous injection of 100 to 500 μg phenylephrine (mix 0.2 mL [200 μg]) of 1% phenylephrine in 9.8 mL of normal saline. 1 mL injections given every 3 to 5 min for ~1 hour before determining if treatment is successful. If this fails, consider shunts.
- Distal shunts
  - Percutaneous: Ebbehoj, Winter, or T-shunt (8–10)
  - Open: Al-Ghorab or corporal snake (11,12)
- Proximal shunts
  - Open: Quackles or Sacher (13,14)
  - Saphenous vein shunt (15)
  - Deep dorsal vein shunt (16)

ONGOING CARE

FOLLOW-UP RECOMMENDATIONS
Bed rest until priapism resolves

Patient Monitoring
Close follow-up with a urologist is required after surgical treatments for priapism.

PATIENT EDUCATION
- Information about long-term outlook, referral for counseling
- Reduction of vasoactive drug therapy if responsible for priapism, and elimination of offending drugs if causal

PROGNOSIS
- Even with excellent treatment for a prolonged priapism, detumescence may require several weeks secondary to edema (1).
- Impotence due to irreversible corporal fibrosis is likely in ischemic priapism and is up to 90% if the priapism lasts >24 hours.
- Despite early intervention, ischemic priapism is likely to result in impotence in up to 50% of men.

COMPLICATIONS
Erectile dysfunction (i.e., impotence)

REFERENCES

1. Huang YC, Harraz AM, Shindel AW, et al. Evaluation and management of priapism: 2009 update. *Nat Rev Urol*. 2009;6(5):262–271.
2. Chrouser KL, Ajiboye OB, Oyetunji TA, et al. Priapism in the United States: the changing role of sickle cell disease. *Am J Surg*. 2011;201(4):468–474.
3. Eland IA, van der Lei J, Stricker BH, et al. Incidence of priapism in the general population. *Urology*. 2001;57(5):970–972.
4. Champion HC, Bivalacqua TJ, Takimoto E, et al. Phosphodiesterase-5A dysregulation in penile erectile tissue is a mechanism of priapism. *Proc Natl Acad Sci U S A*. 2005;102(5):1661–1666.
5. Montague DK, Jarow J, Broderick GA, et al. American Urological Association guideline on the management of priapism. *J Urol*. 2003;170(4, Pt 1):1318–1324.
6. Hoeh MP, Levine LA. Prevention of recurrent ischemic priapism with ketoconazole: evolution of a treatment protocol and patient outcomes. *J Sex Med*. 2014;11(1):197–204.
7. Muneer A, Minhas S, Arya M, et al. Stuttering priapism—a review of the therapeutic options. *Int J Clin Pract*. 2008;62(8):1265–1270.
8. Ebbehoj J. A new operation for priapism. *Scand J Plast Reconstr Surg*. 1974;8(3):241–242.
9. Winter CC. Cure of idiopathic priapism: new procedure for creating fistula between glans penis and corpora cavernosa. *Urology*. 1976;8(4):389–391.
10. Brant WO, Garcia MM, Bella AJ, et al. T-shaped shunt and intracavernous tunneling for prolonged ischemic priapism. *J Urol*. 2009;181(4):1699–1705.
11. Borrelli M, Mitre AI, Alfer Júnior W, et al. Surgical treatment of priapism using Al-Ghorab's technic [in Portuguese]. *Rev Paul Med*. 1983;101(1):27–28.
12. Burnett AL, Pierorazio PM. Corporal "snake" maneuver: corporoglanular shunt surgical modification for ischemic priapism. *J Sex Med*. 2009;6(4):1171–1176.
13. Quackels R. Treatment of a case of priapism by cavernospongious anastomosis [in French]. *Acta Urol Belg*. 1964;32:5–13.
14. Sacher EC, Sayegh E, Frensilli F, et al. Caverno-spongiosum shunt in the treatment of priapism. *J Urol*. 1972;108(1):97–100.
15. Grayhack JT, McCullough W, O'Conor VJ Jr, et al. Venous bypass to control priapism. *Invest Urol*. 1964;1:509–513.
16. Barry JM. Priapism: treatment with corpus cavernosum to dorsal vein of penis shunts. *J Urol*. 1976;116(6):754–756.

ADDITIONAL READING

- Burnett AL. Pathophysiology of priapism: dysregulatory erection physiology thesis. *J Urol*. 2003;170(1):26–34.
- Pryor J, Akkus E, Alter G, et al. Priapism. *J Sex Med*. 2004;1(1):116–120.
- Salonia A, Eardley I, Giuliano F, et al. European Association of Urology guidelines on priapism. *Eur Urol*. 2014;65(2):480–489.

SEE ALSO

Anemia, Sickle Cell; Erectile Dysfunction

CODES

ICD10
- N48.30 Priapism, unspecified
- N48.39 Other priapism
- N48.31 Priapism due to trauma

CLINICAL PEARLS

- Priapism is a prolonged penile erection that lasts >4 hours and is unrelated to sexual stimulation.
- In evaluating priapism, the clinician must distinguish ischemic from nonischemic priapism by history and physical exam, as well as blood gas and possibly ultrasound, if needed.
- Ischemic priapism is an emergent condition that requires immediate urologic evaluation and treatment.
- The most common causes of ischemic priapism are idiopathic, related to treatments for erectile dysfunction, or related to use of substances (medicinal or recreational).
- If an underlying medical condition is identified (sickle cell anemia), proper concomitant treatment is necessary to increase the efficacy of treatment.

PROSTATE CANCER

Jason K. Frankel, MD • Gregory Murphy, MD • Joseph R. Wagner, MD

BASICS

DESCRIPTION
- The prostate is a male reproductive organ that contributes seminal fluid to the ejaculate.
- The prostate gland is about the size of a walnut, averaging 20 to 25 g in volume in an adult male; tends to enlarge after age 50
- Three distinct zones delineate the functional anatomy of the prostate: peripheral zone (largest, neighbors rectal wall, palpable on DRE, most common location for prostate cancer), central zone (contains the ejaculatory ducts), and transition zone (located centrally, adjacent to the urethra).
- Prostatic epitheilial cells produce prostate specific antigen (PSA), which is used as a tumor marker and in screening.

EPIDEMIOLOGY
Incidence
According to the National Cancer Institute, an estimated 220,800 men in the United States will be newly diagnosed with carcinoma of the prostate (CaP) in 2015.

Prevalence
- About 2.8 million men are living with CaP in the United States
- ~27,540 men in the United States will die of CaP in 2015.
- Mean age at diagnosis is 66 years.
- Prostate cancer is the most commonly diagnosed nonskin cancer in men in the United States (~15.9% lifetime risk) and second leading cause of cancer death in men (only ~3% of all CaP results in CaP-related death).
- Autopsy studies find foci of latent CaP in 50% of men in their 8th decade of life.
- Probability of clinical CaP 10.9% (1 in 9) in men aged ≥70 years

ETIOLOGY AND PATHOPHYSIOLOGY
- Adenocarcinoma: >95%; nonadenocarcinoma: <5% (most common transitional cell carcinoma)
- Cells generally stain positive for PSA and prostatic acid phosphatase (PAP)
- Location of CaP: 70% peripheral zone, 20% transitional zone, 5–10% central zone

Genetics
Elevated risk if first-degree relative diagnosed with CaP suggesting genetic component. Specifics unclear

RISK FACTORS
- Age >50 years
- African American race
- Positive family history
- Poorly understood environmental factors

GENERAL PREVENTION
There are no FDA approved drugs or diet modifications to prevent CaP.

- Finasteride has been studied for this purpose. A moderate risk reduction associated with an increased risk of high-grade disease was encountered. Therefore, it has not been FDA approved for prevention (1)[A].

ALERT
Screening for prostate cancer is controversial:

- U.S. Preventive Services Task Force (USPSTF) recommends against PSA-based screen for prostate cancer, concluding the harm of screening outweighs benefit (2)[A].
- For men ages 55 to 69 years, the AUA panel recommends shared decision making between physician and patient regarding PSA screening.
- PSA screening is not recommended in patients with <10 years of estimated life expectancy.

DIAGNOSIS

HISTORY
- Inquire about family history of CaP, symptoms of bladder outlet obstruction, and other voiding symptoms.
- Anorexia and weight loss, bone pain (with metastasis), hematuria, hematospermia (rare)

PHYSICAL EXAM
- DRE to assess for prostatic masses, firmness, or asymmetry
- Evaluate lumbar spine and lymph nodes for evidence of metastasis.

ALERT
Most patients with CaP are asymptomatic.

DIFFERENTIAL DIAGNOSIS
Benign prostatic hyperplasia, prostatitis, prostatic intraepithelial neoplasia (PIN), prostate stones, atypical small acinar proliferation (ASAP)

- The high predictive value of ASAP for subsequent adenocarcinoma warrants repeat biopsy within 3 months.

DIAGNOSTIC TESTS & INTERPRETATION
Initial Tests (lab, imaging)
PSA, DRE, and clinical history primarily determine need for prostate biopsy:

- In general, total PSA ≥4 ng/mL concerning for CaP (sensitivity 21%, specificity 91%)
  - Other benign conditions can elevate PSA (infection, inflammation, normal growth, natural PSA fluctuations, normally high variants).
  - Rectal manipulation will not elevate PSA.
- Age-/race-adjusted "normal" PSA values (ng/mL):

Age	Asians	Blacks	Whites
40–49	0–2.0	0–2.0	0–2.5
50–59	0–3.0	0–4.0	0–3.5
60–69	0–4.0	0–4.5	0–4.5
70–79	0–5.0	0–5.5	0–6.5

- 5-α-Reductase inhibitors decrease PSA by ~50%.
- Other PSA metrics used to aid in CaP diagnosis: PSA velocity, PSA doubling time, PSA density, percentage free PSA
  - Total PSA velocity: ≥0.75 ng/mL/year or >20% baseline for higher values increases CaP risk
  - Free PSA and age/race-adjusted PSA helpful in evaluating risk
  - PSAD (PSA density) ≥0.15 associated with higher prevalence of CaP
- PSA/free PSA and probability of cancer:

PSA (ng/dL)	Cancer Rate	% Free PSA (for PSA 4–10)	Cancer Rate
0–2	1%	0–10%	56%
2–4	15%	10–15%	28%
4–10	25%	15–20%	20%
>10	>50%	20–25%	16%
		>25%	8%

- Prostate biopsy
  - Decision to biopsy involves PSA, DRE findings, and overall clinical suspicion of CaP.
  - Standard biopsy includes systematic random cores from the peripheral zone-base, mid, and apex, generally 8 to 12 cores.
  - The Gleason Grade is the standard pathologic grading system:
    - Ranks specimens from 1 to 5 based on architectural pattern identified, with 1 being most differentiated and 5 being least.
    - Primary and secondary patterns are identified and reported, and the sum is the Gleason score (e.g., 3 + 4 = 7).
    - Most prostate cancer is scored 6 to 10 with 10 having the worst prognosis.
- Staging
  - TNM (tumor, node, and metastasis) staging is used to generate a clinical and pathological stage, which primarily directs treatment. Clinical staging is as follows:
    - T1: cancer found incidentally on TURP or found on biopsy for elevated PSA
    - T2: cancer found on DRE but confined to the prostate
    - T3: cancer found to be extended locally outside of the prostate and/or the seminal vesicle
    - T4: invading adjacent organs
    - N1: denotes local lymph node spread
    - M1: distant metastasis

Follow-Up Tests & Special Considerations
- Bone scan and/or CT scan and/or MRI may be indicated for high-risk cancers.
- Biopsy if suspicious nodal findings
- Alkaline phosphatase associated with bony mets
- Genetic testing (e.g., Prolaris, Oncotype Dx, etc.) is emerging as a prognostic modality.

TREATMENT

Treatment options include:
- Watchful waiting: monitoring with expectation to provide palliation with symptoms
- Active surveillance: close monitoring of PSA, DRE, and repeat biopsy at regular intervals (3)
- Radical prostatectomy: ± pelvic lymph node dissection (PLND)
- Radiation therapy: external beam (EBRT)
- Brachytherapy: radioactive implants placed in prostate; option for early clinical stage localized to the prostate
- Androgen deprivation therapy (ADT) may be surgical or nonsurgical:
  - Bilateral orchiectomy (surgical castration)
  - Gonadotropin-releasing hormone (GnRH) agonist, antagonist, or antiandrogen (medical castration)
- Chemotherapy: includes multiple chemotherapeutic agents used to treat castrate resistant prostate cancer

RISK STRATIFICATION

- Treatment options based upon risk: low, intermediate, and high-risk categories; this is based on risk of recurrence after definitive treatment. Must meet all three criteria to be low risk; any one criterion moves patient to a higher risk group (4)[A]:

Risk Category	Clinical Stage	Serum PSA	Gleason Score
Low	T1–T2a	<10 ng/mL	≤6
Intermediate	T2b–T2c	>10 and ≤20 ng/mL	7
High	T3a	>20 ng/mL	8–10

- Localized CaP
  - Low risk:
    ○ Mainstay of therapy is active surveillance.
    ○ Radical prostatectomy and radiation therapy may be offered.
  - Intermediate risk:
    ○ Mainstay of therapy is radical prostatectomy with LND or radiation therapy.
    ○ Radical prostatectomy has shown a survival benefit in intermediate and high risk prostate cancer (5)[A]
  - High Risk:
    ○ Mainstay of therapy is radical prostatectomy or radiation therapy.
    ○ Adjuvant radiation may be considered based on adverse pathologic findings after prostatectomy

ALERT

- Life expectancy determinations as well as educating the patient of the risks and benefits of surveillance and treatment options is critical.

- Locally advanced CaP:
  - Mainstay of therapy is ADT and radiation. Surgery and adjuvant radiation may also play a role.
- Metastatic CaP:
  - Mainstay of therapy is RT and ADT.
  - ADT specifics:
    ○ GnRH agonists include leuprolide or goserelin.
    ○ GnRH antagonists include degarelix: an alternative to GnRH agonists; suppresses testosterone production and avoids flare phenomenon observed with GnRH agonists
    ○ Side effects of ADT: osteoporosis, gynecomastia, erectile dysfunction (ED), decreased libido, obesity, lipid alterations, greater risk of diabetes, and cardiovascular disease
    ○ Flare phenomenon (disease flare: hot flashes, fatigue) can occur owing to transient increase in testosterone levels on initiation of GnRH agonist therapy.
    ○ If spinal cord metastases are present, the concern for cord compression with a testosterone flare can be avoided by starting antiandrogen therapy prior to initiation of a GnRH agonist.
    ○ Combined androgen blockade with GnRH agonist and antiandrogen (e.g., bicalutamide, nilutamide, or flutamide) may be used to prevent flare.
- Castration-resistant prostate cancer (CRPC)
  - CRPC is defined as progression of disease following ADT. Treatment includes the following:
    ○ Nonmetastatic
      ■ Continue ADT, no further treatment has been shown to increase overall survival.
      ■ Antiandrogen or androgen synthesis inhibitor (e.g., ketoconazole) may be added.

○ Asymptomatic metastatic: no previous therapy with docetaxel:
  ■ Abiraterone: inhibitor of CYP17A (adrenal androgen production), used with prednisone
  ■ Enzalutamide: androgen receptor inhibitor
  ■ Docetaxel: chemotherapeutic that inhibits microtubules
  ■ Sipuleucel-T: immunotherapy
○ Symptomatic metastatic: no previous therapy with docetaxel:
  ■ Abiraterone, enzalutamide, docetaxel
  ■ Radium-223 (radiopharmaceutical) for patients with symptomatic bony metastases and no visceral metastasis.
○ Symptomatic metastatic: previous therapy with docetaxel:
  ■ Good performance status: abiraterone, enzalutamide, cabazitaxel
  ■ Poor performance status: Mainstay is palliative care, may attempt further therapy based on patient wishes.

 ONGOING CARE

FOLLOW-UP RECOMMENDATIONS

- Prostatectomy: PSA and DRE are recommended at regular intervals. PSA threshold defining biochemical recurrence is evolving; however, recent data suggests a cutoff of 0.2 ng/mL (4). A CT and bone scan are usually obtained. If the PSA recurrence is thought to be from local disease, salvage radiation is considered. For metastatic disease, androgen deprivation is considered.
- XRT: PSA and DRE are recommended at regular intervals. Biochemical recurrence is defined as PSA increase ≥2 ng/mL above nadir, a CT and bone scan are usually obtained. If the PSA recurrence is thought to be from local disease, salvage prostatectomy or cryosurgery is considered. For metastatic disease, androgen deprivation is considered.

PROGNOSIS

- Localized disease is frequently curable; advanced disease has a favorable prognosis if lesions are hormone-sensitive.
- 5-year CaP survival by stage: local 100%, regional 100%, distant 28%
- Recurrence risk increased if adverse pathologic features are present: extraprostatic extension, seminal vesicle invasion, positive surgical margins

COMPLICATIONS

- Prostatectomy: Urinary incontinence and ED are the most common long-term issues.
- Radiation therapy: urinary incontinence, ED, radiation cystitis, and radiation proctitis
- Treatment options for ED: PDE5 inhibitors, intracavernosal injections, intraurethral suppositories, vacuum pump, penile prosthesis
- Treatment options for incontinence: oral medications, urethral slings, artificial sphincters

REFERENCES

1. Thompson IM, Goodman PJ, Tangen CM, et al. The influence of finasteride on the development of prostate cancer. *N Engl J Med.* 2003;349(3):215–224.
2. Moyer VA; U.S. Preventive Services Task Force. Screening for prostate cancer: U.S. Preventive Services Task Force recommendation statement. *Ann Intern Med.* 2012;157(2):120–134.

3. Klotz L. Active surveillance for low-risk prostate cancer. *F1000 Med Rep.* 2012;4:16.
4. D'Amico AV, Whittington R, Malkowicz SB, et al. Biochemical outcome after radical prostatectomy, external beam radiation therapy, or interstitial radiation therapy for clinically localized prostate cancer. *JAMA.* 1998;280(11):969–974.
5. Wilt TJ, Brawer MK, Jones KM, et al. Radical prostatectomy versus observation for localized prostate cancer. *N Engl J Med.* 2012;367(3):203–213.

ADDITIONAL READING

- Berthold DR, Pond GR, Soban F, et al. Docetaxel plus prednisone or mitoxantrone plus prednisone for advanced prostate cancer: updated survival in the TAX 327 study. *J Clin Oncol.* 2008;26(2):242–245.
- Bolla M, van Poppel H, Tombal B, et al. Postoperative radiotherapy after radical prostatectomy for high-risk prostate cancer: long-term results of a randomised controlled trial (EORTC trial 22911). *Lancet.* 2012;380(9858):2018–2027.
- Klein EA, Thompson IM Jr, Tangen CM, et al. Vitamin E and the risk of prostate cancer: the Selenium and Vitamin E Cancer Prevention Trial (SELECT). *JAMA.* 2011;306(14):1549–1556.
- Lowrance WT, Scardino PT. Predictive models for newly diagnosed prostate cancer patients. *Rev Urol.* 2009;11(3):117–126.
- National Comprehensive Cancer Network. Clinical practice guidelines: prostate cancer. 2015. www.nccn.org. Accessed 2015.
- Nomiya T, Tsuji H, Ioyama S, et al. Management of high-risk prostate cancer: radiation therapy and hormonal therapy. *Cancer Treat Rev.* 2013;39(8):872–878.
- Pastuszak AW, Pearlman AM, Lai WS, et al. Testosterone replacement therapy in patients with prostate cancer after radical prostatectomy. *J Urol.* 2013;190(2):639–644.
- Schröder FH, Hugosson J, Roobol MJ, et al. Screening and prostate cancer mortality: results of the European Randomised Study of Screening for Prostate Cancer (ERSPC) at 13 years of follow-up. *Lancet.* 2014;384(9959):2027–2035.
- Thompson IM Jr, Goodman PJ, Tangen CM, et al. Long-term survival of participants in the prostate cancer prevention trial. *N Engl J Med.* 2013;369(7):603–610.

CODES

ICD10

C61 Malignant neoplasm of prostate

CLINICAL PEARLS

- Prostate cancer is clinically diverse, ranging from low-risk/indolent disease to high-risk/aggressive disease.
- Most men with CaP are asymptomatic.
- The use of PSA for CaP screening is controversial and necessitates an open conversation between medical provider and patient regarding benefits/risks.
- Active surveillance is an important treatment option to consider for low-risk patients.
- In patients taking 5-α-reductase inhibitors, PSA level to estimate actual PSA.

PROSTATIC HYPERPLASIA, BENIGN (BPH)

Sara M. DeSpain, MD • James E. Hougas, III, MD, Maj, USAF, MC

BASICS

- Benign prostatic hyperplasia (BPH) is caused by a proliferation of both the smooth muscle and epithelial cell lines of the prostate which cause increased volume and can cause compression of the urethra and obstructive symptoms.
- Clinically presents with storage and/or voiding symptoms commonly referred to as lower urinary tract symptoms (LUTS). These include difficulty initiating stream, frequency, or dysuria.
- Symptoms do not directly correlate to prostate volume. Estimated that half of all men with histologic evidence of BPH experience moderate to severe LUTS.
- Progression may result in upper and lower tract infections and may progress to direct bladder outlet obstruction and acute renal failure (ARF).

EPIDEMIOLOGY
Near universal development in men; age dependent

Incidence and Prevalence
Incidence increases with age; wide variety of estimates of prevalence ranging from 70% to 90% by the age of 80 (estimated at 8–20% by age 40).

ETIOLOGY AND PATHOPHYSIOLOGY
- Develops in prostatic periurethral or transition zone.
- Hyperplastic nodules of stromal and epithelial components increase glandular components.
- Etiology is unknown but recently there is a theory that it is from a reawakening of the embryonic induction process because of the similarity between BPH and the embryonic morphogenesis.

COMMONLY ASSOCIATED CONDITIONS
- LUTS
  - LUTS can be divided into two groups: filling/storage symptoms and voiding symptoms.
    - Filling/storage symptoms include frequency, nocturia, urgency, and urge incontinence.
    - Voiding symptoms include difficulty initiating stream, incomplete voiding, weak stream.
    - Can lead to acute or chronic obstructive symptoms
- Sexual dysfunction, including erectile dysfunction and ejaculatory disorders
- LUTS can also be secondary to cardiovascular, respiratory, or renal disease (1).

RISK FACTORS
- Most significant risk factor is age.
- Increased risk of BPH with higher free prostate-specific antigen (PSA) levels, heart disease, and use of β-blockers
- Obesity and lack of exercise can cause LUTS to be more significant.
- No evidence of increased or decreased risk with smoking, alcohol, or any dietary factors.
- Low androgen levels from cirrhosis/chronic alcoholism can reduce the risk of BPH.

GENERAL PREVENTION
- The disease appears to be part of the aging process.
- Symptoms can be managed through weight loss, regulation of fluid intake, decreased intake of caffeine, and increased physical activity.

DIAGNOSIS

HISTORY
- Evaluate symptom severity with the American Urological Society Symptom Index or the International Prostate Symptom Score (IPSS).

- Screen for other causes of symptoms such as infection, procedural history, neurologic causes. Evaluate for comorbid conditions which may produce similar symptoms such as diabetes, CHF, or Parkinson disease.
- Review medication list. Pay particular attention to diuretics and anticholinergic medications. Also, decongestants (increased sphincter tone), opiates (impaired autonomic function), or tricyclic antidepressants (anticholinergic effects)
- Review family history for BPH and prostate cancer.
- Screen for gross hematuria. IPSS of LUTS, patient filled survey to follow severity (2)[A]:
  - Questionnaire: Over the past month, how often have you:
    - 1. Had the sensation of not emptying your bladder completely after you finished urinating?
    - 2. Had to urinate again <2 hours after you finished urinating?
    - 3. Found you stopped and started again several times when you urinated?
    - 4. Found it difficult to postpone urination?
    - 5. Had a weak urinary stream?
    - 6. Had to push or strain to begin urination?
    - 7. Been up to urinate from the time you went to bed at night until the time you got up in the morning?
    - 8. How would you feel if you were to spend the rest of your life with your current symptoms?
  - Scoring of the questionnaire:
    - Questions 1 to 6: no symptoms = 0 points, 1 in 5 times = 1 point, less than half = 2 points, about half = 3 points, more than half = 4 points, most of the time = 5 points
    - Question 7: no occurrence = 0 points, 1 time = 1 point, 2 times = 2 points, 3 times = 3 points, 4 times = 4 points, and 5 times or more = 5 points
    - Question 8: 0 = delighted, 1 = pleased, 2 = mostly satisfied, 3 = mixed, 4 = mostly dissatisfied, 5 = unhappy, 6 = terrible
    - Symptoms are classified as mild (total score 0 to 7), moderate (total score 8 to 19), and severe (total score 20 to 35).
- Nocturia >2 times per night, warrants a frequency/volume chart for 2 to 3 days to detect urinary patterns.

PHYSICAL EXAM
- Digital rectal exam (DRE) finding of symmetrically enlarged prostate, but *size does not always correlate with symptoms.*
- Signs of renal failure due to obstructive uropathy (edema, pallor, pruritus, ecchymosis, nutritional deficiencies)
- If DRE is suggestive of prostate cancer, there is hematuria, recurrent infections, concern for stricture, or evidence of neurologic disease, the patient should be referred to urology.

DIFFERENTIAL DIAGNOSIS
- Obstructive
  - Prostate cancer
  - Urethral stricture or valves
  - Bladder neck contracture (usually secondary to prostate surgery)
  - Inability of bladder neck or external sphincter to relax appropriately during voiding
- Neurologic
  - Spinal cord injury
  - Stroke
  - Parkinsonism
  - Multiple sclerosis

- Medical
  - Poorly controlled diabetes mellitus
  - Congestive heart failure (CHF)
- Pharmacologic
  - Diuretics
  - Decongestants
  - Anticholinergics
  - Opioids
  - Tricyclic antidepressants
- Other:
  - Bladder carcinoma
  - Overactive bladder
  - Nocturnal polyuria (>33% of the 24-hour urine volume occurs at night)
  - Bladder calculi
  - UTI
  - Prostatitis
  - Urethritis/sexually transmitted infections
  - Obstructive sleep apnea (OSA) (nocturia)
  - Caffeine
  - Polyuria (either isolated nocturnal polyuria or 24-hour polyuria)

DIAGNOSTIC TESTS & INTERPRETATION
Initial Tests (lab, imaging)
- Urinalysis (UA) in all patients presenting with LUTS, can help rule out other etiologies such as bladder stones, cancer, UTI, or urethral strictures
- PSA should be offered to all men with a life expectancy of 10 years and who would be surgical candidates if prostate cancer was identified.
- PSA levels also correlate with prostate volume which can help guide treatment choice.
- With bladder cancer risk factors (smoking history or hematuria) obtain urine cytology
- If nocturia is the main concern, consider using a frequency volume chart for urine output.
- Sleep study if OSA or primary nocturnal polyuria is suspected.
- Serum creatinine measurement is not recommended. (AUA recommendation).

Follow-Up Tests & Special Considerations
- No further testing that is recommended in uncomplicated LUTS; further testing when symptoms that do not respond to medical management or if initial evaluation suggests underlying disease.
- Uroflow: volume voided per unit time (peak flow <10 mL/s is abnormal)
- Postvoid residual: either with catheterization or bladder ultrasound (>100 mL = incomplete emptying)
- Transrectal ultrasound: assessment of gland size; not necessary in the routine evaluation
- Abdominal ultrasound: can demonstrate increased postvoid residual or hydronephrosis; not necessary in the routine evaluation

Diagnostic Procedures/Other
- Pressure-flow studies (urine flow vs. voiding pressures) to determine etiology of symptoms
  - Obstructive pattern shows high voiding pressures with low flow rate.
- Cystoscopy
  - Demonstrates presence, configuration, cause (stricture, stone), and site of obstructive tissue
  - May help determine therapeutic option
  - Not recommended in initial evaluation unless other factors, such as hematuria, are present.

TREATMENT

GENERAL MEASURES
- Treatment ranges from watchful waiting to lifestyle modifications, medications, or surgical management.
- Mild symptoms (score of <7) or moderate symptoms (score 8 to 15) that are non-bothersome require no treatment. Reevaluate annually.
- For moderate to severe symptoms, try lifestyle interventions regulation of fluid intake, avoidance of alcohol and caffeine, exercise, diet, and eliminating/reducing contributing medications.
- Medical treatment requires interval follow-up of 2 to 4 weeks for α-blockers and 3 months for 5-α-reductase inhibitors until symptoms improved, then annually.
- Patients with complications including obstruction and urinary retention require bladder drainage.

MEDICATION
- Should be used as additive therapy, lifestyle modifications are still encouraged.
- Two main classes of medications: α-adrenergic antagonists and 5-α-reductase inhibitors.
- The combination of these two medication classes is effective for long-term management of BPH and demonstrated large prostates.
  - α-Adrenergic antagonists
    - Are the first line option for moderate to severe bothersome LUTS. Affect contraction of smooth muscle in the prostatic urethra and bladder neck. Show benefit over placebo. Typically take 2 to 4 weeks to show improvement. May affect blood pressure; requires dose titration and blood pressure monitoring. AUA recommends alfuzosin (Uroxatral), doxazosin (Cardura), and tamsulosin (Flomax) as they are thought to be more selective and have less effect on blood pressure. Prazosin (Minipress) and phenoxybenzamine (Dibenzyline) have insufficient evidence and are not recommended. Most common adverse effect is dizziness. May cause orthostatic hypotension
      - Doxazosin (**Cardura**): 1 to 8 mg/day PO. May delay the occurrence of acute urinary retention but does not decrease incidence.
      - Tamsulosin (**Flomax**): 0.4 to 0.8 mg/day PO
      - Alfuzosin (Uroxatral): 10 mg/day PO
      - **Terazosin (Hytrin)**: Start at 1 mg PO daily at bedtime, max 20 mg daily.
    - Contraindications:
      - Use caution in patients who are also using phosphodiesterase type 5 inhibitors for erectile dysfunction.
      - Do not use in men pursuing cataract surgery until they are postoperative due to the risk for perioperative floppy iris syndrome.
  - 5-α-reductase inhibitors
    - Block conversion of testosterone to dihydrotestosterone, gradually reduce prostatic volume therefore are of most benefit when prostate volume exceeds 40 mL. Require 6 months to show clinical benefit. Two equally effective options:
      - Finasteride (Proscar): 5 mg/day PO
      - Dutasteride (Avodart): 0.5 mg/day PO
    - Used in patients with refractory hematuria after other causes have been ruled out
    - Should not be used in patients without evidence of enlarged prostates
    - Show reduced risk of acute urinary retention, less need for surgical intervention and less overall incidence of prostate cancer.
    - Side effects include decreased libido and erectile dysfunction.

- A PSA value in a patient taking a **5-α-reductase inhibitors will be artificially low.**
- Combination therapy of α-blocker plus 5-α-reductase inhibitor is equal to α-blocker therapy, but superior to monotherapy among men with large prostates. Combination therapy is superior to monotherapy to prevent progression but increase risk of drug-related adverse events.
- Anticholinergic agents are appropriate for irritative LUTS without an elevated postvoid residual (PVR). Options include Solifenacin (Vesicare), Tolterodine (Detrol LA), or Oxybutynin (Ditropan XL). Should be avoided in patients with PVR >250 mL
- If patient also experiences erectile dysfunction phosphodiesterase-5 inhibitors have been shown to have mild improvement of LUTS. Can use Tadalafil (Cialis): 5 mg/day PO but avoid use in combination with α-blockers or in those with CrCl <30 mL/min.

Geriatric Considerations
Drugs to use with caution: anticholinergics, antihistamines, sympathomimetics, tricyclic antidepressants, opioids

ISSUES FOR REFERRAL
- Moderate or severe LUTS that does not respond to medical management.
- BPH related complications such as recurrent UTIs or hematuria, renal insufficiency, and urinary retention.
- Abnormal PSA or prostate exam
- Any history of urethral trauma or stricture, or neurologic disease of the bladder/urinary system

SURGERY/OTHER PROCEDURES
- Indications for surgery:
  - Urinary retention due to prostatic obstruction, recurrent, no improvement with medications
  - Intractable symptoms due to prostatic obstruction AUA score >8 and symptoms
  - Obstructive uropathy (renal insufficiency)
  - Recurrent or persistent UTIs due to prostatic obstruction
  - Recurrent gross hematuria due to enlarged prostate
  - Bladder calculi
- Surgical procedures: TURP remains the gold standard of surgical procedures; however for select patient populations, there are other options available.
- Common complications of TURP:
  - Bleeding can be significant.
  - TUR syndrome: hyponatremia secondary to absorption of hypotonic irrigation fluid
  - Retrograde ejaculation
  - Urinary incontinence
- Other options include transurethral needle ablation (TUNA) and transurethral microwave thermo-therapy (TUMT), or transurethral incision of the prostate (TUIP). Open prostatectomy is more common when prostate exceeds 100 g. Transurethral laser ablation is an alternative option for patients on anticoagulants.

COMPLEMENTARY & ALTERNATIVE MEDICINE
Saw palmetto (*Serenoa repens*) has been thoroughly studied in a subject in Cochrane review, and did not improve LUTS. Other agents including pygeum, cernilton, and herbs with beta sitosterols have been studied less however no current evidence to support their use. Acupuncture failed to show improvement in LUTS in one clinical trial as well. There are no recommended complementary or alternative treatments for BPH.

ONGOING CARE

Patient Monitoring
- Symptom index (IPSS) monitored every 3 to 12 months.
- DRE yearly
  - PSA yearly: should not be checked while patient is in retention, recently catheterized, or within a week of any surgical procedure to the prostate
  - Consider monitoring PVR, if elevated.

DIET
Avoid large boluses of oral or IV fluids or alcohol intake, caffeine may exacerbate symptoms as well.

PATIENT EDUCATION
National Kidney and Urologic Diseases Information Clearinghouse, Box NKUDIC, Bethesda, MD 20893; 301-468-6345

PROGNOSIS
- Symptoms improve or stabilize in 70–80% of patients.
- 25% of men with LUTS will have persistent storage symptoms after prostatectomy.
- Of men with BPH, 11–33% have occult prostate cancer.

COMPLICATIONS
- Urinary retention (acute or chronic)
- Bladder stones
- Prostatitis
- Hematuria

REFERENCES
1. McVary KT, Roehrborn CG, Avins AL, et al. Update on AUA guideline on the management of benign prostatic hyperplasia. *J Urol*. 2011;185(5):1793–1803.
2. Pearson R, Williams PM. Common questions about the diagnosis and management of benign prostatic hyperplasia. *Am Fam Physician*. 2014; 90(11):769–774.

ADDITIONAL READING
- American Urological Association Guidelines: guideline on the management of benign prostatic hyperplasia (BPH). Updated 2010. www.auanet.org. Accessed 2015.
- Edwards JL. Diagnosis and management of benign prostatic hyperplasia. *Am Fam Physician*. 2008;77(10):1403–1410.

CODES

ICD10
- N40.0 Enlarged prostate without lower urinary tract symptoms
- N40.1 Enlarged prostate with lower urinary tract symptoms

CLINICAL PEARLS
- Although medical therapy has changed the management of BPH, it has only delayed the need for TURP by 10 to 15 years, not eliminated it.
- Urinary retention, obstructive uropathy, recurrent UTIs, elevated PSA, bladder calculi, hematuria, and failure of medical therapy are indications for surgical management of BPH.

PROSTATITIS

Kyle Stephens, DO, MPH • Vincent Lo, MD, FAAFP

 BASICS

DESCRIPTION

- Painful or inflammatory condition affecting the prostate gland with or without bacterial etiology, often characterized by urogenital pain, voiding symptoms, and/or sexual dysfunction
- Significant impact on quality of life
- <10% bacteria-proven infection
- National Institutes of Health's classification
  - *Class I: Acute bacterial prostatitis*: symptomatic with fever, perineal pain, dysuria, and obstructive symptoms; polymorphonuclear leukocytes (PMNL) and bacteria in urine
  - *Class II: Chronic bacterial prostatitis*: symptomatic chronic or recurrent bacterial infection with pain and voiding disturbances; PMNL and bacteria in expressed prostatic secretions (EPS), or urine after prostate massage, or in semen
  - *Class III: Chronic prostatitis/chronic pelvic pain syndrome (CP/CPPS)*
    ○ Inflammatory (Subtype IIIA): chronic symptoms with PMNL in EPS/urine after prostate massage or in semen
    ○ Noninflammatory (Subtype IIIB): chronic symptoms without presence of PMNL in EPS/ urine after prostate massage or in semen
  - *Class IV: Asymptomatic inflammatory prostatitis*: incidental finding during prostate biopsy for infertility, cancer workup; presence of PMNL and/ or bacteria in EPS/urine after prostatic massage or in semen
- System(s) affected: genitourinary, renal, reproductive

EPIDEMIOLOGY

Incidence

- Two million cases annually in the United States
- Predominant age: 30 to 50 years old, sexually active; chronic is more common in those >50 years.
- Bacterial prostatitis occurs more frequently in patients with HIV.

Prevalence

- Affects approximately 8.2% of males (1)
- Lifetime probability of diagnosis >25% (1)
- Accounts for 8% of visits to urologists and 1% of visits to primary care physicians (2)
- Percentage of cases by class: Class I: <1%, Class II: 5–10%, Class III: 80–90%, Class IV: 10% (3)

ETIOLOGY AND PATHOPHYSIOLOGY

- Acute bacterial prostatitis (Class I)
  - Likely, etiology from ascending urethral infection with intraprostatic reflux of infected urine into prostatic ducts, often associated with cystitis
  - Can occur after instrumentation of prostate
  - Usually gram-negative bacteria (*Escherichia coli* (most common); *Proteus, Klebsiella, Serratia,* and *Enterobacter* species; *Pseudomonas aeruginosa*)
  - Rarely, gram-positive bacteria (*Staphylococcus aureus, Streptococcus,* and *Enterococcus* species).
  - Confirmed *Staphylococcal* prostatitis should warrant evaluation for hematogenous spread, including endovascular source.
  - Atypical bacteria include *Chlamydia trachomatis, Trichomonas vaginalis,* and *Ureaplasma urealyticum.*
  - Consider *Neisseria gonorrhoeae* or *Chlamydia trachomatis* in sexually active men <35 years.

- Chronic bacterial prostatitis (class II)
  - Similar pathogens as discussed earlier
  - Often occurs as recurrent episodes of infection by same organism
  - Progression from acute to chronic prostatitis is poorly understood but could result from inadequate treatment of acute prostatitis.
- CP/CPPS (class III)
  - Unclear etiology, possibly due to difficult-to-culture infection
  - Inciting agent may cause inflammation or neurological damage in or around the prostate and lead to pelvic floor neuromuscular and/or neuropathic pain.

RISK FACTORS

- Urinary tract infections
- HIV infection
- Prostatic calculi
- Urethral stricture
- Urinary catheterization: indwelling, intermittent
- Genitourinary instrumentation including prostate biopsy (especially in patients with prior quinolone intake), transurethral resection of prostate, cystoscopy
- Urinary retention
- Benign prostatic hypertrophy
- Unprotected sexual intercourse
- Trauma (e.g. bicycle, horseback riding)

GENERAL PREVENTION

Antibiotic prophylaxis for genitourinary instrumentation and prostatic biopsy

COMMONLY ASSOCIATED CONDITIONS

- Benign prostatic hypertrophy
- Cystitis
- Urethritis
- Sexual dysfunction

 DIAGNOSIS

HISTORY

- Acute prostatitis (class I):
  - Acutely ill with fever, chills, malaise
  - Low back pain, myalgias
  - Frequency, urgency, dysuria, nocturia
  - Prostatodynia, pelvic pain, perineal pain
  - Cloudy urine
  - Obstructive voiding symptoms: poor stream, hesitancy
- Chronic prostatitis (classes II and III):
  - More insidious presentation than Class I
  - Symptoms for 3 of 6 previous months
  - Low-grade fever (class II only)
  - Prostatodynia, perineal pain
  - Dysuria, frequency, urgency
  - Lower abdominal pain
  - Low back, testicular, and/or penile pain
  - Hematospermia
  - Sexual dysfunction/painful ejaculation

PHYSICAL EXAM

- Vital signs (unstable vitals suggest sepsis)
- Back exam (CVA tenderness)
- Abdominal exam (bladder distension)

- Prostate exam
  - Class I: Prostate is very tender, warm, firm, edematous.
  - Class II: Often normal but enlarged, tender, edematous, nodular prostate also encountered
  - Class III: Often normal prostate

ALERT

Avoid vigorous massage of the prostate in acute bacterial prostatitis; may induce iatrogenic bacteremia, safe if done gently

DIFFERENTIAL DIAGNOSIS

- Lower urinary tract infection
- Pyelonephritis
- Cystitis (bacterial, interstitial)
- Urethritis
- Prostatic abscess
- Acute/chronic urinary retention
- Benign prostatic hypertrophy Malignancy (prostate, bladder)
- Obstructive calculi
- Foreign body

DIAGNOSTIC TESTS & INTERPRETATION

Initial Tests (lab, imaging)

- Suspected acute prostatitis (Class I)
  - Urinalysis; urine Gram stain/culture and sensitivity
  - CBC with differential; blood culture if fever, chills, or signs of sepsis are present
- Suspected chronic bacterial prostatitis (class II)
  - Urinalysis; urine/EPS/semen: Gram stain/culture and sensitivity
  - Review previous urine culture results.
  - National Institute of Health—Chronic Prostatitis Symptom Index (NIH-CPSI): 9-question symptom survey (http://www.prostatitis.org/symptomindex.html)
  - Diagnostic gold standard: Meares-Stamey 4-glass test (not performed often)
  - 2-glass test (pre- and postmassage urine testing) more common and easier with equivalent sensitivity and specificity (4)
    ○ Cultures of mid-stream preprostate massage urine and EPS/postmassage urine
  - Consider urinary flow rate and postvoid residual volume if urinary retention is present.
- Suspected CP/CPPS (class III)
  - Diagnosis of exclusion
  - Urinalysis; urine/EPS/semen: Gram stain/culture and sensitivity
  - Hematuria if present: urine cytology, cystoscopy, CT urography with or without contrast
  - PSA is not indicated unless malignancy is suspected.
  - Concomitant abdominal pain: CT abdomen
  - Testicular pain: scrotal US
  - Sensation of incomplete bladder emptying: postvoid residual volume with bladder US or catheterization
  - Lumbar radiculopathy: MRI spine

Follow-Up Tests & Special Considerations

- Failure to respond to initial antibiotic therapy: US, CT, or MRI to image prostate and urology referral
- US or CT or MRI if prostatic calculi, malignancy, or abscess are suspected
- Acute bacterial: urinalysis and culture 30 days after initiating treatment
- Chronic bacterial: urinalysis and culture every 30 days (may take several months of treatment to clear)

Diagnostic Procedures/Other
- Needle biopsy or aspiration for culture
- Urodynamic testing (prostatodynia) if indicated
- Cystoscopy (in persistent nonbacterial prostatitis to rule out bladder cancer, interstitial cystitis)

TREATMENT

GENERAL MEASURES
- Analgesics/antipyretics/stool softeners
- Hydration
- Sitz baths to relieve pain and spasm
- Suprapubic catheter for urinary retention
- Anxiolytics, antidepressants if anxiety and/or depression are present

MEDICATION
First Line
- Acute bacterial (outpatient) (3)[A]
  - Fluoroquinolone (ciprofloxacin 500 mg PO q12h or levofloxacin 500 mg PO once daily) for 2 to 4 weeks *or*
  - Trimethoprim-sulfamethoxazole 1 double-strength tab PO q12h for 2 to 4 weeks *or*
  - If gram-positive cocci are seen in initial urine Gram stain, start with amoxicillin 500 mg PO q8h. Adjust antibiotics once culture and sensitivities report is available.
  - Local sensitivity pattern should guide therapy.
  - Ceftriaxone 250 mg IM 1 dose plus doxycycline 100 mg PO q12h daily for 1 week or (azithromycin 1 g PO single dose if at risk for sexually transmitted infection (STI) pathogens

- Acute bacterial (inpatient) (3)[A]
  - Ampicillin 2g IV q6h or fluoroquinolone (ciprofloxacin 400 mg IV q12h or levofloxacin 500 mg q24h); begin oral therapy after afebrile for 24 to 48 hours

- Chronic bacterial (class II) (3,5,6)[A],(7)[C]
  - Fluoroquinolone (e.g., levofloxacin 500 mg PO) once daily for 4 weeks or ciprofloxacin 500 mg PO q12h for 4 to 12 weeks
  - Combination therapy with azithromycin may help to eradicate atypical pathogens.
  - Anti-inflammatory agents for pain symptoms and α-blockers for urinary symptoms

- CP/CPPS (class III) (8,9)[A],(7)[C]
  - No universally effective treatment
  - Treatment choice is patient-centered focusing on symptoms relief of four domains: pain, lower urinary tract symptoms (LUTS), psychological stress, and sexual dysfunction.
    - α-Blockers, antibiotics, and combinations of these therapies achieve greatest improvement in clinical symptoms scores compared to placebo.
    - Tamsulosin 0.4 mg PO once daily at bedtime for 4 to 6 weeks. Continue if there is a positive response.

Second Line
- Piperacillin or ticarcillin with aminoglycoside, erythromycin, tetracycline, cephalexin, fluoroquinolones, (dicloxacillin, nafcillin IV, vancomycin IV
- Finasteride (in patients >45 years, class IIIA, and enlarged prostate glands)
- Atypical: may benefit from erythromycin, doxycycline

ISSUES FOR REFERRAL
Urology referral if antibiotic treatment fails, symptoms persist (especially obstructive voiding symptoms), hematuria, elevated PSA, or for surgical drainage if an abscess persists after ≥1 week of therapy

ADDITIONAL THERAPIES
- Psychotherapy if sexual dysfunction is present
- 5-α-reductase inhibitors, nonsteroidal anti-inflammatory medications, pelvic floor physical therapy, transurethral microwave thermotherapy (7)[C]

SURGERY/OTHER PROCEDURES
Surgical resection for intractable chronic disease or to drain an abscess (7)[C]

COMPLEMENTARY & ALTERNATIVE MEDICINE
Class III: Acupuncture, phytotherapies (pollen extract, quercetin), heat therapy, and myofascial release have limited data to support (7)[C],(10)[A].

INPATIENT CONSIDERATIONS
Admission Criteria/Initial Stabilization
- Proven or suspected abscess
- Unstable vital signs (sepsis)
- Immunocompromised
- Failed outpatient treatment

ONGOING CARE

FOLLOW-UP RECOMMENDATIONS
- Negative urine culture at 7 days predictive of cure after completion of treatment course
- Consider prostatic abscess in patients who do not respond well to therapy.

Patient Monitoring
NIH Chronic Prostatitis Symptom Index (NIH-CPSI): 9 questions, which can be used to evaluate severity of patient symptoms and response to treatment within three domains:
- Pain
- Urinary symptoms
- Quality of life

PROGNOSIS
- Fever and dysuria usually resolve in 2 to 6 days.
- Acute infection usually improves in 3 to 4 weeks.
- Course of chronic prostatitis is often prolonged and difficult to cure; 55–97% cure rate depending on population and drug used
- 20% have reinfection or persistent infection.

COMPLICATIONS
- Prostatic abscess (common in HIV-infected)
- Pyelonephritis
- Gram-negative sepsis, bacteremia
- Urinary retention
- Epididymitis
- Infertility
- Chronic bacterial prostatitis (following acute prostatitis)
- Metastatic infection (spinal, sacroiliac)

REFERENCES

1. Krieger JN, Lee SW, Jeon J, et al. Epidemiology of prostatitis. *Int J Antimicrob Agents*. 2008;31(Suppl 1):S85–S90.
2. Collins MM, Stafford RS, O'Leary MP, et al. How common is prostatitis? A national survey of physician visits. *J Urol*. 1998;159(4):1224–1228.
3. Lipsky BA, Byren I, Hoey CT. Treatment of bacterial prostatitis. *Clin Infect Dis*. 2010;50(12):1641–1652.
4. Nickel JC, Shoskes D, Wang Y, et al. How does the pre-massage and post-massage 2-glass test compare to the Meares-Stamey 4-glass test in men with chronic prostatitis/chronic pelvic pain syndrome? *J Urol*. 2006;176(1):119–124.
5. Videčnik Zorman J, Matičič M, Jeverica S, et al. Diagnosis and treatment of bacterial prostatitis. *Acta Dermatovenerol Alp Pannonica Adriat*. 2015;24(2):25–29.
6. Perletti G, Marras E, Wagenlehner FM, et al. Antimicrobial therapy for chronic bacterial prostatitis. *Cochrane Database Syst Rev*. 2013;(8):CD009071.
7. Rees J, Abrahams M, Doble A, et al. Diagnosis and treatment of chronic bacterial prostatitis and chronic prostatitis/chronic pelvic pain syndrome: a consensus guideline. *BJU Int*. 2015;116(4):509–525. doi:10.1111/bju.13101.
8. Zhu Y, Wang C, Pang X, et al. Antibiotics are not beneficial in the management of category III prostatitis: a meta analysis. *Urol J*. 2014;11(2):1377–1385.
9. Anothaisintawee T, Attia J, Nickel JC, et al. Management of chronic prostatitis/chronic pelvic pain syndrome: a systematic review and network meta-analysis. *JAMA*. 2011;305(1):78–86.
10. Anderson RU, Wise D, Sawyer T, et al. 6-day intensive treatment protocol for refractory chronic prostatitis/chronic pelvic pain syndrome using myofascial release and paradoxical relaxation training. *J Urol*. 2011;185(4):1294–1299.

SEE ALSO

- Prostate Cancer; Prostatic Hyperplasia, Benign (BPH); Urinary Tract Infection (UTI) in Males
- Algorithm: Hematuria

CODES

ICD10
- N41.9 Inflammatory disease of prostate, unspecified
- N41.0 Acute prostatitis
- N41.1 Chronic prostatitis

CLINICAL PEARLS

- Vigorous prostatic massage is contraindicated in acute prostatitis.
- Antibiotic therapy is not proven to be effective in CP/CPPS (Class III) (8).
- At least 14 to 30 days of antibiotic therapy is required for acute prostatitis; longer for chronic bacterial prostatitis
- Imaging is often not needed.

PROTEIN C DEFICIENCY

Elie Chalhoub, MD • Dalia Hammoud, MD • Maissaa Janbain, MD

BASICS

DESCRIPTION
- Protein C is a vitamin K–dependent factor made by the liver that becomes activated when thrombin binds to the endothelial receptor thrombomodulin.
- Activated protein C, with protein S as a cofactor, inactivates factors Va and VIIIa.
- Patients with protein C deficiency have a thrombotic disorder that primarily affects the venous system but can also affect the arterial system.
- System(s) affected: cardiovascular, hemic/lymphatic/immunologic, pulmonary

EPIDEMIOLOGY
Prevalence
- 0.3% of normal individuals
- 4–5% of persons with venous thrombosis (VT)
- Predominant age: Mean age of first thrombosis is 45 years.
- Predominant sex: male = female

ETIOLOGY AND PATHOPHYSIOLOGY
- Polymorphisms in the promoter region of the protein C gene can affect antigen levels. At least 150 mutations have been described in the protein C gene that can lead to functional deficiency.
- New mutations have been described associated with late-onset cerebral thrombosis (1).
- Acquired protein C deficiency can occur with liver disease, ARDS, DIC, chemotherapy with L-asparaginase, 5-FU, methotrexate, and cyclophosphamide, as well as postoperative state and severe infections, especially meningococcemia. Also, rare patients can develop inhibitors to activated protein C. Neonates have lower levels of protein C than adults.

Genetics
Patients heterozygous for protein C deficiency who start warfarin without concomitant heparin can develop warfarin-induced skin necrosis because the half-life of other vitamin K–dependent clotting factors, prothrombin, factor IX, and factor X is much longer than that of protein C (4 to 8 hours). These patients develop extremely low levels of protein C and subsequently increased thrombin generation, leading to necrosis of the skin over central areas of the body such as the breast, abdomen, buttocks, and genitalia (2)[A].

GENERAL PREVENTION
Because protein C deficiency is a congenital disease, there are no preventive measures.

COMMONLY ASSOCIATED CONDITIONS
- Deep and superficial venous thrombosis, often spontaneous
- Up to 50% of homozygotes will have thrombosis.
- Homozygosity is associated with catastrophic thrombotic complications at birth (e.g., *purpura fulminans*).
- Sites of thrombosis can be unusual, including the mesentery and cerebral veins, especially when combined with other risk factors such as oral contraceptives.
- Arterial thrombosis is rare.
- Skin necrosis can be seen in patients on warfarin.
- Recurrent pregnancy losses

DIAGNOSIS

HISTORY
- VT at <40 years of age without another etiology
- Thrombosis in unusual locations (e.g., mesentery, sagittal sinus, portal vein)
- Family history of thrombosis or spontaneous abortion

PHYSICAL EXAM
Normal

DIFFERENTIAL DIAGNOSIS
- Factor V Leiden (causes resistance to activated protein C, not a deficiency of protein C)
- Protein S deficiency
- Antithrombin deficiency
- Dysfibrinogenemia
- Dysplasminogenemia
- Homocystinemia
- Prothrombin 20210 mutation
- Elevated factor VIII levels

DIAGNOSTIC TESTS & INTERPRETATION
Initial Tests (lab, imaging)
- For evaluation of new clot in patient at risk (see "History"): CBC with peripheral smear, PT/INR, aPTT, thrombin time, lupus anticoagulant, antiphospholipid antibodies, factor VIII, anticardiolipin antibody, anti-β_2-glycoprotein I antibody, activated protein C resistance, protein S antigen and resistance, antithrombin III assay, fibrinogen, factor V Leiden, prothrombin G20210A, homocysteine
- Protein C activity assay using a snake venom protease to activate protein C
- Immunoassay for quantitative assessment of protein C level
- Drugs that may alter lab results
  - Oral contraceptives can raise protein C levels.
  - Warfarin reduces protein C levels.
  - Patients should be off warfarin for 2 to 3 weeks before reliable testing (3)[C].
- Disorders that may alter lab results
  - Liver disease reduces protein C levels.

ALERT
Acute thrombosis can lower protein C levels. Repeat confirmatory test of low protein C level at a separate time is advisable. If a normal level of protein C is obtained at presentation, then deficiency can be excluded.

TREATMENT

Treat active thrombosis; follow-up.

GENERAL MEASURES
- Routine anticoagulation for asymptomatic patients with protein C deficiency is not recommended (2)[A].
- Anticoagulation for 6 to 12 months is recommended for patients with protein C deficiency and a first thrombosis.
- Some argue for lifetime anticoagulation; data are limited.
- Anticoagulation for life is indicated for patients with protein C deficiency and recurrent thromboses.
- The role of family screening for protein C deficiency is unclear because most patients with this mutation do not have thrombosis. Screening should be considered for women considering using oral contraceptives or pregnancy and who have a family history of protein C deficiency (4)[B].
- Treatment with LMWH is recommended over unfractionated heparin, unless the patient has severe renal failure (5)[B].
- Treat as outpatient, if possible (5)[B].
- Initiate warfarin together with LMWH on the first treatment day, and discontinue LMWH after minimum of 5 days and two consecutive INRs >2 (5)[A].
- For pregnant women with no prior history of venous thromboembolism (VTE), we suggest antepartum and postpartum clinical vigilance. Postpartum prophylaxis for 6 weeks with prophylactic- or intermediate-dose LMWH is reserved only for patients with positive family history of VTE (3)[C],(5).

MEDICATION
First Line
- Low-molecular-weight heparin (LMWH) (2)[A]: initially for a minimum of 5 days and two consecutive INRs between 2 and 3
  - Enoxaparin (Lovenox) 1 mg/kg SC BID or enoxaparin 1.5 mg/kg/day SC
  - Tinzaparin (Innohep): 175 anti-Xa IU/kg/day SC
  - Dalteparin (Fragmin) 200 U/kg/day
- Factor Xa inhibitors
  - Fondaparinux (Arixtra) <50 kg: 5 mg/day SC; 50 to 100 kg: 7.5 mg/day SC; >100 kg: 10 mg/day SC; contraindicated if CrCl <30 mL/min

- Oral vitamin K antagonist: warfarin (Coumadin), per the most recent chest guidelines, 5mg/day PO then adjusted to an INR of 2 to 3 for at least 3 to 6 months (2)[A],(5)
- Novel oral anticoagulants (NOACs):
  - Dabigatran 150 mg PO BID (after 5 to 10 days of parenteral anticoagulation)
  - Rivaroxaban 15 mg PO BID for 21 days then 20 mg PO QD
  - Apixaban 10 mg PO BID for 7 days then 5 mg PO BID
  - Edoxaban 60 mg PO QD (after 5 to 10 days of parenteral anticoagulation)
- Contraindications
  - Active bleeding precludes anticoagulation; risk of bleeding is a relative contraindication to long-term anticoagulation.
  - Warfarin is contraindicated in patients with a prior history of warfarin-induced skin necrosis.
- Precautions
  - Observe patient for signs of embolization, further thrombosis, or bleeding.
  - Avoid IM injections.
  - Periodically, check stool and urine for occult blood; monitor CBC, including platelets.
  - Heparin: thrombocytopenia and/or paradoxical thrombosis with thrombocytopenia
  - Warfarin: necrotic skin lesions (typically breasts, thighs, and buttocks)
  - LMWH: Adjust dose in renal insufficiency.
- Significant possible interactions
  - Agents that intensify the response to oral anticoagulants: alcohol, allopurinol, amiodarone, anabolic steroids, androgens, many antimicrobials, cimetidine, chloral hydrate, disulfiram, all NSAIDs, sulfinpyrazone, tamoxifen, thyroid hormone, vitamin E, ranitidine, salicylates, acetaminophen
  - Agents that diminish the response to oral anticoagulants: aminoglutethimide, antacids, barbiturates, carbamazepine, cholestyramine, diuretics, griseofulvin, rifampin, oral contraceptives

Second Line
- Heparin 80 mg/kg IV bolus followed by 18 mg/kg/hr; adjust dose depending on PPT.
- In patients requiring large daily doses of heparin, measure an anti-Xa level for dose guidance.
- Alternatively, and for outpatients, unfractionated heparin can be given at 333 U/kg then 250 U/kg SC, without monitoring (5)[C].

ISSUES FOR REFERRAL
Patients with suspected protein C deficiency should be seen by a hematologist.

However, screening and therefore prophylactic treatment of asymptomatic family members is not justified (6).

SURGERY/OTHER PROCEDURES
- Anticoagulation must be held for surgical interventions.

- In patients with acute proximal DVT of the leg *and* an absolute contraindication to anticoagulation, inferior vena cava (IVC) filters are recommended; otherwise, the use of an IVC filter in addition to anticoagulants is not recommended in most patients with acute DVT of the leg (2)[B],(5).

INPATIENT CONSIDERATIONS
Admission Criteria/Initial Stabilization
- Life-threatening VT
- Significant bleeding while on anticoagulant therapy

Nursing
Look for signs of bleeding while on anticoagulation therapy.

ONGOING CARE

FOLLOW-UP RECOMMENDATIONS
Patient Monitoring
- Warfarin requires periodic (monthly after initial stabilization) monitoring of the INR to maintain a range of 2 to 3.
- LMWH is the treatment of choice in pregnancy. Periodic monitoring with anti-Xa levels is recommended in these patients.

DIET
Unrestricted (except if on warfarin—avoid food with significant amounts of vitamin K)

PATIENT EDUCATION
- Patients should be educated about the use of oral anticoagulant therapy if taking such.
- Avoid NSAIDs while on warfarin.
- Avoid OCPs, as they increase risk of thrombosis.

PROGNOSIS
- When compared with normal individuals, persons with protein C deficiency have normal life spans.
- By age 45 years, 50% of the people heterozygous for protein C deficiency will have VT; half will be spontaneous.

COMPLICATIONS
Recurrent thrombosis (requires indefinite anticoagulation)

REFERENCES
1. Yang LH, Wang MS, Zheng FX, et al. Different impact of two mutations of a novel compound heterozygous protein C deficiency with late onset thrombosis. *Genet Mol Res*. 2014;13(2):2969–2977.
2. Bick RL. Prothrombin G20210A mutation, antithrombin, heparin cofactor II, protein C, and protein S defects. *Hematol Oncol Clin North Am*. 2003;17(1):9–36.
3. Moll S. Thrombophilias—practical implications and testing caveats. *J Thromb Thrombolysis*. 2006;21(1):7–15.
4. Langlois NJ, Wells PS. Risk of venous thrombo-embolism in relatives of symptomatic probands with thrombophilia: a systematic review. *Thromb Haemost*. 2003;90(1):17–26.
5. Guyatt GH, Akl EA, Crowther M, et al. Executive summary: Antithrombotic Therapy and Prevention of Thrombosis, 9th ed: American College of Chest Physicians Evidence-Based Clinical Practice Guidelines. *Chest*. 2012;141(Suppl 2):7S–47S.
6. Hornsby LB, Armstrong EM, Bellone JM, et al. Thrombophilia screening. *J Pharm Pract*. 2014;27(3):253–259.

CODES

ICD10
D68.59 Other primary thrombophilia

CLINICAL PEARLS
- Asymptomatic patients with protein C deficiency do not need prophylactic anticoagulation because the risk of thrombosis is low (6).
- Patients with protein C deficiency who have DVT should be anticoagulated for at least 6 months.

PROTEIN S DEFICIENCY

Dalia Hammoud, MD • Elie Chalhoub, MD • Maissaa Janbain, MD

 BASICS

DESCRIPTION
- Protein S is a vitamin K–dependent factor made principally by the liver that acts as a cofactor for protein C.
- Protein C becomes activated when thrombin binds to the endothelial receptor, thrombomodulin.
- Activated protein C, with protein S as a cofactor, inactivates clotting factors Va and VIIIa, and it enhances fibrinolysis.
- Protein S is also able to directly inhibit factors Va, VIIa, and Xa independently of activated protein C.
- Patients with protein S deficiency have a thrombotic disorder that primarily affects the venous system.
- System(s) affected: cardiovascular; hematologic/lymphatic/immunologic; pulmonary

EPIDEMIOLOGY
Incidence
- Predominant age: Mean age of first thrombosis is the 2nd decade of life.
- Predominant sex: male = female

Prevalence
- 0.3% of normal individuals
- Found in 3% of persons with VT

ETIOLOGY AND PATHOPHYSIOLOGY
- >131 mutations in the protein S gene leading to an inherited protein S deficiency have been described. Protein S reversibly binds to the C4b-binding protein. Only the free form acts as a cofactor for activated protein C. This leads to conditions in which free protein S is low, but total protein S is normal. These individuals are prone to thrombosis.
- Acquired protein S deficiency from decreased free protein S can occur during pregnancy; in patients taking oral contraceptives or warfarin; and in DIC, liver disease, nephrotic syndrome, inflammation, L-asparaginase chemotherapy, and acute thrombosis.
- Transient autoantibodies can develop to protein S in patients with acute varicella (1)[C].

Genetics
Autosomal dominant. Heterozygotes have an odds ratio (OR) of venous thrombosis (VT) of 1.6 to 11.5. Arterial thrombosis is more frequent in patients with protein S deficiency who smoke. Homozygotes can have a fulminant thrombotic event in infancy, termed *neonatal purpura fulminans*. Homozygosity or compound heterozygosity, if untreated, is usually incompatible with adult life.

RISK FACTORS
- Oral contraceptives, pregnancy, and the use of HRT increase the risk of VT in patients with protein S deficiency (2)[A].
- Patients with protein S deficiency and another prothrombotic state, such as factor V Leiden, have further increased rate of thrombosis (2)[A].
- Patients heterozygous for protein S deficiency who are initiated on warfarin without concomitant heparin can develop warfarin-induced skin necrosis because the half-life of other vitamin K–dependent clotting factors (e.g., prothrombin, factor IX, and factor X) is much longer than the anticoagulant protein S (4 to 8 hours), leading to a transient hypercoagulable state when protein S becomes depleted. These patients develop extremely low levels of protein S and develop necrosis of the skin over central areas of the body such as the breast, abdomen, buttocks, and genitalia (2)[A].

Pregnancy Considerations
Increased thrombotic risk in patients with protein C deficiency

GENERAL PREVENTION
Because protein S deficiency is a congenital disease, there are no preventive measures.

COMMONLY ASSOCIATED CONDITIONS
- Deep and superficial VT, often spontaneous
- Up to 50% of homozygotes will have thrombosis.
- Homozygosity is associated with catastrophic thrombotic complications at birth: *neonatal purpura fulminans*
- Sites of thrombosis can be unusual, including the mesentery, cerebral veins, and axillary veins.
- Arterial thrombosis is rare, but reported in several case reports.
- Skin necrosis can be seen in patients on warfarin.
- Recurrent pregnancy losses (3).

 DIAGNOSIS

HISTORY
Order testing for patients with VT at age <40 years without another etiology; thrombosis in unusual locations (e.g., mesentery, sagittal sinus, portal vein) with a family history of thrombosis or spontaneous abortion

PHYSICAL EXAM
Normal

DIFFERENTIAL DIAGNOSIS
- Factor V Leiden
- Protein C deficiency
- Antithrombin deficiency
- Dysfibrinogenemia
- Dysplasminogenemia
- Homocysteinemia
- Prothrombin 20210 mutation
- Elevated factor VIII levels

DIAGNOSTIC TESTS & INTERPRETATION
Initial Tests (lab, imaging)
- For evaluation of new clot in patient at risk: CBC with peripheral smear, PT/INR, aPTT, thrombin time, lupus anticoagulant, antiphospholipid antibodies, factor VIII, anticardiolipin antibody, anti-β_2-glycoprotein I antibody, activated protein C resistance, protein S antigen and resistance, antithrombin III assay, fibrinogen, factor V Leiden, prothrombin G20210A, homocysteine
- Protein S activity assay (mainly after obtaining APC resistance)
- Immunoassay for quantitative assessment of total and free protein S levels. Test off vitamin K antagonists.
- Disorders that may alter lab results: Liver disease and pregnancy-reduce protein S levels.
- Total protein S levels are markedly decreased in newborns and young infants; use age-adjusted norms.

TREATMENT

GENERAL MEASURES
- Routine anticoagulation for asymptomatic patients with protein S deficiency is not recommended (2)[A].
- Anticoagulation for 6 to 12 months is recommended for patients with protein S deficiency and a first thrombosis.
- Some argue for lifetime anticoagulation; data are limited.
- Anticoagulation for life is indicated for patients with protein S deficiency and recurrent thrombosis.
- The role of family screening for protein S deficiency is unclear because most patients with this mutation do not have thrombosis. Screening should be considered for women considering oral contraceptives or pregnancy, and who have a family history of protein S deficiency (4)[B].
- Treatment of thrombosis with LMWH is recommended over unfractionated heparin, unless the patient has severe renal failure (5)[B].
- Treat as outpatient, if possible (5)[B].
- Initiate warfarin together with LMWH on the first treatment day, and discontinue LMWH after a minimum of 5 days and two consecutive INRs >2 (5)[A].

- For pregnant women with no prior history of VTE, we suggest antepartum and postpartum clinical vigilance. Postpartum prophylaxis is reserved for patients with positive family history only; in that case, we suggest prophylactic- or intermediate-dose LMWH for 6 weeks (1)[C],(5).

MEDICATION

First Line

- Low-molecular-weight heparin (LMWH) (2)[A] initially for a minimum of 5 days and two consecutive INRs between 2 and 3, at which time it can be stopped

  – Enoxaparin (Lovenox) 1 mg/kg SC BID:
    ○ Alternatively, 1.5 mg/kg/day SC
  – Tinzaparin (Innohep) 175 anti-Xa IU/kg/day SC
  – Dalteparin (Fragmin) 200 IU/kg/day
- Factor Xa Inhibitor
  – Fondaparinux (Arixtra) <50 kg: 5 mg/day SC; 50 to 100 kg: 7.5 mg/day SC; >100 kg: 10 mg/day SC; contraindicated if CrCl <30 mL/min
- Oral anticoagulant: warfarin (Coumadin): 5 mg/day PO then adjusted to an INR of 2 to 3 for at least 6 months (5)[A]
- Novel oral anticoagulants (NOACs) (6):
  – Dabigatran 150 mg po BID (after 5 to 10 days of parenteral anticoagulation)
  – Rivaroxaban 15 mg po BID for 21 days then 20 mg PO QID
  – Apixaban 10 mg PO BID for 7 days then 5 mg PO BID
  – Edoxaban 60 mg PO QID (after 5 to 10 days of parenteral anticoagulation)
- Contraindications
  – Active bleeding precludes anticoagulation; risk of bleeding is a relative contraindication to long-term anticoagulation.
  – Warfarin is contraindicated in patients with a prior history of warfarin-induced skin necrosis.
- Precautions
  – Observe patient for signs of embolization, further thrombosis, or bleeding.
  – Avoid IM injections.
  – Periodically, check stool and urine for occult blood; monitor CBC, including platelets.
  – Heparin: thrombocytopenia and/or paradoxical thrombosis with thrombocytopenia
  – Warfarin: necrotic skin lesions (typically breasts, thighs, and buttocks)
  – LMWH: Adjust dose in renal insufficiency.
- Significant possible interactions
  – Agents that intensify the response to oral anticoagulants: alcohol, allopurinol, amiodarone, anabolic steroids, androgens, many antimicrobials, cimetidine, chloral hydrate, disulfiram, all NSAIDs, sulfinpyrazone, tamoxifen, thyroid hormone, vitamin E, ranitidine, salicylates, acetaminophen

  – Agents that diminish the response to oral anticoagulants: aminoglutethimide, antacids, barbiturates, carbamazepine, cholestyramine, diuretics, griseofulvin, rifampin, oral contraceptives

Second Line

Heparin 80 mg/kg IV bolus, followed by 18 mg/kg/hr; adjust dose depending on aPTT:

- In patients requiring large daily doses of heparin, measure an anti-Xa level for dose guidance.
- Alternatively, in outpatients, unfractionated heparin can be given at 333 units/kg then 250 units/kg SC, without monitoring (5)[C].
- It does not alter plasma protein S concentration.

ISSUES FOR REFERRAL

- Patients with suspected protein S deficiency should be seen by a hematologist.
- Screening and prophylactic treatment of asymptomatic family members is not justified (7).

SURGERY/OTHER PROCEDURES

- Anticoagulation must be held for surgical interventions.
- For most patients with DVT, recommendations are against routine use of vena cava filter in addition to anticoagulation; IVC filter is only recommended in case of contraindication to anticoagulation (5)[A].

INPATIENT CONSIDERATIONS

Admission Criteria/Initial Stabilization

- Life-threatening VT
- Significant bleeding while on anticoagulant therapy

Nursing

Look for signs of bleeding while on anticoagulation therapy.

ONGOING CARE

FOLLOW-UP RECOMMENDATIONS

Patient Monitoring

- Warfarin requires periodic (monthly after initial stabilization) monitoring of the INR.
- Periodic measurement of INR to maintain a range of 2 to 3.
- LMWH is the treatment of choice in pregnancy. Periodic monitoring with anti-Xa levels is recommended in some cases, such as overweight and borderline renal failure.

DIET

Unrestricted

PATIENT EDUCATION

- Patients should be educated about use of oral anticoagulant therapy if taking such.
- Patients undergoing warfarin therapy should avoid drinking alcohol on a daily basis.
- Avoid NSAIDs while on warfarin.

PROGNOSIS

- Persons with protein S deficiency have normal lifespan.
- By age 45 years, 50% of the people heterozygous for protein S deficiency will have VT; half will be spontaneous.

COMPLICATIONS

Recurrent thrombosis (requires indefinite anticoagulation)

REFERENCES

1. Moll S. Thrombophilias—practical implications and testing caveats. *J Thromb Thrombolysis*. 2006;21(1):7–15.
2. Bick RL. Prothrombin G20210A mutation, antithrombin, heparin cofactor II, protein C, and protein S defects. *Hematol Oncol Clin North Am*. 2003;17(1):9–36.
3. Parand A, Zolghadri J, Nezam M, et al. Inherited thrombophilia and recurrent pregnancy loss. *Iran Red Crescent Med J*. 2013;15(12):e13708.
4. Langlois NJ, Wells PS. Risk of venous thromboembolism in relatives of symptomatic probands with thrombophilia: a systematic review. *Thromb Haemost*. 2003;90(1):17–26.
5. Guyatt GH, Akl EA, Crowther M, et al. Executive summary: Antithrombotic Therapy and Prevention of Thrombosis, 9th ed: American College of Chest Physicians Evidence-Based Clinical Practice Guidelines. *Chest*. 2012;141(2)(Suppl):7S–47S.
6. Agnelli G, Buller HR, Cohen A, et al. Oral apixaban for the treatment of acute venous thromboembolism. *N Engl J Med*. 2013;369(9):799–808.
7. Hornsby LB, Armstrong EM, Bellone JM, et al. Thrombophilia screening. *J Pharm Pract*. 2014;27(3):253–259.

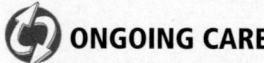 **CODES**

ICD10

D68.59 Other primary thrombophilia

CLINICAL PEARLS

- Asymptomatic patients with protein S deficiency do not require prophylactic anticoagulation because the risk of thrombosis is low; asymptomatic patients do not require anticoagulation (6).
- Patients with protein S deficiency and DVT should be anticoagulated for at least 6 months, especially if first episode.

PROTEINURIA

Andrew S. Allegretti, MD

 BASICS

DESCRIPTION
Urinary protein excretion of >150 mg/day
- Nephrotic-range proteinuria: urinary protein excretion of >3.5 g/day; also called *heavy proteinuria*
- Three pathologic types:
  - Glomerular proteinuria: increased permeability of proteins across glomerular capillary membrane
  - Tubular proteinuria: decreased proximal tubular reabsorption of proteins
  - Overflow proteinuria: increased production of low-molecular-weight proteins

Pediatric Considerations
- Proteinuria: Normal is daily excretion of up to 100 mg/m^2 (body surface area).
- Nephrotic-range proteinuria: daily excretion of >1,000 mg/m^2 (body surface area)

Pregnancy Considerations
- Proteinuria in pregnancy beyond 20 weeks' gestation is a hallmark of preeclampsia/eclampsia and demands further workup.
- Proteinuria in pregnancy before 20 weeks' gestation is suggestive of underlying renal disease.

ETIOLOGY AND PATHOPHYSIOLOGY
- Glomerular proteinuria: increased filtration/larger proteins (albumin) due to the following:
  - Increased size of glomerular basement membrane pores and
  - Loss of proteoglycan negative charge barrier
- Tubular proteinuria: Tubulointerstitial disease prevents proximal tubular reabsorption of smaller proteins (β_2-microglobulin, immunoglobulin [Ig] light chains, retinol-binding protein, amino acids).
- Overflow proteinuria: proximal tubular reabsorption overwhelmed by increased production of smaller proteins
- Glomerular proteinuria
  - Primary glomerulonephropathy
    ○ Minimal-change disease
    ○ Idiopathic/primary membranous glomerulonephritis
    ○ Focal segmental glomerulonephritis
    ○ Membranoproliferative glomerulonephritis
    ○ IgA nephropathy
  - Secondary glomerulonephropathy
    ○ Diabetic nephropathy
    ○ Autoimmune/collagen vascular disorders (e.g., lupus nephritis, Goodpasture syndrome)
    ○ Amyloidosis
    ○ Preeclampsia
    ○ Infection (HIV, hepatitis B and C, poststreptococcal, endocarditis, syphilis, malaria)
    ○ Malignancy (GI, lung, lymphoma)
    ○ Renal transplant rejection
    ○ Structural (reflux nephropathy, polycystic kidney disease)
    ○ Drug-induced (NSAIDs, penicillamine, lithium, heavy metals, gold, heroin)

- Tubular proteinuria
  - Hypertensive nephrosclerosis
  - Tubulointerstitial disease (uric acid nephropathy, hypersensitivity, interstitial nephritis, Fanconi syndrome, heavy metals, sickle cell disease, NSAIDs, antibiotics)
  - Acute tubular necrosis
- Overflow proteinuria
  - Multiple myeloma (light chains; also tubulotoxic)
  - Hemoglobinuria
  - Myoglobinuria (in rhabdomyolysis)
  - Lysozyme (in acute monocytic leukemia)
- Benign proteinuria
  - Functional (fever, exercise, cold exposure, stress, CHF)
  - Idiopathic transient
  - Orthostasis (postural)

RISK FACTORS
- Hypertension
- Diabetes
- Obesity
- Strenuous exercise
- CHF
- UTI
- Fever

Genetics
No known genetic pattern

GENERAL PREVENTION
Control of weight, BP, and blood glucose reduces the risk of proteinuria.

COMMONLY ASSOCIATED CONDITIONS
- Hypertension (common)
- Diabetes mellitus (common)
- Preeclampsia (common)
- Multiple myeloma (rare)

DIAGNOSIS

HISTORY
- Frothy/foamy urine
- Change in urine output
- Blood- or cola-colored urine
- Recent weight change
- Swelling
- Rule out systemic illness: diabetes, heart failure, autoimmune, poststreptococcal infection

PHYSICAL EXAM
- BP
- Weight
- Peripheral edema
- Periorbital/facial edema
- Ascites
- Palpation of kidneys
- Check lungs, heart for signs of CHF

DIFFERENTIAL DIAGNOSIS
Includes all causes listed under "Etiology and Pathophysiology"

DIAGNOSTIC TESTS & INTERPRETATION
Screening for proteinuria is not cost-effective unless directed at groups with hypertension/diabetes, older persons, and so forth.

Initial Tests (lab, imaging)
- Urinalysis (UA) quantitatively estimates proteinuria:
  - Only sensitive to albumin; will not detect smaller proteins of overflow/tubular etiologies
  - False-positive finding if urine pH >7, highly concentrated (specific gravity [SG] >1.015), gross hematuria, mucus, semen, leukocytes, iodinated contrast agents, penicillin analogues, sulfonamide metabolites
  - False-negative finding if urine is dilute (SG 1.005), albumin excretion <20 to 30 mg/dL, protein is nonalbumin
  - Sensitivity, 32–46%; specificity, 97–100%
  - Also can perform sulfosalicylic acid test to detect nonalbumin protein
- If UA positive, perform urine microscopy. Refer to nephrologist if positive for signs of glomerular disease.
- If UA shows trace to 2+ protein, rule out transient proteinuria with repeat UA at another visit:
  - More common than persistent proteinuria
  - Causes include exercise, fever, CHF, UTI, and cold exposure
  - Reassure patient that transient proteinuria is benign and requires no further workup.
- If initial UA shows 3+ to 4+ protein or repeat UA is positive, measure creatinine clearance and quantify proteinuria with 24-hour urine collection (gold standard) or spot urine protein-to-creatinine (P/C) ratio (acceptable practice) (1)[A]:
  - Numerical P/C ratios correlate with total protein excreted in grams per day (i.e., ratio of 0.2 correlates with 0.2 g during a 24-hour collection).
  - Patients age <30 years with 24-hour urine excretion of <2 g/day and normal creatinine clearance should be tested for orthostatic proteinuria:
    ○ Benign condition is present in 2–5% of adolescents.
    ○ Diagnosed with a normal urine P/C ratio in first morning void and an elevated urine P/C ratio in a second specimen taken after standing for several hours
- If protein excretion >2 g/day, consider nephrology referral and begin workup for systemic/renal disease.
- Patients with persistent proteinuria not explained by orthostatic changes should undergo renal ultrasound to rule out structural abnormalities (e.g., reflux nephropathy, polycystic kidney).

Follow-Up Tests & Special Considerations
Renal/systemic disease workup can include the following:
- CBC, ferritin, ESR, serum iron
- Electrolytes, LFTs
- Lipid profile (ideally, fasting)
- Prothrombin time/international normalized ratio
- Anti-phospholipase A2 receptor antibody: positive in ~70% of primary membranous nephropathy
- Antinuclear antibodies: elevated in lupus
- Antistreptolysin O titer: elevated after streptococcal glomerulonephritis

- Complement C3/C4: low in most glomerulonephritis
- HIV, syphilis, and hepatitis serologies: all associated with glomerular proteinuria
- Serum and urine protein electrophoresis: abnormal in multiple myeloma
- Blood glucose: elevated in diabetes
- All patients with diabetes should be screened for microalbuminuria.
- Patients with nephrotic-range proteinuria are at increased risk for hypercholesterolemia and thromboembolic events (~25% of adult patients) with highest risk in membranous nephropathy. Optimal duration of prophylactic anticoagulation is unknown but may extend for the duration of the nephrotic state (2).
- Proteinuric pregnant patients beyond 20 weeks' gestation should be examined for other signs/symptoms of preeclampsia (e.g., hypertension, thrombocytopenia, elevated liver transaminases).

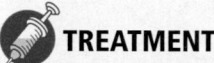 **TREATMENT**

- BP goals for both diabetic and nondiabetic adults is ≤140/90 mm Hg (3)[C].
- Proteinuria goal is <0.5 g/day (4)[A].

GENERAL MEASURES

- Limit protein intake to 0.8 g/kg/day in adults with DM or without DM and glomerular filtration rate (GFR) <30 mL/min/1.73 m^2. Soy protein may be renoprotective. Monitor protein intake with 24-hour urine urea excretion (4)[A].
- Limit sodium chloride intake to <2 g/day to optimize antiproteinuric medications (3)[B]. Effect on BP is further protective (4)[A].
- Limit fluid intake for urine output goal of <2 L/day. Larger urine volumes are associated with increased proteinuria and later GFR decline (4)[B].
- Smoking cessation: Smoking is associated with increased proteinuria and faster kidney disease progression (4)[B].
- Encourage supine posture (up to 50% reduction vs. upright) (4)[B].
- Discourage severe exertion (4)[B].
- Encourage weight loss (4)[B].

MEDICATION
First Line

- ACE inhibitors: first choice; use maximally tolerated doses; use even if normotensive (4)[A]
- Angiotensin receptor blockers (ARBs): proven antiproteinuric and renoprotective; ARBs are first choice if ACE inhibitors are not tolerated (4)[A].
- Combination ACE inhibitor and ARB should not be used. Although shown to reduce proteinuria, combination does not reduce poor CV outcomes and does increase risk of adverse drug reactions (5)[A].

Second Line

- β-Blockers: antiproteinuric and cardioprotective (4)[A]
- Dihydropyridine calcium channel blockers (DHCCBs): should be avoided unless needed for BP control; not antiproteinuric (4)[A]
- Non-DHCCB: antiproteinuric, may be renoprotective (4)[B]
- Aldosterone antagonists: antiproteinuric independent of BP control (4)[B]

- NSAIDs: antiproteinuric, but also nephrotoxic; generally should be avoided (4)[C]

ISSUES FOR REFERRAL
Consider nephrology referral for possible renal biopsy if

- Impaired creatinine clearance
- Nephrotic-range proteinuria
- Unclear etiology of non-nephrotic-range proteinuria
- Diabetics with microalbuminuria

COMPLEMENTARY & ALTERNATIVE MEDICINE

- Corticosteroids: No proven benefit in mortality or need for renal replacement in adults with nephrotic syndrome, although steroids are recommended in some patients who do not respond to conservative treatment. Classically, children with nephrotic syndrome respond better than adults, especially those with minimal-change disease (6)[A].
- Estrogen/progesterone replacement: may be renoprotective in premenopausal women but should be avoided in postmenopausal women (4)[B]

- Antioxidant therapy: may be antiproteinuric in diabetic nephropathy (4)[C]
- Sodium bicarbonate: not antiproteinuric but may block tubular injury caused by proteinuria; correcting metabolic acidosis may decrease protein catabolism (4)[C].
- Avoid excessive caffeine consumption: antiproteinuric in diabetic rat models (4)[C]
- Avoid iron overload (4)[C].
- Pentoxifylline: prevents progression of renal disease by unclear mechanisms (4)[C]
- Mycophenolate mofetil: antiproteinuric and renoprotective in animal models (4)[C]

 ONGOING CARE

FOLLOW-UP RECOMMENDATIONS
Patient Monitoring
All patients with persistent proteinuria should be followed with serial BP checks, UA, and renal function tests in the outpatient setting. Intervals depend on underlying etiology.

PROGNOSIS
- Transient and orthostatic proteinuria are benign conditions that do not convey a poor prognosis.
- Clinical significance of persistent proteinuria varies greatly and depends on underlying etiology.
- Degree of proteinuria is associated with disease progression in chronic kidney disease.

- Independent of GFR, higher levels of proteinuria likely convey an increased risk of mortality, myocardial infarction, and progression to kidney failure (7).

COMPLICATIONS
- Progression to chronic renal failure and the need for dialysis/renal transplant
- Hypercholesterolemia
- Hypercoagulable state

REFERENCES

1. National Kidney Foundation. K/DOQI clinical practice guidelines for chronic kidney disease: evaluation classification, and stratification: guideline 5. Assessment of proteinuria. http://www2.kidney.org/professionals/KDOQI/guidelines_ckd/toc.htm.
2. Kerlin BA, Ayoob R, Smoyer WE. Epidemiology and pathophysiology of nephrotic syndrome-associated thromboembolic disease. *Clin J Am Soc Nephrol*. 2012;7(3):513–520.
3. James PA, Oparil S, Carter BL, et al. 2014 evidence-based guideline for the management of high blood pressure in adults: report from the panel members appointed to the Eighth Joint National Committee (JNC 8). *JAMA*. 2014;311(5):507–520.
4. Wilmer WA, Rovin BH, Hebert CJ, et al. Management of glomerular proteinuria: a commentary. *J Am Soc Nephrol*. 2003;14(12):3217–3232.
5. Fried LF, Emanuele N, Zhang JH, et al. Combined angiotensin inhibition for the treatment of diabetic nephropathy. *N Engl J Med*. 2013;369(20):1892–1903.
6. Kodner C. Nephrotic syndrome in adults: diagnosis and management. *Am Fam Physician*. 2009;80(10):1129–1134.
7. Tonelli M, Muntner P, Lloyd A, et al. Using proteinuria and estimated glomerular filtration rate to classify risk in patients with chronic kidney disease: a cohort study. *Ann Intern Med*. 2011;154(1):12–21.

CODES

ICD10
- R80.9 Proteinuria, unspecified
- R80.2 Orthostatic proteinuria, unspecified
- R80.1 Persistent proteinuria, unspecified

CLINICAL PEARLS

- Transient and orthostatic proteinuria are benign conditions that do not convey a poor prognosis.
- Proteinuria >2 g/day likely represents glomerular malfunction and warrants a nephrology consultation.
- Clinical course varies greatly but, in general, the degree of proteinuria correlates with kidney disease progression.
- First-line therapy for persistent proteinuric patients is a high-dose ACE inhibitor.

PROTHROMBIN 20210 (MUTATION)

Dalia Hammoud, MD • Elie Chalhoub, MD • Maissaa Janbain, MD

BASICS

DESCRIPTION
- Prothrombin 20210 mutation is the second most common inherited risk factor for venous thromboembolism after factor V Leiden mutation.
- Polymorphism (replacement of G by A) in the 3' untranslated end of the prothrombin gene causes increased translation, resulting in elevated synthesis and secretion of prothrombin. This leads to a 2.8-fold increased risk for venous thrombosis.
- Heterozygous carriers have 30% higher plasma prothrombin levels than normal
- System(s) affected: cardiovascular; hemic/lymphatic/immunologic; nervous; pulmonary; reproductive
- Synonym(s): prothrombin G20210A mutation; prothrombin G20210 gene polymorphism; prothrombin gene mutation; FII A^{20210} mutation

EPIDEMIOLOGY
- Found largely in Caucasian population. Found in 2–5% of European and Middle Eastern population, but rarely in nonwhites. Found in 4–8% of persons with venous thromboembolism and in up to 18% of patients with recurrent thrombosis.
- Predominant age: Mean age of first thrombosis is in the 2nd decade of life.
- Predominant gender: male = female

Prevalence
3–5% of the population

ETIOLOGY AND PATHOPHYSIOLOGY
- Replacement of G for A in the 3' untranslated region of the prothrombin gene resulting in relatively higher plasma prothrombin activity, leading to increased risk for venous thrombosis.
- Prothrombin Yukuhashi (Arg596Leu) was described in a Japanese thrombophilic family. The mutant prothrombin had moderately lower, but adequate, activity than wild-type prothrombin. The thrombin molecule generated is resistant to inactivation by antithrombin, thereby conferring an increased susceptibility to thrombosis.
- Gene mutation

Genetics
Autosomal dominant

RISK FACTORS
- Patients with prothrombin 20210 and another prothrombotic state, such as factor V Leiden, have increased rates of thrombosis (1).
- The risk of venous thrombosis in patients with prothrombin 20210 mutation increases when added to the use of oral contraceptives, pregnancy, and the use of hormone replacement therapy as well as any status associated with prolonged immobilization (1).

Pregnancy Considerations
- Increased thrombotic risk in patients with prothrombin 20210.
- A new mutation C20209T has been described recently in women with recurrent pregnancy loss; the clinical and biochemical implications of this mutation are not fully understood yet (2).

GENERAL PREVENTION
Patients with prothrombin 20210 without thrombosis do not require prophylactic anticoagulation (3)[A], except for pregnant women with family history of venous thromboembolism, who require antepartum and 6-week postpartum prophylaxis with LMWH (4)[B].

COMMONLY ASSOCIATED CONDITIONS
Venous thromboembolism

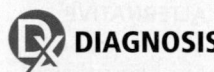

DIAGNOSIS

HISTORY
- Previous thrombosis
- Family history of thrombosis
- Family history of factor prothrombin 20210 mutation

PHYSICAL EXAM
Arterial thrombosis is rare in adults with prothrombin 20210 gene mutation.

DIFFERENTIAL DIAGNOSIS
- Factor V Leiden mutation
- Protein C deficiency
- Protein S deficiency
- Antithrombin deficiency
- Other causes of activated protein C resistance (e.g., antiphospholipid antibodies)
- Dysfibrinogenemia
- Dysplasminogenemia
- Homocystinemia
- Elevated factor VIII levels

DIAGNOSTIC TESTS & INTERPRETATION
Test patients with thrombosis at age <50 years, history of recurrent idiopathic thrombosis, those with thrombosis in unusual locations, or those with strong family history.

Initial Tests (lab, imaging)
- For evaluation of a new clot in patients at risk: CBC with peripheral smear, PT/INR, aPTT, thrombin time, lupus anticoagulant, antiphospholipid antibodies, factor VIII, anticardiolipin antibody, anti-B2 glycoprotein I antibody, activated protein C resistance, protein S antigen and resistance, antithrombin III assay, fibrinogen, factor V Leiden, prothrombin G20210A, homocysteine

- DNA analysis for mutation
- Testing is reliable during acute thrombosis and on any kind of anticoagulation, as is gene analysis (4).
- As appropriate for suspected site of thrombosis: US, CT scan, and V/Q scan

Follow-Up Tests & Special Considerations
Although prothrombin levels are elevated, this is not a sensitive test to make the diagnosis.

Diagnostic Procedures/Other
MR angiography (MRA), venography, or arteriography to detect thrombosis

Test Interpretation
Venous thrombus

TREATMENT
For acute thrombosis

GENERAL MEASURES
- Patients with prothrombin 20210 mutation and a first thrombosis should receive anticoagulation medication initially with heparin or LMWH (1)[A].
- Treatment with LMWH is recommended over unfractionated heparin, unless the patient has severe renal failure (3)[A].
- Treat as outpatient, if possible (3)[B].
- Initiate warfarin on day 1 or 2 of LMWH therapy; discontinue LMWH after minimum of 5 days and 2 consecutive INRs >2 (3)[A].
- Patients should be maintained on warfarin with an INR of 2 to 3 for at least 3 months (4)[A].
- Recurrent thrombosis requires indefinite anticoagulation (1)[B].

MEDICATION
First Line
- Low-molecular-weight heparin (LMWH) (3)[A]
  - Enoxaparin (Lovenox): 1 mg/kg SC BID; tinzaparin (Innohep): 175 anti-Xa IU/kg SC daily; dalteparin (Fragmin): 200 IU/kg SC daily
  - Initiate warfarin on day 1 or 2 of LMWH therapy; continue LMWH for a minimum of 5 days and 2 consecutive INRs >2
  - Fondaparinux (Arixtra): <50 kg: 5 mg SC daily; 50 to 100 kg: 7.5 mg SC daily; >100 kg: 10 mg SC daily
- Oral anticoagulant
  - Warfarin (Coumadin) 5 mg PO daily; then adjusted to an INR of 2 to 3 (4)

- Contraindications
  - Active bleeding precludes anticoagulation (3)[A].
  - Risk of bleeding is a relative contraindication to long-term anticoagulation (3)[A].
  - Warfarin is contraindicated in patients with history of warfarin skin necrosis (3)[A].
  - Fondaparinux: severe renal impairment (CrCl <30 mL/min)
- Precautions
  - Observe patient for signs of embolization, further thrombosis, or bleeding.
  - Avoid IM injections. Periodically check stool and urine for occult blood; monitor CBCs, including platelets.
  - Heparins: thrombocytopenia
  - Warfarin: necrotic skin lesions (typically breasts, thighs, or buttocks)
  - LMWH: Adjust dosage in renal insufficiency.
- Significant possible interactions
  - Agents that intensify the response to oral anticoagulants: alcohol, allopurinol, amiodarone, anabolic steroids, androgens, many antimicrobials, cimetidine, chloral hydrate, disulfiram, all NSAIDs, sulfinpyrazone, tamoxifen, thyroid hormone, vitamin E, ranitidine, salicylates, acetaminophen
  - Agents that diminish the response to anticoagulants: aminoglutethimide, antacids, barbiturates, carbamazepine, cholestyramine, diuretics, griseofulvin, rifampin, oral contraceptives

Second Line
- Heparin 80 mg/kg IV bolus followed by 18 g/kg/hr continuous infusion
- Adjust dose, depending on aPTT.
- In patients requiring large daily doses of heparin, measure an anti-Xa level for dose guidance.
- Alternatively, unfractionated heparin can be given for outpatients at 333 U/kg then 250 U/kg SC (4)[A].

ISSUES FOR REFERRAL
- Recurrent thrombosis on anticoagulation
- Difficulty anticoagulating
- Genetic counseling

SURGERY/OTHER PROCEDURES
- Anticoagulation must be held for surgical interventions.
- For most patients with deep venous thrombosis (DVT), recommendations are against routine use of vena cava filter in addition to anticoagulation, except in case with contraindication to anticoagulation (4)[A].
- Thrombectomy may be necessary in some cases.

INPATIENT CONSIDERATIONS
Admission Criteria/Initial Stabilization
Complicated thrombosis, such as pulmonary embolus; heparin

Discharge Criteria
Stable on anticoagulation

 ONGOING CARE

Compression stockings for prevention

FOLLOW-UP RECOMMENDATIONS
Patient Monitoring
- Warfarin use requires periodic (monthly after initial stabilization) INR measurements, with a goal of 2 to 3 (3)[A].
- Heterozygous prothrombin 20210 mutations increase the risk for recurrent venous thromboembolism (VTE) only slightly once anticoagulation is stopped and should have the same length of anticoagulation as in someone without the mutation.

DIET
- No restrictions
- Food rich in vitamin K may interfere with warfarin anticoagulation.

PATIENT EDUCATION
- Patients should be educated about:
  - Use of oral anticoagulant therapy.
  - Avoidance of NSAIDs while on warfarin
- The role of family screening is unclear, as most patients with this mutation do not have thrombosis. In a patient with a family history of prothrombin 20210, consider screening during pregnancy or if considering oral contraceptive use.

PROGNOSIS
- When compared with normal individuals, persons with prothrombin 20210 have normal lifespan.
- Carriage of the PT20210 mutation has been linked to an increased rate of liver fibrosis in HCV patients (5).

COMPLICATIONS
- Recurrent thrombosis
- Bleeding on anticoagulation

REFERENCES

1. Girolami A, Simioni P, Scarano L, et al. Prothrombin and the prothrombin 20210 G to A polymorphism: their relationship with hypercoagulability and thrombosis. *Blood Rev.* 1999;13(4):205–210.
2. Prat M, Morales-Indiano C, Jimenez C, et al. "20209C-T" a variant mutation of prothrombin gene mutation in a patient with recurrent pregnancy loss. *Ann Clin Lab Sci.* 2014;44(3):334–336.
3. Guyatt GH, Akl EA, Crowther M, et al. Executive summary: Antithrombotic Therapy and Prevention of Thrombosis, 9th ed: American College of Chest Physicians Evidence-Based Clinical Practice Guidelines. *Chest.* 2012;141(2)(Suppl):7S–47S.
4. Moll S. Thrombophilias—practical implications and testing caveats. *J Thromb Thrombolysis.* 2006;21(1):7–15.
5. Maharshak N, Halfon P, Deutsch V, et al. Increased fibrosis progression rates in hepatitis C patients carrying the prothrombin G20210A mutation. *World J Gastroenterol.* 2011;17(45):5007–5013.

ADDITIONAL READING

Seligsohn U, Lubetsky A. Genetic susceptibility to venous thrombosis. *N Engl J Med.* 2001;344(16): 1222–1231.

 SEE ALSO

Antithrombin Deficiency; Deep Vein Thrombophlebitis; Factor V Leiden; Protein C Deficiency; Protein S Deficiency

CODES

ICD10
D68.52 Prothrombin gene mutation

CLINICAL PEARLS

- Prothrombin 20210 mutation is the second most common inherited risk factor for VTE after factor V Leiden mutation.
- Asymptomatic patients with prothrombin 20210 mutation do not need anticoagulation.
- Testing for the prothrombin G20210 mutation may be done while the patient is anticoagulated, as it is a genetic assay.
- For pregnant women homozygous for factor V Leiden, or heterozygous for factor V and prothrombin G20210 mutation, but no prior history of VTE, postpartum prophylaxis with prophylactic or intermediate-dose LMWH or vitamin K antagonists with target INR 2 to 3 for 6 weeks is recommended. Antepartum prophylaxis is added if there is positive family of VTE.

PRURITUS ANI

Jessica Davis, MD • Pia Prakash, MD • Marie L. Borum, MD, EdD, MPH

 BASICS

DESCRIPTION
- Intense, unpleasant anal and perianal itching and/or burning
- Usually acute
- Can be classified as idiopathic (primary) pruritus ani (50–90%) or secondary to anorectal pathology (1)

EPIDEMIOLOGY
Incidence
- 1–5% of the general population (1)
- Predominant age: 30 to 60 years (1)
- Predominant sex: male > female (4:1) (1)

Prevalence
Difficult to estimate as often unreported, one study found present in 2.4% of patients visiting PCPs (2).

ETIOLOGY AND PATHOPHYSIOLOGY
- Perianal itching (primary or secondary) incites itch–scratch cycle that may self-perpetuate, as resulting lichenification worsens pruritus.
- Etiologies of primary pruritus ani
  - Poor anal hygiene
  - Loose or leaking stool that makes hygiene difficult—of note, interestingly, patients with abdominal ostomy bags typically do not complain of pruritus (1).
  - Internal sphincter laxity
  - Idiopathic
- Etiologies of secondary pruritus ani
  - Inflammatory dermatologic disorders
    ○ Allergic contact dermatitis (soaps, perfumes, or dyes in toilet paper, topical anesthetics, oral antibiotics)
    ○ Psoriasis: Lesions tend to be poorly demarcated, pale, and nonscaling.
    ○ Atopic dermatitis ± lichen simplex chronicus: Patients are likely to have asthma and/or eczema.
    ○ Eczema from dietary elements (citrus, vitamin C supplements, milk products, coffee, tea, cola, chocolate, beer, wine)
    ○ Seborrheic dermatitis
    ○ Lichen planus: may be seen in patients with ulcerative colitis and myasthenia gravis
  - Colorectal and anal pathology: rectal prolapse, hemorrhoids, fissures or fistulas, chronic diarrhea/constipation, papillomas, condyloma, polyps, cancer
  - Malignancies: uncommon, but pruritus ani may be presenting symptom of Bowen or Paget disease
  - Infectious etiologies: dermatophytes (*Tinea*), bacteria (*Staphylococcus aureus*, β-hemolytic *Streptococcus*, *Corynebacterium minutissimum* [Erythrasma], gonorrhea, syphilis), viruses (herpes simplex virus [HSV], human papillomavirus [HPV], molluscum), parasites (pinworms, rarely scabies, or pediculosis)
  - Mechanical factors: vigorous cleaning and scrubbing, tight-fitting clothes, synthetic undergarments
  - Systemic diseases: diabetes mellitus (most common), chronic liver disease, renal failure, leukemia or lymphoma, hyperthyroidism, anemia
  - Chemical irritants: chemotherapy, diarrhea (often from antibiotic use)
  - Psychogenic factors: anxiety–itch–anxiety cycle

RISK FACTORS
- Obesity
- Excess perianal hair growth, excessive perspiration
- Underlying anorectal pathology
- Underlying anxiety disorder
- Caffeine intake has been correlated with symptoms.

GENERAL PREVENTION
- Good perianal hygiene
- Avoid mechanical irritation of skin (vigorous cleaning or rubbing, harsh soaps or perfumed products, excessive cleansing with dry toilet paper or "baby wipes," scratching with fingernails, or tight/synthetic undergarments). Minimize moisture in perianal area (absorbent cotton in anal cleft may help keep area dry).
- Avoid laxative use (loose stool is an irritant).

COMMONLY ASSOCIATED CONDITIONS
See earlier listing of conditions causing perianal irritation.

 DIAGNOSIS

HISTORY
- Patient presents with complaint of anal and/or perianal itching, burning, or excoriations.
- Inquire about:
  - Melena or hematochezia
  - Frequency of cleansing and products used on affected area
  - Change in bowel habits
  - Recent antibiotic use
  - Medical history (diabetes in particular)
  - Skin disorders (psoriasis, eczema)
  - Rectal or vaginal discharge
  - Dietary history: focus on the "C"s: Caffeine, coffee, cola, chocolate, citrus, calcium (dairy) (3)
  - Family history of colorectal cancer
  - Anal receptive intercourse
  - Change in toiletry products
  - Household members with itching (possible pinworms)
  - Clothing preference (tight, synthetic) (1)

PHYSICAL EXAM
- Perianal inspection for erythema, hemorrhoids, anal fissures, maceration, lichenification, rashes, warts, excoriations, neoplasia
- Digital rectal exam to check for masses and to evaluate internal sphincter tone, Valsalva to evaluate for prolapse
- Anoscopy to evaluate for hemorrhoids, fissures, other internal lesions
- Classification based on gross appearance
  - Stage 1: erythema, inflamed appearance
  - Stage 2: lichenification
  - Stage 3: lichenification, coarse skin, potential fissures or ulcerations (1)[C]

DIFFERENTIAL DIAGNOSIS
- "ITCHeS" acronym (4)
  - **I**nfection: pinworms, dermatophytes, gram-positive bacteria, HSV, gonorrhea, chlamydia, syphilis, HPV, erythrasma, scabies
  - **T**opical irritant: detergents, garments, deodorants, perfumes, stool leakage
  - **C**utaneous/cancer/colorectal: eczema, psoriasis, lichen planus, lichen sclerosus, seborrheic dermatosis, squamous cell cancer, extramammary Paget disease, Bowen disease, melanoma, fistula, fissure, prolapse, hemorrhoids, colorectal cancer

- **H**ypersensitivity: foods (the "C's" above), medications (colchicine, quinidine, mineral oil)
- e**S**ystemic: diabetes, uremia, cholestasis, hematologic malignancy

DIAGNOSTIC TESTS & INTERPRETATION
Initial Tests (lab, imaging)
Depending on patient's history and exam, consider the following:
- Pinworm tape test; stool for ova and parasites
- CBC, comprehensive metabolic panel, A1c, thyroid studies to identify underlying systemic disease
- Wood lamp examination will show coral-red fluorescence in erythrasma (1).
- Skin scraping with potassium hydroxide (KOH) prep for dermatophytes or candidiasis (as etiology or as superinfection) and mineral oil prep for scabies
- Perianal skin culture (bacterial superinfection)
- Hemoccult testing of stool

Pediatric Considerations
Pinworms are common in children.

Follow-Up Tests & Special Considerations
Anal DNA polymerase chain reaction (PCR) probe for gonorrhea and chlamydia and anal Pap smear for HPV if receptive anal intercourse

Diagnostic Procedures/Other
- Biopsy suspicious lesions (e.g., lichenification, ulcerated epithelium, refractory cases) to exclude neoplasia
- Consider colonoscopy if history, exam, or testing suggests colorectal pathology (family history of colorectal disease, especially if age >40 years, weight loss, rectal bleeding, change in bowel habits).

Geriatric Considerations
- Stool incontinence may be a predisposing factor.
- Consider systemic disease.
- Higher likelihood of colorectal pathology

TREATMENT

GENERAL MEASURES
- Educate patients regarding proper anal hygiene and avoidance of chemical and mechanical irritants (1).
- High-fiber diet and/or bowel regimen to maintain regular bowel movements (1)
- Avoid tight-fitting clothing and use cotton undergarments.
- Talcum powder or cornstarch if excess moisture (1)
- Wear cotton gloves at night to control nocturnal scratching (1).

MEDICATION
First Line
- Treat underlying infections: fungal or dermatophyte infection with topical imidazoles, bacterial infection with topical antibacterials.
- Break itch–scratch cycle with low-potency steroid cream such as hydrocortisone 1% ointment applied sparingly up to 4 times daily (1)[A]. Discontinue when itching subsides. Recommended not to use >12 weeks due to risk of skin atrophy.
- If no response with low-potency steroid, consider high-potency steroid cream.
- Antihistamines may be useful until local measures take effect, particularly sedating antihistamines, which will reduce nighttime itching.

- Some experts suggest a trial of tricyclic antidepressants to reduce nighttime scratching.
- Zinc oxide can be used after completing steroid course for barrier protection (3)[C]; petroleum jelly is another barrier treatment.
- Although trial data are mixed, topical capsaicin cream may be used in combination with steroid cream if refractory itch or hypersensitized skin (1,5)[A].
- A small RCT showed benefit with 0.1% tacrolimus ointment; this may be a good choice in patients with skin thinning at risk for atrophy from prolonged steroid use (6)[C].
- Several small case series have shown symptomatic benefit with methylene blue injection; this may be an additional option for patients with refractory symptoms (7)[C].

Second Line
Radiation may be used to destroy nerve endings (create permanent anesthesia) in intractable cases. This is almost never indicated but is very effective.

ISSUES FOR REFERRAL
- Intractable pruritus: Consider referral to gastroenterology (for colonoscopy) or dermatology (for additional treatment, possibly injections). Refractory or persistent symptoms should signal the possibility of underlying neoplasia, as pruritus ani of long duration is associated with a greater likelihood of colorectal pathology.
- If risks or red flags for colon cancer are present, refer for colonoscopy.

SURGERY/OTHER PROCEDURES
None unless malignancy identified

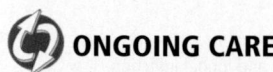 **ONGOING CARE**

FOLLOW-UP RECOMMENDATIONS
See patient in 2 weeks if not improving. Check for persistent lichenification. With refractory pruritus or lichenification that does not resolve, consider underlying malignancy.

DIET
- Trial elimination of foods and beverages known or suspected to exacerbate symptoms: coffee, tea, chocolate, beer, cola, vitamin C tablets in excessive doses, citrus fruits, tomatoes, or spices
- Eliminate foods or drugs contributing to loose bowel movements. Add fiber supplementation to bulk stools and prevent fecal leakage in patients who have fecal incontinence or partially formed stools.

PATIENT EDUCATION
- Review proper anal hygiene:
  - Resist overuse of soap and rubbing.
  - Avoid toiletry products with irritating perfumes and dyes.
  - Avoid use of ointments to the area, including witch hazel.
  - Wear loose, light cotton clothing.
  - If moisture is a problem, unmedicated talcum powder or cornstarch to keep the area dry.
  - Cleanse perianal area after bowel movements with water-moistened cotton.
  - Dry area after bathing by patting with a soft towel or by using a hair dryer (1).
- Avoid medications that cause diarrhea or constipation.
- Avoid foods implicated in pruritus ani: caffeine, cola, chocolate, citrus, tomatoes, tea, beer/wine (3)[C].
- Use barrier protection if engaging in anal intercourse.
- If unable to completely empty rectum with defecation, use small plain-water enema (infant bulb syringe) after each bowel movement to prevent soiling and irritation.

PROGNOSIS
- Conservative treatment is successful in ~90% of patients.
- Idiopathic pruritus ani often is chronic, waxing and waning. Regardless of etiology, however, pruritus ani may be persistent and recurrent.

COMPLICATIONS
- Bacterial superinfection at site of excoriations and potential abscess formation or penetrating infection via self-inoculation with colonic pathogens
- Lichenification

REFERENCES
1. Markell KW, Billingham RP. Pruritus ani: etiology and management. *Surg Clin North Am*. 2010;90(1):125–135.
2. Abramowitz L, Benabderrahmane M, Pospait D, et al. The prevalence of proctological symptoms amongst patients who see general practitioners in France. *Eur J Gen Pract*. 2014;20(4):301–306.
3. Nasseri YY, Osborne MC. Pruritus ani: diagnosis and treatment. *Gastroenterol Clin North Am*. 2013;42(4):801–813.
4. Henderson PK, Cash BD. Common anorectal conditions: evaluation and treatment. *Curr Gastroenterol Rep*. 2014;16(10):408.
5. Gooding SM, Canter PH, Coelho HF, et al. Systematic review of topical capsaicin in the treatment of pruritus. *Int J Dermatol*. 2010;49(8):858–865.
6. Suys E. Randomized study of topical tacrolimus ointment as possible treatment for resistant idiopathic pruritus ani. *J Am Acad Dermatol*. 2012;66(2):327–328.
7. Samalavicius NE, Poskus T, Gupta RK, et al. Long-term results of single intradermal 1% methylene blue injection for intractable idiopathic pruritus ani: a prospective study. *Tech Coloproctol*. 2012;16(4):295–299.

ADDITIONAL READING
- Al-Ghnaniem R, Short K, Pullen A, et al. 1% Hydrocortisone ointment is an effective treatment of pruritus ani: a pilot randomized controlled crossover trial. *Int J Colorectal Dis*. 2007;22(12):1463–1467.
- Handa Y, Watanabe O, Adachi A, et al. Squamous cell carcinoma of the anal margin with pruritus ani of long duration. *Dermatol Surg*. 2003;29(1):108–110.
- Lacy BE, Weiser K. Common anorectal disorders: diagnosis and treatment. *Curr Gastroenterol Rep*. 2009;11(5):413–419.
- Lysy J, Sistiery-Ittah M, Israelit Y, et al. Topical capsaicin—a novel and effective treatment for idiopathic intractable pruritus ani: a randomised, placebo controlled, crossover study. *Gut*. 2003;52(9):1323–1326.
- Rucklidge JJ, Saunders D. Hypnosis in a case of long-standing idiopathic itch. *Psychosom Med*. 1999;61(3):355–358.
- Schubert MC, Sridhar S, Schade RR, et al. What every gastroenterologist needs to know about common anorectal disorders. *World J Gastroenterol*. 2009;15(26):3201–3209.
- Siddiqi S, Vijay V, Ward M, et al. Pruritus ani. *Ann R Coll Surg Engl*. 2008;90(6):457–463.
- Ucak H, Demir B, Cicek D, et al. Efficacy of topical tacrolimus for the treatment of persistent pruritus ani in patients with atopic dermatitis. *J Dermatolog Treat*. 2013;24(6):454–457.
- Weichert GE. An approach to the treatment of anogenital pruritus. *Dermatol Ther*. 2004;17(1):129–133.
- Zuccati G, Lotti T, Mastrolorenzo A, et al. Pruritus ani. *Dermatol Ther*. 2005;18(4):355–362.

 SEE ALSO

Pinworms; Pruritus Vulvae

 CODES

ICD10
L29.0 Pruritus ani

CLINICAL PEARLS
- Pruritus ani is characterized by intense anal and perianal itching and/or burning.
- Usually idiopathic or related to skin irritation with subsequent scratch–itch–scratch cyle
- Conservative treatment with good perianal hygiene and reassurance are successful in 90% of patients.
- Consider trial of dietary elimination of "C's"— citrus, vitamin C supplements, calcium, caffeine, coffee, cola, chocolate.
- Rule out infection in immunosuppressed patients.
- Consider underlying malignancy if refractory

PRURITUS VULVAE

Maeve K. Hopkins, MA, MD • Michael P. Hopkins, MD, MEd

BASICS

DESCRIPTION
- Pruritus vulvae is a symptom, as well as a primary diagnosis:
  - The symptom may indicate an underlying pathologic process.
  - Only when no underlying disease is identified may this be used as a primary diagnosis.
- Pruritus vulvae as a primary diagnosis may also be more appropriately documented as vulvodynia (see "Vulvodynia" topic) or burning vulva syndrome.

EPIDEMIOLOGY
Symptoms may occur at any age during a woman's lifetime.
- Young girls most commonly have infectious or hygiene etiology.
- The primary diagnosis is more common in postmenopausal women.

Incidence
The exact incidence is unknown, although most women complain of vulvar pruritus at some point in their lifetime.

ETIOLOGY AND PATHOPHYSIOLOGY
Vulvar tissue is more permeable than exposed skin due to differences in structure, occlusion, hydration, and susceptibility to friction. It is particularly vulnerable to irritants (1)
- Perfumes
- Soaps
- Laundry detergent
- Douches
- Toilet paper
- Sanitary napkins

RISK FACTORS
- High-risk sexual behavior
- Immunosuppression
- Obesity

GENERAL PREVENTION
- Attention should be paid to personal hygiene and avoidance of possible environmental factors.
- Tight-fitting clothing should be avoided.
- Only cotton underwear should be worn.

COMMONLY ASSOCIATED CONDITIONS
- Infectious etiology
  - Vaginal or vulvar candida
  - *Gardnerella vaginalis*
  - *Trichomonas*
  - Human papillomavirus
  - Herpes simplex virus
- Vulvar vestibulitis
- Lichen sclerosis
- Lichen planus
- Lichen simplex chronicus (squamous cell hyperplasia)
- Malignant or premalignant conditions
- Psoriasis
- Fecal or urinary incontinence
- Dermatophytosis
- Parasites: scabies, phthrius pubis
- Extrammmary Paget's
- Dietary: methylxanthines (e.g., coffee, cola), tomatoes, peanuts
- Autoimmune progesterone dermatitis: perimenstrual eruptions
- Irritant or allergic contact dermatitis
- Atopic dermatitis

DIAGNOSIS

Pruritus vulvae is a diagnosis of exclusion.

HISTORY
- Persistent itching
- Persistent burning sensation over the vulva or perineum
- Change in vaginal discharge
- Postcoital bleeding
- Dyspareunia

PHYSICAL EXAM
- Visual inspection of the vulva, vagina, perineum, and anus
  - Superior surfaces of the labia majora—extending from mons to the anal orifice are most involved.
  - Vulvar skin is leathery or lichenified in appearance.
  - Papillomatosis may be a sign of chronic inflammation.
- Light touch identification of affected areas
- Cotton swab–applied pressure to vestibular glands

DIAGNOSTIC TESTS & INTERPRETATION
- Sodium chloride: *Gardnerella* or *Trichomonas*
- 10% potassium hydroxide: *Candida*
- Viral culture or polymerase chain reaction (PCR): herpes simplex virus
- Directed biopsy: human papillomavirus, lichen, malignancy
- Colposcopy with acetic acid or Lugol solution of vagina and vulva

Follow-Up Tests & Special Considerations
- A patch test may be performed by a dermatologist to assist in identifying a causative agent if contact dermatitis is suspected.
- Exam-directed tissue biopsies are essential in the postmenopausal population to rule out malignancy.

Diagnostic Procedures/Other
Biopsies should be collected from any ulceration, discoloration, raised areas, macerated areas, and the area of most intense pruritus.

Test Interpretation
- Only in the absence of pathologic findings can the primary diagnosis of pruritus vulvae be made.
- In one study, a specific clinicopathologic diagnosis was obtained in 89% of patients by using the most recent 2006 International Society for the Study of Vulvar Diseases (ISSVD) classifications (2).

TREATMENT

Identify the underlying cause or disease to target treatment
- Stop all potential irritants.
- Eliminate bacterial and fungal infection.
- Cool the affected area: Use cool gel packs (not ice packs, which may cause further injury).
- Sitz baths and bland emollients to soothe fissured or eroded skin

MEDICATION

First Line

- 1st-generation antihistamines (3)[C]
  - Hydroxyzine: Initiate with 10 mg before bedtime (slow increase up to 100 mg).
  - Doxepin: Initiate with 10 mg before bedtime (slow increase up to 100 mg).
  - 2nd-generation antihistamines are of little benefit.
- SSRIs (3)[C]
  - Citalopram 20 to 40 mg in the morning may be helpful for daytime symptoms.
- Topical steroids (4)[C]
  - Triamcinolone 0.1% applied daily for 2 to 4 weeks, then twice weekly
  - Hydrocortisone 1–2.5% cream applied 2 to 4 times daily (5)
  - Avoid long-term use due to risk of atrophy.
  - One randomized, controlled trial showed no difference between topical triamcinolone and placebo cream (6).

Second Line

Calcineurin inhibitors such as topical pimecrolimus 1% cream applied BID for 3 weeks (7)[B]

- May lead to an 80% reduction of pruritus

ISSUES FOR REFERRAL

- Persistent symptoms should prompt additional investigation and referral to a gynecologist or gynecologist oncologist.
- Gynecology oncology referral for proven or suspected malignancy
- Dermatology referral for patch testing to evaluate for contact dermatitis

ADDITIONAL THERAPIES

- SC triamcinolone injections (8)[B]
- Alcohol nerve block (9)[B]
- Laser therapy (10)[B]

- GnRH analogue

 ONGOING CARE

- Frequent evaluation, repeat cultures, and biopsies are necessary for cases resistant to treatment.
- Refractory cases may require referral to gynecologist or gynecology oncology for further management.

DIET

Dietary alterations include avoidance of the following:

- Coffee and other caffeine-containing beverages
- Tomatoes
- Peanuts

PATIENT EDUCATION

- American Congress of Obstetricians and Gynecologists: www.acog.org
- National Vulvodynia Foundation: www.nva.org

PROGNOSIS

Conservative measures and short-term topical steroids control most patients' symptoms.

COMPLICATIONS

Malignancy

REFERENCES

1. Farage M, Maibach HI. The vulvar epithelium differs from the skin: implications for cutaneous testing to address topical vulvar exposures. *Contact Dermatitis*. 2004;51(4):201–209.
2. Kelecki KH, Adamhasan F, Gencdal S, et al. The impact of the latest classification system of benign vulvar diseases on the management of women with chronic vulvar pruritus. *Indian J Dermatol Venereol Leprol*. 2011;77(3):294–299.
3. Margesson LJ. Overview of treatment of vulvovaginal disease. *Skin Therapy Lett*. 2011;16(3):5–7.
4. Weichert GE. An approach to the treatment of anogenital pruritus. *Dermatol Ther*. 2004;17(1):129–133.
5. Pincus SH. Vulvar dermatoses and pruritus vulvae. *Dermatol Clin*. 1992;10(2):297–308.
6. Lagro-Janssen AL, Sluis S. Effectiveness of treating non-specific pruritus vulvae with topical steroids: a randomized controlled trial. *Eur J Gen Pract*. 2009;15(1):29–33.
7. Sarifakioglu E, Gumus II. Efficacy of topical pimecrolimus in the treatment of chronic vulvar pruritus: a prospective case series—a non-controlled, open-label study. *J Dermatolog Treat*. 2006;17(5):276–278.
8. Kelly RA, Foster DC, Woodruff JD. Subcutaneous injection of triamcinolone acetonide in the treatment of chronic vulvar pruritus. *Am J Obstet Gynecol*. 1993;169(3):568–570.
9. Woodruff JD, Babaknia A. Local alcohol injection of the vulva: discussion of 35 cases. *Obstet Gynecol*. 1979;54(4):512–514.
10. Ovadia J, Levavi H, Edelstein T. Treatment of pruritus vulvae by means of CO2 laser. *Acta Obstet Gynecol Scand*. 1984;63(3):265–267.

ADDITIONAL READING

- Banerjee AK, de Chazal R. Chronic vulvovaginal pruritus treated successfully with GnRH analogue. *Postgrad Med J*. 2006;82(970):e22.
- Boardman LA, Botte J, Kennedy CM. Recurrent vulvar itching. *Obstet Gynecol*. 2005;105(6): 1451–1455.
- Bohl TG. Overview of vulvar pruritus through the life cycle. *Clin Obstet Gynecol*. 2005;48(4):786–807.
- Caro-Bruce E, Flaxman G. Vulvar pruritus in a post-menopausal woman. *CMAJ*. 2014;186(9):688–689.
- Farage MA, Miller KW, Ledger WJ. Determining the cause of vulvovaginal symptoms. *Obstet Gynecol Surv*. 2008;63(7):445–464.
- Foster DC. Vulvar disease. *Obstet Gynecol*. 2002;100(1):145–163.
- Petersen CD, Lundvall L, Kristensen E, et al. Vulvodynia. Definition, diagnosis and treatment. *Acta Obstet Gynecol Scand*. 2008;87(9):893–901.
- Sener AB, Kuscu E, Seckin NC, et al. Postmenopausal vulvar pruritus—colposcopic diagnosis and treatment. *J Pak Med Assoc*. 1995;45(12):315–317.

 CODES

ICD10

- L29.2 Pruritus vulvae
- N94.819 Vulvodynia, unspecified

CLINICAL PEARLS

- Most women complain of pruritus vulvae at some point in their lifetime.
- Pruritus vulvae is a diagnosis of exclusion once other causes of itching have been ruled out.
- Exam-directed biopsies from any ulceration, discoloration, raised areas, macerated areas, and the area of most intense pruritus are essential to rule out malignancy.
- Initial treatment is conservative.

PSEUDOFOLLICULITIS BARBAE

Maurice Duggins, MD

BASICS

DESCRIPTION
- Foreign-body inflammatory reaction from an ingrown hair resulting in the appearance of papules and pustules. This is found mainly in the bearded area (*barbae*) but may occur in other hairy locations such as the scalp, axilla, or pubic areas where shaving is done (1).
- A mechanical problem: extrafollicular and transfollicular hair penetration
- System(s) affected: skin/exocrine
- Synonym(s): chronic sycosis barbae; pili incarnate; folliculitis barbae traumatica; razor bumps; shaving bumps; tinea barbae; pseudofolliculitis barbae (PFB)

EPIDEMIOLOGY
- Predominant age: postpubertal, middle age (14 to 25 years) (2)
- Predominant sex: male > female (can be seen in females of all races who wax/shave)

Incidence
- Adult male African Americans: unknown
- Adult male whites: unknown

Prevalence
- Widespread in Fitzpatrick skin types IV–VI (darker complexions) who shave
- 45–83% of African American soldiers who shave (1)

ETIOLOGY AND PATHOPHYSIOLOGY
- Transfollicular escape of the low-cut hair shaft as it tries to exit the skin is accompanied by inflammation and often an intraepidermal abscess.
- As the hair enters the dermis, more severe inflammation occurs, with downgrowth of the epidermis in an attempt to sheath the hair.
- A foreign-body reaction forms at the tip of the invading hair, followed by abscess formation.
- Shaving too close
- Plucking/tweezing or wax depilation of hair may cause abnormal hair growth in injured follicles.

Genetics
- People with curly hair have an asymmetric accumulation of acidic keratin hHa8 on hair shaft.
- Single-nucleotide polymorphism (disruption Ala12Thr substitution) affects keratin of hair follicle.

RISK FACTORS
- Curly hair
- Shaving too close or shaving with multiple razor strokes

- Plucking/tweezing hairs
- South Mediterranean/American, Middle Eastern, Asian, or African descent (skin types IV–VI)

GENERAL PREVENTION
- Prior to shaving, rinse face with warm water to hydrate and soften hairs.
- Use adjustable hair clippers that leave very low hair length above skin.
- Shave with either a manual adjustable razor at coarsest setting (avoids close shaves), a single-edge blade razor (e.g., Bump Fighter), a foil-guarded razor (e.g., PFB razor), or electric triple "O-head" razor.
- Empty razor of hair frequently.
- Shave in the direction of hair growth. Do not overstretch skin when shaving.
- Use a generous amount of the correct shaving cream/gel (e.g., Ef-Kay Shaving Gel, Edge Shaving Gel, Aveeno Therapeutic Shave Gel, Easy Shave Medicated Shaving Cream).
- Daily shaving reduces papules/pruritus.
- Regular use of depilatories

COMMONLY ASSOCIATED CONDITIONS
- Keloidal folliculitis
- Pseudofolliculitis nuchae

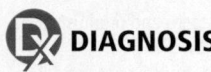

DIAGNOSIS

HISTORY
Pain on shaving; pruritus of shaved areas, irritated "razor bumps"

PHYSICAL EXAM
- Tender, exudative, erythematous follicular papules or pustules in beard area (less commonly in scalp, axilla, and pubic areas); range from 2 to 4 mm
- Hyperpigmented "razor or shave bumps"
- Alopecia
- Lusterless, brittle hair

DIFFERENTIAL DIAGNOSIS
- Bacterial folliculitis
- Impetigo
- Acne vulgaris
- Tinea barbae
- Sarcoidal papules

DIAGNOSTIC TESTS & INTERPRETATION
Initial Tests (lab, imaging)
- Clinical diagnosis
- Culture of pustules: usually sterile; may show coagulase-negative *Staphylococcus epidermidis* (normal skin flora)
- Additional hormonal testing may be indicated in females with hirsutism and/or polycystic ovary syndrome: dehydroepiandrosterone sulfate, luteinizing hormone (LH)/follicle-stimulating hormone (FSH), and free and total testosterone (3)[C].

Test Interpretation
Follicular papules and pustules

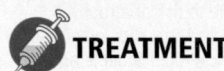

TREATMENT

- Mild cases
  - Stop shaving or avoid close shaving for 30 days while keeping beard groomed and clean (1,2)[C].
  - Consider 5% benzoyl peroxide after shaving and application of 1% hydrocortisone cream at bedtime (or LactiCare HC lotion after shaving) (2)[C].
  - Tretinoin 0.025% cream; apply daily(1)[C]
- Moderate cases
  - Chemical depilatories (barium sulfide; Magic Shave powder); first test on forearm for 48 hours (for irritation) (1–3)[B]
  - Consider eflornithine HCl cream (Vaniqa) to reduce hair growth and stiffness in combination with other therapies (1,4)[B].
- Severe cases
  - Laser therapy: Longer wavelength laser (e.g., neodymium [Nd]:YAG) is safer for dark skin (5)[B].
  - Avoid shaving altogether; grow beard (1–3)[C].

GENERAL MEASURES
Acute treatment
- Dislodge embedded hair with sterile needle/tweezers.
- Discontinue shaving until red papules have resolved (minimum 3 to 4 weeks; longer if moderate or severe); can trim to length >0.5 cm during this time.
- Massage beard area with washcloth, coarse sponge, or a soft brush several times daily.
- Hydrocortisone 1–2.5% cream to relieve inflammation
- Selenium sulfide if seborrhea is present and to help reduce pruritus
- Systemic antibiotics if secondary infection is present

Pregnancy Considerations
Do not use tretinoin (Retin-A), tetracycline, or benzoyl peroxide.

MEDICATION
First Line
- Topical or systemic antibiotic for secondary infection
  - Application of clindamycin (Cleocin T) solution BID or topical erythromycin
  - Low-dose erythromycin or tetracycline 250 to 500 mg PO BID for more severe inflammation
  - Benzoyl peroxide 5%–clindamycin 1% gel BID: Administer until papule/pustule resolves.
- Mild cases: tretinoin 0.025% cream at bedtime; combination of the above therapies
- Moderate disease/chemical depilatories
  - Disrupt cross-linking of disulfide bonds of hair to produce blunt (less sharp) hair tip.
  - Apply no more frequently than every 3rd day: 2% barium sulfide (Magic Shave) or calcium thioglycollate (Surgex); calcium hydroxide (Nair)
- Contraindications
  - Clindamycin: hypersensitivity history; history of regional enteritis or ulcerative colitis; history of antibiotic-associated colitis
  - Erythromycin, tetracycline, tretinoin: hypersensitivity history
- Precautions
  - Clindamycin: colitis, eye burning and irritation, skin dryness; pregnancy Category B
  - Erythromycin: Use cautiously in patients with impaired hepatic function; GI side effects, especially abdominal cramping; pregnancy Category B (erythromycin base formulation).
  - Chemical depilatories: Use cautiously; frequent use and prolonged application may lead to irritant contact dermatitis and chemical burns.
  - Tetracycline: Avoid in pregnancy.
  - Tretinoin: Severe skin irritation; avoid in pregnancy.
  - Benzoyl peroxide: skin irritation and dryness, allergic contact dermatitis
  - Hydrocortisone cream: local skin irritation, skin atrophy with prolonged use, lightening of skin color
- Significant possible interactions
  - Erythromycin: increases theophylline and carbamazepine levels; decreases clearance of warfarin
  - Tetracycline: depresses plasma prothrombin activity

Second Line
Chemical peels with either glycolic acid or salicylic acid

ISSUES FOR REFERRAL
- Worsening or poor response to the above therapies after 4 to 6 weeks should prompt dermatology consultation.
- Occupational demands may also prompt earlier referral to dermatology for more aggressive therapy.

SURGERY/OTHER PROCEDURES
Laser treatment with long-pulsed Nd:YAG is helpful for severe cases.

 ## ONGOING CARE

FOLLOW-UP RECOMMENDATIONS
Patient Monitoring
- As needed
- Educate patient on curative and preventive treatment.

DIET
- No restrictions
- No dietary studies available

PATIENT EDUCATION
- https://medlineplus.com/
- http://www.uptodate.com/home

PROGNOSIS
- Good, with preventive methods
- Prognosis is poor in the presence of progressive scarring and foreign-body granuloma formation.

COMPLICATIONS
- Scarring (occasionally keloidal)
- Foreign body granuloma formation
- Disfiguring postinflammatory hyperpigmentation (use sunscreens; can treat with hydroquinone 4% cream, Retin A, clinical peels)
- Impetiginization of inflamed skin
- Epidermal (erythema, crusting, burns with scarring) and pigmentary changes with laser

REFERENCES
1. Bridgeman-Shah S. The medical and surgical therapy of pseudofolliculitis barbae. *Dermatol Ther*. 2004;17(2):158–163.
2. Perry PK, Cook-Bolden FE, Rahman Z, et al. Defining pseudofolliculitis barbae in 2001: a review of the literature and current trends. *J Am Acad Dermatol*. 2002;46(2)(Suppl):S113–S119.
3. Quarles FN, Brody H, Johnson BA, et al. Pseudofolliculitis barbae. *Dermatol Ther*. 2007;20(3):133–136.
4. Xia Y, Cho S, Howard RS, et al. Topical eflornithine hydrochloride improves the effectiveness of standard laser hair removal for treating pseudofolliculitis barbae: a randomized, double-blinded, placebo-controlled trial. *J Am Acad Dermatol*. 2012;67(4):694–699.
5. Weaver SM III, Sagaral EC. Treatment of pseudofolliculitis barbae using the long-pulse Nd:YAG laser on skin types V and VI. *Dermatol Surg*. 2003;29(12):1187–1191.

ADDITIONAL READING
- Cook-Bolden FE, Barba A, Halder R, et al. Twice-daily application of benzoyl peroxide 5%/clindamycin 1% gel versus vehicle in the treatment of pseudofolliculitis barbae. *Cutis*. 2004;73(6)(Suppl):18–24.
- Daniel A, Gustafson CJ, Zupkosky PJ, et al. Shave frequency and regimen variation effects on the management of pseudofolliculitis barbae. *J Drugs Dermatol*. 2013;12(4):410–418.
- Kindred C, Oresajo CO, Yatskayer M, et al. Comparative evaluation of men's depilatory composition versus razor in black men. *Cutis*. 2011;88(2):98–103.
- Kundu RV, Patterson S. Dermatologic conditions in skin of color: part II. Disorders occurring predominately in skin of color. *Am Fam Physician*. 2013;87(12):859–865.

 ## SEE ALSO

Folliculitis; Impetigo

 ## CODES

ICD10
- L73.1 Pseudofolliculitis barbae
- B35.0 Tinea barbae and tinea capitis
- L73.8 Other specified follicular disorders

CLINICAL PEARLS
- Electrolysis is not recommended as a treatment. It is expensive, painful, and often unsuccessful.
- Combination of laser therapy with eflornithine is more effective than laser alone.
- Use Bump Fighter razor from American Safety Razor Company (http://www.asrco.com/).
- Men may prefer the convenience of the Bump Fighter razor over depilatory products.
- The aversive smell of sulfur could be a problem with some depilatory products.
- Have patient test for skin sensitivity with a small (coin-sized) amount of the depilatory on the bearded area or forearm.

PSEUDOGOUT (CALCIUM PYROPHOSPHATE DIHYDRATE)
Caitlyn M. Rerucha, MD

BASICS

DESCRIPTION
- Autoinflammatory disease triggered by calcium pyrophosphate dihydrate (CPPD) crystal deposition in the joints
- One of many diseases associated with pathologic deposition of crystal, mineralization, and ossification
  - CPPD crystal deposition = chondrocalcinosis, pseudogout
  - Monosodium urate crystal deposition = gout
  - Hydroxyapatite deposition associated with ankylosing spondylitis, osteoarthritis, and vascular calcification
- Suspect pseudogout in arthritis cases with a pattern of joint involvement not usually affected by degenerative joint disease (e.g., metacarpophalangeal joints, wrists)
- Clinical presentation is broad:
  - Asymptomatic CPPD (incidentally identified on radiograph by chondrocalcinosis with or without additional findings of osteoarthritis)
  - Acute CPPD arthritis (acute onset, self-limiting, synovitis)
  - Chronic CPPD crystal inflammatory arthritis (1)[C]
- Chronic CPPD crystal deposition may cause a progressive degenerative arthritis in numerous joints:
  - Primarily affects the elderly
  - Usually involves large joints
- Symptom onset is usually insidious.
- Definitive diagnosis requires the identification of CPPD crystals in synovial fluid.
- System(s) affected: endocrine/metabolic; musculoskeletal
- Synonyms: pseudogout; CPPD; pyrophosphate arthropathy; chondrocalcinosis—when calcification visibly seen within tissues on imaging

EPIDEMIOLOGY
Prevalence
- Predominant age: 80% of patients >60 years
- Predominant sex: male > female 1.4:1
- Prevalence varies on method of identification (chondrocalcinosis on radiograph vs. CPPD crystals in synovial fluid)
- Chondrocalcinosis is present in 1:10 adults age 60 to 75 years and 1:3 by >80 years; however, only a small percentage develop arthropathy.
- 20–43% prevalence of CPPD cyrstals in synovial fluid of osteoarthritic joints at time of joint replacement

ETIOLOGY AND PATHOPHYSIOLOGY
- Arthropathy results from an acute autoinflammatory reaction to CPPD crystals in the synovial cavity.
- CPPD crystal deposition occurs in three general stages:
  - CPPD crystals first develop in the pericellular matrix of the articular cartilage via overproduction of anionic pyrophosphate (PPi).
  - PPi binds calcium to form CPPD crystals that are released from cartilage surface and elicit an inflammatory response. Neutrophils engulf CPPD crystals, inducing the formation of extracellular traps.
  - Increased deposition of CPPD crystals in and around cartilage causes inflammation and damage. Cartilage degeneration is accelerated through mechanical wear and tear of the joint (2)[C].

Genetics
Uncommonly seen in familial pattern with autosomal dominant inheritance (<1% of patients); most cases are sporadic. Mutation in ANKH gene increased risk for calcium crystal formation.

RISK FACTORS
- Advanced age
- Traumatic injury
- CPPD often may occur as a complication in patients hospitalized for other medical and surgical illnesses.

GENERAL PREVENTION
Colchicine 0.6 mg BID may be used prophylactically to reduce frequency of episodes in recurrent CPPD.

COMMONLY ASSOCIATED CONDITIONS
- Hyperparathyroidism
- Hemochromatosis
- Gout
- Hypophosphatasia
- Hypothyroidism
- Ochronosis
- Wilson disease
- Amyloidosis
- Hypomagnesemia
- Familial hypocalciuric hypercalcaemia
- X-linked hypophosphatemic rickets
- Acromegaly

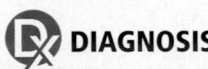

DIAGNOSIS

HISTORY
- Presentation often mimicks gout ("pseudogout").
- Acute CPPD: pain and swelling of ≥1 or more joints; knee involved in 50% of cases; ankle, wrist, toe, and shoulder are also common.
- Can present in proximal joints (mimicking polymyalgia rheumatica), often accompanied by tibiofemoral and ankle arthritis and tendinous calcifications
- Multiple symmetric joint involvement (mimicking RA) in <5% of cases
- May develop after intra-articular injection of hyaluronic acid (Hyalgan, Synvisc)
- Chronic CPPD: progressive degenerative arthritis with superimposed acute inflammatory attacks

PHYSICAL EXAM
- Inflammation (erythema, warmth, tender to touch), joint effusion, decreased range of motion of joint
- 50% associated with fever
- Any synovial joint may be involved.

DIFFERENTIAL DIAGNOSIS
- Illnesses that may cause acute inflammatory arthritis in a single or multiple joint(s):
  - Gout
  - Septic arthritis
  - Trauma
- Other illnesses that may present with an acute inflammatory arthritis:
  - Reiter syndrome
  - Lyme disease
  - Acute RA

DIAGNOSTIC TESTS & INTERPRETATION
Initial Tests (lab, imaging)
Synovial fluid analysis shows an inflammatory effusion:
- Cell count 2,000 to 100,000 WBCs/mL
- Differential predominantly neutrophils (80–90%)
- >50,000 WBC count increases likelihood of septic arthritis, 11% prevalence; number needed to treat (NNT) = 9; >100,000 WBCs/mL, 22% prevalence
- Wet prep with polarized microscopy may demonstrate small numbers of crystals. False-negative rate is high.

ALERT
Rhomboid-shaped weakly positively birefringent crystals in the fluid and within neutrophils is pathognomonic. In contrast, gout crystals are needle-shaped and negatively birefringent.

- Obtain the following metabolic studies in patients <50 years of age and consider in the elderly to exclude underlying disease:
  - Serum calcium, phosphorus, and magnesium
  - Serum alkaline phosphatase
  - Serum parathormone (i-PTH)
  - Serum iron, total iron-binding capacity, and serum ferritin
  - Serum thyroid-stimulating hormone (TSH) level
- Plain radiograph
  - Radiographic findings in pseudogout are neither sensitive nor specific.
  - Punctate and linear calcifications may be visualized in articular hyaline or fibrocartilage (e.g., menisci).
  - Knees, hips, symphysis pubis, and wrists are most commonly affected.
  - Patients with chronic CPPD may demonstrate subchondral cysts and loose bodies (osseous fragmentation with formation of intra-articular radiodense bodies) in joints not typically affected by degenerative joint disease.
- Ultrasound (US)
  - US may be more useful than plain radiography for the diagnosis of pseudogout in peripheral joints, with a positive predictive value of 92% and negative predictive value of 93% (3)[C].
  - US imaging characteristics include joint effusion, synovial thickening, and hyperechoic deposits.
- MRI
  - Chondrocalcinosis may be evident as hypointense lesions on MRI, particularly in association with the menisci of the knee.

Diagnostic Procedures/Other

ALERT
Aspiration of joint fluid with synovial fluid analysis and demonstration of CPPD crystals is required for diagnosis; aspiration may relieve symptoms and speed resolution of the inflammatory process.

Test Interpretation
CPPD crystal deposition in articular cartilage, synovium, ligaments, and tendons

TREATMENT

GENERAL MEASURES
Target symptom relief (reduce inflammation):
- Rest and elevate affected joint(s).
- Apply ice/cool compresses to affected joints.
- Nonweight bearing on affected joint while painful; use crutches or a walker.

MEDICATION
First Line
- A combination of pharmacologic and nonpharmacologic measures is recommended.
- Acute attacks should be treated with cool packs, rest, and joint aspiration with or without steroid injection.
- Chronic inflammatory CPPD arthropathy should be managed prophylactically with oral NSAIDs and/or colchicine (3)[C].
- Oral NSAIDs
  - Ibuprofen 600 to 800 mg PO TID–QID with food; maximum 3.2 g/day
  - Naproxen 500 mg PO BID with food
  - Other NSAIDs at anti-inflammatory doses are effective, although indomethacin has higher complication rates (relative risk [RR] = 2.2) compared with ibuprofen (RR = 1.2).
- Contraindications:
  - History of hypersensitivity to NSAIDs or aspirin
  - Active peptic ulcer disease or history of recurrent upper GI lesions
  - Avoid in renal insufficiency.
  - Serious GI bleeding can occur without warning; patient should be instructed on signs/symptoms. Administer proton pump inhibitor (PPI) or misoprostol 200 μg PO QID in patients at risk for NSAID-induced gastric ulcers.
- Oral colchicine
  - 0.6 mg QID or 0.6 mg hourly until symptoms relieved or vomiting/diarrhea develops; maximum dose per attack 4 to 6 mg; alternatively 0.5 to 1 mg/day may be used; avoid cholchicine with significant renal insufficiency.
- Intra-articular steroid injection
  - Prednisolone–sodium phosphate 4 to 20 mg or triamcinolone diacetate 2 to 40 mg with local anesthetic

ALERT
Significant adverse effects of NSAIDs:
- May elevate BP in patients on antihypertensive therapy
- May blunt antihypertensive effects of ACE inhibitors
- May prolong prothrombin time (PT) in patients taking oral anticoagulants
- Avoid concomitant aspirin use.
- May blunt diuretic effect of furosemide and hydrochlorothiazide
- May increase plasma lithium level in patients taking lithium carbonate

Second Line
- Oral prednisone: 30 to 50 mg/day for 7 to 10 days
- IM triamcinolone acetonide 40 mg; may repeat in 1 to 4 days
- Consider referring patients with large space-occupying tophaceous lesions for surgical removal.

- Alternative therapies for chronic CPPD
  - ACTH, Anakinra (anti-IL1), hydroxychloroquine, infliximab, probenecid, magnesium, ethyldiamine tetracetic acid (EDTA) have all been suggested. Large scale studies are needed to evaluate effectiveness (4)[C].

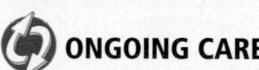 **ALERT**
Recent randomized trial showed no significant effect of methotrexate in chronic-recurrent CPPD (5)[B].

ISSUES FOR REFERRAL
Consider consultation with orthopedist or rheumatologist if septic joint or patient is not responding.

ADDITIONAL THERAPIES
Physical therapy
- Isometric exercises to maintain muscle strength during the acute stage (e.g., quadriceps isometric contractions, leg lifts if knee affected)
- Begin joint range-of-motion (ROM) exercises as inflammation and pain subside.
- Resume weight bearing when pain subsides.

SURGERY/OTHER PROCEDURES
Perform arthrocentesis and joint fluid analysis.

INPATIENT CONSIDERATIONS
Admission Criteria/Initial Stabilization
Consider admission for septic arthritis if:
- Synovial fluid WBC count >50,000/mL
- Treat with appropriate antibiotics pending culture results.

 ONGOING CARE

FOLLOW-UP RECOMMENDATIONS
Patient Monitoring
Reevaluate response to therapy 48 to 72 hours after beginning treatment; reexamine in 1 week then as needed.

DIET
No known relationship to diet

PATIENT EDUCATION
- Rest affected joint.
- Symptoms usually resolve in 7 to 10 days.

PROGNOSIS
- Acute attack usually resolves in 10 days; prognosis for resolution of acute attack is excellent.
- Patients may experience progressive joint damage and functional limitation.

COMPLICATIONS
- Recurrent acute attacks
- Osteoarthritis

Geriatric Considerations
Elderly patients treated with NSAIDs require careful monitoring and are at higher risk for GI bleeding and acute renal insufficiency. No loading dose for colchicine due to high rates of renal insufficiency in elderly patients.

REFERENCES
1. Zhang W, Doherty M, Bardin T, et al. European League Against Rheumatism recommendations for calcium pyrophosphate deposition. Part I: terminology and diagnosis. *Ann Rheum Dis.* 2011;70(4):563–570.
2. Rosenthal AK, Ryan LM. Nonpharmacologic and pharmacologic management of CPP crystal arthritis and BCP arthropathy and periarticular syndromes. *Rheum Dis Clin North Am.* 2014;40(2):343–356.
3. Zhang W, Doherty M, Pascual E, et al. EULAR recommendations for calcium pyrophosphate deposition. Part II: management. *Ann Rheum Dis.* 2011;70(4):571–575.
4. Pascart T, Richette P, Flipo RM. Treatment of nongout joint deposition diseases: an update. *Arthritis.* 2014; 2014:375202.
5. Finckh A, Mc Carthy GM, Madigan A, et al. Methotrexate in chronic-recurrent calcium pyrophosphate deposition disease: no significant effect in a randomized crossover trial. *Arthritis Res Ther.* 2014;16(5):458.

ADDITIONAL READING
- Bruges-Armas J, Bettencourt BF, Couto AR, et al. Effectiveness and safety of infliximab in two cases of severe chondrocalcinosis: nine years of follow-up. *Case Rep Rheumatol.* 2014;2014:536856.
- Daoussis D, Antonopoulos I, Andonopoulos AP. ACTH as a treatment for acute crystal-induced arthritis: update on clinical evidence and mechanisms of action. *Semin Arthritis Rheum.* 2014;43(5):648–653.
- Demertzis JL, Rubin DA. MR imaging assessment of inflammatory, crystalline-induced, and infectious arthritides. *Magn Reson Imaging Clin N Am.* 2011;19(2):339–363.
- Macmullan P, McCarthy G. Treatment and management of pseudogout: insights for the clinician. *Ther Adv Musculoskelet Dis.* 2012;4(2):121–131.
- Richette P, Bardin T, Doherty M. An update on the epidemiology of calcium pyrophosphate dihydrate crystal deposition disease. *Rheumatology (Oxford).* 2009;48(7):711–715.
- Sattui SE, Singh JA, Gaffo AL. Comorbidities in patients with crystal diseases and hyperuricemia. *Rheum Dis Clin North Am.* 2014;40(2):251–278.

CODES

ICD10
- M11.20 Other chondrocalcinosis, unspecified site
- M11.269 Other chondrocalcinosis, unspecified knee
- M11.29 Other chondrocalcinosis, multiple sites

CLINICAL PEARLS
- Suspect CPPD if arthritis case doesn't follow a pattern typical of degenerative joint disease (e.g., metacarpophalangeal joints, wrists).
- Perform arthrocentesis to confirm diagnosis.
- If septic arthritis is considered, treat presumptively with antibiotics until culture results are available.
- NSAID therapy is the preferred treatment for acute flare.
- Oral steroids are useful if NSAIDs are contraindicated.
- Intra-articular steroids can be used *if* septic arthritis has been excluded.

PSORIASIS

Edwin A. Farnell, IV, MD • Michael O. Needham, MD, CPT, MC, USA

BASICS

DESCRIPTION
- A chronic, multisystem inflammatory disorder most commonly characterized by cutaneous erythematous papules and plaques with silvery scale. A complex genetic and immune-mediated disorder with flares related to systemic, psychological, infectious, and environmental factors. Skin disease with multiple different phenotypic variations and degrees of severity.
- Clinical phenotypes
  - Plaque (vulgaris): most common variant (>80% of cases); well-demarcated, scaly, pink-to-red plaques of various sizes; symmetrically distributed on scalp, extensor surfaces of extremities, and trunk
  - Guttate: <2% of psoriasis patients, usually in patients <30 years of age; presents abruptly with 1- to 10-mm droplet-shaped pink papules and fine scale over trunk and extremities; often preceded by group A β-hemolytic streptococcal infection 2 to 3 weeks earlier.
  - Inverse: Affects intertriginous areas and flexural surfaces; pink-to-red plaques with minimal scale; absence of satellite pustules distinguishes it from candidiasis although may coexist.
  - Erythrodermic: ~1–2.25% of psoriasis patients; generalized erythema and scaling, affecting >75% of BSA; associated with desquamation, hair loss, nail dystrophy, and systemic symptoms such as fever, chills, malaise, or high-output cardiac failure; may require hospital admission for management of dehydration, electrolyte abnormalities, and high risk of infection
  - Pustular: sterile pustules; several forms including generalized pustular psoriasis, annular pustular psoriasis, and impetigo herpetiformis; generalized type can result in life-threatening bacterial superinfections, sepsis, and dehydration if left untreated
  - Nail disease: pitting, oil spots, and thickening; nails involved in up to 50% of patients with psoriasis with lifetime incidence of 80–90%
  - Psoriatic arthritis: seronegative inflammatory spondyloarthropathy; mono and assymetrical oligoarthritis

EPIDEMIOLOGY
Incidence
Predominant sex: male = female. Predominant age: two peaks in incidence between the ages of 20 to 30 years and 50 to 60 years.

Prevalence
- 2–4.7%—similar prevalence in all races
- ~80% of patients have mild to moderate disease (1).

ETIOLOGY AND PATHOPHYSIOLOGY
Antigenic triggers activate dendritic cells and T cells; dendritic cells produce type I interferon, and interleukin (IL)-20, which speeds keratinocyte proliferation; myeloid dendritic cells release IL-23 in lymph nodes, recruiting TH1 and TH17 cells to the lesions; T cells produce numerous cytokines, including interferon-γ, IL-17, and IL-22 that stimulate keratinocytes to proliferate and produce proinflammatory antimicrobial peptides and cytokines, which recruit neutrophils to the epidermis and activate dermal fibroblasts.

Genetics
- Genetic predisposition (probably polygenic)
- 40% have psoriasis in a first-degree relative
- Increased incidence of specific human leukocyte antigens (e.g., HLA-Cw6)

- Multiple susceptibility loci contain genes involved in immune system regulation (e.g., psoriasis-susceptibility [PSORS1] locus on chromosome 6p21; polymorphisms in the IL-12/IL-13 receptor, the p40 subunit of IL-12 and IL-23, and the p19 subunit of IL-12) (2)

RISK FACTORS
- Family history
- Local trauma; local irritation (exacerbation)
- HIV; streptococcal infection
- Mental stress (exacerbation)
- Medications (lithium, antimalarials, β-blockers, interferon, withdrawal of steroids)
- Smoking

GENERAL PREVENTION
Avoid triggers, including trauma, sunburns, smoking, and exposure to certain medications (as mentioned earlier), alcohol, and stress; weight loss if obese.

COMMONLY ASSOCIATED CONDITIONS
- Psoriatic arthritis
- Obesity, metabolic syndrome, diabetes, CKD
- Cardiovascular disease; atherosclerotic disease
- Nonalcoholic fatty liver disease (NAFLD)
- Autoimmune: alopecia areata, celiac disease, Crohn disease, systemic sclerosis
- Psychiatric/psychologic: depression, suicide, emotional burden/anxiety, alcohol abuse (3)
- Malignancy: lymphoma, nonmelanoma skin cancer with psoralen-UVA (PUVA) therapy

DIAGNOSIS

HISTORY
- May include sudden onset of clearly demarcated, erythematous plaques with overlying silvery scales; exacerbation of chronic plaques, especially on extensor surfaces and scalp; typically no or mild pruritus; triggers may include streptococcal/viral infection or trauma.
- Family history of similar condition

PHYSICAL EXAM
- Well-demarcated salmon pink-to-red erythematous papules and plaques; silvery scale
- Distribution favors scalp, auricular conchal bowls, and postauricular area; extensor surface of extremities, especially knees and elbows; umbilicus, lower back, intergluteal cleft, and nails
- Nail findings: pitting, oil spots, onycholysis, splinter hemorrhages, subungual hyperkeratosis
- Auspitz sign: underlying pinpoints of bleeding following scraping of plaques
- Koebner phenomenon: new psoriatic lesions arising at sites of skin injury/trauma
- Genitals affected up to 40% of patients (4)
- Sebopsoriasis: Psoriasis can overlap with seborrheic dermatitis as greasy scales on the eyebrows, nasolabial folds, and postauricular and presternal areas.

DIFFERENTIAL DIAGNOSIS
- Plaque: seborrheic dermatitis, nummular eczema, atopic dermatitis, contact dermatitis, lichen planus, lichen simplex chronicus, tinea, pityriasis rubra pilaris, subacute/discoid lupus erythematosus, squamous cell carcinoma in situ
- Guttate: pityriasis rosea, pityriasis lichenoides chronica, lichen planus, secondary syphilis, small plaque parapsoriasis

- Pustular: subcorneal pustulosis, acute generalized exanthematous pustulosis, folliculitis, pemphigus foliaceous
- Erythrodermic: cutaneous T-cell lymphoma, drug-induced erythroderma, ichthyosiform erythroderma

DIAGNOSTIC TESTS & INTERPRETATION
Initial Tests (lab, imaging)
Clinical diagnosis based on history and physical exam. May include negative rheumatoid factor, normal erythrocyte sedimentation rate (ESR), and C-reactive protein (elevated in pustular/erythrodermic variants); uric acid level may be elevated in pustular psoriasis; sterile fluid from pustules with neutrophilic infiltrate; fungal studies in hand and foot psoriasis

Diagnostic Procedures/Other
- Psoriasis Area and Severity Index (PASI) evaluates overall severity and body surface area (BSA) involvement.
- Physicians Global Assessment: Target plaque score and the percentage BSA together; 4-mm punch biopsy from affected skin, if necessary
- Dermatology Life Quality Index (DLQI)

Test Interpretation
Biopsy: thickening of the stratum corneum (hyperkeratosis) with retention of nuclei (parakeratosis); elongation, thickening, and clubbing of rete ridges; dilated tortuous capillary loops in the dermal papillae; perivascular lymphocytic infiltrate, Munro microabscesses: neutrophils in stratum corneum

TREATMENT

GENERAL MEASURES
Adequate topical hydration (emollients), sun exposure (avoid sunburns), stress relief

MEDICATION
First Line
- Mild-to-moderate disease
  - Emollients BID: petrolatum/ointments to maintain skin hydration and minimize pruritus and risk of koebnerization
  - Topical corticosteroids
    ○ Anti-inflammatory, antiproliferative, immunosuppressive, and vasoconstrictive effects; tachyphylaxis develops over time, may alternate to prevent
    ○ Local side effects: skin atrophy, hypopigmentation, striae, acne, folliculitis, and purpura. Systemic side effects: Risk is higher, with higher potency formulations used over a large surface for a prolonged period; pregnancy Category C
    ○ Applications are typically twice daily until lesions flatten/resolve, then taper to PRN use for maintenance.
    ○ Scalp: strong potency in solution/foam vehicle; shampoos and sprays also available
    ○ Face, intertriginous areas, infants: low-potency corticosteroids: 1% hydrocortisone
    ○ Adult initial therapy: medium-potency corticosteroids daily (e.g., 0.1% mometasone or triamcinolone); strong-potency corticosteroids: 0.05% betamethasone or fluocinonide daily; superpotency corticosteroids: clobetasol, halobetasol; limit use to 2 to 4 weeks; avoid occlusive dressings; reserved for recalcitrant plaques

P

- Vitamin D analogues: calcipotriene 0.005% ointment daily to BID; limits keratinocyte hyperproliferation; may be highly effective for short-term control in combination with a superpotent corticosteroid; should not be used with products that can alter pH, such as topical lactic acid; local side effects: burning, pruritus, edema, peeling, dryness, and erythema; pregnancy Category C
- Topical retinoids: tazarotene 0.05% or 0.1% (Tazorac) daily; normalizes abnormal keratinocyte differentiation and diminishes hyperproliferation; may be combined with corticosteroids; side effects: local irritation, photosensitivity; pregnancy Category X
- Topical calcineurin inhibitors: Tacrolimus 0.1% or pimecrolimus 1% may be used as steroid-sparing agents, especially in facial and intertriginous areas.

- Comparison of topical therapies: vitamin D analogues have slower onset of action than topical corticosteroids, but longer disease-free periods for body plaques. For scalp, potent and superpotency steroids more effective (5)[A]
- Combination of superpotent steroids and vitamin D analogs has better efficacy than either as monotherapy or come in combination compounds (6)[A].

• Severe disease: may need combination therapy

- Light therapy: Locally immunosuppressive and antiproliferative. Natural sunlight; UVB (broad/narrow band [BB, NB]) or PUVA: Treatment protocols are skin type dependent: PUVA most effective, followed by NB-UVB, then BB-UVB (7)[A]; well tolerated, but increased risk of nonmelanoma skin cancers with >350 treatments

- Systemic therapies
  ○ Methotrexate: blocks DNA synthesis and inhibits proliferation of lymphoid tissue; start 7.5 to 15 mg/week IV, PO, IM, or SC, then increase 2.5 mg every 2 to 3 weeks, up to 25 mg; contraindicated in pregnancy; supplement with folic acid 1 to 5 mg/day to protect against side effects : hepatotoxicity, pulmonary toxicity, bone marrow suppression; baseline chest x-ray, monitor LFTs, renal function, CBC, testing for latent tuberculosis (TB); consider liver biopsy when cumulative dose reaches 3.5 to 4 g; avoid alcohol and medications that interfere with folic acid metabolism, including Bactrim, sulfamethoxazole, or hepatotoxic agents (e.g., retinoids)
  ○ Cyclosporine: inhibits T-cell activation; start 2.5 mg/kg/day; if insufficient response after 4 weeks, increase by 0.5 mg/kg/day; additional dosage increases every 2 weeks (max dose: 4 mg/kg/day pregnancy Category C; side effects: renal toxicity and hypertension, limit long-term use: monitor renal function, CBC with Mg^{2+} and K^+, and BP
  ○ Acitretin (Soriatane): systemic retinoid; onset ranges from 3 to 6 months; start 25 to 50 mg/day given with the main meal; effective for pustular psoriasis and as a maintenance therapy after stabilization with other agents; sometimes combined with UV-B/PUVA; pregnancy Category X: Pregnancy test before starting; two forms of contraception 1 month before, during, and for at least 3 years after treatment; avoid alcohol (may convert acitretin to etretinate); side effects: alopecia, xerosis, cheilitis, hepatotoxicity, hyperlipidemia, cataracts; monitor LFTs, renal function, lipid profile, CBC, regular eye exams

- Biologics: general guidelines: Screen for latent TB at baseline and yearly, hepatitis panel at baseline, avoid live vaccines; monitor CBC with differential, signs/symptoms of infections, heart failure, malignancy, drug-induced lupus, inflammatory bowel disease, demyelinating disorder. Some concern for "biologic fatigue" phenomenon, or loss of PASI 75 over time though each has been shown to be effective at 24 weeks with a NNT <2. All should be considered effective first-line treatments (7,8)[A]; pregnancy Category B.

  ○ TNF-α inhibitors: etanercept (Enbrel): begin at 50 mg SC twice a week for 3 months then maintenance of 50 mg/week. Adalimumab (Humira): dosing starts at 80 mg SC for 1 week, then 40 mg SC every other week. Infliximab (Remicade): TNF inhibitor: 5 mg/kg IV at weeks 0, 2, and 6; maintenance doses of 5 mg/kg every 8 weeks thereafter; adjust interval, as needed; anaphylaxis-like infusion reaction occurs in <1% of patients.
  ○ IL-12/IL-23 antagonist: ustekinumab (Stelara): patients <100 kg: 45 mg SC at weeks 0 and 4, then every 12 weeks; >100 kg: 90 mg can be given.

Second Line
Immunosuppressives: azathioprine, hydroxyurea, 6-thioguanine, fumaric acid esters, and topicals: salicylic acid; anthralin

ISSUES FOR REFERRAL
Psoriasis >20% of BSA, severe extremity involvement, particularly hands and feet

SURGERY/OTHER PROCEDURES
Psoriasis and psoriatic medications can affect wound healing postoperatively; methotrexate: Monitor for postoperative infections; hold cyclosporine for 1 week before and after; some surgeons may prefer to hold therapy with biologics for up to 1 month before and after surgery.

INPATIENT CONSIDERATIONS
Admission Criteria/Initial Stabilization
Generalized pustular psoriasis/erythrodermic psoriasis: Rule out sepsis; restoration of barrier function of skin with cleaning and bandaging; intensive topical corticosteroid therapy, phototherapy, systemic therapy, particularly medications with a quick onset such as oral cyclosporine; management of electrolytes

 ONGOING CARE

FOLLOW-UP RECOMMENDATIONS
Measure BSA involvement to determine if therapy is working; change therapy or add agent if no improvement is seen.

DIET
Well-balanced diet and exercise to limit cardiovascular risk factors and decrease risk of associated conditions, including obesity, metabolic syndrome, diabetes, and atherosclerosis.

PATIENT EDUCATION
National Psoriasis Foundation: www.psoriasis.org; 800-723-9166

PROGNOSIS
Guttate form may be self-limited and remit after 4 months; chronic plaque type is lifelong, with intermittent spontaneous remissions and exacerbations; erythrodermic and generalized pustular forms may be severe and persistent.

COMPLICATIONS
Psoriatic arthritis, generalized pustular psoriasis, erythrodermic psoriasis

REFERENCES
1. Menter A, Korman NJ, Elmets CA, et al. Guidelines of care for the management of psoriasis and psoriatic arthritis: section 6. Guidelines of care for the treatment of psoriasis and psoriatic arthritis: case-based presentations and evidence-based conclusions. J Am Acad Dermatol. 2011;65(1):137–174.
2. Villaseñor-Park J, Wheeler D, Grandinetti L. Psoriasis: evolving treatment for a complex disease. Cleve Clin J Med. 2012;79(6):413–423.
3. Brenaut E, Horreau C, Pouplard C, et al. Alcohol consumption and psoriasis: a systemic literature review. J Eur Acad Dermatol Venereol. 2013;27(Suppl 3):30–35.
4. Meeuwis KA, de Hullu JA, Massuger LF, et al. Genital psoriasis: a systemic literature review on this hidden skin disease. Acta Derm Venereol. 2011;91(1):5–11.
5. Mason AR, Mason J, Cork M, et al. Topical treatments for chronic plaque psoriasis. Cochrane Database Syst Rev. 2013;(3):CD005028.
6. Hendricks AG, Keijsers RR, de Jong EM, et al. Efficacy and safety of combinations of first-line topical treatments in chronic plaque psoriasis: a systematic literature review. J Eur Acad Dermatol Venereol. 2013;27(8):931–951.
7. Almutawa F, Alnomair N, Wang Y, et al. Systematic review of UV-based therapies for psoriasis. Am J Clin Dermatol. 2013;14(2):87–109.
8. Nast A, Jacobs A, Rosumeck S, et al. Efficacy and safety of systemic long-term treatments for moderate-to-severe psoriasis: a systematic review and meta-analysis [published online ahead of print June 5, 2015]. J Invest Dermatol. 2015;135(11):2641–2648.

ADDITIONAL READING
Galván-Banqueri M, Marín Gil R, Santos Ramos B, et al. Biologic treatments for moderate-to-severe psoriasis: indirect comparison. J Clin Pharm Ther. 2013;38(2):121–130.

 SEE ALSO

Arthritis, Psoriatic

CODES

ICD10
• L40.9 Psoriasis, unspecified
• L40.50 Arthropathic psoriasis, unspecified
• L42 Pityriasis rosea

CLINICAL PEARLS
Chronic lifelong inflammatory skin condition with remissions and exacerbations; set realistic expectations with patient. Disease burden not limited to skin. If one medication does not work, use/combine with another agent.

PSYCHOSIS
Robert A. Baldor, MD, FAAFP

 BASICS

DESCRIPTION
Syndrome seen with schizophrenia, schizoaffective disorder, mood disorder, substance use, medical problems, delirium, and dementia; symptoms include the following:
- Positive symptoms: hallucinations and delusions (fixed false and often paranoid beliefs created as the patient loses the ability to correct errors in thinking)
- Negative symptoms: apathy, avolition, withdrawal
- Disorganized speech/behavior
- Cognition: decreased working memory, difficulty with attention, poor and slow information interpretation

EPIDEMIOLOGY
Prevalence
- Schizophrenia: peak onset 18 to 25 years in men; women peak onset 25 to 35 years
  - 1% of the U.S. population; thought to be similar worldwide
- Delusional disorder: 0.03% of population
- Bipolar type I: 1% of population
- Prevalence in major depression not known

ETIOLOGY AND PATHOPHYSIOLOGY
- Neurodevelopmental predisposition plus 1st/3rd trimester in utero insult (e.g., 1st-trimester infection or 3rd-trimester birth hypoxia) leads to exaggerated neuronal apoptosis in late adolescence with subsequent thalamic sensory overload. Increased dopaminergic mesolimbic transmission may contribute to delusions and hallucinations in schizophrenia. Dopamine deficiency in mesocortical pathways may contribute to frontal lobe hypoactivity often associated with apathy and withdrawal in schizophrenia. Glutamate, neurosteroids, and neurodevelopmental abnormalities are active areas of research.
- Postulated stress-diathesis model: Individuals biologically at risk develop psychosis when under stress.

Genetics
Schizophrenia: 50% concordance for monozygotic twins, little or no shared environmental effect; multiple candidate genes involving disruption of neurodevelopment

RISK FACTORS
Substance abuse (particularly marijuana), family history of psychosis, lower socioeconomic status

GENERAL PREVENTION
Community interventions for early detection and treatment of prodromal symptoms show promise.

COMMONLY ASSOCIATED CONDITIONS
- Serious mental illness is associated with metabolic syndrome, autonomic dysfunction, and sudden cardiac death.
- Cancer mortality: particularly breast and lung cancer
- Substance abuse disorders, including nicotine dependence

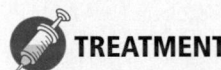 DIAGNOSIS

First, rule out delirium: Psychosis should not have fluctuating consciousness/reduced clarity of awareness.

HISTORY
- Delusions (fixed false beliefs): persecutory (being monitored), bizarre (involving impossible states), somatic (fixed belief in nonexistent serious illness), referential (getting messages from TV, radio, or thoughts inserted/deleted by others), grandiose (belief that one has special powers)
- Hallucinations: auditory, visual, tactile
- Bipolar illness, depression, and dementia are all associated with psychosis, so screen for symptoms of depression, mania, and memory loss.
- Screen for toxidromes of drugs of abuse.
- Screen for history of epileptiform activity.
- Suicidality: higher risk with comorbid depression/mania, previous suicide attempts, drug abuse, agitation/akathisia, poor compliance

PHYSICAL EXAM
- Mental status exam: disorganized idea sequencing and/or error correction, not incorrect thought content, is the *condicio sine qua non* of schizophrenia. Patients often have negative symptoms (e.g., social withdrawal, lack of initiative, poverty of thought) and disorganized behavior.
- Attention to neurologic focalities, antipsychotic-induced parkinsonism, tardive dyskinesia, and akathisia
- May rarely present with catatonia: extreme excitement/lack of movement; posturing, mutism, grimacing, waxy flexibility

DIFFERENTIAL DIAGNOSIS
- Schizophrenia: positive symptoms (psychosis) and negative symptoms (flat affect), prodrome of social withdrawal, cognitive impairment; schizophreniform disorder: psychotic/prodromal symptoms in <6 months; schizoaffective disorder: manic/depressive mood disorder with hallucinations/delusions that persist even when euthymic; schizotypal personality disorder: no true psychosis but distance in relationships and odd beliefs; delusional disorder: nonbizarre delusion (e.g., erotomanic, grandiose, jealous, persecutory, somatic), no negative/mood symptoms
- Mood disorder with psychotic features: can occur in mania/depression. Delusions often mood-congruent; psychosis remits when mood improves.
- Substance-induced psychosis: alcohol and benzodiazepine withdrawal, intoxication with cocaine, bath salts, PCP, cannabis, amphetamines, hallucinogens, and alcohol. May persist beyond acute intoxication
- Borderline personality disorder: During extreme stress, patients often experience auditory/visual hallucinations (psychosis NOS)
- Posttraumatic stress disorder: psychosis associated with traumatic recollections. Often visual hallucinations (vs. more auditory in schizophrenia)
- Psychosis due to general medical condition: delirium, stroke, infection, collagen vascular disease, head injury, tumor, interictal, porphyria, syphilis, and so forth
- Medication-induced psychosis: common causes: steroids, L-dopa, anticholinergic medication, antidepressants in bipolar patients, interferon, digoxin, stimulants

DIAGNOSTIC TESTS & INTERPRETATION
Test for causes of delirium mimicking psychosis, if uncertain.
- Broad screen for medical causes: CBC, metabolic panel, LFTs, thyroid-stimulating hormone (TSH), rapid plasma reagin (RPR), HIV, vitamin B_{12}, U/A, and screens for subclinical infection in elderly
- Screen for drugs of abuse.
- No imaging necessary for diagnosis. Consider MRI/CT to evaluate for medical cause of symptoms, especially if new onset or in elderly. In research studies, schizophrenia is associated with enlarged lateral ventricles and less frontal activity.

Follow-Up Tests & Special Considerations
Because of elevated risk related to schizophrenia and psychotropic medications, screen for metabolic syndrome.
- Consider Wilson disease, porphyria, metachromatic leukodystrophy, inflammatory conditions.
- Consider ECG: Antipsychotics can prolong corrected QT (QTc) interval, particularly ziprasidone, thioridazine, droperidol, IV haloperidol
- Consider lumbar puncture if unable to distinguish from delirium and/or unexplained rapid-onset psychosis.
- Consider electroencephalogram (EEG) for partial complex seizures and psychosis associated with preictal and postictal events.

TREATMENT

Before antipsychotic treatment, lipid profile, fasting blood sugar, LFTs, metabolic panel, weight (1)[B]

MEDICATION
- Antipsychotics are the mainstay of treatment (1)[B].
- Classified as typical versus atypical. Dopamine-2 (D_2) antagonists with varied affinity for the receptor. Atypicals also block serotonin 5-HT2A receptors. Help positive symptoms more than negative. Nonspecific effect on agitation begins early; antipsychotic effect takes 1 to 6 weeks.
- For mania with psychotic features, a mood stabilizer may be used with an antipsychotic.
- For major depression with psychotic features, antidepressant and antipsychotic medications yield better response rate than either medication alone.
- In delirium, must treat underlying cause
- Risks of antipsychotic medications include the following:
  - Acute dystonia: Use 1 to 3 mg IM/IV benztropine initially, then 0.5 to 2 mg BID–TID or diphenhydramine 50 to 100 mg IM/IV BID–TID max 400 mg/day.
  - Parkinsonism: Lower antipsychotic dose; switch to atypical (particularly, quetiapine, olanzapine, or clozapine) or add benztropine 0.5 to 2 mg PO BID–TID, diphenhydramine 25 to 50 mg BID–TID.
  - Akathisia: intense restlessness, especially legs. Lower antipsychotic dose; treat with β-blocker, anticholinergic, or benzodiazepine; may switch to antipsychotic with lower risk for akathisia such as quetiapine, olanzapine, iloperidone, or clozapine.
  - Tardive dyskinesia: 20% of those treated long-term with typicals. Switch to clozapine or quetiapine. If cannot, minimize dose.

– Neuroleptic malignant syndrome: potentially fatal; rigidity, tremor, fever, autonomic instability, mental status changes; discontinue neuroleptic; ICU; volume resuscitation; cooling blankets; no anticholinergics/antihistaminics; consider dantrolene, amantadine, bromocriptine electroconvulsive therapy (ECT).

– Metabolic syndrome, sudden cardiac death (risk higher IM/IV droperidol, IV haloperidol), stroke (elderly), QTc prolonged, pulmonary embolus

First Line

- Benefits of some of the atypical antipsychotics include low risk of extrapyramidal symptoms (quetiapine, olanzapine, iloperidone, or clozapine) and tardive dyskinesia (clozapine, quetiapine); possibly more effective for negative symptoms
- Greater risk of weight gain, new-onset diabetes, and hyperlipidemia with olanzapine and clozapine compared with typicals and some of the other atypicals (ziprasidone, aripiprazole)
- Acute psychotic agitation: olanzapine 5 to 10 mg IM with up to three 10-mg injections over a 24-hour period, care with subsequent benzodiazepines; ziprasidone 10 mg IM q2h or 20 mg q4h; max 40 mg over a 24-hour period; haloperidol/ lorazepam 5 mg/2 mg IM often with 1 mg IM benztropine, max 20 mg haloperidol, and 8 mg lorazepam over a 24-hour period
- Psychosis in schizophrenia
  - Olanzapine: Start 5 to 10 mg at bedtime, target dose 5 to 20 mg/day within 2 days and up to 40 mg/day in treatment-refractory schizophrenia. More likely weight gain, hyperlipidemia, and hyperglycemia than other oral atypicals except clozapine; may have lower rates of discontinuation and rehospitalization than several other atypicals but likely not more efficacy than clozapine. Sedation initially
  - Quetiapine: Start 25 mg BID 25 to 50 mg BID–TID on days 2 and 3, up to 300 to 400 mg in divided doses by day 4. Within 2 weeks, up to 400 to 800 mg/day divided BID–TID; less parkinsonism, useful in Parkinson disease psychosis; more weight gain than aripiprazole, lurasidone, ziprasidone; sedation, restless legs syndrome; more gradual titration tolerated better. Quetiapine XR can start 300 mg/day. Dose increases can be within 1 day and up to 300 mg/day, but slower start and titration may be better; target dose 300 to 800 mg at bedtime
  - Risperidone: Start 1 to 2 mg/day; target dose of 2 to 6 mg/day to be reached over 1 to 2 weeks; doses >6 mg rarely more effective and higher risk of parkinsonism. Higher risk of prolactinemia/ parkinsonism than clozapine, quetiapine, olanzapine
  - Paliperidone: Start 3 to 6 mg/day target dose 6 to 12 mg/day; titrate over 1 to 2 weeks. Higher risk of prolactinemia/parkinsonism than clozapine, quetiapine, olanzapine
  - Ziprasidone: Start 20 to 40 mg PO BID, with target dose of 100 to 200 mg/day in divided doses over 2 weeks; prolongs QTc; less likely to cause weight gain than other atypicals; higher risk of akathisia/parkinsonism than clozapine, quetiapine, olanzapine. Requires meal. Often sedation
  - Aripiprazole: Start 10 to 15 mg/day, may increase up to 30 mg/day over a week or 2; less weight gain but higher rates of akathisia/parkinsonism than clozapine, quetiapine, olanzapine

– Asenapine: Start 5 mg at bedtime or BID sublingually, increase to 10 mg BID if needed over a week or 2; less weight gain than some, higher rates of akathisia/parkinsonism than clozapine, quetiapine, olanzapine; sedation, orthostatic hypotension, numb tongue, nausea, bad taste

– Lurasidone: Start 20 to 40 mg once daily with food (at least 350 calories), increase to 80/120 mg at bedtime if needed over 2 to 4 weeks. Less weight gain than some but higher rates of akathisia/parkinsonism than clozapine, quetiapine, olanzapine; not antihistaminic but α-blocking sedation and serotonergic nausea

– Iloperidone: Start 1 mg BID, may increase by 2 mg BID each day, but slower can be better due to significant orthostasis. Increase to max 12 mg BID. Little akathisia/parkinsonism, less weight gain than olanzapine or clozapine but slower efficacy due to long titration, orthostasis, sedation

Geriatric Considerations

Increased risk of cerebrovascular accident when antipsychotics are used in the elderly with dementia 3[B]

Second Line

- Clozapine: more effective for reducing symptoms, preventing relapse, decreasing tardive dyskinesia, and decreasing suicidality than other antipsychotics but second line given risk of fatal agranulocytosis. National registry for all patients on clozapine, weekly CBC and absolute neutrophil count (ANC) for 6 months then every 2 weeks for 6 months, then every 4 weeks. More weight gain, hyperlipidemia, hyperglycemia, seizures, myocarditis, pulmonary embolus, and sedation but low rate of parkinsonism, tardive dyskinesia. Useful in treatment-refractory psychosis and in Parkinson disease psychosis

- Despite association with more weight gain than other antipsychotics, clozapine and olanzapine do not appear to increase risk of cardiac and all-cause mortality (2,3)[B].

- Long-acting preparations: available for 2 typicals (haloperidol and fluphenazine) and 4 atypicals (risperidone, paliperidone, olanzapine, aripiprazole; olanzapine requires registration due to rare delirium syndrome). Test tolerability with oral medication first. Long-acting antipsychotics promote compliance.
- Long-acting haloperidol, paliperidone, olanzapine, aripiprazole administered every 4 weeks; long-acting risperidone and fluphenazine administered every 2 weeks.

ISSUES FOR REFERRAL

Encourage contact with advocacy groups for families and patients (National Alliance for the Mentally Ill).

ADDITIONAL THERAPIES

Cognitive-behavioral therapy (CBT) is an effective adjuvant to antipsychotics (1)[B].

INPATIENT CONSIDERATIONS

Admission Criteria/Initial Stabilization

At risk for harm to self or others; extreme functional impairment; unable to care for self; new-onset psychosis

Discharge Criteria

No longer a danger to self or others and adequate outpatient treatment in place

 ONGOING CARE

FOLLOW-UP RECOMMENDATIONS

Close follow-up for inpatient discharge (high risk for suicide), use CBT, exercise, teach smoking cessation

PATIENT EDUCATION

National Alliance on Mental Illness: www.nami.org/

PROGNOSIS

Schizophrenia: Fluctuating course, 70% first-episode psychosis patients improve in 3–4 months; 7% will die of suicide; 20–40% will attempt suicide.

REFERENCES

1. National Institute for Health and Care Excellence. Psychosis and schizophrenia in adults: prevention and management. http://www.nice.org.uk/guidance/ cg178. Accessed 2014.
2. Tiihonen J, Lönnqvist J, Wahlbeck K, et al. 11-year follow-up of mortality in patients with schizophrenia: a population-based cohort study (FIN11 study). Lancet. 2009;374(9690):620–627.
3. Strom BL, Eng SM, Faich G, et al. Comparative mortality associated with ziprasidone and olanzapine in real-world use among 18,154 patients with schizophrenia: the Ziprasidone Observational Study of Cardiac Outcomes (ZODIAC). Am J Psychiatry. 2011;168(2):193–201.

ADDITIONAL READING

- McEvoy JP, Lieberman JA, Stroup TS, et al. Effectiveness of clozapine versus olanzapine, quetiapine, and risperidone in patients with chronic schizophrenia who did not respond to prior atypical antipsychotic treatment. Am J Psychiatry. 2006;163(4):600–610.
- van Iersel MB, Zuidema SU, Koopmans RT, et al. Antipsychotics for behavioural and psychological problems in elderly people with dementia: a systematic review of adverse events. Drugs Aging. 2005;22(10):845–858.

 SEE ALSO

Delirium; Schizophrenia

 CODES

ICD10

- F29 Unsp psychosis not due to a substance or known physiol cond
- F20.9 Schizophrenia, unspecified
- F39 Unspecified mood [affective] disorder

CLINICAL PEARLS

- Antipsychotics are the mainstay of treatment; evidence corroborates decreased all-cause mortality in patients who are adherent to these medications.
- Clozapine and long-acting preparations are likely underused in schizophrenia in the United States and may increase adherence, whereas newer atypicals (quetiapine, lurasidone, aripiprazole, olanzapine-fluoxetine combination) may help with depressive symptoms in psychosis.

PULMONARY ARTERIAL HYPERTENSION

Urooj Najm, MBBS • Najm Hasan Siddiqui, MD

 BASICS

DESCRIPTION

- Pulmonary arterial hypertension (PAH) is a category of pulmonary hypertension (PH) characterized by abnormalities in the small pulmonary arteries (precapillary PH) that produce increased pulmonary arterial pressure (PAP) and vascular resistance, eventually resulting in right-sided heart failure. PAH is a progressive disorder associated with increased mortality.
  - Previously, PH was classified as primary PH (without cause: now idiopathic pulmonary arterial hypertension [IPAH]) or secondary PH (with cause or associated condition); now it is clear that some types of secondary PH closely match primary PH (IPAH) in their histology, natural history, and response to treatment. Therefore, WHO classifies PH into five groups based on mechanism, with PAH as group 1 in this classification.
- PAH is diagnosed by right-heart catheterization and defined by:
  - Mean PAP ≥25 mm Hg at rest
  - Pulmonary capillary wedge pressure ≤15 mm Hg (to exclude PH owing to left heart disease; i.e., group 2 PH)
  - Mild or absent chronic lung disease or other causes of hypoxemia (excludes PH owing to lung disease or hypoxemia; i.e., group 3 PH)
  - Absent venous thromboembolic disease (excludes chronic thromboembolic PH; i.e., group 4 PH)
  - Absent systemic disorder (like sarcoidosis), hematologic disorders (like myeloproliferative disease), and metabolic disorders (like glycogen storage disease). Purpose is to exclude group 5 PH.
- PAH is divided into following main categories:
  - Idiopathic: sporadic, with no family history or risk factors
  - Heritable: IPAH with mutations or familial cases with or without mutations
  - Drug- or toxin-induced: mostly associated with anorectics (e.g., fenfluramine), rapeseed oil, L-tryptophan, and illicit drugs such as methamphetamine and cocaine
  - Associated: connective tissue diseases (e.g., systemic lupus erythematosus, rheumatoid arthritis, scleroderma), HIV infection, portal hypertension, congenital heart disease, schistosomiasis, chronic hemolytic anemia (e.g., sickle cell disease)
  - Pulmonary veno-occlusive disease (PVOD) and/or pulmonary capillary hemangiomatosis (PCH) and persistent pulmonary hypertension of the newborn (PPHN) are classified as separate categories due to more differences than similarities with PAH.
    - PVOD and/or PCH: rare cause of PH characterized by extensive diffuse occlusion of the pulmonary veins (unlike PAH which involves the small muscular pulmonary arterioles)
  - PPHN
- System(s) affected: pulmonary, cardiovascular

EPIDEMIOLOGY

- Age: can occur at any age; mean age, 37 years
- Sex (IPAH): female > male (~4:1)

Incidence

- Overall PAH: 5 to 52 cases/million
- IPAH: low, ~2 to 6 per million
- Drug-induced PAH: 1/25,000 with >3 months of anorectic use
- HIV-associated: 0.5/100

- Portal hypertension–associated: 1 to 6/100
- Scleroderma-associated: 6–60%

Prevalence

- PAH: ~15 to 50 cases per million
- IPAH: ~6 cases per million

ETIOLOGY AND PATHOPHYSIOLOGY

- Pulmonary: Inflammation, vasoconstriction, endothelial dysfunction, and remodeling of pulmonary arteries produced by increased cell proliferation and reduced rates of apoptosis lead to obstruction.
- Cardiovascular: right ventricular hypertrophy (RVH), eventually leading to right-sided heart failure
- IPAH: by definition, unknown. True IPAH is mostly sporadic or sometimes familial in nature.
- Pulmonary arteriolar hyperactivity and vasoconstriction, occult thromboembolism, or autoimmune (high frequency of antinuclear antibodies)

Genetics

- 75% of heritable pulmonary arterial hypertension (HPAH) cases and 25% of IPAH cases have mutations in *BMPR2* (autosomal dominant).
- Mutations in *ALK1* and endoglin (autosomal dominant) also are associated with PAH.

RISK FACTORS

- Female sex
- Previous anorectic drug use
- Recent acute pulmonary embolism
- Commonly associated conditions
- First-degree relatives of patient with familial PAH

COMMONLY ASSOCIATED CONDITIONS

See associated PAH, earlier discussed.

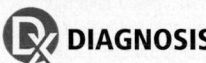 **DIAGNOSIS**

Symptoms of PAH are nonspecific, which can lead to missed or delayed diagnosis of this serious disease.

HISTORY

Dyspnea, weakness, syncope, dizziness, chest pain, palpitations, lower extremity edema

PHYSICAL EXAM

- Pulmonary component of S_2 (at apex in >90% of patients)
- Right ventricular (RV) lift
- Early systolic click of pulmonary valve
- Pansystolic murmur of tricuspid regurgitation
- Diastolic murmur of pulmonic insufficiency (Graham-Steell murmur)
- RV S^3 or S^4
- Edema as jugular vein distention, ascites, hepatomegaly, or peripheral edema

DIFFERENTIAL DIAGNOSIS

Other causes of dyspnea:

- Pulmonary parenchymal disease such as chronic obstructive pulmonary disease
- Pulmonary vascular disease such as pulmonary thromboembolism
- Cardiac disease such as cardiomyopathy
- Other disorders of respiratory function such as sleep apnea

DIAGNOSTIC TESTS & INTERPRETATION

- ECG: RVH and right axis deviation
- Pulmonary function testing and/or arterial blood gas: arterial hypoxemia, reduced diffusion capacity, hypocapnia

- Ventilation–perfusion ratio (V/Q) scan: must rule out proximal pulmonary artery emboli and chronic thromboembolic PH (CTEPH)
- Exercise test: reduced maximal O_2 consumption, high-minute ventilation, low anaerobic threshold, increased PO_2 alveolar–arterial gradient; correlation to severity of disease with 6-minute walk test
- Antinuclear antibody positive (up to 40% of patients)
- LFTs to evaluate for portopulmonary HTN, a complication of chronic liver disease
- HIV test, thyroid function tests, sickle cell disease screening
- Elevated brain natriuretic peptide (BNP) and N-terminal-proBNP may be useful for early detection of PAH in young, otherwise healthy patients with mild symptoms. It can also be used to assess disease severity and prognosis.
- Chest radiograph
  - Prominent central pulmonary arteries with peripheral hypovascularity of pulmonary arterial branches
  - RV enlargement is a late finding.
- Echo Doppler
  - Should be performed with suspicion of PAH; recent studies show some inaccuracy compared with right-sided heart catheterization
  - Most commonly used screening tool
    - Estimates mean PAP and assesses cardiac structure and function, excludes congenital anomalies
    - Echo suggests, but does not diagnose, PAH. Invasive hemodynamic evaluation confirms PAH diagnosis.
- Right atrial and ventricular enlargement; tricuspid regurgitation
- Important to rule out underlying cardiac disease such as atrial septal defect with secondary PH or mitral stenosis
- Cardiac magnetic resonance is not commonly used.

Diagnostic Procedures/Other

- Pulmonary angiography
  - Should be done if V/Q scan suggests CTEPH
  - Use caution; can lead to hemodynamic collapse; use low osmolar agents, subselective angiograms.
- Right-sided cardiac catheterization (gold standard for diagnosis of PAH)
  - Essential first step to confirm diagnosis and determine severity and prognosis by measuring pulmonary arterial pressures and hemodynamics
  - Rule out underlying cardiac disease (e.g., left-sided heart disease) and response to vasodilator therapy.
- Lung biopsy: not recommended unless primary pulmonary parenchymal disease exists
- 6-Minute walk test: classifies severity of PAH and estimates prognosis

Test Interpretation

- Distal arterioles show medial hypertrophy, proliferative/fibrotic intima, complex lesions, and thrombosis.
- Pulmonary veins usually are not affected.

 TREATMENT

- Treat underlying diseases/conditions that may cause PAH to relieve symptoms and improve quality of life and survival.
- PAH-specific treatment has been studied mostly in IPAH.

GENERAL MEASURES

Oxygen supplementation to O_2 >90% is indicated for rest, exercise, or nocturnal hypoxemia.

MEDICATION

- Acute vasodilator test (performed during cardiac catheterization) for all IPAH patients who are potential candidates for long-term oral calcium channel blocker (CCB) therapy
  - Screens for pulmonary vasoreactivity/responsiveness using inhaled nitrous oxide; IV epoprostenol or IV adenosine: Positive response may be a prognostic indicator.
  - Contraindicated in right-sided heart failure or hemodynamic instability
- Chronic vasodilator therapy
  - If IPAH with positive response to acute vasodilator test (a fall in mean PAP of ≥10 mm Hg and to a value <40 mm Hg, with unchanged/increased cardiac output), use CCBs (1)[C]
    - ~13% will initially respond. Long-term clinical response to CCB therapy is small (~7%) (1)[C].
    - CCBs include nifedipine (long-acting), diltiazem, amlodipine.
    - Avoid verapamil due to its significant negative inotropic effect.
    - CCBs are contraindicated in patients with a cardiac index of <2 L/min/m² or a right atrial pressure >15 mm Hg.
  - PAH with negative response to acute vasodilator test or worsening on therapy; specific vasodilator choice based on risk stratification (1)[C].
    - Higher risk (NYHA class III–IV): prostacyclins: improve exercise capacity, cardiopulmonary hemodynamics: epoprostenol (IV) (only drug with demonstrated survival benefit and treatment of choice for most ill; i.e., NYHA functional class IV patients) (1)[B]; treprostinil (IV, SC, or inhaled); iloprost (inhaled); inhaled products associated with bronchospasm
    - FDA recently approved treprostinil extended-release tablets for PAH to improve exercise capacity.
    - Lower risk (NYHA class I–III)
      - Endothelin receptor antagonists: Improve exercise capacity; reducing mortality has been noted (2)[A]: bosentan (PO); ambrisentan (PO). Pregnancy Category X; monitor LFTs monthly.
      - Phosphodiesterase-5 inhibitors: suggested improvement in exercise capacity, cardiopulmonary hemodynamics, and symptoms (1)[C]: sildenafil (PO); tadalafil (PO)
      - Guanylate cyclase stimulant: stimulators of the nitric oxide receptor, improves exercise capacity (3)[B]: riociguat (PO)
      - It is unclear whether any of the above separate classes of drugs significantly reduces mortality; however, pooling all the vasodilators in a recent systematic review shows 39% reduction in mortality (4)[A]; another recent meta-analysis shows that only prostanoid class has survival benefit, particularly IV prostacyclins (1)[B].
      - If one agent fails, vasodilator combination therapy (CT) using two vasodilators (e.g., epoprostenol plus sildenafil) is currently being studied. A recent meta-analysis found CT did not improve outcomes compared with monotherapy (MT). Only 6-minute walk distance was improved when using CT versus MT (5)[A].

- Anticoagulation
  - Improved survival originally suggested in patients with IPAH only. Newer studies show some evidence for favorable effects of anticoagulation on survival in IPAH, HPAH, or PAH associated with anorexigens (1)[B].
  - Warfarin with international normalized ratio of 1.5 to 2.5
    - Contraindications: Avoid in patients with syncope or significant hemoptysis; consider drug interactions.
- Diuretics indicated in patients with RV volume overload (e.g., peripheral edema or ascites) (1)[B]
- Digoxin has little long-term data in PAH: used in RV failure and/or atrial dysrhythmias, increases cardiac output and preserves RV contractility

ISSUES FOR REFERRAL

Refer to a pulmonologist and/or a cardiologist for further evaluation/treatment if PAH is suspected.

SURGERY/OTHER PROCEDURES

- Patients with documented large-vessel thromboembolic disease should be considered for pulmonary thrombectomy.
- Balloon atrial septostomy for severe PAH with right-sided heart failure despite optimized medical therapy to relieve symptoms prior to lung transplant or as a treatment on its own
- Heart–lung or lung transplantation

INPATIENT CONSIDERATIONS

Admission Criteria/Initial Stabilization

- Medical therapy is primarily palliative.
- Hospitalization with invasive monitoring is needed to screen vasodilator responsiveness and initiate vasodilator therapy.
- National registry has been established by the National Heart, Lung, and Blood Institute.

 ONGOING CARE

FOLLOW-UP RECOMMENDATIONS

- Pneumococcal and influenza vaccines
- Exercise: walking or low-level aerobic activity, as tolerated, once stable; respiratory training

Patient Monitoring

Frequently evaluate disease progression and therapeutic efficacy. Objective tests to measure treatment response include 6-minute walk test and cardiopulmonary exercise test.

DIET

Fluid and salt restrictions, especially with RV failure

PATIENT EDUCATION

Discuss disease, prognosis, lifestyle changes, and all therapeutic options (including transplant).

PROGNOSIS

- Median survival is 2 to 3 years from diagnosis; 5-year survival rate is 34% for National Institutes of Health registry; newer studies show 5-year survival near 70% with new treatment.
- Mode of death: right-sided heart failure (most common), pneumonia, sudden death, cardiac death
- Poor prognostic factors
  - Rapid symptom progression
  - Clinical evidence of RV failure
  - WHO functional PAH class 4 (or NYHA functional class III or IV)

- 6-Minute walk distance <300 m
- Peak VO_2 during cardiopulmonary exercise testing <10.4 mL/kg/min
- Echocardiography with pericardial effusion, significant RV enlargement/dysfunction, right atrial enlargement
- Mean right atrial pressure >20 mm Hg
- Cardiac index <2 L/min/m²
- Elevated mean PAP
- Significantly elevated BNP and NT-proBNP; other markers also show promise in predicting survival: RDW, GDF-15, interleukin-6, creatinine
- Scleroderma spectrum of diseases

COMPLICATIONS

- Thromboembolism, heart failure, pleural effusion, and sudden death
- Pregnancy should be avoided due to high maternal mortality (30–50%) and fetal wastage.

REFERENCES

1. Badesch DB, Abman SH, Simonneau G, et al. Medical therapy for pulmonary arterial hypertension: updated ACCP evidence-based clinical practice guidelines. *Chest*. 2007;131(6):1917–1928.
2. Liu C, Chen J, Gao Y, et al. Endothelin receptor antagonists for pulmonary arterial hypertension. *Cochrane Database Syst Rev*. 2009;(3):CD004434.
3. Ghofrani HA, Galiè N, Grimminger F, et al. Riociguat for the treatment of pulmonary arterial hypertension. *N Engl J Med*. 2013;369(4):330–340.
4. Macchia A, Marchioli R, Tognoni G, et al. Systematic review of trials using vasodilators in pulmonary arterial hypertension: why a new approach is needed. *Am Heart J*. 2010;159(2):245–257.
5. Fox BD, Shimony A, Langleben D. Meta-analysis of monotherapy versus combination therapy for pulmonary arterial hypertension. *Am J Cardiol*. 2011;108(8):1177–1182.

 SEE ALSO

Cor Pulmonale; Pulmonary Embolism

CODES

ICD10

- I27.0 Primary pulmonary hypertension
- I27.2 Other secondary pulmonary hypertension

CLINICAL PEARLS

- PAH involves abnormalities in the small pulmonary arteries (precapillary PH) that produce increased PAP and vascular resistance, eventually resulting in right-sided heart failure.
- In patients with PAH, a V/Q scan should be performed to rule out CTEPH; a normal scan effectively excludes a diagnosis of CTEPH.
- CCBs are the first-line agents to manage IPAH.

PULMONARY EDEMA
Timothy R. Takagi, MD

 BASICS

DESCRIPTION
- Pulmonary capillaries leak fluid into the lung interstitium and alveoli, leading to hypoxia and respiratory distress.
- Fluid accumulation results from cardiogenic causes (e.g., heart failure), leading to imbalanced hydrostatic and oncotic pressures within pulmonary capillaries or from noncardiogenic causes (e.g., acute lung injury) that increase alveolar membrane permeability.

EPIDEMIOLOGY
Incidence
- Annual heart failure incidence: 650,000 cases
- Heart failure incidence increases with age.
  - Age 35 to 64 years: 2 cases per 1,000
  - Age 65 to 69 years: 20 cases per 1,000
  - Age >85 years: >80 cases per 1,000
- Disparities in heart failure incidence by race and sex
  - Blacks (16.3/1,000) versus whites (11.9/1,000)
  - Men (15.8/1,000) versus women (11.7/1,000)
- Acute respiratory distress syndrome (ARDS): 190,000 cases annually in United States

Prevalence
Heart failure syndromes: 5.8 million U.S. adults

ETIOLOGY AND PATHOPHYSIOLOGY
- Cardiogenic causes will increase hydrostatic pressure in the pulmonary capillaries, leading to increased transvascular filtration of a protein-poor fluid into lung interstitium.
- Systolic dysfunction is due to decreased contractility of the left ventricle (LV), leading to decreased cardiac output, which in turn stimulates the renin–angiotensin system and increases fluid retention. Diastolic dysfunction is often due to decreased LV compliance secondary to hypertrophy.
- Cardiogenic (left-sided heart failure)
  - Impaired contractility
    - Ischemic heart disease
    - Dilated cardiomyopathy
    - Myocarditis
    - Volume overload
    - Alcoholic cardiomyopathy
  - Increased LV afterload
    - Systemic hypertension (HTN)
    - Aortic stenosis
    - Cocaine abuse
  - Poor diastolic filling
    - LV hypertrophy
    - Hypertrophic cardiomyopathy
    - Mitral stenosis
    - Atrial fibrillation
  - Valvular dysfunction
    - Mitral regurgitation
    - Acute papillary muscle rupture
  - High cardiac output states
    - Thyrotoxicosis
    - Systemic arteriovenous fistulas
    - Anemia
  - Noncompliance with medications or diet
  - Medications with negative inotropic effects
- Noncardiogenic causes will increase permeability of the lung vasculature, leading to accumulation of protein-rich fluid in the lung interstitium and air spaces. Many causes of this vascular permeability are associated with ARDS.

- Noncardiogenic
  - ARDS
  - Acute lung injury
  - Transfusion-related acute lung injury
  - Preeclampsia
  - Rapid ascent to high altitude (>2,500 m)
  - Drug toxicity (salicylates, opiates)
  - Embolism (thrombus, fat, air, amniotic fluid)
  - Neurogenic (after head trauma/surgery)
  - Reexpansion (after pneumothorax/thoracentesis)

Genetics
Multifactorial

RISK FACTORS
- Cardiogenic: HTN, valvular disease, hyperlipidemia, atherosclerosis, diabetes mellitus, obesity, excessive alcohol intake, physical inactivity, dietary choices, and smoking
- Noncardiogenic: sepsis, aspiration, pneumonia, trauma, inhaled toxins, DIC

GENERAL PREVENTION
Early detection and treatment of risk factors, including high blood pressure, diabetes, alcohol intake, obesity, and tobacco abuse (1)[A]

COMMONLY ASSOCIATED CONDITIONS
See "Etiology and Pathophysiology."

 DIAGNOSIS

HISTORY
- Past medical history
  - Underlying comorbidities, including prior heart failure or prior myocardial infarction (MI)
  - Recent trauma
  - Drug or alcohol abuse
  - Dietary or medication noncompliance
  - Recent weight gain or increasing edema
  - Recent use of negative inotropic agents (calcium channel blockers)
  - Recent use of NSAIDs (increase water retention)
- Symptoms
  - Fever or other symptoms of infection
  - Progressive dyspnea
  - Orthopnea and paroxysmal nocturnal dyspnea
  - Cough
  - Fatigue and generalized weakness
  - Pink frothy sputum
  - Chest pain

PHYSICAL EXAM
- Vital signs: tachypnea, tachycardia, and hypoxemia. Patients may be hypotensive or hypertensive.
- General: respiratory distress, diaphoresis
- HEENT (head, eyes, ears, nose, throat): frothy oral secretions, cyanosis
- Cardiac: S_3 or S_4, jugular venous distension, murmurs suggestive of valvular disease
- Pulmonary: crackles or wheezing
- Extremities: edema, cyanosis, mottled skin

DIFFERENTIAL DIAGNOSIS
- COPD
- Pneumonia
- Pulmonary embolism
- Asthma/reactive airway disease
- Pneumothorax
- Cardiac tamponade

- Asphyxiant or toxic gas exposure
- Inhalational burns

DIAGNOSTIC TESTS & INTERPRETATION
Initial Tests (lab, imaging)
- CBC/differential to screen for anemia or infection
- Chemistry panel to screen for acute kidney injury, hyponatremia (associated with severe heart failure), or electrolyte disturbances leading to dysrhythmias
- Troponin may be elevated from recent infarction causing acute heart failure or from myocardial ischemia secondary to elevated ventricular strain. Elevated cardiac enzymes carry a strongly negative prognosis in heart failure.
- In settings of clinical uncertainty, B-type natriuretic peptide (BNP), or N-terminal pro-BNP, can add to clinical judgment in patients with symptoms suggestive of heart failure (1,2)[A]. BNP >500 pg/mL suggests heart failure, and BNP <100 pg/mL suggests alternative causes. BNP may also be elevated due to atrial fibrillation, renal failure, severe valvular disease, or pulmonary HTN.
- Liver function tests (LFTs) to check for elevated transaminases, which can suggest hepatic congestion from heart failure or may indicate heavy alcohol use contributing to cardiomyopathy
- Drug levels (aspirin, opiates, cocaine, alcohol)
- Arterial blood gas to measure PO_2 and A-a gradient
- Serum lipase if suspicious for pancreatitis
- TSH if suspicious for thyrotoxicosis
- Blood/urine cultures and lactic acid if concerned for severe sepsis or septic shock
- Urinalysis to check for nephrotic syndrome or UTI
- Chest x-ray to evaluate for the following:
  - Pneumothorax
  - Cardiomegaly
  - Infiltrate suggestive of pneumonia
  - Increased interstitial markings, perihilar alveolar edema, or pleural effusion
- CT pulmonary angiography if concerned for pulmonary emboli
- ECG to evaluate for ischemia or dysrhythmias
- Echocardiography to assess ventricular function and size, valve function, and for presence of a pericardial effusion or wall motion abnormalities (2)[C].

Follow-Up Tests & Special Considerations
Emergent echocardiography if considering cardiogenic shock, tamponade, or papillary muscle rupture

Diagnostic Procedures
- If cause of pulmonary edema is unknown, a pulmonary artery catheter (or Swan-Ganz) can be inserted to measure the pulmonary artery capillary wedge pressure. A wedge pressure <18 mm Hg favors acute lung injury over cardiogenic pulmonary edema.
- Patients with new-onset or worsening heart failure (without determined cause) should have further evaluation for myocardial ischemia. The pretest probability of underlying ischemic cardiomyopathy should guide the decision on which testing modality to use (1)[C].

 TREATMENT

GENERAL MEASURES
- Guide all treatment based on the suspected cause.
- Start with supplemental oxygen.

MEDICATION
Cardiogenic pulmonary edema

First Line

- Diuretics: reduce preload for acute cardiogenic edema; used in low doses daily for chronic heart failure to manage volume overload. If on chronic diuretics, start IV dose at or above home dose and titrate for acute cardiogenic edema. Onset is 15 to 30 minutes for IV loop diuretics. Monitor for electrolyte derangement and renal dysfunction. Use very carefully in patients with aortic stenosis.
  - Acute: furosemide 40 to 80 mg IV, torsemide 10 mg IV, or bumetanide 1 mg IV
  - Chronic: furosemide 20 to 80 mg q6–8h, torsemide 20 mg/day, or bumetanide 1 mg q12h
- ACE inhibitors or angiotensin receptor blockers (ARBs): reduce afterload for systolic heart failure. Maintenance therapy may be cautiously continued during exacerbation. Avoid in acutely ill patients with hypotension, acute kidney insult, hyperkalemia, or poor diuresis. Use ARBs in patients who are ACE inhibitor-intolerant.
  - Target dose for chronic heart failure: lisinopril 20 to 40 mg/day, enalapril 10 to 20 mg q12h, captopril 50 mg q8h, candesartan 32 mg/day, valsartan 160 mg q12h, losartan 100 mg/day
- β-Blockers: reduce afterload for systolic heart failure. Maintenance therapy may be continued for mild decompensation; hold or reduce dose for moderate to severe decompensation. Avoid if patients are hypotensive or recently received inotropic therapy. Do not initiate until recovery from acute exacerbation of heart failure.
  - Target dose for chronic heart failure: carvedilol 25 mg q12h, metoprolol ER 200 mg/day, bisoprolol 10 mg/day
- Inotropes: Improve contractility in hypotensive patients with severe systolic heart failure and signs of systemic hypoperfusion (2)[B]. Inotropes increase myocardial oxygen demand and may damage the ischemic myocardium.
  - Dobutamine: 5 to 10 μg/kg/min IV, titrate
  - Milrinone: loading dose (optional): 50 μg/kg IV over 10 minutes, then infuse 0.375 to 0.750 μg/kg/min, titrate
  - Dopamine: 5 to 10 μg/kg/min IV, titrate
  - Norepinephrine: 2 to 4 μg/min IV for acute cardiogenic shock following acute MI; not for use in acute decompensated heart failure
- Nitrates: Acute cardiogenic pulmonary edema use IV nitrate vasodilators. Rapid onset. Nitroglycerin IV 5 to 10 μg/min, titrate 5 to 10 μg/min q3–5min to max 200 μg/min until distress resolved or onset of hypotension. For severe HTN, consider IV nitroprusside 5 to 10 μg/min, titrate. Max 400 μg/min. Use <48 hours due to risk of cyanide toxicity.
  - For patients who are not tolerant of ACE inhibitors or ARBs, hydralazine and an oral nitrate should be started (1)[C].
- Precaution: Monitor the additive hypotensive effects of diuretics, nitrates, and afterload reducers.

Second Line

- Thiazide diuretics: hydrochlorothiazide (HCTZ) 25 to 50 mg/day PO, metolazone 2.5 to 10 mg/day PO
- Spironolactone: 25 to 50 mg/day PO; recheck renal function and electrolytes in 7 to 10 days
- Digoxin: 125 μg/day PO, titrate to serum concentration of 0.5 to 0.8 ng/mL
- Noncardiogenic pulmonary edema
  - High-altitude pulmonary edema
    ○ Descent is the single best treatment (3)[A].
    ○ Adjunctive therapy: supplemental oxygen. Consider nifedipine ER 30 mg PO q12h or sildenafil 50 mg PO q8h or tadalafil 10 mg PO q12h (3)[C].

ISSUES FOR REFERRAL

- Cardiology referral for underlying cardiac disease
- Patients with ARDS should be carefully monitored in an ICU setting.

ADDITIONAL THERAPIES

- Noninvasive positive pressure ventilation (NPPV) should be considered early for emergency department patients with acute respiratory distress from cardiogenic pulmonary edema/congestive heart failure (CHF). NPPV decreases preload and afterload, thereby alleviating symptoms and potentially avoiding intubation by allowing time for medications to work. Use cautiously if patients are hypotensive (4)[A].
- Early invasive ventilation should be considered for patients with noncardiogenic pulmonary edema secondary to acute respiratory distress syndrome.

SURGERY/OTHER PROCEDURES

- Extracorporeal membrane oxygenation (ECMO) for severe refractory hypoxia/ARDS
- Intra-arterial balloon pump for cardiogenic shock
- Implantable cardioverter defibrillator (ICD) for sudden cardiac death prevention in patients with prior cardiac arrest or ischemic/dilated cardiomyopathy and LVEF <30% (2)[B]
- Cardiac resynchronization therapy (CRT) may be useful for LVEF ≤35%, sinus rhythm, and QRS >0.15 m/s (2)[B].
- LV assist device (LVAD) for severe systolic dysfunction as bridge to a heart transplant (2)[B].

INPATIENT CONSIDERATIONS

Admission Criteria/Initial Stabilization

- Hypotension
- Acute kidney injury
- Altered mental status
- Dyspnea at rest
- O₂ saturation <90%
- Acute coronary syndromes
- Arrhythmias (i.e., new-onset atrial fibrillation)
- Mild distress: oxygen by nonrebreather mask
- Significant hypoxia
- Intubation for patients with apnea, altered mental status, or hypoxia despite NPPV

IV Fluids

Use crystalloid infusions cautiously. Limit free water.

Nursing

- Daily weights, strict input/output
- Assess for functional improvement.

Discharge Criteria

- Underlying condition treated, fluid status optimized
- Started β-blocker and ACE inhibitor in patients with CHF (1)[B]
- Patient and family educated about diet/medications

 ## ONGOING CARE

FOLLOW-UP RECOMMENDATIONS
Patient Monitoring

- Strict input/output measurement, daily weights
- Posthospitalization appointment in 7 to 10 days

DIET

Low-sodium diet (<2 g/day), fluid restriction (<2 L/day) (2)[C]

PATIENT EDUCATION

- Dietary precautions
- Early signs and symptoms of fluid overload
- Adjust diuretic dose based on recent weight gain.

PROGNOSIS

Mortality: 30–60% for noncardiogenic edema/ARDS; up to 80% for cardiogenic causes

COMPLICATIONS

- Acute hypoxic respiratory failure
- CHF increases long-term risk for dysrhythmias and sudden cardiac death.
- ARDS increases short-term risk for pneumonia and pneumothorax. Long-term complications include risks of pulmonary HTN and fibrosis.

REFERENCES

1. Lindenfeld J, Albert NM, Boehmer JP, et al. HFSA 2010 comprehensive heart failure practice guideline. *J Card Fail.* 2010;16(6): e1–e194.
2. Yancy CW, Jessup M, Bozkurt B, et al. 2013 ACCF/AHA guideline for the management of heart failure: a report of the American College of Cardiology Foundation/American Heart Association Task Force on Practice Guidelines. *J Am Coll Cardiol.* 2013; 62(16):e147–e239.
3. Luks AM, McIntosh SE, Grissom CK, et al. Wilderness Medical Society consensus guidelines for the prevention and treatment of acute altitude illness. *Wilderness Environ Med.* 2010;21(2):146–155.
4. Vital FM, Saconato H, Ladeira MT, et al. Non-invasive positive pressure ventilation (CPAP or bilevel NPPV) for cardiogenic pulmonary edema. *Cochrane Database Syst Rev.* 2008;(3):CD005351.

ADDITIONAL READING

Putensen C, Theuerkauf N, Zinserling J, et al. Meta-analysis: ventilation strategies and outcome of the acute respiratory distress syndrome and acute lung injury. *Ann Intern Med.* 2009;151(8):566–576.

 ## SEE ALSO

Altitude Illness; Congestive Heart Failure: Differential Diagnosis; Respiratory Distress Syndrome, Acute (ARDS)

CODES

ICD10

- J81.1 Chronic pulmonary edema
- J81.0 Acute pulmonary edema

CLINICAL PEARLS

- Diagnosis of the underlying etiology is essential.
- Initial treatment of acute cardiogenic edema among hypertensive/normotensive patients includes IV diuretics, IV nitrates, and NPPV.
- Hypotensive patients with pulmonary edema due to CHF will require careful use of inotropes and vasopressor to improve hemodynamic stability.
- Pulmonary edema from ARDS has very high mortality and requires ICU-level care. Home dietary and medication management are critical for long-term treatment of CHF.

PULMONARY EMBOLISM

Karla A. Oliveros, MD • Alfonso Tafur, MD, MS, RPVI

 BASICS

DESCRIPTION
- Pulmonary embolism (PE) is the most serious presentation of venous thromboembolism (VTE).
- Mortality exceeds 15% during the first 3 months. In 25% of patients, first manifestation is sudden death.

EPIDEMIOLOGY
Case fatality rate 1–60%. For patients with intermediate risk, mortality rate is 3–15% if right ventricular (RV) dilation or dysfunction. If hemodynamically unstable, mortality is >15% due to worsening RV failure and cardiogenic shock.

Incidence
- Approximately 60 to 70 per 100,000, with >100,000 cases annually in the United States.
- Incidence increases with age, most occurring at 60 to 70 years of age.
- 250,000 hospitalizations per year in the United States, 10–60% in hospitalized patients.
  - Highest risk for orthopedic patients
  - 1:1,000 pregnancies (including postpartum)

ETIOLOGY AND PATHOPHYSIOLOGY
- Venous stasis, endothelial damage, and changes in coagulation properties trigger formation of thrombus (1).
- Causes increased pulmonary vascular resistance, impaired gas exchange, and decreased pulmonary compliance. RV failure due to pressure overload is usually the primary cause of death (1).
- DVT in the proximal veins is the most common source of PE, up to 85% of the cases.

Genetics
- Factor V Leiden: Most common thrombophilia. +5.5% in Caucasian, 2.2% in Hispanics, 1.2% in African American, 0.5% in Asian. Associated with 20% of all VTE
- Prothrombin G20210A: 3% of Caucasians, rare in African American, Asian, and Native American; 6% in patients with VTE
- Deficiencies in protein C, S, and antithrombin

RISK FACTORS
- Acquired: age, immobilization, surgery, major trauma, lower limb fractures, joint replacement, spinal cord injury, cancer, hormonal replacement therapy, pregnancy/puerperium, previous thrombosis, paroxysmal nocturnal hemoglobinuria, antiphospholipid syndrome, prolonged travel
- Oral contraceptives is the most frequent medication (1).
- Inherited: Antithrombin deficiency, protein C or S deficiency, factor V Leiden, prothrombin gene mutation G20210A (1)

GENERAL PREVENTION
- Mechanical thromboprophylaxis: early ambulation after surgery, compression stockings, and intermittent pneumatic compression
- Intermediate risk: general, gynecologic, or urologic surgery; prophylaxis is recommended with low-molecular-weight heparin (LMWH), unfractionated heparin (UFH), or fondaparinux.
- High risk: 10 or more days prophylaxis in hip or knee arthroplasty, with LMWH, fondaparinux, apixaban, dabigatran, rivaroxaban, or low-dose UFH. 28 to 35 days with LMWH, fondaparinux, UFH, or vitamin K antagonists (VKA) in hip fracture surgery. LMWH or UFH in major trauma, spinal cord injury
- Long-distance travel (>8 hours): hydration, walking, avoidance of constrictive clothing and frequent calf exercises; if additional risk factors, then compression stockings below knee
- Patients with factor V Leiden, prothrombin G20210A with no previous thrombosis do not need long-term daily prophylaxis.

 DIAGNOSIS

- Establish a pretest probability based on clinical criteria (2).
  - Wells score
    - Clinical signs and symptoms of DVT +3
    - Alternative diagnosis is less likely than PE +3
    - Heart rate >100 +1.5
    - Immobilization previous 4 weeks +1.5
    - Previous DVT/PE +1.5
    - Hemoptysis +1
    - Malignancy +1
    - <2 points, low clinical probability; 2 to 6 points, moderate; >7 points, high
- Recently, Wells and revised Geneva score were simplified (2).
  - Wells score: Each predictor is +1. PE unlikely if 0 to 1, PE likely if >2.
  - Geneva score: Each predictor is +1 except for heart rate >95 which is +2. PE unlikely if 0 to 2 and PE likely if >3.

HISTORY
- Determine if the presentation is provoked or idiopathic. Approximately 30% of cases develop without identifiable risk factor.
- Presence of risk factors and family history
- Bleeding risk (previous anticoagulation, history of bleeding, recent interventions/surgeries, liver disease)
- Sudden onset dyspnea (>85%), chest pain (>50%), cough (20%), syncope (14%), hemoptysis (7%).

PHYSICAL EXAM
- Dyspnea, syncope, hemoptysis, tachycardia, tachypnea, accentuated S^2. Pleuritic chest pain, pleural friction rub, rales (1)
- Signs of DVT, leg swelling, tenderness, visible collateral veins (1)
- Signs of RV failure: jugular vein distention, third or fourth sound, systolic murmur at left sternal edge, hepatomegaly (1)

ALERT
- Massive PE: mortality rate exceeding 20%. Hemodynamic instability with sustained hypotension, pulselessness, or persistent bradycardia, cardiogenic shock, acute manifesting RV failure (1)
- Submassive PE: hemodynamically stable. Mortality rate of 5–25%. No systemic hypotension but there is either RV dysfunction or myocardial necrosis (1,3).
  - RV dysfunction: RV dilation or systolic dysfunction on echocardiography, RV dilation on CT, elevation of brain natriuretic peptide (BNP) or N-terminal pro-BNP (500 pg/mL), or consistent ECG changes
- Low-risk PE: acute and absence of clinical markers of adverse prognosis

DIFFERENTIAL DIAGNOSIS
- Pulmonary: pneumonia, bronchitis, pneumothorax, pneumonitis, chronic obstructive pulmonary disease (COPD) exacerbation, pulmonary edema, pneumothorax
- Cardiac/vascular: myocardial infarction, pericarditis, congestive heart failure (CHF), aortic dissection
- Musculoskeletal: rib fracture(s), musculoskeletal chest wall pain

DIAGNOSTIC TESTS & INTERPRETATION
- D-dimer ELISA: In patients with low pretest probability, it can rule out PE if it is negative (high negative predictive value [NPV]) (1)[A]. It is not diagnostic if positive (low positive predictive value [PPV]) and it is not helpful if pretest probability is intermediate or high (1)[B].
- CBC, creatinine, aPTT and PT, ABG: In young patients with idiopathic, recurrent, or significant family history of VTE, consider testing for hypercoagulable tests.
  - Do not test for protein C, S, factor VIII, or antithrombin in the acute setting or while on treatment, as may be falsely abnormal.
  - Patients with intermediate or high pretest probability and low probability with elevated D-dimer need further diagnostic testing.
- Chest x-ray (CXR): Westermark sign (lack of vessels in an area distal to the embolus), Hampton hump (wedge-shaped opacity with base in pleura), Fleischner sign (enlarged pulmonary arteries), atelectasis, pleural effusion, pulmonary infarct, hemidiaphragm elevation (1)
- ECG: right heart strain, nonspecific rhythm abnormalities, S1Q3T3
- CT pulmonary angiography: sensitivity 96–100%, specificity 86–89%; NPV 99.8%. If normal, it safely excludes PE if low or intermediate clinical probability (1)[A].
- Ventilation/perfusion scintigraphy (V/Q scan): safe with few allergic reactions. Use if CT angiography is not available or contraindicated. A high-probability V/Q scan makes the diagnosis of PE; normal V/Q scan excludes PE (1)[B].
- Pulmonary angiography: gold standard but invasive and technically difficult: 2% morbidity and <0.01 mortality risk (1)[C]
- Echocardiogram: Assess RV function, found in 25% of patients with PE.
- Magnetic resonance angiography: lower sensitivity and specificity than CT angiography
- Compression venous ultrasound (CUS): noninvasive. Sensitivity >90%, specificity approximately 95%. It confirms the diagnosis of PE in patients with clinical suspicion (1)[B].
- CT venography: can be done at the same time as CT angiography; increases diagnostic yield (1)

ALERT
If your preclinical probability is intermediate or high and the patient has a low bleeding risk, start treatment while waiting for the diagnostic results (3)[C].

Follow-Up Tests & Special Considerations
Elevated troponin I or T and elevated BNP are markers for higher risk patients.

TREATMENT

MEDICATION
- If clinical suspicion is high and no contraindications, start treatment immediately.
- Start LMWH, fondaparinux, UFH, as initial therapy for first 5 to 10 days. VKA can be started the 1st day and must overlap with parenteral treatment for minimum of 5 days, until international normalized ratio (INR) is 2 to 3 for 24 hours.
- Following 5 to 10 days of parenteral therapy, dabigatran or edoxaban are also approved (1).

- An oral option for initial and long-term treatment is rivaroxaban or apixaban (1).
- Patients with massive PE with low bleeding risk: Consider systemic thrombolytics if no contraindications. Also in patients <75 years old with submassive PE. Greater benefit if initiated within 48 hours of symptoms onset (1)

First Line

- UFH (3)[A]:
  - IV bolus of 80 U/kg or 5,000 U followed by continuous infusion (initially 18 U/kg/hr or 1,300 U/hr) with dose adjustments to maintain aPTT that corresponds to anti-Xa levels of 0.3 to 0.7
  - SC injection: 2 options:
    ○ Monitored: 17,500 U or 250 U/kg BID with dose adjustments to maintain an aPTT that corresponds to anti-Xa levels of 0.3 to 0.7 measured 6 hours after a dose
    ○ Fixed dose: 333 U/kg initial dose, followed by 250 U/kg BID

- LMWH: preferred due to lower risk of major bleeding and heparin-induced thrombocytopenia (HIT) (1),(3)[A]

  - Enoxaparin (Lovenox) 1 mg/kg/dose SC q12h
  - Dalteparin (Fragmin 200 U/kg SC q24h
  - Fondaparinux (Arixtra): 5 mg (body weight <50 kg), 7.5 mg (body weight 50 to 100 kg), or 10 mg (body weight >100) SC q24h
- Maintenance therapy: Warfarin on day 1, if possible; 5 mg/day for 3 days in hospitalized or older patients, and at a dose of 10 mg in <60 years of aged patients; adjust dose to maintain an INR of 2 to 3. Needs to overlap with UFH, LMWH, or fondaparinux: 5 to 7 days, until 2 consecutive days of therapeutic INR (1).

- Rivaroxaban: 15 mg BID for 3 and then 20 mg once daily to complete treatment. Compared to warfarin, it has less major bleeding side effects while having same efficacy (1)[B].
- Edoxaban: 60 mg once daily (reduced to 30 mg once daily if CrCl 30 to 50 mL/min or body weight <60 kg). Patients require initial treatment with LMWH at least 5 days before starting edoxaban. Less bleeding risk compared to warfarin (1)[B]
- Apixaban: 10 mg BID for 7 days, followed by 5 mg once daily was compared to conventional therapy. Compared to warfarin, noninferior against recurrent symptomatic VTE or death related to VTE, with less frequently major bleeding episodes (1)[B]
- Dabigatran: Require initial treatment with LMWH. Compared to warfarin, 150 mg BID had noninferior efficacy and no differences in major bleeding and fewer episodes of any bleeding (1)[B].

ALERT
Contraindications

- Active bleeding.
- Heparin: HIT
- LMWH: HIT, renal failure
- Warfarin: pregnancy

- Rivaroxaban and Fondaparinux: renal failure (1)[A]
- Edoxaban: severe kidney or liver failure (1)[A]
- Apixaban: renal impairment and nonvalvular atrial fibrillation (1)[A]

- Dabigatran: severe kidney problems. Use of dronedarone or ketoconazole increase risk.

Pregnancy Considerations
- Warfarin is teratogenic and should not be used in pregnant patients (especially in 1st trimester); safe while breastfeeding

- **LMWH**: Dalteparin, enoxaparin, and fondaparinux are Category B; heparin is Category C, use if the benefit overweight risks.
- **UFH**: Require aPTT monitoring. Can cause osteoporosis if used for prolonged period
- Rivaroxaban is Category C.
- Edoxaban and Apixaban: Category B; increases risk of hemorrhage
- Dabigatran: Category C; use it only if benefit overweight side effects.

Second Line

Massive PE: Consider thrombolytics if the patient has hemodynamic compromise and low bleeding risk, intracranial hemorrhage risk: 0.7 to 6.4%: (1),(3)[B]

- Tissue plasminogen activator (tPA) 100 mg infused over 2 hours. Absolute contraindications:
  - Intracranial hemorrhage, known intracranial cerebrovascular or malignant disease, ischemic stroke within 3 months, suspected aortic dissection, bleeding diathesis, active bleeding, recent neurosurgery, or major trauma

SURGERY/OTHER PROCEDURES

- Inferior vena cava (IVC) filter placement if absolute contraindication for anticoagulation or recurrent PE despite adequate anticoagulation treatment (3)[B].

- PREPIC2 trial showed that retrievable IVC filters at 3 months plus anticoagulation compared to anticoagulation alone among patients with severe PE had no benefit reducing the risk of symptomatic recurrent PF (3%, 95% CI, 1.1–6.5% vs. 1.5%, 95% CI, 0.3–4.3%) (3)[C].
- Emergency embolectomy can be considered in patients with massive PE with contraindications for thrombolysis (3)[C].
- Consider catheter-based interventions if massive PE and thrombolytic contraindications (3)[C].
- Consider ultrasound-assisted catheter-directed thrombolysis (USAT) in patients with intermediate risk of death or submassive PE, superior than heparin alone in reversing RV dilation at 24 hours without increase in bleeding complications (1).

INPATIENT CONSIDERATIONS

Admission Criteria/Initial Stabilization
ICU-level care if hemodynamically unstable

⚕ ONGOING CARE

Duration of anticoagulation

- Provoked PE (trigger no longer present): 3 months (1)[B]
- Unprovoked PE: Minimum of 3 months, consider long-term or prolonged secondary prophylaxis if bleeding risk is low (1)[B].
- Cancer-related PE: LMWH first 3 to 6 months. Consider secondary prophylaxis as long as the patient has active cancer (1)[B].

- Recurrent PE: long-term anticoagulation

FOLLOW-UP RECOMMENDATIONS
- If concomitant DVT, knee-height compression stockings, 30 to 40 mm Hg knee height
- If an IVC filter was placed, follow-up for retrieval.

Patient Monitoring
- INR should be checked regularly; target is 2 to 3 (1).
- aPTT needs to be monitored in SC UFH (1).
- Anti-Xa can be checked in special circumstances if treated with LMWH, including pregnancy, younger patients, renal disease.

DIET
Warfarin use; recommend a vitamin K diet.

PROGNOSIS
- Massive PE 50% versus nonmassive PE 8–14%

- Simplified Pulmonary Embolism Severity Index score predicts acute mortality (any one of the following defines high-risk: age >80 years, history of cancer, chronic cardiopulmonary disease, heart rate 110/min, systolic blood pressure <100 mm Hg, O_2 saturation <90%) (1)[B].

- High early mortality risk: shock or hypotension, +SPESI index >1+ RV dysfunction signs by imaging and cardiac laboratory biomarkers (1)
- Intermediate high early mortality risk: no shock or hypotension + SPESI >1 + RV dysfunction signs by imaging and cardiac laboratory biomarkers (1)
- Intermediate low early mortality risk: no shock or hypotension + SPESI >1 + either RV dysfunction by imaging or cardiac laboratory biomarkers (1)
- Low early mortality risk: no shock or hypotension, no SPESI; imaging is optional (if assessed is negative) (1).

COMPLICATIONS
- 1 in 25 patients will develop chronic thromboembolic pulmonary hypertension, recurrent DVT, or PE.
- Younger age, previous PE, and larger perfusion defect were significantly associated with increased risk of CTPH found in 5.2% of 58 patients with previous DVT, and 33.3% of 24 patients with previous PE.
- Incidence of major hemorrhage associated with thrombolytics is 8%; intracerebral bleed is 2% (fatal in 1/2 of cases).

REFERENCES
1. Konstantinides SV, Torbicki A, Agnelli G, et al. 2014 ESC guidelines on the diagnosis and management of acute pulmonary embolism. *Eur Heart J.* 2014;35(43):3033–3069, 3069a–3069k.
2. El Wahsh R, Agha M. Clinical probability of pulmonary embolism: comparison of different scoring systems. *Egypt J Chest Dis Tuberc.* 2012;61(4):419–424.
3. Jaff MR, McMurtry MS, Archer SL, et al. Management of massive and submassive pulmonary embolism, iliofemoral deep vein thrombosis, and chronic thromboembolic pulmonary hypertension: a scientific statement from the American Heart Association. *Circulation.* 2011;123(16):1788–1830.

🔢 CODES

ICD10
- I26.99 Other pulmonary embolism without acute cor pulmonale
- I27.82 Chronic pulmonary embolism

CLINICAL PEARLS

- PE can be excluded in patients who have low pre-test probability and negative D-dimer testing.
- Perform cancer-oriented review of systems and age/gender-appropriate cancer screening in patients >40, recurrent VTE, upper extremity DVT (not related to catheter or lines), bilateral lower extremity DVT, intra-abdominal DVT, resistance to treatment.
- In patients with prolonged baseline aPTT, adjust heparin dose with anti-Xa levels (therapeutic range 0.3 to 0.7).

PULMONARY FIBROSIS

Anna Rudnicki, MD

 BASICS

DESCRIPTION
- Characterized by fibrosis of the lung parenchyma
- Chest CT shows reticular pattern and honeycombing, with subpleural and lower lobe predominance.
- Lung biopsy shows "usual interstitial pneumonia" pattern.
- Classified based on etiology
  - Idiopathic
  - Nonidiopathic

EPIDEMIOLOGY
Incidence
- Incidence of IPF is 7 to 16/100,000 person-years
- Idiopathic pulmonary fibrosis (IPF) is more common in men.
- Most patients with IPF are >60 years.
- Incidence of nonidiopathic pulmonary fibrosis is unknown.

Prevalence
- Prevalence of IPF is 2 to 39 cases/100,000 people.
- Prevalence of nonidiopathic pulmonary fibrosis is unknown.

ETIOLOGY AND PATHOPHYSIOLOGY
- Postulated that microinjury to alveolar epithelial cells causes release of cytokines that activates fibroblasts, which in turn leads to excess production of extracellular matrix.
- Causes of the nonidiopathic form include:
  - Occupational exposure
  - Environmental exposure
  - Drugs
  - Systemic connective tissue diseases
  - Granulomatous diseases

Genetics
- <5% of IPF is familial and may involve mutations in surfactant protein A2 and C and/or abnormal telomere shortening.
- Most likely mode of transmission is autosomal dominant with variable penetrance.

RISK FACTORS
- Family history of pulmonary fibrosis
- Gastroesophageal reflux disease (GERD)
- Smoking
- Exposure to birds, livestock, dust from metals or wood, solvents

GENERAL PREVENTION
Avoid the risk factors mentioned earlier, such as smoking, certain occupational exposures, or drugs that induce pulmonary fibrosis.

COMMONLY ASSOCIATED CONDITIONS
- Pulmonary hypertension: occurs in 30–80% of patients with IPF, likely as a result of hypoxemic vasoconstriction
- GERD
- Nonidiopathic pulmonary fibrosis may be associated with connective tissue diseases (e.g., rheumatoid arthritis and scleroderma).

 DIAGNOSIS

HISTORY
- Slowly progressive dyspnea
- Dry cough

PHYSICAL EXAM
- Tachypnea
- Fine inspiratory crackles
- Possible clubbing

DIFFERENTIAL DIAGNOSIS
- Asbestosis
- Berylliosis
- Coal worker's pneumoconiosis
- Chronic hypersensitivity pneumonitis
- Sarcoidosis
- Silicosis

DIAGNOSTIC TESTS & INTERPRETATION
Initial Tests (lab, imaging)
- High-resolution chest computed tomography (HRCT) is required to make diagnosis. Characteristic findings include a reticular pattern, traction bronchiectasis, and honeycombing. There is a subpleural and lower lobe predominance. There is minimal to no evidence of active inflammation (1,2).
- If the patient has characteristic findings of pulmonary fibrosis on chest CT, then lung biopsy may not necessarily be required (1).
- HRCT is needed as part of initial workup (as above).

Follow-Up Tests & Special Considerations
- Surgical lung biopsy should be considered if clinical presentation and HRCT are not entirely characteristic of pulmonary fibrosis (1).

- Blood work to rule out associated collagen vascular disease (1)
- Bronchoscopy with bronchoalveolar lavage may help rule out other types of interstitial lung disease and concurrent infection (1).

Diagnostic Procedures/Other
- Pulmonary function testing (PFT): initially, may see only decrease in diffusing capacity; later in disease, may develop decrease in lung volumes as well
- Echocardiogram to evaluate for concomitant pulmonary hypertension
- Resting and exercise pulse oximetry to determine need for supplemental oxygen

Test Interpretation
Usual interstitial pneumonitis: shows interstitial scarring, honeycombing, and fibroblastic foci. There is temporal heterogeneity, meaning, there may be areas of normal lung adjacent to fibrosed or inflamed lung.

TREATMENT

GENERAL MEASURES
- Pulmonary rehabilitation (1)[C]
- Consider treating for GERD, even if asymptomatic (1)[B].
- Consider lung transplant evaluation.

MEDICATION
First Line
Supplemental oxygen, if needed (1)[C]

ISSUES FOR REFERRAL
- Patients should be evaluated and cared for longitudinally by a pulmonologist.
- If any uncertainty in diagnosis, then consider referral to thoracic surgery for lung biopsy (3,4).
- Depending on patient age, comorbidities, and preference, may consider referral for lung transplant.

ADDITIONAL THERAPIES
- A recent study showed an increase in mortality in patients treated with a combination of prednisone, azathioprine, and N-acetylcysteine when compared with those receiving placebo or N-acetylcysteine alone (3).

- Recent studies have shown a benefit with the antifibrotic agent pirfenidone and the tyrosine kinase inhibitor nintedanib for slowing the progression of IPF (4,5). These drugs were approved by the FDA in 2014.
- Many other clinical trials are currently under way. Some of the targets being studied include TGF-β, connective tissue growth factor; IL-13; CCL2; CXCR4; and CXCL12, ACE, and angiotensin II (6).

SURGERY/OTHER PROCEDURES
Lung transplant carries a 5-year survival of 50–56%.

COMPLEMENTARY & ALTERNATIVE MEDICINE
None

INPATIENT CONSIDERATIONS
Admission Criteria/Initial Stabilization
Worsening shortness of breath and/or increased oxygen requirements:

- Provide adequate supplemental oxygen.
- Workup for other possible causes of respiratory decompensation
- If no other cause for respiratory decompensation is found, then consider administration of high-dose steroids.

Nursing
Supplemental oxygen to keep saturations >90%

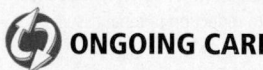 ONGOING CARE

FOLLOW-UP RECOMMENDATIONS
Patient should follow-up with a pulmonologist

Patient Monitoring
Disease progression can be monitored by periodic PFTs and HRCT.

DIET
No specific dietary requirements

PATIENT EDUCATION
- Patients should be counseled extensively regarding the prognosis of this diagnosis and given as much support as possible. Information about support groups in the local community and online may be helpful.
- American Lung Association: http://www.lung.org/lung-health-and-diseases/lung-disease-lookup/pulmonary-fibrosis/

- Pulmonary Fibrosis Foundation: http://www.pulmonaryfibrosis.org/ which includes information about active pulmonary fibrosis clinical trials

PROGNOSIS
- Median survival time was thought to be 2 to 3 years from time of diagnosis. However, recent data from clinical trials suggest that this may be an underestimate.
- Some patients may deteriorate quickly, whereas others can remain stable for an extended period of time. Acute exacerbations carry a high mortality, and ICU treatment (mechanical ventilation) is mostly unsuccessful.
- A higher extent of fibrosis increases the risk of death, whereas a higher percentage-predicted diffusing capacity of lung for carbon monoxide reduced the risk of death.

COMPLICATIONS
- Respiratory failure
- Infection
- Pulmonary hypertension
- Rib fractures secondary to prolonged coughing (especially in elderly patients with decreased bone density)

REFERENCES
1. Raghu G, Collard HR, Egan JJ, et al. An official ATS/ERS/JRS/ALAT statement: idiopathic pulmonary fibrosis: evidence-based guidelines for diagnosis and management. *Am J Respir Crit Care Med*. 2011;183(6):788–824.
2. Lynch DA, Godwin JD, Safrin S, et al. High-resolution computed tomography in idiopathic pulmonary fibrosis: diagnosis and prognosis. *Am J Respir Crit Care Med*. 2005;172(4):488–493.
3. Raghu G, Anstrom KJ, King TE Jr, et al. Prednisone, azathioprine, and N-acetylcysteine for pulmonary fibrosis. *N Engl J Med*. 2012;366(21):1968–1977.
4. King TE Jr, Bradford WZ, Castro-Bernardini S, et al. A phase 3 trial of pirfenidone in patients with idiopathic pulmonary fibrosis. *N Engl J Med*. 2014;370(22):2083–2092.
5. Richeldi L, du Bois RM, Raghu G, et al. Efficacy and safety of nintedanib in idiopathic pulmonary fibrosis. *N Engl J Med*. 2014;370(22):2071–2082.
6. Rafii R, Juarez MM, Albertson TE, et al. A review of current and novel therapies for idiopathic pulmonary fibrosis. *J Thorac Dis*. 2013;5(1):48–73.

ADDITIONAL READING
- Castriotta RJ, Eldadah BA, Foster WM, et al. Workshop on idiopathic pulmonary fibrosis in older adults. *Chest*. 2010;138(3):693–703.
- Covvey JR, Mancl EE. Recent evidence for pharmacological treatment of idiopathic pulmonary fibrosis. *Ann Pharmacother*. 2014;48(12):1611–1619.
- Coward WR, Saini G, Jenkins G. The pathogenesis of idiopathic pulmonary fibrosis. *Ther Adv Respir Dis*. 2010;4(6):367–388.
- Hoo ZH, Whyte MK. Idiopathic pulmonary fibrosis. *Thorax*. 2012;67(8):742–746.
- Lee JS, McLaughlin S, Collard HR. Comprehensive care of the patient with idiopathic pulmonary fibrosis. *Curr Opin Pulm Med*. 2011;17(5):348–354.
- O'Connell OJ, Kennedy MP, Henry MT. Idiopathic pulmonary fibrosis: treatment update. *Adv Ther*. 2011;28(11):986–999.
- Rafii R, Juarez MM, Albertson TE, et al. A review of current and novel therapies for idiopathic pulmonary fibrosis. *J Thorac Dis*. 2013;5(1):48–73.
- Ryu JH, Moua T, Daniels CE, et al. Idiopathic pulmonary fibrosis: evolving concepts. *Mayo Clin Proc*. 2014;89(8):1130–1142.
- Spagnolo P, Del Giovane C, Luppi F, et al. Nonsteroid agents for idiopathic pulmonary fibrosis. *Cochrane Database Syst Rev*. 2010;(9):CD003134.

 CODES

ICD10
- J84.10 Pulmonary fibrosis, unspecified
- J84.112 Idiopathic pulmonary fibrosis

CLINICAL PEARLS
- Pulmonary fibrosis can usually be diagnosed based on characteristic chest CT findings, which include a reticular pattern, traction bronchiectasis, and honeycombing with a peripheral and basilar predominance.
- There are idiopathic and nonidiopathic forms of pulmonary fibrosis.
- Treatment options for pulmonary fibrosis are very limited and, at best, serve to slow the progression of disease.

PYELONEPHRITIS

Katelin M. Lisenby, PharmD • Dana G. Carroll, PharmD, BCPS, CDE • Catherine Scarbrough, MD

 BASICS

DESCRIPTION
- Acute pyelonephritis is a syndrome caused by an infection of the renal parenchyma and renal pelvis, often producing localized flank/back pain combined with systemic symptoms, such as fever, chills, and nausea. It has a wide spectrum of presentation, from mild illness to septic shock.
- Chronic pyelonephritis is the result of progressive inflammation of the renal interstitium and tubules, due to recurrent infection, vesicoureteral reflux, or both.
- Pyelonephritis is considered uncomplicated if the infection is caused by a typical pathogen in an immunocompetent patient who has normal urinary tract anatomy and renal function.
- System(s) affected: renal; urologic
- Synonym: acute upper urinary tract infection (UTI)

Geriatric Considerations
- May present as altered mental status; absence of fever is common in this age group.
- Elderly patients with diabetes and pyelonephritis are at higher risk of bacteremia, longer hospitalization, and mortality.
- The high prevalence of asymptomatic bacteriuria in the elderly makes the use of urine dipstick less reliable in diagnosing UTI in this population (1)[A].

Pregnancy Considerations
- Most common medical complication requiring hospitalization
- Affects 1–2% of all pregnancies. Morbidity does not differ between trimesters.
- Urine culture as test of cure 1 to 2 weeks after therapy

Pediatric Considerations
- UTI is present in ~5% of patients age 2 months to 2 years with fever and no apparent source on history and physical exam.
- Treatment (oral or IV; inpatient or outpatient) should be based on the clinical situation and patient toxicity.

EPIDEMIOLOGY
Incidence
Community-acquired acute pyelonephritis: 28/10,000/year

Prevalence
Adult cases: 250,000/year, with 200,000 hospitalizations

ETIOLOGY AND PATHOPHYSIOLOGY
- *Escherichia coli* (>80%)
- Other gram-negative pathogens: *Proteus, Klebsiella, Serratia, Clostridium, Pseudomonas,* and *Enterobacter*
- *Enterococcus*
- *Staphylococcus: Staphylococcus epidermis, Staphylococcus saprophyticus* (number 2 cause in young women), and *Staphylococcus aureus*
- *Candida*

RISK FACTORS
- Underlying urinary tract abnormalities
- Indwelling catheter/recent urinary tract instrumentation
- Nephrolithiasis
- Immunocompromise, including diabetes
- Elderly, institutionalized patients (particularly women)
- Prostatic enlargement
- Childhood UTI

- Acute pyelonephritis within the prior year
- Frequency of recent sexual intercourse/spermicide use
- New sex partner within the prior year
- Stress incontinence in the previous 30 days
- Pregnancy
- Hospital-acquired infection
- Symptoms >7 days at time of presentation

COMMONLY ASSOCIATED CONDITIONS
- Indwelling catheters
- Renal calculi
- Benign prostatic hyperplasia

 DIAGNOSIS

HISTORY
- In adults
  - Fever
  - Flank pain
  - Nausea ± vomiting
  - Malaise, anorexia
  - Myalgia
  - Dysuria, urinary frequency, urgency
  - Suprapubic discomfort
  - Mental status changes (elderly)
- In infants and children
  - Fever
  - Irritability and poor feeding
  - GI symptoms

PHYSICAL EXAM
- In adults
  - Fever: ≥38°C (100.4°F)
  - Costovertebral angle tenderness
  - Presentation ranges from no physical findings to septic shock.
  - Mental status changes common in the elderly
  - A pelvic exam may be necessary in female patients to exclude pelvic inflammatory disease.
- In infants and children
  - Sepsis
  - Fever
  - Poor skin perfusion
  - Inadequate weight gain/weight loss
  - Jaundice to gray skin color

DIFFERENTIAL DIAGNOSIS
- Obstructive uropathy
- Acute bacterial pneumonia (lower lobe)
- Cholecystitis
- Acute pancreatitis
- Appendicitis
- Perforated viscus; aortic dissection
- Pelvic inflammatory disease; ectopic pregnancy
- Kidney stone
- Diverticulitis

DIAGNOSTIC TESTS & INTERPRETATION
Initial Tests (lab, imaging)
- Urinalysis: pyuria ± leukocyte casts, hematuria, nitrites (sensitivity 35–85%; specificity 92–100%), and mild proteinuria
- Urine leukocyte esterase positive (sensitivity 74–96%; specificity 94–98%)
- Urine Gram stain; urine culture (>100,000 colony-forming units/mL or >100 colony forming units/mL + symptoms) and sensitivities

- CBC, BUN, Cr, GFR, and pregnancy test (if indicated)
- C-reactive protein levels have been shown to correlate with prolonged hospitalization and recurrence; serum albumin <3.3 g/dL also associated with risk for hospital admission.
- Imaging not necessary in routine cases
- Pediatrics: Recent guidelines recommend renal/bladder US, (not voiding cystourethrogram) after first UTI.

Follow-Up Tests & Special Considerations
- Catheterization/suprapubic aspirate should be used to obtain samples from non–toilet-trained children.
- In some geriatric patients catheterization may also be necessary.
- Blood culture(s): indicated in diagnostic uncertainty, immunosuppression, or a suspected hematogenous source
- Recent antibiotic use may alter lab results.
- If patient's condition does not improve within 72 hours or if obstruction/anatomic abnormality suspected, consider:
  - CT scan of abdomen and pelvis ± contrast
  - US of kidneys, ureter, bladder
  - Cystoscopy with ureteral catheterization

Test Interpretation
- Acute: abscess formation with neutrophil response
- Chronic: fibrosis with reduction in renal tissue

 TREATMENT

- 7 days or less of treatment is equivalent to longer treatment regimens in adult patients (including those with bacteremia) without urogenital abnormalities (2)[A].
- IV antibiotics are indicated for inpatients who are toxic or unable to tolerate oral antibiotics.

GENERAL MEASURES
- Broad-spectrum antibiotics initially, tailor therapy to culture and sensitivity results
- Analgesics and antipyretics
- Consider urinary analgesics (e.g., phenazopyridine 200 mg q8h) for dysuria.

MEDICATION
- For empiric oral therapy, a fluoroquinolone is recommended. Should fluoroquinolone resistance exceed 10% or the patient have nausea/vomiting, a single initial IV dose of a long-acting antibiotic such as ceftriaxone 1 g is additionally recommended.
- For parenteral therapy, fluoroquinolone, aminoglycoside ± ampicillin, an extended-spectrum cephalosporin or an extended-spectrum penicillin with or without an aminoglycoside, or a carbapenem are recommended.
- Contraindications:
  - Known drug allergy
  - Fluoroquinolones are not recommended in children, adolescents, and pregnant women unless other alternatives are not available.
  - Nitrofurantoin does not achieve reliable tissue levels for treatment of pyelonephritis.
- Precautions:
  - Most antibiotics require adjustments in dosage for patients with renal insufficiency.
  - Monitor aminoglycoside levels and renal function.

– If *Enterococcus* is suspected based on Gram stain, ampicillin ± gentamicin is a reasonable empiric choice, unless patient is penicillin-allergic; then use vancomycin. If outpatient, add amoxicillin to fluoroquinolone, pending culture results and sensitivity. Do not use a third generation cephalosporin for suspected/proven enterococcal infections.
– >20% *E. coli* strains are resistant to ampicillin and TMP-SMX in community-acquired infections.

First Line
• Adults
  – Oral (initial outpatient treatment)
    ○ Ciprofloxacin: 500 mg q12h for 7 days
    ○ Ciprofloxacin XR: 1,000 mg/day for 7 days
    ○ Levofloxacin: 750 mg/day for 5 days
  – Trimethoprim-sulfamethoxazole (TMP-SMX) (160/800 mg): 1 tab q12h for 14 days provided uropathogen known to be susceptible ± ceftriaxone 1 g initial IV dose given IV (assuming normal creatinine clearance [CrCl])
    ○ Ciprofloxacin: 400 mg q12h
    ○ Levofloxacin: 750 mg/day
    ○ Cefotaxime: 1 g q8–12h up to 2 g q4h
    ○ Ceftriaxone: 1 to 2 g/day
    ○ Cefepime: 1 to 2 g q12h
    ○ Gentamicin: 5 to 7 mg/kg of body weight daily
    ○ Ampicillin: 2 g q6h ± gentamicin for *Enterococcus*
  – Severe illness: IV therapy until afebrile 24 to 48 hours and tolerating oral hydration and medications, then oral agents to complete up to a 2-week course.
• Pediatric
  – Oral: cefdinir: 14 mg/kg/day for 10 to 14 days; ceftibuten 9 mg/kg/day for 10 to 14 days; cefixime 8 mg/kg/day for 10 to 14 days
  – IV (general indication for IV therapy is age <2 months or clinical concern in other ages)
    ○ Ceftriaxone: 75 mg/kg/day (also can be used IM in outpatient setting)
    ○ Cefotaxime: 150 mg/kg/day divided in 3 to 4 doses
    ○ Ampicillin: 100 mg/kg/day divided in 4 doses + gentamicin 7.5 mg/kg/day divided in 3 doses

Second Line
Adults
• Oral
  – Oral β-lactams should be used with caution to treat pyelonephritis due to inferior efficacy and higher relapse rates; if used, provide an initial IV dose of ceftriaxone or a consolidated 24-hour dose of an aminoglycoside and longer courses of therapy (10 to 14 days) recommended.
  – Cefpodoxime (Proxetil): 200 mg q12h
  – Amoxicillin–clavulanate: 875/125 mg q12h or 500/125 mg q8h
• IV
  – Piperacillin–tazobactam: 3.375 g q6–8h
  – Ticarcillin–clavulanate: 3.1 g q4–6h
  – Meropenem: 500 mg q12h

Pediatric Considerations
• Children <2 years of age and children with febrile or recurrent UTI are usually treated for 10 to 14 days.

• Initial empiric antibiotic choice should cover *E. coli*. Add ampicillin if *Enterococcus* is suspected.
  – Oral antibiotics (ceftibuten, cefixime, and amoxicillin/clavulanic acid) may be used alone, *or*
  – IV antibiotics (single daily dosing if an aminoglycoside is chosen) for 2 to 4 days, followed by oral antibiotics for a total of 10 to 14 days (3)[A]
• Complete outpatient antibiotic course in entirety

ISSUES FOR REFERRAL
• Acute pyelonephritis unresponsive to therapy
• Chronic pyelonephritis
• Abnormal urogenital anatomy

SURGERY/OTHER PROCEDURES
Perinephric abscess may require surgical drainage.

INPATIENT CONSIDERATIONS
Admission Criteria/Initial Stabilization
• Inpatient therapy for severe illness (e.g., high fevers, severe pain, marked debility, intractable vomiting, inability to tolerate oral intake, possible sepsis), risk factors for complicated pyelonephritis, pregnancy, or extremes of age
• Outpatient therapy if mild to moderate illness (not pregnant, no nausea/vomiting; fever and pain not severe), uncomplicated, and tolerating oral hydration and medications. Many patients can be treated as outpatients.

IV Fluids
As indicated for dehydration or renal calculi

Discharge Criteria
Discharge on oral agent after patient is afebrile 24 to 48 hours to complete up to 2 weeks of therapy.

ONGOING CARE

FOLLOW-UP RECOMMENDATIONS
• Women: Routine follow-up cultures not recommended unless symptoms recur after 2 weeks; then, urologic evaluation is necessary.
• Men, children, adolescents, patients with recurrent infections, patients with risk factors: repeat cultures 1 to 2 weeks after completing therapy; urologic evaluation after first episode of pyelonephritis and with recurrences

Patient Monitoring
• No response within 48 hours (5% of patients): Reevaluate and review cultures, CT scan, or US to review anatomy; adjust therapy as needed; urologic consult. The two most common causes of failure to respond are a resistant organism and nephrolithiasis.
• Work with parents to monitor response in children.

DIET
Encourage fluid intake.

PROGNOSIS
95% of treated patients respond within 48 hours.

COMPLICATIONS
• Kidney abscess
• Metastatic infection: skeletal system, endocardium, eye, meningitis with subsequent seizures
• Septic shock and death
• Acute/chronic renal failure

REFERENCES
1. Ninan S, Walton C, Barlow G. Investigation of suspected urinary tract infection in older people. *BMJ*. 2014;349:g4070.
2. Eliakim-Raz N, Yahav D, Paul M, et al. Duration of antibiotic treatment for acute pyelonephritis and septic urinary tract infection—7 days or less versus longer treatment: systematic review and meta-analysis of randomized controlled trials. *J Antimicrob Chemother*. 2013;68(10):2183–2191.
3. Strohmeier Y, Hodson EM, Willis NS, et al. Antibiotics for acute pyelonephritis in children. *Cochrane Database Syst Rev*. 2014;(7):CD003772.

ADDITIONAL READING
• Beetz R, Westenfelder M. Antimicrobial therapy of urinary tract infections in children. *Int J Antimicrob Agents*. 2011;38(Suppl):42–50.
• Colgan R, Williams M, Johnson JR. Diagnosis and treatment of acute pyelonephritis in women. *Am Fam Physician*. 2011;84(5):519–526.
• Gupta K, Hooton TM, Naber KG, et al. International clinical practice guidelines for the treatment of acute uncomplicated cystitis and pyelonephritis in women: a 2010 update by the Infectious Diseases Society of America and the European Society for Microbiology and Infectious Diseases. *Clin Infect Dis*. 2011;52(5):e103–e120.
• Hooton TM. Clinical practice. Uncomplicated urinary tract infection. *N Engl J Med*. 2012;366(11):1028–1037.
• Kang C, Kim K, Lee SH, et al. A risk stratification model of acute pyelonephritis to indicate hospital admission from the ED. *Am J Emerg Med*. 2013;31(7):1067–1072.
• Roberts KB. Urinary tract infection: clinical practice guideline for the diagnosis and management of the initial UTI in febrile infants and children 2 to 24 months. *Pediatrics*. 2011;128(3):595–610.
• Takhar SS, Moran GJ. Diagnosis and management of urinary tract infection in the emergency department and outpatient settings. *Infect Dis Clin North Am*. 2014;28(1):33–48.
• Wang A, Nizran P, Malone MA, et al. Urinary tract infections. *Prim Care*. 2013;40(3):687–706.

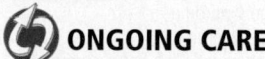

CODES

ICD10
• N12 Tubulo-interstitial nephritis, not spcf as acute or chronic
• N10 Acute tubulo-interstitial nephritis
• N11.9 Chronic tubulo-interstitial nephritis, unspecified

CLINICAL PEARLS
• Pyelonephritis can present with isolated confusion or mental status changes (no fever) in the elderly.
• The most common causes of poor response to treatment are antibiotic resistance and coexisting nephrolithiasis.
• Fluoroquinolones are the initial drugs of choice for treating pyelonephritis. Oral β-lactams are less effective.

PYLORIC STENOSIS

Joshua Scott Will, DO • Jennifer M. Cornwell, DO • Rachel M. Jones, DO

 BASICS

DESCRIPTION

- Progressive narrowing of the pyloric canal, occurring in infancy
- Synonym(s): infantile hypertrophic pyloric stenosis (IHPS)

EPIDEMIOLOGY

- Predominant age: infancy
  - Onset usually at 3 to 6 weeks of age; rarely in the newborn period or as late as 5 months of age
- Considered the most common condition requiring surgical intervention in the 1st year of life
- A recent decline in its incidence has been reported in a number of countries.
- Predominant sex: male > female (4 to 5:1)

Incidence

In Caucasian population, 2 to 5:1,000 babies; less common in African American and Asian populations

Prevalence

National prevalence level is 1 to 2:1,000 infants, ranging from 0.5 to 4.21:1,000 live births.

ETIOLOGY AND PATHOPHYSIOLOGY

- Abnormal relaxation of the pyloric muscles leads to hypertrophy.
- Redundant mucosa fills the pyloric canal.
- Gastric outflow is obstructed, leading to gastric distension and vomiting.
- The exact cause remains unknown, but multiple genetic and environmental factors have been implicated (1,2)[B].
- Breast versus bottle feeding—increased vasoactive intestinal peptide in breast milk may mediate pyloric relaxation and increase gastric emptying while bottle feeding may cause higher serum levels associated with pylorospasm (3)[C].

Genetics

Recent studies have identified linkage to chromosome 11 and multiple loci and chromosome 16 (1,2)[B].

RISK FACTORS

- Incidence higher in firstborn Caucasian boys (lower incidence in African Americans and Asians)
- 5 times increased risk with affected first-degree relative
- Strong familial aggregation and >80% heritability
- Multiple gestation—200 fold increased risk if monozygotic twin diagnosed and 20 fold increased risk if dizygotic twin diagnosed
- Breast feeding protective versus bottle feeding risk increased
- Postnatal macrolide use (i.e., erythromycin, azithromycin)—erythromycin agonist of motilin which might cause continuous contraction of the pyloric muscle (2)[B],(3)[C]
- A recent surveillance study of a population-based birth defects registry identified association between pyloric stenosis and the use of fluoxetine in the 1st trimester, even after adjustment for maternal age and smoking. The adjusted odds ratio was 9.8 (95% CI 1.5–62) (4)[B].

COMMONLY ASSOCIATED CONDITIONS

Associated anomalies present in ~4–7% of infants with pyloric stenosis.

- Hiatal and inguinal hernias (most commonly)
- Other anomalies include the following:
  - Congenital heart disease
  - Esophageal atresia
  - Tracheoesophageal fistula
  - Renal abnormalities
  - Turner syndrome and trisomy 18
  - Cornelia de Lange syndrome
  - Smith-Lemli-Opitz syndrome
- A common proposed genetic link between breast cancer, endometriosis, and pyloric stenosis has been observed in families.

 DIAGNOSIS

HISTORY

- Nonbilious projectile vomiting after feeding, increasing in frequency and severity
- Emesis may become blood-tinged from vomiting-induced gastric irritation.
- Hunger due to inadequate nutrition
- Decrease in bowel movements
- Weight loss

PHYSICAL EXAM

- Firm, mobile ("olivelike") mass palpable in the right upper quadrant (historically 70–90% of the time)
- However, this finding has decreased in occurence to about 13% due to earlier diagnosis with US (3)[C]
- Epigastric distention
- Visible gastric peristalsis after feeding
- Late signs: dehydration, weight loss
- Rarely, jaundice when starvation leads to decreased glucuronyl transferase activity resulting in indirect hyperbilirubinemia

DIFFERENTIAL DIAGNOSIS

- Inexperienced or inappropriate feeding
- GERD
- Gastritis
- Congenital adrenal hyperplasia, salt-losing
- Pylorospasm
- Gastric volvulus
- Antral or gastric web

DIAGNOSTIC TESTS & INTERPRETATION

Metabolic disturbances are late findings and are uncommon in present era of early diagnosis and intervention.

- If prolonged vomiting, then check electrolytes for the following:
  - Hypokalemia
  - Hypochloremia
  - Metabolic alkalosis
- Elevated unconjugated bilirubin level (rare)
- Paradoxical aciduria: The kidney tubules excrete hydrogen to preserve potassium in face of hypokalemic alkalosis.
- Abdominal US is the study of choice.
  - US shows thickened and elongated pyloric muscle and redundant mucosa.
- Upper GI series reveals strong gastric contractions; elongated, narrow pyloric canal (string sign); and parallel lines of barium in the narrow channel (double-tract sign or railroad track sign).

Test Interpretation

Concentric hypertrophy of pyloric muscle

TREATMENT

SURGERY/OTHER PROCEDURES
- Ramstedt pyloromyotomy is curative. The entire length of hypertrophied muscle is divided, with preservation of the underlying mucosa.
- Surgical approaches include open (traditional right upper quadrant transverse) incision, more contemporary circumumbilical incision, and laparoscopic techniques.
- A recent review concluded that the laparoscopic approach results in less postoperative pain and can be performed with no increase in operative time or complications (5)[A].
- Conservative approach
  - Conservative management of infantile hypertrophic pyloric stenosis with atropine can be effective in approximately six out of seven cases but has a lower success rate and longer duration of therapy than surgery (6)[B].
  - Atropine therapy may be considered as an alternative to pyloromyotomy for patients unsuitable or at high risk for surgery and in areas of the world where surgery on small infants is unavailable or unsafe (6)[B].

INPATIENT CONSIDERATIONS
Admission Criteria/Initial Stabilization
- Prompt treatment to avoid dehydration and malnutrition
- Correct acid–base and electrolyte disturbances. Surgery should be delayed until alkalosis is corrected.
- Patients need pre- and postop apnea monitoring. They have a tendency toward apnea to compensate with respiratory acidosis for their metabolic alkalosis.

IV Fluids
To correct dehydration and metabolic abnormalities. For optimal resuscitation in infants, use D5 1/2NS with 20 meq of KCl (3)[C].

ONGOING CARE

FOLLOW-UP RECOMMENDATIONS
Patient Monitoring
- Routine pediatric health maintenance
- Postoperative monitoring, including monitoring for pain, emesis, apnea
- If significant emesis present after 1 to 2 weeks, then upper GI studies needed to rule out incomplete pyloromyotomy or duodenal leak (3)[C]

DIET
- No preoperative feeding
- Initiate feeding 4 hours after surgery with adlib feedings thereafter (7)[A].

PROGNOSIS
Surgery is curative.

COMPLICATIONS
- No long-term morbidity
- Incomplete pyloromyotomy
- Mucosal perforation
- Wound infections
- Delayed feeding due to postoperative vomiting
- Serosal tear
- Subcutaneous emphysema
- 4.6–12% complication rate (3)[C]

REFERENCES
1. Feenstra B, Geller F, Carstensen L, et al. Plasma lipids, genetic variants near APOA1, and the risk of infantile hypertrophic pyloric stenosis. JAMA. 2013;310(7):714–721.
2. Krogh C, Fischer TK, Skotte L, et al. Familial aggregation and heritability of pyloric stenosis. JAMA. 2010;303(23):2393–2399.
3. Peters B, Oomen MW, Bakx R, et al. Advances in infantile hypertrophic pyloric stenosis. Expert Rev Gastroenterol Hepatol. 2014;8(5):533–541.
4. Bakker MK, De Walle HE, Wilffert B, et al. Fluoxetine and infantile hypertrophic pylorus stenosis: a signal from a birth defects-drug exposure surveillance study. Pharmacoepidemiol Drug Saf. 2010;19(8):808–813.
5. Oomen MW, Hoekstra LT, Bakx R, et al. Open versus laparoscopic pyloromyotomy for hypertrophic pyloric stenosis: a systematic review and meta-analysis focusing on major complications. Surg Endosc. 2012;26(8):2104–2110.
6. Mercer AE, Phillips R. Question 2: can a conservative approach to the treatment of hypertophic pyloric stenosis with atropine be considered a real alternative to surgical pyloromyotomy? Arch Dis Child. 2013;98(6):474–477.
7. Graham KA, Laituri CA, Markel TA, et al. A review of postoperative feeding regimens in infantile hypertrophic pyloric stenosis. J Pediatr Surg. 2013;48(10):2175–2179.

ADDITIONAL READING
- Ein SH, Masiakos PT, Ein A. The ins and outs of pyloromyotomy: what we have learned in 35 years. Pediatr Surg Int. 2014;30(5):467–480.
- Everett KV, Capon F, Georgoula C, et al. Linkage of monogenic infantile hypertrophic pyloric stenosis to chromosome 16q24. Eur J Hum Genet. 2008;16(9):1151–1154.
- Everett KV, Chioza BA, Georgoula C, et al. Genome-wide high-density SNP-based linkage analysis of infantile hypertrophic pyloric stenosis identifies loci on chromosomes 11q14–q22 and Xq23. Am J Hum Genet. 2008;82(3):756–762.
- Georgoula C, Gardiner M. Pyloric stenosis a 100 years after Ramstedt. Arch Dis Child. 2012;97(8):741–745.
- National Birth Defects Prevention Network. Selected birth defects data from population-based birth defects surveillance programs in the United States, 2003–2007. Birth Defects Res A Clin Mol Teratol. 2010;88(12):1062–1174.
- Owen RP, Almond SL, Humphrey GM. Atropine sulphate: rescue therapy for pyloric stenosis [published online ahead of print August 2, 2012]. BMJ Case Rep.
- Sommerfeld T, Chalmers J, Youngson G, et al. The changing epidemiology of infantile hypertrophic pyloric stenosis in Scotland. Arch Dis Child. 2008;93(12):1007–1011.
- Wyrick DL, Smith SD, Dassinger MS. Surgeon as educator: bedside ultrasound in hypertrophic pyloric stenosis. J Surg Educ. 2014;71(6):896–898.

 CODES

ICD10
Q40.0 Congenital hypertrophic pyloric stenosis

CLINICAL PEARLS
- Pyloric stenosis is the most common condition requiring surgical intervention in the 1st year of life.
- The condition classically presents between 1 and 5 months of life, with projectile vomiting after feeds and a firm, mobile mass in the right upper quadrant.
- Abdominal US is the study of choice.
- Surgery (laparoscopic Ramstedt pyloromyotomy is the preferred method) is curative.

RABIES

Alan M. Ehrlich, MD

 BASICS

DESCRIPTION
- A rapidly progressive CNS infection caused by a ribonucleic acid (RNA) rhabdovirus affecting mammals, including humans
- Generally considered to be 100% fatal once symptoms develop
- System(s) affected: nervous
- Synonym(s): hydrophobia (inability to swallow water)

EPIDEMIOLOGY
Incidence
- Most cases are in developing countries.
- Estimated 55,000 deaths worldwide per year
- Typically only 1 to 3 cases per year in the United States, with 1/3 of those being due to exposure outside of the United States
- Predominant age: any
- Predominant sex: male = female

ETIOLOGY AND PATHOPHYSIOLOGY
Lyssavirus, an RNA virus in the family *Rhabdoviridae*
- Rabies virus is a neurotropic virus present in saliva of infected animals.
- Transmission occurs via bites from infected animals or when saliva from an infected animal comes in contact with an open wound or mucous membranes.
- Bats are most common reservoir in the United States.

RISK FACTORS
- Professions or activities with exposure to potentially infected (wild or domestic) animals (e.g., animal handlers, lab workers, veterinarians, cave explorers)
- Most U.S. cases are associated with bat exposure.
- Internationally, rabies is widespread in both domestic and feral dogs.
- Human-to-human transmission has occurred through transplantation of cornea, solid organs, and other tissues.
- Travel to countries where canine rabies is endemic.

GENERAL PREVENTION
- Preexposure vaccination for high-risk groups (veterinarians, animal handlers, and certain laboratory workers)
- Consider preexposure vaccination for travelers to areas (such as North Africa) that have increased risk of rabies from domestic animals.
- Immunization of dogs and cats
- Contact animal control and avoid approaching or handling wild (or domestic) animals exhibiting strange behaviors.
- Avoid wild and unknown domestic animals.
- Seek treatment promptly if bitten, scratched, or in contact with saliva from potentially infected animal.
- Prevent infection by prompt postexposure treatment.

- Consider postexposure prophylaxis for individuals in direct contact with bats, unless it is known that an exposure did not occur.
- Hospital contacts of patients infected with rabies do not require postexposure prophylaxis unless there has been exposure through mucous membranes or an open wound (including a bite) to saliva, CSF, or brain tissue from the infect patient.

 DIAGNOSIS

HISTORY
- History of animal exposure
- Most patients do not recall exposure.
- Five stages (may overlap)
  - Incubation period: time between bite and first symptoms: usually 10 days to 1 year (average of 20 to 60 days). Incubation is shortest in patients with extensive bites in the head or trunk.
  - Prodrome: lasts 1 to 14 days; symptoms include pain or paresthesia at bite site and nonspecific flulike symptoms, including fever and headache.
  - Acute neurologic period: lasts 2 to 10 days. CNS symptoms dominate; generally 1 of 2 forms: (i) furious rabies: brief (~5 minute) episodes of hyperactivity with hydrophobia, aerophobia, hyperventilation, hypersalivation, and autonomic instability; (ii) paralytic rabies: Paralysis dominates; may be ascending (as in Guillain-Barré syndrome) or may affect ≥1 limbs differentially
  - Coma: lasts hours to days; may evolve over several days following acute neurologic period; may be sudden, with respiratory arrest
  - Death: usually occurs within 3 weeks of onset as result of complications

PHYSICAL EXAM
Findings range from normal exam to severe neurologic findings, including paralysis and coma, depending on the stage of rabies at the time of presentation.

DIFFERENTIAL DIAGNOSIS
- Any rapidly progressive encephalitis; important to exclude treatable causes of encephalitis, especially herpes
- Transverse myelitis

DIAGNOSTIC TESTS & INTERPRETATION
Initial Tests (lab, imaging)
- Lumbar puncture. WBC count is normal or shows moderate pleocytosis; protein normal or moderately elevated
- Skin biopsy to detect rabies antigen in hair follicles
  - Available through state and federal reference labs
- Rabies antibody titer of serum and CSF
- Skin biopsy from nape of neck for direct fluorescent antibody examination
- Viral isolation from saliva or CSF
- Corneal smear stains are positive by immunofluorescence in 50% of patients.

- Hyponatremia is common.
- Head CT scan: normal or nonspecific findings consistent with encephalitis
- MRI can help rule out other forms of encephalitis.

Follow-Up Tests & Special Considerations
Submit brain of the biting animal for testing if possible.

Test Interpretation
Encephalitis may be found on brain biopsy. Other abnormal findings (e.g., brainstem, midbrain, cerebellum) often found only postmortem.

TREATMENT

Thorough wound cleansing with soap and water is first line of treatment. Irrigate wound with virucidal agent, such as povidone-iodine, if available.

GENERAL MEASURES
- Evaluate risk based on exposure and consult public health officials about the need for rabies prophylaxis.
- In the United States, raccoons, skunks, bats, foxes, and coyotes are the animals most likely to be infected. Any carnivore can carry the disease.
- Before initiating antirabies treatment, consider:
  - Type of exposure (bite or nonbite)
  - Epidemiology of rabies in species involved
  - Circumstances surrounding exposure (provoked vs. unprovoked bite)
  - Vaccination status of offending animal

MEDICATION

ALERT
- Immunosuppression alters immunity after vaccination. Immunosuppressive drugs should be avoided during postexposure prophylaxis if possible. If postexposure prophylaxis is given to an immunosuppressed patient, check serum samples for the presence of rabies virus–neutralizing antibody to assess response to vaccination (1)[C].
- Clean wounds thoroughly, regardless of postexposure prophylaxis status.
- Assess need for postexposure prophylaxis based on circumstances of possible exposure.
- Increased risk:
  - Bites involving skin puncture are high risk; saliva exposure is a risk only if it comes in contact with an open wound or mucous membranes.
  - Wild or domestic animals unavailable for quarantine
  - Bat exposure
  - Hybrid animals of wild and domestic species (e.g., wolf-dog)
  - Unprovoked attack (Feeding a wild animal is considered a provoked attack.)

- Management:
  - Bites from cats, dogs, and ferrets that can be watched for 10 days do not require prophylaxis unless animal shows signs of illness.
  - Skunks, foxes, bats, raccoons, and most carnivores are high risk, and prophylaxis should begin promptly unless animal can be captured and euthanized for pathologic evaluation.
  - For rodents or livestock, consult local public health authorities before initiating prophylaxis.
- Postexposure prophylaxis (2)[B]
  - Passive vaccination: rabies immunoglobulin (RIG, HyperRAB) 20 IU/kg administered once. Infiltrate RIG around the wound if possible. Administer remaining RIG IM. Do not administer RIG using the same syringe or into the same anatomic site as vaccine.
  - Active vaccination: rabies vaccine, human diploid cell vaccine (HDCV) or rabies vaccine adsorbed (RVA) or purified chick embryo cell vaccine IM in the deltoid. Give the first dose, 1 mL, as soon as possible after exposure. The day of the first dose is designated day 0. Give additional 1-mL doses on days 3, 7, and 14. If immunocompromised, give fifth dose on day 28. For children, use the anterolateral aspect of the thigh and avoid the gluteal area.
- For previously vaccinated patients, administer an initial 1-mL IM dose of vaccine immediately and an additional 1-mL dose 3 days later. RIG is not necessary in these patients (2)[B].
- Preexposure vaccination: for people in high-risk groups, such as veterinarians, animal handlers, certain laboratory workers, and those spending time in foreign countries where rabies is enzootic (3)[B]:
  - Primary preexposure: three IM 1-mL injections of HDCV or RVA in deltoid area on days 0, 7, and 21, or 28
  - Preexposure boosters: For people at risk of exposure to rabies, test serum every 2 years. Administer preexposure booster of 1-mL IM if immunity is waning. If titer cannot be obtained, a booster can be administered instead.
- Contraindications: none for postexposure treatment

Pregnancy Considerations
- Pregnancy is not a contraindication to postexposure prophylaxis.
- Rabies vaccination is not associated with a higher incidence of spontaneous abortion, premature births, or fetal abnormalities.

INPATIENT CONSIDERATIONS
Admission Criteria/Initial Stabilization
Clinical rabies
- Comfort care and sedation for all patients.
- Milwaukee protocol: experimental treatment using ketamine, midazolam, and amantadine (originally included ribavirin but no longer recommended) (1,4)[C]. One patient who did not receive pre- or postexposure prophylaxis recovered from clinical rabies in 2004 after being treated with medically induced coma and amantadine I (1)[C].

- Control cerebral artery vasospasm (with an agent such as nimodipine) (4,5)[C].
- Fludrocortisone and hypertonic saline if needed to maintain normal sodium level (5)[C]

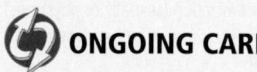 **ONGOING CARE**

FOLLOW-UP RECOMMENDATIONS
After primary vaccination, serologic testing is necessary only if the patient has a disease or takes immunosuppresive medication.

PATIENT EDUCATION
Use screens over ventilation areas in the roof to secure from bats. Avoid exposure to wild mammalian species known to carry rabies and report potential exposures immediately.

PROGNOSIS
- No postexposure failures in the United States since the 1970s.
- If untreated, rabies has the highest case fatality rate of any infectious disease; generally considered to be 100% fatal once symptoms develop.
- There have only been a small number of cases of successful recovery from rabies. Almost all received some form of pre- or postexposure immunization.

COMPLICATIONS
0.6% of people develop mild serum sickness reaction following HDCV boosters. Mild local and systemic reactions are common following vaccination. Do not interrupt immunization series with mild reactions.

REFERENCES

1. Willoughby RE Jr, Tieves KS, Hoffman GM, et al. Survival after treatment of rabies with induction of coma. *N Engl J Med*. 2005;352(24):2508–2514.
2. Rupprecht CE, Briggs D, Brown CM, et al. Use of a reduced (4-dose) vaccine schedule for postexposure prophylaxis to prevent human rabies: recommendations of the Advisory Committee on Immunization Practices. *MMWR Recomm Rep*. 2010;59(RR-2):1–9.
3. Manning SE, Rupprecht CE, Fishbein D, et al. Human rabies prevention—United States, 2008: recommendations of the Advisory Committee on Immunization Practices. *MMWR Recomm Rep*. 2008;57(RR-3):1–28.
4. Aramburo A, Willoughby RE, Bollen AW, et al. Failure of the Milwaukee protocol in a child with rabies. *Clin Infect Dis*. 2011;53(6):572–574.
5. Hu WT, Willoughby RE Jr, Dhonau H, et al. Long-term follow-up after treatment of rabies by induction of coma. *N Engl J Med*. 2007;357(9):945–946.

ADDITIONAL READING
- Centers for Disease Control and Prevention. http://www.cdc.gov/rabies/
- Centers for Disease Control and Prevention. Recovery of a patient from clinical rabies—California, 2011. *MMWR Morb Mortal Wkly Rep*. 2012;61(4):61–65.
- Crowcroft NS, Thampi N. The prevention and management of rabies. *BMJ*. 2015;350:g7827.
- De Serres G, Skowronski DM, Mimault P, et al. Bats in the bedroom, bats in the belfry: reanalysis of the rationale for rabies postexposure prophylaxis. *Clin Infect Dis*. 2009;48(11):1493–1499.
- Eckerle I, Rosenberger KD, Zwahlen M, et al. Serologic vaccination response after solid organ transplantation: a systematic review. *PLoS One*. 2013;8(2):e56974.
- Hemachudha T, Ugolini G, Wacharapluesadee S, et al. Human rabies: neuropathogenesis, diagnosis, and management. *Lancet Neurol*. 2013;12(5):498–513.
- Vora NM, Basavaraju SV, Feldman KA, et al. Raccoon rabies virus variant transmission through solid organ transplantation. *JAMA*. 2013;310(4):398–407.

 SEE ALSO

Bites, Animal and Human

 CODES

ICD10
- A82.9 Rabies, unspecified
- Z20.3 Contact with and (suspected) exposure to rabies

CLINICAL PEARLS
- Rabies is rare in the United States but more common in other areas of the world.
- Seek immediate treatment if exposed to scratch, bite, or saliva of potentially infected animal (e.g., feral dog, bat, fox, raccoon, or other wild mammals).
- Postexposure prophylaxis consists of three steps: local wound cleansing, passive immunization with rabies immunoglobulin, and active immunization with HDCV.
- Consider postexposure prophylaxis for those reporting direct contact with bats, unless it can be verified that an exposure did not occur.

RAPE CRISIS SYNDROME

Ravin V. Patel, MD • Dustin Creech, MD

BASICS

DESCRIPTION
- Definitions (legal definitions may vary from state to state)
  - Sexual contact: intentional touching of a person's intimate parts (including thighs) or the clothing covering such areas, if it is construed as being for the purpose of sexual gratification
  - Sexual conduct: vaginal intercourse between a male and female, or anal intercourse, fellatio, or cunnilingus between persons, regardless of sex
  - Rape (which is a legal term, physician should use the phrase alleged sexual assault): any sexual penetration, however slight, using force or coercion against the person's will
  - Sexual imposition: similar to rape but without penetration or the use of force (i.e., nonconsensual sexual contact, stalking)
  - Gross sexual imposition: nonconsensual sexual contact with the use of force
  - Corruption of a minor: sexual conduct by an individual age ≥18 years with an individual <16 years of age
- Most states have expanded rape statutes to include marital rape, date rape, and shield laws.
- System(s) affected: nervous; reproductive; GI

EPIDEMIOLOGY
- In the United States, 25% of women and 7.6% of men report being target of the definition of rape crisis syndrome listed above. The cost of this are estimated to exceed $5.8 billion annually.
- Anyone can be sexually assaulted, but some populations are especially vulnerable.
  - Adolescents and young children
  - People with disabilities
  - Elderly
  - Low socio-economic status and homeless people
  - Sex workers
  - Those living in institutions/areas of conflict
- Predominant age
  - The incidence of sexual assault peaks in those 16 to 19 years of age, with the mean occurring at 20 years of age
    - Adolescent sexual assault has a greater frequency of anogenital injuries.
- Predominant sex: female > male
  - For males
    - 69% of male victims were first raped before age 18 years.
    - 41% of male victims were raped before age 12 years.

INCIDENCE
- In the United States, approximately 1.5 million women and 834,700 men are sexually assaulted annually (1).
- Estimated that only a fraction of sexual assaults are reported to law enforcement.
- 18% of American women will be sexually assaulted during their lifetime (2).
  - Between 20% and 25% of females will experience rape/attempted rape during their college years.
- 2–3% of American men will be sexually assaulted during their lifetime.
- Most rape victims either know or have some acquaintance with their attacker.

RISK FACTORS
- Chronologic age of adolescent and young adults 16 to 24 years incur sexual assault. Children living in household of sexual assault are increase risk of maltreatment and lifelong poor health.
- Previous history of victimization (sexually or physically)
- Alcohol consumption is estimated to be involved in 1/2 of sexual assault.
- Illicit drug may also contribute to sexual assault.

GENERAL PREVENTION
- The public health approach should include both prevention and avoidance of vulnerability factors and implementation of protective factors.
- Females may benefit from assertiveness training and self-defense training.
- U.S. Preventive Services Task Force found insufficient evidence to support general screening in all their patient (no evidence of harm in screening), but physician should discuss sexual assault and family violence with their patient in nonjudgement manner.

DIAGNOSIS

- In adults
  - History of sexual penetration
  - Sexual contact/conduct without consent and/or with the use of force
- In children
  - Actual observation/suspicion of sexual penetration, sexual contact, or sexual conduct
  - Signs include evidence of the use of force and/or evidence of sexual contact (e.g., presence of semen and/or blood).

HISTORY
- Avoid questioning that implies the patient is at fault.
- Record answers in patient's own words insofar as possible. Include date, approximate time, and general location as best as possible. Document physical abuse other than sexual. Describe all types of sexual contact, whether actual/attempted. Take history of alcohol and/or drug use before or after alleged incident; note that some states require specific forms for documenting history.
- Document time of last activity that could possibly alter specimens (e.g., bath, shower, douche).
- Thorough gynecologic history is mandatory, including last menstrual period, last consenting sexual contact, contraceptive practice, and prior gynecologic surgery (3)[C].

PHYSICAL EXAM
- Use of drawings and/or photographs is encouraged; note that some states require specific forms for documenting physical exam.
- Document all signs of trauma/unusual marks.
- Document mental status/emotional state.
- Use UV light (Wood lamp) to detect seminal stains on clothing/skin.
- Obtaining the patient's consent at each step of examination helps the patient regain a sense of control.

ALERT
- A forensic kit or "rape kit" contains swabs that are collected from the vagina and rectum, and instructions are given with the kit regarding proper collection.
- Many states and emergency departments across the country are using a Sexual Assault Nurse Examiner (SANE) when available. This has led to more consistent and more accurate collection of evidence in alleged rape cases.

- Complete genital–rectal exam, including evidence of trauma, secretions, or discharge.
  - Use of a nonlubricated, water-moistened speculum is mandatory because commonly used lubricants may destroy evidence.
  - Testing and/or specimen collection, as indicated, and in compliance with state requirements (4)

DIFFERENTIAL DIAGNOSIS
Consenting sex among adults

DIAGNOSTIC TESTS & INTERPRETATION
- In females, obtain a serum or urine pregnancy test.
- Record results of wet mount, screening for vaginitis, but also note the presence/absence of sperm and, if present, whether it is motile/immotile.
- Drug/alcohol testing as indicated by history and/or physical findings

TREATMENT

GENERAL MEASURES
- Providing health care to victims of sexual assault/abuse requires special sensitivity and privacy.
- All such cases *must* be reported immediately to the appropriate law enforcement agency.
- With the victim's permission, enlist the help of personnel from local support agencies (e.g., rape crisis center). When available, use of in-house social services is extremely helpful to victim and family.
- SANE programs have been shown to be beneficial, especially in large cities and metropolitan areas with multiple emergency departments of varying capability and staff training/experience.
- Give sedation and tetanus prophylaxis when indicated.
- Discuss possible pregnancy and pregnancy termination with the victim. If hospital policy precludes such as discussion, then information about this option should be offered to the victim via follow-up mechanisms.
- Discuss suspected HIV and hepatitis B exposure and testing with the victim in accordance with hospital, regional, and state policies/protocols. The initial HIV test should be completed within 7 days of the suspected exposure.

MEDICATION

First Line
- Controversy exists regarding empiric antibiotic prophylaxis for victims of sexual assault. However, the Centers for Disease Control and Prevention (CDC) recommends empiric antibiotic prophylaxis of potential sexually transmitted infections (specifically, gonorrhea, chlamydia, trichomoniasis, and potentially syphilis), as many patients will not return for a follow-up visit and many patients prefer immediate treatment (5)[C].
- Cultures are *not* required before initiating treatment but can be considered as part of routine evidence collection.
- Gonorrhea: ceftriaxone 250 mg IM once. Note: Be aware that drug resistance is on the rise in several major cities. Quinolones are no longer recommended for treatment of gonorrhea.
- Chlamydia: azithromycin 1 g PO single dose, or doxycycline 100 mg PO BID for 7 days, *or* erythromycin base 500 mg PO QID for 7 days, *or* erythromycin ethylsuccinate 800 mg PO QID for 7 days
- Syphilis: benzathine penicillin G 2 to 4 million units IM once, or doxycycline 100 mg PO BID for 14 days.

Some suggest ceftriaxone 1 g/day, either IM/IV, for 8 to 10 days, but treatment failures have been reported in several geographic areas.

- Trichomoniasis and bacterial vaginosis, if present (if cultures/wet mount were collected): metronidazole 2 g PO once, *or* metronidazole 500 mg PO BID for 7 days (consider single dose to maximize compliance), *or* metronidazole gel 0.75% 1 full applicator (5 g) intravaginally every day for 5 days; *or* clindamycin cream 2% 1 full applicator (5 g) intravaginally at bedtime for 7 days (considered less efficacious than PO metronidazole)
- If pregnancy prophylaxis is indicated, use levonorgestrel 1.5 mg once (Plan B, progestin-only), efficacious for up to 5 days after the incident.
  - Levonorgestrel alone has proved more effective than the Yuzpe regimen, a method of emergency contraception.
  - *Alternatively*, ethinyl estradiol/levonorgestrel (Yuzpe) 100 μg/0.5 mg once and repeated in 12 hours can be used.
  - Alternatively, ulipristal acetate (Ella) 30 μg once can be used.
  - Alternatively, a copper intrauterine device can be inserted up to 5 days after the earliest predicted date of ovulation in that cycle (6)[C].
- HIV: Currently, there is a low likelihood of HIV transmittance, but the CDC still recommends postexposure prophylaxis (PEP) for victims of sexual assault. Regimen is PEP for 3 to 7 days, with short-term follow-up for further counseling, with a specialist familiar with PEP regimens.
  - Most effective if started within 4 hours and could reduce transmission by as much as 80%; unlikely to be beneficial if started after 72 hours.
- Hepatitis B: if prevalent in area or assailant known to be high risk: hepatitis B immunoglobulin 0.06 mL/kg IM, single dose, and initiate 3-dose hepatitis B virus immunization series. No treatment if the victim has had a complete hepatitis B vaccine series, with documented levels of immunity (7)[C].

Second Line
Pregnancy Considerations
Conduct baseline pregnancy test; discuss pregnancy prevention and termination with patient.

Pediatric Considerations
Assure the child that she or he is a good person and was not the cause of the incident.

INPATIENT CONSIDERATIONS
Admission Criteria/Initial Stabilization
- Contact appropriate social services agency.
- Most adult victims can be treated as outpatients, unless associated trauma (physical/mental) requires admission.
- Most pediatric sexual assault/abuse victims will require admission/outside placement until appropriate social agency can evaluate home environment (8)[C].

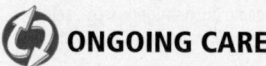 ONGOING CARE

FOLLOW-UP RECOMMENDATIONS
Patient Monitoring
- Patient should be seen in 7 to 10 days for follow-up care, including pregnancy testing and counseling.
- Close exam for vaginitis and treatment if necessary
- Follow-up test for gonorrhea should occur in 1 to 2 weeks.
- Follow-up testing for syphilis, HIV, and hepatitis B should occur at 6 weeks, 3 months, and 6 months.

- Provide telephone numbers of counseling agency(ies) that can provide counseling/legal services to the patient.
- Strongly consider SANE, if available (9)[C].

PATIENT EDUCATION
- Local rape crisis support organizations
- National Sexual Violence Resource Center, 123 Enola Drive, Enola, PA 17025; (877) 739-3895; www.nsvrc.org
- National Domestic Violence Hotline at (800) 799-SAFE(7233) or TTY (800) 787-3224 or www.thehotline.org

PROGNOSIS
- Acute phase (usually 1 to 3 weeks following rape): shaking, pain, wound healing, mood swings, appetite loss, crying. Also feelings of grief, shame, anger, fear, revenge, or guilt
- Late/chronic phase (also called "reorganization"): Female victim may develop fear of intercourse, fear of men, anxiety or increase discomfort during Pap smears, nightmares, sleep disorders, daytime flashbacks, fear of being alone, loss of self-esteem, anxiety, depression, posttraumatic stress syndrome, and somatic complaints (e.g., nonspecific abdominal pain).
- Recovery may be prolonged. Patients who are able to talk about their feelings seem to have a faster recovery. It is unclear if pharmaco- or psychotherapy results in better outcomes.

COMPLICATIONS
Sequelae include the following:
- Trauma (physical and or mental)
- STIs, including HIV
- Unwanted pregnancy (with the possibility of abortion)
  - The rape-related pregnancy rate in the United States is 5% per rape among victims of reproductive age, resulting in >32,000 unwanted pregnancies each year.
  - Adolescents are at highest risk of pregnancy.
- Medical: chronic pain, fibromyalgia, headaches, irritable bowel syndrome, sexual dysfunction
- Psychological: anxiety, depression, posttraumatic stress disorder, eating disorder, substance abuse

REFERENCES
1. Cronholm PF, Fogarty CT, Ambuel B, et al. Intimate partner violence. *Am Fam Physician*. 2011;83(10):1165–1172.
2. Tjaden P, Thoennes N. *Extent, Nature, and Consequences of Rape Victimization: Findings from the National Violence Against Women Survey*. Washington, DC: National Institute of Justice and the Centers for Disease Control and Prevention; 2006.
3. Linden JA. Clinical practice. Care of the adult patient after sexual assault. *N Engl J Med*. 2011;365(9):834–841.
4. U.S. Department of Justice, Office on Violence Against Women. *A National Protocol for Sexual Assault Medical Forensic Examinations (Adults/Adolescents)*. 2nd ed. Washington, DC: U.S. Department of Justice; 2013.
5. Workowski KA, Berman S; Centers for Disease Control and Prevention. Sexually transmitted diseases treatment guidelines, 2010. *MMWR Recomm Rep*. 2010;59(RR-12):1–110.
6. Cheng L, Che Y, Gülmezoglu AM. Interventions for emergency contraception. *Cochrane Database Syst Rev*. 2012;(8):CD001324.

7. Mast EE, Weinbaum CM, Fiore AE, et al. A comprehensive immunization strategy to eliminate transmission of hepatitis B virus infection in the United States: recommendations of the Advisory Committee on Immunization Practices (ACIP) part II: immunization of adults. *MMWR Recomm Rep*. 2006;55(RR-16):1–33; quiz CE1–CE4.
8. DeVore HK, Sachs CJ. Sexual assault. *Emerg Med Clin North Am*. 2011;29(3):605–620.
9. ACOG educational bulletin. Sexual assault. Number 242, November 1997 (replaces no. 172, September 1992). American College of Obstetricians and Gynecologists. *Int J Gynaecol Obstet*. 1998;60(3):297–304.

ADDITIONAL READING
- Centers for Disease Control and Prevention. *Sexual Violence: Facts at a Glance*. Atlanta, GA: Centers for Disease Control and Prevention; 2012.
- *National Consensus Guidelines of Identifying and Responding to Domestic Violence*. San Franscisco, CA: Family Voilence Prevention Fund; 2002.

 SEE ALSO

Chlamydia Infection (Sexually Transmitted); Gonococcal Infections; Hepatitis B; Hepatitis C; HIV/AIDS; Posttraumatic Stress Disorder; Syphilis

 CODES

ICD10
- T74.21XA Adult sexual abuse, confirmed, initial encounter
- T74.22XA Child sexual abuse, confirmed, initial encounter
- Z04.41 Encounter for exam and obs following alleged adult rape

CLINICAL PEARLS
- *Rape* is a legal term, and the examining physician is encouraged to use terminology such as *alleged rape* or *alleged sexual conduct*.
- Marital rape is a federal offense in all 50 states and the District of Columbia; in some states, also applies to unmarried cohabiting couples.
- Because "consent defense" is common, documentation of evidence supporting the use of force or the administration of drugs/alcohol is imperative.
- Use of a protocol is encouraged to assure every victim a uniform, comprehensive evaluation, regardless of the expertise of the examiner. The protocol must ensure that all evidence is properly collected and labeled, chain of custody is maintained, and the evidence is sent to the most appropriate forensic laboratory.
- All medical records must be well documented and legible.
- All medical personnel must be willing and able to testify on behalf of the patient.

The views expressed in this chapter are those of the author and do not reflect the official policy or position of the Department of the Army, Department of Defense, or the U.S. government. Opinions, interpretations, conclusions, and recommendations herein are those of the author and are not necessarily endorsed by the U.S. Army.

RAYNAUD PHENOMENON

Herbert L. Muncie, Jr., MD • Kelsey E. Phelps, MD

 BASICS

DESCRIPTION

- Idiopathic intermittent episodes of vasoconstriction of digital arteries, precapillary arterioles, and cutaneous arteriovenous shunts in response to cold, emotional stress, or blunt trauma
  - A triphasic color change of the fingers (occasionally the toes, rarely nipples) is the principal physical manifestation.
    - The initial color is *white* from extreme pallor, then *blue* from cyanosis, and finally with warming and vasodilatation the skin appears *red*.
    - Thumbs are rarely involved.
  - Swelling, throbbing, and paresthesias are associated symptoms.
  - Primary
    - 80% of patients have primary disease.
    - Episodes are bilateral and nonprogressive.
    - Diagnosis confirmed if after 2 years of symptoms, no underlying connective tissue disease develops.
  - Secondary
    - Progressive and asymmetric
    - Vascular spasm is more frequent and more severe over time. Ulceration is rare; gangrene does not develop; 13% progress to digital fat pad atrophy and ischemic changes of the fingertips.
    - Typically associated with an underlying connective tissue disorder
- System(s) affected: hematologic, lymphatic, immunologic, musculoskeletal, dermatologic, exocrine

Pregnancy Considerations
- Raynaud phenomenon can appear as breast pain in lactating women (1).
- Positive breast milk bacterial culture distinguishes mastitis from Raynaud phenomenon.

Geriatric Considerations
Initial appearance of Raynaud phenomenon after age 40 years often indicates underlying connective tissue disease.

Pediatric Considerations
Associated with systemic lupus erythematosus (SLE) and scleroderma

EPIDEMIOLOGY

Incidence
- Primary
  - Predominant age: 14 years; ~1/4 begin >40 years
  - Predominant sex: female > male (4:1)
- Secondary
  - Predominant age: >40 years
  - Predominant sex: no gender predilection

Prevalence
- Primary: 3–12.5% of men; 6–20% of women (based on clinical history)
- Secondary: ~1% of population

ETIOLOGY AND PATHOPHYSIOLOGY
Unknown. Dysregulation of vascular control mechanisms leads to imbalance between vasodilation and vasoconstriction. There is a reduced endothelin-dependent vasodilation activity and an increased vasoconstriction in peripheral vessels by overproduction of endothelin-1. $5-HT_2$ serotonin receptors may be involved in secondary Raynaud phenomenon. Platelet and blood viscosity abnormalities in secondary contribute to ischemic pathology.

Genetics
Some studies suggest dominant inheritance pattern. ~1/4 of primary patients have a first-degree relative with Raynaud phenomenon.

RISK FACTORS
- Existing autoimmune or connective tissue disorder
- End-stage renal disease with hemodialysis may increase risk if a steal phenomenon associated with the arterial-venous shunt develops.
- Primary and secondary disease associated with elevated homocysteine levels.
- Smoking is not associated with increased risk of Raynaud phenomenon but may worsen symptoms.

GENERAL PREVENTION
- Avoid cold exposure.
- Tobacco cessation
- No relationship has been established between Raynaud phenomenon and vibratory tool use.

COMMONLY ASSOCIATED CONDITIONS
Secondary Raynaud
- Scleroderma; SLE; polymyositis
- Sjögren syndrome; occlusive vascular disease
- Cryoglobulinemia

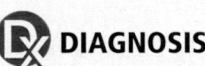 DIAGNOSIS

HISTORY
- Primary
  - Symmetric attacks involving fingers
  - Family history of connective tissue disorder
  - Absence of tissue necrosis, ulceration, or gangrene
  - If after ≥2 years of symptoms, no abnormal clinical or laboratory signs have developed, secondary disease is highly unlikely.
- Secondary
  - Onset typically after 40 years of age
  - Asymmetric episodes more intense and painful
  - Arthritis, myalgias, fever, dry eyes and/or mouth, rash, or cardiopulmonary symptoms
  - History of medication and/or recreational drug use
  - Exposure to toxic agents
  - Repetitive trauma

PHYSICAL EXAM
Pallor (whiteness) of fingertips with cold exposure, then cyanosis (blue), then redness and pain with warming
- Ischemic attacks evidenced by demarcated or cyanotic skin limited to digits; usually starts on one digit and spreads symmetrically to remaining fingers of both hands. The thumb is typically spared.
- May rarely involve other peripheral tissues (e.g., tongue) (2).

- Beau lines: transverse linear depressions in nail plate on most or all fingernails that occurs after exposure to cold or any insult that disrupts normal nail growth.
- Livedo reticularis: mottling of the skin of the arms and legs; benign and reverses with warming
- Primary
  - Normal physical exam
  - Nail bed capillaries have normal appearance: Place 1 drop of grade B immersion oil on skin at base of fingernail and view capillaries with hand-held ophthalmoscope at 10 to 40 diopters.
- Secondary
  - Skin changes, arthritis, and abnormal lung findings suggest connective tissue disease,
  - Ischemic skin lesions: ulceration of finger pads (autoamputation in severe, prolonged cases)
  - Nail bed capillary distortion including giant loops, avascular areas, and increased tortuosity
  - Abnormal Allen test: conducted by having the patient open and close his or her hand several times and then squeezing his or her hand tightly into a fist. The examiner sequentially occludes the ulnar and radial arteries while the patient opens his or her hand to reveal the return of color as a measure of circulation.

DIFFERENTIAL DIAGNOSIS
- Thromboangiitis obliterans (Buerger disease): primarily affects men; smoking-related
- Rheumatoid arthritis (RA)
- Progressive systemic sclerosis (scleroderma): Raynaud phenomenon precedes other symptoms.
- SLE
- Carpal tunnel syndrome; thoracic outlet syndrome
- Hypothyroidism
- CREST syndrome (calcinosis cutis, Raynaud phenomenon, esophageal dysmotility, sclerodactyly, and telangiectasias)
- Cryoglobulinemia; Waldenström macroglobulinemia
- Acrocyanosis
- Polycythemia
- Occupational (e.g., especially from vibrating tools, masonry work, exposure to polyvinyl chloride)
- Drug-induced (e.g., clonidine, ergotamine, methysergide, amphetamines, bromocriptine, bleomycin, vinblastine, cisplatin, cyclosporine)

DIAGNOSTIC TESTS & INTERPRETATION
Provocative test (e.g., ice water immersion) unnecessary
- Primary
  - Antinuclear antibody: negative
  - ESR: normal
- Secondary
  - Tests for secondary causes (e.g., CBC, ESR)
  - Positive autoantibody has low positive predictive value for connective tissue disease (30%).
  - Antibodies to specific autoantigens (e.g., scleroderma with anticentromere or antitopoisomerase antibodies)
  - Videocapillaroscopy is gold standard (200 times magnification).

Follow-Up Tests & Special Considerations
Periodic assessments for a connective tissue disorder

Diagnostic Procedures/Other
Diagnosis is determined by history and physical exam.

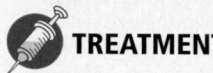

TREATMENT
Assess using a Raynaud Condition Score.

GENERAL MEASURES
- Dress warmly, wear gloves, and avoid cold temperatures.
- During attacks, rotate the arms in a windmill pattern or placing the hands under warm water or in a warm body fold to alleviate symptoms.
- Tobacco cessation
- Avoid β-blockers, amphetamines, ergot alkaloids, and sumatriptan.
- Temperature-related biofeedback may help patients increase hand temperature. 1-year follow-up is no better than control.
- Finger guards to protect ulcerated fingertips

MEDICATION
First Line
- Calcium channel blockers (CCBs). Nifedipine is the best studied and most frequently used.
- Nifedipine: 30 to 180 mg/day (sustained-release form); seasonal (winter) use is effective with up to 75% of patients experiencing improvement.
- Is compatible with breastfeeding
- Contraindications: allergy to drug, pregnancy, CHF
- Precautions: may cause headache, dizziness, light-headedness, edema, or hypotension
- Significant possible interactions
  – Increases serum level of digoxin

Second Line
- Amlodipine (5 to 10 mg/day) and nicardipine are effective and may have fewer adverse effects.
- No data exist to support switching CCB if initial drug is ineffective.
- Small studies support benefit from losartan and fluoxetine.
- Phosphodiesterase type-5 inhibitors (sildenafil, vardenafil) may reduce symptoms without increasing blood flow.
- Parenteral iloprost, a prostacyclin, in low doses (0.5 ng/kg/min over 6 hours), has improved ulcerations with severe Raynaud phenomenon when CCBs failed. Oral prostacyclin has not proven useful.
- Nitroglycerin patches may be helpful, but use is limited by the incidence of severe headache. Nitroglycerin gel has shown promise as a topical therapy.
- Prazosin (1 to 2 mg TID) is the only well-studied α_1-adrenergic receptor blocker with modest effect, but adverse effects may outweigh any benefit.
- ACE inhibitors are no longer recommended.

ISSUES FOR REFERRAL
If an underlying disease is suspected, consider rheumatology consultation for evaluation and treatment.

ADDITIONAL THERAPIES
- Botulinum toxin has shown some effect in reducing vasospastic episodes, frequency of attacks, rest pain, and helping to promote digital ulcer healing (3)[C].

- Aspirin
- Digital or wrist block with lidocaine or bupivacaine (without epinephrine) for pain control
- Short-term anticoagulation with heparin if persistent critical ischemia, evidence of large-artery occlusive disease, or both

SURGERY/OTHER PROCEDURES
Surgical intervention is rarely indicated or used for Raynaud phenomenon. Effect of cervical sympathectomy is transient; symptoms return in 1 to 2 years. Digital fat grafting is a novel modality that has shown improved symptomatology and evidence of measurably increased perfusion in several cases; further study is needed (4)[C].

COMPLEMENTARY & ALTERNATIVE MEDICINE
- *Ginkgo biloba* may reduce the frequency of attacks.
- Well-designed studies have not been done yet (5)[B].

- Fish oil supplements may increase digital systolic pressure and time to onset of symptoms after exposure to cold; not proven in controlled trials
- Vitamin D supplementation led to improvement in self-reported symptoms in vitamin D–deficient patients with Raynaud phenomenon (6)[B].
- Evening primrose oil reduced severity of attacks in one study.
- Oral arginine is no better than placebo.
- Biofeedback is not helpful.

ONGOING CARE

FOLLOW-UP RECOMMENDATIONS
Avoid exposure to cold; reassess for secondary causes.

Patient Monitoring
Manage fingertip ulcers and rapidly treat infection.

DIET
No special diet.

PATIENT EDUCATION
- Tobacco cessation.
- Avoid triggers (e.g., trauma, vibration, cold).
- Dress warmly; wear gloves.
- Warm hands when experiencing vasospasm.

PROGNOSIS
- Attacks may last from several minutes to a few hours.
- 2/3 of attacks resolve spontaneously.
- ~13% of Raynaud patients develop a secondary disorder, typically connective tissue diseases.

COMPLICATIONS
- Primary: very rare
- Secondary: gangrene, autoamputation of fingertips

REFERENCES
1. Barrett ME, Heller MM, Stone HF, et al. Raynaud phenomenon of the nipple in breastfeeding mothers: an underdiagnosed cause of nipple pain. *JAMA Dermatol.* 2013;149(3):300–306.
2. Lioger B, Diot E. Raynaud's phenomenon of the tongue: uncommon presentation of a classical sign. *QJM.* 2013;106(6):583–584.
3. Neumeister MW, Webb KN, Romanelli M. Minimally invasive treatment of Raynaud phenomenon: the role of botulinum type A. *Hand Clin.* 2014;30(1):17–24.
4. Bank J, Fuller SM, Henry GI, et al. Fat grafting to the hand in patients with Raynaud phenomenon: a novel therapeutic modality. *Plast Reconstr Surg.* 2014;133(5):1109–1118.
5. Bredie SJ, Jong MC. No significant effect of Ginkgo biloba special extract EGb 761 in the treatment of primary Raynaud phenomenon: a randomized controlled trial. *J Cardiovasc Pharmacol.* 2012;59(3):215–221.
6. Hélou J, Moutran R, Maatouk I, et al. Raynaud's phenomenon and vitamin D. *Rheumatol Int.* 2013;33(3):751–755.

ADDITIONAL READING
- Herrick AL. Contemporary management of Raynaud's phenomenon and digital ischaemic complications. *Curr Opin Rheumatol.* 2011;23(6):555–561.
- Huisstede BM, Hoogvliet P, Paulis WD, et al. Effectiveness of interventions for secondary Raynaud's phenomenon: a systematic review. *Arch Phys Med Rehabil.* 2011;92(7):1166–1180.
- Malenfant D, Catton M, Pope JE. The efficacy of complementary and alternative medicine in the treatment of Raynaud's phenomenon: a literature review and meta-analysis. *Rheumatology (Oxford).* 2009;48(7):791–795.
- Maverakis E, Patel F, Kronenberg DG, et al. International consensus criteria for the diagnosis of Raynaud's phenomenon. *J Autoimmun.* 2014; 48–49:60–65.

 ## SEE ALSO

Algorithm: Raynaud Phenomenon

 ## CODES

ICD10
- I73.00 Raynaud's syndrome without gangrene
- I73.01 Raynaud's syndrome with gangrene

CLINICAL PEARLS
- The diagnosis of Raynaud phenomenon is based on clinical symptoms.
- Provocative testing is not recommended.
- Initial presentation of Raynaud phenomenon after age 40 years suggests underlying (secondary) disease.
- Raynaud phenomenon is a cause of breast pain in lactating women.
- Primary Raynaud phenomenon is symmetric; secondary Raynaud phenomenon is asymmetric.
- Primary Raynaud phenomenon is treated with handwarming and avoiding cold exposure.
- Digital ulcers are not normal and always merit a workup for secondary disease.

REACTIVE ARTHRITIS (REITER SYNDROME)

Douglas W. MacPherson, MD, MSc–CTM, FRCPC

 BASICS

Reiter syndrome is a seronegative, multisystem, inflammatory disorder classically involving joints, the eye, and the lower genitourinary (GU) tract. Axial joint (e.g., spine, sacroiliac joints) and dermatologic manifestations are common (1)[C].

DESCRIPTION

The classic triad include arthritis, conjunctivitis/iritis, and either urethritis or cervicitis ("can't see; can't pee; can't bend my knee").

- The epidemiology is similar to other reactive arthritides, characterized by sterile joint inflammation associated with infections originating at nonarticular sites. A fourth feature (dermatologic involvement) may include buccal ulceration, balanitis, or a psoriaform skin eruption. (Having only two features does not rule out the diagnosis.)
- Two forms of Reiter syndrome:
  - Sexually transmitted: Symptoms emerge 7 to 14 days after exposure to *Chlamydia trachomatis* and other sexually acquired pathogens.
  - Postenteric infection (including traveler's diarrhea)
- In individuals with new or frequent sexual partners, the triggering infection is likely sexually transmitted (rather than enteric).
- In individuals with a history of recent enteric illness, the triggering event is more likely to be a bacterial enteric infection than sexually transmitted.
- System(s) affected: musculoskeletal, renal/urologic, dermatologic/exocrine
- Synonym(s): idiopathic blennorrheal arthritis; arthritis urethritica; urethro-oculosynovial syndrome; Fiessinger-Leroy-Reiter disease; reactive arthritis

Pediatric Considerations
Juvenile rheumatoid arthritis has many of the same clinical features as Reiter syndrome.

Pregnancy Considerations
No special considerations; usual drug precautions

EPIDEMIOLOGY

Incidence
- Predominant age: 20 to 40 years
- Predominant sex: male > female
- 0.24–1.5% incidence after epidemics of bacterial dysentery
- Complicates 1–2% of nongonococcal urethritis cases

ETIOLOGY AND PATHOPHYSIOLOGY

- The pathophysiology of all the seronegative reactive arthritis syndromes and the immunologic role of infectious diseases as precipitants for clinical illness are incompletely understood.
- Avoiding precipitant infections and early management of multiorgan inflammation is important. Antibiotic treatment following onset of syndrome does not appear to benefit inflammatory joint, eye, or urinary tract symptoms.
- *C. trachomatis* is the most common sexually transmitted infection associated with Reiter syndrome.
- Dysentery-associated Reiter syndrome follows infection with *Shigella, Salmonella, Yersinia,* and *Campylobacter* spp. Enteric-associated Reiter syndrome is more common in women, children, and the elderly than the postvenereal form.

Genetics
HLA-B27 tissue antigen present in 60–80% of patients, suggesting a genetic predisposition.

RISK FACTORS
- New or high-risk sexual contacts 7 to 14 days before the onset of clinical presentation; the primary infection may be subclinical and undiagnosed.
- Food poisoning or bacterial dysentery

GENERAL PREVENTION
- The immune-response characteristics of this syndrome make specific avoidance of infectious precipitants the most important general precaution (and potentially the most difficult to achieve).
- Safe sexual practices; proper food and water hygiene

COMMONLY ASSOCIATED CONDITIONS
- Enteric disease
  - Shigellosis; Salmonellosis; Campylobacteriosis
  - Enteric infection with *Yersinia* spp.
- Urogenital infection
  - *Chlamydia* urethritis/cervicitis (2)[C]
  - *Mycoplasma* or *Ureaplasma* spp.
- HIV/AIDS

 DIAGNOSIS

- Based on clinical presentation with joint, eye, and GU inflammation ("classic triad") and negative serologic testing for rheumatoid factor
- Classic symptoms not always present at the same time
- HLA-B27 testing is not required for diagnosis.

HISTORY
The presence of the clinical syndrome plus
- Diarrhea, dysentery, urethritis, or genital discharge and appropriate exposure history
- Exposure risks, including travel or migration history and potential infectious exposure
- Arthritis associated with urethritis for >1 month (84% sensitive; 98% specific for diagnosis)
- Urethritis occurs 1 to 15 days after sexual exposure.
- Reiter syndrome onset within 10 to 30 days of either enteric infection or STI
- Mean duration of symptoms is 19 weeks.

PHYSICAL EXAM
- Musculoskeletal
  - Asymmetric arthritis (especially knees, ankles, and metatarsophalangeal joints)
  - Enthesopathy (inflammation at tendinous insertion into bone, such as plantar fasciitis, digital periostitis, and Achilles tendinitis)
  - Spondyloarthropathy (spine and sacroiliac joint involvement)
- Urogenital tract
  - Urethritis; prostatitis; cystitis (rare)
  - Balanitis
  - Cervicitis: usually asymptomatic
- Eye
  - Conjunctivitis of one or both eyes
  - Occasionally, scleritis, keratitis, and corneal ulceration
  - Rarely, uveitis and iritis

- Skin
  - Mucocutaneous lesions (small, painless superficial ulcers on oral mucosa, tongue, or glans penis)
  - Keratoderma blennorrhagica (hyperkeratotic skin lesions of palms and soles and around nails—can be mistaken for psoriasis)
- Cardiovascular: occasionally, pericarditis, murmur, conduction defects, and aortic incompetence
- Nervous system: rarely, peripheral neuropathy, cranial neuropathy, meningoencephalitis, and neuropsychiatric changes
- Constitutional
  - Fever, malaise, anorexia, and weight loss
  - Patient can appear seriously ill (e.g., fever, rigors, tachycardia, and exquisitely tender joints).

DIFFERENTIAL DIAGNOSIS
- Rheumatoid arthritis (RA)
- Ankylosing spondylitis
- Arthritis associated with inflammatory bowel disease
- Psoriatic arthritis
- Juvenile RA
- Bacterial arthritis, including gonococcal

DIAGNOSTIC TESTS & INTERPRETATION
- Blood
  - Negative rheumatoid factor
  - Leukocyte count: 10,000 to 20,000 cells/mm^3
  - Neutrophil predominance
  - Elevated ESR and/or CRP
  - Moderate normochromic anemia
  - Hypergammaglobulinemia
- Synovial fluid
  - Leukocyte count: 1,000 to 8,000 cells/mm^3
  - Bacterial culture negative
- Supportive tests
  - Cultures, antigens, or PCR positive for *Chlamydia trachomatis* or stool test positive for *Salmonella, Shigella, Yersinia,* or *Campylobacter* species
  - HIV serology positive (acute retroviral syndrome)
  - HLA-B27-positive (*not required for diagnosis*)
  - Drugs that may alter lab results: Antibiotics may affect isolation of the bacterial pathogens.
- X-ray
  - Periosteal proliferation, thickening
  - Articular bony spurs; erosions at articular margins
  - Residual joint destruction
  - Syndesmophytes (spine); sacroiliitis

Diagnostic Procedures/Other
HLA-B27 histocompatibility antigen: positive result in 60–80% of cases in non–HIV-related Reiter syndrome; HLA testing is not required or recommended for diagnosis. Rheumatoid factor is negative.
- Screen for STI if clinically indicated.
- Screening for enteric infections is rarely useful and generally not indicated.

Test Interpretation
- Seronegative spondyloarthropathy (similar to ankylosing spondylitis, enteric arthritis, and psoriatic arthritis)
- Villous formation within joints; hyperemia, and inflammation
- Prostatitis and seminal vesiculitis
- Skin biopsy similar to psoriasis

TREATMENT

GENERAL MEASURES
Treatment is determined by symptoms.
- Conjunctivitis does not require specific treatment.
- Iritis requires treatment.
- Mucocutaneous lesions do not require treatment.
- Physical therapy (PT) aids recovery.
- Arthritis may become prominent and disabling during the acute phase.

MEDICATION
First Line
- Symptomatic management: NSAIDs, including indomethacin, naproxen, and others; intra-articular or systemic corticosteroids for refractory arthritis and enteritis
  - Contraindications
    - GI bleeding
    - Peptic ulcer, gastritis, or ulcerative colitis
    - Renal insufficiency
- Specific treatment of isolated microorganism (3)[A]:
  - *C. trachomatis*: doxycycline 100 mg PO BID for 7 to 14 days (*Note*: All STIs should be treated whether associated with Reiter syndrome or not.)
  - *Salmonella, Shigella, Yersinia,* and *Campylobacter* infections: ciprofloxacin 500 mg PO BID for 5 to 10 days (*Note*: Emerging antimicrobial resistance may limit the effectiveness of ciprofloxacin. Antibiotic treatment does not reduce GI symptoms or duration of infection or prevent carrier state.)
  - Trials of antibiotic treatment for reactive arthritis have produced mixed results, rendering the efficacy of antibiotics uncertain.
- GI upset: antacids
- Iritis: intraocular steroids
- Keratitis: topical steroids

Second Line
- Aspirin or other NSAIDs
- Sulfasalazine is promising but not approved by the FDA for this indication.
- Methotrexate or azathioprine in severe cases (experimental, not approved or known to be effective); immunosuppressive therapy is relatively contraindicated in HIV-related Reiter syndrome.
- Consultation with specialist is recommended, particularly when considering immunomodulatory agents such as sulfasalazine, methotrexate, or azathioprine or for treatment with anti-TNF medications (etanercept and infliximab) which have shown benefit in isolated case reports.
- Role of antibiotics under investigation—currently unproven effectiveness in seronegative arthritides.
- No published evidence supports the beneficial effect of antibiotics on the long-term outcome in patients with Reiter syndrome.

ISSUES FOR REFERRAL
Joint and eye complications; complex cases—consider reconsultation with rheumatology; ophthalmology

INPATIENT CONSIDERATIONS
Admission Criteria/Initial Stabilization
- Based on severity of disease and associated complications
- Inpatient care may be needed during acute phase.

ONGOING CARE

FOLLOW-UP RECOMMENDATIONS
Activity modification until joint inflammation subsides

Patient Monitoring
Monitor clinical response to anti-inflammatory drugs. Observe for complications, particularly with sulfasalazine and immunosuppressive drugs.

PATIENT EDUCATION
- Educate on risk factors for exposure and recurrence.
- Home physical therapy
- Arthritis Foundation, 1314 Spring Street NW, Atlanta, GA 30309, 404-872-7100
- National Institute of Arthritis and Musculoskeletal and Skin Diseases: http://www.niams.nih.gov/

PROGNOSIS
Prognosis is poor in cases involving the heel, eye, or heart.

COMPLICATIONS
- Chronic or recurrent disease in 5–50% of patients
- Ankylosing spondylitis develops in 30–50% of patients who test positive for HLA-B27 antigen.
- Urethral strictures
- Cataracts and blindness
- Aortic root necrosis

REFERENCES
1. Selmi C, Gershwin ME. Diagnosis and classification of reactive arthritis. *Autoimmun Rev*. 2014; 13(4–5):546–549.
2. Zeidler H, Hudson AP. New insights into *Chlamydia* and arthritis. Promise of a cure? *Ann Rheum Dis*. 2014;73(4):637–644.
3. Barber CE, Kim J, Inman RD, et al. Antibiotics for treatment of reactive arthritis: a systematic review and metaanalysis. *J Rheumatol*. 2013;40(6):916–928.

ADDITIONAL READING
- Carter JD, Inman RD. *Chlamydia*-induced reactive arthritis: hidden in plain sight? *Best Pract Res Clin Rheumatol*. 2011;25(3):359–374.
- Contini C, Grilli A, Badia L, et al. Detection of *Chlamydophila pneumoniae* in patients with arthritis: significance and diagnostic value. *Rheumatol Int*. 2011;31(10):1307–1313.
- Curry JA, Riddle MS, Gormley RP, et al. The epidemiology of infectious gastroenteritis related reactive arthritis in U.S. military personnel: a case-control study. *BMC Infect Dis*. 2010;10:266.
- Kim PS, Klausmeier TL, Orr DP. Reactive arthritis: a review. *J Adolesc Health*. 2009;44(4):309–315.
- Mathew AJ, Ravindran V. Infections and arthritis. *Best Pract Res Clin Rheumatol*. 2014;28(6):935–959.
- National Guideline Clearinghouse. British Association of Sexual Health and HIV (BASHH) United Kingdom national guideline on management of sexually acquired reactive arthritis. 2009:13596. http://www.bashh.org/BASHH/Guidelines/Guidelines/BASHH/Guidelines/Guidelines.aspx. Accessed August 21, 2015.
- Porter CK, Thura N, Riddle MS. Quantifying the incidence and burden of postinfectious enteric sequelae. *Mil Med*. 2013;178(4):452–469.
- Wilson G, Folzenlogen DD. Spondyloarthropathies: new directions in etiopathogenesis, diagnosis and treatment. *Mo Med*. 2012;109(1):69–74.

SEE ALSO

Ankylosing Spondylitis; Arthritis, Psoriatic; Behçet Syndrome

CODES

ICD10
- M02.30 Reiter's disease, unspecified site
- M02.39 Reiter's disease, multiple sites

CLINICAL PEARLS
- Diagnosis of Reiter syndrome is based on the clinical presentation of the classic triad of joint, eye, and GU inflammation and negative serologic testing for rheumatoid factor (signs and symptoms may not all be present at the same time).
- Screen for STI (including HIV) if sexually acquired. Enteric studies are rarely clinically indicated.
- Refer patients with a chronic or recurrent course or those who have clinical complications.

REFRACTIVE ERRORS

Robert M. Kershner, MD, MS, FACS

 BASICS

DESCRIPTION
- Refraction is the bending of a wave of light as it passes through the optical system of the eye. The degree of bending is dependent on the index of refraction through the air, cornea, and lens and is described quantitatively by Snell law. A refractive error refers to the inability of the eye to produce a focused image on the fovea or central part of the retina.
- Emmetropia: When light rays are in perfect focus, the image being viewed is seen clearly.
- Ametropia: any refractive error of the eye that prevents normal focusing of the image
- Hyperopia: When the cornea of the eye is too flat or the eye is too short, light rays fall in focus behind the retina, and the individual is "farsighted."
- Myopia: When the cornea is too steep or the length of the eyeball is too long, the focal point for light rays lies short of the retina, and the individual is "nearsighted."
- Presbyopia: The natural tendency of the crystalline lens to harden/become sclerotic with age, limiting the focusing of the eye on near objects (accommodation). By the age of 40 years, most people do not have enough room within the eye to allow normal excursion of the lens and accommodation; viewing of near objects is blurred, and reading glasses are required.
- Astigmatism: When the cornea is steeper in one meridian more than the other or the globe is not round (i.e., is oval or almond shaped), visual blurriness occurs due to the absence of a single point of focus.
- Anisometropia: an unequal refractive error between the two eyes
- System(s) affected: nervous

Geriatric Considerations
Presbyopia occurs after the age of 40 years.

Pediatric Considerations
Refractive errors can be detected early in life.

EPIDEMIOLOGY
- Predominant age: Refractive errors may be present at birth and can increase in magnitude with age until the eye is fully developed. Often they are not detected until puberty.
- Predominant gender: male = female
- Individuals >40 years of age are more likely to experience presbyopia/the normal loss of accommodation that occurs with age, necessitating the use of reading glasses for close work.

Prevalence
Of the general U.S. population, 70% have some form of ametropia.

ETIOLOGY AND PATHOPHYSIOLOGY
- Developmental (most common)
- Ocular trauma
- Iatrogenic (e.g., post refractive surgery or cataract removal)

Genetics
Inherited

GENERAL PREVENTION
No exercises; optical lenses can correct the refractive error.

COMMONLY ASSOCIATED CONDITIONS
- Patients with diabetes mellitus have fluctuating myopia as a result of poorly controlled blood glucose and concomitant swelling of the crystalline lens.
- Those who have a pathologic steepening of the cornea due to structural weakness (keratoconus) may have increasing myopia and astigmatism throughout life.

 DIAGNOSIS

HISTORY
- Difficulty seeing objects at a distance
- Difficulty focusing on near objects
- Difficulty reading
- Squinting
- Headaches (from squinting)
- In children:
  - Rubbing of the eyes
  - Sitting close to TV/computer screen
  - Problems in sports, particularly declining performance
  - Declining grades
  - Preference for front-row seating
  - Covering of an eye while reading

PHYSICAL EXAM
Snellen eye chart (developed by Dr. Hermann Snellen in 1862)
- Test each eye separately.
- The smallest row of letters that the patient can read determines visual acuity in the uncovered eye.
- The standard convention is visual acuity measured at 20 feet with a Snellen chart. A person with "normal" acuity will see letters clearly at 20 feet as recorded 20/20 (6/6 in meters). A person with 20/200 vision would be considered legally blind and able only to see a letter at 20 feet that a person with normal vision could see clearly at 200 feet.

DIAGNOSTIC TESTS & INTERPRETATION
- Pinhole vision test: To distinguish a refractive error from an organic cause of visual blurring, have the patient look through a pinhole in a card without a corrective lens.
- Patients with a pure refractive error have improved vision because the pinhole blocks nonparallel and unfocused rays of light.
- There are no lab tests for measuring visual acuity.
- A number of digital imaging systems exist for measuring refractive error.
  - Ultrasound or Laser Interferometry can determine the length of the eye (A-Scan or Laser Biometry).
  - Autorefractors can measure myopia, hyperopia, and astigmatism using a projected light into the eye and measuring the quality of its image upon its return.
  - Corneal topography or Orbscan quantitatively and qualitatively measures the amount of curvature on the surface of the cornea that affects the bending and focusing of light on the retina.
  - Wavefront corneal analysis measures the reflected rays of light as they pass into and out of the entire optical system (cornea, lens, and retina).
- Most corneal and refractive imaging techniques are reserved for individuals who are contemplating refractive surgical correction (intraocular lenses or excimer laser surgery "LASIK").

Follow-Up Tests & Special Considerations
Corneal and refractive imaging are used to monitor changing refractive errors postsurgically and to follow pathologic changes such as in keratoconus.

Diagnostic Procedures/Other
- Methods
  - Objective streak retinoscopy may be used to measure the degree of refractive error in spherocylinder correction for the proper spectacle/contact lens.
  - Antimuscarinic agents, such as cyclopentolate (Cyclogyl) or tropicamide (Mydriacyl), applied topically paralyze the ciliary body, preventing accommodation. Cycloplegic refraction can then be performed.
  - α-Adrenergic agents, such as phenylephrine (Neo-Synephrine), can be used concomitantly to stimulate and dilate the pupillary dilator muscle, making measurements easier. They have no effect on cycloplegia.
- Age-related testing
  - Newborns should be examined for general eye health; ophthalmologic evaluation is indicated for any problems discovered.
  - Vision screening should occur at each well-child visit.
  - Visual acuity testing and motility testing should be performed at ~3 to 5 years of age or at any time that a malposition of the eyes, squinting, or difficulty following objects is observed.
  - Visual acuity must be performed by age 5 years or prior to the child entering school to screen for and pick up refractive errors early before they lead to amblyopia.
  - Visual acuity should be retested prior to obtaining a driver's license, at age 40 years, and every 2 to 4 years until age 65 years, after which age evaluations are recommended every 1 to 2 years.

DIFFERENTIAL DIAGNOSIS
- Corneal disease
- Cataract
- Retinal abnormalities
- Diseases of the optic nerve
- Neuromuscular disorders
- Neurologic impairment

TREATMENT

GENERAL MEASURES
- Spectacle lenses (glasses)
- Soft/hard contact lenses
- Surgery

MEDICATION
Precaution: Antimuscarinic agents may induce acute glaucoma via acute-angle closure in susceptible individuals. The elderly and those with high hyperopia or a history of angle closure should not be tested with these agents.

First Line
No medical treatment for refractive error exists.

Second Line
Cycloplegia is sometimes used to "fog/blur" the better seeing eye in cases of amblyopia.

ISSUES FOR REFERRAL
Any individual who fails a basic screening visual acuity test should be promptly referred to an eye care professional for evaluation. Children do not outgrow refractive errors. Left untreated, refractive errors can lead to permanent visual loss.

ADDITIONAL THERAPIES

Eye exercises and visual training may improve hand-to-eye coordination and visual awareness but do not treat refractive error.

SURGERY/OTHER PROCEDURES

- Astigmatic keratotomy with a surgical diamond blade has been performed either as an isolated procedure or as a part of the cataract surgical procedure to effectively flatten the steep corneal meridian (1,2)[C].
- Manual astigmatic keratotomy is being superseded by the femtosecond laser whereby the surgeon applies the laser to perform the limbal corneal relaxing incisions (LRIs) instead of the surgical diamond blade (3)[C].
- Laser-assisted in-situ keratomileusis (LASIK) was approved by the FDA in 1997. A superficial corneal flap is created with a mechanical keratome/femtosecond laser, under which the excimer laser removes a small amount of tissue corresponding to the correction of refractive error, thus reshaping the cornea. LASIK can be used for all refractive errors but not in all patients. Healing is rapid because reepithelialization is not required. Surgery is reserved for those with a stable refractive error and a cornea that is thick enough to allow safe removal of tissue. The procedure is permanent.
- Implantable contact lens (ICL): A thin plastic lens is permanently implanted either in the anterior chamber and anchored to the iris (FDA approved in 2005, VERISYSE) or in the posterior chamber (Visian ICL, FDA approved in 2006) between the iris and the human crystalline lens. All refractive errors can be corrected. Risks include damage to the natural lens during surgery, cataract formation, and intraocular inflammation/infection.
- Excimer laser photorefractive keratectomy: The laser photoablates corneal tissue from the central visual axis, flattening it. Following the procedure, the cornea must reepithelialize. Healing takes several months, during which there is a mild haze and blurring of vision; FDA approved in October 1995.
- Other modifications:
  - LASIK (laser in-situ keratomileusis), which involves removing of the superficial epithelium before laser application (Epi-LASIK).
  - IntraLASIK is a femtosecond laser that is used to create the flap as an alternative to a mechanical keratome.
  - Custom ablation: uses the information from a wavefront map of the cornea and eye to tailor the ablation to remove higher orders of refractive errors
- Older methods now superseded by LASIK:
  - Radial keratotomy: With topical anesthesia, a surgical keratome is used to incise multiple (4 to 8) radial incisions into the peripheral cornea to a depth of ≥85%. The incisions cause gaping and thus flatten the central, optical zone of the cornea. Radial keratotomy is safe and effective, corrects nearsightedness and astigmatism, but has been replaced by excimer laser surgery for its improved accuracy and stability of correction.
  - Photorefractive keratectomy: Surface corneal tissue is removed with the excimer laser to reshape the cornea, correcting nearsightedness, farsightedness, or astigmatism. Risks and disadvantages include pain, keratitis, and potential scarring. Healing requires 3 months with topical antibiotics and steroids, with associated risks of glaucoma, cataract, chronic inflammation, and scarring.
- Several scleral expansion procedures have been under investigation to attempt to increase the space within the ciliary body by surgical means to restore lens movement and accommodation. The results have been unsatisfactory.
- Bifocal intraocular lenses (several types have been approved by the FDA: AcrySof IQ ReSTOR, ReZOOM-AMO, TECNIS-AMO) are implanted in the posterior chamber. They increase the depth of field to allow viewing objects both at near and at distance. Side effects include decreased contrast, glare, ghosting of images, and problems with night vision.
- Accommodative intraocular lenses (Crystalens): first FDA-approved intraocular lens; several others under clinical investigation. The accommodative intraocular lens moves in response to ciliary body movement to allow focusing at different focal lengths. Side effects are minimal. Present lenses have limited range of focus.

ONGOING CARE

FOLLOW-UP RECOMMENDATIONS

Patient Monitoring

- Exams recommended when starting school, entering college, with any change in vision quality, and at the age of onset of presbyopia (the need for reading glasses)
- Individuals with any of the known risks of eye disease or conditions that could affect the eyes (e.g., diabetes, thyroid disease, hypertension, macular degeneration) need annual ocular examinations.
- Family history of eye diseases/refractive errors necessitates annual reexam.

DIET

Although refractive error is unaffected by diet, diet has been shown to be important for retinal health. Diets high in fats, cholesterol, along with cigarette smoking or diabetes can lead to an increased risk of age-related macular degeneration (AMD), a potentially blinding disease of the retina. Diets high in vegetables, low in meats, and high in antioxidants (e.g., lutein, β-carotene, vitamins A, C, and E, zinc, and omega-3 fatty acids) have been shown to be protective for retinal degeneration. The age-related eye disease study (AREDS) formulation, which has been proven effective in numerous clinical trials, includes a specific daily amount of 500-mg vitamin C, 400 IU of vitamin E, 15 mg of β-carotene (often labeled as the equivalent of 25,000-IU vitamin A), 80 mg of zinc as zinc oxide, and 2 mg of copper as cupric oxide to prevent copper deficiency anemia and is taken with meals in two equally divided doses in the morning and evening. This therapy has been superseded by the AREDS2 formulation, which eliminated vitamin E due to its associated increased risk of lung cancer in smokers and replacing β-carotene with lutein and zeaxanthin.

PATIENT EDUCATION

- All patients should have their eyes examined when starting school and periodically thereafter.
- The options of eyeglasses, contact lenses, and permanent surgical correction of refractive errors can be considered.
- Encourage aggressive control of diabetes mellitus and annual exams by an ophthalmologist. These individuals are at increased risk of blindness from their disease and should not undergo refractive corrective surgery.

PROGNOSIS

- Good, if discovered early and corrected appropriately.
- It is not unusual for refractive errors to be temporarily worsened during pregnancy because of hormonal changes in tear function and corneal swelling.

- It is common that refractive errors worsen as a child ages until complete adult growth has been achieved (this is around age 18 to 20 years for girls and 20 to 25 years for boys). This is a common source of concern for parents. Reassurance that refractive change is often seen with growth spurts, especially at puberty, is advised.
- Any refractive change that is increasing/worsening each year should prompt further investigation by an ophthalmologist.

COMPLICATIONS

- Amblyopia or permanent loss of vision that is not correctable with glasses or contact lenses
- Poor school performance
- Inability to pass a drivers license examination

REFERENCES

1. Kershner RM. Keratolenticuloplasty. In: Gills JP, Martin RG, Thornton SP, et al, eds. *Surgical Treatment of Astigmatism*. Thorofare, NJ: Slack; 1994: 143–155.
2. Grabow HB. Intraocular correction of refractive errors. In: Kershner RM, ed. *Refractive Keratotomy for Cataract Surgery and the Correction of Astigmatism*. Thorofare, NJ: Slack; 1994:141.
3. Abbey A, Ide T, Kymionis GD, et al. Femtosecond laser-assisted astigmatic keratotomy in naturally occurring high astigmatism. *Br J Ophthalmol*. 2009;93(12):1566–1569.

ADDITIONAL READING

- American Academy of Ophthalmology. *Policy Statement: Frequency of Ocular Exams*. San Francisco, CA: American Academy of Opthalmology; 2009.
- American Academy of Ophthalmology, American Academy of Pediatrics, American Association for Pediatric Ophthalmology and Strabismus. *Joint Policy Statement: Vision Screening for Infants and Children*. San Francisco, CA: American Academy of Ophthalmology; 2007. http://www.aao.org/clinical-statement/vision-screening-infants-children--2013.
- Fax-on-Demand service of American Academy of Ophthalmology for policy statement and patient education materials: (908) 525-2761.
- National Eye Institute. *Facts About Refractive Errors*. Bethesda, MD: National Eye Institute; 2009. http://www.nei.nih.gov/health/errors/errors/.asp.

 CODES

ICD10

- H52.7 Unspecified disorder of refraction
- H52.00 Hypermetropia, unspecified eye
- H52.10 Myopia, unspecified eye

CLINICAL PEARLS

- Vision screening should occur at each well-child visit.
- Visual acuity testing should be performed at ~3.5 years of age or at any time that the physician or parent is concerned about the child's eye movements, ability to see, or track objects.
- Children *never* grow out of a refractive error. All suspected refractive errors should be referred to the appropriate eye care professional for evaluation to prevent permanent loss of vision from amblyopia.

RENAL TUBULAR ACIDOSIS

Jason Kurland, MD

 BASICS

DESCRIPTION

- Renal tubular acidosis (RTA) is composed of a group of disorders characterized by an inability of the kidney to resorb bicarbonate/secrete hydrogen ions, resulting in normal anion gap metabolic acidosis. Renal function (glomerular filtration rate [GFR]) must be normal or near normal.
- Several types have been identified:
  - Type I (distal) RTA: inability of the distal tubule to acidify the urine due to impaired hydrogen ion secretion, increased back leak of secreted hydrogen ions, or impaired sodium reabsorption (interfering with the generation of negative luminal charge required for hydrogen/potassium secretion). Urine pH >5.5.
  - Type II (proximal) RTA: defect of the proximal tubule in bicarbonate (HCO_3) reabsorption. Proximal tubular HCO_3 reabsorption is absent; plasma HCO_3 concentration stabilizes at 12 to 18 mEq/L due to compensatory distal HCO_3 reabsorption. Urine pH <5.5 unless plasma HCO_3 brought above reabsorptive threshold.
  - Type III RTA: extremely rare autosomal recessive syndrome due to carbonic anhydrase II deficiency; causes mixed type I and type II RTA, osteopetrosis, cerebral calcification, mental retardation
  - Type IV RTA (hypoaldosteronism): due to aldosterone resistance/deficiency that results in hyperkalemia. Urine pH usually is <5.5.

EPIDEMIOLOGY

Incidence
- Predominant age: all ages
- Predominant sex: male > female (with regard to type II RTA with isolated defect in bicarbonate reabsorption)

ETIOLOGY AND PATHOPHYSIOLOGY
- Type I RTA
  - Genetic: autosomal dominant, autosomal recessive associated with sensorineural deafness
  - Sporadic
  - Other familial disorders: Ehlers-Danlos syndrome, glycogenosis type III, Fabry disease, Wilson disease
  - Autoimmune diseases: Sjögren syndrome, rheumatoid arthritis (RA), systemic lupus erythematosus (SLE), thyroiditis (1)
  - Hematologic diseases: sickle cell disease (hyperkalemic), hereditary elliptocytosis
  - Medications: amphotericin B, lithium, ifosfamide, foscarnet, amiloride, triamterene, trimethoprim, pentamidine
  - Toxins: toluene, glue
  - Hypercalciuria, diseases causing nephrocalcinosis
  - Vitamin D intoxication
  - Medullary cystic disease
  - Obstructive uropathy (hyperkalemic)
  - Hypergammaglobulinemic syndrome
  - Chronic pyelonephritis
  - Chronic renal transplant rejection
  - Leprosy
  - Chronic active hepatitis, primary biliary cirrhosis
  - Malnutrition

- Type II RTA
  - Familial (cystinosis, tyrosinemia, hereditary fructose intolerance, galactosemia, glycogen storage disease type I, Wilson disease, Lowe syndrome, inherited carbonic anhydrase deficiency)
  - Sporadic
  - Multiple myeloma, other dysproteinemic states
  - Amyloidosis
  - Heavy metal poisoning (e.g., cadmium, lead, mercury, copper)
  - Medications: acetazolamide, ifosfamide, tenofovir, sulfanilamide, outdated tetracycline, topiramate (2), aminoglycosides
  - Interstitial renal disease
  - Paroxysmal nocturnal hemoglobinuria
  - Defects in calcium metabolism (hyperparathyroidism)
- Type IV RTA
  - Medications: NSAIDs, ACE inhibitors, ARBs, heparin/low-molecular-weight heparin, ketoconazole, calcineurin inhibitors (tacrolimus, cyclosporine—by decreasing expression of mineralocorticoid receptor [3])
  - Diabetic nephropathy
  - Tubulointerstitial nephropathies
  - Primary adrenal insufficiency
  - Markedly decreased distal Na^+ delivery
  - Pseudohypoaldosteronism (PHA) (end-organ resistance to aldosterone)
    - PHA type 1
    - PHA type 2 (Gordon syndrome)

Genetics
- Type I RTA: Hereditary forms due to mutations affecting intercalated cells in collecting tubules (4). May occur in association with other genetic diseases (e.g., Ehlers-Danlos syndrome, hereditary elliptocytosis, or sickle cell nephropathy). The autosomal recessive form is associated with sensorineural deafness.
- Type II RTA: Autosomal dominant form is rare. Autosomal recessive form is associated with ophthalmologic abnormalities and mental retardation. Occurs in Fanconi syndrome, which is associated with several genetic diseases (e.g., cystinosis, Wilson disease, tyrosinemia, hereditary fructose intolerance, Lowe syndrome, galactosemia, glycogen storage disease, metachromatic leukodystrophy)
- Type IV RTA: Some cases are familial, such as PHA type I (autosomal dominant).

GENERAL PREVENTION
Careful use/avoidance of causative agents

COMMONLY ASSOCIATED CONDITIONS
- Type I RTA in children: hypercalciuria leading to rickets, nephrocalcinosis
- Type I RTA in adults: autoimmune diseases (Sjögren syndrome, RA, SLE), hypercalciuria
- Type II RTA: Fanconi syndrome (generalized proximal tubular dysfunction resulting in glycosuria, aminoaciduria, hyperuricosuria, phosphaturia, bicarbonaturia)
- Type II RTA in adults: multiple myeloma, carbonic anhydrase inhibitors (acetazolamide) (5)
- Type IV RTA: diabetic nephropathy

 DIAGNOSIS

HISTORY
- Often asymptomatic (particularly type IV)
- In children: failure to thrive, rickets
- Anorexia, nausea/vomiting, constipation
- Weakness or polyuria (due to hypokalemia)
- Polydipsia
- Osteomalacia in adults

DIFFERENTIAL DIAGNOSIS
- Plasma anion gap should be normal. If not, evaluate for causes of anion-gap metabolic acidosis. (MUDPILES: **m**ethanol, **u**remia, **d**iabetic ketoacidosis, **p**ropylene glycol/paraldehyde, **i**ron/isoniazid ingestion, **l**actic acidosis, **e**thylene glycol, **s**alicylates)
- Extrarenal HCO_3 losses
  - Diarrhea
  - Small bowel, pancreatic, or biliary fistulas
  - Urinary diversion (e.g., ureterosigmoidostomy, ileal conduit)
- Acidosis of chronic renal failure (develops when GFR ≤20 to 30 mL/min)
- Excessive administration of acid load via chloride salts (NaCl, HCl, NH_4Cl, lysine HCl, $CaCl_2$, $MgCl_2$)

DIAGNOSTIC TESTS & INTERPRETATION
- Electrolytes reveal hyperchloremic metabolic acidosis.
- Plasma anion gap normal (anion gap = Na − [Cl + HCO_3]). Normal values (in mEq/L) depend on analyzer used: infants/children 5 to 15; adolescents/adults 4 to 12) (6). Must increase calculated anion gap by 2.5 mEq/L for each 1 g/dL decrease in **albumin** below 4 g/dL
- Plasma K+: Low in type I (if due to impaired distal H^+ secretion/increased H^+ back leak), type II; high in type IV, type I (if due to impaired distal Na^+ reabsorption)
- Plasma HCO_3 (in untreated RTA): type I: <10 to 20 mEq/L; type II: 12 to 18 mEq/L (1); type IV: >17 mEq/L
- BUN/Cr normal or near normal (rules out renal failure as cause of acidosis)
- Urinalysis: Urine pH inappropriately alkaline (>5.5) despite metabolic acidosis in type I; also in type II if HCO_3 above reabsorptive threshold (12 to 18 mEq/L)
- Urine culture: Rule out UTI with urea-splitting organism (may elevate pH) and chronic infection.
- Urine anion gap (UAG; urine [Na^+ + K^+] − Cl^- on a random specimen): reflects unmeasured urine anions, so inversely related to urine NH_4^+ (or acid) excretion. Positive UAG in an acidemic patient indicates impaired renal acid excretion. Urine Na^+ >25 mEq/L required for accurate interpretation of UAG. Results tend to be
  - Negative in HCO_3 losses due to diarrhea, UTI caused by urea-splitting organisms, and other extrarenal causes of nonanion gap metabolic acidosis
  - Variable in type II RTA
  - Positive in type I RTA (7), type IV RTA
  - Positive in impaired acid excretion due to renal failure

- Urine calcium
  - High in type I
  - Typically normal in type II
- Drugs that may alter lab results
  - Diuretics
  - Sodium bicarbonate (and other alkali)
  - Cholestyramine

Initial Tests (lab, imaging)
Serum electrolytes; consider urinalysis, urine culture.

Diagnostic Procedures/Other
- Helpful to measure urine pH on fresh sample with pH meter for increased accuracy instead of dipstick. Pour film of oil over urine to avoid loss of CO_2 if pH cannot be measured quickly.
- Urine NH_4^+ excretion (anion gap only provides a qualitative estimate)
- Urinary acidification (impaired in type I RTA) can be assessed by oral administration of furosemide and fludrocortisone; patients with type I RTA unable to reduce urine pH to <5.3 (8)
- Fractional excretion of HCO_3 >15% during HCO_3 infusion (type II RTA) (1)

Test Interpretation
- Nephrocalcinosis
- Nephrolithiasis
- Rickets
- Osteomalacia, osteopenia
- Findings of an underlying disease causing RTA

TREATMENT

MEDICATION
First Line
- Provide oral alkali to raise serum HCO_3 to normal. Start at a low dose and increase until HCO_3 is normal. Give as sodium bicarbonate (7.7 mEq $NaHCO_3$/650 mg tab), sodium citrate (oral solution, 1 mEq HCO_3 equivalent/mL), sodium/potassium citrate (oral solution), or potassium citrate (tablet, powder, or oral solution: 2 mEq K/mL, 2 mEq HCO_3/mL), depending on need for potassium.
- Type I RTA: Typical doses 1 to 2 mEq/kg/day (in adults), 3 to 4 mEq/kg/day (in children) PO alkali divided 3 to 4 times per day (require much higher doses if HCO_3 wasting is present). May require K^+ supplementation
- Type II RTA: Typical doses 10 to 15 mEq/kg/day alkali, divided 4 to 6 times per day. Very difficult to restore plasma HCO_3 to normal, as renal HCO_3 losses increase once plasma HCO_3 is corrected above resorptive threshold. Exogenous HCO_3 increases K^+ losses, requiring supplemental K^+. Often need supplemental PO_4 and vitamin D due to proximal PO_4 losses. May add thiazide diuretic to induce mild hypovolemia, which increases proximal Na^+/HCO_3^- reabsorption
- Type IV RTA: Avoid inciting medications; restrict dietary K^+. May augment K^+ excretion with loop diuretic, thiazide diuretic, or Kayexalate. Correcting hyperkalemia increases activity of the urea cycle, augmenting renal ammoniagenesis and adding substrate for renal acid excretion. If necessary, 1 to 5 mEq/kg/day alkali divided 2 to 3 times per day. If mineralocorticoid deficiency, fludrocortisone: 0.1 to 0.3 mg/day

- Precautions
  - Sodium-containing compounds will increase urinary calcium excretion, potentially increasing the risk of nephrolithiasis.
  - Mineralocorticoids and sodium-based alkali may lead to hypertension and/or edema.
  - Aluminum-containing medications (antacids, sucralfate) should be avoided if solutions containing citric acid are prescribed because citric acid increases aluminum absorption.
  - Sodium bicarbonate may cause flatulence because CO_2 is formed, whereas citrate is metabolized to HCO_3 in the liver, avoiding gas production.

Second Line
Thiazide diuretics may be used as adjunctive therapy in type II RTA (after maximal alkali replacement) but are likely to further increase urinary K^+ losses.

SURGERY/OTHER PROCEDURES
If distal RTA is due to obstructive uropathy, surgical intervention may be required.

INPATIENT CONSIDERATIONS
Admission Criteria/Initial Stabilization
Generally managed as outpatient; inpatient if acidosis severe, patient unreliable, emesis persistent, or infant with severe failure to thrive

ONGOING CARE

FOLLOW-UP RECOMMENDATIONS
Patient Monitoring
- Electrolytes 1 to 2 weeks following initiation of therapy, monthly until serum HCO_3 corrected to desired range, then as clinically indicated
- Monitor underlying disease as indicated.
- Poor compliance common due to 3 to 6 times per day alkali dosing schedule

DIET
Varies based on serum K^+ level and volume status

PATIENT EDUCATION
- National Kidney & Urologic Diseases Information Clearinghouse, Box NKUDIC, Bethesda, MD 20893, 301-468-6345: http://www.kidney.niddk.nih.gov/
- National Kidney Foundation: https://www.kidney.org/

PROGNOSIS
- Depends on associated disease; otherwise, good with therapy
- Transient forms of all types of RTA may occur.

COMPLICATIONS
- Nephrocalcinosis, nephrolithiasis (type I)
- Hypercalciuria (type I)
- Hypokalemia (type I, type II if given bicarbonate)
- Hyperkalemia (type IV, some causes of type I)
- Osteomalacia (type II due to phosphate wasting), osteopenia (due to buffering of acid in bone)

REFERENCES
1. Reddy P. Clinical approach to renal tubular acidosis in adult patients. *Int J Clin Pract*. 2011;65(3): 350–360.
2. Liamis G, Milionis HJ, Elisaf M. Pharmacologically-induced metabolic acidosis: a review. *Drug Saf*. 2010;33(5):371–391.
3. Heering PJ, Kurschat C, Vo DT, et al. Aldosterone resistance in kidney transplantation is in part induced by a down-regulation of mineralocorticoid receptor expression. *Clin Transplant*. 2004;18(2):186–192.
4. Batlle D, Haque SK. Genetic causes and mechanisms of distal renal tubular acidosis. *Nephrol Dial Transplant*. 2012;27(10):3691–3704.
5. Casaletto JJ. Differential diagnosis of metabolic acidosis. *Emerg Med Clin North Am*. 2005;23(3): 771–787.
6. Lolekha PH, Vanavanan S, Teerakarnjana N, et al. Reference ranges of electrolyte and anion gap on the Beckman E4A, Beckman Synchron CX5, Nova CRT, and Nova Stat Profile Ultra. *Clin Chim Acta*. 2001;307(1–2):87–93.
7. Goswami RP, Mondal S, Karmakar PS, et al. Type 3 renal tubular acidosis. *Indian J Nephrol*. 2012;22(6):466–468.
8. Walsh SB, Shirley DG, Wrong OM, et al. Urinary acidification assessed by simultaneous furosemide and fludrocortisone treatment: an alternative to ammonium chloride. *Kidney Int*. 2007;71(12):1310–1316.

CODES

ICD10
N25.89 Oth disorders resulting from impaired renal tubular function

CLINICAL PEARLS
- Consider RTA in cases of normal anion gap metabolic acidosis with normal/near-normal renal function.
- Type I RTA: urine pH >5.5 in setting of acidemia; positive urine anion gap; acidemia can be severe.
- Type II RTA: urine pH <5.5 unless HCO_3 raised above reabsorptive threshold (12 to 18 mEq/L)
- Type IV RTA: most common subtype; hyperkalemia; urine pH < 5.5; acidemia usually mild
- Treatment includes avoidance of inciting causes, provision of oral alkali (HCO_3 or citrate), and measures to supplement (type II, many type I) or restrict (type IV) potassium.

RESPIRATORY DISTRESS SYNDROME, ACUTE (ARDS)

Muhammad Imran Khan, MD • Najm Hasan Siddiqui, MD

BASICS

DESCRIPTION
- ARDS is an acute, diffuse, inflammatory lung injury that leads to increased pulmonary vascular permeability, increased lung weight, and a loss of aerated tissue (1) with clinical hallmarks of severe hypoxemia and bilateral pulmonary infiltrates.
  - Absence of left atrial hypertension (HTN)
  - By consensus, $PaO_2/FiO_2 < 200$
  - Most severe form of acute lung injury
- System(s) affected: pulmonary; cardiovascular
- Synonym(s): shock lung; wet lung; noncardiac pulmonary edema

EPIDEMIOLOGY
Incidence
ARDS: 10.1 to 86.2 cases/100,000 annually (2)

ETIOLOGY AND PATHOPHYSIOLOGY
Three phases
- Acute exudative phase: characterized by profound hypoxia and associated with inflammation with infiltration of inflammatory and proinflammatory mediators and diffuse alveolar damage
- Fibrosing alveolitis phase: coincides with recovery or after ~1 to 2 weeks; patients continue to be hypoxic and have increased dead space and decreased compliance
- Resolution may require 6 to 12 months.
- Several mediators are involved in the initiation and perpetuation of ARDS.
  - Cytokines
  - Complement activation
  - Coagulation activation
  - Platelet-activating factor
  - Oxygen free radicals
  - Lipoxygenase pathways
  - Neutrophil proteases
  - Nitric oxide
  - Endotoxin
  - Cyclooxygenase pathway products
- Systemic inflammatory response with activation of the previous mediators can occur with direct or indirect injury to the lung.
  - Direct
    ○ Aspiration
    ○ Pulmonary infections
    ○ Air, fat, or amniotic fluid emboli
    ○ Near-drowning
    ○ Pulmonary contusion
    ○ Inhalation of toxic gases and dusts
  - Indirect
    ○ Sepsis
    ○ Shock
    ○ Transfusion
    ○ Trauma
    ○ Overdose
    ○ Pancreatitis, severe
    ○ Eclampsia

RISK FACTORS
- Severe infection (localized or systemic) most common
- Aspiration of gastric contents
- Shock
- Infection
- Trauma with or without lung contusion
- Pneumonia
- Toxic inhalation
- Pancreatitis

- Fat embolism
- Near drowning
- Multiple blood transfusions

GENERAL PREVENTION
No effective measures have been identified.

COMMONLY ASSOCIATED CONDITIONS
- Severe sepsis
- Trauma
- Shock

DIAGNOSIS

HISTORY
- No history of heart disease
- Precipitating event (see "Commonly Associated Conditions"): abrupt onset of respiratory distress

PHYSICAL EXAM
- Tachypnea and tachycardia during the first 12 to 24 hours; respiratory distress
- Lethargy, obtundation
- Flat neck veins
- Hyperdynamic pulses
- Physiologic gallop
- Absence of edema
- Moist, cyanotic skin
- Manifestations of underlying disease

DIFFERENTIAL DIAGNOSIS
- Left ventricular failure
- Interstitial and airway diseases
- Hypersensitivity pneumonitis
- Veno-occlusive disease
- Mitral stenosis: intravascular volume overload
- Toxic shock syndrome

DIAGNOSTIC TESTS & INTERPRETATION
Initial Tests (lab, imaging)
- Arterial blood gases (ABGs) show evidence of severe hypoxemia.
- $PaO_2/FiO_2 < 200$
- ECG: sinus tachycardia; nonspecific ST-T–wave changes
- Pulmonary artery wedge pressure (PAWP) <15 mm Hg
- Cardiac index >3.5 $L/min/m^2$
- Chest x-ray (CXR): normal heart size; fluffy, bilateral infiltrates; air bronchograms common
- Chest CT scan: diffuse interstitial opacities and bullae

Follow-Up Tests & Special Considerations
- Serial blood gases
- Monitor for and treat multisystem organ failure when it occurs.
- Serial CXRs

Diagnostic Procedures/Other
Invasive monitoring of vital signs, cardiac output, and PAWP has been questioned by large clinical trials.

Test Interpretation
- Lungs show exudative, early proliferative or late proliferative phases.
- Interstitial and alveolar edema is present.
- Inflammatory cells and erythrocytes spill into the interstitium and the alveolus.
- Type 1 cells are destroyed, leaving a denuded basement membrane.
- Protein-rich fluid fills the alveoli.
- Type 2 alveolar cells initially appear unaltered.

- Type 2 cells begin to proliferate within 72 hours of initial insult and cover the denuded basement membrane.
- Aggregates of plasma proteins, cellular debris, fibrin, and surfactant remnants form hyaline membranes.
- Over the next 3 to 10 days, alveolar septum thickens by proliferating fibroblasts, leukocytes, and plasma cells.
- Capillary injury begins to occur.
- Hyaline membranes begin to reorganize.
- Fibrosis becomes apparent in respiratory ducts and bronchioles.

TREATMENT

GENERAL MEASURES
- Ensure adequate oxygenation.
- Ventilatory support generally requires endotracheal intubation and use of positive end-expiratory pressure (PEEP) (3)[A].
- Provide appropriate cardiorespiratory monitoring.
- Fluid management

MEDICATION
- No single drug or combination of drugs prevents or treats full-blown ARDS. Treatment is supportive while addressing the underlying cause.
- Supplemental oxygen
- Ventilatory support
  - Most often requires endotracheal intubation with emphasis on lower tidal volumes per weight and optimization of PEEP
  - High-frequency oscillation ventilation seems not to increase the risk of barotrauma or hypotension and reduces the risk of oxygenation failure, it does not improve survival in adult ARDS patients (4)[A].

ISSUES FOR REFERRAL
- All patients with ARDS should be cared for in an ICU with appropriately trained staff.
- Pregnant patients with ARDS also should be followed by a high-risk perinatologist or obstetrician.

ADDITIONAL THERAPIES
- Inotropic agents: dobutamine to maintain adequate cardiac output after appropriate fluid resuscitation fails to restore perfusion
- Corticosteroids: Short-term use during the acute phase has not been shown to be effective. However, prolonged methylprednisolone treatment accelerates the resolution of ARDS, improving a broad spectrum of interrelated clinical outcomes and decreasing hospital mortality and healthcare utilization (5)[A].
- Vasodilators: Inhaled nitric oxide (INO) is not recommended for patients with ARDS. INO results in a transient improvement in oxygenation but does not reduce mortality and may be harmful (6)[A].
- Pulmonary surfactant: successful in neonatal respiratory distress syndrome; investigational outside this age group
- Inhaled β^2-agonists may be helpful during the resolution phase.

904

- There is no current evidence to support or refute the routine use of aerosolized prostacyclin for patients with ARDS (7)[A].
- There is no effect on mortality with granulocyte-macrophage colony–stimulating factor, neutrophil elastase inhibitors, intravenous salbutamol, surfactant, or N-acetylcysteine (8)[A].
- Early use of neuromuscular-blocking agent treatment of patients with severe sepsis and severe ARDS cannot only improve the severity but also reduce 21-day mortality (9)A].

- Antioxidants (e.g., Procysteine) have produced conflicting results.
- Activated protein-C may be helpful in patients with sepsis.
- Deep vein thrombosis (DVT) prophylaxis
- Ulcer prophylaxis

Pregnancy Considerations
Supportive care while identifying the underlying cause of ARDS continues to be important in the management of pregnant women with ARDS. However, fetal well-being, possible need for delivery, and physiologic changes associated with pregnancy must be considered.

INPATIENT CONSIDERATIONS
Admission Criteria/Initial Stabilization
All patients with ARDS should be managed in an ICU setting.
- Consider prone positioning.
- Identify and treat underlying condition.
- Circulatory support, adequate fluid volume, and nutritional support
- Supplemental oxygen
- Monitoring blood gases, pulse oximetry, bedside pulmonary function test
- Support ventilation using lung-protective strategies and PEEP.
- Monitor for systemic hypotension and hypovolemia without fluid overload.
- BP support, if necessary
- Vasopressor agents
- Fluid management with IV crystalloid solutions while monitoring pulmonary status
- Pulmonary catheter pressure monitoring
- Treat underlying disease process.
- Prevent complications.

IV Fluids
- Maintain the intravascular volume at the lowest level consistent with adequate perfusion (assessed by metabolic acid–base balance and renal function).
- If perfusion is inadequate after restoration of intravascular volume (e.g., septic shock), vasopressor therapy is indicated.
- Increase oxygen content with packed erythrocyte transfusions as necessary.
- Provide appropriate nutritional support with enteral or parenteral nutrition.
- Steroid therapy

Nursing
May include any or all of the following:
- Skin, eye, and mouth care
- DVT prophylaxis
- GI prophylaxis
- Suctioning
- Ensure adequate level of sedation and/or paralysis while on mechanical ventilation.
- Oxygen supplementation
- Nebulizer therapy

- Chest physiotherapy
- Tracheostomy care
- Explain all procedures to patient and family; reduce anxiety.

Discharge Criteria
- Supplemental oxygen
- Nutrition counseling
- Family monitoring of signs and symptoms of respiratory distress

 ONGOING CARE

FOLLOW-UP RECOMMENDATIONS
Patient Monitoring
- Vital capacity and static lung compliance are important measures of lung mechanics.
- Daily labs are needed until the patient is no longer critical.
- CXRs to assess endotracheal tube placement, the presence of progressing infiltrates, catheter placement, and complications of mechanical ventilation (e.g., air leaks)
- A Swan-Ganz catheter to assess oxygen delivery, oxygen consumption, and cardiac output may be helpful but has not been shown to improve survival.

DIET
- Nutritional support
- Conservative fluid management shortens ventilator and ICU time but does not affect survival.

PATIENT EDUCATION
ARDS support center and brochure titled "Learn About ARDS": www.ards.org

PROGNOSIS
- Mortality rate is 43% (10).
- Survivors may have pulmonary sequelae with mild abnormalities in oxygenation, diffusion, and lung mechanics, as well as some pulmonary symptoms of cough and dyspnea.
- The prognosis worsens with elevated cardiac troponin-T levels in ARDS patients (11).

COMPLICATIONS
- Permanent lung disease
- Oxygen toxicity
- Barotrauma
- Superinfection
- Multiple organ dysfunction syndrome
- Death

REFERENCES
1. Ranieri VM, Rubenfeld GD, Thompson BT, et al. Acute respiratory distress syndrome: the Berlin definition. *JAMA*. 2012;307(23):2526–2533.
2. Riviello ED, Kiviri W, Twagirumugabe T, et al. Hospital incidence and outcomes of ARDS using the Kigali modification of the Berlin definition [published online ahead of print September 9, 2015]. *Am J Respir Crit Care Med*.
3. Petrucci N, Iacovelli W. Ventilation with lower tidal volumes versus traditional tidal volumes in adults for acute lung injury and acute respiratory distress syndrome. *Cochrane Database Syst Rev*. 2004;(2):CD003844.

4. Gu XL, Wu GN, Yao YW, et al. Is high-frequency oscillatory ventilation more effective and safer than conventional protective ventilation in adult acute respiratory distress syndrome patients? A meta-analysis of randomized controlled trials. *Crit Care*. 2014;18(3):R111.
5. Meduri GU, Bridges L, Shih MC, et al. Prolonged glucocorticoid treatment is associated with improved ARDS outcomes: analysis of individual patients' data from four randomized trials and trial-level meta-analysis of the updated literature [published online ahead of print October 27, 2015]. *Intensive Care Med*.
6. Afshari A, Brok J, Møller AM, et al. Inhaled nitric oxide for acute respiratory distress syndrome (ARDS) and acute lung injury in children and adults. *Cochrane Database Syst Rev*. 2010;(7):CD002787.
7. Afshari A, Brok J, Møller AM, et al. Aerosolized prostacyclin for acute lung injury (ALI) and acute respiratory distress syndrome (ARDS). *Cochrane Database Syst Rev*. 2010;(8):CD007733.
8. Duggal A, Ganapathy A, Ratnapalan M, et al. Pharmacological treatments for acute respiratory distress syndrome: systematic review. *Minerva Anestesiol*. 2015;81(5):567–588.
9. Lyu G, Wang X, Jiang W, et al. Clinical study of early use of neuromuscular blocking agents in patients with severe sepsis and acute respiratory distress syndrome [in Chinese]. *Zhonghua Wei Zhong Bing Ji Jiu Yi Xue*. 2014;26(5):325–329.
10. Zambon M, Vincent JL. Mortality rates for patients with acute lung injury/ARDS have decreased over time. *Chest*. 2008;133(5):1120–1127.
11. Rivara MB, Bajwa EK, Januzzi JL, et al. Prognostic significance of elevated cardiac troponin-T levels in acute respiratory distress syndrome patients. *PLoS One*. 2012;7(7):e40515.

ADDITIONAL READING
- Cole DE, Taylor TL, McCullough DM, et al. Acute respiratory distress syndrome in pregnancy. *Crit Care Med*. 2005;33(10)(Suppl):S269–S278.
- Wheeler AP, Bernard GR. Acute lung injury and the acute respiratory distress syndrome: a clinical review. *Lancet*. 2007;369(9572):1553–1564.

 CODES

ICD10
J80 Acute respiratory distress syndrome

CLINICAL PEARLS
- ARDS is a syndrome characterized by an abrupt onset of diffuse lung injury with severe hypoxemia and bilateral pulmonary infiltrates.
- Treatment of ARDS requires aggressive supportive care in an ICU setting while also addressing the underlying cause.
- The benefit of invasive monitoring of vital signs, cardiac output, and PAWP has been questioned by large clinical trials.

RESPIRATORY DISTRESS SYNDROME, NEONATAL

Mary Cataletto, MD, FAAP, FCCP • Margaret J. McCormick, MS, RN

BASICS

DESCRIPTION
- Neonatal respiratory distress syndrome (NRDS) is a serious disorder of prematurity with a clinical manifestation of respiratory distress.
- Pulmonary surfactants that are deficient at birth and an overly compliant chest wall cause diffuse lung atelectasis.
- System(s) affected: pulmonary
- Synonym(s): hyaline membrane disease; surfactant deficiency

ALERT
A disorder of the neonatal period

EPIDEMIOLOGY
Incidence
- Predominant age: 93% incidence in infants born at or before 28 weeks' gestational age
- Inversely proportional to gestational age and birth weight
- Predominant sex: slight male predominance
- Eighth leading cause of infant death in United States in 2013: 13.3 infant deaths per 100,000 live births (1)
- Despite advances, survival of infants born before 25 weeks' gestation is rare (2).

Prevalence
Common disorder in premature infants, especially those born <28 weeks' gestation

ETIOLOGY AND PATHOPHYSIOLOGY
- Structurally immature lungs and surfactant deficiency lead to diffuse atelectasis.
- Exposure to high FiO_2 and barotrauma associated with mechanical ventilation trigger proinflammatory cytokines that further damage alveolar epithelium.
- Decreased lung compliance leads to alveolar hypoventilation and ventilation–perfusion mismatch.
- Impaired surfactant synthesis and secretion

Genetics
No known genetic pattern

RISK FACTORS
- Premature birth
- Infants of diabetic mothers
- Perinatal asphyxia
- History of RDS in a sibling

GENERAL PREVENTION
- Prevention of premature birth with education and regular prenatal care
- Antenatal corticosteroids
- Manage any medical issues appropriately.
- Healthy behaviors including diet and exercise
- Avoid exposure to tobacco smoke, alcohol, and illegal drugs.

DIAGNOSIS

HISTORY
Preterm neonates with worsening respiratory distress beginning shortly after birth and progressing over first few hours of life.

PHYSICAL EXAM
- Tachypnea
- Grunting
- Nasal flaring
- Subcostal and intercostal retractions
- Decreased breath sounds
- Cyanosis

DIFFERENTIAL DIAGNOSIS
- Early-onset group B streptococcal pneumonia and/or sepsis
- Transient tachypnea of newborn
- Meconium aspiration pneumonia

DIAGNOSTIC TESTS & INTERPRETATION
- CBC and blood culture to rule out sepsis and pneumonia
- Electrolytes: Monitor for hypoglycemia and hypocalcemia.
- Arterial blood gases (ABGs)
  – Hypoxemia (which responds to supplemental oxygen)
  – Features of respiratory and metabolic acidosis

- Chest x-ray (CXR):
  – Diffuse reticulogranular pattern (ground-glass appearance)
  – Air bronchograms
  – Low lung volumes

Diagnostic Procedures/Other
Echocardiogram: Consider if murmur is present to evaluate for patent ductus arteriosus (PDA) and contribution to lung disease due to L → R shunting.

Test Interpretation
- Macroscopically: uniformly ruddy, airless appearance of lungs
- Microscopically: diffuse atelectasis and hyaline membranes (eosinophilic and fibrinous membrane lining air spaces)

TREATMENT

- Along with antenatal steroids, surfactants improve survival for preterm infants.
- Surfactants are now recommended routinely as early in the course of RDS as possible.

GENERAL MEASURES
- Warm, humidified, oxygen-enriched gases if the neonate is ventilating effectively
- Continuous positive airway pressure (CPAP) if infant is active and breathing spontaneously (3)[A]
- Positive-pressure ventilation per ETT via conventional mechanical ventilator (CMV) or high-frequency oscillation ventilator (HFOV) if respiratory failure occurs (i.e., respiratory acidosis, apnea, or hypoxia despite nasal CPAP) (3)[A]
- Transcutaneous monitors to measure CO_2 tension as necessary
- Pulse oximetry
- Umbilical artery catheter placement for continuous BP monitoring and sampling ABGs

MEDICATION
- Pulmonary surfactant (3)[A]
- Side effects: Bradycardia, hypotension, airway obstruction/endotracheal tube blockage with administration; rapid changes in tidal volume due to increased compliance can cause a pneumothorax and small risk of pulmonary hemorrhage.

- Precautions: Transient adverse effects seen with the administration of surfactant may require stopping administration and alleviating situation; may proceed with dosing when stable
- Contraindications: presence of congenital anomalies incompatible with life beyond neonatal period; infant with laboratory evidence of lung maturity
- Perform frequent clinical and laboratory checks so that oxygen and ventilatory support can be modified to respond to respiratory changes (3)[A].

ISSUES FOR REFERRAL
Comorbid conditions associated with prematurity may require consultation during the course of the infant's NICU admission, including PDA (cardiology consult), necrotizing enterocolitis (NEC) (gastroenterology), retinopathy of prematurity (ROP) (ophthalmology), etc.

ADDITIONAL THERAPIES
Treat associated problems of prematurity.

INPATIENT CONSIDERATIONS

Admission Criteria/Initial Stabilization
All neonates with respiratory distress require evaluation, monitoring, and treatment in a NICU; treatment may be required in the delivery room.

IV Fluids
- To maintain blood pressure and perfusion, when necessary
- To provide optimal fluid balance, provide nutritional support.

Nursing
- Supportive care
- Thermoneutral environment
- Respiratory monitoring
- Establish relationship with family to provide education and emotional support.

Discharge Criteria
- Should have stable vital signs and pulse oximetry before discharge
- Medical home and support services should be in place.

ONGOING CARE

FOLLOW-UP RECOMMENDATIONS
Following discharge, infants should be followed closely by their physicians to monitor growth and respiratory symptomatology.

DIET
As clinically indicated

PATIENT EDUCATION
- Educate parents regarding the risks in subsequent pregnancies.
- Advise parents regarding potential issues with chronic lung disease.
- For patient education materials favorably reviewed on this topic, go to Boston Children's Hospital Web site (http://www.childrenshospital.org) and search for respiratory distress syndrome in the "My Child Has" window.

PROGNOSIS
Prognosis and outcome are highly dependent on gestational age and birth weight. Almost half of the infants in Jarjour study who were born at or <25 weeks' gestation had significant neurodevelopmental disabilities on short- and long-term follow-up.

COMPLICATIONS
- Complications specific to NRDS
  - Pneumothorax
  - Chronic lung disease, bronchopulmonary dysplasia (BPD)
  - Pulmonary interstitial edema (PIE)
- Additional complications may occur related to therapeutic interventions and comorbid conditions.

REFERENCES
1. Kochanek KD, Murphy SL, Xu J, et al. Mortality in the United States, 2013. National Center for Health Statistics Data Brief No. 178. http://www.cdc.gov/nchs/data/databriefs/db178.pdf. Accessed 2015.
2. Ancel PY, Goffinet F. Survival and morbidity of preterm children born at 22 through 34 weeks' gestation in France in 2011: results of the EPIPAGE-2 cohort study. *JAMA Pediatr*. 2015;169(3): 230–238.
3. Sweet DG, Carnielli V, Greisen G, et al. European consensus guidelines on the management of neonatal respiratory distress syndrome in preterm infants–2013 update. *Neonatology*. 2013;103(4):353–368.

ADDITIONAL READING
- Finer NN, Carlo WA, Walsh MC, et al. Early CPAP versus surfactant in extremely preterm infants. *N Engl J Med*. 2010;362(21):1970–1979.
- Hamrick SE, Hansmann G. Patent ductus arteriosus of the preterm infant. *Pediatrics*. 2010;125(5):1020–1030.
- Jarjour IT. Neurodevelopmental outcome after extreme prematurity: a review of the literature. *Pediatr Neurol*. 2015;52(2):143–152.
- Stoll BJ, Hansen NI, Bell EF, et al. Trends in care practices, morbidity, and mortality of extremely preterm neonates, 1993-2012. *JAMA*. 2015;314(10): 1039–1051.

 CODES

ICD10
P22.0 Respiratory distress syndrome of newborn

CLINICAL PEARLS
- Surfactants are used routinely as early in the course of RDS as possible.
- If an infant has a murmur, consider an echocardiogram to rule out PDA and shunting.
- Prognosis and outcome are highly dependent on gestational age and birth weight.

RESPIRATORY SYNCYTIAL VIRUS INFECTION

Elizabeth C. McKeen, MD

 BASICS

Respiratory syncytial virus (RSV) is a medium-sized, membrane-bound ribonucleic acid (RNA) virus that causes acute respiratory tract illness in all ages, with the most clinically significant disease occurring in infants and young children.

DESCRIPTION
A major cause of respiratory illness, either of the upper respiratory tract (URT) or of the lower respiratory tract (LRT/bronchiolitis)
- In adults, RSV causes URT infections (URTIs).
- In infants and children, RSV causes URTIs and LRT infections (bronchiolitis and pneumonia).

Pediatric Considerations
- 90–95% of children are infected at least once by the age of 24 months; reinfection is common.
- Leading cause of pediatric bronchiolitis (50–90%)
- Premature infants are at increased risk for severe acute RSV infection.

EPIDEMIOLOGY
- Seasonality: Highest incidence of RSV in the United States occurs between December and March.
- Morbidity: RSV infection leads to over 100,000 annual hospitalizations.
- Mortality: Deaths associated with RSV are uncommon. Children with complex chronic conditions account for the majority of deaths, and the relative contribution of RSV infection to their deaths is unclear (1)[B].

ETIOLOGY AND PATHOPHYSIOLOGY
- RSV-induced bronchiolitis causes acute inflammation, edema, and necrosis of small airway epithelium, air trapping, bronchospasm, and increased mucus production.
- RSV develops in the cytoplasm of infected cells and matures by budding from the plasma membrane.
- Infection spreads through droplets, either airborne or personal contact, that inoculate the nose of a susceptible individual

Genetics
- A genetic predisposition to severe RSV infections may be associated with polymorphisms in cytokine- and chemokine-related genes, including *CCR5*, *IL4*, and affiliated receptors, *IL8*, *IL10*, and *IL13*.
- Infants with transplacentally acquired antibody against RSV are not protected against infection but may have milder symptoms.

RISK FACTORS
- Risk factors for severe disease
  - Prematurity
  - Age <12 weeks
  - Underlying cardiopulmonary disease
  - Immunodeficiency
- Other risk factors
  - Low socioeconomic status
  - Exposure to environmental air pollutants
  - Child care attendance
  - Severe neuromuscular disease
  - Adults: occupational exposure to young children, hospital staff, teachers, and daycare workers

GENERAL PREVENTION
- Hand hygiene is the most important step to prevent the spread of RSV.
  - Alcohol-based rubs are preferred; an alternative is hand washing with soap and water (2)[B].
- Avoid exposure to passive tobacco smoke, especially in infants and children (3)[A].
- Isolate patients with proven or suspected RSV.
- Palivizumab (Synagis), a monoclonal antibody directed against the fushion (F) protein of RSV, is indicated as prophylaxis for:
  - Infants and children <24 months of age with
    ○ Chronic lung disease of prematurity requiring medical therapy within 6 months of the start of RSV season
    ○ Hemodynamically significant congenital heart disease
    ○ Congenital abnormalities of the airway or neuromuscular disease that compromises handling airway secretions
  - Infants born at ≤28 weeks' gestation if they are <12 months of age at the start of the RSV season; prophylaxis should be maintained through the end of the RSV season.
  - Infants born at 29 to 32 weeks' gestation if they are <6 months of age at the start of the RSV season; prophylaxis should be maintained through the end of the RSV season.
  - Infants born at 32 to 35 weeks' gestation who are <3 months of age at the start of the RSV season or who are born during the RSV season if they have one of the following two risk factors:
    ○ Infant attends child care
    ○ ≥1 more siblings or other children <5 years of age living permanently in the child's household
- Dosage: maximum of 5 monthly doses beginning in November or December at 15 mg/kg per dose IM
- Current palivizumab guidelines in the *Red Book*.

COMMONLY ASSOCIATED CONDITIONS
- Asthma
- Otitis media
- Serious bacterial infection (SBI) in infants and children with concurrent RSV infection is rare.

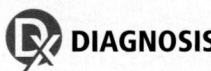 **DIAGNOSIS**

ALERT
In most cases, diagnosis is clinical. Laboratory and radiologic studies are not routinely necessary (2)[B].

HISTORY
- Rhinorrhea and upper respiratory congestion
- Difficulty feeding in infants (due to respiratory effort)
- Increased respiratory rate or signs of increased work of breathing (grunting, flaring, retracting)
- Wheezing
- Cough
- Fever
- History of prematurity, secondhand tobacco exposure, daycare, number and age of siblings
- Immunization history
- Family history of respiratory disease

PHYSICAL EXAM
- Vital signs: fever, signs of increased work of breathing (tachypnea, grunting, flaring, retracting), pulse rate; pulse oximetry ("fifth vital sign") to assess oxygenation
- Ear, nose, throat: rhinorrhea, dry mucous membranes (dehydration)
- Serous otitis or acute otitis; pulmonary: wheezing, crackles
- Skin turgor
- Serial examinations to assess status

Pediatric Considerations
Young infants with bronchiolitis may develop apnea with increased risk of prolonged hospitalization, ICU admission, and mechanical ventilation.

DIFFERENTIAL DIAGNOSIS
- Mild illness/URTI
  - Other respiratory viral infections rhinovirus, human metapneumovirus, influenza virus, human bocavirus
  - Allergic rhinitis
  - Sinusitis
- Severe illness/LRTI
  - Bronchiolitis
  - Asthma
  - Pneumonia
  - Foreign body aspiration

DIAGNOSTIC TESTS & INTERPRETATION
Initial Tests (lab, imaging)
- Routine laboratory testing is not necessary.
  - If obtained, WBC count may be normal or elevated.
  - Virologic tests for RSV, despite high predictive value, rarely change management decisions or outcomes for patients with clinical bronchiolitis.
- Given the low risk of SBI, full septic workups are not necessary unless child appears toxic.
- Chest x-ray (CXR) does not predict disease severity or change patient outcomes but may be helpful if a patient does not improve as expected, if the severity of the disease requires further investigation, or if another diagnosis is suspected.
- When obtained, typical CXR findings include:
  - Hyperinflation and peribronchiolar thickening
  - Atelectasis
  - Interstitial infiltrates
  - Segmental or lobar consolidation

 TREATMENT

GENERAL MEASURES
- Assess hydration status and ability to take fluids orally. Treat dehydration adequately with an oral or IV fluid, particularly in infants.
- Supplemental oxygen is indicated if pulse oximetry falls persistently <90% in previously healthy patients.

MEDICATION
First Line
No first-line medication for RSV infections; treatment is usually supportive; oxygen as needed

Second Line

- Bronchodilators show small, short-term improvements in clinical scores, but this small benefit should be weighed against costs and adverse effects.
  - Bronchodilators do not improve oxygen saturation, reduce hospital admission after outpatient treatment, shorten the duration of hospitalization, or reduce the time to resolution of illness at home.
  - Routine use not recommended
- Nebulized epinephrine is superior to placebo for short-term outcomes for outpatients, particularly in the first 24 hours of care.
  - Epinephrine superior for outpatient clinical outcomes in acute bronchiolitis (4)[A].
- Glucocorticoids do not alter admissions or length of hospitalization (5)[A].
  - Some data suggest that the combination of dexamethasone and epinephrine may reduce outpatient admissions (5)[A].
- A recent study found that montelukast (Singulair) has no effect on the clinical course of acute bronchiolitis (6)[C].
- Ribavirin, a nucleoside analogue and antiviral agent, has not been shown to be efficacious, particularly in immunocompromised patients (7)[A].
- There is no current evidence that nebulized rhDNase changes clinical outcomes in children <24 months of age hospitalized with acute RSV bronchiolitis (8)[B].
- Reserve use of antibacterial agents for patients who have specific findings that suggest a coexisting SBI (9)[B].
- Nebulized 3% saline may reduce the length of stay and improve the clinical severity score in infants hospitalized with acute viral bronchiolitis (10)[A].

ADDITIONAL THERAPIES

- Bulb suctioning of the nares may provide some comfort to infants and allow for easier feeding.
- Efforts are underway to develop a RSV vaccine (11)[C].

Pediatric Considerations

Over-the-counter (OTC) cough and cold medications should not be used in children <6 years due to lack of efficacy and the risk of life-threatening side effects.

COMPLEMENTARY & ALTERNATIVE MEDICINE

No complementary, alternative, or integrative therapies are of proven benefit in the prevention or treatment of RSV bronchiolitis.

INPATIENT CONSIDERATIONS

Admission Criteria/Initial Stabilization

- Clinical judgment of the patient's degree of respiratory distress is the most important consideration. Ill-appearing infants should be hospitalized.
- Significant respiratory distress, an oxygen requirement to keep SpO$_2$ >90%, and the inability to hydrate orally are indications for admission.
- Mechanical ventilation is required in about 5% of infants hospitalized with RSV and 20% of children with underlying congenital heart disease, chronic lung disease, or immunosuppression.

IV Fluids

See "Treatment."

Discharge Criteria

No set criteria for discharge, patients should be recovering and demonstrate:

- Stable respiratory status with no oxygen requirement
- Ability to maintain oral intake and sustain hydration
- Home resources adequate to support necessary home therapies, including caretaker ability to clear the infant's airway with bulb suctioning if needed
- Adequate follow-up and patient education

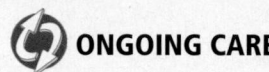 ONGOING CARE

FOLLOW-UP RECOMMENDATIONS

Primary care follow-up to ensure resolution

PATIENT EDUCATION

Bronchiolitis and Your Child, available at http://familydoctor.org/familydoctor/en/diseases-conditions/bronchiolitis.html

PROGNOSIS

Most patients with RSV infection recover fully within 7 to 10 days. Reinfection is common.

COMPLICATIONS

- Infants hospitalized for RSV may be at increased risk for recurrent wheezing and reduced pulmonary function, particularly during the 1st decade of life.
- Overall mortality for infants and children <24 months of age is <1%.
- Although the relationship between RSV and asthma is unclear, RSV bronchiolitis in infancy has been linked to subsequent asthma.

REFERENCES

1. Byington CL, Wilkes J, Korgenski K, et al. Respiratory syncytial virus-associated mortality in hospitalized infants and young children. *Pediatrics.* 2015;135(1):e24–e31.
2. American Academy of Pediatrics Subcommittee on Diagnosis and Management of Bronchiolitis. Diagnosis and management of bronchiolitis. *Pediatrics.* 2006;118(4):1774–1793.
3. DiFranza JR, Masaquel A, Barrett AM, et al. Systematic literature review assessing tobacco smoke exposure as a risk factor for serious respiratory syncytial virus disease among infants and young children. *BMC Pediatr.* 2012;12:81.
4. Hartling L, Fernandes RM, Bialy L, et al. Steroids and bronchodilators for acute bronchiolitis in the first two years of life: systematic review and meta-analysis. *BMJ.* 2011;342:d1714.
5. Fernandes RM, Bialy LM, Vandermeer B, et al. Glucocorticoids for acute viral bronchiolitis in infants and young children. *Cochrane Database Syst Rev.* 2010;(10):CD004878.
6. Amirav I, Luder AS, Kruger N, et al. A double-blind, placebo-controlled, randomized trial of montelukast for acute bronchiolitis. *Pediatrics.* 2008;122(6):e1249–e1255.
7. Hynicka LM, Ensor CR. Prophylaxis and treatment of respiratory syncytial virus in adult immunocompromised patients. *Ann Pharmacother.* 2012;46(4):558–566.
8. Enriquez A, Chu IW, Mellis C, et al. Nebulised deoxyribonuclease for viral bronchiolitis in children younger than 24 months. *Cochrane Database Syst Rev.* 2012;(11):CD008395.
9. Spurling GK, Fonseka K, Doust J, et al. Antibiotics for bronchiolitis in children. *Cochrane Database Syst Rev.* 2007;(1):CD005189.
10. Zhang L, Mendoza-Sassi RA, Wainwright C, et al. Nebulized hypertonic saline solution for acute bronchiolitis in infants. *Cochrane Database Syst Rev.* 2008;(4):CD006458.
11. Poletti P, Merler S, Ajelli M, et al. Evaluating vaccination strategies for reducing infant respiratory syncytial virus infection in low-income settings. *BMC Med.* 2015;13:49.

ADDITIONAL READING

- American Academy of Pediatrics. Section 3: respiratory syncytial virus. In: Pickering LK, Baker CJ, Kimberlin DW, et al, eds. *Red Book: 2012 Report of the Committee on Infectious Diseases.* 29th ed. Elk Grove Village, IL: American Academy of Pediatrics; 2012.
- Gadomski AM, Brower M. Bronchodilators for bronchiolitis. *Cochrane Database Syst Rev.* 2010;(12):CD001266.

 CODES

ICD10

- B97.4 Respiratory syncytial virus causing diseases classd elswhr
- J06.9 Acute upper respiratory infection, unspecified
- J21.0 Acute bronchiolitis due to respiratory syncytial virus

CLINICAL PEARLS

- RSV causes 50–90% of pediatric bronchiolitis.
- Hand sanitation is the primary step for preventing RSV in the general population.
- The diagnosis of RSV is clinical in most cases. Routine lab testing is not necessary.
- Treatment of RSV is usually supportive.
- Palivizumab should be used to prevent RSV in high-risk patients.

RESTLESS LEGS SYNDROME

Donald E. Watenpaugh, PhD • John R. Burk, MD

 BASICS

DESCRIPTION

- Sensorimotor disorder consisting of a strong urge to move the legs, usually with paresthesia (1)[A]
- Symptoms emerge during inactivity.
- Movement relieves symptoms, but they soon recur with inactivity.
- Symptoms occur preferentially in the evening/night.
- Symptoms may involve the arms or be more generalized.
- Patient may also report involuntary leg jerks (1)[A].
- Associated with insomnia and/or functional impairment(s)
- Not solely accounted for by another disorder
- System(s) affected: musculoskeletal; nervous
- Synonym(s): Willis-Ekbom disease

EPIDEMIOLOGY

Incidence
- Onset at any age; increases with age
- Predominant sex: male = female (nulliparous); female (parous) two times > male (2)[B]
- May increase in summer (warm) months

Prevalence
- 4–15% of Caucasian adults; underdiagnosed
- 1–3% in children and adolescents
- Increases with age
- Lower in non-Caucasians

Pregnancy Considerations
10–30% prevalence; exacerbates existing restless legs syndrome (RLS)

ETIOLOGY AND PATHOPHYSIOLOGY

- Primary (early-onset) RLS: subcortical dopamine deficiency/dysmetabolism
- Late-onset (often secondary) RLS:
  - Iron deficiency and associated conditions
  - Chronic extremity tissue pathology/inflammation
  - Medications
    - Most antidepressants (exceptions: bupropion and desipramine)
    - Dopamine-blocking antiemetics (e.g., metoclopramide, prochlorperazine)
    - Some antiepileptic agents (e.g., phenytoin)
    - Phenothiazine antipsychotics; donepezil
    - Theophylline and other xanthines
    - Antihistamines/over-the-counter (OTC) cold preparations (e.g., pseudoephedrine)
    - Adrenergics, stimulants

Genetics
- Early-onset RLS heritability: ~50%
- Genetically heterogenous
  - Susceptibility loci: 2p14, 2q, 6p21.2, 9p, 12q, 14q, 15q23, and 20p
  - Genes: MEIS1, MAP2K5/LBXCOR1, and BTBD9

RISK FACTORS
- Family history (3,4)
- Aging
- Chronic inactivity
- Inadequate sleep
- Associated conditions (see "Commonly Associated Conditions")
- Certain medications (see "Etiology")

GENERAL PREVENTION
- Regular physical activity/exercise
- Adequate sleep
- Avoid evening caffeine, alcohol, tobacco.
- Avoid late-day use of medications that cause RLS.

COMMONLY ASSOCIATED CONDITIONS
- Periodic limb movements of sleep, insomnia, sleep walking, other parasomnias, delayed sleep phase
- Iron deficiency, renal disease/uremia/dialysis, gastric surgery, liver disease
- Parkinson disease, multiple sclerosis, peripheral neuropathy, migraine
- Orthopedic problems, arthritis, fibromyalgia
- Venous insufficiency/peripheral vascular disease, erectile dysfunction
- Pulmonary hypertension, lung transplantation, chronic obstructive pulmonary disease (COPD)
- ADHD, anxiety/depression, "sundowning"
- Pregnancy (especially if Fe- or folate-deficient)

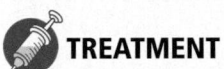 DIAGNOSIS

- Depends on history, yet often "difficult to describe"
- May go undiagnosed for years by multiple doctors

HISTORY
- Signs/symptoms (see also "Description") (1)[A]
  - Limited to evening, night
  - Example descriptions: burning, achy, itching, antsy, "can't get comfortable"
  - Painful in ~35% of patients
  - Discomfort associated with overwhelming urge to move and relieved by movement
  - Urge to move may be the only "discomfort."
  - Movement frequency every 10 to 90 seconds (mean ~25 seconds)
  - Some patients must get up and walk.
  - May involve arms or, rarely, whole body
  - Periodic movements in sleep in ~80% of patients.
  - Insomnia, fatigue, anxiety
- Severity range: from rare, minor problem to daily severe impact on quality of life
- Early-onset RLS (before age 45 years) progresses slowly.
- Late-onset RLS (1)[A]
  - Sometimes secondary to other factors
  - Tends to progress more rapidly
  - May resolve to extent that cause(s) resolve

Pediatric Considerations
Consider child's own words in describing symptoms and these additional supportive findings (1)[A]:
- Insomnia or sleep disturbance
- RLS in immediate biologic relative
- Periodic limb movements during sleep

Geriatric Considerations
For diagnosis in the cognitively impaired
- Rubbing or kneading the legs in evening
- Evening hyperactivity (foot tapping, pacing, fidgeting, tossing/turning in bed)

DIFFERENTIAL DIAGNOSIS
- Claudication: Movement does not relieve pain and may worsen it.
- Motor neuron disease fasciculation/tremor: no discomfort or circadian pattern
- Peripheral neuropathy: usually no circadian pattern; unresponsive to dopamine agonists
- Dermatitis/pruritus: movement only to scratch; no circadian pattern
- Sleep-related leg cramps: isolated and very painful muscle contracture
- Periodic limb movement disorder: no wakeful movements
- Sleep starts: isolated involuntary events
- Rhythmic movement sleep disorder: movement periodicity faster than RLS
- Growing pains: no urge to move or relief by movement; circadian pattern opposite RLS
- ADHD: no sleep disorders or complaints in diagnostic criteria

DIAGNOSTIC TESTS & INTERPRETATION
Serum ferritin to assess for iron deficiency

Diagnostic Procedures/Other
- Sleep study helpful but not required
  - Frequent, periodic movements during wake
- Suggested immobilization test
  - Conducted before nocturnal polysomnography
  - Patient attempts to sit still in bed for 1 hour
  - >40 movements per hour suggests RLS.
- Ankle actigraphy for in-home use
- Electromyography, nerve conduction studies for peripheral neuropathy, radiculopathy

Test Interpretation
- Serum ferritin should be >75 ng/mL.
- Transferrin saturation should be >16%.

TREATMENT

First-line treatments

- Prescribed daily exercise (3)[B]; adequate sleep
- Correct iron deficiency.
- Dopaminergic medications
- For secondary RLS, treat cause(s).
- Multiple possible causes are not mutually exclusive.

GENERAL MEASURES
- If iron deficient, supplement:
  - 325 mg FeSO$_4$ TID
  - Repletion requires months.
- Daily exercise. However, avoid unusual activity that may exacerbate symptoms.
- Regular and replete sleep
- Hot bath and leg massage
- Warm the legs (long heavy socks, electric blanket).
- Intense mental activity (games, puzzles, etc.)
- Avoid exacerbating factors.

MEDICATION
- Use minimum effective dose.
- Preferentially use longer-acting/extended-release options.
- Daytime sleepiness unusual with doses and timing for RLS
- Severe/refractory RLS may require combination therapy (4,5)[A].

First Line

- Dopamine agonists (4,5)[A]; titrate every 3 days to minimum dose necessary to fully control symptoms:
  - Pramipexole (Mirapex): 0.125 to 0.5 mg 1 hour before symptoms; titrate by 0.125 mg
  - Ropinirole (Requip): 0.25 to 4 mg 1 hour before symptoms; titrate by 0.25 mg
  - Divide dose for evening and bedtime symptoms.
  - Transdermal rotigotine (Neupro): 1 to 3 mg/24 hours patch; initiate with 1 mg/day; titrate by 1 mg weekly
  - Avoid dopamine agonists in psychotic patients, particularly if taking dopamine antagonists.
  - Add a different class of medication before exceeding dopamine agonist recommended dose.
- Gabapentin enacarbil (Horizant): 600 mg every day ~5:00 PM (4,5)[A]
- All other medications off-label

Second Line

- Anticonvulsants (for comorbid neuropathy).
  - Pregabalin (Lyrica): 50 to 300 mg/day
  - Carbamazepine: 200 to 800 mg/day
- Opioids (low risk of tolerance/addiction at bedtime)
  - Hydrocodone: 5 to 20 mg/day
  - Tramadol: 50 mg/day
  - Oxycodone: 2.5 to 20 mg/day
- Benzodiazepines and agonists (for associated insomnia or anxiety)
  - Clonazepam (Klonopin): 0.5 to 3 mg/day
  - Temazepam, triazolam, alprazolam, zaleplon, zolpidem, and diazepam
- Dopamine agonists
  - Carbidopa-levodopa (Sinemet or Sinemet CR): 10/100 to 25/250; PRN for sporadic symptoms

Pregnancy Considerations

- Initial approach: nonpharmacologic therapies, assess/correct iron deficiency
- Avoid medications class C or D.
- In 3rd trimester, may consider low-dose clonazepam or opioids (6)[B].

Pediatric Considerations

- First-line treatment: nonpharmacologic therapies, assess/correct iron deficiency
- Low-dose clonidine or clonazepam may be considered.

Geriatric Considerations

- Avoid medications that cause dizziness or unsteadiness.
- Many medications given to elderly cause/exacerbate RLS.

ISSUES FOR REFERRAL

- Severe, intractable symptoms
- Augmentation response to dopaminergic therapy
- Peripheral neuropathy; orthopedic problems
- Peripheral vascular disease; intransigent iron deficiency

ADDITIONAL THERAPIES

- Vitamin, mineral supplements: Ca, Mg, B_{12}, folate
- Clonidine: 0.05 to 0.1 mg/day
- Baclofen: 20 to 80 mg/day
- Methadone: 5 to 10 mg/day
- Oxycodone PR-Naloxone PR: 10 or 5 mg/day
- Prescription or OTC hypnotics

SURGERY/OTHER PROCEDURES

For orthopedic, neuropathic, or leg vascular disease (laser ablation, sclerotherapy, etc.)

COMPLEMENTARY & ALTERNATIVE MEDICINE

- Relaxis leg vibration device (FDA approved; see http://www.sensorymedical.com)
- Sequential pneumatic leg compression
- Enhanced external counterpulsation
- Compression stockings
- Acupuncture
- MicroVas therapy
- Near-infrared light (3)[B]

INPATIENT CONSIDERATIONS

- Control RLS after orthopedic procedures.
- Addition/withdrawal of medications affecting RLS (e.g., narcotics)
- Changes in medical status may require medication changes (e.g., Mirapex contraindicated in renal failure and Requip contraindicated in liver disease).

IV Fluids

- Iron infusion when oral Fe fails or contraindicated.
- When NPO, consider IV opiates.

Nursing

- Evening walks, hot baths, leg massage, and warming
- Sleep interruption risks prolonged wakefulness.

ONGOING CARE

FOLLOW-UP RECOMMENDATIONS

Patient Monitoring

- At 2-week intervals until stable, then annually
- If taking iron, remeasure ferritin.
- If status changes, assess for associated conditions and medications.

DIET

Avoid evening caffeine and alcohol.

PATIENT EDUCATION

- Willis-Ekbom Disease Foundation: www.rls.org
- National Sleep Foundation: sleepfoundation.org
- American Academy of Sleep Medicine: http://sleepeducation.com/

PROGNOSIS

- Early-onset: lifelong condition with no current cure
- Late-onset/secondary: may subside with resolution of precipitating factors
- Current therapies usually control symptoms

COMPLICATIONS

- Vicious cycle between sleep loss from RLS and exacerbation of RLS by sleep loss
- Augmentation of symptoms from prolonged dopaminergic therapy
  - Symptoms increase in severity, occur earlier, and/or spread.
  - Higher doses increase risk.
  - Highest risk from daily levodopa or Sinemet
  - Iron deficiency increases risk.
  - Add alternative medication then slowly downtitrate dopamine agonist.
- Obsessive-compulsive or impulse-control disorders from dopamine agonists
- Iatrogenic RLS (from antidepressants, etc.)

REFERENCES

1. Allen RP, Picchietti DL, Garcia-Borreguero D, et al. Restless legs syndrome/Willis-Ekbom disease diagnostic criteria: updated International Restless Legs Syndrome Study Group (IRLSSG) consensus criteria—history, rationale, description, and significance. *Sleep Med.* 2014;15(8):860–873.
2. Manconi M, Ulfberg J, Berger K, et al. When gender matters: restless legs syndrome. Report of the "RLS and woman" workshop endorsed by the European RLS Study Group. *Sleep Med Rev.* 2012;16(4):297–307.
3. Wilt TJ, MacDonald R, Ouellette J, et al. Treatment for Restless Legs Syndrome. *Agency for Healthcare Research and Quality Comparative Effectiveness Reviews (US).* 2012; Report No.: 12(13)-EHC147-EF.
4. Aurora RN, Kristo DA, Bista SR, et al. The treatment of restless legs syndrome and periodic limb movement disorder in adults—an update for 2012: practice parameters with an evidence-based systematic review and meta-analyses: an American Academy of Sleep Medicine Clinical Practice Guideline. *Sleep.* 2012;35(8):1039–1062.
5. Ferini-Strambi L, Marelli S. Pharmacotherapy for restless legs syndrome. *Expert Opin Pharmacother.* 2014;15(8):1127–1138.
6. Picchietti DL, Hensley JG, Bainbridge JL, et al. Consensus clinical practice guidelines for the diagnosis and treatment of restless legs syndrome/Willis-Ekbom disease during pregnancy and lactation. *Sleep Med Rev.* 2015;22:64–77.

ADDITIONAL READING

- Amos LB, Grekowicz ML, Kuhn EM, et al. Treatment of pediatric restless legs syndrome. *Clin Pediatr (Phila).* 2014;53(4):331–336.
- Garcia-Borreguero D, Benitez A, Kohnen R, et al. Augmentation of restless leg syndrome (Willis-Ekbom disease) during long-term dopaminergic treatment. *Postgrad Med.* 2014;127(7):716–725.

SEE ALSO

- Periodic Limb Movement Disorder
- Algorithm: Restless Legs Syndrome

CODES

ICD10
G25.81 Restless legs syndrome

CLINICAL PEARLS

- Insomnia with frequent tossing/turning and difficulty "getting comfortable" is often RLS.
- Many antidepressants, antipsychotics, antiemetics, and antihistamines cause or exacerbate RLS.
- Titrate medication for RLS, especially dopaminergics, only up to the minimum dose necessary to control symptoms.
- RLS may interfere with use of positive airway pressure to treat obstructive sleep apnea.
- RLS and other sleep disorders may cause ADHD.

RETINAL DETACHMENT

Richard W. Allinson, MD

 BASICS

DESCRIPTION
- Separation of the sensory retina from the underlying retinal pigment epithelium
- Rhegmatogenous retinal detachment (RRD): most common type; occurs when the fluid vitreous gains access to the subretinal space through a break in the retina (Greek *rhegma*, "rent")
- Exudative or serous detachment: occurs in the absence of a retinal break, usually in association with inflammation or a tumor
- Traction detachment: Vitreoretinal adhesions mechanically pull the retina from the retinal pigment epithelium. The most common cause is proliferative diabetic retinopathy.
- System(s) affected: nervous

EPIDEMIOLOGY
Incidence
- Predominant age: Incidence increases with age.
- Predominant sex: male > female (3:2)
- Per year: 1/10,000 in patients who have not had cataract surgery

Prevalence
After cataract surgery, 1–3% of patients will develop a retinal detachment.

ETIOLOGY AND PATHOPHYSIOLOGY
- Traction from a posterior vitreous detachment (PVD) causes most retinal tears. With aging, vitreous gel liquefies, leading to separation of the vitreous from the retina. The vitreous gel remains attached at the vitreous base, in the retinal periphery, resulting in vitreous traction that produces tears in the retinal periphery. There is an ~15% chance of developing a retinal tear from a PVD.
- PVD associated with vitreous hemorrhage has a high incidence of retinal tears.
- Exudative detachment
  – Tumors
  – Inflammatory diseases (Vogt-Koyanagi-Harada disease, posterior scleritis)
  – Miscellaneous (central serous retinopathy, uveal effusion syndrome, malignant hypertension)
- Traction detachment
  – Proliferative diabetic retinopathy
  – Cicatricial retinopathy of prematurity
  – Proliferative sickle-cell retinopathy
- Penetrating trauma

Genetics
- Most cases are sporadic.
- There is an increased risk of RRD if a sibling has been affected by this condition. The risk increases with higher levels of myopia in the family history.

RISK FACTORS
- Myopia (>5 diopters)
- Aphakia or pseudophakia
  – In patients undergoing small-incision coaxial phacoemulsification with high myopia (axial length ≥26 mm), the incidence of retinal detachment is 2.7%.
- PVD and associated conditions (e.g., aphakia, inflammatory disease, and trauma)
- Trauma
- Retinal detachment in fellow eye
- Lattice degeneration: a vitreoretinal abnormality found in 6–10% of the general population

- Glaucoma: 4–7% of patients with retinal detachment have chronic open-angle glaucoma.
- Vitreoretinal tufts: Peripheral retinal tufts are caused by focal areas of vitreous traction.
- Meridional folds: Redundant retina usually is found in the supranasal quadrant.

GENERAL PREVENTION
Patients at risk for retinal detachment should have regular ophthalmologic exams.

Geriatric Considerations
- PVD
- Cataract surgery

Pediatric Considerations
Usually associated with underlying vitreoretinal disorders and/or retinopathy of prematurity

COMMONLY ASSOCIATED CONDITIONS
- Lattice degeneration
- High myopia
- Cataract surgery
- Glaucoma
- History of retinal detachment in the fellow eye
- Trauma

Pregnancy Considerations
Preeclampsia/eclampsia may be associated with exudative retinal detachment. No intervention is indicated, provided hypertension is controlled. Prognosis is usually good.

 DIAGNOSIS

HISTORY
- Sudden flashes (photopsia)
- Shower of floaters
- Visual field loss: "curtain coming across vision"
- Central vision will be preserved if the macula is not detached.
- Poor visual acuity (20/200 or worse), with loss of central vision when macula is detached.

PHYSICAL EXAM
- Slit-lamp exam
- Dilated fundus exam with binocular indirect ophthalmoscopy

DIFFERENTIAL DIAGNOSIS
Retinoschisis (splitting of the retina)
- Vitreous cells and vitreous hemorrhage are found rarely in the vitreous with retinoschisis, whereas they are seen commonly in RRD.
- Retinoschisis usually has a smooth surface and is dome-shaped, whereas RRD often has a corrugated, irregular surface.

DIAGNOSTIC TESTS & INTERPRETATION
Visual field testing: differentiates RRD from retinoschisis. An absolute scotoma is seen in retinoschisis, whereas RRD causes a relative scotoma.

Initial Tests (lab, imaging)
- US can demonstrate a detached retina and may be helpful when the retina cannot be visualized directly (e.g., with cataracts).
- Fluorescein dye leakage can be seen in exudative retinal detachment; caused by central serous retinopathy and other inflammatory conditions

Test Interpretation
- Elevation of the neurosensory retina from the underlying retinal pigment epithelium
- Elevation of retina associated with ≥1 retinal tears in RRD or elevation of the retina without tears in exudative detachment
- In 3–10% of patients with presumed RRD, no definite retinal break is found.
- Tenting of the retina without retinal tears in traction detachment
- Pigmented cells within the vitreous ("tobacco dust")

TREATMENT

GENERAL MEASURES
- Not all retinal tears or breaks need to be treated:
  – Flap or horseshoe tears in symptomatic patients (e.g., patients with flashes or floaters) are treated frequently.
  – Operculated holes in symptomatic patients are treated sometimes.
  – Atrophic holes in symptomatic patients are treated rarely.
- Lattice degeneration with or without holes within the lattice in an asymptomatic patient with prior retinal detachment in the fellow eye may be treated prophylactically.
- Flap retinal tears in asymptomatic patients frequently are treated prophylactically.
- Exudative detachments usually are managed by treating underlying disorder.
- Traction detachments usually are managed by observation. If the fovea is involved, a vitrectomy is needed.

MEDICATION
First Line
- Intraocular gases
  – Air
  – Perfluoropropane (C_3F_8)
  – Sulfur hexafluoride (SF_6)
- Perfluorocarbon liquids
- Silicone oil
- Contraindications to intraocular gas: patients with poorly controlled glaucoma
- Precautions with intraocular gas: Expanding intraocular gas bubble increases intraocular pressure; therefore, avoid higher altitudes.
- Significant possible interactions with intraocular gas: Nitrous oxide used in general anesthesia can expand an intraocular gas bubble.

Second Line
Steroids may cause worsening of central serous retinopathy.

SURGERY/OTHER PROCEDURES
- Timing of repairs
  – Macula attached: within 24 hours. If the detachment is peripheral and does not have features suggestive of rapid progression (e.g., large and/or superior tears), repair can be performed within a few days.
- Macula recently detached: within 10 days of development of a macula-off retinal detachment (1)[B]
  – Old macular detachment: elective repair within 2 weeks

- If a retinal break has led to the development of a retinal detachment, surgery is needed. Surgical options (and combinations) include the following:
  - Demarcation laser treatment
  - Pneumatic retinopexy: Head positioning is required postoperatively.
  - Scleral buckle
  - Vitrectomy
  - Perfluorocarbon liquids for giant tears (circumferential tears ≥90 degrees)
  - Silicone oil for complex repairs
- Anesthesia: local or general
- RRD may have >1 break. If any retinal break is not closed at the time of surgery, the surgery will fail.
- Additional surgery may be required if the retina redetaches secondary to a new retinal break or because of proliferative vitreoretinopathy (PVR).
- Adjuvant combination therapy using 5-fluorouracil (5-FU) and low-molecular-weight heparin (LMWH) may reduce the incidence of PVR in patients undergoing vitrectomy for RRD who are at a greater risk of developing PVR, such as patients with uveitis, but does not seem to be of benefit in cases of established PVR.
- If a vitreous hemorrhage is present, presumably from a retinal tear and the fundus cannot be well visualized, consideration can be given for early vitrectomy (2)[C].
- There is a trend toward primary vitrectomy in the management of RRD. Eyes undergoing pars plana vitrectomy (PPV) for primary RRD repair may not need the addition of a scleral buckle (3)[B].
- There is no statistical difference in the primary reattachment rate between eyes treated with PPV and scleral buckle for RRD in both phakic and pseudophakic/aphakic eyes (4)[A].
- Patients with RRD who are at high risk for PVR (retinal detachment in two or more quadrants, retinal tears >1 clock hour, preoperative PVR, or vitreous hemorrhage). PPV-scleral buckle was associated with higher rates of anatomical success compared to PPV alone (5)[B].
- There is a reduced incidence of intraoperative retinal tear formation using a transconjunctival cannulated PPV system compared to the standard 20-gauge system requiring suture closure.

INPATIENT CONSIDERATIONS

Admission Criteria/Initial Stabilization
- Recognition of condition is key (see "Diagnosis").
- Refer to an ophthalmologist for exam and treatment, if indicated.

ONGOING CARE

FOLLOW-UP RECOMMENDATIONS
- Bed rest prior to surgery.
- Postoperatively, if intraocular gas has been used, the patient may need specific head positioning and should not travel to high altitudes.

Patient Monitoring
- Alert ophthalmologist if there is new onset of floaters or flashes, increase in floaters or flashes, sudden shower of floaters, curtain or shadow in the peripheral visual field, or reduced vision.
- Patients with acute symptomatic PVD should be reexamined by the ophthalmologist in 3 to 4 weeks. The development of a retinal detachment is unlikely if no retinal tears are present on reexamination in 3 to 4 weeks.

- If acute symptomatic PVD is associated with gross vitreous hemorrhage that interferes with complete visualization of the retinal periphery by indirect ophthalmoscopy, the patient should be reexamined at short intervals with indirect ophthalmoscopy until the entire retinal periphery can be observed.
- If the examiner is not certain whether the retina is detached in the presence of opaque medium, US should be performed.

DIET
NPO if surgery is imminent.

PATIENT EDUCATION
American Academy of Ophthalmology, 655 E. Beach Street, San Francisco, CA 94109-1336

PROGNOSIS
- RRD
  - 90% of retinal detachments can be reattached successfully after ≥1 surgical procedures. Postoperative visual acuity depends primarily on the status of the macula preoperatively. Also important is the length of time between the detachment and the repair (75% of eyes with macular detachments of <1 week will obtain a final visual acuity of 20/70 or better).
  - 87% of eyes with a retinal detachment not involving the macula attain a visual acuity of 20/50 or better postoperatively. 37% of eyes with a detached macula preoperatively attain 20/50 or better vision postoperatively.
  - In 10–15% of successfully repaired retinal detachments not involving the macula preoperatively, visual acuity does not return to the preoperative level. This decrease is secondary to complications such as macular edema and macular pucker.

- Risk factors associated with primary RRD repair failure include choroidal detachment, significant hypotony, grade C-1 PVR, four detached quadrants, and large or giant retinal breaks (6)[B]. Additional risk factors associated with primary RRD repair failure include increased number of breaks and inferior location of retinal breaks (7)[B]. Tractional retinal detachment: When not involving the fovea, the patient usually can be observed because it is uncommon for these to extend into the fovea.

- Exudative retinal detachment
  - Management is usually nonsurgical.
  - The presence of shifting fluid is highly suggestive of an exudative retinal detachment. Fixed retinal folds, which are indicative of PVR, are seen rarely in exudative retinal detachment. If the underlying condition is treated, the prognosis generally is good.

COMPLICATIONS
- PVR is the most common cause of failed retinal detachment repair; 10–15% of retinas that reattach initially after retinal surgery will redetach subsequently, usually within 6 weeks, as a result of cellular proliferation and contraction on the retinal surface.
- Partial or total loss of vision due to macular detachment and/or PVR
- Moderate to severe forms of PVR usually are treated with PPV and fluid–gas exchange. If a segmental scleral buckle was placed at the initial procedure, it may need to be revised.
- Primary retinectomy can be used in cases of PVR without a scleral buckle (8)[C].

- Scleral buckles may erode the overlying conjunctiva and lead to an infection.
- Optic neuropathy after PPV for macula-sparing primary RRD

REFERENCES

1. Hassan TS, Sarrafizadeh R, Ruby AJ, et al. The effect of duration of macular detachment on results after the scleral buckle repair of primary, macula-off retinal detachments. *Ophthalmology.* 2002;109(1):146–152.
2. Tan HS, Mura M, Bijl HM. Early vitrectomy for vitreous hemorrhage associated with retinal tears. *Am J Ophthalmol.* 2010;150(4):529–533.
3. Kinori M, Moisseiev E, Shoshany N, et al. Comparison of pars plana vitrectomy with and without scleral buckle for the repair of primary rhegmatogenous retinal detachment. *Am J Ophthalmol.* 2011;152(2):291.e2–297.e2.
4. Soni C, Hainsworth DP, Almony A. Surgical management of rhegmatogenous retinal detachment: a meta-analysis of randomized controlled trials. *Ophthalmology.* 2013;120(7):1440–1447.
5. Storey P, Alshareef R, Khuthaila M, et al. Pars plana vitrectomy and scleral buckle versus pars plana vitrectomy alone for patients with rhegmatogenous retinal detachment at high risk for proliferative vitreoretinopathy. *Retina.* 2014;34(10):1945–1951.
6. Adelman RA, Parnes AJ, Michalewska Z, et al. Clinical variables associated with failure of retinal detachment repair: the European vitreo-retinal society retinal detachment study report number 4. *Ophthalmology.* 2014;121(9):1715–1719.
7. Williamson TH, Lee EJ, Shunmugam M. Characteristics of rhegmatogenous retinal detachment and their relationship to success rates of surgery. *Retina.* 2014;34(7):1421–1427.
8. Tan HS, Mura M, Oberstein SY, et al. Primary retinectomy in proliferative vitreoretinopathy. *Am J Ophthalmol.* 2010;149(3):447–452.

 SEE ALSO

Retinopathy, Diabetic

 CODES

ICD10
- H33.001 Unspecified retinal detachment with retinal break, right eye
- H33.019 Retinal detachment with single break, unspecified eye
- H33.20 Serous retinal detachment, unspecified eye

CLINICAL PEARLS
- If a patient complains of the new onset of floaters or flashes of light, the patient should undergo a dilated eye exam to rule out a retinal tear or retinal detachment.
- There is an increased risk of retinal detachment after cataract surgery.
- PVR can result in redetachment of the retina after an initially successful repair.

RETINOPATHY, DIABETIC

Richard W. Allinson, MD

BASICS

DESCRIPTION
- Noninflammatory retinal disorder characterized by retinal capillary closure and microaneurysms. Retinal ischemia leads to release of a vasoproliferative factor, stimulating neovascularization on retina, optic nerve, or iris.
- Most patients with diabetes mellitus (DM) will develop diabetic retinopathy (DR). It is the leading cause of new cases of legal blindness among residents in the United States between the ages of 20 and 64 years.
- DR can be divided into three stages.
  - Nonproliferative (background)
  - Severe nonproliferative (preproliferative)
  - Proliferative
- System(s) affected: nervous

Geriatric Considerations
Prevalence will increase, as population generally ages and patients with diabetes live longer.

Pregnancy Considerations
- Pregnancy can exacerbate condition.
- Pregnant diabetic women should be examined in 1st trimester, then every 3 months until delivery.

EPIDEMIOLOGY
Incidence
- Peak incidence of type 1, juvenile-onset DM is between the ages of 12 and 15 years.
- Peak incidence of type 2, adult-onset DM is between the ages of 50 and 70 years.
- Incidence of DR is directly related to the duration of diabetes.
- <10 years of age, it is unusual to see DR, regardless of DM duration

Prevalence
- 6.6% of the U.S. population between ages of 20 and 74 years has DM.
- ~25% of the diabetic population has some form of DR.
- Predominant age
  - Risk increases after puberty.
  - 2/3 of juvenile-onset diabetics who have had DM for at least 35 years will develop proliferative DR and will develop macular edema. Proportions are reversed for adult-onset diabetes.
- Predominant sex: male = female (type 1, juvenile-onset DM); female > male (type 2)

ETIOLOGY AND PATHOPHYSIOLOGY
- Related to development of diabetic microaneurysms and microvascular abnormalities
- Reduction in perifoveal capillary blood flow velocity, perifoveal capillary occlusion, and increased retinal thickness at the central fovea in diabetic patients are associated with visual impairment in patients with diabetic macular edema.

RISK FACTORS
- Duration of DM (usually >10 years)
- Poor glycemic control
- Pregnancy
- Renal disease
- Systemic hypertension (HTN)
- Smoking

- Elevated lipid levels associated with increased risk of retinal lipid deposits (hard exudates)
- Myopic eyes (eyes with longer axial length) have a lower risk of DR.

GENERAL PREVENTION
- Monitor and control of blood glucose.
- Schedule yearly ophthalmologic eye exams.

COMMONLY ASSOCIATED CONDITIONS
- Glaucoma
- Cataracts
- Retinal detachment
- Vitreous hemorrhage
- Disc edema (diabetic papillopathy); may occur in type 1/type 2 DM

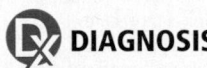

DIAGNOSIS

HISTORY
Diabetic patients should be encouraged to have an annual ophthalmologic exam because early changes are asymptomatic.

PHYSICAL EXAM
- Eye exam: measurement of visual acuity and documentation of the status of the iris, lens, vitreous, and fundus
- Nonproliferative (background) DR
  - Microaneurysms
  - Intraretinal hemorrhage
  - Macular edema causing decrease in central vision
  - Lipid deposits
- Severe nonproliferative (preproliferative) DR
  - Nerve fiber layer infarctions ("cotton wool spots")
  - Venous beading
  - Venous dilatation
  - Intraretinal microvascular abnormalities
  - Extensive retinal hemorrhage
- Proliferative DR
  - New blood vessel proliferation (neovascularization) on the retinal surface, optic nerve, and iris
  - Visual loss caused by vitreous hemorrhage, traction retinal detachment

GENERAL MEASURES
- The Diabetes Control and Complications Trial (DCCT) recommended that for most patients with insulin-dependent DM, blood glucose levels should be as close to the nondiabetic range as is safe to reduce the risk and rate of progression of DR.
  - In the DCCT, insulin-dependent DM patients were randomly assigned into either conventional or intensive insulin treatment. Conventional treatment consisted of one to two daily insulin injections, with daily self-monitoring of urine/blood glucose. Intensive treatment consisted of insulin administered ≥3 times daily by injection/an external pump, with self-monitored blood glucose levels measured at least 4 times per day.
  - The DCCT demonstrated that intensive insulin therapy reduced the risk of macular edema and retinal neovascularization. The benefit of intensive insulin therapy and the reduced risk of DR-associated microvascular complications persist for at least 10 years.
- In the DCCT, intensive insulin therapy was more effective in reducing the risk of progression of DR

in the less advanced stages. However, advanced DR also benefited from the intensive insulin therapy. The Early Treatment Diabetic Retinopathy Study demonstrated that aspirin therapy did not prevent the development of proliferative DR or reduce the risk of visual loss associated with DR.
- Microvascular complications, including proliferative DR, are increased when blood sugar levels are ≥200 mg/dL.
- Poor glycemic control is associated with an increased risk both for development and progression of DR, regardless of the type of DM; that hyperglycemia itself is causative is not established, especially for type 2 DM.
- Cataracts are more common among those with DM. Try to delay cataract surgery in DM patients with retinopathy until the symptoms are severe. Cataract surgery can cause retinopathy to worsen and increase the risk for development of diabetic macular edema.
- HTN has a detrimental effect on DR and must be controlled.

DIFFERENTIAL DIAGNOSIS
Other causes of retinopathy (e.g., radiation, retinal venous obstruction, HTN)

DIAGNOSTIC TESTS & INTERPRETATION
Diagnostic Procedures/Other
- Fluorescein angiography demonstrates retinal nonperfusion, retinal leakage, and proliferative DR.
- Optical coherence tomography (OCT) can be used to help detect diabetic macular edema by measuring retinal thickness.

Test Interpretation
- Increased capillary permeability
- Microaneurysms
- Hemorrhages in retina
- Exudates in retina
- Capillary nonperfusion

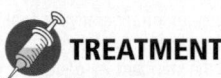

TREATMENT

MEDICATION
- Treatment with the angiotensin-receptor blocker candesartan has been shown to result in regression of DR in some patients (1)[B].

- Nutritional antioxidant intake of vitamins C and E and of β-carotene has no protective effect on DR.
- Atorvastatin may reduce the severity of lipid deposits with clinically significant diabetic macular edema in type 2 DM and dyslipidemia.

SURGERY/OTHER PROCEDURES
- Laser photocoagulation treatment: recommended for patients with proliferative DR and for those with clinically significant macular edema; destroys leaking blood vessels and areas of neovascularization
- The Diabetic Retinopathy Study demonstrated that panretinal photocoagulation reduced overall rate of severe visual loss from 15.9% in untreated eyes to 6.4% in treated eyes. In certain subgroups, the incidence of severe visual loss in untreated eyes was as high as 36.9% within 2 years.
- The Early Treatment Diabetic Retinopathy Study demonstrated that eyes with significant diabetic

macular edema benefited from focal laser treatment. Clinically significant diabetic macular edema (CSDME) is defined as the following:
- Thickening of the retina within 500 μm of the center of the macula
- Hard exudates within 500 μm of the center of the macula associated with thickening of the adjacent retina
- Zone of retinal thickening $\geq$1 disc area within 1 disc diameter of the center of the macula

- Patients with CSDME and high-risk proliferative disease can have simultaneous focal and panretinal photocoagulation without adversely affecting the visual outcome.
- Vitrectomy may benefit some with diffuse macular edema. This may apply especially to eyes with vitreomacular traction found on OCT and with persistent CSDME.
- Intravitreal triamcinolone may be used for DM-related macular edema that fails laser treatment. No long-term benefit of intravitreal triamcinolone relative to focal/grid photocoagulation in patients with CSDME. This is an off-label use (2)[C].

- Ranibizumab, an antibody fragment that binds vascular endothelial growth factor (VEGF), can be used to treat CSDME when injected intravitreally. Ranibizumab 0.3 mg given monthly to treat CSDME resulted in improved vision and reduced central foveal thickness (3)[A]. It is indicated for diabetic macular edema (DME) and for DR in patients with DME.
  - Anti-VEGF therapy is the preferred method of treatment for visual impairment resulting from (DME). Anti VEGF treatment results in superior clinical outcomes compared to laser photocoagulation for DME (4)[A].
  - The 5-year results suggest focal/grid laser treatment at the initiation of intravitreal ranibizumab injection (IRI) is no better than deferring laser treatment for $\geq$24 weeks in eyes with DME involving the central macula with vision impairment (5)[A].
  - Intravitreal ranibizumab treatment for diabetic macular edema may also improve DR severity and reduce the risk of DR progression (6)[A].
  - Monthly (IRI) can slow, but not completely prevent, retinal capillary closure in patients with DME (7)[B].
- Bevacizumab, a full-length antibody that binds VEGF, can be used to treat CSDME when injected intravitreally. This is an off-label use.
  - Intravitreal bevacizumab and ranibizumab have comparable efficacy in treating DME (8)[C].
- Aflibercept, a soluble decoy receptor for VEGF. Aflibercept 2 mg (0.05 mL) injected intravitreally every 4 weeks for the first 5 injections followed by 2 mg (0.05 mL) intravitreally once every 8 weeks. It is indicated for patients with DME and for DR in patients with DME.
  - Intravitreal aflibercept injection (IAI) has demonstrated significant superiority in functional and anatomic endpoints over macular laser photocoagulation (9)[A].
  - At worse levels of initial visual acuity (20/50 or worse) in patients with DME, IAI was more effective in improving vision than ranibizumab or bevacizumab (10)[A]. When the initial vision loss was mild (20/32 to 20/40) in patients with DME, there was no significant difference between aflibercept, ranibizumab, or bevacizumab (10)[A].

- Preoperative bevacizumab can be used as an adjuvant to vitrectomy for complications of proliferative DR. This is an off-label use:
  - At ~10 days after intravitreal injection of bevacizumab, the vascular component of proliferation is markedly reduced, and the contractile components are not yet very significant. Patients with dense fibrovascular proliferation need to be monitored closely for evidence of traction retinal detachment (11)[C].
- Intraocular steroid implants for DME. A dexamethasone implant and a fluocinolone acetonide implant. Complications of these implants include cataract and glaucoma.
- Vitrectomy: recommended for patients with severe proliferative DR, traction retinal detachment involving the macula, and nonclearing vitreous hemorrhage

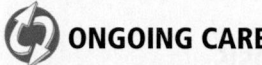 **ONGOING CARE**

FOLLOW-UP RECOMMENDATIONS
Patient Monitoring
Scheduled ophthalmologic eye exams
- Yearly follow-up if no retinopathy
- Every 6 months with background DR
- At least every 3 to 4 months with preproliferative DR
- Every 2 to 3 months with active proliferative DR

DIET
Follow prescribed diet for patients with diabetes.

PATIENT EDUCATION
- Patient education should include regular ophthalmic exams.
- Stress importance of strict blood glucose control through diet, exercise, drugs/insulin, and monitoring of blood glucose.

PROGNOSIS
If the condition is diagnosed and treated early in development, outlook is good. If treatment is delayed, blindness may result.

COMPLICATIONS
- Repeated intravitreal injection of anti-VEGF therapy may increase the risk of sustained intraocular pressure elevation and the possible need for ocular hypotensive treatment (12)[A].
- Blindness

REFERENCES
1. Sjølie AK, Klein R, Porta M, et al. Effect of candesartan on progression and regression of retinopathy in type 2 diabetes (DIRECT-Protect 2): a randomised placebo-controlled trial. *Lancet.* 2008;372(9647):1385–1393.
2. Beck RW, Edwards AR, Aiello LP, et al. Three-year follow-up of a randomized trial comparing focal/grid photocoagulation and intravitreal triamcinolone for diabetic macular edema. *Arch Ophthalmol.* 2009;127(3):245–251.
3. Brown DM, Nguyen QD, Marcus DM, et al. Long-term outcomes of ranibizumab therapy for diabetic macular edema: the 36-month results from two phase III trials: RISE and RIDE. *Ophthalmology.* 2013;120(10):2013–2022.
4. Mitchell P, Wong TY. Management paradigms for diabetic macular edema. *Am J Ophthalmol.* 2014;157(3):505.e8–513.e8.
5. Elman MJ, Ayala A, Bressler NM, et al. Intravitreal ranibizumab for diabetic macular edema with prompt versus deferred laser treatment: 5-year randomized trial results. *Ophthalmology.* 2015;122(2):375–381.
6. Ip MS, Domalpally A, Sun JK, et al. Long-term effects of therapy with ranibizumab on diabetic retinopathy severity and baseline risk factors for worsening retinopathy. *Ophthalmology.* 2015;122(2):367–374.
7. Campochiaro PA, Wykoff CC, Shapiro H, et al. Neutralization of vascular endothelial growth factor slows progression of retinal nonperfusion in patients with diabetic macular edema. *Ophthalmology.* 2014;121(9):1783–1789.
8. Nepomuceno AB, Takaki E, Paes de Almeida FP, et al. A prospective randomized trial of intravitreal bevacizumab versus ranibizumab for the management of diabetic macular edema. *Am J Ophthalmol.* 2013;156(3):502.e2–510.e2.
9. Korobelnik JF, Do DV, Schmidt-Erfurth U, et al. Intravitreal aflibercept for diabetic macular edema. *Ophthalmology.* 2014;121(11):2247–2254.
10. Wells JA, Glassman AR, Ayala AR, et al. Aflibercept, bevacizumab, or ranibizumab for diabetic macular edema. *N Engl J Med.* 2015;372(13):1193–1203.
11. El-Sabagh HA, Abdelghaffar W, Labib AM, et al. Preoperative intravitreal bevacizumab use as an adjuvant to diabetic vitrectomy: histopathologic findings and clinical implications. *Ophthalmology.* 2011;118(4):636–641.
12. Bressler SB, Almukhtar T, Bhorade A, et al. Repeated intravitreous ranibizumab injections for diabetic macular edema and the risk of sustained elevation of intraocular pressure or the need for ocular hypotensive treatment. *JAMA Ophthalmol.* 2015;133(5):589–597.

 SEE ALSO

Diabetes Mellitus, Type 1; Diabetes Mellitus, Type 2

 CODES

ICD10
- E11.319 Type 2 diabetes mellitus with unspecified diabetic retinopathy without macular edema
- E10.319 Type 1 diabetes mellitus with unspecified diabetic retinopathy without macular edema
- E10.329 Type 1 diab w mild nonprlf diabetic rtnop w/o macular edema

CLINICAL PEARLS
- Options for the treatment of diffuse macular edema include focal laser treatment, intravitreal triamcinolone, intravitreal ranibizumab, intravitreal bevacizumab, intravitreal aflibercept, intraocular steroid implants, and vitrectomy.
- High BP should be controlled to reduce the risk of diabetic eye complications.
- Blood glucose levels should be well controlled to help reduce the risk and rate of DR progression.
- Schedule yearly ophthalmologic eye exams.

REYE SYNDROME
Kattie Hoy, MD

 BASICS

DESCRIPTION
- A serious, acute noninflammatory encephalopathy associated with cerebral edema and fatty infiltration of the liver classically noted in children taking aspirin during a viral infection (1,2)
- Occurs primarily in children and adolescents, with an average age of 6 years (2)
- Reye syndrome (RS) is typically biphasic, often initially presenting with symptoms of viral or bacterial infection (i.e., in order of association influenza A or B, varicella, parainfluenza, measles, adenovirus, coxsackieviruses, parechovirus, CMV, EBV, HIV, hepatitis A or B, *Mycoplasma*, and *Chlamydia*), 1 to 5 days without symptoms, followed by onset of severe vomiting, altered mental status, and signs of acute encephalopathy (2,3).
- RS is currently very rare since warning statements by the CDC and American Academy of Pediatrics in 1982 were issues for use of aspirin in children, followed by black box warning in 1986 against use of aspirin in children and teenagers with recent viral illness (4,5).
- System(s) affected: gastrointestinal, nervous, muscular, and cardiac (6)
- Synonym(s): white liver disease

EPIDEMIOLOGY
Incidence
- Predominant age (1,2)
  - 3 months to 12 years, but can occur at any age
  - Peak incidence at 6 years of age
- Predominant sex: male = female (2)
- Currently very rare. In the United States, <0.1/100,000 annually since 1989 (Autret). Prior to issued warnings about aspirin use in children, the United States documented 555 case reports in 1980. Most recent U.S. statistics noted no >2 cases per year between 1994 and 1997 (1).
- Mortality rate 20–40%, male > female (5,7)

ETIOLOGY AND PATHOPHYSIOLOGY
Specific etiology is unknown but appears to be secondary to multiple synergistic factors causing acute mitochondrial injury from significant inhibition of fatty acid oxidation limiting gluconeogenesis causing hypoglycemia, elevated ammonia, acute transaminitis, and hepatic fatty infiltration (1,8).

Genetics
Possible genetic factors that lead to predisposition for development of RS but currently no known genetic pattern (3)

RISK FACTORS
- Pediatric age group
- Prodromal illnesses
  - Viral: influenza A and B, varicella, parainfluenza, measles, adenovirus, coxsackievirus, parechovirus, EBV, CMV, HIV, hepatitis A and B, or rotavirus
  - Bacterial: *Mycoplasma*, *Chlamydia*, *Salmonella*, *Shigella* (3)

- Use of preparations containing aspirin, salicylates, and/or salicylamides (1).
- Other exogenous agents with less significant association: valproic acid, aflatoxin in Thailand, bongkrekate in Indonesia, margosa oil in Southern Asia, unripe ackee fruit in Jamaica, hopentanate in Japan, and insecticides in Canada (1)

GENERAL PREVENTION
- Avoid salicylates in children with viral illnesses because the drug appears to act as a cofactor in susceptible individuals (1).
- A physician should be consulted before giving any child aspirin or antinausea medicines (containing salicylates) during a viral illness, especially influenza A (5).
- Recognize early symptoms of the disease for prompt initiation of supportive treatment (7).

 DIAGNOSIS

RS is a diagnosis of exclusion (1).
- CDC diagnostic criteria (5)
  - Acute noninflammatory encephalopathy with an altered level of consciousness
  - Hepatic dysfunction with liver biopsy showing fatty change or an over 3-fold increase in AST, ALT, and/or ammonia levels
  - No other explanation for cerebral edema or hepatic abnormality
  - Cerebral spinal fluid with white blood cells 8/mm³ of fewer
  - Brain biopsy showing cerebral edema without inflammation
- RS clinical staging system (5)
  - I: vomiting, somnolence, lethargy
  - II: confusion, delirium, combativeness, hyperreflexia, hyperventilation
  - III: obtundation, predominantly flexor motor responses, decorticate, intact pupillary reflex
  - IV: coma, seizures, predominant extensor motor responses, decerebrate posturing, fixed pupils
  - V: coma, flaccid paralysis, loss of deep tendon reflexes, seizures, respiratory arrest, isoelectric EEG, pupils unresponsive

HISTORY
- Recent aspirin use
- Recent prodromal illness
- Sleepiness, lethargy, or confusion
- Sudden onset protracted vomiting

PHYSICAL EXAM
- Hyperpnea, somnolence, altered mental status
- Various stages of neurologic deficits pending stage of syndrome
- Hepatomegaly usually present; icterus absent or only seen moderately; sometimes intracranial pressure elevation (3)[A]

DIFFERENTIAL DIAGNOSIS
- Acute encephalopathy without hepatic abnormalities
  - Encephalitis
  - Meningitis
  - Drug overdose
  - Poisoning
  - Psychiatric illness
  - Diabetes mellitus
- Reye-like syndrome: acute toxic encephalopathy with hepatic abnormalities due to either metabolic disorders or drug or toxin ingestions, including the following (3):
  - Inherited metabolic disorders: organic acidurias with defects in hepatic fatty acid oxidation; fatty acid metabolism defects
  - Acyl-CoA dehydrogenase, carnitine deficiency
    - Urea cycle defects
    - Carbamoyl phosphate synthetase, ornithine transcarbamylase
    - Fructosemia
  - The most commonly diagnosed metabolic disorder in association with RS is medium-chain acyl-coenzyme A dehydrogenase deficiency.
  - Toxin ingestions

DIAGNOSTIC TESTS & INTERPRETATION
- Over 3-fold elevations of AST, ALT, and/or ammonia (5)
- Hypoglycemia (8)
- Possible coagulopathy with abnormal bleeding time, PT, PTT, and/or platelet count (7)
- Mixed respiratory alkalosis and metabolic acidosis (3)
- MRI findings of cerebral edema with signal alteration in many areas including brainstem, thalami, temporal lobe, parasagittal cortex, cerebellar, and subcortical white matter (9)[C]

Follow-Up Tests & Special Considerations
Usually complete resolution of lesions on T2-weighted images except in areas of thalamus, which can take many months to resolve (9)[C]

Diagnostic Procedures/Other
- Lumbar puncture with CSF pressure measurement (5)
- Liver biopsy (5,7)
- Brain biopsy (5)

Test Interpretation
- Liver biopsy notes variably sized multiple intracellular and extracellular vacuoles representing microvesicular steatosis. Hepatocytes also display nuclear pyknosis and fragmentation. The mitochondria are distorted with destroyed cristae (10).
- Brain biopsy with cerebral edema without inflammation (5)
- Increased CSF pressure without pleocytosis (<8 leukocytes/mm³) (5)

Pediatric Considerations
- It is essential to make the diagnosis as early as possible and start appropriate supportive measures immediately as progression to more severe stage is associated with higher mortality (7).
- Must investigate for inborn errors of metabolism in any patient suspected to have RS as well as other etiology due to RS being a diagnosis of exclusion (1).

TREATMENT

GENERAL MEASURES

- Supportive care dictated by the severity of illness (5)[A]
- IV glucose and frequent monitoring of serum glucose to treat hypoglycemia (7)[B].
- Hyperventilation, mannitol, glycerol, and corticosteroids to control intracranial pressure (7)[B]
- Vitamin K, fresh frozen plasma, and platelets as needed for treatment of coagulopathy (7)[B]
- Mechanical ventilation as needed
- Dialysis to remove toxins and toxic metabolites (7)[B]

MEDICATION

- All treatment is supportive and may include the following (7)[B]:
  - Glucose 10–15% IV
  - Vitamin K
  - For increased intracranial pressure
    - Mannitol
    - Dexamethasone
    - Glycerol
- Contraindications: NSAIDs such as diclofenac and mefenamic acid may complicate clinical picture so should not be used (3)[A].
- Precautions: Mannitol and poor renal output may result in vascular overload and pulmonary edema.
- Resveratrol used in animals studies showed protection against the oxidative stress occurring in RS but has yet been researched in clinical practice (10).

SURGERY/OTHER PROCEDURES
Liver transplant (11)[C]

INPATIENT CONSIDERATIONS
Admission Criteria/Initial Stabilization
Medical emergency requiring immediate hospitalization and frequent monitoring, often in an intensive care setting (3)[A]

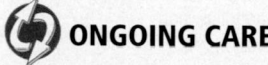 ## ONGOING CARE

FOLLOW-UP RECOMMENDATIONS
Complete bed rest until recovery is noted and able to return to normal activity as tolerated.

Patient Monitoring
Depends on specific residual effects. may require care of physicians; nurses; psychologists; and/or physical, occupational, and/or speech therapists (7)[B]

DIET
NPO during the acute phase

PATIENT EDUCATION
- National Reye Syndrome Foundation, P.O. Box 829, Byron, OH 43506-0829 (800) 233-7393; www.reyessyndrome.org
- National Institutes of Health: http://www.ninds.nih.gov/disorders/reyes_syndrome/reyes_syndrome.htm

PROGNOSIS

- Overall prognosis is related to degree of cerebral edema and ammonia level on admission, correlated with severity of stage (7)[B].
- Outcomes range from a mild illness without progression and complete resolution to a critical illness with significant lasting sequelae or death (7)[B].
- Possible neurologic sequelae include brain damage and disability, problems with attention, concentration, speech, language, and fine and gross motor skills.
- Sequelae are more common with higher stages.

COMPLICATIONS
- Aspiration pneumonia
- Respiratory failure
- Cardiac dysrhythmia/arrest
- Inappropriate vasopressin excretion
- Diabetes insipidus
- Cerebral edema
- Seizures
- Death

REFERENCES

1. Glasgow JF. Reye's syndrome: the case for a causal link with aspirin. Drug Saf. 2006;29(12):1111–1121.
2. Autret-Leca E, Jonville-Béra AP, Llau ME, et al. Incidence of Reye's syndrome in France: a hospital-based survey. J Clin Epidemiol. 2001;54(8):857–862.
3. Pugliese A, Beltramo T, Torre D. Reye's and Reye's-like syndromes. Cell Biochem Funct. 2008;26(7):741–746.
4. Bennett CL, Starko KM, Thomsen HS, et al. Linking drugs to obscure illnesses: lessons from pure red cell aplasia, nephrogenic systemic fibrosis, and Reye's syndrome. A report from the Southern Network on Adverse Reactions (SONAR). J Gen Intern Med. 2012;27(12):1697–1703.
5. Degnan LA. Reye's syndrome: a rare but serious pediatric condition. US Pharm. 2012;37(3):HS6–HS8.
6. Gosalakkal JA, Kamoji V. Reye syndrome and Reye-like syndrome. Pediatr Neurol. 2008;39(3):198–200.
7. Wulur H, Kho LK. Treatment of Reye's syndrome at Sumber Waras Hospital. Acta Paediatr Jpn. 1990;32(4):435–442.
8. Tein I. Impact of fatty acid oxidation disorders in child neurology: from Reye syndrome to Pandora's box. Dev Med Child Neurol. 2015;57(4):304–306.
9. Singh P, Goraya JS, Gupta K, et al. Magnetic resonance imaging findings in Reye syndrome: case report and review of the literature. J Child Neurol. 2011;26(8):1009–1014.
10. Abdin A, Sarhan N. Resveratrol protects against experimental induced Reye's syndrome by prohibition of oxidative stress and restoration of complex I activity. Can J Physiol Pharmacol. 2014;92(9):780–788.
11. Cağ M, Saouli AC, Audet M, et al. Reye syndrome and liver transplantation. Turk J Pediatr. 2010;52(6):662–664.

ADDITIONAL READING

- Belay ED, Bresee JS, Holman RC, et al. Reye's syndrome in the United States from 1981 through 1997. N Engl J Med. 1999;340(18):1377–1382.
- Fischer H. Aspirin and Reye's syndrome. Pediatrics. 2001;107(1):214.
- Glasgow JF, Middleton B. Reye syndrome—insights on causation and prognosis. Arch Dis Child. 2001;85(5):351–353.
- Monto AS. The disappearance of Reye's syndrome—a public health triumph. N Engl J Med. 1999;340(18):1423–1424.
- Schrör K. Aspirin and Reye syndrome: a review of the evidence. Paediatr Drugs. 2007;9(3):195–204.
- Whitten R, Milner DA Jr, Yeh MM, et al. Liver pathology in Malawian children with fatal encephalopathy. Hum Pathol. 2011;42(9):1230–1239.

 ### SEE ALSO

Encephalitis, Viral; Hepatic Encephalopathy

 ### CODES

ICD10
G93.7 Reye's syndrome

CLINICAL PEARLS

- RS is a rare, acute noninflammatory encephalopathy largely affecting children and adolescents.
- Associations include antecedent viral/bacterial infection and aspirin use.
- Most current cases of RS are actually Reye-like syndromes, caused by an inborn error of metabolism or a toxin exposure.
- All current treatment is supportive.
- Acetaminophen is first choice to treat fever followed by ibuprofen, in children.
- Prognosis is related to the degree of cerebral edema and ammonia level on admission and ranges from complete resolution to persistent neurologic sequelae or death.

RH INCOMPATIBILITY

Kirsten A. Winnie, MD • Jennifer G. Chang, MD

BASICS

DESCRIPTION
- Antibody-mediated destruction of red blood cells (RBCs) that bear Rh surface antigens in individuals who lack the antigens and have become isoimmunized (sensitized) to them
  - System(s) affected: hematologic/lymphatic/immunologic
  - Synonym(s): Rh isoimmunization; Rh alloimmunization; Rh sensitization

EPIDEMIOLOGY
Incidence
Predominant age and sex: affects fetuses/neonates of isoimmunized, childbearing females

ETIOLOGY AND PATHOPHYSIOLOGY
- Circulating antibodies to Rh antigens (transplacentally transferred antibodies in the case of a fetus/newborn) attach to Rh antigens on RBCs.
- Immune-mediated destruction of RBCs leads to hemolysis, anemia, and increased bilirubin production.
- Transfusion of Rh-positive blood to Rh-negative recipient
- Maternal exposure to fetal Rh antigens, either antepartum or intrapartum
- Most commonly seen in the Rh-positive fetus or infant of an Rh-negative mother

Genetics
- Complex autosomal inheritance of polypeptide Rh antigens; three genetic loci with closely related genes carry an assortment of alleles: Dd, Cc, and Ee.
- Individuals who express the D antigen (also called *Rho* or *Rho[D]*) are considered Rh-positive. Individuals lacking the D antigen are Rh-negative.
- Variant D alleles (weak D and partial D) are heterogenous, altered forms of the D antigen. Some D variants are at risk of formation of anti-D antibodies, whereas others are not. With current blood typing procedures, certain D variants likely to produce alloimmunization are typed as D-negative, although this does not include all genetic subtypes at risk of isoimmunization (1).
- Another variant D antigen, DEL, has been identified in some individuals (predominantly Asians) who are classified as Rh-negative by the usual assays. Although testing Rh-negative, these individuals are not likely to be sensitized by exposure to Rh-D antigens through pregnancy or transfusion and should be considered clinically Rh-positive (2).
- Antibodies may be produced to C, c, D, E, or e in individuals lacking the specific antigen; only D is strongly immunogenic (3).
- Isoimmunization to Rh antigens in susceptible individuals is acquired, not inherited.

RISK FACTORS
- ~15% of the white population and smaller fractions of other races are Rh-negative and susceptible to sensitization (4).
- Any Rh-positive pregnancy in an Rh-negative woman can result in sensitization.
- Weak D and partial D women are a heterogenous group. Although previously reported to be Rh positive and treated as such, alloimmunization has been reported and can result in HDFN or fatal hydrops fetalis (5).
- Native risk of isoimmunization after Rh-positive pregnancy had been estimated at ≤15% but seems to be decreasing.
- The risk of isoimmunization antepartum is only 1–2%.
- The risk of isoimmunization is 1–2% after spontaneous abortion and 4–5% after induced abortion (6).
- Use of Rho(D) immunoglobulin prophylaxis has reduced incidence of isoimmunization to <1% of susceptible pregnancies (7)[A].

GENERAL PREVENTION
- Blood typing (ABO and Rh) on all pregnant women and prior to blood transfusions
- Antibody screening early in pregnancy
- Rh immunoglobulin prevents only sensitization to the D antigen.
- For prophylaxis, Rho(D) immunoglobulin (RhIG, RhoGAM, HyperRHO, Rhophylac) given to unsensitized, Rh-negative women after the following:
  - Spontaneous abortion
  - Induced abortion
  - Ectopic pregnancy
  - Antepartum hemorrhage
  - Trauma to abdomen
  - Amniocentesis
  - Chorionic villus sampling
  - Within 72 hours of delivery of an Rh-positive infant
  - Given routinely at 28 weeks' gestation
- Prophylaxis is to prevent sensitization affecting a subsequent pregnancy and has little effect on the current pregnancy.
- Dose for prophylaxis
  - 50-μg dose for events up to 12 weeks' gestation
  - 300-μg dose for events after 12 weeks' gestation
  - Higher doses may be required in the event of a large fetal–maternal hemorrhage (>30 mL of whole blood).

COMMONLY ASSOCIATED CONDITIONS
- Hemolytic disease of newborn
- Hydrops fetalis
- Neonatal jaundice
- Kernicterus
- See "Erythroblastosis Fetalis" topic.

DIAGNOSIS

PHYSICAL EXAM
- Jaundice of newborn
- Kernicterus
- Fetal hydrops or fetal death in utero if severe (see "Erythroblastosis Fetalis" topic)

DIFFERENTIAL DIAGNOSIS
- ABO incompatibility
- Other blood group (non-Rh) isoimmunization
- Nonimmune fetal hydrops
- Hereditary spherocytosis
- RBC enzyme defects

DIAGNOSTIC TESTS & INTERPRETATION
Initial Tests (lab, imaging)
- Positive indirect Coombs test (antibody screen) during pregnancy
- Paternal blood type
- Kleihauer-Betke (fetal hemoglobin acid elution, Hb F slide elution) test to quantify an acute fetal–maternal bleed
- Flow cytometry using antibody to hemoglobin F is emerging as an alternative to the Kleihauer-Betke test to detect or quantify fetal–maternal bleed (8).
- Congenital or fetal anemia
- Blood type, direct Coombs test in newborn
- Cell-free fetal DNA (Cff DNA) test (see "Clinical Pearls")

Follow-Up Tests & Special Considerations
Prior administration of Rho(D) may lead to weakly (false-) positive indirect Coombs test in mother and direct Coombs test in infant.

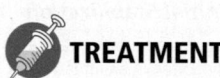

TREATMENT

GENERAL MEASURES
- Depending on severity of involvement, treatment of fetus may include the following:
  - Intrauterine transfusion (9)[C]
  - Early delivery
- Treatment of newborn may include the following:
  - Exchange transfusion
  - Transfusion after delivery
  - Phototherapy
- Inconclusive evidence on efficacy of IVIG to reduce need for exchange transfusion (10)[A]

ISSUES FOR REFERRAL

Because of the specialized, somewhat hazardous treatment measures involved, pregnancies in Rh-sensitized women are usually managed at tertiary-care facilities with maternal fetal medicine specialists.

INPATIENT CONSIDERATIONS

Admission Criteria/Initial Stabilization

Initial monitoring of the newborn is inpatient or in special care nursery if treatment interventions are needed.

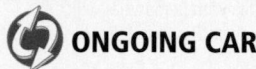 ONGOING CARE

FOLLOW-UP RECOMMENDATIONS

Patient Monitoring

- In most cases, outpatient ambulatory management is appropriate during the antepartum period.
- Antibody titer measured at 20 weeks and every 4 weeks thereafter during pregnancy; a titer of ≥1:16 indicates the need for further testing (5).
- If the patient had a previously affected infant, an Rh-positive fetus in the current pregnancy should be considered at risk regardless of antibody titers (11).
  - Fetal heart rate testing/US to assess fetal status
  - Doppler US measurement of cerebral blood flow is now a suitable alternative to invasive tests (amniocentesis, cordocentesis) for diagnosing fetal anemia (11).
  - Umbilical blood sampling (cordocentesis) for fetal blood type, hematocrit, reticulocyte count, and presence of erythroblasts (5)
  - Amniocentesis for amniotic fluid bilirubin levels (5)
  - Amniocentesis for fetal lung maturity if early delivery is a treatment option (5).

PROGNOSIS

- With appropriate monitoring and treatment, infants born of severely affected pregnancies have a survival rate of >80% (11).
- Even with severe disease, the neurologic outcome of survivors is generally good (8)[C].
- Fetuses with hydrops have a higher mortality rate and higher risk of neurologic impairment (8)[C].
- Disease is likely to be more severe in affected subsequent pregnancies.

COMPLICATIONS

- Pregnancy loss from umbilical blood sampling
- Pregnancy loss from intrauterine transfusion
- Fetal distress requiring emergent delivery (12)

REFERENCES

1. Flegel WA. Molecular genetics and clinical applications for RH. *Transfus Apher Sci*. 2011;44(1):81–91.
2. Shao CP, Xu H, Xu Q, et al. Antenatal Rh prophylaxis is unnecessary for "Asia type" DEL women. *Transfus Clin Biol*. 2010;17(4):260–264.
3. Agre P, Cartron JP. Molecular biology of the Rh antigens. *Blood*. 1991;78(3):551–563.
4. Bianchi DW, Avent ND, Costa JM, et al. Noninvasive prenatal diagnosis of fetal Rhesus D: ready for Prime(r) Time. *Obstet Gynecol*. 2005;106(4):841–844.
5. American College of Obstetricians and Gynecologists. ACOG Practice Bulletin No. 75: management of alloimmunization during pregnancy. *Obstet Gynecol*. 2006;108(2):457–464.
6. Bowman J. Thirty-five years of Rh prophylaxis. *Transfusion*. 2003;43(12):1661–1666.
7. Crowther CA, Middleton P, McBain RD. Anti-D administration in pregnancy for preventing Rhesus alloimmunisation. *Cochrane Database Syst Rev*. 2013;(2):CD000020.
8. Kim YA, Makar RS. Detection of fetomaternal hemorrhage. *Am J Hematol*. 2012;87(4):417–423.
9. Lindenburg IT, Smits-Wintjens VE, van Klink JM, et al. Long-term neurodevelopmental outcome after intrauterine transfusion for hemolytic disease of the fetus/newborn: the LOTUS study. *Am J Obstet Gynecol*. 2012;206(2):141.e1–141.e8.
10. Louis D, More K, Oberoi S, et al. Intravenous immunoglobulin in isoimmune haemolytic disease of newborn: an updated systematic review and meta-analysis. *Arch Dis Child Fetal Neonatal Ed*. 2014;99(4):F325–F331.
11. Moise KJ Jr, Argoti PS. Management and prevention of red cell alloimmunization in pregnancy: a systematic review. *Obstet Gynecol*. 2012;120(5):1132–1139.
12. Elalfy MS, Elbarbary NS, Abaza HW. Early intravenous immunoglobulin (two-dose regimen) in the management of severe Rh hemolytic disease of newborn—a prospective randomized controlled trial. *Eur J Pediatr*. 2011;170(4):461–467.
13. Tiblad E, Tuane Wikman A, Ajne G, et al. Targeted routine antenatal anti-D prophylaxis in the prevention of RhD immunization—outcome of a new antenatal screening and prevention program. *PLoS One*. 2013;8(8):e70984.
14. Hawk AF, Chang EY, Shields SM, et al. Costs and clinical outcomes of noninvasive fetal RhD typing for targeted prophylaxis. *Obstet Gynecol*. 2013;122(3):579–585.

ADDITIONAL READING

American College of Obstetricians and Gynecologists. ACOG Practice Bulletin No. 4: prevention of Rh D alloimmunization. *Int J Gynaecol Obstet*. 1999;66(1): 63–70.

 SEE ALSO

Anemia, Autoimmune Hemolytic; Erythroblastosis Fetalis; Jaundice

 CODES

ICD10

- P55.0 Rh isoimmunization of newborn
- O36.0990 Maternal care for other rhesus isoimmunization, unspecified trimester, not applicable or unspecified
- T80.40XA Rh incompat react due to tranfs of bld/bld prod, unsp, init

CLINICAL PEARLS

- If paternity is certain, determining that the father does not carry the Rh(D) blood group antigen eliminates the need to give RhIG prophylaxis during pregnancy or the need for special fetal surveillance if the mother is already sensitized.
- Cell-free fetal DNA (Cff DNA) testing has evolved as the standard practice in many European countries; it is available in the United States but is not a widely covered benefit. It allows detection of fetal Rh genotype with accuracy of 97.1%, sensitivity of 97.2%, and specificity of 96.8% (11).
- Cff DNA testing with selective administration of Rh immunoglobulin when the fetus tests Rh positive has been shown to be as effective at preventing new Rh sensitization when compared to routine administration of Rh-immunoglobulin to all Rh-negative women. Such an approach avoids unnecessary use of Rh immunoglobulin (13). Currently, routine administration of Rh immune globulin is more cost effective than use of Cff DNA testing in the United States (14).
- The dose of RhIG for prophylaxis is affected by gestational age. The fetal blood volume is only a few milliliters at 12 weeks' gestation. Therefore, a 50-μg dose of RhIG may be used for threatened, spontaneous, or induced abortions up to 12 weeks' gestation, instead of the standard 300-μg dose.

RHABDOMYOLYSIS

Caroline Tschibelu, MD • Chirag N. Shah, MD

BASICS

DESCRIPTION
- Breakdown of skeletal muscle cells and release of intracellular contents into the circulation
- Rhabdomyolysis typically manifests with muscle aches, pains and weakness, and reddish brown (tea-colored) urine, but up to 50% of patients are asymptomatic.

EPIDEMIOLOGY
Incidence
Annually in the United States: 26,000 hospitalized cases

ETIOLOGY AND PATHOPHYSIOLOGY
- Direct muscle trauma (most common cause)
  - Crush injuries
  - Extended periods of muscle pressure (during surgery, unconscious from alcohol ingestion)
  - Burns, electrocution, lightning strike
- Muscle exertion
  - Intense and/or prolonged physical exercise (marathon runners, athletes, contact sports)
  - Seizures
  - Delirium tremens
- Drugs and toxins
  - Alcohol
  - Cocaine (most common recreational drug), methamphetamine, phencyclidine
  - Antipsychotics (due to neuroleptic malignant syndrome, malignant hyperthermia, and severe dystonia)
  - Zidovudine
  - Antimalarials
  - Heroin
  - HMG-CoA reductase inhibitors (statins) (risk <0.01%), higher with high dose and in combination with fibrates
  - Fibrates
  - Colchicine
  - Corticosteroids
  - Carbon monoxide
  - Snake envenomation
  - Bath salts (1)[B]
  - Synthetic cannabinoid: Abuse of synthetic marijuana has been associated with severe rhabdomyolysis (2)[C].
- Muscle ischemia
  - Thrombosis, embolism, sickle cell disease
  - Compartment syndrome
  - Tourniquets
- Infections
  - Viral: influenza A and B, coxsackievirus, HIV, varicella
  - Bacterial: *Streptococcus* or *Staphylococcus* sepsis, gas gangrene, necrotizing fasciitis, *Salmonella*, *Legionella*
  - Malaria
- Hypothermia
- Hyperthermia
- Autoimmune and genetic disorders
  - Polymyositis, dermatomyositis
  - Muscular dystrophies
  - Disorders of lipid metabolism (e.g., carnitine palmitoyltransferase deficiency)
  - Disorders of carbohydrate metabolism (i.e., phosphofructokinase deficiency, phosphoglycerate mutase, myophosphorylase deficiency, aka McArdle disease/deficiency)
  - Glycogen storage diseases (e.g., phosphorylase B kinase deficiency) and others (e.g., lactate dehydrogenase A deficiency)
- Metabolic and endocrinologic:
  - Hypothyroidism or thyrotoxicosis
  - Electrolyte imbalances (e.g., hyponatremia, hypernatremia, hypokalemia, hypocalcemia, hypophosphatemia)
  - Diabetic ketoacidosis
  - Hyperosmolar state

Genetics
- Hereditary causes of rhabdomyolysis are rare but should be suspected for children, patients with recurrent attacks, or patients who have attacks after minimal exertion, mild illness, or starvation.
- The main inherited disorders are described earlier in "Etiology and Pathophysiology."

RISK FACTORS
See "Etiology and Pathophysiology."

GENERAL PREVENTION
- Avoid excessive exertional muscle injury. Preventing hypovolemia is important to prevent renal hypoperfusion, acidemia, and subsequent renal failure.
- Avoid precipitating drugs, metabolic and electrolyte abnormalities.

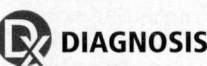

DIAGNOSIS

HISTORY
- Crush injury: direct trauma, prolonged compression/immobility. Causes include motor vehicle accidents (MVA) and entrapment in collapsed buildings. The elderly are more susceptible to crush injury due to immobility and falls. Rhabdomyolysis usually occurs after 1 hour of immobilization, but cases reported with compression lasting <20 minutes.
- Possible history of overexertion or use of drug/toxin (e.g., cocaine, amphetamine, statins)
- Patient may complain of muscle aches, cramps, or fatigue.
- Agitation while patients are in restraints

PHYSICAL EXAM
- May have obvious muscle tenderness/injury and swelling on exam, or muscle exam may be completely normal
- Tea-colored urine is indicative of myoglobinuria.
- Decreased urine output may indicate renal failure.

DIFFERENTIAL DIAGNOSIS
- For acute renal failure with rhabdomyolysis: Any disease that causes acute tubular necrosis may be confused with rhabdomyolysis.
- Renal pigment injury from hemoglobin resembles pigment injury from myoglobin.

DIAGNOSTIC TESTS & INTERPRETATION
Initial Tests (lab, imaging)
- Creatine kinase (CK) is the most important diagnostic enzyme: Elevated >5 times the upper limit of normal or >1,000 U/L. CK levels >5,000 U/L are causally related to acute renal failure (ARF) (3)[A] and should prompt aggressive fluid resuscitation.
- CK levels peak at ~24 hours and return to normal after 3 to 5 days, making it a more sensitive marker than myoglobin. CK is also a cheaper and an easier surrogate than myoglobin. Myoglobin is the enzyme responsible for kidney failure (3)[A].

- Serum myoglobin levels peak within a few hours and return to normal after ~24 hours, as it is cleared quickly from the circulation. Urine/serum myoglobin levels may be useful markers early on, but normal levels do not rule out rhabdomyolysis because of its rapid clearance.
- Urinalysis: Dipstick test positive for blood without erythrocytes in sediment is suggestive of injury from either hemoglobin or myoglobin. However, rhabdomyolysis often presents with hematuria, which is a limitation to using dipstick due to false-positive results.
- Marked elevations of potassium from the muscle injury sometimes are compounded by ARF.
- Initial hypocalcemia: Calcium enters the injured muscle cells and precipitates as calcium phosphate, leading to calcification of ischemic muscle cells. Only correct initial hypocalcemia if patient is symptomatic or has ECG changes; it will self-resolve during the renal recovery phase.
- Hypercalcemia during renal recovery phase: Unique to rhabdomyolysis-induced ARF for 20–30% of patients (3)[A]. As renal function improves, there is mobilization of the precipitated calcium, increase in calcitriol, and hyperphosphatemia resolves.
- Extreme hyperuricemia may be present and can cause acute uric acid nephropathy in the setting of rhabdomyolysis.
- Elevations in BUN and creatinine are indicative of acute renal failure.
- Reversible hepatic dysfunction can occur. However, elevations in alanine aminotransferase (ALT), aspartate aminotransferase (AST), and lactic dehydrogenase may be due to muscle injury and may not indicate any hepatic injury.
- Disseminated intravascular coagulation (DIC) can occur, with increase in coagulation times, fibrin degradation products, and D-dimer; decreases in platelets and fibrinogen.
- Place patient on a 12-lead ECG if rhabdomyolysis is suspected because hyperkalemia can induce fatal arrhythmias.

Follow-Up Tests & Special Considerations
- Delayed renal failure/electrolyte abnormalities despite normal initial levels
- Ongoing muscle injury is manifested by rising creatine phosphokinase (CPK).
- Any renal imaging is similar to other evaluations of acute renal failure.

Diagnostic Procedures/Other
Muscle compartment pressures if compartment syndrome is suspected

Test Interpretation
- Muscle necrosis
- Myoglobin-related renal injury may resemble acute tubular necrosis from other causes.

TREATMENT

GENERAL MEASURES
- Aggressive hydration is often necessary. With severe muscle trauma (crush injuries), up to 12 L of fluid may be sequestered in the muscles, leading to intravascular volume depletion and explaining the low urine output despite fluid resuscitation, which increase the risk for renal failure.

- Monitor CK levels to ensure that rhabdomyolysis has ended.
- Monitor renal function and electrolytes.
- Continuous monitoring of potassium levels to prevent hyperkalemic arrhythmias and potential hypokalemia and arrhythmias.
- If DIC/hepatic dysfunction occurs, patients will need treatment and monitoring appropriate to these conditions.

MEDICATION

First Line
- When rhabdomyolysis is identified, appropriate intervention may prevent renal failure.
- Aggressive fluid resuscitation is the most important intervention: normal saline (NS) and 5% glucose solution with a target urine output of 200 mL/hr. Alternating NS and 5% glucose is recommended to prevent volume overload. Infusion rate should be 500 mL/hr (4)[C].
- Alkalinization of the urine is thought to decrease myoglobin-induced nephrotoxicity in the tubules (sodium bicarbonate to increase urine pH >6.5):
  - Use is controversial without strong evidence of efficacy.
  - Side effects include worsening hypocalcemia.
  - Sodium bicarbonate may be of use in patients with very high CK levels, an acidotic state, or coexisting hyperkalemia.
  - Place 150 mEq (3 ampules) NaHCO3 in 1 L of D5W and infuse at 200 mL/hr.

Second Line
- IV mannitol as a bolus if urine output remains low, 1 to 2 g/kg, not to exceed 200 g in 24 hours and cumulative dose up to 800 g. It is used to prevent ARF (5)[C]. Plasma osmolality should be closely monitored and stopped if diuresis is not adequate (>20 mL/hr).
  - Increases prostaglandins production leading to renal vasodilation and diuresis, making the kidneys less susceptible to myoglobin injury. Also an osmotic agent, filtered but not reabsorbed by the tubules, it increases sodium delivery and diuresis. This may remove necrotic cell debris and fluids trapped in damaged muscle cells preventing rise in compartment pressure and compartment syndrome.
  - Use of mannitol is controversial in this setting because no good evidence indicates that it improves outcomes more than aggressive IV hydration. It is a free-radical scavenger and has renal protective effects when used early, before tubular occlusion.
  - Consider adding furosemide to force diuresis if necessary (40 to 120 mg/day).
  - Diuresis should not be used in anuric renal failure. Customize the regimen for elderly and patients with heart disease.
- Hyperkalemia can result from massive release of intracellular potassium stores or ARF. Severe hyperkalemia may be life-threatening. Treatment is warranted when ECG changes are present (tall, thin T waves; PR prolongation; QRS widening; P wave flattening).
- Treatments aiming at resolving hyperkalemia:
  - Calcium gluconate: to stabilize the cardiac membrane. IV 1 to 2 ampules (0.5 mL 10% Calcium gluconate = 4 mg elemental calcium; give 4 mg/kg/hr for 4 hours)
  - If acidosis is present: 1 to 2 ampules (2 to 3 mL/kg) sodium bicarbonate IV. Remember that sodium bicarbonate administration worsens hypocalcemia.

- If tolerated: Oral sodium polystyrene sulfonate (Kayexalate) as much as 20 g (1 g/kg) can be given via enema.
  - Insulin and albuterol will transiently drive potassium into the cells. Administration of glucose can prevent the hypoglycemic effects of insulin.
  - Precautions: See "Etiology and Pathophysiology," especially drug combinations. Continuous monitoring of potassium levels to prevent overcorrecting with potential hypokalemia and arrhythmias.
  - Indications for dialysis include resistant and symptomatic hyperkalemia (ECG), oliguria (<0.5 mL/kg over 12-hour period), anuria, volume overload, or persistent acidosis (pH <7.1).

ISSUES FOR REFERRAL
- Usually managed as an inpatient
- Diagnosis of muscle entrapment/compartment syndromes may require surgical intervention (fasciotomy) to stop rhabdomyolysis.
- Early escharotomy for compartment syndrome related to burn
- Renal dialysis may be indicated in ARF.

ADDITIONAL THERAPIES
During the oliguric phase, symptomatic hypocalcemia is possible but rare and may benefit from IV calcium gluconate.

SURGERY/OTHER PROCEDURES
For muscle entrapment/compartment syndrome

INPATIENT CONSIDERATIONS

Admission Criteria/Initial Stabilization
- Patients with significant elevations of CK should be admitted for IV hydration and serial laboratory monitoring.
- Usually required for symptomatic patients or other complications

IV Fluids
Volume expansion with normal saline to increase urine output to at least 150 mL/hr

Nursing
Monitoring of vital signs and urine output

Discharge Criteria
CK usually peaks 24 to 36 hours after muscle injury, so monitoring should confirm that the CK is trending down. Renal function should be stable/improving. Electrolytes should be normal. Patients with mild CK elevation, trending down, and normal renal function may be discharged after observation phase.

 ## ONGOING CARE

FOLLOW-UP RECOMMENDATIONS
Outpatient assessment within a few days to recheck CPK, electrolytes, and renal function

Patient Monitoring
- Contingent on disease: essential for metabolic myopathies
- Myotoxic drugs should be discontinued/monitored closely.

DIET
- With renal failure, restrict protein intake to lower BUN level.
- Limit potassium intake.
- With anuria, essential to restrict volume intake

PROGNOSIS
Contingent on primary cause of rhabdomyolysis and on recovery from ARF without complications

COMPLICATIONS
- Death, especially from hyperkalemia/renal failure
- With dialysis and supportive care, the prognosis is very good.

REFERENCES

1. Murphy CM, Dulaney AR, Beuhler MC, et al. "Bath salts" and "plant food" products: the experience of one regional US poison center. *J Med Toxicol*. 2013;9(1):42–48.
2. Durand D, Delgado LL, de la Parra-Pellot DM, et al. Psychosis and severe rhabdomyolysis associated with synthetic cannabinoid use: a case report. *Clin Schizophr Relat Psychoses*. 2015;8(4):205–208.
3. Parekh R, Care DA, Tainter CR. Rhabdomyolysis: advances in diagnosis and treatment. *Emerg Med Pract*. 2012;14(3):1–15.
4. Petejova N, Martinek A. Acute kidney injury due to rhabdomyolysis and renal replacement therapy: a critical review. *Crit Care*. 2014;18(3):224.
5. Cervellin G, Comelli I, Lippi G. Rhabdomyolysis: historical background, clinical, diagnostic and therapeutic features. *Clin Chem Lab Med*. 2010;48(6):749–756.

ADDITIONAL READING

- Bosch X, Poch E, Grau JM. Rhabdomyolysis and acute kidney injury. *N Engl J Med*. 2009;361(1):62–72.
- Shawkat H, Westwood MM, Mortimer A. Mannitol: a review of its clinical uses. *Contin Educ Anaesth Crit Care Pain*. 2012;12(2):82–85.

 ## SEE ALSO

Algorithm: Acute Kidney Injury (Acute Renal Failure)

CODES

ICD10
- M62.82 Rhabdomyolysis
- T79.6XXA Traumatic ischemia of muscle, initial encounter
- T79.6XXD Traumatic ischemia of muscle, subsequent encounter

CLINICAL PEARLS
- Acute CPK elevation into the thousands (often tens of thousands) is necessary before one sees myoglobinuric renal failure.
- The cornerstone of treatment of rhabdomyolysis is aggressive fluid administration.
- Frequent monitoring of potassium, calcium, and creatinine is necessary in the acute period.

RHABDOMYOSARCOMA

Olusola Fasusi, MD • E. James Kruse, DO

BASICS

DESCRIPTION
- Rhabdomyosarcoma (RMS) is the most common soft tissue sarcoma in children <20 years of age. (It is exceedingly rare in adults, representing 3% of all soft tissue sarcomas.)
  - 50% occur in the 1st decade of life.
- Overall, it is an uncommon malignancy that arises from myoblasts.
- Common anatomic sites
  - Head and neck (most common primary site in children)
  - Genitourinary
  - Musculoskeletal (Extremities are the most common primary sites in adults.)
- Subtypes
  - Alveolar (ARMS): 23% of cases
    - More common in the trunk and extremities; clinically more aggressive
  - Embryonal (ERMS): early onset; 57% of cases (most common subtype in children)
    - More likely to occur in the head, neck, and genitourinary areas
      - Classic: comprises 50% of cases
      - Botryoid: Sarcoma botryoids is typically seen in girls <4 years of age, 6% of cases.
      - Spindle cell: 3% of cases pleomorphic: usually occurs in adults, 1% of cases
- Sarcoma (not otherwise specified): comprises 11% of all cases of RMS (most common subtype in adults, reflects inability for pathologists to characterize tumor)
- Undifferentiated: comprises 8% of all cases of RMS
- Associated term(s): soft tissue sarcoma

EPIDEMIOLOGY

Incidence
- 4.5 cases of RMS per 1 million patients <20 years old per year
  - 50% occur within 1st decade of life.
- In adults, RMS represents 3% of all soft tissue sarcomas in adults.

Prevalence
- RMS comprises 3% of all childhood cancers.
- Predominant sex: male > female (1.37:1)

Genetics
- Alveolar: *PAX3-FOXO1* or *PAX7-FOXO1* fusion genes as a result of t(2;13) and t(1;13), respectively; found in 75% of ARMS
- Embryonal: Loss of alleles on chromosome 11 may be seen.

RISK FACTORS
Smoking, advanced maternal age, in utero x-ray exposure, maternal recreational drug use, and history of stillbirths

COMMONLY ASSOCIATED CONDITIONS
- Neurofibromatosis (NF1) 1: 20-fold increased risk of RMS in patients with NF1
- Li-Fraumeni syndrome: p53 mutations predispose to multiple tumors, including RMS.

DIAGNOSIS

HISTORY
- Presents as a progressive painless mass of the head and neck, genitourinary tissue, trunk, or extremities
- RMS of genitourinary tissue may present as vaginal bleeding in females.

- Other symptoms may be noted due to mass effect of the primary or metastatic lesions.
- Family history of genetic syndromes (i.e., NF1, Li-Fraumeni syndrome)

PHYSICAL EXAM
- Painless, enlarging mass
- Polypoid mass protruding from vagina (botryoid)
- Exophthalmos and chemosis (orbital involvement)
- Abdominal pain
- Compression symptoms (i.e., seizures, visual field defects, nerve palsy, headaches)

DIAGNOSTIC TESTS & INTERPRETATION

Initial Tests (lab, imaging)
- Ultrasound: used for differentiation of cystic versus solid mass
- MRI/CT: used to evaluate tumor
- Staging tests: chest x-ray, CT thorax, fluorodeoxyglucose (FDG)-PET
  - Most common site of metastasis is lung; evaluated by CT
  - FDG-PET scans may be useful to detect lymph node or distant metastases; not readily evident on CT or MRI scans

Diagnostic Procedures/Other
- Core needle biopsy, incisional biopsy, or excisional biopsy (based on size of mass)
  - The presence of rhabdomyoblast indicates the diagnosis.
- Immunohistochemical markers
  - Myogenin: commonly expressed in ARMS
  - Desmin: associated with multiple subtypes of RMS
- Pathology
  - Alveolar: rhabdomyoblasts arranged in what grossly appears to mimic pulmonary alveoli
  - Embryonal
  - Classic: rhabdomyoblasts configured in sheets without alveolar pattern
  - Botryoid: "grape-like" appearance of rhabdomyoblasts with notable clustering in the subepithelium forming the cambium layer
  - Spindle cell: rhabdomyoblasts with a spindle-like appearance
- Undifferentiated: rhabdomyoblast arrangement that cannot be classified as any other subtype
- Staging
  - Based on site, size, regional nodal involvement, and distance spread
  - See table.

Stage	Site	T	Tumor diameter	N	M
1	Orbit; head and neck (excluding parameningeal); genitourinary—nonbladder and nonprostate; biliary tract	T1 or T2	a or b	N0 or N1 or NX	M0
2	Bladder or prostate; extremity; cranial parameningeal; other (includes trunk, retroperitoneum, etc.)	T1 or T2	a	N0 or NX	M0
3	Bladder or prostate; extremity; cranial parameningeal; other (includes trunk, retroperitoneum, etc.)	T1 or T2	a	N1	M0
			0 or N1 or NX	M0	
4	All sites	T1 or T2	a or b	N0 or N1	M1

Note: a, ≤5 cm in diameter; b, >5 cm in diameter; T1, confined to site of origin; T2, extension and/or fixation to surrounding tissue; N0, regional nodes not clinically involved; N1, regional nodes clinically involved by neoplasm; Nx, clinical status of regional nodes unknown; M0, no distant metastasis present; M1, metastasis present.

TREATMENT

The three tenets of treatment for adults and children are composed of surgical resection, radiation therapy, and chemotherapy. Patients should be referred to a multidisciplinary treatment team with expertise in oncology for definitive treatment.

SURGERY/OTHER PROCEDURES

- Wide local resection of tumor. If possible, resect metastasis as well.
- However, wide resection may not be feasible in cases where grossly impaired functionality results.
  - All children receive chemotherapy (1)[B].
  - In North America, the three-drug combination of vincristine, dactinomycin, and cyclophosphamide (VAC) is the standard regimen:
    - Vincristine
      - Adverse reactions: alopecia, constipation, peripheral neuropathy
    - Actinomycin-D
      - Adverse reactions: pancytopenia, hepatotoxicity
    - Cyclophosphamide
      - Adverse reactions: hemorrhagic cystitis (mesna for prophylaxis), sterility, transitional cell carcinoma
- In addition, ifosfamide, topotecan, doxorubicin, etoposide, and irinotecan may also be used.
- Duration of chemotherapy depends on risk stratification and ranges from 6 to 12 months.
- Chemotherapy has been less commonly used in adults, who generally undergo treatment with resection and radiation therapy.
- Radiotherapy is currently used for those whose tumor cannot be completely resected.

 ONGOING CARE

FOLLOW-UP RECOMMENDATIONS

Patients should follow up with their multidisciplinary treatment team. Long-term follow-up is necessary for detection of recurrence, metastatic disease, and development of secondary malignancies. Follow-up is composed of physical exam, chest x-ray, and imaging of the primary tumor site every 3 to 6 months for the first 3 years.

PROGNOSIS

- RMS (all cases): 62% 5-year survival
- ARMS: 48% 5-year survival
- ERMS: 73% 5-year survival
- Prognosis in adults is worse; it is unclear whether this is related to subtype of tumor or lack of clear guidelines for adults; this is a rare presentation in adults.

COMPLICATIONS

- Recurrence
- Secondary neoplasm
- Growth abnormalities
- Treatment side effects

REFERENCES

1. Ray A, Huh WW. Current state-of-the-art systemic therapy for pediatric soft tissue sarcomas. *Curr Oncol Rep.* 2012;14(4):311–319.

ADDITIONAL READING

- Arndt CA, Rose PS, Folpe AL, et al. Common musculoskeletal tumors of childhood and adolescence. *Mayo Clin Proc.* 2012;87(5):475–487.
- Hawkins DS, Spunt SL, Skapek SX. Children's Oncology Group's 2013 blueprint for research: soft tissue sarcomas. *Pediatr Blood Cancer.* 2013;60(6):1001–1008.
- Kapoor G, Das K. Soft tissue sarcomas in children. *Indian J Pediatr.* 2012;79(7):936–942.

- Klem ML, Grewal RK, Wexler LH, et al. PET for staging in rhabdomyosarcoma: an evaluation of PET as an adjunct to current staging tools. *J Pediatr Hematol Oncol.* 2007;29(1):9–14.
- Malempati S, Hawkins DS. Rhabdomyosarcoma: review of the Children's Oncology Group (COG) Soft-Tissue Sarcoma Committee experience and rationale for current COG studies. *Pediatr Blood Cancer.* 2012;59(1):5–10.
- Ognjanovic S, Linabery AM, Charbonneau B, et al. Trends in childhood rhabdomyosarcoma incidence and survival in the United States, 1975-2005. *Cancer.* 2009;115(18):4218–4226.
- Parham DM, Ellison DA. Rhabdomyosarcomas in adults and children: an update. *Arch Pathol Lab Med.* 2006;130(10):1454–1465.
- Sultan I, Qaddoumi I, Yaser S, et al. Comparing adult and pediatric rhabdomyosarcoma in the surveillance, epidemiology and end results program, 1973 to 2005: an analysis of 2,600 patients. *J Clin Oncol.* 2009;27(20):3391–3397.

 CODES

ICD10

- C49.9 Malignant neoplasm of connective and soft tissue, unsp
- C49.0 Malignant neoplasm of connective and soft tissue of head, face and neck
- C49.5 Malignant neoplasm of connective and soft tissue of pelvis

CLINICAL PEARLS

- RMS is the most common soft tissue sarcoma in children.
- They can arise at any site and in any tissue except bone.
- All persistent soft tissue masses should be evaluated with imaging (ultrasound to rule out cystic vs. solid, then MRI/CT).
- Fine-needle aspiration may be helpful but core needle versus incisional/excisional biopsy for confirmation.

RHEUMATIC FEVER
Jonathan Schimmel, MD • Achyut B. Kamat, MD

BASICS

DESCRIPTION
- Acute rheumatic fever (ARF) is a delayed inflammatory sequela of group A *Streptococcus* (GAS) tonsillopharyngitis that affects multiple organ systems.
- Can lead to rheumatic heart disease (RHD)
- Recurrence in adults and children is common if antibiotic prophylaxis is withheld.
- Systems affected: cardiovascular, nervous, hematologic/lymphatic/immunologic, skin/exocrine, musculoskeletal

Pediatric Considerations
Can affect any age but most common ages 5 to 15 years

EPIDEMIOLOGY
- ARF and RHD are now largely restricted to developing countries and some poor populations of wealthy countries.
- Male = female, but females more likely to develop chorea.
- Can occur as an epidemic

Incidence
- Worldwide, incidence (new cases) has been declining for decades, attributed to increasing antibiotic use and improved living conditions. Most new cases are in developing countries.
- In early studies, ARF developed in 3% of children with untreated GAS pharyngitis.
- Incidence of ARF in the United States in the 1960s was 13.3/100,000 and is currently <1/100,000.
- 95% of cases currently occur in developing countries.

Prevalence
Worldwide, more than 15 million people have RHD, and prevalence has been rising due to improved medical care and longer survival (despite decreasing incidence of ARF).

ETIOLOGY AND PATHOPHYSIOLOGY
- Preceded by tonsillopharyngitis of GAS, also known as *Streptococcus pyogenes*, a gram–positive organism
- Molecular mimicry: Antibodies against M protein on GAS cross-reacts with cardiac and vessel endothelial proteins, leading to an inflammatory cascade.

Genetics
- Susceptibility is associated with certain genetic polymorphisms, including toll-like receptors, cytokines, and human leukocyte antigen genes. Not fully understood
- Increased susceptibility in certain populations, including Australian aborigines, New Zealand Maori, and Pacific Islanders

RISK FACTORS
Genetic susceptibility and possible increased risk with iron deficiency or low serum albumin.

GENERAL PREVENTION
- Primary prevention: Antibiotics are effective at reducing incidence of ARF after known or suspected GAS pharyngitis. Number needed to treat is 100 (1)
- Secondary prevention: long-term antibiotic prophylaxis to prevent recurrence

DIAGNOSIS

- Requires laboratory evidence of preceding GAS infection (see "Initial Tests (lab, imaging)").
- Revised Jones criteria
- Initial ARF: 2 major OR 1 major + 2 minor
- Recurrent ARF: 2 major OR 1 major + 2 minor OR 3 minor

Major Criteria	Minor Criteria
• Carditis/valvulitis	• Low-risk: fever ≥38.5°C
	• Mod-high risk: fever ≥38°C
• Low-risk: polyarthritis	• Low-risk: polyarthralgia
• Mod-high risk: mono/polyarthritis	• Mod-high risk: monoarthralgia
• Sydenham chorea	• ↑PR interval
• Erythema marginatum	• CRP ≥3 mg/dL, and/or
	• Low-risk: ESR ≥60 mm/hr
	• Mod-high risk: ESR ≥30 mm/hr
• Subcutaneous nodules	

- The revised criteria distinguish between patients with low-risk versus moderate-high risk of having ARF. Patients can be considered low-risk if they are from and among a low incidence group (2)[C].

HISTORY
- ARF presents 1 to 4 weeks following GAS tonsillopharyngitis.
- Polyarthritis is often first, affecting the knees, ankles, elbows, and wrists. Each resolves in days, thus seems to "migrate." Usually self-limited <1 month. Mod-high risk patients may develop monoarthritis. Use of NSAID or aspirin may mask the arthritis.
- Fever
- Erythema marginatum rash
- Pancarditis or valvulitis (50–70%) can be subclinical (asymptomatic without auscultatory findings) or clinically apparent (symptomatic or auscultatory findings).
- Sydenham chorea (clinical diagnosis, in 10–30%)
  - 1 to 6 months after infection, so lab evidence of preceding infection may be absent.
  - More common in 5 to 15 years old, more common in females
  - Improves or ceases during sleep.
  - Psychiatric symptoms may have onset prior to chorea, with emotional lability and obsessive-compulsive symptoms.
  - Usually self-resolves over several months and can relapse

PHYSICAL EXAM
- Neuro: Sydenham chorea: Involuntary movements may be general or unilateral and may involve the face. "Milkmaid grip" is intermittent hypotonia appreciated on test of grip strength.
- Cardiac: pericardial friction rub, blowing holosystolic murmur, rarely diastolic, or new or changing murmur; rarely evidence of heart failure
- Skin
  - Subcutaneous nodules (<10%): firm, painless, up to 2 cm, over bony surfaces or tendons, usually extensor surfaces. More common in severe ARF, persists up to several weeks
  - Erythema marginatum (5–13%): nonpruritic, blanching, evanescent, pale pink macular transitions to central clearing, found on trunk and occasionally limbs, accentuated by warming the skin

DIFFERENTIAL DIAGNOSIS
- Systemic lupus erythematosus
- Poststreptococcal reactive arthritis
- Juvenile rheumatoid arthritis
- Infectious arthritis
- Viral myocarditis
- Innocent cardiac murmur
- Tourette syndrome
- Kawasaki syndrome
- Pediatric autoimmune neuropsychiatric disorders associated with streptococcal infections (PANDAS)

DIAGNOSTIC TESTS & INTERPRETATION
Initial Tests (lab, imaging)
- Bacteriologic/serologic evidence of GAS infection (2)[B]:
  - Rapid streptococcal antigen test with high pre-test probability
  - Throat culture (sensitivity 25% by time of ARF)
  - Elevated or rising antistreptolysin O (ASO) titer; peaks ~1 month postinfection.
- If ASO negative, check anti-DNAse B (peaks ~2.5 months, remains elevated up to 9 months), streptokinase, and antihyaluronidase (3).
- Bacteriologic/serologic evidence may be negative in chorea or chronic indolent rheumatic carditis.
- ESR and CRP are acute-phase reactants that almost always increase in ARF.
- CBC with differential: leukocytosis, possible normocytic anemia
- Complement levels normal (do not need to check)
- ECG: PR prolongation, AV block, signs of pericarditis
- Arthrocentesis of affected joints shows sterile inflammatory fluid with 10 to 100,000 WBC/mm³.
- Chest x-ray: may have cardiomegaly from myocarditis
- Echocardiogram: Assess chamber size and function, pericardial effusion, and valve disease.
- All cases of confirmed or suspected ARF should have an echocardiogram (2)[B], due to the 18% prevalence of subclinical carditis.
- Antimyosin scintigraphy can detect carditis (nonspecific).

Follow-Up Tests & Special Considerations
- ESR and CRP are useful to monitor rebound inflammation.
- Repeat echocardiograms to monitor evolution of carditis, even if not initially present (2)[C].
- Household contacts should be screened with throat culture even if asymptomatic and treated with antibiotics if positive.

Test Interpretation
Prior treatment with aspirin or steroids may lead to falsely normal lab results.

 TREATMENT

GENERAL MEASURES
- Antibiotic
- Anti-inflammatory agent (aspirin or naproxen)
- Manage cardiac manifestations as needed in addition to standard ARF treatment (e.g. dysrhythmia, pericarditis, myocarditis, valvular disease, or heart failure).

MEDICATION
First Line
- Eradication: Treat initially as if active GAS infection, then begin prophylaxis.
- If no penicillin allergy
  - Penicillin VK PO BID for 10 days, or benzathine penicillin G IM for 1, or amoxicillin PO for 10 days (preferred in children) (4)[A]
- If penicillin allergy
  - Cephalosporin 1st generation PO for 10 days (4)[A], azithromycin PO for 5 days, or clindamycin PO for 10 days, or clarithromycin PO for 10 days (4)[B]
- If there is heart failure, AV block third degree, or other severe manifestations of carditis, appropriate traditional management should be initiated.
- Aspirin high-dose is effective for treatment of arthritis and fever (5)[B], but has not been shown to reduce or improve cardiac manifestations (6)[B]. High-dose aspirin for prolonged periods risks salicylate toxicity and if used, consider following salicylate levels.
- If severe carditis is present, consider prednisone, although not shown to prevent or reduce cardiac manifestations (6)[B].
- Chorea generally self-resolves and does not require treatment, but if symptoms are severe, can use valproic acid, carbamazepine, or an antipsychotic if still resistant (3)[B]. If symptoms persist, consider prednisone, which unlike cardiac disease has been shown effective for Sydenham chorea (3)[B].

Second Line
- If penicillin allergy is present, erythromycin is preferred by the New Zealand guidelines, but not by the Infectious Diseases Society of America.
- Naproxen is a reasonable alternative to aspirin (see "Pediatric Considerations").

ISSUES FOR REFERRAL
A cardiologist should be involved in management of ARF.

SURGERY/OTHER PROCEDURES
Valve stenosis is a late sequela that can result from fibrosis and calcification; it may require surgical correction (valve repair preferred over replacement) (7).

INPATIENT CONSIDERATIONS
Admission Criteria/Initial Stabilization
- Initial hospitalization may be helpful for diagnosis and to ensure stability.
- Heart failure requires prompt hospitalization.

IV Fluids
Only if signs of dehydration or to augment preload; use caution if heart failure present.

Nursing
Consider bedrest if severe symptoms, with gradual return to ambulation as tolerated (8)[C].

 ONGOING CARE

FOLLOW-UP RECOMMENDATIONS
- ARF patients should be on a prophylactic antibiotic throughout childhood until age 21 years and possibly indefinitely depending on cardiac damage because recurrence can worsen prognosis (9)[C].
  - First-line prophylaxis is **long-acting** benzathine penicillin G monthly IM injections (9)[A].
  - Penicillin V PO 250 mg BID is an alternative but has risk of nonadherence (9)[B].
  - If penicillin allergy, treat with sulfadiazine (9)[B].
  - If penicillin and sulfa drug allergy, treat with azithromycin (9)[C].
- If diagnostic uncertainty exists, consider 1 year of secondary antibiotic prophylaxis followed by reassessment and echocardiogram (2)[C].
- Routine antibiotic prophylaxis for dental procedures is no longer recommended by the American Heart Association for patients with RHD (7).
- Have low threshold to test and treat episodes of acute tonsillopharyngitis.

Patient Monitoring
Initially weekly, then every 6 months

Pediatric Considerations
- Use aspirin with caution in children given the risk of Reye syndrome.
- Naproxen (10 to 20 mg/kg/day) has been found noninferior to aspirin with fewer risks in ARF, in a small study (5)[B].

Pregnancy Considerations
May exacerbate valve disease, particularly mitral stenosis. Refer pregnant patients to a cardiologist.

DIET
Regular diet, or low-sodium if heart failure present.

PATIENT EDUCATION
American Heart Association: http://www.heart.org

PROGNOSIS
Sequelae are generally limited to the heart and depend on the severity of carditis during an acute attack.

COMPLICATIONS
- Recurrence of ARF due to GAS reinfection
- RHD can occur 10 to 20 years after ARF, with mitral more common than aortic regurgitation, can lead to stenosis. Heart failure is worst complication.
- Jaccoud arthropathy is chronic and involves painless deformities of hands/feet.

REFERENCES

1. Del Mar CB, Glasziou PP, Spinks AB. Antibiotics for sore throat. *Cochrane Database Syst Rev.* 2006;(4):CD000023.
2. Gewitz MH, Baltimore RS, Tani LY, et al. Revision of the Jones criteria for the diagnosis of acute rheumatic fever in the era of Doppler echocardiography: a scientific statement from the American Heart Association. *Circulation.* 2015;131(20):1806–1818.
3. Oosterveer DM, Overweg-Plandsoen WC, Roos RA. Sydenham's chorea: a practical overview of the current literature. *Pediatr Neurol.* 2010;43(1):1–6.
4. Shulman ST, Bisno AL, Clegg HW, et al. Clinical practice guideline for the diagnosis and management of group A streptococcal pharyngitis: 2012 update by the Infectious Diseases Society of America. *Clin Infect Dis.* 2012;55(10):e86–e102.
5. Hashkes PJ, Tauber T, Somekh E, et al. Naproxen as an alternative to aspirin for the treatment of arthritis of rheumatic fever: a randomized trial. *J Pediatr.* 2003;143(3):399–401.
6. Cilliers AM, Manyemba J, Saloojee H. Anti-inflammatory treatment for carditis in acute rheumatic fever. *Cochrane Database Syst Rev.* 2003;(2):CD003176.
7. Webb RH, Grant C, Harnden A. Acute rheumatic fever. *BMJ.* 2015;351:h3443.
8. The Cardiac Society of Australia and New Zealand. *New Zealand Guidelines for Rheumatic Fever: Diagnosis, Management and Secondary Prevention of Acute Rheumatic Fever and Rheumatic Heart Disease: 2014 Update.* Auckland, New Zealand: Heart Foundation of New Zealand; 2014.
9. Gerber MA, Baltimore RS, Eaton CB, et al. Prevention of rheumatic fever and diagnosis and treatment of acute Streptococcal pharyngitis: a scientific statement from the American Heart Association Rheumatic Fever, Endocarditis, and Kawasaki Disease Committee of the Council on Cardiovascular Disease in the Young, the Interdisciplinary Council on Functional Genomics and Translational Biology, and the Interdisciplinary Council on Quality of Care and Outcomes Research: endorsed by the American Academy of Pediatrics. *Circulation.* 2009;119(11):1541–1551.

 CODES

ICD10
- I00 Rheumatic fever without heart involvement
- I01.9 Acute rheumatic heart disease, unspecified
- I01.0 Acute rheumatic pericarditis

CLINICAL PEARLS
- ARF is an inflammatory disease that affects multiple organ systems including the heart.
- Modified Jones criteria for diagnosis include 2 major or 1 major + 2 minor manifestation in the context of a preceding documented GAS infection.
- Treatment involves aspirin and antibiotic eradication followed immediately by long-term antibiotic prophylaxis.

RHINITIS, ALLERGIC

Naureen Bashir Rafiq, MBBS, MD

BASICS

Allergic rhinitis is the collection of symptoms, involving mucous membranes of nose, eyes, ears, and throat after an exposure to allergens like pollen, dust, or dander.

DESCRIPTION
- IgE-mediated inflammation of the nasal mucosa following exposure to an extrinsic protein; an immediate symptomatic response is characterized by sneezing, congestion, and rhinorrhea followed by a persistent late phase dominated by congestion and mucosal hyperreactivity.
- Allergic rhinitis can be classified into seasonal or perennial and can be intermittent or persistent.
- Seasonal responses are usually due to outdoor allergens like tree pollen, flowering shrubs in spring, grasses and flowering plants in summer, and ragweed and mold in fall.
- Perennial responses, or year-round symptoms, are usually associated with indoor allergens like dust mites, mold, and animal dander.
- Occupational allergic rhinitis is caused by allergens at the workplace and can be sporadic or year-round.
- Nonallergic rhinitis (e.g., vasomotor, rhinitis of pregnancy, and rhinitis medicamentosa) can occur.

Pediatric Considerations
Chronic nasal obstruction can result in facial deformities, dental malocclusions, and sleep disorders.

Pregnancy Considerations
Physiologic changes during pregnancy may aggravate all types of rhinitis, frequently in the 2nd trimester.

EPIDEMIOLOGY
- Onset usually in first 2 decades, rarely before 6 months of age, with tendency declining with advancing age.
- The mean age of onset is 8 to 11 years, and about 80% of cases have established allergic rhinitis by age 20 years.

Prevalence
- ~10–25% of the U.S. adult population and 9–42% of the U.S. pediatric population are affected.
- 44–87% of patients with allergic rhinitis have mixed allergic and nonallergic rhinitis, which is more common than either pure form (1).
- Scandinavian studies have demonstrated cumulative prevalence rate of 14% in men and 15% in women.

ETIOLOGY AND PATHOPHYSIOLOGY
- Aeroallergen-driven mucosal inflammation due to resident and infiltrating inflammatory cells, as well as vasoactive and proinflammatory mediators (e.g., cytokines)
- Inhalant allergens:
  – Perennial: house dust mites, indoor molds, animal dander, cockroach/insect detritus
  – Seasonal: tree, grass, and weed pollens; outdoor molds
  – Occupational: latex, plant products (e.g., baking flour), sensitizing chemicals, and certain animals for people working in farms and vet clinics

Genetics
Complex but strong genetic predilection present (80% have family history of allergic disorders)

RISK FACTORS
- Family history of atopy, with a greater risk if both parents have atopy
- Higher socioeconomic status
- Tobacco smoke can exacerbate symptoms and increase risk of developing asthma in patients with allergic rhinitis.
- Having other allergies like asthma
- Unclear evidence regarding risk due to early, repeated exposure to offending allergen and early introduction of solid food.
- Pets in house and houses infested with cockroaches can cause perennial allergic rhinitis.

GENERAL PREVENTION
- Primary prevention of atopic disease has not been proven effective by maternal diet or maternal allergen avoidance (2).
- Exclusive breastfeeding to 6 months of age lowers risk of some atopic disorders
- Symptomatic control by environmental avoidance is the "first-line treatment."
- No evidence to support use of acaricides with mite-proof mattress and pillow covers, carpet and drape removal, removal of plants in the home, and pet control (2,3)[B].
- Air conditioning and limited outside exposure during allergy season (1)[B]
- HEPA air cleaners and vacuum bags of unclear efficacy
- Close doors and windows during allergy season.
- Use a dehumidifier to reduce indoor humidity.

COMMONLY ASSOCIATED CONDITIONS
Other IgE-mediated conditions: asthma, atopic dermatitis, allergic conjunctivitis, food allergy

DIAGNOSIS

Diagnosis is made primarily by history and physical exam.

HISTORY
- Evaluation of nature, duration, and time course of symptoms
- History of atopic dermatitis and/or food allergies
- History of nasal congestion; rhinorrhea; pruritus of nose, eyes, ears, and/or palate; sneezing; itching; and watering eyes
- Family history of allergic diseases
- History of environmental and occupational exposure and various nasal stimuli can help differentiate between allergic and vasomotor rhinitis.

PHYSICAL EXAM
Many findings are suggestive of but not specific for allergic rhinitis:
- Dark circles under eyes, "allergic shiners" (infraorbital venous congestion)
- Transverse nasal crease from rubbing nose upward; typically seen in children
- Rhinorrhea, usually with clear discharge
- Pale, boggy, blue-gray nasal mucosa
- Postnasal mucus discharge
- Oropharyngeal lymphoid tissue hypertrophy

DIFFERENTIAL DIAGNOSIS
- Infectious rhinitis: usually viral, commonly with secondary bacterial infection
  – Usually associated with sinusitis and is known as rhinosinusitis
  – Viral rhinitis averages 6 episodes/year from ages 2 to 6 years.
  – IgA deficiency with recurrent sinusitis
  – Rhinitis medicamentosa:
    ○ Rebound effect associated with continued use of topical decongestant drops and sprays
    ○ ACE inhibitors, reserpine, β-blockers, oral contraceptive pills (OCPs), guanethidine, methyldopa
    ○ Aspirin, NSAIDs
  – Vasomotor (idiopathic) rhinitis caused by numerous nasal stimuli like warm or cold air, scents and odors, light or particulate matter
  – Hormonal: pregnancy, thyroid, OCPs
  – Nonallergic rhinitis with eosinophilia syndrome (NARES)
  – Gustatory: watery rhinorrhea in response to alcohol or food
  – "Skier's nose": watery rhinorrhea in response to cold air
- Conditions associated with rhinitis:
  – Nasal polyps, tumor
  – Septal/anatomic obstruction
    ○ Adenoidal hypertrophy, particularly in children
    ○ Septal abnormality or deflected nasal septum (DNS) in adults

DIAGNOSTIC TESTS & INTERPRETATION
- Lab tests rarely needed
- Skin testing is done to identify the allergen for immunotherapy.

Initial Tests (lab, imaging)
- Testing is rarely indicated.
- If diagnosis implies other causes, consider the following:
  – CBC with differential may show elevated eosinophils.
  – Increased total serum IgE level
  – Nasal probe smear may show elevated eosinophils.
- Medications that may alter lab results
  – Corticosteroids may decrease eosinophilia.
  – Antihistamines suppress reactivity to skin tests; stop antihistamines 7 days before testing.
- CT scan of sinuses is not routinely done but can be used to check for complete opacity, fluid level, and mucosal thickening.

Diagnostic Procedures/Other
- Consider testing in only those cases where allergic symptoms do not respond to treatment and/or considering immunotherapy.
- Specific allergen sensitivity with allergen skin testing or radioallergosorbent testing (RAST); clinical correlation based on history is essential in interpreting results.
- Diagnostic allergen prick tests are used to select agent to determine appropriate environmental control measures, as well as to direct immunotherapy:
  – Prick or puncture: superficial injury to epidermis with application of test antigen
  – Intradermal
- RAST: more expensive and less sensitive than skin testing; typically used in patients in whom skin testing is not practical or a severe reaction is possible
- Rhinoscopy: useful to visualize intranasal anatomy and posterior pharyngeal structures, including adenoids, polyps, and larynx

Test Interpretation

- Nasal washing/scraping: Eosinophils predominate but may see basophils, mast cells.
- Nasal mucosa: submucosal edema but without destruction; eosinophilic infiltration; congested mucous glands and goblet cells

TREATMENT

There are three mainstays of treatment of allergic rhinitis:
- Allergen avoidance
- Medication
- Allergy immunotherapy

GENERAL MEASURES

- Establish specific cause(s) by history and appropriate testing.
- Limit exposure to offending allergen.
- Allergen immunotherapy (desensitization)
  - Reserved when symptoms are uncontrollable with medical therapy or have a comorbidity (e.g., asthma)
  - Specific allergen extract is injected SC in increasing doses to induce patient tolerance.

MEDICATION

Oral medication and intranasal sprays are commonly used.

First Line

- Mild symptoms: 2nd-generation nonsedating antihistamines are the first-line therapy for mild to moderate allergic rhinitis (1,4).
- Adverse effects: mild sedation, mild anticholinergic effects
- Generic (cetirizine, fexofenadine, loratadine; most to least effective)
  - Levocetirizine is a new 2nd-generation nonsedating antihistamine that is effective but costly.
- Intranasal corticosteroids are the first-line therapy for moderate to severe allergic rhinitis (1,4)[A]:
  - Most effective drug class for symptoms of allergic rhinitis
  - Use nasal sprays after showering and direct spray away from septum to improve deposition on mucosal surface.
  - May be used as needed; however, less effective than regular use (1)
  - Adverse effects: nosebleed, nasal septal perforation, and systemic corticosteroid effects
- Systemic steroids should be considered only in urgent cases and only for short-term use.

Second Line

1st-generation antihistamines, such as the following:
- Brompheniramine: 12 to 24 mg PO BID
- Chlorpheniramine: 4 mg PO q4–6h PRN
- Clemastine: 1 to 2 mg PO BID PRN
- Diphenhydramine: 25 to 50 mg PO q4–6h PRN:
  - May precipitate urinary retention in men with prostatism and/or hypertrophy
  - Adverse effects: sedation, prolonged QT interval, performance impairment, and anticholinergic effect

- Nasal antihistamines effective but may be systemically absorbed and thus cause sedation: azelastine, olopatadine
- Decongestants
  - Phenylephrine: 10 mg PO q4h PRN
  - Pseudoephedrine: 60 mg PO q4–6h PRN
  - Oxymetazoline nasal spray (Afrin): 2 to 3 sprays per nostril q10–12h PRN (max 3 days). Intranasal agents should not be used for >3 days due to rebound rhinitis. Discourage use in patients with hypertension (HTN) or cardiac arrhythmia.
- Intranasal anticholinergics such as ipratropium nasal spray 2 sprays per nostril BID to TID
  - Intranasal anticholinergics can increase efficacy in combination with steroid use.
- Leukotriene antagonists such as montelukast 10 mg/day PO
  - Should generally be used as an adjunct, not monotherapy
  - May be first line in those with concomitant asthma
- Mast cell stabilizers such as cromolyn nasal spray 1 spray per nostril TID to QID
  - May take 2 to 4 weeks of therapy for optimal efficacy
  - May be ineffective in patients with nonallergic rhinitis and nasal polyps

ISSUES FOR REFERRAL

Refer to allergist for consideration of immunotherapy.

ADDITIONAL THERAPIES

- Immunotherapy, either by injection (5)[A] or sublingually, which may be better tolerated by children (6)[A]
- Nasal saline use has evidence of efficacy as sole agent or as adjunctive treatment (1,7)[A].

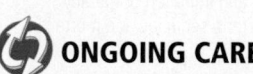
ONGOING CARE

FOLLOW-UP RECOMMENDATIONS

No specific restrictions on activity; emphasize avoiding activity where exposure to the allergen is likely.

Patient Monitoring

Initiation of patient education is critical.

DIET

- No special diet unless concomitant food reactions are suspected and evaluated
- Some patients with severe sensitivity to seasonal pollens may have oral allergy syndrome, which is associated with itching in the mouth with the ingestion of fresh fruits that may cross-react with the allergens.

PATIENT EDUCATION

- Asthma & Allergy Foundation of America, 1717 Massachusetts Ave., Suite 305, Washington, DC 20036; (800) 7-ASTHMA: http://www.aafa.org/
- Other helpful information available at http://acaai.org/ and http://www.aaaai.org/home.aspx

PROGNOSIS

- Acceptable control of symptoms is the goal.
- Treatment is helpful to reduce the risk of comorbidities, such as sinusitis and asthma.

COMPLICATIONS

- Secondary infection such as otitis media or sinusitis
- Epistaxis
- Nasopharyngeal lymphoid hyperplasia
- Airway hyperreactivity with allergen exposure
- Asthma
- Facial changes, especially in children who are mouth breathers
- Sleep disturbance

REFERENCES

1. Wallace DV, Dykewicz MS, Bernstein DI, et al. The diagnosis and management of rhinitis: an updated practice parameter. *J Allergy Clin Immunol*. 2008;122 (2 Suppl):S1–S84.
2. Kramer MS, Kakuma R. Maternal dietary antigen avoidance during pregnancy or lactation, or both, for preventing or treating atopic disease in the child. *Cochrane Database Syst Rev*. 2012;(9):CD000133.
3. Sheikh A, Hurwitz B, Nurmatov U, et al. House dust mite avoidance measures for perennial allergic rhinitis. *Cochrane Database Syst Rev*. 2010;(7):CD001563.
4. Plaut M, Valentine MD. Clinical practice. Allergic rhinitis. *N Engl J Med*. 2005;353(18):1934–1944.
5. Calderon MA, Alves B, Jacobson M, et al. Allergen injection immunotherapy for seasonal allergic rhinitis. *Cochrane Database Syst Rev*. 2007;(1):CD001936.
6. Wilson DR, Lima MT, Durham SR. Sublingual immunotherapy for allergic rhinitis: systematic review and meta-analysis. *Allergy*. 2005;60(1):4–12.
7. Harvey R, Hannan SA, Badia L, et al. Nasal saline irrigations for the symptoms of chronic rhinosinusitis. *Cochrane Database Syst Rev*. 2007;(3):CD006394.

 SEE ALSO

Conjunctivitis, Acute

 CODES

ICD10
- J30.9 Allergic rhinitis, unspecified
- J30.1 Allergic rhinitis due to pollen
- J30.2 Other seasonal allergic rhinitis

CLINICAL PEARLS

- Nasal saline irrigation (flushing 6 to 8 oz) may be very helpful in clearing upper airway of secretions and may precede the use of nasal corticosteroids.
- 2nd-generation antihistamines and intranasal corticosteroids are first-line therapies for allergic rhinitis.
- Referral to allergist is appropriate for identification of offending allergens and consideration of immunotherapy for inadequate symptom control.

R

ROCKY MOUNTAIN SPOTTED FEVER

Ginny H. Lee, MD • Alison Southern, MD, MS, FACEP

BASICS

DESCRIPTION
- Rocky Mountain spotted fever (RMSF) is a potentially fatal tick-borne systemic small vessel vasculitis caused by the bacterium *Rickettsia rickettsii*.
- RMSF is the most common and lethal rickettsial disease in the United States.
- Typically characterized by fever, headache, and myalgias followed by a centripetal (moving inward from the extremities toward the trunk) rash
- System(s) affected: cardiovascular, musculoskeletal, skin, CNS, renal, hepatic, and pulmonary

EPIDEMIOLOGY
Incidence
- In the United States, the incidence of RMSF increased from <2 cases per million persons in 2000 to >8 per million in 2008 (1).
- Reported in all states except Hawaii, Alaska, and Maine
- North Carolina, Tennessee, Oklahoma, Arkansas, and Missouri account for ~60% of cases. RMSF also found in areas of Canada and in Central and South America (2).
- Predominant age: All ages are susceptible; highest prevalence in children 5 to 9 years of age (2,3).
- Predominant sex: male > female, likely due to increased outdoor exposures (3,4).
- Peak incidence occurs with tick exposure, typically in late spring and summer (3).

Prevalence
In the United States, about 2,000 cases are reported annually (2).
- <0.1% of ticks carry virulent Rickettsial species.

ETIOLOGY AND PATHOPHYSIOLOGY
- Infected ticks include the American dog tick, *Dermacentor variabilis* in the eastern United States; the Rocky Mountain wood tick, *Dermacentor andersoni* in the western United States; and the Brown dog tick, *Rhipicephalus sanguineus* in the southwest (1,2).
- An adult tick releases *Rickettsia rickettsii* from its salivary glands after 6 to 10 hours of feeding (1).
- Rickettsiae proliferate inside endothelial cells by binary fission and invade contiguous vascular endothelial cells, causing a small-vessel vasculitis and the characteristic rash.
- Increased vascular permeability leads to edema, hypovolemia, and hypoalbuminemia, with subsequent end-organ injury.
- Platelets are consumed locally due to vascular injury, but coagulopathy or disseminated intravascular coagulation (DIC) is rare (4).
- Incubation time: 2 to 14 days; median 4 to 7 days
- Transplacental transmission of infection has not been demonstrated.
- RMSF can rarely be caused by direct inoculation of tick blood into open wounds or conjunctivae.

RISK FACTORS
- Known tick bite, engorged tick, or presence of tick for >20 hours; *likelihood of infection increases with duration of tick attachment*
- Crushed tick during its removal
- Accumulated outdoor exposure or residence in a wooded area
- Contact with outdoor pets or wild animals

GENERAL PREVENTION
In known tick-prone areas (2,4,5)
- Limit time spent in tall grasses, open areas of low bushy vegetation, and wooded areas.
- Cover exposed skin; wear a hat, long sleeves, pants and closed-toed shoes.
- Use DEET-containing insect repellents on exposed skin. Permethrin can be used on clothing.
- "Tick checks": Carefully inspect the entire body after possible exposure, especially the scalp, neck, and axillae. Ticks are commonly hidden by hair. Closely inspect legs, groin, external genitalia, and waistlines.
- Remove attached ticks in their entirety with fine-tipped tweezers. Grasp the tick close to the skin and gently pull upward. If mouth-parts separate, try to remove gently. Nail polish, petrolatum jelly, and heating do not aid in tick removal. Wear gloves if possible.
- Wash hands and site of bite thoroughly after tick removal to avoid potential mucosal inoculation.
- Prophylactic antibiotic treatment is not recommended.

DIAGNOSIS

Delay in presentation and initiation of therapy increases risk of long-term sequelae and mortality.

HISTORY
Consider RMSF in acute febrile illness, especially with history of potential tick exposure within previous 14 days, travels to an endemic area, and presentation in the late spring or summer. *The painless tick bite goes unnoticed 30–50% of the time. Many patients do not report a bite* (2,4).
- Early disease (days 1 to 3) presents like a viral illness with frontal headache, fever, malaise, body aches, nausea, and vomiting. RMSF is easily mistaken for gastroenteritis, pharyngitis, or mononucleosis.
- Signs and symptoms associated with RMSF with frequency of occurrence
  - Fever, usually >102°F (99–100%)
  - Rash, macular/maculopapular/petechial, blanching (88–90%)
  - Headache (79–91%)
  - "Classic triad" of headache, fever, and rash (50–60%)
  - Myalgias (72–83%)
  - Nausea/vomiting (56–60%)
  - Abdominal pain, particularly in children (35–52%)
  - Cough, nonproductive (33%)
  - CNS dysfunction, stupor/confusion/coma/focal abnormalities (10–30%)
  - Patients may also have malaise, restlessness, arthralgia, conjunctivitis, and peripheral or periorbital edema.

PHYSICAL EXAM
On days 3 to 4, a centripetal rash usually forms (80% of adults), involving the palms and soles, spreading centrally to arms, legs, and trunk. The rash typically starts as an erythematous, macular, or maculopapular exanthem; 50% become petechial or purpuric; blanchable.
- 20% never develop the "classic" rash, delaying diagnosis and resulting in a more severe outcome. Rash can be difficult to visualize on dark-skinned patients.
- Rash may be variable in appearance. *Do not rely solely on the presence or absence of the typical rash for diagnosis*.
- In severe cases, the rash can involve the entire body and mucosal membranes and may progress to necrotic or gangrenous lesions.
- The rash is not associated with pruritus or urticaria; when present, this makes RMSF less likely.
- Hepatosplenomegaly (12–16%)
- Lymphadenopathy (27%)

DIFFERENTIAL DIAGNOSIS
- Viral exanthems (e.g., measles, rubella, roseola)
- Meningoencephalitis (viral meningitis or encephalitis, bacterial meningitis)
- Meningococcemia
- Typhus
- Ehrlichiosis
- Lyme disease
- Leptospirosis
- Toxic shock syndrome
- Adenovirus infection
- Drug reaction or serum sickness
- Mononucleosis
- Kawasaki disease

DIAGNOSTIC TESTS & INTERPRETATION
Diagnosis is often clinical in patients with exposure history in an endemic area. Retrospective confirmation by serology. Do not delay treatment awaiting serology.

Initial Tests (lab, imaging)
- Specific laboratory diagnosis
  - Serum indirect fluorescent antibody (IFA): Titer of >1:64 is diagnostic. A 4-fold increase of acute and convalescent titers confirms an active case of RMSF (1).
  - Antibodies usually develop 7 to 10 days after onset of symptoms; optimal time for testing, therefore, is 14 to 21 days after symptom onset. *Do not delay treatment*.
  - Early treatment may limit antibody formation.
  - Seropositivity increases with age in endemic states. Positive spotted fever group *Rickettsia* antibody does not necessarily signify an acute infection.
- Nonspecific laboratory changes (incidence) (4)
  - WBC count: variable and frequently normal
  - Thrombocytopenia (32–52%)
  - Hyponatremia, mild (19–56%)

- Anemia, mild (5–24%)
- Azotemia (12–14%)
- Elevated AST (36–62%)
- Coagulation derangements are uncommon, despite vascular damage.
- CSF is usually normal; some patients may have mononuclear pleocytosis, elevated protein, and normal glucose.
- Other than occasional nonspecific pneumonic infiltrates on chest radiograph, imaging procedures are rarely helpful.

Diagnostic Procedures/Other
Skin biopsy can offer definitive diagnosis. A 3-mm punch biopsy is sufficient to perform a rapid direct fluorescent antibody (DFA) test (sensitivity 70%, specificity 100%). Electron microscopy (EM) can also identify rickettsiae within endothelial cells. Western immunoblotting confirms the specific spotted fever group species (1,2,4).

Test Interpretation
- Rickettsiae can be demonstrated within endothelial cells by DFA or EM.
- Petechiae due to the vasculitis may be seen on various organ surfaces (e.g., liver, brain, or epicardium).
- Secondary thromboses and tissue necrosis may be seen.

TREATMENT

MEDICATION
First Line
Doxycycline is the treatment of choice in both adults and children (1–4).

- Untreated rickettsial infections have a high rate of morbidity and mortality. Other antibiotics are considerably less effective.
- The ONLY contraindication to doxycycline is severe allergy.
- For adults: 100 mg PO or IV q12h for 7 to 10 days, treat for at least 3 days after the fever resolves.
- For children weighing <45 kg (100 lbs): 2.2 mg/kg/dose (max 200 mg) q12h for 7 to 10 days, treating for at least 3 days after fever resolves; those ≥45 kg, refer to adult dosing (4)
- Fever should subside within 24 to 72 hours with early treatment; may take longer if patient is severely ill.
- If patient has no response to doxycycline, consider an alternate diagnosis. Rickettsial resistance to doxycycline has NOT been documented.
- Side effects of doxycycline
  - Dyspepsia. Take medication with food and water. Avoid dairy products, iron preparations, or antacids, as they may inhibit drug absorption.
  - Photosensitivity may occur. Minimize sun exposure and use sunscreen.
  - Risk of dental staining in children <8 years old is minimal if short courses are administered.

Second Line
- Chloramphenicol: 50 mg/kg/day IV divided q6h (4 g/day max); same dose in renal failure
  - Associated with aplastic anemia and an increased case mortality

- Fluoroquinolones have not been evaluated clinically in RMSF, but they have shown in vitro activity against *R. rickettsii*.
- Sulfa-containing drugs may worsen tick-borne infections and are contraindicated.

Pregnancy Considerations
- Doxycycline is appropriate for this life-threatening infection in pregnancy if suspicion is high, despite the potential risk to fetal bones/teeth.
- Chloramphenicol may be considered during the first 2 trimesters but should be avoided in the 3rd trimester due to potential for gray baby syndrome.

ISSUES FOR REFERRAL
- Consider infectious disease consult.
- Report cases of RMSF to public health authorities.

ADDITIONAL THERAPIES
Patients with neurologic injury or loss of limbs caused by gangrene may require prolonged physical and cognitive therapy.

INPATIENT CONSIDERATIONS
Admission Criteria/Initial Stabilization
- CNS dysfunction
- Nausea/vomiting preventing oral antibiotic therapy
- Immunocompromised patients
- Specific acute organ failure
- Failure of oral pain management
- ICU placement for acutely ill patients with shock

IV Fluids
Aggressive fluid resuscitation and electrolyte management may be required in critically ill patients.

Discharge Criteria
- Resolution of fever
- Ability to take oral therapy and nutrition

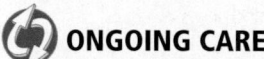 ONGOING CARE

FOLLOW-UP RECOMMENDATIONS
- Hospitalize patients with moderate to severe disease
- Patients with mild disease may be treated as outpatients. Close follow-up is important to identify complications.
- Infection does not confer lifelong immunity.

Patient Monitoring
- Outpatients should be seen every 2 to 3 days until symptoms resolve.
- Follow up CBC, electrolytes, LFTs if clinically indicated.

DIET
Consider nutritional supplementation if intake is poor.

PROGNOSIS
- Prognosis is closely related to timely administration of appropriate antibiotics. Treatment before day 5 of illness can prevent morbidity and mortality (6).
- When treated promptly, prognosis is usually excellent with resolution of symptoms over several days and no sequelae.

- If complications develop, course may be more severe and long-term sequelae (especially neurologic sequelae) more likely (6).
- Children aged 5 to 9 years and elderly >70 years are at higher risk of morbidity and/or mortality (4,6).
  - Black males with G6PD deficiency are at highest risk for fulminant RMSF, in which death can occur within 5 days (4).

COMPLICATIONS
- Encephalopathy (30–40%); most commonly transient impaired level of consciousness or meningismus
- Seizures, focal neurologic deficit (10%)
- Renal injury (10%)
- Hepatitis (10%)
- Congestive heart failure (CHF) (5%)
- Respiratory failure (5%)
- Proximal muscle weakness, changes in personality, paresthesias, distal necrosis, and deafness

REFERENCES
1. Lin L, Decker CF. Rocky Mountain spotted fever. *Dis Mon.* 2012;58(6):361–369.
2. Pujalte GG, Chua JV. Tick-borne infections in the United States. *Prim Care.* 2013;40(3):619–635.
3. Dahlgren FS, Holman RC, Paddock CD, et al. Fatal Rocky Mountain spotted fever in the United States, 1999–2007. *Am J Trop Med Hyg.* 2012;86(4): 713–719.
4. Woods CR. Rocky Mountain spotted fever in children. *Pediatr Clin North Am.* 2013;60(2):455–470. doi:10.1016/j.pcl.2012.12.001.
5. Minniear TD, Buckingham SC. Managing Rocky Mountain spotted fever. *Expert Rev Anti Infect Ther.* 2009;7(9):1131–1137.
6. Botelho-Nevers E, Raoult D. Host, pathogen and treatment-related prognostic factors in rickettsioses. *Eur J Clin Microbiol Infect Dis.* 2011;30(10):1139–1150.

 CODES

ICD10
A77.0 Spotted fever due to Rickettsia rickettsii

CLINICAL PEARLS
- Diagnosis of RMSF requires a high index of clinical suspicion. Painless tick bites often go unnoticed, and some patients may never develop a rash.
- Treatment should begin immediately in suspected cases. Doxycycline is indicated for treatment of RMSF in both adults AND children. The only absolute contraindication is severe allergy to the drug.
- Lab testing is nonspecific and frequently normal.
- Although prevalence is highest in central and southeastern United States, cases have been reported in almost all states.

ROSEOLA

Jeffrey D. Quinlan, MD, FAAFP

 BASICS

Omnipresent infection occurring in infancy and childhood. Majority of cases are caused by human herpesvirus 6 (HHV-6). May be associated with other diseases including encephalitis

DESCRIPTION
- Acute infection of infants or very young children (1)
- Causes a high fever followed by a skin eruption as the fever resolves (1)
- Transmission via contact with salivary secretions or respiratory droplet (1)
- Incubation period of 9 to 10 days (2)
- System(s) affected: skin/exocrine, metabolic, gastrointestinal, respiratory, neurologic
- Synonym(s): roseola infantum, exanthem subitum; pseudorubella; sixth disease; 3-day fever (3)

Pediatric Considerations
A disease of infants and very young children (4)

EPIDEMIOLOGY
- Predominant age
  - HHV-6
    - Infants and very young children (<2 years old) (5)
    - Peak age infection 6 to 9 months, rarely congenital or perinatal infection (1)
    - 95% of children have been infected with HHV-6 by 2 years of life.
  - HHV-7
    - Later childhood
    - Mean age of infection 26 months
    - >90% population with HHV-7 by 10 years (1)
- Predominant sex: male = female (1)
- No seasonal variance

Incidence
Common—accounts for 20% ED visits for febrile illness among children 6 to 8 months (6)

Prevalence
- Peak prevalence is between 9 and 21 months (5).
- Nearly 100% population carrying HHV-6 by 3 years (1)
- Approximately 20% patients with primary HHV-6 have roseola (6).

ETIOLOGY AND PATHOPHYSIOLOGY
- HHV-6 and HHV-7 (4)
- Majority of cases (60–74%) due to HHV-6
  - HHV-6B > HHV-6A (4)
  - HHV-6A seen in children in Africa
  - HHV-6 binds to CD46 receptors on all nucleated cells (4).
- Primary infection typically through respiratory droplets or saliva

- Congenital infection/vertical transmission occurs in 1% of cases (1).
  - Transplacental transmission
  - Chromosomal integration (clinical significance unknown)
- Lifelong latent or persistent asymptomatic infection occurs after primary infection (1).
  - 80–90% population intermittently sheds HHV-6/HHV-7 in saliva (4).
  - Patients are viremic from 2 days prior to fever until defervescence and onset of rash.
  - HHV-6 latency is also implicated in CSF (6).

Genetics
HHV-6 is integrated into the chromosomes of 0.2–3.0% of the population. This leads to vertical transmission of the virus. Clinical significance of this is unknown (1).

RISK FACTORS
- Female gender (5)
- Having older siblings (5)
- At-risk adults: immunocompromised (7)
  - Renal, liver, other solid organ, and bone marrow transplant (BMT) (5)
  - HHV-6 reactivation can occur in 1st week post-transplant (7). HHV-6 viremia occurs in 30–45% of BMT within the first several weeks after transplantation (6).
    - Usually asymptomatic (6)
    - Up to 82% of HHV-6 reactivation/reinfection in solid organ transplant (7)
- Nonrisk factors (5)
  - Child care attendance
  - Method of delivery
  - Breastfeeding (HHV does not appear to pass through breast milk)
  - Maternal age
  - Season

 DIAGNOSIS

HISTORY
- 3 to 5 days abrupt fever 102.2–104.0°F (39–40°C) not associated with a rash (1)
- The child may be fussy during this prodrome (1,6).
- Sudden drop of fever associated with appearance of rash (1)
  - Rash on trunk then spreads centrifugally mainly to neck, possibly also to peripheral extremities, and face.
- Diarrhea (5)
- Mild upper respiratory symptoms (5)
- Rhinorrhea (5)
- Febrile seizure occurs in 13% of cases (1).

PHYSICAL EXAM
- Rash (exanthem subitum) (1)
  - Rose-pink macules and/or papules that blanch
  - First appears on the trunk then peripherally
  - May occur up to 3 days after fever resolves (1)
  - Fades within 2 days
  - Occurs in approximately 20% of patients in the United States (1)
- Mild inflammation of tympanic membrane, pharynx, and/or conjunctiva (1,6)
- Ulcers on soft palate and uvula (Nagayama spots) (1)
- Cervical lymphadenopathy (1)
- Periorbital edema (4)

DIFFERENTIAL DIAGNOSIS
- Enterovirus infection (8)
- Adenovirus infection (1)
- Epstein-Barr virus
- Fifth disease—parvovirus B19 (8)
- Rubella (8)
- Scarlet fever (8)
- Drug eruption (1)
- Measles (1)

DIAGNOSTIC TESTS & INTERPRETATION
- Primarily a clinical diagnosis not requiring laboratory or radiologic testing (1)
- Tests often cannot differentiate latent or active disease (9).
- Specific diagnosis only necessary in severe cases, unclear diagnosis where more serious disease needs to be ruled out, or if considering antiviral therapy (1).

Initial Tests (lab, imaging)
- HHV-6 and HHV-7 by PCR (1,7)
  - Serum, whole blood, CSF, or saliva
  - Becoming more widely available
- HHV-6 IgM immunofluorescence (1)
  - Diagnostic for acute infection
  - Spike seen in 1st week of illness
- HHV-6 IgG immunofluorescence (1)
  - Check at diagnosis and then 2 weeks later.
  - Use with IgM to show primary infection.
  - Negative initial test and rise on follow-up suggests primary infection.
- Viral culture (7)
  - Rarely done
  - No clinical use (very time consuming)
- Other laboratory findings (1)
  - Decreased total leukocytes, lymphocytes, and neutrophils
  - Elevated transaminases
  - Thrombocytopenia

Diagnostic Procedures/Other
- Urine culture: to rule out UTI as source of fever (2)
- Chest x-ray (CXR): if a child has respiratory symptoms

TREATMENT

No treatment necessary, resolves without sequelae (1)[C].

GENERAL MEASURES
- Symptomatic relief including antipyretics (1)[C]
- Hydration (1)[C]

MEDICATION
First Line
- No specific first-line treatment in immunocompetent hosts beyond supportive measures (4)[C]
  - Antivirals are not recommended in immunocompetent.
- No approved antiviral treatment in immunocompromised (4).
- Second-line IV ganciclovir, cidofovir, foscarnet tested in vitro studies in stem cell transplant patients
  - HHV-6B susceptible: ganciclovir and foscarnet (7)[C]
  - HHV-6A and HHV-7 are more resistant to ganciclovir (7).
- Antivirals suggested in individual cases of encephalitis (associated with reactivation of HHV-6) (7)
- In bone marrow and stem cell transplant recipients receiving immunosuppression, ganciclovir prophylaxis is effective in preventing reactivation of HHV-6 (10)[B].

ONGOING CARE

FOLLOW-UP RECOMMENDATIONS
Patient Monitoring
- During febrile prodrome, monitor for dehydration.
- None after typical rash appears and fever resolves
- Mean duration of illness is 6 days (6).
- If febrile seizures occur, they will cease after fever subsides and will not likely recur (6).
- Symptomatic reactivation in immunocompromised (1)

DIET
Encourage fluids.

PATIENT EDUCATION
- Parental reassurance that this is usually a benign, self-limited disease (1).
- There is no specific recommended period of exclusion from out-of-home care for affected children.
- Patient is viremic a few days prior to fever until time of defervescence and rash onset.

PROGNOSIS
- Course: acute, complete recovery without sequelae (1)
- Reactivation in immunocompromised patients is common (6).

COMPLICATIONS
- Febrile seizures
  - 13% patients with roseola (1,6)
  - Accounts for 1/3 of primary seizures in children <2 years old (1)

- Medication hypersensitivity syndromes (drug reaction with eosinophilia and systemic symptoms) (4)
- Reactivation can occur in transplant patients, HIV-1 infection, and other immunocompromised individuals (6).
- Meningoencephalitis occurs in immunocompetent and in immunosuppressed patients (6). Poor association with multiple sclerosis (6)
- Pityriasis rosea (1)
- Possible association with progressive multifocal leukoencephalopathy (6)

REFERENCES

1. Stone RC, Micali GA, Schwartz RA. Roseola infantum and its causal human herpesviruses. *Int J Dermatol*. 2014;53(4):397–403.
2. Watkins J. Diagnosing rashes, part 4: generalized rashes with fever. *Practice Nursing*. 2013;24: 335–340.
3. Ely JW, Seabury Stone M. The generalized rash: part I. Differential diagnosis. *Am Fam Physician*. 2010;81(6):726–734.
4. Wolz MM, Sciallis GF, Pittelkow MR. Human herpesviruses 6, 7, and 8 from a dermatologic perspective. *Mayo Clin Proc*. 2012;87(10):1004–1014.
5. Zerr DM, Meier AS, Selke SS, et al. A population-based study of primary human herpesvirus 6 infection. *N Engl J Med*. 2005;352(8):768–776.
6. Caserta MT, Mock DJ, Dewhurst S. Human herpesvirus 6. *Clin Infect Dis*. 2001;33(6):829–833.
7. Le J, Gantt S. Human herpesvirus 6, 7 and 8 in solid organ transplantation. *Am J Transplant*. 2013;13(Suppl 4):128–137.
8. Ely JW, Seabury Stone M. The generalized rash: part II. Diagnostic approach. *Am Fam Physician*. 2010;81(6):735–739.
9. Dreyfus DH. Herpesviruses and the microbiome. *J Allergy Clin Immunol*. 2013;132(6):1278–1286.
10. Tokimasa S, Hara J, Osugi Y, et al. Ganciclovir is effective for prophylaxis and treatment of human herpesvirus-6 in allogeneic stem cell transplantation. *Bone Marrow Transplant*. 2002;29(7): 595–598.

ADDITIONAL READING

- Ablashi DV, Devin CL, Yoshikawa T, et al. Review part 3: human herpesvirus-6 in multiple non-neurological diseases. *J Med Virol*. 2010;82(11): 1903–1910.
- Caselli E, Di Luca D. Molecular biology and clinical associations of Roseoloviruses human herpesvirus 6 and human herpesvirus 7. *New Microbiol*. 2007;30(3):173–187.
- Dockrell DH, Smith TF, Paya CV. Human herpesvirus 6. *Mayo Clin Proc*. 1999;74(2):163–170.

- Dyer JA. Childhood viral exanthems. *Pediatr Ann*. 2007;36(1):21–29.
- Evans CM, Kudesia G, McKendrick M. Management of herpesvirus infections. *Int J Antimicrob Agents*. 2013;42(2):119–128.
- Fölster-Holst R, Kreth HW. Viral exanthems in childhood—infectious (direct) exanthems. Part 1: classic exanthems. *J Dtsch Dermatol Ges*. 2009;7(4): 309–316.
- Huang CT, Lin LH. Differentiating roseola infantum with pyuria from urinary tract infection. *Pediatr Int*. 2013;55(2):214–218.
- Leach CT. Human herpesvirus-6 and -7 infections in children: agents of roseola and other syndromes. *Curr Opin Pediatr*. 2000;12(3):269–274.
- Lowry M. Roseola infantum. *Pract Nurse*. 2013;43:40–42.
- Stoeckle MY. The spectrum of human herpesvirus 6 infection: from roseola infantum to adult disease. *Annu Rev Med*. 2000;51:423–430.
- Vianna RA, de Oliveira SA, Camacho LA, et al. Role of human herpesvirus 6 infection in young Brazilian children with rash illnesses. *Pediatr Infect Dis J*. 2008;27(6):533–537.

CODES

ICD10
- B08.20 Exanthema subitum [sixth disease], unspecified
- B08.21 Exanthema subitum [sixth disease] due to human herpesvirus 6
- B08.22 Exanthema subitum [sixth disease] due to human herpesvirus 7

CLINICAL PEARLS

- Roseola infection should be suspected if an infant or young child presents with a high temperature without other clinical findings.
- As the fever abates, a macular rash will be seen on the trunk, with eventual spread to the face and extremities in 20% of patients.
- Roseola is a clinical diagnosis, and laboratory testing is not necessary for most children with classic presentation.
- For atypical presentations, complications, and immunocompromised hosts, several laboratory tools are available, including serologic testing for antibody, viral PCR testing, and viral culture.
- Infection is typically self-limiting and without sequelae.
- Usually only symptomatic treatment is needed.
- Consider prophylaxis in patients undergoing bone marrow or stem cell transplant and receiving immunosuppressive therapy.

ROTATOR CUFF IMPINGEMENT SYNDROME

Faren H. Williams, MD, MS • Minjin Fromm, MD

 BASICS

DESCRIPTION

- Compression of rotator cuff tendons and subacromial bursa between the humeral head and the structures that makes up the coracoacromial arch and proximal humerus
- Most common cause of atraumatic shoulder pain in patients >25 years of age
- Primary symptom is pain that is most severe when the arm is abducted between 60 and 120 degrees (the "painful arc").
- Classically divided into three stages
  - Stage I: acute inflammation, edema, or hemorrhage of the underlying tendons due to overuse (typically in those age <25 years)
  - Stage II: progressive tendinosis that leads to partial rotator cuff tear along with underlying thickening or fibrosis of surrounding structures (commonly, ages 25 to 40 years)
  - Stage III: full-thickness tear (typically in patients age >40 years)

EPIDEMIOLOGY

Incidence
- Shoulder pain accounts for 1% of all primary care visits.
- Peak incidence of 25/1,000 patients/year occurs in patients aged 42 to 46 years.
- Impingement responsible for 18–74% of shoulder pain diagnoses.

Prevalence
Prevalence of shoulder pain in general population ranges from ~7% to 30%.

RISK FACTORS
- Repetitive overhead motions (throwing, swimming)
- Glenohumeral joint instability or muscle imbalance
- Acromioclavicular arthritis or osteophytes
- Thickened coracoacromial ligament
- Shoulder trauma
- Increasing age
- Smoking

GENERAL PREVENTION
- Proper throwing and lifting techniques
- Proper strengthening to balance rotator cuff and scapula stabilizer muscles

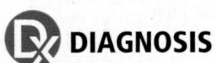 **DIAGNOSIS**

HISTORY
- Gradual increase in shoulder pain with overhead activities (sudden onset of sharp pain suggests a tear)
- Night pain is common, exacerbated by lying on the affected shoulder or sleeping with the affected arm above the head.
- Anterolateral shoulder pain with overhead activities

- May progress to weakness and decreased range of motion if shoulder is not used through full range of motion

PHYSICAL EXAM
- Examine patient for atrophy/asymmetry. Observe how the patient takes off his or her shirt as part of the exam.

- Neer impingement test: Examiner stabilizes the scapula and moves the affected upper extremity through a flexion arc. Patient reports pain with flexion of the shoulder. Sensitivity: 78%. Specificity: 58% (1)[A]
- Hawkins-Kennedy impingement test: Examiner places the arm in 90 degrees of forward flexion and then gently internally rotates the arm. End point for internal rotation is when the patient feels pain or when the rotation of the scapula is felt or observed by the examiner. Test is positive when patient experiences pain during the maneuver. Sensitivity: 74%. Specificity: 57% (1)[A]
- Empty can test (supraspinatus): Examiner asks the patient to elevate and internally rotate the arm with thumbs pointing downward in the scapular plane. Elbow should be fully extended. Examiner applies downward pressure on upper surface of the arm. Test is positive when patient complains of pain with resistance. Sensitivity: 69%. Specificity: 62% (1)[A]
- Lift-off test (subscapularis): Patient internally rotates the shoulder, placing the hand on ipsilateral buttock, then lifts hand off buttock against resistance. A tear in the subscapularis muscle produces weakness of this action. Sensitivity: 42%. Specificity: 97% (1)[A]
- Drop-arm test: Patient fully elevates arm and then slowly reverses the motion. If the arm is dropped suddenly or the patient has extreme pain, the test is positive for a possible rotator cuff tear. Sensitivity: 21%. Specificity: 92% (1)[A]

- Resisted external rotation: weakness suggestive of infraspinatus and/or teres minor tendon involvement
- Examine cervical spine to rule out cervical pathology as source of shoulder pain.
- Neurovascular exam of the upper extremity

DIFFERENTIAL DIAGNOSIS
- Labral injury
- Acromioclavicular arthritis (more common in older patients; positive cross-arm test—pain when affected arm is fully adducted across the chest in the horizontal plane)
- Adhesive capsulitis (rotator cuff tendonitis leads to decreased use and atrophy of rotator cuff muscles, followed by contracture; linked to diabetes and may be related to prior trauma)
- Anterior shoulder instability (prior trauma; more common in patients <25 years old)
- Multidirectional instability
- Biceps tendonitis or rupture (perform Speed and Yergason tests and look for visible or palpable defect of biceps—"Popeye sign")

- Calcific tendonitis
- Cervical radiculopathy (spinal or foraminal stenosis, can test with Spurling maneuver)
- Glenohumeral arthritis (evaluate with plain films)
- Suprascapular nerve entrapment (look for focal muscle atrophy of supra- or infraspinatus)
- Traumatic rotator cuff tear

DIAGNOSTIC TESTS & INTERPRETATION

Initial Tests (lab, imaging)
- Plain-film radiographs of the shoulder (three views): anteroposterior, axillary, scapular Y views
- Plain films may reveal:
  - Osteoarthritis of the acromioclavicular and glenohumeral joints
  - Superior migration of the humeral head (indicative of a large rotator cuff tear)
  - Cystic change of the humeral head and sclerosis of the inferior acromion (indicative of chronic rotator cuff disease)
  - Calcific tendonitis
- MRI is used to definitively assess rotator cuff tendinopathy, partial tears, and complete tears.
- MR arthrogram is preferred for labral pathology.
- Ultrasound is sensitive and specific for rotator cuff tears but is highly operator-dependent.
- CT scan is preferred for bony pathology or for those unable to undergo MRI.

Diagnostic Procedures/Other
- Lidocaine injection test
  - Inject lidocaine into the subacromial space:
    - Repeat impingement tests; if pain is completely relieved and range of motion is improved, likely impingement syndrome (rather than cuff tear).
  - Allows for more accurate strength testing on physical examination:
    - If strength is intact, rule out rotator cuff tear.
    - If range of motion does not improve in any plane, more likely adhesive capsulitis
  - Some pain relief and improved range of motion occurs after lidocaine injection with
    - Glenoid labral tear
    - Capsular strain
    - Glenohumeral osteoarthritis
    - Glenohumeral instability
- A lack of any pain relief suggests other sources or inappropriate placement of injection.

Test Interpretation
May have tendinosis, tendonitis, or muscle/tendon tear

 TREATMENT

Anti-inflammatory agents plus aggressive rehabilitation can improve and fully resolve rotator cuff tendonitis in most patients.

GENERAL MEASURES

- Rest
- Ice or heat for symptom relief
- Activity modification, with avoidance of aggravating activities, particularly overhead motions
- Range-of-motion exercises
- Rotator-cuff and adjacent muscle strengthening to enhance stability and prevent further injuries

MEDICATION

First Line

NSAIDs or other analgesic, often for 6 to 12 weeks

ISSUES FOR REFERRAL

Failure of conservative treatment, persistent pain, weakness, or complete tear of rotator cuff

ADDITIONAL THERAPIES

- Supervised- or home-exercise regimens provide clinically significant pain reduction and improve function (2)[A].
- Physical therapy is effective for short-term and long-term recovery of function (3)[A]:
  – Initial goal is to restore range of motion.
  – After pain resolves, gradually strengthen rotator cuff muscles in internal rotation, external rotation, and abduction.

COMPLEMENTARY & ALTERNATIVE MEDICINE

Acupuncture is of potential benefit to reduce pain and improve function, particularly when used with physical therapy (4)[A].

SURGERY/OTHER PROCEDURES

- Steroid injections may have a significant benefit on pain and function in the short term but do not appear to have a significant long-term effect (5)[A]:
  – Risk for rotator cuff tears not significantly increased in those receiving subacromial steroid injections (6)[C].
- No evidence that surgery is superior to conservative management, or that one surgical technique is superior to another for impingement syndrome (7)[A].
- Platelet-rich therapies for musculoskeletal soft tissue injuries are increasingly common.
  – No apparent effect of platelet-rich plasma injection during arthroscopic rotator cuff repair on overall retear rates or shoulder-specific outcomes (8)[A],(9).
- Extracorporeal shock wave therapy is currently under study as an emerging treatment for calcific tendonitis (10).

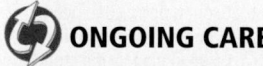 ONGOING CARE

PATIENT EDUCATION

- Physical rehabilitation is necessary, both in conservative course of treatment (i.e., NSAIDs, physical therapy, home exercises) and with surgical intervention. An aggressive trial of rehabilitation should be encouraged prior to extensive testing or surgical intervention. Providing pain relief prior to beginning a program of physical therapy improves adherence and outcomes.
- Symptoms often recur if not fully addressed.

PROGNOSIS

- Variable, depends on underlying pathology
- Most patients improve with conservative management. Recovery can be slow.
- Patients with more severe symptoms—those with symptoms for >1 year—are less likely to respond well with conservative therapies.

COMPLICATIONS

- Progression of injury
- Tendon retraction in complete rotator cuff tear

REFERENCES

1. Alqunaee M, Galvin R, Fahey T. Diagnostic accuracy of clinical tests for subacromial impingement syndrome: a systematic review and meta-analysis. *Arch Phys Med Rehabil*. 2012;93(2):229–236.
2. Kuhn JE. Exercise in the treatment of rotator cuff impingement: a systematic review and a synthesized evidence-based rehabilitation protocol. *J Shoulder Elbow Surg*. 2009;18(1):138–160.
3. Green S, Buchbinder R, Hetrick S. Physiotherapy interventions for shoulder pain. *Cochrane Database Syst Rev*. 2003;(2):CD004258.
4. Vas J, Ortega C, Olmo V, et al. Single-point acupuncture and physiotherapy for the treatment of painful shoulder: a multicentre randomized controlled trial. *Rheumatology (Oxford)*. 2008;47(6):887–893.
5. Gaujoux-Viala C, Dougados M, Gossec L. Efficacy and safety of steroid injections for shoulder and elbow tendonitis: a meta-analysis of randomised controlled trials. *Ann Rheum Dis*. 2009;68(12):1843–1849.
6. Bhatia M, Singh B, Nicolaou N, et al. Correlation between rotator cuff tears and repeated subacromial steroid injections: a case-controlled study. *Ann R Coll Surg Engl*. 2009;91(5):414–416.
7. Gebremariam L, Hay EM, Koes BW, et al. Effectiveness of surgical and postsurgical interventions for the subacromial impingement syndrome: a systematic review. *Arch Phys Med Rehabil*. 2011;92(11):1900–1913.
8. Chahal J, Van Thiel GS, Mall N, et al. The role of platelet-rich plasma in arthroscopic rotator cuff repair: a systematic review with quantitative synthesis. *Arthroscopy*. 2012;28(11):1718–1727.
9. Moraes VY, Lenza M, Tamaoki MJ, et al. Platelet-rich therapies for musculoskeletal soft tissue injuries. *Cochrane Database Syst Rev*. 2013;(12):CD010071. doi:10.1001/14651858. CD010071.pub2.
10. Ioppolo, F, Tattoli M, Di Sante L, et al. Clinical improvement and resorption of calcifications in calcific tendinitis of the shoulder after shock wave therapy at 6 months' follow-up: a systemic review and meta-analysis. *Arch Phys Med Rehabil*. 2013;94(9):1699–1706.

ADDITIONAL READING

- Baumgarten KM, Gerlach D, Galatz LM, et al. Cigarette smoking increases the risk for rotator cuff tears. *Clin Orthop Relat Res*. 2010;468(6): 1534–1541.
- Burbank KM, Stevenson JH, Czarnecki GR, et al. Chronic shoulder pain: part I. Evaluation and diagnosis. *Am Fam Physician*. 2008;77(4):453–460.
- Burbank KM, Stevenson JH, Czarnecki GR, et al. Chronic shoulder pain: part II. Treatment. *Am Fam Physician*. 2008;77(4):493–497.
- Cumpston M, Johnston RV, Wengier L, et al. Topical glyceryl trinitrate for rotator cuff disease. *Cochrane Database Syst Rev*. 2009;(3):CD006355.
- Hanchard NC, Lenza M, Handoll HH, et al. Physical tests for shoulder impingements and local lesions of bursa, tendon or labrum that may accompany impingement. *Cochrane Database Syst Rev*. 2013;(4):CD007427.
- Hegedus EJ, Goode A, Campbell S, et al. Physical examination tests of the shoulder: a systematic review with meta-analysis of individual tests. *Br J Sports Med*. 2008;42(2):80–92.
- Kennedy DJ, Visco CJ, Press J. Current concepts for shoulder training in the overhead athlete. *Curr Sports Med Rep*. 2009;8(3):154–160.

 CODES

ICD10

- M75.40 Impingement syndrome of unspecified shoulder
- M75.110 Incmpl rotatr-cuff tear/ruptr of unsp shoulder, not trauma
- M75.120 Complete rotatr-cuff tear/ruptr of unsp shoulder, not trauma

CLINICAL PEARLS

- Consider impingement syndrome in patients involved with repetitive overhead activities (e.g., swimming, throwing) who present with shoulder pain.
- Atraumatic shoulder pain in middle age often represents rotator cuff tendonitis.
- Supraspinatus tendon is most commonly affected in impingement syndrome.
- Neer and Hawkins tests specifically check for shoulder impingement.
- The empty can maneuver tests for weakness of supraspinatus muscle.
- The drop-arm test is specific for rotator cuff tear.
- Physical therapy over 6 to 12 weeks promotes return to function
- Most patients with shoulder impingement respond well to conservative management. Those who don't should be referred for surgical evaluation.

SALIVARY GLAND CALCULI/SIALADENITIS

Jason E. Cohn, DO, MS • Mark Weitzel, DO • Seth Zwillenberg, MD

 BASICS

DESCRIPTION
- Inflammation and/or infection involving one or more salivary gland
- Sialolithiasis is the cause of ~90% of all obstructive salivary gland diseases.
- Salivary obstruction is usually characterized by a painful swelling of the affected gland when eating, known as "mealtime syndrome."
- The submandibular gland is more commonly affected (80–90% of cases) by sialolithiasis and infection than the parotid gland. Submandibular stones occur more commonly due to higher mucinous content of saliva, longer course of Wharton duct, slow salivary flow, and saliva flow against gravity.
- Can be acute or chronic
  – Types: infectious, obstructive (sialolithiasis), and autoimmune

EPIDEMIOLOGY
Incidence
- Predominant age: Peak incidence is 30 to 60 years.
- Most common in debilitated and dehydrated patients
- 49% men and 51% women, average age 47.5 years; 82% submandibular stones and 18% parotid stones, 44% had a positive smoking history, and 20% of patients were taking diuretics.

Prevalence
- Salivary calculi can be found in 1.2% of the adult population.
- Only 5% of all cases occur in the pediatric population.
- In those with sialographic evidence of benign intraductal obstruction, the obstruction is caused by salivary calculi in >73% of cases.

ETIOLOGY AND PATHOPHYSIOLOGY
- Decreased salivary outflow from anticholinergics, dehydration, or radiation is thought to allow bacterial infection of salivary glands.
- Salivary calculi form by deposition of calcium phosphate. Predisposing factors include salivary stasis, retrograde bacterial contamination from the oral cavity, increased alkalinity of saliva, and physical trauma to salivary duct or gland.
- Gout is a well-known systemic disease known to be associated with salivary stone development. In gout, sialoliths are composed of uric acid.
- Sialadenitis occurs by recurrent inflammatory reactions that result in progressive acinar destruction with fibrous replacement and sialectasis.
- Bacterial sialadenitis: *Staphylococcus aureus*, *Streptococcus viridans*, *Streptococcus pyogenes*, *Haemophilus influenzae*, *Escherichia coli*, *Pseudomonas aeruginosa*, and group B streptococci (neonates and prepubescent children)
- Viral sialadenitis: mumps, cytomegalovirus (CMV), Epstein-Barr virus (EBV), HIV, and enteroviruses

Pediatric Considerations
The two most common causes of sialadenitis in children are mumps and idiopathic juvenile recurrent parotitis.

Genetics
Polygenic cause, with several loci under investigation

RISK FACTORS
- Dehydration
- Anticholinergic use
- Antihistamine use
- Diuretic use
- Poor oral hygiene
- Malnutrition
- Head/neck radiation
- Tuberculosis (TB)
- HIV
- Failure to immunize (mumps)
- Gout
- Diabetes mellitus
- Hypothyroidism
- Renal failure
- Duct strictures
- Previous intraoral procedures

GENERAL PREVENTION
- Adequate hydration
- Maintain proper oral care and hygiene.
- Avoid antihistamines, anticholinergics, and other causes of xerostomia, especially if other risk factors are present.

COMMONLY ASSOCIATED CONDITIONS
- Postoperative dehydration
- Radiation-induced xerostomia
- Drug-induced xerostomia
- Sjögren syndrome
- Hypercalcemia

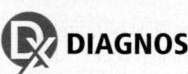 **DIAGNOSIS**

HISTORY
- Acute onset of pain and swelling over the affected salivary gland, especially postprandial
- Dental pain, discharge, foul breath (halitosis), and pain with chewing
- Fever, unintentional weight loss
- Xerostomia
- Recent dental work, surgery
- Immunization history
- Radiation, TB, and HIV exposure
- History of alcoholism, bulimia, and malnutrition (suggest sialadenosis)

PHYSICAL EXAM
- Palpate all salivary glands, floor of mouth, tongue, and neck to assess symmetry, tenderness, induration, edema, presence of stones, and lymphadenopathy.
- Examine duct openings for purulent discharge and saliva.
- Palpate gland gently to express purulent material.
- Examine eyes for interstitial keratitis.
- Note lingual papillary atrophy and/or loss of tooth enamel.

Pediatric Considerations
Stones in children are traditionally smaller in size, within the duct distally, and present with a shorter symptom duration.

DIFFERENTIAL DIAGNOSIS
- Acute bacterial parotitis
- Chronic bacterial parotitis
- Idiopathic juvenile recurrent parotitis

- Dental abscess
- Mumps
- TB
- HIV (in pediatric populations)
- EBV, CMV, enteroviruses
- Tularemia
- Cystic fibrosis
- Lupus
- Sjögren syndrome
- Alcoholism
- Bulimia
- Hypothyroidism
- Pleomorphic adenoma
- Lymphoma
- Sarcoidosis
- Collagen vascular disease
- Metal poisoning

DIAGNOSTIC TESTS & INTERPRETATION
Initial Tests (lab, imaging)
- CBC, electrolytes
- Culture and sensitivity of any expressed pus
- CT scan with IV contrast is the preferred imaging modality.
- Ultrasound can localize abscesses as well as stones. Stones appear hyperechoic with posterior shadowing (1)[B].
- Sonopalpation (concurrent ultrasound with transoral palpation) proved to have a sensitivity and specificity of 96.6% and 90% in finding a calculi (2)[B].
- Minor salivary gland biopsy.

Follow-Up Tests & Special Considerations
- If autoimmune process is suspected, consider ordering appropriate labs, such as autoantibody titers: Sjögren syndrome A (SS-A) and Sjögren syndrome B (SS-B), rheumatoid factor (RF), and antinuclear antibodies (ANAs). Erythrocyte sedimentation rate (ESR) may also be conducted.
- Consider serial CT scans with contrast to evaluate disease resolution.
- Ultrasound can identify indicators of persistent obstruction in patients undergoing sialolithotomy (1)[B].

Diagnostic Procedures/Other
- Sialography to evaluate sialolithiasis and other obstructive lesions
- Sialendoscopy to find and remove sialoliths. In one study, sialendoscopy confirmed 221 (79%) parotid and 812 (93%) submandibular stones (3)[A].
- One study revealed that sonography, cone beam CT and sialendoscopy all had excellent specificity and positive predictive value in diagnosing stones. However, sialendoscopy was superior in sensitivity and negative predictive value (4)[B].
- When sialendoscopy fails, a novel ultrasound-guided needle localization approach has been proposed (5)[B].
- Technetium 99m pertechnetate scintigraphy showed decreased gland excretion and decreased uptake in patients with sialolithiasis (6)[B].

Test Interpretation
In chronic sialadenitis, loss of acini, fibrosis, and periductal lymphocytosis are evident; degree indicates chronicity.

TREATMENT

GENERAL MEASURES
- Maintain hydration.
- Apply warm compresses with massage.
- Maintain good oral hygiene.
- Antibiotics if indicated by diagnosis

MEDICATION

First Line
- Antistaphylococcal penicillins (nafcillin, dicloxacillin) are indicated in areas where methicillin-resistant *Staphylococcus aureus* (MRSA) is not predominant.
- Penicillin-allergic: Use clindamycin 300 mg PO q8h
- Gram negative: third-generation cephalosporin or fluoroquinolone
- Anaerobic: metronidazole or clindamycin
- Antibiotic coverage should be narrowed once culture and sensitivity are available.
- Continue antibiotic therapy for 10 to 14 days.

Second Line
- 1st-generation cephalosporin (cephalexin or cefazolin) or clindamycin is also indicated for empiric coverage.
- If MRSA than Vancomycin.

ISSUES FOR REFERRAL
In the case of poor dentition and dental abscess, refer patient to a dentist.

ADDITIONAL THERAPIES
In the case of chronic sialadenitis with strictures, consider sialostent placement.

SURGERY/OTHER PROCEDURES
- Submandibular stones found in the anterior floor of the mouth can be excised intraorally (sialodochoplasty), whereas those in the hilum require gland excision. Parotid stones usually require parotidectomy (7)[A].
- Good results in patient symptom relief, quality of life and safety have been reported in sialadenitis and sialolithiasis using sialendoscopy (7–10)[A]. However, one study revealed a complication rate of 3.23%. Complications include strictures, ranulas, and lingual nerve injury (11)[C].
- Incision and drainage of parotid abscess is indicated after failing 3 to 5 days of medical management.
- Sialoliths and stenoses can be successfully treated by radiologically or fluoroscopically controlled or sialendoscopically based methods in ~80% of cases. Extracorporeal shock wave lithotripsy (ESWL) is successful in up to 50% of cases.
- Transoral duct slitting is an important method for extraparenchymal submandibular stones, with a success rate of 90%.
- Recent evidence shows that larger stones can be successfully and safely treated with holmium: YAG laser lithotripsy (12,13)[B].

Pediatric Considerations
The most effective diagnostic and therapeutic modality for children with sialadenitis is sialendoscopy with stone retrieval (14)[B].

COMPLEMENTARY & ALTERNATIVE MEDICINE
Consider lemon drops or other sialogogues to promote salivation. In one study, postoperative use of sialogogues nearly halved rates of sialadenitis (15)[C].

INPATIENT CONSIDERATIONS

Admission Criteria/Initial Stabilization
- Parotid abscess
- Sepsis
- Inability to tolerate PO intake
- Airway, breathing, circulation
- Check vital signs, with particular attention to blood pressure, as patient may be septic secondary to abscess formation.
- Evaluate airway patency.

Nursing
Responsibilities may include ensuring excellent oral hygiene and avoiding administration of drugs that cause decreased production or flow of saliva.

Discharge Criteria
- Exclude abscess or sepsis.
- Ensure ability to tolerate PO intake.
- Stable vital signs

ONGOING CARE

FOLLOW-UP RECOMMENDATIONS
- Provide regular follow-up visits for patients with chronic sialadenitis.
- Avoid prescribing medications that cause xerostomia.

Patient Monitoring
Continue to monitor patients with chronic sialadenitis, as decreased salivary gland function due to fibrosis and loss of acini can lead to acute exacerbations.

DIET
- Avoid sialogogues during acute attacks.
- Maintain adequate hydration on an outpatient basis.

PATIENT EDUCATION
- Educate patients on maintaining excellent oral hygiene.
- Educate patients on maintaining good hydration.

PROGNOSIS
- Generally excellent, with acute symptoms resolving in about a week with appropriate treatment
- Patients with autoimmune etiology may have prolonged course due to systemic involvement.

COMPLICATIONS
Abscess, dental caries, recurrent sialadenitis, facial nerve impingement, Ludwig angina

REFERENCES

1. Joshi AS, Lohia S. Ultrasound indicators of persistent obstruction after submandibular sialolithotomy. *Otolaryngol Head Neck Surg.* 2013;149(6):873–877.
2. Patel NJ, Hashemi S, Joshi AS. Sonopalpation: a novel application of ultrasound for detection of submandibular calculi. *Otolaryngol Head Neck Surg.* 2014;151(5):770–775.
3. Zenk J, Koch M, Klintworth N, et al. Sialendoscopy in the diagnosis and treatment of sialolithiasis: a study of more than 1000 patients. *Otolaryngol Head Neck Surg.* 2012;147(5):858–863.
4. Schwarz D, Kabbasch C, Scheer M, et al. Comparative analysis of sialendoscopy, sonography, and CBCT in the detection of sialolithiasis. *Laryngoscope.* 2015;125(5):1098–1101.
5. Joshi AS, Sood AJ. Ultrasound-guided needle localization during open parotid sialolithotomy. *Otolaryngol Head Neck Surg.* 2014;151(1): 59–64.
6. Wu CB, Xi H, Zhou Q, et al. The diagnostic value of technetium 99m pertechnetate salivary gland scintigraphy in patients with certain salivary gland diseases. *J Oral Maxillofac Surg.* 2015;73(3):443–450.
7. Wilson KF, Meier JD, Ward PD. Salivary gland disorders. *Am Fam Physician.* 2014;89(11): 882–888.
8. Atienza G, López-Cedrún JL. Management of obstructive salivary disorders by sialendoscopy: a systematic review. *Br J Oral Maxillofac Surg.* 2015;53(6):507–519.
9. Gillespie MB, O'Connell BP, Rawl JW, et al. Clinical and quality-of-life outcomes following gland-preserving surgery for chronic sialadenitis. *Laryngoscope.* 2014;125(6):1340–1344.
10. Meier BA, Holst R, Schousboe LP. Patient-perceived benefit of sialendoscopy as measured by Glasgow Benefit Inventory. *Laryngoscope.* 2015;125(8):1874–1878.
11. Nahlieli O. Complications of sialendoscopy: personal experience, literature analysis, and suggestions. *J Oral Maxillofac Surg.* 2015;73(1): 75–80.
12. Sionis S, Caria RA, Trucas M, et al. Sialendoscopy with and without holmium: YAG laser-assisted lithotripsy in the management of obstructive sialadenitis of major salivary glands. *Br J Oral Maxillofac Surg.* 2014;52(1):58–62.
13. Phillips J, Withrow K. Outcomes of holmium laser-assisted lithotripsy with sialendoscopy in treatment of sialolithiasis. *Otolaryngol Head Neck Surg.* 2014;150(6):962–967.
14. Francis CL, Larsen CG. Pediatric sialadenitis. *Otolaryngol Clin North Am.* 2014;47(5):763–778.
15. Nakada K, Ishibashi T, Takei T, et al. Does lemon candy decrease salivary gland damage after radioiodine therapy for thyroid cancer? *J Nucl Med.* 2005;46(2):261–266.

ADDITIONAL READING

Koch M, Zenk J, Iro H. Algorithms for treatment of salivary gland obstructions. *Otolaryngol Clin North Am.* 2009;42(6):1173–1192.

CODES

ICD10
- K11.5 Sialolithiasis
- K11.20 Sialoadenitis, unspecified
- K11.21 Acute sialoadenitis

CLINICAL PEARLS
- Sialadenitis occurs mainly in debilitated patients who lack ability to control hydration.
- Sialadenitis is associated with conditions that predispose patient to xerostomia.
- Mainstay of treatment is hydration, good oral hygiene, sialogogues, and possible surgical excision.
- Many cases are now being successfully and safely treated with sialendoscopy.

S

SALMONELLA INFECTION

Justin Thomas Ertle, BS, MD • Marie L. Borum, MD, EdD, MPH

 BASICS

DESCRIPTION
- Infection caused by any serotype of the bacterial genus *Salmonella*, a gram-negative anaerobic bacillus
- Nontyphoidal *Salmonella* typically causes gastroenteritis via foodborne infection and sporadic outbreaks. Less commonly causes infection outside the gastrointestinal tract

Clinical syndromes
- Enteric fever (see "Typhoid Fever")
- Nontyphoidal gastroenteritis
  - Chronic carrier state (>1 year)
- Nontyphoidal invasive disease
  - Bacteremia
    ○ Endovascular complications
    ○ Localized infection outside GI tract

Geriatric Considerations
Patients >65 years old have increased risk of developing invasive disease with bacteremia and endovascular complications due to comorbidities (atherosclerotic endovascular lesions, prostheses, etc.) that increase risk of seeding (1).

Pediatric Considerations
Neonates (<3 months) are more susceptible to invasive disease and complications (1).

EPIDEMIOLOGY
Incidence
- Global incidence of nontyphoidal *Salmonella* enteritidis estimated to be 93.8 million per year in 2009 (2).
  - Wide variation by region from 40 to 3,980 estimated cases per 100,000 in 2009 (2)
- Global incidence of invasive nontyphoidal *Salmonella* infection estimated to be 2.1 to 6.5 million in 2010 (2).
  - Wide variation by region from 0.8 to 227 estimated cases per 100,000 in 2010 (2)
- Most commonly identified foodborne illness in the United States and a common cause of traveler's diarrhea (3)
- Second most common bacteria isolated from stool cultures in diarrheal illness (following *Campylobacter*) in the United States (3)
- Highest incidence in children <5 years old
- Hospitalization rates higher in patients >50 years old
- Peak frequency: July to November

ETIOLOGY AND PATHOPHYSIOLOGY
- *Salmonella enterica*
  - Most pathogenic species in humans
  - 2,500 different serotypes

Etiology
- ~95% of cases are foodborne (3).
- Majority of the other 5% of cases are due to direct or indirect fecal–oral contact with animals or human carriers.
- Iatrogenic contamination (e.g., blood transfusion, endoscopy) is possible, although rare.

Pathophysiology
- Typical infectious dose in immunocompetent patients is ingestion of one million bacteria (3).
- Bacteria ingested invade the distal ileal and proximal colonic mucosa to produce an inflammatory and cytotoxic response.
- Bacteria can enter the mesenteric lymphatic system and then into systemic circulation to cause disseminated/invasive disease.

RISK FACTORS
- Recent travel
- Consumption of undercooked meat, egg, or unpasteurized dairy products. Nonanimal products have also been implicated in outbreaks.
- Contact with live reptiles or poultry.
- Contact with human carrier who has *Salmonella* fecal shedding.
- Impaired gastric acidity: H_2 receptor blockers, antacids, proton pump inhibitors (PPIs), gastrectomy, achlorhydria, pernicious anemia, infants
- Recent antibiotic use
- Reticuloendothelial blockade: sickle cell disease, malaria, bartonellosis
- Immunosuppression: HIV, diabetes, corticosteroid or other immunosuppressant use, chemotherapy
- Iron overload, chronic granulomatous disease
- Age <5 years or >50 years

GENERAL PREVENTION
- Proper hygiene in production, transport, and storage of food (e.g., refrigeration during food storage and thoroughly cooking food prior to consumption)
- Control of animal reservoirs: Avoid contact with high-risk animals, animal feces, and polluted waters.
- Hand hygiene
- CDC Web site (http://www.cdc.gov/salmonella/) tracks outbreaks

COMMONLY ASSOCIATED CONDITIONS
- Gastroenteritis
- Bacteremia: immunocompromised patients or those with underlying medical conditions (e.g., cholelithiasis, prostheses)
- Osteomyelitis: higher incidence in sickle cell disease
- Abscesses: higher incidence with malignant tumors
- Reactive arthritis

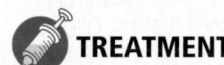 **DIAGNOSIS**

HISTORY
- *Salmonella* infections are typically asymptomatic or result in mild, self-limited gastroenteritis (1)[C].
- Exposure history: travel; contact with infected human, reptile, or poultry; improper food preparation
- Host factors: age, immune status, other risk factors
- Symptoms typically begin 12 to 72 hours after ingestion and resolve within 4 to 10 days (4)[A].
- Acute uncomplicated illness
  - Sudden onset of nausea, vomiting, diarrhea (1)[C]
  - Abdominal cramping (1)[C]
  - Headache (1)[C]
  - Myalgias (1)[C]
  - Fever (1)[C]

PHYSICAL EXAM
- Fever (1)[A]
- Evidence of hypovolemia (1)[C]
- Abdominal tenderness (1)[C]
- Heme-positive stool in some patients (1)[C]
- Hepatosplenomegaly in some patients (3)[C]

DIFFERENTIAL DIAGNOSIS
- Viral gastroenteritis
- Bacterial enteritis due to other organisms
- Pseudomembranous colitis
- Inflammatory bowel disease

DIAGNOSTIC TESTS & INTERPRETATION
Initial Tests (lab, imaging)
- Gastroenteritis
  - Stool culture for *Salmonella*, *Escherichia coli*, *Shigella*, and *Campylobacter* (1)[C]
  - Indications for stool culture include:
    ○ Severe diarrhea (≥6 loose stools daily) (1)[C]
    ○ Diarrhea >1 week in duration (1)[C]
    ○ Fever (1)[C]
    ○ Diarrhea containing blood or mucous (1)[C]
    ○ Multiple cases suggesting an outbreak (1)[C]
  - Fecal leukocytes: positive
- Bacteremia
  - Blood cultures (1)[C]
  - Stool cultures: may also be positive (1)[C]
- Endovascular infection
  - Consider angiography in patients >50 years of age with bacteremia if aortic or vascular source is suspected (4)[A].
- Local infections
  - Wound culture
  - Consider CT or MRI for soft tissue or bone infections (3)[C].
- Chronic carrier state
  - Stool culture positive for >1 year (3)[C]
  - Urine culture may be positive in chronic carriers.

Follow-Up Tests & Special Considerations
- Diarrhea lasting >10 days should prompt investigation for other causes.
- Asymptomatic excretion of *Salmonella* may occur for weeks after infection; follow-up fecal cultures are generally not indicated for patients with uncomplicated gastroenteritis (3,4)[C].
- Follow-up blood cultures are suggested for patients with bacteremia (3)[C].

Test Interpretation
Intestinal biopsies (if taken) may show mucosal ulceration, hemorrhage, and necrosis seen on along with reticuloendothelial hypertrophy/hyperplasia.

TREATMENT

- Treatment for nonsevere nontyphoidal *Salmonella* gastroenteritis in immunocompetent patients is supportive. The illness is typically self-limited. There is no proven benefit to treatment of mild disease. Treatment can suppress the host immunologic, and higher rates of relapse have been reported (1)[C],(5)[A].
- Consider antibiotics in immunocompetent hosts with severe diarrhea, high fever, or in those requiring hospitalization (1)[C].
- Some patients are at increased risk of bacteremia and benefit from antibiotics:
  - Infants <3 months of age (1)[C]
  - Persons >50 years old especially >65 years old (1,3)[C]
  - Patients with hemoglobinopathies, atherosclerotic lesions, and prosthetic valves, grafts, or joints or any immunosuppressed state (1,3)[C],(4)[A]
- Chronic carriage of nontyphoidal *Salmonella*
  - 4 to 6 weeks of antimicrobial therapy
  - Prophylactic therapy in immunocompromised patients (4)[A]

GENERAL MEASURES

- Hydration and electrolyte replacement
- Hand washing and barrier precautions for inpatients
- Avoid antimotility drugs in patients with fever or dysentery. Antimotility drugs may increase contact time of the enteropathogen in the gut mucosa (1)[C].

MEDICATION

First Line

- Gastroenteritis, uncomplicated: No specific medications are necessary. Supportive care (1)[A]
- Gastroenteritis, complicated (due to illness severity or host risk factors such as immunocompromise)
  - Adults (treat for 14 days if immunocompromised)
    ○ Levofloxacin (or other fluoroquinolone) 500 mg/day PO for 7 to 10 days (1)[C]; or
    ○ Trimethoprim-sulfamethoxazole: 160/800 mg PO BID for 7 to 10 days or
    ○ Amoxicillin: 500 mg PO TID for 7 to 10 days or
    ○ Ceftriaxone: 1 to 2 g/day IV for 7 to 10 days or
    ○ Azithromycin: 500 mg/day PO for 7 days (1)[C]
  - Children
    ○ Ceftriaxone: 100 mg/kg/day IV or IM in 2 equally divided doses for 7 to 10 days (1)[C]; or
    ○ Azithromycin: 20 mg/kg/day PO daily for 7 days (1)[C]
  - HIV patients
    ○ Increased duration of antimicrobial therapy and/or zidovudine may decrease relapse (4)[C].
- Bacteremia: Due to resistance trends, treat life-threatening infections in adults with a fluoroquinolone and a 3rd-generation cephalosporin until susceptibilities are determined (4)[A].
  - Adults
    ○ Ciprofloxacin (or other fluoroquinolone): 400 mg IV BID for 10 to 14 days; plus
    ○ Ceftriaxone: 1 to 2 g/day IV for 10 to 14 days; or
    ○ Cefotaxime: 2 g IV q8h for 10 to 14 days
  - Children
    ○ Ampicillin: 200 mg/kg/day in 4 divided doses for 10 to 14 days; or
    ○ Trimethoprim-sulfamethoxazole: 8 to 12 mg/kg/day of trimethoprim component in 2 divided doses for 10 to 14 days; or
    ○ Ceftriaxone: 50 to 75 mg/kg/day (max 1 g) once per day for 10 to 14 days
- Localized infection (e.g., septic arthritis, osteomyelitis, cholangitis, and pneumonia)
  - Same treatment as for bacteremia
  - In sustained bacteremia, prolonged local infection, or immunocompromised patients, give antibiotics PO for 4 to 6 weeks (4)[A].
- Chronic carrier state (shedding >1 year duration)
  - Amoxicillin: 1 g PO TID for 12 weeks; or
  - Trimethoprim-sulfamethoxazole 160 mg/800 mg PO BID for 12 weeks; or
  - Ciprofloxacin: 500 mg PO BID for 4 weeks, or
  - Levofloxacin 500 mg/day for 4 weeks; or
  - Norfloxacin 400 mg PO BID for 4 weeks if gallstones are present.

ALERT

Antimicrobial resistance

- Strains resistant to ampicillin, chloramphenicol, and trimethoprim-sulfamethoxazole have been reported (6)[B].
- Fluoroquinolone resistance is increasing, perhaps due to increasing use in livestock (6)[B].
- Extended-spectrum cephalosporin resistance has been reported with increasing frequency (6)[B].

Second Line

- Aztreonam is an alternative agent that may be useful in patients with multiple allergies or organisms with unusual resistance patterns (4)[A].
- Fluoroquinolones are now routinely given to children for 5 to 7 days in areas of the world where multidrug-resistant Salmonella typhi is common (4)[A].

SURGERY/OTHER PROCEDURES

- Surgical excision and drainage for infected tissue sites, followed by a minimum of 2 weeks of antibiotic therapy (4)[A]
- If biliary tract disease is present, a preoperative 10- to 14-day course of parenteral antibiotics is recommended prior to cholecystectomy.

 ONGOING CARE

FOLLOW-UP RECOMMENDATIONS

Patient Monitoring

- Asymptomatic shedding of Salmonella may occur for weeks after infection. Follow-up fecal cultures are generally not indicated for patients with uncomplicated gastroenteritis. Requirements may differ during a Salmonella outbreak (4)[A].
- Criteria may vary by state and local regulations. Some public health departments require negative stool cultures for health workers and food handlers prior to returning to work. Shedding may last 4 to 8 weeks (4)[A].
- Serotyping of isolates can be performed at public health laboratories.

DIET

Easily digestible foods (1)[C]

PATIENT EDUCATION

- Meticulous hand hygiene; caution handling raw meat, poultry, and eggs
- Fruits and vegetables should be thoroughly washed prior to consumption.
- Thoroughly cooking meats eliminates Salmonella.
- Caution when handling animals with high fecal carriage rates
- www.cdc.gov/salmonella/general/prevention.html

PROGNOSIS

- Most cases of Salmonella gastroenteritis are self-limited and have an excellent prognosis.
- Increased mortality is seen in the young (<3 months), elderly (>65 years), and immunocompromised (1–3).
- Increased mortality is seen with bacteremia and other invasive infections (2,5).
- Mortality is increased in multidrug-resistant strains (5).

COMPLICATIONS

Toxic megacolon, hypovolemic shock, metastatic abscess formation, endocarditis, infectious endarteritis, meningitis, septic arthritis, reactive arthritis, osteomyelitis, pneumonia, appendicitis, cholecystitis (1,3,4)

REFERENCES

1. DuPont HL. Clinical practice. Bacterial diarrhea. N Engl J Med. 2009;361(16):1560–1569.
2. Ao TT, Feasey NA, Gordon MA, et al. Global burden of invasive nontyphoidal Salmonella disease, 2010. Emerg Infect Dis. 2015;21(6).
3. Crum-Cianflone NF. Salmonellosis and the gastrointestinal tract: more than just peanut butter. Curr Gastroenterol Rep. 2008;10(4):424–431.
4. Hohmann EL. Nontyphoidal salmonellosis. Clin Infect Dis. 2001;32(2):263–269.
5. Onwuezobe IA, Oshun PO, Odigwe CC. Antimicrobials for treating symptomatic non-typhoidal Salmonella infection. Cochrane Database Syst Rev. 2012;(11):CD001167.
6. Crump JA, Medalla FM, Joyce KW, et al. Antimicrobial resistance among invasive nontyphoidal Salmonella enterica isolates in the United States: National Antimicrobial Resistance Monitoring System, 1996 to 2007. Antimicrob Agents Chemother. 2011;55(3):1148–1154.

ADDITIONAL READING

- Chen HM, Wang Y, Su LH, et al. Nontyphoid Salmonella infection: microbiology, clinical features, and antimicrobial therapy. Pediatr Neonatol. 2013;54(3):147–152.
- Guerrant RL, Van Gilder T, Steiner TS, et al. Practice guidelines for the management of infectious diarrhea. Clin Infect Dis. 2001;32(3):331–351.
- Hurley D, McCusker MP, Fanning S, et al. Salmonella–host interactions—modulation of the host innate immune system. Front Immunol. 2014;5:481.
- Lee MB, Greig JD. A review of nosocomial Salmonella outbreaks: infection control interventions found effective. Public Health. 2013;127(3):199–206.
- Odey F, Okomo U, Oyo-Ita A. Vaccines for preventing invasive salmonella infections in people with sickle cell disease. Cochrane Database Syst Rev. 2015;(6):CD006975.

 SEE ALSO

Gastroenteritis; Typhoid Fever

 CODES

ICD10

- A02.9 Salmonella infection, unspecified
- A02.0 Salmonella enteritis
- A02.1 Salmonella sepsis

CLINICAL PEARLS

- Nontyphoidal Salmonella infection is typically a foodborne infection associated with a self-limited gastroenteritis.
- Clinical syndromes include gastroenteritis, bacteremia, endovascular infection, localized infection outside the GI tract, and a chronic carrier state.
- Those at greatest risk of complications from Salmonella infection include the young, the elderly, and immunocompromised patients.
- Uncomplicated gastroenteritis in healthy patients can be treated with supportive care.
- Antibiotics should be used in infants, the elderly, immunocompromised patients, and for invasive infections such as bacteremia outside the GI tract.

SARCOIDOSIS

Donnah Mathews, MD, FACP

BASICS

DESCRIPTION
- Sarcoidosis is a noninfectious, multisystem granulomatous disease of unknown cause, commonly affecting young and middle-aged adults.
  - Frequently presents with hilar adenopathy, pulmonary infiltrates, ocular and skin lesions
  - In ~50% of cases, it is diagnosed in asymptomatic patients with abnormal chest x-rays (CXRs).
  - Almost any organ may be involved.
- System(s) affected: primarily pulmonary but also cardiovascular, gastrointestinal, hematologic/lymphatic, endocrine, renal, neurologic, dermatologic, ophthalmologic, musculoskeletal
- Synonym(s): Löfgren syndrome (erythema nodosum, hilar adenopathy, fever, arthralgias); Heerfordt syndrome (uveitis, parotid enlargement, facial palsy, fever); Besnier-Boeck disease; Boeck sarcoid; Schaumann disease (1–3)[C]

EPIDEMIOLOGY
Incidence
Estimated 6/100 person-years (4)

Prevalence
- Estimated 10 to 20/100,000 persons
- <15% of patients with active disease >60 years of age
- Rare in children (4)

ETIOLOGY AND PATHOPHYSIOLOGY
- Despite extensive research, mostly unknown
- Thought to be due to exaggerated cell-mediated immune response to unknown antigen(s)
- In the lungs, the initial lesion is CD4+ T-cell alveolitis, causing noncaseating granulomata, which may resolve or may undergo fibrosis.
- "Immune paradox" with affected organs showing an intense immune response and yet anergy exists elsewhere (1,5)[C].

Genetics
- Reports of familial clustering, with genetic linkage to a section within MHC on short arm of chromosome 6
- 3 to 4 times more common in African Americans
- Although worldwide in distribution, increased prevalence in Scandinavians, Japanese, African Americans, and women (4)

RISK FACTORS
Exact etiology and pathogenesis remain unknown.

GENERAL PREVENTION
None

COMMONLY ASSOCIATED CONDITIONS
None

DIAGNOSIS

HISTORY
- Patients may be asymptomatic.
- Patients may have nonspecific complaints, such as the following:
  - Nonproductive cough
  - Shortness of breath
  - Fever
  - Night sweats
  - Weight loss
  - General fatigue

- Eye pain
- Chest pain/palpitations
- Skin lesions
- Polyarthritis
- Renal calculi
- Facial droop due to Bell palsy
- Encephalopathy, seizures, hydrocephalus (rare)
- Patients >70 years old more likely to have systemic symptoms (5)

PHYSICAL EXAM
- Many patients have a normal physical exam.
- Lungs may reveal wheezing/fine interstitial crackles in advanced disease.
- ~30% of patients have extrapulmonary manifestations (2), which may include the following:
  - Uveitis
  - Other eye findings: conjunctival nodules, lacrimal gland enlargement, cataracts, glaucoma, papilledema
  - Cranial nerve palsies
  - Salivary gland swelling
  - Lymphadenopathy
  - Arrhythmias
  - Hepatosplenomegaly
  - Polyarthritis
  - Rashes (6)[A]

    ○ Maculopapular of nares, eyelids, forehead, base of neck at hairline, and previous trauma sites
    ○ Waxy nodular of face, trunk, and extensor surfaces of extremities
    ○ Plaques (lupus pernio) of nose, cheeks, chin, and ears
    ○ Erythema nodosum (component of Löfgren syndrome)
    ○ Atypical lesions

DIFFERENTIAL DIAGNOSIS
- Infectious granulomatous disease, such as tuberculosis and fungal infections
- Hypersensitivity pneumonitis
- Lymphoma
- Other malignancies associated with lymphadenopathy
- Berylliosis (1)[A]

DIAGNOSTIC TEST & INTERPRETATION
No definitive test for diagnosis, but diagnosis is suggested by the following:
- Clinical and radiographic manifestations
- Exclusion of other diagnoses
- Histopathologic detection of noncaseating granulomas

Initial Tests (lab, imaging)
- CBC: Anemia/leukopenia ± eosinophilia can be seen.
- Hypergammaglobulinemia can exist.
- LFTs: Abnormal liver function and increased alkaline phosphatase can be encountered with hepatic involvement.
- Calcium: Hypercalciuria occurs in up to 10% of patients, with hypercalcemia less frequent.
- Serum ACE inhibitors elevated in >75% of patients but is not diagnostic or exclusionary.
  - Drugs may alter lab results: Prednisone will lower serum ACE and normalize gallium scan. ACE inhibitors will lower serum ACE level.
  - Disorders may alter lab results: Hyperthyroidism and diabetes will increase serum ACE level.

- CXR or CT scan may reveal granulomas/hilar adenopathy. Routine CXRs are staged using Scadding classification.
  - Stage 0 = normal
  - Stage 1 = bilateral hilar adenopathy alone
  - Stage 2 = bilateral hilar adenopathy + parenchymal infiltrates
  - Stage 3 = parenchymal infiltrates alone (primarily upper lobes)
  - Stage 4 = pulmonary fibrosis (7)
- Chest CT scan may enhance appreciation of lymph nodes.
- High-resolution chest CT scan may reveal peribronchial disease.
- Gallium scan will be positive in areas of acute disease/inflammation but is not specific.
- Positron emission tomography (PET) scan can indicate areas of disease activity in lungs, lymph nodes, and other areas of the body but does not differentiate between malignancy and sarcoidosis.
- Cardiac PET scan may detect cardiac sarcoidosis (8)[B].

Diagnostic Procedures/Other
- Pulmonary function tests (PFTs) may reveal restrictive pattern with decreased carbon monoxide diffusing capacity (DLCO).
- Characteristically in active disease, bronchioalveolar lavage fluid has an increased CD4-to-CD8 ratio.
- Ophthalmologic examination may reveal uveitis, retinal vasculitis, or conjunctivitis.
- ECG
- Tuberculin skin test
- Biopsy of lesions should reveal noncaseating granulomas.
- If lungs are affected, bronchoscopy with biopsy of central and peripheral airways is helpful. Endobronchial US (EBUS)–guided transbronchial needle aspiration may potentially have a better diagnostic yield.
- Kveim test (ongoing research): suspension of sterilized splenic cells from a patient with sarcoidosis is injected in an intradermal skin test to evoke a sarcoid granulomatous response over 3 weeks, similar to a tuberculin skin test.

ALERT
If signs indicate Löfgren syndrome (acute sarcoid with bilateral hilar lymphadenopathy, erythema nodosum [EN] and diffuse arthritis/arthralgias), it is not necessary to perform a biopsy because prognosis is good with observation alone, and biopsy would not change management.

Test Interpretation
Noncaseating epithelioid granulomas without evidence of fungal/mycobacterial infection

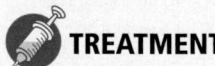

TREATMENT

- Many patients undergo spontaneous remission. It is difficult to assess disease activity and severity, however, making it challenging to develop guidelines.
- No treatment may be necessary in asymptomatic individuals, but treatment may be needed for specific indications, such as cardiac, CNS, renal, or ocular involvement.
- No treatment is indicated for asymptomatic patients with stage I–III radiographic changes with normal/mildly abnormal lung function, although close follow-up is recommended.

- Treatment of pulmonary and skin manifestations is done on the basis of impairment. The symptoms that necessitate systemic therapy remain controversial.
  – Worsening pulmonary symptoms
  – Deteriorating lung function
  – Worsening radiographic findings

MEDICATION
Systemic therapy is clearly indicated for hypercalcemia, cardiac disease, neurologic disease, and eye disease not responding to topical therapy. Most patients with pulmonary sarcoidosis do not require treatment with medications, as many are asymptomatic or have a spontaneous remission.

First Line
- Systemic corticosteroids in the symptomatic individual (dyspnea, cough, hemoptysis) or in the individual with worsening lung function or radiographic findings
  – The optimal dose of glucocorticoids is not known.
  – Usually prednisone initially, 0.3 to 0.6 mg/kg ideal body weight (20 to 40 mg/day) for 4 to 6 weeks.
  – If stable, taper by 5 mg/week to 10 to 20 mg/day over the next 6 weeks.
  – If no relapse, 10 to 20 mg/day for 8 to 12 months
  – Relapse is common.
  – Higher doses (80 to 100 mg/day) may be warranted in patients with acute respiratory failure, cardiac, neurologic, or ocular disease.
- In patients with skin disease, topical steroids may be effective.
- Inhaled steroids (budesonide 800 to 1,600 μg BID) may be of some clinical benefit in early disease with mild pulmonary symptoms.
  – Contraindications: patients with known problems with corticosteroids
  – Precautions: careful monitoring in patients with diabetes mellitus and/or hypertension
  – Significant possible interactions: Refer to the manufacturer's profile of each drug.

Second Line
- All alternative agents to glucocorticoids carry substantial risk for toxicity, including myelosuppression, hepatotoxicity, and opportunistic infection.
- Methotrexate: initially 7.5 mg/week, increasing gradually to 10 to 15 mg/week
- Azathioprine: 50 to 100 mg/day
- Leflunomide: 20 mg/day
- Use of immunosuppressants, such as methotrexate or azathioprine, will require regular monitoring of CBC and LFTs.
- Antimalarial agents, such as chloroquine or hydroxychloroquine
- Tumor necrosis factor antagonists, such as infliximab, have been useful in refractory cases (9)[C].

ISSUES FOR REFERRAL
May be followed by a pulmonologist, with referrals to other specialists as dictated by involvement of other organ systems. If requiring a second-line therapy, should be followed by a specialist.

SURGERY/OTHER PROCEDURES
Lung transplantation in severe, refractory cases; long-term outcomes are unknown.

COMPLEMENTARY & ALTERNATIVE MEDICINE
None known to be effective

ONGOING CARE

FOLLOW-UP RECOMMENDATIONS
There is limited data on indications for the specific tests and optimal frequency of monitoring of disease activity. Suggestions follow.

Patient Monitoring
- Patients on prednisone for symptoms should be seen q1–2mo while on therapy.
- Patients not requiring therapy should be seen regularly (q3mo) for at least the first 2 years after diagnosis, obtaining a thorough history and physical exam, laboratory testing tailored to sites of disease activity, PFTs, and ambulatory pulse oximetry.
- If active disease
  – Every 6 to 12 months, obtain ophthalmologic exam if on hydroxychloroquine.
  – Annually, CBC, creatinine, calcium, LFTs, ECG, 25-hydroxy vitamin D and 1,25 dihydroxy vitamin D, CXR, ophthalmologic examination
- Other testing per individual patient's symptoms, including HRCT, echocardiogram, Holter monitoring, urinalysis (UA), thyroid-stimulating hormone (TSH), bone density, MRI of brain
- The serum ACE level is used by some physicians to follow the disease activity. In patients with an initially elevated ACE level, it should fall toward normal while on the therapy or when the disease resolves.
- If inactive disease, follow annually with history and physical exam, PFTs, ambulatory pulse oximetry, CBC, creatinine, calcium, liver enzymes, 1,25 dihydroxy vitamin D, EKG, ophthalmologic exam.

DIET
No special diet

PATIENT EDUCATION
- The American Lung Association at www.lungusa.org/lung-disease/sarcoidosis/?gclid=CPX6zuipm6MCFQxW2godISFepQ
- Sarcoidosis by Medline Plus at www.nlm.nih.gov/medlineplus/sarcoidosis.html

PROGNOSIS
- 50% of patients will have spontaneous resolution within 2 years.
- 25% of patients will have significant fibrosis, but no further worsening of the disease after 2 years.
- 25% of patients (higher in some populations, including African Americans) will have chronic disease.
- Patients on corticosteroids for >6 months have a greater chance of having chronic disease.
- Overall death rate: <5%

COMPLICATIONS
- Patients may develop significant respiratory involvement, including cor pulmonale.
- Pulmonary hemorrhage from infection with aspergillosis in the damaged lung is possible.
- Other organs, especially the heart (congestive heart failure, arrhythmias), eyes (rarely blindness), and CNS, can be involved with serious consequences. Cardiac, ocular, and CNS involvement usually manifests early on in patients with these complications of the disease.

REFERENCES
1. Baughman RP, Culver DA, Judson MA. A concise review of pulmonary sarcoidosis. *Am J Respir Crit Care Med*. 2011;183(5):573–581.
2. Holmes J, Lazarus A. Sarcoidosis: extrathoracic manifestations. *Dis Mon*. 2009;55(11):675–692.
3. King CS, Kelly W. Treatment of sarcoidosis. *Dis Mon*. 2009;55(11):704–718.
4. Rybicki BA, Iannuzzi MC, Frederick MM, et al. Familial aggregation of sarcoidosis. A case-control etiologic study of sarcoidosis (ACCESS). *Am J Respir Crit Care Med*. 2001;164(11):2085–2091.
5. Dempsey OJ, Paterson EW, Kerr KM, et al. Sarcoidosis. *BMJ*. 2009;339:b3206.
6. Lodha S, Sanchez M, Prystowsky S. Sarcoidosis of the skin: a review for the pulmonologist. *Chest*. 2009;136(2):583–596.
7. Statement on sarcoidosis. Joint Statement of the American Thoracic Society (ATS), the European Respiratory Society (ERS) and the World Association of Sarcoidosis and Other Granulomatous Disorders (WASOG) adopted by the ATS Board of Directors and by the ERS Executive Committee, February 1999. *Am J Respir Crit Care Med*. 1999;160(2):736–755.
8. Tremblay A, Stather DR, Maceachern P, et al. A randomized controlled trial of standard vs endobronchial ultrasonography-guided transbronchial needle aspiration in patients with suspected sarcoidosis. *Chest*. 2009;136(2):340–346.
9. Iannuzzi MC, Fontana JR. Sarcoidosis: clinical presentation, immunopathogenesis, and therapeutics. *JAMA*. 2011;305(4):391–399.

ADDITIONAL READING
- Hoang DQ, Nguyen ET. Sarcoidosis. *Semin Roentgenol*. 2010;45(1):36–42.
- Polychronopoulos VS, Prakash UB. Airway involvement in sarcoidosis. *Chest*. 2009;136(5):1371–1380.

CODES

ICD10
- D86.9 Sarcoidosis, unspecified
- D86.0 Sarcoidosis of lung
- D86.86 Sarcoid arthropathy

CLINICAL PEARLS
- Sarcoidosis is a noninfectious, multisystem granulomatous disease of unknown cause, typically affecting young and middle-aged adults.
- Any organ can be affected.
- Diagnosis is based on clinical findings, exclusion of other disorders, and pathologic detection of noncaseating granulomas.
- Most patients do not need systemic treatment and the disease resolves spontaneously; a few will have life-threatening progressive organ dysfunction.

SCABIES

Kaelen C. Dunican, PharmD • Brandi Hoag, DO

BASICS

DESCRIPTION
- A contagious parasitic infection of the skin caused by the mite *Sarcoptes scabiei*, var. *hominis*
- System(s) affected: skin/exocrine
- Synonym(s): sarcoptic mange

EPIDEMIOLOGY
Incidence
Predominant age: children and young adults

Prevalence
- Global prevalence is estimated at 300 million cases per year.
- May be more prevalent in urban areas and areas of overcrowding

ETIOLOGY AND PATHOPHYSIOLOGY
Itching is a delayed hypersensitivity reaction to the mite saliva, eggs, or excrement.

S. scabiei, var. *hominis*
- An obligate human parasite
- Female mite lays eggs in burrows in the stratum corneum and epidermis.
- Primarily transmitted by prolonged human-to-human direct skin contact
- Infrequently transmitted via fomites (e.g., bedding, clothing, or furnishings)

RISK FACTORS
- Personal skin-to-skin contact (e.g., sexual promiscuity, crowding, nosocomial infection)
- Poor nutritional status, poverty, and homelessness
- Hot, tropical climates
- Seasonal variation: Incidence may be higher in the winter than in the summer (may be due to overcrowding).
- Immunocompromised patients, including those with HIV/AIDS, are at increased risk of developing severe (crusted/Norwegian) scabies.

GENERAL PREVENTION
Prevent outbreaks by prompt treatment and cleansing of fomites (see "Additional Therapies").

DIAGNOSIS

HISTORY
- Generalized itching is often severe and worse at night.
- Determine any contact with infected individuals.
- Initial infection may be asymptomatic.
- Symptoms may develop after 3 to 6 weeks.

PHYSICAL EXAM
- Lesions (inflammatory, erythematous, pruritic papules) most commonly located in the finger webs, flexor surfaces of the wrists, elbows, axillae, buttocks, genitalia, feet, and ankles

- Burrows (thin, curvy, elevated lines in the upper epidermis that measure 1 to 10 mm in length) may be seen in involved areas—a pathognomic sign of scabies.
- Secondary erosions or excoriations from scratching
- Pustules (if secondarily infected)
- Pruritic nodules in covered areas (buttocks, groin, axillae) resulting from an exaggerated hypersensitivity reaction
- Crusted scabies (Norwegian scabies) is a psoriasiform dermatosis occurring with hyperinfestation with thousands of mites (more common in immunosuppressed patients).

Geriatric Considerations
The elderly often itch more severely despite fewer cutaneous lesions and are at risk for extensive infestations, perhaps related to a decline in cell-mediated immunity. There may be back involvement in those who are bedridden.

Pediatric Considerations
Infants and very young children often present with vesicles, papules, and pustules and have more widespread involvement, including the hands, palms, feet, soles, body folds, and head (rare for adults).

DIFFERENTIAL DIAGNOSIS
- Atopic dermatitis
- Contact dermatitis
- Folliculitis/impetigo
- Tinea corporis
- Dermatitis herpetiformis
- Eczema
- Insect bites
- Papular urticaria
- Pediculosis corporis
- Pityriasis rosea
- Prurigo
- Psoriasis (crusted scabies)
- Pyoderma
- Seborrheic dermatitis
- Syphilis

DIAGNOSITC TEST & INTERPRETATION
- Definitive diagnosis is based on microscopic identification of mites, eggs, or fecal pellets (scybala) but diagnosis may be based on history and physical exam (1–4)[C].
- A failure to find mites does not rule out scabies.

Initial Tests (lab, imaging)
CBC is rarely needed but may show eosinophilia.

Diagnostic Procedures/Other
- Examination of skin with magnifying lens
  - Look for typical burrows in finger webs and on flexor aspect of the wrists and on the penis.
  - Look for a dark point at the end of the burrow (the mite).

- Presumptive diagnosis based on clinical presentation, skin lesions, and identification of burrow (1–3).
- Skin scraping
  - Place a drop of mineral oil over a nonexcoriated lesion or burrow.
  - Scrape the lesion with a surgical blade.
  - Examine under a microscope for mites, eggs, egg casings, or feces (1,2)[C].
  - Scraping from under fingernails often may be positive.
  - When mite is not found with scraping, biopsy may reveal mite, eggs, or feces (1,3).
- Potassium hydroxide (KOH) wet mount not recommended because it can dissolve mite pellets.
- Burrow ink test
  - If burrows are not obvious, apply gentian violet or India ink to an area of rash. Wash off the ink with alcohol. A burrow should remain stained and become more evident.
  - Then apply mineral oil, scrape, and observe microscopically, as noted previously (1,3)[C].

Test Interpretation
Skin biopsy of a nodule (although performed rarely) will reveal portions of the mite in the corneal layer.

TREATMENT

GENERAL MEASURES
- Treat all intimate contacts and close household and family members.
- Wash all clothing, bed linens, and towels in hot (60°C) water and dry in hot dryer.
- Personal items that cannot be washed should be sealed in a plastic bag for at least 3 to 5 days.
- Some itching and dermatitis may persist for up to 6 weeks and can be treated with oral antihistamines and/or topical or oral corticosteroids.

MEDICATION
First Line

Permethrin 5% cream (Elimite) is generally accepted as first-line therapy (1–3,5)[A].

- After bathing or showering, apply cream from the neck to the soles of the feet paying particular attention to areas that are most involved; then wash off after 8 to 14 hours and repeat in 1 week.
- The adult dose is usually 30 g per treatment.
- Side effects include itching and stinging (minimal absorption).
- Crusted scabies may require more frequent application (q2–3d for 1 to 2 weeks) in combination with repeated doses of PO ivermectin on days 1, 2, 8, 9, and 15 (2,3,5)[C].

Pediatric Considerations
Permethrin may be used on infants >2 months of age. In children <5 years of age, the cream should be applied to the head and neck as well as to the entire body.

Second Line
- Ivermectin (Stromectol)
  - Not FDA approved for scabies
  - 200 to 250 μg/kg PO as single dose; repeated in 1 week
  - Take with food to improve bioavailability and enhance penetration into the epidermis.
  - May need higher doses or may need to use in combination with topical scabicide for HIV-positive patients
- Crotamiton (Eurax) 10% cream
  - Apply from the neck down for 24 hours, rinse off, then reapply for an additional 24 hours, and then thoroughly wash off.
  - Nodular scabies: Apply to nodules for 24 hours, rinse off, reapply for an additional 24 hours, then thoroughly wash off.
- Precipitated sulfur 2–10% in petrolatum
  - Not FDA approved for scabies
  - Apply to the entire body from the neck down for 24 hours, rinse by bathing, then repeat for 2 more days (3 days total). It is malodorous and messy but is thought to be safer than lindane, especially in infants <6 months of age, and safer than permethrin in infants <2 months of age.
- Lindane (γ-benzene hexachloride, Kwell) 1% lotion
  - Apply to all skin surfaces from the neck down and wash off 6 to 8 hours later.
  - Two applications 1 week apart are recommended but may increase the risk of toxicity.
  - 2 oz is usually adequate for an adult.
    - Side effects: neurotoxicity (seizures, muscle spasms), aplastic anemia
    - Contraindications: uncontrolled seizure disorder, premature infants
    - Precautions: Do not use on excoriated skin, on immunocompromised patients, in conditions that may increase risk of seizures, or with medications that decrease seizure threshold.
    - Possible interactions: concomitant use with medications that lower the seizure threshold

ALERT
Lindane: FDA black box warning of severe neurologic toxicity; use only when all other agents have failed.

Pediatric Considerations
- The FDA recommends caution when using lindane in patients who weigh <50 kg. It is not recommended for infants and is contraindicated in premature infants.
- PO ivermectin should be avoided in children <5 years and in those weighing <15 kg.

Pregnancy Considerations
- Permethrin is pregnancy Category B, and lindane, ivermectin, and crotamiton are Category C.
- Permethrin is considered compatible with lactation, but if permethrin is used while breastfeeding, the infant should be bottlefed until the cream has been thoroughly washed off.

ADDITIONAL THERAPIES
- Crusted scabies may require use of keratolytics to improve penetration of permethrin.
- Benzyl benzoate lotion (not available in the United States but used widely in developing countries)
  - Not FDA approved for scabies.
  - Dose for adults is 25–28%; dilute to 12.5% for children and 6.25% for infants
  - After bathing, apply lotion from the neck to soles of feet for 24 hours.
- Topical ivermectin 1% lotion (investigational, not available for use in the United States) (4)
  - Not FDA approved for scabies.
  - Apply to affected sites and wash off 8 hours later.

COMPLEMENTARY & ALTERNATIVE MEDICINE
Herbal products such as tea tree oil, clove oil, neem oil, and aloe vera require additional evidence to establish efficacy (4).

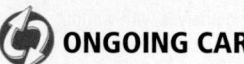 ONGOING CARE

FOLLOW-UP RECOMMENDATIONS
Patient Monitoring
Recheck patient at weekly intervals only if rash or itching persists. Scrape new lesions and retreat if mites or products are found.

PATIENT EDUCATION
- Patients should be instructed on proper application and cautioned not to overuse the medication when applying it to the skin.
- A patient fact sheet is available from the CDC: http://www.cdc.gov/parasites/scabies/

PROGNOSIS
- Lesions begin to regress in 1 to 2 days, along with the worst itching, but eczema and itching may persist for up to 6 weeks after treatment.
- Nodular lesions may persist for several weeks, perhaps necessitating intralesional or systemic steroids.
- Some instances of lindane-resistant scabies have now been reported. These cases do respond to permethrin.

COMPLICATIONS
- Poor sleep due to pruritus
- Social stigma
- Secondary bacterial infection (group A streptococci and Staphylococcus aureus)
- Sepsis
- Glomerulonephritis
- Eczema
- Pyoderma
- Postscabetic pruritus
- Nodules (nodular scabies) may persist for weeks to months after treatment.

REFERENCES
1. Hicks MI, Elston DM. Scabies. *Dermatol Ther.* 2009;22(4):279–292.
2. Gunning K, Pippitt K, Kiraly B, et al. Pediculosis and scabies: treatment update. *Am Fam Physician.* 2012;86(6):535–541.
3. Markova A, Kam SA, Miller DD, et al. In the clinic. Common cutaneous parasites. *Ann Intern Med.* 2014;161(5).
4. Rosamilia LL. Scabies. *Semin Cutan Med Surg.* 2014;33(3):106–109.
5. Currie BJ, McCarthy JS. Permethrin and ivermectin for scabies. *N Engl J Med.* 2010;362(8):717–725.

SEE ALSO

Arthropod Bites and Stings; Pediculosis (Lice)

CODES

ICD10
B86 Scabies

CLINICAL PEARLS
- Prior to diagnosis, use of a topical steroid to treat pruritic symptoms may mask symptoms and is termed *scabies incognito*.
- Environmental control is recommended. All linens, towels, and clothing used in the previous 4 days should be washed in hot water or dry-cleaned. Personal items that cannot be washed or dry-cleaned should be sealed in a plastic bag for 3 to 5 days.
- All members of the affected household may require treatment, especially close contacts (those sharing the same bed or who have intimate contact).
- Eczema and itching may persist for up to 6 weeks after treatment, causing many patients to falsely believe that they have failed treatment or are being reinfected.
- In patients with actual reinfection, either the patient has not applied the medication properly or, more likely, the index patient has not been identified and treated.

SCARLET FEVER

John C. Huscher, MD

 BASICS

DESCRIPTION

- A disease (typically in childhood) characterized by fever, pharyngitis, and rash caused by group A β-hemolytic *Streptococcus pyogenes* (GAS) that produces erythrogenic toxin
- Incubation period: 1 to 7 days
- Duration of illness: 4 to 10 days
- Rash usually appears on the second day of illness.
- Rash first appears on the upper chest and flexural creases and then spreads rapidly all over the body.
- Rash clears at the end of the 1st week and is followed by several weeks of desquamation.
- System(s) affected: head, eyes, ears, nose, throat, skin/exocrine
- Synonym(s): scarlatina

EPIDEMIOLOGY

Incidence
- Rare in infancy because of maternal antitoxin antibodies
- Predominant age: 6 to 12 years
- Peak age: 4 to 8 years
- Predominant sex: male = female
- Rare in the United States in persons >12 years because of high rates (>80%) of lifelong protective antibodies to erythrogenic toxins
- Increased rates are noted in United Kingdom in 2013.

Prevalence
- 5–30% of cases of pharyngitis in children are due to GAS.
- <10% of children with streptococcal pharyngitis develop scarlet fever.

ETIOLOGY AND PATHOPHYSIOLOGY
- Erythrogenic toxin production is necessary to develop scarlet fever.
- Three toxin types: A, B, C
- Toxins damage capillaries (producing rash) and act as superantigens, stimulating cytokine release.
- Antibodies to toxins prevent development of rash but do not protect against underlying infection.
- Primary site of streptococcal infection is usually within the tonsils, but scarlet fever may also occur with infection of skin, surgical wounds, or uterus (puerperal scarlet fever).

RISK FACTORS
- Winter/spring seasonal increase
- More common in school-aged children
- Contact with infected individual(s)
- Crowded living conditions (e.g., lower socioeconomic status, barracks, child care, schools)

GENERAL PREVENTION
- Spread by contact with airborne respiratory droplets
- Asymptomatic contacts do not require cultures/prophylaxis.
- Symptomatic contacts may be treated with or without culture.
- Children should not return to school/daycare until they have received 24 hours of antibiotic therapy.

COMMONLY ASSOCIATED CONDITIONS
- Pharyngitis
- Impetigo
- Rheumatic fever
- Glomerulonephritis

 DIAGNOSIS

HISTORY
Prodrome 1 to 2 days
- Sore throat
- Headache
- Myalgias
- Malaise
- Fever (>38°C [100.4°F])
- Vomiting
- Abdominal pain (may mimic acute abdomen)
- Rash—scarlatiniform erythematous punctate eruption
- Cough, conjunctivitis, hoarseness, and rhinorrhea are more commonly associated with viral infections.

PHYSICAL EXAM
- Oral exam
  - Beefy red tonsils and pharynx with/without exudate
  - Petechiae on palate
  - White coating on tongue: White strawberry tongue appears on days 1 to 2. This sheds by days 4 to 5, leaving a red strawberry tongue, which is shiny and erythematous with prominent papillae.
- Exanthem (appears within 1 to 5 days)
  - Scarlet macules with generalized erythema; blanches when pressed
  - Orange-red punctate skin eruption with sandpaper-like texture, "sunburn with goose pimples"
  - Coarse "sandpaper" rash—helpful in dark-skinned individuals
  - Initially, rash appears on chest and axillae. It then spreads to abdomen and extremities; prominent in skin folds, flexural surfaces (e.g., axillae, groin, buttocks), with sparing of palms and soles.
  - Flushed face with circumoral pallor, red lips
  - Pastia lines: transverse red streaks in skin folds of abdomen, antecubital space, and axillae
  - Desquamation begins on face after 7 to 10 days and proceeds over trunk to hands and feet; may persist for 6 weeks.
  - In severe cases, small vesicular lesions (miliary sudamina) may appear on abdomen, hands, and feet.

DIFFERENTIAL DIAGNOSIS
- Viral exanthem: measles; rubella; roseola
- Infectious mononucleosis
- *Mycoplasma* pneumonia
- Secondary syphilis
- Toxic shock syndrome
- Staphylococcal scalded-skin syndrome
- Kawasaki disease
- Drug hypersensitivity
- Severe sunburn

DIAGNOSTIC TESTS & INTERPRETATION
- Test for GAS pharyngitis by rapid antigen detection test (RADT) and/or culture with pharyngeal swab because clinical features alone do not reliably discriminate between GAS and viral pharyngitis.
- Testing for GAS pharyngitis is *not recommended* for patients with symptoms suggesting a viral etiology (e.g., cough, rhinorrhea, hoarseness, oral ulcers).

Initial Tests (lab, imaging)
- RADT: diagnostic if positive, 95% specific; sensitivity approaches that of culture. Negative RADT should be confirmed by throat culture. Positive RADTs do not require backup culture (1)[C].
- Throat culture: β-hemolytic colonies that are catalase negative and sensitive to bacitracin; culture is the gold standard for confirming streptococcal infection (99% specific, 90–97% sensitive; 5–10% of healthy individuals are carriers) (1).
- Serologic tests (antistreptolysin O titer and streptozyme tests, antihyaluronidase): Confirm recent GAS infection; not helpful or recommended for diagnosis of acute disease.
- Gram stain: gram-positive cocci in chains
- CBC may show elevated WBC count (12,000 to 16,000/mm³); eosinophilia later (second week).
- Follow-up (posttreatment) throat cultures or RADT not routinely recommended
- Diagnostic testing and empiric treatment of asymptomatic household contacts of patients with acute streptococcal pharyngitis is not routinely recommended (2)[B].
- Appropriately symptomatic patients >3 years old with a family member recently diagnosed with laboratory-confirmed GAS pharyngitis may be treated without screening or confirmatory testing (3)[C].

Follow-Up Tests & Special Considerations
- Recent antibiotic therapy may impact culture results.
- Within 5 days of symptoms, antibiotics can delay/abolish antistreptolysin O response.

Test Interpretation
Skin lesions reveal characteristic inflammatory reaction, specifically hyperemia, edema, and polymorphonuclear cell infiltration.

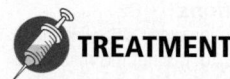 **TREATMENT**

GENERAL MEASURES
Supportive care; analgesic/antipyretic such as acetaminophen or an NSAID, for treatment of moderate to severe symptoms or control of fever

MEDICATION
First Line
The main reason for treating GAS is to decrease the risk of acute rheumatic fever. Early treatment decreases duration of symptoms by 1 to 2 days and decreases the period of contagiousness (3)[B].

- Penicillin (PO; penicillin V and others) for 10 days
  - 250 mg PO BID or TID for ≥27 kg (60 lb); 500 mg BID or TID for >27 kg (60 lb) adolescents and adults(1,4,5)[A]
  - If compliance is questionable, use penicillin G, benzathine: single IM dose 600,000 U for ≥27 kg (60 lb); 1.2 mU for those >27 kg.
- Amoxicillin (PO) 50 mg/kg once daily or 25 mg/kg twice daily for 10 days (use only for definitive GAS because it can induce rash with some viral infections) (6)[A]
  - Contraindications: penicillin allergy
- Acetaminophen for fever and pain
- Precautions: Avoid in patients with penicillin allergy (anaphylaxis).

Second Line
- For patients allergic to penicillin
  - Azithromycin (Zithromax, Z pack): 12 mg/kg/day (max 500 mg) for 5 days (4)[A]
  - Clarithromycin (Biaxin): children >6 months: 7.5 mg/kg BID for 10 days; adults: 250 mg BID for 10 days
- Oral cephalosporins: Many are effective, but first-generation cephalosporins are less expensive:
  - Cephalexin 25 to 50 mg/kg/day divided every 12 hours for 10 days; max 500 mg every 12 hours (1)[A]
  - Cefadroxil 30 mg/kg/day divided BID; max 500 mg BID for 10 days (1)
- Clindamycin 20 mg/kg/day divided TID for 10 days (4)[B]
- Tetracyclines and sulfonamides should not be used.

ALERT
Avoid aspirin in children due to risk of Reye syndrome.

ISSUES FOR REFERRAL
Peritonsillar abscess; shock symptoms: hypotension, disseminated intravascular coagulation (DIC), cardiac, liver, renal dysfunction

SURGERY/OTHER PROCEDURES
- Tonsillectomy is recommended with recurrent bouts of pharyngitis (≥6 positive strep cultures in 1 year).
- While children still may get streptococcal pharyngitis ("strep throat") after a tonsillectomy, the procedure reduces the frequency and severity of infections.

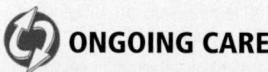 ONGOING CARE

FOLLOW-UP RECOMMENDATIONS
Follow-up throat culture is not needed unless the patient is symptomatic.

Patient Monitoring
GAS is uniformly susceptible to penicillin, treatment failures are typically due to:
- Poor adherence to recommended antibiotic therapy
- β-Lactamase oral flora hydrolyzing penicillin
- GAS carrier state and concurrent viral rash (requires no treatment)
- Repeat exposure to carriers in family: Streptococci persist on nonrinsed toothbrushes and orthodontic appliances for up to 15 days.
- Recurrent GAS pharyngitis after a recent oral antibiotic course can be retreated with the same agent, an alternative oral agent, or IM penicillin G.

DIET
No special diet

PATIENT EDUCATION
- A brief delay in initiating treatment awaiting culture results does not increase the risk of rheumatic fever.
- Complete the entire course of antibiotics.
- Children should not return to school/daycare until they have received >24 hours of antibiotic therapy.
- Can spread person to person: attend to personal hygiene (wash hands, don't share utensils)
- "Recurring strep throat: When is tonsillectomy useful?" (http://www.mayoclinic.org/diseases-conditions/strep-throat/expert-answers/recurring-strep-throat/faq-20058360)

PROGNOSIS
- Symptoms are shortened by 12 to 24 hours with penicillin.
- Recurrent attacks are possible (different erythrogenic toxins).

COMPLICATIONS
- Suppurative
  - Sinusitis
  - Otitis media/mastoiditis
  - Cervical adenitis
  - Peritonsillar abscess/retropharyngeal abscess
  - Pneumonia
  - Bacteremia with metastatic infectious foci: meningitis, brain abscess, osteomyelitis, septic arthritis, endocarditis, intracranial venous sinus thrombosis, necrotizing fasciitis
- Nonsuppurative
  - Rheumatic fever: Therapy prevents rheumatic fever when started as long as 10 days after onset of acute GAS infection.
  - Glomerulonephritis: due to nephritogenic strain of Streptococcus; prevention even after adequate treatment of GAS is less certain
  - Streptococcal toxic shock syndrome: fever; hypotension; DIC; and cardiac, liver, and/or kidney dysfunction related to other toxin-mediated sequelae
  - Cellulitis
  - Weeks to months later, may develop transverse grooves in nail plates and hair loss (telogen effluvium)

REFERENCES
1. Choby BA. Diagnosis and treatment of streptococcal pharyngitis. Am Fam Physician. 2009;79(5):383–390.
2. Shulman ST, Bisno AL, Clegg HW, et al. Clinical practice guideline for the diagnosis and management of group A streptococcal pharyngitis: 2012 update by the Infectious Diseases Society of America. Clin Infect Dis. 2012;55(10):1279–1282.
3. University of Michigan Health System. Pharyngitis. Ann Arbor, MI: University of Michigan Health System; 2013. National Guideline Clearinghouse Guideline Summary NGC-9967.
4. Gerber MA, Baltimore RS, Eaton CB, et al. Prevention of rheumatic fever and diagnosis and treatment of acute streptococcal pharyngitis: a scientific statement from the American Heart Association Rheumatic Fever, Endocarditis, and Kawasaki Disease Committee of the Council on Cardiovascular Disease in the Young, the Interdisciplinary Council on Functional Genomics and Translational Biology, and the Interdisciplinary Council on Quality of Care and Outcomes Research: endorsed by the American Academy of Pediatrics.. Circulation. 2009;119(11):1541–1551.
5. van Driel ML, De Sutter AI, Keber N, et al. Different antibiotic treatments for group A streptococcal pharyngitis. Cochrane Database Syst Rev. 2013;(4):CD004406.
6. Lennon DR, Farrell E, Martin DR, et al. Once-daily amoxicillin versus twice-daily penicillin V in group A beta-haemolytic streptococcal pharyngitis. Arch Dis Child. 2008;93(6):474–478.

 SEE ALSO
- Pharyngitis
- Algorithm: Pharyngitis

 CODES

ICD10
- A38.9 Scarlet fever, uncomplicated
- J02.0 Streptococcal pharyngitis
- A38.0 Scarlet fever with otitis media

CLINICAL PEARLS
- Consider scarlet fever in the differential diagnosis of children with fever and an exanthematous rash.
- Key clinical findings include strawberry tongue, circumoral pallor, and a coarse sandpaper rash.
- Desquamation (7 to 10 days after symptom onset) may last for several weeks following acute illness in scarlet fever.
- Throat culture remains the diagnostic test of choice to document streptococcal illness.
- Penicillin is the drug of choice for treatment.

SCHIZOPHRENIA

Maja Skikic, MD • Jeffrey G. Stovall, MD

BASICS

Schizophrenia is a chronic, severe, and disabling psychiatric condition characterized by neurocognitive changes and impairment in reality testing.

DESCRIPTION
- Major psychiatric disorder characterized by prodrome, active, and residual psychotic symptoms involving disturbances in appearance, speech, behavior, perception, and thought that last for at least 6 months.
- DSM-5 has eliminated subcategories of schizophrenia (1).
- System(s) affected: central nervous system

EPIDEMIOLOGY
Incidence
- 7.7 to 43/100,000 (2)
- Predominant sex: male-to-female ratio = 1.4:1.0
- Age of onset: typically <30 years, earlier in males (early to mid-20s) than females (late 20s), with a smaller peak that occurs in women >45 years (3)

Prevalence
- Lifetime (1%): highest prevalence in lower socio-economic classes and urban settings (2-fold higher risk) (2)
- 1.1% of the population >18 years old; similar rates in all countries

ETIOLOGY AND PATHOPHYSIOLOGY
- Stems from a complex interaction between genetic and environmental factors; higher incidence if prenatal infection or hypoxia, winter births, first-generation immigrants, advanced paternal age, drug use, and genetic (velocardiofacial) syndromes
- Overstimulation of mesolimbic dopamine D_2 receptors, deficient prefrontal dopamine, and aberrant prefrontal glutamate (NMDA) activity results in perceptual disturbances, disordered thought process, and cognitive impairments (4).

Genetics
If first-degree biologic relative has schizophrenia, risk is 8–10%; a 10-fold increase (5).

GENERAL PREVENTION
- Currently, no known preventive measures decrease the incidence of schizophrenia.
- Interventions to improve long-term outcome and associated comorbid conditions are employed during management.

COMMONLY ASSOCIATED CONDITIONS
- Substance use disorders and nicotine dependence are common and lead to significant long-term medical and social complications (6).
- Metabolic syndrome, diabetes mellitus, obesity, and certain infectious diseases, including HIV, hepatitis B, and hepatitis C all occur in higher-than-expected rates in individuals with schizophrenia.

DIAGNOSIS

Focus on identifying an insidious social and functional decline per history with the onset of ≥2 of the following characteristic symptoms on mental status exam:
- Delusions (fixed, false beliefs)
- Hallucinations (auditory > visual perceptual disturbances)
- Disorganized thought (derailed or incoherent speech)
- Grossly disorganized/catatonic behavior (hyper- or hypoactive movements that are often repetitive)
- Negative symptoms (affective flattening, amotivation, avolition, asociality) (1)

PHYSICAL EXAM
No physical findings characterize the illness; however, chronic treatment with neuroleptic agents may result in parkinsonism, tardive dyskinesia, and other extrapyramidal symptoms.

DIFFERENTIAL DIAGNOSIS
- Psychotic disorder due to another medical condition
  - Disorientation, in particular, indicates delirium.
  - Possible medical illnesses include porphyria, TBI, infection, tumor, metabolic, endocrine, and intoxication, including withdrawal states and disorders that affect the CNS (i.e., epilepsy, Huntington disease, Wilson disease, lupus cerebritis, anti-NMDA limbic encephalitis, metachromatic leukodystrophy).
- Substance-induced psychosis: secondary to substance use/abuse, such as cocaine, hallucinogens (amphetamines, LSD, phencyclidine), cannabis (including synthetic), bath salts, alcohol, or prescribed medications including steroids, anticholinergics, and opiates
- Personality disorders (paranoid, schizotypal, schizoid, borderline personality disorder)
- Mood disorders: bipolar disorder, major depressive disorders with psychotic features, or schizoaffective disorder
- Delusional disorder
- Posttraumatic stress disorder
- Cultural belief system

DIAGNOSTIC TESTS & INTERPRETATION
- No tests are available to indicate schizophrenia.
- Imaging and laboratory tests are needed to rule out other causes.

Initial Tests (lab, imaging)
These are needed to rule out a medical etiology of psychotic symptoms and when starting antipsychotic medications; these may include the following:
- Brain MRI, EEG, LP (as clinically indicated)
- CBC, blood chemistries
- Thyroid-stimulating hormone (TSH)
- Blood glucose level, preferably fasting
- Hemoglobin A1C
- Fasting lipid panel
- Vitamin levels (thiamine, vitamin D, B_{12})
- Drug/alcohol screen of blood and urine
- Urinalysis
- Urine pregnancy test
- Rapid plasma reagin (RPR), HIV
- Heavy-metal exposure: lead, mercury
- Ceruloplasmin, urine porphobilinogen as indicated
- ECG, for baseline QTc

Follow-Up Tests & Special Considerations
Clinical and laboratory tests for routine monitoring, at least yearly, if using antipsychotic medications (7)[A]
- Blood pressure, weight, and waist circumference
- CBC, blood chemistries
- Fasting blood glucose level, hemoglobin A1C
- Lipid panel
- TSH
- Pregnancy test and prolactin level, if indicated
- ECG, monitoring for QTc prolongation

Diagnostic Procedures/Other
- Psychological: not a routine part of assessment
- MRI and EEG to rule out seizure/neurologic disorder
- Lumbar puncture if indicated by clinical presentation

Test Interpretation
No diagnostic pathologic findings; however, ventriculomegaly is frequently seen on MRI with whole brain grey matter loss and white matter loss in medial temporal lobe structures preferentially (8)[A].

TREATMENT

MEDICATION
First Line
- Two classes of antipsychotic medications: typical and atypical. First-line treatment is with an atypical antipsychotic given lower potential for extrapyramidal side effects.
  - Atypical (2nd generation)
    - Risperidone, olanzapine, ziprasidone, aripiprazole, quetiapine, paliperidone, iloperidone, asenapine, lurasidone, clozapine
  - Typical (1st generation)
    - Haloperidol, chlorpromazine, fluphenazine, trifluoperazine, perphenazine, thioridazine, thiothixene, loxapine
- Medication choice is based on clinical and subjective response and side effect profile (7)[A].

- Sensitivity to extrapyramidal adverse effects: atypical
- For least risk of tardive dyskinesia: quetiapine, clozapine
- For least risk of metabolic syndrome: aripiprazole, ziprasidone, lurasidone
- For poor compliance/high risk of relapse: injectable form of long-acting antipsychotic such as haloperidol, fluphenazine, risperidone, olanzapine, aripiprazole, or paliperidone
- Usual oral daily dose (initial dose may be lower)
  - Chlorpromazine: 200 mg BID
  - Aripiprazole: 10 to 30 mg/day
  - Asenapine: 5 mg BID (sublingual)
  - Fluphenazine: 5 mg BID
  - Haloperidol: 5 mg BID
  - Lurasidone: 40 to 80 mg/day
  - Olanzapine: 15 to 30 mg/day
  - Paliperidone: 3 to 12 mg/day
  - Perphenazine: 24 mg/day divided BID or TID
  - Quetiapine: 200 to 300 mg BID
  - Risperidone: 3 mg/day
  - Ziprasidone: 60 to 80 mg BID (with meal)
  - Clozapine: 200 mg BID
    - Start 12.5 mg/day and increase daily by 25 mg until dose of 300 mg/day split into BID dosing; do not exceed 900 mg/day.
    - Effective in treatment of refractory or suicidal patients (7)[A]
    - Serious risk of agranulocytosis mandates registration with National Clozapine Registry and monitoring regular periodic CBC with differential (weekly to once monthly).
    - Significant risk of seizure at higher doses
    - Side effects can include myocarditis, DVT, sialorrhea, tachycardia, and weight gain.

ALERT
All antipsychotics are associated with weight gain and carry the risk of metabolic SE and tardive dyskinesia.

- Managing adverse effects of antipsychotics
  - Dystonic reaction (especially of head and neck): Give diphenhydramine 25 to 50 mg IM or benztropine 1 to 2 mg IM.
  - Akathisia: propranolol 10 mg BID or lorazepam 0.5 mg BID
  - Pseudoparkinsonism: trihexyphenidyl 2 mg BID (may be increased to 15 mg/day if needed) or benztropine 0.5 BID (range 1 to 4 mg/day)
  - Akathisia (restlessness): propranolol (30 to 60 mg in divided doses) or lorazepam (range 1 to 2 mg/day)
  - Neuroleptic malignant syndrome: hyperthermia, autonomic dysfunction, and extrapyramidal symptoms; requires hospitalization and supportive management (IVF and cessation of offending neuroleptic)
- Geriatric considerations: All antipsychotics carry a black box warning for increased mortality risk in elderly dementia patients.
- Adjunctive treatments
  - Benzodiazepines
    ○ May be effective adjuncts to antipsychotics during acute phase of illness
    ○ Useful for the treatment of catatonia
    ○ Withdrawal reactions with psychosis or seizures
  - Mood stabilizers (valproic acid, lithium, lamotrigine, carbamazepine): may be effective adjuncts for those with agitated/violent behavior (7,9)[A]
  - Antidepressants: if prominent symptoms of depression are present
  - Metformin: helps minimize risk of metabolic SE with use of AP (10)[A]

ISSUES FOR REFERRAL
- Consider in cases of suicidality, coexistence of an addiction, difficulty in engagement, or poor self-care.
- Patients with schizophrenia should receive multidisciplinary care from both a primary care physician and a psychiatrist.
- Family members often benefit from referral to family advocacy organizations such as NAMI (11)[A].

ADDITIONAL THERAPIES
Family and patient education and psychotherapy. These include specific treatments to reduce the impact of psychotic symptoms and to enhance social functioning. Cognitive-behavioral therapy has been shown to be effective for specific symptoms of schizophrenia (12)[C].

COMPLEMENTARY & ALTERNATIVE MEDICINE
No alternative therapies are validated.

SURGERY/OTHER PROCEDURES
- Electroconvulsive therapy (ECT): For patients presenting with catatonic features, the option of ECT should be considered early when insufficient response to benzodiazepines is observed (7)[B].
- Surgical interventions are not available.

INPATIENT CONSIDERATIONS
Initial stabilization focuses on maintaining a safe environment and reducing acute psychotic symptoms and agitation through the initiation of pharmacologic treatment.

Admission Criteria/Initial Stabilization
The decision to admit is usually based on the patient's risk of self-harm or harm to others and the inability to care for self as governed by local legal statute.

Nursing
Monitor for safety concerns and establish a safe and supportive environment.

Discharge Criteria
Based on the patient's ability to remain safe in the community. It reflects a combination of suicide risk, level of psychotic symptoms, support systems, and the availability of appropriate outpatient services.

 ONGONG CARE

FOLLOW-UP RECOMMENDATIONS
- Long-term symptom management and rehabilitation depend on engagement in ongoing pharmacologic and psychosocial treatment.
- Monitoring is based on evaluation of symptoms (including safety and psychotic symptoms), looking for the emergence of comorbidities, medication side effects, and prevention of complications.

DIET
- Newer atypical antipsychotics confer a higher risk of metabolic side effects such as diabetes, hypercholesterolemia, and weight gain.
- Although there are no specific dietary requirements, attention should be paid to the high risk of development of obesity and metabolic syndrome in individuals with schizophrenia.

PATIENT EDUCATION
- National Institute of Mental Health: *Schizophrenia*, at www.nimh.nih.gov/health/topics/schizophrenia/index.shtml
- *Helping a Family Member with Schizophrenia*: www.aafp.org/afp/20070615/1830ph.html
- National Alliance on Mental Illness (NAMI): www.NAMI.org

PROGNOSIS
- Typical course is one of remissions and exacerbations. Although uncommon, there are known cases of complete remission and of refractory illness.
- Negative symptoms are often most difficult to treat.
- Excessive mortality occurs due to suicide, accidents, coronary artery disease, pulmonary disease, or substance use disorders; guarded prognosis

COMPLICATIONS
- Side effects from antipsychotic medications including tardive dyskinesia, orthostatic hypotension, QTc prolongation, and metabolic syndrome
- Self-inflicted trauma and suicide
- Combative behavior toward others
- Comorbid addictions, including nicotine (13)[A]

REFERENCES

1. American Psychiatric Association. *Diagnostic and Statistical Manual of Mental Disorders*, 5th ed. Arlington, VA: American Psychiatric Association;2013.
2. McGrath JJ. Variations in the incidence of schizophrenia: data versus dogma. *Schizophr Bull*. 2006;32(1):195–197.
3. Riecher-Rössler A, Häfner H. Gender aspects in schizophrenia: bridging the border between social and biological psychiatry. *Acta Psychiatr Scand Suppl*. 2000;102(407):58–62.
4. Laruelle M, Kegeles LS, Abi-Dargham A. Glutamate, dopamine, and schizophrenia: from pathophysiology to treatment. *Ann N Y Acad Sci*. 2003;1003:138–158.
5. Norman RM, Manchanda R, Malla AK, et al. The significance of family history in first-episode schizophrenia spectrum disorder. *J Nerv Ment Dis*. 2007;195(10):846–852.
6. Fagerström K, Aubin HJ. Management of smoking cessation in patients with psychiatric disorders. *Curr Med Res Opin*. 2009;25(2):511–518.
7. Hasan A, Falkai P, Wobrock T, et al. World Federation of Societies of Biological Psychiatry (WFSBP) guidelines for biological treatment of schizophrenia, part 1: update 2012 on the acute treatment of schizophrenia and the management of treatment resistance. *World J Biol Psychiatry*. 2012;13(5):318–378.
8. Shenton ME, Dickey CC, Frumin M, et al. A review of MRI findings in schizophrenia. *Schizophr Res*. 2001;49(1–2):1–52.
9. Essali A, Al-Haj Haasan N, Li C, et al. Clozapine versus typical neuroleptic medication for schizophrenia. *Cochrane Database Syst Rev*. 2009;(1):CD000059.
10. Mizuno Y, Suzuki T, Nakagawa A, et al. Pharmacological strategies to counteract antipsychotic-induced weight gain and metabolic adverse effects in schizophrenia: a systematic review and meta-analysis. *Schizophr Bull*. 2014;40(6): 1385–1403.
11. Mojtabai R, Nicholson RA, Carpenter BN. Role of psychosocial treatments in management of schizophrenia: a meta-analytic review of controlled outcome studies. *Schizophr Bull*. 1998;24(4):569–587.
12. Grant PM, Huh GA, Perivoliotis D, et al. Randomized trial to evaluate the efficacy of cognitive therapy for low-functioning patients with schizophrenia. *Arch Gen Psychiatry*. 2012;69(2):121–127.
13. Saha S, Chant D, McGrath J. A systematic review of mortality in schizophrenia: is the differential mortality gap worsening over time? *Arch Gen Psychiatry*. 2007;64(10):1123–1131.

ADDITIONAL READING

Saks E. *The Center Cannot Hold: My Journey Through Madness*. New York, NY: Hyperion; 2007.

 SEE ALSO

Algorithm: Delirium

 CODES

ICD10
- F20.9 Schizophrenia, unspecified
- F20.0 Paranoid schizophrenia
- F20.1 Disorganized schizophrenia

CLINICAL PEARLS
- A debilitating chronic mental illness that affects all cultures
- Schizophrenia is characterized by positive symptoms, including hallucinations such as voices that converse with/about the patient, delusions that are often paranoid, and negative symptoms, including flattened affect, loss of a sense of pleasure, loss of will/drive, and social withdrawal.
- Multidisciplinary teams to enhance patient and family coping with serious and persistent mental illness, to prevent and treat comorbidities, and to promote recovery

S

SCIWORA SYNDROME (SPINAL CORD INJURY WITHOUT RADIOLOGIC ABNORMALITY)

Patrick M. Carey, DO • Jason B. Alisangco, DO, FAAFP

BASICS

Also called spinal cord injury without radiographic evidence of trauma (SCIWORET), spinal cord injury without CT evidence of trauma (SCIWOCTET), or spinal cord injury without neuroimaging abnormality (SCIWONA)

DESCRIPTION
- SCIWORA occurs after trauma; it is an acute spinal cord injury (SCI) and nerve root trauma resulting in transient or permanent sensory, motor, or combined sensorimotor deficits.
- Neural injuries occur without a fracture or misalignment visible on radiographic imaging (x-ray, CT).
- SCIWORA has a broad presentation, from minor neurologic symptoms to complete quadriplegia.

EPIDEMIOLOGY
Incidence
- Variable: reported to be 19–34% of pediatric spinal cord injuries (1)
- Occurs in all populations but is primarily observed in pediatric patients (90%) (1)
- Bimodal: affects children <8 years old and adults >60 years old; rarely occurs between 16 and 36 years (2)
- There is no association between Chiari malformation type 1 and SCIWORA.

ETIOLOGY AND PATHOPHYSIOLOGY
- Trauma (3)
  – Motor vehicle collision (MVC) (most common cause); either unrestrained passengers, pedestrians, or bicyclists struck by motor vehicles
  – Sports-related injury
  – Significant fall
  – Child abuse
- Mechanism
  – Traumatic neural (edema, hematomyelia, cord disruption) and extraneural (disc injury or ligament disruption) injury occurs after (2,4,5) the following:
    ○ Hyperextension
    ○ Hyperflexion
    ○ Longitudinal distraction
    ○ Ischemic damage
    ○ Secondary injury from inflammatory response to tissue damage

- Age: Pediatric patients have a higher incidence of SCIWORA than adults due to anatomic differences and increased mobility and flexibility (1,4,6).
  – Horizontally oriented facet joints permit more translational motion in the coronal (AP) plane.
  – Anterior wedging of vertebral bodies
  – Elasticity of ligaments and joint capsules permits increased intersegmental movement and disc protrusion.
  – In patients age <8 years, head size-to-trunk ratio is disproportionately large.
  – Weaker nuchal musculature
  – Uncovertebral joints are absent.
  – Pseudosubluxation of C2 to C3
- Location
  – Cervical: upper > lower
  – Thoracic: protected and splinted by ribs, preventing forced flexion and extension
  – Lumbar: rare, usually fatal (1)

RISK FACTORS
- History of trauma
- Age <8 years
- Male: female
  – Adult; 4.5:1 (3,7), Children; 2:1 (3)
- Improper wear of seatbelt

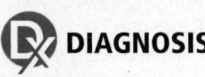
DIAGNOSIS

HISTORY
- MVA
- Sports-related injury
- Fall
- Child abuse

PHYSICAL EXAM
- Assess for sensorimotor deficit.
- Abnormal neurologic findings are not accounted for by known/visible injuries.
- Abnormalities on musculoskeletal exam increases risk of SCI.

DIFFERENTIAL DIAGNOSIS
- End-plate cartilage fracture
- Transverse myelitis
- Intramedulllary hemorrhage
- Anterior spinal artery syndrome
- Disseminated encephalomyelitis
- Atlantoaxial dislocation
- Central cord syndrome
- Brown-Sequard syndrome

DIAGNOSTIC TESTS & INTERPRETATION
- Radiographic screening with CT of the entire spinal column is recommended (5)[C].
- MRI of the region of suspected neurologic injury (5)[C]
- MRI within 24 hours of injury and consider repeat if normal (7)[C]
- Assessment of spinal stability in a SCIWORA patient is recommended with flexion–extension radiographs in the acute setting and at late follow-up, even in the presence of a magnetic resonance imaging (MRI) negative for extraneural injury (5)[C].
- Neither spinal angiography nor myelography is recommended in the evaluation of patients with SCIWORA (5)[C].
- CT scan can reliably rule out fracture.

Follow-Up Tests & Special Considerations
- Adult considerations: Adults are less prone to SCIWORA due to decreased flexibility and mobility in comparison to pediatric patients, although SCIWORA is possible in the setting of acute trauma or cervical spondylosis.
- A normal MRI does not rule out SCIWORA (1,2,7).
- MRI abnormalities correlate closely with neurologic injury and prognosis (3)[C].
- MRI may be able to demonstrate neural and extra-neural injuries: cartilaginous end-plate fracture, edema, herniation, and interspinous ligamentous injury (1,2)

Diagnostic Procedures/Other
- Diagnosis is based on clinical findings of neurologic dysfunction or MRI abnormality.
- Consider diffusion-weighted MRI and somatosensory-evoked potentials (SSEPs) in cases of suspected SCIWORA with normal MRI (5,8)[C].

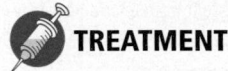
TREATMENT

GENERAL MEASURES
- Immobilize unconscious patients until plain x-ray and CT radiographs are obtained.
- Immobilize until neurologic and pain assessment can be made.
- Transient findings, such as numbness, and a history of trauma should be treated with immobilization following SCI protocol.
- Supportive care and serial neurologic and musculoskeletal exams
- Blood pressure support (5)[C]
- Corticosteroid use is controversial and is not considered standard practice for pediatric cases (6)[C].

ADDITIONAL THERAPIES

- Rigid external immobilization of the spinal segment for 12 weeks (day and night) (1)
- Immobilization for 12 weeks even after the return of normal neurologic function to minimize SCIWORA recurrence (1,2,5)[C]
- Avoidance of "high-risk" activities for up to 6 months following SCIWORA (2,5)[C]
- Initially, treatment is nonoperative. Surgery may be required for spinal cord compression or spine instability secondary to extraneural injury (1,2).
- Surgery for adults is often warranted as disc and ligamentum flavum pathology is common (2)[C].
- Early discontinuation of external immobilization is recommended for patients who become asymptomatic, and spinal stability is confirmed with flexion and extension radiographs (5)[C].

INPATIENT CONSIDERATIONS

Admission Criteria/Initial Stabilization

- Unexplained neurologic findings (2)[C]
- Neurologic injury found via MRI (2)[C]
- Suspected ligamentous lesion (2)[C]
- Trauma and spinal injury protocol
- Rigid immobilization
- Consultation with a spine surgeon

Discharge Criteria

- Neurologic exam without any deficits
- Resolution of transient neurologic symptoms

 ## ONGOING CARE

- SCIWORA can present with no initial symptoms after trauma followed by subsequent neurologic deterioration.
- Reassess neurologic function within 24 to 48 hours if patient presents with no initial symptoms after a traumatic event, as there may be a latency period and secondary injury.
- Clinical symptoms may take as long as 10 days to develop (3).
- Follow-up MRI before discharge

PROGNOSIS

- Initial clinical instability, injury severity, MRI findings, neurologic features, injury location, patient age, and persistence of symptoms have a direct correlation with prognosis.

- Favorable
  - Initial mild to moderate injury
  - Normal or mild edema on initial MRI (1)
  - Resolution of changes as evidenced by follow-up MRI
- Unfavorable
  - Initial severe neural injury
  - MRI findings of spinal cord transection and significant hemorrhage
  - Intramedullary hemorrhage seen on MRI is predictive of complete cord injury (1).
  - Follow-up MRI findings of persistent SCI
  - Higher cervical injuries
  - Patients age <8 years (1)
  - Concominant traumatic brain injury (concussion)

COMPLICATIONS

Iatrogenic, delayed, and recurrent SCIWORA have been reported; therefore, careful handling of trauma patients and close follow-up is warranted.

REFERENCES

1. Launay F, Leet AI, Sponseller PD. Pediatric spinal cord injury without radiographic abnormality: a meta-analysis. *Clin Orthop Relat Res.* 2005;(433):166–170.
2. Kasimatis GB, Panagiotopoulos E, Megas P, et al. The adult spinal cord injury without radiographic abnormalities syndrome: magnetic resonance imaging and clinical findings in adults with spinal cord injuries having normal radiographs and computed tomography studies. *J Trauma.* 2008;65(1):86–93.
3. Boese CK, Oppermann J, Siewe J, et al. Spinal cord injury without radiologic abnormality in children: a systematic review and meta-analysis. *J Trauma Acute Care Surg.* 2015;78(4):874–882.
4. Trigylidas T, Yuh SJ, Vassilyadi M, et al. Spinal cord injuries without radiographic abnormality at two pediatric trauma centers in Ontario. *Pediatr Neurosurg.* 2010;46(4):283–289.
5. Rozzelle CJ, Aarabi B, Dhall SS, et al. Spinal injury without radiographic abnormality (SCIWORA). *Neurosurgery.* 2013;72(Suppl 2):227–233.
6. Easter JS, Barkin R, Rosen CL, et al. Cervical spine injuries in children, part II: management and special considerations. *J Emerg Med.* 2011;41(3):252–256.
7. Boese CK, Lechler P. Spinal cord injury without radiologic abnormalities in adults: a systematic review. *J Trauma Acute Care Surg.* 2013;75(2): 320–330.
8. Shen H, Tang Y, Huang L, et al. Application of diffusion-weighted MRI in thoracic spinal cord injury without radiographic abnormality. *Int Orthop.* 2007;31(3):375–383.

ADDITIONAL READING

- Parikh RN, Muranjan M, Karande S, et al. Atlas shrugged: cervical myelopathy caused by congenital atlantoaxial dislocation aggravated by child labor. *Pediatr Neurol.* 2014;50(4):380–383.
- Piatt JH Jr, Campbell JW. Spinal cord injury without radiographic abnormality and the Chiari malformation: controlled observations. *Pediatr Neurosurg.* 2012;48(6):360–363.
- Shah LM, Zollinger LV. Congenital craniocervical anomalies pose a vulnerability to spinal cord injury without radiographic abnormality (SCIWORA). *Emerg Radiol.* 2011;18(4):353–356.

 ## CODES

ICD10

- S14.109A Unsp injury at unsp level of cervical spinal cord, init
- S14.2XXA Injury of nerve root of cervical spine, initial encounter
- S14.102A Unsp injury at C2 level of cervical spinal cord, init encntr

CLINICAL PEARLS

- If a patient presents with a history of trauma and neurologic symptoms but has negative x-ray and CT findings, consider SCIWORA.
- Spinal cord appearance on MRI provides prognostic information (3)[C].
- Treat SCIWORA with early immobilization, continue for 12 weeks, and avoid high-risk activities for an additional 12 weeks (2)[C].
- Immobilization for 12 weeks is superior to 8 weeks (1)[C].
- Consider serial scans or short-interval follow-up MRI to assess for delayed presentation of pathology (3)[C].

S

SCLERITIS

Matthew J. Schear, DO, MS • Anne Steiner, MD

 BASICS

DESCRIPTION
- Scleritis is a painful, inflammatory process of the sclera, part of the eye's outer coat.
  - Categorized into anterior or posterior and diffuse, nodular, or necrotizing
  - Commonly associated with systemic disorders
  - Frequently requires systemic anti-inflammatory therapy
  - Potentially vision-threatening
- In contrast, episcleritis is a self-limited inflammation of the eye with only mild discomfort.
- System(s) affected: ocular

EPIDEMIOLOGY
- Predominant age: most frequently occurs in 4th and 6th decades; mean age for all types of scleritis is 52 years.
- Predominant sex: female > male (1.6:1)

Incidence
- Anterior scleritis, about 94% of cases (1)[B]
  - Diffuse anterior scleritis (most common)
- Remaining 6% have posterior scleritis

Prevalence
Estimated to be 6 cases/100,000 people in the general population

ETIOLOGY AND PATHOPHYSIOLOGY
- Frequently associated with a systemic illness (1)[B]
  - Most commonly associated with rheumatoid arthritis
  - In about 38% of cases, scleritis is the presenting manifestation of an underlying systemic disorder.
  - Necrotizing scleritis has the highest association with systemic disease.
- Other etiologies
  - Proposed pathogenesis is dependent on type of scleritis. In necrotizing scleritis, the predominant mechanism is likely due to the activity of matrix metalloproteinases.
  - Drug-induced scleritis has been reported in patients on bisphosphonate therapy.
  - Surgically induced necrotizing scleritis is exceedingly rare and occurs after multiple surgeries.
  - Infectious scleritis occurs most commonly after surgical trauma, and *Pseudomonas aeruginosa* in poorly controlled diabetic patients is the most common causative organism (2)[B].

RISK FACTORS
Individuals with autoimmune disorders are most at risk.

COMMONLY ASSOCIATED CONDITIONS
- Rheumatoid arthritis
- Sjögren syndrome
- Granulomatosis with polyangitis
- Ankylosing spondylitis
- Systemic lupus erythematosus
- Reactive arthritis
- Relapsing polychondritis
- Polyarteritis nodosa
- Sarcoidosis
- Inflammatory bowel disease
- Herpes zoster
- Herpes simplex
- HIV
- Syphilis
- Lyme disease
- Tuberculosis

 DIAGNOSIS

HISTORY
- Redness and inflammation of the sclera
  - Can be bilateral in about 40% of cases (1)[B]
- Decrease in visual acuity of two or more Snellen lines occurred in about 16% of patients (1)[B].
- Photophobia and tearing
- Pain ranging from mild discomfort to extreme localized tenderness
  - May be described as constant, deep, boring, or pulsating
  - Pain may be referred to the eyebrow, temple, or jaw.
  - Pain may awaken patient from sleep in early hours of morning.
  - Severe pain is most commonly associated with necrotizing scleritis (1)[B].

PHYSICAL EXAM
- Examine sclera in all directions of gaze by gross inspection.
  - A bluish hue may suggest thinning of sclera.
  - Inspect for breadth and degree of injection.
- Check visual acuity.

- Slit-lamp exam using red-free light
  - Episcleritis: conjunctival and superficial vascular plexuses displaced anteriorly
  - Scleritis: Deep episcleral plexus is the maximum site of vascular congestion, displaced anteriorly d/t edema of underlying sclera. Characteristic blue or violet color, absent in patients with episcleritis
- Ocular tenderness
- Dilated fundus exam to rule out posterior involvement
- A complete physical exam, particularly of the skin, joints, heart, and lungs, should be done to evaluate for associated conditions.

DIFFERENTIAL DIAGNOSIS
- Conjunctivitis
- Episcleritis
- Iritis (anterior uveitis)
- Blepharitis
- Trauma
- Ocular rosacea
- Herpes zoster

DIAGNOSTIC TESTS & INTERPRETATION
- Consider further tests if warranted by history and physical.
- Routine tests to exclude systemic disease
  - CBC, serum chemistry, urinalysis, ESR, and/or C-reactive protein
- Specific tests for underlying systemic illness
  - Rheumatoid factor, anticyclic citrullinated peptide antibodies, antineutrophil cytoplasmic antibody, and antinuclear antibody may aid in the diagnosis.
- Other tests:
  - Fluorescent treponemal antibody absorption (FTA-ABS), rapid plasma reagin, and Lyme titers
- Further imaging studies, such as a chest x-ray and sacroiliac joint films, may be useful if a specific systemic illness is suspected.
- B-scan US to detect posterior scleritis and thickness of sclera
- If indicated, MRI/CT scan to detect orbital disease

Diagnostic Procedures/Other
Biopsy is not routinely required unless diagnosis remains uncertain after above investigations.

Test Interpretation
Different subtypes of scleritis are associated with varying presentations and distinct findings.
- Diffuse anterior scleritis: widespread inflammation
- Nodular anterior scleritis: immovable, inflamed nodule

- Necrotizing anterior scleritis
  - "With inflammation": Sclera becomes transparent.
  - Scleromalacia perforans without inflammation: painless and often associated with rheumatoid arthritis
- Posterior scleritis: associated with retinal and choroidal complications, adjacent swelling of orbital tissues may occur

 TREATMENT

GENERAL MEASURES
If scleral thinning, glasses/eye shield should be worn to prevent perforation.

MEDICATION
- First-line therapies for noninfectious scleritis (3)[C]
  - Oral NSAID therapy, choice based on availability, example is ibuprofen 600 to 800 mg PO TID–QID provided no contraindications exists. About 37% successful (4)[B]
  - Topical steroids as adjunct; prednisolone acetate 1% ophthalmic suspension
  - Subconjunctival triamcinolone acetonide injection only for nonnecrotizing, 40 mg/mL, 97% improvement after one injection. Increased risk of ocular HTN, cataract, and globe perforation (5)[B]
  - Systemic steroids (initial if necrotizing scleritis and preferentially IV if vision threatening, otherwise use if failure of NSAIDs), prednisone 40 to 60 mg PO QD, taper over 4 to 6 weeks
  - Antimetabolites including methotrexate, azathioprine, mycophenolate mofetil, cyclophosphamide, and cyclosporine may be used as steroid-sparing agents. They are generally recommended if steroids cannot be tapered below 10 mg PO QD (4)[C].
- Second-line therapies (4)[C],(5)[B],(6)[A]
  - Immunomodulatory agents, infliximab, and adalimumab can be used if patient has failed or is not a candidate for antimetabolites or calcineurin inhibitors. These agents are preferred over etanercept due to higher treatment success.
- Necrotizing anterior scleritis and posterior scleritis
  - May require immunosuppressive therapy in addition to systemic steroids
  - Treat aggressively due to possible complications if left untreated. May need patch grafting to maintain globe integrity
- Infectious
  - Antibiotic therapy resolves about 18% of cases, whereas the remaining often requires surgical intervention such as débridement (2)[B].

ISSUES FOR REFERRAL
- All patients with scleritis should be managed by an ophthalmologist familiar with this condition.
- Rheumatology referral for coexistent systemic disease is helpful for long-term success.

ADDITIONAL THERAPIES
Immunosuppressants used for autoimmune and collagen vascular disorders may be of help in active scleritis.

SURGERY/OTHER PROCEDURES
- In rare cases, scleral biopsy may be indicated to confirm infection or malignancy.
- Ocular perforation requires scleral grafting.

 ONGOING CARE

Follow-Up Tests & Special Considerations
- No restrictions
- Avoid contact lens—wear only if there is corneal involvement, which is rare.

Patient Monitoring
- Patient in the active stage of inflammation should be followed very closely by an ophthalmologist to assess the effectiveness of therapy.
- Medication use mandates close surveillance for adverse effects.

DIET
No special diet

PATIENT EDUCATION
Scleritis at PubMed Health: http://www.ncbi.nlm.nih.gov/pubmedhealth/PMHT0024411/

PROGNOSIS
Scleritis is indolent, chronic, and often progressive.
- Diffuse anterior scleritis (best prognosis)
- Necrotizing anterior scleritis (worst prognosis)
- Recurrent bouts of inflammation may occur.
- Scleromalacia perforans has the highest risk of perforation of the globe.

COMPLICATIONS
- Decrease in vision, anterior uveitis, ocular hypertension, and peripheral keratitis (1)[B]
- Cataract and glaucoma can result from disease or treatment with steroids.
- Ocular perforation can occur in severe stages.

REFERENCES

1. Sainz de la Maza M, Molina N, Gonzalez-Gonzalez LA, et al. Clinical characteristics of a large cohort of patients with scleritis and episcleritis. *Ophthalmology.* 2012;119(1):43–50.
2. Hodson KL, Galor A, Karp CL, et al. Epidemiology and visual outcomes in patients with infectious scleritis. *Cornea.* 2013;32(4):466–472.
3. Beardsley RM, Suhler EB, Rosenbaum JT, et al. Pharmacotherapy of scleritis: current paradigms and future directions. *Expert Opin Pharmacother.* 2013;14(4):411–424.

4. Sainz de la Maza M, Molina N, Gonzalez-Gonzalez LA, et al. Scleritis therapy. *Ophthalmology.* 2012;119(1):51–58.
5. Sohn EH, Wang R, Read R, et al. Long-term, multicenter evaluation of subconjunctival injection of triamcinolone for non-necrotizing, noninfectious anterior scleritis. *Ophthalmology.* 2011;118(10):1932–1937.
6. Levy-Clarke G, Jabs DA, Read RW, et al. Expert panel recommendations for the use of anti-tumor necrosis factor biologic agents in patients with ocular inflammatory disorders. *Ophthalmology.* 2014;121(3):785–796.e3.

ADDITIONAL READING

- Doctor P, Sultan A, Syed S, et al. Infliximab for the treatment of refractory scleritis. *Br J Ophthalmol.* 2010;94(5):579–583.
- Iaccheri B, Androudi S, Bocci EB, et al. Rituximab treatment for persistent scleritis associated with rheumatoid arthritis. *Ocul Immunol Inflamm.* 2010;18(3):223–225.
- Rachitskaya A, Mandelcorn ED, Albini TA. An update on the cause and treatment of scleritis. *Curr Opin Ophthalmol.* 2010;21(6):463–467.
- Wakefield D, Di Girolamo N, Thurau S, et al. Scleritis: challenges in immunopathogenesis and treatment. *Discov Med.* 2013;16(88):153–157.
- Wakefield D, Di Girolamo N, Thurau S, et al. Scleritis: immunopathogenesis and molecular basis for therapy. *Prog Retin Eye Res.* 2013;35:44–62.

 CODES

ICD10
- H15.009 Unspecified scleritis, unspecified eye
- H15.019 Anterior scleritis, unspecified eye
- H15.039 Posterior scleritis, unspecified eye

CLINICAL PEARLS
- Episcleritis is a self-limited inflammation of the eye with mild discomfort. Scleritis is a painful, severe, and potentially vision-threatening condition. Both conditions can be associated with underlying inflammatory diseases.
- About 35% of all cases of scleritis are associated with a systemic disease such as rheumatoid arthritis. Necrotizing scleritis has the highest association.

S

SCLERODERMA

Ann M. Lynch, PharmD, RPh, AE-C • Deborah M. DeMarco, MD, FACP

 BASICS

DESCRIPTION

- Scleroderma (systemic sclerosis [SSc]) is a chronic disease of unknown cause characterized by diffuse fibrosis of skin and visceral organs and vascular abnormalities.
- Most manifestations have vascular features (e.g., Raynaud phenomenon), but frank vasculitis is rarely seen.
- Can range from a mild disease, affecting the skin, to a systemic disease that can cause death in a few months
- The disease is categorized into two major clinical variants (1).
  - Diffuse: distal and proximal extremity and truncal skin thickening
  - Limited
    - Restricted to the fingers, hands, and face
    - CREST syndrome (calcinosis, Raynaud phenomenon, esophageal dysmotility, sclerodactyly, telangiectasia)
- System(s) affected: include, but not limited to skin; renal; cardiovascular; pulmonary; musculoskeletal; gastrointestinal

Geriatric Considerations
Uncommon >75 years of age

Pediatric Considerations
Rare in this age group

Pregnancy Considerations
- Safe and healthy pregnancies are common and possible despite higher frequency of premature births.
- High-risk management must be standard care to avoid complications, specifically renal crisis.
- Diffuse scleroderma causes greater risk for developing serious cardiopulmonary and renal problems. Pregnancy should be delayed until disease stabilizes.

EPIDEMIOLOGY

Incidence
- In the United States: 1 to 2/100,000/year
- Predominant age
  - Young adult (16 to 40 years); middle-aged (40 to 75 years), peak onset 30 to 50 years
  - Symptoms usually appear in the 3rd to 5th decades.
- Predominant sex: female > male (4:1)

Prevalence
In the United States: 1 to 25/100,000

ETIOLOGY AND PATHOPHYSIOLOGY
Pathophysiology involves both a vascular component and a fibrotic component. Both occur simultaneously. The inciting event is unknown, but there is an increase in certain cytokines after endothelial cell activation that are profibrotic (TGF-β and PDGF).

- Unknown
- Possible alterations in immune response
- Possibly some association with exposure to quartz mining, quarrying, vinyl chloride, hydrocarbons, toxin exposure
- Treatment with bleomycin has caused a scleroderma-like syndrome, as has exposure to rapeseed oil.

Genetics
Familial clustering is rare, but has been seen.

RISK FACTORS
Unknown

 DIAGNOSIS

HISTORY

- Raynaud phenomenon is generally the presenting complaint (differentiated from Raynaud disease, generally affecting younger individuals and without digital ulcers).
- Skin thickening, "puffy hands," pruritus, and gastro-esophageal reflux disease (GERD) are often noted early in the disease process.

PHYSICAL EXAM

- Skin
  - Digital ulcerations
  - Digital pitting
  - Tightness, swelling, thickening of digits
  - Hyperpigmentation/hypopigmentation
  - Narrowed oral aperture
  - SC calcinosis
- Peripheral vascular system
  - Telangiectasia
- Joints, tendons, and bones
  - Flexion contractures
  - Friction rub on tendon movement
  - Hand swelling
  - Joint stiffness
  - Polyarthralgia
  - Sclerodactyly
- Muscle
  - Proximal muscle weakness
- GI tract
  - Dysphagia
  - Esophageal reflux due to dysmotility (most common systemic sign in diffuse disease)
  - Malabsorptive diarrhea
  - Nausea and vomiting
  - Weight loss
  - Xerostomia
- Kidney
  - Hypertension
  - May develop scleroderma renal crisis: acute renal failure (ARF)
- Pulmonary
  - Dry crackles at lung bases
  - Dyspnea
- Nervous system
  - Peripheral neuropathy
  - Trigeminal neuropathy
- Cardiac (progressive disease)
  - Conduction abnormalities
  - Cardiomyopathy
  - Pericarditis
  - Secondary cor pulmonale

DIFFERENTIAL DIAGNOSIS

- Mixed connective tissue disease/overlap syndromes
- Scleredema
- Nephrogenic systemic fibrosis
- Toxic oil syndrome (Madrid, 1981, affecting 20,000 people)
- Eosinophilia–myalgia syndrome
- Diffuse fasciitis with eosinophilia
- Scleredema of Buschke

DIAGNOSTIC TESTS & INTERPRETATION

Initial Tests (lab, imaging)
- Nail fold capillary microscopy—drop out is most significant finding
- CBC
- Creatinine
- Urinalysis (albuminuria, microscopic hematuria)
- Antinuclear antibodies (ANA): positive in >90% of patients
- Anti–Scl-70 (anti-topoisomerase [ATA]) antibody is highly specific for systemic disease and confers a higher risk of interstitial lung disease (ILD).
- Anticentromere antibody usually associated with CREST variant
- Chest radiograph
  - Diffuse reticular pattern
  - Bilateral basilar pulmonary fibrosis
- Hand radiograph
  - Soft tissue atrophy and acro-osteolysis
  - Can see overlap syndromes such as rheumatoid arthritis
  - SC calcinosis

Follow-Up Tests & Special Considerations
- Pulmonary function tests (PFTs)
  - Decreased maximum breathing capacity
  - Increased residual volume
  - Diffusion defect
- Antibodies to U3-RNP—higher risk for scleroderma-associated pulmonary hypertension
- Anti–PM-Scl antibodies (for myositis) (2)[B]
- Anti–RNA polymerase III—higher risk for diffuse cutaneous involvement and renal crisis (3)[A]
- ECG (low voltage): possible nonspecific abnormalities, arrhythmia, and conduction defects
- Echocardiography: pulmonary hypertension or cardiomyopathy
- Nail fold capillary loop abnormalities
- Upper GI
  - Distal esophageal dilatation
  - Atonic esophagus
  - Esophageal dysmotility
  - Duodenal diverticula
- Barium enema
  - Colonic diverticula
  - Megacolon
- High-resolution CT scan for detecting alveolitis, which has a ground-glass appearance or fibrosis predominant in bilateral lower lobes

Diagnostic Procedures/Other
- Skin biopsy
  - Compact collagen fibers in the reticular dermis and hyalinization and fibrosis of arterioles
  - Thinning of epidermis, with loss of rete pegs, and atrophy of dermal appendages
  - Accumulation of mononuclear cells is also seen.
- Right-sided heart catheterization: Pulmonary hypertension is an ominous prognostic feature.

Test Interpretation
- Skin
  - Edema, fibrosis, or atrophy (late stage)
  - Lymphocytic infiltrate around sweat glands
  - Loss of capillaries
  - Endothelial proliferation
  - Hair follicle atrophy
- Synovium
  - Pannus formation
  - Fibrin deposits in tendons
- Kidney
  - Small kidneys
  - Intimal proliferation in interlobular arteries
- Heart
  - Endocardial thickening
  - Myocardial interstitial fibrosis
  - Ischemic band necrosis
  - Enlarged heart
  - Cardiac hypertrophy
  - Pulmonary hypertension
- Lung
  - Interstitial pneumonitis
  - Cyst formation
  - Interstitial fibrosis
  - Bronchiectasis
- Esophagus
  - Esophageal atrophy
  - Fibrosis

TREATMENT

GENERAL MEASURES
- Treatment is symptomatic and supportive.
- Esophageal dilation may be used for strictures.
- Avoid cold; dress appropriately in layers for the weather; be wary of air conditioning.
- Avoid smoking (crucial).
- Avoid finger sticks (e.g., blood tests).
- Elevate the head of the bed during sleep to help relieve GI symptoms.
- Use softening lotions, ointments, and bath oils to help prevent dryness and cracking of skin.
- Dialysis may be necessary in renal crisis.

MEDICATION
First Line
- ACE inhibitors (ACEIs): for preservation of renal blood flow and for treatment of hypertensive renal crisis
- Corticosteroids: for disabling myositis, pulmonary alveolitis, or mixed connective tissue disease (not recommended in high doses due to increased incidence of renal failure)
- NSAIDs: for joint or tendon symptoms. Caution with long-term concurrent use with ACEIs (potential renal complications)
- Antibiotics: for secondary infections in bowel and active skin infections
- Antacids, proton pump inhibitors: for gastric reflux
- Metoclopramide: for intestinal dysfunction
- Hydrophilic skin ointments: for skin therapy
- Topical clindamycin, erythromycin, or silver sulfadiazine: for prevention of recurrent infectious cutaneous ulcers
- Consider immunosuppressives for treatment of life-threatening or potentially crippling scleroderma or interstitial pneumonitis such as cyclophosphamide for ILD (4)[B].

- Nitrates and dihydropyridine calcium-channel blockers for Raynaud phenomenon
- Avoidance of caffeine, nicotine, and sympathomimetics may ease Raynaud symptoms.
- PDE-5 antagonists (e.g., sildenafil), prostanoids, and endothelin-1 antagonists are changing the management of pulmonary hypertension (5).
- Alveolitis: immunosuppressants and alkylating agents (e.g., cyclophosphamide)

ADDITIONAL THERAPIES
- Anti–TNF-α therapy: Preliminary suggestion is that these may reduce joint symptoms and disability in inflammatory arthritis, but small sample sizes and observational biases lend to the need for further well-designed, adequately powered, longitudinal clinical trials.
- Physical therapy to maintain function and promote strength
- Heat therapy to relieve joint stiffness

SURGERY/OTHER PROCEDURES
- Some success with gastroplasty for correction of GERD
- Limited role for sympathectomy for Raynaud phenomenon
- Lung transplantation for pulmonary hypertension and ILD

ONGOING CARE

FOLLOW-UP RECOMMENDATIONS
Patient Monitoring
- Monitor every 3 to 6 months for end-organ and skin involvement and medications. Provide encouragement.
- Echocardiology and PFTs yearly

DIET
Drink plenty of fluids with meals.

PATIENT EDUCATION
- Stay as active as possible, but avoid fatigue.
- Printed patient information available from the Scleroderma Federation, 1725 York Avenue, No. 29F, New York, NY 10128; (212) 427-7040
- Advise the patient to report any abnormal bruising or nonhealing abrasions.
- Assist the patient about smoking cessation, if needed.

PROGNOSIS
- Possible improvement but incurable
- Prognosis is poor if cardiac, pulmonary, or renal manifestations present early.

COMPLICATIONS
- Renal failure
- Respiratory failure
- Flexion contractures
- Disability
- Esophageal dysmotility
- Reflux esophagitis
- Arrhythmia
- Megacolon
- Pneumatosis intestinalis
- Obstructive bowel
- Cardiomyopathy
- Pulmonary hypertension
- Possible association with lung and other cancers
- Death

REFERENCES
1. van den Hoogen F, Khanna D, Fransen J, et al. 2013 classification criteria for systemic sclerosis: an American College of Rheumatology/European League against rheumatism collaborative initiative. *Arthritis Rheum.* 2013;65(11):2737–2747.
2. D'Aoust J, Hudson M, Tatibouet S, et al. Clinical and serologic correlates of anti-PM/Scl antibodies in systemic sclerosis: a multicenter study of 763 patients. *Arthritis Rheumatol.* 2014;66(6):1608–1615.
3. Sobanski V, Dauchet L, Lefèvre G, et al. Prevalence of anti-RNA polymerase III antibodies in systemic sclerosis: new data from a French cohort and a systematic review and meta-analysis. *Arthritis Rheumatol.* 2014;66(2):407–417.
4. Roth MD, Tseng CH, Clements PJ, et al. Predicting treatment outcomes and responder subsets in scleroderma-related interstitial lung disease. *Arthritis Rheum.* 2011;63(9):2797–2808.
5. Volkmann ER, Saggar R, Khanna D, et al. Improved transplant-free survival in patients with systemic sclerosis-associated pulmonary hypertension and interstitial lung disease. *Arthritis Rheumatol.* 2014;66(7):1900–1908.

ADDITIONAL READING
- Herrick AL. Contemporary management of Raynaud's phenomenon and digits ischaemic complications. *Curr Opin Rheumatol.* 2011;23(6):555–561.
- Kowal-Bielecka O, Landewé R, Avouac J, et al. EULAR recommendations for the treatment of systemic sclerosis: a report from the EULAR Scleroderma Trials and Research group (EUSTAR). *Ann Rheum Dis.* 2009;68(5):620–628.
- Phumethum V, Jamal S, Johnson SR. Biologic therapy for systemic sclerosis: a systematic review. *J Rheumatol.* 2011;38(2):289–296.
- Steen VD. Pregnancy in scleroderma. *Rheum Dis Clin North Am.* 2007;33(2):345–358, vii.
- Valerio CJ, Schreiber BE, Handler CE, et al. Borderline mean pulmonary artery pressure in patients with systemic sclerosis. *Arthritis Rheum.* 2013;65(4):1074–1084.

 SEE ALSO

Morphea

 CODES

ICD10
- M34.9 Systemic sclerosis, unspecified
- M34.1 CR(E)ST syndrome
- L94.0 Localized scleroderma [morphea]

CLINICAL PEARLS
- Raynaud phenomenon is frequently the initial complaint.
- Skin thickening, "puffy hands," and GERD are often noted early in disease.
- Patients must be followed proactively for development of pulmonary hypertension or ILD.

S

SEASONAL AFFECTIVE DISORDER

Christopher White, MD, JD, MHA

 BASICS

DESCRIPTION
- Seasonal affective disorder (SAD) is a heterogeneous mood disorder with depressive episodes usually occurring in winter months, with full remissions in the spring and summer.
- Ranges from a milder form (winter blues) to a seriously disabling illness
- Must separate out patients with other mood disorders (such as major depressive disorder and bipolar affective disorder) whose symptoms persist during spring and summer months

EPIDEMIOLOGY
Incidence
- Affects up to 500,000 people every winter
- Up to 30% of patients visiting a primary care physician (PCP) during winter may report winter depressive symptoms.
- Predominant age: occurs at any age; peaks in 20s and 30s
- Predominant sex: female > male (3:1)

Prevalence
- 1–9% of the general population
- 10–20% of patients identified as having mood symptoms will have a seasonal component.

ETIOLOGY AND PATHOPHYSIOLOGY
The major theories currently involve the interplay of phase-shifted circadian rhythms, genetic vulnerability, and serotonin dysregulation.
- Melatonin produced by the pineal gland at increased levels in the dark has been linked to depressive symptoms; light therapy on the retina acts to inhibit melatonin secretion.
- Serotonin dysregulation because it is secreted less during winter months, must be present for light therapy to work, and treatment with SSRIs appears to reverse SAD symptoms
- Decreased levels of vitamin D, often occurring during low-light winter months, may be associated with depressive episodes in some individuals experiencing SAD symptoms.

Genetics
- Some twin studies and a preliminary study on GPR50 melatonin receptor variants have suggested a genetic component.
- Recent studies indicate an association with the melanopsin gene (OPN4).
- Increased incidence of depression, ADHD, and alcoholism in close relatives

RISK FACTORS
- Most common during months of January and February: Patients frequently visit PCP during winter months complaining of recurrent flu, chronic fatigue, and unexplained weight gain.
- Working in a building without windows or other environment without exposure to sunlight

GENERAL PREVENTION
- Consider use of light therapy at start of winter (if prior episodes begin in October), increase time outside during daylight, or move to a more southern location.
- Bupropion (Wellbutrin) is an FDA-approved antidepressant for the prevention of SAD.

COMMONLY ASSOCIATED CONDITIONS
Some individuals with SAD have a weakened immune system and may be more vulnerable to infections.

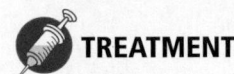 DIAGNOSIS

- Carefully document the presence or absence of prior manic episodes.
- Screen for the existence of any suicidal ideation and safety risk factors.
- Remission of symptoms during spring and summer
- Symptoms have occurred for the past 2 years.
- Seasonal episodes associated with winter months substantially outnumber any nonseasonal depressive episodes.
- Under *DSM-5*, SAD is denoted by adding the "with seasonal pattern" specifier to a diagnosis of major depressive disorder, recurrent.

HISTORY
- Symptoms of depression meeting the criteria for major depressive disorder are the following:
  – Sleep disturbance: either too much or too little
  – Lack of interest in life and absence of pleasure from hobbies/activities
  – Guilt: feelings of guilt or worthlessness
  – Energy: fatigue or constantly feeling tired
  – Concentration: difficulty with concentration and memory
  – Appetite: changes in appetite and weight
  – Psychomotor retardation: Patients feel slowed down with decreased activity.
  – Suicidal thoughts: Patients report thoughts of suicide.
- In SAD, hypersomnia, hyperphagia (craving for carbohydrates and sweets), and weight gain usually predominate. Despite sleeping more, patients report daytime sleepiness and fatigue. Cravings may lead to binge eating and weight gains >20 lb.
- Obtain collateral history if patient is unable to provide insight into the seasonal component.

PHYSICAL EXAM
Use exam to exclude other organic causes for symptoms. Focal neurologic deficits, signs of endocrine dysfunction, or stigmata of substance abuse should prompt further testing.

DIFFERENTIAL DIAGNOSIS
- Similar to that of major depression, meaning that organic causes of low energy and fatigue, such as hypothyroidism, anemia, and mononucleosis (or other viral syndromes), need to be considered.
- Other mood disorders without a seasonal component such as major depression, bipolar disorder, adjustment disorder, or dysthymia

- Symptoms should not be better accounted for by seasonal psychosocial stressors, which often accompany the winter holiday seasons.
- Substance abuse

DIAGNOSTIC TESTS & INTERPRETATION
- Thyroid-stimulating hormone to rule out hypothyroidism
- CBC to rule out anemia
- Rule out electrolyte and glucose dysregulation.
- 25-OH vitamin D level
- Pregnancy test for women of childbearing potential
- Urine toxicology screen if substance abuse is a concern
- Imaging is not useful unless focal neurologic finding or looking to exclude an organic cause.

TREATMENT

MEDICATION
Lack of evidence to determine whether light therapy or medication should be the first-line agent. Both supported by the literature and in some studies have equal efficacy. Medications have more side effects. Adherence to both remains a critical issue. The ultimate choice depends on the acuity of the patient and the comfort level of the prescribing clinician with each treatment modality (1)[B].
- SSRIs such as sertraline (Zoloft), paroxetine (Paxil), fluoxetine (Prozac), citalopram (Celexa), and escitalopram (Lexapro) in their traditional antidepressant doses (2)[B]
- Bupropion (Wellbutrin) is the only antidepressant currently approved by the FDA for the prevention of SAD (3)[B].

ISSUES FOR REFERRAL
- Patients with a history of ocular disease should be referred for an ophthalmologic exam before phototherapy and for serial monitoring.
- Patients who fail to respond or who develop manic symptoms or suicidal ideation once treatment is initiated should be considered for psychiatric referral.

ADDITIONAL THERAPIES
- Phototherapy using special light sources has been shown to be effective in 60–90% of patients, often providing relief with a few sessions (2,4)[B].
- Variables that can regulate effect are the following:
  – Light intensity: Although the minimum light source intensity is under investigation, at least 2,500 lux is suggested (domestic lights emit, on average, 200 to 500 lux). There is good evidence for 10,000 lux as the recommended source (2)[B].

- Treatment duration: Exposure time varies based on intensity of light source, with daily sessions of 30 minutes to a few hours.
- Time of treatment: Most patients respond better by using the light therapy early in the morning.
- Color of light source: Emerging data suggest that shorter sessions of lower intensity light-emitting diodes enriched in the blue spectrum have equal efficacy to the traditional white light treatment and possibly capable of being delivered in a transcranial manner (5)[B].

- Light box is placed on table several feet away, and the light is allowed to shine onto the patient's eyes (sunglasses should be avoided). Ensure that the light box has an ultraviolet filter.
- Most common side effects are eye strain and headache. Insomnia can result if the light box is used too late in the day. Light boxes also can precipitate mania in some patients.
- Dawn simulation machines gradually increase illumination while the patient sleeps, simulating sunrise while using a significantly less intense light source.

COMPLEMENTARY & ALTERNATIVE MEDICINE
- Work to reduce stress levels through meditation, progressive relaxation exercises, and/or lifestyle modification.
- The potential role of vitamin D supplementation is under investigation. Currently, there is a lack of consistent research to satisfactorily demonstrate that treatment improves SAD symptoms. Reported doses vary widely but typically are between 400 and 800 IU/day (6)[B].

INPATIENT CONSIDERATIONS
Admission Criteria/Initial Stabilization
If the patient develops suicidal ideation as part of his or her depression or mania after treatment is initiated

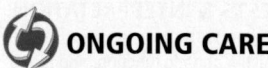 ONGOING CARE

FOLLOW-UP RECOMMENDATIONS
Regular monitoring by PCP or psychiatrist for response to treatment; patients may become manic when treated with SSRIs or light therapy.

Patient Monitoring
Patients should be seen in the outpatient clinic weekly to biweekly when initiating light or pharmacotherapy to monitor treatment results, side effects, and any increased suicidal thoughts if using SSRIs.

DIET
No specific diet modification needed

PATIENT EDUCATION
- Increase time outdoors during daylight.
- Rearrange home or work environment to get more direct sunlight through windows.

PROGNOSIS
Symptoms, if untreated, generally remit within 5 months with exposure to spring light, only to return in subsequent winters. If treated, patients usually respond within 3 to 6 weeks.

COMPLICATIONS
Development of suicidal ideation and mania are two outcomes the clinician needs to monitor.

REFERENCES
1. Lam RW, Levitt AJ, Levitan RD, et al. The Can-SAD study: a randomized controlled trial of the effectiveness of light therapy and fluoxetine in patients with winter seasonal affective disorder. *Am J Psychiatry.* 2006;163(5):805–812.
2. Kurlansik SL, Ibay AD. Seasonal affective disorder. *Am Fam Physician.* 2012;86(11):1037–1041.
3. Niemegeers P, Dumont GJ, Patteet L, et al. Bupropion for the treatment of seasonal affective disorder. *Expert Opin Drug Metab Toxicol.* 2013;9(9):1229–1240.
4. Terman M, Terman JS. Light therapy for seasonal and nonseasonal depression: efficacy, protocol, safety, and side effects. *CNS Spectr.* 2005;10(8):647–663.
5. Jurvelin H, Takala T, Nissilä J, et al. Transcranial bright light treatment via the ear canals in seasonal affective disorder: a randomized, double-blind dose-response study. *BMC Psychiatry.* 2014;14:288.
6. Frandsen TB, Pareek M, Hansen JP, et al. Vitamin D supplementation for treatment of seasonal affective symptoms in healthcare professionals: a double-blind randomised placebo-controlled trial. *BMC Research Notes.* 2014;7:528.

ADDITIONAL READING
- Gordijn MC, 't Mannetje D, Meesters Y. The effects of blue-enriched light treatment compared to standard light treatment in seasonal affective disorder. *J Affect Disord.* 2012;136(1–2):72–80.
- Howland RH. Vitamin D and depression. *J Psychosoc Nurs Ment Health Serv.* 2011;49(2):15–18.
- Mårtensson B, Petterson A, Berglund L, et al. Bright white light therapy in depression: a critical review of the evidence. *J Affective Disorders.* 2015;182:1–7.

- Pail G, Huf W, Pjrek E, et al. Bright-light therapy in the treatment of mood disorders. *Neuropsychobiology.* 2011;64(3):152–162.
- Thaler K, Delivuk M, Chapman A, et al. Second-generation antidepressants for seasonal affective disorder. *Cochrane Database Syst Rev.* 2011;(12): CD008591.

 SEE ALSO

- Bipolar I Disorder; Bipolar II Disorder; Depression
- Algorithm: Depressive Episode, Major

 CODES

ICD10
- F33.9 Major depressive disorder, recurrent, unspecified
- F33.0 Major depressive disorder, recurrent, mild
- F33.1 Major depressive disorder, recurrent, moderate

CLINICAL PEARLS
- SAD is a subtype of major depressive disorder. Once the patient has a diagnosed mood disorder, such as depression or bipolar, ask whether the symptoms vary in a seasonal pattern to qualify for the diagnosis of SAD. Generally, these patients will report sleeping too much, eating too much (especially carbs and sweets), and gaining weight during winter months.
- As with all psychiatric diagnoses, ensure that the symptoms are not due to an organic process or better explained by substance abuse.
- Lack of good evidence to decide whether light therapy or SSRIs should be the first-line agent. Guidelines suggest using SSRIs first if the patient is more acute or has contraindications to light therapy or the clinician is not comfortable with light therapy.
- Light therapy boxes are available from numerous online suppliers but are not extensively regulated; practitioners should take care to ensure that patients are using devices from reputable suppliers.
- If using SSRIs, recent studies indicate that some patients may begin to experience increased suicidal thoughts on therapy; these patients need to be monitored closely as outpatients every 1 to 2 weeks. Patients on light therapy also should be monitored closely initially in order to adjust treatment. Once stabilized, both groups of patients can be seen every 4 to 8 weeks during the winter months.
- All patients who demonstrate suicidal ideation or symptoms of mania should be referred for consideration of hospitalization.

SEIZURE DISORDER, ABSENCE

Felicia Chu, MD

 BASICS

DESCRIPTION

An absence seizure is a generalized epileptic seizure characterized by a brief lapse of awareness.

Absence Seizure Types

Absence seizure types according to the International League Again Epilepsy (ILAE) 2010 classification include (1):

- Typical absence
  - Formerly called *petit mal seizures*
  - Abrupt-onset behavioral arrest, loss of awareness, and blank staring, sometimes with mild upward eye deviation, repetitive blinking
  - May include automatisms, tonic or atonic features, eyelid or facial clonus, autonomic features
  - Lasts 5 to 30 seconds
  - Immediate return to normal consciousness
  - Associated with genetic generalized epilepsies, namely, childhood absence epilepsy, juvenile absence epilepsy, and juvenile myoclonic epilepsy
- Atypical absence
  - Onset and offset less abrupt than typical absence seizures
  - Lasts 10 to 45 seconds
  - Impairment of consciousness often incomplete with continued purposeful activity.
  - Postictal confusion sometimes occur.
  - Associated clinical features more pronounced and frequent than in typical absence; atonia is most common.
  - Associated with syndromic epilepsies, such as Lennox-Gastaut and nonsyndromic epilepsies in patients with developmental delay
- Absence with special features
  - Myoclonic absence:
    - Rhythmic clonic jerking at 2 to 4 Hz which lasts 5 to 10 seconds.
    - Unlike myoclonic seizures with no impairment of consciousness, brief lapses of awareness are characteristic of myoclonic absence.
  - Eyelid myoclonia:
    - Rhythmic clonic jerking of the eyelids at 5 to 6 Hz which lasts 3 to 5 seconds
    - Eyelid myoclonia with absence associated with an impairment of consciousness

Epilepsy Diagnoses

Specific diagnoses according to ILAE (2010):

- Childhood absence epilepsy (CAE)
  - Also known as *pyknolepsy*
  - Typical absence seizures are the only seizure type in 90% of children.
  - 10% develop additional generalized tonic–clonic seizures.
  - Seizures last ~10 seconds and often occur hundreds of times per day.
  - Normal neurologic state and development
  - Spontaneous remission occurs in 65–70% of patients during adolescence.
- Juvenile absence epilepsy (JAE)
  - Typical absence seizures are the main seizure type.
  - Seizures last longer than in CAE and occur usually less than once a day.
  - Generalized tonic–clonic seizures occur in most patients, often in the first 1 to 2 hours after awakening.
  - Seizures often persist into adulthood.

EPIDEMIOLOGY

- Predominant age
  - CAE: onset ages 4 to 10 years, with peak at ages 5 to 8 years
  - JAE: onset ages 9 to 16 years, with peak at ages 10 to 12 years
- Predominant gender
  - Female > male (3:2 to 2:1)
  - Absence epilepsy with myoclonus has male predominance.

Incidence

6 to 8/100,000 per year

Prevalence

5 to 50/100,000

ETIOLOGY AND PATHOPHYSIOLOGY

- Corticoreticular theory implicates abnormal activity in thalamocortical circuits.
- Thalamic reticular nucleus is responsible for both normal sleep spindles and pathologic slow-wave discharges; contains inhibitory gamma-aminobutyric acid-ergic (GABAergic) neurons
- These neurons affect low-threshold calcium currents.
- These circuits can fire in oscillatory/rhythmic fashion:
  - Normally, activation of $GABA_A$ receptors causes 10-Hz oscillations in sleep spindle frequency.
  - If $GABA_B$ receptors are strongly activated, oscillation frequency will be 3 to 4 Hz, similar to spike-and-wave typical absence seizure frequency.

Genetics

- 70–85% concordance occurs in monozygotic twins; 82% share EEG features.
- 33% concordance among first-degree relatives
- 15–45% have a family history of epilepsy.
- Complex multifactorial inheritance
- For childhood absence, genes/loci implicated include 6q, 8q24, and 5q14.
- Mutations of $GABA_A$ receptor and voltage-gated Ca^{2+} channel are implicated.

COMMONLY ASSOCIATED CONDITIONS

- 3–8% of CAE cases evolve into juvenile myoclonic epilepsy.
- Associated with difficulties in visual attention and visuospatial skills, verbal learning and memory, and reduced language abilities.
- Children with CAE have elevated rates of behavioral and psychiatric comorbidities including attentional deficits, anxiety, depression, isolation, and low self-esteem.
- A large study in 2010 detected overall normal cognition, but 35% of subjects had pretreatment attentional deficits that did not resolve with seizure control.

DIAGNOSIS

Seizures are often so brief that untrained observers are not aware of the occurrence.

HISTORY

- Frequently diagnosed in children being evaluated for poor school performance
- Teachers report that child seems to daydream or zone out frequently.
- Child will forget portions of conversations.
- Child with normal IQ underperforms in school.

PHYSICAL EXAM

- Unless a child has another genetic or acquired abnormality, a neurologic exam usually is normal.
- Seizures may be frequent enough to be observed during physical exam:
  - Manifest by behavioral arrest: Child will stop speaking in midsentence, stare blankly, and so forth
  - Automatisms (repetitive stereotyped behaviors) may be present.
  - Child resumes previous activity.
  - Absence seizures can have a variable effect on respiratory rate, but bradypnea is common.
- Seizures may be induced by hyperventilation:
  - Have the child blow on a pinwheel or similar exercise to provoke seizure.
  - Alternatively, ask the patient to perform hyperventilation with eyes closed and count. Patient will open eyes at onset of seizure and stop counting.
- Patient manifests unresponsiveness but retains postural tone in a typical absence seizure.

DIFFERENTIAL DIAGNOSIS

- Complex partial seizures
- Psychogenic nonepileptic seizures
- Attention deficit hyperactivity disorder (ADHD)
- Confusional states and acute memory disorders
- Migraine variants
- Panic/anxiety attacks
- Breath-holding spells
- Nonepileptic staring spells: Suggestive features include:
  - Events do not interrupt play.
  - Events are first noticed by professional such as school teacher, speech therapist, occupational therapist, or physician (rather than parent).
  - During a staring spell, child is responsive to touch or other external stimuli.

DIAGNOSTIC TESTS & INTERPRETATION

- No specific hematologic workup
- Follow blood chemistry, hepatic function, and blood counts specific to drug regimen.
- Drug levels are useful in evaluating symptoms of toxicity or for breakthrough seizures.

Initial Tests (lab, imaging)

- EEG is standard for diagnosis
  - Typical absence features: 3-Hz spike-and-wave activity on normal EEG background
  - Seizures feature bursts of 34-Hz spike-and-wave activity, which may slow to 2.5- to 3-Hz during seizure.
  - Seizure usually is evident clinically if bursts last >3 seconds, subtle changes of transient cognitive impairment may be evident with briefer seizures.
  - Hyperventilation and occasionally photic stimulation may induce seizure, thus confirming diagnosis of typical absence epilepsy. In contrast, atypical absence seizures are not susceptible to induction by hyperventilation or photic stimulation.
- Imaging is not routinely indicated in children with typical absence and normal neurologic exam and IQ.
  - Brain MRI is indicated in atypical absence and in children with mixed seizure types when combined with abnormal neurologic exam or low IQ.
  - If imaging is performed, MRI is preferable to CT scan due to higher sensitivity for anatomic abnormalities.
  - A review of the brain MRIs of 134 patients with idiopathic generalized epilepsy in 2006 showed 24% with structural abnormalities, 88% of which were nonspecific (2)[B].

TREATMENT

GENERAL MEASURES
- Review seizure precautions with every patient diagnosed with or suspected to have epilepsy.
- Seizure precautions include bathroom, kitchen, home, driving, outdoors, and sports safety topics, as well as special considerations for parents.

MEDICATION
Concern regarding generic medications allowing more breakthrough seizures has not been supported in evidence-based studies (3)[A].

ALERT
Certain common anticonvulsants may exacerbate absence including carbamazepine, oxcarbazepine, phenytoin, phenobarbital, tiagabine, vigabatrin, pregabalin, and gabapentin.

First Line
- Ethosuximide blocks T-type calcium channels:
  - First-line, except in absence patients with tonic–clonic seizures (lacks efficacy)
  - High efficacy (4)[A], fastest onset of efficacy (5) [B], and fewer adverse attentional effects compared to valproic acid (4)[A]
  - Side effects: vomiting, diarrhea, abdominal discomfort, hiccups, headache, sedation
  - Adverse effects: rare blood dyscrasias (monitor CBC)
- Valproic acid has multiple mechanisms:
  - First choice in absence patients with tonic–clonic, myoclonic, mixed seizure types
  - Very effective but has highest rate of adverse events leading to treatment discontinuation, including negative attentional effects (4)[A]
  - Side effects: tremor, drowsiness, dizziness, weight gain, alopecia, sedation, vomiting
  - Adverse effects: teratogenicity, pancreatitis, thrombocytopenia, rare fulminant hepatic failure (especially in children <2 years)

Second Line
- Lamotrigine affects sodium channels:
  - Controls seizures but may be less efficacious than ethosuximide or valproic acid (4)[A]
  - May be equally as efficacious for new-onset CAE (5)[B]
  - Side effects: rash, diplopia, headache, insomnia, dizziness, nausea, vomiting, diarrhea
  - Adverse effects: rare Stevens-Johnson rash, more often when coadministered with valproic acid
- Topiramate affects GABA and excitatory neurotransmission:
  - FDA-approved for Lennox-Gastaut syndrome
  - Side effects: psychomotor slowing
  - Adverse effects: weight loss, renal stones, myopia, glaucoma (rare), anhidrosis
- Levetiracetam is used off-label:
  - Has been used as both monotherapy and adjunct therapy for absence seizures
  - A small multicenter randomized controlled trial (RCT) showed modest efficacy but not statistically significant versus placebo (6)[C].
- Zonisamide is also used off-label.
- Clonazepam, nitrazepam, and clobazam may be effective in the short-term but are not recommended for long-term management due to development of tolerance (few months to a year) and side effects.

Pregnancy Considerations
Anticonvulsants, especially valproic acid, are associated with an increase in fetal malformations. Use of valproic acid in women who are or are likely to become pregnant generally is contraindicated. Obtain specialty consultation.

ADDITIONAL THERAPIES
- Most absence seizure patients respond to a single medication.
- Male sex and an early age at diagnosis are associated with the need for two medications to control the disease (7)[B].
- Vagal nerve stimulator (VNS) may be considered as an option for medically refractory absence epilepsy (8)[C].

INPATIENT CONSIDERATIONS
Admission Criteria/Initial Stabilization
- Absence epilepsy rarely requires admission.
- Status epilepticus requires inpatient management.

Discharge Criteria
Resolution of status epilepticus

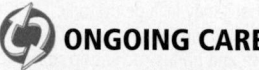 **ONGOING CARE**

FOLLOW-UP RECOMMENDATIONS
- Patients with associated tonic–clonic seizures should avoid high places and swimming alone.
- Absence rarely persists into adulthood, but affected adults may be restricted from driving, working over open flames, and so forth, as with other generalized and partial epilepsy subtypes.
- Patients should be monitored periodically by a neurologist for evolution of absence epilepsy into tonic–clonic or other seizure types.

PROGNOSIS
- Patients whose shortest pretreatment EEG seizures are >20 seconds in duration are more likely to achieve seizure freedom, regardless of treatment (9)[A].
- Of those with CAE without tonic–clonic seizures, 90% remit by adulthood.
- 35% of patients with tonic–clonic seizures experience complete remission of absence seizures.
- 15% of patients develop juvenile myoclonic epilepsy.

COMPLICATIONS
Reported frequencies of typical absence status epilepticus range from 5.8% to 9.4% of patients with CAE.

REFERENCES

1. Berg AT, Berkovic SF, Brodie MJ, et al. Revised terminology and concepts for organization of seizures and epilepsies: report of the ILAE Commission on Classification and Terminology, 2005–2009. *Epilepsia.* 2010;51(4):676–685.
2. Betting LE, Mory SB, Lopes-Cendes I, et al. MRI reveals structural abnormalities in patients with idiopathic generalized epilepsy. *Neurology.* 2006;67(5):848–852.
3. Kesselheim AS, Stedman MR, Bubrick EJ, et al. Seizure outcomes following the use of generic versus brand-name antiepileptic drugs: a systematic review and meta-analysis. *Drugs.* 2010;70(5): 605–621.
4. Glauser TA, Cnaan A, Shinnar S, et al. Ethosuximide, valproic acid, and lamotrigine in childhood absence epilepsy: initial monotherapy outcomes at 12 months. *Epilepsia.* 2013;54(1):141–155.
5. Hwang H, Kim H, Kim SH, et al. Long-term effectiveness of ethosuximide, valproic acid, and lamotrigine in childhood absence epilepsy. *Brain Dev.* 2012;34(5):344–348.
6. Fattore C, Boniver C, Capovilla G, et al. A multicenter, randomized, placebo-controlled trial of levetiracetam in children and adolescents with newly diagnosed absence epilepsy. *Epilepsia.* 2011;52(4):802–809.
7. Nadler B, Shevell MI. Childhood absence epilepsy requiring more than one medication for seizure control. *Can J Neurol Sci.* 2008;35(3):297–300.
8. Arya R, Greiner HM, Lewis A, et al. Vagus nerve stimulation for medically refractory absence epilepsy. *Seizure.* 2013;22(4):267–270.
9. Dlugos D, Shinnar S, Cnaan A, et al. Pretreatment EEG in childhood absence epilepsy: associations with attention and treatment outcome. *Neurology.* 2013;81(2):150–156.

ADDITIONAL READING

- Matricardi S, Verrotti A, Chiarelli F, et al. Current advances in childhood absence epilepsy. *Pediatr Neurol.* 2014;50(3):205–212.
- Vrielynck P. Current and emerging treatments for absence seizures in young patients. *Neuropsychiatr Dis Treat.* 2013;9:963–975.

 CODES

ICD10
- G40.409 Other generalized epilepsy and epileptic syndromes, not intractable, without status epilepticus
- G40.419 Oth generalized epilepsy, intractable, w/o stat epi
- G40.401 Oth generalized epilepsy, not intractable, w stat epi

CLINICAL PEARLS
- If parents are unable to determine the cause of a staring spell, try suggesting that parents mention something exciting or unexpected like "ice cream" during a spell to get the child's attention rather than calling his or her name.
- To help aid with diagnosis during an exam, try having the child blow repetitively on a pinwheel (causing hyperventilation) to attempt to trigger absence seizure.
- Ethosuximide and valproic acid are first-line agents in treatment of absence seizures. Valproic acid and lamotrigine are recommended for absence patients with tonic–clonic and mixed seizure types.

S

SEIZURE DISORDER, PARTIAL

Noel Dunn, MD • David Haight, MD

BASICS

DESCRIPTION
- Seizures occur when abnormal synchronous neuronal discharges in the brain cause transient cortical dysfunction.
- Generalized seizures involve bilateral cerebral cortex from the seizure's onset.
- Partial seizures originate from a discrete focus in the cerebral cortex.
- Partial seizures are further divided into simple and complex subtypes:
  – If consciousness is impaired during a partial seizure, it is classified as complex.
  – If consciousness is preserved, it is a simple partial seizure.

EPIDEMIOLOGY
Prevalence
Partial seizures occur in 20/100,000 persons in the United States.

ETIOLOGY AND PATHOPHYSIOLOGY
- Partial seizures begin when a localized seizure focus produces an abnormal, synchronized depolarization that spreads to a discrete portion of the surrounding cortex.
- The area of cortex involved in the seizure determines the symptoms; for example, an epileptogenic focus in motor cortex produces contralateral motor symptoms.
- In some cases, etiology is related to structural abnormalities that are susceptible to epileptogenesis. Most common etiologies vary by life stage:
  – Early childhood: developmental/congenital malformation, trauma
  – Young adults: developmental, infection, trauma
  – Adults 40 to 60 years of age: cerebrovascular insult, infection, trauma
  – Adults >60 years of age: cerebrovascular insult, trauma, neoplasm
- Complex partial seizures: A common cause is mesial temporal sclerosis.

Genetics
Benign rolandic epilepsy, a form of partial seizure disorder, has an autosomal dominant inheritance pattern with penetrance depending on multiple factors.

RISK FACTORS
- History of traumatic brain injury (1)[B]
- Children exposed to a thiamine-deficient formula (2)[C].

COMMONLY ASSOCIATED CONDITIONS
Epilepsy patients have a higher incidence of depression than the general population.

DIAGNOSIS

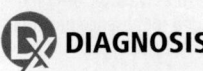

- Seizure activity usually stereotyped.
- Duration: Seconds to minutes, unless status epilepticus develops; status epilepticus may present as focal/generalized convulsions/altered mental status without convulsions.
- Simple partial seizures
  – Simple partial seizures are characterized by localized symptoms. The patient is conscious. Symptoms may involve motor, sensory, or psychic systems.

– Motor: Seizure activity in motor strip causes contraction (tonic) or rhythmic jerking (clonic) movements that may involve one entire side of body or may be more localized (i.e., hands, feet, or face).
  ○ Jacksonian march: As discharge spreads through motor cortex, tonic–clonic activity spreads in predictable fashion (i.e., beginning in hand and progressing up arm and to the face).
– Sensory/psychic
  ○ Todd paralysis: after motor seizure, residual, temporary weakness in the affected area
  ○ Parietal lobe: sensory loss/paresthesias, dizziness
  ○ Temporal lobe: déjà vu, rising sensation in epigastrium, auditory hallucinations/forced memories, unpleasant smell/taste
– Occipital: visual hallucinations
- Complex partial seizures
  – Impaired consciousness by definition
  – May have aura; this is start of seizure.
- Amnesia for the event, postictal confusion
  – Most often, focus in complex partial seizures is temporal/frontal.
  – Motor manifestations may include dystonic posturing/automatisms (i.e., simple, repetitive movements of face and hands such as lip smacking, picking, or more complex actions such as purposeless walking).
  – Frontal lobe seizure is characterized by brief, bilateral complex movements, vocalizations, often with onset during sleep.

HISTORY
- A detailed description of the seizure should be obtained from an observer.
- Review medication list for drugs that lower seizure threshold (e.g., tramadol, bupropion, theophylline).
- Obtain history of drugs of abuse (e.g., cocaine), as they may lower seizure threshold.
- Review history of any prior traumatic brain injury.

PHYSICAL EXAM
Include neurologic exam, with attention to lateralizing signs suggestive of structural lesion.

DIFFERENTIAL DIAGNOSIS
- Nonepileptic seizure
- Syncope/postanoxic myoclonus
- Hypoglycemia
- For hemiparesis following event
  – Transient ischemic attack
  – Hemiplegic migraine

DIAGNOSTIC TESTS & INTERPRETATION
EEG: spikes/sharp waves over seizure focus
- Yield of EEG is increased by being obtained in the first 24 hours following seizure and by sleep deprivation.
- Frontal lobe seizure focus may be difficult to detect by routine EEG.
- If difficulty with diagnosis, continuous video–EEG monitoring may be appropriate.
- Serum electrolytes, including calcium, magnesium, phosphorus; hepatic function panel; CBC; drugs of abuse urine drug screen
- Elevated prolactin, if measured within 10 to 20 minutes of suspected seizure, or elevated creatine phosphokinase; if measured within 6 to 24 hours, may help to differentiate generalized/complex partial seizure from psychogenic seizure (3)[B].
- CSF exam if infection is suspected.
- Urinalysis, chest x-ray, levels of antiepileptic drugs for breakthrough seizure

- Technologic advances in neuroimaging are usually directed at the diagnosis and prognosis for seizure control (4)[C].
- Emergency evaluation of new seizure: CT scan to screen for hemorrhage and stroke
- After emergency evaluation, MRI with thin cuts through area of interest
- If planning epilepsy surgery, positron emission tomography (PET) scan and/or interictal single-photon emission computed tomography (SPECT) may be of value.
- Magnetoencephalography (MEG) is an evolving technology for localizing seizure focus.

TREATMENT

GENERAL MEASURES
- Ask the patient to maintain a seizure diary.
- Note potential triggers, such as stress, sleep deprivation, drug use, discontinuation of alcohol/benzodiazepines, menses.

MEDICATION
- Current guidelines do not recommend for or against starting an antiepileptic drug (AED) after a single unprovoked seizure. Patients should be counseled that AEDs will reduce risk of repeat seizure over 2 years but have no effect on long-term remission (5)[C].
- AEDs act on voltage-gated ion channels, affect neuronal inhibition via enhancement of γ-aminobutyric acid (GABA, an inhibitory neurotransmitter), or decrease neuronal excitation. End result is to decrease the abnormal synchronized firing and to prevent seizure propagation.
- 50% of those with newly diagnosed partial seizures respond to, and tolerate, first AED trial. Up to 50% of those who fail the first AED trial will also fail a second AED trial (6)[B].
- Choose AED based on seizure type, side effect profile, and patient characteristics. Increase dose until seizure control is obtained/side effects become unacceptable.
- Attempt monotherapy, but many patients will require adjunctive agents.
- *Refractory to medications* is defined as failure of at least three anticonvulsants to achieve adequate control.
- AEDs may prevent seizures after a traumatic brain injury (TBI) in the short-term, although they provide no efficacy in long-term prevention (7)[B].
- Several AEDs induce/inhibit cytochrome P450 enzymes (watch for drug interactions).

First Line
- Carbamazepine: Affects sodium channels; side effects include GI distress, hyponatremia, diplopia, dizziness, rare pancytopenia/marrow suppression, and exfoliative rash.
- Oxcarbazepine: Affects sodium channels; side effects include dizziness, diplopia, hyponatremia, and headache.
- Lamotrigine: Affects sodium channels.
  – Side effects include insomnia, dizziness, and ataxia.
  – Risk of Stevens-Johnson reaction (potentially fatal exfoliative rash), especially when given with valproate, requires slow titration.
- Levetiracetam: multiple mechanisms; side effects include sedation, ataxia, and irritability.

Second Line
- Phenytoin: Affects sodium channels; side effects include ataxia, dizziness, diplopia, tremor, GI upset, gingival hyperplasia, and fever.
- Phenobarbital: multiple mechanisms; side effects include sedation and withdrawal seizures.
- Valproate: multiple mechanisms; side effects include GI upset, weight gain, alopecia, and tremor; less common, thrombocytopenia, hepatitis, pancreatitis
- Topiramate: multiple mechanisms; side effects include anorexia, cognitive slowing, sedation, nephrolithiasis, and anhidrosis.
- Gabapentin: multiple mechanisms; side effects include sedation, dizziness, and ataxia.
- Pregabalin: Affects calcium channels; side effects include sedation, dizziness, and weight gain.
- Zonisamide: Affects sodium channels.
  - Side effects include sedation, anorexia, nausea, dizziness, ataxia, anhidrosis, and nephrolithiasis.
  - Cross-reaction with sulfa allergy

Pregnancy Considerations
- Folate should be prescribed for all women of childbearing age who are taking AEDs. AED therapy during the 1st trimester is associated with doubled risk for major fetal malformations (6% vs. 3%).
- Phenytoin in pregnancy may result in fetal hydantoin syndrome.
- Valproate is associated with neural tube defects.
- Fetal insult from seizures following withdrawal of therapy also may be severe. Risk-to-benefit balance should be evaluated with high-risk pregnancy and neurology consultations. Most patients remain on anticonvulsants.
- Consider vagal nerve stimulator during pregnancy (8)[B].

ISSUES FOR REFERRAL
For refractory seizures, consider referral to an epilepsy specialist (9)[B].

ADDITIONAL THERAPIES
- Vagal nerve stimulator provides periodic stimulation to vagus nerve; may induce hoarseness, cough, and dysphagia. High-frequency stimulation in adults provides greater reduction in seizure frequency than low-frequency stimulation but also has greater rates of side effects (10)[B].
- Deep brain stimulation may decrease seizure frequency in medically refractive epilepsy but its efficacy varies by seizure source location (11)[B].
- Repetitive magnetic transcranial stimulation may reduce the frequency of seizures in individuals with refractory focal seizures (12)[B].

SURGERY/OTHER PROCEDURES
- For refractory partial complex seizures with identifiable focus
- Preoperative testing, such as Wada test, should be done to decrease likelihood of inducing aphasia and memory loss.
- 34–74% will be seizure-free after temporal lobe surgery. Prognosis varies for surgical resection of extratemporal foci (13)[B].
- Goal of surgical intervention is to reduce reliance on medications; most patients remain on anticonvulsants postoperatively.

INPATIENT CONSIDERATIONS
Admission Criteria/Initial Stabilization
Admit for unremitting seizure (partial/secondary generalized status epilepticus).

 ONGOING CARE

FOLLOW-UP RECOMMENDATIONS
- Most states have restrictions on driving for those with seizure disorders.
- Depending on seizure manifestation, may also recommend against activities such as swimming, climbing to heights, or operating heavy machinery

Patient Monitoring
AED levels if concern over toxicity, noncompliance, or for breakthrough seizures

DIET
Ketogenic or low-glycemic index diet may improve seizure control in some patients but is not well-tolerated (14)[B].

PATIENT EDUCATION
Avoid potential triggers such as alcohol or drug use and sleep deprivation.

PROGNOSIS
- Risk of seizure recurrence: ~30% after first seizure; of these, 50% will occur in the first 6 months; 90% in the first 2 years.
- Depends on seizure type; rolandic epilepsy has a good prognosis; temporal lobe epilepsy is more likely to be persistent.
- ~25–30% of all seizures are refractory to current medications.
- AEDs initiated after an initial seizure have been shown to decrease the risk of seizure over the first 2 years but are not demonstrated to reduce long-term risk of recurrence.
- The potential for AEDs to confer neuroprotection is under investigation.
- The risk of developing seizure after mild TBI remains high for a long period (>10 years) (1)[B].

COMPLICATIONS
- Risk of accidental injury
- Up to 50–60% of individuals with epilepsy will also have a mood disorder, the most common being depression and anxiety.
- 20–30% of individuals with epilepsy will have memory impairment.

REFERENCES
1. Christensen J, Pedersen MG, Pedersen CB, et al. Long-term risk of epilepsy after traumatic brain injury in children and young adults: a population-based cohort study. Lancet. 2009;373(9669):1105–1110.
2. Fattal-Valevski A, Bloch-Mimouni A, Kivity S, et al. Epilepsy in children with infantile thiamine deficiency. Neurology. 2009;73(11):828–833.
3. Brigo F, Igwe SC, Erro R, et al. Postictal serum creatine kinase for the differential diagnosis of epileptic seizures and psychogenic non-epileptic seizures: a systematic review. J Neurol. 2015;262(2):251–257.
4. Gaillard WD, Cross JH, Duncan JS, et al. Epilepsy imaging study guideline criteria: commentary on diagnostic testing study guidelines and practice parameters. Epilepsia. 2011;52(9):1750–1756.
5. Krumholz A, Wiebe S, Gronseth GS, et al. Evidence-based guideline: management of an unprovoked first seizure in adults: report

of the Guideline Development Subcommittee of the American Academy of Neurology and the American Epilepsy Society. Neurology. 2015;84(16):1705–1713.
6. Bonnett LJ, Smith CT, Donegan S, et al. Treatment outcome after failure of a first antiepileptic drug. Neurology. 2014;83(6):552–560.
7. Thompson K, Pohlmann-Eden B, Campbell LA, et al. Pharmacological treatments for preventing epilepsy following traumatic head injury. Cochrane Database Syst Rev. 2015;(8):CD009900.
8. Houser MV, Hennessy MD, Howard BC. Vagal nerve stimulator use during pregnancy for treatment of refractory seizure disorder. Obstet Gynecol. 2010;115(2, Pt 2):417–419.
9. Hemb M, Velasco TR, Parnes MS, et al. Improved outcomes in pediatric epilepsy surgery: the UCLA experience, 1986–2008. Neurology. 2010;74(22):1768–1775.
10. Panebianco M, Rigby A, Weston J, et al. Vagus nerve stimulation for partial seizures. Cochrane Database Syst Rev. 2015;(4):CD002896.
11. Sprengers M, Vonck K, Carrette E, et al. Deep brain and cortical stimulation for epilepsy. Cochrane Database Syst Rev. 2014;(6):CD008497.
12. Sun W, Mao W, Meng X, et al. Low-frequency repetitive transcranial magnetic stimulation for the treatment of refractory partial epilepsy: a controlled clinical study. Epilepsia. 2012;53(10): 1782–1789.
13. Jobst BC, Cascino GD. Resective epilepsy surgery for drug-resistant focal epilepsy: a review. JAMA. 2015;313(3):285–293.
14. Levy RG, Cooper PN, Giri P. Ketogenic diet and other dietary treatments for epilepsy. Cochrane Database Syst Rev. 2012;(3):CD001903.

ADDITIONAL READING
- Walker LE, Mirza N, Yip VL, et al. Personalized medicine approaches in epilepsy. J Intern Med. 2015;277(2):218–234.
- Wilden JA, Cohen-Gadol AA. Evaluation of first nonfebrile seizures. Am Fam Physician. 2012;86(4): 334–340.

 CODES

ICD10
- G40.109 Local-rel symptc epi w simp prt seiz,not ntrct, w/o stat epi
- G40.209 Local-rel symptc epi w cmplx prt seiz,not ntrct,w/o stat epi
- G40.119 Local-rel symptc epi w simple part seiz, ntrct, w/o stat epi

CLINICAL PEARLS
- It is controversial whether AED treatment is indicated after a first seizure. Treatment should be strongly considered when a clear structural cause is identified/risk of injury from seizure is high (e.g., osteoporosis, anticoagulation).
- Consider vagus nerve stimulation in pregnancy and in patients with medically refractory seizures.
- Postictal elevation in prolactin and CPK levels can help distinguish physiologic from psychogenic seizures.

SEIZURES, FEBRILE

Brigitte N. Ngo, DO • Swati Avashia, MD, FAAP

 BASICS

DESCRIPTION
- By definition, febrile seizures occur in pediatric patients aged 6 months to 5 years with fever ≥100.4°F (38°C). Evidence of an underlying neurologic abnormality, metabolic condition, or intracranial infection excludes this diagnosis.
- Distinguished as simple or complex based on multiple criteria (1):
  - Simple (65–90%; must meet all criteria)
    - Generalized clonic or tonic–clonic seizure activity without focal features
    - Duration <15 minutes
    - Does not recur within 24 hours
    - Resolves spontaneously
    - No history of previous afebrile seizure or seizure disorder
  - Complex (20–30%; only one criterion must be met)
    - Partial seizure, focal activity
    - Duration >15 minutes
    - Recurs within 24 hours

EPIDEMIOLOGY
Incidence
- Approximately 500,000 febrile seizures occur in the United States annually.
- Most occur in children 6 months to 3 years old; only 6–15% occur in patients ≥4 years
- Peak incidence is 18 months of age.
- Risk of recurrence is 30–50% (2).
- Follows a bimodal seasonal pattern that mirrors peaks of febrile respiratory (November to January) and gastrointestinal infections (June to August).

Prevalence
- 2–5% of children in United States and Western Europe have at least one febrile seizure.
- Cumulative incidence varies in other populations (0.5–14%), with higher prevalence in Asia (3).

ETIOLOGY AND PATHOPHYSIOLOGY
A variety of mechanisms have been proposed:
- A lower baseline seizure threshold in the age group affected by febrile seizures.
- Familial genotypes may result in lower seizure thresholds.
- Fever may alter ion channel activity, resulting in increased circuit excitability.
- Cytokines released secondary to infection, specifically interleukin (IL)-1β, increase neuronal activity.

Genetics
- Evidence for genetic association:
  - Greater concordance in monozygotic than dizygotic twins
  - Risk of febrile seizure with a previously affected sibling is increased.
  - Having two affected parents doubles a child's risk of febrile seizure.
  - Positive family history can be seen in 25–40% of cases (4).
- Several rare familial epileptic syndromes present with febrile seizure.

RISK FACTORS
- Family history of febrile seizures; risk increases with the number of affected first-degree relatives.
- Any condition causing fever

- Recent vaccination
  - As febrile seizures are a benign entity, the benefits of vaccination outweigh the risk.
  - Risk increases after the administration of all measles-containing vaccines; peak incidence occurs 7 to 10 days after vaccination.
  - Risk increases on the day of DTaP-IPV-Hib combination vaccine administration, as fever rate increases by 70% compared to giving them separately.
  - Absolute vaccination-associated risk is very low.
- Prenatal exposure to alcohol and tobacco, iron deficiency anemia, daycare attendance, developmental delay, premature birth, and prolonged NICU stay
- Children with iron deficiency anemia may have increased risk for febrile seizures. Consider checking for anemia if the history suggests a risk for iron deficiency (5)[C].

GENERAL PREVENTION
Prevention is not usually indicated given the benign nature of this condition, lack of effective interventions, and side effects of prophylactic medications.

COMMONLY ASSOCIATED CONDITIONS
- Viral infections: Frequently implicated pathogens include human herpesvirus 6, influenza, parainfluenza, adenovirus, and respiratory syncytial virus (RSV).
- Bacterial infections: Frequently associated infections include otitis media, pharyngitis, urinary tract infection (UTI), pneumonia, and gastroenteritis.

DIAGNOSIS

HISTORY
- History of present illness:
  - Description of seizure:
    - Febrile seizures are generalized with clonic or tonic–clonic activity.
    - Absence, myoclonic, atonic, and focal seizures are atypical of febrile seizures and warrant further evaluation.
  - Seizure duration
  - Presence of postictal state (consistent with febrile seizure)
  - Number of seizures in previous 24 hours
  - Lethargy, irritability, or decreased level of consciousness as reported by the caretaker
  - Symptoms of underlying infection
  - Symptoms concerning for neurologic deficits
- Past medical history:
  - Existing conditions, including developmental delay, cerebral palsy, and metabolic disorders
  - Recent antibiotic course
  - History of febrile seizures
  - History of afebrile seizures or seizure disorder
  - History of head injury
  - Vaccination status, recent immunization
- Family history: febrile seizures, afebrile seizures, epilepsy, metabolic disorders, and other neurologic conditions
- Social history: factors concerning for child abuse

PHYSICAL EXAM
- Vital signs should be stable and consistent with intercurrent febrile illness; unstable vital signs or toxic appearance warrant further evaluation.
- Identify the presence or absence of focal deficits on a complete neurologic exam.
- Assess for signs of meningitis, including decreased level of consciousness, irritability, meningeal signs, bulging fontanelle, papilledema, and petechiae.

- Identify cause of fever.
- Assess thoroughly for manifestations of child abuse with a careful skin exam, inspection and palpation for occult trauma, and retinal exam if possible.

DIFFERENTIAL DIAGNOSIS
- Seizures due to an etiology other than febrile seizure:
  - Meningitis, encephalitis
  - Primary epilepsy
  - Neonatal seizure
  - Dravet syndrome
  - Intracranial mass
  - Nonaccidental trauma
  - Electrolyte abnormality
  - Hypoglycemia
  - Metabolic disorder
- Conditions presenting similarly to seizure:
  - Rigors
  - Crying
  - Benign myoclonus of infancy
  - Breath-holding spell
  - Choking episode
  - Tic disorder
  - Parasomnia
  - Arrhythmia
  - Metabolic disorder
  - Dystonic reaction

DIAGNOSTIC TESTS & INTERPRETATION
- Routine laboratory tests are not recommended to identify an underlying cause of a simple febrile seizure (1)[C].
- Rates of UTI in children with simple febrile seizures and in febrile children without seizure are comparable; consider obtaining urinalysis for susceptible patients (2)[B].
- Blood glucose if the patient is convulsing or is obtunded on presentation (2)[B].

- Lumbar puncture
  - In studies of patients with simple febrile seizures conducted since the initiation of routine infant vaccination against *Haemophilus influenzae*, rates of acute bacterial meningitis were very low (0–0.8%).
  - Seizure is unlikely to be the only presenting symptom of meningitis. Symptoms indicating increased likelihood of meningitis include toxic appearance, altered level of consciousness, meningeal signs, focal neurologic deficits, bulging fontanelle, and petechiae.
  - Cases of bacterial meningitis in children with febrile seizures who return to baseline or in the absence of other signs or symptoms are rare (6).
  - Recommendations:
    - Lumbar puncture should be performed in a child with fever and seizure if meningeal signs are present or if there is concern for meningitis or other intracranial pathology based on history and exam (7)[B].
    - In infants aged 6 to 12 months, consider lumbar puncture if the child has not been vaccinated against *H. influenzae* or *Streptococcus pneumoniae* according to schedule (7)[C].
    - Consider lumbar puncture for children with fever and seizure who have recently been treated with antibiotics, as antibiotics may mask meningeal signs and symptoms (7)[C].
    - The yield of lumbar puncture in children with complex febrile seizure is very low; however, some recommend considering a lumbar puncture in these patients (6)[B].

- Neuroimaging is not routinely recommended for the purposes of identifying the cause of a simple febrile seizure (7)[B].
- Studies have demonstrated limited use of emergent imaging in patients who meet criteria for complex febrile seizure based on multiple episodes in 24 hours; however, imaging may be indicated for focal findings or concerning history or exam. There are no current guidelines regarding imaging with complex febrile seizures (8)[B].

Diagnostic Procedures/Other

- EEG is not recommended in neurologically normal children presenting with simple febrile seizure (7)[B].

- There is mixed evidence for use of EEG after complex febrile seizures; some recommend outpatient EEG on follow-up.

TREATMENT

GENERAL MEASURES

- Acute seizure management
  - Airway: Position the patient laterally, suction secretions, and place a nasopharyngeal airway if necessary.
  - Breathing: Administer oxygen for cyanosis; consider bag-mask ventilation or intubation for inadequate ventilation.
  - Circulation: Establish IV access if first-line buccal or nasal midazolam is not effective.

- Antipyretics are helpful for patient comfort but do not prevent seizure recurrence during the initial febrile episode (1)[A].

- Provide supportive care and treat underlying infection if necessary.

MEDICATION

First Line

Treat seizures of ≥5 minutes duration with anticonvulsants:

- Buccal midazolam 0.5 mg/kg or nasal midazolam 0.2 mg/kg (3)
- IV or IM lorazepam 0.1 mg/kg

Second Line

Rectal diazepam is less effective and more commonly associated with respiratory depression than first-line treatments (1)[B].

ISSUES FOR REFERRAL

Simple febrile seizures do not require referral to a pediatric neurologist.

INPATIENT CONSIDERATIONS

Admission Criteria/Initial Stabilization

- Unstable vital signs
- Concerning findings on history or physical exam
- Prolonged seizure requiring anticonvulsants
- Persistent change in mental status
- Inpatient management of underlying condition is required.

ONGOING CARE

FOLLOW-UP RECOMMENDATIONS

- Anticonvulsant prophylaxis during subsequent febrile episodes (1)[B]:

  - The American Academy of Pediatrics recommends against prophylaxis with anticonvulsants due to an unacceptable risk–benefit ratio.

- Phenobarbital is effective but can have serious side effects, including lowering IQ.
- Prophylaxis with valproic acid may be effective but can cause hepatotoxicity and/or hyperammonemia.
- Prophylaxis with phenytoin and carbamazepine is ineffective.
- Oral and rectal diazepam are effective but are not recommended due to the benign nature of febrile seizures.

- Antipyretic prophylaxis during subsequent febrile episodes (1)[A]:

  - No study has demonstrated that fever management will prevent recurrence.
  - Ibuprofen and acetaminophen are no more effective than placebo in preventing recurrence.

PATIENT EDUCATION

There is frequently a high degree of parental anxiety associated with febrile seizures. Suggested anticipatory guidance:

- Febrile seizures do not cause brain damage and are associated with a low risk for sequelae.

- Parents should be reassured after a simple febrile seizure that there is no negative impact on intellect, behavior, or risk of death (1)[B].

- Parents should be prepared for a high probability of recurrence.
- If seizure recurs, position the child safely and do not intervene inappropriately.
- Time the seizure; call rescue if the child turns blue, has difficulty breathing, or the seizure lasts >5 minutes.
- If the seizure spontaneously resolves in <5 minutes and the child is well but sleepy, seek immediate attention, but calling rescue is not necessary.

PROGNOSIS

- Recurrence:
  - Estimates of recurrence rates vary (30–50%).
  - Factors associated with seizure recurrence include age <12 months at time of first episode, first-degree relative with history of febrile seizure, and history of complex febrile seizures.
- Intellectual and behavioral outcomes (2)
  - Febrile seizures do not impact IQ, behavioral abnormalities, academic performance, or neuro-cognitive inattention.
  - Outcomes in children with single and multiple febrile seizures are similar.
- Subsequent development of epilepsy (2)
  - Risk of epilepsy after a simple partial seizure is approximately 1% compared to the general population.
  - Risk is 2.4% in those with multiple simple febrile seizures, age <12 months at time of initial episode and a family history of epilepsy.
  - Factors associated with increased risk include presenting with complex febrile seizure, family history of epilepsy or febrile seizures, cerebral palsy, developmental delay, low birth weight, and prematurity.
- Mortality (2):
  - A slight increase in mortality is attributable in part to underlying neurodevelopmental abnormalities and to the subsequent development of epilepsy.
  - There is not an increased risk for SIDS in siblings of children who have febrile seizures.

COMPLICATIONS

Seizure-related injury, aspiration pneumonia, side effects of prescribed medications or diagnostic procedures, and subsequent parental perception of the child as being vulnerable, especially during subsequent fevers.

REFERENCES

1. Graves RC, Oehler K, Tingle LE. Febrile seizures: risks, evaluation, and prognosis. *Am Fam Physician*. 2012;85(2):149–153.
2. Steering Committee on Quality Improvement and Management, Subcommittee on Febrile Seizures American Academy of Pediatrics. Febrile seizures: clinical practice guideline for the long-term management of the child with simple febrile seizures. *Pediatrics*. 2008;121(6):1281–1286.
3. Farrell K, Goldman R. The management of febrile seizures. *B C Med J*. 2011;53(6):268–273.
4. Syndi Seinfeld D, Pellock J. Recent research on febrile seizures: a review. *J Neurol Neurophysiol*. 2013;4(165):19519.
5. King D, King A. Question 2: should children who have a febrile seizure be screened for iron deficiency? *Arch Dis Child*. 2014;99(10):960–964.
6. Najaf-Zadeh A, Dubos F, Hue V, et al. Risk of bacterial meningitis in young children with a first seizure in the context of fever: a systematic review and meta-analysis. *PLoS One*. 2013;8(1):e55270.
7. Subcommittee on Febrile Seizures, American Academy of Pediatrics. Neurodiagnostic evaluation of the child with a simple febrile seizure. *Pediatrics*. 2011;127(2):389–394.
8. Kimia A, Ben-Joseph EP, Rudloe T, et al. Yield of lumbar puncture among children who present with their first complex febrile seizure. *Pediatrics*. 2010;126(1):62–69.

 CODES

ICD10

- R56.00 Simple febrile convulsions
- R56.01 Complex febrile convulsions
- G40.901 Epilepsy, unsp, not intractable, with status epilepticus

CLINICAL PEARLS

- Febrile seizures are generally benign, and families can be reassured that children are at low risk of death, subsequent development of epilepsy, and learning or behavioral abnormalities.
- History and physical exam are important tools in identifying children presenting with febrile seizure who may be at greater risk for meningitis or other intracranial pathology.
- For simple febrile seizures, routine labs, lumbar puncture, neuroimaging studies, and EEG are not recommended in the absence of clinical suspicion of serious underlying pathology.
- Prophylaxis with anticonvulsants or antipyretics during subsequent febrile episodes is not recommended due to their lack of effectiveness and the risk of medication-associated side effects.

SEPSIS

Patricia Martinez Quinones, MD • Jin Sol Oh, MD • Steven B. Holsten, Jr., MD, FACS

 BASICS

DESCRIPTION
- A systemic inflammatory response secondary to known or suspected infection
- Synonym(s): septicemia
- Systemic inflammatory response syndrome (SIRS)
  - Temperature >38°C (100.4°F) or <36°C (96.8°F)
  - Heart rate (HR) >90 beats/min
  - Respiratory rate (RR) >20 breaths/min
  - WBC >12,000 cells/mm^3, or <4,000 cells/mm^3
- Sepsis signs and symptoms (1)[C]
  - General variables
    ○ Temperature >38.3°C (100.9°F) or <36°C (96.8°F); HR >90 beats/min or >2 standard deviations (SD) above normal for age
    ○ Tachypnea (RR >20 breaths/min or PCO$_2$ <32 mm Hg)
    ○ Acute altered mental status (AMS)
    ○ Significant edema or positive fluid balance (>20 mL/kg over 24 hours)
    ○ Hyperglycemia (plasma glucose >140 mg/dL or 7.7 mmol/L) in the absence of diabetes
  - Inflammatory variables
    ○ Leukocytosis (WBC >12,000 cells/mm^3), or leukopenia (<4,000 cells/mm^3), or normal WBC with >10% bands
    ○ Plasma C-reactive protein (CRP) >2 SD above normal
    ○ Plasma procalcitonin >2 SD above normal
  - Hemodynamic variables
    ○ Arterial hypotension (SBP <90 mm Hg, MAP <70, or SBP decrease of >40 mm Hg in adults or <2 SD below normal for age)
  - Organ dysfunction variables
    ○ Arterial hypoxemia (PaO$_2$/FIO$_2$ <300)
    ○ Acute oliguria (urine output <0.5 mL/kg/hr for at least 2 hours with or without adequate resuscitation)
    ○ Creatinine increase >0.5 mg/dL or 44.2 μmol/L
    ○ Coagulation abnormalities (INR >1.5 or aPTT >60 seconds)
    ○ Ileus (absent bowel sounds)
    ○ Thrombocytopenia (platelet <100,000)
    ○ Hyperbilirubinemia (plasma total bilirubin >4 mg/dL or 70 μmol/L)
  - Tissue perfusion variables
    ○ Elevated serum lactate (>1 mmol/L)
    ○ Decreased capillary refill or skin mottling
- Severe sepsis: sepsis-induced hypoperfusion or acute organ dysfunction
- Septic shock: refractory hypotension, unexplained by other causes, and despite adequate fluid resuscitation:
  - Hypotension is defined as SBP <90 mm Hg, MAP <70 mm Hg, and reduction in SBP >40 mm Hg from baseline.

Pediatric Considerations
- Continuum from sepsis to multisystem organ failure (MSOF) is affected by age-specific physiologic variables in children.
- SIRS in pediatric population requires that abnormality in temperature or WBC be present (2)[C].
- Drug metabolism is reduced in children with severe sepsis. Monitor drug toxicity labs to prevent adverse effects.

Geriatric Considerations
Often more difficult to diagnose; change in mental status/behavior may be the only early manifestation.

EPIDEMIOLOGY
Incidence
- 3/1,000 population
- Increasing incidence; 750,000 new cases annually in the United States
- 2% of hospitalized patients

ETIOLOGY AND PATHOPHYSIOLOGY
- Multifactorial: Widespread endothelial dysfunction, dysregulation of nitric oxide production, and activation of coagulation cascade leads to maldistribution of blood flow, tissue hypoperfusion, and resulting to organ dysfunction.
- An imbalance between proinflammatory and anti-inflammatory mediators leads to systemic tissue damage and significant immunosuppression.
- Causative organisms:
  - Gram-positive bacteria (most common): *Staphylococcus* sp., *Streptococcus* sp., *Enterococcus* sp.
  - Gram-negative: *Escherichia coli*, *Klebsiella* sp., *Proteus* sp., *Pseudomonas* sp. and anaerobic bacteria
  - Fungi: *Candida* sp. (incidence increased 207% from 1976 to 2000)
  - Causative organism not identified in 50–75% of cases
- Common sites of infection: respiratory tract (most common), urinary tract, gastrointestinal tract, skin/soft tissue, CNS, bacteremia

RISK FACTORS
- Extremes of age (very young or age >60 years)
- Ethnicity: African American
- Comorbidities: COPD, congestive heart failure (CHF), cancer, diabetes, and renal insufficiency/failure
- Immunosuppression
- Bacteremia
- Community-acquired pneumonia
- Complicated labor and delivery: premature labor and/or premature rupture of membranes, untreated maternal group B strep colonization
- Nosocomial factors: surgical site infections, indwelling catheters

GENERAL PREVENTION
- Vaccination: pneumococcal vaccine in children and also adults who are ≥65 years or with comorbidities placing them at high risk for disease. *Haemophilus influenzae* type B (infants, young children), influenza (H1N1 in pregnant women), meningococcal vaccine
- γ-Globulin for hypo- or agammaglobulinemia
- Treat group B strep carriers during labor.
- Regular hand washing, sterile technique for catheter placement, appropriate glove use
- Antibiotic prophylaxis for recommended surgical procedures

COMMONLY ASSOCIATED CONDITIONS
- Immunologic: neutropenia, HIV, hypo/agammaglobulinemia, complement deficiency, splenectomy, immunosuppressants (corticosteroids, chemotherapy, TNF-α antagonists)
- Diabetes, alcoholism, malignancy, cirrhosis, burns, multiple trauma, IV drug abuse, malnutrition

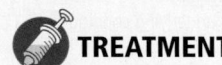 **DIAGNOSIS**

HISTORY
- Past medical, surgical, social, occupational, and travel history to identify risk factors and potential source

- General symptoms
  - Fever, chills, rigors, myalgias
  - Mental status changes: restlessness, agitation, confusion, delirium, lethargy, stupor, coma
- Specific symptoms (relative to primary source)
  - Respiratory: cough, sputum production, dyspnea, pleuritic chest pain
  - Urinary: dysuria, frequency, urgency, flank pain
  - Intra-abdominal: nausea, vomiting, diarrhea, constipation, abdominal pain
  - CNS: stiff neck, headache, photophobia, focal neurologic signs

PHYSICAL EXAM
- Assess vital signs: hyper/hypothermia, tachycardia, tachypnea, hypotension
- Signs of poor perfusion: central venous hypoxia, delayed capillary refill, cyanosis, mottled skin
- Signs of target organ involvement: jaundice, skin lesions (erythema, petechiae, embolic lesions, purpura)

DIFFERENTIAL DIAGNOSIS
- Bacteremia without sepsis
- Viral, rickettsial, spirochetal, and protozoal diseases
- Collagen vascular diseases, vasculitides, pancreatitis, myocardial infarction, CHF, pulmonary embolism, thrombotic thrombocytopenic purpura (TTP), hemolytic uremic syndrome (HUS), thyrotoxicosis, adrenal insufficiency, poisoning, drug reaction

DIAGNOSTIC TESTS & INTERPRETATION
Initial Tests (lab, imaging)
- Two sets of blood cultures to document presence of bacteremia (not required for diagnosis; 50% of blood cultures are negative in severe sepsis/septic shock). Obtain cultures before antibiotic therapy. Do not delay the start of antibiotic therapy (1)[B].
- Cultures/Gram stains from potential sites of infection (sputum, urine, pleural fluid, ascites, CSF, wound)
- CBC with differential, CRP, coagulation profile, comprehensive metabolic profile, lactic acid level, arterial blood gas, urinalysis
- Radiographic studies (plain films, ultrasound, CT, or MRI) to confirm source of infection

Diagnostic Procedures/Other
- Aspiration, biopsy, and/or drainage of potentially infected body sites (pleural cavity, peritoneal cavity, biliary tree, CSF, abscess). Interventional radiology techniques to aid in specimen collection as needed
- Echocardiogram if concern for endocarditis

Test Interpretation
- Common findings: leukocytosis, bandemia (>10%), hyperglycemia, metabolic acidosis, mild hyperbilirubinemia, hypoxemia, respiratory alkalosis, proteinuria
- Less common findings (more severe disease): leukopenia, anemia, thrombocytopenia, coagulopathy, azotemia, hypoglycemia, acidosis

TREATMENT

GENERAL MEASURES
- Assess oxygenation and supplement as needed. Intubate for respiratory failure.
- Invasive monitoring for management of hemodynamic instability using goal-directed therapy.

- Adequate volume resuscitation (30 mL/kg crystalloid for hypotension) within 3 hours of presentation and vasopressors for refractory hypotension (within 6 hours of presentation). Targets are:
  - Central venous pressure (CVP) 8 to 12 mm Hg, MAP ≥65 mm Hg, urine output ≥0.5 mL/kg/hr (1)[A]
  - Central/mixed venous O₂ saturation ≥70%/65%
    ○ If goals not met with fluid resuscitation and/or vasopressor, transfuse PRBCs to achieve hematocrit >30%; if still <70%, add dobutamine (1)[C].
- Identify source of infection and remove septic foci:
  - Early surgical consultation for acute abdomen, empyema, necrotizing fasciitis
  - Interventional radiology consultation for guided drainage
- Transfuse PRBCs, platelets, and/or fresh frozen plasma for coagulopathic complications or in association with planned procedures.
  - Transfuse PRBC if Hgb <7.0 to target Hgb of 7.0 to 9.9 g/dL in absence of tissue hypoperfusion, ischemic coronary artery disease, or acute hemorrhage (1)[B]
- Stress ulcer and DVT prophylaxis (1)[B]
- Glucose control (≥180 mg/dL) (1)[A]

MEDICATION
First Line
- Fluid management
  - Initial therapy: 30 mL/kg of crystalloids (1)[B]
  - Consider adding albumin for patients requiring large volumes of crystalloid (1)[C],(3)[B].
- Vasopressors
  - Norepinephrine 0.01 to 3 μg/kg/min (1,4)[B].
  - Low-dose dopamine for renal protection is not recommended (1)[C].
- Initiate broad-spectrum antibiotic within an hour of recognizing severe sepsis or septic shock (1,4)[A]:
  - Adult (*Pseudomonas* not suspected): vancomycin (loading dose 25 mg/kg) + Gram-negative coverage (3rd-generation cephalosporin, β-lactam/β-lactamase inhibitor, or carbapenem)
  - Adult (*Pseudomonas* suspected): vancomycin + two agents aimed at resistant Gram-negative bacteria ceftazidime/cefepime/carbapenem/piperacillin–tazobactam + either fluoroquinolone (ciprofloxacin) *or* aminoglycoside (gentamicin/amikacin) depending on local hospital sensitivities
  - Nonimmunocompromised child: 3rd-generation cephalosporin
  - Neonate (<7 days old): ampicillin and gentamicin (5)[B]
  - Consider narrowing antibiotic regimen at 48 to 72 hours based on culture results. Anticipate antibiotic course to last 7 to 10 days (1)[B].
- Antifungals if fungal infection suspected: long-term antibiotic use, TPN, GI surgery
  - Adjuvant intravenous immunoglobulins (IVIGs) may reduce mortality in adults (6)[B].

- Possible interactions
  - Aminoglycosides: increase in nephrotoxicity with enflurane, cisplatin, and possibly vancomycin; ototoxicity with loop diuretics; paralysis with neuromuscular-blocking agents
  - Adjust doses for renal and/or hepatic impairment.
- The European Society of Intensive Care Medicine statement in critically ill patients
  - Hydroxyethyl starches (HESs) with MW ≥200 kDA and/or degree of substitution >0.4 are not recommended in severe septic patients (1)[C].
  - Hyperoncotic solutions should not be used in fluid resuscitation.

Pregnancy Considerations
β-Lactam antibiotics, macrolides, and metronidazole generally are considered safe.

Second Line
- Vasopressors: epinephrine, vasopressin
- Consider IV hydrocortisone 200 mg per day if the patient is poorly responsive to both IV fluid resuscitation and vasopressors (1)[C].
- Inotropic therapy with dobutamine may benefit patients with myocardial dysfunction or ongoing hypoperfusion despite adequate intravascular volume and MAP (1)[C].

ADDITIONAL THERAPIES
Intermittent hemodialysis or continuous veno-venous hemofiltration for renal failure

SURGERY/OTHER PROCEDURES
Debride necrotic tissues: Drain or remove abscesses or other foci of infection.

INPATIENT CONSIDERATIONS
Admission Criteria/Initial Stabilization
ICU care

IV Fluids
Aggressive fluid resuscitation with normal saline can result in nongap metabolic acidosis. Not likely with lactated Ringer solution.

ONGOING CARE

FOLLOW-UP RECOMMENDATIONS
Patient Monitoring
- Place arterial line and central venous catheter in unstable patients
- Chem–7 and CBC daily; lactate, mixed venous oxygen saturation q2–4h in initial resuscitation period, and daily INR/PTT if DIC is a concern.
- Follow antibiotic drug levels (vancomycin, gentamicin).
- Foley catheter placement to monitor urine output

DIET
NPO if intubation considered; otherwise, enteral feeds are preferred to preserve GI mucosal integrity (1)[C].

PATIENT EDUCATION
www.nlm.nih.gov/medlineplus/sepsis.html

PROGNOSIS
Mortality is 10–50% overall. Poor prognostic factors include the inability to mount a fever (>40°C), nonurinary source of infection, nosocomial infection, inappropriate antibiotic coverage, and certain comorbidities (AIDS, cancer, immunosuppression).

COMPLICATIONS
GI hemorrhage, DIC, hyperglycemia, de novo embolic foci of infection, ARDS, multiorgan failure, death

REFERENCES
1. Dellinger RP, Levy MM, Rhodes A, et al. Surviving sepsis campaign: international guidelines for management of severe sepsis and septic shock: 2012. *Crit Care Med*. 2013;41(2):580–637.
2. Goldstein B, Giroir B, Randolph A. International pediatric sepsis consensus conference: definitions for sepsis and organ dysfunction in pediatrics. *Pediatric Critical Care Medicine*. 2005;6(1):2–8.
3. Raghunathan K, Shaw A, Nathanson B, et al. Association between the choice of IV crystalloid and in-hospital mortality among critically ill adults with sepsis. *Crit Care Med*. 2014;42(7):1585–1591.
4. De Backer D, Biston P, Devriendt J, et al. Comparison of dopamine and norepinephrine in the treatment of shock. *N Engl J Med*. 2010;362(9):779–789.
5. Paul M, Lador A, Grozinsky-Glasberg S, et al. Beta lactam antibiotic monotherapy versus beta lactam-aminoglycoside antibiotic combination therapy for sepsis. *Cochrane Database Syst Rev*. 2014;(1):CD003344.
6. Stockmann C, Spigarelli MG, Campbell SC, et al. Considerations in the pharmacologic treatment and prevention of neonatal sepsis. *Paediatr Drugs*. 2014;16(1):67–81.

ADDITIONAL READING
- Alejandria MM, Lansang MA, Dans LF, et al. Intravenous immunoglobulin for treating sepsis, severe sepsis and septic shock. *Cochrane Database Syst Rev*. 2013;(9):CD001090.
- Levy MM, Fink MP, Marshall JC, et al. 2001 SCCM/ESICM/ACCP/ATS/SIS International Sepsis Definitions Conference. *Crit Care Med*. 2003;31(4):1250–1256.
- Venkataraman R, Kellum JA. Sepsis: update in the management. *Adv Chronic Kidney Dis*. 2013;20(1):6–13.
- Wiener RS, Wiener DC, Larson RJ. Benefits and risks of tight glucose control in critically ill adults: a meta-analysis. *JAMA*. 2008;300(8):933–944.

CODES

ICD10
- A41.9 Sepsis, unspecified organism
- R65.10 SIRS of non-infectious origin w/o acute organ dysfunction
- R65.20 Severe sepsis without septic shock

CLINICAL PEARLS
- Treat sepsis aggressively with fluid support (with hemodynamic monitoring and pressor support if necessary) early use of broad-spectrum antimicrobial therapy and removal/drainage of foci of infection.
- Despite aggressive treatment, overall mortality is high (10–50%) in patients with severe sepsis/septic shock.

SEROTONIN SYNDROME

Neela Bhajandas, PharmD • Michael C. Barros, PharmD, BCPS, BCACP • Paul N. Williams, MD, FACP

 BASICS

DESCRIPTION

- A potentially life-threatening adverse drug reaction that results from excessive stimulation of peripheral and CNS serotonergic receptors
- It is a concentration-dependent toxicity that can develop in any individual who has ingested drug combinations that synergistically increase synaptic 5-HT.
- Serotonin toxicity occurs in three main settings: (i) therapeutic drug use, which often results in mild to moderate symptoms; (ii) intentional overdose of a single serotonergic agent, which typically leads to moderate symptoms; and (iii) as the result of a drug interaction between numerous serotonergic agents (most commonly, selective serotonin reuptake inhibitors [SSRIs] and monoamine oxidase inhibitors [MAOIs]), most often associated with severe serotonin toxicity.
- Classically characterized by a triad of symptoms that include mental status change, neuromuscular abnormalities, and autonomic hyperactivity
- Onset is usually within 24 hours with 60% of cases occurring within 6 hours of exposure to, or change in, dosing of a serotonergic agent. Rarely, cases have been reported weeks after discontinuation of serotonergic agents.

Geriatric Considerations
Elderly are at increased risk given use of multiple meds.

Pediatric Considerations
- Serotonin syndrome has similar manifestations in children and adults.
- General management is unchanged in children, other than medication dosing.

Pregnancy Considerations
- 3rd-trimester exposure to SSRIs has been associated with transient neonatal complications that may reflect either acute drug withdrawal or serotonergic toxicity.
- Symptoms in neonates may include tremors, increased muscle tone, jitteriness, shivering, feeding/digestive disturbances, irritability, agitation, sleep disturbances, increased reflexes, excessive crying, and respiratory disturbances.

EPIDEMIOLOGY
Seen in about 14–16% of SSRI overdose patients

Incidence
- In 2008, there were 106,336 adverse events reported with antidepressant use including 28 deaths. Most of these were associated with SSRIs, either alone or in combination with other drugs. SSRIs alone were responsible for adverse events in 18.8% of cases, with 55.7% due to intentional causes, 39.5% unintentional, and remainder of causes unknown. Of patients reporting adverse effects with SSRIs, 46.6% had symptoms requiring hospitalization, and significant toxic effects occurred in 90 patients with 2 resultant deaths (1)[A].
- The incidence of serotonin syndrome is rising because serotonergic agents are increasingly used in clinical practice and in combination with other serotonergic agents.

- Predominant age: affects all age groups
- Predominant sex: male = female

ETIOLOGY AND PATHOPHYSIOLOGY
- The result of excessive stimulation in peripheral and CNS serotonergic receptors
- Risk is mediated in a dose-related manner to the action of 5-HT/5-HT agonists on 5HT-1a and/or 5HT-2a receptors. The development mechanism of the syndrome is unknown.
- It is hypothesized that the degree of serotonin elevation in blood plasma has to be 10–15% times above baseline levels to result in serotonin toxicity (2)[A].
- A number of drugs are associated with the serotonin syndrome, which usually involves combination with an SSRI. These include SSRIs (e.g., citalopram, escitalopram, fluoxetine, fluvoxamine, paroxetine, sertraline); MAOIs; SNRIs (duloxetine, venlafaxine, desvenlafaxine); tricyclic antidepressants (e.g., amitriptyline); other antidepressants (buspirone, nefazodone, trazodone); lithium; triptans; anticonvulsants (Depakote); analgesics (fentanyl, meperidine, pentazocine, tramadol); antibiotics (linezolid [weak MAOI], ritonavir); over-the-counter (OTC) cough medications (dextromethorphan); some antipsychotics (risperidone, olanzapine); antiemetics (ondansetron, granisetron); other medications, such as metoclopramide, cyclobenzaprine, L-dopa; dietary supplements (tryptophan); herbal supplements (St. John's wort, nutmeg); methylene blue; and drugs of abuse (e.g., methylenedioxymethamphetamine [MDMA], cocaine, D-lysergic acid diethylamide [LSD], and amphetamine).
- Initially, patients can develop a peripheral tremor, confusion, and ataxia; systemic signs are next (e.g., agitation, diaphoresis, hyperreflexia, and shivering). If it worsens, the severe signs of fever, jerking, and diarrhea may develop. Serotonin syndrome can last from hours to days after the offending agents are stopped and supportive care is initiated.
- Drug interactions are most often the cause of severe cases of serotonin syndrome. Many of the same classes of medications listed earlier are involved, especially MAOIs (including linezolid) with SSRIs.

Genetics
Unknown

RISK FACTORS
- Serotonergic agents
- Reported following ingestion of a single agent. However, the greatest number of adverse events has been shown to be associated with SSRIs in combination with other substances, and the combination of SSRIs and MAOIs carries the greatest risk for developing serotonin toxicity.

GENERAL PREVENTION
- Consider drug–drug interactions when a multidrug regimen is required and avoid if possible.
- Caution patients about taking SSRIs with OTC medications (e.g., dextromethorphan) or herbal supplements (e.g., St. John's wort) prior to consulting a physician.
- Clinician education
- Continual improvement in use of health information technology

 DIAGNOSIS

- Serotonin syndrome is a clinical diagnosis.
- Epidemiologic data suggest that up to 85% of practitioners are unaware of serotonin syndrome.
- *Hunter Toxicity Criteria Decision Rules* aid in the diagnosis of clinically significant serotonin toxicity (sensitivity, 84%; specificity, 97%).
- To fulfill Hunter criteria, a patient must have taken a serotonergic agent and have one of the following:
  - Spontaneous clonus
  - Inducible clonus plus agitation/diaphoresis
  - Ocular clonus plus agitation/diaphoresis
  - Tremor and hyperreflexia
  - Hypertonia
  - Temperature >38°C plus ocular clonus/inducible clonus (3)[A]

HISTORY
- Obtain a thorough drug history, including prescription medications, OTC remedies, dietary supplements, herbal supplements, and illicit drugs. Ask about dose, formulation, and recent changes.
- Address possibility of drug overdose, and obtain collateral information if intentional overdose is suspected.
- Elicit description of symptoms, including their onset and progression.

PHYSICAL EXAM
- Vital signs: tachycardia, hypertension, and hyperthermia (severe cases)
- Neuromuscular findings (seen in over half of patients with serotonin syndrome)
  - Hyperreflexia (greater in lower extremities)
  - Clonus (involuntary muscle contractions, most commonly tested by flexing foot upward rapidly; includes ocular)
  - Myoclonus (greater in lower extremities)
  - Tremor (greater in lower extremities)
  - Hypertonia
  - Bilateral Babinski sign
  - Akathisia
  - Tonic–clonic seizures (severe cases)
  - Autonomic signs
    ○ Diaphoresis
    ○ Mydriasis
    ○ Flushing
    ○ Dry mucous membranes
    ○ Vomiting, diarrhea, increased bowel sounds
    ○ Mental status changes: anxiety, disorientation, delirium (4)[A]
    ○ Severe cases have led to altered level of consciousness, rhabdomyolysis, metabolic acidosis, and disseminated intravascular coagulation (DIC).

DIFFERENTIAL DIAGNOSIS
- Neuroleptic malignant syndrome (NMS)
- Anticholinergic fever (e.g., benztropine, diphenhydramine, oxybutynin, nifedipine, famotidine, atropine, scopolamine; plant poisoning from belladonna/"deadly nightshade," datura, henbane, mandrake, brugmansia)
- Malignant hyperthermia
- Heat stroke

- CNS infection (meningitis, encephalitis)
- Sympathomimetic toxicity
- Nonconvulsive seizures
- Hyperthyroidism
- Tetanus
- Acute baclofen withdrawal

DIAGNOSTIC TESTS & INTERPRETATION
- Serum serotonin levels do not correlate with clinical findings.
- Nonspecific lab findings that may develop include the following:
  - Elevated WBC count
  - Elevated creatine phosphokinase (CK or CPK)
  - Decreased serum bicarbonate
  - Elevated hepatic transaminases
- In severe cases, the following complications may develop:
  - DIC
  - Metabolic acidosis
  - Rhabdomyolysis
  - Renal failure
  - Myoglobinuria
  - Acute respiratory distress syndrome (ARDS) (4)[A]

TREATMENT

- Discontinue all serotonergic agents.
- Supportive care is the mainstay of therapy. This includes administration of oxygen and aggressive IV fluids, continuous cardiac monitoring, and correction of vital signs.
  - Benzodiazepines may be effective for the management of agitation in patients with serotonin syndrome.
  - Administration of serotonin antagonists: Cyproheptadine (histamine and serotonin antagonist) may be useful if supportive measures and sedation (benzodiazepines) are unable to control agitation and correct vital signs.
- Mild cases (afebrile, tachycardia, shivering, diaphoresis, mydriasis, hyperreflexia, intermittent tremor or myoclonus)
  - Discontinue precipitating agent(s).
  - Supportive care
  - Sedation
- Moderate cases (temperature >38°C, autonomic instability, mydriasis, hyperactive bowel sounds, diarrhea, diaphoresis, ocular clonus, hyperreflexia, tremor, mild agitation, or hypervigilance)
  - Discontinue precipitating agent(s).
  - Supportive care
  - Sedation
  - Aggressive treatment of autonomic instability
  - Treatment with cyproheptadine should be initiated if agitation and vital sign abnormalities are unimproved with benzodiazepines and supportive care.
  - Hypotension from MAOI interactions should be treated with low doses of direct-acting sympathomimetics (e.g., norepinephrine, phenylephrine, epinephrine); indirect serotonin agonists, such as dopamine, should be avoided.
  - Severe hypertension and tachycardia should be treated with short-acting agents, such as nitroprusside or esmolol.
  - Avoid use of longer acting agents, such as propranolol.

- Severe cases (temperature >41.1°C, autonomic instability, delirium, muscular rigidity, and hypertonicity)
  - Discontinue precipitating agent(s).
  - Immediate sedation
  - Endotracheal intubation as clinically indicated
  - Paralysis as clinically indicated (maintained with nondepolarizing continuous paralytic agents such as vecuronium, cisatracurium, rocuronium)
  - Antipyretic medications are not effective (4)[A]; the increased body temperature is due to muscle activity, not an alteration in the hypothalamic set point.

MEDICATION
- Activated charcoal: may be used in patients who intentionally overdose on serotonergic agents (3)[A]
- Benzodiazepines: may be used to manage agitation in serotonin syndrome and also may correct mild increases in BP and heart rate. Use with caution in patients with delirium, given the known paradoxical effect of exacerbating delirium.
- Cyproheptadine (Periactin): Consider use if benzodiazepines and supportive measures are unable to control agitation and correct vital signs:
  - Adults: initial dose 12 mg PO (can also be crushed and given via nasogastric [NG] tube) followed by 2 mg q2h until clinical response observed; 12 to 32 mg of drug may be required in a 24-hour period.
  - Children
    - <2 years: 0.06 mg/kg q6h
    - 2 to 6 years: 2 mg q6h
    - 7 to 14 years: 4 mg q6h
  - Unlikely to be effective in patients who have received activated charcoal.
- Use of antipsychotics with 5-HT$_{2A}$ antagonist activity, such as olanzapine and chlorpromazine, is not recommended (4)[A].

ISSUES FOR REFERRAL
- Psychiatry: for assistance with medication management and follow-up care (inpatient psychiatric care vs. outpatient psychiatric follow-up)
- Toxicology/clinical pharmacology service
- Poison control center

INPATIENT CONSIDERATIONS
Patients with known/suspected serotonin syndrome should be admitted to a medical inpatient unit for observation.

Discharge Criteria
- Mental status has returned to baseline.
- Stable vital signs
- No increase in clonus
- Close patient follow-up is ensured.

ONGOING CARE

FOLLOW-UP RECOMMENDATIONS
- In mild cases of serotonin toxicity, address risks and benefits of restarting offending agents. Serotonergic medications need to be titrated slowly, and patients must have close outpatient follow-up with physician.

- If patient developed severe serotonin syndrome, the offending agent should likely not be resumed unless precipitant for serotonin syndrome is found (e.g., combination with another serotonin agonist); the patient can be carefully monitored, or there is clear benefit versus risk of restarting the medication.

PROGNOSIS
- Generally favorable with early recognition of the syndrome and prompt initiation of treatment
- Most cases resolve within 24 hours of discontinuation of serotonergic agents; this can be longer depending on the drug's half-life:
  - MAOIs can result in toxicity for several days.
  - SSRIs can result in toxicity for up to several weeks after discontinuation.
- ICU admission is often indicated in severe cases.

COMPLICATIONS
- Adverse outcomes, including death, are usually the consequence of poorly treated hyperthermia.
- Nonhyperthermic patients who survive typically do not have long-term sequelae.

REFERENCES
1. Bronstein AC, Spyker DA, Cantilena LR Jr, et al. 2008 Annual report of the American Association of Poison Control Centers' National Poison Data System (NPDS): 26th annual report. *Clin Toxicol (Phila)*. 2009;47(10):911–1084.
2. Ables AZ, Nagubilli R. Prevention, recognition, and management of serotonin syndrome. *Am Fam Physician*. 2010;81(9):1139–1142.
3. Dunkley EJ, Isbister GK, Sibbritt D, et al. The Hunter Serotonin Toxicity Criteria: simple and accurate diagnostic decision rules for serotonin toxicity. *QJM*. 2003;96(9):635–642.
4. Boyer EW, Shannon M. The serotonin syndrome. *N Engl J Med*. 2005;352(11):1112–1120.

ADDITIONAL READING
- Isbister GK, Buckley NA, Whyte IM. Serotonin toxicity: a practical approach to diagnosis and treatment. *Med J Aust*. 2007;187(6):361–365.
- McAllen KJ, Schwartz DR. Adverse drug reactions resulting in hyperthermia in the intensive care unit. *Crit Care Med*. 2010;38(6 Suppl):S244–S252.

 CODES

ICD10
G25.79 Other drug induced movement disorders

CLINICAL PEARLS
Consider serotonin syndrome in patients with recent use of a serotonergic agent (particularly if multiple proserotonergic agents are involved) presenting with unexplained tachycardia, hypertension, hyperthermia, clonus, hyperreflexia, and change in mental status.

SEXUAL DYSFUNCTION IN WOMEN

Amanda M. Carnes, MD • Lisa M. Harris, DO

BASICS

- Very common: ~40% of women surveyed in the United States have sexual concerns.
- May present as a lack of sexual desire, impaired arousal, pain with sexual activity, or inability to achieve orgasm, and may be lifelong or acquired

DESCRIPTION

- Female sexual interest or arousal disorder—lack of or significantly reduced sexual interest or arousal as manifested by three of the following:
  - Absent or reduced interest in sexual activity
  - Absent or reduced sexual or erotic thoughts or fantasies
  - No or reduced initiation of sexual activity and unreceptive to partner's attempts to initiate
  - Absent or reduced sexual excitement or pleasure during sexual activity in almost all (75–100%) of sexual encounters
  - Absent or reduced sexual interest or arousal in response to any internal or external sexual or erotic cues
  - Absent or reduced genital or nongenital sensation during sexual activity in almost all (75–100%) of sexual encounters
- Female orgasmic disorder—presence of either of the following in almost all (75–100%) occasions of sexual activity:
  - Marked delay in, marked infrequency of, or absence of orgasm
  - Markedly reduced intensity of orgasmic sensations
- Genitopelvic pain or penetration disorder—persistent or recurrent difficulties with one or more of the following:
  - Vaginal penetration during intercourse
  - Marked vulvovaginal or pelvic pain during intercourse or penetration attempts
  - Marked fear or anxiety about vulvovaginal or pelvic pain in anticipation of, during, or because of vaginal penetration
  - Marked tensing or tightening of pelvic floor muscles during attempted vaginal penetration

ALERT

- Symptoms must be present for ≥6 months; cause clinically significant distress or impairment; and not be caused by another condition (psychiatric or medical), substance/medication, relationship distress, or other stressor.
- System(s) affected: nervous; reproductive; genitourinary; psychiatric
- Synonym(s): hypoactive sexual desire disorder; sexual aversion disorder; female sexual arousal disorder; inhibited female orgasm

EPIDEMIOLOGY

In two large studies, approximately 40% of women reported sexual problems.

Incidence

Sexual problems are highest in women aged 45 to 64 years, then declines secondary to changes in sexual-related personal distress.

Prevalence

Low sexual desire is the most common manifestation, followed by difficulty with orgasm, difficulty with arousal, and sexual pain.

ETIOLOGY AND PATHOPHYSIOLOGY

The pathophysiology of sexual dysfunction is complex and multifactorial because it can be the result of any etiology that interferes with the nonlinear model of female sexual response cycle (emotional intimacy, sexual stimuli, psychological factors, and relationship satisfaction).

- Physiologic
  - Prescription medications
    - SSRIs, MAOIs, and TCAs
    - β-Blockers, ACE inhibitors, and calcium channel blockers
    - GNRH agonists
    - Injectable progestins
    - Antiepileptics
    - Gabapentin
- Endocrine
  - Disorders of the hypothalamic-pituitary-adrenal system, hormonal imbalance/disorders of ovarian function, menopause (surgical or natural)
  - Thyroid disease
  - Diabetes
- Neurologic
  - Spinal cord damage
- Psychologic
  - Maladaptive thoughts/behaviors
  - Interrelational difficulties
  - Body image issues
  - Drug and alcohol abuse
  - Sexual abuse

RISK FACTORS

- Advancing age/menopause
- Previous sexual trauma
- Lack of knowledge about sexual stimulation and response
- Chronic medical problems
  - Depression, anxiety, chronic pain syndromes, and other psychiatric disorders
  - Cardiovascular disease
  - Endocrine disorders
  - Dermatologic disorders
  - Neurologic disorders
  - Cancer
- Gynecologic issues
  - Childbirth
  - Pelvic floor or bladder dysfunction
  - Endometriosis
  - Uterine fibroids
  - Chronic vulvovaginal candidiasis/vaginal infections
  - Female genital mutilation
- Relationship factors such as couple discrepancies in expectations and/or cultural backgrounds and attitudes toward sexuality in family of origin
- Medications or substance abuse

COMMONLY ASSOCIATED CONDITIONS

- Marital/relationship discord
- Depression

DIAGNOSIS

- Female sexual dysfunction is diagnosed by utilizing a validated sexual function screening instrument and a structured interview, including detailed medical and sexual history, to confirm diagnosis.
  - Female Sexual Function Index
  - Brief Index of Sexual Functioning for Women
  - Brief Sexual Symptoms Checklist
  - Decreases Sexual Desire Screener

- The diagnosis requires that the sexual problem be recurrent or persistent and cause personal distress rather than be due solely to partner or relationship issues.

HISTORY

- Detailed sexual history (1)[C].
  - Degree of personal distress
  - Lifelong versus acquired problem
  - Situational versus generalized problem
  - Cultural/societal beliefs regarding sexuality
  - History of sexual trauma
  - Concerns about safety, pregnancy, or STIs
  - Concerns regarding privacy
- Interpersonal relationship factors
  - Current relationship status
  - Family dysfunction
- Physiologic/biologic history
  - Urinary/anal incontinence
  - Medications (including herbal and OTC)
  - Pregnancy/childbirth history
  - Infertility
  - Menopausal status (natural, surgical, or postchemotherapy)
  - STIs and vaginitis
  - Pelvic surgery, injury, or cancer
  - Chronic pelvic pain
  - Abnormal genital tract bleeding
- Psychologic History
  - Low self-image
  - Anxiety
  - Depression
  - Negative past sexual experiences
  - Substance misuse/abuse

PHYSICAL EXAM

- Most commonly, patients have a normal physical exam (1)[C].
  - Assess for anatomic abnormalities.
  - Assess for scars or evidence of trauma.
  - Assess for vaginal atrophy, adequate estrogenization.
  - Assess for infection.
  - Recognize signs of anxiety, apprehension, and pain during the speculum and pelvic exam.
- General physical exam, signs of chronic disease

DIFFERENTIAL DIAGNOSIS

- Medication side effects
- Vaginitis
- Decreased vaginal lubrication secondary to hormonal imbalance
- Decreased sensation secondary to nerve injury
- Multiple sclerosis
- Anatomic abnormalities
- Abdominal surgery (which can interfere with pelvic innervation)
- Depression
- Marital dysfunction, including domestic violence
- Pregnancy
- Pseudodyspareunia (use of complaint of pain to distance self from partner)

DIAGNOSTIC TESTS & INTERPRETATION

Laboratory studies are rarely helpful. There are no reliable correlations between serum hormone levels and sexual dysfunction.

Initial Tests (lab, imaging)

As needed to identify infections and other medical causes (1)[C]

TREATMENT

- Set realistic goals and expectations (2)[C].
- Address underlying medical and psychiatric conditions (3)[C].
- Review basic sex education, sexual response, heterogeneity of normal response, and sexual activity other than intercourse (2,4)[C].
- Education on communication (4)[C]
- Educate on healthy lifestyle, including diet, exercise, sleep, avoidance of tobacco, and reduced alcohol use (2,4)[C].
- Vaginal moisturizers and lubricants (5)[C]
- Cognitive-behavioral therapy (CBT) (individual or couples) to target maladaptive thoughts and behaviors and to disrupt the dysfunctional cycle (3,4)[C]
- Mindfulness-based CBT (2,4)[C]
- Sex therapy: sensate focus, systematic desensitization exercises, homework exchanging physical touch with partner, or directed masturbation alone (3,4)[C]
- Physical therapy/biofeedback (4)[C]

MEDICATION
Sexual dysfunction is often a multifactorial psychosocial condition. Using medications does not usually address the cause of the problem and can, in some cases, make the condition worse.

- Bupropion (2,4)[C]: adjunct for SSRI-induced sexual dysfunction. Improves sexual arousal and orgasm but not desire. Dose: bupropion SR 150 mg orally once or twice daily.
- Flibanserin (3)[C]: possible improvement in sexual desire. Mechanism of action: 5-HT$_{1A}$ agonist and 5-HT$_{2A}$ antagonist.
- Estrogen replacement with or without progestins (2,5)[C],(6)[A]: may improve sexual desire, vaginal atrophy, and clitoral sensitivity. Vaginal estrogen therapy is available in cream, vaginal tablet, or ring form.
- Ospemifene (2)[C]: selective estrogen receptor modulator FDA approved for dyspareunia due to vulvo or vaginal atrophy in postmenopausal women. Dose: ospemifene 60 mg orally once daily.
- Testosterone (2–4)[C]
  - Use in premenopausal women not supported by data.
  - In naturally or surgically postmenopausal women, adding short-term testosterone to hormone replacement may increase desire.
  - Use >6 months contingent on clear improvement and no adverse effects.
  - Side effects: hirsutism, androgenic alopecia, acne, decreased HDL, liver dysfunction; not FDA approved for sexual dysfunction in women
  - Contraindicated in breast or endometrial cancer, thromboembolic disease, or coronary artery disease
  - Dose: oral methyltestosterone 1.25 to 2.5 mg/day (1/10 of men's dose) or topical (patch, gel)
- DHEA and tissue-selective estrogen complexes (TSECs) (3–5)[C]: may improve vaginal atrophy, dryness, and dyspareunia. Not FDA approved. Additional studies needed
- PDE-5 inhibitors (4)[C]: not recommended

ISSUES FOR REFERRAL
Consider referral for CBT, marriage/couples counseling, or sex therapy.

ADDITIONAL THERAPIES
- Smoking cessation and reduction of alcohol intake
- For childhood trauma: scripting, psychotherapy, cognitive restructuring
- For prescription-drug causes: reduced dosages or change to different medication

COMPLEMENTARY & ALTERNATIVE MEDICINE
- Zestra for Women botanical feminine massage oil: Small trial showed increased arousal, desire, genital sensation, ability to have orgasm, and sexual pleasure.
- Yohimbine: not recommended, potentially dangerous
- Ginseng and St. John's wort: No evidence to support treatment of sexual dysfunction.

ONGOING CARE

DIET
Weight reduction if overweight or obese

PATIENT EDUCATION
- American Association of Sex Educators, Counselors, and Therapists: www.aasect.org.
- National Women's Health Resource Center: www.healthywomen.org
- North American Menopause Society: www.menopause.org
- National Vulvodynia Association: www.nva.org

PROGNOSIS
Lack of desire is most difficult type to treat with <50% success.

REFERENCES

1. Latif E, Diamond MP. Arriving at the diagnosis of female sexual dysfunction. *Fertil Steril*. 2013;100(4):898–904.
2. Kingsberg SA, Woodard T. Female sexual dysfunction: focus on low desire. *Obstet Gynecol*. 2015;125(2):477–486.
3. Kingsberg SA, Rezaee RL. Hypoactive sexual desire in women. *Menopause*. 2013;20(12):1284–1300.
4. Basson R, Wierman ME, van Lankveld J, et al. Summary of the recommendations on sexual dysfunctions in women. *J Sex Med*. 2010;7(1, Pt 2):314–326.
5. Tan O, Bradshaw K, Carr BR. Management of vulvovaginal atrophy-related sexual dysfunction in postmenopausal women: an up-to-date review. *Menopause*. 2012;19(1):109–117.
6. Nastri CO, Lara LA, Ferriani RA, et al. Hormone therapy for sexual function in perimenopausal and postmenopausal women. *Cochrane Database Syst Rev*. 2013;(6):CD009672.

ADDITIONAL READING

- American Psychiatric Association. *Diagnostic and Statistical Manual of Mental Disorders*. 5th ed. Arlington, VA: American Psychiatric Association; 2013.
- Basson R. Women's sexual function and dysfunction: current uncertainties, future directions. *Int J Impot Res*. 2008;20(5):466–478.
- Buster JE. Managing female sexual dysfunction. *Fertil Steril*. 2013;100(4):905–915.

- Carey JC. Pharmacological effects on sexual function. *Obstet Gynecol Clin North Am*. 2006;33(4):599–620.
- Meston CM, Bradford A. Sexual dysfunctions in women. *Annu Rev Clin Psychol*. 2007;3:233–256.
- Palacios S. Hypoactive sexual desire disorder and current pharmacotherapeutic options in women. *Womens Health (Lond Engl)*. 2011;7(1):95–107.
- Safarinejad MR. Reversal of SSRI-induced female sexual dysfunction by adjunctive bupropion in menstruating women: a double-blind, placebo-controlled and randomized study. *J Psychopharmacol*. 2011;25(3):370–378.
- Safarinejad MR, Hosseini SY, Asgari MA, et al. A randomized, double-blind, placebo-controlled study of the efficacy and safety of bupropion for treating hypoactive sexual desire disorder in ovulating women. *BJU Int*. 2010;106(6):832–839.
- Shifren JL, Davis SR, Moreau M, et al. Testosterone patch for the treatment of hypoactive sexual desire disorder in naturally menopausal women: results of the INTIMATE NM1 study. *Menopause*. 2006;13(5):770–779.
- Shifren JL, Monz BU, Russo PA, et al. Sexual problems and distress in United States women: prevalence and correlates. *Obstet Gynecol*. 2008;112(5):970–978.
- Silverstein RG, Brown AH, Roth HD, et al. Effects of mindfulness training on body awareness to sexual stimuli: implications for female sexual dysfunction. *Psychosom Med*. 2011;73(9):817–825.
- Simonelli C, Eleuteri S, Petruccelli F, et al. Female sexual pain disorders: dyspareunia and vaginismus. *Curr Opin Psychiatry*. 2014;27(6):406–412.
- Sungur MZ, Gündüz A. A comparison of DSM-IV-TR and DSM-5 definitions for sexual dysfunctions: critiques and challenges. *J Sex Med*. 2014;11(2):364–373.
- Taylor MJ, Rudkin L, Bullemor-Day P, et al. Strategies for managing sexual dysfunction induced by antidepressant medication. *Cochrane Database Syst Rev*. 2013;(5):CD003382.
- Woodis CB, McLendon AN, Muzyk AJ. Testosterone supplementation for hypoactive sexual desire disorder in women. *Pharmacotherapy*. 2012;32(1):38–53.

CODES

ICD10
- R37 Sexual dysfunction, unspecified
- F52.0 Hypoactive sexual desire disorder
- N94.1 Dyspareunia

CLINICAL PEARLS

- Female sexual dysfunction is a common, complex, multifactorial problem.
- Usually patients with sexual dysfunction have a normal physical exam.
- Symptoms of sexual dysfunction peak during perimenopause between the ages of 45 and 64 years.
- Several therapies exist for treating sexual dysfunction in women, including behavioral therapy and medications.

SHOULDER PAIN

Daniel L. Jones, MD • J. Herbert Stevenson, MD

 BASICS

DESCRIPTION
- Shoulder pain is common and affects patients of all ages. Causes include acute trauma or overuse during sports and activities of everyday living.
- Age plays an important role in determining the etiology of shoulder pain.
- Onset and characteristics of pain, weakness, mechanism of injury, and functional limitation help guide an accurate diagnose.

EPIDEMIOLOGY
- Shoulder pain accounts for 16% of all musculoskeletal complaints.
- The lifetime prevalence of shoulder pain is ~70%.
- Predominant etiology varies with age:
  - <30 years: shoulder instability
  - >30 years: rotator cuff (RTC) disorder
    - 30 to 50 years: tendinopathy
    - 40 to 60 years: partial tear
    - >60 years: full-thickness tear
  - >60 years: glenohumeral osteoarthritis (OA)

Incidence
The incidence of shoulder pain is 7 to 25 cases/1,000 patients, with a peak incidence in the 4th to 6th decades.

ETIOLOGY AND PATHOPHYSIOLOGY
Pathology varies with cause:
- Trauma (fracture, dislocation, ligament/tendon tear, acromioclavicular [AC] separation)
- Overuse (RTC pathology, biceps tenosynovitis, bursitis, muscle strain, apophyseal injuries)
  - RTC disorders most commonly result from repetitive overhead activity, leading to RTC impingement with a 3 stage progression:
    - Stage I: tendinopathy
    - Stage II: partial RTC tear
    - Stage III: full-thickness RTC tear
  - Subacromial bursitis can occur with RTC disorders but is rarely an isolated diagnosis.
- Age-related: AC and glenohumeral joint OA, adhesive capsulitis, RTC tear with increasing age; pediatric athletes instability and physeal injuries are more common.
- Rheumatologic (rheumatoid arthritis, polymyalgia rheumatica, fibromyalgia)
- Referred pain (neck, gallbladder)

RISK FACTORS
- Repetitive overhead activity
- Overhead and upper extremity weight-bearing sports (baseball, softball, swimming, tennis, volleyball)
- Weight lifting: AC disorders
- Rapid increases in training frequency or load (often associated with improper technique)
- Muscle weakness or imbalance

- Trauma or fall onto the shoulder
- Diabetes, thyroid disorders, female gender, and age 40 to 60 years are risk factors for adhesive capsulitis.

GENERAL PREVENTION
- Maintain strength and range of motion (ROM).
- Avoid repetitive overhead activities (pitch counts).
- Proper technique (pitching, weight lifting)

 DIAGNOSIS

HISTORY
- Pain characteristics
  - Superior shoulder pain: AC pathology, trapezius strain
  - Lateral/deltoid pain: RTC pathology (RTC pain typically does not extend past elbow.)
  - Diffuse pain: RTC pathology, adhesive capsulitis, glenohumeral OA
  - Posterior (scapular) pain: scapulothoracic dyskinesis
  - Night pain: RTC pathology (pain laying on affected side), adhesive capsulitis, glenohumeral OA
  - Stiff shoulder: adhesive capsulitis
  - Pain with cross-body activities: AC pathology
  - Pain with abduction/external rotation (reaching behind): shoulder instability
  - Pain with overhead activity: RTC pathology, AC pathology, labrum pathology
  - Pain with turning neck, pain past elbow: cervical pathology
- Mechanism of injury
  - Fall on outstretched hand: traumatic shoulder instability/dislocation
  - Fall directly onto shoulder: AC joint sprain, clavicular fracture
  - Repetitive overhead activity: RTC pathology
- Age
  - Shoulder instability (subluxation, dislocation, multidirectional instability) is the most common cause of shoulder pain in young athletes (<30 years old).
  - RTC disorders are the most common cause of shoulder pain in patients >30 years old. Severity of RTC disorder increases with age.
  - Older patients (>60 years old) commonly have OA.
  - Trauma in a young person <40 years is more commonly associated with dislocation/subluxation. In patients >40 years, trauma is more commonly associated with RTC tear.

PHYSICAL EXAM
- Observe face and shoulder movements as patient disrobes, moves arm, and shakes hand.
- Inspect for malalignment, muscle atrophy, asymmetry, erythema, ecchymosis and swelling. Scapular winging suggests long thoracic nerve or muscular (trapezius, serratus anterior) dysfunction. Prominent scapular spine with scalloped infraspinatus fossa suggests infraspinatus atrophy.

- Palpate for tenderness, warmth, bony step-offs.
- Evaluate active and passive ROM and flexibility:
  - Decreased active AND passive ROM are more common with adhesive capsulitis.
  - Mildly decreased active and/or passive ROM may also indicate glenohumeral OA.
- Decreased active, full passive ROM: RTC pathology
- Evaluate for muscle strength including grip, biceps, triceps, and deltoid. Test RTC strength: supraspinatus (empty can test), infraspinatus/teres minor (resisted external rotation, external lag test), subscapularis (lift-off test, belly press, resisted internal rotation). Pain with RTC strength testing indicates RTC pathology. Weakness could suggest tear.
- Special tests
  - Neer, Hawkin tests: RTC impingement
  - Drop-arm test: RTC tear
  - Cross-arm adduction test: AC joint arthritis
  - Speed, Yergason tests: biceps tendinopathy
  - Apprehension, relocation test: anterior glenohumeral joint instability
  - Sulcus sign: inferior glenohumeral joint instability
  - O'Brien, clunk test: labral pathology
  - Spurling test: cervical pathology

DIFFERENTIAL DIAGNOSIS
- Fracture (clavicle, humerus, scapula), contusion
- RTC disorder: impingement, tear, calcific tendonitis
- Subacromial bursitis
- Scapulothoracic dyskinesis
- AC joint pathology (AC separation/OA, osteolysis)
- Biceps tenosynovitis or tear
- Acromial apophysitis or os acromiale
- Glenohumeral joint OA
- Glenohumeral joint instability (acute dislocation or chronic multidirectional instability)
- Adhesive capsulitis
- Labral tear or associated bony pathology
- Muscle strain (trapezius, deltoid, biceps)
- Cervical radiculopathy
- Other: autoimmune, rheumatologic, referred pain, septic joint (biliary/splenic, cardiac, pneumonia/lung mass)

DIAGNOSTIC TESTS & INTERPRETATION
- Shoulder pain can be accurately diagnosed with a careful history and physical exam:
  - Adults with nontraumatic shoulder pain of <4 weeks duration may not require initial imaging.
- History of significant trauma, prolonged symptoms, or red flags (older age, fever, rest pain) suggest need for imaging.
- Plain radiographs are first-line:
  - Assess for fracture, degenerative changes, signs of dislocation (Bankart, Hill-Sachs deformity), signs of large RTC tear (sclerosis, proximal migration of humeral head), anatomic deformities contributing to impingement, and occult tumor.
  - Standard views: anteroposterior, scapular Y, axillary

- EMG study of the upper extremity may help differentiate referred cervical pain from a primary shoulder disorder.
- Obtain ECG if any suspicion for cardiac etiology.
- Serologic tests if autoimmune etiology is suspected.

Follow-Up Tests & Special Considerations
- CT scan can rule out occult fracture.
- MRI is gold standard for noninvasive soft tissue imaging, including RTC, biceps tendon.
- MR arthrogram may be necessary to assess for labral tears or small/partial RTC tears.
- Ultrasound (US) helps assess RTC tears, biceps tendinopathies, and AC joint disorders.

Diagnostic Procedures/Other
Diagnostic arthroscopy after noninterventional means have been exhausted if structural injury is suspected.

Test Interpretation
Depends on underlying diagnosis
- Tendinosis rather than tendonitis is common with stage I impingement.
- Capsular scarring is the hallmark of adhesive capsulitis.
- RTC tendon calcifications with calcific tendonitis

 ## TREATMENT

Treatment is based on underlying diagnosis. In general, conservative therapy includes activity modification, analgesics, and/or anti-inflammatory medicines in association with appropriate rehabilitative programs.

MEDICATION
First Line
- Analgesics and anti-inflammatory medications for symptomatic relief:
  – Ibuprofen: 200 to 800 mg TID
  – Naproxen: 250 to 500 mg BID
  – Acetaminophen: not to exceed 3 g/day

- Corticosteroid injections (subacromial, glenohumeral, AC, subscapular bursa) acutely relieve pain due to RTC pathology, adhesive capsulitis, OA, or scapulothoracic dyskinesis (1)[A]. This improves ability to engage in rehabilitative activities.
- US guidance improves accuracy of anatomic placement of corticosteroid injections (2)[A].

ISSUES FOR REFERRAL
Refer if etiology remains unclear, patient is not responsive to conservative care, for complicated or displaced fractures, or full thickness RTC tears >1 cm acute or chronic in patients <65 years old or any tear with significant changes in functional status. These tears have a high rate of progression, fatty infiltration, or retraction with nonoperative care (3).

ADDITIONAL THERAPIES
- Physical therapy benefits persistent RTC disorders, adhesive capsulitis, and shoulder instability.

- Physical therapy/exercise may improve nonspecific shoulder pain, but it does not generally improve ROM or function (4)[A].

- Manual manipulative therapy (MMT) by chiropractors, osteopathic physicians, or physical therapists improves pain with adhesive capsulitis, RTC, and soft tissue disorders (5)[A]. MMT is generally less effective than glucocorticoid injections at 6 weeks with similar long-term outcomes in adhesive capsulitis (6)[A].

SURGERY/OTHER PROCEDURES

- Surgery is necessary for shoulder pain caused by acute displaced fractures, large RTC tears (criteria as above), shoulder dislocation in patients <20 years of age. Surgery may be necessary for shoulder pain unresponsive to conservative measures >3 to 6 months. Surgery is not more effective than active nonsurgical treatment in impingement syndrome (7)[A].
- Platelet-rich therapies need more conclusive evidence before routine use in treatment of MSK soft tissue injuries (8)[A].

COMPLEMENTARY & ALTERNATIVE MEDICINE
Acupuncture may help with acute shoulder pain. There is no conclusive evidence for the effectiveness of acupuncture.

 ## ONGOING CARE

FOLLOW-UP RECOMMENDATIONS
Limit overhead activity to reduce impingement symptoms.

PATIENT EDUCATION
Refer to specific diagnosis for shoulder pain.

PROGNOSIS
Shoulder pain generally has a favorable outcome with conservative care, but recovery can be slow, with 40–50% of patients complaining of persistent pain or recurrence at 12 months.

REFERENCES

1. Gross C, Dhawan A, Harwood D, et al. Glenohumeral joint injections: a review. *Sports Health*. 2013;(5)2:153–159.
2. Soh E, Li W, Ong KO, et al. Image-guided versus blind corticosteroid injections in adults with shoulder pain: a systematic review. *BMC Musculoskelet Disord*. 2011;12:137.
3. Armstrong A. Evaluation and management of adult shoulder pain: a focus on rotator cuff disorders, acromioclavicular joint arthritis, and glenohumeral arthritis. *Med Clin North Am*. 2014;98(4):755–775.
4. van den Dolder PA, Ferreira PH, Refshauge KM. Effectiveness of soft tissue massage and exercise for the treatment of non-specific shoulder pain: a systematic review with meta-analysis. *Br J Sports Med*. 2014;48(16):1216–1226.
5. Brantingham JW, Cassa TK, Bonnefin D, et al. Manipulative therapy for shoulder pain and disorders: expansion of a systematic review. *J Manipulative Physiol Ther*. 2011;34(5):314–346.
6. Page MJ, Green S, Kramer S, et al. Manual therapy and exercise for adhesive capsulitis (frozen shoulder). *Cochrane Database Syst Rev*. 2014;(8):CD011275.
7. Coghlan JA, Buchbinder R, Green S, et al. Surgery for rotator cuff disease. *Cochrane Database Syst Rev*. 2008;(1):CD005619.
8. Moraes VY, Lenza M, Tamaoki MJ, et al. Platelet-rich therapies for musculoskeletal soft tissue injuries. *Cochrane Database Syst Rev*. 2014;(4):CD010071.

ADDITIONAL READING

- Cadogan A, Laslett M, Hing WA, et al. A prospective study of shoulder pain in primary care: prevalence of imaged pathology and response to guided diagnostic blocks. *BMC Musculoskelet Disord*. 2011;12:119.
- Celik D, Sirmen B, Demirhan M. The relationship of muscle strength and pain in subacromial impingement. *Acta Orthop Traumatol Turc*. 2011;45(2):79–84.
- Littlewood C, Ashton J, Chance-Larsen K, et al. Exercise for rotator cuff tendinopathy: a systematic review. *Physiotherapy*. 2012;98(2):101–109.
- Sipola P, Niemitukia L, Kröger H, et al. Detection and quantification of rotator cuff tears with ultrasonography and magnetic resonance imaging—a prospective study in 77 consecutive patients with a surgical reference. *Ultrasound Med Biol*. 2010;36(12):1981–1989.

 ## CODES

ICD10
- M25.519 Pain in unspecified shoulder
- S43.429A Sprain of unspecified rotator cuff capsule, init encntr
- M19.019 Primary osteoarthritis, unspecified shoulder

CLINICAL PEARLS

- RTC disorders (tendinopathy, tears) are the most common cause of shoulder pain in individuals >30 years of age.
- Shoulder instability (acute dislocation/subluxation or chronic instability) is the most common source of shoulder pain in individuals <30 years of age.
- Patients with diabetes are at increased risk for adhesive capsulitis.

S

SINUSITIS

Chirag N. Shah, MD • Patrick J. Rogers, DO

BASICS

DESCRIPTION
- Acute sinusitis is a symptomatic inflammation of ≥1 paranasal sinuses of <4 weeks' duration resulting from impaired drainage and retained secretions accompanied by obstruction, facial pain/pressure/fullness, or both. Because rhinitis and sinusitis usually coexist, "rhinosinusitis" is the preferred term.
- Disease is subacute when symptomatic for 4 to 12 weeks, recurrent acute when ≥4 annual episodes without persistent symptoms in between and chronic when symptomatic for >12 weeks.
- Uncomplicated rhinosinusitis has no extension of inflammation beyond paranasal sinuses and nasal cavity.
- System(s) affected: head/eyes/ears/nose/throat (HEENT), pulmonary

EPIDEMIOLOGY
- Affects one in eight adults accounting for >30 million individuals in the United States each year diagnosed with rhinosinusitis
- Diagnosis of acute bacterial rhinosinusitis remains the fifth leading reason for prescribing antibiotics.
- 0.5–2% of viral rhinosinusitis episodes have a bacterial superinfection.
- Viral cause in 90–98% of cases

Incidence
Incidence is highest in early fall through early spring (related to incidence of viral upper respiratory infection [URI]). Adults have two to three viral URIs per year; 90% of these colds are accompanied by viral rhinosinusitis. It is the fifth most common diagnosis made during family physician visits.

ETIOLOGY AND PATHOPHYSIOLOGY
- Important features
  - Inflammation and edema of the sinus mucosa
  - Obstruction of the sinus ostia
  - Impaired mucociliary clearance
- Secretions that are not cleared become hospitable to bacterial growth.
- Inflammatory response (neutrophil influx and release of cytokines) damages mucosal surfaces.
- Viral: vast majority of cases (rhinovirus; influenza A and B; parainfluenza virus; respiratory syncytial; adeno-, corona-, and enteroviruses)
- Bacterial (complicates 0.5–2% of viral cases)
  - More likely if symptoms worsen within 5 to 6 days after initial improvement
  - No improvement within 10 days of symptom onset
  - >3 to 4 days of fever >102°F and facial pain and purulent nasal discharge
  - *Streptococcus pneumoniae, Haemophilus influenzae,* and *Moraxella catarrhalis* are the most common bacterial pathogens.
  - Often overdiagnosed, which leads to overuse of and increasing resistance to antibiotics
  - Methicillin-resistant *Staphylococcus aureus* present in 0–15.9% of patients.
- Fungal: seen in immunocompromised hosts (uncontrolled diabetes, neutropenia, use of corticosteroids) or as a nosocomial infection

Genetics
No known genetic pattern

RISK FACTORS
- Viral URI
- Allergic rhinitis
- Asthma
- Cigarette smoking
- Dental infections and procedures
- Anatomic variations
  - Tonsillar and adenoid hypertrophy
  - Turbinate hypertrophy, nasal polyps
  - Cleft palate
- Immunodeficiency (e.g., HIV)
- Cystic fibrosis (CF)

GENERAL PREVENTION
- Hand washing to prevent transmission of viral infection
- Childhood vaccinations up to date
- Avoid close contacts with symptomatic individuals.
- Avoid smoking and exposure to second hand smoke.

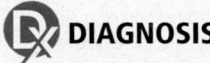

DIAGNOSIS

- History and physical exam suggest and establish the diagnosis but are rarely helpful in distinguishing bacterial from viral causes.
- Use a constellation of symptoms rather than a particular sign or symptom in diagnosis.

HISTORY
- Symptoms somewhat predictive of bacterial sinusitis (1)[C]
  - Worsening of symptoms >5 to 6 days after initial improvement
  - Persistent symptoms for ≥10 days
  - Persistent purulent nasal discharge
  - Unilateral upper tooth or facial pain
  - Unilateral maxillary sinus tenderness
  - Fever
- Associated symptoms
  - Headache
  - Nasal congestion
  - Retro-orbital pain
  - Otalgia
  - Hyposomia
  - Halitosis
  - Chronic cough
- Symptoms requiring urgent attention
  - Visual disturbances, especially diplopia
  - Periorbital swelling or erythema
  - Altered mental status

PHYSICAL EXAM
- Fever
- Edema and erythema of nasal mucosa
- Purulent discharge
- Tenderness to palpation over sinus(es)
- Pain localized to sinuses when bending forward
- Transillumination of the sinuses may confirm fluid in sinuses (helpful if asymmetric; not helpful if symmetric exam).

Pediatric Considerations
- Sinuses are not fully developed until age 20 years. Maxillary and ethmoid sinuses, although small, are present from birth.
- Because children have an average of six to eight colds per year, they are at risk for developing sinusitis.
- Diagnosis can be more difficult than in adults because symptoms are often more subtle.

DIFFERENTIAL DIAGNOSIS
- Dental disease
- CF
- Wegener granulomatosis
- HIV infection
- Kartagener syndrome
- Neoplasm
- Headache, tension, or migraine

DIAGNOSTIC TESTS & INTERPRETATION
Diagnostic tests are not routinely recommended; no diagnostic tests can adequately differentiate between viral and bacterial rhinosinusitis (2)[C].
- None indicated in routine evaluation
- Routine use of sinus radiography discouraged because of the following:
  - ≥3 clinical findings have similar diagnostic accuracy as imaging.
  - Imaging does not distinguish viral from bacterial etiology.
- Limited coronal CT scan can be useful in recurrent infection or failure to respond to medical therapy.

Diagnostic Procedures/Other
Sinus CT if signs suggest extrasinus involvement or to evaluate chronic rhinosinusitis

Test Interpretation
- Inflammation, edema, thickened mucosa
- Impaired ciliary function
- Metaplasia of ciliated columnar cells
- Relative acidosis and hypoxia within sinuses
- Polyps

TREATMENT

Most cases resolve with supportive care (treating pain, nasal symptoms). Antibiotics should be reserved for symptoms that persist >10 days, onset with severe symptoms (high fever, purulent nasal discharge, facial pain) for at least 3 to 4 consecutive days, or worsening signs/symptoms that were initially improving (1,2)[C].

GENERAL MEASURES
- Hydration
- Steam inhalation 20 to 30 minutes TID
- Saline irrigation (Neti pot) or nose drops
- Sleep with head of bed elevated.
- Avoid exposure to cigarette smoke or fumes.
- Avoid caffeine and alcohol.
- Antibiotics are indicated only when findings suggest bacterial infection.
- Analgesics, NSAIDs
- Acute viral sinusitis is self-limiting; antibiotics should not be used.

MEDICATION
First Line
- Decongestants
  - Pseudoephedrine HCl
  - Phenylephrine nasal spray (limited use)
  - Oxymetazoline nasal spray (e.g., Afrin) (not to be used >3 days)
- Analgesics
  - Acetaminophen
  - Aspirin
  - NSAIDs

- Antibiotics
  - Antibiotics have a slight advantage over placebo at 7 to 14 days (3)[A], yet most improve without therapy.
  - Reserve antibiotic use for patients with moderate to severe disease.
  - Choice should be based on understanding of antibiotic resistance in the community.
  - Infectious Disease Society of America recommends the following (1)[C]:
    ○ Start antibiotics as soon as clinical diagnosis of acute bacterial sinusitis is made.
    ○ Use amoxicillin-clavulanate rather than amoxicillin alone.
    ○ Amoxicillin-clavulanate 875/125 mg q12h; 2 g orally BID in geographic regions with high rates of resistant *S. pneumoniae*
    ○ Doxycycline: 100 mg PO BID an alternative to amoxicillin-clavulanate for initial therapy (adults only)
    ○ Trimethoprim-sulfamethoxazole (TMP/SMX) and 3rd generation cephalosporins not recommended due to high rate of resistance (1)[C]
    ○ Treat for 5 to 7 days in adults if uncomplicated bacterial rhinosinusitis (IDSA low-moderate-quality evidence). Treat for 10 to 14 days in children if uncomplicated bacterial rhinosinusitis (IDSA low-moderate-quality evidence).
  - American Academy of Pediatrics recommends the following (1)[C]:
    ○ Amoxicillin: 45 to 90 mg/kg/day in 2 divided doses if uncomplicated acute bacterial sinusitis in children
    ○ Amoxicillin-clavulanate: 80 to 90 mg/6.4 mg/kg/day in 2 divided doses for children with severe illness, recent antibiotics, or attending daycare
    ○ Levofloxacin: 10 to 20 mg/kg/day max 750mg/day if history of type 1 hypersensitivity to PCN (1)[C]
    ○ Clindamycin (30 to 40 mg/kg/day) + cefixime (8mg/kg/day in 2 divided doses) or cefpodoxime (10 mg/kg/day in 2 divided doses) (1)[C] for non-type 1 PCN allergy
    ○ Ceftriaxone: 50 mg/kg IM single dose if not able to tolerate oral meds (4)[C]
- Because allergies may be a predisposing factor, some patients may benefit from use of the following agents:
  - Oral antihistamines
    ○ Loratadine (Claritin), fexofenadine (Allegra), cetirizine (Zyrtec), desloratadine (Clarinex), or levocetirizine (Xyzal)
    ○ Chlorpheniramine (Chlor-Trimeton)
    ○ Diphenhydramine (Benadryl)
  - Leukotriene inhibitors (Singulair, Accolate), especially in patients with asthma
  - Nasal steroids (i.e., fluticasone [Flonase])

Second Line
- Levofloxacin (Levaquin): 750 mg/day for 5 days or moxifloxacin 400 mg/day for 5 to 7 days (adults only) (1)[C]
- If no response to first-line therapy after 72 hours
  - Broaden antibiotic coverage or switch to a different class, evaluate for resistant pathogens or other causes for treatment failure (i.e., noninfectious etiology) fluoroquinolones as above.
- *Note*: Bacteriologic failure rates of up to 20–25% are possible with use of azithromycin and clarithromycin.
- If lack of response to 3 weeks of antibiotics, consider the following:
  - CT scan of sinuses
  - Ear/nose/throat (ENT) referral

ISSUES FOR REFERRAL
Complications or failure of treatment

ALERT
- Meta-analyses have demonstrated no benefit of newer antibiotics over amoxicillin or doxycycline.
- Antibiotics recommendations vary with different guidelines. Patients seen by specialists are different from those in a primary care setting. Patients usually do not have complicated sinusitis in primary care setting.
  - American Academy of Otolaryngology—Head and Neck Surgery Foundation (2)[C] recommends the following:
    ○ Consider watchful waiting without antibiotics in patients with uncomplicated mild illness (mild pain and temperature <101°F) with assurance of follow-up within 7 days.
- PCV-13 pneumococcal vaccine can be helpful in reducing chronic sinusitis in children (5)[B].
- Use of intranasal steroids small but significant improvement in symptoms when used alone or in combination with antibiotics (6)[A].
- Precautions
  - Decongestants can exacerbate hypertension.
  - Intranasal decongestants should be limited to 3 days to avoid rebound nasal congestion.

Pregnancy Considerations
- Nasal irrigation with saline, pseudoephedrine, most antihistamines, and some nasal steroids are safe during pregnancy and lactation.
- Antibiotics safe in pregnancy and lactation
  - Amoxicillin, amoxicillin-clavulanate, cephalosporins
- Antibiotic contraindicated: doxycycline, fluoroquinolones
- Antibiotic safe in lactation but not pregnancy: levofloxacin

SURGERY/OTHER PROCEDURES
- If medical therapy fails, consider sinus irrigation.
- Functional endoscopic sinus surgery is the preferred treatment for medically recalcitrant cases.
- Absolute surgical indications
  - Massive nasal polyposis
  - Acute complications: subperiosteal or orbital abscess, frontal soft tissue spread of infection
  - Mucocele or mucopyocele
  - Invasive or allergic fungal sinusitis
  - Suspected obstructing tumor
  - CSF rhinorrhea

INPATIENT CONSIDERATIONS
Hospitalization for complications (e.g., meningitis, orbital cellulitis or abscess, brain abscess)

ONGOING CARE

FOLLOW-UP RECOMMENDATIONS
Return if no improvement after 72 hours or no resolution of symptoms after 10 days of antibiotics.

PATIENT EDUCATION
- http://familydoctor.org/familydoctor/en.html
- https://www.nlm.nih.gov/medlineplus/

PROGNOSIS
Alleviation of symptoms within 72 hours with complete resolution within 10 to 14 days

COMPLICATIONS
- Serious complications are rare.
- Meningitis, orbital cellulitis, brain abscess
- Cavernous sinus thrombosis
- Osteomyelitis, subdural empyema

REFERENCES
1. Chow AW, Benninger MS, Brook I, et al. IDSA clinical practice guideline for acute bacterial rhinosinusitis in children and adults. *Clin Infect Dis*. 2012;54(8):e72–e112.
2. Rosenfeld RM, Piccirillo JF, Chandrasekhar SS, et al. Clinical practice guideline (update): adult sinusitis. *Otolaryngol Head Neck Surg*. 2015;152(2 Suppl): S1–S39.
3. Ahovuo-Saloranta A, Rautakorpi UM, Borisenko OV, et al. Antibiotics for acute maxillary sinusitis in adults. *Cochrane Database Syst Rev*. 2014;(2):CD000243.
4. Wald ER, Applegate KE, Bordley C, et al. Clinical practice guideline for the diagnosis and management of acute bacterial sinusitis in children aged 1 to 18 years. *Pediatrics*. 2013;132(1):e262–e280.
5. Olarte L, Hulten KG, Lamberth L, et al. Impact of the 13-valent pneumococcal conjugate vaccine on chronic sinusitis associated with *Streptococcus pneumoniae* in children. *Pediatr Infect Dis J*. 2014; 33(10):1033–1036.
6. Hayward G, Heneghan C, Perera R, et al. Intranasal corticosteroids in management of acute sinusitis: a systematic review and meta-analysis. *Ann Fam Med*. 2012;10(3):241–249.

ADDITIONAL READING
- Aring AM, Chan MM. Acute rhinosinusitis in adults. *Am Fam Physician*. 2011;83(9):1057–1063.
- Centers for Disease Control and Prevention. Get Smart: homepage. http://www.cdc.gov/getsmart/.
- Williams JW Jr, Aguilar C, Cornell J, et al. Antibiotics for acute maxillary sinusitis. *Cochrane Database Syst Rev*. 2003;(2):CD000243.
- Wilson JF. In the clinic. Acute sinusitis. *Annal Intern Med*. 2010;153(5):ITC3-1–ITC3-15.

CODES

ICD10
- J01.90 Acute sinusitis, unspecified
- J01.00 Acute maxillary sinusitis, unspecified
- J01.20 Acute ethmoidal sinusitis, unspecified

CLINICAL PEARLS
- When bacterial infection is present, patients recover somewhat more quickly with antibiotics, but the majority will recover with symptomatic treatment alone, and accurate diagnosis of bacterial sinusitis is very difficult.
- Multiple meta-analyses have demonstrated *no* benefit of newer antibiotics over amoxicillin or doxycycline.
- Overall NNT to prevent 1 persistent case at follow-up = 15; harm due to antibiotic-associated diarrhea is similar.
- Significant patient symptom relief with nasal saline spray or drops or irrigation (Neti pot)

SJÖGREN SYNDROME

Mariya Milko, DO, MS • Rubaiya Mallay, DO, FACOI, ACR

 BASICS

- Chronic inflammatory disorder characterized by lymphocytic infiltrates in exocrine organs
- Typically presents with diminished salivary and lacrimal gland function, resulting in sicca symptoms such as dry eyes (xerophthalmia), dry mouth (xerostomia), and parotid enlargement
- Extraglandular manifestations: arthralgia, myalgia, Raynaud phenomenon, pulmonary disease, GI disease, leukopenia, anemia, lymphadenopathy, vasculitis, renal tubular acidosis, lymphoma, CNS involvement with longitudinal transverse myelitis (>4 vertebral segments), and optic neuritis associated with anti-aquaporin-4 antibodies, PNS involvement with small fiber neuropathy
- Primary Sjögren: Not associated with other diseases; *HLA-DRB1*0301* and *HLA-DRB1*1501* are the most common.
- Secondary Sjögren: complication of other rheumatologic conditions, most commonly rheumatoid arthritis; associated with HLA-DR4
- First described by Swedish ophthalmologist Henrik Sjögren (1899–1986)

EPIDEMIOLOGY
Incidence
Annual incidence: ~4/100,000. Primary SS is one of the most common autoimmune diseases, affecting 1–4% of population.
- All races are affected
- Predominant sex: female > male (9:1)
- Predominant age: can affect patients of any age but is most common in the elderly; onset typically in the 4th to 5th decades of life

Prevalence
Sjögren syndrome (SS) affects 1 to 4 million people in the United States.

ETIOLOGY AND PATHOPHYSIOLOGY
- Multifactorial systemic autoimmune process characterized by infiltration of glandular tissue by CD4 T-lymphocytes
- Theorized that glandular epithelial cells present antigen to the T cells. Cytokine production then occurs. There is also evidence for B-cell activation, resulting in autoantibody production and an increased incidence of B-cell malignancies.
- Etiology is unknown. Estrogen may play a role because SS is more common in women. Exogenous factors such as viral proteins (EBV, HCV, HTLV-1) have also been implicated.

Genetics
- A familial tendency suggests a genetic predisposition.
- Associations in the HLA regions *HLA-DQA1*0501*, *HLA-DQB1*0201*, and *HLA-DRB*0301* are the strongest genetic risk factors for SS.

RISK FACTORS
There are no known modifiable risk factors.

GENERAL PREVENTION
- No known prevention. Complications can be prevented by early diagnosis and treatment.
- Oral health providers play a key role in early detection and management of symptoms resulting from salivary dysfunction (1)[C].

COMMONLY ASSOCIATED CONDITIONS
Secondary SS associated with rheumatoid arthritis, scleroderma, systemic lupus erythematosus (SLE), polymyositis, HIV, hepatitis C, MCTD, PBC, hypergammaglobulinemic purpura, necrotizing vasculitis, autoimmune thyroiditis, chronic active hepatitis, mixed cryoglobulinemia

Pregnancy Considerations
Pregnant SS patients with anti-SSA Abs have increased risk of delivering fetus with skin rash and 3rd-degree heart block.

 DIAGNOSIS

- American College of Rheumatology Diagnostic Criteria (2)[A]: Individuals with signs/symptoms that may be suggestive of SS, who have at least two of the following three objective features:
  – Positive serum anti-SSA/Ro and/or anti-SSB/La or (positive rheumatoid factor and ANA titer—1:320)
  – Labial salivary gland biopsy exhibiting focal lymphocytic sialadenitis with a focus score 1 focus/4 mm^2
  – Keratoconjunctivitis sicca with ocular staining score >3 (assuming that individual is not currently using daily eye drops for glaucoma and has not had corneal surgery or cosmetic eyelid surgery in the last 5 years)
- Ocular signs and symptoms
  – Troublesome dry eyes daily for >3 months
  – Recurrent sandy/gritty ocular sensation
  – Use of tear substitute >3 times per day
- Oral signs and symptoms
  – Daily symptoms of dry mouth for ≥3 months
  – Recurrent feeling of swollen salivary glands
  – Need to drink liquid to help swallow dry foods
- Other manifestations: chronic arthritis, type 1 RTA, tubular interstitial nephritis, rheumatoid arthritis, vasculitis, vaginal dryness, pleuritis, pancreatitis

HISTORY
- Decreased tear production; burning, scratchy sensation in eyes
- Difficulty speaking/swallowing, dental caries, xerotrachea
- Enlarged parotid glands or intermittent swelling (bilateral)
- Dyspareunia; vaginal dryness

PHYSICAL EXAM
Common physical exam findings include:
- Eye exam: dry eyes (keratoconjunctivitis sicca), decreased tear pool in the lower conjunctiva, dilated conjunctival vessels, mucinous threads, and filamentary keratosis (slit-lamp examination)
- Mouth exam: dry mouth (xerostomia); decreased sublingual salivary pool (tongue may stick to the tongue depressor); frequent oral caries (sometimes in unusual locations such as the incisor surface and along the gum line); dark red tongue from prolonged xerostomia
- Ear, nose, and throat exam: parotid enlargement, submandibular enlargement
- Skin exam: nonpalpable or palpable vasculitic purpura (typically 2 to 3 mm in diameter and on the lower extremities)

DIFFERENTIAL DIAGNOSIS
- Causes of ocular dryness: hypovitaminosis A, decreased tear production unrelated to autoimmune process, chronic blepharitis or conjunctivitis, impaired blinking (i.e., due to Parkinson disease or Bell palsy), infiltration of lacrimal glands (i.e., amyloidosis, lymphoma, sarcoidosis), low estrogen levels
- Causes of oral dryness: anticholinergic medications, sialadenitis due to chronic obstruction, chronic viral infections (i.e., hepatitis C or HIV), radiation of head/neck
- Causes of salivary gland swelling: unilateral: obstruction, chronic sialadenitis, bacterial infection, neoplasm; bilateral (asymmetric): IgG4-related disease, HIV bilateral (symmetric): hepatic cirrhosis, DM, anorexia/bulimia, acromegaly, alcoholism, hypolipoproteinemia, chronic pancreatitis, acute or chronic viral infection (i.e., mumps, Epstein-Barr virus [EBV], coxsackievirus, echovirus, granulomatous diseases (i.e., tuberculosis, sarcoidosis)

DIAGNOSTIC TESTS & INTERPRETATION
The following tests can be used to support diagnosis:
- Schirmer test (<5-mm wetness after 5 minutes)
- Rose Bengal test (slit lamp)
- Minor salivary gland biopsy (gold standard)
- Auto antibodies: +ANAs (95%), +RF (75%)
- In primary SS: +anti-Ro (anti-SSA, 56%) and +anti-La (anti-SSB, 30%)

Initial Tests (lab, imaging)
Preliminary lab workup
- Basic labs: CBC with differential, BUN/creatinine (Cr), AST/ALT, ESR, C-reactive protein (CRP), urinalysis (UA)
- Special labs: ANA, rheumatoid factor (RF), anti-Ro/SSA, anti-La/SSB, ESR, CRP
- Anti-SSA and anti-SSB antibodies present in 33–74% and 23–52% of SS patients, respectively.
- Other auto antibodies-muscarinic receptor type 3 (M3R) and anti-α-fodrin are being explored with good specificity (3)[A].
- Initial imaging studies may include:
  – Imaging for xerostomia: salivary gland scintigraphy (insensitive but highly specific)
  – Parotid gland sialography (should not be used in acute parotitis)
  – MRI (correlates well with salivary gland biopsy)
- A novel diagnostic tool is Salivary Gland US (SGUS) which is noninvasive and highly specific for salivary gland involvement in SS (4)[A].

Diagnostic Procedures/Surgery
- Salivary gland biopsy: used to confirm suspected diagnosis of SS or to exclude other causes of xerostomia and bilateral glandular enlargement
- Parotid biopsy if malignancy is suspected
- Lymph node biopsy to rule out pseudolymphoma or lymphoma if suspected

Test Interpretation
- Salivary gland histology shows focal collections of lymphocytes; immunocytology shows CD4+ T cell lymphocyte predominance.
- SGUS parameters include:
  - Parenchymal nonhomogeneity—the most useful diagnostic marker with high specificity and good sensitivity (4)[A].
  - US inflammatory findings include hypoechoic and hyperechoic bands (4)[A].
  - Real-time sonoelastography (RTS) to quantify tissue rigidity and assess glandular damage (4)[A]

TREATMENT
- Treatment is primarily supportive.
- Treat sicca symptoms—dry eyes, dry mouth
- Avoid medications that may worsen oral dryness (i.e., anticholinergics).
- Promote good oral hygiene.
- Treat systemic manifestations.
- Address fatigue and pain.

MEDICATION
- Therapy for sicca symptoms: artificial tears and ocular lubricants (5)[C]
- Topical therapy for dry mouth: can be as simple as liberally drinking sips of water, trying sugar-free lemon drops or artificial saliva preparations such as Salivart, Saliment, Xero-Lube, MouthKote
- Immunosuppressive therapy such as hydroxychloroquine can be used for systemic symptoms; however, it has not shown any benefit in relieving refractory sicca symptoms.
- Evoxac (Cevimeline) may be prescribed for SS-associated xerostomia. It works by stimulating muscarinic cholinergic receptors to increase salivary gland secretion.
- Dry eyes are graded by severity of symptoms, conjunctival injection and staining, corneal damage, tear quality, and lid involvement. Artificial tears may be used; however, artificial tears with hydroxyethylcellulose or dextran are more viscous and can last longer.
- Acetaminophen or NSAIDs for arthralgias

First Line
- Xerostomia: sugar-free lozenges, especially malic acid, artificial saliva; pilocarpine 5 mg PO QID or cevimeline 30 mg PO TID
- Keratoconjunctivitis sicca: artificial tears and ocular lubricants for symptomatic relief, topical cyclosporine (Restasis), or autologous tears

Second Line
- Xerostomia: Interferon-alfa lozenges may enhance salivary gland flow.
- Keratoconjunctivitis sicca: topical glucocorticoids or topical NSAIDs (use with caution)
- Immunosuppressive therapy: antimalarials (e.g., hydroxychloroquine) for arthralgias, lymphadenopathies, and skin manifestations; may then consider methotrexate or cyclosporine, which showed subjective improvement but no significant objective improvement
- Early studies show improvement in fatigue with rituximab (6)[B].
- For life-threatening extraglandular manifestations, cyclophosphamide (PO or IV), mycophenolate mofetil, and azathioprine are often used.

ISSUES FOR REFERRAL
- A rheumatologist can help with management of systemic manifestations or resistant symptoms.
- Oral health
- Ophthalmology, for grading of severity and management of xerophthalmia

ADDITIONAL THERAPIES
- Patients should use vaginal lubricants, such as Replens, for vaginal dryness. Vaginal estrogen creams can help in postmenopausal women. Be alert for and treat vaginal yeast infections.
- Xerostomia: small sips of water, good dental care
- Keratoconjunctivitis sicca: Conserve tears with side shields or ski/swim goggles, humidifiers, and moist washcloths.
- Dehydroepiandrosterone (DHEA) does not offer improvement in fatigue and well-being above placebo.

SURGERY/OTHER PROCEDURES
Keratoconjunctivitis sicca: If refractory to artificial tears, punctal occlusion is the treatment of choice.

COMPLEMENTARY & ALTERNATIVE MEDICINE
- Some studies show acupuncture benefits saliva production and symptoms of xerostomia.
- There is insufficient evidence to determine the effects of electrostimulation devices on dry mouth symptoms or saliva production in patients with Sjögren syndrome.

INPATIENT CONSIDERATIONS
May be required for extraglandular manifestations, such as cardiopulmonary disease, renal involvement, and CNS manifestations (e.g., optic neuritis, transverse myelitis, vasculitis, or ischemic stroke)

 ONGOING CARE

FOLLOW-UP RECOMMENDATIONS
Frequency of follow-up depends on severity

Patient Monitoring
- Monitor for complications, systemic manifestations, and relief of symptoms.
- Medicolegal pitfalls: Monitor for parotid tumor or lymphoma.

PATIENT EDUCATION
In most cases, simple measures are adequate: humidifiers, sips of water, chewing gum, or artificial tears.

PROGNOSIS
- Hypocomplementemia is an independent risk factor for premature death.
- Primary SS is associated with increased risks of malignancy, non-Hodgkin lymphoma, and thyroid cancer.

COMPLICATIONS
Complications include dental caries, gum disease, dysphagia, salivary gland calculi, keratitis, conjunctivitis, and scarring of the ocular surface.

REFERENCES
1. Mays JW, Sarmadi M, Moutsopoulos NM. Oral manifestations of systemic autoimmune and inflammatory diseases: diagnosis and clinical management. *J Evid Based Dent Pract.* 2012;12(3 Suppl):265–282.
2. Shiboski SC, Shiboski CH, Criswell L, et al. American College of Rheumatology classification criteria for Sjögren's syndrome: a data-driven, expert consensus approach in the Sjögren's International Collaborative Clinical Alliance cohort. *Arthritis Care Res (Hoboken).* 2012;64(4):475–487.
3. Deng C, Hu C, Chen S, et al. Meta-analysis of anti-muscarinic receptor type 3 antibodies for the diagnosis of Sjögren syndrome. *PLoS One.* 2015;10(1):e0116744.
4. Luciano N, Valentini V, Calabrò A, et al. One year in review 2015: Sjögren's syndrome. *Clin Exp Rheumatol.* 2015;33(2): 259–271.
5. Aragona P, Spinella R, Rania L, et al. Safety and efficacy of 0.1% clobetasone butyrate eyedrops in the treatment of dry eye in Sjögren syndrome. *Eur J Ophthalmol.* 2013;23(3):368–376.
6. Meijer JM, Meiners PM, Vissink A, et al. Effectiveness of rituximab treatment in primary Sjögren's syndrome: a randomized, double-blind, placebo-controlled trial. *Arthritis Rheum.* 2010;62(4): 960–968.

 CODES

ICD10
- M35.00 Sicca syndrome, unspecified
- M35.02 Sicca syndrome with lung involvement
- M35.09 Sicca syndrome with other organ involvement

CLINICAL PEARLS
- Many symptoms of SS can be treated with simple interventions such as artificial tears and sugar-free lozenges.
- Consider lacrimal duct plugs for dry eyes.
- Consider SS in patients with unexplained lung disease and +ANA.
- Patients with primary SS may have an increased incidence of celiac disease because both disease share similar genetics.

SLEEP APNEA, OBSTRUCTIVE

Sonya Shipley, MD

 BASICS

DESCRIPTION
- Obstructive sleep apnea (OSA) is defined as repetitive episodes of cessation of airflow (apnea) at the nose and mouth during sleep due to obstruction at the level of the pharynx.
  - Apneas often terminate with a snort/gasp.
  - Repetitive apneas produce sleep disruption, leading to excessive daytime sleepiness.
  - Associated with oxygen desaturation and nocturnal hypoxemia
  - Usual course is chronic.
- System(s) affected: cardiovascular; nervous; pulmonary
- Synonym(s): Pickwickian syndrome; sleep apnea syndrome; nocturnal upper airway occlusion

EPIDEMIOLOGY
Incidence
- Predominant age: middle-aged men and women
- Predominant sex: male > female (2:1)

Prevalence
- Up to 4% in men, 2% in women
- Prevalence is higher in obese/hypertensive patients.

ETIOLOGY AND PATHOPHYSIOLOGY
OSA occurs when the naso- or oropharynx collapses passively during inspiration. Anatomic and neuromuscular factors contribute to pharyngeal collapse.
- Anatomic abnormalities such as increased soft tissue in the palate, tonsillar hypertrophy, macroglossia, and craniofacial abnormalities, predispose the airway to collapse by decreasing the area of the upper airway or increasing the pressure surrounding the airway.
- During sleep, decreased muscle tone in the naso- or oropharynx contributes to airway obstruction and collapse.
- Upper airway narrowing may be due to the following:
  - Obesity, redundant tissue in the soft palate
  - Enlarged tonsils/uvula
  - Low soft palate
  - Large/posteriorly located tongue
  - Craniofacial abnormalities
  - Neuromuscular disorders
  - Alcohol/sedative use before bedtime

RISK FACTORS
- Obesity
- Age >40 years
- Alcohol/sedative intake before bedtime
- Smoking
- Nasal obstruction (due to polyps, rhinitis, or deviated septum)
- Anatomic narrowing of nasopharynx (e.g., tonsillar hypertrophy, macroglossia, micrognathia, retrognathia, craniofacial abnormalities)
- Acromegaly
- Hypothyroidism
- Neurologic syndromes (e.g., muscular dystrophy, cerebral palsy)

GENERAL PREVENTION
Weight control and avoidance of alcohol and sedatives at night can help to prevent airway collapse.

COMMONLY ASSOCIATED CONDITIONS
- Common
  - Hypertension
  - Obesity
  - Daytime sleepiness
  - Metabolic syndrome
- Rare
  - Cardiac arrhythmias
  - Cardiovascular disease
  - Congestive heart failure
  - Pulmonary hypertension
  - Nasal obstructive problems

 DIAGNOSIS

HISTORY
- Elicit a complete history of daytime and nighttime symptoms. Symptoms can be insidious and present for years.
- Daytime symptoms
  - Excessive daytime sleepiness (EDS) or fatigue (cardinal symptom) (1)[A]
    - Mild symptoms occur during quiet activities (e.g., reading, watching television).
    - Severe symptoms occur during dynamic activities (e.g., work, driving).
  - Tired on morning awakening
  - Sore/dry throat
  - Poor concentration, memory problems, irritability, mood changes
  - Morning headaches
  - Decreased libido
  - Depression
- Nighttime symptoms
  - Loud snoring (present in 60% of people with OSA)
  - Snort/gasp that arouses patient from sleep
  - Disrupted sleep
  - Witnessed apneic episodes at night

PHYSICAL EXAM
- OSA is commonly associated with obesity. It is unlikely to be found in those with normal body weight who do not snore (1)[A].
- Focused head and neck exam
  - Short neck with large circumference
  - Oropharynx
    - Narrowing of the lateral airway wall
    - Tonsillar hypertrophy
    - Macroglossia
    - Micrognathia/retrognathia
    - Soft palate edema
    - Long/thick uvula
    - High, arched hard palate
  - Nasopharynx
    - Deviated nasal septum
    - Poor nasal airflow

DIFFERENTIAL DIAGNOSIS
- Other causes of EDS such as the following:
  - Narcolepsy
  - Idiopathic daytime hypersomnolence
  - Inadequate sleep time
  - Depressive episodes with EDS
  - Periodic limb movements disorder
- Respiratory disorders with nocturnal awakenings such as the following:
  - Asthma
  - Chronic obstructive pulmonary disease
  - Congestive heart failure
- Central sleep apnea
- Sleep-related choking/laryngospasm
- Gastroesophageal reflux
- Sleep-associated seizures (temporal lobe epilepsy)

DIAGNOSTIC TESTS & INTERPRETATION
Initial Tests (lab, imaging)
- When clinically indicated
  - Thyroid-stimulating hormone to evaluate hypothyroidism
  - CBC to evaluate anemia and polycythemia, which can indicate nocturnal hypoxemia.
  - Fasting glucose in obesity to evaluate for diabetes
  - Rare: arterial blood gases to evaluate daytime hypercapnia
- Cephalometric measurements from lateral head and neck radiographs aid in surgical treatment.

Diagnostic Procedures/Other
- The gold standard for OSA is polysomnography (PSG), a nighttime sleep study (1)[A].
  - Demonstrates severity of hypoxemia, sleep disruption, and cardiac arrhythmias associated with OSA and elevated end-tidal CO_2
  - Shows repetitive episodes of cessation/marked reduction in airflow despite continued respiratory efforts
  - Apneic episodes must last at least 10 seconds and occur 10 to 15 times per hour to be considered clinically significant.
  - Complete PSG is expensive, and health insurance may not cover the cost.
- Multiple sleep latency testing is a diagnostic tool used to measure the time it takes from the start of a daytime nap period to the first signs of sleep (sleep latency). It provides an objective measurement of daytime sleepiness.
- The apnea-hypopnea index (AHI) is defined as the total number of apneas and hypoapneas divided by the total sleep time.
  - Mild OSA: AHI = 5 to 15
  - Moderate OSA: AHI = 15 to 30
  - Severe OSA: AHI >30
- Drugs that may alter the test results include benzodiazepines and other sedatives that can amplify the severity of apnea seen during the sleep study.
- Early data suggest that home-based diagnosis using portable monitoring devices may be an alternative to laboratory-based PSG if the test is of sufficient duration (2)[B].

TREATMENT

- Lifestyle modification is the most frequently recommended treatment for mild to moderate OSA. This includes weight loss, exercise, and avoidance of alcohol, smoking, and sedatives, especially before bedtime. Weight loss has been shown to decrease the severity of symptoms in obese patients. Lifestyle modifications should be seen as adjunctive rather than curative therapy (3)[A], and a lack of improvement of symptoms with lifestyle modification should not preclude patients from receiving other therapy such as continuous positive airway pressure (CPAP).
- If OSA is present only when supine, keep the patient off his/her back when sleeping (e.g., tennis ball worn on back of nightshirt or using a sleep position trainer) (4)[B].

- The most effective therapy for mild, moderate, or severe OSA is CPAP (5)[B]. Treatment with CPAP uses a mask interface and a flow generator to prevent airway collapse, thus helping to prevent apnea, hypoxia, and sleep disturbance. Compared with inactive controls, CPAP significantly improves both objective (24-hour systolic and diastolic blood pressures) and subjective measures (Epworth Sleepiness Scale) in OSA patients with symptoms of daytime sleepiness (6)[A]. CPAP may also decrease the risk for atherosclerosis (7)[A] as well as improves insulin resistance in nondiabetic patients (8)[A]. Early data show that these benefits may not be seen in patients who do not have symptoms of daytime sleepiness (9)[B].
- Several types of mask interfaces, including nasal masks, oral masks, and nasal pillows exist for CPAP therapy. Short-term data suggest that nasal pillows are the preferred interface in almost all patients. In patients with compliance difficulty, a different choice of interface may be appropriate (10)[A].
- Oral appliances to treat OSA are available and often subjectively preferred by patients. Although oral appliances have been shown to improve symptoms compared with inactive controls, they are not as effective for reduction of respiratory disturbances as CPAP over short-term data. Treatment with oral appliances may be considered in patients who fail to comply with CPAP therapy (11)[A].

MEDICATION
Medications are yet to be proven effective in treating OSA (12)[A]. Further studies in this area are needed.

First Line
Some short-term data found fluticasone nasal spray, mirtazapine, physostigmine, and nasal lubricant of some benefit; longer-term studies needed.

ISSUES FOR REFERRAL
If sleep apnea is suspected, patient should be referred to a sleep specialist/neurologist for a sleep study evaluation.

SURGERY/OTHER PROCEDURES
Surgical corrections of the upper airway include alteration of the uvula and/or palate such as uvulopalato-pharyngoplasty (UPPP), tracheostomy, and craniofacial surgery. Currently no evidence supports the use of surgery for the treatment of OSA (13)[A].

INPATIENT CONSIDERATIONS
On admission, patients should continue to use CPAP/dental devices if they do so at home. They should bring in their own appliance and know their CPAP settings.

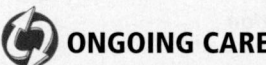 ONGOING CARE

Lifelong compliance with weight loss or CPAP is necessary for successful OSA treatment.

DIET
Overweight and obese patients should be encouraged to lose weight, and all patients must avoid weight gain. Weight loss alone could reduce symptoms of OSA (14)[A].

PATIENT EDUCATION
- Weight loss and avoidance of alcohol and sedatives may reduce OSA symptoms particularly in severe cases (15)[A].

- Significantly sleepy patients should not drive a motor vehicle/operate dangerous equipment.

PROGNOSIS
- EDS is reduced dramatically with appropriate apnea control.
- Lifelong compliance with weight loss or CPAP is necessary for effective treatment of OSA.
- If untreated, OSA is progressive.
- Significant morbidity and mortality with OSA usually are due to motor vehicle accidents or are secondary to cardiac complications, including arrhythmias, cardiac ischemia, and hypertension.

COMPLICATIONS
Untreated OSA may increase the risk for development of hypertension, stroke, myocardial infarction, diabetes, cardiovascular disease, and work-related and driving accidents.

Pediatric Considerations
- The prevalence of pediatric OSA is 1–2% in children 4 to 5 years of age, and the peak incidence is between 3 and 6 years of age.
- Predominant sex: male = female
- Etiology: The most common cause is tonsillar hypertrophy. Additional causes are obesity and craniofacial abnormalities. OSA is also seen in children with neuromuscular diseases, such as cerebral palsy and spinal muscular atrophy, due to abnormal pharyngeal muscle control.
- Signs and symptoms
  – Nighttime: loud snoring, restlessness, and sweating
  – Daytime: hyperactivity and decreased school performance
  – EDS is not a significant symptom.
- Diagnosis: Gold standard is PSG (PSG may be an even better tool in children due to lessened night-to-night variation. There is a lack of studies showing efficacy of home-based diagnostic studies vs. PSG in children). Abnormal AHI is different in children: >1 to 2/hr is abnormal.

- Treatment: Surgery is the first-line treatment in cases due to tonsillar enlargement (reduces symptoms in 70%). Some data suggest improved academic performance if tonsillectomy is performed for OSA. For cases due to obesity/craniofacial abnormalities, patients can use CPAP treatment (16)[A].

Geriatric Considerations
The presence of sleep apnea in the geriatric population may be associated with earlier onset of mild cognitive impairment as well as Dementia at an earlier age. The rate of decline of cognitive function may be slowed by the usage of CPAP (17)[B].

REFERENCES
1. Myers KA, Mrkobrada M, Simel DL. Does this patient have obstructive sleep apnea?: the rational clinical examination systematic review. *JAMA*. 2013;310(7):731–741.
2. Wittine LM, Olson EJ, Morgenthaler TI. Effect of recording duration on the diagnostic accuracy of out-of-center sleep testing for obstructive sleep apnea. *Sleep*. 2014;37(5):969–975.
3. Anandam A, Akinnusi M, Kufel T, et al. Effects of dietary weight loss on obstructive sleep apnea: a meta-analysis. *Sleep Breath*. 2013;17(1):227–234.
4. van Maanen JP, de Vries N. Long-term effectiveness and compliance of positional therapy with the sleep position trainer in the treatment of positional obstructive sleep apnea syndrome. *Sleep*. 2014;37(7):1209–1215.
5. Weaver TE, Mancini C, Maislin G, et al. Continuous positive airway pressure treatment of sleepy patients with milder obstructive sleep apnea: results of the CPAP Apnea Trial North American Program (CATNAP) randomized clinical trial. *Am J Respir Crit Care Med*. 2012;186(7): 677–683.
6. Giles TL, Lasserson TJ, Smith BH, et al. Continuous positive airways pressure for obstructive sleep apnoea in adults. *Cochrane Database Syst Rev*. 2006;(3):CD001106.
7. Drager LF, Polotsky VY, Lorenzi-Filho G. Obstructive sleep apnea: an emerging risk factor for atherosclerosis. *Chest*. 2011;140(2):534–542.
8. Yang D, Liu Z, Yang H, et al. Effects of continuous positive airway pressure on glycemic control and insulin resistance in patients with obstructive sleep apnea: a meta-analysis. *Sleep Breath*. 2013;17(1):33–38.
9. Barbé F, Durán-Cantolla J, Sánchez-de-la-Torre M, et al. Effect of continuous positive airway pressure on the incidence of hypertension and cardiovascular events in nonsleepy patients with obstructive sleep apnea: a randomized controlled trial. *JAMA*. 2012;307(20):2161–2168.
10. Chai CL, Pathinathan A, Smith B. Continuous positive airway pressure delivery interfaces for obstructive sleep apnoea. *Cochrane Database Syst Rev*. 2006;(4):CD005308.
11. Lim J, Lasserson TJ, Fleetham J, et al. Oral appliances for obstructive sleep apnoea. *Cochrane Database Syst Rev*. 2006;(1):CD004435.
12. Mason M, Welsh EJ, Smith I. Drug therapy for obstructive sleep apnoea in adults. *Cochrane Database Syst Rev*. 2013;(5):CD003002.
13. Sundaram S, Bridgman SA, Lim J, et al. Surgery for obstructive sleep apnoea. *Cochrane Database Syst Rev*. 2005;(4):CD001004.
14. Shneerson J, Wright J. Lifestyle modification for obstructive sleep apnoea. *Cochrane Database Syst Rev*. 2001;(1):CD002875.
15. Mason M, Cates CJ, Smith I. Effects of opioid, hypnotic and sedating medications on sleep-disordered breathing in adults with obstructive sleep apnoea. *Cochrane Database Syst Rev*. 2015;(7):CD011090.
16. Marcus CL, Brooks LJ, Draper KA, et al. Diagnosis and management of childhood obstructive sleep apnea syndrome. *Pediatrics*. 2012;130(3): e714–e755.
17. Osorio RS, Gumb T, Pirraglia E, et al. Sleep-disordered breathing advances cognitive decline in the elderly. *Neurology*. 2015;84(19):1964–1971.

 CODES

ICD10
G47.33 Obstructive sleep apnea (adult) (pediatric)

CLINICAL PEARLS
- OSA is characterized by repetitive episodes of apnea at the pharynx, often terminating in a snort/gasp.
- Laboratory PSG is the key to diagnosis.
- CPAP is the most effective form of treatment for both mild to moderate and moderate to severe OSA.
- Central sleep apnea may mimic OSA.

S

SLEEP DISORDER, SHIFT WORK

Ronald G. Chambers Jr., MD, FAAFP • Cindy J. Chambers, MD, MAS, MPH

 BASICS

DESCRIPTION
- The human system fundamentally relies on a natural circadian rhythm coordinated by the suprachiasmatic nucleus (SCN), an endogenous clock or pacemaker of the hypothalamus, which is responsible for linking the nervous system to the endocrine system (1).
- A shift in work schedule can desynchronize this circadian pacemaker with peripheral cells.
- The major environmental factor that can disrupt or reset the circadian rhythm is light at night (LAN) (1).
- Shift work disorder (SWD), also classified as circadian rhythm sleep disorder, shift work is a sleep disorder caused by a misalignment between the internal circadian rhythm and the required sleep-wake schedule resulting from erratic or nighttime shift work (2).
- Diagnostic criteria for SWD requires that all criteria for circadian rhythm disorders be met in addition to specific SWD criteria (see below).
- Criteria for circadian rhythm disorder:
  - A persistent/recurrent sleep disruption due to either an alteration in the circadian (24-hour) timekeeping system or due to a misalignment between endogenous circadian rhythm and exogenous factors that affect sleep
  - A complaint of insomnia/excessive daytime sleepiness or both
  - An impairment in occupational, educational, or social functioning
  - Insomnia or excessive sleepiness temporarily associated with a recurring work schedule that overlaps with the usual time for sleep
  - Symptoms associated with shift work schedule are present for at least 1 month
  - Sleep log or actigraphy monitoring (with sleep diaries) for at least 7 days demonstrates disturbed sleep (insomnia) and circadian and sleep time misalignment
  - Sleep disturbance is not due to another current sleep disorder, substance use disorder, or medication use.

EPIDEMIOLOGY
Prevalence
- Shift workers include those who work night shifts, evening shifts, or rotating shifts, and comprise approximately 15–25% of the workforce in the United States (2).
- SWD has been estimated to affect 10–23% of the presently 22 million American shift workers, with a prevalence estimate of approximately 2–5% of the general population (14.1% night shift workers and 8.1% of rotating shift workers) (3).

PATHOPHYSIOLOGY
- Circadian rhythms are evident in multiple biologic functions, including body temperature, hormone levels, blood pressure, metabolism, cellular regeneration, sleep/wake cycles, and DNA transcription and translation (2).

- Transcription factors involved in circadian rhythm generation collectively referred to as the "molecular clock," control production of the many proteins that are expressed within a period of approximately 24 hours. This molecular clock is self-sustaining but requires resetting daily or it may become out of sync with environmental cues also called "zeitgebers" (2).
- The most powerful *zeitgeber*, or timekeeper, is light. Light transmitted from the retinohypothalamic tract of the eye to the SCN of the hypothalamus upregulates the production of the "clock gene" (PER) (2).
- Periods of darkness cause the SCN to induce the release of melatonin from the pineal gland, which can also help to reset the molecular clock (2).
- A dysynchrony between the endogenous molecular clock and external cues (most notably light/dark cycles) is responsible for the development of circadian rhythm disorders and can have a severe impact on both physical and mental health (2).

RISK FACTORS
- Shift work, including night shifts, early morning shifts, or rotating shifts
- Younger age and "eveningness" (a.k.a. "night owls" rather than "morning larks") may provide some protection from the development of SWD (2).

Genetics
No genetic predisposition has been described.

GENERAL PREVENTION
- Limit rotating shifts.
- Use of bright light during shifts
- Scheduling brief, strategic 10- to 20-minute naps during shifts, if suitable

COMMONLY ASSOCIATED CONDITIONS
- Shift workers in general have impaired immediate free recall, decreased processing speed, and selective attention, impairments that may worsen with longer duration of shift work (2).
- Shift workers also have been shown to have a much higher risk of vehicular accidents, job-related injuries, absenteeism, and quality control errors (2).
- SWD has been associated with GI disease, specifically peptic ulcer disease, cardiovascular disease (CVD), infertility, mood disorders, and pregnancy complications (2).
- There is also evidence for possible increased risk of breast and prostate cancer. As such, the International Agency for Research on Cancer (IARC) has classified shift work that involves a circadian disruption as a probable carcinogen (1).

DIAGNOSIS

This is primarily a clinical diagnosis. However, there are some useful diagnostic aids.

HISTORY
- A careful history is critical to assess sleep disturbance including difficulty falling asleep, staying asleep, or nonrestorative sleep.
- Special attention should be paid to the following (4)[C]:
  - Sleep/wake habits
  - Degree of alertness or sleepiness

  - Sleep environment
  - Light exposure before, during, and after the shift
  - Job-related factors: length of shift, number of consecutive shifts, commute after shift.
  - Medications as well as over-the-counter (OTC) stimulants such as caffeine and energy drinks
  - Impact on social and domestic responsibilities (including drowsy driving)
- It is also essential to evaluate for symptoms of other sleep disorders, which often coexist and can exacerbate SWD such as the following:
  - Snoring (obstructive sleep apnea [OSA])
  - Sudden sleep attacks and leg symptoms (restless legs syndrome [RLS])
  - Falling asleep at inappropriate times, drop attacks, and daytime fatigue (narcolepsy)

PHYSICAL EXAM
Evaluate for depression, GI, CV, and potential cancer risk as well as signs of OSA such as obesity, a large neck, and a tight oropharynx (4)[C].

DIFFERENTIAL DIAGNOSIS
- Other primary sleep disorders: OSA, RLS, narcolepsy, and psychophysiologic insomnia.
- Other circadian rhythm sleep disorder such as delayed sleep phase disorder or jet lag syndrome. Distinguishing among these is challenging even for sleep specialists.

DIAGNOSTIC TESTS & INTERPRETATION
Given possible increased risk for CVD and cancer among shift workers, consider appropriate screenings.

Initial Tests (lab, imaging)
Fasting lipid panel, fasting glucose, age-appropriate cancer screenings

Diagnostic Procedures/Other
- Evaluation of a sleep/wake diary that records the patient's sleep/wake habits including amount of sleep, naps during the waking hours, and mood (1 to 2 weeks) (4)[C].
- Consider actigraphy (a mechanical device, often worn on the arm/leg, to measure movement): serves as a gross measure of time and amount of activity and rest (4)[C]
- Polysomnography, a measure of sleep duration and quality is not typically used to diagnose SWD but may be helpful in ruling out other sleep/wake disorders such as sleep apnea and narcolepsy (2)[C].
- Several diagnostic tools are available including the Multiple Sleep Latency Test (MSLT), the Morningness-Eveningness Questionnaire (MEQ), and the Epworth Sleepiness Scale (ESS) to help determine circadian misalignment (2)[C].

Test Interpretation
Typically, sleep diaries and actigraph data reveal the following:
- Increased sleep latency
- Decreased total sleep time
- Frequent awakenings
- Notably, most people revert to nocturnal sleeping on their days off, meaning that every workweek, they start fresh in their attempt to shift their circadian rhythms to align with work schedules.

TREATMENT

- The only therapeutic modality deemed as "standard" by the American Academy of Sleep Medicine is planned (or prescribed) sleep schedules (5)[C].
- Other commonly used treatment strategies include optimizing sleep hygiene, bright light, melatonin, caffeine and other stimulants as well as hypnotics and other medication sleep aids (discussed below).

GENERAL MEASURES

- Sleep hygiene: An important first step in approaching the treatment of sleep disorders is to educate the patient on proper sleep hygiene including minimizing exposure to bright light before and during scheduled sleep periods (maintain a dark sleeping space, wear dark sunglasses following work shift, wearing eye mask to sleep), maintaining a quiet sleep environment (wearing ear plugs to sleep, disconnecting phone, doorbell), retraining core body temperature to shifted sleep/wake schedule (maintain cool sleeping quarters), and avoiding use of stimulants during second half of work shift (2)[C].
- Sleep time: Educate on need of protected time for sleep prior to and following work shifts with strategic use of naps when possible (4)[C].
- Address work/social/domestic factors: Treat psychosocial stress, depression, encourage healthy eating habits, limit substance use, increase exercise to at least 30 minutes 5 times per week (not within 2 to 4 hours of bedtime) (4)[C].
- Work-related interventions: If possible, reduce number of consecutive shifts (<4) or reduce shift duration (<12 hours), allow adequate time between shifts (>11 hours), and move heavy workload outside circadian nadir (04:00 to 07:00) (4)[C].
- Bright light: Several studies have demonstrated that timed bright light and darkness can promote adaptation to night work (6)[C].
- Bright light therapy with conventional light/light boxes (10,000 lux preferable, but >1,000 lux will help) should be given 30 min/day during the night/early morning shift prior to the nadir of the core body temperature rhythm (6)[C].

MEDICATION

- Melatonin may help shift circadian rhythms and can increase the quality and duration of sleep as well as increase alertness during the work shift.
- Ramelteon (Rozerem), a melatonin receptor agonist, is not FDA-approved for the treatment of SWD but may be helpful in improving daytime sleep (2)[C].
- Antidepressants: Doxepin (tricyclic) and trazodone are FDA-approved for the treatment of insomnia. Given at low doses, doxepin and trazodone can improve sleep without residual daytime impairment (2)[C].
- Intermediate-acting hypnotics zolpidem (Ambien) or eszopiclone (Lunesta) may be used (see below) but can cause postsleep sedation (2)[C].
- Wakefulness-promoting medications are as follows:
  - Modafinil and armodafinil are FDA approved for excessive sleepiness in patients with SWD and can reduce daytime sleepiness and improve cognitive performance (2)[C].
  - Prophylactic caffeine use (200 mg) immediately prior to work shift and during work shift (4)[C].

First Line
Circadian shift/sleep promoting: Melatonin, 3 mg PO or sublingual, 30 minutes before daytime sleep period. It should be taken only when the patient is home and able to go to bed if the hypnotic effects begin (2)[C].

Second Line
- Wakefulness-promoting:
  - Modafinil (Provigil) 100 to 200 mg PO 60 minutes before the shift begins
  - Armodafinil (Nuvigil) 150 to 250 mg is long-acting (12 to 16 hours, depending on food intake) and should be used judiciously in SWD as not to impede a patient's ability to sleep after the shift.
- Sleep promoting:
  - Nonbenzodiazepine hypnotics
    - Zolpidem (Ambien) 5 to 10 mg or eszopiclone (Lunesta) 2 to 3 mg 30 minutes before desired sleep period. Eszopiclone is the only hypnotic approved for use over 35 days.
  - Antidepressants: Doxepin (1 to 6 mg) and trazodone (25 to 50 mg), 1 to 2 hours prior to bed (2)[C]
- Benzodiazepines: Estazolam, flurazepam, quazepam, temazepam, and triazolam are FDA-approved for the treatment of insomnia; however, they have high risk of tolerance and withdrawal, and should be used cautiously for short-term treatment of insomnia (2)[C].
- In general, hypnotics may improve daytime sleep; however, they do not appear to improve sleep maintenance, nighttime alertness, and may cause residual sedation during the work hours, potentially worsening SWD symptoms (2)[C].

ISSUES FOR REFERRAL
Refer to a sleep specialist if there is suspicion of other primary sleep disorders; dependence on hypnotics, alcohol, or stimulants

ONGOING CARE

PATIENT EDUCATION
- Health care providers should discuss good sleep hygiene and recommend on how to optimize the sleep environment.
- Shift workers who need to sleep in the daytime must take serious measures to ensure that their sleep environment is cool, dark, and quiet.
- Reserve bedroom for sleeping and intimacy only. Remove all televisions and telephones from bedroom.
- When going to sleep, turn clock away from bed; discourage prolonged reading in bed.
- Blackout shades are usually necessary in order to achieve the proper darkness.

REFERENCES

1. Stevens RG, Hansen J, Costa G, et al. Considerations of circadian impact for defining "shift work" in cancer studies: IARC Working Group Report. *Occup Environ Med.* 2011;68(2):154–162.
2. Morrissette DA. Twisting the night away: a review of the neurobiology, genetics, diagnosis, and treatment of shift work disorder. *CNS Spectr.* 2013;18(Suppl 1):45–53.
3. Roth T. Appropriate therapeutic selection for patients with shift work disorder. *Sleep Med.* 2012;13(4):335–341.
4. Wright KP Jr, Bogan RK, Wyatt JK. Shift work and the assessment and management of shift work disorder (SWD). *Sleep Med Rev.* 2013;17(1):41–54.
5. American Academy of Sleep Medicine. *The International Classification of Sleep Disorders: Diagnostic and Coding Manual.* 2nd ed. Westchester, IL: American Academy of Sleep Medicine; 2005.
6. Bjorvatn B, Pallesen S. A practical approach to circadian rhythm sleep disorders. *Sleep Med Rev.* 2009;13(1):47–60.

ADDITIONAL READING

- Morgenthaler TI, Lee-Chiong T, Alessi C, et al. Practice parameters for the clinical evaluation and treatment of circadian rhythm sleep disorders. An American Academy of Sleep Medicine report. *Sleep.* 2007;30(11):1445–1459.
- Sack RL, Auckley D, Auger RR, et al. Circadian rhythm sleep disorders: part I, basic principles, shift work and jet lag disorders. An American Academy of Sleep Medicine review. *Sleep.* 2007;30(11):1460–1483.
- Sleep Diary: http://www.helpguide.org/life/pdfs/sleep_diary.pdf.

 CODES

ICD10
G47.26 Circadian rhythm sleep disorder, shift work type

CLINICAL PEARLS

- SWD is associated with shortened and disturbed sleep, fatigue, decreased alertness, cognitive decrements, increased injuries and accidents, reproductive problems, and risks to cardiovascular and gastrointestinal health, and has been classified as a carcinogen given possible association with breast and prostate cancer.
- The most important first diagnostic step in SWD is to obtain and evaluate a sleep diary.

SMELL AND TASTE DISORDERS

Beth Mazyck, MD • Daniel B. Kurtz, PhD

 BASICS

DESCRIPTION
- The senses of smell and taste allow a full appreciation of the flavor and palatability of foods and also serve as a warning system against toxins, polluted air, smoke, and spoiled food.
- Physiologically, the chemical senses aid in normal digestion by triggering GI secretions. Smell/taste dysfunction may have a significant impact on quality of life.
- Loss of smell occurs more frequently than loss of taste, and patients frequently confuse the concepts of flavor loss (as a result of smell impairment) with taste loss (an impaired ability to sense sweet, sour, salty, or bitter).
- Smell depends on the functioning of CN I (olfactory nerve) and CN V (trigeminal nerve).
- Taste depends on the functioning of CNs VII, IX, and X. Because of these multiple pathways, total loss of taste (ageusia) is rare.
- Systems affected: nervous, upper respiratory

EPIDEMIOLOGY
Incidence
There are ~200,000 patient visits a year for smell and taste disturbances.

Prevalence
- Predominant sex: male > female. Men begin to lose their ability to smell earlier in life than women.
- Predominant age: Chemosensory loss is age dependent:
  - Age >80 years: 80% have major olfactory impairment; nearly 50% are anosmic.
  - Ages 65 to 80 years: 60% have major olfactory impairment; nearly 25% are anosmic.
  - Age <65 years: 1–2% have smell impairment.
- Estimated >2 million affected in the United States

ETIOLOGY AND PATHOPHYSIOLOGY
- Smell and/or taste disturbances:
  - Nutritional factors (e.g., malnutrition, vitamin deficiencies, liver disease, pernicious anemia)
  - Endocrine disorders (e.g., thyroid disease, diabetes mellitus, renal disease)
  - Head trauma
  - Migraine headache (e.g., gustatory aura, olfactory aura)
  - Sjögren syndrome
  - Toxic chemical exposure
  - Industrial agent exposure
  - Aging
  - Medications (see below)
  - Neurodegenerative diseases (e.g., multiple sclerosis, Alzheimer disease, cerebrovascular accident, Parkinson disease)
  - Infections (e.g., upper respiratory infection [URI], oral and perioral infections, candidiasis, coxsackievirus, AIDS, viral hepatitis, herpes simplex virus)
- Possible causes of smell disturbance:
  - Nasal and sinus disease (e.g., allergies, rhinitis, rhinorrhea)
  - Cigarette smoking
  - Cocaine abuse (intranasal)
  - Hemodialysis
  - Radiation treatment of head and neck
  - Congenital conditions
  - Neoplasm (e.g., brain tumor, nasal polyps, intranasal tumor)
  - Systemic lupus erythematosus (SLE)
  - Bell palsy
  - Oral/perioral skin lesion
  - Damage to CN I/V
  - Possible association with psychosis and schizophrenia
- Possible causes of taste loss:
  - Oral appliances
  - Dental procedures
  - Intraoral abscess
  - Gingivitis
  - Damage to CN VI, IX, or X
  - Stroke (especially frontal lobe)
- Selected medications that reportedly alter smell and taste:
  - Antibiotics: amikacin, ampicillin, azithromycin, ciprofloxacin, clarithromycin, doxycycline, griseofulvin, metronidazole, ofloxacin, tetracycline, terbinafine, β-lactamase inhibitors
  - Anticonvulsants: carbamazepine, phenytoin
  - Antidepressants: amitriptyline, doxepin, imipramine, nortriptyline
  - Antihistamines and decongestants: zinc-based cold remedies (Zicam)
  - Antihypertensives and cardiac medications: acetazolamide, amiloride, captopril, diltiazem, hydrochlorothiazide, nifedipine, propranolol, spironolactone
  - Anti-inflammatory agents: auranofin, gold, penicillamine
  - Antimanic drugs: lithium
  - Antineoplastics: cisplatin, doxorubicin, methotrexate, vincristine
  - Antiparkinsonian agents: levodopa, carbidopa
  - Antiseptic: chlorhexidine
  - Antithyroid agents: methimazole, propylthiouracil
  - Lipid-lowering agents: statins

Genetics
May be related to underlying genetically associated diseases (Kallmann syndrome, Alzheimer disease, migraine syndromes, rheumatologic conditions, endocrine disorders)

RISK FACTORS
- Age >65 years
- Poor nutritional status
- Smoking tobacco products

GENERAL PREVENTION
- Eat a well-balanced diet, with appropriate vitamins and minerals.
- Maintain good oral and nasal health, with routine visits to the dentist.
- Do not smoke tobacco products.
- Avoid noxious chemical exposures/unnecessary radiation.

Geriatric Considerations
- Elders are at particular risk of eating spoiled food or inadvertently being exposed to natural gas leaks owing to anosmia from aging.
- Anosmia also may be an early sign of degenerative disorders and has been shown to predict increased 5-year mortality (1)[B].

Pediatric Considerations
- Smell and taste disorders are uncommon in children in developed countries.
- In developing countries with poor nutrition (particularly zinc depletion), smell and taste disorders may occur.
- Delayed puberty in association with anosmia (± midline craniofacial abnormalities, deafness, or renal abnormalities) suggests the possibility of Kallmann syndrome (hypogonadotropic hypogonadism).

Pregnancy Considerations
- Pregnancy is an uncommon cause of smell and taste loss or disturbances.
- Many women report increased sensitivity to odors during pregnancy as well as an increased dislike for bitterness and a preference for salty substances.

COMMONLY ASSOCIATED CONDITIONS
URI, allergic rhinitis, dental abscesses

 DIAGNOSIS

Smell and taste disturbances are symptoms; it is essential to look for possible underlying causes.

HISTORY
- Symptoms of URI, environmental allergies
- Oral pain, other dental problems
- Cognitive/memory difficulties
- Current medications
- Nutritional status, ovolactovegetarian
- Weight loss or gain
- Frequent infections (impaired immunity)
- Worsening of underlying medical illness
- Increased use of salt and/or sugar to increase taste of food
- Neurodegenerative disease

PHYSICAL EXAM
Thorough HEENT exam

DIFFERENTIAL DIAGNOSIS
- Epilepsy (gustatory aura)
- Epilepsy (olfactory aura)
- Memory impairment
- Psychiatric conditions

DIAGNOSTIC TESTS & INTERPRETATION
Initial Tests (lab, imaging)
Consider (not all patients require all tests):
- CBC
- Liver function tests
- Blood glucose
- Creatinine
- Vitamin B_{12} level
- Thyroid-stimulating hormone (TSH)
- Serum IgE

- CT scanning is the most useful and cost-effective technique for assessing sinonasal disorders and is superior to an MRI in evaluating bony structures and airway patency. Coronal CT scans are particularly valuable in assessing paranasal anatomy (2)[B].

Follow-Up Tests & Special Considerations
Diagnosis of smell and taste disturbances is usually possible through history; however, the following tests can be used to confirm:

- Olfactory tests

  - Smell identification test: evaluates the ability to identify 40 microencapsulated scratch-and-sniff odorants (3)[B]
  - Brief smell identification test (4)[B]

  - Taste tests (more difficult because no convenient standardized tests are presently available): Solutions containing sucrose (sweet), sodium chloride (salty), quinine (bitter), and citric acid (sour) are helpful.
  - An MRI is useful in defining soft tissue disease; therefore, a coronal MRI is the technique of choice to image the olfactory bulbs, tracts, and cortical parenchyma. Possible placement of an accessory coil (TMJ) over the nose to assist in imaging.

 TREATMENT

GENERAL MEASURES
- Appropriate treatment for underlying cause

- Quit smoking (5)[B].
- Treatment of underlying nasal congestion with nasal decongestants and/or nasal/oral steroids (6–9)[B]
- Surgical correction of nasal blockage/nasal polyps (10)[B]
- Some drug-related smell or taste loss or dysgeusias can be reversed with cessation of the offending medication, but it may take many months (11–14)[B].

- Stop repeated oral trauma (e.g., appliances, tongue-biting behaviors).
- Proper nutritional and dietary assessment (2)[C]
- Formal dental evaluation

MEDICATION
- Treat underlying causes as appropriate. Idiopathic cases will often resolve spontaneously.

- Consider trial of corticosteroids topically (e.g., fluticasone nasal spray daily to BID) and/or systemically (e.g., oral prednisone 60 mg daily for 5 to 7 days) (6)[B].
- Zinc and vitamins (A, B complex) when deficiency is suspected (15)[B]

ISSUES FOR REFERRAL
- Consider referral to an otolaryngologist or neurologist for persistent cases.
- Referral to a subspecialist at a regional smell and taste center when complex etiologies are suspected

SURGERY/OTHER PROCEDURES
If needed for treatment of underlying cause

 ONGOING CARE

DIET
- Weight gain/loss is possible because the patient may reject food or may switch to calorie-rich foods that are still palatable.
- Ensure a nutritionally balanced diet with appropriate levels of nutrients, vitamins, and essential minerals.

PATIENT EDUCATION
- Caution patients not to overindulge as compensation for the bland taste of food. For example, patients with diabetes may need help in avoiding excessive sugar intake as an inappropriate way of improving food taste.
- Patients with chemosensory impairments should use measuring devices when cooking and should not cook by taste.
- Optimizing food texture, aroma, temperature, and color may improve the overall food experience when taste is limited.
- Patients with permanent smell dysfunction must develop adaptive strategies for dealing with hygiene, appetite, safety, and health.
- Natural gas and smoke detectors are essential; check for proper function frequently.
- Check food expiration dates frequently; discard old food.

PROGNOSIS
- In general, the olfactory system regenerates poorly after a head injury. Most patients who recover smell function following head trauma do so within 12 weeks of injury.
- Patients who quit smoking typically recover improved olfactory function and flavor sensation.
- Many taste disorders (dysgeusias) resolve spontaneously within a few years of onset.
- Phantosmias that are flow-dependent may respond to surgical ablation of olfactory mucosa.
- Conditions such as radiation-induced xerostomia and Bell palsy generally improve over time.

COMPLICATIONS
- Permanent loss of ability to smell/taste
- Psychiatric issues with dysgeusias and phantosmia

REFERENCES

1. Pinto JM, Wroblewski KE, Kern DW, et al. Olfactory dysfunction predicts 5-year mortality in older adults. *PLoS One.* 2014;9(10):e107541.
2. Malaty J, Malaty IA. Smell and taste disorders in primary care. *Am Fam Physician.* 2013;88(12):852–859.
3. Doty RL, Shaman P, Dann M. Development of the University of Pennsylvania smell identification test: a standardized microencapsulated test of olfactory function. *Physiol Behav.* 1984;32(3):489–502.
4. Jackman AH, Doty RL. Utility of a three-item smell identification test in detecting olfactory dysfunction. *Laryngoscope.* 2005;115(12):2209–2212.
5. Frye RE, Schwartz BS, Doty RL. Dose-related effects of cigarette smoking on olfactory function. *JAMA.* 1990;263(9):1233–1236.
6. Seiden AM, Duncan HJ. The diagnosis of a conductive olfactory loss. *Laryngoscope.* 2001;111(1):9–14.
7. Deems DA, Doty RL, Settle RG, et al. Smell and taste disorders, a study of 750 patients from the University of Pennsylvania Smell and Taste Center. *Arch Otolaryngol Head Neck Surg.* 1991;117(5):519–528.
8. Apter AJ, Gent JF, Frank ME. Fluctuating olfactory sensitivity and distorted odor perception in allergic rhinitis. *Arch Otolaryngol Head Neck Surg.* 1999;125(9):1005–1010.
9. Mott AE, Cain WS, Lafreniere LG, et al. Topical corticosteroid treatment of anosmia associated with nasal and sinus disease. *Arch Otolaryngol Head Neck Surg.* 1977;123(4):367–372.
10. Olsson P, Stjärne P. Endoscopic sinus surgery improves olfacton in nasal polyposis, a multicenter study. *Rhinology.* 2010;48(2):150–155.
11. Naik BS, Shetty N, Maben EV. Drug-induced taste disorders. *Eur J Intern Med.* 2010;21(3):240–243.
12. Ackerman BH, Kasbekar N. Disturbances of taste and smell induced by drugs. *Pharmacotherapy.* 1997;17(3):482–496.
13. Cowart BJ. Taste dysfunction: a practical guide for oral medicine. *Oral Dis.* 2011;17(1):2–6.
14. Tuccori M, Lapi F, Testi A, et al. Drug-induced taste and smell alterations: a case/non-case evaluation of an Italian database of spontaneous adverse drug reaction reporting. *Drug Saf.* 2011;34(10):849–859.
15. Henkin RI, Martin BM, Agarwal RP. Efficacy of exogenous oral zinc in treatment of patients with carbonic anhydrase VI deficiency. *Am J Med Sci.* 1999;318(6):392–405.

 CODES

ICD10
- R43.9 Unspecified disturbances of smell and taste
- R43.1 Parosmia
- R43.2 Parageusia

CLINICAL PEARLS
- Smell disorders are often mistaken as decreased taste by patients.
- Most smell loss is due nasal passage obstruction.
- Actual taste disorders are often related to dental problems or medication side effects.
- Gradual smell loss is very common in the elderly; extensive workup in this population may not be indicated if no associated signs/symptoms are present but may be predictive of 5-year mortality.

SOMATIC SYMPTOM (SOMATIZATION) DISORDER

William G. Elder, PhD

 BASICS

DESCRIPTION

- A pattern of one or more somatic symptoms recurring or persisting for >6 months that are distressing or result in significant disruption of daily life (1)
- Conceptualization and diagnostic criteria for somatic symptom presentations were significantly modified with the advent of *DSM-5*. Somatic symptom disorder (SSD) is similar in many aspects to the former somatization disorder, which required presentation with multiple physical complaints, no longer based on symptoms counts; current diagnosis is based on the way the patient presents and perceives his or her symptoms.
- SSD now includes most presentations that would formerly be considered hypochondriasis. Hypochondriasis has been replaced by illness anxiety disorders, which is diagnosed when the patient presents with significant preoccupation with having a serious illness in the absence of illness-related somatic complaints.
- Somatization increases disability independent of comorbidity and individuals with SSD have health-related functioning that is two standard deviations below the mean (1,2).
- Symptoms may be specific (e.g., localized pain) or relatively nonspecific (e.g., fatigue).
- Symptoms sometimes may represent normal bodily sensations or discomfort that does not signify serious disease.
- Suffering is authentic. Symptoms are not intentionally produced or feigned.

EPIDEMIOLOGY

Incidence
- Usually, first symptoms appear in adolescence.
- Predominant sex: female > male (10:1) (1)
- Type and frequency of somatic complaints may differ among cultures, so symptom reviews should be adjusted based on culture. More frequent in cultures without western/empirical explanatory models (3).

Prevalence
- Expected 2% among women and <0.2% among men (4)
- Somatization seen in up to 29% of patients presenting to primary care offices (3)
- Somatic concerns may increase, but other features of the presentation decrease such that prevalence declines after age 65 years (5).

ETIOLOGY AND PATHOPHYSIOLOGY
Unknown

Genetics
Consanguinity studies and single nucleotide polymorphism genotyping indicate that both genetic and environmental factors contribute to the risk of SSD (6).

RISK FACTORS
- Child abuse, particularly sexual abuse, has been shown to be a risk factor for somatization.
- Symptoms begin or worsen after losses (e.g., job, close relative, or friend).
- Greater intensity of symptoms often occurs with stress.

COMMONLY ASSOCIATED CONDITIONS
Comorbid with other psychiatric conditions is yet to be determined but is likely to be 20–50% with anxiety, depression, or personality disorders.

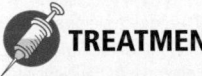 **DIAGNOSIS**

- Determining that a somatic symptom is medically unexplained is unreliable, and it is inappropriate to diagnose a mental disorder solely because a medical diagnosis is not demonstrated. Rely on symptoms and presentation rather than ruling out medical causes in making the SSD diagnosis.
- Illness anxiety and somatic distress are independent but often co-occur.

HISTORY
- One or more somatic complaints, with sometimes a grossly positive review of symptoms
- SSD involves patient excessive thoughts, feelings, or behaviors associated with symptoms or associated health concerns manifested by at least one of the following:
  - Disproportionate and persistent thoughts about the seriousness of the symptoms
  - Persistent high level of anxiety about health or symptoms
  - Excessive time or energy devoted to symptoms or health concerns.
- Diagnoses no longer relies on symptom counts, but common symptoms include:
  - Pain symptoms related to different sites such as head, abdomen, back, joints, extremities, chest, or rectum, or related to body functions such as menstruation, sexual intercourse, or urination.
  - GI symptoms such as nausea, bloating, vomiting (not during pregnancy), diarrhea, intolerance of several foods
  - Sexual symptoms such as indifference to sex, difficulties with erection or ejaculation, irregular menses, excessive menstrual bleeding, or vomiting throughout all 9 months of pregnancy
  - Pseudoneurologic symptoms such as impaired balance or coordination, weak or paralyzed muscles, lump in throat or trouble swallowing, loss of voice, retention of urine, hallucinations, numbness (to touch or pain), double vision, blindness, deafness, seizures, amnesia or other dissociative symptoms, loss of consciousness (other than with fainting); none of these is limited to pain.

- Patients with SSD frequently use alternative treatments, which should be explored for their effects on health and physical functioning (2).

PHYSICAL EXAM
Physical exam remarkable for absence of objective findings to explain the many subjective complaints

DIFFERENTIAL DIAGNOSIS
- Other psychiatric illnesses must be ruled out:
  - Depressive disorders
  - Anxiety disorders
  - Schizophrenia
  - Other somatic disorders: illness anxiety disorder, conversion disorder
  - Factitious disorder
  - Body dysmorphic disorder
- Malingering
- General medical conditions, with vague, multiple, confusing symptoms, must be ruled out.
  - Systemic lupus erythematosus
  - Hyperparathyroidism
  - Hyper- or hypothyroidism
  - Lyme disease
  - Porphyria

DIAGNOSTIC TESTS & INTERPRETATION
Several screening tools are available that help to identify symptoms as somatic:

- Patient Health Questionnaire (PHQ)-15 (screens and monitors symptoms) (7)[B]
- Minnesota Multiphasic Personality Inventory (MMPI) (identifies somatization) (8)[B]

Initial Tests (lab, imaging)
- Laboratory test results do not support the subjective complaints.
- Imaging studies do not support the subjective complaints.

Test Interpretation
None are identified.

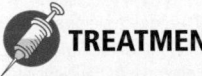 **TREATMENT**

GENERAL MEASURES

- The goal of treatment is to help the person learn to control the symptoms (9)[B].
- A supportive relationship with a sympathetic health care provider is the most important aspect of treatment:
  - Regular scheduled appointments should be maintained to review symptoms and the person's coping mechanisms (at least 15 minutes once a month).
  - Acknowledge and explain test results.

- The involvement of a single provider is important because a history of seeking medical attention and "doctor shopping" is common.
- Antidepressant or antianxiety medication and referral to a support group or mental health provider can help patients who are willing to participate in their treatment.
- Patients usually receive the most benefit from primary care providers who accept the limitations of treatment, listen to their patient's concerns, and provide reassurance.
- It is not helpful to tell patients that their symptoms are imaginary.

MEDICATION

Antidepressants (e.g., SSRIs) help to treat comorbid depression and anxiety (10)[C].

ISSUES FOR REFERRAL

- Discourage referrals to specialists for further investigation of somatic complaints.
- Referrals to support groups or to a mental health provider may be helpful.

ADDITIONAL THERAPIES

Treatments have not been evaluated for this recently reformulated disorder. However, there are numerous studies with positive outcomes for patients with various forms of somatization or medically unexplained symptoms.

- Treatment typically includes long-term therapy, which has been shown to decrease the severity of symptoms.
- Individual or group cognitive-behavioral therapy addressing health anxiety, health beliefs, and health behaviors has been shown to be the most efficacious treatment for somatoform disorders. Cognitive processes modified in therapy include patient tendencies to ruminate and catastrophize (11–13)[A].

ONGOING CARE

FOLLOW-UP RECOMMENDATIONS

Patients should have regularly scheduled follow-up with a primary care doctor, psychiatrist, and/or therapist.

PATIENT EDUCATION

Encourage interventions that decrease stressful elements of the patient's life:

- Psychoeducational advice
- Increase in exercise
- Pleasurable private time

PROGNOSIS

- Chronic course, fluctuating in severity
- Full remission is rare.

- Individuals with this disorder do not experience any significant difference in mortality rate or significant physical illness.
- Patients with this diagnosis do experience substantially greater functional disability and role impairment than nonsomatizing patients.

COMPLICATIONS

- May result from invasive testing and from multiple evaluations that are performed while looking for the cause of the symptoms
- A dependency on pain relievers or sedatives may develop.

REFERENCES

1. American Psychiatric Association. *Diagnostic and Statistical Manual of Mental Disorders.* 5th ed. Arlington, VA: American Psychiatric Publishing; 2013.
2. Harris AM, Orav EJ, Bates DW, et al. Somatization increases disability independent of comorbidity. *J Gen Intern Med.* 2009;24(2):155–161.
3. Elder WG. Somatoform disorders. In: South-Paul J, Matheny SC, Lewis EL, eds. *Current Diagnosis and Treatment in Family Medicine.* 4th ed. New York, NY: Lange-McGraw Hill; 2015.
4. Roca M, Gili M, Garcia-Garcia M, et al. Prevalence and comorbidity of common mental disorders in primary care. *J Affect Disord.* 2009;119(1–3):52–58.
5. Hilderink PH, Collard R, Rosmalen JG, et al. Prevalence of somatoform disorders and medically unexplained symptoms in old age populations in comparison with younger age groups: a systematic review. *Ageing Res Rev.* 2013;12(1):151–156.
6. Koh KB, Choi EH, Lee YJ, et al. Serotonin-related gene pathways associated with undifferentiated somatoform disorder. *Psychiatry Res.* 2011;189(2):246–250.
7. Kroenke K, Spitzer RL, Williams JB. The PHQ-15: validity of a new measure for evaluating the severity of somatic symptoms. *Psychosom Med.* 2002;64(2):258–266.
8. Wetzel RD, Brim J, Guze SB, et al. MMPI screening scales for somatization disorder. *Psychol Rep.* 1999;85(1):341–348.
9. Heijmans M, Olde Hartman TC, van Weel-Baumgarten E, et al. Experts' opinions on the management of medically unexplained symptoms in primary care. A qualitative analysis of narrative reviews and scientific editorials. *Fam Pract.* 2011;28(4):444–455.
10. Somashekar B, Jainer A, Wuntakal B. Psychopharmacotherapy of somatic symptoms disorders. *Int Rev Psychiatry.* 2013;25(1):107–115.
11. Herzog A, Voigt K, Meyer B, et al. Psychological and interactional characteristics of patients with somatoform disorders: Validation of the Somatic Symptoms Experiences Questionnaire (SSEQ) in a clinical psychosomatic population. *J Psychosom Res.* 2015;78(6):553–562.
12. Allen LA, Woolfolk RL, Escobar JI, et al. Cognitive-behavioral therapy for somatization disorder: a randomized controlled trial. *Arch Intern Med.* 2006;166(14):1512–1518.
13. Moreno S, Gili M, Magallón R, et al. Effectiveness of group versus individual cognitive-behavioral therapy in patients with abridged somatization disorder: a randomized controlled trial. *Psychosom Med.* 2013;75(6):600–608.

ADDITIONAL READING

- Elder WG Jr, King M, Dassow P, et al. Managing lower back pain: you may be doing too much. *J Fam Pract.* 2009;58(4):180–186.
- Sharma MP, Manjula M. Behavioural and psychological management of somatic symptom disorders: an overview. *Int Rev Psychiatry.* 2013;25(1):116–124.

CODES

ICD10

- F45.9 Somatoform disorder, unspecified
- F45.20 Hypochondriacal disorder, unspecified
- F45.22 Body dysmorphic disorder

CLINICAL PEARLS

- With the advent of *DSM-5*, diagnosis is now based on a pattern of symptoms rather than an absence of medical explanation.
- A clue is accumulation of several diagnoses with >13 letters (e.g., chronic fatigue syndrome, fibromyalgia syndrome, reflex sympathetic dystrophy, temporomandibular joint syndrome, carpal tunnel syndrome, mitral valve prolapse).
- Inability of more than three physicians to make a meaningful diagnosis suggests somatization.
- Acknowledge the patient's pain, suffering, and disability.
- Do not tell patients the symptoms are "all in their head."
- Emphasize that this is not a rare disorder.
- Discuss the limitations of treatment while providing reassurance that there are interventions that will lessen suffering and reduce symptoms.

SPINAL STENOSIS

N. Wilson Holland, MD, FACP, AGSF • Birju B. Patel, MD, FACP, AGSF

BASICS

DESCRIPTION
Narrowing of the spinal canal and foramen:
- Spondylosis or degenerative arthritis is the most common cause of spinal stenosis, resulting from compression of the spinal cord by disc degeneration, facet arthropathy, osteophyte formation, and ligamentum flavum hypertrophy.
- The L4–L5 level is most commonly involved.

EPIDEMIOLOGY
The prevalence of spinal stenosis increases with age due to "wear and tear" on the normal spine.

Incidence
Symptomatic spinal stenosis affects up to 8% of the general population.

Prevalence
- The prevalence of spinal stenosis can be very high if assessed solely by imaging in elderly patients. Not all patients with radiographic spinal stenosis are symptomatic. The degree of radiographic stenosis does not always correlate with patient symptoms. Lumbar MRI showed significant abnormalities in one study in 22% of asymptomatic patients <60 years and in 57% of patients >60 years. T2-weighted imaging showed a 98% prevalence of disc degeneration in asymptomatic patients >60 years (1)[C].
- Predominant age: Symptoms develop in 5th to 6th decades (congenital stenosis is symptomatic earlier) (2)[A].

ETIOLOGY AND PATHOPHYSIOLOGY
- Spinal stenosis can result from congenital or acquired causes. Degenerative spondylosis is the most common cause.
- Disc dehydration leads to loss of height with bulging of the disc annulus and ligamentum flavum into the spinal canal, increasing facet joint loading.
- Facet loading leads to reactive sclerosis and osteophytic bone growth, further compressing spinal canal and foraminal elements.
- Other causes of acquired spinal stenosis include:
  - Trauma
  - Neoplasms
  - Neural cysts and lipomas
  - Postoperative changes
  - Rheumatoid arthritis
  - Diffuse idiopathic skeletal hyperostosis
  - Ankylosing spondylitis
  - Metabolic/endocrine causes-osteoporosis, renal osteodystrophy, and Paget disease (3)[A]

Genetics
No definitive genetic links

RISK FACTORS
Increasing age and degenerative spinal disease

GENERAL PREVENTION
There is proven prevention for spinal stenosis. Symptoms can be alleviated with flexion at the waist:
- Leaning forward while walking
- Pushing a shopping cart
- Lying in flexed position
- Sitting
- Avoiding provocative maneuvers (back extension, ambulating long distances without resting)

DIAGNOSIS

HISTORY
- The history helps distinguish spinal stenosis from other causes of back pain and peripheral vascular disease.
  - Insidious onset and slow progression are typical. Discomfort with standing, paresthesias and weakness (often bilateral) (4)[C].
  - Symptoms *worsen with extension* (prolonged standing, walking downhill, or down stairs).
  - Symptoms *improve with flexion* (sitting, leaning forward while walking, walking uphill or upstairs, lying in a flexed position).
- Neurogenic claudication (i.e., pain, tightness, numbness, and subjective weakness of lower extremities) may mimic vascular claudication.
- Nocturnal leg cramps may relate to the severity of lumbar spinal stenosis (5)[C].

PHYSICAL EXAM
Neurologic exam may be normal. Key exam areas:
- Examine gait (rule out cervical myelopathy or intracranial pathology).
- Loss of lumbar lordosis
- Evaluate range of motion of lumbar spine.
- Pain with extension of the lumbar spine is typical.
- Straight-leg raise test may be positive if nerve root entrapment is present.
- Muscle weakness is usually mild and involves the L4, L5, and (rarely) S1 nerve roots.
- About half of patients with symptomatic stenosis have a reduced or absent Achilles reflex. Some have reduced or absent patellar reflex.

DIFFERENTIAL DIAGNOSIS
- Vascular claudication. Symptoms of vascular claudication do not improve with leaning forward and usually do not persist with standing or rest.
- Disc herniation
- Cervical myelopathy

DIAGNOSTIC TESTS & INTERPRETATION
Generally a clinical diagnosis. Imaging (MRI is best) is used to stage severity and plan treatment.

Initial Tests (lab, imaging)
- CBC, ESR, C-reactive protein (if considering infection or malignancy)
- New back pain lasting >2 weeks or back pain accompanied by neurologic findings in patients >50 years generally warrants neuroimaging.
- MRI is the modality of choice for the diagnosis of spinal stenosis.
- CT myelography is an alternative to MRI but is invasive and has higher risk of complications.
- Plain radiography helps exclude other causes of new back pain (e.g., malignant lytic lesions) but does not reveal the underlying pathology.
- Radiologic abnormalities in general do not correlate with the clinical severity (6)[C].

Diagnostic Procedures/Other
Surgical decompression is the definitive option for patients who are symptomatic after nonoperative treatment:
- Spinal stenosis generally does not lead to neurologic damage.
- Surgery may be required for pain relief, allowing patients to become more mobile and improving overall health and quality of life.

Test Interpretation
Common radiographic findings include decreased disc height, facet hypertrophy, and spinal canal and/or foraminal narrowing.

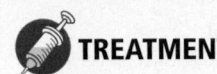

TREATMENT

- In general, nonoperative interventions are preferred unless there are progressive or debilitating neurologic symptoms:
  - Physical therapy, exercise, weight management, lumbar epidural steroid injections, and medications are all options. There is not enough evidence in the current literature to guide definitive clinical practice.
  - Patients considering surgery should understand that the benefits of surgery may diminish over time (7)[A].
  - Rule out other neuropathies and peripheral vascular disease.
- Spinal decompression and physical therapy yield similar effects (8)[A].
- There is some controversy about whether a fusion should be performed with the decompression because of risk of future spondylolisthesis (7)[A],(9)[C],(10)[A].

MEDICATION
First Line
- Acetaminophen: caution in those with preexisting liver disease; increased warnings for hepatotoxicity; limit daily dosing in the elderly.
- NSAIDs: Consider potential for GI side effects, fluid retention, and renal failure.

Second Line
- Tramadol—currently a schedule IV controlled substance. Has the potential to cause confusion, dizziness, lower seizure threshold, and increase fall risk in the elderly; should be used with caution
- There is limited evidence for long-term efficacy of lumbar epidural steroid and/or anesthetic injections. Injections maybe less effective in those with more severe stenosis and those with stenosis involving >3 lumbar levels.
- Use opioids judiciously and only when other treatments have failed to control severe pain.

Geriatric Considerations
- Anti-inflammatory medications should be used with caution in the elderly due to the risks of GI bleeding, fluid retention, renal failure, and cardiovascular risks.

- Side effects of opioids, include constipation, confusion, urinary retention, drowsiness, nausea, vomiting, and the potential for dependence.
- >10% of elderly lack Achilles reflexes.

ISSUES FOR REFERRAL
Refer to a spine surgeon when patients are in unremitting pain or have a neurologic deficit.

ADDITIONAL THERAPIES
- Patients with spinal stenosis are typically able to ride a bicycle because leaning forward tends to relieve symptoms.
- Aquatic therapy (helpful for muscle training and general conditioning)
- Strengthening of abdominal and back extensor muscles
- Gait training
- A brace or corset may help in the short term but is not recommended for prolonged periods due to development of paraspinal muscle weakness.
- Encourage physical activity to prevent deconditioning.

SURGERY/OTHER PROCEDURES
- Surgery is indicated when symptoms persist despite conservative measures (7)[A].
- Age alone should not be an exclusion factor for surgical intervention. Cognitive impairment, multiple comorbidities, and osteoporosis may increase the risk of perioperative complications in the elderly.
- Lumbar decompressive laminectomy is the mainstay of treatment. The traditional approach is laminectomy and partial facetectomy.
- Controversy exists about whether the decompression should be supplemented by a fusion procedure:
  – There is evidence that fusion (simple or complex), as opposed to decompression procedure alone, may be associated with higher risk of major complications, increased mortality, and increased resource use in the elderly.
- A less-invasive alternative, known as interspinous distraction (X STOP implant), is an option (11)[B].
- The evidence for use of the Aperius interspinous implant device is inconclusive (12,13)[C].
- A unilateral partial hemilaminectomy combined with transmedial decompression may adequately treat stenosis with less morbidity in the elderly (14)[C].
- Transforaminal balloon treatment may be a viable option for resistant spinal stenosis pain and functional impairment (15)[B].

INPATIENT CONSIDERATIONS
Admission Criteria/Initial Stabilization
Acute or progressive neurologic deficit

Discharge Criteria
Improved pain or after neurologic deficit has been addressed.

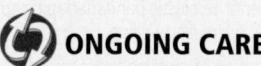 ONGOING CARE

FOLLOW-UP RECOMMENDATIONS
- Follow up based on progression of symptoms.
- No limitations to activity; patients may be as active as tolerated. Exercise should be encouraged.

Patient Monitoring
Patients are monitored for improvement of symptoms and development of any complications.

DIET
Optimize nutrition for weight management and surgery.

PATIENT EDUCATION
- Activity as tolerated, if no other pathology is present (e.g., fractures).
- Patients should present for care if they develop progressive motor weakness and/or bladder/bowel dysfunction.
- Patients should know the natural history of the condition and how best to relieve symptoms.

PROGNOSIS
- Spinal stenosis is generally benign, but the pain can lead to limitation in ADLs and progressive disability.
- Surgery usually improves pain and symptoms in patients who fail nonoperative treatment.
- Surgical outcomes are similar in terms of pain relief and functional improvement for patients of all ages.

COMPLICATIONS
- Severe spinal stenosis can lead to bowel and/or bladder dysfunction.
- Surgical complications include infection, neurologic injury, chronic pain, and disability.

REFERENCES
1. Baker ADL. Abnormal magnetic resonance scans of the lumbar spine in asymptomatic subjects. A prospective investigation. In: Banaszkiewicz P, Kader DF, eds. *Classic Papers in Orthopedics*. London, England: Springer London; 2014: 245–247.
2. Ammendolia C, Stuber K, de Bruin LK, et al. Nonoperative treatment of lumbar spinal stenosis with neurogenic claudication: a systematic review. *Spine Spine (Phila Pa 1976)*. 2012;37(10):E609–E616.
3. Katz JN, Harris MB. Clinical practice. Lumbar spinal stenosis. *N Engl J Med*. 2008;358(8): 818–825.
4. Suri P, Rainville J, Kalichman L, et al. Does this older adult with lower extremity pain have the clinical syndrome of lumbar spinal stenosis? *JAMA*. 2010;304(23):2628–2636.
5. Ohtori S, Yamashita M, Murata Y, et al. Incidence of nocturnal leg cramps in patients with lumbar spinal stenosis before and after conservative and surgical treatment. *Yonsei Med J*. 2014;55(3):779–784.
6. Li AL, Yen D. Effect of increased MRI and CT scan utilization on clinical decision-making in patients referred a surgical clinic for back pain. *Can J Surg*. 2011;54(2):128–132.
7. Weinstein JN, Tosteson TD, Lurie JD, et al. Surgical versus nonsurgical therapy for lumbar spinal stenosis. *N Engl J Med*. 2008;358(8):794–810.
8. Delitto A, Piva SR, Moore CG, et al. Surgery versus nonsurgical treatment of lumbar spinal stenosis: a randomized trial. *Ann Intern Med*. 2015:162(7):465–473.
9. Deyo RA, Ching A, Matsen L, et al. Use of bone morphogenetic proteins in spinal fusion surgery for older adults with lumbar spinal stenosis: trends, complications, repeat surgery, and charges. *Spine (Phila Pa 1976)*. 2012;37(3):222–230.
10. Deyo RA, Mirza SK, Martin BI, et al. Trends, major medical complications, and charges associated with surgery for lumbar spinal stenosis in older adults. *JAMA*. 2010;303(13):1259–1265.
11. Miller LE, Block JE. Interspinous spacer implant in patients with lumbar spinal stenosis: preliminary results of a multicenter, randomized, controlled trial. *Pain Res Treat*. 2012;2012:823509.
12. Postacchini R, Ferrari E, Cinotti G, et al. Aperius interspinous implant versus open surgical decompression in lumbar spinal stenosis. *Spine J*. 2011;11(10):933–939.
13. Surace MF, Fagetti A, Fozzato S, et al. Lumbar spinal stenosis treatment with Aperius perclid interspinous system. *Eur Spine J*. 2012; 21(Suppl 1):S69–S74.
14. Morgalla MH, Noak N, Merkle M, et al. Lumbar spinal stenosis in elderly patients: is a unilateral microsurgical approach sufficient for decompression? *J Neurosurg Spine*. 2011;14(3):305–312.
15. Kim SH, Choi WJ, Suh JH, et al. Effects of transforaminal balloon treatment in patients with lumbar foraminal stenosis: a randomized, controlled, double-blind trial. *Pain Physician*. 2013;16(3):213–224.

 SEE ALSO

Algorithm: Low Back Pain, Acute

 CODES

ICD10
- M48.00 Spinal stenosis, site unspecified
- M48.06 Spinal stenosis, lumbar region
- M48.04 Spinal stenosis, thoracic region

CLINICAL PEARLS
- Spinal stenosis often presents as neurogenic claudication (pain, tightness, numbness, and subjective weakness of lower extremities). This can mimic vascular claudication.
- Neurogenic claudication (as opposed to vascular claudication) is improved by uphill ambulation and lumbar flexion.
- Flexion of the spine generally relieves symptoms associated with spinal stenosis.
- Spinal extension (prolonged standing, walking downhill, and walking downstairs) can worsen symptoms of spinal stenosis.
- Urgent surgery should be considered for patients with cauda equina/conus medullaris syndrome or progressive bladder dysfunction. Most other patients with lumbar spinal stenosis can begin with conservative management.

SPRAIN, ANKLE

Shane L. Larson, MD

BASICS

DESCRIPTION
The most common cause of ankle injury comprising a significant proportion of sports injuries:
- Types of ankle sprains: lateral, medial, and syndesmotic (or high ankle sprain)
  - Lateral ankle sprains are the most common, accounting for 85% of all ankle sprains:
    - In lateral ankle sprains, the anterior talofibular ligament (ATFL) is most likely to be injured.
    - The calcaneofibular ligament (CFL) is the second most likely ligament to be injured.
    - The posterior talofibular ligament (PTFL) is the least likely to be injured.
  - Medial ankle sprains (5–10%) result from an injury to the deltoid ligament.
  - Syndesmotic (or high ankle) injuries account for 5–10% of ankle sprains.
    - The syndesmosis between the distal tibia and distal fibula bones consists of the anterior, posterior, and transverse tibiofibular ligaments and the interosseous ligament and interosseous membrane.
- Ankle sprains are classified according to the degree of ligamentous disruption:
  - Grade I: mild stretching of a ligament with possible microscopic tears
  - Grade II: incomplete tear of a ligament
  - Grade III: complete ligament tear

Geriatric Considerations
Increased risk of fracture in patients with preexisting bone weakness (osteoporosis/osteopenia)

Pediatric Considerations
- Increased risk of physeal injuries instead of ligament sprain because ligaments have greater tensile strength than physes
- Inversion ankle injuries in children may have a concomitant fibular physeal injury (Salter Harris type I or higher fracture).
- Consider tarsal coalition with recurrent ankle sprains.

EPIDEMIOLOGY

Incidence
- Peak incidence in children (0 to 12 years old), then adolescents (13 to 17 years old), and finally adults (≥18 years old) (1)
- 1/2 of all ankle sprains are sports-related; highest incidence in indoor/court sports (basketball, volleyball, tennis), followed by football and soccer (2)
- Most common sports injury
- More common in males age <30 years and females >30 years old

Prevalence
- 25% of sports injuries in the United States
- 75% of all ankle injuries are sprains.

ETIOLOGY AND PATHOPHYSIOLOGY
- Lateral ankle sprains result from an inversion force with the ankle in plantar flexion.
- Medial ankle sprains are due to forced eversion while the foot is in dorsiflexion.
- Syndesmotic sprains result from eversion stress/extreme dorsiflexion along with internal rotation of tibia.

RISK FACTORS
- The greatest risk factor is a prior history of an ankle sprain (3–34% recurrence rate).
- Postural instability, gait alterations
- Joint laxity and decreased proprioception are not risk factors.

GENERAL PREVENTION
- Improve overall physical conditioning:
  - Training in agility and flexibility
  - Single-leg balancing
  - Proprioceptive training (3)
- Taping and bracing may help prevent primary injury in selected sports (i.e., volleyball, basketball, football) or reinjury (4). Taping and bracing do not reduce sprain severity.

COMMONLY ASSOCIATED CONDITIONS
- Contusions
- Fractures
  - Fibular head fracture/dislocation (Maisonneuve)
  - Fracture of the base of the 5th metatarsal
  - Distal fibula physeal fracture (includes Salter-Harris fractures in pediatric patients; most common type of pediatric ankle fracture)

DIAGNOSIS

HISTORY
- Elicit specific mechanism of injury (inversion vs. eversion)
- Popping/snapping sensation during the injury
- Previous history of ankle injuries
- Ability to ambulate immediately after the injury
- Rapid onset of pain, swelling, or ecchymosis
- Location of pain (lateral/medial)
- Difficulty bearing weight
- Past medical history of systemic disorders

PHYSICAL EXAM
- Timing: Initial assessment for laxity may be difficult due to pain, swelling, and muscle spasm. Repeat exam ~5 days after injury may improve sensitivity.
- Compare to uninjured ankle for swelling, ecchymosis, weakness, and laxity
- Neurovascular exam
- Palpate ATFL, CFL, PTFL, and deltoid ligament for tenderness.
- Palpate lateral and medial malleolus, base of 5th metatarsal, navicular, and entire fibula.
  - High ankle sprain associated with fracture of proximal fibula
- Grade I sprain: mild swelling and pain; no laxity; able to bear weight/ambulate without pain
- Grade II sprain: moderate swelling and pain; mild laxity with firm end point noted; weight bearing/ambulation painful
- Grade III sprain: severe swelling, pain, and bruising; laxity with no end point; significant instability and loss of function/motion; unable to bear weight/ambulate
  - Swelling less sensitive for grade of tear in pediatric patient
- Special tests:
  - Anterior drawer test to check for ATFL laxity
  - Talar tilt test to check laxity in CFL (with inversion) or deltoid ligament (eversion)

- Squeeze test: Compress tibia and fibula midcalf to check for syndesmotic injury; sensitivity 30%, specificity 93.5%.
- Dorsiflexion/external rotation test: Positive test is pain at syndesmosis with rotation; sensitivity 20%, specificity 85%.

DIFFERENTIAL DIAGNOSIS
- Tendon injury
  - Tendinopathy/tendon tear
- Fracture and/or dislocation of the ankle/foot
- Hindfoot/midfoot injuries
- Nerve injury
- Contusion

DIAGNOSTIC TESTS & INTERPRETATION
- Ottawa Ankle Rules (nearly 100% sensitive, 30–50% specific) determine need for radiographs to rule out ankle fractures (patient must be 18 to 55 years; certain patients, e.g., diabetics with diminished sensation, may still need radiographs):
  - Pain in malleolar zone
  - Inability to bear weight (walk ≥4 steps) immediately and in the exam room
  - Bony tenderness at tip/posterior edge of the lateral/medial malleolus
    - Note: Ottawa rule for foot imaging series (reported pain in the midfoot zone AND pain with palpation of navicular or base of 5th metatarsal, OR inability to bear weight immediately and in the ER/office)
  - Although Ottawa rules are highly sensitive, they should not overrule clinical judgment.
- If radiographs are indicated, obtain anteroposterior, lateral, and mortise views of the ankle.
  - Small avulsion fractures are associated with grade III sprains.
- Consider CT if radiographs are negative but occult fracture is suspected clinically.
- MRI is the gold standard for soft tissue imaging but is expensive and rarely necessary.
  - Syndesmotic ankle sprains: MRI is more sensitive.
- US is a good second line imaging option with a sensitivity comparable to MRI.

Follow-Up Tests & Special Considerations
If patient condition does not improve in 6 to 8 weeks, consider CT, MRI, or US.

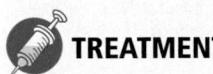

TREATMENT

GENERAL MEASURES
- Most grade I, II, and III lateral ankle sprains can be managed conservatively.
- Conservative therapy: PRICE (protection, relative rest, ice, compression, elevation)
- Protection/compression: For grade I/II sprains, lace-up bracing is superior to air-filled/gel-filled ankle brace, which is superior to elastic bandage/taping to provide support and decrease swelling.
  - Note: The combination of air-filled brace and compression wrap is superior to each individual for return to preinjury joint function at 10 days and 1 month for grades I and II sprains (5)[A].

– Grade III sprains should have short-term immobilization (10 days) with below-the-knee cast, followed by a semirigid brace (air cast). If a patient refuses casting, a 10-day period of strict non–weight-bearing with air cast splint and elastic bandage is a comparable alternative if non–weight-bearing is maintained.

• Rest: Initially, activity as tolerated. Early mobilization and physical therapy speed recovery/reduce pain:
– Weight bearing, as tolerated
– Consider crutches if unable to bear weight.
– Exercises should be initiated as early as tolerated and limited to pain-free range of motion.
– Patients can start mobilization by tracing the alphabet with the foot in the air.
– Resistance exercises with an elastic band

• Ice: Ice for first 3 to 7 days for pain reduction and decrease recovery time

• Elevation: Elevate ankle to decrease swelling.

MEDICATION

• NSAIDs: preferably oral; topical forms (e.g., diclofenac 1% gel) may be used to minimize GI side effects. PRN NSAID dosing has similar outcomes to scheduled dosing with improved safety profile.
– Example: Naproxen 500 mg BID PRN

• Acetaminophen 650 mg q4–6h (max outpatient therapy dose: 3,250 mg/day)

• Opioids if severe pain

ISSUES FOR REFERRAL

• Malleolar/talar dome fracture
• Syndesmotic sprain
• Dislocation/subluxation
• Tendon rupture
• Ongoing instability
• Uncertain diagnosis

ADDITIONAL THERAPIES

Physical therapy:

• After the acute phase of the injury, patients with grade II or III sprain should start physical therapy as soon as possible to increase range of motion, strength, flexibility, and improve proprioceptive balance (wobble board/ankle disk).

• Functional rehabilitation prevents chronic instability and speeds healing.

• Athletes should undergo sports-specific rehabilitation before returning to play.

SURGERY/OTHER PROCEDURES

• Surgery is typically reserved for treatment of complicated recurrent sprains and certain syndesmotic sprains.

• Patients with chronic ankle instability who fail functional rehabilitation or with poor tissue quality may need anatomic repair/reconstructive surgery.

 ONGOING CARE

FOLLOW-UP RECOMMENDATIONS

• After an ankle sprain, ankle-stabilizing orthoses (air stirrup braces, lace-up supports, athletic taping, etc.) should be worn for high-risk sports to prevent future ankle sprains.

• Moderate and severe sprains require ankle orthoses for ≥6 months during sports participation.

• Gradual return to play for athletes with a grade I lateral ankle sprain can generally be accomplished in 1 to 2 weeks; grade II sprain return to play time is 2 to 3 weeks; grade III sprain is approximately 4 weeks.

• Syndesmotic sprains take longer (approx. 8 to 9 weeks) to heal than lateral ankle sprains.

Patient Monitoring

If athletes continue to have symptoms when they return to play or if a patient has pain for 6 to 8 weeks after injury, repeat examination and imaging.

PATIENT EDUCATION

• Crutch training
• Provide training on proper use of elastic bandages, brace, and/or orthoses
• Demonstrate mobilization exercises (alphabet trace, towel grab).

PROGNOSIS

• Earlier physical therapy and mobilization with bracing allows for faster return to daily living and/or sports.

• Higher grade sprains, older patient age, and initial non–weight-bearing status have poorer prognosis and longer recovery.

• Ligamentous strength does not return for months after the injury.

COMPLICATIONS

• Joint instability
• Intermittent swelling/pain if not properly treated
• Accumulation of cartilage damage, leading to degenerative changes
• 5–33% continue to have pain 1 year postinjury.

REFERENCES

1. Doherty C, Delahunt E, Caulfield B, et al. The incidence and prevalence of ankle sprain injury: a systematic review and meta-analysis of prospective epidemiological studies. *Sports Med*. 2014;44(1):123–140.
2. Waterman BR, Owens BD, Davey S, et al. The epidemiology of ankle sprains in the United States. *J Bone Joint Surg Am*. 2010;92(13):2279–2284.
3. McGuine TA, Keene JS. The effect of a balance training program on the risk of ankle sprains in high school athletes. *Am J Sports Med*. 2006;34(7):1103–1111.
4. Pedowitz DI, Reddy S, Parekh SG, et al. Prophylactic bracing decreases ankle injuries in collegiate female volleyball players. *Am J Sports Med*. 2008;36(2):324–327.
5. Beynnon BD, Renström PA, Haugh L, et al. A prospective, randomized clinical investigation of the treatment of first-time ankle sprains. *Am J Sports Med*. 2006;34(9):1401–1412.

ADDITIONAL READING

• Bleakley CM, O'Connor SR, Tully MA, et al. Effect of accelerated rehabilitation on function after ankle sprain: randomised controlled trial. *BMJ*. 2010;340:c1964.
• Farwell KE, Powden CJ, Powell MR, et al. The effectiveness of prophylactic ankle braces in reducing the incidence of acute ankle injuries in adolescent athletes: a critically appraised topic. *J Sport Rehabil*. 2013;22(2):137–142.
• Hiller CE, Nightingale EJ, Lin CW, et al. Characteristics of people with recurrent ankle sprains: a systematic review with meta-analysis. *Br J Sports Med*. 2011;45(8):660–672.
• Kerkhoffs GM, van den Bekerom M, Elders LA, et al. Diagnosis, treatment and prevention of ankle sprains: an evidence-based clinical guideline. *Br J Sports Med*. 2012;46(12):854–860.
• Massey T, Derry S, Moore RA, et al. Topical NSAIDs for acute pain in adults. *Cochrane Database Syst Rev*. 2010;(6):CD007402.
• Pedowitz DI, Reddy S, Parkeh SG, et al. Prophylactic bracing decreases ankle injuries in collegiate female volleyball players. *Am J Sports Med*. 2008;32(2):324–327.
• Raymond J, Nicholson LL, Hiller CE, et al. The effect of ankle taping or bracing on proprioception in functional ankle instability: a systematic review and meta-analysis. *J Sci Med Sport*. 2012;15(5):386–392.

 CODES

ICD10

• S96.919A Strain of unsp msl/tnd at ank/ft level, unsp foot, init
• S93.499A Sprain of other ligament of unspecified ankle, init encntr
• S93.419A Sprain of calcaneofibular ligament of unsp ankle, init

CLINICAL PEARLS

• Children are at an increased risk of physeal injuries because ligaments are stronger than physes.
• Conditioning, including proprioceptive training, before participating in sports and throughout the season helps to prevent ankle sprains.
• Functional rehabilitation, rather than total immobilization, is recommended for quicker return to sport and work.
• If patient's condition is not improving in 6 to 8 weeks, consider advanced imaging with CT, MRI, or US.

SPRAINS AND STRAINS

Daniel L. Jones, MD • J. Herbert Stevenson, MD

BASICS

DESCRIPTION

- *Sprains* are complete or partial ligamentous injuries either within the body of the ligament or at the site of attachment to bone.
  - Classified as grade 1, 2, or 3 (AMA Ligament Injury Classification)
    - Grade 1: stretch injury without ligamentous laxity
    - Grade 2: partial tear with increased ligamentous laxity but firm endpoint on exam
    - Grade 3: complete tear with increased ligamentous laxity and no firm endpoint on exam
  - Usually secondary to trauma (e.g., falls, twisting injuries, motor vehicle accidents)
  - Physical exam is the key to accurate diagnosis.
- *Strains* are partial or complete disruptions of the muscle, muscle-tendon junction, or tendon
  - Classified as
    - First degree: minimal damage to muscle, tendon, or musculotendinous unit
    - Second degree: partial tear to the muscle, tendon, or musculotendinous unit
    - Third degree: complete disruption of the muscle, tendon, or musculotendinous unit
  - Often associated with overuse injuries

Geriatric Considerations
More likely to see associated bony injuries due to decreased joint flexibility and increased prevalence of osteoporosis and osteopenia

Pediatric Considerations
- Sprains and strains account for 24% of pediatric injuries.
- 3 million pediatric sports injuries occur annually.
- Must be concerned about physeal/apophyseal injuries in the skeletally immature patient

EPIDEMIOLOGY

Incidence
~80% of all U.S. athletes experience a sprain or strain at some point.

Prevalence
- Ankle sprains are among the most common injuries in primary care, accounting for ~30% of sports medicine clinic visits. Most ankle sprains are due to inversion injuries (lateral sprains) involving the anterior talofibular ligament. Account for 650,000 annual ER visits in the United States (1)
- Predominant age
  - Sprains: any age in physically active patient
  - Strains: usually 15 to 40 years of age
- Predominant sex: male > female for most; female > male for sprain of acromioclavicular ligament

ETIOLOGY AND PATHOPHYSIOLOGY
- Trauma, falls, motor vehicle accidents
- Excessive exercise; poor conditioning
- Improper footwear
- Inadequate warm-up and stretching before activity
- Prior sprain or strain

RISK FACTORS
- Prior history of sprain or strain is greatest risk factor for future sprain/strain.
- Change in or improper footwear, protective gear, or environment (e.g., surface)
- Sudden increase in training schedule or volume.
- Tobacco use

GENERAL PREVENTION
- Appropriate warm-up and cool-down exercises
- Use proper equipment and footwear.
- Balance training programs improve proprioception and reduce the risk of ankle sprains (2)[B].
- Semirigid orthoses or air casts may prevent ankle sprains during high-risk sports, especially in athletes with history of sprain (3)[A].
- Proprioception and strength training decrease injury risk, stretching does not (4)[A].

COMMONLY ASSOCIATED CONDITIONS
- Effusions, hemarthrosis
- Stress, avulsion, or other fractures
- Syndesmotic injuries
- Contusions
- Dislocations/subluxations

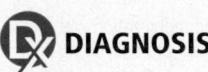

DIAGNOSIS

HISTORY
- Obtain thorough description of mechanism of injury including activity, trauma, baseline conditioning, and prior musculoskeletal injuries.
- May describe feeling or hearing pop or snap

PHYSICAL EXAM
- Inspect for swelling, asymmetry, ecchymosis and gait disturbance.
- Palpate for tenderness.
- Evaluate for decreased range of motion (ROM) of joint and joint instability.
- Evaluate for strength.
- Sprains
  - Grade 1: tenderness without laxity; minimal pain; swelling; little ecchymosis; can bear weight
  - Grade 2: tenderness with increased laxity on exam but firm endpoint; more pain, swelling; often ecchymosis; some difficulty bearing weight
  - Grade 3: tenderness with increased laxity on exam and no firm end point; severe pain, swelling; obvious ecchymosis; difficulty bearing weight

DIFFERENTIAL DIAGNOSIS
- Tendonitis
- Bursitis
- Contusion
- Hematoma
- Fracture
- Osteochondral lesion
- Rheumatologic process

DIAGNOSTIC TESTS & INTERPRETATION
- Ankle
  - Anterior drawer test assesses integrity of anterior talofibular ligament.
  - Talar tilt test assesses integrity of calcaneofibular ligament.
  - Squeeze test assesses for syndesmotic injury.
  - Palpate fibular head.
- Knee
  - Lachman test assesses integrity of anterior cruciate ligament. Posterior drawer assesses integrity of posterior cruciate ligament.
  - Valgus/varus stress tests assess integrity of medial and lateral collateral ligaments, respectively.
- Shoulder
  - Positive apprehension test may indicate glenohumeral ligament sprain.
- Radiographs help rule out bony injury; stress views may be necessary. Obtain bilateral radiographs in children to rule out growth plate injuries.
- Use Ottawa foot and ankle rules (age 18 to 55 years) to determine if radiographs are necessary (5)[A].
- Ankle films: required if pain in the malleolar zone *and*
  - Bone tenderness in posterior aspect distal 6 cm of tibia *or* fibula *or*
  - Unable to bear weight immediately or in emergency department
- Foot films: required if midfoot zone pain is present *and*
  - Bone tenderness at base of 5th metatarsal *or*
  - Bone tenderness at navicular *or*
  - Inability to bear weight immediately or in emergency department

Follow-Up Tests & Special Considerations
- CT scan if occult fracture is suspected
- MRI is the gold standard for imaging soft tissue structures, including muscle, ligaments, and intra-articular structures. If tibiofibular syndesmotic disruption is suspected, MRI is highly accurate for diagnosis.

Diagnostic Procedures/Surgery
Surgery may be required for some partial and complete sprains depending on location, mechanism, and chronicity.

TREATMENT

GENERAL MEASURES
- Acute: *Protection, relative rest* (activity modification), *ice, compression, elevation, medications, modalities* (PRICEMM) therapy
- Ankle sprains: Compression stockings didn't affect pain, swelling, or time to pain-free walking but did show decreased time to return to sport (6)[B].
- Grade 1, 2 ankle sprain: functional treatment with brace, orthosis, taping, elastic bandage wrap
  - Ankle braces (lace-up, stirrup-type, air cast) are a more effective functional treatment than elastic bandages or taping (7)[A].

- Grade 3 ankle sprain: Short period of immobilization may be needed.
- Refer for early physical therapy (8)[A].
- For high-level athletes with more extensive damage (e.g., biceps or pectoralis disruption), consider surgical referral.

MEDICATION

First Line
- Acetaminophen: not to exceed 3 g/day
- NSAIDs
  - Ibuprofen: 200 to 800 mg TID
  - Naproxen: 250 to 500 mg BID
  - Diclofenac: 75 mg BID
- Opioids may be needed acutely for severe pain.

- Acetaminophen and NSAIDs have similar efficacy in reducing pain after soft tissue injuries with less GI side effects, NSAIDs were better than narcotics (9)[B].
- Topical diclofenac, ibuprofen, ketoprofen are effective for pain related to strains and sprains, especially in gel form or patch (10)[A].
- Platelet-rich plasma injections may aid recovery in treatment of muscle strains, but more studies are needed.

ISSUES FOR REFERRAL
- ACL sprain in athletes/physically active
- Salter-Harris physeal fractures
- Joint instability especially chronic
- Tendon disruption (i.e., Achilles, biceps, ACL)
- Lack of improvement with conservative measures

ADDITIONAL THERAPIES
- Physical therapy is a useful adjunct after a sprain, particularly if early mobilization is crucial.
  - Proprioception retraining
  - Core strengthening
  - Eccentric exercises
  - Thera-Band exercises

- After hamstring strain, frequent daily stretching and progressive agility and trunk stabilization exercises may speed recovery and reduce risk of reinjury (11)[A]. Rehab protocols emphasizing eccentric/lengthening exercises are more effective than conventional exercises (12)[B].

SURGERY/OTHER PROCEDURES
- Casting and surgery are reserved for select partial and complete sprains. Need for surgery depends on the neurovascular supply to the injured area as well as the ability to attain full ROM and stability of the affected joint. The need for surgery also depends on activity level and patient preference.

- For primary management of acute lateral ankle sprains, there is no difference between surgical versus conservative therapy. Risks are increased with surgical intervention (1)[A].

ONGOING CARE

FOLLOW-UP RECOMMENDATIONS
If the affected joint has full strength and ROM, the patient can advance activity as tolerated using pain as a guide for return to activity.

Patient Monitoring
After initial treatment, consider early rehabilitation. Limit swelling and provide pain-free, full ROM.

DIET
Weight loss if obese

PATIENT EDUCATION
- Injury prevention through proprioceptive training and physical therapy
- ROM and strengthening exercises to restore functional capacity

PROGNOSIS
Favorable with appropriate treatment and rest. Duration of recovery depends on the severity of injury.

COMPLICATIONS
- Chronic joint instability
- Arthritis
- Muscle contracture

REFERENCES

1. Kerkhoffs GM, Handoll HH, de Bie R, et al. Surgical versus conservative treatment for acute injuries of the lateral ligament complex of the ankle in adults. *Cochrane Database Syst Rev*. 2007;(2):CD000380.
2. Sefton JM, Yarar C, Hicks-Little CA, et al. Six weeks of balance training improves sensorimotor function in individuals with chronic ankle instability. *J Orthop Sports Phys Ther*. 2011;41(2):81–89.
3. Handoll MM, Rowe BH, Quinn KM, et al. Withdrawn: interventions for preventing ankle ligament injuries. *Cochrane Database Syst Rev*. 2011;(5):CD000018.
4. Lauersen JB, Bertelsen DM, Andersen LB. The effectiveness of exercise interventions to prevent sports injuries: a systematic review and meta-analysis of randomised controlled trials. *Br J Sports Med*. 2014;48(11):871–877.
5. Bachmann LM, Kolb E, Koller MT, et al. Accuracy of the Ottawa ankle rules to exclude fractures of the ankle and mid-foot: a systematic review. *BMJ*. 2003;326(7386):417.
6. Bendahou M, Khiami F, Saïdi K, et al. Compression stockings in ankle sprain: a multi-center randomized study. *Am J Emerg Med*. 2014;32(9):1005–1010.
7. Lardenoye S, Theunissen E, Cleffken B, et al. The effect of taping versus semi-rigid bracing on patient outcome and satisfaction in ankle sprains: a prospective, randomized controlled trial. *BMC Musculoskelet Disord*. 2012;13:81.
8. Bleakley CM, O'Connor SR, Tully MA, et al. Effect of accelerated rehabilitation on function after ankle sprain: randomised controlled trial. *BMJ*. 2010;340:c1964.
9. Jones P, Dalziel SR, Lamdin R, et al. Oral non-steroidal anti-inflammatory drugs versus other oral analgesic agents for acute soft tissue injury. *Cochrane Database Syst Rev*. 2015;(7):CD007789.
10. Derry S, Moore RA, Gaskell H, et al. Topical NSAIDs for acute musculoskeletal pain in adults. *Cochrane Database Syst Rev*. 2015;(6):CD007402.
11. Mason DL, Dickens VA, Vail A. Rehabilitation for hamstring injuries. *Cochrane Database Syst Rev*. 2012;(12):CD004575.
12. Askling CM, Tengvar M, Tarassova O, et al. Acute hamstring injuries in Swedish elite sprinters and jumpers: a prospective randomised controlled clinical trial comparing two rehabilitation protocols. *Br J Sports Med*. 2014;48(7):532–539.

ADDITIONAL READING
- Hamilton BH, Best TM. Platelet-enriched plasma and muscle strain injuries: challenges imposed by the burden of proof. *Clin J Sport Med*. 2011;21(1):31–36.
- Seah R, Mani-Babu S. Managing ankle sprains in primary care: what is the best practice? A systematic review of the last 10 years of evidence. *Br Med Bull*. 2011;97:105–135.

SEE ALSO

Tendinopathy

CODES

ICD10
- S93.409A sprain of unsp ligament of unspecified ankle, init encntr
- S96.919A Strain of unsp msl/tnd at ank/ft level, unsp foot, init
- S43.50XA Sprain of unspecified acromioclavicular joint, initial encounter

CLINICAL PEARLS

For acute injury, remember PRICEMM:
- Protection of the joint
- Relative rest (activity modification)
- Apply ice
- Apply compression
- Elevate joint
- Medications for pain
- Other modalities as needed

SQUAMOUS CELL CARCINOMA, CUTANEOUS

Mercedes E. Gonzalez, MD, FAAD • Herbert P. Goodheart, MD

BASICS

- Squamous cell carcinoma (SCC) is a malignant epithelial tumor arising from epidermal keratinocytes. Cutaneous (nonmucous membrane) SCC is the second most common form of skin cancer.
- Lesions most frequently occur on sun-exposed sites of elderly, fair-skinned individuals. Most SCCs arise in actinic keratoses (*solar keratoses*). SCCs that develop from actinic keratoses are slow-growing, minimally invasive, and unaggressive. Thus, the prognosis of an SCC arising from an actinic keratosis is usually excellent because distant metastases are extremely rare.
- An SCC may also appear de novo without a preceding actinic keratosis or emerge from a preexisting human papillomavirus (HPV) infection (*verrucous carcinoma*).
- SCCs may develop from causes other than sun exposure such as within an old burn scar or on sites previously exposed to ionizing radiation.
- Metastases are more likely to occur in thicker tumors >6-mm deep (1). Other risk factors for metastases include lesions that arise on the ears, the vermilion border of the lips, or on mucous membranes. An SCC located on sites that received ionizing radiation on the skin of organ transplant recipients, in chronic inflammatory lesions (e.g., discoid lupus erythematosus), in long-standing scars or cutaneous ulcers (e.g., venous stasis ulcers), or other nonhealing wounds, also have an increased rate of metastasis.
- System(s) affected: skin/exocrine
- Synonym(s): squamous cell carcinoma of the skin; epidermoid carcinoma; prickle cell carcinoma

EPIDEMIOLOGY
- Predominant age: elderly population
- Predominant sex: males > females
- In the United States, >700,000 new cases each year

Incidence
- The escalating incidence in the United States is due to an increase in sun exposure in the general population, aging of the population, earlier and more frequent diagnosis of SCC, and the increase of immunosuppressed patients.
- The incidence is highest in Australia and in the Sun Belt of the United States.

ALERT
Bowen disease (SCC in situ) and frank SCC are two of the few skin cancers that should be considered in African Americans. Such non–sun-related SCCs tend to arise on the extremities de novo, in an old scar, or in a lesion of discoid lupus erythematosus.

ETIOLOGY AND PATHOPHYSIOLOGY
- Exact mechanisms are not established; however, SCC is thought to arise from a multistep process that begins with a single mutated keratinocyte.
- UV radiation damages skin cell nucleic acids (DNA), resulting in a mutant clone of the tumor suppressor gene, *p53*. This leads to an uncontrolled growth of skin cells containing a mutated *p53* gene. Additional mutations in genes controlling cellular proliferation and/or death lead to squamous cell dysplasia, which then progresses to SCC in situ and later invasive SCC that has the potential for metastasis.
- Cumulative UV radiation (including tanning salons, and psoralen-UV-A [PUVA] phototherapy) over a lifetime is the major etiologic factor in SCC (2)[A].

- A high prevalence of HPV DNA from SCC tissue has been noted in immunocompromised as well as immunocompetent specimens of SCC tissue (3).
- Other causative agents: ionizing radiation exposure, inorganic arsenic exposure, coal tar, and other oil derivatives
- Immunosuppression by medications or disease such as HIV/AIDS

Genetics
- Persons of Irish or Scottish ancestry have the highest prevalence of SCC.
- Caucasians with the red hair/fair skin phenotype (associated with certain variant alleles of the human melanocortin-1 receptor [MC1R]) are predisposed to SCC.
- SCC is rare in people of African and Asian descent, although it is the most common form of skin cancer in these populations.

RISK FACTORS
- Older age
- Male sex: However, incidence is increasing in females due to lifestyle changes (e.g., suntan parlors, shorter dresses).
- Chronic sun exposure: SCC is noted more frequently in those with a greater degree of outdoor activity (e.g., farmers, sailors, gardeners).
- Patients with multiple actinic keratoses
- Personal or family history of skin cancer
- Northern European descent
- Fair complexion, fair hair, light eyes
- Poor tanning ability, with tendency to burn
- Organ transplant recipients, chronic immunosuppression
- Exposure to chemical carcinogens (e.g., arsenic, tar) or ionizing radiation
- Smoking (4)
- Therapeutic UV and ionizing radiation exposure
- Defects in cell-mediated immunity related to lymphoproliferative disorders (chronic lymphocytic leukemia [CLL], lymphoma)
- HPV infection
- Chronic scarring and inflammatory conditions
- Specific genodermatoses (e.g., xeroderma pigmentosum, oculocutaneous albinism, and dystrophic epidermolysis bullosa)

GENERAL PREVENTION
Sun-avoidance measures: sunscreens, hats, clothing, and sunglasses with UV protection; tinted windshields and side windows in cars; sun-protective garments

COMMONLY ASSOCIATED CONDITIONS
- Some investigators consider an actinic keratosis to be an early SCC, although relatively few ultimately are found to develop into an SCC.
- Actinic cheilitis and leukoplakia of the mucous membranes of the lips
- Cutaneous horn (see following discussion)
- Xeroderma pigmentosum albinism
- Immunosuppression
- Chronic skin ulcers, preexisting scars, burns

DIAGNOSIS

PHYSICAL EXAM
Lesions occur chiefly on chronically sun-exposed areas.
- Face and backs of the forearms and hands
- Bald areas of the scalp and top of ears in men

- The sun-exposed "V" of the neck as well as the posterior neck below the occipital hairline
- In elderly females, lesions tend to occur on the legs and other sun-exposed locations.
- In African Americans, equal frequency in sun-exposed and unexposed areas
- Clinical appearance
  - Generally slow-growing, firm, hyperkeratotic papules, nodules, or plaques
  - Most SCCs are asymptomatic, although bleeding, pain, and tenderness may be noted.
  - Lesions may have a smooth, verrucous, or papillomatous surface.
  - Varying degrees of ulceration, erosion, crust, or scale
  - Color is often red to brown, tan, or pearly (indistinguishable from basal cell carcinoma).
- Clinical variants of SCC
  - Bowen disease (SCC in situ): solitary lesion that resembles a scaly psoriatic plaque
  - Invasive SCC: often a raised, firm papule, nodule, or plaque. Lesions may be smooth, verrucous, or papillomatous, with varying degrees of ulceration, erosion, crust, or scale.
  - Cutaneous horn: SCC with an overlying cutaneous horn. A cutaneous horn represents a thick, hard, fingernail-like keratinization produced by the SCC. Bowen disease may also produce a cutaneous horn on its surface.
  - Erythroplasia of Queyrat refers to Bowen disease of the glans penis, which manifests as one or more velvety red plaques.
  - Subungual SCC appear as hyperkeratotic lesions under the nail plate or on surrounding periungual skin, often mimicking warts (5).
  - Marjolin ulcer: an SCC evolving from a new area of ulceration or elevation at site of a scar or ulcer
  - HPV-associated SCC: virally induced. An SCC most commonly seen as a new or enlarging warty growth on penis, vulva, perianal area, or periungual region
  - Verrucous carcinoma: subtype of SCC that is extremely well differentiated, can be locally destructive, but rarely metastasizes. Lesions are "cauliflower-like" verrucous nodules or plaques.
  - Basaloid SCC: less common than typical SCC; seen more often in men aged 40 to 70 years

ALERT
Subungual SCC: Such lesions typically mimic warts.

DIFFERENTIAL DIAGNOSIS
- Actinic keratosis: Early SCC lesions may be clinically difficult, if not impossible, to distinguish from a precursor actinic keratosis.
- Basal cell carcinoma may be indistinguishable from an SCC, particularly if the lesion is ulcerated.
- Keratoacanthoma: This lesion also may be clinically and histopathologically impossible to differentiate from an SCC; it is considered by some to be a low-grade variant of an SCC.
- Verruca vulgaris: The appearance of common warts is often similar to that of SCC lesions.
- Seborrheic keratosis
- Pyoderma gangrenosum
- Venous stasis ulcer
- Chemical or thermal burn

DIAGNOSTIC TESTS & INTERPRETATION
Initial Tests (lab, imaging)
- Surgical biopsy to ensure diagnosis: shave, punch, excisional, or incisional biopsy

- Sentinel lymph node biopsy rarely is used to identify micrometastases in patients with high-risk SCC and clinically negative nodes. Whether the early detection of lymph node metastasis leads to enhanced survival in SCC is unknown.
- Patients with lymphadenopathy should be evaluated for metastases with CT scanning, MRI, US, or PET.

Test Interpretation
- Noninvasive SCC is characterized by an intraepidermal proliferation of atypical keratinocytes. Hyperkeratosis, acanthosis, and confluent parakeratosis are seen within the epidermis. Cellular atypia, including pleomorphism, hyperchromatic nuclei, and mitoses are prominent. Atypical keratinocytes may be found in the basal layer and often extend deeply down the hair follicles, but they do not invade the dermis.
- In the in situ type of SCC (Bowen disease), atypia involves the full thickness of the epidermis but the basement membrane remains intact.
- An invasive SCC penetrates through the basement membrane into the dermis. It has various levels of anaplasia and may manifest relatively few to multiple mitoses and display varying degrees of differentiation, such as keratinization.
- Poorly differentiated tumors are clinically more aggressive. SCCs proliferate first by local invasion. Metastases, when they do occur, spread via local lymph ducts to local lymph nodes.

ALERT
Melanoma: An amelanotic melanoma and ulcerated melanoma may also be impossible to distinguish from an SCC.

TREATMENT

MEDICATION
First Line
- Total excision: preferred method for SCCs, permitting histologic diagnosis of the tumor margins
- Electrodesiccation and curettage (ED&C)
  - Best for small lesions (generally <1 cm) on flat surfaces (e.g., forehead, cheek) and SCC in situ (Bowen disease). ED&C may be used to treat superficially invasive SCCs that lack high-risk characteristics, but it is not appropriate for certain high-risk anatomic locations.
- Cryosurgery with LN_2 in selected lesions, such as SCC in situ
- Micrographic (Mohs) surgery is a microscopically controlled method of removing skin cancers that allows for controlled excision and maximum preservation of normal tissue. It has the highest cure rate (94–99%) of all surgical treatments. Mohs surgery may be indicated for the following:
  - Large, recurrent or invasive SCCs (e.g., to bone or cartilage)
  - Lesions with a poorly delineated clinical border
  - Locations where preservation of normal tissue is extremely important (e.g., tip of the nose, eyelids, ala nasi, ears, lips, and glans penis)
- Radiation therapy is a primary treatment option that is generally restricted to older patients who are physically debilitated or are unable to undergo or refuse to undergo excisional surgery.

Second Line
- Immunotherapy with topical imiquimod (Aldara) 5% cream has been successfully used for the treatment of SCC in situ (Bowen disease), actinic keratoses, genital warts, and superficial basal cell carcinoma (6)[A].
- Topical chemotherapy: topical formulations of 5-fluorouracil (5-FU) (6)[A]

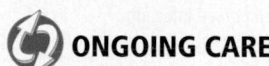

- Intralesional 5-FU and bleomycin has also been used successfully to treat SCCs.
- Photodynamic therapy (PDT): PDT involves application of a photosensitizer (given topically or systemically) followed by exposure to a light source. Used primarily to treat large numbers of solar keratoses and is not recommended for treatment of invasive SCCs.
- In patients with multiple or recurrent SCCs or those at high risk, such as organ transplant recipients, chemoprevention with systemic retinoids, such as acitretin, may be effective for reducing the number of new SCCs, treating existing SCCs, and reducing the risk of recurrence.

ADDITIONAL THERAPIES
For metastatic SCC, oral 5-FU has been used alone or in combination with SC interferon. More recently, epidermal growth factor receptor (EGFR) inhibitors, such as cetuximab (7)[C], are used in combination with systemic chemotherapy for metastatic disease.

SURGERY/OTHER PROCEDURES
- Complete lymphadenectomy of the draining nodal basin for high-risk tumors
- Metastatic disease requires aggressive management by a multidisciplinary team, involving plastic, ENT/maxillofacial, general and onchologic surgeons.

 ONGOING CARE

FOLLOW-UP RECOMMENDATIONS
Patient Monitoring
Skin exam every month for 3 months, 6 months after treatment, and then yearly

PATIENT EDUCATION
Skin self-exam: Encourage sun-avoidance techniques, protective clothing, sunscreens, and so forth. Artificial tanning devices should be avoided.

PROGNOSIS
- For low-risk SCCs: a 90–95% cure rate with appropriate treatment
- Overall, head and neck lesions have better prognosis; however, lip and ear lesions metastasize more frequently when compared with other sites.
- The ability to produce scale (keratinization) indicates a tendency for a lesion to be more differentiated and less likely to metastasize.
- Softer, nonkeratinizing lesions are not as well differentiated and thus are more likely to spread.
- Lesions ≥2 cm are more likely to recur.
- SCCs that arise in areas of non–sun-exposed skin or have a greater tendency to metastasize
- An SCC arising on a mucous membrane or in a chronic ulcer should be regarded as potentially metastatic.
- Recurrence rate and mortality is greater in immunosuppressed patients, especially solid-organ transplant recipients.
- SCCs that are deeply invasive (≥6 mm in SC fat), or have perineural involvement, are more likely to metastasize.
- When SCC does metastasize, it usually occurs within several years from the time of diagnosis and involves draining lymph nodes.
- Once nodal metastasis of cutaneous SCC has occurred, the overall 5-year survival rate has historically been in the range of 25–35%.

COMPLICATIONS
- Untreated, an SCC becomes indurated, with a tendency to ooze, ulcerate, or bleed.
- Local recurrence
- Metastatic disease

REFERENCES
1. Brantsch KD, Meisner C, Schönfisch B, et al. Analysis of risk factors determining prognosis of cutaneous squamous-cell carcinoma: a prospective study. *Lancet Oncol.* 2008;9(8):713–720.
2. Archier E, Devaux S, Castela E, et al. Carcinogenic risks of psoralen UV-A therapy and narrowband UV-B therapy in chronic plaque psoriasis: a systematic literature review. *J Eur Acad Dermatol Venereol.* 2012;26(Suppl 3):22–31.
3. Karagas MR, Nelson HH, Sehr P, et al. Human papillomavirus infection and incidence of squamous cell and basal cell carcinomas of the skin. *J Natl Cancer Inst.* 2006 Mar 15;98(6):389–95.
4. Leonardi-Bee J, Ellison T, Bath-Hextall F. Smoking and the risk of nonmelanoma skin cancer: systematic review and meta-analysis. *Arch Dermatol.* 2012;148(8):939–946.
5. Riddel C, Rashid R, Thomas V. Ungual and periungual human papillomavirus-associated squamous cell carcinoma: a review. *J Am Acad Dermatol.* 2011;64(6):1147–1153.
6. Micali G, Lacarrubba F, Nasca MR, et al. Topical pharmacotherapy for skin cancer: part II. Clinical applications. *J Am Acad Dermatol.* 2014;70(6):979.e1–979.e12.
7. Miller K, Sherman W, Ratner D. Complete clinical response to cetuximab in a patient with metastatic cutaneous squamous cell carcinoma. *Dermatol Surg.* 2010;36(12):2069–2074.

ADDITIONAL READING
- Martorell-Calatayud A, Sanmartín Jimenez O, Cruz Mojarrieta J, et al. Cutaneous squamous cell carcinoma: defining the high-risk variant [in English, Spanish]. *Actas Dermosifiliogr.* 2013;104(5):367–379.
- Wang J, Aldabagh B, Yu J, et al. Role of human papillomavirus in cutaneous squamous cell carcinoma: a meta-analysis. *J Am Acad Dermatol.* 2014;70(4):621–629.

CODES

ICD10
- C44.92 Squamous cell carcinoma of skin, unspecified
- C44.320 Squamous cell carcinoma of skin of unspecified parts of face
- C44.42 Squamous cell carcinoma of skin of scalp and neck

CLINICAL PEARLS
- SCCs that develop from actinic keratoses are generally unaggressive.
- Unlike most basal cell carcinomas, SCCs of the skin are associated with a risk of metastasis, especially those arising on mucous membranes, chronic ulcers, or in immunocompromised patients.
- A subungual SCC can easily be mistaken for a wart.

STEVENS-JOHNSON SYNDROME

Matthew A. Silva, PharmD, RPh, BCPS • Pablo I. Hernandez Itriago, MD, MS, FAAFP

BASICS

DESCRIPTION
- A generalized hypersensitivity reaction, usually to a drug, in which skin and mucous membrane lesions are an early manifestation
- A severe form of erythema multiforme in which >1 mucosal surface is involved; many now consider it to be a different disease with a more difficult course and a more ominous prognosis.
- Stevens-Johnson syndrome (SJS) exists on a continuum with toxic epidermal necrolysis (TEN).
- SJS presents with characteristic targetoid cutaneous lesions when <10% of the body surface area (BSA) is involved.
- Targetoid cutaneous lesion involvement of 10–30% of BSA is considered an overlap between SJS and TEN. Involvement of >30% of BSA is TEN, which has a high morbidity and up to 70% mortality.
- System(s) affected: cardiovascular, hematologic, lymphatic/immunologic, nervous, renal/urologic, skin/exocrine
- Synonym(s): ectodermosis erosiva pluriorificialis; febrile mucocutaneous syndrome; herpes iris; erythema polymorphe; toxic epidermal necrolysis (TEN)

ALERT
Patients with discrete skin lesions and >10% epidermal detachment are at risk of rapid progression to TEN.

Geriatric Considerations
TEN has a greater mortality in older patients.

Pediatric Considerations
Rare in children <3 years of age, more common in years 3 to young adult

Pregnancy Considerations
Pregnancy is a possible predisposing condition.

EPIDEMIOLOGY
Incidence
- Incidence/prevalence of SJS in the United States is difficult to estimate because there is no universally accepted definition of SJS.
- 1.1 to 7.1 and 0.4 to 1.2 cases/1 million person-years for SJS and TEN, respectively

Prevalence
- Predominant sex: male > female (2:1)
- Sex (females): 33–62% for SJS and 61.3–64.3% for TEN
- Age (average range): 25 to 47 years for SJS and 46 to 63 years for TEN, <10% of cases are children.

ETIOLOGY AND PATHOPHYSIOLOGY
- 50% of cases are idiopathic; cross-reactivity between drug classes is suspected (1).
- Associated with abnormal metabolism and clearance of drugs and metabolites (2)
- Slow intrinsic acetylation rates

- 75% of cases involving SJS/TEN including those with overlap associated with a recent medication:
  - 50% of cases occur within 4 weeks and 90% of cases occur within 8 weeks of an offending agent (1).
- Algorithm-based approach is helpful for assessing probability of drug causality in SJS, TEN, or overlap (3)[B],(4).
- Frequently associated with upper respiratory tract infection and recent use of antibiotics
- Sulfonamides are the drugs most strongly associated with SJS and TEN. Then:
  - Cephalosporins
  - Quinolones
  - Aminopenicillins
  - Tetracyclines
  - Macrolides
  - Imidazole antifungals
  - Antiretrovirals (e.g., protease inhibitors, efavirenz, abacavir, amprenavir, telaprevir, fosamprenavir, atazanavir, darunavir, etravirine)
  - Anticonvulsants, especially carbamazepine
  - NSAIDs, especially oxicam
  - Allopurinol, especially in patients of European/Israeli heritage
  - Acetaminophen
  - Vaccines: DPT, BCG, oral polio
  - *Mycoplasma pneumoniae* infection
- Erythematous papular lesions and keratinocyte necrosis are a consequence of cell-mediated immunity.
- Occurs 1 to 2 weeks after initial exposure to offending drugs and within 48 hours on rechallenge
- Accumulation and binding of reactive drug metabolites to mucocutaneous epithelial cells as haptens (3)
- Drug haptens signal drug-specific CD8+ T-lymphocyte and macrophages, which infiltrate and express interleukin 2 (IL-2), tumor necrosis factor-α (TNF-α), and interferon-γ, leading to keratinocyte activation.
- Cytokines enhance keratinocyte expression of soluble Fas ligand and Fas receptors, leading to apoptosis.

Genetics
Associations with *HLA-A*3101* in Northern Europeans; *HLA-B*1501, HLA-B*1502, HLA-B*1511, HLA-B*5801* in patients of Asian ancestry, *HLA-Bw44, HLA-B12,* and *HLA-DQB1*0601*

RISK FACTORS
- Previous history of SJS
- Immunocompromised status, including chronic viral infections with Epstein-Barr virus and HIV (5)
- Patients with HIV infection may be predisposed to developing SJS in response to their medications:
  - HLA allele subtypes A, B, and D
  - Diseases that cause immune compromise (e.g., deficiencies, malignancy)
  - Possibly radiation therapy/ultraviolet light

GENERAL PREVENTION
Secondary prevention possible by avoiding exposure to offending medications/chemical agents.

COMMONLY ASSOCIATED CONDITIONS
- SJS progressing to TEN is ominous prognostically.
- *M. pneumoniae* may be an infectious precursor.

DIAGNOSIS

HISTORY
- Usually a preceding illness for which the medication was given 1 to 3 weeks before initial cutaneous manifestations
- Sudden onset with rapidly progressive pleomorphic rash that includes petechiae, vesicles, bullae
- Considered to be SJS if epidermal detachments affect <10% of the skin
- Classified as TEN if epidermal detachments affect >30% or >10% in the absence of discrete skin lesions
- Discrete skin lesions and 10–30% epidermal detachment are an overlap between SJS/TEN.
- Burning sensation of the skin and sometimes of the mucous membranes
- Usually no pruritus
- Fever 39–40°C (102–104°F)
- Headache, malaise, arthralgias
- Cough productive of thick, purulent sputum

PHYSICAL EXAM
- Recognized by the presence of several of the following features:
  - Vesicles and ulcers on the mucous membranes, especially the mouth and throat
  - Confluent erythematous macules with purpuric, necrotic centers and overlying blistering (1)
  - Epidermal detachment with light lateral pressure (Nikolsky sign)
  - Fever 39–40°C (102–104°F)
  - Crusted nares
  - Conjunctivitis and/or corneal ulcerations
  - Erosive vulvovaginitis/balanitis
  - Cough productive of thick, purulent sputum
  - Tachypnea/respiratory distress
  - Arrhythmias
  - Pericarditis
  - Congestive heart failure (CHF)
  - Mental status changes
  - Seizures
  - Coma
- Sepsis:
  - May be seen in SJS when epidermal detachment affects <10% of the skin
  - Seen in TEN if epidermal detachment >30% or >10% in the absence of discrete skin lesions

DIFFERENTIAL DIAGNOSIS
- Erythema multiforme major
- Exfoliative dermatitis
- Linear IgA bullous dermatosis
- Staphylococcal scalded skin syndrome
- Pemphigus (paraneoplastic)
- Generalized fixed drug eruption
- Burns
- Pressure blisters (coma, barbiturates)

DIAGNOSTIC TESTS & INTERPRETATION
Initial Tests (lab, imaging)
- Culture/serologic tests for suspected sources of infection
- Electrolytes and creatinine
- Urine for albuminuria/hematuria

Follow-Up Tests & Special Considerations
Skin biopsy

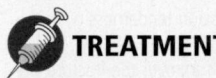 **TREATMENT**

GENERAL MEASURES
- Withdraw all suspected medications, and treat any underlying disease.
- Meticulous care of damaged skin
- Supportive care, including moisture-retentive ointment, petroleum jelly, and sterile saline compresses
- Catheter changing and culturing
- Reverse isolation and temperature control with extensive epidermal loss
- Maintenance of fluid, electrolyte, and protein balance
- Plasmapheresis
- Adequate calorie intake; parenteral nutrition, if necessary
- Mouthwashes of warm saline or a solution of diphenhydramine, lidocaine, and kaolin suspension
- Ophthalmologic consultation and monitoring for corneal damage
- Venous thromboembolism prophylaxis with unfractionated heparin or low-molecular-weight heparin

MEDICATION
First Line
- Corticosteroids are controversial. Early high-dose IV steroids may attenuate disease progression, reduce skin detachment, decrease inflammatory cytokine activity, and improve patient comfort. Withdraw if no benefit is seen in the 1st few days.
- Experimental treatments that appear to have been useful include:
  - Recombinant granulocyte colony-stimulating factor
  - Cyclophosphamide
  - Cyclosporine (6)
  - Intravenous immunoglobulin (IVIG) in HIV-positive patients; IVIG is considered beneficial treatment and prophylaxis, although not approved by the FDA (5). Interferes with Fas ligand-induced apoptosis.
- Contraindications: Avoid steroids in diabetic/immunosuppressed patients/those with chronic infections.

Second Line
- Acyclovir for herpetic infections
- Erythromycin or related antibiotic for *Mycoplasma* infections (empirical use of antibiotics is not recommended)

ADDITIONAL THERAPIES
In severe ocular surface and eyelid inflammation due to acute SJS and TEN, amniotic membrane transplantation is an effective treatment for severe ocular surface and eyelid inflammation, greatly decreasing the risk of significant ocular and visual sequelae.

SURGERY/OTHER PROCEDURES
- Sterile débridement of areas of extensive epidermal loss
- Application of biosynthetic dressings, such as Biobrane to denuded areas
- Damage to the vulva, vagina, or cornea: Consider surgical repair.

INPATIENT CONSIDERATIONS
Admission Criteria/Initial Stabilization
- This disease progresses rapidly; all patients should be admitted.
- Admission to a burn unit greatly improves the outcome for any patient who has sloughed skin over ≥10% of the BSA.
- ICU for bronchiolitis, acute respiratory distress syndrome (ARDS), or multiorgan damage

IV Fluids
Fluid management with saline and macromolecules is necessary in the first 24 hours with decreasing IV fluid requirements as oral intake proceeds with nasogastric tube.

Nursing
- Bed rest until clinically stabilized
- Avoid administration of topical silver sulfadiazine owing to association with sulfonamide and SJS.
- Use a coordinated approach involving critical care, wound care, and burn specialists (1).

 ONGOING CARE

FOLLOW-UP RECOMMENDATIONS
- Extensive documentation of all offending/suspected medications/chemical agents
- Education to limit exposure to offending/suspected medications/chemical agents

DIET
IV nutritional support with increased protein requirements; may need insulin for glycoregulation in this hypercatabolic state

PATIENT EDUCATION
Plan to prevent exposure to offending/suspected medications/agents.

PROGNOSIS
- Rapid onset or evolve over 1 to 2 weeks with resolution over 4 to 6 weeks.
- Often skin/mucous membrane scarring occurs, especially of the vulva
- Blindness/corneal opacities occur in 7–20% of patients.
- Risk of recurrence is as high as 37%.

COMPLICATIONS
- Secondary infections, sepsis, pneumonia, ARDS
- Bronchiolitis obliterans in children
- Dehydration/electrolyte disturbance, acute tubular necrosis
- Corneal ulceration/iritis, urethral erosions, and genitourinary strictures
- Arrhythmias
- Venous thromboembolism, disseminated intravascular coagulation DIC
- Death occurs in 5–15% of the patients with SJS, up to 30% in patients with SJS/TEN overlap, and in up to 50% of patients with TEN (7).

REFERENCES
1. Struck MF, Hilbert P, Mockenhaupt M, et al. Severe cutaneous adverse reactions: emergency approach to non-burn epidermolytic syndromes. *Intensive Care Med*. 2010;36(1):22–32.
2. Gerull R, Nelle M, Schaible T. Toxic epidermal necrolysis and Stevens-Johnson syndrome: a review. *Crit Care Med*. 2011;39(6):1521–1532.
3. Pichler WJ, Naisbitt DJ, Park BK. Immune pathomechanism of drug hypersensitivity reactions. *J Allergy Clin Immunol*. 2011;127(3 Suppl): S74–S81.
4. Sassolas B, Haddad C, Mockenhaupt M, et al. ALDEN, an algorithm for assessment of drug causality in Stevens-Johnson Syndrome and toxic epidermal necrolysis: comparison with case-control analysis. *Clin Pharmacol Ther*. 2010;88(1):60–68.
5. Hazin R, Ibrahimi OA, Hazin MI, et al. Stevens-Johnson syndrome: pathogenesis, diagnosis, and management. *Ann Med*. 2008;40(2):129–138.
6. Reese D, Henning JS, Rockers K, et al. Cyclosporine for SJS/TEN: a case series and review of the literature. *Cutis*. 2011;87(1):24–29.
7. Mockenhaupt M. The current understanding of Stevens-Johnson syndrome and toxic epidermal necrolysis. *Expert Rev Clin Immunol*. 2011;84(6): 803–813.

 SEE ALSO

Burns; Cutaneous Drug Reactions; Dermatitis Herpetiformis; Erythema Multiforme; Pemphigoid, Bullous; Pemphigus Vulgaris; Respiratory Distress Syndrome, Acute (ARDS)

 CODES

ICD10
- L51.1 Stevens-Johnson syndrome
- L51.3 Stevens-Johnson synd-tox epdrml necrolysis overlap syndrome

CLINICAL PEARLS
- Corticosteroid treatment is controversial. If chosen and no response within 1st few days, discontinue.
- Recurrences are possible. Etiologic agents should be identified if possible and avoided indefinitely.

STRESS FRACTURE

Nandhini Veeraraghavan, MD, CAQSM

 BASICS

DESCRIPTION
- Overuse injuries caused by cumulative microdamage from repetitive bone loading.
- Stress fractures occur in different situations:
  - Fatigue fracture: abnormal stress applied to normal bone (e.g., young college athletes or new military recruits with increased physical activity demands and inadequate conditioning)
  - Insufficiency fracture: normal stress applied to structurally abnormal bone (e.g., femoral neck fracture in osteopenic bone)
  - Combination fracture: abnormal stress applied to abnormal bone (e.g., female long-distance runners with premature osteoporosis from female athletic triad)
- Weight-bearing bones of the lower extremity are most commonly affected at the following sites:
  - Tibia
  - Metatarsal bones
  - Fibula
  - Navicular
  - Femoral neck
  - Pars interarticularis
- Less commonly affected sites:
  - Pelvis
  - Calcaneus
  - Ribs
  - Ulna
- High-risk stress fractures occur in zones of tension or areas with poor blood supply and are more likely to result in fracture displacement and/or nonunion. High-risk sites include the following:
  - Tension side of femoral neck
  - Anterior tibial diaphysis
  - Sesamoids
  - Pars interarticularis of lumbar spine (L4, L5)
  - 5th metatarsal at metaphyseal–diaphyseal junction
  - Proximal 2nd metatarsal
  - Medial malleolus
  - Tarsal navicular
  - Patella
  - Talar neck
- Synonym(s): march fracture; fatigue fracture

EPIDEMIOLOGY
Incidence
- Greatest incidence in 15- to 27-year-olds
- Females more commonly affected than males
- Affects 9–21% of track and field athletes annually
- Accounts for as many as 8% of visits to sports medicine and orthopedic clinics
- Occurs in <1% of general population

Prevalence
- Affects 5% of military recruits
- Affects 1–3% of college athletes

ETIOLOGY AND PATHOPHYSIOLOGY
- Bone is a dynamic tissue that is constantly remodeling in response to applied physiologic stress.
- Repetitive loading or overuse causes microfractures that can't heal due to imbalance between bone resorption and bone formation.
- If microdamage accumulates in excess of reparation, bony fatigue leads to stress fracture.

RISK FACTORS
- Intrinsic
  - Female athlete triad (low energy availability with or without disordered eating, menstrual dysfunction, and low bone mineral density)
  - History of previous stress fracture
  - History of osteoporosis, osteomalacia, rheumatoid arthritis, corticosteroid therapy
  - Skeletal malalignment: pes cavus, pes planus, leg length discrepancies, excessive forefoot varus, tarsal coalitions, prominent posterior calcaneal process, tight heel cords
  - Increased vertical loading rate (e.g., heel-to-toe running instead of forefoot striking)
  - Muscle fatigue and decreased lean muscle mass
  - Extremes of body size and composition
  - Previous inactivity or low aerobic fitness
- Extrinsic
  - Type of exercise—running, track and field, basketball, gymnastics, soccer, and dance are highest risk.
  - Rapid increase in mileage, running pace, or training volume
  - Inappropriate footwear
  - Hard training surface
  - Inadequate recovery or rest and training with fatigued muscle
- Tobacco use

GENERAL PREVENTION
- Avoid abrupt increases in physical activity (no more than 10% increase in load per week).
- Reduce intensity and duration of activity if new-onset pain.
- Proper footwear
- Increasing dynamic physical activity (jumping; plyometric training) increases bone density and resistance to mechanical stress.
- Decrease vertical loading rate either by switching to forefoot strike running or (if continuing with heel-to-toe strike) by using a heel pad insert.
- Shock-absorbing foot inserts may help.
- Increasing calcium and vitamin D intake may reduce stress fracture rates in female runners and military recruits.

COMMONLY ASSOCIATED CONDITIONS
- Osteoporosis/osteopenia
- Female athlete triad
- Metabolic bone disorders

DIAGNOSIS

HISTORY
- Insidious onset of vague bony pain over period of weeks worsened with physical activity
- Rest initially relieves pain.
- If untreated, pain progresses and may occur earlier during training sessions or even at rest. Pain also becomes more localized.
- History of recent change in training intensity, alteration in training terrain, and/or footwear
- Assess dietary practices: energy availability, disordered eating, and weight fluctuations, calcium and vitamin D intake
- Assess menstrual history: menarche, oligomenorrhea, or amenorrhea

PHYSICAL EXAM
- Height, weight, BMI, and any stigmata of disordered eating (cold extremities, hypercarotenemia, lanugo hair, calluses on back of fingers, poor oral hygiene, parotid gland hypertrophy, bradycardia, or orthostatic hypotension)
- Antalgic gait
- Point tenderness or percussion tenderness over injury site
- Placing a vibrating tuning fork over the fracture site may intensify pain.
- Swelling may be present.
- Specific tests:
  - Hop test for tibial stress fracture: cannot hop on one leg 10 times; if able to perform test, consider shin splints (medial tibial stress syndrome).
  - Fulcrum test for femoral stress fracture: With patient seated, provoke pain by applying downward force on the distal femur while other hand uses the midthigh as fulcrum on femoral shaft (use with caution to avoid completing a femoral neck stress fracture if clinical suspicion is high).
  - Single-leg hyperextension (Stork) test for pars interarticularis fracture of lumbar spine: Stand on leg of symptomatic side and extend lumbar spine. Positive if painful.
- Anatomic malalignment may be present (leg length discrepancy, pes planus/cavus).

DIFFERENTIAL DIAGNOSIS
- Shin splints (medial tibial stress syndrome—pain resolves with rest; stress fracture pain does not)
- Infection (osteomyelitis)
- Soft tissue injury (sprain, tendonitis, and periostitis)
- Compartment syndrome
- Bony fracture
- Neoplasm (osteoid osteoma)
- Entrapment syndromes
- Intermittent claudication

DIAGNOSTIC TESTS & INTERPRETATION
- None unless clinically indicated for suspected disease (e.g., female athlete triad, hyperparathyroidism, and vitamin D deficiency)
- Plain films:
  - First line in suspected stress fracture
  - Findings typically seen 2 to 8 weeks after onset of pain.
  - Sensitivity during early stages (1 to 2 weeks) may be as low as 10%.
  - May see periosteal callus, "gray cortex sign" (region of decreased cortical intensity), osteopenia, endosteal reaction, or ill-defined cortical margin
  - Severe cases may show discrete fracture.

Follow-Up Tests & Special Considerations
- MRI:
  - Gold standard for imaging stress fractures
  - Very sensitive
  - Better evaluation of exact anatomic location and extent of injury
- Bone scan:
  - Sensitive but nonspecific for stress fracture
  - Should not be used to assess healing process

- CT scan:
  – Less sensitive than MRI or bone scan for early stress fractures but has an important role in evaluating occult fractures of foot, tibia, carpal scaphoid, and pars interarticularis
  – Can distinguish diseases (osteoid osteoma, malignancy, and osteomyelitis) that mimic stress fracture on bone scan
  – Bony detail provided by CT scan allows differentiation of complete versus incomplete fracture, especially when MRI is equivocal.
- US:
  – Not routinely used but may be of particular help in the evaluation of metatarsal stress fracture to distinguish from other causes of metatarsalgia (e.g., Morton neuroma)
- Classification by radiographic grading (1)
- Grade I: normal x-ray, positive short time inversion recovery (STIR) MRI
- Grade II: normal x-ray, positive STIR + positive T2-weighted MRI
- Grade III: discrete line or discrete periosteal reaction on x-ray, positive T1/T2-weighted MRI but with no definite cortical break
- Grade IV: fracture or periosteal reaction on x-ray, positive T1/T2-weighted fracture line.

 TREATMENT

- Protection, rest, ice, compression, and elevation (PRICE) for acute pain and edema
- Decrease activity to the level of pain-free functioning.
- Pain at rest or with gentle range of motion (ROM) may require temporary immobilization.
- Painful ambulation requires patients use crutches with periodic walking trial to assess readiness for nonaided ambulation.
- Pneumatic leg brace is effective in decreasing the return-to-play time for tibial shaft stress fracture (2)[C].
- For low-risk stress fracture, slowly increase impact loading once ambulation and daily activities are pain free. Progression of activity depends on the individual and should be modified according to symptoms (3,4).
- High-risk fractures often require immediate immobilization and a period of non–weight-bearing. Many patients will require early surgical intervention to avoid nonunion and facilitate earlier return to sport (5,6).
- In bisphosphonate-associated femoral stress fracture, prophylactic nail fixation may avoid fracture completion, shorten hospital stay, and decrease subsequent morbidity (7)[C].

MEDICATION
First Line
- Calcium and vitamin D supplementation should be initiated when dietary intake is inadequate or deficiencies are found.
- Acetaminophen
- NSAIDs are beneficial for pain and inflammation but may adversely affect fracture healing and should, therefore, be used only sparingly.

- Bisphosphonates theoretically could treat stress fractures by suppressing bone remodeling. There is no conclusive evidence to prove that this improves fracture healing in humans. Currently, only case reports have shown benefit (8)[A].

ISSUES FOR REFERRAL
Orthopedic consultation for high-risk fractures, failure to improve with standard treatment, evidence of nonunion within 3 to 4 weeks, or inability to tolerate rehabilitation

ADDITIONAL THERAPIES
- Electrical stimulation may be an adjunct for delayed union and nonunion.
- Extracorporeal shock wave therapy (ESWT) and pulsed US may have some potential benefits but require additional study (9)[A].
- Physical therapy:
  – Correct training errors and inappropriate mechanics predisposing to stress fracture.
  – Strengthen muscles around the site of stress fracture.
  – Encourage cross-training to maintain fitness.
  – Correct anatomic variations.
  – Antigravity treadmills

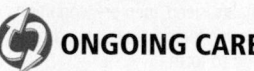 ONGOING CARE

FOLLOW-UP RECOMMENDATIONS
- Once the patient is pain free, low-impact training can start and be advanced gently as tolerated.
- Once running has resumed, increase mileage slowly.

Patient Monitoring
Radiographs every 4 to 6 weeks to document healing progress

PATIENT EDUCATION
- Gradually increase activity as long as pain free
- Rest and reevaluate if there is a recurrence of pain.
- Correct mechanical and training errors.
- Strengthen core muscles.

PROGNOSIS
- Stress fractures in young people have a good prognosis.
- Older patients or those with metabolic bone disease often develop insufficiency fractures in other bones.
- Time to return to full activity:
  – Grade I: 3+ weeks
  – Grade II: 5+ weeks
  – Grade III: 11+ weeks
  – Grade IV: 14+ weeks

COMPLICATIONS
- Completion of fracture
- Delayed union
- Nonunion
- May require surgery with internal fixation

REFERENCES
1. Beck BR, Bergman AG, Miner M, et al. Tibial stress injury: relationship of radiographic, nuclear medicine bone scanning, MR imaging, and CT severity grades to clinical severity and time to healing. Radiology. 2012;263(3):811–818.
2. Matheson GO, Brukner P. Pneumatic leg brace after tibial stress fracture for faster return to play. Clin J Sport Med. 1998;8(1):66.
3. Mayer SW, Joyner PW, Almekinders LC, et al. Stress fractures of the foot and ankle in athletes. Sports Health. 2014;6(6):481–491. doi:10.1177/1941738113486588.
4. Pegrum J, Crisp T, Padhiar N. Diagnosis and management of bone stress injuries of the lower limb in athletes. BMJ. 2012;344:e2511. doi:10.1136/bmj.e2511.
5. Shindle MK, Endo Y, Warren RF, et al. Stress fractures about the tibia, foot, and ankle. J Am Acad Orthop Surg. 2012;20(3):167–176.
6. Behrens SB, Deren ME, Matson A, et al. Stress fractures of the pelvis and legs in athletes: a review. Sports Health. 2013;5(2):165–174.
7. Ward WG Sr, Carter CJ, Wilson SC, et al. Femoral stress fractures associated with long-term bisphosphonate treatment. Clin Orthop Relat Res. 2012;470(3):759–765.
8. Shima Y, Engebretsen L, Iwasa J, et al. Use of bisphosphonates for the treatment of stress fractures in athletes. Knee Surg Sports Traumatol Arthrosc. 2009;17(5):542–550.
9. Griffin XL, Smith N, Parsons N, et al. Ultrasound and shockwave therapy for acute fractures in adults. Cochrane Database Syst Rev. 2012;(2):CD008579. doi:10.1002/14651858.CD008579.pub2.

ADDITIONAL READING
- Chen YT, Tenforde AS, Fredericson M. Update on stress fractures in female athletes: epidemiology, treatment, and prevention. Curr Rev Musculoskelet Med. 2013;6(2):173–181. doi:10.1007/s12178-013-9167-x.
- Ross AC, Manson JE, Abrams SA, et al. The 2011 report on dietary reference intakes for calcium and vitamin D from the Institute of Medicine: what clinicians need to know. J Clin Endocrinol Metab. 2011;96(1):53–58.

 SEE ALSO

Algorithm: Foot Pain

 CODES

ICD10
- M84.38XA Stress fracture, other site, initial encounter for fracture
- M84.369A Stress fracture, unsp tibia and fibula, init for fx
- M84.376A Stress fracture, unspecified foot, init encntr for fracture

CLINICAL PEARLS
- The diagnosis of stress fractures requires a high index of suspicion. X-rays are often negative initially.
- Identify and treat female athletic triad to prevent stress fractures.
- Progress activity levels gradually and avoid sudden increases in activity or running mileage to help prevent stress fractures.
- High-risk fractures often require immobilization and surgery.

STROKE REHABILITATION

Aaron Hauptman, MD • Jordan Eisenstock, MD • Robert A. Baldor, MD, FAAFP

 BASICS

DESCRIPTION

- Stroke is a compromise in blood supply to an area of the nervous system, secondary to hemorrhage or occlusion, with resultant infarction of nervous tissue.
- 3rd leading cause of death and the leading cause of long-term disability in the United States (1)
- Rehabilitation refers to the process of restoring a debilitated person toward baseline functionality.
- Specific rehabilitation techniques should be used depending on the individual and based on particular deficits and brain regions impacted.
- Rehabilitation involves cycling through the following (2):
  – Assessment of patient with the goal of identification and quantification needs of the individual
  – Setting of objectives that are realistic, concrete, and attainable
  – Repetition of assessment to gauge changes in status, with subsequent alteration of techniques as necessary
- Motor impairment is the most commonly recognized impairment secondary to stroke.
- Speech and language, swallowing, vision, sensation, and cognition are also commonly impaired.

EPIDEMIOLOGY

Incidence

- Each year, ~795,000 people suffer stroke; ~610,000 are first attacks, and 185,000 are recurrent attacks (3).
- ~14% of stroke survivors reach full recovery in physical function; 25–50% need assistance poststroke (1).
- According to the WHO, 15 million people suffer stroke worldwide each year. Of these, 5 million die and another 5 million are permanently disabled.

Prevalence

- ~7 million Americans ≥20 years old have had a stroke (~3%) (3).
- ~50 million stroke survivors worldwide (4)
- >1/2 of strokes in people <65 years result in death within 8 years (1).

ETIOLOGY AND PATHOPHYSIOLOGY

Stroke involves a compromise in blood supply to an area, usually by either rupture or blockage of a vessel. Of all strokes, 87% are ischemic, 10% intracerebral hemorrhage, and 3% subarachnoid hemorrhage (3).

Neural Mechanisms of Remodeling

Poststroke remodeling changes provide some degree of recovery that varies considerably between individuals. Outcomes are greatest when remodeling mimics normal organization to the greatest degree possible. Neurophysiologic changes involved in spontaneous recovery include the following (5)[B]:

- Augmented excitability in areas of cortex functionally connected to injured brain
- Increased activity contralateral to traumatized cortex
- Changes in somatotopic map in other regions

Research suggests a critical window for neurophysiologic changes, further understanding of which may facilitate neurorehabilitation by augmenting endogenous healing. Animal studies suggest promising strategies for enhancing rehabilitative efforts including growth factors, hormones, proteins, cytokines, stem cells, and so forth. Studies are ongoing exploring

combinations of plasticity-promoting factors, rehabilitative training, and imaging/biomarker modalities together with carefully timed neurorehabilitation that takes advantage of endogenous plasticity timing. Such work is complicated by the vast heterogeneity of stroke insults but offers promising options for future multimodal treatments.

RISK FACTORS

Risk factors for stroke are discussed in the topics "Stroke, Acute" and "Atherosclerosis."

GENERAL PREVENTION

See "Stroke, Acute."

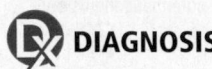 DIAGNOSIS

HISTORY

- For acute stroke symptoms, see "Stroke, Acute."
- A wide variety of systems and functions are commonly impacted by stroke, depending on type, severity, location, and so forth including the following (2):
  – Consciousness and psychological functions
    ○ Orientation, arousal, alertness, attention, intellect, personality, sleep, memory, cognition, perception, behavior, temperament, psychomotor functions, and so forth
  – Perceptual functions, most commonly
    ○ Vision, proprioception, touch sensation
  – Communication, excretory, and sexual functions
    ○ Vocal control and articulation; intake of food (chewing, swallowing), urinary and bowel functions; sexual function
  – Neuromuscular and ADLs
    ○ Muscle strength, stability, endurance, reflexes, tone, gait, voluntary movement

PHYSICAL EXAM

- Neurologic manifestations should be examined based on location of stroke when known but should include investigation of the following:
  – Sensory or motor deficits, especially unilaterally (i.e., hemiparesis/hemiplegia)
  – Dysarthria or aphasia
  – Visual field deficits (i.e., hemianopsia)
  – Dysphagia
  – Apraxia
  – Unilateral facial palsy
- Neuropsychiatric evaluation should be undertaken to assess cognitive, intellectual, personality, memory, psychomotor, and other system changes that may benefit from treatment during rehabilitation.

DIFFERENTIAL DIAGNOSIS

- Differential diagnosis in stroke rehabilitation should take into account acute changes that are inconsistent with general trend in the individual patient's status.
- New changes in motor function, mental status, and so forth could represent new stroke.
- Subacute changes could include a wide range of neuromuscular, neuropsychiatric, or psychiatric diseases that could be related or unrelated to the initial stroke event.

DIAGNOSTIC TESTS & INTERPRETATION

A wide range of standardized, quantifiable scales have been used to track outcomes in stroke rehabilitation. These include the following (2):

- Neurologic scales
  – Glasgow Coma scale, Mini-Mental State Examination, NIH stroke scale among others

- Global ADL scales
  – Including, but not limited to, Barthel index, functional independence measure, modified Rankine scale, Frenchay activities index, Trunk Control Test, timed up-and-go test, Stair Climb Test, Toronto Bedside Swallowing Screening Test, and so forth.
- Family and caretaker contextual factors are very important to stroke rehabilitation and have been shown to impact outcomes, so thorough assessment should include testing such as the following:
  – Caregiver Strain Index, Family Assessment Device
See topic "Stroke, Acute."

Follow-Up Tests & Special Considerations
Monitor the coagulation profile of patients on anticoagulants.

 TREATMENT

- Tailor to specific stroke-related sequelae.
- The three major stroke rehabilitation goals are as follows (1):
  – Prevent/treat prolonged inactivity complications.
  – Prevent recurrent stroke and cardiovascular events.
  – Increase aerobic fitness.

GENERAL MEASURES

Prevention and/or treatment of the complications associated with stroke (4)[C]

- Aspiration
  – Immediately after stroke, up to 50% of patients have dysphagia; this improves in many.
  – Remain NPO until bedside swallow assessment.
  – Prevention of aspiration involves postural changes, increased sensory input, swallowing maneuvers, active exercise programs, diet modifications, nonoral feeding (if indicated), psychological support, and supportive nursing
- Pulmonary embolism/deep venous thrombosis
  – Risk is highest during the first 3 to 120 days poststroke.
  – Pneumatic compression devices and compression stockings
  – Ambulation as soon as possible
- Skin breakdown
  – Increased risk due to loss of sensation, impaired circulation, older age, decreased level of consciousness, inability to move due to paralysis, and incontinence of urine or stool
  – Frequent repositioning (at least q2h) with special care to avoid excessive friction
  – Keep skin clean and dry.
- Spasticity
  – Occurs in ~35% of stroke survivors; treat with combination of modalities:
    ○ Range-of-motion exercises
    ○ Heat, cold, or electric stimulation
    ○ Splinting
    ○ Oral medications for spasticity of cerebral origin (e.g., dantrolene, tizanidine); phenol or botulinum toxin injections for targeting specific muscles or muscle groups
- Malnutrition
  – Nutritional assessment with a diet history and monitoring by a dietician
- Seizures
  – More common after hemorrhagic stroke (11%) than after ischemic stroke (9%)
  – Antiepileptic drugs and elimination of disturbances (i.e., toxins, metabolic) that may lower seizure threshold

- Falls
  - Lifestyle changes
    - Avoid loose rugs; maintain a clear path without obstruction.
    - Avoid slippery surfaces (such as wet floors).
    - Maintain good lighting.
    - Shoes with nonskid soles
    - Slow down movements for transfers or walking.
- Severe sleep apnea
  - Lifestyle changes
    - Stop smoking; lose weight.
    - Sleep on side versus back.
    - Mouthpieces and breathing devices (CPAP)
    - Surgery
- Neurocognitive (6)
  - Wide range of deficit patterns that can be focal (e.g., aphasia) or diffuse (general cognitive slowing)
    - Most broadly effected are orientation, language, attention, and memory.
    - Common particular deficits: aphasia, neglect, cognitive slowing, memory/executive deficits
    - Assessment, treatment, and outcomes vary markedly based on stroke type, location, severity, timing, and additional factors.
    - Cognitive rehabilitation has some success in focal deficits but less in diffuse changes.
    - Pharmacology: evidence of efficacy for escitalopram and rivastigmine
    - Additional modalities under investigation: Therapies such as repetitive transcranial magnetic stimulation and prism adaptation have sown some benefit in driving plasticity and functional brain changes.
- Depression
  - May be organic secondary to stroke or reactive to the stroke itself
  - Poststroke depression has been found to cause higher mortality, poorer functional recovery, and less activity socially (1)[C].
  - Treat with a combination of pharmacotherapy and psychotherapy:
    - Evidence suggests heterocyclic antidepressants are effective in the setting of poststroke depression but must be closely monitored in older adults due to side effects.
    - SSRIs are also effective in treating poststroke depression.
    - All stroke patients should be assessed for depression and treated with the appropriate antidepressant for 6 months.

MEDICATION

First Line

- Management of controllable risk factors, including BP reduction, diabetes, and cholesterol (Initiate statin therapy, if history of TIA or stroke with evidence of atherosclerosis, LDL ≥100, and no CHD.)
- Anticoagulation with warfarin for patients with mechanical prosthetic heart valves and ischemic stroke or TIA (dosage varies depending on optimum INR for patient in setting of comorbidities)
- Note potential medication interactions (e.g., warfarin and SSRIs due to liver enzyme metabolism).
- Antiplatelet drugs (aspirin, aspirin/dipyridamole, clopidogrel) decrease relative risk of stroke, MI, or death by ~22% (7)[C].

ISSUES FOR REFERRAL

For stroke survivors who require 24-hour care of medical comorbidities, close physician supervision, and specialized nursing care (RN with specialized training or rehabilitation experience), an inpatient rehabilitation facility (IRF) can offer hospital-level care.

ADDITIONAL THERAPIES

Physical, occupational, speech, and recreational therapy

INPATIENT CONSIDERATIONS

Admission Criteria/Initial Stabilization

- For stroke survivors requiring 24-hour care, close physician supervision, and specialized nursing care (RN with specialized training or rehabilitation experience), an inpatient rehabilitation facility (IRF) can offer hospital-level care.
- Such patients must also require and receive a minimum of 3 hours daily occupational or physical therapy for no <5 days each week; this can be combined with other skilled modalities, such as speech–language or prosthetic–orthotic services) to meet the 3-hr/day requirement.
- Either the aforementioned is required or an IRF is the only reasonable setting in which a low-intensity rehab program may be executed.
- An alternative setting is a skilled nursing facility for residents needing daily rehabilitation or nursing care on an inpatient basis.

See "Stroke, Acute."

IV Fluids

Avoid D5W in acute setting to avoid hyperglycemia and its secondary effects.

Nursing

An alternative inpatient setting is a skilled nursing facility that provides nursing care or rehabilitation to residents needing daily rehabilitation or nursing care on an inpatient basis.

 ONGOING CARE

FOLLOW-UP RECOMMENDATIONS

Patient should follow-up regularly with primary care physician for management of risk factors for stroke.

Patient Monitoring

Continue to monitor risk factors. Lab studies monitored periodically may include hemoglobin A1c (and finger-stick glucose testing in diabetics), lipid panel, CBC including platelets, lipid profile, coagulation studies (PT/INR—of special importance in patients on anticoagulation).

DIET

Low salt, low calorie, low saturated and trans fat, low cholesterol

PATIENT EDUCATION

National Stroke Association: http://www.stroke.org/

PROGNOSIS

- Strong evidence suggests an organized, interdisciplinary stroke care team of physicians, nurses, therapists, family, and patient can reduce mortality rates and the likelihood of institutional care and long-term disability. It can also enhance recovery and increase ADL independence.
- Aggressive rehabilitation beyond the time window of the 1st poststroke months, including treadmill with or without body weight support, can increase aerobic capacity and sensorimotor functionality.

COMPLICATIONS

- Aspiration
- Pulmonary embolism/deep venous thrombosis
- Muscle atrophy
- Osteoporosis
- Skin breakdown
- Spasticity
- Malnutrition
- Seizures
- Severe sleep apnea

REFERENCES

1. Gordon NF, Gulanick M, Costa F, et al. Physical activity and exercise recommendations for stroke survivors: an American Heart Association scientific statement from the Council on Clinical Cardiology, Subcommittee on Exercise, Cardiac Rehabilitation, and Prevention; the Council on Cardiovascular Nursing; the Council on Nutrition, Physical Activity, and Metabolism; and the Stroke Council. *Circulation*. 2004;109(16):2031–2041.
2. Langhorne P, Bernhardt J, Kwakkel G. Stroke rehabilitation. *Lancet*. 2011;377(9778):1693–1702.
3. Roger VL, Go AS, Lloyd-Jones DM, et al. Heart disease and stroke statistics—2011 update: a report from the American Heart Association. *Circulation*. 2011;123(4):e18–e209.
4. Miller EL, Murray L, Richards L, et al. Comprehensive overview of nursing and interdisciplinary rehabilitation care of the stroke patient: a scientific statement from the American Heart Association. *Stroke*. 2010;41(10):2402–2448.
5. Wahl AS, Schwab ME. Finding an optimal paradigm after stroke: enhancing fiber growth and training of the brain at the right moment. *Front Hum Neurosci*. 2014;8:381.
6. Cumming TB, Marshall RS, Lazar RM. Stroke, cognitive deficits, and rehabilitation: still an incomplete picture. *Int J Stroke*. 2013;8(1):38–45.
7. Furie KL, Kasner SE, Adams RJ, et al. Guidelines for the prevention of stroke in patients with stroke or transient ischemic attack: a guideline for healthcare professionals from the American Heart Association/American Stroke Association. *Stroke*. 2011;42(1):227–276.

 SEE ALSO

- Traumatic Brain Injury (TBI)—Long Term Care; Stroke, Acute; Dementia; Delirium
- Algorithm: Stroke

 CODES

ICD10

- I63.9 Cerebral infarction, unspecified
- I69.10 Unsp sequelae of nontraumatic intracerebral hemorrhage
- I69.11 Cognitive deficits following nontraumatic intcrbl hemorrhage

CLINICAL PEARLS

- Stroke is the third leading cause of death and the leading cause of long-term disability in the United States.
- An essential part of poststroke management is the treatment of controllable risk factors, including BP reduction and cholesterol control (initiate statin therapy, if history of TIA or stroke with evidence of atherosclerosis, LDL ≥100).
- Strong evidence suggests an organized, interdisciplinary stroke care team of physicians, nurses, therapists, family, and patient can reduce mortality rates and the likelihood of institutional care and long-term disability. It can also enhance recovery and increase ADL independence.

S

STROKE, ACUTE
Scott A. Drummond, Jr., DO, DABR

BASICS

A cerebrovascular accident (CVA) is an infarction or hemorrhage in the brain.

DESCRIPTION
Stroke is the sudden onset of a focal neurologic deficit(s) resulting from either infarction or hemorrhage within the brain.

- Two broad categories: ischemic (thrombotic or embolic; 87%) and hemorrhagic (13%)
- Hemorrhage can be intracerebral or subarachnoid.
- System(s) affected: neurologic; vascular
- Synonym(s): CVA; cerebral infarct; brain attack
- Related terms: transient ischemic attack (TIA), a transient episode of neurologic dysfunction due to focal ischemia without permanent infarction on imaging (see topic "Transient Ischemic Attack [TIA]")

Pediatric Considerations
- Cardiac abnormalities (congenital heart disease, paradoxical embolism, rheumatic fever, bacterial endocarditis)
- Metabolic: homocystinuria, Fabry disease

EPIDEMIOLOGY
Incidence
Annual incidence in the United States is ~795,000.

Prevalence
- Prevalence in the United States: 550/100,000
- Predominant age: Risk increases >45 years of age and is highest during the 7th and 8th decades.
- Predominant sex: male > female at younger age, but higher incidence in women with age ≥75 years

ETIOLOGY AND PATHOPHYSIOLOGY
- 87% of stroke is ischemic, three main subtypes for etiology: thrombosis, embolism, and systemic hypoperfusion. Large vessel atherothrombotic strokes are commonly related to the origin of the internal carotid artery. Small vessel lacunar strokes are commonly due to lipohyalinotic occlusion. Embolic strokes are largely from a cardiac source (due to left atrial thrombus, atrial fibrillation, recent MI, valve disease, or mechanical valves) or ascending aortic atheromatous disease (>4 mm).
- 13% of stroke is hemorrhagic; most commonly due to HTN. Other causes include intracranial vascular malformations (cavernous angiomas, AVMs), cerebral amyloid angiopathy (lobar hemorrhages in elderly), and anticoagulation.
- Other causes include fibromuscular dysplasia (rare), vasculitis, or drug use (cocaine, amphetamines).

Genetics
Stroke is a polygenic multifactorial disease, with some clustering within families.

RISK FACTORS
- Uncontrollable: age, gender, race, family history/genetics, prior stroke or TIA
- Controllable/modifiable/treatable
  - Metabolic: diabetes, dyslipidemia
  - Lifestyle: smoking, cocaine use, amphetamine use
  - Cardiovascular: hypertension, atrial fibrillation, valvular heart disease, endocarditis, recent MI, severe carotid artery stenosis, hypercoagulable states, and patent foramen ovale

GENERAL PREVENTION
Smoking cessation, regular exercise, weight control to maintain nonobese BMI and prevent type 2 diabetes,

use alcohol in moderation, control BP, and manage hyperlipidemia; use of antiplatelet agent, such as aspirin, in high-risk persons; treatment of nonvalvular atrial fibrillation with dose-adjusted warfarin or dabigatran, apixaban, and rivaroxaban

COMMONLY ASSOCIATED CONDITIONS
Coronary artery disease is the major cause of death during the first 5 years after a stroke.

DIAGNOSIS

HISTORY
Acute onset of focal arm/leg weakness, facial weakness, difficulty with speech or swallowing, vertigo, visual disturbances, diminished consciousness; presence of vomiting and severe headache favor diagnosis of hemorrhagic stroke.

PHYSICAL EXAM
- Assess airway, breathing, and circulation (ABC).
- Anterior (carotid) circulation: hemiparesis/hemiplegia, neglect, aphasia, visual field defects
- Posterior (vertebrobasilar) circulation: diplopia, vertigo, gait and limb ataxia, facial paresis, Horner syndrome, dysphagia, dysarthria, alternating sensory loss

DIFFERENTIAL DIAGNOSIS
- Migraine (complicated)
- Postictal state (Todd paralysis)
- Systemic infection, including meningitis or encephalitis (infection also may uncover or enhance previous deficits)
- Toxic or metabolic disturbance (hypoglycemia, acute renal failure, liver failure, drug intoxication)
- Brain tumor, primary or metastases
- Head trauma, encephalopathy
- Other types of intracranial hemorrhage (epidural, subdural, subarachnoid)
- Trauma, septic emboli

DIAGNOSTIC TESTS & INTERPRETATION
Primarily used to narrow differential and identify etiology of stroke

Initial Tests (lab, imaging)
- Serum glucose level, including fingerstick testing (REQUIRED to exclude hypo- and hyperglycemia) (1)[B]
- ECG
- CBC, including platelets
- Electrolytes, including BUN and creatinine
- Coagulation studies: PT, PTT, INR
- Markers of cardiac ischemia
- Emergent brain imaging with noncontrast CT (or brain MRI with diffusion weighted [DW-MRI]) to exclude hemorrhage can be lifesaving (1)[A].
- Subsequent multimodal CT (perfusion CT, CTA, unenhanced CT) or MRI to improve diagnosis of acute ischemic stroke

Follow-Up Tests & Special Considerations
Consider LFT, tox screen, blood alcohol, ABG, lumbar puncture if suspected subarachnoid hemorrhage (SAH), EEG if suspect seizures, blood type and cross.

- DW-MRI is more sensitive than CT for acute ischemic stroke; however, MRI also is better than CT for diagnosis of posterior fossa lesions (2)[B].

- Emergent treatment (IV thrombolysis) should NOT be delayed to obtain advanced imaging studies.
- Follow-up imaging of carotid vessels with Doppler ultrasound, CTA, or MRA of head and neck should be completed.

Diagnostic Procedures/Other
Echocardiogram (transthoracic and/or transesophageal) in patients with increased suspicion for cardioembolic source. In cryptogenic stroke patients, prolonged ECG monitoring should be performed with a 30-day event monitor.

Test Interpretation
Early CT findings: hyperdense MCA sign (increased attenuation of proximal portion of the MCA; is associated with thrombosis of MCA), loss of gray-white matter differentiation, sulcal effacement, loss of insular ribbon

TREATMENT

- BP closely monitored in the first 24 hours (1)[A]
  - Antihypertensives should be withheld unless systolic BP >220 mm Hg or diastolic BP >120 mm Hg, with a goal to lower BP by ~15% during first 24 hours if treatment is indicated. If thrombolytic therapy is to be initiated, BP must be <185/110 mm Hg prior to thrombolytics.
  - In acute spontaneous intracranial hemorrhagic stroke, goal for BP control is 160/90 mm Hg or target MAP 110 (see topic, "Subarachnoid Hemorrhage" for details on BP management). With suspicion for elevated ICP, BP should be reduced with goal to keep cerebral perfusion pressure between 61 mm Hg and 80 mm Hg.
  - Antihypertensive medications should be restarted 24 hours after stroke onset for patients with a history of hypertension who are neurologically stable.

ALERT
Thrombolysis: IV thrombolysis should be started in patients with measurable neurologic deficits that do not clear spontaneously, presenting within 3 to 4.5 hours of stroke symptom onset.

- Exclusion criteria for thrombolysis within 3 hours of onset include:
  - Symptoms suggestive of SAH
  - Head trauma or prior stroke within 3 months
  - MI within 3 months
  - GI or gastric ulcer hemorrhage within 21 days
  - Major surgery within 14 days
  - Arterial puncture at noncompressible site within 7 days
  - Any history of intracranial hemorrhage
  - Elevated BP (systolic >185 mm Hg and diastolic >110 mm Hg)
  - Active bleeding or acute trauma on examination
  - Taking anticoagulant and INR ≥1.7
  - Activated PTT not in normal range if heparin received during previous 48 hours; platelet count <100,000 mm^3
  - Blood glucose concentration <50 mg/dL
  - Seizure with postictal residual neurologic impairment
  - Multilobar infarction on CT (hypodensity >1/3 cerebral hemisphere)
  - Patient or family members not able to weigh and understand potential risks and benefits of treatment

- Extended exclusion criteria for thrombolysis within 4.5 hours include per AHA/ASA guidelines:
  – Age >80 years
  – All patients taking oral anticoagulants regardless of INR
  – National Institute of Health (NIH) Stroke Scale >25
  – History of stroke and diabetes
- Antiplatelet agents: Oral aspirin (initial dose, 325 mg) should be started within 24 to 48 hours (1)[A].

MEDICATION
First Line
- BP management (parameters under "Treatment") options include:
  – Labetalol 10 to 20 mg IV over 1 to 2 minutes, which may be repeated once
  – Nicardipine infusion 5 mg/hr, titrate up by 2.5 mg/hr at 5- to 15-minute intervals to maximum of 15 mg/hr; reduce to 3 mg/hr when target BP is reached
- Thrombolysis, IV administration of rtPA: Infuse 0.9 mg/kg, maximum dose 90 mg over 60 minutes with 10% of dose given as bolus over 1 minute.
  – Admit to ICU or stroke unit, with neurologic exams every 15 minutes during infusion, every 60 minutes for next 6 hours, then hourly until 24 hours after treatment.
  – Discontinue infusion and obtain emergent CT scan if severe headache, angioedema, acute hypertension, or nausea and vomiting develop.
  – Measure BP every 15 minutes for first 2 hours, every 30 minutes for next 6 hours, then every hour until 24 hours after treatment. Maintain BP <185/105. Follow-up CT at 24 hours before starting anticoagulants or antiplatelet agents.
- Antiplatelet: aspirin 325 mg/day within 48 hours, or 24 to 48 hours after thrombolytic therapy (1)[A]

Second Line
Carotid endarterectomy (CEA) for carotid artery stenosis rarely is indicated emergently. CEA is indicated for stenosis >70% ipsilateral to TIA or incomplete stroke lesion and may be indicated for 50–69% stenosis in carefully selected patients, depending on risk factors.

ISSUES FOR REFERRAL
Follow-up with neurologist 1 week after discharge, with subsequent follow-up based on individual circumstances

ADDITIONAL THERAPIES
- Prophylactic antibiotics are *not* recommended.
- Deep vein thrombosis (DVT) prophylaxis should be instituted for immobilized patients.
- Corticosteroids are *not* recommended for cerebral brain edema.
- Statin use should be continued without interruption following acute stroke (1)[B].
- At discharge, patient should be referred for physical therapy, occupational therapy, and speech therapy, as necessary.

SURGERY/OTHER PROCEDURES
- Ventricular drain may be placed for patients with acute hydrocephalus secondary to stroke (most commonly due to cerebellar stroke).
- Decompressive surgery is recommended for major cerebellar infarction; it should be considered for malignant middle cerebral artery infarction, especially if the patient is <60 years of age.

- Consider mechanical embolus removal with a cerebral infarction device in carefully selected patients, with evidence of potentially salvageable tissue on advanced imaging.

COMPLEMENTARY & ALTERNATIVE MEDICINE
Acupuncture starting within 30 days from stroke onset may improve neurologic functioning.

INPATIENT CONSIDERATIONS
Admission Criteria/Initial Stabilization
- Observe closely within first 24 hours for neurologic decline, particularly due to cerebral edema.
- Keep head of bed at least 30 degrees when elevated ICP is suspected. Patients with ischemic stroke may benefit from a horizontal bed position during the acute phase.
- Monitor cardiac rhythm for at least first 24 hours to identify any arrhythmias.
- Airway support and ventilatory assistance may be necessary due to diminished consciousness or bulbar involvement; supplemental oxygen should be reserved for hypoxic patients. Consider elective intubation for patients with malignant edema.
- Correct hypovolemia with normal saline.
- All patients should be kept NPO until a formal swallow evaluation has been performed; to reduce risk of aspiration pneumonia, maintain elevated head of bed to 30 degrees.
- Hypoglycemia can cause neurologic dysfunction; rapidly correct during initial evaluation.
- Hyperglycemia within first 24 hours after stroke is associated with poor functional outcomes and AHA/ASA guidelines: Insulin treatment for patients with glucose levels >140 to 180 mg/dL (1)[C].
- In patients with ICH secondary to anticoagulant use, correction of an elevated INR is necessary with use of IV vitamin K and fresh frozen plasma or prothrombin concentrate complex. Factor VII infusion should be used in patients needing urgent surgical intervention (i.e., those with cerebellar hemorrhage who are neurologically deteriorating).
- DVT prophylaxis (1)[B]
- Maintain oxygen saturation >94% (1)[C].
- Early use of physical therapy and discharge planning for rehabilitation need and placement

IV Fluids
IV hydration with maintenance amounts of normal saline until swallowing status is assessed; monitor fluid balance closely.

Nursing
- Regular neurologic exams more frequent in first 24 hours (every 1 to 2 hours)
- Fall precautions; frequent repositioning to prevent skin breakdown

Discharge Criteria
Medically stable, adequate nutritional support, neurologic status stable or improving

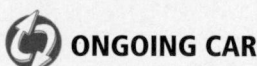 ONGOING CARE

FOLLOW-UP RECOMMENDATIONS
- Secondary prevention of stroke with aggressive management of risk factors
- Platelet inhibition using aspirin, clopidogrel, or aspirin plus extended-release dipyridamole (Aggrenox) based on physician and patient preference

Patient Monitoring
Follow-up every 3 months for 1st year, then annually.

DIET
Patients with impaired swallowing should receive nasogastric or percutaneous endoscopic gastrostomy feedings to maintain nutrition and hydration.

PATIENT EDUCATION
National Stroke Association (800-STROKES or http://www.stroke.org)

PROGNOSIS
Variable, depends on subtype and severity of stroke; NIH stroke scale may be used for prognosis.

COMPLICATIONS
- Acute: brain herniation, hemorrhagic transformation, MI, congestive heart failure, dysphagia, aspiration pneumonia, UTI, DVT, pulmonary embolism, malnutrition, pressure sores
- Chronic: falls, depression, dementia, orthopedic complications, contractures

REFERENCES
1. Jauch EC, Saver JL, Adams HP Jr, et al. Guidelines for the early management of patients with acute ischemic stroke: a guideline for healthcare professionals from the American Heart Association/American Stroke Association. *Stroke*. 2013;44(3): 870–947.
2. Chalela JA, Kidwell CS, Nentwich LM, et al. Magnetic resonance imaging and computed tomography in emergency assessment of patients with suspected acute stroke: a prospective comparison. *Lancet*. 2007;369(9558):293–298.

ADDITIONAL READING
Yew KS, Cheng EM. Diagnosis of acute stroke. *Am Fam Physician*. 2015;91(8):528–536.

 ## CODES
ICD10
- I63.9 Cerebral infarction, unspecified
- I61.9 Nontraumatic intracerebral hemorrhage, unspecified
- I63.50 Cereb infrc due to unsp occls or stenos of unsp cereb artery

CLINICAL PEARLS
- Unless stroke is hemorrhagic or patient is undergoing thrombolysis, BP should not be lowered acutely to maintain perfusion of penumbra region.
- IV thrombolysis should be considered in eligible patients with neurologic deficits that do not clear spontaneously within 3 to 4.5 hours of symptom onset.
- DW-MRI is more sensitive than conventional CT for acute ischemic stroke. MRI is also better than CT for diagnosis of posterior fossa lesions.

SUBCONJUNCTIVAL HEMORRHAGE

Cara Marshall, MD

 BASICS

DESCRIPTION
- Subconjunctival hemorrhage (SCH) is bleeding from small blood vessels underneath the conjunctiva, the thin clear skin covering the sclera of the eye.
- SCH is diagnosed clinically:
  - Flat, well-demarcated areas of extravasated blood can be seen just under the surface of the conjunctiva of the eye (red patch of blood sign).
  - SCH is more common in the inferior and temporal regions (1).
- Typically, SCH resolves spontaneously within 1 to 2 weeks.

EPIDEMIOLOGY
- Male = female; no gender predilection found
- Common; 3% rate of diagnosis in outpatient eye clinic (2)

Incidence
Incidence increases
- With increasing age
- In contact lens wearers (5% of cases) (3)
- With systemic diseases such as diabetes, hypertension (HTN), and coagulation disorders
- During summer months, possibly due to trauma (2)

ETIOLOGY AND PATHOPHYSIOLOGY
- Direct trauma to the blood vessels of the conjunctiva from blunt or penetrating trauma
- Direct trauma to the conjunctiva from improper contact lens placement or improper cleaning
- Increased BP in the vessels of the conjunctiva from HTN or from the temporary increase in BP from a Valsalva type maneuver (e.g., vomiting)
- Damaged vessels from diabetes and atherosclerotic disease
- Increased bleeding tendencies from either thrombocytopenia or elevated PT/elevated INR (4)
- Trauma to the eye

- Valsalva maneuvers causing sudden severe venous congestion such as coughing, sneezing, vomiting, straining, severe asthma or COPD exacerbation, weightlifting or childbirth/labor (1)
- HTN
- Atherosclerotic disease and diabetes
- Bleeding factors such as thrombocytopenia or elevated PT (from either disease or medication side effects)
- In patients age >60 years, HTN is the most common etiology.
- In patients age <40 years, trauma/Valsalva and contact lens use are the most common etiologies.
- In patients age >40 years, conjunctivochalasis (redundant conjunctival folds) and presence of pinguecula are strongly associated (3).

RISK FACTORS
- Age
- Contact lens wearer
- Systemic diseases
- Bleeding disorders (2)
- Recent cataract surgery

GENERAL PREVENTION
- Correct cleaning and maintenance of contact lenses.
- Protective eyewear in sports and hobbies
- Control of high BP
- Optimizing control of systemic diseases such as diabetes and atherosclerotic disease
- Control of prothrombin time (PT)/international normalized ratio (INR) in patients on Coumadin therapy (5)

 DIAGNOSIS

HISTORY
- Generally asymptomatic; usually the patient notices the redness in the mirror or another person mentions it to the patient.
- There should be little to no pain involved (5)[C].
- Obtain history of trauma. SCH can occur 12 to 24 hours after orbital fracture (1).

- Obtain history of contact lens usage or recent cataract, laser-assisted in situ keratomileusis (LASIK), or other ocular surgery (2)[C].
- Comprehensive past medical history to evaluate if at risk for systemic diseases or taking medications that might increase risk
- Obtain history for current systemic symptomatology.

PHYSICAL EXAM
- Evaluate BP to assess control (2)[C].
- Measure visual acuity; this should be normal in a simple SCH (5)[C].
- Verify that the pupils are equal and reactive to light and accommodation; this should be normal with an SCH (5)[C].
- There should be no discharge or exudate noted (5)[C].
- Look at sclera for a bright red demarcated patch.
  - Demarcated area is most often on inferior aspect of eye due to gravity (3)[C].
- If penetrating trauma is a consideration, do a gentle digital assessment of the integrity of the globe (4)[C].
- Slit-lamp exam should be performed if there is a history of trauma (1).

Geriatric Considerations
In older adults, the area of SCH will be more widespread across the sclera (3). Elastic and connective tissues are more fragile with age, and underlying conditions such as HTN and diabetes may contribute.

DIFFERENTIAL DIAGNOSIS
- Viral, bacterial, allergic, or chemical conjunctivitis (enterovirus and coxsackie virus most common) (1)[B]
- Foreign body to conjunctiva
- Penetrating trauma
- Acute angle glaucoma
- Iritis
- Recent ocular surgery
- Contact lens induced
- Child abuse (particularly if bilateral in an infant or toddler) (1)
- May occur in newborns after vaginal delivery

DIAGNOSTIC TESTS & INTERPRETATION

- Typically no testing is indicated; SCH is a clinical diagnosis. If a foreign body is suspected, perform a fluorescein exam.
- Fluorescein exam of a patient with a SCH should show no uptake of staining (5)[C].
- If an orbital fracture is suspected, may obtain plain facial bone films or CT scan (4)[C]

Follow-Up Tests & Special Considerations
If history and physical exam suggest a bleeding etiology (5)[C]
- CBC
- PT/INR

ALERT
If a penetrating injury is suspected, may obtain a CT scan of the orbits but not an MRI (if object may be metal) (4)[C]

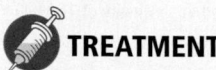

TREATMENT

GENERAL MEASURES
- Control BP.
- Control blood glucose.
- Control INR.
- Wear protective eyewear.

MEDICATION
No prescription medications are useful in treatment of SCH.

ISSUES FOR REFERRAL
- If a penetrating eye injury is suspected, send the patient to the emergency room for emergent ophthalmology consultation.
- If the patient complains of any decreased visual acuity or visual disturbances, refer to an ophthalmologist as soon as possible.
- If there is no resolution of SCH within 2 weeks, patient may need referral to an ophthalmologist.

ADDITIONAL THERAPIES
- Warm compresses
- Eye lubricants (5)[C]

ONGOING CARE

FOLLOW-UP RECOMMENDATIONS
- Follow up only if the area does not resolve within 2 weeks.
- If SCH recurs, then work up patient for systemic sources such as bleeding disorders (5)[C].

PATIENT EDUCATION
- Reassurance of the self-limited nature of the problem and typical time frame for resolution
- Education to return to clinic if the area does not heal or recurs.
- Correct cleaning and maintenance of contact lenses.
- Instructions on causes, self-care, and warning signs are available at PubMed Health: Subconjunctival Hemorrhage at www.ncbi.nlm.nih.gov/pubmedhealth /PMH0002583/.

PROGNOSIS
Excellent

COMPLICATIONS
Rare

REFERENCES

1. Tarlan B, Kiratli H. Subconjunctival hemorrhage: risk factors and potential indicators. *Clin Ophthalmol*. 2013;7:1163–1170.
2. Mimura T, Usui T, Yamagami S, et al. Recent causes of subconjunctival hemorrhage. *Ophthalmologica*. 2010;224(3):133–137.
3. Mimura T, Yamagami S, Mori M, et al. Contact lens-induced subconjunctival hemorrhage. *Am J Ophthalmol*. 2010;150(5):656–665.e1.
4. Wirbelauer C. Management of the red eye for the primary care physician. *Am J Med*. 2006;119(4): 302–306.
5. Cronau H, Kankanala RR, Mauger T. Diagnosis and management of red eye in primary care. *Am Fam Physician*. 2010;81(2):137–144.

ADDITIONAL READING

- Mimura T, Usui T, Yamagami S, et al. Subconjunctival hemorrhage and conjunctivochalasis. *Ophthalmology*. 2009;116(10):1880–1886.
- Mimura T, Yamagami S, Usui T, et al. Location and extent of subconjunctival hemorrhage. *Ophthalmologica*. 2010;224(2):90–95.

CODES

ICD10
- H11.30 Conjunctival hemorrhage, unspecified eye
- H11.31 Conjunctival hemorrhage, right eye
- H11.32 Conjunctival hemorrhage, left eye

CLINICAL PEARLS

- SCH is a clinical diagnosis. The condition is typically asymptomatic and will resolve spontaneously in 1 to 2 weeks.
- Always check BP in a patient with SCH, as HTN is a risk factor.
- Indications for immediate referral to an ophthalmologist are eye pain, change in vision, lack of pupil reactivity, and/or penetrating eye trauma.
- Reassurance and comfort measures are key.
- Contact lens wearers should not wear contacts until the SCH resolves completely.

S

SUBSTANCE USE DISORDERS

S. Lindsey Clarke, MD, FAAFP

 BASICS

DESCRIPTION

A substance use disorder manifests as any pattern of substance use causing significant physical, mental, or social dysfunction.

- Substances of abuse include the following:
  - Alcohol
  - Tobacco
  - Cannabinoids (marijuana)
  - Synthetic cannabinoids (Spice, K2, Mojo, Cloud 9, Relax, Crown); note: Increasingly, these are sold as liquid in eyedropper bottles for use with vaporizing devices (vape/hookah pens).
  - Prescription medications
    - CNS depressants (barbiturates, benzodiazepines, hypnotics)
    - Opioids and morphine derivatives (codeine, fentanyl, hydrocodone, hydromorphone, oxymorphone [Opana], meperidine, methadone, morphine, oxycodone)
    - Stimulants (amphetamines, methylphenidate)
    - Dextromethorphan
  - Stimulants (cocaine, amphetamines, methamphetamines, Khat)
  - Club drugs (MDMA [ecstasy, Molly], PMMA [Superman], flunitrazepam, γ-hydroxybutyrate [GHB])
  - Opioids (heroin, opium, desomorphine [Krokodil])
  - Dissociative drugs (ketamine, phencyclidine [PCP])
  - Hallucinogens (lysergic acid diethylamide [LSD], salvia)
  - Synthetic cathinones (bath salts, Flakka/α-PVP)
  - Inhalants (glue, paint thinners, nitrous oxide)
  - Anabolic steroids
- See also www.drugabuse.gov/drugs-abuse.
- System(s) affected: cardiovascular, endocrine/metabolic, CNS
- Synonym(s): drug abuse; drug dependence; substance abuse

Geriatric Considerations
- Alcohol is the most commonly abused substance, and abuse often goes unrecognized.
- Higher potential for drug interactions

Pregnancy Considerations
Substance abuse may cause fetal abnormalities, morbidity, and fetal or maternal death.

EPIDEMIOLOGY

Incidence
- Predominant age: 16 to 25 years
- Predominant sex: male > female

Prevalence
- 24.6 million (9.4%) Americans reported current illicit drug use in 2013.
- 8.8% for age 12 to 17 years; 21.5% for age 18 to 25 years
- Nearly one in five young adult men use marijuana.

ETIOLOGY AND PATHOPHYSIOLOGY
Multifactorial, including genetic, environmental

Genetics
Substances of abuse affect dopamine, acetylcholine, γ-aminobutyric acid, norepinephrine, opioid, and serotonin receptors. Variant alleles may account for susceptibility to disorders.

RISK FACTORS
- Male gender, young adult
- Depression, anxiety
- Other substance use disorders
- Family history
- Peer or family use or approval
- Low socioeconomic status
- Unemployment
- Accessibility of substances of abuse
- Family dysfunction or trauma
- Antisocial personality disorder
- Academic problems, school dropout
- Criminal involvement

GENERAL PREVENTION
- Early identification and aggressive early intervention improve outcomes.
- Universal school-based interventions are modestly effective for preventing drug use among adolescents.

COMMONLY ASSOCIATED CONDITIONS
- Depression
- Personality disorders
- Bipolar affective disorder

ALERT
Prescription narcotic overdose is the leading cause of accidental death between the ages of 25 and 45 years in the United States; this correlates with increased prescribing of long-acting oxycodone (see www.cdc .gov/injury/wisqars/pdf/leading_causes_of_death_by_ age_group_2013-a.pdf).

 DIAGNOSIS

Substance use disorder (*DSM-5* criteria): ≥2 of the following in past year, with severity based on number of criteria present:

- Missed work or school
- Use in hazardous situations
- Continued use despite social or personal problems
- Craving
- Tolerance (decreased response to effects of drug due to constant exposure)
- Withdrawal upon discontinuation
- Using more than intended
- Failed attempts to quit
- Increased time spent obtaining, using, or recovering from the substance
- Interference with important activities
- Continued use despite health problems

HISTORY
- History of infections (e.g., endocarditis, hepatitis B or C, TB, STI, or recurrent pneumonia)
- Social or behavioral problems, including chaotic relationships and/or employment
- Frequent visits to emergency department
- Criminal incarceration
- History of blackouts, insomnia, mood swings, chronic pain, repetitive trauma
- Anxiety, fatigue, depression, psychosis

PHYSICAL EXAM
- Abnormally dilated or constricted pupils
- Needle marks on skin

- Nasal septum perforation (with cocaine use)
- Cardiac dysrhythmias, pathologic murmurs
- Malnutrition with severe dependence

DIFFERENTIAL DIAGNOSIS
- Depression, anxiety, or other mental states
- Metabolic delirium (hypoxia, hypoglycemia, infection, thiamine deficiency, hypothyroidism, thyrotoxicosis)
- ADHD
- Medication toxicity

DIAGNOSTIC TESTS & INTERPRETATION

ALERT
Screening: a single question: "How many times in the past year have you used an illegal drug or used a prescription medication for nonmedical reasons?": in primary care setting, resulted in sensitivity of 100% and specificity of ~75% (1)[B]

- CRAFFT questionnaire is superior to cut down, annoyed by criticism, guilty about drinking, eye-opener drinks (CAGE) for identifying alcohol use disorders in adolescents and young adults; sensitivity is 94% with ≥2 "yes" answers.
  - C: Have you ever ridden in a *car* driven by someone (including yourself) who was "high" or who had been using alcohol or drugs?
  - R: Do you ever use alcohol or drugs to *relax*, feel better about yourself, or fit in?
  - A: Do you ever use alcohol or drugs while you are *alone*?
  - F: Do you ever *forget* things you did while using alcohol or drugs?
  - F: Do your family or *friends* ever tell you that you should cut down on your drinking or drug use?
  - T: Have you gotten into *trouble* while you were using alcohol or drugs?
- Blood alcohol concentration
- Urine drug screen (UDS) (order qualitative UDS, and if specific drug is in question, a quantitative analysis for specific drug; order confirmatory serum tests if you suspect false positive)
- Approximate detection limits
  - Alcohol: 6 to 10 hours
  - Amphetamines and variants: 2 to 3 days
  - Barbiturates: 2 to 10 days
  - Benzodiazepines: 1 to 6 weeks
  - Cocaine: 2 to 3 days
  - Heroin: 1 to 1.5 days
  - LSD, psilocybin: 8 hours
  - Marijuana: 1 day to 4 weeks
  - Methadone: 1 day to 1 week
  - Opioids: 1 to 3 days
  - PCP: 7 to 14 days
  - Anabolic steroids: oral, 3 weeks; injectable, 3 months; nandrolone, 9 months
- Liver transaminases
- HIV, hepatitis B and C screens
- Echocardiogram for endocarditis
- Head CT scan for seizure, delirium, trauma

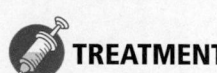 TREATMENT

Determine substances abused early (may influence disposition).

GENERAL MEASURES

- Nonjudgmental, medically oriented attitude
- Motivational interviewing and brief interventions can overcome denial and promote change.
- Behavioral and cognitive therapy
- Community reinforcement
- Interventional counseling
- Self-help groups to aid recovery (Alcoholics Anonymous, other 12-step programs)
- Support groups for family (Al-Anon and Alateen)

MEDICATION

- Alcohol withdrawal: See "Alcohol Abuse and Dependence" and "Alcohol Withdrawal."
- Benzodiazepine or barbiturate withdrawal
  - Gradual taper preferable to abrupt discontinuation
  - Substitution of long-acting benzodiazepine or phenobarbital
- Nicotine withdrawal: See "Tobacco Use and Smoking Cessation."
- Opioid withdrawal
  - Methadone: 20 mg/day PO; use restricted to inpatient settings and specially licensed clinics (2)[A]
  - Clonidine: 0.1 to 0.2 mg PO TID for autonomic hyperactivity (3)[A]
  - Buprenorphine: 8 to 16 mg/day sublingually; may precipitate a more severe withdrawal if initiated too soon; use restricted to licensed clinics and certified physicians (4)[A]
- Stimulant withdrawal
  - No agent with clear benefit for cocaine
  - Anti-cocaine vaccine in development
  - Naltrexone: 50 mg PO twice weekly reduces amphetamine use in dependent patients (5)[B].
  - Methylphenidate ER: titrated up to 54 mg/day PO might enhance abstinence in amphetamine-dependent patients
- Adjuncts to therapy
  - Use all medications in conjunction with psychosocial behavioral interventions.
  - Antiemetics, nonaddictive analgesics for opioid withdrawal
  - Nonhabituating antidepressants, mood stabilizers, anxiolytics, and hypnotics for comorbid mood and anxiety disorders and insomnia that persist after detoxification
- Contraindications
  - Buprenorphine in lactation
  - Naltrexone in pregnancy, liver disease
- Precautions: Clonidine can cause hypotension.
- Significant possible interactions
  - Buprenorphine and ketoconazole, erythromycin, or HIV protease inhibitors
  - Naltrexone and opioid medications (may precipitate or exacerbate withdrawal)

ISSUES FOR REFERRAL

- Consider addiction specialist, especially for opioid and polysubstance abuse.
- Maintenance therapy for opioid dependence (e.g., methadone) only in licensed clinics.
- Psychiatrist for comorbid psychiatric disorders
- Social services

INPATIENT CONSIDERATIONS

Admission Criteria/Initial Stabilization

- Indications for inpatient detoxification
  - History of withdrawal symptoms (e.g., seizures)
  - Disorientation
  - Hallucinations or psychotic features
  - Threat of harm to self or others
  - Obstacles to close monitoring (follow-up)
  - Comorbid medical illness
  - Pregnancy
- For narcotic addiction and withdrawal
- Look for signs of severe infection (e.g., bacterial endocarditis).

IV Fluids

Maintenance until patient is taking fluids well by mouth

Nursing

- Take frequent vital signs during withdrawal.
- Monitor for signs of drug use in the hospital.

Discharge Criteria

- Detoxification complete
- Rehabilitation plan in place

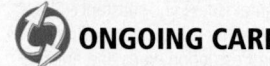 ONGOING CARE

FOLLOW-UP RECOMMENDATIONS

Initially frequent visits to monitor for medical stability and adherence, then progressive follow-up intervals

Patient Monitoring

Verify patient's compliance with the substance abuse treatment program.

DIET

Patients often are malnourished.

PATIENT EDUCATION

- Substance Abuse and Mental Health Services Administration: http://www.samhsa.gov/ or 800-662-HELP for information, treatment facility locator
- National Institute on Drug Abuse: http://www.drugabuse.gov/patients-families and http://www.drugabuse.gov/nidamed-medical-health-professionals/tool-resources-your-practice/patient-materials
- Alcoholics Anonymous: http://www.aa.org/
- Narcotics Anonymous: http://www.na.org.za/

PROGNOSIS

- Patients in treatment for longer periods (≥1 year) have higher success rates.
- Behavioral therapy and pharmacotherapy are most successful when used in combination.

COMPLICATIONS

- Serious harm to self and others: accidents, violence
- Overdoses resulting in seizures, arrhythmias, cardiac and respiratory arrest, coma, death
- Hepatitis, HIV, tuberculosis, syphilis
- Subacute bacterial endocarditis
- Malnutrition
- Social problems, including arrest
- Poor marital adjustment and violence
- Depression, schizophrenia
- Sexual assault (alcohol, flunitrazepam, GHB)

REFERENCES

1. Smith PC, Schmidt SM, Allensworth-Davies D, et al. A single-question screening test for drug use in primary care. *Arch Intern Med*. 2010;170(13):1155–1160.
2. Amato L, Davoli M, Minozzi S, et al. Methadone at tapered doses for the management of opioid withdrawal. *Cochrane Database Syst Rev*. 2013;(2):CD003409.
3. Gowing L, Farrell MF, Ali R, et al. Alpha2-adrenergic agonists for the management of opioid withdrawal. *Cochrane Database Syst Rev*. 2014;(3):CD002024.
4. Mattick RP, Breen C, Kimber J, et al. Buprenorphine maintenance versus placebo or methadone maintenance for opioid dependence. *Cochrane Database Syst Rev*. 2014;(2):CD002207.
5. Jayaram-Lindström N, Hammarberg A, Beck O, et al. Naltrexone for the treatment of amphetamine dependence: a randomized, placebo-controlled trial. *Am J Psychiatry*. 2008;165(11):1442–1448.

ADDITIONAL READING

- Patterson DA, Morris GW Jr, Houghton A. Uncommon adverse effects of commonly abused illicit drugs. *Am Fam Physician*. 2013;88(1):10–16.
- Shapiro B, Coffa D, McCance-Katz EF. A primary care approach to substance misuse. *Am Fam Physician*. 2013;88(2):113–121.
- Standridge JB, Adams SM, Zotos AP. Urine drug screening: a valuable office procedure. *Am Fam Physician*. 2010;81(5):635–640.
- Substance Abuse and Mental Health Services Administration. *Results from the 2013 National Survey on Drug Use and Health: Summary of National Findings*, NSDUH Series H-48, HHS Publication No. (SMA) 14-4863. Rockville, MD: Substance Abuse and Mental Health Services Administration; 2014. http://store.samhsa.gov/home.

 SEE ALSO

Alcohol Abuse and Dependence; Alcohol Withdrawal; Tobacco Use and Smoking Cessation

 CODES

ICD10

- F19.10 Other psychoactive substance abuse, uncomplicated
- F10.10 Alcohol abuse, uncomplicated
- F12.10 Cannabis abuse, uncomplicated

CLINICAL PEARLS

- Substance use disorders are prevalent, serious, and often unrecognized in clinical practice. Comorbid psychiatric disorders are common.
- Substance abuse is distinguished by family, social, occupational, legal, or physical dysfunction that is caused by persistent use of the substance.
- Dependence is characterized by tolerance, withdrawal, compulsive use, and repeated overindulgence.
- Motivational interviewing, brief interventions, and a nonjudgmental attitude can help to promote a willingness to change behavior. Research shows the benefit of referring patients with alcohol dependence to an addiction specialist or treatment program.

SUICIDE

Irene C. Coletsos, MD • Harold J. Bursztajn, MD

 BASICS

DESCRIPTION

Suicide and attempted suicide are significant causes of morbidity and mortality.

EPIDEMIOLOGY

- Predominant sex
  - Women *attempt* suicide 1.5 times more often than men. Men *complete* suicide 4 times more often than women. Men are more likely to choose a means with high lethality.
- Predominant age: adolescent (2nd leading cause of death, 10th leading cause of death overall, per 2013 CDC statistics [latest available]);
- Predominant race: 84% of people who complete suicides are white, non-Hispanic. Native Americans have the next highest rate in the United States. Whites have twice the risk of suicide compared with African Americans.
- Marital status: single > divorced; widowed > married
- Worldwide, in of all countries, youths (ages 10 to 24 years) are the highest risk group.

Incidence

- In 2013, 10th leading cause of death in adults in the United States. Military service (not specifically active duty) is associated with increased risk. In 2009, 2010, 2012, and 2013, more soldiers died of suicide than in active duty, according to a congressional study and the National Center for Veterans.
- Worldwide, the 3rd leading cause of death.

RISK FACTORS

- "Human understanding is the most effective weapon against suicide. The greatest need is to deepen the awareness and sensitivity of people to their fellow man" (Shneidman, American Association of Suicidology).
- Be alert to a combination of "perturbation" (increased emotional disturbance) and "lethality" (having the potential tools to cause death).
- 80% who complete suicides had a previous attempt.
- 90% who complete suicide meet *Diagnostic and Statistical Manual* criteria for Axis I or II disorders: major depression, bipolar disorder, anorexia nervosa, panic disorder, borderline, and antisocial personality disorders. Schizophrenia or acute onset of psychosis are also risk factors, due to command hallucinations or even the negative affect or hopelessness that can accompany these states.
- Substance use (alcohol, hallucinogens, opioids)
- Family history of suicide
- Physical illness
- Despair: feeling unendurable emotional pain *and* has "given up" on self, feels without hope and, consciously or unconsciously, unworthy of help
- Among teenagers: not feeling "connected" to their peers or family; being bullied; poor grades
- Psychosocial: recent loss: What may seem to be a small loss (to a medical provider) may be a devastating loss to the patient. *Patient-specific* factors need to be taken into account: social isolation, anniversaries, and holidays. Patients who attempt suicide also seem to have impaired decision-making skills and risk awareness, and increased impulsivity, compared with patients who have never attempted suicide (1).

- If a patient is incompetent (e.g., too delusional) to inform providers about the potential for suicide, that puts the patient at increased risk, consider hospitalization.
- Access to lethal means: firearms, poisons (including prescription and nonprescription drugs)

GENERAL PREVENTION

- Know how to access resources 24/7 within and outside of the health care institution.
- Screen for risk factors, and consider the overall clinical picture. Screening instruments include the Patient Health Questionnaire-2 (PHQ-2), the PHQ-9, the Columbia Suicide Severity Rating Scale, Beck's Scale for Suicidal Ideation, Linehan's Reasons for Living Inventory, and Risk Estimator for Suicide.
- Treat underlying mental illness and substance abuse. Screen for possession of means of harm, including prescription and nonprescription drugs and firearms (encourage these patients to remove guns from their homes and to relinquish gun licenses).
- Women being treated for cancer, chronic obstructive pulmonary disease (COPD), heart disease, osteoporosis, or stroke were found to be at higher risk for suicide (even without a history of depression).
- Create a safety plan for patients at risk for suicide and their families, including education about how to access emergency care 24 hours a day.
- Public education about how to help others access emergency psychiatric care. Suicidal people may first confide in those they trust outside health care (e.g., family members, religious leaders, community elders, "healers," hairdressers, and bartenders).
- For the military: multiple resources: www.realwarriors.net. Suggested treatments include cognitive restructuring techniques (that their experience with adversity can be a sources of strength) and help with problem-solving (so the service member does not feel like a "burden") therapeutic martial arts training; focus on Vets' helping others: "Power of 1" initiative (any "one" helpful contact could save a life).
- For teens, young adults, and their educators: suggestions and advice for students/families and educators: www.cdc.gov/healthyyouth/adolescenthealth; http://www.stopbullying.gov
- In developing world countries, pesticide ingestion is a common method of suicide. Limiting free access has led to reduced suicide rates.

 DIAGNOSIS

HISTORY

- Depressed patients should be asked about ideation and about a plan:
  - "Have you ever felt that life isn't worth living? Do you ever wish you could go to sleep and not wake up? Are you having thoughts about killing yourself?"
- Use psychodynamic formulation, which combines mental-state exam (i.e., behavior, mood, mental content, judgment), past history (i.e., what resources has the patient used in the past for support and are they currently available?), and history of current illness. If the patient is experiencing a loss, is under stress, and does not have access to a previously sustaining resource (e.g., a significant other, a pet, sports ability, a job), that patient is under increased risk for suicide.

- Prior attempts: precipitants, lethality, intent to die, precautions taken to avoid being rescued, reaction to survival (a patient who is upset that the suicide was not completed is at increased risk)
- History of psychiatric symptoms, substance abuse. Also note strengths, such as reasons to live, hopes for future, social supports. A patient without these is at increased risk.
- Collateral history is important (from friends, family, physicians). It may be appropriate to break confidentiality if patient is at imminent risk of suicide.

PHYSICAL EXAM

- Medical conditions: delirium, intoxication, withdrawal, medication side effects
- Psychosis: Observe for signs of/ask about command auditory hallucinations to kill oneself, delusional guilt, and persecutory delusions.
- In adults: Observe for signs of hopelessness/despair (see "Risk Factors").
- In teens: Screen for risk factors: substance abuse, bullying and social isolation (both common via electronic media), poor grades, because teens may not appear depressed.

DIFFERENTIAL DIAGNOSIS

Differentiate between patients and pseudopatients (i.e., those who are using suicide threats and gestures to manipulate others).

DIAGNOSTIC TESTS & INTERPRETATION

Diagnostic Procedures/Other

Brief tests that could be part of any medical/mental health assessment:

- PHQ-9: http://www.med.umich.edu/1info/FHP/practiceguides/depress/phq-9.pdf
- Columbia Suicide Severity Rating Scale, clinical instructions accessed at: http://www.cssrs.columbia.edu/scales_practice_cssrs.html
- Suicide Trigger Scale version 3 (STS-3), which measures a patient's "ruminative flooding" (self-critical, repetitive thoughts) and "frantic hopelessness" (feeling trapped, suicide is the only choice): http://www.ncbi.nlm.nih.gov/pmc/articles/PMC3443232/

TREATMENT

GENERAL MEASURES

- Patients expressing active suicidal thoughts or who made an attempt require immediate evaluation for risk factors, mental status, and capacity (to determine if they are able/or willing to inform treaters about suicidal intentions), as well as a formal psychiatric consultation. Careful primary care screening can be as effective at identifying risk as a psychological assessment.

- Cognitive therapy decreased reattempt rate in prior suicide attempters by half. (i) Establish therapeutic alliance. Have patient tell a story about recent suicidal thought or action. (ii) Help patient develop the skills needed to deal with the thoughts or feelings that trigger suicidal crises. (iii) Have patient imagine being in the situation that brought on the earlier crisis, but this time, guide that patient to practice problem-solving strategies—reinforcing the use of coping skills, rather than suicidal actions (2)[B],(3).

- Psychotherapy with suicidal patients is a challenge even for the most experienced clinicians. The countertransference, a clinician's feelings toward a patient, can evolve into wanting to be rid of the patient. If the patient detects this, the risk of suicide is heightened. The clinician can avoid this by recognizing countertransference and bearing it within so that the patient remains unaware (4).

- Among military personnel: ACE campaign: Ask about suicidal thoughts; care for the person, including removing access to lethal weapons; "escort" the soldier for help: an emergency room, to calling 911, or a support hotline such as (800) 273-TALK (8255); text: 838255

MEDICATION

- Psychopharmacology "is not a substitute for getting to know the patient" (5)[A].

- Patients are at increased risk of suicide at the outset of antidepressant treatment and when it is discontinued. Consider tapering/switching medical therapies rather than sudden discontinuation. Monitor carefully at these times.

- Anxiety, agitation, and delusions increasing in intensity are risk factors for suicide and should be treated aggressively.

- In patients with mood disorders, a meta-analysis of randomized, controlled trials found that lithium reduced the risk of death by suicide by 60% (5)[A].

- Agitated or combative patients may require sedation with IV or IM benzodiazepines and/or antipsychotics. Clinical response is typically seen within 20 to 30 minutes if given IM/IV.

Pediatric Considerations
FDA posted black box warning for antidepressant use in the pediatric population after increased suicidality was noted. If risk of untreated depression is sufficient to warrant treatment with antidepressants, children must be monitored closely for suicidality.

First Line
ECGs before prescribing or continuing antidepressants or antipsychotics to look for QT prolongation

ISSUES FOR REFERRAL
Consider a psychiatric consult. All decisions regarding treatment must be carefully documented and communicated to all involved health care providers.

INPATIENT CONSIDERATIONS

Admission Criteria/Initial Stabilization
- Inpatient hospitalization, if patient is suicidal with a plan to act or is otherwise at high risk; if immediate risk for self-harm, may be hospitalized involuntarily

- Immediately after a suicide attempt, treat the medical problems resulting from the self-harm before attempting to initiate psychiatric care.

- Order lab work (e.g., solvent screen, blood and urine toxicology screen, aspirin and acetaminophen levels). Patients may not disclose ingestions if they wish to succeed in their attempt or if they are undergoing mental status changes.

- Risk for self-harm continues even in hospital setting. Immediate search for and remove potentially dangerous objects, one-to-one constant observation, medication. Mechanical restraints only if necessary for patient safety.

- The period after transfer from involuntary to voluntary hospitalization is also a time of high risk.

Discharge Criteria
- No longer considered a danger to self/others
- Clinicians should be aware that a patient may *claim* that he or she is no longer suicidal in order to

facilitate discharge—and complete the act. Look for clinical and behavioral signs that the patient truly is no longer in despair and is hopeful, such as improved appetite, sleep, engagement with staff, and group therapy. Clinicians should check with family and ancillary staff because patients may share more information with them than with doctors.

- Provide information about 24/7 resources.

 ONGOING CARE

FOLLOW-UP RECOMMENDATIONS
Patient Monitoring
- Increase monitoring at the beginning of treatment, when changing medications, and on discharge.

- Educate family members and other close contacts/confidants to the warning signs of suicidality. For adults: despair/hopelessness, isolation, discussing suicide, stating that the world would be a "better place" without them, losses in areas key to the patient's self-worth. For youths: may exhibit the same signs and symptoms, but one should be aware of these additional risks: history of abuse (e.g., sexual, physical), bullying in person or via electronic media (e.g., text messages or social Web sites), family stress, changes in eating and sleeping patterns, suicidality of friends, and giving away treasured items

- Make sure that the patient is willing to accept the type of follow-up offered. Do not assume that just setting it up is sufficient protection.

- Curtail access to firearms.

- Limiting the number of pills may be appropriate for an impulsive patient. However, clinicians may believe that by simply limiting the number of pills they prescribe, they are preventing further suicide attempts, an example of "magical thinking." Clinicians who find themselves thinking this way can take it as a warning sign that their patients may actually be at increased risk of suicide.

PATIENT EDUCATION
Patients who feel they are in danger of hurting themselves should consider one or several of these options:
- Call 911.
- Go directly to an emergency room.
- If already in counseling, contact that therapist immediately.
- Call the National Suicide Prevention Hotline at (800) 273-TALK (8255).
- Servicemen and servicewomen and their families can call (800) 796-9699; if there is no immediate answer, call (800) 273-TALK (8255); text 838255.

PROGNOSIS
The key to a favorable course and prognosis is early recognition of risk factors, early diagnosis and treatment of a psychiatric disorder, and appropriate intervention and follow-up.

COMPLICATIONS
- According to the American Association of Suicidality (AAS), the grief process for significant others of suicide victims can be lifelong and can be expressed in emotions ranging from anger to despair. Survivors often attempt to shoulder the burden on their own because of the added guilt and shame of the nature of the attempted death or death.

- The AAS recommends the following:
  – Counseling: could include short-term behavioral therapy as well as psychotherapy; some therapy should focus on the survivors' relationships

to their current and future significant others. Survivors often seek out life partners as "replacements" for those they lost—could interfere with mourning (6).
  – Sympathetic listening by friends
  – Support during holidays
  – More self-help strategies: www.survivorsofsuicide.com

REFERENCES
1. Jollant F, Bellivier F, Leboyer M, et al. Impaired decision making in suicide attempters. *Am J Psychiatry*. 2005;162(2):304–310.
2. Brown GK, Ten Have T, Henriques GR, et al. Cognitive therapy for the prevention of suicide attempts: a randomized controlled trial. *JAMA*. 2005;294(5):563–570.
3. Ghahramanlou-Holloway M, Neely L, Tucker J. A cognitive behavioral strategy for preventing suicide. *Current Psychiatry*. 2014;13(8):19–28.
4. Maltsberger JT, Buie DH. Countertransference hate in the treatment of suicidal patients. *Arch Gen Psychiatry*. 1974;30(5):625–633.
5. Cipriani A, Pretty H, Hawton K, et al. Lithium in the prevention of suicidal behavior and all-cause mortality in patients with mood disorders: a systematic review of randomized trials. *Am J Psychiatry*. 2005;162(10):1805–1819.
6. Massicotte WJ. Faculty, Canadian Institute of Psychoanalysis; Chair, National Scientific Program Committee. Correspondence, April 24, 2009.

ADDITIONAL READING
- Bryan CJ, Jennings KW, Jobes DA, et al. Understanding and preventing military suicide. *Arch Suicide Res*. 2012;16(2):95–110.
- O'Connor E, Gaynes BN, Burda BU, et al. Screening for and treatment of suicide risk relevant to primary care: a systematic review for the U.S. Preventive Services Task Force. *Ann Intern Med*. 2013;158(10):741–754.

 CODES

ICD10
- R45.851 Suicidal ideations
- T14.91 Suicide attempt
- Z91.5 Personal history of self-harm

CLINICAL PEARLS
- Key preventative measure is to listen to a patient and take steps to keep him or her safe. This could include immediate hospitalization. Questions to explore include, "Are you thinking of killing yourself?," "Who do you have to live for?," and "What should change so that you could live with your suffering?"

- Clozapine, lithium, and cognitive-behavioral therapy are associated with a reduction in the risk of suicide.

- Family members and contacts of people who have attempted or committed suicide suffer from reactions ranging from rage to despair. Their grief is often longer lasting and less well-treated because of the shame and guilt associated with the act. Encourage them to discuss this and consider counseling.

- Resources for clinicians: www.suicidology.com; www.suicideassessment.com

SUPERFICIAL THROMBOPHLEBITIS

Emily M. Culliney, MD, FAAFP

 BASICS

DESCRIPTION
- Superficial thrombophlebitis is venous inflammation with secondary thrombosis of a superficial vein.
- Most common in the lower extremities (60–80%), but can occur in the upper extremities/neck.
- Generally a benign and self-limiting process, but can be painful
- Traumatic thrombophlebitis types:
  – Injury
  – IV catheter related
  – Intentional (i.e., sclerotherapy)
- Aseptic thrombophlebitis types:
  – Primary hypercoagulable states: disorders with measurable defects in the proteins of the coagulation and/or fibrinolytic systems
  – Secondary hypercoagulable states: clinical conditions with a risk of thrombosis (venous stasis, pregnancy)
- Septic (suppurative) thrombophlebitis types:
  – Iatrogenic, long-term IV catheter use
  – Infectious, mainly syphilis and psittacosis
- Mondor disease
  – Rare presentation of anterior chest/breast veins of women
- System(s) affected: cardiovascular
- Synonym(s): phlebitis; phlebothrombosis

Geriatric Considerations
Septic thrombophlebitis is more common; prognosis is poorer.

Pediatric Considerations
Subperiosteal abscesses of adjacent long bone may complicate the disorder.

Pregnancy Considerations
- Associated with increased risk of aseptic superficial thrombophlebitis, especially during postpartum
- NSAIDs are contraindicated during pregnancy.

EPIDEMIOLOGY
- Predominant age
  – Traumatic/IV related has no predominate age/sex.
  – Aseptic primary hypercoagulable state
    ○ Childhood to young adult
- Aseptic secondary hypercoagulable state
  – Mondor disease: women, ages 21 to 55 years
  – Thromboangiitis obliterans onset: ages 20 to 50 years
- Predominant sex
  – Suppurative: male = female
  – Aseptic
    ○ Spontaneous formation: female (55–70%)
    ○ Mondor: female > male (2:1)

Incidence
- Septic
  – Incidence of catheter-related thrombophlebitis is 88/100,000 persons.
  – Develops in 4–8% if cutdown is performed

- Aseptic primary hypercoagulable state: antithrombin III and heparin cofactor II deficiency incidence is 50/100,000 persons.
- Aseptic secondary hypercoagulable state
  – In pregnancy, 49-fold increased incidence of phlebitis
  – Superficial migratory thrombophlebitis in 27% of patients with thromboangiitis obliterans

Prevalence
- Superficial thrombophlebitis is common.
- 1/3 of patients in a medical ICU develop thrombophlebitis that eventually progresses to the deep veins.

ETIOLOGY AND PATHOPHYSIOLOGY
- Similar to deep venous thrombosis. Virchow triad of vessel trauma, stasis, and hypercoagulability (genetic, iatrogenic, or idiopathic)
- Varicose veins play a primary role in etiology of lower extremity phlebitis
- Mondor disease pathophysiology not completely understood
- Less commonly due to infection (i.e., septic)
  – *Staphylococcus aureus, Pseudomonas, Klebsiella, Peptostreptococcus* sp.
  – *Candida* sp.
- Aseptic primary hypercoagulable state
  – Due to inherited disorders of hypercoagulability
- Aseptic secondary hypercoagulable states
  – Malignancy (Trousseau syndrome: recurrent migratory thrombophlebitis): most commonly seen in metastatic mucin or adenocarcinomas of the GI tract (pancreas, stomach, colon, and gallbladder), lung, prostate, and ovary
  – Pregnancy
  – Estrogen based oral contraceptives
  – Behçet, Buerger, or Mondor disease

Genetics
Not applicable other than hypercoagulable states

RISK FACTORS
- Nonspecific
  – Varicose veins
  – Immobilization
  – Obesity
  – Advanced age
  – Postoperative states
- Traumatic/septic
  – IV catheter (plastic > coated)
  – Lower extremity IV catheter
  – Cutdowns
  – Cancer, debilitating diseases
  – Burn patients
  – AIDS
  – IV drug use
- Aseptic
  – Pregnancy
  – Estrogen-based oral contraceptives
  – Surgery, trauma, infection
  – Hypercoagulable state (i.e., factor V, protein C or S deficiency, others)

- Thromboangiitis obliterans: persistent smoking
- Mondor disease
  – Breast cancer or breast surgery

GENERAL PREVENTION
- Avoid lower extremity cannulations/IV.
- Insert catheters under aseptic conditions, secure cannulas, and replace every 3 days.
- Avoid stasis and use usual deep vein thrombosis (DVT) prophylaxis in high-risk patients (i.e., ICU, immobilized)

COMMONLY ASSOCIATED CONDITIONS
- Frequently seen with concurrent DVT (6–53%)
- Symptomatic pulmonary embolism can also be seen concurrently (0–10%)
- Both DVT/PE can occur up to 3 months after onset of phlebitis.

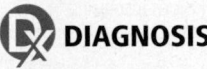 **DIAGNOSIS**

HISTORY
Pain along the course of a vein

PHYSICAL EXAM
- Swelling, tenderness, redness along the course of a vein or veins
- May have a palpable cord along the course of the vein
- May look like localized cellulitis or erythema nodosum
- Fever in 70% of patients in septic phlebitis
- Sign of systemic sepsis in 84% of suppurative cases

DIFFERENTIAL DIAGNOSIS
- Cellulitis
- DVT
- Erythema nodosum
- Cutaneous polyarteritis nodosa
- Lymphangitis

DIAGNOSTIC TESTS & INTERPRETATION
Initial Tests (lab, imaging)
Often none necessary if afebrile, otherwise healthy
- Small or distal veins (i.e., forearms or below the knee): no recommended imaging
- If concern for more proximal extension: venous Doppler US to assess extent of thrombosis and rule out DVT

Follow-Up Tests & Special Considerations
- If suspicious for sepsis
  – Blood cultures (bacteremia in 80–90%)
  – Consider culture of the IV fluids being infused.
  – CBC demonstrates leukocytosis.
- Aseptic: evaluation for coagulopathy if recurrent or without another identifiable cause (e.g., protein C and S, lupus anticoagulant, anticardiolipin antibody, factor V and VIII, homocysteine)

- In migratory thrombophlebitis, have a high index of suspicion for malignancy.
- Repeat venous ultrasound to assess effectiveness of therapy.
  – If thrombosis is extending, more aggressive therapy required.

Test Interpretation
The affected vein is enlarged, tortuous, and thickened with endothelial damage and necrosis.

TREATMENT

GENERAL MEASURES
- Suppurative: consultation for urgent surgical venous excision
- Local, mild
  – Conservative management, antibiotics not useful
  – For varicosities
    ○ Compression stockings, maintain activities
  – Catheter/trauma associated
    ○ Immediately remove IV and culture tip.
    ○ Elevate with application of warm compresses.
    ○ If slow to resolve, consider LMWH.
- Large, severe, or septic thrombophlebitis
  – Inpatient care or bed rest with elevation and local warm compress
  – When the patient is ambulating, then start compression stockings or Ace bandages.

MEDICATION
First Line
- Best medication(s) and duration of treatment are not well-defined (1)[A].
- Localized, mild thrombophlebitis (usually self-limited)
  – NSAIDs and ASA for inflammation/pain to reduce symptoms and local progression.
  – Use of compression stockings can also provide symptomatic relief (2).

Second Line
- Septic/suppurative
  – May present or be complicated by sepsis
  – Requires IV antibiotics (broad spectrum initially) and anticoagulation
- Increasing evidence shows that LMWH/fondaparinux treatment can prevent extension of superficial venous thrombosis in addition to VTE prevention.
- Consider if thrombus present in the large veins or involving the long saphenous vein
  – To prevent venous thromboembolism (VTE), 4 weeks of LMWH; such as enoxaparin
  – 45 days of fondaparinux was found to reduce DVT and VTE by 85% (relative risk reduction) in one large study (3)[B].
- Superficial thrombophlebitis related to inherited or acquired hypercoagulable states is addressed by treating the related disease.

ISSUES FOR REFERRAL
Severely inflamed or very large phlebitis should be evaluated for excision.

SURGERY/OTHER PROCEDURES
- Septic
  – Surgical consultation for excision of the involved vein segment and involved tributaries
  – Drain contiguous abscesses.
  – Remove all associated cannula and culture tips.
- Aseptic: Manage underlying conditions.
  – Evaluate for saphenous vein ligation to prevent deep vein extension after acute phase resolved.
  – Consider referral for varicosity excision.

INPATIENT CONSIDERATIONS
Admission Criteria/Initial Stabilization
- Septic: inpatient
- Aseptic: outpatient

ONGOING CARE

FOLLOW-UP RECOMMENDATIONS
Patient Monitoring
- Septic: routine WBC count and differential. Target treatment based on culture results.
- Severe aseptic
  – Repeat venous Doppler US in 1 to 2 weeks to ensure no DVT and assess treatment effectiveness: Do not expect resolution, just nonprogression.
  – Repeat clotting studies.
- Local, mild thrombophlebitis typically resolves with conservative therapy and does not require specific monitoring unless there is a failure to resolve.

DIET
No restrictions

PATIENT EDUCATION
Review local care, elevation, and use of compression hose for acute treatment and prevention of recurrence.

PROGNOSIS
- Septic/suppurative
  – High mortality (50%) if untreated
  – Depends on treatment delay or need for surgery
- Aseptic
  – Usually benign course; recovery in 2 to 3 weeks
  – Depends on development of DVT and early detection of complications
  – Aseptic thrombophlebitis can be isolated, recurrent, or migratory.
  – Recurrence likely if related to varicosity or if severely affected vein not removed

COMPLICATIONS
- Septic: systemic sepsis, bacteremia (84%), septic pulmonary emboli (44%), metastatic abscess formation, pneumonia (44%), subperiosteal abscess of adjacent long bones in children
- Aseptic: DVT (6–53%), VTE (up to 10%), thromboembolic phenomena

REFERENCES

1. Di Nisio M, Wichers IM, Middeldorp S. Treatment for superficial thrombophlebitis of the leg. *Cochrane Database Syst Rev.* 2013;(4):CD004982.
2. Decousus H, Epinat M, Guillot K, et al. Superficial vein thrombosis: risk factors, diagnosis, and treatment. *Curr Opin Pulm Med.* 2003;9(5):393–397.
3. Di Nisio M, Middeldorp S. Treatment of lower extremity superficial thrombophlebitis. *JAMA.* 2014;311(7):729–730.

ADDITIONAL READING

- Decousus H, Leizorovicz A. Superficial thrombophlebitis of the legs: still a lot to learn. *J Thromb Haemost.* 2005;3(6):1149–1151.
- Decousus H, Quéré I, Presles E, et al. Superficial venous thrombosis and venous thromboembolism: a large, prospective epidemiologic study. *Ann Intern Med.* 2010;152(4):218–224.
- Wichers IM, Di Nisio M, Büller HR, et al. Treatment of superficial vein thrombosis to prevent deep vein thrombosis and pulmonary embolism: a systematic review. *Haematologica.* 2005;90(5):672–677.

 SEE ALSO

Deep Vein Thrombophlebitis

 CODES

ICD10
- I80.9 Phlebitis and thrombophlebitis of unspecified site
- I80.00 Phlbts and thombophlb of superfic vessels of unsp low extrm
- I80.8 Phlebitis and thrombophlebitis of other sites

CLINICAL PEARLS
- Mild superficial thrombophlebitis is typically self-limiting and responds well to conservative care.
- Lower extremity disease involving large veins or proximal saphenous vein may benefit from anticoagulation to prevent DVT.
- Septic thrombophlebitis requires admission for antibiotics and anticoagulation. If severe, consider surgical consultation for venous excision.

SYNCOPE

Santiago O. Valdes, MD, FAAP

BASICS

DESCRIPTION
- Transient loss of consciousness characterized by unresponsiveness, loss of postural tone, and spontaneous recovery; usually caused by cerebral hypoxemia
- System(s) affected: cardiovascular, nervous

EPIDEMIOLOGY

Incidence
- Up to 20% of adults will have ≥1 episode by age 75 years; 15% of children <18 years of age
- Accounts for 1–6% of hospital admissions and ~3% of emergency room visits
- Annually prevalence of fainting spells resulting in medical evaluation was 9.5/1,000 inhabitants (1).

Prevalence
In institutionalized elderly (>75 years of age) is 6%

ETIOLOGY AND PATHOPHYSIOLOGY
- In some cases, vagal response leads to decreased heart rate.
- Systemic hypotension secondary to decreased cardiac output and/or systemic vasodilation leads to a drop in cerebral perfusion and resulting loss of consciousness.
- Cardiac (obstruction to outflow)
  - Aortic stenosis
  - Hypertrophic cardiomyopathy
  - Pulmonary embolus
- Cardiac arrhythmias
  - Sustained ventricular tachycardia (VT)
  - Supraventricular tachycardia (SVT) (atrial fibrillation, atrial flutter, reentrant SVT)
  - 2nd- and 3rd-degree AV block
  - Sick sinus syndrome
- Noncardiac
  - Reflex-mediated vasovagal (neurocardiogenic/neurally mediated), situational (micturition, defecation, cough, hair combing)
  - Orthostatic hypotension
  - Drug induced
  - Neurologic: seizures; transient ischemic attack (can in theory cause syncope but presentation usually markedly clinically different from pure syncope)
  - Carotid sinus hypersensitivity
  - Psychogenic

Genetics
Specific cardiomyopathies and arrhythmias may be familial (i.e., long QT syndrome, catecholaminergic polymorphic VT, Brugada syndrome, hypertrophic cardiomyopathy).

RISK FACTORS
- Heart disease
- Dehydration
- Drugs
  - Antihypertensives
  - Vasodilators (including calcium channel blockers, ACE inhibitors, and nitrates)
  - Phenothiazines
  - Antidepressants
  - Antiarrhythmics
  - Diuretics

GENERAL PREVENTION
See "Risk Factors."

COMMONLY ASSOCIATED CONDITIONS
See "Etiology."

DIAGNOSIS

HISTORY
- Careful history, physical exam, and an ECG are more important than other investigations in determining the diagnosis (2)[A]. Syncope associated with physical exertion suggests a potential cardiac etiology.
- Make sure that the patient or witness (if present) is not talking about vertigo (i.e., sense of rotary motion, spinning, and whirling), seizure, or causes of fall without loss of consciousness.
- Even after careful evaluation, including diagnostic procedures and special tests, the cause will be found in only 50–60% of the patients.
- Onset of syncope is usually rapid, and recovery is spontaneous, rapid, and complete. Duration of episodes are typically brief (<60 seconds). The presence of underlying cardiac or neurologic conditions provides the key to diagnosis.
- Ask for family history of long QT syndrome, hypertrophic cardiomyopathy, or unexplained sudden cardiac death in young family members.

PHYSICAL EXAM
- BP and pulse, both lying and standing
- Check for cardiac murmur or focal neurologic abnormality.

DIFFERENTIAL DIAGNOSIS
- Drop attacks
- Coma
- Vertigo
- Seizure disorder

DIAGNOSTIC TESTS & INTERPRETATION
History and physical examination should guide laboratory testing.

Initial Tests (lab, imaging)
Consider (not all indicated in all individuals) the following:
- CBC
- Electrolytes, BUN, creatinine, glucose (rarely helpful: <2% have hyponatremia, hypocalcemia, hypoglycemia, or renal failure causing seizures)
- Cardiac enzymes (only if history suggestive of cardiac ischemia)
- D-dimer (for pulmonary embolism workup)
- hCG
- Lung scan or helical CT scan of thorax if history and physical exam suggest pulmonary embolism (PE)

Follow-Up Tests & Special Considerations
- If history and physical suggest ischemic, valvular, or congenital heart disease (3)

  - ECG (3)[A]

  - Exercise stress test (if syncope with exertion) (3)[C]

  - Echocardiogram (3)[B]

  - Cardiac catheterization

- If CNS disease suspected (3)[C]
  - EEG
  - Head CT scan
  - Head MRI/MRA when vascular cause is suspected
  - Do not order these tests without hints of CNS disease on history or physical exam.
- ECG monitoring, either in hospital or ambulatory (Holter) (3)[C]
  - Useful in 4–15% of patients
  - Should be done in patients with heart disease or recurrent syncope
  - Arrhythmias frequently documented but not always associated with syncope
- Electrophysiologic studies (3,4)[C]
  - Have been positive in 18–75% of patients
  - Induction of VT and dysfunction of His-Purkinje system are the two most common abnormalities.
  - Should be done in patients with heart disease and recurrent syncope, although they may not show whether arrhythmia noted or induced during study is cause of syncope
- Carotid hypersensitivity evaluation (3,4)[C]
  - Carotid hypersensitivity should be considered in patients with syncope during head turning, especially while wearing tight collars, and with neck tumors and neck scars.
  - The technique is not standardized; one side at a time is compressed gently for 20 seconds with constant monitoring of pulse and BP/ECG.
  - Atropine should be readily available.
- Tilt-table testing ± isoproterenol infusion (3)[B],(4)[C]

  - Provocative test for vasovagal syncope
  - Perform if cardiac causes have been excluded; role in workup of patients with syncope of unknown origin
  - Protocol is not standardized but has been reported positive (symptomatic hypotension and bradycardia) in 26–87% of patients; also positive in up to 45% of control subjects.
- Psychiatric evaluation (3)[C]: Anxiety, depression, and alcohol and drug abuse can be associated with syncope.

Diagnostic Procedures/Other
Patient-activated implantable loop recorders can record 4 to 5 minutes of retrograde ECG rhythm. Helpful in selective patients with recurrent syncope, with yield of 32–80% (3,4)[B].

Test Interpretation
Depends on etiology and presence of underlying cardiac or neurologic conditions

TREATMENT

Maintaining good hydration status and normal salt intake are initial therapy. Educate patients of the premonitory signs of syncope (5)[B].

GENERAL MEASURES
- Elderly patients without previously recognized heart disease should be admitted if the physician thinks that the cause of syncope is likely cardiac.
- Patients without heart disease, especially young patients (age <60 years), can be worked up safely as outpatients.

- Prescribe antiarrhythmics for documented arrhythmias occurring simultaneously with syncope or symptoms of presyncope. Asymptomatic arrhythmias do not necessarily require treatment.
- The decision to treat patients on basis of arrhythmias or conduction abnormalities provoked or detected during EPS is even more problematic: Does the arrhythmia or conduction abnormality have anything to do with the patient's symptoms?
- Most would treat patients with provoked sustained VT with an antiarrhythmic drug that suppressed arrhythmia during study.
- Rationale for such treatment: Recurrent syncope is less frequent in patients with positive EPS who are treated than it is in those who have negative EPS.

MEDICATION

First Line
- Geared toward specific underlying cardiac or neurologic abnormalities
- In cases of recurrent vasovagal/neurocardiogenic/ neurally mediated syncope (6)[B]
  - α-Adrenergic agonists (midodrine)
  - Mineralocorticoids (fludrocortisone)
  - β-Adrenergic blockers

Second Line
- SSRIs (paroxetine, sertraline, fluoxetine)
- Vagolytics (disopyramide)

ISSUES FOR REFERRAL
When cardiac or neurologic etiologies are suspected, obtain appropriate consultation, as indicated.

ADDITIONAL THERAPIES
For vasovagal/neurocardiogenic/neurally mediated syncope
- Counterpressure maneuvers, orthostatic training, and exercise have improved vasovagal symptoms and recurrence (3,5)[C].
- Head-up tilt sleeping (3)[C]
- Abdominal binders and/or support stockings (3)[C]

SURGERY/OTHER PROCEDURES
- Implantable cardioverter-defibrillator (ICD) placement for patients with cardiac conditions with high risk of sudden death and/or recurrent syncope on medications (i.e., long QT syndrome, catecholaminergic polymorphic VT, hypertrophic cardiomyopathy) (3)[B]
- Many recommend pacemaker implantation in patients with the following:
  - 2nd- (Mobitz type II) and 3rd-degree heart block
  - HV intervals >100 ms
  - Pacing-induced infranodal block
  - Sinus node recovery time ≥3 seconds

INPATIENT CONSIDERATIONS

Admission Criteria/Initial Stabilization
Patients with benign etiologies of syncope with negative ED workups are associated with benign outcomes, even in the presence of other risk factors (7)[B].

Patients with suspected cardiac or neurologic cause for syncope should be admitted to the hospital for evaluation.
- Support ABCs.
- Stabilize heart rate and BP, typically with IV fluids.

IV Fluids
Use isotonic crystalloid fluids for fluid resuscitation, if needed.

Nursing
Close monitoring of BP and heart rate during initial presentation

Discharge Criteria
- Attainment of hemodynamic stability
- Satisfactory completion of workup for etiology
- Adequate control of specific arrhythmia or seizure, if present

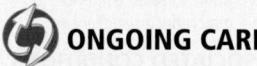 ONGOING CARE

FOLLOW-UP RECOMMENDATIONS

Patient Monitoring
- Frequent follow-up visits for patients with cardiac causes of syncope, especially patients on antiarrhythmics
- Patients with an unknown cause of syncope rarely (5%) are diagnosed during the follow-up.

DIET
- No specific diet unless the patient has heart disease
- Increased fluid and salt intake to maintain intravascular volume in cases of recurrent vasovagal syncope

PATIENT EDUCATION
- Reassure the patient that most cardiac causes of syncope can be treated, and patients with noncardiac causes do well, even if the cause of syncope is never discovered.
- Physical counterpressure maneuvers can prevent recurrences of vasovagal syncope.
- Physician and patient should carefully consider whether the patient should continue to drive while syncope is being evaluated. Physicians should be aware of pertinent laws in their own states.

PROGNOSIS
- Cumulative mortality at 2 years
  - Low: young patients (<60 years of age) with noncardiac or unknown cause of syncope
  - Intermediate: older patients (>60 years of age) with noncardiac or unknown cause of syncope
  - High: patients with cardiac cause of syncope
- Independent predictors of poor short-term outcomes (8,9)[B]
  - Abnormal ECG
  - Shortness of breath
  - Systolic BP <90 mm Hg
  - Hematocrit <30%
  - Congestive heart failure

COMPLICATIONS
- Trauma from falling
- Death (see "Prognosis")

REFERENCES

1. Malasana G, Brignole M, Daccarett M, et al. The prevalence and cost of the faint and fall problem in the state of Utah. *Pacing Clin Electrophysiol.* 2011;34(3):278–283.
2. Kessler C, Tristano JM, De Lorenzo R. The emergency department approach to syncope: evidence-based guidelines and prediction rules. *Emerg Med Clin North Am.* 2010;28(3):487–500.
3. Moya A, Sutton R, Ammirati F, et al. Guidelines for the diagnosis and management of syncope (version 2009). *Eur Heart J.* 2009;30(21):2631–2671.
4. Brignole M, Hamdan MH. New concepts in the assessment of syncope. *J Am Coll Cardiol.* 2012;59(18):1583–1591.
5. Romme JJ, Reitsma JB, Go-Schön IK, et al. Prospective evaluation of non-pharmacological treatment in vasovagal syncope. *Europace.* 2010;12(4):567–573.
6. Kuriachan V, Sheldon RS, Platonov M. Evidence-based treatment for vasovagal syncope. *Heart Rhythm.* 2008;5(11):1609–1614.
7. Grossman SA, Fischer C, Kancharla A, et al. Can benign etiologies predict benign outcomes in high-risk syncope patients? *J Emerg Med.* 2011;40(5):592–597.
8. Quinn JV, Stiell IG, McDermott DA, et al. Derivation of the San Francisco Syncope Rule to predict patients with short-term serious outcomes. *Ann Emerg Med.* 2004;43(2):224–232.
9. Saccilotto RT, Nickel CH, Bucher HC, et al. San Francisco Syncope Rule to predict short-term serious outcomes: a systematic review. *CMAJ.* 2011;183(15):E1116–E1126.

ADDITIONAL READING

- Parry SW, Tan MP. An approach to the evaluation and management of syncope in adults. *BMJ.* 2010;340:c880.
- Reed MJ, Newby DE, Coull AJ, et al. The ROSE (risk stratification of syncope in the emergency department) study. *J Am Coll Cardiol.* 2010;55(8):713–721.
- Strickberger SA, Benson DW, Biaggioni I, et al. AHA/ACCF scientific statement on the evaluation of syncope: from the American Heart Association Councils on Clinical Cardiology, Cardiovascular Nursing, Cardiovascular Disease in the Young, and Stroke, and the Quality of Care and Outcomes Research Interdisciplinary Working Group; and the American College of Cardiology Foundation in Collaboration with the Heart Rhythm Society. *J Am Coll Cardiol.* 2006;47(2):473–484.
- Puppala VK, Dickinson O, Benditt DG. Syncope: classification and risk stratification. *J Cardiol.* 2014;63(3):171–177.
- Sheldon RS, Grubb BP II, Olshansky B, et al. 2015 Heart Rhythm Society expert consensus statement on the diagnosis and treatment of postural tachycardia syndrome, inappropriate sinus tachycardia, and vasovagal syncope. *Heart Rhythm.* 2015;12(6):e41–e63.

 SEE ALSO

- Aortic Valvular Stenosis; Atrial Septal Defect (ASD); Carotid Sinus Hypersensitivity; Patent Ductus Arteriosus; Pulmonary Arterial Hypertension; Pulmonary Embolism; Seizure Disorders; Stokes-Adams Attacks
- Algorithms: Syncope; Transient Ischemic Attack and Transient Neurologic Defects

 CODES

ICD10
R55 Syncope and collapse

CLINICAL PEARLS
- A careful history and physical exam are key to a diagnosis.
- Use the ECG/event-recorder to evaluate for cardiac conditions.
- True neurologic causes of syncope are very rare; by far, cardiac causes are more common.
- <2% of cases are caused by hyponatremia, hypocalcemia, hypoglycemia, or renal failure causing seizures.

SYNCOPE, REFLEX (VASOVAGAL SYNCOPE)

Melinda Y. Kwan, DO, MPH • Norton Winer, MD

 BASICS

Syncope is a reversible loss of consciousness and postural tone secondary to systemic hypotension and cerebral hypoperfusion due to vasodilation and/or bradycardia (rarely, tachycardia) with spontaneous recovery and no neurologic sequelae. The term syncope excludes seizures, coma, shock, or other states of altered consciousness.

DESCRIPTION
- Derived from the Greek term *syncopa*, meaning "to cut short"
- Sudden, transient loss of consciousness characterized by unresponsiveness, falling, and spontaneous recovery
- Common cause of syncope in all age groups, especially in patients with no evidence of neurologic or cardiac disease
- Four main types: vasovagal or neurocardiogenic syncope, situational syncope, orthostatic hypotension, carotid sinus hypersensitivity, and glossopharyngeal/trigeminal neuralgia syncope (uncommon) (1)

EPIDEMIOLOGY
- Mortality: cardiac-related syncope 20–30% and 5% in idiopathic syncope
- Age: any age

Incidence
- Ranges from 7.5% in children aged <18 years and 15% in adults aged >70 years
- 36–62% of all syncopal episodes
- 30% recurrence rate

Prevalence
22% in the general population

ETIOLOGY AND PATHOPHYSIOLOGY
Cause: an abnormal interaction of the normal mechanisms for maintaining BP and upright posture
- In normal individuals, upright posture results in venous pooling and transient decrease in BP.
- Neurally induced syncope may result from a cardio-inhibitory response, a vasodepressor response, or a combination of the two.
- Increased cardiovagal tone leads to bradycardia or asystole and decreased peripheral sympathetic activity leads to venodilation and hypotension (2).
- Vasovagal syncope usually has a precipitating event, often related to fright, pain, panic, exercise, noxious stimuli, or heat exposure (2).
- Carotid sinus syncope is precipitated by position change, turning head, or wearing a tight collar (possible neck tumors or surgical scarring).
- Situational syncope is related to micturition, defecation, postexercise, cough, or swallow (3).
- Glossopharyngeal syncope is related to throat or facial pain (4).

Genetics
Vasovagal syncope: strong heritable component to the etiology of >20% of cases

RISK FACTORS
- Low-resting BP
- Age: older age
- Prolonged supine position with resulting deconditioning of autonomic control

GENERAL PREVENTION
Avoidance of precipitating events or situations. Optimization of diabetes mellitus (DM) control, elastic stockings, adequate hydration. Limited evidence suggests that polydipsia may reduce recurrences.

COMMONLY ASSOCIATED CONDITIONS
- Cardiopulmonary disorders: CHF, MI, arrhythmias, hypertrophic obstructive cardiomyopathy, HTN, PE pulmonary embolism
- Neurologic disorders: autonomic dysfunction, Shy-Drager, Parkinson disease, multiple system atrophy, transient ischemic attack, vertebrobasilar insufficiency, peripheral neuropathy
- Psychiatric disorders:
  – Generalized anxiety disorder
  – Panic disorder
  – Major depression
  – Alcohol dependence

 DIAGNOSIS

HISTORY
- Evaluation of syncope and presyncope are the same.
- Important first to rule out cardiac syncope
- Neurally mediated syncope is preceded by blurred vision, palpitations, nausea, warmth, diaphoresis, or light-headedness, or there may be history of nausea, warmth, diaphoresis, or fatigue *after* syncope (5)[C].
- Vasovagal syncope
  – Three phases: prodrome, loss of consciousness, and postsyncope
  – Precipitating event or stimulus is usually identified, such as panic, fright, pain, or exercise.
  – Athletes may have after exertion (diagnosis of exclusion).
  – Position: *can be preceded by prolonged standing but can occur from any position; generally resolves when the patient becomes supine*
    ○ Preceding events: as discussed above
    ○ Prodrome: as listed above for neurally mediated syncope
  – Duration: generally brief (seconds to minutes)
  – Recovery: may be prolonged with persistent nausea, pallor, and diaphoresis but without neurologic change or confusion
- Carotid sinus syncope is precipitated by position change, after turning head, or wearing a tight collar.
- Situational syncope is related to micturition, defecation, or coughing.
- Glossopharyngeal syncope (less common) is related to throat or facial pain (4)[C]
  – Precipitating events or situations may include panic, pain, exercise, micturition, defecation, coughing, or swallowing.

PHYSICAL EXAM
- Vital signs, including orthostatics and bilateral BP
- Cardiac exam: volume status, murmurs, rhythm, carotid bruits
- Neurologic exam: signs of focal deficit
- Assess for occult blood loss, including guaiac.
- Dix-Hallpike to rule out benign paroxysmal vertigo

DIFFERENTIAL DIAGNOSIS
- Seizure
- Arrhythmia
- Hypoglycemia
- Cardiac syncope
- Cerebrovascular syncope
- Orthostatic hypotension
- Drop attacks
- Psychiatric illness

DIAGNOSTIC TESTS & INTERPRETATION
As indicated by history and physical, includes basic tests to rule out the three main reasons for syncope: hypoglycemia, arrhythmia, and anemia

Initial Tests (lab, imaging)
- Blood sugar
- ECG should be ordered for all patients. Abnormal ECG findings are common in patients with cardiac syncope.
- CBC to rule out anemia
- Head CT, MRI/MRA, carotid ultrasound only in patients whose history or physical exam suggests a neurologic cause of syncope
  – The 2007 American College of Emergency Physicians (ACEP) Guidelines for diagnostic testing for syncope are as follows (6):
    ○ *Level A recommendations*: standard 12-lead ECG
    ○ *Level B recommendations*: none specified
    ○ *Level C recommendations*: laboratory testing and investigations, including echocardiography or head CT, to be performed only if indicated by specific findings in the history or physical examination

Follow-Up Tests & Special Considerations
- 24-hour Holter monitoring only in patients with a high probability of cardiac cause of syncope and/or abnormal ECG findings
- A low hemoglobin without obvious cause of bleed would warrant a guaiac, CT head to rule out subarachnoid hemorrhage (SAH), CT abdomen to rule out retroperitoneal bleed.
- Negative imaging will prompt workup for alternative causes.
- Stroke, bleed, or carotid stenosis will require appropriate disease-oriented management.
- EEG only when history or physical exam is very suggestive of seizure activity
- Implantable loop recorder

Diagnostic Procedures/Other
- Head-up tilt table testing:
  – Contraindicated in patients with known cardiac or neurovascular disease or in pregnancy
  – Indicated for recurrent syncope or single episode accompanied by injury or risk to others (e.g., pilots, surgeons)
  – Uses positional changes to reproduce symptoms
  – Positive tests are diagnostic for vasovagal syncope.
- Carotid sinus massage, only in a monitored setting (i.e., BP and HR monitoring, IV access):
  – Contraindicated in patients with carotid disease (careful auscultation prior to massage is essential)

– Pressure at the angle of the jaw for 5 seconds with simultaneous ECG monitoring
– Positive tests (causing syncope or cardiac pause >3 seconds) are diagnostic of carotid sinus syncope.
• Psychiatric evaluation: to rule out anxiety, depression, and alcohol abuse

TREATMENT

Therapy is primarily for recurrent syncope. Situational syncope will not warrant any treatment.

GENERAL MEASURES
Recognition and avoidance of precipitating events or situations; medical management is based on small, nonrandomized clinical trials.

First Line
• Nonpharmacologic treatment
– Includes patient counseling
  ○ Development of coping skills
  ○ Increased salt and fluid intake
– Moderate exercise training
  ○ Isometric muscle contractions
    ▪ Leg crossing and buttocks clenching
    ▪ Intense gripping of the hands and tensing of the arms
    ▪ These maneuvers increase cardiac output and arterial blood pressure (7).
– Tilt-table training
  ○ Progressively prolonged periods of enforced upright posture

Second Line
• α-Agonists are mainly used for orthostatic hypotension.
– Midodrine is commonly used. It increases peripheral vascular resistance and venous return. Side effects include HTN, paresthesia, urinary retention, "goose bumps," hyperactivity, dizziness, tremor, and nervousness.
• SSRIs: Paroxetine and fluoxetine are SSRIs useful in treating neurocardiogenic/vasovagal syncope.
– Serotonin affects BP and HR via the central nervous system. Serotonin decreases a sympathetic withdrawal response to rapid increases in serotonin levels.
– Side effects include weight gain, nausea, anxiety, sexual dysfunction, and insomnia.
• Mineralocorticoids: Fludrocortisone has been found helpful mainly in orthostatic hypotension.
– Helpful in renal sodium absorption and increasing the vasoconstrictive peripheral vascular response
– Adverse reactions include fluid retention, HTN, CHF, peripheral edema, and hypokalemia.
• β-Blockers: Metoprolol, atenolol, or pindolol are mainly used for postural tachycardia syndrome (POTS).
– Block peripheral vasodilators and ventricular mechanoreceptor stimulation.
– Stabilization of HR and BP
– Side effects: hypotension and bradycardia (with worsening of syncope), fatigue, depression, and sexual dysfunction
– Contraindicated in asthma

ISSUES FOR REFERRAL
Neurology or cardiology, as needed

ADDITIONAL THERAPIES
Use of support/pressure stockings

COMPLEMENTARY & ALTERNATIVE MEDICINE
These include treatments for underlying heart disease or precipitating factors like anxiety. None of these are proven therapies.
• Nutrition and supplements: omega-3 fatty acids, multivitamin, CoQ10, acetyl-L-carnitine, α-lipoic acid, and L-arginine
• Herbs: Green tea (Camellia sinensis), bilberry (Vaccinium myrtillus), ginkgo (Ginkgo biloba)
• Homeopathy: Carbo vegetabilis, opium, sepia
• Acupuncture: It may precipitate fainting.

SURGERY/OTHER PROCEDURES
Pacemaker placement may be of use in patients with frequent neurocardiogenic/vasovagal syncope that is refractory to other therapies (3)[C].
• Prevents prolonged bradycardia or asystole during syncopal episodes
• Long-term effect
• Invasive placement procedure

INPATIENT CONSIDERATIONS

Admission Criteria/Initial Stabilization
2007 ACEP guidelines mandate that the patient be admitted if (6):
• Level B recommendations
– Admit patients with syncope and evidence of heart failure or structural heart disease.
– Admit patients with syncope and high-risk factors.
• High-risk stratification is based on the following factors:
– Older age and associated comorbidities
– Abnormal ECG, hematocrit (Hct) 30 (if obtained)
– History or presence of heart failure, coronary artery disease, or structural heart disease
• Additional causes to admit
– Syncope occurring during exercise
– Syncope causing severe injury
– Family history of sudden death
• IV fluids to stabilize HR and BP

IV Fluids
Isotonic crystalloids, as needed

Nursing
Vital sign monitoring

Discharge Criteria
Hemodynamically stable and workup satisfactory

 ONGOING CARE

DIET
• Increased salt intake may be helpful if not contraindicated (2)[C].
• Maintain fluid intake.

PATIENT EDUCATION
• To identify and avoid precipitating events or situations
• Avoid dehydration, alcohol consumption, warm environments, tight clothing, and long periods of standing motionless.
• Recognize presyncopal symptoms.
• Use behaviors, such as lying down, to avoid syncope.

PROGNOSIS
May be recurrent but not life-threatening

COMPLICATIONS
May result in injury from fall

REFERENCES

1. Angaran P, Klein GJ, Yee R, et al. Syncope. Neurol Clin. 2011;29(4):903–925.
2. Raj SR, Coffin ST. Medical therapy and physical maneuvers in the treatment of the vasovagal syncope and orthostatic hypotension. Prog Cardiovasc Dis. 2013;55(4):425–433.
3. Walsh K, Hoffmayer K, Hamdan M. Syncope: diagnosis and management. Curr Probl Cardiol. 2015;40(2):51–86.
4. Chen-Scarabelli C, Scarabelli TM. Neurocardiogenic syncope. BMJ. 2004;329(7461):336–341.
5. Chen LY, Benditt DG, Shen WK. Management of syncope in adults: an update. Mayo Clin Proc. 2008;83(11):1280–1293.
6. Huff JS, Decker WW, Quinn JV, et al. Clinical policy: critical issues in the evaluation and management of adult patients presenting to the emergency department with syncope. Ann Emerg Med. 2007;49(4):431–444.
7. Coffin ST, Raj SR. Non-invasive management of vasovagal syncope. Auton Neurosci. 2014;184: 27–32.

ADDITIONAL READING
• Lelonek M. Genetics in neurocardiogenic syncope. Przegl Lek. 2006;63(12):1310–1312.
• Márquez MF, Urias-Medina K, Gómez-Flores J, et al. Comparison of metoprolol vs clonazepam as a first treatment choice among patients with neurocardiogenic syncope. Gac Med Mex. 2008;144(6): 503–507.

 SEE ALSO

Algorithms: Syncope; Transient Ischemic Attack and Transient Neurologic Defects

 CODES

ICD10
R55 Syncope and collapse

CLINICAL PEARLS
• History should include a careful analysis of the events preceding the attack.
• It is important to rule out cardiologic or neurologic pathology.
• Prodrome is often present.
• Recovery may be prolonged, with persistent symptoms but no neurologic deficit or confusion.
• Patient counseling to avoid precipitating situations or events is the first-line treatment.
• Pregnant females can have reflex syncope when moving from supine to lateral decubitus or upright positions.

S

SYNDROME OF INAPPROPRIATE ANTIDIURETIC HORMONE SECRETION (SIADH)

Elise J. Barney, DO

 BASICS

DESCRIPTION
- A syndrome of abnormal production of antidiuretic hormone (ADH), despite low serum osmolality, leading to hyponatremia and inappropriately elevated urine osmolality
  - Resulting abnormal urinary free water retention leads to dilutional hyponatremia (total body sodium levels may be normal or near normal, but the patient's total body water is increased).
  - Often secondary to medications but may be associated with an underlying disorder, such as neoplasm, pulmonary disorder, or CNS system disease
- Synonym(s): syndrome of inappropriate secretion of ADH

EPIDEMIOLOGY
Incidence
- Often found in the hospital setting, where incidence can be as high as 35%
- Predominant age: elderly
- Predominate sex: females > males

ETIOLOGY AND PATHOPHYSIOLOGY
- Drugs:
  - Antidepressants (e.g., monoamine oxidase inhibitors [MAOIs], tricyclics, SSRIs)
  - Antineoplastic drugs (e.g., vincristine, vinblastine, cisplatin, cyclophosphamide)
  - Antipsychotic agents (e.g., phenothiazines, thioridazine, haloperidol)
  - Analgesics (e.g., NSAIDs)
  - Antiepileptics (e.g., carbamazepine, oxcarbazepine, valproic acid)
  - Oral hypoglycemics (e.g., chlorpropamide, metformin)
  - Others (e.g., vasopressin, DDAVP, oxytocin, ciprofloxacin, α-interferon, ecstasy)
- Neoplasms (ectopic ADH production):
  - Bronchogenic carcinoma
  - Hodgkin disease
  - Mesothelioma
  - Oat cell carcinoma of the lung
  - Pancreatic carcinoma
  - Small cell carcinoma of the lung
  - Thymoma
- Pulmonary conditions:
  - Asthma/COPD
  - Atelectasis
  - Cystic fibrosis
  - Positive pressure mechanical ventilation
  - Pneumonia
  - Pulmonary tuberculosis (TB)
  - Sarcoidosis
- Neurological causes:
  - Acute porphyria
  - CNS injury (i.e., SAH, trauma, stroke)
  - CNS lupus
  - Encephalitis
  - Epilepsy
  - Guillain-Barré syndrome
  - Meningitis
  - Multiple sclerosis
- Other:
  - HIV infection
  - Hypothyroidism, myxedema
  - Rocky Mountain spotted fever
- Idiopathic

Genetics
- 10% of patients have X-linked mutation of V2R (1)
- Polymorphisms in TPRV4 gene (2)

RISK FACTORS
- Use of predisposing drugs
- Advanced age
- Postoperative status
- Institutionalization

GENERAL PREVENTION
- Search for cause, if unknown.
- Reduce/change medications, if drug-induced.
- Lifelong restriction of fluid intake

COMMONLY ASSOCIATED CONDITIONS
See "Etiology."

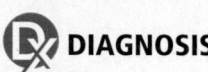 **DIAGNOSIS**

HISTORY
Symptoms:
- Fatigue
- Anorexia
- Nausea
- Vomiting
- Diarrhea
- Headaches
- Unsteady gait
- Falls
- Myalgias/weakness
- Increased thirst
- Confusion
- Seizures, coma

PHYSICAL EXAM
- Euvolemic state
- Mild/moderate hyponatremia (serum Na 125 to 135 mEq/L)
  - Slow cognition and reaction times
  - Hyporeflexia
  - Ataxia
- Severe hyponatremia (serum Na <125 mEq/L) (3)
- Altered mental status
- Lethargy
- Seizures
- Psychosis
- Coma
- Death

DIFFERENTIAL DIAGNOSIS
- Intravascular volume depletion and thiazide-induced
- Appropriate ADH secretion secondary to decreased effective arterial blood volume (e.g., congestive heart failure [CHF], nephrotic syndrome, liver cirrhosis)
- Low solute intake hyponatremia
  - "Tea and toast" diet
  - Beer potomania
- Psychogenic polydipsia
  - Intake usually >10 L/day
  - Diuresis occurs when intake is stopped.
- Endocrinopathies
  - Addison disease
  - Hypothyroidism
- Translocational hyponatremia: caused by hyperglycemia, mannitol, sucrose, glycine
- Pseudohyponatremia
  - Lab artifact caused by hyperlipidemia, paraproteinemias, administration of IVIG
  - Labs using flame photometry or indirect potentiometry susceptible
- Postoperative complications:
  - Caused by nonosmotic release of ADH, probably mediated by pain afferents
  - ADH stimulated by pain, nausea, vomiting, and hypotension
- Cerebral salt-wasting syndrome (hyponatremia, extracellular fluid depletion, CNS insult)

DIAGNOSTIC TESTS & INTERPRETATION
- Serum Na level: low
- Serum urea level: normal to low
- Serum osmolality: low
- Urine osmolality: high; urine osmolality >100 mOsm/kg H_2O (4)
- Urine Na concentration: high; urine Na >30 mEq/L (4)
- Fractional excretion of Na >0.5 % (4)
- Serum ADH level: high (not clinically useful)
- Not usually required for diagnosis but to assess for other concerns:
  - Serum uric acid
  - Serum glucose; creatinine
  - Thyroid function
  - Morning cortisol

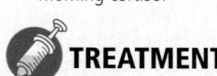 **TREATMENT**

GENERAL MEASURES
- Treatment of the underlying cause is essential.
- Requires frequent monitoring (see "Patient Monitoring")
- Fluid restriction (<1,000 mL/day) is the main form of treatment (5)[C].
- Mildly symptomatic (serum Na >125 mEq/L [>125 mmol/L]): Restrict fluid to <1,000 mL/day.

- Acute (<48 hours duration) or symptomatic (altered mental status, seizure, coma)
  - Hypertonic saline (3% normal saline) bolus
  - Diuresis with loop diuretics
  - Restrict oral free water intake.
  - Increase oral solute intake.
  - Calculate serum Na deficit (mEq Na deficit = [desired Na − actual Na] × 0.5 × body weight [kg]).
  - Increase serum Na slowly with hypertonic saline by 4 to 6 mEq/L over 4 to 6 hours (not to exceed 10 mEq/L in a 24-hour period) (3,6,7).

MEDICATION

- If severe or neurological symptoms: IV 3% sodium chloride to increase serum Na cautiously (8)[B]:
  - If serum Na <120 mEq/L or severe neurologic symptoms; consider bolus of hypertonic saline to increase serum Na by 4 to 6 mEq/L over the first 4 to 6 hours.
- Sodium chloride (NaCl) oral tablets
- Oral urea is an option, but limited due to bitter taste.
- Loop diuretics: furosemide (Lasix) + KCl replacement
- Vasopressin-2 receptor antagonist (the vaptans: tolvaptan, conivaptan) (8),(9)[C]
  - Good efficacy and safety profiles in the treatment of moderate hyponatremia due to SIADH
  - Liberal fluid intake encouraged.
  - Must be initiated in hospital setting.
  - Cost may limit long-term use.
  - Avoid tolvaptan in patients with liver disease.
- Demeclocycline (second line) (10)[C]
  - Blocks ADH at renal tubule; produces nephrogenic diabetes insipidus
  - Dosage for long-term management: 300 to 600 mg PO BID
  - Onset of action within 1 week; therefore, not best for acute management.
- Contraindications: Avoid fluids in CHF, nephrotic syndrome, or cirrhosis. Avoid tolvaptan in patients with cirrhosis due to possible liver injury.
- Precautions: Overly rapid correction (>10 mEq/L/day) can increase risk for osmotic demyelination syndrome:
  - Permanent CNS damage in pons leading to quadriplegia and pseudobulbar palsy.
  - Increased risk in women, alcoholics, malnutrition, hypoxia, and hypokalemia

ALERT
Increase Na levels slowly, no more than 10 mEq/L/24 hr, to prevent complications such as central pontine myelinolysis (CPM) (3)[C].

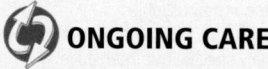

ONGOING CARE

FOLLOW-UP RECOMMENDATIONS
Patient Monitoring
- Careful continuous clinical and laboratory monitoring of hyponatremic state during acute phase:
  - Hourly urine output
  - Urine Na

- Serum Na and potassium (K) every 4 to 6 hours if moderate/severe, then daily once stable
- Goal sodium increase is <10 mEq/L in first 24-hour period, then 8 mEq/L in subsequent 24-hour periods until Na reaches 130 mEq/L (3)[C].
- Chronic management: Treat underlying cause; continue fluid restriction and NaCl tablets as needed.

DIET
Increase protein/solute intake and decrease water intake.

PATIENT EDUCATION
Diet and fluid restrictions

PROGNOSIS
- Depends on underlying cause; in general, higher morbidity and mortality in hospitalized patients with hyponatremia
- If symptomatic (seizure, coma): high mortality due to cerebral edema if serum Na <120 mEq/L (<120 mmol/L)

COMPLICATIONS
- Falls and hip fractures
- Cerebral edema (see "Prognosis")
- Osmotic demyelination with overcorrection (see "Treatment" precautions): central pontine and extrapontine irreversible myelinolysis (6,11)
- Chronic hyponatremia
- Chronic hyponatremia is associated with osteoporosis (12)[C].

REFERENCES

1. Feldman BJ, Rosenthal SM, Vargas GA, et al. Nephrogenic syndrome of inappropriate antidiuresis. *N Engl J Med*. 2005;352(18):1884–1890.
2. Tian W, Fu Y, Garcia-Elias A, et al. A loss-of-function nonsynonymous polymorphism in the osmoregulatory TRPV4 gene is associated with human hyponatremia. *Proc Natl Acad Sci U S A*. 2009;106(33):14034–14039.
3. Spasovski G, Vanholder R, Allolio B, et al. Clinical practice guideline on diagnosis and treatment of hyponatraemia. *Nephrol Dial Transplant*. 2014;29(Suppl 2):i1–i39.
4. Decaux G, Musch W. Clinical laboratory evaluation of the syndrome of inappropriate secretion of antidiuretic hormone. *Clin J Am Soc Nephrol*. 2008;3(4):1175–1184.
5. Ellison DH, Berl T. Clinical practice. The syndrome of inappropriate antidiuresis. *N Engl J Med*. 2007;356(20):2064–2072.
6. Adrogué HJ, Madias NE. The challenge of hyponatremia. *J Am Soc Nephrol*. 2012;23(7):1140–1148.
7. Sterns RH, Nigwekar SU, Hix JK. The treatment of hyponatremia. *Semin Nephrol*. 2009;29(3):282–299.
8. Esposito P, Piotti G, Bianzina S, et al. The syndrome of inappropriate antidiuresis: pathophysiology, clinical management and new therapeutic options. *Nephron Clin Pract*. 2011;119(1):c62–c73.
9. Friedman B, Cirulli J. Hyponatremia in critical care patients: frequency, outcome, characteristics, and treatment with the vasopressin V2-receptor antagonist tolvaptan. *J Crit Care*. 2013;28(2):219.e1–e12.
10. Sherlock M, Thompson CJ. The syndrome of inappropriate antidiuretic hormone: current and future management options. *Eur J Endocrinol*. 2010;162(Suppl 1):S13–S18.
11. Fleming JD, Babu S. Images in clinical medicine. Central pontine myelinolysis. *N Engl J Med*. 2008;359(23):e29.
12. Verbalis JG, Barsony J, Sugimura Y, et al. Hyponatremia-induced osteoporosis. *J Bone Miner Res*. 2010;25(3):554–563.

 SEE ALSO

Hyponatremia

 CODES

ICD10
E22.2 Syndrome of inappropriate secretion of antidiuretic hormone

CLINICAL PEARLS

- Treatment of the underlying cause is a key. Review all medications for potential culprits.
- Consultation is recommended in moderate to severe hyponatremia or if hypertonic saline indicated.
- Fluid restriction is the mainstay of treatment in SIADH. Fluid restriction fails to correct hyponatremia and Na wasting in salt-losing renal disease.
- Cerebral salt wasting is a controversial disease entity and is similar to SIADH. However, patients with SIADH are euvolemic, whereas patients with cerebral salt wasting are hypovolemic. The only real way to establish the diagnosis is through fluid restriction. Serum urate and fractional excretion of urate will be corrected with fluid restriction in SIADH, but will not correct in cerebral salt wasting.
- CPM is a cerebral demyelination syndrome that causes quadriplegia, pseudobulbar palsy, seizures, coma, and death. It is caused by an overly rapid rate of Na correction.
- Safe correction of hyponatremia is important. Online calculators are available: www.medcalc.com/sodium.html.

S

SYPHILIS

Melissa Badowski, PharmD • Mahesh C. Patel, MD

BASICS

DESCRIPTION

- A chronic, systemic infectious disease caused by *Treponema pallidum*
- Transmitted sexually, vertically (maternal–fetal) by direct contact with an active lesion, and via blood transfusions
- Untreated disease includes four overlapping stages.
  - Primary: single (usually) painless chancre at point of entry; appears in 10 to 90 days; chancre heals without treatment in 3 to 6 weeks
  - Secondary: appears 2 to 8 weeks after primary chancre. Nonpruritic rash on palms or soles of feet, mucous membrane lesions, headache, fever, lymphadenopathy, alopecia
  - Latent: seroreactive without evidence of disease
    ○ Early latent: acquired within the last year
    ○ Late latent: exposure >12 months prior to diagnosis
  - Tertiary (late): Serology may be negative (fluorescent treponemal antibody absorption [FTA-ABS] test typically positive).
    ○ Gumma, cardiovascular, and late neurosyphilis; may be fatal
  - Neurosyphilis: *any* type of CNS involvement; can occur at *any* stage
    ○ Psychosis, delirium, dementia
- Syphilis can affect nearly every organ/tissue in the body leading to moniker "the great imitator."

Pediatric Considerations
In noncongenital cases, consider child abuse.

Pregnancy Considerations

- All pregnant patients should be screened with VDRL or rapid plasma reagin (RPR) test early in pregnancy. If high exposure risk, repeat at 28 weeks and at delivery (1,2)[A].
- The same nontreponemal test used for initial screening should be used for follow-up (1,2)[A].

EPIDEMIOLOGY

Incidence

- Syphilis rate decreased until 2000; has increased (primarily in men) since then (3)[A].
- In 2013: 5.3/100,000. Highest for men aged 25 to 29 years and women aged 20 to 24 years (3)[A]

  - Men: 9.8/100,000
  - Women: 0.9/100,000

- Congenital: 8.7 cases/100,000 live births (4)[A]
- Race/ethnicity (3)[A]

  - Male (per 100,000 population)
    ○ White, non-Hispanic: 5.4
    ○ Black, non-Hispanic: 27.9
    ○ Hispanic: 11.6
    ○ Asian/Pacific Islander: 4.6
    ○ American Indian/Alaska native: 4.7
  - Female (per 100,000 population)
    ○ White, non-Hispanic: 0.3
    ○ Black, non-Hispanic: 4.0
    ○ Hispanic: 0.8
    ○ Asian/Pacific Islander: 0.2
    ○ American Indian/Alaska native: 1.0

Prevalence

- Predominant sex: male (91%) > female (9%) (3)[A]
- Greatest increase in men having sex with men (MSM) (3)[A]

ETIOLOGY AND PATHOPHYSIOLOGY

T. pallidum subspecies *pallidum*, spirochete: can enter through intact mucous membranes or breaks in skin. Highly infectious; exposure to as few as 60 spirochetes is associated with ~50% chance of infection

RISK FACTORS

MSM, multiple sexual partners, exposure to infected body fluids, IV drug use, transplacental transmission, adult inmates, high-risk sexual behavior, HIV positive

GENERAL PREVENTION

Education regarding safe sex; condoms reduce but do not eliminate transmission (5)[A]

COMMONLY ASSOCIATED CONDITIONS

HIV infection, hepatitis B, other STIs

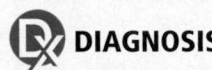

DIAGNOSIS

HISTORY

- Previous sexual contact with partner with known infection or high-risk sexual behavior
- Genital lesions (chancre—primary syphilis)
- Rash, alopecia, malaise, headache, anorexia, nausea, fatigue (secondary syphilis)
- Mental status changes (tertiary syphilis)

PHYSICAL EXAM

Signs/symptoms depend on stage

- Primary: single (occasionally multiple), usually painless ulcer (chancre) in groin or at other point of entry. Regional adenopathy.
- Secondary
  - Rash: skin/mucous membranes
    ○ Rough, red-brown macules, usually on palms and soles
    ○ May appear with chancre or after it has healed
    ○ Condyloma lata
    ○ Alopecia
  - Nonspecific symptoms: fever, adenopathy, malaise, headache, hair loss
- Tertiary
  - Focal neurologic findings (hearing loss, visual loss)
  - Gummas (skin, mucous membranes, other organ systems)

DIFFERENTIAL DIAGNOSIS

- Primary: chancroid, lymphogranuloma venereum, granuloma inguinale, condyloma acuminata, herpes simplex, Behçet syndrome, trauma, carcinoma, mycotic infection, lichen planus, psoriasis, fungal infection
- Secondary: pityriasis rosea, drug eruption, psoriasis, lichen planus, viral exanthema, Stevens-Johnson syndrome
- Positive serology, asymptomatic: previously treated syphilis/other spirochetal disease (yaws, pinta)

DIAGNOSTIC TESTS & INTERPRETATION

Initial Tests (lab, imaging)

- Dark-field microscopy demonstrating *T. pallidum* spirochetes in lesion exudate/tissue biopsy: gold standard but difficult and not very sensitive (6)[A]
- Nontreponemal tests (VDRL/RPR) (3,6)[A]

  - Primary screening test: positive within 7 days of exposure
  - Nonspecific, false-positive results common; must confirm diagnosis with treponemal tests

- Positive test should be quantified and titers followed regularly after treatment.
  ○ Titers usually correlate with disease activity; 4-fold change is clinically significant.
  ○ Titers decrease with time/treatment; following adequate treatment for primary/secondary disease, a 4-fold decline is typically seen after 6 to 12 months.
  ○ Absence of a 4-fold decline suggests potential treatment failure.
  ○ ~15% of appropriately treated patients do not have a 4-fold decline in titer 12 months after treatment. Management is unclear, repeat HIV testing and/or CSF examination and continue to follow titers.
  ○ With appropriate treatment, titers should become negative (see serofast reaction).
  ○ Titers of patients treated in latent stages decline more gradually.
  - Prozone phenomenon: negative results from high titers of antibody; test with diluted serum
  - Serofast reaction: persistently positive results years after successful treatment; new infection diagnosed by 4-fold rise in titer
  - Conditions that may alter treponemal testing (all stages of syphilis can have a false-negative RPR result, especially in primary syphilis)
    ○ Pregnancy, autoimmune disease, mononucleosis, malaria, leprosy, viral pneumonia, cardiolipin antigens, injection drug use, acute febrile illness, HIV infection; elderly can have false-positive results.

- Treponemal tests (*confirmatory test after positive nontreponemal screening test*): FTA-ABS, TP-PA (*T. pallidum* particle agglutination) (6)[A]:

  - Confirmatory test; not used for screening
  - Usually positive for life after treatment
  - Titers of no benefit
  - 15–25% of patients treated during primary stage revert to serologic nonreactivity after 2 to 3 years.

- Lumbar puncture indicated for (6)[A]:

  - Neurologic, ocular, or auditory manifestations
  - Some experts advise in all secondary and early latent cases—even without neurologic symptoms
  - HIV-positive patients with late latent/latent of unknown duration
  - In patients with late latent/latent of unknown duration if nonpenicillin therapy planned
  - In treatment failures
  - If other evidence of active tertiary syphilis is present (e.g., aortitis, gumma, iritis)
  - In children to rule out neurosyphilis
  - VDRL, not RPR, used on CSF; may be negative in neurosyphilis; highly specific but insensitive
  - Send CSF for protein, glucose, and cell count.
  - Monitor resolution by cell count at 6 months along with serologies (see "Patient Monitoring").
  - Negative FTA-ABS or microhemagglutination (MHA)-TP on CSF excludes neurosyphilis (highly sensitive).
  - Positive FTA-ABS or MHA-TP on CSF is not diagnostic because of high false-positive rate.
  - Traumatic tap, tuberculosis (TB), pyogenic/aseptic meningitis can all result in false-positive VDRL.

TREATMENT

GENERAL MEASURES

- Advise patients to avoid intercourse until treatment is complete, and notify partners (6)[A].
- Test for HIV (3,6)[A].
- Management of sexual contacts (6)[A]

  - Presumptively treat partners exposed within 90 days of diagnosis.
  - Treat those exposed >90 days before diagnosis presumptively if serologic results are not available immediately and follow-up is uncertain.
  - Presumptively treat those exposed to a patient diagnosed with syphilis of unknown duration who have high treponemal titers (>1:32).
  - Long-term sex partners of patients with latent infection should be evaluated clinically and serologically and treated accordingly.

MEDICATION

ALERT
Bicillin L-A should be used instead of Bicillin C-R (combination benzathine–procaine penicillin) when penicillin G benzathine is indicated.

First Line
Parenteral penicillin G is the drug of choice. The particular formulation is determined by the disease stage and clinical presentation.

- Primary, secondary, and early latent <1 year (6)[A]

  - Benzathine penicillin G 2.4 million U IM × 1 dose
  - Penicillin-allergic patients: doxycycline 100 mg PO BID for 2 weeks, or tetracycline 500 mg PO QID for 2 weeks, or ceftriaxone 1 to 2 g IM or IV daily for 10 to 14 days
    ○ Azithromycin 2 g PO × 1 dose (early syphilis only; should not be used in HIV, MSM, or pregnancy)
    ○ Resistance and treatment failures have been noted in several U.S. regions.

- Late latent/latent of unknown duration and tertiary without evidence of neurosyphilis (6)[A]

  - Benzathine penicillin G 2.4 million U IM weekly × 3 doses
  - Penicillin-allergic patients: Attempt desensitization and treatment with penicillin or doxycycline 100 mg PO 2 BID for 28 days, or tetracycline 500 mg PO QID for 28 days; compliance may be an issue.

- Ocular or neurosyphilis (6)[A]

  - Aqueous crystalline penicillin G 3 to 4 million U IV q4h as continuous infusion for 10 to 14 days
  - Alternative: Procaine penicillin G 2.4 million U IM daily in conjunction with probenecid 500 mg PO QID for 10 to 14 days (if compliance can be ensured)
  - Penicillin-allergic patients: Attempt desensitization and treat with penicillin; ceftriaxone 2 g/day IM or IV for 10 to 14 days.
  - If late latent, latent of unknown duration, or tertiary in addition to neurosyphilis, consider also treating as recommended for late latent after completion of neurosyphilis treatment.

- Congenital (6)[A]

  - Aqueous crystalline penicillin G 50,000 U/kg/dose IV q12h for the first 7 days of life and q8h thereafter for a total of 10 days, or procaine penicillin G 50,000 U/kg/dose IM daily for 10 days
  - If negative CSF serologies, normal physical exam, and titer: Maternal titer, then 50,000 U/kg benzathine penicillin G IM in single dose is also an alternative.
  - If >1 day of drug is missed, restart course.

  - Children (after newborn period): aqueous crystalline penicillin G 50,000 U/kg/dose IV q4–6h for 10 days; late latent, 50,000 U/kg IM as 3 doses at 1-week intervals
  - For contacts without symptoms: Treat as primary after serologies are obtained.
  - HIV-infected and pregnant patients may show poor response to recommended IM doses. Use IV therapy for all treatment failures in these patients.
  - Do not give benzathine or procaine penicillins IV.

- Children (after newborn period) (6)[A]: aqueous crystalline penicillin G 50,000 U/kg/dose IV q4–6h for 10 days; late latent, 50,000 U/kg IM as 3 doses at 1-week intervals
- Pregnancy (6)[A]

  - Treatment is the same as for nonpregnant patients
  - Some recommend 2nd dose of 2.4 million units benzathine penicillin G 1 week after initial dose in 3rd trimester or with primary, secondary, or early latent syphilis.
  - Penicillin sensitivity: No proven alternatives to penicillin available for treatment during pregnancy.
  - Penicillin-allergic patients: Desensitize and treat with penicillin.
  - HIV-infected pregnant patients may show poor response to recommended IM doses. Use IV therapy for all treatment failures in these patients.
- Treat contacts without symptoms as primary after serologies.
- History of penicillin allergy:
  - Confirmed IgE-mediated reaction: desensitization
  - Questionable history of IgE-mediated hypersensitivity: penicillin skin testing *if* major and minor penicillin determinants available

- Precautions (6)[A]

  - HIV-infected and pregnant patients may show poor response to recommended IM doses. Use IV therapy for all treatment failures in these patients.
  - Do not give benzathine or procaine penicillins IV.

ONGOING CARE

FOLLOW-UP RECOMMENDATIONS

- Clinical and serologic evaluation between 6 and 12 months after treatment; if >1 year duration, check at 24 months (6)[A].
- In HIV-infected persons, clinical and serologic evaluation at 3, 6, 9, 12, and 24 months after therapy (6)[A]

Patient Monitoring

- Use VDRL or RPR test to monitor therapy: 4-fold rise (two dilutions) in titer indicates new infection, whereas failure to decrease 4-fold (two dilutions) in 6 to 12 months may indicate treatment failure (although definitive criteria for cure not established); always use same test (preferably same lab) for initial screening (6)[A].

- Strongly consider retreatment for persistent clinical signs or recurrence, 4-fold rise in titers, or failure of initially high titer to decrease 4-fold by 6 to 12 months.

- Neurosyphilis: repeat lumbar puncture every 6 months to check for normalization of CSF cell count (± CSF-VDRL and protein evaluation) (6)[A]

PATIENT EDUCATION
No intimate contacts until 4-fold titer drop

PROGNOSIS

- Excellent in all cases except patients with late syphilis complications and with HIV infection
- Syphilis in HIV-infected patient
  - Treatment same as for HIV-negative patients
  - More often false-negative treponemal and non-treponemal tests or unusually high titers
  - Response to therapy less predictable
  - Early syphilis: increased risk of neurosyphilis and higher rates of treatment failure
  - Late neurosyphilis: harder to treat; can occur up to 20+ years after infection

COMPLICATIONS

- Membranous glomerulonephritis
- Paroxysmal cold hemoglobinemia
- Meningitis and tabes dorsalis
- Cardiovascular aneurysms; valvular damage
- Irreversible organ damage
- Jarisch-Herxheimer reaction
  - Fever, chills, headache, myalgias, new rash
  - Common when starting treatment (of primary/secondary disease; less common with tertiary) owing to lysis of treponemes
  - Should not be confused with drug reaction
  - Managed with analgesics and antipyretics

REFERENCES

1. Gomez GB, Kamb ML, Newman LM, et al. Untreated maternal syphilis and adverse outcomes of pregnancy: a systematic review and meta-analysis. *Bull World Health Organ.* 2013;91(3):217–226.
2. U.S. Preventive Services Task Force. Screening for syphilis infection in pregnancy: U.S. Preventive Services Task Force reaffirmation recommendation statement. *Ann Intern Med.* 2009;150(10):705–709.
3. Patton ME, Su JR, Nelson R, et al. Primary and secondary syphilis—United States, 2005-2013. *MMWR Morb Mortal Wkly Rep.* 2014;63(18): 402–406.
4. Centers for Disease Control and Prevention. *Sexually Transmitted Disease Surveillance 2012.* Atlanta, GA: U.S. Department of Health and Human Services; 2013.
5. Koss CA, Dunne EF, Warner L. A systematic review of epidemiologic studies assessing condom use and risk of syphilis. *Sex Transm Dis.* 2009;36(7):401–405.
6. Workowski KA, Berman S. Sexually transmitted diseases treatment guidelines, 2010. *MMWR Recomm Rep.* 2010;59(RR-12):1–110.

 SEE ALSO

Chlamydia Infection (Sexually Transmitted); Gonococcal Infections

 CODES

ICD10
- A53.9 Syphilis, unspecified
- A51.0 Primary genital syphilis
- A53.0 Latent syphilis, unspecified as early or late

CLINICAL PEARLS

- Screen all HIV-positive patients and patients with high-risk sexual behaviors for syphilis.
- Penicillin remains the treatment of choice for syphilis.
- Syphilis rates are rising—particularly among MSM.

TARSAL TUNNEL SYNDROME

Jeff Wang, MD, MPH • J. Herbert Stevenson, MD

 BASICS

DESCRIPTION

A compression neuropathy of the posterior tibial nerve as it passes behind the medial malleolus and under the flexor retinaculum (laciniate ligament) in the medial ankle (the tarsal tunnel)

Pregnancy Considerations
- Tarsal tunnel syndrome can occur during pregnancy, typically secondary to local compression caused by fluid retention and volume changes (1).
- Care is supportive. Most cases resolve after pregnancy.

EPIDEMIOLOGY
- Women are slightly more affected than men (56%).
- All postpubescent ages are affected.

ETIOLOGY AND PATHOPHYSIOLOGY
- The posterior tibial nerve passes through the tarsal tunnel, which is formed by three osseus structures—sustentaculum tali, medial calcaneus, and medial malleolus—covered by the laciniate ligament.
- Compression of the posterior tibial nerve within the tarsal tunnel results in decreased blood flow, ischemic damage, and resultant symptoms (1).
- Chronic compression can destroy endoneurial microvasculature, leading to edema and (eventually) fibrosis and demyelination (2).
- Increased pressure in the tarsal tunnel is caused by a variety of mechanical and biochemical mechanisms. The specific cause for compression is identifiable in only 60–80% of patients (1).
- Three general categories: trauma, space-occupying lesions, deformity (1)
  - Trauma including displaced fractures, deltoid ligament sprains, or tenosynovitis
  - Varicosities
  - Hindfoot varus or valgus
  - Fibrosis of the perineurium
- Other causes:
  - Osseous prominences
  - Ganglia; lipoma; neurolemmoma
  - Inflammatory synovitis
  - Pigmented villonodular synovitis
  - Tarsal coalition
  - Accessory musculature
- In patients with systemic disease (e.g., diabetes), the "double crush" syndrome refers to the development of a second compression along the same nerve at a site of anatomic narrowing in patients with previous proximal nerve damage (3).
- Tarsal tunnel decompression may improve sensory impairment and restore protective sensation in diabetic peripheral neuropathies if there is nerve entrapment at the tarsal tunnel.

RISK FACTORS
- Tarsal tunnel syndrome is associated with certain occupations and activities involving repetitive weight bearing on the foot and ankle (jogging, dancing).
- Other possible risk factors include (4):
  - Diabetes
  - Systemic inflammatory arthritis
  - Connective tissue disorders
  - Obesity
  - Varicosities
  - Heel varus or valgus
  - Bifurcation of the posterior tibial nerve into medial and lateral plantar nerves proximal to the tarsal tunnel

 DIAGNOSIS

Tarsal tunnel syndrome is largely a clinical diagnosis, characterized by pain and paresthesias in a predictable distribution along the medial aspect of the ankle and plantar surface of the foot (1).

HISTORY
- History of trauma (may be trivial) to the foot precipitating pain
- Pain behind medial malleolus radiating to the longitudinal arch and plantar aspect of foot including the heel
- Tightness, burning, tingling, and numbness (1)
- Pain usually worsens during standing or activity.
- Pain radiates proximally up the medial leg (Valleix phenomenon) in 33% of patients with severe compression.
- Some patients have substantial night pain (may be related to venostasis).
- Symptoms improve with rest, wearing loose footwear, and elevation.
- In advanced nerve compression, motor involvement may cause weakness, atrophy, and digital contractures of the intrinsic foot muscles (4).

ALERT
Other systemic neuropathies (diabetes, alcoholism, HIV, drug reactions) present with similar symptoms.

PHYSICAL EXAM
- Foot alignment
  - Examine for hindfoot varus or valgus deformity.
  - Exaggerating heel dorsiflexion, inversion, or eversion may reproduce symptoms by stretching or compressing the posterior tibial nerve.
- Palpate the tarsal tunnel and the course of the tibial nerve for tenderness and swelling.
- Tinel sign: Percussion over the the tibial nerve may reproduce paresthesias that radiate distally.

- Valleix sign: Percussion over the tibial nerve may produce paresthesias that radiate proximally.
- Cuff test: Inflating a pneumatic cuff engorges varicosities and reproduces symptoms.
- Compression test: Applying pressure to the tarsal tunnel for 60 seconds may reproduce symptoms.
- Sensory examination
  - The medial calcaneal nerve usually is spared, but numbness and altered sensation may be present in the distribution of the medial or lateral plantar nerves.
  - Vibratory sensation and two-point discrimination are decreased early in the disease process.
- Motor examination
  - Intrinsic foot muscle weakness (difficult to assess)
  - Rarely, weakness of toe plantar flexion may be present.
  - Atrophy of the abductor hallucis or abductor digiti minimi may be seen late in the disease process.

DIFFERENTIAL DIAGNOSIS
- Peripheral neuropathies (diabetes, alcoholism, HIV, or drug related)
- Inflammatory arthritis (rheumatoid arthritis)
- Morton neuroma
- Metatarsalgia
- Subtalar joint arthritis
- Tibialis posterior tendinitis/dysfunction
- Plantar fasciitis
- Plantar callosities
- Peripheral vascular disease
- Lumbar radiculopathy
- Proximal injury or compression of the tibial branch of the sciatic nerve

DIAGNOSTIC TESTS & INTERPRETATION
Initial Tests (lab, imaging)
Routine lab tests help rule out other conditions that may mimic tarsal tunnel syndrome, including diabetic neuropathy, rheumatoid arthritis, thyroid dysfunction, or other systemic illnesses (5).

- Routine weight-bearing radiographs, followed by CT (if necessary) to assess for fracture or structural abnormality
- Consider evaluation of lumbar spine x-ray if double crush (injury to lumbar nerve results in compensatory injury to posterior tibial nerve) is suspected (5).
- MRI: helps assess the tarsal tunnel for soft tissue masses or other sources of nerve compression before surgery (1)
- Ultrasound: Gaining importance and with several advantages over MRI (6); can assess for tenosynovitis, ganglia, varicose veins, or lipomas (1)

Pediatric Considerations
MRI is recommended for evaluating pediatric tarsal tunnel syndrome to exclude neoplastic mass.

Diagnostic Procedures/Other
Electrodiagnostic studies

- Electromyography (EMG) of the intrinsic muscles of the foot can confirm the diagnosis of tarsal tunnel syndrome (7). A normal EMG does not exclude the diagnosis (false-negative rate is ~10%) (1).
- Nerve conduction studies may reveal slowed conduction of the tibial nerve.
- Evaluate for proximal nerve compression, including a lumbar radiculopathy or a double crush phenomenon.

 TREATMENT

Conservative management is recommended, except for acute onset tarsal tunnel syndrome or in the setting of a known space-occupying lesion (excluding synovitis).

MEDICATION
First Line
- Analgesics and anti-inflammatory medications
- Local corticosteroid injection
- Medications that alter neurogenic pain (tricyclic antidepressants, antiepileptic drugs, nerve blockers)

ADDITIONAL THERAPIES
- Rest/immobilization
- Taping and bracing
- Orthotics or shoe modification
- Physical therapy to strengthen the intrinsic and extrinsic muscles of the foot and to restore the medial longitudinal arch
- Other modalities (stretching, US, massage, icing)
- Compression stockings to decrease swelling
- Weight loss for obese patients

SURGERY/OTHER PROCEDURES
- Surgery is indicated (1,2,8).
  - If nonoperative measures fail following a 3- to 6-month trial
  - In the setting of acute tarsal tunnel syndrome
  - If a space-occupying lesion is identified
- The surgical outcome is dependent on technique and postoperative management. 50–95% of cases have good to excellent outcomes.
- At the time of surgery, assess focal swelling, scarring, or nerve abnormalities and look for a pathologic source of compression.
- Postoperative management includes:
  - Non–weight-bearing splint until incision heals (2 to 3 weeks), followed by progressively increased weight-bearing and range of motion exercises
  - Rest, ice, compression, elevation to limit swelling

 ONGOING CARE

PATIENT EDUCATION
- Discuss conservative and surgical options based on individual patient circumstance and preference.
- A decision about surgical intervention should be made with a clear understanding risks, benefits, and potential adverse outcomes.

PROGNOSIS
Surgery is most helpful for:
- Patients with a positive Tinel sign (3)[B]
- Young patients
- Short period between occurrence of symptoms and surgery <1 year (9)[B].
- Localized space-occupying lesion (1)
- No motor neuron involvement

COMPLICATIONS
- The main adverse outcome is an unsuccessful surgical intervention characterized by lack of improvement or recurrence of symptoms (1).
- Causes for a failed tarsal tunnel release include (10):
  - Incorrect diagnosis
  - Incomplete release
  - Adhesive neuritis (external scar formation)
  - Intraneural damage (systemic disease, direct nerve injury)
  - Failure to treat all sources of nerve compression in a double crush phenomenon
- Electrodiagnostic studies are rarely helpful in determining the cause of a failed tarsal tunnel release.
- Results with surgical revision are poorer than those for the primary surgical release.

REFERENCES
1. Ahmad M, Tsang K, Mackenney PJ, et al. Tarsal tunnel syndrome: a literature review. *Foot Ankle Surg.* 2012;18(3):149–152.
2. Dellon AL. The four medial ankle tunnels: a critical review of perceptions of tarsal tunnel syndrome and neuropathy. *Neurosurg Clin N Am.* 2008;19(4):629–648.
3. Dellon AL, Muse VL, Scott ND, et al. A positive Tinel sign as predictor of pain relief or sensory recovery after decompression of chronic tibial nerve compression in patients with diabetic neuropathy. *J Reconstr Microsurg.* 2012;28(4):235–240.
4. Franson J, Baravarian B. Tarsal tunnel syndrome: a compression neuropathy involving four distinct tunnels. *Clin Podiatr Med Surg.* 2006;23(3):597–609.
5. Fantino O. Role of ultrasound in posteromedial tarsal tunnel syndrome: 81 cases. *J Ultrasound.* 2014;17(2):99–112.
6. Patel AT, Gaines K, Malamut R, et al. Usefulness of electrodiagnostic techniques in the evaluation of suspected tarsal tunnel syndrome: an evidence-based review. *Muscle Nerve.* 2005;32(2):236–240.
7. Sung KS, Park SJ. Short-term operative outcome of tarsal tunnel syndrome due to benign space-occupying lesions. *Foot Ankle Int.* 2009;30(8):741–745.
8. Reichert P, Zimmer K, Wnukiewicz W, et al. Results of surgical treatment of tarsal tunnel syndrome. *Foot Ankle Surg.* 2015;21(1):26–29.
9. Gould JS. Recurrent tarsal tunnel syndrome. *Foot Ankle Clin.* 2014;19(3):451–467.

ADDITIONAL READING
- Abouelela AA, Zohiery AK. The triple compression stress test for diagnosis of tarsal tunnel syndrome. *Foot (Edinb).* 2012;22(3):146–149.
- Allen JM, Greer BJ, Sorge DG, et al. MR imaging of neuropathies of the leg, ankle, and foot. *Magn Reson Imaging Clin N Am.* 2008;16(1):117–131.
- Gondring WH, Tarun PK, Trepman E. Touch pressure and sensory density after tarsal tunnel release in diabetic neuropathy. *Foot Ankle Surg.* 2012;18(4):241–246.
- Imai K, Ikoma K, Imai R, et al. Tarsal tunnel syndrome in hemodialysis patients: a case series. *Foot Ankle Int.* 2013;34(3):439–444.

 SEE ALSO

Algorithm: Foot Pain

 CODES

ICD10
- G57.50 Tarsal tunnel syndrome, unspecified lower limb
- G57.51 Tarsal tunnel syndrome, right lower limb
- G57.52 Tarsal tunnel syndrome, left lower limb

CLINICAL PEARLS
- Tarsal tunnel syndrome typically presents with pain and tingling of the medical ankle and plantar foot.
- Tinel sign is the most sensitive and specific physical examination test for diagnosing tarsal tunnel.
- EMG cannot independently diagnose tarsal tunnel syndrome; it is used to confirm a clinical diagnosis.
- Conservative management is recommended, except for patients with an acute onset tarsal tunnel syndrome or known space-occupying lesion.

T

TEETHING

Dana Nguyen, MD, FAAFP • Katrina E. Walters, MD, FAAFP, FM

BASICS

DESCRIPTION
- Teething is the eruption of the primary or deciduous teeth, which most children experience without difficulty. It is a natural, gradual, and predictable process, with normal variation among infants (1,2).
- Primary (deciduous) teeth
  - Primary tooth eruption usually begins at 5 to 7 months of age.
  - The order of primary tooth eruption and average age is the following:
    - Central mandibular incisors (5 to 7 months)
    - Central maxillary incisors (6 to 8 months)
    - Lateral mandibular incisors (7 to 10 months)
    - Lateral maxillary incisors (8 to 11 months)
    - Cuspids (16 to 20 months)
    - 1st molars (10 to 16 months)
    - 2nd molars (20 to 30 months)
  - Delayed eruption may be familial or due to systemic syndromes or nutritional deficiencies. Delayed eruption may also be seen with cleft palate and lower birth weight (3–5).
  - Tooth eruption in premature infants occurs according to postconceptual age rather than age since birth (chronologic age) (2).
  - Natal/neonatal teeth
    - Natal teeth (present at birth) occur in 1/2,000 neonates.
    - Neonatal teeth erupt in the 1st month of life.
    - Natal/neonatal teeth are most often prematurely erupted primary (deciduous) teeth but may be supernumerary.
    - 15–20% of cases are familial; also may be secondary to a syndrome or congenital anomalies of the head and neck.
    - Natal/neonatal teeth may be loose, but most are the normal deciduous lower central incisors and can persist.
    - Natal/neonatal teeth may be removed if there is an aspiration risk or if they cause trauma to the infant or to the mother (breastfeeding) (2).

EPIDEMIOLOGY
Incidence
Predominant age: birth to 3 years of age

ETIOLOGY AND PATHOPHYSIOLOGY
Teething symptoms are more common with eruption of the primary incisors (6).

Genetics
Both premature and delayed tooth eruption may be familial. Primary failure of eruption has been linked to mutations of the *PTHR1* gene (5).

COMMONLY ASSOCIATED CONDITIONS
Teething may be coincident with other common childhood conditions, causing local or systemic signs and symptoms (e.g., fever, GI disturbance, fussiness, drooling, rash, and sleep disturbance). No pattern of symptoms that distinguishes teething from any other cause. Other possible causes of systemic symptoms should be ruled out prior to attributing them to teething (7).

DIAGNOSIS

HISTORY
- Biting
- Drooling
- Rubbing of gingivae
- Sucking
- Irritability
- Wakefulness
- Ear rubbing
- Facial rash
- Decreased appetite for solid foods
- Loose stools
- Temperature elevation <38.3°C
- Many infants do not have any symptoms.

- Symptoms most often occur 4 days before eruption and resolve by 3 days after eruption and are more common in ages 4 to 24 months (6,8–10)[B].

PHYSICAL EXAM
- Infants may have no signs or symptoms of teething, although symptoms are present in most children.
- Excessive drooling and chewing on fingers begins at 3 to 4 months of age. This is also the time that normal hand to mouth stimulation increases salivation.

- Discomfort may be observed more commonly with the eruption of the first tooth, the molars, and/or with the simultaneous eruption of multiple teeth (11)[B].
- Minor signs and symptoms of biting or chewing, drooling, irritability, facial rash, and low-grade fever (<101.9°F; 38.9°C) have been reported in association with teething, although no evidence identifies specific signs/symptoms caused by teething (9)[B].
- Serious signs and symptoms (e.g., fever >101.9°F; 38.9°C, dehydration) are not caused by teething and warrant evaluation for organic disease (7)[A].

- A small red or white spot may appear over the swollen gingivae just prior to tooth eruption.

- Local inflammation, swelling, or hematoma (bluish swelling) can be found on the involved gingivae overlying the erupting tooth. Gingival irritation was present in 96% of infants in one study (11)[B].

DIFFERENTIAL DIAGNOSIS
Herpetic gingivostomatitis: Infants with fever, irritability, sleeplessness, and difficulty feeding may have underlying infection caused by herpes simplex virus. Some infants with positive culture may not have evidence of inflammation or ulceration expected in gingivostomatitis.

DIAGNOSTIC TESTS & INTERPRETATION
Initial Tests (lab, imaging)
Radiographs can distinguish prematurely erupted primary teeth from supernumerary teeth.

TREATMENT

GENERAL MEASURES
- Education of parents regarding common symptoms of teething and management options resulted in decreased use of pharmacologic treatment and increased use of other methods such as rubbing the gums (12)[B].
- Prospective trials show the strongest effectiveness evidence supporting teething rings, followed by cuddle therapy, followed by rubbing the gums to reduce symptoms (13)[B].
- Provide the infant with a safe, one-piece teething ring, clean cloth, or pacifier for gumming.
- Apply pressure over involved swollen gingivae with a clean finger or piece of wet gauze.
- May use cool (but not frozen) fluids, cold teething rings, or cold vegetables such as a peeled cucumber
- Avoid the use of alcohol (historically rubbed on gingivae for an analgesic effect).
- Gingival hematomas that erupt appear as blue cysts. Most do not require medical intervention. Be sure there are no other signs of a bleeding disorder.
- Avoid the following:
  - Dipping a pacifier or teething ring in sugar or honey
  - Giving an infant a bottle in bed
  - Using fluid-filled teething rings (contents may leak)
  - Using frozen foods or teething rings (these could cause thermal damage to the tissues)
  - Tying a teething ring around infant's neck (14)[C]

MEDICATION
First Line
- Initial treatment with medications is not recommended.
- For an infant with low-grade fever, irritability, and/or inflamed gingivae (where other comforting measures have not been of help); acetaminophen in proper doses (15 mg/kg/dose q4–6h PRN) can be used.

Second Line

ALERT
Over-the-counter preparations for teething, such as lidocaine (Xylocaine 2%), or benzocaine (Baby Ora-Gel, Num-Zit Gel, Num-Zit Liquid, Baby Anbesol) should be AVOIDED. Misuse, overuse, toxicity, and sensitivity have been reported.

- These are of questionable benefit because they are washed off quickly by saliva, and the benefit may be due in part to the pressure placed on the gingivae when applied.

  - FDA issued a warning about possible serious harm, to include death (15)[A].

ISSUES FOR REFERRAL

- Parents should establish a dental home for infants by 12 months of age. Dental caries remain the most prevalent infectious disease in children in the United States. Preventative care and anticipatory guidance offered in a dental home help prevent early childhood caries (16)[A].

- Other medical problems may delay tooth eruption. It is reasonable to refer a child who has not erupted a tooth by 18 months of age to a dentist, if he or she is not seeing one already (5)[C].

ADDITIONAL THERAPIES

Infants who bite or chew while breastfeeding can be trained not to bite by withdrawing the child from the breast for a moment, and then resume. Resist urge to startle the infant.

COMPLEMENTARY & ALTERNATIVE MEDICINE

Homeopathy is used to treat teething. Chamomilla is one reported treatment, but no efficacy or safety studies have been published (17)[C].

INPATIENT CONSIDERATIONS

Admission Criteria/Initial Stabilization

Outpatient

 ONGOING CARE

FOLLOW-UP RECOMMENDATIONS

No restrictions

DIET

Breastfeeding can continue during and after teething. Otherwise, no special diet required.

PATIENT EDUCATION

- Parents should be cautioned not to misinterpret teething as the cause of any systemic manifestation. The health provider should be consulted for any systemic complaints.
- American Dental Association, Mouth Healthy Web site: http://www.mouthhealthy.org/en/babies-and-kids/
- Teething Tots: http://kidshealth.org/parent/pregnancy_newborn/common/teething.html

PROGNOSIS

Normal progression through the teething process without illness

COMPLICATIONS

Dental caries are a common childhood illness and can be prevented with fluoride use. Current guidelines recommend the following:

- Use of fluoridated toothpaste for all children beginning with first tooth eruption.
- Use of fluoride varnish every 3 to 6 months after first tooth eruption.
- Dietary fluoride supplements if fluoride is not present in the drinking water (18)[A]

REFERENCES

1. Aktoren O, Tuna EB, Guven Y, et al. A study on neonatal factors and eruption time of primary teeth. *Community Dent Health*. 2010;27(1):52–56.
2. Cunha RF, Boer FA, Torriani DD, et al. Natal and neonatal teeth: review of the literature. *Pediatr Dent*. 2001;23(2):158–162.
3. Kobayashi TY, Gomide MR, Carrara CF. Timing and sequence of primary tooth eruption in children with cleft lip and palate. *J Appl Oral Sci*. 2010;18(3):220–224.
4. Sajjadian N, Shajari H, Jahadi R, et al. Relationship between birth weight and time of first deciduous tooth eruption in 143 consecutively born infants. *Pediatr Neonatol*. 2010;51(4):235–237.
5. Stellzig-Eisenhauer A, Decker E, Meyer-Marcotty P, et al. Primary failure of eruption (PFE)—clinical and molecular genetics analysis [in English, German]. *J Orofac Orthop*. 2010;71(1):6–16.
6. Noor-Mohammed R, Basha S. Teething disturbances: prevalence of objective manifestations in children under age 4 months to 36 months. *Med Oral Patol Oral Cir Bucal*. 2012;17(3):e491–e494.
7. Tighe M, Roe MF. Does a teething child need serious illness excluding? *Arch Dis Child*. 2007;92(3):266–268.
8. Feldens CA, Faraco IM, Ottoni AB, et al. Teething symptoms in the first year of life and associated factors: a cohort study. *J Clin Pediatr Dent*. 2010;34(3):201–206.
9. Macknin ML, Piedmonte M, Jacobs J, et al. Symptoms associated with infant teething: a prospective study. *Pediatrics*. 2000;105(4, Pt 1):747–752.
10. Wake M, Hesketh K, Lucas J. Teething and tooth eruption in infants: a cohort study. *Pediatrics*. 2000;106(6):1374–1379.
11. Kiran K, Swati T, Kamala BK, et al. Prevalence of systemic and local disturbances in infants during primary teeth eruption: a clinical study. *Eur J Paediatr Dent*. 2011;12(4):249–252.
12. Plutzer K, Spencer AJ, Keirse MJ. How first-time mothers perceive and deal with teething symptoms: a randomized controlled trial. *Child Care Health Dev*. 2012;38(2):292–299.
13. Memarpour M, Soltanimehr E, Eskandarian T. Signs and symptoms associated with primary tooth eruption: a clinical trial of nonpharmacological remedies. *BMC Oral Health*. 2015;15:88–95.
14. McIntyre GT, McIntyre GM. Teething troubles? *Br Dent J*. 2002;192(5):251–255.
15. U.S. Food and Drug Administration. FDA Drug Safety Communication: FDA recommends not using lidocaine to treat teething pain and requires new Boxed Warning. http://www.fda.gov/Drugs/DrugSafety/ucm402240.htm. Published June 26, 2014. Updated October 9, 2014.
16. American Academy of Pediatric Dentistry. Clinical Affairs Committee—Infant Oral Health Subcommittee. Guideline on infant oral health care. *Pediatr Dent*. 2012;34(5):148–152.
17. Thompson EA, Bishop JL, Northstone K. The use of homeopathic products in childhood: data generated over 8.5 years from the Avon Longitudinal Study of Parents and Children (ALSPAC). *J Altern Complement Med*. 2010;16(1):69–79.
18. Clark MB, Slayton RL, Segura A, et al. Fluoride use in caries prevention in the primary care setting. *Pediatrics*. 2014;134(3):626–633.

ADDITIONAL READING

- American Academy of Pediatrics. Children's Oral Health Web site: http://www2.aap.org/commpeds/dochs/oralhealth/index.html.
- American Academy of Pediatrics Oral health initiative. Protecting all children's teeth (PACT): a pediatric oral health training program: http://www2.aap.org/oralhealth/pact/pact-home.cfm.
- Williams GD, Kirk EP, Wilson CJ, et al. Salicylate intoxication from teething gel in infancy. *Med J Aust*. 2011;194(3):146–148.

 CODES

ICD10

K00.7 Teething syndrome

CLINICAL PEARLS

- Parents and caregivers should follow the American Academy of Pediatrics' recommendations for treating teething pain.
  - Use a teething ring chilled in the refrigerator (not frozen).
  - Gently rub or massage the child's gums with your finger to relieve the symptoms.
  - Topical pain relievers and medications that are rubbed on the gums are not necessary or even useful because they wash out of the baby's mouth within minutes, and they can be harmful.
- Teething may cause discomfort but does not cause significant fevers.
- Teething babies can still breastfeed. Babies can be taught not to bite, and breastfeeding may continue past 12 months of age without difficulty.

TELOGEN EFFLUVIUM

Quratulanne H. Jan, MD • Arham K. Barakzai, MD

BASICS

Diffuse hair loss or hair thinning; most often an acute self-limited process

DESCRIPTION

Telogen effluvium (TE) is a transient condition in which there is a premature conversion of a significant proportion of anagen (growth phase) hairs into telogen (resting phase) hairs resulting in increased shedding of these resting hair follicles and the clinical appearance of moderate to severe hair thinning.

- Five proposed types of TE (1)
  - Immediate anagen release: a highly common form, lasting 3 to 4 weeks, in which follicles meant to remain in anagen phase enter telogen prematurely due to a signal, including high fever, drug induced, or stress
  - Delayed anagen release: occurs most often post-partum, in which a large group of hair follicles that have remained in the anagen phase for an extended period all together enter the telogen phase, resulting in hair loss
  - Short anagen: a somewhat speculative type, in which at least 50% of the hair follicles have an idiopathic shortening of the anagen phase, resulting in a corresponding doubling of the follicles in the telogen phase
  - Immediate telogen release: Normal resting club hairs remain within the hair follicle until an unknown signal causes their release, initiating the anagen stage to begin. In this type, the resting club hairs are prematurely released, ending the telogen phase abruptly and causing diffuse shedding.
  - Delayed telogen release: in this type, the presence of increased visible light, whether it be a seasonal or environmental change, is thought to end a prolonged telogen phase and initiate the anagen phase, resulting in diffuse shedding of hair follicles.

EPIDEMIOLOGY

Incidence
Second most common cause of alopecia

Prevalence
Unknown

ETIOLOGY AND PATHOPHYSIOLOGY

- The hair cycle consists of two predominant phases. The anagen (growth phase) and the telogen (resting phase), lasting ~3 years and 3 months, respectively. On the scalp, ~10–15% of hairs are in the telogen phase normally. Due to the presence of some types of external/internal stress, there may be an increase in the percentage of telogen hairs. As new anagen hairs emerge, these telogen hair follicles are forced out. The preceding event usually occurs 2 to 3 months prior to the appearance of hair loss.
- It is hypothesized that substance P plays a key role in the pathogenesis of TE through various mechanisms (2,3). Studies have been conducted on human hair follicles in vitro and mice hair follicles in vivo, which support this theory.
- Role of substance P includes the following (4):
  - Upregulation of substance P receptor, NK1, at the gene and protein level, leading to premature catagen development and hair growth inhibition
  - Upregulation of nerve growth factor (NGF) and subsequently its hair apoptosis–producing receptor, p75NTR
  - Downregulation of hair growth–promoting receptor, TrkA
  - Upregulation of major histocompatibility class (MHC) I and β_2-microglobulin resulting in loss of hair follicle immune-privilege
  - Increase in tumor necrosis factor-α release by mast cells resulting in hair keratinocyte apoptosis
- Decreased cortisol levels in chronic stress states may also enhance the effects of substance P (5).

RISK FACTORS

- Infection
- Trauma
- Major surgery
- Thyroid disorder
- Febrile illness
- Malignancy
- Allergic contact dermatitis (6)
- Iron deficiency anemia (7,8)
- Excess vitamin A (1)
- Protein-calorie restriction (1)

- End-stage liver or renal disease
- Hormonal changes (including pregnancy, delivery, and estrogen-containing medications) (1)
- Chronic stress
- Drug induced (β-blockers, anticonvulsants, antidepressants, anticoagulants, retinoids, ACE-inhibitors, etc.) (1)
- Immunizations

DIAGNOSIS

HISTORY
- Commonly, an inciting event 2 to 6 months previous
- Fear of becoming bald
- Patients often present with bags of hair to emphasize the severity of their hair loss.

PHYSICAL EXAM
- Decreased density of hair on the scalp, most commonly involving the crown
- In rare cases of chronic TE, there is hair loss of eyebrows and pubic region.
- May be able to demonstrate diffuse shedding of hair when running fingers through scalp
- Shed hairs are telogen hairs, which have a small bulb of unpigmented or pigmented keratin on the root end.
- May affect nail growth, resulting in the appearance of Beau lines, which are transverse grooves on the nails of the hands and feet

DIFFERENTIAL DIAGNOSIS
- Hypothyroidism
- Hyperthyroidism
- Alopecia areata (diffuse pattern)
- Androgenetic alopecia
- Drug-induced alopecia
- Systemic lupus erythematosus
- Secondary syphilis
- Trichotillomania

DIAGNOSTIC TESTS & INTERPRETATION

Most often, TE is a clinical diagnosis of exclusion. Blood work may be collected primarily to rule out other possible causes of hair loss and/or to identify a possible cause for TE.

Initial Tests (lab, imaging)

If indicated:

- CBC, ferritin
- TSH
- Creatinine
- Consider hepatic enzymes.
- Consider RPR/VDRL.

Diagnostic Procedures/Other

- Hair pull test: unreliable; performed by gently pulling 25 to 30 hairs from various sites on a patient's scalp. Each pull should elicit <5 normal club hairs; increased quantity may indicate possibility of TE (1).
- Hair clip test: Performed by cutting 25 to 30 hairs from the patient's scalp and examining them under a microscope. A negative test (not indicative of TE) will demonstrate <10% of hair shafts of small diameter. A positive test will demonstrate >10% of hair shafts of small diameter (1).
- Trichogram: ~50 hairs are plucked from the patient's scalp, and the number of telogen and anagen hairs present are counted. In TE, there will be >10% of hairs in the telogen phase.
- Scalp biopsy: rarely needed; it is recommended that several 4-mm punch biopsies be obtained, all horizontally embedded to determine an accurate anagen-to-telogen ratio. Histologically, catagen-to-telogen hairs have numerous apoptotic cells in the outer sheath epithelium. >12–15% of hair follicles in telogen phase is consistent with TE (1,9).

TREATMENT

TE is a benign, self-limited process. Identify and correct underlying cause. Patient should be reassured that full hair growth will occur in ~6 months to 1 year. No treatment is required.

MEDICATION

- Minoxidil stimulates hair regrowth via arteriolar smooth muscle vasodilation; not effective in TE
- Oral zinc therapy: New medication that may have benefits for patients with TE through various mechanisms all essential to hair growth, including the following (10)[C]:
  - Cofactor for enzymes needed in nucleic acid and protein synthesis and cell division
  - Inhibition of the catagen phase by blocking certain enzymes involved in hair apoptosis
  - Involved in hair growth regulation via hedgehog signaling

COMPLEMENTARY & ALTERNATIVE MEDICINE

Nigella Sativa (black cumin) essential oil has also been studied and may be beneficial (11).

REFERENCES

1. Headington JT. Telogen effluvium. New concepts and review. *Arch Dermatol.* 1993;129(3):356–563.
2. Grover C, Khurana A. Telogen effluvium. *Indian J Dermatol Venereol Leprol.* 2013;79(5):591–603.
3. Hadshiew IM, Foitzik K, Arck PC, et al. Burden of hair loss: stress and the underestimated psychosocial impact of telogen effluvium and androgenetic alopecia. *J Invest Dermatol.* 2004;123(3):455–457.
4. Peters EMJ, Liotiri S, Bodó E, et al. Probing the effects of stress mediators on the human hair follicle: substance P holds central position. *Am J Pathol.* 2007;171(6):1872–1886.
5. Katayama I, Bae SJ, Hamasaki Y, et al. Stress response, tachykinin, and cutaneous inflammation. *J Investig Dermatol Symp Proc.* 2001;6(1):81–86.
6. Tosti A, Piraccini BM, van Neste DJ. Telogen effluvium after allergic contact dermatitis of the scalp. *Arch Dermatol.* 2001;137(2):187–190.
7. Trost LB, Bergfeld WF, Calogeras E. The diagnosis and treatment of iron deficiency and its potential relationship to hair loss. *J Am Acad Dermatol.* 2006;54(5):824–844.
8. Karadağ AS, Ertugrel DT, Tutal E, et al. The role of anemia and vitamin D levels in acute and chronic telogen effluvium. *Turk J Med Sci.* 2011;41(5):827–833.
9. Sinclair R, Jolley D, Mallari R, et al. The reliability of horizontally sectioned scalp biopsies in the diagnosis of chronic diffuse telogen hair loss in women. *J Am Acad Dermatol.* 2004;51(2):189–199.
10. Karashima T, Tsuruta D, Hamada T, et al. Oral zinc therapy for zinc deficiency-related telogen effluvium. *Dermatol Ther.* 2012;25(2):210–213.
11. Rossi A, Priolo L, Iorio A, et al. Evaluation of a therapeutic alternative for telogen effluvium: a pilot study. *J Cosmet Dermatol Sci Appl.* 2013;3(3-A):9–16.

ADDITIONAL READING

Mounsey AL, Reed SW. Diagnosing and treating hair loss. *Am Fam Physician.* 2009;80(4):356–362.

CODES

ICD10
L65.0 Telogen effluvium

CLINICAL PEARLS

- TE is a self-limited form of nonscarring alopecia; most often acute.
- TE is due to a premature conversion of a significant proportion of anagen (growth phase) hairs into telogen (resting phase) hairs, resulting in increased shedding of these resting hair follicles and the clinical appearance of moderate to severe hair thinning and loss when growth resumes.
- There are many potential causes of TE, both emotional and physiologic. Often it is hard to determine the etiology, but eliminating the stressor often is the key to resolving TE and stimulating new hair growth.
- No treatment is needed. Patient should be reassured that complete hair regrowth will occur in 6 months to 1 year.

T

TEMPOROMANDIBULAR JOINT DISORDER (TMD)

Benjamin N. Schneider, MD • Jessica Johnson, MD, MPH

BASICS

DESCRIPTION
- Syndrome characterized by
  - Pain and tenderness involving the muscles of mastications and surrounding tissues
  - Sound, pain, stiffness, or grating in the temporomandibular joint (TMJ) with movement
  - Limitation of mandibular movement with possible locking or dislocation
  - Recent research suggests that TMD is a complex disorder with multiple causes consistent with a biopsychosocial model of illness (1)[B].
- System(s) affected: musculoskeletal
- Synonym(s): TMJ syndrome; TMJ dysfunction; myofascial pain–dysfunction syndrome; bruxism; orofacial pain

EPIDEMIOLOGY
Incidence
- Symptoms more common in ages 30 to 50 years
- Predominant sex: female > male (4:1)

Prevalence
General prevalence is 6–12% in both adults and older children. Up to 1/2 the population has at least one sign or symptom of TMD, but most are not limited by symptoms, and <1:4 seek medical or dental treatment.

ETIOLOGY AND PATHOPHYSIOLOGY
- Pathophysiology is multifactorial, involving anatomic, behavioral, emotional, and cognitive factors.
- The American Academy of Orofacial Pain categorizes TMD according to three anatomic origins of pain and the change in name from TMJ to TMD emphasizes that many patients suffer from muscular and not articular pain.
- Cranial bone disorder including the mandible
  - Congenital and developmental disorders
  - Acquired disorders (fracture, neoplasm)
- Articular disorders of the joint
  - Congenital disorders
  - Inflammatory disorders: synovitis, arthritides, capsulitis, ankyloses
  - Avascular necrosis (rare)
  - TMJ disk derangement, osteoarthritis
  - Hyper- or hypomobile TMJ
  - TMJ trauma: condylar fractures, dislocation
- Muscle disorders involving the muscles of mastication
  - Occlusomuscular dysfunction (bruxism)
  - Masticatory muscle spasm
  - Myositis
  - Myofibrosis
  - Poorly fitting oral devices (dentures, splints, etc.)
  - Contracture
  - Neoplasia

Genetics
Research is ongoing in gene polymorphisms associated with TMD and other pain disorders. These include the catechol O-methyltransferase gene (COMT), which is thought to be associated with changes in pain responsiveness.

RISK FACTORS
- Macrotrauma to the face, jaw, and neck, including cervical whiplash injuries and hyperextension of jaw
- Rheumatologic and degenerative conditions involving the TMJ
- Psychosocial stress and poor adaptive capabilities
- Repetitive microtrauma from dental malocclusion, including inappropriate dental treatment.
- Link with bruxism and jaw/teeth clenching is inconsistent.

GENERAL PREVENTION
- Elimination of tension-causing oral habits
- Reduction in overall muscle tension

COMMONLY ASSOCIATED CONDITIONS
Craniomandibular disorders, somatization disorder, somatoform pain disorder, other chronic pain syndromes, fibromyalgia, juvenile idiopathic arthritis, tension headache, sleep disturbance, tobacco use

DIAGNOSIS
- TMD is a clinical diagnosis, and localized pain is the unifying feature.
- Several research classification systems exist. Most share several of the history and physical findings listed below.

HISTORY
- Facial and/or TMJ pain
- Locking/catching of jaw; decreased range of motion
- TMJ noises: clicking, grinding, popping
- Headache, earache, neck pain

PHYSICAL EXAM
- Facial symmetry, muscle hypertrophy, intraoral exam
- Palpation of muscles of mastication may reproduce pain.
- Test jaw range of motion (opening, closing, lateral, protrusive) and masticatory muscle strength.
  - Maximal (pain-free) jaw opening with interincisal distance <40 mm is suggestive of joint rather than muscle pathology if accompanied by other signs and symptoms (normal 35 to 55 mm).
  - Deviation to the affected side is common.
- Muscle tenderness and restricted pain-free opening are most consistent distinguishing signs.
- There may be tenderness over the TMJ.
- Clicking or crepitus of jaw with opening

DIFFERENTIAL DIAGNOSIS
- Condylar fracture/dislocation
- Trigeminal neuralgia
- Dental or periodontal conditions
- Neoplasm of the jaw, orofacial muscles, or salivary glands
- Acute, nondental infection: parotitis, sialadenitis, otitis, mastoiditis
- Jaw claudication: giant cell arteritis
- Migraine or tension type headache
- Ramsay-Hunt syndrome (zoster auricular syndrome)

DIAGNOSTIC TESTS & INTERPRETATION
- There are no labs to rule in TMD.
- Blood work may be useful to rule out other conditions (CBC, CMP, ESR, CRP).

Initial Tests (lab, imaging)
- TMD is a clinical diagnosis based primarily on history and physical exam.
- Often, a poor correlation is found between pain severity and pathologic changes seen in joint or muscle tissues. Consider the following for severe or treatment-resistant cases, with MR or CT more useful as part of surgical workup:
  - Panoramic dental radiographs are a good first-line screen.
  - CT scan allows fine detail of bony structures, preferred for trauma.
  - US: Effusion and findings correlate with MRI and subjective pain.
  - MRI: noninvasive study for disc position; more sensitive than US; can help determine need for surgical management

Diagnostic Procedures/Other
- Local anesthetic nerve block can differentiate orofacial pain of articular versus muscular origins.
- Arthroscopy can be diagnostic for cartilage and bony pathology.

Test Interpretation
Positive findings include:
- Condylar head displacement
- Anterior disc displacement
- Posterior capsulitis
- Loosening of disc and capsular attachments
- Chondroid metaplasia of disc leading to disc perforation and degeneration

TREATMENT

Signs and symptoms will abate without intervention in most patients. 50% report improvement in 1 year and 85% by 3 years. With conservative therapy, symptoms resolve in 75% of cases within 3 months.

- Therapeutic exercises, especially if displacement is present, including formal physical therapy.
- Psychosocial interventions, including cognitive-behavioral therapy with or without biofeedback (2)[A]
- Behavior modification to eliminate tension-relieving oral habits (2)[A]
- Occlusal adjustment cannot be recommended for the management or prevention of TMD, as there is an absence of evidence from RCTs that occlusal adjustment treats or prevents TMD (3)[A].
- Insufficient evidence exists either for or against the use of stabilization splint therapy for the treatment of TMD (4)[A].

TESTICULAR MALIGNANCIES

Huy Tan Tran, MD, LCDR, MC, USN • Moses H. Cheng, MAJ, MC, USA

BASICS

DESCRIPTION
- Testicular cancer accounts for 1% of all cancers in men; it is the most common solid malignancy in men aged 15 to 34 years (1).
- An estimated 8,430 new cases were diagnosed, and an estimated 380 deaths occurred in the United States in 2015 (2).
- Treatment produces an overall 5-year survival of 95.3%; for African American patients, this 5-year survival rate is alarmingly lower but has improved from 86% to 90% (2).

ETIOLOGY AND PATHOPHYSIOLOGY
95% of all malignant tumors arising in the testes are germ cell tumors (GCTs), which are subclassified as follows:
- Seminomatous GCTs: most common type overall
- Nonseminomatous GCTs (NSGCTs): These include embryonal cell carcinoma, choriocarcinoma, yolk sac tumor, teratomas, or often multiple cell types; these are more clinically aggressive tumors.

RISK FACTORS
- Cryptorchidism is the most firmly established risk factor: Relative risk of testicular cancer in all patients with cryptorchidism is 3 to 8, with a lower relative risk of 2 to 3 in those undergoing orchiopexy by age 12 years; in patients with unilateral cryptorchidism, the relative risk of testicular cancer in the contralateral normally descended testis is negligible (3).
- Personal history of testicular cancer
- Use of muscle building supplements
- Positive family history for testicular cancer
- Testicular dysgenesis
- Klinefelter syndrome
- Caucasian race
- HIV infections

GENERAL PREVENTION
No evidence that screening for testicular cancer is effective (4).

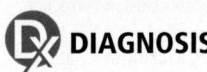

DIAGNOSIS

HISTORY
- A painless solid testicular mass is pathognomonic for testicular cancer.
- Clinical symptoms of epididymitis or orchitis that do not respond to treatment warrant further evaluation.
- Gynecomastia can be a rare systemic endocrine manifestation of testicular neoplasm.

PHYSICAL EXAM
- Testicular exam: Palpate for size, consistency, and nodules; masses do not transilluminate; a firm, hard, or fixed area should be considered suspicious.
- Lymph node and abdominal exam
- Gynecomastia

DIAGNOSTIC TESTS & INTERPRETATION
Initial Tests (lab, imaging)
- α-Fetoprotein (AFP), β-human chorionic gonadotropin (β-hCG), lactate dehydrogenase (LDH), creatinine, chemistry profile, complete blood count, liver enzymes, chest x-ray (CXR), and testicular ultrasound (US)

- Tumor markers AFP, β-hCG, and LDH are used to assist with diagnosis, prognosis, assessing treatment outcome, and monitoring for relapse:
  - AFP
    - Produced by nonseminomatous testicular cancer and is therefore associated with this histologic type
    - Those with a histologically "pure" testicular seminoma and an elevated AFP are assumed to possess an undetected focus of nonseminoma tumor.
  - β-hCG
    - May be associated with both seminomatous or nonseminomatous tumors
    - Hypogonadism and marijuana use may cause benign elevations of β-hCG.
- LDH is less specific than AFP.
- Testicular US is the initial study.
- If an intratesticular mass is identified, measure serum AFP, LDH, and β-hCG and order a CXR.
- CT scan of the abdomen/pelvis, positron emission tomography (PET) scan, MRI of the brain, and bone scan are used for staging and metastases evaluation as clinically indicated.

Diagnostic Procedures/Other
- Radical inguinal orchiectomy is the primary procedure for diagnosis and treatment.
- Testicular biopsy may be rarely considered if a suspicious intratesticular abnormality is identified on US; however, testicular microcalcification on US without any other abnormality can simply be observed and does not demand a biopsy.
- For those with unilateral testicular cancer, contralateral testicular biopsy is not routinely performed but should be considered when there is a cryptorchid testis, marked testicular atrophy, or a suspicious US for intratesticular abnormalities.

Test Interpretation
Clinical staging (5):
- Stage 0: carcinoma in situ
- Stage IA: tumor limited to testis and epididymis without vascular/lymphatic invasion; tumor may invade into the tunica albuginea but not the tunica vaginalis; normal serum tumor markers
- Stage IB: tumor limited to testis and epididymis with vascular/lymphatic invasion or tumor extending through tunica albuginea with involvement of tunica vaginalis; tumor invades the spermatic cord with or without vascular/lymphatic invasion; tumor invades the scrotum with or without vascular/lymphatic invasion; no lymph node involvement or distant metastasis; normal serum tumor markers
- Stage IS: any tumor with elevated serum tumor markers but no nodal involvement or metastasis
- Stage IIA: any tumor with lymph node mass/masses <2 cm
- Stage IIB: any tumor with lymph node mass/masses 2 to 5 cm
- Stage IIC: any tumor with lymph node mass >5 cm
- Stage IIIA: any tumor/lymph node presence; with nonregional nodal or pulmonary metastasis; either serum tumor markers normal or with mild elevation
- Stage IIIB: any tumor/lymph node presence; no distant metastasis or nonregional nodal involvement or pulmonary metastasis; with moderately elevated serum tumor markers
- Stage IIIC: any tumor/lymph node presence; with or without any metastasis; with greatly elevated serum tumor markers

DIFFERENTIAL DIAGNOSIS
Epidermoid cyst, epididymitis, hernia, hydrocele, hematoma, lymphoma, orchitis, spermatocele, testicular torsion, varicocele

TREATMENT

GENERAL MEASURES
- Seminoma: Specifics are noted in the National Comprehensive Cancer Network guidelines (1):
  - Stages IA, IB: Options may include surveillance (preferred) (for low tumor load malignancy, i.e., pT1–pT3), single-agent carboplatin, or radiotherapy (2)[A].
  - Stage IS: Repeat elevated serum tumor marker and abdominal/pelvic CT scan (2)[A].
  - Stage IIA: radiotherapy to include para-aortic and ipsilateral iliac lymph nodes (preferred) or primary chemotherapy (2)[A]
  - Stage IIB: primary chemotherapy (preferred) or radiotherapy in select nonbulky cases to include para-aortic and ipsilateral iliac lymph nodes (2)[A]
  - Stages IIC, III
    - Good risk (any primary site and no nonpulmonary visceral metastases and normal AFP with any β-hCG or LDH): primary etoposide and cisplatin (EP) or bleomycin, etoposide, and cisplatin (BEP) chemotherapy (1)
    - Intermediate risk (any primary site and nonpulmonary visceral metastases and normal AFP with any β-hCG or LDH): primary BEP chemotherapy (1)
- Nonseminoma: Tumors with both seminomatous and nonseminomatous histology are managed as nonseminomatous. See "National Comprehensive Cancer Network guidelines" (1):
  - Stage IA: nonseminomatous surveillance protocol (preferred) or nerve-sparing retroperitoneal lymph node dissection (RPLND) (2)[A]
  - Stage IB: nerve-sparing RPLND or primary BEP chemotherapy (2)[A]; for T2 only can enter nonseminomatous surveillance protocol (2)[B]
  - Stage IS: primary chemotherapy followed by response evaluation:
    - Complete response, negative tumor markers: nonseminomatous surveillance protocol (2)[A]
    - Partial response, negative tumor markers: surgical resection of all residual masses (2)[A]
    - Incomplete response: Consider second-line therapy (2)[A].
  - Stage IIA
    - Negative tumor markers: nerve-sparing RPLND (2)[A] or primary chemotherapy (2)[B]
    - Persistent marker elevation: primary chemotherapy followed by response evaluation
      - Complete response, negative tumor markers: nonseminomatous surveillance protocol (2)[A] or bilateral RPLND +/− nerve-sparing in select cases (2)[B]
      - Partial response, negative tumor markers: surgical resection of all residual masses (2)[A]
      - Incomplete response: Consider second-line therapy (2)[A].
  - Stage IIB
    - Negative tumor markers: primary chemotherapy or nerve-sparing RPLND in highly selected cases (2)[A]

○ Persistent marker elevation: primary chemotherapy followed by response evaluation

- Complete response, negative tumor markers: nonseminomatous surveillance protocol (2)[A] or bilateral RPLND +/− nerve-sparing in selected cases (2)[B]
- Partial response, negative tumor markers: surgical resection of all residual masses (2)[A]
- Incomplete response: Consider second-line therapy (2)[A].
– Stage IIC: primary chemotherapy followed by response evaluation as per stages IIA and IIB (2)[A]
– Stages IIIA, IIIB, and IIIC: primary chemotherapy depending on risk profile, which is based on tumor, metastases, and postorchiectomy serum tumor markers (2)[A]

- Brain metastases: primary chemotherapy +/−radiotherapy, +/− surgery, as clinically indicated

MEDICATION

First Line
Primary chemotherapy regimens for GCTs:

- EP: Etoposide 100 mg/m^2/day IV on days 1 to 5, cisplatin 20 mg/m^2/day IV on days 1 to 5; repeat every 21 days (1)[A].
- BEP: Etoposide 100 mg/m^2/day IV on days 1 to 5, cisplatin 20 mg/m^2/day IV on days 1 to 5; bleomycin 30 U/dose IV weekly on days 1, 8, and 15 or days 2, 9, and 16; repeat every 21 days (1)[A].
- VIP: Etoposide 75 mg/m^2/day IV on days 1 to 5; mesna 120 mg/m^2 slow IV push before ifosfamide on day 1, then mesna 1,200 mg/m^2 IV continuous infusion on days 1 to 5; ifosfamide 1,200 mg/m^2/day on days 1 to 5; cisplatin 20 mg/m^2/day IV on days 1 to 5, repeat every 21 days (1)[A].

Second Line
- These agents are considered in patients who do not respond to first-line therapy or those who experience a recurrence: carboplatin, cisplatin, etoposide, ifosfamide, mesna, paclitaxel, and vinblastine (1)[A].
- Gemcitabine, oxaliplatin, and paclitaxel are used in palliative chemotherapy regimens (1)[A].

ADDITIONAL THERAPIES
Consider sperm banking before treatment that may compromise fertility; rarely covered by insurance.

SURGERY/OTHER PROCEDURES
- Radical inguinal orchiectomy: primary treatment for testicular cancer for all patients; prosthesis can be inserted at this time.
- RPLND identifies nodal metastases and provides accurate pathologic staging of the retroperitoneum.

 ONGOING CARE

FOLLOW-UP RECOMMENDATIONS
- Pure seminoma: Specifics are noted in the National Comprehensive Cancer Network guidelines (1),(2)[A]:

– Stages IA, IB: in general, H&P, optional tumor markers, every 3 to 6 months for 1 years, every 6 to 12 months for years 2 to 33, then annually for years 4 to 5; abdominal/pelvic CT at 3, 6 and 12 months then every 6 to 12 months for years 2 to 3, every 12 to 24 months for years 4 to 5; CXR, as clinically indicated; less frequent if adjuvant therapy is given

– Stage IS: repeat elevated serum tumor marker and assess with abdominal/pelvic CT scan for evaluable disease
– Stages IIA, IIB (select): in general, H&P, optional tumor markers every 3 months for year 1, every 6 months for years 2 to 5; abdominal/pelvic CT at 3 and 6 to 12 months, then annually for years 2 to 3, then as clinically indicated; CXR every 6 months for years 1 to 2
– Stages IIB (select), IIC, and III: Check all serum tumor markers along with chest, abdominal, and pelvic CT:
  ○ Residual mass 0 to 3 cm and normal serum tumor markers: H&P, AFP, β-hCG, LDH, CXR every 2 months for year 1, every 3 months for year 2, every 6 months for years 3 to 4, then annually; abdominal/pelvic CT scan at 3 to 6 months then as clinically indicated, PET scans as clinically indicated
  ○ Residual mass >3 cm and normal serum tumor markers: PET scan 6 weeks after chemotherapy:
    - Negative PET scan: abdominal/pelvic CT scans every 6 months for year 1, then annually for 5 years
    - Positive PET scan: Consider RPLND or second-line chemotherapy or radiotherapy
– Any recurrence: Treat according to extent of disease at relapse.
- Nonseminoma: Specifics are noted in the National Comprehensive Cancer Network guidelines (1):
– Stages IA and IB on surveillance only: H&P, AFP, β-hCG, LDH, every 2 months for year 1, every 3 months for year 2, every 4 to 6 months for year 3, every 6 months for year 4, annually thereafter; CXR and abdominal/pelvic CT depending on IA or IB
– Follow-up after complete response to chemotherapy and RPLND in general: H&P, AFP, β-hCG, LDH every 2 to 3 months for years 1 to 2, every 6 months for years 3 to 5, annually thereafter; abdominal/pelvic CT every 6 months for year 1, annually for year 2, as clinically indicated thereafter
– Follow-up after RPLND only: H&P, AFP, β-hCG, LDH, CXR every 2 months for year 1, every 3 months for year 2, every 4 to 6 for year 3, every 6 months for year 4, annually thereafter; abdominal/pelvic CT at 3 to 4 months and, as clinically indicated, thereafter; CXR every 2 to 4 months year 1, 3 to 6 months year 2, annually thereafter

PROGNOSIS
>90% of patients diagnosed are cured, including 70–80% with advanced tumors (1).

COMPLICATIONS
- Surgical: hematoma, hemorrhage, infection, and infertility
- Radiotherapy: radiation enteritis and infertility
- Late complications (6):
  – Cardiovascular toxicity and second malignancies each have a 25-year risk of about 16% in those treated with chemotherapy and/or radiotherapy.
  – Risk for secondary malignancies remains increased for at least 35 years after treatment.
  – Increased incidence of metabolic syndrome occurs and is likely associated with lower testosterone levels.
  – Other late complications associated with chemotherapy, depending on the regimen, include chronic neurotoxicity, ototoxicity, renal function impairment, and pulmonary fibrosis.

- The incidence of late relapse in treated testicular cancer is now estimated to be 2–6%; the time to late relapse ranges from 2 to 32 years, with a median of 6 years (6).

REFERENCES

1. Motzer RJ, Jonasch E, Agarwal N, et al. Testicular cancer, Version 2.2015. *J Natl Compr Canc Netw*. 2015;13(6):772–799.
2. Howlader N, Noone AM, Krapcho M, et al, eds. SEER Cancer Statistics Review, 1975–2012. Bethesda, MD: National Cancer Institute. http://seer.cancer.gov/csr/1975_2012/. Accessed 2015.
3. Lip SZ, Murchison LE, Cullis PS, et al. A meta-analysis of the risk of boys with isolated cryptorchidism developing testicular cancer in later life. *Arch Dis Child*. 2013;98(1):20–26.
4. Ilic D, Misso ML. Screening for testicular cancer. *Cochrane Database Syst Rev*. 2011;(2):CD007853.
5. Testis. In: Edge SB, Byrd DR, Compton CC, et al, eds. *AJCC Cancer Staging Manual*. 7th ed. New York, NY: Springer; 2010:469–478.
6. Efstathiou E, Logothetis CJ. Review of late complications of treatment and late relapse in testicular cancer. *J Natl Compr Canc Netw*. 2006;4(10): 1059–1070.

ADDITIONAL READING

- Hanna NH, Einhorn LH. Testicular cancer—discoveries and updates. *N Engl J Med*. 2014;371(21):2005–2016.
- Marcell AV, Bell DL, Joffe A, et al. The male genital examination: a position paper of the Society for Adolescent Health and Medicine. *J Adolesc Health*. 2012;50(4):424–425.
- U.S. Preventive Services Task Force. Screening for testicular cancer: U.S. Preventive Services Task Force reaffirmation recommendation statement. *Ann Intern Med*. 2011;154(7):483–486.
- Wood HM, Elder JS. Cryptorchidism and testicular cancer: separating fact from fiction. *J Urol*. 2009;181(2):452–461.

 CODES

ICD10
- C62.90 Malig neoplasm of unsp testis, unsp descended or undescended
- C62.00 Malignant neoplasm of unspecified undescended testis
- C62.10 Malignant neoplasm of unspecified descended testis

CLINICAL PEARLS
- Testicular cancer is the most common solid organ tumor in men aged 15 to 34 years.
- Testicular US is initial imaging of choice for testicular pathology.
- Radical inguinal orchiectomy is used for both diagnosis and treatment, with possible radiotherapy or chemotherapy as adjuvant treatment.
- 96% overall survival at 10 years after diagnosis and treatment

T

TESTICULAR TORSION

Jonathan Green, MD • Michael P. Hirsh, MD

 BASICS

DESCRIPTION
- Twisting of testis and spermatic cord, resulting in acute ischemia and loss of testis if unrecognized.
  - Intravaginal torsion: occurs within tunica vaginalis, only involves testis and spermatic cord
  - Extravaginal torsion: involves twisting of testis, cord, and processus vaginalis as a unit. Typically seen in neonates
- System(s) affected: reproductive

Geriatric Considerations
Very rare in this age group

Pediatric Considerations
Peak incidence is at 14 years of age (1)

EPIDEMIOLOGY
Incidence
- ~1/4,000 males before age 25 years
- Predominant age
  - Occurs from newborn period to 7th decade of life
  - 65% of cases occur in 2nd decade, with peak at age 14 years (1).
  - 2nd peak in neonates (in utero torsion usually occurs around week 32 of gestation) (1)

ETIOLOGY AND PATHOPHYSIOLOGY
- Twisting of spermatic cord causes venous obstruction, edema of testis, and arterial occlusion.
- "Bell clapper" deformity is most common anatomic anomaly predisposing to intravaginal torsion.
  - High insertion of the tunica vaginalis on the spermatic cord, results in increased testicular mobility within tunica vaginalis (2)
  - Bilateral in ~80% of patients (1,2)
- No clear anatomic defect is associated with extravaginal testicular torsion.
  - In neonates, the tunica vaginalis is not yet well attached to scrotal wall, allowing torsion of entire testis including tunica vaginalis (1).
- Usually spontaneous and idiopathic (1)
- 20% of patients have a history of trauma.
- 1/3 have had prior episodic testicular pain.
- Contraction of cremasteric muscle or dartos may play a role and is stimulated by trauma, exercise, cold, and sexual stimulation.
- Increased incidence may be due to increasing weight and size of testis during pubertal development.

- Possible alterations in testosterone levels during nocturnal sex response cycle; possible elevated testosterone levels in neonates (1)
- Testis must have inadequate, incomplete, or absent fixation within scrotum (1,2).
- Torsion may occur in either clockwise or counter-clockwise direction (3).

Genetics
- Unknown
- Familial testicular torsion, although previously rarely reported, may involve as many as 10% of patients (4).

RISK FACTORS
- May be more common in winter
- Paraplegia
- Previous contralateral testicular torsion

 DIAGNOSIS

HISTORY
- Acute onset of pain, often during period of inactivity.
- Onset of pain usually sudden but may start gradually with subsequent increase in severity (1–3).
- Nausea and vomiting are common.
  - Presence may increase the likelihood of testicular torsion versus other differential diagnoses (1,2,5).
- Prior history of multiple episodes of testicular pain with spontaneous resolution in an episodic crescendo pattern may indicate intermittent testicular torsion (6).

PHYSICAL EXAM
- Scrotum is enlarged, red, edematous, and painful (1,2).
- Testicle is swollen and exquisitely tender (1,2).
- Testis may be high in scrotum with a transverse lie.
- Absent cremasteric reflex (1–3)

DIFFERENTIAL DIAGNOSIS
- Torsion appendix testis (this may account for 35–67% of acute scrotal pain cases in children) (2)
- Epididymitis (8–18% of acute scrotal pain cases) (2)
- Orchitis
- Incarcerated or strangulated inguinal hernia
- Acute hydrocele
- Traumatic hematoma
- Idiopathic scrotal edema
- Acute varicocele

- Epididymal hypertension (venous congestion of testicle or prostate due to sexual arousal that does not end in orgasm)
- Testicular tumor
- Henoch-Schönlein purpura
- Scrotal abscess
- Leukemic infiltrate

DIAGNOSTIC TESTS & INTERPRETATION
- Doppler US may confirm testicular swelling, but is diagnostic by demonstrating lack of blood flow to the testicle; positive predictive value (PPV) of 89.4% (5,7)[B].
- In boys with intermittent, recurrent testicular torsion, both Doppler US and radionuclide scintigraphy findings will be normal (7)[B].

Diagnostic Procedures/Other
- Doppler US flow detection demonstrates absent or reduced blood flow with torsion and increased flow with inflammatory process (reliable only in first 12 hours) (7)[B].
- Radionuclide testicular scintigraphy with technetium-99m pertechnetate demonstrates absent/decreased vascularity in torsion and increased vascularity with inflammatory processes (including torsion of appendix testes) (8)[C].

Test Interpretation
- Venous thrombosis
- Tissue edema and necrosis
- Arterial thrombosis
- Decreased Doppler flow also seen in hydrocele, abscess, hematoma, or scrotal hernia (7).
- Sensitivity of radionuclide testicular scintigraphy is decreased relative to ultrasonography because hyperemia in the torsed testicle can mimic flow (8).

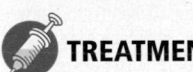 **TREATMENT**

- Manual reduction: Best performed by experienced physician; may be successful, facilitated by lidocaine 1% (plain) injection at level of external ring
  - Difficult to determine success of manual reduction, especially after giving local anesthesia.
  - Manual reduction might require sedation, and the entire process may delay definitive treatment.
  - Even if successful, must always be followed by surgical exploration, urgently but not emergently (6)[C]

- Surgical exploration via scrotal approach at the median raphe allows for exposure of both testes, detorsion, evaluation of testicular viability, orchidopexy of viable testicle, and orchiectomy of nonviable testicle (5)[B].
- In boys with a history of intermittent episodes of testicular pain, scrotal exploration is warranted with testicular fixation if abnormal testicular attachments are confirmed (5)[B].

GENERAL MEASURES

Early exam is crucial because necrosis of the testicle can occur after 6 to 8 hours (1,9)[C].

SURGERY/OTHER PROCEDURES

- Operative testicular fixation of the torsed testicle after detorsion and confirmation of viability. At least 3- or 4-point fixation with nonabsorbable sutures between the tunica albuginea and the tunica vaginalis (5)[B]
- Excision of window of tunica albuginea with suture to dartos fascia (5,10)[B]
- Any testis that is not clearly viable should be removed (5)[B].
- Testes of questionable viability that are preserved and pexed invariably atrophy (5)[B]
- Bilateral testicular fixation is recommended by many surgeons (5)[B].
- Contralateral testicle frequently has similar abnormal fixation and should be explored (5)[B],(6)[C].

 ONGOING CARE

FOLLOW-UP RECOMMENDATIONS

Patient Monitoring

- Postoperative visit at 1 to 2 weeks
- Yearly visits until puberty may be needed to evaluate for atrophy.

DIET

Regular

PATIENT EDUCATION

Possibility of testicular atrophy in salvaged testis with depressed sperm counts. Importantly, fertility rates in patients with one testicle remain excellent.

PROGNOSIS

- Testicular salvage
  - Salvage is related directly to duration of torsion (85–97% if within 6 hours, 20% after 12 hours <10% if >24 hours) (9).
  - The degree of torsion is related to testicular salvage.
    - The median degree of torsion is <360 in patients who are explored and orchidopexy performed.
    - The median degree of torsion is 540 in patients who undergo exploration and require orchiectomy (3).
- 80–94% may have depressed spermatogenesis related to duration of ischemic injury (possibly related to autoimmune-mediated injury) (9).
- Up to 45% of patients undergoing orchiopexy for testicular torsion will develop atrophy of testicle.

COMPLICATIONS

- Possible testicular atrophy
- Decreased or abnormal spermatogenesis
- Infertility
  - Fertility rates with one testicle remain excellent.
  - Nearly, 36% of patients who experience torsion have sperm counts <20 million/mL (8).

REFERENCES

1. Boettcher M, Bergholz R, Krebs TF, et al. Clinical predictors of testicular torsion in children. *Urology*. 2012;79(3):670–674.
2. Edelsberg JS, Surh YS. The acute scrotum. *Emerg Med Clin North Am*. 1988;6(3):521–546.
3. Sessions AE, Rabinowitz R, Hulbert WC, et al. Testicular torsion: direction, degree, duration and disinformation. *J Urol*. 2003;169(2):663–665.
4. Cubillos J, Palmer JS, Friedman SC, et al. Familial testicular torsion. *J Urol*. 2011;185(6)(Suppl): 2469–2472.
5. Van Glabeke E, Khairouni A, Larroquet M, et al. Acute scrotal pain in children: results of 543 surgical explorations. *Pediatr Surg Int*. 1999;15(5–6): 353–357.
6. Eaton SH, Cendron MA, Estrada CR, et al. Intermittent testicular torsion: diagnostic features and management outcomes. *J Urol*. 2005;174 (4, Pt 2):1532–1535.
7. Yagil Y, Naroditsky I, Milhem J, et al. Role of doppler ultrasonography in the triage of acute scrotum in the emergency department. *J Ultrasound Med*. 2010;29(1):11–21.
8. Saleh O, El-Sharkawi MS, Imran MB. Scrotal scintigraphy in testicular torsion: an experience at a tertiary care centre. *Int Med J Malaysia*. 2012;11(1):9–14.
9. Kapoor S. Testicular torsion: a race against time. *Int J Clin Pract*. 2008;62(5):821–827.
10. Figueroa V, Pippi Salle JL, Braga LH, et al. Comparative analysis of detorsion alone versus detorsion and tunica albuginea decompression (fasciotomy) with tunica vaginalis flap coverage in the surgical management of prolonged testicular ischemia. *J Urol*. 2012;188(4)(Suppl): 1417–1422.

 CODES

ICD10

- N44.00 Torsion of testis, unspecified
- N44.03 Torsion of appendix testis
- N44.01 Extravaginal torsion of spermatic cord

CLINICAL PEARLS

- The diagnosis of testicular torsion is usually made on physical exam. Patients with suspected torsion should be taken to the OR without delay. If diagnosis is in question, a testicular Doppler US may be done to evaluate blood flow.
- Although testicular necrosis may be present within 6 to 8 hours of torsion, this is highly variable.
- Infertility can be a problem even if the testicle is viable. Autoimmune antibodies may be produced, and they may affect subsequent fertility.

TESTOSTERONE DEFICIENCY

Michael Lao, MD • Gregory Murphy, MD • Stanton C. Honig, MD

 BASICS

DESCRIPTION

- Testosterone (T) is a critical anabolic hormone involved in various key metabolic pathways.
- It is the principle circulating androgen in males.
- Critical in modulating bodily processes of the cardiovascular, reproductive, hematologic, central nervous, and musculoskeletal systems
- Testosterone deficiency (TD), or hypogonadism, is characterized by low levels of T, often in addition with signs and symptoms attributed to low T levels.
- No universally accepted threshold of T concentration to distinguish eugonadal from hypogonadal men, but the FDA definition is T <300 ng/dL.
- Clinically, TD is divided into primary and secondary.
- T levels can be affected by medical conditions that influence the hypothalamic–pituitary–testis axis, age, and medical comorbidities.
- T levels correlates with overall health and may be associated with sexual function
- T levels decline by 1% per year after age 40.
- Special consideration is needed for men with low T who desire future fertility.
- Synonym(s): hypogonadism; hypoandrogenism; androgen deficiency; and low T

EPIDEMIOLOGY

Incidence
- Overall incidence increases with age
- Symptomatic TD in men in United States ages 30 to 79 years is 5.6%
- 481,000 new cases in the United States in men 40 to 69 years

Prevalence
- Estimates of TD vary widely, but typically 20% of men over 60, 30% over 70, and 50% over 80 years of age.
- 2 to 4 million men in United States

ETIOLOGY AND PATHOPHYSIOLOGY

- Normal hypothalamic–pituitary–testis axis:
  – Hypothalamus produces GnRH, which stimulates pituitary to produce follicle-stimulating hormone (FSH) and luteinizing hormone (LH).
  – LH stimulates the leydig cells to produce T; responsible for 90% of the body's T.
  – T inhibits LH and GnRH through negative feedback at level of hypothalamus and pituitary.
- Primary hypogonadism: Testes produces insufficient amount of T, FSH/LH levels are elevated.
- Secondary hypogonadism: low T from inadequate production of LH
- Mixed hypogonadism: low to normal LH in combination with reduced production of T
- Normal aging process
- Congenital syndromes: cryptorchidism, Klinefelter
- Acquired: cancer, trauma, orchiectomy, prior anabolic steroid abuse
- Infectious: mumps orchitis, HIV, tuberculosis
- Systemic: Cushing syndrome, hemochromatosis, autoimmune, severe illness (e.g., renal disease, cirrhosis), metabolic syndrome, obesity, obstructive sleep apnea, hypogonadotropic hypogonadism
- Drugs and medications: LHRH agonists (leuprolide), corticosteroids, ethanol, ketoconazole, spironolactone, marijuana, opioids, cimetidine
- Elevated prolactin: prolactinoma, dopamine antagonists (e.g., neuroleptics and metoclopramide)

Genetics
- Usually normal
- Klinefelter: XXY karyotype
- Kallmann: abnormal GnRH secretion due to abnormal hypothalamus development

RISK FACTORS
- Obesity, diabetes, COPD, depression, hypothyroid, malnutrition, alcohol, stress
- Chronic infections or inflammatory diseases
- Medications that affect T production or metabolism
- Undescended testicles
- Trauma, testicular radiation, chemotherapy, disorders of the pituitary and/or hypothalamus

GENERAL PREVENTION
General health maintenance and treatment of obesity

COMMONLY ASSOCIATED CONDITIONS
- Infertility, erectile dysfunction, low libido
- Poorer health outcomes
- Osteopenia/osteoporosis and fractures
- Diabetes and insulin resistance, metabolic syndrome
- Increased body weight, adiposity
- Sleep disturbance and depressed mood, poor concentration, irritability

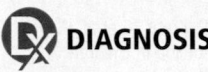 **DIAGNOSIS**

HISTORY
Check for
- Congenital and developmental abnormalities
- Infertility, loss of libido, erectile dysfunction (1)[A]
- Depression, fatigue, difficulty with concentration
- Decreased muscle strength, energy level
- Increase in body fat, development of diabetes
- Bone fractures from relatively minor trauma
- Testicular trauma, infection, radio- or chemotherapy
- Decrease in testicle size or consistency
- Headaches or vision changes suggesting pituitary dysfunction
- Medications

PHYSICAL EXAM
- Infancy: ambiguous genitalia
- Puberty
  – Impaired growth of penis, testicles
  – Lack of secondary male characteristics
  – Gynecomastia, eunuchoid habitus
- Adulthood
  – Decreased muscular development, visceral fat distribution; body habitus changes to suggest corticosteroid excess
  – Presence of gynecomastia
  – Skin changes to suggest hemochromatosis
  – Eunuchoid habitus
- Genitourinary exam
  – Small and/or soft testicles

DIFFERENTIAL DIAGNOSIS
- Delayed puberty
- Obesity
- Normal aging
- Prior anabolic steroid abuse

DIAGNOSTIC TESTS & INTERPRETATION
- T levels vary widely, they are subject to diurnal, seasonal, and age-related variations. There are multiple assays, each with unique characteristics.

Measurement should be obtained between 6 to 10 AM. Confirmation with a second measurement may be necessary. Whether total T or free T most closely correlates with symptomatic deficiency is unclear. Free T with total T is generally preferred. Measurements should not be obtained during acute or subacute illness. T circulates in blood primary bound to SHBG or to albumin. Only 2–3% of total T is found free. Free and albumin-bound T is considered bioavailable. Laboratory findings must be interpreted in the appropriate clinical setting. Bioavailable T is considered most important, but assays are not readily available and calculated bioavailable T is not reliable.
- Lower limit of normal in most reference laboratories for total testosterone is 280 to 300 ng/dL (9.8 to 10.4 nmol/L). The lower limit of normal for free testosterone is 5 to 9 pg/mL (0.17 to 0.31 nmol/L).

Initial Tests (lab, imaging)
- In symptomatic individuals, morning T level is the initial test. Morning timing is more important for younger men in whom there is more diurnal variation. If initial morning testosterone is low and confirmed on repeat test, further evaluation is appropriate (2)[A].
- Endocrine evaluation should include LH and FSH to differentiate between primary versus secondary hypogonadism.
- If primary hypogonadism of unknown origin, consider obtaining karyotype (e.g., Klinefelter) if severe testis atrophy exists.
- If secondary hypogonadism, evaluation may consist of prolactin, iron saturation, pituitary function testing, and/or MRI of pituitary.
- Imaging is not helpful in the initial diagnosis of TD.
- No evidence to support screening for TD in the general population

Follow-Up Tests & Special Considerations
- Routine blood work to measure T response to interventions
- Dual-emission x-ray absorptiometry (DEXA) to measure bone mineral density in men with severe TD or fracture from minimal trauma.
- Pituitary MRI: if there is elevation of prolactin more than twice the upper limit of normal or LH/FSH below normal range

 TREATMENT

T replacement is recommended for symptomatic men (e.g., low libido and/or erectile dysfunction, low energy level, constitutional symptoms, etc.) with low T levels ≤300 ng/dL obtained in the morning. Not recommended for older men with low T levels in absence of signs or symptoms.

GENERAL MEASURES
- Confirm suspicion.
- Obtain hematocrit, prostate-specific antigen (PSA) in men > 40 years, prolactin, LH/FSH, SHBG, estradiol.
- Baseline physical exam including digital rectal exam, and International Prostate Symptom Score (IPSS)
- Correction of underlying cause
- Is future fertility an issue? Different treatment strategies are used in men of reproductive age and/or interest.

- Current evidence fails to demonstrate that higher serum T is associated with greater prostate cancer risk.
- Safety of T therapy in prostate cancer is still uncertain and contraindicated in package insert.
- 2010 Endocrine Guidelines: Patients with organ-confined prostate cancer who have undergone radical prostatectomy and have been disease free for ≥2 years after surgery with undetectable PSA may be considered for T replacement on an individualized basis. Lack of data from randomized trials precludes a general recommendation.

- T therapy should not be used in men with hematocrit >50%, untreated obstructive sleep apnea, and severe lower urinary tract symptoms with an IPSS >19 (3)[A].
- T therapy is not recommended for: mood or strength improvement in otherwise healthy men, or asymptomatic men with low T measurements (3)[A].
- Carefully weigh risks and benefits in men at elevated cardiovascular risk (3,4)[A].

- Clinicians can consider starting short-term T therapy as an adjunctive in men with HIV and low T to promote weight maintenance and gains in lean body mass and strength.

MEDICATION

ALERT
- Avoid contact with females or children (see package insert) in patients applying gel preparations.

- Oral therapy is not recommended due to significant hepatotoxicity.
- The FDA has cautioned that testosterone is approved for men with confirmed low testosterone by laboratory testing and caused by certain medical conditions, NOT just due to aging.
- Despite prior data showing no clear association between testosterone replacement therapy (TRT) and CV disease, there have been several recent papers suggesting that TRT use puts patients at an increased risk for CV disease. These papers have been criticized widely for being flawed due to comparison of unequal groups, short and inaccurate endpoints, flawed laboratory testing, erroneous exclusion criteria, and atypical statistical analysis. Despite this, an FDA panel concluded that there is a possible increased CV risk associated with testosterone use.
- Testosterone replacement therapy (FDA approved)
  - Topical gels/solutions
    - Multiple FDA-approved formulations
    - Most frequently prescribed in United States
    - Mimics normal daily circadian rhythm
    - Good absorption, but 15–20% are nonresponders
    - Transfer concern to children and women
    - Dosage adjustments to obtain optimal results
    - Gel application: arms, back, axilla, and groin
  - Testosterone pellets (Testopel)
    - Minor office procedure with mild discomfort
    - Long-acting formulation, 3 to 4 months
    - 1–2% risk of infection or pellet extrusion
  - Transdermal patch (Androderm)
    - Achieves less robust levels
    - Convenient over gels, no risk of transference
    - High incidence of skin irritation
  - Testosterone cypionate and enanthate (short acting)
    - Injectable (IM), inexpensive
    - Inconvenient: injections every 1 to 3 weeks
    - Starting dose: 100 mg/week, or 200 mg/2 weeks
    - Roller coast effect: levels rise and fall

- Testosterone undecanoate (long acting)
  - Injectable, expensive, convenient
  - Small risk of oil embolism, needs observation in office for 30 minutes postinjection
  - Given approximately every 8 to 12 weeks
- Buccal application (Striant)
  - Adheres to gum line, irritation in 16.3%
  - Poor compliance, every 12 hours application
- Nasal gel (Natesto)
  - Levels overdosing schedule are variable.
  - TID dosing, nasal irritation
- OFF LABEL TREATMENT
  - Human chorionic gonadotropin (hCG)
    - Structure similar to LH, mimics its actions
    - Frequent, 3 times per week starting at 1,500 IU SC
    - Poor compliance
    - Maintenance of testicular volume and fertility
    - Used in men wanting to preserve fertility
  - Clomiphene citrate: oral agent
    - Increases T by interfering with negative feedback, resulting in increased LH and FSH
    - Starting dose of 25 mg daily 3 to 7 times weekly
    - Used in men wanting to preserve fertility
  - Aromatase inhibitors (Arimidex): oral agent
    - Blocks conversion of T to estradiol
    - Does not negatively impact spermatogenesis and testicular volume
    - Utilized in cases of low T/estradiol ratio

ISSUES FOR REFERRAL
- Elevated PSA and/or abnormal prostate exam should be referred to urology.
- Worsening symptoms of BPH or increasing IPSS

ONGOING CARE

FOLLOW-UP RECOMMENDATIONS
Patient Monitoring
- Necessary to monitor effectiveness of therapy as well as for adverse effects: Initially 3 to 6 months after treatment initiation and then annually
- Measure hematocrit at baseline, at 3 to 6 months, and then annually. If hematocrit >54% or symptomatic, stop therapy until hematocrit decreases to a safe level. Treatment includes phlebotomy, blood donation, or adjustment of dose.
- Evaluate patient for hypoxia or sleep apnea.
- Monitor bone mineral density after 1 to 2 years of therapy in these men with osteoporosis or low trauma fracture.
- Changes in voiding symptoms
- Prostate exam done regularly every 6 to 12 months.
- Refer to urology when increase in PSA >0.7 ng/mL within any 12-month period of T treatment or detection of prostatic abnormality on prostate exam.

DIET
Healthy diet and weight reduction if obese

PATIENT EDUCATION
- TD is chronic and likely to need lifelong therapy.
- T replacement comes with many risks, and it is very important to regularly monitor outcomes.
- Women and children must not be allowed to come in contact with T-replacement gel products.

PROGNOSIS
- Sustained reversal of symptoms can be achieved when serum levels of T fall in the normal range.
- Adverse health effects seen in many with chronically low levels of T

COMPLICATIONS
Complications of testosterone replacement
- Decreased testicular volume and azoospermia
- Fluctuations in mood or libido
- Gynecomastia and growth of breast cancer
- Acne and oily skin
- Erythrocytosis (increased hemocrit)
- Exacerbation of sleep apnea
- Hepatotoxicity with prolonged oral use
- Possible prostate enlargement with or without worsening symptoms of BPH
- Unknown cardiovascular risks

REFERENCES
1. Conners WP III, Morgentaler A. The evaluation and management of testosterone deficiency: the new frontier in urology and men's health. *Curr Urol Rep.* 2013;14(6):557–564.
2. Paduch DA, Brannigan RE, Fuchs EF, et al. The laboratory diagnosis of testosterone deficiency. *Urology.* 2014;83(5):980–988.
3. Bhasin S, Cunningham GR, Hayes FJ, et al. Testosterone therapy in men with androgen deficiency syndromes: an Endocrine Society clinical practice guideline. *J Clin Endocrinol Metab.* 2010;95(6):2536–2559.
4. Jenkins LC, Mulhall JP. Editor's comment—how dangerous is testosterone supplementation? *Int Braz J Urol.* 2015;41(2):195–198.

ADDITIONAL READING
- Buvat J, Maggi M, Guay A, et al. Testosterone deficiency in men: systematic review and standard operating procedures for diagnosis and treatment. *J Sex Med.* 2013;10(1):245–284.
- Vigen R, O'Donnell CI, Barón AE, et al. Association of testosterone therapy with mortality, myocardial infarction, and stroke in men with low testosterone levels. *JAMA.* 2013;310(17):1829–1836.

CODES

ICD10
- E29.1 Testicular hypofunction
- E89.5 Postprocedural testicular hypofunction

CLINICAL PEARLS
- Testosterone deficiency is common and prevalence increases with age.
- Testosterone deficiency can have negative adverse impact on many bodily systems.
- Symptomatic men with sexual dysfunction, obesity, and metabolic diseases should be tested for testosterone deficiency and treated.
- Initial test of choice is a morning total and free testosterone; if low, repeat measurements.
- Testosterone replacement therapy in the appropriately selected population can increase lean mass, reduce fat mass, increase bone density, improve libido, and improved erections.

T

THALASSEMIA

Herbert L. Muncie, Jr., MD • Garland Edward Anderson, II, MD

BASICS

DESCRIPTION
- A group of inherited hematologic disorders that affect the synthesis of adult hemoglobin tetramer (HbA) (1,2)[C]
- α-Thalassemia is due to a deficient synthesis of α-globin chain, whereas β-thalassemia is due to a deficient synthesis of β-globin chain:
  - The synthesis of the unaffected globin chain proceeds normally.
  - This unbalanced globin chain production causes unstable hemoglobin tetramers, which leads to hypochromic, microcytic RBCs, and hemolytic anemia.
- α-Thalassemia is more common in persons of Mediterranean, African, and Southeast Asian descent, whereas β-thalassemia is more common in patients of African and Southeast Asian descent.
- Types
  - Thalassemia (minor) trait (α or β): absent or mild anemia with microcytosis and hypochromia
  - α-Thalassemia major with hemoglobin Barts usually results in fatal hydrops fetalis (fluid in $\geq$2 fetal compartments secondary to anemia and fetal heart failure).
  - α-Thalassemia intermedia with hemoglobin H (hemoglobin H disease): results in moderate hemolytic anemia and splenomegaly
  - β-Thalassemia major: results in severe anemia, growth retardation, hepatosplenomegaly, bone marrow expansion, and bone deformities. Transfusion therapy is necessary to sustain life.
  - β-Thalassemia intermedia: Milder disease; transfusion therapy may not be needed or may be needed later in life.
- Other variants include hemoglobin E/β-thalassemia in Southeast Asians, which often mimics the severity of α-thalassemia major; delta thalassemia; hemoglobin H Constant Spring.
- System(s) affected: hematologic/lymphatic/immunologic, cardiac, hepatic
- Synonym(s): Mediterranean anemia; hereditary leptocytosis; Cooley anemia

Pediatric Considerations
- β-Thalassemia major causes symptoms during early childhood, usually starting at 6 months of age, and requires periodic transfusions to sustain life.
- Newborn's cord blood or heel stick should be screened for hemoglobinopathies with hemoglobin electrophoresis or comparably accurate test, although this primarily detects sickle cell disease.

Pregnancy Considerations
- Preconception genetic counseling is advised for couples at risk for having a child with thalassemia and for parents or other relatives of a child with thalassemia (3)[A].

- Once pregnant, a chorionic villus sample at 10 to 11 weeks' gestation or an amniocentesis at 15 weeks' gestation can be done to detect point mutations or deletions with polymerase chain reaction (PCR) technology.

EPIDEMIOLOGY
Incidence
- Occurs in ~4.4/10,000 live births
- Predominant age: Symptoms start to appear 6 months after birth with β-thalassemia major.
- Predominant sex: male = female

Prevalence
- Worldwide, ~200,000 people are alive with β-thalassemia major and <1,000 patients are in the United States.
- In the worldwide population, an estimated 1.5% are β-thalassemia carriers and 5% α-thalassemia carriers (4).

ETIOLOGY AND PATHOPHYSIOLOGY
Unknown; it is unclear how the imbalance of β-globulin in α-thalassemia and α-globin in β-thalassemia results in ineffective red blood cell genesis and hemolysis.

Genetics
- Inherited in an autosomal recessive pattern.
- α-Thalassemia results from a deletion of $\geq$1 of the 4 genes, 2 on each chromosome 16, responsible for α-globin synthesis. 1-gene deletion is a silent carrier state, 2-gene deletion is the trait, 3-gene deletion results in hemoglobin H, and 4-gene deletion results in hemoglobin Bart, causing fatal hydrops fetalis.
- Nondeletional forms do occur rarely. Hemoglobin H Constant Spring is the most common nondeletional form.
- β-Thalassemia is caused by any of >200-point mutations and, very rarely, deletions on chromosome 11; 20 alleles account for >80% of the mutations.
- Significantly disparate phenotype with the same genotype occurs because β-globin chain production can range from near-normal to absent.

RISK FACTORS
Family history of thalassemia

GENERAL PREVENTION
- Prenatal information: genetic counseling regarding partner selection and information on the availability of diagnostic tests during the pregnancy
- Complication prevention
  - For offspring of adult thalassemia patients, an evaluation for thalassemia by 1 year of age
  - Severe forms
    ○ Avoid exposure to sick contacts.
    ○ Keep immunizations up to date.
  - Promptly treat bacterial infections. (After splenectomy, patients should maintain a supply of an appropriate antibiotic to take at the onset of symptoms of a bacterial infection.)
  - Dental checkups every 6 months
  - Avoid activities that could increase the risk of bone fractures.

COMMONLY ASSOCIATED CONDITIONS
See "Complications."

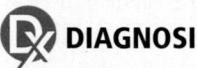

DIAGNOSIS

Thalassemia (minor) trait has no signs or symptoms.

HISTORY
- Poor growth
- Excessive fatigue
- Cholelithiasis
- Pathologic fractures
- Shortness of breath

PHYSICAL EXAM
- Pallor
- Splenomegaly
- Jaundice
- Maxillary hyperplasia/frontal bossing due to massive bone marrow expansion
- Dental malocclusion

DIFFERENTIAL DIAGNOSIS
- Iron deficiency anemia
- Other microcytic anemias: lead toxicity, sideroblastic
- Other hemolytic anemias
- Other hemoglobinopathies

DIAGNOSTIC TESTS & INTERPRETATION
Special tests
- Bone marrow aspiration to evaluate for causes of microcytic anemia is rarely needed.
- Multiple indices have been evaluated to discriminate β-thalassemia trait from iron deficiency anemia, yet none is sensitive enough to exclude β-thalassemia.
- Hemoglobin: usual range 10 to 12 g/dL with thalassemia trait and 3 to 8 g/dL with β-thalassemia major before transfusions.
- Hematocrit
  - 28–40% in thalassemia trait
  - May fall to <10% in β-thalassemia major
- Peripheral blood
  - Microcytosis (MCV <70 fl)
  - Hypochromia (MCH <20 pg)
  - High percentage of target cells
  - Reticulocyte count is elevated.
- Red cell distribution width (RDW)
  - A normal RDW with a microcytic hypochromic anemia is almost always thalassemia trait.
  - The RDW can be elevated in ~50% of thalassemia trait patients. This is in contrast to iron deficiency anemia, where the RDW is almost always elevated (90%).
- Hemoglobin electrophoresis
  - In α-thalassemia trait, no recognizable electrophoretic pattern occurs in adults.
  - However, in the neonatal period, 3–10% of trait patients will have hemoglobin H or hemoglobin Bart at birth, which would confirm α-thalassemia.
  - If HbA_2 is below normal (<2.5%) with a normal HbF level, the diagnosis is α-thalassemia intermedia (HbH disease).
  - In the neonatal period with β-thalassemia trait, the electrophoresis is normal. However, in adults, elevated HbA_2 levels (>4%) may be present but are usually normal (5)[C].
  - β-Thalassemia major or intermedia has elevated HbA_2, elevated HbF, and reduced or absent HbA.
- DNA analysis
  - α-Thalassemia can definitively be diagnosed with genetic testing of hemoglobin A1 and A2 (for deletions and point mutations), but this is not routinely done due to the high cost.
  - High-performance liquid chromatography
  - Cost-effective primary screening tool for children and adolescents (6)[C]
  - Equivocal results should be confirmed with DNA analysis.

Pediatric Considerations
For children, calculate Mentzer index (mean corpuscular volume/RBC count).
- <13: suggests thalassemia
- >13: suggests iron deficiency anemia
- Liver iron concentrations can be assessed with MRI (FerriScan).

TREATMENT

- Outpatient for mild cases
- Inpatient for transfusion therapy

GENERAL MEASURES
- Mild cases (trait or minor) require no therapy.
- Thalassemia intermedia: No therapy is necessary unless hemoglobin falls to a level that causes symptoms; then transfusion therapy is needed. Decision is based on patient's quality of life.
- Iron supplements should not be given unless iron deficiency occurs and is confirmed with low ferritin. Supplements increase the risk of iron overload.
- Thalassemia major
  - A regular transfusion schedule to increase post-transfusion hemoglobin to 13.0 to 14.0 g/L and maintain a mean hemoglobin level of at least 9.3 g/dL (1.4 mmol/L)
  - Patients require >8 transfusion events per year. An event may be multiple transfused units.
  - Iron overload (7)[C]
    - Patients receiving transfusion therapy increase total body iron 4 times the normal amount.
    - Therapy is iron chelation. (See "Medication.")

MEDICATION
Thalassemia intermedia and major: folic acid supplements (1 mg/day)

First Line
β-Thalassemia major
- Iron chelation with deferoxamine (Desferal)
  - Usually continuous SC or IV infusion
  - Acute toxicity: initial—1,000 mg IV, may be followed by 500 mg every 4 hours for 2 doses; subsequent doses of 500 mg every 4 to 12 hours based on response (max 6,000 mg/day)
  - Chronic: 20 to 40 mg/kg over 8 to 12 hours daily
  - Usually started by 5 to 8 years of age
  - Treatment lasts 3 to 5 years to reach serum ferritin <1,000 mg/mL.
- Deferasirox (Exjade): 20 to 30 mg/kg/day PO acceptable alternative; approved for transfusion and non–transfussion-dependent patients with hepatic iron concentrations ≥5 mg/g of dry weight and serum ferritin >300 μg/L; renal and hepatic monitoring is recommended.

Second Line
Chelation with deferiprone (Ferriprox) 25 mg/kg TID PO initially is an acceptable alternative for patients who have not responded to deferoxamine; may provide more cardioprotection. A drawback is weekly CBC because ~1% of patients develop agranulocytosis.

ISSUES FOR REFERRAL
Thalassemia major usually requires hematology consult.

ADDITIONAL THERAPIES
β-Thalassemia intermedia
- Hydroxyurea may improve hemoglobin 1 to 2 g/dL.
- Psychological support seems appropriate for this chronic disease. However, no conclusions can be made regarding specific psychological therapies.

SURGERY/OTHER PROCEDURES
- Splenectomy
  - May be needed if hypersplenism causes an increase in the transfusion requirements (>180 to 200 mL/kg/year) (8)[C]
  - Defer surgery until patient is at least 4 years of age (due to increased infection risk).
  - Administer pneumococcal polyvalent-23 vaccine 1 month before splenectomy. Children should complete their pneumococcal conjugate vaccine series before surgery.
  - Daily penicillin prophylaxis, 250 mg BID, after splenectomy for 2 years for all patients and for children until age 16 years.

- Bone marrow transplantation with HLA-identical related donor stem cells in children before developing hepatitis or iron overload has high likelihood of remission but may impair fertility.

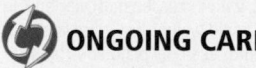 ONGOING CARE

FOLLOW-UP RECOMMENDATIONS
- Thalassemia trait requires no restrictions.
- β-Thalassemia major
  - Avoid strenuous activities (e.g., football, soccer).
  - Acceptable activity levels will be determined on an individual basis depending on the severity of the disorder.

Patient Monitoring
- Thalassemia-trait patients require no special follow-up.
- For β-thalassemia major, lifelong monitoring is necessary because the therapy and disease progression have numerous potential complications.

DIET
- Thalassemia trait requires no restrictions.
- β-Thalassemia major
  - Limit intake of iron-rich foods (e.g., red meats such as liver and some cereals).

PATIENT EDUCATION
Printed patient information available from Cooley Anemia Foundation, 330 7th Ave. Suite 900, New York, NY 10001; http://www.thalassemia.org or http://www.cooleysanemia.org

PROGNOSIS
- Outlook varies depending on type.
- Thalassemia-trait patients live a normal lifespan.
- β-Thalassemia major patients live an average of 17 years and usually die by age 30 years.
- Iron overload causes most of the morbidity and mortality:
  - Cardiac events are the primary cause of death.
  - Myocardial iron deposition is best assessed with MRI T2 (9)[C].
  - Effective iron chelation improves longevity.

COMPLICATIONS
- Chronic hemolysis
- Susceptibility to infections after splenectomy
- Infections from blood transfusion
- Jaundice
- Leg ulcers
- Cholelithiasis
- Osteoporosis and low-trauma fractures
- Impaired growth rate
- Delayed or absent puberty
- Hypogonadism
- Hepatic siderosis
- Splenomegaly
- Cardiac disease from iron overload
- Thromboembolic phenomenon
- Aplastic and megaloblastic crises
- Increased risk of hematologic and abdominal cancer (10)
- Increased risk of dementia (11)

REFERENCES
1. Muncie HL Jr, Campbell J. Alpha and beta thalassemia. *Am Fam Physician*. 2009;80(4):339–344.
2. Higgs DR, Engel JD, Stamatoyannopoulos G. Thalassaemia. *Lancet*. 2012;379(9813):373–383.
3. Tamhankar PM, Agarwal S, Arya V, et al. Prevention of homozygous beta thalassemia by premarital screening and prenatal diagnosis in India. *Prenat Diagn*. 2009;29(1):83–88.
4. Peters M, Heijboer H, Smiers F, et al. Diagnosis and management of thalassaemia. *BMJ*. 2012; 344:e228.
5. Mosca A, Paleari R, Ivaldi G, et al. The role of haemoglobin A(2) testing in the diagnosis of thalassaemias and related haemoglobinopathies. *J Clin Pathol*. 2009;62(1):13–17.
6. Abdel-Messih IY, Youssef SR, Mokhtar GM, et al. Clinical to molecular screening paradigm for β-thalassemia carriers. *Hemoglobin*. 2015; 39(4):240–246.
7. Fleming RE, Ponka P. Iron overload in human disease. *N Engl J Med*. 2012;366(4):348–359.
8. Galanello R, Origa R. Beta-thalassemia. *Orphanet J Rare Dis*. 2010;5:11.
9. Pennell DJ, Udelson JE, Arai AE, et al. Cardiovascular function and treatment in β-thalassemia major: a consensus statement from the American Heart Association. *Circulation*. 2013;128(3):281–308.
10. Chung WS, Lin CL, et al. Thalassaemia and risk of cancer: a population-based cohort study. *J Epidemiol Community Health*. 2015;69(11): 1066–1070.
11. Chen YG, Lin TY, Chen HJ, et al. Thalassemia and risk of dementia: a nationwide population-based retrospective cohort study. *Eur J Intern Med*. 2015;26(7):554–559.

ADDITIONAL READING
- Paulson RF. Targeting a new regulator of erythropoiesis to alleviate anemia. *Nat Med*. 2014;20(4): 334–335.
- Piel FB, Weatherall DJ. The α-thalassemias. *N Engl J Med*. 2014;371(20):1908–1916.

 ## CODES

ICD10
- D56.9 Thalassemia, unspecified
- D56.1 Beta thalassemia
- D56.0 Alpha thalassemia

CLINICAL PEARLS
- Thalassemia (group of inherited hematologic disorders that affect the synthesis of adult hemoglobin tetramer) is a genetic condition; hemoglobin will not improve over time.
- α-Thalassemia is due to a deficient synthesis of the α-globin chain, whereas β-thalassemia is due to a deficient synthesis of the β-globin chain.
- Hemoglobin electrophoresis is needed for genetic counseling but not to make the diagnosis of thalassemia minor when evaluating a patient with mild hypochromic, microcytic anemia, and normal serum ferritin.
- Anemia from thalassemia minor is not due to inadequate iron availability or iron storage. Therefore, iron supplements will not improve the anemia and could be harmful due to GI distress and iron overload. If coexisting iron deficiency is proven, then iron therapy is appropriate.

THORACIC OUTLET SYNDROME

Muhammad Imran Khan, MD • Najm Hasan Siddiqui, MD

BASICS

DESCRIPTION
- A constellation of symptoms that affects the head, neck, shoulders, and upper extremities caused by compression of the neurovascular structures (i.e., brachial plexus and subclavian vessels) at the thoracic outlet, specifically in the area superior to the 1st rib and posterior to the clavicle
- Three forms of thoracic outlet syndrome (TOS) have been described: neurogenic, vascular (containing venous and arterial symptoms), and nonspecific (includes traumatic and secondary to certain provocative movements).
- Synonym(s): scalenus anticus syndrome; cervical rib syndrome; costoclavicular syndrome

Pregnancy Considerations
Generalized tissue fluid accumulations and postural changes may aggravate symptoms.

EPIDEMIOLOGY
Incidence
- Predominant age
  - Neurogenic type (95%): 20 to 60 years
  - Venous type (4%): 20 to 35 years
  - Arterial type (1%; atherosclerosis): young adult or >50 years
- Predominant sex
  - Neurogenic type: female > male (3.5:1)
  - Venous type: male > female
  - Arterial type: male = female
- No objective confirmatory tests are available to measure true incidence.
- Estimated 3 to 8/1,000 cases for neurogenic type
- Incidence of other TOS types is unclear.

ETIOLOGY AND PATHOPHYSIOLOGY
The interscalene triangle area is reduced in TOS and may become smaller during certain shoulder and arm movements. Fibrotic bands, cervical ribs, and muscle variations may further narrow the triangle. Trauma or provocative movements affecting the lower brachial plexus have strong implications in TOS pathogenesis.

- Three known causes of TOS: anatomic, traumatic/repetitive movement activities, and neurovascular entrapment
  - Anatomic: Variations in the anatomy of the neck scalene muscles may be responsible for presentations of the neurologic type of TOS and may involve the superior border of the 1st rib. Cervical ribs also have been implicated as a cause of neurologic TOS, with subsequent neuronal fibrosing and degeneration associated with arterial hyalinization in the lower trunk of the brachial plexus. Fibrous bands to cervical ribs are often congenital.
  - Trauma or repetitive movement activities: Motor vehicle accidents with hyperextension injury and resulting fibrosis, including fibrous bands to the clavicle; musicians who maintain prolonged positions of shoulder abduction or extension may be at increased risk.
  - Neurovascular entrapment: occurring in the costoclavicular space between the 1st rib and the head of the clavicle

RISK FACTORS
- Trauma, especially to the shoulder girdle
- Presence of a cervical rib

- Posttraumatic, exostosis of clavicle or 1st rib, postural abnormalities (e.g., drooping of shoulders, scoliosis), body building with increased muscular bulk in thoracic outlet area, rapid weight loss with vigorous physical exertion and/or exercise, pendulous breasts
- Occupational exposure: computer users; musicians; repetitive work involving shoulders, arms, hands
- Young, thin females with long necks and drooping shoulders

GENERAL PREVENTION
Consider observation or further evaluation in patients with cervical ribs.

COMMONLY ASSOCIATED CONDITIONS
- Paget–von Schrötter syndrome: thrombosis of subclavian vein
- Gilliatt-Sumner hand: neurogenic atrophy of abductor pollicis brevis

DIAGNOSIS

HISTORY
- Neurologic type, upper plexus (C4–C7)
  - Pain and paresthesias in head, neck, mandible, face, temporal area, upper back/chest, outer arm, and hand in a radial nerve distribution
  - Occipital and orbital headache
- Neurologic type, lower plexus (C8–T1)
  - Pain and paresthesias in axilla, inner arm, and hand in an ulnar nerve distribution, often nocturnal
  - Hypothenar and interosseous muscle atrophy
- Venous type: arm claudication, cyanosis, swelling, distended arm veins
- Arterial type: digital vasospasm, thrombosis/embolism, aneurysm, gangrene

PHYSICAL EXAM
- Positive Adson maneuver (head rotation to the affected side with cervical extension and then deep inhalation); test is positive if paresthesias occur or if radial pulse is not palpable during maneuver.
- Tenderness to percussion or palpation of supraclavicular area
- Worsening of symptoms with elevation of arm, overhead extension of arms, or with arms extended forward (e.g., driving a car, typing, carrying objects); prompt disappearance of symptoms with arm returning to neutral position
- Morley test
  - Brachial plexus compression test in the supraclavicular area from the scalene triangle
  - Positive with reproduction of an aching sensation and typical localized paresthesia
- Hyperabduction test: diminishment of radial pulse with elevation of arm above the head
- Military maneuver (i.e., costoclavicular bracing): When patient elevates chin and pushes shoulders posteriorly in an extreme "at-attention" position, symptoms are provoked.
- 1-minute Roos test
  - A thoracic outlet shoulder girdle stress test
  - Shoulders and arms are braced in a 90-degree abducted and externally rotated position; patient is required to clench and relax fists repetitively for 1 minute.
  - A positive test reproduces the symptom.

DIFFERENTIAL DIAGNOSIS
- Cervical disk or carpal tunnel syndrome
- Orthopedic shoulder problems (shoulder strain, rotator cuff injury, tendonitis)
- Cervical spondylitis
- Ulnar nerve compression at elbow and hand
- Multiple sclerosis
- Spinal cord tumor/disease
- Angina pectoris
- Migraine
- Complex regional pain syndromes
- C3–C5 and C8 radiculopathies

DIAGNOSTIC TESTS & INTERPRETATION
Initial Tests (lab, imaging)
CBC, ESR, and C-reactive protein (CRP) determination may rule out underlying inflammatory conditions.
- Radiograph (chest, C-spine, shoulders) (1)[C] may reveal elongated C7 transverse process or a cervical rib, Pancoast tumor, or healed clavicle fracture.
- Nerve conduction studies and electromyography (EMG)
- CT scan or MRI, although MRI is the method of choice when searching for nerve compression
- Improved high-resolution MRN and tractography are valuable tools for identifying the source of nerve compression in patients with neurogenic TOS and can augment current diagnostic modalities for this syndrome (2)[B].
- Contrast-enhanced 3D MRA using provocative arm positioning allows excellent imaging of the arteries and veins on both sides and thus provides a non-invasive imaging alternative to digital subtraction angiography in patients with suspected vascular TOS (3)[B].
- Doppler and duplex US if vascular obstruction is suspected
- Arteriogram and venogram have limited roles; useful when symptoms suggestive of arterial insufficiency or ischemia, or in planning surgical intervention (4)[C].

Diagnostic Procedures/Other
No indicated procedures; anesthetic anterior scalene block may relieve pressure by scalene muscles on the brachial plexus, making this type of block diagnostic and potentially therapeutic, but it poses the risk of procedural damage to the brachial plexus.

Test Interpretation
Systematic results of biopsy have not been reported. There is no indication for biopsy unless to investigate another underlying condition.

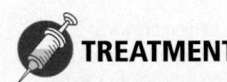

TREATMENT

GENERAL MEASURES
- Conservative management usually involves approaches to reduce and redistribute pressure and traction through the use of physiotherapy or prosthesis.
- Interscalene injections of botulinum toxin have been shown to decrease symptoms of TOS (5)[C]. A single, CT-guided Botox injection into the anterior scalene muscle may offer an effective, minimally invasive treatment for NTOS (6)[A].
- Physical therapy will develop strength in pectoral girdle muscles and achieve normal posture (1)[C].

- Severe cases may use taping, adhesive elastic bandages, moist heat, TENS, or US but should not substitute active exercise and correction of posture and muscle imbalance (7)[B].

MEDICATION

- No firm evidence exists for any approach to the four types of TOS.

- Physical therapy is the first-line treatment (7)[B].

- Anti-inflammatory (ibuprofen)
  – Adult dose: 400 to 800 mg PO q8h; not to exceed 3,200 mg/day
  – Pediatric dose
    ○ <12 years: 10 mg/kg/dose every 6 to 8 hours
    ○ >12 years: as in adults
  – Contraindications: documented hypersensitivity, active PUD, renal or hepatic impairment, recent use of anticoagulants, hemorrhagic conditions
- Neuropathic pain: Tricyclic antidepressants, carbamazepine, gabapentin, phenytoin, pregabalin; muscle relaxants such as baclofen, metaxalone, or tizanidine may be helpful.
- Severe pain: Consider opiates for brachial plexus nerve block, steroid injections.

ISSUES FOR REFERRAL

- Neurologic, anesthesiologic, orthopedic, vascular surgery referral(s) may be indicated depending on the type of pathologic condition.
- Physical and rehabilitation physicians

SURGERY/OTHER PROCEDURES

- Operative if vascular involvement is present and/or loss of function or lifestyle occurs secondary to severity of symptoms and if conservative therapy fails after 2 to 3 months (1)[C]

- Resection of 1st rib or cervical ribs via transaxillary (preferred with good to excellent outcome 80% of patients), supraclavicular (good to excellent outcome 80% of patients), posterior approaches (reserved for complicated TOS due to necessity of large muscle incision). Excellent results were seen in patients who underwent first rib resection in all three forms of TOS (8)[A].

- Transaxillary 1st rib resection (TFRR) may provide better pain relief than supraclavicular neuroplasty of the brachial plexus (SNBP); although, overall, both treatment options have generally positive outcomes (9)[B].

- Transaxillary approach provides a good exposure and cosmetics in patients with TOS. It should be considered as the gold standard in the management of TOS (10)[B].

- Supraclavicular scalenectomy (11)[C]

- Isolated pectoral minor tenotomy (PMT) is a low-risk outpatient procedure that is effective for the treatment of selected patients with disabling NTOS, with early outcomes similar to supraclavicular decompression + PMT (12)[A].

- Excision of adhesive bands, anterior scalenectomy (13)[B]

INPATIENT CONSIDERATIONS
Admission Criteria/Initial Stabilization

Conservative, outpatient, nonpharmacologic treatment is reasonable first-line therapy except in cases of thromboembolic phenomena and acute ischemia, symptoms of chronic vascular occlusion, stenosis, arterial dilatation, or progressive neurologic deficit (7)[B].

 ## ONGOING CARE

FOLLOW-UP RECOMMENDATIONS

Correct improper posture, practice proper posture, exercises to strengthen shoulder elevator and neck extensor muscles, stretching exercises for scalene muscles, support bra for women with pendulous breasts, breast reduction surgery in selected cases; sleep with arms below chest level, avoid/reduce prolonged hyperabduction.

Patient Monitoring
Office follow-up visits every 3 to 4 weeks

PATIENT EDUCATION
Physical therapy, postural exercises, ergonomic workstation

PROGNOSIS
Follow-up from surgery at mean of 7.5 years showed that functional results were excellent, good, fair, and poor in 87 (49.4%), 61 (34.6%), 14 (8%), and 14 (8%) procedures, respectively (14).

Durable long-term functional outcomes can be achieved predicated on a highly selective approach to the surgical management of patients with TOS. A majority of operated patients will not require adjunctive procedures or chronic narcotic use (15).

COMPLICATIONS
- Postoperative shoulder, arm, hand pain, and paresthesias in 10%
- Patients who will have symptomatic recurrences at 1 month to 7 years postoperatively (usually within 3 months): 1.5–2%
- Patients who will have brachial plexus injury, probably due to intraoperative traction: 0.5–1%
- Reoperation is indicated for symptomatic recurrence with long posterior remnant of 1st rib (posterior approach) or with disrupted fibrous adhesions (transaxillary approach).
- Venous obstruction or arterial emboli; usually responds to thrombolytics

REFERENCES

1. Huang JH, Zager EL. Thoracic outlet syndrome. *Neurosurgery.* 2004;55(4):897–902.
2. Magill ST, Brus-Ramer M, Weinstein PR, et al. Neurogenic thoracic outlet syndrome: current diagnostic criteria and advances in MRI diagnostics. *Neurosurg Focus.* 2015;39(3):E7.
3. Ersoy H, Steigner ML, Coyner KB, et al. Vascular thoracic outlet syndrome: protocol design and diagnostic value of contrast-enhanced 3D MR angiography and equilibrium phase imaging on 1.5- and 3-T MRI scanners. *AJR Am J Roentgenol.* 2012;198(5):1180–1187.
4. Sanders RJ, Hammond SL, Rao NM. Diagnosis of thoracic outlet syndrome. *J Vasc Surg.* 2007;46(3):601–604.
5. Lee GW, Kwon YH, Jeong JH, et al. The efficacy of scalene injection in thoracic outlet syndrome. *J Korean Neurosurg Soc.* 2011;50(1):36–39.
6. Christo PJ, Christo DK, Carinci AJ, et al. Single CT-guided chemodenervation of the anterior scalene muscle with botulinum toxin for neurogenic thoracic outlet syndrome. *Pain Med.* 2010;11(4):504–511.
7. Vanti C, Natalini L, Romeo A, et al. Conservative treatment of thoracic outlet syndrome. A review of the literature. *Eura Medicophys.* 2007;43(1):55–70.
8. Orlando MS, Likes KC, Mirza S, et al. A decade of excellent outcomes after surgical intervention in 538 patients with thoracic outlet syndrome. *J Am Coll Surg.* 2015;220(5):934–939.
9. Sheth RN, Campbell JN. Surgical treatment of thoracic outlet syndrome: a randomized trial comparing two operations. *J Neurosurg Spine.* 2005;3(5):355–363.
10. Lattoo MR, Dar AM, Wani ML, et al. Outcome of trans-axillary approach for surgical decompression of thoracic outlet: a retrospective study in a tertiary care hospital. *Oman Med J.* 2014;29(3):214–216.
11. Glynn RW, Tawfick W, Elsafty Z, et al. Supraclavicular scalenectomy for thoracic outlet syndrome—functional outcomes assessed using the DASH scoring system. *Vasc Endovascular Surg.* 2012;46(2):157–162.
12. Vemuri C, Wittenberg AM, Caputo FJ, et al. Early effectiveness of isolated pectoralis minor tenotomy in selected patients with neurogenic thoracic outlet syndrome. *J Vasc Surg.* 2013;57(5):1345–1352.
13. Urschel HC, Kourlis H. Thoracic outlet syndrome: a 50-year experience at Baylor University Medical Center. *Proc (Bayl Univ Med Cent).* 2007;20(2):125–135.
14. Degeorges R, Reynaud C, Becquemin JP. Thoracic outlet syndrome surgery: long-term functional results. *Ann Vasc Surg.* 2004;18(5):558–565.
15. Scali S, Stone D, Bjerke A, et al. Long-term functional results for the surgical management of neurogenic thoracic outlet syndrome. *Vasc Endovascular Surg.* 2010;44(7):550–555.

ADDITIONAL READING

Povlsen B, Belzberg A, Hansson T, et al. Treatment for thoracic outlet syndrome. *Cochrane Database Syst Rev.* 2010;(1):CD007218.

 ## CODES

ICD10
G54.0 Brachial plexus disorders

CLINICAL PEARLS

- Consider breast reduction for patients with pendulous breasts.
- Avoid opiate dependence.
- Consider pain clinic referral if there are nonsurgical causes.

T

THROMBOPHILIA AND HYPERCOAGULABLE STATES

Kirsten Vitrikas, MD

 BASICS

DESCRIPTION
- An inherited or acquired disorder of the coagulation system predisposing an individual to thromboembolism (the formation of a venous, or less commonly, an arterial blood clot) (1)
- Venous thrombosis typically manifests as deep venous thrombosis (DVT) of the lower extremity in the legs or pelvis and pulmonary embolism (PE) (1).
- System(s) affected: cardiovascular, nervous, pulmonary, reproductive, hematologic
- Synonym(s): hypercoagulation syndrome; prothrombotic state

EPIDEMIOLOGY
- An inherited thrombophilic defect or risk can be detected in up to 50% of patients with venous thromboembolism (VTE).
- Factor V Leiden is the most common inherited thrombophilia (1/2 of all currently characterizable inherited thrombophilia cases involve the factor V Leiden mutation), and it is present in its heterozygous form in up to ~20% of patients with a first VTE.
- Heterozygous prothrombin G20210A mutation, the second most common inherited thrombophilia, is present in up to ~8% of patients with VTE.

Incidence
First-time thromboembolism
- ~100/100,000/year among the general population
- <1/100,000/year in those age <15 years
- ~1,000/100,000/year in those age ≥85 years

Prevalence
- 40–80% of lower extremity orthopedic procedures can result in DVT if prophylaxis is not used.
- VTE accounts for ~1.2 to 4.7 deaths per 100,000 pregnancies.

ETIOLOGY AND PATHOPHYSIOLOGY
- Virchow triad as a cause of VTE includes blood stasis, vascular endothelial injury, and abnormalities in circulating blood constituents (i.e., hypercoagulability).
- An imbalance between the hemostatic and fibrinolytic pathways leads to thrombus formation.
- VTE is considered to be the result of genetic tendencies with other acquired risks.
- Upper extremity DVT: >60% are associated with venous catheters. Malignancy is an additional significant risk (2).

Genetics
- The most common genetic thrombophilias (factor V Leiden, prothrombin G20210A, proteins C and S, and antithrombin III deficiency) are inherited in an autosomal dominant pattern.
- Homozygous mutations generally have a higher risk of VTE.
- Factor V Leiden/activated protein C (aPC) resistance is the most common inherited thrombophilia.
  - 2–5% prevalence among Caucasians; rare in African Americans or Asians
  - aPC does not cleave factor Va, so thrombin formation continues.
  - Other acquired risks are synergistic (3).
- Prothrombin gene mutation G20210A: prevalence 6% among Caucasians. Heterozygous carriers have increased risk of thrombosis.
- Hyperhomocysteinemia: 5–6% among the general population; increases risk of coronary artery disease/

myocardial infarction, cerebrovascular accident, and DVT/PE; acquired in those with folate, vitamin B_{12}, and vitamin B_6 deficiencies
- Antithrombin deficiency: <0.2% among the general population; produced in the liver; acquired deficiency in disseminated intravascular coagulation (DIC), sepsis, liver disease, nephrotic syndrome
- Protein C and S deficiencies: 0.5% and 1% incidences, respectively, among the general population. Homozygotes and heterozygotes are hypercoagulable. Vitamin K–dependent, produced in the liver. Protein C inactivates Va and VIIIa. Protein C may become an acquired deficiency in liver disease, sepsis, DIC, acute respiratory distress syndrome, and after surgery. Protein S is a cofactor for protein C, and it may become an acquired deficiency with oral contraceptive pill (OCP) use, pregnancy, liver disease, sepsis, DIC, HIV, and nephrosis.

RISK FACTORS
- Acquired risk factors
  - Immobilization or prolonged travel
  - Trauma
  - Surgery, especially orthopedic
  - Malignancies (especially pancreatic, ovarian, brain, and lymphoma)
  - Pregnancy
  - Acute medical illness
  - Exogenous female hormones/oral contraceptives
  - Obesity
  - Nephrotic syndrome
  - Antiphospholipid syndrome (APS) and lupus anticoagulant
  - Myeloproliferative disorders (polycythemia vera, essential thrombocythemia)
  - Hyperviscosity syndromes (sickle cell, paraproteinemias)
  - Hyperhomocysteinemia secondary to vitamin deficiencies (B_6, B_{12}, folic acid)
  - Tamoxifen, thalidomide, lenalidomide, bevacizumab, L-asparaginase, erythropoietic stimulating agents
  - Previous thromboembolism
- Established genetic factors
  - Factor V Leiden
  - Prothrombin G20210A mutation
  - Protein C deficiency
  - Protein S deficiency
  - Antithrombin III deficiency
- Rare genetic factors
  - Dysfibrinogenemia
  - Hyperhomocysteinemia (methylene tetrahydrofolate reductase mutation)
- Indeterminate factors
  - Elevated factor VIII
- Age: >60 years
- Gender: men
- Race: Incidence is higher among African Americans.

GENERAL PREVENTION
- Consider prophylaxis with medications in any hospitalized patient with VTE risk factors; hospitalized patients should be encouraged to ambulate as soon as possible (4)[A].
- Consider mechanical prophylaxis in patients at increased risk for VTE in whom anticoagulation may be contraindicated (4)[A].
- Consider prophylaxis with low-molecular-weight heparin (LMWH) plus aspirin in pregnant patients with APS or other thrombophilia.

- Consider prophylaxis using LMWH in patients with solid tumors who have additional risk factors for VTE.
- Prophylaxis with unfractionated heparin (UFH) or LMWH should be considered in patients with genetic or acquired risks of thrombosis and an anticipated additional risk, such as the immobilization associated with surgery.
- Use caution with procoagulant medicines (e.g., OCPs) in asymptomatic individuals who have a known hereditary predisposition.

COMMONLY ASSOCIATED CONDITIONS
Advanced age, cancer, pregnancy, obesity, prior history of thrombosis, surgery, immobilization

 DIAGNOSIS

HISTORY
Consider prothrombotic assessment for the following:
- Unprovoked thrombosis at age <45 to 50 years
- Thrombosis at an unusual anatomic site or recurrent thromboses
- Family history suggesting multiple individuals affected with VTE
- Recurrent pregnancy loss or thrombosis with OCP use

PHYSICAL EXAM
- DVT: swelling, pain, warmth, and redness, usually of one extremity
- PE: dyspnea, pleurisy, hemoptysis, hypoxia, tachycardia
- Superficial phlebitis: red, painful cord palpable along the path of thrombosed vein
- Postthrombotic syndrome: pain, swelling, pigmentation, and/or ulceration

DIAGNOSTIC TESTS & INTERPRETATION
Testing for heritable thrombophilia in all patients with a first episode of VTE is not required (2,5)[B].

Initial Tests (lab, imaging)
- CBC
- aPC profile: ≤2.0 implies factor V Leiden mutation; 95–100% are factor V Leiden-positive; false-positive finding in pregnancy or with use of OCPs, confirm with factor V Leiden mutation testing or consider Factor V Leiden mutation testing up front.
  - aPC resistance may be unreliable while taking LMWH or UFH.
- Prothrombin G20210A genetic assay
- ATIII functional assay
  - Will be low with acute thrombosis and on heparin therapy
- Protein C functional assay
  - May be low with acute thrombosis; will be lower on warfarin
- Protein S antigen and functional assay and free S
  - May be low with acute thrombosis; will be lower on warfarin
- Antiphospholipid antibodies: phospholipid-dependent tests and anticardiolipin antibodies, lupus anticoagulant
  - May be unreliable on heparin
- Consider evaluation for subclinical malignancy in an unprovoked thrombosis in those >40 years of age or at greater risk.
- Consider homocysteine level, although treatment of hyperhomocysteinemia (vitamins B_{12} and B_6, folate) does not alter the thrombophilic risk.

Follow-Up Tests & Special Considerations
Dysfibrinogenemia and plasminogen deficiency are
very rare causes of thrombophilia.

 TREATMENT

MEDICATION

First Line
- Parenteral anticoagulation: LMWH has largely
replaced UFH as first-line therapy for VTE.
  - Enoxaparin (Lovenox): 1 mg/kg SC BID for at least
5 days (with concomitant warfarin) until international normalized ratio (INR) has reached 2 for at
least 24 hours; adjust dose for renal disease.
    ○ Enoxaparin is preferred in patients with active
cancer for a minimum of 6 months (can dose at
1.5 mg/kg SC daily), after which time the patient can be reevaluated to continue enoxaparin
or transition to warfarin (4).
    ○ Adverse reactions: bleeding, heparin-induced
thrombocytopenia (HIT) <0.5% incidence, bone
loss (uncommon)
    ○ Reversal: Stop LMWH.
  - UFH: 80 U/kg or 5,000 U IV bolus, then
18 U/kg/hr or 1,000 U/hr to target the activated
partial thromboplastin time (aPTT) to a corresponding anti-Xa level of 0.3 to 0.7 U/mL.
The first aPTT should be checked 6 hours after
initial therapy and adjusted per standard heparin
nomograms, aiming for an adequate level within
24 hours. Transition to warfarin is similar to the
recommendations for enoxaparin.
    ○ SC UFH is an alternative and can be given as
5,000 U IV (once) followed by 250 U/kg SC BID,
or 250 U/kg bolus followed by 250 U/kg BID
(monitored as for IV UFH), or 333 U/kg once
followed by 250 U/kg SC BID (unmonitored).
    ○ Adverse reactions: bleeding, HIT 3% incidence,
bone loss (long-term use)
    ○ Reversal: Stop heparin, protamine.
- Oral anticoagulation
  - Warfarin (Coumadin): 10 mg/day initially and adjust to INR 2 to 3 for at least 3 months, potentially
indefinitely in those with high risk of recurrence,
recurrent or unprovoked VTE
    ○ Warfarin requires careful and frequent monitor-
ing because of many drug–drug and drug–diet
(e.g., vitamin K) interactions.
    ○ Adverse reactions: bleeding, skin necrosis (rare
and early in course)
    ○ Reversal: four-factor prothrombin complex
concentrate (PCC); fresh frozen plasma and/or
vitamin K
- Pregnancy (controversial): Low-dose aspirin and/or
LMWH or UFH; warfarin is contraindicated.
- Several other newly approved anticoagulant medications are indicated for acute management. Their
main benefit is the decreased need for frequent
testing. However, most of the new medications do
not have a reversal agent.

Second Line
Usually indicated when contraindication to heparin
or LMWH, such as heparin-associated thrombosis
and thrombocytopenia, if there is an inability to use
IV drugs, or renal failure. Direct oral anticoagulants
may become first line as more clinical experience is
developed.
- Factor Xa inhibitors
  - Fondaparinux: acute VTE/PE. Weight <50 kg:
5 mg/day SC; weight 50 to 100 kg: 7.5 mg/day

SC; weight >100 kg: 10 mg/day SC; use for 5 to
9 days until oral anticoagulation is therapeutic.
    ○ Prophylaxis: 2.5 mg/day SC
    ○ Dose adjustments: needed for renal insuf-
ficiency; if creatinine clearance is <30 mL/min,
use is contraindicated.
- Oral factor Xa inhibitors
  - Rivaroxaban: FDA-approved for postoperative
thromboprophylaxis after hip/knee replacement,
treatment of DVT/PE, and for thromboembolic
prophylaxis in patients with nonvalvular atrial
fibrillation (6)[C]
  - Apixaban: can be used without need for preceding heparin therapy, less renal clearance than
other oral anticoagulants
  - Edoxaban: requires treatment with heparin
prior to initiation, needs adjustment for renal
impairment
- Direct thrombin inhibitors: most commonly used for
anticoagulation in HIT. Representative drugs include
the following:
  - Lepirudin: excreted by kidneys, crosses the
placenta; dosing based on creatinine clearance;
therapeutic dose based on aPTT
  - Argatroban: liver metabolized; may be dose-
adjusted in liver dysfunction; therapeutic dose
based on aPTT
  - Dabigatran: oral direct thrombin inhibitor, FDA-
approved for treatment of DVT/PE after parenteral
anticoagulant and for thromboembolic prophylaxis in patients with nonvalvular atrial fibrillation
(noninferior to warfarin). Reversal agent newly
available. May be dialyzable (6)[C]

SURGERY/OTHER PROCEDURES
- Catheter extraction/thrombectomy or thrombolysis for unstable cases (e.g., massive PE with
hypotension)
- Inferior vena cava filter
  - Reduces short-term risk of PE in those with
contraindications to anticoagulation (e.g., GI
bleeding, cerebral hemorrhage)
  - May increase long-term risk of recurrent DVT
  - Used for patients with multiple episodes of recurrent thromboembolism despite therapeutic anticoagulation and contraindication to anticoagulation

 ONGOING CARE

FOLLOW-UP RECOMMENDATIONS
Avoid significant risk for trauma (e.g., contact sports,
climbing a ladder).

Patient Monitoring
Monitor warfarin as frequently as needed to maintain
an INR goal of 2 to 3.

DIET
Vitamin K–stable diet if patient is taking warfarin

PATIENT EDUCATION
- Assume that any drug may enhance or attenuate
the warfarin effect.
- Increase the frequency of monitoring following any
medication change to ensure therapeutic anticoagulation and to avoid overanticoagulation, especially
with antibiotics.
- Many drugs may modulate warfarin effect: alcohol,
antibiotics, aspirin, NSAIDs, acetaminophen.

PROGNOSIS
- Anticoagulation should be continued for 3 months
and consideration of longer in those with unprovoked VTE.

- Patients with a provoked VTE (i.e., surgery, hospitalization) not receiving chronic anticoagulation have
a risks of recurrence of 7% (year 1), 16% (year 5),
and 23% (year 10).
- Patients with an unprovoked VTE not receiving
chronic anticoagulation have risks of recurrence of
15% (year 1), 41% (year 5), and 53% (year 10).
- Currently, there are no data from randomized
controlled trials or controlled clinical trials about the
benefits of thrombophilia testing to decrease the
risk of recurrent VTE (1).

COMPLICATIONS
Venous or arterial thrombosis; bleeding in anticoagulated patients

REFERENCES

1. Cohn DM, Vansenne F, de Borgie CA, et al.
Thrombophilia testing for prevention of recurrent
venous thromboembolism. *Cochrane Database
Syst Rev*. 2012;(12):CD007069.
2. Baglin T, Gray E, Greaves M, et al. Clinical guidelines for testing for heritable thrombophilia. *Br J
Haematol*. 2010;149(2):209–220.
3. Anderson JA, Weitz JI. Hypercoagulable states. *Clin
Chest Med*. 2010;31(4):659–673.
4. Hill J, Treasure T. Reducing the risk of venous
thromboembolism in patients admitted to hospital:
summary of NICE guidance. *BMJ*. 2010;340:c95.
5. National Institute for Health and Care Excellence.
*Venous Thromboembolic Diseases: Diagnosis,
Management and Thrombophilia Testing* (NICE
Clinical Guidelines No. 144). London, United
Kingdom: National Institute for Health and Care
Excellence; 2012.
6. Bacchus F, Schulman S. Clinical experience with the
new oral anticoagulants for treatment of venous
thromboembolism. *Arterioscler Thromb Vasc Biol*.
2015;35(3):513–519.

ADDITIONAL READING

Guyatt GH, Akl EA, Crowther M, et al. Executive
summary: antithrombotic therapy and prevention
of thrombosis, 9th ed: American College of Chest
Physicians evidence-based clinical practice guidelines.
Chest. 2012;141(2)(Suppl): 7S–47S.

 CODES

ICD10
- D68.59 Other primary thrombophilia
- D68.51 Activated protein C resistance
- D68.2 hereditary deficiency of other clotting factors

CLINICAL PEARLS
- Factor V Leiden (resistance to aPC) is the most common inherited thrombophilia, with a prevalence of
2–7% in the U.S. Caucasian population.
- Test patients <50 years of age with a history of
venous thrombosis, and consider testing first-degree
relatives.
- Rule out malignancy, especially in those >50 years
of age.

THROMBOTIC THROMBOCYTOPENIC PURPURA

Hedy Smith, MD, PhD • Kellie A. Sprague, MD

BASICS

DESCRIPTION
- An acute syndrome of microangiopathic hemolytic anemia (MAHA) and consumptive thrombocytopenia with deposition of hyaline thrombi in terminal arterioles and capillaries leading to ischemic multiorgan damage
- Thrombotic thrombocytopenic purpura (TTP) is characterized by MAHA and thrombocytopenia, with or without the following signs and symptoms (1):
  - Neurologic symptoms
  - Renal dysfunction
  - Fever
  - Most patients do not show the historic pentad of MAHA, thrombocytopenia, renal dysfunction, neurologic abnormalities, and fever because treatment is initiated before the pentad can develop.

EPIDEMIOLOGY
Incidence
- Predominant age: 18 to 49 years
- Predominant sex: female > male (3:1)
- Incidence ratio in blacks to whites is 7:1
- The age–sex–race standardized incidence of clinically suspected TTP is 8 million/year and 2 million/year in those with ADAMTS13 levels <10% (2).

ETIOLOGY AND PATHOPHYSIOLOGY
- In TTP, the aggregating agent responsible for platelet thrombi is unusually large von Willebrand factor (UL vWF) multimers, which are far larger than those found in normal plasma.
- A metalloproteinase, ADAMTS13, which normally enzymatically cleaves UL vWF multimers to prevent clumping within vessels, is deficient, defective, or absent, allowing UL vWF to react with platelets. This leads to the endothelial cell damage and disseminated thrombi characteristic of TTP.
- Arterioles most often affected are in the brain, kidney, pancreas, heart, and adrenal glands. Lungs and liver are relatively spared.
- In familial TTP, patients have an inherited deficiency of ADAMTS13 (1).
- In acquired idiopathic TTP, autoantibodies are directed against the metalloproteinase ADAMTS13 (1,3).
- Endothelial injury, either directly from a drug/toxin or indirectly via platelet/neutrophil activation has been proposed as a cause of secondary TTP especially in those without ADAMTS13 deficiency.
  - Drug-induced (see "Risk Factors")
  - Hematopoietic cell transplantation

Genetics
TTP is most often an acquired disorder. A congenital form of inherited TTP (Schulman-Upshaw syndrome) is due to a mutation at the ADAMTS13 metalloproteinase gene locus on chromosome 9q34. This rare form of TTP has an autosomal-recessive pattern of inheritance (4).

RISK FACTORS
- Pregnancy and oral contraceptives
- AIDS and early symptomatic HIV infection
- Autoimmune disease
  - Antiphospholipid antibody syndrome
  - Systemic lupus erythematosus
  - Scleroderma
- Cancer

- Hematopoietic stem cell transplantation
- Drug toxicity
  - Cancer chemotherapy
    ○ Mitomycin C and gemcitabine
    ○ Bleomycin and cisplatin
    ○ Bevacizumab
  - Calcineurin inhibitors
    ○ Tacrolimus and cyclosporine
  - Immune-mediated
    ○ Quinine and quinidine
    ○ Ticlopidine and clopidogrel

COMMONLY ASSOCIATED CONDITIONS
- TTP/HUS/atypical HUS (hemolytic uremic syndrome) have similar presentations with MAHA and thrombocytopenia and multiorgan involvement.
- TTP generally presents with minimal renal involvement and may have neurologic abnormalities, whereas the opposite is more characteristic of HUS/atypical HUS.
- However, patients with HUS and TTP may have both prominent renal and neurologic manifestations, often making the diagnosis unclear, hence the historical hybrid name "TTP-HUS."
- ADAMTS13 levels are diminished in adults with familial or acquired idiopathic TTP but are normal in children diagnosed with HUS following infection with Escherichia coli (particularly type O157:H7), so-called Shiga toxin-HUS, and in "atypical HUS," is also called complement mediated thrombotic microangiopathy reflecting the pathophysiology which is related to complement dysregulation.

DIAGNOSIS

- Most common symptoms are nonspecific: nausea, vomiting, weakness, abdominal pain, fatigue, fever
- Related to thrombocytopenia
  - Easy bruising, purpura, or petechiae
  - Epistaxis, menorrhagia, bleeding gums
  - GI bleeding
  - Intracranial hemorrhage
  - Visual symptoms due to retinal hemorrhage
- Related to hemolytic anemia (MAHA): jaundice, fatigue
- Related to end-organ ischemia
  - Neurologic: CNS symptoms occur in 50%.
    ○ Often fluctuating symptoms
    ○ Headache
    ○ Altered mental status: Spectrum runs from behavioral/personality changes to obtundation/stupor/coma.
    ○ Seizures
    ○ Stroke
  - Renal: hematuria, oliguria, or anuria
  - Cardiac: arrhythmia, myocardial infarction, heart failure

HISTORY
- Generally acute onset of symptoms but subacute in about 1/4 of patients
- It is important to assess for potential underlying causes or risk factors (see discussion earlier).

PHYSICAL EXAM
- Fever
- Mental status/neurologic: confusion, coma, stupor, weakness

- HEENT: retinal hemorrhage, scleral icterus, epistaxis
- Abdomen/GI: nonspecific tenderness
- Skin: jaundice, petechiae, purpura, ecchymoses

DIFFERENTIAL DIAGNOSIS
- HUS and atypical HUS: See "Commonly Associated Conditions."
- Antiphospholipid antibody syndrome: prolonged partial thromboplastin time (PTT) and presence of lupus anticoagulant
- Systemic lupus erythematosus
- Malignant hypertension (HTN): diastolic >130 mm Hg, papilledema, retinal hemorrhages
- Pregnancy-associated preeclampsia/eclampsia or hemolysis, elevated liver enzyme levels, and low platelet HELLP levels: low ATIII levels
- Disseminated intravascular coagulation
  - Prolonged prothrombin time (PT)/PTT, low fibrinogen
  - Low factors V and VIII
  - Secondary to sepsis/shock or widely disseminated malignancy
- Idiopathic thrombocytopenic purpura (ITP)
  - No hemolysis, normal lactate dehydrogenase (LDH) and bilirubin
  - Presence of antiplatelet antibodies
- Malignancy-associated microangiopathy
- Evan syndrome (autoimmune hemolytic anemia and thrombocytopenia): positive direct Coombs test
- Sclerodermal kidney

DIAGNOSTIC TESTS & INTERPRETATION
Initial Tests (lab, imaging)
- CBC
  - Hemoglobin (decreased): average is 8 to 10 g/dL
  - Platelets decreased: typically in the 10 to 30,000 range
- Reticulocyte count (increased)
- Haptoglobin decreased (hemolysis)
- Peripheral smear
  - Schistocytes (prominent, >1% of RBCs)
  - Helmet cells, RBC fragments
  - Nucleated RBCs
  - Polychromasia (reticulocytosis)
- Coagulation studies
  - Normal in most; mild elevation in 15%
  - Fibrinogen normal
- Coombs test: negative direct Coombs test
- Electrolytes, BUN/creatinine: mild elevation of BUN and creatinine (creatinine <3 mg/dL)
- Liver function studies: increased indirect bilirubin (hemolysis)
- LDH: 5 to 10 times normal
- Urinalysis
  - Proteinuria, microscopic hematuria
  - Positive dipstick for large blood, but minimal RBCs on microscopic exam
- ECG: sinus tachycardia, heart block
- Troponin: increased if cardiac involvement
- HIV, hepatitis A, B, C testing: Exclude underlying viral precipitant.
- Pregnancy test
- Pretreatment ADAMTS13 activity level of <10% is useful in distinguishing acquired or familial TTP from other disorders.
- Head CT/MRI scan: performed if mental status changes are present to rule out possible intracranial hemorrhage or ischemic changes

Test Interpretation

Biopsy of affected organs shows platelet thrombi within or beneath damaged endothelium. However, biopsy is rarely obtained because the diagnosis is made on clinical grounds and laboratory findings.

 TREATMENT

- Prompt treatment of TTP is necessary due to the high mortality (90%).
- In the absence of another apparent cause, the dyad of MAHA and thrombocytopenia is sufficient to begin treatment for TTP while the workup proceeds (1,3):
  - Plasma exchange transfusion (PEX) is the cornerstone of treatment of classic TTP (3)[A].
  - PEX replaces deficient or defective metalloproteinase (ADAMTS13) and removes UL vWF and antimetalloproteinase antibodies.
  - PEX should begun immediately and continued daily.
  - Optimal PEX duration is variable. Convention is to continue for 2 days after platelet count is ≥150,000, then consider tapering (5)[C].
  - Fresh frozen plasma: temporary measure until PEX can be initiated (3)[B]

MEDICATION
First Line
- Glucocorticoids may be of benefit in some patients. British guidelines recommend its use for all patients (5)[B].
  - Steroids may work by suppressing the autoantibodies inhibiting ADAMTS13 activity.
  - Use may be in patients with severe ADAMTS13 deficiency, in the setting of exacerbation when PEX is stopped or in relapse after remission.
  - Little benefit of steroids when used as monotherapy
  - Doses: prednisone 1 mg/kg/day and taper once in remission or methylprednisolone 1 g/day IV for 3 days
- Rituximab, an anti-CD20 antibody that deletes B cells, may reduce relapse when given in conjunction with PEX and steroids (6).
  - Dose: 375 mg/m^2 IV weekly for 4 weeks

Second Line
The following medications are used in refractory cases:
- Rituximab (5)[B]
- Vincristine, cyclophosphamide cyclosporine
- Intravenous immunoglobulin (IVIG) (3)
- Bortezomib (7)[C],(8)

ISSUES FOR REFERRAL
- Hematology or blood bank for PEX
- Nephrology for dialysis
- Cardiology for presence of significant heart block or ischemia
- Neurosurgery for intracranial hemorrhage

SURGERY/OTHER PROCEDURES
Splenectomy is reserved for severe, refractory cases (9).

INPATIENT CONSIDERATIONS
Admission Criteria/Initial Stabilization
- ABCs, oxygen, IV access, telemetry
- Volume resuscitation if hypotensive/actively bleeding

- Packed RBCs can be transfused safely.
- Platelet transfusion may be used for the treatment of hemorrhage.

Discharge Criteria
On normalization and stabilization of neurologic symptoms, LDH, platelets, and renal function

 ONGOING CARE

FOLLOW-UP RECOMMENDATIONS
- No maintenance therapy is required. After PEX is discontinued, blood counts should be monitored over a few months. If testing results remain normal, testing interval can be lengthened.
- Promptly evaluate any symptoms of relapse.

PATIENT EDUCATION
- On discharge, advise patients to self-monitor for signs of relapse (e.g., fever, headache, bruising).
- Patients should be advised about prolonged periods of fatigue following the acute phase.
- See National Heart, Lung, and Blood Institute Web site: http://www.nhlbi.nih.gov/health/health-topics/topics/ttp

PROGNOSIS
- Most patients recover fully from idiopathic TTP when treated promptly:
  - 30-day mortality is 10% in those who receive PEX.
  - 70% respond within 14 days; 90% respond within 28 days.
  - 80% survival in patients with idiopathic TTP treated with PEX (10)
- Initial LDH and platelet counts are not predictive of the patient's response to treatment.
- Final platelet count and LDH or the length or intensity of treatment does not predict relapse.
- Low levels of ADAMTS13 activity during remission are associated with higher risk of relapse (11).
- In patients with severe ADAMTS13 deficiency, the risk of relapse is estimated to be 41% at 7.5 years, with the greatest risk being in the first year.

COMPLICATIONS
- Patients may experience mild cognitive impairments in attention, concentration, and memory following ≥1 episodes of TTP.
- Complications of PEX include the following:
  - Central line infections and hemorrhage
  - Citrate toxicity
  - Hypersensitivity reactions to frequent plasma exposure
  - Electrolyte abnormalites

REFERENCES

1. Sadler JE. Von Willebrand factor, ADAMTS13, and thrombotic thrombocytopenic purpura. *Blood*. 2008;112(1):11–18.
2. Reese JA, Muthurajah DS, Kremer Hovinga JA, et al. Children and adults with thrombotic thrombocytopenic purpura associated with severe, acquired Adamts13 deficiency: comparison of incidence, demographic and clinical features. *Pediatr Blood Cancer*. 2013;60(10):1676–1682.
3. George JN. Clinical practice. Thrombotic thrombocytopenic purpura. *N Engl J Med*. 2006;354(18): 1927–1935.
4. Levy GG, Nichols WC, Lian EC, et al. Mutations in a member of the ADAMTS gene family cause thrombotic thrombocytopenic purpura. *Nature*. 2001;413(6855):488–494.
5. Scully M, Hunt BJ, Benjamin S, et al. Guidelines on the diagnosis and management of thrombotic thrombocytopenic purpura and other thrombotic microangiopathies. *Br J Haematol*. 2012;158(3): 323–335.
6. Scully M, McDonald V, Cavenagh J, et al. A phase 2 study of the safety and efficacy of rituximab with plasma exchange in acute acquired thrombotic thrombocytopenic purpura. *Blood*. 2011;118(7):1746–1753.
7. Sarode R, Bandarenko N, Brecher ME, et al. Thrombotic thrombocytopenic purpura: 2012 American Society for Apheresis (ASFA) consensus conference on classification, diagnosis, management, and future research. *J Clin Apher*. 2014;29(3):148–167.
8. Yates S, Matevosyan K, Rutherford C, et al. Bortezomib for chronic relapsing thrombotic thrombocytopenic purpura: a case report. *Transfusion*. 2014;54(8):2064–2067.
9. Beloncle F, Buffet M, Coindre JP, et al. Splenectomy and/or cyclophosphamide as salvage therapies in thrombotic thrombocytopenic purpura: the French TMA Reference Center experience. *Transfusion*. 2012;52(11):2436–2444.
10. Kremer Hovinga JA, Vesely SK, Terrell DR, et al. Survival and relapse in patients with thrombotic thrombocytopenic purpura. *Blood*. 2010;115(8):1500–1511.
11. Peyvandi F, Lavoretano S, Palla R, et al. ADAMTS13 and anti-ADAMTS13 antibodies as markers for recurrence of acquired thrombotic thrombocytopenic purpura during remission. *Haematologica*. 2008;93(2):232–239.

ADDITIONAL READING

George JN, Nester CM. Syndromes of thrombotic microangiopathy. *N Engl J Med*. 2014;371(7):654–666.

 CODES

ICD10
- M31.1 Thrombotic microangiopathy
- D69.42 Congenital and hereditary thrombocytopenia purpura
- D69.3 Immune thrombocytopenic purpura

CLINICAL PEARLS

- The diagnosis of TTP is made clinically; common symptoms are nonspecific: nausea, vomiting, weakness, abdominal pain, fatigue, fever, and easy bruising, purpura, or petechiae.
- The historical pentad of fever, neurologic symptoms, renal dysfunction, MAHA, and thrombocytopenia is not present in most patients.
- The dyad of MAHA and thrombocytopenia is sufficient to initiate treatment with PEX.
- Do not wait for results of ADAMTS13 determination to initiate therapy.

THYROID MALIGNANT NEOPLASIA

James P. Miller, MD

BASICS

DESCRIPTION
Thyroid malignant neoplasia is an autologous growth of thyroid nodules with potential for metastases.

- Papillary carcinoma
  - Most common variety, 60–70% of thyroid tumors
  - Peak incidence in the 3rd to 4th decades
  - 3 times more common in women
  - May be associated with radiation exposure
  - Tumor contains psammoma bodies, 50%
  - Metastasizes by lymphatic route (30% at time of diagnosis)
  - Multicentric in ≥20%, especially in children
  - Higher risk in patients with Hashimoto thyroiditis
- Follicular carcinoma
  - 10–20% of thyroid tumors
  - Peak incidence in 5th decade of life
  - Incidence has been decreasing because of the addition of dietary iodine
  - Metastasizes by the hematogenous route
- Hürthle cell carcinoma (variant of follicular with poorer prognosis)
  - 2–3% of thyroid malignancies
  - Usually in patients >60 years old
  - No gender difference
  - Radioresistant
  - Composed of distinct large eosinophilic cells with abundant cytoplasmic mitochondria
  - Variant of follicular carcinoma with worse prognosis
- Medullary thyroid carcinoma (MCT)
  - Arises from parafollicular cells, C cells
  - Multiple endocrine neoplasia (MEN) syndromes (MEN2A, MEN2B, FMTC). Prevalence of MEN2 is 1:30,000.
  - MCT associated with MEN2B occur in childhood, those with MEN2A occur in young adults, and those with FMTC occur at middle age.
  - 3–4% of all thyroid tumors
  - 25–35% are associated with MEN syndromes (2A more common than 2B), which can be familial or sporadic.
  - Calcitonin is a chemical marker.
  - *RET* proto-oncogene mutation is screened; family members who carry the *RET* gene should consider early prophylactic thyroidectomy.
- Anaplastic carcinoma
  - 3% of thyroid tumors
  - Most aggressive form of thyroid neoplasia
  - More common in females
  - Usually in patients >60 years old
- Other: lymphoma, sarcoma, or metastatic (renal, breast, or lung)
- System(s) affected: endocrine/metabolic
- Synonym(s): follicular carcinoma of the thyroid; papillary carcinoma of the thyroid; Hürthle cell carcinoma of the thyroid; anaplastic cell carcinoma of the thyroid

Geriatric Considerations
Risk of malignancy increases at >60 years old.

Pediatric Considerations
- >60% of thyroid nodules are malignant.
- <2% of thyroid malignancies occur in children and adolescents.

EPIDEMIOLOGY
Incidence
- 12.9/100,000 per year in the United States
- Deaths: 0.5/100,000 per year in the United States
- In 2015, estimated 62,450 new cases and 1,950 deaths from thyroid cancer in the United States
- Predominant age: usually >40 years old
- Predominant sex: female > male (2.6:1) prevalence
- Lifetime risk of developing thyroid cancer is 1.1%
- In 2011, 566,708 patients living with thyroid cancer in the United States

ETIOLOGY AND PATHOPHYSIOLOGY
Unknown

Genetics
- Familial polyposis of the colon, Turcot syndrome, and Gardner syndrome with the *APC* gene (5q21)
- Medullary: autosomal dominant with MEN syndrome
- *BRAF* mutation (rare in children)
- *RET* oncogene (more common in children)

RISK FACTORS
- Family history
- Neck irradiation (6 to 2,000 rads): papillary carcinoma
- Iodine deficiency: follicular carcinoma
- MEN2: medullary carcinoma; autosomal dominant
- Previous history of subtotal thyroidectomy for malignancy: anaplastic carcinoma
- Asian race
- Female gender

GENERAL PREVENTION
- Physical exam in high-risk group
- Calcium infusion or pentagastrin stimulation test screening in high-risk MEN patients
- Screen for *RET* proto-oncogene in groups at-risk for MCT.

COMMONLY ASSOCIATED CONDITIONS
Medullary carcinoma: pheochromocytoma, hyperparathyroidism, ganglioneuroma of the GI tract, neuromata of mucosal membranes

DIAGNOSIS

HISTORY
- Change in voice (hoarseness)
- Positive family history
- Neck mass
- Dysphagia
- Dyspnea
- Cough
- Difficulty swallowing

PHYSICAL EXAM
- Neck mass: If fixed to surrounding tissue, this finding suggests advanced disease.
- Cervical adenopathy

DIFFERENTIAL DIAGNOSIS
- Multinodular goiter
- Thyroid adenoma
- Thyroglossal duct cyst
- Thyroiditis
- Thyroid cyst
- Ectopic thyroid
- Dermoid cyst

DIAGNOSTIC TESTS & INTERPRETATION
- Medullary carcinoma: calcitonin level (normal <30 pg/mL [300 ng/L]), pentagastrin stimulation test, and *RET* proto-oncogene
- Thyroglobulin (TG) level: postoperative tumor marker
- DNA content of tumors from biopsy specimen: Diploid content has a better prognosis.
- Thyroid function tests usually normal
- Thyroid scan: 12–15% of cold nodules are malignant; rate is higher in patients <40 years of age and those with microcalcifications on US.
- US: Solid mass and microcalcifications are more suspicious of malignancy.
- CT scan and MRI can be useful to evaluate large substernal masses and recurrent soft tissue masses.
- ^{18}F-FDG positron-emission tomographic scan can help if the cytology is inconclusive; helpful with recurrent disease when patient has a negative ^{131}I scan and an elevated TG level

Diagnostic Procedures/Other
- Fine-needle aspiration (FNA)
- Surgical biopsy/excision
- Laryngoscopy if vocal cord paralysis is suspected.

Test Interpretation
- Papillary: psammoma bodies, anaplastic epithelial papillae
- Follicular: anaplastic epithelial cords with follicles
- Hürthle cell: large eosinophilic cells with granular cytoplasm
- Medullary: large amounts of amyloid stroma
- Anaplastic: small cell and giant cell undifferentiated tumors

TREATMENT

MEDICATION
Postoperatively, will require thyroid hormone replacement: Goal is to keep TSH <0.1 mU/L.
- Levothyroxine (T$_4$, Synthroid) 100 to 200 μg/day
- Liothyronine (T$_3$, Cytomel) 50 to 100 μg/day

GENERAL MEASURES
- Papillary/follicular: [131]I thyroid remnant ablation
- Medullary: Vandetanib has been tried in patients with advanced disease (1)[B].
- Anaplastic: Doxorubicin and cisplatin have achieved partial remission in some patients (2)[B].
- Recurrent tumor: Sorafenib has been used in patients with recurrent disease.

ADDITIONAL THERAPIES
- External beam radiation for advanced disease
- [131]I is used in high-risk patients with papillary and follicular tumors. The role is to ablate remnant thyroid tissue to improve specificity of future TG assays (3)[C].

SURGERY/OTHER PROCEDURES
- Papillary carcinoma: lobectomy with isthmectomy (if lesion <1 cm) or total thyroidectomy and removal of suspicious lymph nodes. Total thyroidectomy for tumors >1 cm (4)[B]
- Follicular carcinoma and Hürthle cell: total thyroidectomy and removal of suspicious lymph nodes
- Medullary carcinoma: total thyroidectomy with central node dissection; unilateral or bilateral modified radical neck dissection if lateral nodes are histologically positive
- Anaplastic carcinoma: aggressive en bloc thyroidectomy; tracheostomy often required; not responsive to [131]I

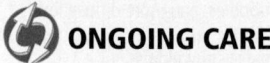 ONGOING CARE

FOLLOW-UP RECOMMENDATIONS
Patient Monitoring
- 10–30% of initially disease-free patients will develop recurrence and/or metastases. 80% recur in neck and 20% with distant metastases. Lung is most common site of distant metastases.
- Thyroid scan at 6 weeks and administration of ^{131}I for any visible uptake; any evidence of residual thyroid tissue (after total thyroidectomy) or lymph node disease noted on scan is treated with radioactive iodine.
- At 6 months and then yearly, the patient should have a thyroid scan and chest x-ray.
- Papillary and follicular: a TG level should be done yearly. Recombinant human thyroid-stimulating hormone (rhTSH)–stimulated TG level may be more sensitive.
- Medullary: Calcitonin level should be done yearly with pentagastrin stimulation.
- The thyroid scan and TG level should be done with the patient in the hypothyroid state induced by 6-week withdrawal of levothyroxine or 2- to 3-week withdrawal of liothyronine.
- Decreased incidence of recurrence when TSH is suppressed.

DIET
Avoid iodine deficiency.

PATIENT EDUCATION
National Cancer Institute: (301) 496-5583; http://www.cancer.gov

PROGNOSIS
- Taken together: 5-year survival of thyroid cancer is 97.8%.
- Favorable factors: female, multifocality, regional LN involvement
- Adverse factors: age >45 years, follicular histology, primary tumor >4 cm, extrathyroid extension, distant metastases
- Papillary carcinoma: 10-year overall survival is 93%; 30-year cancer-related death rate of 6%
- Follicular carcinoma: 10-year overall survival is 85%; histologically, microinvasive tumors parallel papillary tumor results, whereas grossly invasive tumors do far worse; 30-year cancer-related death rate of 15%
- Hürthle cell carcinoma: 93% 5-year survival rate and 83% survival rate overall; grossly invasive tumor survival <25%
- Medullary carcinoma: negative nodes, 90% 5-year survival rate and 85% 10-year survival rate; with positive nodes, 65% 5-year survival rate and 40% 10-year survival rate. Prognosis worse for MEN2B compared to MEN2A. Overall 10-year survival is 75%.
- Anaplastic carcinoma: survival unexpected. Long-term survivors should have original pathology reexamined.

COMPLICATIONS
- Recurrence of tumor is 10–30%; 80% recur in neck, and 20% recur distally
- Hoarseness from tumor invasion or operative injury to recurrent laryngeal nerve
- Hypoparathyroidism from operative injury to parathyroid glands

REFERENCES
1. Wells SA Jr, Robinson BG, Gagel RF, et al. Vandetanib in patients with locally advanced or metastatic medullary thyroid cancer: a randomized, double-blind phase III trial. *J Clin Oncol.* 2012; 30(2):134–141.
2. Shimaoka K, Schoenfeld DA, DeWys WD, et al. A randomized trial of doxorubicin versus doxorubicin plus cisplatin in patients with advanced thyroid carcinoma. *Cancer.* 1985;56(9):2155–2160.
3. Mazzaferri EL, Jhiang SM. Long-term impact of initial surgical and medical therapy on papillary and follicular thyroid cancer. *Am J Med.* 1994; 97(5):418–428.
4. Bilimoria KY, Bentrem DJ, Ko CY, et al. Extent of surgery affects survival for papillary thyroid cancer. *Ann Surg.* 2007;246(3):375–381.

ADDITIONAL READING
- Blamey S, Barraclough B, Delbridge L, et al. Using recombinant human thyroid-stimulating hormone for the diagnosis of recurrent thyroid cancer. *ANZ J Surg.* 2005;75(1–2):10–20.
- Burns WR, Zeiger MA. Differentiated thyroid cancer. *Semin Oncol.* 2010;37(6):557–566.
- Cox AE, LeBeau SO. Diagnosis and treatment of differentiated thyroid carcinoma. *Radiol Clin North Am.* 2011;49(3):453–462, vi.
- Haugen BR, Pacini F, Reiners C, et al. A comparison of recombinant human thyrotropin and thyroid hormone withdrawal for the detection of thyroid remnant or cancer. *J Clin Endocrinol Metab.* 1999; 84(11):3877–3885.
- Marsh DJ, Gimm O. Multiple endocrine neoplasia: types 1 and 2. *Adv Otorhinolaryngol.* 2011;70:84–90.
- Pitt SC, Moley JF. Medullary, anaplastic, and metastatic cancers of the thyroid. *Semin Oncol.* 2010; 37(6):567–579.
- Wang W, Larson SM, Fazzari M, et al. Prognostic value of [18F]fluorodeoxyglucose positron emission tomographic scanning in patients with thyroid cancer. *J Clin Endocrinol Metab.* 2000;85(3):1107–1113.

 ## SEE ALSO

Multiple Endocrine Neoplasia (MEN) Syndromes

 ## CODES

ICD10
C73 Malignant neoplasm of thyroid gland

CLINICAL PEARLS
- Standard workup for a patient suspected of having a thyroid cancer is a physical exam, TSH level, neck US, and FNA.
- TG levels can be elevated in several thyroid disorders. Its usefulness comes once the diagnosis of cancer has been made. It serves as a better marker for recurrent disease.
- ~2% of the normal population will have a positive [18F]-FDG positron-emission tomographic scan, so it is more useful for postresection follow-up.
- FNA results will be benign, malignant, indeterminate, or nondiagnostic. More helpful in planning initial surgical approach.

T

THYROIDITIS

Robert A. Baldor, MD, FAAFP

 BASICS

DESCRIPTION

Inflammation of the thyroid gland that may be painful or painless

- Thyroiditis with thyroid pain
  - Subacute granulomatous thyroiditis (nonsuppurative thyroiditis, de Quervain thyroiditis, or giant cell thyroiditis): self-limited; viral URI prodrome, symptoms and signs of thyroid dysfunction (variable)
  - Infectious/suppurative thyroiditis
    - Bacterial, fungal, mycobacterial, or parasitic infection of the thyroid
    - Most commonly associated with *Streptococcus pyogenes, Staphylococcus aureus,* and *Streptococcus pneumoniae*
  - Radiation-induced thyroiditis: from radioactive iodine therapy (1%) or external irradiation for lymphoma and head/neck cancers
- Thyroiditis with no thyroid pain
  - Hashimoto (autoimmune) thyroiditis (chronic lymphocytic thyroiditis): most common etiology of chronic hypothyroidism; autoimmune disease; 90% of patients with high-serum antithyroid peroxidase (TPO) antibodies
  - Postpartum thyroiditis: episode of thyrotoxicosis, hypothyroidism, or thyrotoxicosis followed by hypothyroidism in the 1st year postpartum or after spontaneous/induced abortion in women who were without clinically evident thyroid disease before pregnancy
  - Painless (silent) thyroiditis (subacute lymphocytic thyroiditis): mild hyperthyroidism, small painless goiter, and no Graves ophthalmopathy/pretibial myxedema
  - Riedel (fibrous) thyroiditis: rare inflammatory process involving the thyroid and surrounding cervical tissues; associated with various forms of systemic fibrosis; presents as a firm mass in the thyroid commonly associated with compressive symptoms (dyspnea, dysphagia, hoarseness, and aphonia) caused by local infiltration of the advancing fibrotic process with hypocalcemia and hypothyroidism
  - Drug-induced thyroiditis: interferon-α, interleukin-2, amiodarone, or lithium

EPIDEMIOLOGY

- Subacute granulomatous thyroiditis: most common cause of thyroid pain; peaks during summer; incidence: 3/100,000/year; female > male (4:1); peak age: 40 to 50 years
- Suppurative thyroiditis: commonly seen with preexisting thyroid disease/immunocompromise
- Hashimoto thyroiditis: peak age of onset, 30 to 50 years; can occur in children; primarily a disease of women; female > male (7:1)
- Postpartum thyroiditis: Female only; occurs within 12 months of pregnancy in 8–11% of pregnancies; occurs in 25% with type 1 diabetes mellitus; incidence is affected by genetic influences and iodine intake.
- Painless (silent) thyroiditis: female > male (4:1) with peak age 30 to 40 years; common in areas of iodine sufficiency
- Riedel thyroiditis: female > male (4:1); highest prevalence age 30 to 60 years

ETIOLOGY AND PATHOPHYSIOLOGY

- Hashimoto disease: Antithyroid antibodies may be produced in response to an environmental antigen and cross-react with thyroid proteins (molecular mimicry). Precipitating factors include infection, stress, sex steroids, pregnancy, iodine intake, and radiation exposure.
- Subacute granulomatous thyroiditis: probably viral
- Postpartum thyroiditis: autoimmunity-induced discharge of preformed hormone from the thyroid
- Painless (silent) thyroiditis: autoimmune

Genetics

Autoimmune thyroiditis is associated with the CT60 polymorphism of cytotoxic T-cell lymphocyte–associated antigen 4. Also associated with HLA-DR4, -DR5, and -DR6 in whites

RISK FACTORS

- Hashimoto disease: family history of thyroid/autoimmune disease, personal history of autoimmune disease (type 1 diabetes, celiac disease), high iodine intake, cigarette smoking, selenium deficiency
- Subacute granulomatous thyroiditis: recent viral respiratory infection
- Suppurative thyroiditis: congenital abnormalities (persistent thyroglossal duct/piriform sinus fistula), greater age, immunosuppression
- Radiation-induced thyroiditis: high-dose irradiation, younger age, female sex, preexisting hypothyroidism
- Postpartum thyroiditis: smoking, history of spontaneous/induced abortion
- Painless (silent) thyroiditis: iodine-deficient areas

GENERAL PREVENTION

Selenium may decrease inflammatory activity in pregnant women with autoimmune hypothyroidism and may reduce postpartum thyroiditis risk in those positive for TPO antibodies.

COMMONLY ASSOCIATED CONDITIONS

Postpartum thyroiditis: family history of autoimmune thyroid disease; HLA-DRB, -DR4, and -DR5

DIAGNOSIS

HISTORY

- Hypothyroid symptoms (e.g., constipation, heavy menstrual bleeding, fatigue, weakness, dry skin, hair loss, cold intolerance)
- Hyperthyroid symptoms (e.g., irritability, heat intolerance, increased sweating, palpitations, loose stools, disturbed sleep, and lid retraction)
- Subacute granulomatous thyroiditis: Sudden/gradual onset, with preceding upper respiratory infection/viral illness (fever, fatigue, malaise, anorexia, and myalgia are common); pain may be limited to thyroid region or radiate to upper neck, jaw, throat, or ears.
- Classic triphasic course (thyrotoxic, hypothyroid, recovery) but variable in the following: subacute, silent, and postpartum thyroiditis (1)[C]

PHYSICAL EXAM

- Examine thyroid size, symmetry, and nodules.
  - Hashimoto disease: 90% have a symmetric, diffusely enlarged, painless gland, with a firm, pebbly texture; 10% have thyroid atrophy.

- Postpartum thyroiditis: painless, small, nontender, firm goiter (2 to 6 months after delivery)
- Riedel thyroiditis: rock-hard, wood-like, fixed, painless goiter, often accompanied by symptoms of esophageal/tracheal compression (stridor, dyspnea, a suffocating feeling, dysphagia, and hoarseness)
- Signs of hypothyroid: delayed relaxation phase of deep tendon reflexes, nonpitting edema, dry skin, alopecia, bradycardia
- Signs of hyperthyroid: moist palms, hyperreflexia, tachycardia/atrial fibrillation

DIFFERENTIAL DIAGNOSIS

Simple goiter; iodine-deficient/lithium-induced goiter; Graves disease; lymphoma; acute infectious thyroiditis; oropharynx and trachea infections; thyroid cancer; amiodarone; contrast dye; amyloid

DIAGNOSTIC TESTS & INTERPRETATION

- Thyroid-stimulating hormone (TSH), anti-TPO antibodies
- Hashimoto disease
  - High titers of anti-TPO antibodies
  - New subtype: IgG4 thyroiditis, which is histopathologically characterized by lymphoplasmacytic infiltration, fibrosis, increased numbers of IgG4-positive plasma cells, and high serum IgG4 levels; more closely associated with rapid progress, subclinical hypothyroidism, higher levels of circulating antibodies, and more diffuse low echogenicity (2)[C]
- Subacute granulomatous thyroiditis
  - High T_4, T_3; low TSH during early stages and elevated later; TSH varies with phase (1)[C].
  - High thyroglobulin; normal levels of anti-TPO and antithyroglobulin antibodies (present in 25%, usually low titers)
  - Elevated erythrocyte sedimentation rate (ESR) (usually >50 mm/hr) and C-reactive protein; mild anemia and slight leukocytosis; LFTs are frequently abnormal during initial hyperthyroid phase and resolve over 1 to 2 months.
- Suppurative thyroiditis
  - In the absence of preexisting thyroid disease, thyroid function is normal but hyper-/hypothyroidism may occur.
  - Elevated ESR and WBC with marked increase in left shift
  - Fine-needle aspiration (FNA) of the lesion with Gram stain and culture is the most useful diagnostic test.
- Postpartum thyroiditis (3)[B]
  - Anti-TPO antibody positivity is the most useful marker for the prediction of postpartum thyroid dysfunction.
  - Women known to be anti-TPO-Ab+ should have TSH measured at 6 to 12 weeks' gestation and at 6 months postpartum or as clinically indicated.
  - Thyrotoxic phase occurs 1 and 6 months postpartum (most commonly at 3 months) and usually lasts only 1 to 2 months.
  - Hypothyroidism occurs between 3 and 8 months (most commonly at 6 months).
  - Most patients (80%) have normal thyroid function at 1 year; 30–50% of patients develop permanent hypothyroidism within 9 years.
  - High thyroglobulin, normal ESR

- Painless (silent) thyroiditis
  - Hyperthyroid state in 5–20%: averages 3 to 4 months, and total duration of illness is <1 year, followed by hypothyroidism and then a return to normal state; some have primary/subclinical hypothyroidism.
  - ~50% have anti-TPO antibodies (1)[C].
- Reidel thyroiditis (4)[C]
  - Hypothyroidism due to extensive replacement of the gland by scar tissue. Anti-TPO antibodies are present in 2/3 of patients along with low radioactive iodine uptake (RAIU).
- Drug-induced thyroiditis
  - Hyper-/hypothyroidism, low RAIU, and variable presence of anti-TPO antibodies
- US: shows variable heterogeneous texture, hypoechogenic in subacute, painless (silent), and postpartum thyroiditis
- Thyroid RAIU scan: decreased in all forms of thyroiditis but not helpful in establishing diagnosis of Hashimoto disease. High RAIU in hashitoxicosis, Graves disease
- Random urine iodine measurement may be helpful to distinguish from other causes of low RAIU.
  - Urine iodine <500 μg/L (subacute granulomatous thyroiditis)
  - Urine iodine >1,000 μg/L (in patients with exposure to excess exogenous iodine/radiocontrast material)

Diagnostic Procedures/Other
- Hashimoto with a dominant nodule should have FNA to rule out thyroid carcinoma.
- Open biopsy is necessary for a definitive diagnosis of Reidel thyroiditis.

Test Interpretation
- Hashimoto disease: lymphocytic infiltration with formation of Askanazy (Hürthle) cells, oxyphilic changes in follicular cells, fibrosis, thyroid atrophy
- Subacute granulomatous thyroiditis: giant cells, mononuclear cell (granulomatous) infiltrate
- Postpartum thyroiditis: lymphocytic infiltration, occasional germinal centers, disruption and collapse of thyroid follicles
- Painless (silent) thyroiditis: lymphocytic infiltration, but without fibrosis, Askanazy cells, and extensive lymphoid follicle formation

TREATMENT

GENERAL MEASURES
Analgesics for pain; corticosteroids for severe granulomatous thyroiditis

MEDICATION
- Hashimoto disease (2)[C]
  - If hypothyroid/goitrous: levothyroxine (1.7 μg/kg/day for adults <50 years of age). If no cardiac complications and no adrenal insufficiency, 1/2 replacement dose and increase to full replacement in 10 days.
    - If >50 years of age or heart disease and/or adrenal insufficiency, begin with 25 μg/day and titrate to TSH of lower limit normal range.
- If thyrotoxic and symptomatic: propylthiouracil and propranolol
- An elevated TSH level in a woman who is pregnant or attempting to become pregnant is an indication for thyroid replacement.
- Subacute granulomatous thyroiditis
  - Anti-inflammatory agents for 2 to 8 weeks (NSAIDs or aspirin)

- Pain with no improvement in 2 to 3 days after NSAID use: Prednisone 40 mg/day; should result in pain relief in 1 to 2 days; if not, question diagnosis.
  - Severe pain: prednisone 40 to 60 mg/day discontinued over 4 to 6 weeks. If pain recurs, increase dose for several weeks and then taper.
  - Symptomatic hyperthyroidism: β-blockers while thyrotoxic (propranolol 40 to 120 mg/day)
  - Symptomatic hypothyroid phase: Levothyroxine, as mentioned earlier, target TSH in the normal range.
- Suppurative thyroiditis
  - Parenteral empiric, broad-spectrum antibiotics, and surgical drainage
- Painless (silent) thyroiditis
  - No treatment needed.
  - If symptomatic during hyperthyroid state, treat with β-blocker (propranolol 40 to 120 mg/day).
  - Prednisone shortens the period of hyperthyroidism. Monitor TSH every 4 to 8 weeks to confirm resolution.
  - Treat hypothyroid symptoms and asymptomatic patients with TSH >10 mU/L with levothyroxine (50 to 100 μg/day), to be discontinued after 3 to 6 months.
- Postpartum thyroiditis (5)[C]
  - Treat symptomatic hyper-/hypothyroid state. Most do not need treatment.
  - Caution in breastfeeding mothers because β-blockers are secreted into breast milk.
  - For symptomatic hypothyroidism, treat with levothyroxine. Otherwise, remonitor in 4 to 8 weeks. Taper replacement hormone after 6 months if thyroid function has normalized.
- Reidel thyroiditis (4)[C]
  - Corticosteroids in early stages but controversial thereafter. Prednisone 10 to 20 mg/day for 4 to 6 months, possibly continued thereafter if effective
  - Long-term anti-inflammatory medications to arrest progression and maintain a symptom-free course
  - Tamoxifen 10 to 20 mg twice daily as monotherapy or in conjunction with prednisone reduces mass size and clinical symptoms.
  - Methotrexate is used with some success.
  - Reduction of goiter seen with a combination of mycophenolate mofetil (1 g BID) and 100 mg/day prednisone
  - Debulking surgery is limited to isthmusectomy to relieve constrictive pressure when total thyroidectomy is not possible.
- Drug-induced thyroiditis
  - Discontinue offending drug.

SURGERY/OTHER PROCEDURES
Enlarged painful thyroid or tracheal compression

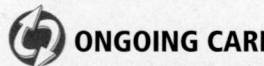

ONGOING CARE

FOLLOW-UP RECOMMENDATIONS
Patient Monitoring
- Hashimoto disease: Repeat thyroid function tests every 3 to 12 months.
- Subacute granulomatous thyroiditis: Repeat thyroid function tests every 3 to 6 weeks until euthyroid, then every 6 to 12 months.
- Postpartum thyroiditis: Check TSH annually.
- Reidel thyroiditis: CT of cervical mediastinal region is recommended.
- TSH every 6 months in patients on amiodarone

Pregnancy Considerations
- Avoid radioisotope scanning if possible.
- Keep TSH maximally suppressed.
- If using RAIU scan, discard breast milk for 2 days because RAI is secreted in breast milk.

PROGNOSIS
- Hashimoto disease: persistent goiter; eventual thyroid failure
- Subacute granulomatous thyroiditis: 5–15% hypothyroid beyond a year: Some with eventual return to normal; remission may be slower in the elderly; recurrence rate: 1–4% after a year
- Painless (silent) thyroiditis: 10–20% hypothyroid beyond a year; recurrence rate 5–10% (much higher in Japan)
- Postpartum thyroiditis: 15–50% hypothyroid beyond a year; women may be euthyroid/continue to be hypothyroid at the end of 1st postpartum year. 70% recurrence rate in subsequent pregnancies; substantial risk exists for later development of hypothyroidism/goiter.

REFERENCES
1. Samuels MH. Subacute, silent, and postpartum thyroiditis. *Med Clin North Am.* 2012;96(2):223–233.
2. Li Y, Nishihara E, Kakudo K. Hashimoto's thyroiditis: old concepts and new insights. *Curr Opin Rheumatol.* 2011;23(1):102–107.
3. De Groot L, Abalovich M, Alexander EK, et al. Management of thyroid dysfunction during pregnancy and postpartum: an Endocrine Society clinical practice guideline. *J Clin Endocrinol Metab.* 2012;97(8):2543–2565. doi:10.1210/jc.2011-2803
4. Hennessey JV. Clinical review: Riedel's thyroiditis: a clinical review. *J Clin Endocrinol Metab.* 2011;96(10):3031–3041.
5. Reid SM, Middleton P, Cossich MC, et al. Interventions for clinical and subclinical hypothyroidism in pregnancy. *Cochrane Database Syst Rev.* 2010;(7):CD007752.

ADDITIONAL READING

Duntas LH. Selenium and the thyroid: a close-knit connection. *J Clin Endocrinol Metab.* 2010;95(12):5180–5188.

 SEE ALSO

Hyperthyroidism; Hypothyroidism, Adult

 CODES

ICD10
- E06.9 Thyroiditis, unspecified
- E06.1 Subacute thyroiditis
- E06.0 Acute thyroiditis

CLINICAL PEARLS

- TSH elevation above the normal range indicates a hypothyroid state; suppressed TSH indicates hyperthyroid state. Follow up with free T_3/T_4 determination.
- Follow patients on thyroid replacement with periodic TSH level.

TINEA (CAPITIS, CORPORIS, CRURIS)

Elisabeth L. Backer, MD

 BASICS

DESCRIPTION

- Superficial fungal infections of the skin/scalp; various forms of dermatophytosis; the names relate to the particular area affected (1).
  - Tinea cruris: infection of crural fold and gluteal cleft
  - Tinea corporis: infection involving the face, trunk, and/or extremities; often presents with ring-shaped lesions, hence the misnomer *ringworm*.
  - Tinea capitis: infection of the scalp and hair; affected areas of the scalp can show characteristic black dots resulting from broken hairs.
- Dermatophytes have the ability to subsist on protein, namely keratin.
- They cause disease in keratin-rich structures such as skin, nails, and hair.
- Infections result from contact with infected persons/animals
  - Zoophilic infections are acquired from animals.
  - Anthropophilic infections are acquired from personal contact (e.g., wrestling) or fomites.
  - Geophile infections are acquired from the soil.
- System(s) affected: skin; exocrine
- Synonym(s): jock itch; ringworm

EPIDEMIOLOGY

Incidence

- Tinea cruris
  - Predominant age: any age; rare in children
  - Predominant sex: male > female
- Tinea corporis
  - Predominant age: all ages
  - Predominant sex: male = female
- Tinea capitis
  - Predominant age: 3 to 9 years; almost always occurs in young children
  - Predominant sex: male = female

Prevalence

Common worldwide

Pediatric Considerations

- Tinea cruris is rare prior to puberty.
- Tinea capitis is common in young children.

Geriatric Considerations

Tinea cruris is more common in the geriatric population due to an increase in risk factors.

Pregnancy Considerations

Tinea cruris and capitis are rare in pregnancy.

ETIOLOGY AND PATHOPHYSIOLOGY

Superficial fungal infection of skin/scalp

- Tinea cruris: Source of infection is usually the patient's own tinea pedis, with agent being transferred from the foot to the groin via the underwear when dressing; most common causative dermatophyte is *Trichophyton rubrum*; rare cases caused by *Epidermophyton floccosum* and *T. mentagrophytes*.

- Tinea corporis: most commonly caused by *T. rubrum*; *T. tonsurans* most often found in patients with tinea gladiatorum.
- Tinea capitis: *T. tonsurans* found in 90% and *Microsporum* sp. in 10% of patients

Genetics

Evidence suggests a genetic susceptibility in certain individuals.

RISK FACTORS

- Warm climates; summer months and/or copious sweating; wearing wet clothing/multiple layers (tinea cruris)
- Daycare centers/schools/confined quarters (tinea corporis and capitis)
- Depression of cell-mediated immune response (e.g., individuals with atopy or AIDS)
- Obesity (tinea cruris and corporis)
- Direct contact with an active lesion on a human, an animal, or rarely, from soil; working with animals (tinea corporis)

GENERAL PREVENTION

- Avoidance of risk factors, such as contact with suspicious lesions
- Fluconazole or itraconazole may be useful in wrestlers to prevent outbreaks during competitive season.

COMMONLY ASSOCIATED CONDITIONS

Tinea pedis, tinea barbae, tinea manus

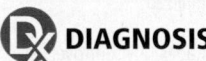 **DIAGNOSIS**

HISTORY

- Lesions range from asymptomatic to pruritic.
- In tinea cruris, acute inflammation may result from wearing occlusive clothing; chronic scratching may result in an eczematous appearance.
- Previous application of topical steroids, especially in tinea cruris and corporis, may alter the overall appearance causing a more extensive eruption with irregular borders and erythematous papules. This modified form is called *tinea incognito*.

PHYSICAL EXAM

- Tinea cruris: well-marginated, erythematous, half-moon–shaped plaques in crural folds that spread to upper thighs; advancing border is well defined, often with fine scaling and sometimes vesicular eruptions. Lesions are usually bilateral and do not include scrotum/penis (unlike with *Candida* infections) but may migrate to perineum, perianal area, and gluteal cleft and onto the buttocks in chronic/progressive cases. The area may be hyperpigmented on resolution.
- Tinea corporis: scaling, pruritic plaques characterized by a sharply defined annular pattern with peripheral activity and central clearing (ring-shaped lesions); papules and occasionally pustules/vesicles present at border and, less commonly, in center.

- Tinea capitis: commonly begins with round patches of scale (alopecia less common). In its later stages, the infection frequently takes on patterns of chronic scaling with either little/marked inflammation or alopecia. Less often, patients will present with multiple patches of alopecia and the characteristic black-dot appearance of broken hairs. Extreme inflammation results in kerion formation (exudative, pustular nodulation).

DIFFERENTIAL DIAGNOSIS

- Tinea cruris
  - Intertrigo: inflammatory process of moist-opposed skin folds, often including infection with bacteria, yeast, and fungi; painful longitudinal fissures may occur in skin folds.
  - Erythrasma: diffuse brown, scaly, noninflammatory plaque with irregular borders, often involving groin; caused by bacterial infection with *Corynebacterium minutissimum*; fluoresces coral red with Wood lamp
  - Seborrheic dermatitis of groin
  - Psoriasis of groin ("inverse psoriasis")
  - Candidiasis of groin (typically involves the scrotum)
  - Acanthosis nigricans
- Tinea capitis
  - Psoriasis
  - Seborrheic dermatitis
  - Pyoderma
  - Alopecia areata and trichotillomania
  - Aplasia cutis congenital
- Tinea corporis
  - Pityriasis rosea
  - Eczema (nummular)
  - Contact dermatitis
  - Syphilis
  - Psoriasis
  - Seborrheic dermatitis
  - Subacute systemic lupus erythematosus (SLE)
  - Erythema annulare centrifugum
  - Erythema multiforme; erythema migrans
  - Impetigo circinatum
  - Granuloma annulare

DIAGNOSTIC TESTS & INTERPRETATION

Wood lamp exam reveals no fluorescence in most cases (*Trichophyton* sp.); 10% of infections, those caused by *T. rubrum* will fluoresce with a green light.

Initial Tests (lab, imaging)

- Potassium hydroxide (KOH) preparation of skin scrapings from dermatophyte leading border shows characteristic translucent, branching, rod-shaped hyphae.
- Arthrospores can be visualized within hair shafts. Spores and/or hyphae may be seen on KOH exam.

Follow-Up Tests & Special Considerations

- Reevaluate to assess response, especially in resistant/extensive cases
- Fungal culture using Sabouraud dextrose agar/dermatophyte test medium

Test Interpretation

- Skin scrapings show fungal hyphae in epidermis.
- Arthrospores found in hair shafts; spores and/or hyphae seen on KOH exam.

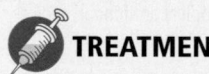

TREATMENT

GENERAL MEASURES

- Careful handwashing and personal hygiene; laundering of towels/clothing of affected individual; no sharing of towels/clothes/headgear
- Evaluate other family members, close contacts, or household pets.
- Avoid predisposing conditions such as hot baths and tight-fitting clothing (boxer shorts are better than briefs).
- Keep area as dry as possible (talcum/powders may be beneficial).
- Itching can be alleviated by OTC preparations such as Sarna or Prax.
- Topical steroid preparations should be avoided (see "Tinea Incognito"), unless absolutely needed to control itching and only after definitive diagnosis and initiation of antifungal treatment.
- Nystatin should be avoided in tinea infections but is indicated for cutaneous candidal infections.
- Avoid contact sports (e.g., wrestling) temporarily while starting treatment.

MEDICATION

First Line

- Tinea cruris/corporis (2)[C]
  - Topical azole antifungal compounds
    - Terbinafine 1% (Lamisil): OTC inexpensive and effective compound; can be applied once or BID for 1 to 2 weeks
    - Econazole 1% (Spectazole), ketoconazole (Nizoral): usually applied BID for 2 to 3 weeks
    - Butenafine 1% (Mentax): applied once daily for 2 weeks; also very effective. To prevent relapse, use for 1 week after resolution.

- Tinea capitis (3)[A]

  - PO griseofulvin for *Trichophyton* and *Microsporum* sp.; microsized preparation available; dosage 10 to 20 mg/kg/day (max 1,000 mg); taken BID or as a single dose daily for 6 to 12 weeks
  - PO terbinafine can be used for *Trichophyton* sp. at 62.5 mg/day in patients weighing 10 to 20 kg; 125 mg/day if weight 20 to 40 kg; 250 mg/day if weight >40 kg; use for 4 to 6 weeks.
  - PO itraconazole can be used for *Microsporum* sp. and matches griseofulvin efficacy while being better tolerated. Dosage of 3 to 5 mg/kg/day, but most studies have used 100 mg/day for 6 weeks in children >2 years of age.

Second Line

Tinea cruris/corporis

- Oral antifungal agents are effective but not indicated in uncomplicated tinea cruris/corporis cases. They can be used for resistant and extensive infections or if the patient is immunocompromised. If topical therapy fails, consider possible oral therapy. Griseofulvin can be given 500 mg/day for 1 to 2 weeks.
- The following oral regimens have been reported in medical literature as being effective but currently are not specifically approved by FDA for tinea cruris:
  - PO terbinafine (Lamisil): 250 mg/day for 1 week
  - PO itraconazole (Sporanox): 100 mg BID once and repeated 1 week later
  - PO fluconazole (Diflucan): 150 mg once per week for 4 weeks
- Topical terbinafine 1% solution has been studied recently and appears effective as a once-daily application for 1 week.
- Oral antifungals have many interactions including warfarin, OCPs, and alcohol; advise checking for drug interactions prior to use; contraindicated in pregnancy. Monitor for liver toxicity when using oral antifungals.

ISSUES FOR REFERRAL

Refer if disease is nonresponsive/resistant, especially in immunocompromised host.

ADDITIONAL THERAPIES

Treatment of secondary bacterial infections

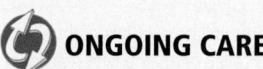

ONGOING CARE

FOLLOW-UP RECOMMENDATIONS

Reevaluate response to treatment.

Patient Monitoring

Liver function testing prior to therapy and at regular intervals during course of therapy for patients requiring oral terbinafine, fluconazole, itraconazole, and griseofulvin.

PATIENT EDUCATION

Explain the causative agents, predisposing factors, and prevention measures.

PROGNOSIS

- Excellent prognosis for cure with therapy in tinea cruris and corporis.
- In tinea capitis, lesions will heal spontaneously in 6 months without treatment but scarring is more likely.

COMPLICATIONS

- Secondary bacterial infection
- Generalized, invasive dermatophyte infection
- Secondary eruptions called dermatophytid reactions may occur at distant sites.

REFERENCES

1. Ameen M. Epidemiology of superficial fungal infections. *Clin Dermatol*. 2010;28(2):197–201.
2. Gupta AK, Cooper EA. Update in antifungal therapy of dermatophytosis. *Mycopathologia*. 2008;166(5–6):353–367.
3. Gupta AK, Drummond-Main C. Meta-analysis of randomized, controlled trials comparing particular doses of griseofulvin and terbenafine for the treatment of tinea capitis. *Pediatr Dermatol*. 2013;30(1):1–6.

ADDITIONAL READING

- Akinwale SO. Personal hygiene as an alternative to griseofulvin in the treatment of tinea cruris. *Afr J Med Med Sci*. 2000;29(1):41–43.
- Bonifaz A, Saúl A. Comparative study between terbinafine 1% emulsion-gel versus ketoconazole 2% cream in tinea cruris and tinea corporis. *Eur J Dermatol*. 2000;10(2):107–109.
- González U, Seaton T, Bergus G, et al. Systemic antifungal therapy for tinea capitis in children. *Cochrane Database Syst Rev*. 2007;(4):CD004685.
- Lesher JL Jr, Babel DE, Stewart DM, et al. Butenafine 1% cream in the treatment of tinea cruris: a multicenter, vehicle-controlled, double-blind trial. *J Am Acad Dermatol*. 1997;36(2, Pt 1):S20–S24.
- Nozickova M, Koudelkova V, Kulikova Z, et al. A comparison of the efficacy of oral fluconazole, 150 mg/week versus 50 mg/day, in the treatment of tinea corporis, tinea cruris, tinea pedis, and cutaneous candidosis. *Int J Dermatol*. 1998;37(9):703–705.
- Seebacher C, Bouchara JP, Mignon B. Updates on the epidemiology of dermatophyte infections. *Mycopathologia*. 2008;166(5–6):335–352.
- Tey HL, Tan AS, Chan YC. Meta-analysis of randomized, controlled trials comparing griseofulvin and terbinafine in the treatment of tinea capitis. *J Am Acad Dermatol*. 2011;64(4):663–670.

 CODES

ICD10

- B35.0 Tinea barbae and tinea capitis
- B35.4 Tinea corporis
- B35.6 Tinea cruris

CLINICAL PEARLS

- Tinea corporis is characterized by scaly plaque, with peripheral activity and central clearing.
- Tinea cruris is characterized by erythematous plaque in crural folds usually sparing the scrotum. Treatment of concomitant tinea pedis is advised.
- Tinea capitis is a fungal infection of the scalp affecting hair growth. Topical therapy is ineffective for this infection.

TINEA PEDIS

Elisabeth L. Backer, MD

BASICS

DESCRIPTION
- Superficial infection of the feet caused by dermatophytes
- Most common dermatophyte infection encountered in clinical practice
- Often accompanied by tinea manuum, tinea unguium, and tinea cruris
- Two clinical forms: acute and chronic; both are contagious
- System(s) affected: skin/exocrine
- Synonym(s): athlete's foot

EPIDEMIOLOGY
- Predominant age: 20 to 50 years, although can occur at any age (1)[C]
- Predominant gender: male > female

Prevalence
4% of population

Pediatric Considerations
Rare in younger children; common in teens

Geriatric Considerations
Elderly are more susceptible to outbreaks because of immunocompromise and impaired perfusion of distal extremities.

ETIOLOGY AND PATHOPHYSIOLOGY
Superficial infection caused by dermatophytes that thrive only in nonviable keratinized tissue.
- *Trichophyton mentagrophytes* (acute)
- *Trichophyton rubrum* (chronic)
- *Trichophyton tonsurans*
- *Epidermophyton floccosum*

Genetics
No known genetic pattern

RISK FACTORS
- Hot, humid weather
- Sweating
- Occlusive/tight-fitting footwear
- Immunosuppression
- Prolonged application of topical steroids

GENERAL PREVENTION
- Good personal hygiene
- Wearing rubber or wooden sandals in community showers, bathing places, locker rooms
- Careful drying between toes after showering or bathing; blow-drying feet with hair dryer may be more effective than drying with towel.
- Changing socks and shoes frequently
- Applying drying or dusting powder
- Applying topical antiperspirants
- Putting on socks before underwear to prevent infection from spreading to groin

COMMONLY ASSOCIATED CONDITIONS
- Hyperhidrosis
- Onychomycosis
- Tinea manuum/unguium/cruris/corporis

DIAGNOSIS

HISTORY
- Itchy, scaly rash on foot, usually between toes; may progress to fissuring/maceration in toe web spaces.
- May be associated with onychomycosis and other tinea infections

PHYSICAL EXAM
- Acute form: self-limited, intermittent, recurrent; scaling, thickening, and fissuring of sole and heel; scaling or fissuring of toe webs; or pruritic vesicular/bullous lesions between toes or on soles
- Chronic form: most common; slowly progressive, pruritic erythematous erosion/scales between toes, in digital interspaces; extension onto soles, sides/dorsum of feet (moccasin distribution); if untreated, may persist indefinitely
- Other features: strong odor, hyperkeratosis, maceration, ulceration
- Tinea pedis may occur unilateral or bilateral.
- Seconday eruptions called dermatophytid reactions may occur at distant sites.

DIFFERENTIAL DIAGNOSIS
- Interdigital type: erythrasma, impetigo, pitted keratolysis, candidal intertrigo
- Moccasin type: psoriasis vulgaris, eczematous dermatitis, pitted keratolysis
- Inflammatory/bullous type: impetigo, allergic contact dermatitis, dyshidrotic eczema (negative KOH examination of scrapings), bullous disease

DIAGNOSTIC TESTS & INTERPRETATION
Wood lamp exam will not fluoresce unless complicated by another fungus, which is uncommon: *Malassezia furfur* (yellow to white), *Corynebacterium* (red), or *Microsporum* (blue-green).

Initial Tests (lab, imaging)
Testing is not needed in typical presentation.
- Direct microscopic exam (potassium hydroxide) of scrapings of the lesions
- Culture (Sabouraud medium)

Test Interpretation
- Potassium hydroxide preparation: septate and branched mycelia
- Culture: dermatophyte

TREATMENT

Treatment is generally with topical antifungal medications for up to 4 weeks and is more effective than placebo:
- Acute treatment
  - Aluminum acetate soak (Burow solution; Domeboro, one pack to one quart warm water) to decrease itching and acute eczematous reaction
  - Antifungal cream of choice BID after soaks
- Chronic treatment:
  - Antifungal creams BID, continuing for 3 days after the rash is resolved: terbinafine 1% (possibly most effective topical), clotrimazole 1%, econazole 1%, ketoconazole 2%, tolnaftate 1%, etc. (2)[A]
  - May try systemic antifungal therapy; see below (consider if concomitant onychomycosis or after failed topical treatment)

GENERAL MEASURES
- Soak with aluminum chloride 30% or aluminum subacetate for 20 minutes BID.
- Careful removal of dead/thickened skin after soaking or bathing
- Treatment of shoes with antifungal powders
- Avoidance of occlusive footwear
- Chronic or extensive disease or nail involvement requires oral antifungal medication and systemic therapy.

MEDICATION
For use when topical therapy has failed

First Line
- Systemic antifungals (3)[A]:
  - Itraconazole (Sporanox): 200 mg PO BID for 7 days (cure rate >90%)
  - Terbinafine (Lamisil): 250 mg/day PO for 14 days
- If concomitant onychomycosis:
  - Itraconazole: 200 mg PO BID for first week of month for 3 months. Liver function testing is recommended.
  - Terbinafine: 250 mg/day PO for 12 weeks, or pulse dosing: 500 mg/day PO for first week of month for 3 months. Not recommended if creatinine clearance is <50 mL/min.
- Pediatric dosing options:
  - Griseofulvin: 10 to 15 mg/kg/day or divided
  - Terbinafine:
    - 10 to 20 kg: 62.5 mg/day
    - 20 to 40 kg: 125 mg/day
    - >40 kg: 250 mg/day
- Itraconazole: 5 mg/kg/day
- Fluconazole: 6 mg/kg/week
- Contraindications: itraconazole, pregnancy Category C

- Precautions: All systemic antifungal drugs may have potential hepatotoxicity.
- Significant possible interactions: Itraconazole requires gastric acid for absorption; effectiveness is reduced with antacids, H_2 blockers, proton pump inhibitors, etc. Take with acidic beverage such as soda if on antacids.

Second Line
- Systemic antifungals: griseofulvin 250 to 500 mg of microsize BID daily for 21 days
- Contraindications (griseofulvin):
  – Patients with porphyria, hepatocellular failure
  – Patients with history of hypersensitivity to griseofulvin
- Precautions (griseofulvin):
  – Should be used only in severe cases
  – Periodic monitoring of organ-system functioning, including renal, hepatic, and hematopoietic
  – Possible photosensitivity reactions
  – Lupus erythematosus, lupus-like syndromes, or exacerbation of existing lupus erythematosus has been reported.
- Significant possible interactions (griseofulvin):
  – Decreases activity of warfarin-type anticoagulants
  – Barbiturates usually depress griseofulvin activity.
  – May potentiate effect of alcohol, producing tachycardia and flush

ISSUES FOR REFERRAL
If extensive or resistant disease, especially in immuno-compromised host

ADDITIONAL THERAPIES
- Treatment of secondary bacterial infections
- Treatment of eczematoid changes

ONGOING CARE

FOLLOW-UP RECOMMENDATIONS
Avoid sweating feet.

Patient Monitoring
Evaluate for response, recognizing that infections may be chronic/recurrent.

DIET
No restrictions

PATIENT EDUCATION
See "General Prevention."

PROGNOSIS
- Control but not complete cure
- Infections tend to be chronic with exacerbations (e.g., in hot weather).
- Personal hygiene and preventive measures such as open-toed sandals, careful drying, and frequent sock changes are essential.

COMPLICATIONS
- Secondary bacterial infections (common portal of entry for streptococcal infections, producing lymphangitis/cellulitis of lower extremity)
- Eczematoid changes

REFERENCES

1. Ameen M. Epidemiology of superficial fungal infections. *Clin Dermatol*. 2010;28(2):197–201.
2. Crawford F, Hollis S. Topical treatments for fungal infections of the skin and nails of the foot. *Cochrane Database Syst Rev*. 2007;(3):CD001434.
3. Bell-Syer SE, Khan SM, Torgerson DJ. Oral treatments for fungal infections of the skin of the foot. *Cochrane Database Syst Rev*. 2012;(10):CD003584.

ADDITIONAL READING

- Gupta AK, Cooper EA. Update in antifungal therapy of dermatophytosis. *Mycopathologia*. 2008; 166(5–6):353–367.
- Rotta I, Sanchez A, Gonçalves PR, et al. Efficacy and safety of topical antifungals in the treatment of dermatomycosis: a systematic review. *Br J Dermatol*. 2012;166(5):927–933.

SEE ALSO

Dermatitis, Contact; Dyshidrosis

CODES

ICD10
B35.3 Tinea pedis

CLINICAL PEARLS

- Treatment is generally with topical antifungal medications for up to 4 weeks.
- Tinea pedis is often recurrent/chronic in nature.
- Careful drying between toes after showering or bathing helps prevent recurrences. (Blow drying feet with hair dryer may be more effective than drying with towel.)
- Socks should be changed frequently. Put on socks before underwear to prevent infection from spreading to groin (tinea cruris).
- Dusting and drying powders (containing antifungal agents) may prevent recurrences.

T

TINEA VERSICOLOR
Elisabeth L. Backer, MD

 BASICS

DESCRIPTION
- Rash due to a common superficial mycosis with a variety of colors and changing shades of color, predominantly present on trunk and proximal upper extremities; macules are usually hypopigmented, light brown, or salmon-colored; fine scale is often apparent. It is not a dermatophyte infection.
- System(s) affected: skin/exocrine
- Synonym(s): pityriasis versicolor

EPIDEMIOLOGY
Incidence
- Common, occurs worldwide, especially in tropical climates, where prevalence can reach 50%
- Predominant age: teenagers and young adults
- Predominant sex: male = female

Pediatric Considerations
Usually occurs after puberty (except in tropical areas); facial lesions are more common in children.

Geriatric Considerations
Not common in the geriatric population

ETIOLOGY AND PATHOPHYSIOLOGY
Inhibition of pigment synthesis in epidermal melanocytes, leading to hypomelanosis; in the hyperpigmented type, the melanosomes are large and heavily melanized (1).
- Saprophytic yeast: *Pityrosporum orbiculare* (also known as *P. ovale*, *Malassezia furfur*, or *M. ovalis*), which is a known colonizer of all humans
- Development of clinical disease associated with transformation of *Malassezia* from yeast cells to pathogenic mycelial form due to host and/or external factors.
- Not linked to poor hygiene

Genetics
Genetic predisposition may exist.

RISK FACTORS
- Hot, humid weather
- Use of topical skin oils
- Hyperhidrosis
- HIV infection/immunosuppression

- High cortisol levels (Cushing, prolonged steroid administration)
- Pregnancy
- Malnutrition
- Oral contraceptives

GENERAL PREVENTION
- Recheck and treat again each spring prior to tanning season.
- Avoid skin oils.

 DIAGNOSIS

HISTORY
- Asymptomatic scaling macules on trunk
- Possible mild pruritus
- More prominent in summer
- Sun tanning accentuates lesions because infected areas do not tan.
- Periodic recurrences are common.

PHYSICAL EXAM
- *Versicolor* refers to the variety and changing shades of colors. Color variations can exist between individuals and also between lesions.
- Sun-exposed areas: Lesions are usually white/hypopigmented.
- Covered areas: Lesions are often brown or salmon-colored.
- Distribution (sebum-rich areas): chest, shoulders, back (also face and intertriginous areas)
  – Face is more likely to be involved in children.
- Appearance: small individual macules that frequently coalesce
- Scale: fine, more visible with scraping

DIFFERENTIAL DIAGNOSIS
Other skin diseases with discolored macules and plaques, including the following:
- Pityriasis alba/rosea ("Christmas tree-like" distribution visible in *P. rosea*)
- Vitiligo (presents without scaling)

- Seborrheic dermatitis (more erythematous; thicker scale)
- Nummular eczema
- Secondary syphilis
- Erythrasma
- Mycosis fungoides

DIAGNOSTIC TESTS & INTERPRETATION
Wood lamp: yellow to yellow-green fluorescence or pigment changes

Initial Tests (lab, imaging)
- Direct microscopy of scales with 10% potassium hydroxide (KOH) preparation to visualize hyphae and spores ("spaghetti and meatballs" pattern)
- Routine lab tests are usually not necessary.
- Fungal culture is not useful.

Test Interpretation
- Short, stubby, or Y-shaped hyphae
- Small, round spores in clusters on hyphae

 TREATMENT

GENERAL MEASURES
- Apply prescribed topical medications to affected skin with cotton balls.
- Pigmentation may take months to fade or fill in.
- Repeat treatment each spring prior to sun exposure; some may require repeated treatment during the summer as prophylaxis.
- Patients who fail topical treatment can be treated with an oral/systemic medication.

MEDICATION
Topical antifungal therapy is the treatment of choice in limited disease. Evidence is generally of poor quality, but data suggest that longer durations of treatment and higher concentrations of active agents produce greater cure rates (2)[A].

First Line
- Ketoconazole 2% shampoo applied to damp skin and left on for 5 minutes for 1 to 3 days *or*
- Selenium sulfide shampoo 2.5% (Selsun):
  – Allowed to dry for 10 minutes prior to showering: daily for 1 week *or*
  – Allowed to remain on body for 12 to 24 hours prior to showering: once a week for 4 weeks *or*

- Clotrimazole 1% topical (Lotrimin) BID for 2 to 4 weeks *or*
- Miconazole 2% (Micatin, Monistat) BID for 2 to 4 weeks *or*
- Ketoconazole 2% (Nizoral) cream BID for 2 to 4 weeks *or*
- Terbinafine (Lamisil) 1% solution BID for 1 week *or*
- Terbinafine (Lamisil Derm Gel) once daily for 1 week
- Cure rates of topical antiyeast preparations typically 70–80%; healing continues after active treatment. Resumption of even pigmentation may take months.
- Contraindications: Ketoconazole is contraindicated in pregnancy.
- Newer preparations: 2.25% selenium sulfide foam; ketoconazole 2% gel

Second Line
- Use for extensive disease or nonresponders
- Oral fluconazole 300 mg once weekly for 2 weeks (3)[A]
- Itraconazole 200 mg/day PO for 1 week; cure rate >90% (3)[A]
- Oral ketoconazole is no longer recommended by FDA due to risks of hepatotoxicity, adrenal insufficiency, and drug–drug interactions.
- Oral terbinafine or griseofulvin is not effective.
- Pramiconazole has been studied but is not yet available for clinical use.

ISSUES FOR REFERRAL
- If resistant to treatment
- If extensive disease occurs in immunocompromised host

 ONGOING CARE

- Ketoconazole 2% or selenium sulfide 2.5% shampoo can be used weekly for maintenance or monthly for prophylaxis.
- Itraconazole 400 mg once monthly during the warmer months of the year can also reduce recurrences.

FOLLOW-UP RECOMMENDATIONS
Warn patients that whiteness will remain for several months after treatment.

Patient Monitoring
- Recheck and treat again each spring prior to tanning season.
- Failure to respond should prompt reassessment or dermatology referral.
- Resistance to treatment, frequent recurrences, or widespread disease may point to immunodeficiency.

PATIENT EDUCATION
For patient education materials favorably reviewed on this topic, contact American Academy of Dermatology, 930 N. Meacham Road, P.O. Box 4014, Schaumberg, IL 60168-4014; (708) 330-0230.

PROGNOSIS
- Duration of lesions months/years
- Recurs almost routinely because this yeast is a known human colonizer
- Pigmentary changes may take months to resolve.

REFERENCES
1. Morishita N, Sei Y. Microreview of pityriasis versicolor and *Malassezia* species. *Mycopathologia.* 2006;162(6):373–376.
2. Hu SW, Bigby M. Pityriasis versicolor: a systematic review of interventions. *Arch Dermatol.* 2010;146(10):1132–1140.
3. Gupta AK, Lane D, Paquet M. Systematic review of systemic treatments for tinea versicolor and evidence-based dosing regimen recommendations. *J Cutan Med Surg.* 2014;18(2):79–90.

ADDITIONAL READING
- Bhogal CS, Singal A, Baruah MC. Comparative efficacy of ketoconazole and fluconazole in the treatment of pityriasis versicolor: a one year follow-up study. *J Dermatol.* 2001;28(10):535–539.
- Faergemann J, Todd G, Pather S, et al. A double-blind, randomized, placebo-controlled, dose-finding study of oral pramiconazole in the treatment of pityriasis versicolor. *J Am Acad Dermatol.* 2009;61(6):971–976.
- Güleç AT, Demirbilek M, Seçkin D, et al. Superficial fungal infections in 102 renal transplant recipients: a case-control study. *J Am Acad Dermatol.* 2003;49(2):187–192.
- Gupta AK, Batra R, Bluhm R, et al. Pityriasis versicolor. *Dermatol Clin.* 2003;21(3):413–429.
- Köse O, Bülent Taştan H, Riza Gür A, et al. Comparison of a single 400 mg dose versus a 7-day 200 mg daily dose of itraconazole in the treatment of tinea versicolor. *J Dermatolog Treat.* 2002;13(2):77–79.

 CODES

ICD10
B36.0 Pityriasis versicolor

CLINICAL PEARLS
- Noncontagious macules of varying colors, with fine scale
- Recurrence in summer months
- More apparent after tanning. Skin areas with fungal infection do not tan; thus, hypopigmented areas become more visible.
- Warn patients that whiteness will remain for several months after treatment.

TINNITUS

Donna I. Meltzer, MD

BASICS

DESCRIPTION
- Tinnitus is a perceived sensation of sound in the absence of an external acoustic stimulus; often described as a ringing, hissing, buzzing, or whooshing
- Derived from the Latin word *tinnire*, meaning "to ring" (1)
- May be heard in one or both ears or centrally within the head (2)
- Two types: subjective (most common) and objective tinnitus
- Subjective tinnitus: perceived only by the patient; can be continuous, intermittent, or pulsatile
- Objective tinnitus: audible to the examiner; usually pulsatile; <1% cases (3)

EPIDEMIOLOGY
Prevalence
- Tinnitus reported by 35 to 50 million adults in United States; although underreported, 12 million seek medical care (4).
- Affects 10–15% of adults
- Prevalence increases with age and peaks between ages of 60 and 69 years (5).
- Prevalence of 13–53% in general pediatric population (6)
- Ethnic: whites > blacks and Hispanics (4)
- Gender: males > females

Incidence
- Incidence increasing in association with excessive noise exposure
- Higher rates of tinnitus in smokers and hypertensives (5)

ETIOLOGY AND PATHOPHYSIOLOGY
- Precise pathophysiology is unknown; numerous theories have been proposed. Cochlear damage from ototoxic agents or noise exposure damage hair cells so that the central auditory system compensates, resulting in hyperactivity in cochlear nucleus and auditory cortex. Animal models have identified brain abnormalities resulting in increased firing and synchrony in auditory cortex (7).
- Causes of subjective tinnitus are the following:
  - Otologic: hearing loss, cholesteatoma, cerumen impaction, otosclerosis, Ménière disease, vestibular schwannoma
  - Ototoxic medications: anti-inflammatory agents (aspirin, NSAIDs); antimalarial agents (quinine, chloroquine); antimicrobial drugs (aminoglycosides); antineoplastic agents, loop diuretics, miscellaneous drugs (antiarrhythmics, antiulcer, anticonvulsants, antihypertensives, psychotropic drugs; anesthetics (3,5)
  - Somatic: temporomandibular joint (TMJ) dysfunction, head or neck injury
  - Neurologic: multiple sclerosis, spontaneous intracranial hypertension, vestibular migraine, type I Chiari malformation
  - Infectious: viral, bacterial, fungal
- Causes of objective tinnitus: patulous eustachian tube
  - Vascular: aortic or carotid stenosis, venous hum, arteriovenous fistula or malformation, vascular tumors, high cardiac output state (anemia)
  - Neurologic: palatal myoclonus, idiopathic stapedial muscle spasm

Genetics
Minimal genetic component

RISK FACTORS
- Hearing loss (but can have tinnitus with normal hearing)
- High level noise exposure
- Advanced age
- Use of ototoxic medications
- Otologic disease (otosclerosis, Ménière disease, cerumen impaction)

GENERAL PREVENTION
- Avoid loud noise exposure and wear appropriate ear protection to prevent hearing loss.
- Monitor ototoxic medications and avoid prescribing more than one ototoxic agent concurrently.

COMMONLY ASSOCIATED CONDITIONS
- Sensorineural hearing loss caused by presbycusis (age associated hearing loss) or prolonged loud noise exposure
- Conductive hearing loss due to cerumen, otosclerosis, cholesteatoma
- Psychological disorders: depression, anxiety, insomnia, suicidal ideation
- Despair, frustration, interference with concentration and social interactions, work hindrance

DIAGNOSIS

HISTORY
- Onset gradual (presbycusis) or abrupt (following loud noise exposure)
- Timing: can be continuous (hearing loss) or intermittent (Ménière disease)
- Pattern: nonpulsatile > pulsatile (often vascular cause)
- Location: bilateral > unilateral (vestibular schwannoma, cerumen, Ménière disease)
- Pitch: high pitch (with sensorineural hearing loss) > low pitch (Ménière disease)
- Associated symptoms: hearing loss, headache, noise intolerance, vertigo, TMJ dysfunction, neck pain
- Exacerbating factors: loud noise; jaw, head, or neck movements
- Alleviating factors: hearing aid, position change, medications
- Medication use (prescription, OTC, supplements)
- Hearing and past noise exposure (occupational, military, recreational)
- Psychosocial history (depression, sleep habits)
- Impact of tinnitus: Tinnitus Handicap Inventory, Tinnitus Functional Index

PHYSICAL EXAM
- HEENT, neck, neurologic, and vascular examinations
- Ear: cerumen impaction, effusion, cholesteatoma
- Check hearing; air and bone conduction testing with 512- or 1,024-Hz tuning fork (Weber and Rinne tests)
- Eye: funduscopic exam for papilledema (intracranial hypertension) or visual field change (mass)
- TMJ: Palpate for tenderness and crepitus with movement.
- Cranial nerve, Romberg test (equilibrium), finger to nose, gait
- Auscultate for bruits or murmurs over ear canal, periauricular areas, orbit, neck, chest

DIFFERENTIAL DIAGNOSIS
Pulsatile tinnitus: carotid stenosis, aortic valve disease, AV malformation, high cardiac output state (anemia, hyperthyroidism), paraganglioma (glomus tumor)
Nonpulsatile tinnitus: auditory hallucinations (8)

DIAGNOSTIC TESTS & INTERPRETATION
- Tinnitus is a symptom; no objective test to confirm diagnosis
- Pure tone audiometry (air and bone conduction)
- Speech discrimination testing
- Tympanometry
- Auditory brainstem response (ABR); less sensitive and specific than MRI for diagnosis of vestibular schwannoma (3)
- Carotid Doppler ultrasonography (neck bruit)

Initial Tests (lab, imaging)
Little evidence to support lab testing other than targeted lab studies based on history and physical exam. Lab investigation is not indicated in all patients; use clinical judgment. Consider the following:
- CBC
- BUN/creatinine, fasting glucose, lipid panel
- Thyroid-stimulating hormone
- Clinical evaluation should precede radiologic studies.
- Nonpulsatile tinnitus: MRI with or without contrast
- Pulsatile tinnitus: Contrast-enhanced temporal bone CT, MRI, MRA/MRV, CTA/CTV, carotid ultrasound, and conventional angiography all have been used to work up pulsatile tinnitus.
- CTA/CTV; CTA evaluates middle ear and arterial causes (carotid artery stenosis, aberrant ICA, persistent stapedial artery); CTV evaluates venous causes (sinus thrombosis, sinus stenosis, dehiscent jugular bulb) (9)[C].
- No studies have compared sensitivity and specificity of MRA/V with CTA/V in the evaluation of pulsatile tinnitus.
- Cerebral angiography is gold standard for diagnosis of suspected dural arteriovenous fistula.

Follow-Up Tests & Special Considerations
Consider HIV, RPR, autoimmune panel, Lyme test, vitamin B_{12} level.

Diagnostic Procedures/Other
Electronystagmography (vestibular testing for Ménière disease)

TREATMENT

GENERAL MEASURES
- Individualize treatment based on the severity of tinnitus and impact on function
- Reassure patient.
- Manage treatable pathology.
- Education, relaxation therapy, cognitive-behavioral therapy (CBT)
- Hearing aids (corrects hearing and might mask tinnitus); can be tried even if there is minimal hearing loss; no evidence to support or refute the use of hearing aids (10)[B]
- Protect hearing against future loud noise.
- Masking sound devices or generators on discontinuation might have decreased tinnitus (residual inhibition).
- Discontinue ototoxic medications.

MEDICATION
No pharmacologic agent has been shown to cure or consistently alleviate tinnitus.

First Line
- Antidepressants (SSRIs or TCAs): probably help with psychological distress. Newer review states insufficient evidence that antidepressant drug therapy improves tinnitus (11)[B].
- Melatonin decreases tinnitus intensity and improves sleep quality; most effective in men, those without depression or prior treatment, and those with more severe bilateral tinnitus (12)[B].

Second Line
- Anticonvulsants are used to treat tinnitus for years. Recent studies indicate that they may have a small effect (of doubtful clinical significance) on tinnitus (13)[A].
- Benzodiazepines help reduce tinnitus distress, but regular use discouraged.
- No difference between gabapentin and control group in patients with isolated tinnitus (14)[B].
- Higher caffeine intake associated with lower incidence of tinnitus in women (15)[B]

ISSUES FOR REFERRAL
- Audiologist for comprehensive hearing evaluation and management
- Otolaryngologist, neurologist, or neurosurgeon depending on pathology
- Dental referral for TMJ treatment and dental orthotics (splint, night guard)
- Therapists for cognitive-behavioral therapy (CBT), biofeedback, education, and relaxation techniques

ADDITIONAL THERAPIES
- Sound therapy (masking): Patients wear low-level noise generators to mask the tinnitus noise; commonly used, but no strong evidence for its efficacy (16)[B].
- CBT employs relaxation exercises, coping strategies, and deconditioning techniques to reduce arousal levels and reverse negative thoughts about tinnitus. Depression and severity of tinnitus improved with CBT (17)[A].
- Tinnitus retraining therapy (TRT) combines counseling, education, and acoustic therapy (soft music, sound machine) to minimize bothersome nature of tinnitus; often requires a team approach and up to 2 years of therapy; might be more effective than sound masking (18)[B].
- Transcranial magnetic stimulation (TMS): A noninvasive method to stimulate neurons in the brain by rapidly changing magnetic fields; insufficient data to support long-term safety of repetitive TMS (19)[B]
- Neurofeedback: a method to help patients regulate abnormal oscillatory brain activity and reduce intensity of tinnitus
- Hyperbaric oxygen therapy: no beneficial effect on tinnitus (20)[A]

SURGERY/OTHER PROCEDURES
- Cochlear implants (for severe sensorineural hearing loss)
- Ablation of cochlear nerve (destroys hearing)
- Epidural stimulation of secondary auditory cortex with implanted electrodes suppressed tinnitus in small subset of patients.
- Otosclerosis: stapedectomy surgery with implantation of ossicular prosthesis
- Severe Ménière disease not alleviated by medications: installation of endolymphatic shunt, labyrinthectomy, or vestibular neurectomy

- Auditory neoplasms: surgical resection/radiation
- Pulsatile tinnitus due to atherosclerotic carotid artery disease: carotid endarterectomy

COMPLEMENTARY & ALTERNATIVE MEDICINE
- Zinc supplements might improve tinnitus in those with zinc deficiency. One study in elderly did not demonstrate effectiveness of zinc treatment (21)[B].
- Ginkgo biloba has potential benefit but recent reviews question the effectiveness (22)[B].
- One evidence-based practice guideline does not recommend Ginkgo biloba, melatonin, zinc, or other dietary supplements for treatment of persistent, bothersome tinnitus (23)[C].
- Botulinum toxin (for palatal myoclonus)
- Acamprosate (used to treat alcohol dependence): Small studies noted improvement in tinnitus severity.
- Hypnosis (unknown effectiveness)
- Acupuncture (unknown effectiveness)

INPATIENT CONSIDERATIONS
Admission Criteria/Initial Stabilization
Not applicable

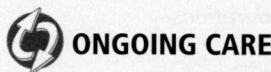 ONGOING CARE

FOLLOW-UP RECOMMENDATIONS
- Audiologist: for hearing evaluation and therapy
- Counseling as needed for psychological distress
- Family physician: as needed for support and guidance

PATIENT EDUCATION
- Help patients understand the relatively benign nature of tinnitus.
- Self-help groups
- American Tinnitus Association: (800) 634-8978; http://www.ata.org/
- National Institute on Deafness and Other Communication Disorders: (800) 241-1044; http://www.nidcd.nih.gov/Pages/default.aspx
- American Academy of Family Physicians: http://familydoctor.org

PROGNOSIS
- Tinnitus persisted in 80% of older patients and increased in severity in 50% (3).
- Focus on managing tinnitus and reducing severity, not curing.

REFERENCES
1. Baguley D, McFerran D, Hall D. Tinnitus. *Lancet.* 2013;382(9904):1600–1607.
2. Langguth B, Kreuzer PM, Kleinjung T, et al. Tinnitus: causes and clinical management. *Lancet Neurol.* 2013;12(9):920–930.
3. Yew KS. Diagnostic approach to patients with tinnitus. *Am Fam Physician.* 2014;89(2):106–113.
4. Shargorodsky J, Curhan GC, Farwell WR. Prevalence and characteristics of tinnitus among US adults. *Am J Med.* 2010;123(8):711–718.
5. Zimmerman E, Timboe A. Tinnitus: steps to take, drugs to avoid. *J Fam Pract.* 2014;63(2):82–88.
6. Bae SC, Park SN, Park JM, et al. Childhood tinnitus: clinical characteristics and treatment. *Am J Otolaryngol.* 2014;35(2):207–210.
7. Galazyuk AV, Wenstrup JJ, Hamid MA. Tinnitus and underlying brain mechanisms. *Curr Opin Otolaryngol Head Neck Surg.* 2012;20(5):409–415.
8. Smith GS, Romanelli-Gobbi M, Gray-Karagrigoriou E, et al. Complementary and integrative treatments: tinnitus. *Otolaryngol Clin North Am.* 2013;46(3):398–408.
9. Sajisevi M, Weissman JL, Kaylie DM. What is the role of imaging in tinnitus? *Laryngoscope.* 2014;124(3):583–584.
10. Hoare DJ, Edmondson-Jones M, Sereda M, et al. Amplification with hearing aids for patients with tinnitus and co-existing hearing loss. *Cochrane Database Syst Rev.* 2014;(1):CD010151.
11. Baldo P, Doree C, Molin P, et al. Antidepressants for patients with tinnitus. *Cochrane Database Syst Rev.* 2012;(9):CD003853.
12. Hurtuk A, Dome C, Holloman CH, et al. Melatonin: can it stop the ringing? *Ann Otol Rhinol Laryngol.* 2011;120(7):433–440.
13. Hoekstra CE, Rynja SP, van Zanten GA, et al. Anticonvulsants for tinnitus. *Cochrane Database Syst Rev.* 2011;(7):CD007960.
14. Dehkordi MA, Abolbashari S, Taheri R, et al. Efficacy of gabapentin on subjective idiopathic tinnitus: a randomized, double-blind, placebo-controlled trial. *Ear Nose Throat J.* 2011;90(4):150–158.
15. Glicksman JT, Curhan SG, Curhan GC. A prospective study of caffeine intake and risk of incident tinnitus. *Am J Med.* 2014;127(8):739–743.
16. Hobson J, Chisholm E, El Refaie A. Sound therapy (masking) in the management of tinnitus in adults. *Cochrane Database Syst Rev.* 2012;(11):CD006371.
17. Martinez-Devesa P, Perera R, Theodoulou M, et al. Cognitive behavioural therapy for tinnitus. *Cochrane Database Syst Rev.* 2010;(9):CD005233.
18. Phillips JS, McFerran D. Tinnitus retraining therapy (TRT) for tinnitus. *Cochrane Database Syst Rev.* 2010;(3):CD007330.
19. Meng Z, Liu S, Zheng Y, et al. Repetitive transcranial magnetic stimulation for tinnitus. *Cochrane Database Syst Rev.* 2011;(10):CD007946.
20. Bennett MH, Kertesz T, Perleth M, et al. Hyperbaric oxygen for idiopathic sudden sensorineural hearing loss and tinnitus. *Cochrane Database Syst Rev.* 2012;(10):CD004739.
21. Coelho C, Witt SA, Ji H, et al. Zinc to treat tinnitus in the elderly: a randomized placebo controlled cross-over trial. *Otol Neurotol.* 2013;34(6):1146–1154.
22. Hilton MP, Zimmermann EF, Hunt WT. Ginkgo biloba for tinnitus. *Cochrane Database Syst Rev.* 2013;(3):CD003852.
23. Tunkel DE, Bauer CA, Sun GH, et al. Clinical practice guideline: tinnitus. *Otolaryngol Head Neck Surg.* 2014;151(Suppl 2):S1–S40.

 CODES

ICD10
- H93.19 Tinnitus, unspecified ear
- H93.11 Tinnitus, right ear
- H93.12 Tinnitus, left ear

CLINICAL PEARLS
- People have different levels of tolerance to tinnitus. It may affect sleep, concentration, and emotional state. Many patients with chronic tinnitus have depression.
- To keep tinnitus from worsening, avoid loud noises and minimize stress.
- Optimal management may involve multiple strategies.

TOBACCO USE AND SMOKING CESSATION

Felix B. Chang, MD, DABMA, FAAMA

BASICS

DESCRIPTION
- Use of tobacco of any form
- *Smokeless tobacco* refers to tobacco products that are sniffed, sucked, or chewed.
- Nicotine sources: cigars, pipes, waterpipes, hookahs, and cigarettes

EPIDEMIOLOGY
Incidence
- 2.4 million new smokers annually in the United States (2.6% initiation rate)
- 58.8% of new smokers are <18 years of age (5.8% initiation rate for teens).

Prevalence
- 443,000 deaths annually in the United States
- Cigarette smoking among adults in the United States: 21.3% of adults in 2012 to 2013
- Highest among those aged 18 to 25 (40.8%)
- Adults aged >25 years (28.5%)
- Race: highest among whites (22.1%) and African Americans (21.3%) and is lower among Hispanics (14.6%) and Asians (12%)
- Gender: male > female (21.5% vs. 17.3%)
- Inversely proportional to education level
- 31% in men >15 years old from 187 countries in 2012

ETIOLOGY AND PATHOPHYSIOLOGY
- Addiction due to nicotine's rapid stimulation of the brain's dopamine system (teenage brain especially susceptible)
- Atherosclerotic risk due to adrenergic stimulation, endothelial damage, carbon monoxide, and adverse effects on lipids
- Direct airway damage from cigarette tar
- Carcinogens in all tobacco products

RISK FACTORS
- Presence of a smoker in the household
- Easy access to cigarettes
- Perceived parental approval of smoking
- Comorbid stress and psychiatric disorders
- Low self-esteem/self-worth
- Poor academic performance
- Boys: high levels of aggression and rebelliousness
- Girls: preoccupation with weight and body image

GENERAL PREVENTION
- Most first-time tobacco use occurs before high school graduation, so educational interventions should target students in grade and middle schools and must address health consequences and psychosocial aspects of smoking.
- The AAFP's Tar Wars program has targeted 4th and 5th graders successfully.
- Other helpful measures include the following:
  - Smoking bans in public areas and workplaces
  - Restriction of minors' access to tobacco
  - Restrictions on tobacco advertisements
  - Raising prices through taxation
  - Media literacy education
  - Tobacco-free sports initiatives

COMMONLY ASSOCIATED CONDITIONS
- Coronary artery disease
- Cerebrovascular disease
- Peripheral vascular disease
- Abdominal aortic aneurysm (AAA)
- COPD
- Cancer of the lip, oral cavity, pharynx, larynx, lung, esophagus, stomach, pancreas, kidney, bladder, cervix, and blood
- Pneumonia
- Osteoporosis
- Periodontitis
- Alcohol use
- Depression and anxiety
- Reduced fertility

Pregnancy Considerations
Women who smoke or are exposed to 2nd-hand smoke during pregnancy have increased risks of miscarriage, placenta previa, placental abruption, premature rupture of membranes, preterm delivery, low-birth-weight infants, and stillbirth.

Pediatric Considerations
- 2nd-hand smoke increases the risk of the following in infants and children:
  - Sudden infant death syndrome
  - Acute upper and lower respiratory tract infections
  - More frequent and more severe exacerbations of asthma
  - Otitis media and need for tympanostomies
- Nicotine passes through breast milk, and its effects on the growth and development of nursing infants are unknown.

DIAGNOSIS

HISTORY
- Ask about tobacco use and 2nd-hand smoke exposure at every physician encounter.
- Type and quantity of tobacco used
- Pack years = packs/day × years
- Awareness of health risks
- Assess interest in quitting.
- Identify triggers for smoking.
- Prior attempts to quit: method, duration of success, reason for relapse

PHYSICAL EXAM
- General: tobacco smoke odor
- Skin: premature face wrinkling
- Mouth: nicotine-stained teeth; inspect for suspicious mucosal lesions
- Lungs: crackles, wheezing, increased or decreased volume
- Vessels: carotid or abdominal bruits, abdominal aortic enlargement, peripheral pulses, stigmata of peripheral vascular disease

DIAGNOSTIC TESTS & INTERPRETATION
- CXR for patients with pulmonary symptoms or signs of cancer but not for screening
- The USPSTF recommends one-time screening US for AAA in men ≥65 years of age who ever smoked (number needed to screen to prevent 1 AAA = 500).

Diagnostic Procedures/Other
PFTs for smokers with chronic pulmonary symptoms, such as wheezing and dyspnea

TREATMENT
Both behavioral counseling and pharmacotherapy benefit patients who are trying to quit smoking especially when use in combination.

ALERT
Provider recommending smoking cessation at *every clinical visit* improves cessation rates. Nonpharmacologic approaches are appropriate for pregnant women and patients who smoke <10 cigarettes/day.

GENERAL MEASURES
- Behavioral counseling includes the 5 As of promoting smoking cessation:
  - Ask about tobacco use at every office visit.
  - Advise all smokers to quit.
  - Assess the patient's willingness to quit.
  - Assist the patient in his or her attempt to quit.
  - Arrange follow-up.
- Patients ready to quit smoking should set a quit date within the next 2 weeks. No difference in success rates between patients who taper prior to their quit date and those who stop abruptly.
- Success increased with a quitting partner, such as a spouse, friend, or coworker, to provide mutual encouragement.
- Patients desiring to quit should dispose of all smoking paraphernalia (such as lighters) on their quit dates to make relapse more difficult.
- Patients must anticipate and avoid social/environmental triggers for smoking and should have a plan for dealing with the urge to smoke.

MEDICATION
First Line
- Varenicline (Chantix): 0.5 mg/day PO for 3 days, then 0.5 mg BID for 4 days, then 1 mg BID for 11 weeks (1)[A]:
  - Start 1 to 4 weeks prior to smoking cessation and continue for 12 to 24 weeks.
  - Superior to placebo and to bupropion; number needed to treat = 7
  - May be combined with nicotine replacement therapy
  - S/E: nausea, insomnia, headache, depression, suicidal ideation; safety not established in adolescents or patients with psychiatric or cardiovascular disease; pregnancy Category C
- Bupropion SR (Zyban): 150 mg PO for 3 days, then 150 mg BID:
  - Start 1 week prior to smoking cessation, and continue for 7 to 12 weeks.
  - Twice as effective as placebo
  - Drug of choice for patients with depression or schizophrenia
  - May be combined with varenicline and NRT in men who smoke >1 PPD
  - S/E: tachycardia, headache, nausea, insomnia, dry mouth; contraindicated in patients who have seizure disorders or anorexia/bulimia; pregnancy Category C (1),(2)[A]
- Nicotine replacement therapy (NRT) (e.g., patch, gum, lozenge, inhaler, nasal spray) (1),(2)[A]:
  - Improves quit rates by 50–70% versus placebo
  - Over-the-counter

- Patch (NicoDerm CQ 21, 14, and 7 mg):
  - 1 patch q24h
  - Start with 21 mg if smoking ≥10 cigarettes/day; otherwise, start with 14 mg.
  - 6 weeks on initial dose, then taper
  - 2 weeks each on subsequent doses
  - No proven benefit beyond 8 weeks
- E-cigarettes
  - Contain less nicotine than cigarette
  - Considered less "dangerous" than tobacco but not as well studied as other NRT (3)[B]
  - Conflicting data on whether teen use increases or decreases risk to cigarette progression
- Gum (Nicorette, 2 and 4 mg):
  - Use 4 mg if smoking ≥25 cigarettes/day
  - Chew 1 piece q1–2h for 6 weeks, then 1 piece q2–4h for 3 weeks, then 1 piece q4–8h for 3 weeks.
- May use in combination with bupropion; monitor for hypertension
- S/E: headache, pharyngitis, cough, rhinitis, dyspepsia; all mainly with inhaler and spray forms
- Pregnancy Category D

Second Line
- Nortriptyline: 25 to 75 mg/day PO or in divided doses:
  - Start 10 to 14 days prior to smoking cessation and continue for at least 12 weeks.
  - Efficacy similar to bupropion, but side effects more common; pregnancy Category D
  - The antidepressants bupropion and nortriptyline aid long-term smoking cessation (4)[A].
- Clonidine: 0.1 mg PO BID or 0.1 mg/day transdermal patch weekly (1):
  - Side effects: hypotension, bradycardia, depression, fatigue; pregnancy Category C

ADDITIONAL THERAPIES
The following interventions have been shown to be effective in helping patients quit smoking:
- Advice from nurses, especially in hospital
- Individual counseling/group therapy
- Telephone counseling/web-based cessation programs
- Exercise (not conclusive, ineffective) (5)[A]
- Acupuncture: short-term effects (6)[A]
- Naltrexone. No evidence (7)[A]
- Opiates antagonist. No evidence (1)[A]

COMPLEMENTARY & ALTERNATIVE MEDICINE
Acupuncture, aversive therapy, and hypnosis have not been proven to enhance long-term smoking cessation.

 ONGOING CARE

FOLLOW-UP RECOMMENDATIONS
- Follow up 3 to 7 days after scheduled quit date and at least monthly for 3 months thereafter.
- Telephone follow-up if office visits not feasible
- Refraining from tobacco products for first 2 weeks is critical to long-term abstinence.

- Encourage patients who relapse to try again. Most smokers experience ≥1 failed attempts before quitting permanently. Reinforce behavioral interventions (8)[A].

Patient Monitoring
- Short-term withdrawal symptoms include dysphoria, depressed mood, irritability, anxiety, insomnia, increased appetite, and poor concentration.
- Longer term risks of smoking cessation include weight gain (4 to 5 kg on average) and depression.
- Quitting also is associated with exacerbations of ulcerative colitis and worsening of cognitive function in patients with schizophrenia.
- Nicotine withdrawal syndrome: dysphoric or depressed mood, insomnia, irritability, frustration, or anger; anxiety, difficulty concentrating, restlessness, and increased appetite or weight gain
- Lung cancer risk by smoking status: heavy smokers 1.00, light smokers 9.44 (0.35 to 0.56), ex-smokers 0.17 (0.13 to 0.23), never smoker 0.09 (0.06 to 0.13); adjusted hazard ratio (95% CI) (9)

DIET
Healthy eating for limiting weight gain following smoking cessation

PATIENT EDUCATION
1-800-QUIT-NOW: free counseling, resources, and support for quitting

PROGNOSIS
- Measurable cardiovascular benefits of smoking cessation begin as early as 24 hours after quitting and continue to mount until the risk is reduced to that of nonsmokers by 5 to 15 years.
- People who quit smoking after a heart attack or cardiac surgery reduce their risk of death by 1/3.
- Relapse rates initially >60% but decrease to 2–4% per year after completing 2 years of abstinence (8)[A].

COMPLICATIONS
- Disability and premature death due to heart attack, stroke, cancer, COPD
- Smoking more than doubles the risk of coronary artery disease and doubles the risk of stroke.
- Smokers are 12 to 22 times more likely than non-smokers to die from lung cancer.

REFERENCES

1. Cahill K, Stevens S, Perera R, et al. Pharmacological interventions for smoking cessation: an overview and network meta-analysis. *Cochrane Database Syst Rev.* 2013;(5):CD009329.
2. Thomsen T, Villebro N, Møller AM. Interventions for preoperative smoking cessation. *Cochrane Database Syst Rev.* 2014;(3):CD002294.
3. Bhatnagar A, Whitsel LP, Ribisl KM, et al. Electronic cigarettes: a policy statement from the American Heart Association. *Circulation.* 2014;130(16):1418–1436.
4. Hughes JR, Stead LF, Hartmann-Boyce J, et al. Antidepressants for smoking cessation. *Cochrane Database Syst Rev.* 2014;(1):CD000031. doi:10.1002/14651858.CD000031.pub4.
5. Ussher MH, Taylor AH, Faulkner GE. Exercise interventions for smoking cessation. *Cochrane Database Syst Rev.* 2014;(8):CD002295. doi:10.1002/14651858.CD002295.pub5.
6. White AR, Rampes H, Liu JP, et al. Acupuncture and related interventions for smoking cessation. *Cochrane Database Syst Rev.* 2014;(1):CD000009. doi:10.1002/14651858.CD000009.pub4.
7. David SP, Lancaster T, Stead LF, et al. Opioid antagonist for smoking cessation. *Cochrane Database Syst Rev.* 2013;(6):CD003086.
8. Agboola S, McNeill A, Coleman T, et al. A systematic review of the effectiveness of smoking relapse prevention interventions for abstinent smokers. *Addiction.* 2010;105(8):1362–1380.
9. Godtfredsen NS, Prescott E, Osler M. Effect of smoking reduction on lung cancer risk. *JAMA.* 2005;294(12):1505–1510.

ADDITIONAL READING
- Larzelere MM, Williams DE. Promoting smoking cessation. *Am Fam Physician.* 2012;85(6):591–598.
- Quitnet: www.quitnet.com

 SEE ALSO

Nicotine Addiction; Substance Use Disorders

 CODES

ICD10
- F17.210 Nicotine dependence, cigarettes, uncomplicated
- F17.213 Nicotine dependence, cigarettes, with withdrawal
- F17.211 Nicotine dependence, cigarettes, in remission

CLINICAL PEARLS
- Every patient who uses tobacco should be offered smoking cessation.
- Use the 5 As: ask, advise, assess, assist, and arrange
- Behavioral counseling and medication are most effective for helping patients to quit smoking when they are used in combination.
- Depression with suicidal ideations is a contraindication to use varenicline.
- Even brief advice to quit has been shown to increase quit rates.
- Following relapse, smokers should be encouraged to make another attempt to stop smoking.

T

TOURETTE SYNDROME

Ravin V. Patel, MD • Dustin Creech, MD

BASICS

DESCRIPTION
- Tourette syndrome (TS) is a movement disorder most commonly seen in school-age children. A childhood-onset neurobehavioral disorder characterized by the presence of multiple motor and at least one phonic tic (see "Physical Exam").
  - Tics are sudden, brief, repetitive, stereotyped motor movements (motor tics) or sounds (phonic tics) produced by moving air through the nose, mouth, or throat.
  - Tics tend to occur in bouts.
  - Tics can be simple or complex.
    - Motor tics precede vocal tics.
    - Simple tics precede complex tics.
  - Tics often are preceded by sensory symptoms, especially a compulsion to move.
  - Patients are able to suppress their tics, but voluntary suppression is associated with an inner tension that results in more forceful tics when suppression ceases.
  - System(s) affected: nervous

EPIDEMIOLOGY
Incidence
- The onset occurs before 18 years of age.
- Predominant age
  - Average age of onset: 7 years (3 to 8 years)
  - Tic severity is greatest at ages 7 to 12 years.
    - 96% present by age 11 years
  - Of children with TS, 50% will experience complete resolution of symptoms by age 18 years (based on self-reporting).
- Predominant sex: male > female (3:1)
- Predominant race/ethnicity: clinically heterogeneous disorder, but non-Hispanic whites (2:1) compared with Hispanics and/or blacks

Prevalence
0.77% overall in children
- 1.06% in boys
- 0.25% in girls

ETIOLOGY AND PATHOPHYSIOLOGY
Abnormalities of dopamine neurotransmission and receptor hypersensitivity, most likely in the ventral striatum, play a primary role in the pathophysiology.
- Abnormality of basal ganglia development
- Thought to result from a complex interaction between social, environmental, and multiple genetic abnormalities.
- Mechanism is uncertain; may involve dysfunction of basal ganglia–thalamocortical circuits, likely involving decreased inhibitory output from the basal ganglia, which results in an imbalance of inhibition and excitation in the motor cortex
- Controversial pediatric autoimmune neuropsychiatric disorder association with *Streptococcus* (PANDAS)
  - TS/OCD cases linked to immunologic response to previous group A β-hemolytic streptococcal infection (GABHS)
  - Thought to be linked to 10% of all TS cases
  - Five criteria
    - Presence of tic disorder and/or OCD
    - Prepubertal onset of neuropsychosis
    - History of sudden onset of symptoms and/or episodic course with abrupt symptom exacerbation, interspersed with periods of partial/complete remission

    - Evidence of a temporal association between onset/exacerbation of symptoms and a prior streptococcal infection
    - Adventitious movements during symptom exacerbation (e.g., motor hyperactivity)

Genetics
- Predisposition: frequent familial history of tic disorders and OCD
- Precise pattern of transmission and genetic origin unknown. Recent studies suggest polygenic inheritance with evidence for a locus on chromosome 17q; sequence variants in *SLITRK1* gene on chromosome 13q also are associated with TS.
- Higher concordance in monozygotic compared with dizygotic twins; wide range of phenotypes

RISK FACTORS
- Risk of TS among relatives: 9.8–15%
- First-degree relatives of individuals with TS have a 10- to 100-fold increased risk of developing TS.
- Low birth weight, maternal stress during pregnancy, severe nausea and vomiting in 1st trimester

COMMONLY ASSOCIATED CONDITIONS
- OCD (28–67%)
- ADHD (50–60%)
- Conduct disorder
- Depression/anxiety including phobias, panic attacks, and stuttering
- Learning disabilities (23%)
- Impairments of visual perception, sleep disorders, restless leg syndrome, and migraine headaches

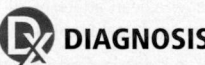

DIAGNOSIS

HISTORY
Diagnosis of TS is based on history and clinical presentation (i.e., observation of tics with/without presence of coexisting disorders). Identify comorbid conditions.

PHYSICAL EXAM
- Typically, the physical exam is normal.
- Motor and vocal tics are the clinical hallmarks.
- Tics fluctuate in type, frequency, and anatomic distribution over time.
- Multiple motor tics include facial grimacing, blinking, head/neck jerking, tongue protruding, sniffing, touching, and burping.
- Vocal tics include grunts, snorts, throat clearing, barking, yelling, hiccupping, sucking, and coughing.
- Tics are exacerbated by anticipation, emotional upset, anxiety, or fatigue.
- Tics subside when patient is concentrating/absorbed in activities.
- Motor and vocal tics may persist during all stages of sleep, especially light sleep.
- Blink-reflex abnormalities may be observed.
- No known clinical measures reliably predict children who will continue to express tics in adulthood; severity of tics in late childhood is associated with future tic severity.
- *Diagnostic and Statistical Manual of Mental Disorders* (5th ed.; *DSM-5*) criteria (1)[C]:
  - A. Both multiple motor and one or more vocal tics have been present at some time during the illness, although not necessarily concurrently.
  - B. The tics may wax and wane in frequency but have persisted for more than 1 year since first tic onset.
  - C. Onset is before age 18 years.

  - D. The disturbance is not attributable to the physiologic effects of a substance (e.g., cocaine) or another medical condition (e.g., Huntington disease, postviral encephalitis)

DIFFERENTIAL DIAGNOSIS
- Chorea/Huntington disease
- Myoclonus
- Seizure
- Ischemic or hemorrhagic stroke
- Essential tremor
- Posttraumatic/head injury
- Headache
- Dementia
- Wilson disease
- Sydenham chorea
- Multiple sclerosis
- Postviral encephalitis
- Toxin exposure (e.g., carbon monoxide, cocaine)
- Drug effects (e.g., dopamine agonists, fluoroquinolones)

DIAGNOSTIC TESTS & INTERPRETATION
Initial Tests (lab, imaging)
- No definitive lab tests diagnose TS. Based on clinical features, particularly the presence of multiple motor and vocal tics.
- Thyroid-stimulating hormone (TSH) should be measured because of association of tics with hyperthyroidism.
- No imaging studies diagnose TS
- EEG shows nonspecific abnormalities; useful only to differentiate tics from epilepsy.

Test Interpretation
- Smaller caudate volumes in patients with TS
- Striatal dopaminergic terminals are increased, as is striatal dopamine transporter (DAT) density.

TREATMENT

GENERAL MEASURES
- Treatment assessment
  - Yale Global Tic Severity Score
  - Tourette-Syndrome Severity Scale
  - Global Assessment of Functioning Scale
  - Gilles de la Tourette Syndrome-Quality of Life Scale
- A detailed history is crucial to management, because tics and comorbidities are interrelated. Goal of treatment should be to improve social functioning, self-esteem, and quality of life.
- Educate that tics are neither voluntary nor psychiatric.
- Many patients require no treatment; patient should play an active role in treatment decisions.
- Educate patient, family, teachers, and friends to identify and address psychosocial stressors and environmental triggers.
- No cure for tics: Treatment is purely symptomatic, and multimodal treatment usually is indicated.
- Neurologic and psychiatric evaluation may be useful for other primary disorders and comorbid conditions (especially ADHD, OCD, and depression).
- TS clusters with several comorbid conditions; each disorder must be evaluated for associated functional impairment because patients often are more disabled by their psychiatric conditions than by the tics; choice of initial treatment depends largely on worst symptoms (tics, obsessions, or impulsivity).

- Nonpharmacologic therapy—reassurance and environmental modification, identification and treatment of trigger, and cognitive behavior therapy
- When pharmacotherapy is employed, monotherapy is preferred to polytherapy.

MEDICATION
First Line
- Atypical antipsychotics
  - Risperidone: now recommended for standard therapy (2)[A]
    - Initiate 0.25 BID; titrate to 0.25 to 6 mg/day
    - As effective as haloperidol and pimozide for tics with fewer side effects
    - Effective against comorbidities such as OCD
    - Side effects may limit use: sedation, weight gain, and fatigue.
- α_2-Adrenergic receptor agonists (2)[B]
  - Historically first-line agents due to favorable side-effect profile, but suboptimal efficacy in limited clinical trials
  - Side effects: sedation and hypotension common
    - Initiate therapy gradually and taper when discontinuing to avoid cardiac adverse events.
  - Clonidine 0.1 to 0.3 mg/day given BID–TID
    - Maximum dose: 0.5 mg/day
    - 25–50% of patients report at least some reduction in tics.
  - Guanfacine 1 to 3 mg/day given daily or BID
    - Less sedating and longer duration of action compared with clonidine
    - Improves motor/vocal tics by 30% in some studies; no better than placebo in others

Second Line
- Neuroleptics
  - Typical antipsychotics
    - High risk for extrapyramidal symptoms (EPS)
    - Haloperidol: initiate 0.5 mg/day and titrate 0.5 mg/week up to 1 to 4 mg at bedtime (3)[B]
      - FDA-approved for treating tics
      - Considered last option of typical antipsychotics due to lower efficacy and increased side effects compared to similar medications
    - Pimozide: initiate 0.5 mg/day and titrate 0.5 mg/week up to 1 to 4 mg at bedtime (4)[A]
      - FDA-approved for treating tics
      - Risk of cardiac toxicity (prolonged Q–T interval and arrhythmias); must be given under ECG monitoring; long-term use may induce sedation, weight gain, depression, pseudoparkinsonism, and akathisia.
      - Found to work better in long-term control of tics versus acute exacerbations
    - Fluphenazine: 2.5 to 10 mg/day
      - Effective but less favored due to side effects
  - Atypical antipsychotics (3)[C]
    - Olanzapine: initiate 2.5 to 5.0 mg/day; titrate up to 20 mg/day
      - Equally effective as haloperidol and pimozide
      - May cause metabolic disturbances and weight gain
    - Quetiapine: initiate 100 to 150 mg/day; titrate to 100 to 600 mg/day
      - Well tolerated but limited data exists
    - Ziprasidone: 5 to 40 mg/day
    - Aripiprazole: initiate 2 mg/day; titrate up to 20 or 30 mg/day
      - Few studies but favorable side-effect profile

- Alternative treatments
  - Topiramate: 25 to 200 mg/day (2)[A]; promising data but not sufficient efficacy so far to recommend as first or second line
  - Tetrabenazine
  - Baclofen
- Treatment of ADHD in patients with tics (5)[A]
  - Stimulants
    - Comorbid tic disorder is not a serious contraindication, as previously held; exacerbation of tics is neither clinically significant nor common.
    - Methylphenidate: 2.5 to 30 mg/day
    - Dextroamphetamine: 5 to 30 mg/day
  - α_2-Adrenergic agonists
    - Guanfacine
    - Clonidine
      - The combination of methylphenidate and clonidine has shown superior efficacy in treating both ADHD and tic symptoms compared to monotherapy with either agent in one trial.
  - Other medications
    - Atomoxetine
    - Desipramine
- Treatment of OCD in patients with tics (6)[B]
  - SSRIs
    - First-line treatment of OCD; can be used in TS as well
    - Side effects include nausea, insomnia, sexual dysfunction, headache, and agitation.
    - Comorbid tic disorder not a contraindication; exacerbation of tics neither clinically significant nor common.
    - Black box warning for suicidality with SSRIs
    - Fluoxetine: 10 to 80 mg/day
    - Fluvoxamine: 50 to 300 mg/day
    - Sertraline: 50 to 200 mg/day
  - Tricyclic antidepressants
    - Clomipramine: 25 to 200 mg/day
      - Can be used in patients refractory to SSRIs or to augment SSRIs in partial responders
      - Side effects: weight gain, dry mouth, lowered seizure threshold, and constipation; ECG changes, including Q–T prolongation and tachycardia

ADDITIONAL THERAPIES
- Botulinum toxin injections in severe cases or where chronic medication therapy is not preferred.
- Habit-reversal training provides a viable tic suppression treatment: Works equally for motor and vocal tics.

SURGERY/OTHER PROCEDURES
Thalamic ablation and deep brain stimulation have been used experimentally (7)[C].

COMPLEMENTARY & ALTERNATIVE MEDICINE
Nonpharmacologic therapy
- Reassurance and environmental modification
- Identification and treatment of triggers
- Behavioral therapy: awareness/assertiveness training, relaxation therapy, habit-reversal therapy, and self-monitoring has shown to significantly decrease tic severity.
- Hypnotherapy
- Biofeedback
- Acupuncture
- Cannabinoids: insufficient evidence to recommend; small trials show small positive effects in some parameters (8)[A].

 ONGOING CARE

FOLLOW-UP RECOMMENDATIONS
Patient Monitoring
Observe for associated psychiatric disorders.

PATIENT EDUCATION
- Reassurance that many patients with tics do not need medication; often education and/or therapy is all that is required.
- National Tourette Syndrome Association: http://www.tsa-usa.org

PROGNOSIS
- Symptoms will fluctuate throughout illness.
- Tic severity typically stabilizes by age 25 years.
- 60–75% of young adults show some improvement in symptoms.
- 10–40% of patients will exhibit full remission.

REFERENCES
1. Kenney C, Kuo SH, Jimenez-Shahed J. Tourette's syndrome. *Am Fam Physician*. 2008;77(5):651–658.
2. Huys D, Hardenacke K, Poppe P, et al. Update on the role of antipsychotics in the treatment of Tourette syndrome. *Neuropsychiatr Dis Treat*. 2012;8:95–104.
3. American Psychiatric Association. *Diagnostic and Statistical Manual of Mental Disorders*. 5th ed. Arlington, VA: American Psychiatric Association; 2013.
4. Roessner V, Plessen KJ, Rothenberger A, et al. European clinical guidelines for Tourette syndrome and other tic disorders. Part II: pharmacological treatment. *Eur Child Adolesc Psychiatry*. 2011; 20(4):173–196.
5. Pringsheim T, Marras C. Pimozide for tics in Tourette's syndrome. *Cochrane Database Syst Rev*. 2009;(2):CD006996.
6. Pringsheim T, Steeves T. Pharmacological treatment for attention deficit hyperactivity disorder (ADHD) in children with comorbid tic disorders. *Cochrane Database Syst Rev*. 2011;(4):CD007990.
7. Lombroso PJ, Scahill L. Tourette syndrome and obsessive-compulsive disorder. *Brain Dev*. 2008;30(4):231–237.
8. Savica R, Stead M, Mack KJ, et al. Deep brain stimulation in Tourette syndrome: a description of 3 patients with excellent outcome. *Mayo Clin Proc*. 2012;87(1):59–62.

ADDITIONAL READING
Curtis A, Clarke CE, Rickards HE. Cannabinoids for Tourette's syndrome. *Cochrane Database Syst Rev*. 2009;(4):CD006565.

 CODES

ICD10
F95.2 Tourette's disorder

CLINICAL PEARLS
- TS is diagnosed by history and witnessing tics; have parent video patient's tics if not present on exam in your office.
- Nearly 50% of children with tics also have ADHD. Stimulants may be used as first-line treatment for ADHD (tics are not a contraindication, as previously believed).

TOXOPLASMOSIS

Jonathan MacClements, MD, FAAFP

BASICS

- *Toxoplasma gondii* is an obligate intracellular protozoan parasite.
- Most common latent protozoan infection
- Clinically significant disease typically manifests only in pregnancy or in an immunocompromised patient.

DESCRIPTION

- Acute self-limited infection in immunocompetent
- Acute symptomatic or reactivated latent infection in immunocompromised persons
- Congenital toxoplasmosis (acute primary infection during pregnancy)
- Ocular toxoplasmosis

Pediatric Considerations

- The earlier fetal infection occurs, the more severe.
- Risk of perinatal death is 5% if infected in 1st trimester.

Pregnancy Considerations

- Pregnant immunocompromised and HIV-infected women should undergo serologic testing.
- Seronegative pregnant women should receive preventive counseling.
- Serologic testing during pregnancy remains controversial.

EPIDEMIOLOGY

Incidence

- Prevalence of congenital toxoplasmosis in the United States: 10 to 100/100,000 live births
- Predominant sex: male > female

Prevalence

- Present in every country. Seropositivity rates range from <10% to >90% (1)[A].
- In the United States, 11% of individuals aged 6 to 49 years are seropositive. Age-adjusted prevalence in the United States is 22.5%.
- Seroprevalence among women in the United States is 15%.

ETIOLOGY AND PATHOPHYSIOLOGY

Transmission to humans

- Ingestion of raw or undercooked meat, food, or water containing tissue cysts or oocytes; usually from soil contaminated with feline feces
- Transplacental passage from infected mother to fetus; risk of transmission is 30% on average.
- Blood product transfusion and solid-organ transplantation
- Ingested *T. gondii* oocysts enter host's gastrointestinal tract where bradyzoites/tachyzoites are released, penetrate contiguous cells, replicate and are transported to susceptible tissues where clinical disease manifests.

Genetics

Human leukocyte antigen (HLA) DQ3 is a genetic marker of susceptibility in AIDS.

RISK FACTORS

- Immunocompromised states, including HIV infection with CD4 cell count <100/μL
- Primary infection during pregnancy; risk of fetal transmission increases with gestational age at seroconversion. Transmission in the 1st trimester is associated with more severe consequences.

- Chronically infected pregnant women who are immunocompromised have an increased risk of transmitting congenital toxoplasmosis.

GENERAL PREVENTION

Prevention is important in seronegative pregnant women and immunodeficient patients.

- Avoid eating undercooked meat: Cook to 152°F (66°C) or freeze for 24 hours at ≤−12°C.
- Avoid drinking unfiltered water.
- Wash produce thoroughly.
- Strict hand hygiene after touching soil
- Wear gloves and wash hands after handling raw meat or cat litter.
- Avoid shellfish (*Toxoplasma* cysts).

COMMONLY ASSOCIATED CONDITIONS

- Chorioretinitis; self-limiting, febrile lymphadenopathy; mononucleosis-like illness
- An unclear association exists between schizophrenia and several infectious agents including *T. gondii*.

DIAGNOSIS

HISTORY

- Congenital toxoplasmosis
  - Clinical presentation varies widely; 80% of patients are asymptomatic at birth.
  - Classic triad (*uncommon*): chorioretinitis, hydrocephalus, cerebral calcifications
  - Manifestations may include prematurity, intrauterine growth retardation (IUGR).
  - Jaundice, rash accompanying a mononucleosis-like illness
  - Mental retardation, seizures, visual defects, spasticity, sensorineural hearing loss
- Ocular toxoplasmosis
  - Chorioretinitis: focal necrotizing retinitis
  - Yellowish-white elevated cotton patch
  - Congenital disease usually bilateral; acquired is more often unilateral.
  - Symptoms include blurred vision, scotoma, pain, and photophobia.
- Acute toxoplasmosis (immunocompetent host)
  - ~90% of patients are asymptomatic.
  - Most common manifestation is bilateral, symmetric, nontender cervical lymphadenopathy.
  - Constitutional symptoms such as fever, chills, and sweats are usually mild.
  - Headaches, myalgias, pharyngitis, hepatosplenomegaly, and diffuse nonpruritic maculopapular rash may occur.
  - Pregnant women are often asymptomatic.
  - Most common site is CNS with toxoplasmic encephalitis.
  - Headache; focal neurologic deficits and seizures
  - Fever usually present
  - Extracerebral toxoplasmosis: pneumonitis; chorioretinitis; rarely: GI system, liver, musculoskeletal system, heart, bone marrow, bladder, and orchitis

PHYSICAL EXAM

- In adults: fever, lymphadenopathy, nonpruritic rash
- In newborns: hydrocephalus, neurologic abnormalities, hepatosplenomegaly, chorioretinitis, microcephaly, mental retardation

DIFFERENTIAL DIAGNOSIS

Syphilis, lymphoma, progressive multifocal leukoencephalopathy, cryptococcal meningitis, congenital TORCH infections, *Listeria* infection, tuberculosis (TB), erythroblastosis fetalis

DIAGNOSTIC TESTS & INTERPRETATION

- CBC: atypical lymphocytosis, anemia, thrombocytopenia
- Serology interpretation
  - In acute infection, IgM antibodies appear within the 1st week.
  - Diagnosis can be made if initial test demonstrates positive IgM and negative IgG, with both tests being positive 2 weeks later.
  - If follow-up IgG remains negative 2 to 4 weeks later but IgM is still positive, it is likely a false positive.
  - Negative IgG rules out prior infection (IgG remains detectable for life).
- Types of serologic tests
  - ELISA: most commonly used
  - Sabin-Feldman dye test: Gold standard against which all other serologic assays are compared.
  - IFA test: more available in commercial labs
  - ISAGA: widely available commercially; more sensitive and specific than IFA for detecting IgM
  - Avidity testing: confirmatory test to establish whether positive IgM/IgG reflects recent or chronic infection
- PCR: *T. gondii* DNA amplification in blood or amniotic fluid; used for diagnosis of fetal infection
- Culture (rarely necessary): Organism can be isolated either by cell culture or by mouse inoculation.

Initial Tests (lab, imaging)

- Diagnosis of primary infection is typically based on history and confirmed by serology.
- Serum *Toxoplasma*-specific IgG and IgM are first step.
- According to the result of IgM test, determine IgG avidity.
- Diagnosis of maternal infection and congenital toxoplasmosis
  - Pregnant women who have mononucleosis-like illness but negative heterophile test should be tested for toxoplasmosis.
  - Maternal infection accurately diagnosed when based on two blood samples at least 2 weeks apart showing seroconversion
  - High avidity of IgG during 1st trimester argues against maternal primary infection.
  - Real-time PCR analysis for *T. gondii* in amniotic fluid predicts fetal infection and helps guide appropriate treatment and surveillance.
  - Fetal ultrasound is useful for prognosis.
  - Routine screening for toxoplasmosis is not recommended.
- Diagnosis of congenital toxoplasmosis after birth
  - Serology requires several serum samples for IgM and IgA antibodies.
  - Sampling of the cord or peripheral blood should be done within the first 2 weeks.
  - Ophthalmologic, auditory, and neurologic examinations; lumbar puncture; and head CT should be performed.
- Diagnosis of toxoplasmic encephalitis
  - Serology for IgG
  - Imaging: MRI is more sensitive than CT scan for identification of characteristic ring-enhancing brain lesions.

- MRI: for identifying multiple ring-enhancing brain lesion in AIDS patients with cerebral toxoplasmosis
- SPECT and PET scans: can help distinguish toxoplasmosis from CNS lymphoma

Diagnostic Procedures/Other
- Lymph node biopsy
- Brain biopsy in CNS disease
- Amniocentesis with PCR (risk of false negatives and false positives)
- Placental isolation of *Toxoplasma* is diagnostic.

Test Interpretation
- Confirmatory, meningocerebritis ± abscesses with necrosis, Giemsa
- Lymph node histology shows triad of:
  - Reactive follicular hyperplasia
  - Irregular clusters of epithelioid histiocytes on and blurring margins of germinal centers
  - Distension of sinuses with monocytoid cells
- Sensitivity of triad 62.5%, specificity 91.3%

TREATMENT

GENERAL MEASURES
Immunocompetent patients usually require no treatment.

MEDICATION
First Line

ALERT
Important: All pyrimethamine-containing regimens should include leucovorin (folinic acid 10 to 25 mg/day PO) during and 1 week after completion of pyrimethamine to prevent drug-induced hematologic toxicity (2)[A].

- Treatment in immunocompromised hosts
  - Initial regimen of choice is pyrimethamine 200 mg loading dose PO, followed by 50 mg/day plus sulfadiazine 4 to 6 g/day PO in 4 divided doses; for those intolerant or allergic to sulfadiazine, clindamycin 600 to 1,200 mg IV or 450 mg PO QID can be used instead.
  - Alternative regimens for patients intolerant to sulfadiazine and clindamycin include the following:
    - Pyrimethamine: 200 mg loading dose PO, followed by 50 mg/day plus azithromycin 900 to 1,200 mg PO once daily
    - Pyrimethamine: 200 mg loading dose PO, then 50 mg/day plus atovaquone 1,500 mg PO BID
    - Sulfadiazine: 1,000 to 1,500 mg QID plus atovaquone 1,500 mg BID
    - Trimethoprim-sulfamethoxazole: 10/50 mg/kg/day PO or IV divided BID (for 30 days) may be a cost-effective alternative.
  - Duration of therapy: typically 6 weeks, lower doses for secondary prophylaxis (2)[A]
  - Use adjunctive steroids should in patients with signs of increased intracranial pressure.
  - Anticonvulsants, if there is a history of seizures
- Prophylaxis in immunocompromised patients
  - Primary prophylaxis: indicated for patients with HIV infection and CD4 count <100 cells/μL who are *T. gondii* IgG–positive
    - Trimethoprim-sulfamethoxazole-DS: 1 tablet PO daily. Alternative for sulfa allergy is dapsone 50 mg/day PO *plus* pyrimethamine 50 mg PO weekly *plus* leucovorin 25 mg PO weekly *or* atovaquone 1,500 mg PO daily.

- Secondary prophylaxis: Following 6 weeks of therapy, administer lower doses of drugs:
  - Sulfadiazine 2 to 4 g/day in two to four divided doses *plus* pyrimethamine 25 to 50 mg/day is the first choice.
  - Alternative regimens include clindamycin 600 mg PO q8h *plus* pyrimethamine 25 to 50 mg/day PO *or* atovaquone 750 mg PO BID to QID ± pyrimethamine 25 mg PO daily.

- Pregnant women (3)[A]
  - There is a lack of evidence on whether antenatal treatment reduces congenital transmission; however, prenatal treatment is usually offered.
  - <18 weeks' gestation: Spiramycin 1 g PO q8h without food until delivery if amniotic fluid PCR is negative. Does not treat infection in the fetus
  - >18 weeks' gestation: Pyrimethamine and sulfadiazine should be considered only if fetal infection is documented by positive amniotic fluid PCR (pyrimethamine is teratogenic):
    - Pyrimethamine: 50 mg PO q12h for 2 days, then 50 mg/day plus sulfadiazine 75 mg/kg PO × 1 dose, then 50 mg/kg q12h (max 4 g/day)
- Treat infected newborns regardless of clinical manifestations:
  - Pyrimethamine 2 mg/kg/day (max 50 mg) for 2 days; then 1 mg/kg/day (max 25 mg) for 2 to 6 month; then 1 mg/kg (max 25 mg) on Monday, Wednesday, and Friday; sulfadiazine 100 mg/kg/day divided BID; and leucovorin 10 mg three times per week during pyrimethamine and 1 week after discontinuation
- Immunocompetent nonpregnant patients generally do not require treatment unless symptoms are severe or prolonged; 1 of 2 regimens can be used:
  - Pyrimethamine: 100 mg loading dose PO, followed by 25 to 50 mg/day *plus* sulfadiazine 2 to 4 g/day in four divided doses
  - Pyrimethamine: 100 mg loading dose PO, followed by 25 to 50 mg/day *plus* clindamycin 300 mg PO QID

Second Line
- Clindamycin: 900 to 1,200 mg TID IV used for ocular and CNS toxoplasmosis alone and in combination with pyrimethamine; as effective as the sulfadiazine-pyrimethamine with fewer adverse effects
- Corticosteroids (prednisone 1 to 2 mg/kg/day) are added for macular chorioretinitis or CNS infection.
- Alternatives: atovaquone (Mepron), azithromycin (Zithromax), clarithromycin (Biaxin), or dapsone *plus* pyrimethamine and leucovorin
- Trimethoprim-sulfamethoxazole appears to be equivalent to pyrimethamine-sulfadiazine in AIDS patients with CNS disease.

ONGOING CARE

FOLLOW-UP RECOMMENDATIONS
Patient Monitoring
Precautions
- Monitor for bone marrow, renal, or liver toxicity.
- Good hydration: Sulfadiazine is poorly soluble and may crystallize in the urine.
- Watch for antibiotic-associated diarrhea.
- Sulfonamides may alter phenytoin and warfarin levels or interfere with oral hypoglycemic agents.

PATIENT EDUCATION
- http://www.aafp.org/afp/2003/0515/p2145.html
- http://familydoctor.org/familydoctor/en/diseases-conditions/toxoplasmosis.html

PROGNOSIS
- Immunodeficient patients often relapse if treatment or suppression therapy is stopped.
- Treatment may prevent the development of untoward sequelae in infants with congenital toxoplasmosis.

REFERENCES
1. Torgerson PR, Mastroiacovo P. The global burden of congenital toxoplasmosis: a systematic review. *Bull World Health Organ*. 2013;91(7):501–508.
2. Montoya JG, Liesenfeld O. Toxoplasmosis. *Lancet*. 2004;363(9425):1965–1976.
3. Montoya JG, Remington JS. Management of *Toxoplasma gondii* infection during pregnancy. *Clin Infect Dis*. 2008;47(4):554–566.

ADDITIONAL READING
- Arantes TE, Silveira C, Holland GN, et al. Ocular involvement following postnatally acquired *Toxoplasma gondii* infection in Southern Brazil: a 28-year experience. *Am J Ophthalmol*. 2015; 159(6):1002.e2–1012.e2.
- Bodaghi B, Touitou V, Fardeau C, et al. Toxoplasmosis: new challenges for an old disease. *Eye (Lond)*. 2012; 26(2):241–244.
- Garweg JG, Stanford MR. Therapy for ocular toxoplasmosis—the future. *Ocul Immunol Inflamm*. 2013;21(4):300–305.
- Kaplan JE, Benson C, Holmes KH, et al. Guidelines for prevention and treatment of opportunistic infections in HIV-infected adults and adolescents: recommendations from CDC, the National Institutes of Health, and the HIV Medicine Association of the Infectious Diseases Society of America. *MMWR Recomm Rep*. 2009;58(RR–4):1–207.
- Wallon M, Franck J, Thulliez P, et al. Accuracy of real-time polymerase chain reaction for *Toxoplasma gondii* in amniotic fluid. *Obstet Gynecol*. 2010;115(4):727–733.

CODES

ICD10
- B58.9 Toxoplasmosis, unspecified
- P37.1 Congenital toxoplasmosis
- B58.2 Toxoplasma meningoencephalitis

CLINICAL PEARLS
- Toxoplasmosis is often asymptomatic in immunocompetent patients, who often don't need treatment for clinical disease.
- Primary prevention is important, particularly for pregnant women and immunodeficient patients.
- The most common manifestation of acute toxoplasmosis in immunocompetent host is bilateral, symmetric, nontender cervical lymphadenopathy.
- Universal screening for congenital toxoplasmosis is not currently recommended.

TRACHEITIS, BACTERIAL

Mary Cataletto, MD, FAAP, FCCP

 BASICS

DESCRIPTION
- Acute, potentially life-threatening infraglottic bacterial infection following a primary viral infection, usually parainfluenzae or influenza viruses
  - Direct laryngoscopy reveals marked subglottic edema and thick mucopurulent secretions, sometimes causing pseudomembranes.
- System(s) affected: pulmonary
- Synonym(s): laryngotracheobronchitis; pseudomembranous croup; bacterial croup

EPIDEMIOLOGY
Incidence
- Estimated incidence: 4 to 8 per 1,000,000 (1)
- First cases described prior to 1950; resurgence of cases has been noted since 1979.
- Peak incidence in children: fall and winter
- Mean age: 5 years (1)
- Infections in adolescents and adults have been reported.
- Predominant sex: male > female (2:1)
- Accounts for 5–14% of upper airway obstruction in children requiring critical care services

Prevalence
- Rare illness
- Most common potentially life-threatening upper airway infection in children
- Methicillin-resistant *Staphylococcus aureus* (MSRA) may contribute to changing epidemiology and virulence.

ETIOLOGY AND PATHOPHYSIOLOGY
- *Staphylococcus aureus* (most common pediatric cause): Consider MRSA.
- *Haemophilus influenzae* type B
- *Streptococcus pyogenes* group A
- *Streptococcus pneumoniae*
- *Moraxella catarrhalis* (associated with higher intubation rate; more frequent in younger children)
- Often polymicrobial

Genetics
No known genetic predisposition

RISK FACTORS
- Periods of increased seasonal activity of respiratory viruses
- Reports following adenoidectomy, with chronic tracheal aspiration, with evidence of other concurrent infections, including sinusitis, otitis, pneumonia, or pharyngitis

GENERAL PREVENTION
- Standard precautions, with scrupulous attention to hand washing, especially when caring for tracheostomy patients
- Vaccination against viruses that may predispose to bacterial tracheitis

COMMONLY ASSOCIATED CONDITIONS
- Consider anatomic abnormalities or foreign body as well as recent pharyngeal or laryngeal surgery.
- Predisposing: Down syndrome, immunodeficiency, subglottic hemangioma, tracheoesophageal fistula repair, tracheobronchomalacia
- Viral coinfection may occur.

 DIAGNOSIS

- May present with fever and systemic toxicity or as more localized disease
- Careful history and physical exam are the best methods to distinguish bacterial tracheitis from croup and other rare causes of upper airway obstruction.

HISTORY
- Prodromal upper respiratory tract symptoms
- Gradual progression of mild upper airway symptoms over 1 hour to 6 days to acute, febrile phase of rapid respiratory decompensation
- No drooling
- No response to aerosolized epinephrine and/or systemic corticosteroids (1)

PHYSICAL EXAM
FEVER >38°C (100.4°F)
- Toxic appearance
- Variable degree of respiratory distress (2)
  - Tachypnea
  - Inspiratory stridor (2)
- Voice and cry usually normal
- Drooling uncommon

DIFFERENTIAL DIAGNOSIS
- Severe croup (viral)
- Spasmodic croup
- Diphtheria in nonvaccinated patients
- Retropharyngeal abscess
- Epiglottitis
- Pneumonia
- Foreign body aspiration

DIAGNOSTIC TESTS & INTERPRETATION
- Routine laboratory studies are not required to make the diagnosis.
- Radiographs are neither definitive nor diagnostic.
- Tracheal endoscopy provides a definitive diagnosis (1,3)[C].

Initial Tests (lab, imaging)
- Bacterial cultures of tracheal secretions are required for culture isolates and sensitivities.
- Rapid antigen or polymerase chain reaction (PCR)–based testing for respiratory viruses may be helpful.

- Routine laboratory studies may not be helpful.
- Blood cultures rarely positive
- CBC results may vary.
  - WBC count may show marked leukocytosis or may be normal.
  - Increased band cell count
- Radiographs may be normal, but exudates may mimic the findings in foreign body aspiration.
- Pneumonic infiltrates are common.
- Anteroposterior (AP) and lateral neck x-rays show subglottic and tracheal narrowing (i.e., steeple sign on AP film) with haziness and radiopaque linear or particulate densities (crusts).
- In patients with risk of acute respiratory obstruction, either do not obtain x-rays or monitor carefully.

Follow-Up Tests & Special Considerations
Follow chest film if suspect pneumonia.

Diagnostic Procedures/Other
- Direct laryngoscopy and tracheoscopy is diagnostic and demonstrates
  - Normal supraglottic structures
  - Marked subglottic erythema and edema
  - Ulcerations
  - Epithelial sloughing
  - Copious mucopurulent secretions ± plaques or pseudomembranes
- Obtain Gram stain and aerobic, anaerobic, and viral cultures of tracheal secretions during the procedure.

Test Interpretation
- Tracheal biopsy is rarely indicated but may be considered in immunodeficient child or child with ulcerative colitis.
- Diffuse inflammation of larynx, trachea, and bronchi
- Mucopurulent exudate; microabscesses may be present.
- Semiadherent membranes (containing numerous neutrophils and cellular debris) may be identified within the trachea.

TREATMENT

- Treat as potentially life-threatening airway emergency.
- Children with suspected or actual bacterial tracheitis should be cared for in a pediatric ICU (1)[C].
- Assess and monitor respiratory status; supplemental oxygen may be required.
- Airway protection and support, as necessary (at least 50% require intubation; some studies report up to 100%)
- Ventilatory support may be required.
- Suctioning
- Different clinical course in previously healthy children compared with those with artificial airway

MEDICATION

- Empiric therapy should cover the most common pathogens until sensitivities are available: antistaphylococcal agent (vancomycin or clindamycin) and a 3rd-generation cephalosporin (e.g., ceftriaxone or cefotaxime) (1,3)[C].
- In the case of technology-dependent children with tracheostomy, make initial antibiotic choices based on previous tracheal culture.
- Narrow regimen when pathogens and sensitivities available (1,3)[C]
- Contraindications: Refer to the manufacturer's literature for each drug.
- Precautions: Refer to the manufacturer's literature for each drug. Avoid aminoglycosides in patients with previous hearing loss.
- Significant possible interactions: Refer to the manufacturer's literature for each drug.

ISSUES FOR REFERRAL

All children with suspected or actual bacterial tracheitis should be cared for in a pediatric ICU by a pediatric critical care team that may include the following subspecialists: pediatric intensivist, infectious disease specialist, pulmonologist, and/or otolaryngologist.

ADDITIONAL THERAPIES

- At present, evidence is lacking to establish the effect of heliox inhalation in the treatment of croup in children.
- For technology-dependent children with artificial airway:
  - Initial antibiotic choices should cover most recent tracheal aspirate isolates and then be refined according to culture and sensitivity results.
  - Adjunctive aerosol therapy may be helpful, particularly when multidrug-resistant organisms are present.

SURGERY/OTHER PROCEDURES

- Tracheostomy is usually not necessary.
- Therapeutic bronchoscopy may be necessary to facilitate removal of inspissated secretions.
- Tracheal membranes may require removal.

INPATIENT CONSIDERATIONS

- Aggressive supportive care and airway protection are paramount.
- Initial treatment of choice for bacterial tracheitis is broad-spectrum antibiotic coverage.
- Children with tracheitis and artificial airways present unique challenges: Tracheoscopy is important in establishing diagnosis in this population.
- Be vigilant for possible MRSA.

Pediatric Considerations

- True pediatric emergency

- Admission to ICU
- Maintain airway: often difficult due to copious secretions
  - Endotracheal or nasotracheal intubation usually needed, especially in infants and children <4 years of age
  - Much less likely to need intubation if child >8 years of age
  - Advantage of intubation is the ability to clear trachea and bronchi of secretions and pseudomembranes.
- Vigorous pulmonary toilet to clear airway of secretions
- Hydration, humidification, antibiotics

Admission Criteria/Initial Stabilization

- Suspected or confirmed diagnosis of tracheitis
- Respiratory distress
- Artificial airway

Nursing

- Provide calm, quiet environment for child once endoscopy and cultures are done.
- Airway monitoring
- Frequent suctioning
- Monitor fluid balance.
- Establish and maintain open lines of communication with child and parents.

Discharge Criteria

No longer in need of acute care

 ONGOING CARE

FOLLOW-UP RECOMMENDATIONS

Patient Monitoring

Children with artificial airways will require ongoing follow-up.

DIET

Varies with clinical situation

PATIENT EDUCATION

Keep immunizations up to date.

PROGNOSIS

- Intubation generally 3 to 11 days
- Usually requires 3 to 7 days of hospitalization
- With effective early recognition and management, complete recovery can be expected.
- Cardiopulmonary arrest and death have occurred.

COMPLICATIONS

- Cardiopulmonary arrest
- Hypotension
- Acute respiratory distress syndrome (ARDS)
- Pneumonia
- Formation of pseudomembranes

REFERENCES

1. Kuo CY, Parikh SR. Bacterial tracheitis. *Pediatr Rev.* 2014;35(11):497–499.
2. Tebruegge M, Pantazidou A, Thorburn K, et al. Bacterial tracheitis: a multi-centre perspective. *Scand J Infect Dis.* 2009;41(8):548–557.
3. American Academy of Pediatrics. *Pediatric Pulmonology.* Elk Grove Village, Illinois, IL: American Academy of Pediatrics; 2011:955.

ADDITIONAL READING

- Hopkins A, Lahiri T, Salerno R, et al. Changing epidemiology of life-threatening upper airway infections: the reemergence of bacterial tracheitis. *Pediatrics.* 2006;118(4):1418–1421.
- Huang YL, Peng CC, Chiu NC, et al. Bacterial tracheitis in pediatrics: 12 year experience at a medical center in Taiwan. *Pediatr Int.* 2009;51(1):110–113.
- Loftis L. Acute infectious upper airway obstructions in children. *Semin Pediatr Infect Dis.* 2006;17(1):5–10.
- Shah S, Sharieff GQ. Pediatric respiratory infections. *Emerg Med Clin North Am.* 2007;25(4):961–979.
- Vorwerk C, Coats T. Heliox for croup in children. *Cochrane Database Syst Rev.* 2010;(2):CD006822.

 SEE ALSO

Croup (Laryngotracheobronchitis); Epiglottitis

 CODES

ICD10

- J04.10 Acute tracheitis without obstruction
- J04.11 Acute tracheitis with obstruction
- J05.0 Acute obstructive laryngitis [croup]

CLINICAL PEARLS

- Bacterial tracheitis is an acute, potentially life-threatening, infraglottic bacterial infection following a primary viral infection that accounts for 5–14% of upper airway obstructions in children requiring critical care services.
- Children with suspected or actual bacterial tracheitis should be cared for in a pediatric ICU.
- Endoscopy provides a definitive diagnosis (2).
- Initial treatment of choice for bacterial tracheitis is broad-spectrum antibiotic coverage, aggressive airway protection, and supportive care (2).

T

TRANSIENT ISCHEMIC ATTACK (TIA)

Emilio A. Russo, MD • G. Daud Noaz, MD, MSBME

BASICS

DESCRIPTION

- A transient episode of neurologic dysfunction due to focal brain, retinal, or spinal cord ischemia without acute infarction
- No longer diagnosed based on timeframe of symptoms
- Most important predictor of stroke: 7–40% of patients with stroke report previous TIA.
- Synonym(s): ministroke

EPIDEMIOLOGY

- Incidence of TIA underestimated because some patients do not report symptoms.
- 200,000 to 500,000 new TIA cases reported each year
  - 83 cases/100,000 people/year in the United States
  - 400 to 800 cases/100,000 persons aged 50 to 59 years
- Prevalence of TIA in general population: ~2.3%
- Predominant age: risk increases >60 years; highest in 7th and 8th decades
- Predominant sex: male > female (3:1)
- Predominant race/ethnicity: African Americans > Hispanics > Caucasians. The difference in African Americans is exaggerated at younger ages.

ETIOLOGY AND PATHOPHYSIOLOGY

Temporary reduction/cessation of cerebral blood flow adversely affecting neuronal function

- Carotid/vertebral atherosclerotic disease
  - Artery-to-artery thromboembolism
  - Low-flow ischemia
- Small, deep vessel disease associated with HTN
  - Lacunar infarcts
- Cardiac diseases
  - 1–6% of patients with MI develop stroke.
- Embolism secondary to the following:
  - Valvular (mitral valve) pathology
  - Mural hypokinesias/akinesias with thrombosis (acute anterior MI/congestive cardiomyopathies)
  - Cardiac arrhythmia (atrial fibrillation accounts for 5–20% incidence)
- Hypercoagulable states
  - Antiphospholipid antibodies
  - Deficiency of protein S, protein C
  - Presence of antithrombin III
  - Oral contraceptives
  - Pregnancy and parturition
- Arteritis
  - Noninfectious necrotizing vasculitis
  - Drugs
  - Irradiation
  - Local trauma
- Sympathomimetic drugs (e.g., cocaine)
- Other causes: spontaneous and posttraumatic (e.g., chiropractic manipulation) arterial dissection
- Fibromuscular dysplasia

Genetics

Inheritance is polygenic, with tendency to clustering of risk factors within families.

RISK FACTORS

- Hypertension (HTN)
- Cardiac diseases (A-fib, MI, valvular disease)
- Diabetes
- Hyperlipidemia
- Atherosclerotic disease (carotid/vertebral stenosis)
- Cigarette smoking
- Thrombophilias

GENERAL PREVENTION

- Lifestyle changes: smoking cessation, diet modification, weight loss, regular aerobic exercise, and limited alcohol intake
- Use of ASA and statins as primary prevention may be considered in certain populations.
- Strict control of medical risk factors: *diabetes* (glycemic control), *HTN* (thiazide and/or ACE/ARB), *hyperlipidemia* (statins), anticoagulation when high risk of cardioembolism (e.g., atrial fibrillation, mechanical valves)

ALERT

10–20% of patients with TIA have CVA within 90 days; 25–50% of those occur within the first 48 hours.

Geriatric Considerations

- Older patients have a higher mortality rate than younger patients—highest in 7th and 8th decades.
- Atrial fibrillation is a frequent cause among the elderly.

Pediatric Considerations

- Congenital heart disease is a common cause among pediatric patients.
- Other causes include the following:
  - Metabolic: homocystinuria, Fabry disease
  - Central nervous system (CNS) infection
  - Clotting disorders
  - Marfan syndrome
  - Moyamoya disease

Pregnancy Considerations

- Preeclampsia, eclampsia, and HELLP
- TTP and hemolytic uremic syndrome
- Postpartum angiopathy
- Cerebral venous thrombosis
- Hypercoagulable states related to pregnancy

COMMONLY ASSOCIATED CONDITIONS

- Atrial fibrillation
- Uncontrolled HTN
- Carotid stenosis

DIAGNOSIS

HISTORY

- Obtain witness accounts with emphasis on symptom onset, progression, and recovery.
- Carotid circulation (hemispheric): monocular visual loss, hemiplegia, hemianesthesia, neglect, aphasia, visual field defects (amaurosis fugax); less often, headaches, seizures, amnesia, confusion
- Vertebrobasilar (brain stem/cerebellar): bilateral visual obscuration, diplopia, vertigo, ataxia, facial paresis, Horner syndrome, dysphagia, dysarthria; also headache, nausea, vomiting, and ataxia
- Past medical history, baseline functional status
- ABCD2 score: predicts risk of CVA within 48 hours (1)[A]

  - Score of 0 to 1: 0%; 2 to 3: 1.3%; 4 to 5: 4.1%; 6 to 7: 8.1%
  - **A**ge >65 years: 1 point
  - **B**P 140/90 mm Hg: 1 point
  - Symptoms of focal weakness: 2 points
  - Speech impaired without weakness: 1 point
  - **D**uration >60 minutes: 2 points
  - **D**uration 10 to 59 minutes: 1 point
  - **D**iabetes: 1 point

PHYSICAL EXAM

- Vital signs, oxygen saturation
- Thorough neurologic and cardiac exams

DIFFERENTIAL DIAGNOSIS

- Evolving stroke
- Migraine (hemiplegic)
- Focal seizure (Todd paralysis)
- Hypoglycemia
- Bell palsy
- Neoplasm of brain
- Subarachnoid hemorrhage
- Intoxication
- Electrolyte abnormalities

DIAGNOSTIC TESTS & INTERPRETATION

Initial Tests (lab, imaging)

- Patients with TIA should undergo neuroimaging evaluation within 24 hours of symptom onset.
- MRI, including diffusion-weighted imaging, is the preferred brain diagnostic modality; if not available then noncontrast head CT (2)[B].
- Noninvasive imaging of the cervicocephalic vessels should be performed routinely as part of the evaluation of suspected TIA (2)[A].
- Initial assessment of the extracranial vasculature may involve carotid US/TCD, MRA, or CTA depending on the availability and expertise and characteristics of the patient (2)[B].
- Routine blood tests (CBC, chemistry, PT/PTT, UPT, and fasting lipid panel) are reasonable in evaluation of patient with TIA (2)[B].

Follow-Up Tests & Special Considerations

- If only noninvasive testing is performed prior to CEA, it is reasonable to pursue two concordant noninvasive findings; otherwise, catheter angiography should be considered (2)[B].
- Echo is reasonable in evaluation of patients with suspected TIA especially when no other cause is noted (2)[B].
- TEE is useful in identifying PFO, aortic arch atherosclerosis, and valvular disease and is reasonable when this will alter management (2)[B].
- Prolonged cardiac monitoring is useful in patients with an unclear etiology after initial brain imaging and ECG (2)[B].
- EEG: if seizure suspected
- After TIA, all patients should be screened for DM with either fasting plasma glucose or hemoglobin A1C.
- Consider a sleep study due to the high prevalence of sleep apnea among TIA patients; treatment with CPAP has shown to improve patient outcomes (3)[B].

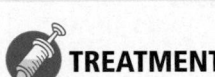

TREATMENT

GENERAL MEASURES

- TIA is a neurologic emergency. Immediate medical attention should be sought within 24 hours of symptom onset.
- Current evidence suggests that patients with high-risk TIAs require rapid referral and 24-hour admission (see ABCD2 scoring).
- Acute phase
  - Inpatient for surgery and high-risk groups
  - Outpatient investigations may be considered based on patient's stroke risk, arrangement of follow-up, and social circumstances.
- Antiplatelet therapy to prevent recurrence or future CVA
- Treatment/control of underlying associated conditions

MEDICATION

- For patients with TIA, the use of antiplatelet agents rather than oral anticoagulation is recommended to reduce risk of recurrent stroke and other cardiovascular events, with the exception of cardioembolic etiologies (2)[A].
- *Uncertain* if switching agent in patients who have additional ischemic attacks while on antiplatelet therapy is beneficial (4)[C].

First Line

- Enteric-coated aspirin: 160 to 325 mg/day in the acute phase (5)[A] followed by long-term antiplatelet therapy for noncardioembolic TIA and anticoagulation for cardioembolic etiology
- Antiplatelet therapy
  - ER dipyridamole–ASA (Aggrenox): 25/200 mg BID (4,6)[B]
  - Combined therapy with dipyridamole and ASA is better than ASA alone (5,7)[A].
  - More expensive than ASA alone and may have more side effects
  - Aspirin 50 to 325 mg/day (4)[A]
    - Contraindications: active PUD and hypersensitivity to ASA or NSAIDs
    - Precautions: may aggravate preexisting peptic ulcer disease; may worsen symptoms of asthma
    - Significant possible interactions: may potentiate effects of anticoagulants and sulfonylurea analogues
  - Clopidogrel 75 mg/day (4)[B]
    - Can be used in patients who are allergic to ASA (4)[B]
    - Precautions: Thrombotic thrombocytopenic purpura (TTP) can occur and increases risk of bleeding when combined with aspirin.
    - May be very slightly more effective than aspirin alone (5)[B]; more expensive and more side effects than aspirin
- Combined aspirin and clopidogrel therapy has been demonstrated to reduce the incidence of subsequent stroke by 21% without increased risk of bleeding when used for a duration of 1 month or less immediately following TIA or CVA (6)[A].
- Anticoagulation therapy
  - Factor Xa inhibitors (rivaroxaban, apixaban), direct thrombin inhibitor (dabigatran)
    - Noninferior to warfarin in nonvalvular A-fib
    - Precautions: avoid in CKD (CrCl <30 mL/min)
    - Expensive
  - Warfarin (INR-adjusted dose) (4)[A]
    - Contraindications: intolerance/allergy, active liver disease, active bleeding, pregnancy
    - Significant possible interactions: antibiotics, antiepileptics, antifungals, and many others
  - ASA 325 mg/day or ASA 81 mg/day and clopidogrel 75 mg/day (4)[A]
    - Patients who cannot take anticoagulation for reasons other than bleeding risk

Second Line

Ticlopidine (Ticlid): 250 mg PO BID

- For patients who cannot tolerate other agents
- Contraindications: hypersensitivity, presence of hematopoietic/hemostatic disorders, conditions associated with bleeding, severe liver dysfunction
- Precautions: neutropenia (0.8% severe), which is reversible with cessation of the drug. Monitor blood counts every 2 weeks for first 3 months. TTP can occur.
- Significant possible interactions: Digoxin plasma levels decreased 15%; theophylline half-life increased from 8.6 to 12.2 hours.

ISSUES FOR REFERRAL

- Neurology for ongoing workup and treatment
- Cardiology if cardiac cause suspected
- Vascular surgery if carotid endarterectomy appropriate

ADDITIONAL THERAPIES

- Secondary prevention of TIA should be initiated; venous thromboembolism (VTE) prophylaxis
- Patients with TIA or ischemic stroke should be started on a statin.
- BP should be reduced when appropriate after 24 hours. ACE inhibitors/thiazide have shown to be of benefit.
- Patients with DM or pre-DM should be advised to follow ADA guidelines to maintain tight glycemic control (3)[A].

SURGERY/OTHER PROCEDURES

- Consider carotid endarterectomy in patients with a high degree of carotid artery stenosis.
- When carotid endarterectomy is indicated for patients with TIA, surgery within 2 weeks is reasonable if there are no contraindications to early revascularization.

INPATIENT CONSIDERATIONS

Admission Criteria/Initial Stabilization

- Symptoms <72 hours and the following:
  - ABCD2 score of ≥3
  - ABCD2 score of 0 to 2 and uncertainty that dx workup can be completed within 2 days as outpatient.
  - ABCD2 score of 0 to 2 and evidence that indicates the patient's event was caused by focal ischemia.
- Correct fluid and electrolyte imbalances.

Discharge Criteria

Consider safety at home if another incident occurs.

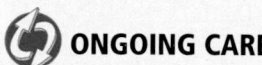 ONGOING CARE

FOLLOW-UP RECOMMENDATIONS

Patient Monitoring

- Follow-up every 3 months for 1st year then annually
- Close attention to recurrent or subsequent CVA

DIET

As appropriate for underlying medical problems

PROGNOSIS

- The risk of stroke on the ipsilateral side within 90 days and cumulative thereafter is 10–20%.
- Frequency increases with the addition of multiple risk factors and severity of carotid stenosis.
- Patients with larger artery occlusion or cardioembolic etiology are at increased risk of recurrence.
- The major cause of death in the first 5 years is cardiac disease.

COMPLICATIONS

- Stroke
- Functional impairment

REFERENCES

1. Tsivgoulis G, Stamboulis E, Sharma VK, et al. Multicenter external validation of the ABCD2 score in triaging TIA patients. *Neurology*. 2010;74(17):1351–1357.
2. Adams RJ, Albers G, Alberts MJ, et al. Update to the AHA/ASA recommendations for the prevention of stroke in patients with stroke and transient ischemic attack. *Stroke*. 2008;39(5):1647–1652.
3. Kernan WN, Ovbiagele B, Black HR, et al. Guidelines for the prevention of stroke in patients with stroke and transient ischemic attack: a guideline for healthcare professionals from the American Heart Association/American Stroke Association. *Stroke*. 2014;45(7):2160–2236.
4. Lansberg MG, O'Donnell MJ, Khatri P, et al. Antithrombotic and thrombolytic therapy for ischemic stroke: Antithrombotic Therapy and Prevention of Thrombosis, 9th ed: American College of Chest Physicians Evidence-Based Clinical Practice Guidelines. *Chest*. 2012;141(2 Suppl):e601S–e636S.
5. Albers GW, Amarenco P, Easton JD, et al. Antithrombotic and thrombolytic therapy for ischemic stroke: American College of Chest Physicians Evidence-Based Clinical Practice Guidelines (8th edition). *Chest*. 2008;133(6 Suppl):630S–669S.
6. Chen S, Shen Q, Tang Y, et al. Efficacy and safety of adding clopidogrel to aspirin on stroke prevention among high vascular risk patients: a meta-analysis of randomized controlled trials. *PLoS One*. 2014;9(8):e104402. doi:10.1371/journal.pone.0104402.
7. De Schryver EL, Algra A, van Gijn J. Dipyridamole for preventing stroke and other vascular events in patients with vascular disease. *Cochrane Database Syst Rev*. 2007;(3):CD001820.

ADDITIONAL READING

Adams HP Jr, del Zoppo G, Alberts MJ, et al. Guidelines for the early management of adults with ischemic stroke: a guideline from the American Heart Association/American Stroke Association Stroke Council, Clinical Cardiology Council, Cardiovascular Radiology and Intervention Council, and the Atherosclerotic Peripheral Vascular Disease and Quality of Care Outcomes in Research Interdisciplinary Working Groups: the American Academy of Neurology affirms the value of this guideline as an educational tool for neurologists.. *Circulation*. 2007;115(20):e478–e534.

 SEE ALSO

Algorithms: Stroke; Transient Ischemic Attack and Transient Neurologic Defects

 CODES

ICD10

- G45.9 Transient cerebral ischemic attack, unspecified
- G45.1 Carotid artery syndrome (hemispheric)
- G45.0 Vertebro-basilar artery syndrome

CLINICAL PEARLS

- Primary/secondary prevention is important, stressing smoking cessation, exercise, weight loss, limited ETOH intake, and control of HTN, hyperlipidemia, and diabetes.
- Antiplatelet therapy (e.g., aspirin or clopidogrel or aspirin-dipyridamole) should be initiated.
- Warfarin should be initiated in patients with atrial fibrillation or cardioembolic risk factors.
- A 30% risk of stroke exists within 5 years of a TIA.

TRANSIENT STRESS CARDIOMYOPATHY

Timothy P. Fitzgibbons, MD, PhD • Gerard P. Aurigemma, MD

 BASICS

DESCRIPTION

- Transient stress cardiomyopathy (TSC) is a unique cause of reversible left ventricle (LV) dysfunction with a presentation indistinguishable from the acute coronary syndromes (ACS), particularly ST-segment elevation myocardial infarction (MI) (1).
- Typically, the patient is a postmenopausal woman who presents with acute chest pain or dyspnea after an identifiable "trigger" (i.e., an acute emotional or physiologic stressor).
- First reported by authors from Japan, TSC was known initially as the *takotsubo syndrome* because the typical LV morphology (i.e., apical ballooning) resembled that of a Japanese octopus trap or *takotsubo* (2)[B].
- Presenting clinical features include the following:
  - Chest symptoms and/or dyspnea
  - ECG changes, including ST-segment elevations or diffuse T-wave inversions
  - Mild elevation in cardiac biomarkers (creatine kinase [CK], troponin)
  - Transient wall motion abnormalities that may involve the base, midportion, and/or lateral walls of the LV.
  - The apex of the right ventricle (RV) may be affected in up to 25% of cases (3)[B].
- Clinical features may vary on a case-by-case basis, and formal diagnostic criteria have not been established.
- Authors from the Mayo Clinic have proposed that 3 of the 4 following criteria establish the diagnosis (1)[A]:
  - Transient akinesis or dyskinesis of the LV apical and midventricular segments with regional wall motion abnormalities extending beyond a single epicardial vascular distribution
  - Absence of obstructive coronary artery disease (CAD) or angiographic evidence of acute plaque rupture
  - New ECG abnormalities, either ST-segment elevation or T-wave inversion
  - Absence of
    - Recent significant head trauma
    - Intracranial bleeding
    - Pheochromocytoma
    - Obstructive epicardial CAD
    - Myocarditis
    - Hypertrophic cardiomyopathy
- Synonym(s): takotsubo cardiomyopathy; apical ballooning syndrome; stress cardiomyopathy; broken heart syndrome; ampulla cardiomyopathy

EPIDEMIOLOGY

Incidence
- TSC accounts for a small percentage (1–3%) of ACS.
- In a recent prospective evaluation of patients admitted to the ICU, as many as 28% had apical ballooning, often in association with sepsis.
- Predominant sex: 82–100% of cases occur in women.
- Predominant age: Mean age of patients is 62 to 75 years.

Prevalence
2.2% of patients presenting to a referral hospital with ST-segment MIs were found to have TSC.

ETIOLOGY AND PATHOPHYSIOLOGY
- The exact pathophysiology is not known.
- A perturbation in the brain-heart axis, originating in the insular cortex, may be the inciting event (4).
- Subsequent overwhelming activation of the sympathetic nervous system initiates a cascade of events, including the following:
  - Catecholamine-induced LV dysfunction: "biased agonism" of epinephrine for β_2-adrenergic receptors, located predominantly at the cardiac apex (5)
  - Endothelial dysfunction and vasospasm
  - Cellular metabolic injury
    - Myocardial norepinephrine release
    - Calcium overload
    - Contraction band necrosis

Genetics
No genetic associations have been described to date.

RISK FACTORS
- Female sex
- Postmenopausal state
- Emotional stress (i.e., argument, death of family member)
- Physiologic stress (i.e., acute medical illness)
- Chronic neurologic or psychiatric disease (4)

COMMONLY ASSOCIATED CONDITIONS
Death from TSC is rare, and most cases resolve rapidly, within 2 to 3 days. Reported complications include:
- Left-sided heart failure
- Pulmonary edema
- Cardiogenic shock and hemodynamic compromise
- Dynamic LV outflow tract gradient complicated by hypotension
- Mitral regurgitation
- Ventricular arrhythmias
- LV thrombus formation
- LV free wall rupture
- Death (rare, 0–8%)

DIAGNOSIS

Because TSC often is indistinguishable from an ACS, it should be treated initially as such:
- Activate emergency medical services or report to emergency department.
- Oxygen, IV access, and ECG monitoring
- Urgent cardiology consultation

HISTORY
- In 2/3 of patients, there is exposure to a "trigger event."
  - Emotional stress: argument, death of family member, divorce, public speaking, and so forth
  - Physiologic stress: acute medical condition such as head trauma, asthma attack, seizure, and so forth
- In 1/3 of patients, there is no identifiable trigger (4).
- Acute onset of dyspnea or chest pain
- Palpitations
- Syncope

PHYSICAL EXAM
Exam may be unremarkable or may include any of the following:
- Tachypnea
- Tachycardia
- Hypotension
- Jugular venous distension
- Bibasilar rales
- S_3 gallop
- Systolic ejection murmur due to dynamic LV outflow tract gradient
- Holosystolic murmur of mitral regurgitation

DIFFERENTIAL DIAGNOSIS
- Acute ST-segment elevation MI
- Pulmonary embolism
- Myopericarditis
- Pheochromocytoma
- Hypertrophic cardiomyopathy
- Subarachnoid hemorrhage or stroke

DIAGNOSTIC TESTS & INTERPRETATION
- ECG should be done urgently and may show the following:
  - Diffuse ST-segment elevations
  - Diffuse and often dramatic T-wave inversions
  - QTc interval prolongation (6)[B]
  - Q waves
- Laboratory tests typically reveal a mild elevation in cardiac biomarkers such as
  - CK (rarely >500 U/mL)
  - Troponin I
  - B-type natriuretic peptide (BNP)
  - Markers of high filling pressures (e.g., BNP) tend to be higher than markers of necrosis (e.g., CK, troponin).
  - TSC can be distinguished from AMI with 95% specificity using a BNP/TnT ratio ≥1,272 (sensitivity 52%) (7)[B].
- Chest radiograph
  - Cardiomegaly
  - Pulmonary edema
- Echocardiogram
  - Reduced LV systolic function
  - Abnormal diastolic function, including evidence of increased filling pressures
  - Regional wall motion abnormalities in one of the following patterns:
    - Classic or "takotsubo-type" ballooning of the apex with a hypercontractile base
    - "Reverse takotsubo": apical hypercontractility with basal akinesis
    - "Midventricular" akinesis with apical and basal hypercontractility
    - Focal or localized akinesis of an isolated segment
  - Dynamic intracavitary LV gradient
  - Mitral regurgitation
  - Variable involvement of the RV
- Cardiac MRI
  - Reduced LV function
  - Wall motion abnormalities as described for transthoracic echocardiography
  - Absence of delayed hyperenhancement with gadolinium

Diagnostic Procedures/Other
- Because ST-segment elevation MI is the diagnosis of exclusion, patients typically are referred for urgent cardiac catheterization.
- Coronary angiography
  - Nonocclusive CAD
  - Rarely, epicardial coronary spasm
  - Endothelial dysfunction as measured by fractional flow reserve or TIMI frame counts
- Left-sided heart catheterization: increased LV end-diastolic pressure to a similar degree as AMI (8)[B]
- Ventriculography: wall motion abnormalities as described for transthoracic echocardiography
- Right-sided heart catheterization
  - Increased pulmonary capillary wedge pressure
  - Secondary pulmonary hypertension
  - Increased right ventricular filling pressures
  - Reduced cardiac output or cardiogenic shock (cardiac index <2 and mean arterial pressure [MAP] <60 mm Hg)

Test Interpretation
Characteristic pathologic findings of involved myocardium have not been described.

TREATMENT

- Activation of emergency medical services
- Advanced cardiac life support therapies as needed
- Oxygen
- IV access
- ECG monitoring

MEDICATION
After diagnostic cardiac catheterization, empirical treatment goals are as follows:
- Management of hypotension: differentiation between cardiogenic shock and dynamic LV cavity gradient
- Management of increased filling pressures and congestive states
- Attenuation of sympathetic drive

First Line
- There are no evidence-based treatment recommendations for TSC.
- Although β-blockers are of theoretical benefit, their use has not been associated with improved outcomes in observational cohorts (4)[B].
- If there is evidence of left ventricular systolic dysfunction or pulmonary edema, consider the following:
  - Furosemide: 20 to 40 mg IV/PO BID as needed to reduce LV filling pressures and dyspnea (9)
  - ACE inhibitors or angiotensin receptor blockers: Lisinopril 10 to 40 mg/day PO or equivalent or valsartan 80 to 160 mg PO BID have been associated with improved outcomes in observational cohorts (4)[B].

Second Line
Short-term anticoagulation should be considered in patients with severely reduced LV function to prevent LV thrombus formation. Unfractionated heparin 80 U/kg IV bolus followed by 18 U/kg/hr IV or Lovenox 1 mg/kg SC BID.

ISSUES FOR REFERRAL
All patients with TSC generally should be comanaged with cardiology while inpatient and referred to cardiology as an outpatient.

ADDITIONAL THERAPIES
- Urgent cardiology consultation and consideration of cardiac catheterization
- Hypotension may require the following:
  - Vasopressors (e.g., dopamine or Levophed) if there is no LV outflow tract gradient (9)[C]
  - Phenylephrine and IV fluids to increase afterload in the presence of an LV outflow tract gradient (9)[C]
  - Cardiogenic shock that is not due to an LV outflow tract gradient may require placement of an intra-aortic balloon pump.

INPATIENT CONSIDERATIONS
Admission Criteria/Initial Stabilization
- 12-lead ECG
- Chest radiograph
- Laboratory testing
- Echocardiography
- Patients with TSC usually are admitted for observation because the differential diagnosis includes ACS.

IV Fluids
Normal saline infusion to support BP, if necessary, and no evidence of heart failure

Discharge Criteria
Generally considered after exclusion of ACS and resolution of
- Congestive state
- Hypotension
- Profound impairments of systolic function

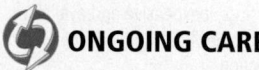 ONGOING CARE

FOLLOW-UP RECOMMENDATIONS
- Impairments in systolic function typically resolve in 2 to 3 days but may last as long as 1 month.
- Patients should follow up with cardiology and serial echocardiography to document improved LV function.

PROGNOSIS
- Prognosis is excellent. Inpatient mortality is rare and ranges from 0% to 8%.
- Recurrence is rare; it also has been reported in 0–8% of patients.

REFERENCES
1. Bybee KA, Prasad A. Stress-related cardiomyopathy syndromes. *Circulation*. 2008;118(4):397–409.
2. Dote K, Sato H, Tateishi H, et al. Myocardial stunning due to simultaneous multivessel coronary spasms: a review of 5 cases [in Japanese]. *J Cardiol*. 1991;21(2):203–214.
3. Fitzgibbons TP, Madias C, Seth A, et al. Prevalence and clinical characteristics of right ventricular dysfunction in transient stress cardiomyopathy. *Am J Cardiol*. 2009;104(1):133–136.
4. Templin C, Ghadri JR, Diekmann J, et al. Clinical features and outcomes of takotsubo (stress) cardiomyopathy. *N Engl J Med*. 2015; 373(10): 929–938.
5. Paur H, Wright PT, Sikkel MB, et al. High levels of circulating epinephrine trigger apical cardiodepression in a β2-adrenergic receptor/Gi-dependent manner: a new model of takotsubo cardiomyopathy. *Circulation*. 2012;126(6): 697–706.
6. Madias C, Fitzgibbons TP, Alsheikh-Ali AA, et al. Acquired long QT syndrome from stress cardiomyopathy is associated with ventricular arrhythmias and torsades de pointes. *Heart Rhythm*. 2011;8(4):555–561.
7. Randhawa MS, Dhillon AS, Taylor HC, et al. Diagnostic utility of cardiac biomarkers in discriminating takotsubo cardiomyopathy from acute myocardial infarction. *J Card Fail*. 2014;20(1):2–8.
8. Medeiros K, O'Connor MJ, Baicu CF, et al. Systolic and diastolic mechanics in stress cardiomyopathy. *Circulation*. 2014;129(16):1659–1667.
9. Hunt SA, Abraham WT, Chin MH, et al. 2009 focused update incorporated into the ACC/AHA 2005 guidelines for the diagnosis and management of heart failure in adults: a report of the American College of Cardiology Foundation/American Heart Association Task Force on Practice Guidelines developed in collaboration with the International Society for Heart and Lung Transplantation. *J Am Coll Cardiol*. 2009;53(15):e1–e90.

 SEE ALSO

Algorithm: Chest Pain/Acute Coronary Syndrome

 CODES

ICD10
I51.81 Takotsubo syndrome

CLINICAL PEARLS
- TSC is a cause of reversible LV dysfunction with a clinical presentation indistinguishable from the ACS, particularly ST-segment elevation MI.
- Echocardiography may strongly suggest the diagnosis.
- Treatment is supportive and should include diuretics and ACE inhibitors in patients with CHF.

TRICHOMONIASIS

Michael Arnold, MD, CDR, MC • Joshua R. Beer, DO

BASICS

DESCRIPTION
- Sexually transmitted urogenital infection caused by a pear-shaped, parasitic protozoan
- Causes vaginitis/urethritis in women, nongonococcal urethritis in men
- In pregnancy, increases risk of preterm labor, preterm premature rupture of membranes, small for gestational age infant, and possibly stillbirth
- Synonym(s): trich; trichomonal urethritis

EPIDEMIOLOGY
Incidence
- Affects >120 million women worldwide. The most common curable sexually transmitted infection (STI) worldwide (1).
- Estimated 1.1 million new cases annually in the United States
- 10–25% of vaginal infections
- 1–17% of cases of NGU in males; reported prevalence among men without urethritis ranges from 0% to 8%
- Predominant age: middle-aged adults
  - Rare until onset of sexual activity
  - Common in postmenopausal women; age is not protective and long-term carriage is possible.
- Women have higher prevalence (1.5 to 4.4 times more than men) and are more commonly symptomatic (2).

Pediatric Considerations
Rare in prepubertal children; diagnosis should raise concern of sexual abuse.

Prevalence
- 3.1% of all U.S. women age 25 to 49 years; 1.5% of U.S. women age 15 to 24 years
- Racial disparity demonstrated
  - 1.3% of white, non-Hispanic women
  - 1.8% of Mexican American women
  - 13.3% of black, non-Hispanic women (2)

ETIOLOGY AND PATHOPHYSIOLOGY
- *Trichomonas vaginalis*: a pear-shaped, flagellated, parasitic protozoan
- Grows best at 35–37°C in anaerobic conditions at pH of 5.5 to 6.0
- STI, but nonsexual transmission is possible because organism can survive several hours in moist environment.

Genetics
No known genetic considerations

RISK FACTORS
- Multiple sexual partners
- Unprotected intercourse
- Lower socioeconomic status
- Other STIs
- Untreated partner with previous infection
- Use of douching or feminine powders

GENERAL PREVENTION
- Use of male or female condoms
- Limiting numbers of sexual partners
- Male circumcision may be protective (3)[B].

COMMONLY ASSOCIATED CONDITIONS
- Other STIs, including HIV
- Bacterial vaginosis

DIAGNOSIS

HISTORY
- Women
  - Yellow-green, malodorous vaginal discharge
  - Vulvovaginal pruritus
  - Dysuria
  - 70–85% are symptomatic.
- Men
  - Dysuria
  - Urethral discharge
  - 80% are asymptomatic.

PHYSICAL EXAM
- Women
  - Vaginal erythema
  - Yellow-green, frothy, malodorous vaginal discharge
  - Cervical petechiae (strawberry cervix; seen in ~10% of patients)
- Men: penile discharge, spontaneous and with expression

DIFFERENTIAL DIAGNOSIS
- Women (other vaginitides)
  - Bacterial vaginosis
  - Vaginal candidiasis
  - Chlamydial infection
  - Gonorrheal infection
- Men (other urethritides)
  - Chlamydial infection
  - Gonorrheal infection

DIAGNOSTIC TESTS & INTERPRETATION
Initial Tests (lab, imaging)
- Wet mounts of vaginal or urethral discharge: direct visualization of motile trichomonads. Most common diagnostic method since inexpensive and available
  - Sensitivity: 60–70%; declines rapidly within 1 hour from collection
  - Specificity: 99.8%
- Culture: sensitivity: >95%, specificity >99%; takes 4 to 7 days for growth
- Nucleic acid amplification test (NAAT)
  - Gold standard for diagnosis (4)
  - Sensitivity and specificity 95–99%
  - FDA approved for vaginal, endocervical, or female urine specimens
  - Results in 1 hour
  - Limited clinical availability
- Antigen detection
  - ELISA and direct fluorescent antibody tests: sensitivity of 80–90%
  - Limited clinical availability

Follow-Up Tests & Special Considerations
Detection on cervical Papanicolaou smear
- Treat since highly specific (97–99%)
- Not effective trichomonas screening test given sensitivity as low as 60%

Diagnostic Procedures/Other
Detection on self-obtained sample with DNA probe assay with specificity >98%

TREATMENT

- Symptomatic individuals require treatment.
- Sexual partners should be treated presumptively.
- Patients should abstain from sexual intercourse during treatment and until they are asymptomatic.

GENERAL MEASURES
The nitroimidazole class is only known effective antimicrobial treatment. If metronidazole resistance is suspected, use tinidazole (5)[A].

MEDICATION
First Line
- Metronidazole: 2 g PO, 1 dose (6)[A]
  - FDA pregnancy risk Category B
  - Cure rate: 84–98%
- Tinidazole: 2 g PO, 1 dose (6)[A]
  - FDA pregnancy risk Category C
  - Abstain from breastfeeding during treatment and for 3 days after the dose.
  - More expensive
  - Reaches higher levels in genitourinary tract
  - Cure rate: 92–100%

Second Line
- Metronidazole: 500 mg PO BID for 7 days
  - Only if still symptomatic after initial treatment
  - Considered first line in HIV-positive individuals
- Can dose with metronidazole or tinidazole 2 g daily for 7 days if infection persists
- May consider IV dosing of metronidazole based on case report that demonstrated cure after multiple failed oral regimens

Pregnancy Considerations
Metronidazole is effective for trichomoniasis infection during pregnancy but may increase the risk of preterm and low-birth-weight babies.
- Studies showed risk in patients receiving four times the standard dosing.
- Trichomoniasis is also associated with prematurity.

ISSUES FOR REFERRAL
- Multidrug-resistant organism
- Patient allergy to metronidazole: Desensitization to metronidazole is recommended.

ADDITIONAL THERAPIES
- Limited clinical trials assessing effectiveness of alternative therapies (4)
- Intravaginal metronidazole gel is not effective.
- Suggested alternative therapies based on small number of case reports
  - Paromomycin 6.25% cream
  - Povidone-iodine douche
  - Boric acid intravaginally
  - Furazolidone intravaginally

COMPLEMENTARY & ALTERNATIVE MEDICINE
See "Additional Therapies."

ONGOING CARE

FOLLOW-UP RECOMMENDATIONS
- If symptoms persist after initial treatment, repeat wet mount or other testing.
- Retest women for *T. vaginalis* recommended within 3 months of treatment. Data insufficient for retesting men (6)[A]
- HIV-positive patients should be screened for trichomonas at time of HIV diagnosis and at least annually (6)[A].

DIET
Abstain from alcohol during treatment and for 24 hours following last dose of metronidazole or 48 to 72 hours following last dose of tinidazole due to disulfiram-like reaction.

PATIENT EDUCATION
Educate about the sexually transmitted aspect.
- Advise patient to notify sexual partner to be treated.
- Discuss STI prevention—condom use can prevent recurrence.
- Abstain from intercourse while undergoing treatment; use condoms if abstention is not feasible.
- Avoid alcohol during treatment with metronidazole or tinidazole.

PROGNOSIS
- Excellent
- Usually eliminated after one course of antibiotics

COMPLICATIONS
Pregnancy Considerations
Linked to low birth weight, preterm premature rupture of membranes, and preterm birth

REFERENCES
1. World Health Organization. Prevalence and incidence of selected sexually transmitted infections, *Chlamydia trachomatis*, *Neisseria gonorrhoeae*, syphilis and *Trichomonas vaginalis*. Methods and results used by WHO to generate 2005 estimates. World Health Organization Web site. http://www.who.int/reproductivehealth/publications/rtis/9789241502450/en/. Accessed December 10, 2015.
2. Sutton M, Sternberg M, Koumans EH, et al. The prevalence of *Trichomonas vaginalis* infection among reproductive-age women in the United States, 2001-2004. *Clin Infect Dis*. 2007;45(10): 1319–1326.
3. Sobngwi-Tambekou J, Taljaard D, Nieuwoudt M, et al. Male circumcision and *Neisseria gonorrhoeae*, *Chlamydia trachomatis* and *Trichomonas vaginalis*: observations after a randomised controlled trial for HIV prevention. *Sex Transm Infect*. 2009;85(2): 116–120.
4. Muzny CA, Schwebke JR. The clinical spectrum of *Trichomonas vaginalis* infection and challenges to management. *Sex Transm Infect*. 2013;89(6): 423–425.
5. Seña AC, Bachmann LH, Hobbs MM. Persistent and recurrent *Trichomonas vaginalis* infections: epidemiology, treatment and management considerations. *Expert Rev Anti Infect Ther*. 2014;12(6):673–685.
6. Workowski KA, Bolan GA. Sexually transmitted diseases treatment guidelines, 2015. *MMWR Recomm Rep*. 2015;64(RR-03):1–137.

ADDITIONAL READING
- Allsworth JE, Ratner JA, Peipert JF. Trichomoniasis and other sexually transmitted infections: results from the 2001-2004 National Health and Nutrition Examination Surveys. *Sex Transm Dis*. 2009;36(12):738–744.
- Fastring DR, Amedee A, Gatski M, et al. Co-occurrence of *Trichomonas vaginalis* and bacterial vaginosis and vaginal shedding of HIV-1 RNA. *Sex Transm Dis*. 2014;41(3):173–179.
- Forna F, Gülmezoglu AM. Interventions for treating trichomoniasis in women. *Cochrane Database Syst Rev*. 2003;(2):CD000218.
- Gülmezoglu AM, Azhar M. Interventions for trichomoniasis in pregnancy. *Cochrane Database Syst Rev*. 2011;(5):CD000220.
- Hale T. *Medications and Mothers' Milk: A Manual of Lactational Pharmacology*. 14th ed. Amarillo, TX: Hale Publishing; 2010.
- Hawkins I, Carne C, Sonnex C, et al. Successful treatment of refractory *Trichomonas vaginalis* infection using intravenous metronidazole. *Int J STD AIDS*. 2015;26(9):676–678.
- Helms DJ, Mosure DJ, Secor WE, et al. Management of *Trichomonas vaginalis* in women with suspected metronidazole hypersensitivity. *Am J Obstet Gynecol*. 2008;198(4):370.e1–370.e7.
- Kirkcaldy RD, Augostini P, Asbel LE, et al. *Trichomonas vaginalis* antimicrobial drug resistance in 6 US cities, STD Surveillance Network, 2009-2010. *Emerg Infect Dis*. 2012;18(6):939–943.
- Klebanoff MA, Carey JC, Hauth JC, et al. Failure of metronidazole to prevent preterm delivery among pregnant women with asymptomatic *Trichomonas vaginalis* infection. *N Engl J Med*. 2001;345(7): 487–493.
- McClelland RS, Sangare L, Hassan WM, et al. Infection with *Trichomonas vaginalis* increases the risk of HIV-1 acquisition. *J Infect Dis*. 2007;195(5): 698–702.
- Meites E. Trichomoniasis: the "neglected" sexually transmitted disease. *Infect Dis Clin North Am*. 2013;27(4):755–764.
- Miller M, Liao Y, Gomez AM, et al. Factors associated with the prevalence and incidence of *Trichomonas vaginalis* infection among African American women in New York City who use drugs. *J Infect Dis*. 2008; 197(4):503–509.
- Saperstein AK, Firnhaber GC. Clinical inquiries. Should you test or treat partners of patients with gonorrhea, chlamydia, or trichomoniasis? *J Fam Pract*. 2010;59(1):46–48.
- Satterwhite CL, Torrone E, Meites E, et al. Sexually transmitted infections among US women and men: prevalence and incidence estimates, 2008. *Sex Transm Dis*. 2013;40(3):187–193.
- Silver BJ, Guy RJ, Kaldor JM, et al. *Trichomonas vaginalis* as a cause of perinatal morbidity: a systematic review and meta-analysis. *Sex Transm Dis*. 2014;41(6):369–376.
- Wendel KA, Workowski KA. Trichomoniasis: challenges to appropriate management. *Clin Infect Dis*. 2007;44(Suppl 3):S123–S129.
- Wiese W, Patel SR, Patel SC, et al. A meta-analysis of the Papanicolaou smear and wet mount for the diagnosis of vaginal trichomoniasis. *Am J Med*. 2000;108(4):301–308.

CODES

ICD10
- A59.9 Trichomoniasis, unspecified
- A59.03 Trichomonal cystitis and urethritis
- A59.01 Trichomonal vulvovaginitis

CLINICAL PEARLS
- Both partners need to be treated for trichomoniasis.
- Retest women within 3 months of treatment.
- Avoid alcohol during treatment with standard agents.
- Treatment does not reduce risk of adverse pregnancy outcomes.
- Male circumcision may be protective.
- Annual screening recommended for HIV-positive patients.
- Not a nationally notifiable condition

T

TRICHOTILLOMANIA

Carol Hustedde, PhD • William G. Elder, PhD

 BASICS

- Trichotillomania (TTM) is a hair-pulling disorder characterized by self-induced, repeated, and often noticeable hair loss. It can become severe and difficult to control.
- TTM is currently conceptualized as a compulsive behavior related to obsessive-compulsive disorder (OCD). Tension or boredom typically play a significant role, and the individual may be conscious or unconscious that they are pulling hair.

DESCRIPTION

- TTM causes uncontrollable hair pulling from anywhere on the body, although the scalp is the most common area followed by the eyelashes, eyebrows, pubic/perirectal area, axilla, and face. It usually results in variable degrees of alopecia.
- TTM usually presents in childhood or early adolescence.
- Denial and hiding of hair pulling is common.
- Recurrence or worsened hair pulling is associated with increased stress/anxiety, but TTM can also occur at times of relaxation and distraction, such as when reading.
- The three subtypes of TTM: early onset, automatic, and focused
- When TTM is associated with trichophagia, it may also result in GI complaints secondary to bezoars
- TTM has frequent comorbidity with other psychiatric diagnoses

EPIDEMIOLOGY

- It is difficult to assess the exact number of individuals affected by TTM because of the social stigma associated with it. Small studies have estimated a range of 1–3.5% for late adolescents and young adults.
- It is possible that up to 1 of 50 individuals are affected by TTM at least once in their lifetime.
- The mean age of onset is at 13 years.
- During childhood, males and females are equally affected by TTM. During adulthood, females are far more affected than males.

ETIOLOGY AND PATHOPHYSIOLOGY

- Serotonin deficiency
- Tension relief
- Habitual behavior
- There is currently a significant flux in the conceptualizations of the mechanisms and causes of impulse control, behavior, anxiety, and OCDs. Brain imaging and biochemical and neuropsychological studies should help to resolve this issue. It can be expected that there will be increased differentiation as well as redefinitions of disorders that are based on neurophysiology and brain circuitry.

Genetics

Genetics appears to contribute to the development of TTM as demonstrated by a higher rate of concordance in monozygotic twins (38.1%) versus dizygotic twins (0%). Genetic involvement is multifaceted and not clearly understood at this time.

RISK FACTORS

- Positive family history
- Other psychiatric disorders: depression, OCD, anxiety, posttraumatic stress disorder (PTSD), eating disorders, nail biting, skin picking

COMMONLY ASSOCIATED CONDITIONS

- Depression
- Anxiety
- OCD
- Eating disorders

Dx **DIAGNOSIS**

- TTM may be difficult to diagnose because individuals may deny it because of the social stigma and embarrassment.
- Several TTM-specific assessment tools have been developed that further understands about psychopathology of TTM.
- Assessment should include multiple sources of information to provide understanding of TTM in context.

HISTORY

- TTM most commonly manifests as hair pulling from any part of the body, resulting in alopecia of variable severity.
- The scalp is the most common area from which hair is pulled but can also involve other parts of the body, such as eyebrows and eyelashes.
- Individuals will conceal hair pulling because of embarrassment. However, when asked about it by a medical professional, they will divulge extent of problem and their efforts to control it.

- TTM may also cause social isolation because individuals may withdraw from friends and family to engage in hair-pulling behavior.
- If TTM is associated with trichophagia (compulsive eating of hair), it may present with various GI symptoms with variable severity, from acute generalized abdominal pain to a bowel obstruction secondary to a trichobezoar.
- TTM is not always associated with anxiety and stress, but it is commonly precipitated by highly stressful situations. The action of hair pulling may be associated with tension relief.

PHYSICAL EXAM

- The most common manifestation of TTM is alopecia.
- The severity of the alopecia is variable, from isolated areas of hair loss to complete baldness.
- Hair loss can be from any part of the body.
- The Friar Tuck sign may be seen, which consists of hair loss seen in a circular pattern with varying lengths of broken hairs.
- There is also a lack of dermatologic abnormalities associated with the hair loss.
- In addition to the hair loss, hair abnormalities consisting of damaged hair follicles, broken hairs of varying lengths
- When TTM is associated with trichophagia and, consequently, trichobezoars, there may be symptoms of abdominal pain, nausea, vomiting, obstructive jaundice, bowel obstruction symptoms, and anemia.
- Patients with TTM may also pull hairs from other people and pets, sometimes surreptitiously. They may also pull fibers from carpets and fabrics.

DIFFERENTIAL DIAGNOSIS

- Alopecia areata
- Tinea capitis
- Traction alopecia
- Loose anagen syndrome
- OCD
- Schizophrenia or other psychotic disorders
- Stereotypic movement disorders
- Factitious behaviors

DIAGNOSTIC TESTS & INTERPRETATION

US or CT scan for trichobezoar detection

Diagnostic Procedures/Other

- Trichotillomania Scale for Children
- Trichotillomania Diagnostic Interview
- National Institute of Mental Health Trichotillomania Questionnaire
- Premonitory Urge for Tics Scale

Test Interpretation

- Punch biopsy: high frequency of telogen hairs; deformed, noninflamed catagen hairs; melanin pigment casts
- Trichogram
- Referrals
  - Some diagnostic procedures may require a dermatology referral. In the presence of missing hair follicles or other hair disorder, a dermatology consult will allow for visual and/or microscopic (trichogram) analysis to determine structure and cycle of the hair disorder.
  - A referral to a psychiatrist, psychologist, or psychopharmacologist who specializes in impulse control and OCD may be helpful. He or she will have access to the specialized symptoms scales described above and also is likely to have professional relationships with psychotherapists who can provide specific therapies, such as habit reversal training. Such referral may also allow for stepped treatment including aggressive use of SSRIs and other antidepressants with combinations of second-line pharmacologic options sometimes tried for impulse control and OCD disorders.

TREATMENT

- Treatment of TTM involves both psychological methods that include specific psychotherapies, pharmacologic treatment, and combined approaches.
- Psychological treatment of TTM may be the primary treatment and is almost always needed in addition to medications.
  - Habit reversal training (HRT) has the strongest empirical support in adults (1)[B]:
    - HRT is a behavioral therapy that is effective in reducing troublesome behaviors associated with TTM. It consists of four main components: awareness training, development of a competing response, building motivation, and generalization of skills.
  - Principles of cognitive-behavior therapy (CBT) can be adjusted to developmental age to treat young children (2)[B].
  - Relaxation training (when stress is high)
  - Support groups to deal with stigma and denial
  - Treatment of comorbid psychiatric condition
  - Unlikely to be helpful
    - Undifferentiated, nonspecific psychotherapy
    - Hypnosis
    - Acupuncture
  - A nutritional supplement, N-acetylcysteine (1,200 to 2,400 mg/day), shows some benefit for adults but not for children and adolescents.

MEDICATION

- Previous RCT studies evaluate pharmacotherapy across various classes of medications had small sample sizes and did not indicate benefit (3).
- SSRIs have not demonstrated efficacy and most studies reported findings on subjects with little comorbidity. These medications may be options in concert with CBT.
  - Fluoxetine (Prozac): 20 to 80 mg/day
  - Sertraline (Zoloft): 50 to 200 mg/day
  - Paroxetine (Paxil): 10 to 50 mg/day
  - Citalopram (Celexa): 20 to 40 mg/day
  - Escitalopram (Lexapro): 10 to 20 mg/day
- Glutamate modulators (e.g., N-acetylcysteine) may reduce TTM in adults; however, benefit has not been demonstrated for children (4).

SURGERY/OTHER PROCEDURES
Surgery is only warranted for removal of trichobezoars.

INPATIENT CONSIDERATIONS
Inpatient admission is usually not due to TTM itself but either treatment of comorbid psychiatric conditions or a bowel obstruction secondary to trichobezoar.

ONGOING CARE

DIET
No special diet required for TTM

PATIENT EDUCATION
- TTM is a multifactorial condition. Not only do medications aid in the treatment of TTM, but also psychological therapies may have a significant benefit as well.
- Online resources: www.trich.org; www.stoppulling.com

PROGNOSIS
TTM tends to be a chronic disorder; however, it can be transient in childhood.

COMPLICATIONS
- Trichobezoars
- Alopecia

REFERENCES

1. Morris SH, Zickgraf HF, Dingfelder HE, et al. Habit reversal training in trichotillomania: guide for the clinician. *Expert Rev Neurother*. 2013;13(9): 1069–1077.
2. Tompkins M. Cognitive-behavior therapy for pediatric trichotillomania. *J Rat-Emo Cognitive-Behav Ther*. 2014;32:98–109.
3. Rothbart R, Stein DJ. Pharmacotherapy of trichotillomania (hair pulling disorder): an updated systematic review. *Expert Opin Pharmacother*. 2014;15(18):2709-2719.
4. Grant JE, Odlaug BL, Kim SW. N-acetylcysteine, a glutamate modulator, in the treatment of trichotillomania: a double-blind, placebo-controlled study. *Arch Gen Psychiatry*. 2009;66(7):756–763.

ADDITIONAL READING

- Chattopadhyay K. The genetic factors influencing the development of trichotillomania. *J Genet*. 2012;91(2):259–262.
- Duke DC, Keeley ML, Geffken GR, et al. Trichotillomania: a current review. *Clin Psychol Rev*. 2010;30(2):181–193.
- Franklin ME, Zagrabbe K, Benavides KL. Trichotillomania and its treatment: a review and recommendations. *Expert Rev Neurother*. 2011;11(8):1165–1174.
- Harrison JP, Franklin ME. Pediatric trichotillomania. *Curr Psychiatry Rep*. 2012;14(3):188–196.
- Trichotillomania Learning Center. Expert consensus guidelines on treatment of trichotillomania, skin picking and other body-focused repetitive behaviors. www.trich.org/dnld/ExpertGuidelines_000.pdf. Accessed 2014.

CODES

ICD10
F63.3 Trichotillomania

CLINICAL PEARLS

- Etiology of TTM is multifactorial and differs among individuals. It is important to distinguish between different etiologies.
- TTM may occur in the presence of comorbid conditions.
- Patients may benefit from psychotherapy and selected medications.
- It is important to realize that TTM is underreported and underdiagnosed because of the social stigma.
- TTM can have a significant impact on psychological, social, academic, and occupational functions.

TRIGEMINAL NEURALGIA

Noah M. Rosenberg, MD

 BASICS

DESCRIPTION
- Disorder of the sensory nucleus of the trigeminal nerve (cranial nerve [CN] V) that produces episodic, paroxysmal, severe, lancinating facial pain lasting seconds to minutes in the distribution of ≥1 divisions of the nerve
- Often precipitated by stimulation of well-defined, ipsilateral trigger zones: usually perioral, perinasal, and, occasionally, intraoral (e.g., by washing, shaving)
- System(s) affected: nervous
- Synonym(s): tic douloureux; Fothergill neuralgia; trifacial neuralgia; prosopalgia

EPIDEMIOLOGY
Incidence
- Women: 5.9/100,000/year
- Men: 3.4/100,000/year
- >70 years of age: ~25.6/100,000/year
- Predominant age:
  - >50 years; incidence increases with age
  - Rare: <35 years of age (consider another primary disease; see "Etiology")
- Predominant sex: female > male (~2:1)

Prevalence
16/100,000

Pediatric Considerations
Unusual during childhood

Pregnancy Considerations
Teratogenicity limits therapy for 1st and 2nd trimesters.

ETIOLOGY AND PATHOPHYSIOLOGY
- Demyelination around the compression site seems to be the mechanism by which compression of nerves leads to symptoms.
- Demyelinated lesions may set up an ectopic impulse generation causing erratic responses: hyperexcitability of damaged nerves and transmission of action potentials along adjacent, undamaged, unstimulated sensory fibers
- Compression of trigeminal nerve by anomalous arteries or veins of posterior fossa, compressing trigeminal root
- Etiologic classification:
  - Idiopathic (classic)
  - Secondary: cerebellopontine angle tumors (e.g., meningioma); tumors of CN V (e.g., neuroma, vascular malformations), trauma, demyelinating disease (e.g., multiple sclerosis [MS])

RISK FACTORS
Unknown

COMMONLY ASSOCIATED CONDITIONS
- Sjögren syndrome; rheumatoid arthritis
- Chronic meningitis
- Acute polyneuropathy
- MS
- Hemifacial spasm
- Charcot-Marie-Tooth neuropathy
- Glossopharyngeal neuralgia

 DIAGNOSIS

HISTORY
Paroxysms of pain in the distribution of the trigeminal nerve

PHYSICAL EXAM
All exam findings typically are negative due to the paroxysmal nature of the disorder.

DIFFERENTIAL DIAGNOSIS
- Other forms of neuralgia usually have sensory loss. Presence of sensory loss nearly excludes the diagnosis of TN (if younger patient, frequently MS).
- Neoplasia in cerebellopontine angle
- Vascular malformation of brain stem
- Demyelinating lesion (MS is diagnosed in 2–4% of patients with trigeminal neuralgia.)
- Vascular insult
- Migraine, cluster headache
- Giant cell arteritis
- Postherpetic neuralgia
- Chronic meningitis
- Acute polyneuropathy
- Atypical odontalgia
- SUNCT syndrome (short-lasting, unilateral, neuralgiform pain with conjunctival injection, and tearing)

DIAGNOSTIC TESTS & INTERPRETATION
- The International Headache Society diagnostic criteria for classic trigeminal neuralgia (TN) are as follows:
  - Paroxysmal attacks of pain lasting from a fraction of 1 second to 2 minutes, affecting ≥1 divisions of the trigeminal nerve
  - Pain has at least an intense, sharp, superficial, or stabbing characteristic; or is precipitated from trigger areas or by trigger factors.
  - Attacks are stereotyped in the individual patient.
  - No clinically evident neurologic deficit found.
  - Not attributed to another disorder
- Secondary TN is characterized by pain that is indistinguishable from classic TN but is caused by a demonstrable structural lesion other than vascular compression.
  - Indicated in all first-time-presenting patients to rule out secondary causes
- MRI versus CT scan: MRI, with and without contrast, offers more detailed imaging and is preferred, if not contraindicated.
- Routine head imaging identifies structural causes in up to 15% of patients.
- No positive findings are significantly correlated with diagnosis.

Test Interpretation
- Trigeminal nerve: inflammatory changes, demyelination, and degenerative changes
- Trigeminal ganglion: hypermyelination and microneuromata

 TREATMENT

GENERAL MEASURES
- Outpatient
- Drug treatment is first approach.
- Invasive procedures are reserved for patients who cannot tolerate, fail to respond to, or relapse after chronic drug treatment.
- Avoid stimulation (e.g., air, heat, cold) of trigger zones, including lips, cheeks, and gums.

MEDICATION
First Line
- Carbamazepine (Tegretol) (1)[A]: Start at 100 to 200 mg BID; effective dose usually 200 mg QID; max dose 1,200 mg/day:
  - 70–90% of patients respond initially.
  - By 3 years, 30% are no longer helped (number needed to treat [NNT] = 1.7) (1)[A]
  - Most common side effect: sedation
- Contraindications: concurrent use of monoamine oxidase inhibitors (MAOIs)
- Precautions: caution in the presence of liver disease
- Significant possible medication interactions: macrolide antibiotics, oral anticoagulants, anticonvulsants, tricyclics, oral contraceptives, steroids, digitalis, isoniazid, MAOIs, methyprylon, nabilone, nizatidine, other H_2 blockers, phenytoin, propoxyphene, benzodiazepines, and calcium channel blockers
- Oxcarbazepine (Trileptal): Start at 150 to 300 mg BID; effective dose usually 375 mg BID; max dose 1,200 mg/day:
  - Efficacy similar to carbamazepine
  - Faster, with less drowsiness and fewer drug interactions than carbamazepine
  - May cause hyponatremia
  - Most common side effect: sedation

Second Line
- Antiepileptic drugs: Insufficient evidence from randomized, controlled trials to show significant benefit from antiepileptic drugs in TN (2)[A].
- Phenytoin (Dilantin): 300 to 400 mg/day (synergistic with carbamazepine):
  - Potent P450 inducer (enhanced metabolism of many drugs)
  - Various CNS side effects (sedation, ataxia)
- Baclofen (Lioresal): 10 to 80 mg/day; start at 5 to 10 mg TID with food (as an adjunct to phenytoin or carbamazepine); side effects: drowsiness, weakness, nausea, vomiting
- Gabapentin (Neurontin): Start at 100 mg TID or 300 mg at bedtime; can increase dose up to 300 to 600 mg TID–QID. Can be used as monotherapy or in combination with other medications and reduces the cost of illness.
- Lamotrigine: Titrate up to 200 mg BID over weeks; side effect: 10% experience rash

- Antidepressants, including amitriptyline, fluoxetine, trazodone:
  - Used especially with anticonvulsants
  - Particularly effective for atypical forms of TN
- Clonazepam (Klonopin) frequently causes drowsiness and ataxia.
- Sumatriptan (Imitrex) 3 mg SC reduces acute symptoms and may be helpful after failure of conventional medical therapy.
- Capsaicin cream topically
- Botulinum toxin injection into zygomatic arch
- Valproic acid (Depakene, Depakote)

ISSUES FOR REFERRAL
Initial treatment failure or positive findings on imaging studies

ADDITIONAL THERAPIES
- Radiotherapy
- Stereotactic radiosurgery, such as gamma knife radiosurgery, has been shown to be effective after drug failure:
  - Produces lesions with focused gamma knife radiation
  - Therapy aimed at the proximal trigeminal root
  - Minimal clinically effective dose: 70 Gy
  - ~60–80% of patients achieve complete relief within 1 year; by 3 years, ~30–40% maintain complete relief (3)[B].
  - Most common side effect: sensory disturbance (facial numbness)
  - Failure rates are higher in patients with past TN-related invasive procedures.

SURGERY/OTHER PROCEDURES
- Microvascular decompression of CN V at its entrance to (or exit from) brain stem:
  - 98% of patients achieve initial pain relief; by 20 months, 86% maintain complete relief (NNT = 2) (4)[B].
  - Surgical mortality across studies was 0.3–0.4%.
  - Most common side effect: transient facial numbness and diplopia, headache, nausea, vomiting
  - Pain relief after procedure strongly correlates with the type of TN pain: Type 1 (shocklike pain) results in better outcomes than type 2 (aching pain between paroxysms).
- Peripheral nerve ablation (multiple methods):
  - Higher rates of failure and facial numbness than decompression surgery
  - Radiofrequency thermocoagulation
  - Neurectomy
  - Cryotherapy: high relapse rate
  - Partial sensory rhizotomy
- 4% tetracaine dissolved in 0.5% bupivacaine nerve block (only a few case reports to date; ropivacaine)
- Alcohol block or glycerol injection into trigeminal cistern: unpredictable side effects (dysesthesia and anesthesia dolorosa); temporary relief

- Peripheral block or section of CN V proximal to Gasserian ganglion
- Balloon compression of Gasserian ganglion
- Evidence supporting destructive procedures for benign pain conditions remains limited (5)[A].

COMPLEMENTARY & ALTERNATIVE MEDICINE
Acupuncture, moxibustion (herb): weak evidence for efficacy (6)[B]

 ## ONGOING CARE

FOLLOW-UP RECOMMENDATIONS
Regular outpatient follow-up to monitor symptoms and therapeutic failure.

Patient Monitoring
- Carbamazepine and/or phenytoin serum levels
- If carbamazepine is prescribed: CBC and platelets at baseline, then weekly for a month, then monthly for 4 months, then every 6 to 12 months if dose is stable (regimens for monitoring vary)
- Reduce drugs after 4 to 6 weeks to determine whether condition is in remission; resume at previous dose if pain recurs. Withdraw drugs slowly after several months, again to check for remission or if lower dose of drugs can be tolerated.

DIET
No special diet

PATIENT EDUCATION
- Instruct patient regarding medication dosage and side effects, risk-to-benefit ratios of surgery, or radiation therapy.
- Support organizations:
  - The Facial Pain Association (formerly the Trigeminal Neuralgia Association): www.fpa-support.org
  - Living with Trigeminal Neuralgia: www.livingwithtn.org

PROGNOSIS
- 50–60% eventually fail pharmacologic treatment.
- After having microvascular decompression surgery, most patients wish they had undergone the procedure sooner.
- Of those, relapse is seen in ~50% of stereotactic radiosurgeries and ~27% of surgical microvascular decompressions.

COMPLICATIONS
- Mental and physical sluggishness; dizziness with carbamazepine
- Paresthesias and corneal reflex loss with stereotactic radiosurgery
- Surgical mortality and morbidity associated with microvascular decompression

REFERENCES
1. Wiffen PJ, Derry S, Moore RA, et al. Carbamazepine for chronic neuropathic pain and fibromyalgia in adults. *Cochrane Database Syst Rev.* 2014;(4):CD005451.
2. Zhang J, Yang M, Zhou M, et al. Non-antiepileptic drugs for trigeminal neuralgia. *Cochrane Database Syst Rev.* 2013;(12):CD004029.
3. Karam SD, Tai A, Wooster M, et al. Trigeminal neuralgia treatment outcomes following Gamma Knife radiosurgery with a minimum 3-year follow-up. *J Radiat Oncol.* 2014;3:125–130.
4. Sekula RF Jr, Frederickson AM, Jannetta PJ, et al. Microvascular decompression for elderly patients with trigeminal neuralgia: a prospective study and systematic review with meta-analysis. *J Neurosurg.* 2011;114(1):172–179.
5. Zakrzewska JM, Akram H. Neurosurgical interventions for the treatment of classical trigeminal neuralgia. *Cochrane Database Syst Rev.* 2011;(9):CD007312.
6. Liu H, Li H, Xu M, et al. A systematic review on acupuncture for trigeminal neuralgia. *Altern Ther Health Med.* 2010;16(6):30–35.

ADDITIONAL READING
- Attal N, Cruccu G, Baron R, et al. EFNS guidelines on the pharmacological treatment of neuropathic pain: 2010 revision. *Eur J Neurol.* 2010;17(9):1113–e88.
- Gronseth G, Cruccu G, Alksne J, et al. Practice parameter: the diagnostic evaluation and treatment of trigeminal neuralgia (an evidence-based review): report of the Quality Standards Subcommittee of the American Academy of Neurology and the European Federation of Neurological Societies. *Neurology.* 2008;71(15):1183–1190.

 ## CODES

ICD10
- G50.0 Trigeminal neuralgia
- B02.22 Postherpetic trigeminal neuralgia

CLINICAL PEARLS
- Patients with TN typically have a normal physical exam.
- The long-term efficacy of pharmacotherapy for TN is 40–50%.
- If pharmacotherapy fails, stereotactic radiosurgery or surgical microvascular decompression often is successful.

TRIGGER FINGER (DIGITAL STENOSING TENOSYNOVITIS)
Alan M. Ehrlich, MD • Robert A. Yood, MD

BASICS

DESCRIPTION
A clicking, snapping, or locking of a finger/thumb with extension movement (after flexion) ± associated pain

EPIDEMIOLOGY
Incidence
- Adult population: 28/100,000/year
  - Rare in children
- 4 times increased risk in diabetics (1)[B].
- Predominant age
  - Childhood form typically involves thumb.
  - Adult form typically presents in the 5th and 6th decades of life and involves thumb/digits.
- Predominant sex
  - Children: female = male
  - Adults: female > male (6:1)

Prevalence
Lifetime prevalence in the general population is 2.6%.

Pediatric Considerations
- The thumb is more commonly involved in children.
- Surgery is often more complicated for children with a trigger finger (as opposed to a trigger thumb).
- Release of the A1 pulley alone is often insufficient, other procedures may be necessary.

ETIOLOGY AND PATHOPHYSIOLOGY
- Narrowing around the A1 pulley from inflammation, protein deposition, or thickening of the tendon itself. Prolonged inflammation leads to fibrocartilaginous metaplasia of the tendon sheath.
- If the flexor tendon become nodular, the triggering phenomenon is worse because the nodule has difficulty passing under the A1 pulley.
- Because intrinsic flexor muscles are stronger than extensors, the finger can stick in the flexed position.
- No clear association with repetitive movements

RISK FACTORS
- Diabetes mellitus
- Rheumatoid arthritis
- Hypothyroidism
- Mucopolysaccharide disorders
- Amyloidosis

GENERAL PREVENTION
Most cases are idiopathic, and no known prevention exists. No clear association with repetitive movements

COMMONLY ASSOCIATED CONDITIONS
- De Quervain tenosynovitis
- Carpal tunnel syndrome
- Dupuytren contracture
- Diabetes mellitus
- Rheumatoid arthritis
- Hypothyroidism
- Amyloidosis

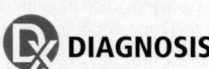

DIAGNOSIS

Diagnosis is based on clinical presentation.

HISTORY
Clicking, snapping, or locking of a digit while attempting to extend; with or without associated pain

PHYSICAL EXAM
- A palpable nodule may be present.
- Snapping/locking may be present but neither is necessary for the diagnosis.
- Tenderness to palpation is variable.

DIAGNOSTIC TESTS & INTERPRETATION
Test Interpretation
- Thickening of the A1 pulley with fibrocartilaginous metaplasia
- Thickening/nodule formation of flexor tendon

TREATMENT

- Splinting the metacarpophalangeal (MCP) joint at 10 to 15 degrees of flexion for 6 weeks with the distal joints free to move:
  - Splinting is more effective for fingers than thumbs (70% vs. 50%).
  - Splinting is less effective with severe symptoms, symptoms >6 months, or if multiple digits are involved (1)[B].
- Injection of long-acting corticosteroid may provide symptom relief. Subsequent injections are less likely to help.
- Surgery often successful for patients unresponsive to splinting/corticosteroid injections.

GENERAL MEASURES
Attempt splinting/steroid injection prior to surgery. Splinting may be more effective for preventing recurrence than as initial treatment (2)[B].

MEDICATION
First Line
- Steroid injection of the tendon sheath/surrounding SC tissue has 57–90% success rate.
- Injection in surrounding tissues is as efficacious as injecting into the tendon sheath (1,3)[B]. Injection into the palmar surface at the midproximal phalanx is associated with less pain than injection of tendon sheath at MCP joint (4)[B].
- Injection using ultrasound guidance does not improve success rate compared to standard injection technique (5)[A]. Corticosteroid injection has higher success rate than splinting (2)[B].

Second Line
- Oral NSAIDs may reduce pain and discomfort but have not been shown to alter underlying disease. NSAIDs do not reduce symptoms of snapping/locking.

- Injection with diclofenac may be an alternative to corticosteroid for patients with diabetes mellitus if increase in blood sugar is a concern (6)[A].
- Corticosteroids are more effective than diclofenac during the first 3 weeks postinjection. Efficacy is similar to other modalities by 3 months postinjection (6)[B].

- In one randomized trial, hyaluronic acid (HA) injections were as effective as corticosteroid injections. The optimal frequency, dosage, and molecular weight of HA injections has yet to be adequately studied.

ISSUES FOR REFERRAL
Refer to a hand surgeon for release if the patient is not responding to splinting and/or steroid injections.

ADDITIONAL THERAPIES
Physiotherapy is helpful, particularly in children.

SURGERY/OTHER PROCEDURES
- Surgical release can be done as an open procedure or percutaneously.

- No apparent differences in success or rates of complications between surgical approaches (6)[A].
- Surgery has a lower rate of recurrence than corticosteroid injection (6)[A].

- Most hand surgeons prefer open release because of concern about nerve injury.

INPATIENT CONSIDERATIONS
Admission Criteria/Initial Stabilization
Day surgery for trigger finger release

Discharge Criteria
Absence of complications

 ONGOING CARE

FOLLOW-UP RECOMMENDATIONS
- Follow up is needed only if symptoms persist or if complications develop after surgery.

- Splinting of the affected digit to minimize flexion/extension of the MCP joint helps symptom resolution (1)[B],(7)[C].

PROGNOSIS
Prognosis is excellent with conservative treatment or surgical intervention. Recurrence following corticosteroid injection is more likely for patients with type 1 diabetes mellitus, younger patients, involvement of multiple digits, and patients with a history of other upper extremity tendinopathies (8)[B].

COMPLICATIONS
- Complications from surgery include infection, bleeding, digital nerve injury, persistent pain, and loss of range of motion of the affected finger. The rate of major complications is low (3%). The rate of minor complications (including loss of range of motion) is higher (up to 28%).
- Injury to the A2 pulley may result in bowstringing, (bulging of the flexor tendon in the palm with flexion). This can be painful.
- Diabetic patients may have increased blood sugar levels for up to 5 days following steroid injection.

REFERENCES
1. Akhtar S, Bradley MJ, Quinton DN, et al. Management and referral for trigger finger/thumb. *BMJ*. 2005;331(7507):30–33.
2. Salim N, Abdullah S, Sapuan J, et al. Outcome of corticosteroid injection versus physiotherapy in the treatment of mild trigger fingers. *J Hand Surg Eur Vol*. 2012;37(1):27–34.
3. Kazuki K, Egi T, Okada M, et al. Clinical outcome of extrasynovial steroid injection for trigger finger. *Hand Surg*. 2006;11(1–2):1–4.
4. Pataradool K, Buranapuntaruk T. Proximal phalanx injection for trigger finger: randomized controlled trial. *Hand Surg*. 2011;16(3):313–317.
5. Cecen GS, Gulabi D, Saglam F, et al. Corticosteroid injection for trigger finger: blinded or ultrasound-guided injection? *Arch Orthop Trauma Surg*. 2015;135(1):125–131.
6. Shakeel H, Ahmad TS. Steroid injection versus NSAID injection for trigger finger: a comparative study of early outcomes. *J Hand Surg Am*. 2012; 37(7):1319–1323.
7. Ryzewicz M, Wolf JM. Trigger digits: principles, management, and complications. *J Hand Surg Am*. 2006;31(1):135–146.
8. Rozental TD, Zurakowski D, Blazar PE. Trigger finger: prognostic indicators of recurrence following corticosteroid injection. *J Bone Joint Surg Am*. 2008;90(8):1665–1672.

ADDITIONAL READING
- Fleisch SB, Spindler KP, Lee DH. Corticosteroid injections in the treatment of trigger finger: a level I and II systematic review. *J Am Acad Orthop Surg*. 2007;15(3):166–171.
- Guler F, Kose O, Ercan EC, et al. Open versus percutaneous release for the treatment of trigger thumb. *Orthopedics*. 2013;36(10):e1290–e1294.
- Huisstede BM, Hoogvliet P, Coert JH, et al. Multidisciplinary consensus guidelines for managing trigger finger: results from the European HANDGUIDE Study. *Phys Ther*. 2014;94(10):1421–1433.
- Wang J, Zhao JG, Liang CC. Percutaneous release, open surgery, or corticosteroid injection, which is the best treatment method for trigger digits? *Clin Orthop Relat Res*. 2013;471(6):1879–1886.
- Will R, Lubahn J. Complications of open trigger finger release. *J Hand Surg Am*. 2010;35(4):594–596.

 CODES

ICD10
- M65.30 Trigger finger, unspecified finger
- M65.319 Trigger thumb, unspecified thumb
- M65.329 Trigger finger, unspecified index finger

CLINICAL PEARLS
- Trigger finger is caused by narrowing of the A1 flexor tendon pulley.
- Splinting the MCP joint at 10 to 15 degrees flexion for 6 weeks is the preferred initial conservative treatment.
- Splinting is more effective for fingers as opposed to thumbs (70% vs. 50%). Splinting is less effective with severe symptoms, longstanding symptoms (>6 months), or if multiple digits are involved.
- Long-acting corticosteroid injections are effective for treatment of trigger finger.
- Open and percutaneous surgical release has high success rates for patients not responsive to splinting or injections.

TROCHANTERIC BURSITIS (GREATER TROCHANTERIC PAIN SYNDROME)

David W. Kruse, MD • Joann Y. Chang, MD

BASICS

Trochanteric bursitis is the historical term referring to lateral hip pain and tenderness over the greater trochanter. Because many patients lack an inflammatory process within the trochanteric bursa, this condition has been more recently referred to as *greater trochanteric pain syndrome* (GTPS) (1).

DESCRIPTION
- Bursae are fluid-filled sacs found primarily at tendon attachment sites with bony protuberances:
  - Multiple bursae are in the area of the greater trochanter of the femur.
  - These bursae are associated with the tendons of the gluteus muscles, iliotibial band (ITB), and tensor fasciae latae.
  - The subgluteus maximus bursa is implicated most commonly in lateral hip pain (1).
- Other structures of the lateral hip include the following:
  - ITB, tensor fasciae latae, gluteus maximus tendon, gluteus medius tendon, gluteus minimus tendon, quadratus femoris muscle, vastus lateralis tendon, piriformis tendon
- *Bursitis* refers to bursal inflammation.
- *Tendinopathy* refers to any abnormality of a tendon, inflammatory or degenerative. *Enthesopathy* refers to abnormalities of the zones of attachment of ligaments and tendons to bones.

EPIDEMIOLOGY
Incidence
- 1.8/1,000 persons/year
- Peak incidence in 4th to 6th decades

Prevalence
- Predominant sex: female > male
- More common in running and contact athletes
  - Football, rugby, soccer

ETIOLOGY AND PATHOPHYSIOLOGY
- Acute: abnormal gait or poor muscle flexibility and strength imbalances lead to bursal friction and secondary inflammation
  - Tendon overuse and inflammation
  - Direct trauma from contact or frequently lying with body weight on hip can cause an inflammatory response ("hip pointer") as well.
- Chronic
  - Fibrosis and thickening of bursal sac due to chronic inflammatory process
  - Tendinopathy due to chronic overuse and degeneration: gluteus medius and minimus most commonly involved (1,2)

Genetics
No known genetic factors

RISK FACTORS
Multiple factors have been implicated (1,3):
- Female gender
- Obesity
- Tight hip musculature (including ITB)
- Direct trauma
- Total hip arthroplasty
- Abnormal gait or pelvic architecture
  - Leg length discrepancy
  - Sacroiliac (SI) joint dysfunction
  - Knee or hip osteoarthritis
  - Abnormal foot mechanics (e.g., pes planus, overpronation)
  - Neuromuscular disorder: Trendelenburg gait

GENERAL PREVENTION
- Maintain ITB, hip, and lower back flexibility and strength.
- Avoid direct trauma (use of appropriate padding in contact sports).
- Avoid prolonged running on banked or crowned surfaces.
- Wear appropriate shoes.
- Appropriate bedding and sleeping surface
- Maintain appropriate body weight loss.

COMMONLY ASSOCIATED CONDITIONS
- Biomechanical factors (1)
  - Tight ITBs, leg length discrepancy, SI joint dysfunction, pes planus
  - Width of greater trochanters greater than width of iliac wings (4)[B]
- Other associated pathology (1):
  - Low back pain
  - Knee and hip osteoarthritis
  - Obesity

DIAGNOSIS

HISTORY
General history (1)
- Pain localized to the lateral hip or buttock
- Pain may radiate to groin or lateral thigh (pseudoradiculopathy).
- Pain exacerbated by:
  - Prolonged walking or standing
  - Rising after prolonged sitting
  - Sitting with legs crossed
  - Lying on affected side
- Other historical features:
  - Direct trauma to affected hip
  - Chronic low back pain
  - Chronic leg/knee/ankle/hip pain
  - Recent increase in running distance or intensity
  - Change in running surfaces

PHYSICAL EXAM
- Observe gait.
- Point tenderness with direct palpation over the lateral hip is characteristic of GTPS (1)[B].
- Other exam features have lower sensitivity (1)[B]:
  - Pain with extremes of passive rotation, abduction, or adduction
  - Pain with resisted hip abduction and external or internal rotation
  - Trendelenburg sign
- Other tests to rule out associated conditions:
  - Patrick-FABERE (flexion, abduction, external rotation, extension) test for SI joint dysfunction
  - Ober test for ITB pathology
  - Flexion and extension of hip for osteoarthritis
  - Leg length measurement
  - Foot inspection for pes planus or overpronation
  - Lower extremity neurologic assessment for lumbar radiculopathy or neuromuscular disorders
  - Hip lag sign (5)

DIFFERENTIAL DIAGNOSIS
- ITB syndrome
- Piriformis syndrome
- Osteoarthritis or avascular necrosis of the hip
- Lumbosacral osteoarthritis/disc disease with nerve root compression
- Fracture or contusion of the hip or pelvis—particularly in setting of trauma
- Stress reaction/fracture of femoral neck—particularly in female runners
- Septic bursitis/arthritis

DIAGNOSTIC TESTS & INTERPRETATION
No routine lab testing is recommended.

Initial Tests (lab, imaging)
- Diagnosis can be made by history and exam (6).
- If imaging is ordered:
  - US can aid in diagnosis and guide aspiration and/or injection.
  - Anteroposterior and frog-leg views of affected hip to rule out specific bony pathology (OA, stress fracture, etc).
  - Consider lumbar spine radiographs if back pain is thought to be a contributing factor.
  - MRI is image of choice in recalcitrant pain or to formally exclude stress fracture.

Follow-Up Tests & Special Considerations
- If there is a concern for a septic bursitis, then aspiration or incision and drainage may be necessary.
- Advanced imaging rarely necessary; detection of abnormalities on MRI is a poor predictor of GTPS (7)[B].

TREATMENT

GENERAL MEASURES

- Physical therapy to address underlying dysfunction and rebuild atrophic muscle
- Correct pelvic/hip instability.
- Correct lower limb biomechanics.
- Low-impact conditioning and aquatic therapy
- Gait training
- Weight loss (if applicable)
- Minimize aggravating activities such as prolonged walking or standing.
- Avoid lying on affected side.
- Runners
  - May need to decrease distance and/or intensity of runs during treatment. Some need to stop running. Amount of time is case specific but may range from 2 to 4 weeks.
  - Avoid banked tracks or roads with excessive tilt.

MEDICATION

First Line

- NSAIDs (1)[B]: Treat for 2 to 4 weeks.
  - Naproxen: 500 mg PO BID
  - Ibuprofen: 800 mg PO TID
- Corticosteroid injection is effective for pain relief (8)[C] and can be considered first-line therapy for selected cases:
  - Dexamethasone: 4 mg/mL or
  - Kenalog: 40 mg/m, useL 1 to 2 mL
  - Consider adding a local anesthetic (short- and/or long-acting) for more immediate pain relief.
  - Can be repeated with similar effect if original treatment showed a strong response
  - Goal is pain relief (9)[A].

ISSUES FOR REFERRAL

- Septic bursitis
- Recalcitrant bursitis

ADDITIONAL THERAPIES

- Ice
- Low-energy shock wave therapy has been shown to be superior to other nonoperative modalities (8)[A].
- Focus on achieving flexibility of hip musculature, particularly the ITB.
- Address contributing factors:
  - Low back flexibility
  - If leg length discrepancy, consider heel lift.
  - If pes planus or overpronation, consider arch supports or custom orthotics.

SURGERY/OTHER PROCEDURES

- Surgery rare but effective in refractory cases (10)[A]
- If surgery is indicated, potential options include:
  - Arthroscopic bursectomy
  - ITB release
  - Gluteus medius tendon repair

COMPLEMENTARY & ALTERNATIVE MEDICINE

- Acupuncture
- Prolotherapy
- Growth factor injection techniques
- Platelet-rich plasma injection

ONGOING CARE

FOLLOW-UP RECOMMENDATIONS

4 weeks posttreatment, sooner if significant worsening

PATIENT EDUCATION

- Maintain hip musculature flexibility, including ITB.
- Correct issues that may cause abnormal gait:
  - Low back pain
  - Knee pain
  - Leg length discrepancy (heel lift)
  - Foot mechanics (orthotics)
- Gradual return to physical activity

PROGNOSIS

Depends on chronicity and recurrence, with more acute cases having an excellent prognosis

COMPLICATIONS

Bursal thickening and fibrosis

REFERENCES

1. Williams BS, Cohen SP. Greater trochanteric pain syndrome: a review of anatomy, diagnosis and treatment. *Anesth Analg.* 2009;108(5):1662–1670.
2. Domb BG, Carreira DS. Endoscopic repair of full-thickness gluteus medius tears. *Arthrosc Tech.* 2013;2(2):e77–e81.
3. Farmer KW, Jones LC, Brownson KE, et al. Trochanteric bursitis after total hip arthroplasty: incidence and evaluation of response to treatment. *J Arthroplasty.* 2010;25(2):208–212.
4. Viradia NK, Berger AA, Dahners LE. Relationship between width of greater trochanters and width of iliac wings in trochanteric bursitis. *Am J Orthop (Belle Mead NJ).* 2011;40(9):E159–E162.
5. Kaltenborn A, Bourg CM, Gutzeit A, et al. The hip lag sign—prospective blinded trial of a new clinical sign to predict hip abductor damage. *PLoS One.* 2014;9(3):e91560.
6. Chowdhury R, Naaseri S, Lee J, et al. Imaging and management of greater trochanteric pain syndrome. *Postgrad Med J.* 2014;90(1068):576–581.
7. Blankenbaker DG, Ullrick SR, Davis KW, et al. Correlation of MRI findings with clinical findings of trochanteric pain syndrome. *Skeletal Radiol.* 2008;37(10):903–909.
8. Stephens MB, Beutler AI, O'Connor FG. Musculoskeletal injections: a review of the evidence. *Am Fam Physician.* 2008;78(8):971–976.
9. Brinks A, van Rijn RM, Willemsen SP, et al. Corticosteroid injections for greater trochanteric pain syndrome: a randomized controlled trial in primary care. *Ann Fam Med.* 2011;9(3):226–234.
10. Lustenberger DP, Ng VY, Best TM, et al. Efficacy of treatment of trochanteric bursitis: a systematic review. *Clin J Sport Med.* 2011;21(5):447–453.

ADDITIONAL READING

- Baker CL Jr, Massie RV, Hurt WG, et al. Arthroscopic bursectomy for recalcitrant trochanteric bursitis. *Arthroscopy.* 2007;23(8):827–832.
- Barnthouse NC, Wente TM, Voos JE. Greater trochanteric pain syndrome: endoscopic treatment options. *Oper Tech Sports Med.* 2012;20:320–324.
- Hugo D, de Jongh HR. Greater trochanteric pain syndrome. *SA Orthopaedic Journal.* 2012;11(1):28–33.
- McMahon SE, Smith TO, Hing CB. A systematic review of imaging modalities in the diagnosis of greater trochanteric pain syndrome. *Musculoskeletal Care.* 2012;10(4):232–239.
- Pretell J, Ortega J, García-Rayo R, et al. Distal fascia lata lengthening: an alternative surgical technique for recalcitrant trochanteric bursitis. *Int Orthop.* 2009;33(5):1223–1227.

CODES

ICD10

- M70.60 Trochanteric bursitis, unspecified hip
- M70.62 Trochanteric bursitis, left hip
- M70.61 Trochanteric bursitis, right hip

CLINICAL PEARLS

- Patients with GTPS often present with an inability to lie on the affected side.
- Femoral neck stress fractures are a do-not-miss diagnosis, particularly in young female runners.
- Corticosteroid injection helps as an initial therapy, particularly for pain relief to allow for aggressive physical therapy.
- Physical therapy is treatment mainstay for correcting biomechanical imbalances and restoring proper function.

T

TUBERCULOSIS

Carlos Atore, MD • Swati Avashia, MD, FAAP

 BASICS

DESCRIPTION
- Active tuberculosis
  - Occurs from primary infection or reactivation of latent infection
  - Affects 10% of infected individuals without preventive therapy
  - Risk increases with immunosuppression: Highest risk is in the first 2 years after infection.
  - Well-described forms: pulmonary (85% of cases), miliary (disseminated), meningeal, abdominal
- Usually acquired by inhalation of airborne bacilli from an individual with active tuberculosis (TB). Bacilli multiply in alveoli and spread via macrophages, lymphatics, and blood. Three possible outcomes:
  - Eradication: Tissue hypersensitivity halts infection within 10 weeks.
  - Primary infection
  - Latent infection (See "Tuberculosis, Latent [LTBI].")

Pediatric Considerations
- In children, there is a faster rate of progression to disease, the risk of progression to disease is higher, and severe disease is more common.
- Most children with pulmonary TB are asymptomatic.
- Treatment of pediatric TB should involve four drugs and be directly observed (DOT).

EPIDEMIOLOGY
Incidence
- Worldwide (2013): 9 million (13% HIV coinfected)
- United States (2013): 9,582 (3.0/100,000), 82 MDR, and 75 of those were foreign born (1).

Prevalence
Worldwide (2013): 157 cases/100,000 population (41% decrease since 1990); highest in Asia and Africa (1)

ETIOLOGY AND PATHOPHYSIOLOGY
- *Mycobacterium tuberculosis*, *Mycobacterium bovis*, or *Mycobacterium africanum* are causative organisms.
- Cell-mediated response by activated T lymphocytes and macrophages forms a granuloma that limits bacillary replication. Destruction of the macrophages produces early "solid necrosis." In 2 to 3 weeks, "caseous necrosis" develops and latent tuberculosis infection (LTBI) ensues. In immunocompetent, granuloma undergoes "fibrosis" and calcification. In immunocompromised patients, primary progressive TB develops.

RISK FACTORS
- For infection: homeless, ethnic minorities, close quarters (correctional facilities, nursing homes, barracks); close contact with infected individual; persons from areas with high incidence of active TB (Asia, Africa, Latin America, former Soviet Union states); health care workers; medically underserved, low income, substance abuse
- For development of disease once infected: HIV; lymphoma; silicosis; diabetes mellitus; chronic renal failure; cancer of head, neck, or lung; children <5 years of age; malnutrition; systemic corticosteroids, immunosuppressive drugs; IV drug abuse, alcohol abuse, cigarette smokers; <2 years since infection with *M. tuberculosis*; history of gastrectomy or jejunal bypass; <90% of ideal body weight

GENERAL PREVENTION
- Screening and treatment of LTBI. Active cases must be reported to health department for identification; test and treat all close contacts.

- Bacille Calmette-Guérin (BCG) vaccine: Live attenuated *M. bovis* prevents 50% of pulmonary disease and 80% of meningitis and miliary disease in children. Use is more common in countries with endemic TB. In the United States, consider BCG for high-risk children with negative PPD and HIV tests or for health workers at risk for drug-resistant infection.

COMMONLY ASSOCIATED CONDITIONS
Immunosuppression; HIV-coinfection; malignancy

 DIAGNOSIS

HISTORY
- Known exposure to individual with active TB
- Immunosuppression
- Tobacco use; recreational drug use
- Signs and symptoms
  - General: fever, night sweats, weight loss, malaise, painless lymph node swelling
  - Pulmonary TB: cough, hemoptysis
  - Abdominal TB: presents acutely as surgical abdomen; chronic abdominal TB varies in presentation, vague abdominal symptoms, abdominal mass, "doughy" abdomen
  - Meningitis: See "Tuberculosis, CNS."
  - Miliary: See "Tuberculosis, Miliary."

PHYSICAL EXAM
- Often entirely normal. Specific findings depend on organs involved: adenopathy, rales, or hepatosplenomegaly.
- Late findings: renal, bone, or CNS disease

DIFFERENTIAL DIAGNOSIS
- Pulmonary TB: pneumonia (bacterial fungal, atypical), malignancy, tularemia, actinomycosis
- Extrapulmonary TB: syphilis, cat-scratch disease, leishmaniasis, leprosy; rheumatoid disease; erythema nodosum, erythema induratum, syphilis, other mycobacterial infections

DIAGNOSTIC TESTS & INTERPRETATION
Initial Tests (Immunogenesis)
To determine immune response to mycobacterium
- Tuberculin skin test (TST) (e.g., PPD): 5 U (0.1 mL) intermediate-strength intradermal injection into volar forearm. Measure induration at 48 to 72 hours:
  - PPD positive if induration
    - >5 mm and HIV infection, recent TB contact, immunosuppressed, disease on x-ray
    - >10 mm and age <4 years or other risk factors
    - >15 mm and age >4 years and no risk factors
    - Two-step test if no recent PPD, age >55 years, nursing home resident, prison inmate, or health care worker. Second test 1 to 3 weeks after initial test; interpret as usual.
  - Context of PPD results:
    - False positive: BCG (unreliable, should not affect decision to treat)
    - False negative: HIV, steroids, gastrectomy, alcoholism, renal failure, sarcoidosis, malnutrition, hematologic or lymphoreticular disorder, very recent exposure
    - If positive once, no need to repeat.
    - No need for control with *Candida*/other

- Interferon-γ release assays (IGRAs) measure interferon release after stimulation in vitro by *M. tuberculosis* antigens (2)[A]:

  - Lack of cross-reaction with BCG and most nontuberculous mycobacteria

    - IGRA is preferred (better specificity) for testing persons who have had BCG (vaccine or for cancer therapy) and for homeless persons, drug abusers and other groups with historically low rates of returning to have TST's interpreted (2)[A].
    - TST is still preferred if age <5 years (3)[A].
    - Either TST or IGRA may be used as periodic screening for persons in high-risk occupations and for recent contacts of persons with known or suspected active TB (2)[A].
    - Cotesting with TST and IGRA may be indicated when the initial test is negative but the risk for poor prognosis is increased (e.g., HIV-infected persons or children <5 years old) (2)[A].

Initial Tests-Active TB (lab, imaging)
- Three consecutive sputum samples (8- to 24-hour intervals with at least one in early in the morning) for acid-fast bacilli (AFB) stain and culture by aerosol induction, gastric aspirate (children), or bronchoalveolar lavage
- Positive AFB: Treat immediately. Culture and sensitivity ultimately guide treatment.
- Chest radiograph
  - Primary TB: infiltrate with or without effusion, atelectasis, or adenopathy. Ghon lesion: calcified tuberculous caseating granuloma (tuberculoma); if associated with calcified ipsilateral hilar lymph node then Ghon (or Ranke) complex
  - Recrudescent TB: cavitary lesions and upper lobe disease with hilar adenopathy
  - HIV: atypical findings with primary infection, right upper lobe atelectasis
- CT chest: good sensitivity, tree-in-bud (centrilobular nodules with branching linear opacities)

Follow-Up Tests & Special Considerations
- Baseline CBC, creatinine, AST, ALT, bilirubin, alkaline phosphatase, visual acuity, and red–green color discrimination (regimens involving ethambutol)
- HIV: If positive, get baseline CD4 count.
- High risk: Check hepatitis B and C (injection drug users, Africa or Asia born, HIV infected).
- Extrapulmonary: urine, CSF, bone marrow, and liver biopsy for culture as indicated
- Nonspecific laboratory findings: anemia, monocytosis, thrombocytosis, hypergammaglobulinemia, SIADH, sterile pyuria

Diagnostic Procedures/Other
- Culture: takes several weeks for definitive results

- Xpert MTB/RIF: The World Health Organization endorses use as the initial test for diagnosis of pulmonary TB and detection of rifampicin resistance in adults and children presumed to have MDR-TB, HIV-associated TB, or TB meningitis (4)[A].

  - Results are available within 2 hours (5).

 TREATMENT

GENERAL MEASURES
- If clinical suspicion, treat immediately. Prescribing physician is responsible for treatment completion.
- Respiratory and droplet precautions
- Not infectious if favorable clinical response after 2 to 3 weeks of therapy and three negative AFB smears

MEDICATION
Use ideal body weight for dosing. Directly observed therapy (DOT) strongly recommended for all, but required for children, institutionalized patients, nonadherent patients, and nondaily regimens.

First Line
- LTBI

  - Isoniazid (INH) for 9 months at 5 mg/kg/day (max of 300 mg) *or* 15 mg/kg (max of 900 mg) 2 times per week (6)[A] *or*
  - INH 15 mg/kg + rifapentine 300 to 900 mg weekly for 12 weeks by DOT for patients age ≥12 years (6)[A]

- Active TB infection

  - Regimen 1 (preferred) (6)[A]
    - ○ Initial phase:
      - ▪ INH 5 mg/kg, rifampin (RIF) 10 mg/kg (max 600 mg), pyrazinamide (PZA) 15 to 30 mg/kg, and ethambutol (EMB) 15 to 20 mg/kg daily for 8 weeks *or*
      - ▪ INH/RIF/PZA/EMB 5 days/week for 8 weeks
    - Continuation phase:
      - ○ INH/RIF daily for 18 weeks; or, if DOT, INH/RIF 5 days/week for 18 weeks (recommended for HIV positive with CD4 <100 cells/mm³ due to increased risk of resistance) *or*
      - ○ INH/RIF 2 to 3 times per week for 18 weeks (not used if HIV positive with CD4 <100 cells/mm³; may have increased risk of relapse) *or*
      - ○ INH/rifapentine once weekly for 18 weeks (acceptable only for HIV patients without cavitary disease, may have increased risk of relapse) (6)[A]

  - Regimen 2
    - ○ Initial phase:
      - ▪ INH/RIF/PZA/EMB daily for 2 weeks, then twice weekly for 6 weeks *or*
      - ▪ INH/RIF/PZA/EMB 5 days/week for 2 weeks, then twice weekly for 6 weeks
    - ○ Continuation phase:
      - ▪ INH/RIF 2 to 3 times per week for 18 weeks (not recommended if HIV positive with CD4 <100 cells/mm³; may have increased risk of relapse) *or*
      - ▪ INH/rifapentine once weekly for 18 weeks (acceptable only for HIV patients without cavitary disease; may have increased risk of relapse) (6)[A]
      - ▪ Treat TB in pregnancy with INH, RIF, and EMB; add pyridoxine 25 mg/day.

Pregnancy Considerations
- Streptomycin: ototoxic and nephrotoxic; do not use in pregnancy. Pyrazinamide is not used in pregnant women in the United States.
- Congenital infection: from maternal miliary or endometrial TB. PPD, CXR, lumbar puncture, and culture placenta. Start treatment promptly if suspected.
- Breastfeeding: OK while taking TB drugs; supplement with pyridoxine 25 mg/day.

Pediatric Considerations
- Children: Ethambutol is not used.
- Children on medication may attend school.

ALERT
- Maximum drug doses: RIF 600 mg all regimens, PZA 2,000 mg/day or 4,000 mg 2 times per week, EMB, 600 mg/day or 4,000 mg 2 times per week
- If patient does not receive PZA during entire first 2 months, extend treatment to 9 months.
- *M. bovis* is resistant to PZA; must be treated 9 months
- Continue EMB until organism susceptibility to INH plus RIF is determined (6)[A].

Second Line
Fluoroquinolones and injectable aminoglycosides. Use when MDR is suspected or patient intolerance.

ISSUES FOR REFERRAL

ALERT
Notify public health authorities for all cases of active TB. Consult infectious disease specialist for cases of drug-resistant TB and for cases involving HIV-positive patients on antiretroviral therapy.

ADDITIONAL THERAPIES
- Pyridoxine: 50 mg may prevent INH-associated peripheral neuropathy, especially for patients who are malnourished or have comorbidities that increase risk of neuropathy (7)[A].
- Steroids: recommended for TB meningitis (8)[A] or pericarditis (8)[B], with concomitant anti-TB therapy

SURGERY/OTHER PROCEDURES
For extrapulmonary complications (spinal cord compression, bowel obstruction, constrictive pericarditis)

COMPLEMENTARY & ALTERNATIVE MEDICINE
Vitamin D deficiency may increase susceptibility to TB and development of active TB (9)[C]. There is conflicting evidence regarding the utility of vitamin D supplementation in TB treatment.

INPATIENT CONSIDERATIONS
- Negative pressure isolation with personal respirators and droplet precautions
- Three consecutive negative sputum AFB smears are necessary for release from isolation.

Discharge Criteria
Once TB has been excluded or the patient has effective therapy, is clinically improving, and is not an infectious risk, arrange outpatient follow-up with a provider comfortable managing TB and coordinate case management with local public health authorities.

 ONGOING CARE

FOLLOW-UP RECOMMENDATIONS
Patient Monitoring
- Monthly visits to assess treatment adherence and adverse medication effects; CXR at 3rd month
- For HIV positive: CD4 count, CBC, and liver enzymes q3mo
- Liver enzymes monthly if chronic liver disease, alcohol use, pregnant, or postpartum. Temporarily halt medications if asymptomatic and enzymes ≥5 times normal or if symptomatic and enzymes ≥3 times normal.
- Visual acuity and red–green color monthly if on ethambutol >2 months or doses >20 mg/kg/day
- If culture-positive after 2 months of therapy, reassess drug sensitivity, initiate DOT, coordinate care with public health authorities, and consider infectious disease consultation (if not already involved).

PATIENT EDUCATION
- Emphasize medication adherence.
- Screen and treat close contacts.
- Alert patient that health authorities must be notified.
- http://www.cdc.gov/tb/publications/factsheets/general/tb.htm

PROGNOSIS
Few complications and full resolution of infection if medications are taken for full course as prescribed

COMPLICATIONS
- Cavitary lesions can become secondarily infected.
- Risk for drug resistance increases with HIV positive, treatment nonadherence, or residence in area with high incidence of resistance.

- MDR-TB: resistance to INH and rifampicin
- XDR-TB: resistant to fluoroquinolones (9% of MDR)

REFERENCES
1. World Health Organization. *WHO global tuberculosis report 2014*. http://www.who.int/tb/publications/global_report/en/. Accessed August 23, 2015.
2. Mazurek GH, Jereb J, Vernon A, et al. Updated guidelines for using interferon gamma release assays to detect *Mycobacterium tuberculosis* infection—United States. *MMWR Recomm Rep*. 2010;59(RR-5):1–25.
3. Centers for Disease Control and Prevention. National shortage of purified-protein derivative tuberculin products. *MMWR Morb Mortal Wkly Rep*. 2013;62(16):312.
4. World Health Organization. Tuberculosis diagnostics: Xpert MTB/RIF test. http://www.who.int/tb/publications/Xpert_factsheet.pdf. Accessed 2015.
5. Lawn, SD. Diagnosis of pulmonary tuberculosis. *Curr Opin Pulm Med*. 2013,19(3):280–288.
6. Hall RG, Leff RD, Gumbo T. Treatment of active pulmonary tuberculosis in adults: current standards and recent advances. Insights from the Society of Infectious Diseases Pharmacists. *Pharmacotherapy*. 2009;29(12):1468–1481.
7. Centers for Disease Control and Prevention. Recommendations for use of an isoniazid-rifapentine regimen with direct observation to treat latent *Mycobacterium tuberculosis* infection. *MMWR Morb Mortal Wkly Rep*. 2011;60(48):1650–1653.
8. World Health Organization. *The Treatment of Tuberculosis: Guidelines*. 4th ed. Geneva, Switzerland: World Health Organization; 2010.
9. Luong Kv, Nguyen LT. Impact of vitamin D in the treatment of tuberculosis. *Am J Med Sci*. 2011;341(6):493–498.

ADDITIONAL READING

Centers for Disease Control and Prevention. Trends in tuberculosis—United States, 2012. *MMWR Morb Mortal Wkly Rep*. 2013;62(11):201–205.

 SEE ALSO

- Tuberculosis, CNS; Tuberculosis, Latent (LTBI); Tuberculosis, Miliary
- Algorithm: Weight Loss, Unintentional

CODES

ICD10
- A15.9 Respiratory tuberculosis unspecified
- A15.0 Tuberculosis of lung
- A19.9 Miliary tuberculosis, unspecified

CLINICAL PEARLS
- Consider TB in patients with chronic cough and one additional risk factor.
- TB is fully curable when diagnosed and treated appropriately.
- Children and elderly clinically exhibit fewer classic features of TB.
- Involve public health authorities early in the diagnostic and treatment process for suspected cases of TB.

TUBERCULOSIS, LATENT (LTBI)

Kay A. Bauman, MD, MPH

 BASICS

DESCRIPTION

- Latent tuberculosis infection (LTBI) is an asymptomatic, noninfectious condition that follows exposure to an active case of tuberculosis. It is usually detected by a positive skin test (i.e., purified protein derivative [PPD]), positive interferon-γ release assay (IGRA) test. In LTBI, acid-fast bacilli smear and culture are negative, and chest x-ray (CXR) does not suggest active TB.
- Tuberculosis (TB) is a common infection transmitted by inhaling airborne bacilli from a person with active TB. The bacilli multiply in the alveoli and are carried by macrophages, lymphatics, and blood to distant sites (e.g., lung, pleura, brain, kidney, bone).
- Active TB occurs in 5–10% of infected individuals not receiving preventive therapy. Chance of active TB increases with immunosuppression and is highest for all individuals within 2 years of infection; 85% of the cases are pulmonary, which spreads person-to-person via an aerosol route.
- The majority (66% in 2014) of active TB cases in the United States occur in foreign-born persons. Most are as the result of reactivation of LTBI (1). Active TB cases continue to decline but at a slower rate than in previous years.
- LTBI treatment is a key component of the TB elimination strategy of the United States.

ALERT
Test for LTBI (PPD or IGRA), and treat latent infection in high-risk populations (1).

EPIDEMIOLOGY
- High-risk groups include immigrants from Asia, Latin America, Africa, and the Pacific basin; homeless persons; persons with a history of drug use or history of incarceration; HIV-infected individuals; and health care workers.
- Also at high risk are those who are newly exposed (particularly children). In 2014, there were 9,412 new cases of TB in the United States (1).
- In 2014, Asians had the highest active TB case rate of all groups, 28.5 times the rate in whites. The rate of TB in Hispanics and in non-Hispanic blacks is 8 times higher than for whites (1).
- Of active TB cases in 2013 in ethnic minorities, 95% of Asian cases, 75% of Hispanic cases, 40% of black cases, and 23% of white cases were foreign-born (1). This highlights the need to screen foreign-born persons for latent TB and treat those with positive screening tests.
- In 2014, 55.3% of foreign-born persons with TB came from five countries: Mexico (20.6%), Philippines (12.1%), Vietnam (8.1%), India (7.7%), and China (6.8%) (1).
- In 2014, 6% of active TB cases in the United States were in HIV-positive individuals, 5% were homeless, 4% were incarcerated, and 2% in long-term care facilities (1).

Prevalence
- 4% of the U.S. population has LTBI.
- 1/3 of the world's population is estimated to harbor latent TB.
- Predominant gender: male > female

ETIOLOGY AND PATHOPHYSIOLOGY
Mycobacterium tuberculosis, Mycobacterium bovis, and *Mycobacterium africanum*

RISK FACTORS
- HIV infection, immunosuppression
- Immigrants (from Asia, Africa, Latin America, Pacific Islands, or area with high rate of TB), including migrant workers
- Close contact with infected individual
- Institutionalization (e.g., prison, nursing home)
- Use of illicit drugs
- Lower socioeconomic status or homeless
- Health care workers
- Chronic medical disease such as diabetes mellitus (DM), end-stage renal disease, cancer, or silicosis; organ transplant (immunosuppression)
- Persons with fibrotic changes on CXR consistent with previous TB infection (2)
- Recent TB skin test (TST) converters (2)
- Laboratory personnel working with mycobacteria

GENERAL PREVENTION
Screen for LTBI and treat individuals with positive tests.

COMMONLY ASSOCIATED CONDITIONS
- HIV infection (see "Initial Tests (lab, imaging)")
- Immunosuppression

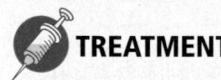 **DIAGNOSIS**

HISTORY
LTBI: Assess risk. History of immigration from a high-risk area, history of IV drug use and/or drug treatment, HIV, homelessness, recent incarceration, immunosuppression

PHYSICAL EXAM
No active signs of infection on exam in patients with LTBI

DIFFERENTIAL DIAGNOSIS
Fungal infections; atypical mycobacteria or *Nocardia*

DIAGNOSTIC TESTS & INTERPRETATION
Initial Tests (lab, imaging)
- None routinely recommended
- In higher risk patients: liver profile, hepatitis C virus (HCV), and hepatitis B virus (HBV) screening
- HIV test recommended to assess risk for active TB in men who have sex with men or persons with a history of IV drug use
- CXR to rule out active TB
- CT scan of the chest has good sensitivity (rarely needed).

Diagnostic Procedures/Other
- Tuberculin Skin Test (TST): PPD: 5 U (0.1 mL) intermediate-strength intradermal volar forearm. Measure induration at 48 to 72 hours:
  - Positive if induration is
    - >5 mm and patient has HIV infection (or suspected) (2), is immunosuppressed, had recent close TB contact, or has clinical evidence of active or old disease on CXR
    - >10 mm and patient age <4 years or has other risk factors noted earlier
    - >15 mm and patient age >4 years and has no risk factors (2)
  - Negative if induration <5 mm on initial test and, if indicated, on second test
  - Use the two-step test (administer a second intradermal test 1 to 3 weeks after initial test; measure and interpret as usual) if patient has had no recent PPD and is age >55 years or is a nursing home resident, prison inmate, or health care worker.
  - Preferred for children <5 years.
- The interferon gamma release assays (IGRA) QuantiFERON-TB and QuantiFERON-TB GOLD; T-SPOT measure the release of interferon by sensitized lymphocytes when exposed to antigens of *M. tuberculosis*. It is unaffected by prior BCG vaccination, requires only one visit, and has improved sensitivity and specificity but is costly (3).
- Special considerations
  - Steroids: false-negative skin test
  - Measles vaccine: May suppress tuberculin activity; simultaneous PPD and measles vaccine recommended; if not simultaneous, defer PPD 4 to 6 weeks after measles vaccine.
  - The multiple-puncture tine test is not recommended.
  - Do not use history of BCG vaccination to ignore a positive PPD in adults and forego treatment.
  - Disorders that may alter results and give a false-negative skin test:
    - Recent viral infection
    - New (<10 weeks) infection
    - Severe malnutrition; HIV; anergy
    - Age <6 months
    - Overwhelming TB

 TREATMENT

GENERAL MEASURES
- Must exclude active TB
- Treatment for LTBI is crucial to control and eliminate TB disease in the United States. LTBI treatment decreases the risk of active TB in those treated and decreases risks of potential spread to others (2).
- Treat LTBI at any age if patient has HIV, has had close TB contact, is a recent converter (<2 years), is an IV drug user, has an abnormal CXR, has a high-risk medical condition, or is in another high-risk group.
- Directly observed therapy (DOT) is recommended if patient adherence is not assured.
  - Use isoniazid (INH) (for 9 months).
  - Acceptable alternative: INH for 6 months
  - Use INH 900 mg and rifapentine 900 mg weekly for 12 weeks.

- Treat LTBI during pregnancy if patient has recent infection or is HIV positive (use INH with pyridoxine, and monitor liver enzymes); otherwise, treatment may be postponed until after delivery (2).
- Consult with public health or ID for HIV infection and suspected INH resistance (2).
- *Note:* Because of severe side effects associated with rifampin and pyrazinamide, these medications are less often recommended for LTBI treatment (2).
- Exclusions: cirrhosis, active hepatitis, history of excessive alcohol consumption (2)

MEDICATION

- INH alone
  - INH-scored tablets: 100 mg, 300 mg, or syrup 10 mg/mL
    - Daily: adult 300 mg; pediatric 10 to 15 mg/kg (maximum 300 mg)
    - Twice weekly: adult 900 mg; pediatric 20 to 30 mg/kg (maximum 900 mg)
    - Treatment for 9 months; typical completion rates of ≤60%
    - Precautions
      - Follow liver function if the patient has history of alcoholism, HBV, HCV, or other liver dysfunction or new signs of liver injury.
      - INH: Peripheral neuritis and hypersensitivity are possible. Consider pyridoxine.
      - INH: An idiosyncratic drug reaction that results in INH-associated severe liver injury was reported by the CDC in 17 patients from 2004 to 2008. Monitoring patients on treatment is recommended, looking for symptoms of liver injury (4).
- INH and rifapentine
  - Patients >12 years: rifapentine, a rifampin-like drug can be used to treat LTBI. 900 mg weekly (if patient >50 kg) and INH, 15 to 25 mg/kg weekly (rounded to nearest 50 or 100 mg; 900 mg max) for 12 weeks given as direct observation therapy. This new and shorter treatment has increased rates of completion compared with 9 months of INH (82% compared with 69% in one trial), slightly more adverse effects (4.9% vs. 3.7%), and is more costly.
    - Contraindications to INH/rifapentine: HIV patients receiving antiretroviral therapy, pregnancy. Rifapentine may cause hyperuricemia and hematuria (5).
- Alternative: rifampin alone
  - Adults 600 mg/day for 4 months; children 10 to 20 mg/kg/day for 6 months (max 600 mg/day). Fewer data exist for efficacy of this regimen but can be considered for contacts of INH-resistant TB or patient with INH contraindications. In one study, the 4-month course increased compliance from 62.6% with INH to 71.6% with rifampin (6).

ADDITIONAL THERAPIES

Pediatric Considerations

- Follow public health recommendations for assessing and treating newborn with mother/household contact with infection or disease.
- If mother or household contact has LTBI, skin test all household contacts, and treat any with positive PPD.

- If contact has abnormal CXR, separate infant until infectious status is known; if not contagious, monitor infant PPD (7).
- If mother has disease and is possibly contagious, evaluate infant for congenital TB and test for HIV; separate newborn until mother is noninfectious (7).
- Treat suspected congenital TB.
- If no congenital disease, start INH and repeat PPD after 3 to 4 months. If positive, reassess infant and finish 9 months of INH. If PPD is negative and source is noninfectious, stop INH and monitor infant (7).
- BCG vaccine, live-attenuated *M. bovis:* used more commonly in developing countries in children to prevent complications of TB

INPATIENT CONSIDERATIONS

Geriatric Considerations

- Before entering a chronic care facility, patients should have a PPD using two-step protocols.
- INH side effects are more pronounced.

Discharge Criteria

- Activity, as tolerated
- No isolation required.

 ONGOING CARE

FOLLOW-UP RECOMMENDATIONS

Patient Monitoring

- During preventive therapy for LTBI: initial monthly visits to assess adherence to regimen and to monitor for hepatitis and neuropathy; if stable, can monitor less frequently
- If patient remains asymptomatic, repeat of CXR is not needed.
- Check liver enzymes if patient is symptomatic, is HIV positive, has chronic liver disease, uses alcohol, or is pregnant or postpartum, and modify drugs, if needed.

DIET

Regular. Consider pyridoxine, 10 to 50 mg/day.

PROGNOSIS

- Generally, there are few complications and treatment is effective if medications are taken as prescribed.
- Retreatment is not necessary.

COMPLICATIONS

Recrudescent TB

REFERENCES

1. Scott C, Kirkling HL, Jeffries C, et al. Tuberculosis trends—United States, 2014. *MMWR Morb Mortal Wkly Rep.* 2015;64(10):265–269.
2. Jensen PA, Lambert LA, Iademarco MF, et al. Guidelines for preventing the transmission of *Mycobacterium tuberculosis* in health-care settings, 2005. *MMWR Recomm Rep.* 2005;54(RR-17):1–141.

3. Campos-Outcalt D. When, and when not, to use the interferon-gamma TB test. *J Fam Pract.* 2005;54(10):873–875.
4. Centers for Disease Control and Prevention. Severe isoniazid-associated liver injuries among persons being treated for latent tuberculosis infection—United States, 2004–2008. *MMWR Morb Mortal Wkly Rep.* 2010;59(8):224–229.
5. Centers for Disease Control and Prevention. Recommendations for use of an isoniazid-rifapentine regimen with direct observation to treat latent *Mycobacterium tuberculosis* infection. *MMWR Morb Mortal Wkly Rep.* 2011;60(48):1650–1653.
6. Page KR, Sifakis F, Montes de Oca R, et al. Improved adherence and less toxicity with rifampin vs isoniazid for treatment of latent tuberculosis: a retrospective study. *Arch Intern Med.* 2006;166(17):1863–1870.
7. American Academy of Pediatrics. *Red Book: 2003 Report of the Committee on Infectious Diseases.* 26th ed. Elk Grove Village, IL: American Academy of Pediatrics; 2003.

ADDITIONAL READING

- Latent Tuberculosis Infections: A guide for primary health care providers. http://www.cdc.gov/tb/publications/ltbi/treatment.htm. Accessed 2015.
- Young DB, Gideon HP, Wilkinson RJ. Eliminating latent tuberculosis. *Trends Microbiol.* 2009;17(5):183–188.

 SEE ALSO

Tuberculosis; Tuberculosis, Miliary

 CODES

ICD10

R76.11 Nonspecific reaction to skin test w/o active tuberculosis

CLINICAL PEARLS

- An estimated 4% of the U.S. population have LTBI. Treatment of LTBI is crucial to control and eliminate TB disease in the United States.
- Test household contacts of PPD-positive patients.
- History of BCG vaccination, especially >10 years before PPD testing, should not be considered as the cause of a positive PPD. The interferon-γ blood test is unaffected by prior BCG vaccination.
- Treat all HIV-positive patients with LTBI with a prophylactic regimen.
- Screen foreign-born persons for latent TB, and treat those who are positive.

TYPHOID FEVER

Douglas W. MacPherson, MD, MSc–CTM, FRCPC

 BASICS

- A common enteric bacterial disease transmitted by ingestion of contaminated food or water
- Most cases in the United States are imported from endemic areas of South or Southeast Asia and Latin America.

DESCRIPTION
- Typhoid fever is an acute systemic illness in humans caused by *Salmonella typhi*.
  – Classic example of enteric fever caused by *Salmonella* bacterium
- Enteric fevers due to *Salmonella paratyphi* can present in a manner similar to classic typhoid fever.
- Typhoid is endemic in developing nations with poor sanitation. Most cases in North America and other developed nations are acquired after travel to disease-endemic areas.
- Travelers visiting family or friends may be at greater risk of typhoid.
- Mode of transmission is fecal–oral through ingestion of contaminated food (commonly poultry or milk) or water.
- Incubation period varies from 7 to 21 days.
- System(s) affected: gastrointestinal; pulmonary; skin/exocrine
- Synonym(s): typhoid; typhus abdominalis; enteric fever; nervous fever; slow fever

Geriatric Considerations
Disease is more serious in the elderly.

Pediatric Considerations
Disease is more serious in infants but may be milder in children.

EPIDEMIOLOGY
Although typhoid outbreaks have been described in the United States, most cases are reported in international travelers returning from endemic transmission areas.
- Predominant age: all ages
- Predominant sex: male = female

Incidence
In the United States, 300 to 500 new cases per year

ETIOLOGY AND PATHOPHYSIOLOGY
- Historically, typhoid fever (untreated) occurs in several week-long stages.
- The initial infection is transmitted via the fecal–oral route, with resultant bacteremia and sepsis. Involvement of the bowel wall (Peyer patch) rarely may be associated with bleeding from the bowel or bowel perforation.
- The first stage involves fluctuations in temperature with relative bradycardia (Faget sign). Other symptoms include headache, cough, malaise, epistaxis, and abdominal pain.
- The second stage involves higher fever (with persistent relative bradycardia). Mental status changes are possible (agitation—"nervous fever"). Rose spots appear on the chest and abdomen. In some patients, abdominal pain is common as is constipation or diarrhea (with characteristic malodorous "pea soup" appearance).
- The third week is when most complications occur due to intestinal hemorrhage or encephalitis.

- The final week is characterized by defervescence and recovery.
- A chronic carrier state may occur with *S. typhi* shedding in the stools. Potential person-to-person transmission may occur. In a chronic carrier state, *S. typhi* resides in the biliary tract and gallbladder. Chronic suppressive antimicrobials may clear the carrier state. In extreme cases, cholecystectomy has been performed as an attempt to clear carriage of *S. typhi*.

RISK FACTORS
Consider in patients presenting with fever after tropical travel or exposure to a chronic carrier.

GENERAL PREVENTION
- Food and water precautions help prevent all enteric infections, including typhoid fever.
- Avoid tap water, salad/raw vegetables, unpeeled fruits, and dairy products in tropical travel.
- Avoid undercooked poultry or poultry products left unrefrigerated for prolonged periods.
- Wash hands before and after food preparation.
- For high-risk travel to an endemic area, consider vaccination against typhoid (1)[A].
  – Parenteral ViCPS or capsular polysaccharide typhoid vaccine (Typhim Vi) *or*
  – Ty21a or live oral typhoid vaccine (Vivotif Berna), particularly if traveler will be at prolonged risk (>4 weeks)
- Consider vaccination for workers exposed to *S. typhi* or those with household or intimate exposure to a carrier of *S. typhi*.
- Occupational health and safety precautions, including screening of domestic and commercial food handlers, may be considered in some situations.

 DIAGNOSIS

Assess the clinical presentation and exposure history, including travel and known exposures to chronic *S. typhi* carriers.

HISTORY
- Travel history to an endemic region and exposure to contaminated food or water
- Exposure to a chronic *S. typhi* carrier
- Fever, headache
- Malaise
- Abdominal discomfort/bloating/constipation
- Diarrhea (less common)
- Dry cough
- Confusion/lethargy

PHYSICAL EXAM
- Fever
- Relative bradycardia
- Cervical adenopathy
- Conjunctivitis
- Rose spot (transient erythematous maculopapular rash in anterior thorax or upper abdomen)
- Splenomegaly
- Hepatomegaly

DIFFERENTIAL DIAGNOSIS
- Malaria
- "Enteric fever–like" syndrome caused by *Yersinia enterocolitica*, pseudotuberculosis, and *Campylobacter* spp.
- Enteric fever caused by nontyphoid *Salmonella* spp.
- Infectious hepatitis
- Dengue
- Atypical pneumonia
- Infectious mononucleosis
- Subacute bacterial endocarditis
- Tuberculosis
- Brucellosis
- Q fever
- Toxoplasmosis
- Typhus
- Viral infections: Epstein-Barr virus (EBV), cytomegalovirus (CMV), viral hemorrhagic agents

DIAGNOSTIC TESTS & INTERPRETATION
Due to the rarity of enteric fevers/typhoid syndromes in the United States, a high level of clinical suspicion is required.
- Definitive diagnosis is by culture of *S. typhi* from blood or other sterile body fluid.
- Isolation of *S. typhi* in sputum, urine, or stool leads to a presumptive diagnosis.
- Serology is nonspecific and typically not useful.
- If there are multiple negative blood cultures or in patients with prior antibiotic therapy, diagnostic yield is better with bone marrow culture.
- Anemia, leukopenia (neutropenia), thrombocytopenia, or evidence of disseminated intravascular coagulopathy. Elevated liver enzymes are common.
- Have a high clinical suspicion for intestinal perforation, or consider serial plain abdominal films looking for evidence of perforation in ill patients complaining of persistent abdominal tenderness.

Diagnostic Procedures/Other
- Bone marrow aspirate for culture of *S. typhi* is more sensitive than blood cultures but rarely indicated as a primary investigation.
- Bone marrow aspiration may be done for evaluation of a fever of unknown origin.

Test Interpretation
Classically, pathology of the bowel shows mononuclear proliferation involving lymphoid tissue of intestinal tract, especially Peyer patches of the terminal ileum.

 TREATMENT

- Treatment of typhoid disease and chronic carrier states must be determined on an individual basis. Factors to be considered include age, public health and occupational health risk (e.g., food handler, chronic care facilities, medical personnel), intolerance to antibiotics, and evidence of biliary tract disease.
- Awareness of emerging drug-resistant *S. typhi* strains and the epidemiology of the patient's exposure help direct primary therapy. Knowledge of local resistance patterns for presumptive treatment or laboratory sensitivity also guide therapy. Fluoroquinolone-resistant *S. typhi* is common in Asia.

GENERAL MEASURES
- Fluid and electrolyte support
- Strict isolation of patient's linen, stool, and urine
- Consider serial plain abdominal films for evidence of perforation, usually in the 3rd to 4th week of illness.
- For hemorrhage: blood transfusion and management of shock

MEDICATION
First Line
- Chloramphenicol: pediatric 50 mg/kg/day PO QID for 2 weeks; adult dose 2 to 3 g per day PO divided q6h for 2 weeks *or*
- Ampicillin: pediatric 100 mg/kg/day (max 2 g) QID PO for 2 weeks; adults 500 mg q6h for 2 weeks *or*
- Ciprofloxacin: 500 mg PO BID for 2 weeks, *indicated in multiple-drug-resistant typhoid*
  - Has been used safely in children; WHO recommends as first line in areas with drug resistance to older first-line antibiotics.
  - Fluoroquinolones may prevent clinical relapse better than chloramphenicol (2)[A].
- Ceftriaxone: pediatric 100 mg/kg/day for 2 weeks; adult dose: 1 to 2 g IV once daily for 2 weeks *or*
- Azithromycin: pediatric 10 to 20 mg/kg (max 1 g) PO daily for 5 to 7 days; adult dose: 1 g PO once followed by 500 mg PO daily for 5 to 7 days
- Chronic carrier state
  - Ampicillin: 4 to 5 g/day plus probenecid 2 g/day QID for 6 weeks (for patients with normal gallbladder function and no evidence of cholelithiasis)
  - Ciprofloxacin: 500 mg PO BID for 4 to 6 weeks is also efficacious. Chloramphenicol resistance has been reported in Mexico, South America, Central America, Southeast Asia, India, Pakistan, Middle East, and Africa.
- Contraindications: Refer to manufacturer's profile.
- Precautions: Rarely, Jarisch-Herxheimer reaction appears after antimicrobial therapy.
- Significant possible interactions: Refer to manufacturer's profile for each drug.

Second Line
- Trimethoprim–sulfamethoxazole one double-strength tablet twice a day for 10 days (Note: Drug resistance is common, local resistance patterns and expert knowledge should guide choice of treatment agent.)
- Furazolidone: 7.5 mg/kg/day PO for 10 days; in uncomplicated multidrug-resistant typhoid; safe in children; efficacy >85% cure

Pregnancy Considerations
Ciprofloxacin therapy is relatively contraindicated in children and in pregnant patients.

ISSUES FOR REFERRAL
Complications of sepsis, bowel perforation

SURGERY/OTHER PROCEDURES
- Complications: bowel perforation
- Cholecystectomy may be warranted in carriers with cholelithiasis, relapse after therapy, or intolerance to antimicrobial therapy.

INPATIENT CONSIDERATIONS
Admission Criteria/Initial Stabilization
- Inpatient if acutely ill
- Outpatient for less ill patient or for carrier

Nursing
Observe enteric precautions.

 ONGOING CARE

FOLLOW-UP RECOMMENDATIONS
Bed rest initially, then activity as tolerated

Patient Monitoring
See "General Measures."

DIET
NPO if abdominal symptoms are severe. With improvement, begin normal low-residue diet, with high-calorie supplementation if malnourished.

PATIENT EDUCATION
- Discuss chronic carrier state and its complications.
- For family members, travelers, or workers at risk, educate about food/water hygiene and provide vaccination.
- Educate patients that the typhoid vaccines do not protect against *S. paratyphi* infection.
- Typhoid vaccines protect 50–80% of recipients (not 100%) with diminishing effectiveness over 2 to 4 years.
- CDC patient handout: http://www.cdc.gov/vaccines/hcp/vis/vis-statements/typhoid.html

PROGNOSIS
Overall prognosis is good with therapy, <2% mortality rate, 15% relapse rate with some antibiotic treatments, and 3% bowel perforation.

COMPLICATIONS
- Intestinal hemorrhage and perforation in distal ileum
- Patients (up to 3%) may become chronic carriers-persistent stool excretor of *S. typhi* for >1 year.
- Seeding of the biliary tract may become a focus for relapse of typhoid fever: most common in females and older patients (>50 years of age)
- Osteomyelitis is more common in patients with sickle cell anemia, systemic lupus erythematosus, and hematologic neoplasms, as well as in immuno-suppressed hosts.
- Endovascular infection in the elderly and in patients with a history of bypass operation or aneurysm
- Rarely, endocarditis or meningitis

REFERENCES

1. Roggelin L, Vinnemeier CD, Fischer-Herr J, et al. Serological response following re-vaccination with *Salmonella typhi* Vi-capsular polysaccharide vaccines in healthy adult travellers. *Vaccine.* 2015;33(33):4141–4145.
2. Thaver D, Zaidi AK, Critchley J, et al. A comparison of fluoroquinolones versus other antibiotics for treating enteric fever: meta-analysis. *BMJ.* 2009; 338:b1865.

ADDITIONAL READING

- Basnyat B. Typhoid fever in the United States and antibiotic choice. *JAMA.* 2010;303(1):34; author reply 34–35.
- Butler T. Treatment of typhoid fever in the 21st century: promises and shortcomings. *Clin Microbiol Infect.* 2011;17(7):959–963.
- Centers for Disease Control and Prevention. National Center for Emerging and Zoonotic Infectious Diseases. Typhoid fever. http://www.cdc.gov/nczved/divisions/dfbmd/diseases/typhoid_fever/. Accessed October 11, 2015.
- Chalya PL, Mabula JB, Koy M, et al. Typhoid intestinal perforations at a University teaching hospital in Northwestern Tanzania: a surgical experience of 104 cases in a resource-limited setting. *World J Emerg Surg.* 2012;7:4.
- Clark TW, Daneshvar C, Pareek M, et al. Enteric fever in a UK regional infectious diseases unit: a 10 year retrospective review. *J Infect.* 2010;60(2):91–98.
- Crump JA, Mintz ED. Global trends in typhoid and paratyphoid fever. *Clin Infect Dis.* 2010;50(2):241–246.
- Date KA, Bentsi-Enchill A, Marks F, et al. Typhoid fever vaccination strategies. *Vaccine.* 2015;33 (Suppl 3):C55–C61.
- Effa EE, Lassi ZS, Critchley JA, et al. Fluoroquinolones for treating typhoid and paratyphoid fever (enteric fever). *Cochrane Database Syst Rev.* 2011;(10):CD004530.
- Kaurthe J. Increasing antimicrobial resistance and narrowing therapeutics in typhoidal salmonellae. *J Clin Diagn Res.* 2013;7(3):576–579.
- Newton AE, Routh JA, Mahon BE. Chapter 3. Infectious diseases related to travel. Typhoid and paratyphoid fever. http://wwwnc.cdc.gov/travel/yellowbook/2016/infectious-diseases-related-to-travel/typhoid-paratyphoid-fever. Accessed October 11, 2015.
- Sánchez-Vargas FM, Abu-El-Haija MA, Gómez-Duarte OG. Salmonella infections: an update on epidemiology, management, and prevention. *Travel Med Infect Dis.* 2011;9(6):263–277.

 ## CODES

ICD10
- A01.00 Typhoid fever, unspecified
- Z22.0 Carrier of typhoid
- A01.03 Typhoid pneumonia

CLINICAL PEARLS
- Consider typhoid (along with malaria, dengue, and other travel-associated infections) in febrile travelers returning from endemic areas such as Latin America, sub-Saharan Africa, or South Asia.
- Routine blood cultures detect *S. typhi* but may be negative if antibiotics are administered prior to testing.
- A history or documentation of vaccination against *S. typhi* does not exclude the diagnosis of typhoid fever.

TYPHUS FEVERS

Douglas W. MacPherson, MD, MSc–CTM, FRCPC

 BASICS

Typhus is an infectious disease syndrome caused by several rickettsial bacterial organisms resulting in acute, chronic, and recurrent disease (1)[C].

DESCRIPTION
- Acute infection caused by three species of *Rickettsia*
  - Epidemic typhus: human-to-human transmission by body louse; primarily in setting of refugee camps, war, famine, and disaster. Recurrent disease occurs years after initial infection and can be a source of human outbreak. Flying squirrels are a reservoir.
  - Endemic (murine) typhus: spread to humans by rat flea bite
  - Scrub typhus: infection and infestation of chiggers and of rodents to humans by the chigger; primarily in Asia and western Pacific areas
- System(s) affected: endocrine/metabolic; hematologic/lymphatic/immunologic; pulmonary; skin/exocrine
- Synonym(s): louse-borne typhus; Brill-Zinsser disease; murine typhus

EPIDEMIOLOGY
- Epidemic and endemic typhus: rare in the United States (outside of South Texas)
- Scrub typhus: travelers returning from endemic areas only (rare)

Incidence
Endemic typhus: <100 cases annually, primarily in states around the Gulf of Mexico, especially South Texas; underreporting suspected

ETIOLOGY AND PATHOPHYSIOLOGY
- Epidemic typhus by *Rickettsia prowazekii*
- Endemic typhus by *Rickettsia typhi*
- Scrub typhus by *Rickettsia tsutsugamushi*

RISK FACTORS
- Vector exposure
- Travel to endemic countries

Geriatric Considerations
Elderly may have more severe disease.

GENERAL PREVENTION
Vector control:
- Scrub typhus: Wear protective clothing and use insect repellents.
- Endemic typhus: Practice ectoparasite and rodent control.
- Epidemic typhus: delousing and cleaning of clothing; vaccine for those at high risk of exposure (typhus vaccine production has been discontinued in the United States)

 DIAGNOSIS

Typhus syndromes are rare in the United States. A high level of clinical suspicion is necessary.

HISTORY
Travel or other risk exposure
- Fever, chills
- Intractable headache
- Myalgias, malaise
- Cough, rash, ocular pain

PHYSICAL EXAM
- General
  - Fever
  - Relative bradycardia (scrub typhus)
- Epidemic typhus
  - Incubation period ~1 week
  - Macular or maculopapular rash beginning on trunk ~5th day of illness
  - Nonproductive cough
  - Pulmonary infiltrates
- Endemic typhus
  - Incubation period 1 to 2 weeks
  - Macular or maculopapular rash beginning on trunk 3rd to 5th day of illness
- Scrub typhus
  - Incubation period 1 to 3 weeks
  - Eschar at bite site
  - Regional lymphadenopathy
  - Generalized lymphadenopathy
  - Splenomegaly
  - Macular or maculopapular rash beginning on trunk approximately 5th day of illness
  - Relative bradycardia early in disease
  - Ocular pain
  - Conjunctival injection

DIFFERENTIAL DIAGNOSIS
- Other rickettsial disease: Rocky Mountain spotted fever; ehrlichiosis; Mediterranean spotted fever (boutonneuse fever) (*Rickettsia conorii*)
- Bacterial meningitis; meningococcemia
- Measles, rubella
- Toxoplasmosis
- Leptospirosis
- Typhoid fever
- Dengue, malaria
- Relapsing fever
- Secondary syphilis
- Viral syndromes: mononucleosis, acute retroviral syndrome

DIAGNOSTIC TESTS & INTERPRETATION
- Specific serologies with rising antibody titer
- If suspected, isolate *Rickettsia* in qualified laboratory to minimize the risk of laboratory-acquired infection.
- CDC Rickettsial Zoonoses Branch 404-639-1075.

Initial Tests (lab, imaging)
- CBC often normal
- Weil-Felix serologic reaction may be positive; test value hampered by low sensitivity and nonspecificity; epidemic and endemic typhus, 4-fold titer rise or titer >1/320 to OX-19; scrub typhus, 4-fold rise in titer to OX-K
- Hyponatremia in severe cases
- Hypoalbuminemia in severe cases
- Recent antibiotic exposure may alter lab results.

Test Interpretation
Diffuse vasculitis on skin biopsy

 TREATMENT

Initiate treatment based on epidemiologic risk and clinical presentation.

GENERAL MEASURES
- Skin and mouth care
- Supportive care for the severely ill, directed at complications

MEDICATION

First Line
- Begin treatment when diagnosis is likely and continue until clinically improved and the patient is afebrile for at least 48 hours; usual course is 5 to 7 days.
- Children ≥8 years of age and adults
  - Doxycycline IV/PO: adults 100 mg q12h, children ≤45 kg: 5 mg/kg/day divided twice daily (max of 200 mg/day); >45 kg: adult dosing
  - Children ≤8 years of age: Risk of dental staining from tetracyclines is minimal with short courses of therapy.
  - Tetracycline: 25 mg/kg PO initially, then 25 mg/kg/day in equally divided doses q6h
- Children ≤8 years of age, pregnant women, or if typhoid fever is suspected
  - Chloramphenicol: 50 mg/kg PO initially, then 50 mg/kg/day in equally divided doses q6h
  - If severely ill, chloramphenicol sodium succinate: 20 mg/kg IV initially, infused over 30 to 45 minutes, then 50 mg/kg/day infused in equally divided doses q6h until orally tolerable
  - Azithromycin, fluoroquinolones, and rifampin may be alternatives depending on the clinical scenario.
- Precautions: Refer to the manufacturer's profile for each drug.
- Significant possible interactions: Refer to the manufacturer's profile for each drug.

Second Line
- Doxycycline: single oral dose of 100 or 200 mg orally for those in refugee camps, victims of disasters, or in the presence of limited medical services
- Isolated reports indicate that erythromycin and ciprofloxacin are effective.
- Azithromycin 1,000 mg orally once a day for 3-day course is effective for scrub typhus; better tolerated than doxycycline but more expensive
- Rifampin may be effective in areas where scrub typhus responds poorly to standard antirickettsial drugs.

ISSUES FOR REFERRAL
Infectious disease consultation is recommended. Contact CDC and local public health authorities.

INPATIENT CONSIDERATIONS

Admission Criteria/Initial Stabilization
- Outpatient care unless severely ill
- Severely ill or constitutionally unstable (e.g., shock)

 ONGOING CARE

FOLLOW-UP RECOMMENDATIONS

Patient Monitoring
- Admit severely ill patients.
- If treated as an outpatient, ensure regular follow-up to assess clinical improvement and resolution.

DIET
As tolerated

PATIENT EDUCATION
Travel advice (minimize exposure risks, vector avoidance, vaccination as appropriate)

PROGNOSIS
- Recovery is expected with prompt treatment.
- Relapses may follow treatment, especially if initiated within 48 hours of onset (this is *not* an indication to delay treatment). Treat relapses the same as primary disease.
- Without treatment, the mortality rate of typhus is 40–60% for epidemic, 1–2% for endemic, and up to 30% for scrub disease.
- Mortality is higher among the elderly.

COMPLICATIONS
Organ-specific complications (particularly in the second week of illness): azotemia, meningoencephalitis, seizures, delirium, coma, myocardial failure, hyponatremia, hypoalbuminemia, hypovolemia, shock, and death

REFERENCES

1. Centers for Disease Control and Prevention. McQuiston J. Rickettsial (spotted and typhus fevers) and related infections (anaplasmosis and ehrlichiosis). http://wwwnc.cdc.gov/travel/yellowbook/2016/infectious-diseases-related-to-travel/rickettsial-spotted-typhus-fevers-related-infections-anaplasmosis-ehrlichiosis. Accessed 2015.

ADDITIONAL READING

- Botelho-Nevers E, Raoult D. Host, pathogen and treatment-related prognostic factors in rickettsioses. *Eur J Clin Microbiol Infect Dis*. 2011;30(10): 1139–1150.

- Botelho-Nevers E, Rovery C, Richet H, et al. Analysis of risk factors for malignant Mediterranean spotted fever indicates that fluoroquinolone treatment has a deleterious effect. *J Antimicrob Chemother*. 2011;66(8):1821–1830.
- Botelho-Nevers E, Socolovschi C, Raoult D, et al. Treatment of Rickettsia spp. infections: a review. *Expert Rev Anti Infect Ther*. 2012;10(12):1425–1437.
- Chikeka I, Dumler JS. Neglected bacterial zoonoses. *Clin Microbiol Infect*. 2015;21(5):404–415.
- Graham J, Stockley K, Goldman RD. Tick-borne illnesses: a CME update. *Pediatr Emerg Care*. 2011;27(2):141–147.
- Green JS, Singh J, Cheung M, et al. A cluster of pediatric endemic typhus cases in Orange County, California. *Pediatr Infect Dis J*. 2011;30(2):163–165.
- Hendershot EF, Sexton DJ. Scrub typhus and rickettsial diseases in international travelers: a review. *Curr Infect Dis Rep*. 2009;11(1):66–72.
- Molina N. Borders, laborers, and racialized medicalization Mexican immigration and US public health practices in the 20th century. *Am J Public Health*. 2011;101(6):1024–1031.
- Panpanich R, Garner P. Antibiotics for treating scrub typhus. *Cochrane Database Syst Rev*. 2002;(3):CD002150.

 CODES

ICD10
- A75.9 Typhus fever, unspecified
- A75.0 Epidemic louse-borne typhus fever d/t Rickettsia prowazekii
- A75.2 Typhus fever due to Rickettsia typhi

CLINICAL PEARLS
- Consider typhus (along with malaria and dengue) in febrile travelers returning from endemic areas.
- Rickettsial infections typically present within 2 to 14 days. Febrile illnesses presenting with onset >18 days after travel are unlikely to be rickettsial.
- Routine blood cultures do not detect *Rickettsia*.
- Prior vaccination does not exclude the diagnosis of typhus.

ULCER, APHTHOUS

Jay A. Brieler, MD

 BASICS

DESCRIPTION
- Self-limited, painful ulcerations of the nonkeratinized oral mucosa, which are often recurrent
- Synonyms: canker sores; aphthae; aphthous stomatitis
  - Comes from *aphth* meaning "ulcer" in Greek; first used by Hippocrates between 460 and 370 BC to categorize oral disease (1)
- Categorization
  - Minor aphthous ulcers (2)
    - Usually <10 mm in diameter
    - Self-limited, healing within 4 to 14 days
    - Rarely affect the dorsum of the mouth
    - Nonscarring
  - Major aphthous ulcers (Sutton disease) (2)
    - Usually >10 mm in diameter
    - Can affect the dorsum of the mouth
    - May take weeks to months to heal
    - Generally more painful than minor aphthous ulcers
    - May cause scarring
  - Herpetiform ulcers (2)
    - Usually 2 to 3 mm in diameter, may coalesce to form larger ulcerations
    - Unrelated to viral-caused herpetic stomatitis
    - Occur in small clusters numbering 10s to 100s, lasting 1 to 4 weeks
    - Generally more painful than minor aphthous ulcers
    - May cause scarring

EPIDEMIOLOGY
- Most frequent chronic disease of the oral cavity, affecting 5–25% of the population (3)
- More common in patients between 10 and 40 years of age, women, Caucasians, nonsmokers, professional students, and those of higher socioeconomic status (3)
- Less frequent with advancing age (4)
- Minor aphthous ulcers
  - Most common: 70–85% of all aphthae
- Major aphthous ulcers
  - 10–15% of all aphthae
- Herpetiform
  - Least common: 10% of all aphthae

Prevalence
Lifetime prevalence of 5–60% (3)

ETIOLOGY AND PATHOPHYSIOLOGY
Likely multifactorial; association with stress-induced rise in salivary cortisol, multiple HLA antigens, cell-mediated immunity; exact etiology unknown (4)

RISK FACTORS
- Genetic factors: Offspring of those with recurrent aphthous ulcers have a 90% chance of developing recurrent aphthous stomatitis (RAS) (5)[C].
- Local trauma: sharp teeth, dental treatments, or mucosal injury secondary to toothbrushing

- Increased stress and anxiety
- Nutritional deficiencies: iron, zinc, vitamin B complex, and folate
- Homocysteinemia (6)[B]
- Immunodeficiency
- Recent cessation of tobacco use
- Food sensitivity: to benzoic acid/cinnamaldehyde
- Medications
  - NSAIDS
  - β-Blockers
  - Alendronate
  - Methotrexate
- Neutropenia
- Anemia
- Endocrine alterations (i.e., menstrual cycle) (2)
- Psychosocial stress

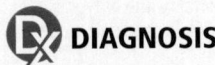 **DIAGNOSIS**

Diagnosis is made by history and clinical presentation. Lab work is rarely helpful to diagnose aphthous ulcers (2)[A].

HISTORY
- May experience prodrome of burning sensation of oral mucosa 2 to 48 hours prior to appearance of ulcers
- Patients typically complain of oral ulcerations, which are painful and exacerbated by movement of the mouth. Exacerbation may also be reported with certain foods (hot, spicy, acidic, or carbonated foods or drinks) (2)[A].
- Ask about ulcerative lesions of other anatomic areas, family history, or prior history of aphthous ulcers (2)[A].

PHYSICAL EXAM
- Round or ovoid ulcerations generally <10 mm in size. Covered with a grayish-white pseudomembrane surrounded by an erythematous halo (3)[A]
- Ulcers are typically found in the buccal or lip mucosa, ventral tongue, soft palate, or oral vestibule. Rarely on the dorsum of the mouth/lips
- Evaluate for signs of secondary infection: elevated temperature, increased surrounding edema, or pus drainage

DIFFERENTIAL DIAGNOSIS
- Oral trauma
  - Biting
  - Dentures
- Infection
  - Herpes virus (herpetic stomatitis): vesicular lesions on keratinized tissue (dorsal tongue, vermillion border). Generally not present on mucosa (5)[C]
  - HIV: Ulcerations have lengthened healing time and tend to be more painful (5)[C].

- Mucocutaneous disease; especially if chronic or nonhealing
  - Lichen planus
  - Pemphigus
- Malignancy: Investigate and closely monitor nonhealing lesions, especially those with ipsilateral cervical lymphadenopathy.
- Important to evaluate for underlying systemic disease, causing aphthous-like ulcerations
  - Highest suspicion in adult patients with their initial episode or in individuals with additional lesions elsewhere in the body (3)[A],(4)[C]
  - Behçet syndrome: autoimmune systemic vasculitis usually involving mucous membranes
    - Genital and oral ulceration
    - Uveitis
  - Reiter syndrome: reactive arthritis, preceded by infection, usually of the genital tract (2)[A]
    - Uveitis
    - Urethritis
    - HLA-B27–associated arthritis
  - Sweet syndrome: acute neutrophilic dermatitis (5)[C]
    - Fever, sudden onset
    - Erythematous skin plaques/papules, well-demarcated
    - Leukocytosis
    - 50% of patients have an associated malignancy
    - Most often in middle-aged females
  - Inflammatory bowel disease (IBD): Crohn disease, ulcerative colitis
    - 10% of patients with Crohn disease experience recurrent oral ulcers (5)[C].
    - Bloody or persistent diarrhea
    - Weight loss
  - Cyclic neutropenia (5)[C]
    - Recurrent fevers associated with infections, occasionally occurring intraorally.
    - Begins in childhood
  - Systemic lupus erythematosus (SLE): autoimmune vascular collagen disease
    - Oral lesions have great variability, including recurrent ulceration.
  - Gluten-sensitive enteropathy (celiac disease)
    - Weight loss and signs of malabsorption
    - Bloating and diarrhea

DIAGNOSTIC TESTS & INTERPRETATION
May consider complete blood count, folic acid, ferritin, vitamin B_{12} to evaluate for systemic causes based on presentation (2)[A]

Follow-Up Tests & Special Considerations
- HIV is associated with increased amount of ulcers and increased healing time.
- Biopsy and viral cultures for nonhealing ulcers or atypical presentations
- Rheumatologic serology if underlying systemic disease is suspected.

TREATMENT

GENERAL MEASURES

- Management is symptomatic. Goal is to reduce inflammation and relieve pain.
- Avoid potentially irritating food or drink:
  - Spicy
  - Acidic
  - Hot
  - Carbonated beverages.
  - Abrasive/hard foods (i.e., chips, nuts, etc.)
- Behavior modification to reduce dental trauma with toothbrush or bruxism

MEDICATION

In general, the goals of treatment depend on the extent of ulceration and frequency of outbreaks.

First Line

- Topical corticosteroids (to improve healing time and symptoms) (2)[A]

  - Adverse effects: may increase risk of oral candidiasis (more likely with higher potency formulations)
  - Preparations
    o Triamcinolone 0.1% dental paste
      ▪ Apply sparingly to ulcers three times daily for up to 2 weeks or until ulcer resolution.
    o Fluocinonide 0.05% gel or ointment
      ▪ Apply sparingly to ulcer four times daily for up to 2 weeks or until ulcer resolution.
    o Dexamethasone 5 mg/5 mL elixir
      ▪ Rinse for 3 minutes and spit four times daily until ulcer resolution.

- Topical anesthetics (to reduce symptoms only) (2)[A]

  - Adverse effects: may cause initial stinging
  - Preparations
    o Lidocaine 2% gel
      ▪ Apply four times daily or prior to eating as needed for pain, for up to 2 weeks or until ulcer resolution.
- Antimicrobial mouth rinses (improve healing time, decrease pain, and may prevent recurrence)
  - Preparations
    o Chlorhexidine aqueous mouthwash 0.12% or 0.2%
      ▪ Use four times daily for up to several months.
      ▪ May cause superficial tooth staining
- Topical immunomodulators (improves healing time, reduces symptoms, and prevents recurrence when used in prodromic phase) (2)[A]

  - Adverse effects: may cause stinging sensation
  - Preparation
    o Amlexanox 5% oral paste
      ▪ Apply to ulcers four times daily for up to 2 weeks or until ulcer resolution.

Second Line

- Systemic corticosteroids—rescue therapy in acute, severe, recurrent outbreaks (2,3)[A]
  - Prednisone 25 mg/day, then tapered over 2 months (3)[A]
- Colchicine, pentoxifylline, thalidomide, and dapsone have been used with variable success but should be used with caution due to side effects (2–4)[A].

ISSUES FOR REFERRAL

Otolaryngology or dental referral if lesions have not resolved as expected.

ADDITIONAL THERAPIES

Vitamin B$_{12}$ supplementation has been shown to decrease burden of outbreaks and recurrence, independent of preexisting deficiency in one small study (7)[B]. Multivitamins have not been shown to be effective (8)[B].

SURGERY/OTHER PROCEDURES

Chemical cautery with silver nitrate (reduces ulcer pain but not healing time) (9)[B]

COMPLEMENTARY & ALTERNATIVE MEDICINE

Some small cohort studies show clinical improvement with minimal side effects of several herbal and alternative treatments (3)[A].

- *Glycyrrhiza* (licorice) (10)[B]
- *Myrtus communis* (myrtle) (11)[B]
- Bee propolis (3)[A]

REFERENCES

1. Preeti L, Magesh K, Rajkumar K, et al. Recurrent aphthous stomatitis. *J Oral Maxillofac Pathol*. 2011;15(3):252–256.
2. Belenguer-Guallar I, Jiménez-Soriano Y, Claramunt-Lozano A. Treatment of recurrent aphthous stomatitis. A literature review. *J Clin Exp Dent*. 2014;6(2):e168–e174.
3. Brocklehurst P, Tickle M, Glenny AM, et al. Systemic interventions for recurrent aphthous stomatitis (mouth ulcers). *Cochrane Database Syst Rev*. 2012;(9):CD005411.
4. Akintoye SO, Greenberg MS. Recurrent aphthous stomatitis. *Dent Clin North Am*. 2014;58(2):281–297.
5. Chavan M, Jain H, Diwan N, et al. Recurrent aphthous stomatitis: a review. *J Oral Pathol Med*. 2012;41(8):577–583.
6. Sun A, Chen HM, Cheng SJ, et al. Significant association of deficiencies of hemoglobin, iron, vitamin B12, and folic acid and high homocysteine level with recurrent aphthous stomatitis. *J Oral Pathol Med*. 2015;44(4):300–305.
7. Carrozzo M. Vitamin B12 for the treatment of recurrent aphthous stomatitis. *Evid Based Dent*. 2009;10(4):114–115.
8. Lalla RV, Choquette LE, Feinn RS, et al. Multivitamin therapy for recurrent aphthous stomatitis: a randomized, double-masked, placebo-controlled trial. *J Am Dent Assoc*. 2012;143(4):370–376.
9. Soylu Özler G. Silver nitrate cauterization: a treatment option for aphthous stomatitis. *J Craniomaxillofac Surg*. 2014;42(5):e281–e283.
10. Martin MD, Sherman J, van der Ven P, et al. A controlled trial of a dissolving oral patch concerning glycyrrhiza (licorice) herbal extract for the treatment of aphthous ulcers. *Gen Dent*. 2008;56(2):206–210; quiz 211–212, 224.
11. Babaee N, Mansourian A, Momen-Heravi F, et al. The efficacy of a paste containing *Myrtus communis* (myrtle) in the management of recurrent aphthous stomatitis: a randomized controlled trial. *Clin Oral Investig*. 2010;14(1):65–70.

ADDITIONAL READING

- Liu C, Zhou Z, Liu G, et al. Efficacy and safety of dexamethasone ointment on recurrent aphthous ulceration. *Am J Med*. 2012;125(3):292–301.
- Pakfetrat A, Mansourian A, Momen-Heravi F, et al. Comparison of colchicine versus prednisolone in recurrent aphthous stomatitis: a double-blind randomized clinical trial. *Clin Invest Med*. 2010;33(3):e189–e195.

 CODES

ICD10

K12.0 Recurrent oral aphthae

CLINICAL PEARLS

- Aphthous ulcers are the most common chronic disease of the oral cavity.
- Most cases are mild, self-limited episodes.
- Appropriate treatment should be aimed at symptom control and promotion of healing.
- If lesions are nonhealing, simultaneously occur elsewhere in the body, or when patients present with a sudden initial episode in adulthood, it is imperative to rule out secondary causes.

U

ULCERATIVE COLITIS

Jason E. Domagalski, MD, FAAFP

BASICS

DESCRIPTION
- Chronic idiopathic inflammatory disease of the colonic mucosa that can affect any section of the colon starting at the rectum with variable extension towards the cecum
- >95% of patients have rectal involvement, 50% have disease limited to rectum and sigmoid; 20% have pancolitis.

EPIDEMIOLOGY

Incidence
- United States: 9 to 12 new cases/100,000 persons/year
- Incidence stable over the past 5 decades
- Predominant age: 15 to 35 years; second and smaller peak in the 7th decade
- Predominant sex: female > male (slight)

Prevalence
205 to 240/100,000 persons

Pregnancy Considerations
- Increased risk of preterm delivery and small for gestational age birth
- 30% with inactive disease relapse in pregnancy
- Patients should delay pregnancy until disease is inactive for at least 3 months.

ETIOLOGY AND PATHOPHYSIOLOGY
Unknown; hypotheses include allergy to dietary components and abnormal immune responses to bacterial or "self" antigens; final common path is mucosal inflammation secondary to immune cell infiltration.

Genetics
- Family history in 5–10% in population surveys and 20–30% in referral-based studies
- 50–60% concordance rate in identical twin studies
- Associations with interleukin 23/Th17 pathway, interleukin 10, and interferon gamma genes

RISK FACTORS
- Better sanitation, indoor work environments, and fatty foods increase risk.
- NSAID use >15 days per month associated with increased risk
- Appendectomy protects against late disease onset.
- Negative association with smoking: Relative risk of smokers is 40% of nonsmokers.

GENERAL PREVENTION
- Increased risk for colon cancer w/o colectomy
- Aspirin (≥300 mg/day) and ursodeoxycholic acid (10 mg/kg/day) are preventive.

Pediatric Considerations
- Breastfeeding may protect against pediatric inflammatory bowel disease (IBD).
- More likely pancolonic at onset and shorter time from diagnosis to colectomy (median 11.1 years)

COMMONLY ASSOCIATED CONDITIONS
- Extracolonic manifestations in 10–15%
- Arthritides, including large joint arthritis, sacroiliitis, and ankylosing spondylitis
- Pyoderma gangrenosum
- Episcleritis and uveitis
- Asymptomatic fatty liver (common)
- Primary sclerosing cholangitis: 1–4%
- Cirrhosis of liver: 1–5%
- Bile duct carcinoma
- Thromboembolic disease: 1–6%

DIAGNOSIS

HISTORY
- Bloody diarrhea; tenesmus; abdominal pain; rectal urgency, occasional fecal incontinence; weight loss; arthralgias
- Grading: Mild (rectal bleeding with <4 bowel movements/day); Moderate (rectal bleeding with >4 bowel movements/day); Severe (rectal bleeding with >4 bowel movements/day and systemically ill [albumin <30g/L])

PHYSICAL EXAM
- Arthralgias and arthritis: 15–40%
- Spondylitis: 3–6%
- Ocular: 4–10%; includes uveitis, cataracts, keratopathy, and central serous retinopathy
- Dermatologic: erythema nodosum, pyoderma gangrenosum
- Pulmonary: pleuritis
- Aphthous ulcers of mouth: 5–10%

DIFFERENTIAL DIAGNOSIS
- Hemorrhoids, neoplasms, colonic diverticula, arteriovenous malformation, Crohn disease
- Infectious diarrhea, including bacterial (enterotoxigenic *Escherichia coli*), *Clostridium difficile* colitis, and parasitic (*Entamoeba histolytica*)
- Herpes simplex, *Chlamydia trachomatis*, *Cryptosporidium*, *Isospora belli*, cytomegalovirus
- Radiation proctitis; ischemic colitis

DIAGNOSTIC TESTS & INTERPRETATION
- Anemia (chronic disease ± iron deficiency)
- Leukocytosis during exacerbation
- Elevated ESR and CRP
- Electrolyte abnormalities, especially hypokalemia
- Hypoalbuminemia, elevated LFTs
- Perinuclear antineutrophil cytoplasmic antibody (pANCA) is elevated in 60–70% of cases, also found in 40% of patients with Crohn disease. Sensitivity 33%, specificity 97%

Initial Tests (lab, imaging)
- Plain abdominal films
  - Obtain immediately if significant abdominal tenderness, fever, and leukocytosis for early diagnosis of toxic megacolon and perforation.
- Upper GI series with small bowel follow-through to rule out Crohn disease.
- Ultrasound, MRI, scintigraphy, and CT may have similar accuracy in diagnosis of IBD (1)[A].
- Stool culture and stool testing for parasites to rule out infectious colitis (2)[C]
- *C. difficile* antigen if recent antibiotics

Diagnostic Procedures/Other
- Sigmoidoscopy (may include biopsy) is often sufficient to make initial diagnosis.
- Colonoscopy (may include biopsy)
  - Evaluate premalignant features; differentiate from Crohn disease; investigate stricture/mass; define extent and location of disease.
- Full colonoscopy contraindicated in severe, active disease/colonic dilatation (risk of perforation)

Test Interpretation
Inflammation of the colonic mucosa with ulcerations:
- Ulcerations are hyperemic and hemorrhagic.
- Mucosal separation, distortion, and atrophy of the crypts on histology (2)[C]

- Extends proximally, without skips
- May affect terminal ileum, so-called backwash ileitis

TREATMENT

Management involves acute treatment of inflammatory symptoms, followed by maintenance of remission; therapeutic approach is determined by symptom severity and the extent of colonic involvement.

- 5-aminosalicylic acid (5-ASA) is effective for inducing remission in mild to moderate disease (NNT = 6) and preventing relapse in quiescent disease (NNT = 4) (3)[A]:
  - Topical mesalamine is superior to oral aminosalicylates and topical steroids for proctitis (3)[A].
  - Combination of oral and topical aminosalicylates is more effective than either alone.
- Corticosteroid therapies are effective for inducing remission in active disease (NNT = 3) (3)[A].
- Azathioprine or 6-mercaptopurine (6-MP) reduce relapse in patients with quiescent disease (NNT = 4) (3)[A].
- Maintenance of remission in mild to moderate distal disease with the following: mesalamine suppositories for proctitis or enemas for distal colitis, sulfasalazine, balsalazide, or combination oral and topical mesalamine (3)[A]
- Maintain remission in mild to moderate extensive disease with sulfasalazine, olsalazine, mesalamine, and balsalazide (3)[A].
- Infliximab is effective at inducing remission in ambulatory patients with moderate to severely active disease (NNT = 4) (3)[A].

GENERAL MEASURES
Control inflammation, prevent complications, and replace nutritional losses and blood volume.

MEDICATION

First Line
- Sulfasalazine
  - Uncoated tablets. Adults: initial: 1 g PO q6–8h; maintenance: 500 mg PO q6h; children ≥6 years: initial: 40 to 60 mg/kg/day PO in 3 to 6 divided doses; maintenance: 30 mg/kg/day PO divided q6h (max 2 g/day)
  - Enteric-coated tablets. Adults: initial: 3 to 4 g/day PO in divided doses q6–8h; maintenance: 2 g/day PO in divided doses; children ≥6 years: initial: 40 to 60 mg/kg/day PO in 3 to 6 divided doses; maintenance: 30 mg/kg/day PO in 4 divided doses (max 2 g/day)
- Mesalamine
  - Oral delayed-release tablets (Asacol HD) to induce remission; adults: 800 mg PO TID for 6 weeks
  - Oral controlled-release tablets (Pentasa) for maintenance of remission; adults: 1 g PO QID
  - Single daily dose available for mesalamine (Lialda; acute therapy 4.8 g once daily or 2.4 g once daily for maintenance) and (Apriso; 1.5 g once daily; approved in the United States ONLY for maintenance)
  - Once daily dosing is as effective as conventional TID dosing for mild to moderately active UC treatment and to maintain remission (4)[A]
- 5-ASA (e.g., mesalamine) enemas and suppositories to treat proctitis/proctosigmoiditis:
  - Suppositories: (Canasa) adults: 1,000 mg per rectum at bedtime for 3 to 6 weeks

- Enemas: adults: 4 g per rectum, retained for 8 hours each night; use for 3 to 6 weeks or until remission is achieved.
- Balsalazide: adults: 2.25 g PO TID for total daily dose of 6.75 g for 8 to 12 weeks; children/adolescents: 2.25 g PO TID for total daily dose of 6.75 g or 750 mg PO TID for total daily dose of 2.25 g for 8 weeks
- Olsalazine: adults: 500 mg PO BID (up to 3 g/day); children >2 years old: 30 mg/kg/day in 2 divided doses (up to 2 g/day), primarily used for maintenance

Second Line
- Prednisone for severe exacerbations: adult dosage: initial: 40 to 60 mg/day PO (max 1 mg/kg/day) for 7 to 10 days; taper over 2 to 3 months; can be given IV in hospitalized patients
- Infliximab is effective in patients whose disease is refractory to conventional treatment (3,5)[A]:
  - Adult dose: 5 mg/kg IV at weeks 0, 2, and 6 for induction, then maintenance of 5 mg/kg IV is given every 8 weeks
- Adalimumab: for moderate to severe ulcerative colitis refractory to steroids and azathioprine/6-MP. Initial dose: 160 mg SC (given as four injections on day one or two injections daily over 2 consecutive days; limit injections to 40 mg per injection); 2nd dose 2 weeks later: 80 mg, and maintenance: 40 mg every other week thereafter; should only be continued if evidence of remission by 8 weeks (5)

Pediatric Considerations
- Infliximab can increase the risk of cancer in children; weigh risks versus benefits.
- Immunomodulators can be used in children unresponsive to steroids and aminosalicylates or who cannot be weaned from high-dose steroids:
  - Daily abdominal plain films until improvement
  - If dilatation of colon increases or treatment has failed to attain reversal in 72 hours, surgical consultation for emergency colectomy is indicated.

SURGERY/OTHER PROCEDURES
- Indicated for medically refractory disease (particularly with high-dose steroids)
- May be emergent for massive hemorrhage, perforation, and toxic dilatation of the colon. The emergency surgery of choice is total or subtotal abdominal colectomy with end ileostomy.
- Surgery is also indicated for cancer/multisite mucosal dysplasia.
- Total colectomy with ileostomy is *curative*.
- Total proctocolectomy with ileal pouch anal anastomosis (IPAA) is the most common surgery and an appropriate alternative to ileostomy. Common complications include pouchitis (50%) and need for reoperation in up to 30% (2)[C].
- Regular proctoscopic surveillance is required if a colonic mucosal cuff is retained.

COMPLEMENTARY & ALTERNATIVE MEDICINE
- Insufficient evidence supports the efficacy of probiotics for maintaining remission (6)[A].
- Encouraging results in limited studies for aloe vera gel, wheat grass juice, *Andrographis paniculata* extract (HMPL-004), topical Xilei-san, curcumin, *Boswellia serrata* gum resin, *Plantago ovata* seeds, evening primrose oil, wormwood, and *Tripterygium wilfordii* (7)[A]
- Fecal microbiota transplant associated with nonsignificant increase in remission rate (8)[B].

INPATIENT CONSIDERATIONS
Admission Criteria/Initial Stabilization
- Obtain imaging studies to assess disease activity.
- Initiate IV corticosteroids and rule out infectious etiologies (*C. difficile*, cytomegalovirus, shigella/amoeba).

 ONGOING CARE

FOLLOW-UP RECOMMENDATIONS
Patient Monitoring
- Surveillance colonoscopy. Recommendations vary. Most begin a surveillance program after 8 years of disease with involvement beyond the splenic flexure with colonoscopy every 1 to 2 years including multiple random biopsies or targeted biopsies using chromoendoscopy.
- Initiate annual surveillance immediately in patients with primary sclerosing cholangitis.
- Magnification chromoendoscopy may detect significantly more intraepithelial neoplasias than conventional colonoscopy.
- Nonadenomatous dysplastic lesions or masses are associated with cancer in 33–83% of cases and warrant total colectomy.
- Annual LFTs and cholangiography for cholestasis
- Annual BUN/creatinine for patients on long-term mesalamine

Pediatric Considerations
Cancer surveillance is important because cumulative risk of cancer increases with duration of disease.

DIET
- NPO during acute exacerbations
- Lactose-free diet is often recommended.
- Omega-3 fatty acids, seal and cod liver oil, dietary lactulose, wheat grass juice, vitamin D, and diets with decreased meat and alcohol have been recommended to reduce relapses and improve systemic symptoms (inconsistent evidence) (7)[A].

PATIENT EDUCATION
- Adherence to drug therapy is important to induce and maintain remission.
- Crohn and Colitis Foundation of America (CCFA): http://www.ccfa.org/

PROGNOSIS
- Variable; mortality for initial attack is ~5%; 75–85% experience relapse; up to 20% require colectomy.
- Colon cancer risk is the single most important factor affecting long-term prognosis.
- Primary sclerosing cholangitis increases the risk of colon cancer in patients with ulcerative colitis.
- Left-sided colitis and ulcerative proctitis have favorable prognoses with probable normal lifespan.

Geriatric Considerations
- Increased mortality if first presentation occurs after 60 years of age.
- Consider lower medication dosages and slower titration due to risks of polypharmacy.

COMPLICATIONS
Perforation (2–3% of hospitalized patients); obstruction; hemorrhage; fulminant colitis; toxic megacolon; liver disease; stricture formation (<Crohn disease); colon cancer

REFERENCES
1. Horsthuis K, Bipat S, Bennink RJ, et al. Inflammatory bowel disease diagnosed with US, MR, scintigraphy, and CT: meta-analysis of prospective studies. *Radiology.* 2008;247(1):64–79.
2. Kornbluth A, Sachar DB. Ulcerative colitis practice guidelines in adults: American College of Gastroenterology, Practice Parameters Committee. *Am J Gastroenterol.* 2010;105(3):501–523.
3. Talley NJ, Abreu MT, Achkar JP, et al. An evidence-based systematic review on medical therapies for inflammatory bowel disease. *Am J Gastroenterol.* 2011;106(Suppl 1):S2–S25.
4. Feagan BG, MacDonald JK. Once daily oral mesalamine compared to conventional dosing for induction and maintenance of remission in ulcerative colitis: a systematic review and meta-analysis. *Inflamm Bowel Dis.* 2012;18(9):1785–1794.
5. Sandborn WJ, van Assche G, Reinisch W, et al. Adalimumab induces and maintains clinical remission in patients with moderate-to-severe ulcerative colitis. *Gastroenterology.* 2012;142(2):257.e3–265.e3.
6. Jonkers D, Penders J, Masclee A, et al. Probiotics in the management of inflammatory bowel disease: a systematic review of intervention studies in adult patients. *Drugs.* 2012;72(6):803–823.
7. Ng SC, Lam YT, Tsoi KK, et al. Systematic review: the efficacy of herbal therapy in inflammatory bowel disease. *Aliment Pharmacol Ther.* 2013;38(8):854–863.
8. Moayyedi P, Surette MG, Kim PT, et al. Fecal microbiota transplantation induces remission in patients with active ulcerative colitis in a randomized controlled trial. *Gastroenterology.* 2015;149(1):102.e6–109.e6.

ADDITIONAL READING
- Huang X, Lv B, Jin HF, et al. A meta-analysis of the therapeutic effects of tumor necrosis factor-α blockers on ulcerative colitis. *Eur J Clin Pharmacol.* 2011;67(8):759–766.
- Racine A, Cuerq A, Bijon A, et al. Isotretinoin and risk of inflammatory bowel disease: A French nationwide study. *Am J Gastroenterol.* 2014;109(4):563–569.

 SEE ALSO

Algorithm: Hematemesis (Bleeding, Upper Gastrointestinal)

 CODES

ICD10
- K51.90 Ulcerative colitis, unspecified, without complications
- K51.919 Ulcerative colitis, unspecified with unspecified complications
- K51.80 Other ulcerative colitis without complications

CLINICAL PEARLS
- UC always involves the colon and has continuous areas of inflammation with shallow mucosal ulcerations, and crypt granulomas are not seen on biopsy (differentiating features from Crohn colitis).
- Treat proctitis with 5-ASA suppositories.
- Colectomy is curative.
- Routine surveillance colonoscopy is recommended every 1 to 2 years after patients have had UC for 8 years.

U

UPPER RESPIRATORY INFECTION (URI)

Lisa M. Schroeder, MD • Vu D. Tran, MD

BASICS

Upper respiratory infections (URIs) are one of the most common medical diagnoses, contributing to ~30 million office visits annually and resulting in significant lost productivity through missed days from work/school.

DESCRIPTION
- Inflammation of nasal passages resulting from infection with multiple respiratory viruses
- Most cases are mild to moderate in severity, self-limited, and amenable to self-treat.
- System(s) affected: ENT; pulmonary

EPIDEMIOLOGY
- Each virus has different seasonal peaks (e.g., rhinovirus: late spring, fall); most infections occur during the winter months.
- Symptoms usually peak in 1 to 3 days and can last up to 2 weeks.
- Transmission:
  - Contact with contaminated skin/surface followed by contact with mucous membranes (hand-to-face contact)
  - Aerosolized particles from sneezing and coughing
- Viruses may last up to 2 hours on skin and even longer on environmental surfaces.

Incidence
- Predominant age: children > adults
  - Preschool children: 5 to 7 URI/year
  - Kindergarten: 12 URI/year
  - Schoolchildren: 7 URI/year
  - Adolescents/adults: 2 to 3 URI/year
- Predominant sex: male = female

ETIOLOGY AND PATHOPHYSIOLOGY
Rhinoviruses infect the ciliated epithelial mucosa of the upper airway, resulting in edema, hyperemia, and mucous production.
- Histology: edema of subepithelial connective tissue and a scanty cellular infiltrate containing neutrophils, plasma cells, lymphocytes, and eosinophils with exudation of serous and mucinous fluid
- Rhinovirus causes a "nondestructive" inflammation of the mucous membranes.
- Influenza and parainfluenza viruses denude respiratory epithelium to the basement membrane.
- Several hundred viral strains from different families; spread within geographic region and groups with close contact
  - Rhinovirus (>100 serotypes): 30–50%; incubation period 1 to 5 days
  - Influenza virus types A, B, C: 10–15%; incubation period 1 to 4 days
  - Coronaviruses: 10–15%
  - Parainfluenza, respiratory syncytial virus (RSV): 5%; more common in children; incubation period 1 week
  - Enteroviruses, adenoviruses: <10%
- In many cases, no specific pathogen is identified.

RISK FACTORS
- Exposure to infected people
- Touching one's face with contaminated fingers
- Allergic disorders
- Smoking
- Immunosuppression
- Stress

GENERAL PREVENTION
- Frequent hand washing, especially in children (1,2)[A]
- Limiting exposure to infected persons/children
- Probiotic milk (with live culture lactobacillus) may reduce respiratory infections in children age <7 (3)[A].

COMMONLY ASSOCIATED CONDITIONS
- Pharyngitis
- Sinusitis
- Otitis media
- Bronchitis
- Bronchiolitis
- Pneumonia
- Croup
- Asthma

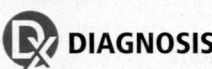

DIAGNOSIS

HISTORY
- Nasal congestion: 80–100%
- Sneezing: 50–70%
- Throat irritation: 50%
- Cough: 40%
- Hoarseness: 30%
- Malaise: 20–25%
- Headache: 25%
- Fever >100°F (37.7°C): 0–1%

PHYSICAL EXAM
- Low-grade temperature; mild tachycardia common with fever; tachypnea if significant respiratory involvement
- Rhinorrhea (clear, yellow, or green)
- Mucosal edema and/or inflammation
- Postnasal drainage
- Pharyngeal erythema
- Dull tympanic membranes

DIFFERENTIAL DIAGNOSIS
- Allergic rhinitis
- Acute sinusitis
- Strep pharyngitis
- Epiglottitis
- Infectious mononucleosis
- Pneumonia
- Influenza
- Pertussis
- Otitis media

DIAGNOSTIC TESTS & INTERPRETATION

Initial Tests (lab, imaging)
- No routine lab testing is typically needed, as diagnosis is based on clinical findings.
- In cases of pharyngitis, rapid streptococcal antigen testing with reflex culture can be used to rule out group A streptococcal infection if clinically suspected.
- Rapid influenza antigen testing if influenza is suspected.
- Heterophile antibody testing if infectious mononucleosis is suspected.
- Imaging not routinely indicated

Follow-Up Tests & Special Considerations
Patients should consider contacting a physician's office for fever >101°F associated with systemic symptoms, difficulty breathing, or purulent drainage >2 days.

TREATMENT

GENERAL MEASURES
- Smoking cessation
- Vaporizer/humidifier: no consistent benefit proven
- Cold preparations do not change course
- Antibiotics not indicated
- Avoid cough and cold preparations under age of 2 years.

MEDICATION
Most cases of URI resolve spontaneously without specific intervention. Treatment is symptom-driven and for patient comfort.

First Line
- Saline nasal irrigation is safe for adults and children.
- *Antibiotics are not recommended. They produce minimal to no reduction in symptoms or duration, with greater risk of side effects from usage (4)[A].*
- Analgesics: acetaminophen, and NSAIDs for relieving aches and pains associated with URI (5,6)[A]

Second Line
- Many mouthwashes, gargles, and lozenges are promoted to relieve the pain of sore throat. The demulcent effects of hard candy, gargling with warm saline, and products with anesthetics (benzocaine/phenol) may provide pain relief.
- Aromatic oils (menthol, camphor, eucalyptus), produce a sensation of increased airflow without a significant change in airflow resistance.
- Topical decongestants (sympathomimetics) reduce nasal mucosa swelling and airflow resistance and promote drainage. Sprays preferred over drops in patients >6 years of age:
  - *Limit use to 3 days*, as rebound congestion may occur after 72 hours of use with resultant rhinitis medicamentosa.
    - Oxymetazoline
      - Adults and children aged 6 to 12 years: 0.05% solution, 2 to 3 sprays in each nostril BID

- Oral decongestants (sympathomimetic) have some advantages over topical decongestants: longer duration of action, lack of local irritation, and no risk of rebound congestion (7)[B].
  - Pseudoephedrine: potential for abuse/misuse or diversion for methamphetamine production
  - Use with caution for patients with cardiovascular disease, HTN, and BPH:
    ○ Adults: 60 mg q4–6h (120 mg sustained-release q12h) superior to placebo in short-term use (7)
    ○ Children aged 6 to 12 years: 30 mg q4 to 6h; 2 to 5 years: 15 mg q4 to 6h
- Acute cough, postnasal drip, and throat clearing associated with the common cold can be treated with a first-generation antihistamine/decongestant preparation (brompheniramine and sustained-release pseudoephedrine) (8)[A].
- Antihistamines: minimal benefit when used as monotherapy. Only first-generation (sedating) antihistamines show any symptomatic relief, but sedation may be worse than relief (9)[B]:
  - Chlorpheniramine
    ○ Adults: 4 mg QID, 8 mg TID, 12 mg BID
    ○ Children age 6 to 12 years: 2 mg q4–6h
  - Diphenhydramine
    ○ Adults: 25 to 50 mg q4–6h PRN
    ○ Children age 6 to 12 years 12.5 to 25 mg q4–6h PRN

Pediatric Considerations
In 2007, the FDA issued a warning to limit the use of all cough and cold preparations for children age ≤2 years due to risk of overdose (10,11)[A].

COMPLEMENTARY & ALTERNATIVE MEDICINE
- Zinc prevents viral replication in vitro:
  - Avoid intranasal preparations of zinc: risk of potential permanent loss of smell (12)[C]
  - Has shown moderate benefit in reducing symptoms and duration, but proper dosing has not been determined
- Echinacea has not proven consistently effective for treatment of common cold symptoms (12)[C].
- Probiotics may decrease severity and duration of URIs and possibly reduce episodes (3,13)[B].
- Vitamin C (ascorbic acid) (14)[C]
  - Regular supplementation trials have shown that vitamin C may reduce the duration of colds.
  - Vitamin C prophylaxis *not* recommended for general use but may be beneficial in those exposed to severe physical exertion and cold environments.

Geriatric Considerations
Cold medications, especially decongestants and antihistamines, commonly produce adverse effects in older patients and should not be used routinely.

Pregnancy Considerations
- Decongestants: Most are Category B or C.
- Antihistamines: Most are Category B or C.

 ONGOING CARE

FOLLOW-UP RECOMMENDATIONS
Contact a physician's office for prolonged fever, difficulty breathing, or concern for secondary complications.

DIET
Encourage fluids and adequate hydration.

PATIENT EDUCATION
- Discuss the difference between viral and bacterial infections; instruct about appropriate antibiotic use.
- Good hand hygiene
- Symptomatic treatment; no cure
- Reinfection is possible with reexposure.
- Patient information: www.niaid.nih.gov/factsheets/cold.htm

PROGNOSIS
- Excellent; expect full recovery. Usual duration 5 to 7 days but may last up to 2 weeks. For smokers, 3 to 4 additional days
- Cough may persist after other symptoms have resolved.

COMPLICATIONS
Small percentage may develop worsening symptoms leading to secondary otitis media, sinusitis, bronchitis, or pneumonia.

REFERENCES

1. Centers for Disease Control and Prevention. http://www.cdc.gov/getsmart/community/materials-references/index.html.
2. Jefferson T, Del Mar CB, Dooley L, et al. Physical interventions to interrupt or reduce the spread of respiratory viruses. *Cochrane Database Syst Rev.* 2011;(7):CD006207.
3. Hatakka K, Savilahti E, Pönkä A, et al. Effect of long term consumption of probiotc milk on infections in children attending day care centres: double blind, randomised trial. *BMJ.* 2001;322(7298):1327.
4. Kenealy T, Arroll B. Antibiotics for the common cold and acute purulent rhinitis. *Cochrane Database Syst Rev.* 2013;(6):CD000247.
5. Li S, Yue J, Dong BR, et al. Acetaminophen (paracetamol) for the common cold in adults. *Cochrane Database Syst Rev.* 2013;(7):CD008800.
6. Kim SY, Chang YJ, Cho HM, et al. Non-steroidal anti-inflammatory drugs for the common cold. *Cochrane Database Syst Rev.* 2013;(6):CD006362.
7. Horak F, Zieglmayer P, Zieglmayer R, et al. A placebo-controlled study of the nasal decongestant effect of phenylephrine and pseudoephedrine in the Vienna Challenge Chamber. *Ann Allergy Asthma Immunol.* 2009;102(2):116–120.
8. Pratter MR. Cough and the common cold: ACCP evidence-based clinical practice guidelines. *Chest.* 2006;129(1)(Suppl):72S–74S.
9. Sutter AI, Lemiengre M, Campbell H, et al. Antihistamines for the common cold. *Cochrane Database Syst Rev.* 2003;(3):CD001267.
10. Centers for Disease Control and Prevention. Infant deaths associated with cough and cold medications—two states, 2005. *MMWR Morb Mortal Wkly Rep.* 2007;56(1):1–4.
11. Singh M, Das RR. Zinc for the common cold. *Cochrane Database Syst Rev.* 2013;(6):CD001364.
12. Linde K, Barrett B, Wölkart K, et al. Echinacea for preventing and treating the common cold. *Cochrane Database Syst Rev.* 2006;(1):CD000530.
13. Hao Q, Lu Z, Dong BR, et al. Probiotics for preventing acute upper respiratory tract infections. *Cochrane Database Syst Rev.* 2011;(9):CD006895.
14. Hemilä H, Chalker E. Vitamin C for preventing and treating the common cold. *Cochrane Database Syst Rev.* 2013;(1):CD000980.

ADDITIONAL READING

Wald ER, Applegate KE, Bordley C, et al. Clinical practice guideline for the diagnosis and management of acute bacterial sinusitis in children aged 1 to 18 years. *Pediatrics.* 2013;132(1):e262–e280.

 SEE ALSO

Bronchitis, Acute; Pharyngitis; Rhinitis, Allergic

 CODES

ICD10
- J06.9 Acute upper respiratory infection, unspecified
- J11.1 Influenza due to unidentified influenza virus with other respiratory manifestations
- B97.4 Respiratory syncytial virus causing diseases classd elswhr

CLINICAL PEARLS

- Supportive therapy is mainstay for most upper respiratory tract infections.
- Point of care testing can rule out group A *Streptococcus* infection in the appropriate clinical setting
- Limit unnecessary use of antibiotics.
- URI symptoms last 3 to 4 more days in smokers.

U

URETHRITIS

Maria Harsha Wusu, MD, MSEd • Joanne Wilkinson, MD, MSc

 BASICS

DESCRIPTION
- Inflammation of the urethra
- Common manifestation of sexually transmitted infection
- Frequently associated with dysuria, pruritus, and/or urethral discharge; classified as gonococcal (caused by *Neisseria gonorrhoeae*) and nongono-coccal (caused by other bacteria, or less commonly autoimmune disorders [Reiter syndrome], trauma, or chemical irritation)

EPIDEMIOLOGY
Incidence
- In 2013, there were >330,000 reported cases of gonorrhea, with a rate of 106.1 cases per 100,000 population (0.6% decrease since 2012) (1)
- In 2013, there were >1.4 million reported cases of *Chlamydia trachomatis* infection, or 446.6 cases per 100,000 population (1.5% decrease since 2012) (2)
- Rate of chlamydial infection in U.S. women was more than twice that of men, reflecting higher rates of screening (1).
- Highest incidences of gonorrhea and chlamydia among young men and women, ages 15 to 24 years (1)

ETIOLOGY AND PATHOPHYSIOLOGY
- Most common cause is infection via sexual transmission of *N. gonorrhoeae*, a gram-negative diplococcus.
- *N. gonorrhoeae* interacts with nonciliated epithelial cells→ cellular invasion→ inflammation, neutrophil production, bacterial cell phagocytosis (2)
- Sexually transmitted *C. trachomatis* infection is the most common cause of nongonococcal urethritis.
- Other established pathogens
  - *Mycoplasma genitalium*
  - *Trichomonas vaginalis*
  - *Ureaplasma urealyticum*
  - Herpes simplex virus (rare)
  - Adenovirus (rare)
- Noninfectious causes (generally rare)
  - Chemical irritants (i.e., soaps, shampoos, douches, spermicides)
  - Foreign bodies
  - Urethral instrumentation

RISK FACTORS
- One or more sex partner(s)
- New sex partner
- History of or coexisting STI
- Sex partner with concurrent partner(s)
- Inconsistent condom use outside of a mutually monogamous relationship
- Exchanging sex for money or drugs
- Member of population with increased prevalence of infection, including incarcerated populations, military recruits, black and Hispanic persons

GENERAL PREVENTION
- Use of male condoms, female condoms, or cervical diaphragms
- Abstinence or reduction in the number of sex partners
- Behavioral counseling

COMMONLY ASSOCIATED CONDITIONS
ALERT
Annual chlamydia and gonorrhea screening is recommended for all sexually active women <25 years, women >25 years with risk factors, and all men who have sex with men (3).

DIAGNOSIS

- Chief complaint
  - Urethral discharge (mucopurulent suggestive of *N. gonorrhoeae*)
  - Dysuria
  - Erythema of the urethral meatus
  - Symptom onset 2 to 8 days following exposure
- History
  - Sexual history, including condom use, number of partners, sexual behaviors
  - Previous STIs
  - Substance abuse
  - Recent travel
  - Symptoms indicative of complications or additional sites of infection (i.e., men: testicular pain and swelling, anal itching, rectal pain or bleeding; women: lower abdominal pain, dyspareunia, irregular vaginal bleeding)
- Male GU exam (possible findings)
  - Urethral discharge
  - Meatal erythema
  - Testicular tenderness
  - Palpate scrotum to check for epididymitis or orchitis.
  - Check for ulcers.
  - Check for inguinal lymphadenopathy.
- Female GU exam (possible findings)
  - Vaginal discharge
  - Endocervical discharge, hyperemia, and/or friability

Pediatric Considerations
Pediatric infections with gonorrhea and chlamydia after the neonatal period strongly suggest sexual contact. If indicated, investigations should be initiated promptly (3).

DIFFERENTIAL DIAGNOSIS
- Other genitourinary tract diseases
  - Cystitis/urinary tract infection
  - Epididymitis
  - Prostatitis
  - PID
  - Pyelonephritis
- Vaginal atrophy, especially in postmenopausal women
- Stevens-Johnson syndrome
- Reiter syndrome: uveitis, urethritis, arthritis
- Wegener granulomatosis

DIAGNOSTIC TESTS & INTERPRETATION
ALERT
Health care providers are required to report all gonorrhea and chlamydia infections in accordance with local and state requirements.

Initial Tests (lab, imaging)
- Gram-stain diagnosis of urethritis if: urethral secretions with ≥2 WBC per oil immersion field, mucopurulent or purulent discharge, or first void urine sediment with ≥10 WBC per high-power field (hpf) (3)
- Gonorrhea
  - Nucleic acid amplification test (NAAT): in men: first void urine preferred (90–100% sensitivity, 97–100% specificity for gonorrhea); in women: vaginal swab preferred (patient or clinician collected), end cervical swab acceptable, first void urine may detect 10% fewer infections (3)[A]
  - Culture: traditional gold standard—most commonly used in cases of suspected treatment resistance (3)
- Chlamydia
  - NAAT: in men: first catch urine equal to urethral swab (85–95% sensitivity, 93–99% specificity); in women: vaginal swab preferred (patient or clinician collected), end cervical swab acceptable, first void urine may detect 10% fewer infections (3)[A]
  - Tissue cultures: traditional gold standard, but currently NOT recommended (3)
  - If concern for trichomonas: NAAT (urine, urethral, vaginal, or endocervical swab), wet mount, or culture
  - There is no FDA-approved diagnostic test available for *M. genitalium*.

ALERT
Due to the similarity in clinical symptoms and high rates of coinfection, cotesting for gonorrhea and chlamydia infection is recommended. In addition, given that risk factors for gonorrhea and chlamydia indicate risks for other STIs, screening for HIV, RPR, Hepatitis C, and Hepatitis B may also be indicated.

Follow-Up Tests & Special Considerations
- Test of cure for chlamydia and gonorrhea is recommended in pregnant women or when treatment noncompliance is suspected (3).
- Repeat testing in 3 months recommended due to rates of reinfection (3)
- HIV infection: Persons with HIV infection should receive the same treatment as patients without HIV infection (3).

Diagnostic Procedures/Other
Urethrocystoscopy for cases with suspected foreign body, intraurethral warts, urethral stricture

Test Interpretation
Urethral strictures (untreated gonorrhea), intraurethral lesions (venereal warts, congenital anomalies), PID, or tubo-ovarian abscesses are possible.

URINARY TRACT INFECTION (UTI) IN FEMALES

TREATMENT

GENERAL MEASURES
- Most cases can be treated in the outpatient setting.
- Single-dose regimens with direct observation preferred (3)

MEDICATION

First Line
- Gonorrhea
  - Ceftriaxone 250 mg IM plus either: azithromycin 1 g PO × 1 dose (preferred) *OR* doxycycline 100 mg PO BID for 7 days (if azithromycin allergy) (3)[A]
  - For children ≤45 kg: ceftriaxone 25 to 50 mg/kg (max 125 mg) IM × 1 dose. For children >45 kg: use adult dosing.
- Chlamydia
  - Azithromycin: 1 g PO × 1 dose *OR*
  - Doxycycline: 100 mg PO BID for 7 days (3)[A]
  - Alternative regimens (all for 7 days): erythromycin base 500 mg PO QID, erythromycin ethylsuccinate 800 mg PO QID, levofloxacin 500 mg daily, *OR* ofloxacin 300 mg PO BID
- Trichomonas
  - Metronidazole: 2 g PO × 1 dose
- Recurrent and resistant urethritis
  - Metronidazole: 2 mg PO single dose *OR* tinidazole 2 g PO single dose plus azithromycin 1 g PO × 1 dose
- Contraindications: sensitivity to any of the indicated medications
- Precautions: Patients taking tetracyclines may have increased photosensitivity.
- Significant possible interactions
  - Tetracyclines should not be taken with milk products or antacids.
  - Oral contraceptives may be rendered less effective by oral antibiotics. Patients and partners should use a back-up method of birth control for the remainder of the cycle.

Pregnancy Considerations
- Chlamydia: All pregnant women <25 years and older women at increased risk should be screened for chlamydia at their first prenatal visit and again in the 3rd trimester. Women with chlamydia infections should be treated, have a documented TOC 3 to 4 weeks after treatment, and retested in 3 months (3).
- Gonorrhea: All pregnant women under <25 years and older women at increased risk should be screened for gonorrhea at their first prenatal visit and again in the third trimester. Women with gonorrhea infections should be treated and be retested in 3 months (3).
- Tetracyclines and quinolones are contraindicated.
- Avoid erythromycin estolate because of an increased risk of cholestatic jaundice.
- Single-dose therapy is recommended.

Second Line
- Gonorrhea: If ceftriaxone is not an option, cefixime 400 mg PO × 1 dose plus either: azithromycin 1 g PO × 1 dose OR doxycycline 100 mg PO BID for 7 days (if azithromycin allergy); followed by a TOC in 1 week (3).

- Chlamydia alternative regimens (all for 7 days): erythromycin base 500 mg PO QID, erythromycin ethylsuccinate 800 mg PO QID, levofloxacin 500 mg daily, OR ofloxacin 300 mg PO BID (3)

ONGOING CARE

FOLLOW-UP RECOMMENDATIONS
- Sexual activity should be avoided for 7 days following administration of single-dose therapy or until completion of multiday regimen.
- All sexual partners who came in contact with the patient within 60 days should be referred for evaluation, testing, and presumptive treatment (3).
- Expedited partner therapy (EPT) is an acceptable alternative. EPT—the practice of treating the diagnosed patient's sex partner(s) for chlamydia or gonorrhea by providing medications or prescriptions to the patient to provide to the partner(s) without clinical evaluation (3).

Patient Monitoring
- Instruct patients to return if symptoms persist or recur after completing treatment.
- Test of cure in 3 to 4 weeks in pregnant women suspected of nonadherence, reinfection, persistent symptoms
- Screen for reinfection in all patients at 3 months.

DIET
Avoid alcohol when taking metronidazole.

PATIENT EDUCATION
- Behavioral counseling interventions are recommended. Evidence of benefit increase with intensity of intervention (4).
- Successful approaches include basic information about STIs and transmission, assess risk for transmission, include training skills (i.e., condom use, communication about safe sex, problem solving, goal setting) (4).

PROGNOSIS
If the diagnosis is firmly established, appropriate medications are prescribed and the patient is compliant with treatment; relief of symptoms occurs within days and the problem will resolve without squeal.

COMPLICATIONS
- Stricture formation
- Epididymitis
- Prostatitis
- PID in women
- Disseminated gonococcal infection
- Gonococcal meningitis
- Gonococcal endocarditis
- Perinatal transmission (chlamydial conjunctivitis, chlamydial pneumonia, ophthalmia neonatorum)
- Reiter syndrome

REFERENCES

1. Centers for Disease Control and Prevention. *Sexually Transmitted Disease Surveillance, 2013*. Atlanta, GA: U.S. Department of Health and Human Services; 2014.
2. LeFevre ML. Screening for chlamydia and gonorrhea: U.S. Preventive Services Task Force recommendation statement. *Ann Intern Med*. 2014;161(12):902–910.
3. Workowski KA, Bolan GA. Sexually transmitted diseases treatment guidelines, 2015. *MMWR Recomm Rep*. 2015;64(RR-03):1–137.
4. O'Connor EA, Lin JS, Burda BU, et al. Behavioral sexual risk-reduction counseling in primary care to prevent sexually transmitted infections: a systematic review for the U.S. Preventive Services Task Force. *Ann Intern Med*. 2014;161(12):874–883.

ADDITIONAL READING

U.S. Preventive Services Task Force. Final Recommendation Statement. Gonorrhea and Chlamydia. Screening 2014. http://www.uspreventiveservicestaskforce.org/Page/Document/RecommendationStatementFinal/chlamydia-and-gonorrhea-screening. Accessed 2015.

SEE ALSO

- Chlamydia Infection (Sexually Transmitted); Epididymitis; Gonococcal Infections; Pelvic Inflammatory Disease (PID); Prostatitis; Urinary Tract Infection (UTI) in Females; Urinary Tract Infection (UTI) in Males; Vulvovaginitis, Estrogen Deficient; Vulvovaginitis, Prepubescent
- Algorithms: Dysuria; Genital Ulcers; Urethral Discharge

CODES

ICD10
- N34.2 Other urethritis
- A56.01 Chlamydial cystitis and urethritis
- A54.01 Gonococcal cystitis and urethritis, unspecified

CLINICAL PEARLS

- Inflammation of the urethra, frequently associated with dysuria, pruritus, and/or urethral discharge
- Common manifestation of STI
- Classified as gonococcal (caused by *N. gonorrhoeae*) and nongonococcal
- Nucleic acid amplification test (NAAT) preferred method of diagnosis for men and women
- Single-dose regimens with direct observation preferred
- In cases of gonorrhea or chlamydia infection, in person or expedited partner therapy (EPT) recommended for all partners of patients within the last 60 days
- Given that risk factors for gonorrhea and chlamydia indicate risk for other STIs, screening for HIV, RPR, Hepatitis C, and Hepatitis B may also be indicated.
- Repeat testing for gonorrhea and chlamydia in 3 months recommended due to rates of reinfection.
- Special considerations in pediatric and pregnant populations
- Treatment in persons with HIV infection is the same as in patients without HIV infection.
- Health care providers are required to report all gonorrhea and chlamydia infections in accordance with local and state requirements.

URINARY TRACT INFECTION (UTI) IN FEMALES
Akhil Das, MD, FACS

 BASICS

DESCRIPTION
- Urinary tract infection (UTI) is the presence of pathogenic microorganisms within the urinary tract with concomitant symptoms.
- This topic refers primarily to infectious cystitis; other complicated UTIs, such as pyelonephritis, are discussed elsewhere.
- Uncomplicated UTI: occurs in patients who have a normal, unobstructed urinary tract, who have no history of recent instrumentation, and whose symptoms are confined to the lower urinary tract. Uncomplicated UTIs are most common in young, sexually active women.
- Complicated UTI: an infection of the lower or upper urinary tract in the presence of an anatomic abnormality, a functional abnormality, or a urinary catheter
- Recurrent UTI: symptomatic UTIs that follow resolution of an earlier episode, usually after appropriate treatment
  - No single definition of the frequency of recurrent UTI exists, but a pragmatic definition is ≥3 infections per year.
  - Most recurrences are thought to represent reinfection rather than relapse.
  - No evidence indicates that recurrent UTIs lead to health problems such as hypertension or renal disease in the absence of anatomic or functional abnormalities of the urinary tract (1)[A].
- System(s) affected: renal/urologic
- Synonym(s): cystitis; infectious cystitis

EPIDEMIOLOGY
Incidence
- Accounts for 8 million doctor visits and 1 million emergency room visits, and contributes to >100,000 hospital admissions each year
- 11% of women have UTIs in any given year.
- Predominant age: young adults and older
- Predominant sex: female > male

Prevalence
- >50% of females have at least one UTI in their lifetime.
- One in four women have recurrent UTIs.

ETIOLOGY AND PATHOPHYSIOLOGY
- Bacteria and subsequent infection in the urinary tract arise chiefly via ascending bacterial movement and propagation (1).
- Pathogenic organisms (*Escherichia coli*) possess adherence factors and toxins that allow initiation and propagation of genitourinary infections:
  - Type 1 and *P. pili* (*pyelonephritis-associated pili*)
  - Lipopolysaccharide
- Most UTIs are caused by bacteria originating from bowel flora:
  - *E. coli* is the causative organism in 80% of cases of uncomplicated cystitis.
  - *Staphylococcus saprophyticus* accounts for 15% of infections.
  - Enterobacteriaceae (i.e., *Klebsiella, Proteus, Enterobacter,* and *Pseudomonas)* also contribute.
- *Candida* is associated with nosocomial UTI (2).

Genetics
Women with human leukocyte antigen 3 (HLA-3) and nonsecretor Lewis antigen have an increased bacterial adherence, which may lead to an increased risk in UTI.

RISK FACTORS
- Previous UTI
- Diabetes mellitus (DM)
- Pregnancy
- Sexual activity
- Use of spermicides or diaphragm
- Underlying abnormalities of the urinary tract such as tumors, calculi, strictures, incomplete bladder emptying, urinary incontinence, neurogenic bladder
- Catheterization
- Recent antibiotic use
- Poor hygiene
- Estrogen deficiency
- Inadequate fluid intake

GENERAL PREVENTION
- Maintain good hydration.
- Women with frequent or intercourse-related UTI should empty bladder immediately before and following intercourse; consider postcoital antibiotic.
- Avoid feminine hygiene sprays and douches.
- Wipe urethra from front to back.
- Cranberry juice (not cranberry juice cocktail) consumption may prevent recurrent infections.

COMMONLY ASSOCIATED CONDITIONS
See "Risk Factors."

Geriatric Considerations
- Elderly patients are more likely to have underlying urinary tract abnormality.
- Acute UTI may be associated with incontinence or mental status changes in the elderly.

 DIAGNOSIS

HISTORY
Note: Any or all may be present:
- Burning during urination
- Pain during urination (dysuria)
- Urgency (sensation of need to urinate often)
- Frequency
- Sensation of incomplete bladder emptying
- Blood in urine
- Lower abdominal pain or cramping
- Offensive odor of urine
- Nocturia
- Sudden onset of urinary incontinence
- Dyspareunia

PHYSICAL EXAM
- Suprapubic tenderness
- Urethral and/or vaginal tenderness
- Fever or costovertebral angle tenderness indicates upper UTI.

DIFFERENTIAL DIAGNOSIS
- Vaginitis
- Asymptomatic bacteriuria
- STDs causing urethritis or pyuria
- Hematuria from causes other than infection (e.g., neoplasia, calculi)
- Interstitial cystitis
- Psychological dysfunction

DIAGNOSTIC TESTS & INTERPRETATION
Initial Tests (lab, imaging)
- No lab testing is necessary in women with high likelihood of lower UTI based on classic symptoms.
- Urinalysis
  - Pyuria (>10 neutrophils/high-power field [HPF])
  - Bacteriuria (any amount on unspun urine, or 10 bacteria/HPF on centrifuged urine)
  - Hematuria (>5 RBCs/HPF)
- Dipstick urinalysis
  - Leukocyte esterase (75–96% sensitivity, 94–98% specificity, when >100,000 colony-forming units [CFU])
  - Nitrite tests are useful with nitrite-reducing organisms (e.g., enterococci, *S. saprophyticus, Acinetobacter*).
- Urine culture: *only* indicated if diagnosis is unclear or patient has recurrent infections and resistance is suspected. It is neither cost-effective nor usually helpful for lower-tract, uncomplicated UTI.
  - Presence of 100,000 CFU/mL of organism indicates infection.
  - Identification of a single organism at lower CFU per milliliter likely also represents infection in the presence of appropriate symptoms.
  - Suspect a contaminated specimen when culture shows multiple types of bacteria.
- Imaging studies are often not required in most cases of UTI.

Follow-Up Tests & Special Considerations
- In nonpregnant, premenopausal women with symptoms of UTI, positive urinalysis, and no risks for complicated infection, empirical treatment may be given without obtaining a urine culture.
- Dipstick urinalysis may be helpful but not necessary in patients with characteristic symptoms (i.e., high pretest probability).
- Imaging may be indicated for UTIs in men, infants, immunocompromised patients, febrile infection, signs or symptoms of obstruction, failure to respond to appropriate therapy, and in patients with recurrent infections.
- CT scan and MRI provide the most complete anatomic data in adults.

Pediatric Considerations
For infants and children, obtain US; if ureteral dilatation is detected, obtain either voiding cystourethrogram or isotope cystogram to evaluate for reflux.

Diagnostic Procedures/Other
- Urethral catheterization maybe necessary to obtain a urine specimen from children and adults if the voided urine is suspected of being contaminated.
- Suprapubic bladder aspiration or urethral catheterization techniques can be used to obtain specimens from infants.
- Cystourethroscopy can be used for patients with recurrent UTIs and previous anti-incontinence surgery or hematuria (3)[A].

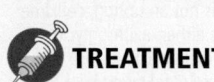 **TREATMENT**

GENERAL MEASURES
- Maintain good hydration.
- Maintain good hygiene.
- 1/4 of women with uncomplicated UTI experience a second UTI within 6 months and 1/2 at some time during their lifetime.

MEDICATION

First Line

- The urinary tract topical analgesic phenazopyridine 100 to 200 mg TID produces rapid relief of symptoms and should be offered to patients with more than minor discomfort; it is available over the counter. This medication is not a substitute for definitive treatment. This medication also may alter urinalysis but not the urine culture.
- Uncomplicated UTI (adolescents and adults who are nonpregnant, nondiabetic, afebrile, immunocompetent, and without genitourinary anatomic abnormalities)
  - Trimethoprim-sulfamethoxazole (TMP-SMZ; Bactrim): 160/800 mg PO BID for 3 days, best where resistance of *E. coli* strains <20%
  - 5-day course of nitrofurantoin or 3-day fluoroquinolone course should be used in patients with allergy to TMP-SMZ and in areas where *E. coli* resistance to TMP-SMZ >20% (3)[A].
  - Fosfomycin (Monurol): 3 g PO single dose (expensive)
- Lower UTI in pregnancy
  - Nitrofurantoin (Macrobid): 100 mg PO BID for 7 days
  - Cephalexin (Keflex): 500 mg PO BID for 7 days
- Postcoital UTI: single-dose TMP-SMX or cephalexin may reduce frequency of UTI in sexually active women.
- Complicated UTI (pregnancy, diabetes, febrile, immunocompromised patient, recurrent UTIs): Extend course to 7 to 10 days of treatment with antibiotic chosen based on culture results; may begin with fluoroquinolone, TMP-SMX, or cephalosporin while awaiting results (avoid using nitrofurantoin for complicated UTI)
  - Fluoroquinolones are not safe during pregnancy and are usually avoided in treatment of children.
  - TMP-SMX use in pregnancy is not desirable (especially in 3rd trimester) but is appropriate in some circumstances (3)[A].

Second Line

- Uncomplicated UTI
  - Ciprofloxacin: 250 mg PO BID for 3 days; should be reserved for complicated UTIs
  - β-Lactams (amoxicillin/clavulanate, cefdinir, cefpodoxime proxetil) for 3 to 7 days
- Chronic UTIs
  - Women with recurrent symptomatic UTIs can be treated with continuous or postcoital prophylactic antibiotics. Treatment duration guided by the severity of patient symptoms and by physician and patient preference: Consider 6 months of therapy, followed by observation for reinfection after discontinuing prophylaxis.
    - Continuous antimicrobial prophylaxis involves daily administration of low-dose TMP-SMX 40/200 mg or nitrofurantoin 50 to 100 mg, among others.
- Another treatment option is self-started antibiotics.

Pediatric Considerations

Long-term antibiotics appear to reduce the risk of recurrent symptomatic UTI in susceptible children, but the benefit is small and must be considered together with the increased risk of microbial resistance.

ISSUES FOR REFERRAL

Men with uncomplicated UTI and most other patients with complicated UTI should be referred to a urologist for evaluation.

Pediatric Considerations

UTI in children, especially <1 year of age, should prompt workup for urinary tract anomalies.

SURGERY/OTHER PROCEDURES

- Urinary tract obstruction with urosepsis requires urgent drainage of the obstructed system.
- Patients with emphysematous pyelonephritis or pyonephrosis may need immediate surgical intervention.

COMPLEMENTARY & ALTERNATIVE MEDICINE

- Preliminary studies indicate that *Vaccinium macrocarpon* (cranberry) juice may help to prevent and treat UTIs by inhibiting bacterial adherence to the bladder epithelium.
- Cranberry juice may decrease the number of symptomatic UTIs over a 1-year period, particularly for women with recurrent UTIs. The optimal dosage or method of administration (e.g., juice, tablets, or capsules) is still unclear.

INPATIENT CONSIDERATIONS

Inpatient evaluation is reserved for patients with complicated or upper tract UTIs. Majority of UTIs are managed in an outpatient setting.

 ## ONGOING CARE

FOLLOW-UP RECOMMENDATIONS

- First or rare UTI: Young or middle-aged, nonpregnant adult females require no follow up if UTI is clinically cured after 3-day therapy.
- If symptoms persist after 2 to 3 days of therapy, obtain culture/sensitivity and change antibiotic accordingly.

Pregnancy Considerations

- UTI during pregnancy always requires culture/sensitivity and usually requires a 7- to 14-day treatment.
- Following the treatment of acute infection, pregnant women warrant surveillance urine cultures every trimester. They may receive prophylactic antibiotics for the remainder of pregnancy for recurrent or upper tract disease.

PATIENT EDUCATION

- Although no controlled studies support this intervention, postcoital voiding is commonly advised.
- FamilyDoctor Web site: http://familydoctor.org/familydoctor/en/diseases-conditions/urinary-tract-infections.html

PROGNOSIS

Symptoms resolve within 2 to 3 days of antibiotic treatment in almost all patients.

COMPLICATIONS

- Pyelonephritis or sepsis
- Renal abscess
- Acute urinary outlet obstruction

Pregnancy Considerations

Pregnant females, infants, and young children with cystitis are at higher risk of pyelonephritis.

REFERENCES

1. Kodner CM, Thomas Gupton EK. Recurrent urinary tract infections in women: diagnosis and management. *Am Fam Physician*. 2010;82(6):638–643.
2. Hooton TM. Clinical practice. Uncomplicated urinary tract infection. *N Engl J Med*. 2012;366(11):1028–1037.
3. Zalmanovici Trestioreanu A, Green H, Paul M, et al. Antimicrobial agents for treating uncomplicated urinary tract infection in women. *Cochrane Database Syst Rev*. 2010;(10):CD007182.

ADDITIONAL READING

- Gupta K, Hooton TM, Naber KG, et al. International clinical practice guidelines for the treatment of acute uncomplicated cystitis and pyelonephritis in women: a 2010 update by the Infectious Diseases Society of America and the European Society for Microbiology and Infectious Diseases. *Clin Infect Dis*. 2011;52(5):e103–e120.
- Jepson RG, Craig JC. Cranberries for preventing urinary tract infections. *Cochrane Database Syst Rev*. 2008;(1):CD001321.
- Litza JA, Brill JR. Urinary tract infections. *Prim Care*. 2010;37(3):491–507.
- Mehnert-Kay SA. Diagnosis and management of uncomplicated urinary tract infections. *Am Fam Physician*. 2005;72(3):451–456.
- Mody L, Juthani-Mehta M. Urinary tract infections in older women: a clinical review. *JAMA*. 2014;311(8):844–854.
- Stapleton A, Stamm WE. Prevention of urinary tract infection. *Infect Dis Clin North Am*. 1997;11(3):719–733.
- Williams G, Craig JC. Long-term antibiotics for preventing recurrent urinary tract infection in children. *Cochrane Database Syst Rev*. 2011;(3):CD001534.

 ## SEE ALSO

Algorithm: Dysuria

CODES

ICD10

- N39.0 Urinary tract infection, site not specified
- N30.90 Cystitis, unspecified without hematuria
- N30.91 Cystitis, unspecified with hematuria

CLINICAL PEARLS

- Uncomplicated UTIs cause significant morbidity but generally do not cause renal damage.
- Treatment of uncomplicated UTIs reduces morbidity, but the risk of recurrence stays the same.
- Bacteria originating from intestinal tract cause most UTIs, especially *E. coli*.
- Imaging studies are not required for most women with UTIs.
- Uncomplicated UTIs should be treated for 3 days (TMP-SMX) or 5 days (nitrofurantoin). All pregnant women with bacteriuria should be treated.

URINARY TRACT INFECTION (UTI) IN MALES

Amy L. Wiser, MD

 BASICS

DESCRIPTION

- Cystitis is an infection of the lower urinary tract, usually resulting from a single gram-negative enteric bacteria. (See also "Prostatitis," "Pyelonephritis," and "Urethritis.")
- System(s) affected: renal/urologic
- Synonym(s): urinary tract infection (UTI); cystitis
- Conventional consideration of UTI in male newborn, infant, and elderly men is complicated, with associated functional/structural mechanisms.
- In otherwise healthy males ages 15 to 50 years, UTI is uncommon and considered uncomplicated.

EPIDEMIOLOGY

Incidence
- Approximately 20% of UTIs occur in men (1).
- Predominant age: increases with age
- Uncommon in men <50 years of age
- 6 to 8 infections/10,000 men aged 21 to 50 years (2)

Prevalence
Lifetime prevalence approximately 14% (1)

ETIOLOGY
- *Escherichia coli* (majority of infections)
- *Klebsiella*
- *Enterobacter*
- *Enterococcus*
- *Proteus*
- *Serratia*
- *Citrobacter*
- *Providencia*
- *Streptococcus faecalis* and *Staphylococcus* sp.
- *Pseudomonas* and *Morganella* (more common in elderly and catheterized patients)
- Pathogenesis—bacterial entry into urinary tract via ascension or bladder instrumentation

Genetics
Not applicable

RISK FACTORS
- Age
- Obesity (3)
- History of prior UTI
- Outlet obstruction
  - Benign prostatic hypertrophy (BPH)—incidence of 33% of men with UTIs (4)
  - Urethral stricture
  - Calculi
- Cognitive impairment
- Fecal incontinence
- Urinary incontinence
- Anal intercourse
- Recent urologic surgery
- Infection of the prostate/kidney
- Urinary tract instrumentation, catheterization
- Immunocompromised host
- Diabetes
- Bladder diverticula
- Neurogenic bladder
- Institutionalization
- Uncircumcised
- Engaging in sex with an infected female partner (2)

GENERAL PREVENTION
- Prompt treatment of predisposing factors
- Use a catheter only when necessary; if needed, use aseptic technique and closed system and remove as soon as possible.
- Currently, cranberry products are not recommended for preventing UTIs in men (5).

COMMONLY ASSOCIATED CONDITIONS
- Acute bacterial pyelonephritis
- Chronic bacterial pyelonephritis
- Urethritis
- Prostatitis
- Prostatic hypertrophy
- Prostate cancer

Geriatric Considerations
Bacteriuria is common among the elderly; may be related to functional status and usually is transient. Of men older than 65 years of age, 5–10% have asymptomatic bacteriuria (ASB). If ASB is noted, no treatment is needed (6,7).

Pediatric Considerations
Can be associated with obstruction to normal flow of urine, such as vesicoureteral reflux. Unique diagnostic criteria and evaluation recommendations exist (see below) (8).

 DIAGNOSIS

HISTORY
- Urinary frequency
- Urinary urgency
- Dysuria
- Hesitancy
- Slow urinary stream
- Dribbling of urine
- Nocturia
- Suprapubic discomfort or perineal pain
- Low back pain
- Hematuria
- Systemic symptoms (chills, fever) or flank pain, nausea, vomiting present with concomitant pyelonephritis or prostatitis (9).

PHYSICAL EXAM
- Suprapubic tenderness
- Costovertebral angle (CVA) tenderness and/or fever may be present with concomitant pyelonephritis/prostatitis/epididymitis.

DIFFERENTIAL DIAGNOSIS
- Anatomic/functional pathology of the urinary tract
- Urethritis/STIs
- Infections in other sites of the genitourinary tract (e.g., epididymis, prostatitis). More than 90% of men with febrile UTI have concomitant prostate infection (9).

DIAGNOSTIC TESTS & INTERPRETATION
- Urine dipstick/manual microscopy of clean catch midstream void showing the following:
  - Pyuria (>10 WBCs)
  - Bacteriuria
  - Positive leukocyte esterase (in males: sensitivity, 78%; specificity, 59%; positive predictive value [PPV], 71%; negative predictive value [NPV], 67%)
  - Positive nitrite (in males: sensitivity, 47%; specificity, 98%; PPV, 96%; NPV, 59%)
  - In general, leukocyte esterase is more sensitive and nitrite is more specific in detecting UTI (10).
- Automated microscopy/flow cytometry that measures cell counts and bacterial counts can be used to improve screening characteristics (sensitivity, 92%; specificity, 55%; PPV, 47%; NPV, 97%). The high NPV of these screening tests allows for more judicious use of urine culture (11).
- Urine culture: >100,000 colony-forming units (CFU; $>10^5$ CFU) of bacteria/mL of urine confirm diagnosis.
- Lower counts, such as $>10^3$ CFU, also may be indicative of infection, especially in the presence of pyuria.
- Diagnosis in infants and children <24 months made on the basis of both pyuria and 50,000 CFU on culture.
- Renal and bladder ultrasound recommended in infants and young children after first confirmed UTI.

Follow-Up Tests & Special Considerations
- Consider assessing for risk factors for STIs, as chlamydial/gonococcal urethritis can mimic a UTI. If risk factors are present, use urine nucleic acid amplification tests to identify gonococcal and *Chlamydia* infections and treat as necessary.
- Further urologic evaluation is warranted to rule out other disorders in men with recurrent UTI, febrile UTI, or pyelonephritis. This may include the following:
  - Ultrasound
  - Cystoscopy
  - Urodynamics
  - IV pyelography
- Value of a urologic evaluation in a single uncomplicated UTI has not been determined (9).
- Antibiotics prior to culture or phenazopyridine prior to urine dipstick can alter results.

Test Interpretation
Depends on site of infection

TREATMENT

GENERAL MEASURES
- Hydration
- Analgesia, if required
- Patient with indwelling catheters
  - If asymptomatic bacterial colonization, no need to treat (sterilization of urine is not possible, and resistant organisms may take up residence).
  - If symptomatic of acute infection, institute treatment.

MEDICATION
First Line
- Acute, uncomplicated cystitis

  - Treat empirically; strongly consider if nitrite positive, using local resistance patterns or based on culture and sensitivity results for 7 days (9)[B]. For empirical therapy, a fluoroquinolone or trimethoprim-sulfamethoxazole DS usually used to treat the most likely pathogens (9).

- Complicated, febrile, or recurrent infection

  - Prescribe a minimum of 2 weeks antibiotics based on antimicrobial sensitivities with repeat urine check after the treatment. In men with febrile UTI or pyelonephritis, prostatic involvement also has to be considered. Treatment of concomitant prostatitis requires antimicrobials with good prostatic tissue and fluid penetration (fluoroquinolones) (9)[B].

Second Line
According to culture and sensitivity results and patient's history

ISSUES FOR REFERRAL
Further urologic evaluation and referral are warranted to rule out other disorders in men with recurrent UTI, febrile UTI, or pyelonephritis.

INPATIENT CONSIDERATIONS
Admission Criteria/Initial Stabilization
- Inability to tolerate oral medications
- Acute renal failure
- Suspected sepsis

ONGOING CARE

FOLLOW-UP RECOMMENDATIONS
Patient Monitoring
Close follow-up until clinically well

DIET
Encourage adequate fluid intake.

PATIENT EDUCATION
For patient education materials about this topic that have been reviewed favorably, contact the National Kidney Foundation, 30 E. 33rd Street, Suite 1100, New York, NY 10016; 212-889-2210.

PROGNOSIS
Clearing of infections with appropriate antibiotic treatment

COMPLICATIONS
- Pyelonephritis
- Ascending infection
- Recurrent infection
- Prostatitis

REFERENCES

1. Griebling TL. Urologic diseases in America project: trends in resource use for urinary tract infections in men. *J Urol*. 2005;173(4):1288–1294.
2. Wagenlehner FM, Weidner W, Pilatz A, et al. Urinary tract infections and bacterial prostatitis in men. *Curr Opin Infect Dis*. 2014;27(1):97–101.
3. Semins MJ, Shore AD, Makary MA, et al. The impact of obesity on urinary tract infection risk. *Urology*. 2012;79(2):266–269.
4. Drekonja DM, Rector TS, Cutting A, et al. Urinary tract infection in male veterans: treatment patterns and outcomes. *JAMA Intern Med*. 2013;173(1):62–68.
5. Jepson RG, Williams G, Craig JC. Cranberries for preventing urinary tract infections. *Cochrane Database Syst Rev*. 2012;(10):CD001321.
6. Rowe TA, Juthani-Mehta M. Diagnosis and management of urinary tract infection in older adults. *Infect Dis Clin North Am*. 2014;28(1):75–89.
7. Matthews SJ, Lancaster JW. Urinary tract infections in the elderly population. *Am J Geriatr Pharmacother*. 2011;9(5):286–309.
8. Roberts KB, Downs SM, Finnell SM, et al. Urinary tract infection: clinical practice guideline for the diagnosis and management of the initial UTI in febrile infants and children 2 to 24 months. *Pediatrics*. 2011;128(3):595–610.
9. Grabe M, Bishop MC, Bjerklund-Johansen TE, et al. Uncomplicated urinary tract infections in adult. In: *Guidelines on Urological Infections*. Arnhem, The Netherlands: European Association of Urology; 2013:15–25.
10. Koeijers JJ, Kessels AG, Nys S, et al. Evaluation of the nitrite and leukocyte esterase activity tests for the diagnosis of acute symptomatic urinary tract infection in men. *Clin Infec Dis*. 2007;45(7):894–896.
11. Evans R, Davidson MM, Sim LR, et al. Testing by Sysmex UF-100 flow cytometer and with bacterial culture in a diagnostic laboratory: a comparison. *J Clin Pathol*. 2006;59(6):661–662.

ADDITIONAL READING

- Coupat C, Pradier C, Degand N, et al. Selective reporting of antibiotic susceptibility data improves the appropriateness of intended antibiotic prescriptions in urinary tract infections: a case-vignette randomised study. *Eur J Clin Microbiol Infect Dis*. 2013;32(5):627–636.
- Foxman B. Urinary tract infection syndromes: occurrence, recurrence, bacteriology, risk factors, and disease burden. *Infect Dis Clin North Am*. 2014;28(1):1–13.
- Gerber GS, Brendler CB. Evaluation of the urologic patient: history, physical examination, and urinalysis. In: Walsh PC, Retik AB, Vaughn ED Jr, et al, eds. *Campbell's Urology*. 8th ed. Philadelphia, PA: Saunders; 2002:107.
- Koeijers JJ, Verbon A, Kessels AG, et al. Urinary tract infection in male general practice patients: uropathogens and antibiotic susceptibility. *Urology*. 2010;76(2):336–340.

 SEE ALSO

- Prostate Cancer; Prostatic Hyperplasia, Benign (BPH); Prostatitis; Pyelonephritis; Urethritis
- Algorithms: Dysuria; Urethral Discharge

 CODES

ICD10
- N39.0 Urinary tract infection, site not specified
- N30.90 Cystitis, unspecified without hematuria
- N30.91 Cystitis, unspecified with hematuria

CLINICAL PEARLS

- Cystitis is an infection of the lower urinary tract, usually resulting from a single gram-negative enteric bacteria.
- Risk factors/causes: age, history of UTI, obesity, BPH, cognitive impairment, fecal incontinence, urinary incontinence, anal intercourse, recent urologic surgery, catheterization, infection of the prostate/kidney, urinary tract instrumentation, immunocompromised host, diabetes, neurogenic bladder, outlet obstruction, sex with infected female partner
- Evaluation: urinalysis, urine culture, STI testing (e.g., gonorrhea, *Chlamydia* by culture/DNA probe)
- Treat empirically with fluoroquinolones or trimethoprim-sulfamethoxazole DS for 7 days.

U

UROLITHIASIS
Phillip Fournier, MD

BASICS

DESCRIPTION
- Stone formation within the urinary tract: Urinary crystals bind to form a nidus which grows to form a calculus (stone).
- Range of symptoms: asymptomatic to obstructive; febrile morbidity if result of infection

EPIDEMIOLOGY
- The worldwide epidemiology differs according to both geographic area (higher prevalence in hot, arid, or dry climates) and socioeconomic conditions (dietary intake and lifestyle). Radiolucent stones and stones secondary to infection are less influenced by environmental conditions.
- Vesical calculosis (bladder stones) due to malnutrition during early life is frequent in Middle East and Asian countries.
- Incidence in industrialized countries seems to be increasing, probably due to improved diagnostics as well as to increasingly rich diets.
- Increased incidence in patients with surgically induced absorption issues, such as Crohn disease and gastric bypass surgery (1)[B]

Incidence
- In industrialized countries: 100 to 200/100,000/year (2)
- Predominant age: Mean age is 40 to 60 years.
- Predominant sex: male > female (~2:1) (3)

ETIOLOGY AND PATHOPHYSIOLOGY
- Supersaturation and dehydration lead to high salt content in urine which congregates.
- Stasis of urine
  - Renal malformation (e.g., horseshoe kidney, ureteropelvic junction obstruction)
  - Incomplete bladder emptying (e.g., neurogenic bladder, prostate enlargement, multiple sclerosis)
- Crystals may form in pure solutions (homogeneous) or on existing surfaces, such as other crystals or cellular debris (heterogeneous).
- Balance of promoters and inhibitors: organic (Tamm-Horsfall protein, glycosaminoglycan, uropontin, nephrocalcin) and inorganic (citrate, pyrophosphate)
- Calcium oxalate and/or phosphate stones (80%)
  - Hypercalciuria
    ○ Absorptive hypercalciuria: increased jejunal calcium absorption
    ○ Renal leak: increased calcium excretion from renal proximal tubule
    ○ Resorptive hypercalciuria: mild hyperparathyroidism
  - Hypercalcemia
    ○ Hyperparathyroidism
    ○ Sarcoidosis
    ○ Malignancy
    ○ Immobilization
    ○ Paget disease
- Hyperoxaluria
  - Enteric hyperoxaluria
    ○ Intestinal malabsorptive state associated with irritable bowel disease, celiac sprue, or intestinal resection
    ○ Bile salt malabsorption leads to formation of calcium soaps.
  - Primary hyperoxaluria: autosomal recessive, types I and II
  - Dietary hyperoxaluria: overindulgence in oxalate-rich food

- Hyperuricosuria
  - Seen in 10% of calcium stone formers
  - Caused by increased dietary purine intake, systemic acidosis, myeloproliferative diseases, gout, chemotherapy, Lesch-Nyhan syndrome
  - Thiazides, probenecid
- Hypocitraturia
  - Caused by acidosis: renal tubular acidosis, malabsorption, thiazides, enalapril, excessive dietary protein
- Uric acid stones (10–15%): hyperuricemia causes as discussed earlier
- Struvite stones (5–10%): infected urine with urease-producing organisms (most commonly *Proteus* sp.)
- Cystine stones (<1%): autosomal recessive disorder of renal tubular reabsorption of cystine
- Bladder stones: seen with chronic bladder catheterization and some medications (indinavir)
- In children: usually due to malnutrition

Genetics
- Up to 20% of patients have a family history. However, spouses of those who form stones have higher calcium excretion rates than controls, suggesting strong dietary–environmental factors.
- Autosomal dominant: idiopathic hypercalciuria
- Autosomal recessive
  - Cystinuria, Lesch-Nyhan syndrome, hyperoxaluria types I and II
  - Ehlers-Danlos syndrome, Marfan syndrome, Wilson disease, familial renal tubular acidosis

RISK FACTORS
- White > African American in regions with both populations
- Family history
- Previous history of nephrolithiasis
- Diet rich in protein, refined carbohydrates, and sodium, carbonated drinks
- Occupations associated with a sedentary lifestyle or with a hot, dry workplace
- Incidence rates peak during summer secondary to dehydration.
- Obesity
- Surgically/medically induced malabsorption (Crohn disease, gastric bypass, celiac)

GENERAL PREVENTION
- Hydration (4)[A]
- Decrease salt and meat intake
- Avoid oxalate-rich foods.

Pediatric Considerations
Rare: more common in men with low socioeconomic status

Pregnancy Considerations
- Pregnant women have the same incidence of renal colic as do nonpregnant women.
- Most symptomatic stones occur during the 2nd and 3rd trimesters, heralded by symptoms of flank pain/hematuria.
- Most common differential diagnosis is physiologic hydronephrosis of pregnancy. Use ultrasound to avoid irradiation. Noncontrast-enhanced CT scan also is diagnostic.
- Treatment goals
  - Control pain and avoid infection, and preserve renal function until birth or stone passage.
  - 30% require intervention, such as stent placement.

DIAGNOSIS

HISTORY
- Pain
  - Renal colic: acute onset of severe groin and/or flank pain
  - Distal stones may present with referred pain in labia, penile meatus, or testis.
- Microscopic/gross hematuria occurs in 95% of patients.
- Nonspecific symptoms of nausea, vomiting, tachycardia, diaphoresis
- Low-grade fever without signs of infection
- Infectious origin: associated with high-grade fevers require more urgent treatment (see the following text)
- Frequency and dysuria especially occur with stones at the vesicoureteric junction (VUJ).
- Asymptomatic: nonobstructing stones within the renal calyces

PHYSICAL EXAM
Tender costovertebral angle with palpation/percussion and/or iliac fossa

DIFFERENTIAL DIAGNOSIS
- Appendicitis
- Ruptured aortic aneurysm
- Musculoskeletal strain
- Pyelonephritis (upper UTI)
- Pyonephrosis (obstructed upper UTI; emergency)
- Perinephric abscess
- Ectopic pregnancy
- Salpingitis

DIAGNOSTIC TESTS & INTERPRETATION
- Urinalysis for RBCs, leukocytes, nitrates, pH (acidic urine <5.5 is associated with uric acid stones; alkaline >7 with struvite stones)
- Midstream urine for microscopy, culture, and sensitivity
- Blood: urea, creatinine, electrolytes, calcium, and urate; consider CBC.
- Parathyroid hormone only if calcium is elevated
- Stone analysis if/when stone passed

Initial Tests (lab, imaging)
- Noncontrast-enhanced helical CT scan of the abdomen and pelvis has replaced IV pyelogram as the investigation of choice (5)[A].
  - Stone is found most commonly at levels of ureteric luminal narrowing: pelviureteric junction, pelvic brim, and VUJ.
  - Acute obstruction: Proximal ureter and renal pelvis are dilated to the level of obstruction, and perinephric stranding is possible on imaging.
- Renal ultrasound may be as effective with lower radiation at diagnosis as well as identifying obstruction (6)[B].
- X-ray of kidneys, ureter, and bladder to determine if stone is radiopaque or lucent
  - Calcium oxalate/phosphate stones are radiopaque.
  - Uric acid stones are radiolucent.
  - Staghorn calculi (that fill the shape of the renal calyces) are usually struvite and opaque.
  - Cystine stones are faintly opaque (ground-glass appearance).
- Ultrasound has low sensitivity and specificity but is often the first choice for pregnant women.

TREATMENT

GENERAL MEASURES

- 75% of patients are successfully treated conservatively and pass the stone spontaneously.
- Stones that do not pass usually require surgical intervention.
- 30–50% of patients will have recurrent stones.
- Increase fluid intake; eliminate carbonated drinks.

MEDICATION

- Medical expulsive therapy: α_1-antagonists (e.g., tamsulosin) and calcium channel blockers (e.g., nifedipine) improve likelihood of spontaneous stone passage with a number needed to treat (NNT) of ~5 (7).
- Category C in pregnancy

ISSUES FOR REFERRAL

- Urgent referral of patients with UTI/sepsis or acute renal failure/solitary kidney
- Early referral of pregnant patients, large stones (>8 mm), chronic renal failure, children
- Refer patients if no passage at 2 to 4 weeks or poorly controlled pain.

ADDITIONAL THERAPIES

- Uric acid stone dissolution therapy
  - Alkalinize urine with potassium citrate; keep pH >6.5.
  - Allopurinol 100 to 300 mg/day PO (for those who continue to form stones despite alkalinization of urine)
- Cystine stone dissolution/prevention
  - Alkalinize urine with potassium citrate; keep pH >6.5.
  - Chelating agents: captopril, α-mercapto propionylglycine, D-penicillamine
- Consider altering medications that increase risk of stone formation: probenecid, loop diuretics, salicylic acid, salbutamol, indinavir, triamterene, acetazolamide.
- Vitamin D supplementation has not been proven to induce stone formation.
- Treat hypercalciuria with thiazides on an acute basis only
- Treat hypocitraturia with potassium citrate and high-citrate juices (e.g., orange, lemon).
- Treat enteric hyperoxaluria with oral calcium/magnesium, cholestyramine, and potassium citrate.

SURGERY/OTHER PROCEDURES

- Immediate relief of obstruction is required for patients with the following conditions:
  - Sepsis
  - Renal failure (obstructed solitary kidney, bilateral obstruction)
  - Uncontrolled pain, despite adequate analgesia
- Emergency surgery for obstruction
  - Placement of a retrograde stent (i.e., endoscopic surgery, usually requires an anesthetic)
  - Radiologic placement of a percutaneous nephrostomy tube
- Elective surgery for stone treatment
  - Extracorporeal shock wave lithotripsy
  - Ureteroscopy with basket extraction/lithotripsy (laser/pneumatic)
  - Percutaneous nephrolithotomy
- Open surgery is uncommon.

INPATIENT CONSIDERATIONS

Admission-Criteria/Initial Stabilization

- Analgesia
  - Combination of NSAIDs (ketorolac 30 to 60 mg) and oral opiate
  - Parenteral opioid if vomiting or if preceding fails to control pain (morphine 5 to 10 mg IV or IM q4h)
  - Antiemetic if required or prophylactically with parenteral narcotics
- Septic patients with urosepsis or pyonephrosis may require IV antibiotics (once blood and urine cultures are taken), IV fluids, and, in severe cases, cardiorespiratory support in intensive care during recovery.

ONGOING CARE

FOLLOW-UP RECOMMENDATIONS

- Patients with ureteric stones who are being treated conservatively should be followed until imaging is clear or stone is visibly passed.
  - Strain urine and send stone for composition.
  - Tamsulosin and nifedipine in selected patients to speed passage
  - Present to the hospital if pain worsens/signs of infection.
  - If pain management is suboptimal or stone does not progress or pass within 2 to 4 weeks, patient should be referred to a urologist and imaging should be repeated.
- Patients with recurrent stone formation should have follow-up with a urologist for metabolic workup: 24-hour urine for volume, pH, creatinine, calcium, cystine, phosphate, oxalate, uric acid, and magnesium.

DIET

ALERT

- Increased fluid intake for life cannot be overemphasized for decreasing recurrence. Encourage intake of 2 to 3 L/day; advise patient to have clear urine rather than yellow.

- Decrease or eliminate carbonated drinks.
- Patients who form calcium stones should minimize high-oxalate foods such as green leafy vegetables, rhubarb, peanuts, chocolates, and beer.
- Decrease protein and salt intake.
- Lowering calcium intake is inadvisable and even may increase urine calcium excretion.
- Increase phytate-rich foods such as natural dietary bran, legumes and beans, whole cereal (8).
- Avoid excessive vitamin C and\or vitamin D.

PROGNOSIS

- Spontaneous stone passage depends on stone location (proximal vs. distal) and stone size (<5 mm, 90% pass; >8 mm, 10% pass).
- Stone recurrence: 50% of patients at 10 years

REFERENCES

1. Matlaga BR, Shore AD, Magnuson T, et al. Effect of gastric bypass surgery on kidney stone disease. *J Urol*. 2009;181(6):2573–2577.
2. Tiselius HG. Epidemiology and medical management of stone disease. *BJU Int*. 2003;91(8):758–767.
3. Scales CD Jr, Curtis LH, Norris RD, et al. Changing gender prevalence of stone disease. *J Urol*. 2007;177(3):979–982.
4. Qiang W, Ke Z. Water for preventing urinary calculi. *Cochrane Database Syst Rev*. 2004;(3):CD004292.
5. Worster A, Preyra I, Weaver B, et al. The accuracy of noncontrast helical computed tomography versus intravenous pyelography in the diagnosis of suspected acute urolithiasis: a meta-analysis. *Ann Emerg Med*. 2002;40(3):280–286.
6. Luyckx F. Who wants to go further has to know the past: a comment upon: ultrasonography versus computed tomography for suspected nephrolithiasis-R. Smith-Bindman et al. N Engl J Med. 2014 Sep 18;371(12):1100-1110. *World J Urol*. 2015;33(10):1371–1372.
7. Hollingsworth JM, Rogers MA, Kaufman SR, et al. Medical therapy to facilitate urinary stone passage: a meta-analysis. *Lancet*. 2006;368(9542);1171–1179.
8. Grases F, Costa-Bauza A, Prieto RM. Renal lithiasis and nutrition. *Nutr J*. 2006;5:23.

ADDITIONAL READING

- Penniston KL, Jones AN, Nakada SY, et al. Vitamin D repletion does not alter urinary calcium excretion in healthy postmenopausal women. *BJU Int*. 2009;104(10):1512–1516.
- Qaseem A, Dallas P, Forciea MA, et al. Dietary and pharmacologic management to prevent recurrent nephrolithiasis in adults: a clinical practice guideline from the American College of Physicians. *Ann Intern Med*. 2014;161(9):659–667.

SEE ALSO

Algorithms: Dysuria; Renal Calculi; Urethral Discharge

CODES

ICD10

- N20.9 Urinary calculus, unspecified
- N20.0 Calculus of kidney
- N20.1 Calculus of ureter

CLINICAL PEARLS

- Incidence in industrialized countries seems to be increasing, probably due to improved diagnostics as well as to increasingly rich diets.
- Vesical calculosis (bladder stones) due to malnutrition during early life is frequent in Middle East and Asian countries.
- Medical expulsive therapy: α_1-Antagonists (e.g., terazosin) and calcium channel blockers (e.g., nifedipine) improve likelihood of spontaneous stone passage with NNT of ~5.
- Increased fluid intake for life cannot be overemphasized for decreasing recurrence. Encourage 2 to 3 L/day intake; advise patient to have clear urine rather than yellow.
- Patients who form calcium stones should minimize high-oxalate foods such as green leafy vegetables, rhubarb, peanuts, chocolates, and beer.
- Decrease protein and salt intake.
- Lowering calcium intake is inadvisable and even may increase urine calcium excretion.

U

URTICARIA
Irina Pechenko, MD • Katie L. Westerfield, DO

BASICS

DESCRIPTION
- A cutaneous lesion involving edema of the epidermis and/or dermis presenting with acute onset and pruritis, returning to normal skin appearance within 24 hours
- Pathophysiology is primarily mast cell degranulation and subsequent histamine release.
- Angioedema may occur with urticaria although angioedema is characterized by sudden pronounced erythematous edema of the lower dermis and subcutis; may take up to 72 hours to remit.
- Pruritus and burning are more commonly associated with urticaria; pain more often with angioedema.
  - Spontaneous urticaria: acute: persists <6 weeks
- Specific extrinsic triggers drugs, foods, infections, envenomation, allergens, and autoimmune
- Underlying etiology may be difficult to pinpoint.
  - Chronic spontaneous urticaria: persists >6 weeks with >2 episodes/week off-treatment
- Recurrent acute urticaria: if symptoms occur <2 times a week.
- For those with chronic urticaria, 40% have concurrent angioedema.
- Chronic infection, pseudoallergy, malignancy including mastocytosis, autoimmunity (especially thyroid), and medications may underlie the remaining 20% (1).
- Inducible urticaria
  - Dermatographism: "skin writing" or the appearance of linear wheals at the site of any type of irritation. This is the most common physical urticaria.
  - Cold urticaria: Wheals occur within minutes of rewarming after cold exposure; 95% idiopathic but can be due to infections (mononucleosis, HIV), neoplasia, or autoimmune diseases.
  - Delayed pressure urticaria: Urticaria occurs 0.5 to 12 hours after pressure to skin (e.g., from elastic or shoes), may be pruritic and/or painful, and may not subside for several days.
  - Solar urticaria: from sunlight exposure, usually UV; onset in minutes; subsides within 2 hours
  - Heat urticaria: from direct contact with warm objects or air; rare
  - Vibratory urticaria/angioedema: very rare; secondary to vibrations (e.g., motorcycle)
  - Cholinergic urticaria: due to brief increase of core body temperature from exercise, baths, or emotional stress; small pin-sized (5 to 10 mm) wheals surrounded by an erythema but also can have larger wheals. This is the second most common form.
  - Adrenergic urticaria: also caused by stress; extremely rare; vasoconstricted, blanched skin around pink wheals as opposed to cholinergic's erythematous surrounding
  - Contact urticaria: wheals at sites where chemical substances contact the skin, may be either IgE-dependent (e.g., latex) or IgE-independent (e.g., stinging nettle)
  - Aquagenic and solar urticaria: small wheals after contact with water of any temperature or UV light, respectively; rare

- System(s) affected: integumentary
- Synonym(s): hives; wheals

EPIDEMIOLOGY

Incidence
- Equally distributed across all ages: female > male (2:1 in chronic urticaria)
- In 20% of patients, chronic urticaria lasts >10 years (1).

Prevalence
- 5–25% of the population
- Of people with urticaria, 40% have no angioedema, 40% have urticaria and angioedema, and 20% have angioedema with no urticaria.
- Up to 3% of the population has chronic idiopathic urticaria.

ETIOLOGY AND PATHOPHYSIOLOGY
- Mast cell degranulation with release of inflammatory reactants, which leads to vascular leakage, inflammatory cell extravasation, and dermal (angioedema) and/or epidermal (wheals/hives) edema
- Histamine, cytokines, leukotrienes, and proteases are main active substances released.
- Spontaneous acute urticaria
  - Bacterial infections: strep throat, sinusitis, otitis, urinary tract
  - Viral infections: rhinovirus, rotavirus, hepatitis B, mononucleosis, herpes
  - Foods: peanuts, tree nuts, seafood, milk, soy, fish, wheat, and eggs; tend to be IgE-mediated; pseudoallergenic foods such as strawberries, tomatoes, preservatives, and coloring agents contain histamine.
  - Drugs: IgE-mediated (e.g., penicillin and other antibiotics), direct mast cell stimulation (e.g., aspirin, NSAIDs, opiates)
  - Inhalant, contact, ingestion, or occupational exposure (e.g., latex, cosmetics)
  - Parasitic infection; insect bite/sting
  - Transfusion reaction
- Spontaneous chronic urticaria
  - Chronic subclinical allergic rhinitis, eczema, and other atopic disorders
  - Chronic indolent infections: *Helicobacter pylori*, fungal, parasitic (*Anisakis simplex*, strongyloidiasis), and chronic viral infections (hepatitis)
  - Collagen vascular disease (cutaneous vasculitis, serum sickness, lupus)
  - Thyroid autoimmunity, especially Hashimoto
  - Hormonal: pregnancy and progesterone
  - Autoimmune antibodies to the IgE receptor α chain on mast cells and to the IgE antibody
  - Chronic medications (e.g., NSAIDs, hormones, ACE inhibitors). NSAID sensitivity demonstrated almost in half of adults with chronic urticaria and presents with a worsening of symptoms 4 hours after ingestion (2)[A].
  - Malignancy
  - Physical stimuli (cold, heat, vibration, pressure) in physical urticaria

Genetics
No consistent pattern known: Chronic urticaria has increased frequency of HLA-DR4 and HLA-D8Q MHC II alleles.

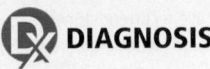

DIAGNOSIS

HISTORY
Fast onset; resolves in <24 to 48 hours, pruritis

PHYSICAL EXAM
- Single/multiple raised, polymorphic indurated plaques with central pallor and edema with an erythematous flare
- Evaluate for underlying conditions including thyroid abnormalities (nodules), bacterial, viral, or fungal infection (e.g., fever).

DIFFERENTIAL DIAGNOSIS
- Anaphylaxis (may present with urticaria)
- Morbilliform or fixed drug eruptions
- Erythema multiforme
- Systemic lupus erythematous (SLE), vasculitis, and polyarteritis
- Angioedema without urticaria
- Urticaria pigmentosa/systemic mastocytosis
- Bullous pemphigoid (urticarial stage)
- Arthropod bite
- Atopic/contact dermatitis
- Viral exanthem

DIAGNOSTIC TESTS & INTERPRETATION
- Directed by clinical suspicion of underlying cause:
  - Allergy skin tests and radioallergosorbent test (RAST) for inhaled allergens, insects, drugs, or foods
  - Infection: Consider pharyngeal culture, LFTs, mononucleosis test, urinalysis in appropriate setting.
- Chronic urticaria (idiopathic or spontaneous CIU/CSU) (3): Extensive lab testing is not indicated and has not proven to improve outcome nor is it cost-effective. Limit lab testing according to clinical history and indication. Skin or IgE testing should be limited to specific history of provoking allergen (4)[C].
  - CBC, ESR, and CRP is recommended by most guidelines.
  - Thyroid function tests, LFTs, and urinalysis are recommended by several guidelines.
  - Consider allergy skin tests and RAST for inhaled allergens, insects, drugs, or foods; total IgE level.
  - Autoimmune: ESR, ANA, RF, complement (e.g., CH50, C3, C4), cryoglobulins in urticarial vasculitis
  - Tests for *H. pylori* (e.g., antibodies) in dyspeptic patients. Consider stool for ova and parasites in at-risk individuals.
  - Autologous serum skin testing: injection of serum under skin to test for presence of IgE receptor–activating antibodies
  - Consider malignancy workup, including serum protein electrophoresis and immunofixation in the proper setting.

- Use the Urticaria Activity Score (UAS7) for assessing CSU.
- Recently was developed Urticaria Control Test (UCT)
  - The tool to assess disease control in patients with chronic urticaria (spontaneous and inducible) (5)[A].

Diagnostic Procedures/Other
- Food and drug reactions: elimination of (or challenges with) suspected agents
- Physical and special forms of urticaria: challenge tests:
  - Dermatographism: Stroke skin lightly with rounded object and observe for surrounding urticaria.
  - Cold urticaria: ice cube test: Place ice cube on skin for 5 minutes; observe for 10 to 15 minutes.
  - Cholinergic: Exercise to the point of sweating/partial immersion in 42°C bath for 10 minutes.
  - Solar: exposure to different wavelengths of light
  - Delayed pressure: Apply 5-lb sandbag to back for 20 minutes; observe 6 hours later.
  - Aquagenic: Apply water at various temperatures.
  - Vibratory: Apply vibration 4 to 5 minutes with a lab mixing device; observe.
- Skin biopsy with lesions lasting >24 hours

 TREATMENT

ISSUES FOR REFERRAL
Referral to an allergist, immunologist, or dermatologist for recalcitrant cases

MEDICATION
First Line
- 2nd generation antihistamine (H_1) blockers are the first-line treatment of any urticaria in which avoidance of stimulus is impossible or not feasible (6,7)[A]:
  - Fexofenadine (Allegra): 180 mg/day
  - Loratadine (Claritin): 10 mg/day, increasing to 30 mg/day if needed; only medication studied for safe use in pregnancy
  - Desloratadine (Clarinex): 5 mg/day (8)[A]
  - Cetirizine (Zyrtec): 10 mg/day, increasing to 30 mg per day if needed
  - Levocetirizine (Xyzal): 5 mg/day; requires weight-based dosing in children (8)[A]
  - Rupatadine: novel H_1 antagonist with antiplatelet-activating factor activity
- 1st-generation antihistamines (H_1; for patients with sleep disturbed by itching):
  - Older children and adults: hydroxyzine or diphenhydramine 25 to 50 mg q6h
  - Children <6 years of age: diphenhydramine 12.5 mg q6–8h (5 mg/kg/day) or hydroxyzine (10 mg/5 mL) 2 mg/kg/day divided q6–8h
- Precautions and notes: Drowsiness and dry mouth and eyes in 1st-generation H_1 blockers (elderly)

Second Line
Doubling the typical 2nd-generation H_1 blocker dosages should be attempted before adding 1st-generation H_1 or H_2 blockers (6,7,8)[A].

- H_2-specific antihistamines (beneficial as adjuvants): cimetidine, ranitidine, nizatidine, famotidine

Third Line
- Corticosteroids: prednisolone 20 to 50 mg/day for max of 10 days; best used only for exacerbations; avoid chronic use (6,7)[C].
- Doxepin: tricyclic antidepressant with strong H_1- and H_2-blocking properties; 10 to 30 mg at bedtime; sedation limits usefulness (6)[C].
- Leukotriene antagonists (montelukast, zileuton, and zafirlukast): safe and worth trying in chronic, unresponsive cases; useful alone but best used in addition to antihistamines; limited data on use in treating acute urticaria (2)[A]
- Refractory symptoms
  - Omalizumab: anti-IgE; effective, expensive. 150 to 300 mg SQ q2–4wk. Restricted to allergists and those who can manage acute anaphylaxis (3,6,9,11)[A], significantly reduce the urticarial symptoms of CIU/CSU at 12 weeks. The best effects is reached with omalizumab dose 300 mg (3)[A]. Omalizumab is currently the only licensed treatment for H_1-antihistamine-refractory chronic spontaneous urticaria, has a favorable risk/benefit ratio, and was well tolerated in clinical studies (2).
  - Cyclosporine: well-studied, effective (2.5 to 5 mg/kg/day); best used in combination with antihistamines; significant renal side effects (6,7)[C]
  - Methotrexate: antifolate; proven useful in recalcitrant cases; GI upset most common complaint; long-term requires LFT monitoring
  - UV therapy decreases number of mast cells; has shown promise in the treatment of mastocytosis-induced urticaria (7)[C].
- Adding Vitamin D 4,000 U/day for 12 weeks may decrease the symptoms and USS score (10)[C].

INPATIENT CONSIDERATIONS
Admission Criteria/Initial Stabilization
Educating patient on use of EpiPen as pathophysiology similar. If the airway is threatened, immediate consult to evaluate for laryngeal edema and need for airway access.

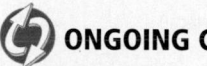 ONGOING CARE

PROGNOSIS
Resolution of acute symptoms: 70% <72 hours. chronic urticaria: 35% symptom-free in a year; another 30% will see symptom reduction

REFERENCES
1. Leru P. Urticaria—an allergologic, dermatologic or multidisciplinary disease? Rom J Intern Med. 2013;51(3–4):125–130.
2. Cavkaytar O, Arik Yilmaz E, Buyuktiryaki B, et al. Challenge-proven aspirin hypersensitivity in children with chronic spontaneous urticaria. Allergy. 2015;70(2):153–160.
3. Saini SS, Bindslev-Jensen C, Maurer M, et al. Efficacy and safety of omalizumab in patients with chronic idiopathic/spontaneous urticaria who remain symptomatic on H1 antihistamines: a randomized, placebo-controlled study. J Invest Dermatol. 2015;135(1):67–75.
4. Choosing Wisely initiative of ABIM: American Academy of Allergy, Asthma & Immunology recommendation. http://www.choosingwisely.org/wp-content/uploads/2015/02/AAAAI-Choosing-Wisely-List.pdf.
5. Weller K, Groffik A, Church MK, et al. Development and validation of the Urticaria Control Test: a patient-reported outcome instrument for assessing urticaria control. J Allergy Clin Immunol. 2014;133(5):1365–1372, 1372.e1–1376.e1.
6. Zuberbier T, Aberer W, Asero R, et al. The EAACI/GA(2)LEN/EDF/WAO guideline for the definition, classification, diagnosis, and management of urticaria: the 2013 revision and update. Allergy. 2014;69(7):868–887.
7. Bernstein JA, Lang DM, Khan DA, et al. The diagnosis and management of acute and chronic urticaria: 2014 update. J Allergy Clin Immunol. 2014;133(5):1270–1277.
8. Staevska M, Popov TA, Kralimarkova T, et al. The effectiveness of levocetirizine and desloratadine in up to 4 times conventional doses in difficult-to-treat urticaria. J Allergy Clin Immunol. 2010;125(3):676–682.
9. Maurer M, Rosén K, Hsieh HJ, et al. Omalizumab for the treatment of chronic idiopathic or spontaneous urticaria. N Engl J Med. 2013;368(10):924–935.
10. Rorie A, Goldner WS, Lyden E, et al. Beneficial role for supplemental vitamin D3 treatment in chronic urticaria: a randomized study. Ann Allergy Asthma Immunol. 2014;112(4):376–382.
11. Zuberbier T, Maurer M. Omalizumab for the treatment of chronic urticaria. Expert Rev Clin Immunol. 2015;11(2):171–180.

ADDITIONAL READING
- Maurer M, Weller K, Bindslev-Jensen C, et al. Unmet clinical needs in chronic spontaneous urticaria. A GA²LEN task force report. Allergy. 2011;66(3):317–330.
- Poonawalla T, Kelly B. Urticaria: a review. Am J Clin Dermatol. 2009;10(1):9–21.
- Zuberbier T, Balke M, Worm M, et al. Epidemiology of urticaria: a representative cross-sectional survey. Clin Exp Dermatol. 2010;35(8):869–873.

 CODES

ICD10
- L50.9 Urticaria, unspecified
- L50.1 Idiopathic urticaria
- L50.8 Other urticaria

CLINICAL PEARLS
- "Chronic urticaria" with <2 episodes/week should be approached as acute.
- Antihistamines are the best studied and most efficacious therapy but may require higher-than-normal doses for efficacy.
- Lesions lasting >24 hours should be evaluated for urticarial vasculitis.

U

UTERINE AND PELVIC ORGAN PROLAPSE

Maryse A. Pedoussaut, MD • John Delzell, Jr., MD, MSPH • Suzanne Minor, MD, FAAFP

BASICS

DESCRIPTION
- Symptomatic descent of one or more of (1,2)
  - The anterior vaginal wall (bladder or cystocele)
  - The posterior vaginal wall (rectum or rectocele)
  - The apex of the vagina (uterine cervix descent and prolapse)
  - The vault (cuff) after hysterectomy (vault prolapse)
- Prolapses above or to the hymen are not symptomatic (2).
- Associated symptoms (2)
  - Feeling of vaginal or pelvic pressure
  - Heaviness
  - Bulging
  - Bowel or bladder symptoms
- Cost associated with treatment is more than $1 billion annually (~200,000 surgeries/year) (2).

EPIDEMIOLOGY
Incidence
Pelvic organ prolapse (POP) is common but not always symptomatic. It does not always progress with time. In a 3-year prospective cohort study of 249 women, prolapse increased by at least 2 cm in 11% and regressed by 2 cm in 3% (2).

Prevalence
- A national survey of 7,924 women (over 20 years of age) found a prevalence of 25% for one or more pelvic floor disorders (including urinary incontinence, fecal incontinence, and POP). Prevalence of POP was 2.9% (3).
- The prevalence of lower urinary tract symptoms is as high as 50% in parous women. 11% of all women have surgery for POP or lower urinary tract symptoms by 80 years old (4).
- 3–6% of women who present for gynecologic care have a prolapse beyond hymen (2).

ETIOLOGY AND PATHOPHYSIOLOGY
- Insidious process begins long before symptoms develop.
- There is a complex interaction between the pelvic floor musculature, connective tissue, and the vaginal wall, which provides support from the perineum to the sacrum (2). Integrity of levator ani is essential to this support system by providing a platform on which the pelvic organs rest (2).
- Symptomatic women typically have multiple defects, including laxity of supporting tissue and damage to the levator ani (2).
- Half of anterior prolapse can be attributed to apical descent of the vagina (2).

RISK FACTORS
- Vaginal childbirth (2): Women who have delivered two children vaginally have a relative risk of 8.4 and every additional child (up to five deliveries) increases the risk of prolapse by 10–20% (2).
- Age: Every 10 years of age increases the risk of prolapse by 40% (2). POP will become more prevalent, as the elderly population is expected to double by 2030 (5).
- Obesity: BMI >25 may increase the risk of developing prolapse (2).

- Constipation: independent risk factor in a survey of more than 2,000 women (2)
- Race: White and Hispanic women may be at higher risk than black or Asian women (2).
- Occupation (heavy lifting): variable support in the literature (2)
- Hysterectomy: variable support in the literature (2)
- Obstetric factors (operative delivery, infant weight, length of pushing in second stage of labor): variable support in the literature (2)

GENERAL PREVENTION
There is some evidence that pelvic floor muscle training ("Kegel exercises") may decrease the risk of symptomatic POP (6)[B]. Weight loss and proper management of conditions that cause increase in intra-abdominal pressure may help prevent the problem.

COMMONLY ASSOCIATED CONDITIONS
- Urinary incontinence
- Other urinary symptoms (4)
  - Urgency
  - Frequency

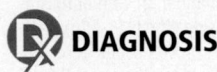

DIAGNOSIS

HISTORY
- Less than half of women discuss symptoms with PCP. Only 10–12% seek medical attention. Barriers include embarrassment, social stigma, ability to cope, belief that POP is part of the aging process, belief that treatment options are limited, and fear of surgery (4).
- Common symptoms include the following:
  - Feeling a bulge in vagina
  - Something "falling out" of vagina
  - Pelvic pressure
  - Difficulty with voiding or defecation
  - Urgency
  - Frequency
  - Incontinence (urinary or fecal)
  - Constipation
- Document the presence, duration, and severity of urinary, bowel, or prolapse symptom. Assess impact on sexual function and quality of life with validated questionnaires (PISQ 9 OR 12) (1,7).
- Assess past medical history.
  - Gravity and parity/obstetric history
  - History of ascites
  - Chronic constipation
  - Document physical impairment (mobility, dexterity, or visual acuity), as this may affect management (1).
  - Document the patient's desire, goals, and expectation (1).

PHYSICAL EXAM
- Abdominal examination to document any distention or masses
- Complete pelvic and rectal examination. Have patient cough or strain, particularly in an upright (standing) position while examining the distal vagina.

- The GOLD STANDARD is to measure vaginal descent using the Pelvic Organ Prolapse Quantification (POPQ) scale, which is a scale that describes the prolapse in relationship to the vaginal hymen (2). The validated simplified version has four measurements with classification in four stages. Patient is supine with the head of the bed at 45 degrees, performing Valsalva.
  - Stage 1: prolapse in which the distal point is superior or equal to 1 cm above hymen
  - Stage 2: prolapse in which the distal point is between 1 cm above and 1 cm below hymen
  - Stage 3: prolapse in which the distal point is superior or equal to 1 cm below the hymen, but some vaginal mucosa is not everted
  - Stage 4: complete vaginal vault eversion ("procidentia"). Entire vaginal mucosa everted (2)
- A split speculum can be used to observe anterior, posterior, and apical parts of the vagina successively.
- Patient should be standing for maximum descent (2).

DIFFERENTIAL DIAGNOSIS
- Rectal prolapse
- Hemorrhoids
- Bartholin cyst
- Cervical elongation

DIAGNOSTIC TESTS & INTERPRETATION
Initial Tests (lab, imaging)
- Urinalysis if symptomatic POP (1)
- Renal function (serum creatinine) if urinary incontinence and probability of renal impairment (1)
- Imaging: not routinely recommended (1)

Follow-Up Tests & Special Considerations
- Postvoid residual if patient has urinary incontinence
- Urodynamic testing prior to invasive treatment or after treatment failure to plan further therapy (1)
- Imaging of upper urinary tract if hematuria or back pain (1)
- Cystoscopy recommended if patient has hematuria, pain, or discomfort suggesting bladder lesion (1)
- Colonoscopy or sigmoidoscopy if patient has fecal incontinence (1)
- Colonoscopy, air contrast barium enema, and/or computed tomography if change in bowel habits or rectal bleeding (1)

TREATMENT

GENERAL MEASURES
- Treatment should take into account type and severity of symptoms, patient's age, other comorbid conditions, sexual function, infertility, and risk of recurrence.
- Treatment for asymptomatic patients
  - Stage 1 or 2: clinical observation (2)
  - Stage 3 or 4: regular follow-up and evaluation (every 6 to 12 months) (2)
- Treatment is indicated when there is urinary/bowel obstruction or hydronephrosis regardless of the degree of prolapse (2).

- A vaginal pessary should be considered in all women presenting with symptomatic prolapse (8)[B].
  - There are more than 13 types of silicone devices that may be inserted into the vagina to support the pelvic organs.
  - The most commonly used pessaries are the ring pessary and Gellhorn (8).
  - They may prevent prolapse progression and may prove to be an appropriate prevention strategy in the future because the surgical failure rate is around 30% (2).
  - Most women can be successfully fitted with a pessary (8)[B].
  - Satisfaction rate for patients using pessaries is very high (8)[B].
- Complications may be seen with neglected pessaries, such as erosions, abrasions, ulcerations, and vaginal bleeding. Minor complications such as vaginal discharge and odor can be treated without discontinuing pessary use (8)[B]. Vaginal erosion can be treated by removal of pessary and optional vaginal estrogen supplementation.

MEDICATION
First Line
- Treatment of vaginal atrophy with topical estrogens may be beneficial for symptomatic POP (9)[B] if there are no contraindications. Suggested to use in conjunction with pelvic floor muscle training (9)
- Vaginal creams
  - Estradiol cream 0.01% (Estrace)
  - Conjugated estrogens 0.625 mg/day (Premarin)
- Vaginal tablet
  - Estradiol 10 μg (Vagifem)
- Vaginal ring
  - Estradiol 2 mg (Estring)

ISSUES FOR REFERRAL
Referral when pessary or surgery is necessary

ADDITIONAL THERAPIES
Pelvic floor muscle training may reduce the symptoms of POP (1). Pelvic floor muscle training does not affect the degree of prolapse, only the symptoms (1).

SURGERY/OTHER PROCEDURES
- Reconstructive procedures are done with the goal of restoration of vaginal anatomy.
- Reconstructive surgery is associated with a high rate of failure (1 in 3 lifetime risk of repeat surgery). New procedures, using surgical mesh and graft material, have higher success rates but limited follow-up or comparative data (2).

- Abdominal procedures such as sacral colpopexy using graft material have a higher success rate but a longer operating time, longer time to return to normal activity levels, and an increased cost (10)[B]. There may be resulting problems with sexual function and bladder/bowel complaints (2).

 ONGOING CARE

PATIENT EDUCATION
- Patients should be educated about pessary complications and possible symptoms of POP if they are still asymptomatic.
- Limit caffeine product and bladder irritants if urinary symptoms.
- Using insoluble fibers may help patients with bowel complaints such as constipation.

COMPLICATIONS
- There is a risk of vaginal mesh extrusion, erosions, dyspareunia, and pelvic pain after surgical repair (11).
- Delays in diagnosis (4)[B]
  - 61% reported POP symptoms to a physician.
  - 65.9% blamed themselves for the delay (fear of surgery, embarrassment).
  - 1/3 of women blame their physician for the delay in diagnosis.

REFERENCES
1. Abrams P, Andersson KE, Birder L, et al. Fourth International Consultation on Incontinence recommendations of the International Scientific Committee: evaluation and treatment of urinary incontinence, pelvic organ prolapse, and fecal incontinence. *Neurourol Urodyn.* 2010;29(1):213–240.
2. Abed H, Rogers RG. Urinary incontinence and pelvic organ prolapse: diagnosis and treatment for the primary care physician. *Med Clin North Am.* 2008;92(5):1273–1293.
3. Wu JM, Vaughan CP, Goode PS, et al. Prevalence and trends of symptomatic pelvic floor disorders in U.S. women. *Obstet Gynecol.* 2014;123(1):141–148.
4. Krissi H, Eitan R, Peled Y. The role of primary physicians in the diagnostic delay of lower urinary tract and pelvic organ prolapse symptoms. *Eur J Obstet Gynecol Reprod Biol.* 2012;161(1):102–104.
5. Chow D, Rodríguez LV. Epidemiology and prevalence of pelvic organ prolapse. *Curr Opin Urol.* 2013;23(4):293–298.
6. Hagen S, Stark D. Conservative prevention and management of pelvic organ prolapse in women. *Cochrane Database Syst Rev.* 2011;(12): CD003882.
7. Aschkenazi S, Rogers R, Beaumont J, et al. The modified short pelvic organ prolapse/urinary incontinence sexual questionnaire, the PISQ-9, for use in a general female population. http://www.ics.org/Abstracts/Publish/46/000201.pdf. Accessed 2014.
8. Robert M, Schulz JA, Harvey MA, et al. Technical update on pessary use. *J Obstet Gynaecol Can.* 2013;35(7):664–674.
9. Ismail SI, Bain C, Hagen S. Oestrogens for treatment or prevention of pelvic organ prolapse in postmenopausal women. *Cochrane Database Syst Rev.* 2010;(9):CD007063.
10. Maher C, Feiner B, Baessler K, et al. Surgical management of pelvic organ prolapse in women. *Cochrane Database Syst Rev.* 2013;(4):CD004014.
11. Chermansky CJ, Winters JC. Complications of vaginal mesh surgery. *Curr Opin Urol.* 2012; 22(4):287–291.

 CODES

ICD10
- N81.9 Female genital prolapse, unspecified
- N81.10 Cystocele, unspecified
- N99.3 Prolapse of vaginal vault after hysterectomy

CLINICAL PEARLS
- Many women do not discuss POP with their doctor—ask routinely.
- Vaginal pessary should be considered in all patients with symptomatic prolapse.
- Traditional surgical treatment has a high long-term failure rate (1 in 3).

U

UTERINE MYOMAS

Jessica M. Schechtman, DO • Michael P. Hopkins, MD, MEd

 BASICS

DESCRIPTION
- Uterine leiomyomas are well-circumscribed, pseudo-encapsulated, benign monoclonal tumors composed mainly of smooth muscle with varying amounts of fibrous connective tissue (1,2).
- Three major subtypes
  - Subserous: common; external; may become pedunculated
  - Intramural: common; within myometrium; may cause marked uterine enlargement
  - Submucous: ~5% of all cases; internal, evoking abnormal uterine bleeding and infection; occasionally protruding from cervix
- Rare locations: broad, round, and uterosacral ligaments
- System affected: reproductive
- Synonym(s): fibroids; myoma; fibromyoma; myofibroma; fibroleiomyoma

EPIDEMIOLOGY
Incidence
- Cumulative incidence up to 80%
  - 60% in African American women by age 35 years; 80% by age 50 years
  - 40% in Caucasian women by age 35 years; 70% by age 50 years (1,3,4)
- Incidence increases with each decade during reproductive years.
- Rarely seen in premenarchal females
- Predominant sex: females only

ETIOLOGY AND PATHOPHYSIOLOGY
- Enlargement of benign smooth muscle tumors that may lead to symptoms affecting the reproductive, GI, or genitourinary system
- Complex multifactorial process involving transition from normal myocyte to abnormal cells and then to visibly evident tumor (monoclonal expansion)
  - Hormones (1): Increases in estrogen and progesterone are correlated with myoma formation (i.e., rarely seen before menarche). Estrogen receptors in myomas bind more estradiol than normal myometrium (2).
  - Growth factors (1)
    - Increased smooth muscle proliferation (transforming growth factor β [TGF-β], basic fibroblast growth factor [bFGF])
    - Increase DNA synthesis (epidermal growth factor [EGF], platelet-derived growth factor [PDGF], activin, myostatin)
    - Stimulate synthesis of extracellular matrix (TGF-β)
    - Promote mitogenesis (TGF-β, EGF, insulin-like growth factor [IGF], prolactin)
    - Promote angiogenesis (bFGF, vascular endothelial growth factor [VEGF])
  - Vasoconstrictive hypoxia (1): proposed, but not confirmed, mechanism of myometrial injury during menstruation

Genetics
- A variety of somatic chromosomal rearrangements have been described in 40% of uterine myomas.
  - Mutations in the gene encoding mediator complex subunit 12 (MED12) on the X chromosome were found in 70% of myomas in one study (3).
- Higher levels of aromatase and therefore estrogen have been found in myomas in African American women (3).

RISK FACTORS
- African American heritage
  - 2.9 times greater risk than Caucasian women; occur at a younger age, are more numerous, larger, and more symptomatic (1,4)
- Early menarche (<10 years)
- Oral contraceptive use before 16 years old (4)
- Nulliparous
- Hypertension
- Familial predisposition
  - 2.5 times more likely in women with a first-degree relative with myomas (1)
- Obesity
  - Risk increases by 21% with each 10 kg of weight gain (1).
- Alcohol
- Risk decreased by: parity, progesterone only contraceptives, diet (fruits, veggies, low fat dairy) (4)

COMMONLY ASSOCIATED CONDITIONS
Endometrial and breast cancer also associated with high, unopposed estrogen stimulation

 DIAGNOSIS

HISTORY
- Usually asymptomatic; 30% present with abnormal symptoms—usually enlarged uterus or heavy bleeding (2,4).
- Symptoms include the following:
  - Abnormal uterine bleeding: usually heavy/prolonged menses
  - Pain: infrequent; usually associated with torsion of pedunculated myoma, degeneration, or cervical dilation by submucous myoma near cervical os
  - Pressure on bladder: suprapubic discomfort, urinary frequency/obstruction
  - Pressure on rectosigmoid: may cause low back pain, constipation
  - Infertility: rare, estimated 1–2.5% (2); usually from submucous myoma distorting the uterine cavity or interference with implantation

ALERT
Rapid growth, particularly in perimenopausal/postmenopausal patients; may indicate sarcoma. Extremely rare, 0.1–0.3% of cases (2)

PHYSICAL EXAM
- Usually incidental finding on abdominal and pelvic exam
- Firm, smooth nodules/masses arising from uterus
- Masses are mobile without tenderness.

DIFFERENTIAL DIAGNOSIS
- Intrauterine pregnancy
- Cancer, including ovarian, uterine, or leiomyosarcoma
- Cecal/sigmoid tumor
- Appendiceal abscess
- Diverticulitis
- Pelvic kidney
- Urachal cyst

DIAGNOSTIC TESTS & INTERPRETATION
Initial Tests (lab, imaging)
- Pregnancy test
- Hemoglobin
- Pelvic ultrasound: standard confirmatory test; shows characteristic hypoechoic appearance (4,5)

- Saline infusion hysterosonography: helps to distinguish submucosal myomas
- Hysterosalpingogram: evaluates the contour of the endometrial cavity (5)
- CT scan or MRI: provides info on degeneration and special relationships (4); may help to differentiate complex cases or used when uterine artery embolization is planned (5)[B]

Follow-Up Tests & Special Considerations
Consider cancer antigen 125 (CA-125): may be slightly elevated in some cases of uterine myoma but generally more useful in differentiating myomas from various gynecologic adenocarcinomas
- IV pyelogram: if suspect ureteral distortion (5)
- Barium enema

Diagnostic Procedures/Other
- Fractional dilation and curettage: aids in ruling out cervical/uterine carcinomas when clinically suspicious
- Hysteroscopy: helps to diagnose submucosal/intracavitary myomas
- Laparoscopy: useful in complex cases and to rule out other pelvic diseases/disorders

Test Interpretation
- Myomas are usually multiple and vary in size and location; have been reported up to 100 lb
- Gross pathology: firm tumors with characteristic whorl-like trabeculated appearance; a thin pseudocapsular layer is present.
- Microscopic: bundles of smooth muscle mixed with varying amounts of connective tissue elements running in different directions
- Cellular variant has a preponderance of muscle cells. Mitoses are rare.
- May undergo various types of degeneration
  - Hyaline degeneration: very common
  - Calcification: late result of circulatory impairment to myomas
  - Infection and suppuration: most common with submucosal myomas
  - Necrosis: most common with pedunculated myomas secondary to torsion

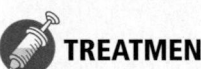 TREATMENT

- Treatment must be individualized and based on symptoms, fertility desires, and time until menopause.
- Medical therapy may be of benefit.
- Patients with minimal symptoms may be treated with iron preparations and analgesics.
- Conservative management of asymptomatic myomas
  - Pelvic exams and ultrasounds at ≥3-month intervals if size remains stable
  - Substantial regression usually occurs after menopause.
- Surgical options should be considered if symptomatic or worrisome myomas are unresponsive to conservative/medical management.

GENERAL MEASURES
Patients not desiring pharmacologic therapy or surgery may consider the following:

- Uterine artery embolization: averages 50% shrinkage of myomas (6)[A]; painful and may cause ovarian failure (1–2%), amenorrhea, postembolization syndrome, or other complications; shorter hospital stay and quicker recovery but no difference in satisfaction compared with hysterectomy (2,4)[B]; high reintervention rate (15–32% by 2 years) compared to hysterectomy/myomectomy (7% by 2 years) (6)

- MR-guided focused ultrasound (MRgFUS): noninvasive, ultrasound transducer passes through abdominal wall and causes coagulative necrosis of fibroid; up to 98% reduction in myoma volume and symptoms. Not appropriate for some types of myomas (2)[B]. Efficacy may be comparable with other hysterectomy-sparing procedures (7)[B]. Fertility has been shown to be preserved (4)[A] although risks and outcomes data is limited (4).

MEDICATION

- Progestins may reduce overall uterine size (5)[B].
  - Norethindrone 10 mg/day
  - Medroxyprogesterone 200 mg IM monthly
  - Levonorgestrel intrauterine device (2)[B]
- Combination oral contraceptives: may help prevent development of new fibroids and control bleeding
  - Contraindications: history of thromboembolic events
- Gonadotropin-releasing hormone agonists
  - Nafarelin (nasal spray), goserelin acetate, and leuprolide
  - Induces abrupt artificial menopause; may reduce myoma symptoms dramatically; induces atrophy of myomas by up to 40% in 2 to 3 months (5)[B]
  - May be valuable as preoperative adjunct to myomectomy/hysterectomy by allowing recovery of anemia, donation of autologous blood, and possibly converting abdominal to vaginal hysterectomy (4,5,8)[B]
  - Not recommended for use >6 months because of osteoporosis risk
  - Following discontinuation, myomas return within 60 days to pretherapy size.
- Antiprogesterones
  - Mifepristone
    - Shown to have similar reduction in myoma size as gonadotropin-releasing hormone agonists (7)[B]
    - Decreases heavy bleeding and increases quality of life (9)[A]
  - Selective progesterone receptor modulator (SPRM)
    - Ulipristal acetate: may be as effective as gonadotropin-releasing hormones with fewer side effects (4)[B]

ISSUES FOR REFERRAL

- Medical therapy may be initiated by a primary care physician/gynecologist after adequate pelvic examination.
- Surgical considerations may be pursued with gynecologic consultation.
- Uterine embolization may be discussed with an interventional radiologist.

SURGERY/OTHER PROCEDURES

- Surgical management is indicated in the following situations (5)[B]:
  - Excessive uterine size or excessive rate of growth (except during pregnancy)
  - Submucosal myomas when associated with hypermenorrhea
  - Pedunculated myomas that are painful or undergo torsion, necrosis, and hemorrhage.
  - If a myoma causes symptoms from pressure on bladder/rectum
  - If differentiation from ovarian mass is not possible

- If associated pelvic disease is present (endometriosis, pelvic inflammatory disease)
- If infertility/habitual abortion is likely due to the anatomic location of the myoma
- Surgical procedures
  - Preliminary pelvic examination, Pap smear, and endometrial biopsy should be performed to rule out malignant/premalignant conditions.
  - Hysterectomy: may be performed vaginally, laparoscopically, robotically, or by laparotomy
    - Effective in relieving symptoms and improving quality of life (4,7)[B]
    - Similar fertility and live birth rates between laparoscopic and abdominal myomectomy (2)[B]
    - FDA discourages the use of laparoscopic power morcellation during hysterectomy or myomectomy for uterine fibroids given the risk of spreading an occult malignancy and all patient should be counseled preoperatively of risk (4).
  - Abdominal, laparoscopic, robotic, or hysteroscopic myomectomy may be performed in younger women who want to maintain fertility (5,10)[B].
  - Hysteroscopic/laparoscopic cautery/laser myoma resection can be performed in selected patients.
  - Endometrial ablation: for small submucosal myomas

INPATIENT CONSIDERATIONS

Admission Criteria/Initial Stabilization
- Usually outpatient
- Inpatient for some surgical procedures

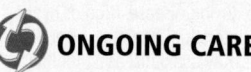 ONGOING CARE

FOLLOW-UP RECOMMENDATIONS
Patient Monitoring
- Pelvic examination and ultrasound: every 2 to 3 months for newly diagnosed symptomatic/excessively large myomas
- Hemoglobin and hematocrit: if uterine bleeding is excessive
- Once uterine size and symptoms stabilize, monitor every 6 to 12 months although no high quality evidence exists (4).

DIET
No restrictions

PATIENT EDUCATION
- Society of Interventional Radiology: http://sirweb.org/patients/uterine-fibroids/
- U.S. Department of Health and Human Services: http://www.womenshealth.gov/publications/our-publications/fact-sheet/uterine-fibroids.html?from=AtoZ
- American Congress of Obstetricians and Gynecologists: http://www.acog.org

PROGNOSIS
- Resection of submucosal fibroids has been associated with increased fertility (7)[B].
- At least 10% of myomas recur after myomectomy; however, only 25% require further treatment (4,7)[B].

COMPLICATIONS
- May mask other gynecologic malignancies (e.g., uterine sarcoma, ovarian cancer)
- Degenerating fibroids may cause pain and bleeding.
- May rarely prolapse through the cervix

Pregnancy Considerations
- Rapid growth of fibroids is common.
- Pregnant women may need additional fetal testing if placenta is located over or near fibroid.

- Complications during pregnancy: abortion, premature labor, 2nd-trimester rapid growth leading to degeneration/pain, 3rd-trimester fetal malpresentation, and dystocia during labor and delivery
- Cesarean section is recommended if the endometrial cavity was entered during myomectomy due to increased risk of uterine rupture.

Geriatric Considerations
In postmenopausal patients with newly diagnosed uterine myoma/enlarging uterine myomas have a high suspicion of uterine sarcoma/other gynecologic malignancy.

REFERENCES

1. Parker WH. Etiology, symptomatology, and diagnosis of uterine myomas. *Fertil Steril.* 2007;87(4):725–736.
2. Duhan N, Sirohiwal D. Uterine myomas revisited. *Eur J Obstet Gynecol Reprod Biol.* 2010;152(2):119–125.
3. Bulun SE. Uterine fibroids. *N Engl J Med.* 2013;369(14):1344–1355.
4. Stewart EA. Clinical practice. Uterine fibroids. *N Engl J Med.* 2015;372(17):1646–1655.
5. Wallach EE, Vlahos NF. Uterine myomas: an overview of development, clinical features, and management. *Obstet Gynecol.* 2004;104(2):393–406.
6. Gupta JK, Sinha A, Lumsden MA, et al. Uterine artery embolization for symptomatic uterine fibroids. *Cochrane Database Syst Rev.* 2014;(12):CD005073.
7. Parker WH. Uterine myomas: management. *Fertil Steril.* 2007;88(2):255–271.
8. Lethaby A, Vollenhoven B, Sowter M. Pre-operative GnRH analogue therapy before hysterectomy or myomectomy for uterine fibroids. *Cochrane Database Syst Rev.* 2001;(2):CD000547.
9. Tristan M, Orozco LJ, Steed A, et al. Mifepristone for uterine fibroids. *Cochrane Database Syst Rev.* 2012;(8):CD007687.
10. NICE interventional procedure guidance 522. Hysteroscopic morcellation of uterine leiomyomas (fibroids). June 2015. Available at www.guidance.nice.org.uk/ipg522

ADDITIONAL READING

Laughlin SK, Schroeder JC, Baird DD. New directions in the epidemiology of uterine fibroids. *Semin Reprod Med.* 2010;28(3):204–217.

 CODES

ICD10
- D25.9 Leiomyoma of uterus, unspecified
- D25.2 Subserosal leiomyoma of uterus
- D25.1 Intramural leiomyoma of uterus

CLINICAL PEARLS

- Uterine myomas are benign smooth muscle tumors composed mainly of fibrous connective tissue.
- Usually incidental finding on pelvic exam or ultrasound but may cause pelvic pain and pressure, abnormal uterine bleeding, and/or infertility
- Management ranges from conservative to medical to surgical.

U

UVEITIS

Shailendra K. Saxena, MD, PhD • Mikayla Spangler, PharmD • Laura K. Klug, PharmD

BASICS

DESCRIPTION
- A nonspecific term used to describe any intraocular inflammatory disorder
- Symptoms vary depending on depth of involvement and associated conditions.
- The uvea is the middle layer of the eye between the sclera and retina. The anterior part of the uvea includes the iris and ciliary body. The posterior part of the uvea is the choroid.
  - Anterior uveitis: refers to ocular inflammation limited to the iris (iritis) alone or iris and ciliary body (iridocyclitis)
  - Intermediate uveitis: refers to inflammation of the structures just posterior to the lens (pars planitis or peripheral uveitis)
  - Posterior uveitis: refers to inflammation of the choroid (choroiditis), retina (retinitis), or vitreous near the optic nerve and macula
- System(s) affected: nervous
- Synonym(s): iritis; iridocyclitis; choroiditis; retinochoroiditis; chorioretinitis; anterior uveitis; posterior uveitis; pars planitis; panuveitis. Synonyms are anatomic descriptions of the focus of the uveal inflammation.

Geriatric Considerations
The inflammatory response to systemic disease may be suppressed.

Pediatric Considerations
- Infection should be the primary consideration.
- Allergies and psychological factors (depression, stress) may serve as a trigger.
- Trauma is also a common cause in this population.

Pregnancy Considerations
May be of importance in the selection of medications

EPIDEMIOLOGY
- Predominant age: all ages
- Predominant sex: male = female, except for human leukocyte antigen B27 (HLA-B27) anterior uveitis: male > female, autoimmune etiology: female > male

Incidence
- Overall prevalence is 38 to 714 cases/100,000 annual incidence.
- Anterior uveitis is the most common.

Prevalence
Iritis is 4 times more prevalent than posterior uveitis.

ETIOLOGY AND PATHOPHYSIOLOGY
- Infectious: may result from viral, bacterial, parasitic, or fungal etiologies
- Suspected immune-mediated: possible autoimmune or immune-complex–mediated mechanism postulated in association with systemic (especially rheumatologic) disorders
  - Autoimmune uveitis (AIU) patients should be referred to an ophthalmologist for local treatment.
- Isolated eye disease
- Idiopathic (~25%)
- Some causative medications may cause uveitis. The most causative medications include rifabutin, bisphosphonates, sulfonamides, metipranolol, topical corticosteroids, brimonidine, prostaglandin analogs,

anti–vascular endothelial growth factor (VEGF) agents, bacillus Calmette-Guerin (BCG) vaccination, and systemic and intraocular cidofovir.
- Masquerade syndromes: diseases such as malignancies that may be mistaken for primary inflammation of the eye

Genetics
- No specific pattern for uveitis in general
- Iritis: 50–70% are HLA-B27–positive.
- Predisposing gene for posterior uveitis associated with Behçet disease may include HLA-B51.

RISK FACTORS
- No specific risk factors
- Higher incidence is seen with specific associated conditions.

COMMONLY ASSOCIATED CONDITIONS
- Viral infections: herpes simplex, herpes zoster, HIV, cytomegalovirus
- Bacterial infections: brucellosis, leprosy, leptospirosis, Lyme disease, propionibacterium infection, syphilis, tuberculosis (TB), Whipple disease
- Parasitic infections: acanthamebiasis, cysticercosis, onchocerciasis, toxocariasis, toxoplasmosis
- Fungal infections: aspergillosis, blastomycosis, candidiasis, coccidioidomycosis, cryptococcosis, histoplasmosis, sporotrichosis
- Suspected immune-mediated: ankylosing spondylitis, Behçet disease, Crohn disease, drug or hypersensitivity reaction, interstitial nephritis, juvenile rheumatoid arthritis, Kawasaki disease, multiple sclerosis, psoriatic arthritis, Reiter syndrome, relapsing polychondritis, sarcoidosis, Sjögren syndrome, systemic lupus erythematosus, ulcerative colitis, vasculitis, vitiligo, Vogt-Koyanagi (Harada) syndrome
- Isolated eye disease: acute multifocal placoid pigmentary epitheliopathy, acute retinal necrosis, bird-shot choroidopathy, Fuchs heterochromatic cyclitis, glaucomatocyclitic crisis, lens-induced uveitis, multifocal choroiditis, pars planitis, serpiginous choroiditis, sympathetic ophthalmia, trauma
- Masquerade syndromes: leukemia, lymphoma, retinitis pigmentosa, retinoblastoma

DIAGNOSIS

HISTORY
- Decreased visual acuity
- Pain, photophobia, blurring of vision (1)[C]
  - Usually acute
- Anterior uveitis (~80% of patients with uveitis) (1)[C]
  - Generally acute in onset
  - Deep eye pain
  - Photophobia (consensual)
- Intermediate and posterior uveitis (2)
  - Unresolving floaters
  - Generally insidious in onset
  - More commonly bilateral

PHYSICAL EXAM
Slit-lamp exam and indirect ophthalmoscopy are necessary for precise diagnosis (1)[C].
- Anterior uveitis (~80% of patients with uveitis)
  - Conjunctival vessel dilation
  - Perilimbal (circumcorneal) dilation of episcleral and scleral vessels (ciliary flush)

- Small pupillary size of affected eye
- Hypopyon or hyphema (WBCs or RBCs pooled in the anterior chamber)
- Frequently unilateral (95% of HLA-B27–associated cases); if first occurrence and otherwise asymptomatic, no further diagnostic testing is needed (1)[C].
- Bilateral involvement and systemic symptoms (fever, fatigue, abdominal pain) may be associated with interstitial nephritis (1)[C].
- Systemic disease is most likely to be associated with anterior uveitis (in one study, 53% of patients were found to have systemic disease) (1)[C].
- Intermediate and posterior uveitis
  - More commonly bilateral
  - Posterior inflammation will generally cause minimal pain or redness unless associated with an iritis.

DIFFERENTIAL DIAGNOSIS
- Acute angle-closure glaucoma
- Conjunctivitis
- Episcleritis
- Keratitis
- Scleritis

DIAGNOSTIC TESTS & INTERPRETATION
No specific test for the diagnosis of uveitis. Tests for etiologic factors or associated conditions should be based on history and physical exam (1)[C].

Initial Tests (lab, imaging)
- CBC, BUN, creatinine (interstitial nephritis) (1)[C]
- HLA-B27 typing (ankylosing spondylitis, Reiter syndrome) (1)[C]
- Antinuclear antibody, ESR (systemic lupus erythematosus, Sjögren syndrome) (1)[C]
- Venereal disease research laboratory (VDRL) test, fluorescent titer antibody (syphilis) (1)[C]
- Fluorescent treponemal antibody absorption (FTA-ABS) or microhemagglutination assay for antibodies to *Treponema pallidum* (MHA-TP) (1)[C]
- Purified protein derivative (PPD) tuberculin skin test (TB) (1)[C]
- Lyme serology (Lyme disease) (1)[C]
- Disorders that may alter lab results: immunodeficiency
- Chest x-ray (sarcoidosis, histoplasmosis, TB, lymphoma) (1)[C]
- Sacroiliac radiograph (ankylosing spondylitis) (1)[C]

Diagnostic Procedures/Other
Slit-lamp exam (1)[C]

Test Interpretation
- Keratic precipitates
- Inflammatory cells in anterior chamber or vitreous
- Synechiae (fibrous tissue scarring between iris and lens)
- Macular edema
- Perivasculitis of retinal vessels

TREATMENT

GENERAL MEASURES
- Outpatient care with urgent ophthalmologic consultation
- Medical therapy is best initiated following full ophthalmologic evaluation.

- Treatment of underlying cause, if identified
- Anti-inflammatory therapy

MEDICATION
First Line
- The treatment depends on the etiology, location, and severity of the inflammation.
- Prednisolone acetate 1% ophthalmic suspension: 2 drops to the affected eye q1h initially, tapering to once a day with improvement
  - Contraindications
    - Hypersensitivity to the medication or component of the preparation
    - Topical corticosteroid therapy is contraindicated in uveitis secondary to infectious etiologies, unless used in conjunction with appropriate anti-infectious agents.
  - Precautions
    - Topical corticosteroids may increase intraocular pressure, increase susceptibility to infections, impair corneal or scleral wound healing, or cause corneal epithelial toxicity or crystalline keratopathy. Prolonged use may cause cataract formation and exacerbate existing herpetic keratitis, which may masquerade as iritis.
  - Significant possible interactions
- Systemic corticosteroids are useful for maintenance therapy for patients with noninfectious uveitis. These should always be used with other immunosuppressive medications for steroid-sparing effects; prednisone 5 to 10 mg daily (3,4)[B].
- Cycloplegic agents may be used to dilate the eye and relieve pain. Agents include scopolamine hydrobromide 0.25% (Isopto Hyoscine) or atropine 1% 1 to 2 drops up to QID or homatropine hydrobromide (Isopto) 2% or 5% 1 to 2 drops BID or as often as q3h if necessary (1)[C].
  - Contraindications
    - Cycloplegia is contraindicated in patients known to have, or be predisposed to, glaucoma.
  - Precautions
    - Use extreme caution in infants, young children, and elderly because of increased susceptibility to systemic effects.

Second Line
- Anti-inflammatory: prednisolone sodium phosphate 1%, dexamethasone sodium phosphate 0.1%, dexamethasone suspension, rimexolone 1% (Vexol), and loteprednol etabonate 0.5% (Lotemax), difluprednate (Durezol) 0.05% (1,4)[C]
  - Rimexolone 1% (Vexol) may be equally effective as prednisolone acetate 1% for short-term treatment of anterior uveitis (1)[C].
  - Loteprednol etabonate (Lotemax) may not be as effective as prednisolone acetate 1% but may be less likely to increase intraocular pressure in cases of acute anterior uveitis.
- Periocular corticosteroids may be injected with triamcinolone acetonide being most commonly used; 40 mg/1 mL (5)[C].
- Intravitreous corticosteroid deposits may also be used for long-term maintenance. Fluocinolone acetonide (Retisert) 590 μg released >30 months, dexamethasone (Ozurdex) 0.7 mg released slowly >3 to 6 months (4,5)[B].
  - Retisert has caused all patients to develop cataracts and significant increases in intraocular pressure in about 2/3 of patients, whereas Ozurdex

had only 1/4 of patients require medication for increased intraocular pressure and 15% develop cataracts (5)[C].
- Intravitreal corticosteroid injections are used only in severe cases of recurrence; triamcinolone acetonide 4 to 20 mg/0.1 mL, dexamethasone phosphate 0.4 mg/0.1 mL, dexamethasone implant (Ozurdex)
  - Ozurdex has a longer effect than triamcinolone acetonide.
- Immunosuppressive agents including antimetabolites (methotrexate, azathioprine, and mycophenolate mofetil), T-cell inhibitors (cyclosporine, tacrolimus, and sirolimus), and alkylating agents (cyclophosphamide, chlorambucil) may be employed in cases resistant to initial treatment but close monitoring is required (4,5)[C].
- Although biologic therapy has been used for refractory uveitis, the sparsity of randomized clinical trials as well as high cost and adverse effect potential of these agents limit their use (3,4)[C].
- Systemic and ophthalmic preparations of NSAIDs may provide some symptom relief (1)[C].

ISSUES FOR REFERRAL
Caution should be used when using empiric treatment; referral to an ophthalmologist is recommended in most cases.

SURGERY/OTHER PROCEDURES
Various surgical procedures may be used therapeutically for visual rehabilitation, diagnostically, or to manage complications associated with uveitis (6).

ONGOING CARE

FOLLOW-UP RECOMMENDATIONS
Patient Monitoring
- Complete history and physical to evaluate for associated systemic disease
- Ophthalmologic follow-up as recommended by consultant

PATIENT EDUCATION
- Instruct on proper method for instilling eye drops.
- Wear dark glasses if photophobia is a problem.

PROGNOSIS
- Depends on the presence of causal diseases or associated conditions
- Uveitis resulting from infections (systemic or local) tends to resolve with eradication of the underlying infection.
- Uveitis associated with seronegative arthropathies tends to be acute (lasting <3 months) and frequently recurrent.

COMPLICATIONS
- Cycloplegia: paralysis of the ciliary muscle of the eye, resulting in a loss of accommodation
- Loss of vision as a result of the following:
  - Keratic precipitate deposition on the corneal or lens surfaces (1)
  - Increased intraocular pressure, acute angle-closure glaucoma (1)
  - Formation of synechiae
  - Cataract formation (1)
  - Vasculitis with vascular occlusion, retinal infarction
  - Macular edema (1)
  - Optic nerve damage

REFERENCES
1. American Optometric Association. Optometric clinical practice guideline: care of the patient with anterior uveitis. http://www.aoa.org/documents/CPG-7.pdf. Accessed 2015.
2. Selmi C. Diagnosis and classification of autoimmune uveitis. *Autoimmun Rev.* 2014;13(4–5): 591–594.
3. de Smet MD, Taylor SR, Bodaghi B, et al. Understanding uveitis: the impact of research on visual outcomes. *Prog Retin Eye Res.* 2011;30(6): 452–470.
4. Babu K, Mahendradas P. Medical management of uveitis—current trends. *Indian J Ophthalmol.* 2013;61(6):277–283.
5. Gallego-Pinazo R, Dolz-Marco R, Martínez-Castillo S, et al. Update on the principles and novel local and systemic therapies for the treatment of noninfectious uveitis. *Inflamm Allergy Drug Targets.* 2013;12(1):38–45.
6. Murthy SI, Pappuru RR, Latha KM, et al. Surgical management in patient with uveitis. *Indian J Ophthalmol.* 2013;61(6):284–290.

ADDITIONAL READING
- Levy RA, de Andrade FA, Foeldvari I. Cutting-edge issues in autoimmune uveitis. *Clin Rev Allergy Immunol.* 2011;41(2):214–223.
- Majumder PD, Biswas J. Pediatric uveitis: an update. *Oman J Ophthalmol.* 2013;6(3):140–150.
- Pan J, Kapur M, McCallum R. Noninfectious immune-mediated uveitis and ocular inflammation. *Curr Allergy Asthma Rep.* 2014;14(1):409.
- Yang MM, Lai TY, Luk FO, et al. The roles of genetic factors in uveitis and their clinical significance. *Retina.* 2014;34(1):1–11.

SEE ALSO

Conjunctivitis, Acute; Glaucoma, Primary Closed-Angle; Scleritis

CODES

ICD10
- H20.9 Unspecified iridocyclitis
- H30.90 Unspecified chorioretinal inflammation, unspecified eye
- H20.019 Primary iridocyclitis, unspecified eye

CLINICAL PEARLS
- Symptoms vary depending on depth of involvement and associated conditions but should be suspected when eye pain is associated with visual changes.
- Severe or unresponsive uveitis may require therapy, including periocular injection of corticosteroids, sustained-release corticosteroid implants, systemic corticosteroids, cytotoxic agents, immunosuppressive agents, immunomodulatory agents, or tumor necrosis factor inhibitors.

VAGINAL ADENOSIS
Maeve K. Hopkins, MA, MD • Michael P. Hopkins, MD, MEd

BASICS

DESCRIPTION
- The normal vagina is lined with squamous epithelium. Adenosis is characterized by the presence of columnar epithelium or glandular tissue in the wall of the vagina.
- Around week 15 of embryologic development, the müllerian system, which forms the upper 2/3 of the vagina, fuses with the invaginating cloaca or urogenital sinus to form the lower 1/3 of the vagina. Squamous metaplasia from the cloacal region then produces squamous epithelium within the vagina (1).
- Adenosis occurs when this squamous epithelium fails to epithelialize the vagina completely.
- Three main types of adenosis epithelium described
  - Endocervical
  - Endometrial
  - Tubal
- System(s) affected: reproductive

Geriatric Considerations
- Adenosis is a disorder of the young female. By menopause, the vagina and cervix should be completely epithelialized.
- The presence of glandular epithelium in the postmenopausal patient is an indication for excision and close evaluation for the possibility of a well-differentiated adenocarcinoma.

Pregnancy Considerations
Pregnancy produces a wide eversion of the transformation zone of the cervix. This occasionally will become so widely everted that it will extend onto the vaginal fornices, leading to the impression of adenosis. This will resolve after the pregnancy is completed.

EPIDEMIOLOGY

Incidence
- Although the cumulative incidence of vaginal adenosis is unknown, the incidence of cloacal malformations is 1/20,000 to 1/25,000 live births.
- Although spontaneous vaginal adenosis appears to be fairly common (10% of adult women), it is mostly an insignificant coincidental finding. Widespread symptomatic involvement is rare (2).

Prevalence
- In the United States, adenosis is relatively common; affecting 10–20% of young females studied. As maturation progresses with puberty, epithelialization occurs.

- Predominant age
  - Age <1 month: 15%
  - Prepubertal: typically absent
  - Age 13 to 25 years: 13%
  - Age >25 years: decreasing prevalence, uncommon beyond age 30 years (2)

ETIOLOGY AND PATHOPHYSIOLOGY
- In most young females, the etiology is incomplete squamous metaplasia or epithelialization. This occurs as a natural phenomenon and resolves with age.
- Described as congenital or acquired (2)
  - Congenital: proliferation of the remnant müllerian epithelium in the vagina due to exposure to diethylstilbestrol (DES) in utero (DES daughters)
  - Transformation-related protein 63 (TRP63/p63) marks the cell fate decision of müllerian duct epithelium to become squamous epithelium in the cervix and vagina. DES disrupts the TRP63 expression and induces adenosis lesions (3). It has also been suggested that DES induces vaginal adenosis by inhibiting the BMP4/Activin A-regulated vaginal cell fate decision through a downregulation of RUNX1 (4).
  - Acquired: trauma and inflammation causing spontaneous de novo changes or changes in an acquired lesion in the vaginal epithelium
  - Additional reports have documented adenosis occurring subsequent to sulfonamide-induced Stevens–Johnson syndrome and after treatment of vaginal condylomas with 5-fluorouracil (5).

RISK FACTORS
Adenosis of the vagina/cervix may arise in up to 90% of DES daughters, and there is a 40-fold increased risk of the subsequent development of clear cell adenocarcinoma (6).

GENERAL PREVENTION
None: last DES exposure in the 1970s

COMMONLY ASSOCIATED CONDITIONS
DES exposure
- Adenosis from DES exposure should lead to an evaluation of other DES-related abnormalities.
- Müllerian tract anomalies associated with DES exposure include cervical hood, cervical ridge, shortened cervix, incompetent cervix, and T-shaped uterine cavity.
- Patients with known DES exposure should have their reproductive tract evaluated prior to conception.

- Most patients with adenosis have not been DES-exposed and do not require evaluation of the reproductive system.
- DES is a synthetic, nonsteroidal estrogen that was used to prevent spontaneous abortions or premature deliveries from 1938 to 1971 (6). An estimated 5 million women were prescribed DES during this period (3).
- The FDA issued a drug bulletin in 1971 advising physicians to stop prescribing DES to pregnant women because of its link to vaginal clear cell adenocarcinoma in DES daughters (6).

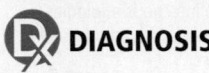

DIAGNOSIS

HISTORY
- Maternal DES exposure
- Complaints of
  - Profuse mucoid vaginal discharge from the glandular epithelium
  - Pruritus
  - Pain/soreness of the vaginal introitus
  - Postcoital bleeding
  - Dyspareunia

PHYSICAL EXAM
On pelvic exam, adenosis appearance is varied: patchy or diffuse red stippling, granularity or nodularity, single or multiple cysts, erosions, ulcers, or warty protuberances that may even extend to the vulva.

DIFFERENTIAL DIAGNOSIS
- Erosive lichen planus
- Fixed drug eruption
- Erythema multiforme
- Bullous skin disease
- Adenocarcinoma
  - A thorough evaluation for adenocarcinoma of the vagina arising in adenosis should be done.
  - A biopsy may be necessary to ensure that the process represents only benign adenosis.

DIAGNOSTIC TESTS & INTERPRETATION
Initial Tests (lab, imaging)
Four-quadrant Pap smear should be used liberally to isolate quadrants of the vagina that may contain abnormalities. No imaging is indicated, unless diagnosed with underlying malignancy.

Follow-Up Tests & Special Considerations
Pap smear can be followed by colposcopy and biopsy.

Diagnostic Procedures/Other
Colposcopy should be used to outline areas of adenosis to ensure that no malignancy is present.

Test Interpretation
- Biopsy will show benign glandular epithelium.
- Biopsies in the areas of ongoing squamous metaplasia are typical (7).

TREATMENT

GENERAL MEASURES
- Unless malignancy is present, conservative treatment is indicated.
- In most young females with this condition, it will resolve with expectant management (2).
- Treatment is warranted in women with severe subjective symptoms that impair the quality of life (8).
- For patients with focal lesions and no history of DES exposure, simple excision appears to be an effective modality of treatment (5)

ISSUES FOR REFERRAL
Malignancy found on biopsy warrants referral to gynecologic oncology specialist.

SURGERY/OTHER PROCEDURES
- Aggressive therapy, such as laser or surgical excision, is necessary if premalignant or malignant changes arise (4).
- Symptomatic treatment with carbon dioxide laser coagulation, unipolar coagulation, or, lastly, vaginal resection (2)

INPATIENT CONSIDERATIONS
Admission Criteria/Initial Stabilization
Outpatient management

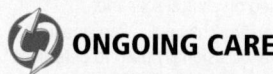

ONGOING CARE

FOLLOW-UP RECOMMENDATIONS
Patient Monitoring
If the initial colposcopy is normal, a yearly four-quadrant Pap smear of the vagina and of the cervix is all that is necessary.

DIET
No special diet

PATIENT EDUCATION
- No limitations
- It is not necessary to avoid intercourse or placing objects in the vagina.
- The patient should be educated to keep normal guideline-recommended pelvic and Pap smear appointments. In most situations, this is benign, and expectant management is all that is necessary.
- http://www.acog.org/

PROGNOSIS
- It is expected that most patients will have squamous metaplasia and epithelialization with complete resolution of the adenosis.
- The rare patient, 1/1,000 to 1/10,000, may develop adenocarcinoma in the adenosis and will require definitive therapy as for vaginal cancer.
  - Cumulative incidence of progression of adenosis to adenocarcinoma is 1.5/1,000 for DES daughters (6).

COMPLICATIONS
- Infertility with DES association
- Adverse pregnancy outcome with DES association
- Adenocarcinoma of vagina
- Clear cell adenocarcinoma with DES association

REFERENCES
1. Reich O, Fritsch H. The developmental origin of cervical and vaginal epithelium and their clinical consequences: a systematic review. *J Low Genit Tract Dis*. 2014;18(4):358–360.
2. Kranl C, Zelger B, Kofler H, et al. Vulval and vaginal adenosis. *Br J Dermatol*. 1998;139(1):128–131.
3. Laronda MM, Unno K, Butler LM, et al. The development of cervical and vaginal adenosis as a result of diethylstilbestrol exposure in utero. *Differentiation*. 2012;84(3):252–260.
4. Larondo M, Unno K, Ishi K, et al. Diethylstilbestrol induces vaginal adenosis by disrupting SMAD/RUNX1-mediated cell fate decision in the Müllerian duct epithelium. *Dev Biol*. 2013;381(1):5–16.
5. Martin AA, Atkins KA, Lonergan CL, et al. Vaginal adenosis as a dermatologic complaint. *J Am Acad Dermatol*. 2013;69(2):e92–e93.
6. National Toxicology Program, Department of Health and Human Services. Diethylstilbestrol. *Report on Carcinogens*. 12th ed. Research Triangle Park: National Toxicology Program, U.S. Department of Health and Human Services. 2011:159–161.
7. Chattopadhyay I, Cruickshan DJ, Packer M. Non diethylstilbestrol induced vaginal adenosis—a case series and review of literature. *Eur J Gynaecol Oncol*. 2001;22(4):260–262.
8. Cebesoy FB, Kutlar I, Aydin A. Vaginal adenosis successfully treated with simple unipolar cauterization. *J Natl Med Assoc*. 2007;99(2):166–167.

ADDITIONAL READING
- Bamigboye AA, Morris J. Oestrogen supplementation, mainly diethylstilbestrol, for preventing miscarriages and other adverse pregnancy outcomes. *Cochrane Database Syst Rev*. 2003;(3):CD004353.
- Sandberg EC. The incidence and distribution of occult vaginal adenosis. *Am J Obstet Gynecol*. 1968;101(3):322–334.

 SEE ALSO

Vaginal Malignancy

 CODES

ICD10
- Q52.4 Other congenital malformations of vagina
- N89.8 Other specified noninflammatory disorders of vagina
- T38.5X5A Adverse effect of other estrogens and progestogens, initial encounter

CLINICAL PEARLS
- Adenosis is characterized by the presence of columnar epithelium or glandular tissue in the wall of the vagina.
- Adenosis is more common among the daughters of women exposed to DES.
- Adenosis is rarely associated with an underlying vaginal malignancy.

V

VAGINAL BLEEDING DURING PREGNANCY

Virginia Van Duyne, MD

 BASICS

DESCRIPTION

- Vaginal bleeding during pregnancy has many causes and ranges in severity from benign with normal pregnancy outcome to life-threatening for both infant and mother.
- Etiology can be from the vagina, cervix, uterus, fetus, or placenta. The differential diagnosis is guided by the gestational age of the fetus.

EPIDEMIOLOGY

Prevalence

- In early pregnancy: 7–25% of patients
- In late pregnancy: 0.3–2% of patients

ETIOLOGY AND PATHOPHYSIOLOGY

- Many times the cause is unknown.
- Anytime in pregnancy:
  - Cervicitis (infectious or noninfectious)
  - Vaginal or cervical trauma (including postcoital)
  - Cervical lesion or neoplasia
  - Hyperemia of cervix (increased blood flow from pregnancy)
- Early pregnancy:
  - For up to 50% of early pregnancy bleeding, no cause is ever found.
  - Ectopic pregnancy: leading cause of 1st-trimester maternal death in the United States. Risk factors: previous ectopic, trauma to fallopian tubes (tubal surgery, infection, tumor), congenital anomaly of tubes, in utero diethylstilbestrol (DES) exposure, current use of IUD, history of infertility, tobacco use
  - Spontaneous abortion: risk factors: advanced maternal age (AMA), alcohol use, tobacco use, anesthetic gas, heavy caffeine use, cocaine use, chronic maternal diseases (poorly controlled diabetes mellitus [DM], celiac disease, autoimmune diseases such as antiphospholipid syndrome), short interconception time (3 to 6 months), current use of IUD, maternal infection (e.g., herpes simplex virus [HSV], gonorrhea, chlamydia, toxoplasmosis, listeriosis, HIV, syphilis, malaria), medications (e.g., retinoids, methotrexate, NSAIDs), multiple previous therapeutic abortions, previous spontaneous abortion, toxins (arsenic, lead, polyurethane), uterine abnormalities (congenital, adhesions, fibroids)
  - Implantation bleeding: benign, about 6 days after fertilization
  - Uterine fibroids
  - Subchorionic bleed: in late 1st trimester
  - Low-lying placenta
  - Gestational trophoblastic disease: hydatidiform mole (most common), choriocarcinoma, or placental-site trophoblastic tumors
- Late pregnancy:
  - Bloody show of labor (mucus plug)
  - Placenta previa: painless bleeding; occurs in 0.4% deliveries in the United States. Risk factors: previous history of placenta previa, previous uterine surgery (cesarean section, D&C), chronic hypertension, multiparity, multiple gestation, tobacco use, AMA

- Placental abruption: painful bleeding; occurs in 1–2% deliveries in the United States. Risk factors: previous placental abruption, 1st-trimester bleeding, hypertension, preeclampsia, multiple gestation, tobacco, cocaine or methamphetamine use, unexplained elevated maternal α-fetoprotein, poly- or oligohydramnios, AMA, trauma to abdomen, premature rupture of membranes, thrombophilia, short umbilical cord, male fetus, chorioamnionitis, nutritional deficiency
- Vasa previa: minimal bleeding with fetal distress; rare (1:2,500 deliveries). Risk factors: in vitro fertilization, multiple gestation, placental abnormalities (low-lying position, bilobate, succenturiate lobe, velamentous insertion of umbilical cord)
- Placenta accreta, increta, percreta: risk factors: uterine scar (e.g., from cesarean section, endometrial ablation or D&C), current placenta previa, AMA, tobacco use, multiparity, uterine anomalies, uterine fibroids, hypertension
- Uterine rupture: vaginal bleeding, abnormal fetal heart rate, and disordered or hypertonic uterine contractions with or without pain. Risk factors: previous cesarean section (most common), trauma, use of oxytocin or prostaglandins, multiparity, external cephalic version, placental abruption, shoulder dystocia, placenta percreta, müllerian duct anomalies, history of pelvic radiation

RISK FACTORS

See specific etiologies in earlier discussion.

GENERAL PREVENTION

- Address modifiable risk factors such as domestic violence and tobacco and drug use.
- If placenta or vasa previa, nothing per vagina

 DIAGNOSIS

HISTORY

- Anytime in pregnancy: quality of pregnancy dating, context (e.g., following bowel movement, during voiding, after intercourse, drug use, or trauma including domestic violence), amount of bleeding, obstetrical history, personal or family history of inherited bleeding disorders
- Early pregnancy: severe nausea/vomiting (can be associated with molar pregnancy); amount of bleeding, pelvic pain, or suprapubic cramping (e.g., spontaneous abortion, ectopic) complications in previous pregnancies (e.g., spontaneous abortion, abruption, 1st-trimester vaginal bleeding)
- Late pregnancy: contractions (labor), abdominal pain especially between contractions (abruption, uterine rupture), presence or absence of fetal movement, rupture of membranes
- See "Etiology and Pathophysiology" for additional pertinent history.

PHYSICAL EXAM

- Vital signs: When present, signs of hemodynamic instability are first tachycardia and tachypnea, then hypotension and thready pulse.

- Abdomen: uterine tenderness, fundal height (increasing fundal height may be associated with placental abruption)
- Speculum: Visualize cervix and identify source of bleeding (from cervical os or from within vagina).
- Cervix: assess for dilation; required to assess for labor but should not be performed until placenta previa ruled out via ultrasound
- Fetal monitoring: Doppler heart tones in early pregnancy; external fetal monitoring for gestational age >26 weeks

DIFFERENTIAL DIAGNOSIS

- Hematuria (UTI, kidney stones)
- Rectal bleeding

DIAGNOSTIC TESTS & INTERPRETATION

Initial Tests (lab, imaging)

- CBC
- Blood type and screen; if significant hemorrhage, type and cross-match
- Quantitative β-human chorionic gonadotropin (β-hCG):
  - Prior to 12 weeks, levels can be followed serially every 2 days with following trends:
    - Doubles or at least 66% rise in 48 hours in normal pregnancy
    - Falls in spontaneous abortion
    - Extremely high in molar pregnancy
    - Rises gradually (<50% in 48 hours) or plateaus in ectopic pregnancy
- Transvaginal ultrasound should be used to confirm an intrauterine pregnancy (IUP) when the quantitative β-hCG >2,000 (1)[A].
- Other lab tests based on clinical scenario:
  - Wet mount, gonorrhea/chlamydia, Pap smear
  - Progesterone level occasionally used to determine viability in threatened abortion (<5 indicates not viable, >25 indicates viability, 5 to 25 is equivocal).
  - Bleeding time, fibrinogen, and fibrin split products: if suspect coagulopathy or abruption
  - Kleihauer-Betke: low sensitivity and specificity for abruption; helpful for dosing Rho(d) immune globulin (RhoGAM)
- Ultrasound is the preferred imaging modality.
  - Early pregnancy:
    - Gestational sac seen at 5 to 6 weeks; fetal heartbeat observed by 8 to 9 weeks
    - Diagnostic of ectopic with nearly 100% sensitivity when β-hCG level 1,500 to 2,000 mIU/mL. If no IUP is present and ultrasound does not confirm ectopic pregnancy, serial quantitative β-hCG values should be followed (2)[C].
  - Late pregnancy:
    - Proceed to rule out placenta previa with ultrasound, labor with serial cervical exams, and abruption with external fetal monitoring.

ALERT

Confirm fetal presentation and placental position prior to cervical exam.

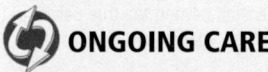 **TREATMENT**

MEDICATION

First Line

- Treat underlying cause of bleeding, if identified.
- If mother is Rh negative, give RhoGAM to prevent autoimmunization. In late pregnancy, dose according to the amount of estimated fetomaternal hemorrhage.
- If cause of bleeding is preterm labor, consider betamethasone for fetal lung maturity if <34 weeks' gestation. Tocolytics may be used to prolong pregnancy to allow for course of steroids.
- If threatened abortion: Consider progesterone (relative risk 0.53) (3)[A].
- If mother has an inherited bleeding disorder or if bleeding is severe, consider recombinant or donor blood products.

SURGERY/OTHER PROCEDURES

- Cesarean section may be indicated for recurrent or uncontrolled bleeding with placenta or vasa previa.
- If ectopic is diagnosed, immediate surgical treatment may be needed. Some early ectopic pregnancies can be treated medically if certain criteria are met (2)[C].
- Surgical uterine evacuation is necessary for molar pregnancy due to malignant potential (4)[C].
- Incomplete or inevitable spontaneous abortion: Management is patient centered. In the absence of infection, patient may elect expectant, medical, or surgical management. If expectant management, typically wait 2 weeks for patient to complete abortion; most complete by 9 days. If at 2 weeks abortion is not completed or medical management has failed, surgical intervention (D&C or aspiration) is generally indicated (5)[A]. May send tissue to pathology to confirm.

INPATIENT CONSIDERATIONS

Admission Criteria/Initial Stabilization

- In early pregnancy: based on quantity of bleeding, need for surgical treatment for ectopic pregnancy, or presence of infection in case of spontaneous abortion
- In late pregnancy, if significant bleeding and/or presence of maternal or fetal compromise
- In late pregnancy with trauma, if ≥2 contractions/10 minutes

Discharge Criteria

- In late pregnancy, may discharge when bleeding has stopped; labor, previa, and abruption have been ruled out; and fetal heart tracing is normal.
- After trauma in late pregnancy, may discharge home if normal fetal heart tracing for ≥4 hours with <2 contractions/10 minutes

 ONGOING CARE

Patient Monitoring

- Patient should be instructed to report any increase in the amount or frequency of bleeding and to seek immediate care if experiencing fever, abdominal pain, or sudden increased bleeding. Patient should save any tissue passed vaginally for examination.
- Frequency of outpatient follow-up as indicated based on etiology of bleeding

PATIENT EDUCATION

- American Academy of Family Physicians (AAFP): www.familydoctor.org
- American College of Obstetricians & Gynecologists (ACOG): www.acog.org

PROGNOSIS

- Prognosis depends on the etiology of vaginal bleeding, severity of bleeding, and rapidity of diagnosis.
- Maternal mortality is 31.9 deaths/100,000 ectopic pregnancies.
- 1/2 of patients with early pregnancy bleeding miscarry. If fetal heart activity (ultrasound) present in 1st-trimester bleed, <10% chance of pregnancy loss.
- Heavy bleeding in early pregnancy, particularly when accompanied by pain, is associated with higher risk of spontaneous abortion. Spotting and light episodes are not, especially if lasting only 1 to 2 days.
- Subchorionic hemorrhage has about 2- to 3-fold increased risk of spontaneous abortion. Smaller hemorrhage and presence of viable fetal heart rate confer lower risk of loss. Most resolve spontaneously.
- Women with early pregnancy bleeding have an increased risk of preterm delivery, premature rupture of membranes, manual removal of placenta, placental abruption, elective cesarean delivery, and term labor induction later in the same pregnancy. These women also have an increased risk of adverse pregnancy outcomes, including hyperbilirubinemia, congenital anomalies, NICU admission, and reduced neonatal birth weight. Finally, there is an increased risk in subsequent pregnancies of recurrence of early pregnancy bleeding.
- Bed rest has not been shown to affect the outcome of bleeding in early pregnancy but may be indicated for bleeding in late pregnancy with placenta or vasa previa or with maternal hypertension.

REFERENCES

1. Crochet JR, Bastian LA, Chireau MV. Does this woman have an ectopic pregnancy? The rational clinical examination systematic review. *JAMA*. 2013;309(16):1722–1729.
2. Deutchman M, Tubay AT, Turok D. First trimester bleeding. *Am Fam Physician*. 2009;79(11):985–994.
3. Wahabi HA, Fayed AA, Esmaeil SA, et al. Progestogen for treating threatened miscarriage. *Cochrane Database Syst Rev*. 2011;(12):CD005943.
4. Snell BJ. Assessment and management of bleeding in the first trimester of pregnancy. *J Midwifery Womens Health*. 2009;54(6):483–491.
5. Nanda K, Lopez LM, Grimes DA, et al. Expectant care versus surgical treatment for miscarriage. *Cochrane Database Syst Rev*. 2012;(3):CD003518.

ADDITIONAL READING

- Chi C, Kadir RA. Inherited bleeding disorders in pregnancy. *Best Pract Res Clin Obstet Gynaecol*. 2012;26(1):103–117.
- Dadkhah F, Kashanian M, Eliasi G. A comparison between the pregnancy outcome in women both with or without threatened abortion. *Early Hum Dev*. 2010;86(3):193–196.

- Griebel CP, Halvorsen J, Golemon TB, et al. Management of spontaneous abortion. *Am Fam Physician*. 2005;72(7):1243–1250.
- Grimes DA. Estimation of pregnancy-related mortality risk by pregnancy outcome, United States, 1991 to 1999. *Am J Obstet Gynecol*. 2006;194(1):92–94.
- Hasan R, Baird DD, Herring AH, et al. Association between first-trimester vaginal bleeding and miscarriage. *Obstet Gynecol*. 2009;114(4):860–867.
- Lykke JA, Dideriksen KL, Lidegaard O, et al. First-trimester vaginal bleeding and complications later in pregnancy. *Obstet Gynecol*. 2010;115(5):935–944.
- Magann EF, Cummings JE, Niederhauser A, et al. Antepartum bleeding of unknown origin in the second half of pregnancy: a review. *Obstet Gynecol Surv*. 2005;60(11):741–745.
- Mercier FJ, Van de Velde M. Major obstetric hemorrhage. *Anesthesiol Clin*. 2008;26(1):53–66.
- Mukul LV, Teal SB. Current management of ectopic pregnancy. *Obstet Gynecol Clin North Am*. 2007;34(3):403–419.
- Oyelese Y, Ananth CV. Placental abruption. *Obstet Gynecol*. 2006;108(4):1005–1016.
- Publications Committee, Society for Maternal-Fetal Medicine, Belfort MA. Placenta accreta. *Am J Obstet Gynecol*. 2010;203(5):430–439.
- Sakornbut E, Leeman L, Fontaine P. Late pregnancy bleeding. *Am Fam Physician*. 2007;75(8):1199–1206.
- Walfish M, Neuman A, Wlody D. Maternal haemorrhage. *Br J Anaesth*. 2009;103(Suppl 1):i47–i56.
- Wijesiriwardana A, Bhattacharya S, Shetty A, et al. Obstetric outcome in women with threatened miscarriage in the first trimester. *Obstet Gynecol*. 2006;107(3):557–562.

 SEE ALSO

Abnormal Pap and Cervical Dysplasia; Abortion, Spontaneous (Miscarriage); Abruptio Placentae; Cervical Malignancy; Cervical Polyps; Cervicitis, Ectropion, and True Erosion; Chlamydia Infection (Sexually Transmitted); Ectopic Pregnancy; Placenta Previa; Preterm Labor; Trichomoniasis; Vaginal Malignancy

CODES

ICD10

- O20.9 Hemorrhage in early pregnancy, unspecified
- O46.90 Antepartum hemorrhage, unspecified, unspecified trimester
- O20.0 Threatened abortion

CLINICAL PEARLS

- Obtain blood type and screen all women presenting with vaginal bleeding in pregnancy and administer RhoGAM to all Rh-negative patients.
- For up to 50% of early pregnancy bleeding, no cause is ever found.
- Always consider ectopic pregnancy in 1st-trimester bleeding.
- Do not perform digital exam in late pregnancy bleeding until placenta has been located on ultrasound.

V

VAGINAL MALIGNANCY

Jay R. Patibandla, MD • Michael P. Hopkins, MD, MEd

BASICS

DESCRIPTION
- Carcinomas of the vagina are uncommon: 3% of gynecologic malignancies, 2,300 new cases annually.
- Vaginal intraepithelial neoplasia (VAIN), defined by squamous cell atypia, is classified by the depth of epithelial involvement:
  - VAIN 1: 1/3 thickness
  - VAIN 2: 2/3 thickness
  - VAIN 3 and carcinoma in situ (CIS): >2/3 with CIS, designating full-thickness neoplastic changes without invasion through the basement membrane
- Invasive malignancies: Vaginal malignancies include squamous cell carcinoma (85–90%), adenocarcinoma (5–10%), sarcoma (2–3%), and melanoma (2–3%). Clear cell carcinoma is a subtype of adenocarcinoma. Invasive squamous cell carcinoma has the potential for metastasis to the lungs and liver.
- To be classified as a vaginal malignancy, only the vagina can be involved. If the cervix or vulva is involved, then the tumor is classified as a primary cancer arising from the cervix or the vulva.
- Most vaginal malignancies are metastatic (e.g., cervix, vulva, endometrium, breast, ovary).

Pregnancy Considerations
This malignancy is not associated with pregnancy.

EPIDEMIOLOGY

Incidence
- An estimated 4,070 new cases will be diagnosed in 2015 with 910 resulting deaths (1).
- Predominant age
  - CIS: mid-40 to 60 years
  - Invasive squamous cell malignancy: mid-60 to 70 years
  - Adenocarcinoma: any age; 50 years is the mean age. Peak incidence is between 17 and 21 years of age.
  - Clear cell adenocarcinoma occurs most often in females <30 years with a history of exposure to diethylstilbestrol (DES) in utero.
  - Mixed müllerian sarcomas and leiomyosarcomas in the adult population: mean age 60 years

Pediatric Considerations
Vaginal tumors are extremely rare. Rhabdomyosarcoma (botryoid and embryonal subtype) is the most common malignant neoplasm of the vagina. Less common entities are germ cell tumor and clear cell adenocarcinoma.

Prevalence
In the United States, it is one of the rarest of all gynecologic malignancies (3%).

ETIOLOGY AND PATHOPHYSIOLOGY
- Women with a history of cervical malignancy have a higher probability of developing squamous cell malignancy in the vagina even after hysterectomy.
- Human papillomavirus (HPV) is found in 80–93% of patients with vaginal CIS and 50–65% of the patients with invasive vaginal carcinoma (2,3).
- HPV-16 is the most common, found in 66% of CIS and 55% of invasive vaginal cancers.
- Smokers have a higher incidence.

- Clear cell adenocarcinoma of the vagina in young women has been associated with DES exposure. The incidence, however, is exceedingly rare, estimated at 1/1,000 to 1/10,000 exposed females.
- Metastatic lesions can involve the vagina, spreading from the other gynecologic organs.
- Although rare, renal cell carcinoma, lung adenocarcinoma, GI cancer, pancreatic adenocarcinoma, ovarian germ cell cancer, trophoblastic neoplasm, and breast cancer can all metastasize to the vagina.

Genetics
No known genetic pattern

RISK FACTORS
- Similar risk factors as cervical cancer
- Age
- African American
- Smoking
- Multiple sex partners, early age of first sexual intercourse
- History of squamous cell cancer of the cervix or vulva
- HPV infection
- Vaginal adenosis
- Vaginal irritation
- DES exposure in utero

COMMONLY ASSOCIATED CONDITIONS
Due to the field effect, patients with vaginal cancer are more likely to develop malignancy in the cervix or vulva and should be followed closely.

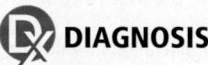

DIAGNOSIS

HISTORY
- Abnormal bleeding is the most common symptom.
- Postcoital bleeding can result from direct trauma to the tumor.
- Vaginal discharge
- Dyspareunia
- Urinary symptoms, including hematuria and increased frequency
- Constipation
- Pain along with symptoms and signs of hydroureter are late findings when the tumor has spread into the paravaginal tissues and extends to the pelvic sidewall.

Pediatric Considerations
In children, sarcomas can present either as a mass protruding from the vagina or as abnormal genital bleeding.

PHYSICAL EXAM
Pelvic examination
- The vagina, uterus, adnexa (fallopian tubes and ovaries), bladder, and rectum should be evaluated for unusual changes.
- Vaginal malignancies are found most commonly on the posterior wall in the upper 1/3 of the vagina.

DIFFERENTIAL DIAGNOSIS
- Premalignant changes: VAIN 1, 2, 3, and CIS
- Adequate biopsies ensure that invasive lesions are not overlooked. Invasive lesions penetrate the basement membrane and cannot be treated conservatively.

- Other malignancies, such as endometrial, cervix, bladder, or colon cancer, can invade directly into the vagina or metastasize to the vagina.
- In the childbearing years, trophoblastic disease should be considered.
  - The vagina is a common site of metastases; however, biopsy should typically be avoided because the implants are very vascular and may hemorrhage if sampled.
  - The clinical presentation is typically obvious so histopathologic confirmation before treatment is not required.

DIAGNOSTIC TESTS & INTERPRETATION

Initial Tests (lab, imaging)
- Pap smear may incidentally detect asymptomatic lesions.
- Biopsy suspicious lesions
- Chest x-ray (CXR): to evaluate for metastatic disease
- CT scan and MRI: to evaluate the liver and retroperitoneum, especially the lymph nodes in the pelvic and periaortic area
- PET scan detects primary and secondary metastatic lesions more often than CT scan.

ALERT
PET scan correlation with CT scan lesions strongly suggests malignancy.

Follow-Up Tests & Special Considerations
- Lymphoscintigraphy (sentinel lymph node mapping) as part of the pretreatment evaluation can result in a change in the radiation fields and improve comprehensive treatment planning in women with vaginal cancer.
- HPV vaccination: Implementation of prophylactic HPV vaccination could prevent ~2/3 of the intraepithelial lesions in the lower genital tract but is yet unproven.

Diagnostic Procedures/Other
- Colposcopy with directed biopsies for small lesions
- Wide excision under anesthesia of superficial disease may be necessary to ensure that invasive cancer is not present.
- Cystoscopy to rule out bladder invasion
- Proctosigmoidoscopy to rule out rectal invasion

Test Interpretation
Tumors are staged clinically:
- Stage 0: VAIN and CIS
- Stage I: carcinoma limited to the vaginal wall (26%)
- Stage II: involves the subvaginal tissues but has not extended to the pelvic wall (37%)
- Stage III: extends to the pelvic wall (24%)
- Stage IV: extends beyond the true pelvis (13%)
  - IVa: Tumor invades bladder and/or rectal mucosa and/or direct extension beyond the true pelvis.
  - IVb: spread to distant organs

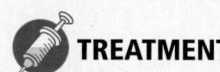

TREATMENT

GENERAL MEASURES
Treatment methods for VAIN and CIS include the following:
- Wide local excision
- Partial or total vaginectomy

- Intravaginal chemotherapy with 5% fluorouracil cream
- Laser therapy
- Intracavitary radiation therapy

MEDICATION
- Imiquimod
  - In a review of the effectiveness of 5% imiquimod cream in the treatment of VAIN, the following results were reported (4)[C]:
    - 26–100% of patients had complete regression.
    - 0–60% of patients had partial regression.
    - 0–37% experienced recurrence.
- Contraindications
  - The diagnosis must be established with certainty prior to treatment.
  - If there is any doubt that a process beyond in situ disease exists, vaginectomy must be performed. These patients are often elderly, and aggressive therapy is limited by the patient's performance status and ability to tolerate radical surgery, chemotherapy, or radiation.

ISSUES FOR REFERRAL
Patients should be treated by a gynecologic oncologist and/or a radiation oncologist.

ADDITIONAL THERAPIES
- Treatment with radiotherapy depends on the stage of disease. This treatment option should be discussed with physicians experienced with this malignancy.
- It is common to use radiotherapy and chemotherapy (chemoradiation) for better cancer control.
- Early-stage primary squamous cell carcinoma treated with radiation alone has shown good results (5)[A].
- Stage III vaginal cancer may benefit from combined radiation and hyperthermia (6)[C].
- Patients with advanced squamous cell carcinoma or adenocarcinoma receive concurrent irradiation and cisplatin-based chemotherapy (7)[B].
- Neoadjuvant chemotherapy followed by radical surgery may benefit select patients (8)[C].
- In most tumor types, metastatic disease from the vagina to other sites is only minimally responsive to chemotherapy.
- With one exception, no chemotherapeutic agents have shown a survival advantage. The exception is childhood sarcomas, which have been treated with combinations of the following:
  - Vincristine
  - Dactinomycin (actinomycin-D)
  - Cyclophosphamide (Cytoxan)
  - Cisplatin
  - Etoposide (VP-16)

SURGERY/OTHER PROCEDURES
- Whenever there is a doubt as to the presence or absence of invasive disease, vaginectomy must be performed.
- Invasive lesions usually are treated by radiation therapy, but stage I lesions can be treated with radical hysterectomy or radical vaginectomy with pelvic lymph node dissection (9)[A].
- If the lesion involves the lower vagina, inguinal node dissection also must be done because cancer involving the lower vagina can metastasize to the groin region.

- Premenopausal women who desire to retain ovarian function are better candidates for radical surgery for early-stage disease, with vaginal reconstruction possible afterward.
- Patients who have not completed their family can occasionally be treated with limited resection and localized radiation to the area.
- Sarcomas are treated by radiation therapy followed by pelvic exenteration if persistent disease is present.

Pediatric Considerations
The treatment of vaginal tumors today mainly consists of neoadjuvant chemotherapy followed by local control with surgery or radiotherapy.

Geriatric Considerations
Older patients, many with a long history of smoking, are at a higher risk for malignancies requiring surgical treatments.

 ONGOING CARE

FOLLOW-UP RECOMMENDATIONS
- Patients are usually ambulatory and able to resume full activity by 6 weeks after surgery.
- Most patients are fully active while receiving chemotherapy and radiation therapy.

Patient Monitoring
- Pelvic examination and Pap smear every 3 months for 2 years, then every 6 months for the next 3 years and then yearly thereafter
- Annual CXR

PATIENT EDUCATION
- Printed patient information available from American College of Obstetricians and Gynecologists, 409 12th St., SW, Washington, DC 20024-2188; 800-762-ACOG: http://www.acog.org
- American Cancer Society: http://www.cancer.gov
- Medline Plus: http://www.nlm.nih.gov/medlineplus/vaginalcancer.html

PROGNOSIS
Stage and 5-year survival (10)
- I: 77.6%
- II: 52.2%
- III: 42.5%
- IVA: 20.5%
- IVB: 12.9%

COMPLICATIONS
- Those typically associated with major abdominal surgery or radiation therapy
- Common complications of treatment include rectovaginal or vesicovaginal fistulas, rectal/vaginal strictures, radiation cystitis, and/or proctitis.

REFERENCES

1. Siegel RL, Miller KD, Jemal A. Cancer statistics, 2015. *CA Cancer J Clin*. 2015;65(1):5–29.
2. Daling JR, Madeleine MM, Schwartz SM, et al. A population-based study of squamous cell vaginal cancer: HPV and cofactors. *Gynecol Oncol*. 2002;84(2):263–270.
3. Smith JS, Backes DM, Hoots BE, et al. Human papillomavirus type-distribution in vulvar and vaginal cancers and their associated precursors. *Obstet Gynecol*. 2009;113(4):917–924.
4. Iavazzo C, Pitsouni E, Athanasiou S, et al. Imiquimod for treatment of vulvar and vaginal intraepithelial neoplasia. *Int J Gynaecol Obstet*. 2008;101(1):3–10.
5. Tran PT, Su Z, Lee P, et al. Prognostic factors for outcomes and complications for primary squamous cell carcinoma of the vagina treated with radiation. *Gynecol Oncol*. 2007;105(3):641–649.
6. Franckena M, van der Zee J. Use of combined radiation and hyperthermia for gynecological cancer. *Curr Opin Obstet Gynecol*. 2010; 22(1):9–14.
7. Dalrymple JL, Russell AH, Lee SW, et al. Chemoradiation for primary invasive squamous carcinoma of the vagina. *Int J Gynecol Cancer*. 2004;14(1):110–117.
8. Benedetti Panici P, Bellati F, Plotti F, et al. Neoadjuvant chemotherapy followed by radical surgery in patients affected by vaginal carcinoma. *Gynecol Oncol*. 2008;111(2):307–311.
9. Tjalma WA, Monaghan JM, de Barros Lopes A, et al. The role of surgery in invasive squamous carcinoma of the vagina. *Gynecol Oncol*. 2001;81(3):360–365.
10. Beller U, Benedet JL, Creasman WT, et al. Carcinoma of the vagina. FIGO 26th Annual Report on the Results of Treatment in Gynecological Cancer. *Int J Gynaecol Obstet*. 2006;95(Suppl 1): S29–S42.

ADDITIONAL READING

- Creasman WT. Vaginal cancers. *Curr Opin Obstet Gynecol*. 2005;17(1):71–76.
- Fernandez-Pineda I, Spunt SL, Parida L, et al. Vaginal tumors in childhood: the experience of St. Jude Children's Research Hospital. *J Pediatr Surg*. 2011;46(11):2071–2075.
- Frumovitz M, Gayed IW, Jhingran A, et al. Lymphatic mapping and sentinel lymph node detection in women with vaginal cancer. *Gynecol Oncol*. 2008;108(3):478–481.
- Gray HJ. Advances in vulvar and vaginal cancer treatment. *Gynecol Oncol*. 2010;118(1):3–5.
- Hampl M, Sarajuuri H, Wentzensen N, et al. Effect of human papillomavirus vaccines on vulvar, vaginal, and anal intraepithelial lesions and vulvar cancer. *Obstet Gynecol*. 2006;108(6):1361–1368.

 CODES

ICD10
- C52 Malignant neoplasm of vagina
- D07.2 Carcinoma in situ of vagina
- N89.3 Dysplasia of vagina, unspecified

CLINICAL PEARLS
- Vaginal cancer is rare; 85–90% of vaginal cancers are squamous cell.
- Vaginal malignancies are found most commonly on the posterior wall in the upper 1/3 of the vagina.
- Most vaginal malignancies are metastatic (from cervix, vulva, endometrium, breast, or ovary).

V

VAGINITIS AND VAGINOSIS

Heather O'Connor Greer, MD • Patricia Beauzile, MD

 BASICS

DESCRIPTION

- "Vaginosis" and "Vaginitis" are broad terms indicating any disease process of the vagina caused by or leading to infection, inflammation, or changes in the normal vaginal flora.
- The difference between vaginitis and vaginosis is the presence (vaginitis) or absence (vaginosis) of inflammation.
- The most common symptoms of vaginitis/vaginosis are vaginal discharge, odor, itching, burning, or pain.
- The most common causes of vaginitis are bacterial vaginosis (BV), vulvovaginal candidiasis (VVC), and trichomoniasis.
- Other causes of vaginitis can be stratified by age and are generally associated with postmenopausal vaginal atrophy or foreign bodies in the pediatric population.
- Lichen planus, lichen sclerosus, and psoriasis, may also cause vaginitis.
- Diagnosis of vaginitis relies on thorough history, physical exam, and clinical assessment. Microscopy, cultures, DNA probes, and tissue biopsy can be helpful in confirming diagnosis.
- BV is the most common cause of vaginal discharge in reproductive-aged women. It is caused by a disturbance in the normal vaginal flora. The normally dominant hydrogen-peroxide producing lactobacilli are overwhelmed by an overgrowth of gram-negative species causing an increase in the vaginal pH, discharge, and odor.
- VVC is the second most common cause of vaginitis in reproductive-aged women. It is caused by invasion of the *Candida* organism into the superficial epithelial cells of the vagina causing mild to severe vaginal inflammation, pruritis, and discharge.

EPIDEMIOLOGY

- Vaginal symptoms are typical and common in the general population and are one of the most frequent reasons women present to their medical care providers accounting for approximately 10 million office visits each year (1).
- About 30% of women with complaint of vaginal discharge or irritation remain undiagnosed despite extensive testing.
- In the United States, BV continues to be the leading cause of vaginal complaints.
- The frequency of VVC is highest among women in their reproductive years (2).
- Neither vaginal candidiasis nor BV is considered to be sexually transmitted diseases.
- Vaginal trichomoniasis is a common sexually transmitted disease with 7.4 million cases diagnosed yearly in the United States (3).

ETIOLOGY AND PATHOPHYSIOLOGY

- BV (4)
  - BV is caused by a change in the normal vaginal flora. Dominant lactobacilli responsible for maintaining the acidic vaginal pH are overcome by an increase of the gram-negative organisms.
  - Change in the vaginal environment leads to an increase in the pH and an overgrowth of vaginal anaerobes causing a malodorous discharge and frothy vaginal discharge.
  - BV is highly prevalent and associated with multiple adverse outcomes, including enhanced HIV transmission.

- The organisms generally implicated in BV infections include:
  - *Gardnerella vaginalis*
  - *Prevotella* species
  - *Porphyromonas* species
  - *Bacteroides* species
  - *Peptostreptococcus* species
  - *Mycoplasma hominis*
  - *Ureaplasma urealyticum*
  - *Mobiluncus* species
  - *Fusobacterium* species
  - *Atopobium vaginae*
- VVC
  - VVC is caused by *Candida albicans* (80–92%) and *C. glabrata* (<10%)
  - Candida organisms can be identified in the lower genital tract in healthy women, and it is thought to gain access via rectal and perianal colonization and migration.
  - Symptoms occur when candidal organisms overwhelm the normal vaginal flora and invade the superficial vaginal epithelial cells causing inflammation, pruritis, and thick vaginal discharge.
- Trichomoniasis
  - Caused by an infection via *Trichomonas vaginalis*, a flagellate protozoan. The organism infects the squamous epithelium of the vagina, as well as the urethra, and paraurethral glands. This infection is primarily transmitted during sexual intercourse.
  - Other sources of vaginitis/vaginosis are usually mediated by disruption of the vaginal squamous epithelium. This disruption can lead to inflammation, pain, and discharge.
  - Other than the three most common causes of vaginitis/vaginosis, menses, sexual activity, contraception, pregnancy, foreign bodies, estrogen levels, STDs, and use of vaginal hygiene products, topical creams, or antibiotics can contribute to vaginal symptoms

RISK FACTORS

- BV:
  - Sexual activity; while BV is not considered an STD, studies show increased rates of BV in women with multiple sex partners
  - Women who have sex with women
  - The presence of STDs such as HSV-2 (5)
- VVC:
  - Diabetes
  - Use of broad-spectrum antibiotics.
  - Immunosuppression
  - Higher estrogen levels have been associated with increased vaginal yeast infection, explaining why it is more commonly diagnosed in reproductive-aged women and in pregnancy.
- Trichomoniasis:
  - Inconsistent use of barrier contraception
  - Multiple sex partners
  - African Americans
  - Limited education and low socioeconomic status
- Other risk factors associated with vaginitis/vaginosis:
  - Decreased estrogen
  - Smoking
  - Use of vaginal douches and creams.
  - Tight fitting clothing
  - Poor hygienic practice
  - Changes in diet

GENERAL PREVENTION

- Vulvar hygiene
- Treatment of sexual partners generally is not recommended but may be considered in recurrent cases.

COMMONLY ASSOCIATED CONDITIONS

- STDs such as gonorrhea, chlamydia, or HSV
- Vaginal intraepithelial neoplasia and cancer can present with symptoms of vaginitis.
- Desquamative inflammatory vaginitis presents with similar symptoms but most commonly occurs in postmenopausal women.

 DIAGNOSIS

HISTORY

- General principles:
  - The key to diagnosis is clarification of the presenting symptoms.
  - Onset, timing, and character of the vaginal symptoms are important questions to ask.
  - Many patients will be asymptomatic, and diagnosis is made on routine physical exam and lab testing.
  - Symptomatic patients generally complain of itching, burning, irritation, and abnormal discharge.
- BV
  - Symptomatic patients complain of abnormal vaginal discharge and a fishy odor.
- VVC
  - Symptomatic women report itching, burning, irritation, dyspareunia, burning with urination, and a white thick discharge.
- Trichomoniasis
  - Symptomatic patients will complain of abnormal discharge, itching, burning, or postcoital bleeding.

PHYSICAL EXAM

- BV
  - Thin watery, sometimes foamy discharge. Can appear beige- or tan-colored. An amine or "fishy" smell may be present on exam.
  - The vaginal epithelium should appear normal and noninflamed.
- VVC
  - Erythema and swelling of the vulva and vaginal mucosa
  - Some patients may have vulvar excoriation and fissures.
  - If discharge is present, it is usually white, thick, and can have a cottage cheese appearance. Some women may have thin white dilute discharge. No odor is present.
- Trichomoniasis
  - Significant erythema of the vulva and vaginal mucosa
  - Greenish discharge with an amine or fishy odor
  - Discharge can also appear purulent in some patients.
  - Occasionally punctate hemorrhages can be seen on the vaginal walls and on the cervix ("strawberry cervix").

DIFFERENTIAL DIAGNOSIS

- Physiologic discharge
- Leukorrhea of pregnancy
- STDs
- Foreign body
- Contact dermatitis
- Cervicitis
- Desquamative inflammatory vaginitis
- Urinary tract infection (UTI)
- Atrophic vaginitis
- Dermatoses: lichen sclerosus, lichen planus, seborrheic dermatitis, psoriasis

DIAGNOSTIC TESTS & INTERPRETATION

- BV
  - Symptomatic patients complain of an abnormal vaginal discharge and a fishy odor.
  - Clinical diagnosis is established with Amsel criteria. A positive diagnosis can be made if 3 out of 4 of the following criteria are present (6)[B].
    - Gray, frothy, or foamy discharge
    - Vaginal pH >4.5
    - A positive amine or "Whiff" test with use of KOH solution added to discharge
    - >20% of the epithelial cells identified as "clue cells"
- VVC
  - Visualization of blastospores or pseudohyphae on saline or 10% KOH microscopy
  - A positive culture in a symptomatic patient
- Trichomoniasis
  - Visualization of motile trichomonads on saline microscopy (7)[B]

TREATMENT

GENERAL MEASURES

- Avoid douching and tight fitting clothing.
- Regular use of condoms and spermicides may help to prevent BV.

MEDICATION

- BV
  - Metronidazole 500 mg orally BID for 7 days, vaginally 0.75% gel 1 applicator daily for 5 days, or clindamycin given vaginally (1 applicator = 100 mg) for 5 days (8)[A]. Recurrent infection may require repeated treatment (e.g., 1 week monthly for 6 months).
- VVC
  - Uncomplicated infections can be treated with a one time dose of fluconazole 150 mg tab. Topical/vaginal suppository antifungal regimens such as butoconazole, clotrimazole, miconazole, terconazole, or nystatin creams. Treatment can range from 3 to 7 days (7)[A].
  - Recurrent or complicated infections may require additional oral dosing of fluconazole 150 mg tab for extended treatment and/or prophylaxis (9)[A].
- Trichomoniasis
  - A one time 2 g oral dose of either tinidazole or metronidazole. Alternatively, 500 mg dose of metronidazole twice daily for 7 days (10)[A].
  - The patient's partner should be treated as well and counseled to abstain from sex until both patients have completed treatment.

ISSUES FOR REFERRAL

Treating male partners does not reduce symptoms or prevent recurrence, but can be considered in patients with recurrent infection.

COMPLEMENTARY & ALTERNATIVE MEDICINE

A Cochrane analysis reviewed the use of probiotics for BV and found inconclusive evidence to recommend probiotics as primary treatment or as a preventive strategy (11)[A]. Further study was recommended.

ONGOING CARE

FOLLOW-UP RECOMMENDATIONS

- Delay sexual relations until symptoms clear/discomfort resolves
- Use of condoms may reduce recurrence of BV.

Patient Monitoring

- No specific follow-up needed; if symptoms persist or recur within 2 months, repeat pelvic exam and culture.
- Consider suppressive therapy for recurrent infection.

PATIENT EDUCATION

American College of Obstetricians and Gynecologists (ACOG), 409 12th St., SW, Washington, DC 20024-2188; 800-762-ACOG: www.acog.org

PROGNOSIS

VVC: 80–90% of uncomplicated cases cured with appropriate treatment; 30–50% of recurrent infections return after discontinuation of maintenance therapy; there is a relatively high spontaneous remission rate of untreated symptoms as well.

COMPLICATIONS

- VVC may occur following treatment of BV.
- BV has been associated with an increased risk of acquisition and transmission of HIV.
- BV has been associated with increased risk of preterm birth, chorioamnionitis, postpartum and postabortal endometritis, and pelvic inflammatory disease.

REFERENCES

1. Sobel JD. Vulvovaginitis in healthy women. *Compr Ther.* 1999;25(6–7):335–346.
2. Kent HL. Epidemiology of vaginitis. *Am J Obstet Gynecol.* 1991;165(4, Pt 2):1168–1176.
3. Weinstock H, Berman S, Cates W Jr. Sexually transmitted diseases among American youth: incidence and prevalence estimates, 2000. *Perspect Sex Reprod Health.* 2004;36(1):6–10.
4. Hill GB. The microbiology of bacterial vaginosis. *Am J Obstet Gynecol.* 1993;169(2, Pt 2):450–454.
5. Esber A, Vicetti Miguel RD, Cherpes TL, et al. Risk of bacterial vaginosis among women with herpes simplex virus type 2 infection: a systematic review and meta-analysis. *J Infect Dis.* 2015;212(1):8–17.
6. Money D. The laboratory diagnosis of bacterial vaginosis. *Can J Infect Dis Med Microbiol.* 2005;16(2):77–79.
7. Sobel JD, Kapernick PS, Zervos M, et al. Treatment of complicated *Candida vaginitis*: comparison of single and sequential doses of fluconazole. *Am J Obstet Gynecol.* 2001;185(2):363–369.
8. Beigi RH, Austin MN, Meyn LA, et al. Antimicrobial resistance associated with the treatment of bacterial vaginosis. *Am J Obstet Gynecol.* 2004;191(4):1124–1129.
9. Sobel JD, Wiesenfeld HC, Martens M, et al. Maintenance fluconazole therapy for recurrent vulvovaginal candidiasis. *N Engl J Med.* 2004;351(9):876–883.
10. Gabriel G, Robertson E, Thin RN. Single dose treatment of trichomoniasis. *J Int Med Res.* 1982;10(2):129–130.
11. Senok AC, Verstraelen H, Temmerman M, et al. Probiotics for the treatment of bacterial vaginosis. *Cochrane Database Syst Rev.* 2009;(4):CD006289.

ADDITIONAL READING

- Donders G. Diagnosis and management of bacterial vaginosis and other types of abnormal vaginal bacterial flora: a review. *Obstet Gynecol Surv.* 2010;65(7):462–473.
- Li J, McCormick J, Bocking A, et al. Importance of vaginal microbes in reproductive health. *Reprod Sci.* 2012;19(3):235–242.
- Pappas PG, Kauffman CA, Andes D, et al. Clinical practice guidelines for the management of candidiasis: 2009 update by the Infectious Diseases Society of America. *Clin Infect Dis.* 2009;48(5):503–535.
- Ray D, Goswami R, Banerjee U, et al. Prevalence of *Candida glabrata* and its response to boric acid vaginal suppositories in comparison with oral fluconazole in patients with diabetes and vulvovaginal candidiasis. *Diabetes Care.* 2007;30(2):312–317.
- Workowski KA, Berman S. Sexually transmitted diseases treatment guidelines, 2010. *MMWR Recomm Rep.* 2010;59(RR-12):1–110.

 SEE ALSO

Algorithm: Discharge, Vaginal

 CODES

ICD10

- N76.0 Acute vaginitis
- B37.3 Candidiasis of vulva and vagina
- N95.2 Postmenopausal atrophic vaginitis

CLINICAL PEARLS

Clinical symptoms, signs, and microscopy have relatively poor performance compared with so-called gold standards such as culture and DNA probe assays, but these more sensitive assays can detect organisms that may not be causing symptoms.

- Most women experience relief of symptoms with therapy chosen without such gold standard tests, even when the treatment does not correspond with the underlying infection.
- Vaginal pH is underused as a diagnostic tool for evaluation of vaginitis.

V

VARICOSE VEINS

Joseph A. Florence, MD • Leigh D. Johnson, MD

BASICS

DESCRIPTION
- Superficial venous disease causing a permanent dilatation and tortuosity of superficial veins, usually occurring in the legs and feet; caused by systemic weakness in the vein wall and may result from congenitally incomplete valves or valves that have become incompetent
- Affects legs where reverse flow occurs when dependent
- Truncal varices involve the great and small saphenous veins; branch varicosities involve the saphenous vein tributaries.
- Categorized as the following:
  – Uncomplicated (cosmetic)
  – With local symptoms (pain confined to the varices, not diffuse)
  – With local complications (superficial thrombophlebitis, may rupture causing bleeding)
  – Complex varicose disease (diffuse limb pain, swelling, skin changes/ulcer)
- System(s) affected: cardiovascular; skin

ALERT
Ulceration of varicose veins has a high rate of infection, which can lead to sepsis.

Geriatric Considerations
- Common; usually valvular degeneration but may be secondary to chronic venous deficiency
- Elastic support hose and frequent rests with legs elevated rather than ligation and stripping

Pregnancy Considerations
- Frequent problem
- Elastic stockings are recommended for those with a history of varicosities or if prolonged standing is involved.

EPIDEMIOLOGY
Incidence
- Predominant age: middle age
- Predominant gender: female > male (2:1)
- National Women's Health Information Center estimates that 50% of women have varicose veins.

ETIOLOGY AND PATHOPHYSIOLOGY
- Varicose veins are caused by venous insufficiency from faulty valves in ≥1 perforator veins in the lower leg, causing secondary incompetence at the saphenofemoral junction (valvular reflux).
- Valvular dysfunction causing venous reflux and subsequently venous hypertension (HTN)
- Failed valves allow blood to flow in the reverse direction (away from the heart), from deep to superficial and from proximal to distal veins.
- Deep thrombophlebitis
- Increased venous pressure from any cause
- Congenital valvular incompetence
- Trauma (consider arteriovenous fistula; listen for bruit)
- Presumed to be due to a loss in vein wall elasticity with failure of the valve leaflets
- An increase in venous filling pressure is sufficient to promote varicose remodeling of veins by augmenting wall stress and activating venous endothelial and smooth muscle cells (1).

Genetics
Autosomal dominant with incomplete penetrance

RISK FACTORS
- Increasing age
- Pregnancy, especially multiple pregnancies
- Prolonged standing
- Obesity
- History of phlebitis (postthrombotic syndrome)
- Family history
- Female sex
- Increased height
- Congenital valvular dysfunction

COMMONLY ASSOCIATED CONDITIONS
- Stasis dermatitis
- Large varicose veins may lead to skin changes and eventual stasis ulceration.

DIAGNOSIS

HISTORY
- Symptoms range from minor annoyance/cosmetic problem to a lifestyle-limiting problem.
- Localized symptoms: pain, burning, itching
- Generalized symptoms
  – Leg muscular cramp, aching
  – Leg fatigue/swelling
- Pain if varicose ulcer develops
- Symptoms often worse at the end of the day, especially after prolonged standing.
- Women are more prone to symptoms due to hormonal influences: worse during menses.
- No direct correlation with the severity of varicose veins and the severity of symptoms

PHYSICAL EXAM
- Inspect lower extremities while the patient is standing. Varicose veins in the proximal femoral ring and distal portion of the legs may not be visible when the patient is supine.
- Varicose veins are the following:
  – Dilated, tortuous, superficial veins, chiefly in the lower extremities
  – Dark purple/blue in color, raised above the surface of the skin
  – Often twisted, bulging, and can look like cords
  – Most commonly found on the posterior/medial lower extremity
- Edema of the affected limb may be present.
- Skin changes may include the following:
  – Eczema
  – Hyperpigmentation
  – Lipodermatosclerosis
- Spider veins (idiopathic telangiectases)
  – Fine intracutaneous angiectasis
  – May be extensive/unsightly
- Neurologic sensory and motor exam
- Peripheral arterial vasculature; pulses
- Musculoskeletal exam for associated rheumatologic/orthopedic issues

DIFFERENTIAL DIAGNOSIS
- Nerve root compression
- Arthritis
- Peripheral neuritis
- Telangiectasia: smaller, visible blood vessels that are permanently dilated
- Deep vein thrombosis
- Inflammatory liposclerosis

DIAGNOSTIC TESTS & INTERPRETATION
Duplex ultrasound: Noninvasive imaging duplex ultrasound will confirm the etiology, anatomy, and pathophysiology of segmental venous reflux. The severity of both symptoms and signs tends to correlate with the degree of venous reflux, which is identified by duplex ultrasound as retrograde or reversed flow of greater than 0.5 second duration (2).

Diagnostic Procedures/Other
Duplex scanning, venous Doppler study, photoplethysmography, light-reflection rheography, air plethysmography, and other vascular testing should be reserved for patients who have venous symptoms and/or large (>4 mm in diameter) vessels or large numbers of spider telangiectasia indicating venous HTN.

Test Interpretation
A clinical classification illustrating the current physical state is useful in clinical practice (1).
- 0: no visible or palpable signs of venous disease
- 1: spider veins or telangiectasias
- 2: varicose veins
- 3: edema
- 4: skin changes (pigmentation, eczema, lipodermatosclerosis, atrophie blanche)
- 5: healed ulcer
- 6: active ulcer

TREATMENT

- Conventional wisdom suggests conservative therapy (e.g., elevation, external compression, weight loss) as being helpful; while compression stockings improve the severity of varicose veins, they do not seem to improve quality of life (3)[B].
- There is insufficient, high-quality evidence to determine whether or not compression stockings are effective as the sole and initial treatment of varicose veins in people without healed or active venous ulceration, or whether any type of stocking is superior to any other type (4)[A].
- All the current modalities of endoluminal and open surgical treatment have similar short-term outcomes and risks (5)[A].
- Appropriate surgical treatment has the best long-term outcomes and evidence base (5)[A].
- Treatment of choice, however, depends on many factors, including local expertise (5)[A].
- When comparing quality of life, pain relief, and long-term relief, surgery is favored (6)[A].
- Endovenous laser ablation (EVLA); radiofrequency ablation, foam sclerotherapy, and surgical stripping for great saphenous varicose veins are all efficacious (7)[A].
- Endovenous ablation (radiofrequency and laser) is at least as effective as surgery in the treatment of great saphenous varicose veins and outcomes remain similar at 2 years (8)[A]; however, ultrasound-guided foam sclerotherapy has insufficient support from available data (8)[A].
- The ambulatory conservative hemodynamic correction of venous insufficiency method (cure conservatrice et hémodynamique de l'insuffisance veineuse en ambulatoire [CHIVA]) is a less-invasive approach based on venous hemodynamics with deliberate preservation of the superficial venous system. The CHIVA method reduces recurrence of varicose veins and produces fewer side effects than vein stripping (9)[A].

GENERAL MEASURES
Patients with unsightly varicose veins often seek treatment for cosmetic reasons.

MEDICATION

Superficial thrombophlebitis is not an infective condition and does not require antibiotic treatment.

ISSUES FOR REFERRAL

- Emergency: bleeding from a varicosity that has eroded the skin
- Urgent: varicosity that has bled and is at risk for bleeding again
- Soon: ulcer that is progressive/painful despite treatment
- Routine
  - Active/healed ulcer/progressive skin changes that may benefit from surgery
  - Recurrent superficial thrombophlebitis
  - Troublesome symptoms attributable to varicose veins or patient and provider feel that the extent, site, and size of the varicosities are having a severe impact on quality of life.

ADDITIONAL THERAPIES

- Apply elastic stockings before lowering legs from the bed.
- Activity
  - Frequent rest periods with legs elevated
  - If standing is necessary, frequently shift weight from side to side.
  - Appropriate exercise routine as part of conservative treatment
  - Walking regimen after sclerotherapy is important to help promote healing.
  - Never sit with legs hanging down.
- Physical therapy

SURGERY/OTHER PROCEDURES

- Surgery
  - Improved quality-adjusted life-years and symptoms compared to conservative management at 2 years (1)[A]
  - Surgery is indicated if there is pain, recurrent phlebitis, or skin changes/ulceration or for cosmetic improvement for severe cases.
  - Minimally invasive techniques include the following:
    - Radiofrequency ablation (RFA): compared with surgery provides a faster return to work; less pain, better short-term quality of life; less bruising and tenderness compared with endovenous laser therapy (1)[A]
    - Endovenous microwave ablation (EMA) is an effective new technique for the treatment of varicose veins and had a more satisfactory clinical outcome than high ligation and stripping (HLS) in the short term (10)[A].
    - EVLA is as effective as conventional surgery (CS) and superior to ultrasound-guided foam sclerotherapy (UGFS), according to occlusion on ultrasound duplex (11)[B].
    - Quality of life improves after treatment in all groups (EVLA, CS, UGFS), significantly (11)[B].
    - There is no significant difference between EVLA and open surgery in patients with great saphenous vein incompetence (12)[A].
- Sclerotherapy is a simple, safe, and particularly effective for smaller, early varicosities and also for residual veins after surgery (13)[C].
- Radiotherapy
  - RFA takes longer to perform but has better early outcome than CS in patients with great saphenous varicose veins.
  - Radiofrequency and laser treatments replace "stripping"; however, most varicosities still require phlebectomy/sclerotherapy.

 ## ONGOING CARE

DIET

- No special diet
- Weight-loss diet is recommended if obesity is a problem.

PATIENT EDUCATION

- Avoid long periods of standing and crossing legs when sitting.
- Exercise (walking, running) regularly to improve leg strength and circulation.
- Maintain an appropriate weight.
- Wear elastic support stockings.
- Avoid clothing that constricts legs.
- Surgery/sclerotherapy may not prevent development of varicosities, and the procedure may need to be repeated in later years.
- National Heart, Lung and Blood Institute, Communications and Public Information Branch, National Institutes of Health, Building 31, Room 41–21, 9000 Rockville Pike, Bethesda, MD 20892; 301-496-4236. http://www.nhlbi.nih.gov/
- JAMA Patient Page| Treatment of Varicose Veins; http://jama.jamanetwork.com/article.aspx?articleid=1672241

PROGNOSIS

- Usual course: chronic
- Favorable with appropriate treatment
- Surgery has a nonsignificant reduction in the risk of varicose vein recurrence compared with liquid sclerotherapy and endoluminal interventions (6)[A].
- Increasing disease severity by venous clinical severity score (VCSS) is associated with reductions in quality of life (14)[B].

COMPLICATIONS

- Complications with sclerotherapy include hyperpigmentation, matting, local urticaria, cutaneous necrosis, microthrombi, accidental intra-arterial injection, phlebitis, deep vein thrombosis, thromboembolism, scintillating scotomas, nerve damage, and allergic reactions.
- Petechial hemorrhages
- Chronic edema
- Superimposed infection
- Varicose ulcers
- Pigmentation
- Eczema
- Recurrence after surgical treatment
- Scarring/nerve damage from stripping technique
- Neurologic complications after sclerotherapy are rare (6)[B].

REFERENCES

1. Hamdan A. Management of varicose veins and venous insufficiency. *JAMA.* 2012;308(24):2612–2621.
2. Coleridge-Smith P, Labropoulos N, Partsch H, et al. Duplex ultrasound investigation of the veins in chronic venous disease of the lower limbs—UIP consensus document. Part I. Basic principles. *Eur J Vasc Endovasc Surg.* 2006;31(1):83–92.
3. Nandhra S, El-sheikha J, Carradice D, et al. A randomized clinical trial of endovenous laser ablation versus conventional surgery for small saphenous varicose veins. *J Vasc Surg.* 2015;61(3):741–746.
4. Shingler S, Robertson L, Boghossian S, et al. Compression stockings for the initial treatment of varicose veins in patients without venous ulceration. *Cochrane Database Syst Rev.* 2013;(12):CD008819.
5. Wright N, Fitridge R. Varicose veins—natural history, assessment and management. *Aust Fam Physician.* 2013;42(6):380–384.
6. Kistner RL, Eklof B, Masuda EM. Diagnosis of chronic venous disease of the lower extremities: the "CEAP" classification. *Mayo Clin Proc.* 1996;71(4):338–345.
7. Nesbitt C, Eifell RK, Coyne P, et al. Endovenous ablation (radiofrequency and laser) and foam sclerotherapy versus conventional surgery for great saphenous vein varices. *Cochrane Database Syst Rev.* 2011;(10):CD005624.
8. Sell H, Vikatmaa P, Albäck A, et al. Compression therapy versus surgery in the treatment of patients with varicose veins: a RCT. *Eur J Vasc Endovasc Surg.* 2014;47(6):670–677.
9. Bellmunt-Montoya S, Escribano JM, Dilme J, et al. CHIVA method for the treatment of chronic venous insufficiency. *Cochrane Database Syst Rev.* 2013;(7):CD009648.
10. Yang L, Wang XP, Su WJ, et al. Randomized clinical trial of endovenous microwave ablation combined with high ligation versus conventional surgery for varicose veins. *Eur J Vasc Endovasc Surg.* 2013;46(4):473–479.
11. Biemans AA, Kockaert M, Akkersdijk GP, et al. Comparing endovenous laser ablation, foam sclerotherapy, and conventional surgery for great saphenous varicose veins. *J Vasc Surg.* 2013;58(3):727–734.e1.
12. Rasmussen L, Lawaetz M, Bjoern L, et al. Randomized clinical trial comparing endovenous laser ablation and stripping of the great saphenous vein with clinical and duplex outcome after 5 years. *J Vasc Surg.* 2013;58(2):421–426.
13. Subbarao NT, Aradhya SS, Veerabhadrappa NH. Sclerotherapy in the management of varicose veins and its dermatological complications. *Indian J Dermatol Venereol Leprol.* 2013;79(3):383–388.
14. Lozano Sánchez FS, Sánchez Nevarez I, González-Porras JR, et al. Quality of life in patients with chronic venous disease: influence of the socio-demographical and clinical factors. *Int Angiol.* 2013;32(4):433–441.

 ## CODES

ICD10

- I83.90 Asymptomatic varicose veins of unspecified lower extremity
- I83.009 Varicose veins of unsp lower extremity w ulcer of unsp site
- I83.10 Varicose veins of unsp lower extremity with inflammation

CLINICAL PEARLS

- Long-term safety and efficacy of surgery for the treatment of varicose veins is supported by low-quality evidence. Less-invasive treatments, which are associated with less periprocedural disability and pain, are supported by short-term studies (4)[A].
- Endovascular treatment of varicose veins is safe and effective and has a rapid recovery (7)[A]. Insufficient evidence exists to prefer sclerotherapy over surgery (6)[A].
- The efficacy of sclerotherapy is not significantly affected by the choice of sclerosant, dose, formulation (foam vs. liquid), local pressure dressing, or degree and length of compression (6)[A].

V

VASCULITIS
Irene J. Tan, MD, FACR

 BASICS

DESCRIPTION
An inflammatory blood vessel disorder
- Clinical features result from the destruction of blood vessel walls with subsequent thrombosis, ischemia, bleeding, and/or aneurysm formation.
- Vasculitis consists of a large, heterogeneous group of diseases classified by the predominant size, type, and the location of involved blood vessels (1).
  - Small-vessel vasculitis
    - Microscopic polyangiitis (MPA)
    - Granulomatosis with polyangiitis (GPA, formerly Wegener granulomatosis)
    - Eosinophilic granulomatosis with polyangiitis (EGPA; formerly Churg-Strauss syndrome)
    - Antiglomerular basement membrane disease (anti-GBM)
    - Cryoglobulinemic vasculitis
    - IgA vasculitis (Henoch-Schönlein purpura [HSP])
    - Hypocomplementemic urticarial vasculitis
  - Medium-vessel vasculitis
    - Polyarteritis nodosa (PAN)
    - Kawasaki disease (KD)
  - Large-vessel vasculitis
    - Takayasu arteritis (TAK)
    - Giant cell arteritis (GCA)
- Vasculitis occurs as a primary disorder or secondary to infection, a drug reaction, malignancy, or connective tissue disease.
  - Variable vessel vasculitis
    - Behçet disease
    - Cogan syndrome
  - Single-organ vasculitis
    - Cutaneous leukocytoclastic angiitis
    - Cutaneous arteritis
    - Primary CNS vasculitis
  - Vasculitis associated with systemic disease
    - Lupus vasculitis
    - Rheumatoid vasculitis
    - Sarcoid vasculitis
  - Vasculitis associated with other etiology
    - Hepatitis C–associated cryoglobulinemic vasculitis
    - Hepatitis B–associated vasculitis
    - Syphilis-associated aortitis
    - Drug-induced immune complex vasculitis
    - Drug-associated antineutrophil cytoplasmic antibodies (ANCA)–associated vasculitis
    - Cancer-associated vasculitis
- Protean features often delay definitive diagnosis.

EPIDEMIOLOGY
Highly variable, depending on the particular syndrome
- Hypersensitivity vasculitis is the most commonly encountered vasculitis in clinical practice.
- KD, IgA vasculitis, and dermatomyositis are more common in children.
- TAK is most prevalent in young Asian women. GPA, MPA, and EGPA are more common in middle-aged males.
- GCA occurs exclusively in those >50 years of age and is rare in the African American population.

Incidence
Annual incidence in adults (unless otherwise specified)
- IgA vasculitis: 200 to 700/1 million in children <17 years of age
- GCA: 170/1 million
- KD: depends on race/age; ~170/1 million
- PAN: 2 to 33/1 million
- GPA: 4 to 15/1 million
- MPA: 1 to 24/1 million
- EGPA: 1 to 3/1 million
- TAK: 2/1 million
- Hypersensitivity vasculitis: depends on drug exposure
- Viral-/retroviral-associated vasculitis: unknown; >90% of cases of cryoglobulinemic vasculitis are associated with hepatitis C.
- Connective tissue disorder–associated vasculitis: variable

ETIOLOGY AND PATHOPHYSIOLOGY
- Three major immunopathogenic mechanisms
  - Immune-complex formation: systemic lupus erythematosus (SLE), IgA vasculitis (HSP), and cryoglobulinemic vasculitis
  - ANCAs: GPA, MPA, and EGPA
  - Pathogenic T-lymphocyte response: GCA and TAK
- Pathophysiology best understood where known drug triggers have been identified (e.g., antibiotics, sulfonamides, and hydralazine)

Genetics
- A number of the vasculitic syndromes have been linked to candidate genes.
- No single gene has been found to cause vasculitis.
- Angiotensin-converting enzyme insertion/deletion polymorphism is associated with susceptibility to vasculitis, especially in Behçet disease and IgA vasculitis.

RISK FACTORS
A combination of genetic susceptibility and environmental exposure likely triggers onset.

GENERAL PREVENTION
Early identification is the key to prevent irreversible organ damage in severe forms of systemic vasculitis.

COMMONLY ASSOCIATED CONDITIONS
Hepatitis C (cryoglobulinemic vasculitis), hepatitis B (PAN), cytomegalovirus (CMV), Epstein-Barr virus (EBV), HIV (viral-/retroviral-associated vasculitis), SLE, rheumatoid arthritis (RA), Sjögren syndrome, mixed connective tissue disease (MCTD), dermatomyositis, ankylosing spondylitis, Behçet disease, relapsing polychondritis (CTD-associated vasculitis), respiratory tract methicillin-resistant *Staphylococcus aureus* (MRSA) (GPA)

Dx **DIAGNOSIS**

HISTORY
- Consider age, gender, and ethnicity.
- Comprehensive medication history
- Family history of vasculitis
- Constitutional symptoms: fever, weight loss, malaise, fatigue, diminished appetite, sweats

- CNS/PNS: mononeuritis multiplex, polyneuropathy, headaches, visual loss, tinnitus, stroke, seizure, encephalopathy
- Heart/lung: myocardial infarction, cardiomyopathy, pericarditis, cough, chest pain, hemoptysis, dyspnea
- Renal: hematuria
- GI: abdominal pain, hematochezia, perforation
- Musculoskeletal: arthralgia, myalgia
- Miscellaneous: unexplained ischemic or hemorrhagic events, chronic sinusitis, and recurrent epistaxis
- Note the organs affected and estimate the size of blood vessels involved.
- Demographics, clinical features, and the predominant vessel size/organ involvement help identify specific type of vasculitis.

PHYSICAL EXAM
- Vital signs: blood pressure (hypertension) and pulse (regularity and rate)
- Skin: palpable purpura, livedo reticularis, nodules, ulcers, gangrene, nail bed capillary changes
- Neurologic: cranial nerve exam, sensorimotor exam
- Ocular exam: visual fields, scleritis, episcleritis
- Cardiopulmonary exam: rubs, murmurs, arrhythmias
- Abdominal exam: tenderness, organomegaly

DIFFERENTIAL DIAGNOSIS
- Fibromuscular dysplasia
- Embolic disease (atheroma, cholesterol emboli, atrial myxoma, mycotic aneurysm with embolization)
- Drug-induced vasospasm (cocaine, amphetamines, ergots)
- Thrombotic thrombocytopenic disorders (disseminated intravascular coagulation [DIC], thrombotic thrombocytopenic purpura [TTP], antiphospholipid syndrome, heparin- or warfarin-induced thrombosis)
- Systemic infection (infective endocarditis, fungal infections, disseminated gonococcal infection, Lyme disease, syphilis, Rocky Mountain spotted fever [RMSF], bacteremia)
- Malignancy (lymphomatoid granulomatosis, angioimmunoblastic T-cell lymphoma, intravascular lymphoma)
- Miscellaneous (Goodpasture syndrome, sarcoidosis, amyloidosis, Whipple disease, congenital coarctation of aorta)

DIAGNOSTIC TESTS & INTERPRETATION

ALERT
- Renal involvement is often clinically silent. Routine serum creatinine and urinalysis with microscopy are needed to identify underlying glomerulonephritis.

- Initial tests to exclude alternate diagnosis and guide appropriate therapy
- Routine tests
  - CBC
  - Liver enzymes
  - Serum creatinine
  - Urinalysis with microscopy

- Specific serology
  - Antinuclear antibodies (ANA)
  - Rheumatoid factor (RF)
  - Rapid plasma reagin/venereal disease reaction level (RPR/VDRL)
  - RMSF titer
  - Lyme titer
  - Complement levels C3, C4
  - ANCA
  - Antiproteinase 3 antibodies (anti-PR3)
  - Antimyeloperoxidase antibodies (anti-MPO)
  - Hepatitis screen for B and C
  - Cryoglobulin
  - Anti-GBM titer
  - HIV
  - Serum and urine protein electrophoresis
- Miscellaneous
  - Drug screen
  - ESR
  - C-reactive protein
  - Creatine kinase (CK)
  - Blood culture
  - ECG
- CXR, CT scan, MRI, and arteriography may be required to delineate extent of organs involved.

Diagnostic Procedures/Other
- Electromyography with nerve conduction can document neuropathy and target nerve for biopsy.
- Biopsy of affected site confirms diagnosis (e.g., temporal artery, sural nerve, renal biopsy).
- If biopsy is not practical, angiography may be diagnostic for large- and medium-vessel vasculitides.
- Bronchoscopy may be required to differentiate pulmonary infection from potentially life-threatening hemorrhagic vasculitis in patients with hemoptysis.

Test Interpretation
Blood vessel biopsy shows immune cell infiltration into vessel wall layers with varying degrees of necrosis and granuloma formation, depending on the type of vasculitis

 TREATMENT

GENERAL MEASURES
- Discontinue offending drug (hypersensitivity vasculitis)
- Simple observation for mild cases of IgA vasculitis
- ANCA-associated vasculitis has 2-phase treatment: initial induction followed by maintenance (steady tapering of corticosteroids with immunosuppressants or immunomodulators)

MEDICATION
First Line
Corticosteroids are initial anti-inflammatory of choice.

Second Line
Cytotoxic medications, immunomodulatory, or biologic agents (e.g., cyclophosphamide (2)[B],(3,4)[A] methotrexate (4,5)[A], azathioprine (4,5)[A], leflunomide (4)[A], mycophenolate mofetil (2)[B],(4)[A], and rituximab (3,4)[A], are often required in combination with corticosteroids for rapidly progressive vasculitis with significant organ involvement or inadequate response to corticosteroids.

ISSUES FOR REFERRAL
- Rheumatology referral for complicated cases where newer or more toxic treatments are required.
- Nephrology referral for persistent hematuria or proteinuria, rising creatinine, or a positive ANCA titer
- Pulmonary referral for persistent pulmonary infiltrate unresponsive to antibiotic therapy or if gross hemoptysis

ADDITIONAL THERAPIES
- IVIG and aspirin for KD, but corticosteroids are contraindicated.
- Plasma exchange appears to improve recovery of patients with severe acute renal failure secondary to vasculitis and pulmonary hemorrhage (4)[A].

SURGERY/OTHER PROCEDURES
Rarely, corrective surgery is required to repair tissue damage as a result of aggressive vasculitis.

INPATIENT CONSIDERATIONS
Admission Criteria/Initial Stabilization
- Hemoptysis, acute renal failure, intestinal ischemia, any organ-threatening symptoms or signs, and/or need for biopsy
- Initial therapy is guided by the organ system involved.
  - If pulmonary hemorrhage is present, life-saving measures may include mechanical ventilation, plasmapheresis, and immunosuppression.
  - If acute renal failure is present, attend to electrolyte and fluid balance and consider plasma exchange and immunosuppression.
  - If signs of intestinal ischemia are present, make NPO and consider plasmapheresis, immunosuppression, and parenteral nutrition.

Discharge Criteria
Stabilization or resolution of potential life-threatening symptoms

 ONGOING CARE

FOLLOW-UP RECOMMENDATIONS
If significant coronary artery disease is involved in KD, moderate activity restriction may be of benefit.

Patient Monitoring
Frequent clinical follow-up supported by patient self-monitoring to identify disease relapse

DIET
Alter diets for patients with renal involvement or hyperglycemia/dyslipidemia

PROGNOSIS
Prognosis is good for patients with vasculitis and limited organ involvement. Relapsing courses, renal, intestinal, or extensive lung involvement have a poorer prognosis.

COMPLICATIONS
- Persistent organ dysfunction may be the result of the disease, medications, or inflammation/scarring in the more serious forms of vasculitis.
- Early morbidity/mortality is due to active vasculitic disease; delayed morbidity/mortality may also be secondary to complications of chronic therapy with cytotoxic medications.

REFERENCES

1. Jennette JC, Falk RJ, Bacon PA, et al. 2012 revised International Chapel Hill Consensus Conference nomenclature of vasculitides. *Arthritis Rheum*. 2013;65(1):1–11.
2. Appel GB, Contreras G, Dooley MA, et al. Mycophenolate mofetil versus cyclophosphamide for induction treatment of lupus nephritis. *J Am Soc Nephrol*. 2009;20(5):1103–1112.
3. Stone JH, Merkel PA, Spiera R, et al. Rituximab versus cyclophosphamide for ANCA-associated vasculitis. *N Engl J Med*. 2010;363(3):221–232.
4. Walters GD, Willis NS, Craig JC. Interventions for renal vasculitis in adults. A systematic review. *BMC Nephrol*. 2010;11:12.
5. Bosch X, Guilabert A, Espinosa G, et al. Treatment of antineutrophil cytoplasmic antibody associated vasculitis: a systematic review. *JAMA*. 2007;298(6):655–669.

ADDITIONAL READING

- Bertsias G, Ioannidis JP, Boletis J, et al. EULAR recommendations for the management of systemic lupus erythematosus. Report of a Task Force of the EULAR Standing Committee for International Clinical Studies Including Therapeutics. *Ann Rheum Dis*. 2008;67(2):195–205.
- Gatto M, Iaccarino L, Canova M, et al. Pregnancy and vasculitis: a systematic review of the literature. *Autoimmun Rev*. 2012;11(6–7):A447–A459.
- Lee YH, Choi SJ, Ji JD, et al. Associations between the angiotensin-converting enzyme insertion/deletion polymorphism and susceptibility to vasculitis: a meta-analysis. *J Renin Angiotensin Aldosterone Syst*. 2012;13(1):196–201.
- National Heart Lung and Blood Institute Diseases and Conditions Index: Vasculitis. www.nhlbi.nih.gov/health/dci/Diseases/vas/vas_whatis.html
- Vasculitis Foundation: www.vasculitisfoundation.org/

 CODES

ICD10
- I77.6 Arteritis, unspecified
- M31.30 Wegener's granulomatosis without renal involvement
- M30.0 Polyarteritis nodosa

CLINICAL PEARLS

- Suspect vasculitis in patients with a petechial rash, palpable purpura, glomerulonephritis, pulmonary-renal syndrome, intestinal ischemia, or mononeuritis multiplex.
- Exclude silent renal involvement by routinely obtaining serum creatinine and urinalysis with microscopy.
- Vasculitis has "skip" lesions, which may complicate diagnostic biopsy.
- In patients with vasculitis, look for a primary underlying process such as infection, thrombosis, or malignancy.

V

VENOUS INSUFFICIENCY ULCERS

Barbara J. Provo, MSN, RN, FNP-BC, CWON • Shahriar Alizadegan, MD

BASICS

- Venous insufficiency disorders include simple spider veins, varicose veins, and leg edema.
- In the United States, 23% of adults have varicose veins, an estimated 22 million women and 11 million men.
- Venous leg ulcers are the most serious consequence of venous insufficiency.
- Venous leg ulcers are a type of chronic wound affecting up to 1% of adults in developed countries at some point during their lives.
- 500,000 people in the United States have chronic venous ulcers, with an estimated treatment cost of >$3 billion per year.

DESCRIPTION

- Full-thickness skin defect with surrounding pigmentation and dermatitis
- Most frequently located in ankle region of lower leg ("gaiter region")
- Present for >30 days and fails to heal spontaneously
- May only have mild pain unless infected
- Other signs of chronic venous insufficiency include edema/brawny edema and chronic skin changes (i.e., hyperpigmentation and/or fibrosis).

EPIDEMIOLOGY

Up to 80% of leg ulcers are caused by venous disease; arterial disease accounts for 10–25%, which may coexist with venous disease.

Incidence

- Overall incidence of venous ulcers is 18/100,000 persons.
- Prevalent sex: women > men (20.4 vs. 14.6 per 100,000 for venous ulcer); increased with age for both sexes

Prevalence

- Seen in ~1% of adult population in industrialized countries, increased to 5% in patients ≥80 years old
- Prevalence studies only available for Western countries
- Point prevalence underestimates the extent of the disease because ulcers often recur.
- 70% of ulcers recur within 5 years of closure.

ETIOLOGY AND PATHOPHYSIOLOGY

- In a diseased venous system, venous pressure in the deep system fails to fall with ambulation, causing venous hypertension.
- Venous hypertension comes from the following:
  - Venous obstruction
  - Incompetent venous valves in the deep or superficial system
  - Inadequate muscle contraction (e.g., arthritis, myopathies, neuropathies) so that the calf pump is ineffective
- Venous pressure transmitted to capillaries leading to venous hypertensive microangiopathy and extravasation of RBCs and proteins (especially fibrinogen)
- Increased RBC aggregation leads to reduced oxygen transport, slowed arteriolar circulation, and ischemia at the skin level, contributing to ulcers.
- Leukocytes aggregate to hypoxic areas and increase local inflammation.
- Factors promoting persistence of venous ulcers
  - Prolonged chronic inflammation
  - Bacterial infection, critical colonization

RISK FACTORS

- History of leg injury
- Obesity
- Congestive heart failure (CHF)
- History of deep venous thrombosis (DVT)
- Failure of calf muscle pump (e.g., ankle fusion, inactivity) is a strong independent predictor of poorly healing wounds.
- Previous varicose vein surgery
- Family history

GENERAL PREVENTION

- Primary prevention after symptomatic DVT: Prescribe compression hose to be used as soon as feasible for at least 2 years (≥20 to 30 mm Hg compression).
- Secondary prevention of recurrent ulceration includes compression, correction of the underlying problem, and surveillance. Circumstantial evidence from two RCTs showed those who stopped wearing compression hose were more likely to recur.
- Compression hose reduces rates of recurrence compared with no compression.
- Because most ulcers develop following some type of trauma, avoiding lower leg trauma may help to prevent ulceration.

COMMONLY ASSOCIATED CONDITIONS

Up to 50% of patients have allergic reactions to topical agents commonly used for treatment.

- Contact sensitivity was more common in patients with stasis dermatitis (62% vs. 38%).

- Avoid neomycin sulfate in particular (including triple antibiotic ointment) (1)[A].

DIAGNOSIS

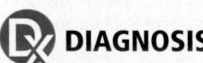

A diagnosis of venous reflux or obstruction must be established by an objective test beyond the routine clinical examination of the extremity.

HISTORY

- Family history of venous insufficiency and ulcers
- Recent trauma
- Nature of pain: achy (better with leg elevation)
- Wound drainage
- Duration of wound and over-the-counter (OTC) treatments already attempted
- History of DVTs (especially factor V Leiden mutation; strongly associated with ulceration)
- History of leg edema that improves overnight
- Edema that does not improve overnight is more likely lymphedema.

PHYSICAL EXAM

- Look for evidence of venous insufficiency:
  - Pitting edema
  - Hemosiderin staining (red and brown spotty or diffuse pigment changes)
  - Stasis dermatitis
  - White skin lesions (atrophie blanche)
  - Lipodermatosclerosis ("bottle neck" narrowing in the lower leg from fibrosis and scarring)
- Look for evidence of significant lymphedema (i.e., dorsal foot or toe edema, edema that does not resolve overnight or with elevation). This may require referral for special comprehensive lymph therapy.
- Examine for palpable pulses.

ALERT

- Examine wound for the following:
  - Length, width, depth, to monitor wound healing rate
  - Presence of necrotic tissue
  - Presence of biofilms or infection: purulent material in the wound, increased amount odorous exudate, spreading cellulitis, fever, and chills
- Get initial and interim girth measurements (at ankle and midcalf) to monitor edema.
- Important to rule out poor arterial circulation:
  - Compression dressings cannot be used in patients with ankle brachial index (ABI) <0.8.

DIFFERENTIAL DIAGNOSIS

- Arterial insufficiency ulcer
- Neuropathic ulcer
- Malignancy
- Sickle cell ulcer
- Vasculitic ulcer
- Calciphylaxis
- Cryoglobulinemia
- Pyoderma gangrenosum
- Collagen vascular disease
- Leishmaniasis
- Cutaneous tuberculosis

DIAGNOSTIC TESTS & INTERPRETATION

- Consider prothrombin time (PT)/international normalization ratio (INR) and partial thromboplastin time (PTT) if patient is anticoagulated.
- Consider biopsy of leg ulcers that fail to heal or have atypical features.
- Consider factor V Leiden mutation; strongly associated with venous ulcers.
- Test for diabetes as necessary with fasting glucose.
- Use duplex imaging to diagnose anatomic and hemodynamic abnormalities with venous insufficiency. It will also identify any DVT present.

Diagnostic Procedures/Other

- Check ABI for evidence of arterial disease.
- An ABI <0.8 is a relative contraindication to compression therapy.
- Duplex imaging for evaluation of superficial and deep venous reflux and incompetent perforator veins
- With concomitant severe arterial insufficiency, refer to a vascular surgeon for revascularization.

Test Interpretation

Strongly consider biopsy on wounds with atypical locations, failure to heal, or any suspicion of malignancy.

TREATMENT

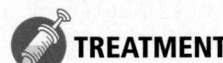

GENERAL MEASURES

Dressings: All wounds need some kind of a dressing underneath the compression system.

- Wound dressings: No single type of dressing proved superior (2)[B].

- Maintain semimoist wound environment: not excessively wet or dry.
- Wounds are often exudative until edema is decreased: Use absorptive dressings (calcium alginate or absorptive pads). Both superabsorbent diapers and female protection pads are cost-effective alternatives.
- Consider using barrier ointment/cream to prevent maceration of surrounding skin.
- If wound tends to be dry, use a hydrogel.
- A hydrocolloid dressing may be used with minimal exudate, if skin adhesive is tolerated.

MEDICATION

- Effective compression management is the cornerstone of therapy.

- Diuretics may help to reduce edema, but compression is the mainstay.
- Routine use of antibiotics for all venous ulcers is not recommended (1)[A],(3).
- Levamisole, not widely available, was the only systemic antibiotic with some evidence of benefit in terms of ulcer healing, versus treatment of infection (2)[B],(3).
- Evidence is insufficient for use of silver-based preparations and honey for healing wounds.
- Pentoxifylline 400 mg PO TID, in addition to local care and compression, improves cure rates. There is some response even without compression. GI side effects are common (4)[A].
- Aspirin 300 mg PO daily; effective when used with compression therapy

ISSUES FOR REFERRAL
- With prominent toe or foot edema, consider lymphedema. Refer to a certified lymphedema therapist (CLT).
- Refer to a wound clinic for complex or poorly healing ulcers.
- Refer to a vein clinic or vascular specialist for recurrent ulcers.
- Use home health nurses to help with immobile patients needing frequent wrapping/dressing changes.

ADDITIONAL THERAPIES
- Edema management: Reduce venous hypertension and improve venous return to reduce inflammation, pain, and improve healing (5)[A].
  - Compression therapy for edema management is the cornerstone of treatment for venous insufficiency with or without ulcers.
  - Short-stretch multilayer bandages are ideal for acute phase, until edema is stable, and the patient can be fitted for compression hose.
  - Long-term compression hose (fit once edema is reduced). Aim for a minimum pressure 20 to 30 mm Hg, preferably 30 to 40 mm Hg.
  - Elevation of legs to heart level for 30 minutes 3 to 4 times per day.
  - Exercise to strengthen calf muscle pump is also effective.
- Infection control
  - Débride necrotic tissue.
  - Treat cellulitis (usually gram-positive bacteria) with bactericidal systemic antibiotics. Suspect local infection when there is pain or no improvement in the wound after 2 weeks of compression. Consider deep quantitative swab, after thorough cleansing, or tissue biopsy for culture.
  - Treat critical colonization with topical antimicrobials, such as cadexomer iodine (silver dressings and honey are widely used, but definitive data are lacking) (3)[B].
- For venous ulcers resistant to healing with wound care and compression, consider adding an intermittent compression pump 1 to 4 hr/day.
- Encourage exercise (e.g., activation of calf muscle pump with ankle flexion and extension) in conjunction with leg compression and elevation.
- Vacuum-assisted closure (VAC) dressings may be beneficial, but no clear benefit over optimal traditional wound care.

SURGERY/OTHER PROCEDURES
- Necrotic tissue impedes healing.
  - Consider sharp débridement.
  - Other methods include enzymatic ointments (collagenase), low-frequency ultrasound, and wet-to-wry dressings.

- Avoid using collagenase with silver dressings because silver inactivates the enzyme.
- Allografts made of synthetic skin bilayered with living keratinocytes and fibroblasts improve healing at 6 months; insufficient evidence to support use of autografts.
- In patients with ulcers refractory to conservative therapy, a variety of endovenous and surgical options exist. Consultation with a vascular surgeon is recommended.
- Endovenous ablation of incompetent superficial and perforator veins has shown to reduce the size and recurrence of ulcers in those who have failed conventional compression therapy (6)[A].
- A subset of patients with nonhealing ulcers have stenosis and obstruction of the deep venous system. Venous angioplasty and stenting is emerging as an important adjunct to compression and other medical therapy (7)[A].

COMPLEMENTARY & ALTERNATIVE MEDICINE
- Chestnut seed extract (50 mg BID) is effective for venous insufficiency but not ulceration.
- Topical medicinal honey used on wounds shows no evidence of improved healing.
- Oral zinc has not been shown to be beneficial

INPATIENT CONSIDERATIONS
For those with acute significant cellulitis

Admission Criteria/Initial Stabilization
Infected wounds requiring IV antibiotics, especially in diabetics

ONGOING CARE

- Venous insufficiency is a lifelong issue.
- After resolution of an ulcer, edema management must be maintained lifelong.

FOLLOW-UP RECOMMENDATIONS
When ulcers are nearly healed and edema is controlled, switch from compression bandages to compression hose.
- Insurance may not reimburse for compression hose unless an ulcer is present.
- Referral for hose fitting must be done just prior to the ulcer being healed.

Patient Monitoring
Monitor the ulcer for healing by measuring its area. Expect at least 10% reduction every 2 weeks.

DIET
- Obese patients may benefit from weight loss.
- Low-salt diets help fluid retention.

PATIENT EDUCATION
Patient education for understanding of underlying mechanism is important for long-term management.
- Develop long-term plan for edema management and instruction on compression therapy.
- Instruct the patient on topical wound therapy.
- Teach early recognition and treatment of new ulcers or cellulitis.

PROGNOSIS
- Ulcers recur frequently. Early identification and immediate treatment are essential.
- Ongoing diligence, with edema control, avoiding infections, and avoiding trauma are important.

REFERENCES
1. Machet L, Couché C, Perrinaud A, et al. A high prevalence of sensitization still persists in leg ulcer patients: a retrospective series of 106 patients tested between 2001 and 2002 and a meta-analysis of 1975-2003 data. Br J Dermatol. 2004;150(5):929–935.
2. Palfreyman SJ, Nelson EA, Lochiel R, et al. WITHDRAWN: dressings for healing venous leg ulcers. Cochrane Database Syst Rev. 2014;(5):CD001103.
3. O'Meara S, Al-Kurdi D, Ologun Y, et al. Antibiotics and antiseptics for venous leg ulcers. Cochrane Database Syst Rev. 2014;(1):CD003557.
4. Jull AB, Arroll B, Parag V, et al. Pentoxifylline for treating venous leg ulcers. Cochrane Database Syst Rev. 2012;(12):CD001733.
5. O'Meara S, Cullum NA, Nelson EA. Compression for venous leg ulcers. Cochrane Database Syst Rev. 2012;(11):CD000265.
6. Harlander-Locke M, Lawrence PF, Alktaifi A, et al. The impact of ablation of incompetent superficial and perforator veins on ulcer healing rates. J Vasc Surg. 2012;55(2):458–464.
7. Raju S, Darcey R, Neglén P. Unexpected major role for venous stenting in deep reflux disease. J Vasc Surg. 2010;51(2):401–408.

ADDITIONAL READING
- Hamdan A. Management of varicose veins and venous insufficiency. JAMA. 2012;308(24):2612–2621.
- Kearon C, Kahn SR, Agnelli G, et al. Antithrombotic therapy for venous thromboembolic disease: American College of Chest Physicians Evidence-Based Clinical Practice Guidelines (8th Edition). Chest. 2008;133(6 Suppl):454S–545S.
- Metcalf DG, Bowler PG. Biofilm delays wound healing: a review of the evidence. Burns Trauma. 2013;1(1);5–12.
- O'Donnell TF Jr, Passman MA, Marston WA, et al. Management of venous leg ulcers: clinical practice guidelines of the Society for Vascular Surgery and the American Venous Forum. J Vasc Surgery. 2014;60(2 Suppl):3S–59S.
- Varatharajan L, Thapar A, Lane T, et al. Pharmacological adjuncts for chronic venous ulcer healing: a systematic review [published online ahead of print June 1, 2015]. Phlebology.

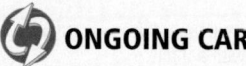 CODES

ICD10
- I87.2 Venous insufficiency (chronic) (peripheral)
- I83.009 Varicose veins of unsp lower extremity w ulcer of unsp site
- I89.0 Lymphedema, not elsewhere classified

CLINICAL PEARLS
- Initial diagnostic workup should include venous duplex scan and arterial evaluation.
- Refer patients with ABI <0.8 to vascular surgery specialist.
- Refer patients with recurrent or poor healing venous ulcers to venous specialist or wound specialist.
- Compression is essential for edema management with or without wounds.
- Treat critical colonization with topical antimicrobials (avoid neomycin).
- Make sure that the diagnosis is correct, and biopsy when in doubt.

VENTRICULAR SEPTAL DEFECT

Ian D. Thomas, MD • Brent J. Barber, MD

BASICS

DESCRIPTION
- Congenital or acquired defect of the interventricular septum that allows communication of blood between the left and the right ventricles
- Other than bicuspid aortic valve, it is the most common congenital heart malformation reported in infants and children. It also occurs as a complication of acute myocardial infarction (MI).
- Severity of the defect is correlated with its size, with large defects being the most severe.
- Blood flow across the defect typically is left to right, depending on defect size and pulmonary vascular resistance (PVR).
- Prolonged left to right shunting of blood can lead to pulmonary hypertension (HTN). This may eventually lead to a reversal of flow across the defect and cyanosis (Eisenmenger complex).

Geriatric Considerations
Almost entirely associated with MI

Pediatric Considerations
Congenital defect

ALERT
- Pregnancy may exacerbate symptoms and signs of a ventricular septal defect (VSD).
- Can be tolerated during pregnancy if VSD is small
- May be associated with an increased risk of pre-eclampsia in women with an unrepaired VSD

EPIDEMIOLOGY
Incidence
- Congenital defect: no gender predilection, occurs in ~2/1,000 live births and accounts for 30% of all congenital cardiac malformations
- Post-MI: Males are affected more than females.

Prevalence
In the United States:
- Congenital defect: lowered prevalence in adults due to spontaneous closure
- Post-MI: estimated to complicate 1–3%

ETIOLOGY AND PATHOPHYSIOLOGY
- Congenital
- In adults, complication of MI

Genetics
Multifactorial etiology; autosomal dominant and recessive transmissions have been reported.

RISK FACTORS
- Congenital:
  - Risk of sibling being affected: 4.2%
  - Risk of offspring being affected: 4%
  - Prematurity
- Complication of MI:
  - First MI
  - HTN
  - Most frequently within first week after MI
  - Occurs in 1–3% of MIs, most commonly after anterior MI

GENERAL PREVENTION
Avoid prenatal exposure to known risk factors (ibuprofen, marijuana, organic solvents, febrile illness). For adults, avoid risk factors for MI and obtain evaluation before pregnancy.

COMMONLY ASSOCIATED CONDITIONS
- Congenital:
  - Tetralogy of Fallot
  - Aortic valvular deformities, especially aortic insufficiency and bicuspid aortic valve
  - Down syndrome (trisomy 21), endocardial cushion defect
  - Transposition of great arteries
  - Coarctation of aorta
  - Tricuspid atresia
  - Truncus arteriosus
  - Patent ductus arteriosus
  - Atrial septal defect
  - Pulmonic stenosis
  - Subaortic stenosis
- Adult: coronary artery disease

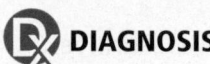

DIAGNOSIS

HISTORY
- Presentation depends on the degree of shunting across the defect; may be completely asymptomatic with small defects
- Respiratory distress, tachypnea, tachycardia
- Diaphoresis with feeds, poor weight gain in infants

PHYSICAL EXAM
- Small defect:
  - Harsh holosystolic murmur loudest at left lower sternal border
  - Detected after PVR drops at 4 to 8 weeks of life
- Moderate defect:
  - Harsh holosystolic murmur at left lower sternal border associated with a thrill
  - Forceful apical impulse with lateral displacement
  - Increased intensity of P_2
  - Diastolic rumble at apex due to increased flow across the mitral valve
- Large defect:
  - Holosystolic murmur heard throughout the precordium with diastolic rumble at apex with precordial bulge and hyperactivity, although large defects may have little or no murmur initially
  - If congestive heart failure (CHF) exists: tachycardia, tachypnea, and hepatomegaly
  - If pulmonary HTN exists: cyanosis with exertion
  - If Eisenmenger complex is present: cyanosis and clubbing

DIFFERENTIAL DIAGNOSIS
- Any defect with left-to-right shunt, such as patent ductus arteriosus, atrial septal defect
- Children: tetralogy of Fallot
- Adults: mitral regurgitation

DIAGNOSTIC TESTS & INTERPRETATION
Initial Tests (lab, imaging)
- A 12-lead ECG may suggest severity of VSD. Initially, left ventricular hypertrophy and left atrial enlargement may be evident. As pulmonary HTN develops, right ventricular hypertrophy and right atrial enlargement may be seen.
- A chest x-ray (CXR) may demonstrate increased pulmonary vascularity and/or cardiomegaly.
- A 2D echocardiogram for visualization of location and size of defect
- Color flow Doppler for direction and velocity of VSD jet; may be used to estimate right ventricular pressure

Follow-Up Tests & Special Considerations
- Weight and hematocrit check
- Cardiac catheterization performed occasionally for perioperative planning or to assess need for closure of defect

Diagnostic Procedures/Other
- Cardiac catheterization (left and right sides of heart) can confirm the diagnosis, document number of defects, quantify ratio of pulmonary blood flow to systemic blood flow (Qp/Qs), and determine PVR.
- Demonstration of an oxygen saturation step up from the right atrium to the distal pulmonary artery

Test Interpretation
- Congenital VSD (four major anatomic types)
  - Membranous (70%)
  - Muscular (20%)
  - Atrioventricular canal type (5%)
  - Supracristal (5%; higher in Asians)
- Post-MI VSD predominantly involves muscular septum.
- After surgical repair, right bundle branch block is common.

TREATMENT

- Start diuretic therapy if overload signs are present (1)[A].
- Minimize IV fluids.
- Consider ACE inhibitor and/or digoxin.
- Nasogastric feeds for neonates
- Correct anemia via iron supplementation or a possible RBC transfusion.

GENERAL MEASURES
- Appropriate health care maintenance
- Outpatient, until surgical repair is indicated
- Inpatient in setting of acute MI
- Inpatient for treatment of severe CHF

MEDICATION
First Line
- Per the 2007 American Heart Association guidelines, endocarditis antibiotic prophylaxis is not recommended for most VSDs. It is recommended for VSDs associated with complex cyanotic heart disease, during the first 6 months after surgical repair, or for residual VSDs located near the patch following surgery (2)[A]. However, recent reports suggest that patients with a left ventricle to right atrium VSD (Gerbode defect) may be at higher risk for endocarditis and thus may also need antibiotic prophylaxis (3)[C].
- Pediatric: Medications aim to control pulmonary edema, decrease work of breathing, and allow for growth:
  - Furosemide 1 to 2 mg/kg PO/IV once to twice a day
  - Spironolactone 1 to 2 mg/kg/day divided BID
  - Captopril
    - Infants: Oral: 0.3–2.5 mg/kg/day divided every 8–12 hours; max 2 mg/kg/day
    - Children and adolescents: Oral: 0.3–6 mg/kg/day divided every 8–12 hours; maximum daily dose: 150 mg/day

– Digoxin: infants <2 years of age, 10 μg/kg/day PO divided BID; children, 2 to 10 years of age, 5 to 10 μg/kg/day PO divided BID; children >10 years of age, 2 to 5 μg/kg/day PO divided BID

- Adults: Digoxin and diuretics may be beneficial in some circumstances (1)[A].

- Side effects:
  – Drugs that increase systemic vascular resistance may increase left-to-right shunting and cause signs and symptoms of pulmonary overcirculation.
  – HTN

Second Line
- Surgical closure is generally indicated if the pulmonic-to-systemic flow is >2:1 or with poorly controlled pulmonary overcirculation despite maximal medical and dietary interventions.
- If an infant with a VSD has persistent pulmonary HTN or failure to grow, surgical repair generally is recommended prior to 6 months of age even if patient is otherwise asymptomatic.
- For post-MI VSDs, afterload reduction, inotropic support, intra-aortic balloon pump, and left ventricular assist device may be used to stabilize the patient prior to surgery. Surgical repair includes septal debridement and patch placement.

ISSUES FOR REFERRAL
Close follow-up of a congenital VSD is necessary until primary intracardiac repair is performed to ensure that significant pulmonary HTN does not develop.

ADDITIONAL THERAPIES
- Infant caloric requirements up to 150 kcal/kg/day or more for adequate weight gain
- Treatment of iron deficiency anemia to increase oxygen-carrying capacity

SURGERY/OTHER PROCEDURES
- Surgical correction with either a VSD patch or repair is commonly used. Postsurgical outcomes for isolated VSD are excellent. Complications are rare and include reoperation for residual VSD, extended hospital stay, arrhythmias, valve injury, depressed ventricular function, and heart block (4)[B].
- Percutaneous transcatheter device closure has become a safe and effective option for some children with small to moderate VSDs. Complications include valvular regurgitation, residual defects, and heart block. There is a greater risk of conduction abnormality with this technique compared to surgical closure. Recent studies have shown steroids may decrease this risk (5)[A].
- Perventricular device closure (hybrid technique) of some subtypes of isolated VSDs without cardiopulmonary bypass is feasible under transesophageal echocardiographic (TEE) guidance. Complications are similar to percutaneous closure (6)[A].

INPATIENT CONSIDERATIONS
Admission Criteria/Initial Stabilization
- Failure to thrive
- Pulmonary overcirculation/CHF
- Stabilize airway
- Reduce temperature stress

Nursing
Frequent vital sign monitoring; daily weight and calorie counts

Discharge Criteria
CHF stabilization, weight gain, or successful repair

ONGOING CARE

FOLLOW-UP RECOMMENDATIONS
- Small VSDs without evidence of CHF or pulmonary HTN generally can be followed every 1 to 5 years after the neonatal period.
- Moderate to large VSDs require more frequent follow-up.
- Potential complications of VSDs include right ventricular outflow obstruction and aortic valve prolapse.

Patient Monitoring
- Physical growth and development monitoring
- Influenza vaccine for children >6 months of age
- Palivizumab to children <12 months of age with hemodynamically significant lesions. Children with small VSDs do not need RSV prophylaxis (7)[A].

DIET
- Low sodium in heart failure
- High calorie in failure to thrive

PATIENT EDUCATION
- No activity restriction in absence of pulmonary HTN
- Parents need support and instructions for prevention of complications until the child is ready for surgery.

PROGNOSIS
- Congenital:
  – Course is variable depending on the size of the VSD.
  – Small VSD: many will close spontaneously by age 3 years. Muscular defects are more likely to close spontaneously.
  – Large VSD: CHF or failure to thrive in infancy necessitating surgical repair.
  – 20-year cumulative survival rate after surgery for isolated VSD is 87%; 40 years is 78% (8).
  – Progressive pulmonary vascular disease and pulmonary HTN are the most feared complications of VSD caused by left-to-right shunting and may eventually lead to reversal of the shunt (Eisenmenger complex). Death usually occurs in the 4th decade of life if untreated.
- Post-MI:
  – With medical management alone, 80–90% mortality in the first 2 weeks
  – Prognosis worse with inferior MI compared with anterior MI

COMPLICATIONS
- CHF
- Aortic insufficiency
- Sudden death
- Hemoptysis
- Cerebral abscess
- Paradoxical emboli
- Cardiogenic shock
- Heart block rarely may accompany surgical closure.
- Pulmonary HTN

REFERENCES

1. Faris RF, Flather M, Purcell H, et al. Diuretics for heart failure. *Cochrane Database Syst Rev*. 2012;(2):CD003838.
2. Wilson W, Taubert KA, Gewitz M, et al. Prevention of infective endocarditis: guidelines from the American Heart Association: a guideline from the American Heart Association Rheumatic Fever, Endocarditis, and Kawasaki Disease Committee, Council on Cardiovascular Disease in the Young, and the Council on Clinical Cardiology, Council on Cardiovascular Surgery and Anesthesia, and the Quality of Care and Outcomes Research Interdisciplinary Working Group. *Circulation*. 2007;116(15):1736–1754.
3. Lax D, Bhatt RD, Klewer SE, et al. Are all ventricular septal defects created equal? *J Am Soc Echocardiogr*. 2010;23(7):791.e5–791.e7.
4. Scully BB, Morales DL, Zafar F, et al. Current expectations for surgical repair of isolated ventricular septal defects. *Ann Thorac Surg*. 2010;89(2):544–549.
5. Yang L, Tai BC, Khin LW, et al. A systematic review on the efficacy and safety of transcatheter device closure of ventricular septal defects (VSD). *J Interv Cardiol*. 2014;27(3):260–272.
6. Yin S, Zhu D, Lin K, et al. Perventricular device closure of congenital ventricular septal defects. *J Card Surg*. 2014;29(3):390–400.
7. American Academy of Pediatrics Committee on Infectious Diseases; American Academy of Pediatrics Bronchiolitis Guidelines Committee. Updated guidance for palivizumab prophylaxis among infants and young children at increased risk of hospitalization for respiratory syncytial virus infection. *Pediatrics*. 2014;134(2):415–420.
8. Menting ME, Cuypers JA, Opić P, et al. The unnatural history of the ventricular septal defect: outcome up to 40 years after surgical closure. *J Am Coll Cardiol*. 2015;65(18):1941–1951.

ADDITIONAL READING

Penny DJ, Vick GW III. Ventricular septal defect. *Lancet*. 2011;377(9771):1103–1112.

 ## SEE ALSO

Down Syndrome; Acute Coronary Syndromes: NSTE-ACS (Unstable Angina and NSTEMI); Tetralogy of Fallot

 ## CODES

ICD10
- Q21.0 Ventricular septal defect
- I23.2 Ventricular septal defect as current comp following AMI
- Q21.3 Tetralogy of Fallot

CLINICAL PEARLS
- A loud 2/6 to 3/6 low-pitched harsh holosystolic murmur at the left lower sternal border is typical.
- A diastolic rumble at the apex indicates moderate to large VSD or Qp:Qs >2:1, which likely will require surgical or percutaneous closure.
- Disappearance of the murmur could be secondary to spontaneous closure of the defect or the development of pulmonary HTN.
- Development of a new murmur of semilunar valve insufficiency should be further evaluated. Pulmonary regurgitation may occur as PVR increases, and the development of aortic regurgitation usually will require early surgery.

V

VERTIGO

Jeremy Raab, MD • James J. Arnold, DO, FAAFP

BASICS

DESCRIPTION
- A symptom, not a disease process. Among the potential causes are several life-threatening conditions. As such, the cause must be identified in order to determine the appropriate treatment.
- Sensation of movement ("room spinning") when no movement is actually occurring; results from peripheral or central causes or may be induced by medications/anxiety disorders
- Important to distinguish between vertigo, presyncope (patient feels like they are going to black out; vision and hearing may become obscured), disequilibrium (off balance), and light-headedness (vague, inconsistent symptoms, no rotational component)
- System(s) affected: nervous
- Synonym(s): dizziness; acute vestibular neuritis; labyrinthitis; benign paroxysmal positional vertigo (BPPV)

EPIDEMIOLOGY
Incidence
- Vertigo accounts for 54% of cases of dizziness reported in primary care; >90% of these patients are diagnosed with peripheral causes such as BPPV (1).
- Predominant sex: Female = male; women are more likely to experience central causes, particularly vertiginous migraine.

Geriatric Considerations
- Elderly patients with risk factors for cerebrovascular disease (CVD) are more likely to experience central causes.
- BPPV is commonly undiagnosed in the elderly and is an important risk factor for falls.

Prevalence
- Ranges from 5 to 10% within the general population
- Lifetime prevalence for BPPV is 2.4%.

ETIOLOGY AND PATHOPHYSIOLOGY
- Dysfunction of the rotational velocity sensors of the inner ear results in asymmetric central processing. This is related to the combination of sensory disturbance of motion and malfunction of the central vestibular apparatus.
- Peripheral causes: Acute labyrinthitis, acute vestibular neuritis, BPPV (posterior canal 85–95%, lateral canal 5–15%), herpes zoster oticus, cholesteatoma, Ménière disease, otosclerosis, perilymphatic fistula, superior canal dehiscence syndrome, motion sickness; (1,2) BPPV, vestibular neuritis, and Ménière disease account for 93% of all vertigo (2).
- Central causes: cerebellar tumor, CVD, migraine, multiple sclerosis (1)
- Drug causes: psychotropic agents (antipsychotics, antidepressants, anxiolytics, anticonvulsants, mood stabilizers), aspirin, aminoglycosides, furosemide (diuretics), amiodarone, α-/β-blockers, nitrates, urologic medications, muscle relaxants, phosphodiesterase inhibitors (sildenafil), excessive insulin, ethanol, quinine, cocaine
- Other causes: cervical, psychological

Genetics
Family history of CVD/migraines may indicate higher risk of central causes.

RISK FACTORS
- History of migraines
- History of CVD/risk factors for CVD
- Use of ototoxic medications
- Trauma/barotrauma
- Perilymphatic fistula
- Heavy weight bearing
- Psychosocial stress/depression
- Exposure to toxins

GENERAL PREVENTION
If due to motion sickness, consider pretreatment with anticholinergics, such as scopolamine.

DIAGNOSIS

HISTORY
- Determine if true vertigo or not by asking, "when you have dizzy spells, do you feel light-headed or do you see the world spin around you?" This reliably differentiates vertigo from nonvertiginous dizziness (1,2)[C].
- Obtain other medical and medication history: recent use of ototoxic medications (e.g., aminoglycosides); history of alcohol, nicotine, and caffeine use; sexual history; history of CVD/risk factors for CVD (1,3).
- Ask about duration of symptoms (2)[C].
  - A few seconds: peripheral cause such as unilateral loss of vestibular function; late stages of Ménière disease
  - Several seconds to a few minutes: BPPV; perilymphatic fistula
  - Several minutes to 1 hour: posterior TIA; perilymphatic fistula
  - Hours: Ménière disease, migraine, acoustic neuroma
  - Days: early acute vestibular neuritis, CVA, migraine, MS
  - Weeks: psychogenic (constant symptoms without improvement)
- Provoking factors that help distinguish different causes of vertigo (2)[C]
  - Changes in head position: acute labyrinthitis, BPPV, cerebellar tumor, MS, perilymphatic fistula
  - Spontaneous episodes/no clear provoking factors: vestibular neuritis, TIA/CVA, Ménière disease, migraine, MS
  - Recent URI: vestibular neuritis
  - Stress: psychogenic causes, migraine
  - Immunosuppression: herpes zoster oticus
  - Changes in ear pressure, trauma, loud noises: perilymphatic fistula
- Symptoms that help distinguish between common causes (does not include all, see differential diagnoses) (2,3)[C]
  - Aural fullness: acoustic neuroma, Ménière disease
  - Ear/mastoid pain: acoustic neuroma, acute middle ear disease (AOM, herpes zoster oticus)
  - Facial weakness: acoustic neuroma, herpes zoster oticus
  - Focal neurologic findings: cerebellar tumor, CVD, MS
  - Headache: acoustic neuroma, migraine
  - Hearing loss: Ménière disease, acoustic neuroma, otosclerosis, labyrinthitis, herpes zoster oticus, transient ischemic attack (TIA), cholesteatoma, perilymphatic fistula
  - Imbalance: acute vestibular neuritis (moderate), cerebellar tumor (severe)
  - Phonophobia/photophobia: migraine
  - Rash: herpes zoster oticus
  - Tinnitus: acute labyrinthitis, acoustic neuroma, Ménière disease

PHYSICAL EXAM
- Neurologic: cranial nerves. Consider the HINTS battery to when evaluating for a central cause (4)[C].
  - Horizontal **H**ead **I**mpulse: Rapidly bring patient's head to midline from 20 degrees. Patients with peripheral vertigo will show rapid saccades to refocus on target. In central vertigo, eyes will stay on target.
  - Direction-changing **N**ystagmus: Nystagmus typically is unidirectional. Nystagmus that changes direction with eye motion indicates a central lesion.
  - **T**est of **S**kew: Vertical eye movement during cover-uncover test indicates a central lesion. A normal test has no movement.
  - A combination of these findings is 96.8% sensitive, 98.5% specific for CVA/other central cause (HINTS positive) (4)[C].
- Balance
  - Peripheral: mild to moderate, able to walk
  - Central: severe, unable to walk
- Dix-Hallpike maneuver (2)[C]: Rapidly move the patient from seated to supine position with the head turned 45 degrees to the right. Observe for nystagmus and ask the patient if he or she is experiencing vertigo. Note: There may be 5 to 20 seconds of latency before nystagmus/vertigo begin. Wait until symptoms resolve, then return the patient to the sitting position. Always repeat on the left side.
  - The presence of extinguishing horizontal nystagmus is a positive test, consistent with peripheral causes and specifically posterior canal BPPV.
  - If induced nystagmus does not subside, consider central causes.
  - Vertical nystagmus always indicates a central cause.
  - In primary care, PPV of 83% for BPPV and NPV of 52%
  - If Dix-Hallpike is negative, check for lateral canal BPPV: With patient supine, rapidly rotate head 90 degrees. If nystagmus induced, wait for it to subside, then return to neutral. Repeat on other side. Nystagmus with this test suggests lateral canal BPPV (5)[C].
- Head and neck: tympanic membranes
  - Vesicles: herpes zoster oticus
  - Cholesteatoma
  - Infection
- Cardiovascular: orthostatic changes in BP, dehydration/autonomic dysfunction

DIFFERENTIAL DIAGNOSIS
- Acoustic neuroma
- Anxiety disorder
- Arrhythmia
- BPPV (posterior or lateral canal)
- Cerebellar degeneration, hemorrhage, or tumor
- Dehydration
- Eustachian tube dysfunction/middle ear effusion
- Hypoglycemia
- Labyrinthitis/labyrinthine concussion
- Ménière disease
- Multiple sclerosis
- Orthostatic hypotension
- Perilymphatic fistula
- Parkinson disease
- Peripheral neuropathy
- Syphilis
- Superior canal dehiscence syndrome
- Vascular ischemia

- Vertiginous migraine
- Vestibular neuritis/ototoxicity

DIAGNOSTIC TESTS & INTERPRETATION

Initial Tests (lab, imaging)

- Labs not routinely necessary and identify a cause in <1% of patients (2)[C]
- Stat MRI if a central cause is suspected to rule out stroke. CT cannot reliably see the posterior fossa and will not show changes in the early stages of an infarct. Vertigo may be the only symptom of acute stroke (4)[C].
- ENT/audiology referral if Ménière disease is suspected for electronystagmography (1,2,4)[C].
- If acoustic neuroma is suspected, either CT or MRI to evaluate internal auditory canal (1,2,4)[C].

Diagnostic Procedures/Other

Audiometry if acoustic neuroma or Ménière disease is suspected

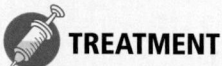 **TREATMENT**

GENERAL MEASURES

Treatments depend on cause.

- BPPV: Epley maneuver (1,3,5)[A] and modified Epley maneuver (1)[B] (Epley maneuver–YouTube)
- Vestibular neuritis and labyrinthitis
  - Vestibular-suppressant medications (1)[C],(3)
  - Vestibular rehabilitation exercises (1)[B],(3)
  - No evidence to support improvement of symptoms with corticosteroid use (6)[B]
- Ménière disease (see separate topic) (1)[B],(3):
  - Low-salt diet (<1 to 2 g/day)
  - Diuretics such as hydrochlorothiazide
- Vascular ischemia: prevention of future events through BP reduction, lipid lowering, smoking cessation, antiplatelet therapy, and anticoagulation, if necessary. MRI or CT if suspected (1,4)[C],(3)
- Vertiginous migraines: dietary and lifestyle modifications, vestibular rehab, prophylactic and abortive medications (1)[B],(3)
- Psychological: SSRIs are better than benzodiazepines for anxiety related vertigo. Use slow titration to avoid worsening symptoms (1)[B].

MEDICATION

Avoid use of medication in mild cases. Use for acute phase only (few days at most), as longer term use may impair adaptation/compensation by the brain (1). Medications not recommended for BPPV (1,3,5)[C]

- Meclizine: 12.5 to 50 mg PO q4–8h (1)
  - Dimenhydrinate: 25 to 100 mg PO, IM, or IV q4–8h (1) Precautions: prostatic hyperplasia, glaucoma
  - Adverse effects: sedation, xerostomia
  - Interactions: CNS depressants
- Prochlorperazine: 5 to 10 mg PO or IM q6–8h; 25 mg rectally q12h; 5 to 10 mg by slow IV over 2 minutes (1)
  - Contraindications: blood dyscrasias, age <2 years, hypotension
  - Precautions: acutely ill children, glaucoma, breast cancer history, impaired cardiac function, prostatic hyperplasia
  - Adverse effects: sedation, extrapyramidal effects
  - Interactions: phenothiazines, tricyclic antidepressants

- Metoclopramide: 5 to 10 mg PO q6h, 5 to 10 mg slow IV q6h (1)
  - Contraindications: concomitant use of drugs with extrapyramidal effects, seizure disorders
  - Precautions: history of depression, Parkinson disease, hypertension
  - Adverse effects: sedation, fluid retention, constipation
  - Interactions: linezolid, cyclosporine, digoxin, levodopa
- Psychiatric causes (1)
  - SSRIs for depression/anxiety (1)[B]
  - Lorazepam (Ativan) 0.5 to 2 mg orally, IM, or IV q4–8h for short-term relief of more severe anxiety
  - Diazepam (Valium) 2 to 10 mg orally or IV q4–8h for short-term relief of more severe anxiety

Geriatric Considerations

Use vestibular-suppressant medications with caution due to increased risk of falls and urinary retention.

Pregnancy Considerations

Meclizine and dimenhydrate are pregnancy Category B.

ISSUES FOR REFERRAL

Consider referral to otolaryngologist, ENT specialist, vestibular rehabilitation therapist, or neurologist if patient requires further care.

ADDITIONAL THERAPIES

- Epley maneuver/modified Epley maneuver for BPPV to displace calcium deposits in the semicircular canals (1,3,5)[A]
  - Effective for short-term symptomatic improvement and for converting patient from positive to negative Dix-Hallpike maneuver (1)[A] and some studies suggest long term relief (1)[C]
  - Contraindications: carotid stenosis, unstable cardiac disease, severe neck disease
- Lateral canal BPPV may respond to barbecue roll maneuvers (5)[C].
- Vestibular rehabilitation exercises: ball toss, lying-to-standing, target-change, thumb-tracking, tightrope, walking turns (1)[B]

 ONGOING CARE

FOLLOW-UP RECOMMENDATIONS

Balance exercises should be adhered to for symptom reduction and return to normal activities of daily living (ADLs).

Patient Monitoring

After 1 to 2 weeks, assess for the following:

- Recurrence of symptoms
- New-onset symptoms
- Medication-related adverse effects
- Relief from vestibular rehabilitation exercises

DIET

- Restricted salt intake for Ménière disease
- Dietary modifications for vertiginous migraine

PATIENT EDUCATION

- Reduce sodium intake (Ménière disease).
- Avoid triggers such as caffeine/alcohol (vertiginous migraine).

PROGNOSIS

Depends on diagnosis and response to treatment

COMPLICATIONS

- Anxiety
- Depression
- Disability
- Injuries from falls

REFERENCES

1. Swartz R, Longwell P. Treatment of vertigo. *Am Fam Physician*. 2005;71(6):1115–1122.
2. Labuguen RH. Initial evaluation of vertigo. *Am Fam Physician*. 2006;73(2):244–251.
3. Post RE, Dickerson LM. Dizziness: a diagnostic approach. *Am Fam Physician*. 2010;82(4):361–368.
4. Yew KS, Cheng EM. Diagnosis of acute stroke. *Am Fam Physician*. 2015;91(8):528–536.
5. Bhattacharyya N, Baugh RF, Orvidas L, et al. Clinical practice guideline: benign paroxysmal positional vertigo. *Otolaryngol Head Neck Surg*. 2008;139(5 Suppl 4):S47–S81.
6. Fishman JM, Burgess C, Waddell A. Corticosteroids for the treatment of idiopathic acute vestibular dysfunction (vestibular neuritis). *Cochrane Database Syst Rev*. 2011;(5):CD008607.

ADDITIONAL READING

- Fife TD, Iverson DJ, Lempert T, et al. Practice parameter: therapies for benign paroxysmal positional vertigo (an evidence–based review): report of the Quality Standards Subcommittee of the American Academy of Neurology. *Neurology*. 2008;70(22):2067–2074.
- Hilton M, Pinder D. The Epley (canalith repositioning) maneuver for benign paroxysmal positional vertigo. *Cochrane Database Syst Rev*. 2014;(12):CD003162.

 SEE ALSO

- Ménière Disease; Motion Sickness, Vertigo, Benign Paroxysmal Positional (BPPV)
- Algorithm: Dizziness

CODES

ICD10

- R42 Dizziness and giddiness
- H81.10 Benign paroxysmal vertigo, unspecified ear
- H81.49 Vertigo of central origin, unspecified ear

CLINICAL PEARLS

- Risk factors include migraines, CVD/CVD risk factors, ototoxin exposure/meds, trauma/barotrauma, perilymphatic fistula, heavy weight bearing, psychosocial stress.
- Acute vertigo with a normal horizontal head impulse, direction-changing nystagmus, and skew deviation (HINTS positive) is highly sensitive and specific for CVA.
- Nystagmus indicates a positive Dix-Hallpike test implies a peripheral cause. If nystagmus persists, investigate a central cause.
- The Epley maneuver is recommended for the treatment of BPPV; the modified Epley can be performed at home.
- Medications are not recommended for BPPV.

V

VERTIGO, BENIGN PAROXYSMAL POSITIONAL (BPPV)

Chirag N. Shah, MD • Kyung In Yoon, MD

BASICS

DESCRIPTION
- Benign paroxysmal positional vertigo (BPPV) is a mechanical disorder of the inner ear characterized by a brief period of vertigo experienced when the position of the patient's head is changed relative to gravity.
- The brief period of vertigo is caused by abnormal stimulation of ≥1 of the 3 semicircular canals of the inner ear, with the posterior canal most commonly affected.
- BPPV is the single most common cause of vertigo.

EPIDEMIOLOGY
- The lifetime prevalence of BPPV is 2.4%, and the 1-year incidence is 0.6%. The age of onset is most commonly between the 5th and 7th decades of life, and the incidence of BPPV increases with each decade of life, peaking in the 6th and 7th decades.
- Prevalent sex: female > male
- BPPV affects the quality of life of elderly patients and is associated with reduced activities of daily living scores, falls, and depression.

Prevalence
- Common
- 2.4% with one year incidence 0.6%

ETIOLOGY AND PATHOPHYSIOLOGY
- In BPPV, calcite particles (otoconia) that normally weight the sensory membrane of the maculae become dislodged and settle into the semicircular canal, changing the dynamics of the canal. Reorientation of the canal relative to gravity causes the otoconia to move to the lowest part of the canal, causing displacement of the endolymph, deflection of the cupula, and activation of the primary afferent. This results in the generation of nystagmus and the associated sensation of vertigo.
- BPPV may be idiopathic, posttraumatic, or associated with viral neurolabyrinthitis.

DIAGNOSIS

- The diagnosis is established based on history and findings on positional testing, clarified by Dix and Hallpike in 1952 (1,2)[A].
- Positional tests place the plane of the canal being tested into the plane parallel with gravity.

HISTORY
- Brief episodes of vertigo (sensation that the room is spinning) associated with
  - Rolling over in bed
  - Getting out of bed
  - Looking up (referred to as "top-shelf syndrome")
  - Bending forward
  - Quick head movements

- Patients may also complain of light-headedness or feeling "off balance."
- Frequently, patients complain of nausea and, if severe enough, vomiting.

PHYSICAL EXAM
- The Dix-Hallpike Test (DHT) is used to diagnose BPPV (1)[A]. The test provokes the characteristic nystagmus associated with the symptoms of vertigo. For the DHT, the estimated sensitivity is 79% (95% CI 65–94) and specificity is 75% (95% CI 33–100) (3)[B].

- To perform the DHT, the patient is positioned in long-sitting on the exam table with the knees extended. The head is then rotated 45 degrees toward the side to be tested. The patient is then lowered quickly to supine with the head 30 to 40 degrees below the horizontal, over the edge of the exam table. The position is maintained for a minimum of 45 to 60 seconds.
- For each position, the clinician notes the direction of the fast phase of the nystagmus and the latency and duration of the nystagmus.

Posterior canal BPPV:
- In the head-hanging position, the otoconia move away from the ampullary organ resulting in upward ipsi-torsional nystagmus.
- The superior poles of the eyes beat up toward the forehead and rotate toward the lower-most ear, the involved ear
- On return to the seated position, the otoconia move toward the ampullary organ resulting in the nystagmus reversing direction.
- The latency of onset of nystagmus is 1 to 45 seconds, and the duration is usually <1 minute.
- The nystagmus fatigues (reduction in the severity of symptoms) with repeated positioning.

Horizontal canal BPPV
- Directional-changing positional nystagmus is observed in the test positions; the eyes will beat linear-horizontal toward the ground (geotropic nystagmus) or beat toward the sky (apogeotropic nystagmus).
- One position may illicit a stronger nystagmus response. The side with great intensity indicates the side involved with geotropic lateral canal BPPV and the uninvolved side with apogeotropic lateral canal BPPV.

Anterior canal BPPV
- In the head-hanging position, the nystagmus is downbeating and torsional, with the top of the eye torting away from the lower ear.

- Usually caused by "canal switching" from canalith repositioning procedure (CRP) maneuvers
- No further testing is indicated unless the diagnosis is uncertain, or there are additional symptoms and signs unrelated to BPPV that warrant testing.

DIFFERENTIAL DIAGNOSIS
- Orthostatic hypotension and other disorders that cause low BP; symptoms usually occur when the patient stands up.
- Damage to the brainstem or cerebellum can cause positional vertigo but is accompanied by other neurologic signs and usually has a different pattern of nystagmus.
- Low spinal fluid pressure may cause positional symptoms that are better when the patient lies down.
- Migraine-associated vertigo
- Traumatic brain injury

TREATMENT

- The CRP or Epley maneuver is effective in the treatment of posterior canal BPPV (1)[A]. Using a particle repositioning maneuver, the clinician moves the patient through a series of positions. With each position, the otoconia settles to the lowest part of the canal. The debris is moved around the arc of the canal into the vestibule. In randomized controlled trials, the average short-term success rate of the CRP following one treatment session is 80 ± 9% (1)[A].
- The clinician moves the patient through a series of four provoking positions:
  - 1) Placement of the right posterior canal (involved canal) in the right head-hanging position of the DHT
  - 2) The head is then rotated a total of 90 degrees toward the left (uninvolved side) into 45 degrees of left head rotation.
  - 3) Maintaining 45 degrees of left head rotation, the patient is rolled onto the left side (uninvolved side) with the head slightly elevated from the supporting surface.
  - 4) The patient then sits up and flexes the neck 36 degrees. Each position is maintained for a minimum of 45 seconds or as long as the nystagmus lasts. The procedure is repeated three times.

- CRP is the best maneuver for posterior BPPV and should be offered to all age groups (4)[A].
- Semont maneuver is also another maneuver, less superior when performed alone (4)[A].
- Contraindications are carotid stenosis, unstable cardiac disease, and severe neck disease. If the CRP is ineffective, self-administered CRP is performed at home (1)[A]. The patient performs the CRP on the bed with the head extended over the edge of a pillow. Better outcomes are achieved with a combination of CRP with self-administered CRP (1)[A].
- CRP and Semont are ineffective for horizontal BPPV; variations of the Lempert maneuver, barbecue roll, or Gufoni maneuver are widely used treatment methods for horizontal BPPV.
- Postmaneuver activity restrictions were previously advocated but in controlled trials it did not differ in clinical outcomes, which suggests that restrictions do not appear to affect the efficacy of positional maneuvers (2,4)[A].

MEDICATION

- Vestibular suppressant medications are not recommended for treatment of BPPV, other than for the short-term management of vegetative symptoms (3)[A].
- Antiemetics such as ondansetron (Zofran) may be considered for prophylaxis for patients who have had severe nausea or vomiting with the DHT.
- Vestibular suppressants such as benzodiazepines and antihistamine anticholinergics such as meclizine should be avoided because they may suppress nystagmus during the DHT and treatment.

ISSUES FOR REFERRAL

Consider a referral to a specialist if BPPV is unresponsive to treatment or if the patient is diagnosed with atypical BPPV involving the anterior or lateral canal. Other maneuvers are available for treatment of typical and atypical BPPV. Consider referring to a physical therapist, otolaryngologist, or neurologist.

ADDITIONAL THERAPIES

- Brandt-Daroff exercises and habituation exercises are not as effective as self-administered CRP. At 1 week, the average success rate for the Brandt-Daroff exercise is 23–24% compared with 90% for self-administered CRP (1,5)[A].
- Surgical intervention is rarely indicated, except for refractory BPPV, and includes posterior canal occlusion and singular neurectomy.

ONGOING CARE

FOLLOW-UP RECOMMENDATIONS
The patient should follow up within a week after treatment to ensure resolution.

PATIENT EDUCATION
A number of illustrative videos are available at www.youtube.com for education and self-CRP maneuvers.

PROGNOSIS
80% cure rate with CRP maneuvers, with a 30% recurrence rate at 1 year (6)[A], and 44% redevelop BPPV within 2 years (1)[A]

COMPLICATIONS
During the maneuvers, a canal conversion may occur. The debris from the canal being treated may reflux into another canal.

REFERENCES

1. Helminski JO, Zee DS, Janssen I, et al. Effectiveness of particle repositioning maneuvers in the treatment of benign paroxysmal positional vertigo: a systematic review. *Phys Ther.* 2010;90(5):663–678.
2. Devaiah AK, Andreoli S. Postmaneuver restrictions in benign paroxysmal positional vertigo: an individual patient data meta-analysis. *Otolaryngol Head Neck Surg.* 2010;142(2):155–159.
3. Halker RB, Barrs DM, Wellik KE, et al. Establishing a diagnosis of benign paroxysmal positional vertigo through the dix-hallpike and side-lying maneuvers: a critically appraised topic. *Neurologist.* 2008;14(3):201–204.
4. Fife TD, Iverson DJ, Lempert T, et al. Practice parameter: therapies for benign paroxysmal positional vertigo (an evidence-based review): report of the Quality Standards Subcommittee of the American Academy of Neurology. *Neurology.* 2008;70(22):2067–2074.
5. Amor-Dorado JC, Barreira-Fernández MP, Aran-Gonzalez I, et al. Particle repositioning maneuver versus Brandt-Daroff exercise for treatment of unilateral idiopathic BPPV of the posterior semicircular canal: a randomized prospective clinical trial with short- and long-term outcome. *Otol Neurotol.* 2012;33(8):1401–1407.
6. Smouha EE. Time course of recovery after Epley maneuvers for benign paroxysmal positional vertigo. *Laryngoscope.* 1997;107(2):187–191.

ADDITIONAL READING

- Epley JM. The canalith repositioning procedure: for treatment of benign paroxysmal positional vertigo. *Otolaryngol Head Neck Surg.* 1992;107(3):399–404.
- Mandalà M, Santoro GP, Asprella Libonati G, et al. Double-blind randomized trial on short-term efficacy of the Semont maneuver for the treatment of posterior canal benign paroxysmal positional vertigo. *J Neurol.* 2012;259(5):882–885.
- Radtke A, von Brevern M, Tiel-Wilck K, et al. Self-treatment of benign paroxysmal positional vertigo: Semont maneuver vs Epley procedure. *Neurology.* 2004;63(1):150–152.
- Strupp M, Dieterich M, Brandt T. The treatment and natural course of peripheral and central vertigo. *Dtsch Arztebl Int.* 2013;110(29–30):505–515.

CODES

ICD10
- H81.10 Benign paroxysmal vertigo, unspecified ear
- H81.12 Benign paroxysmal vertigo, left ear
- H81.11 Benign paroxysmal vertigo, right ear

CLINICAL PEARLS

- The diagnosis of BPPV is based on history and findings on positional testing (DHT).
- The typical presentation is reports of transient episodes of vertigo (sensation that the room is spinning) associated with a change in position of the head relative to gravity.
- BPPV may be treated effectively with particle-repositioning maneuvers in the office and at home.
- Vestibular suppressant medications and antiemetics are not recommended for treatment of BPPV, other than for the short-term management of symptoms.

V

VINCENT STOMATITIS

Steven A. House, MD, FAAFP, FAAHPM, HMDC

BASICS

DESCRIPTION

- Inflammatory oral infection of the gingiva, characterized by gingival necrosis, bleeding, and pain
- Disease caused by *Fusobacterium*, *Prevotella intermedia*, spirochetes, and heavy growth of oral flora
- Concomitant infection with Epstein-Barr virus, herpes simplex virus, and type 1 human cytomegalovirus is common.
- Organisms invade gingiva and oral papillae with the formation of a pseudomembranous exudate.
- Clinical presentation includes ulceration, halitosis, pain, bleeding, and necrosis. It is differentiated from other periodontal diseases in that onset is rapid, papillae are ulcerated and appear "punched out," and there is interdental necrosis (1).
- Synonym(s): Vincent angina; trench mouth; acute necrotizing ulcerative gingivitis

EPIDEMIOLOGY

Incidence

- Predominant age: 18 to 30 years in developed countries
- 3 to 14 years of age among malnourished children

Prevalence

- A Chilean study of 9,203 students aged 12 to 21 years revealed a prevalence of 6.7%.
- Overall prevalence decreases with age.

ETIOLOGY AND PATHOPHYSIOLOGY

- Impaired host immunologic response due to immunocompromise or malnutrition
- Loss of integrity of the oral mucosa
- Increased bacterial attachment with herpesvirus active infection

RISK FACTORS

- Poor oral hygiene
- Orthodontics (2)
- Infrequent or absent dental care
- Malnutrition
- Tobacco use
- Herpesvirus infection
- Immunosuppression
- Psychological stress
- Diabetes, especially if uncontrolled (3)
- Down syndrome
- Pregnancy (3)

GENERAL PREVENTION

- Regular dental care
- Proper oral hygiene
- Appropriate nutrition
- Prompt recognition and institution of therapy
- Stress management

COMMONLY ASSOCIATED CONDITIONS

- Bacteremia
- Osteomyelitis
- Tooth loss
- Noma/cancrum oris, which can be life-threatening.
- Aspiration pneumonia

DIAGNOSIS

HISTORY

- Acute onset of gingival ulcer
- Halitosis
- Painful, bleeding, and inflamed gingiva
- Fever
- Malaise
- History of immunosuppression chemotherapy, HIV infection
- History of herpesvirus infection

PHYSICAL EXAM

- Ulceration of the oral papillae
- Inflamed, erythematous gingiva
- Formation of gray, pseudomembranous exudate
- Necrotic tissue on gingiva and surrounding structures
- Cervical lymphadenopathy

DIFFERENTIAL DIAGNOSIS

- Herpes simplex virus
- Periodontitis
- Pericoronitis
- Medication side effects
- Oral malignancy
- Xerostomia
- Diphtheria
- Lymphoma/leukemia
- Primary syphilis
- Ascorbic acid deficiency
- Gingivitis
- Behçet disease

DIAGNOSTIC TESTS & INTERPRETATION

Initial Tests (lab, imaging)

- Diagnosis is primarily based on clinical exam, but if systemic illness or localized spread to surrounding tissues is suspected, the following studies should be considered:
  - Aerobic and anaerobic cultures of inflamed or debrided tissue
  - Group A strep rapid antigen detection assay
  - Group A strep throat culture
  - Blood cultures if systemic involvement
  - Dental radiographs
  - Facial radiographs or CT of the neck and sinuses if infection has progressed

TREATMENT

MEDICATION
- Decision regarding locus of treatment (outpatient or inpatient) and route (PO or IV) depends on the degree of systemic illness present and on the involvement of structures in the neck.
- Medication regimens provided below are for outpatient treatment.

First Line
- Penicillin V K 500 mg q6h for 7 to 10 days (4)[C] *or*
- Amoxicillin 500 mg TID for 7 days *or*
- Amoxicillin-clavulanate 875 mg q12h for 7 to 10 days if more concerned regarding complications

Second Line
- Metronidazole 500 mg q8h for 7 to 10 days *or*
- Erythromycin 500 mg BID for 7 days (if PCN allergy) (4)[C] *or*
- Clindamycin 450 mg q8h for 7 to 10 days (if PCN allergy) (1)[C]

ISSUES FOR REFERRAL
Patients can be evaluated and treated by oral surgeon, dentist/periodontist, or ear, nose, and throat specialist depending on patient preference and severity of infection.

ADDITIONAL THERAPIES
- Chlorhexidine gluconate 0.12% BID or salt water rinses (2)[C]
- Pain management with NSAIDs (5)[C]

SURGERY/OTHER PROCEDURES
- Débridement of inflamed and necrotic tissue
- Dental extraction

INPATIENT CONSIDERATIONS
Admission Criteria/Initial Stabilization
- Failure of oral antibiotics and disease progression
- Need for parenteral antibiotics and analgesia
- Inability to meet nutritional and/or hydration needs

IV Fluids
May be required if patient is unable to tolerate oral fluids

Discharge Criteria
- Arrest of disease progression and improvement at site
- Ability to tolerate oral antibiotics and fluids
- Oral analgesia is effective

 ONGOING CARE

FOLLOW-UP RECOMMENDATIONS
Frequent dental cleanings and examinations

DIET
- Proper nutrition
- Multivitamin supplementation

PATIENT EDUCATION
- Proper nutrition
- Appropriate oral hygiene
- Tobacco cessation
- Stress management

COMPLICATIONS
- Malnutrition
- Pain
- Poor dentition, tooth loss
- Systemic infection
- Involvement of soft tissues and structures of the neck

REFERENCES

1. Atout RN, Todescan S. Managing patients with necrotizing ulcerative gingivitis. *J Can Dent Assoc.* 2013;79:d46.
2. Sangani I, Watt E, Cross D. Necrotizing ulcerative gingivitis and the orthodontic patient: a case series. *J Orthod.* 2013;40(1):77–80.
3. Silk H. Diseases of the mouth. *Prim Care.* 2014;41(1):75–90.
4. Edwards PC, Kanjirath P. Recognition and management of common acute conditions of the oral cavity resulting from tooth decay, periodontal disease, and trauma: an update for the family physician. *J Am Board Fam Med.* 2010;23(3):285–294.
5. Hodgdon A. Dental and related infections. *Emerg Med Clin North Am.* 2013;31(2):465–480.

ADDITIONAL READING

- Carlson JA, Dabiri G, Cribier B, et al. The immunopathobiology of syphilis: the manifestations and course of syphilis are determined by the level of delayed-type hypersensitivity. *Am J Dermatopathol.* 2011;33(5):433–460.
- Lopez R, Fernandez O, Jara G, et al. Epidemiology of necrotizing ulcerative gingival lesions in adolescents. *J Periodontal Res.* 2002;37(6):439–444.
- Marik PE. Pulmonary aspiration syndromes. *Curr Opin Pulm Med.* 2011;17(3):148–154.
- Porter SR. Diet and halitosis. *Curr Opin Clin Nutr Metab Care.* 2011;14(5):463–468.
- Slots J. Herpesviral-bacterial synergy in the pathogenesis of human periodontitis. *Curr Opin Infect Dis.* 2007;20(3):278–283.

 CODES

ICD10
A69.1 Other Vincent's infections

CLINICAL PEARLS
- Poor oral hygiene and immunosuppression are key factors in infection.
- Early recognition and institution of therapy decrease complications.
- Penicillin is the drug of choice for patients not systemically ill.

VITAMIN B₁₂ DEFICIENCY

Justin D. Chaltry, DO • Katie L. Westerfield, DO

BASICS

- Vitamin deficiency related to inadequate intake or absorption of cobalamin (vitamin B_{12})
- Cobalamin is critical for CNS myelination and normal functioning.
- Deficiency can cause a multitude of symptoms and disorders including megaloblastic anemia, bone marrow dysfunction, and diverse and potentially irreversible neuropsychiatric changes.
- Neuropsychiatric disorders are due to demyelination of cervical, thoracic dorsal, and lateral spinal cords; demyelination of white matter; and demyelination of cranial and peripheral nerves (1)[C].
- Low vitamin B_{12} level can lead to elevated methylmalonic acid (MMA) and homocysteine levels.
- Elevated MMA causes abnormality in fatty acid synthesis affecting neuronal membrane.
- Elevated homocysteine is neurotoxic through overstimulation of the *N*-methyl-D-aspartate (NMDA) receptor and toxic to vasculature through activation of coagulation system and effects on endothelium.

DESCRIPTION

Normal B_{12} absorption

- B_{12} present in animal-source foods (meat, fish, eggs, milk) and foods fortified with B_{12}
- Dietary vitamin B_{12} (cobalamin) bound to food is cleaved by acids in stomach and bound to haptocorrin (commonly known as R-factor).
- Duodenal proteases cleave B_{12} from haptocorrin.
- In duodenum, B_{12} uptake depends on binding to intrinsic factor (IF) secreted by gastric parietal cells.
- B_{12}-IF complex is absorbed by terminal ileum into portal circulation.
- Body's B_{12} stored in liver = 50–90%
  - B_{12} secreted into bile from liver recycled via enterohepatic circulation
  - Delay 5 to 10 years from onset of B_{12} deficiency to clinical symptoms due to hepatic stores and enterohepatic circulation
- Typical Western diet: 5 to 30 μg/day; however, only 1 to 5 μg/day is effectively absorbed.
  - Recommend 2.4 μg/day for adults and 2.6 μg/day during pregnancy and 2.8 μg/day during lactation (most prenatal vitamins contain B_{12})

EPIDEMIOLOGY

Prevalence

- Endemic area: Northern Europe, including Scandinavia; more common in those of African ancestry
- Increasing recognition in breastfed-only infant populations with vitamin B_{12} deficient mothers
- Prevalence 5–20% in developed countries
  - 12% in elderly living in community
  - 30–40% in elderly in institutions, sick, or malnourished
  - 5% patients in tertiary reference hospitals
- Prevalence by age group
  - 20 to 39 years old: prevalence 3%
  - 40 to 59 years old: prevalence 4%
  - >70 years old: prevalence 6%

ETIOLOGY AND PATHOPHYSIOLOGY

- Decreased oral intake
  - Vegetarians and vegans: B_{12} is found in animal-source foods; however, strict vegetarians uncommonly develop deficiency because only 1 mg/day is needed, with adequate amounts present in legumes.
- Decreased IF
  - Pernicious anemia (PA): can be associated with autoantibodies directed against gastric parietal cells and/or IF
  - Chronic atrophic gastritis: autoimmune attack on gastric parietal cells causing autoimmune gastritis and leading to decreased IF production
  - Gastrectomy: Removal of entire or part of stomach decreases amount of parietal cells.
- Decreased ileal absorption
  - Crohn disease: Terminal ileal inflammation decreases body's ability to absorb B_{12}.
  - Chronic alcoholism: decreases body's ability to absorb B_{12}
  - Ileal resection
  - Pancreatic insufficiency: Pancreatic proteases are required to cleave the vitamin B_{12}-haptocorrin bond to allow vitamin B_{12} to bind to intrinsic factor.
  - *Helicobacter pylori* infection impairs release of B_{12} from bound proteins.
- Medications: Proton pump inhibitors (PPIs), H_2 antagonists, and antacids decrease gastric acidity, inhibiting B_{12} release from dietary protein; metformin
- Hereditary (rare)
  - Imerslund-Grasbeck disease (juvenile megaloblastic anemia)
  - Congenital deficiency of transcobalamin
  - Severe methylene tetrahydrofolate reductase deficiency
  - Abnormalities of methionine synthesis

Causes:

- Food-cobalamin malabsorption syndrome
  - As many as 60–70% of cases
  - Primary cause in elderly
  - Pathophysiology: inability to release cobalamin from food or binding protein, especially if in the setting of hypochlorhydria
  - Seen in atrophic gastritis, long-term ingestion of antacids and biguanides, possible relationship to *H. pylori* infection
- PA
  - 15–30% of all cases; most frequent cause of severe disease. Neurologic disorders are common presenting complaints.
  - Common in elderly, as high as 20%, with mild atrophic gastritis, hypochlorhydria, and impaired release of dietary vitamin B_{12}
  - Autoimmune disease with destruction of gastric fundal mucosa cells via a cell-mediated process
  - Anti-gastric parietal cell antibodies: sensitivity >90%, specificity 50%; use for screening test
  - Anti-intrinsic factor antibodies: sensitivity 50%
  - Associated with other autoimmune diseases
- Insufficient dietary intake: 2% of cases; vegans or long-standing vegetarians
- Infants born to vitamin B_{12}-deficient mothers may have deficiency or develop it if breastfed exclusively.

- Intestinal causes:
  - 1% of cases; prevalence depends on risk factors, such as surgical conditions
  - Gastrectomy: due to decreased production of intrinsic factor
  - Gastric bypass: appears 1 to 9 years after surgery, prevalence 12–33%
  - Ileal resection or disease
  - Fish tapeworm
  - Severe pancreatic insufficiency
- Undetermined etiology
  - 1/10 of cases

Genetics

Imerslund-Grasbeck disease (juvenile megaloblastic anemia) caused by mutations in the amnionless (AMN) or cubilin (CUBN) genes with autosomal recessive pattern of inheritance; inadequate ileal uptake of B_{12}-IF complex and B_{12} renal protein reabsorption

GENERAL PREVENTION

Risk factors: vegan diet, age >65 years, female, chronic atrophic gastritis, Crohn disease or other ileal disorders, chronic medication use including PPI, metformin, H_2 antagonists

DIAGNOSIS

Symptoms and physical exam findings:

- Asymptomatic patients may be diagnosed by the incidental finding of anemia or an elevated mean corpuscular volume (MCV) during routine testing or evaluation of unassociated disorders.
- Hematologic
  - Frequent: macrocytosis, neutrophil hypersegmentation, spinal cord medullar megaloblastosis (blue spinal cord)
  - Rare: isolated thrombocytopenia and neutropenia, pancytopenia
    Very rare: hemolytic anemia, thrombotic microangiopathy with schistocytes
- Neuropsychiatric
  - Frequent: sensory polyneuritis, paresthesias, positive Babinski sign, weakness, gait unsteadiness, loss of proprioception (impaired vibratory sensation, positive Romberg, ataxia, hyperreflexia)
  - Classic, but uncommon: subacute combined degeneration of spinal cord associated with PA; myelin degeneration in the lateral and posterior columns; ataxia, proprioception and vibration loss, bowel and bladder incontinence, orthostatic hypotension, decreased memory, mania, delirium, psychosis, depression
- Digestive
  - Classic: Hunter glossitis, jaundice, and high lactate dehydrogenase and bilirubin
  - Possible: abdominal pain, dyspepsia, nausea, vomiting, diarrhea
  - Rare: mucocutaneous ulcers
- Other
  - Frequent: pallor, edema, jaundice
  - Under investigation: chronic vaginal and urinary infections, atrophy of vaginal mucosa, hypofertility, venous thromboembolism, angina, miscarriages
  - Commonly insidious and nonspecific; thus, delay in diagnosis is common.

HISTORY

- Underlying disease associated with vitamin B$_{12}$ deficiency
- Fatigue, anorexia
- Depression
- Falls (due to diminished proprioception)
- Loss of sensation in "stocking-glove" distribution
- Glossitis/loss of sense of taste, and other subtle, nonspecific neurologic symptoms

DIAGNOSTIC TESTS & INTERPRETATION

- Measurement of vitamin B$_{12}$, CBC (MCV)
- Measurement of B$_{12}$ may be low or low normal depending on institution's cutoff value.
  - 65–95% sensitivity levels <200 pg/mL
  - May need additional tests such as MMA and homocysteine if vitamin B$_{12}$ level is low normal (<350 pg/mL) and no evidence of anemia depending on clinical suspicion
- If high suspicion on normal B$_{12}$ with high/normal MCV, consider testing MMA and homocysteine levels.
- MCV often increased
- Measurement of MMA
  - More sensitive and specific than homocysteine
  - Levels increased in renal failure and volume depletion
- Measurement of homocysteine
  - Levels increased in folate deficiency, renal failure, and homocystinuria
- MMA and homocysteine levels only reliable in an untreated patient, as levels fall with supplementation
- Other tests: folate and other markers of anemia (iron studies)
- MCV may be normal, decreased, or increased if vitamin B$_{12}$ deficiency coexists with other forms of anemia, such as iron deficiency or hemolysis. Thus, RBCs may be normochromic, normocytic, or hypochromic microcytic.

ALERT

- Low levels of vitamin B$_{12}$ are seen in folate deficiency, HIV, and multiple myeloma.
- Elevated levels of vitamin B$_{12}$ are seen in renal disease, occult malignancy, and alcoholic liver disease and as a result of technical error.
- Macrocytosis may be due to folate deficiency, reticulocytosis, medications, bone marrow dysplasia, and hypothyroidism or be masked by concomitant microcytic anemia.
- Serum homocysteine and MMA
  - Elevated in B$_{12}$ deficiency secondary to decreased metabolism
  - If both are normal, B$_{12}$ deficiency is effectively ruled out.
  - If MMA is normal and homocysteine is increased, think folate deficiency.
- PA
  - Check antibody to intrinsic factor; positive test is confirmatory for PA, but sensitivity is only 50–70%.
  - Anti-parietal cell antibody positivity indicates PA.
  - For patients who are antibody positive, consider screening for autoimmune thyroid disease.

Pregnancy Considerations

- Because B$_{12}$ crosses the placenta, pregnant women with low levels of B$_{12}$ are at higher risk of having children with neural tube defects, congenital heart defects, developmental delay, and failure to thrive.
- Exclusively breastfed infants of mothers who are B$_{12}$ deficient are at risk of developing B$_{12}$ deficiency. Infants breastfed from B$_{12}$-deficient mothers might not show signs or symptoms until 4 to 6 months of age, which may include developmental regression, feeding difficulties, lethargy, or hypotonia.

Diagnostic Procedures/Other

- Bone marrow exam is usually unnecessary in the evaluation of B$_{12}$ deficiency because of the inability to differentiate from folate deficiency.
- Spinal cord imaging is not standard; MRI in selected cases, especially with severe myelopathy

 TREATMENT

MEDICATION

- Parenteral cyanocobalamin replacement recommended in patients with severe neurologic symptoms: IM cyanocobalamin (2)[C]
  - 1,000 μg/day for 7 days, *then*
  - 1,000 μg weekly for 4 weeks, *then*
  - 1,000 μg monthly for life

- High-dose, daily oral cyanocobalamin at doses of 1,000 to 2,000 μg are as effective as monthly intramuscular injection and is the preferred route of initial therapy in most circumstances because it is cost-effective and convenient (3)[A]. Requires greater patient compliance. Transnasal and buccal preparations of cyanocobalamin are also available; however, further study is needed.

ALERT

Folic acid without vitamin B$_{12}$ in patients with PA is contraindicated; it will not correct neurologic abnormalities.

INPATIENT CONSIDERATIONS

Admission Criteria/Initial Stabilization

- Consider blood transfusion for severe anemia.
- Draw blood for hematologic parameters before transfusing.

 ONGOING CARE

FOLLOW-UP RECOMMENDATIONS

Patient Monitoring

- Hematologic
  - Reticulocytosis in 1 week
  - Rise in hemoglobin beginning at 10 days; usually will return to normal in 6 to 8 weeks
  - Monitor potassium in profoundly anemic patients (hypokalemia due to potassium use).
  - Serum MMA decreases with replacement therapy.
- Neurologic: can note improvement within 3 months of treatment; however, maximum improvement noticed at 6 to 12 months. Some symptoms may be irreversible.

DIET

Meat, animal protein, and legumes unless contraindicated

REFERENCES

1. Lachner C, Steinle NI, Regenold WT. The neuropsychiatry of vitamin B12 deficiency in elderly patients. *J Neuropsychiatry Clin Neurosci.* 2012;24(1):5–15.
2. Stabler SP. Clinical practice. Vitamin B12 deficiency. *N Engl J Med.* 2013;368(2):149–160.
3. Vidal-Alaball J, Butler CC, Cannings-John R, et al. Oral vitamin B12 versus intramuscular vitamin B12 for vitamin B12 deficiency. *Cochrane Database Syst Rev.* 2005;(3):CD004655.

ADDITIONAL READING

- Allen LH. How common is vitamin B-12 deficiency? *Am J Clin Nutr.* 2009;89(2):693S–696S.
- Bizzaro N, Antico A. Diagnosis and classification of pernicious anemia. *Autoimmun Rev.* 2014; 13(4–5):565–568.
- Fernández-Bañares F, Monzón H, Forné M. A short review of malabsorption and anemia. *World J Gastroenterol.* 2009;15(37):4644–4652.
- Langan RC, Zawistoski KJ. Update on vitamin B12 deficiency. *Am Fam Physician.* 2011;83(12):1425–1430.
- Mazokopakis EE, Starakis IK. Recommendations for diagnosis and management of metformin-induced vitamin B12 (Cbl) deficiency. *Diabetes Res Clin Pract.* 2012;97(3):359–367.
- Oberley MJ, Yang DT. Laboratory testing for cobalamin deficiency in megaloblastic anemia. *Am J Hematol.* 2013;88(6):522–526.

 CODES

ICD10

- E53.8 Deficiency of other specified B group vitamins
- D51.0 Vitamin B12 defic anemia due to intrinsic factor deficiency
- D51.3 Other dietary vitamin B12 deficiency anemia

CLINICAL PEARLS

- Consider screening for B$_{12}$ deficiency in high-risk patients including the elderly and monitoring B$_{12}$ levels annually if on metformin or **on chronic PPIs.**
- Correcting folate deficiency without treating with cyanocobalamin in megaloblastic anemia may correct hematologic but not neurologic disorders.
- Vitamin B$_{12}$ deficiency can coexist with other causes of anemia, including iron deficiency or hemolysis; thus, MCV can be normal, decreased, or increased.
- For patients with PA, cyanocobalamin replacement must be lifelong.
- Patients with PA are at increased risk for other autoimmune conditions as well as gastric malignancy.

V

VITAMIN D DEFICIENCY

Marissa Hamrick, MD • Frank J. Domino, MD • Samir Malkani, MD, MRCP–UK

 BASICS

This topic covers the commonly acquired vitamin D deficiency and not type II vitamin D–resistant rickets/type I pseudovitamin D–resistant rickets (both rare autosomal recessive disorders).

DESCRIPTION
- Vitamin D is both a hormone and a vitamin.
- Cholecalciferol (D_3) is synthesized in the skin by exposure to ultraviolet B (UV-B) radiation. Ergocalciferol (D_2) and D_3 are present in foods.
- D_2 and D_3 are hydroxylated in the liver to 25 vitamin D (calcidiol), its major circulating form.
- Calcidiol is further hydroxylated in the kidney to the active metabolite 1,25 vitamin D (calcitriol).
- Hypocalcemia stimulates parathyroid hormone (PTH) to be secreted, which prompts the increased conversion of 25 vitamin D to 1,25 vitamin D.
  - 1,25 vitamin D decreases renal calcium and phosphorus excretion, increases intestinal calcium and phosphorus absorption, and increases osteoclast activity. These effects increase serum calcium.

EPIDEMIOLOGY
- Unclear in general population
- In the community, a cohort study of asymptomatic adolescents in Boston found 24.1% were deficient, with 4.6% severely deficient.
- A study of hospitalized patients in Massachusetts found 57% vitamin D–deficient (VDD).
- Women with history of osteoporosis/osteoporotic fracture have high prevalence of vitamin D deficiency.
- A cohort study in Arizona found >25% of adults were VDD; highest rates among African Americans and Hispanics
- A study of about 56,000 individuals across Europe found 13% to have vitamin D deficiency.

Pediatric Considerations
NHANES data found 70% of children did not have sufficient 25-OH vitamin D serum levels (9% deficient and 61% insufficient), which was associated with an increase in BP and decrease in high-density lipoprotein (HDL) cholesterol.

ETIOLOGY AND PATHOPHYSIOLOGY
- Insufficient dietary intake of vitamin D and/or lack of UV-B exposure (in sunlight) results in low levels of vitamin D.
  - This limits calcium absorption, causing excess PTH to be released.
- PTH stimulates osteoclast activity, which helps to normalize calcium and phosphorous, but results in osteomalacia.
- Dietary deficiency
  - Inadequate vitamin D intake

- Inadequate sunlight exposure
  - Institutionalized/hospitalized patients
- Chronic illness: liver/kidney disease
- Malabsorptive states

Genetics
Vitamin D–dependant rickets type 1 occurs due to inactivating mutation of the 1 alpha hydroxylase gene; as a result, calcidiol is autosomal recessive not hydroxylated to calcitriol.

RISK FACTORS
- Inadequate sun exposure
- Female
- Dark skin
- Immigrant populations
- Low socioeconomic status
- Latitudes higher than 38 degrees
- Elderly
- Institutionalized
- Depression
- Medications (phenobarbital, phenytoin)
- Gastric bypass surgery
- Obesity

GENERAL PREVENTION
- Adequate exposure to sunlight and dietary sources of vitamin D (plants, fish); many foods are fortified with vitamin D_2 and D_3.
- Recommended minimum daily requirement from the 2010 Institute of Medicine Report is minimally 600 IU/day for those 1 to 70 years of age and 800 IU/day for those >70 years of age. Up to 4,000 IU/day is safe in healthy adults without risk of toxicity.
- Higher intake of vitamin D recommended for age >50 years
- 2005 and 2009: Meta-analysis demonstrated for ages 51 to 70 years, minimally recommended supplementation is 800 IU/day to prevent nonvertebral fractures.

Pediatric Considerations
The American Academy of Pediatrics recommends all breast-fed babies receive 400 IU/day of vitamin D beginning "within the first few days of life."

Pregnancy Considerations
ACOG recommends data insufficient to screen all pregnancies; only those "at risk" and states it is safe to take 1,000 to 2,000 IU/day during pregnancy (1)[B].

Geriatric Considerations
U.S. Preventive Services Task Force recommends seniors take at least 800 IU/day vitamin D to reduce risk of falls in community-dwelling older adults (2)[A].

COMMONLY ASSOCIATED CONDITIONS
- Osteomalacia, osteoporosis
- Premenstrual syndrome
- Rickets
- Celiac disease

- Gastric bypass
- Chronic renal disease
- Bacterial vaginosis in pregnant women
- Hypertension

ALERT
VDD is associated with risk of myocardial infarction (MI) and all-cause mortality (3)[A].

 DIAGNOSIS

- Nonspecific musculoskeletal complaints
- Weak antigravity muscles
- Fracture with minimal trauma

HISTORY
- Senior citizens at risk of falling
- Renal disease
- GI (malabsorption) disorders
- Liver dysfunction
- Immigration from tropical to colder climates
- Dark-skinned/veiled individuals
- Housebound patients
- Women at perimenopause

PHYSICAL EXAM
- Vague neurologic signs: numbness, proximal myopathy, paresthesias, muscle cramps, laryngospasm
- Chvostek sign: contraction of the facial muscles by tapping along the facial nerve
- Trousseau phenomenon: carpal spasms and paraesthesia produced by pressure on nerves and vessels of the upper arm, by inflation of a BP cuff
- Tetany, seizures

DIAGNOSTIC TESTS & INTERPRETATION
Initial Tests (lab, imaging)
- 25-OH vitamin D (most sensitive measure of vitamin D status)
- Vitamin D deficiency
  - <20 ng/mL
- PTH elevation: not routinely obtained unless severe deficiency
- Low-normal/low calcium and phosphorous
- Elevated alkaline phosphatase (in later disease)
- Plain radiographs: If atypical fracture, radiographs may show osteomalacia (pseudofractures/looser zones) in pelvis, femur, and fibula.
- Osteoporosis screen
  - Women ≥65 years with no risk factors
  - Women ≥60 years at risk: body weight <70 kg (best predictor)
  - Less evidence: smoking, low body mass index, family history, decreased activity, alcohol or caffeine use
  - African American women have higher bone density than Caucasians.

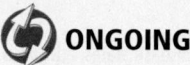 **TREATMENT**

- Treatment goals remain unclear, but current "normal" 25-OH vitamin D levels are based on suppression of PTH.

- Obesity: Treatment of VDD in obesity, especially those who are obese and depressed, improves depressive symptoms and may improve weight loss (4)[B].

ALERT

All-cause mortality: Cochrane Systematic Review found vitamin D supplementation lowers all-cause mortality (5)[A].

Geriatric Considerations

In senior citizens, serum 25-OH vitamin D of 20 ng/mL resulted in improved physical performance scores; recent data suggests supplementation may not improve fracture risk and remains unclear about a true benefit.

MEDICATION

- Vitamin D sufficient (25-OH vitamin D $\geq$20 ng/mL)

  – Vitamin D 800 to 4,000 IU/day D_2/D_3 (6)[A]

  – D_3 (animal derived) may be slightly more effective than D_2 (plant derived), but clinical significance is uncertain.

  – Calcium supplementation: Unclear benefit and may increase some CHD risk in patients. No supplementation currently required (see below).

- Vitamin D deficiency (25-OH vitamin D <20 ng/mL)

  – D_2 50,000 IU/week for 8 to 12 weeks, followed by 800 to 2,000 IU/day of vitamin D_3 (6)[A]

- Calcium: meta-analysis data support

  – Dietary intake of ~700 mg/day leads to best outcomes; higher doses did NOT decrease risk of osteoporotic fractures.

  – Dietary calcium may be more beneficial than calcium supplementation.

  – Supplementary calcium associated with an increased risk of MI, especially in women (7)[A], but this data remains controversial (8)[C].

ISSUES FOR REFERRAL

Endocrinology if no response to treatment

ADDITIONAL THERAPIES

Aggressive calcium in ICU patients with ionized calcium <3.2 mg/dL or if symptomatic (tetany, seizures, QT prolongation, bradycardia, or hypotension, or ventilated patient with decreased diaphragmatic function)

INPATIENT CONSIDERATIONS

Admission Criteria/Initial Stabilization

- Symptoms of severe hypocalcemia *or*
- Malabsorption syndromes

 ONGOING CARE

FOLLOW-UP RECOMMENDATIONS

Follow-up of abnormal 25-OH vitamin D not required

DIET

- Cod liver oil is most potent source of vitamin D and has ~1,300 IU vitamin D/tablet/tablespoon.
- Fatty fish (tuna, salmon)
- Fortified milk (100 IU/8 oz), cereal, and foods

PROGNOSIS

- Systematic review of 63 observational studies found adequate 25-OH vitamin D levels correlate with lower rates of colon, breast, and prostate cancer.
- Cohort study found that vitamin D deficiency is correlated with increased risk of all-cause mortality.

ALERT

Meta-analysis data support supplementation of >500 IU/day lowered the risk of all-cause mortality (5,9)[A] but remains controversial.

REFERENCES

1. ACOG Committee on Obstetric Practice. ACOG Committee Opinion no. 495: vitamin D: screening and supplementation during pregnancy. *Obstet Gynecol*. 2011;118(1):197–198.
2. Moyer VA; U.S. Preventive Services Task Force. Prevention of falls in community-dwelling older adults: U.S. Preventive Task Force recommendation statement. *Ann Intern Med*. 2012;157(3):197–204.
3. Correia LC, Sodré F, Garcia G, et al. Relationship of severe deficiency of vitamin D to cardiovascular mortality during acute coronary syndromes. *Am J Cardiol*. 2013;111(3):324–327.
4. Vimaleswaran KS, Berry DJ, Lu C, et al. Causal relationship between obesity and vitamin D status: bi-directional Mendelian randomization analysis of multiple cohorts. *PLoS Med*. 2013;10(2):e1001383.
5. Bjelakovic G, Gluud LL, Nikolova D, et al. Vitamin D supplementation for prevention of mortality in adults. *Cochrane Database Syst Rev*. 2011;(7): CD007470.
6. Holick MF, Binkley NC, Bischoff-Ferrari HA, et al. Evaluation, treatment, and prevention of vitamin D deficiency: an Endocrine Society clinical practice guideline. *J Clin Endocrinol Metab*. 2011;96(7): 1911–1930.
7. Bolland MJ, Avenell A, Baron JA, et al. Effect of calcium supplements on risk of myocardial infarction and cardiovascular events: meta-analysis. *BMJ*. 2010;341:c3691.
8. Chrysant SG, Chrysant GS. Controversy regarding the association of high calcium intake and increased risk for cardiovascular disease. *J Clin Hypertens (Greenwich)*. 2014;16(8):545–550.
9. Chowdhury R, Kunutsor S, Vitezova A, et al. Vitamin D and risk of cause specific death: systematic review and meta-analysis of observational cohort and randomised intervention studies. *BMJ*. 2014; 348:g1903.

CODES

ICD10

- E55.9 Vitamin D deficiency, unspecified
- M83.8 Other adult osteomalacia

CLINICAL PEARLS

- Risk factors for VDD: senior citizen, renal disease, GI (malabsorption) disorders, liver dysfunction, immigration from tropical to colder climates, dark-skinned/veiled individuals, housebound patients, perimenopause
- Diagnosis: 25-OH vitamin D (most sensitive measure of vitamin D status)
- Vitamin D deficiency: <20 ng/mL
- Up to 4,000 IU/day is safe in healthy adults without risk of toxicity.
- 2005 and 2009: Meta-analysis demonstrated for ages 51 to 70 years minimally recommended supplementation is 800 IU/day to prevent nonvertebral fractures.
- The American Academy of Pediatrics recommends all breast-fed babies receive 400 IU/day of vitamin D beginning within a few days of birth.

V

VITAMIN DEFICIENCY

Michelle E. Szczepanik, MD • Christopher D. Meyering, DO

 BASICS

DESCRIPTION

- Vitamins are essential micronutrients required for normal metabolism, growth, and development.
- Deficiencies are less common in the Western world but certain populations are at increased risk.
- Regulations mandating vitamin supplementation in food products, adequate food supply, and availability of vitamin supplements all make vitamin deficiencies in the Western world lower.
- Toxicity is rare in water-soluble vitamins; however, is possible with fat-soluble vitamins (A, D, E, K).

EPIDEMIOLOGY

Incidence
- Predominant age
  - Geriatric population, pregnant women, exclusively breastfed infants, and individuals with certain chronic disease states
- Individuals from Africa and Southeast Asia are at increased risk.
- True incidence is unknown as most vitamin deficiencies are asymptomatic.

Prevalence
- Varies by age groups, comorbid conditions, geography, and setting (i.e., urban, rural)
- The prevalence of vitamin B_{12} deficiency is around 6% in those <60 years of age but increases to around 20% after the age of 60 (1).
- Vitamin D deficiency has become increasingly recognized and its prevalence is increased in individuals with darker skin pigmentation, obesity, low dietary intake of vitamin D, or low sunlight exposure.

ETIOLOGY AND PATHOPHYSIOLOGY
- Deficiencies usually related to disease can develop under healthy conditions and generally occur due to 1 of 5 mechanisms:
  - Reduced intake
  - Diminished absorption
  - Increased use
  - Increased demand
  - Increased excretion
- Chronic disease states: HIV, malabsorption (such as celiac sprue and short bowel syndrome), chronic liver and kidney disease, alcoholism, malignancies, pernicious anemia, and rare inborn errors of metabolism
- Bariatric surgeries: gastric bypass, gastrectomy, small or large bowel resection
- Predisposition related to certain drugs: prednisone, phenytoin, isoniazid, protease inhibitors, methotrexate, phenobarbital, alcohol, nitrous oxide, H_2 receptor antagonists, metformin, colchicine, cholestyramine, 5-fluorouracil, 6-mercaptopurine, azathioprine, chloramphenicol, proton pump inhibitors, chronically used antibiotics, penicillamine, and hydralazine
- Malnutrition, imbalanced nutrition, obesity, fad diets, extreme vegetarianism, total parenteral nutrition, bulimia/anorexia, and other eating disorders
- Dialysis
- Parasitic infestation

Genetics
- Cystic fibrosis
- Hartnup disease
- Rare genetic predisposition
  - Autoimmune disease (e.g., pernicious anemia)
  - Congenital enzyme deficiencies (e.g., biotinidase or holocarboxylase synthetase deficiency)

- Transcobalamin II deficiency
- Ataxia and vitamin E deficiency (AVED)
- A-β-lipoproteinemia

RISK FACTORS
Poverty, malnutrition, chronic disease states, advanced age, dietary restrictions, bariatric surgery, and exclusively breastfed infants

GENERAL PREVENTION
- Ingesting large and varied amounts of vitamins increases risk of toxicity and drug–drug interactions.
- Antioxidant supplement use has not been shown to impact cancer incidence and, in some studies, has *increased* risk of death (2).
- Avoidance of restrictive diets decreases the likelihood of vitamin deficiency.
- In particular age groups or with certain risk factors, vitamin supplementation may be recommended.
- U.S. Preventive Services Task Force (USPSTF) recommends vitamin D supplementation in community-dwelling adults aged 65 years or older who are at increased risk for falls (3)[B].
- USPSTF recommends against low-dose supplementation with vitamin D (<400 IU) and calcium (<1,000 mg) to reduce fracture risk in noninstitutionalized populations and concluded that data on the effects of higher doses were insufficient (3).
- USPSTF recommends that all women planning or capable of pregnancy take a daily supplement containing 0.4 to 0.8 mg of folic acid (4)[A].
- USPSTF recommends against the use of beta carotene or vitamin E supplements for the prevention of cardiovascular disease or cancer (2).
- The American Academy of Pediatrics recommends that all infants and children, including adolescents, have a minimum daily intake of 400 IU of vitamin D beginning soon after birth (5).

COMMONLY ASSOCIATED CONDITIONS
Anemia, neuropathies, dermatitis, visual disturbances

DIAGNOSIS

HISTORY
- Review dietary intake (6)
- Decreased visual acuity or night blindness (7)
- Poor wound healing or easy bruising (8)
- Skin changes or new rash (8)
- Neuropathy (6)
- Abnormal food cravings (pica)
- Osteomalacia or history of low-energy fracture (9)
- Previous birth of a child with spina bifida
- Previous GI or bariatric surgery (1)
- Recurrent or persistent vomiting or diarrhea
- Prior or current medical conditions
  - Tuberculosis (TB), HIV infection, hepatitis, cancer
  - Hypermetabolic state
    ○ Thyrotoxicosis
    ○ 2nd- or 3rd-degree burns
    ○ Extensive or chronic wound
    ○ Any systemic infection
- Chronic disease requiring steroids, disease-modifying antirheumatic drugs (DMARDs), or immunosuppressants
- Malabsorptive or chronic GI disorder: celiac disease, sprue, Crohn disease, ulcerative colitis, GERD
- Parenteral or enteral nutrition via tube feeding
- Pregnancy

- Amenorrhea or infertility issues (10)
- Medications, supplements
- Food allergies or intolerances, fad or restrictive diet

PHYSICAL EXAM
- Neurologic exam: gait, memory/cognitive impairment, reflexes, sensory or motor impairment, peripheral neuropathy (1,6)
- Oropharyngeal exam to look for glossitis, bleeding gums, hyperemic pharynx, stomatitis, cheilitis (1)
- Skin exam to look for maculosquamous dermatitis, photosensitive pigmented dermatitis, ecchymosis and/or petechiae (6)
- Visual assessment

DIFFERENTIAL DIAGNOSIS
Many conditions may mimic signs and symptoms of vitamin deficiencies.
- Diabetes mellitus (DM), thyroid disorders, hyperparathyroidism, heart failure, Alzheimer disease, multiple sclerosis, substance abuse, toxic ingestions, and hematologic disorders/malignancies

DIAGNOSTIC TESTS & INTERPRETATION

Initial Tests (lab, imaging)
- No routine screening indicated.
- Test if symptomatic or history indicates at high risk. If clinical characteristics are present, consider the following:
  - 25-OH vitamin D (5)
  - Prothrombin time (PT)/partial thromboplastin time (PTT)
  - Vitamin B_{12} and folate levels (1)
  - Serum homocysteine and methylmalonic acid levels if high suspicion of vitamin B_{12} deficiency with normal serum B_{12} level (6)
  - Retinol serum level, retinol binding protein
- Ancillary tests include the following:
  - BUN, calcium, phosphorus, magnesium
  - Albumin, liver function tests
  - CBC
  - Parathyroid hormone
- Bone densitometry indicated in the following (11)[A]:
  - Women 65 years of age or older without previous known fractures or risk factors
  - Women <65 years old whose 10-year fracture risk is equal to that of a 65-year-old white woman without additional risk factors.
  - According to the United States fracture risk assessment tool (FRAX), the 10-year fracture risk for a 65-year-old white woman without risk factors is 9.3%.
- Give bariatric surgery patients additional consideration as they are at risk for deficiencies. Laparoscopic gastric banding is less frequently associated with vitamin deficiencies (10).
- Cyanocobalamin, thiamine, vitamin A
- Disease states from vitamin deficiency
  - Vitamin A (retinol): night blindness, complete blindness, xerophthalmia
  - Vitamin B_1 (thiamine)
    ○ Wernicke encephalopathy: acute syndrome with memory disturbance, truncal ataxia, nystagmus, ophthalmoplegia
    ○ Korsakoff syndrome: anterograde and retrograde amnesia, confabulation
    ○ Dry beriberi: symmetric motor and sensory peripheral neuropathy, paresthesias, loss of reflexes
    ○ Wet beriberi: neuropathy with cardiovascular symptoms of peripheral vasodilation, high-output failure, dyspnea, and tachycardia

○ Infantile beriberi: loud piercing cry, cyanosis, tachycardia, cardiomegaly, dyspnea, vomiting, seizures
- Vitamin B_2 (riboflavin): glossitis, stomatitis, cheilitis, hyperemia of the pharyngeal mucosal membranes, normocytic-normochromic anemia
- Vitamin B_3 (niacin): pellagra: photosensitive pigmented dermatitis, dementia, and diarrhea
- Vitamin B_5 (pantothenic acid): paresthesias and dysthesias, anemia
- Vitamin B_6 (pyridoxine): dermatitis, cheilosis, atrophic glossitis, stomatitis, neuropathy
- Vitamin B_9 (folate): megaloblastic anemia, rarely manifest neurologic symptoms
- Vitamin B_{12} (cobalamin): pernicious anemia, shuffling broad-based gait, atrophic glossitis, loss of vibration and position sense, cognitive impairment
- Vitamin C (ascorbic acid): scurvy: ecchymoses, bleeding gums, petechiae, hyperkeratosis, arthralgias, impaired wound healing
- Vitamin D (calciferol): rickets, osteomalacia
- Vitamin E: neuromuscular disorders and hemolysis
- Vitamin K: easy bruising, mucosal bleeding, melena, hematuria
- Biotin: changes in mental status, dysesthesias, nausea, maculosquamous dermatitis of the extremities

TREATMENT

MEDICATION
- Ask patients about any herbal or dietary supplements and encourage them to bring in vitamin and supplement bottles for review.
- Assess for potential adverse drug effects/reactions. Patients with alcohol dependence should receive thiamine, folic acid, and MVI.
- Treat patients with suspected thiamine deficiency with 100 mg thiamine prior to IV fluids containing glucose to prevent precipitation of Korsakoff psychosis (10).
- If there is concomitant B_{12} and folate deficiency, then start B_{12} first to avoid precipitating subacute combined degeneration of the spinal cord (1).
- Consider obtaining prealbumin/albumin levels and a dietary consult for malnourished patients.
- Bariatric surgery patients will need lifelong vitamin supplementation; there are no consensus practice guidelines for supplement dosing regimens (12)

Geriatric Considerations
- Vitamin B_{12} deficiency exists in around 20% of the general population ≥60 years of age. Treat symptomatic or severe deficiency with an intramuscular (IM) injection of cyanocobalamin 1,000 μg/day 3 times a week for 2 weeks. If there are neurologic symptoms then give the same dose of cyanocobalamin every other day for 3 weeks or until symptoms have resolved. To prevent recurrence or treat mild deficiency, use a regimen of oral B_{12} 1,000 μg/day or an IM injection of B_{12} 1,000 μg every month (6). Low-dose oral therapy with 50 to 150 μg/day may be considered for mild cases (1). High-dose (1,000 to 2,000 μg/day) oral treatment is as effective as monthly IM injections, but use caution in patients with malabsorption or compliance issues (1,6)[C].

- >40% of elderly in United States are vitamin D deficient. Deficiency is defined as a serum 25-OH vitamin D level of <20 ng/mL. Treatment of vitamin D deficiency is 50,000 IU of oral ergocalciferol weekly for 8 weeks (3,10,13)[B].

Pediatric Considerations
- Vitamin K deficiency bleeding (9)
  - Neonates may exhibit signs of vitamin K deficiency because they require 1 week of life to establish intestinal flora which manufactures vitamin K.
  - Condition peaks 2 to 10 days after birth: bleeding from the umbilical stump and/or circumcision site, generalized bruising, and GI hemorrhage
  - Infrequent in developed countries due to routine injection of newborns with vitamin K (1 mg)

- Vitamin D deficiency: Vitamin D supplementation (400 IU/day) is recommended in all exclusively breastfed infants starting in the first few days of life (5)[A].

- All nonbreastfed infants and older children drinking <1,000 mL/day of vitamin D-fortified formula or milk should receive a vitamin D of 400 IU/day (5).

- Adolescents may receive a vitamin D supplement of 400 IU/day (5).

- Morbidly obese and minority children are at increased risk for vitamin D deficiency (14).

- In children age >6 months in developing countries, vitamin A supplementation has been shown to decrease mortality (7)[B].

- Vitamin deficiency associated with developmental delay.

Pregnancy Considerations
All pregnant women and women of childbearing age considering pregnancy are strongly encouraged to take a multivitamin containing at least 0.4 mg folic acid daily to prevent neural tube defects (4)[A].

ONGOING CARE

DIET
Vitamins are best utilized by the body from food intake. Supplements should be used where it is not feasible to ingest the recommended amount of a particular vitamin.

PATIENT EDUCATION
- In healthy adults, multivitamins have no value in a patient with an adequate diet and may increase risk of some cancers.
- Drug–drug interactions may occur between vitamins and some medications. Patients should report all supplements along with medications to their health care provider.
- Risk of vitamin toxicity occurs most commonly with the fat-soluble vitamins (A, D, E, K).

PROGNOSIS
Most vitamin deficiencies are fully reversible if treated without undue delay.

COMPLICATIONS
- Vitamin toxicities
- Liver failure (vitamins A, D, E, K)
- Desquamation of skin (vitamin A)
- Neuropathy (vitamin B_6)
- Kidney stones (vitamin C, vitamin D)
- Hypercoagulability (vitamin K)
- Pseudohyperparathyroidism (vitamin D)
- Masking of pernicious anemia (folic acid)

REFERENCES

1. Hunt A, Harrington D, Robinson S. Vitamin B12 deficiency. *BMJ*. 2014;349:g5226.
2. Vitamin, mineral, and multivitamin supplements for the primary prevention of cardiovascular disease and cancer: recommendation statement. *Am Fam Physician*. 2015;91(1):52D–52F.
3. LeBlanc ES, Zakher B, Daeges M, et al. Screening for vitamin D deficiency: a systematic review for the U.S. Preventive Services Task Force. *Ann Intern Med*. 2015;162(2):109–122.
4. Wolff T, Witkop CT, Miller T, et al. Folic acid supplementation for the prevention of neural tube defects: an update of the evidence for the U.S. Preventive Services Task Force. *Ann Intern Med*. 2009;150(9):632–639.
5. Wagner CL, Greer FR; American Academy of Pediatrics Section on Breastfeeding, et al. Prevention of rickets and vitamin D deficiency in infants, children, and adolescents. *Pediatrics*. 2008;122(5):1142–1152.
6. Stabler SP. Clinical practice. Vitamin B12 deficiency. *N Engl J Med*. 2013;368(2):149–160.
7. World Health Organization. *Guideline: Vitamin A Supplementation in Infants and Children 6–59 Months of Age*. Geneva, Switzerland: World Health Organization; 2011.
8. Lauer B, Spector N. Vitamins. *Pediatr Rev*. 2012; 33(8):339–351.
9. Schulte R, Jordan LC, Morad A, et al. Rise in late onset vitamin K deficiency bleeding in young infants because of omission or refusal of prophylaxis at birth. *Pediatr Neurol*. 2014;50(6):564–568.
10. Tack J, Deloose E. Complications of bariatric surgery: dumping syndrome, reflux and vitamin deficiencies. *Best Pract Res Clin Gastroenterol*. 2014;28(4):741–749.
11. U.S. Preventive Services Task Force. Screening for osteoporosis: recommendation statement. *Am Fam Physician*. 2011;83(10):1197–1200.
12. Pournaras DJ, le Roux CW. After bariatric surgery, what vitamins should be measured and what supplements should be given? *Clin Endocrinol*. 2009;71(3):322–325.
13. Forrest KY, Stuhldreher WL. Prevalence and correlates of vitamin D deficiency in US adults. *Nutr Res*. 2011;31(1):48–54.
14. Turer CB, Lin H, Flores G. Prevalence of vitamin D deficiency among overweight and obese US children. *Pediatrics*. 2013;131(1):e152–e161.

CODES

ICD10
- E56.9 Vitamin deficiency, unspecified
- E56.0 Deficiency of vitamin E
- E55.9 Vitamin D deficiency, unspecified

CLINICAL PEARLS
- Obtain a thorough dietary history.
- Specifically ask patients about supplement use.
- Vitamin D supplementation is recommended in community-dwelling adults aged 65 years or older who are at increased risk for falls (3). All women planning or capable of pregnancy should take a daily supplement containing 0.4 to 0.8 mg of folic acid (4). All infants and children, including adolescents, should have a minimum daily intake of 400 IU of vitamin D beginning soon after birth (5).

V

VITILIGO

Sonia Rivera-Martinez, DO, FACOFP • Karen Sheflin, DO

BASICS

DESCRIPTION
- An acquired depigmentation of the skin, which correlates with a loss of epidermal melanocytes. There are three clinical variants, each with subtypes.
- Localized: often in childhood, rapid onset then stabilizes. Involvement of hair is common early in the course. Lacks associated autoimmune diseases.
  – Focal: few lesions, random distribution
  – Segmental: Lesions occur within a dermatome (mostly trigeminal) or may follow Blaschko lines. Lesions usually stop abruptly at the midline (1).
  – Mucosal: Only mucosal surfaces involved
- Generalized/nonsegmental (most common variant): progressive, with flares, commonly associated with autoimmunity. Common locations are acral, periorificial, and in sites sensitive to pressure/friction (Koebner phenomenon) (1).
  – Vulgaris: most common subtype; scattered macules; often symmetric, wide distribution; mostly hands, axillae, and groin
  – Acrofacial: on distal extremities and face
  – Mixed: coexistence of above
- Universal: involves >80% of the body surface area (BSA). Most likely to have family history; comorbidities are common and associated with poorest quality-of-life (QOL) scores.
- Other rare variants
  – Ponctué: discrete confetti-like macules (1)
  – Inflammatory: peripheral erythematous rim (1)
  – Trichrome: Tan zone is present between normal and depigmented skin (1).
  – Quadrichrome: as above but with marginal/perifollicular hyperpigmentation (1)
  – Blue: Dermal melanophages give blue hue, in areas affected by prior postinflammatory hyperpigmentation (1).
- System(s) affected: skin, mucous membranes
- Synonym(s): leukoderma

EPIDEMIOLOGY
- 50% begin before age 20 years, peak in females: 1st decade; males: 5th decade. Onset earlier with positive family history; can appear as early as 6 weeks (1).
- Predominance: male = female; however, females are more likely to seek treatment (1).
- No race or socioeconomic predilection

Prevalence
~1% in the United States and Europe; 0.1–8% in the world; highest in Gujarat, India, at 8.8% (1)

ETIOLOGY AND PATHOPHYSIOLOGY
Most likely a spectrum of disorders with a common phenotype and multiple mechanisms contribute to the pathology (convergence theory).
- Genetic: see above.
- Autoimmune: humoral autoantibodies and skin-homing T cells (1)
- Neural: local or systemic dysregulation leading to excess neurotransmitters (1)
- Viral: direct melanocyte toxicity, cytomegalovirus (CMV), hepatitis C, and Epstein-Barr virus (EBV) found in lesional biopsies (1)
- Oxidative stress from elevated H_2O_2 and NO and decreased catalase and erythrocyte glutathione (1)

Genetics
- Polygenic/multifactorial inheritance
- 20% of patients report affected relative, but monozygotic twins have only 23% concordance.

- HLA haplotypes, small nucleotide polymorphisms, and specific genes are all possible contributors (1).

RISK FACTORS
- Family history of vitiligo/autoimmune disorders
- Personal history of associated conditions

COMMONLY ASSOCIATED CONDITIONS
- Most common
  – Endocrine: thyroid disease (hypo-/hyperthyroidism), hypoparathyroidism, Addison disease, insulin-dependent diabetes
  – Dermatologic: psoriasis, atopic dermatitis, alopecia areata, chronic urticaria, halo nevi, ichthyosis
  – Pernicious anemia
  – Hypoacusis, rheumatoid arthritis
  – Ocular abnormalities in up to 40%
  – Elevated antinuclear antibodies in up to 40%
  – Elevated thyroperoxidase antibodies in 50%
- Less common
  – Systemic lupus erythematosus
  – Inflammatory bowel disease
  – Melanoma (may be a sign of positive outcome of melanoma) and other skin cancers
  – Syndromes: Alezzandrini; mitochondrial encephalomyopathy, lactic acidosis, and stroke-like episodes (MELAS); Schmidt; and autoimmune polyendocrinopathy candidiasis ectodermal dysplasia (APCED)
- Age >50 years at onset should prompt investigation for associated conditions.

Pediatric Considerations
Associated with Hashimoto thyroiditis in a significant portion of children. Screening at onset and possibly annually may be beneficial.

DIAGNOSIS

HISTORY
- Inquire about recent history of sunburns, pregnancy, skin trauma, or emotional stress (1).
- Family history of premature graying, vitiligo, and autoimmune disorders
- Review of systems for related associated conditions
- Ascertain psychological impact on QOL, Dermatology Life Quality Index (DLQI).

PHYSICAL EXAM
- Full-body skin exam with Wood lamp to accentuate lesions and distinguish depigmentation from hypopigmentation (1)
- Lesions are well-demarcated, uniform white macules and patches.
- Look for evidence of repigmentation (most commonly around hair follicles).

DIFFERENTIAL DIAGNOSIS
- Infectious: tinea versicolor, leprosy, leishmaniasis, onchocerciasis, treponematoses (pinta/syphilis)
- Postinflammatory hypopigmentation: psoriasis, atopic dermatitis, pityriasis alba, systemic lupus erythematosus, scleroderma
- Inherited hypomelanoses: piebaldism, tuberous sclerosis, Waardenburg, hypomelanosis of Ito, Vogt-Koyanagi-Harada
- Malformations: nevus anemicus, nevus depigmentosus
- Paraneoplastic: mycosis fungoides, melanoma-associated leukoderma
- Occupational and chemical induced
  – Occupational: phenolic/catechol derivatives and arsenic-containing compounds

– Chemical: numerous, including cosmetics, cleansers, insecticides, and even medications (imatinib, potent topical corticosteroids [TCS]) (1)
- Melasma: Normal skin may be confused as vitiligo in the setting of surrounding hyperpigmentation.
- Halo nevi
- Lichen sclerosus et atrophicus
- Idiopathic guttate hypomelanosis
- Progressive-acquired macular hypomelanosis

DIAGNOSTIC TESTS & INTERPRETATION

Initial Tests (lab, imaging)
- TSH, CBC, ANA (1)
- Consider antithyroid peroxidase, antithyroglobulin antibodies, hemoglobin, vitamin B_{12} levels if family/patient history of autoimmune disease (1).

Follow-Up Tests & Special Considerations
- Monitor for disease progression/flares.
- Monitor for symptoms of related conditions.

Diagnostic Procedures/Other
- Skin biopsy is rarely needed. Highest yield is with comparison of lesional/perilesional biopsies.
- Consider ophthalmologic and audiologic evaluation.

Test Interpretation
Few or no epidermal melanocytes. At margins, melanocytes may be larger, vacuolated, and dendritic. Early lesions show inflammation and later, degeneration, including of adnexa and nerves.

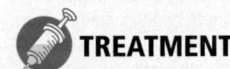

TREATMENT

The variant of vitiligo may affect response.
- If untreated, progression is the natural course for those with mucosal involvement, family history, koebnerization, and nonsegmental variants.
- Lesions that respond best are on the face, of recent onset, in darker skin type, and in younger patients.

GENERAL MEASURES
- Sunscreen to decrease sunburn and prevent accentuation of uninvolved skin
- Corrective camouflage as coverup (Cover FX, Dermablend)

MEDICATION
- Individualize therapy depending on age, extent, distribution, and rate of progression.
- Many therapies are considered "off-label" and not FDA-approved for vitiligo, although they are often considered first-line therapy.

- Corticosteroids: Mid-potency topical corticosteroids (mometasone furoate, fluticasone propionate) applied daily as monotherapy are considered first-line treatments. Do not use on face/axilla/groin; do not occlude except under close monitoring. Pediatric: as above, for children >12 years of age. Consider decreased potency. Local side effects including atrophy, telangiectasia, hypertrichosis, acneiform eruptions, and striae limit treatment; regular steroid holidays are recommended (2). The combination of light therapy and TCS is the most effective treatment overall (3). Most efficacious on sun-exposed areas: face/neck, dark-skinned patients, newer lesion (3). Addition of tretinoin 0.025–0.05% BID is effective and can decrease potential skin atrophy (4). Systemic corticosteroids can be helpful, but dosage and safety parameters have not been fully evaluated (2,5)[A].

- Topical calcineurin inhibitors: slightly inferior to TCS as monotherapy but better side effect profile (3,6,7)[B]; can be used as adjunctive to light therapy; carries a controversial black box warning for a theoretical risk of lymphoma or skin cancer. Extensive safety profiling has not revealed any evidence for this in children or adults using topical calcineurin inhibitors. Local reactions include burning sensation, pruritus, erythema, and rare transient hyperpigmentation (3).

  – Tacrolimus 0.03% or 0.1% ointment BID (2). Pediatric: 0.03% ointment BID, for children >2 years of age (7)
  – Pimecrolimus 1% cream BID (2). Pediatric: as adults, for children >2 years of age (7)

- Topical vitamin D_3 analogs: less effective than TCS alone, but in combination with TCS or phototherapy can shorten time until, and improve stability of, repigmentation (5,7)[B].

  – Calcipotriene ointment 1 to 2 times per day. Pediatric: not defined.
  – Available as a combination formulation, betamethasone dipropionate 0.064%/calcipotriene 0.005% ointment daily, max dose of 100 g/week for 4 weeks, not for >30% BSA, and not for face/axilla/groin. Pediatric: not defined.

- Oral vitamin D_3: reported to induce repigmentation. Oral vitamin D_3 35,000 U once daily plus low-calcium diet for 6 months. Pediatric: not defined.

- Phototherapy: Narrow band UVB (NBUVB) is superior to UVA and indicated for lesions involving more than 15–20% BSA (5,7,8)[A]. Psoralen and khellin enhance the effect of light. Psoralen plus UVA (PUVA) may increase the incidence of skin cancers. Khellin may have reduced cross-linking of DNA and may be less carcinogenic; however, it is associated with increased liver toxicity (8). L-phenylalanine can be used topically and orally as a photosensitizer for natural or artificial light. Pediatric: Oral PUVA is contraindicated.

- Laser therapy: Excimer laser (308 nm) is superior to other light therapy. Helium–neon laser works for segmental vitiligo (7)[A].

- Antioxidants: may have protective role in preventing melanocyte degradation from reactive oxygen species. Options include vitamin C, vitamin E, Vitix, *Polypodium leucotomos* extracts, and *Ginkgo biloba* (6)[B].

- Surgical therapy: See later discussion.

- New concepts: Tumor necrosis factor-α inhibitors, cyclosporine, cyclophosphamide, azathioprine, minocycline, and immunosuppressants are currently being evaluated (8).

First Line

- Recommended: avoidance of triggering factors plus TCS alone or in combination with NBUVB
- Alternatively
  – Topical calcineurin inhibitors (preferred for face, neck, axilla, and groin)
  – NBUVB
  – PUVA in adults
  – Camouflage and psychotherapy should be offered to all patients at any stage (8).

Second Line

- Recommended: photochemotherapy with psoralens or vitamin D analogues
- Alternatively
  – Topical vitamin D analogues
  – Targeted phototherapy

- 308-nm laser in combination with topical steroids, topical calcineurin inhibitors, or vitamin D analogues
- Oral corticosteroids (pulse therapy)
- Surgical treatments indicated for stable 2- to 3-cm lesions, refractory to other treatments
  - Mini-punch graft (pretreat with cryotherapy/dermabrasion or posttreat with phototherapy) (9)[B]
  - Suction blister graft (9)[B]
  - Autologous melanocyte suspension transplant (6)[B]

ISSUES FOR REFERRAL

- Dermatologist: for facial/widespread vitiligo or when advanced therapy is necessary
- Ophthalmologist: for ocular symptoms or monitoring of TCS near eyes
- Endocrinologist: evaluation/management of associated conditions
- Psychologist: for severe distress
- Medical geneticist for associated conditions

ADDITIONAL THERAPIES

- Depigmentation therapy with monobenzone, hydroquinone, or Q-switched ruby laser: for extensive vitiligo recalcitrant to therapy (9)
- Pseudocatalase with addition of NBUVB (2)[B]
- Prostaglandin E for short-duration disease and localization to face and scalp (2)[B]
- Cosmetic tattooing for localized stable vitiligo

SURGERY/OTHER PROCEDURES

- Goal is to transport melanocytes from other areas of the skin. Methods include punch, blister, or split-thickness skin grafting, or transplantation of autologous melanocytes.
- Dermabrasion and curettage alone or in combination with 5-fluorouracil may induce follicular melanocyte reservoirs (7)[A].
- Patients who koebnerize or form keloids may be worse, and permanent scarring is a risk for all patients.

COMPLEMENTARY & ALTERNATIVE MEDICINE

- *Ginkgo biloba* 60 mg PO daily may significantly improve extension and spreading of lesions (8)[B].
- *Polypodium leucotomos* may help with repigmentation with NBUVB and aid in reducing phototoxic reactions (7,8)[B].

 ONGOING CARE

FOLLOW-UP RECOMMENDATIONS

- Monitor for symptoms of related conditions.
- With topical steroids, follow at regular intervals to avoid steroid atrophy, telangiectasia, and striae distensae.

DIET
No restrictions

PATIENT EDUCATION

- Discussion of disease course, progression, and cosmesis
- Education regarding trauma/friction and Koebner phenomenon

PROGNOSIS

- Vitiligo may remain stable or slowly or rapidly progress.

- Spontaneous repigmentation is uncommon.
- Generalized vitiligo is often progressive, with flares. Focal vitiligo often has rapid onset, then stabilizes.

COMPLICATIONS

- Adverse effects of each treatment modality
- Psychiatric morbidity: depression, adjustment disorder, low self-esteem, sexual dysfunction, and embarrassment in relationships (1)
  – Different cultures may have different perceptions/social stigmas about vitiligo. Some believe it to be contagious or related to infection. Women with vitiligo may have difficulty finding a marriage partner and have low self-esteem.

REFERENCES

1. Alikhan A, Felsten LM, Daly M, et al. Vitiligo: a comprehensive overview Part I. Introduction, epidemiology, quality of life, diagnosis, differential diagnosis, associations, histopathology, etiology, and work-up. *J Am Acad Dermatol*. 2011;65(3):473–491.
2. Colucci R, Lotti T, Moretti S. Vitiligo: an update on current pharmacotherapy and future directions. *Expert Opin Pharmacother*. 2012;13(13):1885–1899.
3. Felsten LM, Alikhan A, Petronic-Rosic V. Vitiligo: a comprehensive overview Part II: treatment options and approach to treatment. *J Am Acad Dermatol*. 2011;65(3):493–514.
4. Kwon HB, Choi Y, Kim HJ, et al. The therapeutic effects of a topical tretinoin and corticosteroid combination for vitiligo: a placebo-controlled, paired-comparison, left-right study. *J Drugs Dermatol*. 2013;12(4):e63–e67.
5. Bacigalupi RM, Postolova A, Davis RS. Evidence-based, non-surgical treatments for vitiligo: a review. *Am J Clin Dermatol*. 2012;13(4):217–237.
6. Lepe V, Moncada B, Castanedo-Cazares JP, et al. A double-blind randomized trial of 0.1% tacrolimus vs 0.05% clobetasol for the treatment of childhood vitiligo. *Arch Dermatol*. 2003;139(5):581–585.
7. Whitton ME, Pinart M, Batchelor J, et al. Interventions for vitiligo. *Cochrane Database Syst Rev*. 2015;(2):CD003263.
8. Taieb A, Alomar A, Böhm M, et al. Guidelines for the management of vitiligo: the European Dermatology Forum consensus. *Br J Dermatol*. 2013;168(1):5–19.
9. Patel NS, Paghdal KV, Cohen GF. Advanced treatment modalities for vitiligo. *Dermatol Surg*. 2012;38(3):381–391.

CODES

ICD10
L80 Vitiligo

CLINICAL PEARLS

- Vitiligo can be a psychologically devastating skin disease.
- Screen for associated diseases, particularly if onset occurs later in life.
- Treatment should be individualized based on BSA, skin type, and patient goals.
- Dermatology consultation when extensive disease, facial involvement, and when advanced treatments are considered.

VOCAL CORD DYSFUNCTION

Daniel A. Cieslak, MD • Emily M. Culliney, MD, FAAFP

 BASICS

DESCRIPTION

- Vocal cord dysfunction (VCD): a breathing disorder in which vocal cords adduct inappropriately primarily on inspiration, producing airflow obstruction that may result in dyspnea, wheezing, and stridor
- Synonym(s): paradoxical vocal fold motion (PVFM)

EPIDEMIOLOGY

Incidence
Not well defined

Prevalence
- Unknown; likely uncommon in the general population
- Most frequently diagnosed in patients evaluated for asthma and exercise-induced dyspnea
- Female predominance, 2:1 (1)
- 71% of patients are adults and 29% of patients <18 years of age. Also has been diagnosed in young children/infants (1)
- Suspect occurrence in approximately 3% of intercollegiate athletes with exercise-induced asthma (2).

ETIOLOGY AND PATHOPHYSIOLOGY

- Exact etiology is unclear—both organic and nonorganic causes have been identified.
- Possible laryngeal hyperresponsiveness to irritants, such as smoke, dust, postnasal drip, gastroesophageal reflux disease (GERD), URI, or other irritants (3)
- Noncompetitive and competitive exercises—unknown mechanism (4)
- Psychological factors such as anxiety, severe social stresses (e.g., competitive sports), history of sexual abuse (2)

Genetics
None defined

RISK FACTORS
See "Commonly Associated Conditions."

COMMONLY ASSOCIATED CONDITIONS

- Asthma
- GERD
- Rhinosinusitis
- Psychological conditions such as posttraumatic stress disorder, anxiety, depression, and panic disorder

 DIAGNOSIS

HISTORY

- Recurrent episodes of "difficulty breathing in," wheezing, throat or chest tightness, choking sensation, stridor, panic, and agitation
- Stridulous sounds that are loudest above the throat, less audible throughout the chest wall.
- Some patients (typically elite athletes) experience inspiratory stridor that resolves spontaneously when activity ceases.
- The stridor is often mistaken for wheezing, leading to misdiagnosis of asthma or exercise-induced asthma.
- Dysphonia or aphonia is possible between attacks.
- History of multiple ED visits, possibly multiple intubations
- The symptoms tend to be relatively mild but can be prolonged and severe.
- Patients may report their asthma medications do not help their symptoms.

PHYSICAL EXAM

- Inspiratory stridor
- Cough
- Wheezing (especially if unresponsive to bronchodilators)
- Mild respiratory distress

DIFFERENTIAL DIAGNOSIS

- Asthma: primary differential diagnosis because wheezing is a big component—although VCD can coexist with asthma (1,2). The key differences between the two are the following:
  - Asthma typically has wheeze on expiration, VCD on inspiration.
  - Asthma symptoms associated with nocturnal awakenings, uncommon in VCD
  - Asthma is not typically associated with a sensation of choking.
  - Asthma symptoms usually improve with albuterol use (3).
  - VCD causes more difficulty with inspiration rather than expiration.
  - VCD is not responsive to asthma treatment (unless coexisting) (2).
- Anaphylaxis
- Foreign body
- Laryngeal angioedema
- Chronic obstructive pulmonary disease
- Epiglottitis
- Vocal cord polyps/tumor
- Vocal cord paralysis
- Croup
- Tracheal stenosis or masses
- Laryngomalacia (1)
- Neurologic cause: vagus or recurrent laryngeal nerve injury, amyotrophic lateral sclerosis (3)

DIAGNOSTIC TESTS & INTERPRETATION

Initial Tests (lab, imaging)
- Flexible laryngoscopy—gold standard (2)[C]
  - Allows for direct visualization of abnormal adduction of the vocal cords
  - May allow for diagnosis in more than half of asymptomatic patients; however, provocation tests such as methacholine (5), exercise (4), and histamine may be needed for diagnosis (4,5)[C].

- Pulmonary function testing with flow volume loop
  - Most commonly used test
  - Positive findings consist of normal expiratory volume loop with a flattened inspiratory volume loop. This is consistent with extrathoracic upper airway obstruction (6)[C].
  - May require exercise testing for patients in whom exercise is the trigger
  - Useful for distinguishing from asthma, which may show a scooped expiratory loop
- Imaging
  - Chest radiographs to rule out other causes of dyspnea (2)
  - High-resolution CT of upper airways to evaluate for stenosis, masses (if not able to visualize trachea during laryngoscopy) (7)
- Arterial blood gases
  - Useful to rule out other causes of severe respiratory distress

 TREATMENT

GENERAL MEASURES
- Short term
  - Asthma control/treatment with appropriate meds, if coexisting (3)[C]
  - Reassurance and relaxation techniques:
    - Pursing lips
    - Panting (rapid, shallow breathing)
    - Diaphragmatic breathing
    - Breathing through the nose or a straw
    - Exhaling with a hissing sound
  - Continuous positive airway pressure (CPAP)
  - Intermittent CPAP with heliox (helium-oxygen) mixture may reduce airway resistance in some patients (1,2)[C].
  - Anxiolytics if associated with anxiety attack (must confirm normal oxygen saturation prior to administration)
  - Intubation with severe symptoms (3)[C]
- Long term
  - Avoid triggers.
  - Behavioral speech/voice therapy (8)[B]
  - Treat underlying conditions.

MEDICATION
First Line
No medications are specifically helpful. Exercise-induced VCD may respond to anticholinergics in addition to speech therapy; thus, consider a trial of ipratropium if symptoms are exercise-induced (9)[C].

ISSUES FOR REFERRAL
- Diagnosis and treatment may require assistance of pulmonologist, otolaryngologist, allergist, psychiatrist, and/or psychologist.
- Speech therapy is the mainstay of long-term treatment for patients with ongoing symptoms. It helps reduce recurrence.

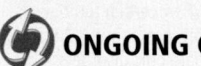 **ONGOING CARE**

PROGNOSIS
Spontaneous resolution is common.

REFERENCES
1. Morris MJ, Allan PF, Perking PJ. Vocal cord dysfunction: etiologies and treatment. *Clin Pulm Med*. 2006;13(2):73–86.
2. Ibrahim WH, Gheriani HA, Almohamed AA, et al. Paradoxical vocal cord motion disorder: past, present and future. *Postgrad Med J*. 2007;83(977):164–172.
3. Gimenez LM, Zafra H. Vocal cord dysfunction: an update. *Ann Allergy Asthma Immunol*. 2011;106(4):267–274.
4. Chiang T, Marcinow AM, deSilva BW, et al. Exercise-induced paradoxical vocal fold motion disorder: diagnosis and management. *Laryngoscope*. 2013;123(3):727–731.
5. Perkins PJ, Morris MJ. Vocal cord dysfunction induced by methacholine challenge testing. *Chest*. 2002;122(6):1988–1993.
6. Mobeireek A, Alhamad A, Al-Subaei A, et al. Psychogenic vocal cord dysfunction simulating bronchial asthma. *Eur Respir J*. 1995;8(11):1978–1981.
7. Lee KS, Boiselle PM. Update on multidetector computed tomography imaging of the airways. *J Thorac Imaging*. 2010;25(2):112–124.
8. Sullivan MD, Heywood BM, Beukelman DR. A treatment for vocal cord dysfunction in female athletes: an outcome study. *Laryngoscope*. 2001;111(10):1751–1755.
9. Doshi DR, Weinberger MM. Long-term outcome of vocal cord dysfunction. *Ann Allergy Asthma Immunol*. 2006;96(6):794–799.

ADDITIONAL READING
- Deckert J, Deckert L. Vocal cord dysfunction. *Am Fam Physician*. 2010;81(2):156–159.
- Jain S, Bandi V, Zimmerman J, et al. Incidence of vocal cord dysfunction in patients presenting to emergency room with acute asthma exacerbation. *Chest*. 1997;116(Suppl 2):243S.
- Newsham KR, Klaben BK, Miller VJ, et al. Paradoxical vocal-cord dysfunction: management in athletes. *J Athl Train*. 2002;37(3):325–328.
- Pargeter NJ, Mansur AH. The effectiveness of speech and language therapy in vocal cord dysfunction. *Thorax*. 2006;61(Suppl 2):ii126.
- Weir M. Vocal cord dysfunction mimics asthma and may respond to heliox. *Clin Pediatr (Phila)*. 2002;41(1):37–41.

 CODES

ICD10
- J38.3 Other diseases of vocal cords
- J38.00 Paralysis of vocal cords and larynx, unspecified
- J38.1 Polyp of vocal cord and larynx

CLINICAL PEARLS
- Always consider VCD in poorly controlled asthmatics.
- A multidisciplinary approach may be required for diagnosis and treatment.
- Speech therapy is the mainstay of long-term treatment.

VON WILLEBRAND DISEASE

Aneel A. Ashrani, MD, MS • Ewa M. Wysokinska, MD

BASICS

DESCRIPTION
- von Willebrand disease (vWD) is a bleeding disorder caused by deficiency or a defect of *von Willebrand factor* (vWF) protein.
- vWF is critical to the initial stages of blood clotting, acting as a bridge for platelet adhesion; it also acts as a carrier for factor VIII (FVIII).
- vWD primarily manifests as mucocutaneous or perioperative bleeding or menorrhagia.
- vWD is an inherited condition but rarely can be acquired (1–3).

EPIDEMIOLOGY
Prevalence
- Prevalence of the inherited forms of vWD is 1 in 100 to 10,000 of the general population with 2:1 female-to-male ratio (1).
- Exact prevalence of the acquired forms of vWD (AvWD) is unknown but is estimated to be up to 0.1% of the general population.

Pediatric Considerations
Many cases of vWD are diagnosed in childhood, often during initial years of menstruation. vWD may be difficult to diagnose before 6 months of age.

Pregnancy Considerations
Although levels of vWF increase during pregnancy, women with vWD are more likely to experience an increased incidence of obstetric complications that manifest with bleeding.

ETIOLOGY AND PATHOPHYSIOLOGY
- vWF is a large, multimeric protein that is released from endothelial cells and is also carried within platelets in α-granules.
- vWF binds to collagen at sites of vascular injury and creates a surface for platelet adhesion through GP1b receptor. This results in platelet plug formation.
- vWF is also a carrier for FVIII and stabilizes this factor from degradation. A deficiency in vWF may result in lower levels of FVIII.
- When vWF is deficient or dysfunctional, primary hemostasis is compromised, resulting in increased mucocutaneous and postprocedural bleeding.
- Three major categories of vWD exist
  - Type 1, the most common and mildest form, represents 60–80% of cases.
    ○ Mild to moderate quantitative deficiency of vWF and concordant deficiency of FVIII
    ○ Generally, a mild bleeding disorder
  - Type 2 caused by qualitative defect in vWF accounts for 10–30% of cases and is divided into the following multiple subtypes.
    ○ Type 2A is noted for loss of hemostatically active large multimers with low ristocetin cofactor/vWF activity.
    ○ Type 2B, noted for increased binding affinity for platelets, is associated with thrombocytopenia, low ristocetin cofactor/vWF activity, abnormal ristocetin-induced platelet aggregation (RIPA), and loss of large multimers.
    ○ Type 2M is noted for defective platelet or collagen binding without loss of large multimers.
    ○ Type 2N demonstrates defective binding to FVIII, which results in increased clearance of Factor VIII and hemophilia A–like picture

- Type 3 represents 1–5% of cases.
  ○ Most severe form characterized by markedly decreased-to-undetectable levels of vWF and FVIII
  ○ Manifests as hemophilia A with hemarthroses (1–4)
- Acquired form of vWD (AvWD) may be due to cardiovascular, hematologic, or autoimmune conditions, as well as tumors and medications.
- The pathophysiology of AvWD is related to the underlying cause and may result from shear induced cleaving of vWF in cardiovascular conditions, increased adsorption of vWF by certain tumor cells or activated platelets, or presence of anti-vWF auto-antibodies detected in hematologic disorders.

Genetics
- The 175-kb gene for vWF is located on short arm of chromosome 12.
- Type 1 follows an autosomal dominant inheritance pattern, with variable expressivity.
- Type 2 varies but primarily follows an autosomal dominant inheritance pattern.
- Type 3 follows an autosomal recessive inheritance pattern (4).

COMMONLY ASSOCIATED CONDITIONS
AvWD may be found in patients with hematologic disorders such as MGUS and myeloproliferative neoplasms. Commonly associated cardiovascular conditions include aortic stenosis and LVAD placement.

DIAGNOSIS

HISTORY
- Most patients with vWD have a positive family history of bleeding disorder; however, patients with mild forms of vWD and their families may be unaware of their disease. Those with acquired vWD usually have no family history of this disorder.
- The most important component of diagnosis is the hemostatic history often aided by specifically designed bleeding questionnaires.
- Common symptoms are those of mucocutaneous (recurrent epistaxis, menorrhagia, ecchymosis) or postprocedural bleeding. Hemarthroses are a rare presentation, mostly associated with types 2N and 3.

PHYSICAL EXAM
- Physical exam may be entirely normal, although there may be some ecchymoses.
- Findings suggestive of other causes of increased bleeding should be sought (liver disease, skin laxity, or telangiectasias).

DIFFERENTIAL DIAGNOSIS
- Primary hemostatic disorders: congenital thrombocytopenia or qualitative platelet defects, coagulation factor deficiencies
- Secondary hemostatic disorders: liver disease, uremia, connective tissue disorders, coagulation factor inhibitors

DIAGNOSTIC TESTS & INTERPRETATION
Initial Tests (lab, imaging)
- The specific tests for vWD include vWF antigen (vWF:Ag), vWF activity/ristocetin cofactor activity (vWF:RCo) (if available: collagen-binding activity [vWF:CB]) and FVIII activity; these tests should be ordered when suspicion for vWD is high. Additional specific tests include RIPA, vWF multimer analysis, vWF propeptide (vWFpp), and genetic testing.

- Other tests include CBC, PT/INR, aPTT, platelet function analyzer assay (PFA-100).
  - Platelet count is often normal, except in type 2B or in AvWD when there is an underlying myeloproliferative disorder.
  - Platelet function assays via PFA-100 (i.e., collagen/epinephrine and collagen/ADP closure time) are usually prolonged but may be normal in mild disease.
  - PT/INR is normal, unless there is concurrent liver disease or warfarin/Coumadin use.
  - Activated PTT may be prolonged if a decrease in FVIII accompanies vWD.
- Specific tests for vWD
  - vWF antigen testing is done via immunologic methods
    ○ vWF antigen testing has a positive predictive value (PPV) of 33% for detecting significant FVIII deficiency and a PPV of 80% for detecting ristocetin cofactor activity abnormalities.
    ○ vWF antigen may be normal in type 2 vWD.
  - Ristocetin cofactor activity is a functional assessment of vWF. Ristocetin promotes binding of platelets to vWF, and this activity is disproportionately reduced compared to vWF antigen in most forms of type 2 vWD.
  - Ratio of vWF:RCo to vWF:Ag <0.5 to 0.7 may be used to differentiate type 1 from type 2 vWD.
  - Alternatively, latex particle–enhanced immunoassay may be used to quantify vWF activity. A specific monoclonal anti-vWF antibody directed against platelet GP1b–binding site of vWF adsorbed onto the latex reagent reacts with plasma vWF proportional to the vWF activity.
  - Collagen-binding activity, another functional assessment of vWF, is reduced in most forms of vWD.
  - FVIII activity may be normal or mildly decreased in most types of vWD (in 2N and type 3, levels are markedly decreased).
  - vWFpp is useful in accelerated clearance variants of vWD.
  - vWF multimer analysis is performed by electrophoresis on agarose gel. This test differentiates patients with type 2 vWD.
  - RIPA is useful in diagnosing type 2B vWD.
  - FVIII-vWF binding assay activity is low in patients with type 2N vWD.
  - Genotype testing may also be used especially for types 2 and 3 (1–4).

Follow-Up Tests & Special Considerations
- Unless patients have severe forms of vWD or are undergoing treatment, follow-up laboratory studies are not usually obtained.
- Patients with blood group O have 20–30% baseline lower levels of vWF antigen and ristocetin cofactor activity.
- vWF is an acute-phase reactant, so elevations may be seen in inflammatory conditions, liver disease, pregnancy (which may correct mild deficits), or with estrogen use.

TREATMENT

GENERAL MEASURES
- Most patients with type 1 vWD do not require activity restrictions.
- Patients with type 3 vWD should avoid contact sports.
- An emergency ID bracelet may be useful.

MEDICATION

First Line

- Desmopressin (DDAVP)
  - Enhances release of vWF from endothelial cells
  - Primarily effective for type 1 vWD; not to be used in type 2B
  - Typically raises vWF by 2- to 3-fold from baseline levels (5)[B]
  - Not effective in severe deficiencies, in types of vWD with defective vWF, or for prophylaxis prior to major procedures
  - Dosed 0.3 μg/kg (max 20 mg) IV/SC; intranasal (high concentration) spray: <50 kg: 150 μg/day; >50 kg: 300 μg/day (Stimate)
  - Common side effects: flushing, tachycardia, water retention, hyponatremia
  - Obtain repeat testing of ristocetin cofactor activity and FVIII 1 and 4 hours after infusion to evaluate peak response and clearance of DDAVP.
  - Tachyphylaxis may develop with prolonged dosing; limit use to administering DDAVP once every 24 to 48 hours for 3 to 5 days.
- vWF and FVIII concentrates
  - Plasma-derived vWF and FVIII concentrates of various purity such as Humate-P, Alphanate, Wilate, or Fandhi (not available in United States) are commercial concentrates of vWF and FVIII that are given in doses of 25 to 60 IU/kg/day based on clinical situation (6,7)[B]
    - Administration of 1 IU/kg vWF:RCo concentrate raises the plasma RCo activity by approximately 2%.
    - Dose of vWF concentrate may be adjusted for FVIII levels and ristocetin cofactor activity.
    - FVIII levels should be monitored to avoid supranormal levels and possible venous thromboembolism (VTE).
    - Contraindicated if patient develops alloantibodies to vWF
  - New recombinant form of vWF concentrate is effective in clinical trials but not yet available for clinical use (8)[B].
  - In patients with severe bleeding phenotype, prophylactic treatment is used.
- Cryoprecipitate
  - Cryoprecipitate contains FVIII, fibrinogen, vWF, factor XIII, and fibronectin.
  - Not considered as safe as the virus-inactivated plasma concentrates listed above and should not be used unless those are unavailable
- Antifibrinolytics
  - Useful for mucosal bleeding
  - Contraindicated in patients with hematuria due to risk of retention of large blood clots in the renal collecting system
  - Given as adjunct to DDAVP
  - Aminocaproic acid may be given at 50 to 70 mg/kg (max: 5 g; lower doses may be effective) q4–6h IV or PO.
  - Tranexamic acid may be given at 10 to 15 mg/kg IV or 25 mg/kg (1,300 mg) PO q8–12h.
- Recombinant FVIIa/Novoseven
  - Used for patients who develop alloantibodies to vWF
  - Given as IV bolus of 90 μg/kg q2h or 20 μg/kg every hour until hemostasis is achieved

Second Line

- Oral contraceptives raise vWF/FVIII levels and have a role in the treatment of chronic menorrhagia.
- Platelets may be given as an adjunct to factor concentrates if hemostasis has not been achieved.

- IVIG has been useful in some patients with AvWD associated with monoclonal gammopathy (9).
- Recombinant FVIIa has been used effectively in patients with type 3 vWD.

ISSUES FOR REFERRAL
The diagnosis and management of vWD is not always straightforward; consider consultation with hematologist.

SURGERY/OTHER PROCEDURES
Valve replacement or correction may be curative for patients with AvWD associated with underlying cardiovascular conditions.

INPATIENT CONSIDERATIONS

Admission Criteria/Initial Stabilization

- For patients with major bleeding or those undergoing major surgical procedures, levels of ristocetin cofactor/vWF activity and FVIII need to be restored to 80 to 100 IU/dL for first 2 days and then maintained >50 IU/dL for 5 to 7 days.
- For patients undergoing minor surgical procedures, maintain FVIII levels >50 IU/dL for 5 to 7 days.
- For patients delivering or in need of epidural anesthesia, obtain FVIII levels >50 IU/dL.

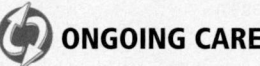 ONGOING CARE

FOLLOW-UP RECOMMENDATIONS
Patients should be seen by a hematologist prior to invasive procedures for determination of perioperative management or advice regarding delivery.

Patient Monitoring
Patients with mild disease do not require monitoring.

DIET
No dietary restrictions are recommended. However, aspirin and other NSAIDs should be avoided due to their antiplatelet effects, which can exacerbate the bleeding phenotype.

PATIENT EDUCATION
National Hemophilia Foundation: www.hemophilia.org/NHFWeb/MainPgs/MainNHF.aspx?menuid=182&contentid=47&rptname=bleeding

PROGNOSIS
Most patients with vWD have a normal life expectancy.

COMPLICATIONS

- Significant perioperative bleeding may occur.
- Patients with type 3 vWD and type 2N can have bleeding complications similar to patients with hemophilia A such as hemarthrosis and intracranial hemorrhage.
- Patients with aortic stenosis and AvWD are known to have higher rates of GI bleeding.
- Multiple transfusions may result in alloantibodies against vWF.
- Venous thromboembolism may result from supranormal levels of FVIII.

REFERENCES

1. Ng C, Motto DG, Di Paola J. Diagnostic approach to von Willebrand disease. *Blood*. 2015;125(13):2029–2037.
2. Lillicrap D. von Willebrand disease: advances in pathogenetic understanding, diagnosis, and therapy. *Blood*. 2013;122(23):3735–3740.
3. Nichols WL, Hultin MB, James AH, et al. von Willebrand disease (VWD): evidence-based diagnosis and management guidelines, the National Heart,

Lung, and Blood Institute (NHLBI) Expert Panel report (USA). *Haemophilia*. 2008;14(2):171–232.
4. Laffan MA, Lester W, O'Donnell JS, et al. The diagnosis and management of von Willebrand disease: a United Kingdom Haemophilia Centre Doctors Organization guideline approved by the British Committee for Standards in Haematology. *Br J Haematol*. 2014;167(4):453–465.
5. Hanebutt FL, Rolf N, Loesel A, et al. Evaluation of desmopressin effects on haemostasis in children with congenital bleeding disorders. *Haemophilia*. 2008;14(3):524–530.
6. Mannucci PM, Chediak J, Hanna W, et al. Treatment of von Willebrand disease with a high-purity factor VIII/von Willebrand factor concentrate: a prospective, multicenter study. *Blood*. 2002;99(2):450–456.
7. Thompson AR, Gill JC, Ewenstein BM, et al. Successful treatment for patients with von Willebrand disease undergoing urgent surgery using factor VIII/VWF concentrate (Humate-P). *Haemophilia*. 2004;10(1):42–51.
8. Mannucci PM, Kempton C, Millar C, et al. Pharmacokinetics and safety of a novel recombinant human von Willebrand factor manufactured with a plasma-free method: a prospective clinical trial. *Blood*. 2013;122(5):648–657.
9. Tiede A, Rand JH, Budde U, et al. How I treat the acquired von Willebrand syndrome. *Blood*. 2011; 117(25):6777–6785.

ADDITIONAL READING

- Kessler CM. Diagnosis and treatment of von Willebrand disease: new perspectives and nuances. *Haemophilia*. 2007;13(Suppl 5):3–14.
- Kumar S, Pruthi RK, Nichols WL. Acquired von Willebrand disease. *Mayo Clin Proc*. 2002;77(2):181–187.
- Lippi G, Franchini M, Salvagno GL, et al. Correlation between von Willebrand factor antigen, von Willebrand factor ristocetin cofactor activity and factor VIII activity in plasma. *J Thromb Thrombolysis*. 2008;26(2):150–153.
- Mannucci PM. Treatment of von Willebrand's disease. *N Engl J Med*. 2004;351(7):683–694.
- Robertson J, Lillicrap D, James PD. Von Willebrand disease. *Pediatr Clin North Am*. 2008;55(2):377–392.
- Sciscione AC, Mucowski SJ. Pregnancy and von Willebrand disease: a review. *Del Med J*. 2007;79(10):401–405.

 SEE ALSO

Algorithms: Bleeding Gums; Ecchymosis

 CODES

ICD10
D68.0 Von Willebrand's disease

CLINICAL PEARLS

- vWD varies from a minor to severe bleeding disorder; affects 1–2% of the U.S. population.
- It is important to determine the exact type of vWD (1, 2, or 3) to guide treatment.
- AvWD should be considered in patients with acquired bleeding disorder if they have underlying predisposing conditions.

VULVAR MALIGNANCY

Jay R. Patibandla, MD • Michael P. Hopkins, MD, MEd

 BASICS

DESCRIPTION

- Premalignant lesions of the vulva are collectively known as vulvar intraepithelial neoplasia (VIN). Exposure to human papillomavirus (HPV) has been linked to >70% of VIN (1).
- Invasive squamous cell carcinoma is the most common malignancy involving the vulva (90% of patients); can be well, moderately, or poorly differentiated and derives from keratinized skin covering the vulva and perineum.
- Melanoma is the second most common type of vulvar malignancy (8%) and sarcoma is the third (1).
- Other invasive cell types include basal cell carcinoma, Paget disease, adenocarcinoma arising from Bartholin gland or apocrine sweat glands, adenoid cystic carcinoma, small cell carcinoma, verrucous carcinoma, and sarcomas.
- Sarcomas are usually leiomyosarcoma and probably arise at the insertion of the round ligament in the labium major; however, sarcoma can arise from any structure of the vulva, including blood vessels, skeletal muscle, and fat.
- Rarely, breast carcinoma has been reported in the vulva and is thought to arise from ectopic breast tissue.
- System(s) affected: reproductive

Geriatric Considerations
- Older patients with associated medical problems are at high risk from radical surgery. The surgery, however, is usually well tolerated.
- Patients who are not surgical candidates can be treated with combination chemotherapy and/or radiation.
- In the very elderly, palliative vulvectomy provides relief of symptoms for ulcerating symptomatic advanced disease.

EPIDEMIOLOGY
Incidence
- In 2015, 5,150 women were diagnosed with vulvar cancer and 1,080 women died from vulvar cancer in the United States (2).
- Ethnic distribution: more common in Caucasian women than in any other race
- Surveillance, epidemiology, and end result (SEER) data showed that the incidence of in situ vulvar carcinoma increased by >400% between 1973 and 2000.
- Mean age at diagnosis 65 years; in situ disease: mean age 40 years; invasive malignancy: mean age 60 years (3)

ETIOLOGY AND PATHOPHYSIOLOGY
- Patients with cervical cancer are more likely to develop vulvar cancer later in life, secondary to "field effect" phenomenon with a carcinogen involving the lower genital tract (3).
- HPV has been associated with squamous cell abnormalities of the cervix, vagina, and vulva; 55% of vulvar cancers are attributable to oncogenic HPV, predominantly HPV 16 and 33; 92% of VIN 2/3, vaginal intraepithelial neoplasia (VAIN) 2/3, and anal intraepithelial neoplasia (AIN) are attributable to HPV.
- Squamous cell carcinoma
  - The warty basaloid type, also known as bowenoid type, is related to HPV infection and occurs in younger women. Although traditionally graded in a three-level system, the International Society for the Study of Vulvovaginal Disease voted not to use a grading system for VIN in 2004.

This system eliminated VIN 1 and combined VIN 2 and VIN 3. This is based on the fact that VIN 1 is not reproducible. VIN 2 and VIN 3 were combined because VIN 2 is rare and carries the same risk of progression to malignancy as VIN 3 (1).
  - The more common variant is simplex or differentiated and does not appear to be related to HPV, occurs in older age groups, and associated with lichen sclerosus and chronic venereal diseases; it is thought to carry a higher risk of progression to malignancy.
  - Melanoma, second most common histology, often identified in postmenopausal women; often pigmented but can be amelanotic, arising de novo, often found on clitoris or labia minora.
- Cases not associated with HPV infection are typically associated with vulvar dystrophies, such as lichen sclerosus or squamous cell hyperplasia.
- Smoking is associated with squamous cell disease of the vulva, possibly from direct irritation of the vulva by the transfer of tars and nicotine on the patient's hands or from systemic absorption of carcinogen.

Genetics
No known genetic pattern

RISK FACTORS
- VIN or cervical intraepithelial neoplasia (CIN)
- Smoking
- Lichen sclerosus (vulvar dystrophy)
- HPV infection, condylomata or sexually transmitted diseases (STD) in the past
- Low economic status
- Autoimmune processes
- Immunodeficiency syndromes or immunosuppression
- Northern European ancestry

GENERAL PREVENTION
- HPV vaccination has the potential to decrease vulvar cancer by 60% (3–5).
- Abstinence from smoking/smoking cessation counseling (1)

COMMONLY ASSOCIATED CONDITIONS
- Patients with invasive vulvar cancer are often elderly and have associated medical conditions.
- High rate of other gynecologic malignancies

 DIAGNOSIS

HISTORY
Complaints of pruritus or raised lesion in the vaginal area

PHYSICAL EXAM
- In situ disease: a small raised area associated with pruritus, single vulvar plaque, ulcer, or mass on labia majora, perineum, clitoris
- Vulvar bleeding, dysuria, enlarged lymph nodes less common symptomatology
- Invasive malignancy: an ulcerated, nonhealing area; as lesions become large, bleeding occurs with associated pain and foul-smelling discharge; enlarged inguinal lymph nodes indicative of advanced disease.

DIFFERENTIAL DIAGNOSIS
- Infectious processes can present as ulcerative lesions and include syphilis, lymphogranuloma venereum, and granuloma inguinale.
- Disorder of Bartholin gland, seborrheic keratosis, hidradenomas, lichen sclerosus, epidermal inclusion cysts
- Crohn disease can present as an ulcerative area on the vulva.
- Rarely, lesions can metastasize to the vulva.

DIAGNOSTIC TESTS & INTERPRETATION
Initial Tests (lab, imaging)
- Hypercalcemia can occur when metastatic disease is present.
- Squamous cell antigen can be elevated with invasive disease.

Follow-Up Tests & Special Considerations
- Upon examination, any suspicious lesions should be biopsied.
- Diagnosis based on histologic findings following vulvar biopsy (6)
- The vulva can be washed with 3% acetic acid to highlight areas and visualized with a colposcope, allows for visualization of acetowhite lesions and vascular lesions (6).
- For patients with new onset of pruritus, the area of pruritus should be biopsied.
- Liberal biopsies must be used to diagnose in situ disease prior to invasion and to diagnose early invasive disease.
- The patient should not be treated for presumed benign conditions of the vulva without full exam and biopsy, including Pap smear and colposcopy of cervix, vagina, and vulva.
- When symptoms persist, reexamine and rebiopsy.
- Treatment of benign condyloma of the vulva has not been shown to decrease the eventual incidence of in situ or invasive disease of the vulva.
- CT scan to evaluate pelvic and periaortic lymph node status if tumor >2 cm or if suspicion of metastatic disease (6)[A].

Diagnostic Procedures/Other
Office vulvar biopsy is done to establish the diagnosis.

Test Interpretation
A surgical staging system is used for vulvar cancer (International Federation of Obstetrics and Gynecology Classification).

- Stage I: tumor confined to the vulva
  - Stage IA: lesions ≤2 cm in size, confined to the vulva or perineum and with stromal invasion ≤1 mm, no node metastasis
  - Stage IB: lesions >2 cm in size or with stromal invasion >1 mm, confined to the vulva or perineum, with negative nodes
- Stage II: tumor of any size with extension to adjacent perineal structures (lower 1/3 urethra, lower 1/3 vagina, anus) with negative nodes
- Stage III: tumor of any size with or without extension to adjacent perineal structures (lower 1/3 urethra, lower 1/3 vagina, anus) with positive inguinofemoral lymph nodes
  - Stage IIIA
    - With 1 lymph node metastasis (≥5 mm), or
    - 1 to 2 lymph node metastases (<5 mm)
  - Stage IIIB
    - With ≥2 lymph node metastases (≥5 mm), or
    - ≥3 lymph node metastases (<5 mm)
  - Stage IIIC: with positive nodes with extracapsular spread
- Stage IV: tumor invades other regional (upper 2/3 urethra, upper 2/3 vagina) or distant structures
  - Stage IVA: tumor invades any of the following:
    - Upper urethral and/or vaginal mucosa, bladder mucosa, rectal mucosa, or fixed to pelvic bone
    - Fixed or ulcerated inguinofemoral lymph nodes
  - Stage IVB: any distant metastasis, including pelvic lymph nodes (7)[B]

TREATMENT

GENERAL MEASURES

- Wide excision can be performed for carcinoma in situ, and any suspicious lesion should be excised for definitive diagnosis.
- Cystoscopy and sigmoidoscopy should be performed if there is a question of invasion into the urethra, bladder, or rectum.

MEDICATION

- As an adjuvant therapy, fluorouracil (Efudex) cream for in situ disease can produce occasional results but is not well tolerated because of irritation of the vulva (8)[A].
- Chemoradiotherapy with cisplatin and 5-fluorouracil (5-FU) has been successful in advanced or recurrent disease, although local morbidity is increased (8)[A].
- Contraindications: elderly patients: If chemotherapeutic agents are used, pay close attention to the patient's performance status and ability to tolerate aggressive chemotherapy.

ISSUES FOR REFERRAL

Patients may need care from a gynecologic oncologist and/or a radiation oncologist.

ADDITIONAL THERAPIES

- Preoperative radiation therapy can be used in those with advanced vulvar cancer (6)[B].
- Adjuvant radiation should be considered with tumor size >4 cm, evidence of lymphovascular invasion, positive surgical margins, or lymph node involvement.
- Preoperative chemoradiation allows for a less radical surgical procedure in patients who are not surgical candidates (8)[A].
- Postoperative radiation decreases recurrence frequency and may improve survival (8)[A].
- Radiation is contraindicated with verrucous carcinoma because it induces anaplastic transformation and increases metastases.

SURGERY/OTHER PROCEDURES

- In situ disease can be treated with wide excision or laser vaporization of the affected area. Laser vaporization is preferable in the younger patient, whereas wide excision is preferable in the elderly patient, in whom the risk of invasive disease is also higher (6)[A].
- If tumor extension within <1 cm from structures that will not be removed, preoperative radiation to prevent inadequate surgical margins prior to excision
- Inguinofemoral lymphadenectomy removal of superficial inguinal and deep femoral lymph nodes
- 1 cm tumor-free margin is required because smaller margin would increase risk of recurrence (8)[A].
- Stage IA: radical local excision without lymph node dissection
- Stage IB: radical local excision with either sentinel lymph node biopsy (SLNB) or ipsilateral inguinofemoral lymph node dissection because the risk of metastases is >8%
- Stage II: modified radical vulvectomy and/or chemoradiation and groin node dissection
- Stages III and IV: neoadjuvant chemoradiation and less radical surgery
- Pelvic exenteration after radiation provides effective therapy for advanced or recurrent malignancies involving the bladder or rectum.

- More limited surgery
  - Has been undertaken for early invasive lesions, especially in young patients, to preserve the clitoris and sexual function
  - Sentinel lymph node biopsy (SLNB) also has been advocated for early invasive lesion (stage IB or higher). It has shown to accurately diagnose groin metastases in women with early vulval cancer and unknown groin node status. This will limit the surgical morbidity associated with inguinofemoral lymphadenectomy (IFL) in those with early stage disease (9)[A].
  - Radical vulvectomy with bilateral groin node dissection through separate incisions provides better cosmetic results than en bloc technique.
  - Unilateral lymphadenectomy should be considered when lesion <2 cm, lateral lesion >2 cm from vulvar midline, or no palpable groin nodes (7)[B].

INPATIENT CONSIDERATIONS

Typically inpatient for treatment

Admission Criteria/Initial Stabilization

In advanced malignancy involving the urethra and rectum, concomitant cisplatin/5-FU chemotherapy with radiation produces a significant decrease in size of the primary tumor, usually obviating the need for pelvic exenteration.

ONGOING CARE

FOLLOW-UP RECOMMENDATIONS

Patient Monitoring

- Early stage, treated with surgery alone: clinical exam of the groin nodes and vulvar area every 6 months for 2 years; then annually
- Following chemoradiation, assessment for further treatment within 6 to 12 weeks of therapy completion
- Advance stage, clinical exam of the groin nodes and vulvar area every 3 months for 2 years; then every 6 months for 3 years, and then annually (10)[B]
- Cervical and/or vaginal cytology annually
- Majority of relapses occur within 1st year.

DIET

As tolerated and according to comorbid conditions

PATIENT EDUCATION

- American College of Obstetricians and Gynecologists (ACOG), 409 12th St. SW, Washington, DC 20024-2188; (800) 762-ACOG; http://www.acog.org/
- American Cancer Society: http://www.cancer.org/

PROGNOSIS

The 5-year survival is based on stage:

- Stage I: 78.5%
- Stage II: 58.8%
- Stage III: 43.2%
- Stage IV: 13.0%
- Inguinal and/or femoral node involvement is the most important determinant of survival (11)[A].

COMPLICATIONS

- The major complications from radical vulvectomy and groin node dissection are wound breakdown, lymphedema, urinary stress incontinence, and psychosexual consequences.
- Two common complications with radical vulvectomy and bilateral groin node dissection
  - In the immediate postoperative period, ~50% of patients experience breakdown of the wound.

This requires aggressive wound care by visiting nurses as often as twice a day. The wounds usually granulate and heal over a period of 6 to 10 weeks.
  - ~15–20% of patients experience some form of mild to moderate lymphedema after the groin node dissection. These patients should be instructed in the use of leg elevation and support hose. <1% of patients experience severe, debilitating lymphedema.

REFERENCES

1. Crosbie EJ, Slade RJ, Ahmed AS. The management of vulval cancer. *Cancer Treat Rev.* 2009;35(7):533–539.
2. Siegel RL, Miller KD, Jemal A. Cancer statistics, 2015. *CA Cancer J Clin.* 2015;65(1):5–29.
3. U.S. Cancer Statistics Working Group. *United States Cancer Statistics: 1999–2010 Incidence and Mortality Web-based Report.* Atlanta, GA: Department of Health and Human Services, Centers for Disease Control and Prevention, and National Cancer Institute; 2013.
4. Hampl M, Sarajuuri H, Wentzensen N, et al. Effect of human papillomavirus vaccines on vulvar, vaginal, and anal intraepithelial lesions and vulvar cancer. *Obstet Gynecol.* 2006;108(6):1361–1368.
5. Markowitz LE, Dunne EF, Saraiya M, et al. Quadrivalent human papillomavirus vaccine: recommendations of the Advisory Committee on Immunization Practices (ACIP). *MMWR Recomm Rep.* 2007;56(RR–2):1–24.
6. de Hullu JA, van der Zee AG. Surgery and radiotherapy in vulvar cancer. *Crit Rev Oncol Hematol.* 2006;60(1):38–58.
7. Radziszewski J, Kowalewska M, Jedrzejczak T, et al. The accuracy of the sentinel lymph node concept in early stage squamous cell vulvar carcinoma. *Gynecol Oncol.* 2010;116(3):473–477.
8. Shylasree TS, Bryant A, Howells RE. Chemoradiation for advanced primary vulval cancer. *Cochrane Database Syst Rev.* 2011;13(4):CD003752.
9. Lawrie TA, Patel A, Martin-Hirsch PP, et al. Sentinel node assessment for diagnosis of groin lymph node involvement in vulval cancer. *Cochrane Database Syst Rev.* 2014;(6):CD010409.
10. Stuckey A, Schutzer M, Rizack T, et al. Locally advanced vulvar cancer in elderly women: is chemoradiation beneficial? *Am J Clin Oncol.* 2013;36(3):279–282.
11. Salani R, Backes FJ, Fung MF, et al. Posttreatment surveillance and diagnosis of recurrence in women with gynecologic malignancies: Society of Gynecologic Oncologists recommendations. *Am J Obstet Gynecol.* 2011;204(6):466–478.

CODES

ICD10

- C51.9 Malignant neoplasm of vulva, unspecified
- D07.1 Carcinoma in situ of vulva
- C51.0 Malignant neoplasm of labium majus

CLINICAL PEARLS

- 60% of vulvar cancers are attributable to oncogenic HPV, and 92% of all VIN 2/3, VAIN 2/3, and AIN are attributable to HPV. Therefore, HPV vaccination has the potential to decrease vulvar cancer by 1/3.
- Biopsy all suspicious or nonhealing vulvar lesions.

V

VULVODYNIA

Jessica Johnson, MD, MPH • Amy L. Wiser, MD

 BASICS

DESCRIPTION
- Vulvar pain lasting 3 months or more. Occurs in the absence of relevant visible findings, relevant lab abnormalities, or a clinically identifiable neurologic disorder
- Classification by ISSVD is based on whether pain is generalized or localized and whether it is provoked (by physical contact), spontaneous, or mixed.
  – Generalized: involvement of majority of the vulva; usually persistent or spontaneous pain
  – Localized: severe pain of certain vulvar areas such as the vestibule (formerly known as *vestibulodynia*), usually provoked with touch or attempted vaginal entry; thought to be the leading cause of painful intercourse among premenopausal women
    ○ Primary: introital dyspareunia from first episode of intercourse or first insertion of tampon or vaginal speculum
    ○ Secondary: introital dyspareunia developing after a period of painless intercourse, tampon use, or speculum exams

EPIDEMIOLOGY
- Most women diagnosed between age 20 and 80 years
- Nearly half of woman opt not to seek treatment (1).
- Patients are psychologically comparable with asymptomatic controls and have similar marital satisfaction.

Incidence
- Recent retrospective study estimates annual rate of new onset vulvodynia to be 1.8% (2).
- Evidence indicates lifetime cumulative incidence approaches 15%, suggesting nearly 14 million U.S. women will experience persistent vulvar discomfort at some point in their lives (3).

Prevalence
- Reports between 8.3% and 16%; non–clinical-based studies approximate a prevalence of 7% with validation by exam (1).
- Studies show Hispanics are 80% more likely to present with vulvar pain compared with Caucasians and African Americans.

ETIOLOGY AND PATHOPHYSIOLOGY
- Vulvodynia is likely to be neuropathically mediated:
  – Allodynia and hyperalgesia are thought to result from neurogenic inflammation, leading to sensitization of primary afferents by inflammatory peptides, prostaglandins, and cytokines. Impulses transmitted to the CNS, where reinforcing signals sustain pain loop
  – In recent investigations of vulvar biopsy specimens, increased neuronal proliferation and branching in vulvar tissue are evident when compared with tissue of asymptomatic women.
- Pelvic floor pathology also should be considered: In one study, the vulvodynia group showed an increase in pelvic floor hypertonicity at the superficial muscle layer, less vaginal muscle strength with contraction, and decreased relaxation of pelvic floor muscles after contraction (3).
- No cause of vulvodynia has been established. It is most likely a neuropathic pain caused by a combination of the following:
  – Recurrent vulvovaginal candidiasis or other infections
  – Immune-mediated chronic neuro-inflammatory process within vulvar tissues
  – Chemical exposure (trichloroacetic acid) or physical trauma
  – Reduced estrogen receptor expression/changes in estrogen concentration
  – CNS etiology, similar to other regional pain syndromes

RISK FACTORS
- Vulvovaginal infections, specifically candidiasis. Unclear if infection, treatment, or underlying hypersensitivity is the cause (1). Multiple infections compound this risk.
- Hormonal factors: Controversial evidence proposes increased risk with use of oral contraception pills (OCPs); early age at first use of OCPs and longer duration of use has been associated with increased risk.
- Pelvic floor dysfunction: Increased instability of pelvic floor muscles may perpetuate vulvar tissue inflammation, leading to vascular changes and histamine release.
- Comorbid interstitial cystitis and painful bladder syndrome; potentially related to common embryologic origin of structures
- Abuse: increased risk of vulvodynia if childhood had physical or sexual abuse by a primary family member; causal relationship remains unclear (3).
- Depression and anxiety (1)
- Other neuropathic disorders, including regional pain syndrome

Genetics
Proposed genetic deficiency impairing one's ability to stop the inflammatory response triggered by infection or chemicals; homozygosity of the two alleles of the IL-1 receptor antagonist occurs in 25–50% of vestibulodynia patients, compared with <10% in controls (4).

GENERAL PREVENTION
- Wear 100% cotton underwear in the daytime and no underwear to sleep.
- Avoid douching and other vulvar irritants such as perfumes, dyes, and detergents.
- Avoid abrasive activities and tight, synthetic clothing.
- Avoid panty liners.
- Clean the vulva with water only and pat area dry after bathing.
- Avoid use of hair dryers in the vulvar area.

COMMONLY ASSOCIATED CONDITIONS
Higher incidence of chronic pain syndromes associated with vulvodynia, including chronic cystitis, irritable bowel syndrome, fibromyalgia, migraines, depression, endometriosis, low back pain. Women with vulvodynia have a higher incidence of depression and anxiety both preceding and resulting from their symptoms (1).

℞ DIAGNOSIS

- Vulvodynia is a clinical diagnosis and it should be suspected in any women with chronic pain at the introitus and vulva (4)[B].

- Pain should be characterized using a standard measure such as the McGill Pain Questionnaire; duration and nature of the pain should be established. Use physical exam to rule out other causes of vulvovaginal pain. Negative fungal culture, along with relevant history and positive cotton swab test, confirm diagnosis.

HISTORY
Adequate sexual, social, and pain history should be taken to assess degree of symptoms. Visual pain scales and pain diaries may be helpful (5)[B]:
- Onset of vulvodynia often sudden and without precedents
- Pain often described as generalized, unprovoked.

- Quality of pain is burning, stinging, irritating, or rawness (1).
- Specifically ask about bowel and bladder habits, history of trauma or abuse, history of infections including herpes, and personal hygiene.
- Specific skin complaints may suggest alternate diagnosis; a history of allergies may suggest vulvar dermatitis.
- Assess for precipitants of vulvar pain: tight garments, bicycle riding, tampon use, prolonged sitting, perfumed or deodorant soaps, douching (1)
- Assess for complaints of dyspareunia:
  – Presence of vaginismus (involuntary vaginal muscle spasm), adequate lubrication, anorgasmia, partner problems, abuse
  – Psychosexual morbidity significantly higher in patients with vulvodynia; counseling may complement medical interventions.

PHYSICAL EXAM
- Ask patient to show where pain is localized or most painful.
- Mouth and skin exams to assess for lesions suggestive of lichen planus or lichen sclerosus
- Vaginal exam should be done to exclude other causes of vulvovaginal pain, including external inspection; palpation; and single digit, speculum, and bimanual exams:
  – The vulva may be erythematous, especially at the vestibule. Discomfort with separation of the labia minora is common.
  – Spontaneous or elicited pain at the lower 1/2 of anterior vaginal wall suggests bladder etiology.
- Bulbocavernosus and anal wink reflexes should be checked to assess for peripheral neuropathy.

DIFFERENTIAL DIAGNOSIS
- Infections: candidiasis, herpes, human papillomavirus (HPV), bacterial vaginosis, trichomoniasis, dermatophytes
- Inflammation: lichen planus, immunobullous disorder, allergic vulvitis, lichen sclerosus, atrophic vaginitis
- Neoplasia: Paget disease, vulvar or vaginal intraepithelial neoplasia, squamous cell carcinoma
- Neurologic/muscular: herpes neuralgia, spinal nerve compression, vaginismus

DIAGNOSTIC TESTS & INTERPRETATION
- Cotton swab or Q-tip test: Vulva tested for localized areas of pain beginning at thighs and continuing medially toward vestibule using the soft end and broken sharp end of the cotton swab. Five distinct positions (2, 4, 6, 8, and 10 o'clock) surveyed using light palpation. Pain rated on a scale from 0 (none) to 10 (most severe). Posterior introitus and posterior hymenal remnants most common sites of increased sensitivity.
- Test for concurrent vaginismus: Apply pressure with a gloved finger to levator ani and obturator internus muscles to assess for tenderness, pain, or contracture.

Initial Tests (lab, imaging)
- Vaginal pH, wet mount, and yeast culture are recommended to rule out vaginitis.
- Gonorrhea and chlamydia testing done at physician's discretion
- HPV screening is unnecessary; no association has been identified between HPV and vulvodynia.

Follow-Up Tests & Special Considerations
- Varicella-zoster and herpes simplex virus should be considered if ulcers or vesicular eruptions are present.
- Consider biopsy if concerned for neoplasm or dermatophyte infection or if the patient is resistant to treatment.

Diagnostic Procedures/Other
Colposcopy can be helpful if epidermal abnormalities are present. This should be done with caution because acetic acid worsens vulvar pain.

Test Interpretation
No specific histologic features are associated with vulvodynia, although reactive squamous atypia has been observed. Biopsies are unnecessary for diagnosis. Presence of rash/altered mucosa is not consistent with vulvodynia; this requires further evaluation (5)[C].

 TREATMENT

A trial of several medications for at least 3 months is usually needed.

GENERAL MEASURES
Combining treatments should be encouraged when treating women with vulvodynia (5)[C]: Various reports on use of a combination of medical treatments, psychotherapy, and dietary intervention reveal women on these combinations do significantly better compared with those who receive medication only.

MEDICATION
- Oral therapies
  - Tricyclic antidepressants (TCAs): first-line treatment for unprovoked vulvodynia (5)[B]; do not stop use abruptly; contraindicated in patients with cardiac abnormalities and those taking MAOIs; fatigue, constipation, sweating, palpitations, and weight gain are most common side effects
    - Amitriptyline, nortriptyline: most widely studied; start at 10 mg daily; dose should be titrated to pain control. Average effective dose is 60 mg daily. In one study, a 47% complete response rate was recorded (6)[B]. Nortriptyline may be preferred due to less anticholinergic adverse effects.
  - Anticonvulsant therapies:
    - Gabapentin: Started at 300 mg daily at HS and increased by 300 mg every 3 days. Maximum recommended dose is 3,600 mg daily divided into 3 doses. Dosing regimen limits popularity.
    - Topiramate and lamotrigine have been recommended if other therapies are not effective.
  - SSNRIs: not commonly used; however, have been helpful in those who cannot tolerate TCAs
    - Venlafaxine or duloxetine have also been used; evidence is limited.
  - Opioids/NSAIDs: not consistently helpful in relieving vulvar pain
- Topical therapies
  - A trial of local anesthetics may be recommended for all patients who present with vulvodynia. Use judiciously to avoid increased irritation (5)[C].
  - Lidocaine 5% ointment: for provoked vestibulodynia; application advised 15 to 20 minutes prior to intercourse. Penile numbness and possible toxicity with ingestion can occur.
    - In one study, lidocaine 5% ointment was left in vestibule overnight (average of 8 hours) for a period of 6 to 8 weeks; at follow-up, up to 76% of women reported no discomfort with intercourse (3)[C].

- Cromolyn 4% cream: decreases mast cell degranulation in vulvar tissue; recommended application TID (1)[C]
- Capsaicin 0.025%: decreases in discomfort and increases in frequency of intercourse with 20-minute daily application (3)[B]
- Topical amitriptyline 2% combined with baclofen 2% is helpful in patients with comorbid vaginismus.
- Topical corticosteroids and testosterone creams have not been shown to alleviate symptoms of vulvodynia.
- Gabapentin 3–6% ointment (must be compounded)
- Topical nitroglycerin may be helpful but may cause headaches.
- Topical estrogen
- Injectable therapies
  - Triamcinolone acetonide: no more than 40 mg should be injected monthly; is best when combined with 0.25–0.5% bupivacaine
  - Submucosal methylprednisone and lidocaine: reports of up to 68% response rate with weekly injections (5)[B]
  - Interferon-α: useful in treatment of vestibulodynia. Side effects (myalgias, fever, malaise) limit its use.
  - Botulinum toxin A injectable is being studied.

ISSUES FOR REFERRAL
A team approach is recommended for most effective management. Triage to psychosexual medicine, psychology, partner therapy, and pain management teams should be strongly considered (5)[B].

ADDITIONAL THERAPIES
- Cognitive-behavioral therapy (CBT): One randomized trial revealed that CBT is associated with a 30% decrease in vulvar discomfort with sexual intercourse. CBT is the recommended treatment for patients who present with dyspareunia as a main complaint (4)[B].
- Biofeedback/physical therapy: useful with concomitant vaginismus. Treats both generalized and localized vulvar pain; treatment value for unprovoked pain remains unclear. Most studies report an average of 12- to 16-week treatment time.
- Vaginal dilators
- Surface electromyography (sEMG): efficacious for pelvic floor rehabilitation. Patients are more likely to experience pain-free sexual intercourse after sEMG. Significant reductions seen on pain measures at long-term follow-up.

COMPLEMENTARY & ALTERNATIVE MEDICINE
Acupuncture: Small studies of women with unprovoked vulvodynia who did not respond to conventional treatment reported significant decreases in pain severity with acupuncture; treatment value with provoked pain is unknown (5)[C].

SURGERY/OTHER PROCEDURES
- Surgery may be considered for patients with localized symptoms who have failed to respond to other measures. Not recommended for generalized vulvodynia (5)[B]
- 60–80% of women who undergo surgery report a significant reduction in pain symptoms; however, when surveyed, patients prefer behavioral therapies than surgical intervention.
- All patients who are considering surgical intervention should be tested and treated for vaginismus. Vestibulectomy is less successful in this subgroup.

- Surgical approaches
  - Local excision: precise localization of painful areas; tissue closed in elliptical fashion
  - Total vestibulectomy: Tissue is removed from Skene ducts to perineum. The vagina is then brought down to cover defect.
  - Perineoplasty: vestibulectomy plus removal of perineal tissue; incision usually terminated above the anal orifice; reserved for severe cases (4)[B]

 ONGOING CARE

PATIENT EDUCATION
Patients should be reassured that this condition is neither infectious, nor does it predispose to cancer (5)[C]. Emphasize self-hygiene. Encourage treatment with home remedies, including ice packs, sitz baths with baking soda, olive oil, and barrier cream to preserve moisture after bathing.

PROGNOSIS
Traditionally viewed as a chronic pain disorder, new evidence of remission has been documented; recent 2-year follow-up study revealed 1 in 10 vulvodynia patients reported remission regardless of treatment (7).

REFERENCES
1. Shah M, Hoffstetter S. Vulvodynia. *Obstet Gynecol Clin North Am*. 2014;41(3):453–464.
2. Reed BK, Haefner HK, Sen A, et al. Vulvodynia incidence and remission rates among adult women: a 2-year follow-up study. *Obstet Gynecol*. 2008;112(2, Pt 1):231–237.
3. Boardman LA, Stockdale CK. Sexual pain. *Clin Obstet Gynecol*. 2009;52(4):682–690.
4. Reed BD. Vulvodynia: diagnosis and management. *Am Fam Physician*. 2006;73(7):1231–1238.
5. Nunns D, Mandal D, Byrne M, et al. Guidelines for the management of vulvodynia. *Br J Dermatol*. 2010;162(6):1180–1185.
6. Stockdale CK, Lawson HW. 2013 vulvodynia guideline update. *J Low Genit Tract Dis*. 2014;18(2): 93–100.
7. Davis SN, Bergeron S, Binik YM, et al. Women with provoked vestibulodynia experience clinically significant reductions in pain regardless of treatment: results from a 2-year follow-up study. *J Sex Med*. 2013;10(12):3080–3087.

 CODES

ICD10
- N94.819 Vulvodynia, unspecified
- N94.818 Other vulvodynia
- N94.810 Vulvar vestibulitis

CLINICAL PEARLS
- Vulvodynia is a clinical diagnosis; it should be suspected in any woman with chronic pain at the introitus and vulva.
- A decrease in pain may take weeks to months and may not be complete.
- No single treatment is proven in all women; improvement over time is common even without treatment.

V

VULVOVAGINITIS, ESTROGEN DEFICIENT

Maria De La Luz Nieto, MD

BASICS

DESCRIPTION
- Vaginal atrophy is due to decreased blood flow to vaginal epithelium, resulting in thinning of the female genital tissues.
- Estrogen deficiency affects all tissues in the female body; however, the genital tissues are especially hormone-responsive and are most affected, leading to atrophy.
- Patients with estrogen-deficient vulvovaginitis may present with urinary incontinence, vaginal burning and itching, dyspareunia, increased urinary frequency, or recurrent UTIs.
- System(s) affected: reproductive

EPIDEMIOLOGY
Incidence
- Predominant age: postmenopausal females. The average age of menopause in the United States is 51.3 years but ranges from 45 to 55 years old.
- May affect lactating women
- Predominant sex: female only
- May occur in younger women with premature ovarian failure

Prevalence
- Most postmenopausal women are affected to some degree.
- Up to 40% of postmenopausal women experience symptoms severe enough to seek treatment.

ETIOLOGY AND PATHOPHYSIOLOGY
- Decreased estrogen levels in the vagina and vulva result in decreased blood flow and decreased lubrication of vaginal and vulvar tissue.
- Vaginal and vulvar tissues become thin secondary to decreased vaginal cell maturation.
- Decreased cellular maturation results in decreased glycogen stores, which affects the normal vaginal flora and pH.
- Estrogen deficiency due to the following:
  - Menopause (surgical or natural)
  - Premature ovarian failure (chemotherapy, irradiation, autoimmune, anorexia, genetic)
  - Postpartum, lactation

- Medications that alter hormonal concentration, such as gonadotropin-releasing hormone agonists, and antiestrogens, such as tamoxifen and danazol
- Elevated prolactin from hypothalamic–pituitary disorders

Genetics
No known pattern

RISK FACTORS
Estrogen-deficient states

COMMONLY ASSOCIATED CONDITIONS
- Urge and stress urinary incontinence
- Pelvic organ prolapse
- Frequent UTIs
- Bacterial vaginosis or yeast infections

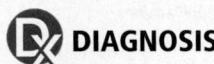

DIAGNOSIS

HISTORY
- All female patients should be asked about symptoms because many women are embarrassed to discuss these issues with their health care providers (1)[C].
  - Vaginal dryness
  - Dyspareunia
  - Pruritus
  - Burning
  - Pressure
  - Tenderness
  - Malodorous discharge
  - Urinary symptoms: dysuria, hematuria, frequency, infections, stress, and urge urinary incontinence
- Ask about self-treatment and products used.
- Determine exposure to irritants (e.g., soaps, feminine sprays, lotions, lubricants, constant pad use).

PHYSICAL EXAM
Evidence for the diagnosis includes the following:
- Loss of pubic hair
- Decreased vulvar and vaginal fullness
- Decreased vulvar subcuticular fat and moisture
- Pale-appearing, shiny, smooth vaginal and urethral epithelium
- Vaginal shortening, intolerance to speculum exams

- Loss of vaginal rugation
- Pelvic organ prolapse
- Shorten urethra

DIFFERENTIAL DIAGNOSIS
- Malignancy
- Dermatologic conditions of vulva and vagina:
  - Dermatitis
  - Lichen sclerosis
  - Lichen planus
- Bacterial or yeast vulvovaginitis

DIAGNOSTIC TESTS & INTERPRETATION
Because vulvovaginitis is a clinical diagnosis, labs are not always necessary, but if suspect dermatologic or oncologic condition, biopsy is recommended (2)[A].

Initial Tests (lab, imaging)
However, the following labs may be obtained as corroborative of clinical impression:
- Check follicle-stimulating hormone (FSH) and estrogen levels. FSH rises and estrogen drops with menopause.
- Evaluate for infections via wet preparation and vaginal pH (usually >5).
- Urine dip and urinalysis if suspected concomitant UTI
- Perform cytology for maturation index: Higher proportion of parabasal cells and lower proportion of intermediate and superficial cells indicate decreased maturation index.

Follow-Up Tests & Special Considerations
Drugs that may alter lab results:
- Estrogen therapy will alter the maturation index.
- Digoxin has estrogen-like properties.
- Tamoxifen may produce menopausal-type symptoms but also may act on genital tissues as a weak estrogen agonist.
- Progestins, danazol, and gonadotropin-releasing hormone agonists may produce a reversible pseudo-menopause state.

Test Interpretation
- Thinning of the cornified squamous layer of both the vulva and the vagina
- Increased parabasal cells
- Compact underlying collagenous tissue

TREATMENT

GENERAL MEASURES
- Wear loose-fitting, undyed cotton underwear.
- Avoid prolonged pad use, especially scented pads.
- Avoid feminine deodorant sprays and douching.
- Use over-the-counter water-based lubricants, as needed.
- Symptomatic relief, if needed (e.g., cool baths or compresses)

MEDICATION
- Vaginal estrogen can reverse atrophic changes and help to alleviate symptoms (3)[A].
  - Vaginal cream 1 g (conjugated equine estrogens or estradiol cream): Insert via applicator each night for 14 days and then 2 to 3 times per week.
  - Vaginal estradiol 10-μg tablet: Insert via pre-loaded applicator each night for 14 days and then 2 to 3 times per week.
  - Estradiol-containing vaginal ring 2 mg: Insert into vagina, and replace every 3 months.
- Estrogen therapy should be used in the lowest possible dose for the shortest duration of time (4)[B].
- Long-term therapy may be necessary owing to the chronic nature of estrogen-deficient vulvovaginitis (5)[A].
- Systemic therapy typically is used as hormonal treatment of vasomotor symptoms and not for the primary treatment of estrogen-deficient vulvovaginitis.
- Contraindications
  - Breast or estrogen-dependent carcinoma
  - Undiagnosed vaginal bleeding
  - Thromboembolic disorders
  - Thrombophlebitis
  - Pregnancy
- Precautions: Any abnormal vaginal bleeding must be evaluated.
- Nonestrogen therapy: estrogen agonist/antagonist (6)[B]

  - Ospemifene (Osphena) 60-mg tablet daily
- Contraindications
  - Breast or estrogen-dependent carcinoma
  - Undiagnosed vaginal bleeding

  - Thromboembolic disorders
  - Thrombophlebitis
  - Hepatic impairment
- Precautions: Any abnormal vaginal bleeding must be evaluated, monitor for DVT and stroke.

ISSUES FOR REFERRAL
- Refer to urogynecologist for evaluation if symptomatic due to pelvic organ prolapse and/or stress and urge urinary incontinence.
- Recurrent UTIs should be referred to urogynecology and/or urology for evaluation.

INPATIENT CONSIDERATIONS
Admission Criteria/Initial Stabilization
Outpatient treatment

ONGOING CARE

FOLLOW-UP RECOMMENDATIONS
No restrictions

Patient Monitoring
Instruct the patient that symptoms should improve within 30 to 60 days. If they do not, reevaluate and reexamine for other causes.

DIET
No special diet

PATIENT EDUCATION
- American College of Obstetricians and Gynecologists (ACOG), 409 12th St., SW, Washington, DC 20024-2188; 800-762-ACOG: http://www.acog.org/
- Lactating postpartum women with high levels of prolactin are in a hypoestrogenic state. These women should be instructed to use lubrication for symptoms of dyspareunia and reassured that the symptoms will resolve when they are no longer breastfeeding.

PROGNOSIS
The prognosis is excellent. Most symptoms will be alleviated with vaginal estrogen replacement therapy.

COMPLICATIONS
- Recurrent UTIs may occur in women with vaginal atrophy.
- Vaginal atrophy predisposes patients to vaginal infections.

REFERENCES

1. Mehta A, Bachmann G. Vulvovaginal complaints. *Clin Obstet Gynecol.* 2008;51(3):549–555.
2. Johnston SL, Farrell SA, Bouchard C, et al. The detection and management of vaginal atrophy. *J Obstet Gynaecol Can.* 2004;26(5):503–515.
3. Farquhar CM, Marjoribanks J, Lethaby A, et al. Long term hormone therapy for perimenopausal and postmenopausal women. *Cochrane Database Syst Rev.* 2005;(3):CD004143.
4. Ibe C, Simon JA. Vulvovaginal atrophy: current and future therapies (CME). *J Sex Med.* 2010;7(3):1042–1050.
5. Suckling J, Lethaby A, Kennedy R. Local oestrogen for vaginal atrophy in postmenopausal women. *Cochrane Database Syst Rev.* 2006;(4):CD001500.
6. Constantine G, Graham S, Portman DJ, et al. Female sexual function improved with ospemifene in postmenopausal women with vulvar and vaginal atrophy: results of a randomized, placebo-controlled trial. *Climacteric.* 2015;18(2):226–232.

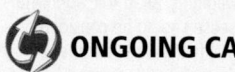

CODES

ICD10
- N95.2 Postmenopausal atrophic vaginitis
- E28.39 Other primary ovarian failure

CLINICAL PEARLS
- Estrogen-deficient vulvovaginitis affects virtually all postmenopausal women to some degree.
- This disorder is often associated with urinary incontinence, increased urinary frequency, and recurrent UTIs.
- Lab tests are generally unnecessary to make the diagnosis.
- Vaginal estrogen preparations, rather than systemic preparations, should be the first-line therapy in a woman whose primary complaint is associated with vaginal atrophy.

V

VULVOVAGINITIS, PREPUBESCENT

Sarah Parrott, DO

BASICS

DESCRIPTION
- Vulvitis is inflammation of the external genitals.
- Vaginitis, often associated with vaginal discharge, is inflammation involving the vaginal mucosa.
- In premenarchal girls, vulvitis is usually primary with secondary extension into the vagina.
- System(s) affected: reproductive, skin/exocrine
- Synonym(s): vaginitis; vulvitis

EPIDEMIOLOGY
Incidence
Unknown

Prevalence
Most common gynecologic problem in prepubertal girls

ETIOLOGY AND PATHOPHYSIOLOGY
- In the prepubertal child, the levels of estrogen are low.
- Due to the low levels of estrogen, the vaginal epithelium is thin, immature, and fragile.
- Absence of pubic hair and a well-developed labia as well as close proximity of the anus and vagina, make contamination more likely.
- The prepubertal child also has an absence of lactobacilli, creating a neutral to alkaline vaginal pH.
- Neutral pH, atrophic mucosa, and moist environment of the vagina increase the risk of infection.
- Most cases of pediatric vulvovaginitis are nonspecific inflammation.
- Specific infections that occur are typically respiratory, enteric, or sexually transmitted.
- Nonspecific vulvovaginitis
- Poor perineal hygiene
- Nonspecific chemical irritants (bubble baths, scented soaps, shampoos)
- Tight-fitting clothing
- Etiology
  - Bacterial: The most common bacteria are introduced from respiratory and GI tracts.
    - The most common respiratory pathogen is *Streptococcus pyogenes* (1)[B]. Vulvitis may occur in the absence of respiratory symptoms.
    - Urinary tract infections are common in children with vulvovaginitis (2)[B].
    - *Escherichia coli* is the most common fecal pathogen.
    - *Shigella* vaginitis is associated with mucopurulent bloody discharge and likewise, is not always accompanied by a history of diarrhea.

- *Enterobius vermicularis* (pinworms)
  - Very common in young children and certain populations
  - Should be considered in children with vaginal itching and irritation
  - Most common symptom is nocturnal perineal itching.
  - Foreign body
    - Presents with foul-smelling, bloody, or brown discharge from the vagina
    - Should be considered with recurrent vulvovaginitis where other causes have been eliminated
  - Other
    - With chronic vulvovaginitis, anatomic abnormalities or systemic disease should be considered:
      - Anatomic abnormalities include double vagina with fistula, ectopic ureter, and urethral prolapse.
  - Systemic disease (inflammatory diseases)
  - Other conditions, such as lichen sclerosus, vitiligo, psoriasis, and atopic dermatitis, should be considered.

Genetics
Understudied

RISK FACTORS
- Prepubertal girls are particularly susceptible due to behavioral and anatomic reasons:
  - Inadequate hand washing or perineal cleansing after urination and defecation
  - Tight-fitting clothing
  - Proximity of the vagina to the anus, lack of protective hair, and labial fat pads
  - Trauma
- Obese girls are also susceptible to nonspecific vulvovaginitis (3)[A].

GENERAL PREVENTION
- Good perineal hygiene (including wiping from front to back)
- Urination with legs spread apart and labia separated
- Avoidance of tight-fitting clothing and nonabsorbent underwear
- Avoidance of irritants such as harsh/perfumed soaps and bubble baths

ALERT
Cultures of sexually transmitted organisms in prepubertal children warrant investigations of sexual abuse.

DIAGNOSIS

HISTORY
- Irritation and erythema of vulva
- Itching
- Bleeding
- Vaginal discharge
- Unpleasant odor
- Dysuria
- Soreness

PHYSICAL EXAM
- Look for evidence of chronic illness or dermatologic disease.
- Look for trauma or other signs that may correlate with abuse.
- Inspect the genital area in the supine position:
  - Excoriation of the genital area
  - Inflammation (erythema, swelling) of the introitus
  - Inspect the vagina and cervix in the knee–chest position or frog leg position.
  - Perform rectal exam if vaginal bleeding or abdominal pain.

DIFFERENTIAL DIAGNOSIS
- Contact dermatitis
- Eczema
- Psoriasis
- Lichen sclerosus

DIAGNOSTIC TESTS & INTERPRETATION
Initial Tests (lab, imaging)
- Culture for bacteria, fungi (yeast), or viruses (herpes)
- Urinalysis, urine culture, and urine for STI (via nucleic acid amplification test)
- Tape exam for pinworms
- Potassium hydroxide and saline smears of vaginal discharge, if present
- If an anatomic abnormality is suspected, imaging may be necessary to confirm.
- Consider consultation with a pediatric or adult gynecologist to determine the most appropriate imaging study.

Follow-Up Tests & Special Considerations
Exploration of the vagina for a foreign body may be necessary in cases of persistent, recurrent vulvitis.

Diagnostic Procedures/Other

If blood or foul-smelling discharge is present, visualization is mandatory:

- Place the child in the knee–chest position for best results. Hold the buttocks apart and slightly upward.
- Visualization of the vagina may be necessary by using a nasal speculum or infant laryngoscope.
- If available, consider referral to a provider with specific training/experience in this specialized exam.

TREATMENT

- The definitive diagnosis of bacterial vulvitis requires a culture of vulva and vaginal secretions.
- The typical colony count and bacterial mix are unknown in prepubescent girls. Antibiotic use should be directed against the species with the highest colony count.
- General hygiene should always be recommended, particularly in cases of a retained foreign body (e.g., toilet paper).
- When no cause is identified, treatment should focus on hygiene as well as minimizing soap exposure and tight-fitting clothes (1).

GENERAL MEASURES

- Appropriate health care: outpatient (except where systemic illness requires hospital care)
- Soak the vulva/perineum in a small amount of clear, warm water for 15 minutes BID.
- If smegma is present in the labial folds, clean the area gently with a mild soap.

MEDICATION

First Line

- To break the itching–scratching–infection cycle, use a low-dose topical hydrocortisone cream for a limited time.
- Estrogen deficiency with labial adhesion/agglutination: estrogen cream 0.625 mg to fused area nightly for 2 weeks
- Emollients or protective creams may offer symptomatic relief.
- Antibiotic use should be restricted to cases of bacterial infection only (4)[A].
- Specific organisms on culture
  - Group A *Streptococcus*, *S. pneumoniae*: penicillin V (Pen Vee K) 250 mg PO BID–TID for 10 days
  - *Haemophilus influenzae*: amoxicillin, 20 to 40 mg/kg/day PO divided TID for 7 days
  - *Staphylococcus aureus*: cephalexin, 25 to 50 mg/kg/day PO divided QID for 7 to 10 days *or* dicloxacillin, 25 mg/kg/day divided QID for 7 to 10 days *or* amoxicillin-clavulanate, 20 to 40 mg/kg/day PO divided BID for 7 to 10 days

- *S. pyogenes*: amoxicillin, 50 mg/kg/day PO divided into 3 doses/day for 10 days
- *Candida* sp.: topical nystatin (Mycostatin), miconazole, clotrimazole, or terconazole
- *Shigella*: trimethoprim/sulfamethoxazole or ampicillin for 5 days
- Pinworms: mebendazole, 100 mg PO, repeated in 2 weeks
- *Chlamydia trachomatis*: ≤45 kg: erythromycin, 50 mg/kg/day QID for 14 days; ≥45 kg and <8 years old: azithromycin, 1 g PO single dose; ≥45 kg and ≥8 years old: azithromycin, 1 g PO single dose or doxycycline 100 mg BID for 7 days
- *Neisseria gonorrhoeae*: ≤45 kg: ceftriaxone, 125 mg IM plus medication for chlamydia; >45 kg: ceftriaxone, 250 mg IM × 1 plus medication for chlamydia
- *Trichomonas*: metronidazole, 15 mg/kg/day PO divided TID (max 250 mg TID) for 7 days
- Contraindications: allergy to proposed treatment
- Precautions: Avoid potential allergens and topical sensitizers if possible.

ISSUES FOR REFERRAL

- Suspected sexual abuse
- Suspected anatomic abnormality (except minor labial agglutination)
- Persistent, severe, or recurrent infections

ONGOING CARE

FOLLOW-UP RECOMMENDATIONS

Patient Monitoring

Monitor for fever, pruritus, and vaginal discharge.

DIET

- Healthy balanced diet, high in fiber to prevent constipation
- Adequate fluid intake

PATIENT EDUCATION

Hygiene

- Wipe front to back after elimination.
- Avoid bubble baths and other irritating products.
- Clean daily with mild soap and water and dry gently with soft towel or cool hair dryer.
- Apply bland ointments for skin protection, if necessary.

PROGNOSIS

Excellent

COMPLICATIONS

- If an STI is identified and not treated effectively, the patient is at risk for pelvic inflammatory disease (PID).
- Vaginismus

REFERENCES

1. Gorbachinsky I, Sherertz R, Russell G, et al. Altered perineal microbiome is associated with vulvovaginitis and urinary tract infection in preadolescent girls. *Ther Adv Urol.* 2014;6(6):224–229.
2. Stricker T, Navratil F, Sennhauser FH. Vulvovaginitis in prepubertal girls. *Arch Dis Child.* 2003;88(4):324–326.
3. Van Eyk N, Allen L, Giesbrecht E, et al. Pediatric vulvovaginal disorders: a diagnostic approach and review of the literature. *J Obstet Gynaecol Can.* 2009;31(9):850–862.
4. Dei M, Di Maggio F, Di Paolo G, et al. Vulvovaginitis in childhood. *Best Pract Res Clin Obstet Gynaecol.* 2010;24(2):129–137.

ADDITIONAL READING

- Delago C, Finkel MA, Deblinger E. Urogenital symptoms in premenarchal girls: parents' and girls' perceptions and associations with irritants. *J Pediatr Adolesc Gynecol.* 2012;25(1):67–73.
- Joishy M, Ashtekar CS, Jain A, et al. Do we need to treat vulvovaginitis in prepubertal girls? *BMJ.* 2005;330(7484):186–188.
- Velander MH, Mikkelsen DB, Bygum A. Labial agglutination in a prepubertal girl: effect of topical oestrogen. *Acta Derm Venereol.* 2009;89(2):198–199.

CODES

ICD10

- N76.0 Acute vaginitis
- N77.1 Vaginitis, vulvitis and vulvovaginitis in dis classd elswhr

CLINICAL PEARLS

- Vulvovaginitis is the most common gynecologic problem in prepubescent girls.
- The hypoestrogenic state and prepubescent anatomy may increase susceptibility to vulvar and vaginal infection.
- Treatment is typically supportive (avoid scratching, warm soaks) but may require antibiotics if a bacterial infection is suspected.
- Isolating an infection with known sexual transmission should prompt further investigation.
- Recurrent or persistent vulvitis, especially with foul-smelling discharge, should prompt a skilled exam of the vagina for a retained foreign body.
- Good perineal hygiene will limit this condition.

V

WARTS
Mercedes E. Gonzalez, MD, FAAD • Herbert P. Goodheart, MD

BASICS

- Warts (verrucae) are benign growths that are confined to the epidermis. All warts are caused by the human papillomavirus (HPV). Warts can appear on any area of the skin or mucous membranes. Common warts are predominantly seen in children and young adults.
- Clinically, warts are rather arbitrarily described as the following:
  - Common warts (verrucae vulgaris)
  - Plantar warts (verrucae plantaris)
  - Flat warts (verrucae plana)
  - Venereal warts (condyloma acuminatum)
  - Epidermodysplasia verruciformis is a rare, lifelong hereditary disorder characterized by chronic infection with HPV.
- System(s) affected: skin/exocrine

DESCRIPTION

- Common warts are most often found at sites subject to frequent trauma, such as the hands and feet. Because warts often vary widely in shape, size, and appearance, the various descriptive names for them generally reflect their clinical appearance, location, or both.
- For example, filiform (fingerlike) warts are threadlike, planar warts are flat, and plantar warts are located on the plantar surfaces (soles) of the feet.
- Genital warts, or condyloma acuminata, may be large and cauliflower-like, or they may consist of small papules.
- Warts on mucous membranes (mucosal papillomas), such as those in the mouth or vagina, tend to be white in color due to moisture retention.

EPIDEMIOLOGY

Incidence
- Predominant age: young adults and children
- Predominant sex: female = male

Prevalence
- ~7–10% of the U.S. population
- Common warts appear 2 times as frequently in whites as in blacks or Asians.

ETIOLOGY AND PATHOPHYSIOLOGY

- HPV is a double-stranded, circular, supercoiled DNA virus.
- The virus infects epidermal keratinocytes, stimulating cell proliferation.
- Various strains of DNA HPV: To date, >150 different subtypes have been identified.
- Common warts: HPV types 2 and 4 (most common), followed by types 1, 3, 27, 29, and 57
- Palmoplantar warts: HPV type 1 (most common), followed by types 2, 3, 4, 27, 29, and 57
- Flat warts: HPV types 3, 10, and 28
- Butcher warts: HPV type 7
- The virus is passed primarily through skin-to-skin contact or from the recently shed virus kept intact in a moist, warm environment.

RISK FACTORS

- HIV/AIDS and other immunosuppressive diseases (e.g., lymphomas)
- Immunosuppressive drugs that decrease cell-mediated immunity (e.g., prednisone, cyclosporine, and chemotherapeutic agents)
- Pregnancy

- Handling raw meat, fish, or other types of animal matter in one's occupation (e.g., butchers)
- Previous wart infection

GENERAL PREVENTION
There is no known way to prevent warts.

DIAGNOSIS

- Most often made on clinical appearance
- Skin biopsy, if necessary

PHYSICAL EXAM

- Distribution of warts is generally asymmetric, and lesions are often clustered or may appear in a linear configuration due to scratching (autoinoculation).
- Common wart: rough-surfaced, hyperkeratotic, papillomatous, raised, skin-colored to tan papules, 5 to 10 mm in diameter; several may coalesce into a larger cluster (mosaic wart); most frequently seen on hands, knees, and elbows; usually asymptomatic but may cause cosmetic disfigurement or tenderness
- Filiform warts: These are long, slender, delicate, fingerlike growths, usually seen on the face around the lips, eyelids, or nares.
- Plantar warts often have a rough surface and appear on the plantar surface of the feet in children and young adults.
  - Can be tender and painful; extensive involvement on the sole of the foot may impair ambulation, particularly when present on a weight-bearing surface.
  - Most often seen on the metatarsal area, heels, and toes in an asymmetric distribution (pressure points)
  - Pathognomonic "black dots" (thrombosed dermal capillaries); punctate bleeding becomes more evident after paring with a no. 15 blade.
  - Both common and plantar warts generally demonstrate the following clinical findings:
    - A loss of normal skin markings (dermatoglyphics) such as finger, foot, and hand prints
    - Lesions may be solitary or multiple, or they may appear in clusters (mosaic warts).
- Flat warts: slightly elevated, flat-topped, skin-colored or tan papules, small (1 to 3 mm) in diameter
  - Commonly found on the face, arms, dorsa of hands, shins (women)
  - Sometimes exhibit a linear configuration caused by autoinoculation
  - In men, shaving spreads flat warts.
  - In women, they often occur on the shins, where leg shaving spreads lesions.
- Epidermodysplasia verruciformis (rare): Widespread flat, reddish brown pigmented papules and plaques that present in childhood with lifelong persistence on the trunk, hands, upper and lower extremities, and face are characteristics.

DIFFERENTIAL DIAGNOSIS

- Molluscum contagiosum
- Seborrheic keratosis
- Epidermal nevus
- Acrochordon (skin tag)
- Solar keratosis and cutaneous horn
- Acquired digital fibrokeratoma
- Squamous cell carcinoma (SCC)
- Keratoacanthoma

- Subungual SCC can easily be misdiagnosed as a subungual wart or onychomycosis.
- Corns/calluses
  - Corns (clavi) are sometimes difficult to distinguish from plantar warts. Like calluses, corns are thickened areas of the skin and most commonly develop at sites subjected to repeated friction and pressure, such as the tops and the tips of toes and along the sides of the feet.
    - Corns are usually hard and circular, with a polished or central translucent core, like the kernel of corn from which they take their name.
    - Corns do not have "black dots," and skin markings are retained except for the area of the central core.

ALERT
- A melanoma on the plantar surface of the foot can mimic a plantar wart.
- Verrucous carcinoma, a slow-growing, locally invasive, well-differentiated SCC, also may be easily mistaken for a common or plantar wart.

DIAGNOSTIC TESTS & INTERPRETATION
Diagnosis
- HPV cannot be cultured and lab testing is rarely necessary.
- Definitive HPV diagnosis can be achieved by the following:
  - Electron microscopy
  - Viral DNA identification employing Southern blot hybridization is used to identify the specific HPV type present in tissue.
  - Polymerase chain reaction may be used to amplify viral DNA for testing.

Follow-Up Tests & Special Considerations
Skin biopsy if unusual presentation or if diagnosis is unclear

Test Interpretation
- Histopathologic features of common warts include digitated epidermal hyperplasia, acanthosis, papillomatosis, compact orthokeratosis, hypergranulosis, dilated tortuous capillaries within the dermal papillae, and vertical tiers of parakeratotic cells with entrapped red blood cells above the tips of the digitations.
- In the granular layer, HPV-infected cells may have coarse keratohyaline granules and vacuoles surrounding wrinkled-appearing nuclei. These koilocytic (vacuolated) cells are pathognomonic for warts.

TREATMENT

- The abundance of therapeutic modalities described below is a reflection of the fact that none of them is uniformly or even clearly effective in trials. Placebo treatment response rate is significant and quality of evidence in general is poor. Beyond topical salicylates, there is no clear evidence-based rationale for choosing one method over another (1)[A].
- The choice of method of treatment depends on the following:
  - Age of the patient
  - Cosmetic and psychological considerations
  - Relief of symptoms

– Patient's pain threshold
– Type of wart
– Location of the wart
– Experience of the physician

GENERAL MEASURES
• There is no ideal treatment.
• In children, most warts tend to regress spontaneously.
• In many adults and immunocompromised patients, warts are often difficult to eradicate.
• Painful, aggressive therapy should be avoided unless there is a need to eliminate the wart(s).
• For surgical procedures, especially in anxious children, pretreat with anesthetic cream such as EMLA (emulsion of lidocaine and prilocaine).

MEDICATION
First Line
• Self-administered topical therapy
  – Keratolytic (peeling) agents: The affected area(s) should be hydrated first by soaking in warm water for 5 minutes before application. Most over-the-counter agents contain salicylic acid and/or lactic acid; agents such as Duofilm, Occlusal-HP, Trans-Ver-Sal, and Mediplast.
• Office-based
  – Cantharidin 0.7%, an extract of the blister beetle that causes epidermal necrosis and blistering
  – Combination cantharidin 1%, salicylic acid 30%, and podophyllin resin 5% in flexible collodion; applied in a thin coat, occluded 4 to 6 hours, then washed off.

Second Line
Home-based
• Imiquimod 5% (Aldara) cream, a local inducer of interferon, is applied at home by the patient. It is approved for external genital and perianal warts and is used off-label and may be applied to warts under duct tape occlusion. It is applied at bedtime and washed off after 6 to 10 hours. Applied to flat warts without occlusion.
• Topical retinoids (e.g., tretinoin 0.025–0.1% cream or gel) for flat warts
Office-based
• Immunotherapy: induction of delayed type hypersensitivity with the following:
  – Diphenylcyclopropenone (DCP) (2)[B]
  – Dinitrochlorobenzene (DNCB)
  – Squaric acid dibutylester (SADBE): There is possible mutagenicity and side effects with this agent.
• Intralesional injections
  – Mumps or *Candida* antigen
  – Bleomycin: Intradermal injection is expensive and usually causes severe pain.
  – Interferon-α-2b
• Oral therapy
  – Oral high-dose cimetidine: possibly works better in children
  – Acitretin (an oral retinoid)
• Other treatments (all have all been used with varying results)
  – Dichloroacetic acid, trichloroacetic acid, podophyllin, formic acid, aminolevulinic acid in combination with blue light, 5-fluorouracil, silver nitrate, formaldehyde, levamisole, topical cidofovir (3)[B] or IV cidofovir for recalcitrant warts in the setting of HIV, and glutaraldehyde
• The quadrivalent HPV vaccine has cleared recalcitrant, chronic oral, and cutaneous warts (4)[C].

COMPLEMENTARY & ALTERNATIVE MEDICINE
• Duct tape: Cover wart with waterproof tape (e.g., duct tape). Leave the tape on for 6 days, and then soak, pare with emery board, and leave uncovered overnight; then reapply tape cyclically for eight cycles; 85% resolved compared with 60% efficacy with cryotherapy (5)[A].
• Hyperthermia: safe and inexpensive approach; immerse affected area into 45°C water bath for 30 minutes 3 times per week
• Hypnotherapy
• Raw garlic cloves have demonstrated some antiviral activity.
• Vaccines are currently in development.

Pregnancy Considerations
The use of some topical chemical approaches may be contraindicated during pregnancy or in women who are likely to become pregnant during the treatment period.

SURGERY/OTHER PROCEDURES
• Cryotherapy with liquid nitrogen (LN_2) may be applied with a cotton swab or with a cryotherapy gun (Cryogun). Aggressive cryotherapy may be more effective than salicylic acid (6)[A], but it is associated with increased adverse effects (blistering and scarring):
  – Best for warts on hands; also during pregnancy and breastfeeding
  – Fast; can treat many lesions per visit
  – Painful; not tolerated well by young children
  – Freezing periungual warts may result in nail deformation.
  – In darkly pigmented skin, treatment can result in hypo- or hyperpigmentation.
• Light electrocautery with or without curettage
  – Best for warts on the knees, elbows, and dorsa of hands
  – Also good for filiform warts
  – Tolerable in most adults
  – Requires local anesthesia
  – May cause scarring
• Photodynamic therapy: Topical 5-aminolevulinic acid is applied to warts followed by photoactivation (7)[B].
• CO_2 or pulse-dye laser ablation: expensive and requires local anesthesia
• For filiform warts: Dip hemostat into LN_2 for 10 seconds, then gently grasp the wart for 10 seconds and repeat. Wart sheds in 7 to 10 days.

 ONGOING CARE

FOLLOW-UP RECOMMENDATIONS
Patient Monitoring
1/3 of the warts of epidermodysplasia may become malignant.

PROGNOSIS
• More often than not (especially in children), warts tend to "cure" themselves over time.
• In many adults and immunocompromised patients, warts often prove difficult to eradicate.
• Rarely, certain types of lesions may transform into carcinomas.

COMPLICATIONS
• Autoinoculation (pseudo-Koebner reaction)
• Scar formation
• Chronic pain after plantar wart removal or scar formation
• Nail deformity after injury to nail matrix

REFERENCES
1. Kwok CS, Gibbs S, Bennett C, et al. Topical treatments for cutaneous warts. *Cochrane Database Syst Rev*. 2012;(9):CD001781.
2. Choi Y, Kim do H, Jin SY, et al. Topical immunotherapy with diphenylcyclopropenone is effective and preferred in the treatment of periungual warts. *Ann Dermatol*. 2013;25(4):434–439.
3. Fernández-Morano T, del Boz J, González-Carrascosa M, et al. Topical cidofovir for viral warts in children. *J Eur Acad Dermatol Venereol*. 2011;25(12):1487–1489.
4. Cyrus N, Blechman AB, Leboeuf M, et al. Effect of quadrivalent human papillomavirus vaccination on oral squamous cell papillomas. *JAMA Dermatol*. 2015;151(12):1359–1363.
5. Wenner R, Askari SK, Cham PM, et al. Duct tape for the treatment of common warts in adults: a double-blind randomized controlled trial. *Arch Dermatol*. 2007;143(3):309–313.
6. Kwok CS, Holland R, Gibbs S. Efficacy of topical treatments for cutaneous warts: a meta-analysis and pooled analysis of randomized controlled trials. *Br J Dermatol*. 2011;165(2):233–246.
7. Ohtsuki A, Hasegawa T, Hirasawa Y, et al. Photodynamic therapy using light-emitting diodes for the treatment of viral warts. *J Dermatol*. 2009;36(10):525–528.

ADDITIONAL READING
• Dasher DA, Burkhart CN, Morrell DS. Immunotherapy for childhood warts. *Pediatr Ann*. 2009;38(7):373–379.
• Simonart T, de Maertelaer V. Systemic treatments for cutaneous warts: a systematic review. *J Dermatolog Treat*. 2012;23(1):72–77.

 CODES

ICD10
• B07.9 Viral wart, unspecified
• B07.0 Plantar wart
• A63.0 Anogenital (venereal) warts

CLINICAL PEARLS
• No single therapy for warts is uniformly effective or superior; thus, treatment involves a certain amount of trial and error.
• Because most warts in children tend to regress spontaneously within 2 years, benign neglect is often a prudent option.
• Conservative, nonscarring, least painful, least expensive treatments are preferred.
• Freezing and other destructive treatment modalities do not kill the virus but merely destroy the cells that harbor HPV.

W

WILMS TUMOR

John K. Uffman, MD, MPH

 BASICS

DESCRIPTION

- An embryonal renal neoplasm containing blastemal, stromal, or epithelial cell types, usually affecting children <5 years of age
- Most common renal tumor in children; fifth most common pediatric malignancy
- Staging: In the United States, National Wilms Tumor Study Group (NWTSG) staging is done pretreatment based on radiographic imaging and surgery, whereas in Europe/Asia, Société Internationale d'Oncologie Pédiatrique (SIOP) staging is done *after* neoadjuvant chemotherapy is administered (1):
  - I: tumor limited to kidney; completely excised
  - II: tumor extends beyond kidney; completely excised
  - III: residual nonhematogenous tumor confined to abdomen (lymph nodes positive, spillage of tumor, peritoneal implants, extension beyond resection region)
  - IV: hematogenous metastases
  - V: bilateral renal involvement
- System(s) affected: renal/urologic
- Synonym(s): nephroblastoma

Pediatric Considerations
- Occurs only in children
- Most common renal malignancy in childhood

EPIDEMIOLOGY

Incidence
- Frequency rare in East Asian populations than Whites
- Frequency higher in black children than in whites
- Predominant age: median age of 36.5 months
- Predominant sex: female > male (1.1:1)
- Represents 6–7% of all childhood cancers
  - >80% are diagnosed before 5 years of age (median age is 3.5 years at diagnosis).
  - Wilms tumor makes up 95% of all renal cancers in children <15 years (2).

Prevalence
United States: 0.69/100,000; 7.6 cases/1 million children <15 years old

ETIOLOGY AND PATHOPHYSIOLOGY
- Hereditary or sporadic forms of genetic mutation
- Familial form: autosomal dominant trait with incomplete penetrance (1%)
- Potential of parental occupational exposure (machinists, welders, motor vehicle mechanics, auto body repairmen)

Genetics
- Several congenital anomalies are known to be associated with Wilms tumor. A 2-stage mutational model has been proposed: occurrence in either hereditary form or sporadic form. Patients with aniridia have a deletion of the short arm of chromosome 11 (11p13).
- Abnormalities of chromosome 11 at the 11p15 locus are associated with Beckwith-Wiedemann syndrome. Wilms tumor-suppressor gene (*WT1*) has been identified as well as additional candidates for another suppressor gene (*WT2*). Chromosome band 17q12–17q21 has been linked to two kindreds with Wilms tumor, and other kindred are associated with a Wilms tumor predisposition gene at 19q13.3–19q13.4. Loss of heterozygosity at chromosomes 16q and 1p is associated with adverse outcome (1).
- p53 is associated with anaplastic Wilms tumors (2).

RISK FACTORS
- Familial occurrence (5%) (2)
  - These patients tend to have earlier age of onset.
  - Familial patients have greater risk of bilateral disease.
- Parental occupation (machinists, welders, motor vehicle mechanics, auto body repairmen)
- Maternal exposure to pesticides prior to child's birth (3)
- High birth weight or preterm birth (3)
- Compared with firstborn, being a second or later birth may be associated with significantly decreased risk of Wilms tumor (3).

GENERAL PREVENTION
- Routine surveillance in patients with syndromes associated with Wilms tumor
- Routine screening with serial renal US at 3- to 4-month intervals has been recommended in children who have syndromes associated with an incidence of Wilms tumor >5% (4)[C].
- Routine screening with serial renal US is also recommended for infants born to kindreds with familial Wilms (every 3 to 4 months until age 7 years) (4)[C].

COMMONLY ASSOCIATED CONDITIONS
- Aniridia (partial or complete absence of iris) 600 times normal risk
- Hemihypertrophy (100 times normal risk)
- Cryptorchidism
- Hypospadias
- Duplicated renal collecting systems
- Denys-Drash syndrome (nephropathy, renal failure, male pseudohermaphroditism, Wilms tumor)
- Klippel-Trenaunay syndrome
- Wilms tumor, aniridia, genitourinary malformations, and mental retardation (WAGR) complex
- Beckwith-Wiedemann syndrome (visceromegaly, macroglossia, omphalocele, hyperinsulinemic hypoglycemia)

 DIAGNOSIS

- Symptoms of pain, anorexia, vomiting, malaise in 30% (1)
- >90% present with asymptomatic abdominal mass (5)

HISTORY
- History of increasing abdominal size
- Usually asymptomatic; may have fever, abdominal pain

PHYSICAL EXAM
- Palpable upper abdominal mass
- Fever, hepatosplenomegaly
- Rarely, signs of acute abdomen with free intraperitoneal rupture
- Cardiac murmur
- Ascites, prominent abdominal wall veins, varicocele
- Gonadal metastases
- Aniridia (present in 1.1% of Wilms tumor patients)
- Hypertension (20–65%) (1)

DIFFERENTIAL DIAGNOSIS
- Neuroblastoma
- Hepatic tumor
- Sarcoma
- Rhabdoid tumor
- Cystic nephroma
- Renal cell carcinoma (generally occurs in older children)

- Mesoblastic nephroma: distinguished only by histology. Age usually <6 months, essentially benign, although metastases have been reported; tend to be locally invasive
- Nephroblastomatosis: considered premalignant; may present as nodularity of one or both kidneys

DIAGNOSTIC TESTS & INTERPRETATION
- Urinalysis (occasional hematuria, proteinuria)
- CBC (anemia)
- Lactate dehydrogenase
- Plasma renin (rarely helpful)
- Urine catecholamines
- Serum creatinine and calcium
- Coagulation factors
- Chest radiograph
- Abdominal US (with Doppler imaging): best initial test. Gives best information about tumor and extension into inferior vena cava
- CT scan (with IV and oral contrast material) of chest and abdomen. Allows anatomic visualization and excludes synchronous bilateral disease with a high degree of sensitivity (2)
- CT may have high sensitivity and specificity for atriocaval thrombus and obviate the needs for US (2).
- Chest lesions only identified on CT have improved event-free survival with three drug treatment regimens (6)[B].

Diagnostic Procedures/Other
Occasionally, bone marrow aspiration is necessary to distinguish from neuroblastoma.

Test Interpretation
- Favorable findings (mortality of 7%)
  - Bulky lesion, well encapsulated
  - Focal areas of hemorrhage and necrosis
  - Absence of anaplasia and sarcomatous cell types
  - Presence of blastemal, stromal, and epithelial elements (5)
    - Predominance of epithelial elements usually are less aggressive when diagnosed early but tend to be resistant to treatment when diagnosed late.
    - Predominance of blastemal elements indicate more aggressive tumors.
- Unfavorable histology (mortality rate of 57%)
  - Anaplasia: markedly enlarged and multipolar mitotic figures, 3-fold enlargement of nuclei in comparison with adjacent similar nuclei, hyperchromasia of enlarged nuclei; anaplasia may be diffuse or focal.
  - Sarcomatous changes: now considered to be separate from Wilms, not subtypes (mortality 64%)
  - Rhabdoid tumor of the kidney: now considered to be separate tumor from Wilms
- Nephroblastomatosis: considered premalignant
- Nephrogenic rests (5): These are precursor lesions found in 25–40% of Wilms; found in 1% of infants at autopsy, but most do not develop into malignancy.

 TREATMENT

GENERAL MEASURES
- Appropriate health care: inpatient workup and treatment until stable postoperatively and induction chemotherapy completed

- Chemotherapy; some recommend pretreatment with neoadjuvant chemotherapy (1).
  - May decrease incidence of intraoperative tumor rupture (debatable)
  - May result in inappropriate treatment with chemotherapeutic agents of non-Wilms tumors (5%) or benign lesions (1.6%)
  - Results in the inability to directly compare treatment results worldwide
- Radiation therapy in stage II (unfavorable histology), stage III, and stage IV

MEDICATION

First Line

- Children typically treated with protocols based on staging, histology, and other variables as part of a multimodal therapy approach (chemotherapy, radiation, surgery). The following medications may be used as part of a protocol:
- Dactinomycin (Actinomycin-D)
- Vincristine
- Doxorubicin
- Cyclophosphamide (Cytoxan)
- Ifosfamide
- Etoposide
- Topotecan
- Irinotecan

Second Line

- Doxorubicin (Adriamycin)
- Cyclophosphamide

SURGERY/OTHER PROCEDURES

- Exploration of contralateral kidney no longer required if adequate CT done preoperatively
- Radical nephroureterectomy and lymph node sampling is needed to provide precise staging information.
- Renal-sparing resection
  - Tumors are usually too large, but 10–15% may be amenable to partial nephrectomy if given preoperative chemotherapy (4)[C].
  - May be recommended for patients with high risk of bilateral disease or renal failure (4)[C]
- Sampling of any enlarged lymph nodes (absence of any lymph nodes in the surgical specimen mandates treatment as stage III disease) (5)[B]
- Identification of any retained tumor with titanium clips
- Tumor should be given to pathologist fresh, not in formalin.
- Vertical midline incision if tumor extension to right atrium—increased morbidity (2)
- Bilateral Wilms tumors (represent 4–6% of Wilms) (5)[B]
  - Preoperative chemotherapy with reevaluation by CT or MRI after 6 weeks (some are biopsied prior to chemotherapy)
  - Renal-sparing operation at 6 weeks if good response to chemotherapy:
    ○ Partial nephrectomy or wedge excision of tumor is preferred but only if it does not compromise tumor resection.
    ○ Kidney with lowest tumor burden is addressed first. If successful resection is accomplished, radical nephrectomy can be done on the contralateral kidney. Bilateral partial nephrectomy may be possible in some cases.

- Preoperative treatment also generally is accepted in a solitary kidney, horseshoe kidneys, intravascular extension of tumor above the intrahepatic vena cava, and in the case of respiratory distress from extensive metastatic tumor.
- Treatment of patients with relapsed Wilms (7)[B]: Current treatment is either with chemotherapy with or without radiation therapy alone or high-dose chemotherapy followed by autologous stem cell rescue.

 ONGOING CARE

FOLLOW-UP RECOMMENDATIONS

Patient Monitoring

- Multidrug chemotherapy every 3 to 4 weeks for 16 weeks to 15 months depending on stage
- Every 4 months for 1 year, every 6 months for second to third year; yearly after that
- CBC, CT of chest and abdomen with each visit
- Patients at high risk for developing Wilms tumor should be monitored with renal US every 3 to 4 months until 5 years of age. Patients with Beckwith-Wiedemann syndrome or Simpson-Golabi-Behmel syndrome should have yearly US until 7 years of age (8)[C].

PATIENT EDUCATION

- Possibility of second malignancy (up to 12% by age 50 years)
- Side effects of chemotherapy, radiation therapy

PROGNOSIS

- With favorable histology (1)
  - Children <2 years of age and stage I, favorable histology: 98% survival in NWTSG 1 to 3 studies
  - Children with stage III, favorable histology tumor: overall survival of 89% in NWTSG 3 to 4 studies
- With diffuse anaplasia (1)
  - Children with stage I, diffuse or focal anaplasia: overall survival 82.6%
  - Stage II tumors with anaplasia: overall survival 81.5%
  - Stage III tumors with anaplasia: overall survival 66.7%
  - Stage IV tumors with anaplasia: overall survival 33.3%
- With bilateral involvement (stage V): 4-year survival 81.7% (1)
- With rhabdoid features: 19% 3-year survival
- Survival of patients with relapsed Wilms tumor is 40–70% (8)[B]:
  - Patients with pulmonary relapse only had higher 4-year survival rate (77.7%) compared to other sites (41.6%).

COMPLICATIONS

- Complication rate of 6–10%
- 1–2% will develop second malignant neoplasms (leukemia, lymphoma, hepatocellular carcinoma, soft tissue sarcoma): 12.2% by 50 years of age
- High risk of delivering low-birth-weight infants, perinatal mortality in offspring of female survivors of Wilms tumor
- Chest is usual site of recurrence.
- Occurrence of second malignant neoplasms in 2% of patients 7 to 34 years after treatment
  - Bone and soft tissue sarcomas, breast cancer, hepatocellular carcinoma, lymphoma, gastrointestinal tract tumors, melanoma, leukemias

- Surgical complications
  - Postoperative small bowel obstruction (5–7%)
  - Tumor rupture with spillage in 15.3% according to NWTSG-5; this may be spontaneous or surgical and results in upstaging the tumor. Only 2.7% of spills are considered avoidable. Incidence of tumor spillage is reported at 2.2% by SIOP following preoperative neoadjuvant chemotherapy (5)[B].
- Local tumor recurrence
  - Abdominal tumor recurrence after tumor spillage is reduced by radiation therapy (10 or 20 Gy).
- Renal failure
- Cardiomyopathy (usually related to doxorubicin and radiation therapy)
- Impaired pulmonary function (radiation therapy)

REFERENCES

1. Sonn G, Shortliffe LM. Management of Wilms tumor: current standard of care. Nat Clin Pract Urol. 2008;5(10):551–560.
2. Davidoff AM. Wilms tumor. Adv Pediatr. 2012;59(1):247–267.
3. Chu A, Heck JE, Ribeiro KB, et al. Wilms' tumour: a systematic review of risk factors and meta-analysis. Paediatr Perinat Epidemiol. 2010;24(5):449–469.
4. Nakamura L, Ritchey M. Current management of Wilms' tumor. Curr Urol Rep. 2010;11(1):58–65.
5. Ko EY, Ritchey ML. Current management of Wilms' tumor in children. J Pediatr Urol. 2009;5(1):56–65.
6. Grundy PE, Green DM, Dirks AC, et al. Clinical significance of pulmonary nodules detected by CT and not CXR in patients treated for favorable histology Wilms tumor on national Wilms tumor studies-4 and -5: a report from the Children's Oncology Group. Pediatr Blood Cancer. 2012;59(4):631–635.
7. Presson A, Moore TB, Kempert P. Efficacy of high-dose chemotherapy and autologous stem cell transplant for recurrent Wilms' tumor: a meta-analysis. J Pediatr Hematol Oncol. 2010;32(6):454–461.
8. Scott RH, Walker L, Olsen ØE, et al. Surveillance for Wilms tumor in at-risk children: pragmatic recommendations for best practice. Arch Dis Child. 2006;91(12):995–999.

CODES

ICD10

- C64.9 Malignant neoplasm of unsp kidney, except renal pelvis
- C64.1 Malignant neoplasm of right kidney, except renal pelvis
- C64.2 Malignant neoplasm of left kidney, except renal pelvis

CLINICAL PEARLS

- Wilms is the most common renal tumor in children; it is an embryonal renal neoplasm containing blastemal, stromal, or epithelial cell types, usually affecting children <5 years of age.
- Nephrectomy performed as soon as possible after completing radiographic evaluation is the major component in tumor staging.
- Sampling regional lymph nodes or specifically mentioning "No nodes present" in the operative report is necessary or the tumor will automatically be considered stage III.

W

ZOLLINGER-ELLISON SYNDROME

Douglas S. Parks, MD

BASICS

DESCRIPTION
- Zollinger-Ellison syndrome (ZES) triad
  - Markedly elevated gastric acid secretion
  - Peptic ulcer disease
  - A gastrinoma or non-β islet cell tumor of the pancreas or duodenal wall that produces gastrin
    - Gastrinomas (at the time of diagnosis) may be single or multiple (1/2 to 2/3), large or small, benign or malignant (2/3), sporadic (70–75%) or associated with *multiple endocrine neoplasia type 1* (MEN1) (25–30%).
- System(s) affected: endocrine/metabolic, gastrointestinal
- Synonym(s): Z-E syndrome; pancreatic ulcerogenic tumor syndrome; multiple endocrine neoplasia, partial; ulcerogenic islet cell tumor

EPIDEMIOLOGY
Incidence
- 1 to 3 per million per year in the United States
- Predominant age: middle age (30 to 65 years). Mean age of onset is 43 years. Presents a decade earlier in patients with ZES/MEN1.
- Predominant sex: male > female (1.3:1)

Pediatric Considerations
Aggressive cases have been reported in teenagers.

Pregnancy Considerations
Rare, pregnancy alters medication choices and surgical timing.

ETIOLOGY AND PATHOPHYSIOLOGY
- Gastrinoma is equally distributed between the head of the pancreas and the first or second portion of the duodenum; if in the pancreas, the lesion is more likely to metastasize to the liver.
- Hypergastrinemia results in gastric mucosal hypertrophy and increased acid production. Increased acid production causes mucosal ulceration. Diarrhea and malabsorption are also common in ZES.
- Also may be found rarely in the mesentery, peritoneum, spleen, skin, or mediastinum (possibly metastasis with primary not identified)

Genetics
~25–30% of cases occur in association with the MEN1 syndrome—tumors of pancreas, pituitary, and parathyroid.

RISK FACTORS
- MEN1
- Family history of ulcer disease

GENERAL PREVENTION
Screen first-degree relatives of patients with MEN1.

COMMONLY ASSOCIATED CONDITIONS
- MEN1
- Insulinoma
- Carcinoid tumors

DIAGNOSIS

HISTORY
Average of 5 years of symptoms, including recurrent ulcers before diagnosis is made
- Abdominal pain is the most common symptom (80%).
- Diarrhea (postprandial and fasting) (70%)
- Heartburn (60%)
- Nausea (30%)
- Reflux esophagitis
- Vomiting that is unresponsive to standard therapy
- Weight loss

PHYSICAL EXAM
- Hepatomegaly with metastasis
- Conjunctival pallor if anemic
- Jaundice (tumor compressing common bile duct)
- Epigastric tenderness
- Dental erosions
- Heme + stools on rectal exam
- Complications of severe peptic ulcer disease, including hemorrhage, perforation, and obstruction
- Signs of MEN1 are hypercalcemia, hyperparathyroidism, and Cushing syndrome.

Geriatric Considerations
Consider the diagnosis in a patient with persistent or recurring peptic ulcer disease; it is a less aggressive disease if it appears after 65 years.

DIFFERENTIAL DIAGNOSIS
- Elevated serum gastrin with hypochlorhydria/achlorhydria
  - Atrophic gastritis
  - Drug-induced (associated with proton pump inhibitors [PPIs])
  - Gastric cancer
  - Pernicious anemia
  - Postvagotomy
- Elevated serum gastrin with normal or increased gastric acid
  - Antral G-cell hyperfunction
  - Chronic renal failure
  - *Helicobacter pylori* infection
  - Gastric outlet obstruction
  - Retained gastric antrum
- Consider gastrinoma in all patients with the following symptoms:
  - Recurrent or refractory ulcer disease
  - Gastric hypertrophy and ulcers
  - Duodenal and jejunal ulcers
  - Ulcers and diarrhea
  - Ulcers and kidney stones
  - Hypercalcemia and ulcers
  - Pituitary disease
  - Family history of ulcer disease or endocrine tumors suggestive of MEN1

DIAGNOSTIC TESTS & INTERPRETATION
- Preferred test is secretion stimulation test: gastrin level >100 pg/mL (>100 ng/L) (1,2)[A].
- Some gastrin assays undermeasure serum gastrin. If have strong index of suspicion but gastrin levels low, may need to repeat with a different lab (3)[B].
- Gastric secretory studies: basal acid output

- Alternative test is calcium infusion test: gastrin level >400 pg/mL (test is less specific and more dangerous because of IV calcium infusion)
- Elevated serum gastrin fasting level: >1,000 pg/mL with ulcers diagnostic; >200 pg/mL with ulcers is suggestive.
- Elevated basal gastric acid output: >15 mEq/hr (>15 mmol/hr)
- Gastric pH <2 with elevated gastrin
- Check serum calcium, phosphorus, cortisol, and prolactin to rule out MEN1.
- Drugs may alter lab results:
  - Histamine (H_2) blockers and PPIs may increase gastric pH and serum gastrin.
  - Hold PPIs 7 days and H_2 blockers 2 days prior to drawing gastrin level.
- Endoscopic US: finds 24–38% of primary tumors
- Endoscopic findings include esophagitis, duodenal ulceration with multiple ulcers, and prominent gastric and duodenal folds.
- Used to localize tumor for possible resection
- Much more likely to find tumors >3 cm (95%) than <1 cm (<15%) (4)[B]
- Abdominal CT scan: most useful for pancreatic tumors and metastasis >3 cm
- Abdominal US, MRI, and angiography are not typically useful except in large tumors.
- Somatostatin receptor scintigraphy (SRS): more sensitive than radiologic studies, still only finds 30% of small tumors
- Portal venous sampling and selective venous sampling for gastrin can localize the area of tumor and metastasis (80–90% sensitivity).
- Brain imaging (MRI) and serum calcium are useful if MEN1 is suspected.
- Because pancreatic tumors are most likely to be large and to metastasize to the liver (worse prognosis), SRS and an abdominal CT scan are suggested to look for resectable tumors. Surgical resection may improve prognosis (5)[B].

Diagnostic Procedures/Other
Endoscopy may reveal tumors in the duodenal wall; multiple ulcers, including jejunal ulcers; and prominent gastric and duodenal folds.

Test Interpretation
- 90% of gastrinomas are found in the gastric triangle (the borders are the bile duct, the junction of second and third portions of the duodenum, and the junction of the head and body of pancreas).
- ~50% of gastrinomas are in the head of the pancreas (more likely >3 cm, metastasis to liver).
- ~50% of gastrinomas are in the wall of the first or second portion of duodenum (more likely to be small, solitary).
- 2/3 of gastrinomas are malignant.
- 50% of gastrinomas stain positive for adrenocorticotropic hormone (ACTH), vasoactive intestinal polypeptide, insulin, or neurotensin.
- 1/3 of patients have metastasis on presentation: regional nodes > liver > bone, > peritoneum, spleen, skin, and mediastinum.
- Biopsy shows hyperplasia of antral gastrin-producing cells, and histology is similar in appearance to carcinoid.

TREATMENT

GENERAL MEASURES
- Goals are to control acid hypersecretion and resect the tumor.
- Advanced imaging initially to evaluate for resection
- Surgical removal when primary tumor can be identified and as adjunct to control symptoms
- Medical treatment for symptom control when primary tumor is not found or metastasis on initial diagnosis

MEDICATION
- PPIs are the first-line treatment; add H_2 blockers.
- Medications heal 80–85% of ulcers, most of which recur. Lifelong medication use should be anticipated.
- 4- to 8-fold higher PPI dose often necessary
  - Start at a lower dose, and titrate to symptoms (or maximum recommended dosage).
- If hyperparathyroidism is present (MEN1), correct hypercalcemia.

First Line
- PPIs
  - Omeprazole 60 to 120 mg/day
  - Lansoprazole 60 to 180 mg/day (doses >120 mg need to be divided BID)
  - Rabeprazole 60 to 100 mg/day up to 60 mg BID
  - Pantoprazole 40 to 240 mg/day PO; 80 to 120 mg q12h IV
- H_2 blockers
  - Cimetidine 300 mg q6h up to 2.4 g/day
  - Ranitidine 150 mg q12h up to 6 g/day
  - Famotidine 20 mg q6h; up to 640 mg/day
- Contraindications
  - Known hypersensitivity to the drug
  - H_2 blockers: antiandrogen effects, drug interactions due to cytochrome P450 inhibition
  - PPIs: none
- Precautions
  - Adjust doses for geriatric patients and patients with renal insufficiency.
  - Gynecomastia has been reported with high-dose cimetidine (>2.4 g/day).
  - PPIs may induce a profound and long-lasting effect on gastric acid secretion, thereby affecting the bioavailability of drugs depending on low gastric pH (e.g., ketoconazole, ampicillin, iron).
- Significant possible interactions: Consider drug–drug interactions and consult prescribing materials accordingly.

Second Line
- Octreotide may slow growth of liver metastases, or (occasionally) promote regression. Octreotide LAR can be given every 28 days (4)[B].
- Chemotherapy regimens using streptozocin, 5-fluorouracil, and doxorubicin shows limited response.
- Interferon shows a limited response but may be useful in combination with octreotide.

SURGERY/OTHER PROCEDURES
- Laparotomy may be necessary to search for resectable tumors unless patient has liver metastasis on presentation or MEN1; surgery improves outcomes (6)[B].
- Definitive therapy: removal of identifiable gastrinomas (95% of tumors are found at the time of surgery; 5-year cure is 40% when all are removed)

- Total gastrectomy is rarely indicated.
- In MEN1, parathyroidectomy, by lowering calcium, may also decrease acid production and decrease antisecretory drug use. Gastrinomas in MEN1 are generally small, benign, and multiple, and surgery is not usually curative in this situation.

INPATIENT CONSIDERATIONS
Admission Criteria/Initial Stabilization
- Titrate medication to symptom control
- Appropriate surveillance postoperatively to look for metastasis

ONGOING CARE

FOLLOW-UP RECOMMENDATIONS
Patient Monitoring
- Longitudinal follow-up to evaluate for metastases
- Titrate medical therapy to control symptoms.

- Advise patients of potential danger of stopping antisecretory treatment. Rare cases have been reported of severe adverse outcomes within 2 days of stopping PPIs (7)[B]. Gastric acid analysis can help guide medical therapy to maintain basal gastric acid output at <10 mEq/hr (<2 mEq/hr if patient has complications such as perforation or esophagitis).

DIET
Restrict foods that aggravate symptoms.

PATIENT EDUCATION
Inform patients as to the nature of disease and prognosis.

PROGNOSIS
- Overall survival rate: 5 to 10 years: 69–94%
- The prognosis improves with complete surgical removal of the tumor.
- If liver metastasis is present on initial surgery, 5-year survival is 30–40%; 10-year survival is 25%.
- Mortality is directly related to liver metastasis tumor size and presence of pancreatic tumors (4,5)[B].

COMPLICATIONS
- Complications of peptic ulcer disease (bleeding, perforation, obstruction)
- 2/3 of gastrinomas are malignant with metastasis.
- Paraneoplastic phenomena (e.g., production of ACTH with resulting Cushing syndrome) is possible.
- Decrease in vitamin B_{12} levels is possible with long-term PPI use (8)[A].

REFERENCES

1. Berna MJ, Hoffmann KM, Long SH, et al. Serum gastrin in Zollinger-Ellison syndrome: II. Prospective study of gastrin provocative testing in 293 patients from the National Institutes of Health and comparison with 537 cases from the literature. Evaluation of diagnostic criteria, proposal of new criteria, and correlations with clinical and tumoral features. *Medicine (Baltimore)*. 2006;85(6):331–364.
2. Kuiper P, Biemond I, Masclee AA, et al. Diagnostic efficacy of the secretin stimulation test for the Zollinger-Ellison syndrome: an intra-individual comparison using different dosages in patients and controls. *Pancreatology*. 2010;10(1):14–18.
3. Rehfeld JF, Bardram L, Hilsted L, et al. Pitfalls in diagnostic gastrin measurements. *Clin Chem*. 2012;58(5):831–836.
4. Hoffmann KM, Furukawa M, Jensen RT. Duodenal neuroendocrine tumors: classification, functional syndromes, diagnosis and medical treatment. *Best Pract Res Clin Gastroenterol*. 2005;19(5):675–697.
5. Jensen RT. Gastrinomas: advances in diagnosis and management. *Neuroendocrinology*. 2004;80(Suppl 1): 23–27.
6. Morrow EH, Norton JA. Surgical management of Zollinger-Ellison syndrome; state of the art. *Surg Clin North Am*. 2009;89(5):1091–1103.
7. Poitras P, Gingras MH, Rehfeld JF. The Zollinger-Ellison syndrome: dangers and consequences of interrupting antisecretory treatment. *Clin Gastroenterol Hepatol*. 2012;10(2):199–202.
8. Thomson AB, Sauve MD, Kassam N, et al. Safety of the long-term use of proton pump inhibitors. *World J Gastroenterol*. 2010;16(19):2323–2330.

ADDITIONAL READING

- Hirschowitz BI, Fineberg N, Wilcox CM, et al. Costs and risks in the management of patients with gastric acid hypersecretion. *J Clin Gastroenterol*. 2010;44(1):28–33.
- Mortellaro VE, Hochwald SN, McGuigan JE, et al. Long-term results of a selective surgical approach to management of MEN-1. *Am Surg*. 2009;75(8):730–733.
- Smallfield GB, Allison J, Wilcox CM. Prospective evaluation of quality of life in patients with Zollinger-Ellison syndrome. *Dig Dis Sci*. 2010; 55(11):3108–3112.

CODES

ICD10
E16.4 Increased secretion of gastrin

CLINICAL PEARLS
- Consider ZES if peptic ulcers recur or if high doses of PPI are needed to control symptoms/ulcers.
- ~25–30% of cases of ZES occur in association with MEN1.
- Once ZES is diagnosed, it is important to search for gastrinomas in the head of the pancreas and the first or second portion of the duodenum.
- PPIs heal ZES ulcers. Patients should anticipate lifelong therapy.

INDEX

NOTE: Page numbers preceded by A- indicate Algorithms.